MW00837594

Odze and Goldblum

SURGICAL PATHOLOGY *of the* GI TRACT, LIVER, BILIARY TRACT, and PANCREAS

Odze and Goldblum

SURGICAL PATHOLOGY *of the* GI TRACT, LIVER, BILIARY TRACT, and PANCREAS

Fourth Edition

ROBERT D. ODZE, MD, FRCP(C)
Adjunct Professor of Pathology
Tufts University School of Medicine
President, Dr. Robert Odze Pathology LLC
Boston, Massachusetts

JOHN R. GOLDBLUM, MD
Chairman of Pathology
Cleveland Clinic
Professor of Pathology
Cleveland Clinic Lerner College of Medicine
Cleveland, Ohio

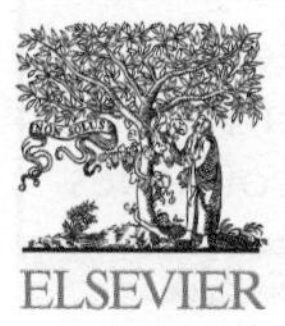

ELSEVIER

ELSEVIER
1600 John F. Kennedy Blvd.
Ste. 1600
Philadelphia, PA 19103-2899

ODZE AND GOLDBLUM SURGICAL PATHOLOGY OF THE GI TRACT, LIVER, BILIARY TRACT, AND PANCREAS
FOURTH EDITION

ISBN: 978-0-323-67988-6

Notices

Knowledge and best practice in this field are constantly changing. As new research and experience broaden our understanding, changes in research methods, professional practices, or medical treatment may become necessary. Practitioners and researchers must always rely on their own experience and knowledge in evaluating and using any information, methods, compounds, or experiments described herein. In using such information or methods they should be mindful of their own safety and the safety of others, including parties for whom they have a professional responsibility. With respect to any drug or pharmaceutical products identified, readers are advised to check the most current information provided (i) on procedures featured or (ii) by the manufacturer of each product to be administered, to verify the recommended dose or formula, the method and duration of administration, and contraindications. It is the responsibility of practitioners, relying on their own experience and knowledge of their patients, to make diagnoses, to determine dosages and the best treatment for each individual patient, and to take all appropriate safety precautions. To the fullest extent of the law, neither the Publisher nor the authors, contributors, or editors, assume any liability for any injury and/or damage to persons or property as a matter of products liability, negligence or otherwise, or from any use or operation of any methods, products, instructions, or ideas contained in the material herein.

The Publisher

Previous editions copyrighted 2015, 2009, 2004 by Elsevier Inc.

Library of Congress Control Number: 2021936449

Executive Content Strategist: Michael Houston
Senior Content Development Manager: Kathryn DeFrancesco
Publishing Services Manager: Catherine Jackson
Senior Project Manager: John Casey
Design Direction: Bridget Hoette

Printed in India

9 8 7 6 5 4 3 2

This book is dedicated to my family, particularly my mother, Natasha, who has always been my inspiration for hard work and dedication to my craft.

RDO

To the love of my life and wife of 32 years, Asmita; to my four amazing and accomplished children, Andrew (and fiancé Audrey), Ryan (and fiancé Jess), Janavi, and Raedan, and my constant companions Luna and Thor; to my late parents, Bette Jean and Raymond; and to the rest of the Goldblum and Shirali families, whom I adore and will always cherish.

JRG

CONTRIBUTORS

N. VOLKAN ADSAY, MD
Professor and Chair
Department of Pathology
Koc University School of Medicine
Koc University Research Center for Translational Medicine (KUTTAM)
Istanbul, Turkey

DANIELA ALLENDE, MD
Director, Gastrointestinal and Hepatobiliary Pathology
Vice-Chair of Research
Pathology and Laboratory Medicine
Cleveland Clinic
Cleveland, Ohioact

KAMRAN BADIZADEGAN, MD
Vice President
Kid Risk, Inc.
Orlando, FL

OLCA BASTURK, MD
Associate Attending Pathologist
Department of Pathology
Memorial Sloan Kettering Cancer Center
New York, New York

PAULETTE BIOULAC-SAGE, MD
Professeur Emeritus
Inserm U1053
Bordeaux University
Bordeaux, France

IAN S. BROWN, MBBS, FRCPA
Histopathologist
Envoi Pathology
Visiting Pathologist
Department of Anatomical Pathology
Royal Brisbane and Women's Hospital
Brisbane, Queensland, Australia

DAVID J. CANGEMI, MD
Senior Associate Consultant
Gastroenterology and Hepatology
Mayo Clinic
Jacksonville, Florida

FÁTIMA CARNEIRO, MD, PhD
Senior Researcher
Department of Pathology
Institute of Molecular Pathology and Immunology of the University of Porto
Professor, Medical Faculty of Porto University
Head of Pathology Department
Centro Hospitalar Universitário São João
Porto, Portugal

BARBARA A. CENTENO, MD
Assistant Chief, Pathology Service
Director of AP QA/Safety
Senior Member
Department of Pathology
H. Lee Moffitt Cancer Center and Research Institute
Professor, Department of Oncologic Sciences
Morsani College of Medicine
University of South Florida
Tampa, Florida

NATALIE CIOMEK, MD
Founder, Digital Creator, and Author
Mededdo LLC
Boston, Massachusetts

TILL S. CLAUDITZ, MD
Associate Professor
Head of Gastrointestinal Pathology Service
Department of Pathology, with Section Molecular Pathology and Cytology
University Medical Center Hamburg-Eppendorf
Hamburg, Germany

MARGARET H. COLLINS, MD
Professor of Pathology
Department of Pathology and Laboratory Medicine
University of Cincinnati College of Medicine
Division of Pathology and Laboratory Medicine
Cincinnati Children's Hospital Medical Center
Cincinnati, Ohio

JAMES M. CRAWFORD, MD, PhD
Professor and Chair
Pathology and Laboratory Medicine
Donald and Barbara Zucker School of Medicine at Hofstra/Northwell
Hempstead, New York;
Senior Vice President of Laboratory Services
Northwell Health
New Hyde Park, New York

MICHAEL W. CRUISE, MD, PhD
Staff, Department of Pathology
Cleveland Clinic
Cleveland, Ohio

ANTHONY J. DEMETRIS, MD
Professor of Pathology
Department of Pathology
University of Pittsburgh
Director, Division of Liver and Transplant Pathology
University of Pittsburgh Medical Center
Pittsburgh, Pennsylvania

VIKRAM DESHPANDE, MD
Professor of Pathology
Harvard Medical School
Pathologist
Massachusetts General Hospital
Boston, Massachusetts

MOHAMED I. EL HAG, MD, MS, FCAP
Assistant Professor
Case Western Reserve University
Staff Pathologist
University Hospitals Cleveland Medical Center
Cleveland, Ohio

FRANCIS A. FARRAYE, MD, MSc
Director, Inflammatory Bowel Disease Center
Mayo Clinic
Professor of Medicine
Mayo Clinic School of Medicine
Jacksonville, Florida

JUDITH A. FERRY, MD
Director of Hematopathology
Department of Pathology
Massachusetts General Hospital
Professor of Pathology
Department of Pathology
Harvard Medical School
Boston, Massachusetts

MILTON J. FINEGOLD, MD
Professor
Departments of Pathology and Immunology and Pediatrics
Baylor College of Medicine
Houston, Texas

CLINTON G. FULMER, MD, PhD
Staff, Department of Pathology
Robert J. Tomsich Pathology and Laboratory Medicine Institute
Cleveland Clinic
Cleveland, Ohio

JOANNA A. GIBSON, MD, PhD
Associate Professor
Department of Pathology
Yale University School of Medicine
New Haven, Connecticut

JONATHAN N. GLICKMAN, MD, PhD
Director of Surgical Pathology
Department of Pathology
Beth Israel Deaconess Medical Center
Associate Professor
Department of Pathology
Harvard Medical School
Boston, Massachusetts

JOHN R. GOLDBLUM, MD
Chairman of Pathology
Cleveland Clinic
Professor of Pathology
Cleveland Clinic Lerner College of Medicine
Cleveland, Ohio

ILYSSA O. GORDON, MD, PhD
Associate Professor of Pathology
Department of Pathology
Cleveland Clinic
Cleveland, Ohio

JASON L. HORNICK, MD, PhD
Director of Surgical Pathology and Immunohistochemistry
Department of Pathology
Brigham and Women's Hospital
Professor of Pathology
Harvard Medical School
Boston, Massachusetts

RALPH H. HRUBAN, MD
Professor
Departments of Pathology and Oncology
The Johns Hopkins University School of Medicine
Baltimore, Maryland

PRODROMOS HYTIROGLOU, MD
Professor
Department of Pathology
Aristotle University Medical School
Thessaloniki, Greece

DHANPAT JAIN, MBBS, MD
Professor, Director of Program in GI and Liver Pathology
Department of Anatomic Pathology
Yale University School of Medicine
New Haven, Connecticut

JOSE JESSURUN, MD
Professor of Pathology
Department of Pathology and Laboratory Medicine
New York-Presbyterian Hospital
Weill Cornell Medical Center
New York, New York

NANCY M. JOSEPH, MD, PhD
Associate Professor
Department of Pathology
University of California, San Francisco
San Francisco, California

SANJAY KAKAR, MD
Professor and Chief of Hepatobiliary Pathology
Department of Anatomic Pathology
University of California, San Francisco
San Francisco, California

DAVID E. KLEINER, MD, PhD
Senior Research Physician
Chief, Post-Mortem Section

DAVID S. KLIMSTRA, MD
Consultant Pathologist
Memorial Sloan Kettering Cancer Center
Chief Medical Officer
Paige.AI
New York, New York

BENCE KŐVÁRI, MD, PhD
Assistant Professor
Department of Pathology
University of Szeged
Albert Szent-Györgyi Medical School
Szeged, Hungary;
Department of Pathology
H. Lee Moffitt Cancer Center & Research Institute
Tampa, Florida

ALYSSA M. KRASINSKAS, MD
Professor
Department of Pathology and Laboratory Medicine
Emory University
Atlanta, Georgia

LAURA W. LAMPS, MD
Godfrey D. Stobbe Professor and Director of Gastrointestinal Pathology
Department of Pathology
University of Michigan Health System
Ann Arbor, Michigan

GREGORY Y. LAUWERS, MD
Senior Member and Director of Gastrointestinal Pathology
Department of Pathology
H. Lee Moffitt Cancer Center & Research Institute
Professor
Departments of Pathology & Cell Biology and Oncologic Sciences
University of South Florida
Tampa, Florida

BRIGITTE LE BAIL, MD, PhD
Professor of Pathology
Staff Pathologist, Unit Chief
Department of Pathology
Pellegrin University Hospital
Bordeaux University Medical School
Bordeaux, France

DAVID N.B. LEWIN, MD
Professor
Department of Pathology and Laboratory Medicine
Medical University of South Carolina
Charleston, South Carolina

KELSEY E. McHUGH, MD
Staff Pathologist
Pathology and Laboratory Medicine Institute
Cleveland Clinic
Cleveland, Ohio

JOSEPH MISDRAJI, MD
Associate Professor
Department of Pathology
Massachusetts General Hospital
Boston, Massachusetts

BITA V. NAINI, MD
Associate Professor
Division Chief, Anatomic Pathology
Chief of Hepatobiliary Pathology
Department of Pathology and Laboratory Medicine
David Geffen School of Medicine at UCLA
Los Angeles, California

AMY E. NOFFSINGER, MD
Vice President and Medical Director, Gastrointestinal Pathology
Inform Diagnostics
Irving, Texas

ROBERT D. ODZE, MD, FRCP(C)
Adjunct Professor of Pathology
Tufts University School of Medicine
President, Dr. Robert Odze Pathology LLC
Boston, Massachusetts

RISH K. PAI, MD, PhD
Professor of Laboratory Medicine and Pathology
Department of Laboratory Medicine and Pathology
Mayo Clinic Arizona
Scottsdale, Arizona

NICOLE C. PANARELLI, MD
Associate Professor of Pathology
Department of Pathology
Albert Einstein College of Medicine
Attending Pathologist
Department of Pathology
Montefiore Medical Center
Bronx, New York

DEEPA T. PATIL, MBBS, MD
Associate Professor of Pathology
Harvard Medical School
Associate Staff
Department of Pathology
Brigham and Women's Hospital
Boston, Massachusetts

MARTHA BISHOP PITMAN, MD
Professor
Department of Pathology
Harvard Medical School
Director of Cytopathology
Department of Pathology
Massachusetts General Hospital
Boston, Massachusetts

THOMAS PLESEC, MD
Assistant Professor of Pathology
Department of Anatomic Pathology
Cleveland Clinic Lerner College of Medicine
Cleveland, Ohio

LIHUI QIN, MD, PhD
Associate Professor of Pathology
Department of Pathology and Laboratory Medicine
New-York Presbyterian Hospital
Weill Cornell Medical Center
New York, New York.

SARANGARAJAN RANGANATHAN, MD
Professor and Division Director
Pathology and Laboratory Medicine
Cincinnati Children's Hospital Medical Center
Cincinnati, Ohio

MICHELLE D. REID, MD, MS
Professor, Director of Cytopathology
Department of Pathology
Emory University
Atlanta, Georgia

MARIE E. ROBERT, MD
Professor
Departments of Pathology and Internal Medicine
Yale University School of Medicine
New Haven, Connecticut

PIERRE RUSSO, MD
Professor
Department of Pathology and Laboratory Medicine
University of Pennsylvania Perelman School of Medicine
Director, Division of Anatomic Pathology
The Children's Hospital of Philadelphia
Philadelphia, Pennsylvania

ERICA C. SAVAGE, MD
Staff Pathologist
Robert J. Tomsich Pathology & Laboratory Medicine Institute
Cleveland Clinic
Cleveland, Ohio

CHANJUAN SHI, MD, PhD
Professor
Department of Pathology
Duke University Medical Center
Durham, North Carolina

MICHAEL TORBENSON, MD
Professor
Department of Laboratory Medicine and Pathology
Mayo Clinic
Rochester, Minnesota

MICHAEL B. WALLACE, MD, MPH
Chief, Division of Gastroenterology and Hepatology
Sheikh Shakhbout Medical City
Fred C. Andersen Professor of Medicine
Mayo Clinic
Abu Dhabi, United Arab Emirates

HELEN H. WANG, MD, DrPH
Staff Pathologist
Department of Pathology
Beth Israel Deaconess Medical Center
Professor
Department of Pathology
Harvard Medical School
Boston, Massachusetts

KAY WASHINGTON, MD, PhD
Professor
Department of Pathology, Microbiology and Immunology
Vanderbilt University Medical Center
Nashville, Tennessee

AILEEN WEE, MBBS, FRCPath, FRCPA
Professor
Department of Pathology
Yong Loo Lin School of Medicine
National University of Singapore
Senior Consultant Pathologist
Department of Pathology
National University Hospital
Singapore

MARIA WESTERHOFF, MD
Professor, Gastrointestinal and Hepatobiliary Pathology
Department of Pathology
University of Michigan
Ann Arbor, Michigan

LAURA D. WOOD, MD, PhD
Associate Professor
Johns Hopkins University School of Medicine
Baltimore, Maryland

MATTHEW M. YEH, MD, PhD
Professor, Director of Gastrointestinal and Hepatic Pathology
Department of Pathology
Adjunct Professor of Medicine
University of Washington School of Medicine
Seattle, Washington

PREFACE

The fourth edition of *Surgical Pathology of the GI Tract, Liver, Biliary Tract, and Pancreas* represents the most clinically relevant and comprehensive textbook of gastrointestinal (and related organs) pathology worldwide. We believe this edition is a significant improvement over the third in a number of ways, as it focuses on the methods and algorithms that pathologists can use to approach and solve difficult differential diagnoses readily. The fourth edition contains one new chapter (Algorithmic Approach to Diagnosis of Pancreatic Disorders). All other chapters have been significantly expanded to include the most recent immunohistochemical and molecular data and a basic approach to diagnostic pathology. For instance, this edition includes many new and updated differential diagnosis tables and summary boxes that pathologists can use at the microscope. We have also separated and significantly expanded the discussion of molecular features of tumors, much of which has only been elucidated in the past 5 years. This book truly merges science and pathology at a practical level. The chapters on algorithmic approach to interpretation of tubal gut, pancreatic, and liver biopsies provide diagnostic algorithms that enable pathologists to navigate the often complex and overlapping inflammatory disorders in a thoughtful and precise manner.

In this edition, the editors have paid extra attention to the quality of the images, which we believe have been improved significantly from previous editions. Overall, more than 800 new photographs have been added. Similar to the previous edition, the fourth edition includes an online version that readers can access from any laptop computer worldwide.

Consistent with our fundamental approach to GI pathology, we have produced this textbook with the goal of providing the most relevant and up-to-date clinical, etiologic, molecular, and therapeutic management information necessary for surgical pathologists to make clinically relevant diagnoses. Ultimately, this is a morphology-based textbook, with particular emphasis on histological features that can differentiate diseases based on evaluation of biopsy, cytology, and resection specimens. However, this book provides abundant clinical correlates and information that would be helpful to gastroenterologists and surgeons as well.

The overall organization of the textbook is similar to prior editions, which have been welcomed widely and have enjoyed great success. We believe it allows readers to obtain information quickly and methodically, according to the thinking process used by pathologists while evaluating cases at the microscope. We are proud to note that the chapters in this edition are written by world-leading pathologists, most of whom have a longstanding special interest and expertise in their particular field. As in the third edition, the editors have paid careful attention to the writing style, structure, and content of each chapter to provide the reader with a consistent and easily readable approach to GI pathology. We, the editors, have not left any stone unturned in this fourth edition. It is a book we hope will be enjoyed by pathologists and clinicians worldwide.

Robert D. Odze, MD, FRCP(C)
John R. Goldblum, MD

ACKNOWLEDGMENTS

As in previous editions, many individuals in both medical and nonmedical fields contributed to the production of this textbook. We are most appreciative of all the technical, administrative, and support staff involved. We would also like to thank Jonathan Alpert for his advice regarding the style of the book cover.

Professionally, I will always be greatly indebted to my longtime friends and mentors, Dr. Donald Antonioli and Dr. Harvey Goldman, for their support, teaching, and guidance both in my personal life and particularly in gastrointestinal pathology. Dr. Goldblum would like to acknowledge his lifelong mentor in gastrointestinal pathology, Dr. Henry Appelman, as well as Kathleen Ranney for secretarial support and Ahmed Bakhshwin for content review and proofing.

Finally, we would like to thank all of the authors of the fourth edition for providing state-of-the-art, comprehensive discussions related to their fields of interest and for their patience required to labor through the long and sometimes cumbersome editorial process. We are very proud of the final product, which is a direct result of the dedication and skill of the authors of this book.

Robert D. Odze, MD, FRCP(C)
John R. Goldblum, MD

CONTENTS

PART 1 GASTROINTESTINAL TRACT

PART 2 GALLBLADDER, EXTRAHEPATIC BILIARY TRACT, AND PANCREAS

PART 3 LIVER

PART 1

GASTROINTESTINAL TRACT

SECTION I

GENERAL PATHOLOGY OF THE GASTROINTESTINAL TRACT

CHAPTER 1

Gastrointestinal Tract Endoscopic and Tissue Processing Techniques and Normal Histology

Michael B. Wallace, Francis A. Farraye, James M. Crawford

Chapter Outline

INTRODUCTION

Endoscopy provides a unique opportunity to visualize the mucosal surface of the gastrointestinal (GI) tract and, through endoscopic imaging techniques, a variety of extraluminal and extraintestinal organs and structures. When considered within the context of a specific clinical picture, endoscopic images may be all that is needed to establish a specific diagnosis or provide sound clinical management.[1] However, endoscopists often must sample tissue and/or obtain specimens for cytology, although optical endomicroscopy methods have rapidly advanced and are now replacing the need for ex vivo microscopy in some situations. Examination by a qualified pathologist of specimens obtained at endoscopy is a routine and critical part of managing disorders of the alimentary tract. The purpose of this chapter is to orient the pathologist to the clinical and technical considerations unique to specimens obtained endoscopically from the alimentary tract and to promote collaboration between endoscopists and pathologists in procurement and processing of tissue samples, and, when appropriate, in endomicroscopy. This is followed by a discussion of the normal anatomy of the tubal gut.

BOWEL PREPARATION

The effectiveness of endoscopy often depends on the quality of the bowel preparation.[2] Preparation of the upper GI tract for endoscopy typically involves, at minimum, a 6-hour fast. Preparation for colonoscopy is achieved by use of oral purging agents, either with or without enemas. Most colonoscopy preparation regimens include the use of a clear liquid or low-residue diet for 1 to 2 days, followed by cleansing with oral polyethylene glycol (PEG)-electrolyte solution or other low-volume, often hypertonic solution combined with water intake. Splitting the dose, or "split prep," between the evening before and the morning of the procedure has been widely shown to improve preparation quality compared with only evening-before dosing[3] (Box 1.1). In general, vomiting is reported more frequently with oral PEG-based high-volume lavage regimens than with other agents.[4,5] PEG lavage regimens reportedly provide more consistent cleansing.[6,7]

Purgative- and laxative-based regimens are more likely to cause flattening of surface epithelial cells, goblet cell depletion, lamina propria edema, mucosal inflammation, and increased crypt cell proliferation, although these effects

BOX 1.1 Common Preparation Methods for Colonoscopy

48-hr clear liquid diet, 240-mL magnesium citrate PO, senna derivative laxative
48-hr clear liquid diet, senna derivative laxative, rectal enema
24-hr clear liquid diet, 240 mL magnesium citrate PO or 4 L PEG-electrolyte lavage
24-hr clear liquid diet, 2 L PEG-electrolyte lavage, cascara-based laxative
24-hr clear liquid diet, 2 L sodium phosphate electrolyte lavage

PEG, Polyethylene glycol; *PO*, per os (by mouth).

occur infrequently. Osmotic electrolyte solutions, such as PEG-based solutions, are better agents for preserving mucosal histology.[8–11] In the most severe form of mucosal damage caused by purgatives such as sodium phosphates, sloughing of the surface epithelium, neutrophilic infiltration of the lamina propria, and hemorrhage may be encountered, and the changes may even resemble pseudomembranous colitis, nonsteroidal antiinflammatory drug–induced injury, or inflammatory bowel disease.[9,12,13] Oral sodium phosphate bowel preparations were removed from the U.S. market in 2008 after their use was associated with renal injury. Chemical-induced colitis, caused by inadequate cleaning of endoscopic instruments, also has been reported but is very rare. Sodium phosphate–based preparations may also cause endoscopically visible aphthoid-like erosions similar in appearance to Crohn's disease.[15] Mucosal changes in this situation may also resemble pseudomembranous colitis, both endoscopically and microscopically.[16]

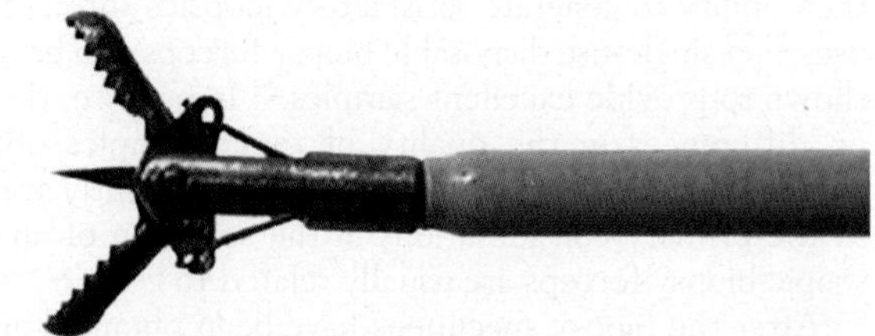

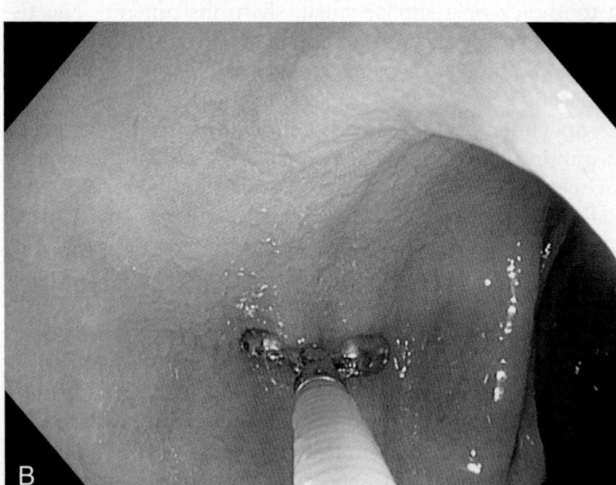

FIGURE 1.1 Endoscopic biopsy forceps. A, The biopsy forceps have been opened, revealing two sets of gripping "teeth" and a central spike used to impale the tissue. **B,** The biopsy forceps in use. The forceps are pressed against the mucosa and subsequently closed to obtain a tissue sample.

METHODS FOR OBTAINING TISSUE SPECIMENS

There are a limited number of methods available for obtaining tissue via GI endoscopy. This section describes several of these methods and the common situations in which they are used. A key issue is whether tissue resection is diagnostic or performed for therapeutic or curative intent. Increasingly, endoscopic removal of superficial carcinoma is being performed by endoscopic mucosal resection (EMR) or endoscopic submucosal dissection (ESD). In these cases, definitive pathologic staging (grade, depth-of-invasion, lymphovascular invasion, margin status) are critical.

Endoscopic Pinch Biopsy

Pinch biopsy, performed with the use of a biopsy forceps during endoscopy, is the most common form of tissue sampling; the biopsy site is usually fully visualized at the time of sampling. Suction capsule biopsy requires fluoroscopic guidance to position a long tube with the biopsy apparatus and is done separately from endoscopy without visualization. Suction capsule biopsy without bowel visualization is still performed in some centers, but it is less successful than endoscopy-guided biopsy in obtaining tissue and therefore has fallen out of favor.[17] Pinch biopsies may be small or large (the latter are referred to as "jumbo" biopsies) and can be obtained with or without the use of electrocautery. Electrocautery has value for hemostasis and destruction of residual tissue but introduces burn artifact into the harvested tissue.

All standard biopsy forceps have a similar design (Fig. 1.1). The sampling portion consists of a pair of small cups that are in apposition when closed. In this manner, they can be passed through the channel of a gastroscope or colonoscope. Some biopsy forceps have a spike at the base of the cup or teeth to help seat the forceps against the mucosa. The spike also helps impale multiple biopsy specimens before the forceps are removed from the endoscope.

After insertion into the endoscope and emergence from the distal end, routine biopsy forceps can be opened to a 4- to 8-mm width. The opened forceps are pressed against the mucosal surface for tissue sampling. Large-cup (jumbo) biopsy forceps have jaws that open to a width of 7 to 9 mm. The biopsy forceps are closed against the mucosal surface, and the endoscopist pulls the forceps away from the mucosa to remove the fragment of tissue. This method often yields samples that include muscularis mucosae, except in regions such as the gastric body, where the mucosal folds are quite thick.[18] The submucosa is sampled occasionally with either standard or jumbo forceps.[19]

The sample size varies according to the amount of pressure the endoscopist applies to the forceps. In addition, application of a fully opened biopsy forceps flush against the mucosa before closure usually yields larger pieces of tissue, compared with tissue obtained by tangential sampling or incomplete opening of the forceps. In general, biopsy specimens are 4 to 8 mm in length.[20,21] The forceps shape does not impart a significant difference in either size or adequacy of biopsy specimens.[20] While reusable biopsy forceps retain their ability to generate satisfactory biopsies through many uses,[21,22] single-use disposable biopsy forceps also have been shown to provide excellent samples.[23] In essence, there are no differences in the quality of tissue samples obtained among the dozen or more biopsy forceps currently available, so the primary considerations in the selection of an endoscopic biopsy forceps are usually related to cost.[24]

After the biopsy specimens have been obtained and the forceps have been removed from the endoscope, an assistant dislodges the tissue fragments from the forceps with a toothpick or a similar small, sharp instrument. The tissue is then placed into a container with appropriate fixative and labeled according to instructions provided by the endoscopist.

Specimens obtained with a jumbo forceps often exceed 6 mm in maximum diameter, but these are not necessarily deeper than standard biopsies. Rather, a jumbo forceps typically provides more mucosa for analysis. This is particularly useful during surveillance tissue sampling, such as in patients with Barrett's esophagus or ulcerative colitis. Jumbo biopsy forceps are as safe as standard biopsy forceps.[25] However, the use of jumbo forceps is limited by their diameter because the instrument cannot fit through a standard endoscope accessory channel. Jumbo forceps require a 3.2-mm–diameter channel, characteristic of therapeutic endoscopes, which may be less comfortable for patients. In addition, although jumbo biopsy specimens are larger than standard biopsy specimens, this does not necessarily mean that they are of greater diagnostic value.[26]

Upper endoscopy or colonoscopy may be performed for clinical indications driven by symptomatology. Colonoscopy, in particular, may also be performed for screening purposes in clinically asymptomatic individuals. Selection of a biopsy site at the time of endoscopy is driven by the need to assess visible mucosal abnormalities. In addition, it is advantageous to establish the inflammatory status of the "background" mucosa by sampling normal-appearing mucosa during the evaluation of conditions such as gastroesophageal reflux disease (GERD), nonulcer dyspepsia, diarrhea, polyps, and nodules and for surveillance of premalignant conditions, including Barrett's esophagus and inflammatory bowel disease. For example, in patients with inflammatory or dysplastic polyps of the stomach, it is essential to sample adjacent nonpolypoid mucosa to help determine the background disorder in the stomach in which the polyp has developed. As a second example, the ampulla of Vater may be biopsied to exclude adenomatous change in patients with familial adenomatous polyposis because the lifetime incidence of ampullary adenomas in these patients exceeds 50%.[27]

Biopsy of biliary or pancreatic strictures may be carried out under fluoroscopic guidance during endoscopic retrograde cholangiopancreatography (ERCP) with the use of either standard or specially designed biopsy forceps.[28] Even gallbladder lesions observed on ERCP may be amenable to endoscopic biopsy, although this is rarely performed clinically.[28] Endoscopy-directed diagnostic biopsies are extremely safe. In one study of 50,833 consecutive patients who underwent upper endoscopy, none had any biopsy-associated complications.[25] The risk of perforation after diagnostic or therapeutic colonoscopy (with polypectomy) is extremely low.[29]

Occasionally, an endoscopist uses a specialized insulated biopsy forceps to sample a small polyp ("hot biopsy"), after which remaining tissue is ablated in situ using electrocautery.[30] Unfortunately, cautery artifact in such small tissue samples often makes histologic interpretation difficult (or impossible).[18,31] In addition, the electrocautery technique carries an excessive risk of perforation resulting from deep tissue burn, particularly in the cecum and ascending colon.[32,33] Finally, destruction of residual dysplastic tissue by electrocautery may be incomplete in as many as 17% of cases.[34] For these reasons, hot biopsies have been largely abandoned by most endoscopists. A rare exception to this is a technique called "hot avulsion," which is used to resect fibrotic tissue within a larger adenoma of the colon. This typically occurs when prior attempts at resection or tattooing have caused fibrosis. Special high-energy cutting electrosurgical currents are used in combination with hot biopsy forceps to preserve tissue architecture and minimize thermal injury.[35]

There is now substantial literature available regarding the approach of the "resect and discard" concept for diminutive colorectal polyps found during screening colonoscopy. This concept suggests that one can safely perform endoscopic removal of diminutive colon polyps (usually by simple pinch biopsy removal using cold forceps or cold snare polypectomy) without the need for pathologic analysis of the polyp. The reasoning is that diminutive polyps have a very low likelihood of harboring either malignancy or advanced adenomatous features such as high-grade dysplasia or villiform change. Therefore discarding these lesions without histologic evaluation should be cost-effective and clinically efficacious,[36-38] with an endoscopic sensitivity for correctly classifying adenomas of 94% and a specificity of 89%.[36] Furthermore, these polyps may be assessed by in situ optical scanning techniques that can help predict polyp histology.[39] For instance, narrow band imaging and other similar image-enhanced methods have a reported negative predictive value of 95%,[40] which further increases physician confidence that the polyps can be discarded without pathologic examination. A recent comprehensive review of the literature by the American Society for Gastrointestinal Endoscopy suggests that prespecified accuracy thresholds have been met in specific circumstances. In this setting, a resect and discard (along with nonremoval of diminutive rectosigmoid hyperplastic polyps) is acceptable.[41] However, the success of applying such endoscopic criteria for optical diagnosis only remains an open question because successful optical identification of adenomas may not be achieved in routine clinical practice outside of academic medical centers.[42]

Endoscopic Polypectomy

Diminutive polyps may be sampled by pinch biopsy at the time of upper endoscopy or colonoscopy. Polyps larger than 0.5 cm are amenable to snare polypectomy, although the size of the polyp that can be excised may be limited by the size of the loop placed around it (and the endoscopist's estimation of perforation risk). During endoscopy, a loop of wire is placed around a polypoid lesion that protrudes into the lumen of the gut for the purpose of removing the polyp (Fig. 1.2). This technique is used primarily for colonic polyps, but polyps throughout the alimentary tract may be excised in this manner.

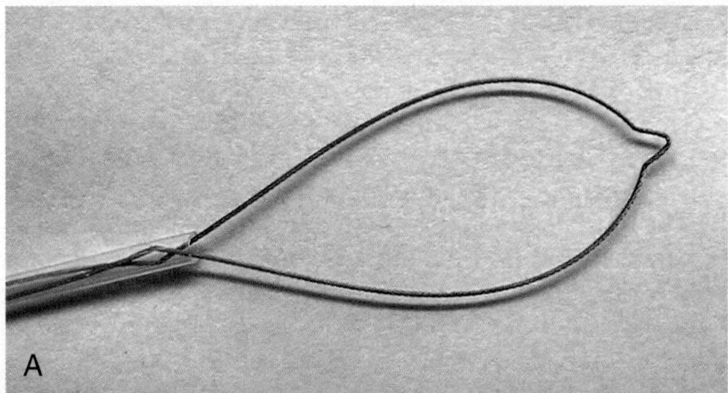

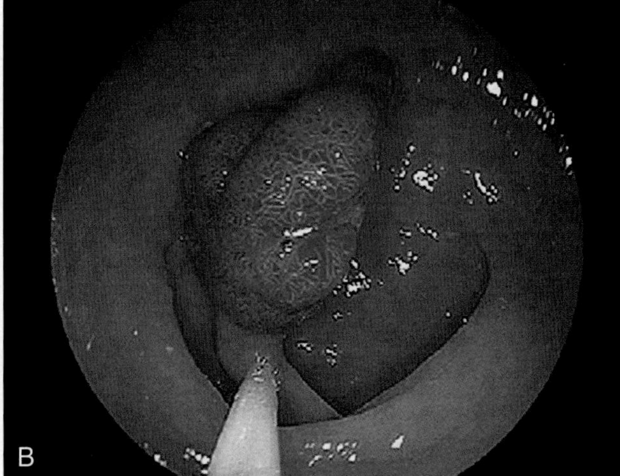

FIGURE 1.2 Endoscopic snare polypectomy. A, An open metal snare extends out of a protective plastic sheath. **B,** A polypectomy snare has been placed over a pedunculated polyp and tightened around the polyp stalk. Electrical current is applied through the metal loop of the snare, which helps cut through the stalk and cauterize blood vessels.

Alternatively, large polyps can be removed in a piecemeal fashion and submitted to pathology in several parts. This technique usually requires multiple transections of the lesion until the entire polyp has been removed.[30] One caveat with the latter technique is that identifiable tissue margins may be lost, so the pathologist is often unable to determine the status of the resection margins.

Snares are available in a variety of shapes and sizes. Some snares can be rotated, which provides the endoscopist with greater control of snare placement. The choice of snare size is usually based on the size of the lesion being removed. The selection of a particular snare shape is a matter of personal choice. Snare polypectomy is performed in a similar fashion regardless of whether colonic, esophageal, gastric, or small bowel lesions are being removed. The ampulla of Vater may be resected by standard snare techniques if an ampullary lesion is discovered.[43] Depending on their size, excised polyps are either retrieved through the suction channel of the endoscope or held by the snare after resection while the colonoscope is removed from the patient.

Historically, snare polypectomy was only rarely performed without electrical current (i.e., cold polypectomy); however, this is now growing rapidly as data suggest that it is of similar efficacy and lower risk. The cold method tends to remove a wider margin of tissue and also a more superficial depth of tissue, but both are highly effective for complete polypectomy.[44] Many endoscopists have reported successful removal of diminutive polyps (<0.5 cm in diameter) during both "hot" (with electrocautery) and "cold" (without electrocautery) snare polypectomy,[45,46] although cold polypectomy may be preferred because of the absence of cautery artefact in the resected small tissue specimens.[47] These endoscopists use small metal snares, termed *mini-snares*, that open to a size of either 1 to 2 cm or 2 to 3 cm.

A hot snare allows the endoscopist to apply modulated electrosurgical current to a metal wire that cuts through pedunculated polyps at the base. This assists tissue cutting and coagulation. Electrocautery also minimizes bleeding from larger blood vessels that are characteristically located in the stalk of a pedunculated polyp. Information on the relative risk of clinically significant hemorrhage after hot polypectomy is limited, but the risk is generally considered to be low (0.4%).[48,49] A higher risk of postpolypectomy hemorrhage occurs in patients with pedunculated polyps larger than 1.7 cm or a stalk diameter larger than 0.5 cm, sessile polyps, or malignant lesions.[50,51] Cold polypectomy (without electrical current) avoids the use of cautery and thereby limits the amount of burn artifact in the specimen and minimizes the risk of perforation. Postprocedure bleeding may actually be less following cold snare polypectomy, possibly because the electrocautery may damage the large vessels and hence impede hemostasis.[52] For smaller polyps (<10 mm), there appears to be no difference in postprocedure bleeding from hot versus cold polypectomy.[53,54]

In general, the risk of perforation from either mechanical or electrical injury is minimal but is greater in portions of the colon that are covered by a free serosal surface, such as the transverse colon. The risk of perforation during snare polypectomy is less than 0.1%,[55,56] and perforation usually results from transmural burn secondary to cautery. One commonly used technique aimed at decreasing the risk of perforation is to pull the snared polyp away from the mucosa so less cautery is applied to the underlying tissue.

For polyps excised in one piece by either hot or cold polypectomy, the polyp base constitutes the surgical margin of resection. This is true for both pedunculated and sessile polyps. For polyps removed by hot snare polypectomy, the cauterized portion of the specimen constitutes the surgical margin. An artificial stalk can be created when large sessile lesions are loop-excised. A true pedunculated polyp, with a stalk, has a narrow base that persists after removal; the base of a sessile polyp is typically as wide as the mucosal surface that is sampled.

Another commonly used method is saline-assisted polypectomy.[57,58] A small needle is passed through the endoscope and inserted into the gut wall adjacent to the polyp. A bolus of normal saline is then injected. Fluid collects within the submucosal plane, lifting the mucosal-based polyp away from the muscularis propria. A standard snare polypectomy is then performed, but the cushion of saline insulates the deeper tissue layers from the electrical current. Saline-assisted polypectomy is usually reserved for large sessile polyps and ampullary polyps and, theoretically, results in a decreased rate of polypectomy-associated perforation.

Endoscopic Mucosal Resection

The use of a liquid cushion to expand the submucosa and minimize transmural cautery damage is a principal feature of EMR. This technique is commonly used to resect premalignant and malignant lesions confined to the mucosa.[59] In general, EMR requires some measure of confidence that a lesion is, in fact, confined to the mucosa or submucosa. Historically, endoscopists relied on endoscopic ultrasonography (EUS) to determine the depth of a particular lesion before EMR. However, this has not been shown to provide high accuracy.[59] Typically, endoscopists attempt to distinguish between lesions that are noninvasive (no submucosal invasion), superficially invasive (typically < 500 to 1000 microns below the submucosa), and deeply invasive (>1000 microns into the submucosa). Standard polypectomy or piecemeal EMR is sufficient for noninvasive lesions, and ESD is preferred to assess depth and margin status for superficially invasive lesions.

Several variations of the EMR technique are currently used. Many rely on submucosal injection of liquid, but there is no agreement regarding the type or quantity of liquid that should be injected[60]; recent evidence suggests that viscous agents improve resection efficiency.[61] There is general agreement that the selected lesion should appear, endoscopically, to be raised by the cushion of liquid before the EMR is performed. Failure to lift the lesion despite generous use of submucosal saline (the so-called *nonlifting sign*) may be a sensitive indicator that a lesion has invaded into the muscularis propria or deeper into the bowel wall.[62]

The most common cap-assisted EMR technique is similar to variceal band ligation but is followed by snare resection of the pseudopolyp created by the band. This is known as *band-ligation EMR* (Fig. 1.3) and is most commonly used in Barrett's esophagus–associated neoplasia.

EMR allows the endoscopist to attempt an en bloc resection and thus, potentially, to completely resect an early malignant lesion. En bloc resection is limited, however, to small lesions (1.5 to 2 cm in largest diameter).[63] If deep margins are positive for neoplasia, surgical resection of the affected region is advocated.[64] Current indications for EMR include superficial carcinoma of the esophagus or stomach in patients who are not candidates for surgery;

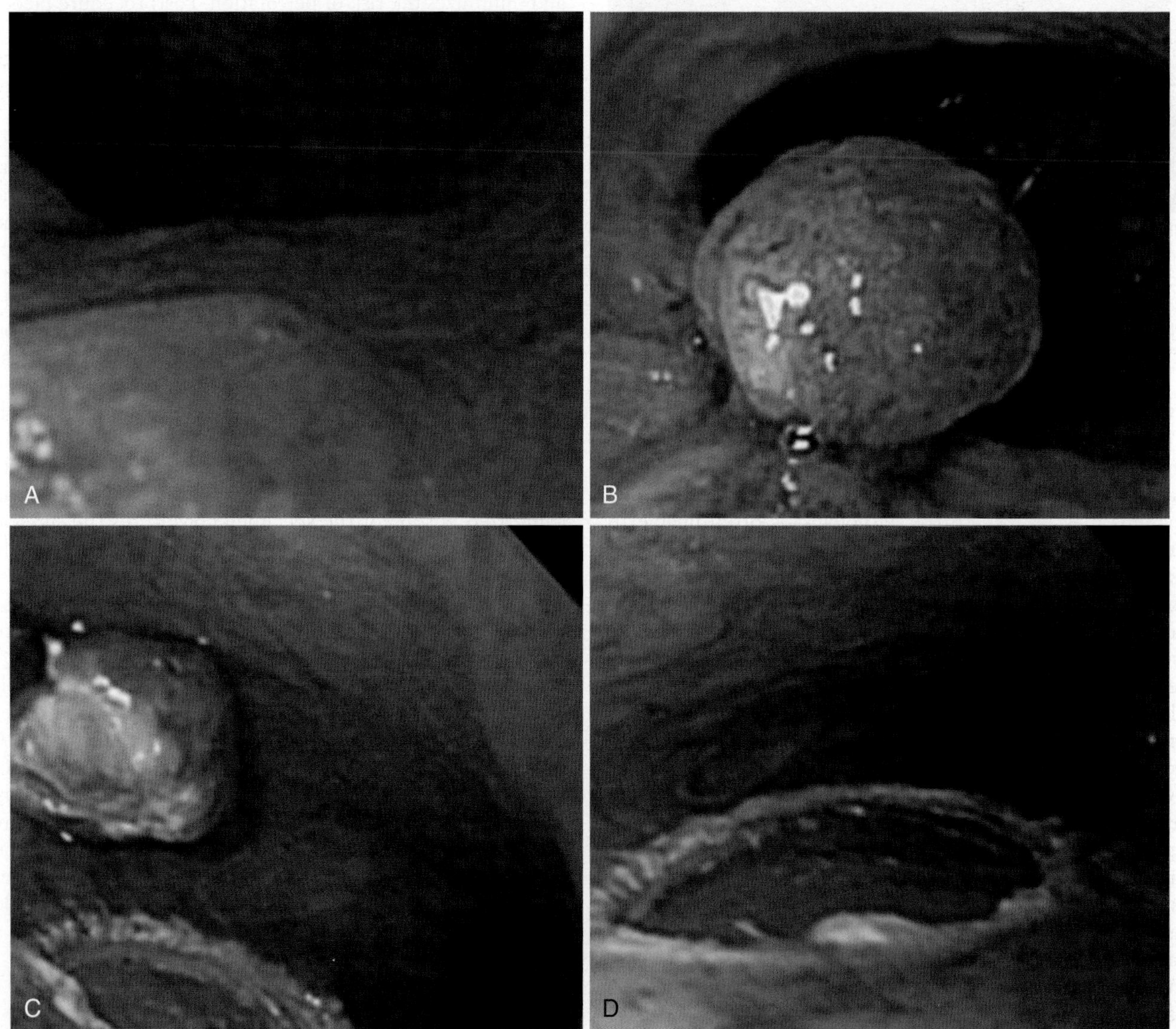

FIGURE 1.3 Band-ligation endoscopic mucosal resection. A, A region of endoscopically visible high-grade dysplasia in the esophagus. **B,** A rubber band ligator has been applied to the base of the lesion after aspiration of the mucosa and submucosa into a cap affixed to the end of the endoscope. The result is a polypoid area containing the dysplastic tissue. **C,** The pseudopolyp has been resected by snare cautery and can be retrieved for tissue processing. **D,** The region where dysplasia was present has been removed, leaving a clean-based ulcer.

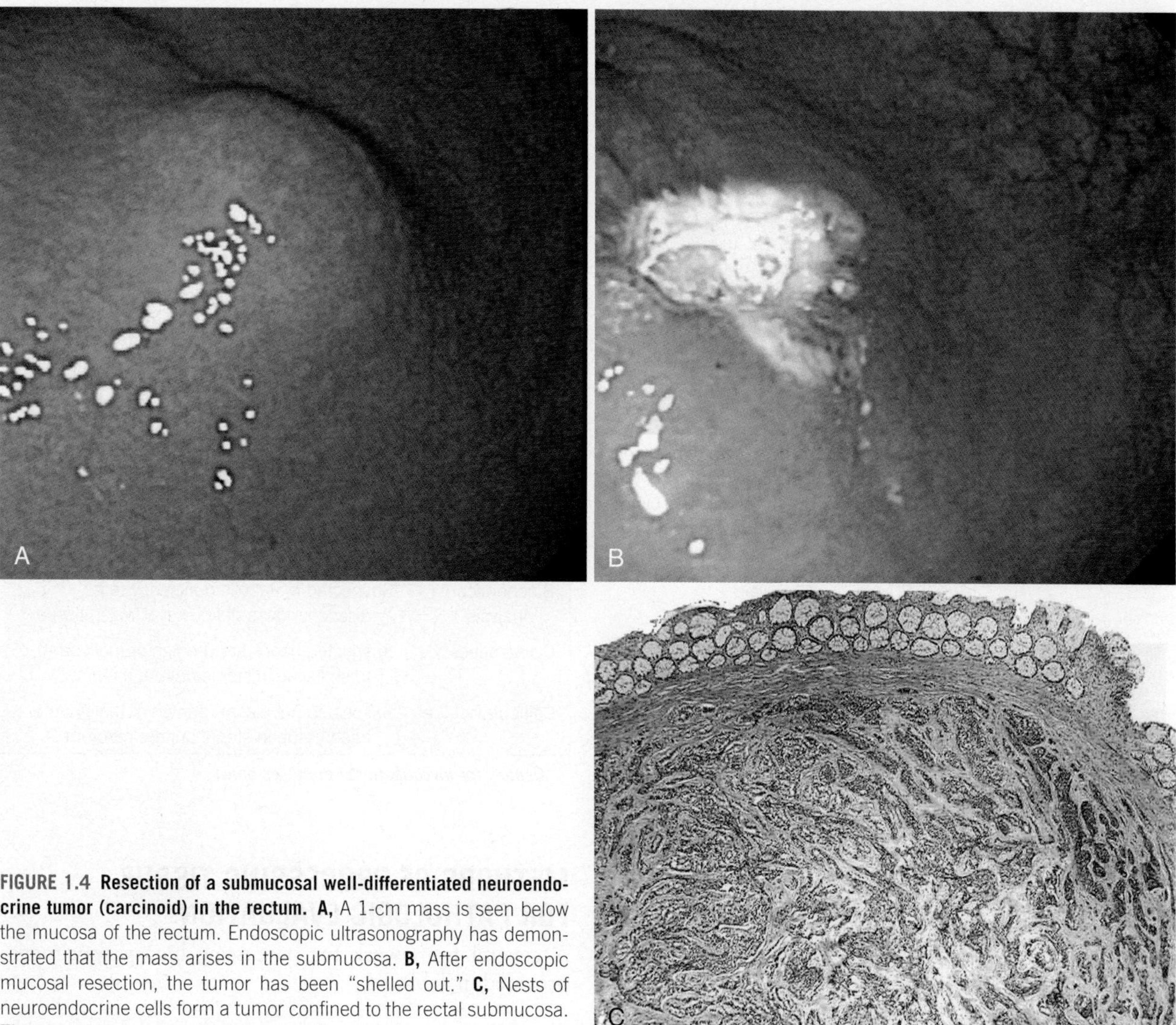

FIGURE 1.4 Resection of a submucosal well-differentiated neuroendocrine tumor (carcinoid) in the rectum. A, A 1-cm mass is seen below the mucosa of the rectum. Endoscopic ultrasonography has demonstrated that the mass arises in the submucosa. **B,** After endoscopic mucosal resection, the tumor has been "shelled out." **C,** Nests of neuroendocrine cells form a tumor confined to the rectal submucosa. There were no tumor cells at the resection margins.

unifocal high-grade (or low-grade) dysplasia in Barrett's esophagus; and large, flat colorectal adenomas (which may otherwise require piecemeal resection), regardless of the degree of dysplasia. EMR as a form of primary therapy for small, superficial cancers has gained increasing popularity in the United States and Europe because of its high level of efficacy and safety.[63-65] EMR is also used as a form of primary therapy for small submucosal lesions such as rectal well-differentiated neuroendocrine tumors (carcinoid) or leiomyomas. In many cases, the submucosal lesion can be completely resected[66] (Fig. 1.4).

Major complications of EMR include bleeding and perforation. Bleeding occurs in fewer than 20% of cases, depending on the size of the lesion and its location, but is typically managed conservatively, or rarely with repeat endoscopy and coagulation.[63,64] Perforation rates are lower than 2% in the hands of experienced operators.[67] A recent recommendation is that the endoscopist should immediately inspect the underside of the resected specimen for the presence of a "target sign" (Fig. 1.5), a pale ring of muscularis mucosa resected with the mucosal lesion. Applying endoscopic clips to the corresponding defect in the resection site is purported to represent an effective method to mitigate the risk of postprocedure bleeding.[68] In the hands of experienced operators, EMR results in large specimens for pathologic analysis, even in the absence of complete resection. Success rates for resection of larger lateral spreading colonic adenomas by EMR approximates 98%,[65] greatly reducing the need for surgical resection.

Endoscopic Submucosal Dissection

ESD is a more advanced method of resection of GI neoplasia. It allows for en bloc resection of lesions larger than 2 cm, thus allowing precise deep and lateral margin assessment and precise histologic assessment of depth of invasion. Like EMR, the technique involves submucosal injection of a lifting agent, but is followed by circumferential incision of the mucosa 5 to 10 mm outside of the lesion margins, and then endoscopic dissection through the submucosa to fully separate the lesion. This method requires special electrosurgical knives, and it is more technically demanding and time-consuming than EMR. Recent European guidelines (U.S. guidelines are not currently available) suggest that ESD is preferred for cancers

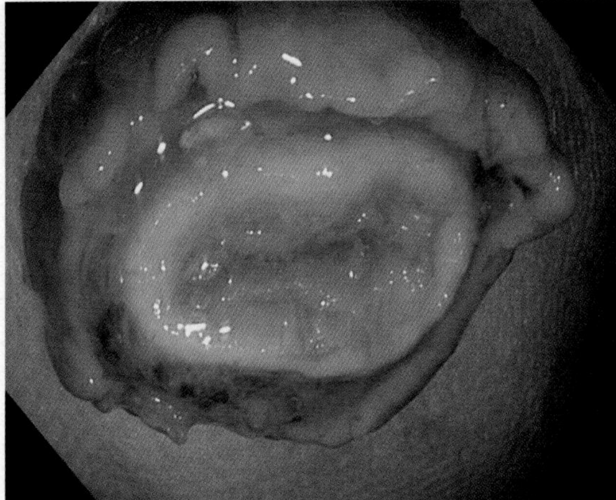

FIGURE 1.5 Ex vivo view of a resected polyp. The *central white ring* corresponds to the muscularis propria and indicates a perforation of the bowel wall. The *blue layer* represents submucosa that is stained by injection of methylene blue during endoscopic mucosal resection. When properly recognized, as was done here, the perforation can be closed immediately by endoscopic clipping.

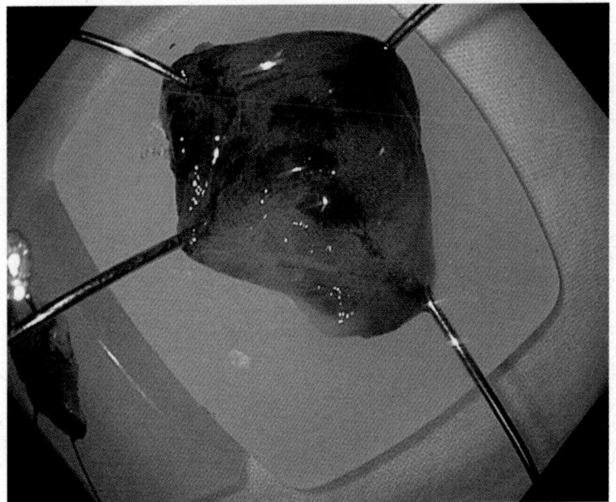

FIGURE 1.6 Barrett's esophagus specimen removed by cap-band endoscopic mucosal resection and pinned to a paraffin block at the bedside with the mucosal side up to facilitate margin and depth assessment.

or suspected cancers limited to the superficial submucosa. Because of variability in lymphatic spread from different organs, current guidelines suggest that esophageal cancers limited to 500 microns or less submucosal invasion, and gastric/colonic cancers limited to 1000 microns invasion are considered potentially curative by ESD. Other factors include histologic features that increase the likelihood of lymphatic/distant spread such as poor differentiation, lymphovascular invasion, and tumor budding.[69] For this reason, it is essential that endoscopists and pathologists collaborate closely to optimize specimen orientation, preparation, and histologic reporting. Both EMR and ESD specimens are typically flattened and pinned in the endoscopy laboratory to enable margin assessment and proper orientation (Fig. 1.6).

To facilitate coordination, it is helpful if the endoscopist indicates that the specimen was resected with curative intent and requests margin status and histologic features associated with curative resection, as noted earlier.

TABLE 1.1 Techniques of Processing Tissue Specimens Obtained by Endoscopy

Technique	Comment
Formalin fixation	Routine processing of all alimentary tract biopsies; immediate immersion in fixative; permits immunohistochemistry and molecular analysis
Flow cytometry	Suspected hematologic malignancy; fresh tissue in sterile culture medium
Electron microscopy	Suspected poorly differentiated malignancy, infection (e.g., Whipple disease, microsporidiosis); immediate immersion in electron microscopy fixative
Electron microscopy fixative only	Suspected systemic mastocytosis for which plastic-embedded thick sections with toluidine blue staining may be used for identification of mast cells
Microbial culture	Suspected viral, fungal, or parasitic infection; sterile tissue
Biochemical analysis	Suspected metabolic deficiency (e.g., disaccharidase deficiency); frozen tissue
Cytogenetics*	Suspected neoplasm (benign or malignant); fresh tissue in sterile culture medium
Cell culture*	Suspected neoplasm (benign or malignant); fresh tissue in sterile culture medium

**Usually for investigational purposes only.*

METHODS OF PROCESSING TISSUE FOR PATHOLOGIC EVALUATION

A general framework for processing biopsy specimens is provided in Table 1.1.

Formalin

Of the many types of fixatives used for human tissue, 10% buffered formalin remains the standard and is well suited for mucosal biopsies of the GI tract. It is inexpensive, harmless to the tissue even after long periods, and compatible with most of the stains commonly used for morphologic assessment. Hollende solution, B5, and Bouin fixative have been used for mucosal biopsies because of better preservation of nuclear morphology compared with formalin. However, the heavy metal content of these fixatives creates biohazard disposal problems that are greater than those of formaldehyde-based fixatives. These fixatives also interfere with isolation of nucleic acid from tissue; the search for substitute fixatives and new tissue processing techniques is an active area of scientific investigation.[70]

On occasion, the formaldehyde in formalin may be irritating to the eyes and upper respiratory tract of laboratory personnel. The level at which formalin is considered carcinogenic is well above the level that causes sensory irritation, which has a threshold of 1.0 ppm.[71] Accordingly, in pathology suites, proper ventilation should be used to maintain exposure below 1.0 ppm, the lowest concentration that may exert a cytotoxic effect in humans.[72,73] A workplace surveillance program for formalin exposure is recommended.[74]

Typical occupational exposure in endoscopy suites is exceedingly brief, so special ventilation is not usually required in that hospital area.

Alimentary tract biopsy specimens should be placed in a volume of formalin fixative that is at least 10 times greater than that of the tissue, and the fixative should surround the specimen completely. These parameters are usually easily met with small endoscopic tissue samples and even with those obtained by EMR, using small tubes of fixative solution. For routine processing, it is a common mistake to place specimens on saline-soaked gauze for delivery to the pathology suite, because severe drying may occur. Complete immersion of these biopsies in formalin should always occur at the bedside. Formaldehyde diffuses into tissue at a rate of approximately 1.0 mm per hour at room temperature.[75] Therefore up to 1 hour is often needed to adequately fix a specimen with a diameter greater than 1.0 mm, and more time is needed for larger specimens. Controlled microwave fixation at 63° to 65°C can greatly speed the process and is useful for rapid processing of specimens.[76]

Orientation of Formalin-Fixed Tissue Obtained at Endoscopy

Esophageal, gastric, and colonic mucosal biopsies do not require precise orientation before tissue processing and embedding. Until the mid-1980s, most peroral small intestinal biopsies were obtained by either a Crosby suction capsule or a Quinton hydraulic assembly.[77,78] These two methods were performed fluoroscopically and therefore did not permit direct visualization of the alimentary tract. Biopsies obtained by these methods were carefully oriented under a dissecting microscope before fixation and embedding. By the late 1980s, fluoroscopy was replaced by a suction capsule biopsy procedure in direct endoscopic biopsy of the small intestine.[79,80] Biopsies obtained by this technique are not usually oriented before immersion in fixative, processing, and embedding. Rather, microscopic examination of multiple tissue sections usually permits identification of portions of the small-intestinal mucosa that are well oriented and therefore can be assessed satisfactorily for tissue architecture.

In contrast, processing of an endoscopic polypectomy specimen in the pathology suite requires diligent effort.[81] The size and surface configuration (bosselated or villiform) of the polyp should be noted, and the base of the polyp should be identified and described as to whether it is sessile or contains a cylindrical stalk. Regardless of the configuration of the stalk, the base of the polyp should always be inked. Ink and cautery artifact on a microscopic slide are valuable landmarks for locating the relevant resection margins. Small polyps (<1 cm in diameter) should be bisected along the vertical plane of the stalk so that the surgical margin is included. Both halves of the specimen can then be submitted in one cassette.

Section levels should be numbered consecutively; the first level is the one usually located closest to the middle of the polyp stalk. Large polyps (≥1 cm in diameter) may be sectioned differently if the polyp head is too wide to fit into a single cassette. First, the polyp is bisected along its long axis and fixed overnight in formalin. Once fixed, the sides of the polyp may be trimmed away from the stalk on a vertical axis and submitted in separate cassettes that are labeled accordingly. The middle of the polyp, including the base, is sectioned vertically and submitted in an appropriate number of cassettes. If a stalk is identified histologically, the status of the margins should be noted in the surgical pathology report.

If the polyp has been excised in a piecemeal fashion, the size, color, surface configuration (bosselated or villiform), and aggregate dimensions of the tissue fragments should be noted. It is important to record the number of tissue fragments received in the pathology suite.

Flow Cytometry

GI lesions suspected of representing a lymphoproliferative process are usually submitted for histology but should also be processed for flow cytometry.[82] Biopsy specimens intended for flow-cytometric analysis, such as gastric biopsies of a mass suspected of being lymphoma, or EUS-guided fine-needle aspiration (FNA) samples from concerning lymph nodes, should be placed in sterile culture medium and delivered as rapidly as possible to the flow cytometry laboratory. Ideally, this should occur within several hours, but storage of specimens at 4°C overnight is an acceptable alternative.

On receipt in the laboratory, the tissue specimen is disaggregated, and a cell suspension is prepared. Cocktails of fluorescently labeled antibodies appropriate to the diagnostic question are applied to the cell suspension. Current flow cytometry machines can analyze 5000 to 10,000 cells per second, measuring multiple wavelengths of laser-induced fluorescence simultaneously and thus permitting rapid and highly efficient analysis of cell populations. This technique cannot be performed on fixed tissue. It is therefore incumbent on the endoscopist to consider the possibility of a lymphoproliferative disorder at the time of endoscopy to ensure that tissue is preserved in a fresh state. Communication between the endoscopist and the pathologist before or immediately after the procedure increases the likelihood that the flow cytometry sample will be received and processed in a timely fashion.

Electron Microscopy

For the rare instances in which electron microscopy of an alimentary tract biopsy is contemplated, tissue samples should be placed directly into the appropriate fixative, which usually consists of a mixture of paraformaldehyde and glutaraldehyde. Unlike formaldehyde-based fixatives, bifunctional glutaraldehyde fixatives penetrate only approximately 0.5 mm into the tissue. Therefore tissue fragments to be placed in fixative for subsequent electron microscopy should, ideally, measure less than 1.0 mm in maximal dimension. Indications for electron microscopy of endoscopic biopsy specimens are now largely limited to examination of unusual tumors.[83] However, this technique is also helpful in cases of diarrhea of unknown cause in children and for detection of parasitic organisms in patients with acquired immunodeficiency syndrome (AIDS).

TABLE 1.2 Endoscopic Events That May Affect Tissue Analysis

Event	Comment
Trauma (tissue hemorrhage)	"Scope trauma" (caused by mechanical damage from the endoscope) or excessive mechanical manipulation for access before biopsy
Cautery artifact	Excessive use of electrical current during "hot" biopsy
Crush artifact	Excessive use of mechanical force during pinch biopsy
Inadequate sampling depth	Absence of submucosa (e.g., evaluate submucosal lesion, rule out amyloid) Absence of submucosa (for evaluation of Hirschsprung disease)
Inadequate sampling location	Insufficient regional sampling (e.g., of "normal-appearing" mucosa)
Chemical colitis	Inadequate rinsing of cleaning solution from the endoscope
Laxative-induced changes	Edema, damage to surface epithelium from exposure to oral and rectal laxatives
Air-drying	Failure to immerse specimen promptly in fixative
Postbiopsy healing	Sampling of a previous biopsy site during subsequent endoscopy
Wrong fixative	Formalin rather than fixative for electron microscopy (suboptimal but not irretrievable)
No fresh tissue	Failure to preserve fresh tissue; precludes flow cytometry, cytogenetics

Data from Bussolati G, Annaratone L, Berrino E, et al. PLoS One. *2017;12(8):e0182965; Arts JH, Rennan MA, de Heer C.* Regul Toxicol Pharmacol. *2006;44:144-160; Bernstein S, Council on Scientific Affairs. Formaldehyde.* JAMA. *1989;261:1183-1187; Conolly RB, Kimbell JS, Janszen DB, et al.* Regul Toxicol Pharmacol. *2002;35:32-43.*

ENDOSCOPY-INDUCED ARTIFACTS

Many types of tissue artifacts may be introduced into tissues as a result of bowel preparation, endoscopic trauma, or tissue handling. Some of these are listed in Table 1.2. Histologic features of artifacts are provided in Table 1.3. The most common type of artifact (or effect) is lamina propria edema and intramucosal hemorrhage, known as *scope trauma* (Fig. 1.7). Other effects include aggregation and clumping of inflammatory cells in the lamina propria, surface flattening, mucin depletion, and even erosion and influx of air into the tissue (pseudolipomatosis).[84-86] The most common histologic artifacts include cautery and crush artifacts occurring as a complication of tissue resection techniques. These may be difficult to avoid in clinical practice given the nature of current endoscopic resection technologies (Fig. 1.8). Cautery artifact as a result of hot biopsy is a normal and expected component of endoscopic polypectomy with electrocautery. Specifically, the region of cauterization may provide a useful landmark of the surgical margin.

TABLE 1.3 Histologic Artifacts Related to Endoscopy

Event	Feature
"Scope trauma"	Mucosal lamina propria hemorrhage or edema
Changes related to bowel preparation	Clumping of inflammatory cells, mucin depletion, epithelial degenerative changes, focal neutrophilic infiltration, hemorrhage, edema, air in mucosa (pseudolipomatosis)
Insufflation of air at endoscopy	Air spaces within mucosa or submucosa (pseudolipomatosis)
Cautery artifact	Coagulated, eosinophilic tissue without cellular or nuclear detail
Crush artifact	Compressed tissue with markedly elongated, wavy nuclear remnants and no identifiable architecture
Chemical colitis from inadequate cleaning of the endoscope	Degenerative damage to or sloughing of surface epithelium, intraepithelial neutrophils and congestion, focal intramucosal hemorrhage
Laxative-induced changes	Lamina propria edema and neutrophilic infiltration, flattening or sloughing of mucosal surface epithelium, decreased goblet cell numbers
Air-drying	Eosinophilic and compressed tissue and loss of nuclear detail at edge of tissue fragment
Postbiopsy healing	See Table 1.4

PATHOLOGIC FEATURES OF A HEALING BIOPSY SITE

After endoscopic biopsy, the tissue healing process begins quickly (Table 1.4). After endoscopic polypectomy involving removal of both mucosa and a portion of submucosa, granulation tissue forms during the first days after biopsy[87] (Fig. 1.9A,B). Routine superficial biopsies that involve only mucosa reepithelialize within 48 hours (see Fig. 1.9C) and heal completely within a few weeks with only mild residual architectural distortion (see Fig. 1.9D). Ulcers that penetrate into the muscularis propria, such as those that form after aggressive EMR, often take 3 to 6 days to reepithelialize (see Fig. 1.9F,G) and as long as 1 month to heal completely.

After routine endoscopic mucosal biopsy during upper or lower endoscopy, there is no increased risk of perforation because of subsequent insufflation (as from repeat endoscopy or from barium enema), even immediately after the biopsy. The risk of perforation after a deep biopsy or EMR that involves the muscularis propria returns to baseline within 3 to 6 days.[87]

Pathologists should be aware of the changes associated with colonic biopsy site repair and not misinterpret focal architectural distortion of the mucosa or focal submucosal scarring as evidence of inflammatory bowel disease. In addition, the finding of muscularis propria in a biopsy specimen in which this depth of sampling is not expected (e.g., in an esophageal biopsy specimen) should be reported to alert the treating physician of the potential risk of perforation.

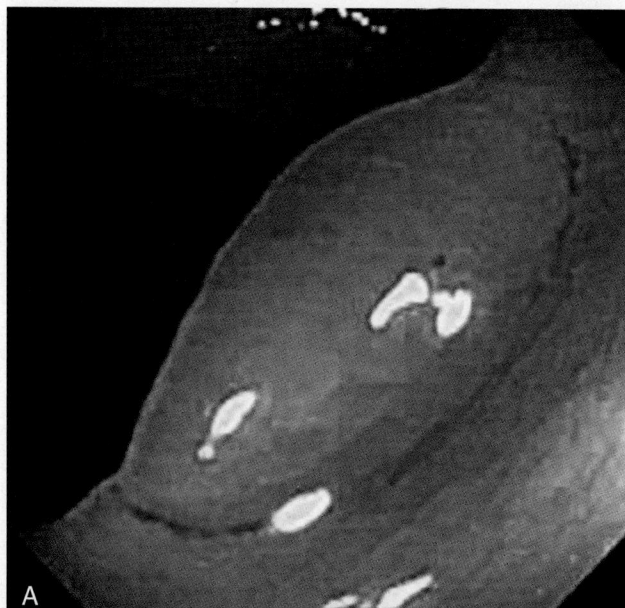

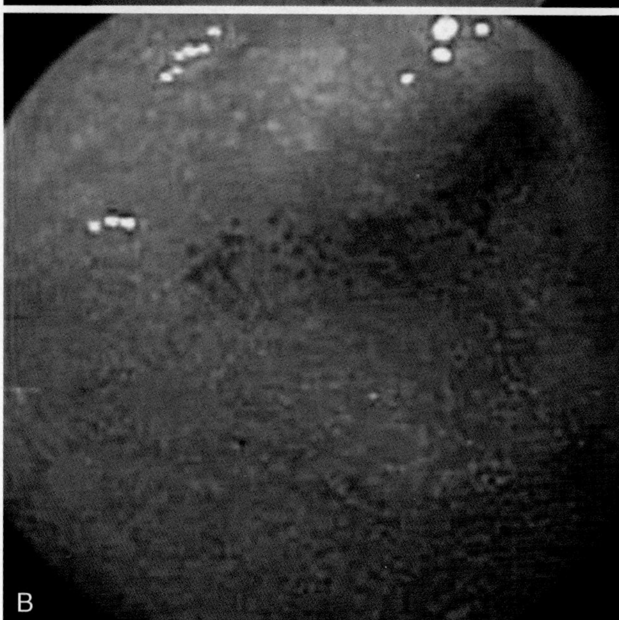

FIGURE 1.7 Endoscopic appearance of "scope trauma." A, A duodenal fold is swollen because of lamina propria edema induced by passage of an endoscope; the region shows a subtle ring of mucosal hemorrhage. **B,** The colonic mucosa demonstrates multifocal areas of mucosal hemorrhage after withdrawal of the colonoscope; these were not present during initial advancement of the colonoscope into the colon. *(Photographs courtesy of Dirk Van Leeuwen, Dartmouth Mary Hitchcock Medical Center, Lebanon, NH.)*

METHODS FOR OBTAINING CYTOLOGY SPECIMENS

See Chapters 3, 36, and 46.

Brush Cytology

Brush cytology is a method used for broad sampling of the mucosal surface.[88,89] Cytology brushes all have a common design: Bristles, usually composed of nylon or metal fibers, branch off a thin metal shaft that runs lengthwise within a protective plastic sheath. The various brushes that are currently available do not seem to vary in terms of performance characteristics.[90] The cytology brush is passed through an accessory channel of an endoscope. The end of the sheath is passed out of the tip of the endoscope, and the bristle portion of the brush is then extended from the sheath. The brush is rubbed back and forth several times along the surface of the lesion or stricture and is then pulled back into the sheath. The sheath is withdrawn from the endoscope, and the brush is pushed out of the sheath, thus exposing the bristles. The bristle portion of the brush may be cut off, placed into fixative, and sent in its entirety to the cytopathology laboratory. Alternatively, the bristles may be rolled against a glass slide in the endoscopy suite. The slides should be immediately sprayed with fixative or submerged within it and subsequently delivered to the cytopathologist. If smears are made in the endoscopy suite, little additional benefit is derived from inclusion of the bristles for cytopathologic analysis.[91] Brush cytology is most often used in the pancreaticobiliary tree to sample strictures in the pancreaticobiliary tract. Another common use is sampling of esophageal plaques or lesions suspected to represent candidiasis.

Fluorescence in situ hybridization (FISH) is an increasingly used technique that can be applied to biliary brush cytology tissue specimens in patients with suspected pancreaticobiliary cancer and in those with primary sclerosing cholangitis (who are at increased risk for cholangiocarcinoma). FISH relies on the fact that a very high percentage of pancreaticobiliary malignancies show chromosomal aneuploidy, typically with chromosomal gains or additions. The presence of these polysomies is strongly associated with malignancy. Commonly used and commercially available probes are used to target the pericentromeric regions of chromosomes 3 (CEP 3), 7 (CEP 7), and 17 (CEP 17) and the chromosomal band 9p21 (LSI 9p21). FISH can be performed on biliary brush cytology specimens. When FISH results are combined with those of routine biliary cytology, the diagnostic yield is much higher.[92,96]

More recently, wide-area transepithelial sampling (WATS) with computer-assisted three-dimensional (3D) analysis has come under consideration for assessment of Barrett's-related dysplasia.[97] This involves sampling of the esophageal mucosa with an abrasive brush that generates a hybrid cytology/histology tissue sample, which is then processed and analyzed by computer-assisted morphologic assessment. Cytologic sampling of the Barrett's mucosa for cytogenetics, FISH, and molecular studies also has gained recognition as a means to identify both dysplasia and risk for progression to adenocarcinoma.[98,99] Endoscopic sampling of gastric tissue for FISH and molecular studies also has become increasingly important in the evaluation of gastric cancer.[100]

Fine-Needle Aspiration

FNA is another widely used method for obtaining tissue for cytology.[101-103] FNA needles may be used during standard endoscopy or EUS. EUS provides endoscopists with the ability to sample tissue from parenchymal lesions and lymph nodes and fluid from cystic lesions. EUS provides real-time imaging to ensure that the intended target is localized and sampled. The needles used for FNA during endoscopy are

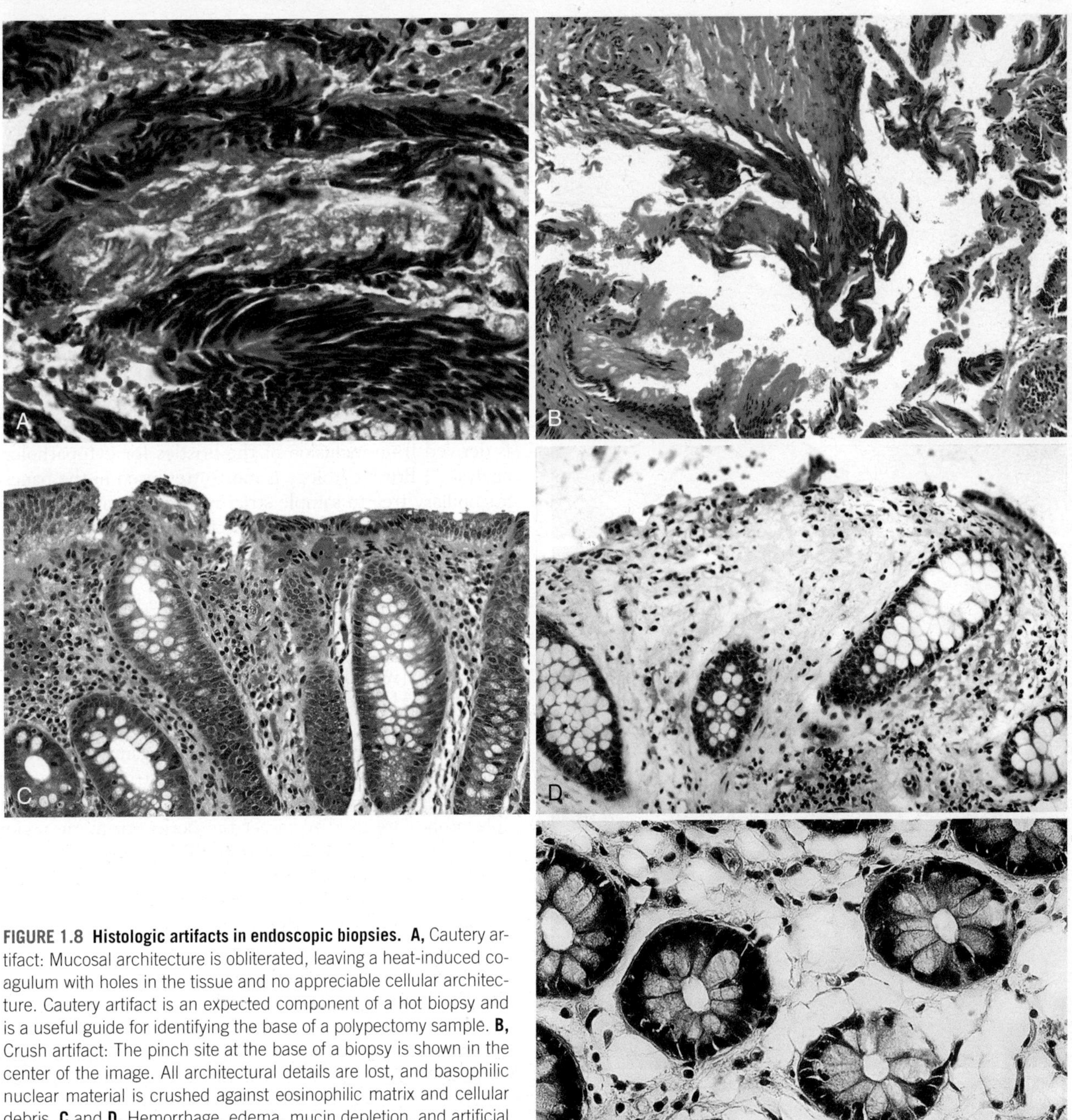

FIGURE 1.8 Histologic artifacts in endoscopic biopsies. A, Cautery artifact: Mucosal architecture is obliterated, leaving a heat-induced coagulum with holes in the tissue and no appreciable cellular architecture. Cautery artifact is an expected component of a hot biopsy and is a useful guide for identifying the base of a polypectomy sample. **B,** Crush artifact: The pinch site at the base of a biopsy is shown in the center of the image. All architectural details are lost, and basophilic nuclear material is crushed against eosinophilic matrix and cellular debris. **C** and **D,** Hemorrhage, edema, mucin depletion, and artificial shearing of the surface epithelium as a result of bowel preparation procedures and endoscopic trauma. **E,** Pseudolipomatosis of the colonic mucosa secondary to insufflation of air at the time of endoscopy.

TABLE 1.4 Pathologic Features of a Healing Mucosal Biopsy Site

Time	Feature
Immediate	Blood clot with coagulum
Hours	Acute inflammation; granulation tissue reaction
2 days*	Reepithelialization of inflamed biopsy site by ingrowth of epithelial cells from adjacent preserved epithelium; early formation of submucosal scar
1-4 weeks	Restoration of mucosa with rudimentary glandular architecture, maturation of submucosal scar
Months	Residual minimal mucosal architectural distortion, submucosal scar

**Longer with deep biopsies that involve the muscularis propria.*

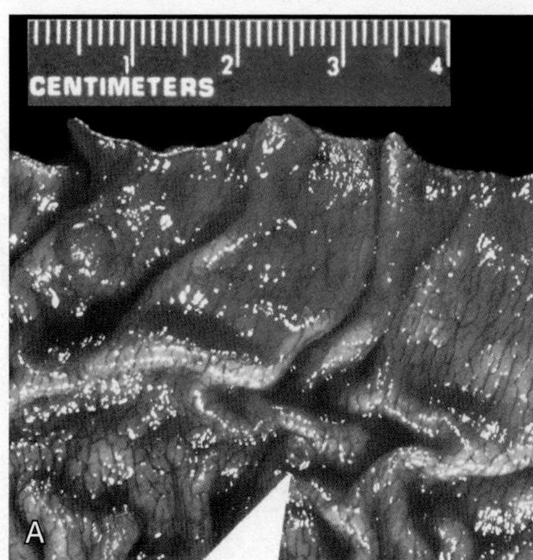

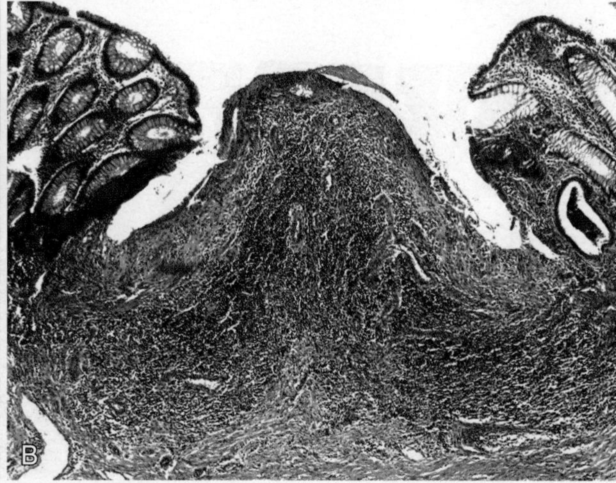

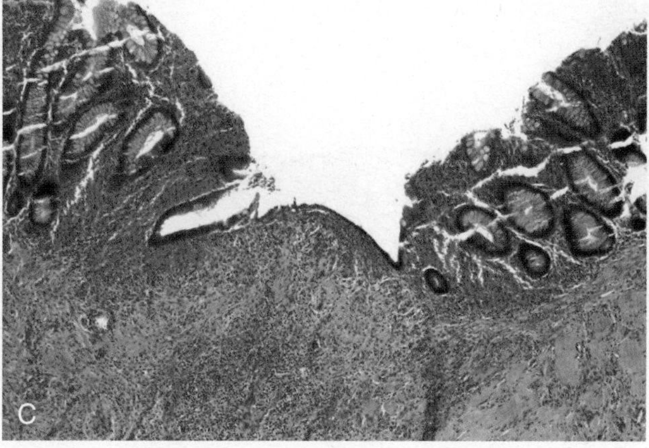

FIGURE 1.9 Healing of the colon after endoscopic biopsy, based on examination of biopsy sites in colonic segmental resections at known intervals after an endoscopic procedure. A, Gross photograph of a resected colon specimen 2 days after endoscopic biopsy of a small pedunculated adenoma. *White arrowhead* at bottom points to the original biopsy site. A small defect is visible and has a protruding knob of granulation tissue. **B,** Photomicrograph of the endoscopic polypectomy site shows ulceration, inflammation, and a granulation tissue reaction. **C,** Two days after simple endoscopic pinch biopsy, there is a smaller mucosal defect. An attenuated layer of epithelium already covers the healing biopsy site.

Continued

hollow 19- to 25-gauge needles and are often fitted with a central stylet to avoid gathering of intervening tissue. Some needles can also obtain a "core" of tissue (which may be analyzed histologically) in addition to samples for cytologic evaluation.

Once the lesion of interest has been identified, the sheath is pushed out of the endoscope, and the needle is advanced into the target tissue under ultrasonographic guidance (during EUS). If a stylet is present, it is removed, and suction is applied to a syringe at the proximal end of the needle. The endoscopist moves the needle forward and backward within the lesion, filling the distal needle lumen with tissue. Some endoscopists use suction during EUS FNA of solid lesions, whereas others do not. Suction is used to aspirate cysts[104] for obvious reasons; there is some disagreement regarding the use of stylets in routine practice.[105] The needle is then withdrawn into the sheath, and the entire apparatus is removed from the endoscope. Complications from FNA biopsy occur in fewer than 2% of cases; they include bleeding and, in the setting of pancreatic mass FNA, acute pancreatitis.

Fine-Needle Biopsy

Over the past decade, there has been substantial improvement in needle design to allow core biopsy via EUS-guided needles. The most significant advance was the utilization of a Franseen-type needle (bi- or tri-pronged) that captures core specimens, even with 25-G needles (available in 19 to 25 G). Recent studies show that these needles allow histologic and molecular assessment in more than 95% of samples.[106]

Optical Techniques

In recent years, there has been an increase in the use of optical techniques to assess in real time the pathologic status of patients with various disease states.[107] Narrow band imaging (NBI) is a technique in which a high-definition videoendoscope is used to allow evaluation of the GI mucosal surface without the use of dyes. NBI is commercially available, and a high percentage of endoscopists have access to this technology. NBI uses different types of optical filters to apply specific wavelengths of light that can achieve deep penetration of the tissue. Specifically, use of red light results in visualization of deeper tissue layers, because red light penetrates more deeply into tissue than blue light does. NBI allows enhanced mucosal and vascular resolution, compared with white-light endoscopy. NBI also allows the endoscopist to evaluate large areas of the GI mucosa without the use of vital dyes. Several other endoscopic manufacturers have developed similar techniques including blue light imaging (BLI), linked color imaging (LCI), and iScan, all of which

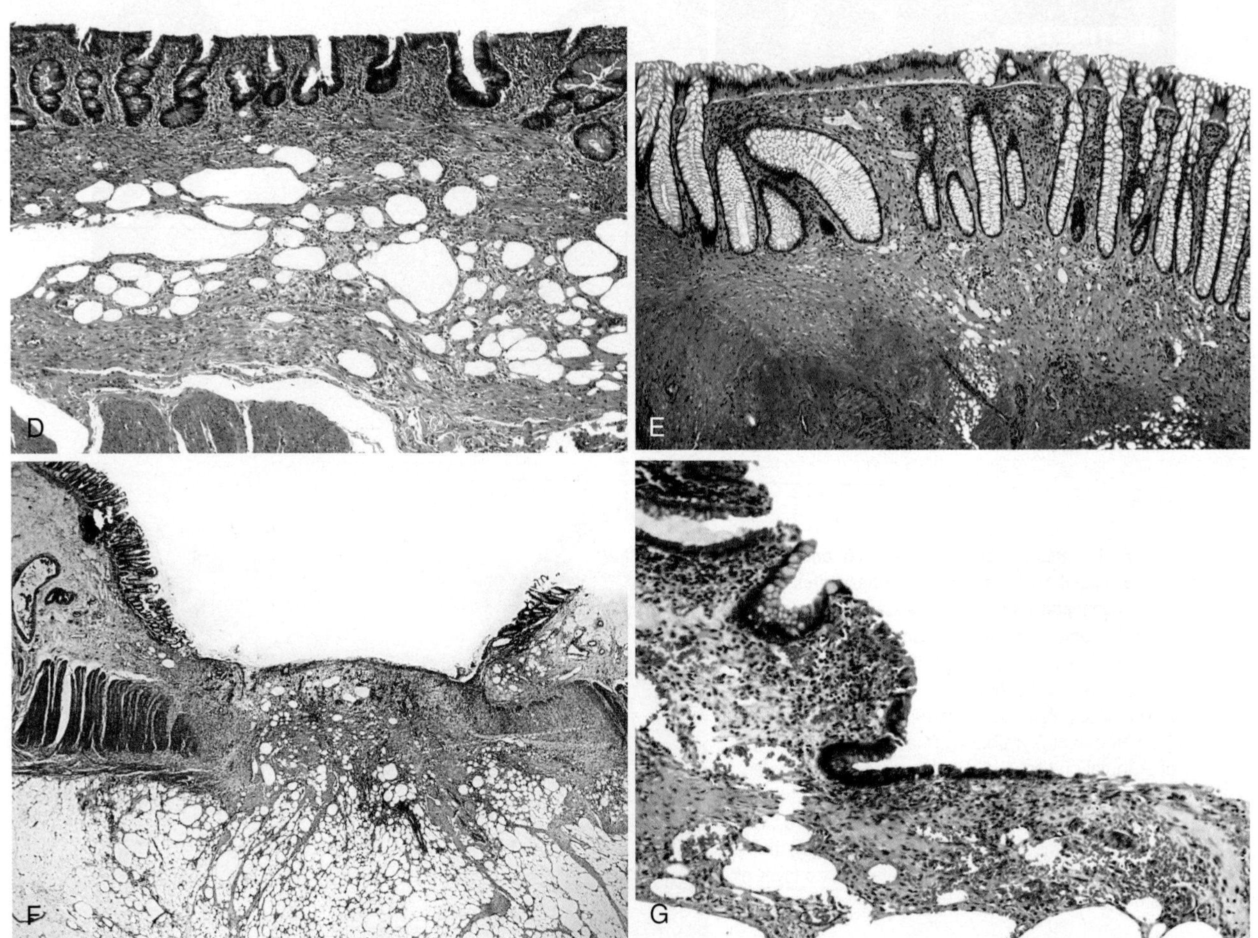

FIGURE 1.9, cont'd **D,** One month after endoscopic biopsy, mucosal integrity is restored, but budding (regenerative) glands, an inflamed lamina propria and submucosa, and disorganized ingrowth of smooth muscle cells in the region of the former muscularis mucosae are present. **E,** Two months after endoscopic biopsy, the mucosa exhibits glandular architectural distortion, no discernible muscularis mucosae, and scarring of the submucosa. **F,** One week after transanal endoscopic mucosal resection that included a substantial sample of muscularis propria, the residual defect is still ulcerated, and there is extensive mural scarring. **G,** High-power image of the margin of the defect shows early reepithelialization of the ulcer from intact adjacent mucosa.

enhance mucosal features and color to create greater contrast between normal and abnormal tissue.[108]

NBI has several clinical uses. In Barrett's esophagus, evaluation with NBI in which the vascular pattern and the mucosal regularity are assessed can be used to identify patients with dysplastic mucosa[108] (Fig. 1.10A,B). NBI has also been used to evaluate gastric and colonic lesions, in attempts to increase the polyp detection rate during screening colonoscopy and to assess for dysplasia or malignancy in endoscopically visible lesions. In its earlier forms, NBI did not appear to increase the adenoma or polyp detection rate during screening colonoscopy[109,110]; however, in more recent improvements, NBI and BLI have been shown to increase adenoma detection.[111] This technology raises the possibility of performing an "optical biopsy" to identify adenomas during endoscopy. As stated earlier, whether diminutive, resected lesions optically identified as adenomas should still be sent for formal pathologic evaluation or simply discarded remains a highly controversial issue.

One other technique related to NBI is confocal laser endomicroscopy (CLE). This technique uses laser technology to illuminate tissue and detect reflected fluorescent light. This technique allows cellular resolution in vivo and in real time. The technique can be performed with special endoscopes (scope-based CLE) or with standard endoscopes using specialized mini-probes that can be passed through the working channel of the endoscope (probe-based CLE). Probes are available for use in the esophagus, stomach, colon, and biliary tree. This technique has not entered mainstream clinical practice but is currently an area of intense research because there is a wide range of potential clinical applications, including the evaluation of Barrett's esophagus, gastric and colonic polypoid lesions, inflammatory bowel disease, and pancreaticobiliary strictures (see Fig. 1.10C–F).[112] Barrett's esophagus may be the most promising area of interest given the desire to target dysplastic or malignant tissue for targeted biopsy and potential ablation.[113-115] Other areas of intense research for CLE include assessment of epithelial integrity (gap function) in patients with inflammatory bowel disease and irritable bowel syndrome.[116,117] However, it is unclear whether CLE will be used routinely in clinical practice in the future.

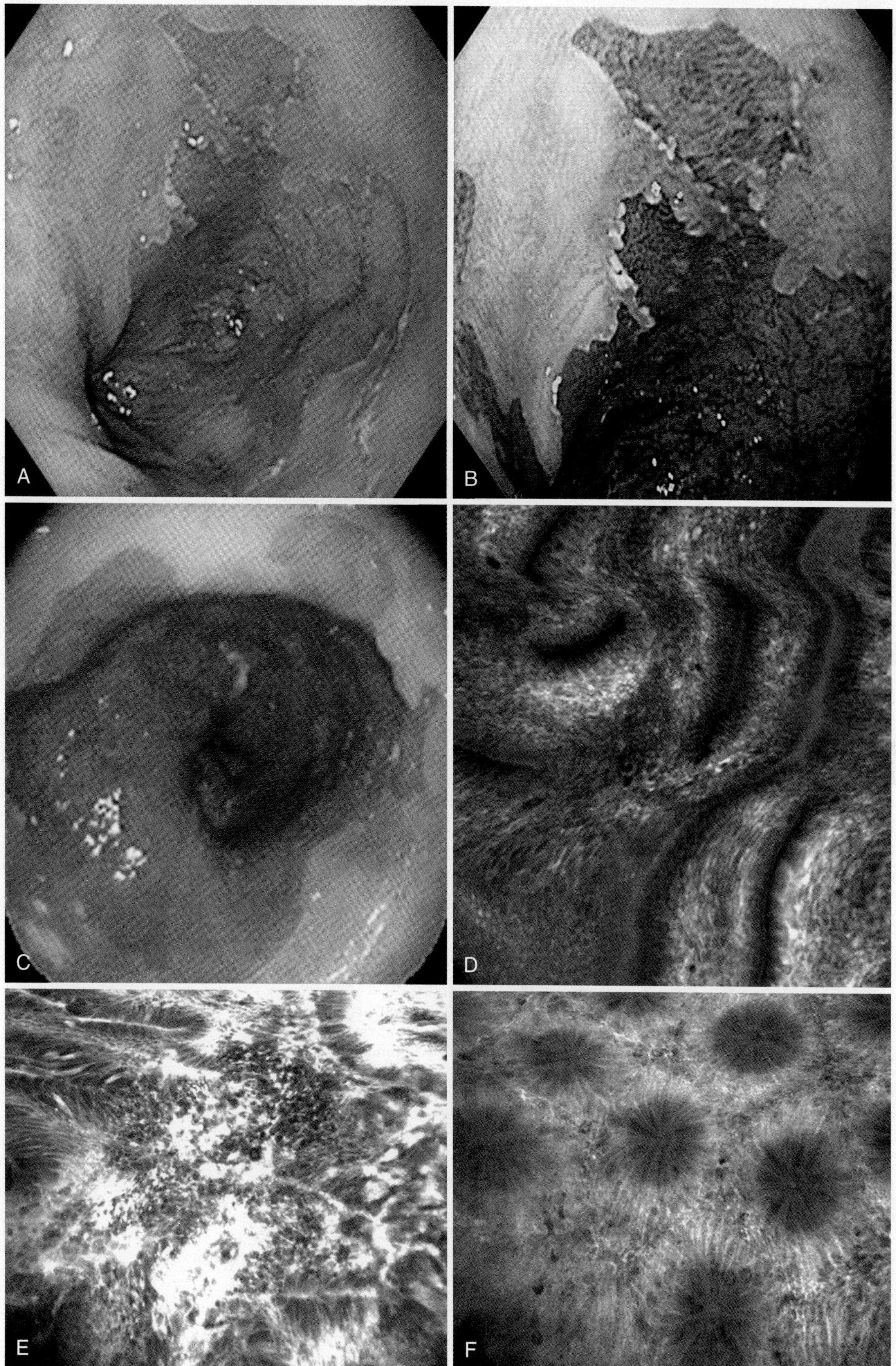

FIGURE 1.10 Optical imaging of the tubal gut. A, Standard white-light image of a segment of Barrett's esophagus. **B,** Narrow band image (NBI) of the same esophagus. **C,** White-light image of Barrett's esophagus and (**D**) confocal laser endomicroscopy (CLE) of the same area. **E,** CLE image of intramucosal adenocarcinoma in Barrett's esophagus after administration of intravenous fluorescein contrast. There is significant loss of glandular architecture and leakage of fluorescein contrast. Large pleomorphic nuclei appear dark with this imaging modality. **F,** Normal colonic mucosa is seen with CLE after intravenous administration of fluorescein dye. Crypts are evenly spaced, and there is uniform distribution of dye within colonocytes. *(Images courtesy of Dr. Sharmila Anandasabapathy, Mount Sinai School of Medicine, New York, NY.)*

NORMAL HISTOLOGY OF THE TUBAL GUT

Esophagus

The adult human esophagus measures approximately 25 cm in length. For the endoscopist, the length of the esophagus is measured as the anatomic distance from the incisors. The esophagus usually begins at 15 cm, and the gastroesophageal junction (GEJ) is typically located at 40 cm. The 3-cm segment of proximal esophagus at the level of the cricopharyngeus muscle (15 to 18 cm from the incisors) is referred to as the *upper esophageal sphincter*. The 2- to 4-cm segment just proximal to the anatomic GEJ (at 36 to 40 cm from the incisors), at the level of the diaphragm, is referred to as the *lower esophageal sphincter*. Both "sphincters" are physiologic because there are no universal anatomic landmarks that outline these high-pressure regions in relation to the underlying esophageal musculature, although they can often be recognized during endoscopy by experienced clinicians.

In keeping with the structural organization of the entire alimentary tract (Fig. 1.11), the wall of the esophagus consists of mucosa, submucosa, muscularis propria, and adventitia.[118] The *mucosa* has a smooth, glistening, pink-tan surface. It has three components: a nonkeratinizing stratified squamous epithelial layer with an underlying lamina propria and muscularis mucosae (Fig. 1.12). The basal cell

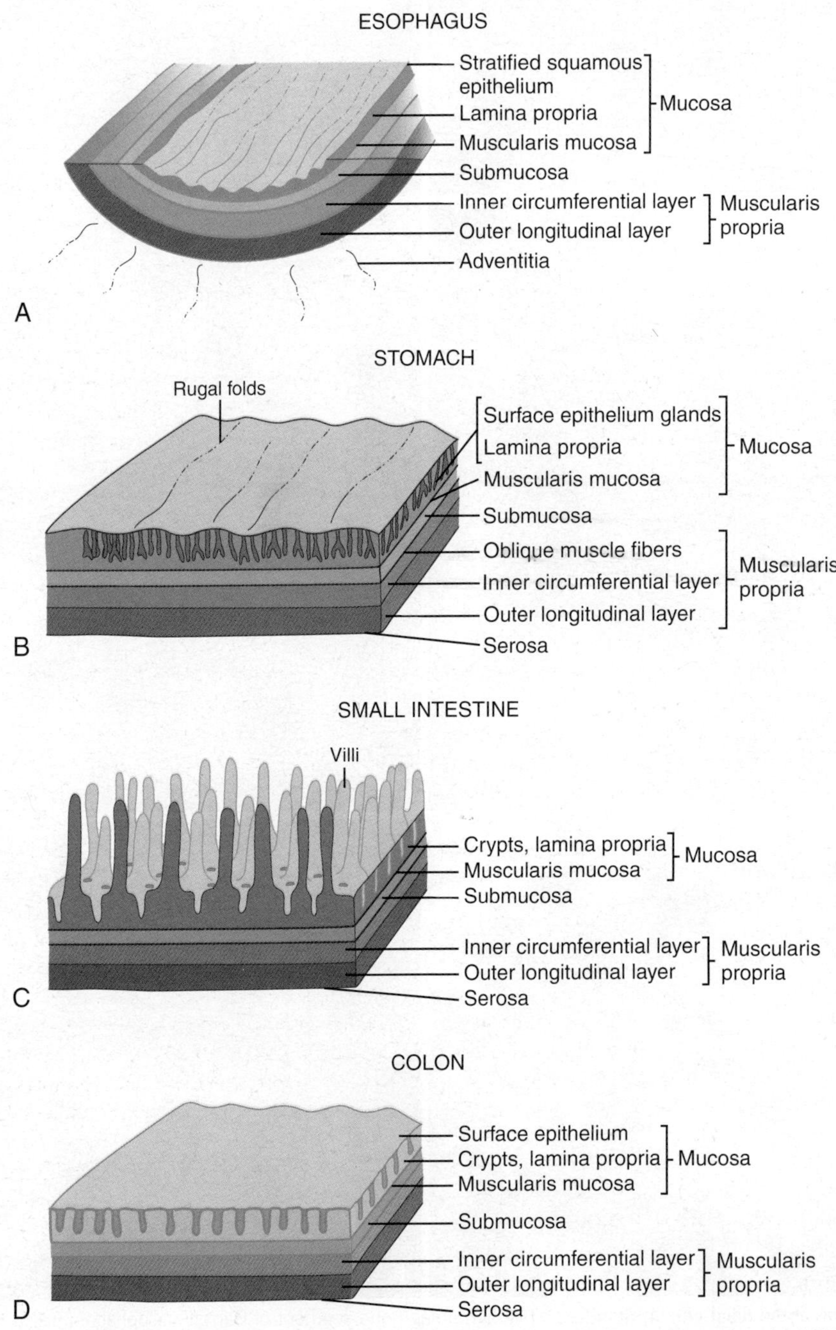

FIGURE 1.11 Microanatomy of the tubal gut. A, Esophagus. **B,** Stomach. **C,** Small intestine. **D,** Colon. *(From Crawford JM. Principles of anatomy. In: Rustgi AK, Crawford JM, eds. Gastrointestinal Cancers: Biology and Clinical Management. Philadelphia: Saunders; 2003:121–131.)*

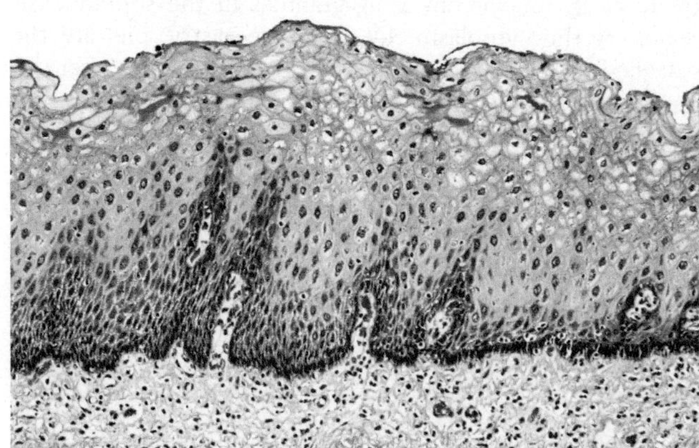

FIGURE 1.12 Normal histology of the esophageal mucosa. Stratified nonkeratinizing squamous mucosa exhibits a basal zone of regenerating cells, rete pegs that extend partially into the epithelial layer, and scattered intraepithelial lymphocytes.

zone of the squamous epithelium occupies 10% to 15% of the total thickness of the epithelial layer. A small number of specialized cell types, such as endocrine cells, Langerhans cells, and lymphocytes, are typically present in the deeper portion of the squamous epithelium. The intraepithelial lymphocytes (IELs) are mainly T cells.[119] Melanocytes may be present in the esophagus in 3% to 8% of normal individuals.[120,121] The lamina propria is the nonepithelial (mesenchymal) portion of the mucosa and is located above the muscularis mucosae. It consists of areolar connective tissue and contains vascular and neural structures and scattered inflammatory cells. Fingerlike extensions of the lamina propria, termed *papillae*, extend into the epithelial layer, usually to between one-third and one-half of its thickness. In esophagitis (e.g., reflux esophagitis), the papillae extend into the upper third of the epithelial layer. The muscularis mucosae is a thick layer of longitudinally oriented smooth muscle bundles.

The *submucosa* consists of loose connective tissue containing blood vessels, a rich network of lymphatics, inflammatory cells, lymphoid follicles, nerve fibers (including the ganglia of the Meissner plexus), and submucosal glands. Submucosal glands, which connect to the lumen of the esophagus by ducts lined with squamous epithelium, are scattered along the entire esophagus but are more concentrated in the upper and lower portions. Submucosal glands are suspended within the delicate mesenchyme of the submucosa. They have a simple acinar structure and resemble salivary glands in that they contain mucous cells surrounding a central lumen in a radial fashion. Their mucin-containing fluid secretions help lubricate the esophagus. Submucosal glands also secrete biologically active peptides such as those from the trefoil factor family 3 (TTF3)[122]; these peptides play a role in mucosal protection and repair. Identification of a squamous duct and submucosal mucous glands is considered a definitive anatomic landmark of the tubular esophagus. In the deep portion of the submucosa, the gland ducts contain two discrete layers of cuboidal cells, which become progressively more squamoid at higher levels of the submucosa and mucosa. A mild, concentric, chronic inflammatory infiltrate surrounding the gland ducts is commonly present.

Endoscopic biopsies of the esophagus usually yield squamous epithelium, lamina propria, and, occasionally, the prominent underlying muscularis mucosae. Sampling of the submucosa is variable. The anatomic landmarks change in patients with Barrett's esophagus. The lamina propria no longer lies underneath the epithelial layer only but is also located between the glands. A newly developed and more delicate muscularis mucosae lies directly underneath the glands. This layer of muscularis mucosae represents the superficial layer of a "double muscularis" in patients with Barrett's esophagus.[123] Other potential landmarks of esophageal origin in Barrett's esophagus include squamous islands[124] and palisade vessels (veins >100 μm in size) in and above the muscularis mucosae.[125]

Stomach

The stomach is a large, saccular organ with a volume of 1.2 to 1.5 L but a potential capacity of more than 3 L. It extends from just left of the midline superiorly, where it is joined to the esophagus, to just right of the midline inferiorly, where it connects to the duodenum. The stomach begins at the GEJ, which is generally considered to represent the most proximal point of the gastric folds. It ends at the pylorus, where the muscularis propria thickens to create the *pyloric sphincter*. The concavity of the right, inner curve of the stomach is termed the *lesser curvature*, and the convexity of the left, outer curve is called the *greater curvature*. The angle along the lesser curve, termed the *incisura angularis*, marks the approximate point at which the stomach narrows before its junction with the duodenum.

The stomach is divided into five anatomic regions. The *cardia* is a narrow (0.1 to 0.4 cm in length), conical portion of the stomach that is located immediately distal to the GEJ. It has no anatomic landmarks and therefore is defined by the presence of mucous glands or mixed mucous and oxyntic glands in the most proximal gastric mucosa. The *fundus* is the dome-shaped portion of the proximal stomach that extends superolateral to the GEJ and is composed exclusively of oxyntic glands. The *body*, or *corpus*, comprises the remainder of the stomach proximal to the incisura angularis. The stomach distal to the incisura, called the *antrum*, contains simple mucous glands and is demarcated from the duodenum by the *pylorus* and its associated sphincter.

The gastric wall consists of mucosa, submucosa, muscularis propria, and serosa. The interior surface of the stomach exhibits coarse *rugae* ("folds"). The rugal folds of mucosa and submucosa extend longitudinally and are most prominent in the proximal stomach. The rugae flatten when the stomach is distended. A finer, mosaic-like pattern is delineated by small furrows within the mucosa. Finally, the delicate texture of the mucosa is punctuated by millions of gastric foveolae, or "pits," which lead to the mucosal glands.

The normal gastric mucosa has two main epithelial compartments: the superficial foveolar ("leaflike") compartment and the deeper glandular compartment. The foveolar compartment is relatively uniform throughout the stomach. In contrast, the glandular compartment exhibits major differences in thickness and composition in different regions of the stomach (Fig. 1.13). The foveolar compartment consists of mucous cells, which line the entire mucosal surface, and gastric pits *(foveolae)*. The tall, columnar, mucin-secreting

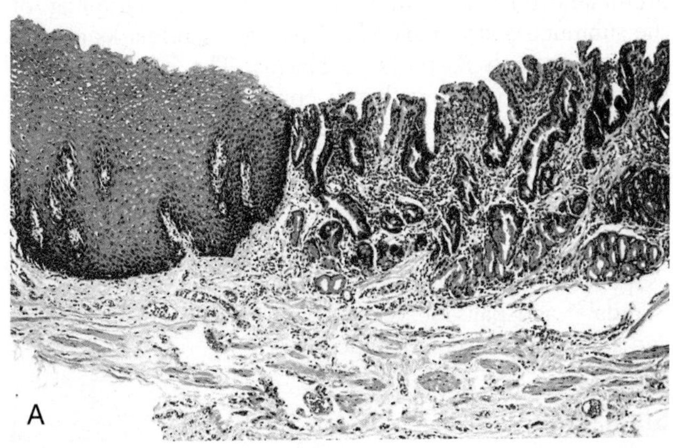

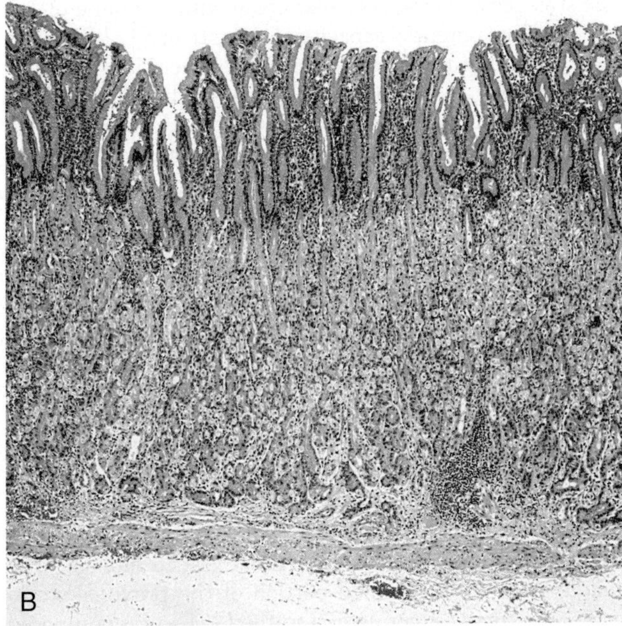

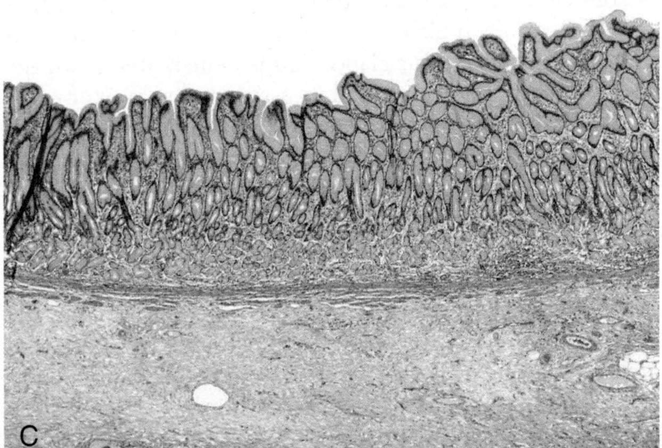

FIGURE 1.13 Normal histology of the stomach. A, Low-power view of the distal esophagus and proximal stomach (cardia); the cardia exhibits simple mucous glands (and some oxyntic glands) underlying the surface and crypt epithelium. **B,** Low-power view of gastric body, showing the robust oxyntic mucosa. **C,** Low-power view of the antral mucosa shows a thinner mucosa, with mucous glands only.

foveolar cells contain basal nuclei and crowded, small, relatively clear, mucin-containing granules in the supranuclear region of the cytoplasm. Deep in the gastric pits are the so-called *mucous neck cells,* which have a lower content of mucin granules and are thought to represent the cell progenitors of both the surface epithelium and the gastric glands. Mitoses may be identified in this region because the entire gastric mucosal surface is usually replaced completely every 2 to 6 days.

The glandular compartment consists of gastric glands, which vary among the different anatomic regions of the stomach.

As noted earlier, in the cardia the mucosal glands contain either pure mucous cells or a mixture of mucous and oxyntic cells for a length of 0.1 to 0.4 cm in most individuals (see Chapter 15). In a small proportion of individuals, a portion of the circumference of the cardia may contain only pure oxyntic glands.

- *Oxyntic glands* (also called *fundic glands*) are found in the fundus and body and contain parietal cells, chief cells, and scattered endocrine cells. The term *oxyntic* is derived from the Greek *oxynein,* meaning "acid-forming."
- *Antral* and *pyloric glands* are identical and contain both mucus-secreting cells and endocrine cells. At the junction of the antrum with the gastric body, the glands usually show a mixture of mucous and oxyntic glands. This histologic junction migrates proximally a few centimeters with age. Distally, where the pyloric mucosa enters the proximal duodenum, the small intestinal mucosa (discussed later) appears to override the mucous glands. In turn, the mucous glands quickly transition to a location below the level of the muscularis mucosae to form the duodenal Brunner glands.

Gastric gland cell types include the following:

- *Mucous cells* populate the mucous glands of the cardia and antral regions and secrete mucus and pepsinogen II. The mucous neck cells in the oxyntic glands of the body and fundus secrete mucus as well as group I and group II pepsinogens.
- *Parietal cells* line mainly the upper half of the oxyntic glands in the fundus and body. They are recognizable by their bright eosinophilia on hematoxylin and eosin (H&E) stain, which is attributable to the abundance of mitochondria. Scattered parietal (and chief) cells can be seen in the antrum as well, particularly in the proximal transition zone within the true antrum.
- *Chief cells* are concentrated at the base of oxyntic glands in the fundus and body and are responsible for secretion of the proteolytic proenzymes *pepsinogen I and II.* Chief cells are notable for their basophilic cytoplasm; ultrastructurally, they are classic protein-synthesizing cells, having an extensive subnuclear rough endoplasmic reticulum, a prominent supranuclear Golgi apparatus, and numerous apical secretory granules.
- *Endocrine* (or *enteroendocrine*) *cells* are scattered among the epithelial cells of the oxyntic and mucous glands. The cytoplasm of these triangle-shaped cells contains small, brightly eosinophilic granules that are concentrated on the basal aspect of the cell. These cells can act in an "endocrine" fashion by releasing their products into the circulation or in a "paracrine" fashion via secretion directed into the local tissue. In antral mucosa, most endocrine

cells consist of gastrin-producing *G cells*. In the body, the endocrine cells produce histamine, which binds the H_2 receptor on parietal cells and leads to increased acid production. These cells are also referred to as *enterochromaffin-like cells*. Other enterochromaffin-like cells in the oxyntic glands include *D cells* (which produce somatostatin) and *X cells* (which produce endothelin). These cells play an important role in modulating acid production.

The aging gastric mucosa is reported to exhibit partial glandular atrophy, with increased connective tissue extracellular matrix in the lamina propria.[126]

The Gastric Cardia

The stomach begins at the most proximal aspect of the gastric folds. The gastric cardia is viewed as an anatomic region of the stomach, approximately 0.1 to 0.4 cm in length, which is located at the proximal cone of the gastric cavity, just distal to the squamocolumnar mucosal boundary (*Z*-line) in normal individuals. Traditionally, the gastric cardia is viewed as having "cardiac" mucosa, which is a mucinous, glandular mucosa typically lacking the oxyntic glands that contain chief and parietal cells (see Fig. 1.13A). However, some individuals show a mixture of both types of glands (mucous and oxyntic) (see later discussion and Chapters 14 and 15).

The strict (physiologic) definition of the GEJ is actually manometric in that the high-pressure zone of the lower esophageal sphincter defines the true distal end of the esophagus. Because manometry is not a normal part of routine endoscopy and the GEJ passes through the diaphragmatic orifice, performing endoscopy on a live, breathing patient makes it difficult to identify precisely the true anatomic location of the GEJ region. The point of flaring of the gastric cavity identified by retroflexion of the endoscope is considered to be a reliable indicator of the beginning of the stomach. However, an axial hiatal hernia or proximal migration of the squamocolumnar mucosal junction in the setting of gastroesophageal reflux (whether physiologic or pathologic) can make it very difficult to identify the anatomic site of the most proximal stomach at the time of endoscopy.

The origin and nature of epithelium in the cardia region of the stomach is controversial. In 1997, Öberg and colleagues[127] found that 26% of endoscopic biopsies obtained at and below the GEJ in 334 patients showed absence of cardia-type mucinous glands. Patients who had cardiac mucosa were also significantly more likely to have GERD. Chandrasoma and coworkers[128] reported that the presence of cardia-type gastric mucosa or "oxyntocardiac mucosa" (combined oxyntic and mucous glands) in the GEJ correlated with acid reflux. They concluded that all cardia-type mucosa in the GEJ region represents metaplastic transformation of the squamous epithelium as a result of reflux. In another autopsy study by the same group,[129] the entire circumference of the GEJ was examined histologically in 18 patients, and cardia-type mucosa was completely absent in 10 (56%). These findings were contradicted by Kilgore and associates,[130] who found cardia-type mucosa at the GEJ in all autopsies of 30 pediatric patients, a population considered to be at low risk for GERD.

Twenty years later, the nature and origin of the cardiac mucosa remains controversial.[131] Increased chronic inflammatory cells are encountered in the cardiac mucosa of 100% of patients with GERD[132] and can even be considered as a baseline normal for the columnar mucosa of the GEJ in the adult population.[133] The extent of cardiac mucosa correlates positively with age, abdominal obesity, and the extent of acid exposure in the distalmost esophagus.[134] The hypothesis has been advanced that GERD reprograms esophageal progenitor cells to first undergo cardiac mucosal metaplasia, which later evolves into intestinal metaplasia.[135] Hence the gastric cardia may be more appropriately conceptualized as a very narrow strip (usually <3 mm) of mucosa at the GEJ which, although present in most apparently normal individuals, may not actually be a normal structure. For a more detailed discussion of the gastric cardia and intestinal metaplasia of the GEJ region, the reader is referred to Chapters 14 and 15.

Small Intestine

The adult *small intestine* is approximately 6 m in length. The *colon* (large intestine) is approximately 1.5 m in length. The first 25 cm of small intestine, the duodenum, is retroperitoneal; the jejunum marks the entry of the small intestine into the peritoneal cavity. The remainder of the small intestine is intraperitoneal until the point at which it enters the colon at the ileocecal valve. The demarcation between the jejunum and ileum is not a clearly defined landmark; the jejunum arbitrarily constitutes the proximal third of the intraperitoneal portion, and the ileum the remainder.

The most distinctive feature of the small intestine is its mucosal lining, which is designed to provide maximal surface area for the purpose of food absorption. The luminal area is enhanced by the presence of circumferentially oriented plica circulares, which protrude into the lumen to impart a corrugated texture to the intestinal surface. When cut in longitudinal section and examined histologically, the plica circulares are seen to provide an undulating substrata for the mucosal lining (Fig. 1.14A). At medium-power magnification, the mucosa consists of innumerable *villi*, which extend into the lumen as finger-like projections covered by epithelial lining cells (see Fig. 1.14B). The central core of lamina propria contains blood vessels, lymphatics, a small population of lymphocytes, eosinophils, mast cells, and scattered fibroblasts and vertically oriented smooth muscle cells. Between the bases of the villi are the pitlike crypts of Lieberkühn, which contain stem cells that replenish and regenerate the epithelium. The crypts extend down to the muscularis mucosae. The muscularis mucosae is a smooth, continuous sheet that serves to anchor the configuration of villi and crypts alike. Villus height is greatest in the duodenum (except in the first portion) and in the proximal jejunum. Figure 1.14C,D represents a tissue sample obtained by a fluoroscopic suction-capsule biopsy technique. In normal individuals, the villus-to-crypt height ratio is between 4:1 and 5:1, but this is variable. In the proximal duodenum, which is exposed to gastric peptic juices to the highest degree, the villus-to-crypt height ratio may reach only 2:1 to 3:1. Within the duodenum are abundant submucosal mucous glands, termed *Brunner glands* (see Fig. 1.14E). They are present immediately distal to the pyloric channel and extend into the second portion of the duodenum. These glands secrete bicarbonate ions (which help neutralize peptic juice as it enters the small intestine), glycoproteins, and

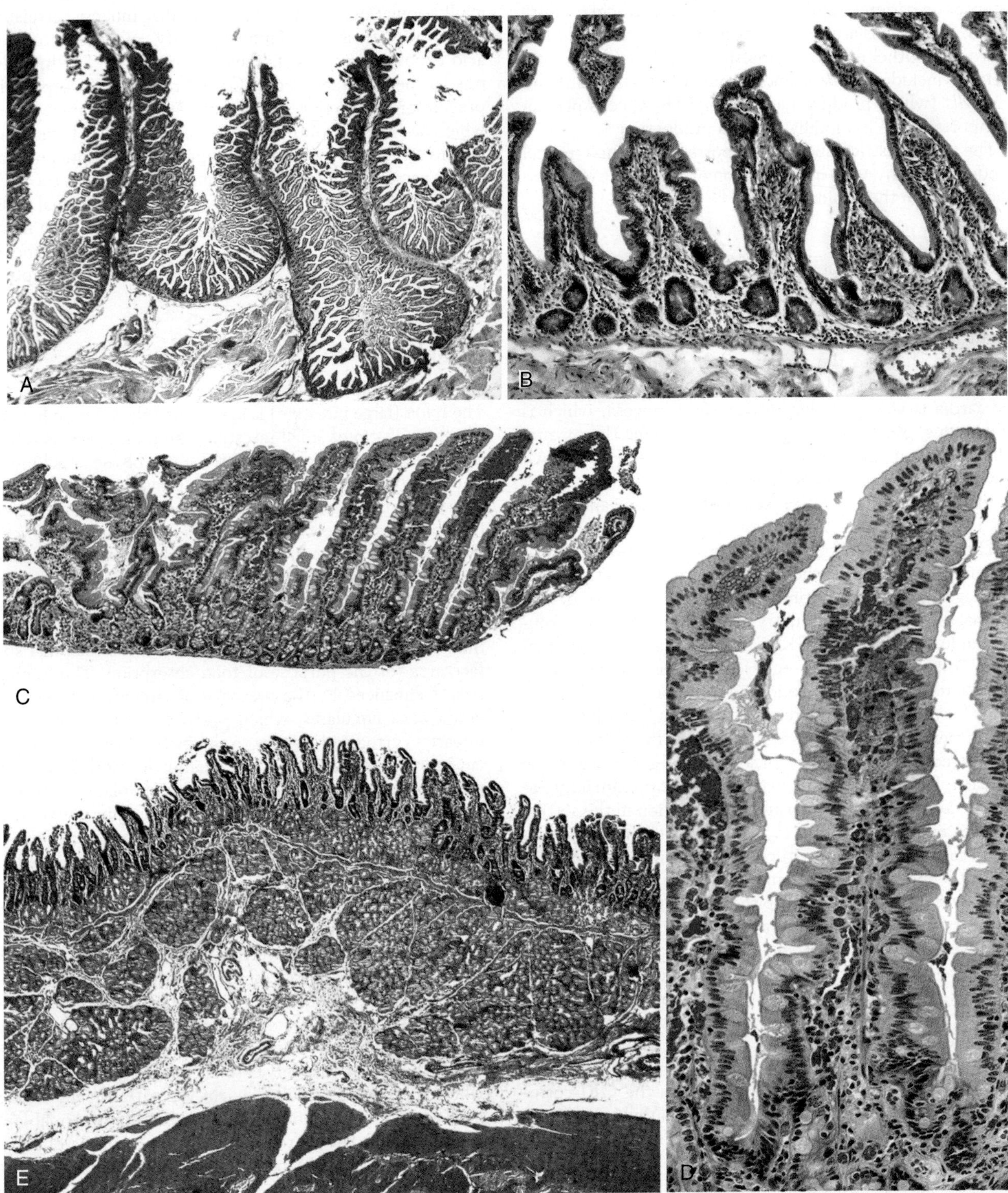

FIGURE 1.14 Normal histology of the small intestine. A, Low-power image of the distal jejunum from a surgical specimen *(longitudinal section).* The mucosa rests on the plica circulares; the muscular layer at the base of the image is the muscularis propria. **B,** Medium-power image shows mucosal villi and short crypts. **C,** Low-power image of a fluoroscopic suction-capsule biopsy of the third portion of the duodenum shows tall villi and short crypts resting on the muscularis mucosa. Vascular congestion is an occasional artefact of the suction technique. **D,** High-power image of a villus shows the vascular stalk and an epithelial layer resting on a basement membrane. Absorptive enterocytes exhibit basal nuclei and an apical "brush border," and there are interspersed goblet cells. Intraepithelial lymphocytes are rare. **E,** Low-power image of the duodenum shows villiform mucosa, a submucosa occupied by Brunner glands, and underlying muscularis propria.

pepsinogen II. Except for their submucosal location, Brunner glands are virtually indistinguishable from the mucous glands of the distal stomach.

The surface epithelium of the small intestinal villi contains three principal cell types. *Columnar absorptive cells* are recognized by the dense array of *microvilli* on their luminal surface (the "brush border") and by an underlying mat of microfilaments (the "terminal web") (see Fig. 1.14D). Interspersed regularly between absorptive cells are mucin-secreting *goblet cells* and a few *endocrine cells*, described later. Goblet cells in the small intestine contain mainly acidic sialated mucins, identifiable by the Alcian blue stain performed at pH 2.5 (acidic). Within the crypts reside stem cells, goblet cells, more abundant endocrine cells, and scattered *Paneth cells*. Paneth cells contain apically oriented, bright eosinophilic granules and help maintain intestinal homeostasis through secretion of growth factors and a variety of antimicrobial proteins (e.g., *defensins*) that play a critical role in mucosal innate immunity against bacterial and viral infection.[136-139] Paneth cells also are implicated in intestinal stem cell regulation and intestinal epithelial cell–immune cell interactions.[140] Paneth cells are located throughout the small intestine and in the proximal portion of the colon, including the cecum, ascending colon, and proximal portion of the transverse colon. They normally are absent from the distal transverse, descending, and sigmoid colon and the rectum.

Enteroendocrine Cells

A diverse population of *enteroendocrine cells* are scattered among the epithelial cells that line the small intestinal villi and small and large intestinal crypts. Comparable cells are present in the epithelium lining the pancreas, biliary tract, lung, thyroid, and urethra. Gut enteroendocrine cells exhibit characteristic morphologic features. In most cells, the cytoplasm contains abundant fine eosinophilic granules that harbor secretory products. Super-resolution microscopy shows that coexpressed hormones may be stored in separate intracellular secretory vesicles[141] or within the same vesicles.[142] The main portion of the cell is located at the base of the epithelium, and the nucleus resides on the luminal side of the cytoplasmic granules. The number of enteroendocrine cells in the small intestine is greater than in the colon. The greatest diversity of enteroendocrine cell types is in the duodenum and jejunum, and they become less diverse distally.[143] 5-Hydroxytryptamine–containing enteroendocrine cells are present in all regions of the small and large intestine and compose the single largest endocrine cell population. A minor proportion of these cells contain substance P. The second largest cell population is that of glicentin cells, which are more numerous in the ileum and colon. Somatostatin cells occur throughout the alimentary tract. Cells that store cholecystokinin, motilin, secretin, or gastric inhibitory polypeptide are more numerous in the duodenum and jejunum compared with the ileum. *Gastrin cells* are few and occur exclusively in the proximal duodenum. Many other peptides and bioactive compounds are released by enteroendocrine cells in the small intestine and colon, including β-endorphin, pro–γ-melanocyte-stimulating hormone (pro–γ-MSH), β-lipotropin, neurotensin, glicentin, glucagon, and pancreatic polypeptide.

Histologic distinction between enteroendocrine cells and Paneth cells is based on the size and color of the eosinophilic cytoplasmic granules. Although both cell types are pyramidal in shape, with broad bases that narrow toward the crypt lumen, enteroendocrine cells are small (approximately 8 μm in height), do not extend to the surface of the epithelial layer, and contain abundant small, deeply eosinophilic granules. These granules may have a basal orientation, with the nucleus displaced apically. Paneth cells are larger (about 20 μm in vertical height), with a luminal apical plasma membrane, and they contain a population of larger, coarse, and brightly eosinophilic granules. Paneth cell granules are always apical relative to the basally located cell nucleus.

The Intestinal Mucosal Immune System

Humans are exposed to an enormous load of environmental antigens through the GI tract, and the ultrastructural surface area of the GI tract exposed to environmental antigens far exceeds that of the skin and pulmonary tract. The immune system must balance antigenic tolerance against immune defense. The function of the intestinal immune system is best addressed on the basis of its anatomy, almost all features of which can be identified by routine light microscopy (Fig. 1.15). Throughout the small intestine and colon are nodules of *lymphoid tissue*, which lie either within the mucosa or within both the mucosa and the submucosa. Lymphoid nodules distort the surface epithelium to produce broad domes rather than villi; within the distal ileum, confluent areas of dense lymphoid tissue become macroscopically visible as *Peyer patches*. The surface epithelium overlying lymphoid nodules contains both columnar absorptive cells and *M (membranous) cells*, the latter found only in the small and large intestinal lymphoid sites. These cells cannot be readily identified by light microscopy. M cells are capable of transporting antigenic macromolecules, intact, from the lumen to the underlying lymphocytes, thus serving as an important afferent limb of the *intestinal immune system*.

Throughout the intestines, T lymphocytes are scattered within the surface epithelium, usually at the base of the epithelial layer. These T cells are referred to as IELs and are generally of the cytotoxic CD8+ phenotype. However, there is remarkable diversity of T-cell subtypes, some unique to the intestine.[144] In normal small intestinal villi, IELs usually decrease in number from the base toward the tip. CD3 immunohistochemistry can aid in detection of IELs, particularly because some lymphocytes have irregular nuclear borders, which make their identification on H&E stain more difficult.[145] In healthy individuals, the duodenum usually contains less than 26 to 29 IELs per 100 epithelial cell nuclei (mean, 11 per 100 in H&E-stained sections, 13 per 100 in CD3-stained sections).[146] The range of IEL counts among healthy individuals can vary widely, from 1.8 to 26 per 100 epithelial nuclei, and there is no correlation between IEL counts and the villus-to-crypt height ratios.[147] The mean number of IELs decreases progressively in the distal small intestine and colon.[148,149] Normal villus IEL counts in the terminal ileum are in the range of 2 IELs per 100 epithelial nuclei.[150] A normal IEL count in the ileum does not preclude abnormality in the duodenum.[151] A modest elevation in IEL counts accompanies many types of inflammatory conditions of the colon.[152]

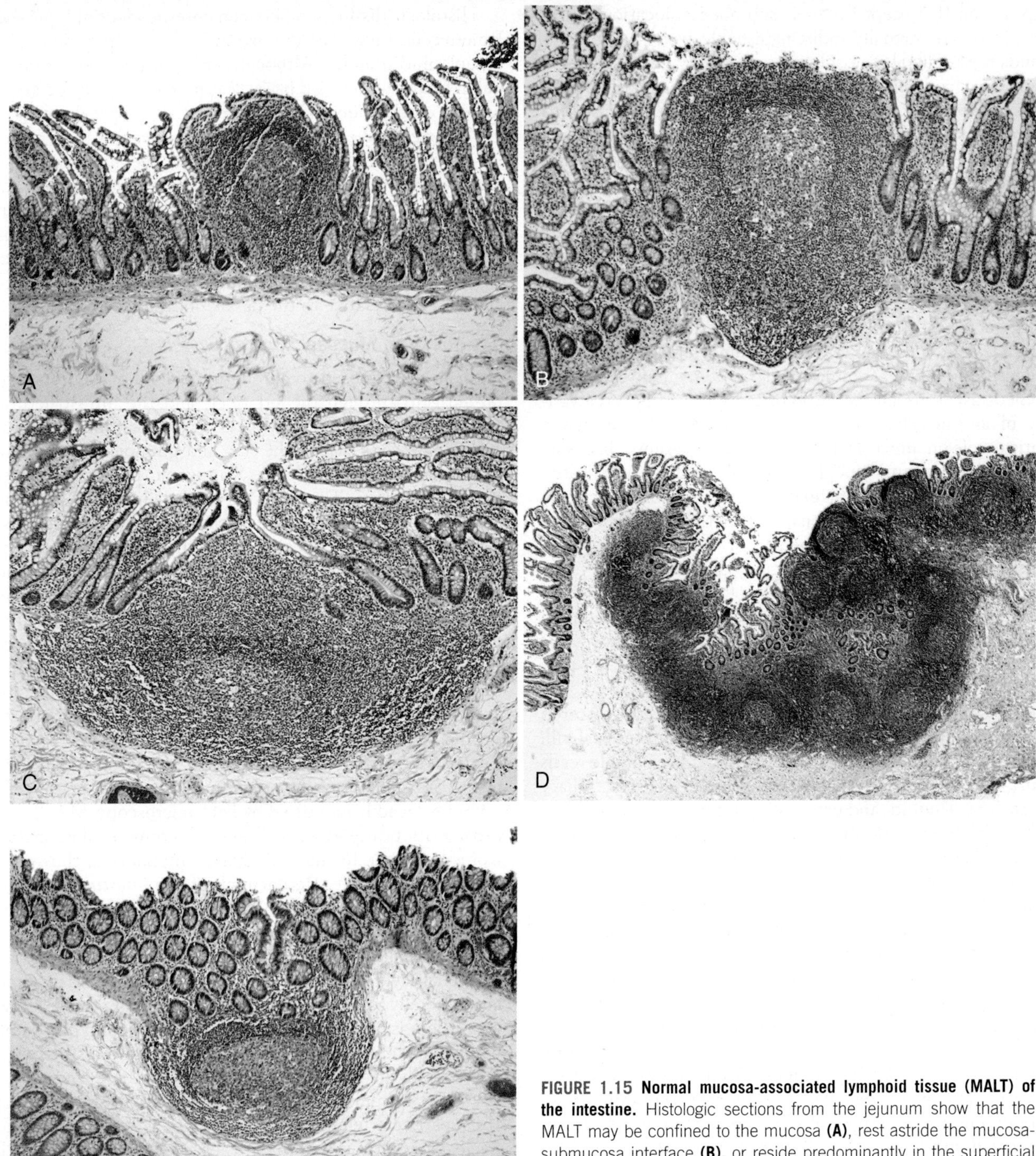

FIGURE 1.15 Normal mucosa-associated lymphoid tissue (MALT) of the intestine. Histologic sections from the jejunum show that the MALT may be confined to the mucosa **(A)**, rest astride the mucosa-submucosa interface **(B),** or reside predominantly in the superficial submucosa **(C).** Peyer patches in the ileum are organized collections of MALT **(D).** A focus of MALT in the colon also is shown **(E).**

The lamina propria contains helper T cells (CD4+), educated B cells, and plasma cells. The lamina propria plasma cells secrete dimeric immunoglobulin A (IgA), IgG, and IgM, which enter into the splanchnic circulation. IgA is transcytosed directly across enterocytes, or across hepatocytes, for secretion into bile; both are mechanisms for delivering IgA into the intestinal lumen. Finally, other antigen-presenting cells located in the lamina propria include macrophages and dendritic cells. The intestinal lymphoid nodules and mucosal lymphocytes, together with isolated lymphoid follicles in the appendix and mesenteric lymph nodes, constitute the mucosa-associated lymphoid tissue (MALT). Although MALT is most prominent in the small intestine, the concept has relevance to both the stomach (as an acquired anatomic compartment) and the colon (in which it also is normally present; see Chapter 31 for details).

Colon

The colon is subdivided into the cecum and the ascending, transverse, and descending colon. Unlike the jejunum and ileum, whose anatomic location and mechanical attachment to the posterior abdomen are entirely dictated by the mesentery, the anatomic locations of the colonic segments are established by other means. The bulbous cecum and the ascending colon constitute the entire portion of the colon on the right side of the abdomen and are fixed in location. Although peritoneal membrane covers their ventral surfaces, the dorsal aspect of both the cecum and the ascending colon adheres directly to the posterior abdominal wall. (The appendix, which inserts into the cecum just below the insertion of the ileum into the cecum, is an intraabdominal viscus that is entirely covered with peritoneum.) The transverse colon begins at the hepatic flexure and swings across the most ventral aspect of the abdominal cavity to reach the splenic flexure. The transverse colon is suspended by the lesser omentum, which reflects off the greater curvature of the stomach. In turn, the greater omentum hangs from the transverse colon. The descending colon is adherent to the left posterior abdominal wall, similar to its counterpart (the ascending colon) on the right side of the peritoneal cavity. The sigmoid colon begins at the pelvic brim and loops ventrally into the peritoneal cavity. The sigmoid colon is the only portion of the colon that is suspended entirely by mesentery. Therefore, it is subject to redundancy that may, rarely, lead to volvulus. Distally, the colon is adherent to the posterior wall of the pelvis beginning at the rectum, at approximately the level of the third sacral vertebra. Halfway along its 15-cm length, the rectum passes between the crura of the peroneal muscles to exit the abdominal cavity.

In normal adults, the length of the colon is quite variable but usually measures in the range of 0.8 to 1.1 m. From the endoscopist's perspective, the rectal canal is approximately 15 cm in length, beginning at the anal verge. The variable length of the sigmoid colon makes identification of further landmarks less reliable, but the splenic flexure is located about 0.4 m proximal to the anal verge, and the hepatic flexure about 0.7 m proximal.

The anatomy of the wall of the colon is unique in that the external layer of the muscularis propria is discontinuous. Instead, three longitudinal strips of smooth muscle lie on top of the inner continuous circumferential smooth muscle layer of the muscularis propria. These longitudinal strips are termed the *tinea coli*. One strip is located at the attachment of the mesentery to the colon. The second and third strips are located equidistant at approximately 120 and 240 degrees around the circumference of the colon. Each strip is approximately 0.5 cm in width, and they become more prominent distally. The tinea coli begin at the cecum, so the bulbous end of the cecum is creased by the outer two tinea coli as they arc to their respective locations on opposite sides of the cecal wall. Notably, throughout the entire length of colon, arteries and veins penetrate through the continuous inner muscle layer at the edges of the tinea coli. These blood vessels constitute the circumferential ramifications of the mesenteric vasculature. Hence there are three double tracks of holes in the inner muscle coat resulting from the orifices created by the penetrating vasculature. It is through these holes that diverticula usually protrude (see Chapter 8). Small tags of adipose tissue, the *epiploic appendages*, also are attached to the colon, at the edges of the nonmesenteric tinea coli 120 and 240 degrees around the circumference of the colon. In this way, two double tracks of intermittent epiploic appendages are created along the entire length of the colon. Protruding diverticula can be difficult to identify because they are in the same circumferential location as the epiploic appendages and may, in fact, protrude *into* epiploic appendages.

The cecum has the widest diameter of the colon, as well as the highest wall tension. Nevertheless, the mural thickness of the normal cecum is only approximately 0.2 cm. The mural thickness increases gradually over the length of the colon and reaches approximately 0.4 cm in the sigmoid colon, which corresponds to the increasingly solid nature of the luminal contents. The lack of a continuous outer longitudinal muscle layer in the muscularis propria implies that the circumferential inner smooth muscle layer dictates the real diameter of the colon. The diameter varies irregularly from mildly pinched constrictions to intervening dilated segments, each approximately 2 to 4 cm in length. From the luminal aspect, the constrictions are termed *haustral folds*, and they are prominent anatomic features notable during endoscopy.

The ileum inserts into the cecum at the *ileocecal valve*. This is a prominent circumferential lip of mucosa and fatty submucosa that extends approximately 0.5 to 1 cm into the cecal lumen. The luminal opening may be slit-shaped or oval. The thickness of the "lip" is approximately 0.3 cm, but it may be thicker in some individuals. The proximal aspect of the ileocecal valve contains small intestinal mucosa, and the distal aspect has colonic mucosa. The mucosal transition occurs at the level of the abrupt luminal convexity of the valve. This structure represents the mechanism that minimizes reflux of cecal contents into the ileum. Whether the "valve" restricts flow of ileal contents into the cecum has never been established; it does not constitute a real muscular sphincter.

The function of the colon is to reclaim luminal water and electrolytes. Unlike the mucosa of the small intestine, the colonic mucosa has no villi and is flat. The mucosa is punctuated by numerous straight, nonbranching, tubular crypts that extend down and touch the muscularis mucosae (Fig. 1.16A). The surface epithelium is composed of columnar absorptive cells, which have shorter and less abundant microvilli than those in the small intestine, and goblet cells. The crypts contain abundant goblet cells, endocrine cells (see the earlier discussion of the small intestine), and undifferentiated crypt cells. Paneth cells are occasionally present at the base of crypts in the cecum and the ascending and proximal transverse colon. IELs are present throughout the colonic mucosal epithelium. Normal counts are less than 5 IELs per 100 epithelial nuclei.[149]

Two sources of potential diagnostic error arise from the normal variation in colonic mucosal microanatomy. First, on occasion, the colonic mucosa exhibits undulation of the surface as a normal anatomic variant (see Fig. 1.16B–D). A particular feature of this variant is that crypts that are located at the base of undulations appear to branch in the upper third of the mucosa (see Fig. 1.16E), akin to the type II crypt branching evident on scanning electron microscopy.[152] Confusion arises when these normal crypts are interpreted

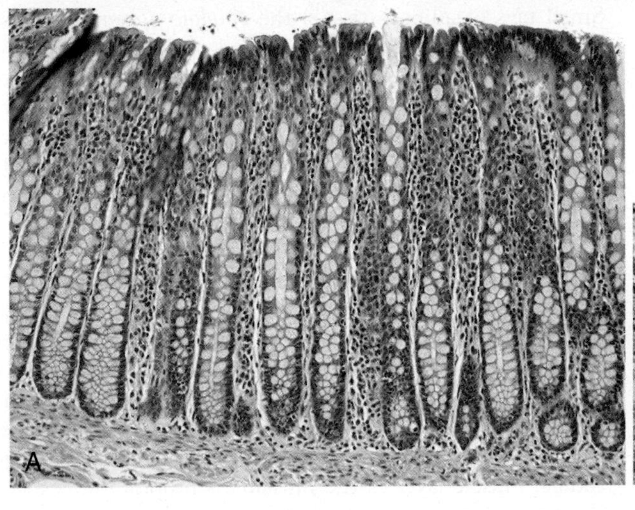

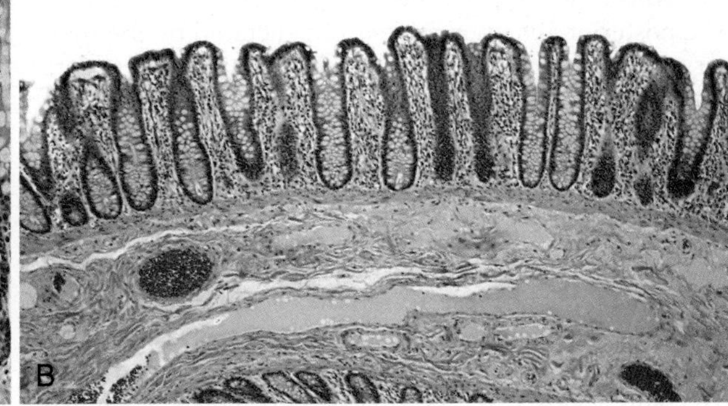

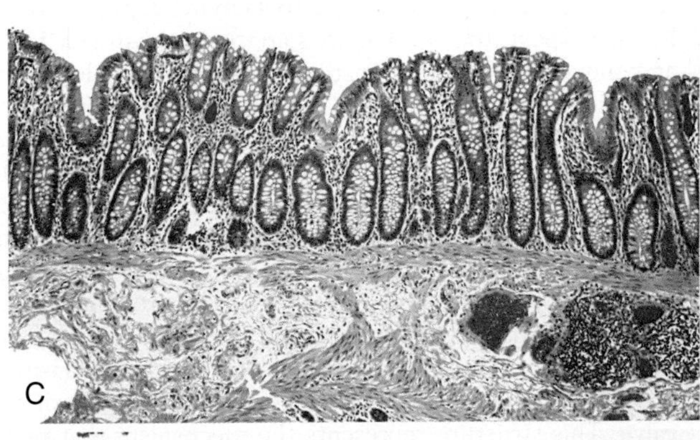

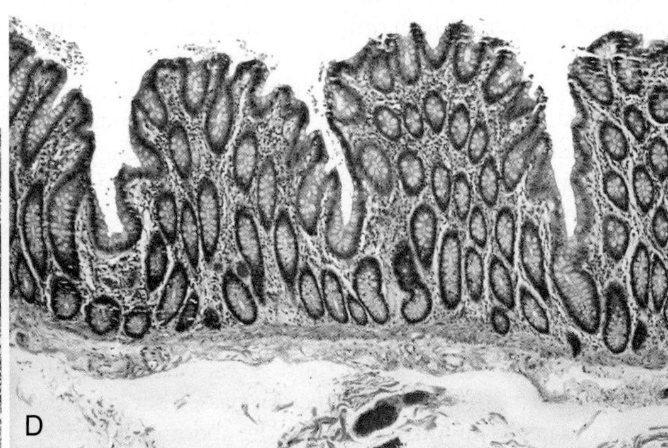

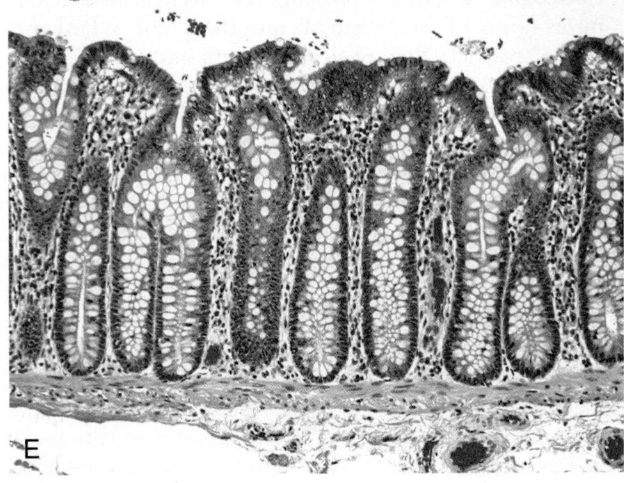

FIGURE 1.16 Normal histology of the colon. A, High-power view shows the characteristic vertically oriented crypts resting on the muscularis mucosae. The delicate lamina propria normally contains a modest population of mononuclear cells, predominantly lymphocytes. **B–D,** Medium-power images of normal colonic mucosa from different portions of the same surgical resection specimen demonstrate variability in the contour of the mucosal surface. **E,** Normal colonic crypts may exhibit branching in the upper third of the mucosal layer.

as evidence of architectural distortion characteristic of chronic colitis. Crypt branching is considered abnormal only when it occurs in the lower two-thirds of the mucosal layer. Second, in the immediate vicinity of a mucosal lymphoid nodule, the crypts are typically distorted.[153] Although this may be obvious if the tissue section transects a lymphoid nodule, a tissue section that passes near but not through a lymphoid nodule will reveal only disorganized crypts. Scanning of multiple serial sections helps identify the lymphoid nodule.

Appendix

The vermiform appendix is a narrow, worm-shaped structure that protrudes from the posteromedial aspect of the cecum, 2 cm (or less) below the insertion of the ileum into the cecum. The appendix is located at the proximal root of the outer tinea coli of the cecum. Because the anterior tinea coli of the cecum is usually prominent, it serves as a guide to locate the appendix. The length of the normal appendix is quite variable, from 2 to 20 cm in length. Its diameter is

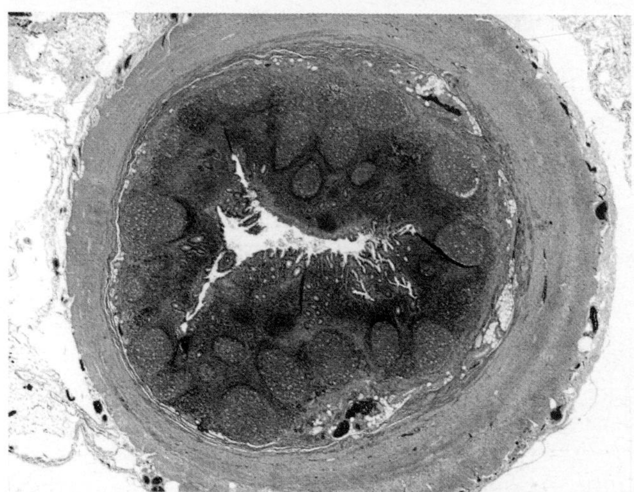

FIGURE 1.17 Normal histology of the appendix. In this low-power view, mucosa-associated lymphoid tissue is visible in the mucosa and submucosa.

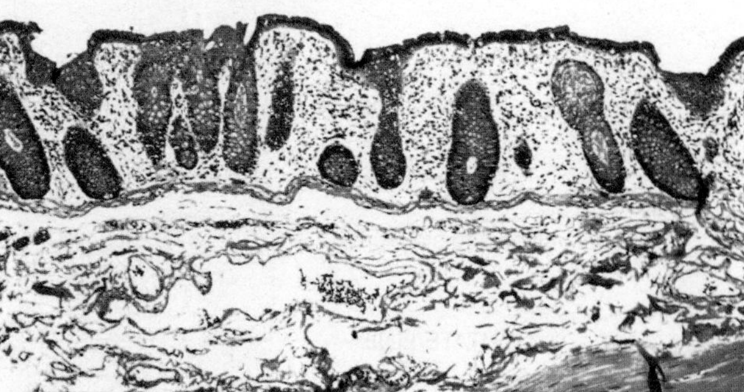

FIGURE 1.18 Normal histology of the rectum, showing the more rudimentary glands, lack of extension down to the muscularis mucosae, and mild crypt distortion.

consistent and uniform along its length, approximately 0.3 to 0.5 cm. It has a rudimentary mesentery only on a portion of its length. The intraperitoneal location of the appendix also is variable. The appendix may lie behind the cecum, hang over the brim of the pelvis, or lie in front or behind the ileum. However, in any individual, the location is relatively fixed.

The appendix is completely invested by peritoneum, and it has both an inner circumferential layer and a fully circumferential outer longitudinal muscle layer of the muscularis propria. The mucosa of the appendix is colonic in type. However, the most prominent feature is the abundance of lymphoid tissue that lies within both the lamina propria and the submucosa (Fig. 1.17). The lymphoid tissue is particularly prominent in younger individuals and dissipates gradually over a person's lifetime. The concept that the appendix undergoes normal "fibrous obliteration" late in life has long been postulated. Alternative proposals include the concepts of subclinical episodes of appendicitis caused by fecaliths[154] or results from stromal proliferation in response to clinically silent mucosal or axial neuromas caused by repeated subclinical attacks of appendiceal inflammation.[155] Regardless, preemptive appendectomy at the time of pancreas transplantation has shown that obliterative fibrosis is present in approximately 30% of specimens.[156]

Rectum and Anus

The rectum begins within the abdominal cavity and tapers rapidly to the base of the pelvis. The discontinuous tinea coli converge and unite, again constituting a complete outer longitudinal smooth muscle layer of the muscularis propria. Where the rectum exits the peritoneal cavity to enter the anal canal, it is completely invested by both inner and outer smooth muscle coats of the muscularis propria and acquires an adventitia rather than a serosal covering.

There are subtle differences in the normal histology of the distal rectal mucosa.[157] Compared with nonrectal colonic mucosa, distal rectal mucosa exhibits crypts that are not as closely spaced and are slightly shorter (Fig. 1.18). Unlike the crypts in the rest of the colon, those in the rectum do not extend directly down to the muscularis mucosae. The crypts may be slightly dilated or tortuous and are somewhat less numerous. The surface epithelium may be slightly cuboidal rather than tall columnar. The intervening lamina propria contains a moderate number of lymphocytes, plasma cells, macrophages, and occasional neutrophils. Scattered muciphages are common in the lamina propria of the rectum, particularly in older adults. Presumably, they represent the vestiges of previous mucosal injury. It is important to recognize the simplified and somewhat distorted mucosal architecture of the distal rectal columnar mucosa as normal and not as indicating true architectural distortion characteristic of chronic inflammatory bowel disease.

The anal canal is a complex anatomic structure that shows considerable individual variation in mucosal histology[157] (see Chapter 32). First, it is critical to understand the macroscopic anatomy of the anal canal (Fig. 1.19). The rectal vault descends into the muscular anal canal, which is composed of the muscularis propria of the anal canal (the internal anal sphincter) and the anorectal skeletal musculature (the external anal sphincter). The external anal sphincter is a complex arrangement of perineal muscle fibers, the most proximal of which is the puborectalis muscle (sling). The puborectalis muscle loops from the pubis bone around the upper portion of the anal canal and back to the pubis, imparting a sharp mucosal angle to the posterior aspect of the rectal vault. As the rectum enters the anal canal, the transverse folds of the colorectal mucosa end, and the mucosa aligns along the long axis into 6 to 10 vertical *anal columns*. The anal columns terminate about halfway down the anal canal, with interconnecting semicircular *anal valves* that delineate discrete mucosal recesses termed the *anal sinuses*. Anal mucin-producing glands empty into the anal sinuses. These anal valves and sinuses are particularly prominent in children but become less pronounced with age. The anal columns may actually protrude into the lumen, earning the name *anal papillae*. The circumferential ring of anal valves and sinuses is termed the *dentate line*. Immediately below the dentate line is a zone of smooth mucosa, which flares at the *anal verge* to become anal skin, which is visible on external examination. The overall distance of the anal canal, in vivo, averages 4.2 cm in normal adults.

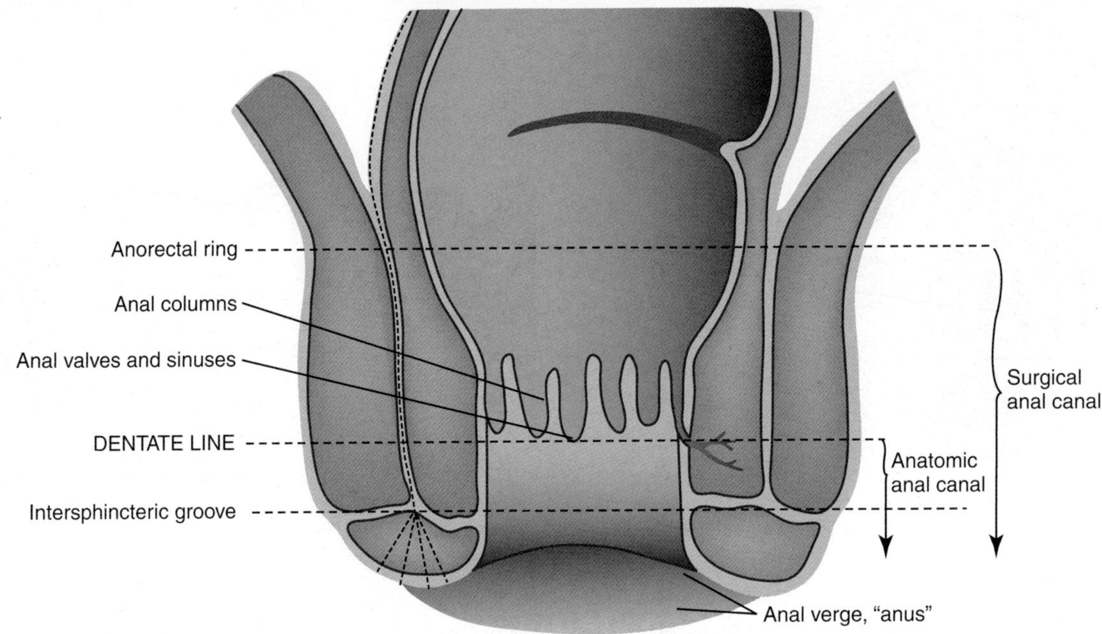

FIGURE 1.19 Macroscopic anatomy of the anal canal; submucosal mucin-producing glands are shown emptying into an anal sinus.

The mucosa of the anal canal is divided into three zones according to the type of epithelial lining. The upper third, above the anal columns, is rectal columnar mucosa. Next is the *anal transitional zone,* which spans the distance of the anal columns down to the dentate line, approximately 1 cm. Distal to the dentate line is a nonkeratinizing stratified squamous mucosa; at the anal verge, this becomes keratinized skin and contains adnexal structures typical of perineal skin.

The mucosa of the anal transitional zone is the most variable (Fig. 1.20). In some instances, nonkeratinizing anal squamous mucosa extends up the anal columns and transitions directly into the columnar rectal mucosa at its most proximal extent. However, in many individuals, a *transitional mucosa* is present that consists of four to nine cell layers that are neither squamous nor columnar but rather stratified cuboidal or polygonal and overlie a basal cell layer. Occasional mucin goblet cells may be present as well. Transitional mucosa may be present, especially in the anal sinuses, extending proximal from the nonkeratinizing squamous mucosa of the lower anal canal and transitioning to rectal columnar mucosa proximally. Regardless of whether the anal canal mucosa is columnar, transitional, or nonkeratinizing squamous, this region retains the designation of the *anal transitional zone.*

LYMPH NODE DRAINAGE AND LYMPHATICS OF THE TUBAL GUT

General principles of lymphatic drainage are straightforward.[158] Lymphatics in the mucosa or submucosa drain through the muscularis propria and then enter either into larger lymphatic channels located in the perivisceral adventitia or into a pedicle or mesentery. However, there are key anatomic features in each segment of the tubal gut that have become increasingly important to understand because of the intraoperative use of sentinel lymph node biopsy to identify lymph nodes that drain invasive carcinomas of the gut and potentially harbor metastatic cancer.[159-161]

Esophagus

The mucosal anatomy of the esophagus bears one key difference from the remainder of the tubal gut: The squamous mucosa overlies a definitive layer of lamina propria, which is supported by the muscularis mucosae and submucosa. In the stomach, small intestine, and colon, the lamina propria is intimately interdigitated with the epithelium, so the bases of epithelial glands or crypts lie directly on the muscularis mucosae. Hence, unlike elsewhere, in the esophagus there is a rich mucosal plexus of lymphatics in the lamina propria oriented predominantly in a longitudinal direction.[162] This plexus connects with less extensive plexuses in the submucosa and muscularis propria and eventually drains to regional lymph nodes. Because of this arrangement, esophageal cancers can display early and extensive intramucosal, submucosal, and mural spread along the axis of the esophagus, well beyond the margins of grossly visible tumor.

Stomach

In the stomach, lymphatic channels are absent from the superficial lamina propria but are present in the interglandular region of the deeper portions of the mucosa.[163] They converge into thicker channels that pierce the muscularis mucosae and enter a submucosal plexus. From there, they drain into the lymphatic plexus between the circular and longitudinal layers of the muscularis propria, which runs along the muscle fibers to form a polygonal meshwork. Valves are present in this intramural network. From there, larger lymphatic channels track along the major arteries and veins into the gastric and colonic mesenteries.

Small Intestine

The lymphatic drainage of the small intestine is distinct.[164] The lamina propria of each villus contain three or more lymphatic channels that run parallel to one another along the

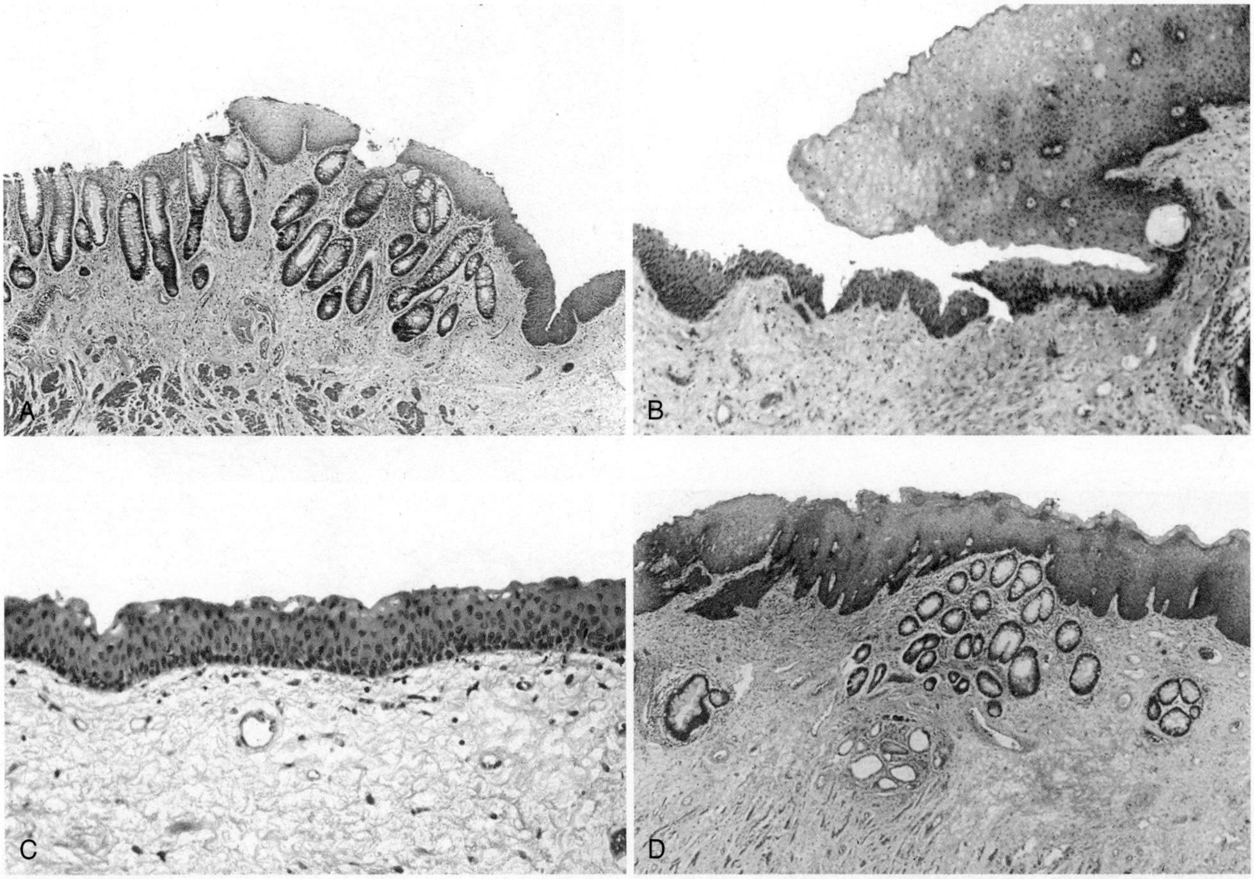

FIGURE 1.20 Normal histology of the anal canal. A, Mucosal squamocolumnar transition at the top of an anal column. **B,** Mucosal transition from transitional mucosa *(left)* to anal squamous mucosa *(right)* at the lip of an anal sinus. **C,** Anal transitional mucosa. **D,** Anal verge, with epidermis overlying dermal sebaceous glands.

long axis. Given the heavy flow of chylomicrons and fatty droplets from the absorptive epithelium to the lymphatic space, the endothelial lining typically contains numerous gaps. These lymphatic channels collect into central lacteals located within the deeper part of the villi, which have a continuous endothelial lining and a reticulin fiber sheath to which smooth muscle fibers attach. The smooth muscle fibers are also oriented longitudinally in the villi, and they intermittently contract to force lymph along the channels. The lacteals anastomose with each other at the base of each villus and form an expanded sinus network, the intravillous lymphatic sinus. Penetrating lymphatic channels then traverse the muscularis mucosae to enter an extensive submucosal lymphatic plexus. This latter plexus drains through lymphatics in the muscularis propria to large conducting lymphatics in the mesentery and, thence, to the major lymphatic ducts located mainly parallel to the larger vascular structures and at the mesenteric root.

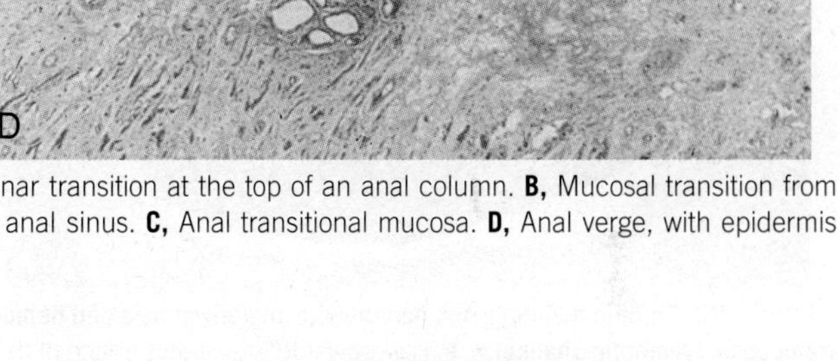

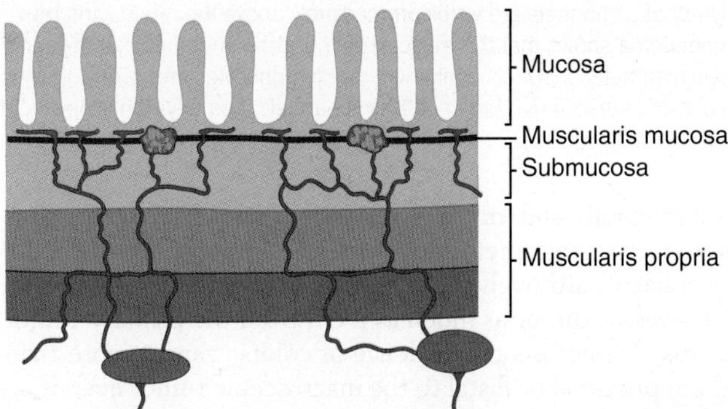

FIGURE 1.21 Diagram of the lymphatic system that drains the colon wall. Terminal twigs of the lymphatics lie just above the muscularis mucosae, at the base of the lamina propria. There are occasional dilated lymphatic spaces that span the muscularis mucosae. There is a limited submucosal lymphatic plexus, and there are plexuses within the muscularis propria. Immediately adjacent to the muscularis propria are epicolic lymph nodes, which drain toward the mesenteric root through paracolic, intermediate, and principal lymph nodes *(not shown)*. (*From Crawford JM. Principles of anatomy. In: Rustgi AK, Crawford JM, eds. Gastrointestinal Cancers: Biology and Clinical Management. Philadelphia: Saunders; 2003:121-131.*)

Colon

In the colon, a lymphatic plexus lies just underneath the muscularis mucosae. This plexus sends small branches into the deep mucosa at the level of the bases of the colonic crypts to form a narrow lymphatic zone located immediately above the muscularis mucosae.[165] The submucosal plexus drains to an intramural lymphatic plexus located between the inner circular and outer discontinuous longitudinal layers of the muscularis propria (Fig. 1.21). As in the small intestine, lymphatic channels that exit the colonic wall enter the mesocolon in a radial pattern of drainage. Intramucosal,

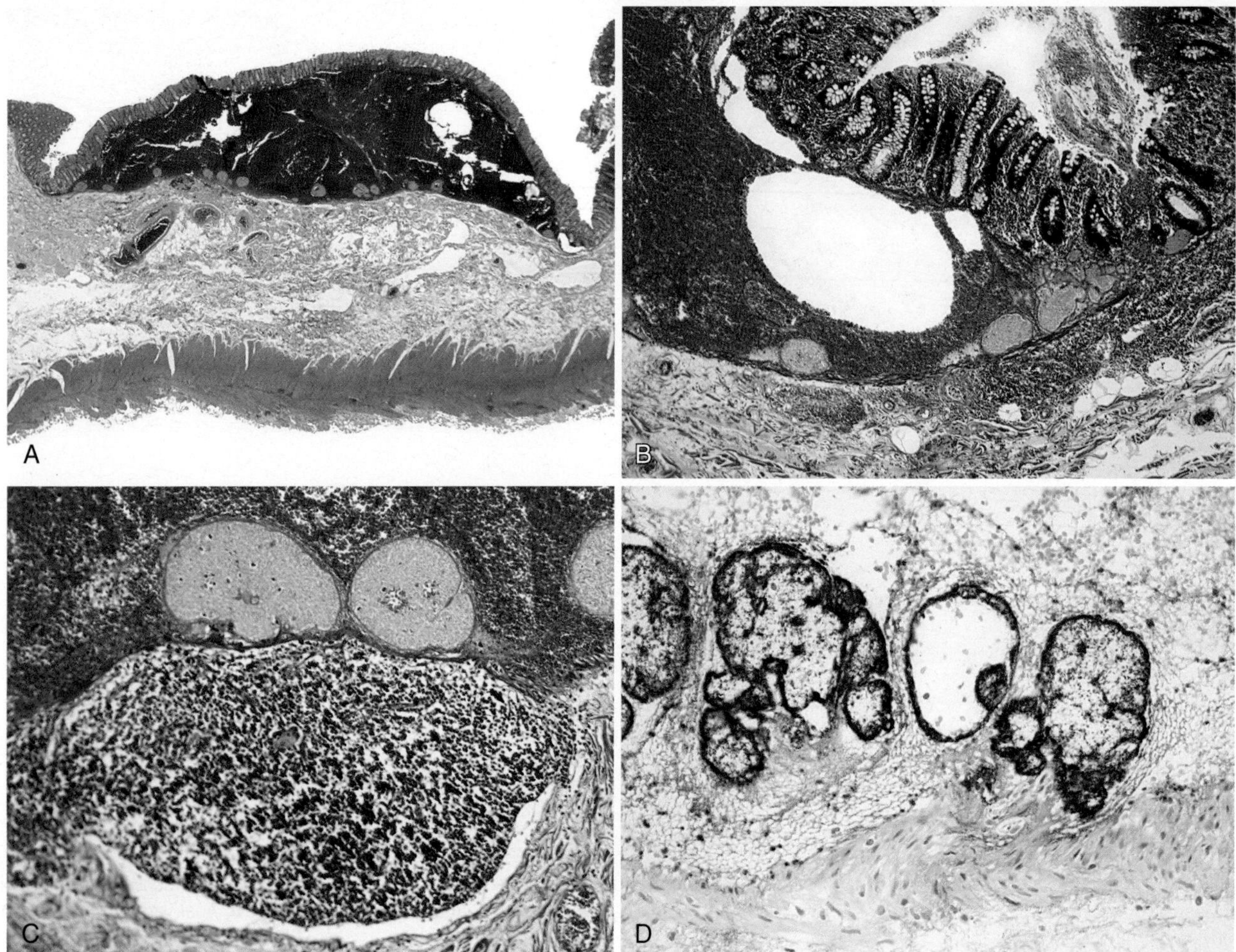

FIGURE 1.22 Colonic histology of a patient with angiodysplasia and hemorrhage into the base of the mucosa, which enables ready visualization of the intramucosal lymphatic channels. A, Low-power full-thickness image of the colon demonstrates an intramucosal hematoma. Lightly eosinophilic-stained lymphatic channels are visible immediately above the muscularis mucosa (hematoxylin and eosin stain). **B,** Medium-power image of the edge of the hematoma shows that the muscularis mucosae underlies both hematoma and lymphatic channels (Trichrome stain). **C,** Higher-power image shows two lymphatic channels containing rare lymphocytes and overlying mucosa-associated lymphoid tissue (trichrome stain). **D,** Factor VIII immunostain confirms the vascular origin of these channels. Some lymphocyte nuclei are evident within the lymphatic space (hematoxylin counterstain).

submucosal, and mural lymphatic channels may be sites for microscopic metastasis. However, in contrast with the esophagus, although there may be intramural lateral spread of invasive tumor as much as 2 cm from the primary tumor focus,[166] microscopic evidence of colonic cancer more than 2 cm proximal or distal to the macroscopic tumor mass is an exceedingly rare occurence.[167]

The existence of lymphatic channels in the colorectal mucosa located immediately above the muscularis mucosae is often overlooked by pathologists, particularly in light of the fact that lymphatic channels are very difficult to identify on routine H&E-stained tissue sections (Fig. 1.22).

The number of intramucosal lymphatics does not increase in inflammatory conditions (e.g., ulcerative colitis) but does increase in association with some pathologic changes such as widening of the muscularis mucosae, hyperplasia of the muscle fibers, filiform changes in the mucosa, and hyperplasia of the MALT.[168] In colonic specimens with epithelial dysplasia (adenomatous change), an association between dysplastic epithelium and ectatic, and quantitatively increased, lymphatics may be present. However, in cases with carcinoma, no relationship between malignant tumor and quantity of intramucosal lymphatics has been identified. Deposits of carcinoma within intramucosal lymphatics typically occur only within the immediate vicinity of the primary tumor mass. Whether intramucosal lymphatics are involved in clinically significant colorectal tumor metastasis remains to be determined. Abundant data suggest that carcinomas confined to the mucosa (intramucosal) are not at significant risk of lymph node metastasis.[169] Invasion of carcinoma into the submucosa remains a biologic requisite for regional or distant cancer metastasis.[170]

Lymph Nodes

The esophagus drains into numerous lymph node groups, including five directly adjacent to the esophagus in paratracheal, peribronchial, paraesophageal, carinal, and posterior mediastinal locations; supraclavicular lymph nodes may also exhibit drainage from the esophageal region (Fig. 1.23). The cervical esophagus also drains into the internal jugular and cervical lymph nodes, the upper tracheal lymph nodes, and, potentially, the supraclavicular lymph nodes. The infradiaphragmatic portion of the esophagus drains into the left gastric nodes along the lesser curvature and into the ring of lymph nodes surrounding the cardia.

Lymphatics from the gastric wall drain into numerous lymph nodes distributed in chains along the greater and lesser curvatures, in the cardia region, and in the splenic hilum (Fig. 1.24). As detailed by Fenoglio-Preiser and colleagues,[162] the drainage patterns are as follows:

- Lesser curvature and lower esophagus: left gastric lymph nodes
- Pylorus: right gastric and hepatic lymph nodes along the course of the hepatic artery
- Cardia: pericardial lymph nodes surrounding the GEJ and left gastric lymph nodes
- Proximal portion of the greater curvature: pancreaticosplenic lymph nodes in the hilum of the spleen
- Distal part of the greater curvature: right gastroepiploic lymph nodes in the greater omentum, and to the pyloric lymph nodes at the head of the pancreas

Effluents from all lymph node groups ultimately pass to the celiac nodes surrounding the main celiac axis.

There are approximately 200 mesenteric lymph nodes in the small and large intestinal mesentery. Small mesenteric lymph nodes lie along the radial and arcuate ramifications of the distal mesenteric vasculature subjacent to the bowel wall (Fig. 1.25). Larger ones lie along the primary arcades and major intestinal arteries, especially near the bifurcation of major vessels. The major lymph node groups are located at the root of the superior and inferior mesenteric arteries. These lymphatics converge in lymph nodes located at the mesenteric root. Lymph fluid passes from there to the *cisterna chyli*, a lymphatic sac that lies in the retroperitoneum behind the aorta and immediately below the diaphragm (Fig. 1.26). The cisterna chyli gives rise to the thoracic duct, which tracks alongside the aorta into the thorax. From there, it runs between the aorta and the azygos vein and receives lymphatic branches from the posterior mediastinal structures, the intercostals, and the jugular, subclavian, and bronchomediastinal ducts before emptying into the angle between the left internal jugular and left subclavian veins.

FIGURE 1.23 Lymph nodes of the esophagus are separated into six regional node systems. (*From Crawford JM. Principles of anatomy. In: Rustgi AK, Crawford JM, eds. Gastrointestinal Cancers: Biology and Clinical Management. Philadelphia: Saunders; 2003:121–131.*)

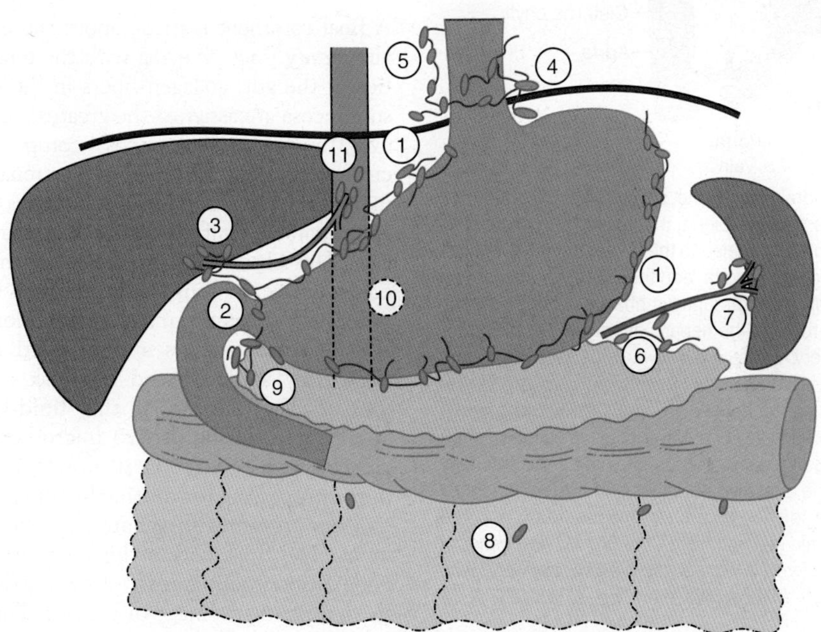

FIGURE 1.24 Lymph nodes that drain the stomach and pancreas are separated into (1) lesser curvature and left gastric lymph nodes, (2) right gastric lymph nodes, (3) hepatic hilar lymph nodes, (4) pericardial lymph nodes, (5) paraesophageal lymph nodes, (6 and 7) pancreaticosplenic lymph nodes, (8) gastroepiploic lymph nodes in the greater omentum, (9) pancreaticoduodenal lymph nodes, (10) paraaortic lymph nodes, and (11) celiac lymph nodes. The celiac lymph nodes drain into the cisterna chyli *(not shown)*, and from there into the thoracic duct. (*From Crawford JM. Principles of anatomy. In: Rustgi AK, Crawford JM, eds. Gastrointestinal Cancers: Biology and Clinical Management. Philadelphia: Saunders; 2003:121–131.*)

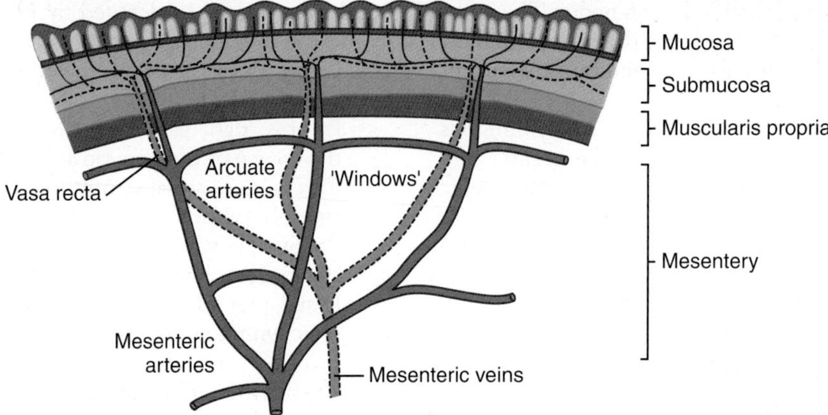

FIGURE 1.25 Vascular supply of the small intestine and colon. Radially oriented mesenteric arteries are interconnected by arcuate arteries, providing extensive anastomoses between regions of the arterial circulation. Terminal arteries penetrate the muscularis propria and ramify in an extensive arteriolar network in the submucosa. Terminal arterioles enter the mucosa to supply intramucosal capillary arcades. Mucosal blood exits through venules back into the submucosa and then by veins through the muscularis propria into the mesenteric venous system. Unlike the mesenteric arterial system, there are only limited anastomotic connections between mesenteric veins, and drainage is essentially linear into the portal venous system. Lymphatic channels accompany the major blood vessels of the mesentery *(not shown)*; the vascular architecture provides orientation for location of small mesenteric lymph nodes lying along the radial and arcuate arteries, especially at the bifurcations of the arteries. (*From Crawford JM. Principles of anatomy. In: Rustgi AK, Crawford JM, eds. Gastrointestinal Cancers: Biology and Clinical Management. Philadelphia: Saunders; 2003:121–131.*)

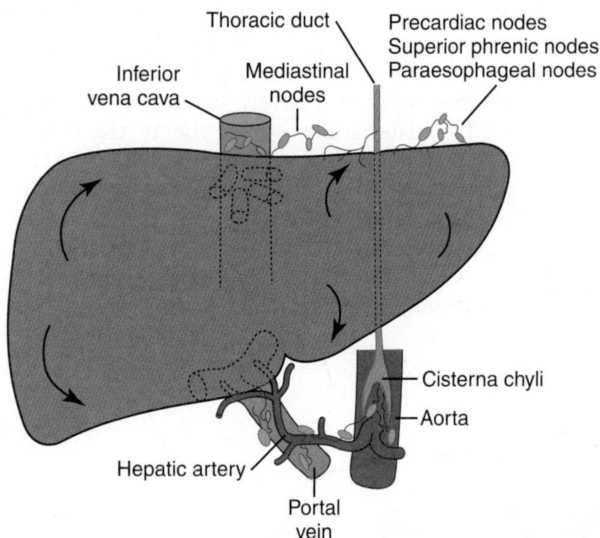

FIGURE 1.26 Lymph node drainage of the splanchnic root and liver. Lymph from the intestines gathers along the mesenteric roots *(not shown)* and travels immediately cephalad to the cisterna chyli, at the celiac root on the ventral aspect of the aorta, and then to the thoracic duct. The hepatic corpus drains primarily through lymphatics in the portal tree *(not shown)* and then exits through the hepatic hilum into lymph nodes adjacent to the hepatic artery. These drain toward the celiac root and cisterna chyli. There is limited lymphatic drainage of the corpus into lymphatics that are situated along the hepatic veins and collect into lymph nodes alongside the inferior vena cava. The liver capsule collects lymph from the superficial portions of the liver corpus, draining anteroinferiorly toward the hilum and hepatic artery lymph nodes and posterosuperiorly toward lymph nodes of the inferior vena cava, mediastinum, and the paraesophageal/diaphragmatic region. (*From Crawford JM. Principles of anatomy. In: Rustgi AK, Crawford JM, eds. Gastrointestinal Cancers: Biology and Clinical Management. Philadelphia: Saunders; 2003:121–131.*)

Distal rectal lymphatics drain laterally along the course of the inferior hemorrhoidal vessels, and from there into paraaortic lymph nodes to end in the hypogastric, obturator, and internal iliac nodes. Alternatively, they follow the superior rectal artery to drain into lymph nodes in the sigmoid mesocolon near the origin of the inferior mesenteric artery. Lymphatic fluid drains from the anus into the endopelvic fascia along the lateral aspect of the ischiorectal space, to the genital femoral sulcus on either side, and ultimately to the inferomedial group of superficial inguinal lymph nodes. Some anal canal lymphatics connect with the rectal lymphatics, whereas others may drain to the common iliac, middle and lateral sacral, lower gluteal, external iliac, or deep inguinal lymph nodes.

The Interstitium

A final comment is made about the interstitial spaces of the alimentary tract. Starting with the tensile mechanical properties of the gut, collagen fibers in the muscularis propria and submucosa are assigned the greatest contribution.[171,172] However, the mucosal-submucosal composite also appears to be a critical contributor to the tensile strength of this tubular organ in both the radial and longitudinal axes.[173] The tensile strength is comparable to, if not higher than, that of the muscularis propria. This observation is particularly notable in the proximal colon, where the muscularis propria is both at its thinnest and potentially subject to massive distension without rupture.

The submucosa is a fluid-filled interstitial space supported by an interlaced network of thick collagen bundles.[174] The volume of this fluid-filled compartment is appreciated during in vivo microscopy (as during endomicroscopy) or endoscopic ultrasonography, but not following tissue processing for routine histology; freezing tissue before fixation preserves the anatomy of this interstitial compartment. The fluid within this compartment drains to lymph nodes, potentially constituting a striking "headwaters" for the lymphatic drainage of the gut. The biology of this tissue space may be of substantive relevance to understanding cancer metastasis, especially from early stage cancers.[175]

The full reference list may be accessed online at Elsevier eBooks for Practicing Clinicians.

BOX 2.2 American Society for Gastrointestinal Endoscopy Recommendations for Surveillance and Management of Dysplasia for Patients with Inflammatory Bowel Disease

We recommend that all patients with ulcerative colitis (UC) or Crohn's disease colitis undergo a screening colonoscopy 8 years after disease onset to (1) reevaluate extent of disease and (2) initiate surveillance for colorectal neoplasia.

We recommend surveillance colonoscopy be performed every 1 to 3 years beginning after 8 years of disease in patients with UC with macroscopic or histologic evidence of inflammation proximal to and including the sigmoid colon and for patients with Crohn's colitis with more than one-third of colon involvement.

We recommend chromoendoscopy with targeted biopsies as the preferred surveillance technique to maximize dysplasia detection.

We suggest that chromoendoscopy-targeted biopsies are sufficient for dysplasia surveillance in patients with inflammatory bowel disease (IBD) and that consideration should be given to taking two biopsies from each colon segment for histologic staging to assess extent and severity of inflammation.

We suggest that random biopsies with targeted biopsies of any suspicious-appearing lesions remain a reasonable alternative for dysplasia surveillance if the yield of chromoendoscopy is reduced by significant underlying inflammation, significant pseudopolyposis, or poor preparation or if chromoendoscopy is not available.

We recommend that patients with IBD whose polypoid dysplastic lesions have been removed completely receive endoscopic surveillance at 1 to 6 months and at 12 months, with yearly surveillance examinations thereafter.

We suggest that patients with IBD whose nonpolypoid dysplastic lesions have been removed completely receive endoscopic surveillance at 1 to 6 months and at 12 months, with yearly surveillance thereafter.

We recommend proctocolectomy in patients with IBD if a detected lesion is not endoscopically resectable, if there is evidence of dysplasia at the base of the lesion, or if endoscopically invisible high-grade dysplasia or multifocal low-grade dysplasia is found in the colon during a high-quality chromoendoscopy examination.

From American Society for Gastrointestinal Endoscopy Standards of Practice Committee, Shergill AK, Lightdale JR, Bruining DH, et al. The role of endoscopy in inflammatory bowel disease. Gastrointest Endosc. *2015;81:1101–1121.*

BOX 2.3 SCENIC International Consensus Summary of Recommendations for Surveillance and Management of Dysplasia in Patients with Inflammatory Bowel Disease

DETECTION OF DYSPLASIA ON SURVEILLANCE COLONOSCOPY

When performing surveillance with white-light colonoscopy, high definition is recommended rather than standard definition.

When performing surveillance with standard-definition colonoscopy, chromoendoscopy is recommended rather than white-light colonoscopy.

When performing surveillance with high-definition colonoscopy, chromoendoscopy is suggested rather than white-light colonoscopy.

When performing surveillance with standard-definition colonoscopy, narrow-band imaging is not suggested in place of white-light colonoscopy.

When performing surveillance with high-definition colonoscopy, narrow-band imaging is not suggested in place of white-light colonoscopy.

When performing surveillance with image-enhanced high-definition colonoscopy, narrow-band imaging is not suggested in place of chromoendoscopy.

MANAGEMENT OF DYSPLASIA DISCOVERED ON SURVEILLANCE COLONOSCOPY

After complete removal of endoscopically resectable polypoid dysplastic lesions, surveillance colonoscopy is recommended rather than colectomy.

After complete removal of endoscopically resectable nonpolypoid dysplastic lesions, surveillance colonoscopy is suggested rather than colectomy.

For patients with endoscopically invisible dysplasia (confirmed by a gastrointestinal pathologist) referral is suggested to an endoscopist with expertise in inflammatory bowel disease surveillance using chromoendoscopy with high-definition colonoscopy

From Laine L, Kaltenbach T, Barkun A, et al. SCENIC international consensus statement on surveillance and management of dysplasia in inflammatory bowel disease. Gastroenterology. *2015;148:639–651.*

The AGA and BSG guidelines previously recommended proctocolectomy in cases of "flat" HGD.[32] More recently, it has been suggested that if LGD or HGD is confirmed on random biopsy (so-called "invisible dysplasia") by an expert GI pathologist, a repeat colonoscopy should be performed with enhanced imaging techniques, such as chromoendoscopy, to assess for the presence of a visible lesion, which may be resected; if a visible lesion is not identified, colectomy should be considered.[30] Recommendations from the ASGE and SCENIC international consensus on the detection and management of dysplasia in patients with IBD are listed in Box 2.2 and Box 2.3, respectively.[19,31]

Studies have demonstrated that the use of chromoendoscopy can greatly increase the detection rate of dysplasia in patients with UC who have been enrolled in a surveillance program.[33] Chromoendoscopy with targeted biopsies revealed significantly more dysplastic lesions than conventional colonoscopy with random biopsies. The overall sensitivity of chromoendoscopy for predicting neoplasia was 93% to 97%.[34-36] Given these findings, consensus guidelines from several organizations have endorsed the use of chromoendoscopy in surveillance colonoscopy by trained endoscopists.[22,24] As more data regarding chromoendoscopy become available and new imaging techniques are developed, guidelines for surveillance endoscopy in patients with IBD will be refined to reflect these advances. It is also likely that molecular biology techniques will play a more important role in the future as an adjunct to endoscopic biopsy.[37]

SCREENING AND SURVEILLANCE GUIDELINES FOR COLON POLYPS

The following is a review of the management of colonic polyps in patients who do not have IBD.[38,39] This summary includes screening for colon polyps, surveillance after polypectomy and resection for CRC, and the approach to the patient with a malignant polyp.

CRC is the second most common cause of cancer death in the United States. The overall mortality rate approaches 60%. Approximately 5% to 6% of individuals born in the United States will develop colon cancer in their lifetime, and 2.5% will die of the disease. The incidence does not vary significantly between men and women. It is estimated that almost 147,950 new cases of CRC will be diagnosed and 53,200 deaths will occur from CRC in the United States in 2020.[40] CRC is a suitable disease for screening because it is a common malignancy with a long, asymptomatic preclinical phase and a high survival rate if detected in its early stage. Prevention of CRC should be achievable by application of screening programs to identify asymptomatic patients with adenomatous polyps and to remove them. In The National Polyp Study, colonoscopic polypectomy decreased the expected incidence of CRC by 53%.[41] Indeed the risk of developing and/or dying from CRC has been decreasing in adults 55 years and older, which has been attributed to many factors, including use of colonoscopy and endoscopic polypectomy.[42]

Definition and Clinical Considerations

Small (<1 cm) tubular adenomas are extremely common and have a low risk of becoming malignant. Only a small proportion of these develop histologic features of HGD or cancer. There has been an increasing appreciation of the concept of the "advanced adenoma" as the target for colonoscopic screening.[43] *Advanced adenoma* is defined as any adenomatous polyp 1 cm or larger in diameter or any polyp, regardless of size, with villous or tubulovillous histology, or with HGD in the absence of invasive CRC. Efforts to reduce colon cancer are now shifting mainly to strategies to reliably detect and resect advanced adenomas before they become malignant rather than focusing on identifying small tubular adenomas. It should also be noted that interobserver variability among pathologists with regard to diagnosis of villous components and HGD in an adenoma is high.[44] Therefore reproducible histologic criteria must be developed by pathologists so that future prospective outcome studies can accurately predict the fate of patients with advanced adenomas. Currently, 70% of polyps removed at colonoscopy are adenomas. It has been estimated that more than 80% of these are tubular, 5% to 15% are tubulovillous, and 5% to 15% are villous adenomas.[45]

Initial Management of Polyps

Colonoscopy is the most accurate method for detecting polyps and allows immediate biopsy and resection. It quickly replaced the fecal occult blood test (FOBT), flexible sigmoidoscopy, and barium enema as the primary screening modality, although flexible sigmoidoscopy, FOBT, and other stool-based tests, such as the fecal immunochemical test (FIT) and stool DNA tests with fecal immunochemical testing (i.e., Cologuard), are also approved methods for screening for CRC in the asymptomatic patient. Computed tomography (CT) colonography, another option, is still considered investigational as a screening modality. It should be reserved for patients with incomplete optical colonoscopies because the test has not been determined to be cost-effective for routine screening and is not reimbursed by most insurance plans.[46] A complete colonoscopy should be performed at the time of every initial polypectomy to detect and resect all synchronous adenomas. Additional colonoscopic examinations may be required after resection of a large sessile adenoma, if there were multiple adenomas or if the quality of the colonic preparation was suboptimal.

Management of Small Polyps

Small polyps (<1 cm), either sessile or pedunculated, can be resected by a number of different techniques, both with and without electrocautery. Cold snare polypectomy has replaced cold biopsy and hot biopsy techniques in removing small polyps.[47] The most recent guidelines put forth by the US Multi-Society Task Force, a group represented by the ACG, AGA, and ASGE, were published in 2020 and recommend that diminutive polyps (≤5 mm in diameter) and small polyps (6 to 9 mm) be removed with cold snare polypectomy. Removal with cold biopsy forceps is not recommended because of high rates of incomplete resection, but can be considered for polyps 2 mm or less if cold snare polypectomy is considered to be technically difficult.[39]

Management of Sessile Serrated Adenomas/ Polyps (Sessile Serrated Lesion)

There is no evidence that small, distally located hyperplastic polyps (HPs) carry an increased risk for CRC, but it is now accepted that certain variants of serrated polyps are precursors to CRC. For example, serrated polyps have been linked to the development of sporadic adenocarcinomas with high-level microsatellite instability, which are associated with the development of "interval cancers" after colonoscopy.[48] Hyperplastic-appearing polyps at risk for such progression are usually large (>5 mm), sessile, covered with a layer of yellow mucus, and found proximally in the colon on colonoscopy. These have been called *sessile serrated polyps* (SSPs), *sessile serrated adenomas* (SSAs), *sessile serrated adenomas/polyps* (SSA/Ps), and most recently by the World Health Organization (WHO) as *sessile serrated lesions* (SSL). These SSLs tend to be found later in life (median age, 61 years), with a slight female predominance.[48] Initially, such lesions are not cytologically dysplastic, but over time, as a result of increased microsatellite instability, they develop cytologic dysplasia and are precursors to CRC, accounting for approximately 15% to 20% of these cancers.[49] Dysplastic serrated polyps are classified as sessile serrated lesions/adenomas with dysplasia (SSAD) or traditional serrated adenomas (TSAs).[50]

Because of their malignant potential, guidelines have recommended that large, proximally located, serrated polyps be managed in the same way as adenomas of similar size. These guidelines recommend that serrated lesions proximal to the sigmoid colon and all lesions larger than 5 mm be completely resected.[48,50] When large lesions are removed piecemeal, a follow-up colonoscopy should be performed in 6 months to ensure that no residual polyp tissue has been left behind. The latest guideline by the U.S. Multi-Society Task Force suggests that patients with 1 or 2 SSLs smaller than 10 mm should have repeat surveillance colonoscopy in 5 to 10 years, patients with 3 or 4 SSLs smaller than 10 mm should have repeat surveillance colonoscopy in 3 to 5

TABLE 2.2 Recommendations for Surveillance and Screening Intervals in Individuals with Serrated Polyps

Baseline Colonoscopy: Most Advanced Finding	Recommended Surveillance Interval (y)
≤20 HPs in rectum or sigmoid colon <10 mm	10
≤20 HPs proximal to the sigmoid colon <10 mm	10
1-2 SSLs <10 mm	5–10
3-4 SSLs <10 mm	3–5
5-10 SSLs <10 mm	3
SSL ≥10mm	3
SSL with dysplasia	3
HP ≥10 mm	3–5
TSA	3
Piecemeal resection of SSL ≥20 mm	6 mo

HP, *Hyperplastic polyp;* SSL, *sessile serrated lesion;* TSA, *traditional serrated adenoma.*
Data from Gupta S, Lieberman D, Anderson JC, et al. Recommendations for follow-up after colonoscopy and polypectomy: a consensus update by the US Multi-Society Task Force on colorectal cancer. Gastroenterology. *2020;158:1131–1153.*

years, and patients with 5 to 10 SSLs should have surveillance colonoscopy in 3 years. Additionally, patients with an SSL 10 mm or larger, an SSL with dysplasia, or TSA should have a surveillance examination in 3 years. However, it is recommended that surveillance examination in 10 years can be performed for HPs measuring less than 10 mm, provided that the total number within the colon is 20 or fewer.[38] See Table 2.2 for a summary of recommendations for the colonoscopic surveillance of serrated polyps.

SERRATED POLYPOSIS SYNDROME

Serrated polyposis syndrome (SPS), formerly known as *hyperplastic polyposis,* is a syndrome characterized by the presence of multiple serrated lesions, either SSLs or hyperplastic polyps. The WHO has defined SPS as a syndrome meeting one of the following criteria: (1) at least five serrated polyps proximal to the sigmoid colon, with two or more larger than 10 mm; (2) any serrated polyps proximal to the sigmoid colon in any patient who has a first-degree relative with SPS; (3) more than 20 serrated polyps of any size in any location throughout the colon.[51] The risk of cancer in SPS is unknown but is thought to be increased, and a retrospective study showed a 7% risk of cancer at 5 years in patients undergoing surveillance.[52] Surveillance colonoscopy is recommended at 1- to 3-year intervals with attempted removal of all polyps larger than 5 mm. Surgical resection is recommended if the number of polyps is too great to be endoscopically managed, there is evidence of HGD in a serrated polyp that cannot be removed in its entirety, or there is development of cancer.[53] Surgery should involve resection of the portion of the colon that contains the cancer and the portion that has the largest polyps; usually, an extended right hemicolectomy or subtotal colectomy is performed. Patients will then need annual surveillance examination of the remaining colon and rectum.

MANAGEMENT OF LARGE PEDUNCULATED POLYPS

Endoscopic resection of large polyps can be challenging because of the risks for hemorrhage, perforation, and incomplete resection. Most endoscopists resect large pedunculated polyps using a hot snare, and, indeed, the latest guidelines by the U.S. Multi-Society Task Force recommend that hot snare polypectomy be used for lesions 10 mm in size and greater.[40] Further, it is recommended that transection should occur at the middle to lower aspect of the stalk, to provide an adequate specimen for histologic assessment. Additionally, it is recommended that large pedunculated polyps be retrieved en bloc and not be divided into smaller fragments to allow for retrieval through the colonoscope, so that proper assessment of resection margins can be performed.

MANAGEMENT OF LARGE SESSILE POLYPS

The prevalence of large sessile polyps is approximately 0.8% to 5.2% in patients undergoing colonoscopy. Malignancy is found in 5% to 22% of these polyps. These polyps tend to recur locally after resection; one study quoted a recurrence rate as high as 46%.[54] This same study found that the recurrence rate could be reduced to 3.8% with repeated endoscopic procedures and the use of argon plasma coagulation. Another investigation found that the use of EMR for resection of large sessile polyps was successful in 90% of cases, with size larger than 40 mm and use of argon plasma coagulation leading to lower success rates.[55]

Cold or hot snare polypectomy, with or without submucosal injection to “lift” the polyp before removal, is recommended for removal of nonpedunculated polyps measuring 10 to 19 mm. EMR is the preferred method for removal of nonpedunculated polyps 20 mm or greater, ideally performed by an endoscopist experienced in advanced polypectomy techniques. Further, the endoscopist is encouraged to resect all grossly visible tissue of a lesion in the safest minimum number of pieces and use of a contrast agent, such as methylene blue, in a submucosal injection before polypectomy is recommended to assist with recognition of the different submucosal layers. EMR techniques are reviewed in Chapter 1.

The endoscopist may tattoo near the polypectomy site with India ink after endoscopic resection to facilitate visualization during a subsequent endoscopic procedure. A patient who has undergone colonoscopic excision of a large sessile polyp in piecemeal fashion should have follow-up colonoscopy in 6 months to verify complete removal. If residual polyp tissue is present, it should be resected with EMR, and the completeness of this resection should be documented within another 6- to 12-month interval. Once complete removal has been established, subsequent surveillance examination is recommended in 1 year and then 3 years.

POSTPOLYPECTOMY SURVEILLANCE

Because a large number of patients with adenomas are being identified by colonoscopy, the burden placed on medical

TABLE 2.3 Recommendations for Post-Colonoscopy Follow-Up in Average Risk Adults with Normal Colonoscopy or Adenomas

Baseline Colonoscopy: Most Advanced Finding	Recommended Surveillance Interval (y)
No polyps	10
1–2 tubular adenomas <10 mm	7–10
3–4 tubular adenomas <10 mm	3–5
5–10 tubular adenomas <10 mm	3
Adenoma >10 mm	3
Adenoma with tubulovillous or villous histology	3
Adenoma with high-grade dysplasia	3
>10 adenomas on single examination	1

Data from Gupta S, Lieberman D, Anderson JC, et al. Recommendations for follow-up after colonoscopy and polypectomy: a consensus update by the US Multi-Society Task Force on colorectal cancer. Gastroenterology. *2020;158:1131–1153.*

resources (i.e., the timely availability of colonoscopy) is increasing dramatically.[56] In 2020 the U.S. Multi-Society Task Force updated their recommendations for surveillance colonoscopy after polypectomy (Table 2.3).[38] After an initial high-quality colonoscopy has been performed with complete polypectomy, surveillance colonoscopy is recommended in 7 to 10 years for patients with 1 or 2 small (<10 mm) tubular adenomas, and 3 to 5 years in patients with 3 or 4 small adenomas. For patients with 5 to 10 small tubular adenomas, surveillance examination is recommended in 3 years. Similarly, 3-year surveillance is recommended for findings of an adenoma 10 mm or greater, an adenoma with tubulovillous or villous histology, or an adenoma with HGD. If more than 10 adenomas are identified, surveillance examination is recommended in 1 year. Finally, a surveillance colonoscopy is recommended in 6 months if an adenoma measuring 20 mm or larger is removed in a piecemeal fashion.

MANAGEMENT OF MALIGNANT POLYPS

A malignant polyp is defined as an adenoma with invasion into the submucosa but not the muscularis propria.[57] Once a malignant polyp is identified, the clinical question often then centers on whether the polyp can be safely and effectively removed endoscopically, or if surgery is needed. The endoscopist can use certain endoscopic features to help predict whether a polyp has deep submucosal invasion (>1-mm invasion into the submucosa), in which case surgery should be considered; these features include ulceration of the lesion surface with destruction of the normal vascular and pit pattern, as well as the stiffness of the lesion and/or colon wall.[58] However, it should be noted that en bloc endoscopic snare resection is still regarded as acceptable for pedunculated polyps with features of deep submucosal invasion in the polyp head.

If a nonpedunculated polyp has no features of deep submucosal invasion, removal with EMR or ESD may be considered,

BOX 2.4 Unfavorable Histologic Features in Malignant and Nonpedunculated Colorectal Lesions

PEDUNCULATED LESIONS
Margin between the tumor and cautery line <2 mm
Poor differentiation
Lymphovascular invasion
Inadequate orientation of the histologic sections

NONPEDUNCULATED LESIONS
Piecemeal resection
Positive resection margins
Invasion depth >1000 μm
Poor differentiation
Lymphovascular invasion
Tumor budding
Inadequate orientation of the histologic sections

From Rex DK, Shaukat A, Wallace MB. Optimal management of malignant polyps, from endoscopic assessment and resection to decisions about surgery. Clin Gastroenterol Hepatol. *2019;17:1428–1437.*

with an aim toward en bloc resection to allow for adequate assessment of histology and submucosal depth. If submucosal invasion is identified in an endoscopically resected polyp, certain important unfavorable histologic features should be noted (Box 2.4), because they portend a higher risk for residual cancer in the bowel wall and/or lymph nodes and therefore warrant surgical referral.[58] Patients with a malignant sessile polyp that shows favorable prognostic criteria should have follow-up colonoscopy within 3 to 6 months to check for residual neoplastic tissue at the polypectomy site. After one negative follow-up examination, the clinician may revert to a standard surveillance regimen.

COLONOSCOPIC SURVEILLANCE AFTER COLON CANCER RESECTION

Patients who have undergone resection for colon cancer should be entered into a surveillance program to detect early recurrence of the initial primary cancer and to detect metachronous colorectal neoplasms. It has also been shown that the annual incidence for metachronous cancers in surveillance groups after cancer resection is 0.35% per year.[59] Furthermore, one study demonstrated that up to 40% of patients with locoregional disease will develop recurrent cancer, 90% of which will occur within 5 years.[60]

On the basis of the available data, patients should undergo a high-quality perioperative clearing by colonoscopy in nonobstructive tumors or within a 3- to 6-month interval after surgery in the case of obstructive CRC. Alternatively, a CT colonography can be considered to exclude synchronous neoplasm in patients with obstructive CRC, which precludes complete colonoscopy. Surveillance endoscopy should be performed in all patients 1 year after resection because of the high yield of detecting early metachronous cancers. If the first surveillance colonoscopy is negative, the next examination needs to be done after a 3-year interval. Recommendations for surveillance in patients after CRC resection are reviewed in Box 2.5.[61]

The full reference list may be accessed online at Elsevier eBooks for Practicing Clinicians.

BOX 2.5 Colonoscopy Recommendations for Surveillance after Cancer Resection

1. We recommend that patients with colorectal cancer (CRC) undergo high-quality perioperative clearing with colonoscopy. The procedure should be performed preoperatively of within a 3- to 6-month interval after surgery in the case of obstructive CRC. The goals of perioperative clearing colonoscopy are detection of synchronous cancer and detection and complete resection of precancerous polyps.
2. We recommend that patients who have undergone curative resection of either colon or rectal cancer receive their first surveillance colonoscopy 1 year after surgery (or 1 year after the clearing perioperative colonoscopy). Additional surveillance recommendations apply to patients with rectal cancer.
3. We recommend that, after the 1-year colonoscopy, the interval to the next colonoscopy should be 3 years, and then 5 years. Subsequent colonoscopies should occur at 5-year intervals, until the benefit of continued surveillance is outweighed by diminishing life expectancy. If neoplastic polyps are detected, the intervals between colonoscopies should be in accordance with the published guidelines for polyp surveillance intervals. These do not apply to patients with Lynch syndrome.
4. Patients with localized rectal cancer who have undergone surgery without total mesorectal excision, those who have undergone transanal local excision (transanal excision or transanal endoscopic microsurgery) or endoscopic submucosal dissection, and those with locally advanced rectal cancer who did not receive neoadjuvant chemoradiation and then surgery using total mesorectal excision techniques are at increased risk for local recurrence. In these situations, we suggest local surveillance with flexible sigmoidoscopy or EUS every 3-6 months for the first 2-3 years after surgery. These surveillance measures are in addition to recommended colonoscopic surveillance for metachronous neoplasia.
5. In patients with obstructive CRC precluding complete colonoscopy, we recommend CTC as the best alternative to exclude synchronous neoplasms. Double-contrast barium enema is an acceptable alternative if CTC is not available.
6. There is insufficient evidence to recommend the routine use of fecal immunochemical test (FIT) or fecal DNA for surveillance after CRC resection.

From Kahi CJ, Boland CR, Dominitz JA, et al. Colonoscopy surveillance after colorectal cancer resection: recommendations from the US Multi-Society Task Force on colorectal cancer. Gastroenterology. *2016;150:758–768.*

CHAPTER 3

Diagnostic Cytology of the Gastrointestinal Tract

Helen H. Wang

Chapter Outline

INTRODUCTION

The popularity of gastrointestinal (GI) cytology for the diagnosis of infection and malignancy has waxed and waned during the past few decades. The ability to distinguish between high-grade dysplasia or carcinoma in situ and invasive carcinoma in biopsy specimens and the more prevalent expertise of surgical pathology cause some to consider cytology an unnecessary duplication of GI mucosal biopsies. However, the combined use of endoscopy, ultrasound guidance, and fine-needle aspiration (FNA) has expanded the horizons of GI cytology.[1] The refined nonendoscopic sampling methods coupled with cellular markers have rekindled interest in screening high-risk populations with cytology for esophageal carcinoma.[2]

Specimen Types

Types of GI tract specimens commonly received in the cytology laboratory include those obtained by endoscopic brushings and ultrasound-guided endoscopic FNA. Endoscopic FNA has enabled endoscopists to reach farther than they can with biopsy forceps to sample mural and extramural lesions, including lesions adjacent to the GI tract. The nonendoscopic specimens obtained with balloon- or mesh-type samplers have been investigated to ascertain their usefulness in the surveillance of populations at high risk for esophageal carcinoma.[3,4]

Specimen Preparations

Direct smears can be made from materials collected on the endoscopic brush, in the needle, or on the balloon and mesh samplers; these can then be either fixed immediately in 95% ethanol and stained with the Papanicolaou method or left to air-dry and stained with Diff-Quik (Dade-Behring, Inc., Deerfield, IL) or Wright-Giemsa stain. Alternatively, the material can be rinsed into a medium such as CytoLyt, CytoRich, or 50% ethanol for liquid-based preparations. The specimen can then be processed by a concentration method, such as ThinPrep Processor (Hologic, Marlborough, MA) or Cytospin (ThermoFisher Scientific, Waltham, MA),[5,6] to make slides that are then stained with the Papanicolaou method. According to a College of American Pathologists Interlaboratory Comparison Program in Nongynecologic Cytology, ThinPrep preparations performed better than non-ThinPrep preparations.[5] However, liquid-based preparations, including ThinPrep, involve altered morphology and artifacts that require adjustment by cytopathologists, such as cleaner background with altered or reduced background and extracellular elements, architectural changes (smaller cell clusters and sheets and more three-dimensional clusters), altered cell distribution (more dyshesion–dissociation of cells at the periphery of cell clusters or as single cells), and changes in cytological morphology (enhanced nuclear features and smaller cell size).[7] Residual material from liquid-based preparations lends itself to cell block making for histological examination and ancillary studies.[8-10]

Value and Accuracy of Specimens

Cytology specimens have some advantages over specimens obtained by endoscopic biopsy. The brush can sample a wider area, and the fine needle can reach deeper lesions than can be reached by biopsy forceps. Also, both the brush and the fine needle are less invasive than biopsy forceps and less likely to cause bleeding. In addition, cytology has a shorter turnaround time than histology. Direct smears can be ready for review within minutes with no compromise of the quality of the preparation (unlike frozen sections of biopsy specimens, which compromise the quality of the final or permanent preparation). However, as mentioned, cytology is limited in its ability to distinguish between high-grade dysplasia or carcinoma in situ and invasive carcinoma.

Despite the potential duplication of cytology and biopsy, the literature has consistently shown that the highest diagnostic yield is obtained with the combined use of these specimens.[11-13] The yield of cytology is significantly higher when the brushing is performed before rather than after the biopsy.[14]

NORMAL MORPHOLOGY

Esophagus

Intermediate-type squamous cells with abundant cytoplasm and vesicular nuclei are seen in the normal esophagus (Fig. 3.1). Superficial-type squamous cells with abundant cytoplasm and small pyknotic nuclei can also be seen in small numbers. Single cells and clusters of ciliated columnar cells from the respiratory tract with no clinical significance may be seen rarely.

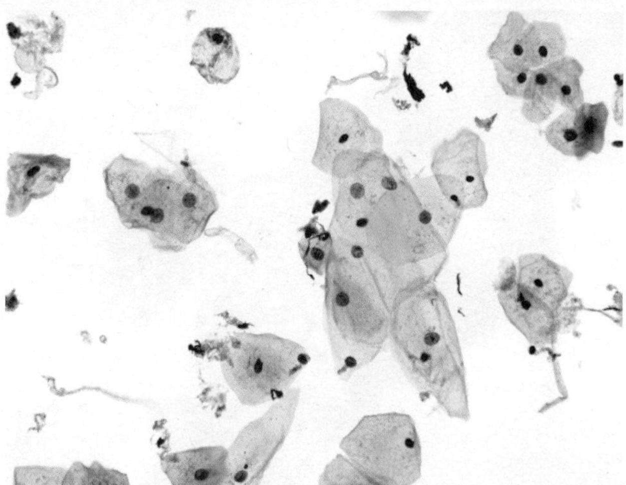

FIGURE 3.1 Brushing specimen from a normal esophagus is composed predominantly of intermediate squamous cells (Papanicolaou stain).

Stomach

Gastric surface foveolar cells can shed as single cells or in sheets. When in sheets, the columnar cells exhibit abundant cytoplasm, regularly spaced nuclei, and open chromatin arranged in a honeycomb or palisaded pattern (Fig. 3.2), depending on the orientation. When they are shed as single cells, they often lose their cytoplasm to become naked nuclei. In endoscopic FNA specimens, the sheets of foveolar cells can mimic cells from a mucinous neoplasm, and the single naked nuclei, because of their small, monomorphic appearance, can mimic cells from a pancreatic endocrine tumor.

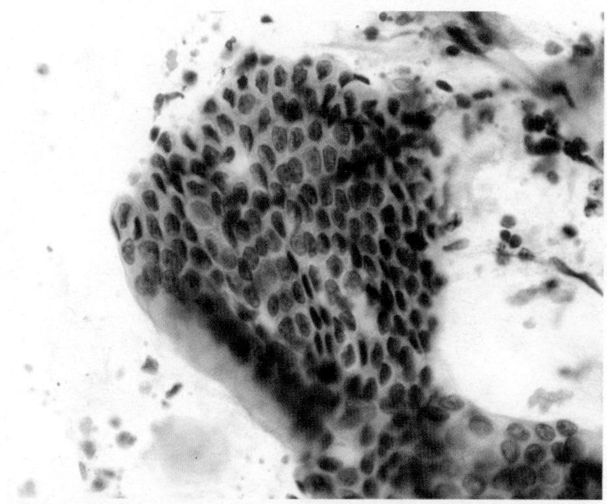

FIGURE 3.2 A sheet of benign gastric foveolar cells in a slightly distorted honeycomb pattern with evident columnar cells in palisading arrangement at the periphery is seen in a gastric brushing specimen. The presence of small nucleoli in some of the cells may indicate reactive change (Papanicolaou stain).

Small Intestine

The lining cells of the small intestine can be easily distinguished from gastric foveolar cells by the presence of goblet cells. On low magnification, the specimen typically has a Swiss cheese appearance, with the "holes" representing either goblet cells or gland openings of the crypts (Fig. 3.3).

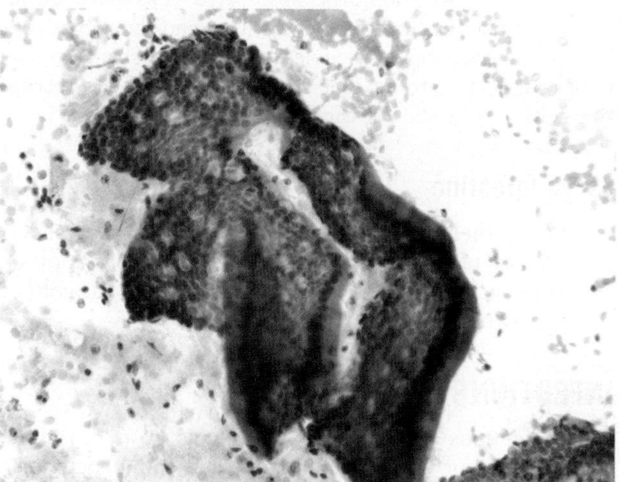

FIGURE 3.3 A complex sheet of small intestinal–type epithelium is seen in a duodenal brushing specimen. It has a Swiss cheese appearance, with the "holes" representing either goblet cells or gland openings of the crypts (Papanicolaou stain).

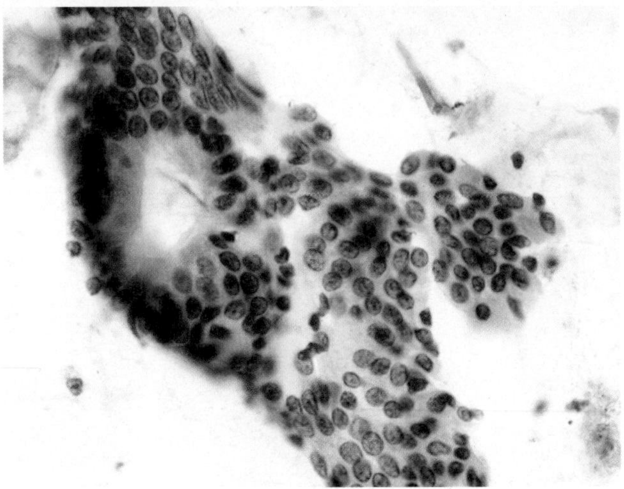

FIGURE 3.4 A sheet of normal colonic columnar epithelial cells is present in a colonic brushing specimen. A gland opening is seen in the left half of the field (Papanicolaou stain).

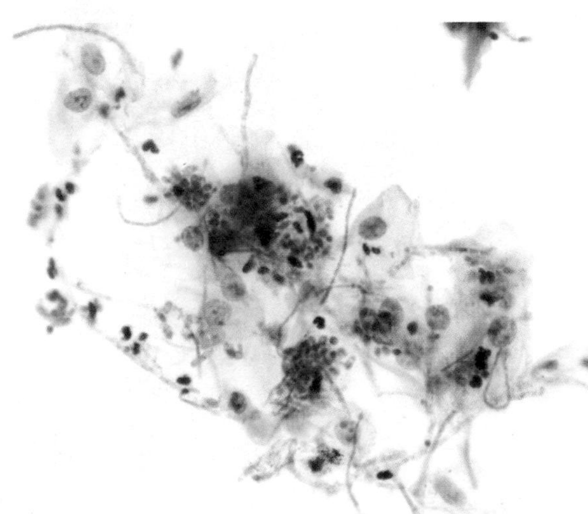

FIGURE 3.5 Pseudohyphae and yeast forms from *Candida* species are seen in an esophageal brushing specimen. Inflammatory cells and debris are in the background (Papanicolaou stain).

On high magnification, the absorptive cells have either finely granular or vacuolated cytoplasm, and the goblet cells have single large mucin vacuoles and crescent-shaped nuclei with rounded contours. The striated border of the absorptive cells may be seen at the periphery of the sheets.

Large Intestine

Normal epithelium is characterized on cytology by sheets or strips of tall columnar cells with abundant cytoplasm and basal nuclei. Partial or complete openings of the colonic crypts may be seen (Fig. 3.4).

INFECTIONS

Most infectious agents that affect human hosts can infect the GI tract of immunocompetent and immunocompromised patients.[15] Some infectious agents have a predilection for the GI tract. The more common ones are discussed in this section.

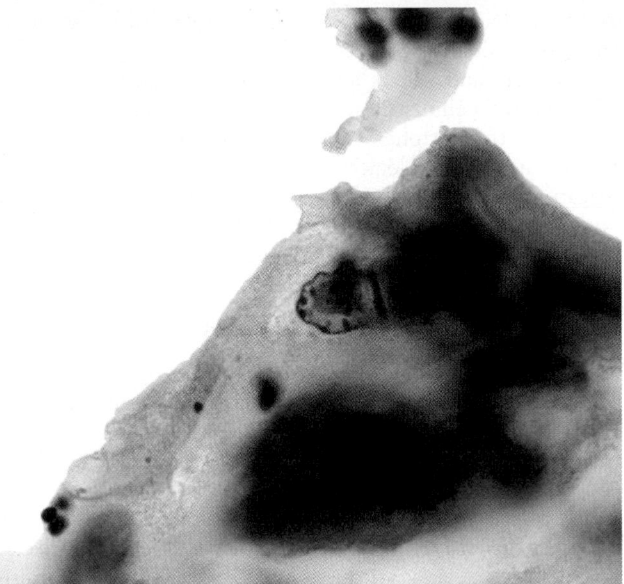

FIGURE 3.6 A Cowdry type A inclusion characterized by an eosinophilic intranuclear body surrounded by a halo is seen in the center of the field in this specimen from an esophageal brushing of herpetic esophagitis (Papanicolaou stain).

Candida

Candida almost exclusively involves the esophageal portion of the GI tract. Brushings are more sensitive than biopsy specimens in the detection of esophageal candidiasis.[13] Contamination by oral *Candida* is usually not a problem because the brush is contained within a sheath when it is passed into and out of the endoscope and is expelled from the sheath only to sample the lesion. The organisms appear as pink to purple pseudohyphae and yeast formations on Papanicolaou stain (Fig. 3.5). Reactive squamous cells and inflammatory cells are often observed in the background.

Herpes Simplex Virus

Herpes simplex virus infection can theoretically affect epithelial cells anywhere along the GI tract, but it is most commonly seen in the esophagus. Multinucleation, nuclear molding, ground-glass chromatin, and eosinophilic intranuclear inclusions are the characteristic features of infected cells (Fig. 3.6).

Cytomegalovirus

Cytomegalovirus infection affects epithelial, stromal, and endothelial cells along the GI tract and is characterized by large cells with a single large basophilic intranuclear inclusion with a perinuclear halo (Fig. 3.7). Intracytoplasmic textured inclusions can occasionally be seen in the affected cells.

Helicobacter pylori

Helicobacter pylori infection occurs exclusively in the stomach and is perhaps the most common infection of the GI tract. These organisms can be demonstrated on imprint smears of gastric biopsies or on brush cytology specimens.[16,17]

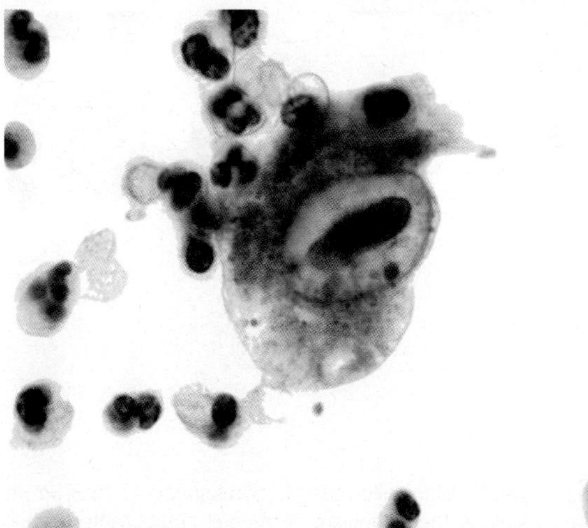

FIGURE 3.7 Both intranuclear and intracytoplasmic inclusions are seen in this cytomegalovirus-infected cell from an esophageal brushing. The intranuclear inclusion is a large amphophilic to basophilic body surrounded by a halo, and the intracytoplasmic inclusion is characterized by small, granular, basophilic to amphophilic bodies (Papanicolaou stain).

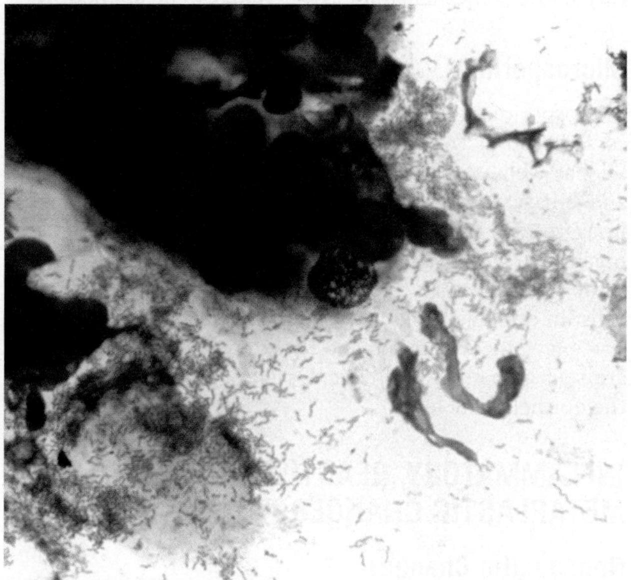

FIGURE 3.8 Numerous *S*-shaped organisms consistent with *Helicobacter pylori* are present in the mucus adjacent to a sheet of epithelial cells on a gastric brushing specimen (Diff-Quik preparation).

Examination of imprint and brushing cytology specimens is comparable, if not superior, in sensitivity (88%) and specificity (61%) to histological examination of sections stained with hematoxylin and eosin (H&E) and modified Giemsa stain.[16,17] The benefits of imprint and brushing cytology are rapid results, high specificity, and low cost. However, the efficacy of cytological detection depends on the extent of colonization by these organisms. When present in large quantity, they are evident even at low magnification, but they can be difficult to identify when present in small numbers. On Papanicolaou stain, *H. pylori* organisms appear as faintly basophilic, *S*-shaped rods admixed with mucus in the vicinity of glandular cell clusters (Fig. 3.8). Special stains, such as a triple stain combining silver, H&E, and Alcian blue at pH 2.5, can enhance their detection by cytology.[18]

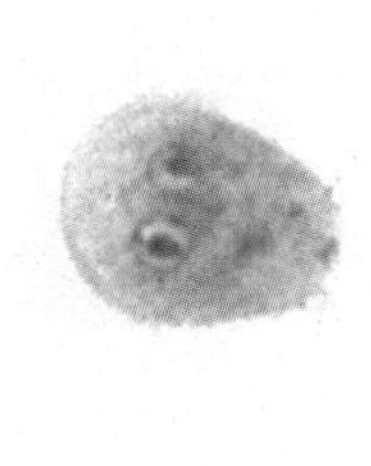

FIGURE 3.9 A pear-shaped, gray, binucleate *Giardia* organism is seen in the center of the field in this duodenal brushing specimen (Papanicolaou stain).

Giardia

Giardia affects the duodenum of both immunocompetent and immunocompromised hosts. Brush cytology is a useful method for detecting *Giardia* because the organisms are on the luminal surfaces of the intestinal epithelial cells. They are flat, gray, pear-shaped, and binucleate, with four pairs of flagella (Fig. 3.9).[19] In addition to brush cytology, they are also nicely visualized on cytological preparations from the residual formalin in the biopsy container; these can be used to enhance biopsy diagnosis.[20] *Giardia lamblia* trophozoites have been found to be immunoreactive for the protooncogene *KIT* (C-*kit*, CD117), which may help to identify the organisms.[21]

Atypical Mycobacteria

Atypical mycobacteria accumulate within macrophages in the lamina propria, and very rigorous brushing is required for the infected macrophages to be included in the cytology sample. The presence of isolated foamy histiocytes on the smear should raise the level of suspicion of an atypical mycobacterial infection (Fig. 3.10). In general, the organisms are present in large numbers. On Diff-Quik–stained smears, the mycobacteria form numerous rod-shaped negative images, either within the histiocytes or in the background (Fig. 3.11).[22] Special stains for acid-fast bacilli are necessary to confirm the diagnosis.

Cryptosporidia

Cryptosporidia can involve any glandular epithelium of the GI tract in patients infected with the human immunodeficiency virus (HIV) and can be detected by examination of stool and cytology specimens.[23] Cryptosporidia are 2- to 5-μm, round, basophilic bodies on the luminal surfaces of the epithelial cells. Therefore they are seen only when the

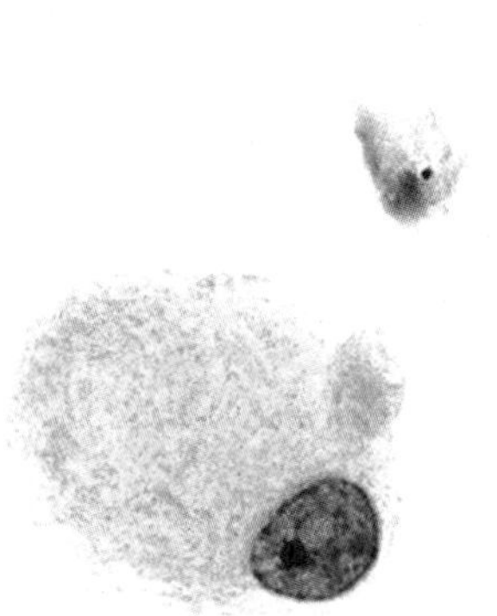

FIGURE 3.10 A histiocyte with abundant granular cytoplasm is present in this duodenal brushing specimen from a man with human immunodeficiency virus (HIV) infection. On special stain, the cell is shown to be filled with acid-fast bacilli, consistent with atypical mycobacteria (Papanicolaou stain).

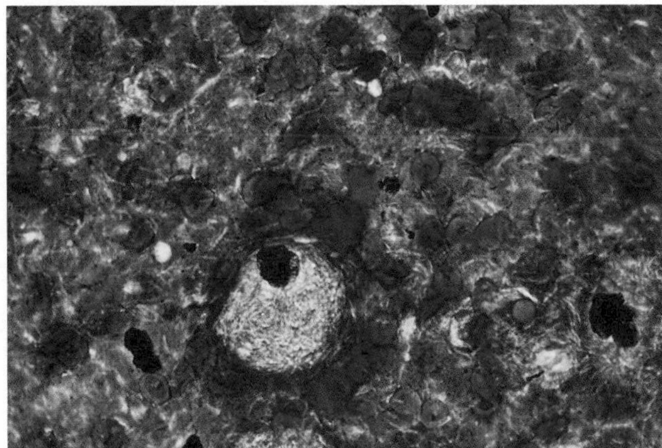

FIGURE 3.11 Numerous negative images of rod-shaped organisms are seen within and outside the histiocyte in the center of the field (from the same case as in Fig. 3.10) (Diff-Quik preparation).

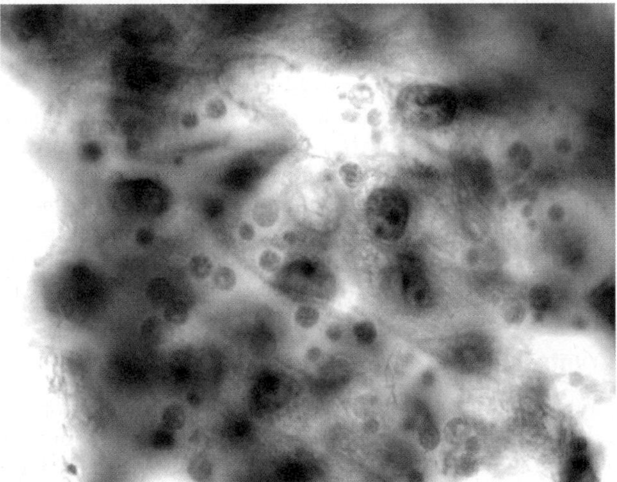

FIGURE 3.12 Many round basophilic bodies of cyclosporidia (2 to 5 μm in diameter) are seen on the surface of this sheet of gastric epithelial cells on a brushing specimen (Papanicolaou stain).

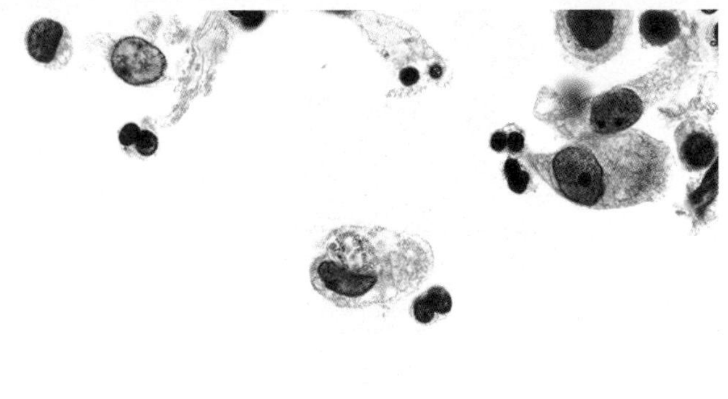

FIGURE 3.13 Several eosinophilic rods of microsporidia (1 to 3 μm in diameter) are visible in the cytoplasm of the cell in the center of this duodenal brushing specimen. They are typically found in the supranuclear portion of the cytoplasm (Papanicolaou stain).

plane of focus is shifted to the surfaces of the cells where the organisms reside (Fig. 3.12). When in doubt, confirmatory Gomori methenamine-silver stain can be applied.

Microsporidia

Microsporidia can be detected on cytological specimens such as stool, nasal secretions, duodenal aspirates, and bile, as well as on brushing specimens from the duodenum and biliary tract.[24-26] On Papanicolaou stain, they appear in aggregates as brightly eosinophilic, rod-shaped or ovoid organisms measuring 1 to 3 μm in diameter (Fig. 3.13). They are present in both epithelial cells and inflammatory cells. In epithelial cells, they are located in the supranuclear portion of the cytoplasm and therefore, like cryptosporidia, are seen at a slightly different plane of focus from that of the epithelial nuclei.

INFLAMMATORY, REACTIVE, AND METAPLASTIC CHANGES

Nonspecific Changes

Any injury to the mucosa can evoke a nonspecific inflammatory or reactive epithelial change. When the injury is sufficient to result in ulceration, the change (i.e., the epithelial repair) can become so extreme that it may mimic a malignancy. It is often difficult to determine whether the reparative epithelium is of glandular or squamous origin. Although epithelial repair is characterized by prominent eosinophilic nucleoli, they are usually neither huge nor numerous (i.e., more than three or four) (Fig. 3.14). The appearance of atypical stromal cells or their stripped nuclei from granulation tissue can also be quite alarming (Fig. 3.15). In spite of striking nuclear enlargement of such cells, hyperchromasia is absent. Instead, they have fine, homogeneous chromatin and thin, smooth nuclear membranes.

Both cellular arrangements and the features of individual cells are useful in distinguishing between severe reactive and neoplastic changes. Cells with reactive or reparative changes are usually arranged in flat sheets without three-dimensionality or prominent cell dyshesion. In contrast,

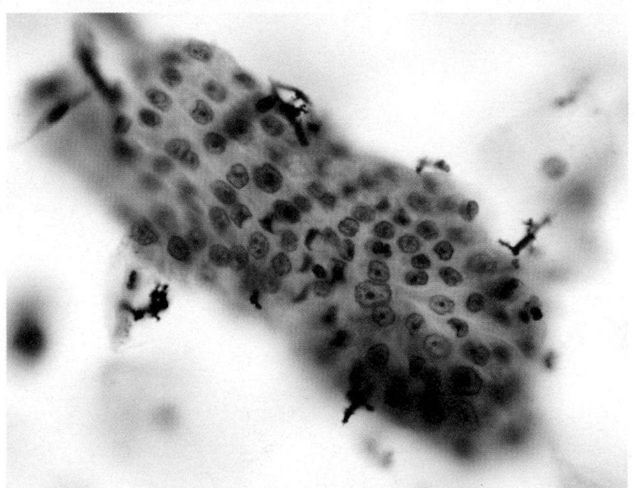

FIGURE 3.14 A sheet of reactive epithelial cells is seen in this esophageal brushing specimen. The cells have sharp cellular borders and are variably enlarged with prominent nucleoli. The nuclear membranes in some cells appear wavy but without sharp angles or indentations. A few inflammatory cells are superimposed on or infiltrating this sheet. It is difficult to be certain whether these cells are squamous or glandular (Papanicolaou stain). (*Courtesy of Dr. Mark Roth of the National Cancer Institute, Rockville, Md.*)

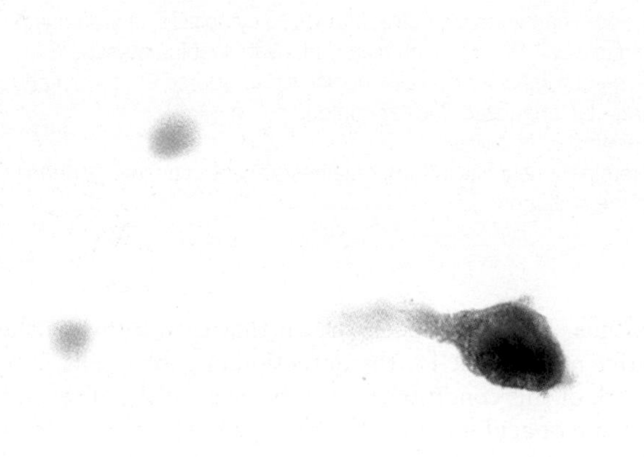

FIGURE 3.15 A single, atypical, ovoid- to spindle-shaped cell with an enlarged, smudged nucleus is seen in a gastric brushing specimen from a patient with resection-proven benign gastric ulcer with abundant granulation tissue at the ulcer bed (Papanicolaou stain).

dyshesion, presented either as "feathering" (dissociation of cells) at the periphery of cell clusters or as the dispersion of numerous isolated cells, is usually evident with neoplasms, as is three-dimensionality. In addition, the enlarged nuclei in reactive or reparative changes usually have uniform size and a similar number of small, prominent nucleoli, in contrast to the variation in nuclear and nucleolar size and shape as well as the chromatin pattern in the neoplastic lesions. Specific types of reactive cells may also be seen, such as those with radiation-induced changes (Fig. 3.16). As in other organs,

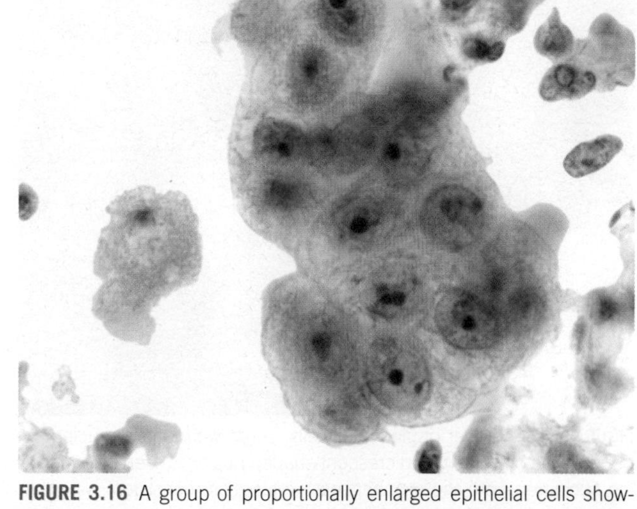

FIGURE 3.16 A group of proportionally enlarged epithelial cells showing prominent nucleoli and finely vacuolated cytoplasm is seen on this esophageal brushing specimen from a patient with previous radiation therapy for squamous cell carcinoma (Papanicolaou stain).

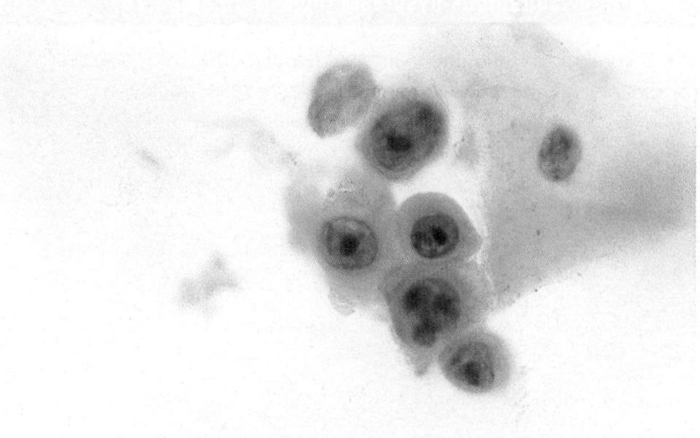

FIGURE 3.17 A loose group of parabasal-sized squamous cells with dense cytoplasm and prominent nucleoli can be seen in this esophageal brushing specimen from a patient known to have pemphigus vulgaris (Papanicolaou stain).

the cells are proportionally enlarged, with metachromatic cytoplasm and nuclear or cytoplasmic vacuoles.

Pemphigus

Rarely, pemphigus vulgaris, an autoimmune disease of the skin and mucous membranes that attacks the intercellular junctions and causes a suprabasilar bleb or blister as well as acantholysis, may affect the esophagus. Numerous acantholytic cells are usually present. The characteristic cells are round to polygonal, uniform, parabasal-sized, and isolated.[27,28] The cytoplasm is dense and may have perinuclear eosinophilic staining or a clear halo. The cells appear atypical because of the high nucleus-to-cytoplasm ratio, the enlarged nuclei, and the prominent multiple, even irregular, nucleoli (Fig. 3.17). A bar- or bullet-shaped nucleolus is characteristic.[29] However, the cells have smooth nuclear membranes, and the chromatin is pale, fine, and even. Normal mitotic figures can be seen. These atypical cells resemble those in repair except for the increased number of single cells.

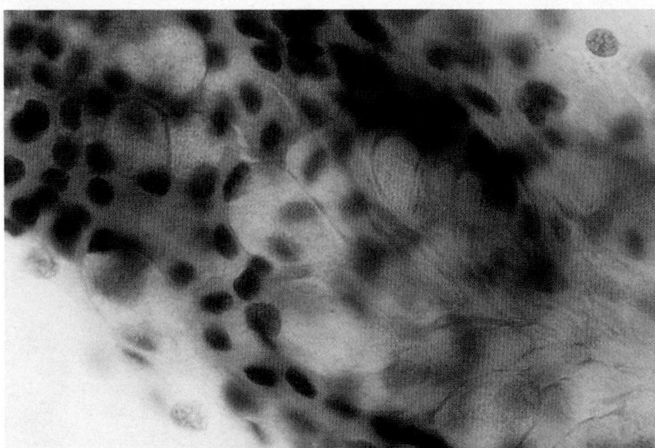

FIGURE 3.18 A sheet of glandular cells, some with large vacuoles expanding the cytoplasm and crescent-shaped nuclei, is seen on a brushing specimen from the esophagogastric junction, consistent with Barrett's esophagus (Papanicolaou stain).

BOX 3.1 Squamous Dysplasia (Figs. 3.19 and 3.20)

- Some but not all of the malignant features to varying degrees, such as increased nucleus-to-cytoplasm ratio, nuclear enlargement, hyperchromasia, irregular nuclear membrane, and aberrant chromatin pattern
- Fewer atypical cells than carcinoma
- Absent tumor diathesis

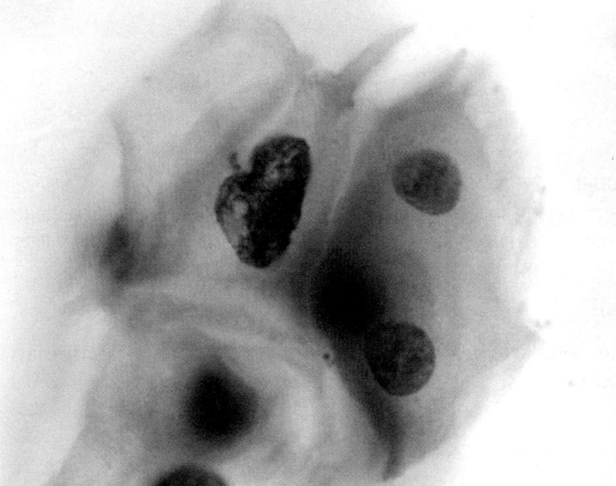

FIGURE 3.19 A dysplastic squamous cell is surrounded by a few reactive-appearing squamous cells. The dysplastic cell shows mild hyperchromasia, nuclear membrane irregularity, and chromatin aberration, but it still has a fair amount of cytoplasm. Therefore it is considered low grade (Papanicolaou stain). (*Courtesy of Dr. Mark Roth of the National Cancer Institute, Rockville, Md.*)

Barrett's Esophagus

Cytology is not the optimal tool for the diagnosis of Barrett's esophagus. When glandular epithelial cells are seen in a cytology specimen, it is difficult to be certain whether they represent cells from the gastric side of the esophagogastric junction or metaplastic glandular cells from the

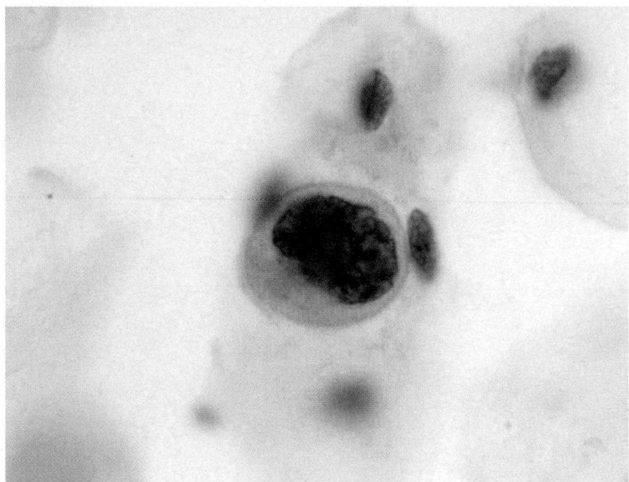

FIGURE 3.20 Compared with the dysplastic cell in Figure 3.19, this dysplastic squamous cell has more pronounced nuclear membrane irregularity and a much higher nucleus-to-cytoplasm ratio. It is, therefore, considered high grade (Papanicolaou stain). (*Courtesy of Dr. Mark Roth of the National Cancer Institute, Rockville, Md.*)

BOX 3.2 Well-Differentiated Squamous Cell Carcinoma (Fig. 3.21)

- Predominantly isolated cells with sharp cytoplasmic borders and variable cell shapes, such as round, oval, or spindle-shaped
- Hyperchromatic or pyknotic nuclei with obscured chromatin and irregular, angulated nuclear contours
- Keratinized cytoplasm
- Prominent necrosis or tumor diathesis and keratinaceous debris in the background

esophagus. It has also been shown that cytology is neither sensitive nor specific for the detection of goblet cells,[30,31] a hallmark of this condition, in part because of the absence of a blue hue of acid mucin with the Papanicolaou stain. However, a long segment of Barrett's esophagus is more readily appreciated by cytology because of the reduced probability of sampling error.[31] Its appearance is similar to that of the lining epithelium of the small intestine, with a Swiss cheese pattern at low magnification and goblet cells with single, large cytoplasmic vacuoles on high magnification (Fig. 3.18). The honeycomb arrangement of the glandular cells in Barrett's esophagus usually tends to be slightly more irregular than that of normal small intestinal epithelium. With liquid-based preparations, they are sometimes isolated cells and may show a pale-bluish color of their mucus to contrast with the yellow-green of foveolar cell mucus.[32] This contrast may be subtle and it is not always appreciated.

NEOPLASTIC LESIONS

Squamous Dysplasia or Carcinoma

Dysplastic squamous cells of the esophagus have morphology similar to that of the dysplastic cells on cervicovaginal Papanicolaou smears (Box 3.1 and Figs. 3.19 and 3.20).[33] The cellular features of squamous cell carcinoma vary with the degree of differentiation (Box 3.2 and Fig. 3.21; Box 3.3 and Fig. 3.22).

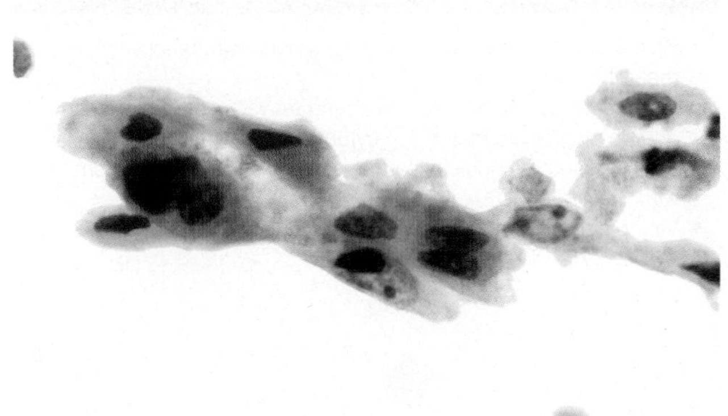

FIGURE 3.21 A keratinized squamous cell with a hyperchromatic nucleus characteristic of well-differentiated squamous cell carcinoma is present in this esophageal brushing specimen along with nonkeratinized tumor cells (Papanicolaou stain).

BOX 3.3 Moderately and Poorly Differentiated Squamous Cell Carcinoma (Fig. 3.22)

- Less striking keratinization of the cytoplasm
- Tumor cells in crowded, haphazardly arranged cell clusters with indistinct cell borders
- Vesicular chromatin with prominent nucleoli

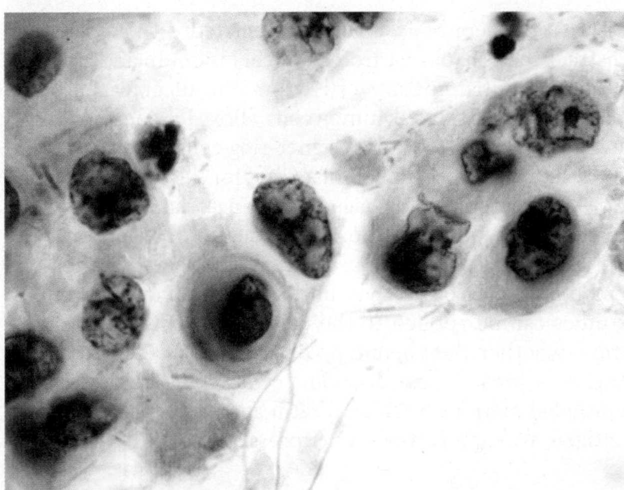

FIGURE 3.22 In contrast to the cells seen in Figure 3.21, tumor cells from a poorly differentiated squamous cell carcinoma have vesicular chromatin and occasional prominent nucleoli. The single-cell pattern, dense basophilic cytoplasm, and endoplasmic and ectoplasmic demarcation in a cell close to the center of the field suggest squamous differentiation (Papanicolaou stain).

Glandular Dysplasia or Carcinoma

Glandular dysplasia and carcinoma in the esophagus usually arise in the setting of Barrett's esophagus. The precursor lesions of adenocarcinoma in the stomach and in the intestine can manifest as either polypoid or flat dysplastic lesions. Adenomas of the stomach and dysplasia of the esophagus or stomach are similar in cytological appearance. Although the few reported studies on this topic were based on very small numbers of cases[30,31,34,35] and were insufficient to provide definitive conclusions on the usefulness of cytological surveillance,[36] the preliminary results appear promising. Low-grade dysplasia may be difficult to distinguish from artifactual crowding, whereas high-grade dysplasia may be confused with either severe reparative change or invasive carcinoma (Box 3.4 and Fig. 3.23; Box 3.5 and Fig. 3.24; Box 3.6 and Fig. 3.25). Because of the difficulties with the morphological diagnosis of dysplasia, molecular alterations have been investigated for risk stratification. Indeed, esophageal brushings, including the nonendoscopic specimens, are suitable for DNA ploidy analysis, fluorescence in situ hybridization, molecular genetics, and biomarker analysis.[37-40] In this regard, DNA content abnormalities (aneuploidy/tetraploidy) and overexpression of p53 are the strongest predictors of disease progression,[41,42] but none of these has yet found widespread, routine application.

BOX 3.4 Low-Grade Glandular Dysplasia (Fig. 3.23)

- Architectural abnormality (e.g., stratification manifested as crowding and overlapping on cytology)
- Elongated nuclei with increased nucleus-to-cytoplasm ratio
- Mild hyperchromasia and absent or inconspicuous nucleoli
- Minimal or negligible dyshesion

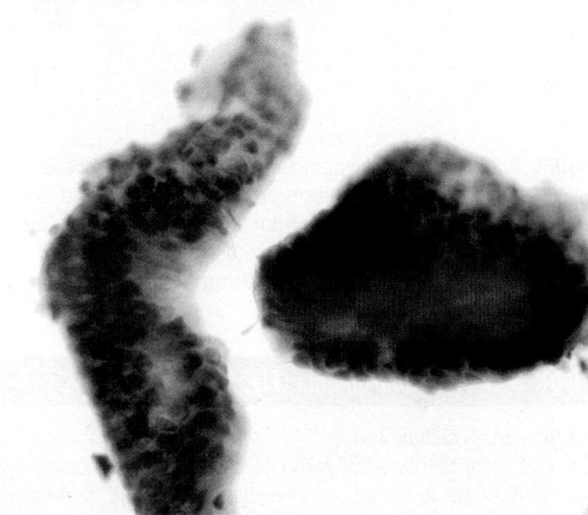

FIGURE 3.23 A strip of stratified columnar cells with slightly enlarged and elongated nuclei is seen in an esophageal brushing specimen from a patient with biopsy-proven low-grade dysplasia in Barrett's esophagus (Papanicolaou stain).

BOX 3.5 High-Grade Glandular Dysplasia (Fig. 3.24)

- Both architectural and cellular abnormalities
- Atypical cells in haphazardly arranged sheets and clusters, or singly as a result of dyshesion
- Cellular abnormalities similar to those seen in invasive adenocarcinoma but less pronounced

The amount and characteristics of the cytoplasm of the tumor cells depend on the degree of differentiation. Appearance varies from abundant vacuolated or granular cytoplasm to scant dense cytoplasm that is difficult to distinguish from that of a poorly differentiated squamous cell carcinoma.

Signet-ring cell carcinoma, a type of adenocarcinoma that occurs most commonly in the stomach, is worthy of

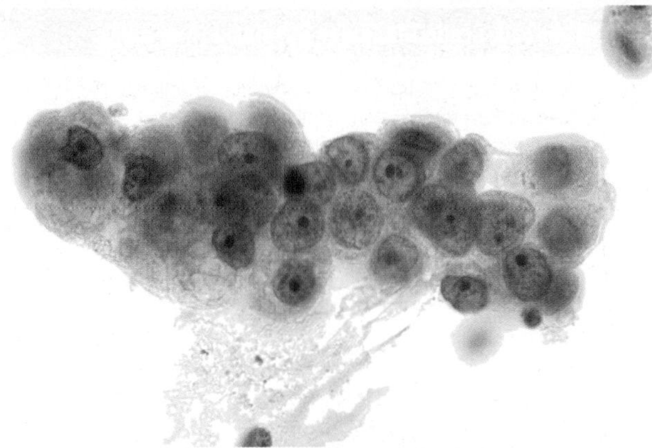

FIGURE 3.24 A sheet of haphazardly arranged and overlapped atypical cells with granular cytoplasm on a clean background is seen in an esophageal brushing specimen from a patient with biopsy-proven high-grade dysplasia in Barrett's esophagus. The nuclei show chromatin aberration and occasional nucleoli, but the cells do not appear to be malignant (Papanicolaou stain).

BOX 3.6 Adenocarcinoma (Fig. 3.25)

- Increased cellularity
- Abnormal cellular arrangements, such as isolated cells, "feathering" at the edges of cellular groups, and haphazard crowding within the groups
- Variable degrees of gland formation by atypical cells
- Atypical cellular features, such as nuclear pleomorphism, high nucleus-to-cytoplasm ratio, nuclear enlargement, chromatin aberration, and irregular nuclear membrane with or without nucleoli
- Possibility of tumor diathesis (old blood and necrotic debris) in the background

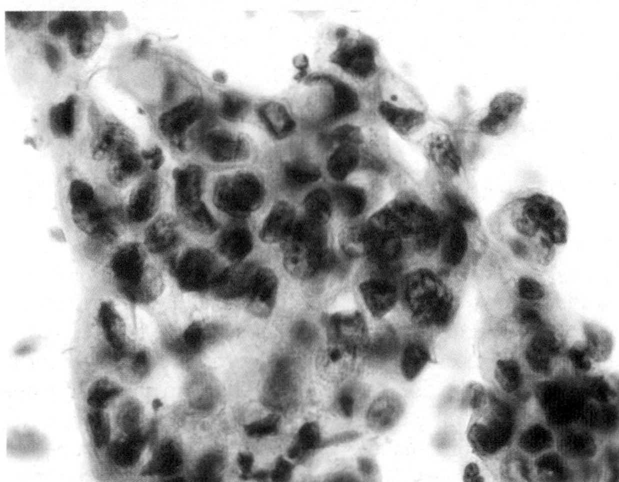

FIGURE 3.25 Compared with the cells in Figure 3.24, the cells in this gastric brushing from a well-differentiated adenocarcinoma show significant three dimensionality and a more pronounced haphazard arrangement. Cytoplasmic vacuolization as well as polarization of cells indicates glandular differentiation. Red blood cells are apparent in the background. The much increased cellularity and marked architectural abnormality indicate an invasive adenocarcinoma (Papanicolaou stain).

special consideration because it can be difficult to detect on both cytological and histological preparations. Because the malignant cells predominantly infiltrate the lamina propria, they are often not included in the brush cytology sample unless mucosal ulceration is present. The reactive

BOX 3.7 Signet-Ring Cell Carcinoma (Fig. 3.26)

- Prominent inflammation in the background with reactive or reparative epithelial changes
- Isolated cells with moderate to abundant vacuolated cytoplasm and no phagocytic material in cytoplasm
- Crescent-shaped nucleus compressed against the cytoplasm with pointed ends
- Variable degrees of nuclear atypia

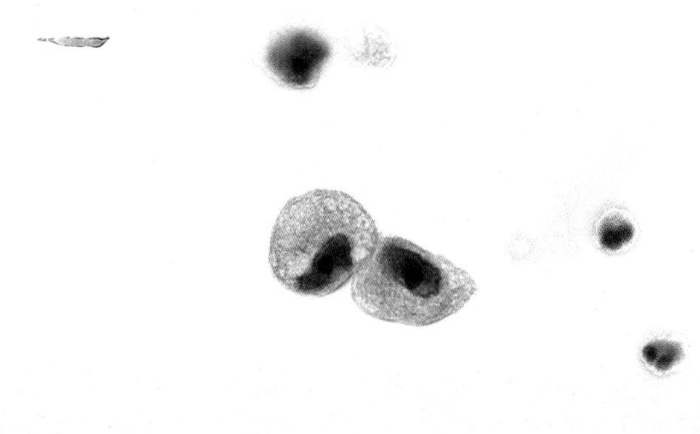

FIGURE 3.26 Two cells with abundant vacuolated cytoplasm and nuclei with slightly irregular nuclear membranes and prominent nucleoli are seen in this gastric brushing specimen of a biopsy-proven signet-ring cell carcinoma. No phagocytic material is seen in the vacuolated cytoplasm (Papanicolaou stain).

or reparative epithelial changes associated with an ulcer can distract the pathologist from the real lesion. In addition, the numerous inflammatory cells from the ulcer can obscure the scattered, isolated tumor cells (Box 3.7 and Fig. 3.26). Even when detected, some signet-ring cells have such bland nuclei that they can be mistaken for histiocytes, which have intracytoplasmic phagocytized material and a very low nucleus-to-cytoplasm ratio. A high degree of suspicion is the best safeguard against failure to detect a signet-ring cell carcinoma by cytology. When in doubt, immunocytochemical studies can be applied to the cytological material to determine whether the phenotype of the cells of interest is epithelial or histiocytic. Carcinoma cells should be positive for epithelial markers, such as keratin and epithelial membrane antigen, whereas histiocytes express CD68 and CD163.

Neuroendocrine Neoplasms

GI neuroendocrine neoplasms are classified into three main categories according to the latest classification from the World Health Organization[43]: (1) well-differentiated neuroendocrine neoplasms: neuroendocrine tumors (NETs)—including low-grade (G1), intermediate-grade (G2), and high-grade (G3); (2) poorly differentiated neuroendocrine neoplasms: neuroendocrine carcinomas—both small cell and large cell; and (3) mixed neoplasms: mixed neuroendocrine–nonneuroendocrine neoplasms, which can be either well or poorly differentiated. In addition to morphology, the distinction between grade 1, grade 2, and grade 3 NET depends on mitoses and the Ki67 proliferation index,[43] which also distinguish NET from neuroendocrine carcinoma.

The prognosis of NET depends on the grade and on features that cannot be evaluated on cytological preparations, including size and site of the lesion, presence of local invasion, angioinvasion, patterns of hormone production, and metastases.[44] Cytological atypia, mitotic index, and the proliferative index obtained by Ki67 immunostaining can be evaluated to some extent on cytological materials. Along the GI tract, the small intestine is the most common site for such tumors, followed by the rectum,[45] with the stomach a distant third. Their incidence appears to have increased in the last five decades, and this increase is most prominent in the small intestine, stomach, and rectum.[45] Cytological specimens from the ileum and rectum are almost never seen. Our experience with cytology of GI NET has primarily involved tumors in the stomach and duodenum (Box 3.8 and Fig. 3.27). The tendency of NET cells to lose their cytoplasm causes them to mimic lymphomas with small cell morphology because of their small size and characteristic monomorphism. Such stripped nuclei can be distinguished from low-grade small cell lymphoma by their complete absence of cytoplasm and their finely granular ("salt-and-pepper") chromatin pattern. Of course, one should always find intact cells to confirm the diagnosis. Small cell neuroendocrine carcinomas (small cell carcinomas) of the GI tract are similar to those seen elsewhere and are characterized by small cells with scant cytoplasm, showing nuclear molding and a finely dispersed chromatin pattern. Mitoses and necrosis are also prominent features of these tumors.

BOX 3.8 Neuroendocrine Tumor (Carcinoid) (Fig. 3.27)

- Dyshesive monomorphic epithelial cells
- Plasmacytoid appearance of the cells with eccentric round to oval nuclei and moderate amount of basophilic dense cytoplasm
- Tendency to lose cytoplasm and to present as stripped nuclei
- "Salt-and-pepper" chromatin pattern

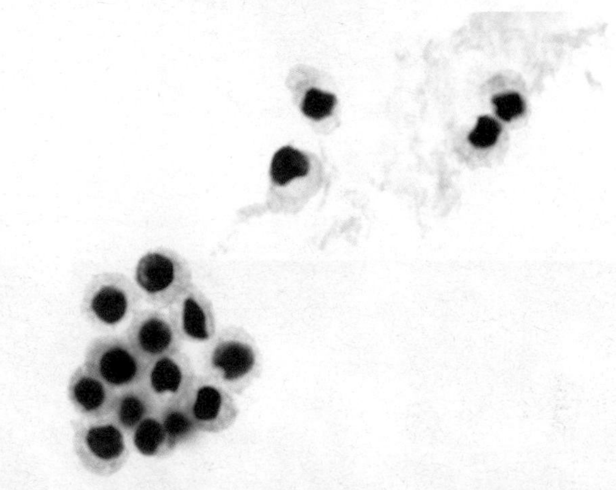

FIGURE 3.27 A loose cluster of epithelial cells and a few single monomorphic epithelial cells are seen in this duodenal brushing specimen from a grade 1 neuroendocrine (carcinoid) tumor. The eccentric nuclei give the cells a plasmacytoid appearance (Papanicolaou stain).

Mesenchymal Tumors

Mesenchymal tumors common in the GI tract include leiomyomas (predominantly of the muscularis mucosae of the esophagus and colorectum), GI stromal tumors, and leiomyosarcomas. Because of their submucosal or mural location, these tumors are not usually accessible by endoscopic brush unless the tumor is ulcerated. Endoscopic FNA with or without ultrasound guidance is the preferred method of sampling. Specimens from leiomyomas usually consist of sparse bland, cohesive spindle cells arranged in parallel lines with evenly spaced nuclei and abundant intercellular fibrillary matrix.[46] However, specimens from GI stromal tumors and leiomyosarcomas are usually cellular with loose and crowded fragments and individual spindle or epithelioid cells (Box 3.9 and Fig. 3.28).

The individual cells of GI stromal tumors have a tendency to lose their cytoplasm to become stripped, spindle-shaped, or round to oval nuclei.[47,48] Perinuclear or paranuclear vacuoles are present in some cells. Delicate cytoplasm and prominent nuclear palisading have also been noted.[49] The tumor cells may appear spindly or epithelioid.[50,51] Although leiomyosarcomas tend to show more significant nuclear pleomorphism and atypia as well as a less prominent vascular pattern than GI stromal tumors,[52,53] immunocytochemistry, polymerase chain reaction (PCR) analysis of *KIT*, or both are needed to make the definitive distinction between the two. Most GI stromal tumors show strong diffuse positivity for CD117 and DOG1, whereas leiomyosarcomas are typically positive for desmin and actin[53,54] and negative for CD117 and DOG1. Although immunocytochemical staining for CD117 and DOG1 is useful in confirming a cytological diagnosis of GI stromal tumor, the diagnosis of malignancy still depends on evaluation of the resected specimen for evaluation of factors (tumor size and mitotic activity) that cannot be assessed on cytological specimens.[55]

BOX 3.9 Gastrointestinal Stromal Tumor (Fig. 3.28)

- Cellular specimen with fascicles, clusters, and sheets of spindle or epithelioid cells or both
- Cell groups spread out thinly on the slide despite their large size
- Prominent small blood vessels
- Possibility of numerous single cells and naked nuclei
- Delicate fibrillary cytoplasm with wispy cytoplasmic extensions and indistinct cell borders
- Ovoid- to spindle-shaped and occasional wavy nuclei
- Uncommon high-grade features, such as marked nuclear atypia, frequent mitoses, and necrosis

Lymphoid Tumors

The GI tract, the stomach in particular, is the most common extranodal site for both diffuse large B-cell lymphoma and extranodal marginal zone lymphoma of mucosa-associated lymphoid tissue (MALT lymphoma), which combined constitute almost 50% of all non-Hodgkin lymphomas.[56,57] The cytological appearance of lymphoma of the GI tract depends on its subtype. With adequate material and a combination of morphology and flow cytometry, a diagnosis of lymphoma can be established on the basis of a cytology specimen.[58] The large cell type usually does not pose any diagnostic difficulty on morphology, because large malignant lymphoid cells are sufficiently atypical to raise the suspicion of a malignancy (Fig. 3.29). The challenge is to recognize them as being lymphoid and to distinguish them from poorly differentiated epithelial or mesenchymal tumors. Their lymphoid nature may in fact be easier to identify on cytology than in a small biopsy specimen. Large cell lymphoma cells shed as isolated, relatively monomorphic, large

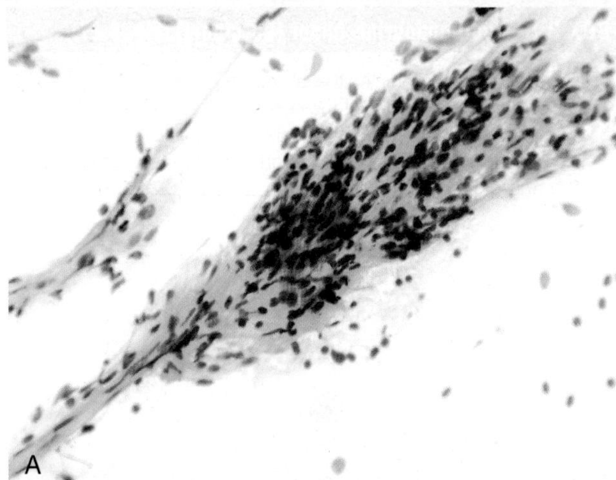

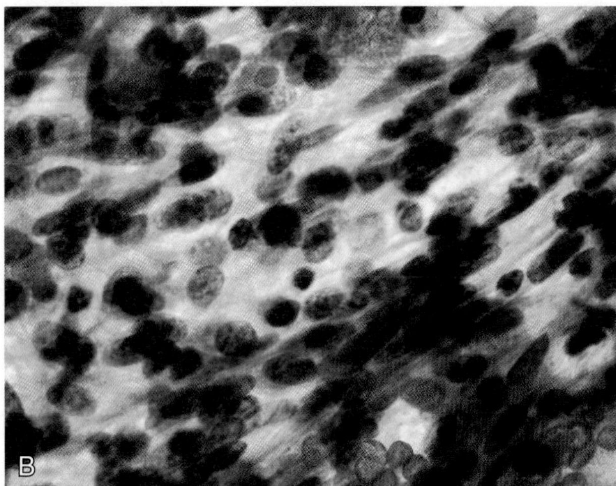

FIGURE 3.28 **A,** A hypercellular fascicle of spindle-shaped cells is seen in this endoscopic gastric fine-needle aspiration specimen of a gastrointestinal stromal tumor (Papanicolaou stain). **B,** On higher magnification, the cells have fibrillary cytoplasm and ovoid- to spindle-shaped bland nuclei (Papanicolaou stain).

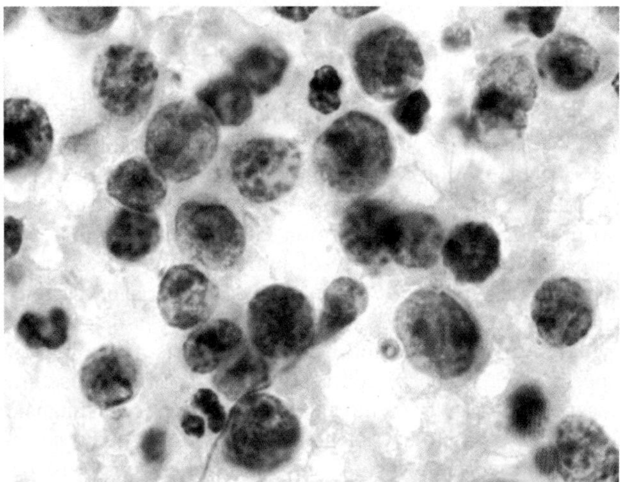

FIGURE 3.29 Gastric brushing from a biopsy-proven large B-cell lymphoma shows a monomorphic population of large atypical cells with scant cytoplasm and central large prominent nucleoli. Apoptotic bodies and a few inflammatory cells are noted in the background (Papanicolaou stain).

BOX 3.10 Lymphoma of the Mucosa-Associated Lymphoid Tissue (MALT lymphoma) (Fig. 3.30)

- Predominance of small- to medium-sized lymphocytes in an apparently inflammatory specimen
- Monomorphism and subtle atypia in the lymphoid population

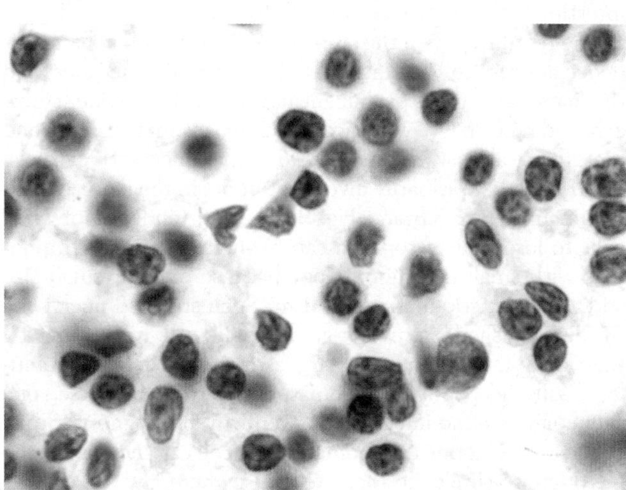

FIGURE 3.30 Endoscopic fine-needle aspiration of a biopsy-proven gastric MALT lymphoma shows a monomorphic population of medium-sized lymphoid cells with slightly irregular nuclear membranes and occasional nucleoli. Each of these cells may be mistaken for a reactive lymphocyte. The presence of many similar-appearing lymphoid cells raises the suspicion of a lymphoma (Papanicolaou stain). (*Courtesy of Dr. Martha Pitman, Massachusetts General Hospital, Boston, Mass.*)

atypical cells with scant cytoplasm, vesicular nuclei, and a single large nucleolus or multiple prominent nucleoli.[59] The absence of any true cohesion is the principal diagnostic feature of a lymphoma. Although a poorly differentiated carcinoma may shed predominantly as single cells, cell clusters can usually be found after a careful search. In addition, a poorly differentiated carcinoma often has more abundant cytoplasm, which may or may not be vacuolated, and a greater degree of nuclear pleomorphism than a large cell lymphoma. Immunocytochemical staining facilitates the distinction between lymphoma and carcinoma.

A low-grade small cell lymphoma, such as MALT lymphoma, can be difficult to diagnose by cytology. It may be mistaken for an inflammatory process (Box 3.10 and Fig. 3.30), because it may contain a polymorphous population of small, intermediate-sized, and large cells.[60,61] The dominant cell population is usually intermediate-sized lymphoid cells that contain a moderate amount of cytoplasm, show slight nuclear membrane irregularities, and have inconspicuous or completely absent nucleoli. These cells may show "plasmacytoid" morphology on air-dried preparations. Diagnosis of MALT lymphoma by cytology is challenging. A definitive diagnosis is usually made by cytology in only 50% of the cases,[60,62] and reactive follicular hyperplasia is often erroneously diagnosed.[61] While brushings may obtain limited materials, endoscopic ultrasound-guided FNA has been shown to yield sufficient materials for immunohistological, flow cytometric, and cytogenetic assessments for diagnosis of lymphoproliferative disorders.[63]

The full reference list may be accessed online at Elsevier eBooks for Practicing Clinicians.

CHAPTER 4

Infectious Disorders of the Gastrointestinal Tract

Nicole C. Panarelli

Chapter Outline

INTRODUCTION

Gastrointestinal (GI) infections are a major cause of morbidity and mortality worldwide. As the number of transplant patients and those with other immunocompromising conditions increases, and as global urbanization and transcontinental travel become more frequent, the surgical pathologist must be familiar with infectious diseases that were once limited to tropical regions of the world or the realm of esoterica.

The goal of the surgical pathologist in evaluating GI specimens for infectious colitis is two-fold. First, acute self-limited processes and infectious processes must be differentiated from chronic idiopathic inflammatory bowel disease (IBD)—ulcerative colitis (UC) or Crohn's disease (CD) (Table 4.1). Second, attempts must be made to identify the specific infecting organisms. In recent years, histochemical stains, immunohistochemistry, and molecular analysis have expanded the surgical pathologist's ability to diagnose infectious processes. As these techniques have evolved, our knowledge of the specific histological patterns of inflammation related to various organisms has also increased.

Most enteric infections are self-limited. Patients who undergo endoscopic biopsies usually have chronic or debilitating diarrhea or systemic symptoms, or they are immunocompromised. A discussion with the gastroenterologist regarding symptomatology and colonoscopic findings, as well as knowledge of the patient's travel history, dietary habits, sexual practices, and immune status, can aid the evaluation of biopsies for infectious diseases.

VIRAL INFECTIONS OF THE GI TRACT

The type of viral infection and the manifestations of disease vary with the site of infection and the immune status of the patient. Viral gastroenteritis results from a host of pathogens; those likely to be encountered in surgical pathology practice are emphasized here.

Cytomegalovirus

Clinical Features

Primary cytomegalovirus (CMV) infections in immunocompetent persons are usually asymptomatic. CMV infection may develop anywhere in the GI tract, from mouth to anus, in both immunocompromised and immunocompetent persons.[1] More than 50% of the adult population is seropositive, but infection is latent in most immunocompetent individuals.[2] CMV is best known as an opportunistic

TABLE 4.1 Morphological Features of CMV, Adenovirus, and HSV Infection

Features	CMV	Adenovirus	HSV
Cell involved	Stromal and endothelial cells, macrophages, rarely epithelial cells of the upper gastrointestinal tract	Epithelial only—either surface epithelial cells or goblet cells in colon	Epithelial cells, usually squamous
Location of inclusion	Nucleus and cytoplasm	Nucleus	Nucleus
Characteristics of inclusion	"Owl's-eye" morphology in nucleus, basophilic or eosinophilic and granular in cytoplasm	Basophilic "smudge cell" replacing nucleus most common, rarely, acidophilic inclusions with halos (Cowdry type A)	Acidophilic with clear halo and peripheral chromatin margination (Cowdry type A) or blue and homogeneous with "ground-glass" appearance (Cowdry type B)
Associated changes	Cellular enlargement, apoptosis, mixed inflammatory infiltrate, vasculitis	Surface cell disarray, loss of orientation, apoptosis, cells not enlarged	Sloughing of epithelial cells, neutrophil and macrophage-rich infiltrate, multinucleated cells common

CMV, Cytomegalovirus; *HSV*, herpes simplex virus.

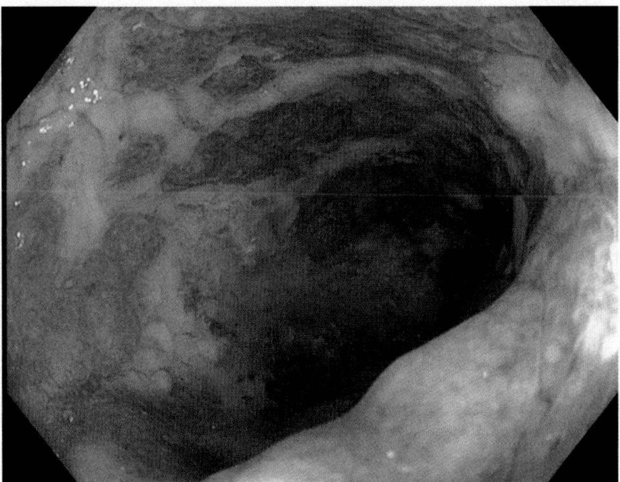

FIGURE 4.1 Cytomegalovirus produces confluent serpentine ulcers in the distal colon of an immunocompromised patient.

pathogen in patients with a suppressed immune system, most commonly in those with the acquired immunodeficiency syndrome (AIDS) and in solid organ or bone marrow transplant recipients.[3]

When symptomatic disease occurs in immunocompetent hosts, it is usually self-limited and produces a mononucleosis-like syndrome. GI involvement is subclinical in most cases. Indeed, symptomatic patients are often elderly and prove to have underlying malignancies or hematological disorders that compromise their immune systems.[4]

Symptoms vary with site of infection. Colitis causes diarrhea (either bloody or watery), abdominal pain, fever, and weight loss. Patients with esophageal infection often have dysphagia and odynophagia.[4] A rare, but important, entity associated with pediatric CMV infection is hypertrophic gastropathy and protein-losing enteropathy resembling Ménétrier's disease.[5] CMV infection is an uncommon but well-characterized cause of segmental intestinal ischemia.[6]

CMV reactivation may be superimposed on chronic GI diseases such as UC and CD. In such cases, CMV superinfection is associated with exacerbations of the underlying disease, steroid-refractory disease, toxic megacolon, and a higher mortality rate.[7] Reactivation is particularly associated with steroid-refractory disease, and, thus, some authorities recommend routine immunohistochemical evaluation for CMV in biopsies from patients with steroid-refractory UC.[8,9]

Pathological Features

CMV causes a remarkable variety of gross lesions. Ulceration is the most common; the ulcers may be single or multiple and superficial or deep. They can be quite large (>10 cm), and often have a well-circumscribed, "punched-out" appearance (Fig. 4.1).[1] Segmental ulcerative lesions and linear ulcers may mimic CD. Other gross lesions include mucosal hemorrhage, pseudomembranes, and inflammatory polyps or masses.[10,11]

The histological spectrum of CMV infection ranges from minimal inflammation to deep ulcers with prominent granulation tissue and necrosis. Frequently observed histological features include mucosal ulceration, a neutrophil-rich mixed inflammatory infiltrate, and cryptitis of glandular epithelium. Crypt abscesses, crypt atrophy and loss, and numerous apoptotic enterocytes may be seen as well. CMV-associated ischemia features vasculitis with numerous endothelial viral inclusions associated with inflammation, necrosis, and thrombosis of the affected vessel.

Infected cells show both nuclear and cytoplasmic enlargement (hence the name, "cytomegalovirus") (Fig. 4.2A). Characteristic "owl's-eye" intranuclear viral inclusions and granular intracytoplasmic inclusions may be seen on routine hematoxylin and eosin (H&E) preparations (see Fig. 4.2B,C). Inclusions are preferentially found in endothelial cells, stromal cells, macrophages, and, rarely, in glandular epithelial cells, particularly in the upper GI tract (Fig. 4.3). In contrast to adenovirus or herpes, CMV inclusions are often found deep within ulcer bases rather than at the edges of ulcers or in the superficial mucosa. Adjacent nuclei may be enlarged, appear smudged, or have a "ground-glass" appearance, but they lack typical inclusions. Characteristic inclusions with virtually no associated inflammatory reaction may occur in severely immunocompromised patients.

Although CMV inclusions are usually readily identifiable in routine sections, rare inclusions can be missed, particularly if exuberant inflammation obscures diagnostic findings (Fig. 4.4A,B). Examination of multiple levels and

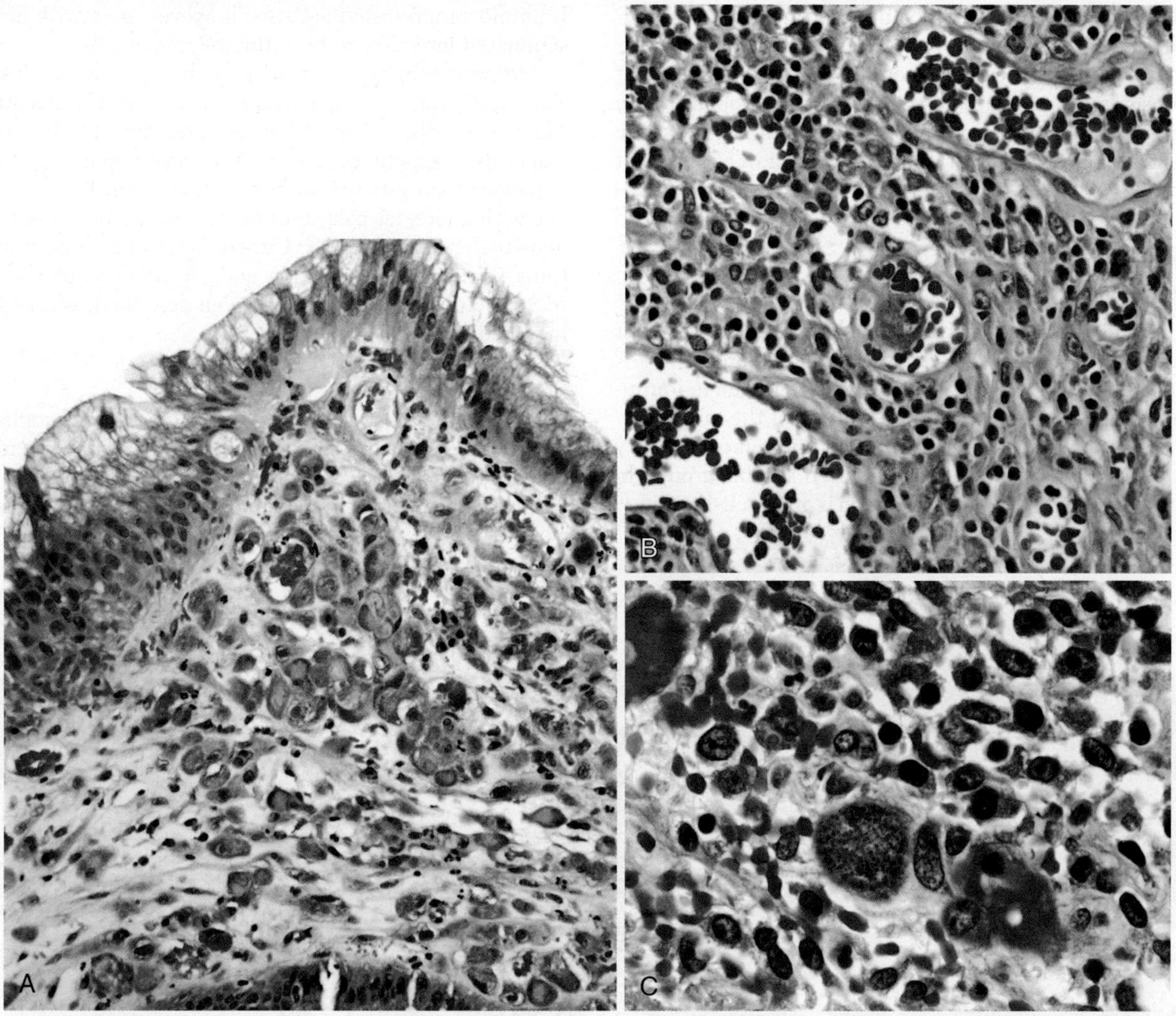

FIGURE 4.2 A, A polyp removed from the gastric antrum contains innumerable cytomegalovirus (CMV) inclusions within endothelial and stromal cells. CMV causes both nuclear enlargement and enlargement of the entire cell. **B,** Characteristic "owl's-eye" nuclear inclusions are seen within an endothelial cell at the base of an ulcer. **C,** Granular, basophilic cytoplasmic inclusions may also be seen.

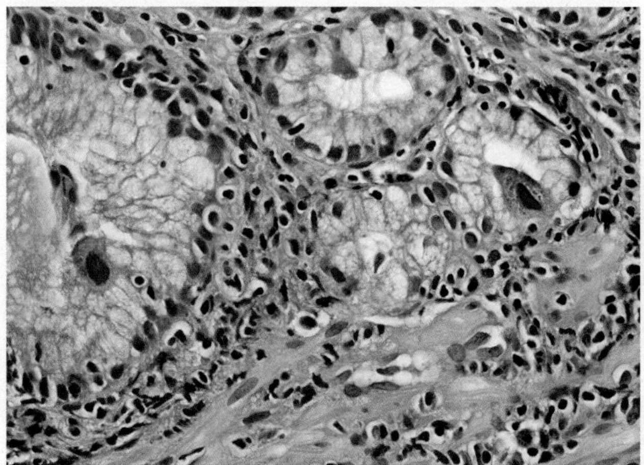

FIGURE 4.3 CMV may infect epithelial cells in the upper gastrointestinal tract. Nuclear and cytoplasmic inclusions are present in Brunner's glands in this duodenal biopsy.

use of immunohistochemistry can aid in detecting scarce inclusions.[8] On the other hand, inclusions are rarely found in uninflamed mucosae, even when immunohistochemistry is employed.[12-14] Because even single CMV inclusions may prove to be clinically important, pathologists should investigate the possibility of CMV infection when other suspicious features are present.[15]

Other diagnostic aids include viral culture, polymerase chain reaction (PCR) assays, in situ hybridization, serological studies, and antigen tests.[16] Serological studies often have limited usefulness because of the persistence of latent CMV infection. In addition, isolation of CMV in culture does not imply active infection, because the virus can be excreted for months to years after a primary infection.

Differential Diagnosis

The differential diagnosis of CMV includes primarily other viral infections (see Table 4.1), particularly adenovirus. Adenovirus inclusions are usually crescent shaped, located in surface epithelium, and only intranuclear in location. CMV inclusions are typically located in either the nucleus or cytoplasm of endothelial or stromal cells. The ballooning degeneration phase of adenovirus infection, just before cell lysis, most closely resembles CMV.

The distinction between CMV infection and graft-versus-host disease in bone marrow transplant recipients can be particularly difficult because the clinical and histological features are similar. Immunohistochemistry should be used to rule out CMV infection in this setting, because failure to identify CMV infection could result in delay of antiviral therapy.[17] Furthermore, these conditions may coexist. Graft-versus-host disease is favored when there is abundant apoptosis associated with crypt necrosis and dropout in the setting of minimal inflammation (Fig. 4.5). The presence of residual nests of endocrine cells favors graft-versus-host disease.

Herpesvirus

Clinical Features

Herpetic infection can occur throughout the GI tract but is most common in the esophagus and anorectum.[18,19] Although herpes infection of the gut is often seen in immunocompromised patients and remains one of the most common infections in patients with human immunodeficiency virus (HIV) infection, it is not limited to this group. In immunocompetent patients, infection is often self-limited.[20] Immunocompromised patients, however, are at risk for disseminated infection and life-threatening illness.

Herpetic esophagitis presents with odynophagia, dysphagia, chest pain, nausea, vomiting, fever, and GI bleeding.[20] Many have disseminated herpes infection at the time of diagnosis. Herpetic proctitis is the most common cause of nongonococcal proctitis in homosexual men. Patients present with anorectal pain, tenesmus, constipation, discharge, hematochezia, and fever.[21] Concomitant neurological symptoms (difficulty in urination and paresthesias of the buttocks and upper thighs) are also well described, as is inguinal lymphadenopathy.

Pathological Features

Ulcers are the most common gross finding in the esophagus, and these are usually associated with an exudate. The ulcers are deep or shallow and often well circumscribed. Some patients have vesicles surrounding the ulcers.[22,23] Many

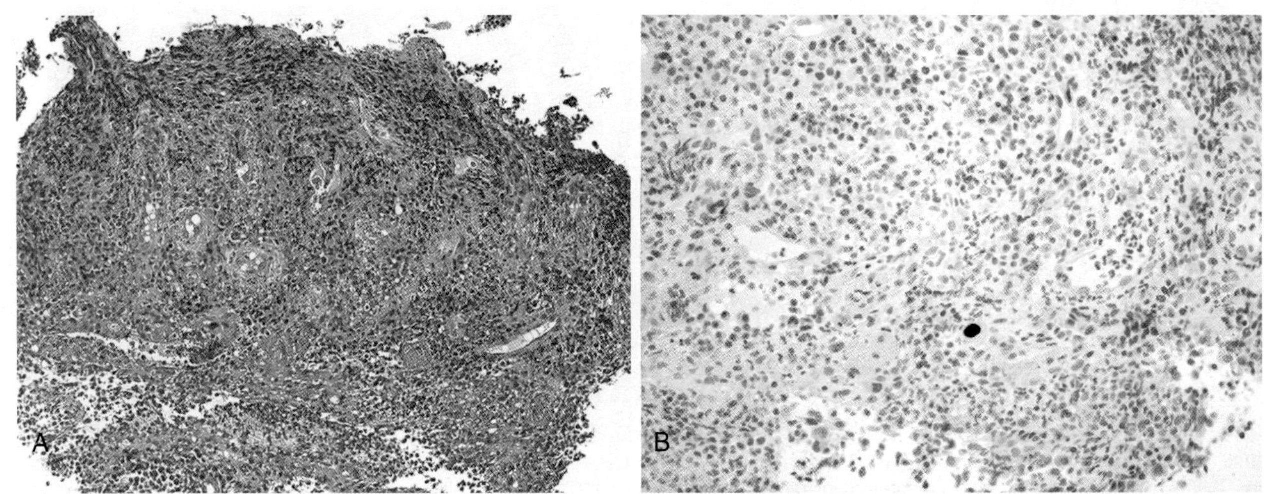

FIGURE 4.4 **A,** Cytomegalovirus inclusions are easily missed in inflamed granulation tissue. **B,** An immunostain highlights rare inclusions.

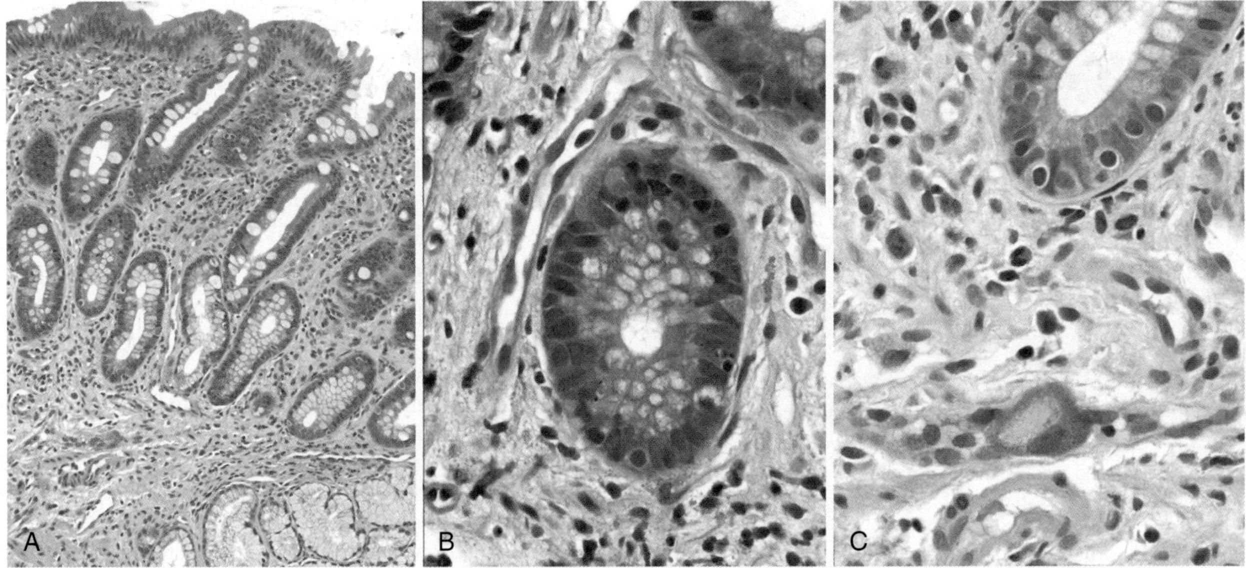

FIGURE 4.5 **A,** Biopsy samples from the duodenum of a patient with graft-versus-host disease do not show increased inflammation. **B,** Numerous apoptotic bodies are present, but are small and inconspicuous, as is typical in the upper gastrointestinal tract. **C,** A single cytomegalovirus inclusion is present in an endothelial cell, but is unassociated with an inflammatory reaction.

patients have a nonspecific erosive esophagitis without discrete ulcers, however.[23] In herpetic proctitis, the presence of perianal vesicles is common, often in association with pustules or shallow ulcers.[24] Proctoscopic findings include ulceration and mucosal friability. Vesicles may extend into the anorectum.

Typical histological findings, regardless of site, include ulceration, neutrophils in the lamina propria, and an inflammatory exudate that often contains sloughed epithelial cells (Fig. 4.6A). Prominent aggregates of macrophages also may be present.[25] In the anorectum, perivascular lymphocytic cuffing and crypt abscesses may be seen as well.

Characteristic viral inclusions and multinucleate giant cells are present in only a minority of biopsy specimens (see Fig. 4.6B,C). The best place to search for viral inclusions is in the squamous epithelium at the edges of ulcers and in sloughed cells in the exudate. Two types of nuclear inclusions may be found: acidophilic inclusions with a surrounding clear halo and peripheral chromatin margination (Cowdry type A inclusions) and homogeneous, powdery, basophilic inclusions that replace the nucleus (Cowdry type B inclusions). Inclusion-bearing cells may be singly nucleated or multinucleated. The histological findings for herpes simplex virus 1 (HSV-1) and HSV-2 are indistinguishable.

Differential Diagnosis

The differential diagnosis predominantly includes other viral infections, including CMV and varicella-zoster, that may infect the GI tract (see Table 4.1). Varicella produces histological findings identical to those of HSV, but patients often have a rash.[26] Mixed infections are common in many situations in which herpetic infection is found. Immunohistochemistry can distinguish the two. Viral culture and PCR are valuable diagnostic aids.[27] Serological studies may be useful if there is a very high or rising antibody titer but have limited use because latent infections can persist for years.[28]

Adenovirus

Adenovirus infection is second only to rotavirus as a cause of childhood diarrhea, and it is associated with a broad spectrum of diseases in both children and adults.[29] It has gained more attention in recent years as a cause of diarrhea in immunocompromised patients, especially those with AIDS and those who have received bone marrow or solid organ transplants.[30] Virtually all patients experience diarrhea, sometimes accompanied by fever, weight loss, and abdominal pain. Adenovirus is also associated with ileal and cecal intussusception in children.[31] Characteristic inclusions may

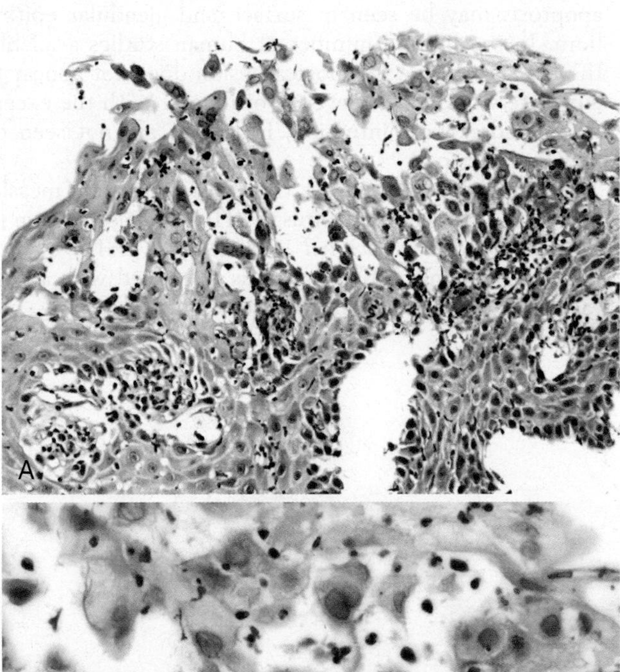

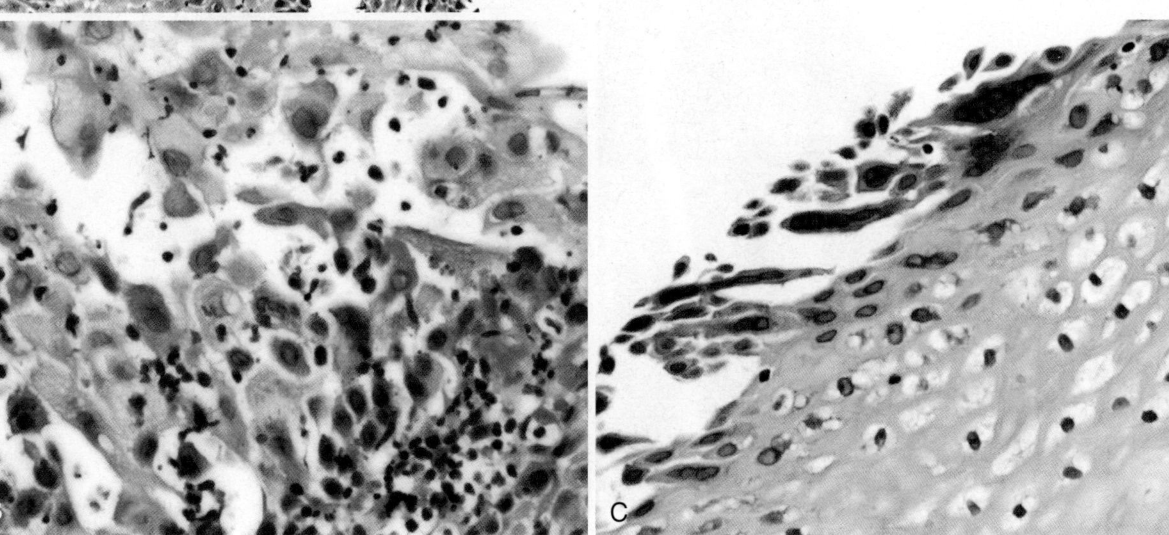

FIGURE 4.6 **A,** Esophageal biopsy shows dyshesion and sloughing of squamous epithelial cells, intraepithelial neutrophils, and herpetic inclusions within squamous cells. **B,** Higher-power view shows the homogeneous basophilic "ground-glass" inclusions of herpes simplex virus with peripherally marginated chromatin. **C,** Multiple inclusions may be present within a single cell, known as a polykaryon.

be seen, especially in immunocompromised patients, in the nuclei of surface epithelial cells (particularly goblet cells); these are often accompanied by apoptotic epithelial cells and degenerative epithelial changes. Cells containing characteristic nuclear inclusions are known as "smudge cells" because of their enlarged, homogeneous, basophilic quality (Fig. 4.7; see Table 4.1). On the other hand, adenovirus inclusions are often quite subtle and may be disregarded as reactive or degenerative cytological atypia. Immunohistochemistry, PCR, and viral serology are useful diagnostic aids (Fig. 4.8).[14] This entity is discussed further and illustrated in Chapter 5.

Other Enteric Viruses

Acute viral gastroenteritis is one of the most common causes of illness worldwide. Although most infections are self-limited, viral gastroenteritis can cause severe dehydration (particularly when caused by rotavirus), as well as chronic diarrhea in children with immunodeficiency syndromes such as severe combined immunodeficiency.[32] Enteric viral infections are a significant cause of diarrhea in patients with AIDS. Rotavirus and enterovirus, like adenovirus, are associated with intussusception in children. Many enteric viruses do not cause disease in humans; others seldom cross the stage of the surgical pathologist because they are detected in stool samples rather than biopsy specimens. Common enteric viruses known to cause diarrhea in humans include, but are not limited to, adenovirus, rotavirus, coronavirus, astrovirus, Norwalk virus, enteric caliciviruses, echovirus, and other enteroviruses.[32] Enteric involvement was documented in the coronavirus-associated severe acute respiratory syndrome (SARS), and diarrhea was a common presenting symptom in that outbreak.[33]

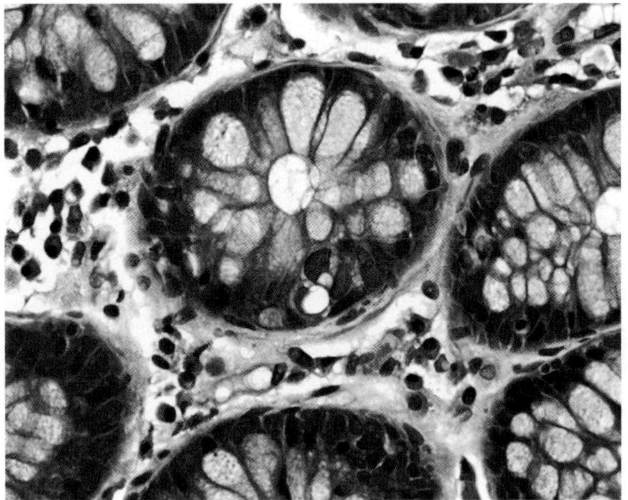

FIGURE 4.7 Multiple adenovirus inclusions, or "smudge cells," are seen within the colonic epithelial cells in this biopsy from a patient with AIDS.

Small bowel biopsy findings include villous fusion, broadening, and blunting; crypt hypertrophy; and an increased mononuclear cell infiltrate within the lamina propria with variably present neutrophils (Fig. 4.9). There also may be an increase in intraepithelial lymphocytes. Reactive and degenerative epithelial changes are usually present, particularly at the surface, including epithelial cell disarray and loss of nuclear polarity.[34,35] Increased apoptosis may be seen in surface and glandular epithelium. In the limited number of human studies available, the severity of the histological lesion does not appear to correlate with clinical severity of illness. With the exception of adenovirus infection, inclusions are not seen on light microscopy.

Other viruses that affect the GI tract include measles (rubeola), human herpesvirus 8 (HHV-8; also known as *Kaposi sarcoma–associated herpesvirus*), HHV-6, and Epstein-Barr virus (EBV), which is associated with a wide variety of lymphoproliferative disorders.[32,36-38]

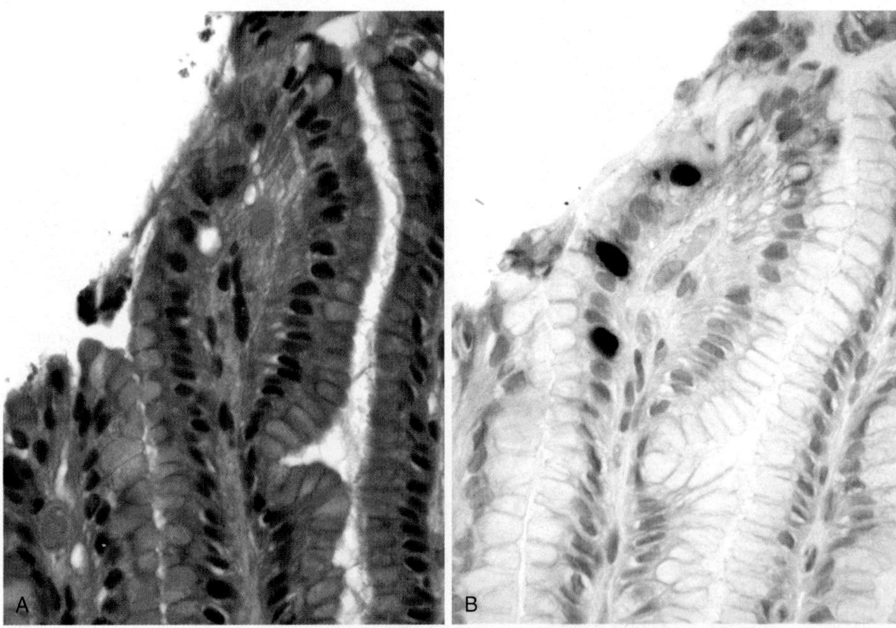

FIGURE 4.8 **A,** Adenovirus inclusions are barely perceptible in the foveolar epithelial cells of this gastric biopsy. **B,** Immunohistochemical stains are necessary to make the diagnosis. (*Courtesy of Dr. Gregory Y. Lauwers, Moffitt Cancer Center.*)

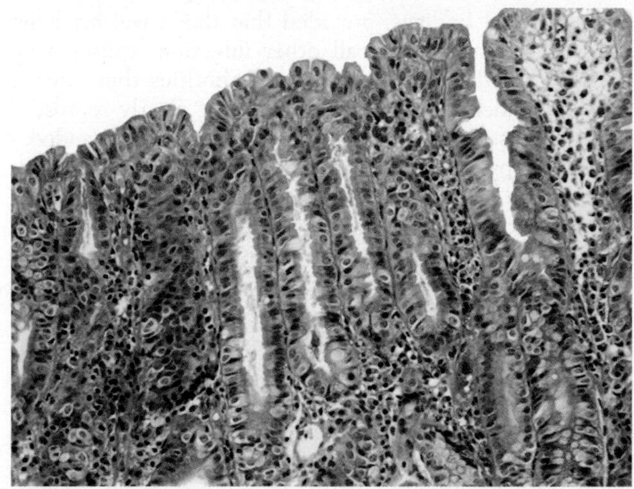

FIGURE 4.9 Villous fusion, surface reactive and degenerative changes, and mononuclear cell infiltrates are nonspecific features that can be seen in biopsies from patients with gastroenteritis caused by enteric viruses.

Human Papillomaviruses

Human papillomavirus (HPV) has been implicated in the pathogenesis of esophageal papillomas, esophageal squamous cell carcinomas, anal condylomas, and anal squamous cell carcinomas. These entities are discussed in detail in Chapters 19, 24, and 32.

Human Immunodeficiency Virus

GI disease is an important cause of morbidity and mortality in patients affected by HIV and in those with AIDS (Table 4.2). Although opportunistic pathogens are often found in these patients, there is a subgroup in whom no pathogens are found despite extensive clinical and pathological evaluation. The two major disease entities associated with HIV in the absence of other demonstrable pathogens are chronic idiopathic esophageal ulcers and AIDS enterocolopathy.

Chronic idiopathic esophageal ulcers reportedly cause approximately 30% of ulcers found in HIV-infected

TABLE 4.2 Gastrointestinal Infections Commonly Encountered by Surgical Pathologists in the HIV-Positive Population

Organism	Main Sites of Involvement	Key Features
Viruses		
Cytomegalovirus	Anywhere in the gastrointestinal tract	Intranuclear and intracytoplasmic inclusions, mainly in fibroblasts and endothelial cells Intranuclear: owl's-eye inclusions Intracytoplasmic: granular inclusions
Herpes simplex	Squamous mucosa (esophagus, anus), may also cause proctitis	Intranuclear inclusions in multinucleated epithelial cells
Bacteria		
Mycobacteria		
M. tuberculosis	Ileocecal region	Large, confluent necrotizing granulomas, concentrated in submucosa Scarce organisms on acid-fast bacilli stain
M. avium intracellulare	Duodenum, rectum	Intracellular acid-fast bacilli inhabit macrophages and distort villous architecture
Intestinal spirochetosis	Throughout colon	Adherent basophilic "fringe" of bacteria No inflammatory response
Malakoplakia	Throughout colon	Mural and mucosal macrophages contain targetoid concretions of mineralized bacterial breakdown products
Fungi		
Candida spp.	Esophagus, disseminated infection in severely immunocompromised	Yeast and pseudohyphae in sloughed squamous epithelial cells and keratin debris
Histoplasmosis	Duodenum	Small budding yeasts in macrophages
Microsporidia spp.	Small intestine	Minute intraepithelial spores, difficult to see without special stains, epithelial cell disarray
Protozoa		
Cryptosporidium parvum	Small intestine and colon	Intracellular organisms at cell apex with "blue bead" appearance
Cyclospora cayetanensis	Small intestine and colon	Round and elongated forms within epithelial cells
Cystoisospora belli	Small intestine and colon	Largest coccidians, ovoid or elliptical intracellular bodies
HIV-associated ulcerative esophagitis	Esophagus	Large ulcers with nonspecific histology; diagnosis of exclusion—requires evaluation for identifiable pathogens
HIV-associated enterocolopathy	Small intestine and colon	Villous blunting and fusion in the small intestine, increased apoptosis, crypt hyperplasia Controversial entity—may be a pattern due to multiple unidentifiable pathogens

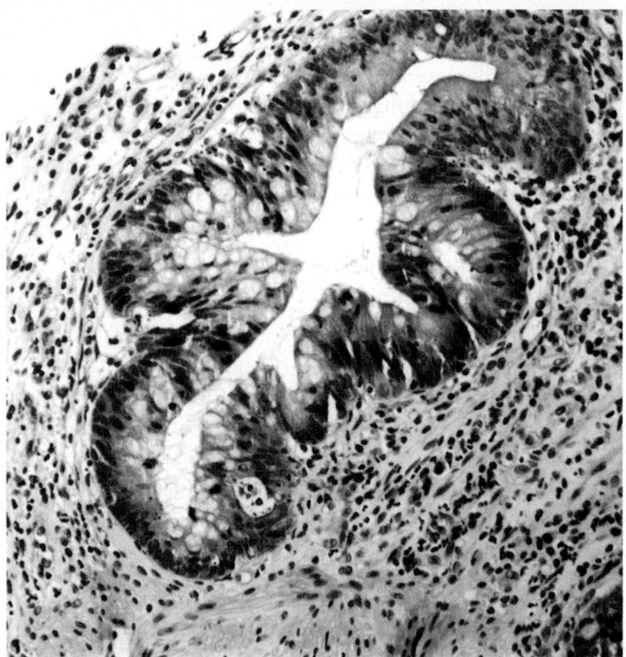

FIGURE 4.10 Increased apoptotic cells in the glands are a prominent feature of HIV-associated enterocolopathy.

patients.[39] The ability of HIV to directly cause these ulcers remains controversial, although evidence of HIV within the ulcerative lesions has been demonstrated by molecular analysis, immunohistochemical studies, and enzyme-linked immunosorbent assays (ELISAs).[40] Patients experience severe odynophagia, chest pain, and weight loss. The middle esophagus is the most common location, followed by the distal esophagus. Endoscopically, the ulcers consist of one or more well-circumscribed lesions of variable depth that can mimic ulcers caused by other infectious agents, particularly viral pathogens. They can be quite large (>3 cm in greatest dimension) and deep, with irregular margins and overhanging, edematous edges. Mucosal bridges and sinus tract formation may occur.[40] Histologically, the ulcers contain granulation tissue with a mixed acute and chronic inflammatory infiltrate that often contains eosinophils. By definition, special histochemical stains and immunohistochemical stains for identifiable pathogens must be negative. This finding is especially important because these ulcers are sometimes treated with steroids. This entity is also discussed in Chapter 5.

HIV/AIDS enteropathy/colopathy is a somewhat controversial entity that has been loosely defined as the morphological changes, such as villous blunting, crypt hyperplasia, and apoptosis, seen in the gut of patients with HIV/AIDS and chronic diarrhea for which no other infectious cause has been identified.[41-43] Controversy arises because asymptomatic patients may have similar morphological findings on biopsy and, conversely, severely symptomatic patients may have normal biopsies.[44] In addition, there is always the added concern that a causative pathogen simply has been missed. Because patients with HIV/AIDS do have severe impairments of GI function, including diarrhea, malabsorption, and weight loss, even in the absence of any demonstrable pathogens, many authors support the use of the term *AIDS enteropathy* (or *colopathy*) to describe the morphological findings, provided that the bowel has been adequately sampled and all other infectious causes have been excluded.[45] However, other authorities think this is a poorly understood term that does not clearly represent a specific disease entity and, therefore, should be avoided.

Endoscopy and colonoscopy findings are usually normal. In the small bowel, the histological features include villous blunting and atrophy, crypt hypertrophy, increased intraepithelial lymphocytes, variably increased mononuclear cells in the lamina propria, increased mitoses within glandular epithelial cells, and increased numbers of apoptotic enterocytes at the surface and in the glands. In the colon, inflammatory changes are similar, but the apoptotic epithelial cells in the glandular epithelium are often very prominent (Fig. 4.10).[41-44] The changes resemble those seen in mild graft-versus-host disease and chemotherapy-related mucosal injury. Other pathogens, particularly other viruses such as CMV and adenovirus that can produce similar histological features, must be rigorously excluded.

Severe Acute Respiratory Syndrome Coronavirus 2 (SARS-CoV-2)

Severe acute respiratory syndrome coronavirus 2 (SARS-CoV-2) causes the illness known as COVID-19. It emerged in the Hubei province of central China in late 2019, triggering a global pandemic.[46] COVID-19 is primarily a lower respiratory tract disease that causes fever, cough, pneumonia, and, in severe cases, respiratory failure and death. Transmission occurs via respiratory droplets. The virus uses cellular serine proteases, such as TMPRSS2, to prime its spike proteins and enters cells via the angiotensin-converting enzyme 2 (ACE2) receptor, located on pneumocytes and some enterocytes.[47-49] Up to 30% of patients with COVID-19 experience digestive symptoms, including abdominal pain, nausea, vomiting, diarrhea, and loss of appetite.[50,51] A smaller proportion first present with GI illness.[52] An association between increased disease severity and GI involvement was found in one study; however, overall mortality is similar to that for those who do not experience GI symptoms.[50,53] There is no specific therapy for COVID-19–related diarrhea, and care is supportive.

Very little is known about the histopathological features of GI SARS-CoV-2 infection. One case of hemorrhagic diarrhea reportedly yielded normal-appearing biopsy samples.[54] Similarly, a case in which the authors detected ACE2 protein expression by immunofluorescence in glandular epithelia appeared essentially normal in routine sections.[55] Intestinal ischemia associated with mesenteric and small vessel thromboses, as well as pneumatosis intestinalis, are increasingly reported.[55a,55b] Viral RNA is detectable in stool samples of approximately half of COVID-19 patients and persists for several weeks after infection; stool samples are positive in a small subset of patients with negative respiratory swab samples.[55] However, strong evidence for fecal-oral transmission is presently lacking.[56]

Mild liver injury, including elevated transaminases, prolong prothrombin time, and hypoproteinemia may also occur in up to 50% of COVID-19 patients. Nonspecific features, including hepatocellular apoptosis, increased mitotic activity, and lobular inflammation are reported. It is not clear whether these findings are related to viral toxicity or effects of polypharmacy in critically ill patients.[57]

BACTERIAL INFECTIONS OF THE GI TRACT

Bacterial diarrhea is a worldwide health problem. Many bacterial infections of the gut are related to ingestion of contaminated water or food and foreign travel to areas of poor sanitation. Although bacterial pathogens are often recovered by microbial culture, surgical pathologists may play a valuable role in diagnosis. Despite the dizzying array of bacterial infections that may affect the GI tract, many produce a similar spectrum of histological features and may be generally categorized as follows (Table 4.3):

1. Organisms that produce mild or no histological changes, such as *Vibrio cholerae* and *Neisseria gonorrhoeae*
2. Organisms that produce the histological features of acute infectious/self-limited colitis (ASLC) or focal active colitis (FAC), such as *Campylobacter*, *Aeromonas*, and some *Salmonella* spp.
3. Organisms that produce specific or characteristic histological features, such as pseudomembranes, granulomas, chronic colitis, or ischemia

Acute Self-Limited Colitis

The ASLC pattern is the most common pattern in enteric infections. Typical histological features include neutrophils in the lamina propria, with or without crypt abscesses and cryptitis; preservation of crypt architecture; and lack of basal plasmacytosis (Fig. 4.11).[58-61] The acute inflammatory component is often most prominent in the middle to upper levels of the crypts. Lack of crypt distortion, Paneth cell metaplasia, and basal lymphoplasmacytosis help to distinguish ASLC from IBD (Table 4.4).[59] The changes may be focal, as in focal active colitis, or diffuse.

Surgical pathologists should be aware of the infections that are most likely to mimic CD, UC, and ischemic colitis (Boxes 4.1 to 4.3, Table 4.5). Because most patients do not present for endoscopy until several weeks after the onset of symptoms, pathologists usually are not exposed to the classic histological features of acute infectious colitis. This is important because the resolving phase of infectious colitis is more challenging to diagnose. At this stage, only occasional foci of neutrophilic cryptitis and only patchy increases in lamina propria inflammation may be found, and these may, in fact, contain abundant plasma cells and increased intraepithelial lymphocytes, features that are also seen in CD or even lymphocytic colitis. It is important to be aware of the patient's symptoms (particularly acute versus chronic onset) and, ideally, the culture results, because the exact diagnosis may be difficult to resolve on histological grounds alone. The pathological details of specific bacterial infections are discussed in the following sections.

Major Causes of Bacterial Enterocolitis

Vibrio cholerae *and Related Species*

V. cholerae (specifically the toxigenic O1 strain) is the causative agent of cholera, an important worldwide cause of watery diarrhea and dysentery that may lead to significant dehydration, electrolyte imbalance, and death within hours.[62] Most infections result from consumption of raw or undercooked seafood, especially shellfish. Other vibrios, including non-O1 strains of *V. cholerae*, *Vibrio vulnificans*, and *Vibrio parahaemolyticus*, also can cause severe gastroenteritis.[63] *Vibrio hollisae*, known to cause severe diarrhea, was recently reclassified as *Grimontia hollisae*.[64] Symptoms of cholera include the abrupt onset of diarrhea, usually profusely watery and rarely bloody, accompanied by abdominal pain, vomiting, muscle cramps, and fever. Disseminated infection is a particularly important risk with immunocompromised patients; patients with underlying liver disease, partial or total gastrectomy, and diseases of iron metabolism are also at risk for more serious *Vibrio* infections.[65]

Despite the severity of the illness, *V. cholerae* O1 is a noninvasive toxin-producing organism that causes minimal or no histological change to the intestinal mucosa. Nonspecific findings such as small bowel mucin depletion, degenerative surface epithelial changes, and a mild increase in lamina propria mononuclear cells have been rarely reported.[66,67] Nontoxigenic O1 and other non-*cholerae Vibrio* spp. may show erosive enterocolitis with active neutrophilic inflammation and associated hemorrhage. Stool and blood cultures are the mainstays of clinical diagnosis.[68,69]

Aeromonas *and Related Species*

Initially thought to be nonpathogenic gram-negative bacteria, *Aeromonas* and related species are increasingly recognized as causes of gastroenteritis in both children and adults, and elaborate toxins similar to those of better-recognized pathogens, such as *Shigella* spp.[70-73] *Aeromonas hydrophila*, *Aeromonas caviae*, and *Aeromonas sobria* most often cause GI disease in humans.[73] Infection usually is caused by exposure to untreated water but also may result from consumption of contaminated foods such as produce, meat, and dairy products. Infections most frequently occur in the late spring, summer, and early fall, and children are most commonly affected. A mild, self-limited diarrheal illness is most common, sometimes accompanied by nausea, vomiting, and cramping abdominal pain. A more severe, dysentery-like illness occurs in 15% to 25% of patients, featuring bloody or mucoid diarrhea and fecal leukocytes.[71] This variant is most likely to mimic chronic idiopathic IBD endoscopically.

Endoscopic findings include mucosal edema, friability, erosions, exudates, and loss of vascular pattern. The distribution is often segmental, either right- or left-sided, and may mimic CD (Table 4.6).[72,74] The histological features are usually those of ASLC, including cryptitis, crypt abscesses, and a neutrophilic infiltrate in the lamina propria. However, ulceration and focal architectural distortion may be seen in some cases (Fig. 4.12).

The differential diagnosis includes other infectious colitides and chronic idiopathic IBD. When architectural distortion is present in a patient with more chronic symptoms or macroscopic features mimicking chronic idiopathic IBD, it may be difficult to resolve the issue of *Aeromonas* infection versus CD or UC. Although there are no histological features specific for *Aeromonas* infection, it is important for the surgical pathologist to realize that this is one of the bacteria that can most closely mimic chronic idiopathic IBD. Stool cultures are critical to diagnosis, and certain selective media may be required.[75]

Escherichia coli

Escherichia coli is the most common gram-negative human pathogen. The diarrheogenic *E. coli* are classified into five

TABLE 4.3 Classification of Bacterial Infections of the Gastrointestinal Tract by Histological Pattern

Inflammatory Pattern	Organism	Disease Distribution	Other Key Pathological Features
Acute self-limited colitis	*Campylobacter* spp.	Ileocecal region, appendix, mesenteric lymph nodes	Occasional crypt architectural distortion
	Salmonella spp., nontyphoidal strains	Ileocecal region	Occasional crypt architectural distortion
	Shigella spp., early stages	Extends proximally from rectum	Inflammatory bowel disease–like pattern in later stages; see below
	Aeromonas spp.	Segmental colitis	Occasional crypt architectural distortion
Inflammatory bowel disease–like	*Yersinia* spp.	Ileocecal region, appendix, mesenteric lymph nodes	Epithelioid granulomas with lymphoid cuffing and central suppurative inflammation
	Salmonella typhi	Ileocecal region	Deep ulcers Reactive lymphoid follicles infiltrated by macrophages Necrosis of Peyer's patches Crypt architectural distortion
	Shigella spp., late stages	Left colon more severely affected, may be patchy	Occasional pseudomembranes
	Mycobacterium tuberculosis	Ileocecal region, mesenteric lymph nodes	Large, confluent centrally necrotic granulomas, concentrated in submucosa
	Mycobacterium avium intracellulare complex	Duodenum, rectum	Diffuse histiocytic inflammation, abundant intracellular organisms (immunocompromised hosts) Necrotizing granulomas, rare organisms (immunocompetent hosts)
	Treponema pallidum (syphilis)	Anorectum	Rare, poorly formed granulomas Proliferative endarteriolitis with perivascular cuffing of plasma cells Subtle architectural distortion Spirochetes subjacent to squamous epithelium or in and around crypt epithelium on immunostains
	Chlamydia trachomatis	Anorectum	Rare, poorly formed granulomas
Ischemic colitis	Enterohemorrhagic *Escherichia coli*	Ascending and transverse colon	Fibrin thrombi Pseudomembranes Superficial necrosis with sparing of deep crypt regions
	Clostridioides difficile	Pancolitis, more severe distally, rectum may be spared	Pseudomembranes Crypt cell apoptosis "Signet ring" morphology of sloughed epithelial cells
	Clostridium septicum	Ileocecal region	Pseudomembranes Absence of neutrophils
	Clostridium perfringens	Jejunum, ileum	Pneumatosis
	Klebsiella oxytoca	Ascending and transverse colon	Usually lacks pseudomembranes
Minimal changes	*Vibrio cholera*	Small intestine	Mucin depletion Degenerative epithelial changes Increased lamina propria mononuclear inflammation
	Brachyspira spp. (spirochetosis)	Any segment of colon	Adherent organisms produce basophilic fringe on mucosal surface
	Neisseria spp.	Anorectum	Focal cryptitis
	Enteroadherent *E. coli*	Ascending colon	Degenerative surface epithelial changes Adherent bacteria at the surface with "brush border" appearance

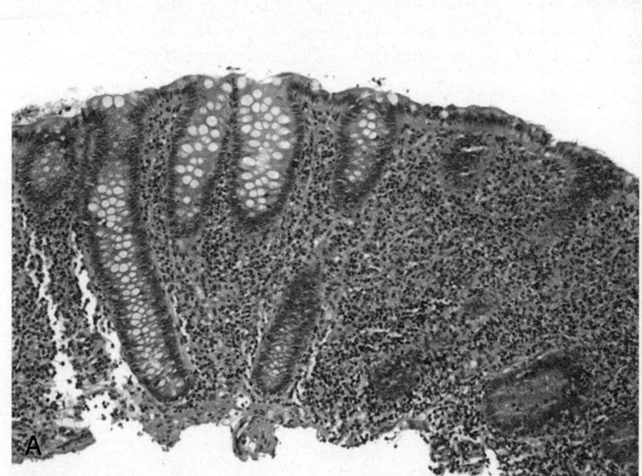
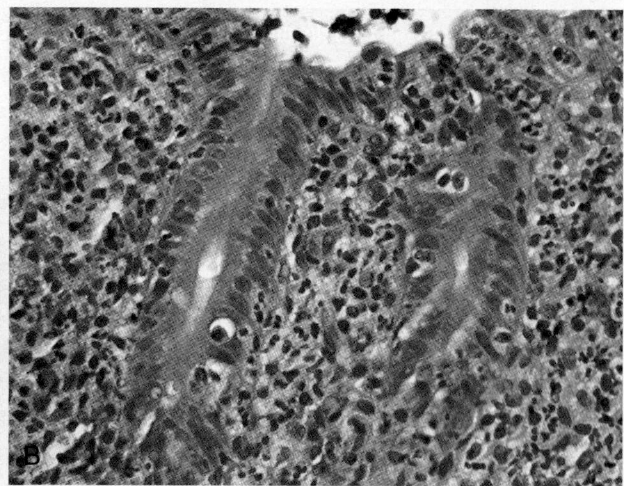

FIGURE 4.11 **A,** Acute self-limited colitis features increased lamina propria inflammation with preserved architecture. **B,** Neutrophil-rich inflammation is present in the lamina propria and infiltrating damaged crypts.

TABLE 4.4 Comparison of Acute Self-Limited Colitis and Inflammatory Bowel Disease Patterns

Features	Acute Self-Limited Colitis	Inflammatory Bowel Disease Pattern
Presentation	Sudden, usually spontaneously resolves	Insidious, worsens progressively
Distribution	Organism dependent, but usually segmental or patchy	Patchy (Crohn's disease) Continuous, extending proximally (ulcerative colitis)
Histological Features		
Lamina propria inflammation	Mixed, neutrophil-rich, evenly or superficially distributed	Basal lymphoplasmacytosis
Cryptitis and crypt abscesses	Present	Present
Architectural distortion	Absent	Present
Paneth cell metaplasia	Absent	Present
Granulomas	Poorly formed, if present, associated with crypt rupture	May be present
Overlapping features	Late stages may feature lymphoplasmacytic inflammation and mild architectural distortion	Early stages may have preserved architecture, lack Paneth cell metaplasia

BOX 4.1 Bacterial Mimics of Crohn's Disease

Yersinia spp.
Mycobacterium tuberculosis
Salmonella typhimurium
Aeromonas spp.
Syphilis
Lymphogranuloma venereum

BOX 4.2 Bacterial Mimics of Ulcerative Colitis

Shigella spp.
Nontyphoid *Salmonella* spp.
Aeromonas spp.
Syphilis
Lymphogranuloma venereum

BOX 4.3 Bacterial Mimics of Ischemic Colitis

Foodborne
- Enterohemorrhagic *Escherichia coli*
- *Clostridium perfringens* (pigbel)

Antibiotic-associated
- *Clostridioidies difficile*
- *Clostridium perfringens*
- *Klebsiella oxytoca*

Neutropenia-associated
- *Clostridium septicum*

groups, based primarily on serotyping (Box 4.4).[76,77] If pathogenic *E. coli* is suspected, the clinical laboratory should be notified to search for it specifically, because it may be missed on routine culture. In addition, because pathogenic *E. coli* strains are often cleared rapidly from stool (often within 4 to 7 days), cultures should be taken as early as possible.

TABLE 4.5 Comparison of Ischemic Colitis with Common Infectious Mimics

Features	Ischemic Colitis	Enterohemorrhagic *Escherichia coli*	*Clostridioides difficile*
Clinical setting	Hemodynamic or mechanical vascular compromise Systemic vasculitis	Consumption of contaminated food, especially beef and produce	Nosocomial, history of antibiotic use May be community acquired
Disease distribution	Watershed areas (splenic flexure, rectosigmoid colon)	Ascending and transverse colon	Pancolitis, more severe distally
Crypt withering	Present	Present	May be present
Crypt dilatation	May be present	May be present	Prominent
Lamina propria hyalinization	Present	Present	Not prominent
Pseudomembranes	Often present	Often present	Present
Cryptitis	Uncommon	Present	Present
Fibrin thrombi	Present	Present	Uncommon
Confirmatory studies	Typical imaging features	Culture	Polymerase chain reaction for toxin-related genes

TABLE 4.6 Features Useful in the Differential Diagnosis of Crohn's Disease and Its Bacterial Infectious Mimics

Features	Crohn's Disease	*Yersinia spp.*	*Mycoplasma tuberculosis*	*Salmonella typhimurium*	*Aeromonas*	Syphilis and Lymphogranuloma venereum
Distribution	Patchy, involves multiple sites	Limited to ileocecal region	Preferentially involves ileocecal region, may involve multiple sites	Limited to ileocecal region	Segmental or pancolitis	Limited to anorectal region
Granulomata	Few, variably present, epithelioid, noncaseating, lack lymphoid cuff	Numerous, confluent, noncaseating with central suppurative inflammation and lymphoid cuff	Numerous, confluent, caseating with lymphoid cuff	Rare	Absent	Rare, crypt rupture associated
Inflammatory pattern	Chronic active colitis involving any segment	Chronic active colitis limited to areas with granulomas	Chronic active colitis limited to areas with granulomas	Chronic colitis with hyperplastic lymphoid follicles infiltrated by macrophages Necrosis of Peyer patches, extending to overlying mucosa	Acute self-limited colitis	Chronic active colitis, Proliferative endarteriolitis with perivascular cuffing of plasma cells
Architectural distortion	Prominent	Prominent	Prominent	Prominent	Focal or absent	Present, but limited

Enterotoxigenic and Enteropathogenic E. coli

These noninvasive organisms cause nonbloody diarrhea. Enterotoxigenic *E. coli* (ETEC) is a major cause of traveler's diarrhea and of outbreaks within industrialized nations.[78] Enteropathogenic *E. coli* (EPEC) is predominantly an infection of infants and neonates.[79] The gross and microscopic pathology of ETEC and EPEC have not been well described in humans.

Enteroinvasive E. coli

Enteroinvasive *E. coli* (EIEC) are very similar to *Shigella* genetically and in their clinical presentation and pathogenesis; therefore, although not well described, the pathology may be expected to be similar as well.[80] Symptoms include diarrhea (typically mucoid and watery, but nonbloody), tenesmus, fever, malaise, and abdominal cramps. EIEC is transmitted by contaminated cheese, water, and person-to-person contact; it is also a cause of traveler's diarrhea.[81] The organisms produce a severe, dysentery-like illness and bacteremia; this can be a particular problem in AIDS patients.[82]

Enteroadherent E. coli

This noninvasive strain of enteroadherent *E. coli* (EAEC) is similar to EPEC. Both have been increasingly recognized as causes of chronic diarrhea and wasting in AIDS patients.[83–85]

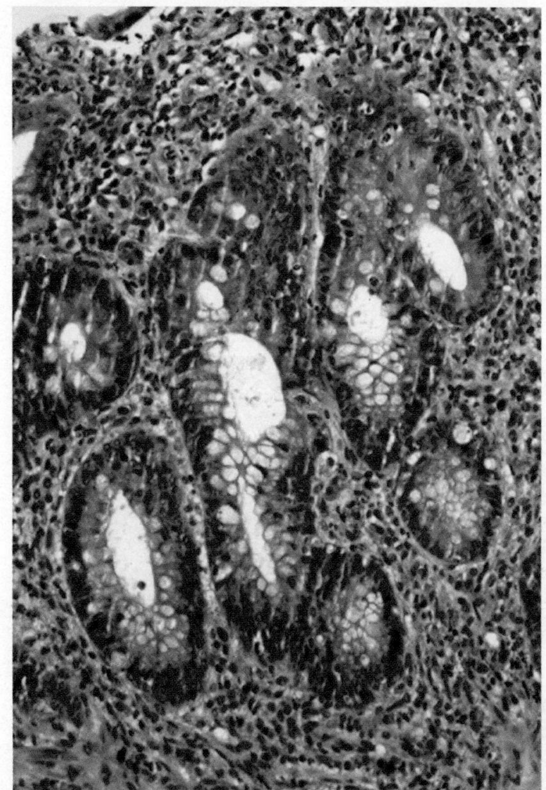

FIGURE 4.12 Focal cryptitis and architectural distortion are seen in a right colon biopsy specimen in a case of culture-proven *Aeromonas* infection that was initially thought to be Crohn's disease based on the endoscopic appearance.

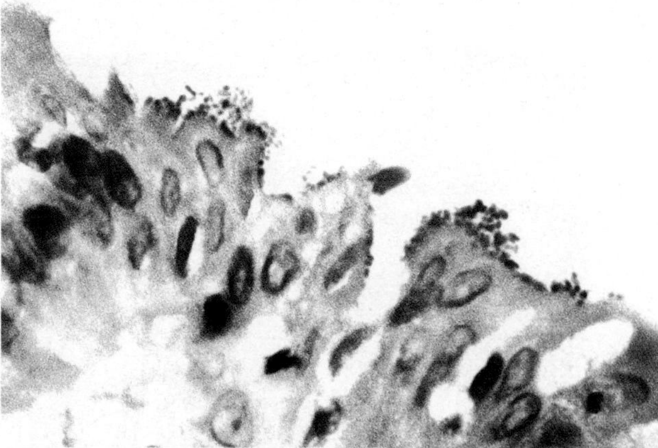

FIGURE 4.13 Enteroadherent *Escherichia coli* in a patient with AIDS. A coating of gram-negative rods with little inflammatory reaction is seen at the surface of the colonic mucosa (Gram stain). (*Courtesy of Dr. Mary Bronner, University of Utah School of Medicine.*)

Although endoscopic findings are usually unremarkable, right colon biopsies more often yield pathological findings. Histological examination shows degenerated surface epithelial cells with associated intraepithelial inflammatory cells. A coating of adherent bacteria on the surface epithelium is the most prominent feature (Fig. 4.13). The bacteria may be tightly or loosely adherent. The histological findings can be patchy and can resemble an exaggerated brush border; they may easily be missed at low power.[86] In addition, specimens from infected patients may show no associated inflammatory reaction whatsoever. The main entities in the differential diagnosis are normal mucosa and spirochetosis; the bacteria in EPEC and EAEC are not spirillar, in contrast to those in spirochetosis.

BOX 4.4 Key Features of *Escherichia* Species Infections of the Gastrointestinal Tract

GENERAL FEATURES
- Foodborne gram negative bacilli
- Most common cause of bacteria-associated diarrhea worldwide
- Cattle are largest reservoir
- Fecal-oral transmission in humans

ENTEROPATHOGENIC AND ENTEROTOXIGENIC *E. COLI*
- Noninvasive, colonize small intestine
- Cause secretory diarrhea
- Affect travelers, and infants
- Pathological features not well described

ENTEROINVASIVE *E. COLI*
- Mucoid, watery, but nonbloody diarrhea
- Affects travelers and AIDS patients
- Pathological features not well described, but may be similar to shigellosis given genetic similarity

ENTEROADHERENT *E. COLI*
- Adherent, but noninvasive, to the right colon
- Diarrhea and wasting in AIDS patients
- Fringe-like bacteria adherent to surface with little inflammation

ENTEROHEMORRHAGIC *E. COLI*
- Shiga toxin–producing strain
- Causes severe bloody diarrhea, hemolytic uremic syndrome, thrombotic thrombocytopenic purpura
- Acute ischemic colitis–like features with fibrin thrombi and relative sparing of deep mucosa

Enterohemorrhagic E. coli

Clinical Features

The most common strain of enterohemorrhagic *E. coli* (EHEC) is O157:H7. This pathogen gained national attention in 1993 when a massive outbreak in the western United States was linked to contaminated ground beef. Although contaminated meat is the most frequent mode of transmission, infection may also occur through contaminated water, milk, and produce and through person-to-person contact. EHEC produces a cytotoxin similar to that of *Shigella dysenteriae*, but there is no invasion.[87] Hemolytic-uremic syndrome or thrombotic thrombocytopenic purpura may develop in affected persons, and children and the elderly are at particular risk for grave illness.[88] In some studies, the use of antibiotics to treat EHEC appears to increase the risk for hemolytic-uremic syndrome.[89] Symptoms usually consist of bloody diarrhea with severe abdominal cramps and mild or no fever.[87]

Pathological Features

Endoscopically, patients typically have severe mural edema with associated hemorrhage. The mucosa is eroded and ulcerated, and ulcers often have an overlying purulent exudate. The edema may be so marked as to cause obstruction, and surgical resection may be required to relieve this or to control bleeding. The right colon is usually most severely affected.[90] The histological features closely resemble ischemic colitis of other causes, including marked edema and hemorrhage in the lamina propria and submucosa with associated mucosal acute inflammation, crypt withering, and lamina propria

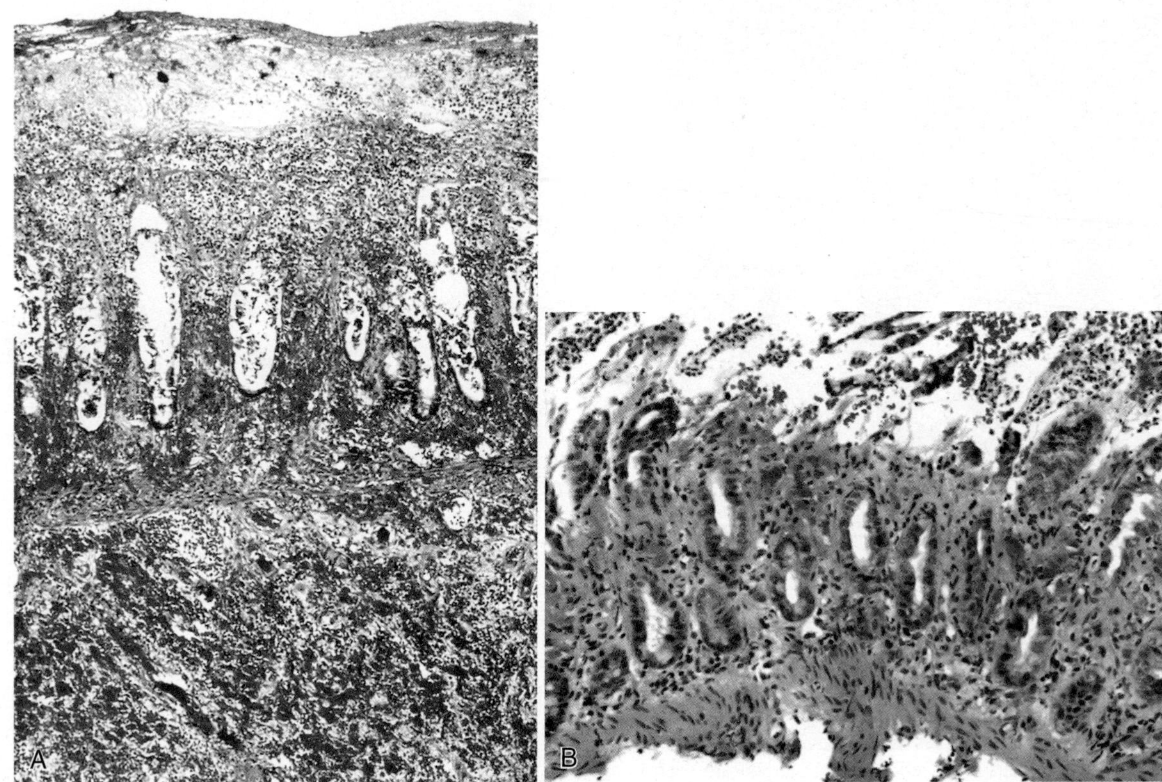

FIGURE 4.14 Enterohemorrhagic *Escherichia coli*. **A,** Transmural hemorrhagic necrosis and an acute inflammatory exudate are seen in this right colon resection from a patient with *E. coli* O157:H7 infection. **B,** The crypt withering and lamina propria hyalinization simulate ischemic colitis.

hyalinization (Fig. 4.14). Microthrombi may be present within small-caliber blood vessels, and pseudomembranes resembling antibiotic-associated pseudomembranous colitis (PMC) are occasionally present as well. Mucosal necrosis is frequently seen, often involving the upper portion of the mucosa but sparing the deeper crypts.[90,91] Stool culture is invaluable in making the diagnosis; however, routine stool cultures cannot distinguish O157:H7 from normal intestinal flora, because microbiological diagnosis requires screening on selective agar. An immunohistochemical stain for the EHEC organism has been described. Fortunately, PCR-based assays are increasingly available.[92]

Differential Diagnosis

The differential diagnosis primarily includes *Clostridioides difficile*–related PMC and ischemic colitis of other causes, from which EHEC may be histologically indistinguishable (see Table 4.5). The clinical history, including the possibility of consumption of contaminated food, the age of the patient, and macroscopic findings may aid in distinguishing ischemia from *E. coli* infection. The C. *difficile* antigen test or PCR assays, or both, may be helpful, if positive.

Antibiotic-associated hemorrhagic colitis has been reported in association with *Klebsiella oxytoca*. This colitis is hemorrhagic, segmental, most common in the right and transverse colon, and lacks pseudomembranes.[93] A history of penicillin therapy is key to distinguishing this infection from EHEC.

Salmonella

Salmonellae are gram-negative bacilli that are transmitted through food and water and are prevalent where sanitation is poor. They are an important cause of both food poisoning and traveler's diarrhea.[94] Human disease is caused by subspecies of *S. enterica*. The subspecies include typhoid and nontyphoid serovars.[95] Enteric (typhoid) fever is usually caused by the serovar *S. typhi* but may also be caused by *S. paratyphi;* the most common nontyphoid species include *S. enteritidis*, *S. typhimurium*, *S. muenchen*, *S. anatum*, and *S. give*. Although historically enteric fever was considered a much more severe disease and nontyphoid salmonellosis a milder one, more recent literature suggests a greater degree of overlap (both clinically and pathologically) than previously thought. Patients with low gastric acidity are at increased risk of salmonellosis, and patients with AIDS have a greater risk of *Salmonella* infection and a greater likelihood of severe infection and septicemia.[96,97]

Typhoid (Enteric) Fever

Typhoid fever typically manifests with abdominal pain, headache, an elevation in fever over several days, and occasionally constipation. An abdominal rash and leukopenia are often seen. Diarrhea, which begins in the second or third week of infection, is initially watery but may progress to severe GI bleeding. Perforation and toxic megacolon may complicate typhoid fever.[98]

Any level of the alimentary tract may be involved, but the characteristic pathology is associated with lymphoid aggregates and Peyer patches and therefore is most prominent in the ileum, appendix, and ascending colon. Grossly, the bowel wall is thickened and raised nodules may be seen corresponding to hyperplastic lymphoid tissue. Aphthous

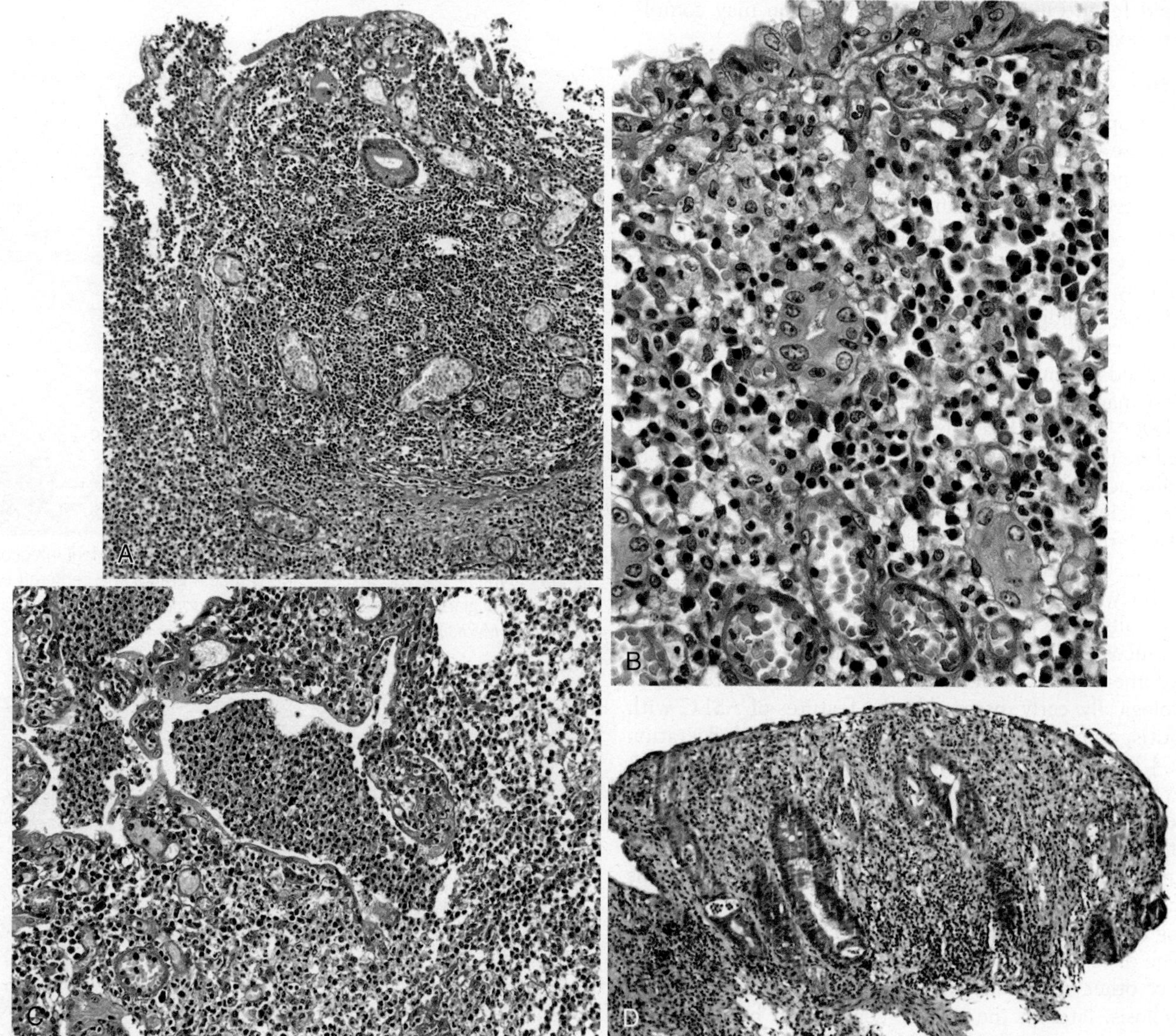

FIGURE 4.15 **A,** The typical histological lesion of typhoid fever is ulceration overlying a lymphoid aggregate or Peyer's patch. **B,** The typical inflammatory infiltrate is predominantly mononuclear, featuring plasma cells, lymphocytes, and histiocytes, with inconspicuous neutrophils. **C,** Architectural distortion can mimic that of chronic idiopathic inflammatory bowel disease. **D,** Nontyphoid *Salmonella* infection often shows features of acute infectious-type colitis but can also exhibit mild architectural disarray and gland loss. (**A** *courtesy of Dr. A. Brian West, Yale University.*)

ulcers overlying lymphoid aggregates, linear ulcers, discoid ulcers, and full-thickness ulceration and necrosis are common as the disease progresses. Associated suppurative mesenteric lymphadenitis may occur. Occasionally, the mucosa is grossly normal or only mildly inflamed and edematous.[99-102]

Macrophages are the predominant inflammatory cell. Hyperplasia of Peyer's patches leads to acute inflammation of the overlying epithelium (Fig. 4.15A,B). Eventually, macrophages infiltrate and obliterate the lymphoid follicles; neutrophils are not prominent. Necrosis then begins in the Peyer's patch and spreads to the surrounding mucosa, which eventually ulcerates. Ulcers are typically deep.[99-102] Architectural distortion that may mimic UC or CD is well described (see Fig. 4.15C). Typhoid fever occasionally shows features more consistent with ASLC, including prominent neutrophils, cryptitis, crypt abscesses, and overlying fibrinous exudate. Granulomas are occasionally seen.

Nontyphoid Salmonella *Species*

Nontyphoid *Salmonella* infection typically manifests as a self-limited gastroenteritis. Endoscopic findings include mucosal redness, ulceration, and exudates; pathological features are those of nonspecific ASLC. Occasionally, significant crypt distortion may be seen (see Fig. 4.15D).[99,100,103]

The differential diagnosis of typhoid fever includes other infections as well as chronic idiopathic IBD (see Box 4.2), and there may be significant histological overlap among these entities. A prominence of neutrophils and granulomas is rare in typhoid fever, and although significant crypt distortion has been reported in some cases of salmonellosis, it is usually more pronounced in chronic idiopathic IBD.[101,102] The differential diagnosis of nontyphoid *Salmonella* infection includes other causes of infectious ASLC, and occasionally chronic idiopathic IBD as well. Clinical presentation and blood and stool cultures can be invaluable to the pathologist in sorting out this differential diagnosis, and bone marrow biopsy culture may be useful in establishing the diagnosis of typhoid fever. Of note, *Salmonella* infection may complicate preexisting idiopathic IBD.[104]

Shigella

Shigella spp. are virulent, invasive, gram-negative bacilli that cause severe watery and bloody diarrhea and are a major cause of infectious diarrhea worldwide. Infection is transmitted by water contaminated with feces, and person-to-person transmission is also possible. It has the highest infectivity rate of the enteric gram-negative bacteria; symptoms may result from ingestion of a very low number of organisms. Children younger than 6 years of age are commonly affected, as are homosexual men and malnourished or debilitated patients.[105,106] Constitutional symptoms are the earliest manifestation and include abdominal pain, malaise, and fever. The diarrhea is often watery initially; this is followed by the onset of bloody diarrhea containing mucus or pus and accompanied by tenesmus. Complications include severe dehydration, sepsis, perforation, toxic megacolon, reactive arthritis, Reiter syndrome, and hemolytic-uremic syndrome.[106] Chronic disease is rare.

Grossly, the large bowel is typically affected (the left side usually more severely), but the ileum may be involved. The mucosa is hemorrhagic, with exudates that may form pseudomembranes. Ulcerations are variably present.[107] Histologically, early disease has the features of ASLC with cryptitis, crypt abscesses (often superficial), and ulceration (Fig. 4.16). Pseudomembranes similar to those of *Clostridioides difficile* (formerly *Clostridium difficile*) infection may be seen, as may aphthous ulcers similar to those seen in CD. As the disease continues, increased mucosal destruction occurs with many neutrophils and other inflammatory cells in the lamina propria. Marked architectural distortion mimicking idiopathic IBD is well described.[108]

The differential diagnosis of early shigellosis is primarily that of other infections, particularly EIEC and C. *difficile*. Shigellosis, later in the disease course, can be extremely difficult to distinguish from UC (see Box 4.2), both endoscopically and histologically. Stool cultures and clinical presentation may be helpful in this instance. Multiple stool cultures may be necessary, because the organism dies rapidly and prolonged transit time may affect culture yield.

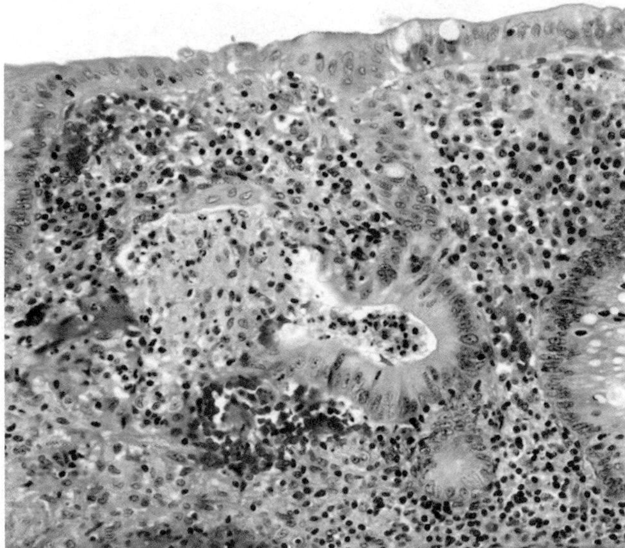

FIGURE 4.16 This biopsy from a patient with *Shigella sonnei* infection shows cryptitis, a crypt abscess, and a mucin granuloma centered on a damaged gland. (*Courtesy of Dr. Mary Bronner, University of Utah School of Medicine.*)

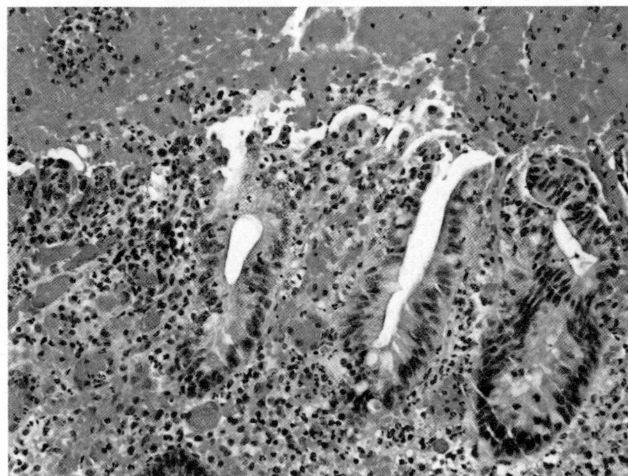

FIGURE 4.17 This case of culture-proven *Campylobacter jejuni* colitis shows a neutrophilic infiltrate with overlying surface mucosal erosion and hemorrhage. The architecture is largely preserved.

Campylobacter

Campylobacter (the name is derived from the Greek for "curved rod") is a genus of gram-negative bacteria that are major causes of diarrhea worldwide.[94] Infection is most commonly associated with consumption of undercooked poultry, raw milk, or untreated water. *Campylobacter jejuni* is more frequently associated with food borne gastroenteritis; *Campylobacter fetus* and the other, less common species are more often seen in immunosuppressed patients and homosexual men.[109,110] *Campylobacter* infects patients of all ages, but infants, children, and young adults are most often affected. The incidence in HIV-positive patients is higher than in the general population, and severe, chronic, recurrent, or disseminated infections are more common in this group. *Campylobacter* infection is associated with the subsequent development of several autoimmune disorders, including Guillain-Barré syndrome, Henoch-Schönlein purpura, and reactive arthropathy.[111] *Campylobacter* infection may also cause exacerbations of underlying chronic idiopathic IBD.[112] Patients typically have fever, malaise, abdominal pain (often severe), and watery diarrhea that may contain blood and fecal leukocytes. Nausea, vomiting, tenesmus, myalgias, and headache are variably present. Symptoms typically resolve within 1 to 2 weeks, but relapse is common.[113]

Endoscopic findings include friable colonic mucosa with associated erythema and hemorrhage.[114,115] Histological examination shows features of ASLC. Mild crypt distortion may occasionally be seen, although the architecture overall is preserved (Fig. 4.17). The differential diagnosis primarily includes other forms of infectious enterocolitis that produce the acute infectious-type colitis or focal active colitis pattern. Occasionally, when crypt distortion is seen, *Campylobacter* colitis can mimic chronic idiopathic IBD. Cultures are useful in resolving the differential diagnosis.[115]

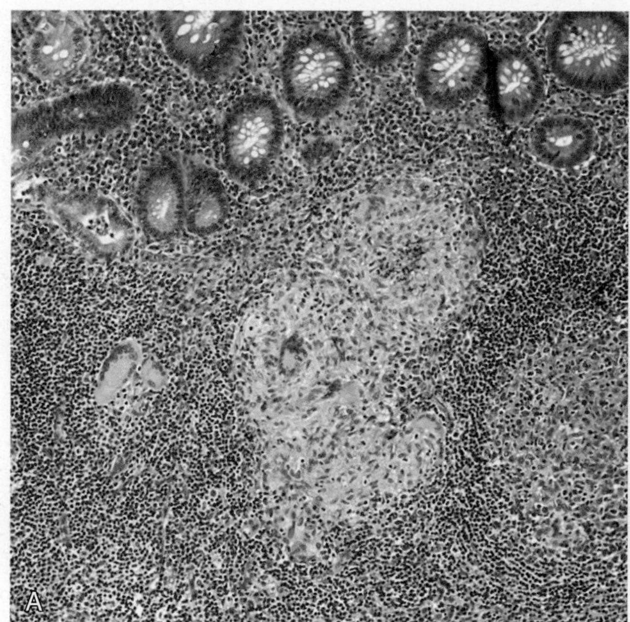
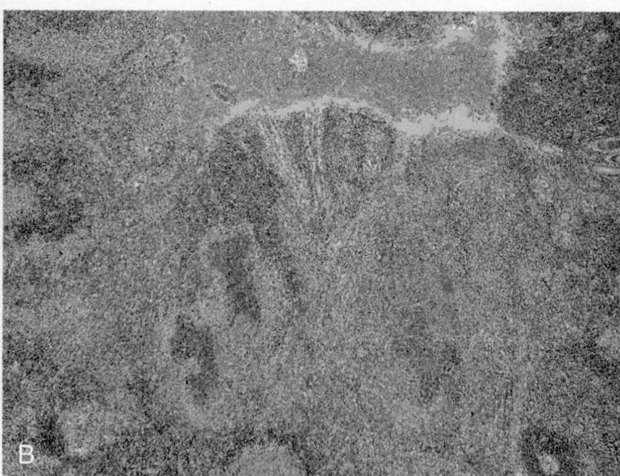

FIGURE 4.18 A, Epithelioid granulomas with prominent lymphoid cuffs are typical of *Yersinia enterocolitica* infection. **B,** Lymphoid hyperplasia with necrotizing granulomatous inflammation and prominent microabscess formation in a case of appendicitis caused by *Yersinia pseudotuberculosis.*

Yersinia

Yersinia are among the most common agents of bacterial enteritis in Western and Northern Europe, and the incidence is rising in both Europe and the United States. These gram-negative coccobacilli may cause appendicitis, ileitis, colitis, and mesenteric lymphadenitis. Although yersiniosis is usually a self-limited process, chronic infections (including chronic colitis) have been well documented.[116] Immunocompromised and debilitated patients, children, and patients who are taking desferrioxamine or have iron overload, are at risk for serious disease.[117-119] *Yersinia enterocolitica* and *Yersinia pseudotuberculosis* are the species that cause human GI disease.[120]

Yersinia organisms preferentially involve the ileum, right colon, and appendix and may cause a pseudoappendicular syndrome. In addition, they are responsible for many cases of isolated granulomatous appendicitis. Grossly, the involved bowel has a thickened, edematous wall with nodular inflammatory masses centered on Peyer's patches. Aphthous and linear ulcers may be seen. Involved appendices are enlarged and hyperemic, as in suppurative appendicitis; perforation is often seen.[121,122] Involved lymph nodes may show gross foci of necrosis.

Both suppurative and granulomatous patterns of inflammation are common, and these are often mixed. Significant overlap is seen between the histological features of infection with either species, and either may show epithelioid granulomas with prominent lymphoid cuffing (Fig. 4.18A), lymphoid hyperplasia, transmural lymphoid aggregates, mucosal ulceration, and lymph node involvement. GI infection with *Y. pseudotuberculosis* has been characteristically described as a granulomatous process with central microabscesses, almost always accompanied by mesenteric adenopathy (see Fig. 4.18B).[121-123] Gram stains are usually not helpful, but cultures, serological studies, and PCR assays may be useful in confirming the diagnosis.

The major differential diagnosis includes other infectious processes, particularly with mycobacteria and *Salmonella* spp. Acid-fast stains and culture results should help distinguish mycobacterial infection; clinical features and the presence of greater numbers of neutrophils, microabscesses, and granulomas may help distinguish yersiniosis from salmonellosis.

CD and yersiniosis may be difficult to distinguish from one another, and they have a long and complicated relationship (see Table 4.6 and Box 4.1). They may show similar histological features, including transmural lymphoid aggregates, skip lesions, and fissuring ulcers. In fact, isolated granulomatous appendicitis has in the past frequently been interpreted as primary CD of the appendix. However, generalized IBD rarely develops in patients with granulomatous inflammation confined to the appendix.[122,124] Features that favor a diagnosis of CD include cobblestoning of mucosa and creeping fat, grossly, and microscopic changes of chronicity, including crypt distortion, thickening of the muscularis mucosae, and prominent neural hyperplasia. However, some cases are indistinguishable on histological grounds alone.

Clostridial Diseases of the Gut

Clostridial organisms are some of the most potent toxigenic bacteria in existence. Members of this group of bacteria are responsible for PMC/antibiotic-associated colitis (usually C. *difficile*); necrotizing jejunitis (usually *Clostridium perfringens* [formerly *Clostridium welchii*]); neutropenic enterocolitis or typhlitis (often *Clostridium septicum*), a serious complication of both chemotherapy-associated and primary neutropenia; and botulism (*Clostridium botulinum*) (Table 4.7).

Clostridioides difficile–*Related Colitis*

Clinical Features

Clostridium difficile was recently renamed *Clostridioides difficile* to reflect substantial genetic differences from other

TABLE 4.7 Key Features of Common *Clostridioides* and *Clostridium* Infections of the Gastrointestinal Tract

Features	*Clostridioides difficile*	*Clostridium perfringens*	*Clostridium septicum*
Source	Spores travel via person-to-person transmission and proliferate in background of antibiotic use and altered intestinal flora	Contaminated food, particularly pork	Opportunistic, may come from contaminated food
Clinical setting	Nosocomial, community acquired	Meat consumption after a period of malnutrition, some cases arise in background of diabetes mellitus	Immunocompromise, particularly chemotherapy (neutropenic enterocolitis/ "typhlitis")
Endoscopic features	Pancolitis, yellow-white pseudomembranes bleed when scraped off, mucosal erythema and friability	Dusky-red with loss of folds and vascular pattern, may have pseudomembranes	Terminal ileum and right colon have multiple ulcers with overlying pseudomembranes
Histological features	Features of acute ischemia, pseudomembranes Ballooned, dilated crypts lined by attenuated epithelium, intercrypt necrosis, superficial epithelial cells slough into the lumen and may mimic signet ring cells	Transmural necrosis with hemorrhage and pneumatosis, pseudomembranes Gram-positive organisms in necrotic mucosa	Transmural mononuclear infiltrate and necrosis with neutrophilic debris at ulcer bases, pseudomembranes, pneumatosis

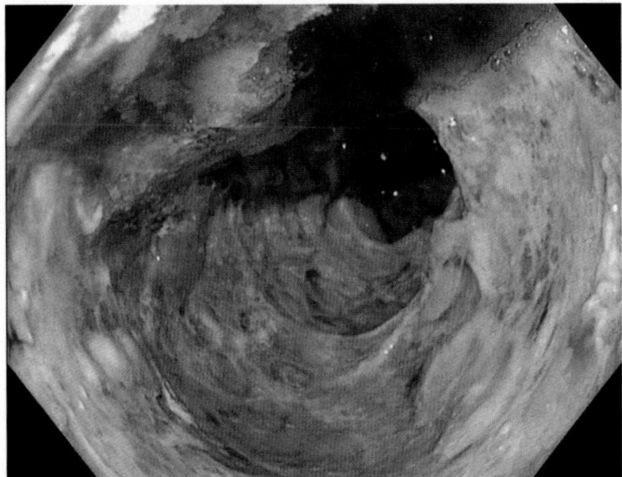

FIGURE 4.19 Yellow-gray pseudomembranes bleed when disrupted in a case of *Clostridioides difficile* colitis.

species of clostridia.[125] C. *difficile* infection is most commonly related to prior antibiotic exposure (especially orally administered antibiotics), because the organism cannot establish infection within the gut in the presence of normal flora.[126] It is the most common nosocomial GI pathogen. Infection occurs via person-to-person transmission of spores. The majority of patients are elderly, although infection is certainly not limited to this group.[127,128] Recurrent disease is seen in up to half of cases, despite successful treatment. Furthermore, the incidence of community-acquired severe or life-threatening C. *difficile* colitis in healthy individuals in North America has increased because of the hypervirulent and antibiotic-resistant BI/NAP1 strain.[129] The range of clinical disease is highly variable, from mild diarrhea to fully developed PMC to fulminant disease with perforation or toxic megacolon. Watery diarrhea is almost always present initially and may be accompanied by abdominal pain, cramping, fever, and leukocytosis. Bloody diarrhea is sometimes seen. Symptoms can occur as long as several weeks after discontinuation of antibiotic therapy.[130,131]

Pathological Features

The entire colon is often involved, but the disease may be patchy or segmental, and any segment of the bowel may be affected, including the small bowel and the appendix. Classic PMC shows yellow-white pseudomembranes, most commonly in the left side of the colon, that bleed when scraped (Fig. 4.19). The rectum may be spared.[132] Atypical findings include mucosal erythema and friability without pseudomembranes, and typical histological findings may be seen in the absence of macroscopically evident pseudomembranes.

Histologically, classic PMC features "volcano" or "mushroom" lesions with intercrypt necrosis and ballooned crypts, giving rise to the laminated pseudomembrane composed of fibrin, mucin, and neutrophils (Fig. 4.20A). Ballooned glands are filled with neutrophils and mucin (see Fig. 4.20B,C), and the superficial epithelial cells are often lost. Degenerated goblet cells may slough and spill into the lumen of degenerated and necrotic crypts (see Fig. 4.20D); it is important to be aware of this reactive morphological change in the context of PMC, because it can mimic signet ring cell adenocarcinoma. Severe and prolonged PMC may lead to full-thickness mucosal necrosis. Less characteristic nonspecific lesions, usually focal active colitis with occasional crypt abscesses but lacking the pseudomembranous feature, have been well described in association with a positive C. *difficile* toxin assay.[133]

Differential Diagnosis

It is important to remember that the term "pseudomembranous colitis" is descriptive, not a specific diagnosis. Although most cases of PMC are related to C. *difficile*, other infectious entities (especially *Shigella* and EHEC), as well as ischemic colitis, can have a similar appearance. A hyalinized lamina propria favors the diagnosis of ischemia; other features, such as crypt withering, pseudomembranes, and mucosal necrosis, may be seen in either entity.[25] Endoscopically, pseudomembrane formation is more frequent in PMC, although it can be seen in ischemia.

A history of antibiotic use may be important in making the diagnosis (see Box 4.3). PCR for C. *difficile* toxin–related

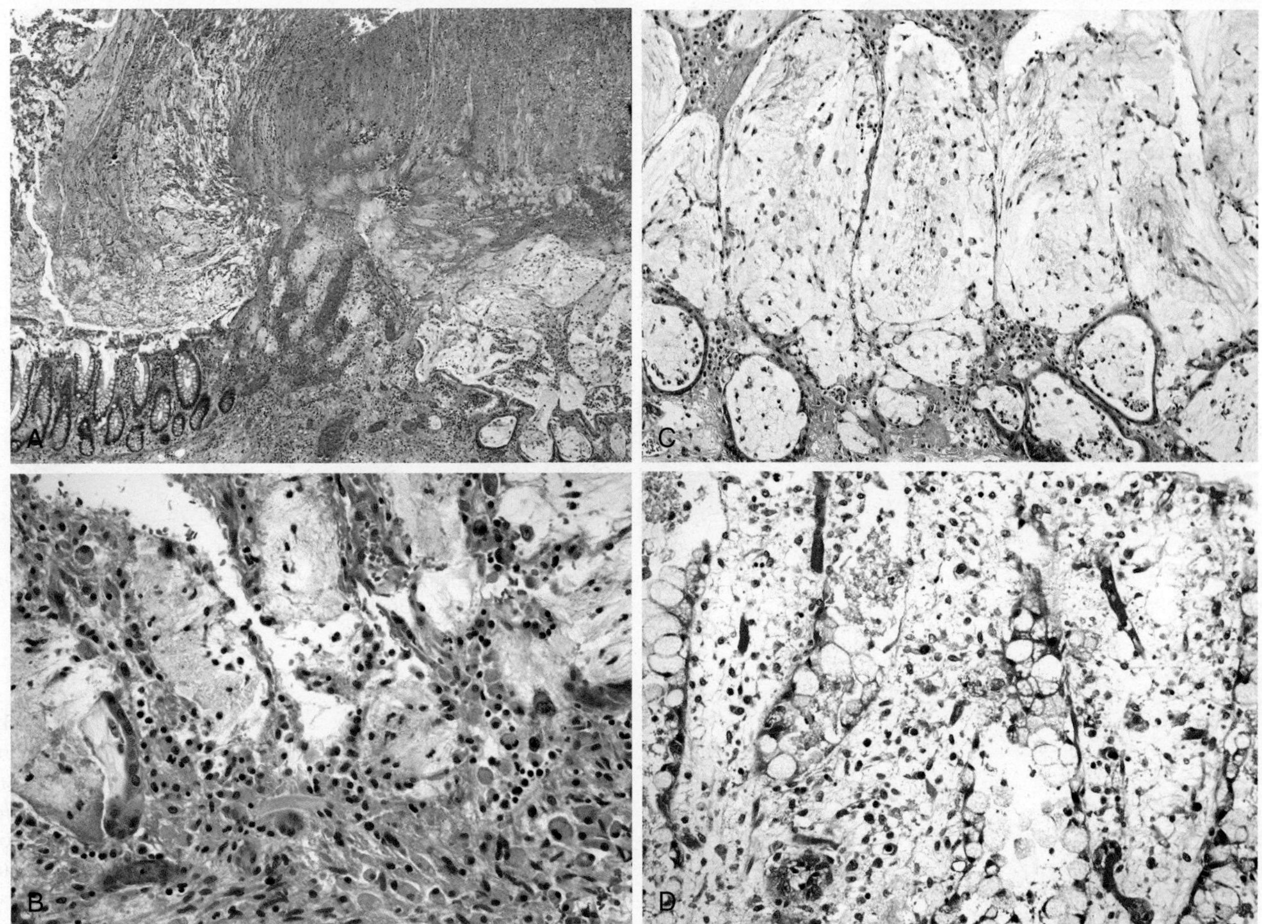

FIGURE 4.20 **A,** Pseudomembranes comprise layers of fibrin, mucin, and inflammatory cells extruded from necrotic crypts in a classic "volcano" configuration. **B,** Dilated crypts are denuded and contain mucin, sloughed epithelial cells, and inflammatory cells. **C,** Intercrypt necrosis ensues and obscures the native mucosal architecture. **D,** Sloughed epithelial cells have a signet ring appearance, but should not be mistaken for malignancy.

genes have recently replaced enzyme immunoassays (EIAs) that detect toxins A and B, owing to their superior sensitivity and specificity.[134] Yet, PCR is still used in conjunction with EIA because the former does not distinguish between biologically active toxins and asymptomatic carrier states.[135] Although stool culture is considered the gold standard, it is technically demanding and requires at least 3 days to produce reliable results.[135]

Clostridium perfringens

Clinical Features

C. *perfringens* causes segmental necrotizing enteritis (also termed *enteritis necroticans* or *pigbel*) related to food poisoning. This bacteria also causes diarrhea unrelated to food poisoning, which is often associated with antibiotic use, diabetes, and hospitalization in elderly patients.[136-141] Food-related infection is most common in Southeast Asia and Papua New Guinea. The onset of disease usually follows a meal rich in infected meat and occurs in persons with malnutrition and those in endemic areas who routinely eat very-low-protein diets and foods that are high in protease inhibitors.[142] Similar cases have been described after eating binges in Western countries.[143] Symptoms include abdominal pain, bloody diarrhea, and vomiting, often with abdominal distention. Complications include perforation, obstruction, bowel gangrene, and septicemia with shock and rapid death. Mild or subacute forms have also been described. Involvement is predominantly seen in the jejunum but is not limited to that site.

Pathological Features

The bowel is often dusky gray-green, as in ischemia. Necrotic areas may be segmental and quite focal, with intervening areas of normal mucosa. The mucosal exudate can be similar to that of PMC, but inflammation and necrosis often become transmural and lead to perforation. Histologically, the mucosa is necrotic and ulcerated, with a heavy acute inflammatory infiltrate at the edges of ulcers (Fig. 4.21A). Small-vessel vasculitis and microthrombi may be seen. Pneumatosis may be present in severe cases, particularly in the mucosa and submucosa (see Fig. 4.21B). Gram-positive bacilli typical of *Clostridium* can be found in the necrotic exudate.[141]

Differential Diagnosis

The major entities in the differential diagnosis of necrotizing enteritis include ischemia and other infections that cause an ischemic-type injury, such as EHEC (see Box 4.3). The clinical history of consumption of large quantities of meat (especially pork or pork products) may be helpful,

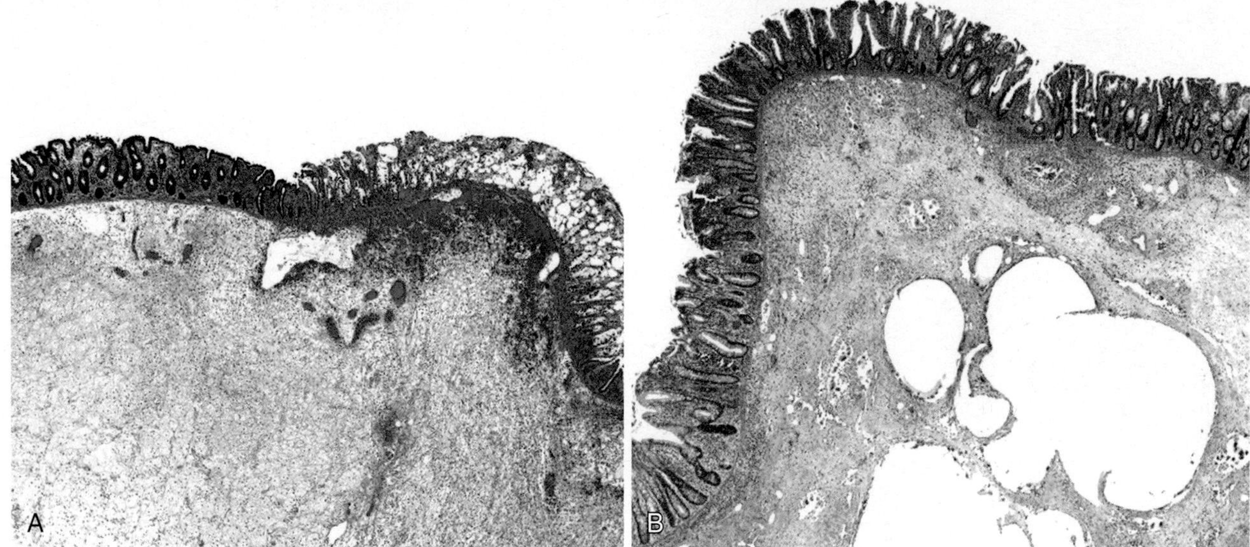

FIGURE 4.21 **A,** Mucosal hemorrhage, necrosis, ulceration, and crypt withering that mimic ischemia are seen in this case of *Clostridium perfringens* infection. **B,** Pneumatosis may also be found in the submucosa. (**A** *courtesy of Dr. Robert D. Odze, Brigham and Women's Hospital.*)

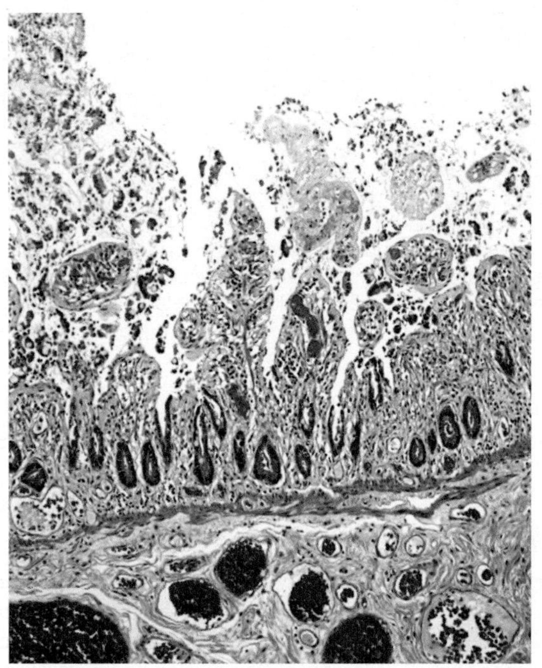

FIGURE 4.22 Typhlitis (neutropenic enterocolitis) in a chemotherapy patient features ulceration with hemorrhage, prominent submucosal edema, mucosal ulceration and necrosis, and almost no neutrophils.

along with exclusion of other possible causes of ischemia. Cultures can help to distinguish C. *perfringens* from other bacteria.

Clostridium septicum

Clinical Features

C. *septicum* is associated with neutropenic enterocolitis (typhlitis), a serious complication of both chemotherapy-related and primary neutropenia. Most patients have received chemotherapy within the month before the onset of colitis.[144] Although C. *septicum* has been frequently reported as a causative agent of typhlitis, especially in adults, other commonly implicated bacteria include other clostridial species, *E. coli*, *Pseudomonas* and *Klebsiella* spp., and enterococci.[145] C. *septicum* infection is also associated with malignancies (particularly adenocarcinoma) in the colon and distal ileum, and infection may be the first indication of such a tumor.[146] Patients usually are seen with the abrupt onset of GI hemorrhage, accompanied by fever, abdominal pain and distention, and diarrhea. The pain often initially localizes to the right lower quadrant but quickly progresses to peritonitis, shock, and sepsis. Perforation is a well-described complication, and infection is often fatal.

Pathological Features

The right colon (especially the cecum) is preferentially involved, although the ileum and other sites in the colon may be affected. Gross findings include diffuse dilatation and edema of the bowel, with varying severity of ulceration and hemorrhage. Exudates and pseudomembranes resembling C. *difficile* colitis are common. Microscopically, changes range from mild hemorrhage to prominent submucosal edema, ulceration, marked hemorrhage, and focal necrosis, often with a striking absence of neutrophils (Fig. 4.22).[145] However, neutrophils may sometimes be found despite peripheral neutropenia. Sometimes organisms can be detected in the wall of the bowel on Gram staining.

Differential Diagnosis

The differential diagnosis includes ischemic colitis and PMC (see Box 4.3). The appropriate clinical setting and dearth of inflammatory cells should favor a diagnosis of neutropenic enterocolitis. Culture is the most helpful technique for confirming the diagnosis of C. *septicum* infection, and isolation of the organism from blood cultures may be helpful in septic patients.

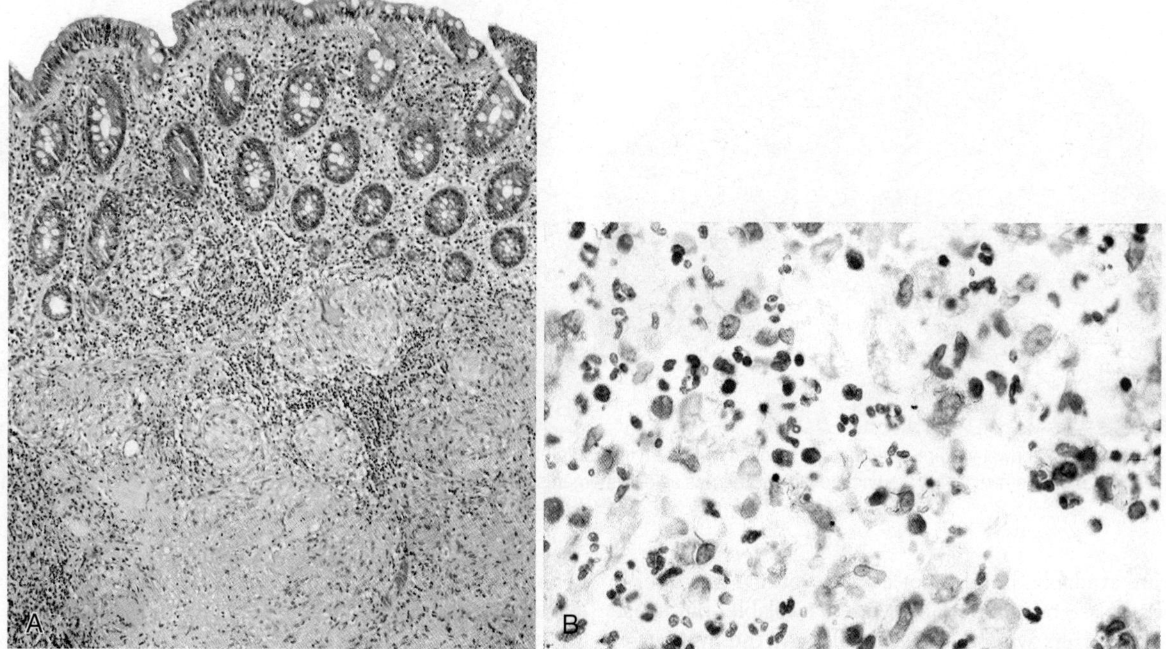

FIGURE 4.23 A, Colonic *Mycobacterium tuberculosis* infection with mucosal and submucosal confluent, caseating granulomas. **B,** Acid-fast organisms are seen in the necroinflammatory infiltrate (Ziehl-Neelsen stain).

Mycobacterial Infections of the GI Tract

Mycobacterium tuberculosis

Clinical Features

There has been a remarkable resurgence of tuberculosis in Western countries, the result in large part to AIDS, but also to institutional overcrowding and immigrant populations. Tuberculosis remains common in developing countries as well.[147,148] GI tuberculosis may be acquired through several mechanisms, including swallowing infected sputum in pulmonary tuberculosis, ingestion of contaminated milk (rare where pasteurization is common), hematogenous spread from pulmonary or miliary disease, and direct extension from adjacent organs.[148,149]

GI symptoms (rather than pulmonary) may be the initial presentation of disease, and extrapulmonary manifestations of tuberculosis are more common in AIDS patients than in immunocompetent persons. In addition, primary GI tuberculosis in the absence of pulmonary infection has been well documented.[150] Symptoms and signs of GI tuberculosis vary with the site or sites of involvement. The ileocecal and jejunoileal areas are most commonly involved, probably because of the abundance of lymphoid tissue at those locations. Associated mesenteric adenopathy is very common. Involvement of the ascending colon, duodenum, or rectum is less frequent. Gastroesophageal, appendiceal, or anal/perianal involvement is rare but is well documented in the literature.[151–153] Peritoneal tuberculosis is slightly more common than GI tuberculosis and may cause ascites as well as clinically significant adhesions.[154]

Regardless of the site of involvement, patients often have nonspecific symptoms, including weight loss, fever, abdominal pain, diarrhea, or a palpable abdominal mass.[155] Other symptoms include night sweats, malaise, anorexia, GI bleeding, and signs of malabsorption. Symptoms have often been present for months.

Pathological Features

Strictures and ulcers (often occurring together) are the most common endoscopic findings, along with thickened mucosal folds and inflammatory nodules.[150,155,156] The ulcers are often circumferential and transverse. Multiple and segmental lesions with skip areas are common and may mimic those of CD (see Table 4.6 and Box 4.1).[151,157] Large inflammatory masses (tuberculomas), usually involving the ileocecum, may be seen, and well-described complications include obstruction, perforation, and hemorrhage. The wall of the bowel is often thickened and edematous, with transmural inflammation, lymphoid hyperplasia, and fibrosis in later stages of the disease. Ulcers may be superficial or deep and may overlie hyperplastic Peyer's patches (aphthoid ulcers). The characteristic histological lesion consists of caseating, often confluent, granulomas (Fig. 4.23A) that may be present at any level of the gut wall but most commonly appear in the submucosa. A rim of lymphocytes is often present at the periphery of the granulomas, and giant cells are variably present. Older lesions are frequently hyalinized and calcified, and well-formed granulomas may be rare and difficult to find.[158-160] Inflammation of submucosal vessels is common, and architectural distortion that mimics chronic idiopathic IBD is frequently seen overlying areas of granulomatous inflammation. Characteristic granulomas are often present within involved lymph nodes.

Acid-fast stains sometimes demonstrate organisms (see Fig. 4.23B), especially within necrotic areas or macrophages, but culture is usually required for definitive diagnosis. The acid-fast bacilli of *Mycobacterium tuberculosis* are typically rod shaped and have a "beaded" morphology. Organisms may be abundant in immunocompromised patients yet rare and difficult to detect in immunocompetent persons, and the number of organisms may vary with the age of the lesion and previous antituberculosis therapy.[161] Immunohistochemical

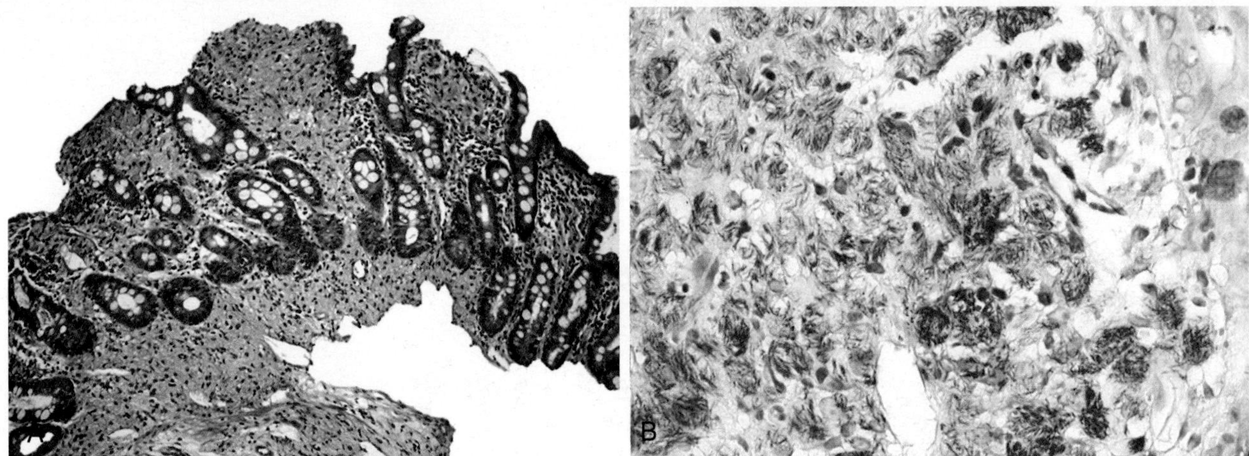

FIGURE 4.24 A, Small bowel villi are distended by clusters of histiocytes containing *Mycobacterium avium-intracellulare*, with little associated inflammatory response. **B,** The histiocytes are packed with numerous acid-fast organisms typical of *Mycoplasma avium-intracellulare* (Ziehl-Neelsen stain).

stains are available, but are not used in routine practice.[162] PCR assays are becoming more widely available, but sensitivity also suffers with this methodology if the number of organisms is low.[163] Purified protein derivative (PPD) tests may be helpful but are unreliable in immunocompromised or debilitated patients, whereas interferon-gamma release assays may be more sensitive.[164] Some atypical mycobacteria, such as *Mycobacterium kansasii* and *Mycobacterium bovis*, may cause similar pathological findings.

Differential Diagnosis

The differential diagnosis includes other granulomatous infectious processes, especially yersiniosis and fungal disease, and noninfectious processes such as sarcoidosis, Behçet's disease, reaction to foreign material, and granulomatous changes secondary to a delayed or interval appendectomy. The granulomas of yersiniosis are typically suppurative, but noncaseating, with striking lymphoid cuffs, but there may be considerable histological overlap.[122] CD may be difficult to distinguish from tuberculosis; features favoring CD are linear rather than circumferential ulcers, transmural lymphoid aggregates, and deep fistulas and fissures. Tuberculosis also commonly lacks mucosal cobblestoning. Granulomata are more numerous and larger in patients with tuberculosis compared with CD. Confluent and centrally necrotic granulomata are typical of tuberculosis, but are not seen in CD.[159,160] CD and tuberculosis may coexist, particularly in patients treated with infliximab, a tumor necrosis factor-α neutralizing agent. The pattern of involvement in these patients is somewhat unusual, with most exhibiting extrapulmonary tuberculosis. The emergence of infection is often associated with initiation of treatment.[165,166]

Mycobacterium avium-intracellulare *Complex*

Clinical Features

Mycobacterium avium-intracellulare complex is the most common mycobacterium isolated from the GI tract. It is typically found in patients with AIDS and other immunocompromising conditions, although it is occasionally seen in immunocompetent persons.[167-170] Symptoms include diarrhea, abdominal pain, fever, and weight loss and often reflect systemic infection. Endoscopy findings are usually normal, although white nodules, small ulcers, or hemorrhages may be seen.

Pathological Features

The small bowel is preferentially involved, but colonic and gastroesophageal involvement may be present, as may mesenteric adenopathy.[169,171] Histological manifestations vary with the site and the immune status of the patient. Small bowel biopsies from immunocompromised patients typically show villi distended by a diffuse infiltration of histiocytes containing bacilli (Fig. 4.24A), with little inflammatory response other than occasional poorly formed granulomas.[172] Immunocompetent patients usually have a well-formed, often epithelioid granulomatous response, either with or without necrosis. The small bowel is most often involved, but similar histiocytic infiltrates may be seen in the colon and other areas of the GI tract. Bacilli stain with acid-fast stains (see Fig. 4.24B), as well as periodic acid–Schiff (PAS) and Gomori methenamine silver (GMS) stain. Mycobacteria (including *M. tuberculosis* and *Mycobacterium leprae*) may also stain for desmin, actin, and keratin. Culture and PCR assays can be extremely helpful in diagnosis. Organisms are usually abundant in the immunocompromised host but may be harder to detect in healthy patients. The differential diagnosis includes Whipple's disease and other organisms that inhabit the mononuclear phagocytic system (Table 4.8).[173-175]

Spirochetal Infections of the GI Tract

Syphilis

Clinical Features

GI syphilis (*Treponema pallidum* infection) predominantly involves the anorectum, although other sites may be involved, particularly the stomach. Many authorities think that syphilis, particularly anorectal syphilis, is markedly underdiagnosed because of the variability of the clinical findings. Once thought to be a disease diminishing in frequency, the rate of syphilis infection doubled in the early part of the 21st century; men who have sex with men are disproportionately affected.[176-178] Patients are often asymptomatic, but pain (often with defecation), constipation, bleeding, and

TABLE 4.8 Infections of the Mononuclear Phagocytic System

Organism	Histological Features	Positive Histochemical Stains
Mycobacterium avium-intracellulare complex	Abundant bacilli distend striated macrophages, which may appear blue-tinged	Acid-fast PAS-D GMS
Tropheryma whipplei	Bacilli and chunks of degraded bacteria within macrophages	PAS-D Gram positive
Rhodococcus equii	Intracellular coccobacilli	PAS-D Gram positive Partially acid-fast
Malakoplakia	Degenerated gram-negative bacteria form targetoid Michaelis-Gutmann bodies	PAS-D von Kossa Prussian blue
Histoplasma capsulatum	2-4 μm intracellular yeast with narrow-based budding	GMS
Leishmania donovani	2-4 μm basophilic amastigotes with oval central nucleus Kinetoplast perpendicular to nucleus creates "double knot" configuration	Giemsa

GMS, Gomori methenamine silver; *PAS-D*, periodic acid–Schiff diastase.

discharge may be present in syphilitic proctitis. Luetic gastritis commonly manifests with upper GI bleeding, which can occur early or late in the course of the disease. Melena and coffee-ground emesis may be present, along with nausea, fever, malaise, anorexia, early satiety, and epigastric pain.

Pathological Features

Gross findings in primary syphilis include anal chancres (indurated, circular lesions as large as 2 cm in diameter that may be single or multiple, with variably present tenderness) that may be associated with a mild proctitis (Fig. 4.25). Signs of secondary syphilis typically manifest 6 to 8 weeks later and include masses, a mucocutaneous rash, or condyloma lata (raised, moist, smooth warts that secrete mucus and are associated with itching and a foul odor). Inguinal adenopathy is typical. Gross signs of primary and secondary infection sometimes coexist. The mass lesions of secondary syphilis may mimic malignancy, and surgical removal without a prior biopsy should be avoided.[179] Gastric involvement may be either an early or a late manifestation of syphilis. The most common presenting sign is upper GI bleeding, and patients typically have antral erosions, ulcers, or features of gastritis endoscopically. Ulcers may have irregular, heaped edges that mimic those of malignancy.[180]

Anorectal syphilis features a dense lymphohistiocytic infiltrate with prominent plasma cells and lymphoid aggregates, although basal lymphoplasmacytosis is not prominent (Fig. 4.26A).[181] Cryptitis and crypt abscesses, architectural distortion, and Paneth cell metaplasia are less prominent. Granulomas are sparse and poorly formed. Proliferative endarteriolitis with reactive endothelial cells and perivascular plasma cells is an important diagnostic clue. Anal squamous mucosa is often ulcerated and hyperkeratotic with submucosal fibrosis and a subepithelial band of lymphocytes, macrophages, and plasma cells (Fig. 4.27).[182] Syphilitic gastritis often features a dense plasmacytic infiltrate with neutrophil-rich gland destruction, proliferative endarteritis, and ill-formed granulomata.[183] The glands may be relatively spared by inflammation. Fibrosis may be prominent as the disease progresses.

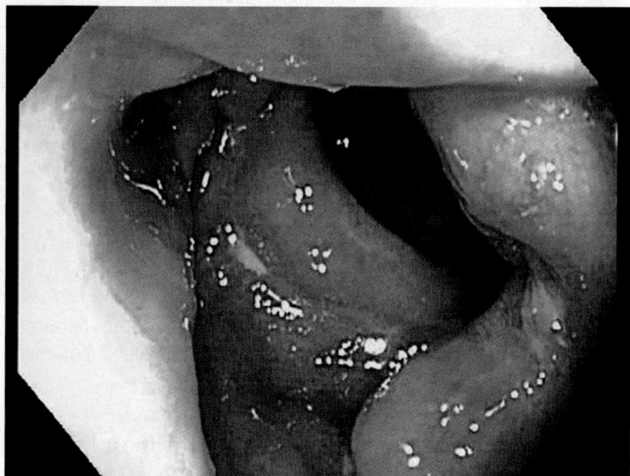

FIGURE 4.25 Syphilitic proctitis on endoscopy produces multiple shallow ulcers on an erythematous background.

Differential Diagnosis

The gross differential diagnosis of chancre includes anal fissures, fistulas, and traumatic lesions. In general, condyloma acuminata are more dry and more keratinized than condyloma lata. As mentioned earlier, both anorectal and gastric syphilis can mimic malignancy. The histological differential diagnosis primarily includes other infectious processes, such as *Helicobacter pylori* infection in the stomach. If the plasma cell infiltrate is prominent and monomorphic and effaces the normal architecture, a hematopoietic neoplasm with plasmacytic differentiation should be considered. Occasional large, bizarre "activated" lymphocytes are also sometime observed as a component of mixed inflammation including eosinophils and neutrophils.[184] *Treponema pallidum* immunohistochemistry may identify the spirochetes, which are often located in the superficial lamina propria of squamous mucosa, near blood vessels (see Fig. 4.27A,B).[185] Silver impregnation stains such as Warthin-Starry, Steiner, and Dieterle are less reliable, but occasionally demonstrate the organisms.[182,184] Darkfield examination of anorectal

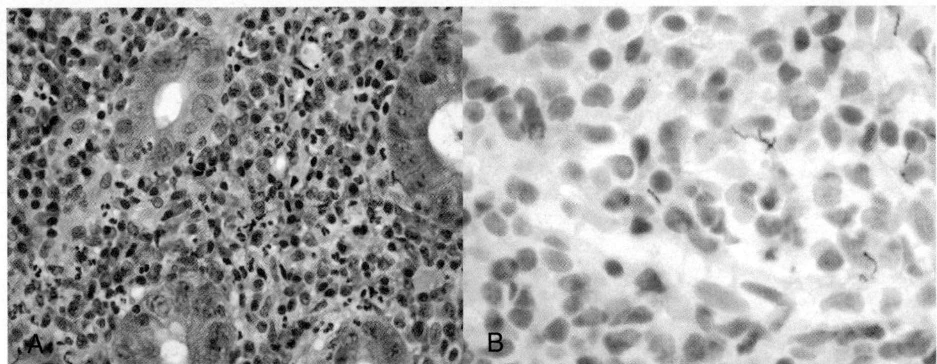

FIGURE 4.26 **A,** Syphilitic proctitis featuring neutrophilic cryptitis and a striking plasmacytic infiltrate in the lamina propria. **B,** Numerous spirochetes are detected with treponeme immunostaining. (*Courtesy of Dr. Ilke Nalbantoglu, Yale School of Medicine.*)

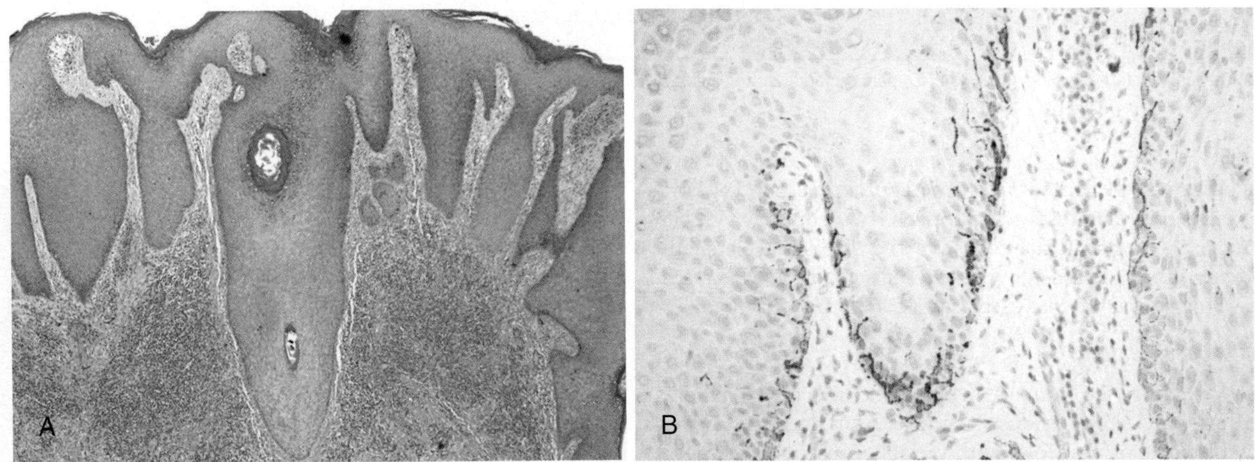

FIGURE 4.27 **A,** Anal syphilis features a dense band of lymphoplasmacytic inflammation subjacent to the squamous epithelium. **B,** Treponeme immunostaining demonstrates the organisms at the epithelial-subepithelial junction. (*Case Courtesy of Dr. Rhonda K. Yantiss, Weill Cornell Medicine.*)

discharge may show organisms, although care must be taken in interpretation, because spirochetes are also present in the normal gut flora as well as in intestinal spirochetosis. Serological studies such as the rapid plasma reagin (RPR), Venereal Disease Research Laboratory (VDRL), and fluorescent treponemal antibody absorption (FTA-ABS) tests can confirm the diagnosis.[177]

Important differential diagnoses of anorectal syphilis include IBD and lymphogranuloma venereum (LGV), as discussed subsequently (see Other Causes of Sexually Transmitted Bacterial Proctocolitis).

Intestinal Spirochetosis

Intestinal spirochetosis is a condition characterized by the presence of spirochetal microorganisms on the luminal surface of the large bowel mucosa. The prevalence of spirochetosis ranges from 2% to 16% in Western nations but is significantly higher in developing countries and among homosexual and HIV-infected patients, in whom the prevalence is reportedly as high as 50% based on both biopsy findings and stool culture.[186] It also has been described in association with a wide variety of conditions, including diverticular disease, chronic idiopathic IBD, hyperplastic polyps, and adenomatous polyps.[187] Spirochetosis represents infection by a heterogeneous group of related organisms, most importantly *Brachyspira aalborgi* and *Brachyspira pilosicoli*, which are genetically unrelated to *T. pallidum*. Patients with spirochetosis may harbor one or both of these species.[186]

Although patients with this histological finding often have symptoms such as diarrhea or anal pain and discharge, it is not clear that spirochetosis causes these symptoms.[187,188] Many patients have other infections (especially gonorrhea) complicating the clinical picture. Any level of the colon may be involved, as may the appendix. Typically, endoscopic abnormalities are mild or absent.

On H&E staining, spirochetosis resembles a fuzzy, "fringed" blue line, resembling a brush border on surface epithelial cells of the colonic mucosa (Fig. 4.28A). Invasion is not seen, and the changes can be focal. Most have no associated inflammatory infiltrate, although occasionally cryptitis is seen. The organisms stain intensely with Warthin-Starry, Dieterle, or similar silver stains (see Fig. 4.28B). They also stain with Alcian blue (pH 2.5) and PAS.[186,188] An immunohistochemical stain is available, and many authorities argue that the immunostain is superior, because the quality of silver impregnation stains varies widely depending on the freshness of the reagents and the ability of the technician.[189] The differential diagnosis consists primarily of a prominent glycocalyx, which should not stain with silver impregnation stains. Occasionally, EAEC can give a similar appearance, but *E. coli* are gram negative and lack spirillar morphology.

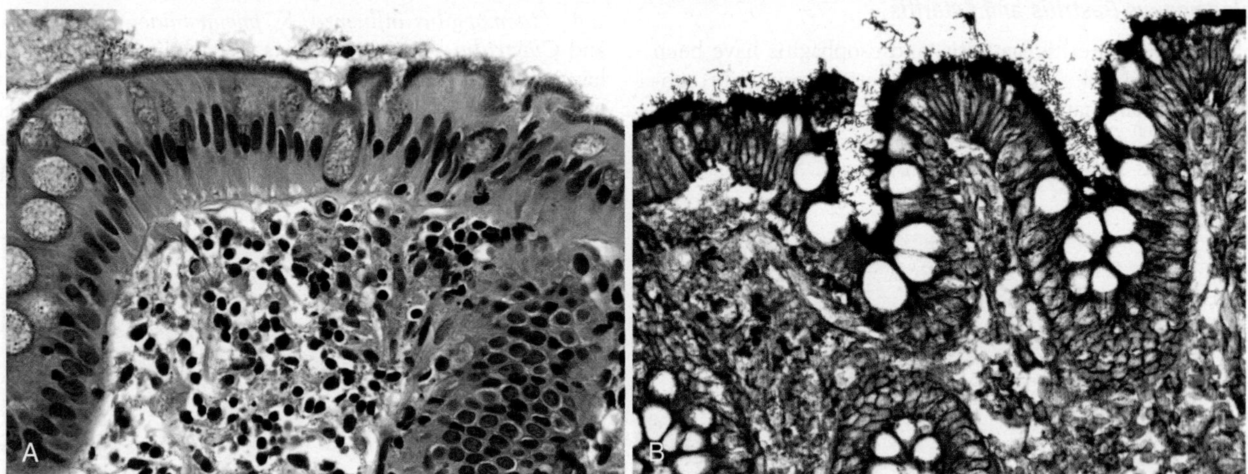

FIGURE 4.28 **A,** Spirochetosis is characterized by a fuzzy, "fringed" blue line at the luminal border of the colonic mucosa. **B,** Organisms stain intensely with silver impregnation staining (Warthin-Starry stain).

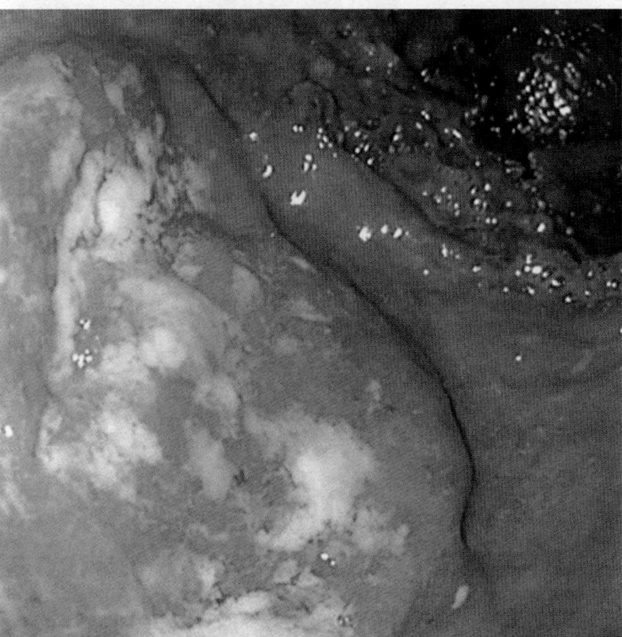

FIGURE 4.29 Ulceration and nodularity may raise concern for malignancy in sexually transmitted proctitis. This case of lymphogranuloma venereum simulated a rectal mass.

Other Causes of Sexually Transmitted Bacterial Proctocolitis

Other causes of sexually transmitted bacterial proctocolitis include *Chlamydia* spp., *Neisseria gonorrhoeae,* and *Calymmatobacterium granulomatis*. Patients typically are seen with anal discharge, pain, diarrhea, constipation, bloody stools, and tenesmus. Proctoscopic findings range from normal to mucosal friability, erosions, and erythema (Fig. 4.29).

Chlamydia trachomatis serotypes L1, L2, and L3 cause LGV. Anal pain is usually severe and accompanied by bloody discharge and tenesmus. The anorectum is the most common site, but LGV has been described in the ileum and colon as well.[190] The inflammatory infiltrate is similar to that seen in syphilitic proctitis and features lymphoplasmacytic mucosal and submucosal infiltrates with foci of neutrophilic cryptitis and rare granulomas (Fig. 4.30).[181] Rectal swabs subjected to culture, direct immunofluorescence studies, and nucleic acid detection are useful clinical assays.[191] Both syphilitic proctocolitis and LGV display striking clinical and histological overlap with IBD (see Fig. 4.30). In fact, IBD is often clinically suspected in patients with both infections. Mucosal biopsies from patients with IBD are more likely to display eosinophil infiltration, crypt destruction and distortion, and Paneth cell metaplasia, whereas submucosal lymphohistiocytic and plasma cell–rich inflammation and proliferative endarteriololitis are more common in sexually transmitted infections.[182]

Granuloma inguinale, caused by C. *granulomatis,* features anal and perianal disease that can appear similar to LGV, although extension into the rectum favors LGV. Warthin-Starry or Giemsa stains may aid in visualization of the Donovan bodies typical of granuloma inguinale.[192]

Anorectal gonococcal infection is reportedly present in more than 40% of both women and men with uncomplicated gonorrhea. Proctoscopic examination is usually unremarkable. Most biopsy findings in rectal gonorrhea are normal; some reveal a mild increase in neutrophils and mononuclear cells or focal cryptitis.[193] Gram-negative cocci can occasionally be seen on Gram staining of anal discharge, and culture can be a valuable diagnostic aid. *Neisseria meningitidis* has also been isolated from the anorectums of homosexual men, but it remains unclear whether this represents colonization or an actual pathogen in this location.

Miscellaneous Bacterial Infections

Bacterial Esophagitis

Bacterial esophagitis is rare and usually is found in immunocompromised or debilitated patients. Implicated bacteria include *Staphylococcus aureus, Lactobacillus acidophilus,* and *Klebsiella pneumoniae.* Endoscopic findings include ulceration, pseudomembrane formation, and hemorrhage. Histological findings include acute inflammation and necrosis with bacteria demonstrable in the wall of the esophagus (Fig. 4.31).[194]

Phlegmonous Gastritis and Enteritis

Phlegmonous enteritis, gastritis, and esophagitis have been well documented. This is a suppurative, primarily submucosal inflammatory process characterized by marked edema.[195-200] The causative organisms vary and include *Streptococcus spp., particularly S. pyogenes, Staphylococcus spp., Haemophilus influenza, K. pneumoniae, Enterococcus,* and *Clostridia.*[198] Most patients are debilitated, and many have cirrhosis or alcoholic liver disease. Affected patients may have nonspecific GI or systemic symptoms, or phlegmonous disease may be found incidentally at autopsy. Patients typically develop an acute abdomen, sometimes

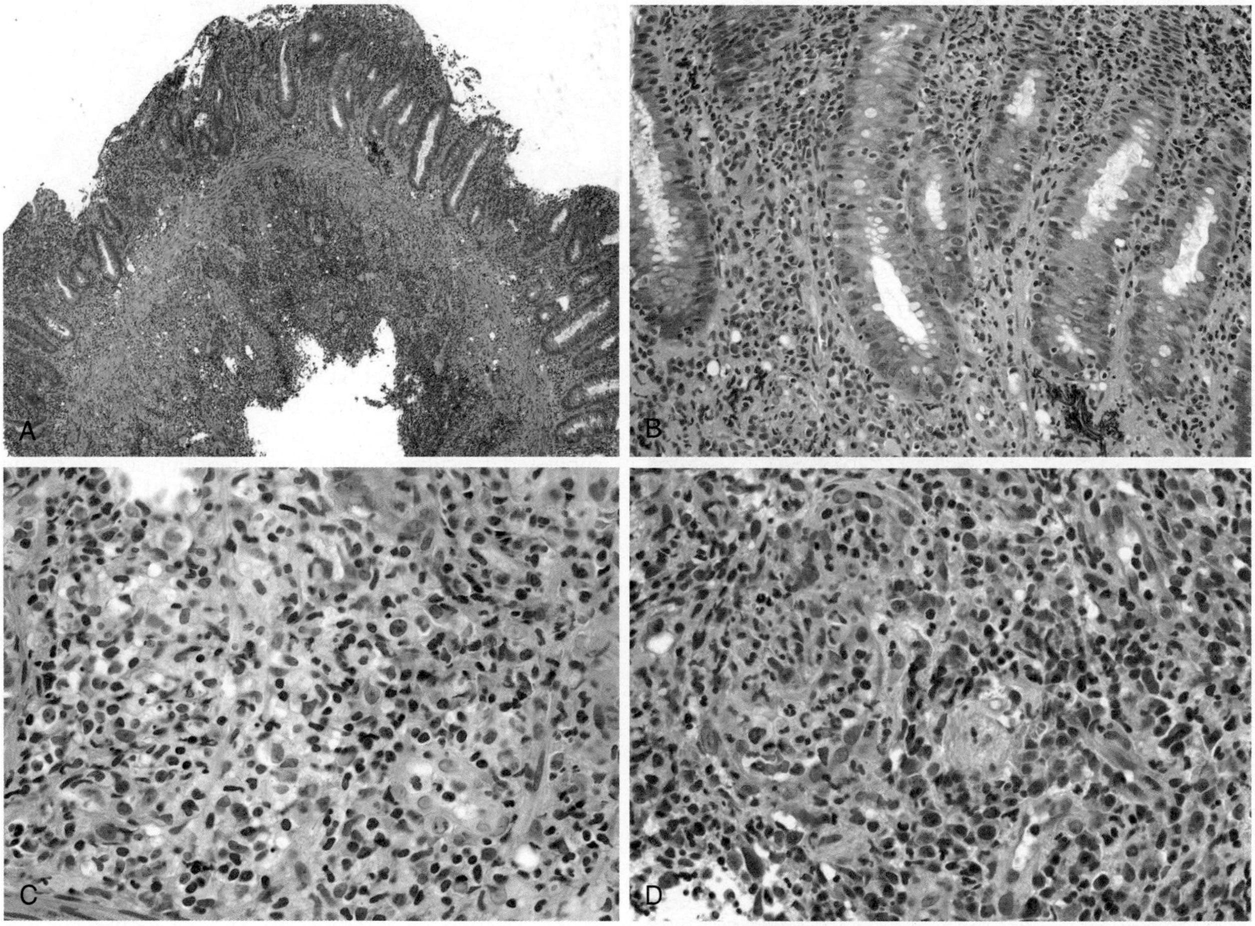

FIGURE 4.30 A, Lymphogranuloma venereum closely mimics inflammatory bowel disease owing to "bottom heavy" lymphoplasmacytic inflammation. **B,** The architecture is better preserved than in inflammatory bowel disease and Paneth cell metaplasia is absent. **C,** Well-formed granulomas are not seen, but loose histiocyte aggregates are common. **D,** Perivascular inflammation is also a diagnostic hallmark and is often plasma cell rich.

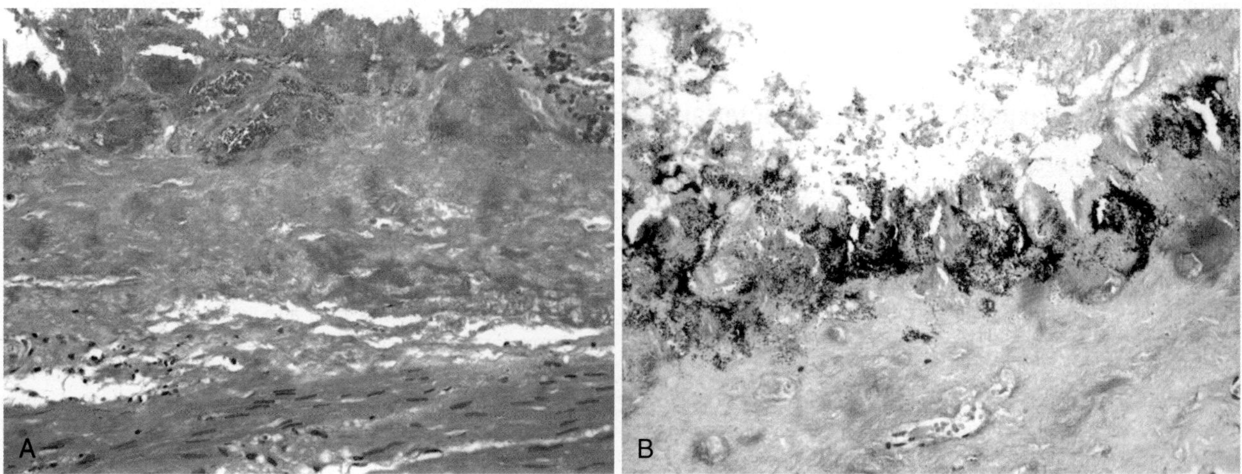

FIGURE 4.31 A, Bacterial esophagitis is characterized by mucosal ulceration and necrosis, with clusters of bacteria at the surface and invading into the wall. **B,** Gram staining highlights the clusters of bacteria within the esophageal wall.

complicated by hematemesis or vomiting of purulent material. Any portion of the alimentary tract may be involved. Typically, the gut wall is markedly thick and edematous.[199] Occasionally, gas-producing organisms such as C. *perfringens* may lead to the formation of gas bubbles in the submucosa ("emphysematous" changes) (Fig. 4.32). Although the mucosa may be red and friable, discrete ulceration is rarely present. Histologically, there is intense edema and acute inflammation located predominantly in the submucosa, and there may be transmural involvement as well.[200] The mucosa may be spared or sloughed entirely, especially in the stomach. Venous thrombosis may complicate the picture, causing ischemic changes. Gram staining may show organisms in the bowel wall, a finding that is diagnostic.

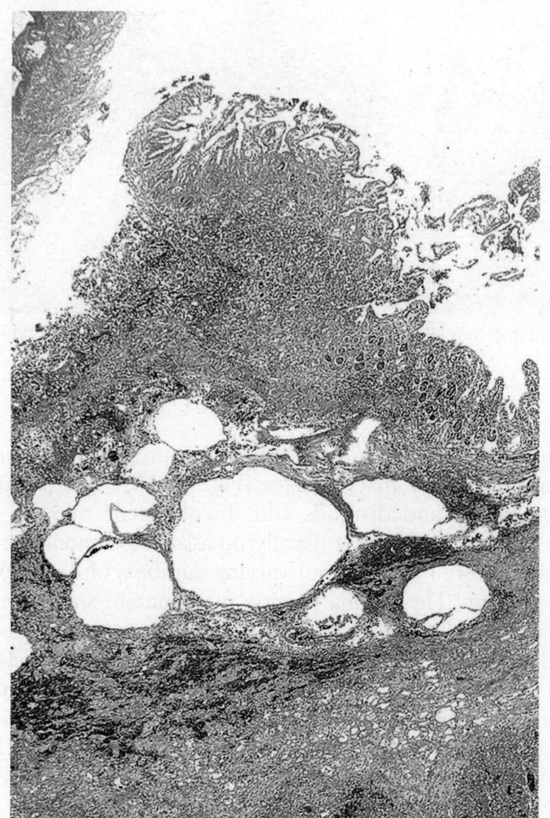

FIGURE 4.32 Emphysematous (phlegmonous) enteritis caused by *Clostridium perfringens*. Notice the transmural necrosis and mucosal sloughing with associated gas bubbles in the gut wall. (*Courtesy of Dr. David Owen, University of British Columbia.*)

Actinomycosis

Clinical Features

The filamentous, anaerobic, gram-positive bacterium *Actinomyces israelii* is a normal inhabitant of the oral cavity and the upper GI tract. Rarely, it produces a chronic, nonopportunistic GI infection.[201-203] Infection is usually in a solitary site, and it may occur at any level of the GI tract. Symptoms include fever, weight loss, abdominal pain, and, occasionally, a palpable mass. Perianal fistulas and chronic (often granulomatous) appendicitis have been described. Actinomycosis is sometimes associated with diverticular disease.

Pathological Features

Grossly, inflammation may produce a large, solitary mass, with or without ulceration, and infiltration into surrounding structures.[202] The organism typically produces actinomycotic ("sulfur") granules, consisting of irregular round clusters of bacteria rimmed by eosinophilic, clublike projections (Splendore-Hoeppli material). The inflammatory reaction is predominantly neutrophilic, with occasional abscess formation (Fig. 4.33A). Palisading histiocytes and giant cells, as well as frank granulomas, often surround the neutrophilic inflammation. There may be an associated fibrotic response. Gram staining reveals the filamentous, gram-positive organisms (Fig. 4.33B). GMS and Warthin-Starry stains are also used to show these organisms. Commensal actinomyces may be present at the luminal surface, and these do not necessarily imply invasive infection, particularly if there is no inflammatory response. Invasive actinomycosis requires several weeks of intravenous antibiotic therapy for treatment; therefore demonstration of the organisms within the

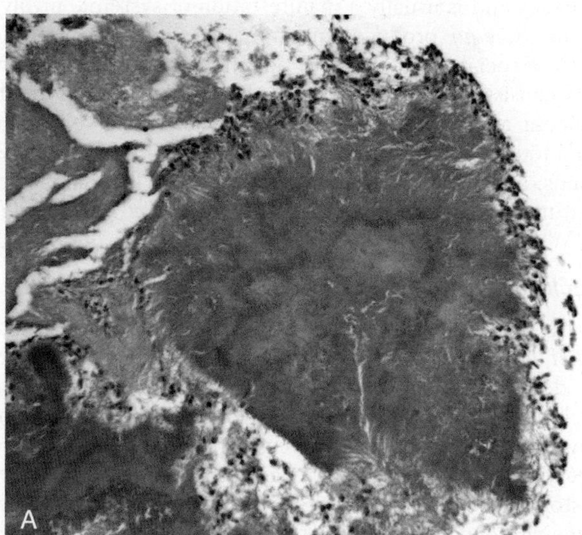

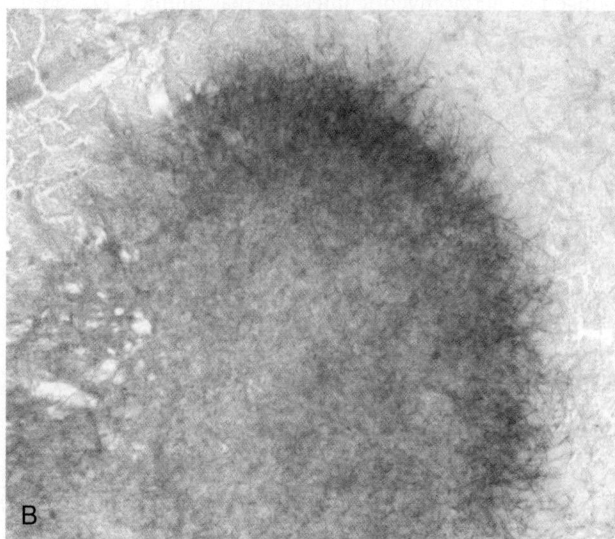

FIGURE 4.33 **A,** Actinomycotic ("sulfur") granule consisting of irregularly rounded clusters of bacteria bordered by Splendore-Hoeppli material and an acute inflammatory exudate. **B,** Gram staining highlights the filamentous gram-positive organisms.

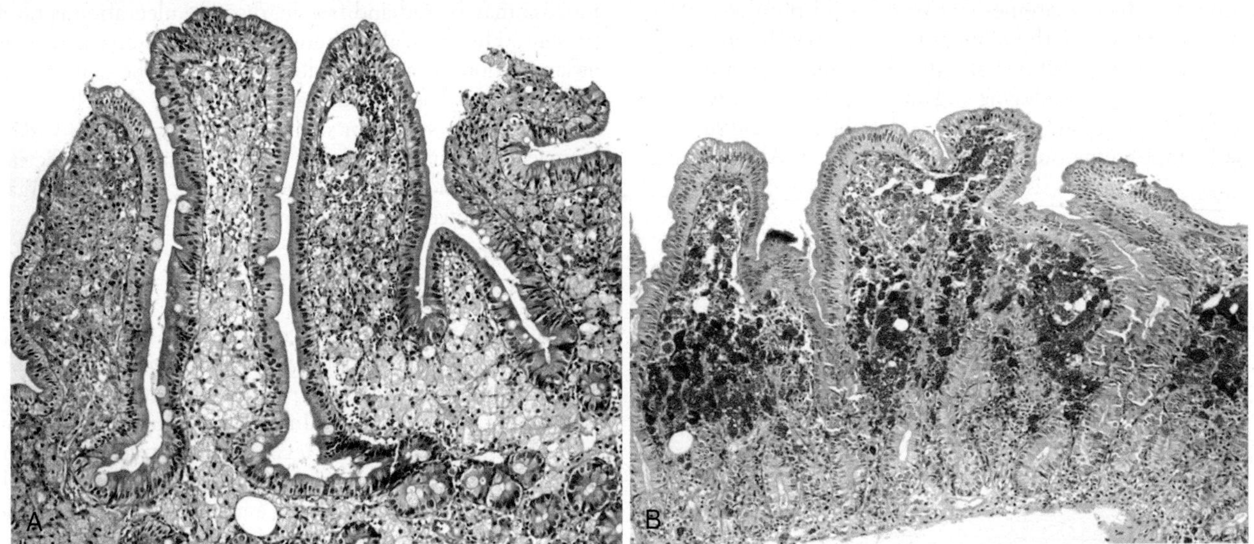

FIGURE 4.34 A, Villi are distended by an infiltrate of foamy macrophages with scattered fat cells and a patchy neutrophilic infiltrate. **B,** The Whipple bacillus stains intensely with periodic acid–Schiff stain.

wall of the bowel with an associated inflammatory response should be present before the diagnosis is suggested. This may require multiple levels of lesional tissue sections.

Differential Diagnosis

The macroscopic differential diagnosis includes peptic ulcer, lymphoma, and carcinoma. The histological differential diagnosis includes primarily other infectious agents, particularly *Nocardia*. *Nocardia* are partially acid-fast and do not form the typical sulfur granules of actinomycosis; however, cultures may be required to distinguish these two filamentous organisms. Even though actinomyces are GMS positive, they have a more slender morphology than fungi and do not bud or produce hyphae. Care should be taken not to confuse actinomycosis with other bacteria that form clusters and chains but are not truly filamentous, such as *Pseudomonas* and *E. coli*. Occasionally, the transmural inflammation, fibrosis, and granulomatous inflammation produced by actinomycotic infection may mimic CD.

Whipple's Disease

Clinical Features

Whipple's disease is caused by the gram-positive bacillus *Tropheryma whipplei* (formerly *Tropheryma whippelii*), a type of acinetobacterium. Classic descriptions of the disorder document its occurrence in middle-aged white men with chronic weight loss, arthritis, malabsorption, lymphadenopathy, and endocarditis. In its advanced stages, the disease causes neuropsychiatric manifestations. More recently, cases affecting women, and familial associations have been recognized. Cultivation of the organism from healthy individuals raises the possibility that it is commensal in some.[204]

Pathological Features

The small bowel is most often affected, although colonic and appendiceal involvement may be seen as well. Endoscopically, mucosal folds are thickened and coated with yellow-white plaques, often with surrounding erythema and friability. Histologically, the characteristic lesion results from massive infiltration of the lamina propria and submucosa with foamy macrophages (Fig. 4.34A). The infiltrate often blunts and distends villi. Involvement may be diffuse or patchy. There is usually no associated mononuclear inflammatory infiltrate, but varying numbers of neutrophils are present. The lamina propria may contain small foci of fat, and overlying vacuolization of enterocytes may occur as well. This bacillus is strongly PAS positive (see Fig. 4.34B); and PCR assays may be diagnostic as well. The differential diagnosis includes predominantly *M. avium-intracellulare* infection. Infection by other intracellular organisms such as *Histoplasma* or *Rhodococcus* may rarely simulate Whipple's disease (see Table 4.8).

Rhodococcus equi

The gram-positive coccobacillus *Rhodococcus equi* may occasionally infect humans, particularly the immunocompromised. GI infection manifests as chronic (often bloody) diarrhea and is usually a manifestation of systemic involvement. *R. equi* produces inflammatory polyps, sometimes with associated mesenteric adenitis. Histologically, polyps consist of organism-laden macrophages that pack the mucosa and submucosa, often with an associated granulomatous response. Organisms stain with PAS and Gram stains, and they may be partially acid-fast. The histological features may mimic infection with *M. avium-intracellulare* or Whipple's disease (see Table 4.8).[205]

Rocky Mountain Spotted Fever

Rocky Mountain spotted fever is caused by *Rickettsia rickettsii*, which is transmitted by the bite of the common wood or dog tick. Many patients have significant GI findings, including nausea, vomiting, diarrhea, pain, and GI bleeding. These manifestations may precede the rash. Involvement of every portion of the GI tract has been documented. Typical histological findings include vasculitis, often with accompanying nonocclusive microthrombi, and hemorrhage. The inflammatory infiltrate is composed of mononuclear cells with occasional lymphocytes, macrophages, and neutrophils.

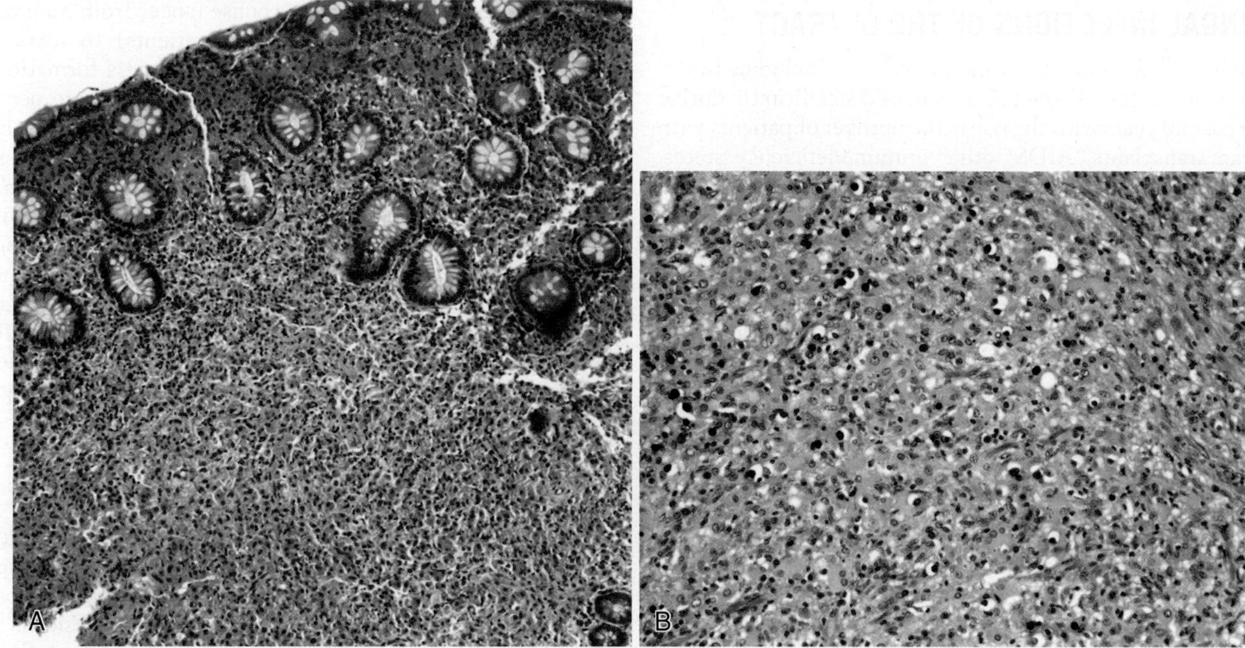

FIGURE 4.35 **A,** This colon biopsy shows the dense histiocytic infiltrate with admixed lymphocytes and plasma cells typical of malakoplakia. **B**, Higher-power view highlights targetoid Michaelis-Gutmann bodies. (*Courtesy of Dr. Joel K. Greenson, University of Michigan.*)

Immunofluorescence staining demonstrates the organism, and serological studies may also be of use.[206]

Malakoplakia

Malakoplakia is a rare disorder caused by incomplete digestion of microbes by mononuclear inflammatory cells.[207,208] Numerous bacteria, including *E. coli, Klebsiella, Yersinia,* mycobacterial organisms, and *R. equi,* have been implicated. Most cases are associated with colorectal adenocarcinoma or some other immunocompromising condition.[209] Soft yellow plaques containing a dense histiocytic infiltrate may be seen in any portion of the GI tract.[210] Macrophages contain targetoid concretions of PAS-positive, diastase-resistant undigested material, called Michaelis-Gutmann bodies (Fig. 4.35). These concretions mineralize over time; thus they are highlighted by von Kossa and Prussian blue stains (see Table 4.7).

Bacillary Angiomatosis

Bacillary angiomatosis comprises pyogenic granuloma-like lesions that occur in immunocompromised patients and mimic Kaposi sarcoma. They are usually associated with *Bartonella quintana.*[211]

Helicobacter pylori *and* Helicobacter heilmannii

These bacteria are discussed in Chapter 15.

Sarcina ventriculi *and Related Organisms*

Sarcina ventriculi and related species are an increasingly recognized group of gram-positive cocci found in gastric biopsy and resection specimens. They are found in patients with delayed gastric emptying of various causes, including prior resection, gastric banding, and obstructing masses. Thus, although patients with *Sarcina* infection often report epigastric pain, bloating, and vomiting, clinical and imaging findings usually reveal other explanations for these symptoms.[212] It is not clear whether these organisms are pathogenic or simply a marker of luminal stasis. Their association with rare cases of emphysematous gastritis raises the possibility that they may be pathogenic in susceptible hosts.[213]

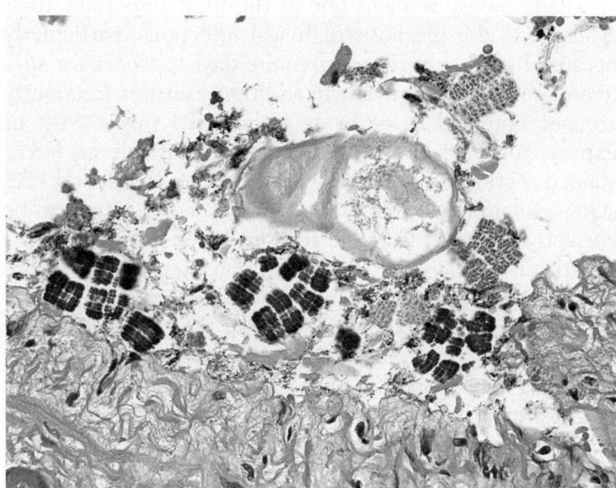
FIGURE 4.36 *Sarcina* spp. form tetrads of spherical organisms within the debris of a gastric ulcer. (*Courtesy of Dr. Raul S. Gonzalez, Beth Israel Deaconess Medical Center*)

Sarcina spp. occur in tetrads or multiples of four, reflecting cell division in multiple planes of growth. They are spherical with refractile cell walls, resembling vegetable matter. They localize to surface foveolar epithelium or luminal ulcer debris (Fig. 4.36).

The main differential diagnosis is *Micrococcus* spp. These are also gram-positive cocci that occur in tetrads, but they are smaller than *Sarcina. Micrococcus* are also commensal organisms, but may cause disease in immunocompromised patients.

FUNGAL INFECTIONS OF THE GI TRACT

The incidence of invasive fungal infections, including fungal infections of the GI tract, has increased significantly during the past 20 years with the rise in the number of patients with organ transplants, AIDS, other immunodeficiency states, or long-term chemotherapy.[214] GI fungal infections occur most commonly in immunocompromised patients, but virtually all have been described in immunocompetent persons as well. Fungal infections of the GI tract can be roughly divided into two categories: those caused by transmucosal invasion and those that disseminate after primary infection of another site (usually pulmonary). In addition, invasive fungal infections are associated with repetitive abdominal surgeries, widespread use of antimicrobial agents, intrusive vascular lines, diabetes, total parenteral nutrition, neonatal prematurity, and advancing age.

In general, signs and symptoms of GI fungal infections are similar regardless of the type of fungus; they include diarrhea, vomiting, melena, frank GI bleeding, abdominal pain, and fever. Esophageal fungal infections usually manifest with odynophagia and dysphagia. Fungal infections of the GI tract are often part of a disseminated disease process, but GI symptoms and signs may be the presenting manifestations.

Tissue biopsy remains one of the most important tools available in the diagnosis of fungal infections, particularly because fungal cultures may require days to weeks for adequate growth and analysis. In addition, cultures frequently are not obtained as often as pathologists might wish or expect. Although organisms may be identifiable on H&E-stained sections in cases of heavy infection, GMS and PAS stains remain invaluable diagnostic aids. Fungi often can be correctly classified in tissue sections based on morphological criteria (Table 4.9). However, fungi exposed to antifungal therapy or ambient air may produce bizarre and unusual forms. Microbiological culture remains the gold standard for speciation, especially because antifungal therapy may vary according to the specific type of fungus isolated. Helpful diagnostic aids, in addition to culture, include serological assays, antigen tests, immunohistochemistry, and molecular assays. Knowledge of the patient's geographic or travel history also can be very helpful in diagnosing fungal infections.

Candida Species

Candida is the most common infection of the esophagus, but it may infect any level of the GI tract. The GI tract is a major portal for disseminated candidiasis, because *Candida* often superinfects ulcers that develop from other causes.[215] *Candida albicans* is the most common species, but *Candida tropicalis* and *Candida (Torulopsis) glabrata* can produce similar manifestations. In addition, other non-*albicans* species (e.g., *Candida krusei, Candida parapsilosis*) are emerging as important causes of invasive fungal infection.[216]

The esophagus typically contains white plaques that can be readily scraped off to reveal ulcerated mucosa underneath. The gross features of candidiasis in the remainder of the GI tract are variable and include ulceration, pseudomembrane formation, and inflammatory masses (Fig. 4.37A). If vascular invasion is prominent, the bowel may appear infarcted. Involvement may be diffuse or segmental. The associated inflammatory response ranges from minimal (especially in immunocompromised patients) to marked with prominent neutrophilic infiltrates, abscess formation, erosion or ulceration, and necrosis. Granulomas are occasionally present as well. Fungi may invade any level of the gut wall. Invasion of mucosal and submucosal blood vessels is sometimes a prominent feature in invasive *Candida* infection. *C. albicans* and *C. tropicalis* produce a mixture of budding yeast forms, hyphae, and pseudohyphae (see Fig. 4.37B). *C. glabrata* features tiny budding yeast forms (similar to those of *Histoplasma*) but does not produce hyphae or pseudohyphae.[217] It is important to morphologically differentiate between invasive candidiasis and superficial colonization, because *Candida* is capable of colonizing benign ulcers and mucosal surfaces without invasion.

Aspergillus Species

Aspergillus infection of the GI tract occurs almost exclusively in immunocompromised patients. Gross findings are similar to those seen with *Candida* infection.[218] Most patients with aspergillosis have coexistent lung lesions.[219] The characteristic lesion of aspergillosis is a nodular infarction consisting of a zone of ischemic necrosis centered on blood vessels containing fungal organisms (Fig. 4.38).[220] Fungal hyphae often extend outward from the infarct, in parallel or radial arrays. The inflammatory response ranges from minimal to marked, with a prominent neutrophilic infiltrate, and granulomatous inflammation may develop as well. Transmural infarction of the bowel wall is common. The typical hyphae of *Aspergillus* are septate, with parallel walls, and they branch at acute angles.

Fusarium is an emerging fungal infection in patients undergoing transplantation that may closely mimic aspergillosis morphologically. Cultures are required to differentiate these fungi.[221]

Mucormycosis

Mucormycosis refers to infections with fungi in the order Mucorales.[222,223] Important human pathogens that infect the GI tract include *Mucor indicus* and *Rhizopus oryzae*.[222,224]

The histological lesions of mucormycosis are remarkably similar to those seen in aspergillosis because it is also an angioinvasive fungus that produces ischemic infarction. In contrast to *Aspergillus*, these organisms have broad, ribbon-like, pauciseptate hyphae that branch at random angles and appear optically clear when sectioned transversely (Fig. 4.39).[225] Ulcers are the most common gross manifestation; they are often large with rolled, irregular edges that may mimic malignancy. These fungi may also superinfect previously ulcerated tissues. Patients with diabetes or other causes of systemic acidosis are at increased risk for mucormycosis.[226]

Basidiobolomycosis

Basidiobolomycosis is caused by *Basidiobolus ranarum*, an organism in the order Entomophthorales. It was originally described in Saudi Arabia and is endemic in Arizona in the United States.[227,228] GI disease may simulate malignancy or IBD because patients present with abdominal pain and,

TABLE 4.9 Morphological Features of Fungi Involving the Gastrointestinal Tract

Organism	Primary Geographical Distribution	Morphological Features	Host Reaction	Major Differential Diagnoses
Aspergillus spp.	Worldwide	Hyphae-septate: uniform width Branching-regular: acute angles Conidial head formation in cavitary lesions	Ischemic necrosis with angioinvasion Acute inflammation Occasionally granulomatous	Mucorales *Fusarium* *Pseudallescheria boydii*
Blastomyces dermatitidis (North American blastomycosis)	Similar to histoplasmosis; rare cases from Africa and Central America	Large pleomorphic (8–15 μm) spherical to ovoid yeast Intracellular or extracellular Broad-based buds Multinucleate	Mixed suppurative and granulomatous reaction	*Histoplasma* spp. *Cryptococcus neoformans* (especially capsule-deficient) *Coccidioides immitis*
Candida albicans *Candida tropicalis*	Worldwide	Mixture of budding yeast and pseudohyphae Occasional septate hyphae	Usually suppurative, with variable necrosis and ulceration Occasionally granulomatous Occasional angioinvasion	*Trichosporon*
Candida (Torulopsis) glabrata	Worldwide	Budding yeast No hyphae No "halo" effect	Similar to other *Candida* spp.	*Histoplasma* *Cryptococcus*
Cryptococcus neoformans	Worldwide	Highly pleomorphic (4–7 μm) Uninucleate Narrow-based buds Usually mucicarmine positive Positive Fontana-Masson	Usually suppurative; may have extensive necrosis Sometimes granulomatous	Histoplasmosis Blastomycosis *Candida glabrata*
Histoplasma capsulatum var. capsulatum	Worldwide, but endemic in Ohio, Mississippi River basins; parts of Central and South America; St. Lawrence River basin in Canada	Uniform small (2–5 μm), uninucleate ovoid yeast Narrow-based buds Intracellular"halo" effect around organism on H&E	Lymphohistiocytic infiltrate with parasitized histiocytes Occasional granulomas	*Cryptococcus* *Penicillium marneffei* *Candida glabrata* *Pneumocystis jiroveci* Intracellular parasites
Pneumocystis jiroveci	Worldwide	Ovoid Cup or crescent-shaped if collapsed No buds Internal enhancing detail	Characteristic foamy casts May have suppurative or granulomatous inflammation as well	Histoplasmosis Small parasites
Mucorales	Worldwide, associated with diabetics more than any other mycosis	Hyphae-pauciseptate: ribbon-like, thin walls Branching-haphazard	Similar to *Aspergillus*	Similar to *Aspergillus*
Basidiobolus ranarum	Middle East Southeastern United States	Thin-walled, broad, pauciseptate hyphae	Tissue eosinophilia, Splendore-Hoeppli material Charcot-Leyden crystals Granulomas	Mucorales *Aspergillus* spp.
Penicillium marneffei	Southeast Asia, China Emerging mycosis in immunocompromised	Intracellular yeast forms Elongated forms with central septation	Diffuse macrophage infiltrates	*Cryptococcus* spp. *Histoplasma* spp. *Candida glabrata*

sometimes, a palpable mass. Young patients, those with peptic ulcer disease, and diabetic patients are at increased risk. Infection is usually seen in immunocompetent hosts.[224]

The morphological features of the fungus are similar to those of mucormycosis, but angioinvasion is rare. The hyphae are thin walled, broad, and pauciseptate, often associated with Splendore-Hoeppli material, Charcot-Leyden crystals, and tissue eosinophilia (Fig. 4.40). The inflammatory reaction may be suppurative or granulomatous, and necrosis is usually prominent.[229]

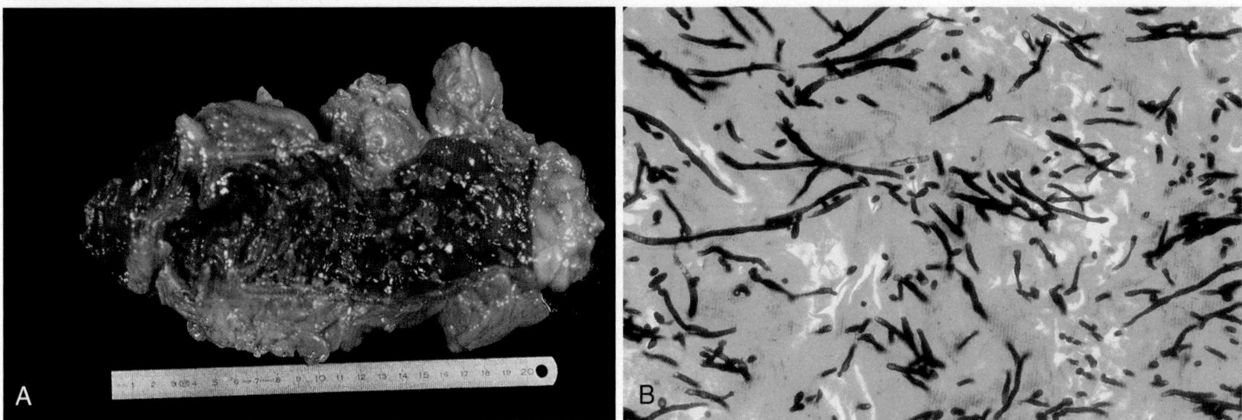

FIGURE 4.37 **A,** Colonic candidiasis featuring yellow-white plaques with associated marked mucosal ulceration. **B,** GMS staining shows the mixture of budding yeast and pseudohyphae typical of *Candida* spp. (**A** *courtesy of Dr. Cole Elliott, Pathology Associates of Albuquerque.*)

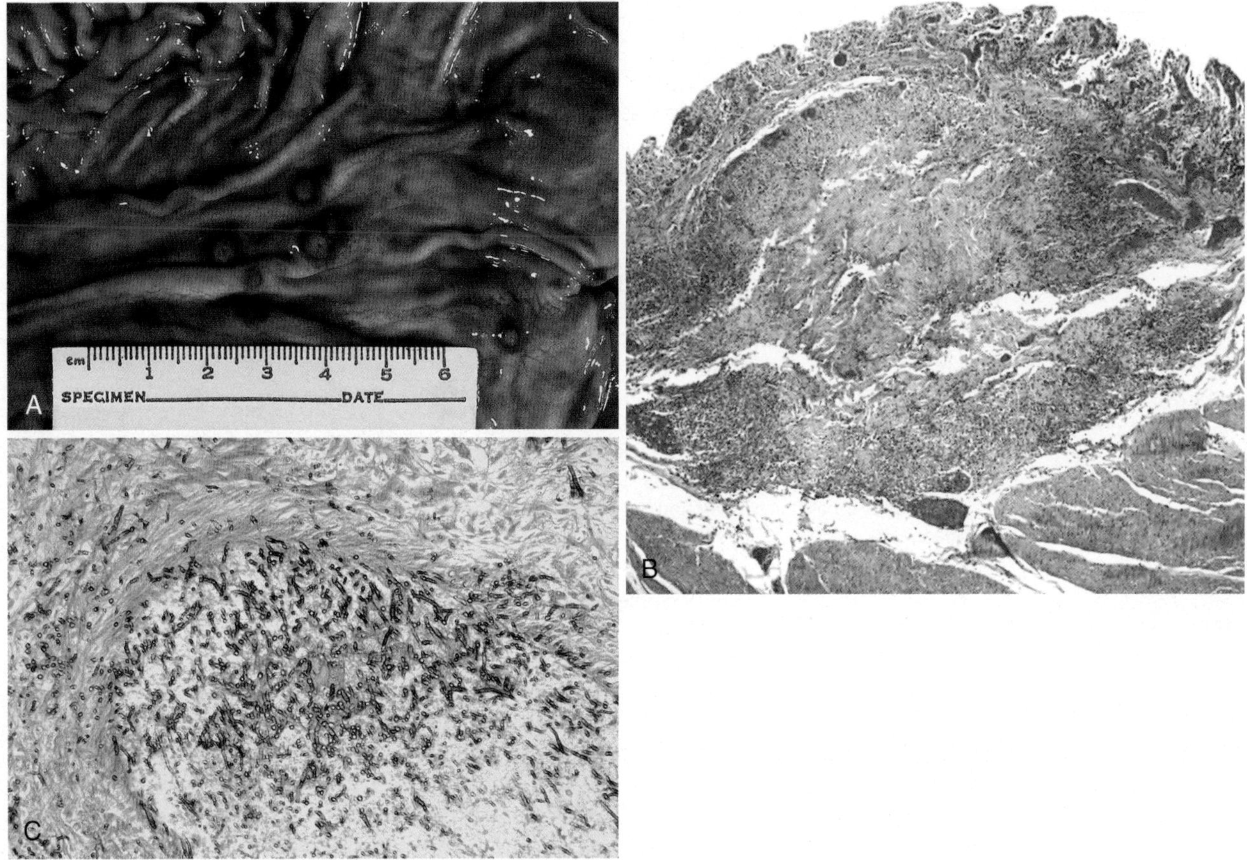

FIGURE 4.38 **A,** Typical macroscopic "target lesion" of aspergillosis, shown here in the stomach, consisting of hemorrhagic infarction and necrosis centered on a blood vessel. **B,** Histologically, this lesion corresponds to a nodular infarction of the mucosa and submucosa caused by occlusion of the vessels by *Aspergillus.* **C,** *Aspergillus* organisms fill and penetrate a vessel in the submucosa (GMS stain).

Histoplasmosis

Histoplasma capsulatum is endemic to the central United States but has been described in many nonendemic areas as well.[230] GI involvement occurs in more than 80% of patients with disseminated infection. Patients may present with signs and symptoms of GI illness, but lack concomitant pulmonary involvement. The ileum is the most common site, but any portion of the GI tract may be involved.[231,232] Gross lesions range from normal to ulcers, nodules, and obstructive masses. Histological findings include diffuse lymphohistiocytic infiltrates and nodules, usually involving the mucosa and submucosa, with associated ulceration (Fig. 4.41). These lesions are usually located over Peyer's patches. Discrete granulomas and giant cells are present in only a minority of cases. In immunocompromised patients, large numbers of organisms may be seen with virtually no tissue reaction. *Histoplasma* organisms are small, ovoid, usually intracellular yeast forms with small buds at the more pointed pole.[233]

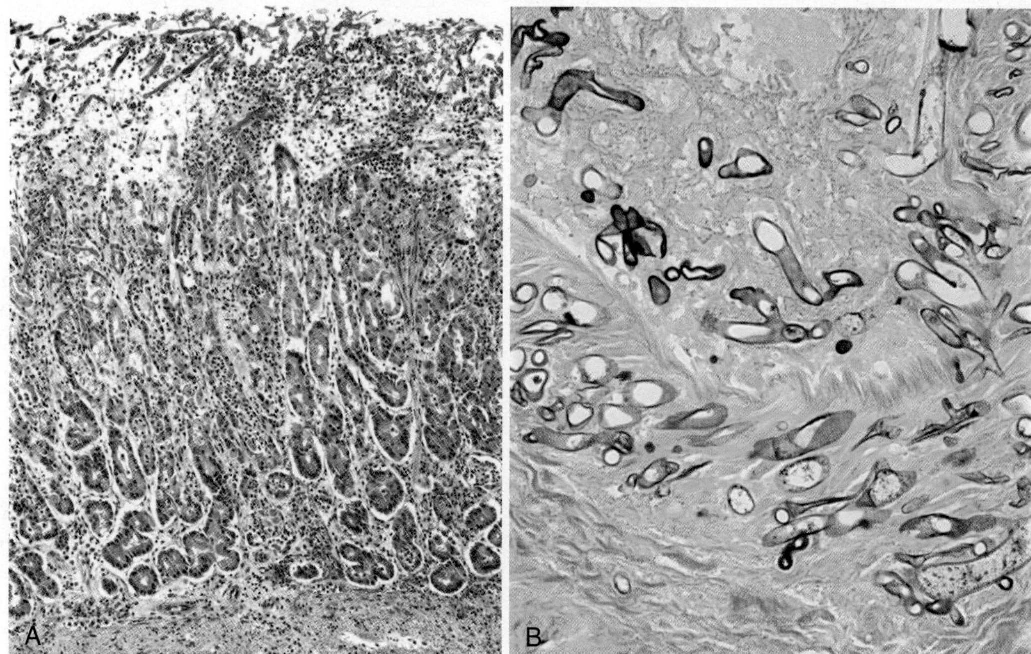

FIGURE 4.39 **A**, Mucormycosis of the stomach, featuring fungi within the mucosa with a surrounding neutrophilic infiltrate and mucosal sloughing. *(Courtesy Dr. Owen Middleton, University of Alabama at Birmingham.)* **B**, GMS stain shows typical broad, ribbon-like, pauciseptate fungi with irregular branching and optically clear centers.

Cryptococcus neoformans

The fungus *Cryptococcus neoformans* is an unusual but important cause of GI infection. Almost all patients with GI cryptococcosis have hematogenously disseminated disease with multisystem organ involvement, and most have associated pulmonary and meningeal disease.[234,235] Grossly, cryptococcal infection may be located anywhere in the GI tract. Endoscopic lesions include nodules and ulcers, sometimes associated with a thick white exudate. However, the mucosa is normal in many cases.[234] Histological features include typical round to oval yeast forms with narrow-based budding, and cryptococci may show considerable variation in size. Occasionally, they produce hyphae and pseudohyphae. Often a halo effect can be seen with H&E staining, representing the capsule of the organism. Both superficial and deep involvement may occur, and lymphatic involvement is not uncommon. The inflammatory reaction is variable and depends on the immune status of the host, ranging from a suppurative, necrotizing inflammatory reaction, often with granulomatous features (Fig. 4.42), to virtually no reaction (e.g., in anergic hosts).[234] The mucopolysaccharide capsule stains with Alcian blue, mucicarmine, Fontana-Masson, and colloidal iron; GMS stains are positive as well. Alcian blue and mucicarmine do not label capsule-deficient cryptococci, but they are positive with Fontana-Masson staining.[234]

Pneumocystis jiroveci

Although the life cycle of *Pneumocystis jiroveci* (formerly *P. carinii*) more closely resembles that of a protozoan, there is convincing molecular evidence that *P. jiroveci* has greater homology with fungi. *P. jiroveci* pneumonia is a major cause of morbidity in the AIDS population, and extrapulmonary (including GI) involvement is not uncommon.[236] In addition to patients with AIDS, *Pneumocystis* infection has been reported rarely in the context of organ transplantation, hematological malignancy, other immunodeficiency states, and steroid therapy. *Pneumocystis* infection has also been reported in association with infliximab therapy.[237] Endoscopically, infection produces a nonspecific, often erosive, esophagogastritis or colitis, sometimes with small polypoid nodules. Microscopically, granular, foamy eosinophilic casts similar to those seen in pulmonary infection may be observed in mucosal vessels or in the lamina propria (Fig. 4.43A).[236] As in the lung, a wide variety of inflammatory responses may occur, including granulomatous inflammation, prominent macrophage infiltrates, and necrosis. The organisms are 5- to 7-μm spherules that have cup or crescent shapes when collapsed (see Fig. 4.43B). Many contain characteristic, single or paired, comma-shaped internal structures. Organisms stain with GMS and toluidine blue.

Penicillium marneffei

Penicillium marneffei is a dimorphic fungus endemic to Southeast Asia, southern China, and Hong Kong. It is increasingly recognized as an emerging cause of invasive mycosis in immunocompromised patients.[238,239] Frequent sites of infection include the lungs and liver, followed by the GI tract. Patients experience abdominal cramping and watery or bloody diarrhea. Dissemination occurs rapidly and may be fatal.

Endoscopic abnormalities, including ulcers, erosions, petechiae, and masses occur in any segment of GI tract.[240] Most cases show diffuse macrophage infiltrates with intracellular yeast forms. Occasional elongated ("pill capsule") forms with central septation can span up to 20 μm. *P. marneffei* reproduce by fission; budding is not seen.[241]

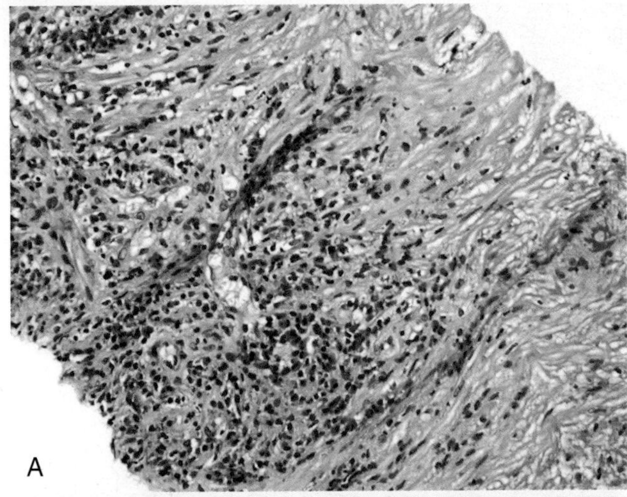

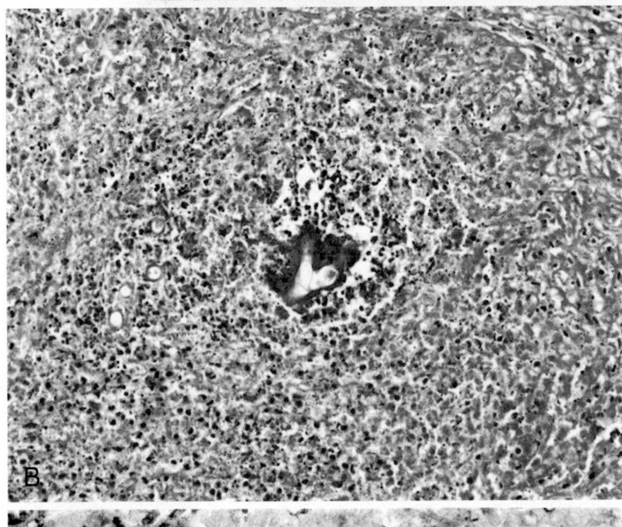

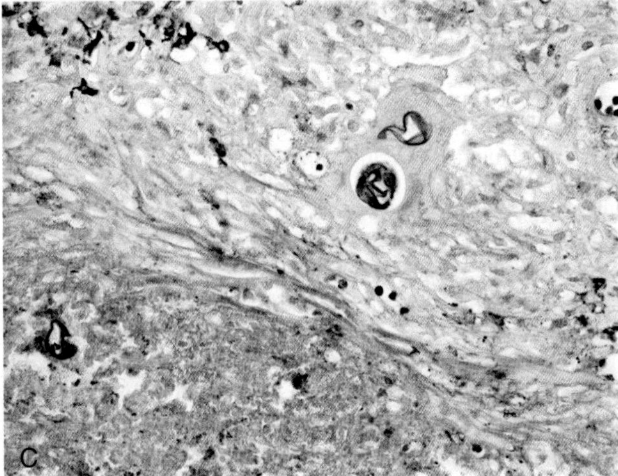

FIGURE 4.40 A, Basidiobolomycosis features prominent necrosis and numerous eosinophils, as seen in this biopsy of a paracolonic mass. **B,** The organisms are broad, have optically clear centers, and are surrounded by a striking Splendore-Hoeppli reaction. **C,** GMS staining shows the optically clear centers and the characteristic "cellophane ball" crumpled appearance of the fungi.

Other fungal infections that occasionally involve the GI tract, but are not discussed in detail here, include *Blastomyces dermatitidis* and *Paracoccidioides brasiliensis* (South American blastomycosis), which can mimic chronic idiopathic IBD both clinically and radiographically.[242,243]

PARASITIC INFECTIONS OF THE GI TRACT

Protozoal Infections

Protozoa are prevalent pathogens in tropical and subtropical countries, and they also cause some of the most common intestinal infections in North America and Europe. Immigration, increasing numbers of immunocompromised patients, use of institutional child care facilities, and the development of improved diagnostic techniques have enhanced understanding and recognition of these protozoa. Many protozoal illnesses are diagnosed by examination of stool samples, but they are also important to the surgical pathologist.

Entamoeba histolytica

Clinical Features

Approximately 10% of the world's population is infected with the *Entamoeba histolytica* parasite, predominantly in tropical and subtropical regions. In Western countries, this infection is most often seen in immigrants, overseas travelers, homosexual males, and institutionalized persons. Infection is usually acquired through contaminated water or food, and it also can be spread by the fecal-oral route.[244,245] Sexual transmission has been reported occasionally. Although some patients suffer a severe, dysentery-like, fulminant colitis, many others are asymptomatic or show only vague GI symptoms.[246] Complications include bleeding and dissemination to other sites, particularly the liver. Rarely, large inflammatory masses (amebomas) may form.[247]

Pathological Features

Colonoscopy findings may be normal in asymptomatic patients and in those with mild disease. The cecum is the most common site of involvement, followed by the right colon, rectum, sigmoid, and appendix. Grossly, small ulcers are seen initially, but these may coalesce to form large, irregular, geographic or serpiginous ulcers (Fig. 4.44). Ulcers may undermine adjacent mucosa to produce classic "flask-shaped" lesions (Fig. 4.45A), and there may be associated inflammation or inflammatory polyps as well.[248] The intervening mucosa is often normal. Fulminant colitis, resembling UC; PMC, resembling that caused by C. *difficile*; and toxic megacolon have all been described in association with *E. histolytica* infection.

Histologically, early lesions show a mild neutrophilic infiltrate. In some cases, numerous organisms are present at the luminal surface with little associated inflammation. In more advanced disease, ulcers are often deep, extending into the submucosa, with undermining of adjacent normal mucosa. There is usually abundant necroinflammatory debris, which in many cases exceeds the amount of associated inflammation. The organisms are usually found in ulcer debris. Invasive amebae are also occasionally present in the bowel wall. Adjacent mucosa is usually normal but may show gland distortion. The organisms may be few in number. They resemble macrophages, with foamy cytoplasm and round, eccentric nuclei. The presence of ingested red blood cells (see Fig. 4.45B,C) is a helpful diagnostic clue. In asymptomatic patients and those with only mild symptoms, histological changes may range from normal to a heavy mixed inflammatory infiltrate. Organisms may be

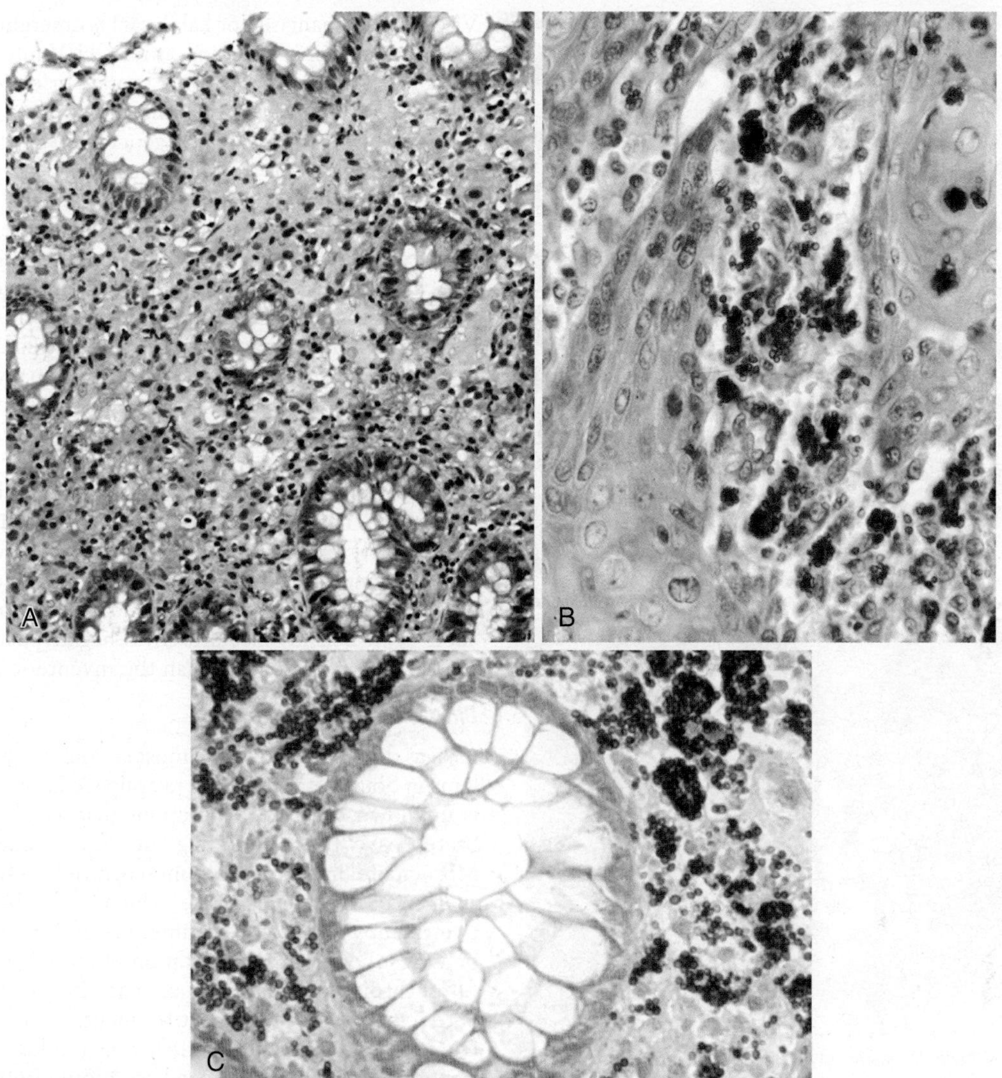

FIGURE 4.41 **A,** A colon biopsy specimen shows numerous histiocytes within the lamina propria in this case of histoplasmosis. **B**, Macrophages within the esophagus are packed with *Histoplasma* with very little associated inflammatory reaction in this esophageal biopsy from an immunocompromised patient (H&E/methenamine silver stain). **C**, On GMS staining, numerous *Histoplasma* organisms are seen distending histiocytes in the lamina propria. (*Courtesy of Dr. Patrick J. Dean, GI Pathology, PLLC.*)

difficult or impossible to detect in these patients. Invasive amebiasis does not usually occur in patients who have only mild or absent symptoms.[249]

Differential Diagnosis

It may be difficult to distinguish amebae from macrophages in inflammatory exudates. However, amebae are trichrome-positive and PAS-positive, and macrophages stain with immunostains such as CD68 and CD163. In addition, amoeba have a much lower nuclear-to-cytoplasmic ratio than macrophages and are usually more round and pale, with a more open nuclear chromatin pattern. The differential diagnosis of amebiasis includes CD, UC, and other types of infectious colitis, particularly when gross skip lesions or significant architectural distortion is present. Although some features of amebiasis may mimic idiopathic IBD, many of the other diagnostic features of CD (e.g., transmural lymphoid aggregates, mural fibrosis, granulomas, neural hyperplasia) and UC (e.g., basal lymphoplasmacytosis, diffuse architectural distortion, pancolitis) are not typically present in amebiasis.

Flagellates

Giardia lamblia

Giardiasis (*Giardia lamblia* infection) is the leading GI protozoal disease in the United States and occurs throughout temperate and tropical regions worldwide. The prevalence rate is higher among children, particularly those who attend day care centers.[250] Patients experience explosive, foul-smelling, watery diarrhea, abdominal pain and distention; nausea; vomiting; malabsorption; and weight loss. The infection may resolve spontaneously, but often persists for weeks or months if left untreated. A proportion of patients go on to develop chronic giardiasis, featuring diarrhea often accompanied by marked weight loss, signs of malabsorption, and anemia. Complications include dehydration, especially in children, and failure to thrive among infants and small children. Many infections are asymptomatic, however. The cyst, which is the infective form, is chlorine resistant and may survive in water for several months. However, the mechanism by which these organisms cause GI illness is poorly understood.[251]

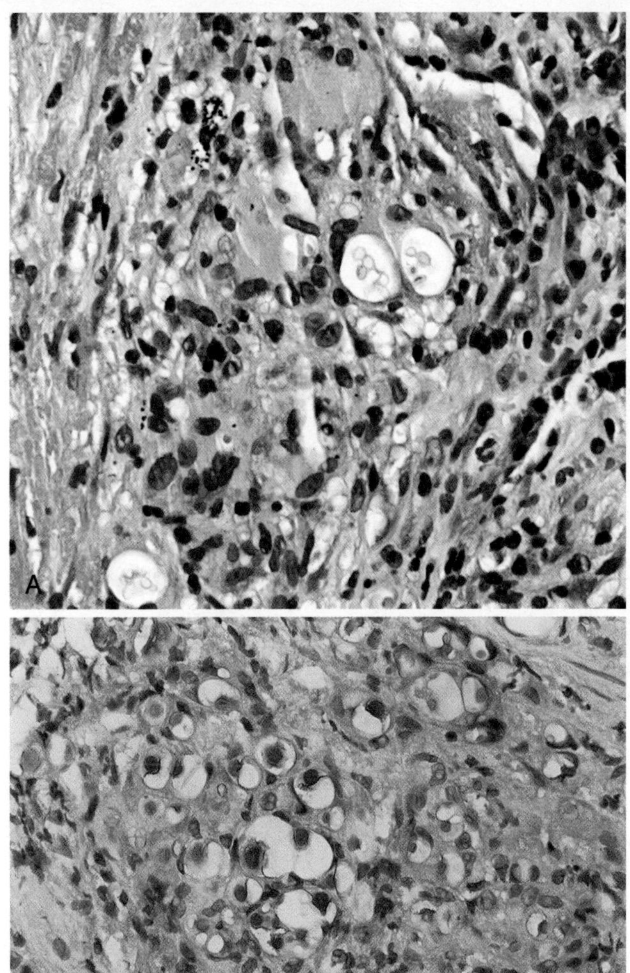

FIGURE 4.42 This case of gastric cryptococcosis features a granulomatous reaction with associated giant cells and acute inflammation. **A**, A halo or "soap-bubble" effect can be seen around the organisms. **B**, The round to oval yeast forms have a mucopolysaccharide capsule that stains with mucicarmine. (*Courtesy of Dr. Kay Washington, Vanderbilt University School of Medicine.*)

Endoscopic examination is generally unremarkable, and small intestinal biopsies are often normal in appearance. Rarely, biopsies may show mild to moderate villous blunting and increased lamina propria inflammatory cells, including neutrophils, plasma cells, and lymphocytes.[252-254] *Giardia* trophozoites resemble pears that are cut lengthwise and contain two ovoid nuclei with a central karyosome (Fig. 4.46). They cluster at the luminal surface; tissue invasion is not a feature of this infection. Although *Giardia* is characteristically described as a small bowel inhabitant, colonization of the stomach and colon has also been reported. Absence or a marked decrease of plasma cells in the lamina propria in a patient with giardiasis should alert the pathologist to the possibility of an underlying immunodeficiency disorder (see Chapter 5).[255]

Leishmania donovani *and Related Species*

Leishmaniasis is endemic in more than 80 countries in Africa, Asia, South and Central America, and Europe. Visceral leishmaniasis (or kala-azar) is emerging as an important opportunistic infection among HIV-infected patients, particularly in southwestern Europe. In endemic areas, it often affects children and young adults.[256,257]

GI involvement is rare and generally part of disseminated disease. Any level of the GI tract may be affected. GI signs and symptoms include fever, abdominal pain, diarrhea, dysphagia, malabsorption, and weight loss. The spectrum of endoscopic findings includes normal mucosa, focal ulceration, and changes of enteritis. Histologically, amastigote-containing macrophages are present in the lamina propria. In large numbers, macrophages may distend and blunt intestinal villi. An associated inflammatory infiltrate is normally absent. The amastigotes are rounded, 2- to 4-μm basophilic organisms with a round to oval central nucleus and a thin external membrane (Fig. 4.47). The kinetoplast lies tangentially or perpendicular to the nucleus, producing a characteristic "double-knot" configuration. They are highlighted by Giemsa staining.

The differential diagnosis primarily includes other parasitic and fungal infections. *Leishmania* may be confused with organisms such as *Histoplasma* and *Trypanosoma cruzi* (see Table 4.4). Leishmaniae are GMS negative, and they affect the lamina propria rather than the myenteric plexus.[258,259]

Chagas Disease

Chagas disease is one of the most serious public health problems in South America. The prevalence in the United States is unknown, and most infections diagnosed in the United States have been in immigrants from endemic areas.[260] Most acute infections go unrecognized. Infected persons then enter the chronic phase, which in the absence of effective therapy lasts for a lifetime. GI dysfunction is the second most common manifestation of chronic Chagas disease (after cardiac involvement), and parasitic involvement of the enteric nervous system most frequently causes an achalasia-like megaesophagus (Fig. 4.48), a megacolon, or both.[261,262] The stomach and small bowel are more rarely affected. GI disease results from damage to intramural neurons. Upper GI symptoms include dysphagia, odynophagia, reflux, aspiration, weight loss, cough, and regurgitation. Imaging studies may show a range of appearances from mild achalasia to megaesophagus. Lower GI symptoms include constipation, stool impaction, and abdominal pain; imaging studies reveal a markedly dilated and elongated megacolon.

Histologically, there is inflammatory destruction of the myenteric plexus, with eventual loss of as much as 95% of neurons. However, the parasite is rarely visible in myenteric plexuses. The inflammatory infiltrate is primarily lymphocytic, with inflammation of the nerve fibers and ganglion cells that extends into the muscular wall. Accompanying findings include degenerative neuronal changes, loss of nerve fibers and ganglion cells, and fibrosis. The differential diagnosis includes idiopathic primary achalasia as well as other visceral neuropathies. However, many of these latter disorders lack inflammation of the myenteric plexus.[261,263] Unlike primary achalasia, Chagas disease usually involves other organ systems (especially the heart) or other areas of the GI tract. Nevertheless, often the differential diagnosis must be resolved clinically. Helpful laboratory tests include PCR assays, serological studies, and culture. Negative laboratory test results do not exclude infection, however, given the frequently low levels of parasitemia.[264]

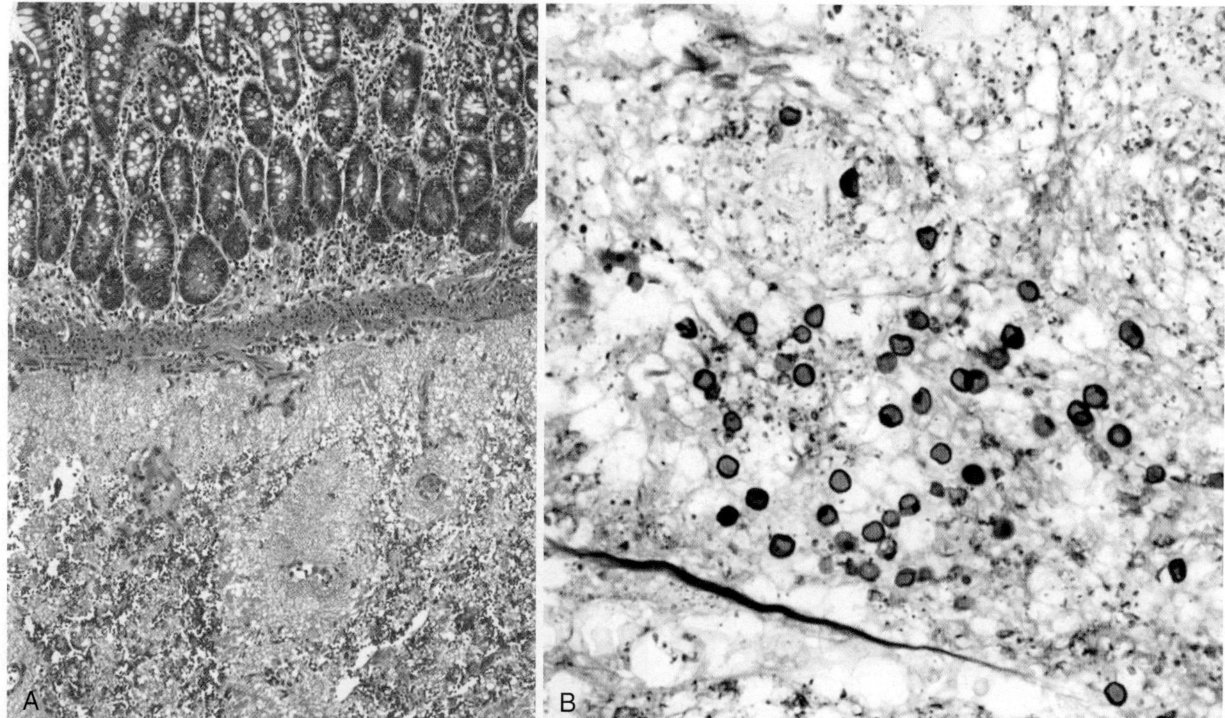

FIGURE 4.43 **A,** Small bowel resection shows the characteristic foamy casts of *Pneumocystis jiroveci* in the submucosa. **B**, GMS stain highlights numerous cyst forms with central enhanced staining. (**B** *courtesy of Dr. Henry Appelman, University of Michigan.*)

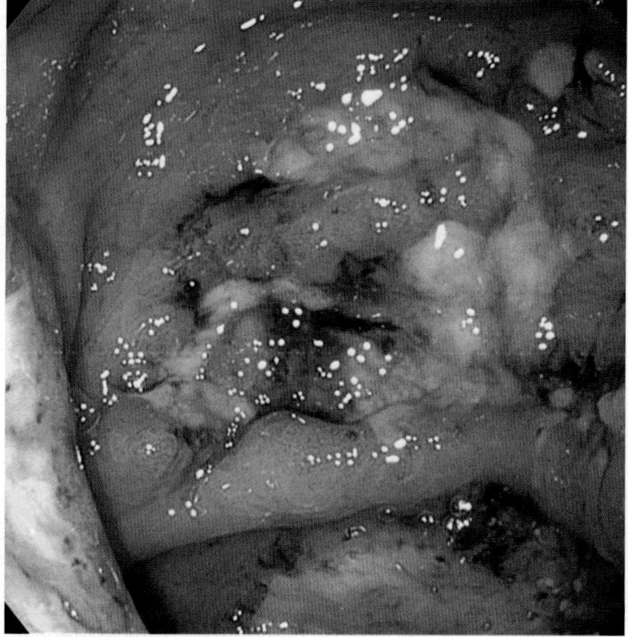

FIGURE 4.44 Early small ulcers coalesce and may appear serpiginous or circumferential in *Entamoeba histolytica* colitis.

Ciliates

Balantidium coli

The ciliate *Balantidium coli* produces a spectrum of clinical and pathological changes similar to those produced by *E. histolytica*. *B. coli* cells are distinguished from amebae by their larger size, kidney bean–shaped nucleus, and, the presence of cilia (Fig. 4.49).[265]

Coccidians and Related Organisms

Some unicellular organisms, namely, *Cryptosporidium parvum*, *C. hominis*, *C. meleagridis*, *Cyclospora cayetanensis*, *Cystoisospora belli*, and *Microsporidia*, cause clinically similar diarrheal illness in immunocompromised and young patients all over the world.[266-270] These organisms were historically all considered coccidians, but have recently been reclassified on the basis of molecular data. *Cryptosporidia* spp. are now classified as gregarines, a subclass of Conoidasida closely related to coccidians.[267] *Cystoisospora belli* (formerly *Isospora belli*) and *Cyclospora cayetanensis* are still classified as coccidians.[268-270] *Microsporidia* was previously classified as a protozoan, but is now considered to be a fungus.[266]

Infection is particularly important when considering the differential diagnosis of diarrhea in patients with AIDS, but it is also seen in healthy persons, including infants and children, in developing countries. Transmission is normally by the fecal-oral route, either directly or via contaminated food and water. These organisms also cause diarrhea (often prolonged) in healthy adults, especially travelers, and institutionalized individuals. Diarrhea may be accompanied by fever, weight loss, abdominal pain, and malaise. In immunocompetent persons, infection is self-limited, but immunocompromised patients are at risk for chronic, severe diarrhea with malabsorption, dehydration, and death. Many infections are asymptomatic. Endoscopic findings are usually absent or mild and include mild erythema, mucosal granularity, mucosal atrophy, and superficial erosions. Although electron microscopy was once considered the gold standard for diagnosis, it is expensive and not widely used. Examination of stool specimens may be very helpful (particularly with special stains), but analysis of mucosal biopsy

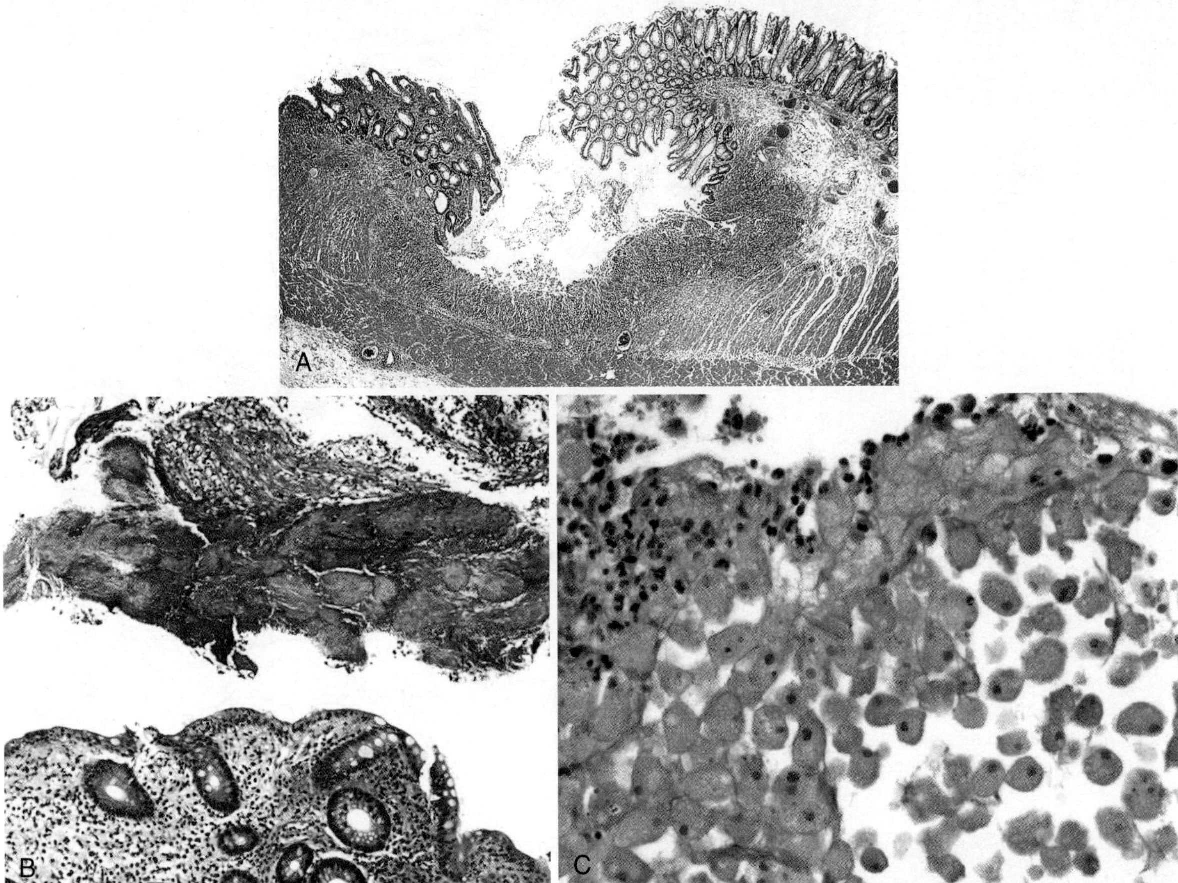

FIGURE 4.45 A, This entamoebic ulcer is deep and flask-shaped, undermining adjacent normal mucosa. **B,** Amoebiasis is often associated with abundant debris that contains more degenerated apoptotic material than intact inflammatory cells. **C,** *Entamoeba histolytica* have pale, round nuclei with foamy cytoplasm and contain ingested erythrocytes.

specimens is more sensitive. A comparison of the morphological features of these organisms is given in Table 4.10. ELISA techniques, immunohistochemistry, and PCR studies are also available for their detection.[270]

Cryptosporidium parvum

Cryptosporidium parvum has a worldwide distribution, and transmission is through contaminated food and water.[271] It is most common in the small bowel, but it may infect any segment of the GI tract. The characteristic appearance is that of a 2- to 5-μm, basophilic, spherical body that protrudes from the apex of the enterocyte within extracytoplasmic vacuoles (Fig. 4.50). The organisms have been referred to as "blue beads" given their round, basophilic appearance. They are found in the crypts or in the surface epithelium. Associated mucosal changes include villous atrophy (occasionally severe), crypt hyperplasia, mixed inflammation, and crypt abscesses. Giemsa and Gram stains may aid in diagnosis, and immunohistochemical antibodies are available. Cryptosporidia may be distinguished from most other coccidians by their size and unique apical location.[272]

Cyclospora cayetanensis

Cyclospora is the most recently discovered enteric coccidian. Infection may be asymptomatic, and *Cyclospora* can infect immunocompromised or immunocompetent patients. This organism most commonly infects the small bowel.[273] Histological changes in mucosal biopsies are similar to those of other coccidians, including mild villous blunting, patchy lamina propria inflammation, and surface epithelial disarray. Intracellular forms of *Cyclospora* include 2- to 3-μm schizonts and 5- to 6-μm, banana-shaped merozoites located within enterocytes (Fig. 4.51). Organisms are often located within the upper third of the enterocyte, within a parasitophorous vacuole. The organisms are acid-fast with modified Kinyoun or similar stains and are also positive with auramine. However, they are GMS, PAS, Gram, and trichrome negative. They exhibit autofluorescence under epifluorescent light.[255]

Cystoisospora belli *and Related Species*

Cystoisospora belli (formerly *Isospora belli*) has a worldwide distribution but is more common in tropical and subtropical regions than temperate climates. It is transmitted by ingestion of food or water contaminated with oocysts. Patients with cystoisosporiasis are more likely to have peripheral eosinophilia than those infected by other coccidians. Infection may be severe and debilitating in immunocompromised patients, and widespread dissemination has been reported rarely.[274] The small bowel is the most common site of *Cystoisospora* infection, but the colon may also be involved. Histological changes include villous blunting, which may be severe; surface epithelial and nuclear disarray; crypt hyperplasia; mixed inflammation, often with

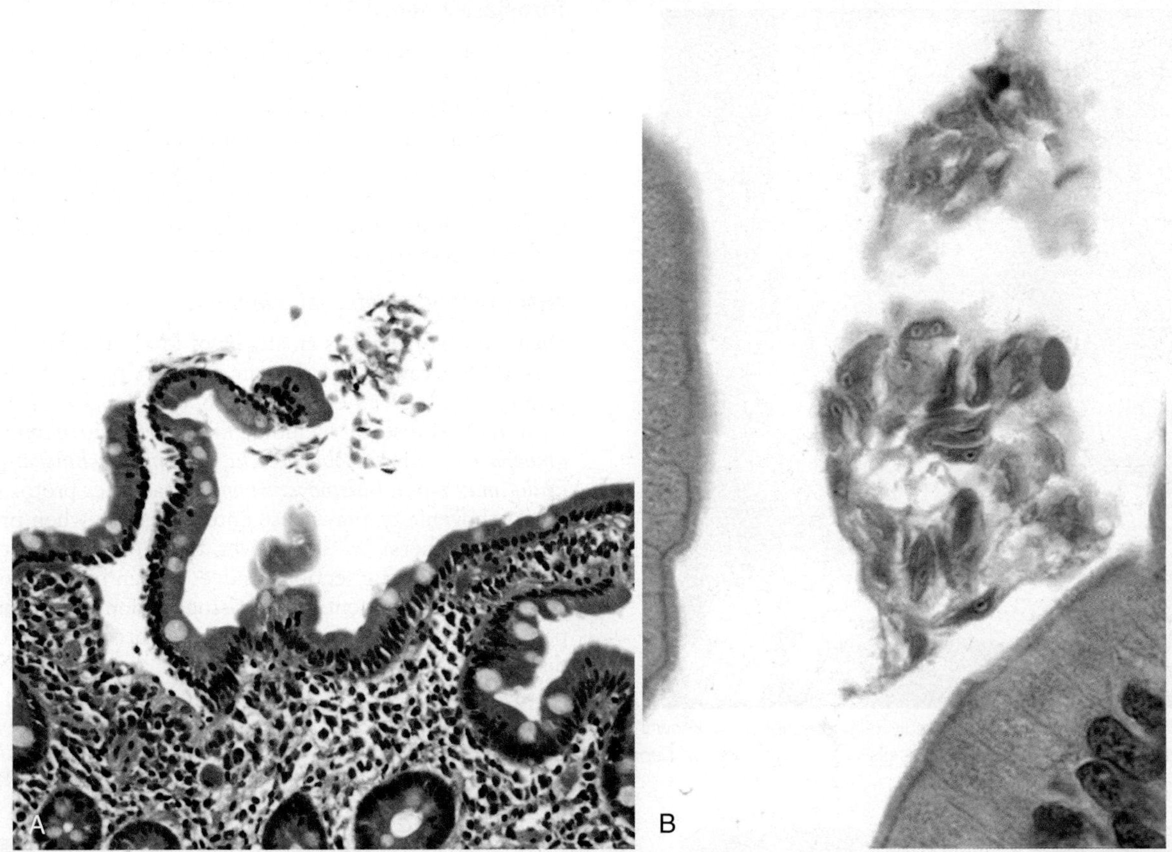

FIGURE 4.46 **A,** Duodenal mucosa with numerous *Giardia* trophozoites at the luminal surface, illustrating the "falling leaves" pattern. **B,** Higher-power view shows the typical pear-shaped morphology with two prominent nuclei. (*Courtesy of Dr. Rodger Haggitt, University of Washington.*)

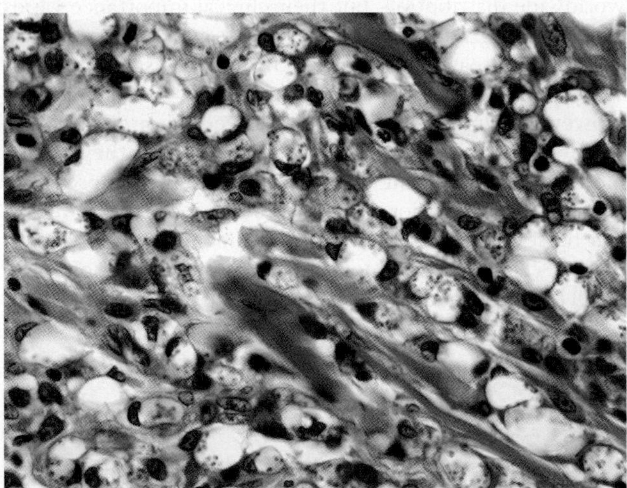

FIGURE 4.47 Macrophages containing numerous *Leishmania* amastigotes. (*Courtesy Dr. Bruce Smoller, University of Arkansas for Medical Science.*)

prominent eosinophils; and, in chronic infections, fibrosis of the lamina propria. *Cystoisospora* is the largest coccidian (15 to 20 μm). Intraepithelial inclusions are present in all stages of infection (Fig. 4.52) and can be found within both epithelial cells and macrophages in the lamina propria. Inclusions are both perinuclear and subnuclear. Schizonts and merozoites (the asexual forms) are crescent or banana shaped; sexual forms are round with a prominent nucleus. The organisms often have an associated loose parasitophorous vacuole. GMS and Giemsa stains are useful to highlight the organism. *Cystoisospora* are PAS-D positive (often with a granular staining pattern). They may be easily confused with goblet cells or hyaline globules (thanatasomes).[274,276] The latter show diffuse staining with PAS-D, GMS, and mucicarmine, whereas C. *belli* are negative for GMS and mucicarmine.[274]

Microsporidia

Microsporidia is the least likely coccidian to affect immunocompetent patients. *Enterocytozoon bieneusi* and *Encephalitozoon intestinalis* are the most common human pathogens in this group. Dissemination may occur, especially with *E. intestinalis* infection.[277,278] The organisms are usually present in the small bowel, but any level of the GI tract may be affected. Microsporidia are difficult to detect in H&E-stained sections. The histological features include patchy villous blunting, vacuolization and disarray of the surface epithelium, and patchy lymphoplasmacytic infiltrates in the lamina propria. A modified trichrome stain can aid greatly in the diagnosis (Fig. 4.53), and the organisms also stain with Warthin-Starry and Brown-Brenn stains. Occasionally, microsporidial organisms in biopsy specimens demonstrate birefringence under polarized light because of their chitin-rich internal polar filament. However, this method is unreliable, because spore birefringence is unpredictable and because microscopes and light sources vary.[279]

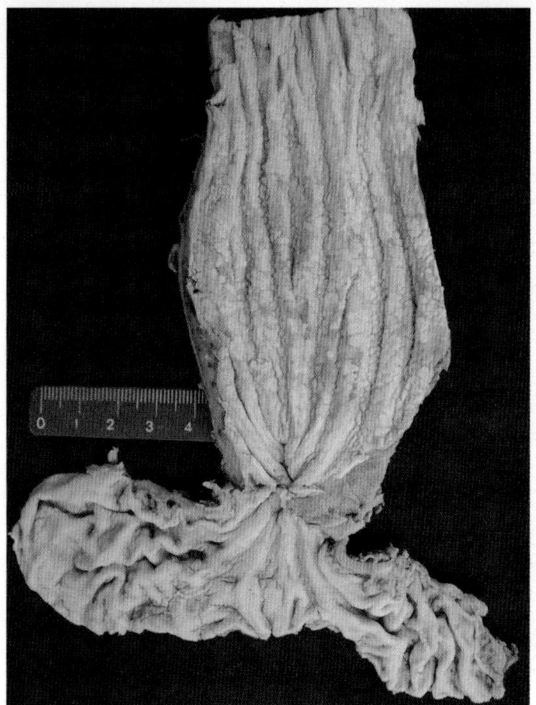

FIGURE 4.48 Elongated and markedly dilated esophagus, known as "megaesophagus," caused by Chagas disease. (*Courtesy of Dr. Dennis Baroni-Cruz, University of Santa Cruz.*)

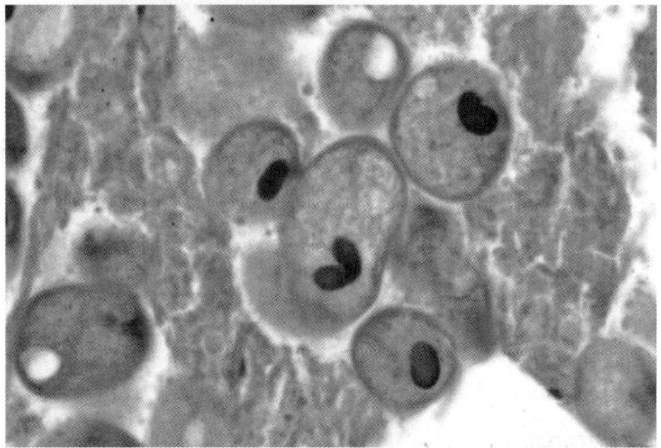

FIGURE 4.49 *Balantidium coli* in the bowel wall. Notice the large size, kidney bean–shaped nucleus, and cilia. (*Courtesy of Dr. David Owen, University of Michigan.*)

Toxoplasma gondii

GI toxoplasmosis is primarily a disease of immunocompromised hosts. Ulcers have been described, and organisms are usually located in the ulcer base. Both crescent-shaped tachyzoites and tissue cysts containing bradyzoites may be present in tissue sections. Immunohistochemistry and PCR assays, as well as serological tests, are useful diagnostic aids; however, serologies may be unreliable in severely immunocompromised patients.[280]

Miscellaneous Protozoal Infections

Dientamoeba fragilis is an ameba of low pathogenicity that occasionally causes diarrhea in affected patients.[281,282] A variety of other amebae are also occasionally associated with mild GI disease, including *Entamoeba hartmanni, Entamoeba coli, Entamoeba polecki, Iodamoeba butschlii,* and *Endolimax nana. Blastocystis hominis*, another protozoan of low pathogenicity, may cause enteric disease when present in large numbers.[283,284] However, these organisms are only rarely seen in tissue sections. Indeed, when protozoa of low pathogenicity are identified in tissue sections, symptomatic patients should be evaluated for alternative causes of GI disease.

Helminthic Infections

Although the most common method of diagnosing GI helminth infections is examination of stool for ova and parasites, these organisms are occasionally detected in biopsy or resection specimens. Hookworms, roundworms (both *Ascaris* and *Enterobius*), and whipworms are the most common helminthic infections in humans.[285-288] GI helminths have a worldwide distribution, but their clinical importance varies with the geographical region. They are more often a cause of serious disease in nations with deficient sanitation systems, poor socioeconomic status, and hot, humid climates. However, helminthic infections are seen in immigrants and in patients who travel to endemic areas, and they are an increasingly important problem in immunocompromised hosts.[288-290] Nutritional problems caused by helminths can be severe and even life-threatening, especially in children.[288] The most common site of anatomic infection is the small bowel, although the stomach and large bowel may also be involved.

TABLE 4.10 Morphological Features of Coccidians and Related Unicellular Organisms

Feature	Microsporidia	Cryptosporidia	*Cyclospora*	*Cystoisospora*
Classification	Fungus	Parasite, gregarines	Parasite, coccidian	Parasite, coccidian
Size	2- to 3-μm spores	2–5 μm	2- to 3-μm schizonts 5- to 6-μm merozoites	15-20 μm (largest coccidian)
Location	Epithelial cells; rarely macrophages	Apical surface of epithelial cells	Upper third of epithelial cell	Epithelial cells and macrophages
Staining properties	Modified trichrome, Giemsa, Gram, Warthin-Starry positive	Giemsa, Gram stain positive	Acid-fast, auramine positive GMS, PAS, Giemsa negative	Giemsa, Gram, PAS positive GMS, mucicarmine negative
Other	May be birefringent under polarized light	Organism bulges from luminal surface of enterocyte apex	Parasitophorous vacuole	Parasitophorous vacuole Eosinophilic infiltrate

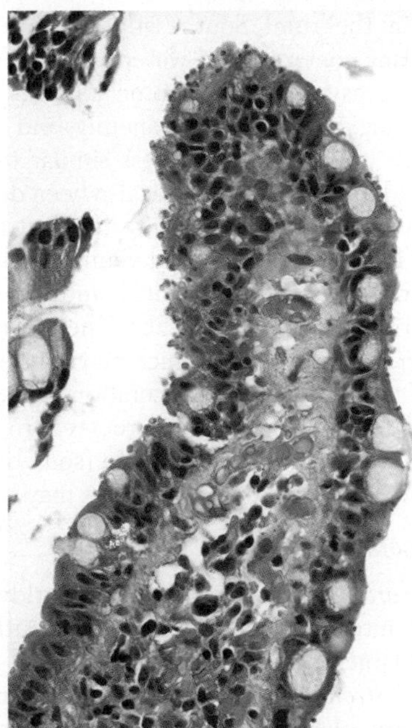

FIGURE 4.50 *Cryptosporidium parvum* infection. The 2- to 5-μm, basophilic, spherical bodies protrude from the apex of the enterocytes, giving a "blue bead" appearance.

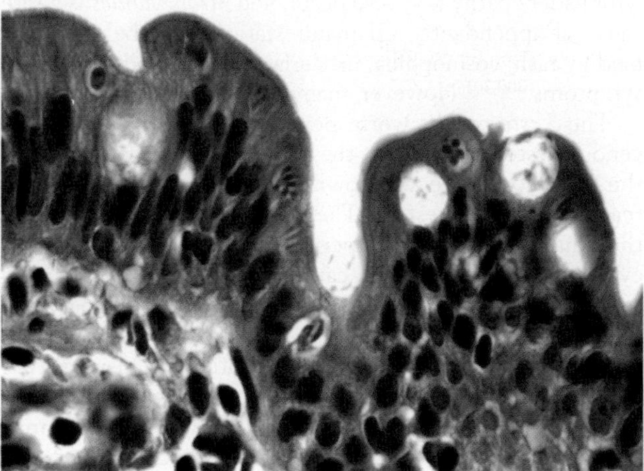

FIGURE 4.51 Both crescent-shaped merozoites and round schizonts are located within surface enterocytes in this case of *Cyclospora* infection. Notice the small parasitophorous vacuole. (*From a case done by Dr. Rhonda K. Yantiss, Weill Cornell Medicine.*)

Nematodes

Enterobius vermicularis

Pinworms (*Enterobius vermicularis*) are among the most common human parasites. They have a worldwide distribution but are more common in cold or temperate climates and in developed countries. They are extremely common in the United States and northwestern Europe.[291,292] The infective egg resides in dust and soil, and transmission is thought to be by the fecal-oral route. The worms live and reproduce in the ileum, cecum, proximal colon, and appendix, and then the female migrates to the anus to lay eggs and die. The eggs and worms produce symptoms of pruritus ani.[291] Although many infections are asymptomatic,

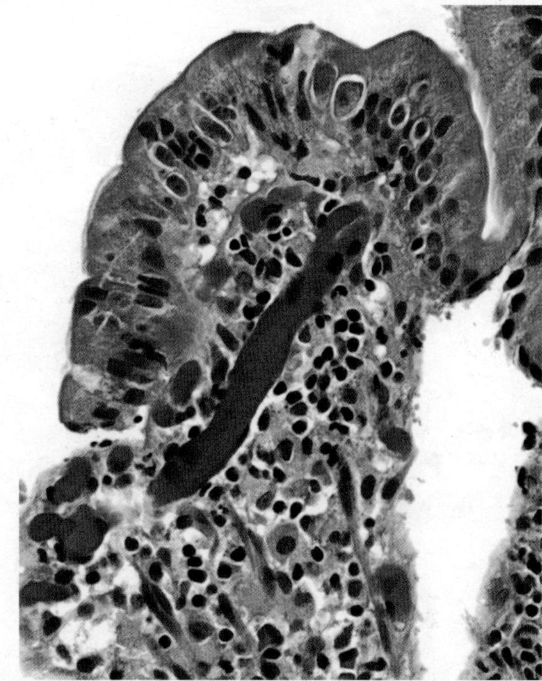

FIGURE 4.52 *Cystoisospora belli* infection. A small bowel villus has surface epithelial disarray and large coccidians typical of *Cystoisospora* within parasitophorous vacuoles. (*Courtesy of Dr. Joel K. Greenson, University of Michigan.*)

appendicitis, vulvovaginitis, colitis, and peritoneal involvement have all been described. Heavy infections may cause abdominal pain, nausea, and vomiting.[287]

The etiological role of *Enterobius* in appendicitis and colitis is controversial. Although pinworms are detected in approximately 0.6% of resected appendices, their ability to cause mucosal damage has been a subject of debate.[293,294] Some think that the lack of inflammation surrounding invasive pinworms indicates that the organism invades only after the appendix has been removed, to escape the decrease in oxygen tension. However, *Enterobius* organisms are, in fact, capable of mucosal invasion, and, like fecaliths, they can obstruct the appendiceal lumen and cause inflammation.[295]

The worms are 2 to 5 mm in length and therefore may be seen with the naked eye (Fig. 4.54). Although the mucosa of the GI tract often appears normal on examination, hemorrhage and ulceration may occur with tissue invasion. Invasive pinworms often incite little or no inflammatory reaction, but an inflammatory infiltrate composed of neutrophils and eosinophils occurs uncommonly. Granulomas, sometimes with necrosis, may develop as a reaction to degenerating worms or eggs. These have been described in the omentum and peritoneum, as well as in the appendix, anus, and colon in rare cases.[296] Primary *Enterobius* infection may be difficult to distinguish from infection complicating a preexisting inflammatory disorder such as an inflamed anal fissure.

Ascaris lumbricoides *(Roundworm)*

Ascaris is one of the most common parasites in humans. It has a worldwide distribution but is most common in tropical regions. The worms are ingested from soil contaminated with feces. Clinical findings are variable and include appendicitis, massive infection with obstruction and

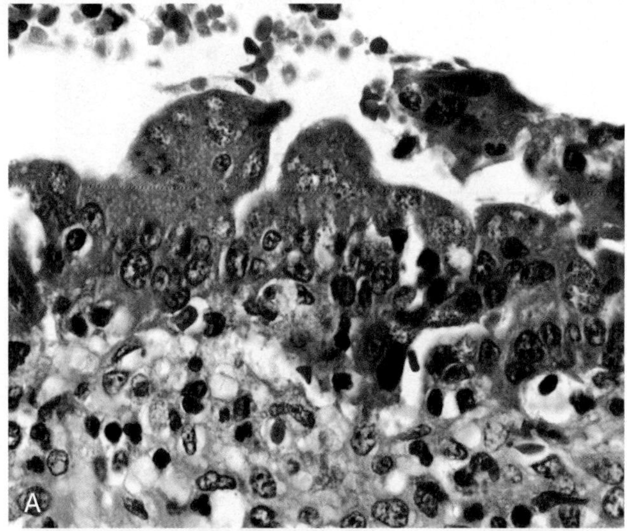

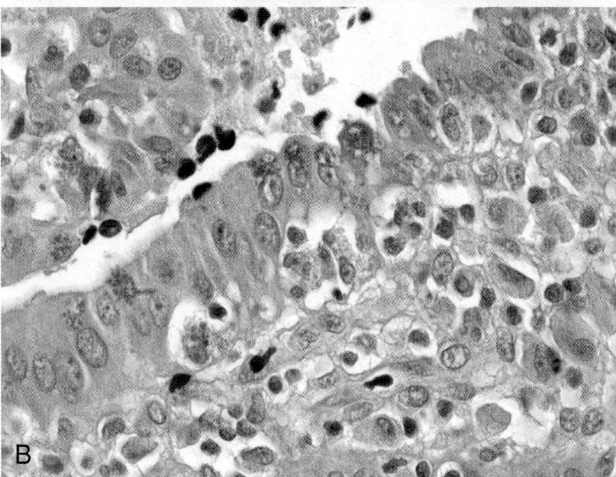

FIGURE 4.53 A, Microsporidiosis featuring surface epithelial disarray and subtle vacuolization with the surface enterocytes. **B,** Modified trichrome stain highlights the organisms.

perforation, childhood growth retardation, and pancreaticobiliary obstruction.[288,289] Giant worms (as large as 20 cm in length) may be identified endoscopically or in resection specimens (Fig. 4.55). Tissue damage occurs primarily at sites of attachment.

Ancylostomiasis (Hookworm)

Hookworm (*Ancylostoma duodenale* and *Necator americanus*) is a common parasite in all tropical and subtropical countries. The worms attach to the intestinal wall and withdraw blood from villous capillaries, which results in anemia. Other clinical symptoms include abdominal pain, diarrhea, hypoproteinemia, and cough with eosinophilia when the worms migrate. Any level of the GI tract may be involved. Endoscopically, the worms (which measure about 1 cm in length) are visible to the naked eye.[288] Histological changes are often minimal but may include villous blunting and eosinophilic infiltration. Pieces of worm are occasionally detected in biopsy specimens.

Trichuris trichiura *(Whipworm)*

Whipworm (*Trichuris trichiura*) is a soil helminth with a worldwide distribution; it is most common in tropical climates. In the United States, it is most often seen among immigrants and in the rural Southeast.[288,297] Infection is acquired by ingesting contaminated water or food. Although most infections are asymptomatic, some patients develop diarrhea, GI bleeding, malabsorption, anemia, and appendicitis. An ulcerative inflammatory process similar to that in Crohn's disease and rectal prolapse have also been described. The worms can live anywhere in the intestine but are most commonly found in the right colon and ileum. Adult worms can span up to 3 cm and have a threadlike anterior segment and a thick posterior segment (Fig. 4.56). They thread their anterior end under the epithelium, which may cause mucosal edema, erythema, hemorrhage, and ulceration at the attachment site (Fig. 4.57). Histologically, enterocyte atrophy with an associated mixed inflammatory infiltrate (sometimes rich in eosinophils) and occasional crypt abscesses may be seen.

Strongyloides stercoralis

Strongyloides stercoralis is a nematode with a worldwide distribution. In the United States, it is endemic in southeastern urban areas with large immigrant populations and in mental institutions.[298] *Strongyloides* occurs primarily in adults, many of whom are hospitalized, suffer from chronic illnesses, or are immunocompromised.[299] Steroids and human T-lymphotropic virus type I (HLTV-I) infection are also associated with strongyloidiasis. Symptoms and signs include diarrhea, abdominal pain and tenderness, nausea, vomiting, weight loss, malabsorption, and GI bleeding. Mesenteric lymphadenopathy may also occur, and *Strongyloides* is a rare cause of appendicitis. GI manifestations may be accompanied by rash, eosinophilia, urticaria, pruritus, and pulmonary symptoms.[300,301] However, many patients are asymptomatic.

The *S. stercoralis* worm penetrates the skin, enters the venous system, travels to the lungs, and then migrates up the respiratory tree and down the esophagus to eventually reach the small intestine. The female lives and lays eggs in the small intestine, thus perpetuating the organism's life cycle. This autoinfective capability allows the organism to reside in the host and produce illness for a long time, upward of 30 years. In addition, widespread dissemination may occur in immunocompromised patients, causing severe and even fatal illness.

Lesions may be seen in the stomach, as well as in the small and large intestine. Endoscopic findings include hypertrophic mucosal folds and ulcers. However, features typical of PMC have also been reported.[302,303] Histologically, both adult worms and larvae may be found in the crypts, but they can be difficult to detect. Adult worms typically have sharply pointed tails that may be curved (Fig. 4.58). Other histological features include villous blunting, ulcers (which may be fissuring), edema, and a dense eosinophilic and neutrophilic infiltrate. Granulomas are occasionally present as well. The presence of larvae with sharply pointed, sometimes curved tails within the glands of the GI mucosa is essentially diagnostic of strongyloidiasis. In the proper clinical and geographical setting, however, *Capillaria* infection is also in the differential diagnosis. Rarely, fulminant intestinal strongyloidiasis may mimic chronic idiopathic IBD. Ancillary diagnostic tests include stool examination for larvae, worms, or eggs and serological tests.

Anisakis simplex *and Related Species*

The *Anisakis simplex* nematode parasitizes fish and sea mammals; humans ingest them by eating raw or pickled fish. The most common clinical manifestations are those of acute

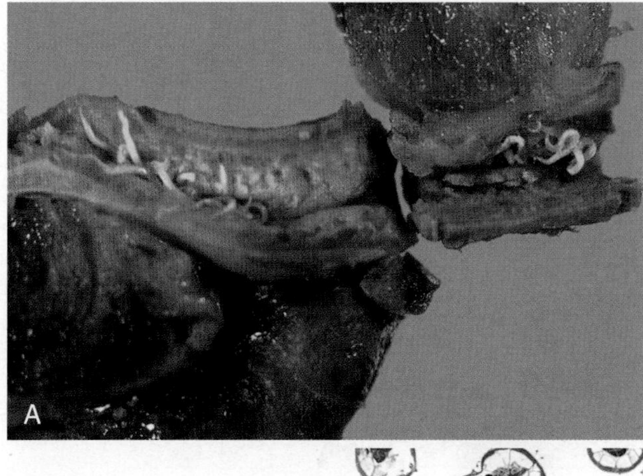

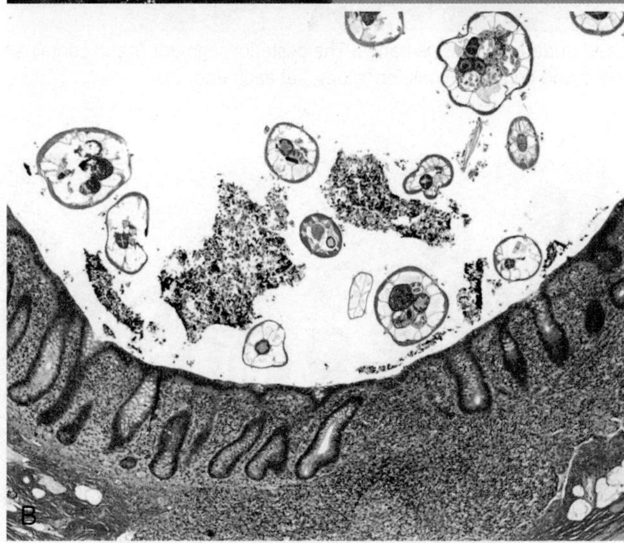

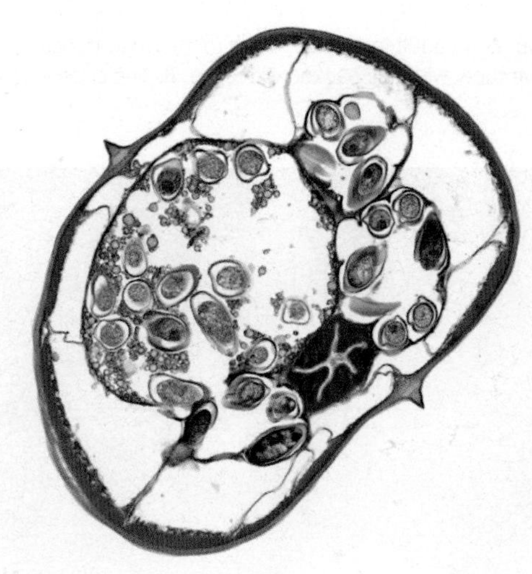

FIGURE 4.54 **A**, Appendix containing numerous pinworms. **B,** Numerous pinworms are present at the surface of the appendix. **C,** Cross-section of worm showing cuticle, typical lateral ala, and numerous eggs characteristic of *Enterobius vermicularis.* (**A** *courtesy of Dr. George F. Gray, Jr., Vanderbilt University Medical Center.*)

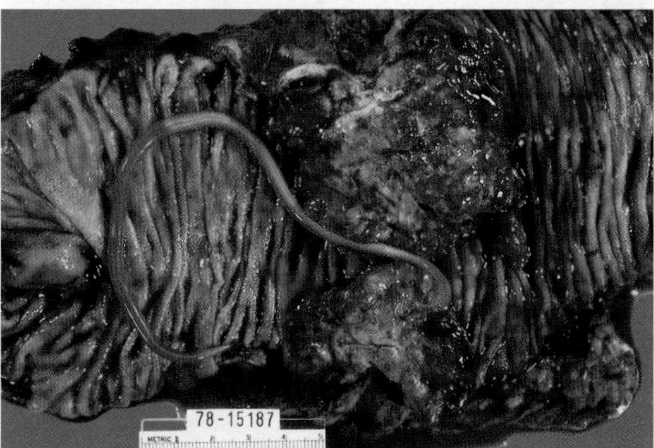

FIGURE 4.55 *Ascaris* atop colon cancer at resection. (*Courtesy of Dr. George F. Gray, Jr., Vanderbilt University Medical Center.*)

gastric anisakiasis, which is characterized by epigastric pain, nausea, and vomiting within 12 hours after ingestion of parasitized food. The symptoms may mimic peptic ulcer disease. The allergenic potential of *Anisakis* spp. has also been recognized, and some patients with gastroallergic anisakiasis manifest both GI effects and hypersensitivity symptoms such as urticaria, angioedema, eosinophilia, and anaphylaxis.[304]

The stomach is the most frequent site of involvement, although the small bowel, colon, and appendix may also be involved. Endoscopic findings include mucosal edema, hemorrhage, erosions, ulcers, and thickened mucosal folds. Occasionally, larvae may be identified and removed endoscopically.[305] Histological findings include an inflammatory infiltrate that is rich in eosinophils and may extend transmurally into serosal and mesenteric tissues (Fig. 4.59). Eosinophilic microabscesses, granulomas, and giant cells may also develop. Inflammatory changes usually surround worms.[306] Larvae (0.5 to 3.0 cm in length) are occasionally seen in tissue sections but very rarely in stool samples.[307]

Capillaria *Species (Intestinal Capillariasis)*

Capillaria infection is most common in the Philippines, Thailand, and other parts of Asia, although cases have been reported in nonendemic areas. The worms are ingested by eating infected raw fish. Clinical signs and symptoms include malabsorption accompanied by diarrhea and abdominal pain.[308,309] The worms measure 2 to 4 cm in length and are most commonly found in the crypts of the small bowel, although they may also invade the lamina propria. There usually is no inflammatory reaction, but villous blunting, mucosal sloughing, and mild inflammatory changes have been described.

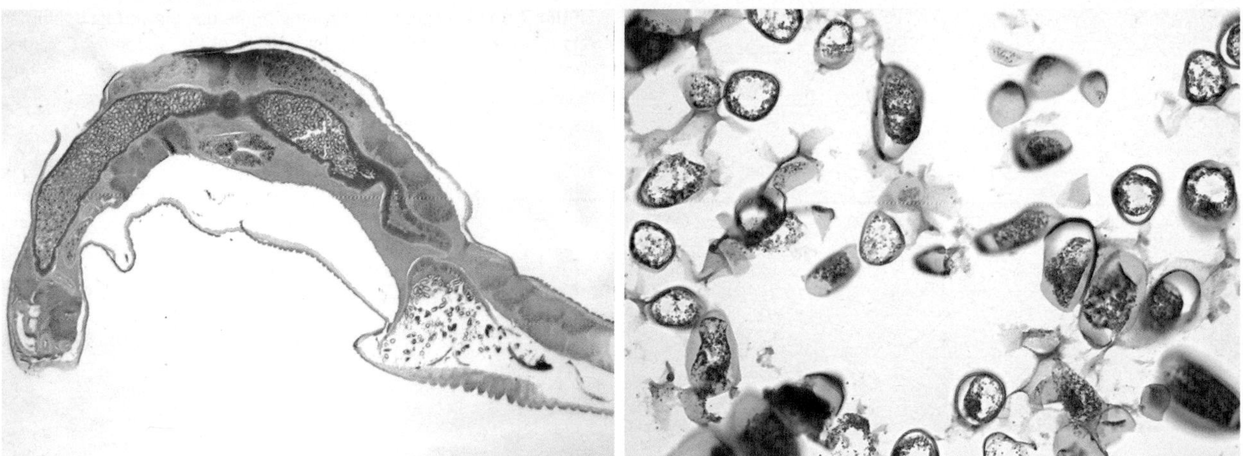

FIGURE 4.56 **A,** An adult female *Trichiuris trichiura* worm has a thick cuticle and underlying muscle bands. The posterior segment *(right)* contains the reproductive tube, which is packed with eggs. **B,** The eggs have refractile shells and condensations, or "plugs," at each end.

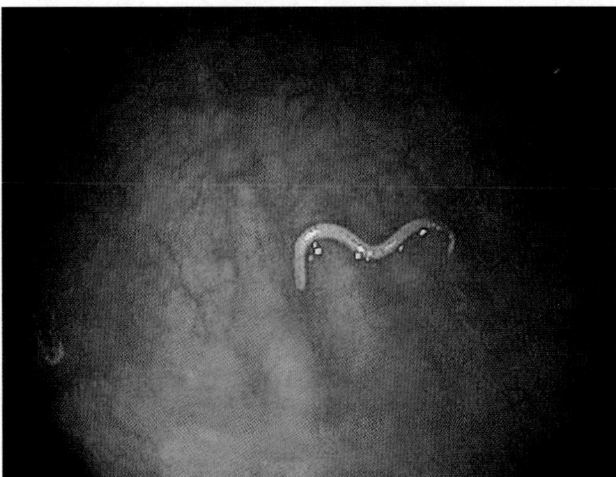

FIGURE 4.57 The wider posterior segment of *Trichiuris trichiura* is visible in the lumen of the colon, whereas the narrow anterior segment is buried in the mucosa.

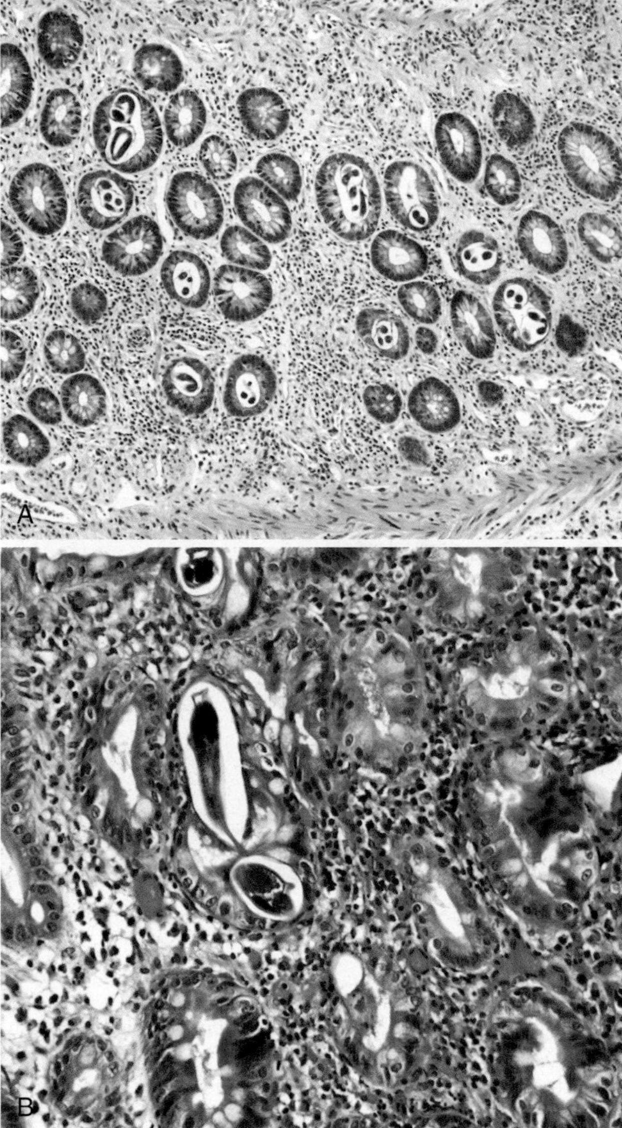

FIGURE 4.58 **A**, Numerous *Strongyloides stercoralis* are seen within the crypts in this case of colonic *Strongyloidiasis* infection. **B**, Typical worms and larvae have curved, sharply pointed tails.

Trematodes

Schistosomiasis

Schistosomiasis is one of the most common diseases in the world. All species of *Schistosoma* that infect humans have the capability to cause significant GI disease, but the gut is a target organ for *Schistosoma mansoni, Schistosoma japonicum, Schistosoma mekongi,* and *Schistosoma intercalatum* infections. These trematodes are endemic in Africa, Asia, and parts of the Americas. In the United States, infected patients are often immigrants, travelers, or persons who have worked abroad. Humans become infected by exposure to contaminated water. Patients usually experience diarrhea (often bloody) accompanied by anemia, weight loss, and protein-losing enteropathy.[310] More dramatic GI presentations have been described, such as profound dysentery-like illness, obstruction, perforation, intussusception, rectal prolapse, fistulae, and perianal abscesses.[311] Schistosomes (most frequently *Schistosoma haematobium*) occasionally cause appendicitis.[312]

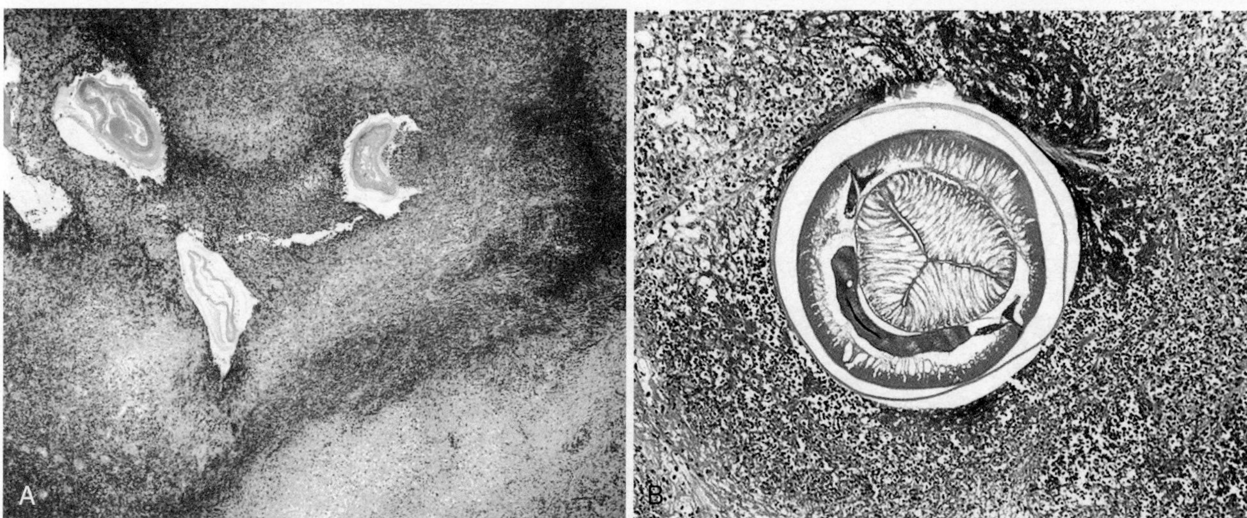

FIGURE 4.59 Gastric anisakiasis. **A**, Areas of geographic necrosis and an inflammatory infiltrate rich in eosinophils surrounds *Anisakis* larvae. **B**, Large Anisakis worm in the center of a submucosal eosinophilic and neutrophilic abscess. (**A** *courtesy of Dr. A. Morgan Wright and Dr. Melissa Upton, University of Washington;* **B** *courtesy of Dr. David Owen, University of Michigan.*)

Any level of the GI tract may be affected. Endoscopically, *Schistosoma* can cause inflammatory polyposis (particularly in the distal colon) with associated mucosal granularity, friability, punctate ulcers, and hemorrhages. Histologically, inflammatory polyps and mucosal ulcers with associated granulomatous inflammation and an eosinophilic infiltrate are typical.[310] Eggs may be detected in histological specimens and are sometimes calcified. As lesions progress, there is increased fibrosis and an increase in macrophages and multinucleated giant cells. Schistosome eggs are variably acid-fast; in H&E-stained sections the calcified eggs are typically dark blue or black and somewhat amorphous (Fig. 4.60). The worms themselves are slender and elongated, measuring approximately 0.5 to 2.5 cm in length, and are occasionally found within veins.

Fasciolopsis buski *and Related Species*

More than 50 species of intestinal flukes have been described in humans, but most clinically significant infections are caused by *Fasciolopsis buski*, *Echinostoma* spp., and *Heterophyes* spp. These flukes are most common in Asia. They are ingested with aquatic plants. After maturation, the adult worm attaches to the proximal small bowel mucosa. The majority of infections are asymptomatic. Symptoms, which usually occur as a result of heavy infection, include diarrhea, often alternating with constipation; abdominal pain; anorexia; nausea and vomiting; and malabsorption. Ileus, obstruction, and GI bleeding have been described.[313] The large worms (approximately 4 cm) may be seen endoscopically, and mucosal ulceration, inflammation, and abscess formation may occur at sites of tissue attachment.[314]

Cestodes

Taenia saginata (beef tapeworm), *Taenia solium* (pork tapeworm), and *Hymenolepis nana* (dwarf tapeworm) may occasionally cause GI disease. They can be several meters long (Fig. 4.61A). They attach to the small intestinal mucosa via a scolex (see Fig 4.61B) and the length of the worm coils within the lumen, causing symptoms of weight loss, nausea, vomiting, and diarrhea. *Diphyllobothrium latum* (fish tapeworm) is a rare cause of vitamin B_{12} deficiency.[315]

Other Helminthic Infections

The Central American nematode, *Angiostrongylus costaricensis*, may cause dramatic, even fatal, ileocecal infection characterized by the presence of large, obstructive inflammatory masses with perforation and mesenteric vessel thrombosis.[316] *Trichinella spiralis* is a rare cause of diarrhea.[317] Oesophagostomiasis, a parasitic disease usually seen in nonhuman primates, may form deep inflammatory masses, predominantly in the right colon and appendix.[318]

The differential diagnosis of helminthic infections usually involves differentiation among the various types of worms. However, other entities to be considered include causes of ulcerative inflammation, eosinophilic infiltration, and granulomatous inflammation, such as tuberculosis, amebiasis, allergic enteritis, and Crohn's disease.

The full reference list may be accessed online at Elsevier eBooks for Practicing Clinicians.

ACKNOWLEDGMENT

The author wishes to thank Dr. Laura W. Lamps for her work on prior editions of the chapter.

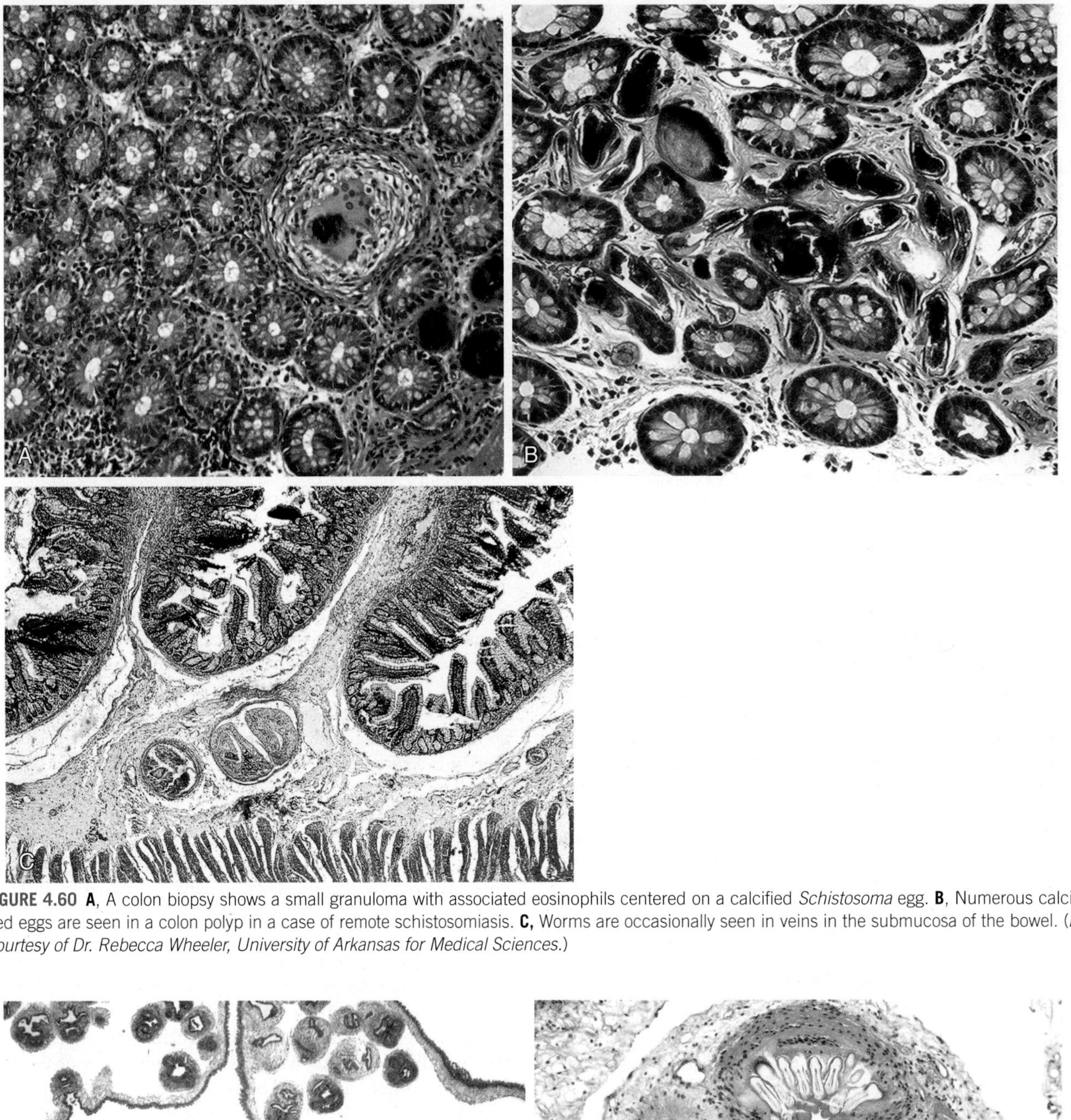

FIGURE 4.60 **A**, A colon biopsy shows a small granuloma with associated eosinophils centered on a calcified *Schistosoma* egg. **B**, Numerous calcified eggs are seen in a colon polyp in a case of remote schistosomiasis. **C,** Worms are occasionally seen in veins in the submucosa of the bowel. (**A** *courtesy of Dr. Rebecca Wheeler, University of Arkansas for Medical Sciences.*)

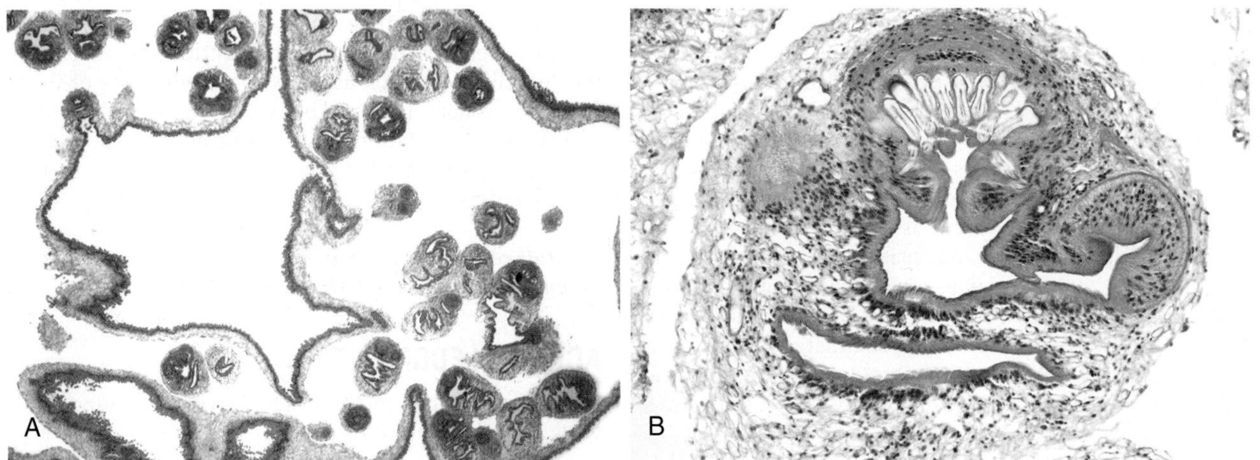

FIGURE 4.61 **A,** Adult *Taenia solium* are large worms with well-developed cardiovascular, gastrointestinal, and reproductive anatomy. **B,** The scolex contains a sucker and hooklets that attach the worm to the intestinal mucosa.

CHAPTER 5

Manifestations of Immunodeficiency in the Gastrointestinal Tract

Kay Washington, Chanjuan Shi

Chapter Outline

PRIMARY IMMUNODEFICIENCIES

Many of the primary immunodeficiencies (Table 5.1) are associated with gastrointestinal (GI) lesions. Manifestations of immune deficiency in the GI tract may be broadly divided into three categories[1]: increased susceptibility to infection,[2] idiopathic chronic inflammatory conditions, and[3] increased risk of neoplasia. Although many GI lesions are infectious (Table 5.2), chronic inflammatory conditions resembling celiac disease and inflammatory bowel disease (IBD) (Table 5.3) are seen in many patients with antibody deficiencies and diseases of immune dysregulation and are probably the result of the inability of dysfunctional mononuclear cells to suppress unwanted immune responses. All patients with primary immunodeficiencies are at increased risk of neoplasia[1] (Table 5.4), most commonly non-Hodgkin lymphoma (NHL), and the GI tract is often the primary site of involvement.[2] In addition to the risk of lymphoma, some of the primary immune deficiencies are associated with increased risk of gastric adenocarcinoma[3] and colorectal carcinoma.[4,5]

Predominantly Antibody Deficiencies

Selective Immunoglobulin A Deficiency

Defined as a serum immunoglobulin A (IgA) concentration of less than 50 μg/mL, selective IgA deficiency is the most common primary immunodeficiency[6]; it occurs in 1 of 600 people of Northern European ancestry.[7,8] The disorder is 20 times more common in white Americans than in African Americans. Defects in antibody production in patients with IgA deficiency represent a continuum with those seen in common variable immunodeficiency (CVID), and 20% to 30% of IgA-deficient patients also have deficits in IgG subclasses. Mutations in the *TNFRSF13B* gene have been identified and associated with IgA deficiency.[9-11] This gene encodes a member of the tumor necrosis factor-receptor (TNFR) superfamily, the transmembrane activator and calcium-modulator and cyclophilin-ligand interactor (TACI), which mediates isotype switching in B lymphocytes (see later discussion). Although the mutational defect remains unknown in many cases, some human leukocyte antigen (HLA) haplotypes have been associated with IgA deficiency. In addition, the pathogenesis of selective IgA deficiency is likely heterogeneous, involving several pathways controlling B-cell functions or regulatory regions of the *IGHA* (Ig heavy constant α) gene.[12]

Clinical manifestations of IgA deficiency range from no symptoms to recurrent infections (typically involving mucosal surfaces), autoimmune disorders, allergic diseases, and malignancy, but they are typically milder than those seen with CVID. Recurrent upper and lower respiratory tract infections are common in both disorders. Similarly, GI manifestations of IgA deficiency are the same as those associated with CVID. Infections are less common than might be expected, possibly because of compensation for lack of mucosal IgA by transport of IgM across the mucosa into the gut lumen, but include acute diarrheal illnesses caused by bacterial enterocolitis and chronic diarrhea caused by persistent *Giardia intestinalis (lamblia)* infection. Chronic strongyloidiasis has also been reported.[13]

Susceptibility to autoimmune disorders such as insulin-dependent diabetes mellitus and celiac disease may be inherited together with IgA deficiency; all three conditions are linked to particular major histocompatibility haplotypes and probably represent genetically linked susceptibilities in certain populations. The prevalence of celiac disease, the most common noninfectious GI complication of IgA deficiency, is 7.7% in children with IgA deficiency, compared with 1:500 in the general population.[14] Antigliadin IgA and endomysial IgA antibodies cannot be used as screening tools

TABLE 5.1 Molecular Basis of Primary Immunodeficiency Disorders

Disease	Proposed Cause
Predominantly Antibody Deficiencies	
Selective IgA deficiency	Impaired IgA synthesis; molecular defect unknown in most cases; mutation in *TNFRSF13B* in ~5%
Common variable immunodeficiency	Impaired B-cell maturation; molecular defect unknown in most cases; mutation in *TNFRSF13B* in ~10%-15%; others include *TNFRSF13C, CD19, CD81, CD21,* and *CD20*
X-linked agammaglobulinemia	Mutation in *BTK* results in absence of BTK in B cells
Hyper-IgM syndrome	Mutation in *CD40L,* leading to absence of CD40 ligand on T cells (CID generally less profound than SCID). Other affected genes reported include *AICDA, UNG, INO80,* and *MSH6*
Combined Immunodeficiencies (CIDs)	
Severe combined immunodeficiency (SCID)	Multiple defects, most commonly in the common γ chain; Others include adenosine deaminase deficiency, IL7Rα deficiency, JAK3 deficiency, and T-cell receptor deficiencies
Omenn's syndrome	Hypomorphic missense mutation in *RAG1* and *RAG2*
Inducible costimulator deficiency (ICOS)	Mutations in *ICOS*
CIDs with Syndromic Features	
Wiskott-Aldrich syndrome	Mutation in *WASP* gene involved in cell trafficking and motility
DiGeorge syndrome	Thymic hypoplasia; microdeletion in 22q11.2
Hyper-IgE syndrome	Mutation in *STAT3* (loss of function) in autosomal dominant form; mutation in *DOCK8* in autosomal recessive form (CID generally less profound than SCID)
Anhidrotic ectodermodysplasia with immunodeficiency	Mutations in *IKBKG* in X-linked dominant form (NEMO deficiency); Mutations in *IKBA* (gain of function) in autosomal dominant form
Disease of Immune Dysregulation	
X-linked inhibitor of apoptosis protein (XIAP) deficiency	Mutations in the *BRIC4* gene (encoding XIAP)
LPS-responsive beige-like anchor (LRBA) protein deficiency	Bi-allelic mutations in *LRBA*
Immune dysregulation, polyendocrinopathy, enteropathy, X-linked syndrome	Mutations in *FOXP3*
Cytotoxic T-lymphocyte antigen 4 (CTLA4) deficiency	Heterozygous mutations in *CTLA4*
Congenital Defects of Phagocytes	
Chronic granulomatous disease	Mutations in gene for component of NADPH oxidase; *CYBB* mutation in X-linked form; mutations in *CYBA, NCF1, NCF2,* or *NCF4* in autosomal recessive forms
Defects in Intrinsic and Innate Immunity	
Chronic mucocutaneous candidiasis	STAT1 gain-of-function mutation

Ig, Immunoglobulin; *NADPH,* reduced nicotinamide adenine dinucleotide phosphate.
From Bousfiha A, Jeddane L, Picard C, et al. The 2017 IUIS Phenotypic Classification for Primary Immunodeficiencies. J Clin Immunol. *2018;38(1):129–143.*

in the IgA-deficient population, but the morphology of celiac disease occurring in the setting of IgA deficiency is similar to that seen in immunocompetent patients. In addition, a spruelike illness characterized by chronic diarrhea with villous atrophy that does not respond to a gluten-free diet may be seen in IgA deficiency, as in CVID. Pernicious anemia complicating chronic atrophic autoimmune gastritis is seen more commonly in IgA deficiency than in CVID, and nodular lymphoid hyperplasia (NLH) in the small bowel is only rarely reported.[15] As with other B-cell disorders, the incidence of Crohn's disease and gastric adenocarcinoma appears to be increased in IgA deficiency.[16]

X-Linked Agammaglobulinemia

The typical patient with X-linked agammaglobulinemia (XLAG) is susceptible to bacterial infections because of the absence of all circulating immunoglobulin subtypes; mature circulating B cells are low to absent. This disorder is characterized by an inability to make antibodies to virtually all antigens. The molecular basis of most cases of XLAG was elucidated in 1993, when a defect in the *BTK* (Bruton tyrosine kinase) gene was found[17,18]; subsequent studies have identified numerous deleterious mutations.[19-21] The *BTK* gene encodes a nonreceptor tyrosine kinase expressed in B-cell and myelomonocytic cell lineages but not in T cells.

TABLE 5.2 Gastrointestinal Infections in Primary Immunodeficiency

Disease	Gastrointestinal Infections
Selective IgA deficiency	*Giardia intestinalis*; strongyloidiasis
Common variable immunodeficiency	*Giardia intestinalis*; *Cryptosporidium*; CMV; *Salmonella* species and *Campylobacter jejuni*
X-linked agammaglobulinemia	*Giardia intestinalis*; *Cryptosporidium* *Salmonella, Campylobacter, mycoplasma,* Rotavirus, coxsackievirus, poliovirus
Hyper-IgM syndrome	*Giardia intestinalis, Cryptosporidium, Entamoeba histolytica, Salmonella, Histoplasma capsulatum*
Severe combined immunodeficiency	*Candida*; *Salmonella* and other bacterial pathogens; CMV, rotavirus, Epstein-Barr virus
Inducible co-stimulator deficiency	*Campylobacter; Salmonella; Cryptosporidium;* CMV; HHV6; norovirus; adenovirus
DiGeorge syndrome	*Candida*
Hyper-IgE syndrome	Candidiasis; infections with *Cryptococcus*; histoplasmosis
Anhidrotic ectodermal dysplasia with immunodeficiency	*Mycobacterial* infection
Chronic mucocutaneous candidiasis	*Candida*; *Histoplasma capsulatum*

CMV, Cytomegalovirus; *Ig,* immunoglobulin.

TABLE 5.3 Inflammatory Gastrointestinal Lesions in Primary Immunodeficiency

Disease	Manifestation
IgA deficiency	Celiac disease Food allergies Crohn's disease–like lesion Nodular lymphoid hyperplasia
Common variable immunodeficiency	Multifocal atrophic gastritis ± intestinal metaplasia Villous atrophy Nodular lymphoid hyperplasia Crohn's disease–like lesion Granulomatous enteropathy Colitis (ulcerative colitis–like; lymphocytic colitis)
X-linked agammaglobulinemia	Crohn's disease–like lesion Perianal fistula and perianal abscess
Hyper-IgM syndrome	Nodular lymphoid hyperplasia Oral and perianal ulcers
Severe combined immunodeficiency	GVHD-like lesion, small bowel and colon Esophageal reflux
Omenn's syndrome	GVHD-like lesion, small bowel and colon
Inducible co-stimulator deficiency	IBD-like lesion
Wiskott-Aldrich syndrome	Crohn's disease–like lesion involving colon
Hyper IgE syndrome	Eosinophilic esophagitis; eosinophilic infiltration of other GI segments
Anhidrotic ectodermal dysplasia with immunodeficiency	Gastric ulcer/erosion; active colitis
X-linked inhibitor of apoptosis deficiency	Crohn's disease
LPS-responsive beige-like anchor protein deficiency	Atrophic gastritis; IBD-like disease; collagenous colitis
Cytotoxic T-lymphocyte antigen 4 insufficiency	Atrophic gastritis; celiac disease; Crohn's disease
Immune dysregulation, polyendocrinopathy, enteropathy, X-linked syndrome	GVHD-like changes; celiac disease; enteropathy with a complete depletion of goblet cells
Chronic granulomatous disease	Esophageal and gastric outlet obstruction; Crohn's disease–like lesion in small bowel; colitis (ulcerative colitis–like and Crohn's disease–like) Pigmented macrophages
Chronic mucocutaneous candidiasis	Atrophic gastritis

GVHD, Graft-versus-host disease; *Ig,* immunoglobulin; *LPS,* lipopolysaccharides; *IBD,* inflammatory bowel disease.

TABLE 5.4 Malignancies Involving the Gastrointestinal Tract in Primary Immunodeficiency

Disease	Gastrointestinal Malignancy
Immunoglobulin A deficiency	Lymphoma Gastric adenocarcinoma
Common variable immunodeficiency	Gastric adenocarcinoma B-cell lymphoma, involving small bowel Adenocarcinoma of the colon, ± neuroendocrine features
X-linked agammaglobulinemia	Non-Hodgkin lymphoma Gastric adenocarcinoma Colorectal adenocarcinoma
Hyperimmunoglobulin M syndrome	Plasma cell proliferation Colorectal carcinoma High-grade neuroendocrine carcinomas of the gastrointestinal tract and biliary tree
Wiskott-Aldrich syndrome	Gastrointestinal lymphoma
Hyper-IgE syndrome	Lymphoma
LPS-responsive beige-like anchor protein deficiency syndrome	Lymphoma; gastric adenocarcinoma
Cytotoxic T-lymphocyte antigen 4 deficiency	Gastric adenocarcinoma

BTK functions in intracellular signaling pathways essential for pre–B-cell maturation, but the exact mechanism by which the defects in *BTK* lead to B-cell maturation arrest remains unclear. XLAG may have more phenotypic diversity than has previously been recognized, because adults with mild or no clinical symptoms but with deficiencies in BTK have been described.[22-24] Age at onset, disease severity, and phenotype are roughly associated with mutation severity (as classified based on structural and functional consequences) in some but not all cohorts.[19,20]

IBD and Crohn's disease are less common in XLAG than in CVID, perhaps because of preserved T-cell function in XLAG,[25] although persistent or recurrent diarrhea is reported in up to 65% of patients.[19,26-28] Age at onset of GI symptoms is younger than in CVID patients, and autoimmune diseases are less common. Small-intestinal and colonic mucosal biopsies in the XLAG patient without GI symptoms are notable only for the lack of plasma cells in the lamina propria, giving the lamina propria an empty appearance. Mucosal architecture is unremarkable, and villous blunting is not seen. Approximately one-third of patients are seen initially with GI complaints, most commonly diarrhea or perirectal abscess, and 10% in one study had chronic GI symptoms, either from persistent infection with *G. intestinalis*, *Campylobacter jejuni*, *Salmonella*, mycoplasma, or enteropathic *Escherichia coli* or secondary to bacterial overgrowth. No cause for chronic diarrhea was found in half of these patients.[29] Chronic infection with rotavirus is also reported in this population.[30] Because biopsies are not routinely performed for this disorder, few descriptions of histopathological findings are available, but moderate blunting of duodenal villi with crypt hyperplasia and an increase in lamina propria inflammatory cells have been reported in acute infections.[31] Degenerative changes may be noted in epithelial cells on the surface of the villus with no increase in crypt apoptosis[32]; crypt cells are spared, and the crypt zone undergoes a compensatory hyperplasia. The histological changes of acute rotavirus infection are reported to resemble celiac disease but are patchier and quickly revert to normal with resolution of infection.[33]

In addition to GI infections, a chronic ulcerating inflammatory condition, clinically similar to Crohn's disease, has been reported that is manifested by recurrent diarrhea, malabsorption, ulcers, and small bowel strictures (Fig. 5.1). IBD and enteritis are relatively more common in XLA patients carrying missense mutations with only partial loss of gene function.[26] A prominent lymphocytic inflammatory infiltrate without plasma cells or granulomas is seen in the affected areas.[34,35] In one case, enterovirus was found by polymerase chain reaction in inflamed ileum and adjacent mesenteric lymph nodes, suggesting that infection may be responsible for these lesions in some XLAG patients.[36]

Patients with XLAG are at increased risk for malignancy, even in childhood. The most common malignancy in this group is NHL, which often involves the GI tract, and many of these cases occur in children younger than 10 years of age.[37] There are rare reported cases of gastric adenocarcinoma[37] and colorectal adenocarcinoma.[5] The increased incidence of colorectal carcinoma for patients with XLAG was calculated as 30-fold in one study,[5] although other registry studies have reported few or no colorectal cancers in their patients with XLAG.[28,38] In most of the reported cases, XLAG patients with colorectal carcinoma are young adults in their twenties who are seen with advanced-stage tumors. In one reported case, multiple colorectal adenomas in addition to carcinoma were found.[5]

Hyperimmunoglobulin M Syndrome

X-linked hyperimmunoglobulin M syndrome (HIMG), the most common form, results from a mutation in the gene for CD40 ligand, which leads to loss of isotype switching. T cells from patients with this disorder lack the CD40 ligand and therefore do not interact with CD40 on the B-cell surface, an event necessary for immunoglobulin class switching. Recessive mutations in CD40 are seen in rare patients with HIMG. X-linked HIMG and HIMG caused by defects in CD40 are generally thought to be a primary B-cell deficiency, but in the 2017 International Union of Immunological Societies (IUIS) Classification, they have been assigned to the category of "combined immunodeficiencies generally less profound than severe combined immunodeficiency."[39] Rare cases of recessive autosomal HIMG have been reported and are ascribed to mutations in other genes, such as *AIDCDA*, *CD40*, *UNG*, and *MSH6*, leading to defects in immunoglobulin class-switch recombination and/or somatic hypermutation.[40,41] Patients with HIMG have very low levels of IgG and IgA and normal or elevated levels of IgM.[42] They are susceptible to pyogenic infections similar to those encountered in XLAG, and in addition are susceptible to *Pneumocystis carinii* pneumonia. A variety of intracellular pathogens such as mycobacterial species, fungi, and viruses (e.g., cytomegalovirus [CMV], adenovirus) are implicated in causing disease in these patients. The most common site of infection is the upper or lower respiratory tract

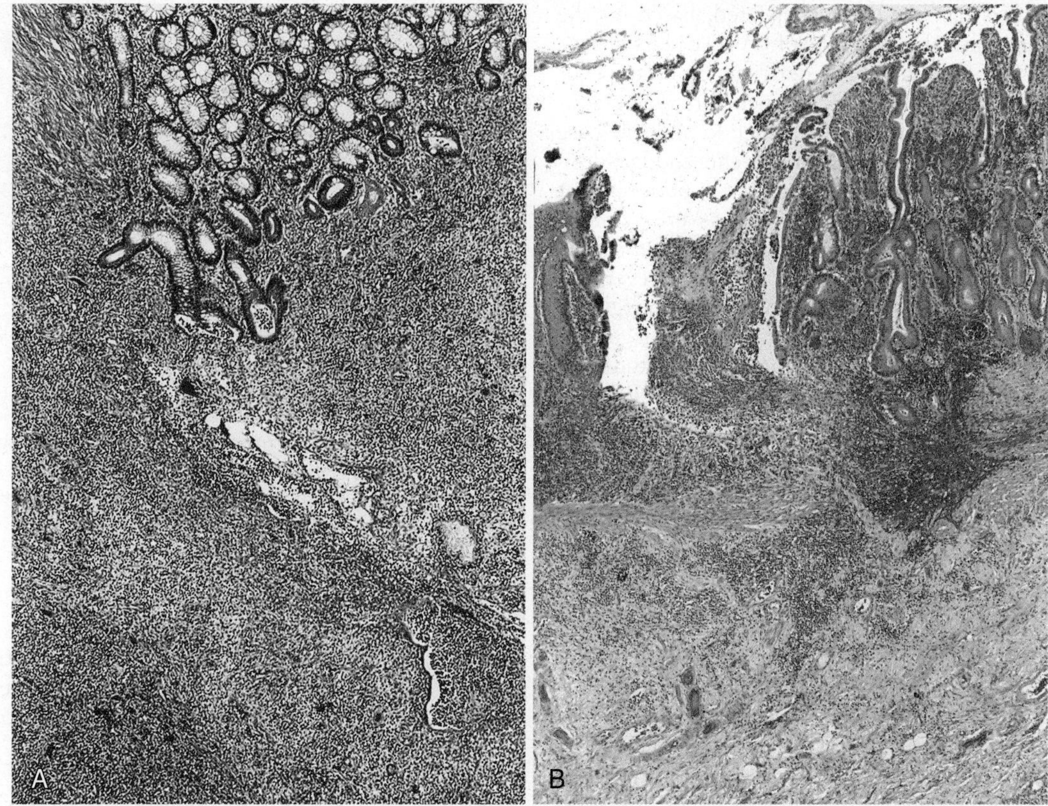

FIGURE 5.1 A–B, A chronic inflammatory disorder with fissuring necrosis and small-intestinal ulcers resembling Crohn's disease occurs in some patients with X-linked agammaglobulinemia. Granulomas are typically absent (H&E stain).

(approximately 50% and 80% of cases, respectively).[42] Disseminated infection[43,44] and esophageal infection with *Histoplasma capsulatum* are also reported in X-linked HIMG.

Diarrhea occurs in one-third to one-half of patients[42,45] and follows a chronic course in most. Chronic watery diarrhea may be caused by *Cryptosporidium* infection; *G. intestinalis*, *Salmonella*, and *Entamoeba histolytica* have also been implicated, although in most patients no pathogen is identified.[42] NLH involving the GI tract is reported in approximately 5% of patients.[45] Lymphoid hyperplasia may also result in hepatosplenomegaly, lymphadenopathy, and enlargement of the tonsils.[46] IBD was reported in a few patients with X-linked HIMG and chronic diarrhea.[45] A phenotype of Crohn's disease and hemophagocytic lymphohistiocytosis was described in a 5-year-old boy with X-linked HIMG.[47] Sclerosing cholangitis is a common and serious complication (affecting about 20% of European patients) and is often related to chronic infection with *Cryptosporidium;* liver transplantation may be necessary.[45] In one European series, three of five patients infected with hepatitis B developed hepatocellular carcinoma.[45]

Patients with XHIM are prone to autoimmune hematological diseases, including cyclic or chronic neutropenia, and oral and perianal ulcers are common during neutropenic episodes.[45] Massive proliferation of IgM-producing plasma cells may involve the GI tract, liver, and gallbladder, usually in the second decade of life, and may prove fatal.[48] High-grade neuroendocrine carcinoma of the small intestine, colon, and pancreas has been reported in this disorder,[49-51] and there is an increased incidence of liver and biliary tract tumors.[50]

Common Variable Immunodeficiency

Although CVID is not a common disorder, it is probably the most common symptomatic primary immunodeficiency, accounting for 12% to 36% of all primary immunodeficiency. Clinical and immunological features are heterogeneous, but most patients are seen with recurrent bacterial infections, usually involving the upper and lower respiratory tracts and leading to chronic lung disease and bronchiectasis. Patients may be seen with CVID at any age from infancy to late adult life with a mean age at diagnosis being around 30 years, and males and females are equally affected. Autoimmune manifestations such as thyroid dysfunction, pernicious anemia, autoimmune hemolytic anemia, autoimmune thrombocytopenia, and rheumatoid arthritis are common, and granulomatous involvement of skin and visceral organs mimicking sarcoidosis may be seen in CVID.[52-54] Chronic GI disorders resulting in malabsorption and weight loss occur in approximately 20% of patients with CVID.

CVID is characterized immunologically by hypogammaglobulinemia involving multiple antibody classes. T-cell abnormalities are common; below-normal proliferative responses to mitogens are found in 40% of patients, and 20% have a relative lack of CD4+ T cells.[55] The common abnormality shared by IgA deficiency and CVID is failure of terminal maturation of B lymphocytes into plasma cells producing various Ig subtypes. A primary B-cell defect is favored in many patients, but in others defective antigen responsiveness in helper T cells may be the underlying basis for the disorder.

A genetic basis has long been suspected, based on the observation that familial inheritance of CVID occurs in 20% of cases[55] and that CVID and IgA deficiency tend to occur in the same family; individual family members may gradually convert from one disorder to the other. In multiple-case families, CVID is often present in the parents and IgA deficiency in the offspring, consistent with the hypothesis that CVID may develop later in life as a more severe manifestation of a common defect involving immunoglobulin class switching. In the majority of CVID patients, however, the underlying genetic basis is unknown. CVID is thought to be a polygenic disease for most patients, with monogenetic defects only identified in a small portion of cases. Studies of isotype switching led to the discovery that the *TNFRSF13B* gene, which encodes the member of the TNFR family, TACI, is mutated in approximately 10% to 15% of patients with CVID and 5% of patients with IgA deficiency.[56] TACI mediates isotype switching in B cells and survival of plasma cells. TACI is also involved in central B-cell tolerance and inhibiting peripheral B-cell expansion,[57] and this may be the basis for the susceptibility of patients with TACI mutations to autoimmune and lymphoproliferative disorders.[56] New gene defects in *BAFFR (TNFRSF13C)*, *CD19*, *CD81*, *CD21*, and *CD20* (now called *MS4A1*) resulting in a CVID phenotype have been described in a small number of patients,[57,58] underscoring the genetic heterogeneity of this disorder, and next-generation sequencing studies have identified numerous candidate causative genes. In addition, genome-wide association studies have demonstrated a strong association of CVID with the major histocompatibility region.[59]

Patients with CVID are at particular risk for chronic inflammatory disorders and malignancies affecting the GI tract. The inflammatory disorders may represent a response to acute or chronic infection, but in some patients the GI lesions are probably a manifestation of autoimmunity and are associated with other disorders of autoimmunity.[35] In one large clinical study of patients with CVID, 22% had one or more autoimmune diseases, most commonly idiopathic thrombocytopenia purpura (6%) and autoimmune hemolytic anemia (5%).[54]

Infections in CVID

Chronic infection with *G. intestinalis (lamblia)* is a common problem in patients with CVID and may or may not cause clinical symptoms. In some cases, malabsorption, steatorrhea, and villous abnormalities can be reversed if *Giardia* is eradicated. Small bowel mucosal abnormalities in giardiasis include villous blunting, increased intraepithelial lymphocytes, and NLH. The trophozoite form of the organism can be identified on small bowel biopsy (Fig. 5.2). The prevalence of *Giardia* infection in this population appears to be decreasing, but giardiasis remains a significant cause of chronic diarrhea in CVID.[16]

Other GI infections are less common in CVID. Cryptosporidiosis is occasionally found. The prevalence of common bacterial intestinal infections (e.g., *Salmonella*, *Campylobacter*) does not appear to be increased. Although prolonged antibiotic use is common in these patients, an increase in pseudomembranous colitis has not been reported.[16] On occasion, viral and fungal organisms infect the GI tract in CVID patients, but such infections are less common in CVID than in acquired immunodeficiency syndrome (AIDS). CMV infection involving the esophagus, stomach, jejunum, and ileocecal area and resulting in multiple ulcers and obstructing strictures has been reported in a patient with CVID.[16]

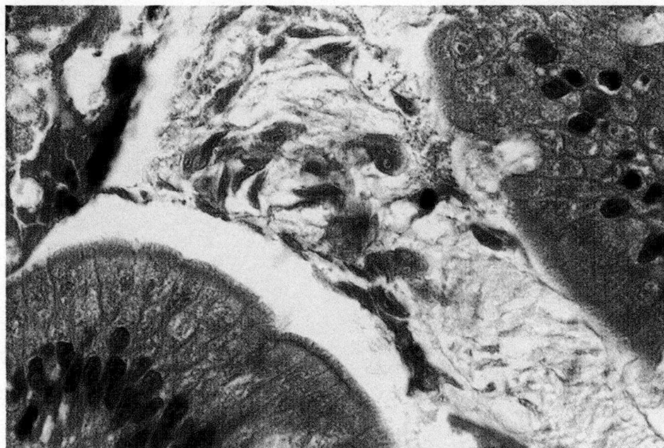

FIGURE 5.2 Giardiasis. Numerous trophozoites in varying orientations are closely associated with the surface of this small bowel biopsy specimen from a patient with common variable immunodeficiency. The underlying epithelium is normal (H&E stain).

Inflammatory Disorders and Malignancy in CVID

Stomach. In the stomach, a nonspecific increase in lamina propria lymphocytes is seen in some patients with CVID (Fig. 5.3A); increased apoptosis of gastric epithelial cells is present in some cases[35,60] (see Fig. 5.3B). In a study of gastric biopsies from 34 patients with CVID and dyspepsia, 41% of patients were infected with *Helicobacter pylori*. All *H. pylori*–positive patients and 20% of *H. pylori*–negative patients had chronic gastritis, and 50% of those infected with *H. pylori* had multifocal atrophic gastritis. In this study, 10% of *H. pylori*–negative patients had multifocal atrophic gastritis.[61] Atrophic gastritis resembling autoimmune atrophic gastritis on clinical and morphological grounds (see Fig. 5.3C) and resulting in pernicious anemia may occur in the absence of demonstrable anti–parietal cell antibodies in these patents. Atrophic gastritis may develop at a very young age in patients with CVID, and it has been reported in a 6-year-old patient who developed multifocal gastric adenocarcinoma at 11 years of age.[62]

Adults with CVID are also at increased risk for gastric adenocarcinoma. It has been estimated that patients with CVID have a 47-fold increase in gastric carcinoma compared with the general population of Great Britain,[63] and gastric carcinoma ultimately develops in 5% to 10% of CVID patients, usually many years after the onset of hypogammaglobulinemia. However, recent data demonstrate a significantly reduced risk of gastric cancer in these patients, likely resulting from the eradication of *H. pylori* infection by antibiotics.[64] Atrophic gastritis and intestinal metaplasia in the gastric body are thought to be the main risk factors for gastric cancer in CVID patients. CVID-associated gastric cancers are usually moderately to poorly differentiated intestinal-type adenocarcinomas with prominent intratumoral lymphocytes.[65]

Small Bowel. In the small bowel, a spruelike lesion with villous blunting occurs in some patients with CVID and is

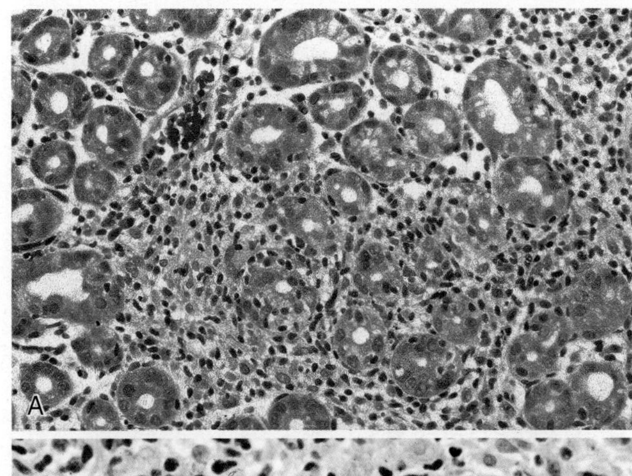

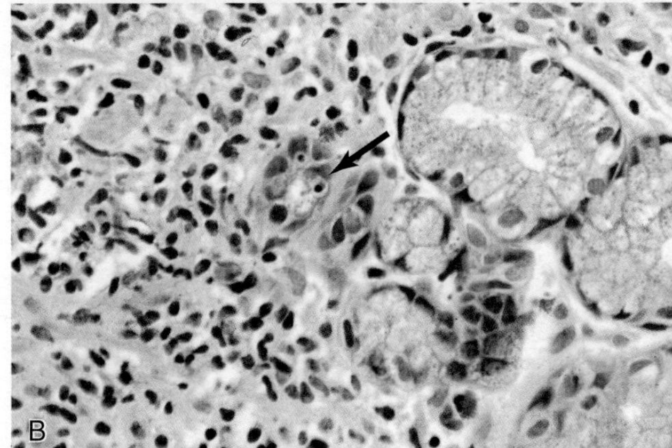

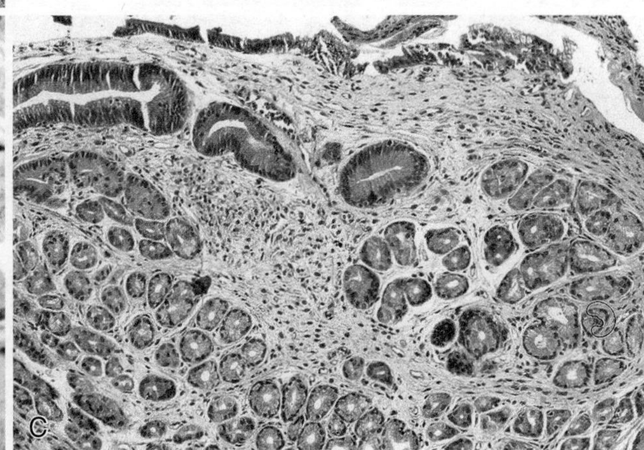

FIGURE 5.3 A, In common variable immunodeficiency (CVID), the gastric mucosa often contains a nonspecific mononuclear cell infiltrate. **B,** Notice the apoptotic body *(arrow)* and the absence of plasma cells. **C,** Loss of gastric glands leads to atrophic gastritis at a young age in patients with CVID. Loss of parietal cells results in pernicious anemia and may occur in the absence of antiparietal cell antibodies (H&E stain).

associated with severe malabsorption, often requiring parenteral nutrition. Villous atrophy associated with CVID generally lacks the degree of crypt hyperplasia seen in celiac disease (Fig. 5.4A), but may be indistinguishable on biopsy. In general, the lamina propria inflammatory infiltrate is not as prominent as in celiac disease, and enterocyte maturation is normal, with preservation of the brush border.[35] Most CVID patients with this small bowel lesion do not respond to a gluten-free diet, although an elemental diet may be beneficial, and most respond to corticosteroids, at least initially.[66] Plasma cells are absent or are found only in very small numbers in the lamina propria. Surface intraepithelial lymphocytes are often markedly increased (see Fig. 5.4B), even in the absence of villous atrophy. In some cases, an increase in apoptotic bodies is found in crypt epithelial cells (see Fig. 5.4C). Clinical autoimmune enteritis with loss of goblet cells has also been reported.[60]

Granulomatous enteropathy has also been reported in patients with CVID and may be associated with protracted diarrhea unresponsive to antibiotic therapy. Poorly formed nonnecrotizing granulomas are found in the lamina propria in multiple sites in the GI tract, including the stomach, small intestine, and colon[60,67]; the diarrhea usually resolves with intravenous immunoglobulin therapy.

NLH in the GI tract is characterized by multiple discrete hyperplastic lymphoid nodules in the lamina propria and submucosa of the small intestine (Fig. 5.5), large intestine, or both, and is probably a result of chronic antigenic stimulation. The germinal centers of the follicles are composed of proliferating B cells with scattered tingible body macrophages; the mantle zones contain mature and immature B cells, and the extramantle zones contain a mixture of cell types including B cells, T cells, and macrophages. NLH is found in as many as 60% of patients with CVID but may be seen in the setting of giardiasis without antibody deficiency. In contrast with NLH in CVID patients, plasma cells are present in the extramantle zones in nonimmunodeficient patients. NLH is not considered a malignant disorder. However, malignant lymphomas of the GI tract in patients with immunodeficiencies often arise in a background of NLH, and clonal immunoglobulin gene rearrangement has been demonstrated in NLH in the GI tract of a child with CVID.[68] Consistent with these observations, the most common malignancy in CVID is NHL, which affects approximately 8% of patients[54]; these lymphomas often originate in extranodal sites, with small bowel the most common GI site. Most of these lymphomas are of B-cell origin; they include diffuse large B-cell lymphoma (DLBCL) and follicular lymphoma.[54]

Chronic inflammatory processes involving small or large bowel that are clinically similar to IBD develop in some patients with CVID. In some patients, the small bowel is the primary site of involvement and the lesions resemble Crohn's disease, with transmural inflammation and small bowel obstruction. Granulomas usually are not present in these Crohn's disease–like disorders.[69]

Large Bowel. The colitis occurring in CVID is variable in morphology. In some patients, the inflammatory process is limited to the colon and clinically mimics ulcerative colitis. Mucosal architectural distortion with crypt destruction is

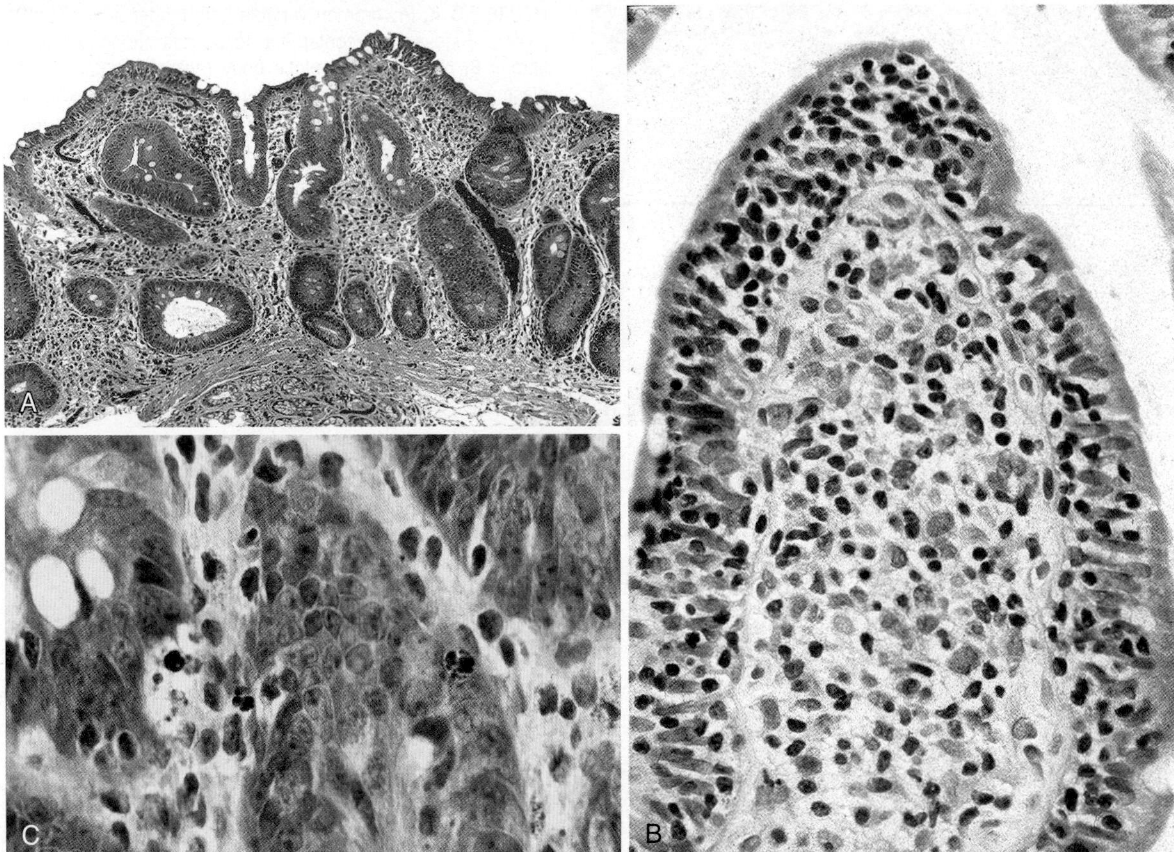

FIGURE 5.4 **A,** Villous atrophy associated with common variable immunodeficiency (CVID) may be severe and may lead to profound malabsorption. Notice the relatively sparse inflammatory infiltrate. **B,** The surface epithelium of the small intestine often contains a marked increase in the number of intraepithelial lymphocytes in CVID. **C,** An increase in crypt cell apoptosis is often found in small bowel biopsies with villous atrophy in CVID (H&E stain).

present, although crypt distortion is less pronounced than in most cases of ulcerative colitis, with less crypt branching (Fig. 5.6A). Neutrophils are present in the lamina propria and crypt epithelium (see Fig. 5.6B). In contrast with ulcerative colitis, plasma cells are not present in the lamina propria in CVID-associated colitis, and an increase in CD8+ T cells (compared with normal controls and those with IBD) has been reported in the colons of CVID patients.[70] In some cases, the crypt destruction and mucosal distortion is accompanied by increased apoptosis, and the histology is similar to that of colonic graft-versus-host disease (GVHD).[35,60] Milder cases of colitis in CVID may resemble lymphocytic colitis, characterized by increased intraepithelial lymphocytes and minimal mucosal distortion,[71] and an atypical form of collagenous colitis with pseudomembranes has been reported in one patient.[72] The etiology and pathogenesis of colitis in these patients remain largely unknown. The association of chronic GI inflammatory disorders and autoimmune disorders in these patients and the resemblance of the lesions to other disorders of immune dysregulation imply that the colitis of CVID may be autoimmune in origin.

Adenocarcinoma of the colon is reported in young patients with CVID. Small cell neuroendocrine carcinoma of the cecum was reported in a 16-year-old boy, who died of liver metastases 5 months after diagnosis.[73] In another case, 9 adenocarcinomas and 20 adenomas were present synchronously in the colon of a 22-year-old man with CVID.[74]

Combined Cellular/Humoral Immunodeficiencies

Severe Combined Immunodeficiency

Severe combined immunodeficiency (SCID) is a heterogeneous group of congenital disorders characterized by defects in both B-cell and T-cell function. Children with SCID typically are seen in the first year of life with severe recurrent bacterial or viral infections. A number of molecular defects may result in SCID. Most are autosomal recessive, including adenosine deaminase deficiency, which accounts for 50% of autosomal recessive SCID; T-cell receptor deficiencies; JAK3 deficiency; and IL-7 receptor deficiency.[75] However, X-linked SCID, resulting from a defect in the common γ chain, is the single most common type of SCID in the United States.[76] It has a characteristic phenotype of absence of T cells and natural killer (NK) cells but normal B-cell numbers, although the B cells are dysfunctional.

GI disorders in SCID are caused by a variety of infectious pathogens. Oral, esophageal, and perianal candidiasis is common, and profound diarrhea may develop in children with SCID early in life. In general, GI biopsy specimens from these patients show a hypocellular lamina propria without plasma cells or lymphocytes. Because these patients are susceptible to viral infections, examination of stool for viral particles may be indicated. In particular, rotavirus, normally a self-limited infection, may cause chronic diarrhea in these children. Although villous blunting has been described

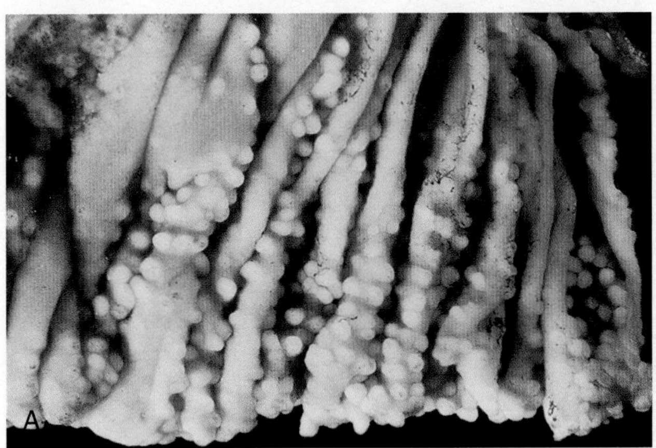

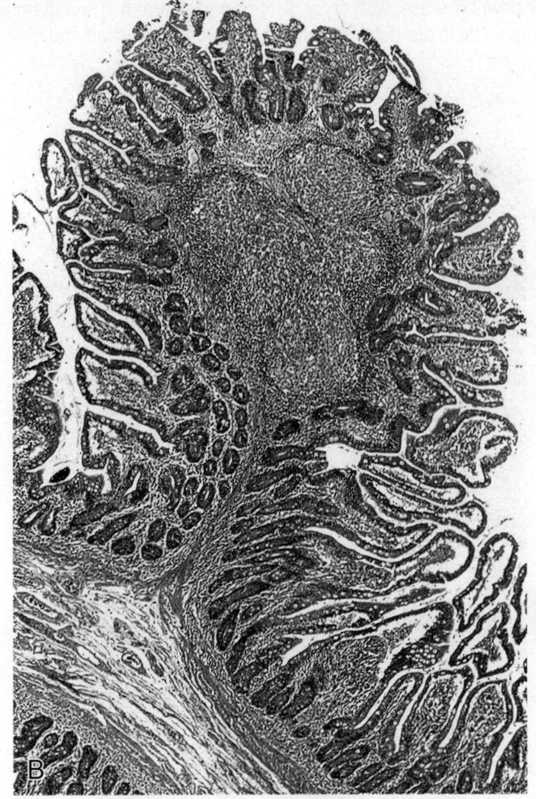

FIGURE 5.5 A, Nodular lymphoid hyperplasia in common variable immunodeficiency. Numerous small mucosal and submucosal nodules are present. **B,** Most of the lymphoid nodules contain enlarged germinal centers. Overlying villi are slightly distorted (H&E stain).

in acute rotavirus infection in normal children[33] and in animal models,[77] the intestinal pathology of chronic rotavirus infection has not been described in SCID patients. Cytopathic viral infections that may be identified on GI biopsy include CMV and adenovirus (Fig. 5.7). *Salmonella* may also cause chronic GI infection in SCID patients. Patients receiving nonirradiated blood products or allogeneic bone marrow transplants are susceptible to GVHD. Furthermore, a GVHD-like process affecting the colon and small intestine has been described in patients with SCID who had not undergone bone marrow transplantation.[78,79] Children with SCID may be a greater risk for reflux esophagitis than the normal population.[80]

Omenn's Syndrome

Omenn's syndrome is an autosomal recessive type of SCID with clinical and pathological features of GVHD. The immunological hallmark of the disease is expansion of an oligoclonal population of T cells and a near absence of B cells.[76] Infants with Omenn's syndrome are seen with diffuse erythroderma, hepatosplenomegaly, lymphadenopathy, and failure to thrive[81]; chronic diarrhea and alopecia are common. Hypereosinophilia and hypogammaglobulinemia are characteristic. Paradoxically, serum IgE levels are increased, although B lymphocytes are not detectable in the circulation, lymph nodes, or skin. Activated circulating T cells are normal to increased in number but constitute an oligoclonal population. The underlying basis for these findings in Omenn's syndrome is impairment but not complete loss of the V(D)J recombination process as a result of mutations in *RAG1* or *RAG2*, the recombination activating genes.[76] Mutations in these genes were first identified in a subset of SCID patients with T^- B^- SCID. The occurrence of this type of SCID and Omenn's syndrome in the same kindred furnished the clue that Omenn's syndrome was caused by mutations in the same genes. Differences between T^- B^- SCID and Omenn's syndrome can be explained by the presence of two entirely defective alleles in SCID and the presence of one marginally functional allele that is capable of establishing the oligoclonal T-cell population in patients with Omenn's syndrome. Infants with SCID with maternal T-cell engraftment may exhibit GVHD symptoms indistinguishable on clinical grounds from Omenn's syndrome,[82] and a diagnosis of Omenn's syndrome depends on excluding this possibility by appropriate human leukocyte antigen typing or molecular analysis. Published accounts of the histopathological changes in Omenn's syndrome are scant, but skin changes resemble those of GVHD,[83,84] and numerous apoptotic crypt cells are found in colonic biopsies in a pattern similar to that of GVHD (unpublished observations). Crypt injury and an increase in lamina propria eosinophils may also be seen (Fig. 5.8).

Inducible Co-stimulator Deficiency

Inducible co-stimulator *(ICOS)* was originally thought to be one of monogenes responsible for CVID. Recent studies, however, demonstrated pronounced T-cell defects in ICOS deficiency (see review by Bogaert and colleagues).[57] Thus ICOS deficiency is classified by the 2017 IUSI classification as combined immunodeficiency generally less profound than SCID.[85] ICOS is involved in germinal center formation, terminal B-cell differentiation, effector T-cell responses, and immune tolerance. ICOS deficiency leads to complete lack of class-switched memory B cells and defective T-cell activation. ICOS deficiency is characterized by a CVID-like clinical presentation, including refractory diarrhea, recurrent sinopulmonary and GI infections, autoimmunity, and neoplasia. In addition, T-cell defects with viral and opportunistic infection are frequently observed.

Patients with ICOS deficiency frequently present with inflammatory bowel disease–like symptoms; although virus is likely the causative agent in most patients, no virus is detected in some patients.[86] Pathologically it has been described as chronic active colitis in some cases. Viral pathogens identified in patients with colitis include CMV and HHV6. Other intestinal infectious agents include

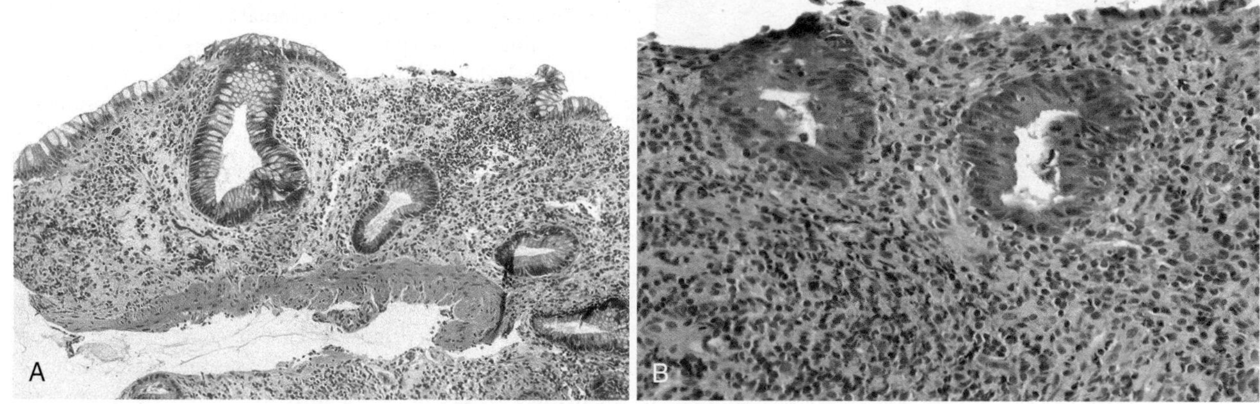

FIGURE 5.6 Colitis in common variable immunodeficiency may mimic inflammatory bowel disease, with crypt distortion and loss. **A,** The inflammatory infiltrate is relatively sparse in some cases, compared with ulcerative colitis, and plasma cells are not present. **B,** Notice crypt shortfall and infiltration of crypts by acute inflammatory cells (acute cryptitis).

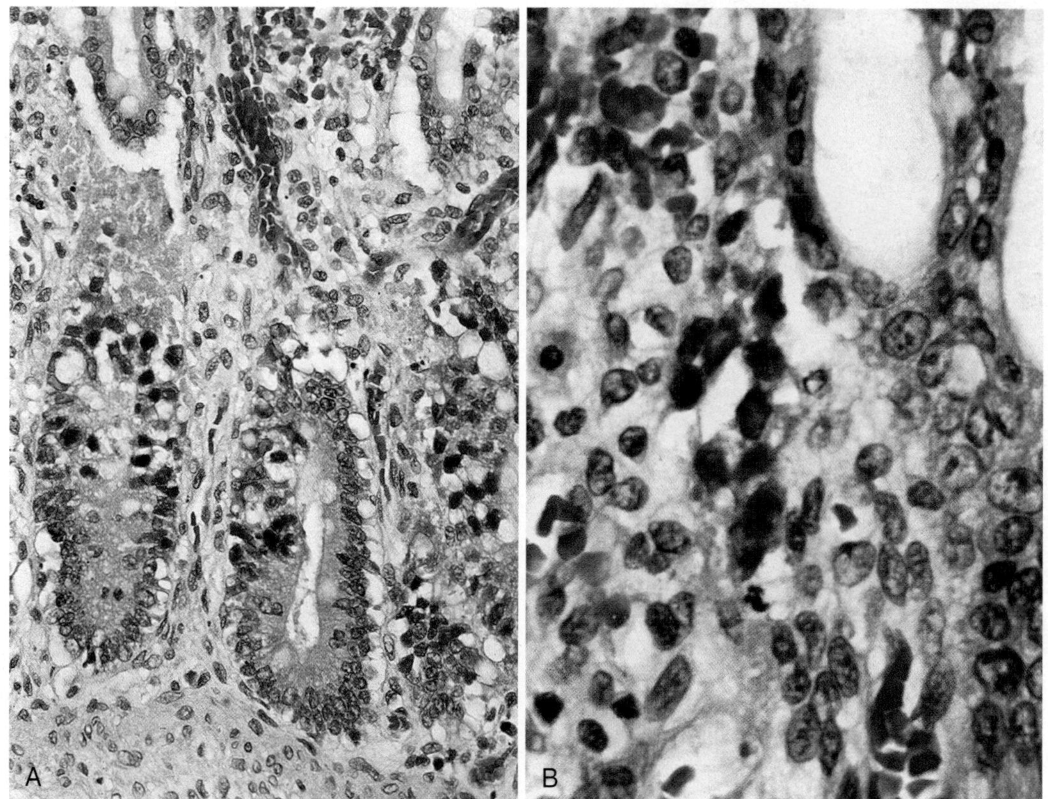

FIGURE 5.7 **A,** Disseminated adenovirus may involve the gastrointestinal tract in patients with severe combined immunodeficiency. Here, the small bowel crypts are involved; in less severe cases, inclusions may be identified only in surface mucosa. **B,** With adenovirus, infected cells are typically not enlarged. Classic "smudge cells" with homogeneous nuclear staining are shown (H&E stain).

Campylobacter, Salmonella, norovirus, adenovirus, and *Cryptosporidium.*[86,87] Squamous cell carcinoma and large granular lymphocyte T cells with clonal expansion have been reported in two patients.

DiGeorge Syndrome

DiGeorge syndrome is caused by a microdeletion in chromosome 22q11.2, which leads to a congenital malformation of the third and fourth pharyngeal pouch, resulting in thymic and parathyroid hypoplasia. This disease is the most common microdeletion syndrome in humans[88] and is estimated to affect 1 of 4000 live births.[89] T cells are markedly reduced in number, but B cells are normal in number and functionality. Midline anomalies affecting the GI tract (e.g., esophageal atresia, imperforate anus) are seen in some cases in association with DiGeorge syndrome, and watery diarrhea and malabsorption have been described but not well characterized.[90] Oral candidiasis is common. Dysphagia and feeding difficulties have been reported in infants with 22q11.2 deletion.[91]

Wiskott-Aldrich Syndrome

Wiskott-Aldrich syndrome, characterized by early onset of profound thrombocytopenia with small platelets, eczema, and recurrent infections, is inherited as an X-linked recessive

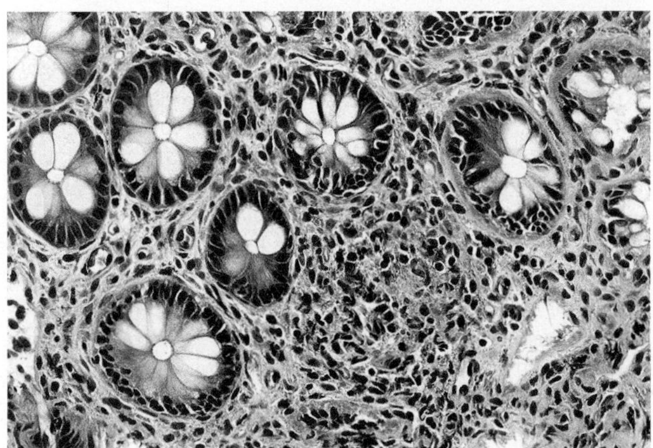

FIGURE 5.8 Omenn's syndrome. Focal crypt destruction with a localized increase in lamina propria eosinophils is seen (H&E stain).

disease. Platelets and T cells are most severely affected. The genetic basis of Wiskott-Aldrich syndrome, described in 1994, is a mutation of the *WASP* gene, which encodes an intracellular protein expressed exclusively in hematopoietic cells.[92] This protein is involved in transduction of signals from cell surface receptors to the actin cytoskeleton and is important in cytoskeletal architecture and cell trafficking and motility. Diarrhea is reported in patients with this disorder but has been poorly characterized.[90] Bloody diarrhea in these patients is often attributed to thrombocytopenia, and biopsies may not be performed because of the risk of hemorrhage. A Crohn's disease–like inflammatory process with cobblestone appearance and inflammatory pseudopolyps involving the descending and transverse colon has been reported in Wiskott-Aldrich syndrome.[93] Massive hemorrhage from aneurysms involving the liver, small bowel mesentery, and kidney has been reported.[94]

Hyperimmunoglobulin E Syndrome

Also known as *Job syndrome*, hyperimmunoglobulin E (hyper-IgE) syndrome is a rare, multisystem disorder characterized by recurrent elevated serum IgE, eczema, and recurrent skin and sinopulmonary infections.[95] Two genetic etiologies have been identified: loss of function of *DOCK8* in the autosomal recessive form of the disorder,[96] and mutations in *STAT3* (loss of function) in the more common autosomal dominant form.[97] Recently mutations in phosphoglucomutase-3 *(PGM3)*, caspase recruiting domain family member 11 *(CARD11)*, and *ZNF431* have been reported in patients with hyper-IgE syndrome. Homozygous truncating mutations in *ZNF431* cause low constitutive levels of STAT3 mRNA. Deficiencies in *STAT3*, *ZNF431*, and *DOCK8* lead to impaired Th17 development/differentiation, antibody deficiency, excessive IgE production, and eczema.[98]

In addition to findings related to the immune system, characteristic facial features and dental and skeletal abnormalities occur in the autosomal dominant form, and severe viral cutaneous infections are seen in the autosomal recessive form.[95] Chronic diarrhea and disorders resembling IBD are not reported in hyper-IgE syndrome. Mucocutaneous candidiasis, tissue-invasive fungal infections with *Cryptococcus* (reported in the esophagus[99] and colon[100]), and ileocecal histoplasmosis mimicking Crohn's disease have been reported in these patients.[101,102] Perforation of the colon, probably related to infection with staphylococcal species, has also been reported,[103] as well as diverticulitis in a young patient.[104] The principal GI manifestations in patients with STAT3-deficient hyper-IgE syndrome are GI dysmotility and significant eosinophilic infiltration throughout the GI tract.[105] The histology in the esophagus is consistent with eosinophilic esophagitis, which is the likely cause of esophageal rings, linear furrows, diverticula, and upper esophageal strictures seen in these patients. Patients with hyper-IgE syndrome do not appear to be at increased risk for primary GI malignancy.

Anhidrotic Ectodermodysplasia with Immunodeficiency

Anhidrotic ectodermodysplasia with immunodeficiency (EDA-ID) or NEMO syndrome results from mutations in two genes: nuclear factor-κN (NF-κB) essential modulator *(NEMO)* for X-linked EDA-ID and *IκBα* for autosomal-dominant EDA-ID. Mutations in these genes cause impaired NF-κB signaling pathway.[106] NF-κB is critical for many signaling pathways, involving the development of cell types and tissues of ectodermal origin, osteoclastogenesis, vascular lymphatic formation, and proinflammatory cytokine production. Clinical manifestations include ectodermal dysplasia, vascular anomalies, and osteopetrosis in addition to combined immunodeficiency with defects in humoral, innate, and cell-mediated immunity, characterized by hypogammaglobulinemia, variable specific antibody function, and variable T-cell counts and functions.[107]

Patients with EDA-ID are susceptible to encapsulated bacterial (e.g., *Streptococcus pneumoniae*, *Haemophilus influenza*, and *Staphylococcus aureus*), mycobacterial, and viral infections, whereas fungal infections are rare.[106,107] Inflammatory and autoimmune diseases are common in these patients.[107] Colitis, panniculitis, retinitis, and arthritis have been reported. Some cases present with autoimmune hemolytic anemia. Liver pathology can show macrophages and/or granulomata, predominantly in the portal tract, with positive acid-fast bacillus (AFB) staining.[107] The most common finding in the GI tract is AFB-positive macrophages in the mucosa in a background of otherwise normal mucosa, within granulomas, or active inflammation. Active colitis with no chronicity but variably prominent intraepithelial and lamina propria eosinophils is seen in some patients. Mycobacterial species (mainly *Mycobacterium avium intracellulare*) were isolated in these lesions.[107] Gastric ulceration, erosive gastritis or chronic gastritis can be present in gastric biopsy, but with no evidence of *H. pylori* organisms. Enterocolitis with possible autoimmune or autoinflammatory etiology (NEMO colitis) has been reported in approximately 25% of cases. It occurs early in childhood, presenting with intractable diarrhea and usually responding to steroid treatments. Microscopically it is characterized by an active colitis with an abundance of neutrophils in the superficial mucosa with no crypt distortion or granulomas.[106]

Diseases of Immune Dysregulation

X-Linked Inhibitor of Apoptosis Protein Deficiency

X-linked inhibitor of apoptosis protein (XIAP) deficiency results from defects in the *BRIC4* gene, which encodes XIAP. XIAP is an anti-apoptotic molecule, but it is also involved in innate immunity and in the negative regulation of inflammation.[108] Clinical features associated with XIAP deficiency include hemophagocytic lymphohistiocytosis usually triggered by Epstein-Barr virus (EBV) infection, recurrent splenomegaly, and IBD.

IBD is observed in 26% of cases and usually occurs in infancy. IBD in patients with XIAP deficiency is associated with NOD2 dysfunction in monocytes,[109] and NOD2 is the first discovered Crohn's disease gene. In addition, the clinical and histological features are similar to those seen in Crohn's disease, but the disease is usually severe and resistant to drug treatments. Focal inflammation can be observed in the stomach, ileum, colon, and anus, and the large bowel is always affected.[109] Skip lesions and focal ulceration is a frequent finding. Microscopically crypt abscess, granulomas, lamina propria neutrophilic infiltration, and transmural inflammation are seen.[108,109]

Lipopolysaccharide-Responsive Beige-Like Anchor Protein Deficiency

Lipopolysaccharide-responsive beige-like anchor protein (LRBA) deficiency is caused by biallelic mutations in the *LRBA* gene. Previously LRBA was considered as CVID, but the new IUIS[85] classifies it as a disease of immune dysregulation with autoimmunity. LRBA deficiency leads to altered B-cell function as well as T-cell abnormalities with a low number of T-regulatory cells and poor suppressive function.[110] It is characterized by autoimmunity, chronic diarrhea, hypogammaglobulinemia, and recurrent infections, with autoimmune disorders the main clinical manifestations, including autoimmune hemolytic anemia and immune thrombocytopenic purpura.[111] Autoimmune GI disorders are common.[110,111] These patients frequently present with chronic diarrhea. Abnormalities can be seen in the stomach (atrophic gastritis), small intestine, and large intestine. Small bowel findings are similar to those seen in celiac disease, with villous blunting, expansion of lamina propria with lymphoplasma cells, and increased intraepithelial lymphocytes.[112] Reported pathological findings in the colon include chronic active colitis and collagenous colitis. Chronic active colitis is described as a remarkable increase in mixed acute and chronic inflammatory cell numbers in the lamina propria, decreased number of crypts, and lamina propria fibrosis.[112] Early-onset Crohn's disease was reported in one case with severe disease.

Other disorders associated with LRBA deficiency include lymphoproliferative disease with splenomegaly, lymphadenopathy, and hepatomegaly. Lymphoma has been reported in three cases.[111] Other reported malignancies are nephroblastoma, squamous cell carcinoma, gastric adenocarcinoma. and melanoma.

Cytotoxic T-Lymphocyte Antigen 4 Deficiency

Cytotoxic T-lymphocyte antigen 4 (CTLA4) is highly expressed on activated and regulatory T cells and plays a critical role in maintenance of tolerance to self-antigens. Heterozygous germline mutations in *CTLA4* cause variable clinical presentations, including various organ-specific autoimmune diseases, hypogammaglobulinemia, recurrent infections, and malignancies.[110,113] In 22% of mutation carriers, presentation mainly includes severe GI symptoms, and 59% present with GI involvement overall. Diarrhea is the most frequent presentation and is severe in some patients with weight loss, wasting, and total parenteral nutrition.[113] Crohn's disease with deep T-cell infiltration in the submucosa to superficial ulcerative lesions or deep-seated inflammatory changes is observed in some patients. Other GI findings include atrophic gastritis, celiac disease, and acute pancreatitis. There are increased plasma cells in the gastric, small intestinal, and colonic mucosa. Four cases of gastric cancer have been reported in these patients.[110,113]

Immune Dysregulation, Polyendocrinopathy, Enteropathy, X-linked Syndrome

Immune dysregulation, polyendocrinopathy, and enteropathy, X-linked (IPEX) syndrome is caused by mutations in the Forkhead box protein 3 *(FOXP3)* gene. FOXP3 is involved in the dominant regulation of immune responses to self-antigens through programming Treg-cell lineage development and function.[114] IPEX syndrome is characterized by the clinical triad of chronic diarrhea secondary to autoimmune enteropathy, autoimmune endocrinopathy, which most commonly affects the pancreas and/or thyroid gland, and eczematous dermatitis.[114]

IPEX usually manifests in affected males with severe watery or bloody-mucoid diarrhea early in life. Failure to thrive is common. The entire GI tract may be involved; the most common site is the small bowel, followed by large bowel, stomach, and esophagus. Anti-enterocyte antibodies are detected in most patients.[115,116] GI pathology primarily shows GVHD-like histological changes with prominent crypt apoptosis (Fig. 5.9). Small bowel disease with villous atrophy mimicking celiac disease has also been

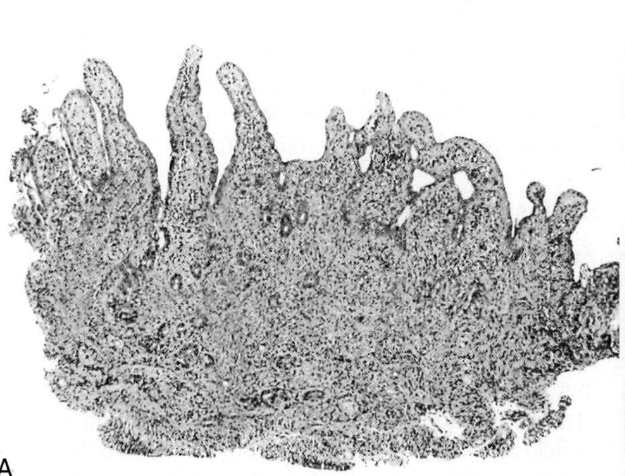

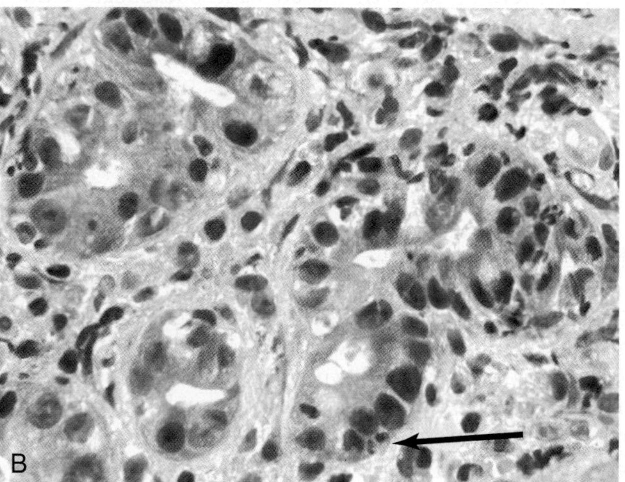

FIGURE 5.9 The GI tract in immune dysregulation, polyendocrinopathy, and enteropathy, X-linked syndrome shows graft-versus-host disease–like changes with villous injury **(A),** and prominent apoptotic bodies (**B,** *arrow*) (H&E stain).

reported in IPEX.[116,117] Additional GI findings include enteropathy with a complete loss of goblet cells and atrophic gastritis.[116,118]

Other Primary Immunodeficiencies

Chronic Granulomatous Disease

In chronic granulomatous disease (CGD), phagocytic cells are unable to reduce molecular oxygen to create the superoxide anion and its metabolites necessary for eradication of certain catalase-positive intracellular microbes. CGD is genetically heterogeneous, resulting from a mutation in any of four components of reduced nicotinamide adenine dinucleotide phosphate (NADPH) oxidase. The most common form of the disease, accounting for 70% of cases, is X-linked recessive with mutations in the *CYBB* gene; four other forms are autosomal recessive with mutations in the *CYBA, NCF1, NCF2,* or *NCF4* gene.[119] As a result of this defect, patients with CGD suffer from recurrent bacterial and fungal infections; abscesses in a variety of sites and pneumonia are common. They are also prone to develop inflammatory and rheumatic diseases, such as an IBD-like condition and a lupus-like syndrome. GI manifestations are seen nearly half of cases, which can be broadly grouped into obstructive and inflammatory categories.

Obstruction can occur in patients with CGD at a number of levels of the GI tract, from esophagus to small bowel. Gastric outlet obstruction is more common in the X-linked form of the disease.[119] In some cases, the obstruction is caused by infiltration of the viscus wall by pigment-laden macrophages (the histological hallmark of CGD) or by granulomatous inflammation. In other cases, the obstruction is reportedly secondary to a functional disturbance in GI motility, although infiltration of the deep layers of the organ by macrophages often cannot be excluded. Esophageal dysmotility and structural abnormalities are observed in 26% of cases.[120] Esophageal obstruction occurs in 1% of CGD patients[119]; biopsies of the esophageal mucosa usually show nonspecific findings or reflux esophagitis[121] but may demonstrate pigmented macrophages. Involvement of the gastric antrum and pylorus is somewhat more common, occurring in 16% of patients, and gastric outlet obstruction may be the first manifestation of CGD. Granulomas, giant cells, and macrophages laden with brown-yellow fine pigment are commonly present in gastric biopsy specimens,[122] but in some cases only nonspecific inflammation is seen.[123] Small bowel obstruction is relatively rare in CGD but is occasionally reported in the context of an inflammatory process.[124] In a review of small bowel and rectal biopsies from nine patients with CGD, pigment-laden macrophages were found in the lamina propria at both sites. In the small bowel, the macrophages were located deep in the mucosa adjacent to crypts, but when numerous, they also extended into the villus core (Fig. 5.10). In rectal biopsies, the number of pigmented histiocytes was quite variable, ranging from rare scattered cells to large numbers of histiocytes accumulating between the base of the crypts and the muscularis mucosae. Granulomas with giant cells were also present in rectal biopsies from some patients. In one of eight cases, distortion of crypt architecture without crypt abscesses was seen.[125]

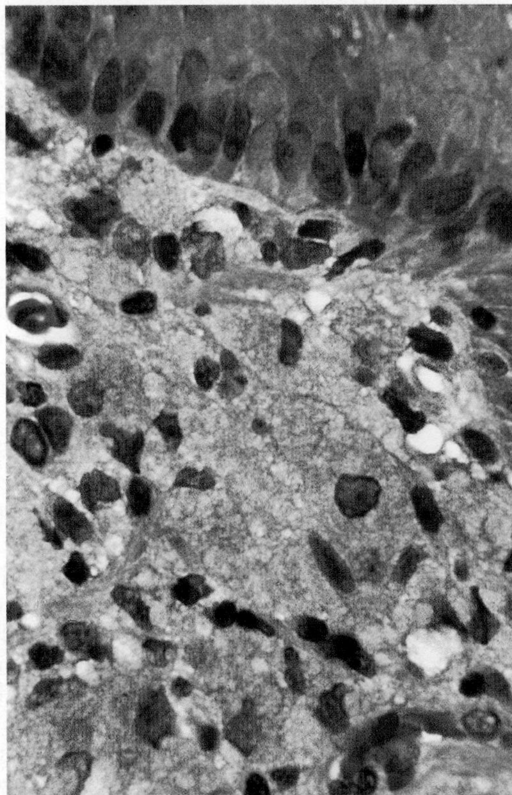

FIGURE 5.10 Chronic granulomatous disease. Accumulation of pigmented macrophages containing light-brown, dusky material in the small intestinal mucosa is seen (H&E stain).

Chronic inflammatory processes that are indistinguishable from IBD affecting the small and large bowel may occur in CGD patients[126]; as with obstructive lesions of the GI tract, these lesions are more common in the X-linked form of the disease.[119] Polymorphisms in genes unrelated to NADPH oxidase may modify the clinical phenotype in CGD; certain polymorphisms in the genes for myeloperoxidase and Fcγ receptors are strongly associated with GI complications.[127] Involvement of the small bowel in CGD may produce fistulas, longitudinal ulcers, stenosis, and nonnecrotizing granulomatous inflammation that can be mistaken for Crohn's disease[128]; discontinuous inflammation and perianal disease may also contribute to the difficulty in distinguishing the two entities.[129] The granulomas seen in intestinal lesions in CGD are often more florid than is usually seen in Crohn's disease, but granulomas are not present in all cases. In a study of colitis in one CGD patient, the presence of an acute and chronic inflammatory infiltrate confined to the colonic mucosa, crypt abscesses, and lack of granulomas were more suggestive of ulcerative colitis than Crohn's disease. Mucosal architectural distortion and ulceration were not as prominent as is usually the case in ulcerative colitis, however, and pigmented macrophages were present in the lamina propria.[126]

Chronic Mucocutaneous Candidiasis

Chronic mucocutaneous candidiasis is a heterogeneous group of disorders characterized by persistent *Candida* infection of the skin, nails, and mucous membranes.

Autoimmune disorders and a polyglandular endocrinopathy syndrome including pernicious anemia are common, occurring in more than 50% of patients. There is a high frequency of association with thymoma and systemic lupus erythematosus.[130] Mutations in *STAT1* have been identified in the autosomal dominant form of the disease,[131,132] and the autosomal recessive form has been linked to deficiency in interleukin-17 receptor A.[133] Immune defects include disorders of T-cell immunity with variable B-cell involvement. The most common GI manifestation is esophageal candidiasis. Although superficial infection with *Candida* is a defining characteristic, infections with other fungi (e.g., *H. capsulatum*) and bacteria are common.[134]

Miscellaneous Immune Deficiency Syndromes

Other rare disorders of immunity occasionally associated with GI manifestations include *leukocyte adhesion deficiency*, in which delayed wound healing and susceptibility to bacterial and fungal infection lead to necrotizing enterocolitis.[135] A chronic inflammatory process with multiple aphthous ulcers involving the gastric antrum, terminal ileum, cecum, and right colon, which resolved with bone marrow transplantation, has also been reported in leukocyte adhesion deficiency,[136] and a case of rectal ulcer resembling Crohn's disease has been reported in a pediatric patient.[137]

IBD and enteropathy have been reported in a number of other rare primary immunodeficiencies, including disorders of immune dysregulation, autoinflammatory disorders, complement deficiencies, and phenocopies of inborn errors of immunity (Table 5.5).

GRAFT-VERSUS-HOST DISEASE (GVHD)

GVHD, most commonly involving GI tract, skin, or liver, develops in as many as 50% of allogeneic bone marrow transplant recipients.[138] Indeed, the most common cause of persistent nausea and anorexia in patients beyond day 20 after transplantation is acute GVHD.[139] Changes identical to those seen in GVHD after allogeneic transplantation may be seen in the GI tract and liver after autologous stem cell transplantation and are considered to be a form of GVHD resulting from a lack of regulation of immune mechanisms by the reconstituting immune system. This syndrome of acute GVHD–like changes in the GI tract after autologous transplantation is rare, occurring in gastric biopsies in only 4% of patients with upper GI tract symptoms[140] and approximately 5% of all autologous transplantation patients.[141] Most reported autologous GVHD is observed in patients transplanted for multiple myeloma.[141] Rarely, GVHD occurs after solid organ transplantation or blood transfusion.[142] Symptoms indicative of GI tract involvement by GVHD include profuse diarrhea, crampy abdominal pain, GI hemorrhage, anorexia, nausea, and vomiting. Severe GI bleeding and peritonitis have also been reported.[143]

Historically, acute GVHD has been defined as occurring less than 100 days after myeloablative stem cell transplantation. However, current clinical practices in stem cell transplantation have rendered this classification inadequate because the use of reduced-intensity regimens, for instance, has led to late occurrence of otherwise typical acute GVHD. Accordingly, recommendations for classification of GVHD as acute or chronic have been developed by an expert panel convened by the National Institutes of Health[144] (Table 5.6). Characteristic skin, GI tract, or liver abnormalities are now classified as *acute GVHD* regardless of time after transplantation. Diagnosis of *chronic GVHD* requires the presence of at least one diagnostic clinical sign or distinctive clinical manifestation confirmed by biopsy or other relevant tests in the same or another organ. In the GI tract, the presence of an esophageal web, stricture, or concentric rings documented by endoscopy or barium contrast radiography is sufficient to establish the diagnosis of chronic GVHD. Distinctive criteria that are, by themselves, insufficient to establish a diagnosis of chronic GI GVHD include pancreatic exocrine insufficiency, anorexia, nausea, vomiting, diarrhea, weight loss, and wasting syndrome.[144]

Acute GVHD

On endoscopic examination, the appearance of the GI mucosa in acute GVHD is variable, ranging from only mucosal edema and erythema to more severe changes such as ulcers and mucosal sloughing.[145] The major histological features of GVHD in the GI tract are epithelial cell apoptosis and a relatively sparse mononuclear inflammatory cell infiltrate (Fig. 5.11A). Apoptotic epithelial cells are found primarily in the regenerative compartment of the mucosa, such as the crypt in the colon and small intestine and the neck area of gastric glands. In the colon, the apoptotic cells are particularly conspicuous and are termed "exploding crypt cells"; these cells contain intracytoplasmic vacuoles filled with karyorrhectic nuclear debris (see Fig. 5.11B). Apoptotic cells are smaller and less conspicuous in the gastric mucosa (Fig. 5.12). In more severe cases of acute GVHD, crypt abscesses may be seen, and destruction and loss of crypts is seen. In the most severe cases, mucosal sloughing and extensive ulceration occur. In the stomach, granular eosinophilic necrotic cellular debris without neutrophils may be present in the lumina of injured gastric glands.[146] Villous blunting is commonly seen in small bowel GVHD. A grading system for acute GVHD affecting the colon has been proposed[147] (Fig. 5.13 and Table 5.7); however, correlations with clinical symptoms and patient outcome are weak.

The changes that occur in the GI tract in acute GVHD are not entirely specific. The differential diagnosis includes drug-related injury, infection, recurrent hematological malignancy, and other causes of immune activation (Table 5.8). In particular, mycophenolate mofetil (MMF) treatment may cause active colitis with ulcers, marked crypt cell apoptosis, and a mixed lamina propria inflammatory infiltrate that can mimic GVHD (Fig. 5.14).[148] Other reported patterns of injury include IBD-like changes and, more rarely, ischemic colitis.[149] Normal biopsy findings in sites distant from these GVHD-like lesions should raise the question of MMF-associated colitis rather than GVHD[150]; improvement after discontinuation of MMF is also good evidence that the injury was drug related. Recently immune

TABLE 5.5 Other Primary Immunodeficiencies with Gastrointestinal Manifestations

Disease	Clinical Features	Gastrointestinal Manifestations
Combined Immunodeficiencies with Associated or Syndromic Features		
ARPC1B deficiency[187]	Platelet abnormalities, recurrent infections, cutaneous vasculitis, eosinophilia, and inflammatory diseases	Intestinal inflammation (crypt distortion with prominent eosinophils)
Dyskeratosis congenital with SAMD9 gain of function[188]	Myelodysplasia, infection, restriction of growth, adrenal hypoplasia, genital phenotypes, and enteropathy (MIRAGE) syndrome	Esophageal achalasia; colon dilation; IBD-like lesions
Diseases of Immune Dysregulation		
STAT3 gain of function[189]	Infantile-onset multisystem autoimmune disease and delayed-onset mycobacterial disease	Autoimmune enteropathy; lymphocytic colitis
Autoimmune polyendocrinopathy-1[190]	Autoimmune polyendocrinopathy, candidiasis, and ectodermal dystrophy (APECED)	Candida esophagitis; autoimmune gastritis; celiac disease; infectious diarrhea; IBD-like lesion
ITCH deficiency[191]	Dysmorphic facies, failure to thrive, hepatosplenomegaly, multisystem autoimmune disease, and delayed motor development	Candida esophagitis; early-onset IBD-like disease; autoimmune hepatitis (very common)
IL-10/IL-10 receptor deficiency[192]	Folliculitis, recurrent infections, arthritis, B-cell lymphoma, and neonatal-onset IBD	Crohn's disease with pronounced perianal disease and fistulas
Autoinflammatory Disorders		
Familial Mediterranean fever[39]	Recurrent fever and acute inflammation of the membranes lining the abdomen, joints, and lungs	Ulcerative colitis–like disease
Mevalonate kinase deficiency[39]	Recurrent febrile attacks with lymphadenopathy, diarrhea, skin lesions, hepatosplenomegaly, and abdominal pain	IBD
Blau syndrome[39]	Granulomatous polyarthritis, dermatitis, and uveitis	Crohn's colitis
Complement Deficiencies		
Ficolin 3 deficiency[39]	Increased susceptibility to infection	Necrotizing enterocolitis in infancy
CD55 deficiency[193]	Early-onset protein-losing enteropathy and thrombosis	Primary intestinal lymphangiectasia; IBD-like lesions
Phenocopies of Inborn Errors of Immunity		
Thymoma with hypogammaglobulinemia[194]	Severe, recurrent bacterial and opportunistic infections, autoimmunity, thymoma, chronic diarrhea, complete absence of B cells	Infectious enterocolitis; autoimmune enteropathy

IBD, Inflammatory bowel disease.

Data from Kahr WH, Pluthero FG, Elkadri A, et al. Loss of the Arp2/3 complex component ARPC1B causes platelet abnormalities and predisposes to inflammatory disease. Nat Commun. *2017;8:14816; Narumi S, Amano N, Ishii T, et al. SAMD9 mutations cause a novel multisystem disorder, MIRAGE syndrome, and are associated with loss of chromosome 7.* Nat Genet. *2016;48(7):792–797; Leppkes M, Neurath MF, Herrmann M, Becker C. Immune deficiency vs. immune excess in inflammatory bowel diseases—STAT3 as a rheo-STAT of intestinal homeostasis.* J Leukoc Biol. *2016;99(1):57–66; Schwimmer D, Glover S. Primary immunodeficiency and the Gut.* Gastroenterol Clin N Am. *2019;48(2):199–220; Lohr NJ, Molleston JP, Strauss KA, et al. Human ITCH E3 ubiquitin ligase deficiency causes syndromic multisystem autoimmune disease.* Am J Hum Genet. *2010;86(3):447–453; Tegtmeyer D, Seidl M, Gerner P, Baumann U, Klemann C. Inflammatory bowel disease caused by primary immunodeficiencies—Clinical presentations, review of literature, and proposal of a rational diagnostic algorithm.* Pediatr Allergy Immunol. *2017;28(5):412–429; Bousfiha A, Jeddane L, Picard C, et al. The 2017 IUIS Phenotypic Classification for Primary Immunodeficiencies.* J Clin Immunol. *2018;38(1):129–143; Ozen A, Comrie WA, Ardy RC, et al. CD55 deficiency, early-onset protein-losing enteropathy, and thrombosis.* N Engl J Med. *2017;377(1):52–61; Kelesidis T, Yang O. Good's syndrome remains a mystery after 55 years: A systematic review of the scientific evidence.* Clin Immunol. *2010;135(3):347–363.*

checkpoint inhibitors, including CTLA-4 inhibitors (e.g., ipilimumab) and PD-1/PD-L1 inhibitors, have been widely used for treatment of various advanced-stage malignancies, which can also cause GI toxicity mimicking GVHD.[151-153] Use of proton pump inhibitor (PPI) therapy has been associated with an increase in apoptotic epithelial cells in the gastric mucosa (Fig. 5.15), mimicking the histological changes seen in GVHD.[154]

Changes similar to GVHD have been reported in colonic biopsies from patients with severe T-cell deficiencies,[79] malignant thymoma,[155] and primary immune disorders such as CVID.[35,60] In patients who have undergone bone marrow transplantation, the effects of cytoreductive therapy (Fig. 5.16) may resemble changes of GI GVHD in the early posttransplantation period; therefore a diagnosis of GVHD must be made with caution before

TABLE 5.6 Classification of Graft-versus-Host Disease

Classification	Time of Onset	Features
"Classic" acute GVHD	≤100 days after HSCT	Maculopapular rash, nausea, vomiting, anorexia, profuse diarrhea, ileus, or cholestatic hepatitis
Persistent, recurrent, or late acute GVHD	>100 days after HSCT	Same as "classic" acute GVHD, without diagnostic or distinctive manifestations of chronic GVHD; often seen after withdrawal of immunosuppression
"Classic" chronic GVHD	No time limit	At least one diagnostic or distinctive manifestation of chronic GVHD without features characteristic of acute GVHD
Overlap syndrome of acute and chronic GVHD	No time limit	Features of acute and chronic GVHD appear together

GVHD, Graft-versus-host disease; *HSCT,* hematopoietic stem cell transplantation.

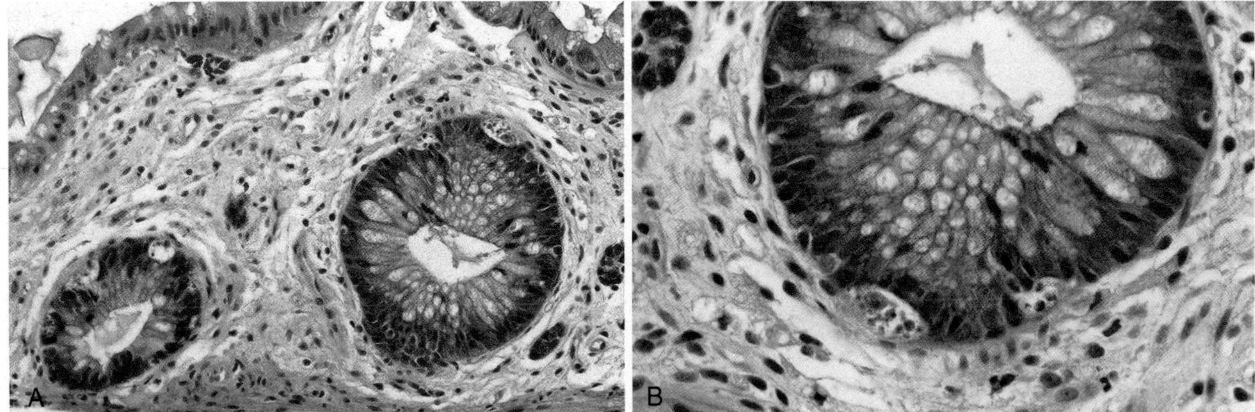

FIGURE 5.11 Acute graft-versus-host disease (GVHD) involving the colon. A, The lamina propria inflammatory infiltrate is relatively sparse; no crypt loss is seen in this example, although crypts are slightly distorted. **B,** Large apoptotic bodies known as *exploding crypt cells* are typical of colonic GVHD.

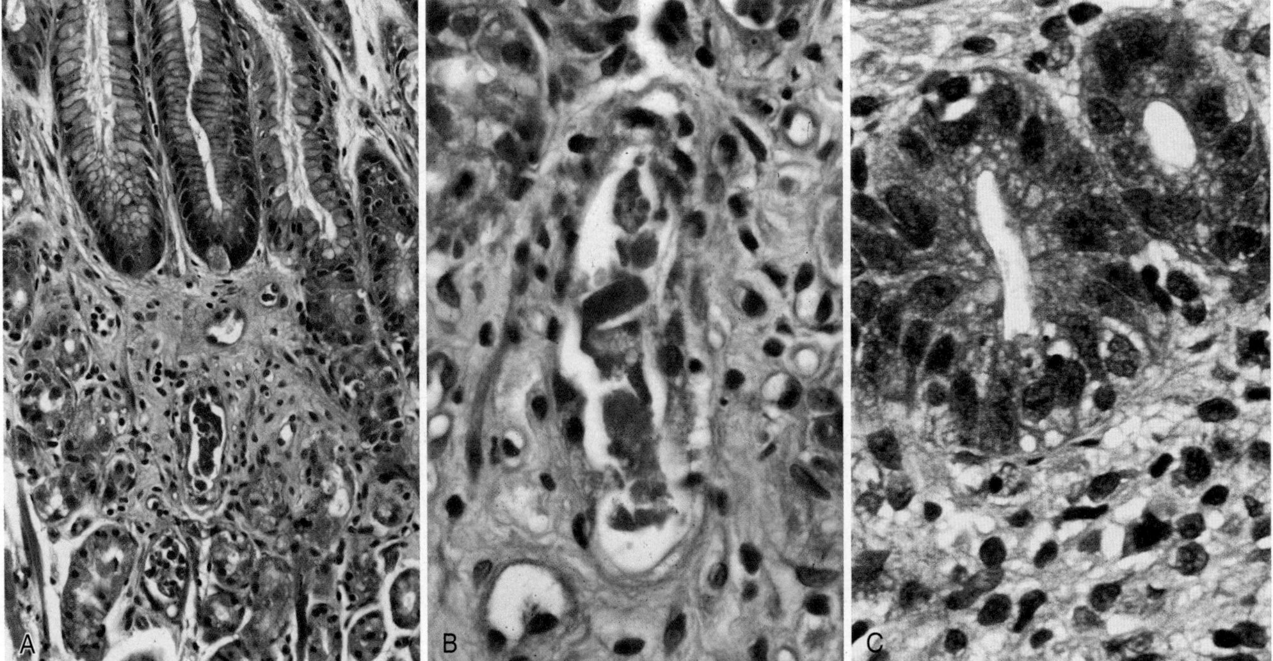

FIGURE 5.12 A, In the gastric body, dilated glands containing granular eosinophilic debris are sometimes found in acute graft-versus-host-disease (GVHD). **B,** As in the colon, the inflammatory infiltrate is relatively sparse. **C,** Apoptotic bodies in glandular epithelium are often small and inconspicuous in acute GVHD in the stomach (H&E stain).

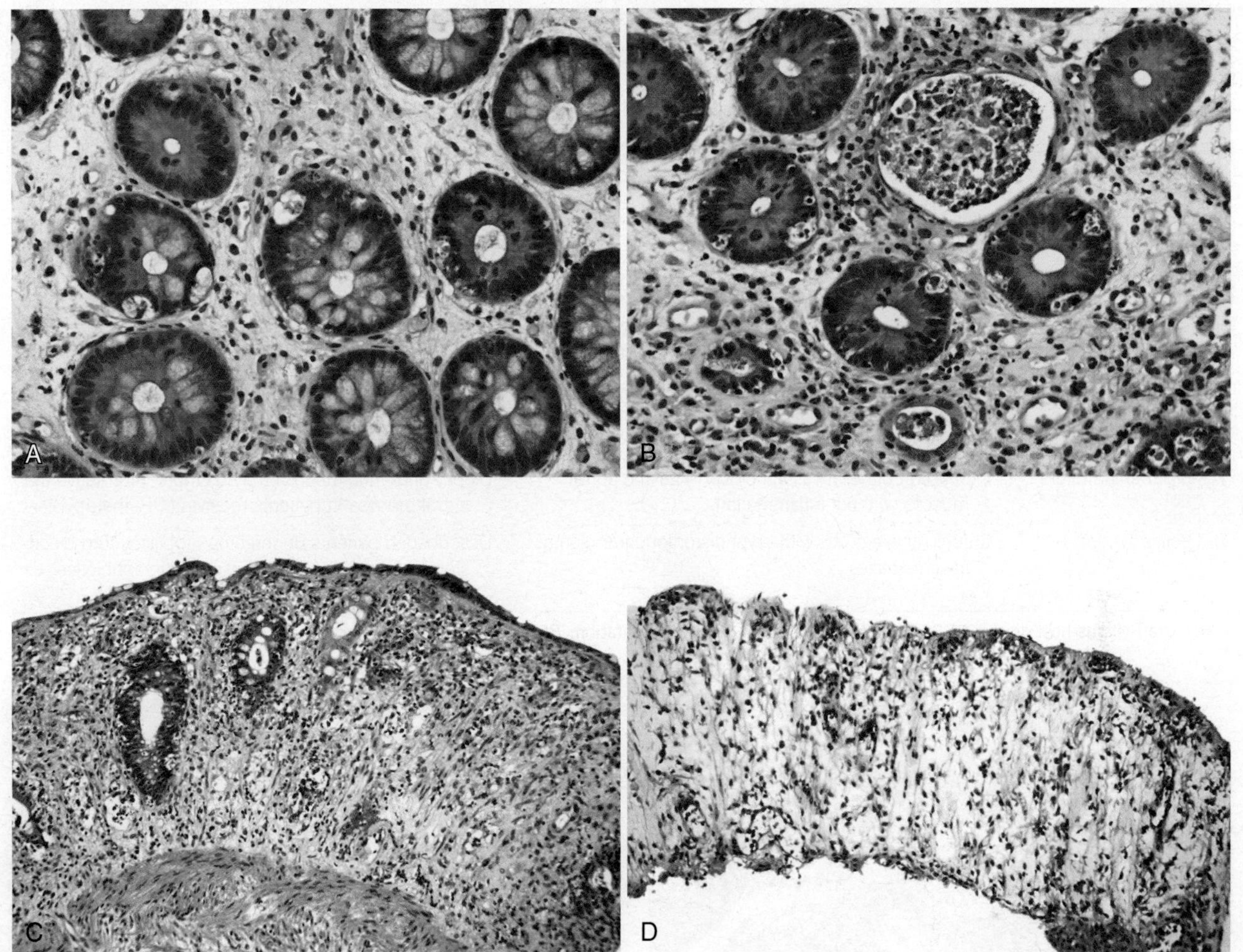

FIGURE 5.13 **A,** An example of grade I acute graft-versus-host-disease (GVHD) in the colon consisting of scattered single-cell apoptotic epithelial cells. **B,** Grade II acute GVHD showing epithelial apoptosis, crypt atrophy, and crypt abscesses. **C,** Grade III acute GVHD with loss of contiguous crypts. **D,** Grade IV acute GVHD with replacement of mucosa by loose granulation tissue (H&E stain).

TABLE 5.7 Grading of Acute Graft-versus-Host Disease of the Colon

Grade	Histological Features
I	Rare apoptotic cells, without crypt loss
II	Loss of individual crypts
III	Loss of two or more contiguous crypts
IV	No identifiable crypts (mucosal ulceration)

From Sale GE, Shulman HM, McDonald GB, Thomas ED. Gastrointestinal graft-versus-host disease in man. A clinicopathologic study of the rectal biopsy. Am J Surg Pathol. *1979;3(4):291–299.*

day 21 after transplantation. Recurrence of hematological malignancies, particularly acute lymphoblastic leukemia, may also mimic acute GVHD.[156] CMV infection may produce mucosal damage characterized by apoptotic epithelial cells, mimicking GVHD; differentiation from GVHD relies on the demonstration of viral inclusions.[146] GVHD and CMV infection may occur simultaneously, making it difficult to separate the effects of each process on the GI tract. Infection with *Clostridium difficile* has also been reported to be associated with GI GVHD and a high nonrelapse mortality rate in this group; it is postulated that C. *difficile* toxin may predispose to increased severity of GVHD.[157]

Chronic GVHD

Chronic GVHD is clinically similar in many ways to some of the collagen vascular diseases and has been compared with autoimmune disorders such as scleroderma, Sjögren's syndrome, and primary biliary cirrhosis. Chronic GVHD involves multiple organs that are not involved by acute GVHD, such as the salivary gland, mouth, eye, and upper respiratory tract.[146]

In chronic GVHD, skin changes of dermal fibrosis may resemble scleroderma, and involvement of the oral squamous mucosa leads to painful ulcers and submucosal fibrosis. Involvement of minor salivary glands results in an oral sicca syndrome. In advanced cases, ulcers and submucosal fibrosis occur in the esophagus (Fig. 5.17), the most commonly affected site in the GI tract.[150] Small bowel involvement is less common; when present,

TABLE 5.8 Differential Diagnosis of Graft-versus-Host Disease

Diagnosis	Features	Comments
Conditioning regimen	Epithelial cell apoptosis; increased mitotic activity; crypt cell regeneration	Found in early period after transplantation (up to day 20); severe injury at day 20 likely represents GVHD because effects of chemotherapy and radiation are typically improving by then
Cytomegalovirus	Increased epithelial cell apoptosis; nuclear inclusions may be sparse	May occur concomitantly with gastrointestinal GVHD
Cryptosporidium	Increased epithelial cell apoptosis	Rarely encountered in biopsies in HSCT population
Mycophenolate mofetil	Colitis with increased crypt cell apoptosis, focal ulcers, mixed lamina propria inflammatory infiltrate	Apoptotic bodies in sites other than colon are suggestive of GVHD[148]
Checkpoint inhibitors	Increased epithelial cell apoptosis in gastric, small-intestinal, and colonic mucosa; crypt dropout/distortion in small and large intestine	Frequent active inflammation (cryptitis, crypt abscess, and lamina propria neutrophilic infiltrates) and lamina propria expansion[152]
Proton pump inhibitors	Increased epithelial cell apoptosis in gastric antral mucosa, without inflammation	Biopsy of oxyntic mucosa may be more informative than antral mucosa in patients receiving PPI therapy[154]
Cord colitis syndrome	Chronic active colitis with crypt distortion; granulomas in some cases	Described in patients undergoing umbilical cord blood stem cell transplantation; response to antibiotics suggests infectious etiology[160]

GVHD, Graft-versus-host disease; *HSCT,* hematopoietic stem cell transplantation; *PPI,* proton pump inhibitor.

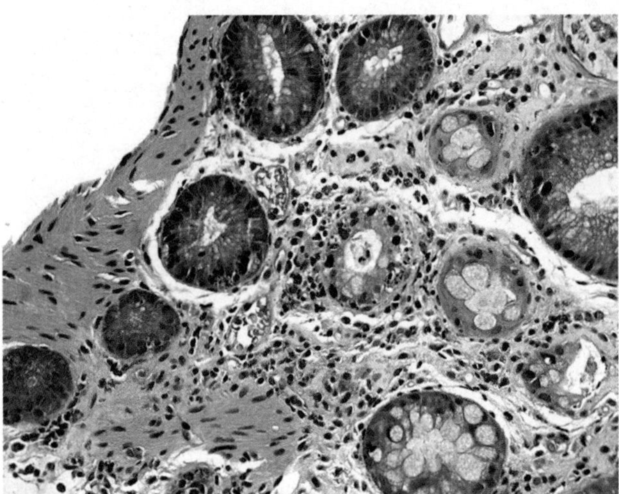

FIGURE 5.14 Mycophenolate mofetil–induced colitis. Prominent crypt cell apoptosis and relatively sparse mononuclear inflammatory infiltrate in the lamina propria may mimic graft-versus-host-disease (GVHD) (H&E stain).

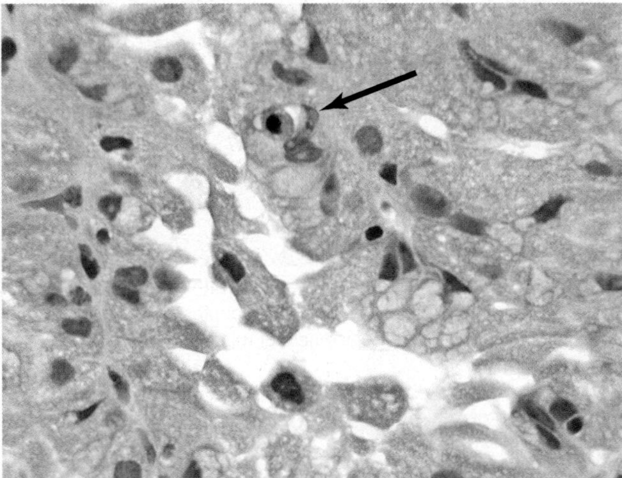

FIGURE 5.15 Increased gastric epithelial cell apoptosis *(arrow)* has been associated with proton pump inhibitor (PPI) use. Notice the apical cytoplasmic protrusions in parietal cells, typical of the PPI effect (H&E stain).

it is associated with diarrhea. Focal fibrosis of the lamina propria and segmental submucosal fibrosis, with minimal mucosal changes, have been reported.[158] In colonic biopsies, chronic colitis similar to that seen in ulcerative colitis has also been reported in allogeneic bone marrow transplant recipients.[159] These changes consist of mild to moderate crypt distortion and crypt atrophy, and it is unclear whether the mucosal architectural distortion is caused by chronic GVHD or by other factors. In one study, similar findings of mild chronic active colitis, with granulomas in some cases (Fig. 5.18), were reported in 10% of patients undergoing umbilical cord blood stem cell transplantation, occurring 88 to 314 days after transplantation. Although patients were culture negative, this "cord colitis syndrome" responded to antibiotic therapy, suggesting an infectious etiology.[160]

NEUTROPENIC ENTEROCOLITIS

Neutropenic enterocolitis (NEC) is a necrotizing inflammatory process that predominantly affects the cecum, terminal ileum, and ascending colon and occurs most commonly in the setting of neutropenia. Hemorrhagic necrosis of the cecum in this setting has also been termed *typhlitis*. Historically, most patients with NEC have had acute leukemia, although NEC has also been reported in patients undergoing stem cell or autologous bone marrow transplantation for solid malignancies.[161] NEC also occurs in patients with aplastic anemia, renal transplant recipients, and those with other hematological malignancies. Incidence varies from less than 1% to almost 7% in children with cancer,[162,163] with a pooled incidence of about 5% in adult patients.[161] Most patients have received chemotherapy in the previous 30 days,[164] and absolute neutrophil counts of less than

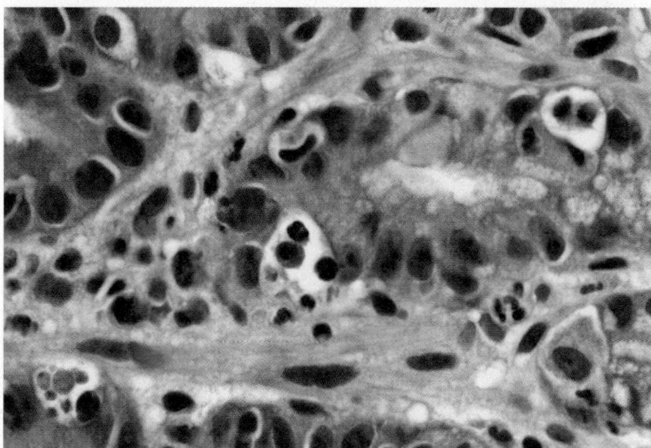

FIGURE 5.16 Pretransplantation cytoreductive therapies can injure gastrointestinal mucosa, resulting in increased apoptotic bodies, seen here in the colon, that mimic graft-versus-host disease (H&E stain).

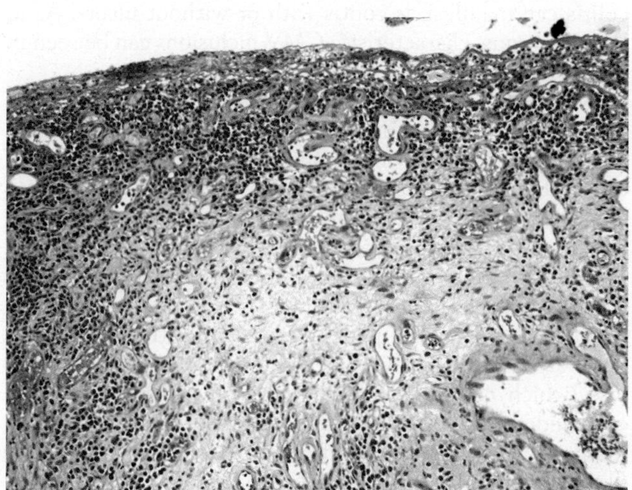

FIGURE 5.17 Nonspecific ulcers with submucosal fibrosis may be seen in the esophagus in patients with chronic graft-versus-host syndrome (H&E stain).

1500 cells/mm^3 are associated with the disease. Patients may be seen with clinical features suggestive of acute appendicitis, such as fever and right lower quadrant pain.[165] One-third are seen with GI hemorrhage,[164] and rarely a palpable right lower quadrant mass is present. The combination of abdominal pain, diarrhea, and fever is the most common presentation; diagnosis is often established by radiographic studies showing a fluid-filled, dilated cecum and inflammatory changes in the abdomen.[165]

On gross examination, the cecum and other affected portions of the GI tract are dilated, edematous, and congested or hemorrhagic. Pneumatosis intestinalis (Fig. 5.19A) may be seen but is relatively rare. The mucosa is hemorrhagic, often necrotic, and covered with granular eosinophilic debris; no significant inflammatory reaction is present (see Fig. 5.19B). The pathogenesis of this disorder is initiated with mucosal injury, primarily related to recent administration of chemotherapeutic agents and augmented by neutropenia. Bacterial invasion of the injured mucosa then occurs, with *Clostridium* spp. implicated as major offenders; fungi such as *Candida* spp. have also been implicated as causative or contributing agents. Toxins produced by organisms invading the gut wall lead to edema and necrosis. Distention of the bowel wall leads to decreased blood flow, adding an element of ischemic injury. Most patients become septicemic. If NEC is left untreated, the prognosis is grave, but patients may survive with optimal medical and surgical management; recovery depends on the restoration of adequate neutrophil counts.

THE GASTROINTESTINAL TRACT IN HIV INFECTION

GI illnesses are common in patients with human immunodeficiency virus (HIV) infection, with presenting symptoms of diarrhea, nausea, vomiting, anorexia, and abdominal pain. Before the use of new, highly active antiretroviral therapy (HAART), opportunistic infections with pathogens such as *Isospora, Mycobacterium avium-intracellulare* complex (MAC), microsporidia, *Cryptosporidium*, and CMV were frequent causes of diarrhea, malabsorption, and wasting

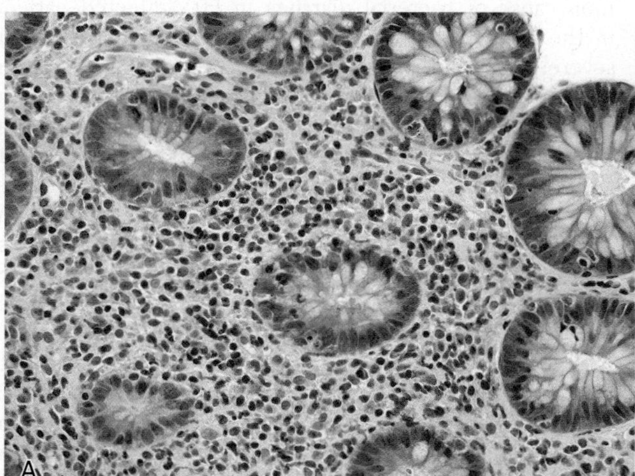

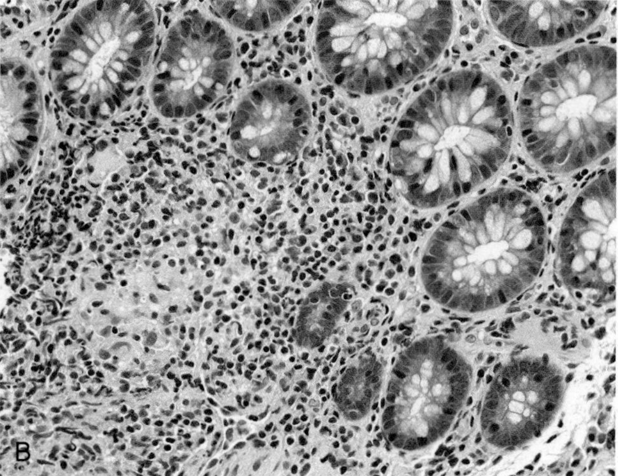

FIGURE 5.18 Increased crypt cell apoptosis **(A)** and loose nonnecrotizing granulomas **(B)** may be seen in "cord colitis syndrome" occurring after umbilical cord blood stem cell transplantation (H&E stain) *(Courtesy of Dr. Jason Hornick, Brigham and Women's Hospital, Boston, MA).*

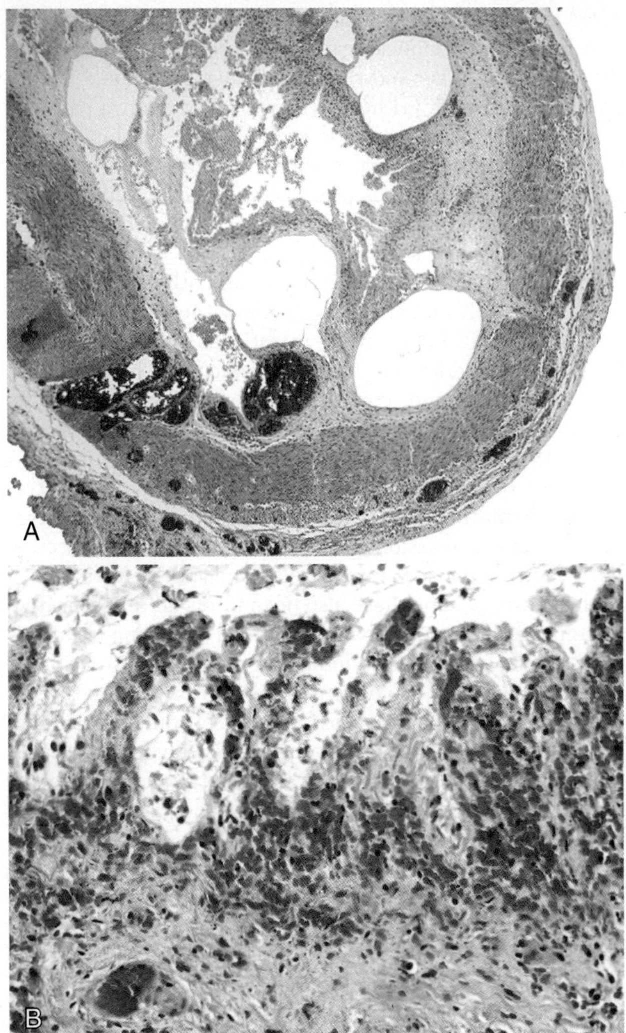

FIGURE 5.19 Neutropenic enterocolitis. A, Clear spaces in the bowel wall represent pneumatosis coli. The mucosa is necrotic, hemorrhagic, and lacks a significant inflammatory response. **B,** Sloughed epithelium is seen in the lumen (H&E stain).

(Table 5.9). Although the prevalence of intestinal pathogens has dramatically decreased since then, from a reported 85% (in men with AIDS and diarrhea) to 12% (found almost exclusively in homosexual men), current studies continue to show a high prevalence of GI dysfunction in HIV-infected patients. Chronic diarrhea is reported in approximately 25% of HIV patients and was not associated with degree of immune suppression in one cohort[166]; clinical trial data suggest that in some cases the diarrhea is linked to the effects of antiretroviral therapy itself.[167]

Infections

CMV remains the most common pathogen in HIV-infected patients, and CMV infection can involve any segment of the GI tract, most commonly the esophagus and colon. CMV esophagitis often manifests with distal esophageal ulceration. CMV primarily infects endothelial cells, followed by macrophages; biopsy specimens obtained from the ulcer bed are, therefore, more likely to demonstrate characteristic CMV cytopathic effects. Endoscopic features in CMV

TABLE 5.9 HIV-Associated Gastrointestinal Diseases

Infection	Neoplasia
Giardia intestinalis	Kaposi's sarcoma
Cryptosporidium parvum	Burkitt lymphoma
Isospora belli	Diffuse large B-cell lymphoma
Microsporidia	Plasmablastic lymphoma
Cytomegalovirus	Anal squamous cell carcinoma
Candida albicans	Hodgkin lymphoma
Listeria monocytogenes	
Strongyloides stercoralis	
Human herpesvirus 8	
Epstein-Barr virus	

gastritis include patchy erythema, erosions, or multiple small ulcers. Unlike other sites in the GI tract, in the stomach the epithelial cells are preferentially infected. CMV colitis can manifest as colitis with or without ulcers. As in the esophagus, characteristic CMV inclusions can be seen in stromal and endothelial cells.

Although GI herpes simplex virus (HSV) infection occurs less frequently than CMV infection, approximately 5% of esophageal ulcerative lesions in HIV-infected patients are caused by HSV infection.[168] HSV esophagitis can manifest as either vesicular or ulcerative lesions. Unlike CMV esophagitis, HSV characteristically infects squamous epithelium.

One of the important differential diagnoses for CMV and HSV esophagitis in HIV-infected patients is idiopathic esophageal ulcer. HIV patients with idiopathic esophageal ulcer always are seen with severe odynophagia and weight loss, which often respond to therapy with corticosteroid or thalidomide or both.[169] Endoscopically, HIV-associated idiopathic esophageal ulceration appears as large, irregular ulcers in the middle or distal esophagus. To diagnose idiopathic esophageal ulcer, exclusion of infectious etiologies is required.

Bacterial pathogens involving the GI tract in the HIV-positive population include C. *difficile*, mycobacteria, and spirochetes. C. *difficile*–associated colitis is the most common cause of bacterial diarrhea in HIV-infected patients in the HAART era.[170] GI MAC infection can be seen in severely immunocompromised patients, involving the stomach, the small intestine (Fig. 5.20A), and, rarely, the colon. Endoscopic presentations include normal-appearing mucosa, friability, multiple raised nodules, or ulceration. Microscopically, the lamina propria of the intestinal mucosa may be stuffed with distended macrophages containing the organisms, which can be confirmed by a special stain for acid-fast bacilli (see Fig. 5.20B). Periodic acid–Schiff (PAS) stain characteristically reveals abundant delicate bacilli in macrophages (see Fig. 5.20C).

Human intestinal spirochetosis has been associated with diarrhea in HIV patients and preferentially infects the surface epithelium of the distal colon and rectum. In addition to HIV-infected individuals, intestinal spirochetosis is also found in the general population. The prevalence of intestinal spirochetosis varies considerably from region to region and is more common in men than in women. For example,

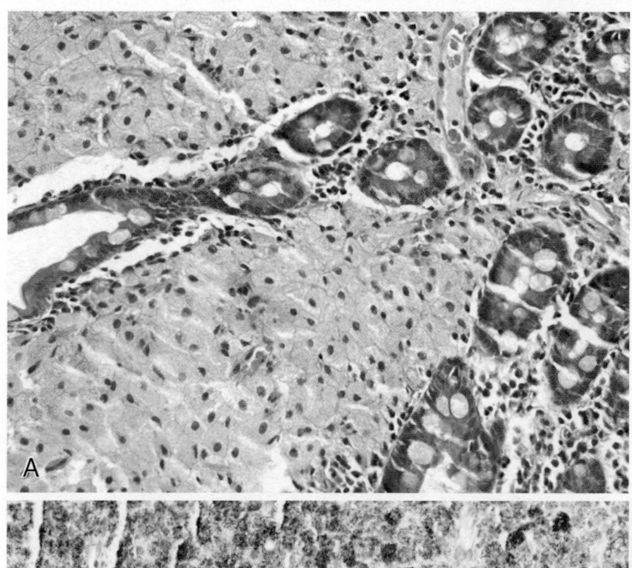
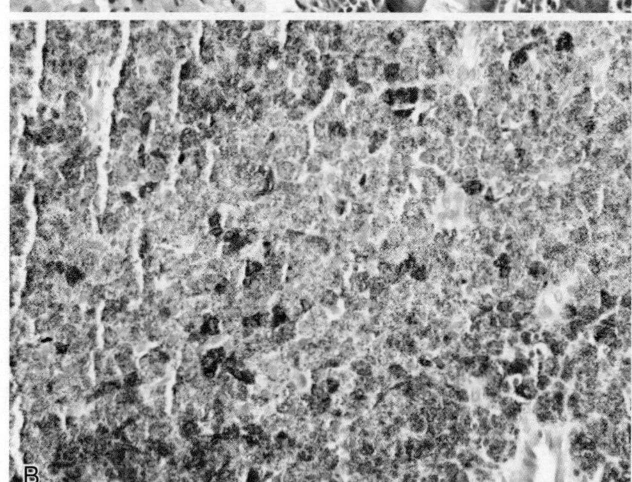
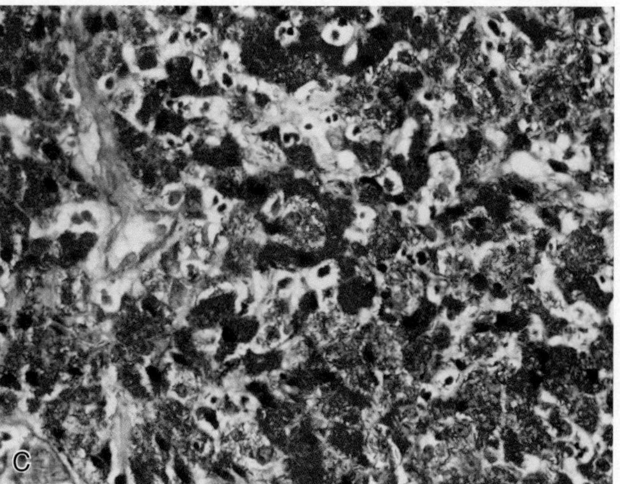

FIGURE 5.20 **A,** *Mycobacterium avium-intracellulare* complex involving the duodenum in HIV infection is manifested as accumulation of macrophages with foamy cytoplasm in the lamina propria. **B,** Acid-fast stain reveals numerous organisms. **C,** Periodic acid–Schiff stain shows abundant delicate bacilli in macrophages.

in Western countries, the prevalence of intestinal spirochetosis in rectal biopsies is 2% to 7%, whereas in developing countries it is much higher, ranging from 11.4% to 32.6%. Among homosexual and HIV-infected men, the rate is even higher, up to 54%. Two strains of *Bachyspira*[171] have been identified as being responsible for intestinal spirochetosis—*Brachyspira aalborgi* and *Brachyspira pilosicoli*—with *B. aalborgi* being the major causative agent in Western countries.

Because many cases of intestinal spirochetosis are asymptomatic, there is debate as to whether intestinal spirochetosis is a pathogen or a commensal. However, accumulating evidence supports the notion that intestinal spirochetosis can be the cause of GI symptoms in a subset of patients, especially in homosexual men, HIV patients, and children.[172-174] Association of intestinal spirochetosis with invasive colitis and hepatitis, rectal discharge, rectal bleeding, and even spirochetemia has been reported. Improvement of symptoms after eradication of the spirochetes is seen in individuals with symptomatic intestinal spirochetosis.[175]

Intestinal spirochetes have long been considered noninvasive. However, some studies have demonstrated invasion of spirochetes beyond the surface epithelium.[176] The presence of spirochetes in epithelial cells, lamina propria, macrophages, and even Schwann cells has been reported. In addition, invasive intestinal spirochetosis is associated with immediate-type immune reaction of the host, featured by a marked increase of IgE-producing plasma cells in the lamina propria and intraepithelial mast cells. Stunting, destruction, and loss of microvilli are seen in invasive cases and can result in reduction of the resorptive surface, leading to diarrhea. Invasive intestinal spirochetosis has been correlated to GI symptoms in the general population, whereas homosexual and HIV-infected men are more likely to be symptomatic regardless of invasion, for unclear reasons.

The most common symptoms associated with intestinal spirochetosis include diarrhea, abdominal pain, altered bowel movement habits, and rectal bleeding.[175] Intestinal spirochetosis can affect the rectum, the colon, or both; the site of densest colonization varies among patients. Appendiceal involvement by intestinal spirochetosis also occurs.[175] The endoscopic appearance of the colon is largely normal; however, some subtle changes (e.g., erythema) may be present. Biopsy reveals long, undulating bacteria vertically attached to the brush border, forming a blue bushy layer on hematoxylin and eosin (H&E) staining (Fig. 5.21A). The organisms stain dark black with Warthin-Starry stain (see Fig. 5.21B). The colonic mucosa is always unremarkable, with no increase in chronic inflammation and no active colitis. However, in a small subset of patients, mild inflammatory changes such as increased intraepithelial lymphocytes can be seen. A severe acute inflammatory reaction with crypt abscesses and ulcers was reported in two patients with advanced HIV infection.[176]

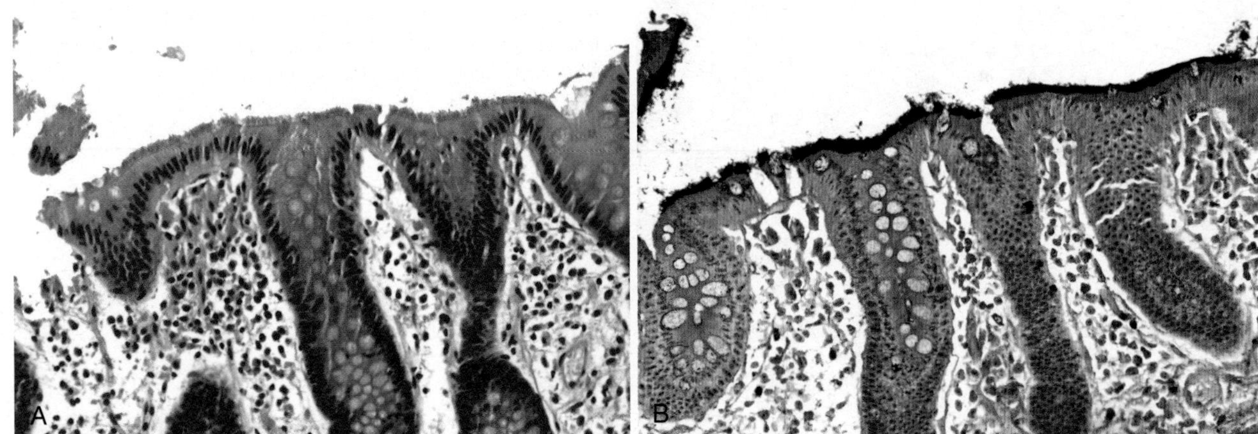

FIGURE 5.21 **A,** Intestinal spirochetosis involving the colon in human immunodeficiency virus infection is characterized by long, undulating bacteria vertically attached to the brush border, forming a bushy layer (H&E stain). **B,** Warthin-Starry stain reveals dark-brown to black spirochetes.

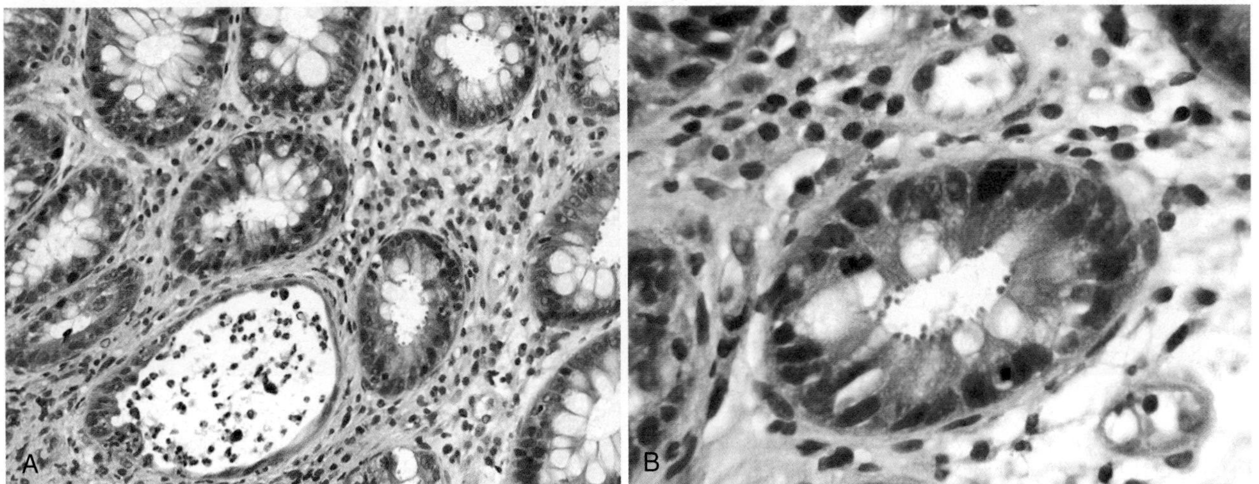

FIGURE 5.22 **A,** Cryptosporidial infection in the colon in HIV infection may produce a relatively mild acute inflammatory infiltrate, with mild cryptitis and a few crypt abscesses. **B,** The organism may be visualized on H&E-stained slides as spherical basophilic forms adherent to the luminal surface of crypt epithelial cells.

In general, no treatment is needed for asymptomatic cases, but if intestinal spirochetosis is identified as the sole intestinal pathology in a symptomatic patient, it is treated with antibiotics to eradicate the spirochetes. Metronidazole is the drug of choice.[175] Most cases treated with metronidazole show symptom improvement with eradication of the bacteria in follow-up biopsies.[173,174]

Candida is the most common HIV-associated fungal pathogen, with the esophagus the site most often involved, although the prevalence in this population is decreasing.[177] Esophageal candidiasis is characterized by white or yellow plaques with surrounding mucosal erythema endoscopically. Biopsy of the plaques reveals necroinflammatory exudates, budding yeast forms, and pseudohyphae. In HIV-infected patients, histoplasmosis is most likely to involve the ileocecal region, occasionally leading to GI bleeding, obstruction, perforation, and stricture. Intestinal mucosal biopsies reveal marked infiltration of the lamina propria by macrophages containing budding yeasts.

GI parasitic infections are uncommon in HIV-infected patients after HAART. They mainly occur in the small intestine. Infecting agents include *Cryptosporidium*, *Microsporidium*, *Isospora*, and *Giardia*. In cryptosporidiosis, the parasite inhabits the microvillous brush border of the intestinal epithelium, causing enfacement of the brush border. The intestinal epithelium may be atrophic and in disarray. A relatively mild active colitis may be seen in the colon, with cryptitis and a few crypt abscesses (Fig. 5.22). *Microsporidium* is difficult to identify on H&E-stained sections; special stains such as Giemsa may be beneficial, and electron microscopy is the gold standard for confirming the presence of the organism in the surface epithelial cells.

HIV Enteropathy

GI dysfunction, as manifested by D-xylose malabsorption, is common, even in early HIV disease. It may be a manifestation of HIV enteropathy, defined as a reduction in small bowel villous surface area associated with chronic diarrhea in the absence of enteric pathogens. The pathogenesis of HIV enteropathy is not well understood. The chronic diarrhea may be caused by an unidentified pathogen, but there

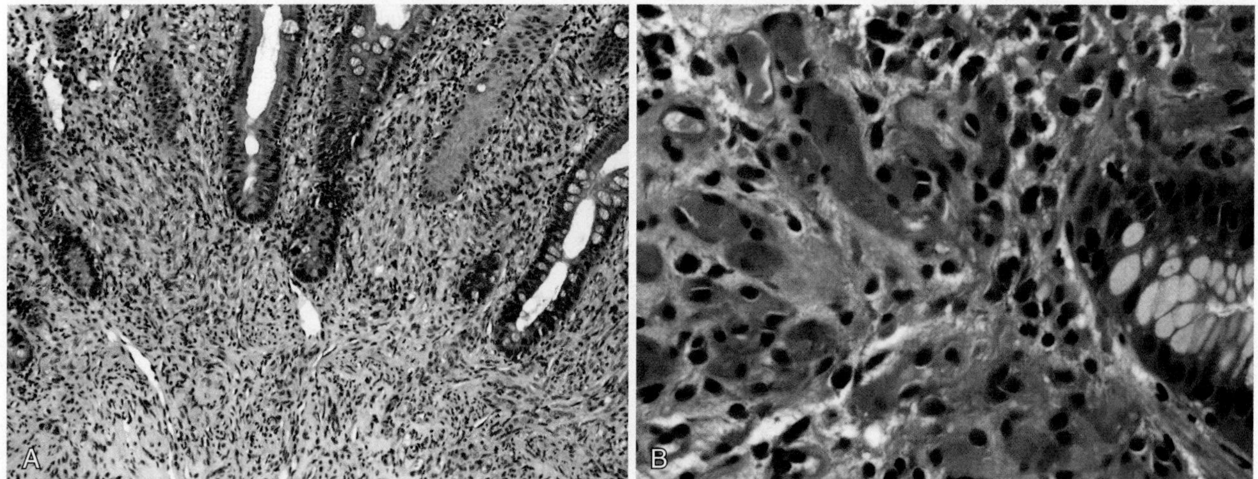

FIGURE 5.23 Kaposi's sarcoma of the colon. A, A proliferation of spindled cells in the mucosa is seen replacing the colonic crypts and muscularis mucosa. **B,** Slitlike spaces containing erythrocytes are present.

is evidence that diarrhea is directly related to local infection by the virus. Studies have shown that HIV-infected patients show improvement in clinical symptoms after initiation of HAART. Studies of intestinal permeability, epithelial cell barrier function, and cytoskeletal integrity have demonstrated changes in HIV-infected subjects after administration of antiviral agents alone.[178] These studies indicate that medications should also be considered as a cause of diarrhea in these patients, and they may account for up to 45% of noninfectious cases[179]; commonly implicated medications are nelfinavir, ritonavir, saquinavir, indinavir, and didanosine.

In small bowel biopsies, HIV enteropathy is characterized by relatively mild villous blunting without well-developed crypt hyperplasia.[180] The degree of villous atrophy is typically less than that seen in celiac disease. The histology of the colon in HIV enteropathy is less well understood. Increased epithelial cell apoptosis has been reported in association with HIV infection[181]; however, it is unclear whether this is related to the presence of the virus, other immune mediators, or antiretroviral therapy. The presence of an opportunistic pathogen, especially *Cryptosporidium, Microsporidium, Isospora,* or *Giardia* in the small intestine and *Salmonella, Shigella, Mycobacterium, Cryptosporidium, E. histolytica,* and CMV in the colon, must always be ruled out in these patients.

Malignancy

The effective use of HAART in the treatment of HIV has led to a gradual decline in infectious diseases and an increase in HIV-associated malignancies (see Table 5.6); it is estimated that about one-third of HIV-positive patients will die from cancer.[182] The most prevalent cancers in this population are Kaposi's sarcoma (KS) and AIDS-related NHL. KS is still a common HIV-associated malignancy, despite a decline in incidence since the advent of HAART. Studies have reported GI involvement in 40% of KS cases at initial presentation and in as many as 80% of cases at autopsy.[183] Endoscopically, KS appears as flat to raised, purple plaques. Microscopically, the lesion is composed of plump spindle cells, which often form fine vascular lumina containing red blood cells (Fig. 5.23). Hemosiderin and eosinophilic hyaline droplets may be present. KS is caused by human herpes virus 8 (HHV-8). Immunohistochemistry for HHV-8 is useful in confirming the diagnosis.

The AIDS-related NHL lymphomas are predominantly of B-cell lineage; the two most common subtypes in this setting are DLBCL (immunoblastic, centroblastic, and anaplastic variants) and Burkitt lymphoma[184] (Fig. 5.24), Primary effusion lymphoma (PEL), and plasmablastic lymphoma occur more specifically in HIV infection than in other immunodeficient states.[184] The GI tract is the most common site of extranodal NHL, including Burkitt lymphoma and DLBCL.[185,186] Classic PEL affects the peritoneal cavity, whereas solid PEL may be seen in extraserous sites such as large intestine and lymph nodes. Plasmablastic lymphoma has been documented in the oral cavity and anorectum.[183] The development of these HIV-associated malignancies is often attributable to co-infection by viruses such as HHV-8 (also called *Kaposi sarcoma–associated herpesvirus*) and Epstein-Barr virus. In addition to these more common HIV-associated cancers, large database studies have shown an association of HIV infection with other GI malignancies, including esophageal, gastric, colorectal, anal, and pancreatic carcinomas; hepatocellular carcinoma; and cholangiocarcinoma.[182]

The full reference list may be accessed online at Elsevier eBooks for Practicing Clinicians.

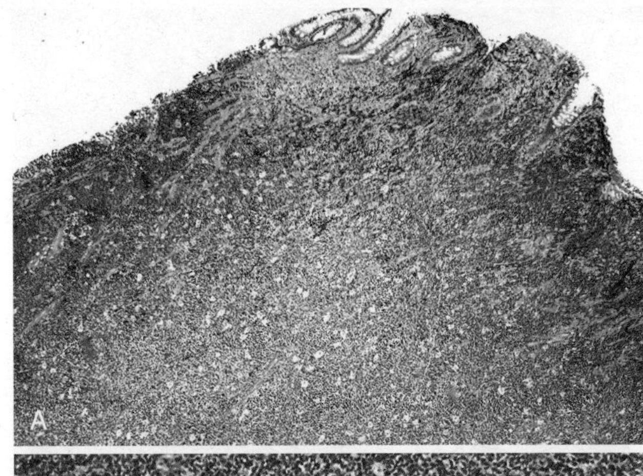

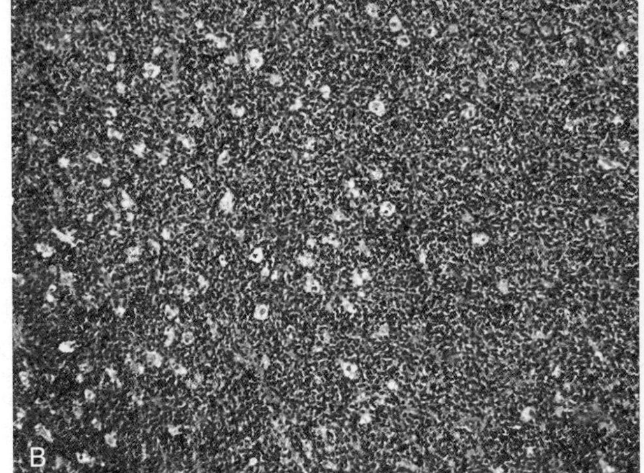

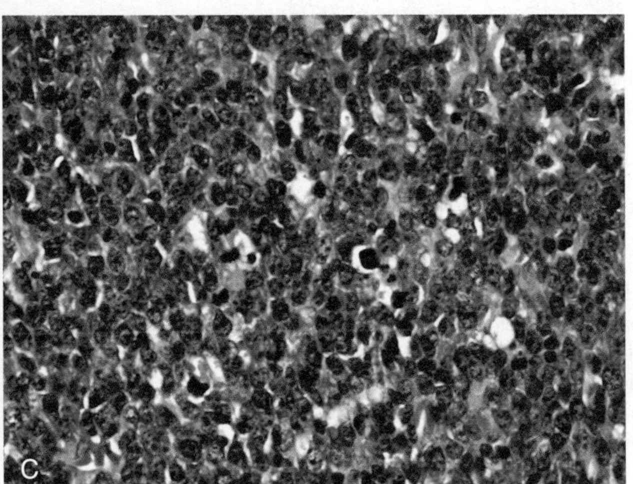

FIGURE 5.24 A–C, Burkitt lymphoma in the rectum in an HIV-infected patient. Diffusely infiltrative, atypical lymphocytes with scattered tingible body macrophages result in the characteristic "starry-sky" appearance (H&E stain).

CHAPTER 6

Autoimmune Disorders of the Gastrointestinal Tract

Vikram Deshpande

Contents

INTRODUCTION

The gastrointestinal (GI) tract is a rich lymphoid organ by virtue of the fact that there are numerous immune cells in the lamina propria as well as abundant lymphoid follicles and Peyer's patches distributed throughout, which is collectively referred to as *mucosa-associated lymphoid tissue* (MALT). Complex interactions between enterocytes, antigen-presenting cells, lymphocytes, and other elements of the immune system occur in this specialized microenvironment.

The GI mucosal immune system plays an important role in homeostasis. It is responsible for regulation of localized immune responses to the numerous antigenic substances that come into contact with the mucosa. The MALT orchestrates an immune response against pathogenic antigens (e.g., infectious microorganisms) while actively suppressing the immune response to nonpathogenic antigens (e.g., symbiotic microorganisms, food). Dysregulation of the molecular and cellular mechanisms that underlie these processes is associated with the development of multiple disease states.

Autoimmune disorders of the GI tract are commonly associated with extraintestinal manifestations, or they rarely manifest as primary gutcentric autoimmune disorders. Autoimmune disorders of the GI tract are rare if diseases such as idiopathic inflammatory bowel disease (IBD) and gluten-sensitive enteropathy (which are related to autoimmune mechanisms in some capacity) are excluded.

Several well-established autoimmune disorders, including gluten-sensitive enteropathy, autoimmune gastritis, and idiopathic IBD, are discussed in other chapters of this book.

In this chapter, two conditions that have been extensively studied during the past few years are covered in detail: autoimmune enteropathy (AIE) in its various forms and immunoglobulin G4 (IgG4)-related disease.

AUTOIMMUNE ENTEROPATHY

General Comments and Classification

AIE is an uncommon disorder with myriad clinical manifestations. It results from immune-mediated injury to the tubular gut and therefore normally responds to various degrees of immunosuppressive therapy. Although characteristic histopathological damage can be recognized, the diagnosis is best made collectively by both the pathologist and the treating physician. This requires a thoughtful review of all available clinical, endoscopic, and histological features. AIE is often misdiagnosed as celiac disease, thus the lack of response to gluten withdrawal often serves as the first clinical diagnostic clue of an inaccurate diagnosis.

AIE was first described in 1982 by Unsworth and colleagues, who reported a 15-month-old child with diarrhea, flattening of small-intestinal villi, and the presence of a circulating autoantibody to gut epithelium.[1] After recognizing six additional pediatric cases, Unsworth and Walker-Smith[2] proposed a four-point definition of AIE: protracted diarrhea and villous atrophy; no response to a gluten-free diet or total parenteral nutrition; circulating autoantibodies to gut epithelium or associated autoimmune diseases (suggesting a predisposition to autoimmunity); and exclusion of severe immunodeficiency. In 1986, Mirakian reported a series of 14 children with protracted diarrhea and evidence of autoimmunity, a condition that was described as an autoimmune variant of idiopathic protracted diarrhea of infancy.[3]

AIE occurs in adults,[4-14] but it more commonly affects infants during the first 6 months of life. The estimated incidence is less than 1 case per 100,000 infants, and it affects both sexes equally.[14] Although traditionally considered a disease of the small intestine, the entire gut, pancreas, and liver may be affected.

Two syndromic forms of AIE are recognized: immune dysregulation, polyendocrinopathy, enteropathy, and X-linked (IPEX) syndrome and autoimmune polyendocrinopathy-candidiasis-ectodermal dystrophy syndrome (APECED), also known as *autoimmune polyendocrine syndrome type 1* (APS-1). Both are monogenetic disorders caused by loss-of-function mutations in a gene that regulates T-cell development and function. The defective gene results in T-cell overactivity.

Syndromic Associations

Immune Dysregulation, Polyendocrinopathy, Enteropathy, and X-linked Syndrome

IPEX syndrome is an X-linked recessive disorder characterized by polyendocrinopathy, various autoimmune conditions, and severe, prolonged diarrhea.[15-17] IPEX syndrome is caused by germline loss-of-function mutations in the forkhead box P3 gene (*FOXP3*, located at Xp11.23-q13.3). FOXP3 is required for normal development and function of regulatory T cells, a small subset of CD4+ helper T cells of critical importance in the regulation of self-tolerance and immune homeostasis.[18] Loss of FOXP3 activity leads to immune overactivity in response to antigen stimulation and cellular injury through CD4+ effector T cells.[19]

IPEX syndrome classically manifests in early infancy with AIE, insulin-dependent diabetes mellitus, and cutaneous manifestations.[14,19] Dermatological involvement may manifest as eczema, atopic dermatitis, psoriasis, alopecia, and pemphigoid nodularis.[14,20] IPEX syndrome may have a wide array of other manifestations of autoimmunity (Box 6.1).[20,21] Patients also may have lymphadenopathy, splenomegaly, and thymic involution. [14] The prognosis is usually grim, with most patients dying within the first year of life. However, milder cases with onset later in life (≤24 years of age) have also been described.[5,22]

Autoimmune Polyglandular Syndrome Type 1

APECED syndrome (i.e., APS-1) is a rare condition that is more prevalent among Finns, Sardinians, and Iranian Jews.[23] This autosomal recessive disease is characterized by a triad of mucocutaneous candidiasis, autoimmune hypoparathyroidism, and Addison's disease, although a wide spectrum of autoimmune abnormalities may be seen.

The syndrome is caused by loss-of-function mutations in the autoimmune regulator *(AIRE)* gene (located at 21q22.3). The *AIRE* gene encodes a transcription factor that regulates expression of self-antigens in the thymus, and it is critical for deletion of self-reactive T cells.[23,24] Defects in AIRE lead to the development of T cells that recognize self-antigen, resulting in autoimmune diseases.

Affected patients are commonly diagnosed soon after birth with mucocutaneous candidiasis affecting the tongue, esophagus, and nails.[14] With time, chronic candidiasis predisposes to oral and esophageal squamous cell carcinoma.[25-27] Autoimmune hypoparathyroidism and adrenocortical failure (Addison's disease) typically develops in the first decade of the patient's life.[14] Enteropathy is diagnosed in approximately 20% of patients.[24] A wide array of other autoimmune diseases may develop (Box 6.2).[14,28] Various ectodermal abnormalities, including keratoconjunctivitis, vitiligo, alopecia, dental enamel hypoplasia, pitted nail dystrophy, and tympanic membrane calcification, may also develop.[24] Splenic atrophy or asplenia may occur.[23] Unlike IPEX syndrome, the onset of APECED syndrome is less fulminant, and the prognosis is significantly more favorable.

BOX 6.1 Diseases Associated with Immune Dysregulation, Polyendocrinopathy, Enteropathy, and X-Linked Syndrome

Thrombocytopenia
Neutropenia
Hypothyroidism
Thyroiditis
Type 1 diabetes
Lymphadenopathy
Coombs-positive hemolytic anemia
Atopic dermatitis
Pemphigoid nodularis
Arthritis
Myositis
Tubulointerstitial nephritis
Membranous glomerulonephritis

BOX 6.2 Diseases Associated with Autoimmune Polyendocrinopathy-Candidiasis-Ectodermal Dystrophy Syndrome

Candida infection
Addison's disease
Keratoconjunctivitis
Vitiligo
Alopecia
Tubulointerstitial nephritis
Hemolytic anemia
Asplenia
Type 1 diabetes
Autoimmune hepatitis
Gonadal dysfunction
Hypopituitarism
Hypoparathyroidism
Autoimmune thyroiditis
Autoimmune gastritis

Clinical Features

The clinical hallmark of AIE is refractory diarrhea, which may be accompanied by malabsorption and weight loss. In infants, low body weight and slow growth may be seen.[14] The disease affects men and women within a broad age range. In the largest series of adult AIE cases reported, most patients were white, both sexes were equally affected, and the median age at diagnosis was 55 years.[4]

This is an uncommon disease in adults, and most patients are initially misdiagnosed with celiac disease.[4] A history of autoimmune disease is obtained in up to 87% of patients.[4] Associated autoimmune conditions include hypothyroidism, rheumatoid arthritis, myasthenia gravis, idiopathic thrombocytopenic purpura, autoimmune gastritis, and

BOX 6.3 Autoantibodies Associated with Autoimmune Enteropathy

Antinuclear
Anti–liver-kidney microsomal
Anti–smooth muscle
Anti–gastric parietal cell
Anti–pancreatic islet cell
Antiinsulin
Antiendoplasmic reticulum
Antireticulin
Antigliadin
Antiadrenal cell
Antithyroglobulin
Anti–55-kDa protein in the jejunum
Antivillin
Anti–AIE-75

polyneuropathy. Another notable association, particularly in children, is the relationship with other immunodeficiency syndromes.[29] Three cases have been associated with thymoma.[12,30]

Because of the association of AIE with other autoimmune diseases, serological testing for autoantibodies is commonly positive.[5,10,14,21] Autoantibody testing was positive in up to 67% of patients in one series.[4] The antibodies, which are directed against a variety of antigens in patients' sera, include ANA, anti-LKM, anti-SMA, anti-parietal cell, and many others (Box 6.3). The relevance of gut epithelial cell antibodies is discussed later.

Other laboratory findings include normal B-lymphocyte and T-lymphocyte counts and complement levels. Some patients may have immunoglobulin A (IgA) deficiency,[4,31] but a broader immunoglobulin deficiency, especially if the albumin level is relatively normal, suggests common variable immunodeficiency (CVID), which can cause an enteropathy similar to celiac disease or AIE.

The small-intestinal endoscopic features, which include duodenal scalloping, erythema, erosions/ulcerations, fissuring, and a mosaic pattern, are generally nonspecific.[4,21] Similarly, there may be endoscopic abnormalities of the colon, including loss of vascular pattern, mucosal friability, contact bleeding, erythema, and ulceration.[13,32] Severe macroscopic colitis (including pancolitis) has been reported in patients with IPEX syndrome.[21] There may be signs and symptoms of extraintestinal involvement. Abdominal CT may reveal mesenteric lymphadenopathy.[4,5]

Serological detection of antibodies directed against the intestinal brush border, and/or detection of cytoplasm of enterocytes and goblet cells, has constituted the mainstay of serological testing for autoimmune enteropathy. In their original series, Unsworth and Walker-Smith reported antienterocyte antibodies in 5 of 6 patients,[2] and antienterocyte antibodies were detected in all 14 patients reported in two overlapping British series.[32,33] Antienterocyte antibodies are identified in 50% to 80% of patients,[4,29,34] and anti–goblet cell antibodies are seen in approximately 30% of patients.[4] However, although these tests aid in the diagnosis of AIE, it has been argued, often persuasively, that these antibodies should not be included as diagnostic criteria for AIE[29] because their direct role in epithelial injury has not been documented. Of greater concern, however, is that these antibodies are not specific (as mentioned earlier) or entirely sensitive for AIE. Antienterocyte antibodies have been noted in HIV infection, and anti–goblet cell antibodies can be detected in patients with IBD,[35] celiac disease,[36,37] autoimmune hepatitis, chronic hepatitis C virus (HCV) infection, insulin-dependent and non–insulin-dependent diabetes, and in healthy controls.[2,3,6,38] The presence of these antibodies may merely reflect epitope spreading and thus represent an epiphenomenon related to destruction of intestinal absorptive and goblet cells. Furthermore, there is no apparent correlation between antibody titer and histological severity.[38]

As a practical matter, the presence of antienterocyte and anti–goblet cell antibodies should only be evaluated in conjunction with the clinical information and the histological findings. Their absence should not necessarily exclude the diagnosis of AIE.

Pathogenesis

Although the precise molecular mechanisms underlying AIE remain unknown, the robust relationship with other immunodeficiency disorders alludes to an alteration of gut immunity as the main mechanism behind this disorder.[16] The intestinal mucosa is a site of complex interactions between the immune system and the environment, including dietary antigens and gut microflora.[14]

The expression of HLA class II molecules, a key component of T-cell activation, is usually restricted to cells of the immune system, where they mediate antigen presentation and induction of the immune response. Although epithelial cells generally do not express HLA class II molecules, mature enterocytes at the tips of small-intestinal villi are an exception in that they constitutively express these molecules under normal physiological conditions and present antigens to autologous CD4+ helper T cells. Antigen presentation by enterocytes could, theoretically, suppress T-cell activity, which presumably allows for tolerance to dietary antigens encountered by small-intestinal epithelium, a phenomenon referred to as *oral tolerance*.

In contrast, enterocytes of AIE patients exhibit aberrant expression of HLA class II molecules, with inappropriate expression of HLA-DR in crypt enterocytes.[31-33,39-41] It has been hypothesized that aberrant HLA class II expression by crypt enterocytes induces CD4+ T-cell overactivity and subsequent T-cell–mediated injury of the intestinal epithelium through direct cytotoxicity or cytokine secretion.[29,31,41] Increased numbers of CD25+ T cells have been documented in small-intestinal biopsies of AIE patie nts,[11,31,41] and CD25+ T cells regressed with therapy in at least one case.[41] Enterocyte injury by overactive T cells is emerging as a possible unifying mechanism to explain AIE.

Pathological Features

The small intestine appears to be the primary organ involved in AIE and the focus of most histological descriptions. However, it is becoming increasingly clear that the disease is rarely restricted to the small bowel because involvement of the stomach and colon are also commonly reported.

Small Intestine

The pathological features of AIE vary, but some patterns of injury may be considered characteristic, particularly in the duodenum, ileum, and jejunum.[11,13,33,42,43] Small-intestinal

AIE can be largely grouped into three general histological patterns: (1) chronic active enteritis, (2) celiac disease–like pattern, and (3) graft-versus-host disease (GVHD)-like pattern. Biopsies that show multiple histological patterns are not uncommon. Although these patterns do not correlate with a specific disease phenotype, they are conceptually useful for the pathologist in generating a differential diagnosis.

The chronic active enteritis pattern is the most common pattern of injury. It consists of a lymphoplasmacytic inflammatory infiltrate with moderate to severe villous blunting and crypt hyperplasia (Fig. 6.1).[44] Neutrophilic inflammation may be prominent and sometimes occurs with crypt abscesses.[45] Apoptosis may be present. Surface erosions and gastric foveolar metaplasia may be present. Eosinophils are typically seen but are not prominent.

The celiac disease pattern features increased intraepithelial lymphocytes, and villous blunting, and may be histologically indistinguishable from celiac disease (Fig. 6.2). The GVHD pattern features increased apoptosis in crypt epithelium with a relative absence of inflammation, similar to acute GVHD. Apoptosis may be a striking feature in terms of the number of cells affected, and partial or total glandular destruction may be present.[21] Other nonspecific reactive or regenerative epithelial changes include mucin depletion, crypt architectural irregularity, and increased mitotic activity.

In addition to the findings noted earlier, small-bowel biopsies may also show loss of multiple cell lineages, including goblet cells, endocrine cells, and Paneth cells (see Fig. 6.2).[4,5,31,46-48] In one study, loss of neuroendocrine cells in the intestinal crypts was observed in 78% of small-bowel and/or colon biopsies in AIE patients; occasional loss (9%) was observed in CVID patients, while neuroendocrine cell density was intact in patients with IBD and IgA deficiency. In this study, loss of goblet cells occurred in 89% of cases, whereas loss of Paneth cells occurred in 78%.[46] In some cases, the absence of goblet cells in biopsies coincided with detection of anti–goblet cell antibodies.[32] An absence of plasma cells in the lamina propria may be an indication of concurrent CVID.[4]

In our experience, the features most helpful in suggesting a diagnosis of AIE are villous blunting, lamina propria expansion by mixed but predominantly mononuclear inflammation, neutrophilic activity, patchy increase in intraepithelial lymphocytes, and loss of one of more cell lineages, most often endocrine and goblet cells.

Colon. Colonic involvement has been reported in a relatively large number of cases.[4,5,8,9] It affects most patients

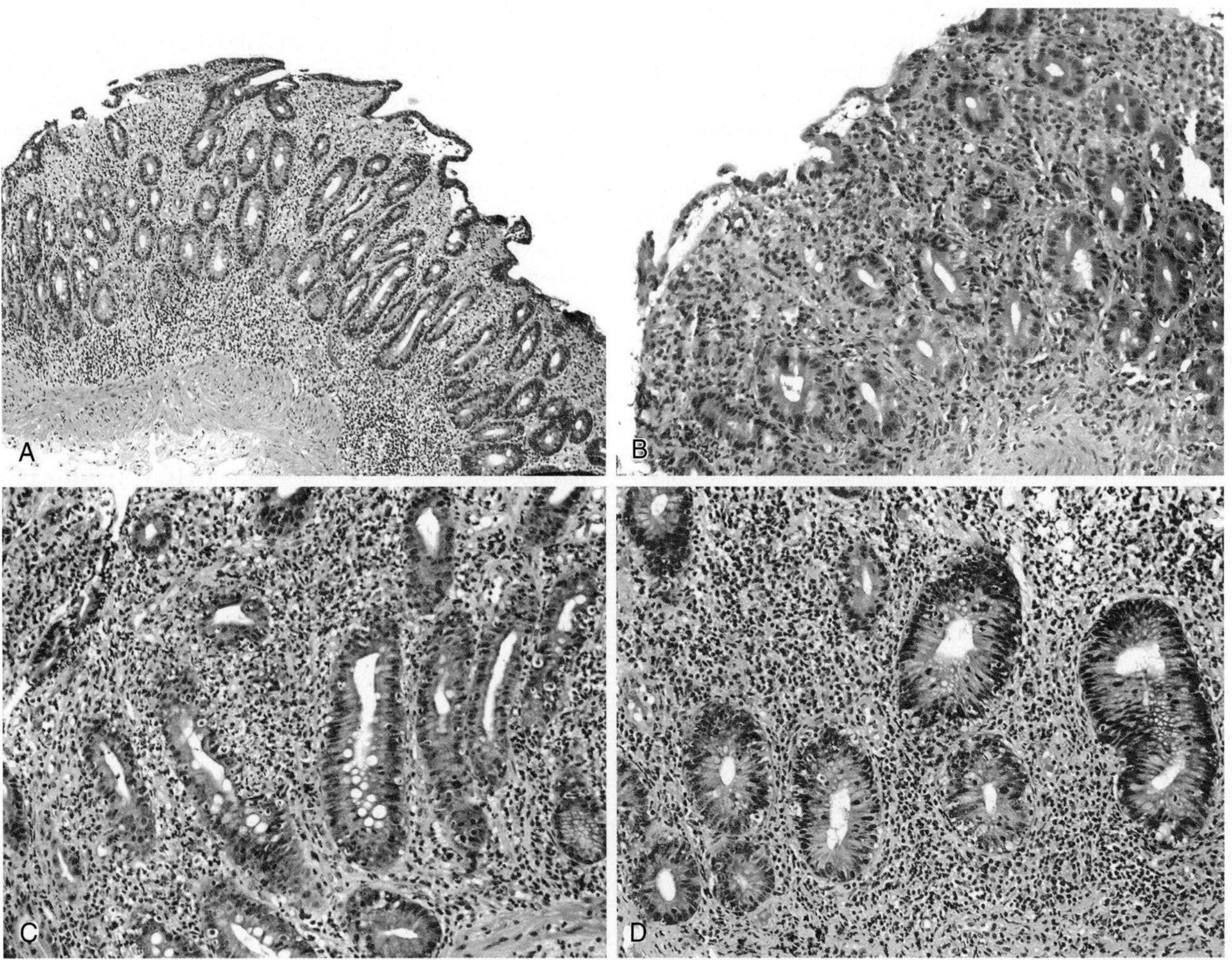

FIGURE 6.1 Histopathological features of autoimmune enteropathy involving the duodenum. A, The duodenal mucosa typically exhibits chronic active enteritis with prominent villous blunting. **B,** The duodenal mucosa shows blunting and severe epithelial injury. **C,** A mixed, predominantly lymphoplasmacytic inflammatory infiltrate and neutrophilic cryptitis are seen within the lamina propria. The amount of crypt epithelial cell apoptosis varies, but apoptotic cells are often readily identifiable. Paneth cells and goblet cells may be decreased in numbers or entirely absent. **D,** Apoptosis may be prominent in some cases, imparting an appearance reminiscent of acute graft-versus-host disease.

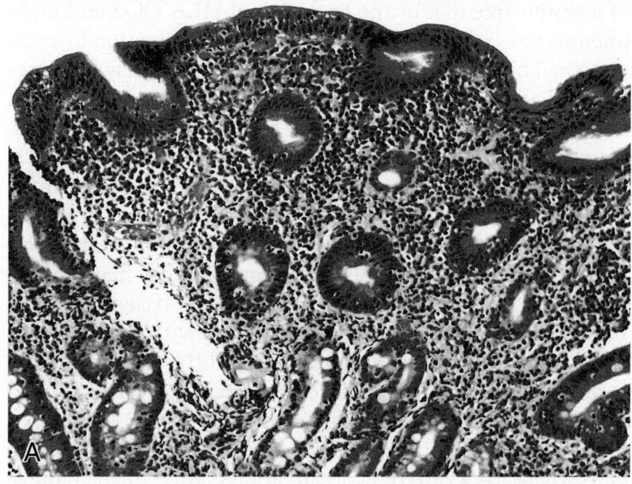

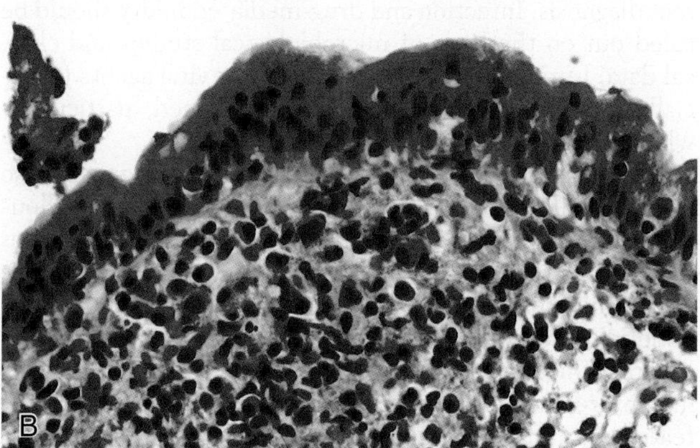

FIGURE 6.2 Autoimmune enteropathy (AIE) with celiac disease–like features. A and **B,** In some instances, AIE may exhibit histopathological features that are indistinguishable from celiac disease. The duodenal biopsy exhibits total villous blunting with crypt hyperplasia, lymphoplasmacytic expansion of the lamina propria, and markedly increased intraepithelial lymphocytes in surface epithelium.

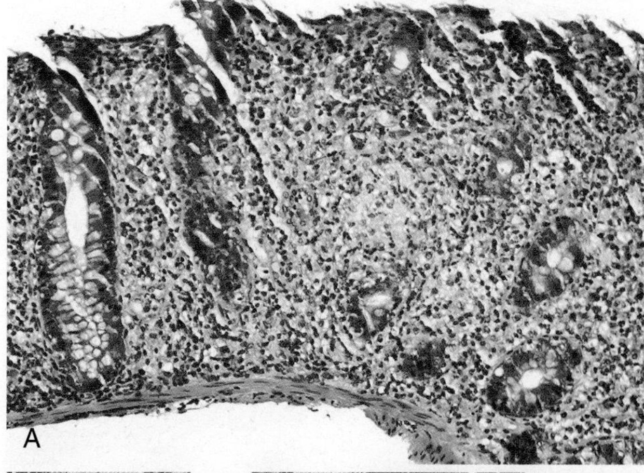

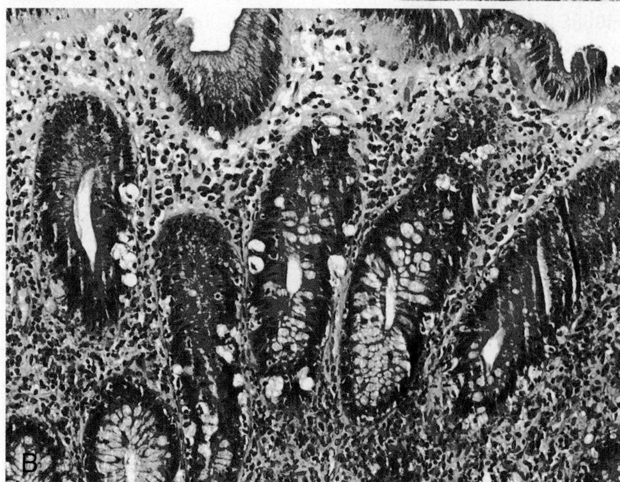

FIGURE 6.3 Autoimmune enteropathy involving the colon. A, Colonic biopsies may exhibit a mixed, predominantly lymphoplasmacytic inflammatory infiltrate within the lamina propria, along with associated neutrophilic cryptitis and crypt injury. **B,** As in the small intestine, crypt epithelial cell apoptosis may be striking, mimicking acute graft-versus-host disease.

with AIE and IPEX syndrome. Histological features include lymphoplasmacytic expansion of the lamina propria; neutrophilic cryptitis, either with or without crypt abscesses; and increased apoptosis in crypt epithelium (Fig. 6.3).[4,21,32] Increased apoptosis may be striking, and the predominant feature may be reminiscent of acute GVHD (Fig. 6.4).[11]

Colonic biopsies may exhibit features that are not immediately identifiable as AIE, such as severe colitis with crypt destruction, pyloric metaplasia, and/or crypt atrophy.[21,32] A lymphocyte-predominant pattern of inflammation that is indistinguishable from lymphocytic colitis may be present as well.[31] One case with thickening of the subepithelial collagen layer in the duodenal mucosa and in the entire colorectal mucosa, which was indistinguishable from collagenous colitis, has also been reported.[49] In our experience, colonic involvement may also be reminiscent of IBD, with crypt architectural irregularities, multinucleated epithelioid giant cells, and Paneth cell metaplasia. However, the full-blown histological features of active chronic colitis of the IBD type are not seen.

Gastric Involvement

Involvement of the stomach may occur in the form of moderate to severe gastritis with expansion of the lamina propria, neutrophils, and apoptotic activity (Fig. 6.5).[4,8,13,21,34] Active gastritis with glandular destruction has been reported.[11] A lymphocytic gastritis-like pattern has also been reported. Some patients exhibit a peculiar form of atrophic gastritis that resembles autoimmune atrophic gastritis but involves the entire stomach and lacks neuroendocrine cell hyperplasia, distinguishing this disease from autoimmune gastritis.[50] In our experience, the stomach may also exhibit an acute GVHD-like appearance, with near-normal mucosa with increased apoptosis in glandular epithelium, with or without glandular atrophy.

Esophagus

The esophagus may show inflammatory infiltrates,[41] and severe ulcerative esophagitis has been reported in one case.[31] We have seen patients with a mild neutrophilic esophagitis and occasional apoptotic cells.

Liver and Pancreas

Chronic sclerosing cholangitis has been reported in patients with elevated transaminase and alkaline phosphatase levels and liver biopsies showing portal mononuclear inflammation and fibrosis.[11,31] Hepatitis with fibrosis has been described in several cases.[41,51,52] Involvement of the exocrine pancreas

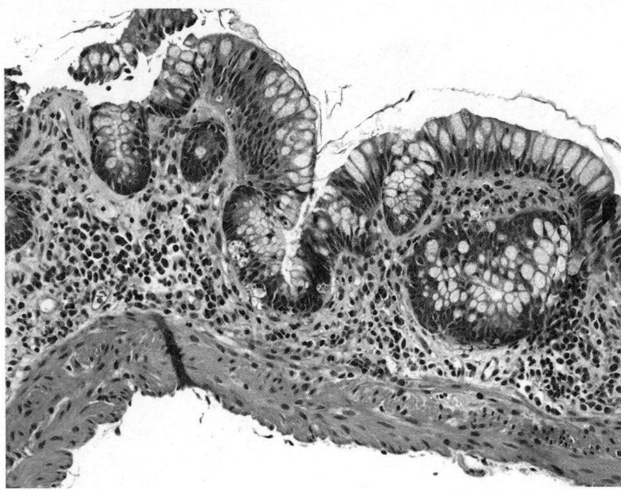

FIGURE 6.4 Autoimmune enteropathy involving the colon. Biopsy shows a marked increase in apoptosis.

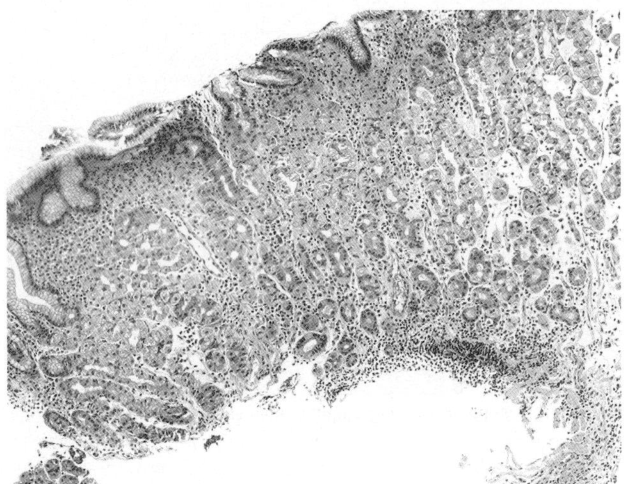

FIGURE 6.5 Autoimmune enteropathy involving the stomach. Stomach biopsies may exhibit various degrees of inflammation. This biopsy of the gastric body shows chronic gastritis involving both superficial and deep portions of the mucosa.

may manifest clinically as elevation of amylase and lipase levels or as evidence of pancreatic exocrine insufficiency.[8,15,53] Histological examination shows various degrees of lymphocytic inflammation.[15,41,51,53] The inflammation may be duct centric and associated with squamous metaplasia of the pancreatic ducts.[41] In one case, postmortem examination revealed marked atrophy of the exocrine pancreas with greatly diminished content of zymogen granules.[53]

Differential Diagnosis

A diagnosis of AIE requires exclusion of celiac disease. This distinction may be difficult in a subset of AIE patients with histological features that mimic celiac disease (see Fig. 6.4) and with positive celiac serology, which may be found in up to 33% of AIE patients. One particularly problematic aspect is that these patients may meet the diagnostic criteria for refractory sprue by virtue of positive celiac serology, but they do not respond to a gluten-free diet.[4] In this setting, awareness of additional clinical, laboratory, and pathological features of AIE may be essential to arrive at the correct diagnosis, despite the problematic aspects of antibody testing. In some cases, exclusion of celiac disease may necessitate trial of a gluten-free diet or the exclusion of HLA DQ2 and DQ8 phenotypes.[10] Significant neutrophilic inflammation in small intestinal biopsies, particularly crypt abscesses, may help suggest a diagnosis of AIE rather than celiac disease. Although neutrophilic inflammation may be seen in some cases of celiac disease, they are rare, occurring in less than 1% of cases.[54]

The spectrum of small intestinal disease resulting in chronic diarrhea is wide and also includes tropical sprue, Whipple's disease, CVID, IBD, and drug-induced enteropathy.[55] Checkpoint inhibitor enteropathy may mimic AIE, with both anti-PD1 and anti-CTLA4–based therapies showing histological features that overlap with AIE.[56] Other drugs that should be considered in the differential diagnosis include olmesartan (an angiotensin II receptor blocker) and idelalisib (a phosphoinositide 3-kinase inhibitor).[57]

Although the differential diagnosis of a chronic active enteritis pattern of AIE is broad, appreciation of the clinical setting combined with detection of involvement of multiple sites in the gut should allow pathologists to suspect the correct diagnosis. Infection and drug-mediated injury should be ruled out on the basis of microbiological studies and clinical data. Immunohistochemical stains for viral agents (especially cytomegalovirus) should be performed, particularly when apoptosis is prominent.

In pediatric patients, the differential diagnosis also includes allergic enteropathy, which may cause villous blunting and involve multiple sites in the GI tract as well. Allergic enteropathy, however, should exhibit an eosinophilic-predominant inflammatory infiltrate.[45] Immunodeficiencies should also be considered. Other pediatric enteropathies, such as microvillus inclusion disease and tufting enteropathy, should be considered, but they classically feature minimal inflammation in biopsies.[45,58]

Histological evaluation of upper and lower endoscopic samples in an attempt to identify the multiple sites of involvement is often diagnostically helpful. However, involvement of multiple sites may bring into question the possibility of IBD as well as checkpoint inhibitors.[56] This may also be the case when neutrophilic inflammation is prominent, with numerous crypt abscesses, or when some features of chronicity (e.g., Paneth cell metaplasia in the distal colon) are identified. In our experience, other pathological features of chronic IBD, such as basal lymphoplasmacytosis, pseudopyloric gland metaplasia, or significant crypt architectural disarray, are not normally seen in AIE. Similarly, granulomas have not been reported in AIE. Assessment of the presence and numbers of endocrine cells, goblet cells, and Paneth cells is helpful because markedly decreased numbers or absence of one of these cells favors a diagnosis of AIE.

Treatment and Prognosis

Immunomodulation remains the mainstay of therapy for AIE patients. High-dose steroids are often needed at the time of presentation to control the patient's diarrhea. Total parenteral nutrition often is needed.[5,28] However, limited response to therapy is common. Many patients require prolonged steroid therapy or subsequent treatment with an immunomodulator (e.g., cyclophosphamide, azathioprine, 6-mercaptopurine, infliximab).[4,28] In one recent study 85% of patients showed a clinical response to budesonide.[55] The prognosis varies and depends on the severity of symptoms, the severity of intestinal damage, and the extent of extraintestinal manifestations.[14] Bone marrow transplantation may be used in patients who do not respond to immunosuppression.[28]

In some patients, pathological findings may significantly improve with therapy[10,31,41,44] or completely resolve,[4] although it appears that this situation is less common than persistence of pathological findings. In some cases, the persistent inflammation may be predominantly eosinophilic.[45] Significant histological improvement may be seen in the absence of clinical improvement,[31] which is a caveat for the role of serial biopsies in the assessment of severity of disease or response to treatment.

It is difficult to ascertain whether patients are at increased risk for neoplasia. However, one case of enteropathy-associated T-cell lymphoma that developed in an adult AIE patient has been described.[59] One case of a diffuse large B-cell lymphoma developing in a patient with IPEX syndrome has also been reported.[60]

IMMUNOGLOBULIN G4–RELATED DISEASE OF THE GASTROINTESTINAL TRACT

IgG4-related disease is a multisystem, mass-forming, inflammatory disorder that often mimics a neoplasm.[61-63] IgG4-related disease has been misclassified in the past, and it is often misinterpreted as a nonspecific inflammatory disorder.[64] Diseases as seemingly diverse as autoimmune pancreatitis, sclerosing cholangitis, retroperitoneal fibrosis, and inflammatory pseudotumor are now believed to be part of the IgG4-related disease spectrum.[61-63,65] Widespread recognition of the disease has, unfortunately, also resulted in overdiagnosis of IgG4-related disease, an error often triggered by excessive reliance on increased numbers of IgG4-positive cells for the diagnosis. Increased numbers of IgG4-positive cells are seen in a diverse set of diseases, one that includes other inflammatory diseases as well as neoplasms. IgG4-related disease most frequently involves the pancreatobiliary system, and although involvement of the tubular gut has been documented, clinically significant disease at this site is uncommon. The hepatic and pancreatic manifestations are discussed in detail in Chapters 40 and 48.

General Comments and Criteria

Although IgG4-related disease affects a wide range of organs and its manifestations are often protean, many aspects suggest a single cohesive entity: tumefactive lesions that mimic malignancy, synchronous or metachronous involvement of a relatively constant group of organs, elevated serum IgG4 levels, characteristic histological appearance, elevated numbers of IgG4-positive plasma cells, and elevated IgG4/IgG ratio.[61-63]

There is no single feature that is pathognomonic of this disease. Instead, a diagnosis of IgG4-related disease requires a multimodal approach that includes: (1) imaging findings, (2) elevated serum IgG4 level, (3) multiple organ involvement, (4) favorable response to immunosuppressive therapy, and (5) histological features.

Elevated Serum Immunoglobulin G4 Level

The frequency of elevated serum IgG4 levels is approximately 70%.[66] An elevated serum IgG4 level, although characteristic of IgG4-related disease, unfortunately also occurs in a variety of other diseases, including neoplastic disorders.[67] Nonetheless, in a patient with characteristic clinical and radiological features, an elevated serum IgG4 level supports a diagnosis of IgG4-related disease. Higher serum levels are more specific for IgG4-related disease; >4 times normal levels is highly suggestive of IgG4-related disease.[68] A normal serum IgG4 level, however, does not exclude a diagnosis of IgG4-related disease. Approximately 20% to 30% of patients, typically those with disease isolated to a single organ, will lack an elevated serum IgG4 level.

Multiple Organ Involvement

Synchronous or metachronous tumefactive enlargement of multiple organs, particularly those frequently affected by this condition, strongly suggests IgG4-related disease. For example, enlarged submandibular salivary glands in a patient suspected to have autoimmune pancreatitis is strongly indicative of the latter disease. Histological evaluation of the gland may show classic features of IgG4-related sialadenitis (i.e., IgG4-related disease of the salivary gland) and may avoid an invasive pancreatic biopsy.[69-71] Similarly, IgG4-related sclerosing cholangitis is frequently associated with autoimmune pancreatitis.[72,73]

Response to Immunosuppressive Therapy

IgG4-related disease shows a swift response to immunosuppressive therapy, with a dramatic decrease in size of the mass and normalization of pancreatic and bile duct strictures in patients with pancreatobiliary manifestations.[74] The absence of a swift response to steroids should prompt reevaluation of the diagnosis, especially to rule out a malignant process.

Pathological Features

Histologically, the disease is characterized by the presence of a dense lymphoplasmacytic infiltrate (Fig. 6.6), dense fibrosis that is invariably arranged in a storiform pattern (see Fig. 6.6), and obliterative phlebitis (Fig. 6.7).[61,62,64] A definitive diagnosis of IgG4-related disease requires at least two of these three features. Although it is the least common feature, obliterative phlebitis is a unique facet of this disease. Medium-sized veins are involved, and the lumen is typically obliterated by a lymphoplasmacytic infiltrate. Occasionally, obliterated arterial channels are also identified.[75]

In addition to the characteristic morphological appearance, a definitive diagnosis of IgG4-related disease requires elevated numbers of IgG4-positive plasma cells (Fig. 6.8). An IgG4/IgG ratio of more than 40% provides additional support of the diagnosis.[61,62,64]

A diagnosis of IgG4-related disease requires a thoughtful review of clinical, radiological, and serological data (specifically serum IgG4) as well as evaluation of all available biopsies. The full spectrum of histological features is often seen on a resection specimen; biopsies may lack storiform fibrosis and/or obliterative phlebitis.[76] Furthermore, an increase in IgG4-positive cells may be patchy, thus a biopsy may not capture foci with the highest number of cells. Finally, increased numbers of IgG4-positive cells are seen in a range of inflammatory and neoplastic diseases. Although elevated numbers of IgG4-positive plasma cells are detected in mucosal biopsies of patients with IgG4-related disease, the involvement is not usually clinically apparent.

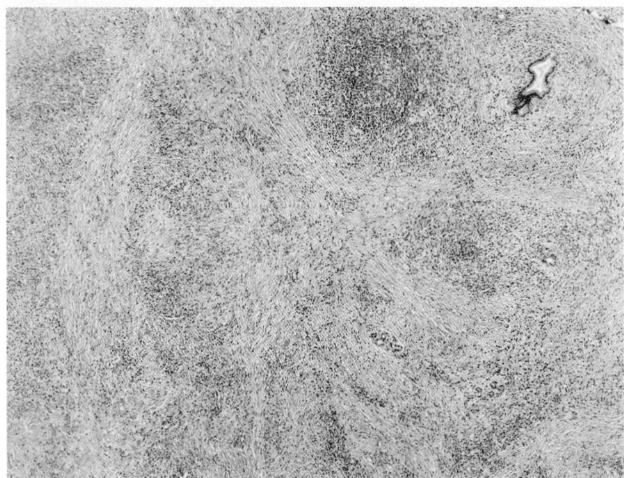

FIGURE 6.6 Immunoglobulin G4–related disease of the pancreas. Low-power view demonstrates the characteristic storiform type of fibrosis seen in this disease. Notice the single duct.

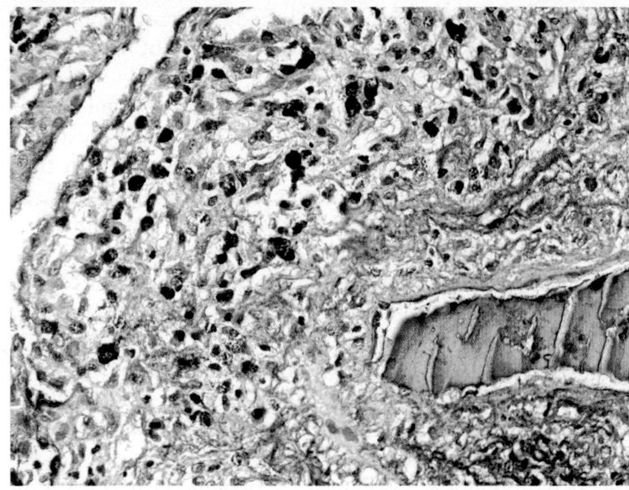

FIGURE 6.8 Immunoglobulin G4 (IgG4)-related disease. The immunohistochemical stain for IgG4 shows elevated numbers of IgG4-positive plasma cells adjacent to a focus of obliterative phlebitis. An unambiguous diagnosis of IgG4-related disease requires elevated numbers of IgG4-bearing plasma cells.

These caveats often preclude an unequivocal diagnosis of IgG4-related disease based solely on needle biopsies. When only some of the histological and/or immunohistochemical features of IgG4-related disease are present, one pragmatic approach would be to provide a descriptive diagnosis, one that raises the possibility of IgG4-related disease. This approach should prompt further investigation for IgG4-related disease and would circumvent the many pitfalls associated with this diagnosis. The ultimate diagnosis of IgG4-related disease rests on a deliberate and comprehensive analysis of all available clinical, radiological, serological, and biopsy material. [66] More recently, these features have been codified into classification criteria for IgG4-related disease, and these features may also assist in the diagnosis.[66]

Stomach

IgG4-related gastropathy has been described only in the context of autoimmune pancreatitis, thus data are lacking on gastric manifestations in patients with systemic IgG4-related disease. The endoscopic features are nonspecific, although chronic gastric ulceration has been reported.[77,78]

The corpus and antral mucosa may show a diffuse transmucosal lymphoplasmacytic infiltrate, a pattern reminiscent of *Helicobacter pylori* gastritis.[77] However, unlike active *H. pylori* gastritis, neutrophils are uncommon. A deep mucosal lymphoplasmacytic infiltrate is also typical of IgG4-related gastropathy (Fig. 6.9). However, IgG4-positive plasma cells are usually easily found, whereas they are absent in *H. pylori* gastritis.[79] IgG4-related gastropathy may also resemble autoimmune gastritis; however, unlike autoimmune gastritis, the antrum is not usually spared. Notably, IgG4-positive plasma cells (>10/high-power field [HPF]) are identified in autoimmune gastritis, although they are absent in other forms of chronic atrophic gastritis and in *H. pylori* gastritis.[79]

Rarely, IgG4-related disease can form a gastric mass and even mimic a gastrointestinal stromal tumor[80]; diffuse

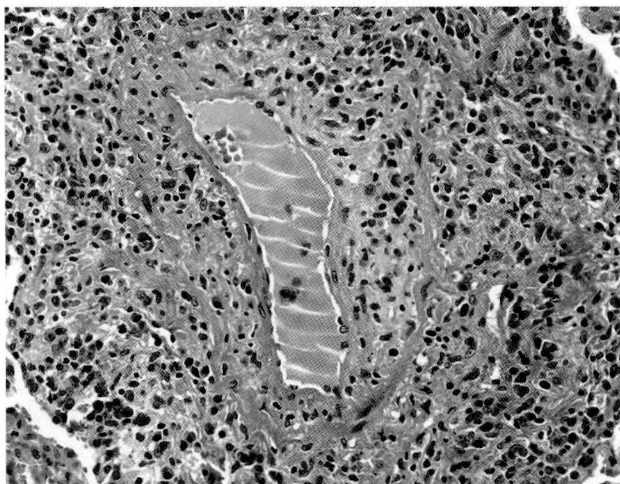

FIGURE 6.7 Focus of obliterative phlebitis in immunoglobulin G4–related disease. The lumen is partially obliterated by a dense lymphoplasmacytic infiltrate.

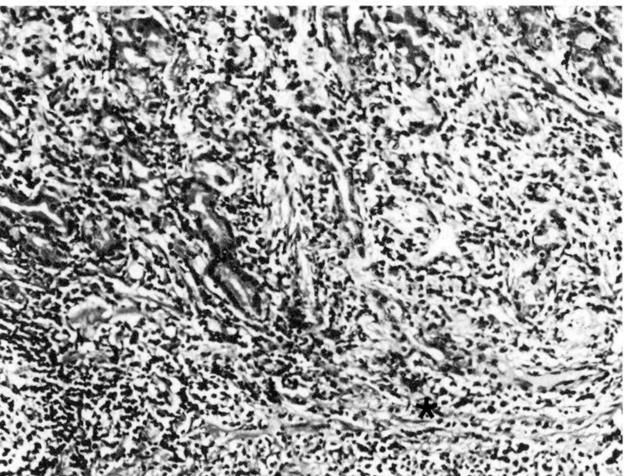

FIGURE 6.9 Immunoglobulin G4 (IgG4)-related gastropathy. The lower half of the gastric mucosa is shown. Note the dense lymphoplasmacytic infiltrate. Immunohistochemical stain *(not shown)* revealed more than 100 IgG4-positive plasma cells per high-power field. *Asterisk* indicates muscularis mucosae.

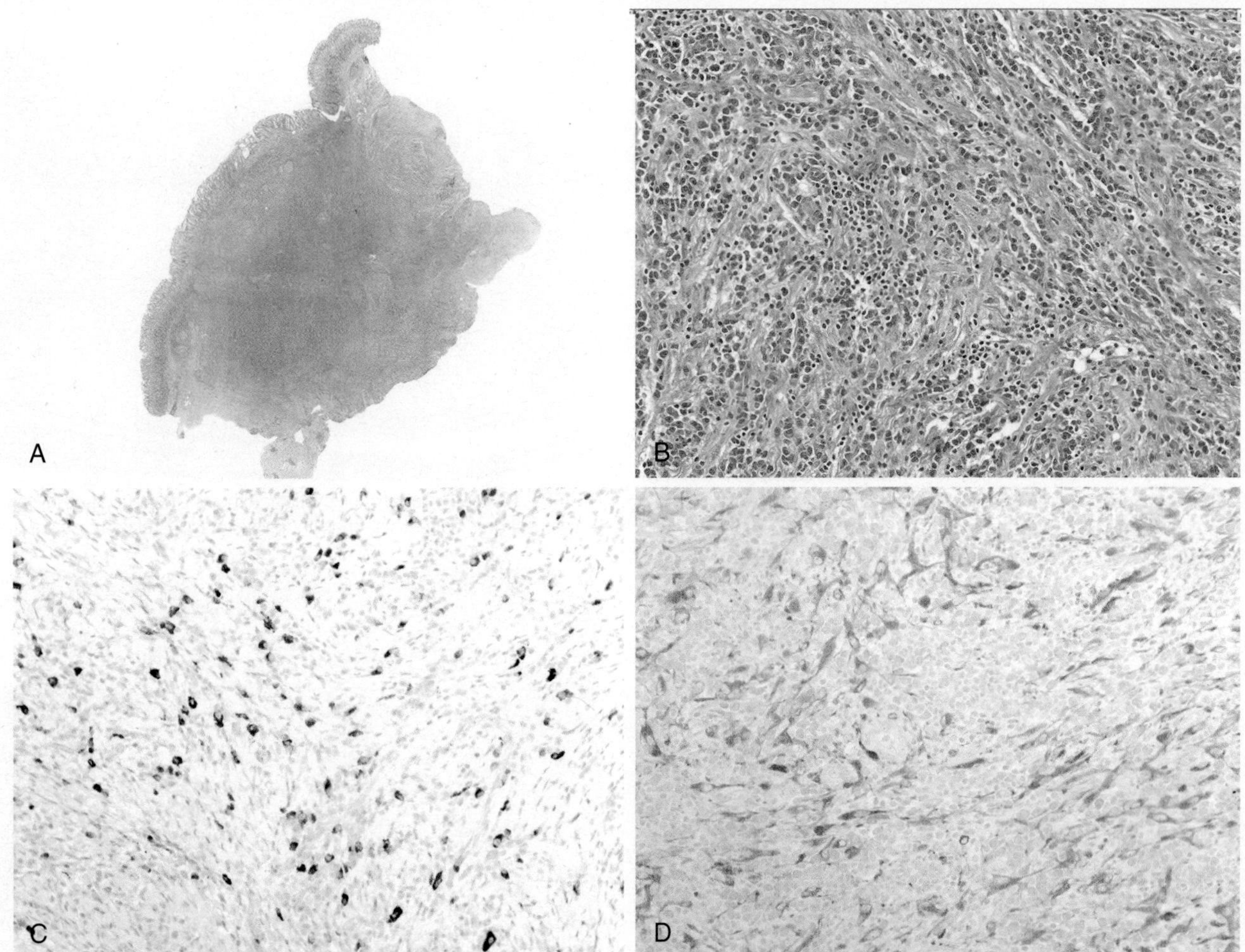

FIGURE 6.10 Gastric inflammatory myofibroblastic tumor mimicking IgG4-related disease. A, Submucosal gastric lesion. **B,** Dense fibroinflammatory infiltrate with numerous plasma cells. The neoplastic spindle cells are inconspicuous and show only mild atypia. **C,** Immunohistochemical stain for IgG4 shows a marked increase in IgG4-positive cells. **D,** Immunohistochemical stain for anaplastic lymphoma kinase (ALK) shows that the stromal cells are diffusely and strongly positive for ALK.

thickening of the gastric wall has also been described.[81,82] However, inflammatory myofibroblastic tumors may closely mimic gastric mass–forming IgG4-related disease (Fig. 6.10).

Ampulla

A biopsy from the ampullary region may assist in differentiating autoimmune pancreatitis from pancreatic carcinoma and in discerning IgG4-related sclerosing cholangitis (a steroid-responsive disease) from primary sclerosing cholangitis. A more detailed discussion is provided in Chapter 40.

Small Bowel and Colon

Involvement of the lower gut is extremely uncommon. When seen in isolation, the finding of elevated numbers of IgG4-positive plasma cells at these locations is more likely to represent one of the myriad of diseases associated with elevated numbers of IgG4-positive cells, such as IBD.[83] Nevertheless, there have been several reports of IgG4-related disease involving the small bowel and colon.[84-87] Histologically, these case reports describe varying degrees of ulceration, transmural inflammation, and obliterative phlebitis and arteritis (Figs. 6.11 and 6.12).[84-86] A diagnosis of IgG4-related enteritis or colitis has relied on elevated numbers of IgG4-positive cells and an elevated IgG4/IgG ratio. It is notable that the disease as documented in these reports lacks many features that would normally support its inclusion in the IgG4 spectrum; specifically, the disease is confined to the bowel, and these patients lacked systemic involvement. In practice, when confronted with small bowel or colonic disease showing histological features of IgG4-related disease combined with elevated numbers of IgG4-positive cells, it would be prudent to exclude a diagnosis of IBD. These features should also prompt a careful analysis to exclude mimics of IgG4-related disease, including inflammatory myofibroblastic tumor and infections such as syphilis.[88,89] Both IBD and infections (e.g., syphilis) may be associated with increased numbers of IgG4-positive cells, figures that exceed the threshold set for IgG4-related disease.[88,89]

Nodular lesions composed of inflamed, but paucicellular, hyalinized fibrous tissue associated with an increase in IgG4-positive cells have been described in the bowel.[87] Although their fibroinflammatory nature resembles IgG4-related disease, it remains unclear if these lesions belong to the spectrum of IgG4-related disease or comprise a unique type of fibroinflammatory disease.[87]

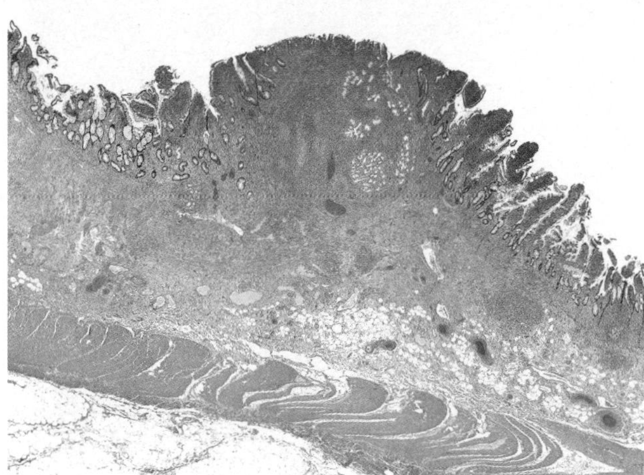

FIGURE 6.11 Small bowel with a dense mucosal and focally submucosal inflammatory infiltrate. Note the pyloric-type metaplasia. The immunohistochemical stain for IgG4 is shown in Fig. 6.12.

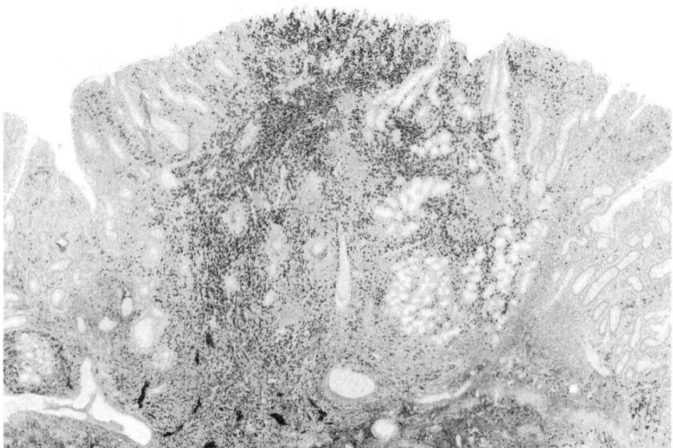

FIGURE 6.12 Immunohistochemical stain for IgG4 performed on the case illustrated in Fig. 6.11 shows a marked increase in IgG4-positive cells. Although this finding raised the possibility of IgG4-related disease, the lack of storiform fibrosis, obliterative phlebitis, elevated serum IgG4, and lack of systemic disease argued against a diagnosis of IgG4-related disease. The underlying cause of the small bowel strictures remains unclear.

Gallbladder

Gallbladder involvement by IgG4-related disease is typically asymptomatic. Nevertheless, examination of the gallbladder may offer diagnostically useful information to support a diagnosis of IgG4-related disease.[90-92] Occasionally, IgG4-related cholecystitis may be mistaken for gallbladder carcinoma on imaging.[93]

Grossly, the gallbladder may be appreciably thickened and fibrotic. Histologically, there is a transmural inflammatory infiltrate with significant involvement of the subserosal tissue, which occasionally forms circumscribed inflammatory nodules (Figs. 6.13 and 6.14).[90] Unlike most forms of cholecystitis, the subserosal infiltrate is significantly more prominent than mucosal-based inflammation. Obliterative phlebitis is frequently identified within the subserosal tissue (see Figs. 6.13 and 6.14). A marked increase in IgG4-positive plasma cells is normally found in both the mucosal compartment and in the subserosal infiltrate. The latter two findings are important to rule out other inflammatory diseases of the gallbladder, including lymphoplasmacytic cholecystitis. Elevated numbers of IgG4 cells have also been reported in xanthogranulomatous cholecystitis and hyalinizing cholecystitis; neither disease is believed to be associated with IgG4-related disease.[94,95]

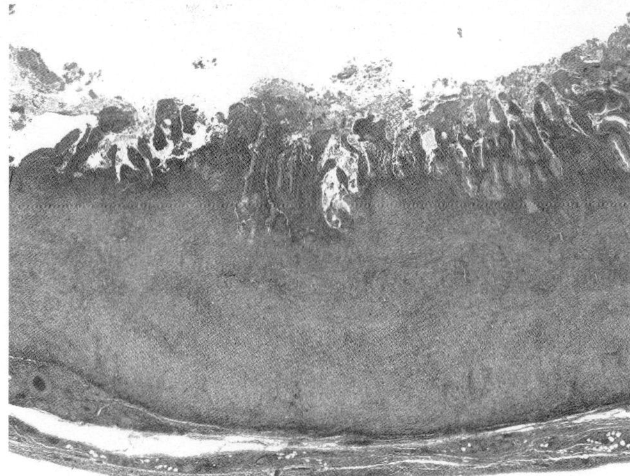

FIGURE 6.13 IgG4-related cholecystitis. Although the mucosa is involved, the serosal dominance is strongly indicative of IgG4-related disease.

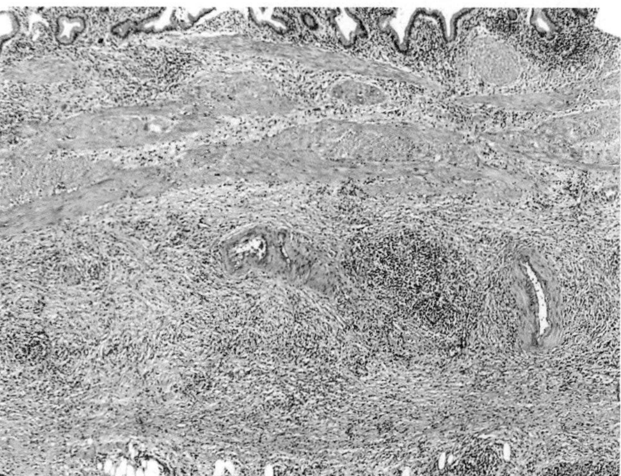

FIGURE 6.14 Immunoglobulin G4–related cholecystitis. The gallbladder shows a dense mucosal- and serosal-based inflammatory infiltrate. The subserosal infiltrate forms a poorly defined inflammatory mass lesion.

Retroperitoneum and Mesentery

Retroperitoneal fibrosis is one of the prototypic manifestations of IgG4-related disease, although IgG4-related disease is likely responsible for only approximately 50% of these cases.[96] Cases of retroperitoneal fibrosis that do not meet the definition for IgG4-related disease continue to be referred to as *idiopathic retroperitoneal fibrosis*.[96] Histological features of IgG4-related retroperitoneal fibrosis include a diffuse lymphoplasmacytic infiltrate that is rich in IgG4-positive plasma cells, fibrosis arranged in a storiform pattern, moderate tissue eosinophilia, and partially or completely obliterated veins (Figs. 6.15 to 6.17).[65,96] However, this classic morphological spectrum may not be represented in a core biopsy.[76] The disease is often long-standing

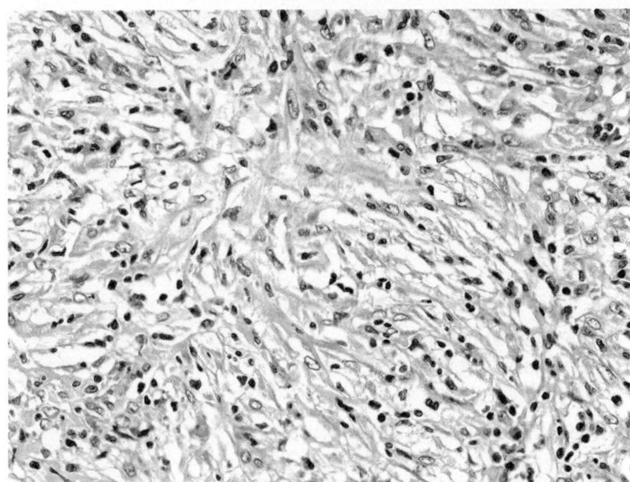

FIGURE 6.15 IgG4-related retroperitoneal disease. Note the storiform-type fibrosis and dense lymphoplasmacytic infiltrate. The fibroblasts/myofibroblasts (spindle cells) are prominent but lack atypia.

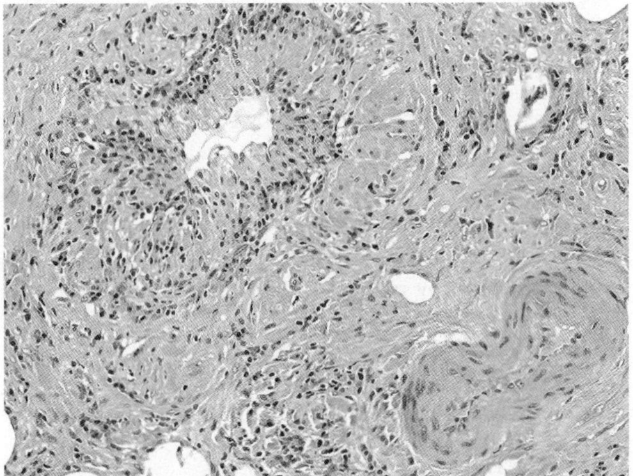

FIGURE 6.16 IgG4-related retroperitoneal fibrosis. Note the focus of phlebitis.

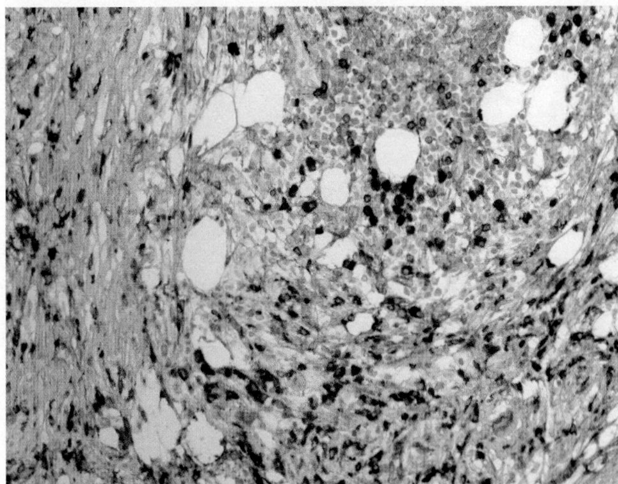

FIGURE 6.17 An IgG4 stain performed on the case illustrated in Figs. 6.15 and 6.16. The increased number of IgG4-positive cells supports a diagnosis of IgG4-related disease.

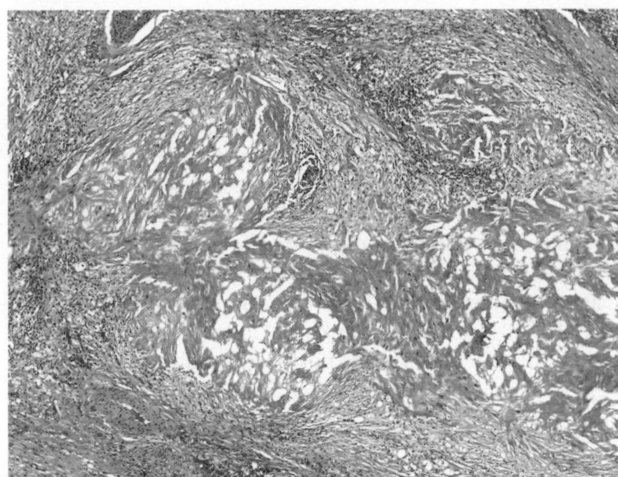

FIGURE 6.18 Sclerosing mesenteritis. Although significant inflammation and fibrosis is present, the presence of fat necrosis argues against a diagnosis of IgG4-related disease.

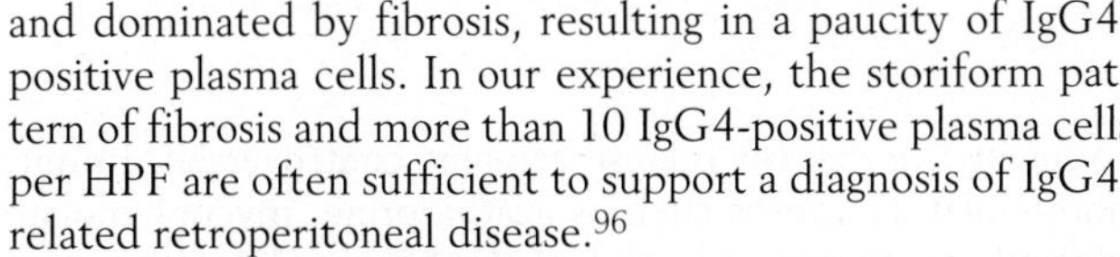

and dominated by fibrosis, resulting in a paucity of IgG4-positive plasma cells. In our experience, the storiform pattern of fibrosis and more than 10 IgG4-positive plasma cells per HPF are often sufficient to support a diagnosis of IgG4-related retroperitoneal disease.[96]

In a recent study of 26 patients with retroperitoneal fibrosis, rituximab was associated with symptom improvement and diminution in the size of lesions in both IgG4-related retroperitoneal fibrosis and idiopathic retroperitoneal fibrosis.[97]

The mesenteric manifestations of IgG4-related disease are less widely recognized, although it has been theorized that some cases previously classified as sclerosing mesenteritis may belong to the IgG4-related disease spectrum.[98-101] Retroperitoneal and mesenteric adipose tissue may be simultaneously involved. Non-IgG4 forms of sclerosing mesenteritis usually show widespread fat necrosis (Figs. 6.18 and 6.19), whereas IgG4-related sclerosing mesenteritis lacks this finding and is characterized by fibrosis, a dense lymphoplasmacytic infiltrate, obliterative phlebitis, and elevated numbers of IgG4-positive plasma cells. Some authors have expressed skepticism about the concept of IgG4-related disease of the mesentery because most cases in the literature lack the cardinal manifestations of IgG4-related disease.[101]

Differential Diagnosis

A wide range of inflammatory and neoplastic diseases are associated with elevated numbers of IgG4-positive cells (Box 6.4) The density of IgG4-positive cells in some diseases, such as granulomatosis with polyangiitis (Wegener's) and rheumatoid arthritis, may be higher than in IgG4-related disease.[82,83] Some inflammatory myofibroblastic tumors may be associated with a dense lymphoplasmacytic infiltrate that is rich in IgG4-positive cells; notably, the stromal cells may be inconspicuous. However, the stromal cells typically show at least mild atypia; stromal cells in IgG4-related disease lack cytological atypia.[88] It is important to reiterate that a mere increase in IgG4-positive cells without characteristic histological features does not constitute evidence of IgG4-related disease.

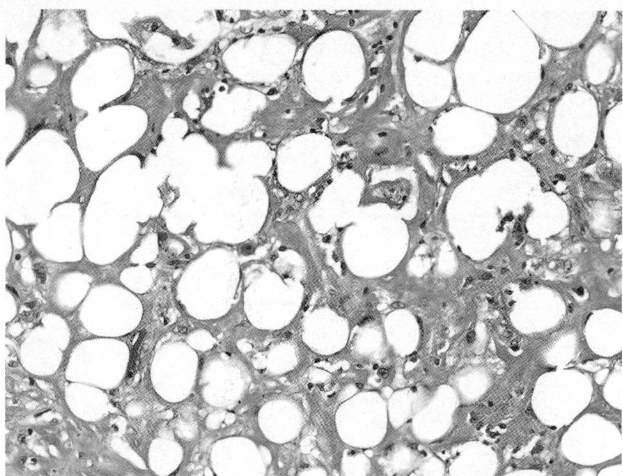

FIGURE 6.19 Sclerosing mesenteritis. Higher-power view of the image shown in Fig. 6.18. Regardless of the number of IgG4-positive cells, the presence of fat necrosis and accompanying histiocytes would argue against a diagnosis of IgG4-related disease.

IgG4-positive plasma cells are also identified in individuals with pouchitis, a finding that appears to have predictive value. Patients with more than 10 IgG4-positive plasma cells per HPF in biopsies from the pouch had higher pouch inflammatory scores as measured by endoscopic evaluation.[102-104] Patients with chronic antibiotic-refractory pouchitis also show elevated serum IgG4 levels.[102,103]

IgG4-positive plasma cells are increased in Cronkhite-Canada syndrome. IgG4 immunostaining was positive (>5 cells/HPF) in 52% of Cronkhite-Canada syndrome polyps but in only 12% of juvenile polyposis syndrome polyps.[86]

Natural History and Treatment

In general, the natural history of IgG4-related disease is variable, ranging from spontaneous improvement to progressive irreversible damage of vital organs. Overall, the risk for death is significantly higher in patients with IgG4-related disease than in the general population, with an estimated odds ratio of 2.07.[105] This increased risk is likely accounted for by disease involving the liver, kidney, heart, aorta, and CNS.

Glucocorticoid therapy represents the first-line treatment for inducing remission.[106] The response to steroids is generally swift, although relapses are noted in almost one-half of cases after glucocorticoid tapering. Rituximab, a monoclonal anti-CD20 antibody, has also been used to induce remission. The use of maintenance low-dose steroids to lower the risk for relapse remains controversial. Immunomodulatory agents such as azathioprine, mycophenolate mofetil, methotrexate, and cyclophosphamide have also been used for maintenance.

BOX 6.4 Pathological Differential Diagnosis of Immunoglobulin G4–Related Disease

INFECTIONS
Bacterial
Mycobacterial
Viral
Spirochetal (e.g., syphilis)
Infections involving specific sites
- Aortitis
- Otitis media/mastoiditis

NEOPLASMS AND TUMORS
Inflammatory myofibroblastic tumors
Inflammatory infiltrate in background of tumors

LYMPHOPROLIFERATIVE DISORDERS
MALT lymphoma with plasmacytic differentiation
Plasma cell neoplasia

EOSINOPHILIC DISORDERS
Eosinophilic angiocentric fibrosis
Kimura's disease
Angiolymphoid hyperplasia with eosinophilia

INFLAMMATORY/AUTOIMMUNE DISORDERS
Inflammatory pseudotumors
Systemic disease
Multicentric Castleman's disease
Rosai-Dorfman disease
Sarcoidosis
ANCA-associated vasculitis
Granulomatosis with polyangiitis
Eosinophilic granulomatosis with polyangiitis

PANCREATOBILIARY TRACT
Primary sclerosing cholangitis
Type 2 AIP
Follicular cholangitis

ORBIT/SALIVARY GLANDS
Sjögren's syndrome
Chronic sialadenitis, not otherwise specified

AIP, *Autoimmune pancreatitis;* ANCA, *antineutrophil cytoplasmic antibodies;* MALT, *mucosa-associated lymphoid tissue.*
From Bledsoe JR, Shinagare SA, Deshpande V. Difficult diagnostic problems in pancreatobiliary neoplasia. Arch Pathol Lab Med. *2015;139(7):848-857.*

The full reference list may be accessed online at *Elsevier eBooks for Practicing Clinicians.*

CHAPTER 7

Systemic Illnesses Involving the Gastrointestinal Tract

David N.B. Lewin

Chapter Outline

INTRODUCTION

Systemic illnesses commonly affect the gastrointestinal (GI) tract. GI symptoms and morphological changes can result from several different pathogenetic mechanisms, such as nonspecific or constitutional symptoms, pathological changes common to intestinal and extraintestinal organs, secondary changes such as opportunistic infections or drug reactions, and metastatic disease. This chapter focuses on morphological alterations in the GI tract resulting from disorders that primarily affect other organ systems.

CARDIOVASCULAR DISORDERS

Cardiac Surgery and Heart Transplantation

GI complications after open heart surgery are uncommon, occurring in approximately 4% of cases; however, the mortality rate can be high (approximately 16% for those with infective endocarditis).[1,2] The most common complication is postoperative ileus (which has the lowest mortality). Other complications typically consist of GI hemorrhage secondary to stress ulceration, vascular insufficiency with ischemic necrosis of bowel, and acute diverticulitis. Additional risk factors for ischemia include end-stage renal disease, female sex, non–coronary artery bypass graft, and long pump times.[2]

In contrast with GI complications after open heart surgery, GI complications after cardiac transplantation have been reported in as many as 20% of patients.[3,4] Complications include all of the hemorrhagic conditions mentioned previously. In addition, the use of steroids and immunosuppressive agents increases the risks of intestinal perforation, fistula formation, and infectious GI diseases. These patients are also at risk for posttransplantation lymphoproliferative disorders[5] (see Chapter 53).

Ischemic Disease

Intestinal ischemic disease can be divided into two major subsets: nonthrombotic (approximately 60% of cases) and thrombotic (approximately 40% of cases).[6] Nonthrombotic causes of ischemic disease include decreased mesenteric blood flow secondary to cardiac failure, shock, atherosclerotic vascular disease, disseminated intravascular coagulation, vasculitis, and fibromuscular dysplasia. Thrombotic causes can be divided into arterial embolism, arterial thrombosis, and venous thrombosis. These are a heterogeneous group of disorders usually seen in older adults.[7] Colonic ischemia, the most common disorder (typically nonthrombotic), has a favorable prognosis. Acute mesenteric ischemia, in contrast, has a poor prognosis, with a survival rate of only 50%.[6] The classic presentation is "pain out of proportion to examination." Histologically, resultant lesions range from epithelial and lymphocytic apoptosis[8] to mucosal necrosis and transmural infarction of the bowel (Fig. 7.1). Specifics concerning histology and pathology are discussed in Chapter 11. The most critical factor influencing outcomes in patients is the speed of diagnosis and intervention.

DERMATOLOGICAL DISORDERS

Both the skin and the GI tract may become involved in a variety of disease processes. These lesions may be divided as follows:

1. Primary dermatological disorders that also involve the GI tract (Box 7.1). These lesions are discussed in this section.
2. Systemic disorders involving both the skin and the GI tract (Box 7.2). These lesions are discussed in other areas of this chapter.
3. Primary GI disorders with skin manifestations. Only skin disorders associated with malignancies of the GI tract are discussed in this chapter. The remaining lesions are discussed elsewhere in this textbook.

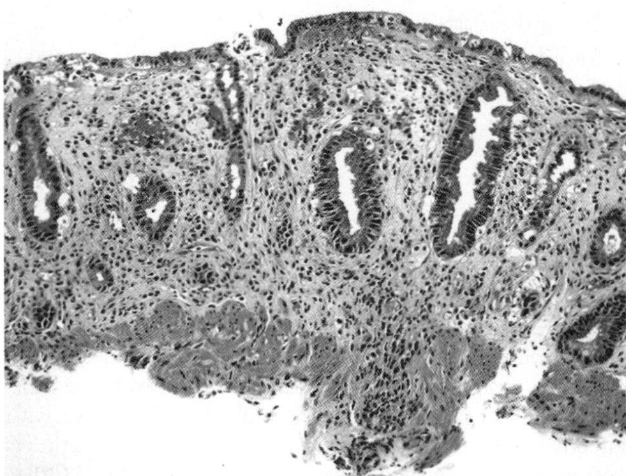

FIGURE 7.1 Early ischemia of the colon. Intermediate magnification reveals atrophy and mucin depletion of the epithelium. A mild acute inflammatory infiltrate is present, as is epithelial apoptosis. The lamina propria has a characteristic light-pink, homogeneous appearance.

Bullous Diseases

The majority of primary dermatological bullous disorders that involve the GI tract occur in conjunction with a skin disorder (excluding dermatitis herpetiformis). These diseases typically involve the upper portion of the esophagus. Patients are seen with symptoms of dysphagia and odynophagia. Histologically, the lesions in esophageal squamous mucosa appear similar to those in the skin. The key distinguishing morphological features are the level of the plane of separation (vesicle formation), the type of inflammatory infiltrate, and the presence or absence of acantholysis.[9] Because the bullae rarely remain intact, diagnosis of

BOX 7.1 Primary Dermatological Diseases Involving the Gastrointestinal Tract

- Bullous diseases
  - Epidermolysis bullosa
  - Pemphigus vulgaris
  - Bullous pemphigoid
  - Erythema multiforme
    - Stevens-Johnson syndrome
    - Hailey-Hailey and Darier's diseases
  - Dermatitis herpetiformis
- Dermatogenic enteropathy
  - Eczema
  - Psoriasis

BOX 7.2 Systemic Diseases Involving the Skin and Gastrointestinal Tract

- Vascular disorders
  - Hereditary hemorrhagic telangiectasia (Rendu-Osler-Weber disease)
  - Kaposi's sarcoma
  - Blue rubber bleb nevus syndrome
  - Necrotizing angiitis
  - Degos disease (malignant atrophic papulosis)
- Metabolic disorders
  - Acrodermatitis enteropathica
  - Fabry's disease (angiokeratoma corporis diffusum)
  - Plummer-Vinson syndrome
- Rheumatological and connective tissue disorders
  - Scleroderma
  - Dermatomyositis
  - Systemic lupus erythematosus
  - Polyarteritis nodosa
  - Pseudoxanthoma elasticum
  - Ehlers-Danlos syndrome
- Miscellaneous disorders
  - Amyloidosis
  - Familial Mediterranean fever
  - Mastocytosis

these lesions on GI biopsy specimens is challenging. The diagnosis is usually made on the basis of appropriate clinical information combined with biopsies of the skin lesions. In the esophagus, lesions often rupture and produce erosions; occasionally, fibrosis and stricture formation are also seen.

Epidermolysis Bullosa

Epidermolysis bullosa, a group of more than 12 genetically determined disorders that involve all organs lined by squamous epithelium,[10] is characterized by the formation of vesiculobullous lesions secondary to minor trauma. The site of cleavage can be in the dermis (dermolytic or dystrophic form), at the dermoepidermal junction (junctional form), or in the epidermis (epidermolytic or simplex form). Involvement of the GI tract occurs in 50% of patients with the dystrophic form and in 33% of those with the junctional or simplex form.[11] Stricture and esophageal webs occur most frequently in the dystrophic form but can also be seen rarely in the junctional or simplex form. In addition, anal and perianal disease and perianal blistering are seen in all types. Histologically, this lesion is characterized by separation of the epithelium and formation of bullae, with little or no inflammatory infiltrate.

Epidermolysis bullosa acquisita is a rare acquired disorder with clinical characteristics similar to those of epidermolysis bullosa except for adult onset, milder skin disease, and lack of family history.[12] It may be associated with systemic diseases such as amyloidosis, multiple myeloma, diabetes mellitus, and inflammatory bowel disease (IBD). A subset of patients have circulating immunoglobulin G (IgG) that recognizes collagen IV. Endoscopic biopsy may show linear deposition of IgG in the basement membrane.

Pemphigus Vulgaris

Pemphigus vulgaris is a bullous disorder that affects middle-aged and older individuals. The bullae are superficial and flaccid. The lesion is an intraepidermal bulla formed by acantholysis (loss of intracellular bridges). Histologically, the cells lose their normal angular contours and become rounded. Basal keratinocytes typically remain attached to the epidermal basement membrane. The inflammatory infiltrate is variable; eosinophils and lymphocytes are the cells most commonly present in the epidermis, both surrounding and within the bullae and within the subjacent lamina propria. Standard biopsy forceps may provide only superficial specimens that are inadequate for diagnosis.[13] Direct immunofluorescence for immunoglobulins and complement component C3 is positive in the epidermal intercellular spaces.[14] The incidence of esophageal involvement is unclear. Some studies report endoscopic lesions in as much as 80% of patients.[15,16] In addition, immunofluorescence performed on esophageal mucosa is usually positive in all patients with active disease.[17]

Bullous Pemphigoid

Bullous pemphigoid is a subepidermal bullous disorder characterized by large, tense blisters on the skin. Mucosal involvement of the GI tract is much less common than in pemphigus vulgaris,[18] although one report described esophageal blisters in 4% of patients with typical bullous pemphigoid.[19] The histology of the bullous lesion has not been described. However, linear deposits of IgG and complement in the basement membrane of the esophagus and occasionally in the stomach, similar to those found in the skin, have been described.[18] A single case of bullae in the colon has also been reported.[20]

Cicatricial pemphigoid (benign mucous membrane pemphigoid) is an autoimmune bullous disease related to bullous pemphigoid. It has similar immunohistochemical linear deposition of C3 and IgG. The circulating autoantibodies recognize bullous pemphigoid antigen 2 (BPAC2). Esophageal involvement has been reported in approximately 4% of patients with the disease.[21]

Erythema Multiforme

Erythema multiforme, as the name implies, is a cutaneous reaction pattern characterized by a combination of skin and mucosal lesions. The mucosal lesions usually occur on the lips or in the oral cavity and conjunctiva. However, the esophagus and, rarely, other regions of the GI tract may be involved.[22] Included in this group of disorders is Stevens-Johnson syndrome (macular trunk lesions with mucosal involvement).[23] Many of these lesions occur secondary to drug reactions (type IV hypersensitivity reactions) or, occasionally, reactions to infectious agents such as mycoplasmae. In the esophagus, lesions have been described as small white patches similar to those caused by *Candida* spp. infection. Histologically, superficial ulceration and marked intraepithelial lymphocytosis are often observed. Individual squamous cell necrosis most often involves the basal cells but may also include the entire thickness of the epithelium. Lesions typically regress and, as such, biopsies from the GI tract are rarely procured.

Hailey-Hailey and Darier's Diseases

Hailey-Hailey disease, also known as *benign familial pemphigus*, is a rare disorder with an autosomal dominant inheritance pattern. Patients typically are seen in the fourth to fifth decade of life with blistering and crusting skin lesions in intertriginous zones. Mucous membrane involvement is rare but may occur. Darier's disease is similar to Hailey-Hailey disease, but its onset is typically in the first to second decade of life. Histological features of both include dyskeratosis, suprabasal acantholysis, papillomatosis, and suprabasal separation with loss of intracellular bridges. Darier's disease more commonly involves the esophagus.[24]

Dermatitis Herpetiformis

Dermatitis herpetiformis is a pruritic vesicular dermatitis with a symmetric distribution on the skin. Unlike the previously discussed bullous disorders of the skin, this disease does not produce bullous lesions in the GI tract. Dermatitis herpetiformis is strongly associated with celiac disease. Approximately 70% of patients with dermatitis herpetiformis show evidence of villous atrophy on small bowel biopsy.[25] However, most patients are asymptomatic. Of patients with dermatitis herpetiformis, 90% are positive for endomysial autoantibodies[26] (typically seen with celiac sprue as well). Human leukocyte antigen associations are similar for both dermatitis herpetiformis and celiac sprue. Both the skin disease and the GI symptoms can be controlled by a gluten-free diet.[27]

Dermatogenic Enteropathy

Many GI symptoms and histological findings have been described in patients with active psoriasis and eczema.

Steatorrhea and malabsorption are not uncommon, and the terms *dermatogenic enteropathy* and *psoriatic enteropathy* have been applied to these syndromes.[28,29] Histologically, the duodenal mucosa shows an increase in the numbers of mast cells and eosinophils. A subset of patients have increased numbers of duodenal intraepithelial lymphocytes and antibodies to gliadin (suggestive of latent celiac sprue).[30] In addition, the colon may show increased lamina propria cellularity, active inflammation, and occasional gland atrophy in mucosal biopsy specimens from patients who have psoriasis without bowel symptoms.[31]

Dermatological Disorders Associated with Malignancies of the GI Tract

Acanthosis Nigricans

Acanthosis nigricans consists of numerous brown, hyperpigmented, velvety skin plaques located in the axillae, groin, and flexural areas. The lesion has two major forms—one associated with internal malignancies and the other associated with insulin resistance. Microscopically, dermal lesions are characterized by diffuse hyperkeratosis and papillomatosis. Epithelial hyperplasia of the esophagus also has been described.

When present, this lesion is usually associated with adenocarcinomas of the stomach and colon. At least one report has suggested that it is caused by the production of transforming growth factor-α by tumor cells.[32]

Tylosis

Focal nonepidermolytic palmoplantar keratoderma (tylosis) is a rare, autosomal dominant, inherited defect of keratinization. It is strongly associated with the development of squamous cell carcinoma of the esophagus, with tumors appearing in 95% of patients.[33] The skin lesion is characterized by thickening of the stratum corneum of the palms and soles. The esophageal mucosa in tylosis is typically affected by papillomatosis, which appears as multiple small protrusions, some with spines as a result of acanthosis. Molecular studies have mapped the defective gene to a small region on chromosome 17q25.[34,35] The same region has been implicated in the development of sporadic squamous cell carcinoma and Barrett's esophagus–associated adenocarcinoma.

Miscellaneous Disorders

Several other nonspecific skin diseases are associated with GI neoplasms.[36] These diseases include generalized dermal pigmentation, migratory thrombophlebitis, and seborrheic keratosis (Leser-Trélat sign).[37]

ENDOCRINE DISORDERS

Alterations in the secretion of endocrine hormones in endocrine disorders may have a variety of GI effects. Most of these produce functional GI symptoms such as vomiting, diarrhea, constipation, and abdominal pain secondary to changes in GI motility (Table 7.1). Most of these diseases do not cause significant morphological or histological abnormalities and are described only briefly here.

Adrenal Gland

Addison's disease (primary chronic adrenocortical insufficiency) may cause common GI disturbances such as anorexia, nausea, vomiting, and diarrhea.[38] Pheochromocytomas are characterized by hypertension resulting from high catecholamine levels. Intestinal pseudo-obstruction, megacolon, and even bowel ischemia have also been described and are thought to be secondary to the vasoconstrictive action of excess catecholamine levels.[39]

Hypothalamus and Pituitary

The hypothalamus and pituitary function as a unit. Disorders of either one infrequently affect the GI tract. Hypopituitarism affects intestinal motility, as does hypothyroidism. Pituitary adenomas are part of multiple endocrine neoplasia

TABLE 7.1 Gastrointestinal Manifestations of Endocrine Disorders

Organ	Endocrine Disorder	Gastrointestinal Manifestation
Adrenal	Addison's disease	Anorexia, weight loss, abdominal pain, diarrhea
	Pheochromocytoma	Watery diarrhea, intestinal ischemia
Hypothalamus and pituitary	Acromegaly	Increased incidence of colonic polyps and neoplasms
Pancreas	Diabetes	Motility disorders, infections, abdominal pain
	Gastrinoma	Peptic ulcers, gastric fundic hyperplasia
	VIPoma	Watery diarrhea
	Somatostatinoma	Diabetes, steatorrhea
	Glucagonoma	Angular stomatitis and glossitis, giant intestinal villi
Parathyroid	Hyperparathyroidism	Nausea, vomiting, abdominal pain
	Hypoparathyroidism	Malabsorption
Thyroid	Hyperthyroidism	Hypermotility: diarrhea or steatorrhea
	Hypothyroidism	Decreased motility: reflux, bezoars, ileus, constipation
	Medullary carcinoma	Watery diarrhea

VIP, Vasoactive intestinal peptide.

(MEN) syndrome, discussed later in this chapter. Of the hyperpituitary lesions, acromegaly is of interest with respect to GI neoplasia. Acromegaly is characterized by chronic hypersecretion of growth hormone and insulin-like growth factor, usually resulting from a pituitary adenoma. It is associated with overgrowth of the musculoskeletal system and all organs, including the GI tract. Acromegaly has been shown to increase epithelial cell proliferation in the colon,[40] and an increased prevalence of colonic adenomas and colonic carcinoma has been observed.[41] An increased risk of gastric carcinoma has also been suggested but is less well established.[42]

Pancreas

Diseases of the exocrine and endocrine pancreas commonly affect the GI tract. These include pancreatic exocrine insufficiency, diabetes, and hormonal effects of functional pancreatic endocrine neoplasms. Pancreatic exocrine insufficiency typically gives rise to steatorrhea and malabsorption and is discussed further in Chapter 40.

Diabetes can involve significant GI symptoms.[43] These result from decreased motility secondary to autonomic nervous system dysfunction. Patients have symptoms such as abdominal pain, bloating, early satiety, nausea, and vomiting. Abdominal bloating appears to correlate best with decreased gastric emptying.[44] The delayed gastric emptying associated with gastric atony and gastric dilation is called *gastroparesis diabeticorum*, and an increased risk of bezoar formation is apparent. Patients can also experience periodic intractable diarrhea and crampy abdominal pain. Because of hypomotility, these patients are at risk for bacterial infection and malabsorption. Patients are also at increased risk for *Candida* infection of the esophagus.[45] Histological features are nonspecific. Neuropathic findings with silver stains have been described,[46] as have periodic acid–Schiff (PAS)–positive vascular deposits in the vessels of the submucosa.[47]

Excess hormonal production from the pancreatic islets of Langerhans can be a result of diffuse hyperplasia (nesidioblastosis) or pancreatic endocrine tumors. Many hormones, such as insulin, glucagon, somatostatin, pancreatic polypeptide, gastrin, adrenocorticotropic hormone, calcitonin, parathormone, and serotonin, can be produced by these lesions. All GI manifestations reflect altered digestive function and motility.[48]

Parathyroid

Both hyperparathyroidism and hypoparathyroidism can cause GI symptoms. GI symptoms occur in one-half of patients with hyperparathyroidism and may be the presenting symptom in 15% of cases.[49] These patients typically have abdominal pain, nausea, vomiting, and constipation. Many of these symptoms are thought to be caused by hypercalcemia, which results in altered neuronal transmission and neuromuscular excitability.[50] Hypoparathyroidism can be associated with malabsorption and steatorrhea. The small intestinal mucosa is typically histologically normal, but rare associations with celiac sprue have been reported.[51]

Thyroid

Both hyperthyroidism and hypothyroidism can cause GI symptoms. Hyperthyroidism produces hypermotility of the gut, and hypothyroidism causes hypomotility. Hyperthyroidism can result in rapid gastric emptying, watery diarrhea, and steatorrhea.[52] No constant structural changes in the mucosa or in the wall of the bowel have been consistently reported. Hypothyroidism can be associated with gastric bezoar formation, ileus, volvulus, constipation, and megacolon.[52] In patients with marked myxedema, dilation and thickening of the bowel wall with microscopic accumulation of mucopolysaccharide substances in the submucosa, muscularis propria, and serosa have been described.[53]

Thyroid neoplasms may also produce GI effects. Medullary carcinoma of the thyroid is a tumor of the calcitonin-producing endocrine C cells of the thyroid gland. Patients may have prominent "explosive" watery diarrhea as the result of ectopic hormone production.[54] Papillary carcinoma of the thyroid also can be associated with Gardner's syndrome.[55]

Multiple Endocrine Neoplasia

The MEN syndromes are a group of autosomal dominant inherited disorders associated with hyperplasia or neoplasms of several endocrine organs. Three main varieties of this syndrome can occur—MEN I, MEN IIa, and MEN IIb (or III). GI manifestations are caused by the products of endocrine proliferations.[56] Each of these syndromes is associated with a mutant gene locus—MEN I with the *MEN1* gene locus, and MEN IIa and IIb with the *RET* gene locus. MEN I is associated with pancreatic endocrine tumors (often gastrinomas) and with the Zollinger-Ellison syndrome, which is associated with gastric and duodenal disease. MEN IIb may be associated with ganglioneuromatosis, ganglion cell hyperplasia, and hypertrophy of the plexuses of Meissner and Auerbach in the GI tract. Chronic constipation, diarrhea, or both may be associated with MEN IIb.[57]

HEMATOLOGICAL DISORDERS

Hemorrhagic Disorders

Patients with bleeding disorders may develop spontaneous hemorrhage in any part of the GI tract. Between 10% and 25% of patients with hemophilia suffer from GI hemorrhage.[58] Von Willebrand's disease,[59] heparin or warfarin overdose, vitamin K deficiencies, platelet deficiency, thrombotic thrombocytopenic purpura, and hemolytic-uremic syndrome (HUS) can all result in hemorrhage of the GI tract. This is most commonly seen in the upper GI tract and typically is most prominent in the submucosa. It can be severe enough to involve the entire thickness of the bowel wall and give rise to an intramural hematoma.[60] More severe lesions can cause luminal narrowing, rigidity with obstruction, and, rarely, intussusception.[58]

Thrombotic Disorders

Sickle cell anemia,[61] polycythemia rubra vera,[62] and other thrombotic disorders[63] can produce thrombosis, leading to infarction and hemorrhage of the intestines. Sickle cell anemia causes sickling of red blood cells and hyperviscosity of the blood and typically produces arterial and capillary obstruction.[61] It involves the watershed areas of the distal transverse colon and splenic flexure, which have the lowest oxygen tension. Sickled red blood cells may be found in the vessels. Polycythemia usually leads to venous obstruction of the portal and mesenteric veins. These lesions involve the deeper parts of the bowel wall, including the muscularis propria. Diagnosis is based on the finding of venous thrombi in the mesenteric and mesocolic tissues not in the field of infarction, which occur in conjunction with appropriate clinical history.

Megaloblastic Anemia

Megaloblastic anemias are associated with deficiencies of folic acid and vitamin B_{12}. These anemias are characterized by megaloblastic proliferation of actively growing cells, as is typically described in bone marrow aspirations but is also seen in the epithelial cells of the GI tract. As a result of impaired DNA synthesis, actively dividing cells in the gastric pits, small bowel, and colonic crypts typically show enlarged, immature-appearing nuclei (Fig. 7.2). The nucleus-to-cytoplasm ratio is decreased. The overall numbers of mitotic figures are also reduced. In addition, PAS-negative, Alcian blue–negative cytoplasmic vacuoles have been described in duodenal enterocytes.[64] Megaloblastic anemia can be caused by pernicious anemia secondary to autoimmune gastritis; therefore gastric findings of atrophic autoimmune gastritis may also be present.

Leukemia and Lymphoma

Involvement of the GI tract is often noted in patients with leukemia and lymphoma. This can occur directly by tumor (primary or secondary), secondary to complications of disease, or secondary to therapy (see Chapter 31 for details).

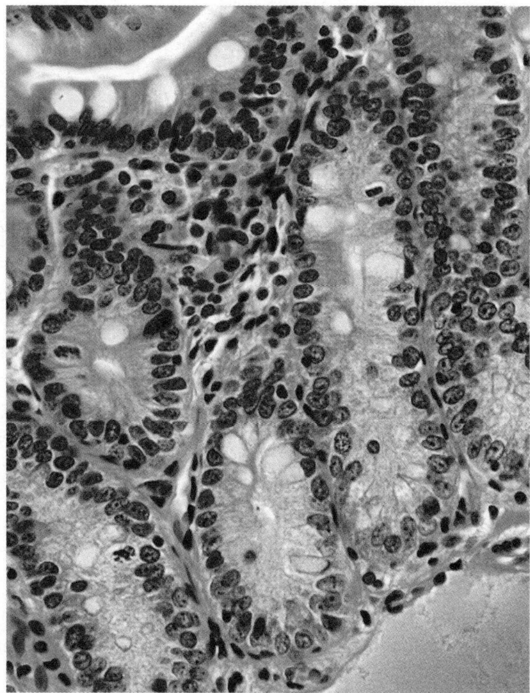

FIGURE 7.2 Nucleomegaly in megaloblastic anemia. In this high-power view, actively dividing cells are evident in crypts of the small intestine. Many enlarged, immature-appearing nuclei can be seen in the upper third of the crypt.

Autopsy studies have revealed GI involvement in 50% of patients with leukemia.[65] In secondary involvement of the GI tract by either leukemia or lymphoma, tumor infiltrates are often multifocal and may be present anywhere from the esophagus to the rectum.[66] These infiltrates can cause aphthous-type ulcers (typical of leukemic infiltrations) or can result in polypoid, masslike, or large ulcers (typical of lymphomatous involvement).[67] The larger mass lesions can occasionally cause obstruction or intussusception.[68] Histological features are those typical of the particular type of leukemia or lymphoma. Malignant cells are typically found in the mucosal and submucosal tissue. Tissue should be collected for molecular and cytogenetic analysis because many leukemias and lymphomas include diagnostic and clinically important changes.[69] Primary lymphomas of the GI tract are often solitary lesions, although diffuse forms do occur (usually in the small bowel).

Secondary effects of tumor overgrowth, or of chemotherapy, resulting in decreased numbers of platelets and inflammatory cells can lead to hemorrhagic lesions of the GI tract and opportunistic infections. In addition, neutropenic colitis, which is a necrotizing inflammatory disorder of the colon that occurs in neutropenic patients, can occur with chemotherapy and, rarely, as a complication of acute leukemia.[70] Finally, patients who have received a bone marrow transplant may develop graft-versus-host disease, which is characterized by apoptotic destruction of the epithelium throughout the GI tract. It typically manifests with diarrhea. Histologically, it is characterized by apoptosis of the epithelial cells, followed by crypt and gland loss and, ultimately, mucosal erosion and ulceration.[71]

METABOLIC DISORDERS

Acrodermatitis Enteropathica

Acrodermatitis enteropathica is a systemic disorder that occurs secondary to zinc deficiency resulting from a congenital defect in absorption of dietary zinc. This disorder has been localized to a gene *(SLC39A4)* that codes for a transmembrane zinc uptake protein (hZIP4).[72] It typically manifests after infancy and weaning (although rare cases have been described in adulthood[73]). It is characterized by chronic diarrhea associated with failure to thrive, periorofacial dermatitis, paronychia, nail dystrophy, alopecia, susceptibility to infection, and behavioral changes. Serum zinc levels are typically decreased. Treatment is provided in the form of oral zinc. Mucosal biopsy of the small bowel can be normal or can show mild, patchy villous lesions. Abnormal inclusion bodies have been described in Paneth cells on electron microscopy.[74] Acrodermatitis may also be caused by zinc deficiency secondary to Crohn's disease[75] or malnutrition.[76]

Plummer-Vinson Syndrome (Paterson–Brown Kelly Syndrome)

The unusual Plummer-Vinson syndrome has shown a recent decrease in incidence.[77] It is characterized by iron deficiency (its presumed cause), dysphagia, and esophageal webs.[78] Dermatological findings of angular stomatitis, atrophic tongue, and brittle nails are also seen. Long-standing disease is associated with an increased incidence of postcricoid carcinoma. Iron repletion improves all lesions.

Vitamin Disorders

In general, vitamin disorders are not associated with specific GI symptoms or lesions. Exceptions are brown bowel syndrome, which is thought to be caused by a deficiency of vitamin E (discussed later), and pellagra, which is associated with niacin deficiency (discussed in this section). Multiple vitamin deficiencies are often noted in malabsorptive disorders. Vitamins, macronutrients, and minerals are thought to have a protective effect with respect to neoplasia of the GI tract, especially for esophageal[79,80] and gastric[81] malignancies. Deficiency in vitamin K or anticoagulation therapy leads to a decrease in coagulation factors and can result in hemorrhagic lesions throughout the body.[82] In the GI tract, these range from focal petechial hemorrhages to frank exsanguination. No specific histological features are associated with these lesions. Similarly, vitamin C deficiency (scurvy) can lead to hemorrhage and delayed wound healing. Deficiencies of folic acid and vitamin B_{12} are associated with megaloblastic anemia and megaloblastic changes in the epithelial cells of the stomach and small intestine.[83] Olestra (a nonabsorbed fat replacement) may decrease the absorption of fat-soluble vitamins.[84]

Pellagra

Pellagra is a vitamin deficiency that has major GI effects. It is caused by a deficiency of niacin, either dietary (deficiency found in developing countries, alcoholics, and older adults) or secondary to impaired absorption (e.g., Crohn's disease,[85] amyloidosis[86]). It is characterized clinically by diarrhea, dermatitis, and dementia. Diarrhea is often bloody. However, patients can have steatorrhea.[87] The vitamin deficiency interferes with the normal renewal of epithelial tissue; hence, the effects on the skin and GI tract. Endoscopically, approximately half of patients have lesions. However, all have microscopic inflammation. Endoscopic lesions range from redness and granularity to focal ulceration and more extensive confluent lesions. Microscopically, the inflammatory infiltrate is nonspecific. In the esophagus, mild to severe esophagitis is seen.[88] The small bowel may be normal or may show mild villous blunting and increased inflammatory cells in the lamina propria.[89] In the large bowel, a mild to moderate inflammatory infiltrate with features of colitis cystica superficialis (cystic dilation of the crypts and crypt abscess formation) has been described. Patients usually respond to niacin replacement therapy.

Lipoprotein Disorders

Abetalipoproteinemia

Abetalipoproteinemia (discussed further in Chapter 10) is an autosomal recessive disorder characterized by a defect in the secretion of plasma lipoproteins that contain apolipoprotein B. Patients have steatorrhea, usually in infancy, with central nervous system symptoms such as disturbance in gait and balance and fatigue.[90] On peripheral smear, acanthocytes are usually prominent (in 50% of red blood cells). Laboratory findings show an absence of very-low-density lipoproteins, the presence of chylomicrons, and a reduction in triglycerides and other lipids. The defect occurs in a microsomal triglyceride transfer protein required for the secretion of plasma lipoproteins containing apolipoprotein B.[91] Normal intraluminal digestion of lipids occurs, along with transport of triglycerides and monoglycerides and their reesterification in enterocytes. However, lipids cannot be excreted on the basal lateral membrane of the enterocytes into blood and lymphatics. Histologically, this translates into prominent accumulation of fine lipid droplets within the basal aspect of the enterocytes (Fig. 7.3). These can be stained with Oil Red O on frozen-section tissue or seen by electron microscopic examination. The overall architecture of the small bowel is normally well maintained. One pitfall in diagnosis is the similar appearance of lipid droplets identified in normal individuals after a recent lipid-rich meal; therefore the diagnosis should be made only in fasting patients.

Tangier Disease

Tangier disease is an autosomal recessive disorder characterized by deposition of cholesteryl esters in the reticuloendothelial system, almost complete absence of high-density lipoprotein in the plasma, and aberrant cellular lipid trafficking.[92] Clinically, patients present with hepatosplenomegaly, enlarged tonsils, peripheral neuropathy, and, occasionally, diarrhea. Laboratory studies reveal low blood levels of high-density lipoprotein and cholesterol (caused by lack of apoprotein A) and high levels of triglycerides. Endoscopically, the lesions are described as tiny yellow nodules or orange-brown spots.[93] Microscopic examination reveals clusters of foamy histiocytes in the lamina propria (Fig. 7.4). Electron microscopic findings include intracytoplasmic vacuoles unbounded by membranes; these are often confluent in appearance[94] (see Chapter 10 for details).

Lysosomal Storage Disorders

Lysosomes, which are a major component of the intracellular digestive tract, contain hydrolytic enzymes made in the endoplasmic reticulum. These enzymes break down a variety of complex macromolecules that are either a component of the cell or are taken up by phagocytosis. Lysosomal storage disorders are inherited disorders (usually autosomal recessive) caused by lack of a functional enzyme or defective enzyme lysosome targeting. Substances typically accumulate within cells at the site where most of the degraded material is found; degradation typically occurs at this location.

Storage disorders can be divided based on the biochemical nature of the accumulated metabolite into glycogenoses, sphingolipidoses (lipidoses), mucopolysaccharidoses, mucolipidoses, and others. Most of these diseases have prominent central or peripheral nervous system effects.[95] Except for Fabry's disease, they do not have significant GI effects. Case reports of malabsorption in GM1 gangliosidosis,[96] diarrhea in Niemann-Pick disease,[97] and diarrhea and vomiting in Wolman's disease have been described.[98]

The importance of these diseases is that depositions can be identified in a variety of cells in the GI tract (Table 7.2), typically in the phagocytic cells (macrophages) in the lamina propria. The histological appearance typically reveals an accumulation of cells with foamy cytoplasm. The material may be positive for fat stains such as Oil Red O or Sudan black on frozen-section tissue or PAS stain, depending on the particular substance that has accumulated. Electron

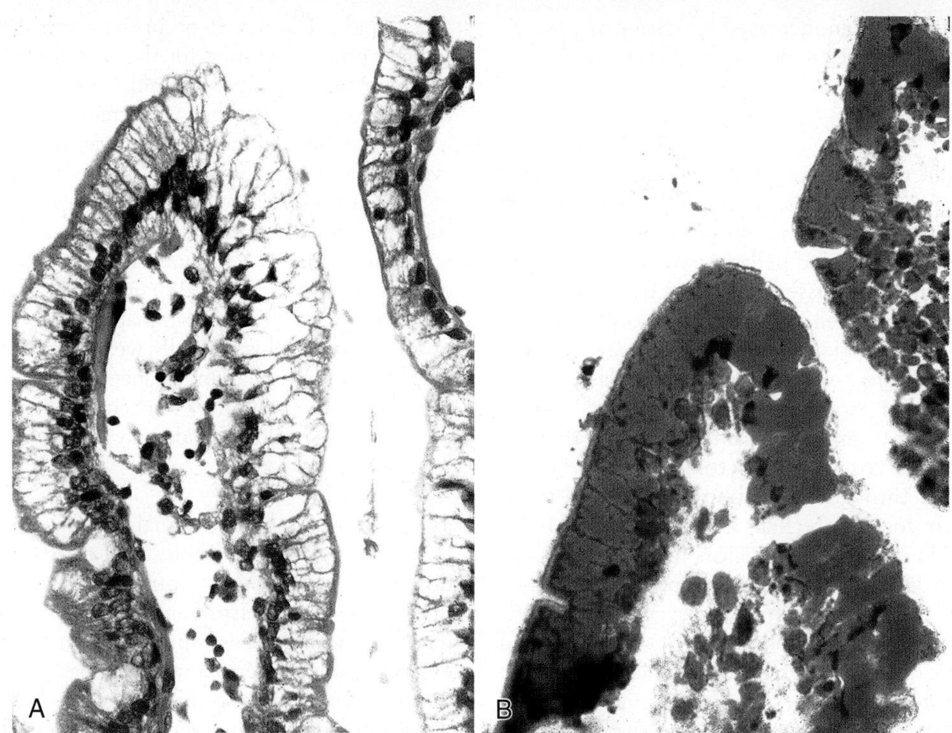

FIGURE 7.3 Abetalipoproteinemia. A, High-power view shows vacuolated epithelial cells that are clear-staining. **B,** Fat stain highlights the fat in the surface epithelial cells. *(From Lewin D, Lewin KJ. Small intestine. In: Weidner N, Cote RJ, Suster S, et al., eds. Modern Surgical Pathology. Philadelphia: Saunders; 2003:742.)*

microscopic examination typically reveals enlarged, unusually shaped lysosomes. Historically, many of these diagnoses have been made on rectal biopsy with histochemical stains and subsequent electron microscopic examination.[99-101] This technique has largely been supplanted by specific enzyme content analysis of circulating lymphocytes or biopsy material. Differentiation among the common mimics of storage disorders is described in the next section.

Fabry's Disease

Fabry's disease is a rare, X-linked lipid storage disorder that is caused by a deficiency of lysosomal α-galactosidase A and results in cellular deposition of glycolipids in many tissues. Clinically, these patients have involvement of multiple organ systems. Symptoms include excruciating pain in the extremities (acroparesthesia), skin vessel ectasia (angiokeratoma), corneal and lenticular opacity, cardiovascular disease, stroke, and renal failure.[102] GI symptoms are seen in 62% of male and 29% of female heterozygotes.[103] Features include vascular ectasia,[104] delayed gastric emptying,[105] diarrhea, and, rarely, ischemic bowel disease with perforation.[106] Histologically, glycolipid deposition is identified in vacuolated ganglion cells in the Meissner plexus and in small blood vessels. By electron microscopy, laminated and amorphous intralysosomal, "zebra-like," osmiophilic deposits occur in ganglion cells, smooth muscle fibers, and endothelial cells.[103]

Common Mimics of Lysosomal Storage Diseases

Common mimics of lysosomal storage diseases are summarized in Table 7.3. These are divided into two general categories: pigmented and nonpigmented. The majority of lesions result from a proliferation of histiocytes with either engulfed infectious organisms or cellular or extracellular material.

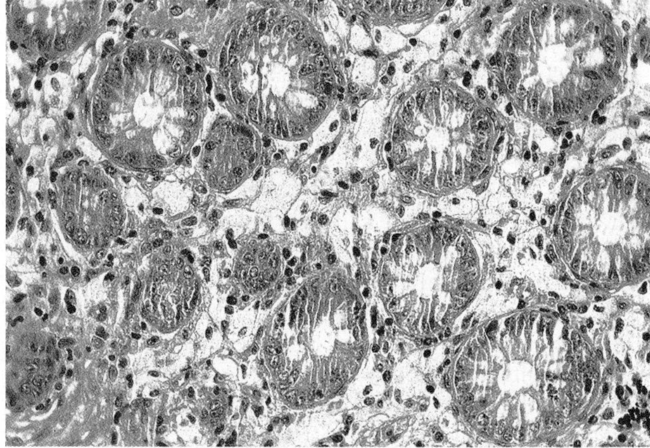

FIGURE 7.4 Tangier disease involving the colon. This condition represents a deposition of cholesterol esters in tissue histiocytes.

Pigmented lesions, which are in the differential diagnosis of neuronal ceroid lipofuscinosis, include melanosis, pseudomelanosis, brown bowel syndrome, hemosiderosis, and barium granuloma. Nonpigmented lesions are in the differential diagnosis of all of the rest of the lysosomal storage diseases and include xanthoma, muciphages, Whipple's disease, *Mycobacterium avium-intracellulare* complex (MAC) infection, pseudolipomatosis, malakoplakia, granular cell tumors, signet ring adenocarcinoma, and malignant histiocytosis.

Pigmented Lesions

Melanosis. Melanosis coli is characterized by pigment deposition in macrophages in the lamina propria. Endoscopically, the bowel mucosa can appear normal or brownish in color,

TABLE 7.2 Lysosomal Storage Diseases

Disease	Enzyme Deficiency	Major Accumulating Metabolite	GI Symptoms	Affected Cells	Histological Features	Electron Microscopic Features
Glycogenoses						
Type 2 Pompe disease	α-1,4-Glucosidase	Glycogen	None	Hepatocytes, cardiac and skeletal muscle cells	Glycogen within sarcoplasm, PAS positive	Glycogen
Sphingolipidoses						
GM1 gangliosidosis	GM1 ganglioside β-galactosidase	GM1 ganglioside	Malabsorption	Neurons	Ballooned neurons, fat stain positive	Whorled configurations
GM2 Gangliosidosis						
Tay-Sachs disease	Hexosaminidase α subunit	GM2 ganglioside	None	Neurons	Ballooned neurons, fat stain positive	Whorled configurations
Sandhoff disease	Hexosaminidase β subunit	GM2 ganglioside	None	Neurons	Ballooned neurons, fat stain positive	Whorled configurations
Variant AB	Ganglioside activator protein	GM2 ganglioside	None	Neurons	Ballooned neurons, fat stain positive	Whorled configurations
Sulfatidoses						
Metachromatic leukodystrophy	Arylsulfatase A	Sulfatide	None	Phagocytic cells	Inclusions stain with toluidine blue or other metachromatic stains	Free lipid bodies without cytosomes
Multiple sulfatase deficiency	Arylsulfatases A, B, C	Sulfatide, heparan sulfate, dermatan sulfate	None	Phagocytic cells	Inclusions stain with toluidine blue and other metachromatic stains	Zebra bodies
Krabbe disease	Galactosylceramidase	Galactocerebroside	None	Phagocytic cells	Globoid PAS-positive cells	Curved tubular inclusions
Fabry's disease	α-Galactosidase A	Ceramide trihexoside	Delayed gastric emptying	Phagocytic, ganglion, and endothelial cells; smooth muscle fibers	Vacuolization, fat stain positive	Zebra bodies
Gaucher disease	Glucocerebrosidase	Glucocerebroside	None	Phagocytic cells	Fibrillary cytoplasm (tissue paper–like), PAS positive	Elongated lysosomes, stacks of bilayers
Niemann-Pick disease	Sphingomyelinase	Sphingomyelin	Diarrhea	Phagocytic cells, axons, Schwann cells	Innumerable small, uniform vacuoles, PAS positive	Zebra bodies
Mucopolysaccharidoses (MPS)						
Hurler's syndrome (MPS I)	α-L-Iduronidase	Dermatan sulfate, heparan sulfate	None	Phagocytic cells, endothelial cells fibroblasts	Balloon cells, PAS positive	Lamellated zebra bodies
Hunter's syndrome (MPS II)	L-Iduronidase sulfatase	Dermatan sulfate, heparan sulfate	None	Phagocytic cells, endothelial cells, intimal cells, fibroblasts	Balloon cells, PAS positive	Lamellated zebra bodies

Continued

TABLE 7.2 Lysosomal Storage Diseases—cont'd

Disease	Enzyme Deficiency	Major Accumulating Metabolite	GI Symptoms	Affected Cells	Histological Features	Electron Microscopic Features
Mucolipidoses (ML)						
I-cell disease (ML2)	Mannose-6-phosphate phosphorylating enzyme	Mucopolysaccharide, glycolipid	None	Gastric chief cells, enterocytes	Vacuolated cells, PAS and fat stain positive	Enlarged lysosomes
Other						
Cystinosis	Cystine	Cystine transported	None	Phagocytic cells	Polarizable crystals, unfixed specimen	Membrane-bound crystals
Mannosidosis	Oligosaccharides	Mannosidase	None	Phagocytic cells, nerve and muscle cells, fibroblasts	Small vacuoles, PAS positive on frozen section only	Small membrane-bound bodies with fibrillar material
Neuronal ceroid lipofuscinosis (Batten's disease and Kufs disease)	Unknown	Ceroid or lipofuscin-like protein	None	Phagocytic cells, some muscle and Schwann cells, endothelial cells	Large, coarse, granular pigment, positive for Sudan black, PAS, acid-fast, yellow autofluorescence	Globules with a granular matrix, "Finnish snowballs"
Wolman's disease	Acid lipase	Cholesterol esters, triglycerides	Diarrhea, vomiting	Phagocytic cells	Large lipid vacuoles, fat stain positive	Membrane-bound lipid droplets

GI, Gastrointestinal; *PAS*, periodic acid–Schiff stain.

depending on the amount of pigment present. Occasionally, the pigment is so prominent that the mucosa shows multiple foci of tiny white polypoid lesions on a brown background. The white lesions represent normal or hyperplastic lymphoid aggregates that do not contain pigment.[107] Histologically, the pigment in macrophages has a dark-brown, granular appearance, and these cells may be located anywhere in the lamina propria (Fig. 7.5A). The pigment in the macrophage contains polymerized glycolipids, glycoproteins, and melanin ("melanized ceroid")[108] and is typically associated with anthraquinone laxative use. However, a number of studies have shown an association with increased apoptosis of epithelial cells[108,109] (caused by laxatives as well as chronic colitis,[110] chronic granulomatous disease,[111] and bamboo leaf extract[112]) and have suggested that melanosis is a nonspecific marker of increased apoptosis.

Pseudomelanosis. This is a rare benign condition characterized by the presence of discrete, flat, small, brown-black spots located typically in duodenal mucosa (speckled duodenum) but also reported in gastric mucosa.[113] It occurs in any age group and appears to be associated with upper GI bleeding, chronic renal failure, hypertension, or diabetes mellitus.[114] Unlike melanosis coli, it is not associated with use of anthraquinone laxatives. Microscopically, the black pigment is located subepithelially in mucosal macrophages, often at the tips of the villi (see Fig. 7.5B). Histochemical studies have revealed that the pigment represents a mixture of iron sulfide, hemosiderin, lipomelanin, and ceroid. It is typically negative or only focally positive with iron stains. Electron microscopic studies have revealed the material to be located in lysosomes.

Brown Bowel Syndrome. This is a rare acquired disorder that is associated with malabsorptive states and vitamin E deficiency. It is characterized by accumulation and deposition of lipofuscin pigment predominantly in the smooth muscle of the bowel, which gives a brown color to the bowel. It occurs most often in the small bowel but can involve the colon or stomach as well. Vitamin E (α-tocopherol) is an antioxidant that prevents peroxidation of unsaturated fatty acids. It is postulated that a deficiency in this vitamin may result in oxidized lipids, which polymerize with polysaccharides to form the brown pigment. Histologically, the pigment is most prominent in the smooth muscle cells of the muscularis mucosae and propria. Some pigmentation of macrophages, nerves, ganglia, and vascular smooth muscle also is usually observed.[115] The distribution of the pigment in conjunction with an appropriate clinical history often helps in differentiation of this lesion from those described earlier. The pigment, which stains positive with PAS, acid-fast, and fat stains on unfixed tissues, also shows the typical bright yellow autofluorescence pattern of lipofuscin. Electron microscopic examination usually reveals mitochondrial damage as well as pigment concentrated in the perinuclear Golgi region.[116] Clinically, the pigment does not have any direct effect on the bowel, although defects in contractility,[117] intussusception,[118] and toxic megacolon have been reported.[119]

Hemosiderosis/Hemochromatosis. In advanced iron overload disorders such as hemosiderosis or hemochromatosis,

TABLE 7.3 Macrophage Infiltrates in the Lamina Propria

Diagnosis	Histology	Histochemical	Immunohistochemical
Pigmented			
Melanosis	Dark brown, granular macrophages	PAS and acid-fast positive	CD68 positive (must bleach pigment)
Pseudomelanosis	Black, subepithelial macrophages	Iron positive	CD68 positive
Brown bowel syndrome	Brown smooth muscle cells	PAS, acid-fast positive Yellow autofluorescence	N/A
Hemosiderosis/ hemochromatosis	Finely granular, brown to black particles in epithelial cells	Iron positive	N/A
Barium granuloma	Gray, finely granular refractile pigment	PAS negative	N/A
Chronic granulomatous disease	Golden-brown macrophages	Fat stain and PAS positive	N/A
Nonpigmented			
Xanthoma	Clear, foamy macrophages	Fat stain positive on unfixed tissue	α_1-Antitrypsin, monocyte chemotactic and activating factor positive
Muciphages	Clear, foamy macrophages	d-PAS, Alcian blue positive	CD68 and lysozyme positive
Pseudolipomatosis	Clear open space with no cell lining	Negative for all stains	Negative for all immunostains
Whipple's disease	Pink, foamy macrophages	d-PAS granular positive	FISH for rRNA positive
Mycobacterium avium	Pink, foamy macrophages	Acid-fast or Fite positive d-PAS diffuse positive	CD68 positive
Malakoplakia	Pink, foamy macrophages with nuclear grooves; Michaelis-Gutmann bodies (MGB)	d-PAS positive MGB positive for calcium and iron	CD68 positive
Granular cell tumor	Pink, granular histiocytic cells	d-PAS positive	S100 positive
Signet ring cell adenocarcinoma	Clear cytoplasm with displaced nucleus	d-PAS-, Alcian blue-, and mucin-positive globules	Cytokeratin positive
Clear cell carcinoid tumor	Clear cells with foamy cytoplasm	d-PAS and mucin negative	Chromogranin positive
Malignant histiocytosis	Granular Langerhans cells with irregular elongate nuclei and nuclear grooves	d-PAS and mucin negative	S100 and CD1a positive

d-PAS, Periodic acid–Schiff with diastase; *FISH,* Fluorescence in situ hybridization; *PAS,* periodic acid–Schiff; *rRNA,* ribosomal ribonucleic acid.

iron is deposited in parenchymal cells throughout the body. In the GI tract, deposits are found most commonly in the parietal cells of the stomach, the Brunner glands in the duodenum, and the epithelial cells of the gut.[120,121] Some minor amounts of pigment can also be seen in macrophages. The pigment appears as finely granular, dark-brown to black particles. It stains positive with iron stains. The pigment must be differentiated from pseudomelanosis duodeni, which is typically larger and located predominantly in macrophages.

Barium Granuloma. This is a complication of barium examination, typically of the colon. It occurs secondary to extravasation of barium into the wall of the bowel as a result of mucosal injury, overinflation of a rectal balloon, or intrinsic inflammatory disease.[122] Endoscopically, it may manifest as a polypoid lesion and may mimic an adenoma or carcinoma. Histologically, one sees a granulomatous reaction surrounding gray, finely granular, refractile, PAS-negative material located in the cytoplasm of histiocytes and in the lamina propria (see Fig. 7.5C). The material is not birefringent. Radiographs of the paraffin block can help reveal the presence of radiopaque material.[123]

Nonpigmented Lesions

Xanthoma. This is a fairly common lesion of the GI tract most commonly found in the stomach. The terms *xanthoma, xanthelasma, lipid island,* and *xanthogranulomatous inflammation* are used synonymously. Endoscopically, xanthomas appear as small yellow nodules or streaks on the mucosa. They represent an accumulation of lipid and cholesterol within macrophages. Microscopically, one sees a collection of macrophages containing foamy cytoplasm positive for fat stains on unfixed tissue (Fig. 7.6A). Immunohistochemical stains for α_1-antitrypsin and monocyte chemotactic and activating factor are also typically positive,[124] whereas cytokeratin and mucin stains are negative. The lesions are typically associated with chronic inflammatory states[125] but can be seen with malignancies.[124]

Muciphages. These are mucin-rich phagocytes that accumulate as a result of mucosal damage. They are most common in the rectum (as many as 40% of all rectal biopsies contain muciphages)[126] and are also commonly found in the lamina propria and in the stalk of adenomatous polyps.[127] Endoscopically, muciphages can appear as polyps

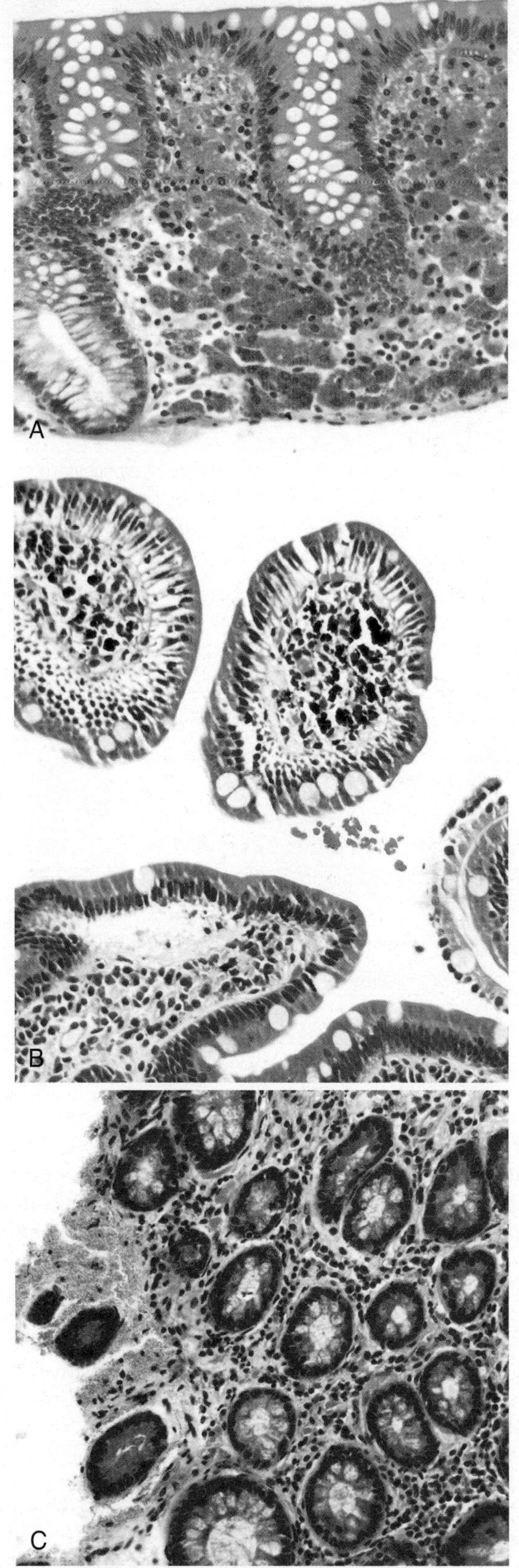

FIGURE 7.5 Pigmented cells mimicking lysosomal storage disease. A, Melanosis coli. Colonic mucosa contains lamina propria macrophages with dark-brown, granular appearance. **B,** Pseudomelanosis. Duodenal mucosa contains macrophages with a black pigment. **C,** Barium. Colonic mucosa contains a gray, finely granular material in the lamina propria.

or nodules. Histologically, foamy histiocytes containing coarse cytoplasmic vacuoles are present in the superficial lamina propria (see Fig. 7.6B). Mild fibrosis and architectural distortion may occur in cases associated with a previous injury.[128] Histochemical stains with d-PAS (PAS with diastase digestion) and Alcian blue at pH 2.5 and with immunohistochemical stains for CD68 and lysozyme are positive in muciphages.

Pseudolipomatosis. This is a common iatrogenic lesion caused by influx of air into the mucosa secondary to endoscopy-related trauma. It is a benign, transient lesion[129] that is characterized histologically by clear open spaces in the lamina propria or submucosa, representing trapped gas, without an epithelial or endothelial cell lining[130] (see Fig. 7.6C). These clear spaces do not stain with any specific immunohistochemical or histochemical reaction.

Whipple's Disease. This is a systemic infection that is caused by a cultivation-resistant bacterium, *Tropheryma whipplei*. In the GI tract, it is primarily found in the small bowel; however, it can involve the stomach,[131] esophagus, and colon as well.[132] Histologically, one sees characteristic abundant, pink-colored, foamy macrophages filling the lamina propria. These macrophages may contain small granules that are positive for d-PAS. Extracellular lipid is often present (see Fig. 7.6D). Electron microscopic examination reveals intracellular and extracellular bacterial rods in various stages of disintegration. These bacteria are also found within IgA-positive plasma cells.[133] With the use of fluorescence in situ hybridization (FISH) for ribosomal RNA, the active organism appears to be most prevalent near the tips of intestinal villi in the lamina propria.[134]

***Mycobacterium avium-intracellulare* Complex Infection.** This is a common pathogen in AIDS that may also be seen in other immunocompromised patients.[135] It typically affects the small bowel and colon. Endoscopically, the mucosa can appear normal or coarsely granular.[136] Histologically, abundant, variably sized sheets of foamy macrophages are seen in the lamina propria and cause widening of the villi (see Fig. 7.6E). Diagnosis is made with acid-fast or Fite stain positivity; numerous elongated organisms are revealed within the macrophages. PAS stain typically reveals a relatively diffuse fibrillary staining pattern in macrophages, as opposed to the granular staining characteristic of Whipple's disease. The organisms are typically intact, unlike the various stages of disintegration that are seen in Whipple's disease.

Malakoplakia. This is a rare bacterial infection that affects patients with an underlying macrophage phagolysosome defect (not typically seen in patients with AIDS).[137] It is usually caused by *Escherichia coli* or *Klebsiella* spp.[138] and is often seen in the urinary tract. However, it can involve any portion of the GI tract. Endoscopically, the mucosa shows numerous soft, yellow plaques on the mucosa. Rarely, a mass lesion composed of macrophages may develop. Histologically, there is infiltration of the lamina propria by neutrophils and abundant macrophages; the latter often contain nuclear grooves (see Fig. 7.6F). Michaelis-Gutmann bodies, which are small, pale, intracytoplasmic concretions that stain for calcium and iron, are diagnostic. Macrophages also stain with d-PAS. Electron microscopic examination reveals degenerated bacilli in phagolysosomes, similar to those seen in Whipple's disease.[139]

Granular Cell Tumor. These tumors are believed to be of neurogenic origin and are typically found in the esophagus, but they can occur anywhere in the GI tract.[140] Rare cases have been described in the small bowel and colon.[141,142] They are mostly benign, but malignant tumors have rarely been described. The tumors typically manifest as nodules in patients with nonspecific GI symptoms. Histologically, these tumors include abundant epithelioid or histiocytic cells with distinct pink granular cytoplasm in the lamina propria or submucosa (see Fig. 7.6G). The cells are positive for d-PAS and are strongly S100 positive. Electron microscopic examination reveals cells filled with giant autophagic vacuoles (lysosomes) that contain myelin-like debris of giant lysosomes.

Signet Ring Cell Adenocarcinoma. This tumor shows an infiltration of malignant cells with clear cytoplasm and

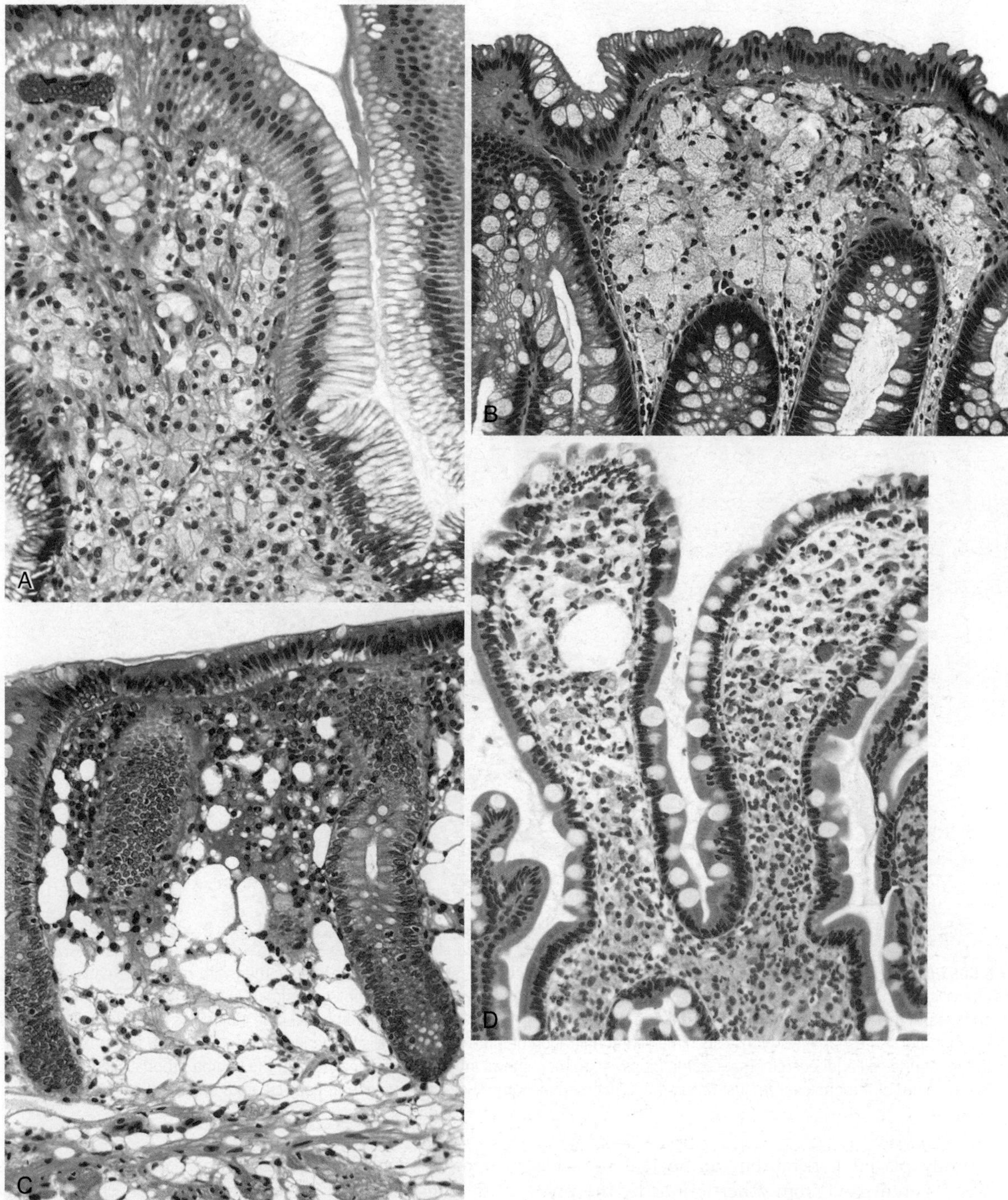

FIGURE 7.6 Nonpigmented cells mimicking lysosomal storage disease. A, Xanthoma. A gastric biopsy specimen with abundant macrophages in the lamina propria is shown. The macrophages have a bland central nucleus with foamy cytoplasm. **B,** Muciphages in the rectum. Rectal biopsy specimen contains foamy macrophages with coarse, large cytoplasmic vacuoles in the superficial lamina propria. **C,** Pseudolipomatosis. Colonic biopsy specimen shows clear, unlined spaces in the lamina propria. **D,** Whipple's disease. A small bowel biopsy specimen shows expansion of the villus by numerous pink macrophages. A single clear space, representing extracellular lipid, is present in the tip of one of the villi.

Continued

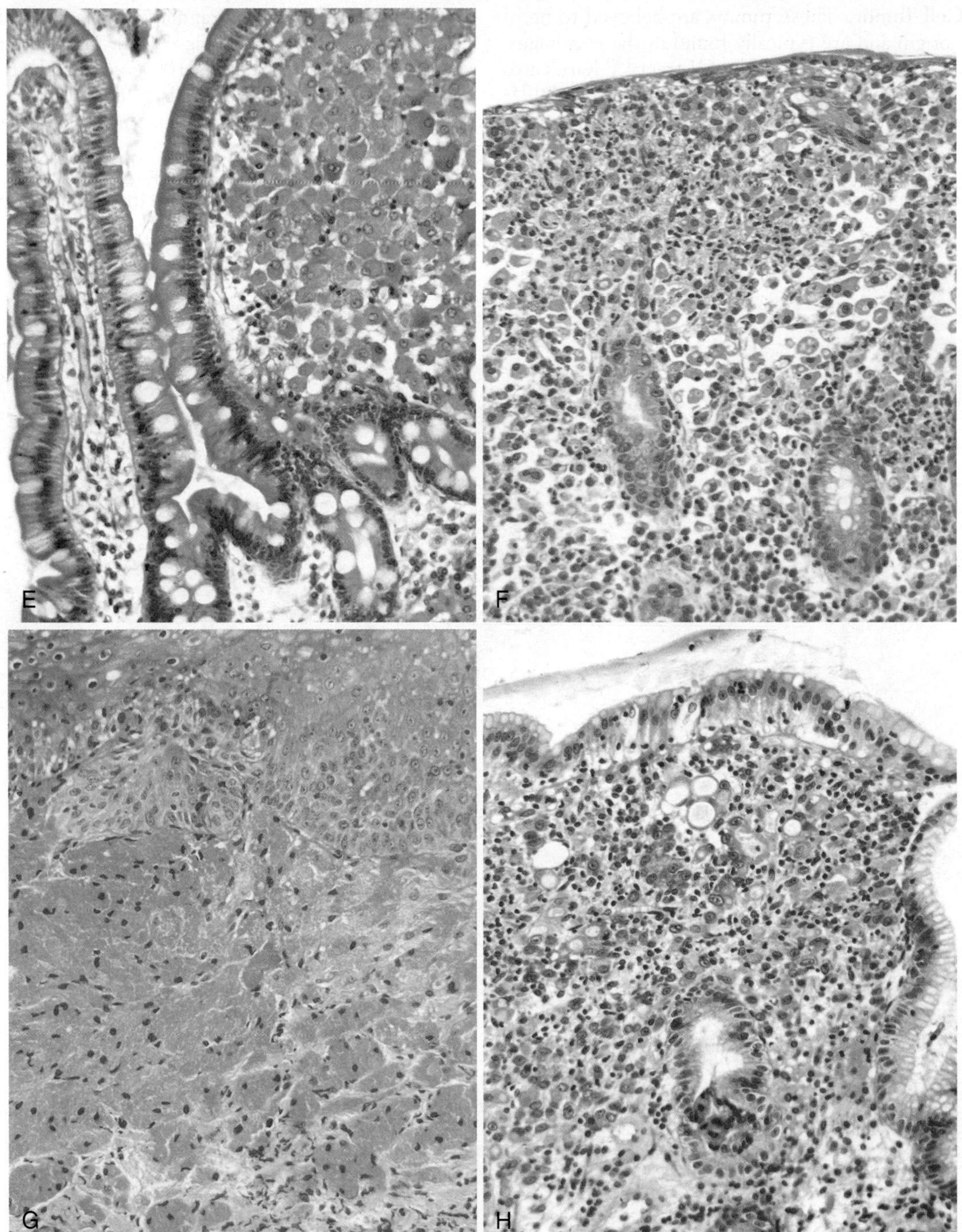

FIGURE 7.6 CONT'D E, *Mycobacterium avium-intracellulare* complex infection. A small bowel biopsy specimen with marked expansion of the lamina propria of the villi by pink, homogeneous macrophages is shown. **F,** Malakoplakia. Colonic biopsy specimen shows infiltration of the lamina propria with macrophages. A marked acute inflammatory infiltrate is also seen. The macrophages contain small blue inclusions (Michaelis-Gutmann bodies). **G,** Granular cell tumor. An esophageal biopsy specimen with infiltration of large granular cells in the lamina propria below the squamous epithelium is shown. **H,** Signet ring cell adenocarcinoma. Gastric biopsy specimen shows infiltration of single cells in the lamina propria. Signet ring cells can be identified in the center of the photograph, just under the surface epithelium. They contain eccentrically located, enlarged, atypical nuclei.

an eccentrically placed hyperchromatic nucleus (see Fig. 7.6H). It is differentiated from other lesions by the presence of highly atypical nuclear features and by positivity with mucin and cytokeratin stains.[143]

Clear Cell Carcinoid Tumor. A rare case has been reported of a gastric carcinoid composed entirely of clear cells with foamy cytoplasm.[144] Immunopositivity for endocrine markers such as chromogranin A or electron microscopic demonstration of dense core granules helps define the lesion.

Langerhans Cell Histiocytosis. Langerhans cell histiocytosis can involve any portion of the GI tract, either as part of generalized disease or as a separate primary entity. Involved areas may manifest as a polypoid or mass lesion. Histologically, one sees a mucosal infiltrate composed of Langerhans cells that have irregular, elongated nuclei and prominent nuclear grooves and folds. The cytoplasm of the tumor cells is abundant and finely granular. These tumors are usually associated with a prominent eosinophilic infiltrate. As with mucosa-associated lymphoid tissue (MALT) lymphoma, invasion and destruction of the epithelium are common.[145] Immunohistochemical stains for S100 and CD1a are intensely positive in tumor cells. Electron microscopic examination reveals Birbeck granules in the cytoplasm of tumor cells.[146]

Amyloidosis

Amyloidosis is not a single disease but the product of a variety of diseases. The common feature of these diseases is extracellular deposition of amyloid proteins that stain with Congo red and show apple-green birefringence under polarized light. The proteins have a typical fibrillary appearance on electron microscopy. All amyloid fibrils are protein complexes with a common tertiary molecular structure, referred to as a *twisted β-pleated sheet pattern.*

Classification

Historically, amyloidosis was classified according to its clinical presentation (localized vs. diffuse) or its underlying cause (primary, secondary, hereditary, or endocrine related); now, the classification is determined on the basis of the biochemical composition of the amyloid fibrils (Table 7.4). The most common types that involve the GI tract are AA, AL, and Aβ2M. In addition to the more common proteins listed in the table, a number of other types of amyloid proteins have been described, such as Aβ (β protein precursor), AApoA1 (apolipoprotein A1), ALys (lysozyme), ACys (cystatin C), and AGel (gelsolin).

TABLE 7.4 Amyloidosis

Etiology	Type	Disease	Amyloid Precursor Protein
Primary	AL	Myeloma, Waldenström macroglobulinemia, plasma cell dyscrasias, B-cell malignancies	Light chains
	AH	Heavy chain disease	Immunoglobulin G1
Secondary	AA	Chronic inflammatory lesions: inflammatory bowel disease, rheumatoid arthritis, chronic infections, familial Mediterranean fever Rare malignancies: gastric and renal carcinoma	Serum amyloid A
	Aβ2M	Long-term kidney dialysis	β_2-Microglobulin
Hereditary	ATTR	Familial amyloid polyneuropathy	Transthyretin (prealbumin)
	AFib		Fibrinogen A α-chain
Endocrine	AIAAP	Endocrine associated	Islet amyloid polypeptide

Clinical Features

GI involvement is common in all types of systemic amyloidosis (primary and secondary), ranging from 85% to 100%.[147-149] In most cases associated with systemic amyloidosis, patchy involvement of the GI tract is seen without associated symptoms. However, a variety of GI symptoms may occur, including bleeding,[150] pseudo-obstruction,[151] decreased motility,[152] and, rarely, perforation.[153] The greater the number of deposits and the more widespread the involvement, the higher the likelihood of clinical symptoms. Vascular involvement by amyloid produces fragility and rupture of affected vessels, which can lead to the development of petechial hemorrhage of the mucosa and ischemic disease and its manifestations. In fact, ulcerating lesions may mimic IBD grossly.[154]

Amyloid infiltration within nerve[155] and muscle fibers[156] can cause motility disorders. Malabsorption may result from stasis and bacterial overgrowth. Finally, amyloidosis can occasionally manifest as a solitary mass lesion or polyp that mimics a malignant tumor.[157] Endoscopically, the mucosa may appear normal or may show a fine granular appearance with erosions, friability, and thickening of the valvulae conniventes.[158,159]

Pathological Features

Microscopically, amyloid deposits are extracellular and have a classic waxy, homogeneous appearance (Fig. 7.7A). Pink hyaline amyloid may contain small, slitlike spaces caused by cracking during tissue processing. Histochemical stains for Congo red (the most specific), toluidine blue, crystal violet, fluorochrome, and thioflavine are usually positive with all types of amyloid (see Fig. 7.7B). Amyloid also stains positive with the PAS reaction and negative with lipid and mineral stains. In general, AA amyloid seems to localize to capillaries, small arterioles, and the mucosa. AL amyloid is often found in the muscularis propria and in medium-size to large vessels. Aβ2M amyloid is found mainly in the muscularis propria and in small arterioles and venules, forming subendothelial nodular lesions.[160] AL and AA forms also can be distinguished by pretreatment with potassium permanganate. This pretreatment abolishes the Congo red affinity of the AA fibrils but not that of the AL fibrils.[161] Immunohistochemical stains with antibodies to amyloid A, immunoglobulins λ and κ light chain amyloid fibril proteins, β_2-microglobulin, and transthyretin characterize the majority of amyloid deposits.[162] Electron microscopy reveals an interlocking meshwork of fibrils that measure 7.5 to 10 nm in diameter with variable length.

Amyloidosis should be differentiated from arteriosclerosis in blood vessels and from collagen in the lamina propria, submucosa, and muscularis (in systemic sclerosis). Congo red stains can help with this differential diagnosis in that neither arteriosclerosis nor collagen stains with Congo red. One study suggested that Congo red stain may not be sensitive enough in patients with early amyloidosis in minute amounts.[163]

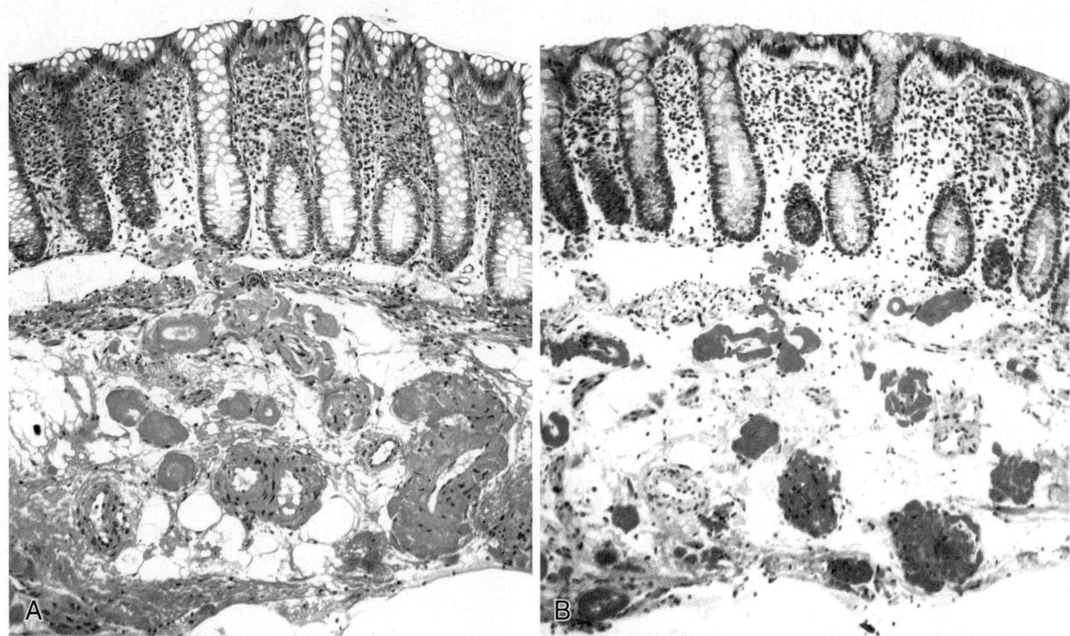

FIGURE 7.7 Amyloidosis. A, Intermediate-power view of a colonic mucosal biopsy specimen. Homogeneous material is present in the vessels in the submucosa and as extracellular deposits. The overlying colonic mucosa is unremarkable. **B,** Same section stained with Congo red. The amyloid deposits have a bright orange-red appearance.

GI biopsy is a procedure commonly used to diagnose amyloidosis. Rectal biopsies have a sensitivity of 85%, compared with a sensitivity of 54% for fat biopsies.[147] In the rectum, amyloid deposits are most commonly seen in small arterioles and veins in the submucosa; therefore a deep suction biopsy is usually required for adequate evaluation. Some studies have suggested that gastric or small bowel biopsies have a sensitivity as high as 100% for the diagnosis of amyloidosis.[156,164]

Familial Mediterranean Fever (Familial Paroxysmal Polyserositis, Recurring Polyserositis)

Familial Mediterranean fever is an inherited autosomal recessive disorder seen almost exclusively in Sephardic Jews, Arabs, Armenians, and people of Turkish descent. It is characterized by recurring and self-limited attacks of fevers and serosal inflammation involving the peritoneal, synovial, and pleural membranes. This disease typically begins in childhood or adolescence and recurs at irregular intervals throughout life.[165] GI involvement consists of acute inflammation limited to the serosal surfaces of the bowel (peritonitis). Repeated episodes can result in the formation of peritoneal adhesions that may cause obstruction. Systemic amyloidosis may also occur in untreated patients. The AA amyloid type is believed to develop as a consequence of recurrent inflammation. Furthermore, amyloid deposits in the lamina propria and the submucosal vessels may occur without symptoms. The disease is often treated with colchicine.

PULMONARY DISORDERS

Hypoxia-producing pulmonary disorders can lead to ischemic injury of the GI tract. An increased incidence of peptic ulcer disease has also been described in patients with chronic obstructive pulmonary disease.[166] This is thought to be the result of hypercapnia, which stimulates gastric acid secretion. Pneumonia, bronchitis, asthma, and idiopathic pulmonary fibrosis are all associated with gastroesophageal reflux disease (GERD).[167] It is also believed that GERD may cause or exacerbate several pulmonary diseases.

REPRODUCTIVE DISORDERS

Effects of Pregnancy and Exogenous Hormones

A number of GI problems may develop during pregnancy. Nausea, vomiting, and heartburn are common in the first trimester. Some studies suggest that these effects are secondary to human chorionic gonadotropin or estrogen secretion,[168] which leads to abnormalities in gastric myoelectrical activity and contractility.[169] Secondary esophagitis may develop as a result of severe vomiting. Reflux, peptic ulcers, *Helicobacter pylori* infection, and cholecystitis are also increased. In addition, constipation is a frequent problem during the late stages of pregnancy. Thrombosed external hemorrhoids, anal fissures, and rectal wall prolapse can occur secondary to vaginal delivery.[170]

Pregnancy outcomes are generally favorable in patients with IBD. Population studies suggest that maternal IBD is associated with increased odds of preterm delivery, low birth weight, smallness for gestational age (Crohn's disease), and congenital malformations (ulcerative colitis).[171-173] The risk of pregnancy-related complications and the disease behavior during pregnancy depend mainly on disease activity at the time of conception. However, pregnancy does not seem to influence the course of IBD. Most drugs used to treat IBD are safe to use in pregnancy and breastfeeding. Biological agents do cross the placenta (mainly in the third trimester)

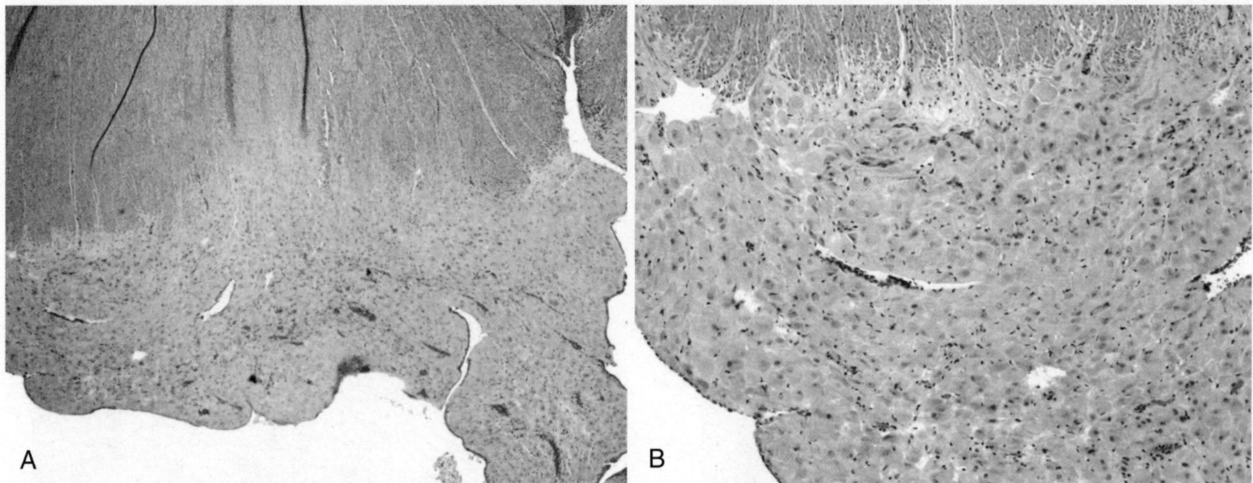

FIGURE 7.8 Decidualization of the peritoneum. A, Low-power view of the serosal aspect of a colonic resection specimen. Muscularis propria is present at the superior portion of the image with marked thickening and decidualization of the subserosal tissue. **B,** High-power view of the plump pink (decidualized) cells present between the muscularis propria (superior) and mesothelial cells (inferior).

and are often held after 30 weeks' gestation and restarted after delivery.[174]

Oral contraceptive pills and exogenous estrogens are associated with nausea and vomiting. They also are associated with thrombosis and, consequently, an increased risk for ischemia of the small bowel and colon.[175]

Decidualization of the Peritoneum

Ectopic decidualization of the peritoneum is a rare lesion. It can yield macroscopic nodules (peritoneal deciduosis or deciduosis peritonei) that mimic peritoneal carcinomatosis.[176] Grossly, multiple light-tan peritoneal masses or nodules typically are identified at the time of caesarean section. Microscopically, plump pink (decidualized) cells are present between the mesothelial cells and muscularis propria (Fig. 7.8). This is a physiological reaction with an excellent prognosis and spontaneous resolution after delivery.

Endometriosis

Clinical Features

Endometriosis is a condition characterized by the presence of endometrial glands or stroma outside of the uterus. It can involve any portion of the GI tract. The most common sites of involvement are organs in the pelvis such as the rectosigmoid colon, appendix, and small bowel. The GI tract is involved in 12% to 37% of cases.[177] Intestinal endometriosis is usually asymptomatic. However, when symptomatic, it typically causes obstructive symptoms as a result of adhesions. Complete obstruction of the bowel lumen occurs in less than 1% of cases.[177] Other atypical presentations include diarrhea and GI bleeding. Symptoms are often temporally associated with the onset of menses.

Pathological Features

Endometriosis may be solitary or multifocal, and it may manifest as a mass lesion or with volvulus, intussusception, luminal narrowing, or adhesions. Endometrial glands or stroma are usually present on the serosal surface but may involve any layer of the bowel wall. On a cut surface, the endometriosis often appears sclerotic with punctate hemorrhagic or brown areas. Microscopically, this disorder is characterized by the presence of endometrial-type glands or stroma (smaller, slightly elongated cells that are packed together, often with intermingled red blood cells) and hemosiderin-laden macrophages (Fig. 7.9). At least two of these three findings should be present for a diagnosis of endometriosis to be established with certainty. In addition, fibrosis and prominent smooth muscle proliferation may surround foci of endometriosis. Fresh hemorrhage may occur. Immunohistochemical staining for estrogen receptors is usually positive in both the glands and stromal cells.[178]

Differential Diagnosis

Most importantly, the differential diagnosis includes invasive adenocarcinoma. This can be extremely problematic to differentiate on fine-needle aspiration specimens. With this sampling procedure, the glandular epithelium is preferentially aspirated and may show nuclear atypia, mimicking an adenocarcinoma. The finding of hemorrhage, hemosiderin-laden macrophages, and stromal cells helps establish a correct diagnosis. On histological section, differentiation from adenocarcinoma depends on the finding of characteristic stroma and hemosiderin-laden macrophages, in addition to glandular epithelium. Endometriosis may occasionally be present in mucosal biopsies[179] and can resemble colitis cystica profunda. If smooth muscle proliferation is prominent, differentiation from a leiomyoma can be achieved by deeper sectioning of the tissue to look for glandular epithelium. In difficult cases, colonic glands are positive for carcinoembryonic antigen, whereas endometrial glands are negative for this peptide.[180]

RHEUMATOLOGICAL DISORDERS

Connective tissue disorders can affect the GI tract in a variety of ways. They can cause hypomotility, secondary to muscle inflammation or atrophy, or ischemic disease, secondary to vasculitis. A variety of lesions may develop secondary to pharmacological therapy for these disorders. Hypomotility is most commonly seen in scleroderma, mixed connective

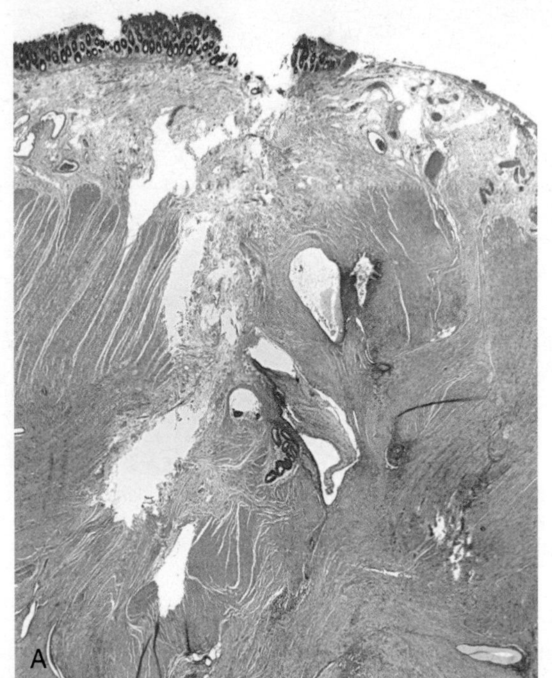

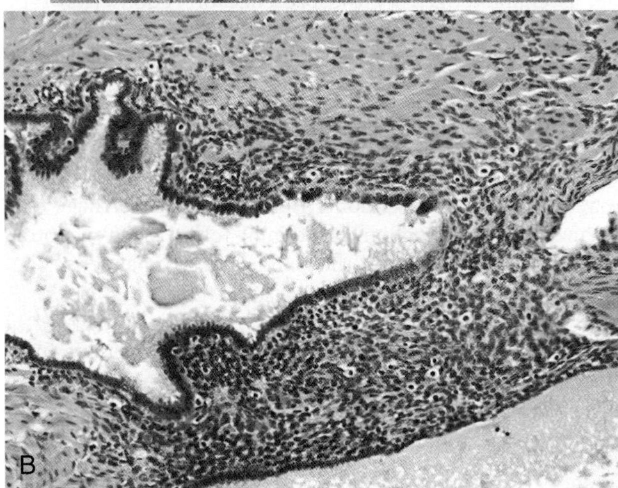

FIGURE 7.9 Endometriosis of the colon. A, Low-power view of the full thickness of the colon. Glandular epithelium containing blue mucin and dark-blue endometrial stroma is identified in the muscularis propria of the colon. Marked muscular hypertrophy is also seen. **B,** High-power view of infiltrating, bland, well-formed glands with characteristic stroma.

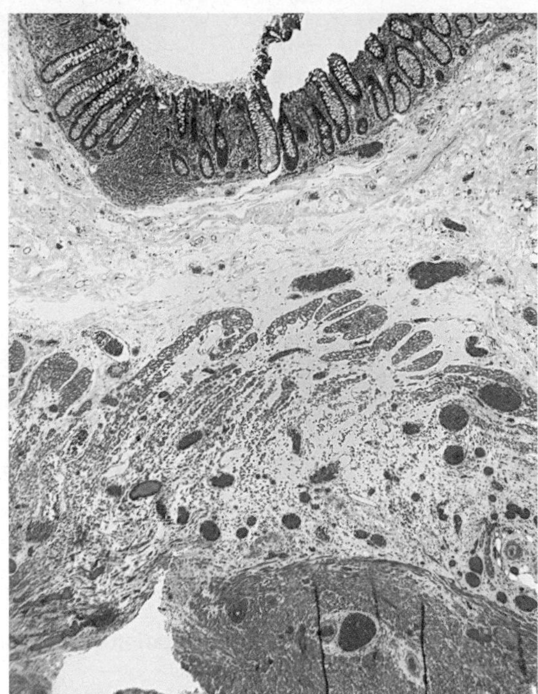

FIGURE 7.10 Scleroderma. Intermediate-power view of the colon stained with trichrome reveals atrophy and increased fibrosis of the inner circular layer of the muscularis propria.

tissue disease, and polymyositis/dermatomyositis. Vasculitis predominates in systemic lupus erythematosus (SLE), rheumatoid arthritis, polyarteritis nodosa, and Behçet's syndrome. The majority of these disorders are treated with antiinflammatory drugs that can have major GI effects. For example, rheumatoid arthritis is typically treated with nonsteroidal antiinflammatory drugs (NSAIDs), which can cause peptic ulceration and bleeding.

Scleroderma

Scleroderma (progressive systemic sclerosis) is a systemic disease of unknown cause characterized by inflammation, fibrosis, upregulated collagen production, and vasculitis. GI involvement is common and is typically characterized by hypomotility (see Chapter 8 for details). Scleroderma can be part of CREST syndrome (*c*alcinosis, *R*aynaud phenomenon, *e*sophageal involvement, *s*clerodactyly, and *t*elangiectases). Scleroderma most commonly involves the esophagus; manometric abnormalities are seen in up to 90% of patients.[181] However, abnormalities of the entire GI tract may also be observed. Colonic dysfunction has been reported in up to 20% of patients.[182]

In the esophagus, lower esophageal sphincter pressure is reduced, and gastric emptying of the stomach is delayed.[183] Both of these factors increase the incidence of GERD, erosive esophagitis, and stricture formation. The small and large intestine may also be involved. Typical features include scattered wide-mouthed diverticula,[184] pseudo-obstruction,[185] and intestinal perforation.[186]

Pathologically, scleroderma is characterized by smooth muscle atrophy and its replacement by collagenized fibrous tissue (Fig. 7.10). The lesion most commonly affects the inner circular muscle layer but can involve the entire muscularis propria on occasion. Fibrous tissue is highlighted by trichrome stain, which reveals atrophy and loss of muscle tissue. Fibrosis may also involve the submucosa to a variable degree.[187] Muscular atrophy results in atony and dilation and produces wide-mouthed pseudodiverticula that can be identified radiographically. In addition, the small vessels of the bowel may show a proliferative endarteritis and mucinous changes of the media.[188] Rarely, ischemic ulcers can occur as a result.

Dermatomyositis and Polymyositis

Dermatomyositis and polymyositis are inflammatory myopathies that primarily involve skeletal muscle. Skin involvement also occurs in dermatomyositis. These disorders may be associated with motor dysfunction of the GI tract.[189] The striated muscle of the cervical esophagus is most frequently affected when delayed esophageal emptying is common.[190] Histological changes include chronic inflammation, edema, and muscle atrophy. Features can mimic scleroderma, but fibrosis is not prominent in these disorders.

Systemic Lupus Erythematosus

SLE is a systemic multisystem autoimmune disease that affects the GI tract in approximately 20% of patients. The development of vasculitis can lead to ischemia[191] and perforation of the GI tract. SLE also has been associated with malabsorption, protein-losing enteropathy,[192] and amyloidosis.[193]

Mixed Connective Tissue Disease

Mixed connective tissue disease has features of scleroderma, SLE, and polymyositis. GI abnormalities are common.[194] GI features are similar to those of scleroderma, with motility dysfunction[195] and vasculitis being the most common complications.

Rheumatoid Arthritis

GI involvement occurs in 25% of patients with long-standing rheumatoid arthritis.[196] Notably, this occurs in the form of a necrotizing vasculitis that affects small to medium-size arteries, similar to polyarteritis nodosa. The condition is usually asymptomatic. However, hemorrhage or even perforation may occur.[197] GI lesions may also be seen in association with long-term use of NSAIDs, and in rare cases, long-standing inflammation can lead to amyloidosis.

Reactive Arthritis

The term *reactive arthritis* refers to a group of inflammatory disorders associated with arthritis (spondyloarthropathy). It includes psoriatic arthritis, Reiter's syndrome, ankylosing spondylitis, and arthritis associated with IBD. Most affected individuals (70%)[198] have chronic active colitis. Interestingly, clinical remission is always associated with normal gut histology.[199]

Sjögren's Syndrome

Sjögren's syndrome is a clinicopathological entity characterized by dry eyes and mouth secondary to immune-mediated destruction of the lacrimal and salivary glands. Patients with Sjögren's syndrome may develop immune-mediated destruction of the pharyngeal and esophageal glands with fissuring and ulceration of the pharynx and esophagus. Esophageal webs have been observed in up to 10% of patients. Atrophic gastritis, atrophy, and chronic inflammation of the esophageal glands have been noted as well.[200] Histologically, the salivary glands of the esophagus show a periductal and perivascular lymphocytic inflammatory infiltrate that can occasionally be quite marked.

Hereditary Connective Tissue Disorders

Hereditary connective tissue disorders, such as Ehlers-Danlos syndrome and pseudoxanthoma elasticum, result from a defect in collagen synthesis or structure. These defects result in thinning of the bowel wall and vascular structures[201]; patients are at increased risk for GI hemorrhage and perforation.[202] Patients with Ehlers-Danlos syndrome also have diaphragmatic hernias and GI diverticula. Upper GI tract hemorrhage occurs in 13% of patients with pseudoxanthoma elasticum.[203] In these cases, submucosal, yellowish, nodular lesions, similar to xanthoma-like skin lesions, may be seen.[204] Histological examination typically reveals superficial mucosal hemorrhage, erosion, and elastic tissue degeneration of small and medium-size arteries with calcified plaque formation.

UROLOGICAL DISORDERS

Acute Renal Failure

Postsurgical or trauma-associated acute renal failure often results in gastric or duodenal erosions, ulceration, and hemorrhage secondary to hypotension, stress, and multiorgan failure.[205]

Hemolytic-Uremic Syndrome

HUS is an acute onset of microangiopathic hemolytic anemia, thrombocytopenia, and renal dysfunction. Cases associated with *E. coli* infection often manifest with a GI prodrome that is difficult to differentiate histologically from an acute colitis.[206] Presentations mimicking intestinal intussusception[207] and ulcerative colitis have also been described.[208] During HUS, an associated colitis is seen in most patients, and there is a 1% to 2% incidence of colonic perforation.[209] Marked mucosal and submucosal edema and hemorrhage of the colon can occur, but inflammation usually is not significant (Fig. 7.11). Microvascular angiopathy

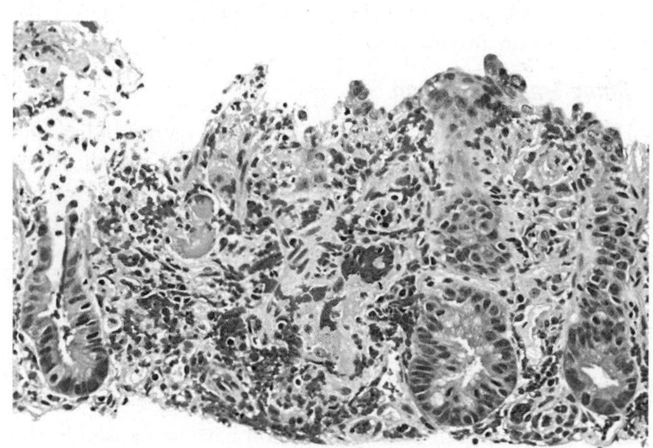

FIGURE 7.11 Hemolytic-uremic syndrome secondary to *Escherichia coli* infection. Intermediate-power view of mucosa shows erosion, hemorrhage, edema, and a paucity of inflammation. Focal endothelial cell damage with thrombi is present. (*Courtesy Dr. Elizabeth Montgomery, The Johns Hopkins University, Baltimore.*)

with endothelial cell damage and overt thrombosis may also be observed.[210]

Chronic Renal Failure

A variety of GI lesions may develop in patients with chronic renal failure. These are mainly associated with uremia, long-term hemodialysis, or kidney transplantation.

Uremia

GI symptoms that are common among patients with uremia include GERD,[211] nausea, vomiting, anorexia, epigastric pain, and upper GI hemorrhage. Early studies suggested an increased incidence of dyspepsia, ulcer disease, and *H. pylori* gastritis. However, studies indicate that the incidence of these conditions is not significantly different from that in the general population.[212] GI hemorrhage occurs in up to 15% of patients, accounts for 15% to 20% of all deaths in patients on long-term dialysis, and is often associated with angiodysplasia. Bleeding abnormalities may also occur as a result of platelet dysfunction. Mucosal abnormalities range from edema to ulceration and occur in 60% of patients who die from uremia.[213] The pathogenesis of uremic syndrome–associated GI tract disease is unclear. However, many manifestations of uremia are relieved by dialysis, which suggests a role for humoral factors. In addition, gastric mucosal calcinosis may be identified in patients with chronic renal failure or uremia and after renal transplantation.[214] Microscopically, calcinosis appears as small, white, flat plaques or nodules that contain amorphous basophilic deposits within the subepithelial compartment of the superficial lamina propria.

Long-Term Hemodialysis

Acute fluid loss during the process of dialysis can lead to hypotension and nonocclusive mesenteric ischemia.[215,216] Peritonitis secondary to bacterial infection and acute bowel obstruction secondary to incarcerated hernia into the catheter tract can also develop in patients undergoing peritoneal dialysis.[217] Patients on dialysis are also susceptible to *Salmonella* spp. enteritis[218] and dialysis-associated β_2-microglobulin amyloidosis.[219]

Kidney Transplantation

GI complications are an important cause of morbidity and mortality in kidney transplant recipients.[220] Complications are mainly related to immunosuppression therapy. Patients are at risk for opportunistic infections, including *Candida* spp., cytomegalovirus, herpesvirus, *Cryptosporidium* spp., and *Strongyloides* spp. These patients also are at increased risk for exacerbation of diverticulitis, for unknown reasons.[221]

Urinary Conduits

Three basic types of urinary diversion have been used in the treatment of congenital or malignant disorders—ureterosigmoidostomy, ileal neobladder, and antirefluxing colonic conduits.

Ureterosigmoidostomy, whereby the ureter is implanted into the sigmoid colon, is associated with a greatly increased risk for colonic neoplasia at or near the site of anastomosis.[222] Hence, this type of diversion is no longer popular. Adenocarcinomas typically arise 15 to 25 years after surgery and are histologically identical to typical colon adenocarcinomas. Endoscopic surveillance biopsies are recommended to screen for epithelial dysplasia.[223] In addition to dysplasia, one may see inflammatory polyps, edema, crypt branching, and Paneth cell metaplasia.[222,224]

Creation of an ileal neobladder (Kock or Charleston pouch) is now the most common procedure performed in patients who require some form of urinary diversion. These pouches are created from a portion of ileum that is separated from the fecal stream, and risk of malignancy has not been associated with these procedures. However, mucosal biopsy of these pouches may reveal histological changes over time. Early changes (over the first year) include shortening of villi with loss of microvilli and decreased numbers of goblet cells.[225] Late changes (after 4 years) consist of marked flattening of the epithelium with epithelial stratification, similar to urothelium.[226] Dysplasia has not been described.

Antirefluxing colonic conduits, using a segment of colon that is isolated from the fecal stream, appear to be associated with a lower degree of retrograde reflux and therefore a decreased incidence of pyelonephritis.

Screening for recurrent malignant urothelial disease is typically done with cytology. These urine specimens typically have classic degenerative epithelial cells (small bowel surface epithelium). One looks for atypical cells with increased nuclear-to-cytoplasmic ratio, cell clusters, and nuclear pleomorphism.[227]

MISCELLANEOUS DISORDERS

Chronic Granulomatous Disease

Chronic granulomatous disease (discussed further in Chapter 10) is a rare X-linked or autosomal recessive inherited disorder of phagocyte function. It is characterized by recurrent infections in infants and children.[228] Affected children suffer from chronic infections, often with abscess formation, in many organs. The GI system is involved in approximately 25% of patients.[229] Patients may present with vitamin B_{12} deficiency and an abnormal Schilling test result that is not corrected by the addition of intrinsic factor, as well as steatorrhea, obstruction, or bleeding. The defect lies in the inability of the body to destroy catalase-positive bacteria and fungi as a result of a lack of hydrogen peroxide production by phagocytic leukocytes. This condition may be diagnosed by the finding of a negative nitroblue tetrazolium assay or by other tests that reveal decreased bactericidal activity of leukocytes.

This disease is characterized by necrosis and abscess and sinus tract formation, which may be seen in the form of gastric outlet obstruction,[229,230] perineal abscess, diffuse colitis,[231] or even esophageal narrowing.[232] Histologically, necrotizing lesions often have sparse and poorly formed granulomas, frequently with marked eosinophilia. Microorganisms usually are not detectable in the lesion. The mucosa of the small and large intestine shows clusters of enlarged macrophages, often located adjacent to the muscularis mucosae in the basal portion of the lamina propria. The macrophages range from 50 to 100 μm in diameter and contain a golden-brown lipofuscin type of pigment (Fig. 7.12). The pigment stains positively with fat stains and the PAS reaction. The pigment is refractile on standard histological section as well. Rectal biopsy may show an increased number of inflammatory cells

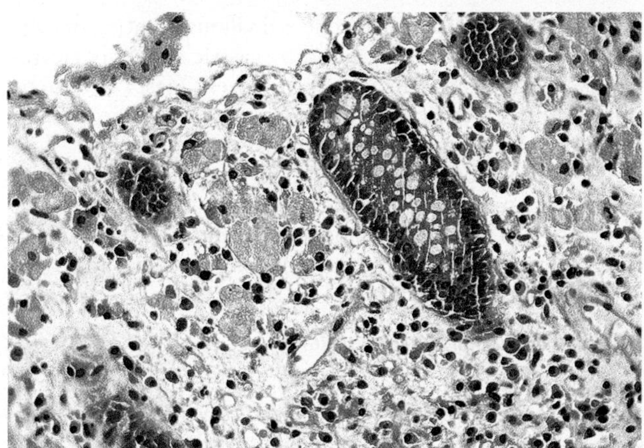

FIGURE 7.12 Chronic granulomatous disease of the colon. Pigmented macrophages are present in the lamina propria and simulate the appearance of melanosis coli.

(including plasma cells, neutrophils, and eosinophils) in the lamina propria.

The differential diagnosis includes other granulomatous disorders, such as mycobacterial and fungal infections, sarcoidosis, and IBD. These lesions can be excluded by stains or cultures and by appropriate clinical history. Pigment-laden macrophages may resemble several storage disorders, such as Batten's disease and brown bowel syndrome. Other storage disorders typically do not involve PAS-positive pigments. Whipple's disease and MAC infection have PAS-positive material but are not typically refractile. Finally, melanosis coli may have a similar pigment, but macrophages in this condition are usually more prominent in the superficial lamina propria and are not usually present in the small intestine.

Sarcoidosis

Sarcoidosis rarely involves the GI tract. The stomach is the most common site of sarcoidosis,[233] although involvement of the entire GI tract has been reported. It occurs in middle-age patients and is usually associated with pulmonary disease, although the GI tract may rarely be the first site of involvement. Sarcoidosis is characterized by an abnormal immune response and the formation of multiple noncaseating granulomas. This condition is also associated with high serum angiotensin-converting enzyme activity.[234] The cause is unknown. In patients with sarcoidosis, a high frequency of humoral autoimmunity (increased incidence of antibodies to H^+,K^+-ATPase, gliadin, and endomysium) is seen.[235] However, there does not appear to be an increased incidence of pernicious anemia or celiac disease.

The pathology of sarcoidosis is variable. The mucosa may show no abnormalities, or it may be severely involved, with a linitis plastica–like appearance of the stomach.[236] Ulceration and bleeding have been reported. Microscopically, the hallmark of sarcoidosis is the presence of noncaseating granulomas. These granulomas are composed of epithelioid histiocytes, with or without giant cells, and are often associated with a rim of lymphocytes at the periphery (Fig. 7.13). They may be present in any layer of the bowel wall and may be associated with tissue damage.

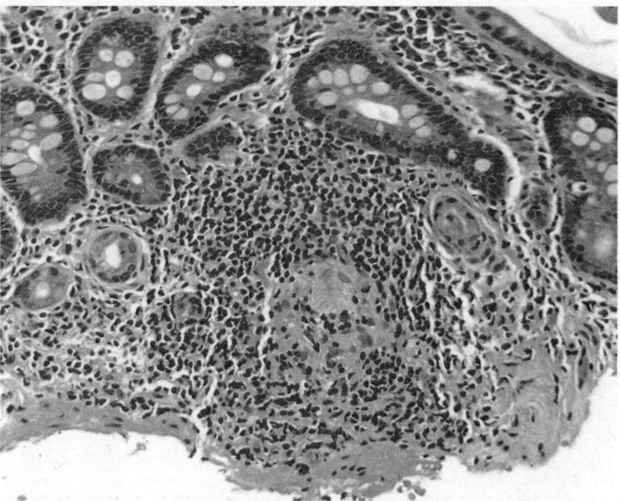

FIGURE 7.13 Sarcoidosis. High-power view of a mucosal granuloma includes epithelioid histiocytes with a rim of lymphocytes. The lesion is present just above the muscularis mucosae in a small-bowel biopsy specimen.

The importance of sarcoidosis lies in its differential diagnosis with other causes of granulomas (which are numerous) and with Crohn's disease. Often, the cause can be ascertained only with an appropriate clinical history. Sarcoidosis is less common than Crohn's disease in the GI tract and is more often seen in black patients. Mycobacterial infections (especially in patients with associated pulmonary disease) should also be considered. Acid-fast stains may be performed on the granulomas in suspected cases, and the purified protein derivative skin test may also help distinguish between the two diseases. Essentially, a diagnosis of sarcoidosis can be established only after other diseases have been excluded.

Mast Cell Disorders

Mastocytosis

Both systemic mastocytosis and urticaria pigmentosa (the cutaneous form of mast cell disease) may have GI involvement by disease or by an increase in the number of mast cells. In systemic mastocytosis, 70% to 80% of patients have GI symptoms when a careful history is obtained.[237] Abnormalities include diarrhea, peptic ulcer pain, GI bleeding, nondyspeptic abdominal pain, urgency, and fecal incontinence.[238] A proportion of patients also have gastric acid hypersecretion caused by hyperhistaminemia. This condition can lead to ulcer disease and may even mimic Zollinger-Ellison syndrome. Gastric erosions, duodenal ulceration or varices secondary to hepatic fibrosis, and portal hypertension can cause GI hemorrhage.[237]

The stomach and duodenum are most commonly involved.[239] A variety of changes can be seen, including focal urticaria-like mucosal lesions, edematous thickening of the mucosal folds, gastric erosions, and peptic-type ulcerations.

Histologically, mastocytosis is characterized by an abnormal proliferation of tissue mast cells. The mast cell infiltrate is usually seen throughout the GI tract but predominantly in the mucosa and submucosa (Fig. 7.14A). It is often associated with other inflammatory cells such as eosinophils (see Fig. 7.14B). The infiltrate can be very

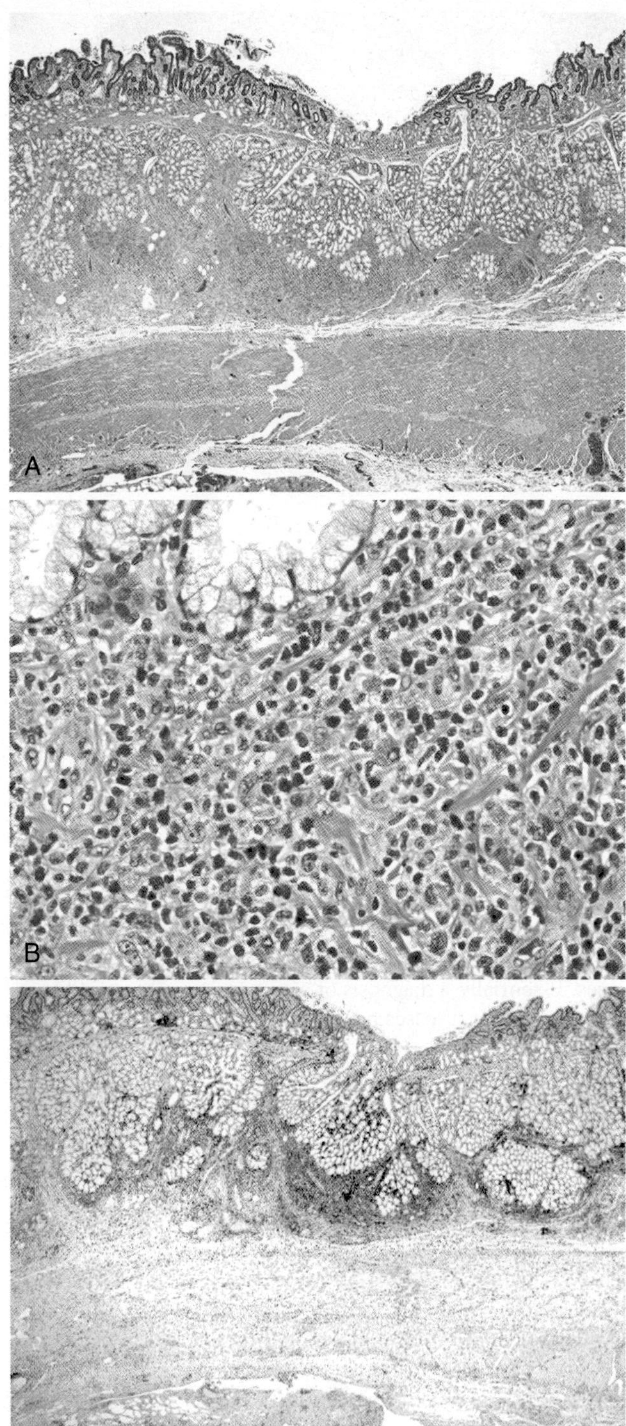

FIGURE 7.14 Mastocytosis. A, Low-power view of the duodenum shows surface erosion and proliferation of mast cells and eosinophils in the submucosa beneath the Brunner glands, just above the muscularis mucosae. **B,** High-power view of mast cells with abundant eosinophils, and adjacent Brunner glands *(top of image).* **C,** Low-power view with CD117 immunohistochemical stain reveals abundant positive mast cells. A greater number of mast cells are present than can be appreciated with hematoxylin and eosin stain.

dense. Associated and mild mucosal villous blunting may be seen. Secondary changes caused by gastric acid hypersecretion, such as erosions, may be seen as well. Mast cells can be stained with chloroacetate esterase stains, with the Giemsa stain, and with immunohistochemical stains for CD117 (see Fig. 7.14C) or for mast cell tryptase. Patients with urticaria pigmentosa may also show increased numbers of mast cells in biopsies of the stomach and duodenum, although mast cell numbers do not correlate with elevated skin mast cell counts in this condition.[240]

Mast Cell Activation Syndrome (MCAS)

Mast cell activation syndrome is a condition with signs and symptoms involving the integumentary, gastrointestinal, cardiovascular, respiratory, and neurological systems. Proposed criteria include episodic symptoms consistent with mast cell mediator release affecting two or more organ systems (in the GI tract: nausea, vomiting, diarrhea, abdominal cramping). Laboratory studies include elevated tryptase levels either above 15 ng/mL or above patient baseline during symptomatic periods. There have been attempts to assess mast cell numbers in the GI tract, however similar to mastocytic enterocolitis (discussed in the next section), a consistent cutoff value cannot be found.[241]

Mastocytic Enterocolitis

Several studies have suggested that increased mast cells are present in patients with irritable bowel syndrome and diarrhea. The term *mastocytic enterocolitis* has been recommended. These studies suggest that the presence of more than 20 mast cells per high-power field (normal, 13 to 15 ± 3 per high-power field) indicates a pathologically increased mast cell number, typically using immunohistochemical staining with CD117. However a meta-analysis did not find a consensus for number of mast cells, and an overlap in range between patients and controls that was too great to be of clinical significance could not justify the routine evaluation of mast cell count.[242-244]

Neoplastic Disease

Neoplastic diseases from other sites may involve the GI tract through tumor invasion of the GI tract or indirectly through paraneoplastic syndromes.

Tumors can invade the GI tract either by direct extension or by metastasis. As many as 20% of extraintestinal tumors metastasize to the bowel.[245,246] The most common neoplasms that directly involve the small or large intestine are carcinomas from the pancreas, prostate gland, urinary bladder, and female genital tract and ovarian tumors through peritoneal seeding. Peritoneal seeding typically involves the serosal surface. Tumors that metastasize relatively frequently to the intestines are melanoma and carcinoma of the breast and lung. Primary carcinoma of the digestive tract may also metastasize to other parts of the GI tract, particularly the diffuse linitis plastica variant of gastric carcinoma.[247] Metastatic breast carcinoma, particularly the lobular type, can mimic primary signet ring cell carcinoma and may even have a linitis plastica appearance[248] (Fig. 7.15). Immunohistochemical stains for estrogen and progesterone receptors, GATA-3, gross cystic fluid protein, and CK5/6 are often positive in breast carcinoma, whereas

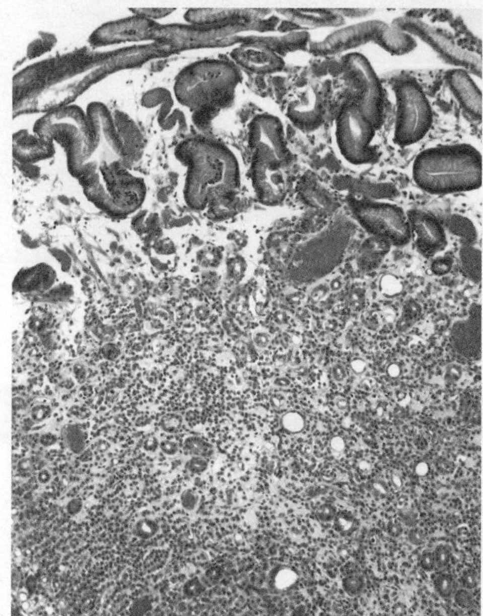

FIGURE 7.15 Metastatic lobular carcinoma involving the stomach. Intermediate-power view of a gastric biopsy specimen shows an infiltrate of numerous small cells in the lamina propria. There is the suggestion of single-cell filing typical of lobular carcinoma of the breast. Signet ring cells are not identified.

CK20, DAS-1, MUC5AC, and MUC6 are often positive in gastric carcinoma.[249] Epithelial malignancies that metastasize to the GI tract are typically differentiated from primary tumors of the GI tract by the lack of epithelial dysplasia or other (adenoma) precursor lesions adjacent to the tumor and by the finding of prominent lymphatic invasion by metastatic lesions. Metastases are often multicentric as well. Furthermore, colonic tumors are usually CK7 negative and CK20 positive, whereas gastric or other foregut tumors are often CK7 positive and CK20 variable.[250]

Paraneoplastic syndromes may develop secondary to release of hormones or antibodies from tumor cells. Typical examples include the watery diarrhea syndrome seen with bronchial carcinoid tumors and small cell carcinoma of the lung. The syndrome is caused by the release of serotonin, which causes hypermotility of the gut.[251] Small cell carcinoma can also lead to gastroparesis secondary to antibody (anti-Hu) production by the tumor.[252] Another example is Zollinger-Ellison syndrome caused by excessive gastrin production from gastrinomas; patients often present with multiple duodenal ulcers secondary to gastrin-induced acid hypersecretion.[253]

The full reference list may be accessed online at Elsevier eBooks for Practicing Clinicians.

CHAPTER 8

Neuromuscular Disorders of the Gastrointestinal Tract

Dhanpat Jain

Chapter Outline

INTRODUCTION

Normal bowel motility depends on smooth muscle, interstitial cells of Cajal (ICC), the intrinsic and extrinsic nerve supply and their supporting cells, and various neuroendocrine peptides. Abnormalities in any one or more of these components may result in bowel dysmotility. In addition, other inflammatory cells such as lymphocytes, eosinophils, and mast cells may act directly, or indirectly, on the neuromuscular apparatus of the bowel wall. The clinical manifestations of motility disorders depend on the extent and specific site of the abnormality. Some of these disorders present with distinct clinical features (e.g., idiopathic hypertrophic pyloric stenosis, Hirschsprung's disease, achalasia), whereas others have nonspecific manifestations. For example, patients with congenital idiopathic hypertrophic pyloric stenosis present with projectile vomiting in the first month of life, often associated with an olive-size abdominal mass. Patients with Hirschsprung's disease manifest with delayed passage of meconium. The pathogenesis of many of these conditions is still poorly understood. In fact, many disorders have no specific pathological features and lack standardized diagnostic criteria. This has led to marked variability in the approach to a diagnostic workup among different laboratories.[1] To address these issues, an international working group was formed in 2007. This group published a comprehensive guideline for handling of most specimens, including biopsies and resections, pertaining to GI motility disorders. The classification proposed by this group is recognized as the London classification of neuromuscular disorders of the GI tract. This classification has placed various primary neuropathies and myopathies into well-delineated categories. However, it includes only a short list of secondary disorders. A modified version of this classification is shown in Box 8.1. It is expected that this will lead to application of uniform criteria, use of standardized terminology, and an improvement in our understanding of gastrointestinal (GI) motility disorders.

Muscle Coats of the Bowel Wall

Knowledge of the basic organization of the neuromuscular apparatus of the bowel is essential to understand and diagnose GI motility disorders. The neuromuscular framework of the bowel is similar throughout the tract. However, there are some minor variations.[2] The bowel smooth muscle is composed of a thin superficial layer that separates mucosa from submucosa (muscularis mucosae) and a thick outer layer (muscularis propria), which has an inner circular and outer longitudinal coat. The muscularis propria is organized into an inner circular and outer longitudinal layer, except for the esophagus, which has only a single longitudinal muscle coat. The proximal part of the muscularis propria of the esophagus is formed entirely of skeletal muscle. The skeletal muscle merges with the smooth muscle of the esophagus in the vicinity of the proximal half of the organ (Fig 8.1). Thus esophageal motility is susceptible to the effects of systemic disorders of both smooth and skeletal muscle. In the

BOX 8.1 Classifications of Neuromuscular Disorders

A. PRIMARY NEUROPATHY

Absent Neurons
- Aganglionosis (Hirschsprung's disease)

Decreased number of neurons
- Hypoganglionosis

Increased number of neurons
- Intestinal neuronal dysplasia, type B
- Ganglioneuromatosis

Degenerative neuropathies

Inflammatory neuropathies
- Lymphocytic ganglionitis
- Eosinophilic ganglionitis

Abnormal content in neurons
- Intraneuronal inclusion disease
- Megamitochondria

Abnormal neuronal coding

Relative immaturity of neurons

Abnormal enteric glia
- Increased number of glia
- Decreased number of glia

B. PRIMARY MYOPATHY

Muscularis propria malformations
- Focal absence of enteric muscle coats
- Segmental fusion of enteric muscle coats
- Presence of additional muscle coats
- Colonic desmosis (absent connective tissue scaffold)

Muscle cell degeneration
- Degenerative leiomyopathy
  - Sporadic
  - Familial
- Inflammatory myopathies
  - Lymphocytic leiomyositis
  - Eosinophilic leiomyositis

Muscle hyperplasia/hypertrophy
- Muscularis mucosae hyperplasia

Abnormal content in myocytes
- Filament protein abnormalities
  - Alpha actin myopathy
  - Desmin myopathy
- Inclusion bodies
  - Polyglucosan bodies
- Amphophilic "M" bodies
- Megamitochondria

C. INTERSTITIAL CELLS OF CAJAL (ICC) ABNORMALITIES (MESENCHYMOPATHIES)

Absent ICC

Increased ICC

Decreased ICC

D. NEUROHORMONAL ABNORMALITIES

E. SECONDARY NEUROPATHY

Systemic disorders
- Paraneoplastic inflammatory neuropathy
- Diabetic neuropathy
- Chagasic neuropathy
- Connective tissue disorder–associated neuropathy
- Storage disease
- Amyloidosis

Local disorders
- Crohn's disease

F. SECONDARY MYOPATHY

Systemic disorders
- Desmin myopathy
- Muscular dystrophies
- Mitochondrial cytopathies
- Metabolic storage disorders
- Amyloidosis
- Progressive systemic sclerosis
- Other collagen vascular disorders
- Cystic fibrosis

Local disorders
- Obstructive/postirradiation muscle failure

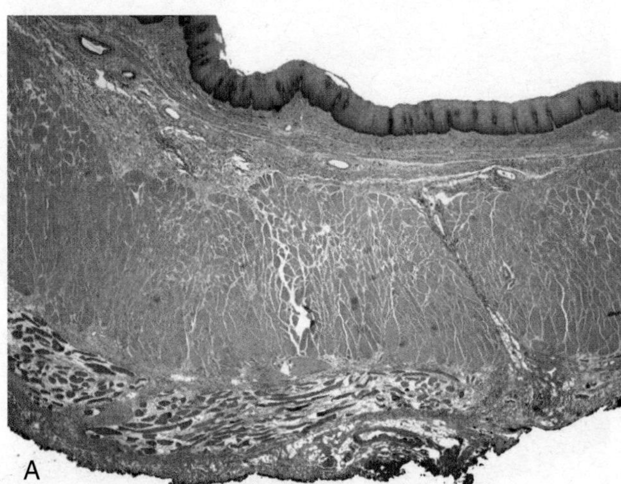

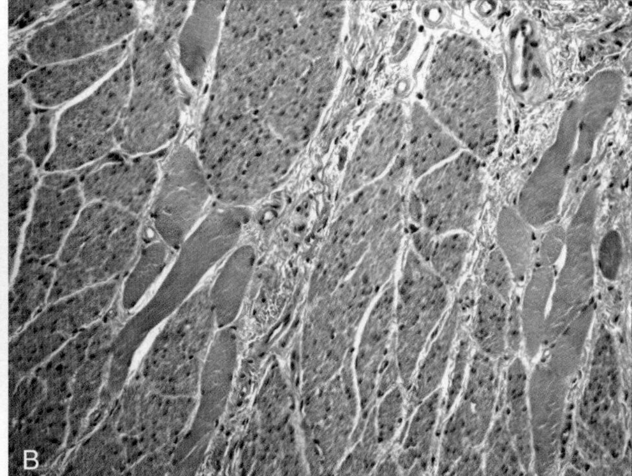

FIGURE 8.1 **A,** Low-magnification view of a section obtained near the proximal margin from an esophagectomy specimen shows skeletal muscle fibers in the outer layer of muscularis propria of the proximal esophagus. **B,** Higher-magnification view of a section obtained from the mid-esophagus shows skeletal muscle fibers merging imperceptibly with smooth muscle fibers of muscularis propria.

stomach, an additional inner oblique muscle layer is also present. In contrast, the outer longitudinal layer in the colon forms thick localized bands of muscle termed *taenia coli*. The muscularis mucosae of the colon continues into the anal canal. The inner circular layer of muscularis propria of the rectum becomes thickened distally to form the internal anal sphincter. The external anal sphincter is formed of skeletal muscle and is connected to the skeletal muscle of the pelvic floor. The outer longitudinal muscle layer of the rectum continues in between the inner and outer anal sphincters and then separates caudally into multiple septa, which then diverge fanwise throughout the subcutaneous part of the external sphincter into the skin. These fibers are responsible for the characteristic corrugated appearance of the perianal skin. In addition, the muscle fibers from the outer longitudinal coat and the internal anal sphincter extend into the submucosa to form a meshwork of fibers surrounding the vascular plexuses (muscularis submucosae ani). The organization of the muscle layers in the appendix is similar to the colon, except that it lacks *taenia coli*.

Neural Network of the Bowel

The organization of the neural network in the bowel is quite complex. The extrinsic nerve supply of the bowel wall consists of both sympathetic and parasympathetic nerve fibers that penetrate the wall and become the intrinsic neural plexus. The sympathetic fibers originate in the prevertebral ganglia and parallel the superior and inferior mesenteric arteries. The parasympathetic fibers are located alongside the posterior branch of the vagus nerve. The intrinsic neural system of the bowel wall is organized into three plexuses: the submucosal plexus (Meissner's plexus), the deep submucosal plexus (Henle's plexus) and the myenteric plexus (Auerbach's plexus) (Fig. 8.2). The most easily identified, and prominent, is the myenteric plexus, which is composed of clusters of ganglion cells connected by an intricate network of nerves located in the space between the inner circular and outer longitudinal muscle layers. The ganglion cells are surrounded by glial cells. Although the ganglion cells and nerve bundles are easily identified within these plexuses (Fig. 8.3A), the intricacy of the neural meshwork of fibers is not easily detectable on hematoxylin and eosin (H&E)–stained tissue sections. Whole-mount specimens, silver stains, and/or immunostains are normally needed to visualize the complexity of the neural network (Fig. 8.3B).[3,4]

In addition to muscle fibers and the neural network, a third population of mesenchymal cells, the ICC, are critical for bowel motility. These cells generate a slow wave of depolarization and represent the "pacemaker cells" of bowel peristalsis.[5,6] Their function is, in turn, modulated by both intrinsic and extrinsic neural inputs. These cells are difficult to detect on routine tissue sections, and most of our initial knowledge regarding the morphology and structural organization of these cells stems from ultrastructural studies.[7-9] Ultrastructurally, these cells show a partial basal lamina, many intermediate filaments, darkly staining cytoplasm, abundant rough endoplasmic reticulum, sublamellar caveolae, oval indented nuclei, and lack of myosin filaments. Many of these features overlap with smooth muscle cells. It was soon realized that these cells express *c-kit* (CD117), a tyrosine kinase receptor. *c-kit* or DOG1 immunostains can be used to visualize these cells.[10-13] It is now recognized that ICC are part of an intricate neural network and have a close association between smooth muscle

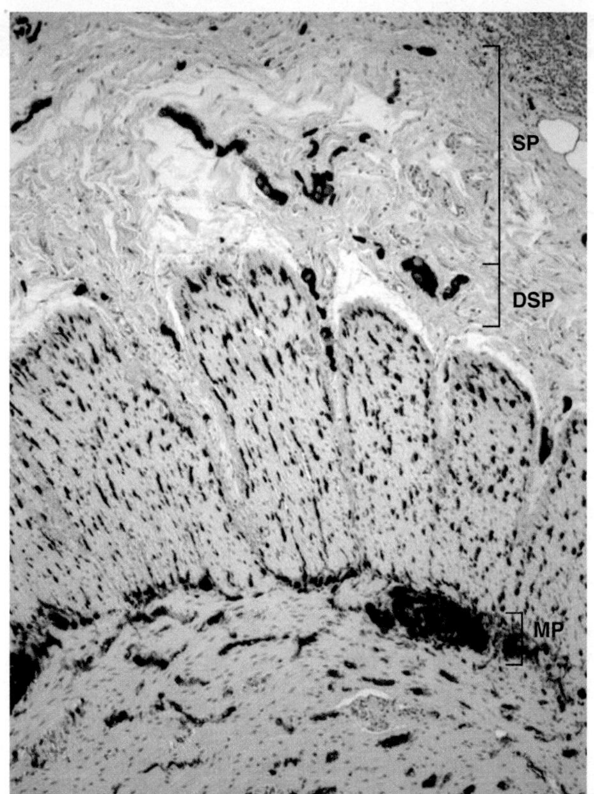

FIGURE 8.2 Section of normal colon shows the neural plexus: submucosal plexus *(SP)*, deep submucosal plexus *(DSP)*, and myenteric plexuses *(MP)* (S100 stain).

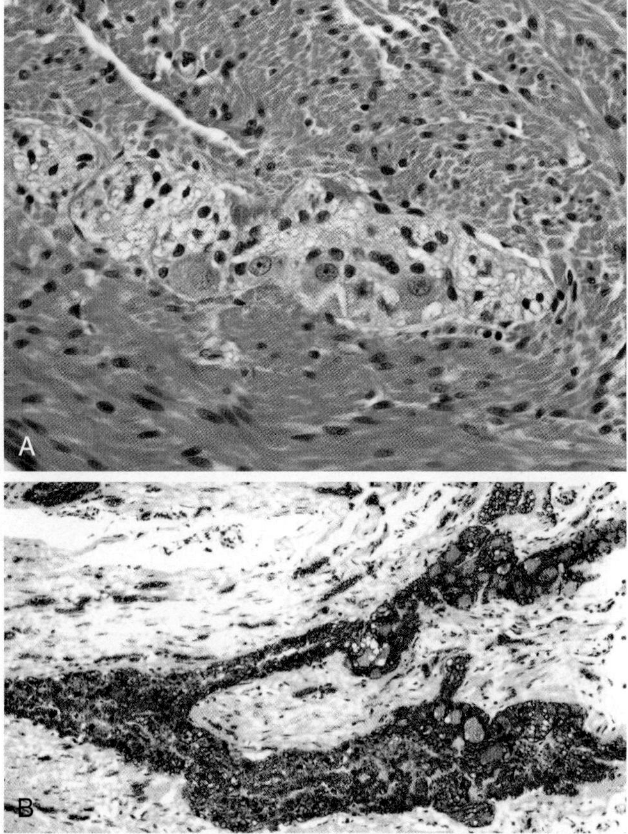

FIGURE 8.3 **A,** Normal ganglion cells (H&E stain). **B,** A tangential section of muscularis propria shows myenteric ganglia in the complex neural network, which is not evident in a well-oriented section (S100 stain).

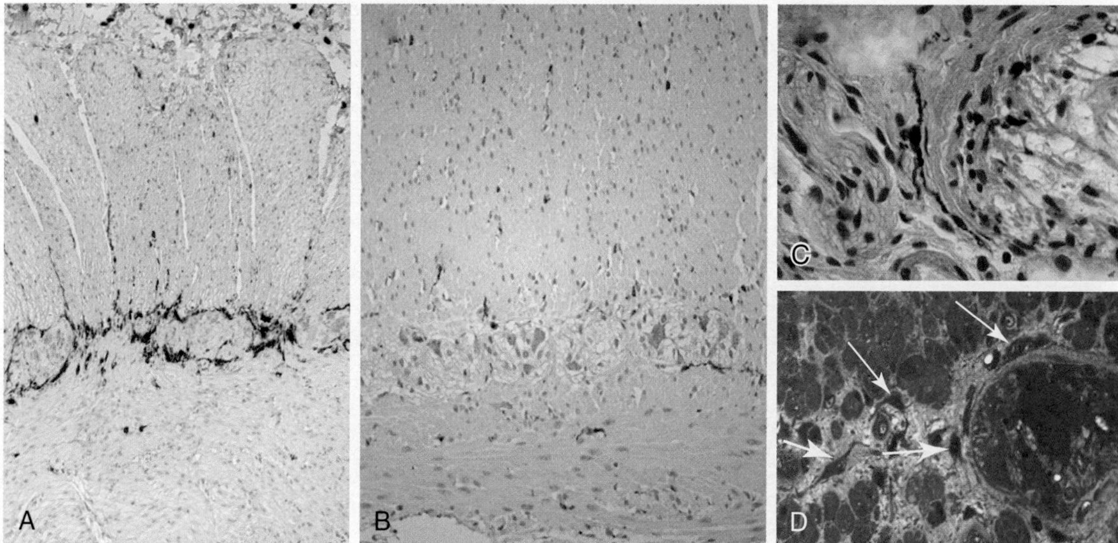

FIGURE 8.4 **A,** Section from a small intestine shows interstitial cells of Cajal (ICC) extending into the inner circular and outer longitudinal layers of the muscularis propria (KIT/CD117 stain). A dense collection of ICC is present around the myenteric plexus. **B,** Section of colon shows distribution of ICC (KIT stain). Compared with the small intestine, fewer KIT-positive ICC are present around the myenteric plexus, which may be difficult to appreciate on low magnification. **C,** High-power view of muscularis propria shows multiple processes of KIT-positive ICC. In well-oriented sections, this morphology is difficult to appreciate. **D,** Semi-thin resin-embedded section shows ICCs *(arrows)* around the myenteric ganglia (toluidine blue stain).

cells and nerve endings. They are most easily identified surrounding the myenteric plexus, especially in the small bowel, where the network of cells extends into the inner and outer muscle coats (Fig. 8.4A–D). In addition, there is also a distinct ICC plexus in the submucosa. The distribution and organization of ICC in the appendix is similar to that in the colon. The structural organization of ICC has been described in the various segments of the GI tract (from esophagus to anus). Minor regional differences within each bowel segment do exist.[14]

The neuromuscular organization of the appendix is similar to the colon and small bowel. However, the ganglia are sometimes embedded deeper into the circular or longitudinal layer (Fig. 8.5A–B). The neural and ICC networks in the appendix are similar to the colon, but with less aggregation of ICC surrounding the myenteric plexus (Fig. 8.5B–C). Understanding the neuromuscular organization of the appendix is helpful because it is sometimes examined intraoperatively to evaluate the extent of aganglionosis.[15]

ESOPHAGUS

Primary Achalasia

Achalasia is a motor disorder of the esophagus characterized by failure of the lower esophageal sphincter to relax in response to swallowing.[16,17] Clinically, achalasia is divided into three subtypes: type I, classic type; type II, achalasia with compression; and type III, spastic achalasia.[18] It is uncommon, as the overall prevalence rate is less than $10/10^5$ population.[19] Its incidence has been fairly stable over the past 50 years. It is a disease of adults mainly older than 60 years of age and affects both sexes equally. Achalasia is more frequent in North America, northwestern Europe, and Australia than in other regions, and it is more common in Caucasians.

Clinical Features

The major clinical manifestations of achalasia differ between children and adults. Younger children (<5 years of age) and infants typically present with a feeding aversion, failure to thrive, choking, recurrent pneumonia, nocturnal cough, aspiration, or nonspecific regurgitation. Older children and adults often manifest with vomiting, chest pain, and dysphagia for solids and liquids. Heartburn is a common symptom (50%), even in untreated patients. However, only a minority of patients have documented gastroesophageal reflux disease.[20] The diagnosis is confirmed with imaging studies and manometry. Barium studies typically reveal reduced peristalsis, a characteristic beaklike deformity of the distal esophagus, and dilation of the proximal esophagus. Manometry studies reveal abnormal peristalsis, increased intraluminal pressure, and incomplete and delayed relaxation of the lower esophageal sphincter. Endoscopy and endoscopic ultrasonography are often performed to rule out coexisting mucosal pathology and to exclude secondary causes of achalasia ("pseudoachalasia").

Pathogenesis

The most significant feature of achalasia is loss of myenteric ganglion cells. However, the cause of ganglion cell loss is unknown. Current data suggest that myenteric inflammation precedes loss of ganglion cells, but the initial inciting events that cause the disease remain unknown.[21] Environmental factors, viral infection, autoimmune mechanisms, and genetic predisposition have all been proposed. In addition, there is some data to suggest familial aggregation. Rare familial forms associated with alacrimia (absence of tears) and adrenocorticotropic hormone (ACTH) insensitivity have been described (Allgrove's syndrome, or "Triple A" syndrome).[22,23] Concordance in monozygotic twins and an association with Down's syndrome has also been reported. A significant association has been found with class II human leukocyte antigen (HLA) DQw1 in Caucasian patients. The alleles identified, *HLA DQB1*0602, DQA1*0101,* and *DRB1*15,* are the same ones that have been found to be associated with other autoimmune disorders, including multiple sclerosis and Goodpasture's syndrome, Graves' disease, myasthenia gravis, polymyositis, autoimmune

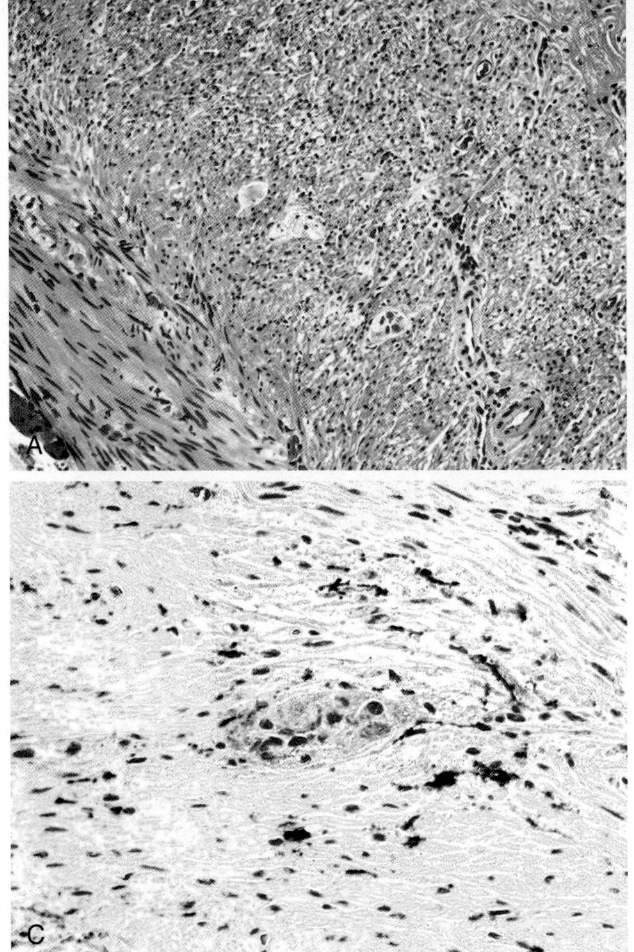

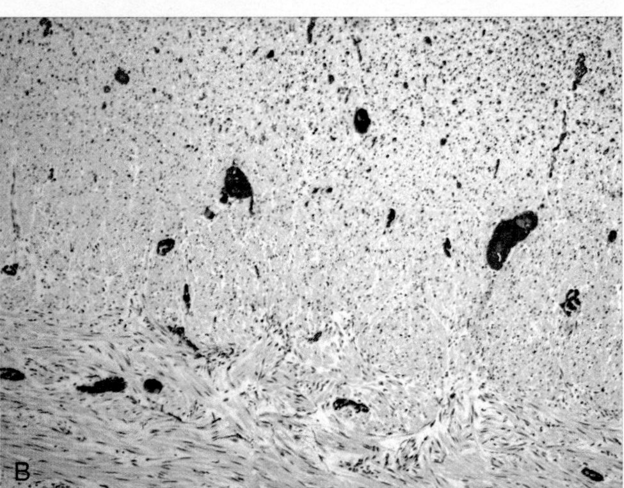

FIGURE 8.5 **A,** Muscularis propria of a normal appendix shows ganglia of the myenteric plexus in the deeper layers of circular and longitudinal muscle, instead of at the junction of the two (H&E stain). **B,** S100 stain highlights the neural plexus in the appendix and the location of the ganglia within the circular and longitudinal layers of muscularis propria. **C,** KIT stain shows the organization of interstitial cells of Cajal in the circular and longitudinal layers of muscularis propria, showing very few cells around the myenteric ganglia, similar to the colon.

polyglandular syndrome, Sjögren's syndrome, and Sicca syndrome. Antimyenteric neuronal antibodies have been identified in some patients.[24-28] It has been shown in an ex vivo model that on exposure to sera from achalasia patients, gastric corpus mucosa shows phenotypic and functional changes that mimic achalasia.[29] A factor in the serum, other than an antineuronal antibody, may be responsible for this phenomenon.[29] Varicella-zoster viral DNA has been identified in the myenteric plexus in rare cases by in situ hybridization.[30] Lymphocytes taken from the lower esophageal sphincter area seem to respond to herpes simplex virus (HSV) exposure by producing gamma interferon and cytotoxic T-cell proliferation, suggesting a role for remote/latent HSV infection, although studies looking for a variety of neurotropic and non-neurotrophic viruses have failed to provide any conclusive evidence for a viral infection.[31,32] Polymorphisms in VIP receptor-1, c-kit, and interleukin 23 receptor *(IL23R)* genes may increase susceptibility to achalasia.[33-35] VIP is responsible for relaxation of esophageal smooth muscle, whereas KIT plays an important role in the function of ICC. The IL23 pathway is important in immune activation and plays an important role in many chronic inflammatory disorders, including inflammatory bowel disease.

As noted previously, the pathogenesis of achalasia is poorly understood. However, progressive inflammatory destruction of myenteric ganglion cells is the most important underlying event. This results in failure of the lower esophageal sphincter to relax in response to swallowing.[36] Esophageal peristalsis is decreased or completely absent. This results in esophageal dilatation, chronic stasis, and reactive hypertrophy of the muscularis propria. There also is a substantial decrease in VIP-containing neurons in the distal esophagus.[37,38] Subsequently, it has been shown that nitric oxide is a primary esophageal inhibitory neurotransmitter. It colocalizes with VIP in ganglion cells. In addition, intrinsic nitrergic ganglion cells are lost, or markedly decreased, in achalasia. In fact, loss of VIP-positive ganglion cells is synonymous with loss of nitrergic ganglion cells.[39,40] Unfortunately, most early studies evaluated specimens only at the time of autopsy or esophagectomy, which showed end-stage disease. However, study of esophagomyomectomy specimens has given some insight into the early sequence of events in this condition.[35] These studies revealed that as the disease progresses, the inflammatory infiltrate decreases in intensity, whereas loss of ganglion cells and degeneration of the myenteric plexus become more prominent features.

Pathological Features

Pathologists often encounter esophagus specimens resulting from an esophagectomy for end-stage achalasia. Grossly, the esophagus shows dilation, and the extent depends on the severity and duration of disease (Fig. 8.6A). It often contains stagnant and foul-smelling partially digested food. The distal end is typically narrowed and stenotic.

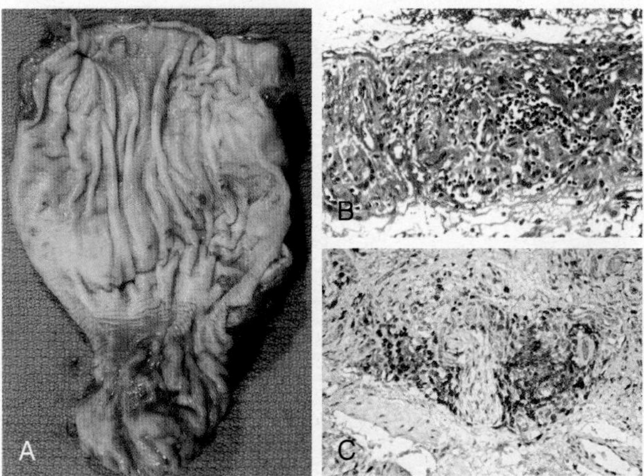

FIGURE 8.6 A, Resection specimen of achalasia shows a dilated proximal segment and a narrow distal segment. **B,** Myenteric plexus in a patient with end-stage achalasia. There are no residual ganglion cells, and the chronic inflammatory cells are seen in and around a fibrotic nerve (H&E stain). **C,** Strong CD8 staining of lymphocytes within the myenteric plexus of a patient with end-stage achalasia. (**A** *courtesy of Dr. Henry Appleman, University of Michigan.*)

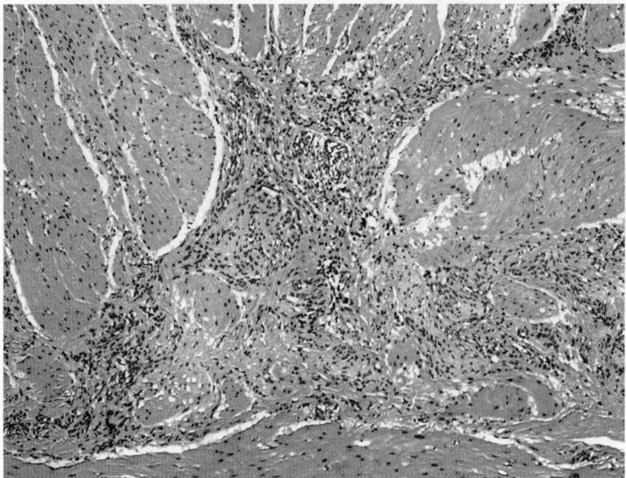

FIGURE 8.7 Specimen from a patient with achalasia shows complete absence of ganglion cells in the myenteric plexus, which appears hyperplastic. There is perineural inflammation with eosinophils (H&E stain).

The main histological abnormality in achalasia is related to the myenteric plexus, although numerous secondary changes are often present, presumably resulting from prolonged stasis and reflux. Widespread, often total, loss of myenteric ganglion cells is the cardinal feature of achalasia (see Fig. 8.6B; Fig. 8.7). Better preservation of the ganglion cells may be present in the more proximal portions of the esophagus.[16] Some degree of neural hyperplasia may accompany neuronal loss (see Fig. 8.7). A variable amount of chronic inflammation often admixed with eosinophils and plasma cells is typical. Mast cells may be noted surrounding the myenteric nerves and residual ganglion cells[41] (see Fig. 8.6B and Fig. 8.7). In end-stage disease, the degree of inflammation may become minimal or disappear completely. One ultrastructural study showed that numerous mast cells are also present within the inflammatory infiltrate closely associated with the nerve fibers.[42] Occasionally, lymphocytes may infiltrate the cytoplasm of ganglion cells (ganglionitis). The majority of chronic inflammatory cells are CD3-positive T cells, most of which are CD8-positive (see Fig. 8.6C), although the relative percentage of these cells decreases with progression of disease.[36,43,44] A large subset of T cells represents either resting or activated cytotoxic cells.

Other changes frequently present are related to distal esophageal obstruction and include muscularis propria hypertrophy, muscularis propria eosinophilia, and dystrophic calcification. Hypertrophied muscle may also show degenerative changes, including cytoplasmic vacuolation and liquefactive necrosis. The branches of the vagus nerve within the adventitia are unremarkable in most cases, although degenerative changes in the vagus nerve and in dorsal motor nuclei have been described as well.[17] These changes may be caused by infection with a neurotrophic virus; however, no specific virus has been identified thus far.[44,45] The squamous mucosa also shows secondary changes, including diffuse hyperplasia, increased intraepithelial lymphocytes ("lymphocytic esophagitis"), papillomatosis, basal cell hyperplasia, and an increase in nonspecific lamina propria inflammation.[46] Some of these changes mimic reflux esophagitis, although sustained lower esophageal pressure does not allow regurgitation of gastric contents in untreated cases.[47] Increased intraepithelial eosinophils, sometimes raising a concern for eosinophilic esophagitis, are seen.[48] Despite symptoms of dysphagia and presence of motor dysfunction, studies show that this is not likely to represent eosinophilic esophagitis, although few cases of eosinophilic esophagitis in achalasia that respond to steroids have also been reported.[49-51] After esophagomyotomy, gastroesophageal reflux develops in up to 50% of patients and can lead to the development of Barrett's esophagus in some cases.[52,53]

Differential Diagnosis

Biopsies are not performed to establish a diagnosis of achalasia. Pathologists encounter this condition when a resection is performed or at autopsy. The role of biopsy in patients with achalasia is largely to exclude Barrett's esophagus (postmyotomy), dysplasia, and malignancy. The differential diagnosis of achalasia, both clinically and pathologically, is pseudo-achalasia, secondary to tumors or paraneoplastic syndrome. These are easily resolved with esophageal manometry and imaging, or with biopsies when a mass is present. Occasionally, strictures at the gastroesophageal junction secondary to reflux, prior surgery, or trauma can mimic achalasia (Fig. 8.8A–B). The esophagus may show muscular hypertrophy and neural hyperplasia similar to achalasia. However, on close examination, ganglion cells are easily identified in the neural plexus, and there is a lack of inflammatory or degenerative changes in the ganglion cells. In postinfectious or autoimmune-mediated ganglion cell loss, lymphocytic inflammation may be present in or around ganglion cells. Residual ganglion cells can often be identified (Fig. 8.8C). In paraneoplastic achalasia, the diagnosis of malignancy is often already known, and despite histological similarity with the idiopathic form, their differentiation is seldom a problem clinically. Chagas' disease, which also causes massive dilation of the esophagus with ganglion cell loss, should be suspected in any patient from an endemic area. By the time achalasia-type features develop, the infectious organisms

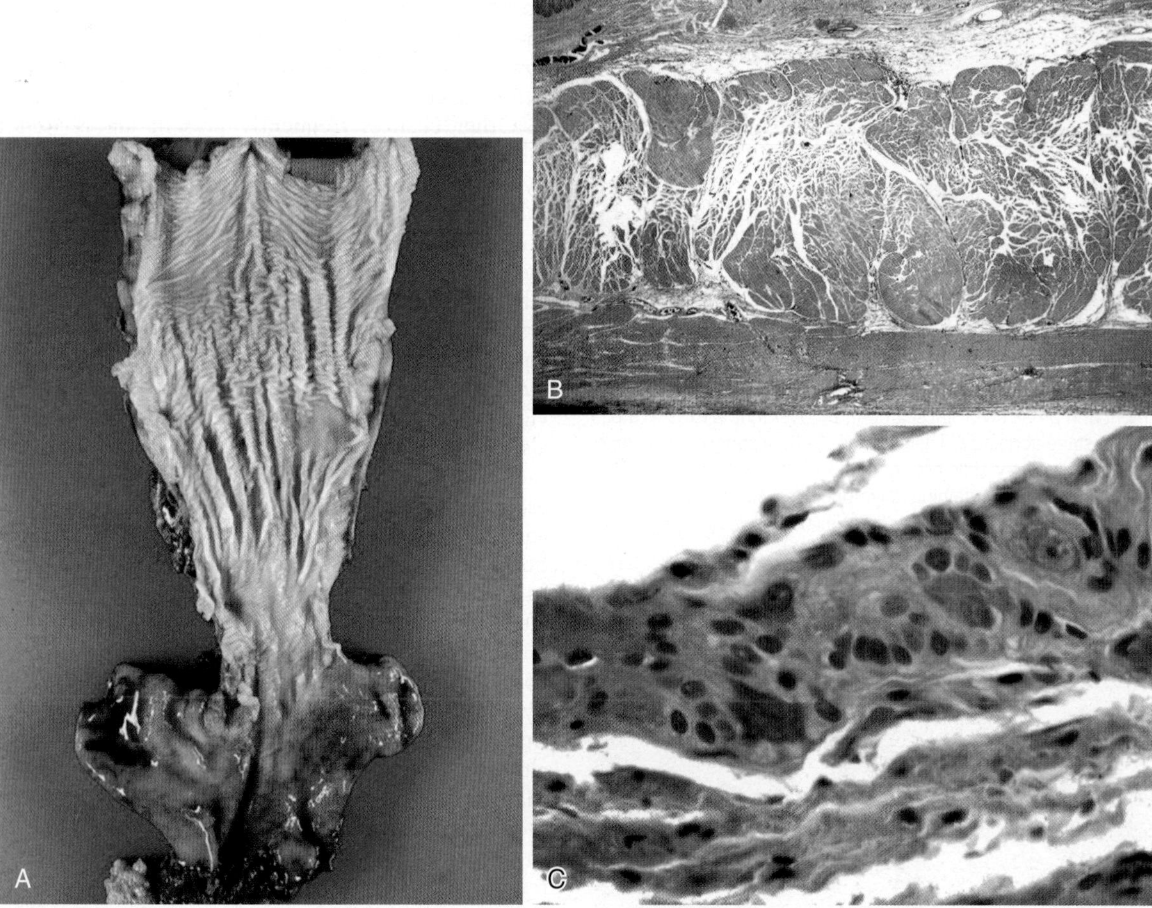

FIGURE 8.8 **A,** Stricture of the distal esophagus near the gastroesophageal junction developed after reflux surgery in this patient and led to proximal dilatation and muscular hypertrophy, mimicking achalasia **(B).** However, microscopy showed a normal population of ganglion cells in the myenteric plexus (H&E stain). **C,** Inflammatory infiltrate and degenerative changes in the ganglion cells can be seen in a wide variety of immune-mediated or postviral cases of ganglion cell loss (H&E stain).

can no longer be demonstrated in the tissues, and thus one has to rely on serological evidence of infection. Patients with Chagas' disease may also show dilatation of other hollow viscera with ganglion cell loss.

Natural History and Treatment

Achalasia is a chronic disorder, and the treatment is largely palliative. Medications such as anticholinergics, nitrates, and calcium channel blockers are used in some circumstances but result in only partial benefit. Pneumatic dilatation and botulinum toxin injection into the lower esophageal sphincter show an initial response, but the results are usually short lasting. The best results are typically obtained with esophagomyotomy of the lower esophageal sphincter, either with or without pneumatic dilatation. Patients with type II achalasia have the most favorable outcome and show better response to treatment. Esophageal resection is usually reserved for end-stage cases. Patients have an increased long-term risk for developing squamous cell carcinoma of the esophagus.[52,54] The risk is about 33-fold higher than in the general population.[55] Studies show that the risk for adenocarcinoma is also higher, although to a lower degree.[56]

Secondary Achalasia

As discussed earlier, signs and symptoms indistinguishable from primary achalasia may be encountered with other conditions such as Chagas' disease or in association with a neoplasm that directly invades the myenteric plexus.[57] In some cases, a paraneoplastic phenomenon may cause secondary achalasia, such as paraneoplastic achalasia associated with small cell carcinoma. Rare associations have been described with other tumors, such as leiomyomatosis of the esophagus and sarcoidosis.[58-60] In sarcoidosis, inflammation surrounding the myenteric plexus has been described, but without granulomas. One of these reported patients showed resolution of symptoms with steroid treatment.[58]

Chagas' disease results from infection with the protozoan *Trypanosoma cruzi*.[61,62] The infection is acquired from the bite of blood-sucking reduviid bugs. The geographical distribution of the disease is limited to certain parts of the world, such as South America, Central America, and Africa. Chagas' disease is uncommon in the United States and occurs almost exclusively in immigrants from endemic countries, such as Brazil. Any part of the GI tract may be affected; however, the esophagus and the sigmoid colon are the most frequent sites. Infection results in dysmotility and often massive dilatation (e.g., megaesophagus, megacolon). In the esophagus, the symptoms closely resemble idiopathic achalasia. Colonic involvement results in constipation and intestinal pseudo-obstruction. These features are seen in the chronic phase of disease, and by the time symptoms are noted, the organisms are usually no longer present in the myenteric plexus.

Idiopathic Muscular Hypertrophy of the Esophagus

This is a poorly understood condition of uncertain etiology and clinical significance. Most of the reported cases with pathological descriptions have been diagnosed at the time of autopsy. The condition can be diagnosed clinically with imaging techniques and esophageal motility studies. New clinical diagnostic criteria have been proposed.[63,64] Some cases are symptomatic, presenting with symptoms such as dysphagia, chest pain, vomiting, and weight loss, whereas others are entirely asymptomatic.[65] Some patients also develop gastroesophageal reflux.[64] Esophageal spasm and increased intraluminal pressure are believed to be the cause of symptoms. The disorder occurs in adults, with no gender or race predilection. Many patients with this disorder also have diabetes. Some cases have shown autosomal dominant inheritance and association with bilateral cataracts and Alport-like nephropathy.[66] Squamous cell carcinoma has also been described in some cases.[67] Pathologically, the muscularis propria is markedly thickened, particularly toward the distal end[65] (Fig. 8.9). Some cases also show a mild degree of lymphocytic infiltration in the myenteric plexus. The vast majority of cases lack evidence of muscle fiber degeneration, fibrosis, ganglion cell abnormalities, or neural plexus abnormalities.

Differential Diagnosis

A variable degree of muscular hypertrophy of the esophageal musculature may be seen in patients with distal obstruction of any cause, including achalasia. However, the cause of the obstruction is often obvious clinically (see Fig. 8.8A). Histologically, the muscle fibers appear normal in idiopathic muscular hypertrophy, and ganglion cells and neural plexus are present. The key is to exclude distal obstruction in the presence of markedly hypertrophic muscularis propria.

STOMACH

Idiopathic Hypertrophic Pyloric Stenosis

Idiopathic hypertrophic pyloric stenosis is a disorder characterized by thickened pyloric musculature and features of gastric outlet obstruction. Infantile, late-onset/adolescent, and adult forms of this disorder have been described. Infants present with projectile vomiting, usually within 2 to 4 weeks of birth, but occasionally presentation is delayed.[68-73] It occurs in approximately 1 in 1000 live births, has a high familial incidence, has a strong male preponderance, and classically occurs in the first-born child. The incidence of this condition is increasing in some countries (Britain and Ireland) but decreasing in others (United States, Germany, Canada, and Denmark).[74-78] Regional variation within countries is also known to occur.[75]

Clinical Features

Infants classically present with progressive, nonbilious vomiting, which gradually assumes a more characteristic projectile pattern. The hypertrophied pylorus may be palpated as an olive-size epigastric mass in some individuals. In fact, gastric peristalsis may be visible to the naked eye

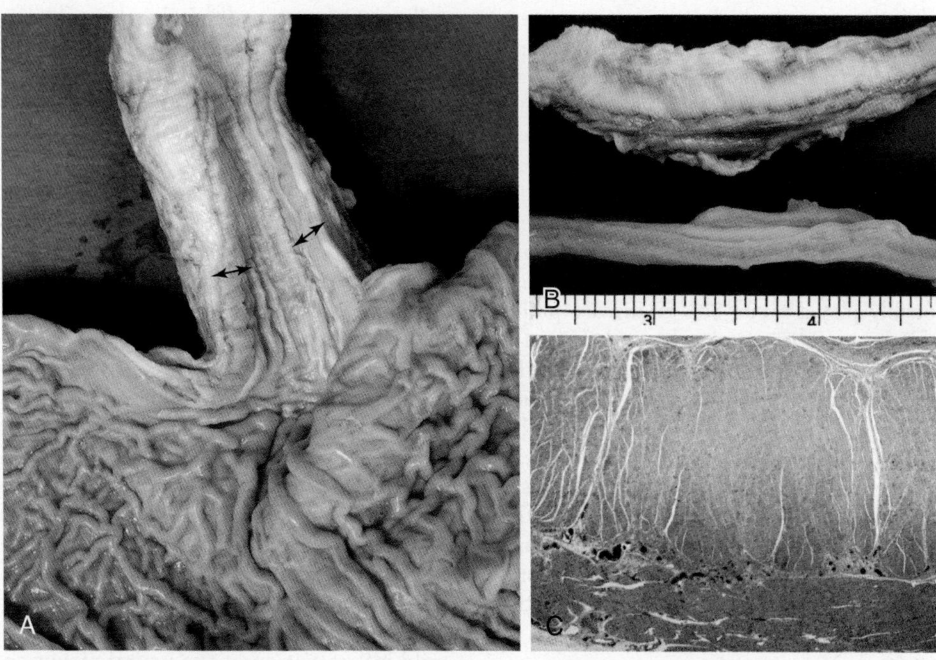

FIGURE 8.9 Idiopathic muscular hypertrophy of esophagus. A, Gross specimen shows marked thickening of the muscularis propria of the esophagus that is more prominent distally, toward the gastroesophageal junction *(arrows)*. Compare this with the normal wall of the stomach and the lack of any gross mucosal abnormalities. **B,** A cross-section of hypertrophic muscle from the same case *(top)* compared with normal esophagus *(bottom)*. **C,** Microscopy shows hypertrophied muscularis propria and a lack of any other associated histological changes, including inflammation, fibrosis, muscle degeneration, or myenteric plexus abnormalities (H&E stain).

on examination of the abdomen. Some patients also have an associated congenital diaphragmatic hernia. More recent studies suggest that presentation with classic symptoms and signs is uncommon. Hence, a higher degree of clinical suspicion is required for establishing an early diagnosis.[79] Idiopathic hypertrophic pyloric stenosis is uncommon in adults, but it has been reported.[80] Most cases in adults are secondary to scarring caused by juxtapyloric peptic ulceration, inflammatory bowel disease, or tumors.[81]

Pathogenesis

The pathogenesis of the disease remains unclear. A genetic predisposition and other environmental precipitating factors have been implicated (e.g., bottle feeding, respiratory distress syndrome).[82] Its incidence appears to be decreasing parallel with an increasing trend toward breastfeeding and young maternal age.[77,83] Prenatal use of erythromycin and various other macrolide antibiotics have also been implicated as risk factors, but the evidence is not conclusive.[84,85] There is no association with *Helicobacter pylori* infection.[86] Rare cases have been associated with esophageal atresia and other types of congenital malformations and syndromes (e.g., Cornelia de Lange syndrome, Smith-Lemli-Opitz syndrome).[87,88]

The disease does not show any evidence of mechanical obstruction. In fact, the pylorus can be easily intubated in affected patients.[89] Uncoordinated peristalsis of the stomach, including the pyloric musculature ("pylorospasm"), is one theory of pathogenesis. Other factors that may play a role include immaturity of the enteric nervous system, hormonal imbalance between gastrin and somatostatin, redundancy of the overlying mucosa, lack of KIT-positive ICC, and lack of nitric oxide synthase (NOS).[90-95] Interestingly, homozygous transgenic mice carrying inactivating genes for NOS develop hypertrophy of the pylorus.[96] In humans, a familial tendency and a high concordance rate in twins has been reported. The incidence is higher in monozygotic twins compared with dizygotic twins.[97] There are at least five genetic loci (IHPS1-5) that have been associated with this disease, of which the strongest association is with IHPS-1, which regulates the *NOS1* gene.[98] Neuronal NOS is a critical enzyme in the production of nitric oxide that mediates relaxation of pyloric smooth muscle. Several *RET* genomic variants associated with the disorder have also been identified.[99] However, unlike Hirschsprung's disease, these variants probably play a minor role in disease pathogenesis.[100] Several linkage analysis studies have identified an association with a loci on chromosomes 2, 3, 5, 6, 7, 11, 12, 16, and X.[99,101,102] Genome-wide association studies have revealed significant risk loci involving several genes that include *NKX2-5*, *EML4-MTA3*, *APOA1*, and *BARX-1*.[103] However, there is tremendous heterogeneity, and thus it is unlikely that a single gene is solely responsible for this disease. Within a single family pedigree, the disease may be linked to a single locus or gene.[104,105] Thus a commonly accepted theory is that environmental factors lead to this condition in genetically predisposed hosts.[88]

Pathological Features

The pathological features are similar in children and adults (Fig. 8.10). Grossly, the pylorus is greatly thickened and fusiform in appearance. The proximal stomach may show dilation depending on the severity and duration of obstruction. Histologically, cases of pyloric stenosis reveal a thick inner circular muscle (up to four times normal). The muscle fibers are disorganized, show increased intercellular collagen, and are sometimes associated with a mild lymphocytic infiltrate. The longitudinal muscle is frequently attenuated as well. The enteric nerve plexus is often hypertrophied and shows a relative increase in the number of Schwann cell nuclei. Glial cells show degeneration, characterized by pyknosis and vacuolation. ICC are markedly reduced or absent in the hypertrophied muscle layers, the myenteric plexus, and the outer longitudinal muscle.

Differential Diagnosis

Biopsies of the pyloric musculature in children are seldom performed. The diagnosis is made entirely on clinical grounds. When it presents in adults, biopsies are obtained to exclude a neoplasm or other lesions that can lead to pyloric stenosis.

Natural History and Treatment

Surgical myotomy is widely considered the definitive method of treatment. Pyloric hypertrophy typically disappears within a few months after the procedure.[106] In fact, histology of the pylorus evaluated several months after myotomy often reveals restoration of abnormalities of the nerve fibers, glial cells, ICC, and neuronal NOS.[107] Thus the long-term outcome of affected patients postsurgery is excellent.[108]

Gastroparesis

Gastroparesis is characterized by food retention in the stomach caused by delayed emptying. In most cases it is associated with another condition (Table 8.1), most commonly diabetes, largely resulting from autonomic dysfunction or following vagotomy.[109] It has been known to rarely occur in patients with cirrhosis.[110] In some cases it truly remains idiopathic. Patients with symptoms that are indistinguishable from gastroparesis but lack delayed gastric emptying have been referred to as having a *gastroparesis-like syndrome*.[111] Most patients remain asymptomatic, however some develop intermittent vomiting that can become very unpleasant and intractable. Such patients invariably have advanced complications of diabetes. The pathophysiological basis for this disorder is poorly understood and disputed. Abnormalities of the vagus nerve are suspected, but findings have not been consistent.[112,113]

Pathological examination of the stomach shows a variety of subtle changes in the neuromuscular apparatus.[114,115] Most cases appear to have normal musculature, but a few show mild atrophy with increased interstitial fibrosis.[115] On H&E stain, amphophilic "M" bodies that are periodic acid-Schiff (PAS)–negative are seen in many cases (Fig. 8.11A–B).[115] These are thought to represent degenerative changes in smooth muscle cells. These are different from the PAS-positive polyglucosan inclusions that are seen in a variety of GI motility disorders (discussed later). In some cases, mild inflammation of the neural plexus and ganglia is present, composed largely of T cells (Fig. 8.11C).[114] Rare cases with marked inflammation of the neural plexus responsive to treatment with steroids have been reported.[116] Some cases show a decreased number of ganglion cells, which includes both NOS-positive and NOS-negative neurons.

A decreased number of ICC in the myenteric plexus and muscular layers has also been documented in some cases, whereas the ICC lose their dendritic processes and acquire a more rounded phenotype in other cases (Fig. 8.11D).[114] Interestingly, animal models of gastroparesis also show loss of ICC.[117] Patients with gastroparesis-like syndrome reveal similar histological changes, but to a much lesser extent.[118] From a practical diagnostic perspective, recognition of muscle atrophy or cytoplasmic inclusion bodies is easy, whereas recognition of a subtle loss of ganglion cells and changes in the ICC network requires morphometry. Of note, about one-half of cases do not show any of these abnormalities, which has led to the speculation that all of these changes may be secondary in nature. Because there are no therapeutic implications linked to specific histological changes, there is no role for extensive morphometric workup in clinical practice.

SMALL AND LARGE INTESTINE

Hirschsprung's Disease

Hirschsprung's disease is a heterogeneous group of disorders characterized by a lack of ganglion cells, which results

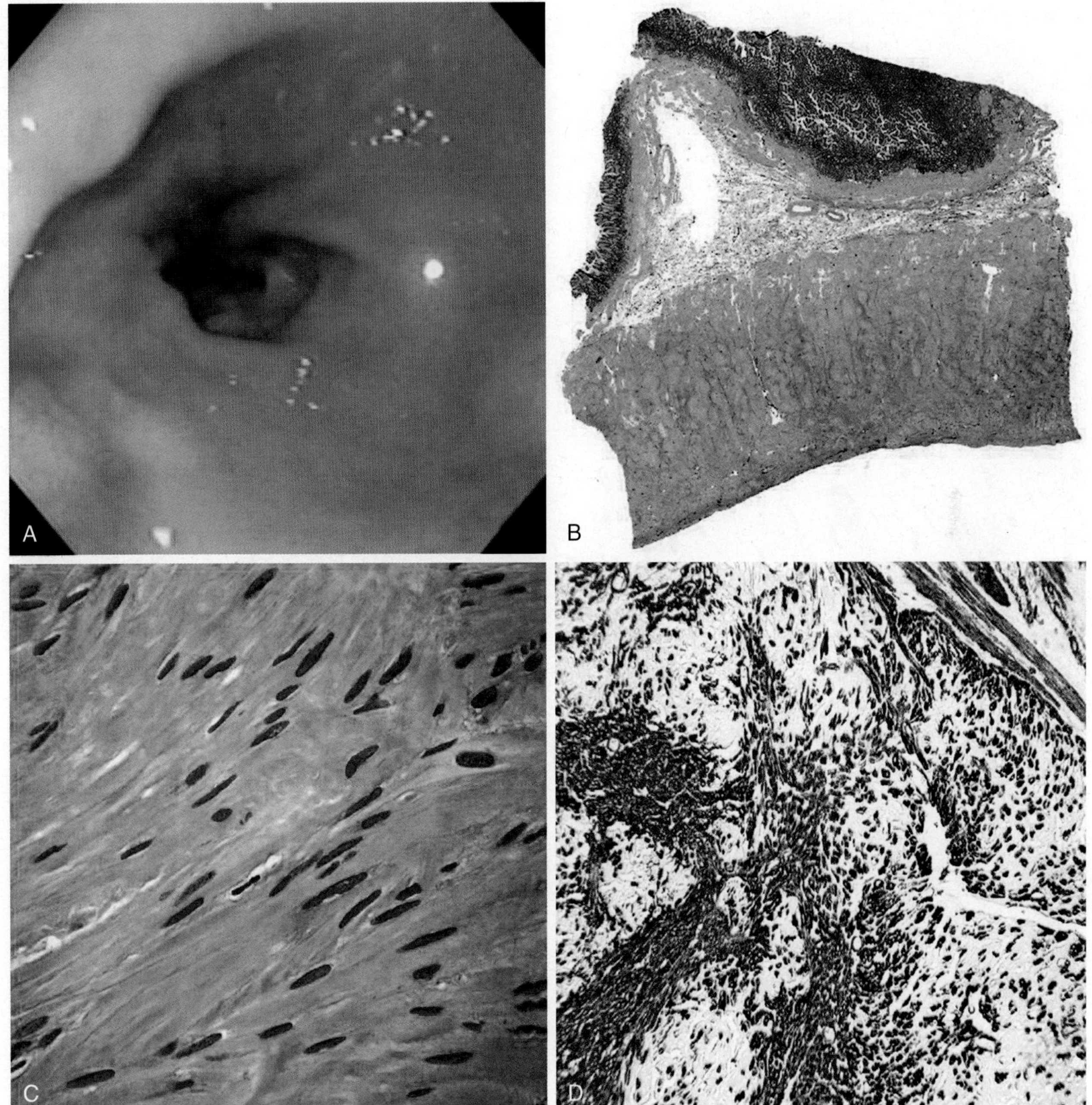

FIGURE 8.10 **A,** Esophagogastroduodenoscopy (EGD) of the pyloric canal shows marked narrowing and failure to relax after dilatation. **B,** Full mount of the pyloric region demonstrates marked thickening of the muscularis propria (scanning magnification). **C,** High magnification shows fascicles of smooth muscle with disorderly stratification. **D,** Immunohistochemical stain for smooth muscle actin confirms the presence of layers of smooth muscles. (*From Zarineh A, Leon ME, Saad RS, Silverman JF. Idiopathic hypertrophic pyloric stenosis in an adult, a potential mimic of gastric carcinoma. Pathol Res Int. 2010;2010:614280.*)

TABLE 8.1 Various Causes of Gastroparesis

Type	Causes
Idiopathic	Unknown etiology
Associated with other disorders	Diabetes mellitus: type 1 and type 2
	Amyloidosis
	Connective tissue disorders (e.g., scleroderma, systemic lupus erythematosus)
	Neurological disorders (e.g., Parkinson disease, dysautonomia)
	Renal insufficiency
	Cirrhosis
Post–viral infection	Norovirus, Epstein-Barr virus, cytomegalovirus, and herpesvirus
Postsurgical	Fundoplication and vagotomy
Paraneoplastic	Small cell carcinoma
Medications	Opioids, antibiotics, antiarrhythmics, and anticonvulsants

in bowel dysmotility.[119] The most common form (75% to 80% of cases) involves the distal sigmoid colon and rectum (short-segment disease or classic Hirschsprung's disease). In a smaller number of cases (10%), the disease (lack of ganglion cells) extends proximal to the splenic flexure (long-segment disease). Rarely (5%), the entire large bowel, with or without proximal small intestine, is devoid of ganglion cells (total bowel aganglionosis). Involvement of ≤ 2 cm of the distal rectum is referred to as *very-short-segment Hirschsprung's disease.* Zonal aganglionosis, in which the absence of ganglion cells is patchy, is extremely rare. Of course, this type may be responsible for surgery failures.[120]

Classic Hirschsprung's disease is a congenital disorder. The worldwide incidence rate varies from 1/5000 to 1/10,000 live births, with a striking male preponderance (3 to 4.5:1), and there are ethnic differences. Rare acquired forms as well as adult cases have also been described.[121,122] Long-segment disease and total bowel aganglionosis show familial aggregation. However, classic Hirschsprung's disease is usually sporadic (70%) in origin. A large number of associated conditions have been reported with Hirschsprung's disease, including Down's syndrome, cardiovascular malformations, neurofibromatosis, Waardenburg-Shah syndrome,

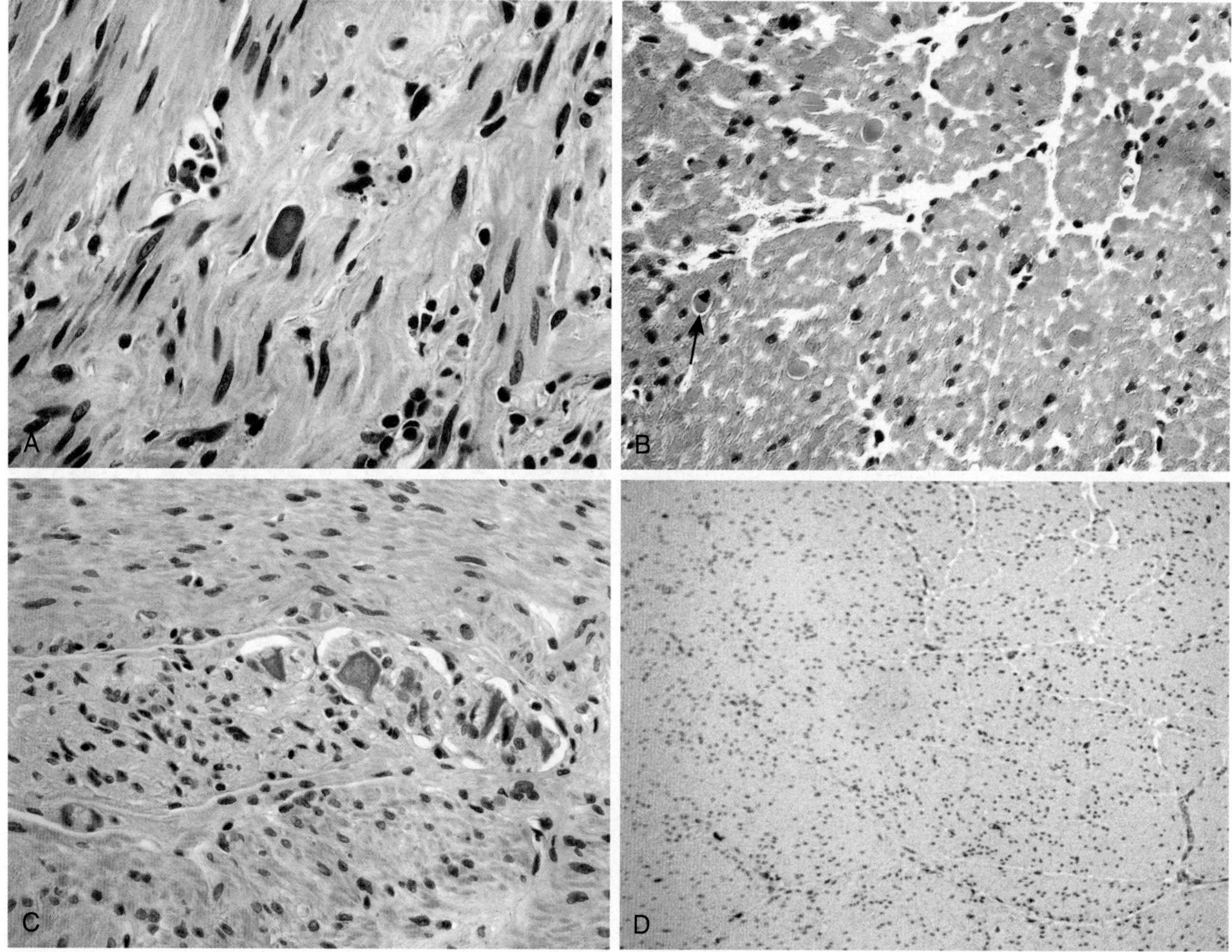

FIGURE 8.11 A, Amphophilic "M" inclusions in the smooth muscle of the muscularis propria of the stomach in a patient with gastroparesis (H&E stain). **B,** Another example shows many such inclusions at lower magnification, one of which exhibits a pyknotic nucleus *(arrow),* suggesting that these may be degenerating smooth muscle fibers (H&E stain). **C,** Mild lymphocytic ganglionitis in a case of gastroparesis (H&E stain). **D,** KIT stain reveals marked reduction in the number of interstitial cells of Cajal, some of which have lost dendritic processes.

Laurence-Monn-Bardet-Biedl syndrome, Ondine's curse (Haddad syndrome), Goldberg-Shprintzen syndrome, Mowat-Wilson syndrome, congenital hypoventilation syndrome, multiple endocrine neoplasia (MEN) and neuroblastoma, total colonic agenesis, and imperforate anus, many of which belong to the category of neural crest disorders ("neurocristopathies").[119,123]

Clinical Features

About 6.5% of patients present in the first week of life, 40% present by 6 months, and 50% present by 1 year of age.[119] Clinical presentation varies by age at presentation and extent of the aganglionosis. The earliest and most common form of clinical presentation is delayed (>48 hours) passage of meconium in the newborn accompanied by feeding intolerance, abdominal distension, and bilious emesis. Sometimes bowel perforation (colon or appendix) may be the presenting feature. Patients with total bowel aganglionosis tend to present with symptoms of intestinal obstruction. Infants and older children tend to present with chronic constipation, often accompanied by abdominal distension and vomiting. Some patients develop compensatory hypertrophy of the normally innervated proximal bowel, which leads to a milder form of disease and, thus diagnosis is delayed until later in adulthood. However, the pathogenesis of adult-onset Hirschsprung's disease remains poorly understood.[124] The clinical diagnosis of Hirschsprung's disease is facilitated with the use of imaging studies (rectal enema) and rectal manometry, which are good screening tools, but the diagnosis is ultimately established on histology (discussed later). Enterocolitis, which is more common in Hirschsprung patients with Down's syndrome, is a serious and occasionally life-threatening complication. The pathogenesis of enterocolitis is unknown. Defects in IgA secretion, infection by toxigenic bacteria, and altered microbiome have all been implicated.[125-128] The prognosis of the enterocolitis has been associated with the extent of aganglionosis and the severity of inflammation.[129,130] A subset of Hirschsprung's patients develop inflammatory bowel disease, Crohn's disease more often than ulcerative colitis, many years postsurgery.[131].

Pathogenesis

The pathogenesis of Hirschsprung's disease involves failure of the neural crest-derived ganglion cell precursors to migrate appropriately, colonize, and survive in the bowel during embryogenesis. The genetics of Hirschsprung's disease, whether nonsyndromic or syndromic, is complex and involves several susceptibility loci. Most of these lead to impaired signal transduction by RET tyrosine kinase. Various genes have either been associated or implicated in the pathogenesis of Hirschsprung's disease, including *RET, SEMA3, EDNRB, EDN3, GDNF, SOX10, ECE1, NTN, ZFHX1B, PHOX2B, L1CAM, KBP, TCF4,* and *NRG1*.[132-141] Approximately 50% of cases are associated with specific genetic abnormalities. In the others, the underlying genetic alterations remain essentially unknown.[140] Mutations of the *RET* proto-oncogene, which are the most frequent, have been identified in 20% to 25% of short-segment cases and 40% to 70% of long-segment cases. Mutations in the other genes occur in less than 10% of cases. Besides mutations, genetic polymorphisms in key genes, such as *RET* or *NRG1*, confer an increased risk for Hirschsprung's disease.[142,143] In addition, gene expression array studies have identified differential expression of a number of other genes *(RELN, GAL, GAP43, NRSN1,* and *GABRG2)* that have been thought to play a role in Hirschsprung's disease.[144] These genes are involved in neuronal migration, nerve growth, nerve stimulation, neurotransmitter receptors, and smooth muscle relaxation.[144] The mode of inheritance of Hirschsprung's disease is variable. Familial forms of long- and short-segment disease are autosomal dominant with incomplete penetrance. However, variants associated with other congenital malformations are mostly autosomal recessive. Sporadic cases are believed to have a variable pattern of inheritance. The genetics of Hirschsprung's disease is complex and explains the varied recurrence rates and incomplete penetrance observed in families.[141] It also explains the varied clinical presentations and outcomes.

Pathological Features

Classic cases of Hirschsprung's disease reveal a distal narrow aperistaltic hypertonic segment, which is aganglionic, and a dilated proximal segment of colon caused by obstruction (Fig. 8.12A). The distal hypertonic segment reveals hypertrophy of Schwannian nerve fibers and a complete lack of ganglion cells in all neural plexuses (Fig. 8.12B). In normal individuals, one to five ganglion cells are present, in clusters, for every 1 mm length of rectum. Each cluster of ganglion cells contains about 2 to 7 cells, each cell being about 20 to 30 μ in diameter. The ganglion cells are scattered and fewer in number in the submucosa compared with the myenteric plexus. Mature ganglion cells are typically large cells, have an eccentric round nucleus with prominent nucleolus, perinuclear cytoplasmic pallor, and amphophilic to basophilic cytoplasmic Nissl granules, mostly aggregated at the periphery (Fig. 8.13A). In newborns, the cells are often smaller in size, and the nucleoli and cytoplasmic granules are not prominent, making their identification in tissue sections difficult (see Fig. 8.13). Their differentiation from endothelial cells, lymphocytes, or plasma cells can be problematic, especially in frozen sections. The normal arrangement of ganglion cells in clusters and their association with nerve fibers facilitates their recognition. At the time of frozen section, toluidine blue, Giemsa, or Diff-Quick stains, in addition to routine stains, may aid in identification of ganglion cells. Immunostains to help identify ganglion cells have been recommended in difficult cases (Fig. 8.14). A variety of antibodies may be useful, such as neuron-specific enolase (NSE), *ret* oncoprotein, bcl-2, cathepsin D, Phox2b, PGP 9.5 HuC and HuC/D, or NeuN.[119,133,145-148] Of these immunomarkers, HuC/D, Phox2b (nuclear), and NeuN are fairly sensitive and thus are the preferred markers (Fig. 8.14A,B). In routine clinical practice, none of the neuronal markers offer a significant advantage over thorough histological examination of H&E sections by an experienced pathologist.[149] In equivocal cases, these neuronal markers can be useful; however, these should still be used with some caution despite claims of high specificity.[149]

Although a full-thickness transmural biopsy specimen offers better assessment of the neural plexuses because it allows visualization of the more prominent Auerbach plexus, it requires general anesthesia and introduces a risk for perforation and the development of stricture. Rectal suction

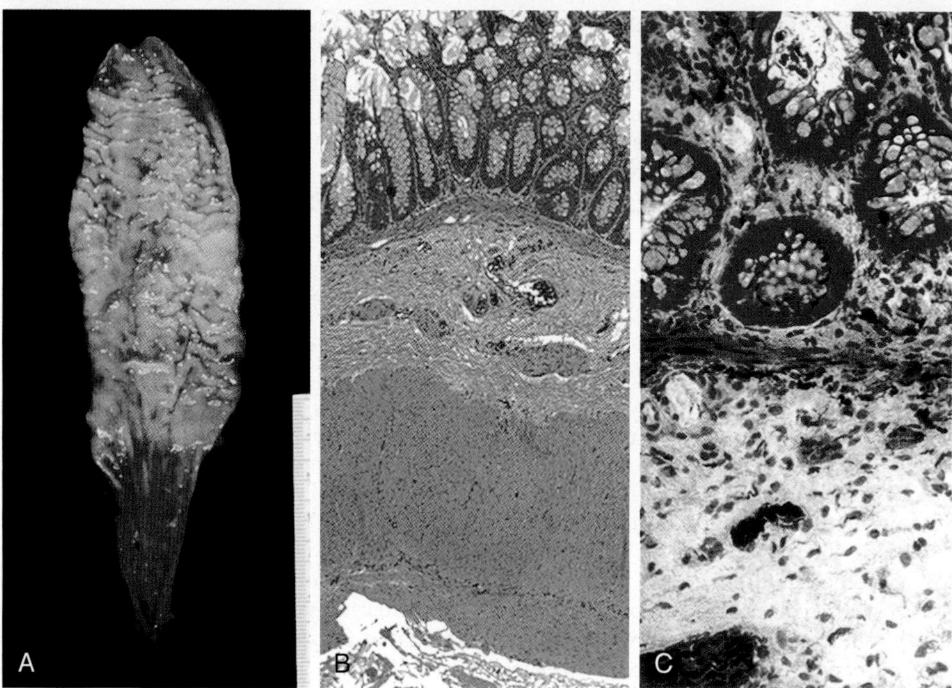

FIGURE 8.12 **A,** Resection specimen in a case of short-segment (classic) Hirschsprung's disease shows a dilated proximal segment and a narrow, aganglionic distal segment. **B,** Section of colon in Hirschsprung's disease shows submucosal neural hyperplasia and lack of ganglion cells (H&E stain). **C,** Acetylcholinesterase *(AChE)* stain performed on a frozen section of a mucosal biopsy specimen of the rectum in a patient with Hirschsprung's disease shows positively stained fibers in the submucosa, muscularis mucosa, and lamina propria. The presence of AChE-positive fibers in the muscularis mucosa and lamina propria supports a diagnosis of Hirschsprung's disease.

biopsies, which do not require general anesthesia and avert the complications associated with full-thickness biopsies, have become the standard of practice. Full-thickness biopsies are now largely restricted to older children (>1 year of age) and patients in whom the results of rectal suction biopsy are equivocal.[119]

To understand the zonal distribution of ganglion cells in the distal rectum and appropriate location of the biopsy site, understanding of the anatomy of the anorectal junction, various landmarks, and terminology is essential.[119] The inner circular muscle layer of the muscularis propria of the rectum continues distally and becomes a thick circular band recognized as the internal anal sphincter. The length of the internal anal sphincter defines the length of anatomic anal canal, which is proximally lined by colonic-type mucosa and distally by squamous mucosa. In the middle is the anal transitional zone that has a mix of colonic, transitional, or squamous mucosa. The anal transitional zone is irregular, and its length varies among individuals. In the anal transition zone, the longitudinal mucosal folds (anal columns) are inferiorly separated by anal valves and sinuses. The imaginary line connecting the base of the anal valves is called the *dentate (pectinate) line.* Distal to this is a groove called *Hilton's white line* that defines the junction of squamous mucosa with the anal skin (mucocutaneous junction) and corresponds to the lower border of the internal anal sphincter. The skin-covered area distal to this mucocutaneous junction overlies the external anal sphincter and is referred to as the *anal verge.* Multiple studies have demonstrated that there is a zone of hypoganglionosis (not aganglionosis) that extends <0.5 cm from the dentate line (not the anal verge).[119] This distance tends to be shorter in neonates (about 10 mm). Thus presence of sparse submucosal ganglion cells in rectal suction biopsies from this area can erroneously lead to a diagnosis of Hirschsprung's disease.[119] As such, biopsies showing a transitional or squamous lining epithelium may represent this hypoganglionic zone and need to be interpreted with caution. To overcome the issue of physiological hypoganglionosis, some authorities advocate obtaining multiple biopsies at 1, 2, and 3 cm above the dentate (pectinate) line. This is increased to 2, 3, and 4 cm in older children.[150] This avoids all biopsies being either too low or too high. Rectal suction biopsies are obtained using devices that allow measurement of the distance from the anal verge, but not from the internal landmarks (e.g., dentate line).[119] Thus a biopsy 2 cm from the anal verge in a neonate would roughly correspond to 1 cm above the dentate line. It is also recognized that the ganglion cells in the myenteric plexus extend further caudally compared with submucosal ganglia, implying that if there are ganglion cells in the submucosa, ganglion cells will also be present in the corresponding underlying myenteric plexus, thus excluding Hirschsprung's disease. A full-thickness biopsy can be obtained closer to the dentate line because the hypoganglionosis zone extends for a shorter distance (about 5 mm) in the myenteric plexus.

Sample adequacy is essential while evaluating a rectal suction biopsy. Ideally, the biopsy should be at least 3 mm in maximum dimension, with submucosa representing about 50% of the tissue.[150] However, in practice, this is not always possible, and inadequacy rates for suction rectal mucosal biopsies range from 9% to 17%, mostly a result of limited submucosa.[150] In practice, biopsies can be considered adequate if they are 2 to 3 mm in greatest dimension, with the majority of sections showing submucosa that is at

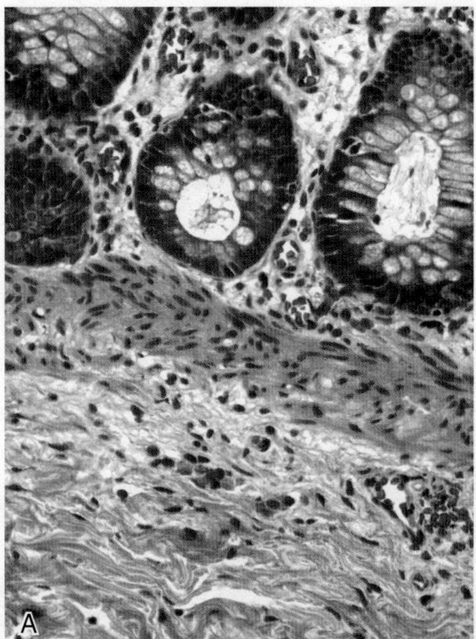

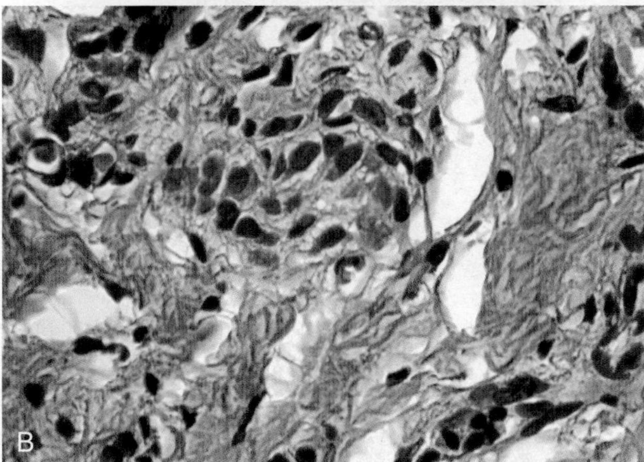

FIGURE 8.13 A, In a newborn, many immature ganglion cells are small, with scant cytoplasm and inconspicuous Nissl granules. These cells can be mistaken for plasma cells on frozen section (H&E stain). **B,** Higher magnification shows that some of the ganglion cells have more typical morphology, whereas some appear immature, and there is a greater number of ganglion cells in each cluster.

least one-third of the total biopsy thickness. The lining epithelium of the tissue in the biopsy should be entirely of the colonic-type. If the biopsy fails to reveal any ganglion cells and the lining epithelium is of squamous or transitional-type, it should be considered inadequate. Inadequate biopsies with equivocal results may necessitate repeat biopsies or full-thickness/seromuscular biopsies, especially in children older than 1 year of age.[119]

The presence of unequivocal ganglion cells (mature or immature) virtually excludes the diagnosis of Hirschsprung's disease. On the other hand, the absence of ganglion cells in the submucosa in an adequate rectal biopsy taken more than 2 cm above the dentate (pectinate) line is indicative of Hirschsprung's disease.[133] However, before committing to this diagnosis, one needs to adequately study the biopsy and use other ancillary tests to support this diagnosis. The presence of hypertrophic nerves (>40 μ thick) in the submucosa is often seen in Hirschsprung's disease (see Fig. 8.12B), although this alone should not be considered sufficient evidence to establish the diagnosis. These nerves have a perineurium that stains with glucose transporter 1 (Glut1) and show ultrastructural and immunohistochemical features similar to peripheral (non-enteric) nerves. These hypertrophic nerves are thought to arise from nonintestinal autonomic ganglia, primarily in the pelvis. Such hypertrophic nerves may be absent in premature neonates, in patients with long-segment disease, and those with total bowel aganglionosis. Once the initial sections fail to reveal ganglion cells, multiple additional serial sections should be examined before a definitive diagnosis of Hirschsprung's disease is rendered. Most laboratories obtain at least 50 to 100 H&E-stained serial sections, while others exhaust the entire block before stating "no ganglion cells identified."[133] In addition, most would also seek supportive evidence by performing histochemical or immunohistochemical stains before rendering a diagnosis of Hirschsprung's disease. Traditionally, histochemistry for acetylcholinesterase on frozen tissue has been used as an ancillary test.[151] In classic cases, abnormally coarse and diffusely acetylcholinesterase-positive nerve fibers are seen in the muscularis mucosae and the lamina propria. These are lacking in biopsy specimens from normal individuals (see Fig. 8.12C). Such fibers are few and difficult to demonstrate in newborns with Hirschsprung's disease, and they tend to increase with age. Some pathologists combine a lactate dehydrogenase stain, which stains ganglion cells, with acetylcholinesterase on frozen sections. An H&E stain should always accompany the histochemical stain for comparison. The residual frozen tissue should then be submitted for routine histology and serial sectioning to ensure that it also lacks ganglion cells before rendering a diagnosis of Hirschsprung's disease. It should be kept in mind that the acetylcholinesterase stain is performed on a separate tissue fragment, and occasionally the results are discrepant compared with the routine biopsy. The limitation of acetylcholinesterase stain is that it requires frozen tissue that is not always available in a given case. It is also a tricky stain to perform and requires substantial experience and expertise on behalf of the laboratory performing the test and the pathologist interpreting the stain. In recent years, calretinin immunostain has emerged as a good alternative to acetylcholinesterase in the diagnostic workup of intestinal dysganglionoses, and it does not require frozen sections.[152-154] In fact, a few studies that compared these stains showed that interpretation of a calretinin stain is easier and superior compared with acetylcholinesterase.[153,154] In these studies, there were no false positives with the calretinin stain and only rare false negatives, the latter mainly a result of either weak staining or inexperience of the pathologist. Normally, calretinin immunostain shows granular immunoreactivity in nerve fibers in the lamina propria, muscularis mucosae, and submucosa. It also stains ganglia (Fig. 8.15A,B). Any positive staining in the nerve fibers, even when ganglia are not seen, excludes the possibility of Hirschsprung's disease, whereas complete absence of staining supports this diagnosis (Fig. 8.15C,D). Calretinin immunoreactivity in mast cells is normal and serves as an internal control. Mast cell positivity can be easily differentiated from neural positivity and seldom causes any diagnostic problems (see Fig 8.15D). Occasionally equivocal acetylcholinesterase staining results

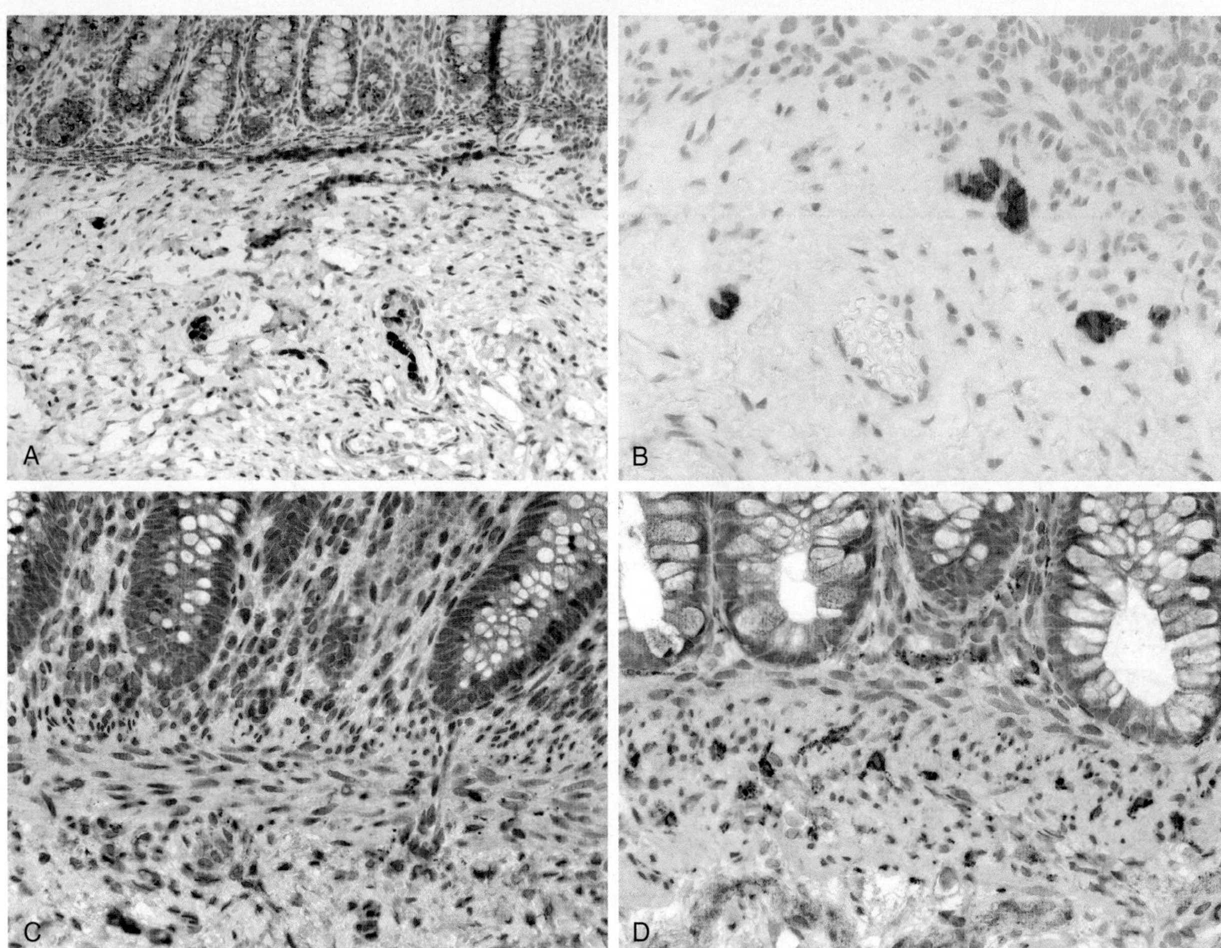

FIGURE 8.14 **A,** Immunostaining with neuN antibody to highlight submucosal ganglion cells in suspected Hirschsprung's disease. **B,** Immunostaining with HuC/D antibody to highlight submucosal ganglion cells in a suspected case of Hirschsprung's disease. **C,** Immunostaining with Choline transporter (Ch T) antibody to show absent to sparse staining in the lamina propria and muscularis mucosae in a normal biopsy. **D,** Immunostaining with Choline transporter (Ch T) antibody showing coarse and intense staining in the mucosal nerves in a case of Hirschsprung's disease (**C** and **D** *courtesy Raj Kapur).*

in the presence of ganglion cells in the biopsies causing confusion, especially in Down's syndrome patients. However, this can be easily resolved by showing positive staining for calretinin. It should be recognized that about 2% to 10% of Down's syndrome patients do have associated Hirschsprung's disease.[155] More recently, immunostaining for Choline transporter (Ch T) has been used as an alternative for acetylcholinesterase stain, and it does not require frozen sections (see Fig 8.14C,D).[119] The Ch T immunostain highlights the abnormal cholinergic nerve fibers in the deep lamina propria and muscularis propria very similar to the acetylcholinesterase stain, although the interpretation can be difficult at times and requires some experience. Abnormalities of ICC in Hirschsprung's disease have also been shown in some studies, although it appears that the changes are likely secondary in nature and of little diagnostic value.[156,157] A rare example of an of extra layer of muscle in a patient with Hirschsprung's disease associated with Mowat-Wilson syndrome has also been reported.[158]

Preoperative biopsies are performed to establish a diagnosis before corrective surgery and remain the gold standard for diagnosis.[119] Each laboratory should establish their own protocol for handling such cases (Fig. 8.16). The need for a piece of tissue to be kept for acetylcholinesterase stain is now considered redundant because, as discussed earlier, a calretinin stain is superior and can be performed on formalin-fixed tissue. However, a diagnosis of Hirschsprung's disease rests on demonstration of an absence of ganglion cells, or lack of staining for calretinin. In practice, it could be difficult at times to determine whether the negative calretinin staining is caused by sampling or technical reasons. Thus some pathologists still use an acetylcholinesterase stain because it may be the only positive finding. Multiple serial sections should be examined before a definitive diagnosis is rendered. Most laboratories obtain at least 50 to 100 serial sections stained with H&E before establishing a definitive diagnosis of Hirschsprung's disease.[133] Unstained sections are used for calretinin. The presence of ganglion cells or appropriate staining for calretinin in nerves in a colonic biopsy rules out the possibility of conventional Hirschsprung's disease. The presence of crush artifact or small size of the biopsy are other reasons that could lead to an incorrect diagnosis. One should not hesitate to request a repeat biopsy in this situation. Some patients with Hirschsprung's disease have zonal aganglionosis or hyperganglionosis with skip areas, involving the small intestine or colon.[159-161] These cases are thought

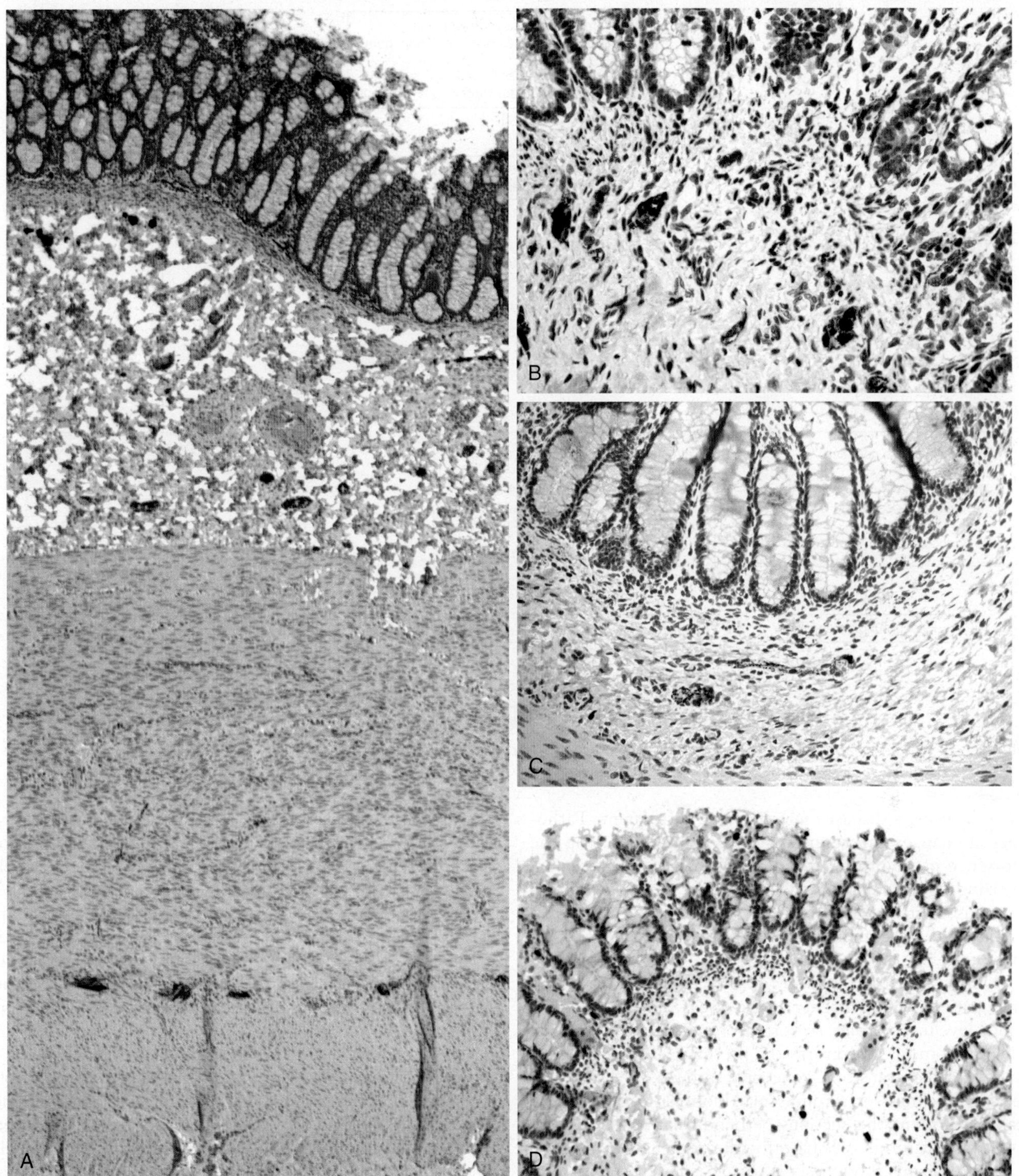

FIGURE 8.15 **A,** Calretinin immunostain in normal colon shows intense staining in ganglion cells in the myenteric and submucosal plexus and nerve bundles. **B,** Higher magnification of a rectal suction mucosal biopsy specimen from a patient with suspected Hirschsprung's disease shows intense staining in the nerve fibers of the submucosa, muscularis mucosae, and lamina propria. This staining pattern excludes Hirschsprung's disease. **C,** In another example, weaker and fewer nerve fibers are shown with granular staining for calretinin, but this is enough to exclude Hirschsprung's disease. **D,** Rectal suction mucosal biopsy specimen from a patient with Hirschsprung's disease shows lack of any staining in the nerve fibers of the submucosa, muscularis mucosae, or lamina propria. Scattered positively stained mast cells are easy to distinguish from nerves and ganglion cells.

to be acquired in nature and of diverse etiology (viral enterocolitis, ischemia, or other forms of injury). Other possibilities include inability of vagal and sacral crest cells to migrate appropriately. Occurrence of segmental aganglionosis, although rare, implies that absence of ganglion cells in the appendix cannot be used as absolute evidence of total bowel aganglionosis, particularly when making a decision regarding the extent of resection during a surgery.

In addition, specific attention should be given to the presence or absence of mucosal inflammation in cases of

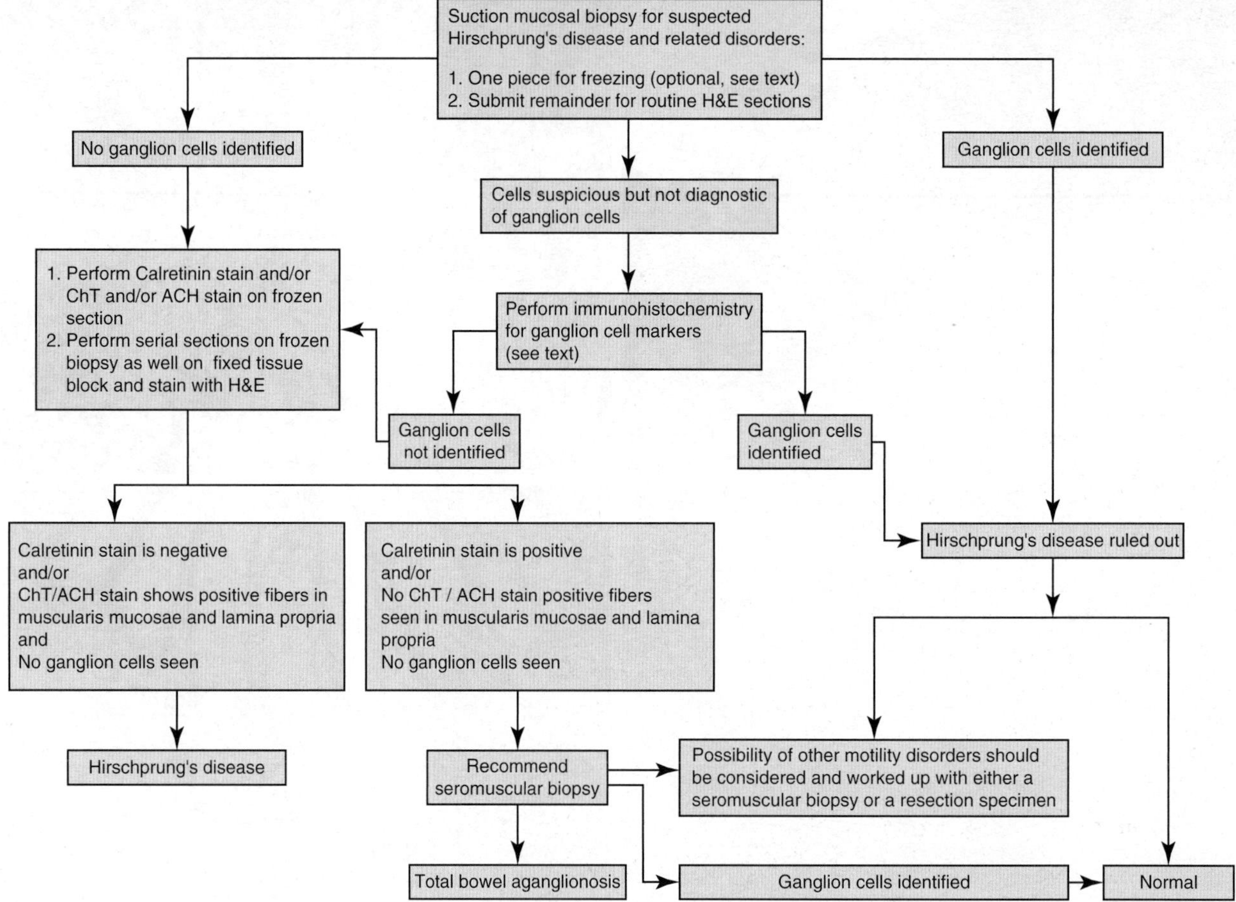

FIGURE 8.16 Diagnostic approach to a suction mucosal biopsy for the workup of Hirschsprung's disease and related disorders.

Hirschsprung's disease, which is not infrequent. Pathological changes can resemble acute colitis, including the presence of cryptitis and crypt abscesses, neonatal necrotizing enterocolitis, ischemic colitis, or pseudomembranous colitis (Fig. 8.17).[125,162,163] Severe cases, with transmural necrotizing inflammation, may progress to perforation.

During surgical resection of the aganglionic segment in a patient with Hirschsprung's disease, frozen sections from leveling biopsies are often obtained before making the anastomosis to confirm the presence of ganglion cells and to avoid transition zone pull-through.[164] These can be full-thickness or seromuscular biopsies. Care must be taken to orient the sections perpendicular to the serosal plane and carefully evaluate for the presence of ganglion cells in the myenteric plexus. An absence of submucosal ganglia in this setting has little significance. Multiple sections (usually 4 to 10) are obtained that are stained with H&E, while some like to use Romanowsky stains (Diff-Quik, Giemsa, or toluidine blue). The goal is to find a level at which normal ganglia (euganglionosis) are found. The anastomosis (for ostomy or proximal to distal) is usually performed at least 5 cm above the euganglionic leveling biopsy to avoid a transitional zone pull-through. Although the transitional zone is reported to be generally <5 cm, rarely it has been reported to be as long as 22.9 cm.[165] It is also recommended that once the site for anastomosis is identified, the entire circumference (donut) of the proximal bowel margin should be submitted for frozen section en-face to ensure normal ganglia throughout the entire circumference.[164] The presence of only 1 to 2 ganglion cell bodies in the ganglia with scant associated neuropils or >2 hypertrophic nerves in greater than one-eighth of the circumference of the margin, even in the presence of normal ganglia elsewhere in the section, should alert one that this may still be the transitional zone. Anastomosis should be attempted only after one has reached a completely euganglionic segment.

Handling of resection specimens in Hirschsprung's disease varies among different laboratories. One may follow the guidelines suggested by the international working group.[150,164] The goals of examining a resection specimen are largely to document and define the extent of aganglionosis and the presence of normal ganglia at the proximal resection margin. One easy way to achieve this is to obtain transverse (en face) sections from the proximal and distal margins and then take a longitudinal strip along the entire length of the specimen. This may be submitted as multiple sequential sections, or as a "swiss roll," in a single block keeping the orientation of the proximal and distal segments. Alternatively, one may submit multiple transverse sections from the entire specimen, at 1-cm intervals with longitudinal strips from the intervening areas. Frozen samples can be obtained from the narrow-involved segment, transitional zone, and proximal normal-appearing colon for histochemical stains.

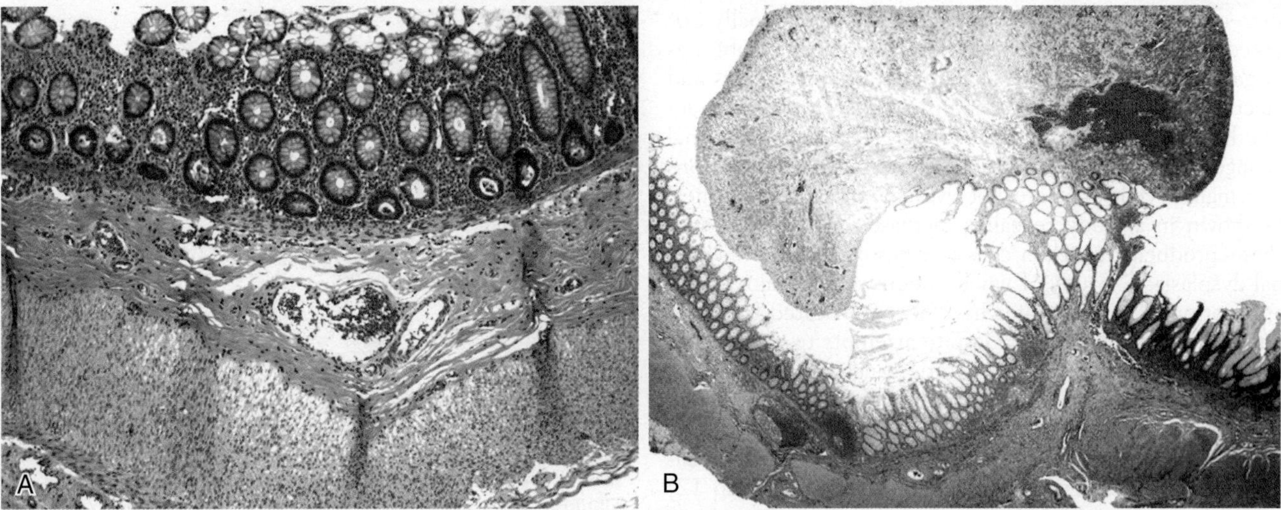

FIGURE 8.17 A, Mild colitis in a patient with Hirschsprung's disease shows a mild increase in lamina propria inflammatory cells and cryptitis, mimicking "self-limited" colitis (H&E stain). **B,** Another case in which Hirschsprung's disease–associated colitis mimics pseudomembranous colitis (H&E stain).

Differential Diagnosis

Establishing a diagnosis of Hirschsprung's disease in suction mucosal biopsies remains a diagnostic challenge, especially in newborns or premature babies. The issue is largely related to reliable identification of ganglion cells. When ganglion cells are not identified, one must ensure that the biopsy is adequate, it is obtained from the correct anatomic area, and special stains support the diagnosis. Patients who present with features suggestive of Hirschsprung's disease but fail to show absence of ganglion cells on biopsies remain a diagnostic challenge. The clinical differential diagnosis for these cases includes other types of dysganglionoses, intestinal pseudo-obstruction, constipation, ileus, toxic megacolon, and hypothyroidism. Once ganglion cells are identified in mucosal biopsies, possibilities include very short (ultrashort)-segment Hirschsprung's disease and other dysganglionoses (hypoganglionosis and intestinal neuronal dysplasia). However, their diagnosis and even existence remains controversial and thus should be entertained only in resection specimens or full-thickness biopsies. Regardless, most of these disorders are managed similarly. Some patients with an acetylcholinesterase staining pattern similar to Hirschsprung's disease and/or hypertrophic nerves, but with ganglion cells in biopsies, are believed to represent very-short-segment Hirschsprung's disease. This remains a controversial entity and likely represents a heterogenous group comprising aganglionosis, hypoganglionosis, and anal achalasia. Because the distal 2 to 3 cm of rectum normally contains only sparse ganglion cells, these diagnoses are difficult to establish.[166]

Treatment and Follow-up

Treatment involves surgical resection of the involved segment of bowel followed by restoration of bowel continuity. This may be performed in two stages in which a definitive anastomosis is performed following an initial colostomy. More commonly, it is performed as a one-stage "endorectal pull-through" procedure.[133] Seromuscular biopsies, obtained laparoscopically, are generally submitted for intraoperative frozen-section evaluation to ensure the presence of ganglion cells at the proximal margin of the resected segment before completion of the anastomosis, and also to confirm a lack of ganglion cells in the affected segment of colon. However, frozen sections performed for evaluation of ganglion cells may be problematic and should not replace a preoperative suction mucosal biopsy.[167] The prognosis of most surgically treated cases is excellent. Most patients are able to achieve continence. Some patients continue to have postoperative dysmotility despite anastomosis of euganglionic segments. This phenomenon has been attributed to immaturity of ganglion cells, which improves with time.[168] About 3% of patients require reoperation. Long-term follow-up studies show that most patients achieve good quality of life into adulthood, with minimal or no problems. However, some patients continue to have incontinence, whereas others have problems with constipation and enterocolitis.[169,170]

Other Developmental Disorders of the Enteric Nervous System

This heterogenous group of disorders includes hypoganglionosis, hyperganglionosis, and abnormal differentiation of ganglion cells. Enteric ganglia may also be involved secondarily by systemic metabolic defects, such as lysosomal storage disorders. Neuropathic forms of familial intestinal pseudo-obstruction (discussed later) are considered another form of developmental abnormality.

Clinically, these disorders resemble Hirschsprung's disease. However, ganglion cells are present. The acetylcholinesterase stain may mimic the pattern seen in Hirschsprung's disease, with strong staining in some cases, and little or no staining in others. Although diagnostic criteria for aganglionosis (Hirschsprung's disease) are well established, objective criteria necessary to define and diagnose other enteric dysganglionoses are poorly established and often impractical to apply.[171-174] This has resulted in the use of many different terms for these disorders, such as *variant Hirschsprung's disease*, *pseudo-Hirschsprung's disease*, or *Hirschsprung's disease allied disorders*. Subtle alterations in the number of ganglion cells are almost impossible to diagnose on routine suction mucosal biopsies. Quantitation of the neural plexuses, neural and glial stroma, and ganglion cells are extremely difficult to perform, even on conventionally oriented transmural biopsies. Alterations in specific subtypes of ganglion cells can be resolved only by special stains and electrophysiological studies, and protocols for clinical practice have not been established.[4] It is likely that functional changes may underlie the subtle morphological alterations of ganglion cells that are not evident on routine studies, as shown in a study revealing increased nitric oxide synthase–producing ganglion cells in cases of intestinal neuronal dysplasia.[175] Study of whole-mount sections along with application of special stains have been advocated to better characterize these lesions. Despite attempts to standardize the counting method for myenteric ganglia using neuronal markers and having better guidelines for establishing the diagnosis, there is marked interobserver variability in this regard.[147,176] The median number of ganglia in the myenteric plexus has been shown to be 8/mm (range 2 to 12) in routine stains and 15/mm (range 2 to 23) with use of special stains.[177] The size of ganglion cells varies from 10 to 40 μ. The median number of neurons per ganglion has been reported to be 3 per ganglion (range, 2 to 6) on H&E stain and 10 per ganglion (range, 4 to 14) using special stains.[177] The numbers are higher in whole-mount thick sections.[177] Variability related to age, site, and among different individuals along with stretching of the tissues during processing make it even more difficult to design criteria that can help differentiate intestinal dysganglionoses based on mild to moderate alterations in ganglion cell numbers.[147] Hence, the criteria suggested by the international working group are very conservative.

It is also unclear if the histological changes described earlier are secondary in nature. This cannot be determined on the basis of evaluation of mucosal biopsies and requires full-thickness biopsies or evaluation of resection specimens. Thus only cases (congenital or acquired) that show severe abnormalities are diagnosed reliably. The diagnostic utility of calretinin stain in mucosal biopsies in these conditions remains unknown.

Hypoganglionosis

This condition refers to a reduction in the number of ganglia in neural plexuses, decreased number of ganglion cells per ganglion, and small size of ganglia.[178] This condition may exist in some segments of the colon in patients with Hirschsprung's disease or as an isolated (primary) condition leading to intestinal pseudo-obstruction. The genetic polymorphic variants, or mutations, associated with Hirschsprung's disease are absent in this condition.

Because of methodological variations, the international working group determined that there are no criteria that can be used uniformly among different laboratories or institutions. It has been suggested that ≤ 1 ganglion (cluster of neuronal cells)/mm or ≤ 2 neurons per ganglion constitutes hypoganglionosis (Fig. 8.18).[150] The acetylcholinesterase stain shows very weak or absent staining in the lamina propria, and hypertrophic nerve twigs associated with Hirschsprung's disease are typically lacking. A review of 92 cases reported in the literature showed that many features are similar to Hirschsprung's disease, including male predominance (M:F 3:1), clinical presentation with severe chronic constipation, pseudo-obstruction, and/or enterocolitis. In contrast, only 32% of patients presented in the neonatal period compared with over 90% in Hirschsprung's disease. This may be a result of difficulty establishing a definitive diagnosis. Hypoganglionosis can be focal, segmental, or diffuse. The hypoganglionic segment is usually narrow and is associated with dilatation of the proximal bowel.[124] However, occasionally one can see fewer numbers of ganglion cells in colonic resections performed for unrelated reasons and in patients without any motility issues. This puts into question the validity of evaluating ganglion cell numbers in motility disorders and the existence of this entity as a clinical disease.[179] The management and long-term outcome and complications are also similar to Hirschsprung's disease.

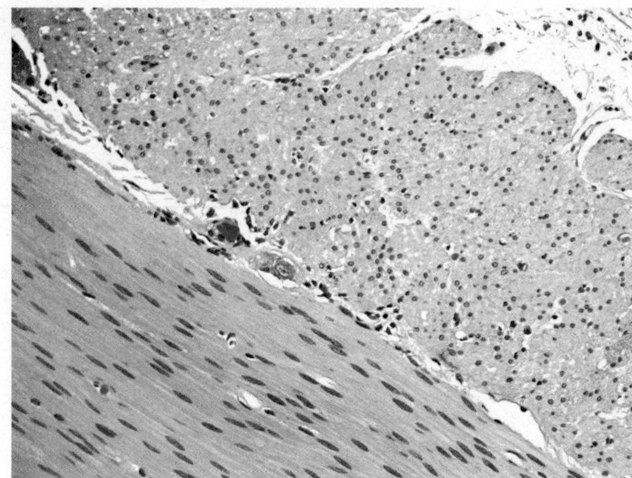

FIGURE 8.18 Section from the jejunum in a 12-year-old boy with total parenteral nutrition dependent pseudo-obstruction shows markedly reduced numbers of ganglion cells in the myenteric plexus, representing hypoganglionosis (H&E stain). (*Courtesy of Raj Kapur, University of Washington, Seattle.*)

Hyperganglionosis

This condition is characterized by an increased number of ganglion cells and neural hyperplasia. This also has been referred to as *intestinal neuronal dysplasia* (IND). Two forms (IND-A and IND-B) are recognized.[180] IND-A is extremely rare, constitutes <5% of all IND, and has been characterized by sympathetic aplasia, myenteric hyperplasia, and colonic inflammation.[181,182] The myenteric plexus shows an increased number of ganglion cells in each ganglion. However, the submucosal ganglia are normal appearing, and ectopic ganglion cells are not present. The clinical presentation includes episodes of intestinal obstruction, bloody stools, and diarrhea. Surgical resection is believed to be curative.

IND-B is a controversial entity that is characterized by marked neural hypertrophy and an increased number of large ganglion cells in the submucosal neural plexuses. It constitutes about 95% of all IND cases.[172,183,184] This is considered an anomaly of the parasympathetic neural system of the bowel. The diagnostic criteria for IND-B have changed over time. Currently, it requires the presence of giant submucosal ganglia, which is defined as >8 ganglion cell cross sections per submucosal ganglion. Such "giant" ganglia should constitute >20% of all ganglia, and at least 25 submucosal ganglia should be evaluated (Fig. 8.19).[174] The myenteric plexus may show hypoganglionosis in some

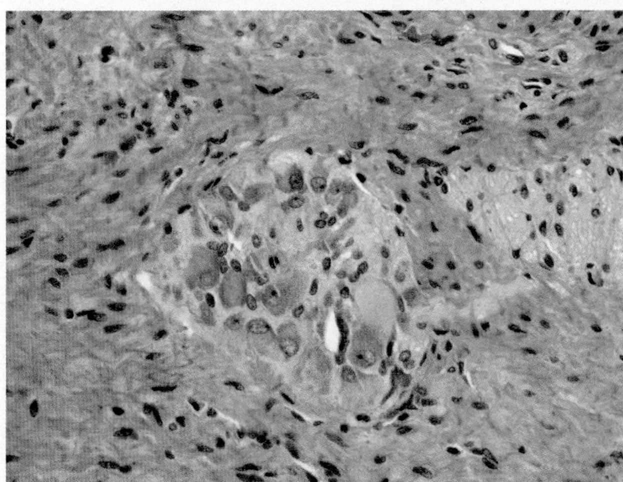

FIGURE 8.19 More than eight large ganglion cells are present in this ganglion, a finding that some would consider suggestive of intestinal neuronal dysplasia (H&E stain).

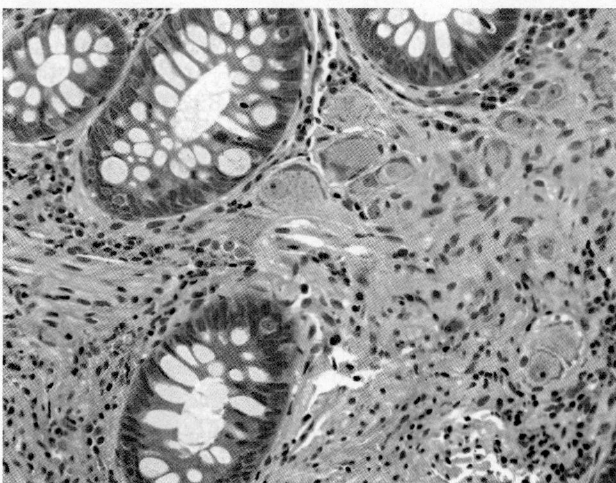

FIGURE 8.20 Presence of ganglion cells and hypertrophic nerve fiber in the lamina propria is suggestive of ganglioneuromatosis (H&E stain). In multiple endocrine neoplasia (MEN 2b) syndrome, this tends to be diffuse and can be seen only in the submucosa.

cases, whereas some are even associated with aganglionosis similar to Hirschsprung's disease.[184] Rare cases that are clinically similar, with increased numbers of ganglion cells only in the myenteric plexus, have been described.[185] The acetylcholinesterase stain reveals increased staining in the lamina propria similar to Hirschsprung's disease, early in the course of disease. Hyperplasia of the myenteric plexus may be evident in some cases. Involvement may be limited to the rectum, or it may be extensive. Small bowel involvement is rare. The clinical presentation is related to chronic constipation. Premature infants and infants younger than 1 year of age normally show higher numbers of ganglion cells per submucosal ganglion (see Fig. 8.13B). Thus it is recommended that a diagnosis of IND-B should be made only in children older than 1 year of age and younger than 4 years of age.[174]

An increase or decrease in the number of ganglia may also be caused by mechanical obstruction. A rare case of mechanical obstruction caused by a Ladd's band, associated with IND-B–type changes, has been reported. This case subsequently developed degeneration of ganglion cells (hypoganglionosis), enteric plexus, and ICC.[186] Such an adaptive response combined with neuronal plasticity has also been shown in animal models of mechanical bowel obstruction.[187,188]

Homozygous mutant mice deficient in Ncx/Hox11L.1 show features similar to IND-B. However, these mutations have not been found in human subjects.[189,190] No specific genetic mutations have been associated with this disorder, although a possible association with *RET* variants has been suggested.[191]

Management of IND-B depends on the extent of the involvement. Conservative treatment is possible in many patients.[192-194] Surgical options are largely similar to Hirschsprung's disease.

Increased ganglion cells and ectopic ganglion cells in the lamina propria can also be seen in patients with intestinal ganglioneuromas. Sporadic lesions are usually single and localized, however these can also be diffuse (ganglioneuromatosis) (Fig. 8.20). Diffuse ganglioneuromatosis is almost always associated with MEN 2B and mutations in the *RET* proto-oncogene. It can manifest as bowel dysmotility. The presence of isolated ganglion cells in the deep lamina propria alone is not considered abnormal.[195]

Despite several reports of IND-B and hypoganglionosis in the literature and many attempts to reach a consensus regarding diagnostic criteria,[174,179,196] these entities remain controversial. Their clinical significance also remains unclear, and even their existence is still in question. IND-B is now considered a histological pattern of disease that does not require surgical treatment. The rarity of these conditions is highlighted by the fact that many experts in the field at major institutions across the world have spent their entire lifetime without ever making a diagnosis of either hypoganglionosis or hyperganglionosis (IND).

Intestinal Pseudo-Obstruction

Intestinal pseudo-obstruction is defined as a clinical syndrome caused by inability of the bowel to propel its contents in the absence of a mechanical obstruction. Both acute and chronic forms are recognized.

Acute Intestinal Pseudo-Obstruction

Paralytic Ileus

Paralytic ileus is the most common cause of intestinal pseudo-obstruction. It occurs after abdominal surgery, after abdominal trauma, or in patients with peritonitis.[197] The entire bowel becomes paralyzed and distended. The diagnosis is made on clinical grounds, and treatment is supportive.[197] No specific histopathological changes are recognized in this condition.

Acute Idiopathic Intestinal Pseudo-Obstruction (Ogilvie's Syndrome)

This is a rare and potentially serious complication in patients who have recently undergone surgery or are ill from other causes.[198] Rare cases following colonic herpes or CMV infections have been described.[199,200] The pathogenesis is poorly understood, although temporary autonomic dysfunction is suspected. Patients demonstrate bowel dilatation, most often confined to the right colon, which may lead to transmural ischemia and perforation, the latter occurring most frequently in the cecum. Pathological changes are nonspecific but mimic ischemia secondary to increased intramural pressure. The condition, in most instances, resolves with supportive care.

Chronic Intestinal Pseudo-Obstruction

Chronic idiopathic intestinal pseudo-obstruction (CIIP) is caused by a variety of disorders that may affect any component of the bowel neuromuscular apparatus.[176,201-203] It most commonly involves the small intestine and/or colon. It may result from primary abnormalities of the neuromuscular apparatus of the gut (primary), be part of a generalized or systemic disorder (secondary), or have an unknown etiopathogenesis (idiopathic). Based on the component of the neuromuscular apparatus involved, four major categories have been recognized: those with abnormalities of the smooth muscle (myopathic form), those with abnormalities of the neural system (neuropathic form), those with ICC abnormalities (mesenchymopathic form), and those with abnormalities of neurohormonal peptides (see Box 8.1). Many disorders show involvement of more than one component, whether they are primary, secondary, or idiopathic in nature.

The clinical features of CIIP vary depending on the etiology and severity of the underlying abnormality. Most primary neuromuscular disorders present at an very early age, and their etiology and clinicopathological features are very different from those presenting in adults (Table 8.2).[204] Many of these features have been shown to be associated with genetic mutations (inherited familial or sporadic) that interfere with the function and/or development of the neuromuscular apparatus. Some are syndromic with multisystemic involvement, while others involve only the GI tract. These syndromes are quite rare. The common ones with associated genes and their key features are shown in Table 8.3.

Symptoms are typical of intestinal obstruction, such as abdominal distention, pain, and vomiting. Distention may be gradual, but it may also become severe, especially when both the small intestine and colon are involved. Generally, these patients show alternating diarrhea and constipation, rather than obstipation. Diarrhea is generally secondary to bacterial overgrowth caused by stasis, and it may result in substantial weight loss. Perforation occurs rarely. The clinical manifestations of CIIP are similar among the various subtypes. Some patients remain asymptomatic until middle age, whereas others are entirely asymptomatic. The diagnosis is often delayed for many years (median 8 years). Many patients end up having had multiple exploratory laparotomies.[205]

Etiopathogenesis

For both myopathic and neuropathic forms, sporadic and familial cases are recognized.[201] In the older literature, these were all classified as types I to IV based on the mode of transmission and associated abnormalities, but genomic analysis has shown that most of the primary forms are associated with specific genetic alterations (inherited or sporadic) and fit in with some of the previously described syndromes/phenotypes.[206] For example, megacystis-microcolon intestinal hypoperistalsis (MMIH) syndrome, previously also known as *Berdon's syndrome,* which is characterized by narrow-caliber hypoperistaltic colon, esophageal dilatation, megacystis, and sometimes uterine inertia, has been shown to be associated with mutations in the Actin G2 gene *(ACTG2)*.[207-210] Abnormalities in this gene and the *RET* promoter have also been identified in

TABLE 8.2 Comparison of Pediatric and Adult Chronic Intestinal Pseudo-Obstruction

	Pediatric	Adult
Etiology	Majority (>80%) appear to be congenital and primary. Secondary forms are rare (<10%).	Secondary forms are common (>50% of cases).
Disease subtype	Neuropathies are more common (about 70%) compared with myopathic forms (about 30%).	Neuropathies (majority inflammatory) are also more common (about 45%) compared with myopathies (about 30%).
Symptoms onset	Onset is prenatal, from birth or early infancy; most patients (65% to 80%) present by 12 months of age.	Median age of onset is 20 to 40 years of age.
Clinical features	Recurrent or continuous episodes of intestinal pseudo-obstruction occur with symptoms present from birth/early life.	Chronic abdominal pain and distention with superimposed acute episodes of pseudo-obstruction occur.
	Pain is infrequent (about 30%).	Pain is a cardinal symptom present in most (about 80%).
	Urological involvement is common (36% to 100%).	Urological involvement is rare.
	Intestinal malrotation occurs in about 30% of cases.	Intestinal malrotation is rare.
	There is a high-risk for colonic and small bowel volvulus.	There is a low risk for colonic and small bowel volvulus.
Natural history	Poor outcomes. There is a risk for mortality in approximately 20% of cases.	Overall mortality is low, but there is a high mortality when the associated disease has a poor prognosis (e.g., neoplasia).
Diagnosis	Diagnosis relies on clinical picture and radiology together with specialized tests (e.g., intestinal manometry, histopathology.	Diagnosis is made on the clinical picture and radiology with variable use of intestinal manometry. Histopathology has a positive yield in the majority of patients but guides treatment only in a minority.

TABLE 8.3 Syndromes with Intestinal Pseudo-Obstruction and Associated Genes and Key Features

Syndrome	Gene Involved	Gene Function	Mode of Inheritance	Age of Onset	Clinical Manifestation	Predominant Phenotype
Megacystis-microcolon intestinal hypoperistalsis (MMIH) syndrome	*ACTG2*	Encodes enteric smooth muscle actin	AD	Prenatal, neonatal to third decade of life	Variable phenotype with visceral myopathy involving GI and genitourinary tracts; prune-belly phenotype, milder involvement with severe constipation	Myopathic
	MYH11	Encodes myosin light chain	AR			
	MYLK	Encodes a kinase required for myosin activation and its interaction with actin	AR			
	LMOD1	Encodes leiomodin in smooth muscle cells, which plays a role in actin cytoskeletal assembly	AR			
	MYL9	Encodes a regulatory myosin light chain	AR			
Multisystemic smooth muscle dysfunction (MSMS) syndrome	*ACTA2*	Encodes smooth muscle actin alpha-2, which is part of the actin family	AD	Childhood to adult	Involvement of CVS (patent ductus arteriosus, aneurysms, vasculopathy), GI (hypoperistalsis/CIIP), weak bladder, congenital mydriasis	Myopathic
Mitochondrial neurogastrointestinal encephalomyopathy (MNGIE)	*TYMP*	A nucleoside that maintains adequate thymidine in mitochondria	AR	Infancy to third decade of life	Involvement of GI and nervous system	Neuropathic
Mungan's syndrome	*RAD21*	Encodes for the rad21 protein, which is part of a cohesion complex that controls chromatid pairing and unpairing in cell replication. Plays an important role in epithelial and neuronal survival and Apolipoprotein B regulation in the GI tract	AR	First to second decade of life	CIIP, megaduodenum, long-segment Barrett's esophagus, and cardiac abnormalities	Myopathic and neuropathic
Chronic atrial and intestinal dysrhythmia (CAID)	*SGOL1*	Encodes Shugoshin-like 1 protein, which is component of the cohesion pathway and plays a role in chromatid pairing and unpairing in cell replication	AR	First to fourth decade of life	Cardiac dysrhythmias and GI involvement	Neuropathic
Waardenburg's syndrome type IV	*Sox 10*	Encodes sox 10 protein, which is important in migration and development of the neural crest and peripheral nervous system	AD	Neonatal period	Peripheral neuropathy with hypomyelination, sensorineural deafness and pseudo-obstruction, and aganglionosis/Hirschsprung's disease	Neuropathic
	EDNRB	Encodes for endothelin receptor type B, which regulates development and function of blood vessels, production of certain hormones, and stimulation of cell growth and division.				
	EDN3	Endothelin 3 interacts with endothelin receptor type B, which together play an important role in development of neural crest cells				

Continued

TABLE 8.3 Syndromes with Intestinal Pseudo-Obstruction and Associated Genes and Key Features—Cont'd

Syndrome	Gene Involved	Gene Function	Mode of Inheritance	Age of Onset	Clinical Manifestation	Predominant Phenotype
Congenital myopathy and gastrointestinal pseudo-obstruction	*POLG1*	Encodes for the catalytic subunit of mitochondrial DNA	AR	Neonatal period	Severe hypotonia and generalized skeletal and smooth muscle weakness, severe abdominal distension and hypoactive bowel	Neuropathic
	FLNA	Encodes large cytoskeletal proteins	X-linked recessive	Neonatal period	CIIP, prune-belly phenotype	Myopathic
Hydrocephalus with stenosis of the aqueduct of Sylvius (HSAS)	*L1CAM*	Encodes a transmembrane glycoprotein involved in neurite outgrowth and neuronal migration	X-linked recessive	Neonatal period	Congenital hydrocephalus, stenosis of aqueduct, corpus callosum dysgenesis, CIIP	Neuropathic
Multiple endocrine neoplasia (MEN) 2B	*RET*	Expressed in the neural crest cells of the enteric ganglia and encodes a member of the receptor tyrosine kinase family of transmembrane receptors	AD	Infancy to third decade of life	Marfanoid habitus, myopathy, medullary carcinoma of the thyroid, pheochromocytoma, ganglioneuroma, and CIIP/chronic constipation	Neuropathic
Piebaldism	*c-Kit*	Encodes for a tyrosine kinase receptor	AD	Birth to adult	Congenital white forelock and multiple symmetrical stable hypopigmented or depigmented macules and chronic constipation	Neuropathic
MELAS (mitochondrial myopathy, epilepsy, l actic acidosis, and strokelike episodes)	*mtDNA*	Encodes tRNA	Mitochondrial pattern	Childhood to adult	Muscle weakness and pain, recurrent headaches, loss of appetite, vomiting, seizures, and lactic acidosis. Strokelike episodes beginning before 40 years of age with temporary muscle weakness (hemiparesis) and vision abnormalities. Progressive brain damage leading to vision loss, movement problems, and dementia	Mixed phenotype
Familial diabetes and recurrent pancreatitis	*mtDNA*	Encodes tRNA	Mitochondrial pattern: disease passed on only by the mother (maternal pattern) to offspring (male or female)	Childhood to adult	Early-onset non–insulin-dependent (type 2) diabetes, sensorineural deafness, chronic constipation, and other GI symptoms	Mixed phenotype

AD, autosomal dominant; AR, autosomal recessive; CIIP, chronic idiopathic intestinal pseudo-obstruction; CVS, cardiovascular; GI, gastrointestinal.

a subset of patients with African degenerative leiomyopathy, which has long been considered an acquired disease with important interaction between environmental factors and patient genetics.[211,212] Other genes associated with MMIH syndrome include *MYH11*, *MYLK*, *LMOD1*, and *MYL19*.[213-217] Rare cases of X-linked intestinal pseudo-obstruction show mutations in the *FLNA* gene.[218] This gene encodes a protein (filamin A) that plays a role in cell shape and motility.[219,220] These children have a variety of associated malformations, including intestinal malrotation and cardiac abnormalities. A rare case with an extra layer of smooth muscle between the inner circular and outer longitudinal muscle coat has also been reported.[218] In other cases reported to have an extra layer of smooth muscle, genetic testing was not available.[221] Multisystemic smooth muscle dysfunction syndrome has been associated with mutations in the actin A2 gene *(ACTA2)* and is characterized by congenital mydriasis, retinal artery tortuosity, livedo reticularis, ascending thoracic aortic aneurysm and dissection, coronary artery disease, patent ductus arteriosus, arteriopulmonary window, cerebral arteriopathy, periventricular white matter lesions, hypotonic bladder, intestinal malrotation and hypoperistalsis, and pulmonary hypertension.[222] Rare cases with desmin abnormalities have also been described in which involvement of systemic skeletal and cardiac muscle is also seen.[223-225] Various syndromes/phenotypes with the associated genes and key features are shown in Table 8.3.

For idiopathic cases with myopathic changes, although smooth muscle degeneration is believed to be responsible for bowel dysmotility, the pathogenesis of most cases remains obscure. Rare cases show a T-cell–rich inflammatory leiomyositis. These are possibly autoimmune in nature.[226] A distinctive type of nonfamilial visceral myopathy has been described in young children from southern, central, and eastern Africa (African degenerative leiomyopathy, also known as *Bantu pseudo-Hirschsprung's disease*).[227] This disorder is associated with progressive degeneration of enteric smooth muscle, predominantly involving the large bowel and leading to CIIP and massive colonic dilatation (megacolon).

Several pathogenetic mechanisms are involved in the neuropathic forms as well. These include altered mitochondrial dysfunction, altered calcium signaling, autoimmunity, and free radical injury.[228,229] It is also likely that there is complex interaction between environmental factors and genetic predisposition. Many genes associated with neuropathic forms of CIIP have also been identified (see Table 8.3). These include thymidine phosphorylase (also known as *endothelial cell growth factor-1* or *ECGF-1*), DNA polymerase–γ gene *(POLG)*, and the transcription factor *SOX10*, some of which are associated with mitochondrial disorders.[230-232] CIIP is an underrecognized manifestation of mitochondrial disorders.[233,234] One study of 63 patients with idiopathic intestinal pseudo-obstruction detected 15 (19%) mitochondrial myopathies that were not clinically suspected.[235] These included five cases with mutations in the DNA polymerase–γ gene, five with mutations in the thymidine phosphorylase gene, and two with mutations in the $tRNA^{leuUUR}$ gene. Mutations in thymidine phosphorylase have been shown to be responsible for familial cases of mitochondrial neurogastrointestinal encephalomyopathy (MNGIE), a disorder characterized by intestinal pseudo-obstruction, progressive external ophthalmoplegia, ptosis, polyneuropathy, and leukoencephalopathy.[236,237] Mutations in the $tRNA^{leuUUR}$ gene are associated with MELAS (mitochondrial myopathy, epilepsy, lactic acidosis, and stroke-like episodes) and with familial diabetes and recurrent pancreatitis.[238,239] Other syndromes associated with CIIP and identified genetic alterations include Mungan's syndrome, chronic atrial and intestinal dysrhythmia (CAID), and hydrocephalus with stenosis of the aqueduct of Sylvius (HSAS)[240,241] (see Table 8.3).

The etiopathogenesis of idiopathic forms also remains poorly understood and likely multifactorial. Decreased ganglion cell survival may be a factor in some cases, as suggested by decreased *Bcl-2* gene product in enteric ganglion cells.[242] Some cases reveal inflammatory neuronal degeneration, which suggests an autoimmune or infectious etiology[243,244]; neuronal autoantibodies are detected in some patients (Table 8.4).[245] One study suggested that antineuronal antibodies may contribute to neuronal dysfunction via activation of autophagy involving the Fas receptor complex.[229] Some cases represent a paraneoplastic manifestation, whereas others remain truly idiopathic.[246] Lack of connective tissue scaffolding for the smooth muscle cells in the muscularis propria has been reported to be associated with CIIP and chronic constipation and referred to as *desmosis coli* (colonic desmosis).[247,248] These cases manifest with colonic dilatation and also reveal hypoganglionosis or dysganglionosis in the small bowel. Lysosomal storage disorders like Fabry's disease may also involve intestinal ganglia.[249]

Mesenchymopathies, characterized by abnormalities of ICC, seem to be a heterogenous group of disorders. ICC function as the pacemaker cells of the bowel and play an important role in gut motility. Steel-mutant mice that lack KIT-positive ICC show marked constipation as well as features suggestive of CIIP.[250,251] Also, blockade of the KIT receptor results in a severe disturbance of bowel motility.[252] Piebaldism in humans, a condition associated with inactivating *KIT* mutations, is associated with lifelong constipation.[253-255] It has been shown that some cases of CIIP show near-total or total loss of KIT-positive ICC.[256-259] Rare cases of ICC hyperplasia without an underlying germline *KIT* mutation presenting as CIIP have been reported.[260,261] Changes in ICC are also seen in a variety of

TABLE 8.4 Antibodies Identified in Paraneoplastic CIIP

Antibody	Target
Type I Anti Hu	Neurons
Type II Anti-Ri	Neurons
Anti-Yo	Anti–Purkinje cell cytoplasmic antibodies
N-type voltage-gated calcium channel antibodies	N-type voltage-gated calcium channels
P/Q-type calcium channel antibodies	P/Q-type calcium channels
Ganglionic and muscle-type nicotinic acetylcholine receptor antibodies	Nicotinic acetylcholine receptors

CIIP, chronic idiopathic intestinal pseudo-obstruction.

other myopathic and neuropathic forms in which these are thought to be secondary in nature.[256]

Another ill-defined group of GI motility disorders includes abnormalities of neurohormonal peptides that affect the GI neuromuscular apparatus. CIIP has been reported in cases of neuroblastoma and ganglioneuroblastoma.[262,263] Vasoactive intestinal polypeptide (VIP) produced by tumors has also been implicated as a cause of intestinal dysmotility. Tumor resection in these cases results in resolution of pseudo-obstruction. Many of these cases can also be considered secondary CIIP, as a part of a paraneoplastic syndrome. A rare case of pancreatic polypeptide cell hyperplasia associated with intestinal pseudo-obstruction has also been reported.[264]

Pathological Features

The morphological changes in different forms of CIIP are varied. Although some show predominantly myopathic, neuropathic, or ICC changes, others show a mixed phenotype. In some cases, no morphological changes can be identified on routine H&E stains and seen only on special stains or ultrastructural examination. In some cases, no significant morphological abnormalities can be identified despite extensive workup.

Grossly, the involved segment of bowel may be dilated, and the wall appears thick, normal, or thin depending on the degree of distention (Fig. 8.21). In cases of primary visceral myopathy, the bowel can be hugely dilated with very thick muscularis propria. Initially, there is an absence of mucosal abnormalities. However, inflammation, ulceration, and ischemia may develop secondary to stasis and extensive dilatation.[201]

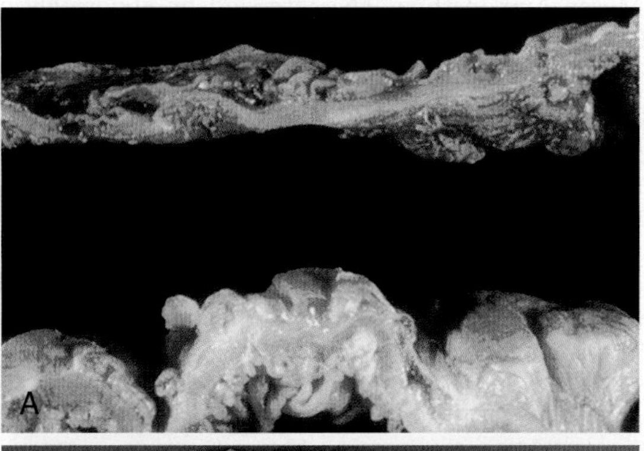

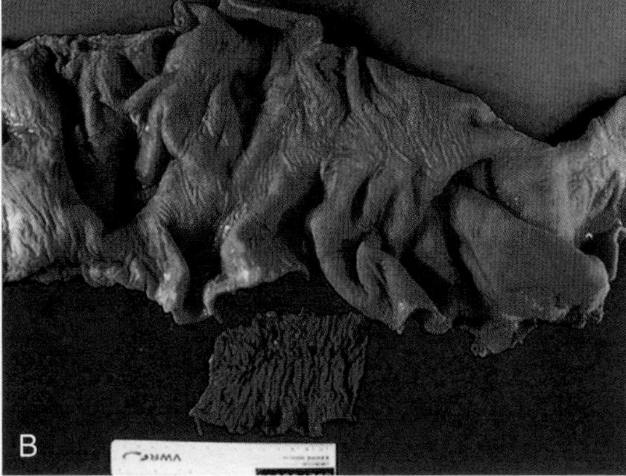

FIGURE 8.21 A, Resection specimen of colon in visceral myopathy shows thinning of the wall *(top)* and thickening of the muscle *(bottom)* in the same patient. **B,** Resection specimen from a patient with visceral myopathy shows massively dilated colon with flattening of the mucosal folds and a thick wall. A short segment of normal colon has been placed below the dilated colon for comparison.

Myopathic Changes. The bowel reveals degeneration and fibrous replacement of the smooth muscle on histology. Degenerative changes are most prominent in the muscularis propria, but they also affect the muscularis mucosae and thus may be occasionally identified in mucosal biopsy specimens.[265] Although the published literature suggests that the outer longitudinal layer tends to be more severely involved in this disorder, in our experience, either both layers are equally involved or the inner circular layer may be involved in isolation. (Fig. 8.22).[201,266] These cases must be differentiated from scleroderma based on other pathological features and clinical findings. Muscle degeneration results in fibrosis, cytoplasmic vacuolation, variation in muscle fiber size, and thinning of the bowel wall (Fig. 8.23A, C). Fibrosis may be subtle and require a trichrome stain to be fully appreciated (Fig. 8.23B, D).[201] The relative thickness of the circular and longitudinal muscle layers varies among individuals, anatomic location, and method of sectioning. Measurement of their ratio has little practical significance. Other changes include variation in nuclear size and increased chromasia, increased mitotic activity, and variation in fiber size. Cytoplasmic inclusions of various types have been described. Amphophilic "M" bodies that are PAS-negative can be seen in the muscularis propria similar to slow transit, constipation, and diabetic gastropathy (see the Gastroparesis section earlier in this chapter and Fig 8.11A,B).[267] These inclusions likely represent degenerating smooth muscle fibers. Similar PAS-positive intracytoplasmic eosinophilic inclusions (5 to 20 μm in size) are seen in polyglucosan body myopathy.[268] These inclusions stain with polyglucosan antibodies, similar to Lafora bodies, and ultrastructurally are composed of nonlysosomal filamentous material located beneath the sarcolemma and between myofibrils.[269] In familial forms of visceral myopathy (e.g., MMIS syndrome) associated with defects in α-actin, PAS-positive cytoplasmic inclusions can be seen that are best highlighted with an α-actin/SMA immunostain.[270]

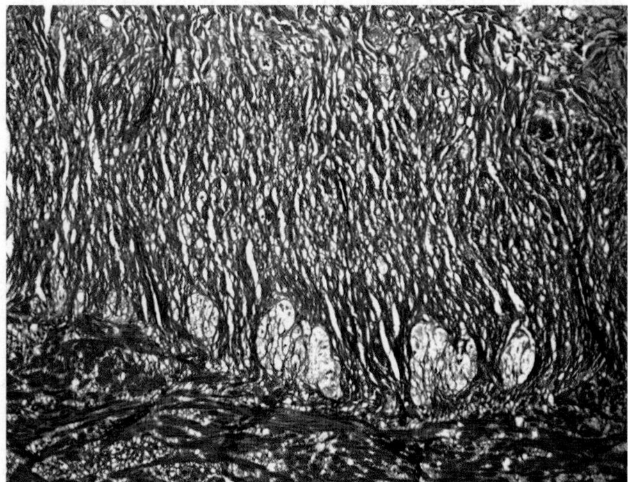

FIGURE 8.22 Visceral myopathy in this case shows preferential atrophy and fibrosis of the inner circular layer of muscularis propria (trichrome stain).

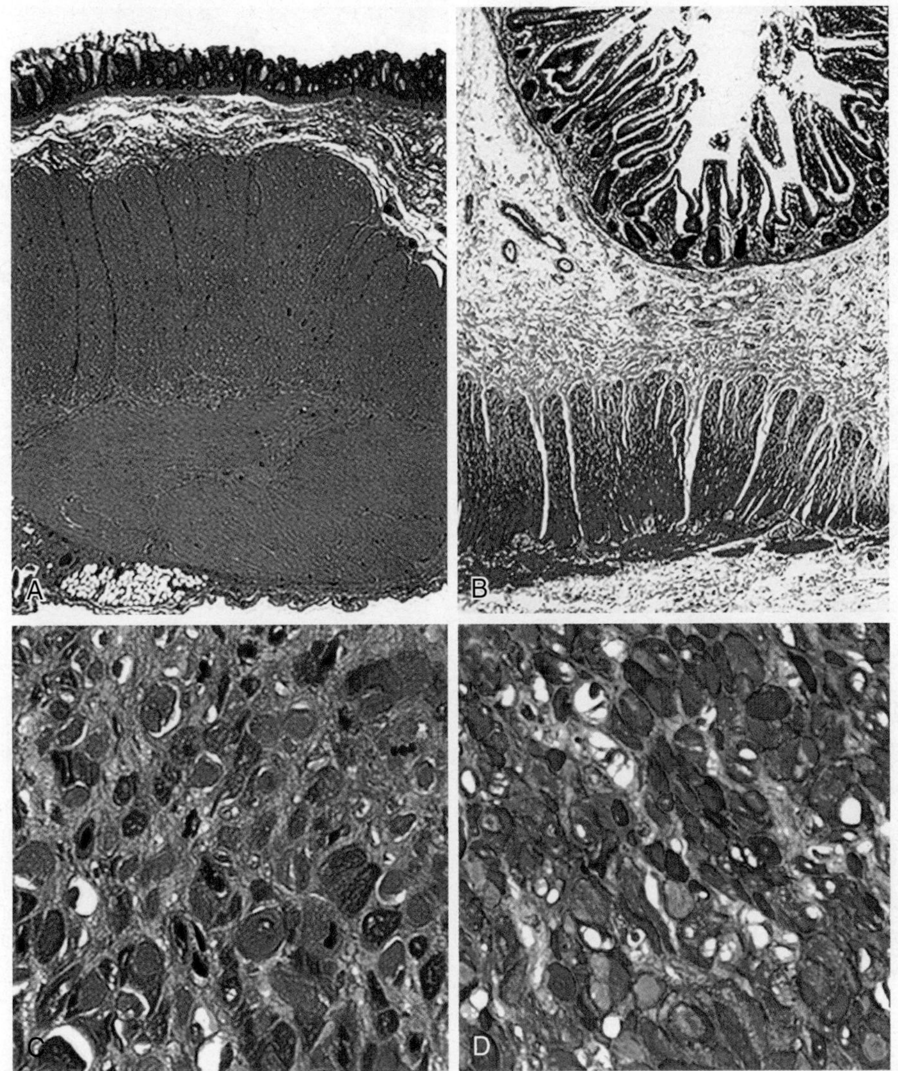

FIGURE 8.23 **A,** Low-power view of a case of visceral myopathy shows marked hypertrophy of both layers of muscularis propria (H&E stain). **B,** A section of small intestine shows delicate interstitial fibrosis in a case of visceral myopathy (trichrome stain). **C,** Higher magnification of the smooth muscle in the muscularis propria shows degenerative changes. **D,** Another view in the same case shows moderate interstitial fibrosis (trichrome stain).

Ultrastructurally, cytoplasmic inclusions represent aggregates of degenerated myofibrils.[268] However, one must be aware of potential artifactual changes in the muscle that are not uncommonly seen in surgical specimens (Fig. 8.24A,B). Artifactual vacuolation, cytoplasmic pseudo-inclusions, and thinning of the muscle layers are not uncommon in colonic resections (see Fig. 8.24). Chronic ischemia and radiation can also cause thinning of the muscularis propria and fibrosis. However, in these cases, fibrosis is patchy, discontinuous, and coarse, sometimes leading to complete extinction of the muscle layer in the involved region (Fig. 8.25). Rare cases with deficient smooth muscle α-actin show an absence of staining with smooth muscle actin antibodies, particularly in the inner circular muscle layer (Fig. 8.26A).[224,271,272] However, similar changes can be limited to the terminal ileum in cases without any evidence of dysmotility. Thus caution is warranted in interpreting this finding (see Fig. 8.26B).[273] Electron microscopy shows nonspecific degenerative changes that include mitochondrial vacuolation, and this may be the only evidence of myopathy in cases in which light microscopy is normal.[201,227,266,274] In cases with actin abnormalities, aggregates of intermediate filaments may be seen on electron microscopy. An extra layer of smooth muscle in the muscularis propria may be found in some cases, either in the large or small intestine.[218,221,275] The extra layer of circular or oblique muscle coat has been typically described between the inner circular and outer longitudinal layers or occasionally outside the outer longitudinal layer.[221] In one example, this was seen as a subserosal layer of longitudinal muscle coat in the small bowel grossly visible as a tenia coli–like band.[221] This phenomenon has also been reported in a case of X-linked intestinal pseudo-obstruction with *FLNA* gene mutation (Fig. 8.27).[218] In this case, in addition to the extra layer of smooth muscle, multinucleated myocytes were also noted in the innermost layer of muscularis propria.[218] Occasionally, one may see abnormal layering of muscle for a short distance, usually near the ileocolonic junction, without any motility issues (Fig. 8.28).

Neuropathic Changes. Neuropathic changes are represented by a variety of qualitative and quantitative changes in ganglion cells, supporting glia, and nerve fibers on histology. The changes can be diffuse or segmental.[276,277]

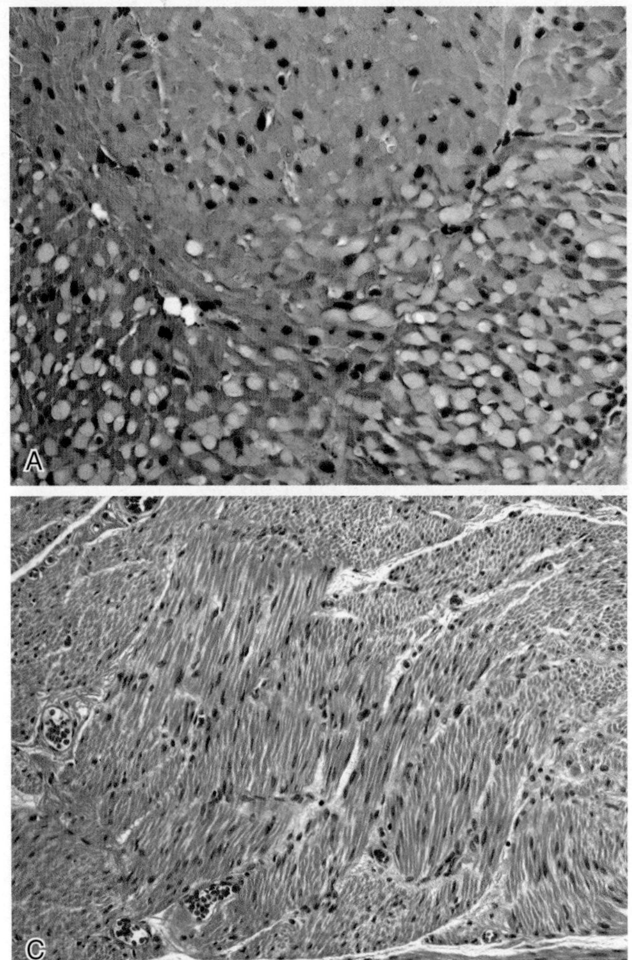
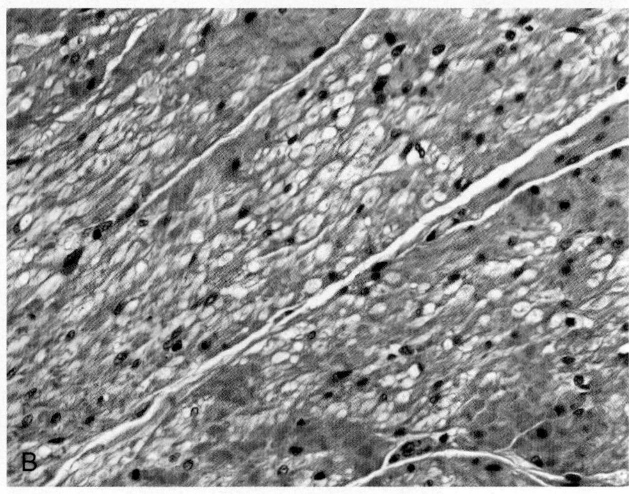

FIGURE 8.24 A, Artifactual cytoplasmic clearing simulating cytoplasmic inclusions is frequently present and should not to be confused with myopathic changes (H&E stain). Other findings associated with myopathic changes (e.g., nuclear pleomorphism, fiber size variation, interstitial fibrosis, increased mitosis, ultrastructural changes) are typically absent. **B,** Artifactual vacuolation in muscularis propria is also often focal and not accompanied by other myopathic changes (trichrome stain). **C,** Nuclear palisading is seen in a section of small bowel muscularis propria (H&E stain). This is often patchy and has no association with bowel dysmotility. It is likely an artifact of unclear nature.

Determination of increased or decreased neuronal density remains a controversial area despite attempts at standardization.[176,177] Stretching of the tissues may result in a decrease in neuronal cell counts, which may also occur as a result of aging. In adults, the mean number of neurons per ganglion is estimated to be four in the myenteric plexus (three in the jejunum and six in the colon) and two in the submucosal plexus.[150,278] There are approximately eight ganglia/cm of bowel. Because there is a lack of standardization, an international working group suggested the use of criteria for patients with hypoganglionosis. This includes ≤1 ganglion/mm length of bowel and ≤2 neurons per ganglion (see also the Hypoganglionosis section earlier in this chapter). A variety of degenerative changes may be present as well. These include cytoplasmic vacuolation, cell swelling, chromatolysis, and nuclear pyknosis and fragmentation (Fig. 8.29A–C). In intranuclear inclusion neuropathy, cytomegalovirus-like (CMV-like) intranuclear inclusions may be identified in neurons (Fig. 8.29D).[279-282] By electron microscopy, these inclusions represent non–membrane-bound osmiophilic proteinaceous material composed of 8-nm curved filaments, not viral particles.[283] Megamitochondria may be seen in some cases, which is indicative of a mitochondrial disorder (Fig. 8.29B). The presence of foamy cytoplasm should make one suspect an underlying lysosomal storage disease like Fabry's disease.[249]

Some cases show inflammation of the ganglia and myenteric plexus consisting of lymphocytes, eosinophils, or mast cells [246] (Fig. 8.30A). Although a few lymphocytes may be present surrounding neural plexus, inflammatory cells are not present within ganglia or directly in contact with ganglion cells under normal circumstances. Lymphocytes are mostly T cells. These can be highlighted and characterized using immunohistochemical markers (CD45, CD3, CD20, CD25, CD4, CD8). However, their precise characterization adds little in clinical practice. Eosinophilic myenteric ganglionitis has been mainly described in children, with only rare reports in adults (see Fig. 8.30B).[244,284-286] Increased mast cells have also been reported in bowel dysmotility and are believed to interact with the neural apparatus causing dysmotility.[287,288] However, enumeration of mast cells or their identification around the neural plexus has unclear significance at present.

In addition, subtle degenerative changes may be present within glia and axons.[201] These changes are best appreciated with a special stain applied to thick en face/tangential embedded sections of the bowel or to whole-mount preparations. The axons may also show swelling and cytoplasmic vacuolation. However, such changes can also be seen in unrelated conditions and thus are etiologically nonspecific (Fig. 8.31A–C). In the past, silver stains were used to identify abnormalities of argyrophobic and argyrophilic ganglion

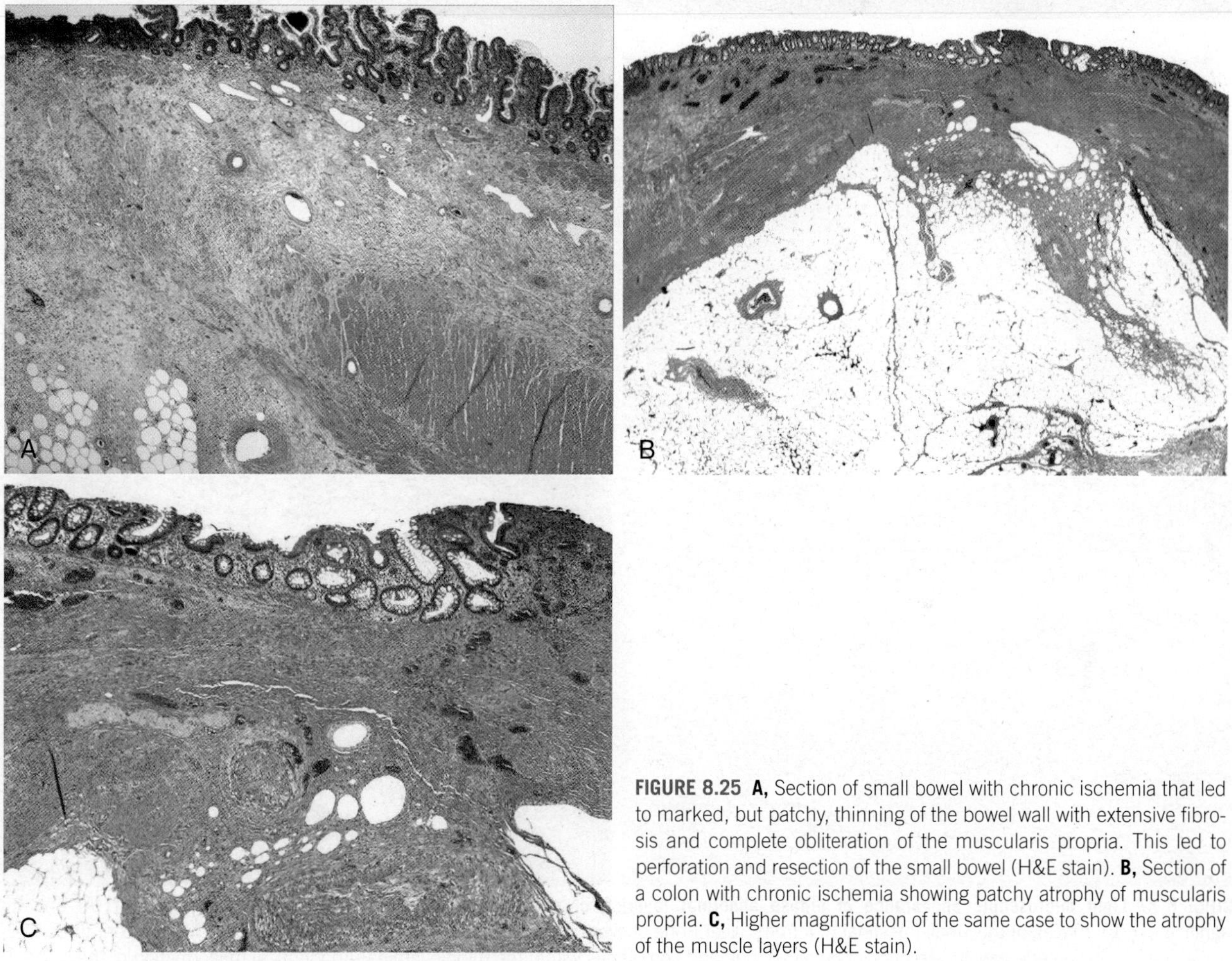

FIGURE 8.25 **A,** Section of small bowel with chronic ischemia that led to marked, but patchy, thinning of the bowel wall with extensive fibrosis and complete obliteration of the muscularis propria. This led to perforation and resection of the small bowel (H&E stain). **B,** Section of a colon with chronic ischemia showing patchy atrophy of muscularis propria. **C,** Higher magnification of the same case to show the atrophy of the muscle layers (H&E stain).

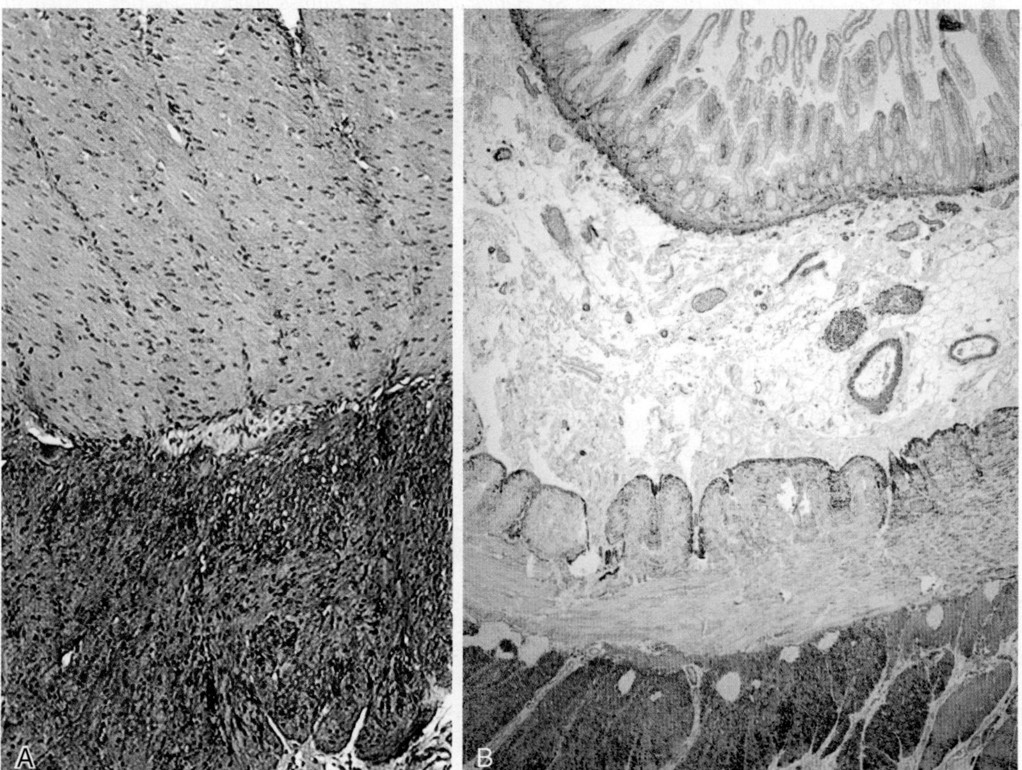

FIGURE 8.26 **A,** Immunostain for α-smooth muscle actin (α-SMA) in a case of visceral myopathy shows lack of staining in the inner circular layer. The outer longitudinal layer appears normal. **B,** Lack of staining for α-SMA is seen in a normal terminal ileum with preserved staining in the thin inner circular layer and in the entire longitudinal layer. This is a not infrequent finding in sections from the terminal ileum of patients without any dysmotility, and it remains of unclear pathogenesis and significance.

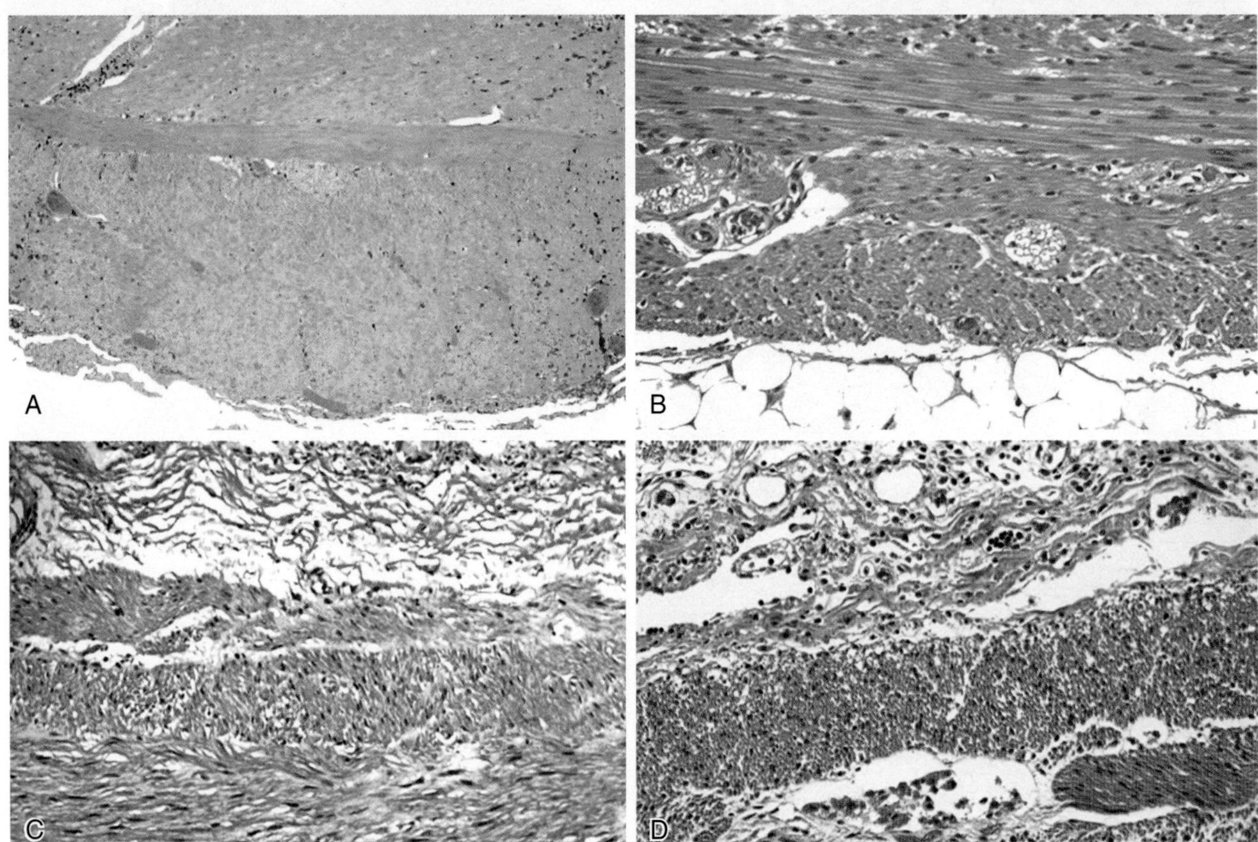

FIGURE 8.27 Light microscopic appearance of diffuse abnormal layering of small-intestinal smooth muscle. Low-magnification **(A)** and high-magnification **(B)** images of the small-intestinal wall from patient one show abnormal layering of the muscularis propria, with at least three distinct muscle laminae. Myenteric ganglia are present on either side and sometimes within the middle lamina. An identical malformation of the muscularis propria was identified in the small intestine of patient two (a nephew of patient one) **(C)**, and in patient five, an unrelated infant **(D)**. (A–C, H&E stain; D, modified Gomori trichrome stain.) (*From Kapur RP, Robertson SP, Hannibal MC, et al. Diffuse abnormal layering of small intestinal smooth muscle is present in patients with FLNA mutations and X-linked intestinal pseudo-obstruction. Am J Surg Pathol. 2010;34:1528–1543.)*)

cells; however, these stains are currently obsolete. S100, PGP9.5, or NSE immunostains can be used to highlight the neural plexus and neuronal cell bodies. A variety of other immunohistochemical markers have been used as well. These include VIP, substance P and related tachykinins, NOS, neuropeptide Y, calcitonin gene–related peptide, and Bcl-2. These show abnormal expression in the enteric nervous system in neuropathic obstruction, but they lack disease specificity and fail to differentiate primary from secondary changes.[205,246] Of these antibodies, Bcl-2 (Fig. 8.32) has been more widely used as a marker of increased neuronal apoptosis and neuropathic changes, although some studies question its utility.[242,289] The glial network surrounding the ganglion cells are best highlighted with S100 or PGP9.5 rather than glial fibrillary acidic protein (GFAP) unlike in the central nervous system. However, quantitation of glia in the GI tract is highly subjective, is difficult to quantify, and lacks diagnostic specificity.

Mitochondrial disorders show both myopathic and neuropathic changes including muscle atrophy and decreased number of ganglion cells. Some disorders may appear unremarkable on routine histology (Fig. 8.33). Rare cases may show complete disappearance of the muscularis propria or one of its layers focally. These changes may be variable among different segments of the GI tract, as reported in one patient with deficiency of complex 1 associated with intestinal pseudo-obstruction.[290] This case showed a decreased number of ganglion cells in the myenteric plexus in both the colon and stomach. In contrast, the small bowel showed a normal myenteric plexus but showed ectopic ganglion cells in the lamina propria and giant ganglia in the

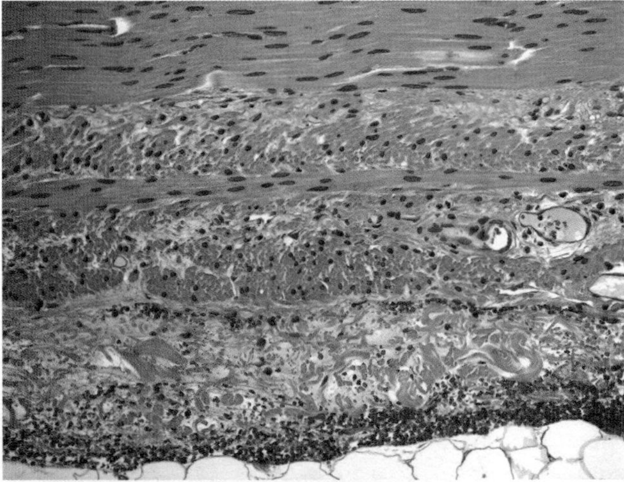

FIGURE 8.28 Abnormal layering of muscle in the ascending colon near the ileocecal valve from a patient without intestinal dysmotility (H&E stain). This finding was focal and was likely an artifact of tangential sectioning.

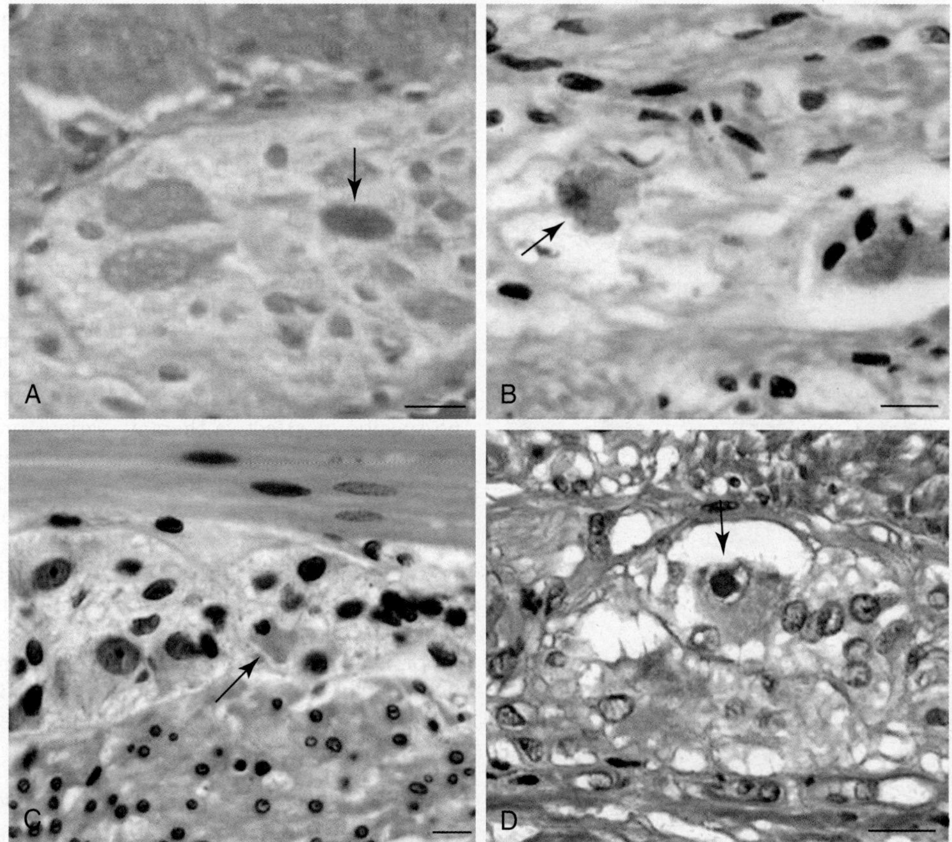

FIGURE 8.29 Examples of the appearance of myenteric ganglion cells in H&E-stained sections. A, Degenerate neuron *(arrow)* with adjacent neurons showing microvacuolation. **B,** Megamitochondria: cytoplasmic eosinophilic inclusions in a ganglion cell *(arrow)* of a child with Alpers' disease representing enlarged mitochondria (scale bar = 25 μm). **C,** Neuronal degeneration: a degenerating neuron *(arrow)* is present in this ganglion from a child who underwent small bowel transplantation for hypoganglionosis and intestinal pseudo-obstruction. **D,** Intranuclear inclusion body: a large eosinophilic inclusion body is present in a ganglion cell *(arrow)* from an infant with hypoganglionosis, intestinal dysmotility, and encephalopathy caused by neuronal intranuclear inclusion disease mitochondrial myopathy. (*From Knowles CH, De Giorgio R, Kapur RP, et al. Gastrointestinal neuromuscular pathology: guidelines for histological techniques and reporting on behalf of the Gastro 2009 International Working Group. Acta Neuropathol. 2009;118:271–301.*)

submucosa, similar to IND-B. Histochemistry on frozen sections showed patchy defects with cytochrome-C oxidase stain, ragged red fibers with modified Gomori trichrome stain, and mitochondrial proliferation with succinate dehydrogenase stain, similar to skeletal muscle. Limited experience with these conditions, necessity of employing fastidious neuron counting techniques, and complex clinical and pathological analysis has limited the study of such cases to only a few highly specialized centers.[176] One must also be aware of artifactual changes in ganglion cells and axons that are frequently encountered in conditions that are not associated with dysmotility or neuropathies (see Fig. 8.31 and Fig. 8.34).

Mesenchymopathic Changes. Abnormalities in ICC network and numbers have been shown in many of these disorders, including Hirschsprung's disease, slow transit constipation, achalasia, and gastroparesis, and they likely contribute to dysmotility.[291] In these conditions, the changes are likely secondary in nature as they revert to normal once the primary abnormality is corrected. In rare cases, abnormalities of ICC are considered the primary abnormality or the only finding.[292] Many of these cases clinicopathologically resemble primary visceral myopathy, while others do not show any other obvious pathological findings (Fig. 8.35A). Study of the ICC network requires immunostains, advanced microscopic techniques (e.g., confocal or three-dimensional [3D] microscopy), and/or electron microscopy.[293-296] With the availability of good immunostains for ICC (KIT and DOG1), electron microscopy is seldom required in clinical practice.[260] Cases with ICC abnormalities reveal near-total or total loss of ICC in the involved segment of bowel (small bowel and/or colon). Some cases may show the presence of ICC, but the neural network may be abnormal. In others, only a subset of ICC (submucosal plexus) may be lacking.[292] However, these abnormalities are difficult to appreciate on routine formalin-fixed tissues and require advanced microscopic techniques to study the tissues in 3D.[295,297] In rare cases, ICC hyperplasia has been identified that can be sporadic or associated with known syndromes, and it is associated with intestinal dysmotility in some patients.[260,298,299] The diffuse form of ICC hyperplasia is difficult to recognize without special stains, while some forms show a distinct band of benign spindle cell proliferation between the two layers of muscularis mucosa seen on H&E stain (see Fig. 8.35B,C). Although marked reduction or total absence of ICC is easy to recognize, subtle changes in their numbers are difficult to identify without detailed morphometry. The criteria used to

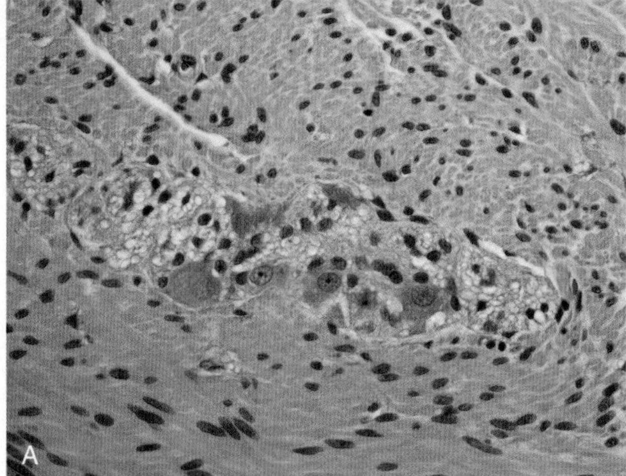

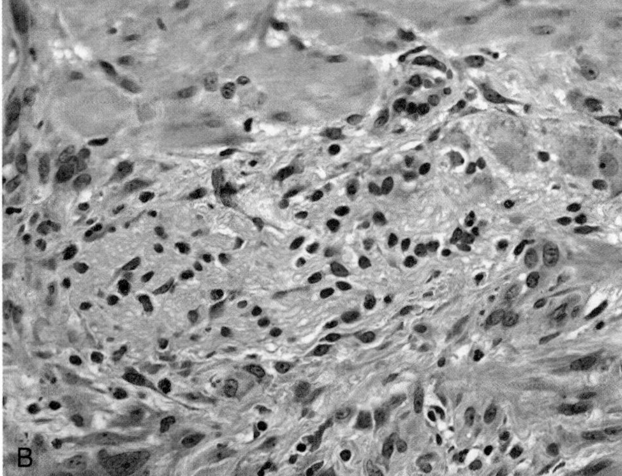

FIGURE 8.30 A, Example of lymphocytic myenteric ganglionitis with few lymphocytes surrounding the ganglion cell cluster (H&E stain). **B,** Case of eosinophilic myenteric ganglionitis showing few eosinophils surrounding the ganglion cells (H&E stain).

document a reduction of ICC also remain poorly standardized. Using a conservative approach, a reduction of >50% of ICC compared with controls has been suggested as a rough threshold.[150,176,278,300] Application of these guidelines in clinical practice must be validated.

Abnormalities of Neurohormonal Peptides. The histological changes in CIIP associated with neurohormonal abnormalities remain poorly studied, and no specific features are described. The changes seen are likely functional and secondary in nature.

Differential Diagnosis

The main pathological differential diagnosis includes mechanical obstruction, which could be intraluminal or extrinsic. Obstruction may not always be obvious clinically. It may be discovered at the time of gross examination of the resection specimen. The common causes of obstruction easily overlooked clinically are internal hernias, adhesions, volvulus, and fibrous bands. One of the confounding factors is that many of these patients undergo multiple laparotomies for a variety of reasons, leading to adhesions. The histological changes secondary to obstruction vary, ranging from normal to marked neuromuscular hypertrophy. The differential diagnosis of secondary causes of intestinal pseudo-obstruction is discussed later, and the key is to recognize the underlying condition and its association with intestinal dysmotility. It is also very important to recognize a variety of artifacts in smooth muscle cells, ganglia, and nerves that can closely mimic myopathic or neuropathic changes (see Figs. 8.24, 8.31, and 8.34).

Treatment and Prognosis

Infants and children tend to have a poorer prognosis and die at a young age.[205,301] CIIP in adults usually has a prolonged course (20 to 30 years).[203] Secondary forms generally follow the course and prognosis of the underlying condition. Treatment is symptomatic and supportive because there is no specific or effective therapy. Various prokinetic agents, such as cisapride, domperidone, metoclopramide, octreotide, and erythromycin, have shown variable success.[203,302] Surgical resection may be performed in resistant cases. A favorable outcome is expected in patients with limited bowel involvement.[302] However, substantial resection of small and/or large bowel may be required, and this results in total parenteral nutrition dependence. Intestinal transplantation is gradually emerging as a possible treatment option in intractable cases.[303,304] The main causes of death in these patients are related to surgery, total parenteral nutrition, or posttransplant complications.[301]

Secondary Chronic Intestinal Pseudo-Obstruction

A variety of systemic disorders and medications/toxins have been associated with intestinal dysmotility. These may have a neuropathic or myopathic phenotype, or they may show mixed features, similar to idiopathic cases. The classification used by the international working group (see Box 8.1) includes only a limited number of conditions. A more extensive list is shown in Box 8.2.

Systemic Disorders

Patients with scleroderma or progressive systemic sclerosis may show significant involvement of the bowel, resulting in a severe motility disorder that often requires surgical resection.[305] Clinically, esophageal involvement usually predominates. The inner circular layer of the bowel wall is often preferentially involved, in contrast with primary visceral myopathy in which the outer longitudinal muscle layer is typically most affected.[201,306] In scleroderma, collagen replacement of the muscle layer tends to be nearly complete, unlike the type of interstitial fibrosis characteristic of primary visceral myopathy, which is usually delicate and incomplete (Fig. 8.36A,B). Fibrosis may cause muscle weakness resulting in diverticula with squared-mouth ostia. Mucosal changes are nonspecific and are secondary to the underlying motility problem (e.g., reflux esophagitis and villous blunting due to bacterial overgrowth in the small bowel).

Pseudo-obstruction, with muscle damage, may occur in patients with dermatomyositis/polymyositis, systemic lupus erythematosus, myotonic dystrophy, and progressive muscular dystrophy.[305,307-311] Patients with amyloid deposition in the muscularis propria (myopathy) or myenteric plexus (neuropathy) may uncommonly present with intestinal pseudo-obstruction. AA-type amyloid is often deposited in the myenteric plexus, whereas AL-type amyloid is more often deposited in the muscularis propria (Fig. 8.37).[312-315]

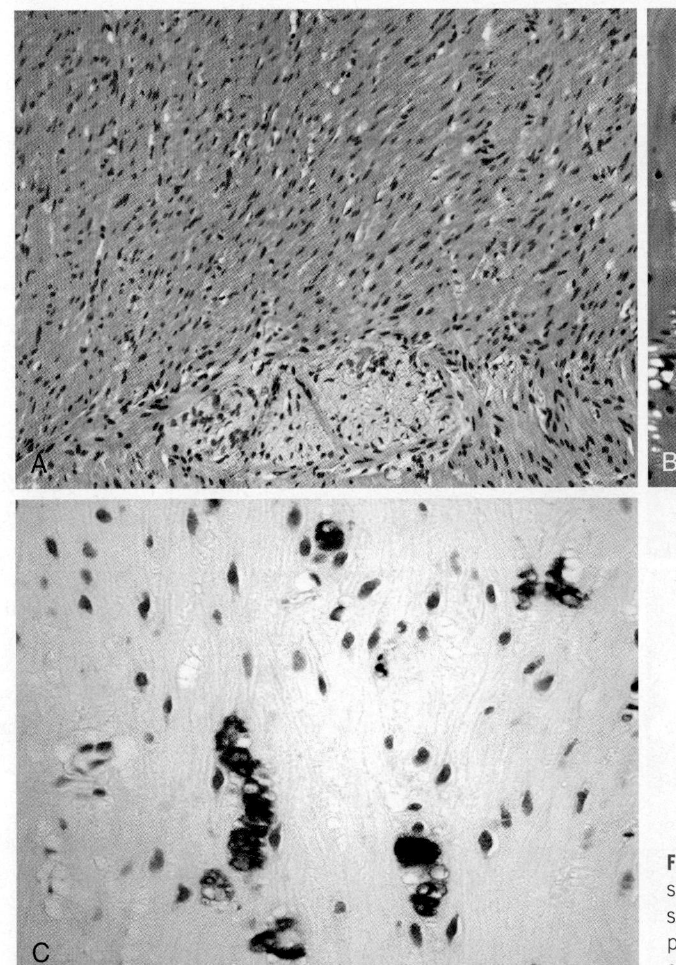
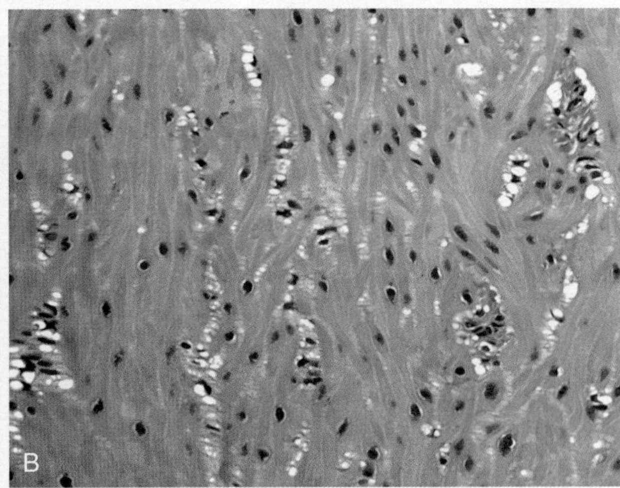
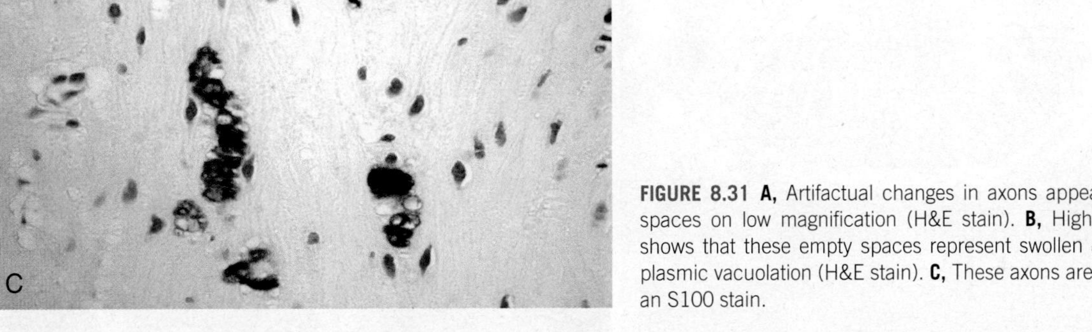

FIGURE 8.31 A, Artifactual changes in axons appear as tiny empty spaces on low magnification (H&E stain). **B,** Higher magnification shows that these empty spaces represent swollen axons with cytoplasmic vacuolation (H&E stain). **C,** These axons are highlighted with an S100 stain.

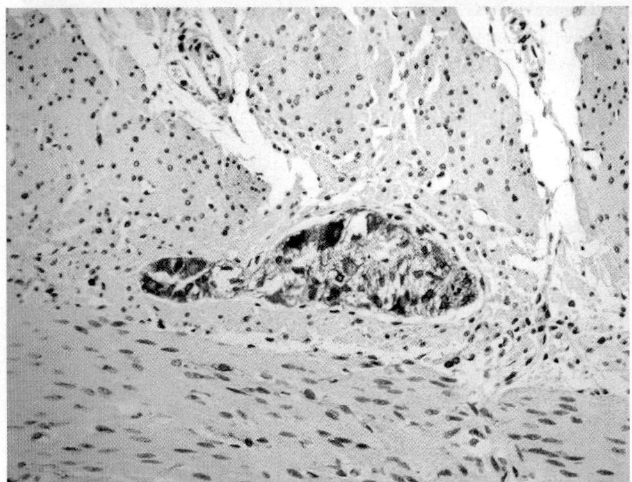

FIGURE 8.32 Bcl-2 immunostain shows a normal staining pattern in neurons. Loss of staining is considered abnormal.

Familial autonomic dysfunction and Shy-Drager syndrome may be associated with dysmotility, but no specific pathological changes have been identified in these conditions. Parkinson disease has also been associated with GI dysmotility, and Lewy bodies have been demonstrated in the enteric ganglion cells, but these are best demonstrated with the immunostain using antibody against phosphorylated alpha-synuclein.[316,317] Whether this finding can be used to prospectively diagnose patients with Parkinson's disease on colonic biopsy has not been adequately studied.[317,318] Spinal cord injury or disrupted communication between the central nervous system and the gut can also lead to intestinal pseudo-obstruction.[319,320] Diffuse polyclonal lymphoid infiltration of the small intestine is another rare condition of uncertain pathogenesis but likely represents inflammatory/autoimmune myopathy.[321] Intestinal pseudo-obstruction may also occur in patients with hypoparathyroidism, hypothyroidism, and pheochromocytoma.[311] However, diabetes is by far the most common endocrine disorder associated with bowel dysmotility. This may result from autonomic dysfunction, electrolyte abnormalities, and/or vasculopathy. Rarely, intestinal pseudo-obstruction associated with relative adrenal insufficiency due to sudden withdrawal of steroids has been reported.[322] Eosinophilic gastroenteritis and radiation enteritis may also result in intestinal pseudo-obstruction. Deep forms of eosinophilic gastroenteritis that involve the muscularis propria are typically associated with dysmotility (Fig. 8.38A,B). Kawasaki's disease can also be rarely associated with intestinal pseudo-obstruction.[323] Destruction of ganglion cells associated with paraneoplastic syndromes has been well described in patients with small cell carcinoma of the lung, and rarely in patients with other types of tumors.[324-326]

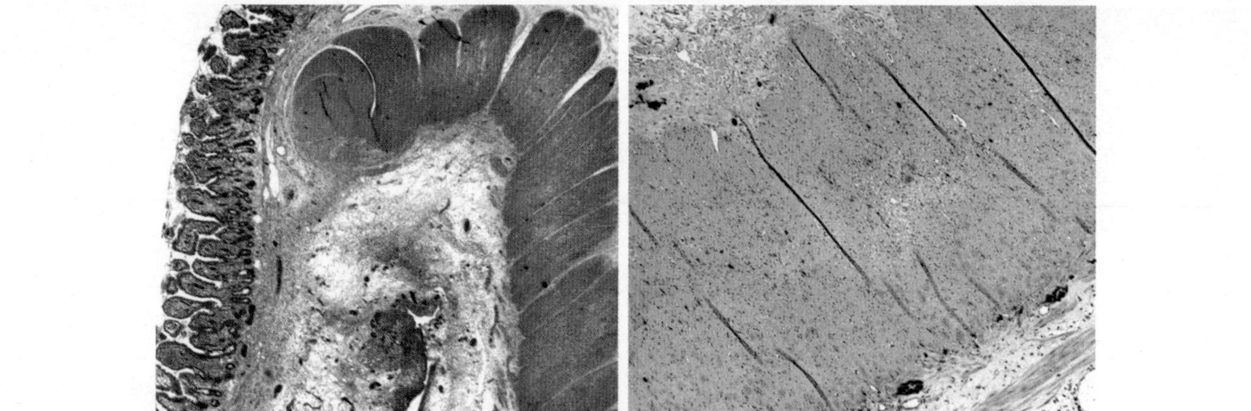

FIGURE 8.33 **A,** Mitochondrial myopathy, showing atrophic longitudinal muscle with extensive fibrosis and, focally, a complete absence of both layers of muscularis propria in the small bowel (trichrome stain). **B,** S100 stain reveals a marked decrease in the nerves in the myenteric plexus and muscular layers; the number of ganglia also appears to be reduced. In an example of pseudo-obstruction in a patient with mitochondrial myopathy with defects in complex 1, H&E staining reveals normal histology **(C)** and normal ganglia and myenteric plexus **(D).** (**A** *and* **B** *courtesy Dr. Robert Riddell.*)

In such cases, neuronal autoantibodies have been detected, suggesting immune-mediated ganglion cell destruction.

Drugs and Toxins

A variety of pharmacological agents (e.g., phenothiazines, tricyclic antidepressants, ganglionic blockers, vincristine, clonidine, and antiparkinsonian medication) may have a marked effect on bowel motility. For instance, use or ingestion of naturally occurring toxins such as *Amanita phalloides* may result in intestinal pseudo-obstruction.[327]

Infections and Postinfection Intestinal Pseudo-Obstruction

Viral infection, particularly the herpes group of viruses, has been associated with systemic autoimmune disturbances and bowel dysmotility. Visceral involvement concurrent with varicella zoster cutaneous involvement has been shown to result in dysmotility of the stomach, small intestine, colon, and anus.[328,329] Bowel dysfunction resolves with improvement of cutaneous disease. CMV

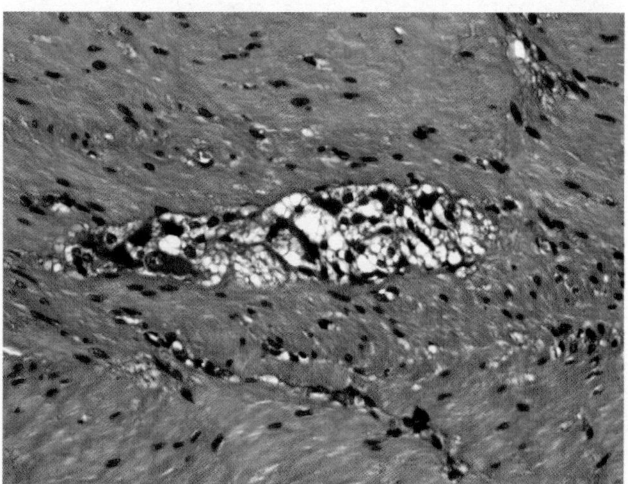

FIGURE 8.34 Artifactual cytoplasmic eosinophilia and pyknotic nuclei in a case of diverticulosis mimicking neuropathic changes (H&E stain).

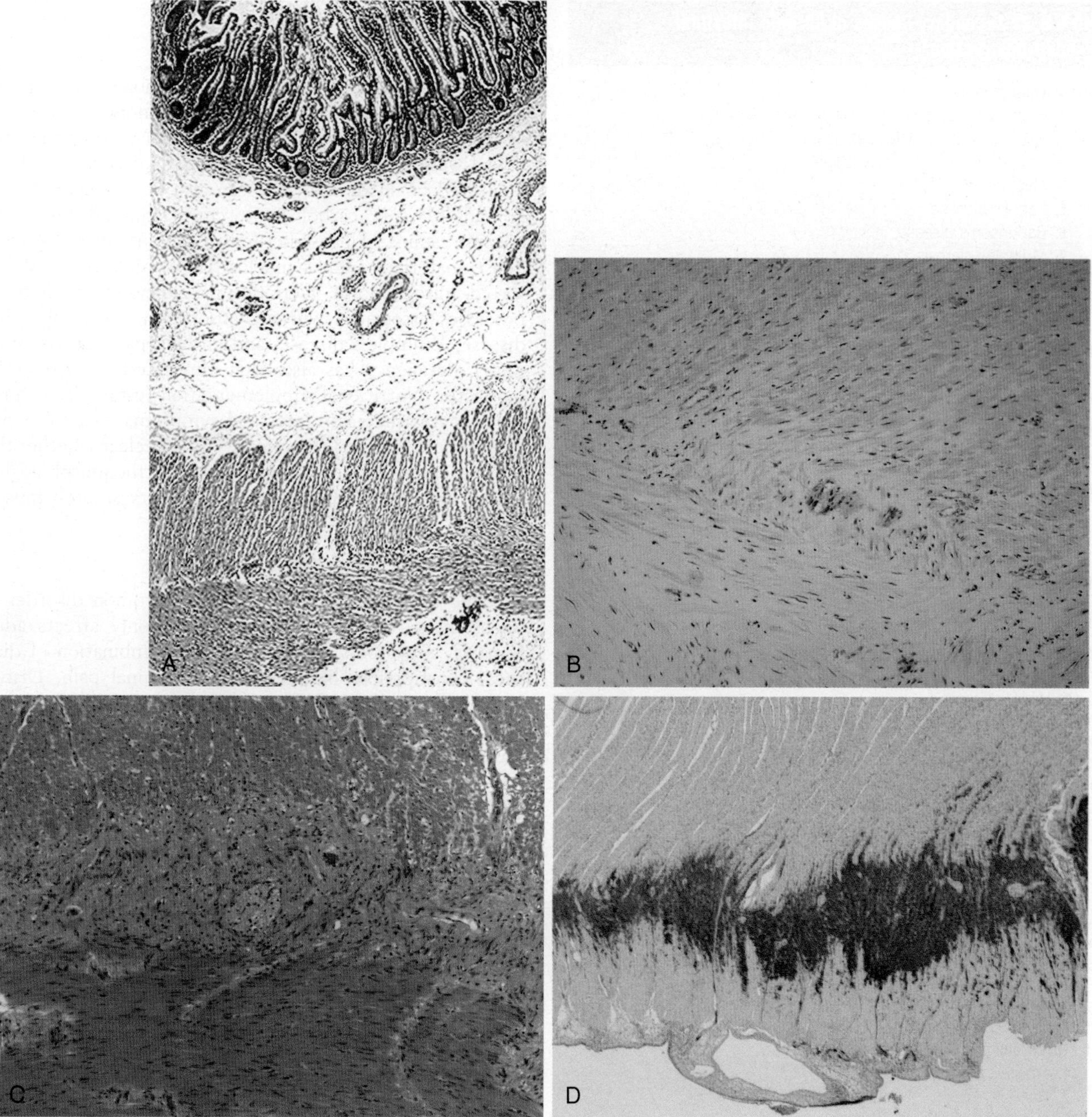

FIGURE 8.35 A, A case of chronic idiopathic intestinal pseudo-obstruction without any significant pathological changes shows a total absence of interstitial cells of Cajal in a section of the small intestine (KIT stain) and in the colon **(B). C,** Hyperplasia of interstitial cells of Cajal easily evident in a section from colon on H&E stain, and very nicely highlighted with KIT immunostain **(D).**

infection has also been implicated in intestinal pseudo-obstruction, especially in immunocompromised individuals.[330,331] In some cases, evidence of Epstein-Barr virus (EBV) infection has been demonstrated by polymerase chain reaction (PCR) and in situ hybridization studies of the myenteric plexus.[332] JC virus has been shown in the myenteric plexus in cases of intestinal pseudo-obstruction. However, the results of this study have not been replicated and thus remain controversial.[333,334] Histologically, the only clue may be the presence of inflammatory cells surrounding ganglia and myenteric plexus, or typical viral inclusions in ganglion cells. Flavivirus has also been recently implicated in intestinal pseudo-obstruction.[335] Lyme disease and Chagas' disease may also involve the small and/or large intestine resulting in intestinal pseudo-obstruction.[62,336,337]

Once the infections resolve, about 3.7% to 36% of patients develop some chronic GI symptoms, including bowel dysmotility and pseudo-obstruction.[338] This can occur secondary to some of the neurotropic viruses discussed earlier. The common bacterial infections leading to postinfection dysmotility are *Salmonella*, *Shigella*, and *Campylobacter*. The infectious organisms have usually disappeared by this time, and pathologically the changes are fairly nonspecific. Besides mild periganglionic lymphocytic infiltrate, one may not see other pathological alterations (Fig. 8.39). It is typically self-limited, although symptoms may last for many months.

BOX 8.2 Secondary Causes of Chronic Intestinal Pseudo-Obstruction

A. **Systemic disorders**
1. Progressive systemic sclerosis/polymyositis
2. Systemic lupus erythematosus
3. Progressive muscular dystrophy
4. Myotonic dystrophy
5. Fabry's disease
6. Parkinson's disease
7. Multiple sclerosis
8. Ehlers-Danlos syndrome
9. Neurofibromatosis
10. Familial dysautonomia

B. **Endocrine and metabolic disorders**
1. Diabetes mellitus
2. Hypothyroidism
3. Hypoparathyroidism
4. Pheochromocytoma
5. Acute intermittent porphyria

C. **Infiltrative disorders**
1. Amyloidosis
2. Diffuse lymphoid infiltration
3. Eosinophilic gastroenteritis

D. **Paraneoplastic**
1. Small cell carcinoma
2. Others

E. **Infections**
1. *Trypanosoma Cruzi* (Chagas' disease)
2. Herpes virus
3. Cytomegalovirus
4. Epstein-Barr virus
5. Lyme disease
6. Flavivirus

F. **Miscellaneous conditions**
1. Ceroidosis (brown bowel syndrome)
2. Small intestinal diverticulosis
3. Radiation enteritis
4. Jejunoileal bypass
5. Celiac disease
6. Gastroschisis
7. Kawasaki's disease
8. Amyloidosis
9. Postneonatal necrotizing enterocolitis

G. **Toxins and pharmacological agents**
1. Tricyclic antidepressants
2. Phenothiazines
3. Ganglionic blockers
4. Clonidine
5. Antiparkinsonism medication
6. Opiates (narcotic bowel syndrome)
7. Amanita phalloides toxin

Treatment and Prognosis

The prognosis and treatment of secondary intestinal pseudo-obstruction vary according to the underlying condition. Patients with progressive systemic sclerosis often die within 5 to 10 years secondary to renal, cardiac, or pulmonary complications. Patients with small cell carcinoma usually die within 1 year of presentation of extraintestinal manifestations. Cases associated with viral infection are generally self-limited. Intestinal pseudo-obstruction caused by systemic diseases, such as systemic lupus erythematosus or amyloidosis, generally follow the course of the underlying disease.

Miscellaneous Conditions

Ceroidosis (Brown Bowel Syndrome)

This condition is characterized by deposition of light-brown, granular, lipofuscin-like pigment within smooth muscle cells of the muscularis mucosae and/or muscularis propria of the bowel wall (Fig. 8.40).[339-342] The pigment is usually easily identified on H&E stain but can also be highlighted with Fontana-Masson, carbol lipofuscin, PAS, and PAS with diastase stains. Ultrastructurally, the granular electron-dense material contains myelin figures and abnormal distorted mitochondria. Ceroidosis has been seen in many processes associated with malabsorption, including celiac disease, Whipple's disease, and chronic pancreatitis. Vitamin E deficiency has also been implicated as an underlying factor. Nutritional supplementation (especially vitamin E) alleviates the gastrointestinal symptoms in some, while most require surgical resection.[343] It is unclear whether this phenomenon represents a purely nonspecific morphological marker of a systemic disease or a primary smooth muscle disorder.

Irritable Bowel Syndrome

Irritable bowel syndrome (IBS) is a common disorder of uncertain pathogenesis. It most commonly affects adult females. Symptoms include one or a combination of diarrhea, constipation, bloating, and abdominal pain. Disturbances of bowel motility and enhanced visceral sensitivity have been implicated as possible etiological factors. Colonoscopy is typically normal, and routine examination of mucosal biopsy specimens does not normally show any pathological abnormalities. However, quantitative histological studies, immunohistochemical analysis, and ultrastructural studies have revealed some subtle alterations, such as an increase in the number of lymphocytes, mast cells, and enterochromaffin cells.[344,345] These changes point to activation of the enteric immune system and neuro-immune interactions, but they have little value in routine diagnostic evaluation of biopsy specimens from affected patients. Biopsies are often performed to rule out other potential causes of the patient's illness.

Small Bowel Diverticulosis

The most common types of small bowel diverticula are congenital in origin and include Meckel's diverticulum and duodenal diverticulosis. Less commonly, acquired cases of small bowel diverticulosis are encountered secondary to neuromuscular abnormalities.[346,347] Extensive diverticulosis involving small and/or large bowel has been reported in the setting of Marfan's syndrome that can sometimes present even in older adults.[348] Diverticula result from mucosal outpouchings secondary to fibrosis-induced mural weakness. In cases with scleroderma-like morphological changes, Raynaud's phenomenon is frequently present, although clinical scleroderma is not evident. Some cases are related to known neurological disease processes such as Fabry's disease. The diverticulosis can be complicated by diverticulitis, bacterial overgrowth, blind loop syndrome, malnutrition, enteroliths, intestinal obstruction, and intestinal perforation.[348-350] In cases with underlying weakness of the bowel wall, the perforation can occur, even in the absence of diverticulosis.[351]

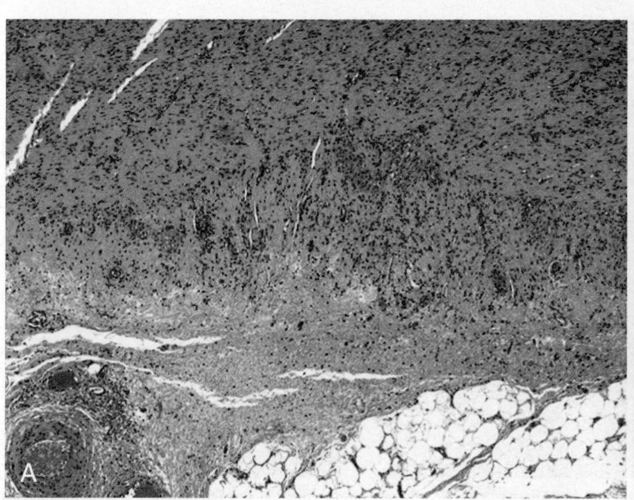

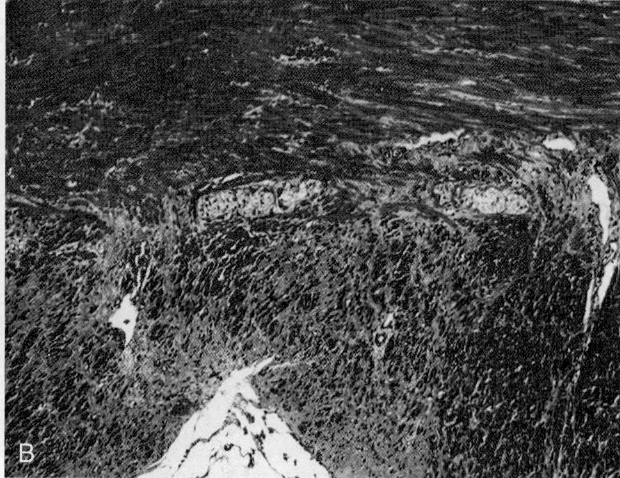

FIGURE 8.36 A, In this case of scleroderma, there is complete replacement of the outer longitudinal layer of the muscularis propria caused by fibrosis (H&E stain). Unlike most cases of scleroderma, the inner circular layer is relatively well preserved. **B,** Another case of scleroderma shows extensive and coarse fibrosis in areas of partially preserved longitudinal layer of muscularis propria (trichrome stain). Compare this with the delicate type of interstitial fibrosis seen in visceral myopathy (see Fig. 8.23B).

Severe Idiopathic Constipation (Slow-transit Constipation, Arbuthnot Lane Disease)

This condition, which is characterized by chronic constipation resulting from reduced colonic propulsive capacity,[352,353] most commonly affects young women. Onset of disease may occur in early childhood or later in adulthood. Symptoms often persist, despite use of laxatives. Melanosis coli is a common histological finding. Such cases have been labeled *cathartic colon*. However, whether laxative abuse is the underlying cause remains controversial. In severe and resistant cases, colectomy may need to be performed. This disease represents a heterogenous group of disorders comprising myopathic, neuropathic, and ICC abnormalities similar to those seen with intestinal pseudo-obstruction. These include hypoganglionosis, intraganglionic neurofilaments, degenerative changes in ganglion cells, neural hyperplasia, decreased glial cells in the neural plexus, increased mast cells, hyaline cytoplasmic inclusions in smooth muscle cells, muscular hypertrophy, abnormal collagen framework in the muscle layer, abnormal staining patterns for various muscle markers, and reduced numbers of ICC.[267,287,288,352,354-357] Of these, reduced numbers of ICC is the only consistent finding in most cases. However, from a clinical perspective, standardized diagnostic criteria are lacking, and all of these changes lack specificity.[358] For example, identification of hypoganglionosis is difficult to recognize, as discussed previously. Similarly, it is difficult to quantify muscle hypertrophy or neural hyperplasia, and it is further unclear if these changes are primary or secondary in nature. Cytoplasmic inclusions in smooth muscle have also been identified in normal small and large bowel, as well in Chagas' disease, thus they lack specificity.[267] Mast cells have also been implicated in bowel dysmotility. However, quantification for clinical purposes remains a controversial issue. Increased mast cells have been associated with both constipation and diarrhea.[288,359] Most of the histological changes have been studied in large bowel, although study of ileum also reveals milder but similar changes.[360] Thus in practice, one can only be descriptive when dealing with such cases. Whether chronic slow-transit constipation represents a mild form of idiopathic intestinal pseudo-obstruction is unknown.

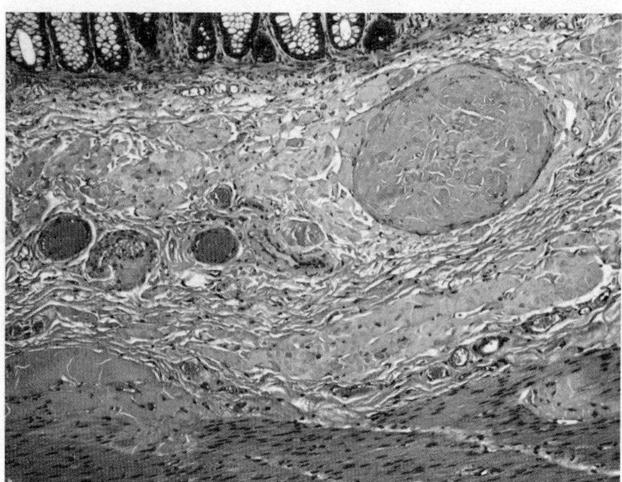

FIGURE 8.37 Amyloidosis with extensive deposition of pale eosinophilic amorphous material in the submucosa, surrounding blood vessels, and muscular propria (H&E stain). Extensive deposition of amyloid can lead to intestinal pseudo-obstruction.

The differential diagnosis of slow-transit constipation is constipation caused by obstructive defecation. This also represents a heterogenous group of disorders that largely result from anorectal dysfunction that leads to functional obstruction. Very few studies have documented the pathological changes in the colon. Some show a global decrease in neural-associated glial cells and a decrease in submucosal ganglia, whereas the myenteric ganglia, muscularis propria, and ICC remain normal.[361]

DIFFERENTIAL DIAGNOSIS AND WORKUP OF PATIENTS WITH INTESTINAL DYSMOTILITY

Diagnosis of motility disorders is challenging for both clinicians and pathologists. Unfortunately, despite many advances, the pathogenesis of many dysmotility conditions

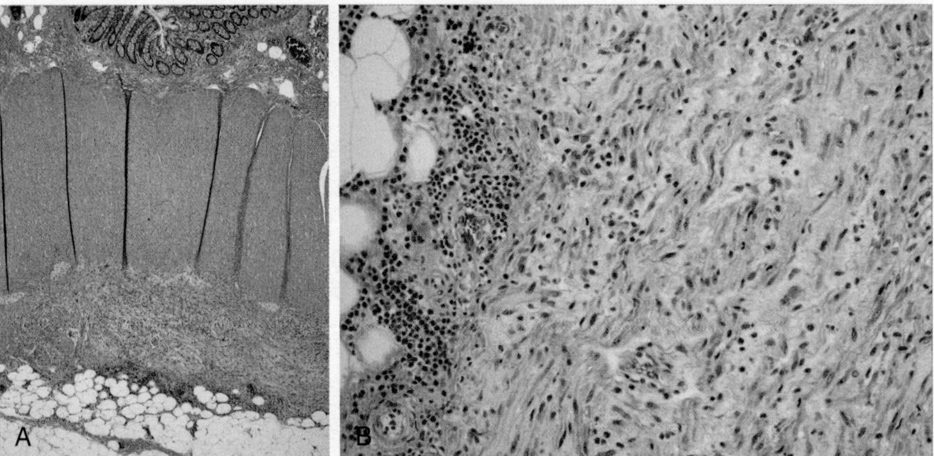

FIGURE 8.38 **A,** Eosinophilic gastroenteritis involving only the muscularis propria inflammation. **B,** Higher magnification of the same case showing that most of the infiltrating cells are eosinophils, and there is associated degenerative changes in the myocytes. (H&E stain).

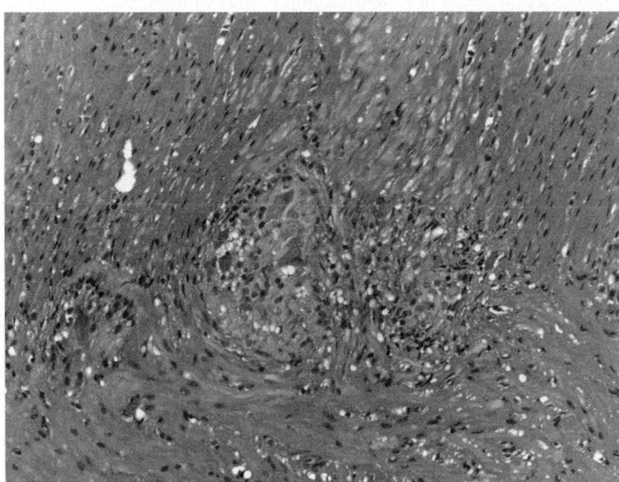

FIGURE 8.39 Lymphocytic inflammation in and around myenteric ganglia in a case of post-varicella intestinal pseudo-obstruction. The patient recovered after 2 months without any treatment.

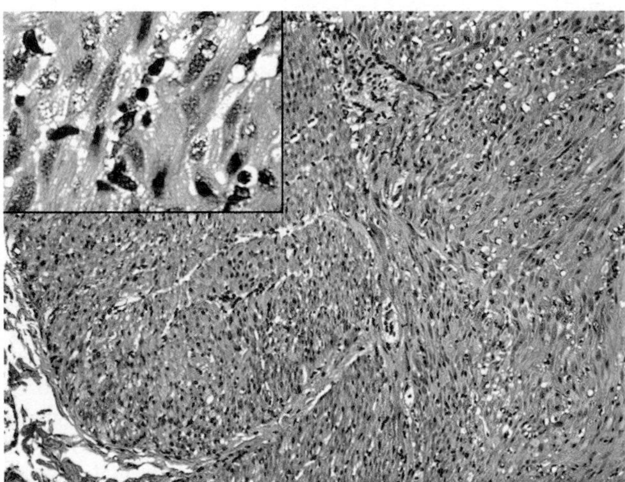

FIGURE 8.40 In brown bowel syndrome, there is brownish discoloration in the smooth muscle cells of muscularis propria at low magnification (H&E stain). At higher magnification, the cytoplasmic pigment appears granular, light brown, and lipofuscin-like. No other abnormalities of the smooth muscle cells or muscularis propria are present. (*Courtesy Dr. Thomas Smyrk, Mayo Clinic, Rochester, Minnesota.*)

is still poorly understood, and many disorders lack specific diagnostic features. Thus the diagnostic approach to patients with intestinal dysmotility requires careful evaluation of the patient's clinical presentation, family history, medication use, exposure to toxins, imaging and physical findings, and pathological features.[362] An international working group has proposed a classification scheme, guidelines for uniform methodologies, and criteria for the diagnosis of GI motility disorders (Tables 8.5 and 8.6).[150,278] However, despite attempts at improving diagnostic uniformity, challenges persist. One of the major problems is to differentiate primary from secondary disorders. The problem is confounded by tissue artifacts, which, at times, can be impossible to differentiate from true pathology.

Clinically, early onset of symptoms in childhood or in the neonatal period suggests a developmental or inherited disorder (primary), whereas the vast majority of motility disorders diagnosed in adults are acquired (secondary). Many disorders, particularly CIIP, have an insidious onset. Thus the chronic nature of the disease may not be overtly obvious. A positive family history is often lacking because the disease may be mild or subclinical, and affected individuals may not seek clinical attention. The presence of other associated abnormalities (e.g., external ophthalmoplegia), developmental defects (malrotation), and dilatation of other segments of GI tract or other viscera (e.g., duodenum, gallbladder, or urinary bladder) helps point toward an inherited form of visceral myopathy. Detailed family history and often genetic analysis are needed for the proper diagnosis. Careful evaluation of associated symptoms or signs can often help determine the primary cause of bowel dysmotility. Occasionally, the underlying systemic disorder may be diagnosed only after pathological evaluation of the bowel specimen, as in some collagen vascular disorders like scleroderma. A positive history of medication use, or exposure to toxin, is often difficult to evaluate because many patients consume multiple drugs, and the impact of specific drugs on bowel motility may not be well known. A positive history of a preceding viral illness may suggest a possible infectious/postinfectious cause of pseudo-obstruction.[328,329] In some cases, serology for circulating antineuronal and anti–smooth muscle antibodies may be helpful.[226,230] Endoscopy, laparotomy, and radiology may help exclude mechanical causes of intestinal obstruction. Gastrointestinal manometry, which helps differentiate mechanical from functional obstruction, is increasingly being used in all specialized centers.[230,362] It also helps differentiate neuropathic from myopathic causes of dysmotility. Other investigations, such as neurological and autonomic tests, may also play a role in the diagnostic workup. The majority of patients with intestinal obstruction have an underlying secondary mechanical cause (e.g., adhesions, extrinsic compression, or internal hernia).

From a pathologist's point of view, careful evaluation of the gross findings of the resection specimen combined with a systematic approach to the histological examination of tissue specimen are essential (Fig. 8.41). The approach suggested here is based on the recommendations of the

TABLE 8.5 Relationship Between Clinical Entities and Pathological Phenotypes

Clinical Entities	Primary Change	Associated Changes
Primary Disorders		
• Hirschsprung's disease	• Aganglionosis of rectosigmoid ± more proximal bowel • Hypoganglionosis or immature ganglia in transitional zone*	• Abnormal ICC networks • Muscular hyperplasia/hypertrophy • IND type B* • Eosinophilic ganglionitis* • Abnormal neurochemical coding*

• Idiopathic achalasia	• Hypoganglionosis or aganglionosis (LES)
	  • ± Degenerative neuropathy
	  • ± Lymphocytic or eosinophilic ganglionitis
	  • ± Abnormal neurochemical coding (deficiency of nNOS-containing myenteric neurons)
		• Abnormal ICC networks

• Idiopathic gastroparesis	• Unknown	• Abnormal neurochemical coding (loss of nNOS expression) • Abnormal ICC networks
• Congenital chronic intestinal pseudo-obstruction	• Aganglionosis • Hypoganglionosis • ± Intraneuronal nuclear inclusions • Degenerative neuropathy • Muscularis propria malformations • Degenerative leiomyopathy	• Abnormal ICC networks • Abnormal neurochemical coding • Neuronal immaturity • IND type B

• Acquired chronic intestinal pseudo-obstruction	• Hypoganglionosis or aganglionosis
	  • ± Degenerative neuropathy
	  • ± Lymphocytic or eosinophilic ganglionitis†
	  • ± Abnormal neurochemical coding (deficiency of one or more subtype of myenteric neuron)
	• Degenerative leiomyopathy ± lymphocytic or eosinophilic leiomyositis†
		• Abnormal ICC networks
		• Filament protein abnormalities
		• Polyglucosan inclusion bodies
		• Increased glia

• Mitochondrial disorder	• Megamitochondria ± abnormal cristae in ganglion cells and/or myocytes‡	• Highly variable histopathology ranging from neuropathic, myopathic to normal appearance

• Slow-transit constipation	• Unknown	• Hypoganglionosis
		  • ± Degenerative neuropathy
		  • ± Abnormal neurochemical coding (deficiency of ChAT and increased in NOS-containing myenteric neurons)
		• IND type B
		• Lymphocytic ganglionitis
		• Abnormal neurochemical coding (other)
		• Abnormal ICC networks
		• Amphophilic "M" inclusion bodies

• Idiopathic megarectum/megacolon	• Unknown	• Hypoganglionosis ± degenerative neuropathy • IND type B • Abnormal neurochemical coding • Degenerative leiomyopathy • Muscularis mucosae hypertrophy • Filament protein abnormalities • Atrophic desmosis

Continued

TABLE 8.5 Relationship Between Clinical Entities and Pathological Phenotypes—cont'd

Clinical Entities	Primary Change	Associated Changes
Secondary (Systemic) Disorders		
• Muscular dystrophy	• Defective myofilaments	• Degenerative leiomyopathy
• MEN 2B	• Ganglioneuromatosis	
• Neurofibromatosis	• Ganglioneuromatosis • ICC hyperplasia	
• Paraneoplastic gastroenteropathy	• Hypoganglionosis or aganglionosis + lymphocytic ganglionitis and/or leiomyositis¶	• Increased glia
• Diabetic gastroenteropathy	• Unknown	• Degenerative neuropathy • Abnormal ICC networks • Amphophilic inclusion bodies • Abnormal neurochemical coding (deficiency of nNOS-containing myenteric neurons)

The placement of these pathologies is still not certain. Filamin A mutations have been identified in an X-linked form of CIPO associated with other syndromic features (short small bowel and malrotation). In these cases, grade 1 is clearly appropriate. However, the pathology reported (degenerative neuropathy) has not been absolutely consistent among publications and is not specific to the syndromic form.

ChAT, choline acetyl transferase; CIPO, chronic intestinal pseudo-obstruction; ICC, interstitial cells of Cajal; IND, intestinal neuronal dysplasia; LES, lower esophageal sphincter; MEN, multiple endocrine neoplasia; NOS, nitric oxide synthase.

**May be present in the transitional zone of Hirschsprung's disease and correlate with persistent obstructive symptoms if incompletely resected.*

†Histopathological diagnosis should be complemented by serum autoimmune markers (e.g., antineuronal antibodies).

‡This histopathological feature is not seen in all cases; definitive diagnosis typically requires other forms of testing (e.g., skeletal muscle biopsy, molecular genetic analysis).

From Knowles CH, De Giorgio R, Kapur RP, et al. The London Classification of gastrointestinal neuromuscular pathology: report on behalf of the Gastro 2009 International Working Group. Gut. *2010;59(7):882–887.*

international working group.[278] The pathological specimens fall into three categories (1) suction mucosal biopsies (largely from the rectum), (2) full-thickness or seromuscular biopsies, and (3) resection specimens.

Suction Mucosal Biopsies

From the preceding discussion of various disorders, it is clear that mucosal biopsies often show only nonspecific findings and thus are of limited value in the workup of GI motility disorders, except Hirschsprung's disease. Their role is largely to exclude a primary mucosal disorder. In some disorders such as IBS, a variety of mucosal changes have been described, but these lack diagnostic specificity, and their evaluation is largely limited to research. On the other hand, suction mucosal biopsies of the rectum, which provide larger and deeper tissue compared with conventional endoscopic biopsies, have become the standard method of practice in the diagnostic workup of Hirschsprung's disease.

Full-Thickness/Seromuscular Biopsies

An appropriate diagnostic workup of GI motility disorders often requires a full-thickness biopsy combined with electron microscopy and special stains (see Fig. 8.41). Utility of full-thickness biopsies with immunohistochemical analysis has been shown to be useful in identifying myopathic or neuropathic changes.[363] However, the appropriate site and number of biopsies to be obtained have not been established. Biopsies can be obtained laparoscopically or by open surgery. In general, for patients with localized disease, samples from the most affected/dilated segment of bowel along with uninvolved areas are considered most helpful. For generalized disease, biopsies from the first available loop of jejunum, about 15 cm distal to the ligament of Treitz, has been suggested because this coincides with the location to measure small bowel motor activity by manometry. Some disorders can be patchy, so multiple samples are recommended. A sample size of 1.5 × 1.5 cm is considered adequate. Whenever feasible, some tissue should be frozen and some immediately fixed in glutaraldehyde for electron microscopy. Frozen sections are useful for performing histochemical stains in patients with mitochondrial myopathies, to demonstrate neurons and neural plexus, and to perform immunofluorescence. The biopsy should then be immediately fixed in neutral buffered formalin and pinned to a cork or sylgard board with the mucosal surface in contact with the board to allow for improved fixation of the muscle layers. Care should be taken not to stretch the biopsy. Ideally, both longitudinal and transverse sections should be obtained from the biopsy. Three sections for H&E stain, at different levels from each block, are ideal. For studying neural networks and ICC, whole-mount or en face sections offer a distinct advantage. However, these studies require special expertise and are largely limited to research.

Resection Specimens

Resections for GI motility disorders performed for treatment provide the best specimens for diagnostic workup (see Fig. 8.41). Handling of the resection specimen for Hirschsprung's disease is discussed earlier in this chapter. The goals are to confirm the presence of aganglionosis, define the extent of aganglionosis, and determine the presence of normal ganglions cells at the anastomosis. Small bowel and large bowel resections are handled similarly. The specimens should be fixed immediately after

TABLE 8.6 Diagnostic Criteria for Histological Phenotypes

Diagnosis	QL/QT	Minimum*	Adjunctive	Findings (Brief)
Aganglionosis	QL, QT	H&E or EH	EH (AChE) IHC (calretinin)†	Complete absence of neurons Hypertrophic submucosal extrinsic nerves
Hypoganglionosis	QL	H&E	IHC (PGP9.5, NSE)†	Severe reduction in ganglia and neurons
Ganglioneuromatosis	QL	H&E	IHC (PGP9.5, NSE, S100)†	Hamartomatous increase in neurons and glia
IND, type B	QT	EH (LDH)		>8 neurons in >20% of 25 submucosal ganglia
Degenerative neuropathy	QL	H&E		Degenerative cytological appearance
Inflammatory neuropathies	QL OT	H&E IHC (CD45, CD3)		Gross infiltrates or eosinophils ≥ 1 intraganglionic and/or >5 periganglionic lymphocytes/ganglion
Abnormal content in neurons	QL	H&E	IHC (SUM01), TEM	Intraneuronal nuclear inclusion bodies Megamitochondria
Abnormal neurochemical coding	QL, QT	IHC‡ IHC‡	IHC (PGP9.5, NSE)†§	Decreased immunostaining vs. controls Reduced defined subsets of neurons
Neuronal immaturity	QL	H&E	EH (LDH, SDH)	Morphologically immature neurons
Abnormal enteric glia	QL	H7E	IHC (S100, GFAP)	Marked increase
Muscularis propria malformations	QL, QT	H&E		Any departure from two muscle layers
Degenerative leiomyopathy	QL	H&E	Tinctorial,¶ IHC (SMA) TEM	Myocyte damage and loss, fibrosis
Inflammatory leiomyopathy	QL	H&E		Inflammatory cell infiltrate
Muscularis mucosae hyperplasia	QL	H&E		Increased thickness muscularis mucosae
Filament protein abnormalities	QL	IHC (SMA)		Absent SMA in circular muscle**
Inclusion bodies	QL, QT	H&E		Smooth muscle amphophilic "M" bodies
		Tinctorial (PAS)		Smooth muscle polyglucosan bodies
		TEM		Megamitochondria in myocytes
Atrophic desmosis	QL	Tinctorial¶		Total or focal lack of connective tissue scaffold
Abnormal ICC networks	QL	IHC (CD117) IHC (Ano 1)		>50% reduced ICC compared with control sections

CD117 *is synonymous with c-kit ;* Ano 1 *is synonymous with DOG1.*

AChE, acetylcholinesterase; EH, enzyme histochemistry; ICC, interstitial cells of Cajal; GFAP, glial fibrillary acidic protein; IHC, immunohistochemistry; IND, intestinal neuronal dysplasia; LDH, lactate dehydrogenase; NSE, neuron-specific enolase; PAS, periodic acid–Schiff; PGP9.5, protein gene product 9.5; QL, qualitative; QT, quantitative; SDH, succinate dehydrogenase; SMA, smooth muscle alpha-actin; TEM, transmission electron microscopy

**As recommended by IWG guidelines,[9] well-oriented sections are required at a minimum of three levels through an appropriately fixed and oriented block.*

†General neural markers used for comparison (Hu C/D, neurofilament are alternatives).

‡As yet undefined; most commonly employed are: NO, ChAT, SP, VIP. Note: although provisionally included, these are not a recommendation of the international working group guidelines for general pathology practice.

§Pan-neuronal markers are used in this context to determine whether absolute numbers of neurons are reduced.

¶Trichrome, Van Gieson, or picrosirius stain.

***Region specificity: this is a normal finding in ileum.*

Modified from Knowles CH, De Giorgio R, Kapur RP, et al. The London Classification of gastrointestinal neuromuscular pathology: report on behalf of the Gastro 2009 International Working Group. Gut. *2010;59(7):882–887.*

cleansing of the lumen. Frozen samples for histochemistry along with tissues fixed in glutaraldehyde for potential electron microscopy should be obtained. From the large bowel, samples should be obtained from the ascending colon, transverse colon, left/sigmoid colon, and rectum. Sections from the intestines should be obtained from the transverse and longitudinal axis, although in general, transverse sections are more informative. Longitudinal sections can produce an erroneous impression of thinning or thickening of the longitudinal muscle layer, depending on whether or not tenia coli have been included in the sections. Resections for achalasia and gastroparesis should be handled similarly. The bowel wall should be carefully evaluated for any thickening or thinning and any extra layer or absence of muscular coat. The presence of square-mouthed diverticula throughout the length of small or large intestine points toward a congenital etiology with underlying muscle weakness, while the presence of narrow-mouthed sigmoid diverticula suggests an acquired etiology with normal muscle contractility.

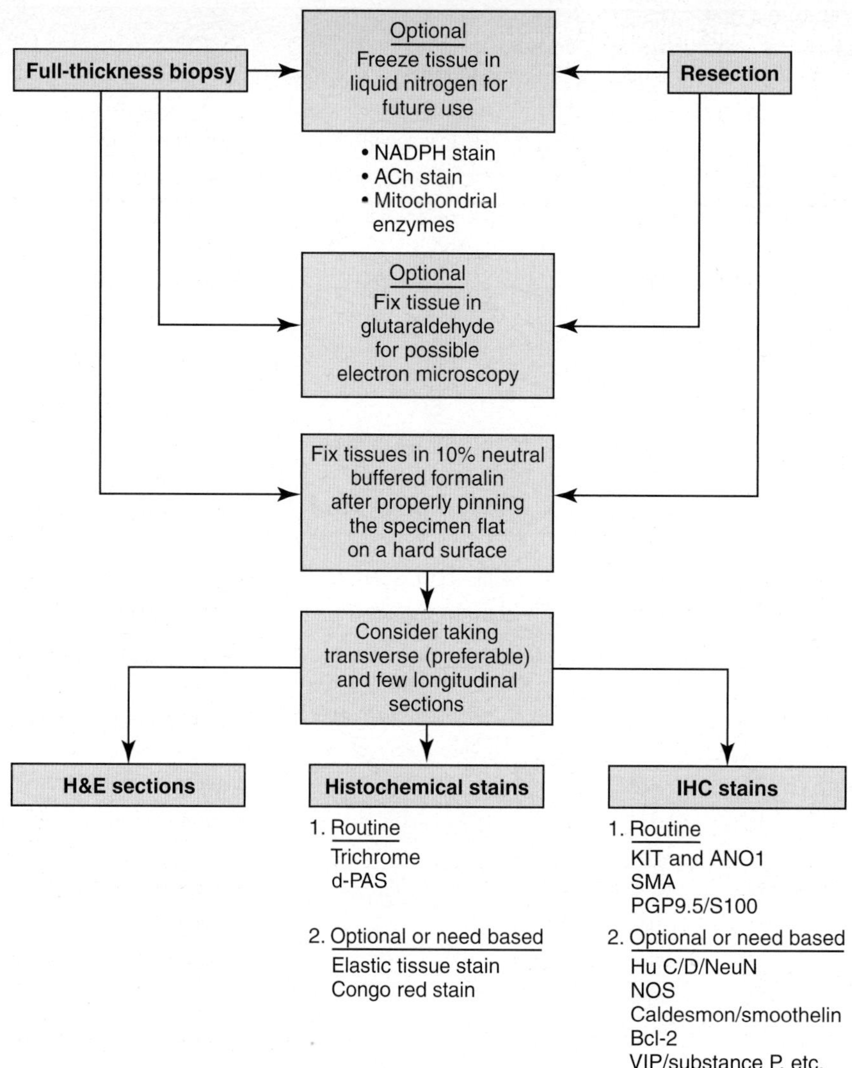

FIGURE 8.41 Handling of tissues for the workup of neuromuscular disorders of the gastrointestinal tract. *ACh,* Acetylcholine; *d-PAS,* periodic acid–Schiff stain with diastase digestion; *H&E,* hematoxylin and eosin stain; *NADPH,* reduced nicotinamide adenine dinucleotide phosphate; *NOS,* nitric oxide synthase; *PGP9.5,* protein gene product 9.5; *SMA,* smooth muscle actin; *VIP,* vasoactive intestinal peptide.)

Microscopy

On routine histology, careful examination of the mucosal changes and the neuromuscular apparatus should be performed. Particular attention should be given to the thickness of the muscle layers, myocyte morphology, pattern of fibrosis, number and morphology of ganglion cells, number and distribution of ICC, presence or absence of neural plexus hypertrophy or atrophy, and presence or absence of inflammation involving the neuromuscular apparatus. Inflammation surrounding the neural plexus along with ganglionitis may point toward an infectious or paraneoplastic/autoimmune neuropathy, whereas dense lymphocytic inflammation limited to the muscular layers may suggest autoimmune leiomyositis.[226,243] However, one should be cautious when evaluating inflammation within the neuromuscular apparatus because secondary involvement (e.g., inflammatory bowel disease) is much more common than primary involvement. Intranuclear inclusions in ganglion cells as well as cytoplasmic inclusions in smooth muscle fibers are associated with certain motility disorders. Neural hypertrophy and atrophy, although nonspecific, may indicate involvement of the neuromuscular apparatus and an underlying motility disorder. Artifactual cytoplasmic vacuolation and nuclear pyknosis in muscle and ganglion cells, which are not uncommon in resection specimens performed for a variety of conditions, should be differentiated from pathological alterations (see Figs. 8.31 and 8.34). True degenerative changes in the muscle are often diffuse extensive, accompanied by thinning or hypertrophy of the muscle and interstitial fibrosis, whereas artifacts tend to be focal.

Histochemical Stains

A panel of histochemical stains are useful in the evaluation of GI motility disorders. Connective tissue stains, such as trichrome or Elastic Van-Gieson, are helpful in delineating the pattern of fibrosis. PAS, both with and without diastase, highlights polyglucosamine inclusion bodies, whereas Congo red is useful for identifying amyloid. In many cases, amyloid deposition is suspected on H&E stain, but in others it is subtle or focal and easily missed. The role of acetylcholinesterase stain in the workup of Hirschsprung's disease was discussed in detail earlier in this chapter. Modified Gomori trichrome, cytochrome C, and succinic dehydrogenase stains are useful to demonstrate mitochondrial abnormalities in patients with mitochondrial myopathies, and they require frozen tissues. Silver staining techniques for studying the neural networks are obsolete, and these have been replaced by immunohistochemical stains. Use of NADPH stain on frozen tissues for highlighting the neural plexus in whole-mount or en face sections is recommended by some authorities.

Immunohistochemical Stains

A variety of immunohistochemical stains are helpful in evaluating cases in which routine histological examination is either normal, nonspecific, or nondiagnostic. These include stains to highlight myofilaments, neural plexus, ganglion cells, ICC, viral infections, and neurohormonal peptides. For highlighting the neural plexus, one can use S100, PGP 9.5, or NSE. Antibodies suggested to be useful for identification of myofilaments include alpha smooth muscle actin (α-SMA), smoothelin, caldesmon, and desmin. Of these, α-SMA staining is the most useful, whereas others such as smooth muscle myosin heavy chain, smoothelin, and histone deacetylase 8 have unclear utility. These stains may show decreased expression in the muscle layers despite normal staining with alpha-SMA.[354] Desmin myopathy is often a systemic disease diagnosed with skeletal muscle biopsies. ICCs are difficult to appreciate on H&E-stained tissue. KIT (CD117) or DOG1(Ano1) immunohistochemistry is useful. DOG1 is superior to KIT because it does not stain mast cells. However, most studies that evaluated ICC (quantitative or qualitative) have been performed using the KIT antibody. Quantitation of ICC and evaluation of their network is difficult on routine tissue sections. It requires experience and appropriate controls.[3,355] Whole-mount and en face sections using immunofluorescence staining and confocal/3D microscopy are important for studying the ICC network. Abnormalities of ICC must be considered in the differential diagnosis, particularly when routine histology is unremarkable. Although the presence or absence of ICC is usually appreciated on routine tissue sections, subtle abnormalities of the deep muscular/submucosal ICC plexus are better evaluated on frozen tissue with immunofluorescence.[297] A more detailed evaluation of the enteric nervous system with an elaborate immunohistochemical antibody panel (VIP, substance P and related tachykinins, nitric oxide synthase, neuropeptide Y, and calcitonin gene–related peptide) has not been validated for routine clinical use.

Electron Microscopy

Electron microscopy can be extremely valuable in some cases, particularly when light microscopy is nondiagnostic. Many degenerative changes in the muscle cells, neurons, or mitochondria are best identified on ultrastructural examination.

Molecular and Genetic Analysis

As discussed earlier in this chapter, the underpinning of many of the primary GI motility disorders has now been elucidated with genomic analysis. Many of the identified genes are involved in the function and development of the GI neuromuscular apparatus. However, despite easy availability of high-throughput sequencing, in current practice their diagnostic utility in GI motility disorders is still limited. For example, Hirschsprung's disease, which has been associated with a variety of genetic alterations, can pose diagnostic challenges, but the molecular diagnosis currently has no role. On the other hand, genetic mutational analysis in some of the primary dysmotility disorders, especially those that present with overlapping phenotypes (MMIHS or MIMM), can be invaluable. Both the patients and their family members must be investigated. This becomes particularly important when the disease phenotype is mild and presentation is atypical. The molecular and genetic tests can also be important in the diagnosis of mitochondrial disorders (e.g., MELAS, MNGIE), especially when presenting with atypical features or when the neuromuscular apparatus fails to show any histological findings.[235] The mutations can be seen in the nuclear or mitochondrial DNA.[364] Serum lactate and thymidine phosphorylase activities, brain MRI, and muscle biopsies are all essential in the diagnosis of mitochondrial disorders.[235]

CONCLUSION AND FUTURE OUTLOOK

Accurate diagnosis of GI motility disorders requires correlation of various clinical and laboratory data to establish diagnosis. For example, one study that looked at 21 cases of intestinal pseudo-obstruction showed myopathic changes in nine cases (43%), neuropathic changes in two cases (9.5%), and mixed changes in two cases (9.5%).[365] Abnormalities of ICC were found in 10 cases (48%). In eight cases, routine histology failed to show any changes, but abnormalities of ICC (2; 9.5%) or ganglion cell numbers (4; 19%) were found on immunohistochemical analysis. Neuropathic forms are more common in some studies, however, validity of many diagnoses based on quantitative changes in ganglia can be questioned. Recent recommendations and guidelines suggested by the international working group are likely to circumvent some of these issues. However, this group of disorders still remains frustrating despite extensive and sometimes expensive workup in many cases. Although a number of changes are sometimes identified, their significance in the pathophysiology and nature (primary vs. secondary) remains unclear. Application of genomic medicine has already led to better understanding of the underlying molecular mechanisms and etiopathogenesis in some of the motility disorders. It is anticipated that with standardization of the methodology, diagnostic criteria, and application of evolving technologies in the field of proteomics and genomics, our understanding of these disorders is likely to advance, leading to better diagnosis and treatment.

The full reference list may be accessed online at Elsevier eBooks for Practicing Clinicians.

CHAPTER 9

Congenital and Developmental Disorders of the Gastrointestinal Tract

Pierre Russo

Chapter Outline

MOLECULAR MECHANISMS OF GASTROINTESTINAL DEVELOPMENT

Recent advances in our understanding of the molecular controls of gut development have flowed from studies of a number of vertebrate and invertebrate models, including *Caenorhabditis elegans* (roundworm), sea urchins, *Drosophila*, zebrafish, and the mouse. These have provided insight into the genetic mechanisms that direct formation and modeling of the gastrointestinal (GI) tract, highlighted the importance of endodermal-mesenchymal interactions, and demonstrated the high degree of phylogenetic conservation of these mechanisms. Gut development is controlled by a number of intercellular signaling pathways in which transcription factors such as *FoxA*, *GataE*, *Xlox*, *Cdx*, and *Hox11/13b* are critical for gut differentiation. A discussion of these studies is beyond the scope of this chapter, and several excellent reviews are available.[1-5] Early development of the endoderm depends on molecular signaling pathways such as that of the Wnt pathway, which acts by stabilizing β-catenin, allowing it to translocate to the nucleus to activate transcription genes. Ablation of β-catenin in the notochord and primitive streak abrogates endoderm formation.[6] In drosophila and in the mouse, there are regional differences in the specific expression of Homeobox *(Hox)* genes along the gut axis.[3,5] For example, hindgut defects in mice can be linked to defective expression of Hoxd-13.[5] Another family of signaling genes critical in cellular cross-talk is the Hedgehog *(Hh)* family, which appears essential to anterior-posterior, dorsal-ventral, and radial patterning. Knockout and transgenic mouse models of various hedgehog components result in a variety of malformed phenotypes, ranging from esophageal atresia to persistent cloaca.[7] Vertebrate homologs of *Hh* exist in three forms: sonic *(Shh)*, Indian *(Ihh)*, and Desert *(Dhh)*, which have different but overlapping expression patterns. For example, $Shh^{-/-}$ mutant embryos die in utero and have overgrown duodenal villi, resulting in occlusion analogous to duodenal stenosis in humans. Selective postnatal blocking of Hh signaling resulted in a wasting and runted phenotype characterized by diarrhea, with disorganized intestinal villi, hyperplastic crypts, and enterocyte vacuolization.[7] Epigenetic factors may also contribute to different phenotypic development as well as disease susceptibility in genetically identical individuals. For example, different degrees of methylation of CpG groups in the agouti mouse, which can vary according to maternal intake of B-group vitamins, may result in variation in coat colors.[8] Epigenetic factors such as diet and the development of the microbiome appear to play a major role, especially in postnatal development of the GI tract.[5]

EMBRYOLOGY AND ANATOMIC DEVELOPMENT OF THE GASTROINTESTINAL TRACT

The development of the GI tract proceeds through three major overlapping steps: formation of the gut tube during blastogenesis, differentiation of the specific segments of the digestive tract and its accessory organs during organogenesis, and histogenesis of the individual organs with their specialized cell types.[3] Major developmental milestones are outlined in Table 9.1. The first two steps, development of the primitive gut tube during blastogenesis followed by organogenesis, take place during the embryonic period, which begins on the day of fertilization and ends on the 56th postconceptual day (8th week). The developing human is more susceptible to teratogenic agents during the embryonic period than at any other period of development. The fetal period, which begins on postconceptual day 57 and ends at birth, is characterized by the final stages of rotation and fixation as well as by continued elongation and histogenesis of the GI tract. By 15 to 20 weeks of gestation, the fetal gut essentially resembles that of the newborn.[2] An overview of these basic processes, especially as pertains to the GI tract, is presented in Table 9.2. The pattern of congenital anomalies of the GI tract varies depending on the developmental period from which they arise (Table 9.3).

Blastogenesis extends from fertilization to day 28. During the first half of blastogenesis, the bilaminar disc and the basic body plan of dorsoventrality, rostrocaudal axis, and laterality are established. During the second half of blastogenesis, the midline developmental field directs the process of gastrulation, which establishes all three germ layers (endoderm, mesoderm, and ectoderm). The mammalian digestive system is derived from each of these layers: the epithelial lining from the endoderm, the muscle layers and supportive elements from the mesoderm, and the neurons of the enteric nervous system from the ectoderm. It is during this period that the basic plan of the GI tract is established through the inductive influences of the notochord, primitive streak, emerging mesoderm, and other anatomic components of the midline developmental field on the primitive endoderm. These inductive influences predetermine the sites of the specific segments of the GI tract and the primordia of its accessory organs of digestion. For example, at the end of gastrulation in mice, further patterning of the endoderm is determined by regional expression of factors such as Sox2 and Hhex in the anterior endoderm, and Cdx2 in the posterior endoderm.[4] Simultaneously, during the third and fourth weeks, cephalocaudad and lateral folding of the embryo converts the trilaminar germ disc into an elongated cylinder. The primitive gut is at that point somewhat arbitrarily divided into three major segments: a cranial foregut, a midgut open to the yolk sac via the vitelline duct, and a hindgut (Fig. 9.1). Each of these segments will give rise to specialized regions of the gut and, as in the case of the foregut, to other organs such as the thyroid, lungs, liver, and pancreas. The blood supply to the primitive gut is derived from the vitelline arteries of the yolk sac. The celiac, superior mesenteric, and inferior mesenteric arteries vascularize the abdominal foregut, midgut, and hindgut, respectively, and by convention determine the boundaries of each (Fig. 9.2).

Organogenesis extends from day 29 to day 56 (weeks 5 to 8). Suddenly, during the fifth week, the entire tubular GI tract, its major divisions, and its accessory organs of digestion, having been predetermined during blastogenesis, emerge from the imprinted primordium of the primitive endodermal tube. The abdominal portion of the foregut is divided into the esophagus, stomach, and proximal duodenum. The common origin of the trachea and esophagus from the foregut results in various forms of fistulae if separation

TABLE 9.1 Developmental Milestones

Event	Time of First Expression
Gastrulation	Week 3
Gut tube largely closed	Week 4
Liver and pancreas buds	Week 4
Growth of intestines into cord	Week 7
Intestinal villus formation	Week 8
Retraction of intestines into abdominal cavity	Week 10
Organ formation complete	Week 12
Parietal cells detectable, pancreatic islets appear, bile secretion, intestinal enzymes detectable	Week 12
Swallowing detectable	Week 16 and 17
Mature motility	Week 36

From Montgomery RK, Mulberg AE, Grand RJ. Development of the human gastrointestinal tract: twenty years of progress. Gastroenterology. *1999;116(3):702–731.*

TABLE 9.2 Overview of Gastrointestinal Development in the First 10 Weeks

	Embryo								Fetus	
Feature	**Blastogenesis**		**Organogenesis**							
Week	**1**	**2**	**3**	**4**	**5**	**6**	**7**	**8**	**9**	**10**
Bilaminar disc, endoderm	X									
Yolk sac, connecting stalk		X								
Trilaminar disc			X							
Early: midline developmental field, induction of gastrointestinal patterning			X							
Late: primitive foregut, midgut, hindgut; respiratory and hepatic primordia				X						
Cylindrical embryo, definitive tubular gastrointestinal tract, umbilical cord					X					
Beginning intestinal rotation						X				
Remodeling, growth, histogenesis; anus completed							X	X	X	X
Return of bowel to abdomen, final rotation and fixation										X
Sexual differentiation of perineum										X

TABLE 9.3 Patterns of Congenital Anomalies Arising During Various Developmental Periods

Developmental Period	Age (Wk)	Developmental Events	Congenital Anomalies
Embryo			
Early blastogenesis	1-2	Basic patterning of body: dorso-ventrality, rostral caudal axis, laterality	Lethal to embryo: empty chorionic sac and global embryonic growth disorganization
Late blastogenesis	3-4	Midline developmental field Right-left–sidedness (visceral situs) Induction of endodermal primordia Basic patterning of the gastrointestinal tract	Lethal to embryo: empty chorionic sac and global embryonic growth disorganization Severe gastrointestinal anomalies as part of extensive, sometimes monstrous maldevelopment of embryo, not necessarily lethal (see Table 9.1)
Organogenesis	5-8	Differentiation of endodermal primordia into specific segments of gastrointestinal tract and accessory digestive organ Histogenesis	Isolated anomalies of the gastrointestinal tract Disruptions and deformations
Fetus			
	9-10	Return and final rotation and fixation of intestinal loop Sexual differentiation of perineum	Isolated abnormalities of rotation and fixation. Disruptions and deformations.
	11-34	Histogenesis, remodeling, growth	

From Huff DS. Developmental anatomy and anomalies of the gastrointestinal tract, with involvement in major malformative syndromes. In: Russo P, Ruchelli E, Piccoli D, eds. Pathology of Pediatric Gastrointestinal and Liver Disease. *New York: Springer; 2004:3–37.*

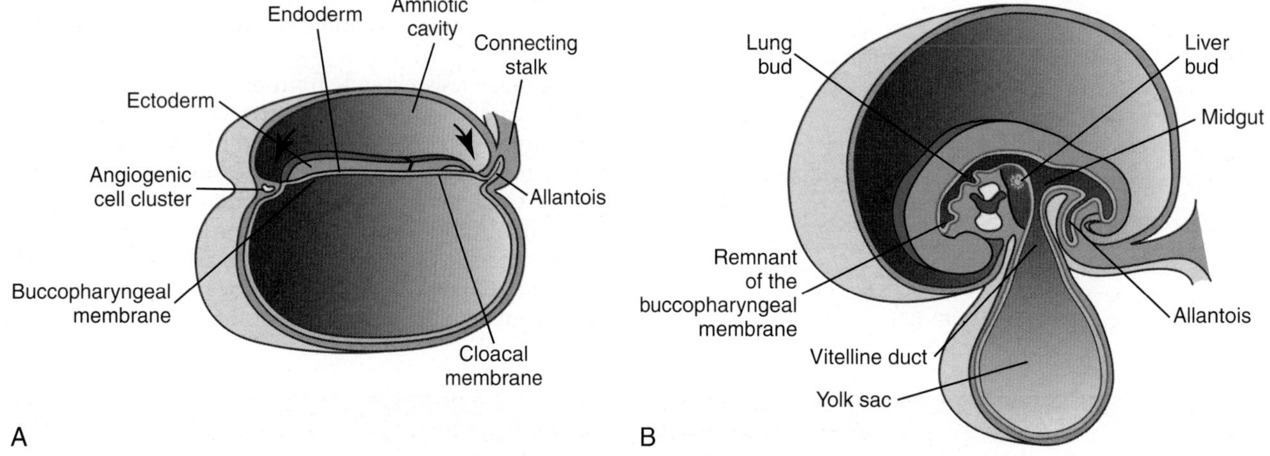

FIGURE 9.1 Sagittal midline sections of the embryo demonstrating cephalocaudal folding and effect on developing gut tube. A, Pre-somite embryo with the flat embryonic disc. **B,** End of the first month. Folding of the embryo has created the gut tube with a foregut, midgut, and hindgut. The midgut communicates with the yolk sac. (*From Sadler TW. Langman's Medical Embryology. 8th ed. Philadelphia: Lippincott Williams & Wilkins; 2000:99.*)

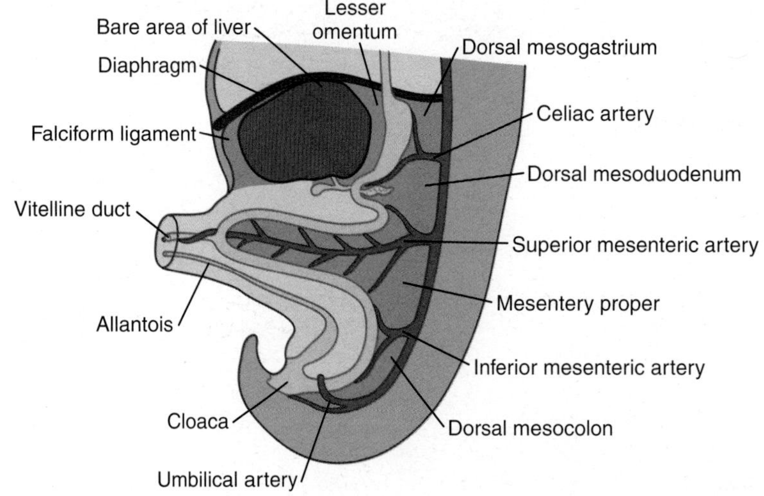

FIGURE 9.2 Primitive dorsal and ventral mesenteries. The celiac artery supplies the foregut. The superior mesenteric artery supplies the midgut, running through the mesentery and continuing toward the yolk sac as the vitelline artery. (*From Sadler TW. Langman's Medical Embryology. 8th ed. Philadelphia: Lippincott Williams & Wilkins; 2000:273.*)

is incomplete. The hepatic diverticulum arises from the proximal duodenum, its cephalic portion budding into the transverse septum (precursor of the diaphragm) to become the liver, and its caudal portion giving rise to the gallbladder and extrahepatic biliary tree. Dorsal and ventral pancreatic buds also emerge from the proximal duodenum. As elongation of the midgut proceeds much faster than growth of the embryo from the sixth week on, the intestine pushes out into the stalk of the yolk sac. As it does so, it rotates 90 degrees counterclockwise (as viewed from the front of the embryo) around the axis of the superior mesenteric artery (SMA), so that the cranial limb ("pre-arterial" in relation to the SMA) moves to the embryo's right, and the caudal limb ("postarterial") moves to the embryo's left (Fig. 9.3A,B). Continued elongation, especially of the pre-arterial segment, results in a series of folds called *jejuno-ileal loops*, the identity of which Keibel believed were retained in the adult.[9] The postarterial loop, most of which will form the colon, remains relatively straight. Around 63 days of life, under largely unknown influences, the intestines suddenly return to the abdominal cavity. As it returns, there is a further anticlockwise 180-degree rotation, which, added to the previous rotation, makes a total of 270 degrees (Fig. 9.3C). As a result, the third portion of the duodenum passes horizontally caudal and dorsal to the artery, and the proximal anchoring point comes to lie near the final position of the ligament of Treitz to the left of the artery. The superior mesenteric artery hangs over the ventral wall of the third portion of the duodenum. As the distal limb then rapidly returns, it swings ventral and rostral to the proximal loop, and the cecum comes to lie in the right abdomen near the liver (Fig. 9.3D). Rotation is completed by the 10th week, and fixation continues throughout fetal life as the mesenteries become adherent to the parietal peritoneum. The cecum and liver then separate by unknown mechanisms, the increasing distance occupied by the lengthening ascending colon, with the final position of the liver being the right upper quadrant and that of the cecum being the right lower

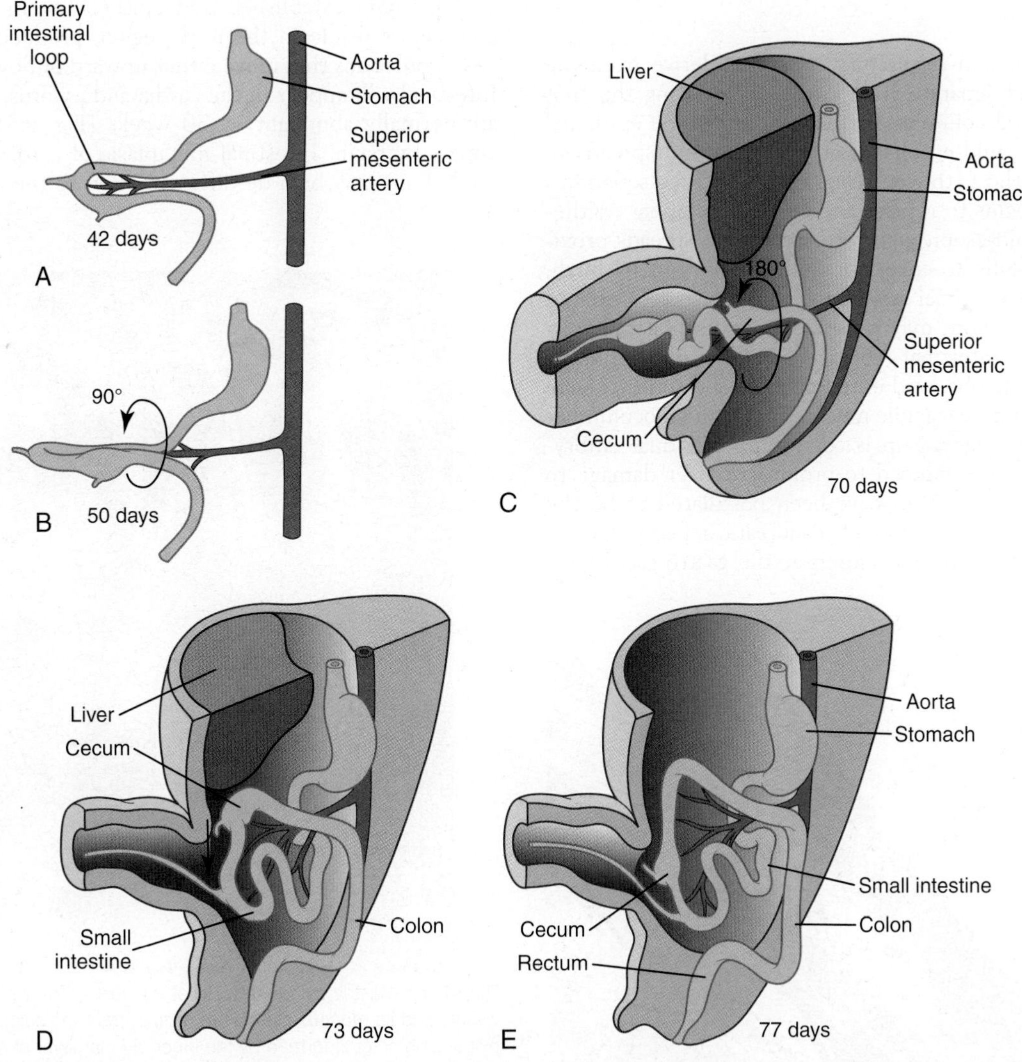

FIGURE 9.3 Intestinal rotation. A and **B,** At the end of the 6th week, the intestinal loop herniates through the umbilicus and rotates 90 degrees counterclockwise. **C,** As the small intestine elongates, it forms the jejuno-ileal loops. During the 10th week, the loops retract into the abdominal cavity and rotate an additional 270 degrees counterclockwise. **D,** As the midgut completes its return, the cecum lies in the right upper quadrant. **E,** Separation of the liver and cecum with the cecum assuming its definitive position in the right lower quadrant. (*From Larsen WJ. Human Embryology. 2nd ed. Hong Kong: Churchill Livingstone; 1997:241.*)

quadrant (Fig. 9.3E). This separation is referred to, probably incorrectly, as *cecal descent*. See Estrada[10] for an extensive review and Kluth et al.[11] for a recent reevaluation of these events.

Mucosal histogenesis transforms the primitive undifferentiated epithelium of the gut tube into the specific epithelia of the final differentiated segments of the digestive tract. Although histogenesis begins in the late embryonic period, most of the histological transformation occurs during fetal life. It begins with a transient phase of epithelial proliferation. The proliferating epithelium completely occludes the lumen of the duodenum, significantly narrows the lumen of the esophagus, and may mildly narrow the lumens of the cardia, pylorus, upper jejunum, and distal ileum. These proliferations may be accompanied by the transient formation of multiple antimesenteric diverticula in the duodenum, upper jejunum, and distal ileum. Some instances of congenital atresia, stenosis, or diverticula may be the result of abnormalities in the formation or resolution of the proliferative phase.

Esophagus

The esophagus and respiratory apparatus derive from the endoderm and separate from each other during the first month. Ciliated columnar epithelium covers the epithelial surface of the mid-esophagus at 10 weeks and spreads to both ends by the 11th week (Fig. 9.4). Stratified squamous epithelium begins to replace the ciliated columnar epithelium in the mid-esophagus at 16 weeks and spreads proximally and distally to cover the entire esophagus by birth, except for the proximal esophagus, where islands of ciliated columnar epithelium may persist. These disappear shortly after birth.[12-14] Intestinal goblet cells in the distal esophagus have been rarely observed in the neonate and fetus, though positive staining with acidic mucins at the squamocolumnar junction in this age group is common.[15] Residual embryonic cells that are induced to proliferate after damage to the squamous epithelium have been postulated to be the source of Barrett's metaplasia.[16] Pancreatic acinar tissue has been observed in young children at the gastro-esophageal junction, independent of Barrett's esophagus, esophagitis, or gastritis.[17] The superficial cardiac glands of the lamina propria appear in the 13th week. The submucosal mucous glands appear in the 27th week. The circular muscle layer is present at 8 weeks, the longitudinal layer at approximately 13 weeks, followed by the muscularis mucosae. The waves of differentiation begin in the esophagus, propagate caudally, and then propagate cranially at the anorectal junction. The two meet at the ileocecal junction.

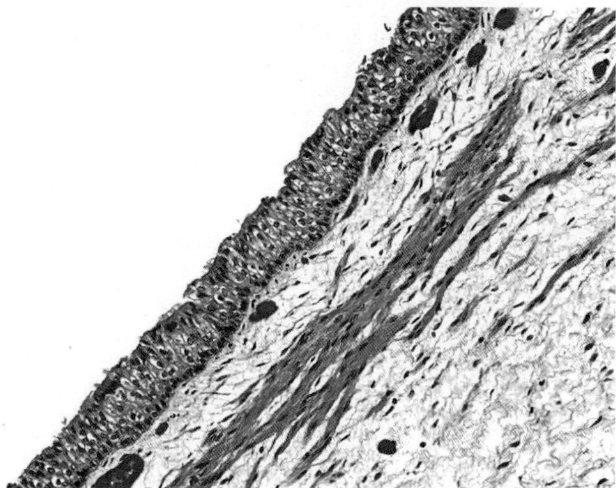

FIGURE 9.4 Stratified focally ciliated columnar epithelium in the esophagus of a 22-week fetus.

Stomach

During the fifth week of life, differential growth of the dorsal wall of the stomach results in the formation of the greater curvature. Subsequent rotation of the stomach 90 degrees along a craniocaudal axis during the seventh week, followed by fixation of the second part of the duodenum to the dorsal body wall forms the lesser sac of the peritoneal cavity. Prenatal ultrasound examinations have shown that the stomach continues to grow in a linear fashion from 13 to 39 weeks. Studies of the development of the mouse stomach have established that epithelial stem cells of the gastric pits reside in the neck region, producing different cell populations that move either upward or downward.[18,19] Intestinal villi appear in the cardia and pylorus, where they are normally abundant by 30 weeks (Fig. 9.5). They disappear by birth. Intestinal metaplasia of cardiac or pyloric epithelium may be a de-differentiation to the normal fetal

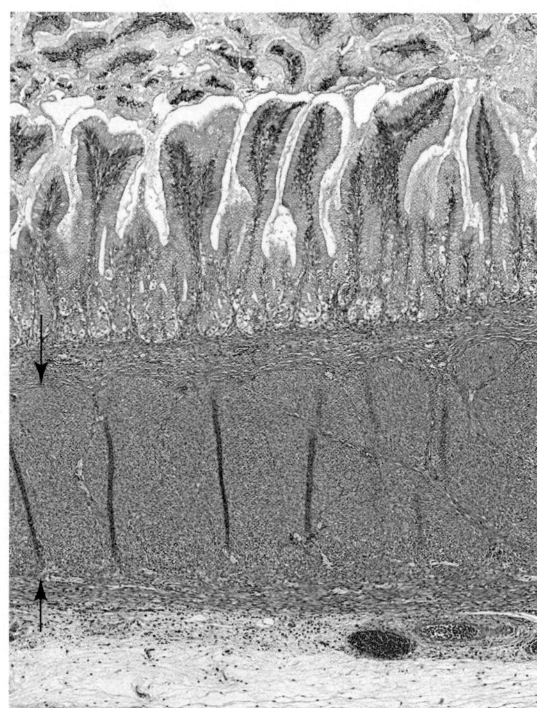

FIGURE 9.5 Gastric pyloric mucosa at 24 weeks. The pyloric mucosa is villous, and its mucous glands are distinct from the gastric glands. The pyloric sphincter is formed by the inner circular layer of the muscularis propria (between the two *arrows*). The outer longitudinal layer is *below*, and Auerbach's plexuses are visible between the two. The inner most oblique layer is not present in the pyloric sphincter (*From Ernst LM, Ruchelli ED, Huff DS. Color Atlas of Fetal and Neonatal Histology. New York: Springer; 2011.*)

condition. The cardiac mucosa is thought to arise from undifferentiated gastric mucosa and not from esophageal metaplasia.[20] The development of the gastric glands occurs early during fetal life. Glandular pits are formed during the 11th to 12th week of fetal life, along with emergence of the first cells of the parietal lineage. By 15 to 17 weeks of gestation, fetal gastric glands are essentially similar to the adult's, with compartmentalization into foveolus, isthmus, neck, and base, containing the various phenotypically differentiated cell types.[2] Further development of the stomach involves thickening of the glandular region with proliferation and maturation of the chief cells, which are relatively fewer in the neonatal stomach than in the adult, and which do not produce pepsin in the newborn.[21] Gastric pH is relatively high in the neonate and becomes comparable to that of adults by 2 years of age. This may partly result from buffering by amniotic fluid, but also from a relative lack of gastrin, levels of which increase in the first few postnatal months.[21]

Small and Large Intestine

Rearrangement of the endodermal epithelium resulting from elongation of the gut tube, rather than epithelial proliferation as previously thought, leads to temporary occlusion of the lumen by the end of the sixth week.[22] Defects in subsequent recanalization of the lumen can result in stenoses or duplication of the digestive tract. As the lumen expands, the epithelium undergoes folding that will eventually lead to the formation of villi. Mesenchymal cells grow toward the lumen to form early villi, and this process is orchestrated by elaborate endodermal-mesodermal cross-talk under the control of signaling pathways including the BMP, Hedgehog, PDGF, TGF-β, and Wnt pathways and the mesenchymal transcription factors *FoxL1*, *FoxF1*, and *FoxF2*.[4] Villi and crypts appear first in the duodenum in the eighth week, spread to the mid–small intestine by the 9th week, and reach the distal ileum by the 12th week. The early intestinal mucosa consists of stratified epithelium, with gradual appearance of columnar epithelium, first at the apices and then along the sides of villi. By the 10th week, only intervillus epithelium remains stratified.[3] By 9 to 10 weeks, absorptive cells of the proximal intestine display a brush border with an array of microvilli.[23] Eosinophilic globules can be frequently observed within the fetal intestinal epithelium (Fig. 9.6); these have been referred to as *thanatosomes* and seem to reflect apoptotic activity.[24] Both Wnt and BMP signaling pathways appear to be involved in the formation of crypts.[4] These crypts contain the stem cells that will serve as the source of the epithelial cells, which are renewed every 4 days.[5] Cytological differentiation of the crypts begins with the appearance of goblet cells in the eighth week followed by Paneth cells and enteroendocrine cells in the ninth week. Clusters of entero-endocrine cells occurring on the top of villi in the duodenum and upper jejunum during the 20th week of gestation have been described as *Segi's cap*.[25] The Notch pathway plays a critical role in epithelial differentiation by regulating the specification of absorptive versus secretory lineages, which is controlled by differences in expression of factors such as *Hes1*, *Atoh1* and *Neurog3*.[4] Atoh1 (also called *Math1*) is a basic loop-helix-loop transcription factor that appears to be a key regulator of secretory cell (goblet, Paneth, and enteroendocrine cells) development, whereas absorptive cells appear to be *Math1*-independent.[26] Neonates have been reported with an absence of gut secretory cells.[27] Patients with mutations in a gene called *Neurogenin 3* have presented with malabsorptive diarrhea and a complete absence of enteroendocrine cells.[28] The time of appearance and electron-microscopic features of 13 enteroendocrine cells have been described in human embryos between 9 and 22 weeks of gestation.[29] Brunner's glands appear in the proximal duodenum in the 12th week. The histological appearance of the small intestine resembles that of a newborn by 20 weeks.[30] In addition, perinatal and postnatal acquisition of the gut microbiome is essential for proper maturation and immune development.[31]

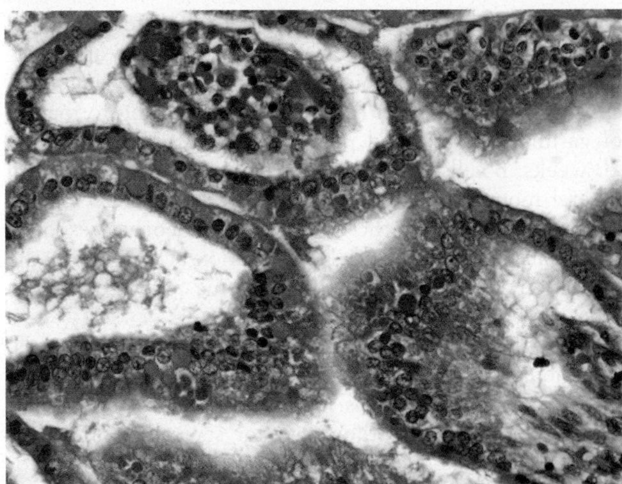

FIGURE 9.6 Small bowel of a 19-week fetus. Brightly eosinophilic globules can be observed in the surface epithelium and appear to correspond to "thanatosomes," which may reflect apoptotic activity.

The enteric nervous system is derived from the neural crest and includes contributions from the sympathetic system, growing along the arterial supply, and from the parasympathetic system, with branches of the vagal nerve innervating the upper GI tract, while the pelvic splanchnic nerves innervate the descending colon and rectum. The ENS contains $> 100 \times 10^6$ neurons comprising four major classes and at least 18 functional subtypes.[32] These enteric neural crest cells (ENCCs) appear in the developing human foregut around 3 weeks, migrate in a craniocaudal direction, and are detected in the hindgut by week 7.[32] The development of the enteric nervous system is beyond the scope of this chapter, and recent references should be consulted.[32-37]

Similar to the intestinal epithelium, the **colonic mucosa** consists of a stratified epithelium beginning around 8 weeks. At approximately the 10th week, villi with developing crypts cover the surface of the large intestine and persist until the 28th week. Therefore intestinal villi are normally seen in the embryo, not only in the small intestine but also in the cardia, pylorus, and colon (Fig. 9.7). The intervillous surface epithelium differentiates into a single layer containing goblet cells by the 13th to 16th week. After birth, a 100-fold increase in the number of intestinal crypts occur, along with an expansion of crypt cells.[21] An outline of the histogenesis of the muscular coats and myenteric plexus is presented in Table 9.4. The development of the **mucosal**

lymphoid system is outlined in Table 9.5. The fetal mucosal lymphoid system has the capacity to respond to an abnormal intrauterine antigenic stimulus with expansion of T cells and B cells within Peyer's patches and the formation of germinal centers and plasma cells, possibly as early as 20 weeks. B cells within patches do not produce IgG until several months postnatally, and the fetus receives its IgG transplacentally from the mother.[31] The neonate responds to the antigenic stimulus of colonization at birth with the formation of germinal centers and plasma cells 2 to 4 weeks after birth.

IgA is the major immunoglobulin of the intestinal mucosa, and though undetectable at birth, it coats the mucosal surface once breastfeeding is initiated and will offer passive immune protection to the infant for several months after birth. Other bioactive compounds in human milk, including oligosaccharides and glycoproteins, also exert protective influences to the developing gut.[31]

CONGENITAL ANOMALIES OF THE GASTROINTESTINAL TRACT

General Aspects

The causes of anomalies of the GI tract include chromosomal abnormalities (numerical and structural); single-gene defects; maternal diseases, especially diabetes; and maternal exposure to drugs, especially hydantoin (pyloric stenosis, duodenal and anal atresia). Causes of disruptions include inherited[38] and noninherited maternal and fetal thrombophilic diseases, intrauterine hypoxic/ischemic events, intrauterine infection including varicella,[39] iatrogenic vascular disruptions,[40] and maternal exposure to vasoactive drugs.[41] Other diseases of the embryo such as cystic fibrosis and epidermolysis bullosa underlie some GI anomalies. Deformations are limited to abnormal shapes of the liver and abnormal rotation and fixation associated with defects of the diaphragm, body wall, and umbilicus. The cause of most anomalies is unknown. Anomalies that arise after completion of organogenesis are often disruptions or deformations; otherwise the causes are not specific to any developmental period.

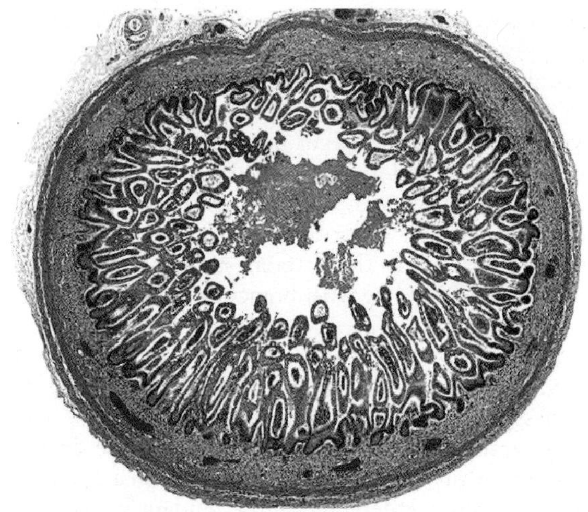

FIGURE 9.7 The large bowel of this 22-week fetus has a villiform epithelium, similar to that of the small bowel.

Esophagus

Short Esophagus

A congenital short esophagus is a rare anomaly that is associated with intrathoracic development of the stomach. It may be difficult to distinguish from the more common

TABLE 9.5 Histogenesis of Mucosal Lymphoid Tissue

Week	Feature
Intrauterine	
7	Intraepithelial lymphocytes
10	T cells with surface recognition
12	PHA-responsive lymphocytes
14	Lymphocytes with PHA cytotoxicity and ability to mediate graft vs. host response
17-20	Mast cells in small intestine
19	Solitary lymphoid follicle in distal ileum, appendix, and colon
24	Peyer's patches in distal ileum
40	Solitary lymphoid follicles in duodenum, rectum, and possibly stomach
Postnatal	
2-4	Germinal centers and plasma cells

PHA, *Phytohemagglutinin.*
From Huff DS. Developmental anatomy and anomalies of the gastrointestinal tract, with involvement in major malformative syndromes. In: Russo P, Ruchelli E, Piccoli D, eds. Pathology of Pediatric Gastrointestinal and Liver Disease. *New York: Springer; 2004:3–37.*

TABLE 9.4 Histogenesis of the Muscular Coats and Myenteric Plexus

			Small Bowel	Colon	
Layer	**Esophagus**	**Stomach**	**Distal**	**Proximal**	**Distal**
Circular	6	7	7	9	8
Longitudinal	8	11	10	26	11
Muscularis mucosae	12	14	21	26	21
Myenteric plexus	6	7	7	8	12
Bidirectional peristalsis			12	12	
Unidirectional peristalsis			30	30	

TABLE 9.6 Occurrence of Atresia and Stenosis of the Gastrointestinal Tract

	Number per Live Births	% of All Intestinal Atresia
Esophagus	1:3000	
Stomach	Rare	
Duodenum	1:1500	50%
Jejunum	1:2000	20%
Ileum	1:2000	25%
Colon	Rare	5%
Rectum, anus	1:5000	
Multiple		15%

Number per live births varies widely from series to series.
From Huff DS. Developmental anatomy and anomalies of the gastrointestinal tract, with involvement in major malformative syndromes. In: Russo P, Ruchelli E, Piccoli D, eds. Pathology of Pediatric Gastrointestinal and Liver Disease. *2nd ed. New York: Springer; 2014:3–37.*

TABLE 9.7 Disorders with Multiple Gastrointestinal Atresias/Stenoses

Familial intestinal polyatresia syndrome
Multiple gastrointestinal abnormalities
Epidermolysis bullosa, lethal and nonlethal
Carmi's syndrome (aplasia cutis)
Congenital immunodeficiency syndrome
Severe combined immunodeficiency syndrome
Other types not specified
Cystic fibrosis
Gastroschisis

congenital hiatal hernia. Features that favor the diagnosis of a congenital short esophagus include early identification of the intrathoracic stomach during the second trimester and the consistent absence of an abdominal stomach bubble on antenatal ultrasound examination.[42] Furthermore, in the congenital short esophagus, the intrathoracic stomach is supplied by segmental arteries from the descending thoracic aorta, rather than by intrathoracic extensions of the gastric artery, as observed in hiatal hernia.[14] Congenital hiatal hernia, by contrast, appears to develop later in gestation and is a result of defective development of the lumbar part of the diaphragm. The differences between these conditions are more than academic as the outcome of repair of a congenital short esophagus is more guarded than that of hiatal hernia.[42]

Esophageal Atresia and Tracheoesophageal Fistula

Atresias and stenoses may occur at any site along the tract, but some sites are more commonly involved than others (Table 9.6). Several disorders associated with multiple atresias/stenoses of the GI tract are listed in Table 9.7. Key distinguishing features of the various types of congenital atresias and stenosis along the GI tract are listed in Table 9.8.

Esophageal atresia is the most common congenital abnormality of the esophagus and occurs in about 1 in 3000 live births; an associated tracheoesophageal fistula is present in 70% to 90% of cases. There is a slight male predominance. A history of polyhydramnios is found in a majority of patients with atresia. Esophageal atresia without a fistula is associated with a small stomach[43] and absence of a GI gas pattern. A fistula from the distal esophageal segment allows passage of gastric contents into the respiratory tract, causing respiratory symptoms. Approximately 50% of patients have associated congenital anomalies, of which the VATER/VACTERL association (consisting of a combination of Vertebral anomalies, Anal atresia, Cardiac defects, Tracheo-Esophageal fistula, Renal and Limb anomalies) is the most common.[44] Conditions associated with esophageal atresia and tracheoesophageal fistula are listed in Box 9.1. Familial forms not associated with hereditary syndromes are probably multifactorial.

Gross[45] and Swenson et al.[46] proposed the most commonly used classifications of types of esophageal atresia and tracheoesophageal fistula. Figure 9.8 schematically depicts five common variations found in many current publications. The most common form, comprising about 85% of cases, consists of a blind-ending proximal pouch with a fistula from the trachea to the distal portion (Fig. 9.9). The tracheal ostium of a fistula to the distal esophageal segment is often at the carina but may be higher in the trachea. Likewise, the ostium of a fistula to the proximal esophageal pouch is often in the upper trachea but is sometimes lower. The length of the distal segment varies. Some may be a short stump barely visible above the diaphragm, and others may be sub-diaphragmatic.[47] Therefore the distance between the upper esophageal pouch and distal esophageal segment may be short or long, depending on these variations. Short-gap lesions are more easily and successfully repaired than long-gap lesions. A fistula from the upper esophageal pouch and/or the distal esophageal segment may arise from one or both bronchi forming a broncho-esophageal fistula(e). The trachea may be absent, in which case the distal trachea or both main bronchi arise from the esophagus. An esophageal stenosis may be present at the site of a tracheoesophageal fistula without esophageal atresia.

The association with a multitude of genetic defects, particularly the VATER/VACTERL association, suggests that multiple genetic pathways may be involved, of which mutations and deletions of the *FOX* gene cluster on chromosome 16q24 appear to be the most significant.[44,48] Adriamycin administered intraperitoneally to pregnant rodents results in esophageal anomalies and tracheoesophageal fistulae in about 50% of the pups. In this model, there appears to be interference with the division of the esophago-tracheal tube into ventral and dorsal components.[49] No such association has been reported in humans. The sonic hedgehog *(SHH)* pathway may also play a role. *Shh*$^{-/-}$ mice have severe tracheoesophageal fistula.[49] SHH regulates the FOXF1 gene, which has recently been shown to be associated with esophageal atresia and the VACTERL association.[50] The occasional coexistence of esophageal atresia and tracheoesophageal fistula with foregut duplications and bronchopulmonary foregut malformations suggests a common pathogenesis.

TABLE 9.8 Congenital Atresias and Stenoses of the Gastrointestinal Tract

Location	Incidence	Key Clinical Features	Key Pathological Features
Esophagus	Atresia 1:3000 Stenosis 1:30,000	>50% associated anomalies; VACTERL association most common Choking and respiratory distress on first day of life Absence of normal gastrointestinal gas pattern Stenoses may present later in life	Atresias associated with tracheo-esophageal fistula in 85% of cases Stenosis in middle one-third; usually membranous Stenosis in distal one-third; usually caused by a tracheobronchial remnant
Stomach	1:100,000	Variable; birth to childhood Prenatal history of polyhydramnios Nonbilious vomiting; single large gastric bubble "Single-bubble" sign on radiographs in cases of complete obstruction	Some cases may be associated with epidermolysis bullosa, aplasia cutis, pancreatic heterotopias, or adenomyoma
Idiopathic hypertrophic pyloric stenosis	1:500	Projectile vomiting in first weeks of life Palpable epigastric mass Associated with several multiple congenital anomalies syndromes	Concentric hyperplasia and hypertrophy of pyloric muscularis propria
Duodenum	1:1500	Most common site of intestinal stenoses Nonbilious vomiting if proximal to ampulla; bilious if distal "double-bubble" gas pattern	Atresias are usually membranous 50% stenoses associated with other anomalies including annular pancreas, or malrotation
Jejunum/ileum	1:1500	85% single; 15% multiple Rare familial forms Abdominal distension; gas-filled loops Meconium ileus is presenting feature in 20% of cases of cystic fibrosis	95% are atresias; 5% are stenoses 50% of atresias are type III with associated mesenteric defect
Anorectal	1:4000	60% associated with other malformations Imperforate anus with abnormal perineum Failure to pass meconium with cutaneous, vesicular, urethral, or vaginal (females) fistulae	High atresias more common in males, low atresias more common in females Most severe form is persistent cloaca

BOX 9.1 Disorders with Esophageal Atresia and Tracheoesophageal Fistula

Single gene disorders
- CHARGE syndrome
- Pallister-Hall syndrome
- Opitz G syndrome
- Fanconi's anemia
- VACTERL + hydrocephalus (multiple single-gene defects)

Chromosomal abnormalities
- Trisomy 13, 18, 21
- 22q11 deletion (DiGeorge's syndrome)
- Opitz syndrome
- 13 q deletion

Associations
- VACTERL association
- Oculo-auriculo-vertebral spectrum (Goldenhar's syndrome)
- Martinez-Frias syndrome

Data from de Jong EM, Felix JF, de Klein A, Tibboel D. Etiology of esophageal atresia and tracheoesophageal fistula: "mind the gap". Curr Gastroenterol Rep. 2010;12(3):215–222.

The prognosis is poorer for babies of low birth weight and with associated anomalies, especially cardiac. Postoperatively, there is risk of anastomotic leaks leading to pneumonitis and mediastinitis.[51] Gastroesophageal reflux, resulting from abnormal peristalsis, is common, occurring in up to 50% of children.[52] Motility abnormalities following successful surgical repair have been attributed to histological abnormalities of the Auerbach plexus in the distal esophagus and stomach.[53] The proximal portion of the distal esophageal segment may lack a muscularis propria. Tracheomalacia and other tracheal anomalies are also common, occurring in 75% of patients, which may, in some cases, be severe enough to require tracheostomy.[52] Ectopic gastric mucosa has been reported at the site of repair of an atresia. Chronic esophagitis and gastric metaplasia are late complications.[54]

Congenital esophageal stenosis has an incidence of about 1 in 50,000 live births and results from a congenital malformation of the esophageal wall caused by a membranous diaphragm or web[55]; intramural tumors such as pancreatic heterotopias,[56] adenomyomas, or leiomyomas[57,58]; or cartilage nodules suggestive of tracheobronchial remnants.[58] Membranous stenosis is most frequent in the middle third of the esophagus[14,51] (Fig. 9.10), and tracheobronchial remnants are most frequent in the distal portion. These are associated with other anomalies in up to one-third of cases, including tracheoesophageal fistula.[51,59] Concomitant atresias of other segments of the GI tract have been reported. Some patients with Hirschsprung's disease have congenital GI atresias and stenoses including esophageal atresia.[60] Associations with congenital pyloric stenosis,[61] duodenal atresia,[62] and biliary and anorectal atresia[63] have been reported. An autosomal recessive syndrome called *multiple gastrointestinal anomalies syndrome* consisting of atresias of the esophagus, duodenum, extrahepatic biliary tree, and anorectal area together with hypoplasia of the pancreas, malrotation of the intestines, and

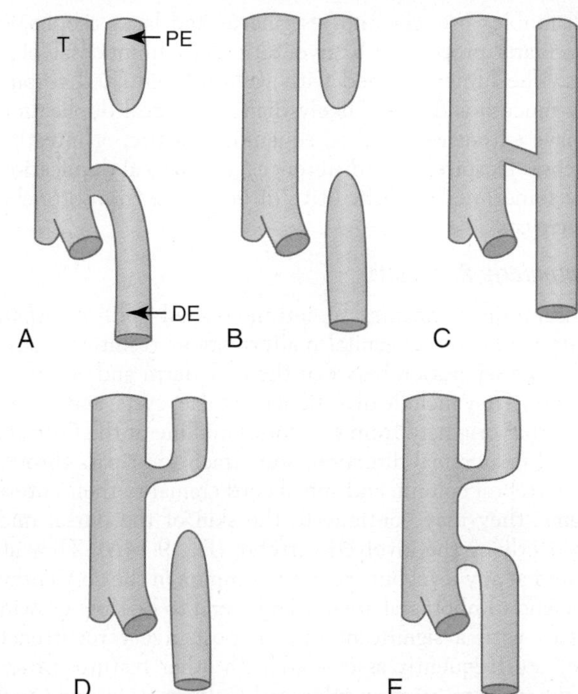

FIGURE 9.8 Types of esophageal atresia and tracheoesophageal fistula. A, Blind proximal esophageal pouch, fistula from distal trachea to distal esophageal segment (85% of cases). **B,** Esophageal atresia without a fistula, "pure esophageal atresia" (8% of cases). **C,** Tracheoesophageal fistula without esophageal atresia, "H type" or "N type" 3 fistula (4% of cases). **D,** Fistula from upper trachea to proximal esophageal pouch, blind distal esophageal segment (1% of cases). **E,** Fistula from upper trachea to proximal esophageal pouch and fistula from distal trachea to distal esophageal segment (1% of cases). *DE,* distal esophageal segment; *PE,* proximal esophageal pouch; *T,* trachea. (**C** *from Skandalakis JE, Gray SW, Ricketts R. The esophagus. In: Skandalakis JE, Gray SW, eds. Embryology for Surgeons. Baltimore: Williams & Wilkins; 1994:65-112.* **E** *data from Stocker JT. The respiratory tract. In: Stocker JT, Dahmer LP, eds. Pediatric Pathology. Philadelphia: Lippincott Williams & Wilkins; 2001:445-517; and Huff DS. Developmental anatomy and anomalies of the gastrointestinal tract, with involvement in major malformative syndromes. In: Russo P, Ruchelli E, Piccoli D, eds. Pathology of Pediatric Gastrointestinal and Liver Disease. New York: Springer; 2004:3-37.*)

hypospadias has been described.[64,65] Associated malformations of the respiratory tract include communicating[66] and noncommunicating bronchopulmonary foregut malformations,[67] abnormal pulmonary lobation, horseshoe lung,[68] pulmonary hypoplasia, and tracheobronchial malacia.[69] Unrecognized associated malformations may be the source of persistent symptoms following successful surgery. The typical symptoms, signs, and imaging features of gastric, duodenal, and jejunal atresia may be masked by a more proximal esophageal atresia.

Esophageal Cysts and Duplications

The GI malformations referred to as *duplications* represent an array of lesions with an equally confusing nomenclature. Other names used include *dorsal enteric remnants, posterior mediastinal cysts, dorsal enteric cysts, enterocysts, enterogenous cysts, neurenteric cysts, persistent neurenteric canal, diverticula, giant diverticula,* and *thoracic duplications of the intestine.* Much of the confusion results from the fact that these cysts may be lined by any type of epithelium

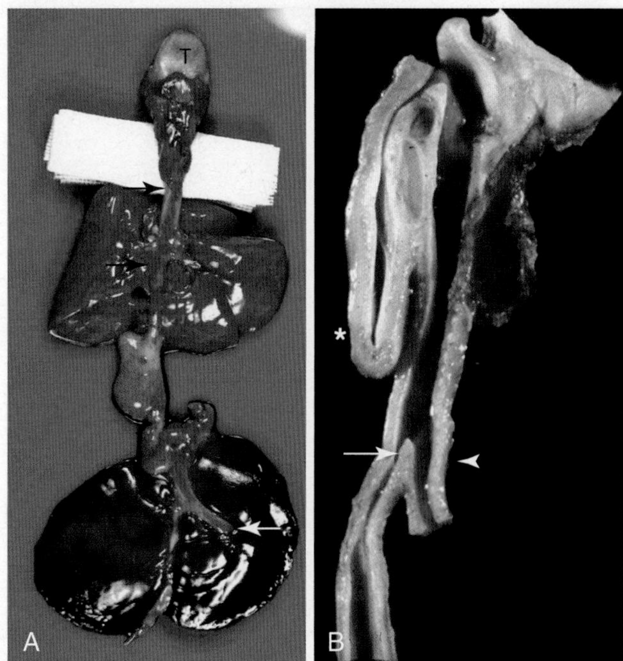

FIGURE 9.9 The most common type of esophageal atresia and tracheoesophageal fistula. A, This is a variation with a blind proximal esophageal pouch *(upper black arrow)* and a wide-mouthed fistula from the carina to the distal esophageal segment *(lower black arrow). T,* tongue. *White arrow* points to the hypoplastic gallbladder. The proximal part of the distal esophageal segment demonstrates agenesis of the muscularis propria. Tracheomalacia is present Same patient as in Figures 9.16 to 9.18. **B,** Median section of another example. The blind proximal pouch is marked with an *asterisk.* The brown structure on the right opposite the proximal pouch is the thyroid gland. The fistula from the distal trachea has a narrow mouth *(white arrow)* and a normal muscularis propria. This is a short gap lesion. *White arrow* points to the distal trachea. (*From Huff DS. Developmental anatomy and anomalies of the gastrointestinal tract, with involvement in major malformative syndromes. In: Russo P, Ruchelli E, Piccoli D, eds. Pathology of Pediatric Gastrointestinal and Liver Disease. New York: Springer; 2004:15.*)

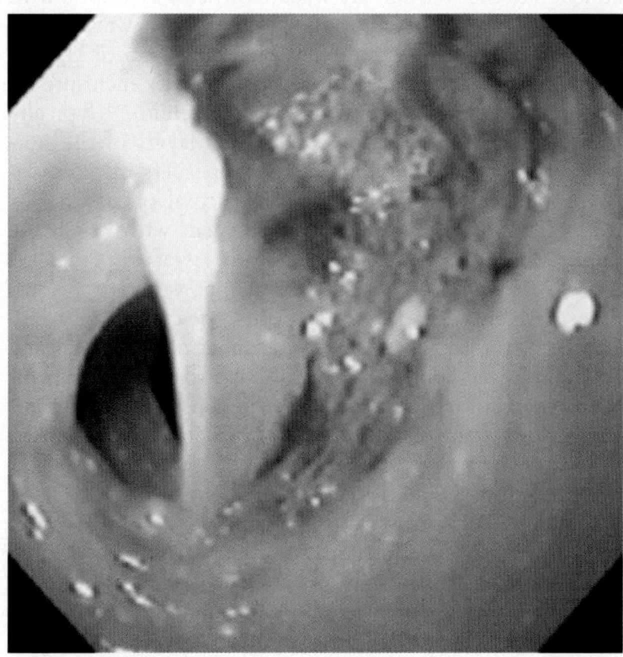

FIGURE 9.10 Esophageal stenosis. Endoscopic view of a membranous web. (*Courtesy of Dr. Petar Mamula, Division of Gastroenterology, The Children's Hospital of Philadelphia.*)

TABLE 9.9 Distributions of Gastrointestinal Duplications

Site	%
Esophageal	20
Thoracoabdominal	4
Gastric	7
Duodenal	5
Jejunoileal	44
Colonic	15
Rectal	5
TOTAL	100

May include neurenteric cysts.
From Bond SJ, Groff DB. Gastrointestinal duplications. In: O'Neill JA, et al., eds. Pediatric Surgery. *St. Louis: Mosby; 1998:1257–1267.*

derived from the alimentary or respiratory tracts. A useful and simple classification proposed by Dimmick and Hardwick[70] divides them into two groups: (1) duplications and (2) neurenteric (dorsal enteric) cysts. *Neurenteric remnant* is a more appropriate term than *neurenteric cyst* because a cyst is only one of several malformations included in this spectrum.

Duplications are cystic or tubular replicas of a segment of the GI tract. They are directly contiguous with the segment with which they are associated. Anomalies of adjacent vertebrae, spinal cord, or dorsal body wall are not present. Any segment from the mouth to the anus may be involved (Table 9.9). Cystic duplications, especially noncommunicating ones, may form an expanding intramural mass and cause stenosis or atresia with signs and symptoms of obstruction appropriate to the site. Upper esophageal duplications often produce respiratory obstruction.

Cystic duplications are partially intramural or are attached to the wall and often share muscularis propria with the involved segment. The lumen of the cyst may communicate with the normal lumen. Histological diagnostic criteria include (1) attachment to the esophagus; (2) enclosure by two muscle layers; and (3) lining by epithelium.[59] Typically the wall of the cyst is composed of all layers of the normal GI tract including inner and outer layers of muscularis propria and myenteric and submucosal plexuses (Fig. 9.11). The mucosa is that of the segment with which the duplication is associated, but heterotopias of any other GI mucosa may be present. Cysts containing various epithelial types have also been referred to as *enteric cysts* (Fig. 9.12). Gastric heterotopias are most common in esophageal and small-intestinal duplications but also may be seen in those of the anorectum. A summary of the key distinguishing characteristics of congenital intestinal cysts and duplications is presented in Table 9.10.

Tracheobronchial foregut duplications result from incomplete separation of the primitive lung bud from the foregut during the fourth to ninth week of gestation. They are located anteriorly and are usually lined by ciliated columnar epithelium; the wall may contain mucous glands and cartilage (Fig. 9.13). The rare **esophageal duplications with intramural cartilaginous heterotopias** are confused with bronchogenic cysts. Bronchogenic cysts are attached to or adjacent to the bronchial tree, not the esophagus. The wall mimics bronchus not esophagus and lacks esophageal muscularis propria with myenteric and submucosal plexuses. The lumen is lined with well-differentiated respiratory mucosa and is less likely than esophageal duplications to have extensive stratified squamous, gastric, or intestinal mucosa. Despite these differences, esophageal duplications may sometimes be difficult to differentiate from bronchogenic cysts.

Neurenteric Remnants

Neurenteric remnants, sometimes called *split notochord syndrome*,[71] are congenital malformations resulting from a failure of separation between the endoderm and ectoderm in utero. They include diverticula, fistulae, cysts, and fibrous cords that originate from the dorsal midline of the GI tract, extend in a cranial direction, and attach to or pass through the vertebral column and spinal cord cranial to their enteric origins; they may continue to the skin of the dorsal midline overlying the involved vertebra (Fig. 9.14A). They are located at any level but are most common in the cervicothoracic and lumbosacral area.[72] They tend to be slow-growing masses with a significant rate of postsurgery recurrence. They are frequently associated with other features of spinal dysraphism, such as split-cord malformations, and with vertebral anomalies.[73] The walls of the fistulae, diverticula, and cysts are composed of all of the normal layers of the gastrointestinal tract. Neuroglial and less likely leptomeningeal tissues are found in and around the lesions close to or involving the vertebra and spinal cord (see Fig. 9.14B). The mucosa may be indigenous to any segment of the GI tract, and several types may coexist. The most severe forms are part of malformation complexes that are lethal to the fetus or neonate and are diagnosed during a perinatal autopsy. Symptoms and signs in living patients relate to the GI tract, central nervous system, or midline of the back. GI manifestations are similar to those of duplications described earlier and include respiratory distress, obstruction of the GI tract, obstruction of the hepatobiliary and pancreatic ducts, and peptic ulceration with GI hemorrhage or perforation. Central nervous system manifestations include abnormal function of the spinal cord associated with its malformations or compression, infectious meningitis associated with fistulae from the GI tract or dorsal cutaneous surface to the meninges, and chemical meningitis from perforation of an intraspinal cyst.

Stomach

Congenital agastria is exceptionally rare; one case documents an esophago-duodenal junction with microscopic evidence of gastric mucosa.[74] Agastria can be part of the complex of anomalies in acephalic-acardiac fetuses. This condition is believed to be caused by an interruption in the normal vascular supply, as in the arterial disruption sequence in monozygotic twins with placental artery-artery shunts, resulting in absence of the head and heart, upper limbs, and foregut derivatives.[75] **Microgastria** is a rare malformation of the stomach that is almost always associated with multiple other congenital anomalies, including limb-reduction anomalies and the VACTERL sequence.[76-80] Children may present with a history of failure to thrive or severe gastroesophageal reflux. Nonvisualization of the stomach on prenatal ultrasound examination

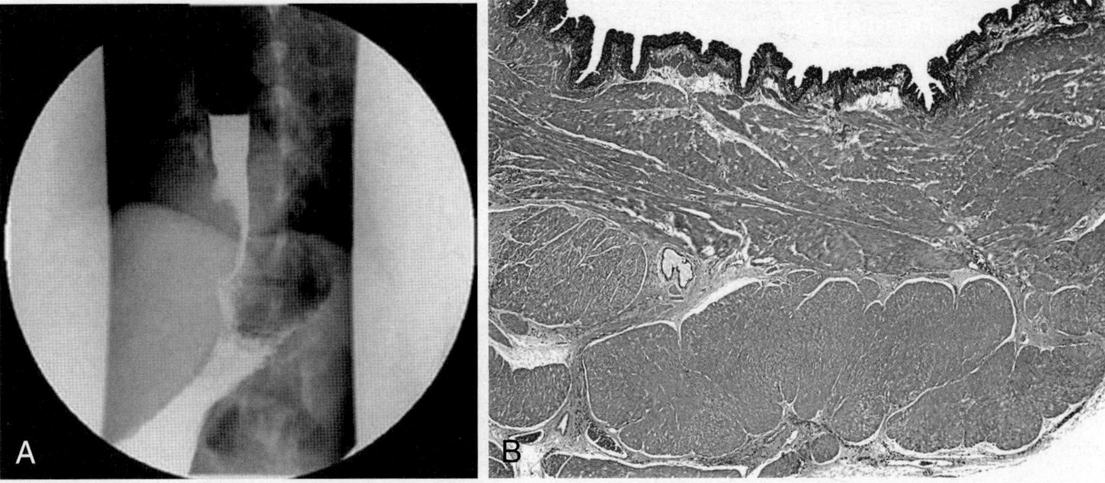

FIGURE 9.11 Esophageal duplication cyst. A, Radiograph showing a large intramural defect in the esophagus. **B,** Microscopic section of an esophageal duplication cyst from a 2-month-old boy. The wall is made up of both circular and longitudinal muscle layers; the epithelium is stratified, columnar, and focally ciliated.

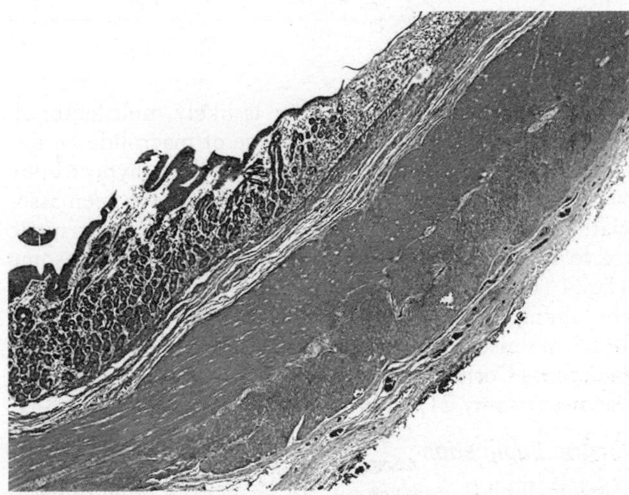

FIGURE 9.12 Microscopic section of an enteric cyst. Posterior mediastinal cyst from an 11-month-old boy is characterized by gastric mucosa and well-formed muscle layers.

may enable early diagnosis.[81] **Isolated microgastria** is extremely rare; case reports document successful treatment by gastric augmentation.[82,83] Cases can present with asplenia, hepatic symmetry, and intestinal malrotation. Microgastria is believed to result from interference with elongation of the posterior wall of the stomach, which during the fifth week grows faster than the anterior wall, forming the greater curvature. **Dextroposition** usually occurs in visceral situs inversus as part of asplenia–bilateral right-sidedness (Ivemark's syndrome). In over 50% of cases, the liver is symmetric, with the gallbladder, stomach, pancreas, and duodenum on the right side.[75] Reviews on the clinical and genetic aspects of laterality syndromes and on the genetic control of left-right symmetry in vertebrate development are available.[84-86] There are reports of isolated dextrogastria.[87,88]

Gastric Atresia and Stenosis

Atresia and stenosis of the stomach are rare. Less than 1% of all atresia and stenosis of the esophago-gastrointestinal tract are gastric.[89] Most involve the prepyloric antrum or the pylorus. The body is rarely involved. Most are membranous. Segmental stenosis of the body may result in an "hourglass" stomach. Pyloric atresia associated with epidermolysis bullosa results from healing of a circumferential mucosal injury by exuberant granulation tissue that fuses the apposed mucosal surfaces, occluding the narrow pyloric channel, and matures into fibrous tissue.[90,91] It is caused by mutations in the *ITGA6* and *ITGB4* genes, which code for the corresponding units of α6β4 integrin, an adhesion molecule expressed in a variety of epithelia, including the epidermis and GI tract, where it forms an integral part of the hemidesmosomes.[92] Rarely a large intramural pyloric pancreatic heterotopia or adenomyoma causes pyloric obstruction.[93]

More than 50% of patients with gastric atresia have a history of polyhydramnios. Patients with atresia or severe stenosis present with persistent nonbilious vomiting following the first feeding. Excessive salivation may mimic that of esophageal atresia. The first stools are less voluminous than usual, and subsequent stools decrease in volume and disappear. A single large gastric gas bubble and absence of an intestinal gas pattern are present at birth. Patients with mild stenosis may have less severe symptoms at birth resulting in delayed diagnosis. The symptoms may be delayed for several years, making differentiation between congenital and acquired stenosis difficult. Most isolated nonsyndromic cases are sporadic, but some are familial with an autosomal recessive inheritance pattern. A few are associated with some of the disorders of multiple GI atresias and stenoses listed in Table 9.7. Pyloric atresia with atresia of the small intestine and colon is a recognized association.[94]

Infantile hypertrophic pyloric stenosis (IHPS) is a clinical-pathological entity distinct from congenital pyloric atresias and stenoses. Some reports may have applied the name *infantile hypertrophic pyloric stenosis* to the congenital pyloric atresias and stenoses discussed earlier, causing confusion between the two.[95] IHPS arises postnatally and is the most common surgical condition causing nonbilious emesis in infancy. The incidence ranges

TABLE 9.10 Congenital Intestinal Cysts and Diverticula

Anomaly	Embryological Origin	Key Clinical Features	Key Pathological Features
Duplication cyst	Unknown	May be cystic or tubular 40% occur in terminal ileum Attached to dorsal or mesenteric side of intestinal segment May be intramural	Composed of normal intestinal muscle layers with nerve plexuses Epithelial lining may be stratified squamous, ciliated columnar, gastric, or enteric
Neurenteric remnant (aka *enteric cyst*)	Persistence of neurenteric canal	Posterior cyst, sinus, or fistula extending to or involving spinal cord Most common in cervical or lumbar area Vertebral anomalies in 50% Overlying cutaneous hyperpigmentation or hypertrichosis	Composed of normal layers of gastrointestinal tract in association with neuroglial tissue
Tracheobronchial foregut duplication cyst	Incomplete separation of lung bud from foregut	Anterior mediastinum	Wall may contain mucous glands or cartilage Epithelial lining is ciliated columnar
Intestinal diverticulum	Remnant of omphalomesenteric duct	Located on antimesenteric portion of intestinal segment Most frequent in terminal ileum (Meckel's diverticulum)	Composed of all layers of the intestinal wall. Mucosa enteric with frequent heterotopias

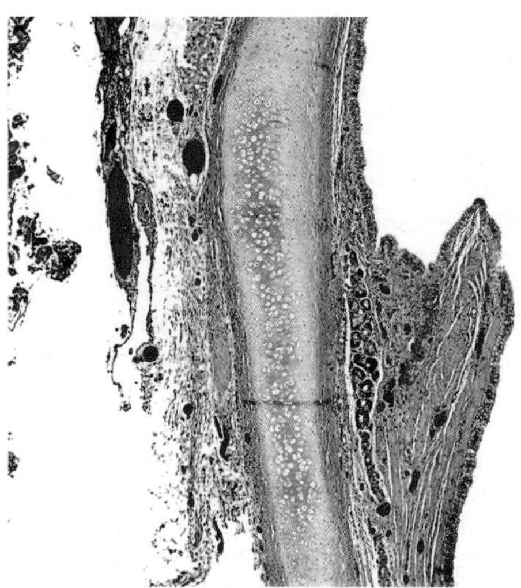

FIGURE 9.13 Microscopic section from a foregut duplication cyst from the anterior mediastinum of an 11-year-old boy is characterized by respiratory epithelium with cartilage and mucous glands in the wall.

from about 0.5 to 4 in 1000 live births, the differences in incidence probably largely related to differences in ascertainment.[96] Intrauterine and neonatal imaging studies detect no pyloric abnormalities in babies who subsequently develop IHPS, and the lesion has been rarely diagnosed in a fetus. The pathology is characterized by concentric hyperplasia, hypertrophy, fibrosis, and elastosis of the pyloric muscularis, especially the circular layer, sometimes with mucosal erosions and inflammation. The clinical presentation is characterized by the onset of projectile vomiting at 3 to 5 weeks of age and visible gastric peristaltic waves. A palpable epigastric mass with the size and consistency of an olive and a distinctive appearance on ultrasound examination is usually present. It is more often familial and has a higher male-to-female ratio than congenital lesions. The disorder is likely multifactorial. Gastric acid hypersecretion and use of macrolide antibiotics producing hyperperistalsis and pyloric hypertrophy have been postulated.[97] Five genetic loci have been associated with IHPS, including the gene coding for nitric oxide synthase (NOS), *IHPS1*, located on chromosome 12q24 (for a review, consult[96]). Abnormalities of NOS-containing neurons had been demonstrated in IHPS.[98] IHPS has also been described in a number of syndromes including Cornelia de Lange's syndrome, Apert's syndrome, trisomy 21, and trisomy 18.

Gastric Duplication

Foregut duplications account for about 35% of all duplications of the GI tract, with gastric duplications accounting for about 7% (see Box 9.1). Gastric duplications involve the greater curvature. They generally do not communicate with the gastric lumen. Gastric duplication cysts are most often lined by gastric or enteric-type epithelium, though respiratory epithelium can be observed.[99] Associated anomalies, including duplications in other parts of the GI tract, are common.[100]

Neonatal Gastric Perforation

Neonatal gastric perforation can be categorized as spontaneous or traumatic. Spontaneous cases are associated with asphyxia, very low birth weight, necrotizing enterocolitis, steroid use, or they are idiopathic. There also appears to be an association with other GI malformations such as midgut volvulus and intestinal atresia.[101] Truly idiopathic cases are rare and appear to be associated with prematurity[102] and infection of the gastric wall with invasive *Candida* or *Staphylococcus*.[103] An abnormal distribution of pacemaker cells in the gastric wall resulting in hypomotility has been postulated in some cases.[104] Traumatic cases are usually the result of gastric intubation. Infants present with abdominal distension, respiratory distress, and pneumoperitoneum.[105]

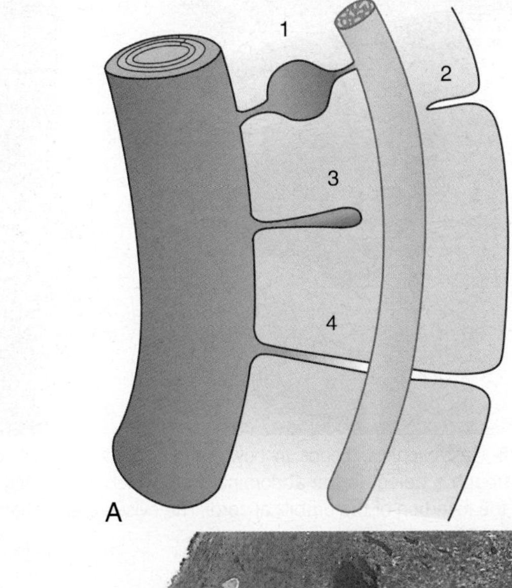

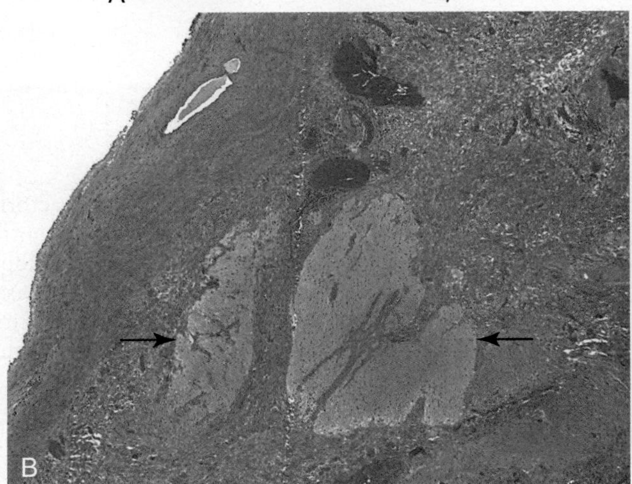

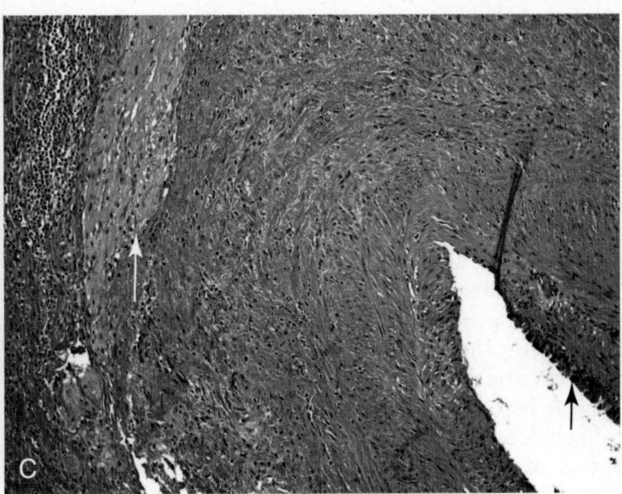

FIGURE 9.14 **A,** Dorsal enteric remnants. **B,** Microscopic section of a neurenteric cyst from a 1-year-old child. The wall of the cyst is that of gastrointestinal tissue with islands of neuroglial tissue *(arrows)*. The epithelial lining has been mostly eroded but consists of a low cuboidal to focally columnar epithelium. **C,** Higher-power view from the remnant shows the enteric lining of the cyst *(black arrow)* next to an island of glial tissue *(white arrow)*. (**A** *from Dimmick JE, Hardwick DF. Gastrointestinal system and exocrine pancreas. In: Dimmick JE, Kalousek DK, eds. Developmental Pathology of the Embryo and Fetus. Philadelphia: JB Lippincott; 1992:509-544.*)

Small and Large Intestine

Hernias and Abdominal Wall Defects

Hernias represent a heterogeneous group of disorders that frequently involve the GI tract (Box 9.2). The first three are discussed here as they are most frequently confused with each other and are particularly relevant to the developing intestinal tract. Recent studies have suggested an increasing prevalence of omphalocele and gastroschisis in the United States and elsewhere, a significant finding given the relatively high mortality rate associated with these conditions.[106]

Omphalocele (Exomphalos)

An *omphalocele* is a defect of the anterior abdominal wall at the insertion of the umbilical cord, occurring in 1 in 5000 to 1 in 20,000 live births, but is probably higher if stillbirths and aborted fetuses are included.[107] The umbilical cord at the site of the defect is replaced by a sac formed of amnion and peritoneum that contains intestinal loops and sometimes parts of the liver (Fig. 9.15). The size of the defect can range in size from a few centimeters to defects that involve a major portion of the anterior abdominal wall. Muscle, fascia, and skin are absent at the site of the defect.[108] It is associated most characteristically with Beckwith-Wiedemann syndrome and with various trisomies as well as numerous single-gene defects.[109,110] The cause is unknown but likely involves failure of abdominal wall closure when the intestines return to the abdominal cavity. An association with maternal smoking during pregnancy has been found.[111,112] Most cases are now diagnosed on prenatal ultrasonography. The prognosis depends on associated malformations. Successful surgical treatment usually involves excision of the membrane and covering of the exposed viscera in a Silastic bag with progressive re-integration of the contents into the

BOX 9.2 Types of Hernias in Children

- Omphalocele (exomphalos)
- Cloacal exstrophy
- Gastroschisis (laparoschisis)
- Congenital diaphragmatic hernia
- Hernia of Morgagni
- Inguinal hernia
- Femoral hernia
- Umbilical hernia
- Epigastric hernia

From Tovar JA. Chapter 33. Hernias. In: Pediatric Gastrointestinal Disease. *Walker AW, et al., eds. 2004, Hamilton, Ontario: BC Decker; 2004:573–588.*

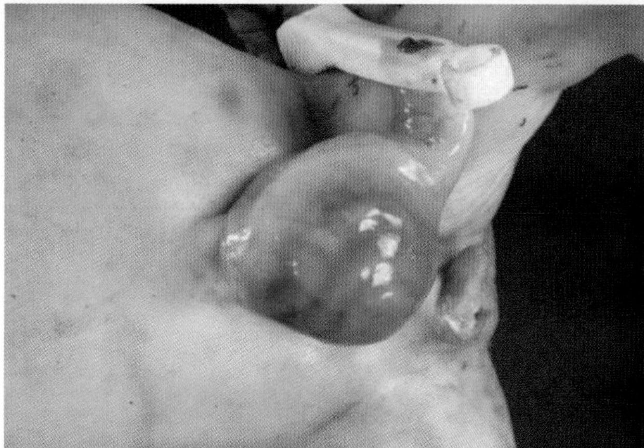

FIGURE 9.15 Omphalocele. The sac is located at the site of insertion of the umbilical cord and is covered by amnion. Loops of bowel can be observed within the sac.

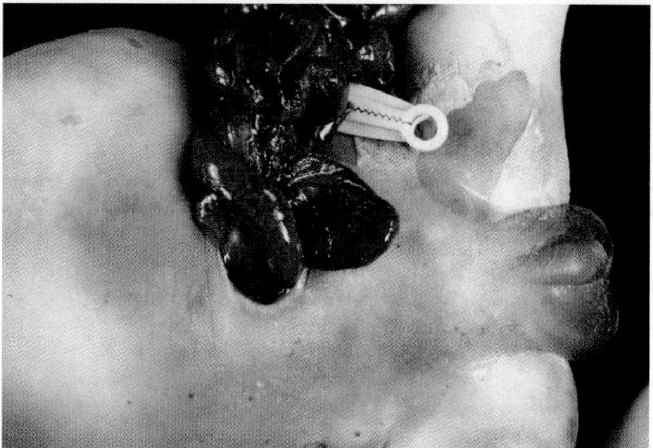

FIGURE 9.16 Gastroschisis. Loops of bowel and a portion of liver extravasate through a defect in the abdominal wall, which lies slightly to the right of the insertion of the umbilical cord. The eviscerated contents are not covered by a sac.

abdominal cavity.[107] Intestinal necrosis resulting in short bowel syndrome is a major complication.

Gastroschisis (Laparoschisis)

Gastroschisis results from a small (generally less than 5 cm) defect of the abdominal wall just to the right of the umbilical cord insertion, allowing evisceration of bowel loops, stomach, and sometimes the gonads (Fig. 9.16). It is distinguished from an omphalocele by the absence of a sac covering the eviscerated contents and by a normal insertion of the cord. The condition has a prevalence of about 1 in 10,000 live births, with an increase in the past 30 years and which is probably higher if stillbirths and aborted fetuses are included.[107] Its etiology is unknown; occlusion or disruption of the right omphalomesenteric artery has been proposed.[113] Exchanges between the fetal internal environment and the amniotic fluid in utero results in fetal malnutrition and growth restriction, and exposes the serosa of the loops to inflammation-generating substances, resulting in edema and thickening of the loops.[107] Associated malformations and abnormal karyotypes are less frequent than those seen in infants with omphalocele. As the majority of cases are now detected by prenatal ultrasonography, prenatal interventions, such as repeated amniotic fluid exchange to remove inflammatory compounds in the amniotic fluid, have been proposed.[114] Elective cesarian delivery by 36 weeks of life with early primary surgical repair appears to be the treatment of choice.[115] Interruption of vascular flow in utero to a portion of the bowel may result in focal atresia. An intraabdominal "compartment" syndrome may develop after surgical repair as a result of to increased intraabdominal pressure and decreased vascular perfusion, leading to necrosis of variable lengths of bowel.[107]

Cloacal Exstrophy

Cloacal exstrophy is a very rare malformation that appears to result from rupture of the cloacal membrane and failure of descent of the urorectal septum.[116] An omphalocele protrudes through a major defect in the abdominal wall, containing an exteriorized bladder and prolapsed ileum. There is an imperforate anus and many other abnormalities, including abnormal and ambiguous genitalia, separated pubic bones, and vertebral anomalies.

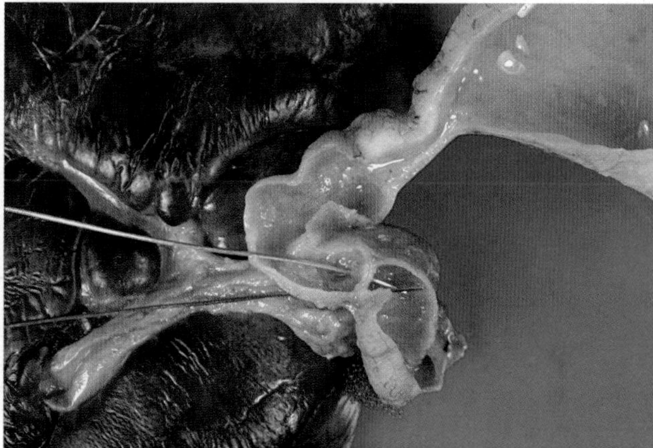

FIGURE 9.17 Membranous duodenal stenosis at the level of the ampulla of Vater. The upper probe goes through a tiny orifice in the membrane. The lower probe is in the ampulla.

Congenital Atresias and Stenoses

Approximately 75% of all intestinal stenoses and 40% of all intestinal atresias are **duodenal** (see Table 9.6). Intrinsic duodenal atresias and stenoses most often involve the first and second portions, the foregut portion of the duodenum, in close proximity to the entrances of the biliary and pancreatic ducts. This explains the association of duodenal atresia with hepatobiliary and pancreatic duct abnormalities.[117] Approximately 75% of duodenal stenoses are immediately distal to the ampulla. The majority are membranous (Fig. 9.17). Those of the third and fourth portions are often at the duodeno-jejunal junction and are associated with malrotation and midgut volvulus. Ladd's bands, resulting from incomplete absorption of the cecal and ascending colon mesenteries, can cause external compression and stenosis of the duodenum; they are usually associated with malrotation, preduodenal portal vein, and superior mesenteric artery syndrome.

Polyhydramnios and prematurity are common in patients with duodenal atresia. Vomiting begins at birth and is nonbilious if the obstruction is proximal to the ampulla of Vater and bilious if the obstruction is distal to the ampulla.

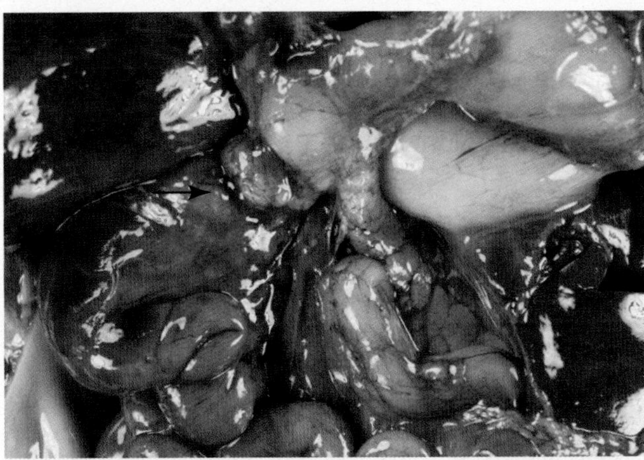

FIGURE 9.18 Annular pancreas in a 17-day-old baby girl who presented with signs of duodenal obstruction. Polyhydramnios was noted during the pregnancy. A ring of pancreas *(arrow)* completely surrounds the second portion of duodenum.

Intrauterine bilious vomiting may be associated with ulcers of the umbilical cord, necrosis of adjacent umbilical vessels, and fatal fetal hemorrhage into the amniotic fluid. The presence of ulcers of the umbilical cord should lead to the suspicion of duodenal or proximal jejunal atresia–stenosis distal to the ampulla.[118] The classic radiographic double-bubble sign, a dilated gas-filled duodenum proximal to the obstruction separated by the pylorus from a dilated gas-filled stomach, may not be seen if atresia of the esophagus or stomach is also present. The symptoms and signs of less severe stenoses may be mild and delayed, leading to delayed diagnosis and confusion with acquired obstruction. Over 50% of patients have additional congenital anomalies.[119] These include annular pancreas in 33% and malrotation in 28%,[120] both of which may be familial.

Annular pancreas is a complete encirclement of the second part of the duodenum by pancreatic tissue (Fig. 9.18). It occurs with a frequency of 1 in 20,000 live births.[121] When manifest in infancy, it is associated with other anomalies in 75% of cases, including trisomy 21, tracheoesophageal fistula, and cardiac anomalies.[122] The age at presentation is determined by the severity of obstruction and by associated anomalies, with one-third of cases presenting in the neonatal period, one-third during infancy, and one-third later in life.[121] Symptoms in older children and adults may include recurrent vomiting caused by partial obstruction as well as pain due to gastritis and peptic ulcers.[121] Peptic symptoms result from gastric overdistension caused by the partial obstruction, with consequent hypergastrinemia, hyperchlorhydria, and ulceration.[123] The histology of the pancreas is unremarkable.

Any type of atresia or stenosis can occur in the **jejunum** and **ileum**. Approximately 95% are atresias, and 5% are stenoses. Type I atresias in which the mucosa and submucosa form an obstructing web or diaphragm account for 19%, type II atresias in which the blind ends are connected by a cord account for 31%, and atresias with no connection between the blind ends and with a defect in the mesentery (type III) account for 46% (Fig. 9.19A,B). Although the jejunum and ileum are approximately equally involved, approximately one-third involve the proximal jejunum, one-third involve the distal ileum, and the remaining one-third involve all other segments. Approximately 85% are single, and 15% are multiple. These figures vary from study to study.[120,124]

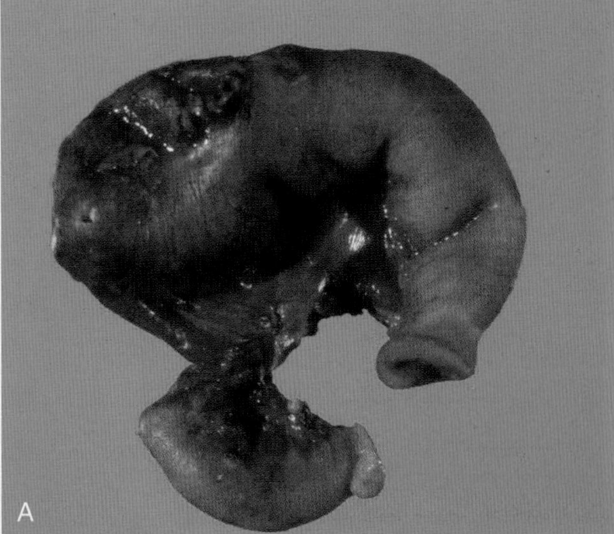

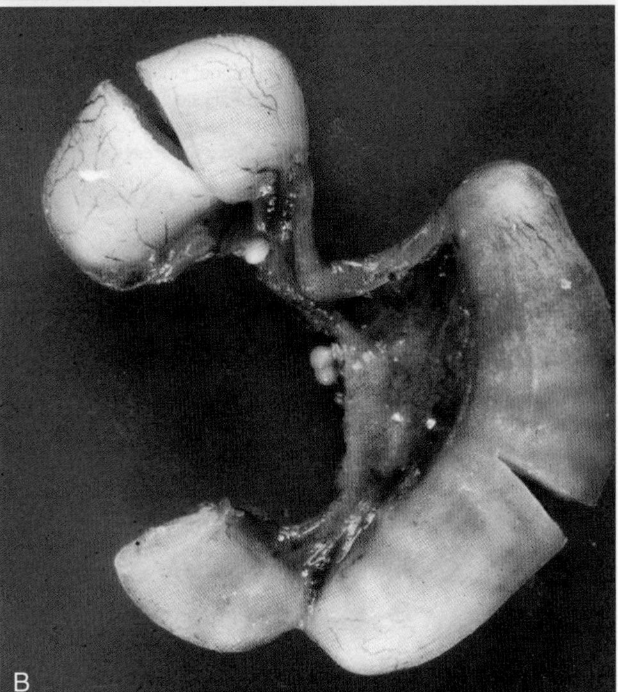

FIGURE 9.19 Intestinal atresia. A, Two blind-ended segments connected by a portion of mesentery. The dilated proximal segment has ruptured. **B,** Multiple intestinal atresias.

Two additional types are unique to the small intestine. The first is multiple atresias with a gross pathological appearance that has been appropriately described as a "string of sausages" or "string of beads" (Fig. 9.20A). The radiographic appearance has been described as a "string of pearls."[125] Histological examination reveals multifocal atresia with a sievelike multiple intestinal lumen caused by multiple mucosal adhesions (Fig. 9.20B). The total length of the small bowel is extremely short. This condition is familial and autosomal recessive in many cases. Some have been associated with severe congenital immunodeficiency.[126,127] Whole-exome sequencing in these

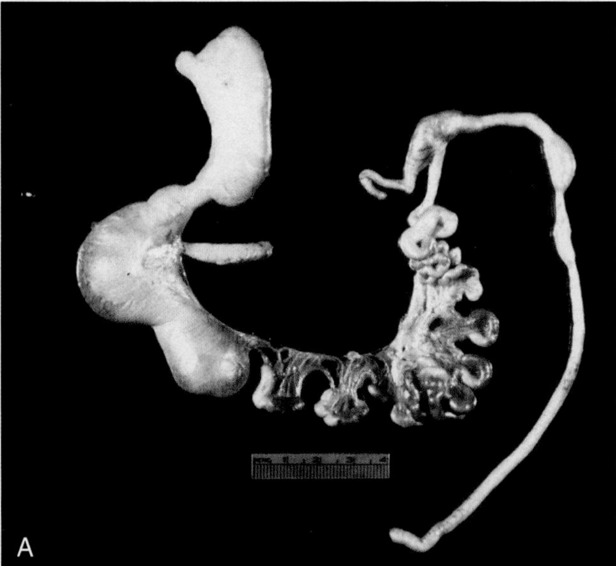

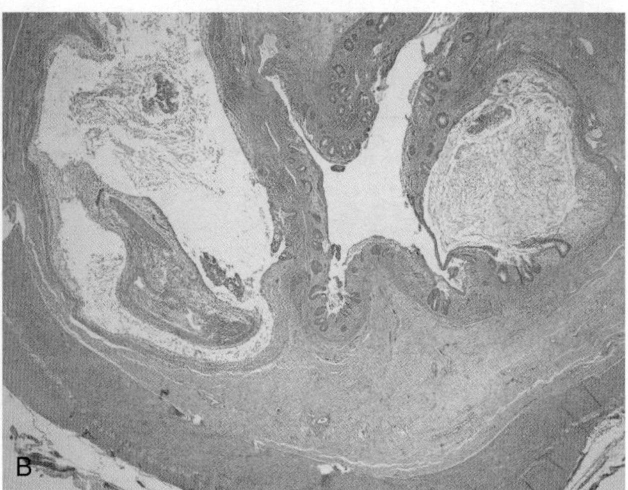

FIGURE 9.20 Multiple intestinal atresias or "string of sausages." A, The gastrointestinal tract from the distal esophagus to the distal rectum is displayed. The first atresia is at the duodenal jejunal junction, and the duodenum is severely dilated. The ends of the atretic segments are connected by fibrous cords. The bowel is extremely short. **B,** Histological section from the bowel of a 4-month-old boy with TTC7A deficiency showing multiple sieve-like lumens. (**A** *from Huff DS. Developmental anatomy and anomalies of the gastrointestinal tract, with involvement in major malformative syndromes. In: Russo P, Ruchelli E, Piccoli D, eds. Pathology of Pediatric Gastrointestinal and Liver Disease. New York: Springer; 2004:3-37.*)

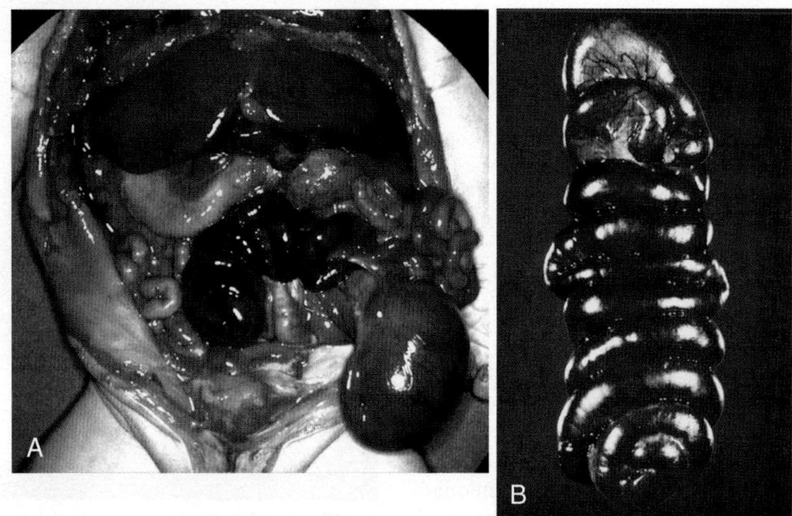

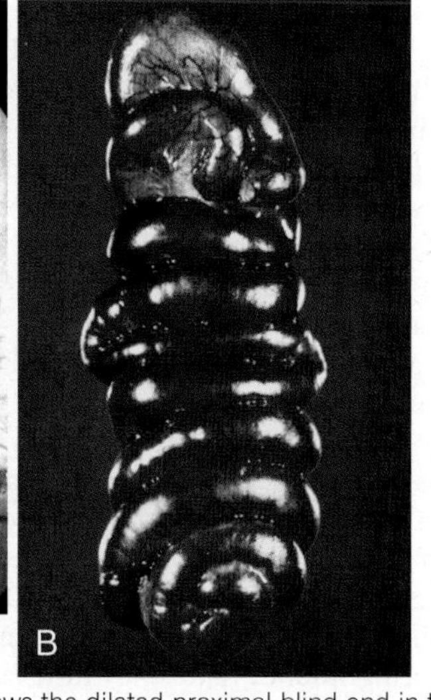

FIGURE 9.21 Apple peel or Christmas tree atresia and heterotaxy. A, In situ view shows the dilated proximal blind end in the left lower abdomen, the spiraled, dusky blind distal end in the lower mid-abdomen, absence of the mesentery between the two blind ends, the stomach on the right, a symmetric liver, a midline gallbladder, and a preduodenal portal vein. **B,** The apple peel. (*From Huff DS. Developmental anatomy and anomalies of the gastrointestinal tract, with involvement in major malformative syndromes. In: Russo P, Ruchelli E, Piccoli D, eds. Pathology of Pediatric Gastrointestinal and Liver Disease. New York: Springer; 2004:3-37.*)

cases has identified a mutation in the gene tetratricopeptide repeat domain-7A *(TTC7A)* located on chromosome 2p21.[128] The second unique type is the apple core or Christmas tree atresia (Fig. 9.21). A long segment of jejunum and ileum is missing between the two blind ends that are not connected by a fibrous chord, and there is a large defect in the mesentery. The dilated proximal blind end is similar to that of any atresia, but the distal blind segment is spiraled like an apple peel around retrograde mesenteric arteries from the ileocolic, right colic, or inferior mesenteric artery. This atresia is also often familial and autosomal recessive[129] and is more frequently associated with other malformations than the usual types of jejunoileal atresia.

The clinical presentation of proximal jejunal atresia–stenosis is similar to that of duodenal atresia–stenosis distal to the ampulla. The more distal the obstruction, the less likely are polyhydramnios, immediate bilious vomiting at birth, and jaundice and the more likely are generalized abdominal distention and early obstipation. Radiographically, proximal lesions are characterized by a few dilated loops of bowel with air-fluid levels, and distal lesions are characterized by numerous such loops. Associated congenital anomalies are less common than with atresia and stenoses in the esophagus, duodenum, rectum, and anus because many are caused by disruptions in fetuses who had normal development during blastogenesis and organogenesis. There are many associated disorders.[130] In Caucasian infants, the risk for cystic fibrosis is more than 210 times higher in those with jejunoileal atresia than in those without the atresia.[131]

Colonic atresia or stenosis is rare. It may be part of any multiple GI atresia syndrome (see Table 9.7). Atresia of the ileum[132] or colon is seen in association with syndromic or nonsyndromic Hirschsprung's disease.[133] The clinical presentation is usually that of rapidly progressive abdominal distension. Failure to pass meconium is common. No meconium is found in the rectum, which instead contains mucus. Radiographs demonstrate numerous loops of distended bowel, some with air-fluid levels and a low cutoff point. The presenting symptoms, signs, and radiographic changes of colonic atresia may be masked by an associated jejunoileal atresia.

Malrotation

Failure of the normal process of rotation and return to the abdomen of the intestinal loops may occur at any stage along the process. Normal rotation is probably a gradual continuous process, except for the return of the intestine to the abdomen and completion of the rotation, which are abrupt. Abnormalities of rotation do not correspond to any position encountered during normal rotation,[11] and each case has a somewhat unique anatomy. Despite this, many authors find that use of a simplification of the thorough classification of Estrada[10] facilitates description of these malformations. The three types frequently listed are nonrotation, mixed rotation, and reverse rotation. The position of the third portion of the duodenum relative to the superior mesenteric artery is crucial in differentiating them from normal and from each other. Complete failure of rotation, or **nonrotation**, results in a right-sided jejunum and ileum, a low mid-abdominal cecum, and a colon residing in the left abdomen. Incomplete or **mixed** rotation, which is more common, results in the small bowel occupying mainly the right side of the abdomen, with the cecum generally residing in the right upper quadrant (Fig. 9.22). All are associated with a short mesenteric attachment and midgut volvulus. With mixed rotation, the volvulus may occur in the first few days of life, while in the others symptoms may be delayed or intermittent. The short mesenteric attachment can lead to twisting of the midgut around the pedicle of the superior mesenteric artery, with consequent bowel obstruction and vascular compromise. An unattached cecum, ascending colon, and hepatic flexure may be associated with Ladd's bands binding the hepatic flexure to the third portion of the duodenum and to the right abdominal wall, sometimes resulting in duodenal obstruction. **Reverse rotation** is the rarest type and occurs consequent to the two following errors of re-entry of the bowel loops following the combined 270-degree counterclockwise rotation outside the abdominal cavity: (1) if the postarterial segment returns first, the small bowel lies ventral to the colon and superior mesenteric artery, and the colon behind. This may result in compression of the mesenteric arterial flow[134]; (2) if the pre-arterial segment returns first, the colon will occupy the right half of the abdomen, and the small bowel will lie in the left side. These cases can be associated with situs anomalies of other organs.[135,136]

Abnormal fixation and abnormal mesenteries of various segments form internal hernias. Right and left mesocolic hernias are two common forms. An unusually long mesentery of an unfixed cecum and ascending colon attached along or to the right of the midline may be so redundant as to form an internal hernia pouch called a *right mesocolic hernia*. If, as in the case of nonrotation, the small bowel is in the right side of the abdomen, then the small bowel can become entrapped in the right mesocolic internal hernia, resulting in obstruction and strangulation. Similarly, an unusually long mesentery of an unfixed descending colon attached along the left side of the abdomen may be so redundant as to form a left mesocolic internal hernia (Fig. 9.23). If the small bowel is located in the left abdomen, it can become entrapped in the left mesocolic hernia, resulting in obstruction and strangulation.

Malrotation occurs in about 3 in 10,000 live births and fetal deaths,[137] and 60% to 90% have associated malformations.[137-139]

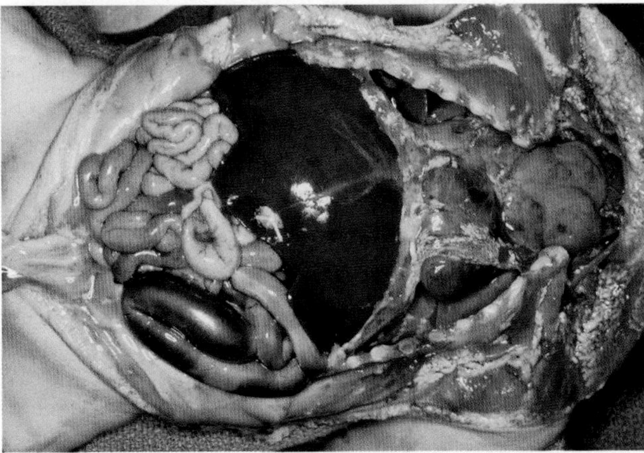

FIGURE 9.22 Malrotation of incomplete or mixed type. The small bowel lies mostly in the right abdomen, and the colon in the left. The cecum and appendix are visible in the right upper quadrant.

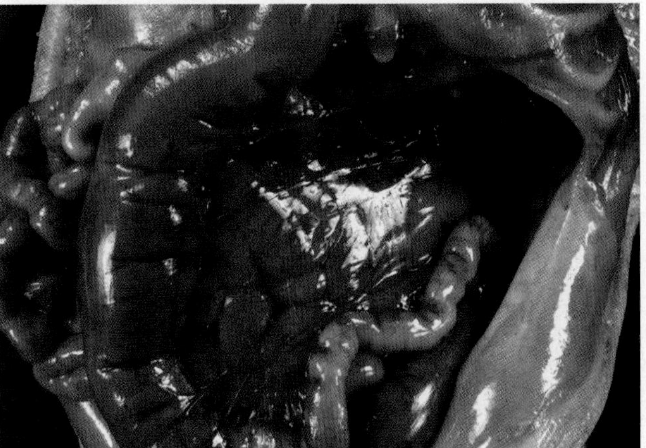

FIGURE 9.23 Term female patient with trisomy 9 and multiple congenital anomalies. She had incomplete rotation of the bowel with the small intestine located mainly in the right portion of the abdomen. The descending colon is unfixed and has a long mesenteric attachment.

Duplications

As with foregut duplications, intestinal duplications are directly contiguous with the segment with which they are associated. They can occur anywhere along the GI tract, although the ileum is the most frequent site.[135] Duplications are dorsal to the intestine, usually mesenteric, and sometimes intramural.[140] Duodenal duplications involve the concave medial border of the second portion adjacent to the hepatobiliary and pancreatic ductal systems. Cystic duodenal duplications may clinically mimic choledochal cysts, cysts of the pancreatic duct, or pancreatic pseudocysts. Jejunal, ileal, and colonic duplications may cause intussusception or volvulus.

Tubular duplications may be short or involve entire segments such as the entire esophagus and stomach combined or the distal ileum, cecum, entire colon, and anus. Most are attached along the dorsal or mesenteric border (Fig. 9.24). Some are attached to the lateral border forming parallel, side-by-side segments referred to as *double barrel duplications*. Rarely the duplication has a separate mesentery and blood supply and is called a *loop duplication*. Communications between the lumen of a tubular duplication and the normal lumen are common and may be located at the proximal or distal end of the duplication or at both ends. Multiple communications may occur. Double-barrel duplications of the colon, rectum, and anus are associated with duplications of part or all of the genitourinary tracts and external genitalia forming symmetrical or asymmetrical right and left GI and genitourinary tracts and perineums. A tubular duplication with a proximal communication and a blind distal end forms an expanding mass that may obstruct the normal lumen or adjacent structures. Similarly, a **cystic** duplication may also cause obstruction of the involved segment

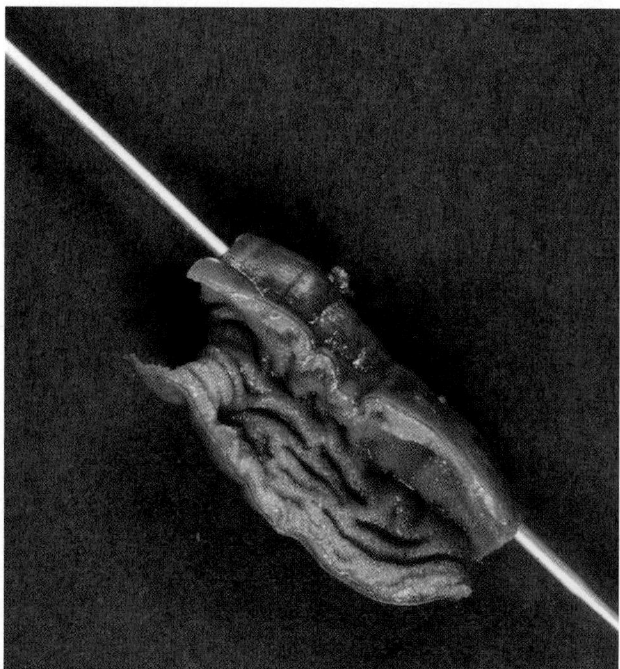

FIGURE 9.24 Tubular duplication, jejunum. The probe passes through a tubular duplication extending along the mesenteric side of the resected segment.

(Fig. 9.25). The wall of a duplication is usually thick with well-formed muscle layers. The epithelial lining may consist of gastric, intestinal, or respiratory-type epithelium and may contain heterotopic pancreatic rests. Complete excision is the treatment of choice. The embryogenesis of duplications is not well understood. An abnormally exuberant proliferative phase, defective resolution of the proliferative phase, and persistence of the normal transient diverticula seen in embryos are some possibilities. Some may be caused by mild abnormalities of development of the notochord, neurenteric canal, and related structures of the midline developmental field, and therefore may be a forme fruste of neurenteric cysts.

Congenital Diverticula, Including Omphalomesenteric Remnants and Meckel's Diverticulum

GI diverticula can be divided into mesenteric and antimesenteric diverticula. Mesenteric diverticula are thought to be primarily related to the neurenteric remnants and duplications discussed earlier. Antimesenteric diverticula are with few exceptions part of the spectrum of omphalomesenteric remnants that includes Meckel's diverticulum and is summarized in Table 9.11 and Figure 9.26.

The omphalomesenteric (vitelline) duct is the last point to close after separation of the intestine from the yolk sac, usually by the 10th week of embryonic life.[108] The entire duct may remain patent and may drain intestinal contents at the umbilicus. The more common **Meckel's diverticulum** results from persistence of the vitelline duct immediately adjacent to the bowel wall; it occurs in approximately 2% of individuals and accounts for approximately 90% of all omphalomesenteric remnants. The other variations are rare and are listed in Table 9.10. The remnants are located from 15 to 167 cm proximal to the ileocecal valve, but most are 40 cm from the valve.[141] Seventy-five percent of diverticula are from 1 to 5 cm long, but some are up to 26 cm long.[142] Meckel's diverticula are composed of all layers of the normal intestinal wall as are most cysts and fistulae. The mucosa is ileal. Heterotopias are common. Gastric mucosa is seen in half of all Meckel's diverticula (Fig. 9.27), in 62% of those with diverticulitis, in one-third of fistulae, and occasionally in umbilical polyps. In diverticula, 94% of the gastric heterotopias are of fundal type; in fistulae and umbilical polyps, 70% are fundal.[143] Pancreatic heterotopias are found in 5% of Meckel's diverticula, where they can often be identified at the tip by gross examination and occasionally in umbilical polyps.[45] Duodenal, colonic, and rarely biliary mucosa can be found. Omphalomesenteric remnants can be distinguished from urachal remnants by the presence of columnar or intestinal epithelium in the former, whereas the latter are lined by transitional epithelium.

Twenty-five percent of omphalomesenteric remnants are symptomatic.[144] Fundal-type gastric mucosa causes ulcers that present with pain, hemorrhage, and perforation leading to peritonitis. Meckel's diverticulitis mimics appendicitis. Intussusception, volvulus around a solid cord or vascular remnant to the umbilicus, incarceration by a fibrous cord or vascular remnant, or a knot formed by a long diverticulum around a loop of intestine will all lead to obstruction. Fistulae may drain intestinal contents and mucus at

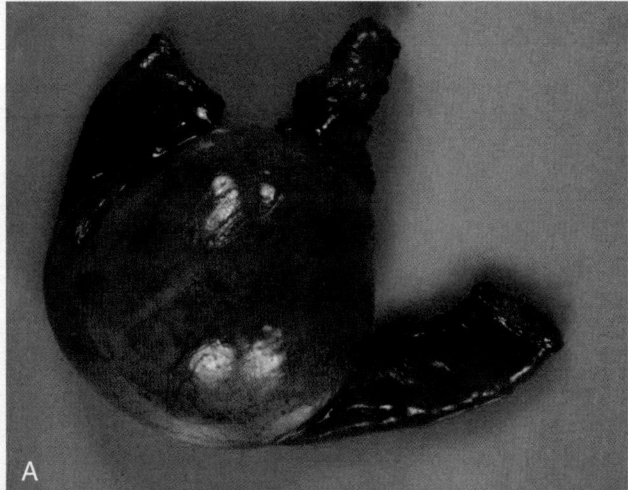

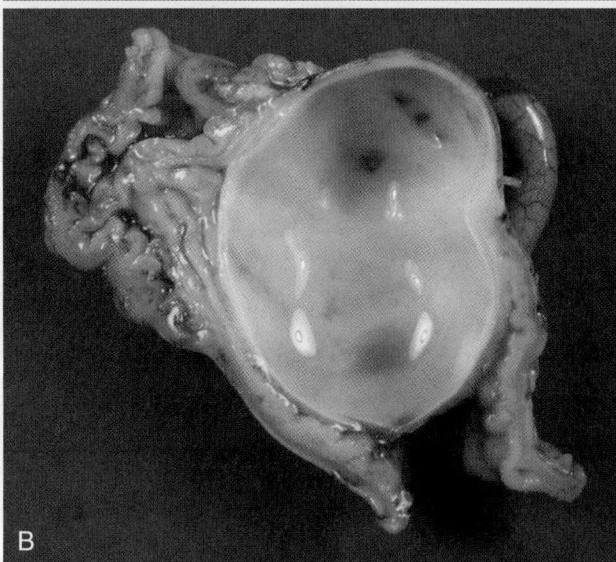

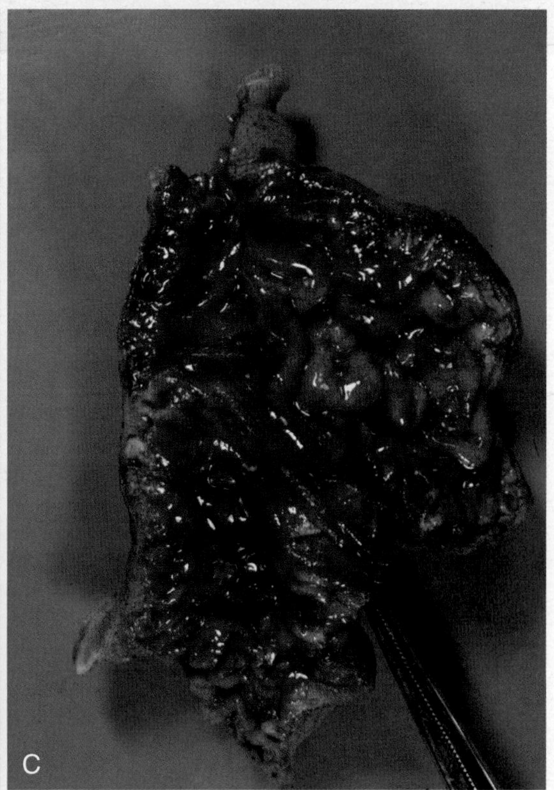

FIGURE 9.25 A, Cystic duplication of the ileum causing obstruction. **B,** Opened cystic duplication with a smooth lining that histologically consisted of a flattened enteric epithelium. **C,** Opened segment of ileum with a communicating duplication containing gastric mucosa with prominent rugal folds.

TABLE 9.11 The Spectrum of Omphalomesenteric Remnants

	%*
Meckel's diverticulum	90
Tip unattached	
Tip attached to umbilicus	
Tip attached to mesentery	
Solid cord	5
Fistula	3
Cyst	1
Intraabdominal within solid cord	
In abdominal wall at umbilicus	
Umbilical remnant	1
Umbilical polyp	
Umbilical sinus	
Total	100
Omphalomesenteric vessel remnants	
From mesentery to umbilicus	
From Meckel's diverticulum to umbilicus	
From Meckel's diverticulum to mesentery	

**Percentages are estimates.*

Data from Huff DS. Developmental anatomy and anomalies of the gastrointestinal tract, with involvement in major malformative syndromes. In: Russo P, Ruchelli E, Piccoli D, eds. Pathology of Pediatric Gastrointestinal and Liver Disease. *2nd ed. New York: Springer; 2014:3–37; Moses WR. Meckel's diverticulum: a report of 2 unusual cases.* N Engl J Med. *1947;182:251–253; Skanalakis JE, Gray SW, et al. The small intestine. In: Skanalakis JE, Gray SW, eds.* Embryology for Surgeons. *Baltimore: Williams and Wilkins; 1994:184–241; Soderland S. Meckel's diverticulum: a clinical and histological study.* ACTA Chir Scand. *1959;118(Suppl):1–233.*

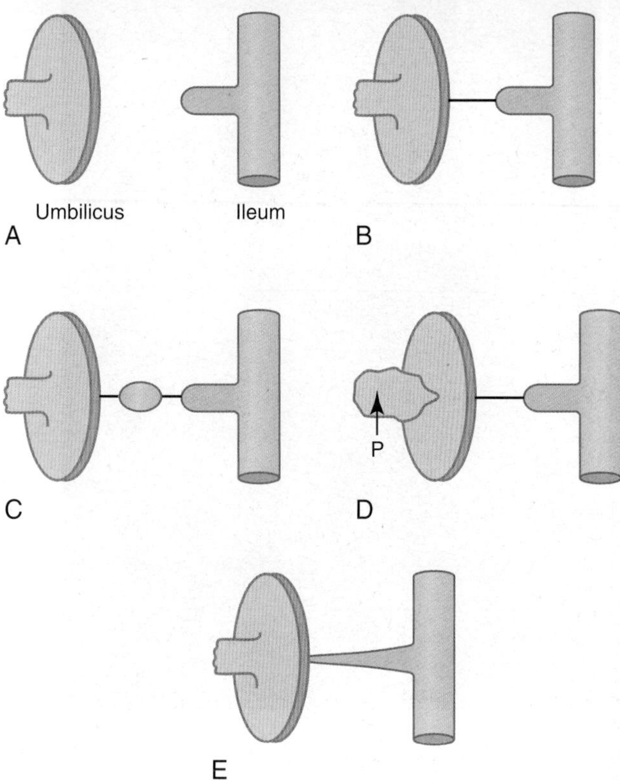

FIGURE 9.26 **The spectrum of omphalomesenteric remnants.** **A,** Meckel's diverticulum. **B,** Meckel's diverticulum attached to the umbilicus by a solid cord. **C,** Omphalomesenteric cyst in a solid cord. **D,** Umbilical polyp *(P)*. An umbilical sinus may be present. **E,** Patent omphalomesenteric fistula. Note: In **B, C,** and **D** a diverticulum may not be present, and in **D** a solid cord may not be present. *(From Huff DS. Developmental anatomy and anomalies of the gastrointestinal tract, with involvement in major malformative syndromes. In: Russo P, Ruchelli E, Piccoli D, eds. Pathology of Pediatric Gastrointestinal and Liver Disease. New York: Springer; 2004:29.)*

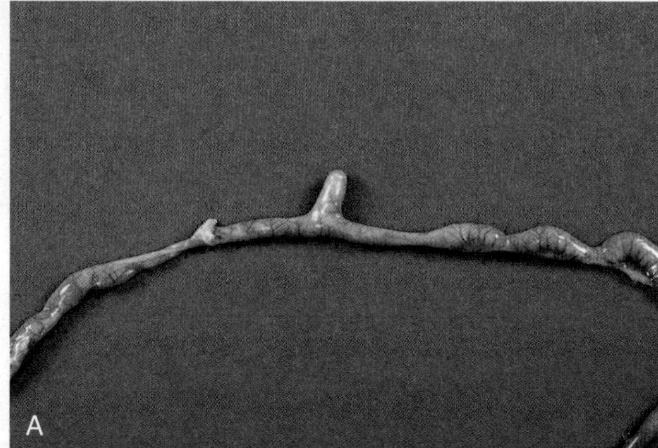

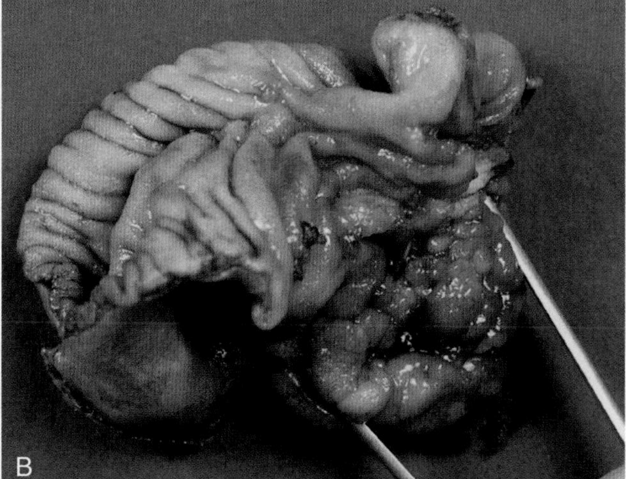

FIGURE 9.27 **A,** Meckel's diverticulum in a 35-week stillborn infant. **B,** Meckel's diverticulum largely lined by gastric mucosa with rugal folds.

the umbilicus. Omphalomesenteric remnants are common in patients with multiple congenital anomalies, but other anomalies are infrequent in otherwise normal patients with Meckel's diverticulum.

Heterotopias

Heterotopic gastric mucosa can occur in duplications and diverticula of the alimentary tract, and more rarely as isolated lesions. They have been documented from the oropharynx to the rectum and can present grossly as nodules, polyps, or erosions.[145] The heterotopias can secrete gastric acid, leading to inflammation, bleeding, perforation, and intussusception.[146] They can be detected by 99mTc pertechnetate scintigraphy. Surgical excision is the treatment of choice. **Heterotopic pancreatic** tissue is most commonly noted in the stomach and proximal small bowel,[147,148] although it can be seen in the liver, spleen, umbilicus, and other sites. Heterotopic pancreatic tissue also affects small bowel stenoses, duplications, and diverticula. The majority of patients are asymptomatic.[148] Rare cases of adenocarcinoma arising in pancreatic heterotopias have been documented.[149] They histologically consist mostly of ducts and acini (Fig. 9.28). A closely related lesion, consisting of ducts in association with smooth muscle hyperplasia and sometimes referred to as *adenomyoma*, is also considered to be a pancreatic heterotopia (see Fig. 9.28D,E).[150]

Anorectal Malformations

Anorectal anomalies constitute an important group of malformations occurring in about 1 in 4000 live births, with one-third being isolated and the rest associated with other anomalies.[151] Approximately 60% occur in males and 40% in females. They have been associated with mutations in almost every chromosome, though trisomy 21 and microdeletion of chromosome 22q11.2 appear to be the most frequent.[151] The pathogenesis and embryological events surrounding these malformations are poorly understood. The early hindgut is the cloaca, a cavity formed at about 21 days of gestation into which the hindgut, tailgut, allantois duct, and mesonephric duct empty. It is generally believed that during the sixth to seventh weeks of gestation, by a process of differential growth and apoptosis, the urorectal septum (which divides the hindgut and the allantois) proliferates caudally toward the cloacal membrane (which forms the junction between endoderm and ectoderm) and fuses with it, resulting in separate urogenital and anorectal sinuses. Perforation of the cloacal membrane occurs at about day 50. Interruptions of any of these steps can result in anorectal anomalies.[152] Some

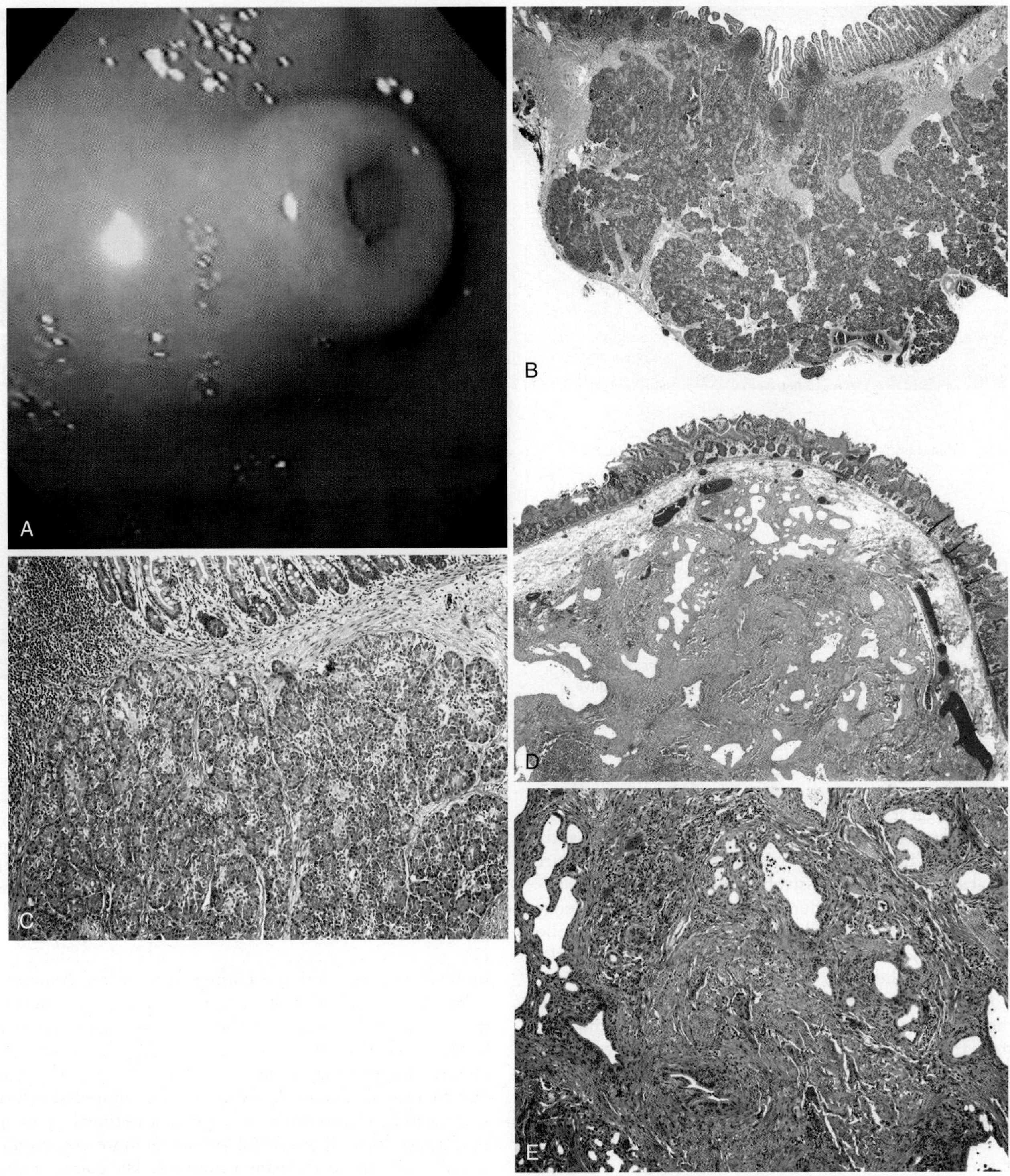

FIGURE 9.28 Pancreatic remnant. A, Endoscopic view of a pancreatic remnant. **B,** Low-power microscopic section of a segmental jejunal excision in a 24-day-old boy reveals pancreatic tissue extending to the serosa. **C,** Higher-power view highlights pancreatic acinar and endocrine tissue. **D,** A section from an adenomyoma is characterized by the presence of ducts with a marked smooth muscle component. No acinar or endocrine tissue is present. **E,** Higher-power view of adenomyoma. (**A** *courtesy Dr. Petar Mamula, The Children's Hospital of Philadelphia.*)

TABLE 9.12 Types of Anorectal Atresias and Fistulae

Atresia	Fistula	
	Male	Female
Anorectal agenesis	Rectocloacal	Rectocloacal
	Rectovesicle	Rectovesicle
	Rectoprostatic urethra	Rectovaginal, high
	Without fistula	Without fistula
Rectal atresia	Without fistula	Without fistula
Anal agenesis	Rectobulbar urethra	Rectovaginal, low rectovestibular
	Without fistula	Without fistula
Imperforated anus	Anoraphe, perineal or scrotal	Anovestibular
	Anocutaneous	Anocutaneous
Anal stenosis	Anocutaneous	Anocutaneous
None	Anterior anus	Anterior anus

From Huff DS. Developmental anatomy and anomalies of the gastrointestinal tract, with involvement in major malformative syndromes. In: Russo P, Ruchelli E, Piccoli D, eds. Pathology of Pediatric Gastrointestinal and Liver Disease. *New York: Springer; 2004:3–37.*

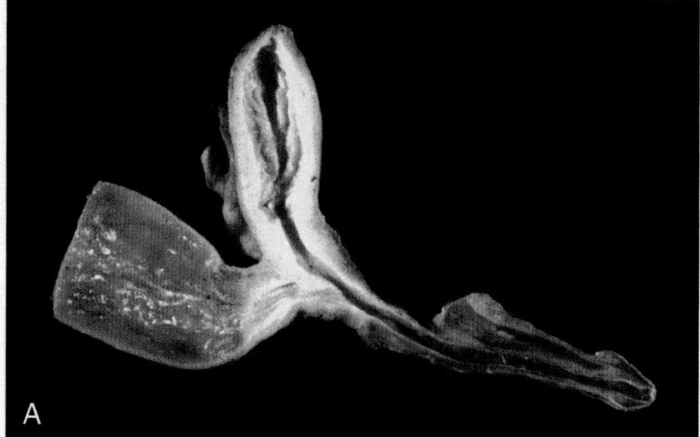

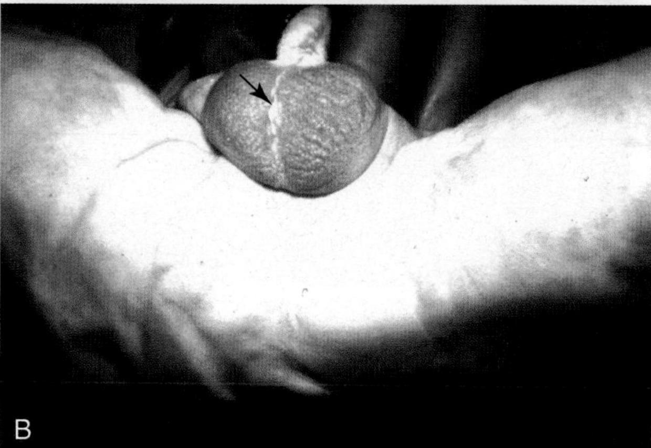

FIGURE 9.29 Two varieties of anorectal atresia with fistulae. A, Median section after perfusion fixation. This is anorectal agenesis with a rectoprostatic urethral fistula at the level of the verumontanum. **B,** External view of the perineum, scrotum, and penis. The patient has a flat perineum, anal agenesis, and an anoscrotal raphe fistula. The raphe is prominent, and water injected into the rectum under pressure distended the raphe and leaked from its widest point at the *arrow.* (*From Huff DS. Developmental anatomy and anomalies of the gastrointestinal tract, with involvement in major malformative syndromes. In: Russo P, Ruchelli E, Piccoli D, eds. Pathology of Pediatric Gastrointestinal and Liver Disease. New York: Springer; 2004:3-37.*)

studies suggest that, contrary to the traditional concepts, urorectal separation is not accomplished by the active caudal growth of the urorectal septum and that the urorectal septum is only passively involved in the process.[153] There is increasing evidence for the role of the Hedgehog gene in these anomalies, particularly Sonic Hedgehog *(Shh)* and homeobox families of genes.[154] Several classifications of the many variations within the spectrum of anorectal atresias and fistulae have been proposed.[155-157] The classification presented in Table 9.12 is modified from the Wingspread classification[157] and the classification of Kiely and Pena.[158] Presumably the higher the lesion, the earlier the time of onset and the more severe the abnormality of development.[159] The list is arranged in descending order of level of the lesion, with the highest at the top and the lowest at the bottom. The interposition of the uterus and vagina between the anorectum and urinary tract during the 9th and 10th weeks explains the difference in the fistulae seen in males and females. Two-thirds are high lesions in males, and two-thirds are low lesions in females.[155] Rectal atresia is a high blind-ending rectum with a normal-appearing perineum, an intact anus, and a blind-ending anal canal. Anorectal agenesis is a high blind-ending rectum and an abnormal perineum, with absence of the anus and anal canal (Fig. 9.29). Anal agenesis is a low blind-ending rectum and an abnormal-appearing perineum, with absence of the anus and anal canal. The most severe form of anorectal atresia is persistent cloaca with or without a perineal opening. It is a rare form of anorectal atresia, is more common in females, and there are many variations. The colon, genital tract, and urinary tract join together to form a common structure (Fig. 9.30). If the perineal outlet is atretic or severely stenotic, the cloaca may be massively cystic.

Patients present with failure to pass meconium. In most cases, the anus is absent, severely abnormal, or displaced anteriorly. Patients with high lesions have a higher incidence

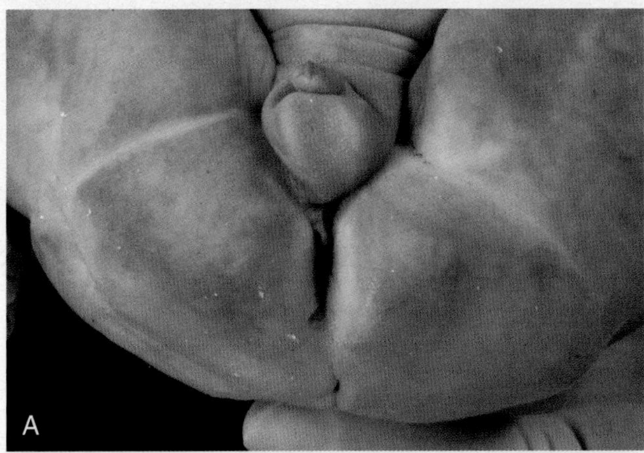

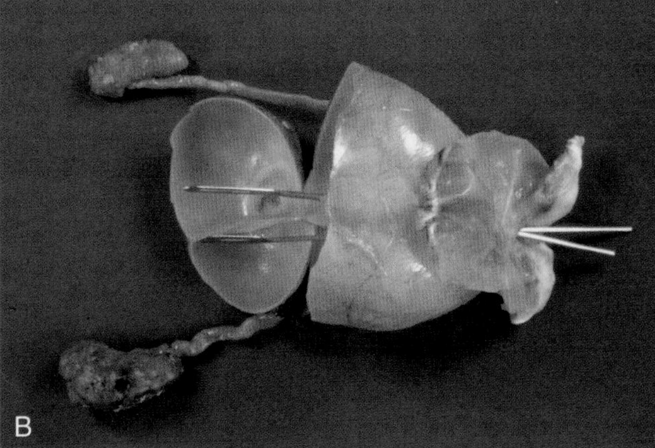

FIGURE 9.30 Cloacal anomaly. A, A 46 XX female neonate with a single perineal opening, fused labial folds, and a prominent phallus. **B,** Excised specimen showing a dilated duplex vagina communicating with the rectum through a single opening. Each probe is in one-half of the duplex vagina; the lower portion of the dividing septum is incomplete. The probes exit through a common opening with the rectum, which has been opened. There was a narrow vesicovaginal fistula *(not shown),* which resulted in bilateral hydroureters and cystic dysplastic kidneys.

of associated malformations than those with low lesions; the incidence is highest in patients with cloacal anomalies. Congenital heart disease, usually tetralogy of Fallot or ventricular septal defect, is seen in approximately 20%. GI anomalies are seen in 10% to 15%. Tracheoesophageal malformations predominate, and duodenal atresia–stenosis, malrotation, small and large intestinal atresia, and Hirschsprung's disease are also found. Urinary tract anomalies are among the most common associated anomalies and have been reported in up to 60% in some series. Vesicoureteral reflux and renal agenesis or dysplasia are among the most common. Genital anomalies are as frequent as urinary anomalies and include cryptorchidism and hypospadias in males and bicornuate or septate uterus and septate vagina in females. Patterns of associated anomalies include multiple intestinal atresias, CHARGE and VACTERL associations, and many others, listed by Huff[130] and Roberts.[108]

The full reference list may be accessed online at Elsevier eBooks for Practicing Clinicians.

CHAPTER 10

Enteropathies Associated with Chronic Diarrhea and Malabsorption in Childhood

Pierre Russo

Chapter Outline

INTRODUCTION AND GENERAL REMARKS

The aims of this chapter are to review the pathological features of the major intestinal disorders of infancy and early childhood, with an emphasis on congenital disorders resulting in chronic diarrhea and malabsorption, and to illustrate their appearance on small-intestinal biopsies and specimens (Box 10.1). Other major categories of disorders that can cause chronic diarrhea, such as infections, immunodeficiencies (primary and secondary), gluten-sensitive enteropathy (GSE) and other food allergies, and motility and pancreatic disorders are discussed in other chapters of this book. Chronic diarrhea occurring in the neonatal period presents particularly difficult diagnostic and therapeutic challenges. *Intractable diarrhea of infancy* is a term that was coined by Avery and colleagues[1] to refer to these cases, most of which remained undiagnosed and were associated with high mortality at that time. Since these initial reports, more precise identification of disorders that cause intractable diarrhea of infancy has led to the use of prolonged parenteral nutrition, immunosuppression, and bowel and hematopoietic stem cell transplantation to improve survival of these children, prompting the need for timely and accurate diagnosis. Investigation of some of these disorders has also led to significant advances in our understanding of gastrointestinal (GI) and immunological functions. For instance, investigation of microvillus inclusion disease has helped identify genes responsible for intracellular vesicular transport. The discovery that mutations in the gene that codes for FOXP3 cause immunodysregulation, polyendocrinopathy and enteropathy (IPEX) syndrome and its animal homologue, the *Scurfy* mouse, has led to recognition of the critical role this gene plays in control of the immune response and in autoimmunity and immune tolerance.

BIOPSY SAMPLING AND INDICATIONS IN CHILDREN

In current pediatric GI practice, intestinal biopsies are most frequently obtained from the duodenum via forceps during endoscopic examination, during which biopsies are also obtained from the esophagus and stomach (esophagogastroduodenoscopy [EGD]). In addition to obtaining biopsies for routine histology, samples may also be snap-frozen (for disaccharidase analysis) or submitted for electron microscopy (for confirmation of microvillus inclusion disease). Biopsies from both proximal and distal duodenum are recommended, including biopsies of endoscopically normal mucosa, as many disorders affecting the duodenum have a focal distribution. In children, for example, the lesions in GSE may be patchy, and villous atrophy may coexist with normal mucosa.[2] Furthermore, villous atrophy may be limited to or most severe in the duodenal bulb at the time of diagnosis.[2,3] As pediatric EGD has evolved into a routine outpatient procedure, the indications for its use have correspondingly changed. At The Children's Hospital of Philadelphia, the first-time EGD rate increased 12-fold in a 20-year interval between 1985 and 2005, with isolated abdominal pain replacing GI bleeding as the most frequent indication.[4] Much of this increase appears to have been driven by the dramatic increase in food allergy–related disorders such as eosinophilic esophagitis, by the increased prevalence of celiac disease and its clinically atypical forms (for which

BOX 10.1 Enteropathies of Infancy and Childhood

- Congenital transport and enzymatic deficiencies
  - Glucose-galactose malabsorption
  - Disaccharidase deficiency
  - Fructose malabsorption
  - Abetalipoproteinemia
  - Chylomicron retention disease
  - Sodium-chloride diarrhea
  - Primary bile acid malabsorption
- Congenital defects of intestinal epithelial differentiation
  - Microvillus inclusion disease
  - Tufting enteropathy
- Enteroendocrine cell dysgenesis
- Autoimmune enteropathy
- Very early onset inflammatory bowel disease
  - Necrotizing enterocolitis–short gut syndrome
  - Lymphangiectasia
- Metabolic diseases and tumors

intestinal biopsy is the "gold standard" for establishing a diagnosis), and by the routine use of EGD in addition to colonoscopy in the evaluation of children with suspected inflammatory bowel disease (IBD). According to one study, the most frequent indications for EGD and colonoscopy in children younger than 1 year of age were diarrhea, failure to thrive, reflux, and rectal bleeding.[5] Histological abnormalities were detected in two-thirds of cases, whereas only 2% of mucosal biopsies were insufficient. Sampling even endoscopically normal-appearing mucosa is recommended, as it may help assess the "background" features of the mucosa, and histological examination may reveal clinically relevant findings unsuspected by the endoscopist (e.g., granulomas).[6,7] A pediatric study found that a routine duodenal biopsy performed for indications such as gastroesophageal reflux, vomiting, abdominal pain, anemia, and during the evaluation of Crohn's disease yielded pathological findings in about 17% of cases.[7]

Intestinal biopsy findings in some entities, such as congenital transport disorders, are associated with a normal biopsy, whereas others, such as autoimmune enteropathy (AIE) or celiac disease, have variable degrees of villous atrophy with or without inflammation. A few disorders, such as abetalipoproteinemia or microvillus inclusion disease, present characteristic findings on intestinal biopsy (Table 10.1).

INTESTINAL DEVELOPMENT IN CHILDREN

Villi appear in the duodenum during the 8th week postfertilization, and crypts of Lieberkuhn are noted during the 9th week, spreading caudally and arriving in the distal ileum by the 14th week. The definitive histological features of the duodenum are established by the 14th week postfertilization, and its histology closely resembles that of the newborn by 20 weeks. The transition from pyloric to duodenal mucosa is gradual in some cases; duodenal-like villi may be found in the distal pylorus, and pyloric-like epithelium may be found in the duodenum. Enteroendocrine and goblet cells appear to differentiate before 14 weeks under the influence of the Notch pathway and transcription factors such as Hes 1 and Atoh1 (Math1).[8] The villus height–crypt depth ratio in the duodenum of a newborn is similar to that of an adult.

TABLE 10.1 Diagnostic Findings on Small-Intestinal Biopsies

Intestinal Biopsy	Differential Diagnosis
Normal	Sucrase-isomaltase deficiency Congenital lactase deficiency Fructose malabsorption Glucose galactose malabsorption Congenital Na^+/Cl^- diarrhea
Inflammatory lesions +/– villous atrophy	Celiac disease Autoimmune enteropathy Protracted infectious diarrhea Immunodeficiency states (most) Bacterial overgrowth Cow's milk or soy protein intolerance Chronic inflammatory bowel diseases
Specific lesions	
Fat-filled enterocytes	Abetalipoproteinemia Anderson's disease
Ectatic lymphatics	Lymphangiectasia
Dense inspissated mucus	Cystic fibrosis
Epithelial abnormalities	Microvillus inclusion disease Tufting enteropathy
Eosinophils	Eosinophilic gastroenteritides
Absence or paucity of inflammatory cells	Severe combined immunodeficiency Agammaglobulinemia

Newborns usually lack plasma cells in the first week of life, gradually acquiring them during the first month of life, with IgM-containing plasma cells predominating. By 3 months of life, IgA plasma cells predominate. Normal numbers of plasma cells and ratios of IgA/IgM/IgG are attained by the first year of life.[9]

CONGENITAL DISORDERS OF INTESTINAL DIGESTION, ABSORPTION, AND TRANSPORT

This group of disorders is among the most common cause of congenital diarrhea. These are conditions in which a defect in one mechanism of digestion or transport leads to chronic diarrhea (Table 10.2). The clinical picture of congenital disaccharidase deficiency and carbohydrate malabsorption, for example, is an osmotic diarrhea due to the unabsorbed solute in the ileum. The more rapid transit through the GI tract in the child results in a more severe diarrhea than in the adult. The diagnosis is obtained by the determination of disaccharidase activities in homogenates of small-bowel biopsies or by breath testing. Intestinal biopsies in these disorders are generally normal or only very slightly abnormal, without ultrastructural anomalies, except for the lipid trafficking disorders, which will be discussed in the next section. Thus a normal-appearing small-bowel mucosa from a patient with prolonged diarrhea, especially a young infant, should alert the clinician to consideration of these entities.

Lipid Trafficking Disorders

Most clinical disorders of fat malabsorption result either from pancreatic disease (such as cystic fibrosis) or ileal

TABLE 10.2 Molecular Basis of Disorders of Digestion, Absorption, and Transport

Disease	Gene	Location	Function
Disaccharidase Deficiency			
Congenital lactase deficiency	*LCT*	2q21	Lactase-phlorizin hydrolase activity
Sucrase-isomaltase deficiency	*SI*	3q25-q26	Isomaltase-sucrase
Maltase-glucoamylase deficiency	*MGAM*	7q34	Maltase-glucoamylase activity
Ion and Nutrient Transport Defects			
Glucose-galactose malabsorption	*SLC5A1*	22q13.1	Na^+/glucose cotransporter
Fructose malabsorption	*SLC2A5*	1p36	Fructose transporter
Fanconi-Bickel syndrome	*SLC2A2*	3q26	Basolateral glucose transporter
Cystic fibrosis	*CFTR*	7q31.2	cAMP-dependent CL^- channel
Acrodermatitis enteropathica	*SLC39A4*	8q24.3	Zn^{2+} transporter
Congenital chloride diarrhea	*SLC26A3*	7q22-q31.1	CL^-/base exchanger
Congenital sodium diarrhea	*SPINT2*	19q13.1	Serine-protease inhibitor
Lysinuric protein intolerance	*SLC7A7*	14q11	Hydrolyzes endopeptidases/exopeptidases Amino acid basolateral transport
Congenital bile acid diarrhea	*SLC10A2*	13q3	Ileal Na^+/bile salt transporter
Pancreatic Insufficiency			
Enterokinase deficiency	*TMPRSS15*	21q21	Proenterokinase
Trypsinogen deficiency	*PRSS1*	7q34	Trypsinogen synthesis
Pancreatic lipase deficiency	*PNLIP*	10q25.3	Hydrolyzes triglycerides to fatty acids
Lipid Trafficking			
Abetalipoproteinemia	*MTTP*	4q23	Transfer lipids to apolipoprotein
Hypobetalipoproteinemia	*APOB*	2p24	Apolipoprotein that forms chylomicrons
Chylomicron retention disease	*SARA2*	5q31.1	Intracellular chylomicron trafficking

From Berni Canani RB, Terrin G, Cardillo G, Tomaiuolo R, Castaldo G. Congenital diarrheal disorders: improved understanding of gene defects is leading to advances in intestinal physiology and clinical management. *J Pediatr Gastroenterol Nutr.* 2010;50(4):360–366.

involvement (as in Crohn's disease) with loss of the enterohepatic circulation of bile acids. Intestinal biopsies play a limited role in the diagnosis of these disorders. However, primary abnormalities involving abnormalities of fat transport within the enterocyte, though much less frequent, can result in a characteristic vacuolization of the enterocyte in intestinal biopsies.

Abetalipoproteinemia

Abetalipoproteinemia is an autosomal recessive disorder characterized by the absence of apo B-containing lipoproteins. The molecular basis for the defect is a mutation of the gene coding for microsomal triglyceride transfer protein (MTP) located on chromosome 4q22 (see Table 10.2).[10] MTP is responsible for assembly of lipoprotein particles and for the proper folding of ApoB, preventing its premature degradation.[11] Fatty acids within intestinal cells thus cannot be exported as chylomicrons. Patients have diarrhea and fat malabsorption, usually appearing within the first few months of life, with acanthocytosis and deficiencies in fat-soluble vitamins that result in retinitis pigmentosa and neurological symptoms. There is clinical heterogeneity, however, with signs and symptoms presenting in older adult patients in a significant proportion of cases. Serum levels of cholesterol and triglycerides are typically low and do not increase after a fatty meal. Small-bowel biopsies typically reveal preserved villous morphology (Fig. 10.1A). Characteristic multivacuolated fat-filled enterocytes are noted in intestinal biopsies of fasting patients, which on electron microscopy are irregular in size and generally non–membrane-bound (see Fig. 10.1B). No lipid is noted in the extracellular space. Hepatic biopsies in these cases typically reveal steatosis, with numerous non–membrane-bound lipid droplets noted in the hepatic cytoplasm.[12] Fibrosis evolving to cirrhosis has been reported in occasional patients.[13]

Hypobetalipoproteinemia

Hypobetalipoproteinemia is an autosomal dominant disorder caused by a mutation in the *APO B* gene located on chromosome 2, leading to truncated apo B protein.[14] Homozygous patients have a clinical and histological phenotype essentially indistinguishable from abetalipoproteinemia, whereas heterozygous patients have only a mild phenotype.

Chylomicron Retention Disease

Chylomicron retention (Anderson's) disease is similar to abetalipoproteinemia in its GI manifestations and impact on growth, though acanthocytosis is usually absent, and neurological and ocular abnormalities are much less severe. Also, in contrast with abetalipoproteinemia, serum fasting triglyceride levels are normal, and hypocholesterolemia is less marked. Apolipoprotein B and MTP are produced, but there

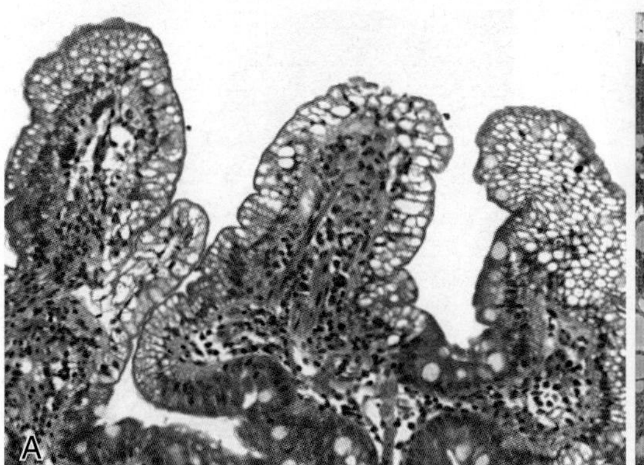

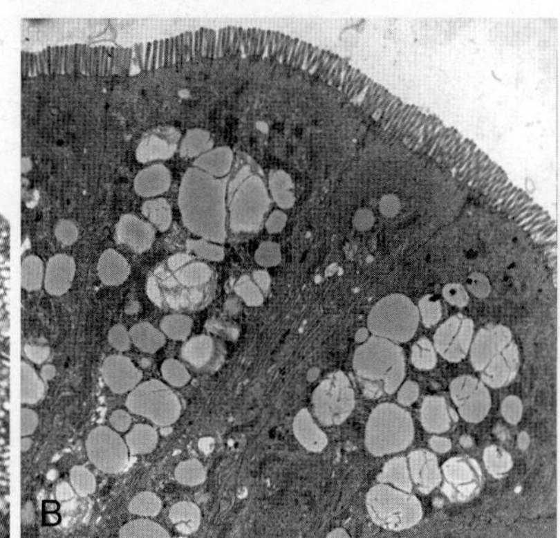

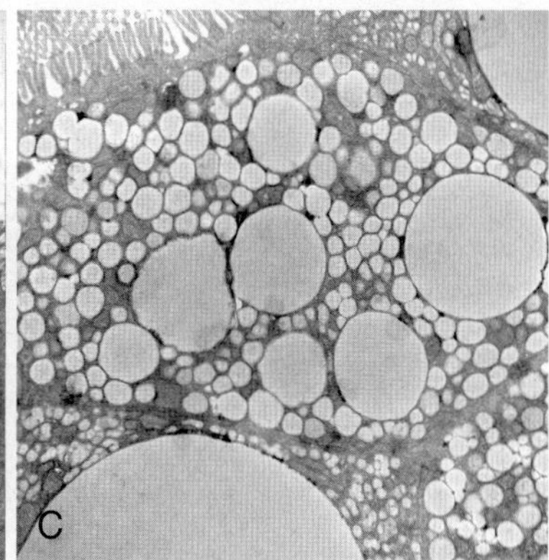

FIGURE 10.1 Lipid transport disorders. A, Abetalipoproteinemia. The intestinal biopsy reveals diffuse vacuolization of the enterocytes with preserved villous morphology. **B,** Ultrastructural appearance is characterized by variable-size lipid droplets filling the enterocytes. **C,** Chylomicron retention disorder. The histological features are identical to abetalipoproteinemia. Electron microscopy reveals numerous lipid vacuoles that appear to be membrane bound by the endoplasmic reticulum.

is failure to secrete the chylomicrons across the enterocyte basolateral membrane. The causative gene, *SARA2*, codes for Sar1b, part of the small guanosine triphosphatase family of proteins associated with intracellular trafficking.[15] The pathological features in small-bowel biopsies are essentially indistinguishable from abetalipoproteinemia.

Minor degrees of enterocyte vacuolization (e.g., caused by a recent feed) are common in intestinal biopsies in infants; in these cases, vacuolation is neither as marked nor as diffuse as in the lipid trafficking disorders. In addition, lipid droplets are present in the intercellular spaces and lacteals after feeding, but they are absent in these spaces in disorders causing impaired lipid transport.

CONGENITAL DEFECTS OF INTESTINAL EPITHELIAL DIFFERENTIATION

Microvillus Inclusion Disease

Initially described by Davidson et al. in 1978[16] and subsequently recognized worldwide, microvillus inclusion disease (MVID) is an autosomal recessive disease characterized by refractory secretory diarrhea, usually occurring within the first week of life, though a late-onset form can manifest in the first few months of life.[17] Investigation of clusters of cases within the Navajo population identified mutations in the *MYO5B* gene.[18] Homozygosity mapping of an extended Turkish kindred allowed Muller and colleagues to locate the gene locus to chromosome 18q21.[19] *MYO5B* codes for myosin Vb (MYO5B), which interacts with RAB small GTPases (RAB8a, RAB10, RAB11), which play a crucial role in maintaining cell polarity, apical trafficking, and development of microvilli.[20] Whole-exome sequencing of patients with a milder phenotype has identified mutations in the *STX3* gene, coding for syntaxin 3, which also acts as a regulator of cellular protein trafficking.[21]

Small-bowel biopsies are usually characterized by severe villus atrophy, mild or moderate crypt hyperplasia, and a variable degree of inflammation in the lamina propria, but without crypt destruction (Fig. 10.2A). The diagnosis may be strongly suspected on paraffin-embedded sections by the absence of a distinct brush border using periodic acid–Schiff (PAS) stain and by the presence of PAS-positive diastase-resistant densities at the apex of the enterocytes (Fig. 10.2B,C). Similar observations are noted using immunohistochemical staining for alkaline phosphatase and anti-CD10. More recently, similar results using antibodies directed against anti-Rab11a, a small guanosine triphosphatase (GTPase) protein on the surface of recycling endosomes, has provided further evidence that MVID is a disorder of apical plasma membrane recycling.[22] The pathognomonic ultrastructural features include absent or small stubby microvilli, vesicular structures located toward the apex of the enterocytes containing microvilli, and granules containing dense amorphous material (Fig. 10.3). Microvillus inclusions have also been reported in the colon, gallbladder, and renal tubular epithelium in these patients.[23] A variety of different ultrastructural features has also been noted in patients with this disorder, and finding the "typical" inclusions may require a prolonged search.[24]

Patients with MVID are dependent on total parenteral nutrition (TPN), though improved survival may require small-bowel transplantation.[25]

Congenital Tufting Enteropathy

First described by Reifen et al.,[26] patients with congenital tufting enteropathy (CTE, epithelial dysplasia) present in the neonatal period with watery diarrhea. Prenatal history is uneventful, and the disease appears to be inherited in an autosomal recessive fashion, as suggested by the finding of other affected siblings and frequent parental consanguinity. The incidence is estimated at 1 in 50,000 to 100,000 live births in Europe, and it appears to be more frequent in patients of Arabic origin.[27] The disorder has been linked to mutations in the *EPCAM* gene located on chromosome 2p21 and coding for the epithelial cell adhesion molecule.[28] This molecule belongs to a family of cell-adhesion receptors, associated with tight-junction proteins, and is responsible for cell-to-cell interaction by recruiting actin filaments to sites of contact.[29] Patients with this mutation appear to have disease limited to the GI tract. A second group of patients with CTE has been described with a syndromic form of the disorder characterized by choanal atresia, other atresia, punctate keratitis, dermatological abnormalities, and bone malformations resulting from mutations in *SPINT2*, which also cause congenital sodium diarrhea.[30-32]

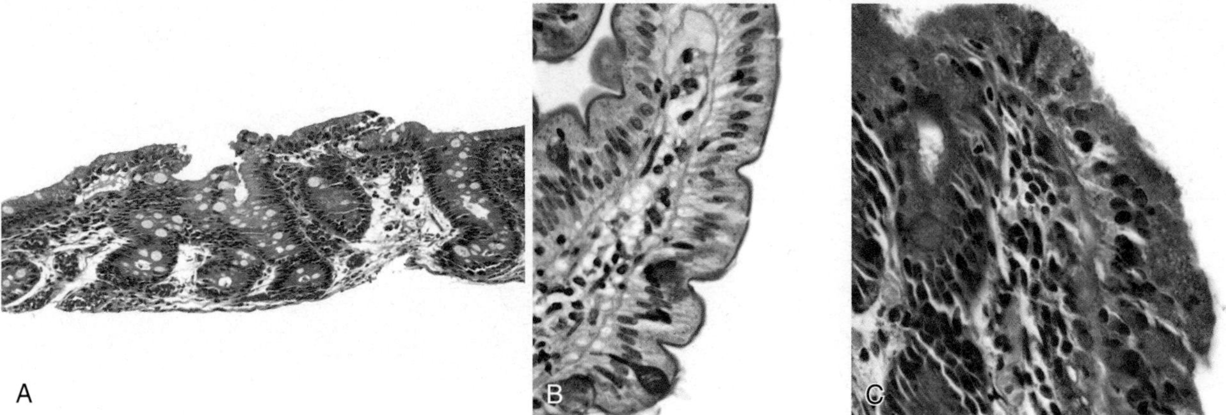

FIGURE 10.2 Microvillus inclusion disease. A, Biopsy from a 2-week-old patient reveals marked villous atrophy, minimal crypt hyperplasia, and no inflammation. **B,** The brush border of the normal intestine is well outlined by PAS stain. **C,** By comparison with B, the intestinal brush border in microvillus inclusion disease is not discerned, and the inclusions appear as an-ill-defined diffuse positivity toward the apex of the enterocytes (PAS stain).

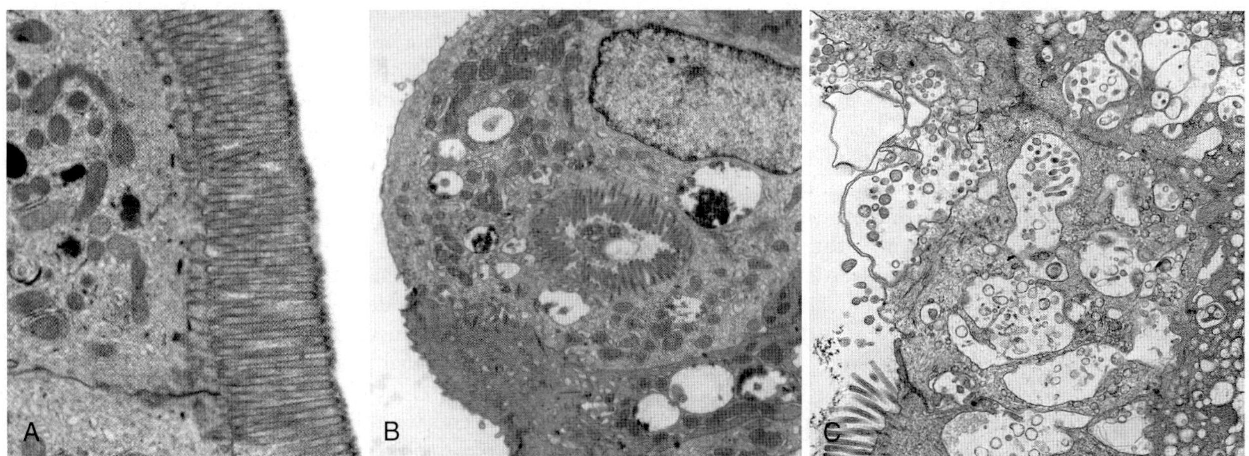

FIGURE 10.3 A, Electron micrograph of a normal enterocyte brush border shows numerous well-formed microvilli. **B,** Microvillus inclusion disease. Microvilli are absent. A large inclusion containing profiles of microvilli is noted in the cytoplasm, with a number of other inclusions containing dense amorphous material. **C,** Microvillus inclusion disease. Dilated spaces containing numerous vesicular structures and a few elongated forms resembling microvilli.

The histological hallmarks are severe villus atrophy with the formation of "tufts" of rounded, teardrop-shaped enterocytes that appear to shed into the lumen. There may be a mild increase in lamina propria inflammatory cells, but intraepithelial lymphocytes do not appear to be significantly increased. The brush border is normal by PAS staining, and electron microscopic findings are nonspecific. Dilated crypts have also been described. Epithelial abnormalities typically vary over time and may be subtle or absent in the first biopsy, making diagnostic confirmation difficult, especially early in presentation (Fig. 10.4). Absence of immunohistochemical staining for MOC31 (an antibody directed against EPCAM) is thus a useful diagnostic feature in patients with CTE and *EPCAM* mutations and should be included in the histological panel of intestinal biopsy evaluation in any infant presenting with prolonged diarrhea.[30,33] Immunohistochemical staining for EPCAM in patients with *SPINT2* mutations, however, is preserved and similar to normal controls, whereas no change in staining intensity or localization for SPINT2 was seen in patients with either *EPCAM* or *SPINT2* mutations.[30]

In most patients, the severity of the malabsorption and diarrhea makes them dependent on long-term parenteral nutrition, and in some cases intestinal transplantation is a therapeutic option with or without liver transplantation because of the associated parenteral nutrition–induced cirrhosis. A more indolent clinical course has also been observed with some patients reported to have been eventually weaned off TPN.[34]

Enteroendocrine Cell Dysgenesis

Enteric anendocrinosis is a recently described autosomal recessive disorder associated with a congenital absence of enteroendocrine cells in the small and large bowel secondary to mutations in the *NEUROG3* gene, located on chromosome 10q21.3, required for differentiation of epithelial cells to the endocrine phenotype.[35] Affected patients are characterized by a congenital diarrheal syndrome with profound malabsorption of all nutrients from birth. Patients also typically develop insulin-dependent diabetes, some during infancy and others later in childhood.[35,36] Pancreatic exocrine function is normal. Neurogenin-3–null mice

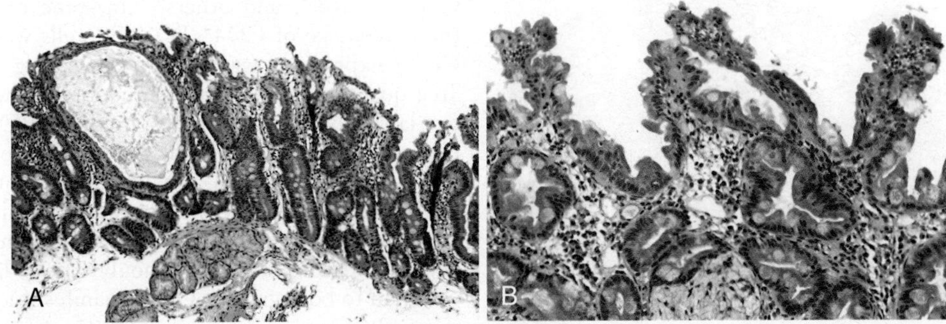

FIGURE 10.4 Tufting enteropathy. A, Biopsy from 4-month-old girl reveals villous atrophy and crypt hyperplasia. Some glands appear cystically dilated. Numerous small tufts are noted along the epithelial surface. **B,** Higher-power view reveals the surface epithelium appearing as characteristic "tufts."

lack enteroendocrine cells[37] and are severely diabetic as neurogenin-3 is also required for pancreatic endocrine development.[38]

Intestinal biopsies may be normal or reveal villous atrophy, the severity of changes perhaps related to different mutations in the *NEUROG 3* gene[36] (Fig. 10.5). The brush border is normal, and goblet and Paneth cells are present. Inflammatory cells in the lamina propria do not appear significantly increased, and there is no crypt-destructive process. Electron microscopy confirms the presence of microvilli and the absence of microvillus inclusions.[39] The characteristic absence of enteroendocrine cells in the small bowel and colon is confirmed by immunohistochemistry for chromogranin A.

Patients with autoimmune polyglandular syndrome I may also have absent or markedly reduced enteroendocrine cells, which may be transient.[40] Loss of enteroendocrine cells may be observed in patients with AIE, along with loss of goblet and Paneth cells.

Mutations in the *PCSK1* gene, which encodes an endoprotease called *proprotein convertase 1/3* (PC1/3), have been associated with malabsorptive diarrhea and other endocrinopathies including adrenal insufficiency, hypothyroidism, and hypogonadism.[41] PC1/3 is responsible for converting prohormones to their biologically active form. In the author's experience with one such case, small-bowel biopsies showed mild, nonspecific changes with retained staining for chromogranin. Only the use of antibody against PC1/3 showed loss of staining. The diagnosis is suspected clinically by the combination of malabsorption with endocrinopathies.

Tricho-Hepato-Enteric Syndrome

Girault et al.[42] described a group of patients with dysmorphic features consisting of a prominent forehead, broad nose, hypertelorism, and wooly, easily removable abnormal hair (trichorrhexis nodosa) in association with intractable diarrhea and immunodeficiency, which they termed *syndromatic intractable diarrhea* because of the constellation of extra-intestinal manifestations. Most of the patients reported were of Middle Eastern origin, and there was parental consanguinity and a history of similarly affected siblings. The immunodeficiency was characterized by impaired T-cell and antibody responses despite normal immunoglobulin levels. Infants with similar clinical features had been previously reported as having tricho-hepato-enteric (THE) syndrome[43,44] in which thin sparse hair (trichomalacia) was seen in association with hypertelorism, chronic diarrhea, a history of premature delivery, and intrauterine growth restriction. In addition, the cases described by Verloes also presented with neonatal hemochromatosis, characterized by liver failure, cirrhosis, and multivisceral iron deposition.[44] THE is caused by *TTC37* gene mutations in 60% of cases and *SKIV2L* mutations in 40% of cases.[45,46] TTC37 protein is expressed in may tissues and is a component of the SKI complex, required for exosome-mediated RNA surveillance.[45] SKIV2L appears to be involved in mRNA decay pathways and may play a role in immune control mechanisms.[47]

Intestinal biopsies have revealed variable villous atrophy without a conspicuous increase in inflammatory cells and without specific features. Serially obtained biopsies suggest that villous atrophy can improve with time and that the inflammatory infiltrate is not consistent. The hair is described as wooly with microscopic features of trichorrhexis nodosa. Hepatic involvement is inconsistent. Hartley et al. also observed platelet abnormalities consisting of reduced α-granules and abnormal lipid inclusions and canalicular system.[48]

DISORDERS OF IMMUNOMODULATION

Autoimmune Enteropathy

AIE is probably the most frequent disorder leading to infantile intractable diarrhea.[49] The main diagnostic criteria are severe protracted diarrhea; intestinal biopsy changes generally characterized by villous atrophy with a usually marked crypt-destructive inflammation, often with a decrease or absence of goblet and Paneth cells, and exclusion of other causes of villus atrophy. Circulating gut autoantibodies are a useful but not necessary diagnostic feature. Most cases occur in infancy or the first year of life, though this entity has also been reported in older children, in girls, and even in adults in whom it may be responsible for a proportion of cases referred to as *refractory sprue*. Thus several clinical types exist and include pediatric and adult forms.[50] Pediatric forms can be further divided into IPEX, IPEX-like, and secondary forms associated with another primary immunodeficiency. The most commonly recognized association is with

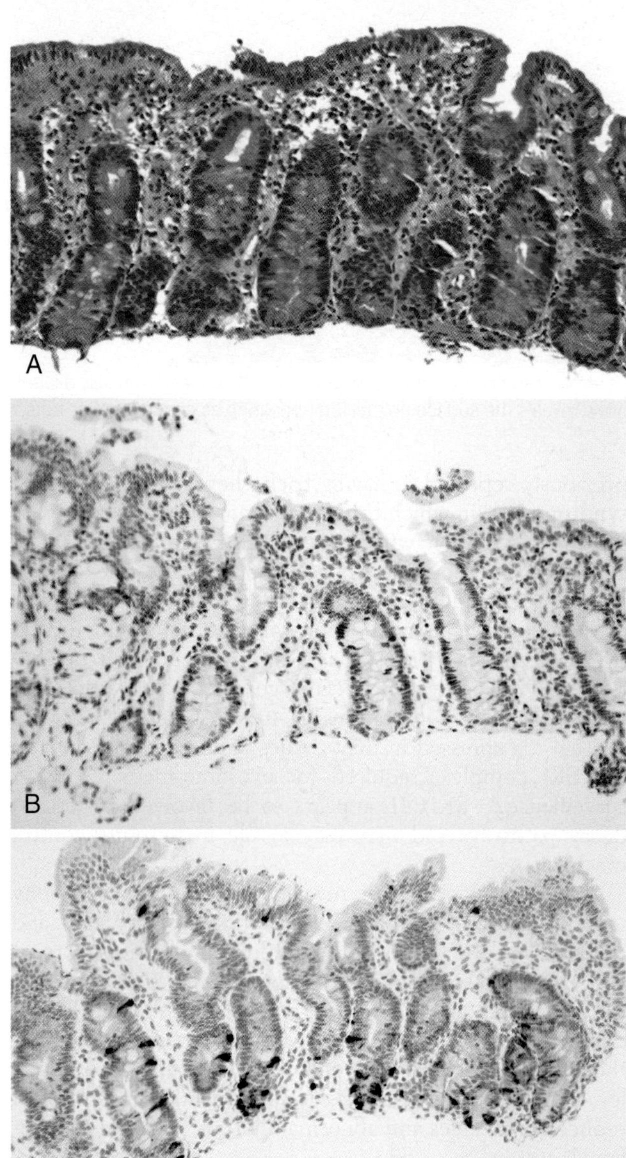

FIGURE 10.5 Enteroendocrine cell deficiency. A, Intestinal biopsy from 10-month-old patient with *NEUROG 3* mutation who presented with severe chronic diarrhea and also developed diabetes. The histological features reveal villous atrophy and some crypt hyperplasia. No significant inflammation is noted. **B,** Immunohistochemical staining for chromogranin reveals absence of enteroendocrine cells. **C,** Chromogranin staining on an age-matched normal small-bowel control.

the X-linked IPEX syndrome, initially described by Powell et al.[51] This syndrome has been related to mutations in the *FOXP3* gene (Xp11.23).[52] These mutations result in lower levels of $CD4^+$ $CD25^+$ regulatory T cells with absence or very low levels of FOXP3 protein expression and consequent impaired suppression of the inflammatory response and extensive autoimmune manifestations.[53-55] Approximately 50% of patients with otherwise typical manifestations of AIE, including females, have no detectable *FOXP3* mutations and have been designated *IPEX-like.* These patients have been found to harbor mutations in a variety of immune regulatory genes, including *STAT5b, STAT1, CTLA4, LRBA,* and others.[55] In some of these patients, the percentage of $CD4^+$ $FOXP3^+$ cells was normal, while CD25 expression was absent, suggesting preservation of Treg quantity but abnormal function.[55] There is extensive overlap in the clinical manifestations of IPEX and IPEX-like patients, the most frequent being enteropathy characterized by watery diarrhea, usually starting in the first year of life in IPEX patients, typically a little later in the IPEX-like group. Eczema, exfoliative dermatitis, and autoimmune endocrinopathies, most commonly type 1 diabetes, are also common to both groups. Other manifestations include anemia, neutropenia, glomerulonephritis, interstitial nephritis, autoimmune hepatitis, and cardiopulmonary disease, seen in various proportions in patients with different mutated genes.[55]

The entire GI tract is often involved in AIE, and histopathological findings in duodenal and small-bowel biopsies are usually characterized by severe villus atrophy, crypt hyperplasia, and a mixed inflammatory infiltrate of the lamina propria. Marked inflammatory destruction of intestinal crypts with extensive apoptosis is a feature noted in many cases, similar to those noted in intestinal graft-versus-host disease, and confirms an abnormal immune-mediated attack against intestinal epithelium[56] (Fig. 10.6A–C). However, there appears to be a marked variation in histological features, with some cases showing milder degrees of intestinal damage. In contrast with cases of GSE with flat villi, intraepithelial lymphocytes tend to be relatively few in number, although some investigators have reported cases with increased intraepithelial lymphocytes, indistinguishable from celiac disease, except for a usually negative celiac serology.[57] A concomitant crypt-destructive colitis and gastritis are present in the majority of cases.

One of the hallmarks of this entity, noted since the first reports of AIE, is the presence of antienterocyte antibodies, detected by indirect immunofluorescence using the patient's serum on frozen sections of normal bowel. Positive fluorescence usually results in a linear pattern along the apex and basolateral border of the enterocyte[23,58-61] (Fig. 10.6D). The antibodies are predominantly IgG and have been described as complement-fixing,[58] though IgM and IgA have also been described.[60,62] Antibodies reacting against mucus or goblet cells have also been described, and intestinal biopsies in these cases have shown a marked depletion of goblet cells.[63,64]

The target of the antienterocyte antibodies is still a matter of investigation, though a 75-kDa antigen reactive with autoantibody in the sera of patients with IPEX syndrome has been reported.[65] This protein is expressed in the epithelial cells of the small bowel, colon, and kidney, and it may play a role in protein-protein interactions in the enterocyte. A 95-kDa antigen identified as *villin* has also been reported in IPEX patients,[66] and more than one antigen is likely involved.

However, the role of these antibodies in the diagnosis of AIE is debatable. These antibodies have been reported to occur after onset of the disease and to disappear before restoration of mucosal integrity,[61] and they may thus represent an epiphenomenon without playing a causative role in mucosal damage. Similar antienterocyte antibodies have also been described in adult AIDS patients without digestive

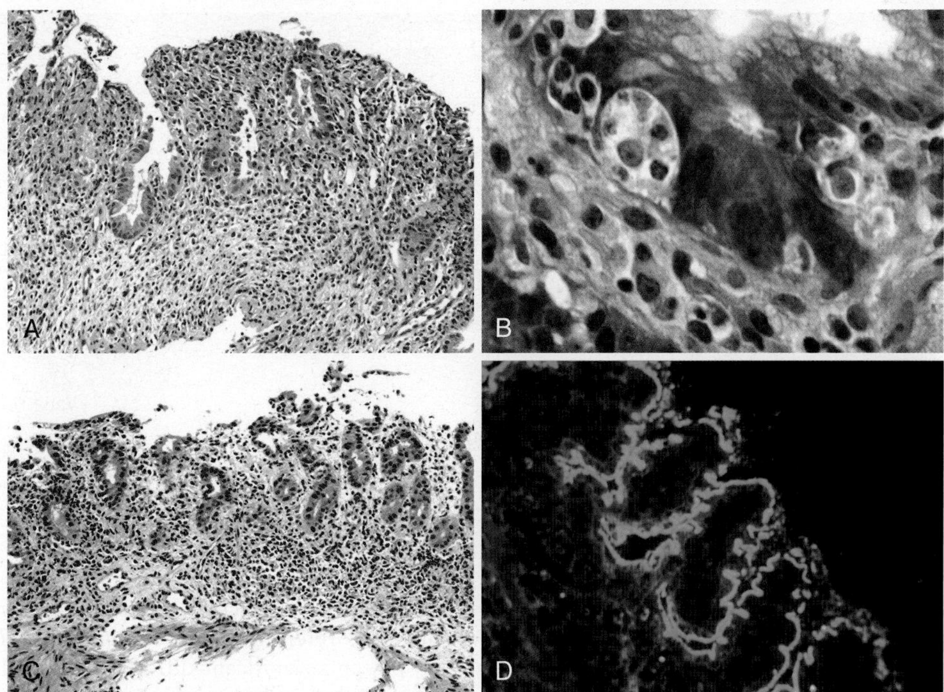

FIGURE 10.6 Autoimmune enteropathy. A, Duodenal biopsy from a 3-month-old patient reveals severe destructive inflammation with marked crypt and villous atrophy. **B,** Numerous foci of apoptosis with lymphocytic "satellitosis" are present at the base of the crypts. **C,** Gastric antral biopsy from the same patient also reveals marked gastritis. **D,** Antienterocyte antibodies. Indirect immunofluorescence using the patient's serum, layered onto normal duodenum, and followed by application of fluorescein-conjugated antihuman IgG reveals positive linear staining along the apex of the enterocytes.

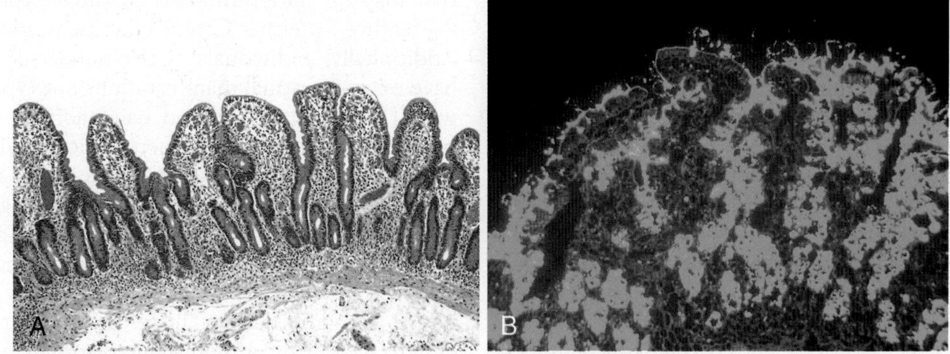

FIGURE 10.7 Autoimmune enteropathy in an adult. A, Duodenal biopsy from an 18-year-old woman with chronic diarrhea unresponsive to a gluten-free diet; the patient also developed thyroiditis. There is moderate villous atrophy and inflammation. Note also the absence of Paneth and goblet cells. **B,** Antienterocyte antibodies. Same technique as described in Figure 10.6D. The positivity in this case is within goblet cells.

symptoms.[67] The specificity of anti–goblet cell antibodies has also been questioned. Anti–goblet cell antibodies have been detected in patients with chronic IBD (Crohn's and ulcerative colitis) and their first-degree relatives[68] and in a series of treated and untreated patients with celiac disease and controls.[69] Finally, the usefulness of these antibodies in the diagnosis of AIE in young infants is also probably limited, given that there is little IgG production in the first 3 months of life and that IgG detected in the infant is likely maternal in origin.[70]

In adults, the clinical picture appears to be that of celiac disease unresponsive to gluten withdrawal.[71-78] Corazza et al. reported four adult women with refractory celiac disease, none of whom had had malabsorptive symptoms in childhood, thus confirming an adult onset.[73] Akram et al. reported on a series of 15 (7 females) patients, 42 to 67 years of age, in whom celiac disease was excluded by lack of response to gluten-free diet or absence of the celiac disease susceptibility HLA genotypes.[71] All patients had protracted diarrhea, weight loss, and malnutrition.

The differential diagnosis of AIE includes, in addition to celiac disease and graft-versus-host disease, enterocolitis associated with various immunodeficiency states, and histological features of AIE with circulating autoantibodies may be observed.[79] A high index of suspicion for AIE should be present when there is a severe inflammatory crypt-destructive process with villous atrophy and increased apoptosis in the base of the crypts, loss of goblet and Paneth cells, or an intestinal inflammatory process in a patient with autoimmune phenomena (Fig. 10.7). Testing for circulating antienterocyte antibodies is useful in older children and adults but may have limited use in young infants. Mortality

TABLE 10.3 Differentiating Features of Severe Diarrhea of Early Infancy

	Microvillus Inclusion Disease	Tufting Enteropathy	Enteroendocrine Cell Dysgenesis	Autoimmune Enteropathy
Presentation	First 2 weeks	First 2 weeks	First 2 weeks	After 1 month
Gene defect	*MYO5b* (18q21)	*EpCAM* (2p21)	*NEUROG 3* (10q21.3)	*FOXP3* (Xp11.23) in IPEX syndrome
Extra-intestinal disease	Low gamma-glutamyltransferase cholestasis post- bowel transplantation	Dysmorphism; autoimmune diseases (arthritis)	Insulin-dependent diabetes	Polyendocrinopathies
Antienterocyte antibodies	No	No	No	Yes
Villous atrophy	Yes	Variable	Variable	Variable
Surface epithelium	Absent brush border	Tufting and desquamation	Normal	Normal or atrophic
Lamina propria inflammation	Minimal	Variable	Minimal	Usually increased

in older reported cases of AIE is high. A combination of immunosuppressants were used in most cases, including steroids, calcineurin inhibitors, and rapamycin, resulting in an overall survival of 65%, while hematopoietic stem cell transplantation in selected patients resulted in similar survival with better disease resolution.[80] Immunosuppression is required in adults.[71]

Major differentiating features between various etiologies of severe diarrhea of early infancy are presented in Table 10.3.

Autoimmune Polyendocrine Syndrome (APS 1)

Autoimmune polyendocrine syndrome 1 (APS 1), also referred to as *autoimmune polyendocrinopathy – candidiasis – ectodermal dystrophy* (APECED), is an autosomal recessive disorder with heterogeneous clinical manifestations. It is caused by mutations in the *AIRE* gene, which codes for a transcription factor primarily expressed in medullary thymic epithelial cells, where negative selection is thought to occur.[81] The type 1 form is characterized by various endocrinopathies of an autoimmune nature, often beginning in childhood or early teenage years, with chronic mucocutaneous candidiasis resulting from a T-cell defect starting soon after birth and dystrophy of ectodermal tissues.[82] Malabsorption can occur in up to 25% of patients and appears to result from destruction of intestinal endocrine cells.[83] A specific deficiency of cholecystokinin-producing enteroendocrine cells has been reported in one patient, with seeming reappearance of the cells when the diarrhea abated.[40] Small-bowel biopsies show mild changes or can even be normal, in contrast with the crypt-destructive inflammation usually seen in AIE.

VERY EARLY ONSET INFLAMMATORY BOWEL DISEASE

Approximately 25% of incident cases of IBD occur during childhood, most commonly diagnosed during the young teenage years. In about 15% of patients, the diagnosis is established before 6 years of age, with up to 6% diagnosed at younger than 3 years of age.[84] For reasons that are unclear, a marked increase in the occurrence of IBD has occurred in this age group in recent decades.[85] This subgroup of IBD patients is referred to as *very early onset IBD* (VEO-IBD) and presents significant differences from IBD occurring in older children and in adults, including more severe clinical disease unresponsive to conventional IBD therapy and a greater proportion of cases featuring an underlying monogenic disorder.[86] In many of these cases, intestinal disease may be the presenting feature of the underlying immunodeficiency. These cases typically feature a diffuse colitis that may be "indeterminate" without typical differentiating features of either Crohn's disease or ulcerative colitis.[87] Additionally, individuals with monogenic disorders may have extra-intestinal manifestations not typically associated with IBD, such as nail and hair anomalies, epidermolysis bullosa, and autoimmune hemolytic anemia.[88] They may also develop significant problems such as immunodeficiency, affecting treatment options, and a greater potential for receiving escalated treatment regimens involving extensive surgery and more intensive medical therapies.[88] Other than the early age of onset and the constellation of extra-intestinal manifestations, histological features that may orient the search for a monogenic disorder in childhood IBD would include particularly severe chronic colitis in an early biopsy, the presence of increased eosinophils with significant crypt architectural changes, associated small-bowel villous blunting, and increased crypt apoptosis.[89]

Recent advances in molecular technology, such as whole-exome sequencing (WES) have allowed the discovery of genes and pathways associated with VEO-IBD.[77,90] These genes are, for the most part, different from the genetic variants found in genome-wide association studies of IBD in older children and adults.[91] The defects that are associated with VEO-IBD include genes involved in intestinal epithelial barrier function, phagocyte bacterial killing, T-cell regulation, hyperimmune or autoimmune inflammatory disorders, and function of the adaptive immune system (Table 10.4).[89,92] As many of these newly described monogenic disorders involve immune regulatory pathways, there is extensive overlap with primary immunodeficiencies such as common variable immunodeficiency (CVID), Wiskott-Aldrich syndrome (WAS), and chronic granulomatous disease, which can also present with features of VEO-IBD.[93,94]

TABLE 10.4 Disorders Associated with Very Early Onset Inflammatory Bowel Disease

Gene	Disease	Pathogenic Inheritance	Phenotypic Features
Defect in Epithelial Barrier Function			
ADAM17		Autosomal recessive	Psoriasiform erythroderma, pustules, broken hair, abnormal nails, small bowel and colonic involvement
IKBKG	NEMO	X-linked	Hypodontia, thin hair, frontal bossing, recurrent infections, enteropathy
COL7A1	Epidermolysis bullosa	Autosomal recessive	Recurrent blistering or erosions, esophageal stricture, anal fissures and stenosis, enteropathy, hair and nail abnormalities
FERMT1	Klinder's syndrome	Autosomal recessive	Recurrent skin blisters, esophageal strictures, colonic involvement
TTC7A	Hereditary multiple intestinal atresia	Autosomal recessive	Intestinal atresia, dermatitis, alopecia, immunodeficiency
GUCY2		Autosomal dominant gain of function	Diarrhea, esophagitis, electrolyte abnormalities, ileal obstruction, dilated small bowel, secretory diarrhea
Defect in NADPH Oxidase Complex			
CYBA *CYBB* *NCF1* *NCF2* *NCF4*	Chronic granulomatous disease	Autosomal recessive X-linked Autosomal recessive Autosomal recessive Autosomal recessive	Life-threatening bacterial and fungal infections, excessive inflammation characterized by granulomas in any organ including small and large intestine, gastric outlet obstruction, perianal disease
NOX1		Autosomal recessive loss of function	Bacterial infections, colonic involvement
Defect in Adaptive Immunity			
IL-10 *IL-10RA* *IL-10RB*	IL-10 deficiency	Autosomal recessive	Neonatal onset, folliculitis, panenteric disease, perianal disease, lymphoma
RAG1 *RAG2* *ZAP70* *IL7R*	Severe combined immunodeficiency (typically T cells and B cells) Omenn's syndrome	Autosomal recessive Autosomal recessive	Recurrent severe infections, chronic diarrhea, failure to thrive, variable intestinal involvement Skin inflammation, variable intestinal involvement
PTEN	PTEN hamartoma tumor syndrome (PHTS)		Thyroiditis, autoimmune hemolytic anemia, hamartomas, adenopathy, adenoid lymphoid hyperplasia, thymic hyperplasia, developmental delay, enteropathy
LRBA	LRBA deficiency	Autosomal recessive	Enteropathy, lymphoproliferation, immune deficiency
WASP *ARPC1B*	Wiskott-Aldrich syndrome	X-linked autosomal recessive loss of function	Thrombocytopenia, eczema, eosinophilia, immune deficiency, colonic involvement
BTK	X-linked agammaglobulinemia	X-linked	Recurrent infections after first few months of life, variable intestinal involvement
DKC1	Dyskeratosis congenita	X-linked	Microcephaly, intrauterine growth restriction, nail dystrophy, abnormal skin pigmentation, leukoplakia of oral mucosa, enteropathy, stricture formation
ITGB2	Leukocyte adhesion deficiency-1	Autosomal recessive	Delayed separation of umbilical cord, recurrent bacterial infections, leukocytosis, lack of pus and impaired wound healing, enteropathy
ICOS	ICOS deficiency		Common variable immunodeficiency, splenomegaly, autoimmune disease, recurrent bacterial infections, enteropathy
DOCK8	Hyper-IgE syndrome	Autosomal recessive	Skin abscesses, eczema, allergic diseases, sinopulmonary infections, broad nasal base and bridge, frontal bossing, deep-set eyes, retained primary teeth, fractures, scoliosis, enteropathy
PIK3CD	Activated PI3K-delta syndrome	Autosomal recessive	Sinopulmonary infections, chronic active viral infections, lymphadenopathy and nodular lymphoid hyperplasia, risk of B-cell lymphoma, enteropathy

TABLE 10.4 Disorders Associated with Very Early Onset Inflammatory Bowel Disease—cont'd

Gene	Disease	Pathogenic Inheritance	Phenotypic Features
Impaired Regulatory T cells			
FOXP3	Immunodysregulation, polyendocrinopathy, enteropathy X-linked syndrome (IPEX)	X-linked	Neonatal-onset secretory diarrhea, growth failure, infection, skin rash, diabetes, thyroiditis, cytopenia, other autoimmune conditions, enteropathy
IL-2RA	IPEX-like	X-linked	Enteropathy, eczema, autoinflammatory disease
STAT1	IPEX-like	Autosomal dominant gain of function	Enteropathy, arthritis
STAT3	STAT3 GOF IPEX-like	Autosomal recessive gain of function	Lymphadenopathy, autoimmune cytopenia, multiorgan autoimmunity, infection, eczema, short stature, enteropathy
STAT5b	STAT5b deficiency	Autosomal recessive	Growth failure, IGF-1 deficiency, chronic pulmonary disease, enteropathy
ITCH	ITCH deficiency	Autosomal recessive	Autoimmune inflammatory cell infiltration of lungs, liver, gut, growth failure, diarrhea, hepatosplenomegaly, enteropathy
IL-21 *IL-21R*		Autosomal recessive	
CTLA4	Complex immune dysregulation syndrome	Autosomal dominant	Enteropathy, autoimmune disease
Autoinflammatory and Hyperinflammatory defects			
MVK	Hyperimmunoglobulin D syndrome	Autosomal recessive	Episodic nausea, fever, abdominal pain, oral ulcers, arthritis, splenomegaly, enteropathy
NLRC4		Autosomal dominant gain of function	Inflammasome activation. hemophagocytic lymphohistiocytosis, episodic inflammation, pan-enteric disease
MEFV	Familial Mediterranean fever	Gain of function	Serositis, periodic fevers, rash, arthritis, enteropathy
HPS1 *HPS4*	Hermansky Pudlak syndrome	Autosomal recessive	Oculocutaneous albinism, pulmonary fibrosis, bleeding disorder, colitis
XIAP	X-linked lymphoproliferative syndrome	X-linked	Infectious mononucleosis or hemophagocytic lymphohistiocytosis secondary to EBV, splenomegaly, abnormal immunoglobulins, lymphoma, enteropathy
TRIM22		Autosomal recessive	Granulomatous colitis, severe perianal disease
SKIV2L		Autosomal recessive	Intrauterine growth restriction, failure to thrive, Trichorrhexis nodosa, frontal bossing, villous atrophy
STXBP2		Autosomal recessive	Hemophagocytic lymphohistiocytosis, enteropathy
CASP8	Caspase-8 deficiency (CEDS)	Autosomal recessive	Lymphadenopathy, splenomegaly, recurrent bacterial and viral infections, especially sinopulmonary infections, hypogammaglobulinemia, enteropathy

Adapted from Conrad MA, Kelsen JR. Genomic and immunologic drivers of very early-onset inflammatory bowel disease. *Pediatr Dev Pathol*. 2019;22(3):183–193.

Genetic variants associated with dysfunction of the intestinal epithelial barrier can result in severe enteropathy. For example, mutations in the *ADAM 17* gene (which result in impaired release of tumor necrosis factor-α [TNF]-α) result in malabsorptive diarrhea with skin and hair abnormalities,[95] whereas mutations in the *IKBKG* gene (which encodes NEMO) result in X-linked ectodermal dysplasia and immunodeficiency.[96] Homozygous mutations in tetratricopeptide repeat domain 7A *(TTC7A)* gene have been associated with several phenotypes including a severe combined immunodeficiency with multiple intestinal atresias and IBD (see Fig. 9.20B).[97,98]

Many defects in adaptive immunity have been associated with severe combined immune deficiency (SCID) and can occur with loss-of-function mutations in recombination activating genes (*RAG1* or *RAG2*), the interleukin (IL)-7 receptor gene *(IL7R)*, which causes Omenn syndrome, and the *PTEN* gene. The landmark discovery of mutations involving the antiinflammatory IL-10 cytokine and its receptors IL-10RA and IL-10RB, resulting in severe infantile

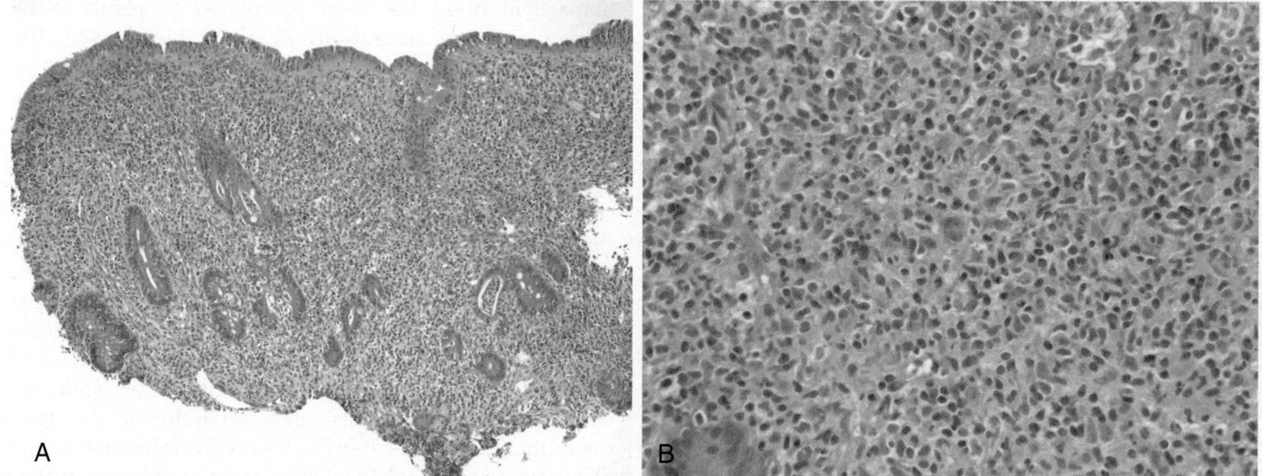

FIGURE 10.8 Colon biopsies from a 10-year-old girl with long-standing colitis and an activating mutation in the *PIK3CD* gene. A, Active chronic colitis with cryptitis and extensive crypt loss with a marked polyphenotypic cellular infiltrate. **B,** Higher-power view shows atypical lymphocytes. Immunohistochemistry confirmed polyclonality, and gene rearrangement studies were negative.

enterocolitis and perianal disease, was the first to demonstrate causal genetic defects in patients with VEO-IBD.[99] The essential role for IL-10 in limiting intestinal inflammation had already been demonstrated by the spontaneous development of severe colitis in IL-10–deficient mice.[100]

Gain-of-function mutations in the *PIK3CD* gene, which encodes the p110δ catalytic subunit of the heterodimer PI3Kδ, cause activated phosphoinositide 3-kinase delta syndrome (APDS) and have been identified in an increasing number of patients who present with a common variable immunodeficiency phenotype associated with a severe enteropathy.[101] These patients have a broad phenotypic presentation including recurrent respiratory infections, enteropathy, failure to thrive, autoimmunity, and lymphoproliferation (Fig. 10.8). The predominant immunological phenotype is hyper-IGM syndrome with decreases in B cells and T cells.

Several autoinflammatory/hyperinflammatory states have been linked with VEO-IBD. These include mevalonate kinase deficiency; mutations in the *NLRC4* gene, which codes for a nucleotide-binding protein activating caspase in the inflammasome complex; familial Mediterranean fever; Hermansky-Pudlak syndrome; and X-linked lymphoproliferative syndrome with loss of function of the X-linked inhibitor of apoptosis (XIAP). XIAP is involved in NOD2-mediated NF-κB signaling. In addition to impaired bacterial sensing, there is impaired apoptosis of activated T cells, resulting in a hyperinflammatory state with increased cytokine production and an IBD-like phenotype (Fig. 10.9). Defects in phagocyte NADP oxidase complex (chronic granulomatous disease) and defects in impaired regulation of T cells (AIE, IPEX, and IPEX-like disorders) are covered in other sections of this chapter and book.

NECROTIZING ENTEROCOLITIS

Neonatal necrotizing enterocolitis (NEC) is the most serious acquired GI disorder of neonates and the most common cause of intestinal perforation and acquired short-gut syndrome among patients in neonatal intensive care units.[102] The severity of disease and its attendant complications is inversely proportional to gestational age, reaching an incidence of 10% and a mortality of 26% among very low birth weight (<1500-g) infants.[103] However, about 10% of cases occur in nearly full-term infants with a variety of risk factors, including cyanotic heart disease, volvulus, aganglionosis, and gastroschisis.

Early signs and symptoms of NEC may be subtle and nonspecific, such as apnea, bradycardia, and lethargy, suggesting sepsis. More specific GI signs include abdominal distension, absent bowel sounds, vomiting, and diarrhea, with radiographic findings such as ileus and pneumatosis intestinalis. More advanced disease is characterized by a perforated viscus in a severely ill child.[104]

The ileocecal region, a vascular "watershed," is most frequently involved, though 25% of children may only have involvement of either the ileum or colon. Disease extending from the ligament of Treitz to the rectum, pan-NEC, may be seen in fatal cases. Continuous and discontinuous involvement occurs in an equal proportion of children. The affected bowel is distended, is grayish or purple (if there is hemorrhage), and the wall is thin and fragile with grossly discernable gas bubbles in cases of pneumatosis (Fig. 10.10). Ischemic hemorrhagic necrosis is the predominant histological manifestation and may be limited to the mucosa or involve the entire thickness of the wall. Inflammatory cell infiltrates occur with progression of the disease and appear to be a response to both the necrosis and the bacterial proliferation. In contradistinction to infectious colitis, crypt microabscesses are uncommon in patients with NEC.[102] Although mesenteric thromboembolism, most frequently resulting from umbilical artery catheterization in neonates, can also cause necrosis of the bowel, occlusion of large vessels is uncommon in patients with NEC, though it may be noted in autopsy cases, where it is believed to be a secondary phenomenon. Intestinal pneumatosis develops as a result of fermentation of intraluminal contents resulting from bacterial overgrowth. Healing changes include re-epithelialization, granulation tissue formation, and fibrosis, which can be associated with stenosis and strictures in surviving infants (Fig. 10.11).

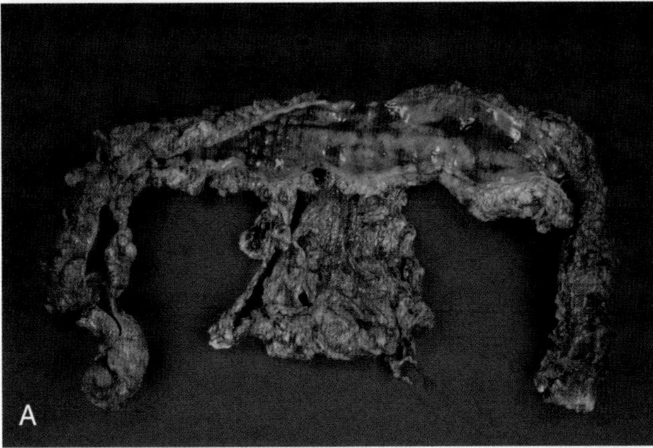

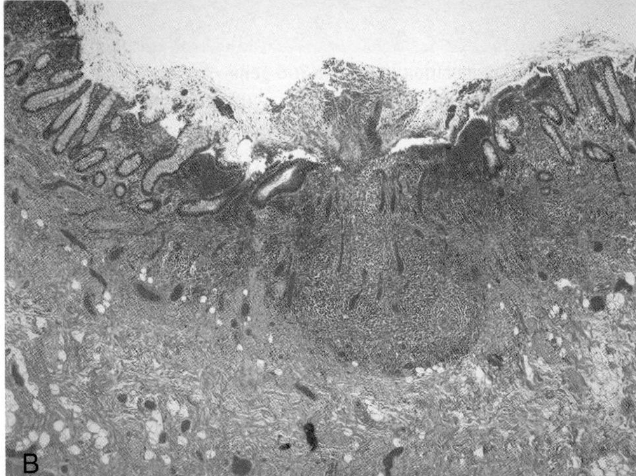

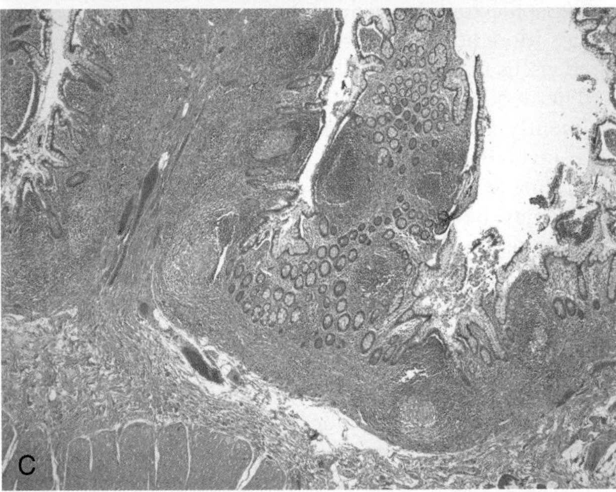

FIGURE 10.9 Terminal ileum and colon from a boy with infantile-onset inflammatory bowel disease, genetically identified as XIAP deficiency at 16 years of age. A, Colon resection from the patient at 10 years of age shows extensive mucosal hemorrhage with cobblestoning and stricture formation. **B,** sections from the colon reveal a diffuse active chronic colitis with ulcers. **C,** Sections from a subsequent partial ileectomy reveals multiple granulomas.

The pathogenesis of NEC is incompletely understood, but is believed to be multifactorial, resulting from a combination of genetic predisposition, intestinal immaturity with inadequate motility, a heightened and inappropriate inflammatory response, abnormal microbial colonization, and an imbalance in microvascular tone.[104] Ischemic damage in NEC has been postulated to result in part from circulatory alterations diverting blood away from the abdominal organs to the heart and brain during episodes of hypoxia (the "diving" reflex). Intramural vessels are hypothesized to be the primary target, resulting from a combination of ischemia and inflammation and mediated by the release of vasoconstrictor agents such as peptide endothelin-1 and free radicals such as nitric oxide.[103] Because NEC usually occurs after the beginning of enteral feeding, enteral alimentation has also been proposed as a contributing factor. Human milk appears to reduce the risk for NEC.[105] A number of different bacterial pathogens have also been associated with NEC as well as various cytokines. Endotoxin, platelet-activating factor, and tumor necrosis factor-α have also induced ischemic damage in experimental models of NEC.[106] Medical therapy includes discontinuing enteral feeds and using antibiotics, intravenous fluids, and parenteral nutrition along with circulatory support. Surgery is indicated in cases of intestinal perforation, when there is progressive clinical deterioration despite optimal medical management, and for resection of strictures and stenoses in convalescing patients. The goal of surgery is to resect only grossly necrotic tissue and to preserve as much bowel as possible. Intraoperative frozen sections for assessment of viability of surgical margins are probably neither indicated or useful.

LYMPHANGIECTASIA

Intestinal lymphangiectasia may be primary or secondary, and it results in protein-losing enteropathy (PLE) (Box 10.2). Primary lymphangiectasia is a rare disorder usually diagnosed in children younger than 3 years of age who present with diarrhea, PLE, hypoalbuminemia, hypogammaglobulinemia, and lymphopenia, resulting in secondary immunodeficiency. Malabsorption may cause deficiencies in fat-soluble vitamins. Primary disorders appear to result from congenital obstruction to lymph flow or abnormal lymphatic structure and may be essentially limited to intestinal lymphatics, as in primary lymphangiectasia,[107,108] or they may involve multiple organs, as in hereditary lymphedema, also known as *Milroy disease,* associated with mutations in the gene encoding vascular endothelial growth factor receptor 3.[109-111] Other disorders may be associated with characteristic congenital anomalies, such as Turner's, Noonan's, and Hennekam's syndromes.[112,113] Intestinal lymphangiectasia has also been reported in premature infants.[114] It has been postulated that congenital hypoplasia of lymphatics may also cause PLE in neonates.[115]

Secondary lymphangiectasia may be "central," resulting from cardiac disease, or from local obstruction to lymphatics due to a variety of causes. In children, secondary immunodeficiency resulting from extensive protein losses in stools has been reported with intestinal malrotation and cavernous hemangioma of the jejunum.[116] Cardiac causes of lymphangiectasia with PLE usually result from obstruction to systemic venous return or from surgical procedures that cause increased systemic venous pressure.[117,118] PLE occurs in up to 10% of patients who have undergone the Fontan operation for correction of tricuspid atresia and other right-sided cardiac malformations, and it carries a poor prognosis, with a 5-year survival of about 50%.[119]

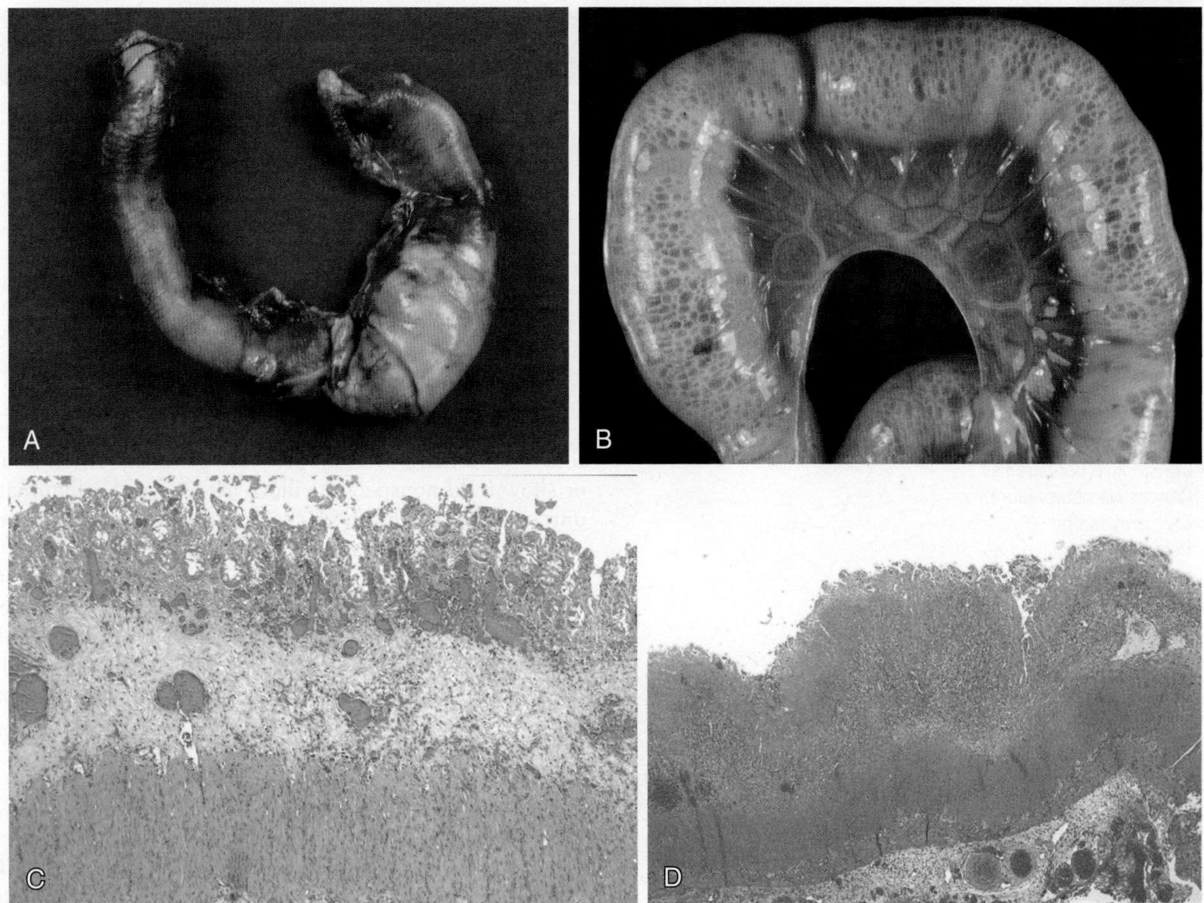

FIGURE 10.10 Necrotizing enterocolitis (NEC). A, segmental small-bowel resection from a 2-month-old patient shows congestion with focal greenish areas of necrosis. **B,** Autopsy specimen from a 1-month-old patient is characterized by extensive pneumatosis. **C,** Early NEC is characterized mainly by mucosal ischemic hemorrhagic necrosis. **D,** Transmural necrosis with extensive inflammatory infiltration. Cystic areas to the right of the micrograph represent early pneumatosis.

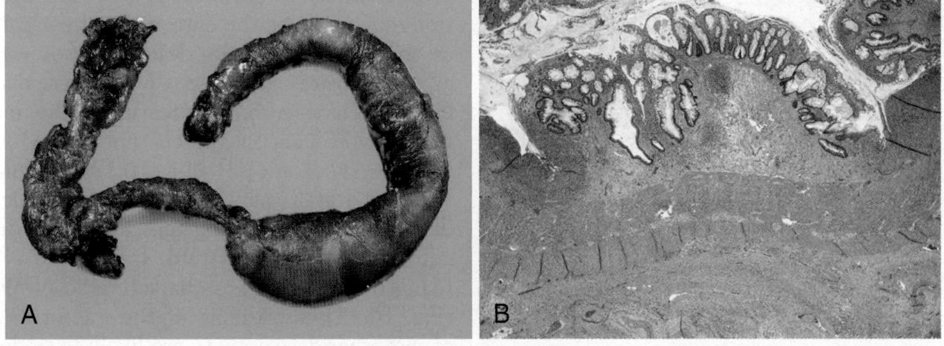

FIGURE 10.11 A, Healed NEC with focal areas of stricturing. **B,** Micrograph from stricture characterized by transmural fibrosis and chronic mucosal architectural changes.

This procedure creates a direct communication between the systemic venous return and the pulmonary arterial system, resulting in chronically sustained increased systemic venous pressure. Associated factors that may contribute to PLE in these patients include inflammatory mediators, decreased enterocyte heparin sulfate synthesis, and chronic mesenteric ischemia.[120]

The endoscopic appearance is usually characteristic, with swollen opaque villi, white nodules, or submucosal elevations.[121,122] Histological examination reveals blunted villi with dilated lacteals (Fig. 10.12). The finding of occasional dilated lymphatics in a biopsy of a patient without significant symptoms is not infrequent and is of no diagnostic value. Conversely, mucosal biopsies may be nondiagnostic when the lesions are focal and will almost always miss lymphangiectasia of deeper layers of the bowel wall. Dietary therapy appears to be a cornerstone of treatment to maintain protein levels.[122] Localized forms of intestinal lymphangiectasia may be amenable to surgical resection.[123]

BOX 10.2 Intestinal Lymphangiectasia

PRIMARY LYMPHANGIECTASIA
- Localized to intestinal lymphatics
  - Waldmann's syndrome
- Associated with other syndromes
  - Milroy's disease
  - Turner's syndrome
  - Noonan's syndrome
  - Hennekam's syndrome
  - Yellow nail syndrome
  - Neurofibromatosis type I
  - Klippel-Trenaunay syndrome
  - Infantile systemic hyalinosis

SECONDARY LYMPHANGIECTASIA
- Cardiac disease
  - Constrictive pericarditis
  - Congestive heart failure
  - Cardiomyopathy
  - Post-Fontan procedure
- Lymphatic obstruction
  - Malrotation
  - Lymphoma
  - Tuberculosis
  - Sarcoidosis
  - Radiation therapy
  - Crohn's disease
  - Retroperitoneal fibrosis

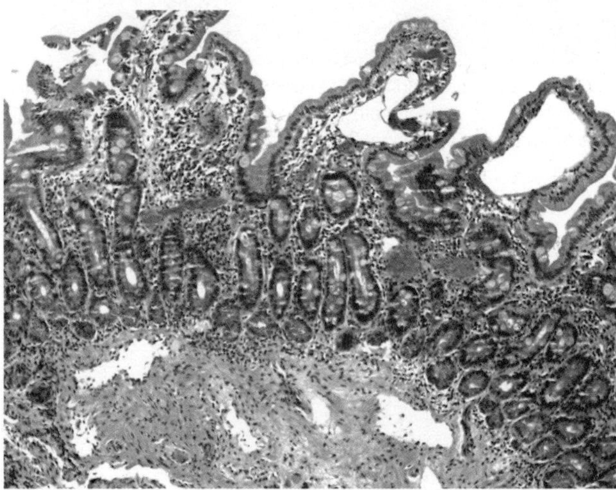

FIGURE 10.12 Lymphangiectasia. A 10-year-old girl with protein-losing enteropathy following the Fontan procedure. Dilated lymphatics are noted in the mucosa and submucosa in this duodenal biopsy.

METABOLIC DISEASES

Metabolic disorders may result in chronic diarrhea and malabsorption (Box 10.3). Several **congenital disorders of glycosylation** (CDG) are associated with prominent GI manifestations. These are part of a large group of disorders that are related to defects in the synthesis and attachment of glycans to proteins and lipids, and they currently comprise about 24 entities, most of which present with neurological manifestations. Failure to thrive with diarrhea, PLE, and hepatic abnormalities have been described mainly in phosphomannose isomerase deficiency (MPI-CDG, formerly CDG type Ib) and ALG6-CDG (formerly CDG type Ic).[124-126] Small-bowel biopsies are generally unremarkable or show mild nonspecific villous atrophy and inflammation unresponsive to gluten or cow's milk withdrawal; electron microscopic changes are characterized by distension of the smooth endoplasmic reticulum with lipid-containing inclusions[127] or insoluble precipitated protein.[128] Absence or marked reduction in the level of enterocyte heparan sulfate may explain the PLE.[129,130] Reported hepatic abnormalities range from mild degrees of steatosis to congenital hepatic fibrosis; congenital hepatic fibrosis, without renal cysts, may be the only feature of MPI-CDG.[125] Dilatation of the crypts of the large intestine has also been observed in some cases[131] (Fig. 10.13). Diagnosis of CDG can be confirmed by isoelectric focusing of serum transferrin; MPI-CDG can be treated with mannose. Murch described three infant boys with massive diarrhea associated with abnormal intestinal glycosaminoglycans with a complete absence of heparan sulfate.[129]

BOX 10.3 Metabolic Disorders Presenting with Severe Diarrhea in Infancy

- Disorders of glycosylation (carbohydrate-deficient glycoprotein syndrome)
- Glycogen storage disease type Ib
- Sialic acid storage disease
- Mucopolysaccharidoses
- Wolman's disease
- Infantile Refsum disease
- Oxidative phosphorylation defect with mitochondrial DNA mutation
- Infantile systemic hyalinosis

According to a report from a consortium of European centers, close to half of patients with **glycogen storage disease type Ib** manifest protracted diarrhea and a clinical profile similar to chronic IBD; defects in neutrophil function may underlie the enteritis in these patients.[132] Several disorders resulting from deficient lysosomal degradation of glycoconjugates can present with severe diarrhea of infancy. Chronic diarrhea can be a feature of the **mucopolysaccharidoses** (MPS) and has been reported with MPS III (Sanfilippo's syndrome)[133] (Fig. 10.14); nodular infiltration of the bowel wall may be noted endoscopically, though the diarrhea is likely most often caused by impairment of the autonomic nervous system. Infiltration of the mucosa by foamy macrophages is characteristic of **Wolman's disease** (Fig. 10.15); shortening of the microvilli and impairment of disaccharidase activity are likely to underlie the diarrhea observed in these patients.[134] **Tangier disease** is a high-density lipoprotein (HDL)-deficiency syndrome characterized by accumulation of cholesterol in tissue macrophages throughout the body and prevalent atherosclerosis, resulting from mutations in the gene coding for ATP-binding cassette transporter 1 (ABCA1). Endoscopic examination reveals characteristic orange nodules in the mucosa, with accumulation of fat noted in the macrophages in the lamina propria and smooth muscle cells.[135]

Glycolipid storage disorders are generally characterized in the GI tract by the presence of lipid deposits in Schwann cells, ganglia, muscle, and endothelial cells,[136,137] usually without symptoms attributable to the deposits.

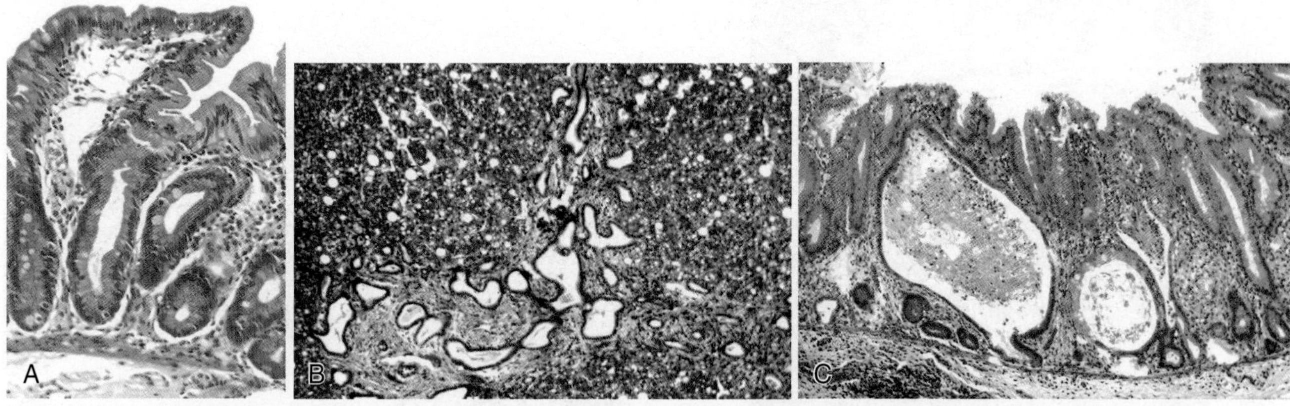

FIGURE 10.13 Congenital disorder of glycosylation, type Ib, phosphomannose-isomerase deficiency. This 4-year-old boy presented with protein-losing enteropathy and hepatomegaly. **A,** Dilated mucosal lymphatics were noted in the small bowel. **B,** Congenital hepatic fibrosis, without evidence of renal disease. **C,** The colon was characterized mainly by dilatation of the crypts.

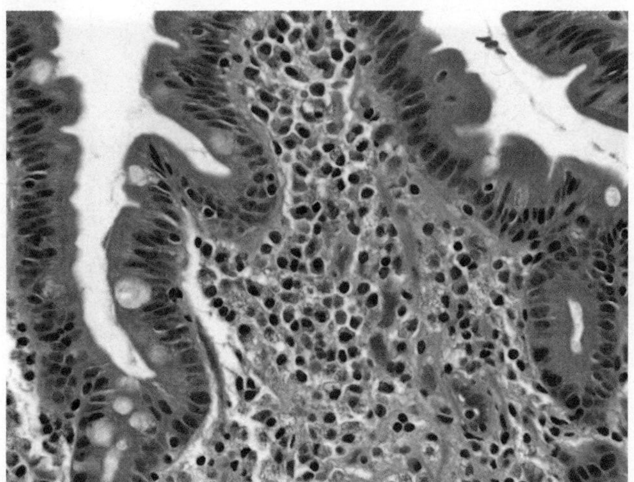

FIGURE 10.14 Mucopolysaccharidosis type III (Sanfilippo's syndrome). Intestinal biopsy in a 16-year-old female shows numerous vacuolated mononuclear inflammatory cells in the lamina propria.

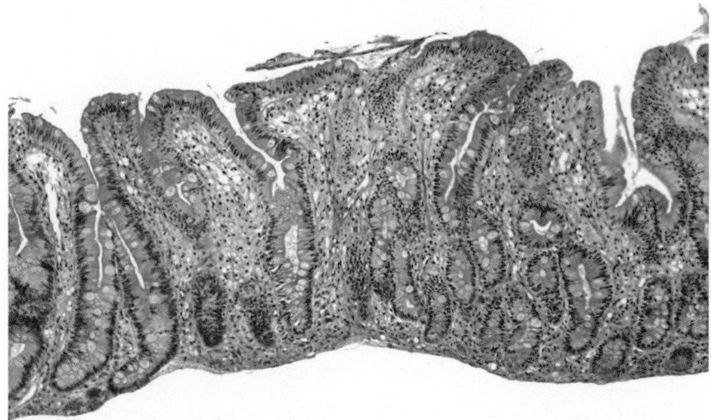

FIGURE 10.15 Wolman's disease. Foamy macrophages fill the lamina propria.

However, more than one-half of patients with **Fabry's disease**, an X-linked disorder resulting in deficiency of α-galactosidase, experience GI symptoms mimicking irritable bowel syndrome. There is accumulation of a lipid, globotriaosylceramide, in the enteric neurons interfering with normal gut motility and resulting in delayed gastric emptying, bacterial overgrowth, and subsequent diarrhea and steatorrhea.[138] Enzyme replacement therapy with agalsidase alfa has improved symptoms in these patients.[139] Severe protracted diarrhea in association with low cholesterol levels in the first month of life are important manifestations of some the more severe forms of peroxisomal disorders such as **infantile Refsum disease**[140]; this clinical presentation must be differentiated from lipid transport disorders such as **abetalipoproteinemia.** Cormier-Daire and colleagues reported two infants with chronic diarrhea and villous atrophy caused by a respiratory chain complex III deficiency associated with mitochondrial DNA mutations[141]; severe diarrhea has been described as a presenting manifestation in other disorders associated with mitochondrial DNA rearrangements.[142] **Infantile systemic hyalinosis** is a rare, apparently autosomal recessive disorder characterized by painful joint contractures and skin nodules resulting from widespread deposits of a hyaline substance in the skin, skeletal muscle, GI tract, and endocrine organs (Fig. 10.16). The disorder was well documented by Landing,[143] though the first description of the disease was probably by Nezelof.[144] PLE resulting from intestinal lymphangiectasia has been described in many of these patients.[145,146] On electron microscopy, floccular amorphous material was observed around blood vessels in the dermis and postulated to interfere with collagen formation.[147] The exact biochemical defect is unknown.

NEOPLASTIC DISORDERS

Neoplasms rarely present as chronic diarrhea in children, especially in infants and toddlers, though diarrhea is occasionally a major or presenting manifestation. Some neoplasms cause symptoms by direct infiltration of the bowel wall or by secretion of a hormone or substance that is active in the GI tract. Diffuse infiltration of the bowel resulting in

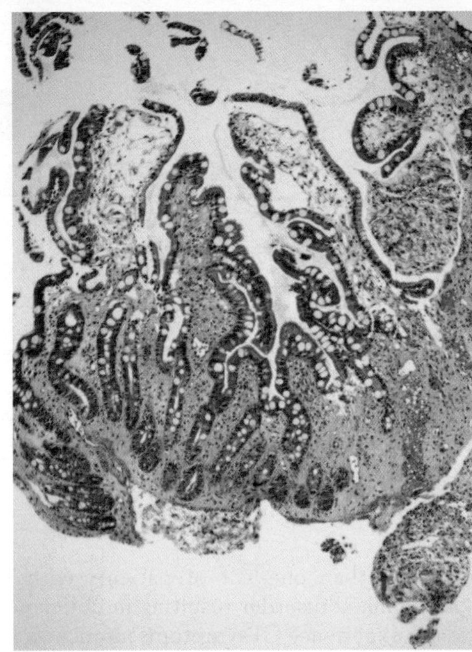

FIGURE 10.16 Infantile systemic hyalinosis. Duodenal biopsy from a 17-month-old boy with protein-losing enteropathy, painful contractures, and gingival hyperplasia. An amorphous acellular material fills the lamina propria (Masson-Trichrome).

severe diarrhea in neonates has been reported with Langerhans cell histiocytosis[148,149] and visceral myofibromatosis[150] (Fig. 10.17). Neuroblastomas and ganglioneuroblastomas presenting with watery diarrhea, hypokalemia, and achlorhydria have been documented in numerous reports.

The full reference list may be accessed online at Elsevier eBooks for Practicing Clinicians.

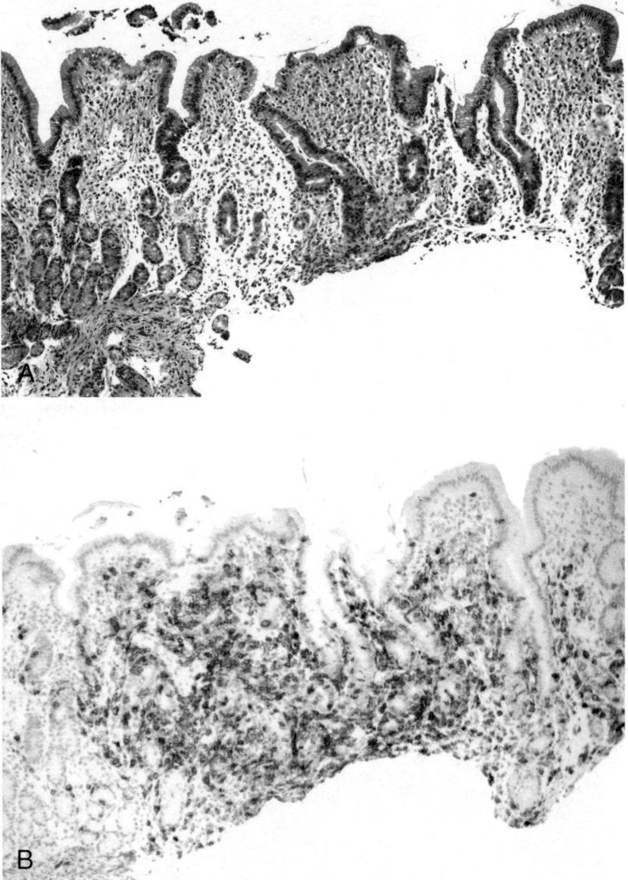

FIGURE 10.17 Langerhans cell histiocytosis. A, Intestinal biopsy from a 2-year-old child reveals blunted and distorted villi by the neoplastic histiocytes. **B,** CD1a immunohistochemical stain.

11 Vascular Disorders of the Gastrointestinal Tract

Daniela Allende

Contents

INTRODUCTION

The gastrointestinal (GI) tract performs energy-demanding functions of digestion and absorption of nutrients while maintaining a critical barrier between the internal milieu and the external (luminal) environment. It also contributes to the activities of the immune system. These functions depend on a reliable blood supply. It is not surprising, therefore, that vascular disorders have important clinical manifestations. Vascular disorders usually manifest clinically as bleeding or ischemia, both of which occur in acute and chronic forms. In this chapter, vascular disorders are discussed in the context of these two types of clinical presentation, although there is considerable overlap between them.

ANATOMY OF THE GI VASCULAR SYSTEM

The proximal esophagus derives its blood supply from the superior and inferior thyroid arteries, the middle esophagus from the bronchial and right intercostal arteries, and the distal esophagus from the left gastric and left inferior phrenic artery with additional supply from the splenic artery and celiac trunk.[1] The middle and lower esophagus also receives arterial blood directly from the aorta. Venous drainage is also segmental. Blood from the proximal esophagus drains into the superior vena cava, that from the middle esophagus into the azygos or hemiazygos veins, and that from the distal esophagus through the left and short gastric veins into the portal vein.[1] Anastomoses among the vessels that supply each of these regions result in complex arterial and venous networks. For instance, the venous network in the mucosa and submucosa of the middle and distal esophagus is the source of esophageal varices in patients with portal hypertension.

The stomach, proximal duodenum, gallbladder, liver, and pancreas are supplied by branches of the celiac trunk. The distal duodenum is supplied by a branch of the superior mesenteric artery. Numerous anastomoses between esophageal and gastric feeding vessels result in a complex vascular network which results in a protective effect against ischemia in these organs. The gastric and duodenal veins drain into the portal system.

The remainder of the small intestine is supplied by the inferior pancreaticoduodenal, jejunal, and ileal branches of the superior mesenteric artery, which also supplies the cecum and ascending and proximal transverse colon through its ileocolic, middle colic, and right colic branches. The inferior mesenteric artery supplies the distal transverse colon to the proximal rectum, whereas the distal rectum is supplied by the internal iliac and pudendal arteries. The arterial supply of the small and large intestines consists of numerous vascular arcades (vasa recta) with abundant anastomoses that result in a rich collateral circulation that helps protect the bowel against damage from pathological processes within individual blood vessels. Certain areas of the large bowel are predisposed to vascular insult, such as the splenic flexure and rectosigmoid colon. The ileocecal region is also predisposed to ischemic injury, but to a lesser extent.[2-4] Venous drainage of the colon and rectum follows the arterial supply. The vascular collaterals in the rectum provide another location in which varices may develop in patients with portal hypertension.

The anus is supplied by the superior, middle, and inferior rectal arteries. Branches of these arteries have multiple small arteriovenous anastomoses with submucosal venous plexuses. Interestingly, the blood flow to the anal canal exceeds its metabolic requirements. Venous drainage of the anus is mainly to the superior rectal vein.

Blood flow to the GI tract is normally under tight physiological regulation through the autonomic nervous system. For example, the blood supply increases by as much as 100% immediately after ingestion of a meal. On the other hand, in states of shock, when it is vital to maintain blood flow to critical organs such as the central nervous system, splanchnic blood flow may be drastically reduced, sometimes beyond the critical level needed to maintain viability of the intestinal mucosa.

SAMPLING OF RESECTION SPECIMENS

In general, surgery is performed for failed medical therapy and/or for perforation and other complications. Appropriate macroscopic inspection and sampling are critical to achieve a correct diagnosis. The serosal or adventitial surface, depending on the location within the GI tract, may reveal hemorrhage, necrosis, and serosal fibrin deposition if a perforation is present. Perforations can be microscopic and, as such, not readily evident on gross examination. However, the presence of external fibrinous membranes is often indicative of the perforation site. Serial sectioning should be performed if the perforation is not immediately evident. Serosal adhesions should also be sampled as they can represent the area most indicative of the underlying injury. Tissue sections should target the areas of worse injury to document the severity of disease and to help identify the underlying etiology. Special attention should be paid to sectioning the vasculature in the mesentery and omentum. In cases of thromboembolic disease and vasculitis, the key histological features often reside in the mesentery. Representative sections of the surgical margins should be obtained to predict viability of the anastomosis and any potential complications. If the specimen is received fresh, tissue may be submitted for culture and even immunofluorescence, if clinically indicated.

UPPER GI BLEEDING

General Comments

Bleeding from the upper GI tract is a frequent indication for endoscopy and is common worldwide. In the United States, acute GI bleeding accounts for 250,000 to 300,000 hospitalizations per year.[5] Up to 14% of patients admitted on an emergency basis and as many as 28% of patients hospitalized die of their acute GI bleeding.[6,7] Upper GI tract bleeding, defined as bleeding proximal to the ligament of Treitz, is four times more common than lower GI tract bleeding.[8] Upper GI bleeds occur most commonly in elderly patients, although in conditions such as hereditary hemorrhagic telangiectasia (HHT), onset of disease may occur as early as the third decade of life.[9] Risk factors for upper GI tract bleeding include older patient age, alcohol use, and concomitant use of drugs such as nonsteroidal antiinflammatory drugs (NSAIDs) and anticoagulants.[10]

Patients often present with direct evidence of a GI bleed, such as hematemesis, melena, heme-positive stools, and, less commonly, hematochezia. They may also present with signs and symptoms of iron-deficiency anemia, such as syncope, chest pain, dizziness, and shortness of breath. In severe, acute, life-threatening hemorrhage, the clinical presentation is usually a result of shock or cardiovascular collapse.

Esophagus

The most important causes of esophageal bleeding are varices that develop as a result of portal hypertension, Mallory-Weiss lacerations, or esophagitis (Table 11.1).

Esophageal Varices

Esophageal varices are dilated, tortuous veins within the lamina propria and submucosa that bulge into the esophageal lumen because of portal hypertension and portosystemic shunting. Esophageal varices may develop in any condition that leads to portal hypertension, but they are most often associated with alcoholic cirrhosis. The demographic features of patients with esophageal varices are similar to those of patients with cirrhosis and portal hypertension. In some parts of the world, hepatic schistosomiasis is a common cause of esophageal varices. Varices are typically asymptomatic until they rupture into the esophageal lumen, which results in hematemesis or melena.

Bleeding varices are most common in the caudal portion of the esophagus. However, a discrete bleeding site is usually difficult to identify pathologically. Varices tend to collapse at the time of autopsy and therefore are best diagnosed endoscopically. In autopsy specimens, eversion and formalin fixation of the esophagus are techniques that can be used to help demonstrate varices. Grossly dilated, tortuous veins may be seen in the distal esophagus, in particular below the aortic arch, protruding into the lumen (Fig. 11.1A). There may be superimposed thrombosis and mucosal erosions.

Histologically, dilated lamina propria and submucosal veins are characteristic. These are usually associated with fresh hemorrhage, organizing thrombi, and hemosiderin deposition (Fig. 11.1B). Surface ulcers, erosions, and reactive epithelial changes in the overlying epithelium may be present as well. In specimens examined after treatment with sclerotherapy or endoscopic ligation, other findings may include thrombosis, ulceration, necrosis, inflammation, and fibrosis as a late event.[11,12] Elastic and/or Movat stains can help highlight obliterated blood vessels.

Although variceal bleeding is the most important cause of hematemesis in patients with portal hypertension, other causes of upper GI bleeding are implicated in approximately 50% of patients who are seen with hematemesis (Table 11.2; see Table 11.1).

TABLE 11.1 Pathological Features of Entities That Cause Esophageal Bleeding

Entity	Key Clinical Features	Key Pathological Features	Treatment
Gastroesophageal reflux disease	Most common symptoms are heartburn, regurgitation, and dysphagia More prevalent after 40 years of age	Typically distal 7 cm of esophagus Background esophagitis: squamous hyperplasia, intraepithelial neutrophils, and increased eosinophils and lymphocytes	Medical options: PPI and H_2 antagonists Surgical options: fundoplication and gastropexy
HSV infection	Main symptom: odynophagia Common in immunocompromised patients, particularly organ and bone marrow transplant recipients Occurs in immunocompetent patients	Vesicles early feature; coalesce to form ulcer Ground-glass nuclear inclusions in squamous cells at edge of shallow, punched-out ulcers HSV immunostain confirms the diagnosis	Antivirals (e.g., acyclovir) May resolve spontaneously in immunocompetent patients
Candida infection	Main symptom: substernal dysphagia More common in immunocompromised patients Often coexists with other etiologies	Patchy white mucosal plaques Neutrophils, yeast, and pseudohyphae in superficial squamous epithelium Usually with desquamation: often detached fragments in biopsies Fungal stains (PAS, GMS) often helpful	Antifungals (e.g., fluconazole, itraconazole)
CMV infection	Main symptom: odynophagia Common in immunocompromised patients In HIV-infected patients, more common than HSV	Ulcers deeper, more linear than in HSV Single large nuclear and multiple amphophilic cytoplasmic inclusions in capillary endothelial or stromal cells in granulation tissue at base Immunostaining may be necessary because inclusions can be rare	Antivirals (e.g., ganciclovir, foscarnet)
NSAIDs	Concomitant illnesses necessitating NSAIDs (e.g., chronic back pain, arthritis) Simultaneous alcohol use common	Shallow, large ulcers with broad base, usually in middle esophagus Usually devoid of background esophagitis	Discontinue medication Supportive therapy
Pill/medication induced	Sudden onset of symptoms Pills swallowed without fluids Can be caused by many medications (e.g., tetracycline, potassium chloride, bisphosphonate, quinidine)	Nonspecific superficial desquamation of squamous epithelium, spongiosis, necrotic keratinocytes Exudate seen commonly with quinidine-induced ulcers	Educate patient to take pills with fluids Discontinue medication, or start liquid therapy if necessary Supportive therapy
Radiation	Usually a history of head and neck, mediastinal, pulmonary, or esophageal malignancy	Fibrinoid necrosis and dilation of blood vessels, vascular intimal proliferation, stromal fibrosis, stellate fibroblasts ± cytological atypia and increased apoptosis	Supportive therapy Surgery if perforation or fistula develops
Foreign-body injury	Most common in children; also seen in elderly, psychiatric patients, and inmates Sudden onset of symptoms; may lead to esophagovascular fistula	Nonspecific necrosis, inflammation, and ulceration; may progress to perforation	Endoscopic or surgical removal Resection or repair of perforation or fistula
Chemical injury	Similar to foreign body injury Alkaline ingestion damages esophagus more commonly	Necrosis more common	Supportive therapy May require resection
Varices*	Occur in portal hypertension (cirrhotic and noncirrhotic) Schistosomiasis and viral hepatitis are common causes worldwide Typically asymptomatic until rupture; rebleeding is common	Most common in distal 3 to 4 cm of esophagus Dilated tortuous veins of lamina propria and submucosa bulging into lumen, fresh hemorrhage and adjacent thrombosis Erosions and ulcers uncommon Thrombosis, ulceration, necrosis, and inflammation more likely after therapy	Sclerosing and banding varices Portosystemic shunting Medical management of portal hypertension
Mallory-Weiss tears*	Strong association with chronic alcoholism; ASA use common Typical history (retching or forceful vomiting) in only 30% Related to upward diaphragmatic movement	Minority involve esophagus; majority in lesser curve of proximal stomach, may be at esophagogastric junction Nonspecific mucosal breach with acute hemorrhage, seldom into submucosa Usually no acute inflammatory response	Usually self-limited If therapy is required: balloon tamponade, embolization, medical management Surgery rare

ASA, *Acetylsalicylic acid;* CMV, *cytomegalovirus;* GMS, *Grocott-Gomori methenamine–silver nitrate*; H_2, *histamine 2;* HIV, *human immunodeficiency virus;* HSV, *herpes simplex virus;* NSAIDs, *nonsteroidal antiinflammatory drugs;* PAS, *periodic acid–Schiff;* PPI, *proton pump inhibitor.*
**Most common causes.*

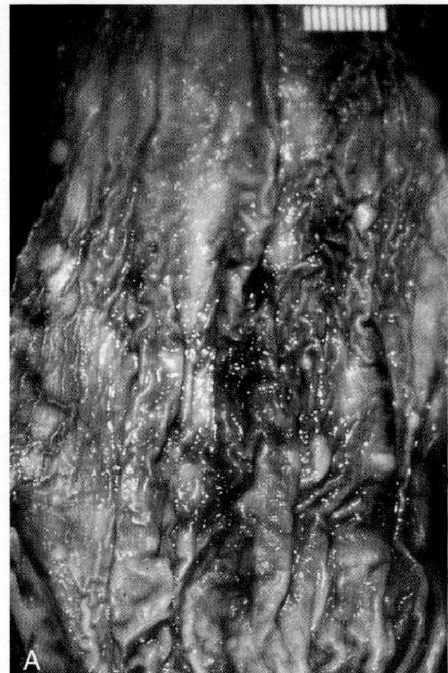

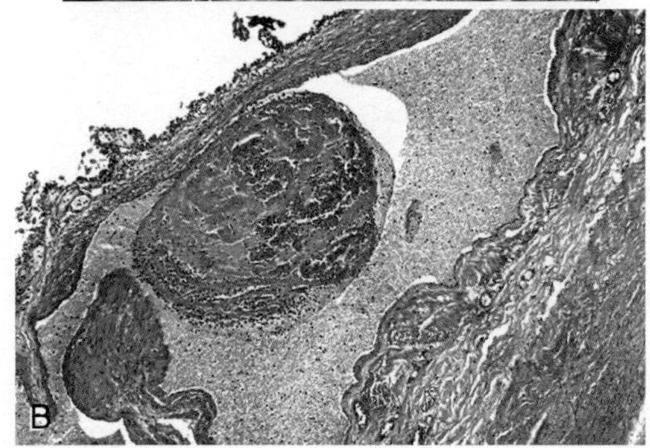

FIGURE 11.1 Esophageal varices. A, Dilated, tortuous veins bulge into the esophageal lumen, where there is focal fresh hemorrhage. **B,** Dilated submucosal veins contain organizing thrombi. (**A** *courtesy of Dr. Dhanpat Jain, Yale University School of Medicine, New Haven, CT.*)

Esophageal varices often rebleed. The risk of dying within 6 weeks of an initial bleed is 20% to 30% in patients with cirrhosis-related portal hypertension.[13] Variceal bleeding may precipitate hepatic encephalopathy in cirrhotic patients. Treatment modalities include sclerosis and banding of individual varices, portosystemic shunting, and pharmacological management of portal hypertension.

Mallory-Weiss Laceration

Mallory-Weiss laceration is a longitudinal tear of the mucosa located in the region of the gastroesophageal junction. These lesions may bleed profusely.[14] A clinical history of retching or forceful vomiting is identified in approximately 30% of patients. Mallory-Weiss lacerations develop mainly in patients with chronic alcoholism and typically occur in the third to fifth decades of life. Concomitant aspirin use has been reported in approximately 30% of patients. Other risk factors include upward diaphragmatic movement related to coughing, heavy lifting, pregnancy, and abdominal trauma.[15] Mallory-Weiss laceration is an uncommon complication of upper GI endoscopy in association with retching and hiatal hernia. In addition, some patients present with melena or iron-deficiency anemia.

The pathogenesis of Mallory-Weiss laceration is related to upward movement of the diaphragm and an increase in intraabdominal pressure, which leads to protrusion of the proximal stomach into the thoracic cavity. This is often preceded by nausea, which causes distention of the stomach and reflux of gastric contents into the esophagus. When protrusion of the distended stomach is forceful, longitudinal lacerations may develop. Lacerations are more likely to occur in patients with a hiatal hernia.

Most Mallory-Weiss lacerations are located on the gastric side of the gastroesophageal junction. Only a minority involve the tubular esophagus.[14] They occur most commonly on the lesser curve of the proximal stomach (Fig. 11.2) but may also occur at the gastroesophageal junction. Histologically, Mallory-Weiss lacerations are characterized by a longitudinal breach of the mucosa that extends into the submucosa, but generally not into the muscularis propria, usually accompanied by hemorrhage, either with or without an acute inflammatory response. Healing Mallory-Weiss lacerations show granulation tissue, fibrosis, epithelial regeneration, and other features of healing ulcers.

Mallory-Weiss lacerations are usually treated supportively. In some patients with persistent bleeding, pharmacological management, balloon tamponade, embolization, and, rarely, surgery may be required to establish hemostasis. Boerhaave's syndrome (acute perforation of the esophagus) is a catastrophic event that is considered a complication of Mallory-Weiss lacerations. However, patients with Boerhaave's syndrome do not typically present with severe acute GI bleeding.[16]

Esophagitis and Esophageal Ulcers

Esophagitis and esophageal ulcers are most commonly caused by gastroesophageal reflux disease (GERD), infection (e.g., herpesvirus, *Candida*, cytomegalovirus), drugs, chemical or physical injury from accidental or intentional ingestion of toxic (alkaline and acidic) substances, or foreign objects. Bleeding from esophagitis is usually occult, and patients commonly present with anemia. Bleeding from esophageal ulcers varies in severity depending on the cause, but it is most often acute. Signs and symptoms include hematemesis, chest or epigastric pain, and odynophagia. Most patients with acute bleeding present initially in the emergency department,[17] and many of them have significant comorbid conditions.

Overall, GERD-associated ulcers are most common, and they occur in all age groups, although they are more prevalent after 40 years of age. Ulcers caused by infections are more likely to occur in immunocompromised patients. Certain drugs are more commonly associated with esophageal mucosal injury, such as doxycycline, amoxicillin, ciprofloxacin, metronidazole, rifaximin, antihypertensive drugs, NSAIDS, bisphosphonates, and warfarin, among many others.[18] Concomitant alcohol use has been reported in a subset of patients with NSAID-induced esophageal ulcers, suggesting that it may have a synergistic effect. Ulcers related to medication injury are common in the elderly, whereas those caused by foreign objects are more common in children. Reflux is less likely to be associated with bleeding than use of NSAIDs, which causes injury by direct mucosal contact.[19]

TABLE 11.2 Pathological Features of Entities That Cause Gastric or Duodenal Bleeding

Entity	Key Clinical Features	Key Pathological Features	Treatment
Helicobacter pylori–induced peptic ulcers	Most common cause Decreasing prevalence rates	Gastritis more common in antrum Typically superficially oriented lymphoplasmacytic gastritis with neutrophil infiltrate and spiral forms of *H. pylori* May have reactive lymphoid follicles, intestinal metaplasia, and mucosal atrophy Ulcers may be located in duodenum	*H. pylori* eradication therapy Antisecretory therapy
Chemical-induced ulcers	NSAID use is a clear predisposing factor to gastric bleeding	Erosions or shallow ulcers More common in fundus and body Usually without background gastritis	Discontinue medication, or significantly reduce dose
		Mucin loss with nuclear enlargement and hyperchromasia in adjacent epithelium	Supportive therapy
Stress-related ulcers	Patients with multiple comorbidities; risk factors include prior PUD, CNS trauma or surgery, sepsis, multiple trauma, liver and kidney failure, and organ transplantation In hospital patients, duodenal ulcers more later in course Curling ulcer: following burns Cushing ulcer: following neurological injury or surgery	Erosions or shallow ulcers Usually without background gastritis More common in fundus and body, may also be seen in duodenum Abrupt erosions or ulcers with interstitial hemorrhage, reactive epithelial atypia Adjacent mucosa with acute hemorrhagic gastritis, diffuse mucosal hyperemia, edema	Supportive therapy; may include blood transfusion. Prophylactic therapy to prevent additional ulcers (includes PPI, antacids, H_2 antagonists, sucralfate, prostaglandin analogues)
Dieulafoy lesions	Most common in middle-aged and elderly men	Most common in proximal stomach on lesser curve Similar lesions reported in distal esophagus and small and large bowel Small mucosal defect with abnormally large, thick-walled artery in base Adjacent mucosa usually lacks inflammation	Therapeutic endoscopy (e.g., clipping, electrocoagulation, injection sclerotherapy, banding) Surgical ligation or resection
Cameron ulcers	Associated with hiatal hernias	Linear ulcers in hiatal hernias Histological features of a benign ulcer	Therapeutic endoscopy to control bleeding Surgical management of hernia
Varices*	Most commonly in continuity with esophageal varix with similar morphology	See Table 11.1	
Portal hypertensive gastropathy and gastric vascular ectasia	See Table 11.3	See Table 11.3	
HHT	Autosomal dominant disease with variable penetrance and expression Telangiectases on skin and mucous membranes Frequently have history of GI bleeding 20% have no family history of symptoms	More common in the stomach, but also seen in the esophagus and duodenum Lesions include telangiectasias, arteriovenous malformations, aneurysms, venous varicosities, and arteriovenous fistulas Classically clusters or tufts of dilated, tortuous arteriolar-venular connections without intervening capillaries	Medical therapy includes danazol, estrogen, aminocaproic acid Therapeutic endoscopy (coagulation, cautery, or laser) Surgical resection
Hemodialysis-associated telangiectasia	Long-term hemodialysis	Morphologically similar to HHT, may appear reddish and fernlike grossly	Therapeutic endoscopy (thermal coagulation)

CNS, *Central nervous system;* GI, *gastrointestinal;* H_2, *histamine 2;* HHT, *hereditary hemorrhagic telangiectasia;* NSAID, *nonsteroidal antiinflammatory drug;* PPI, *proton pump inhibitor;* PUD, *peptic ulcer disease.*
**Most common cause.*

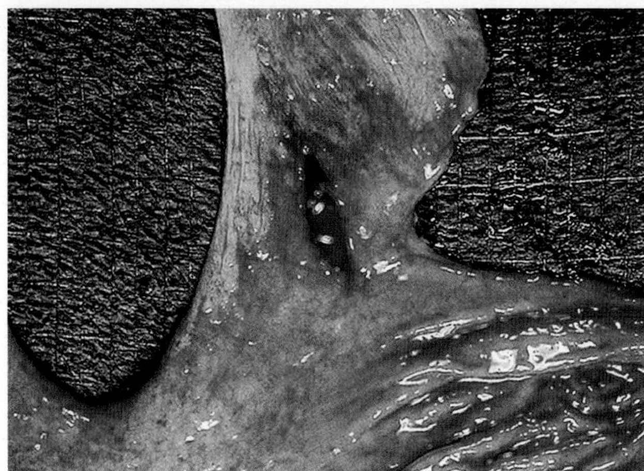

FIGURE 11.2 Mallory-Weiss laceration: a longitudinal mucosal tear, in this case traversing the esophagogastric junction into the lesser curve of the proximal stomach.

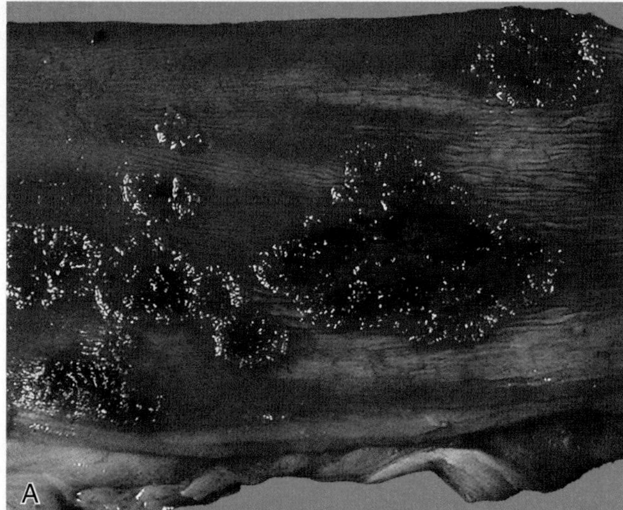

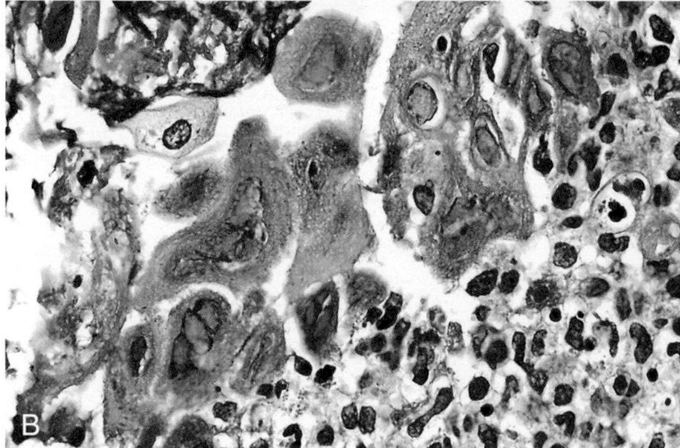

FIGURE 11.3 Herpes esophagitis. A, Multiple ulcers are present in the esophageal mucosa with hemorrhagic bases and erythematous, vesicular borders; notice the separate cluster of small erythematous vesicles. **B,** Characteristic multinucleate cells with Cowdry type A inclusions.

Other causes of esophageal ulcers include Crohn's disease and radiation-induced injury caused by vascular compromise. Injury from chemical agents, such as lye, is caused by their corrosive effect on the mucosa.

Ulcers resulting from GERD occur mainly in the distal third of the esophagus. Adjacent mucosal changes typical of reflux, such as squamous hyperplasia with prominent fibrovascular papillae and intraepithelial inflammation (eosinophils, neutrophils, and/or lymphocytes), are usually present. Herpesvirus inclusions are identified most readily in squamous cells at the edges of herpetic ulcers (Fig. 11.3A,B). In contrast, cytomegalovirus inclusions are most often found in endothelial cells and/or stromal cells at the ulcer base. *Candida* should be considered wherever neutrophils accumulate in the surface epithelium, usually in association with superficial desquamation. Morphological features of radiation injury include dilated and thickened capillaries with deposition of hyaline, prominent endothelial cells, and reactive stroma with atypical stellate fibroblasts. NSAID-induced ulcers are typically large, shallow lesions with a broad base and are most common in the middle esophagus (Fig. 11.4).[19] Pill esophagitis shows superficial epithelial sloughing, keratinocyte necrosis, spongiosis, intraepithelial eosinophils, and associated crystalline birefringent particles (Fig. 11.5A,B). Ulcerating malignant neoplasms may also be a source of bleeding, but this is an unusual presentation of esophageal cancer.[20] However, the most common indication for endoscopy in patients with a secondary malignant neoplasm of the esophagus is GI bleeding.[21] Bleeding from NSAID-induced ulcers is usually active and infrequently complicated by strictures. Rarely, esophageal or gastric ulcers perforate or penetrate into contiguous vascular organs, such as the heart and aorta, leading to massive bleeding[22] (Fig. 11.6). Ulcers resulting from foreign bodies are particularly prone to this type of complication.[20-24]

Acute Esophageal Necrosis

Acute esophageal necrosis (AEN; also known as *black esophagus*) is a rare disease. It develops as a result of multiple factors, such as ischemia (hemodynamic compromise and

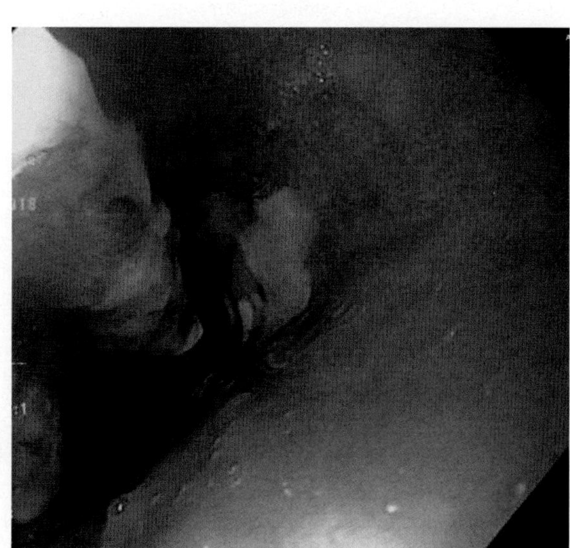

FIGURE 11.4 Endoscopic image of a broad-based esophageal ulcer associated with NSAID use.

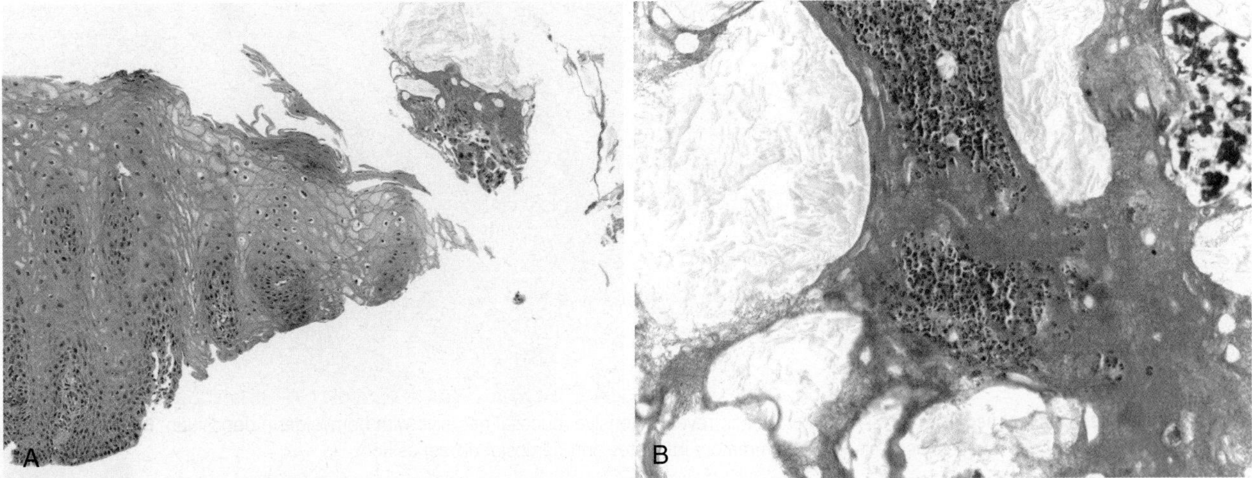

FIGURE 11.5 Pill esophagitis. A, Squamous epithelium with acanthoses and focal parakeratosis. Detached fibrinopurulent membrane with crystalline material. **B,** At higher magnification, the birefringent material consistent with pill-induced injury is noted within the fibrinopurulent membrane.

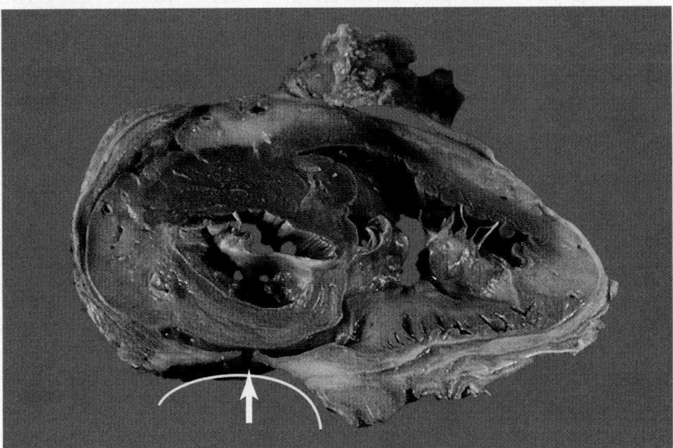

FIGURE 11.6 Ulcer into the heart. Coronal section of the heart with an adherent esophageal ulcer base *(yellow line)* and perforation into coronary sinus *(arrow)* that resulted in massive upper gastrointestinal bleeding.

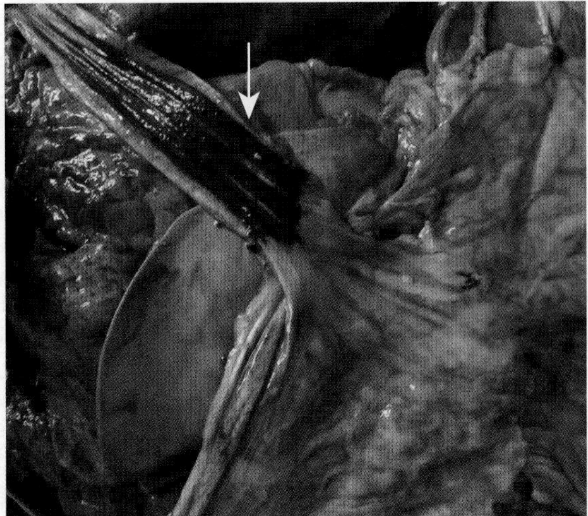

FIGURE 11.7 Acute esophageal necrosis ("black esophagus"). Black discoloration *(arrow)* of the mucosal surface in the esophageal area affected characterizes this entity (*Courtesy of Dr. Kaarina Ristmägi, East-Tallinn Central Hospital, Tallinn, Estonia*)

low-flow states), corrosive injury (such as gastric contents in the setting of esophago-gastroparesis and gastric outlet obstruction), and in patients with decreased protective/reparative mechanisms of the mucosal barrier (which is common in malnourished and debilitated patients).[25] Patients are frequently older-aged males who present with bleeding, epigastric/abdominal pain, vomiting, dysphagia, fever, and syncope. At endoscopy, and on macroscopic examination, there is diffuse circumferential black-colored mucosal discoloration that starts distally and extends proximally (Fig. 11.7). Pathologically, necrosis of the esophageal mucosa, with variable involvement of the submucosa and muscularis propria, are typical features observed (Fig. 11.8A,B). This entity is associated with a mortality rate of approximately 32%.[26] Complications include perforation, mediastinitis, esophageal stricture, and infection.

Esophageal Diverticula

Esophageal diverticula are rare and usually asymptomatic. However, patients with diverticula may occasionally present with upper GI tract bleeding. Bleeding may occur in association with an ulcer, entrapped pills, or use of anticoagulants.[27]

Stomach

Aside from bleeding from varices, which commonly involves both the esophagus and the proximal stomach, gastric bleeding is most often caused by benign ulcers and erosive gastritis (see Table 11.2).

Gastric Varices

Gastric varices have clinical and pathological features similar to those of esophageal varices. They most commonly occur on the lesser curve of the proximal stomach, in continuity with esophageal varices.[28] Reports vary as to whether gastric varices, compared with esophageal varices, are less likely[28] or equally likely[29] to bleed. Bleeding from gastric varices, when it does occur, is usually severe.[28]

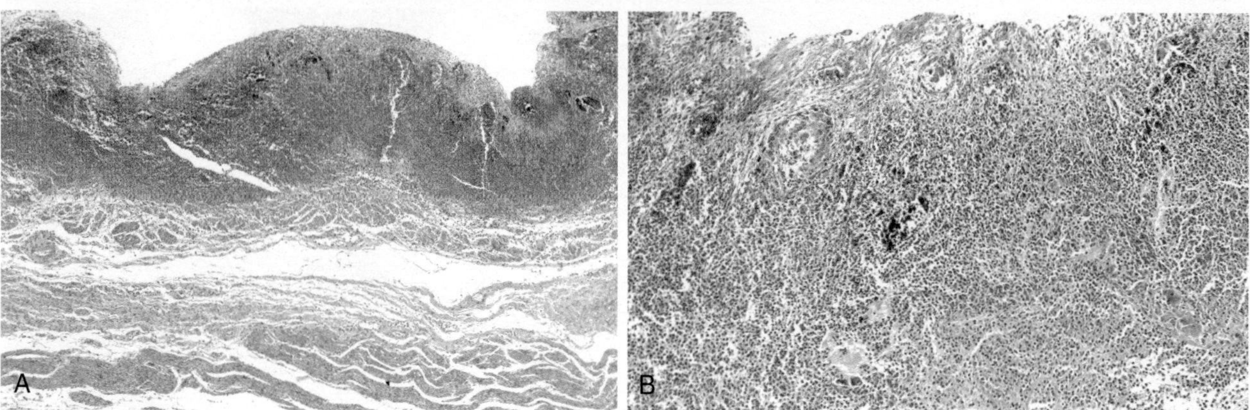

FIGURE 11.8 Acute esophageal necrosis. A, Histological section reveal extensive mucosal necrosis with hemosiderin deposition. **B,** At higher magnification, there is full-thickness mucosal necrosis with inflammatory infiltrates and hemosiderin deposition.

Gastritis and Gastric Ulcers

Clinical Features and Etiology

An estimated 350,000 cases of acute gastric ulcers are diagnosed annually in the United States. There are many causes of acute gastric (and duodenal) ulceration. Overall, gastric ulcers are more common in men than in women, and they most often occur in middle-aged and elderly patients.

Peptic ulcers, both acute and chronic (including those located in the duodenum), account for 20% to 50% of cases of upper GI bleeding.[30] Risk factors for peptic ulcer disease include *Helicobacter pylori* infection, NSAIDs, and alcohol.

Stress ulcers are defined as acute gastric ulcers that develop in patients with shock, sepsis, or trauma.[31] Stress ulcers have multiple synonyms, such as *acute hemorrhagic gastritis*. *Curling ulcers* are those that develop after severe burns. *Cushing ulcers* are those that develop after severe head trauma. *Steroid ulcers* are caused by steroid use. Risk factors for stress ulcers include respiratory failure, coagulopathy, recent major surgery, major trauma, severe burns, hepatic or renal disease, sepsis, and hypotension.[32]

Bleeding from acute gastritis may also occur in long-distance runners and is of uncertain pathogenesis.[33,34] Cocaine can cause gastric erosions and bleeding.[35] Bleeding may also occur when an ulcer erodes into an underlying blood vessel. For instance, Dieulafoy lesions (also called *caliber-persistent artery*) are bleeding ulcers that occur most commonly in the lesser curvature of the stomach in close proximity to the cardia, but they can also occur in the small and large intestine and rarely in the esophagus.[36-38] Dieulafoy lesions are characterized by the presence of a single, unusually largediameter mural arteriole that penetrates into the submucosa (Fig. 11.9A). These large vessels may cause massive bleeding (Fig. 11.9B–D). It has been reported in 1% to 2% of resection specimens and more recently with prior surgery.[39] *Cameron ulcers* are defined as linear ulcers that form in a sliding hiatal hernia; they can cause gastric bleeding.

Mass lesions, located either in the mucosa or deeper within the gastric wall, may erode the overlying mucosa and cause chronic low-grade bleeding (Fig. 11.10). Fundic gland polyps, gastric adenomas, ectopic pancreas, malignant tumors (e.g., primary gastric adenocarcinomas, lymphomas, endocrine tumors), GI stromal tumors, and metastatic tumors (e.g., melanomas, breast carcinomas) can all cause upper GI bleeding. Gastric bleeding may occasionally be iatrogenic in origin, such as in patients postsurgery for obesity.[40]

Pathological Features

Gastric ulcers are loosely defined as full-thickness loss of the gastric mucosa. Gastric erosions, in contrast, are defined by partial loss of mucosa, with preservation of the muscularis mucosae. On gross examination, erosions appear as small, focal, erythematous areas of mucosa. Gastric ulcers are sharply demarcated, usually circular depressions in the mucosal surface. Acute ulcers may have an erythematous base and are usually covered with clotted blood and fibrin. Chronic ulcers have a distinctive gross appearance resulting from scarring of the underlying tissue. It results in the formation of radiating cicatricial folds in the mucosa surrounding the ulcer. Histologically, erosions show loss of superficial mucosa, fibrinopurulent exudate, and reactive changes in the surrounding epithelium (loss of mucin, nuclear hyperchromasia, and increased mitotic activity). Acute ulcers show necrosis, granulation tissue, and hemorrhage. Chronic ulcers have a granulation tissue base with underlying fibrosis that often involves the muscularis propria. In cases of Dieulafoy lesions, the large-sized artery in the submucosa is usually associated with mucosal erosion and evidence of bleeding.

Portal Hypertensive Gastropathy

Portal hypertensive gastropathy occurs in up to 90% of patients with cirrhosis-related typically severe portal hypertension. It is characterized by a mosaic pattern of the mucosa at endoscopy, either with or without petechial hemorrhages, usually in the proximal stomach. Portal hypertensive gastropathy may also occur in patients without cirrhosis. It is most often detected in patients with portal hypertension who are being evaluated for variceal bleeding. Portal hypertensive duodenopathy has been described in 51% of portal hypertensive patients and is an uncommon cause of occult GI bleeding. Endoscopic features include erythema, erosions, ulcers, telangiectases, and duodenal varices. Some authors have described a characteristic "snakeskin" appearance to the gastric mucosa (Fig. 11.11).[41] Endoscopic-pathological correlation of portal hypertensive gastropathy

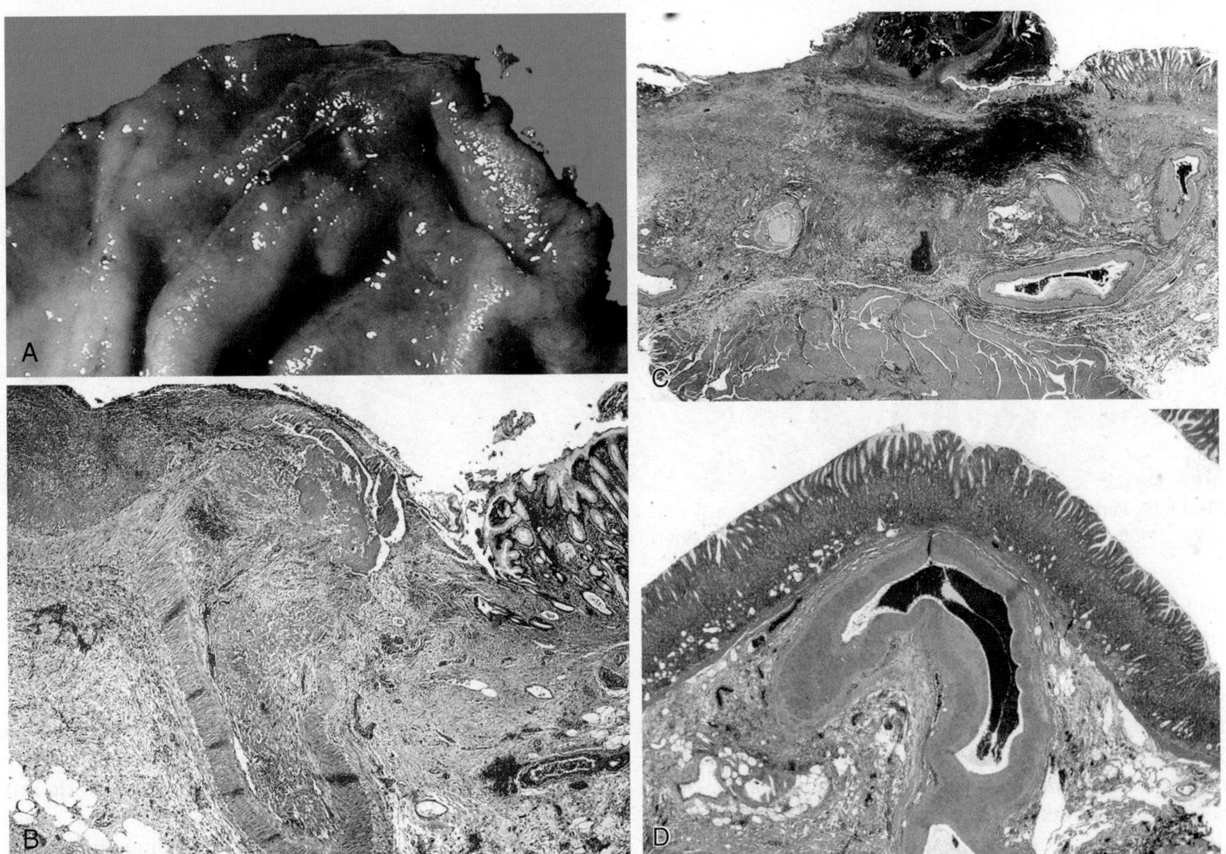

FIGURE 11.9 Dieulafoy lesion. A, Prominent submucosal artery with surgical clip. **B,** Abnormally large submucosal artery eroding through the gastric mucosa. **C,** Large, tortuous submucosal artery with thrombus adherent to ulcer base and submucosal hemorrhage (elastic Van Gieson stain). **D,** An example of more intact overlying mucosa with the characteristic thick-walled submucosal artery almost reaching the surface (**A** and **B** *courtesy of Dr. Dhanpat Jain, Yale University School of Medicine, New Haven, CT.*)

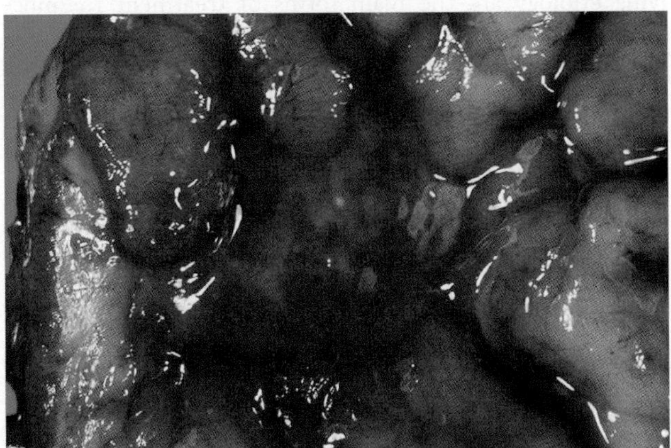

FIGURE 11.10 Centrally ulcerated gastric lymphoma.

is about 67%.[42] Patients can be asymptomatic, or they can have abdominal pain and other symptoms of chronic bleeding.

Altered blood flow has been implicated in the pathogenesis of portal hypertensive gastropathy. Other postulated mechanisms include nitric oxide production, tumor necrosis factor-α synthesis, and sensitivity to prostaglandin inhibition.[43]

Portal hypertensive gastropathy occurs most commonly in the fundus and body of the stomach. Histological features include the presence of numerous ectatic and congested capillaries and venules in otherwise relatively normal-appearing mucosa and submucosa. However, morphological findings classic of "reactive" gastropathy are frequently present as well. Many cases show lamina propria edema below the surface epithelium (Fig. 11.12A,B). Fibrin

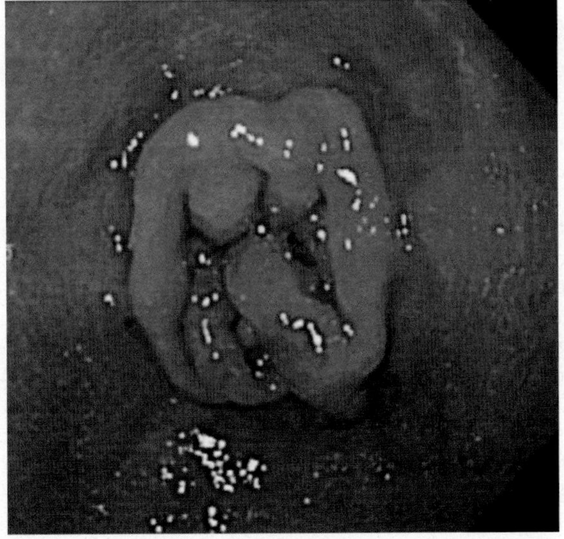

FIGURE 11.11 Endoscopic image of classic "snakeskin" appearance in a case of portal hypertensive gastropathy.

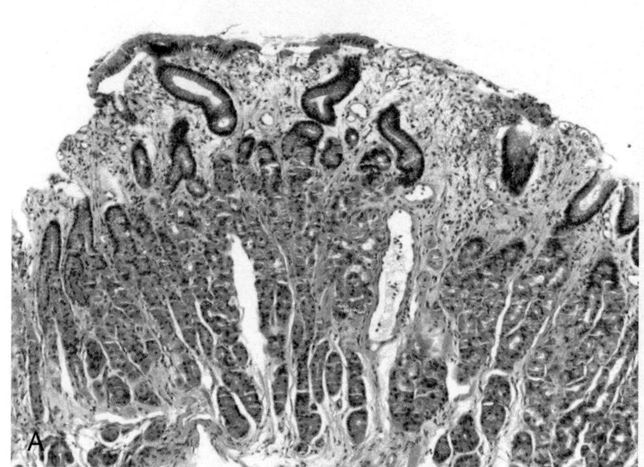

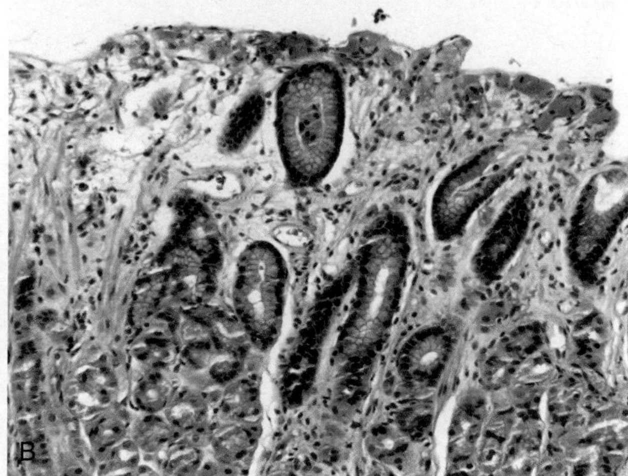

FIGURE 11.12 Portal hypertensive gastropathy. A, A gastric biopsy reminiscent of reactive gastropathy with mild reactive mucin loss and corkscrewing of gastric pits. **B,** At higher magnification, there is typically subepithelial lamina propria edema and congested capillaries.

thrombi, lamina propria inflammation, mucosal fibrosis, and fibrohyalinosis are not common components of portal hypertensive gastropathy, but they do occur in more chronic cases.[43-46] There is no particular association with atrophic gastritis, CREST syndrome (*c*alcinosis, *R*aynaud phenomenon, *e*sophageal involvement, *s*clerodactyly, and *t*elangiectases), or bone marrow transplantation (Table 11.3). Portal hypertensive duodenopathy usually occurs in association with gastropathy; it is characterized by capillary congestion, capillary angiogenesis, and edema in the duodenal lamina propria (Fig. 11.13A–D), but usually only minimal inflammation.[41]

Bleeding from portal hypertensive gastropathy is usually chronic and often controllable by medical or surgical management of the underlying cause of the patient's portal hypertension.

Gastric Antral Vascular Ectasia

Gastric antral vascular ectasia (GAVE) affects mainly women of middle age, frequently causes iron-deficiency anemia, and is associated with portal hypertension/cirrhosis in about 30% to 40% of cases. It is sometimes associated with achlorhydria, atrophic gastritis, and CREST syndrome. Autoimmune disorders are present in approximately 62% of patients with GAVE.[43] At endoscopy, GAVE is characterized by a linear pattern of mucosal hyperemia on the antral rugae that appears similar to the stripes of a watermelon; hence, the synonym, *watermelon stomach* (Fig. 11.14).[47] This endoscopic appearance tends to be more diffuse in cases of cirrhosis but usually involves only the gastric antrum. The pathogenesis of GAVE is believed to be altered gastric motility, but this has never been confirmed.

Histologically, GAVE is characterized by the presence of dilated capillaries in the mucosa and submucosa, often containing microthrombi, which represent the histological hallmark of this entity. Thrombi can be subtle on hematoxylin and eosin (H&E) stain. CD61 immunostain is a helpful diagnostic tool in some cases.[48] Some studies have shown an increased number and caliber of mucosal vessels in GAVE in comparison with portal hypertensive gastropathy.[48] Fibromuscular hyperplasia of the intervening lamina propria and focal hyalinosis are characteristic features, along with edema, congestion, and reactive changes of the foveolar epithelium[45,46,49] (Fig. 11.15A–C). Inflammation is typically minimal. Surface erosion is uncommon.

In mucosal biopsies, both portal hypertensive gastropathy and GAVE should be distinguished histologically from chronic radiation gastritis, which also shows ectatic mucosal capillaries. In contrast, radiation injury is characterized by prominent endothelial cells and hyaline thickening of dilated capillaries and small blood vessels, sometimes associated with thrombosis (Fig. 11.16). Features that differentiate portal hypertensive gastropathy from GAVE are summarized in Table 11.3.

Endoscopic mucosal ablation and treatment of the underlying etiology are the main forms of treatment for most patients with GAVE. Antrectomy is reserved for patients with uncontrollable bleeding.

Hereditary Hemorrhagic Telangiectasia (Rendu-Osler-Weber Disease)

HHT, also referred to as *Rendu-Osler-Weber disease,* is an autosomal dominant condition in which telangiectases involve the mucous membranes of the oral cavity, but also any portion of the GI tract, where they may bleed.[50] The disorder affects both sexes equally and occurs in all races. The typical clinical triad consists of telangiectasia (mucosal and/or visceral) and recurrent epistaxis in a patient with a family history of the disorder, such as in a first-degree relative. About 20% of patients do not reveal a family history of either telangiectasia or recurrent bleeding.[9] Most patients express at least two of the following four manifestations: epistaxis, telangiectasia, visceral lesions (including GI telangiectasia), and a positive family history.[51] At least 600 mutations, involving multiple gene loci (*ENG* 61%, *ACVRL1* 37%, *MADH4* ~2%, rarely *HHT3* and *HHT4*), have been implicated in HHT.[52] GI bleeding is more likely in patients with *HHT1/ENG* mutations.[50] Upper GI bleeding is common and can be difficult to distinguish from epistaxis; the two are the most common manifestations of HHT. GI bleeding is often difficult to control. Blood transfusion requirements in excess of 100 units have been reported in some patients.

TABLE 11.3 Comparative Features of Portal Hypertensive Gastropathy and Gastric Antral Vascular Ectasia

Features	Portal Hypertensive Gastropathy	Gastric Antral Vascular Ectasia
Clinical		
Age	Adults and children	Middle aged to elderly
Gender	Male predominance	Female : male = 4 : 1
Cirrhosis	~95%	~40%
Portal hypertension	100%	~40%
Iron-deficiency anemia	Uncommon	Typical
Atrophic gastritis	Not associated	Associated
CREST syndrome	Not associated	Associated
Bone marrow transplantation	Not associated	Associated
Endoscopic		
Location	Proximal stomach	Antrum
Red spots	Present	Present
Mosaic pattern	Present	Absent
Watermelon pattern	Absent	Often present
Pathological		
Background mucosa*	Oxyntic	Antral
Ectatic mucosal vessels	Present	Present
Fibrin thrombi*	Absent	Present
Spindle cell proliferation*	Absent	Present
Fibrohyalinosis*	Absent	Present
CD61-positive stain in thrombi	Absent	Present
Treatment		
Endoscopic ablation	Not required	Effective
Control of portal hypertension	Effective	May also be necessary

CREST, *Calcinosis, Raynaud phenomenon, esophageal involvement, sclerodactyly, and telangiectases.*
**Most important distinguishing features.*

GI tract lesions include telangiectases, arteriovenous malformations (AVMs), and angiodysplasias. Telangiectases, which are the most common lesions, appear grossly as bright red spots on the mucosa. They frequently involve the stomach and proximal small intestine.[52] These lesions are composed of a tuft of dilated venules and arterioles that communicate directly with one another, thereby bypassing capillaries (Fig. 11.17). The precise vascular architecture is often difficult to appreciate in routine histological sections, but evaluation of serial sections may help.[53]

Telangiectasia may also occur in patients with scleroderma, as part of CREST syndrome. The morphology of telangiectases associated with scleroderma is similar to that in HHT, thus distinction therefore requires clinical and serological correlation (rheumatoid factor, antinuclear antibody, SCL-70 antibody, and anticentromeric protein antibody). Telangiectases may also develop in patients with chronic renal failure after hemodialysis.[54]

Treatment options for GI hemorrhage associated with HHT include drug therapy with estrogen, danazol, or aminocaproic acid; endoscopic coagulation, cautery, or laser therapy; and surgical resection.

LOWER GI BLEEDING

Lower GI tract bleeding refers to any type of bleeding from a source located distal to the ligament of Treitz.[55] Hemodynamically significant bleeding from the lower GI tract is most commonly caused by colonic diverticula and angiodysplasia (angiectasia). Other causes are listed in Table 11.4. Colorectal causes are more prevalent than small-intestinal causes. Chronic low-grade bleeding is often not visible to the patient. It may be detected only by fecal occult blood testing.

Lower GI bleeding occurs most commonly in the seventh decade of life. Although it is five times less common than upper GI bleeding, patients with lower GI bleeding are more likely to require surgery.[56] The most common clinical presentation of patients with lower GI bleeding is passage of bright-red blood per rectum (hematochezia). Similar to upper GI bleeding, lower GI bleeding may result in melena, anemia, or hemodynamic instability. Investigative modalities useful for identification of the source of lower GI bleeding include colonoscopy, angiography, nuclear scan, barium enema, and push enteroscopy.[57]

Diverticulosis

Diverticulosis accounts for 30% to 40% of cases of significant lower GI hemorrhage.[58] Bleeding occurs in up to 15% of patients with diverticular disease, and is often associated with NSAID use, hyperuricemia, or cerebrovascular disease.[56] Left-sided diverticula are defined as acquired outpouchings of the colonic mucosa that protrude through the muscularis propria, typically at the points of entry of the vasa recta (Fig. 11.18A–C). They are usually situated in intimate contact with penetrating blood vessels, where inflammation and ulceration of diverticula can lead to erosion of the vessel wall and bleeding. Diverticular bleeding may be slow and chronic if venous in origin, or acute and severe if an artery is involved. Right-sided diverticula are not usually associated with penetrating vessels. GI bleeding in Meckel's diverticula is usually from foci of gastric heterotopia that cause peptic ulceration of the adjacent mucosa (Fig. 11.19).

Most episodes of bleeding caused by colonic diverticula resolve spontaneously. However, up to one-third of patients require transfusion or therapeutic intervention. Treatment options include contact coagulation, epinephrine injection, hemoclip application, fibrin sealant, and surgical resection.

Angiodysplasia

Angiodysplasia (angiectasia) is the second most common cause of lower GI bleeding in elderly patients (>70 years of age).[59] Angiodysplasia is characterized by the presence of a cluster of abnormally dilated blood vessels in the mucosa and submucosa of the lower GI tract. Bleeding from angiodysplasia is usually chronic and recurrent, but

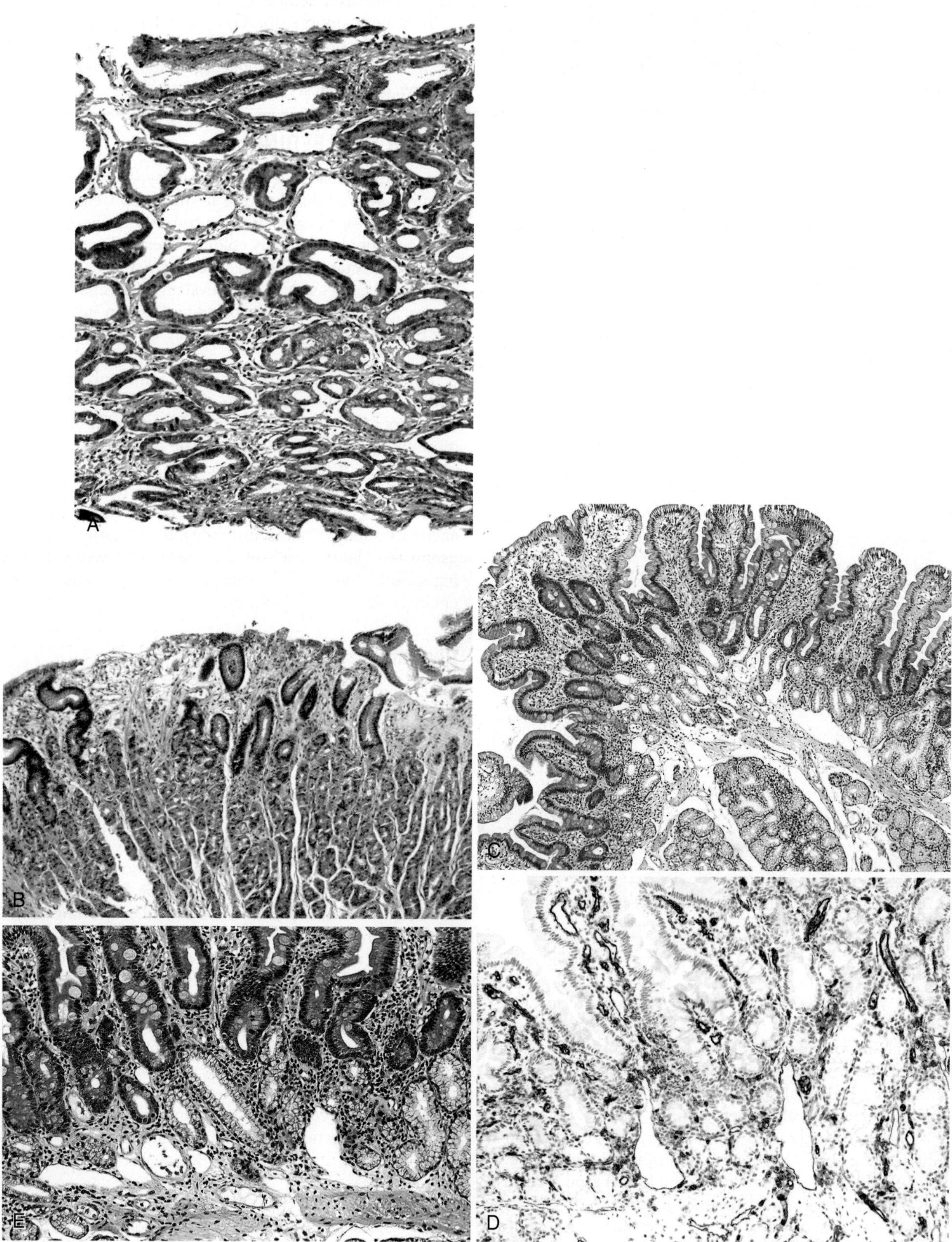

FIGURE 11.13 Portal hypertensive gastropathy. A, Ectatic vessels in the gastric mucosa. Notice the absence of thrombi and fibrohyalinosis. **B,** Although not a specific feature, some cases reveal subepithelial lamina propria edema. **C,** Portal hypertensive duodenopathy: ectatic capillaries in duodenal mucosa. **D,** Immunohistochemical staining for CD31 highlights the dilated duodenal capillaries. **E,** Ectatic capillaries amidst minimal lamina propria lymphoplasmacytic inflammation.

massive hemorrhage occurs in approximately 10% to 15% of affected patients.

Angiodysplasia is an acquired lesion associated with aging. It has an overall incidence of 0.8% in screening populations.[60] Angiodysplasia results from dilated preexisting venules, thus they are not considered true malformations. The majority of cases occur in the right colon (80%), and 10% to 15% occur in the small intestine.[60] Although usually readily seen at colonoscopy and angiography, angiodysplasia is often difficult to detect on gross examination of a resection specimen without the use of specific injection techniques.[61] By performing vascular injection studies of resected colons, Boley and Brandt determined that angiodysplasia develops as a result of intermittent partial obstruction of small veins that drain the colonic mucosa and submucosa as they course through the muscularis propria. They postulated that obstruction is caused by muscle contraction and increased tension within the bowel wall, which is highest in the region of colon with the greatest diameter (i.e., the cecum).[59] With time, obstruction of the penetrating veins in the muscularis propria leads to dilation and tortuosity of the submucosal veins and, consequently, the venules and capillaries that drain them. Dilation of capillaries ultimately leads to loss of capillary sphincter function, which creates arteriovenous fistulas and secondary effects on the structure of the feeding arteries.

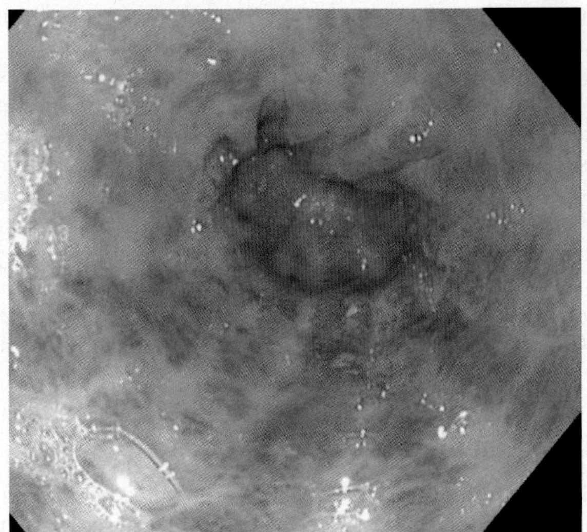

FIGURE 11.14 Watermelon stomach appearance on endoscopy in a case of gastric antral vascular ectasia (GAVE).

Angiodysplasia is often difficult to diagnose in pathological specimens. In resection specimens examined in the fresh state, one may see only small (usually 1 to 5 mm) focus of enhanced vascular markings and erythema, and even these subtle signs may be absent. Lesions can be multiple and be associated with surface erosion. In specimens examined after formalin fixation, the lesions are usually not visible on the mucosal surface. Few laboratories are equipped to perform injection studies, which require processing of fresh specimens. With fixed resection specimens, slicing the bowel wall with a sharp blade at the site of suspected mucosal abnormalities helps reveal the lesion. If a vascular lesion is detected, histological examination usually reveals a discrete cluster of dilated, thin-walled tortuous veins and venules within the submucosa (Fig. 11.20A), and some associated with dilated capillaries in the overlying mucosa as well (Fig. 11.20B–D). In long-standing disease, there may be arterialization of veins. Occasional enlarged arteries may be noted.

Diagnosis of angiodysplasia in biopsy specimens is usually problematic. The main histological component of angiodysplasia is normally situated in the submucosa, which may not be sampled in superficial endoscopic biopsies. When capillary dilation involves the mucosa, biopsy specimens may show only one or two ectatic capillaries, and these may collapse when the specimen is immersed in formalin. In more advanced lesions with more extensive mucosal involvement, clusters of dilated capillaries may distort the architecture of the mucosa, displacing glands and separating the crypts from each other (Fig. 11.21).

In most instances, bleeding can be controlled adequately by medications and therapeutic endoscopy. Angiographic techniques not only enable precise localization of angiodysplasia but also allow for treatment by superselective embolization. Surgical resection is reserved for patients with uncontrolled bleeding.

Arteriovenous Malformation

In contrast with angiodysplasia, which is an acquired lesion that develops mainly in elderly, AVMs develop

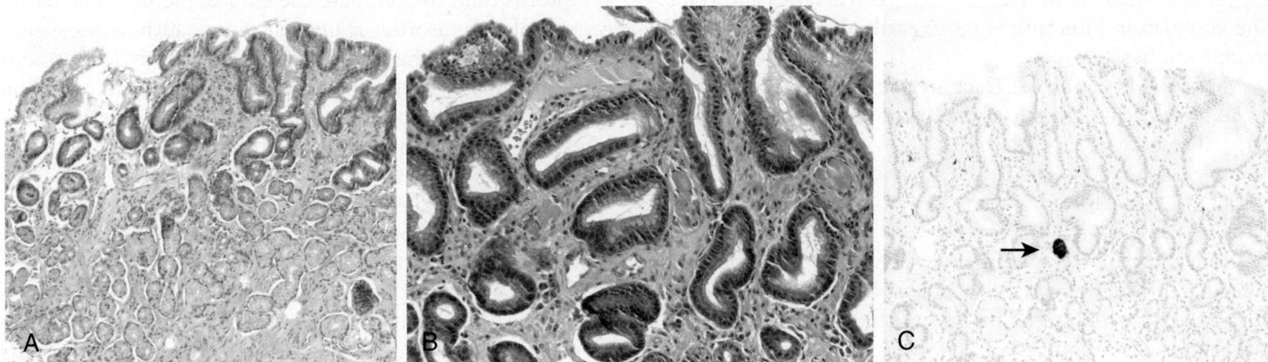

FIGURE 11.15 Gastric antral vascular ectasia. A and **B,** Gastric antral mucosa with fibromuscular hyperplasia of the lamina propria, fibrin thrombi, hyalinosis, capillary ectasia, and reactive foveolar epithelial changes. **C,** CD61-positive expression *(arrow)* can aid in the diagnosis in cases with less obvious thrombi on H&E stain.

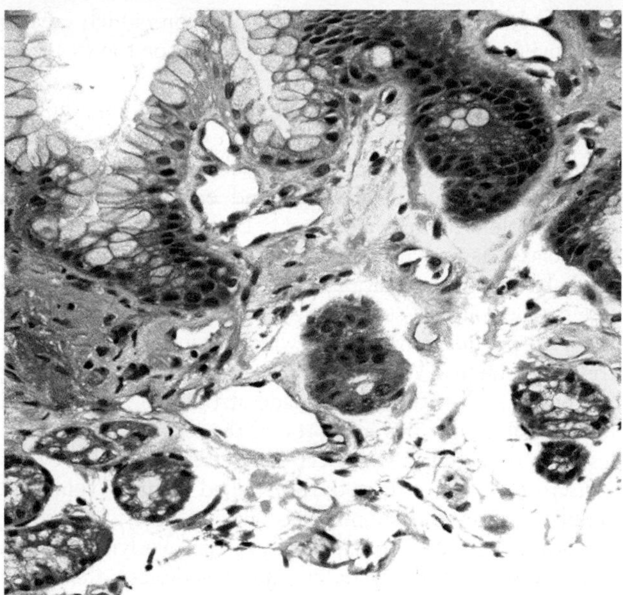

FIGURE 11.16 Chronic radiation gastritis. Notice the ectatic mucosal capillaries with thrombosis *(left side)* and mucosal fibrosis.

during embryological or fetal life and are typically present at birth. AVMs also differ from angiodysplasia in that the former results in an abnormal direct communication between arteries and veins. Because of this communication, arterial blood flows directly into the venous system at higher-than-normal pressures, bypassing the (high-resistance) capillary bed. AVMs can manifest clinically with bleeding at any age.

In the GI tract, AVMs occur most often in the sigmoid colon and rectum, and they are usually located external to the muscularis propria—that is, in the subserosa (Fig. 11.22). The malformation usually consists of a tangled mass of tortuous, variably dilated arteries, veins, and vessels with intermediate characteristics. Veins in AVMs undergo "arterialization" in response to exposure to elevated (arterial) blood pressure. They develop a thick, muscular wall as a result of myointimal hyperplasia (Fig. 11.23). It has been proposed that idiopathic myointimal hyperplasia of the mesenteric veins (discussed later) is an example of venous arterialization as a complication of AVM. Histologically, AVMs are characterized by the presence of a complex cluster of tortuous, dilated vascular channels and vessels that appear intermediate in structure between arteries and veins. The vascular architecture is more easily depicted by angiographic studies.

Most AVMs of the GI tract are treated angiographically by superselective embolization. Large lesions may require surgical resection.

Hemorrhoids

Hemorrhoids are very common. Clinically, most patients present in middle age with anal pain or bleeding.[62-64] Hemorrhoids arise from the anal cushions, which are normal anatomic structures of the anorectal canal. The anal cushions are composed of tufts of anastomosing arterioles and venules in the submucosa; they are embedded within compact, dense, submucosal collagenous and elastic fibrous stroma and covered by anorectal mucosa. Hemorrhoids develop as a result of degenerative changes that occur in the supporting stroma or as a result of locally increased intravascular pressure, or both. The blood vessels become engorged and the cushions prolapse, strangulate, thrombose, ulcerate, and bleed. Histological sections of hemorrhoids show tufts of engorged, dilated veins and arteries often associated with thrombi and hemorrhage, in a dense stroma, covered by anal or rectal mucosa, which is often ulcerated (Fig. 11.24). In case of prolapsed hemorrhoidal tissue, the pathology specimen can include fibers of smooth muscle (part of the rectum muscularis propria and/or internal anal sphincter muscle) without significant clinical implications in most cases. It is extremely rare to see striated muscle in this setting as it denotes portions of external anal sphincter muscle within the specimen and a higher risk for postoperative complications. Treatment options for hemorrhoids include dietary modification, sclerotherapy, photocoagulation, diathermy, banding, laser ablation, cryotherapy, and surgical hemorrhoidectomy.

Anal Fissures

Anal fissures are a linear tearing of anal mucosa resulting from persistent hypertonia and spasm of anal sphincter muscles. They can extend from the dentate line to the anal verge. Patients typically present with pain associated with defecation and bleeding. They commonly present in the posterior midline and in young adults, although fissures can occur in all ages. Lateral fissures ("off midline") have been associated with concomitant conditions such as Crohn's disease, HIV, syphilis, sexual abuse, and carcinoma, among others. Histological changes include mucosal ulceration with prominent granulation tissue, which may develop into fistulas (Fig. 11.25). The squamous epithelium may exhibit reactive epithelial changes, acanthosis, and even hyperkeratosis and parakeratosis. With chronicity, there is fibrosis and hyalinization.

Diaphragm Disease

Diaphragm disease is a rare cause of GI bleeding linked to chronic use of NSAIDs. This entity was first described in the small intestine in 1988.[65,66] Similar abnormalities have been described in the large intestine as well.[67,68] GI bleeding associated with diaphragm disease is usually occult. Obstructive symptoms tend to dominate the clinical picture. The pathogenesis of this disorder is unclear. Some authorities suggest that inhibition of the cyclo-oxygenase pathway leads to erosions in the GI tract, modulation of nuclear factor-κB and peroxisome proliferator–activated receptor-γ, and increased intestinal permeability, which lead to mucosal injury. Alternatively, NSAID-associated circumferential ulceration, followed by the development of submucosal fibrosis and mucosal regeneration, is another possible mechanism that may result in diaphragm formation.

Diaphragms may be single or multiple, but the disease distribution is usually focal. The lumen of the involved segment of bowel is often stenosed. As opposed to Crohn's disease, there is no fat wrapping in diaphragm disease because microperforations are not a component of this disease.[69] The diaphragms are composed exclusively of mucosa and

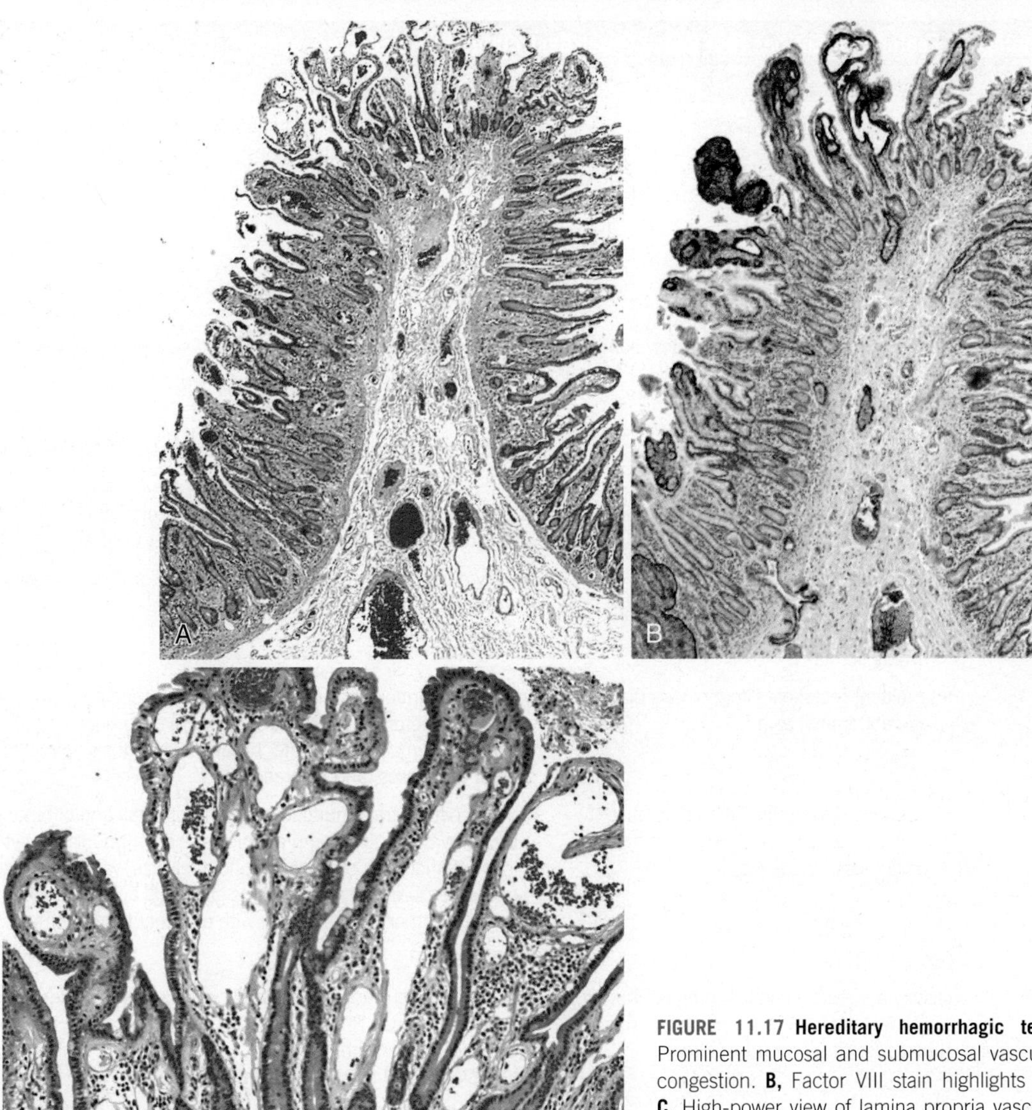

FIGURE 11.17 Hereditary hemorrhagic telangiectasia. A, Prominent mucosal and submucosal vascular dilation and congestion. **B,** Factor VIII stain highlights tufts of vessels. **C,** High-power view of lamina propria vascular ectasia and congestion.

TABLE 11.4 Pathological Features of Entities That Cause Lower Gastrointestinal Bleeding

Entity	Key Clinical Features	Key Pathological Features
Diverticular disease*	Most frequent in elderly Accounts for 30% to 40% of cases of significant lower GI hemorrhage	Most common in the sigmoid colon Thickened muscularis propria, exaggerated mucosal folds Pseudodiverticula extend through muscularis at points of entry of vasa recta Inflammation of diverticula may lead to vascular erosion and bleeding
Angiodysplasia*	Common in elderly patients Chronic and recurrent bleeding Common cause of bleeding in renal failure	Usually in right colon Dilated, tortuous, thin-walled submucosal veins, capillaries, and arterioles with arteriovenous anastomoses Most commonly submucosal; may involve mucosa
Arteriovenous malformation	Developmental defects, but may present at any age	Most common in sigmoid colon and rectum Arterialized veins with thick muscular walls are associated with a knot of tortuous, dilated veins and arteries
Dieulafoy lesion	See Table 11.2	See Table 11.2
Varices (rectal, stomal)	Associated with portal hypertension and mesenteric and splenic vein obstruction	Occur at portosystemic anastomoses in the rectum and at enterocolic-cutaneous stomas Histological features are similar to upper GI varices

Continued

TABLE 11.4 Pathological Features of Entities That Cause Lower Gastrointestinal Bleeding—cont'd

Entity	Key Clinical Features	Key Pathological Features
Portal hypertensive colopathy	Seen in portal hypertension Strong association with cirrhosis, but no correlation with degree	Dilated tortuous mucosal and submucosal capillaries correspond to red spots seen at endoscopy
Hereditary hemorrhagic telangiectasia	See Table 11.2	See Table 11.2
Hemodialysis-associated telangiectasia	See Table 11.2	See Table 11.2
Hemorrhoids	Common in adults, increase in prevalence after third decade	Dilated submucosal and mucosal blood vessels, usually with thrombosis and hemorrhage
Infections	See Table 11.5	See Table 11.5
Mucosal prolapse	History of prior lower GI tract trauma or surgery Diverticular disease	Reactive, hyperplastic mucosa with fibromuscular lamina propria and architectural distortion
Meckel's diverticulum	GI bleed most common presentation in children	True diverticulum on antimesenteric border of ileum Heterotopic oxyntic mucosa with peptic ulcer in 65%
Stercoral ulcers	Acute GI bleed in elderly patients Typically a history of constipation Common in renal patients treated for hyperkalemia	Sharply demarcated ulcers in rectosigmoid, formed as pressure sores caused by hard feces High risk of perforation
Ulcerative colitis	Intermittent rectal bleeding, bloody diarrhea, and abdominal pain	Typically continuous colonic involvement proceeding proximally from the rectum with crypt architectural distortion, lymphoplasmacytic infiltrate, basal plasmacytosis, cryptitis, crypt abscesses, and ulceration
Crohn's disease	More variable symptoms than ulcerative colitis, including abdominal pain, fatigue, weight loss, and fever	Typically patchy transmural involvement of small and/or large bowel by deep ulcers, mural fibrosis and lymphoplasmacytic inflammation with reactive lymphoid follicles, variable degrees of architectural distortion, pyloric gland metaplasia, and cryptitis and crypt abscesses, with or without granulomas
Ischemic enterocolitis	See Table 11.9	See Table 11.9
Radiation enterocolitis	History of prostate cancer common in men; cervical cancer common in women Rare cause of lower GI bleeding	Dilated, tortuous mucosal capillaries with prominent endothelial cells in mucosa Hyalinized vessels with prominent endothelial cells, stellate fibroblasts, and fibrosis in submucosa
Collagenous colitis	Watery diarrhea Female predominance: 4:1 Rare cause of lower GI bleeding	Marked thickening of the subepithelial collagen table with entrapment of inflammatory cells and capillaries; subepithelial collagen may mimic hyalinosis of ischemic colitis
Diversion colitis	History of previous bowel resection with fecal stream diversion May cause bloody rectal discharge	Friable mucosa with normal or distorted architecture, mucin depletion, bandlike lymphoplasmacytic infiltrate most dense in the upper mucosa, rare cryptitis, Paneth cell metaplasia, and prominent reactive lymphoid follicles
Diaphragm disease	History of NSAID use	Transverse stenosing membrane composed of submucosa lined on both sides by mucosa, with central aperture
Ehlers-Danlos syndrome, vascular type	Acute hemorrhage and bowel perforation in young patients resulting from deficiency of collagen type 3	Most commonly affects the sigmoid colon Thinned muscularis propria and diminished submucosa Proliferating fibroblasts surrounding fat Frayed, degenerated vascular and stromal collagen

GI, *Gastrointestinal;* NSAIDs, *nonsteroidal antiinflammatory drugs.*
**Most common causes.*

submucosa, without involvement of the muscularis propria or adventitia. Histologically, the diaphragm represents a disc of submucosa lined by mucosa, usually with a central erosion. There is usually evidence of chronic and/or chronic active mucosal injury, and lamina propria eosinophilia.[69] Typically, the submucosa is fibrotic. In fact, the connective tissue fibers are usually oriented perpendicular to the lumen of the bowel, and these are often associated with haphazardly arranged nerves, blood vessels, and thickened smooth muscle fibers (Fig. 11.26).[66] This pattern of fibrosis is typical of diaphragm disease.

Ehlers-Danlos Syndrome, Vascular Type (Type IV)

Ehlers-Danlos syndrome (EDS) is a heterogeneous group of inherited disorders characterized by defective collagen and

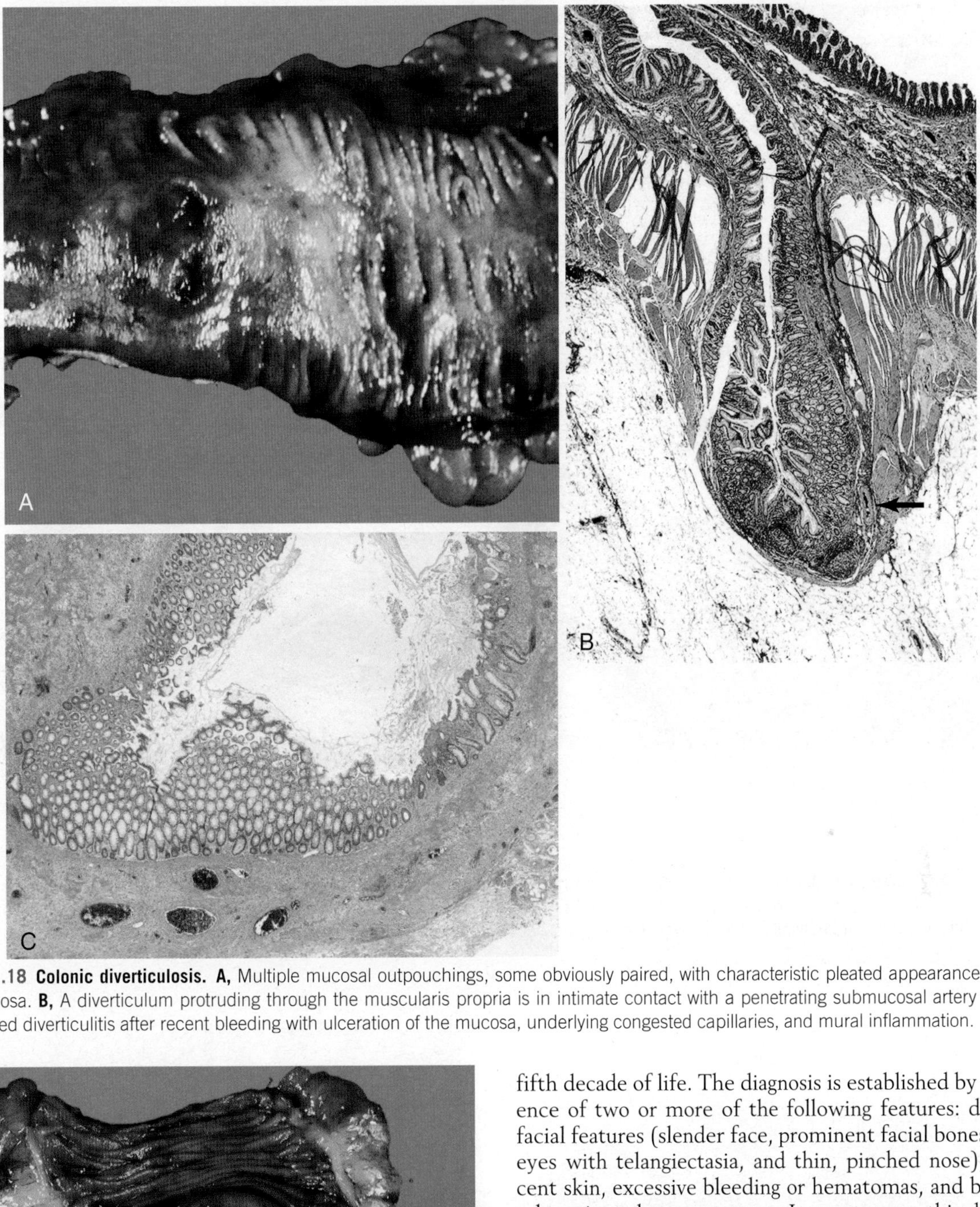

FIGURE 11.18 Colonic diverticulosis. A, Multiple mucosal outpouchings, some obviously paired, with characteristic pleated appearance of the sigmoid mucosa. **B,** A diverticulum protruding through the muscularis propria is in intimate contact with a penetrating submucosal artery *(arrow)*. **C,** Complicated diverticulitis after recent bleeding with ulceration of the mucosa, underlying congested capillaries, and mural inflammation.

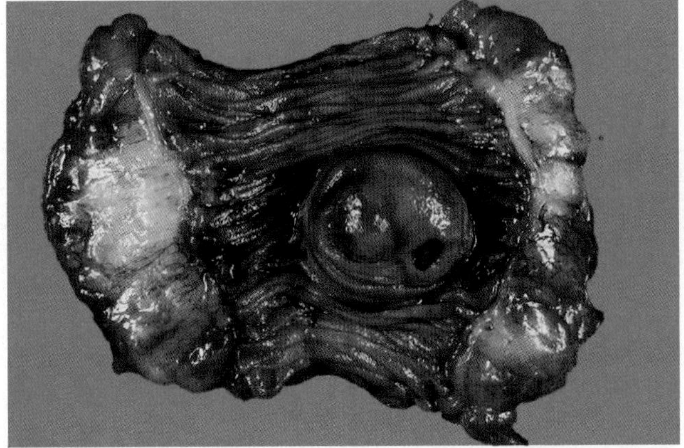

FIGURE 11.19 Everted Meckel's diverticulum with peptic ulcer.

connective tissue synthesis. Of these, EDS type IV (vascular type) causes GI tract pathology and leads to significant complications in up to 25% of patients by 20 years of age and up to 80% by 40 years of age.[70] Patients usually succumb to complications of this disease by the fourth or fifth decade of life. The diagnosis is established by the presence of two or more of the following features: distinctive facial features (slender face, prominent facial bones, bulging eyes with telangiectasia, and thin, pinched nose), translucent skin, excessive bleeding or hematomas, and blood vessel or visceral organ rupture. In most cases, this disorder is inherited in an autosomal dominant manner, although many cases are sporadic. EDS type IV is caused by mutations in the *COL3A1* and *COL1A1* genes, which result in defective synthesis of type III procollagen and diminished extracellular type III and, less commonly, type I collagen. The result is weakening of the supporting connective tissue stroma, including the submucosa and blood vessels.

The sigmoid colon is most commonly affected, but the small bowel, stomach, and even the esophagus may also be involved in rare cases.[71] EDS type IV causes thinning of the muscularis propria and submucosa of the GI tract (Fig. 11.27). Complications include diverticula, perforation, and dissection/rupture of medium to large vessels that leads to hemorrhage. Microscopically, vascular and stromal collagen is often frayed and fragmented. The submucosal

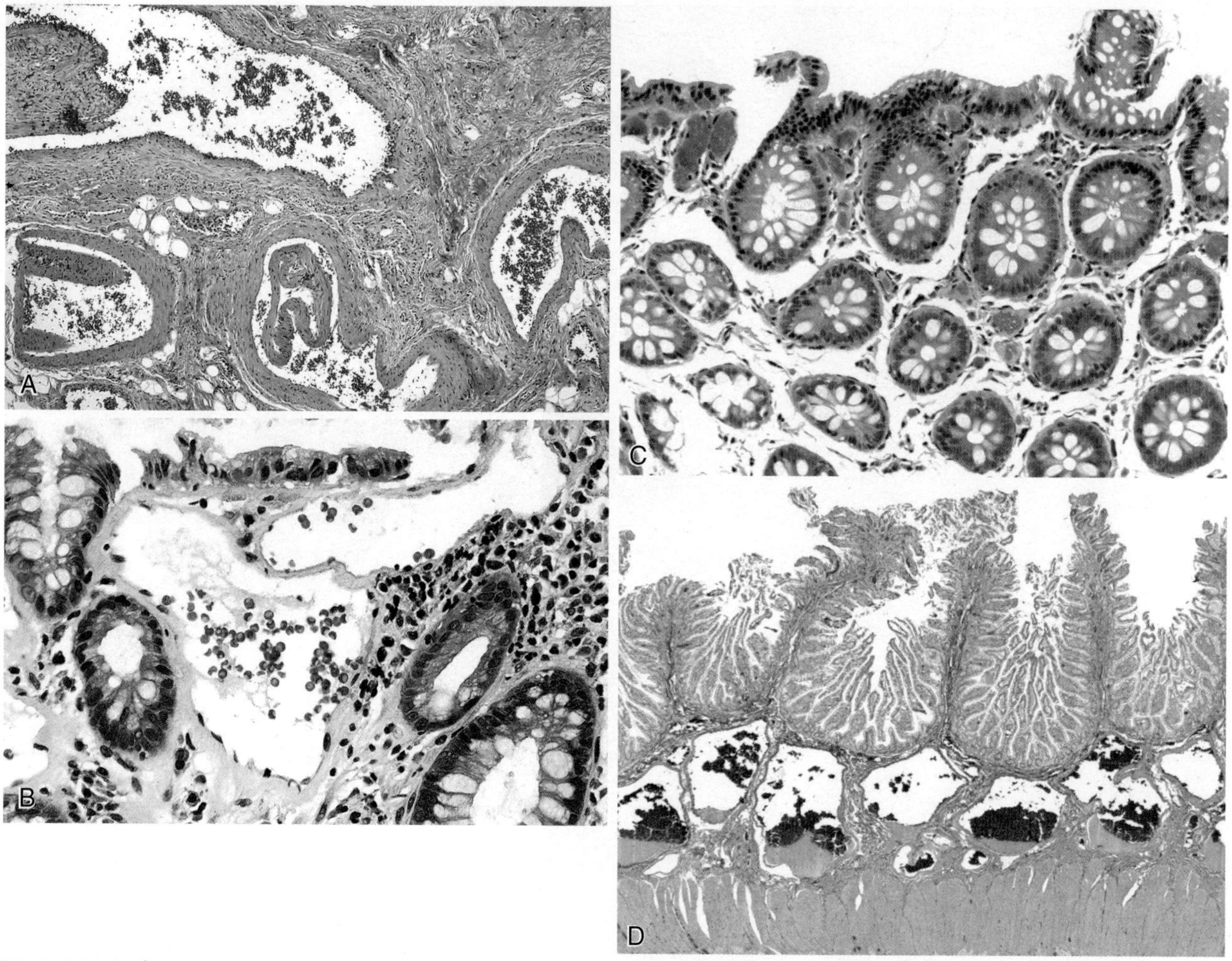

FIGURE 11.20 **Angiodysplasia. A,** Cluster of dilated veins in colonic submucosa. **B,** Secondarily dilated, tortuous capillaries in the lamina propria of overlying mucosa. **C,** A subtle case of angiodysplasia with mucosal clusters of abnormal congested capillaries. **D,** Low-power magnification of a segment of small bowel with markedly dilated and congested submucosal vessels, with smaller capillaries extending into the mucosa.

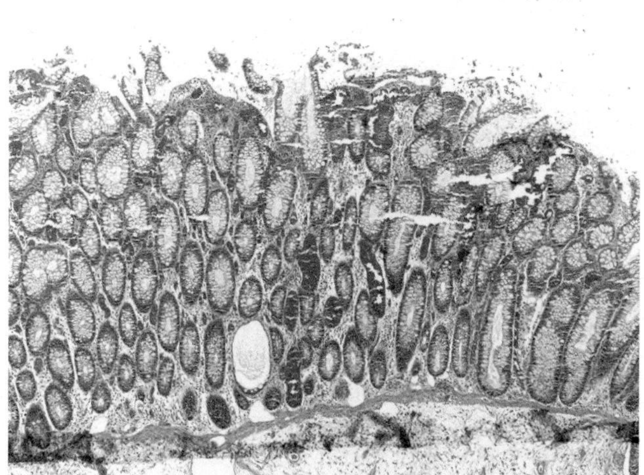

FIGURE 11.21 Angiodysplasia. Capillaries in the lamina propria slightly displacing the adjacent colonic crypts.

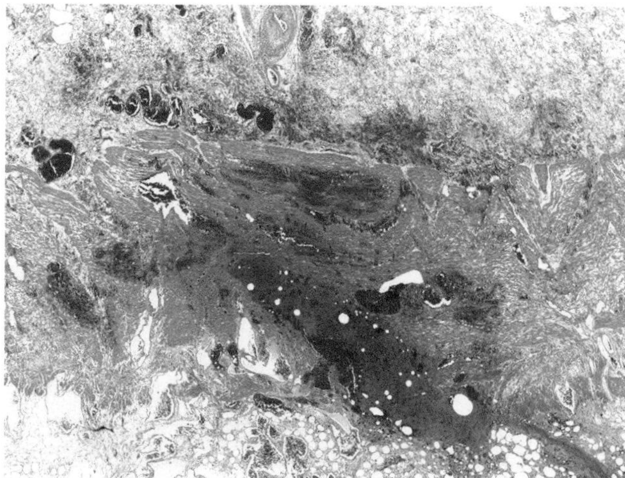

FIGURE 11.22 Arteriovenous malformation of small intestine. Dilated, tortuous subserosal veins with thickened muscular walls and occasional arteries involving the submucosa, muscularis propria, and subserosa.

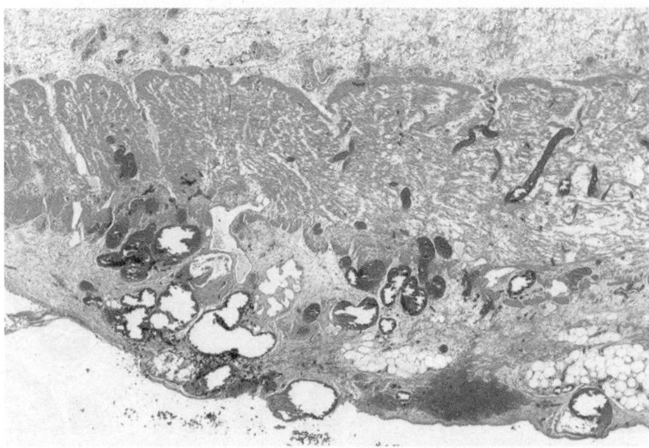

FIGURE 11.23 Arteriovenous malformation of the small intestine. External to the muscularis propria, there are variably dilated subserosal blood vessels, with intermediate characteristics between arteries and veins, and dilated lymphatics.

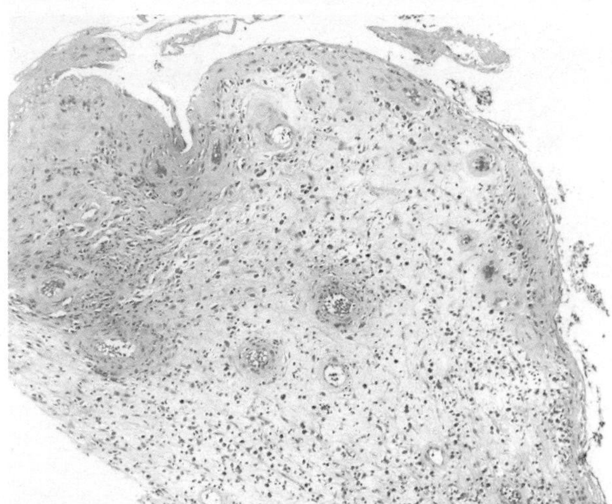

FIGURE 11.25 Anal fissure. Prominent granulation tissue with complete denudation of the epithelial surface in this case.

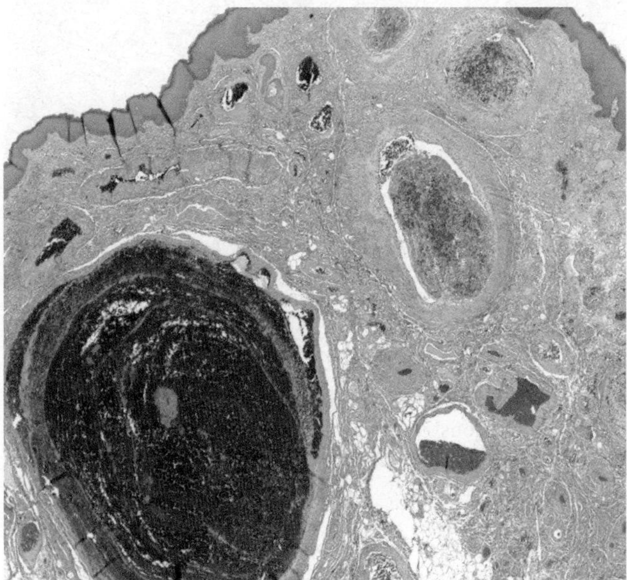

FIGURE 11.24 External partially thrombosed hemorrhoids with dilated and engorged veins.

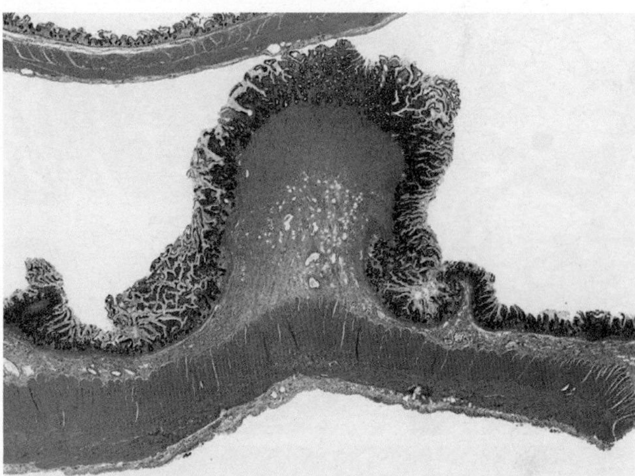

FIGURE 11.26 Diaphragm disease. Segment of small bowel with a "diaphragm" and thickened plicae, with evidence of submucosal fibrosis.

blood vessels may be thin, thick, or nodular in appearance. The outer layers of the blood vessel walls may appear discontinuous. The muscularis propria often shows secondary ischemic changes. Inflammation is uncommon. Diminished expression of type III collagen (vascular and extravascular) can be demonstrated by immunohistochemical staining.

Up to 8% of patients die of bowel rupture and sepsis.[70] Bleeding may occur as a result of ruptured blood vessels in the bowel wall. Treatment is surgical resection of the affected segment. Up to one-third of patients have recurrent perforations.

Miscellaneous Entities

Acute or chronic radiation-induced injury can lead to GI bleeding. In the acute phase, histological changes include reactive changes in epithelial cells, apoptosis, swelling of endothelial cells, capillary dilation and congestion/thrombosis, and even ulcers.[72] Chronic radiation injury in the GI tract is characterized by the presence of dilated, tortuous capillaries with hyaline thickening and prominent capillary endothelial cell nuclei (Fig. 11.28). Subendothelial foam cells can be present in some cases. Dilated capillaries located near the mucosal surface may rupture and cause hemorrhage. Histologically, this condition should be distinguished from portal hypertensive colopathy in patients with portal hypertension. In this condition, the dilated capillaries typically lack hyalinization and prominent endothelial cell nuclei typical of radiation injury (Fig. 11.29). In resection specimens with chronic radiation injury, sclerosis of submucosal and extramural arteries is characteristic. It is associated with fibrosis and stenosis, the presence of atypical stellate fibroblasts, and secondary chronic ischemic changes (Fig. 11.30).

Amyloidosis can affect the GI tract, and in most cases, the small intestine. Symptoms may be vague, but bleeding, ischemia, and perforation have been described. The diagnosis can be established in most cases via rectal biopsy containing submucosal vessels. Histological sections show the characteristic amorphous eosinophilic deposits within vessel

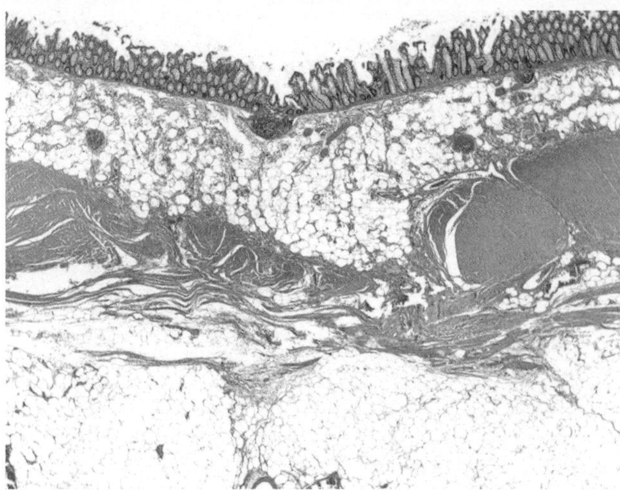

FIGURE 11.27 Ehlers-Danlos syndrome. Marked thinning of the muscularis propria, characteristic of the disease.

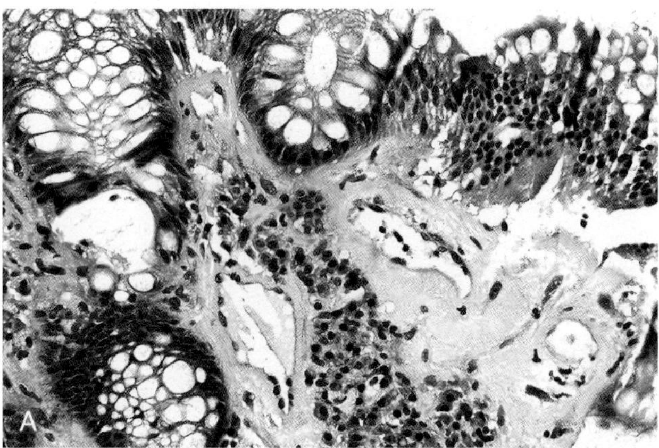

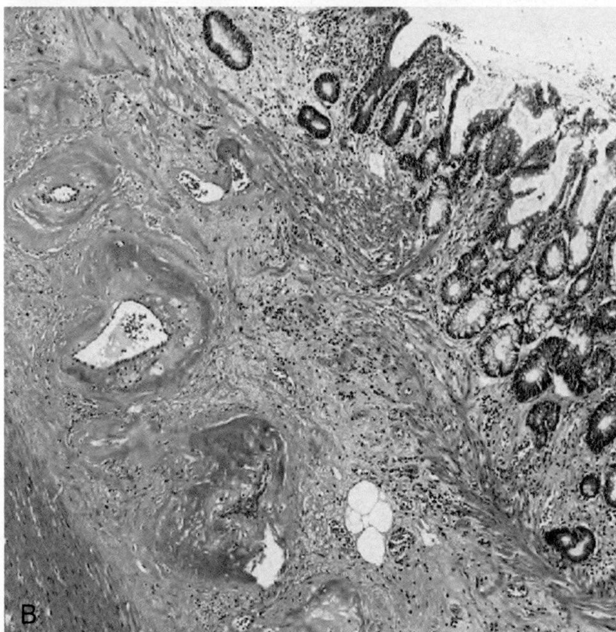

FIGURE 11.28 Chronic radiation proctitis. A, Dilated capillaries of the rectal mucosa have abnormally prominent endothelial cell nuclei and are surrounded by a cuff of hyalinized lamina propria. **B,** Markedly hyalinized submucosal arteries with obliteration of the lumen and foam cell change in the setting of radiation-induced vasculopathy.

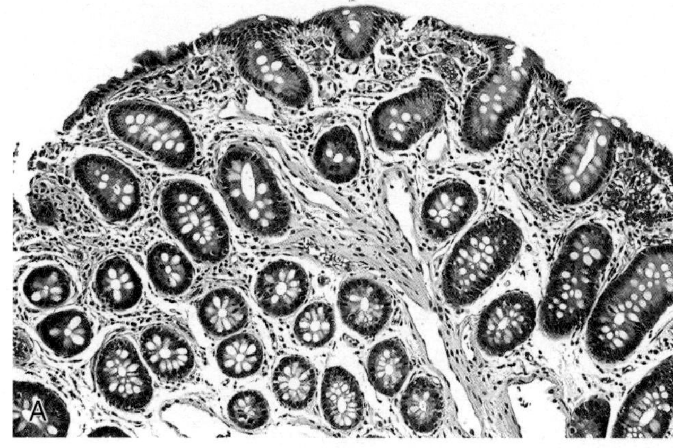

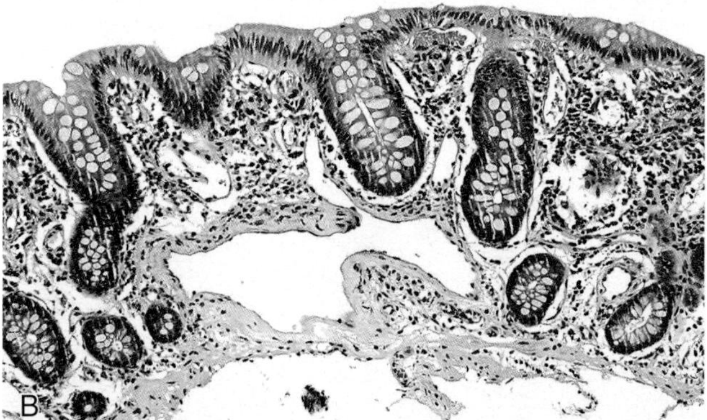

FIGURE 11.29 Portal hypertensive colopathy. A, Dilated capillaries are evident in the colonic lamina propria. **B,** At higher magnification, endothelial cell nuclei do not appear prominent, and there is no hyalinization of the surrounding lamina propria.

walls and/or connective tissue (Fig. 11.31). The eosinophilic material demonstrates apple-green birefringence under polarized light. Specific subtyping of amyloid is performed via mass-spectrometry proteomics analysis with a high degree of accuracy.[72]

Many types of inflammatory conditions can cause lower GI bleeding. Microbial agents that can cause GI bleeding include cytomegalovirus (Fig. 11.32A–C), which predominantly affects immunocompromised patients; *Salmonella; Shigella;* enterohemorrhagic *Escherichia coli* (Fig. 11.33); *Clostridium difficile* (Fig. 11.34); *Clostridium perfringens* (Fig. 11.35); and *Klebsiella oxytoca*[73] (Table 11.5). Certain GI parasites can also cause bleeding, such as *Entamoeba histolytica, Strongyloides,* and hookworms.

Solitary rectal ulcer syndrome is a form of anal and pelvic floor musculature dysfunction. Lesions can be multiple and involve other GI sites as well. Key histological features include architectural distortion of the mucosa associated with fibromuscular hyperplasia of the lamina propria, superficial ischemic changes, and hyperplastic muscularis mucosae (Fig. 11.36). (See Chapter 17 for details.)

Active ulcerative colitis (Fig. 11.37) or Crohn's disease (Fig. 11.38) frequently manifests with bloody diarrhea, in particular during flares. A small subset of patients with collagenous colitis may show deep fissuring linear ulcers along with the classic thickened subepithelial collagen layer. In such cases, the colon is susceptible to tearing of the mucosa, bleeding, and perforation during colonoscopy[74,75]

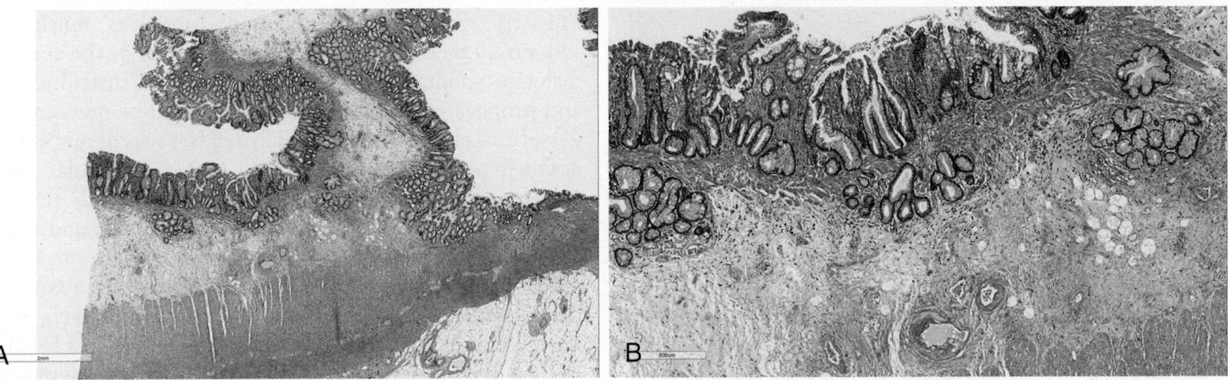

FIGURE 11.30 Chronic radiation. A, Section of bowel wall with a postinflammatory polyp and mural fibrosis. **B,** Chronic mucosal injury with evidence of pyloric gland metaplasia, submucosal fibrosis, and hyalinized vessels.

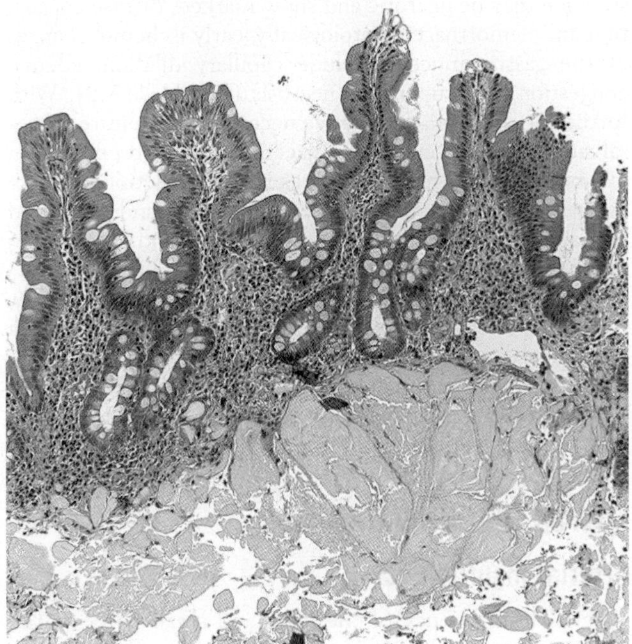

FIGURE 11.31 Amyloidosis. Submucosal and lamina propria eosinophilic amorphous globular deposition of amyloid in a case of ischemic bowel.

(Fig. 11.39). Use of NSAIDs and iatrogenic (such as from endoscopic procedures) and stercoral ulcers in the rectum of elderly patients are a common cause of lower GI bleeding as well (Fig. 11.40).

Ulcerated malignant neoplasms, both primary and metastatic, cause bleeding that is usually chronic and often clinically silent. Primary lymphomas, endocrine tumors, and adenocarcinomas are the major culprits in the small bowel, whereas adenocarcinomas predominate in the large intestine (Fig. 11.41). Other less common causes of bleeding include GI stromal tumors, Kaposi's sarcomas, and malignant melanomas. Polypoid lesions, both nonneoplastic (inflammatory) and neoplastic, can bleed, particularly those with a long stalk that may undergo torsion[76] (e.g., polypoid prolapsing mucosal folds of diverticular disease).

UPPER GI ISCHEMIA

Ischemic injury to the GI tract is common, particularly in elderly individuals. As the percentage of the population older than 50 years of age increases, the incidence of GI ischemia is expected to increase. There are three general clinicopathological patterns of ischemic injury: transient, acute, and chronic. In transient injury, the damage is usually confined to the mucosa and is typically reversible. An example of transient ischemia is that caused by hypotension and hypoperfusion. Acute ischemia is often fulminant. Thus transmural necrosis and perforation may develop if left untreated. Common causes of acute fulminant ischemic injury include sudden thromboembolic occlusion of the mesenteric arteries. Chronic (recurrent) ischemia typically results in the formation of mural fibrosis and strictures combined with chronic or chronic active inflammatory changes in the mucosa. Ischemic injury is uncommon in the esophagus and stomach. It is far more common in the small and large intestines.

Esophagus

Esophageal ischemia is uncommon because of its rich blood supply provided by multiple anastomoses between esophageal blood vessels. However, esophageal ischemia may occur in patients with severe atherosclerosis or vasculitis (e.g., granulomatosis with polyangiitis, Behçet's disease), drugs (such as pill esophagitis and sodium polystyrene [Kayexalate], among others) and, rarely, as a complication of trauma or surgical intervention. Acute necrotizing esophagitis (described earlier in this chapter) has been attributed to ischemia,[77] but its cause is unknown. In fact, recovery rates are higher than one might expect if the disorder were primarily caused by ischemia.[78]

Stomach

As in the esophagus, the presence of multiple anastomoses among blood vessels provides a rich vascular supply to the stomach, and for this reason, ischemia is uncommon. When ischemia does occur in the stomach, there are often multiple contributing factors. Causes of gastric ischemia are listed in Box 11.1.

In most cases, acute gastric ischemia is associated with an underlying abnormal perfusion due to hypovolemic states/hypoperfusion, mechanical problems (volvulus, acute gastric distention), or iatrogenic injury (e.g., sclerotherapy).[79] In gastric volvulus, constriction of the blood vessels leads to venous obstruction. This causes congestion, arterial compromise, and ischemic necrosis.

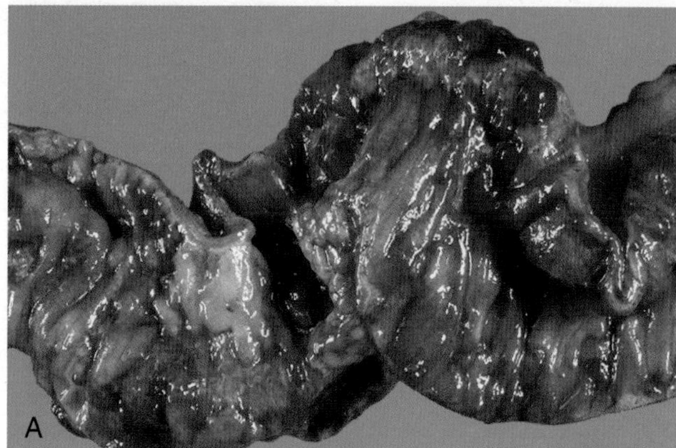

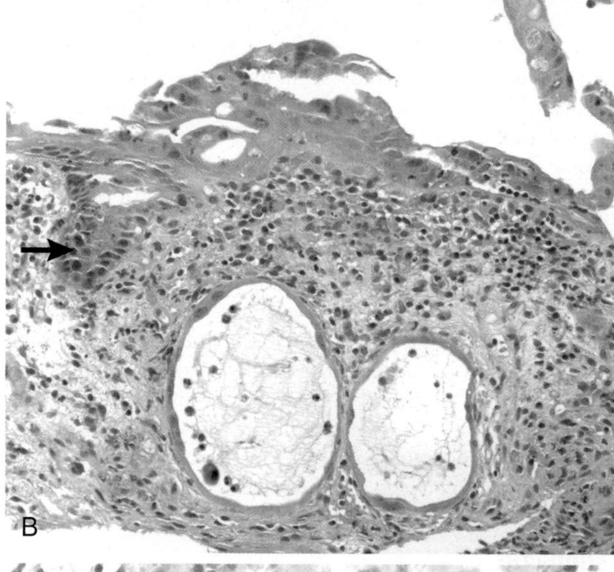

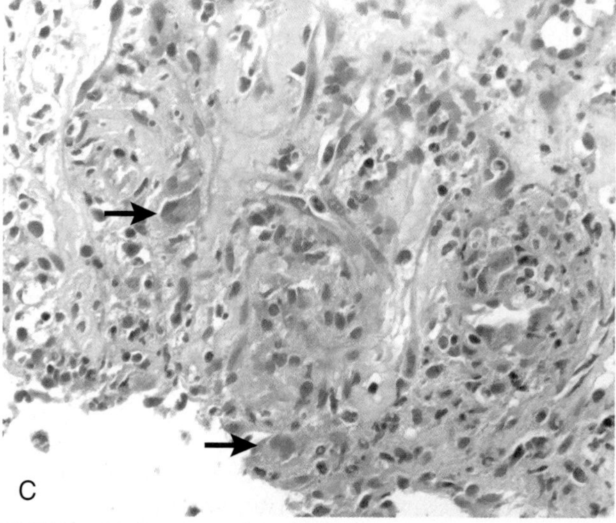

FIGURE 11.32 Cytomegalovirus (CMV) infection. A, Small bowel with multiple CMV ulcers, some of which have hemorrhagic bases, are present. **B,** CMV colitis with marked lamina propria edema, individual crypt injury with attenuated epithelium, neutrophilic infiltrates, and rare intranuclear epithelial inclusion *(arrow).* **C,** Numerous characteristic CMV inclusions in stromal cells *(arrows).*

Chronic gastric ischemia occurs as a result of obstruction of the celiac trunk vessels, which is most often due to atherosclerosis or intrinsic/extrinsic compression of blood vessels (such as those resulting from tumors) but sometimes in the setting of radiation as well. Atherosclerosis may result in gastric necrosis if it is severe and involves multiple vessels simultaneously. Atherosclerotic debris in the aorta may dislodge spontaneously or as a result of instrumentation and propagate into the distal submucosal or mucosal blood vessels as atheroemboli, which leads to ischemic mucosal necrosis and surface erosions.[80] Chronic vascular insufficiency may lead to gastroparesis that is typically reversible if vascular perfusion is reestablished.[81] Acute and chronic ischemic complications of bariatric surgery are not uncommon.[82] Lastly, a broad list of medications and toxins have been associated with ischemic injury in the stomach, including alcohol, Kayexalate, and sevelamer[83,84] (Fig. 11.42).

The gross appearance of ischemic gastritis depends on the severity, extent, and duration of ischemia. Early lesions often reveal mottled mucosa with erythema, erosions, and superficial ulcers. In patients with gastric volvulus, the entire stomach may be necrotic and show marked, diffuse congestion and hemorrhage. Histologically, early ischemic changes of the gastric mucosa include capillary dilation, edema, congestion, and superficial necrosis (Fig. 11.43A,B). With further progression, coagulative necrosis of the entire mucosal surface may occur. The adjacent uninvolved epithelium exhibits reactive changes, such as mucin depletion, reactive nuclear hyperchromasia and enlargement, and increased mitoses. Full-thickness mucosal necrosis and perforation may follow if the patient is not treated (Fig. 11.43C,D).

The gastric mucosa has considerable reparative ability. Ischemic lesions that extend no deeper than the mucosa often heal completely, provided that perfusion is reestablished. Deep lesions may heal, but they usually resolve with fibrous scarring. Chronic ischemia, however, may lead to gastroparesis and mural fibrosis.

LOWER GI ISCHEMIA

Arterial Insufficiency

Arterial insufficiency of the large and small bowel is the most common cause of intestinal ischemia (Table 11.6). Patients with acute mesenteric ischemia commonly present with abdominal pain and hematochezia. Paradoxically, elderly patients (who are the most prone to ischemia from arterial insufficiency) often experience little or no pain until the disease is far advanced, and sometimes this leads to disastrous consequences. Patients with chronic mesenteric ischemia, who constitute fewer than 5% of all those with intestinal ischemia, often suffer from postprandial abdominal pain. This pain usually begins about 30 minutes after a meal, peaks during the following hour, and then typically resolves within 3 hours. Arterial insufficiency may be classified as nonocclusive or occlusive. See Box 11.2 for a list of nonocclusive and occlusive causes of ischemia (Table 11.7).

Nonocclusive Arterial Insufficiency

Nonocclusive, or "central," arterial insufficiency is characterized by failure to deliver sufficient oxygen to the tissues, as a result of inadequate blood flow, in the absence of arterial obstruction. Poor oxygenation of the blood may be an important contributing factor. Common causes of nonocclusive arterial insufficiency are hypotension, shock of any cause (e.g., cardiogenic, hemorrhagic, septic, traumatic), dehydration, and cardiac dysrhythmias. Vasoconstrictor

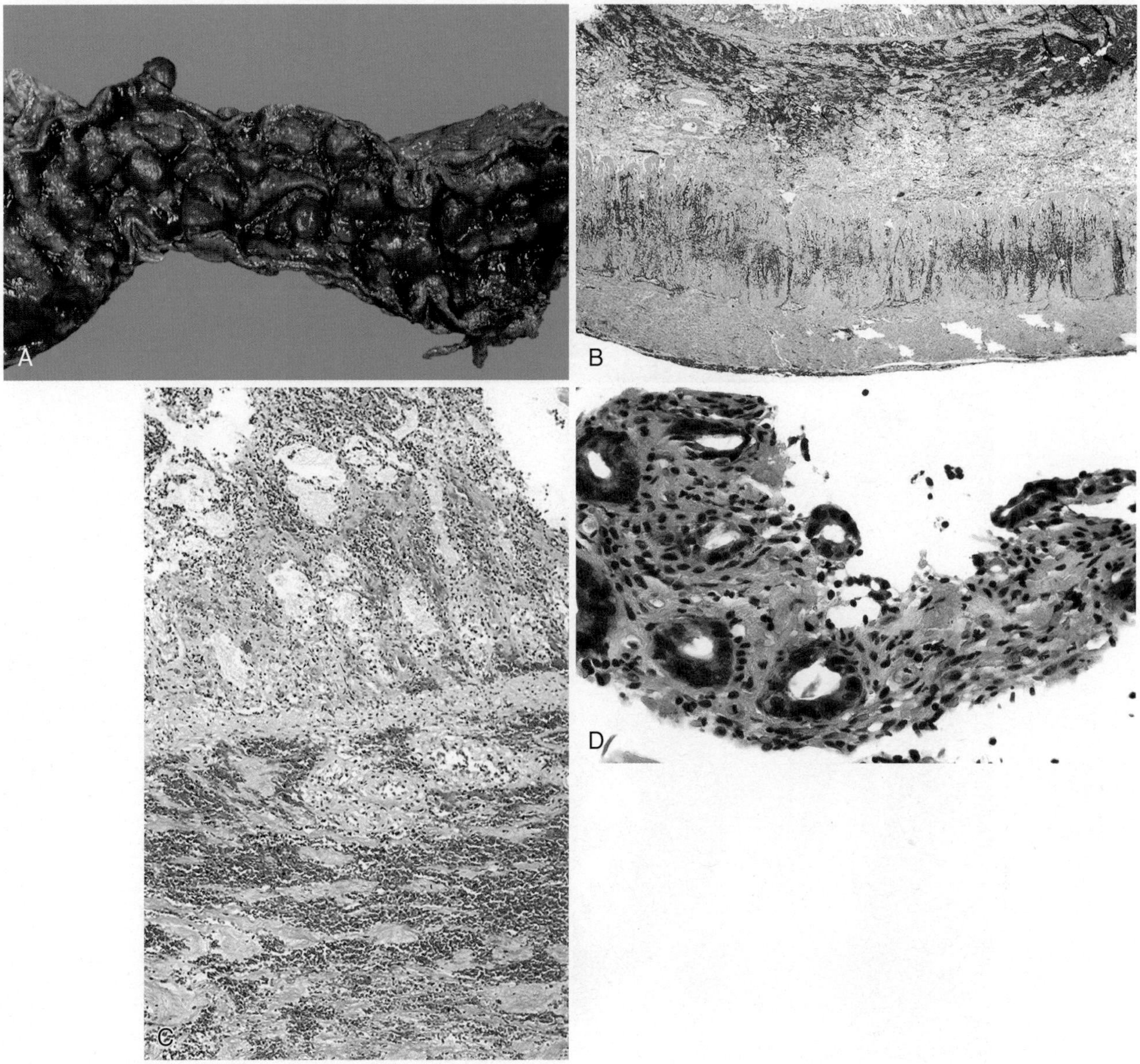

FIGURE 11.33 Enterohemorrhagic *Escherichia coli* enterocolitis. A, Diffuse mucosal hemorrhage and inflammation with gangrenous gross appearance of mucosa. **B,** Transmural hemorrhagic necrosis. **C,** Architecturally normal small-intestinal mucosa with extensive submucosal hemorrhage, ghosts of crypts, and intense intramucosal neutrophil infiltrate. **D,** Ischemic colitis–like mucosal changes of *E. coli* enterocolitis.

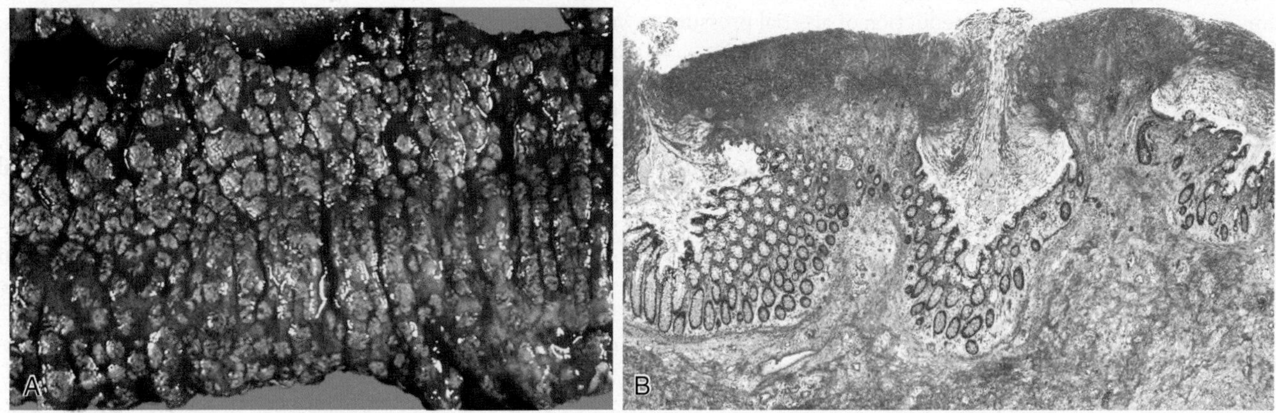

FIGURE 11.34 Pseudomembranous colitis. A, Diffuse mucosal erythema with plaques of yellow exudate. **B,** Characteristic eruptive necroinflammatory exudate with spared adjacent mucosa.

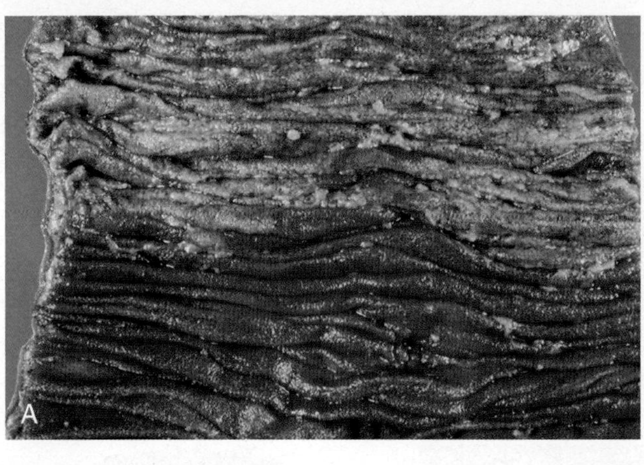

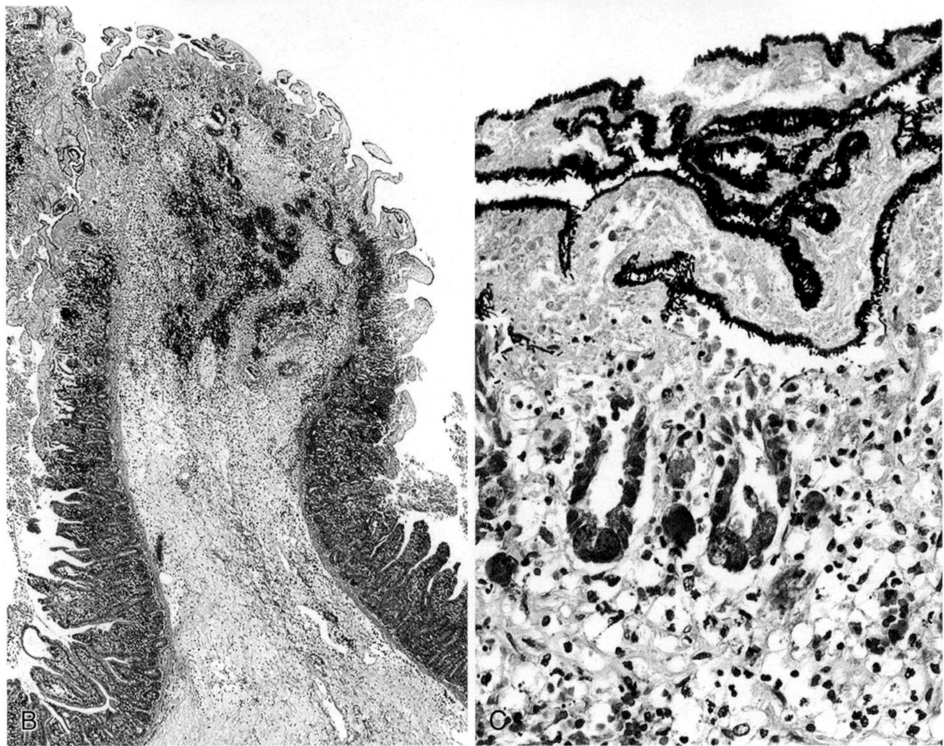

FIGURE 11.35 Enteritis necroticans due to *Clostridium perfringens*. A, Granular surface of small-bowel mucosa with flecks of yellow exudate. **B,** Coagulative necrosis of the mucosa at the tip of the plica. **C,** Dense colonization of the surface of villi by gram-positive bacilli (Brown-Hopps stain).

drugs, such as digitalis, vasopressin, and propranolol, can also cause arterial insufficiency. In elderly patients, atherosclerotic disease often causes nonocclusive stenosis of the major arteries, which increases their susceptibility to ischemic injury if there is a further reduction of arterial pressure (Fig. 11.44).

In nonocclusive ischemia, a critical feature that determines outcome is the duration of arterial insufficiency. The intestinal tract is remarkably tolerant of hypoxia. This property allows for shunting of the splanchnic circulation to the central nervous system in situations of severe shock. Among the layers of the intestinal wall, the mucosa is most susceptible to hypoxia, but it also has the greatest regenerative capacity. Therefore complete recovery from severe mucosal only ischemic damage is quite often possible.

Occlusive Arterial Insufficiency

Occlusive, or "peripheral," arterial insufficiency is characterized by the presence of an obstruction to arterial blood flow; the cause may be intraluminal, intramural, or extramural. Thrombi and emboli are the most common causes of intraluminal occlusion[85] (Fig. 11.45). Radiologically placed coils, beads, and gels are potential iatrogenic causes. Intramural causes include atherosclerosis, dissecting aneurysms, radiation injury, amyloidosis, and diabetes. Mesenteric vascular involvement in polyarteritis nodosa (Fig. 11.46), granulomatosis with polyangiitis, Behçet's disease, rheumatoid arthritis, systemic lupus erythematosus (SLE), scleroderma, syphilis, and other arteritides are considered intramural causes of ischemia as well. Certain drugs and toxins cause arterial occlusion by inducing vasospasm, including potassium salts, cocaine, and some forms of snake and scorpion venom. In addition to causing vasospasm, cocaine may cause fragmentation of the internal elastic lamina and "subelastic" edema, and it may induce thrombosis and platelet aggregation[86,87] (Fig. 11.47). Extramural causes include compression by tumors/masses or adhesion bands, volvulus (Fig. 11.48), torsion, and intussusception.

TABLE 11.5 Infections That May Result in Lower Gastrointestinal Bleeding

Agent	Clinical Presentation	Pathological Findings
Dysentery group: *Shigella* Nontyphoidal *Salmonella* *Campylobacter jejuni* *Yersinia enterocolitica and Yersinia* pseudotuberculosis Enteroinvasive *Escherichia coli*	Dysentery: Small-volume diarrhea with frank or occult bleeding Left lower-quadrant abdominal cramps May be febrile and toxic Extraintestinal manifestations in *Shigella* and *Yersinia*	Normal mucosal architecture with superficial edema Epithelium with mucin depletion and reactive changes Lymphoplasmacytic infiltrate in lamina propria with variable neutrophil content and focal cryptitis Focal erosions or shallow ulcers *Shigella:* Mainly affects distal colon *Salmonella:* May mimic ulcerative colitis *Campylobacter:* May affect jejunum to anus *Yersinia:* Commonly appendix, ileum, and colon; may have necrotizing granulomas; mimics Crohn's disease
Enterohemorrhagic *E. coli*	Bloody diarrhea (acute hemorrhagic colitis) Hemolytic-uremic syndrome Thrombotic thrombocytopenic purpura	Colonic mucosa with normal architecture Lamina propria hemorrhage with minimal inflammation Fibrin thrombi in capillaries Focal mucosal necrosis
Salmonella typhi	Week 1: Fever, headache, abdominal pain, rose-pink rash Week 2: More continuous fever, toxic features Week 3: Disordered mentation, toxemia "pea soup diarrhea," hemorrhage, perforation Week 4: Recovery	Longitudinally oriented oval ulcers overlying Peyer's patches Intense acute inflammation, edema, fibrin exudate, capillary thrombi
Mycobacterium tuberculosis	Nonspecific abdominal pain, weight loss, fever, diarrhea or constipation, blood in stool	Ileocecal involvement most common; multiple erosions or superficial ulcers; may have inflammatory mass with mural hypertrophy and necrotizing granulomas
Clostridium difficile	Fever, leukocytosis, abdominal pain Watery diarrhea with mucus and occult blood Ileus, toxic dilation of the colon	Stage I: Focal superficial mucosal necrosis with plume of necroinflammatory exudate emerging between two crypts Stage II: Groups of type I lesions with confluent exudates Stage III: Complete mucosal necrosis with confluent fibrinopurulent pseudomembrane
Klebsiella oxytoca	Hemorrhagic colitis after antibiotic therapy	Similar changes to other infectious enterocolitides, exudate not as prominent
Lymphogranuloma venereum	Fever, diarrhea, bloody or mucopurulent discharge, lymphadenopathy	Rectal strictures, abscesses, fistulas Neutrophil infiltrates with crypt abscesses, stellate abscesses, ulcers, granulomas
Entamoeba histolytica	Dysentery of gradual onset Acute necrotizing colitis with toxic megacolon (0.5% of cases)	Most common in cecum and ascending colon Flask-shaped ulcer with numerous variable-sized vacuoles containing organisms that engulf red blood cells
Necator americanus and *Ancylostoma duodenale*	Chronic iron-deficiency anemia through blood loss No overt bleeding	Most common in small bowel Multiple superficial erosions with acute inflammation Lamina propria eosinophils with eosinophilic crypt abscesses
Trichuris trichiura	Mucoid diarrhea and occult bleeding in heavy infestations (*Trichuris* dysentery syndrome)	Most commonly seen in cecum, dilated crypts, mucosal necrosis
CMV	Usually in immunocompromised patients	Mucosal erosion or ulcer, may have pseudomembrane; CMV inclusions in endothelial cells, fibroblasts and histiocytes most commonly; may have occlusive vasculitis
EBV	Rare symptomatic GI involvement in absence of a lymphoproliferative disorder	Thickened bowel mucosa with punctate hemorrhage, erosion, or ulcer Lymphoplasmacytic and histiocytic lamina propria infiltrate
Candida species	Usually in immunocompromised patients	Abrupt ulcers, yeast, and pseudohyphae in wispy yellow exudate

CMV, *Cytomegalovirus;* EBV, *Epstein-Barr virus;* GI, *gastrointestinal.*

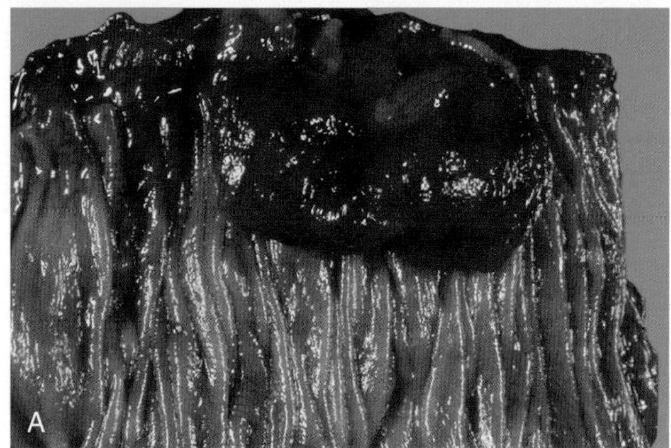

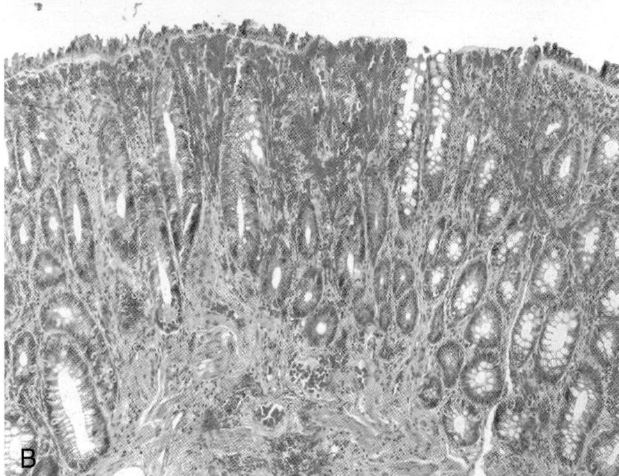

FIGURE 11.36 Mucosal prolapse. A, Gross appearance of mucosal prolapse with erythematous granular mucosa protruding on the surface. **B,** Fibromuscular hyperplasia of the lamina propria with slight architectural distortion of the colonic crypts.

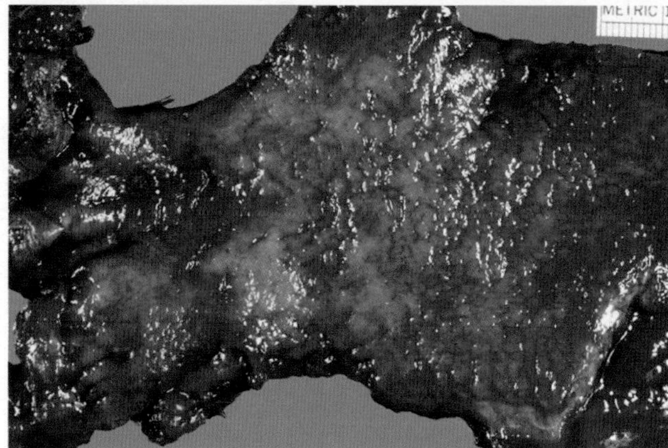

FIGURE 11.37 Ulcerative colitis. Hemorrhagic, granular mucosa involves the rectum *(left)* and extends proximally.

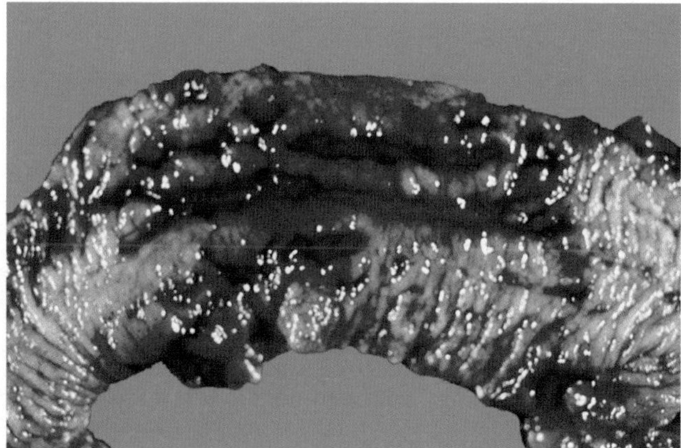

FIGURE 11.38 Crohn's disease. Segmental involvement of the colon by hemorrhagic, longitudinally disposed, linear ulcers ("bear claw" ulcers).

In occlusive disorders, some important considerations that determine outcome are the size of the obstructed vessel and its degree of collateral circulation. Atheroembolic occlusion of terminal arterioles in the intestinal submucosa often leads to focal mucosal ulceration.[88,89] Because the extramural vessels have a richer collateral supply, occlusion or compromise of several of these vessels is usually necessary to induce ischemic damage.

Pathological Features of Arterial Insufficiency

The pathological features of both occlusive and nonocclusive ischemic enteritis, or colitis, are similar, except that in occlusive disease, ischemia is usually segmental in distribution and uniform within the affected region, whereas in nonocclusive cases it is patchy, variable in severity, and often widespread. Segmental ischemic changes may occur anywhere in the large and small bowel but most commonly involve the colon in the vicinity of the splenic flexure. Histological evaluation of ischemic injury should include examination of mesenteric and serosal vessels whenever possible (see Table 11.7).

Transient ischemia occurs mostly as a result of nonocclusive insults. The initial histological changes are similar to those of early acute occlusive ischemia and are typically confined to the mucosa. On restoration of arterial function, mucosal regeneration is typical. Of all intestinal epithelial cells, those in the proliferative zones of the crypts are the most resistant to ischemic injury. If these cells survive an ischemic episode, on restoration of the blood supply they act as a reservoir for epithelial regeneration and contribute to restitution of mucosal morphology, which may be complete. Severe transient ischemia can cause deeper mural injury, perhaps also affecting the submucosa and muscularis propria. This usually results in the development of fibrosis and strictures similar to those seen in patients with chronic ischemia. Of note, once the episode of acute ischemia subsides, the regenerative epithelial changes seen in the recovery phase can be striking and mimic dysplasia (Fig. 11.49).

In early acute ischemia, when examined by endoscopy or in resection specimens, the mucosa is typically friable, swollen (edematous), and erythematous, and it may bleed quite easily on palpation. Histological features of early-stage lesions include surface epithelial degeneration, necrosis and sloughing, loss of epithelium in the superficial portions of the glands (termed *withering crypts*), dilation and congestion of mucosal capillaries, lamina propria hemorrhage, and early hyalinization of the lamina propria caused by leakage of plasma proteins from injured capillaries, which may contain thrombi (Fig. 11.50A–C). Residual viable epithelial cells often show reactive changes with mucin loss, hyperchromatic nuclei, and increased mitoses. Initially, acute inflammation is minimal. In the small intestine, ischemic

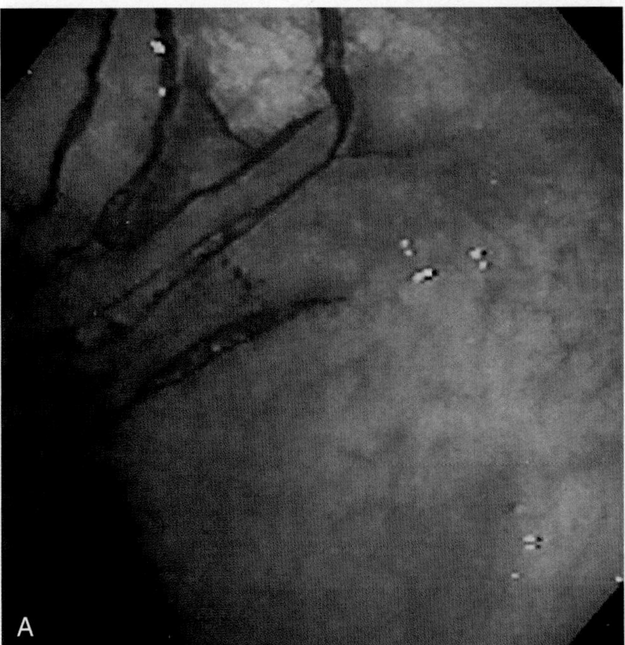

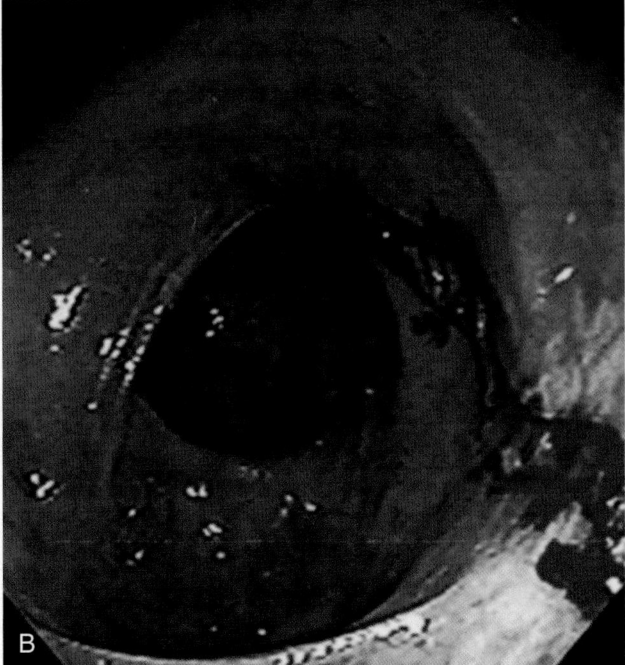

FIGURE 11.39 Collagenous colitis. A–B, Linear mucosal tears that developed and bled when the colon was insufflated during endoscopy.

changes develop initially at the tips of the intestinal villi. With ongoing ischemia, mucosal necrosis extends through the entire length of the villi and then involves the bases of the crypts (Fig. 11.51A). Empty spaces within the mucosa, bounded by viable basement membrane material, may represent the only remnants of intestinal crypts ("crypt ghosts") in ischemic injury (Fig. 11.51B). The submucosa is usually edematous, with engorged veins, either with or without hemorrhage, but the muscularis propria may be viable unless the ischemic insult is near complete or complete and relatively acute in onset. With time, tissue damage and subsequent reperfusion leads to neutrophil infiltration in the mucosa and submucosa, ulceration, and necroinflammatory

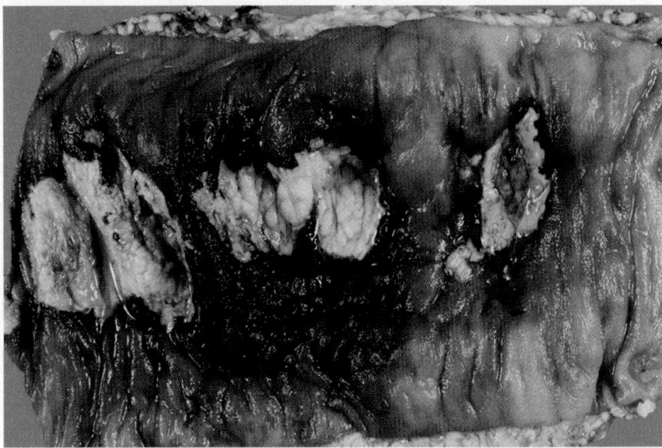

FIGURE 11.40 Stercoral ulcers in the rectum after prolonged constipation. White fibrinous acute inflammatory exudates adhere to the bases of the ulcers and are surrounded by dark patches of hemorrhage.

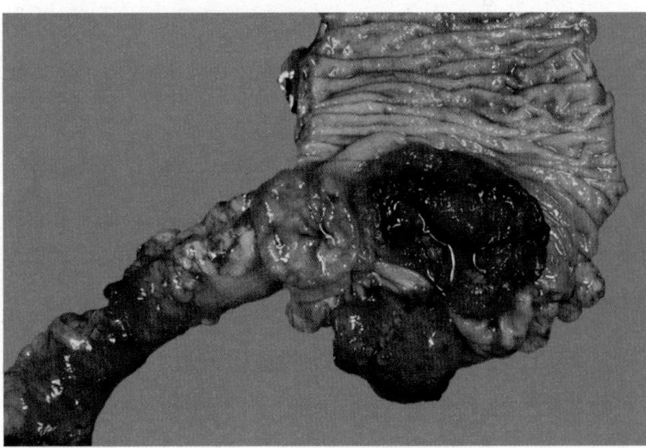

FIGURE 11.41 Ulcerated cecal adenocarcinoma. The patient was seen with iron-deficiency anemia and heme-positive stools.

BOX 11.1 Causes of Gastric Ischemia

CENTRAL CAUSES
Hypotension (shock, trauma, sepsis, head injuries, burns)
Hypoxemia

VASCULAR COMPRESSION
Volvulus

INTRALUMINAL VASCULAR OBSTRUCTION
Emboli
- Atheromatous macroemboli
- Atheromicroemboli
- Iatrogenic emboli (e.g., radiologically placed beads, coils)

Thrombi
- Arterial
- Venous
- Vascular mural processes

Vasculitis
Arteriosclerosis
Chronic radiation injury

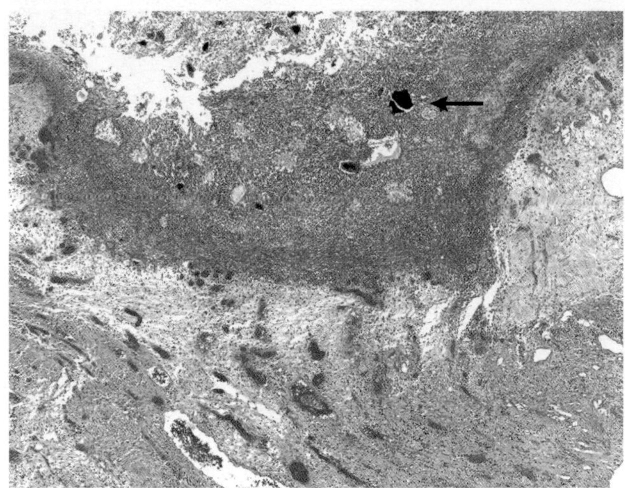

FIGURE 11.42 Sevelamer crystals, displaying an orangeophilic tinge and true fish-scale appearance, associated with full-thickness mucosal necrosis.

membrane debris. Transmural necrosis and perforation occur in patients with sudden complete occlusion of arteries if blood flow to the organ is not restored. This is often referred to as an *infarct*. At this stage, the bowel wall often appears thickened and edematous. Organizing acute serositis and fibrin deposition can be seen at sites of perforation as a response to injury. As the muscularis propria undergoes necrosis, the bowel wall becomes thin, friable, and easily disrupted (Fig. 11.52A–B). In the subacute phase of ischemia, there may be prominent granulation tissue associated with mucosal ulcers and inflammatory polyp formation. There may be a florid fibroblastic proliferation in the ulcer stroma and numerous capillaries. Regenerative epithelial changes can be seen in areas of more preserved mucosa. On occasion, superimposed bacterial infection (e.g., clostridia) may lead to the formation of gas bubbles within the bowel wall, termed *intestinal pneumatosis*.

In contrast, chronic ischemia, which is typically low grade and recurrent, is characterized by fibrosis and chronic

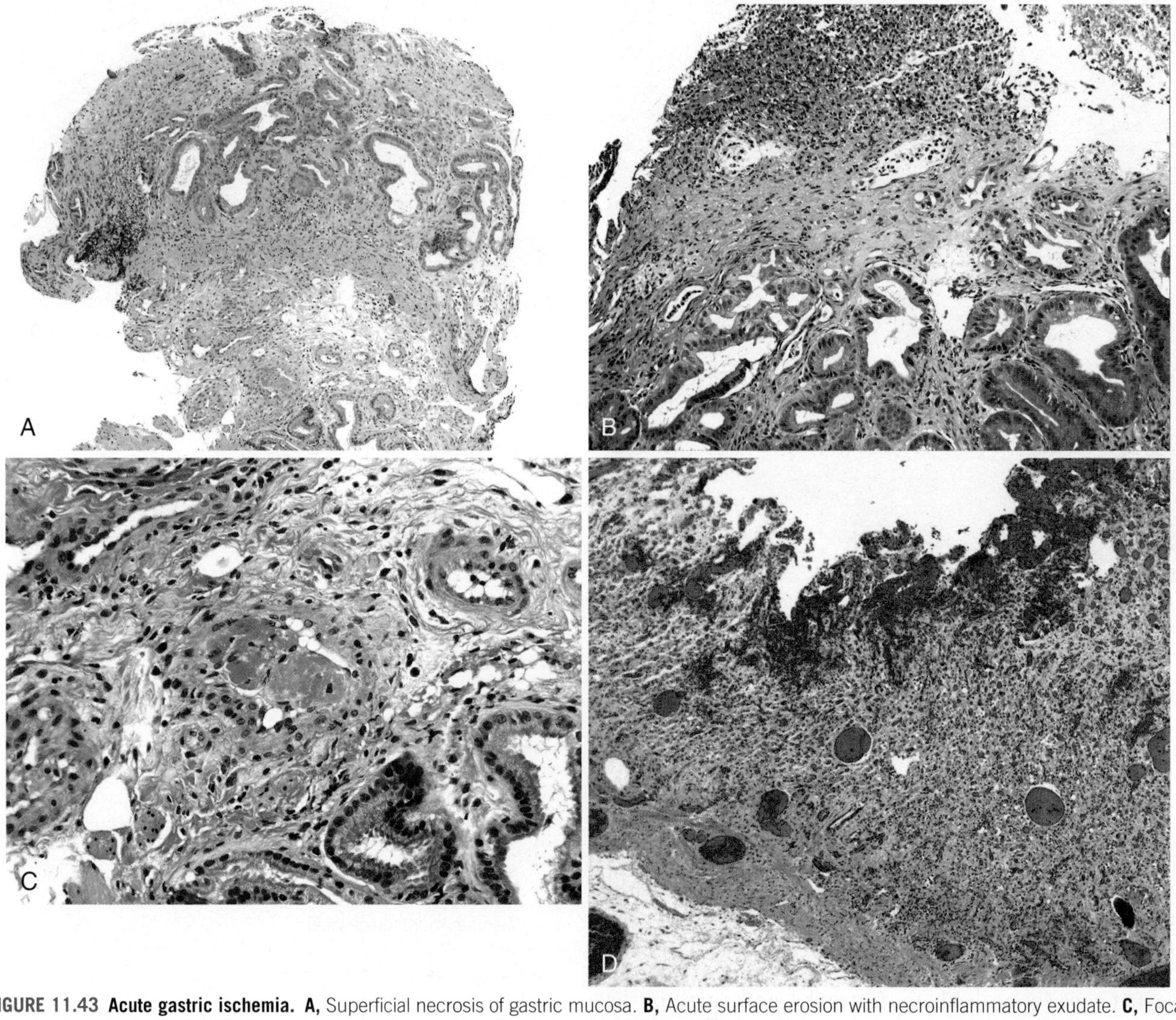

FIGURE 11.43 Acute gastric ischemia. A, Superficial necrosis of gastric mucosa. **B,** Acute surface erosion with necroinflammatory exudate. **C,** Focal vascular thrombosis. **D,** Full-thickness hemorrhagic necrosis with a few residual "withering" deep glands.

TABLE 11.6 Frequency of Different Causes of Acute Mesenteric Ischemia

Cause	Frequency (%)
Mesenteric artery embolism	50
Nonocclusive mesenteric ischemia	25
Mesenteric artery thrombosis	10
Mesenteric venous thrombosis	10
Focal segmental ischemia	5

From Brandt LJ. Intestinal ischemia. In: Sleisenger MH, Feldman M, Friedman LS, Brandt LJ, eds. Sleisenger and Fordtran's Gastrointestinal and Liver Disease: Pathophysiology, Diagnosis, Management. *Philadelphia: Saunders; 2006:2563-2885.*

BOX 11.2 Arterial Causes of Intestinal Ischemia

NONOCCLUSIVE (CENTRAL) ISCHEMIA

- Low flow
  - Systemic hypotension
  - Cardiac failure
  - Shock (cardiogenic, hemorrhagic, septic, traumatic)
  - Dysrhythmias
  - Vasoconstrictor drugs
  - Digitalis, vasopressin, propranolol
  - Dehydration
- Hypoxemia
  - Respiratory compromise
  - Oxygen depletion

OCCLUSIVE (PERIPHERAL) ISCHEMIA

- External
  - Volvulus, torsion, intussusception
  - Compression (e.g., tumor, celiac compression syndrome)
- Luminal
  - Thrombi (hypercoagulable states, atherosclerotic injury)
  - Emboli
  - Macroemboli
  - Atherosclerosis
  - Atrial fibrillation
  - Prosthetic heart valves
  - Rheumatic heart disease
  - Mural thrombi
  - Atheromicroemboli after aortic instrumentation
  - Radiologically placed emboli
- Mural
  - Atherosclerosis (stenosis, occlusion)
  - Dissecting aneurysms
  - Tumor invasion
  - Chronic radiation injury

ARTERITIS AND OTHER ARTERIOPATHIES

See Table 11.8.

mucosal injury. The fibrosis is usually circumferential and involves all layers of the bowel wall, including the mucosa (Fig. 11.53A). At this stage, hemosiderin deposits may be present, indicating previous episodes of hemorrhage. Strictures may cause intestinal obstruction. Linear ulcers are commonly associated with strictures. Chronic mucosal injury includes architectural crypt distortion, pseudopyloric and Paneth cell metaplasia, and many of the other features of inflammatory bowel disease (see Chapter 17) (Fig. 11.53B).

TABLE 11.7 Arterial Insufficiency: Occlusive vs. Nonocclusive Disease

	Occlusive Ischemia	Nonocclusive Ischemia
Clinical associations	Occlusion of arterial vessels resulting from intraluminal, intramural, or extramural causes	Shock, dehydration, cardiac dysrhythmias, drugs (e.g., beta blockers)
Underlying pathogenesis	Obstruction of arterial blood flow	Inadequate oxygen delivery/low blood flow (systemic)
Macroscopic findings	Ischemic changes that are segmental in distribution and uniform in severity	Gross evidence of ischemic injury can be patchy, often widespread, and variable in severity
Microscopic findings	Features of ischemic changes (as described) that are uniform in severity	Features of ischemic injury (as described) with histological variation of severity within a segment

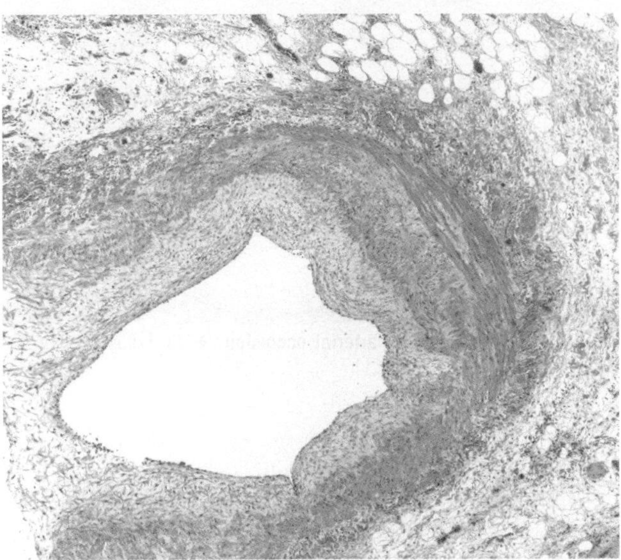

FIGURE 11.44 Nonobstructive atherosclerotic disease. There is marked stenosis of this small subserosal artery.

Venous Insufficiency

Venous insufficiency is less common than arterial insufficiency as a cause of intestinal ischemia. A comparison with arterial insufficiency is summarized in Table 11.8. It accounts for approximately 5% to 15% of cases of intestinal ischemia overall.[90,91] It involves the superior mesenteric vein in most cases (see Tables 11.6 and 11.8). Similar to patients with acute arterial ischemia, those with venous insufficiency usually present with abdominal pain. However, venous insufficiency usually affects younger patients,

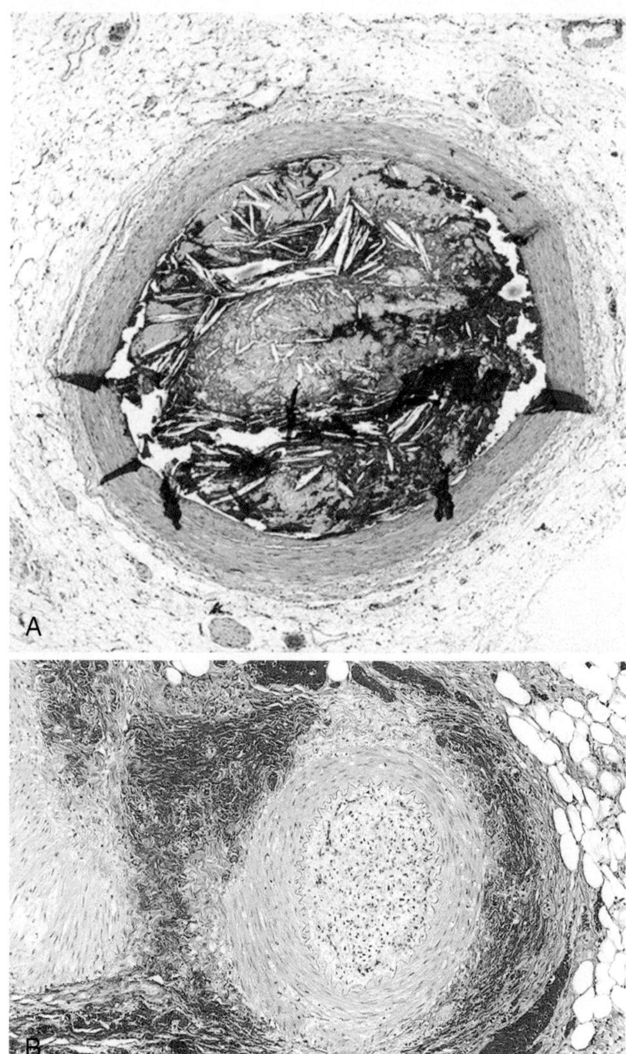

FIGURE 11.45 Intraluminal arterial occlusion. A, Embolus. **B,** Thrombus.

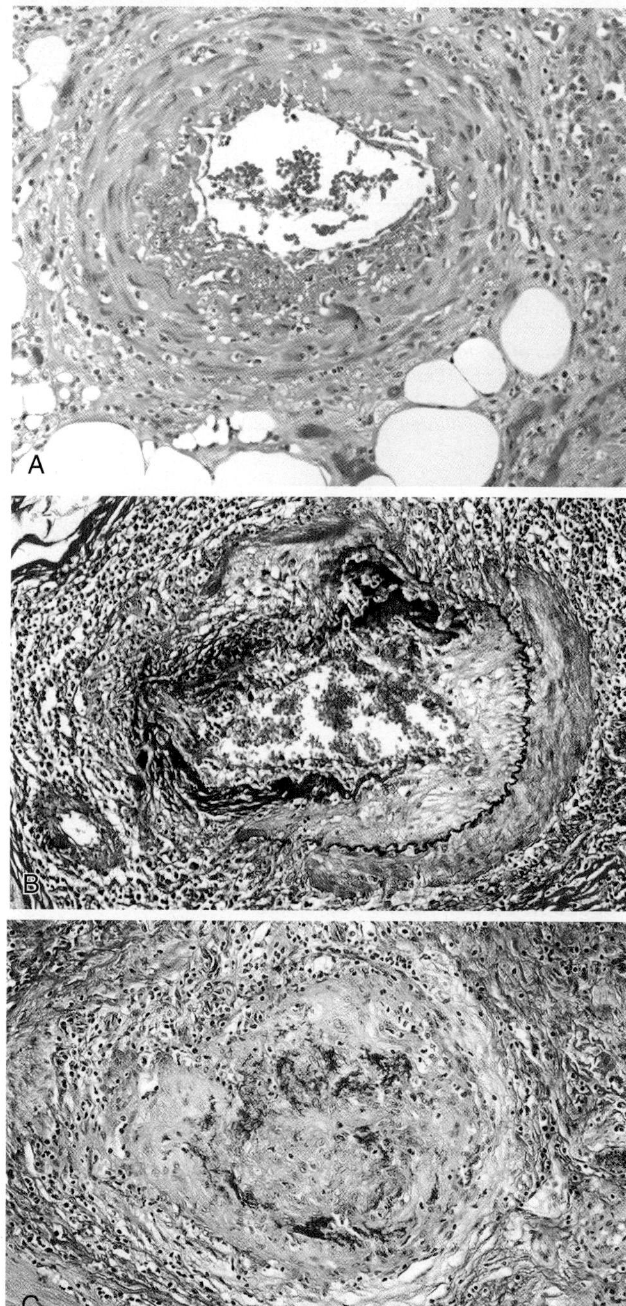

FIGURE 11.46 Polyarteritis nodosa. A, Cross-section of a vessel with fibrinoid necrosis of the wall and mixed inflammation cell infiltrate. **B,** Destruction of left side of arterial wall and elastic lamina with a neutrophil infiltrate (elastic Van Gieson stain). **C,** Fibrinoid necrosis (fibrin staining magenta in the trichrome Martius scarlet blue stain).

including children and young adults, in whom a diagnosis of ischemia may not be suspected initially. The pathogenesis of venous insufficiency may be related to external venous compression, thrombosis (intraluminal), or intramural processes (Box 11.3). External venous compression and mesenteric venous thrombosis are the most common causes. Mural processes include several relatively uncommon but distinctive entities (e.g., idiopathic myointimal hyperplasia of mesenteric veins, enterocolic lymphocytic phlebitis) that are probably underrecognized clinically and pathologically. The histological features and differential diagnoses of these entities are summarized in Table 11.9.

In patients with venous obstruction, arterial flow to the affected segment of the bowel is usually unobstructed; hence, the tissue becomes progressively and severely engorged until either drainage is achieved through unobstructed collateral veins, or the resistance of the tissue exceeds arterial pressure. At this point, arterial flow ceases, and the affected segment of bowel undergoes necrosis in a manner similar to arterial insufficiency. Therefore the initial phase of venous insufficiency is characterized by severe vascular congestion, hemorrhage, and edema, before tissue necrosis develops.

Segmental swelling of the bowel may be quite extreme. The mucosa appears boggy and hemorrhagic, and the plicae circulares or plicae semilunares often appear markedly thickened (Fig. 11.54). On histological examination, one sees intense venous congestion of the bowel wall, dilation of engorged veins, marked tissue edema, and intramural hemorrhage. Evidence of venous thrombi, phlebitis, or

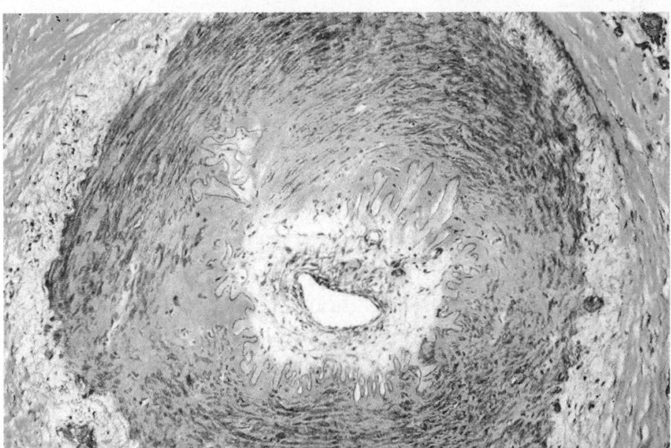

FIGURE 11.47 Cocaine arteriopathy. Fragmented internal elastic lamina with "subelastic" edema (Masson trichrome stain).

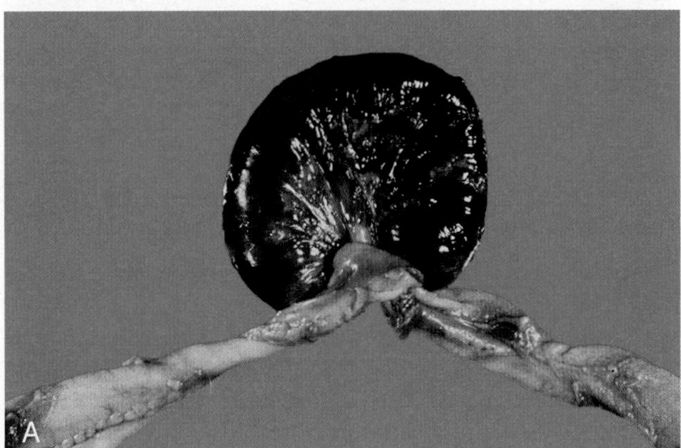

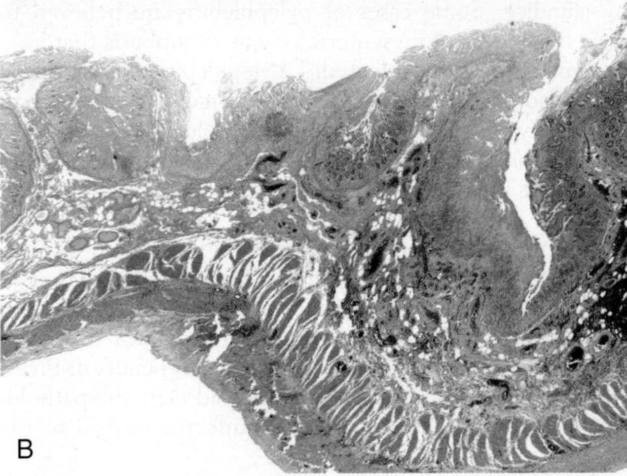

FIGURE 11.48 Volvulus. A, Gangrenous loop of small intestine (closed-loop obstruction). The dark color of the affected loop is caused by intense vascular congestion, and it is distended because of the accumulation of secretions and bacterial fermentation. **B,** Partial necrosis of the wall, mainly involving the mucosa and submucosa, accompanied by hemorrhage.

other forms of venopathy should be considered in all cases in which the etiology is unclear.

External Mesenteric Venous Compression

The most common cause of mesenteric venous insufficiency is external mesenteric venous compression. This is commonly caused by volvulus, torsion, adhesions, intussusception, or trauma. Because of the normal low intraluminal pressure of veins, these structures are easily occluded externally. If the occlusion is of sufficient duration, thrombosis may develop as well. Volvulus, torsion, and bowel entrapment may cause closed-loop obstruction in which the lumen of the bowel is sealed off at the point of compression. As a result, luminal secretions accumulate, which facilitates bacterial proliferation, toxin production, inflammation, and necrosis. Mesenteric venous compression by extraabdominal trauma is rare. It has been attributed to a tight seat belt during prolonged plane travel in some cases[92] (Fig. 11.55).

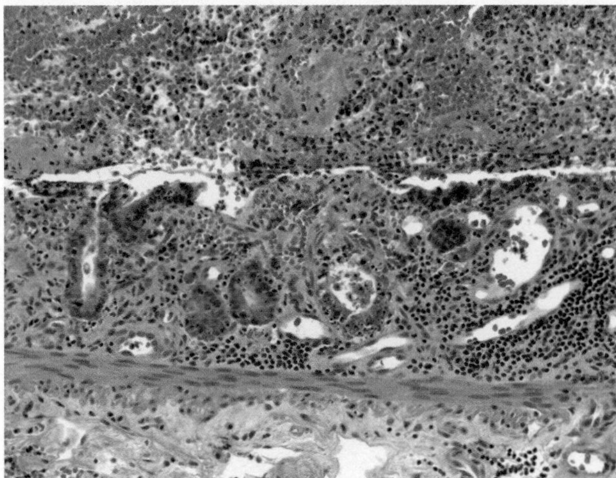

FIGURE 11.49 Ischemic colitis with marked regenerative epithelial changes including nuclear hyperchromasia, prominent nucleoli, and increased apoptosis, mimicking dysplasia.

Mesenteric Venous Thrombosis

Mesenteric venous thrombosis usually manifests as progressive, severe abdominal pain of acute onset. It may occur in individuals of any age, but patients tend to be male and younger (40 to 60 years of age) than those with arterial insufficiency.[93] Until recently, mesenteric venous thrombosis was most often diagnosed at laparotomy, in resection specimens, or at autopsy. However, improved radiological techniques, including computed tomographic angiography and magnetic resonance imaging, now enable many cases to be diagnosed radiologically. Thus increasing numbers of patients are being treated medically with thrombolytic therapy, rather than surgery.[94] Furthermore, as a result of advances in understanding of hypercoagulable states and myeloproliferative disorders, the cause of mesenteric venous thrombosis is now known in as many as 80% of cases.

In the absence of external venous compression, an intramural pathological process, or a localized cause of thrombosis such as an intraabdominal abscess, acute diverticulitis, acute pancreatitis, or venous invasion by tumor (Fig. 11.56), most patients with mesenteric venous thrombosis have an underlying predisposition to thrombosis. Therefore it is important to investigate these patients clinically for predisposing conditions that may lead to recurrence and for relatives who may carry the predisposition to thrombosis. Hypercoagulable states include factor V Leiden mutation, the presence of antiphospholipid antibody, and deficiency of protein C or S (see Box 11.3).

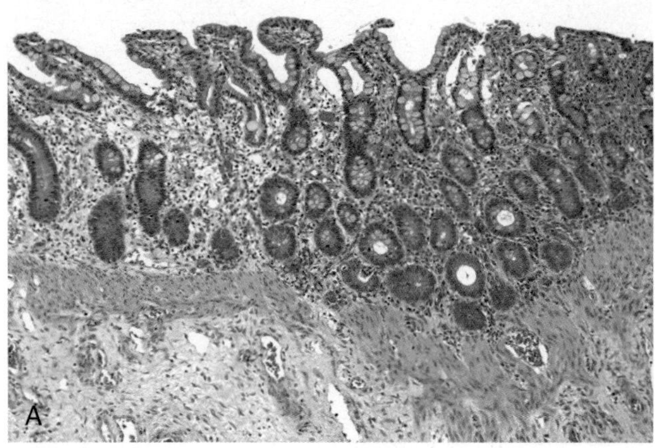

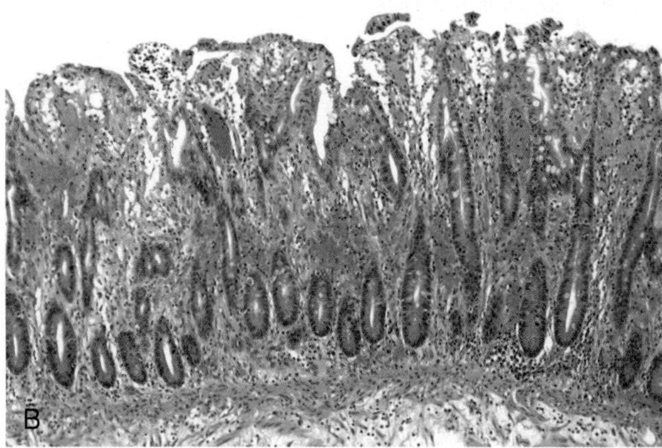

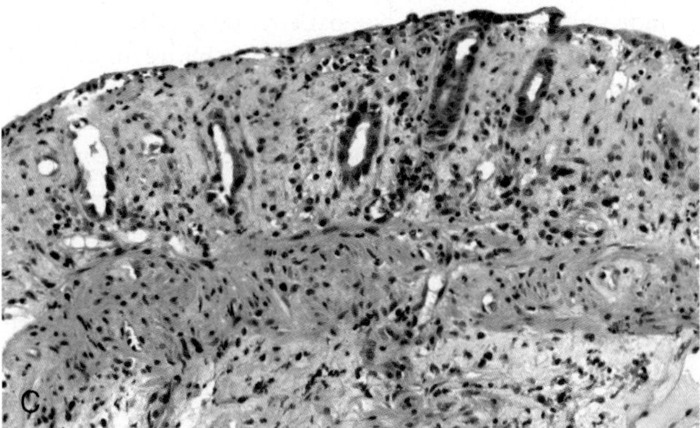

FIGURE 11.50 Early acute ischemia. A, Mild reactive mucin loss in the surface epithelial cells with lamina propria hemorrhage. **B,** More pronounced lamina propria hemorrhagic changes with focal edema and denudation of the surface epithelium. **C,** Withered crypts with prominent hyalinization of the lamina propria and complete attenuation of the surface epithelium.

Myeloproliferative disorders, such as polycythemia vera, have also been found to be causative. The *JAK2* V617F mutation has been detected in some patients with mesenteric venous thrombosis before the development of an overt myeloproliferative disorder.[95]

The gross and microscopic appearances of the affected segment of bowel are similar to those described in cases of mesenteric venous insufficiency. In addition, thrombi are typically found in veins located in the submucosa, adventitia, and mesentery (Fig. 11.57A) and in veins distant from areas of necrosis. The splenic, portal, and hepatic veins may be involved in some cases. Typically, arteries are not affected. Blood vessels located proximal to the area of thrombus are typically engorged and dilated. Mucosal and intramural congestion and hemorrhage, with submucosal edema and extravasation of erythrocytes, are common (Fig. 11.57B–C). Ischemic necrosis of the mucosa may be seen on microscopic examination. When the area of thrombosis is localized, it usually begins within large-sized blood vessels and propagates proximally toward smaller ones. However, if the underlying cause of ischemia is a hypercoagulable state, thrombosis begins in the small-sized vessels and propagates centrally toward the larger ones.[91] Patients may present with acute, subacute, or chronic symptoms and sometimes with Budd-Chiari syndrome. However, even in patients with an acute presentation, it is common to detect thrombi at various stages of organization (Fig. 11.57D).

Intramural Disorders

Portal Pylephlebitis

Pylephlebitis is a form of septic (often suppurative) thrombophlebitis of the portal venous system, usually associated with gram-negative enteric aerobes and anaerobes. Portal pylephlebitis is a condition that develops most commonly as a complication of diverticulitis, perforated appendicitis, and sometimes complicated hemorrhoids. Patients typically present with a high fever that is sometimes accompanied by jaundice. Some cases of pylephlebitis are believed to arise from areas of mesenteric venous thrombosis that have become secondarily infected.[96] Pylephlebitis is most often diagnosed on the basis of clinical and radiological findings, but it may be encountered by the pathologist on evaluation of resection specimens or at autopsy. It may also be inferred in patients with a hepatic abscess and an appropriate clinical history.

The pathognomonic histological lesion is an acutely inflamed vein of the mesenteric/portal system that is associated with bacteria or fungi and either a recent or organized thrombus. Pylephlebitis identified in a surgical resection specimen from a patient with a ruptured appendix or diverticular disease–associated abscess should alert the pathologist to the possibility of spread of infected emboli to the liver.

Pylephlebitis usually requires aggressive antimicrobial therapy. If left untreated, it may lead to the development of septic emboli. Hepatic abscesses occur in up to 50% of cases. The mortality rate exceeds 30%.[94,97] Early diagnosis and therapy improve overall outcome.

Mesenteric Phlebitis

Mesenteric phlebitis occurs in several types of systemic vasculitides that affect both arteries and veins. These disorders include Behçet's disease, Buerger's disease, SLE, rheumatoid arthritis, and granulomatosis with polyangiitis. This condition is discussed more thoroughly in the Vasculitides section later in this chapter.

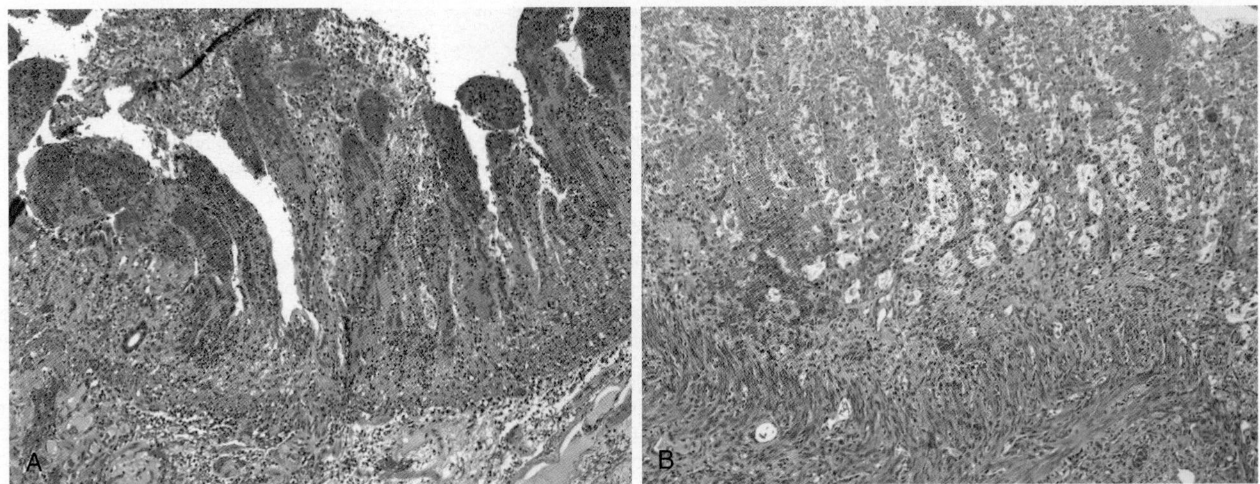

FIGURE 11.51 Severe acute ischemia. A, As the insult persists, there is complete denudation of the epithelial cells lining the villi, with extensive hemorrhagic changes and capillary congestion. **B,** The "ghost" image of prior crypts is still evident in some cases, after mucosal necrosis evolves.

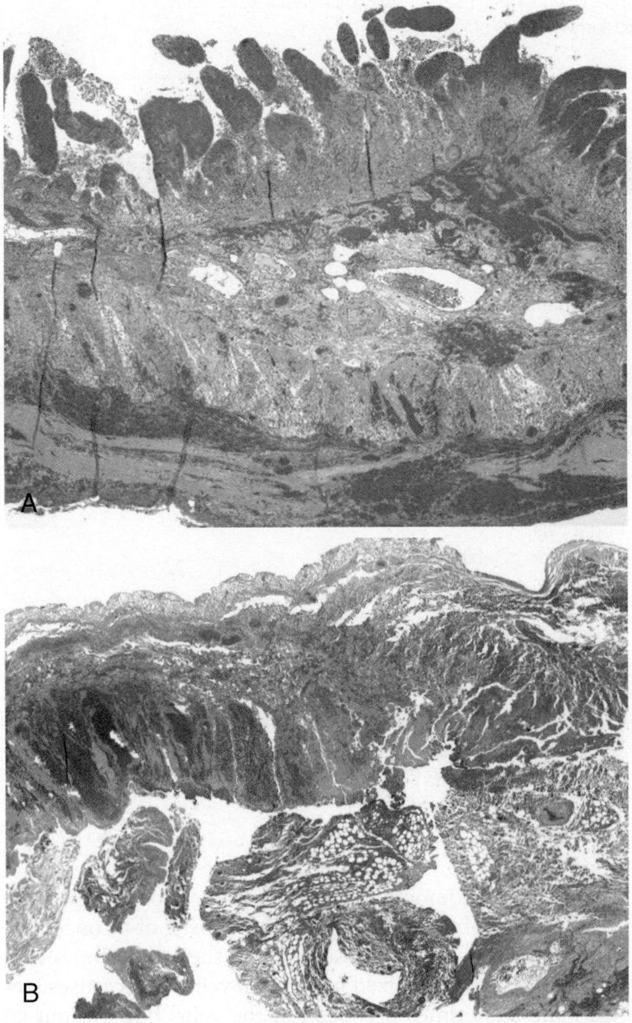

FIGURE 11.52 A, Acute ischemia (later stages) involving the full thickness of the bowel wall, leading to perforation and serositis. **B,** Sections from a perforation site with prominent granulation tissue adjacent to ischemic bowel.

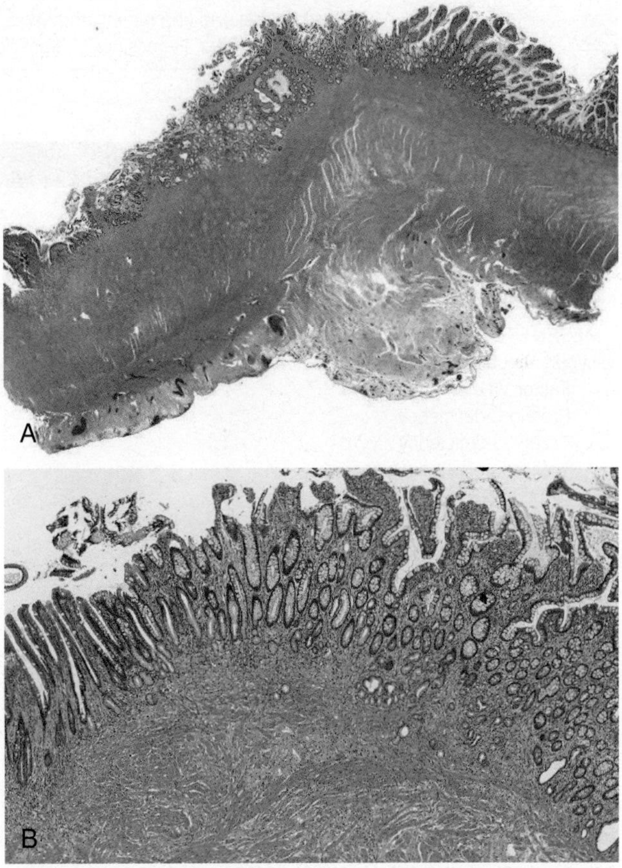

FIGURE 11.53 A, Chronic ischemia can manifest in a variety of ways. In this case, there is architectural distortion and mural fibrosis, mimicking inflammatory bowel disease. **B,** Chronic mucosal injury with focal pyloric gland metaplasia.

TABLE 11.8 Diagnostic Features of Arterial vs. Venous Insufficiency

	Arterial Insufficiency	Venous Insufficiency
Clinical presentation and associations	Tends to occur in older patients. Cardiovascular disease, metabolic syndrome, smoking, hypercholesterolemia, hypertension, and so on.	Tends to occur in younger patients (including children and young adults) Autoimmune diseases, drugs, prothrombotic disorders, and so on.
Macroscopic findings	Typically a segmental process (if occlusive). Erythematous to hemorrhagic friable mucosal changes with attenuated villi or colonic folds. Ulceration. Hemorrhagic changes, thinning of the wall with marked luminal dilation and possibly perforation, with evidence of purulent membranes on the serosal surface.	Marked congestion, swelling, dusky to erythematous mucosa, frank hemorrhage and discoloration (early). Thinning of the bowel wall with luminal dilation. Tissue necrosis, even perforation (late).
Histological findings	Reactive mucin loss on epithelial cells with sloughing of surface epithelium and withered crypts. Congested small lamina propria capillary and red blood cell extravasation into the lamina propria.	Marked venous congestion with engorged vessels, and hemorrhagic changes in mucosa. Reactive mucin loss in epithelial cells. Lamina propria edema that extends into the wall.
Acute phase	There may be evidence of arteritis, arteriopathy, or intraluminal thrombi. Early hyalinization of the lamina propria.	
Subacute phase	More pronounced epithelial changes with ulcers, and necrosis. Prominent granulation tissue and inflammatory polyps. Eventually full-thickness necrosis if ischemia persists. More established hyalinization of lamina propria. In some cases, there may be regenerative epithelial changes in areas that are more preserved.	There may be phlebitis, venopathy, or thrombi. Marked hemorrhagic changes and edema with sloughing of the mucosa lining. Frank necrosis that can extend transmurally.
Chronic phase	Chronic mucosal injury, metaplastic changes (pseudopyloric, left-sided Paneth cells), and/or linear ulcers. Postinflammatory polyps. Mural fibrosis and chronic inflammation, particularly in areas of stenosis/strictures. Hemosiderin deposition.	Much less common but may present similarly to the arterial insufficiency.

BOX 11.3 Venous Causes of Intestinal Ischemia

EXTERNAL VENOUS COMPRESSION
- Volvulus
- Entrapment by adhesion band
- Intussusception

MESENTERIC VENOUS THROMBOSIS
- Hypercoagulable states, genetic
  - Factor V Leiden mutation
  - Protein C deficiency
  - Protein S deficiency
  - Antithrombin III deficiency
  - *G202101A* mutation in prothrombin gene
  - Antiphospholipid antibodies
  - Methyltetrahydrofolate deficiency
  - Hyperhomocysteinemia
- Hypercoagulable states, acquired
  - Dehydration
  - Oral contraceptive use
  - Paraneoplastic states
- Hematological disorders
  - Polycythemia vera
  - Essential thrombocythemia
  - Paroxysmal nocturnal hemoglobinuria
  - *JAK2* V617F mutation
- Other conditions
  - Portal hypertension
  - Intraabdominal inflammation (e.g., diverticulitis, abscess, pancreatitis)
  - Malignant tumors (e.g., renal, hepatic)
  - Sclerotherapy
  - Splenectomy
  - Postoperative state

MURAL PROCESSES
- Portal pylephlebitis
- Mesenteric phlebitis
  - Behçet's disease
  - Buerger's disease
  - Systemic lupus erythematosus
  - Rheumatoid arthritis
  - Granulomatosis with polyangiitis (Wegener's granulomatosis)
- Idiopathic myointimal hyperplasia of mesenteric veins (IMHMV)
- Enterocolic phlebitis (lymphocytic, necrotizing, granulomatous)
- Mesenteric phlebosclerosis

Idiopathic Myointimal Hyperplasia of Mesenteric Veins

Idiopathic myointimal hyperplasia of mesenteric veins (IMHMV) is a rare condition that mimics inflammatory bowel disease clinically. The disease has been reported mainly in young to middle-aged men who present with abdominal pain, diarrhea or constipation, and rectal bleeding. The endoscopic findings of left-sided mucosal erythema, ulceration, friability, granularity, and cobblestoning often result in a presumptive clinical diagnosis of inflammatory bowel disease.

The pathognomonic histological features of IMHMV are seen in the mural blood vessels; they consist of a concentric proliferation of smooth muscle cells in the intima and media of small- to medium-sized intramural veins. This causes stenosis and sometimes occlusion of the veins but without an associated inflammatory infiltrate (Fig. 11.58). The arteries are normal, but the veins become enlarged and muscular, so they can easily be mistaken for arteries.[98] A Van Gieson stain can help distinguish arteries from veins in such

TABLE 11.9 Histological Features and Differential Diagnosis of Disorders That Cause Mesenteric Venous Insufficiency (Excluding Venous Compression)

Entity	Key Clinical Features	Etiology	Key Pathological Features	Treatment
Mesenteric venous thrombosis	Progressive or acute-onset abdominal pain, often in young patients	Hypercoagulable states, hematological disorders, portal hypertension, intraabdominal inflammation	Thrombosis of mesenteric veins, intense transmural vascular engorgement and hemorrhage in affected segment; mucosal congestion, hemorrhage, and ischemic necrosis	Resect affected segment; determine cause; if indicated, anticoagulate
Portal pylephlebitis	High fever and jaundice after diverticulitis or appendicitis with rupture; may seed hepatic abscess	Intestinal gram-negative bacteria or anaerobes	Suppurative thrombophlebitis of the portal venous system; hepatic abscess	Aggressive antibiotic therapy
IMHMV	Left-sided abdominal pain, diarrhea or constipation, rectal bleeding in young to middle-aged men; mucosa friable with ulceration and cobblestoning on endoscopy	Possibly secondary to arteriovenous fistula	Myointimal hyperplasia of mesenteric veins (seen in resection specimens); mild ischemic changes with thick-walled vessels in mucosal biopsies; affects left colon only	Resect affected segment
Enterocolic phlebitis	Abdominal pain, diarrhea and hematochezia, or right-sided abdominal mass in middle-aged to elderly patients	Unknown	Lymphocytic phlebitis with dense cuff of T cells surrounding, infiltrating, and obstructing mesenteric veins, with vascular engorgement and hemorrhage; or necrotizing phlebitis with neutrophil infiltrate and fibrinoid necrosis; or granulomatous phlebitis with giant cell infiltrate and damage to vein wall; mainly affects terminal ileum and cecum	Resect affected segment
Mesenteric phlebosclerosis	Chronic abdominal pain and diarrhea; colonic mucosa dark, edematous	Unknown	Sclerosis and calcification of mesenteric veins; chronic ischemic changes in mucosa	Resect affected segment

IMHMV, *Idiopathic myointimal hyperplasia of mesenteric veins.*

cases. In contrast with acute mesenteric venous ischemia, cases of IMHMV do not show mucosal congestion, vascular engorgement, or hemorrhage within the bowel wall. Rather, the mucosa characteristically shows numerous thick-walled ("arteriolized") dilated capillaries, swollen endothelial cells, subendothelial hyaline deposits, and bright eosinophilic thrombi (Fig. 11.59A–B).[99] The epithelium may reveal mucin depletion, withered crypts, and other features typical of ischemia (i.e., loss of surface epithelium, reactive changes in residual crypt epithelium, and hyalinization of the lamina propria).

The pathogenesis of the disease remains poorly understood. On the basis of a similarity of the pathological changes in the mural and extramural veins to those in saphenous veins that have been used in coronary artery bypass surgery, Genta et al., in the initial description of this entity, postulated that the disorder may be a consequence of arteriovenous fistulization.[100] Subsequent studies have supported this theory.[101] Small, localized foci of pathological changes similar to IMHMV have been demonstrated in intestinal specimens resected for unrelated conditions, but they contained surgical anastomoses or other forms of healed (traumatic) injury, in which arteriovenous communications are expected to occur.[102] An alternative pathogenetic theory suggests that IMHMV represents the end stage of "phlebitis" because lesions morphologically similar to IMHMV have been observed in cases of lymphocytic, granulomatous, and necrotizing phlebitis.[103]

A diagnosis of IMHMV may rarely be suspected on clinical grounds, but it is usually established only on pathological evaluation of a resection specimen. The disorder is localized to the veins of discrete segments of the intestine and therefore is not considered a systemic form of "vasculitis." Resection of the affected segment of bowel is considered curative. Disease recurrences have not been reported.

Enterocolic (Lymphocytic, Granulomatous, or Necrotizing) Phlebitis

Enterocolic phlebitis is a term that was initially introduced to encompass a variety of related disorders termed *lymphocytic, granulomatous,* or *necrotizing* phlebitis. This name was proposed on the basis that granulomatous phlebitis and necrotizing phlebitis almost always occur in association with lymphocytic phlebitis, and not uncommonly all three

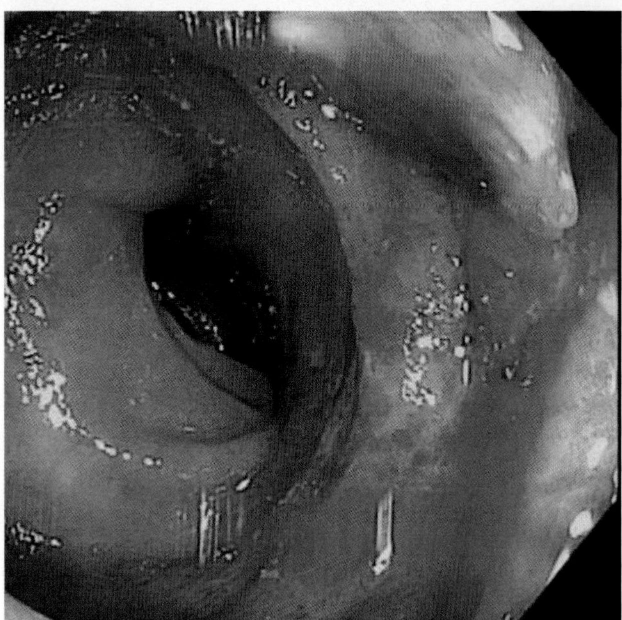

FIGURE 11.54 Endoscopic photograph of ischemic colitis revealing boggy mucosa with erythema and superficial mucosal erosions.

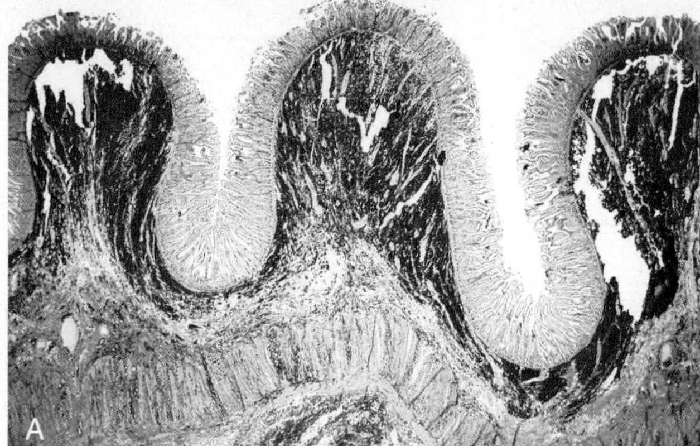

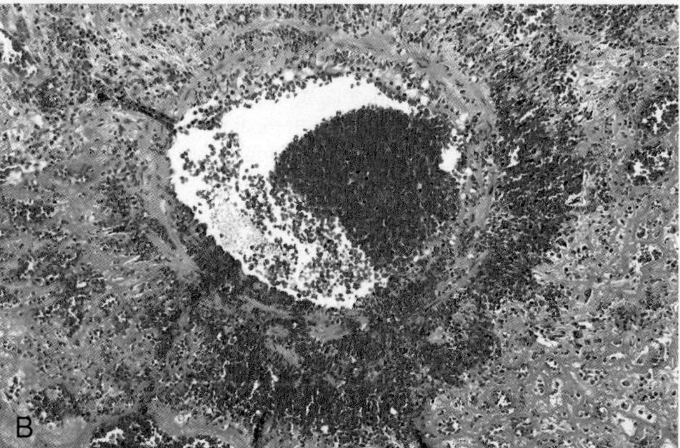

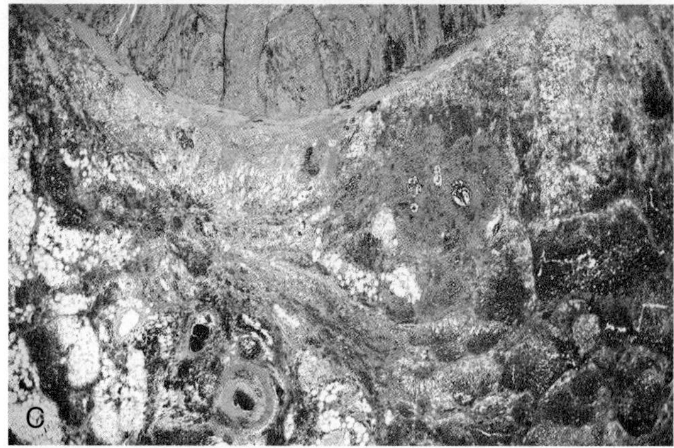

FIGURE 11.55 Acute segmental mesenteric venous obstruction caused by prolonged external compression by a tight seat belt. A, Intense transmural hemorrhage with expansion of the submucosa. **B,** Engorged vein with erythrocyte extravasation through the vein wall. **C,** Engorged blood vessels and hemorrhage in the subserosa.

forms are present together in the same pathological specimen.[103] Saraga et al. included IMHMV within the spectrum of enterocolic phlebitis,[103] but it is considered separately in this chapter, primarily because it occurs predominantly in the left colon, whereas enterocolic phlebitis occurs typically in the right colon and terminal ileum. In addition, the age and sex distributions of patients with these entities differ (see Table 11.9). Furthermore, whereas foci of IMHMV may be seen in association with enterocolic phlebitis and other unrelated forms of intestinal injury, most clinically evident cases of clinical IMHMV show no evidence of enterocolic phlebitis.[102]

The older term *mesenteric inflammatory veno-occlusive disease* (MIVOD) has been largely abandoned. It was originally used to describe seven cases, of which four were lymphocytic phlebitis, two necrotizing phlebitis, and one mixed lymphocytic and granulomatous phlebitis. Three of the seven cases also had foci of IMHMV.[104]

Similar to IMHMV, enterocolic phlebitis is a localized process rather than a systemic disease. Resection of the affected segment of the intestinal tract is considered curative. Patients with lymphocytic phlebitis are typically elderly and present with abdominal pain caused by ischemia of the right colon or terminal ileum, or with a right-sided abdominal mass caused by cecal edema or intussusception.[103,105-107] An association with hypertension, cardiovascular disease, drugs (such as flutamide), tumors, renal insufficiency, and lymphocytic colitis has been described.[72]

The ischemic features of enterocolic phlebitis are typical of mesenteric venous obstruction, showing engorgement of the veins of the bowel wall, mural hemorrhage, edema, and mucosal necrosis (Fig. 11.60A). Histologically, the lymphocytic phlebitis form of enterocolic phlebitis is characterized by a diffuse infiltrate of small lymphocytes within the walls of intramural veins, which also forms dense perivenular cuffs (Fig. 11.60B,C). The lymphocyte cuffs are typically circumferential. However, in tissue sections distant from areas of ischemia, a crescentic pattern of inflammation may be seen.[108] The inflammatory infiltrate is composed of CD3+ CD8+ T cells, some of which have cytotoxic characteristics, admixed with smaller numbers of B cells. Some affected veins may be thrombosed. There is sparing of accompanying arteries.

In enterocolic phlebitis, areas of necrotizing phlebitis (in which the mural infiltrate is composed mainly of neutrophils and is associated with fibrinoid necrosis of the vessel walls) and thrombosis are usually found underlying or adjacent to areas of mucosal necrosis. Granulomatous phlebitis, in which the mural infiltrate contains histiocytes and giant cells associated with damage to the walls of veins

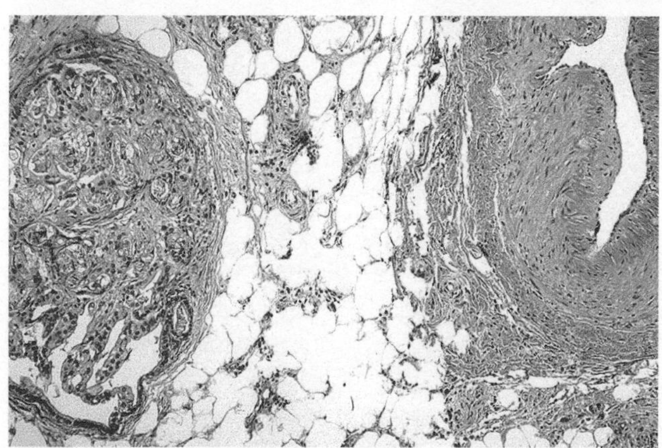

FIGURE 11.56 Occlusion of mesenteric vein by metastatic adenocarcinoma. The paired artery, on the right, is unaffected.

(Fig. 11.60D,E), may also be seen focally.[109] Enterocolic phlebitis has also been reported in association with lymphocytic enteritis and colitis.[107,110] A single report of gastroduodenal lymphocytic phlebitis illustrates that this pattern of inflammatory vasculopathy may not be restricted to the distal small bowel and colon.[90]

The diagnosis can be made on resection specimens only because mucosal biopsies usually only reveal nonspecific features of ischemic-type injury. The lack of arterial involvement, a lymphocytic-rich infiltrate (not neutrophilic or eosinophilic), and its typical segmental nature distinguish these entities from other types of vasculitis that affect the GI tract, such as IgA vasculitis, panarteritis nodosa, eosinophilic granulomatosis with polyangiitis, systemic lupus erythematosus, and Behcet's syndrome.[111]

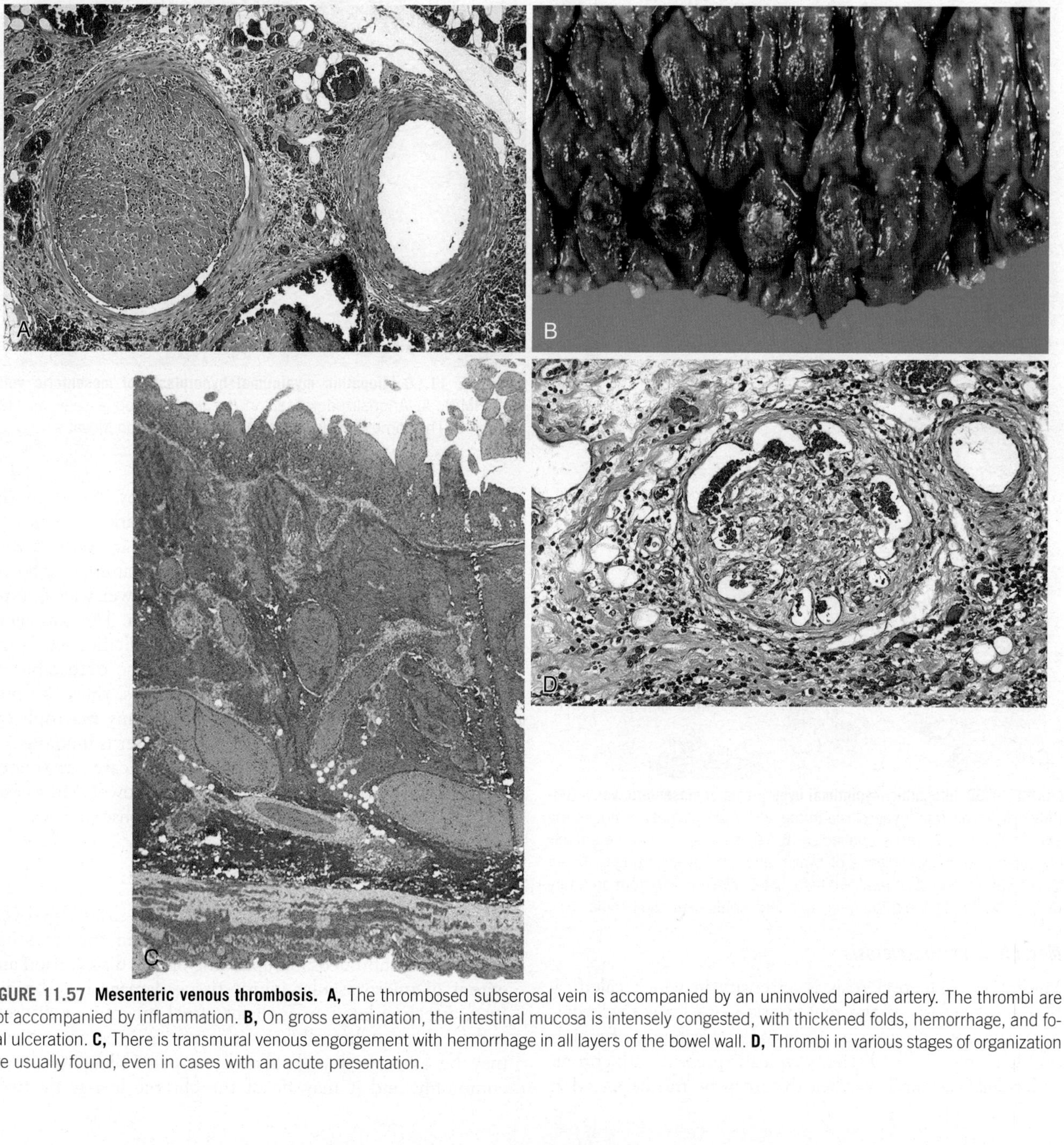

FIGURE 11.57 Mesenteric venous thrombosis. A, The thrombosed subserosal vein is accompanied by an uninvolved paired artery. The thrombi are not accompanied by inflammation. **B,** On gross examination, the intestinal mucosa is intensely congested, with thickened folds, hemorrhage, and focal ulceration. **C,** There is transmural venous engorgement with hemorrhage in all layers of the bowel wall. **D,** Thrombi in various stages of organization are usually found, even in cases with an acute presentation.

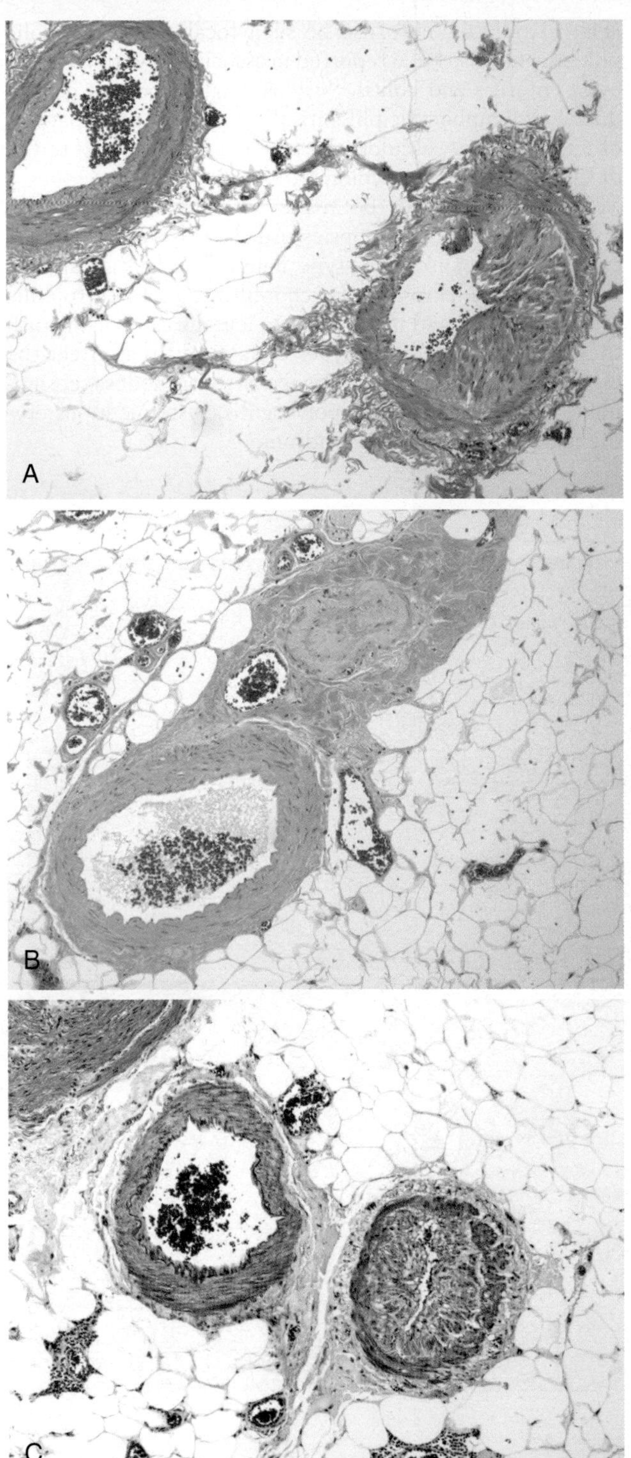

FIGURE 11.58 Idiopathic myointimal hyperplasia of mesenteric veins (IMHMV). A, Myointimal hyperplasia in the vein *(right)* almost occludes the lumen. The artery *(left)* is unaffected. **B,** Veins (superior) can be entirely occluded and show evidence of hyalinization in advance stages. **C,** An elastic Van Gieson stain readily differentiates a vein *(right)* from an artery *(left)* in IMHMV by the absence of an arterial internal elastic lamina.

Mesenteric Phlebosclerosis

Mesenteric phlebosclerosis is an entity in which calcification and sclerosis of the mesenteric veins leads to chronic nonthrombotic progressive occlusion and ischemia of mainly the right colon.[112-114] Patients typically present with chronic abdominal pain and diarrhea that may be misdiagnosed as

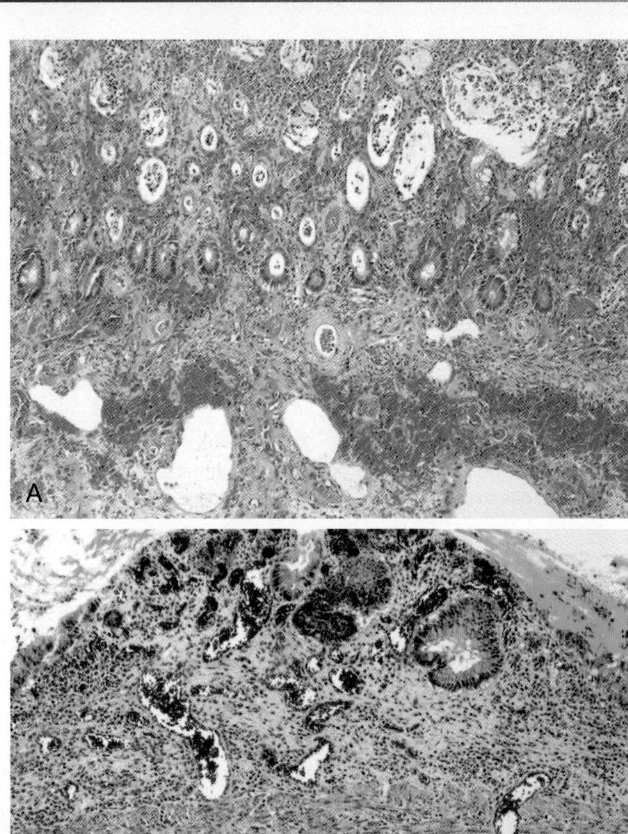

FIGURE 11.59 Idiopathic myointimal hyperplasia of mesenteric veins (IMHMV). A, Arterialized vessels in the lamina propria seen on H&E stain. **B,** The same vessels can be also highlighted on Movat stain.

inflammatory bowel disease. At endoscopy, however, the colonic mucosa appears edematous and dark, with prominent blue-black vessels and shallow ulcers, in contrast with the appearance of the colonic mucosa in inflammatory bowel disease.[115] In resection specimens, the bowel wall is typically fibrotic, causing stenosis of the lumen. The pathognomonic histological feature is sclerosis and calcification of the mesenteric veins (Fig. 11.61), which is also detectable on plain abdominal radiographs. In some cases, there is fibrosis of the mucosa and submucosa with foamy macrophages within the wall. The etiology of this disorder is unknown. It has been primarily reported in Asians. Most cases are treated by resection of the affected region of the bowel. Most cases do not show recurrence or other adverse consequences.

Microvascular Insufficiency

Several disease processes may affect small-sized blood vessels (arterioles, capillaries, and venules) in the intestinal mucosa and submucosa. Depending on the distribution and extent of microvascular injury, tissue damage may be diffuse, affecting large areas of intestinal mucosa, or discrete and localized. Clinically, tissue injury may be silent, or it may be associated with abdominal pain. Bleeding occurs commonly, and it may be of the chronic low-grade type,

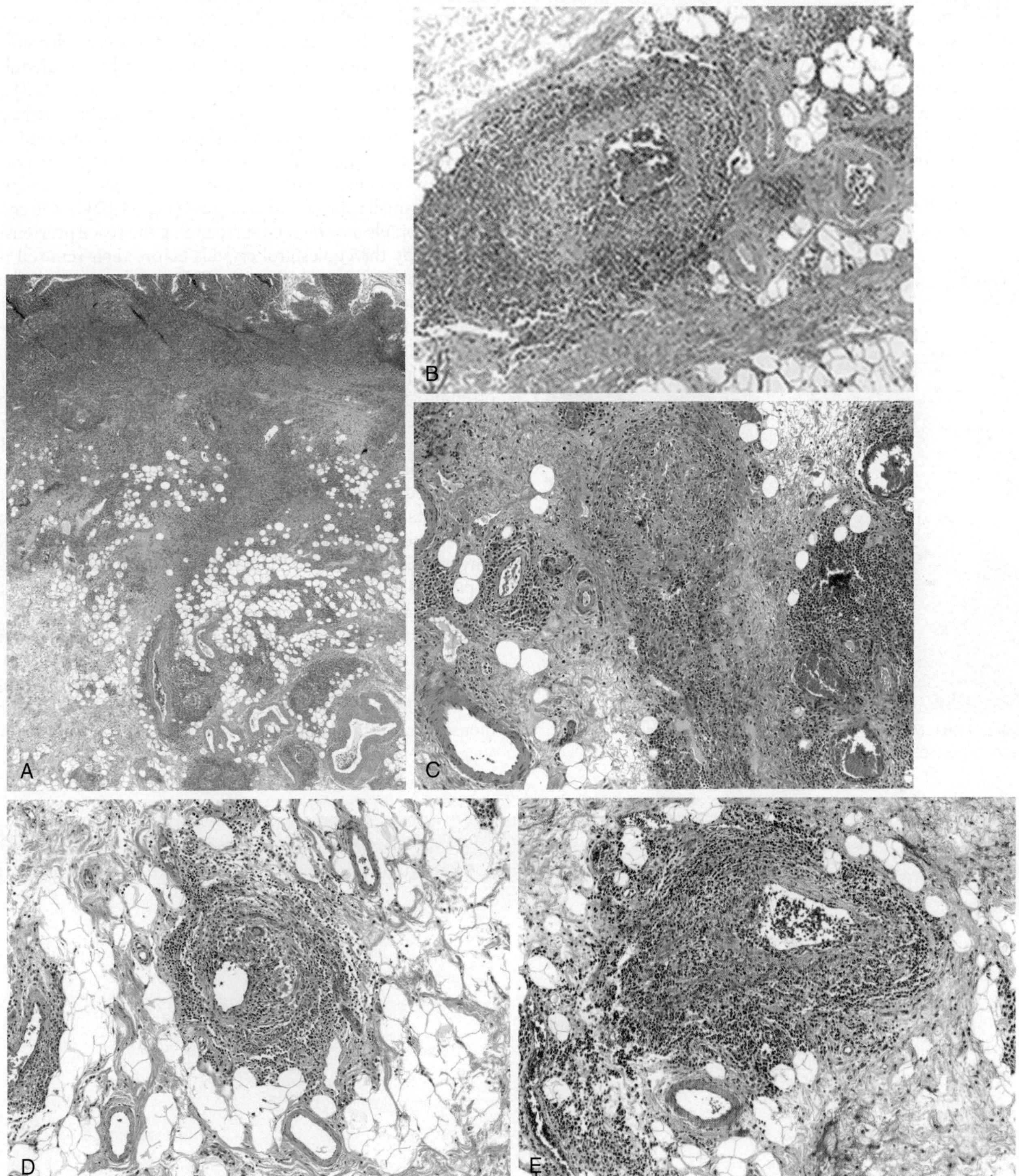

FIGURE 11.60 Enterocolic phlebitis. A, Low-power magnification of an intestine segment with prominent lymphocytic infiltrate centered around the veins. **B,** Submucosal vein with dense lymphocytic infiltrate and perivascular cuffing. **C,** Granulomatous phlebitis with destruction of the wall. **D,** Occasional multinucleated giant cells can be seen. **E,** Movat stain helps differentiate the involved vein from the adjacent spared artery.

leading to anemia. If the process is widespread, there may be extensive mucosal injury and loss, resulting in the development of an acute abdomen clinically.

Common causes of microvascular insufficiency are listed in Table 11.10. In many cases, the pathological features are diagnostic. Capillary lesions, such as thrombi associated with disseminated intravascular coagulation, or thrombotic thrombocytopenic purpura, erythrocyte blockage in sickle cell disease (Fig. 11.62), and ectatic capillaries associated with chronic irradiation injury, may be detected in mucosal biopsies. In contrast, leukocytoclastic vasculitis of IgA vasculitis, as well as angiopathies associated with diabetes mellitus and amyloidosis, may not be evident in the mucosa and are more easily diagnosed in specimens that contain submucosal tissue. Atheromicroemboli may be seen in mucosal biopsies, but they are usually more numerous and more easily detected in the submucosa.

If the mucosal capillaries are obstructed (as in disseminated intravascular coagulation, thrombotic thrombocytopenic purpura, and sickle cell disease), foci of mucosal ischemia, lamina propria hemorrhage, and superficial erosions may be present. If extensive, they may lead to the development of large areas of mucosal necrosis.

Obstruction of arterioles by atheromicroemboli may be extensive, yet without obvious signs of mucosal injury because of the well-developed collateral circulation of the intestinal mucosa. When atheroembolic obstruction of submucosal vessels is sufficient to cause localized mucosal ischemia, punched-out areas of shallow mucosal ulceration may develop, with sharply defined edges and a flat granulation tissue base at the level of the muscularis mucosae (Fig. 11.63A,B). If sufficient tissue sections of the ulcer have been obtained, atheromicroemboli can usually be recognized by the presence of sharp-edged, cigar-shaped spaces surrounded by a few occluding inflammatory cells in the obstructed lumina of small submucosal arterioles (Fig. 11.63C). Often, a few eosinophils may be seen surrounding the space previously occupied by the cholesterol crystals before their removal by histological processing (Fig. 11.63D). Atheromicroembolism frequently results from instrumentation of the aorta in patients with severe atherosclerosis.[88,89]

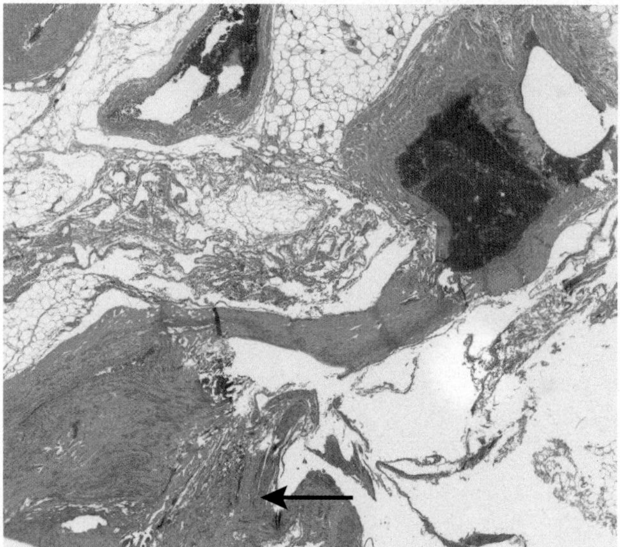

FIGURE 11.61 Mesenteric phlebosclerosis demonstrating a tortuous hyalinized vessel wall with scant calcifications *(arrow)*.

Stenosis of submucosal arterioles as a result of deposition of abnormal products in the vessel walls tends to cause chronic, often progressive, ischemia. However, when this condition is exacerbated by an episode of central hypotension, at which time the systolic pressure is insufficient to irrigate the already compromised intestinal vascular bed, the clinical presentation is frequently acute. Insudation of glycosylation products in patients with diabetes mellitus, deposition of amyloid proteins in the walls of small submucosal vessels in patients with amyloidosis[116] (Fig. 11.64), and progressive vascular fibrosis in patients with chronic radiation injury may all compromise the vascular supply to the mucosa in this manner.

In Behçet's disease, which is a type of vasculitis that affects mainly larger-sized blood vessels, arterioles and venules may also be involved. Because arterioles and venules are most likely to be sampled in mucosal and submucosal biopsies, a diagnosis of intestinal Behçet's disease may be suggested in mucosal biopsy specimens.

TABLE 11.10 Microvascular Causes of Intestinal Ischemia

Causes	Presentation	Main Vessels Affected	Pathological Characteristics	Distribution of Injury
Disseminated intravascular coagulation	Acute	Capillaries	Thrombi	Widespread
Thrombotic thrombocytopenic purpura	Acute	Capillaries	Platelet thrombi	Widespread
Sickle cell disease	Acute, recurrent	Capillaries, venules	Sickle cell blockage	Widespread
IgA vasculitis (Henoch-Schönlein purpura)	Acute	Arterioles, venules	Leukocytoclastic vasculitis, immunoglobulin A deposits	Widespread
Behçet's disease	Acute, recurrent	Arterioles, venules	Vasculitis	Widespread
Diabetes mellitus	Chronic	Arterioles, capillaries	Glycosylation product deposits in walls and basement membranes	Widespread
Amyloidosis	Chronic	Arterioles	Amyloid deposits in walls	Widespread
Chronic radiation injury	Chronic	Arterioles, capillaries	Subendothelial fibrosis, gaping capillaries, hyalinized vessels, and foam cell arteriopathy	Localized
Yttrium microspheres from selective internal radiation therapy	Acute	Arterioles, capillaries	Glass microspheres 15 to 35 mm in diameter eliciting fibrosis, giant cell reaction, erosion, or ulcer	Localized
Atheromicroemboli	Acute	Arterioles	Acicular clefts in obstructed vessels	Localized
Cytomegalovirus infection	Acute	Capillaries	Viral inclusions in endothelial cells at ulcer base	Localized

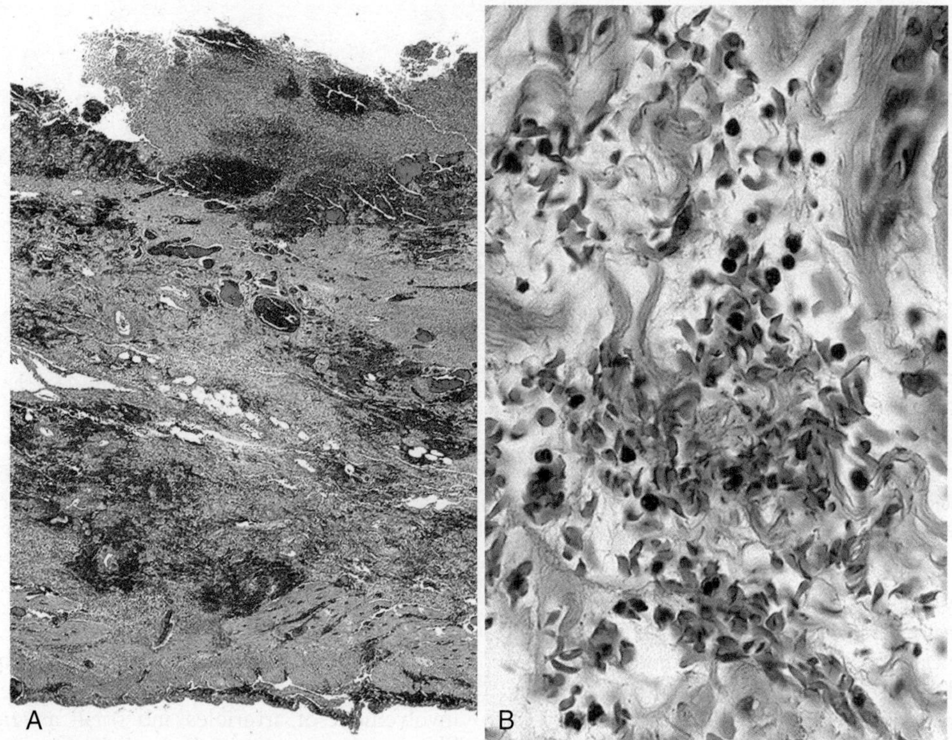

FIGURE 11.62 Sickle cell disease. A, Capillary congestion and hemorrhage are present in all layers of the bowel wall along with ischemic mucosal necrosis. **B,** Intravascular and extravasated sickle cells can be identified on high-power examination.

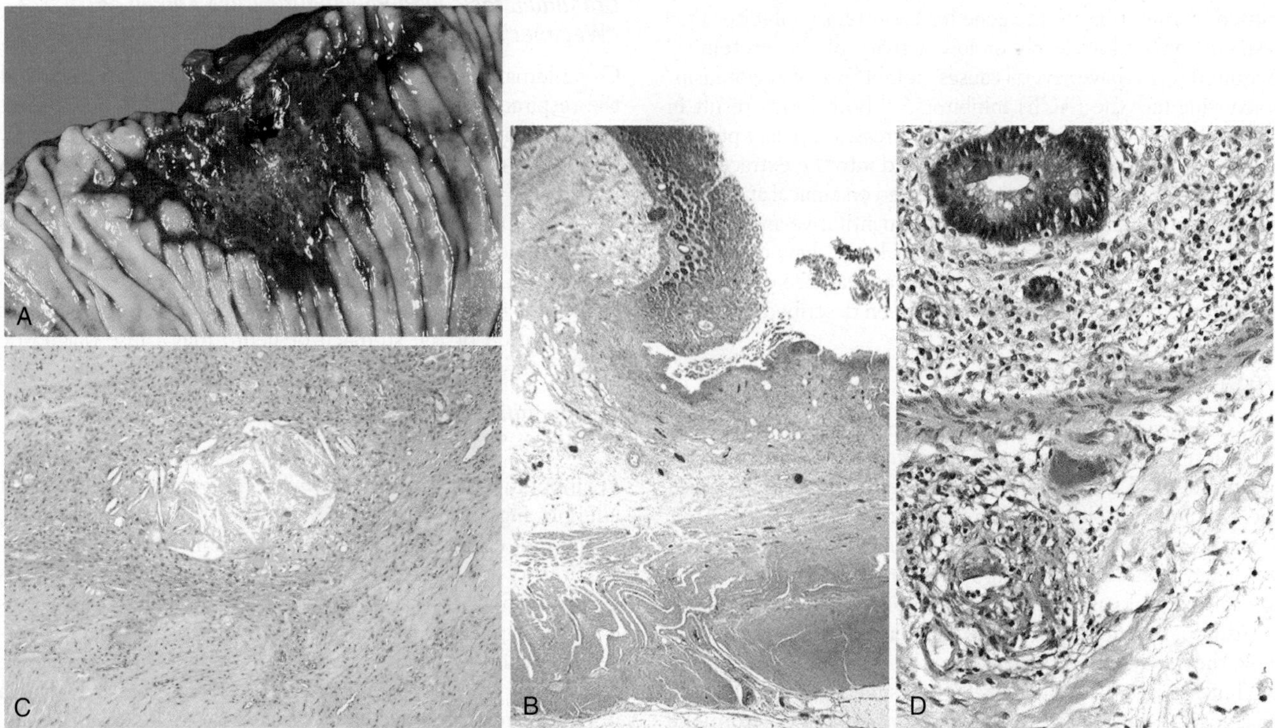

FIGURE 11.63 Ulceration caused by submucosal atheroemboli. A, The ulcers typically have sharply defined edges and a flat base of granulation tissue at the level of the muscularis mucosae. **B,** The deeper layers of the bowel wall are often unaffected. **C,** Obstructed vessels are located in the submucosa and can be identified by the presence of intravascular, cigar-shaped clefts surrounded by an inflammatory infiltrate. **D,** Eosinophils are often present at the edges of the clefts formed by removal of the cholesterol crystals during histological processing.

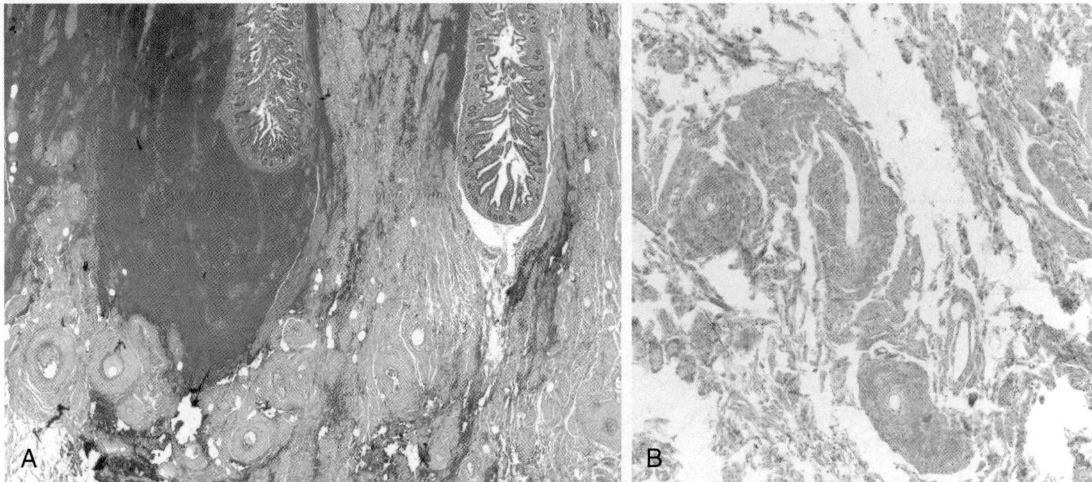

FIGURE 11.64 Amyloidosis. A, Deposits of AA amyloid in the walls of submucosal arteries and veins leads to vascular insufficiency and chronic ischemia. **B,** The diagnosis can be confirmed by positive (orangeophilic) staining with Congo red (as illustrated here) or by immunohistochemistry.

Another entity that falls within the realm of microvascular insufficiency is angioedema of the intestines.[117] In this condition, patients typically present with one or more episodes of otherwise unexplained severe, cramping abdominal pain that may last for several days, and radiological studies show reversible segmental edema of the small or large intestine without evidence of arterial compromise.[118] Although it may be confined to the intestines initially, angioedema commonly involves other organs, including the skin of the mouth and face and the upper respiratory tract. Hereditary forms are commonly caused by mutations in the gene for C1 esterase inhibitor that result in either low levels or low activity of the protein.[119] Acquired forms have several causes, notably use of angiotensin-converting enzyme (ACE) inhibitors.[120] Both forms result in elevated levels of bradykinin, which increases capillary permeability with leakage of intravascular fluid into the extracellular space. The diagnosis is usually established on clinical and radiological grounds and is correlated with quantitative and qualitative evaluation of C1 esterase inhibitor levels. Few cases have been biopsied, thus the morphological appearance of affected areas of the colonic mucosa have not been described.

VASCULITIDES

The classification of vasculitides, many of which affect the GI tract, is controversial and regarded by some as having limited clinical utility.[121-124] Of the several schemes in use, the Chapel Hill classification is the one used here,[123] but with the addition of Behçet's disease and Buerger's disease. The classification scheme and the particular characteristics of each type of vasculitis are summarized in Table 11.11.

Although many types of vasculitis affect the GI tract and liver, they are usually diagnosed on the basis of a combination of clinical features, radiological studies, and serological tests. Diagnostic biopsies are most commonly obtained from the skin or kidney. Small-vessel vasculitis, encountered in mucosal biopsies of the GI tract, and medium-vessel vasculitis, found in specimens resected for intestinal ischemia, should always elicit a more extensive search for possible systemic involvement. The current classifications are devoted solely to primary vasculitis. However, infection, myeloproliferative disorders, and other malignancies are among the other disease associations that should be excluded in this setting.

Small-Vessel Disease

Small-vessel vasculitides are characterized by necrotizing or leukocytoclastic injury to capillaries and venules, with less involvement of arterioles and small arteries. Larger-sized blood vessels are not affected. These disorders fall into two main groups, separated by the presence or absence of immune globulin deposition and antineutrophil cytoplasmic antibodies (ANCAs).

Granulomatosis with Polyangiitis (also known as "Wegener's Granulomatosis")

Granulomatosis with polyangiitis is a granulomatous disease of the respiratory tract that is often accompanied by nasal sinus and renal involvement. It is associated with a paucity of immunoglobulin deposition. Ninety percent of patients are ANCA positive. In addition to the presence of characteristic destructive granulomas, necrotizing small-vessel vasculitis (Fig. 11.65 A,B) is typically present. Granulomatosis with polyangiitis may affect the GI tract, particularly the mesenteric arteries, which can lead to ischemic injury to the intestines.[127] Granulomatous inflammation of the stomach or ileum may cause diagnostic confusion with Crohn's disease.[128]

Eosinophilic Granulomatosis with Polyangiitis (also known as "Churg-Strauss Syndrome")

Eosinophilic granulomatosis with polyangiitis a form of allergic angiitis characterized by the presence of asthma, peripheral eosinophilia, granulomatous inflammation of the respiratory tract, and eosinophil-rich necrotizing vasculitis (Fig. 11.66) that usually responds to steroid therapy. It is an ANCA-positive vasculitis that involves small-sized arteries and veins. Approximately 50% of patients experience abdominal pain and bleeding from GI ischemia, which is a poor prognostic factor.[129]

Examination of pathology specimens may reveal a necrotizing form of granulomatous vasculitis with giant cells and eosinophilia (Fig. 11.67A,B).[124]

Immunoglobulin A (IgA) Vasculitis (also known as "Henoch-Schönlein Purpura")

In immunoglobulin A (IgA) vasculitis, IgA-predominant immune complexes are deposited within small-sized blood

TABLE 11.11 Primary Vasculitides of the Gastrointestinal Tract

Vessel Size	Disorder	Clinical Characteristics, Etiology, and Comments	Key Histological Features
Medium		Affects celiac, mesenteric, and hepatic arteries; no glomerulitis or pulmonary capillaritis	Necrotizing arteritis
	PAN	Often associated with hepatitis B	Transmural fibrinoid necrosis; early neutrophil infiltrate, later monocytes, macrophages, lymphocytes; pseudoaneurysms
	Kawasaki's disease	Febrile disease of children <5years of age; often involves coronaries; mucocutaneous lymph node syndrome	Less fibrinoid necrosis, more mural edema than PAN; infiltrate of monocytes, macrophages, lymphocytes
Small		Affects capillaries and venules; variable involvement of arterioles; no larger-vessel involvement	Necrotizing or leukocytoclastic vasculitis
	Granulomatosis with polyangiitis (Wegener's granulomatosis)	Granulomatous inflammation of respiratory tract; necrotizing glomerulonephritis often present; 90% ANCA positive	Necrotizing vasculitis
	Eosinophilic granulomatosis with polyangiitis (Churg-Strauss syndrome)	Associated with asthma and peripheral eosinophilia; eosinophil-rich and granulomatous inflammation of respiratory tract; commonly ANCA positive	Eosinophil-rich necrotizing vasculitis
	IgA vasculitis (Henoch-Schönlein purpura)	IgA deposits in small vessels; involves skin, gut, glomeruli; arthralgias or arthritis; ANCA negative	Leukocytoclastic angiitis
	Cryoglobulinemic vasculitis	Cryoglobulinemia with deposits in small vessels; skin and glomeruli involved; associated with hepatitis C and hypocomplementemia; ANCA negative	Leukocytoclastic angiitis
	Lupus, rheumatoid, and other immune complex vasculitides	Immune complex deposits in small vessels; ANCA negative	Necrotizing vasculitis
Unclassified			
	Behçet's disease	Onset in twenties or thirties; oral and genital ulceration, ocular inflammation, arthritis	Neutrophil or lymphocyte infiltrate of small veins and arteries; ulcers, transmural inflammation, strictures; may mimic Crohn's disease
	Buerger's disease	Affects tobacco users, most male and <45years of age; generally affects arteries to extremities; GI involvement rare; immune deposits not detected; ANCA negative	Occlusive inflammatory thrombi with neutrophils, microabscesses, giant cells in medium-sized arteries and veins; progressive organization of thrombi; vessel wall and elastic lamina remain intact
	Kohlmeier-Degos disease	Affects all sexes and all ages; systemic manifestations preceded by erythematosus, red or pink papules, mainly on trunk, arms, and legs	Occlusive noninflammatory arteriopathy with intimal hyperplasia, endothelial cell proliferation, and progressive sclerosis with consequent zonal tissue infarction

ANCA, *Antineutrophil cytoplasmic antibodies; GI, gastrointestinal;* IgA, *immunoglobulin A;* PAN, *polyarteritis nodosa.*
Modified from Jennette JC, Falk RJ. The role of pathology in the diagnosis of systemic vasculitis. Clin Exp Rheumatol. *2007;25(1 Suppl 44):S52-S56.*

vessels that exhibit leukocytoclastic angiitis. The process affects small vessels of the skin, kidneys, and joints. In 75% to 85% of cases, the GI tract is involved.[72] Children and young adults are most often affected. The condition usually develops after an upper respiratory tract infection. GI involvement results in ischemia with abdominal pain, bleeding, and intramural hemorrhage, which is the GI counterpart of the palpable purpura commonly observed in skin.[130] Histological features include fibrinoid necrosis of the vessel walls with leukocytoclastic vasculitis, neutrophilic and mononuclear infiltrates, and fibrin thrombi. IgA deposition in the blood vessel basement membrane can be demonstrated by immunofluorescence. Serological tests for ANCA are typically negative. In general, the disease follows a benign clinical course and is self-limited, but complications such as perforation, strictures, and intussusception can occur.

Leukocytoclastic Vasculitis

Although the term *leukocytoclastic vasculitis* is sometimes used to describe a specific disease entity, it simply refers to a pattern of small-vessel inflammation characterized by leukocyte fragmentation and fibrinoid necrosis of arterioles, capillaries, and venules (Fig. 11.68). This pattern of injury may be seen in a variety of vasculitides. The term is also

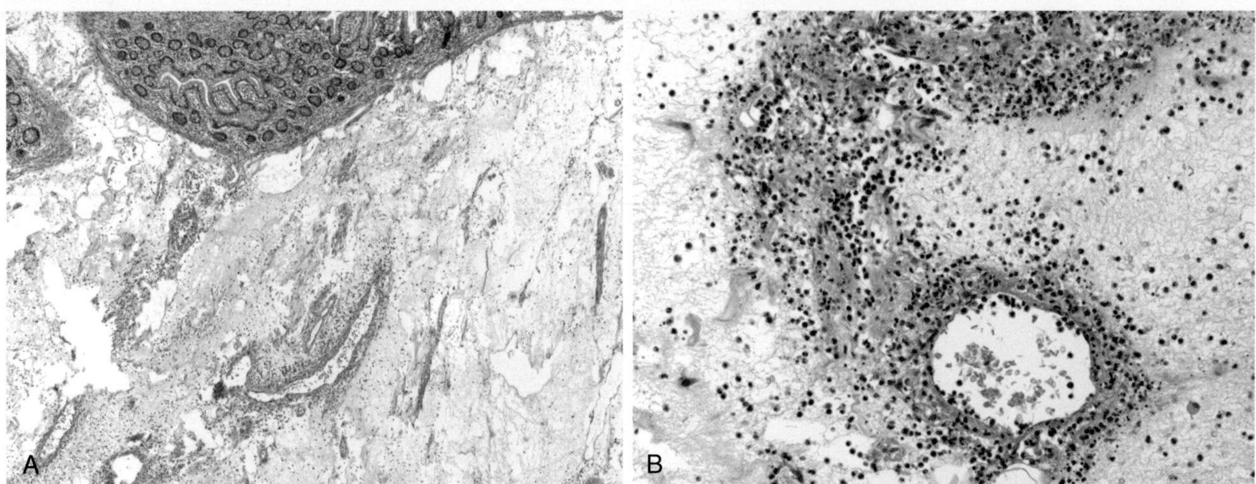

FIGURE 11.65 Granulomatosis with polyangiitis (Wegener's granulomatosis). A, There is necrotizing vasculitis with narrowing of the vascular lumen involving a segment of small bowel. **B,** At higher magnification, there is necrotizing vasculitis with vague histiocytic infiltrate.

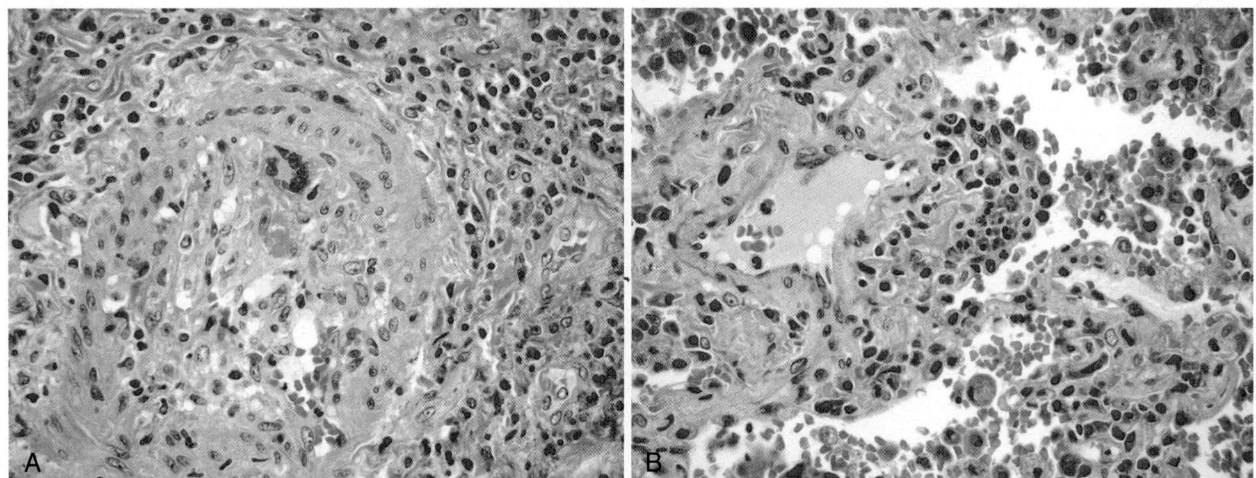

FIGURE 11.66 Eosinophilic granulomatosis with polyangiitis (Churg-Strauss syndrome). A, An infiltrate of mononuclear cells, giant cells, and scattered eosinophils involves a small vessel within which there is focal fibrin thrombosis. **B,** Eosinophil-rich vasculitis characteristic of Churg-Strauss syndrome in a pulmonary biopsy specimen. (*Courtesy of Dr. Robert Homer, Yale University School of Medicine, New Haven, CT.*)

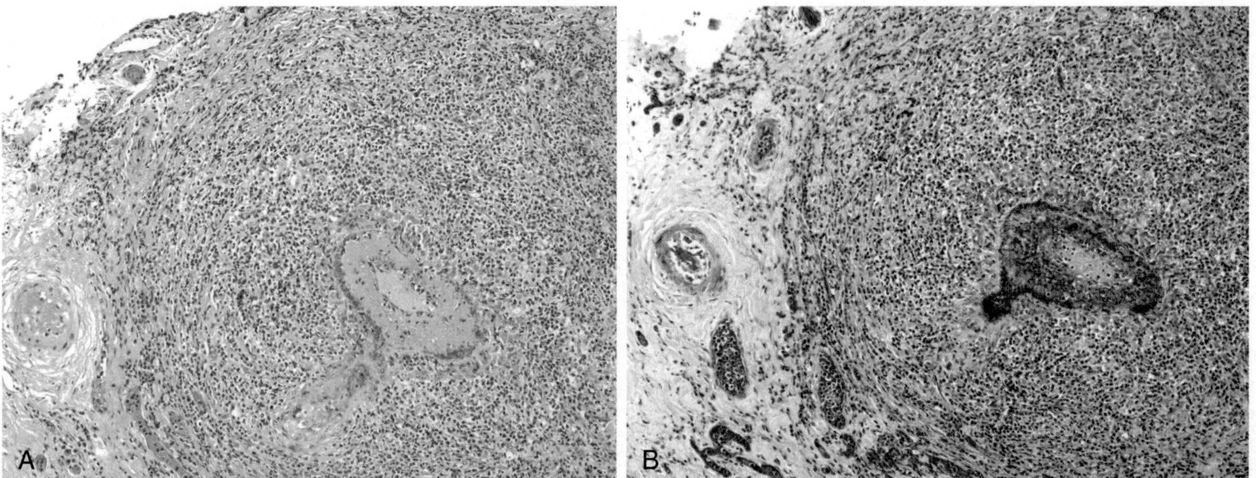

FIGURE 11.67 Churg-Strauss syndrome in the gastrointestinal tract. A, Dense inflammatory infiltrates rich in eosinophils damage small vessels. **B,** Movat stain highlights the vessel wall, many times obscured by the inflammatory infiltrate.

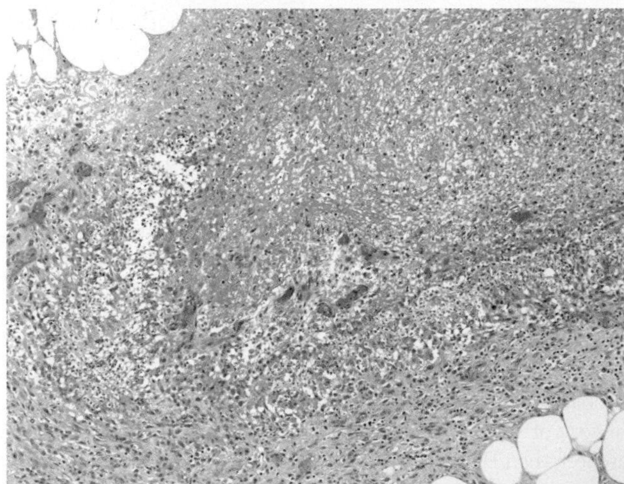

FIGURE 11.68 Leukocytoclastic vasculitis. Well-developed leukocytoclastic vasculitis with mixed inflammatory infiltrate in the vessel wall. (*Courtesy of Dr. Robert Homer, Yale University School of Medicine, New Haven, CT.*)

occasionally used synonymously with *hypersensitivity vasculitis,* which is a disorder of adults associated with skin rash and leukocytoclastic vasculitis. GI involvement in these cases is usually mild and self-limited.[131] Hypersensitivity vasculitis bears morphological similarity to immunoglobulin A vasculitis (Henoch-Schönlein purpura); however, there is some evidence that they are, in fact, two distinct entities.[132]

Cryoglobulinemic Vasculitis

Cryoglobulinemic vasculitis refers to a type of small-vessel immune complex vasculitis that occurs in patients with hepatitis C and cryoglobulinemia. The skin and kidneys are more commonly involved than the intestines, but intestinal ischemic injury has occasionally been reported.[133] Some cases present with ulcers and strictures resembling inflammatory bowel disease. Histological sections show a leukocytoclastic vasculitis with associated thrombi and deposition of IgG, IgM, and complement by immunofluorescence.[72]

Systemic Lupus Erythematosus and Other Immune Complex Diseases

Approximately 50% of patients with SLE show GI involvement by small-vessel immune complex vasculitis. The clinical manifestations are variable. Patients may experience nausea, vomiting, abdominal pain, diarrhea, malabsorption, pancreatitis, protein-losing enteropathy, and segmental ischemic necrosis of the intestines.[134] GI involvement is present in only approximately 10% of patients with rheumatoid arthritis. Symptoms include abdominal pain, nausea, and vomiting. Ischemic injury may lead to bowel necrosis and perforation.[135] Resection specimens may show small-vessel (arteries and veins) necrotizing vasculitis with fibrinoid necrosis, hemorrhage and edema in the mucosa, submucosa, and bowel wall as well as varying degrees of tissue necrosis (Fig. 11.69A–C). C3 complement deposition can be seen on immunofluorescence.[124]

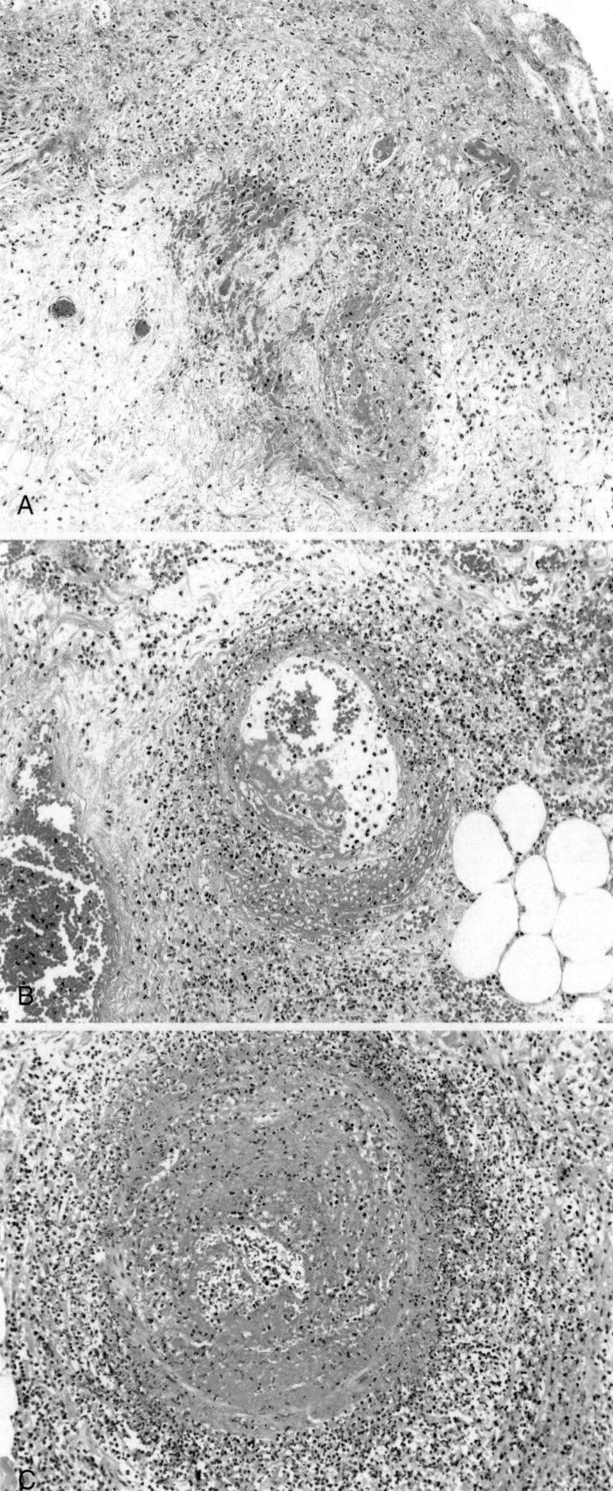

FIGURE 11.69 Systemic lupus erythematosus. A, There is transmural necrosis with neutrophilic inflammation and fibrin thrombi in small blood vessels (leukocytoclastic vasculitis). **B–C,** Fragmented and intact neutrophils infiltrate the vessel wall with fibrinoid medial necrosis and thrombosis. (**C,** *Courtesy of Dr. Michael Kashgarian, Yale University School of Medicine, New Haven, CT.*)

Behçet's Disease

Behçet's disease, which is a vasculitis of unknown etiology, is linked to the presence of human leukocyte antigen (HLA) B51. It is most common in countries situated along the ancient Silk Road, particularly Turkey, but it also occurs elsewhere, especially in Japan.[136] Clinical features, which usually develop in the third or fourth decade of life, are diverse and include oral and genital ulceration, retinitis and uveitis, erythema nodosum and other skin disorders, and arthritis.

GI involvement develops in 3% to 26% of patients and is most common in the terminal ileum and right colon, where it may mimic Crohn's disease or ulcerative colitis (Fig. 11.70).[137] In resection specimens, small-vessel lymphocytic phlebitis, either with or without arteritis, is present in the submucosa, often associated with ulceration. Some authors have proposed that the disease affects the vasa vasorum. Granulomas are not normally part of the histological spectrum of findings in this entity. Ulcers have been reported to be associated with lymphoid follicles and Peyer's patches[138] (aphthous lesions); although small, they have a tendency to penetrate deeply within the bowel wall and cause perforation. Large-sized blood vessels are less commonly involved than small ones, and their involvement may lead to ischemia or infarction. The vascular inflammation in the GI tract may be predominantly lymphocytic[139] or predominantly neutrophilic,[140] possibly reflecting different stages of the disease or a response to immunosuppressive therapy.

GI involvement in Behçet's disease often necessitates resection of the affected segment of bowel. However, disease recurrence is common, and further intervention is required in approximately 50% of cases. The differential diagnosis of GI Behçet's disease includes Crohn's disease, ulcerative colitis, and chronic ischemic enterocolitis, but the diagnosis is usually made on the basis of both clinical and the serological features (Table 11.12).

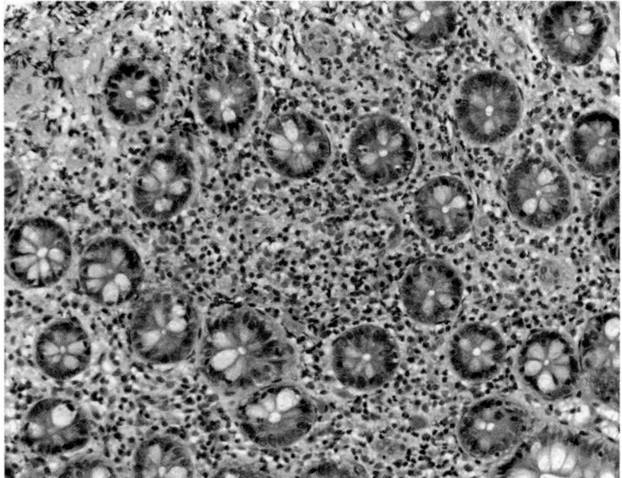

FIGURE 11.70 Behcet's disease showing focal active colitis and focal crypt dropout in the terminal ileum, mimicking Crohn's disease.

In 2009 Cheon et al. proposed an algorithm to distinguish Behçet's disease from Crohn's disease. The basis of the algorithm lies in categorizing the typical (not pathognomonic) Behçet's ulcer as fewer than five oval, deep, discrete ileocecal ulcers.[141] With this definition, patients were classified as "definite Behçet's disease" if they had concurrent systemic Behçet's disease, "probable intestinal Behçet's disease" if they had an oral ulcer only, or "suspected Behçet's disease" if they had neither systemic Behçet's disease nor an oral ulcer. All other ulcers were considered atypical and nondiagnostic in the absence of systemic Behçet's disease, although they were categorized as probable intestinal Behçet's disease if there was a concurrent history of systemic Behçet's disease. This algorithm produced greater than 95% sensitivity and greater than 80% specificity in detecting definite, probable, or suspected Behçet's disease. Although the algorithm has not been validated by others, there appears to be some value in the recognition that Behçet's disease is most often associated with well-defined, discrete, oval, deep ulcers that usually number less than five.

Interestingly, a lymphocytic form of arteritis has been described in patients with Crohn's disease. As opposed to Behçet's disease, arteries, not veins, in the areas of mural inflammation are involved, and granulomas can be seen in up to one-third of cases.

Buerger's Disease

Buerger's disease, also termed *thromboangiitis obliterans,* is a vasculitic disorder that affects mainly men younger than 50 years of age who have a long history of heavy cigarette smoking. The disorder results in impairment of the vascular supply to the lower extremities, which causes claudication and rubor, but occasionally the small mesenteric vessels are involved with acute inflammation and thrombosis, resulting in intestinal ischemia.[142] The thrombi tend to be inflammatory, but the vessel walls usually escape the effects of severe injury. Typically, the internal elastic lamina remains intact, but some patients may show intimal thickening and fibrosis.

Malignant Atrophic Papulosis (Kohlmeier-Degos Disease)

Malignant atrophic papulosis is a rare type of occlusive arteriopathy that occurs in patients of any age and affects both sexes.

TABLE 11.12 Differential Diagnosis Between Behçet's Disease and Crohn's Disease

	Behçet's Disease	Crohn's Disease
Clinical features	Predominantly in male; onset 20-40 years of age Recurrent oral ulcers Uveitis (common) Skin disease (common) Arthritis (common)	Predominantly in male, onset 15-29 years of age Abdominal pain, bloody diarrhea, weight loss, upper gastrointestinal tract Uveitis (uncommon) Arthritis (uncommon)
Pathology findings Macroscopy Microscopy	Ileocecal involvement (common) Colonic disease (less common) Perianal disease (uncommon) Perforation (more common) Stricture/fistula/abscess (less common) Round, deep ulcers Small vessels lymphocytic (or neutrophilic) phlebitis, with or without arteritis No granulomas	Ileocecal involvement (common) Colonic disease (common) Perianal disease (common) Perforation (less common) Stricture/fistula/abscess (common) Longitudinal ulcer in a cobblestone mucosa Can have lymphocytic arteritis rarely Granulomas in up to one-third of cases

The epidemiology of this disorder is unclear. However, familial clustering has been reported, with a young male predisposition.[143] Atrophic papulosis may exist as a purely cutaneous benign form or as a systemic "malignant" form that affects the GI tract and central nervous system. Cutaneous red or pink papules are typically found on the trunk, arms, and legs, and these commonly precede systemic manifestations. Patients may also present with abdominal pain and features of peritonitis or with manifestations of central nervous system involvement.[144] Endoscopic findings include infarcts and ulcers.

Malignant atrophic papulosis may involve any region of the GI tract. However, the small bowel is most commonly involved. Lesions are characterized by progressive sclerosis of small and medium-sized arteries with zonal tissue infarction. Serosal white plaques with red borders may be seen grossly.[145] Characteristic histological features include intimal hypercellularity with endothelial cell proliferation of small and medium-sized submucosal arteries and superimposed arterial thrombosis, but typically with only minimal or no inflammation. Vascular changes are associated with progressive intestinal necrosis, which may be full-thickness. GI manifestations may be similar to other types of vasculitis, particularly SLE, a disease of which malignant atrophic papulosis has been considered a variant.[145]

In patients with systemic involvement, the most common cause of death is intestinal perforation and peritonitis as a consequence of infarction.[145] Enterocutaneous fistulas have also been reported. In addition to surgical management, medical therapy includes anticoagulants, antiplatelet drugs, and immunosuppressive agents.

Segmental Arterial Mediolysis

Segmental arterial mediolysis (SAM) is discussed here, although it is not considered a true vasculitis. SAM is a rare lesion that was initially described in 1976 as *segmental mediolytic arteritis* and is best characterized as a noninflammatory, nonatherosclerotic arteriopathy that predominantly affects the abdominal arteries.[146] In a review of 27 patients,[147] Inada et al. supported the observations of Slavin[146] of partial or total mediolysis of large muscular arteries of the abdomen, most commonly the middle colic artery. In this review, SAM occurred in patients who ranged from 44 to 88 years of age, with a male predisposition, although cases have been reported in younger patients as well.[148] The most common presenting symptom was intraabdominal bleeding. On angiography, lesions may mimic the nodular appearance of PAN.

In addition to the middle colic artery, other involved abdominal arteries may include the gastric, gastroepiploic, inferior pancreaticoduodenal and hepatic[149] arteries. Reportedly, SAM may also affect cerebral, coronary, and pulmonary arteries.[150] Pathologically, these arteries undergo total or partial mediolysis, medial degeneration, and eventually aneurysm formation, hemorrhage, and rupture (Fig. 11.71).

Patients require surgical intervention and may worsen with immunosuppressive therapy, rendering distinction from PAN important.[151] Rarely, SAM may complicate PAN.[152]

Medium-Vessel Disease

Medium-vessel vasculitides affect the main visceral arteries, including the celiac, mesenteric, and hepatic arteries. These disorders are considered to be within the spectrum of necrotizing vasculitis.

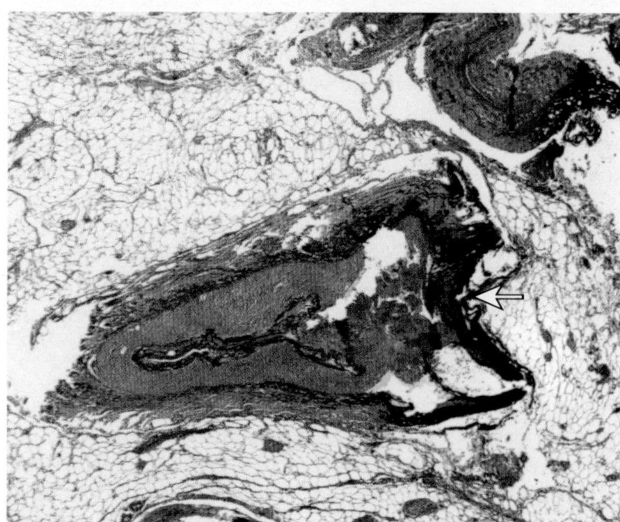

FIGURE 11.71 In segmental arterial mediolysis, the area disruption occurs as a result of mediolysis and can be highlighted in Movat stain.

Polyarteritis Nodosa

Polyarteritis nodosa occurs most frequently in middle-aged males. It has been associated with viral infections such as hepatitis B, hepatitis C, CMV, and parvovirus B19.[124] In approximately 50% of patients with polyarteritis nodosa, the celiac and mesenteric arteries are involved, and this may result in small-intestinal ischemia. The disease process less commonly affects the colon, liver, and pancreas.[125] Histologically, polyarteritis nodosa is characterized by transmural fibrinoid necrosis of arteries, accompanied by a neutrophil infiltrate in the early stages of disease and monocytes, macrophages, and lymphocytes in the later stages (see Fig. 11.46). Pseudoaneurysms are common and are responsible for the characteristic nodularity of the blood vessels, which is implied by the term *nodosa*.

Kawasaki's Disease

Kawasaki's disease usually occurs in children younger than 5 years of age and is characterized by the presence of mucocutaneous lymphadenopathy and coronary artery disease. In the fully developed disorder, patients have fever, skin rash on the palms and soles, cutaneous desquamation, strawberry tongue, and conjunctival congestion.[126] GI involvement by this disease is not rare and may manifest as abdominal pain, nausea, vomiting, diarrhea, small-bowel bleeding, and ischemic perforation. The necrotizing arteritis associated with this condition shows a predilection for the coronary arteries, which may develop aneurysms, thrombosis, or rupture. Histological sections of the GI segment involved may reveal necrotizing vasculitis with luminal ectasia and superimposed thrombosis of submucosal arteries (Fig. 11.72).

Large-Vessel Disease

Giant Cell Arteritis

Giant cell arteritis is considered a large-vessel vasculitis, but it can, rarely, affect medium-sized vessels such as the mesenteric vessels in the GI tract. Patients are usually older females who manifest cranial symptoms, and if there is involvement of mesenteric vessels, patients will also have abdominal symptoms. Some cases of GI disease are entirely asymptomatic.[72,123] The histological hallmark is a patchy granulomatous arteritis of muscular arteries. The infiltrate is lymphohistiocytic with giant cells and accompanies the other classic findings such as thickening of the intima and necrosis of the blood vessel (Fig. 11.73A). An elastic stain can help highlight the presence of internal elastic lamina disruption or duplication (Fig. 11.73B).

Localized Vasculitis of the GI Tract

In a small subset of patients, vasculitis occurs in the GI tract in patients without systemic involvement. Reports have described patients with isolated GI tract involvement by necrotizing vasculitis,[153-155] emphasizing that vasculitis is not always systemic. These patients commonly undergo surgical intervention, but with variable outcomes that are generally more favorable when there is involvement of the gallbladder, pancreas, and appendix.[155]

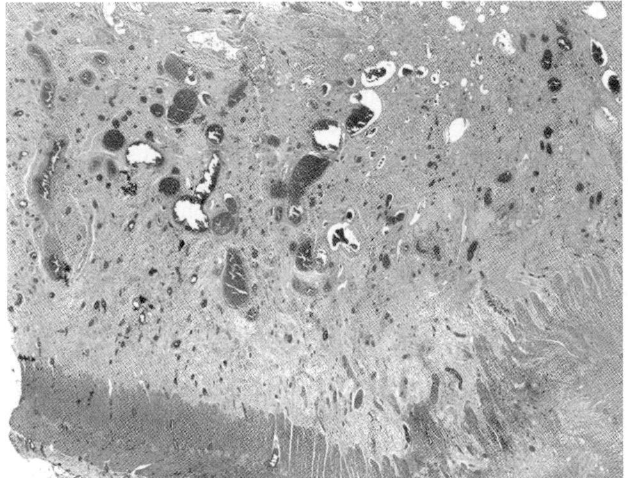

FIGURE 11.72 Kawasaki's disease. Submucosal vessels with marked congestion and luminal ectasia as a result of necrotizing vasculitis.

DIFFERENTIAL DIAGNOSIS OF ISCHEMIA IN LOWER GI TRACT BIOPSIES

The classic features of acute ischemic colitis described in the preceding sections of this chapter are summarized as follows: mucosa of normal architecture with necrosis and sloughing of the surface epithelium, loss of epithelium in the superficial aspects of the crypts (either with or without ghosts of crypts), mucin depletion and reactive changes in the residual crypt epithelium with nuclear hyperchromasia and increased mitoses, paucity or complete absence of acute inflammatory cells in the early stages of the disease, and the presence of hyalinosis in the lamina propria (Fig. 11.74; Table 11.13). However, some of these histological features are not specific for ischemic injury. The differential diagnosis of ischemia in colonic biopsies includes a number of entities, all of which have potential for showing overlapping histological findings (Fig. 11.75).

Certain phases of C. *difficile*–induced pseudomembranous colitis can mimic ischemic colitis. Although early lesions, characterized by the presence of a volcanic (eruptive) inflammatory exudate, are distinctive, late (type II or III) lesions are characterized by mucosal necrosis and the presence of a necroinflammatory pseudomembrane that can mimic severe acute ischemic colitis. The presence of lamina propria hyalinization, attenuated crypts with loss of superficial epithelium, and reactive epithelial changes ("microcrypts") are features supportive of ischemia. Continuous (as opposed to patchy) involvement of mucosa, with pseudomembranes, in the absence of endoscopic evidence of a polyp or mass, is more suggestive of C. *difficile* colitis.[156]

Acute hemorrhagic (infectious) colitis, such as that caused by *E. coli* O157:H7 and certain other bacteria, including *K. oxytoca*,[73] may mimic ischemia by also showing architecturally normal mucosa, intramucosal hemorrhage, and capillary fibrin thrombi, especially in the early stages of infection before significant infiltration of neutrophils has occurred. Abundant acute inflammation and hemorrhage, with relative preservation of mucosal integrity and without withering (attenuated) crypts, are features more indicative of acute hemorrhagic colitis. Furthermore, *E. coli* of this type involves the right colon more than the left. However, clinical, endoscopic, and

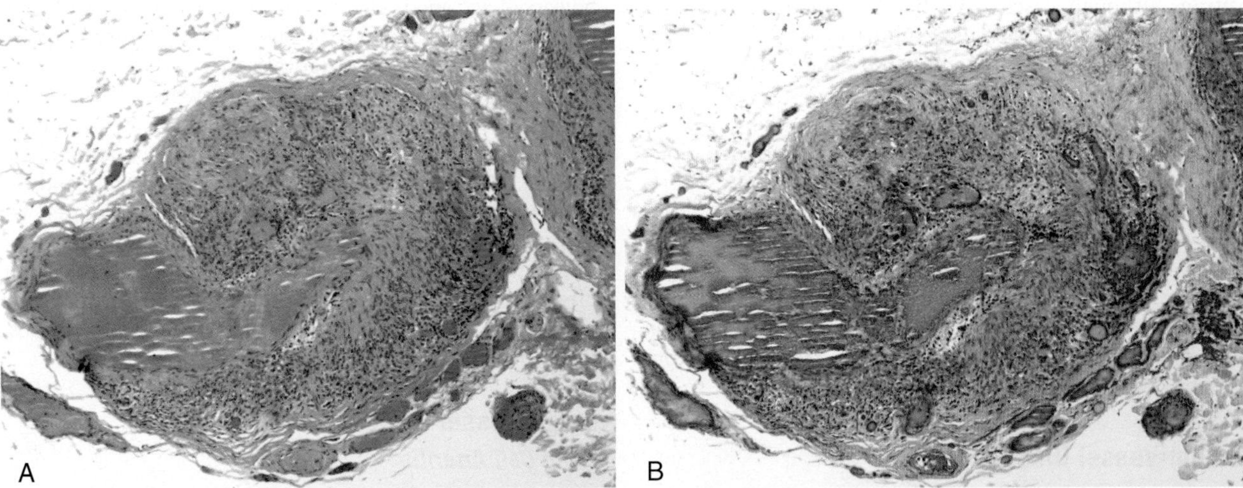

FIGURE 11.73 Giant cell arteritis. A, Muscular artery with prominent granulomatous vasculitis associated with multinucleated giant cells. **B,** Movat stain reveals disruption of the elastic lamina.

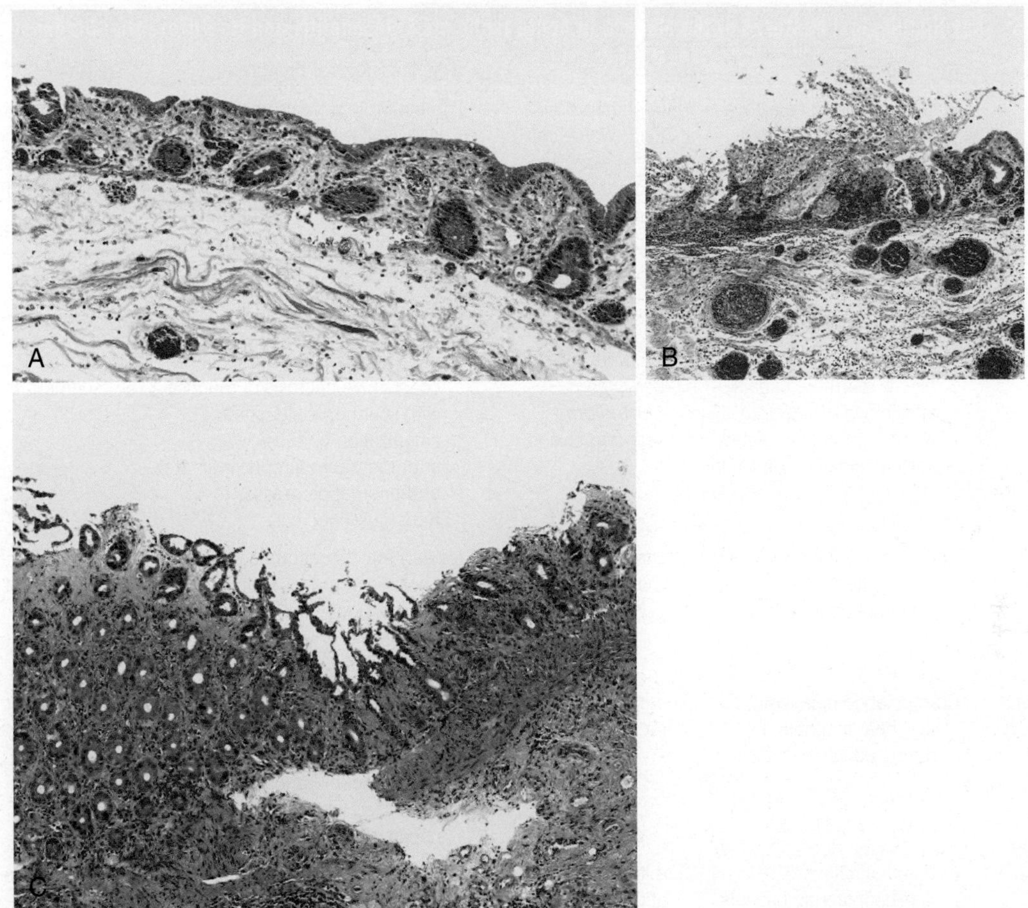

FIGURE 11.74 Histological features of acute ischemia in intestinal mucosa. A, The early stages of ischemic injury show mild surface epithelial injury with reactive mucin loss, lamina propria edema, and reactive epithelial changes. **B,** Further ischemia leads to progressive loss of superficial epithelium. Ghosts of (withered) crypts are seen and eventually full-thickness mucosal necrosis. **C,** In an endoscopic biopsy specimen, the appearance of the mucosa may range from normal to frank ischemic injury (as seen here) with withered crypts and marked hyalinization of the lamina propria.

TABLE 11.13 Key Histological Features of the Mucosa in Acute Ischemic Enterocolitis and Its Differential Diagnosis

Entity	Key Clinical Features	Etiology	Key Pathological Features	Treatment
Acute intestinal ischemia	Acute crampy abdominal pain, followed by bloody or maroon diarrhea	Arterial (occlusive or nonocclusive), venous, or microvascular insufficiency	Loss of surface epithelium with hyalinization of lamina propria; progressive loss of gland epithelium from surface down; mucin depletion, reactive epithelial atypia in crypts, crypt cell mitoses; scant acute inflammation initially	Conservative treatment (parenteral fluids, food restriction, broad-spectrum antibiotics) unless surgical exploration is indicated (perforation or gangrene)
Pseudomembranous enterocolitis	Acute-onset diarrhea with loose, watery stools; or fever, leukocytosis, and crampy abdominal pain	Toxigenic *Clostridium difficile* infection in susceptible host, 2 days to 12 weeks after antibiotic use	Type I lesion: Superficial mucosal necrosis with erupting spray of fibrinopurulent exudate Type II: Desquamated epithelium in groups of crypts with plaques of inflammatory exudate that cover mucosal surface Type III: Full-thickness mucosal necrosis with hemorrhage and overlying confluent pseudomembrane	Stop precipitating antibiotics and treat with metronidazole or vancomycin

Continued

TABLE 11.13 Key Histological Features of the Mucosa in Acute Ischemic Enterocolitis and Its Differential Diagnosis—cont'd

Entity	Key Clinical Features	Etiology	Key Pathological Features	Treatment
Hemorrhagic (infectious) enterocolitis	Watery, nonbloody diarrhea and abdominal cramps, progressing to bloody diarrhea; nausea, vomiting, fever; can cause HUS in children or TTP in adults	Enterohemorrhagic *Escherichia coli, Klebsiella oxytoca;* bacterial toxins damage capillary endothelium	Lamina propria hemorrhage occurs early, followed by superficial mucosal necrosis with loss of surface epithelium and superficial gland epithelium. Neutrophils infiltrate lamina propria and glands. With resolution, lymphocytes and plasma cells infiltrate	Parenteral hydration, rest bowel, avoid antibiotic use (increases risk of HUS and TTP)
Enteritis necroticans	Acute abdominal pain with bloody diarrhea, usually after binge eating; also when high-protein diet is introduced after starvation	*Clostridium perfringens, Clostridium septicum* toxins	Usually affects small bowel; coagulative necrosis of mucosa with scant exudate, surface colonization by *Clostridia,* submucosal neutrophil infiltrate and edema; progresses to transmural necrosis	Resection of affected segment of intestine
Neutropenic enterocolitis	Acute abdominal pain with bloody diarrhea in a setting of neutropenia	*Clostridium septicum, Clostridium perfringens*	Usually affects cecum; coagulative necrosis of mucosa with little or no exudate; paucity of neutrophils at viable edges; progresses to transmural necrosis	Resection of affected segment of intestine
Acute radiation injury	Crampy abdominal pain, diarrhea, and nausea during course of radiation	Therapeutic ionizing radiation	Loss of surface and gland epithelium, increased cellularity of lamina propria, lamina propria edema and hemorrhage, hyalinized vessels, dilated capillaries, atypical fibroblasts	Resolves spontaneously after course of radiation
Kayexalate injury	Abdominal pain and diarrhea; uremic patients particularly susceptible	Sorbitol component of the Kayexalate preparation	Rhomboid or triangular basophilic nonpolarizing crystals adherent to epithelium or in inflammatory exudates; ischemic pattern of mucosal injury; distinguished from cholestyramine by mosaic pattern in H&E stain and red (not pink) color in Ziehl-Neelsen stain	Cease treatment
Glutaraldehyde colitis	Severe acute crampy abdominal pain beginning 3-6 hours after colonoscopy; bloody diarrhea	Glutaraldehyde sterilant retained in endoscope channels and sprayed on mucosa during endoscopy	Identical to those of acute intestinal ischemia	Parenteral fluids if necessary; resolves spontaneously
Collagenous colitis	Chronic watery diarrhea, primarily in middle-aged women; may have associated cramping abdominal pain	Etiology unclear; abnormal collagen metabolism, bacteria, and medication-mediated damage have been implicated	Increased lamina propria lymphoplasmacytic inflammation and intraepithelial lymphocytes; marked subepithelial collagenous deposition that may mimic hyalinosis of ischemic colitis; superimposed acute inflammation and necroinflammatory pseudomembrane may mimic pseudomembranous colitis	Steroid therapy, cholestyramine, bismuth, and 5-aminosalicylate derivatives and immunosuppressives are therapeutic options; surgical management in selected cases (very rarely)
Amyloidosis	Most common with systemic amyloidosis (usually reactive or secondary AA type); diarrhea, steatorrhea, and weight loss; may have gastrointestinal bleeding or motility disorder	Abnormally pleated protein deposited in extracellular tissues	Lamina propria pink, homogenous amyloid deposition, usually with normal crypt or surface epithelium with or without coexisting capillary, venular, and arteriolar amyloid deposits	Treatment of underlying cause; supportive therapy, sometimes steroid therapy

H&E, *Hematoxylin and eosin stain;* HUS, *hemolytic-uremic syndrome;* TTP, *thrombotic thrombocytopenic purpura.*

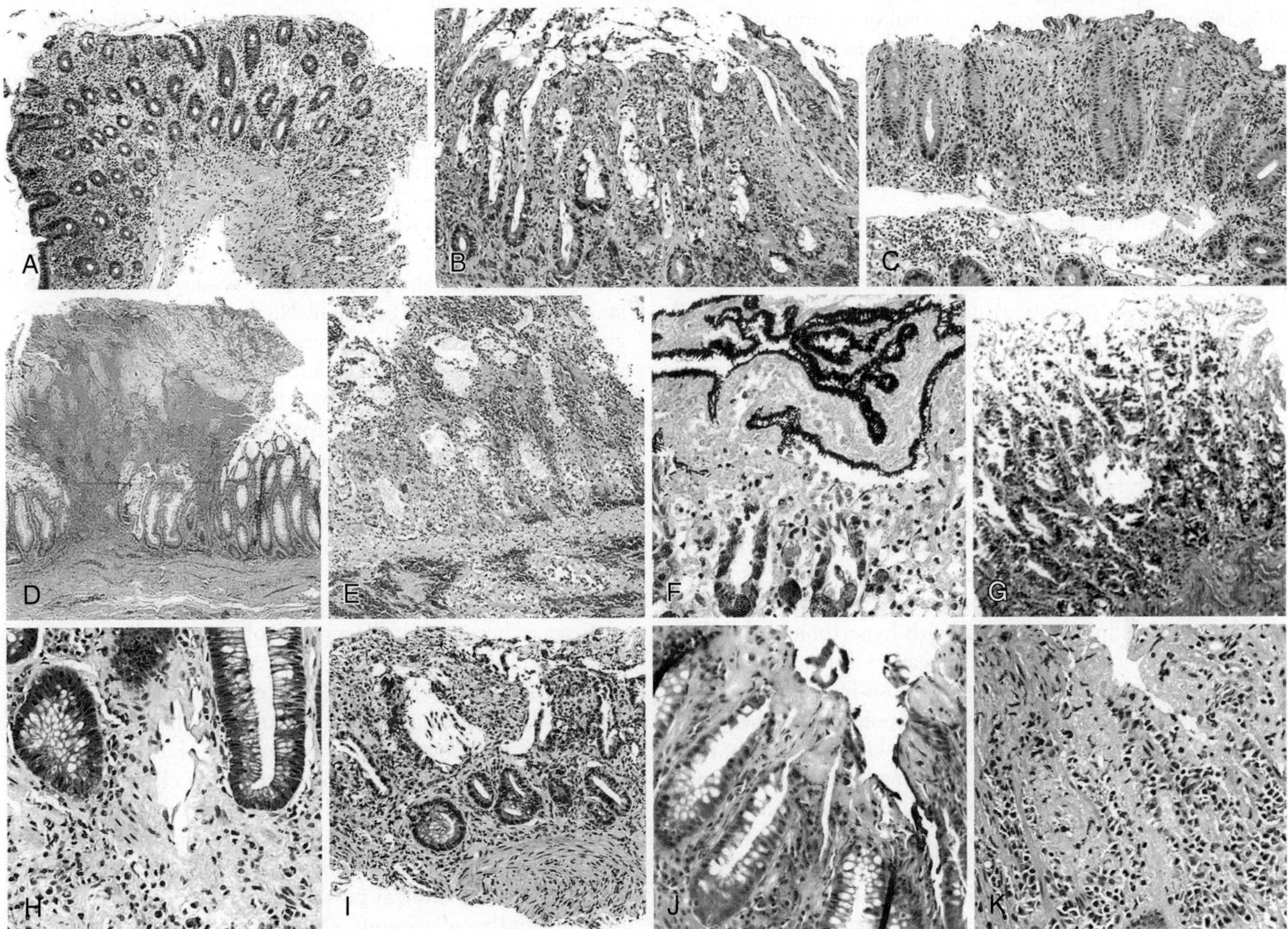

FIGURE 11.75 Entities in the histological differential diagnosis of ischemic colitis. A–C, Ischemic colitis. **A,** There is a relatively abrupt transition from mucosa of normal architecture to focal full-thickness ischemic injury, with reactive changes in adjacent crypts. **B,** Ghosts of crypts, loss of superficial epithelium, mucosal congestion and hemorrhage, and lamina propria hyalinosis. **C,** Deep crypt dropout with superficial epithelial loss and mild hyalinosis. **D,** Pseudomembranous colitis. Eruptive necroinflammatory exudate without hyalinosis or significant lamina propria hemorrhage. **E,** Hemorrhagic colitis. Marked mucosal and submucosal hemorrhage and significant neutrophilic infiltrate. **F,** Enteritis necroticans. Negligible neutrophilic infiltrate with a dense layer of *Clostridium* bacilli on surface epithelium. **G,** Neutropenic enterocolitis. Autolytic-type degenerative appearance of mucosa without significant neutrophilic inflammation. **H,** Radiation colitis. Notice the dilated lamina propria capillaries with prominent endothelial cells and mild hyalinosis. **I,** Glutaraldehyde colitis. This pattern of loss of superficial epithelium, mucosal congestion and hemorrhage, and "withering" crypts is indistinguishable from ischemic colitis. **J,** Collagenous colitis. The denuded surface epithelium with a marked increase in subepithelial collagen may mimic the hyalinosis of ischemia. **K,** Amyloidosis. The detached surface epithelium with lamina propria amyloidosis may also mimic the hyalinosis of ischemia.

bacteriological correlation may be required to distinguish these two entities with complete certainty.

Enteritis necroticans is a rare type of necrotizing enterocolitis usually caused by C. *perfringens*. Toxins produced by the bacteria induce coagulative necrosis of the mucosa that mimics acute ischemia. However, in contrast with ischemia, enteritis necroticans, which typically affects the small bowel, usually shows coagulative necrosis associated with only scant or negligible neutrophilic exudate, exhibits surface colonization by clostridial organisms, and may be associated with intestinal pneumatosis. Clinically, the rapid development of toxemia and multiorgan failure helps distinguish this condition from primary ischemic colitis.

Neutropenic enterocolitis, an infectious disorder most often caused by *Clostridium septicum*, develops in patients who are neutropenic, most commonly because of chemotherapy. Toxins produced by this organism are normally degraded in the presence of neutrophils, but in their absence may cause coagulative necrosis of the mucosa and submucosa, producing ischemia. The mucosa in patients with neutropenic enterocolitis typically reveals coagulative necrosis, marked edema, and hemorrhage in the absence of an acute inflammatory reaction. The diagnosis of neutropenic enterocolitis is often made clinically in patients who are known to be neutropenic as a result of chemotherapy, but it may be unsuspected in patients with other conditions, such as undiagnosed cyclic neutropenia.

Both acute and chronic radiation colitis may cause ischemic colitis and mimic primary ischemic colitis. The histological and pathological effects of radiation therapy vary with the interval between completion of radiation treatment and onset of symptoms.[157] Acute radiation injury (within 2 to 3 days after radiation treatment) is characterized by surface epithelial damage, nuclear atypia with bizarre mitoses, attenuation or loss of crypt epithelium, increased apoptosis, endothelial swelling, capillary thrombosis, and ulcers. In this phase, features of primary ischemic colitis, such as lamina propria hyalinosis, and withering crypts are not normally present. In the chronic phase of radiation injury, superimposed episodes of ischemia or the presence of mucosal or submucosal fibrosis can mimic primary acute or chronic ischemic colitis.[158] However, the presence of dilated, thickened, and hyalinized small and medium-sized blood vessels, prominent reactive or bizarre endothelial cells, myofibroblasts and fibroblasts, and foamy cell plaques within arteries are distinctive features of chronic radiation injury.[159]

There is a long list of drugs and toxins associated with ischemic-type injury of the GI tract (Table 11.14). Common associated drugs that can produce a pattern of injury in the colon that mimics primary acute ischemic colitis include oral contraceptives, potassium chloride, NSAIDs, pseudoephedrine, agonists of 5-hydroxytryptamine, Kayexalate, and even glutaraldehyde, which is used as a sterilizing agent for endoscopic equipment.[160] Cocaine and NSAID-induced injury were previously discussed in this chapter. Oral contraceptives, and other hormonal medications that include estrogen, in particular, can predispose to venous thrombosis leading to ischemic colitis, typically in young females. Kayexalate has been associated with ischemic-type injury, but its actual role in mucosal injury remains controversial. Kayexalate can be administered in a suspension with hypertonic sorbitol to diminish fecal impaction seen in earlier formulas. Several studies reported colonic ischemic necrosis in such a scenario, raising concern that sorbitol may be responsible for the injury instead [84,161,162] In addition, patients taking Kayexalate may have other ischemic-related predisposing factors such as renal failure with hypotension, uremia, and elevated renin. In fact, lower rates of colonic necrosis were demonstrated in non-uremic rats on Kayexalate-sorbitol enemas when compared with uremic counterparts.[161] Similar findings have also been suggested in humans.[162] Interestingly, sorbitol is not visible on histological sections, and, more importantly, Kayexalate has distinct histological features. Despite its unclear role in ischemia, it is important to recognize Kayexalate on histological sections as it may alert clinicians to further investigate the formula that was given. As opposed to other cases of ischemic colitis, the presence of diagnostic triangular or rhomboidal, basophilic, nonpolarizing crystals adherent to the epithelium or within the inflammatory exudate are characteristic findings associated with Kayexalate-induced colitis (Fig. 11.76A–B).[162] Kayexalate crystals should be distinguished from cholestyramine by the presence of a mosaic pattern on H&E stain and a red color on Ziehl-Neelsen stain. Patients with glutaraldehyde colitis often complain of severe lower abdominal pain that develops within a few hours after an endoscopic procedure. Biopsies at this stage may show mucosal necrosis, sloughing of the surface and superficial crypt epithelium (Fig. 11.76C), and hyalinosis of the lamina propria in the absence of a neutrophilic infiltrate—histological features that are virtually indistinguishable from those of primary acute ischemic injury. Sevelamer crystals can also induce similar effects in the mucosa.

Other disorders that may rarely cause confusion with primary ischemia are collagenous colitis and colonic amyloidosis. In biopsy specimens from patients with collagenous colitis, detachment of the surface epithelium and the presence of a thickened and irregular subepithelial collagen band can mimic ischemia-related hyalinization. However, in contrast with ischemia, collagenous colitis is characterized by entrapment of capillaries and inflammatory cells in the lamina propria, increased intraepithelial lymphocytes, and positive immunohistochemical staining for type III collagen (not usually done for clinical purposes). Furthermore, clinically, patients with collagenous colitis usually have nonbloody, watery diarrhea and are overwhelmingly older females. A

TABLE 11.14 Summarized List of Drugs Associated with Ischemic-Type Injury

Antibiotics	Tricyclic antidepressants
Amoxicillin/ampicillin	Phenothiazine derivatives
Tetracycline	**Hormonal agents**
Fluoroquinolone	Estrogen
Macrolide	Oral contraceptives
Cephalosporin	Danazol
Laxatives	Flutamide
Kayexalate	Depot progestogen
Sevelamer	Hormone replacement therapy
Colesevelam	**Illicit agents**
Colestipol	Cocaine
Cholestyramine	Amphetamines
Magnesium citrate	**Immunomodulators/antiinflammatory**
Bisacodyl	Interferon
Glycerin enemas	Azathioprine
Diuretics	Anti–tumor necrosis factor
Furosemide	Nonsteroidal antiinflammatory drugs
Ethacrynic acid	Mycophenolate
Chemotherapeutic agents	**Serotonin agonist/antagonist**
Vinorelbine	Alosetron: 5HT3 antagonist
Paclitaxel	Sumatriptan: 5HT1 agonist
Docetaxel	**Miscellaneous**
Constipation-inducing agents	Digitalis
Opiates	Decongestants
Calcium channel blockers	Ergot alkaloids
Psychotropic medications	Vasopressin
Antiepileptics	Simvastatin
Oxybutynin	Glutaraldehyde

Modified from Uberti G, Goldblum JR, Allende DS. Ischemic enterocolitis and its differential diagnosis. Sem Diagn Pathol. *2014;31(2):152-164.*

trichrome stain can often help distinguish true fibrosis in cases of collagenous colitis (positive) from hyalinosis related to ischemic colitis (negative).

Similarly, amyloid deposition in the lamina propria can mimic ischemia-related hyalinosis.[163] However, in amyloidosis, the mucosa is usually otherwise within normal limits, without crypt or surface epithelial injury. On occasion, vascular involvement by amyloidosis causes superimposed ischemic colitis as a result of the underlying vascular pathological process. A Congo red, Sirius red, or crystal violet stain can be useful in this setting to highlight the presence of amyloid.

It is well established in the literature that morphological overlap exists between chronic ischemia and inflammatory bowel disease, in particular Crohn's disease. In addition, many have argued that ischemia plays a role in the development of Crohn's disease as a result of hypercoagulable states and inflammation leading to occlusion of small vessels in the antimesenteric border of the terminal ileum, for example. Patients with ischemic injury tend to be older, and inflammatory bowel disease frequently occurs in younger patients, but these are not absolutes. Predisposing conditions (e.g., diabetes, medications) and associated conditions (e.g., cardiovascular disease, history of myocardial infarction) should be evaluated as well for an accurate diagnosis. On endoscopy, ischemia can be segmental, causing sharply demarcated areas of injury associated with the corresponding vascular supply. Crohn's disease can have a patchy distribution, commonly affects the ileocecal valve, and the inflammatory process is often not well delineated. These two entities may be indistinguishable on histological sections alone, but the presence of granulomas associated with deeply located vasculature should prompt the diagnosis of Crohn's disease in this differential.

The differential diagnosis between mucosal prolapse and ischemia can be challenging. Mucosal prolapse tends to be a disease of the rectum and sigmoid colon (typically not concentric, affects anterior wall of rectum commonly), while ischemia can occur in any colonic segment in a concentric fashion. In fact, most would argue that ischemia cannot occur in the rectum because of its rich vasculature. There is macroscopic overlap between these two entities as they can present with ulcers, erythematous mucosa, and polypoid lesions. On histological sections, differentiating features that favor mucosal prolapse would include thick muscle bundles surrounding groups of colonic crypts in a "lobular" arrangement. Although there may be superficial erosion, there is no evidence of mucosal necrosis or perforation in cases of prolapse. Ischemic-type injury in younger adults is less common than in older adults but is still not infrequently encountered in clinical practice. Some recurrent etiologies associated with this pattern of injury include medications, hypercoagulable states, collagen vascular diseases and vasculitis, and strenuous exercise/dehydration, among others.

The full reference list may be accessed online at *Elsevier eBooks for Practicing Clinicians*.

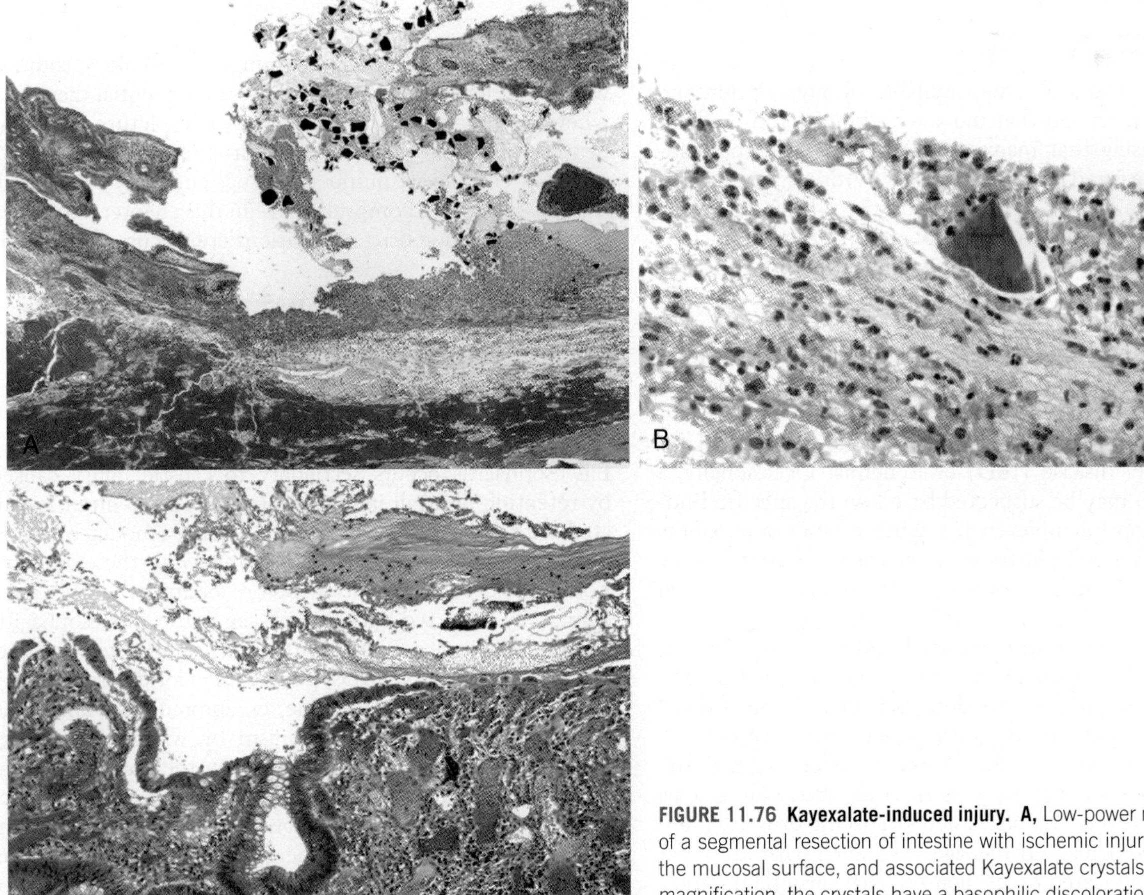

FIGURE 11.76 Kayexalate-induced injury. A, Low-power magnification of a segmental resection of intestine with ischemic injury, necrosis of the mucosal surface, and associated Kayexalate crystals. **B,** At higher magnification, the crystals have a basophilic discoloration and classic fish-scale appearance. **C,** Sloughing of epithelial cells seen as part of the early changes identified in Kayexalate-associated injury.

CHAPTER 12

Drug-Induced Disorders of the Gastrointestinal Tract

Joseph Misdraji

Chapter Outline

INTRODUCTION

Given the plethora of drugs available by prescription and over the counter, and that most are administered orally, it is not surprising that many drugs can cause gastrointestinal (GI) disease. The injury caused by drugs can be due to direct toxic effects of the drug on the GI mucosa, toxic effects to the mesenchymal components of the gut, including the enteric nervous system, systemic effects of the drug, or indirect damage such as in antibiotic-associated pseudomembranous colitis. The patterns of injury associated with drugs include virtually all of the patterns of inflammatory injury described in the GI tract. Thus, in these situations, a medication history is essential to avoid confusion with other common types of inflammatory disorders, such as inflammatory bowel disease (IBD) or ischemia. Occasionally, a drug reaction may be suspected based on the specific findings in the biopsy sample, such as when crystals or pigments are identified. Rarely, histology alone is enough to implicate a specific drug without knowledge of the patient's clinical profile.

In this chapter on drug-induced injury of the GI tract, nonspecific histological injury patterns, and the drugs associated with these patterns, are described first. Some of these patterns are organ specific, such as reactive gastropathy or pill esophagitis, whereas others are more generalizable to the entire GI tract, such as ulcers, strictures, or vasculitis. This section is followed by a discussion of specific drugs that are well known to cause GI damage, beginning with the most commonly implicated drugs, nonsteroidal antiinflammatory drugs (NSAIDs) and proton pump inhibitors (PPIs). Some of these agents produce a wide range of pathology, some of which are nonspecific and generate a differential diagnosis, whereas others produce a characteristic picture that may be more readily recognizable as a drug reaction by pathologists. Given the vast number of drugs currently available, it is impossible to be comprehensive in this chapter. However, the most common drug associations are discussed in detail.

NONSPECIFIC INJURY PATTERNS

Organ-Specific

Esophagus

Pill Esophagitis

Pill esophagitis occurs secondary to caustic injury caused by retention of a pill in the esophagus. This is often associated with failure to swallow an adequate amount of liquid with the tablet or capsule and swallowing these medications in the supine position before bedtime.[1-5] The most commonly reported agents that can cause pill esophagitis include antibiotics (particularly doxycycline, tetracycline, and clindamycin), NSAIDs, potassium chloride, iron supplements, ascorbic acid, quinidine, emepronium bromide, and alendronate.[1,2,5-14] The mechanism by which these drugs cause esophagitis differs depending on the particular agent involved. Tetracyclines, ascorbic acid, and ferrous sulfate produce acidic solutions when dissolved in water, suggesting that they produce acid burns, whereas phenytoin produces an alkaline solution and possibly alkaline burn.[4,9] Production of local hyperosmolarity by potassium chloride and intracellular

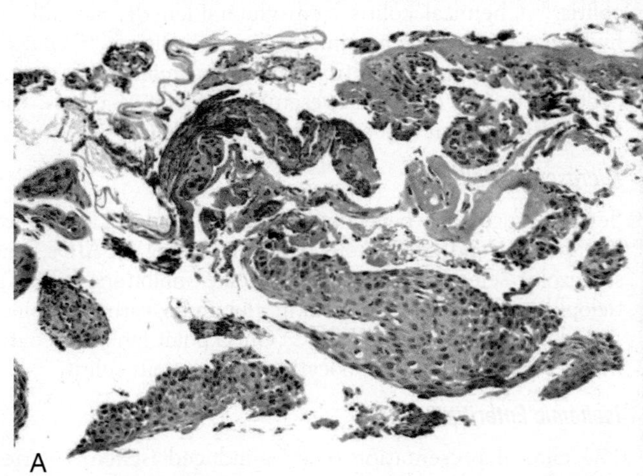
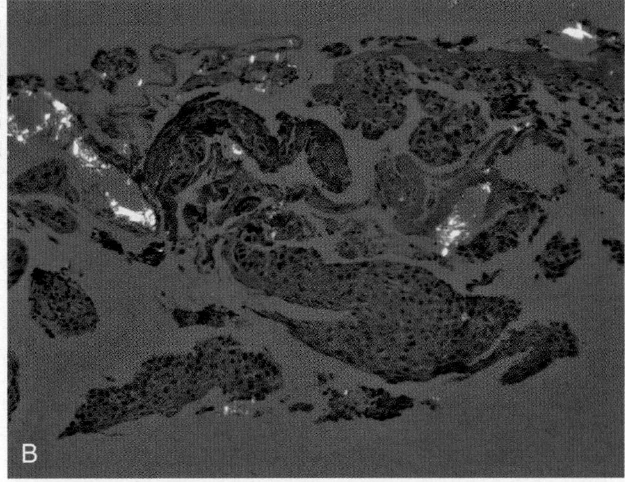

FIGURE 12.1 Pill esophagitis. A, Fragment of reactive squamous epithelium with fibrin and inflammatory cells. **B,** The same slide under polarized light demonstrates the presence of crystalline polarizable material consistent with pill fragments.

poisoning after mucosal uptake by doxycycline and NSAIDs may be the mechanism of injury of these agents.[4,9,15]

Women and older patients are more often affected.[2-5,9,10] However, the age range is wide. Different drugs are consumed by different age groups. In a review of 650 reported cases, the average age of patients who had quinidine-related esophageal injury was 60, whereas the average age of patients injured by oral antibiotics was 30.[12] Most patients present with odynophagia, retrosternal pain, and dysphagia[3-6,8,9] and do not have a history of esophageal dysmotility.[2,4] Complications of pill esophagitis include esophageal strictures, hemorrhage, esophageal perforation, and even death.[3,4,9,13,16]

Endoscopic findings include erythema, mucosal denudation, discrete ulcers or erosions, and strictures.[2,5,6,9,12,13,16,17] The squamous epithelium may exfoliate, forming an intraluminal cast, a condition known as esophagitis dissecans superficialis.[11,18] Sloughing esophagitis with longitudinal sloughing of the middle to distal esophagus is characteristic of esophagitis secondary to dabigatran, a thrombin inhibitor.[19-21] Quinidine-induced esophageal injury occasionally manifests with exuberant exudates that mimic carcinoma.[4,5] Remnants of the pill may also be seen.[1] The usual sites of involvement are the midesophagus at the level of the aortic arch (22 to 24 cm) and, in patients with left atrial enlargement, the distal esophagus at 30 to 35 cm.[1,3-5,8] However, distal involvement with stricture may easily be mistaken for reflux esophagitis.[2,5] Histological evaluation shows the usual features of esophagitis, with acute inflammation, erosions or ulcers, and granulation tissue.[6,8] Polarizable crystalline material may be an important clue to the diagnosis (Fig. 12.1) although it is not present in all cases.[6] Multinucleation of squamous epithelial cells has been reported in association with alendronate-associated esophageal injury.[6,22] Perivascular edema has been described in the ulcers secondary to doxycycline.[23,24] Esophageal strictures have been described in patients taking potassium chloride, doxycycline, tetracycline, acetylsalicylic acid, ascorbic acid, phenytoin, and quinidine.[2]

Stomach

Reactive Gastropathy

Reactive gastropathy was a condition initially thought to be specifically related to gastric mucosal injury caused by reflux of duodenal contents into the stomach and was also known as alkaline gastritis or bile reflux gastritis.[25,26] This distinctive histological entity is now considered a nonspecific response to a variety of gastric irritants, of which bile is only one. NSAIDs and alcohol are also common causes. The features of reactive gastropathy (or "chemical gastritis") include foveolar hyperplasia with a "corkscrew" appearance to the pits, surface epithelial degeneration with cuboidalization of the foveolar glandular cells and mucin depletion, lamina propria edema, vascular congestion, a paucity of inflammatory cells, and smooth muscle hyperplasia in the lamina propria. The muscle fibers are typically oriented perpendicular from the muscularis mucosae toward the mucosal lumen (Fig. 12.2).[25,27] Small foci of atrophy with pseudopyloric or intestinal metaplasia are common and may reflect ulcer repair.[27]

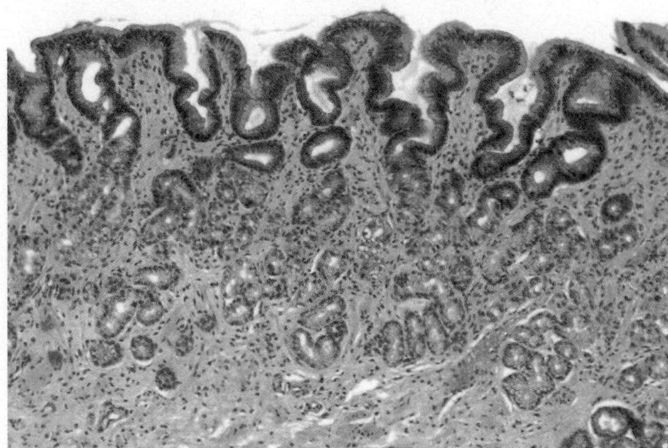

FIGURE 12.2 Chemical gastritis. The antral mucosa shows damage to the foveolar cells characterized by mucin diminution, basophilia, and elongation of the pits, which have an irregular contour. The lamina propria shows mild fibrosis but little inflammation.

Small and Large Intestine

Celiac Disease–Like Enteropathy

Increasingly, a celiac disease–like enteropathy secondary to medications has been reported. Villous atrophy, variable

TABLE 12.1 Patterns of Colitis and Possible Drug-Related Etiologies

Pattern of Colitis	Possible Drug
Eosinophilic colitis	NSAIDs, gold, carbamazepine, antiplatelet agents, estroprogestinic agents
Lymphocytic colitis/ collagenous colitis	NSAIDs, proton pump inhibitors, ticlopidine, ranitidine, simvastatin, flutamide, carbamazepine, sertraline, penicillin V
Focal active colitis	NSAIDs, oral sodium phosphate
Ischemic colitis	NSAIDs, glutaraldehyde, antibiotics, chemotherapy, nasal decongestants, constipation-inducing medications, laxatives, vasopressor agents, cocaine, ergotamine, serotonin agonists/antagonists including sumatriptan, high-dose estrogen and progesterone, amphetamines, digitalis, diuretics, immunomodulators such as interleukin-2
Apoptotic colitis	Bowel prep with oral sodium phosphate, laxatives, chemotherapeutic agents (especially 5-fluorouracil), mycophenolate mofetil, idelalisib, NSAIDs, cyclosporine A
Pseudomembranous colitis	NSAIDs, amoxicillin, levofloxacin, antibiotic associated *Clostridium difficile* colitis
Immune-mediated colitis	Immune checkpoint inhibitors
Neutropenic colitis	Chemotherapy

lymphocytic exocytosis, and variable crypt apoptoses may mimic celiac disease, and clinical circumstances, including onset of symptoms related to initiation of the suspected medication, severe presentation, and absence of response to gluten withdrawal, may be clues to the correct diagnosis. Olmesartan and other sartans are the most widely known agents that cause this, but other agents can produce a similar picture, such as ticlopidine, idelalisib, checkpoint inhibitors, and mycophenolate mofetil.[28-34]

Large Intestine

Colitis

Drugs may cause patterns of injury that mimic virtually every other known type of colitis. The patterns of colitis that suggest particular agents are listed in Table 12.1. Eosinophilic colitis (Fig. 12.3) is associated with numerous drugs, including NSAIDs, gold compounds, and carbamazepine hypersensitivity.[35-37] In one series of patients undergoing colonoscopy for probable drug colitis, increased eosinophils were found in the left colon of patients taking NSAIDs, antiplatelet agents, or estroprogestinic agents, regardless of colonoscopic findings.[38] NSAIDs are associated with increased lymphocytes and scattered neutrophils in the lamina propria, or an appearance similar to that of lymphocytic colitis.[39] Alpha methyldopa and NSAIDs may cause a neutrophilic colitis, mimicking infection.[40] Amoxicillin and levofloxacin have been implicated in cases of pseudomembranous colitis.[36] Chemical colitis from glutaraldehyde, alcohol, or hydrogen peroxide can mimic ischemic colitis.[41-45] Checkpoint inhibitor therapy, rituximab, mesalamine, and etanercept can cause colitis that resembles ulcerative colitis, can trigger IBD, or can exacerbate preexisting IBD.[46-56]

Microscopic Colitis

Several drugs have been implicated in the development of lymphocytic and collagenous colitis, including NSAIDs, lansoprazole, selective serotonin reuptake inhibitors (SSRIs), ticlopidine, ranitidine, simvastatin, flutamide, carbamazepine, sertraline, and penicillin V.[36,57-63] Checkpoint inhibitor colitis may resemble either lymphocytic or collagenous colitis.

Ischemic Enteritis/Colitis

The clinical presentation of drug-induced ischemia varies depending on the offending agent, the mesenteric vessels involved, the interval between exposure of the drug and clinical presentation, and the general status of the patient. Segmental involvement is typical. The histology is identical to that of ischemia due to other causes. It may reveal ulceration, necrosis, edema, and fibrosis, depending on the stage of injury. Drugs associated with ischemic colitis include antibiotics, NSAIDs, chemotherapeutic agents such as the taxanes, nasal decongestants, constipation-inducing medications, laxatives, vasopressor agents, cocaine, ergotamine, serotonin agonists/antagonists including sumatriptan, oral contraceptives, amphetamines, digitalis, diuretics, and immunomodulators such as interleukin-2.[36,64] The mechanisms by which drugs cause ischemia vary. For instance, estrogens may result in vascular thromboses, ergotamine may cause vascular spasm leading to proctitis with the development of shallow ulcers, cocaine is a potent sympathomimetic mesenteric vasoconstrictor that produces severe intestinal ischemia, diuretics may cause extracellular fluid volume changes that favor peripheral circulation over mesenteric circulation, and antibiotics may cause hypersensitivity vasculitis. Chemical colitis, such as from glutaraldehyde or alcohol enemas, can also appear histologically indistinguishable from ischemic colitis.[41-45]

Focal Active Colitis

Focal active colitis (FAC) is defined as cryptitis that involves one or a few crypts, and is associated with epithelial injury and often a surrounding mononuclear infiltrate in an otherwise unremarkable colonic biopsy (Fig. 12.4). It is historically associated with Crohn's disease. In a 1997 study involving patients without a prior history of IBD, Greenson et al.[65] found that most symptomatic patients with FAC had acute self-limited or infectious colitis, whereas FAC in asymptomatic patients carried no clinical significance. None developed Crohn's disease. However, 19 of 42 patients in this study were taking NSAIDs, leaving open the possibility that NSAIDs were the cause of FAC. Subsequently, FAC was reported by Driman et al.[66] in patients given oral sodium phosphate as a bowel prep regimen, and they suggested that the idiopathic cases in Greenson's report may have been due to bowel prep.

Pseudo-obstruction

Drug-induced pseudo-obstruction, or paralytic ileus, rarely comes to the attention of surgical pathologists, because the

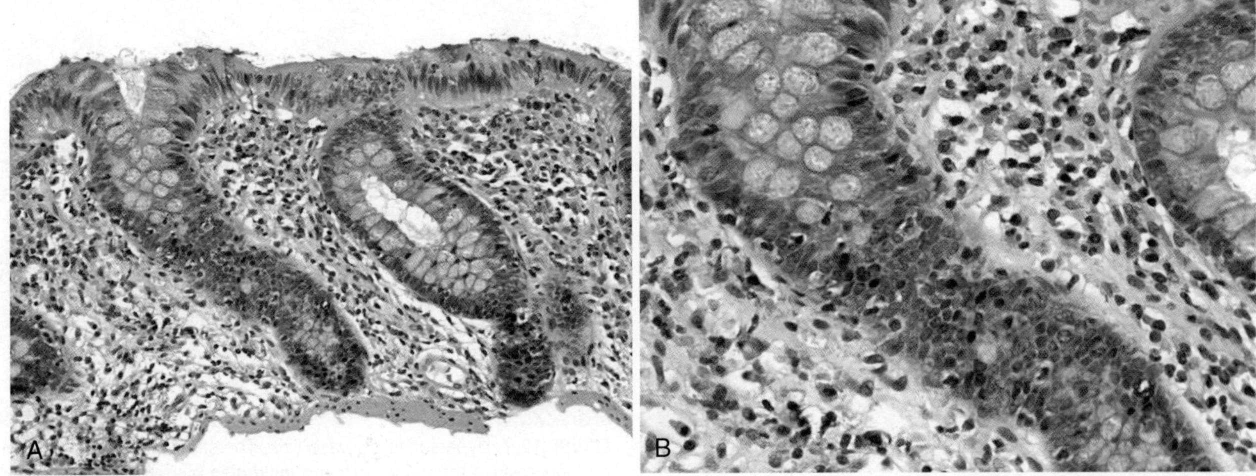

FIGURE 12.3 Eosinophilic colitis. A, The colon biopsy shows increased eosinophils in the lamina propria. **B,** A high-power view shows infiltration of the crypt epithelium by eosinophils.

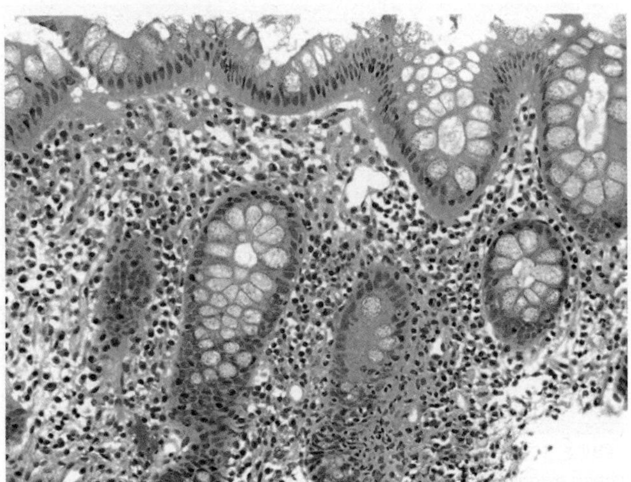

FIGURE 12.4 Focal active colitis. A colon biopsy shows an inflamed crypt with intraepithelial neutrophils and increased inflammation in the lamina propria in this area, in otherwise normal-appearing mucosal biopsy.

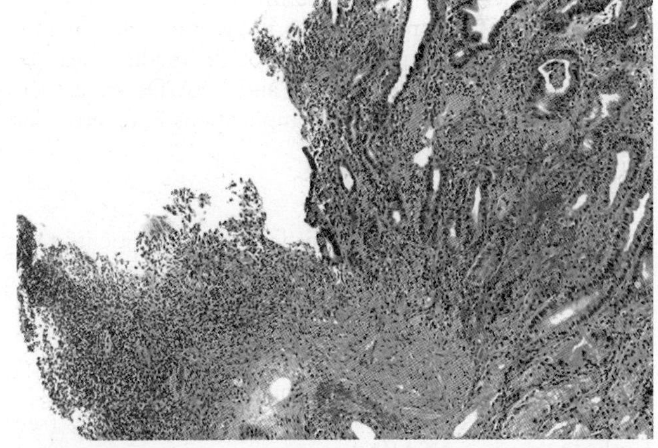

FIGURE 12.5 Duodenal ulcer with fibrinopurulent exudate *(left)* and mucosal inflammation and hemorrhage *(right)* in a patient who attempted suicide by ingesting acetaminophen.

usual treatment is discontinuation of the offending agent. However, complications such as megacolon or perforation may ensue, necessitating surgical intervention. Many drugs can damage the myenteric plexus, causing loss of neurons and schwannosis. Narcotics, phenothiazines, tricyclic antidepressants, anthraquinone laxatives, anti-Parkinson's drugs, clonidine, calcium channel blockers, and vincristine are associated with pseudo-obstruction.

Non–Organ-Specific

Ulcers

Numerous drugs can cause erosions or ulcers in the GI tract. These may be encountered as a single isolated lesion, with nonspecific features, or as part of a more widespread ischemic, cytotoxic, or inflammatory process (Fig. 12.5). Potassium chloride was one of the earliest reported agents implicated in causing ulcers and even strictures in the GI tract, including the stomach.[67,68] Certainly the most common drug to result in gastric and other GI tract ulcers are NSAIDs.[69] These drugs not only damage the mucosa, but they also retard ulcer healing.[70] Other drugs associated with GI ulcers include alendronate, doxycycline, chemotherapeutic agents, corticosteroids, ferrous sulfate, sodium polystyrene sulfonate (Kayexalate), ergot, gold compounds, and colchicine.[1,7,68,71-73]

Perforation

Although drug-induced perforation is uncommon, it may complicate severe ischemic, toxic, or inflammatory colitis of any cause. Intestinal perforation has been reported in cancer patients taking bevacizumab, a monoclonal antibody directed against vascular endothelial growth factor (VEGF) that is used in the treatment of metastatic colon cancer, non–small cell lung cancer, ovarian cancer, renal cell carcinoma, and other cancers.[74-78] From a meta-analysis of the literature, intestinal perforations occur in about 1.1% of patients who have taken bevacizumab, with a mortality rate of 8.8%.[79] Perforations also occur in about 1.3% of patients on VEGF receptor tyrosine kinase inhibitors, with a 28.6% mortality rate.[80] Intestinal perforation has also been

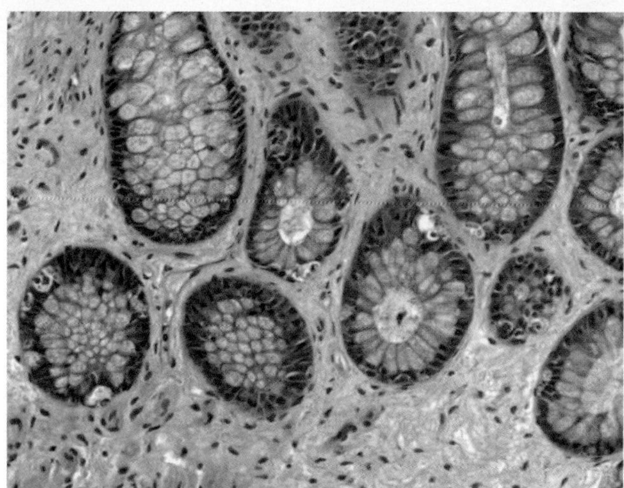

FIGURE 12.6 Apoptotic colopathy. Colonic mucosal biopsy with increased apoptotic bodies in the crypt epithelium.

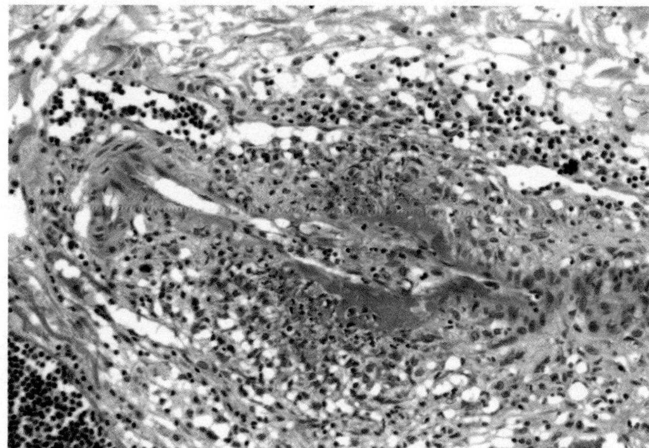

FIGURE 12.7 Hypersensitivity vasculitis. The small arteriole shows fibrinoid necrosis of the vessel wall and infiltration by neutrophils, similar to leukocytoclastic vasculitis in the skin.

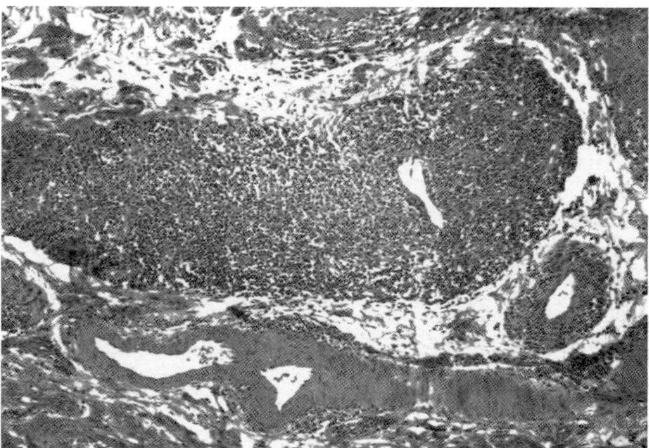

FIGURE 12.8 Lymphocytic enterocolic phlebitis. A medium-size vein shows extensive infiltration by lymphocytes. Notice the uninvolved artery at the bottom of the field.

reported in association with temsirolimus,[81] immunosuppressive medications (steroids, azathioprine), NSAIDs,[82,83] slow-release potassium chloride, flucytosine, neuroleptic medications,[84] tocilizumab,[85] and other medications. In addition, corticosteroids, opioids, and NSAIDs are associated with an increased risk of complications in diverticular disease, including perforation.[86-89]

Strictures

Esophageal strictures have been described in patients taking potassium chloride, doxycycline, tetracycline, acetylsalicylic acid, ascorbic acid, phenytoin, and quinidine.[2] Several drugs have been implicated in intestinal strictures such as potassium chloride and pancreatic enzyme replacement. A dramatic example of intestinal and colonic strictures secondary to drugs is "diaphragm disease" due to NSAIDs (see further section on NSAIDs).

Apoptosis

Several drugs have been associated with increased apoptotic bodies in the crypt epithelium and occasionally associated with dilated crypts containing apoptotic debris. These drugs include penicillin V, mycophenolate mofetil, checkpoint inhibitors, methotrexate, capecitabine, etanercept, and infliximab (Fig. 12.6).[49,50,90-92]

Vasculitis

Drug-induced vasculitis can affect the blood vessels of the GI tract, and result in ischemia. Quinidine, ranitidine, clarithromycin, angiotensin-converting enzyme inhibitors, acetylsalicylic acid, carbidopa/levodopa, ampicillin, chlorpromazine, and ciprofloxacin have all been implicated in Henoch-Schönlein purpura (HSP). GI involvement by HSP can manifest as diarrhea and vomiting and can be complicated by obstruction or perforation. GI involvement is most common in the second part of the duodenum, but it can also affect the esophagus, stomach, colon, and rectum. Discrete coinlike lesions that coalesce or hemorrhagic and ecchymotic lesions have been described.

Biopsy shows granulocytes in the wall of small arterioles or venules with necrosis of the vessel wall similar to findings in leukocytoclastic vasculitis (Fig. 12.7).[93]

Another form of vasculitis that may be related to drugs is lymphocytic enterocolic phlebitis (see Chapter 11 for details), a condition that affects the right colon, small intestine, or sigmoid colon, often with ischemic consequences. In lymphocytic enterocolic phlebitis, veins show perivascular lymphocytic inflammation, with subendothelial aggregation, thickening of the vessel wall, and occasionally fibrinoid necrosis of the blood vessel (Fig. 12.8). In some cases, the inflammation is sparse, and myointimal hyperplasia is more prominent. Rare cases have shown associated lymphocytic infiltrate in the mucosa and epithelium analogous to lymphocytic colitis or collagenous colitis.[94,95] Lymphocytic enterocolic phlebitis was initially described in three patients who had taken rutoside, a phlebotonic drug commonly used in Europe to treat varicose veins.[94] Although another reported case also occurred in a patient on rutoside, subsequent cases have not corroborated an association with this drug. Reports of patients who had taken the antiandrogen drug flutamide and developed this form of vasculitis[95,96] support the notion that a hypersensitivity reaction to drugs explains some cases of lymphocytic enterocolic phlebitis.

Indirect Injury

Secondary Infectious Colitis

Various drugs may promote infections of the GI tract. The association of antibiotics with pseudomembranous colitis caused by *Clostridium difficile* is the most well-known example. Necrotizing enterocolitis, neutropenic enterocolitis, or other infections, including GI candidiasis, may develop in people who have received chemotherapy.[97] Immunosuppressive therapies predispose patients to opportunistic infectious organisms such as cytomegalovirus.[98,99]

Patients with iron overload on deferoxamine therapy are predisposed to develop *Yersinia* infection.[100] Both the iron overload and its treatment contribute to the risk of infection. Iron is an essential growth factor for bacteria, including *Yersinia*. Normally, free iron in the host is too low to support the growth of virulent organisms. For bacterial pathogens, successful infection relies on invading cells, in part to acquire iron. Strains that have the *Yersinia* high-pathogenicity island are able to synthesize the siderophore yersiniabactin, enabling them to acquire iron from host proteins.[101] Transfusion with its resultant iron load increases the amount of iron available to the organism, and iron overload impairs neutrophilic phagocytic activity.[102] Furthermore, the addition of exogenous siderophores, such as deferoxamine, makes iron more available for the organism.[101] The combination of iron overload and deferoxamine therapy increases the risk of *Yersinia* infection; in one study, invasive *Yersinia* infection was diagnosed in 14 patients with β-thalassemia at a frequency 5000-fold greater than that in the general population, and all but two patients were taking deferoxamine at the time of diagnosis of infection.[103]

PPIs may also indirectly predispose to infection. Gastric acid plays a role in the killing of bacteria. Reducing gastric acid may reduce the ability to eliminate bacterial pathogens. An association between PPI use and bacterial gastroenteritis, primarily with *Campylobacter* and *Salmonella*, has also been reported.[104-106] Similarly, the reduced ability to kill bacterial spores may explain a reported association between PPI use and C. *difficile* infection.[107,108]

SPECIFIC AGENTS

Nonsteroidal Antiinflammatory Drugs

Disease Associations

NSAIDs are the most widely prescribed drugs in the world and are associated with numerous patterns of injury to the GI tract. NSAID-induced injury to the upper GI tract injury includes esophagitis, esophageal strictures, gastric, esophageal, and duodenal ulcers, GI bleeding, and perforation. Lower GI tract injury includes enteritis, small intestinal or colonic ulcers, colitis, perforation, and distinctive strictures of the distal small intestine and colon known as *diaphragm disease*. NSAIDs can also, paradoxically, exacerbate preexisting diseases of the colon. The relative risk of developing serious GI complications in patients exposed to NSAIDs is five to six times higher than in the nonexposed population.[109] However, the risk of serious complications seems to be declining somewhat, perhaps due to the introduction of safer NSAIDs, use of PPIs, and a reduction in dose of NSAIDs.[110]

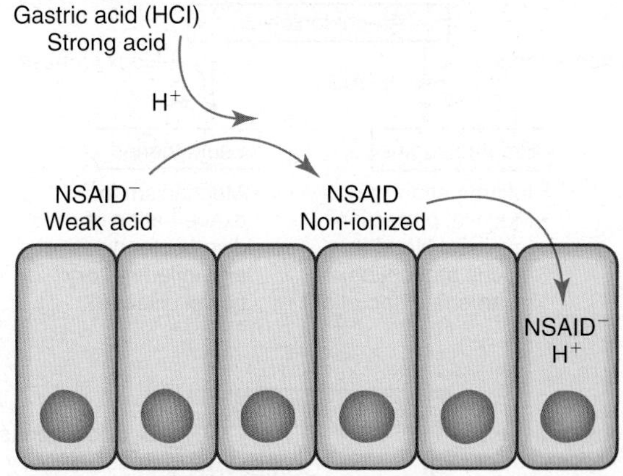

FIGURE 12.9 Mechanism of "ion trapping." NSAIDs are weak acids that, in the gastric environment, accept a proton from hydrochloric acid. As a nonionic molecule, the NSAID can pass through cell membranes. Within cells, the NSAID releases its proton, becoming ionized again, rendering it unable to pass through the membranes. The NSAID is essentially trapped in the cell where it can interrupt cellular processes, including mitochondrial respiration.

Pathogenesis

NSAIDs induce GI injury through various local and systemic mechanisms. Because NSAIDs are weak acids, in the strong acid environment of the stomach, they become un-ionized and pass through cell membranes. Once inside the cell, they are ionized and are trapped within the cell ("ion trapping") (Fig. 12.9).[111,112] Within cells, NSAIDs uncouple oxidative phosphorylation, which depletes the cells of adenosine triphosphate (ATP).[111,112] The insult to epithelial cells results in increased mucosal permeability, which allows gastric acid, bacteria, or bile acids to further damage the mucosa. NSAIDs promote leukocyte-endothelial cell adhesion in the microvasculature, possibly causing ischemic mucosal damage. Significantly, NSAIDs suppress prostaglandin synthesis via inhibition of cyclooxygenase (Fig. 12.10).[111,113] Whereas some prostaglandins are responsible for inflammation, others, in particular PGE_2 and PGI_2, are involved in the regulation of mucosal mucin production, bicarbonate secretion, mucosal blood flow, epithelial cell proliferation, and epithelial restitution, all of which contribute to upper GI tract mucosal protection from acid.[111] Suppression of prostaglandins results in mucosal injury. Cyclooxygenase (COX) exists as two different isoforms, and the ability of NSAIDs to cause damage is related more to their ability to selectively inhibit COX-1 rather than COX-2.[112] COX-1 is abundant in gastric mucosa; COX-2 is expressed at low levels in intact stomach, but is upregulated when COX-1 is inhibited or after injury.[112] The introduction of selective COX-2 inhibitors was viewed as a promising development in reducing GI side effects of NSAIDs. Two major studies, the Celecoxib Long-Term Arthritis Safety Study (CLASS)[114] and the Vioxx Gastrointestinal Outcomes Research Trial (VIGOR)[115] demonstrated that these agents are associated with a significantly lower incidence of upper GI events (perforations, ulcers, bleeding) than nonselective NSAIDs, although these claims are disputed among some authorities.[116] However, because they selectively block prostacyclin production, COX-2 inhibitors leave thromboxane unopposed, which can lead to thrombotic events.

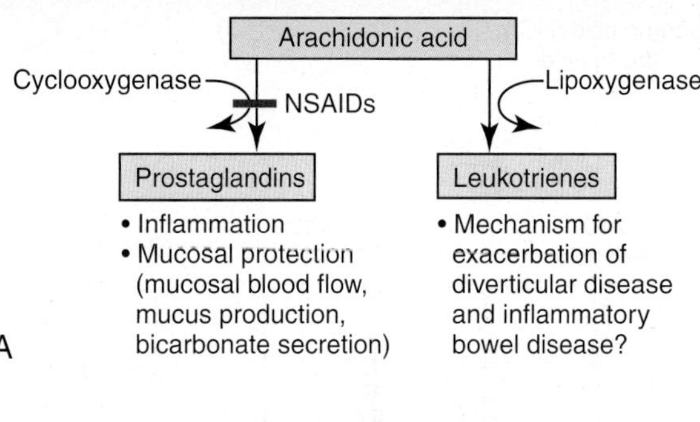

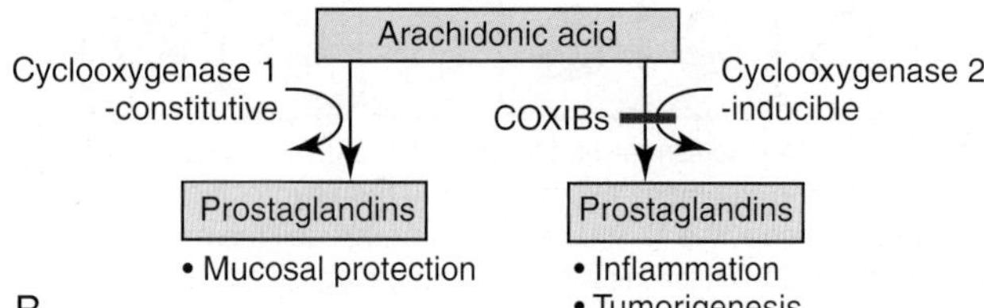

FIGURE 12.10 Mechanism of action of NSAIDs. A, Nonselective NSAIDs interfere with cyclooxygenase metabolism of arachidonic acid, leading to reduction in prostaglandins, some of which are responsible for inflammation. However, some prostaglandins promote mucosal health and the decrease in production of these prostaglandins may enhance NSAID injury to the mucosa. Additionally, by interfering with the cyclooxygenase pathway, NSAIDs shunt more arachidonic acid to the lipoxygenase pathway, with increased production of leukotrienes. The increase in leukotrienes may explain the paradoxical worsening of diverticular disease or inflammatory bowel disease in some patients consuming NSAIDS. **B,** COX-2 selective inhibitors (COXIBs) selectively interfere with the COX-2 isoform relative to the COX-1 isoform. These agents reduce the prostaglandins responsible for inflammation relative to prostaglandins that promote mucosal health and may reduce the incidence of gastrointestinal toxicity associated with NSAIDs.

The mechanisms whereby NSAIDs affect the lower GI tract may be similar to the ones that cause upper GI tract injury. Direct toxic effects on the mucosa, depletion of enterocyte ATP, and increased intestinal permeability have been proposed as having a role in lower GI tract injury.[117] Consistent with this theory is the fact that the ability of an NSAID to enter the enterohepatic circulation correlates with its ability to damage the intestinal tract, presumably by increasing the exposure time of the intestinal mucosa to high concentrations of the agents.[117] However, parenteral administration of NSAIDs may also lead to lower GI tract injury, suggesting a systemic mechanism related to prostaglandin suppression, although oral preparations usually result in a greater degree of injury than parenteral formulations.[117] The diversion of arachidonic acid to the lipoxygenase pathway results in the formation of leukotrienes and other inflammatory mediators, possibly explaining the paradoxical exacerbation of IBD and diverticular disease experienced by some patients who take NSAIDs.[86] Yet another potential mechanism through which NSAIDs may damage the lower GI tract is ischemia. Intravenous indomethacin causes rapid splanchnic vasoconstriction in dogs. This may be sufficient to cause damage at "watershed" sites in the GI tract.

Several factors determine the likelihood of suffering from complications of NSAID use. These include age, alcohol use, smoking, concomitant *Helicobacter pylori* infection, the type of NSAID, and the duration of use. Older age, alcohol use, and smoking are risk factors for complications due to NSAIDs, although the level of risk is difficult to quantify.[82] The role of *H. pylori* is complex. Some evidence suggests that the risk of NSAID injury is paradoxically greater in *H. pylori*–negative patients, perhaps because *H. pylori* infection increases prostaglandin levels in gastric mucosa.[70] Other studies suggest that *H. pylori* significantly increases the risk of ulcer or bleeding in NSAID users, and that eradication of *H. pylori* before starting NSAID therapy markedly reduces the incidence of ulcers or bleeding.[118-120] *H. pylori* has numerous effects on the gastric mucosa, including enhancing prostaglandin production and increasing neutrophilic inflammation, and these may influence NSAID-induced gastric injury in a variety of ways.[118] The duration of NSAID use may affect the types of injury sustained as well. Short-term use is more often seen with gastric erosions or bleeding, whereas long-term use is associated with ileal and colonic strictures. The type of NSAID may also be relevant for certain forms of injury. For example, the small intestine is exposed to higher concentrations of NSAIDs that enter the enterohepatic circulation, increasing the likelihood of intestinal injury with those agents. Other factors that may distinguish NSAIDs and their risk of GI complications include their COX-1 and COX-2 selectivity and plasma half-life.[82]

Esophagitis and Esophageal Strictures

Pill esophagitis can be caused by various NSAIDs (see section on pill esophagitis). Several studies have shown an association between NSAID use and erosive or necrotizing esophagitis, a greater severity of esophagitis, or less improvement of esophagitis at the time of follow-up biopsy,[121-126] but other studies have not shown an association between NSAID use and the presence or severity of esophagitis.[127,128] NSAID usage has also been associated with an increased risk of esophageal strictures.[16,129,130]

Reactive Gastropathy

Up to 45% of patients taking NSAIDs will develop chemical gastritis or reactive gastropathy.[131-133] This pattern of gastritis has not been shown to be a predictor of ulcer or bleeding risk in these patients.[27]

Erosions and Ulcers

NSAID erosions are usually located in the gastric body and typically heal within several days whether or not the NSAID is continued. In contrast, NSAID ulcers are often large and multiple, are more common in the gastric antrum than the duodenum, and are usually painless.[119,134] Lower GI ulcers most commonly involve the ileocecal region or proximal colon.[135] However, examination with double-balloon endoscopy or capsule endoscopy can uncover mucosal breaks or ulcers in segments of the small intestine that are traditionally not amenable to endoscopic examination.[136,137] Histologically, these ulcers are entirely nonspecific and are indistinguishable from other idiopathic benign colonic ulcers. Complications include stenoses/strictures, bleeding, and perforation.[134]

NSAID Colitis

Patients who develop NSAID colitis typically have been taking NSAIDs for a few months, but often less than 1 year, for inflammatory conditions such as arthritis. Implicated

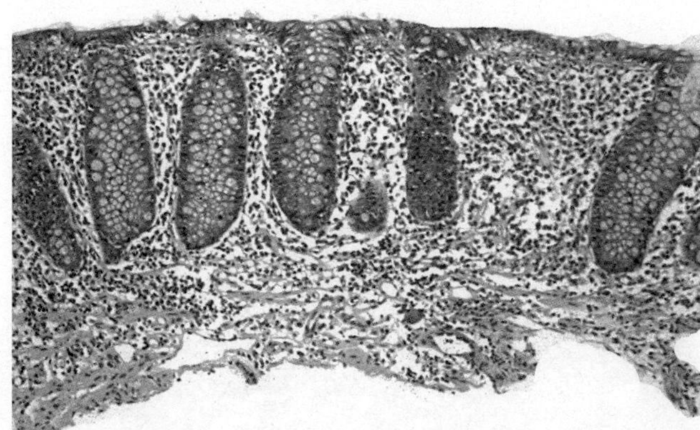

FIGURE 12.11 NSAID colitis. The colonic mucosa shows increased cellularity of the lamina propria with a mixed but predominantly lymphocytic infiltrate. Notice the resemblance to lymphocytic colitis or paucicellular lymphocytic colitis.

most frequently are sustained-release NSAIDs, fenamate NSAIDs, and diclofenac preparations, although it is unclear whether this is a reflection of their popularity. Women outnumber men. Presenting symptoms include bloody diarrhea, weight loss, iron-deficiency anemia, and abdominal pain.[138,139] Colonoscopy may be normal or may show nonspecific inflammatory changes, including erythema, friability, small ulcers, or aphthous ulcers.[139] Any segment of the colon may be affected, including segmental involvement or even pancolonic involvement (pancolitis).[139,140] Cessation of NSAIDs causes resolution of the diarrhea and histological inflammation.[138] In protracted cases, some evidence suggests that patients may respond to steroids, sulfasalazine, or metronidazole.

Goldstein and Cinenza[39] described the histological features of 14 cases of NSAID colitis in 1998. In their series, patchy colitis was present in 13 cases. Histological examination showed an inflammatory infiltrate that was mild in 9 cases and marked in 5, and composed of a mixed infiltrate of lymphocytes, plasma cells, and neutrophils in 8 cases, predominantly neutrophilic inflammation in 4, and predominantly lymphoplasmacytic infiltrate in 2 (Fig. 12.11). Seven cases showed surface erosion. Crypt "disarray" and mildly increased surface intraepithelial lymphocytes were noted in occasional cases, but none had crypt distortion, granulomas, markedly increased surface intraepithelial lymphocytes, thickened subepithelial collagen table, or surface epithelial apoptotic bodies. Therefore they concluded that NSAID colitis is in the differential with other diseases that may show FAC or nonspecific inflammation in the colon, including Crohn's disease and infectious colitis.

Additional series have further defined the possible spectrum of NSAID colitis. In a case-control study of 31 patients with collagenous colitis, Riddell et al.[57] demonstrated a significantly more prevalent use of NSAIDs in patients with collagenous colitis than in controls (19 vs. 4, respectively). In this report, NSAID use preceded the onset of diarrhea in all 19 patients using NSAIDs, the diarrhea improved in 3 patients after cessation of NSAIDs, and rechallenge in 1 patient resulted in a recurrence of diarrhea. The authors suggested that the association between collagenous colitis and arthritis might be, in fact, due to NSAIDs. NSAIDs also have been implicated in lymphocytic colitis. In a study of 40 patients with lymphocytic colitis, half of the patients were using NSAIDs, and patients on NSAIDs had higher surface intraepithelial lymphocyte counts.[59] In 2004, Goldstein and Bhanot[141] described a paucicellular variant of lymphocytic colitis that had similar clinical associations with classic lymphocytic colitis, namely the female predominance, frequent normal appearance endoscopically, and frequent presentation with watery stools. The frequency of NSAID use was similar in this group and the classic lymphocytic colitis group (21% and 24%, respectively). In a third group of 100 asymptomatic patients with descending colonic biopsies obtained during screening colonoscopy, NSAID use was reported in 39% of patients with morphologically normal colonic mucosal biopsies, 50% of patients with paucicellular lymphocytic colitis, and 75% of patients with classic lymphocytic colitis. They concluded that paucicellular lymphocytic colitis should be considered as part of the spectrum of lymphocytic colitis and that NSAIDs are associated with this pattern of colitis. They noted that the pattern of paucicellular lymphocytic colitis is similar to some of the cases in their original description of NSAID colitis. Other reports substantiate the link between NSAID use and microscopic colitis,[139,142,143] although not all studies have confirmed this association.[60-62,144,145]

Other forms of colitis have been reported with NSAIDs. In a report on 11 cases of NSAID colitis, Puspok et al.[139] described a pattern similar to ischemic colitis in 9 cases (Fig. 12.12). A report of eosinophilic colitis with clinical features of hypersensitivity has also been reported.[37] Two cases of acute colitis, with neutrophilic cryptitis and mucin depletion, were reported in patients on etodolac.[40] A case of pseudomembranous colitis was reported in a patient taking diclofenac.[146] Increased apoptosis has been described in patients on NSAIDs. Deshpande et al.[147] reported frequent NSAID use among patients with unexplained chronic colitis, raising the possibility that NSAIDs can cause colitis indistinguishable from IBD.

Diaphragm Disease

A rare but distinctive complication of long-term (longer than 1 year) NSAID use is termed *diaphragm disease*.[148,149] Patients often present with subacute intestinal obstruction, abdominal pain, iron-deficiency anemia, or fecal occult blood,[148,150-153] and in one case[154] the symptoms presented 2 years after cessation of NSAID use. Other presentations include chronic diarrhea, change in bowel habits, or weight loss. The disease has been difficult to recognize in the past, but the introduction of new techniques to visualize remote segments of the small bowel, such as retrograde double-balloon enteroscopy and capsule endoscopy, has aided in identifying the pathological diaphragms. Interestingly, retention of the video capsule behind the strictures is reported.[148,153] The most common radiological findings include strictures and bowel wall thickening, mimicking Crohn's disease.[153] Grossly, the characteristic lesion is a thin concentric mucosal web or diaphragm (Fig. 12.13).[150,155,156] These diaphragms commonly affect the ileum, ascending, or proximal transverse colon.[139,150-153,156] They frequently are numerous (averaging about nine), cluster in the same general region, and are very difficult to detect from inspection of the external surface of the bowel.[148,155,156] Histologically,

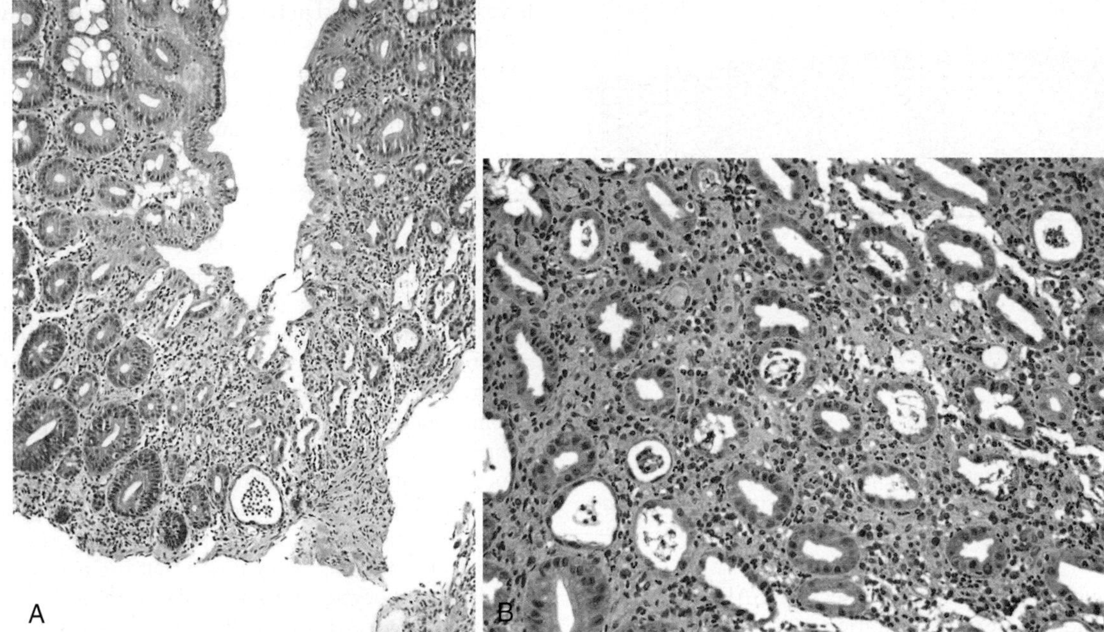

FIGURE 12.12 **NSAID colitis with ischemic pattern. A,** A colonic mucosal biopsy of a patient with clinically proven NSAID colitis shows a pattern resembling ischemic colitis, with withered, degenerate crypts, focal crypt abscess, and sparse inflammation in the lamina propria. **B,** A high-power view shows withered degenerate crypts with mucin depletion, mixed lamina propria infiltrates, and patchy crypt inflammation. (*Courtesy Dr. Laura Lamps.*)

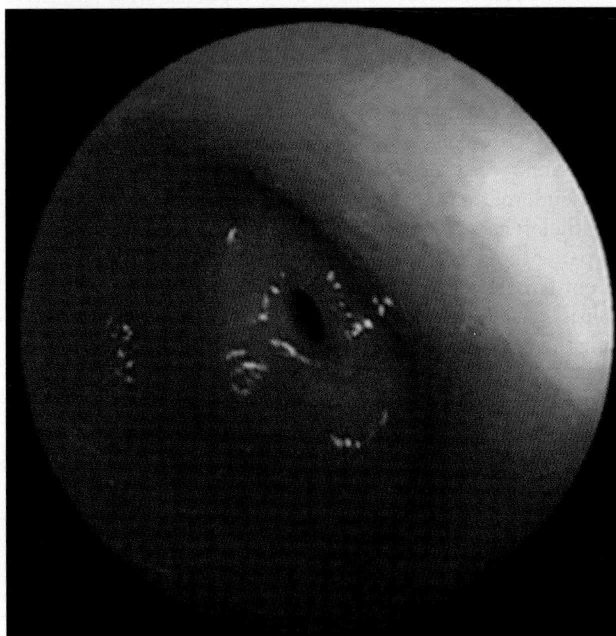

FIGURE 12.13 Diaphragm disease. Endoscopic image of a mucosal diaphragm shows the narrowed lumen with circumferential diaphragm-like mucosal web. (*From Nosho K, Endo T, Yoda Y, et al. Diaphragm disease of small intestine diagnosed by double-balloon enteroscopy. Gastrointest Endosc. 2005;62[1]:187-189.*)

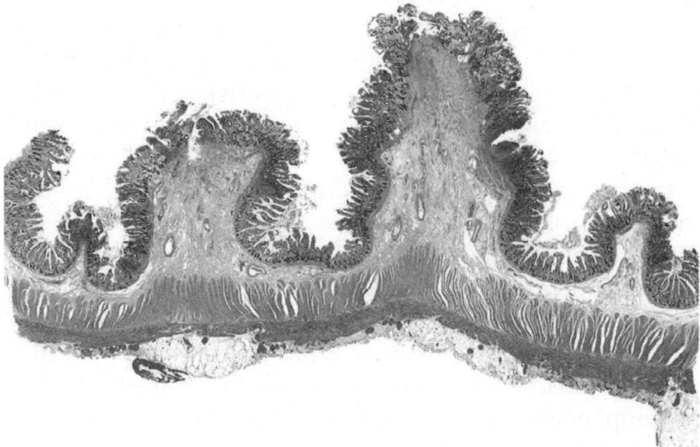

FIGURE 12.14 Diaphragm disease. Histologically, the diaphragms are composed of submucosal fibrosis with erosion or ulceration at the apex. (*From Parfitt JR, Driman DK. Pathological effects of drugs on the gastrointestinal tract: a review. Human Pathol. 2007;38[4]:527-536.*)

submucosal fibrosis and mild mucosal inflammation may be the only findings (Fig. 12.14).[156] A chaotic arrangement of smooth muscle fibers, vascular elements, and neural elements resembling neuromuscular and vascular hamartomas has been described.[148,149,157] Mucosal erosions or ulcers may be seen at the apex of the stricture.[149,156] Other mucosal changes are variable, and include villous blunting, cryptitis, rare crypt abscesses, increased eosinophils, or pseudopyloric metaplasia.[149,156] The presumed mechanism involves the formation of a linear ulcer along the crests of haustral folds, with subsequent repair and fibrosis. The resulting band of fibrosis constricts in a "purse-string" fashion to form a mucosal diaphragm. Endoscopic balloon dilatation has been reported to be successful in the initial management of diaphragms.[158] Otherwise, resection is required. Recurrence has been reported.[156] Although intuitively a direct toxic effect from the NSAIDs on the intestinal mucosa would seem to be the likeliest mechanism of injury, reports of diaphragms in patients treated with suppositories[159] and in bypassed ileal segments suggest a systemic mechanism.[155] In one series, diaphragms were associated with *CYP2C9*3* polymorphism, which causes higher plasma concentrations of NSAIDs in those individuals,[160] also suggestive of a systemic effect.

Perforation

Perforation of the GI tract is usually a complication of ulcer disease or diverticular disease, and NSAID use is associated with an increased risk of this complication,[86,134,161] which carries a higher mortality than other forms of NSAID-induced GI disease. The risk of NSAID-related GI perforation is similar in the upper and lower GI tract.[162] The type of NSAID and its plasma half-life play a role in the risk of perforation.[162]

Exacerbation of Diverticular Disease or Inflammatory Bowel Disease

NSAIDs may exacerbate preexisting colonic disease. Patients on NSAIDs have a relative risk of 1.52 of having symptomatic diverticular disease relative to patients not on these agents.[163] Significantly, diverticular bleeding, perforation, and fistula-formation have been reported with NSAID use.[86,164-167] Several observational studies report that NSAIDs may precipitate relapse in patients with preexisting IBD, particularly in those with ulcerative colitis.[168-170] GI symptoms and flares of IBD have also been described with rofecoxib, a selective COX-2 inhibitor, but symptoms generally resolve with discontinuation of the NSAID.[171,172] Other studies have failed to find an association between NSAIDs and flares in IBD.[173,174] One survey-based study found that low doses of NSAIDs did not affect disease activity, but higher doses (≥5 times/month) were associated with active disease at follow-up in Crohn's patients only.[175]

Differential Diagnosis

NSAID-induced injury is difficult to distinguish from injury related to other agents. In the stomach, NSAID damage is indistinguishable from reactive gastritis from other causes, such as bile or alcohol. NSAID colitis must be considered in any colonic biopsy from a patient with diarrhea that has increased cellularity of the lamina propria with features of lymphocytic or collagenous colitis. Given the wide range of morphology associated with NSAIDs, it may also be necessary to consider NSAIDs in cases of ischemic colitis, pseudomembranous colitis, or colonic perforation. There are no morphological distinguishing features to distinguish NSAIDs from the other causes of these conditions. Diaphragm disease may be difficult to distinguish from other stricturing disorders, and a history of long-term NSAID use may be the most important distinguishing characteristic. NSAID strictures tend to be narrow-based, multiple, and located in the ileum and/or right colon.

Proton Pump Inhibitors

PPIs are frequently used to treat gastroesophageal reflux and peptic ulcer disease. These agents block gastric acid production by binding the H^+, K^+ -ATPase on the canalicular surface of the parietal cell membrane. They are very effective at reducing gastric acidity. However, evidence that they exacerbate corpus gastritis and atrophy, cause endocrine cell hyperplasia and gastric polyps, and are associated with microscopic colitis have caused some concern regarding their long-term safety. They may also confer an increased risk of developing C. *difficile* infection or bacterial gastroenteritis.[104-106,108]

Exacerbation of Corpus Gastritis and Atrophy

One possible consequence of long-term use of PPIs is exacerbation of corpus gastritis and atrophy, precursors of gastric cancer. Typically, *H. pylori* colonizes the gastric antrum more effectively than the corpus, and this is possibly related to acid production by the corpus.[176] Suppression of gastric acidity presumably allows the organisms to colonize the corpus, because it either enables better contact between the organisms and the corpus foveolar epithelium, or reduces buffering of the ammonia produced by the organism, or both.[176] The result may be increased corpus gastritis and atrophy in some patients.[176-184] Some reports found no association between PPI use and the development or progression of gastric atrophy in *H. pylori*–infected patients, even though some authors confirmed that the corpus shows worse gastritis.[185-189] A recent meta-analysis of the literature supports the fact that PPI use is associated with higher rates of gastric atrophy in patients with *H. pylori*, but a lower rate of atrophy in *H. pylori*–negative patients.[190] Even without atrophy, corpus-predominant gastritis in *H. pylori* infection has been shown to place patients at increased risk for the development of gastric cancer.[191] Because treatment of *H. pylori* reverses corpus gastritis,[178] patients should be evaluated for *H. pylori* and treated for the infection before beginning long-term therapy with PPIs.[192]

Endocrine Hyperplasia

Patients given antisecretory drugs show compensatory increased gastrin levels, and the clinical relevance of hypergastrinemia has been explored in numerous studies. Patients treated with H_2 histamine antagonists may have up to a twofold rise in serum gastrin level, but endocrine cell hyperplasia has not been a problem in this patient group.[193] Long-term treatment with omeprazole is also associated with a twofold to fourfold increase in serum gastrin level in a subset of patients.[180,182,183,193,194] Gastrin is trophic for fundic mucosa and the enterochromaffin-like (ECL) cells.[195] Endocrine cell hyperplasia has been documented among patients on long-term proton pump blockade therapy.[179,180,183,194] In the last several years, gastric neuroendocrine tumors occurring in patients on very-long-term PPI therapy have been reported,[196-198] but whether the association is more than coincidental is not clear at this time.

Parietal Cell Hyperplasia and Fundic Gland Polyps

Some patients taking PPIs develop parietal cell hyperplasia of the corpus characterized by enlarged and more numerous parietal cells that protrude into the gland lumen (Fig. 12.15).[199-201] Fundic gland cysts may follow, presumably due to obstruction of acid flow out of the gland by the protruding parietal cells, resulting in an appearance similar to that of fundic gland polyps (FGPs).[199,201] Several early reports in the literature described FGPs (sometimes multiple) in patients subjected to prolonged PPI use.[202-204] Furthermore, some of the reported patients experienced disappearance of the polyps with discontinuation of the PPI, and recurrence with resumed use of the medication.[202] Some authors disputed these findings, however.[205-207] The number of reported patients on PPIs with FGPs is small

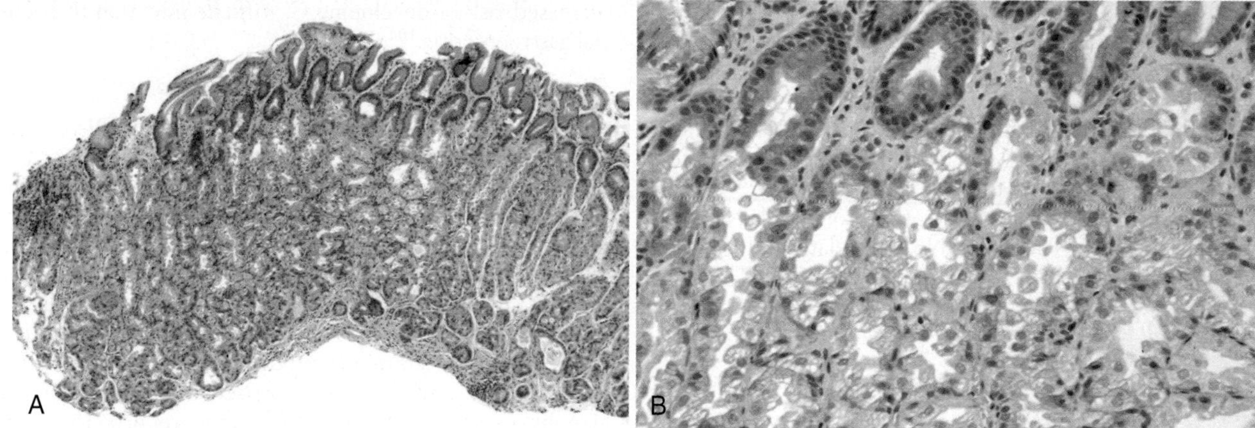

FIGURE 12.15 Parietal cell hyperplasia. A, The oxyntic mucosa shows expansion of the parietal cell mass, with distended parietal cells protruding into the gland lumen. **B,** High-power view showing distended parietal cells with vacuolated cytoplasm protruding into the gland lumen.

relative to the large number of patients currently on PPIs. Also, FGPs occur in patients without *H. pylori*[208] (possibly because the enzymatic degradation of gastric mucus by the organisms facilitates outflow from the gastric glands and protects against mucosal cyst formation), and the role of this infection as a confounding factor has been questioned. In a case-control study limited to patients without *H. pylori* gastritis, the incidence of FGPs among patients taking PPIs was similar to that of a control population,[209] although they included patients who had taken PPIs for only 4 weeks. Since that report, several studies have confirmed that prolonged PPI use is strongly associated with the development of polyps.[210-212] In a prospective study, PPI use was the strongest risk factor for the development of FGPs, with an odds ratio of 9 in multiple logistic regression.[212] A recent meta-analysis of the literature showed that PPI use was associated with an odds ratio of 2.46 for the development of FGPs, and that the risk increased with more than 12 months of exposure.[213]

Microscopic Colitis

Thomson et al.[58] reported a series of six patients who developed either lymphocytic (five cases) or collagenous (one case) colitis secondary to lansoprazole. All of them developed colitis after switching from omeprazole to lansoprazole, and all resolved within a week of cessation of the drug. Case-control studies have corroborated the association between PPI use and microscopic colitis,[61,62] with one study showing a particularly high association with combined PPIs and NSAIDs.[60] However, one study found no association.[145]

Differential Diagnosis

Parietal cell hyperplasia secondary to PPIs can be a mimic of the gastric changes in Zollinger-Ellison syndrome. The latter often has more cystic dilatation of the glands. Also, PPI use is obviously manyfold more likely than Zollinger-Ellison syndrome. Clinical information can help distinguish the two.

Resins

The crystals of various resins have been described in GI tract pathology material, of which the most important is Kayexalate because of its association with colonic necrosis. The characteristics of the crystals and their staining properties using acid-fast stain, periodic acid–Schiff (PAS) with diastase digestion, or Congo red stains can aid in distinguishing among the various resins. The acid-fast bacillus (AFB) stain has been touted as most useful in the distinction of the various crystals (Table 12.2).[214,215] However, specific identification of a resin by its crystals and its staining properties can be unreliable. Reviewing the patient's medication list is the easiest (and most cost-effective) way to identify a resin when crystals are encountered in GI pathology material.

Sodium Polystyrene Sulfonate (Kayexalate)

Hyperkalemia develops in patients with chronic renal insufficiency and is often treated with Kayexalate, a cation-exchange resin administered either orally or as an enema. To reduce the risk of constipation and impaction, sodium polystyrene sulfonate is mixed with a hypertonic solution of sorbitol, a cathartic agent. Several series have been reported of acute colonic necrosis in patients given sodium polystyrene sulfonate in sorbitol with a mortality rate in one series of 36%.[216-222] Most, but not all, cases occurred postoperatively, in patients with end-stage renal disease, or in patients with uremia.[218]

The extent of necrosis has been variable, ranging from the entire colon, rectum, and portions of the terminal ileum to segmental colonic necrosis. Pseudomembranes have been described along with other, nonspecific features of colonic necrosis (dusky discoloration, ulcers, edema, etc.). Histologically, the lesions range from mucosal necrosis to transmural necrosis with perforation, mucosal ulcers, or pseudomembranes. The diagnostic finding is the presence of Kayexalate crystals overlying the necrotic or ulcerated area. Kayexalate crystals are refractile and slightly basophilic, with a "mosaic" pattern. They stain red with either PAS or acid-fast stain (Fig. 12.16).[216,217]

In the initial description of this condition, Lillemoe et al.[223] demonstrated that the culprit is not sodium polystyrene sulfonate, but the sorbitol with which it is administered. However, colonic necrosis in patients administered calcium polystyrene sulfonate (Kalimate) not suspended in sorbitol has been reported, suggesting that polystyrene sulfonate itself may be pathogenic.[224] Patients treated with sodium polystyrene

TABLE 12.2 Comparison of the Histological Characteristics and Staining Properties of the Various Crystals That Can Be Encountered in Gastrointestinal Pathology Material

	H&E Characteristics	Acid-Fast Stain	PAS stain	Congo Red Stain
Kayexalate	Deep violet, with cracks in a mosaic pattern	Magenta to black	Magenta	Unstained
Sevelamer	Two-toned pink and yellow, with curvilinear cracks in fish-scale pattern	Magenta	Violet	
Bile acid sequestrants	Orange to magenta, smooth with infrequent cracks	Dull yellow	Gray to pink	Bright vermillion

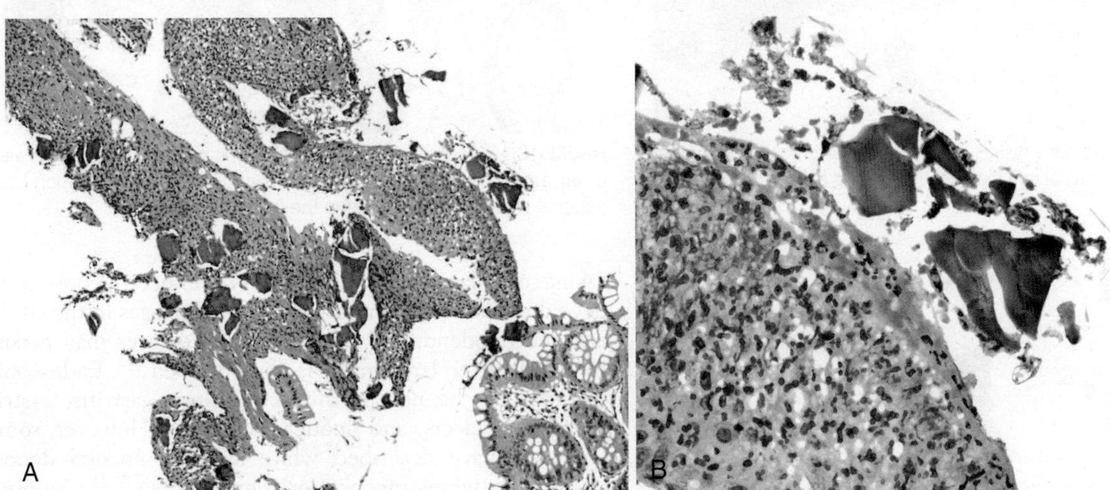

FIGURE 12.16 Colonic ulcer due to Kayexalate. A, A section of the ulcer shows fibrinopurulent exudate with numerous embedded crystals. **B,** High-power view shows the characteristic basophilic crystal of Kayexalate with a mosaic pattern.

sulfonate without sorbitol suffer GI side effects, but compared with patients who received sorbitol, they are more likely to be chronic users, more likely to have had oral administration as opposed to rectal enema, and less likely to have bowel necrosis, suggesting that sorbitol administration induces more severe complications.[225] The mechanism by which sodium polystyrene sulfonate/sorbitol induces colonic necrosis is not known, although uremia, changes in blood volume after dialysis, immunosuppressive therapy, peripheral vascular disease, and thrombocytopenia-related coagulation defects may be contributing factors. It is unclear whether renal failure predisposes patients to this complication, or whether patients with renal failure are simply more likely to be hyperkalemic and thus be given sodium polystyrene sulfonate.

Upper GI tract injury due to Kayexalate in sorbitol is uncommon. One case report describes a patient with serpiginous ulcers in the cecum and gastric antrum associated with Kayexalate crystals.[216] In a subsequent series,[226] 11 patients were found to have Kayexalate crystals in the esophagus only (3 cases), the stomach only (2), the duodenum (2), or the stomach and esophagus (4 patients). The crystals were either adherent to intact mucosa, or in 8 patients (73%) with ulcers or erosions, admixed with exudates. GI bleeding was the most common indication for biopsy (36%). Unlike the patients with lower GI tract injury, the patients with upper GI tract injury did not require surgical intervention.

Differential Diagnosis

Kayexalate-induced necrosis is difficult to distinguish from ischemic colitis or pseudomembranous colitis. The presence of Kayexalate crystals suggests Kayexalate-induced necrosis rather than other causes of ischemic colitis, although it is not conclusive. Kayexalate crystals must be distinguished from sevelamer and cholestyramine crystals, which have different microscopic appearances and staining properties. Also, food material can on occasion resemble Kayexalate crystals. Clinical details and drug ingestion history are imperative.

Sevelamer

Sevelamer is an anion-exchange resin used to treat hyperphosphatemia in patients with chronic renal disease. Sevelamer crystals have been described in the colon, small bowel, and esophagus, associated with a wide range of mucosal injury patterns, including bowel ischemia, necrosis, and colonic and esophageal ulcers.[227-231] They have also been found in colonic biopsies with only crypt disarray and Paneth cell metaplasia, mucosal prolapse, colonic inflammatory polyps, and colonic adenomas,[227] suggesting that in some cases the crystals may be incidental. Currently, it remains unclear whether sevelamer causes mucosal injury or is merely a bystander, although higher doses or impaction of the tablets may cause mucosal ulcers. The crystals differ from Kayexalate crystals in that they have curvilinear cracks that impart a "fish-scale" appearance and a two-tone color pattern of bright pink linear accents superimposed on a gray-yellow background (Fig. 12.17).[227] On PAS with diastase digestion the crystals acquire a violet color, and on AFB stain they acquire a magenta color.[214,227]

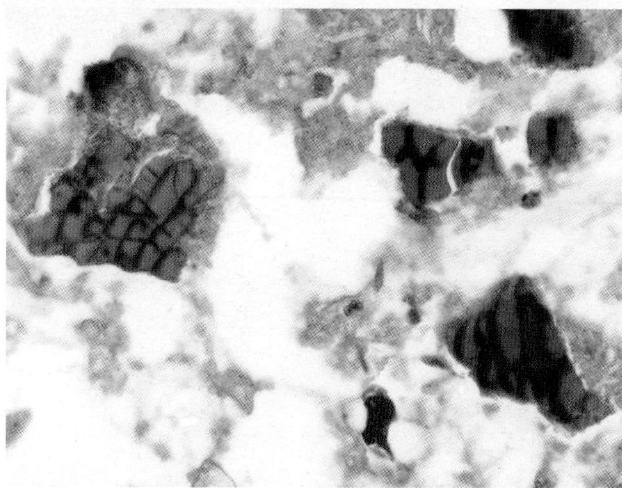

FIGURE 12.17 Sevelamer crystals have curvilineal cracks resembling fish scales. The crystals are yellow, with pink along the cracks.

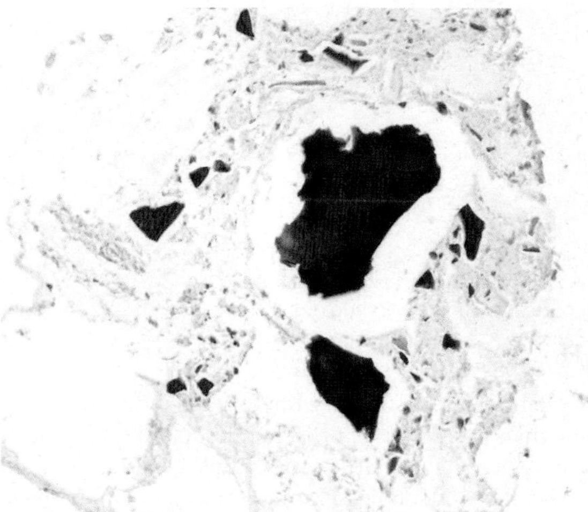

FIGURE 12.18 Cholestyramine crystals are magenta and have relatively few cracks.

Bile Acid Sequestrants

Bile acid sequestrants include cholestyramine, colesevelam, and colestipol. Since the introduction of statins to treat hypercholesterolemia, bile acid sequestrants are more often used to treat bile acid–mediated diarrhea. Crystals of these resins have been reported most often in the colorectum and in both normal and inflamed specimens, including erosions or ulcers.[232] The crystals are polygonal, with variable eosinophilic staining ranging from near black to magenta to orange (Fig. 12.18). One report describes curious round crystals embedded in colonic mucosa in a patient on colestipol.[233] The crystals are generally smooth and glassy, with few fracture lines, although larger crystals can mimic sevelamer. The crystals acquire a dull yellow color on AFB stain.[232] It is unlikely that bile acid sequestrants cause mucosal injury, and the crystals are probably bystanders.

Lanthanum

Lanthanum is a non–calcium-based phosphate binder, used to treat hyperphosphatemia in patients on dialysis. Patients

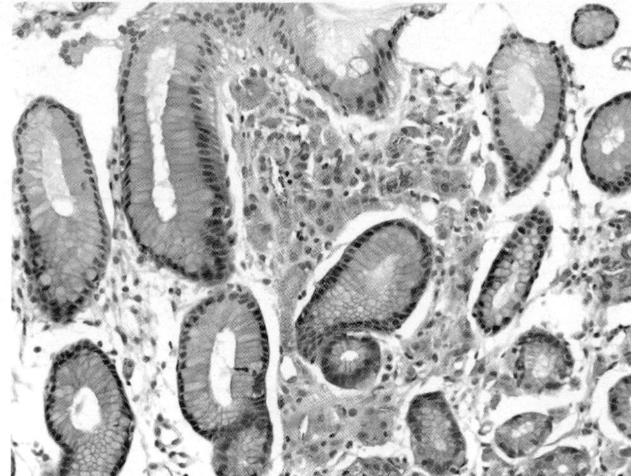

FIGURE 12.19 Lanthanum deposits in gastric mucosa. High-power view of an antral biopsy shows gray-brown and focally purple amorphous material within histiocytes within the lamina propria.

taking oral lanthanum carbonate have been reported to develop deposits of lanthanum in macrophages in the stomach and duodenum,[234-244] which in rare cases may persist for years after lanthanum is discontinued.[234] Endoscopic features can be nonspecific and include gastritis, gastric erosions or ulcers, and duodenal ulcers.[234] However, some observers have described white annular mucosal deposits, diffuse white mucosa, or white spots.[242-244] Biopsies of the stomach or duodenum show mucosal macrophages with amphophilic granular amorphous material with coarse brown to deep purple refractile deposits (Fig. 12.19).[234-238] Iron stains may show weak staining, causing confusion with iron therapy gastritis.[234,236] Energy-dispersive X-ray spectroscopy has confirmed that the deposits contain lanthanum, phosphorus, and calcium.[234,235,237-239]

Iron Therapy

Patients taking iron tablets may sustain injury to esophageal or gastric mucosa. Characteristic brown crystalline material can be found in the lamina propria, in surface exudates, and less often in thrombosed vessels; the deposits are highlighted by Perl's Prussian blue stain (Fig. 12.20).[245-248] In most cases, the iron is associated with erosions or ulcers. A pattern of reactive gastropathy or chronic gastritis may be noted in some cases.[247,249] In the study by Abraham et al.,[249] half of the patients had underlying toxic, mechanical, or infectious conditions that might predispose them to mucosal injury, but others have argued that it is the iron itself that causes the injury.[248] Iron therapy has also been associated with iron in macrophages in the small bowel lamina propria, known as pseudomelanosis (Fig. 12.21).[248,250,251] The patterns of iron deposition seen with iron medication must be distinguished from iron within gastric glandular cells, which is more often seen in patients with hereditary hemochromatosis.

Differential Diagnosis

Reactive Gastropathy. Iron-induced gastric injury is histologically similar to reactive gastritis due to other causes. The

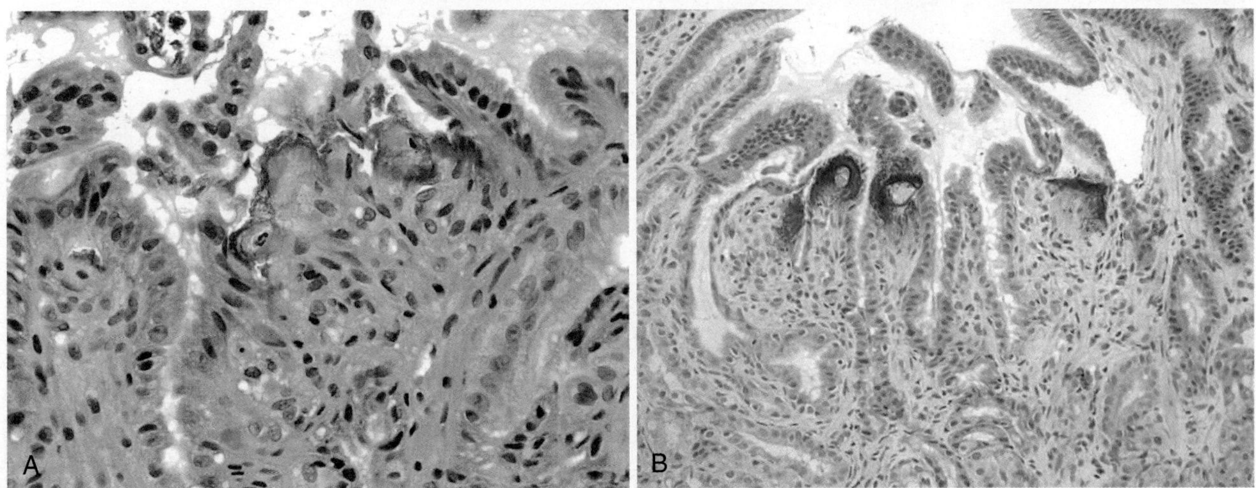

FIGURE 12.20 Iron therapy injury. A, A gray deposition is present in the gastric mucosa, undermining the surface epithelium, which appears injured. **B,** An iron stain confirms that the material is iron.

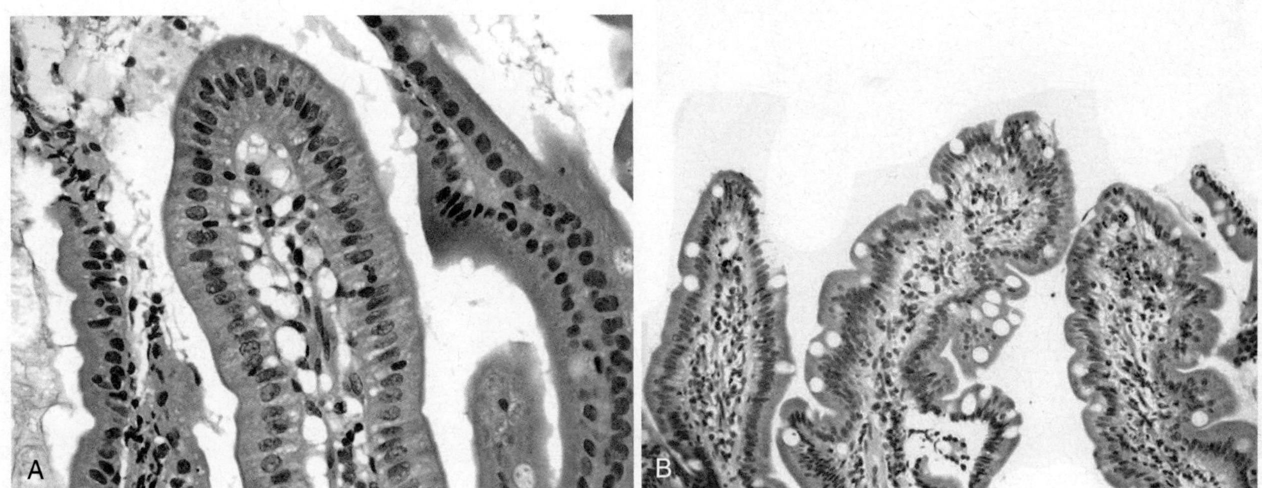

FIGURE 12.21 Pseudomelanosis. A, Pigment is present in macrophages in the lamina propria of this villus. **B,** An iron stain confirms the presence of iron in macrophages.

only distinguishing feature is the presence of iron crystals in the subepithelial lamina propria, which are highlighted by an iron stain.

OsmoPrep-Associated Gastritis. Rarely, patients prescribed OsmoPrep as bowel prep develop a pattern of reactive gastropathy with purple to black deposits in the superficial lamina propria.[252]

Antacids, Sucralfate, and Gastric Mucosal Calcinosis

Gastric mucosal calcinosis refers to small calcifications within the gastric mucosa, typically beneath the surface epithelium, either in the antrum or in the body (Fig. 12.22). They may stain deeply pink or be only partially calcified refractile material, some of which may be rimmed by histiocytes.[253] The gastric mucosa may be otherwise unremarkable, or show changes of reactive gastropathy. This condition is an example of metastatic calcification that occurs in patients with an imbalance of calcium and phosphate. Several conditions can lead to metastatic calcification, including drugs. In a report by Greenson et al.,[253] all patients with this condition were either orthotopic transplant patients or had chronic renal failure, and all were taking either aluminum-containing antacids or sucralfate. The authors suggested that these antacids play a role in the genesis of this condition. Elemental analysis of one case demonstrated that the deposits contained aluminum, phosphorus, calcium, and chlorine. Subsequently, Stroehlein et al.[254] reported six cases in renal transplant patients, none of whom was taking sucralfate and only one was taking low doses of an aluminum-containing antacid (Gelusil). Interestingly, many of these patients were taking H_2-receptor antagonists or PPIs, raising questions about the role of alkalization in precipitating calcium-phosphates in the stomach. Another case report describes gastric calcinosis in a nontransplant patient with dyspepsia and hypoparathyroidism who was taking various medications, including calcium acetate, calcitriol, and metoprolol (which contains small amounts of aluminum as an inactive ingredient).[255]

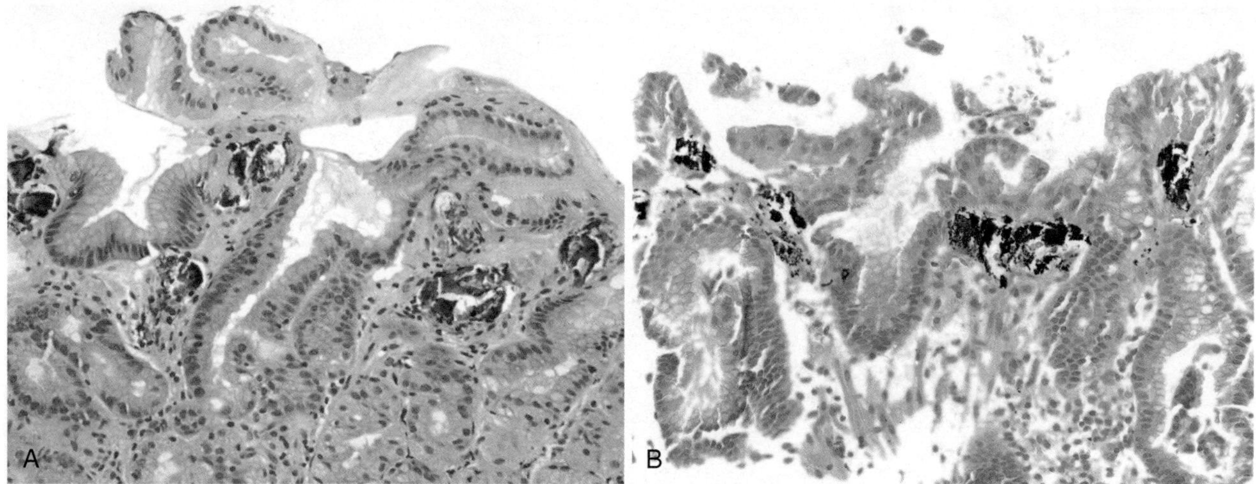

FIGURE 12.22 Gastric mucosal calcinosis. A, Basophilic crystalline material is present in the lamina propria of the stomach. The epithelium is mildly reactive. **B,** von Kossa stain confirms that the material contains calcium.

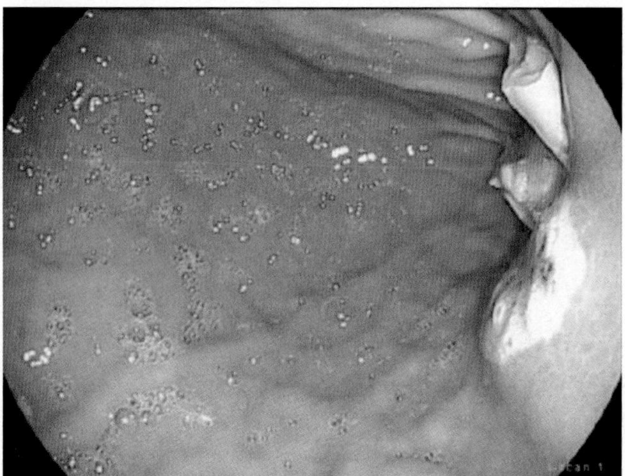

FIGURE 12.23 Endoscopic view of doxycycline injury within the stomach. The antrum shows a white plaquelike lesion *(right)*.

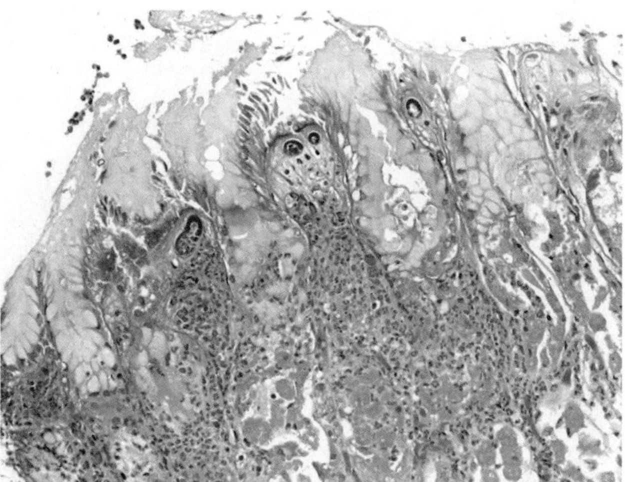

FIGURE 12.24 Doxycycline-induced gastric injury. The surface epithelium in this case is injured and the glands appear necrotic with a neutrophilic infiltrate in the lamina propria. The characteristic feature of doxycycline-induced injury is the eosinophilic degeneration of the subepithelial capillaries.

Doxycycline

In 2013, Xiao et al. reported a peculiar pattern of gastric injury in two patients taking doxycycline.[256] Both patients had white plaquelike lesions in the stomach (Fig. 12.23) that, on histological examination, showed reactive gastropathy with superficial mucosal necrosis and adherent fibrinoid material and curious eosinophilic vascular degeneration of superficial mucosal capillaries with fibrin thrombi (Fig. 12.24). Subsequently, others confirmed these findings in both stomach and duodenum,[23,257,258] and extended the description of vascular injury into the esophagus with descriptions of perivascular edema and endotheliitis in esophageal ulcers related to doxycycline (Fig. 12.25).[23,24]

Olmesartan

Olmesartan is an angiotensin II receptor antagonist used in the treatment of hypertension. In 2012, Rubio-Tapia et al. at the Mayo Clinic reported a series of 22 patients who had a severe enteropathy that required hospitalization in 14 of them.[28] Despite its histological resemblance to celiac disease or to collagenous sprue, olmesartan-induced enteropathy does not respond to gluten withdrawal and serological tests for celiac disease are generally negative. Histological features of olmesartan-induced enteropathy include total or partial villous atrophy, variably thickened subepithelial collagen table, active inflammation, and lymphocytic exocytosis in the superficial epithelium (Fig. 12.26).[28,259] Others have noted loss of goblet cells and increased apoptoses, reminiscent of autoimmune enteropathy.[260] Some patients have lymphocytic or collagenous colitis or gastritis as well.[28,261] Similar findings have also been reported with valsartan,[262] suggesting that other drugs in this class may produce similar pathology.

Mycophenolate Mofetil

Mycophenolate mofetil (MMF) is an immunosuppressive drug mainly used in the management of organ transplant rejection. MMF blocks the de novo pathway of purine

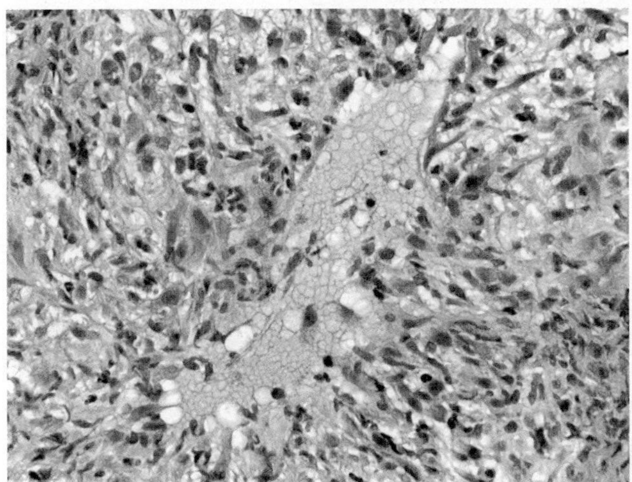

FIGURE 12.25 Doxycycline-induced esophageal ulcer. High-power view of a vessel in the base of the ulcer showing perivascular edema, endothelial injury, and reactive fibroblasts with scattered inflammatory cells.

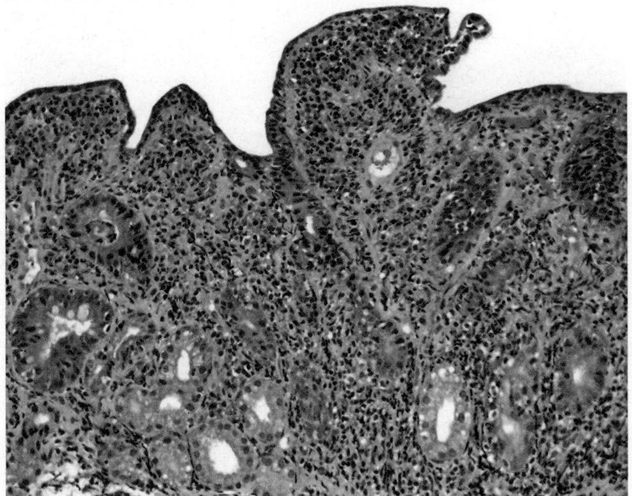

FIGURE 12.26 Duodenal biopsy in olmesartan injury showing villous atrophy with enterocyte injury, modest increase in surface lymphocytes, and expansion of the lamina propria, mimicking celiac disease.

synthesis, and enterocytes are partly dependent on this pathway; GI toxicity is one of the main limitations of the drug. Diarrhea, nausea, vomiting, dysphagia, dyspepsia, melena, and hematemesis are common presenting features of MMF toxicity.[31,34] Endoscopic findings may be relatively subtle, ranging from normal to nonspecific mild changes such as erythema.[33,34] Histological features vary according to the segment of the GI tract involved, but are reminiscent of graft-versus-host disease (GVHD) or Crohn's disease. In the esophagus, erosions or esophagitis may be seen.[31,34] In the stomach, reactive gastropathy, increased epithelial cell apoptoses, and granulomas are described.[31,34] In the small intestine, the villous atrophy, dilated damaged crypts, lamina propria edema, increased crypt apoptoses, and patchy neutrophilic inflammation may resemble GVHD or even celiac disease.[31-34] Colonic biopsies resemble GVHD with crypt architectural disarray, dilated damaged crypts, lamina propria edema, mild inflammation, and increased crypt apoptoses (Fig. 12.27).[34,91,263-266] Less often, the features in the small bowel and colon suggest Crohn's disease with patchy increased lamina propria inflammation, including neutrophils, lymphoid hyperplasia, granulomas, erosions or ulcers, and cryptitis or crypt abscesses.[34,91,265,267]

Differential Diagnosis

GVHD can closely resemble MMF toxicity. Clinical circumstances usually distinguish the two. However, if both are clinical considerations, histological features that suggest GVHD include a greater degree of crypt apoptotic microabscesses, more hypereosinophilic crypts, and residual endocrine cell aggregates, whereas eosinophils tend to be more common in MMF toxicity.[268]

Colchicine

Colchicine is an alkaloid used to treat gout and other medical conditions. Its effects are attributed to its ability to bind tubulin and inhibit its polymerization into microtubules, thereby interfering with neutrophil degranulation, chemotaxis, and mitosis. Patients with either renal or hepatic failure may develop colchicine toxicity, manifested by a

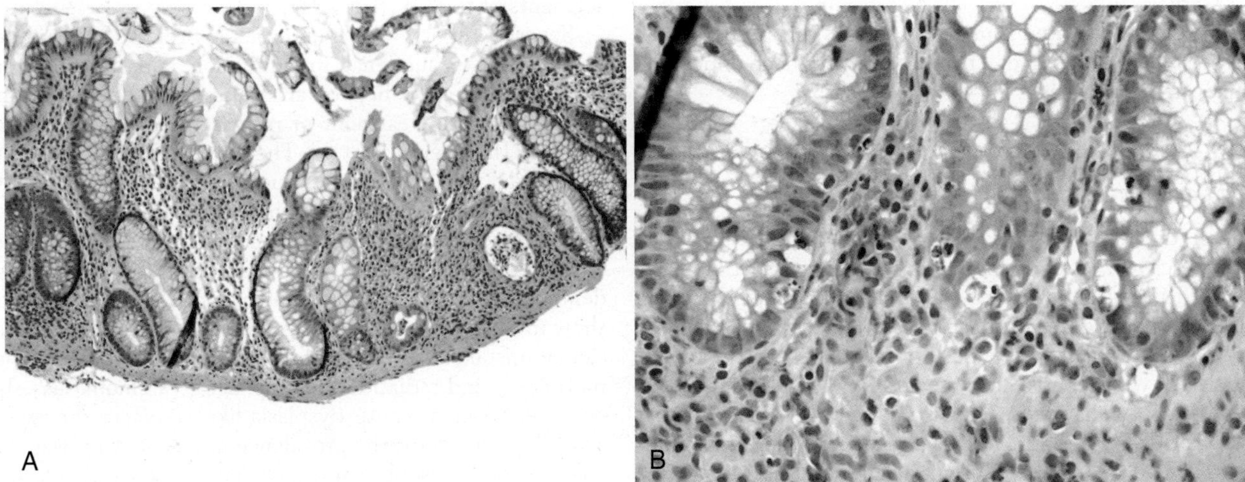

FIGURE 12.27 Mycophenolate mofetil toxicity. A, A low-power view shows features reminiscent of graft-versus-host disease with crypt disarray, crypt dropout, and mild inflammation. **B,** A high-power view shows increased crypt apoptoses.

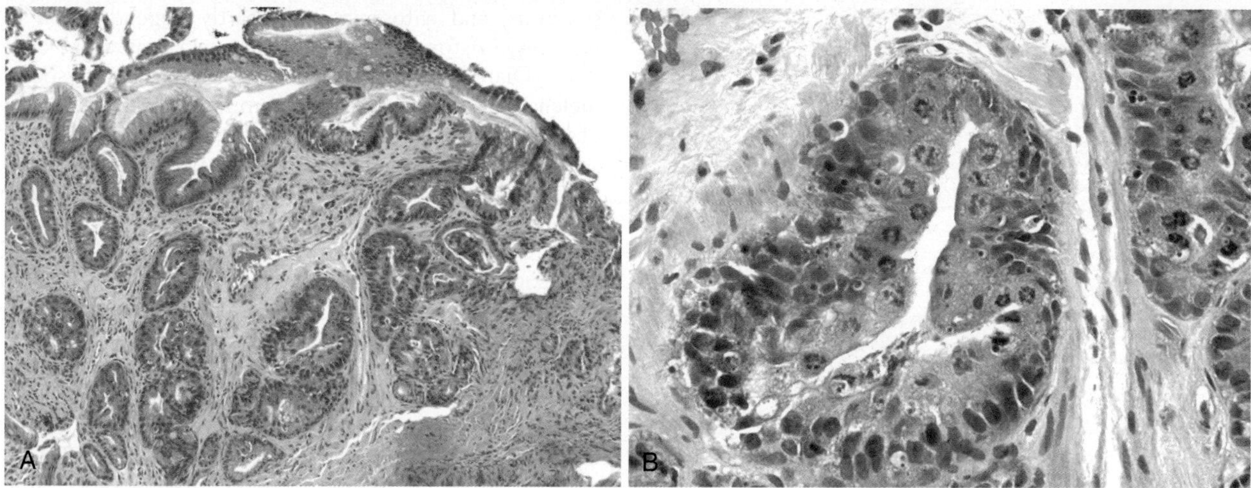

FIGURE 12.28 Colchicine toxicity. A, In this low-power view of a biopsy of the gastroesophageal junction, the glands appear hyperchromatic and disorganized, mimicking dysplasia. **B,** A high-power view demonstrates numerous mitotic figures arrested in metaphase, with several "ring" forms.

cholera-like syndrome associated with dehydration, shock, bone marrow suppression, and acute renal failure.[269] In the GI tract, colchicine toxicity is associated with variable mucosal injury in the esophagus, stomach, and small intestine. Reduced epithelial cell layers, nuclear swelling, and dyskeratosis have been described in the esophagus.[269] In the duodenum, variable villous atrophy, nuclear pseudostratification, loss of polarity, and increased apoptotic bodies have been described.[270] A characteristic finding is the presence of numerous mitoses arrested in metaphase, particularly in the neck cells.[269,270] These may assume a characteristic "ring" pattern (Fig. 12.28).[270] These changes are not observed in patients taking colchicine who do not have clinical evidence of toxicity.

Differential Diagnosis

Dysplasia. Colchicine toxicity can mimic dysplasia, given the nuclear pseudostratification, apoptotic debris, and increased mitotic figures. As with other non-neoplastic conditions that mimic dysplasia, colchicine toxicity shows epithelial maturation that provides evidence of a reactive condition. The ring mitoses are the primary distinguishing feature. Clinical history and drug ingestion history are necessary.

Chemotherapy-Related Injury. Numerous ring mitoses can be seen in the setting of chemotherapy-induced mucosal injury, such as taxanes.

Anticancer Therapies

Traditional Chemotherapy

Several GI complications related to chemotherapy have been described. Esophagitis with stricture formation has occurred in patients receiving combination chemotherapy (often containing doxorubicin [Adriamycin]) and radiation.[1,97,271] Capecitabine and 5-fluorouracil (5-FU) are associated with colitis characterized by crypts lined by flattened epithelial cells, occasional crypt apoptotic bodies, crypt dropout, and cytological atypia in the remaining crypts (Fig. 12.29).[272,273] Taxanes can be associated with mitotic arrest and ring mitoses, similar to colchicine, in the esophagus, gastroesophageal junction (Fig. 12.30), or other segments of the GI tract.[274,275]

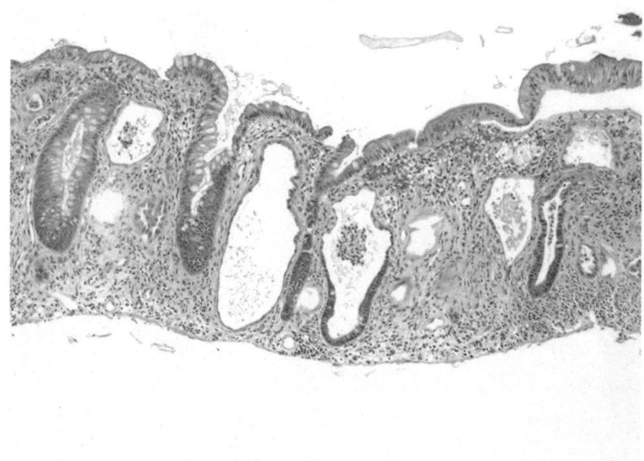

FIGURE 12.29 5-Fluorouracil (5-FU) colitis. The colonic mucosa shows preserved crypts immediately adjacent to dilated damaged crypt lined by attenuated epithelial cells.

Several reports of chemotherapy-related GI injury describe gastroduodenal inflammation and ulceration in patients undergoing hepatic arterial infusion chemotherapy (HAIC) for the treatment of primary or metastatic carcinoma of the liver.[72,73,276-278] The chemotherapeutic agents most often implicated are 5-fluoro-2-deoxuridine (FUDR) and mitomycin C. Patients with upper GI complaints after HAIC may have erosions and ulcers on endoscopy, most often in the antropyloric region, and less often in the duodenum and esophagus.[72,278] Histological examination may show marked epithelial atypia in the region of the ulcer that can be mistaken for early carcinoma.[73,276,277] Systemic chemotherapy and radiation for esophageal carcinoma has also been reported to cause dysplasia-like atypia in the stomach.[279] In one study, the prevalence of gastric dysplasia–like changes in the esophageal cancer population was 7.5%.[279] The authors describe dysplasia-like changes in the foveolar

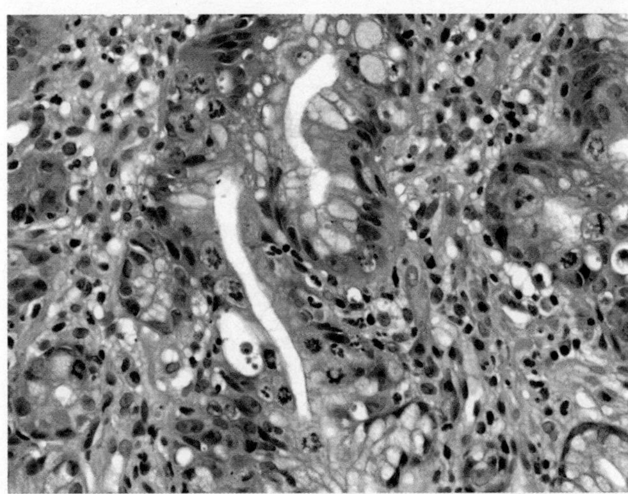

FIGURE 12.30 Taxane-induced injury of the gastroesophageal junction. In biopsies, the atypia of the gland epithelium with numerous ring mitoses can be mistaken for high-grade dysplasia.

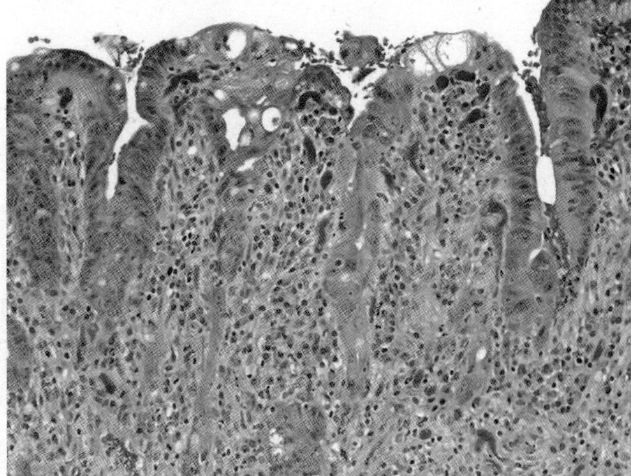

FIGURE 12.31 Chemotherapy-induced atypia of the duodenum in a Whipple specimen. The duodenum shows atrophy of the villi, with marked epithelial atypia characterized by cytoplasmic eosinophilia, vesicular nuclei with prominent nucleoli, and modest nuclear pleomorphism. The changes may be mistaken for dysplasia.

epithelium and atrophic features with microcyst formation in the glands (Fig. 12.31).

Differential Diagnosis

The atypia secondary to chemotherapy can mimic dysplasia or carcinoma. Features of these cases that assist in the distinction with carcinoma include preservation of mucosal architecture; atypia limited to or accentuated toward the basilar aspect of the glands; bizarre atypia exceeding that usually seen in carcinoma; low nuclear-to-cytoplasmic ratio; prominent cytoplasmic eosinophilia, often with vacuolization; few or no mitotic figures; cytological resemblance to radiation effect; similar atypia within fibroblasts and endothelial cells; and, in the stomach, absence of intestinal metaplasia in adjacent gastric epithelium.[277] In addition, in the stomach, chemotherapy atypia often involves both foveolar and gland epithelium.[279]

Immune Checkpoint Inhibitors

Immune checkpoint inhibitors (ICI) are a relatively new class of drugs that inhibit immune cell checkpoints, thereby increasing antitumor responses by T cells. Checkpoint blockade with checkpoint inhibitors has become standard therapy for many types of cancers. The most commonly targeted checkpoints are cytotoxic T lymphocyte–associated antigen 4 (CTLA-4), programmed cell death protein-1 (PD-1), and programmed cell death protein ligand-1 (PD-L1) receptors.

Patients treated with ICIs can develop diarrhea and enterocolitis, which can be life-threatening. CTLA-4 inhibitors are more likely to cause enterocolitis than PD-1 inhibitors. Diarrhea occurs in about 13% of patients on anti–PD-1 and in about 33% for anti–CTLA-4. Colitis occurs in 0.7% to 1.6% for anti–PD-1, 5% to 22% for anti–CTLA-4 and 13.6% for combination therapy.[46,280] Perforation of the colon or small intestine may occur.[55,281,282] In patients with preexisting IBD, the risk of flare is 30% with anti–CTLA-4 therapy, whereas the risk is low with anti–PD-1 therapy.[46] Treatment of ICI-induced colitis involves high-dose corticosteroids and infliximab or other NSAIDs.[49,55,283] Mortality is approximately 5%.[55] Some studies have shown that patients who develop immune-mediated diarrhea or colitis may have improved overall survival and progression-free survival than those who do not, possibly reflecting the magnitude of the immune response.[284]

With anti–CTLA-4 therapy, enterocolitis may develop after 1 to 10 doses of ipilimumab, with a median onset time of 1 month after infusion.[46] Nonbloody diarrhea, nausea and vomiting, and abdominal pain are common complaints.[55] Endoscopic features include edema, erythema, friability, multifocal or large ulcers, and fibrinopurulent exudates, usually involving the distal colon.[50,280,285-288] However, up to two-thirds of patients have extensive involvement of the colon, with endoscopic colitis proximal to the splenic flexure.[46,287,288] A continuous pattern of involvement is described in 45% to 79% of cases.[46,288] Upper GI findings can be normal despite histological changes.[50]

For anti–PD-1 therapy, the time of onset of symptoms is later than anti–CTLA-4 therapy, and is generally 2 to 4 months after treatment.[46] Delayed onset, up to 1 year after treatment, and recurrence after discontinuation of anti–PD-1 therapy have been described.[46] For combination therapy, the median time to onset is about 5 weeks.[46] Endoscopic findings include erythema, erosions, and ulcers, but a patchy distribution is seen in 75% of cases.[46] Two-thirds of patients investigated for GI adverse events secondary to anti–PD-1 therapy have upper GI tract abnormalities, including necrotizing gastritis.[46]

Histological features of ICI-induced colitis include expanded lamina propria with a lymphoplasmacytic and eosinophilic infiltrate, patchy cryptitis, increased apoptosis in crypts, and variably increased intraepithelial lymphocytes. Occasional cases may show more active inflammation, including crypt abscesses or ulcers (Fig. 12.32).[49,50,280,285-288] A pattern of ischemic colitis, lymphocytic colitis, or collagenous colitis has also been reported.[49,289-291] In cases with perforation, background mucosa may show crypt abscesses, inflammatory pseudopolyps, and fissures.[292] Although most cases show only limited crypt disarray,[287,288] recurrent colitis may show crypt distortion reminiscent of ulcerative colitis, but the increased crypt apoptosis distinguishes ICI-induced colitis from typical ulcerative colitis.

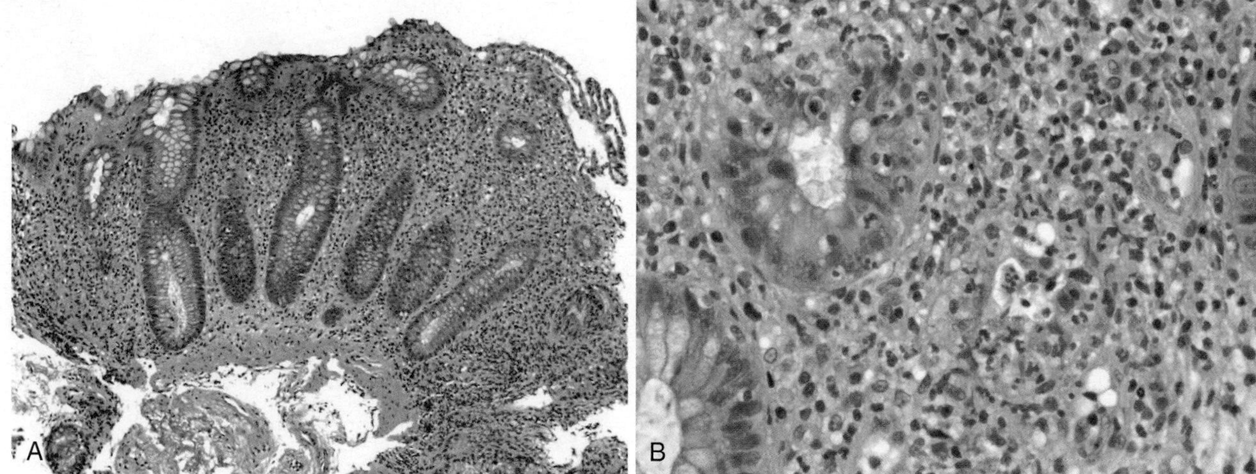

FIGURE 12.32 Inflammatory colitis secondary to cytotoxic T lymphocyte–associated antigen 4 (CTLA-4) antibodies. A, Colonic mucosal biopsy with lamina propria expansion by a mononuclear infiltrate. In this biopsy, crypt architecture is essentially preserved. **B,** High-power view demonstrates mixed infiltrates in the lamina propria, cryptitis *(left)* and crypt destruction *(right)*, mimicking inflammatory bowel disease.

Similar findings can be seen in the stomach and duodenum (Fig. 12.33). Mild changes include expansion of the lamina propria by lymphoplasmacytic inflammation, increased eosinophils, increased intraepithelial lymphocytes, and increased apoptosis.[30,50,55,293] Active gastritis or duodenitis with villous blunting may be seen, and infrequently gland abscesses are present in the stomach.[291] Rarely, the gastritis is severe, with edema, denuded mucosa, fibrinopurulent exudates, and brisk neutrophilic inflammation.[294] Esophagitis with numerous intraepithelial lymphocytes and dyskeratotic keratinocytes has been reported.[295] Ileal biopsies may show villous blunting, apoptosis, expansion of the lamina propria, and neutrophilic villitis.[291]

Differential Diagnosis

Ulcerative Colitis. ICI-induced colitis usually does not show marked crypt architectural distortion or basal plasmacytosis characteristic of ulcerative colitis. Cases of recurrent ICI-induced colitis may have crypt disarray that mimics ulcerative colitis, but often demonstrate increased crypt apoptosis that helps distinguish this disorder from idiopathic IBD.

Graft-Versus-Host Disease. The increased crypt apoptosis, preserved architecture, and crypt dropout may resemble GVHD. The clinical circumstances help differentiate the two.

Autoimmune Enteropathy. Increased crypt apoptosis, goblet cell depletion, and patchy intraepithelial lymphocytes may resemble autoimmune enteropathy. The history of checkpoint inhibitor therapy is essential to making the correct diagnosis.

Microscopic Colitis. A pattern of lymphocytic colitis or collagenous colitis may be seen in ICI-induced colitis. Increased apoptosis is usually a feature of ICI-induced colitis.

Idelalisib

Idelalisib is a selective inhibitor of phosphatidylinositol 3-kinase δ (PI3Kδ) that has antitumor effects against several hematopoietic malignancies, including chronic lymphocytic leukemia/small lymphocytic lymphoma, follicular lymphoma, and other low-grade B-cell lymphomas. About 40% of patients on idelalisib develop diarrhea that can be severe enough to require hospitalization. Colonoscopic features include mucosal erythema, congestion, granularity, erosions, ulcers, or pseudomembranes. In 2015, two groups simultaneously reported the histological features of enterocolitis resulting from idelalisib.[29,296] The colonic features are reminiscent of MMF colitis or GVHD. Intraepithelial lymphocytosis may be the only finding, resembling lymphocytic colitis. A common finding is increased crypt apoptosis, including "exploding" apoptotic epithelial cells in crypts and crypt dropout, strongly resembling GVHD (Fig. 12.34). Neutrophilic infiltration of the crypts, with crypt abscesses and attenuated glands, may be seen, and when this pattern is observed, either with or without the apoptotic crypt epithelial cells, it is important to exclude infectious agents such as cytomegalovirus (CMV), adenovirus, or human herpesvirus-6 (HHV-6).[297] Infrequently, there may be crypt disarray or Paneth cell metaplasia when the interval between the onset of diarrhea and biopsy is prolonged.[296] Small-intestinal biopsies may also show crypt apoptosis, with decreased goblet cells, increased intraepithelial lymphocytes, and villous blunting, mimicking celiac disease.[29] Less often, there may be crypt dropout with apoptosis mimicking GVHD.

Selective Internal Radiation

Selective internal radiation, in which radioactive yttrium-90 microspheres are injected rather than traditional chemotherapeutic agents, can be associated with gastroduodenal ulceration and the presence of black microspheres within mucosal capillaries (Fig. 12.35).[7,298-300]

Neutropenic Colitis

Neutropenic colitis is a clinicopathological syndrome characterized by an inflammatory or septic intraabdominal process in the setting of neutropenia, usually due to chemotherapy for hematological malignancy or solid tumors (or, less often, other causes of neutropenia).[301-304] Chemotherapeutic agents traditionally associated with neutropenic colitis include cytosine arabinoside (ara-C), vincristine,

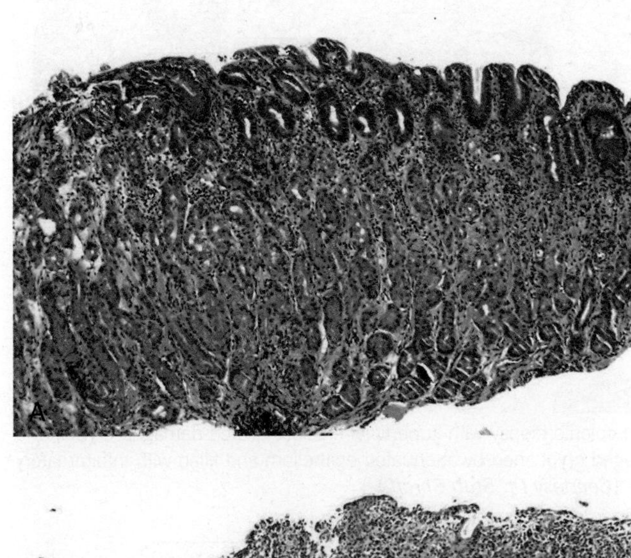

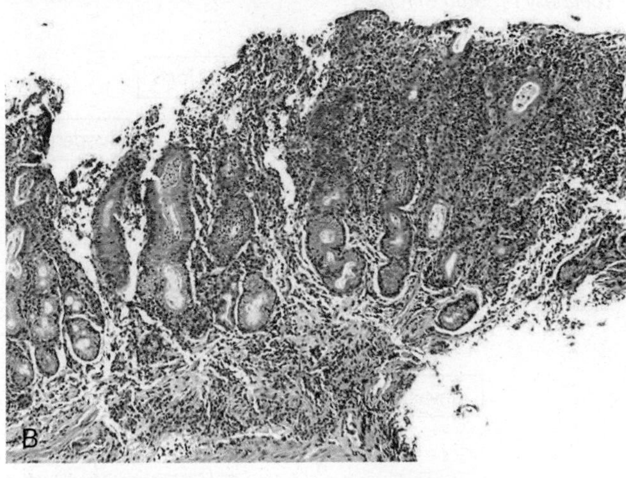

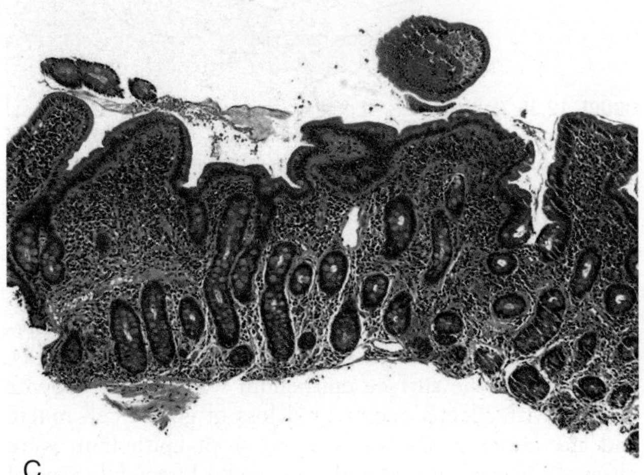

FIGURE 12.33 Spectrum of upper gastrointestinal tract pathology related to immune checkpoint inhibitors. A, In this gastric biopsy, there is a mild inflammatory infiltrate in the lamina propria. **B,** Gastric mucosa with neutrophilic inflammation of the surface foveolar compartment, mimicking *Helicobacter pylori* gastritis. **C,** Duodenal mucosa showing expansion of the lamina propria and villous blunting.

doxorubicin, methotrexate, cyclophosphamide, etoposide (VP-16), daunomycin, and prednisone.[305] It also has been recognized in patients treated with vinorelbine, docetaxel, paclitaxel, carboplatin, gemcitabine, and 5-FU for ovarian, lung, colon, or breast cancer.[305] Its predisposition to involve the ileum, appendix, cecum, or right colon accounts for the alternative names of "necrotizing enteropathy," "typhlitis," and "ileocecal syndrome,"[306] but it can affect other segments of the intestine as well.[305,307] It is characterized by damage to the mucosa with subsequent infection and systemic complications. The mucosal injury is probably drug induced in cases association with chemotherapy; however, other factors may contribute, including local infection, necrosis of leukemic tumor deposits, or ischemia due to sepsis-related hypotension (Fig. 12.36).[306] Regardless of the cause of the damage, once the mucosal barrier has been breached, invasion by enteric and opportunistic organisms is facilitated by the neutropenic status of the host. Tissue necrosis due to the infection may add to the insult.[306] The number of organisms implicated in neutropenic colitis is large and includes *Pseudomonas, Escherichia, Klebsiella, Enterobacter,* and *Candida.* Also, CMV may cause cecal ulcers in patients with malignancies, and produce a similar syndrome.

Classically, the syndrome begins 7 to 10 days after chemotherapy treatment with fever, diarrhea that may be bloody, abdominal pain, nausea, and vomiting.[304-306] Blood cultures most often yield *Clostridium septicum, C. difficile, Pseudomonas, Klebsiella, Enterobacter,* or *Escherichia coli.*[306] Stool cultures, however, are usually negative.[304] CT findings of thickening of the bowel wall or pneumatosis intestinalis support the diagnosis but are not entirely specific.[301,305] Recurrence may occur if the patient is further treated with chemotherapy.[305]

Grossly, the affected segment may appear dilated, edematous, and often hemorrhagic.[305] Microscopic features of neutropenic colitis include edema, hemorrhage, ulcers, thromboses, and mucosal or transmural necrosis with perforation. The epithelium may show changes compatible with chemotherapy effect. Fungal or bacterial organisms may be seen infiltrating necrotic tissue without an appropriate inflammatory response.[305,307] In patients with hematological malignancies, tumor deposits may be found (Fig. 12.37).

The treatment is challenging due to the difficulty in making a diagnosis coupled with the rapid progression to septic shock. Conservative management is initially attempted, with surgical intervention reserved for patients who deteriorate or who have indications for surgery such as perforation, generalized peritonitis, or continued bleeding despite correction of any coagulopathy.[306] In cases necessitating surgery, right hemicolectomy is considered the operation of choice, but the surgical approach depends on the segment involved, with some cases requiring extensive small bowel resection.[301] Recombinant granulocyte colony-stimulating factor may help reverse the neutropenia. Mortality ranges from 40% to 100%.[305-307]

Differential Diagnosis

The histology of neutropenic colitis overlaps with that of pseudomembranous colitis and ischemic colitis, but unlike those entities, neutrophils are absent or rare, which enables a specific diagnosis. The clinical scenario is usually highly suggestive in patients with neutropenic colitis.

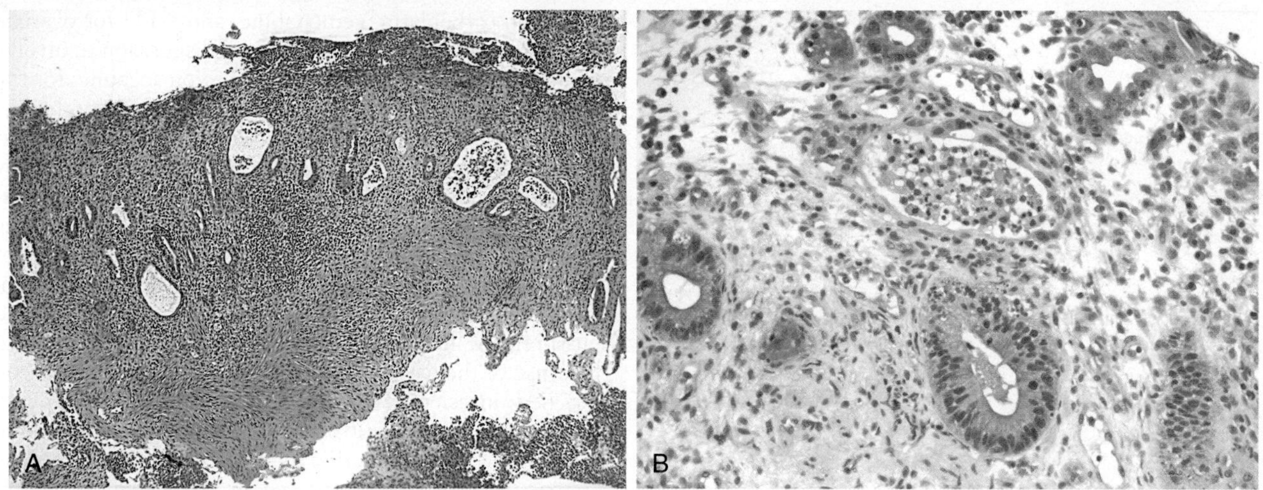

FIGURE 12.34 Idelalisib colitis resembling GVHD. A, Medium-power view of a colonic biopsy with superficial erosion, dilated damaged crypts, and debris with neutrophils within crypts. **B,** High-power view shows dilated damaged crypt lined by attenuated epithelium and filled with inflammatory cells *(top)* and another crypt with increased epithelial cell apoptoses *(bottom)*. (*Courtesy Dr. Stuti Shroff.*)

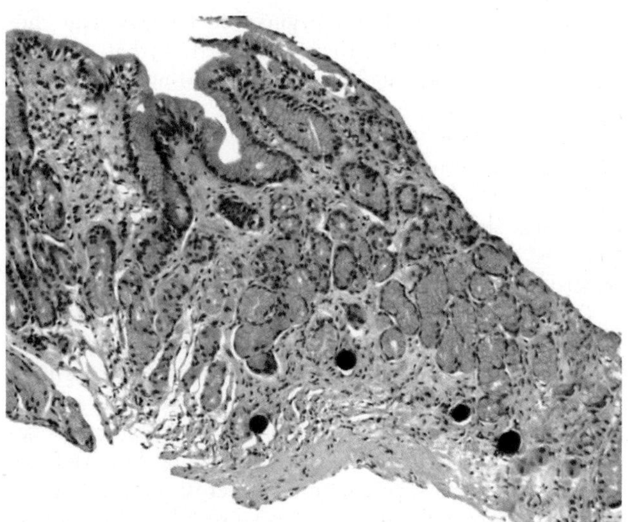

FIGURE 12.35 Yttrium microspheres. A gastric biopsy shows characteristic dark spherules in the small vessels of the lamina propria.

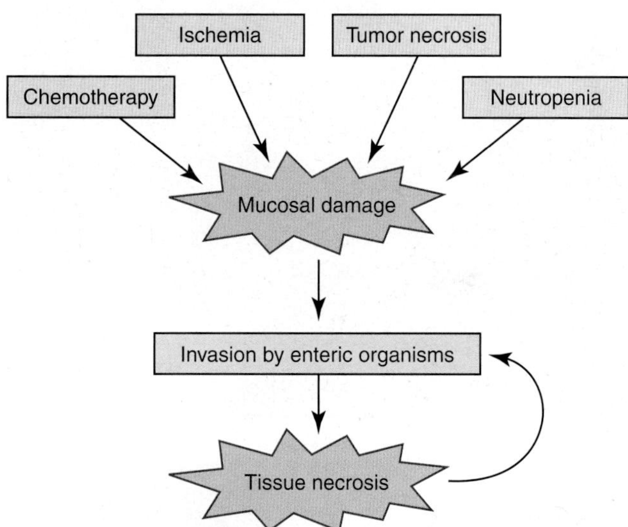

FIGURE 12.36 Pathogenesis of neutropenic colitis. The initial mucosal damage may be related to chemotherapy, but other factors such as ischemia, tumor necrosis, or neutropenia may contribute. The mucosal damage enables enteric organisms to invade into the tissue, which, in the neutropenic patient, causes extensive tissue necrosis, further invasion by organisms, and, often, a catastrophic outcome.

Cathartics

Laxatives can be divided into bulk, osmotic, or irritant (stimulant) types.

Bulk laxatives include derivatives of psyllium seeds (Metamucil) and are poorly absorbed by the colon, thus causing water retention and loose stool. GI damage is not a complication of this group of laxatives.

Osmotic or saline laxatives are either hyperosmotic (sodium phosphate, either oral or as a solution with sodium biphosphate used as an enema, magnesium sulfate, and magnesium citrate) or isosmotic (polyethylene glycol). These agents act by increasing the osmolarity of stool and thus trapping water and reducing stool consistency, or, in the case of isosmotic solutions, by overwhelming the colon's ability to absorb water. They are usually well tolerated and effective; therefore they are often used as bowel preparatory agents for endoscopic procedures.

In 1977, Meisel et al.[308] reported that Fleet's enema and rectal bisacodyl caused endoscopically detectable mucosal abnormalities, including hyperemia, obliteration of the normal vascular pattern, and mucosal friability. Histologically, disruption of the surface epithelium was seen in patients treated with Fleet's enema, and loss of goblet cell mucin and alterations in the surface and crypt epithelium were observed in patients treated with rectal bisacodyl. Several studies have documented colonic pathology in association with oral sodium phosphate (NaP) as well. In 1998, Driman et al.[66] reported aphthous ulcers (Fig. 12.38) in 2.6% of biopsies from patients treated with oral NaP and focal active colitis (FAC) in an additional 3.5%. Furthermore, they noted increased proliferation (as measured by immunohistochemical staining with MIB-1) and increased apoptotic bodies in the crypts in these patients. Other reports have confirmed the association of FAC, erosions, or crypt apoptotic bodies with the administration of oral NaP.[309-312]

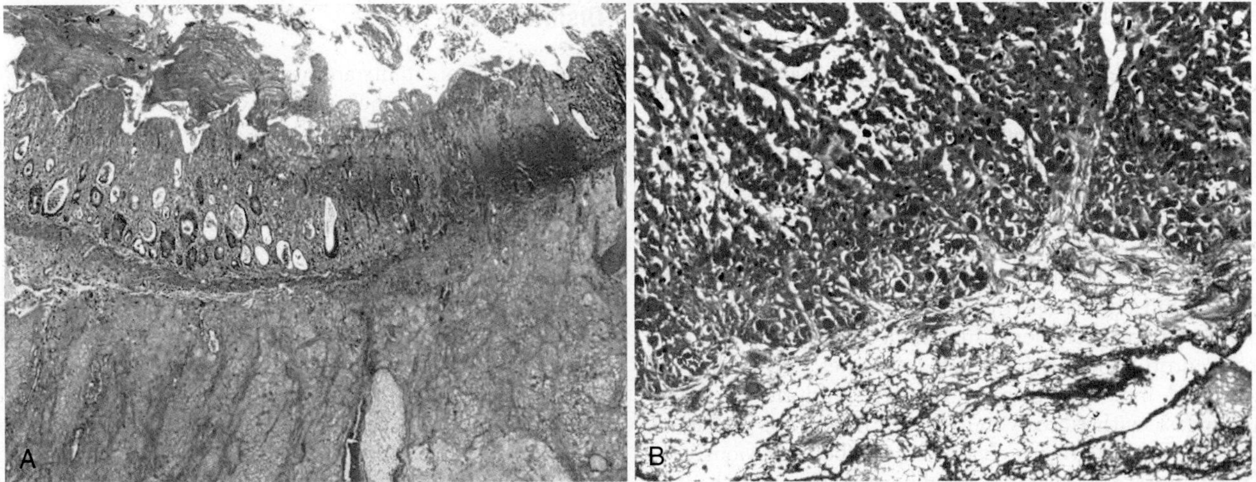

FIGURE 12.37 Neutropenic colitis. A, Low-power view of a segment of colon with neutropenic colitis demonstrates coagulative necrosis of the mucosa and submucosa, with mucosal changes resembling ischemia, including withered atrophic crypts and fibrin in the lamina propria. **B,** The interface between viable muscularis propria *(top)* and necrotic muscularis propria and pericolonic soft tissue *(bottom)* shows a conspicuous absence of neutrophils.

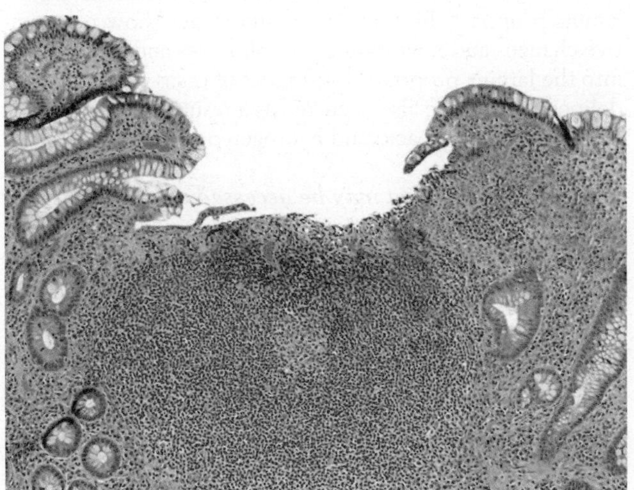

FIGURE 12.38 Aphthous ulcer. An ileal biopsy shows a superficial erosion overlying a reactive lymphoid aggregate, classic for an aphthous ulcer.

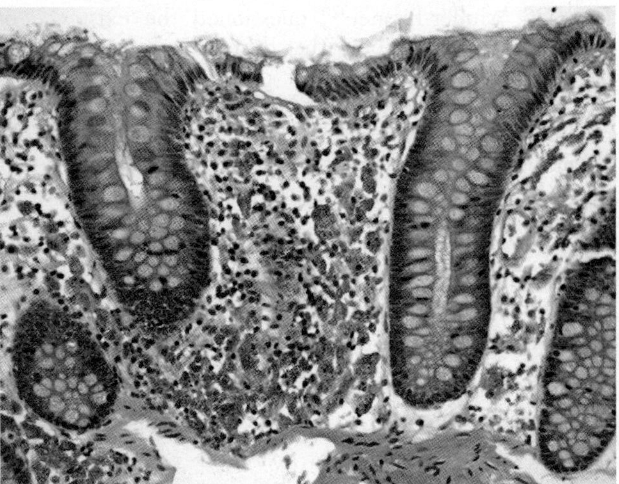

FIGURE 12.39 Melanosis coli. Macrophages within the lamina propria of the colon are heavily pigmented, consistent with melanosis coli.

Another reported GI complication of hyperosmotic saline laxatives is ischemic colitis.[313]

Stimulant or irritant laxatives promote intestinal motility or interfere with colonic mucosal transport of water and electrolytes. They fall into several groups: diphenylmethane derivatives (phenolphthalein, bisacodyl, and sodium picosulfate), anthraquinone derivatives (senna and cascara), ricinoleic acid (castor oil), and surface-acting agents (docusates).

Anthraquinones are plant-derived compounds that undergo bacterial metabolism within the colon, producing the active forms, which induce fluid secretion and increased colonic motility. They are associated with melanosis coli, "cathartic colon," and possibly neoplasia. Melanosis coli refers to the deposition of lipofuscin in macrophages within the lamina propria (Fig. 12.39). The proximal colon is more prominently affected. The formation of lipofuscin is the result of the breakdown of apoptotic colonic epithelial cells.[314] In animal experiments,[315] anthraquinone administration led to a dose-related increase in apoptosis of the colonic surface epithelial cells. Most of the resulting apoptotic bodies were subsequently phagocytosed by macrophages and transported into the lamina propria, where they were transformed into lipofuscin in macrophage lysosomes. Patients with melanosis coli often have increased numbers of apoptotic bodies in the colonic surface epithelium. Although melanosis coli is often attributed to chronic anthraquinone laxative use, a history of laxative use is not always elicited in cases of melanosis coli. An article by Lee[90] describing increased apoptosis in drug-induced colitis (particularly 5-FU and NSAIDs) provides evidence that melanosis might conceivably be seen in other drug-related lesions of the colon. Therefore melanosis coli can be viewed as a marker of increased colonic epithelial cell apoptosis, of which laxatives are one cause. In fact, a triad of melanosis coli, increased crypt apoptoses, and scattered eosinophils may be a sign of a drug reaction.

The evidence for enteric nervous system damage related to chronic laxative use is based on uncontrolled observations in few patients. In 1968, Smith reported the histological findings in a colectomy specimen from a patient who had consumed long-term laxatives,[316] leading to the long-held belief that chronic laxative use caused damage to the enteric nervous system and could lead to loss of function of the colon, a state known as cathartic colon. In that initial description, Smith described reduction in the number of myenteric neurons and axons, with increased Schwann cells. The remaining neurons had irregular, ill-defined margins with one or two swollen processes. Axons were irregular in caliber, and a few traveled randomly, apparently regenerating. Afterward, Riemann and Schmidt described the ultrastructural changes in cathartic colon.[317] They found edematous distention or ballooning of axons, loss of structural elements such as neurosecretory granules and neurotubuli, and increased lysosomes. Other reports described mucosal atrophy and fatty infiltration of the submucosa with fibrosis, but the authors were unable to confirm the neuronal changes described previously.[318] Krishnamurthy et al.[319] found abnormal neuronal changes similar to those described in cathartic colon in patients with severe idiopathic constipation, raising the question of whether the changes were caused by the laxatives or the original condition that led to the patients taking laxatives. In 1996, Muller-Lissner[320] questioned the existence of cathartic colon. He noted that despite increasing laxative use, the incidence of cathartic colon was decreasing. He speculated that a laxative that had fallen out of favor, podophyllin, may have been responsible for the cases of cathartic colon. In aggregate, there is insufficient evidence to determine that laxatives cause long-term neurological damage to the colon.[321,322]

Disinfectants

Chemical disinfectants are used to clean endoscopy instruments, and some of these contain compounds that are toxic to mucosae. Glutaraldehyde at a concentration of 2% is a common disinfectant, and has been reported as a cause of chemical colitis presumably when the agent was retained in the endoscope channels as a result of inadequate flushing after disinfection.[44,323] Patients usually present between a few hours and 2 or 3 days with abdominal pain, tenesmus, and bloody diarrhea.[43,44,323] Endoscopic findings include sharply delineated patches of mucosal erythema, erosions, ulcerations, or mucosal necrosis, usually involving the rectum, sigmoid colon, and descending colon.[44,323,324] Histological examination shows features indistinguishable from those of ischemic colitis or from the injury caused by some toxin-producing bacteria, including mucin depletion, eosinophilia of the superficial lamina propria, and in more injured areas breakdown of the epithelium beginning at the top of the mucosa and progressing toward the crypts, hemorrhage, fibrin deposition, and fibrin thrombi in capillaries within the lamina propria.[44] Biopsies from later stages show regenerative changes and migration of lymphocytes and plasma cells into the lamina propria.[44] Outbreaks of cases of florid pseudolipomatosis have also occurred as a result of disinfectants, including peracetic acid and hydrogen peroxide.[325,326]

***The full reference list may be accessed online at** Elsevier eBooks for Practicing Clinicians.*

SECTION II

INFLAMMATORY DISORDERS OF THE GASTROINTESTINAL TRACT

CHAPTER 13

Algorithmic Approach to Diagnosis of Inflammatory Disorders of the Gastrointestinal Tract

Deepa T. Patil, Robert D. Odze

Contents

INTRODUCTION

The conventional approach to teaching about inflammatory disorders of the gastrointestinal (GI) tract is to describe the clinical and histological features of individual disease entities. Unfortunately, rendering a specific diagnosis is not always possible when evaluating mucosal biopsies of the GI tract. Therefore it is incumbent on the pathologist to evaluate all of the clinical, endoscopic, and histological features in each case to help establish a specific diagnosis. One of the biggest challenges in mucosal biopsy pathology is recognizing a specific morphological pattern of injury. Use of standardized terminology is critical because each discrete morphological pattern of injury has well-defined etiological associations and therapeutic implications. For instance, a diagnosis of *Barrett's esophagus* (BE) or *inflammatory bowel disease* (IBD) leads to lifelong endoscopic surveillance of the patient and imposes a significant burden on patients and on the health care system. Use of nonstandardized terms such as *nonspecific esophagitis*, *nonspecific colitis*, or *colonic mucosa with acute and chronic inflammation* is misleading and therefore not helpful for patient management.

The purpose of this chapter is to outline a simple algorithmic approach to the diagnosis of common inflammatory disorders of the GI tract in mucosal biopsies. The process begins by dividing biopsies into one of several broad categories (e.g., normal, inflammatory, neoplastic) and is followed by a systematic evaluation of morphological features to determine a specific morphological pattern of injury. This approach often implies a fairly standard etiological differential diagnosis.

ESOPHAGUS

Esophageal biopsies can be broadly categorized as normal, inflammatory, or neoplastic (Fig. 13.1). Normal esophageal mucosa is composed of nonkeratinizing squamous epithelium with a basal zone that is typically one to three cell layers thick, papillae that are confined to the lower half of the mucosa, and lamina propria that is composed of loose connective tissue without inflammatory cells (Fig. 13.2). The presence of surface keratinization (hyperkeratosis), parakeratosis, spongiosis, or an abnormal number of inflammatory cells in the epithelium is a sign of mucosal injury and should lead to further evaluation of the biopsy specimen for a specific morphological pattern of injury.

If a biopsy is considered "inflammatory," the next step is to evaluate the dominant inflammatory cell type. Inflammation in the esophagus may be dominated by eosinophils, neutrophils, lymphocytes, or a combination of these cells, and each of these categories has well-defined etiological associations (see Fig. 13.1). Disorders with prominent eosinophilic and/or neutrophilic patterns of inflammation are classified as *active esophagitis*. As illustrated in Fig. 13.1, gastroesophageal reflux disease (GERD) and infections may be associated with more than one pattern of inflammation;

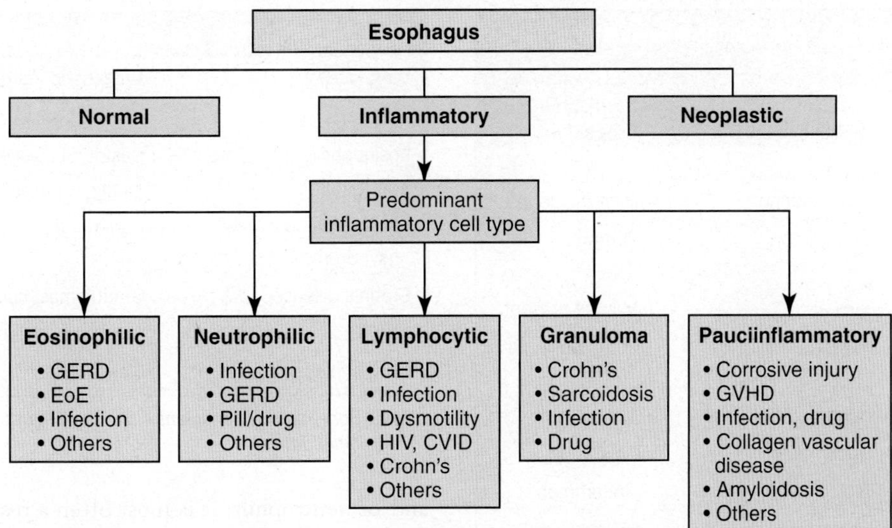

FIGURE 13.1 Algorithmic approach to diagnosis of inflammatory disorders of the esophagus. *CVID*, Common variable immunodeficiency; *EoE*, eosinophilic esophagitis; *GERD*, gastroesophageal reflux disease; *GVHD*, graft-versus-host disease; *HIV*, human immunodeficiency virus.

for this reason, they are always in the differential diagnosis of inflamed (or even near-normal) esophageal biopsies. However, endoscopic or histological evidence of esophagitis is present in only approximately 40% of patients with well-established GERD.

Eosinophil-Predominant Esophagitis

Intraepithelial eosinophilic infiltration is one of the most common patterns of inflammatory injury in esophageal biopsies. GERD and eosinophilic esophagitis (EoE) are the diseases most commonly associated with this pattern of injury. The presence of eosinophils in esophageal mucosa is not necessarily diagnostic of primary EoE (a well-defined clinicopathological disorder that is discussed in detail in Chapter 14). No single clinical, endoscopic, histological, or treatment parameter allows for absolute distinction of GERD from EoE. However, there are a variety of histological features and combinations of features that can certainly help point a pathologist toward a diagnosis of EoE. EoE is a clinicopathological diagnosis and requires correlation with patient symptoms; endoscopic features; the density, pattern, and gradient of eosinophilic infiltration in mucosal biopsies; and treatment response. Some of the salient features that help distinguish GERD from EoE are summarized in Table 13.1 and illustrated in Fig. 13.3. Eosinophilic infiltration in esophageal mucosa may also be present in disorders other than GERD and EoE. A list of these disorders and the clinical or morphological features that are helpful in making these diagnoses is presented in Table 13.2.

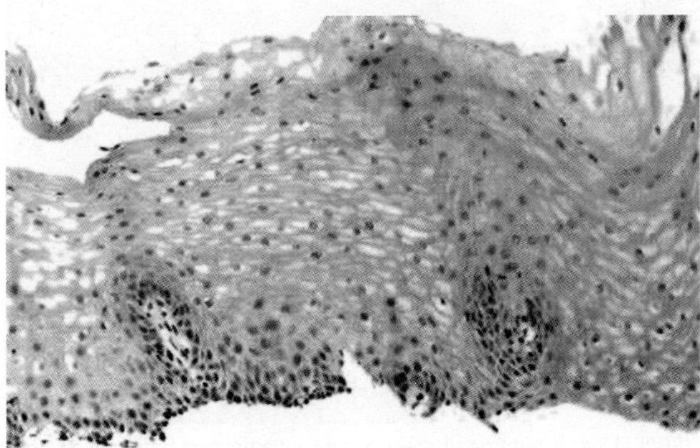

FIGURE 13.2 Normal esophageal squamous mucosa has a basal layer one to two cells thick and papillae restricted to the lower half.

Neutrophil-Predominant Esophagitis

A neutrophil-predominant inflammatory pattern of injury may be associated with infections, GERD, pill esophagitis, or corrosive mucosal injury (Fig. 13.4), among others. The presence of surface hyperkeratosis in association with a neutrophilic infiltrate should always prompt a search for fungi, such as *Candida*. Yeast and pseudohyphae may, at times, be confined to surface keratinous debris and may be associated with either minimal or no inflammation in the epithelium and lamina propria. Cytomegalovirus (CMV) and herpes esophagitis may also be associated with a neutrophil-predominant pattern of inflammation, and these infections may be diagnosed when typical viral inclusions are demonstrated in the biopsy. A diagnosis of pill esophagitis should be considered when the inflammation, or ulcer, is present in the upper and middle levels of the esophagus. The biopsy may show refractile, crystalline particles within necroinflammatory debris that represent pill fragments. This diagnosis requires correlation with the patient's medication history. Similarly, the presence of active esophagitis containing scattered atypical cells with large, hyperchromatic epithelial and/or stromal nuclei may be indicative of radiation esophagitis. Corrosive mucosal injury often leads to necrosis of the upper half of the squamous epithelium, and a band of neutrophils may be present between the superficial necrotic and deeper viable mucosa.

Lymphocyte-Predominant Esophagitis

Intraepithelial lymphocytosis of variable degrees is not an uncommon finding in esophageal biopsies. When it is associated with basal cell hyperplasia and scattered eosinophils

TABLE 13.1 Eosinophil-Predominant Inflammatory Pattern

Features	Reflux Esophagitis	Eosinophilic Esophagitis
Clinical History		
Allergy/asthma	Low incidence	High incidence
Food impaction	Uncommon	Common
Symptoms		
GERD symptoms	Typical	May be present
Dysphagia	May be present	Common
Endoscopy		
Rings	Uncommon	Typical
Linear furrows	Uncommon	Typical
Erosions/ulcers	Typical	Uncommon
pH/impedance	Abnormal	Normal
Pathology		
Inflammation gradient	Distal >> Mid/upper	Mid/upper >> Distal
Eosinophilic Infiltrate		
Maximum number	<10/HPF	>15/HPF
Clusters	No	Yes
Superficial aggregates	No	Yes
Microabscesses	No	Yes
BCH/spongiosis	Mild	Severe
Therapy		
Response to PPIs	Yes	No
Response to steroids	No	Yes

BCH, *Basal cell hyperplasia;* GERD, *gastroesophageal reflux disease;* HPF, *high-power field;* PPIs, *proton pump inhibitors.*

TABLE 13.2 Other Causes of Esophageal Eosinophilia

Diagnosis	Diagnostic Features
Infections	Viral inclusions/parasites on biopsy
Eosinophilic gastroenteritis	Gastric/SI involvement
Achalasia	Motility studies
Hypereosinophilic syndrome	Peripheral blood hypereosinophilia
Crohn's disease	Granulomas, colon/SI involvement
GVHD	Apoptosis, history of BMT
Drug hypersensitivity	Clinical history

BMT, *Bone marrow transplantation;* GVHD, *graft-versus-host disease;* SI, *small intestine.*

and/or neutrophils, it is most often a result of GERD. The presence of hyperkeratosis and scattered neutrophils should always raise suspicion for *Candida* esophagitis. The presence of a pure lymphocytic infiltrate (usually ≥ 20 lymphocytes per high-power field) associated with mucosal injury in the form of edema and basal cell hyperplasia, particularly in the peripapillary epithelium, is consistent with *lymphocytic esophagitis* (Fig. 13.5). Lymphocytic esophagitis is a poorly defined entity with a myriad of etiological associations; the most notable are motility disorders and systemic immune-mediated diseases such as Crohn's disease and connective tissue disorders. Crohn's disease manifests in the esophagus with a lymphocytic esophagitis pattern of injury more often in pediatric patients than in adults. Other disorders that cause intraepithelial lymphocytosis in the esophagus are listed in Box 13.1. When the lymphocytic infiltrate is distributed predominantly at the epithelial lamina propria interface and scattered necrotic keratinocytes along with vacuolization of basal cells are present, the possibility of a dermatological disorder such as lichen planus should be considered.

FIGURE 13.3 An eosinophil-predominant inflammatory infiltrate associated with marked basal cell hyperplasia and lamina propria fibrosis is typically seen in primary eosinophilic esophagitis.

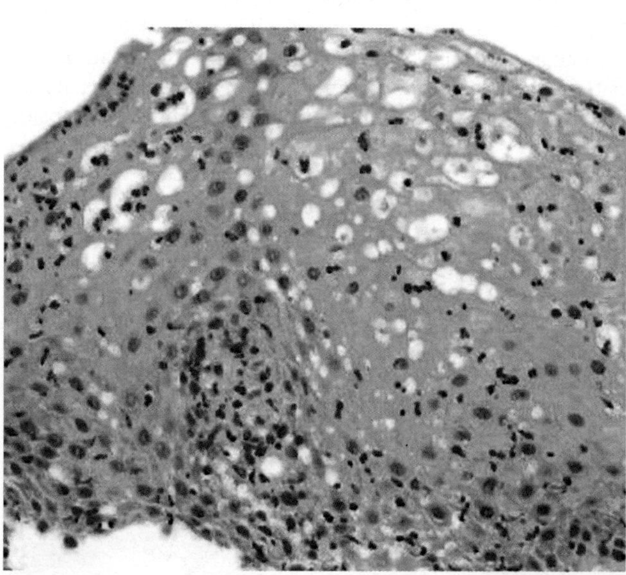

FIGURE 13.4 A neutrophil-predominant inflammatory infiltrate is often associated with infections but may be seen in association with gastroesophageal reflux disease, drugs, or corrosive mucosal injury.

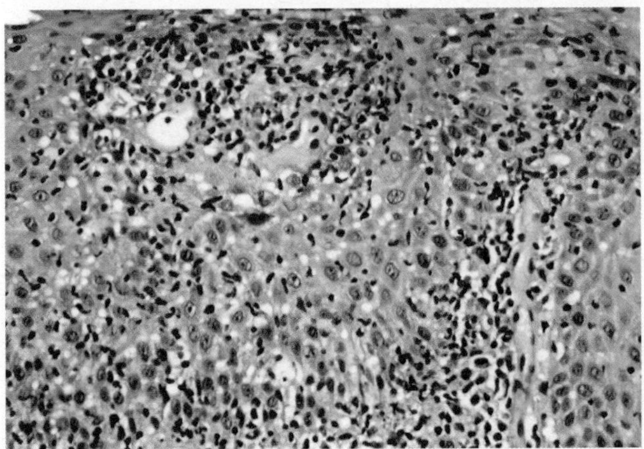

FIGURE 13.5 Lymphocytic esophagitis is a poorly defined entity with many etiological associations. It is characterized by increased intraepithelial lymphocytosis with peripapillary accentuation and spongiosis.

Granulomas

Granulomatous esophagitis (Fig. 13.6) is associated with Crohn's disease or sarcoidosis in almost all cases. Rare causes of granulomatous esophagitis include mycobacterial or fungal infection, vasculitis, and drug-induced mucosal injury.

Pauciinflammatory Esophagitis

A list of pauciinflammatory disorders is shown in Table 13.3. Graft-versus-host disease (GVHD) is the disorder that most frequently manifests with this pattern of mucosal injury (Fig. 13.7). Apoptosis and necrosis in the absence of inflammation, characteristic of GVHD, overlaps with mycophenolate-induced mucosal injury. Infections in immunocompromised patients also may lack an inflammatory response. Amyloidosis is another disorder that may be easily missed because the mucosa is typically completely normal, and the diagnostic changes are subtle, usually confined to the blood vessels in the lamina propria and superficial submucosa.

Ulcers

In some instances, one may see ulcerated granulation tissue, without viable mucosa, in a biopsy of the esophagus. A specific diagnosis cannot be rendered in most of these cases. However, biopsies with this pattern of injury should always be evaluated for viral inclusions, pill fragments, and neoplastic cells before they are dismissed as *nonspecific*.

BOX 13.1 Lymphocytic Esophagitis: Etiological Associations

Crohn's disease (particularly in pediatric age group)
GERD
Infections
Motility disorders
Allergy/asthma
Autoimmune diseases
Immunodeficiency (HIV, CVID)
Celiac disease
Esophageal involvement in dermatological disorders

CVID, *Common variable immunodeficiency;* GERD, *gastroesophageal reflux disease;* HIV, *human immunodeficiency virus.*

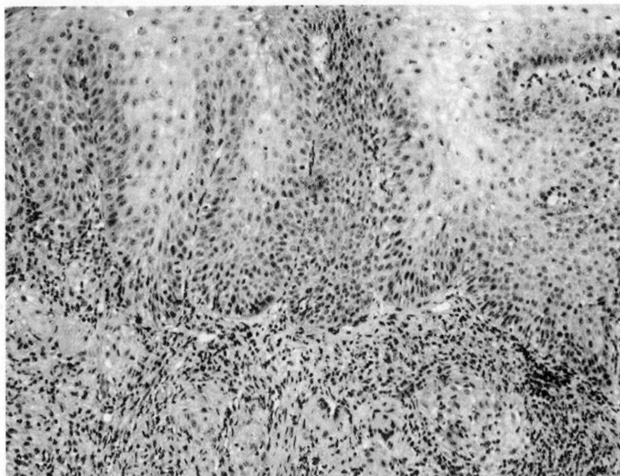

FIGURE 13.6 Granulomatous esophagitis is most commonly a manifestation of Crohn's disease or sarcoidosis.

GASTROESOPHAGEAL JUNCTION

The anatomic gastroesophageal junction (GEJ) is endoscopically defined as the proximal limit of the gastric rugal folds.

TABLE 13.3 Pauciinflammatory Pattern of Mucosal Injury in the Esophagus

Diagnosis	Features
CMV, HSV	Viral inclusions
GVHD, mycophenolate	Increased apoptosis
Corrosive injury	Superficial necrosis
Taxol, colchicine toxicity	Mitotic arrest
Skin disorders (pemphigus)	Vesicles, bullae
Scleroderma	Submucosal fibrosis
Amyloidosis	Perivascular deposits

CMV, *Cytomegalovirus;* GVHD, *graft-versus-host disease;* HSV, *herpes simplex virus.*

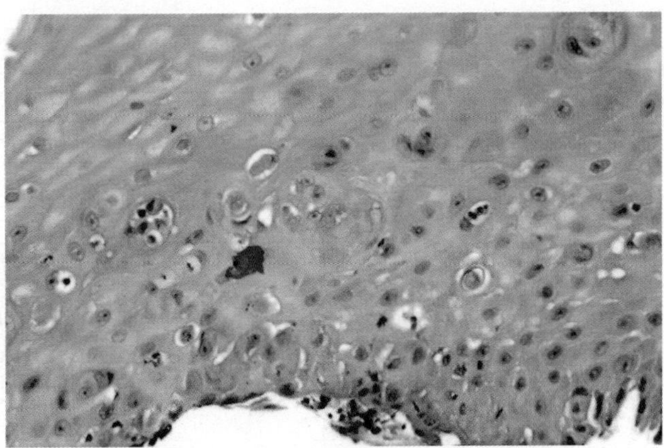

FIGURE 13.7 Graft-versus-host disease is characterized by minimal inflammation and single-cell epithelial necrosis. Similar features can be seen in drug-induced mucosal injury.

The squamocolumnar junction (SCJ) represents the point of transition from pearly-gray squamous mucosa of the esophagus to salmon-red columnar mucosa of the proximal stomach (or distal esophagus in cases of BE). In healthy individuals, the SCJ is located at the GEJ, whereas in patients with BE, the SCJ is located proximal to the anatomic GEJ. When an endoscopic biopsy is submitted with a question of BE, it is imperative for the pathologist to know the precise location of the biopsy, even before histological evaluation is performed. Biopsies labeled as *GEJ*, *SCJ*, or *Z-line* cannot be definitely labeled as BE, even when goblet cells are identified in the biopsy, unless there are morphological features in the biopsy specimen that help determine whether the columnar epithelium was taken from the anatomic esophagus. These features include multilayered epithelium, mucosal or submucosal glands or ducts (Fig. 13.8), subsquamous ("buried") glands, or hybrid epithelium. Additionally, based on current American College of Gastroenterology guidelines, a definitive diagnosis of BE can be rendered only if the biopsies have been obtained at a distance of 1 cm above the GEJ (from and confined to the distal esophagus) and in which goblet cells are identified in the columnar epithelium.

FIGURE 13.8 Intestinal metaplasia in a biopsy obtained from the gastroesophageal junction (GEJ). The presence of esophageal ducts or glands adjacent to foci of intestinal metaplasia indicates that the sample was obtained from the distal esophagus. However, a definitive diagnosis of Barrett's esophagus requires that intestinal metaplasia is documented in a distal esophageal biopsy that is obtained at a distance ≥ 1 cm above the GEJ.

STOMACH

General Comments

Gastric mucosal biopsies may be broadly categorized on morphological evaluation as either normal, inflammatory, or neoplastic. Another category consists of lamina propria infiltrates or pigment depositions in the absence of significant lymphoplasmacytic, neutrophilic, or eosinophilic inflammation (Fig. 13.9). Normal gastric corpus mucosa is composed of closely packed oxyntic glands, whereas the antrum is composed of pure mucus glands arranged in a vague lobular configuration (Fig. 13.10). In the proximal corpus, basally located compact mucosal (mucinous) glands, similar in appearance to those at the SCJ and in the gastric cardia of patients with BE, have recently been described (Fig. 13.11). These glands have been proposed to represent a potential source of stem cells, but this needs further research to define properly. In older children and young adults, both gastric compartments (antrum and corpus) show minimal intervening stroma and either few or no plasma cells in the lamina propria. With advancing patient age, up to 5 to 10 mononuclear cells per high-power field are considered normal, particularly in the antrum. A few lymphocytes or plasma cells in the lamina propria in the absence of epithelial injury or regeneration should not be considered indicative of active or chronic disease. Primary lymphoid follicles without active germinal centers are normally present at the base of the gastric corpus mucosa as well, and these should not be considered a manifestation of chronic gastritis. However, the presence of multiple clusters of plasma cells (at least 3 to 4 clusters, composed of 6 to 8 plasma cells each), lymphoid aggregates in the antrum, lymphoid aggregates with active germinal centers, and a bandlike lymphoplasmacytic infiltrate beneath the surface epithelium are all considered features of chronic gastritis.

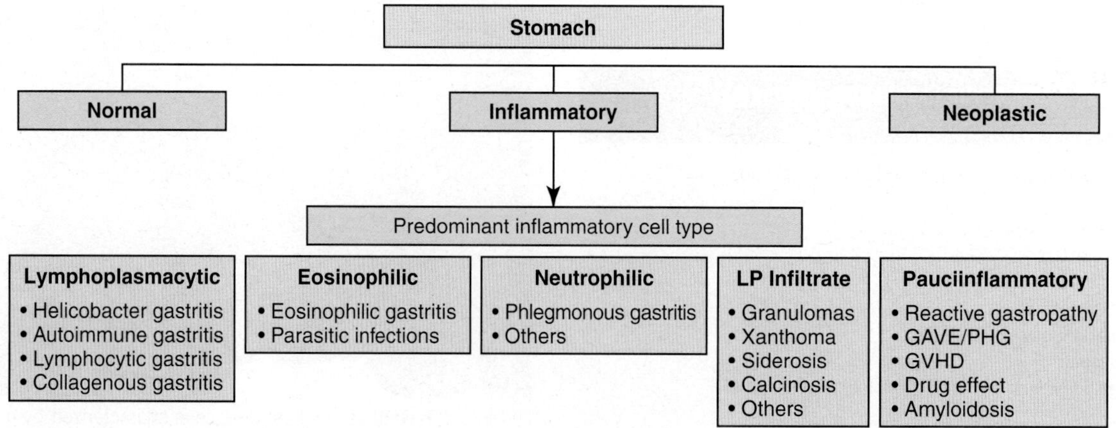

FIGURE 13.9 Algorithmic approach to diagnosis of inflammatory disorders of the stomach. *GAVE*, Gastric antral vascular ectasia; *GVHD*, graft-versus-host disease; *LP*, lamina propria; *PHG*, portal hypertensive gastropathy.

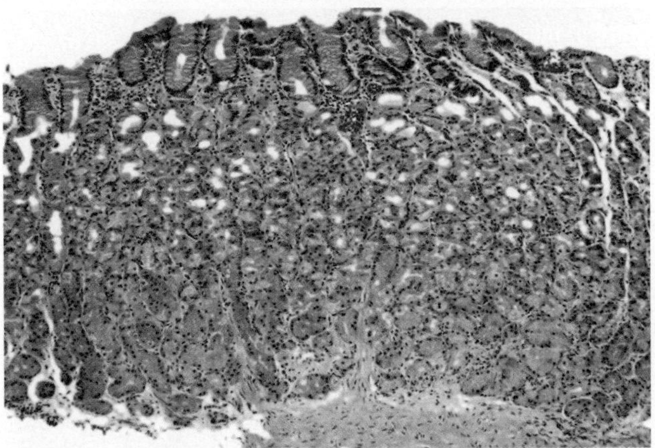

FIGURE 13.10 Normal gastric mucosa is composed of oxyntic glands (corpus) or mucus glands (antrum) covered by surface foveolar epithelium and minimal lymphoplasmacytic infiltrate in the lamina propria.

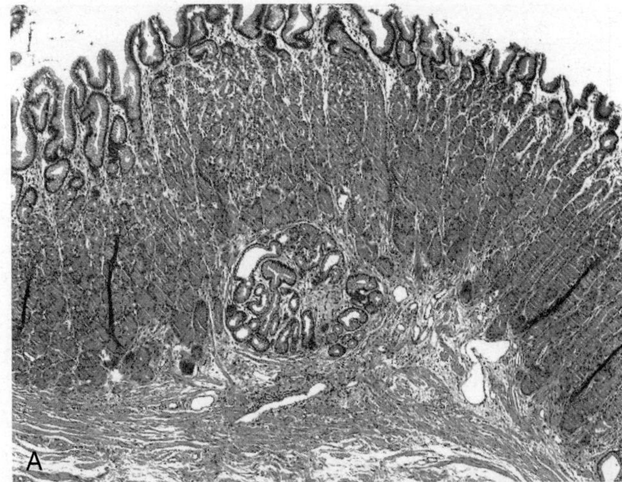

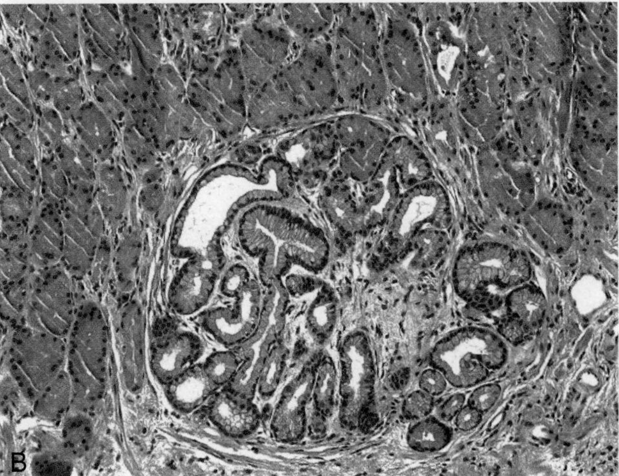

FIGURE 13.11 A and B, Compact mucus glands in the corpus mucosa within the gastric fundus. These gastric compact mucus glands are lined by columnar cells with apical mucin droplets, identical to cardiac mucosa.

Gastritis

Determination of the predominant inflammatory cell type in the lamina propria is the first step in diagnosing gastritis (see Fig. 13.9). A lymphoplasmacytic infiltrate is by far the most common type of inflammatory reaction seen in gastric biopsies in routine practice. This pattern (also broadly referred to as *chronic gastritis*) includes several well-defined clinicopathological entities. This pattern of inflammation should be evaluated for pattern of injury (focal vs. diffuse), region of the stomach predominantly involved (antrum vs. corpus, or both), location in the mucosa (superficial vs. deep), presence or absence of active inflammation, presence or absence of microorganisms, atrophy of oxyntic glands, endocrine cell hyperplasia, intraepithelial lymphocytes (IELs), and quality of the subepithelial collagen layer, among others (Table 13.4).

Focal Gastritis

Focal active gastritis may be a gastric manifestation of IBD, particularly in pediatric patients (Fig. 13.12). The etiological associations of focal active gastritis in adults are diverse, and the association with IBD is weak. Infections such as CMV and adenovirus, *Helicobacter heilmannii*, and drug reactions, especially immune checkpoint inhibitor–induced gastritis, can also cause focal active gastritis.

Diffuse Gastritis

Lymphoplasmacytic

The two diseases most commonly encountered in routine clinical practice in association with diffuse chronic gastritis with lymphoplasmacytic inflammation are *Helicobacter pylori* infection and autoimmune gastritis. The presence of a neutrophilic infiltrate should always raise suspicion of *H. pylori* gastritis, but an active inflammatory component may be present in almost any type of chronic gastritis, such as autoimmune, drug-induced, lymphocytic, or collagenous gastritis. *Helicobacter* gastritis is an antral-predominant gastritis with a superficial bandlike inflammatory infiltrate beneath the surface foveolar epithelium (Fig. 13.13A). It is associated with a variable active (neutrophilic) component. The latter finding may be mild in cases of *H. heilmannii* gastritis. Autoimmune gastritis involves the corpus, causing atrophy of the oxyntic glands (see Fig. 13.13B), and leads to intestinal metaplasia, endocrine cell hyperplasia, and eventually gastric neuroendocrine tumors.

Intraepithelial Lymphocytes

Increased IELs (>25 per 100 epithelial cells) in the absence of other significant pathological changes is suggestive of lymphocytic gastritis (Fig. 13.14). This condition usually manifests as pan-gastritis, but the disease may be patchy in some cases. Common etiological associations of this pattern of mucosal injury include celiac disease, hypersensitivity response to *H. pylori* infection, human immunodeficiency virus (HIV) infection, and drugs (e.g., ticlopidine).

Thick Subepithelial Collagen

Thickening of the subepithelial collagen layer is rarely seen in gastric biopsies, but this pattern of injury encompasses two distinct clinical disorders (Fig. 13.15). Collagenous gastritis in pediatric patients usually involves only the stomach, whereas in adults it typically occurs in association with involvement of the small intestine (collagenous sprue), colon (collagenous colitis), or both. The inflammatory component

TABLE 13.4 Differential Diagnosis of Diffuse Chronic Gastritis Pattern of Injury

Feature	*Helicobacter*	Other Infectious	Autoimmune	Lymphocytic	Collagenous	Eosinophilic
Lymphoplasmacytic infiltrate	Prominent	Present	Present	Present	Present	May be present
Antral predominance	Yes	No	No	May be seen	May be seen	Absent
Superficial bandlike infiltrate	Prominent	May be present	Absent	May be present	May be present	Absent
Microorganisms or viral inclusions	Present	Present	Absent	Absent	Absent	Absent
Oxyntic gland atrophy	May be present	May be present	Prominent	Absent	Absent	Absent
Endocrine cell hyperplasia	Absent	Absent	Prominent	Absent	Absent	Absent
Increased IELs	May be present	Absent	Absent	Prominent	May be present	Absent
Thick subepithelial collagen layer	Absent	Absent	Absent	Absent	Present	Absent
Eosinophil clusters, aggregates, and epithelial damage	Absent	May be present	Absent	Absent	May be present	Prominent

IELs, *Intraepithelial lymphocytes.*

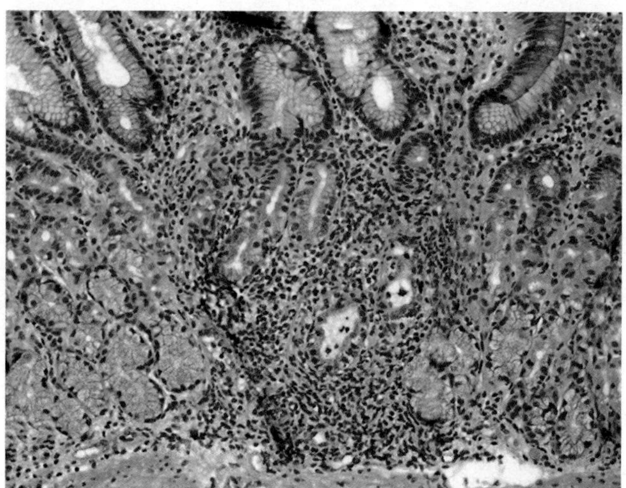

FIGURE 13.12 Focal enhancing gastritis is characterized by a discrete cuff of lymphohistiocytic infiltrate around mucus or oxyntic glands and may be associated with inflammatory bowel disease in children. A similar pattern of injury has also been described in the setting of immune checkpoint inhibitor–induced gastritis.

in collagenous gastritis may be dominated by IELs or eosinophils in the lamina propria, and some cases may be misdiagnosed as *lymphocytic* or *eosinophilic* gastritis if attention is not paid to the character of the subepithelial collagen layer.

Increased Eosinophils

Eosinophilic gastritis is characterized by an eosinophil-predominant infiltrate (Fig. 13.16). It is composed of large clusters and aggregates of eosinophils in the lamina propria associated with epithelial injury in the form of cryptitis or crypt abscesses. A clinical history of asthma, food allergies, connective tissue disorder, or drug intake is typically present. Rarely, parasitic infection may lead to eosinophilic gastritis.

Increased Neutrophils

A pure neutrophilic pattern of inflammation (without lymphocytes or plasma cells) is rare but is characteristic of phlegmonous gastritis. In this condition, severe active inflammation is centered in the submucosa, whereas the overlying mucosa may be normal. This disease has a high mortality rate unless prompt clinical intervention, often in the form of gastrectomy, is instituted.

Pauciinflammatory Gastritis

A pauciinflammatory pattern of gastric mucosal damage is typically associated with injury from noxious stimuli, such as nonsteroidal antiinflammatory drugs (NSAIDs), steroids, alcohol, or bile reflux (Fig. 13.17). It is also a common pattern of repair and regeneration after gastric injury from many causes (e.g., ulcers). The characteristic morphological features include prominent regenerative epithelial changes in the absence of a significant inflammatory infiltrate. Surface erosions or ulcers and prominent lamina propria hemorrhage are features of acute erosive and *acute hemorrhagic* gastritis, respectively, but these are simply severe forms of reactive gastropathy. Use of one or more drugs or bile reflux may lead to erosive or hemorrhagic gastritis. The presence of marked foveolar hyperplasia composed of corkscrew-shaped (regenerative) gastric foveolar epithelium is typical of reactive gastropathy in general.

The morphological clues to the correct diagnosis in diseases that share a pauciinflammatory pattern of injury are summarized in Table 13.5. Prominent apoptotic activity, particularly in the antrum, is typical of GVHD. Blood vessels should always be evaluated for amyloidosis before a biopsy is diagnosed as "normal." Infections in immunocompromised hosts can produce a pauciinflammatory pattern of injury. These include CMV, adenovirus, and even severe fungal infections such as *Aspergillus*.

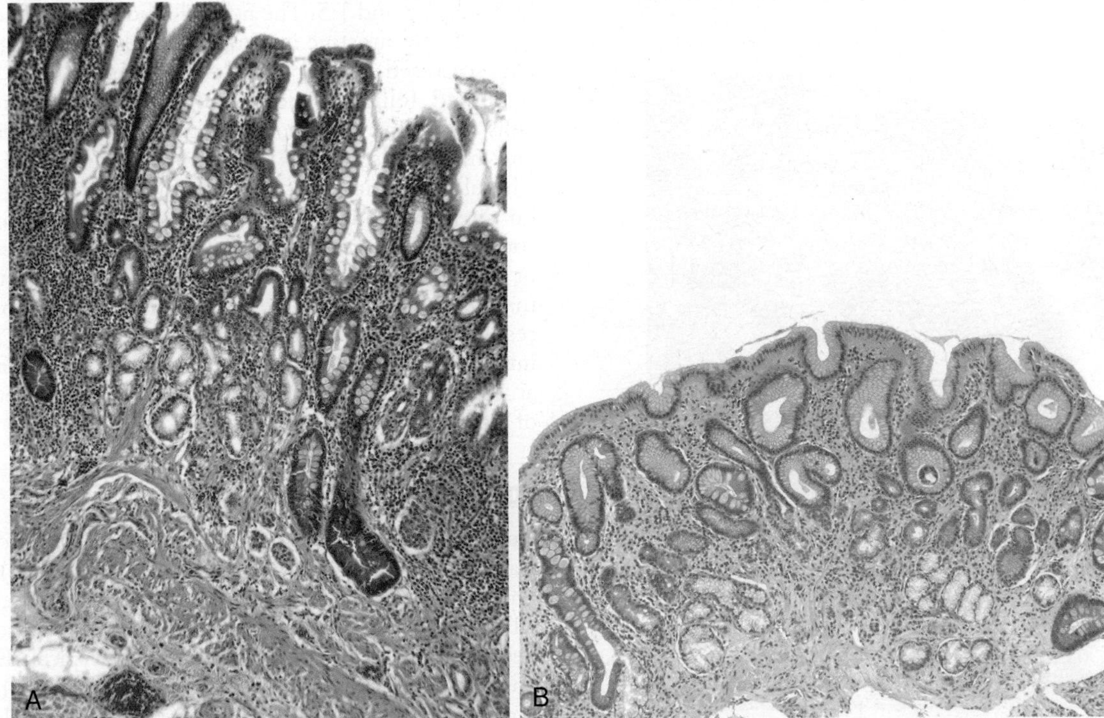

FIGURE 13.13 **A,** Diffuse chronic gastritis shows a bandlike infiltrate of lymphocytes and plasma cells beneath surface foveolar epithelium. In severe cases, the full thickness of the gastric mucosa is involved. This pattern is most commonly associated with *Helicobacter pylori* infection. **B,** Autoimmune gastritis typically shows lymphoplasmacytic inflammation distributed throughout the lamina propria. In this example, there is paucity of oxyntic glands along with intestinal and pseudopyloric gland metaplasia.

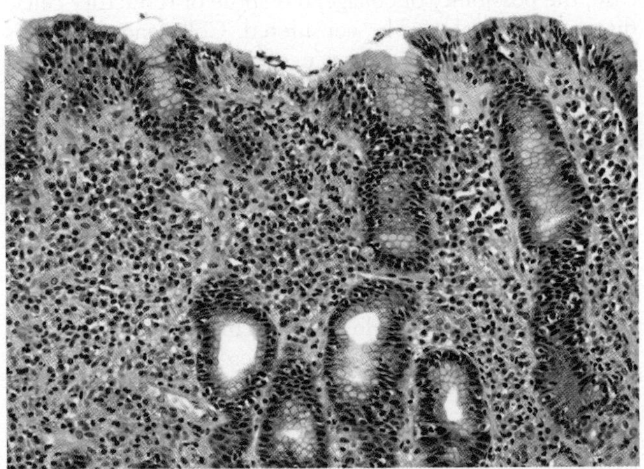

FIGURE 13.14 Lymphocytic gastritis shows markedly increased intraepithelial lymphocytes and in most cases is associated with either celiac disease or *Helicobacter pylori* infection.

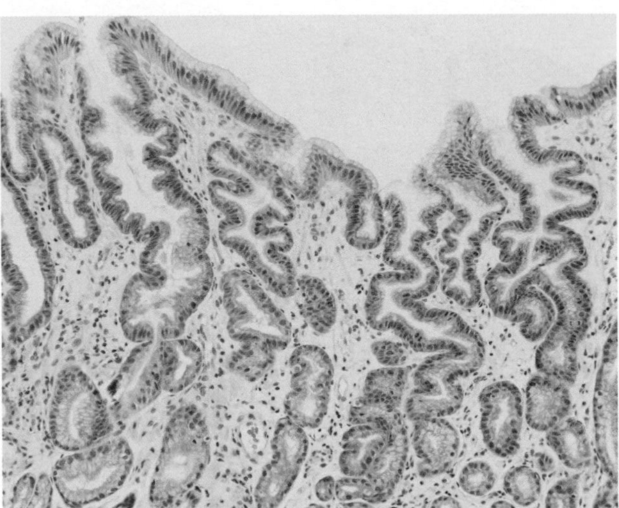

FIGURE 13.15 Collagenous gastritis shows expansion of the lamina propria by lymphocytes, plasma cells, and eosinophils. There is surface epithelial injury with mucin loss and a distinct subepithelial layer of collagen with entrapped stromal cells, inflammatory cells, and capillaries.

Infiltrates

The lamina propria should always be inspected carefully for infiltrates, and in females, metastatic breast cancer should always be considered and ruled out. Metastatic breast cancer not uncommonly mimics inflammatory cells in the deep lamina propria. Thus, even in patients with typical gastritis features, such as that caused by *H. pylori*, one should be careful to exclude covert metastatic cells in biopsies of females (Fig 13.18). Granulomas in the stomach are a manifestation of Crohn's disease or sarcoidosis in most instances. Other infectious and noninfectious causes of granulomatous gastritis are summarized in Table 13.6. Foamy histiocytes with abundant cytoplasm and small, grooved, pale nuclei are typical of mucosal xanthoma (Fig. 13.19). At endoscopy, this may appear as small, white or yellow nodules or plaques. Iron and calcium deposits are the two most common types of pigment deposition in gastric mucosal biopsies. Iron deposition may result from iron pill gastritis or hemochromatosis, among others. (Fig. 13.20). Gastric

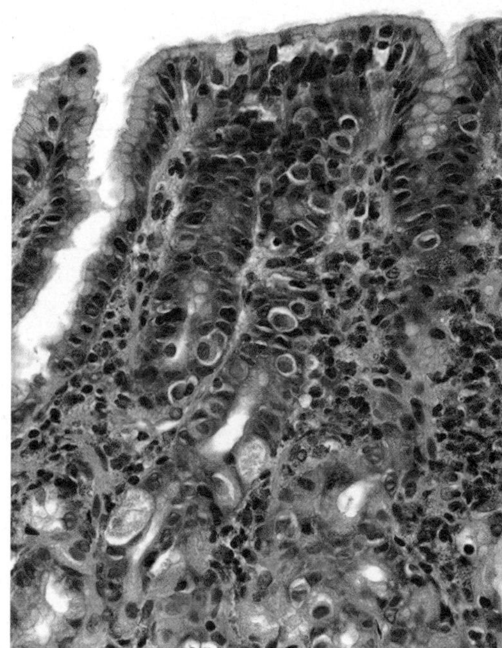

FIGURE 13.16 Eosinophilic gastritis is characterized by large clusters and aggregates of eosinophils in the lamina propria as well as intraepithelial infiltration and damage by eosinophils.

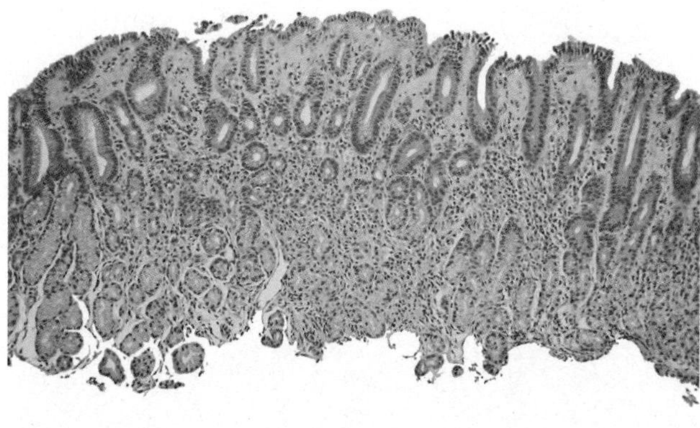

FIGURE 13.17 Reactive or chemical gastropathy shows foveolar hyperplasia, fibromuscular proliferation in the lamina propria, and absence of significant inflammatory infiltrate. It is associated most often with bile reflux or with nonsteroidal antiinflammatory drug- or alcohol-induced surface mucosal injury.

mucosal calcinosis may occur in organ transplant recipients or in patients with end-stage renal failure who are consuming aluminum hydroxide–containing antacids or sucralfate.

SMALL INTESTINE

General Comments

Small-intestinal biopsies may be broadly categorized as *normal, inflamed,* or *neoplastic* (Fig. 13.21). Normal small-intestinal mucosa shows a crypt-to-villus ratio normally between 1:3 and 1:5. The normal mucosal immune system of the small intestine is composed of lymphoid aggregates and scattered IELs, particularly in epithelium overlying lymphoid follicles, and an admixture of inflammatory cells including lymphocytes, plasma cells, eosinophils, and mast cells within the lamina propria (Fig. 13.22). Therefore suspicion of an inflammatory disorder is based on an expansion of the lamina propria with inflammatory cells, the presence of an increased number of IELs, or both. Inflammatory disorders of the small intestine may also show a variable degree of villous atrophy. As a result, inflammatory disorders are also broadly grouped into those that often cause complete loss of normal villous architecture and those in which there is partial or no loss of villous architecture.

Complete Villous Atrophy

Celiac disease is, by far, the most common disorder associated with complete villous atrophy (Fig. 13.23). A systematic approach to small intestine disorders with complete villous atrophy also requires evaluation for the presence and degree of intraepithelial lymphocytosis, atypical IELs, subepithelial collagen thickness, active (neutrophilic) inflammation, eosinophils in the lamina propria, goblet cells, apoptosis, and infectious (often parasitic) organisms. The specific disorders that manifest with these features are summarized in Table 13.7.

Celiac disease is typically associated with a marked increase in IELs (>30 per 100 epithelial cells). In patients with a known history or serological suspicion of celiac disease, the possibility of collagenous sprue or refractory celiac disease should always be considered. Collagenous sprue is characterized by the presence of an irregular, thickened subepithelial collagen layer. Establishing a diagnosis of refractory celiac disease requires additional tests, such as immunohistochemical evaluation of the type of intraepithelial lymphocytic infiltrate, flow cytometry (for loss of surface T-cell antigens), and, in some cases, polymerase chain reaction (for assessment of clonality of lymphocytes). Typically, celiac disease and type 1 refractory celiac disease show increased CD3− and CD8+ IELs, whereas type 2 refractory celiac disease shows loss of CD8 in a significant proportion of the infiltrating T lymphocytes. A diagnosis of type 2 refractory celiac disease is clinically significant because of the high risk for enteropathy-associated T-cell lymphoma (EATL). The salient clinical and pathological differences between type 1 and type 2 refractory celiac disease are summarized in Table 13.8.

Complete villous atrophy with increased IELs may also be seen in other autoimmune or immunodeficiency disorders, including HIV infection, common variable immunodeficiency (CVID), and autoimmune enteropathy (AIE). Patients with AIE reveal circulating antienterocyte and anti–goblet cell antibodies and an absence of goblet cells in the mucosa, either with or without increased apoptotic activity. IELs are also increased, which may lead to a misdiagnosis of celiac disease. In patients with a history of celiac disease unresponsive to gluten withdrawal, the possibility of AIE should be considered strongly, particularly if the symptoms are severe. A similar pattern of mucosal injury may also be seen in some patients with bacterial overgrowth.

TABLE 13.5 Differential Diagnosis of a Pauciinflammatory Pattern of Stomach Injury

Feature	Reactive Gastropathy	GVHD	GAVE	PHG	Amyloidosis
Foveolar hyperplasia	Prominent	Absent	May be present	May be present	Absent
Mucin depletion	Present	Absent	Absent	Absent	Absent
Vascular ectasia	Present	Absent	Prominent	Prominent	Absent
Distribution of injury	Antrum > corpus	Antrum > corpus	Antrum	Corpus	Antrum or corpus
Fibrin thrombi	Absent	Absent	Present	Absent	Absent
Prominent submucosal vessels on endoscopy	Absent	Absent	Absent	Present	Absent
Increased apoptosis	Absent	Present	Absent	Absent	Absent
Perivascular amyloid deposits	Absent	Absent	Absent	Absent	Present

GAVE, *Gastric antral vascular ectasia;* GVHD, *graft-versus-host disease;* PHG, *portal hypertensive gastropathy.*

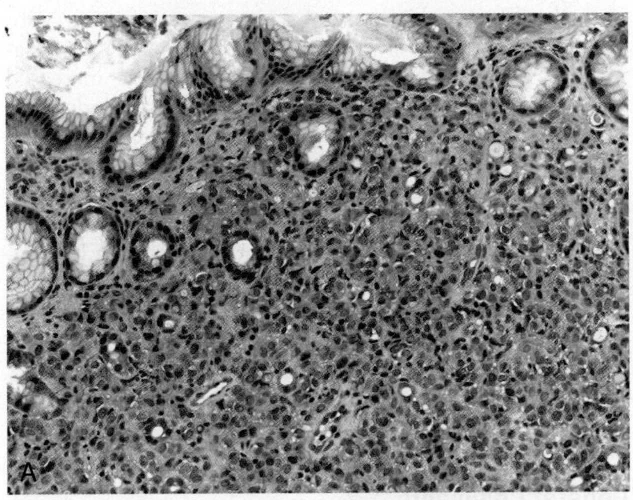

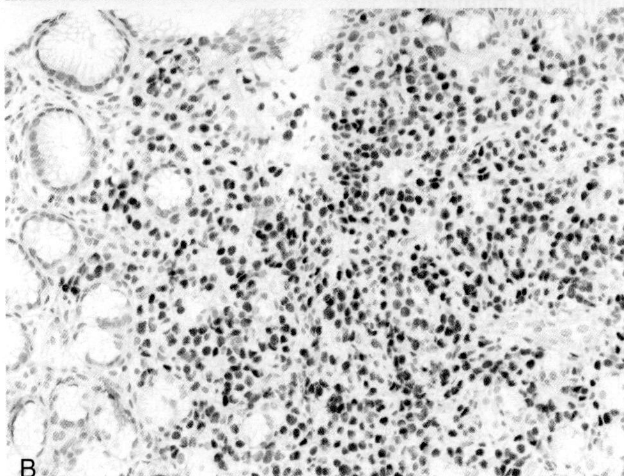

FIGURE 13.18 A, Metastatic lobular carcinoma in a gastric biopsy. The lamina propria shows monotonous epithelioid cells with a moderate amount of eosinophilic cytoplasm and no/minimal nuclear pleomorphism. The nuclear size is ≤ 3 to 4 times the size of a lymphocyte nucleus. Rare cells show single intracytoplasmic lumen. **B,** The neoplastic cells show diffuse expression of estrogen receptor.

TABLE 13.6 Granulomatous Gastritis

Infectious	Noninfectious
Mycobacterial	Crohn's disease
Candida, aspergillosis	Sarcoidosis
Mucormycosis	Foreign body
Histoplasmosis	Cancer
Blastomycosis	Chronic granulomatous disease
Anisakis, *Strongyloides stercoralis*	Idiopathic
Schistosoma mansoni	
Helicobacter pylori	

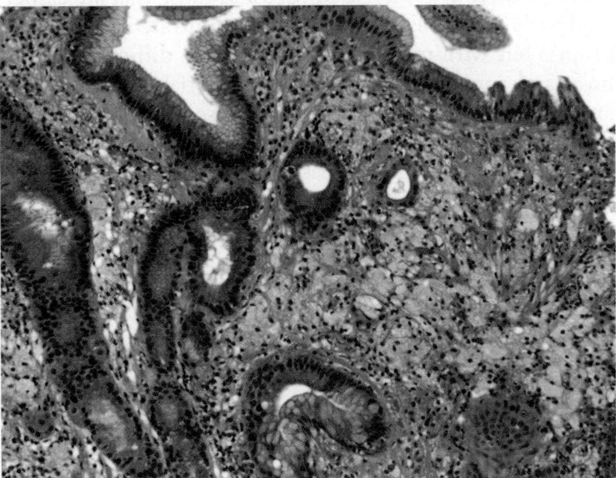

FIGURE 13.19 Histiocytic infiltrate in lamina propria composed of large, foamy, lipid-filled histiocytes is typical of gastric mucosal xanthoma. Mycobacterial infection and signet ring cell carcinoma are possible and should be ruled out.

The nitrogen breath test and evaluation of the patient's response to antibiotics are helpful in diagnosing this condition.

Active inflammation (neutrophils or eosinophils) within the crypt or surface epithelium, is uncommon in patients with celiac disease and should always raise suspicion of an infectious or other inflammatory process such as Crohn's disease. Increased eosinophils in the epithelium and lamina propria, when associated with epithelial injury, are suspicious for eosinophilic gastroenteritis.

Increased apoptosis in patients with complete villous atrophy should prompt an additional workup for AIE. Loss of goblet cells in mucosal biopsies is seen in only approximately

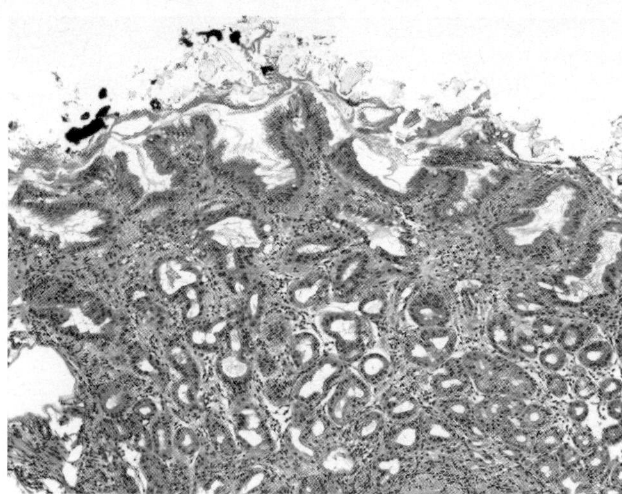

FIGURE 13.20 Iron pill gastritis is characterized by refractile, brown, crystalline material located within the superficial lamina propria and within the foveolar compartment of the gastric mucosa.

50% of cases of AIE, so workup for antienterocyte antibodies is an important step in establishing this diagnosis. If the serological tests are not available, the patient's response to a trial of steroids is also helpful in diagnosing AIE. Increased apoptotic activity may be present in patients with HIV infection, mycophenolate toxicity, or GVHD as well.

Partial Villous Atrophy

The differential diagnosis of inflammatory disorders of the small intestine associated with partial villous atrophy is extensive. Broadly, they are divided into conditions that are associated with increased IELs and those that are associated with an increased inflammatory infiltrate in the lamina propria but with no increase in IELs. The differential diagnosis and approach to patients with partial villous atrophy and increased IELs is similar to that used for patients with complete villous atrophy and increased IELs (discussed earlier). Biopsies showing increased inflammation but with no increase in IELs can be further evaluated according to the type of inflammatory infiltrate.

Lymphoplasmacytic

Increased lymphocytes and plasma cells, associated with partial villous atrophy and an absence of increased IELs, is commonly seen in patients with peptic duodenitis or IBD (Crohn's disease, and, rarely, ulcerative colitis). The presence of mucinous or gastric surface foveolar metaplasia is a sign of previous mucosal injury, and this feature can be seen in these disorders and many others (Fig. 13.24). Involvement with IBD is characterized by a more severe inflammatory infiltrate, a greater degree of active inflammation, granulomas, and concurrent involvement of the ileum, colon, or both. *H. pylori* gastritis and NSAIDs may be associated with peptic duodenitis.

Eosinophils

Increased eosinophils may be seen in parasitic infections, eosinophilic gastroenteritis, drug hypersensitivity reactions, and mastocytosis (Fig. 13.25). Eosinophilic gastroenteritis occurs in mucosal, mural, and serosal forms. However, only the mucosal form can be excluded with certainty in biopsy specimens.

Lamina Propria Infiltrates

Granulomatous inflammation of the small intestine is most commonly a manifestation of Crohn's disease or sarcoidosis (Fig. 13.26). The presence of a diffuse histiocytic infiltrate in the lamina propria should raise concern for atypical mycobacterial infection or Whipple's disease. Histochemical stains demonstrate acid-fast bacilli in the former case, and periodic acid–Schiff stain with diastase digestion (d-PAS) demonstrates typical positive macrophages in Whipple's disease.

Normal Villous Architecture

Many disorders of the small intestine are associated with normal villous architecture. For instance, infection with *Giardia* or *Cryptosporidium* usually does not incite a significant inflammatory response but may cause increased IELs in some circumstances. Other conditions include abetalipoproteinemia (cytoplasmic vacuolation in enterocytes), CVID (absence of plasma cells in lamina propria), and amyloidosis.

The differential diagnosis of small-intestinal biopsies with normal villous architecture and increased IELs (Fig. 13.27) is broad and includes latent celiac disease, nongluten food hypersensitivity, tropical sprue, bacterial overgrowth, immunodeficiency disorders, and, in rare instances, IBD.

COLON

General Comments

The diagnostic approach to interpretation of colon biopsies is similar to that recommended in other portions of the GI tract, with a few exceptions. On initial review, it is helpful to place the colon biopsy in one of four broad categories: *normal, inflammatory, lamina propria infiltrate,* or *neoplasia.* In contrast with biopsies obtained with upper GI endoscopy, those obtained with colonoscopy often show mild pathological abnormalities and artifacts as a result of the bowel preparation procedure (see further discussion later in this chapter).

On initial evaluation of mucosal biopsies of the colon, inflammatory disorders may be separated into four general categories: *chronic, acute, eosinophilic,* and *paucicellular* (Fig. 13.28). In contrast with biopsies obtained from the rest of the tubular gut, the degree of preservation or disturbance of crypt architecture is an important discriminatory feature that helps pathologists distinguish certain categories of inflammatory disorders. Interpretation of colon biopsies should incorporate all clinical (particularly endoscopic) information about the patient, with particular emphasis on the anatomic distribution of endoscopic abnormalities. Clinical information such as the timing and sequence of colonic symptoms and signs, medication history, prior illnesses of the patient and family members, and, most importantly, the type and quality of diarrhea (e.g., bloody versus nonbloody) is helpful when evaluating colon biopsies. For instance, almost all patients with ulcerative colitis have

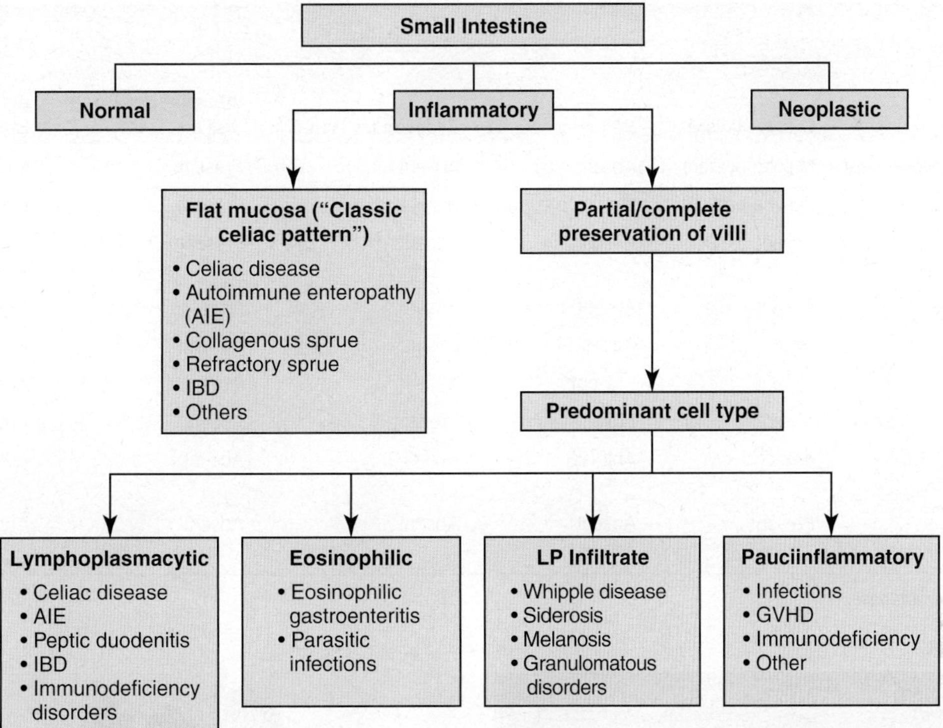

FIGURE 13.21 Algorithmic approach to diagnosis of inflammatory disorders of the small intestine. *GVHD,* Graft-versus-host disease; *IBD,* inflammatory bowel disease; *LP,* lamina propria.

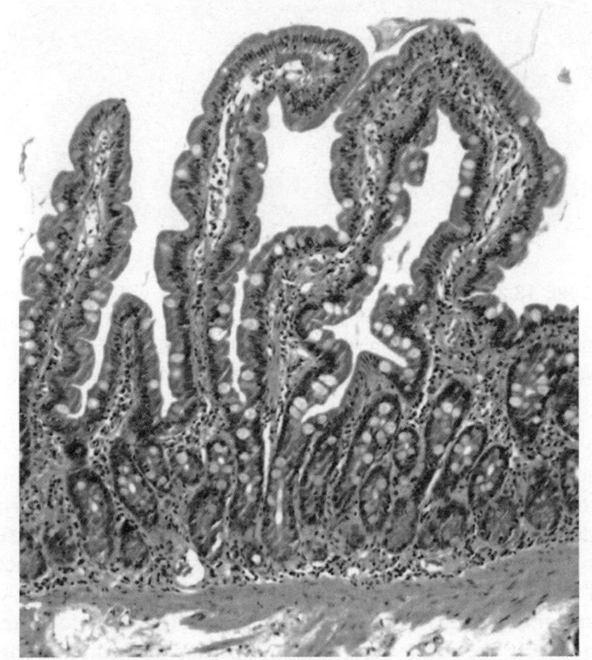

FIGURE 13.22 Normal small-intestinal mucosa is characterized by a crypt-to-villus ratio in the range of 1:3 to 1:5, scattered intraepithelial lymphocytes, lymphoid aggregates, and a mixed inflammatory infiltrate in the lamina propria.

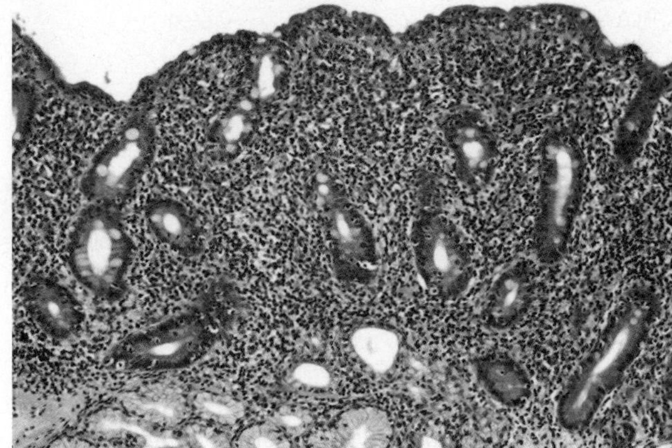

FIGURE 13.23 The celiac-like pattern shows complete villous atrophy, crypt hyperplasia, expansion of lamina propria by a mixed inflammatory infiltrate, and a marked increase in intraepithelial lymphocytes.

bouts of bloody diarrhea, whereas patients with microscopic colitis or an infiltrative disorder have mainly nonbloody ("watery") diarrhea.

In some instances, it is perfectly acceptable to use a broad pattern of *colitis* as a diagnostic term in pathology reports, as is often done with upper GI biopsies. In these instances, it is frequently helpful to offer clinicians a differential diagnosis of common causes of the particular pattern of colitis recognized by the pathologist. Ultimately, it is incumbent on the physician to interpret the diagnostic pattern of colitis in conjunction with the clinical and endoscopic findings to formulate a priority diagnosis. Diagnoses such as *chronic active colitis* or *acute hemorrhagic colitis* are usually sufficient to guide patient management.

Normal versus Abnormal

As mentioned earlier, colon biopsies that do not have an obvious inflammatory component, lamina propria infiltrate,

TABLE 13.7 Differential Diagnosis of Duodenal Mucosa with Complete Villous Atrophy and Increased Intraepithelial Lymphocytes

Feature	Celiac Disease	Refractory Sprue	Collagenous Sprue	Inflammatory Bowel Disease	Autoimmune Enteropathy
Ileal and colonic involvement	May be present	Absent	Absent	Present	May be present
Active inflammation	May be present	May be present	May be present	Present	May be present
Granulomas unrelated to crypt rupture	Absent	Absent	Absent	Present (Crohn's disease)	Absent
Absent goblet cells	Absent	Absent	Absent	Absent	Present
Increased apoptosis	Absent	Absent	Absent	Absent	Present
Abnormal T cells	Absent	Present	Absent	Absent	Absent
Thick subepithelial collagen	Absent	Absent	Present	Absent	Absent
Antibodies	Anti-tTG	Anti-tTG	Anti-tTG	Absent	Antienterocyte; antigoblet cell
Response to gluten withdrawal	Present	Absent	Absent	Absent	Absent

tTG, *Tissue transglutaminase.*

TABLE 13.8 Type 1 versus Type 2 Refractory Celiac Disease

Feature	Type 1	Type 2
Aberrant T cells	Absent	Present
Clonal TCR	Absent	Present
HLA DQ2 homozygous	May be seen	Present
Associated UJ/EATL	Absent	Present
Immunosuppression response	Present	Absent
EATL risk	Low	As much as 60% at 5 years
Mortality	Slight increase	<50% at 5 years

EATL, *Enteropathy-associated T-cell lymphoma;* HLA, *human leukocyte antigen;* TCR, *T-cell receptor;* UJ, *ulcerative jejunitis.*

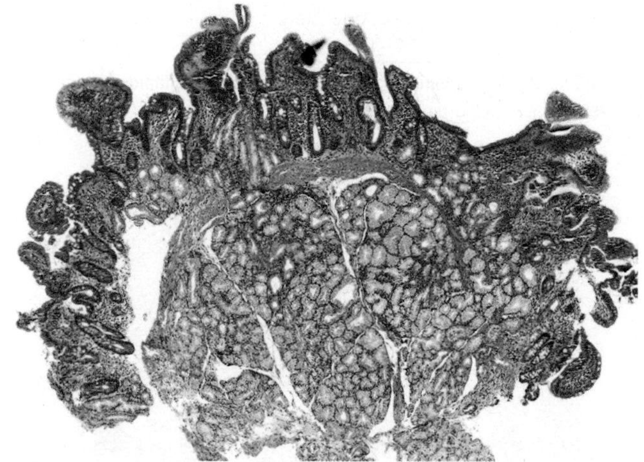

FIGURE 13.24 Gastric surface foveolar metaplasia with mild lymphoplasmacytic expansion of the lamina propria. This pattern of injury suggests prior mucosal injury and is most commonly associated with peptic duodenitis and use of nonsteroidal antiinflammatory drugs.

or neoplastic lesion should be evaluated initially in regard to whether they appear within normal limits given the effects of bowel preparation (Fig. 13.29 and Box 13.2; see also Chapter 1). In terms of normal variations, the distal several centimeters of rectum is an area often subject to chronic and repeated injury. As a result, with advancing age, it often shows a slight degree of crypt atrophy and distortion. This finding should not be overinterpreted as evidence of chronic colitis. Because of the normal undulation of the mucosa in the colon, superficial or tangential biopsies may show branching crypts. If this is present in the superficial portion of the mucosa, it is usually considered normal.

The quantity of lamina propria inflammation, and particularly the number of eosinophils, varies throughout the colon and among people in different geographic regions of the world. For instance, the right colon often shows a slightly greater degree of lamina propria mononuclear inflammation compared with the left colon. In addition, lamina propria eosinophils are typically more numerous in the right colon, but this varies significantly according to geographic region and climate. The osmotic effect of most bowel preparatory agents can result in clumping of lymphocytes and plasma cells within the lamina propria, edema, and even congestion and hemorrhage, the latter possibly related to endoscope trauma as well. Other effects of bowel preparatory procedures include a mild degree of surface epithelial degeneration, crypt regeneration, and apoptosis. In some instances, apoptoses are quite prominent and may lead to a false diagnosis of apoptotic colopathy. Infiltration of the superficial aspects of lymphoid aggregates by neutrophils may also develop as a result of bowel preparation. Insufflation of air at the time of endoscopy can lead to the acquisition of air vacuoles within the mucosa and submucosa, termed *pseudolipomatosis*. However, in contrast with a true lipoma, air vacuoles are not lined by lipocytes; instead, they are bordered by lamina propria or submucosal tissue, and they exhibit substantial variation in size and shape.

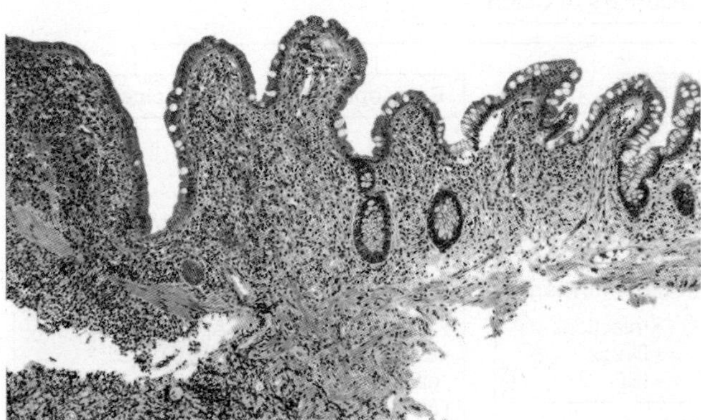

FIGURE 13.25 Eosinophil-predominant inflammatory infiltrate in the lamina propria in small-intestinal biopsies raises the possibility of eosinophilic gastroenteritis, drug-induced injury, or parasitic infestation, but it should also prompt a careful evaluation for mast cell and Langerhans cell infiltration, which is almost always accompanied by a prominent eosinophilic infiltrate.

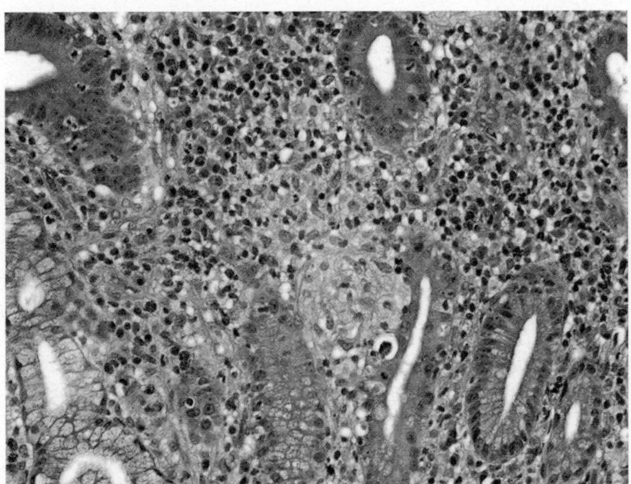

FIGURE 13.26 Epithelioid granulomas infiltrating the lamina propria of the small intestine may be seen in infectious disorders and Crohn's disease. The discrete epithelioid granulomas are distinct from the diffuse infiltrate of foamy histiocytes seen in Whipple's disease.

Inflammatory Disorders

Chronic Colitis

Biopsies of the colon that show increased inflammation (colitis) may be initially classified as either chronic, acute, eosinophilic, or paucicellular for the purpose of determining the most likely pattern of colitis and, ultimately, the etiology of the inflammatory disorder. Separation into acute or chronic type is performed by identifying histological features of chronicity (see Chapter 17). Table 13.9 provides a list of features of chronicity and activity in the colon. The finding of one or more features of chronicity is sufficient to diagnose colitis as chronic, whereas the presence of one or more features of activity indicates an active (acute) phase of disease. Therefore biopsies that show chronicity are best categorized as either *chronic inactive* or *chronic active* (the latter usually graded as *mild, moderate,* or *severe*). Biopsies that show features of activity without features of chronicity are interpreted as *active* or *acute* colitis.

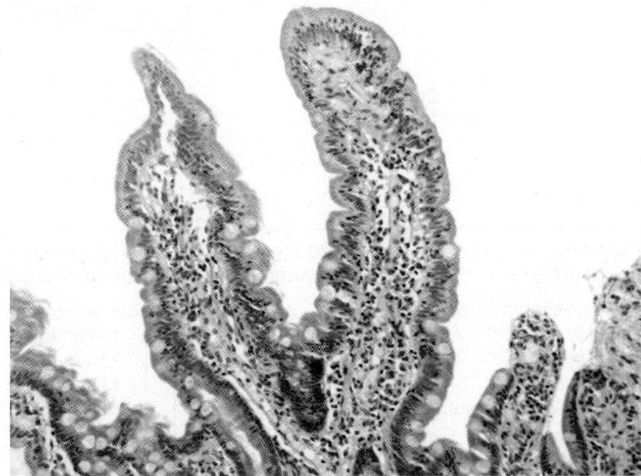

FIGURE 13.27 The differential diagnosis of small-intestinal biopsies with normal villous architecture and diffuse increase in intraepithelial lymphocytes is broad, and a systematic workup should be performed to identify a specific etiological cause.

Chronic Colitis with Preserved Architecture

The next decision point that is helpful in evaluating chronic (or active) colitides is determination of the status of the crypt architecture (normal vs. abnormal). Common disorders that show preserved crypt architecture but also reveal other well-established features of chronicity (Fig. 13.30) are summarized in Fig. 13.31. These include microscopic colitis (both lymphocytic and collagenous colitis), early IBD (both ulcerative colitis and Crohn's disease), post-treatment IBD, drug reactions, diverticulosis, and some forms of infectious colitis. *Shigella* or *Chlamydia* infection can result in the development of features of chronicity, such as basal lymphoplasmacytosis, basal lymphoid aggregates, mild crypt distortion, and granulomas. Biopsies demonstrating chronic colitis but with preserved crypt architecture may be subclassified as predominantly neutrophilic, predominantly lymphoplasmacytic, or pauciinflammatory for the purpose of narrowing the differential diagnosis. The most common forms of chronic colitis with preserved crypt architecture and a prominent neutrophilic inflammation are early-onset IBD, infectious colitis, and drug reactions. Table 13.10 summarizes some of the discriminating features of infectious colitis that may mimic Crohn's disease. This topic is covered in more detail in Chapter 17.

Determination of the anatomic distribution of disease helps one arrive at a more specific etiology. For instance, many types of infectious colitis are segmental rather than diffuse in distribution or involve the right colon more often than the left. In contrast, IBD is either diffuse and continuous and always involves the rectum (ulcerative colitis) or the ileum and colon (Crohn's disease). In general, infectious colitis is characterized by the presence of neutrophils in the lamina propria and superficial crypt epithelium; in contrast, full-thickness mucosal involvement by neutrophils is more typical in IBD.

Biopsies that show chronic colitis with preserved crypt architecture and a predominantly lymphoplasmacytic inflammatory infiltrate occur often in patients with microscopic colitis, early or resolving IBD, drug reactions,

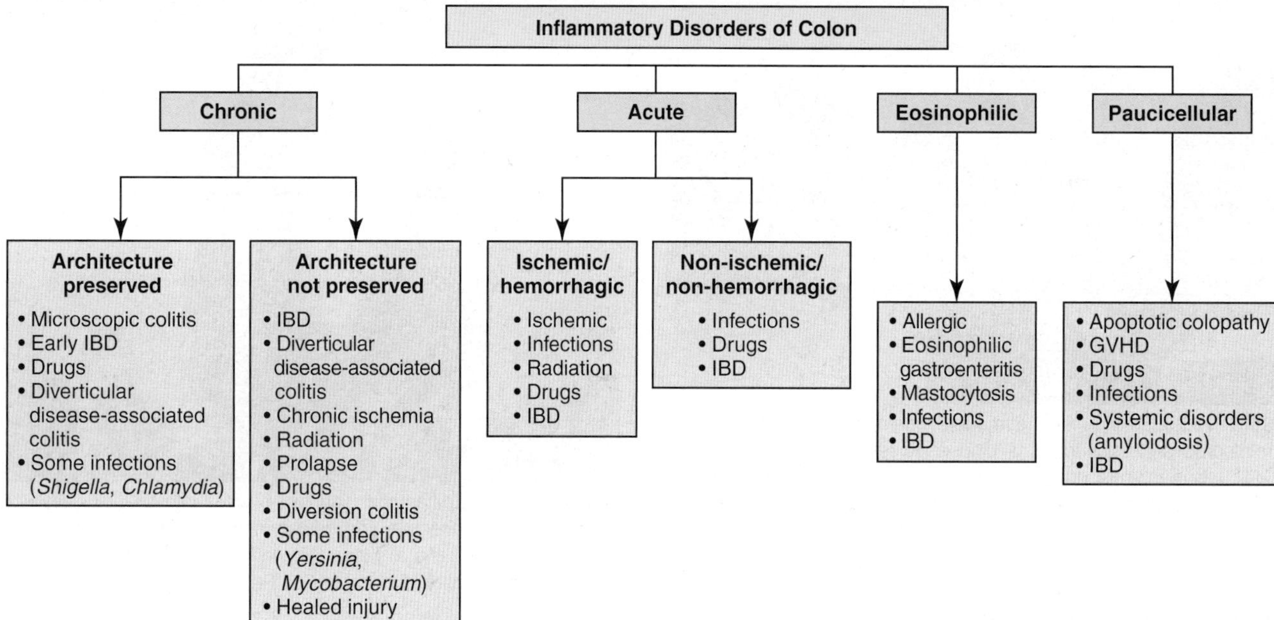

FIGURE 13.28 Algorithmic approach to diagnosis of inflammatory disorders of the colon. *GVHD,* Graft-versus-host disease; *IBD,* inflammatory bowel disease.

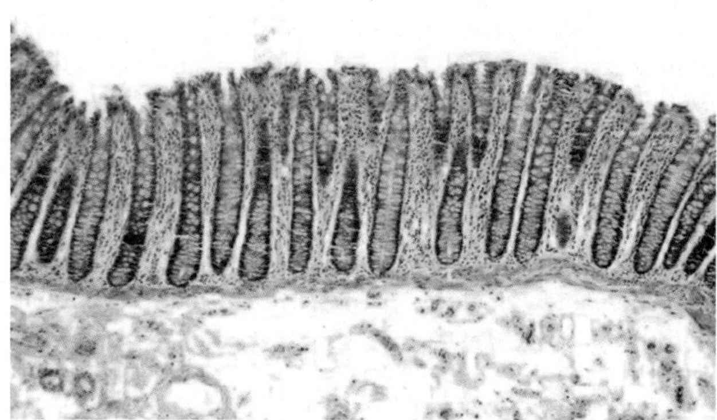

FIGURE 13.29 Normal colon biopsies show straight, tubular crypts that reach all the way to the muscularis mucosae. Cecal and ascending colon biopsies normally show more inflammatory cells in the lamina propria than are seen in the rest of the colon, and mild architectural disarray is normal for rectal biopsies.

TABLE 13.9 Inflammatory Disorders of the Colon

Features of Chronicity (Chronic Colitis)	Features of Activity (Active Colitis)
Crypt distortion/atrophy	Epithelial degeneration
Basal plasmacytosis	Epithelial regeneration
Diffuse mixed inflammation	Edema
Basal lymphoid aggregates	Hemorrhage
Metaplasia (Paneth, pyloric, other)	Necrosis
Paneth hyperplasia	Erosion/ulcer
Fibrosis/collagen	Neutrophils
Granulomas	Eosinophils (intra-epithelial)
	Apoptosis

BOX 13.2 Colon: Normal Variations and Artifacts Associated with Bowel Preparation

Crypt atrophy (rectum)
Branching crypts (superficial)
↑ Inflammation (eosinophils) in right colon
Clumping of lymphocytes/plasma cells
Edema
Congestion/hemorrhage
Surface degeneration
Crypt regeneration
Apoptosis
Few neutrophils (lymphoid aggregates)
Air vacuoles (pseudolipomatosis)
Other

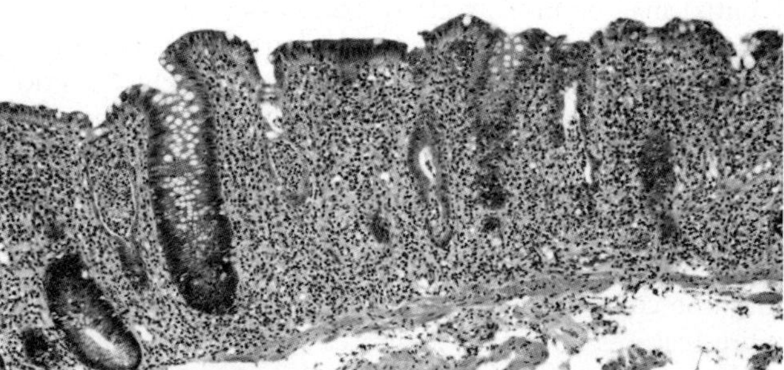

FIGURE 13.30 Chronic colitis with preserved architecture shows full-thickness inflammatory infiltrate and basal lymphoplasmacytosis that separates the base of the crypts from the muscularis mucosae. Architectural features of chronicity (crypt disarray, crypt branching) are not present in this pattern of injury.

diverticulosis, or even some forms of (resolving) infectious colitis. One of the major difficulties in this category of inflammatory disorders involves differentiating microscopic colitis from IBD (Table 13.11). Both the clinical/endoscopic and microscopic features of the biopsies are helpful to distinguish these disorders. For instance, patients with microscopic colitis usually have watery (nonbloody) diarrhea and either normal or only mildly abnormal (erythematous) endoscopic abnormalities. In contrast, patients with IBD usually have recurrent bouts of bloody diarrhea and show more significant endoscopic abnormalities, such as erythema, friability, and ulceration. Biopsies from a small proportion of patients with microscopic colitis may show features of chronicity such as basal plasmacytosis, crypt distortion, basal lymphoid aggregates, and Paneth cell metaplasia; however, in contrast with IBD, these features are typically mild and focal. Rarely, patients with lymphocytic or collagenous colitis develop a bandlike histiocytic infiltrate in the subepithelial lamina propria, which on occasion includes the development of giant cells and granulomas.

Chronic Colitis with Abnormal Crypt Architecture

The most common diseases in this category are IBD, diverticular disease–associated colitis (sometimes referred to as *segmental colitis*), chronic ischemia, chronic radiation colitis, and mucosal prolapse. To narrow the differential diagnosis when evaluating biopsies that reveal chronic colitis and abnormal crypt architecture (Fig. 13.32), it is helpful to distinguish those that show fibrosis or hyaline-like material in the lamina propria from those that do not. Lamina propria fibrosis and deposition of hyaline-like material in the lamina propria are common features in patients with ischemia, radiation injury, or mucosal prolapse. Table 13.12 summarizes some of the characteristics that differentiate these three disorders.

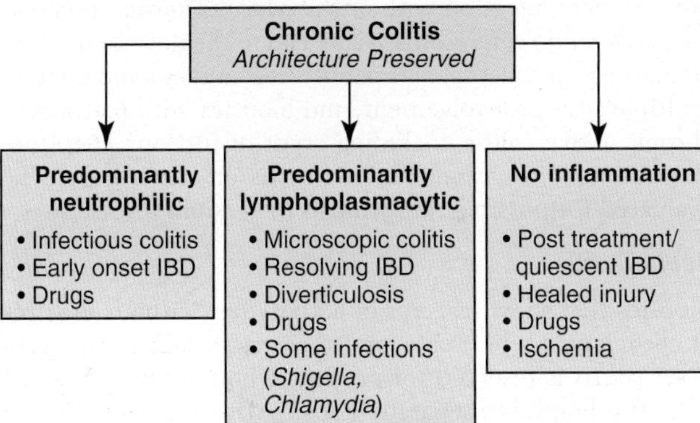

FIGURE 13.31 Algorithmic approach to chronic colitis with normal architecture. *IBD,* Inflammatory bowel disease.

TABLE 13.11 Microscopic Colitis versus Inflammatory Bowel Disease

Feature	Microscopic Colitis	Inflammatory Bowel Disease
Clinical presentation	"Watery" diarrhea	Malabsorptive or bloody diarrhea ± systemic signs
Endoscopic appearance	Normal or mildly abnormal (erythema); rare ulcers	Segmental or diffuse erythema; friability, ulcers common

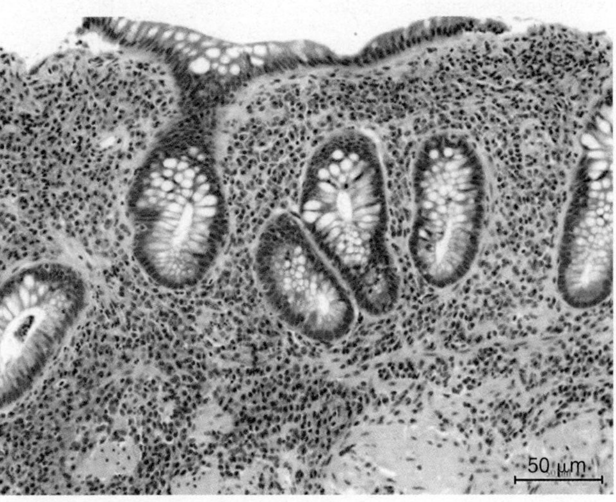

FIGURE 13.32 Cases of chronic colitis with abnormal crypt architecture show architectural features of chronicity (crypt disarray, crypt branching, crypt loss, and crypt shortening) with or without the presence of basal lymphoplasmacytosis.

TABLE 13.10 Chronic Infection versus Crohn's Disease

Feature	*Mycobacterium tuberculosis*	*Yersinia enterocolitica*	Crohn's Disease
Caseating granulomas	Frequent	Rare	Absent
Confluent granulomas	Frequent	Frequent	Absent
Few granulomas	Rare	Rare	Common
Prominent lymphoid cuff	Frequent	Frequent	Uncommon
Ulcers (both aphthous and deep)	Common	Common	Common
Architectural distortion	Common	Common	Common
Changes of chronicity unassociated with sites of granulomatous inflammation	Absent	Absent	Common
Multiple sites of involvement	Common	Rare	Common

In contrast, ulcerative colitis, Crohn's disease, diverticular disease–associated colitis, and diversion colitis are the most frequent disorders that show chronic colitis with crypt architectural distortion but without lamina propria fibrosis or hyaline-like material. Biopsies from patients with ulcerative colitis or Crohn's disease are categorized as *chronic inactive* or *chronic active*. The latter may be subdivided into *mild*, *moderate*, or *severe* depending on the severity of inflammation and the degree of epithelial injury. Distinguishing ulcerative colitis from Crohn's disease in mucosal biopsies is usually not possible, particularly in patients who have had prior medical treatment, in which case portions of the mucosa may show reversion of architectural changes and a normal or near-normal appearance (Table 13.13). Therefore in posttreatment IBD, the principal role of the pathologist is to determine the extent and severity of disease and the presence or absence of dysplasia. Distinguishing ulcerative colitis from Crohn's disease is usually not possible unless biopsies show granulomas unrelated to ruptured crypts, the patient has chronic or chronic active ileal disease (unrelated to "backwash" ileitis, bowel preparation, or drug reaction), or the patient has Crohn's disease–associated anal disease. However, in IBD patients whose biopsies are obtained before treatment, ulcerative colitis can be distinguished from Crohn's disease if the inflammatory changes are segmental or patchy, there is an absence of rectal involvement, granulomas unrelated to ruptured crypts are present, the patient has Crohn's disease–associated anal disease, or there is upper GI or ileal disease. In some cases of ulcerative colitis, there is relative or absolute rectal sparing (initial presentation in children) and/or segmental disease (left-sided colitis with a cecal patch). This subject is discussed in more detail in Chapter 17.

Mucosal biopsies in areas of involvement of diverticular disease–associated colitis are identical to ulcerative colitis. Therefore these two disorders cannot be distinguished by analysis of mucosal biopsies. Absence of rectal involvement and absence of involvement of mucosa proximal to areas of diverticulosis favor diverticular disease–associated colitis.

Many types of drugs, such as mycophenolate, ipilimumab, and other immune checkpoint inhibitors, can mimic IBD. Knowledge of the timing and sequence of symptoms and signs in relation to drug intake is essential for establishing a particular drug as the cause of a patient's colitis.

As mentioned earlier, some types of infectious colitis can develop histological features of chronicity, mimicking IBD. For instance, infection with either *Mycobacterium tuberculosis* or *Yersinia enterocolitica* can lead to the development of granulomas, segmental and patchy ileal and colonic disease, multiple sites of involvement, and biopsies with features of chronic active colitis, including crypt distortion. Therefore all patients with granulomatous ileitis or colitis should be evaluated for possible tuberculosis or *Yersinia* infection.

TABLE 13.12 Differential Diagnosis of Chronic Colitis with Abnormal Crypt Architecture and Lamina Propria Fibrosis or Hyalinization

Feature	Chronic Ischemia (Primary)	Radiation	Prolapse
Polyp/mass formation	Rare	Rare	Present
Primarily rectal involvement	Rare	Present	Present
IBD-like mucosal inflammation	Rare	May be present	Absent
Withering crypts	May be seen	May be seen	May be seen
Pseudomembrane	May be seen	Absent	Absent
Hyalinization	Prominent	Prominent	Absent
Fibromuscular hyperplasia	May be seen	Absent	Prominent
Vascular dilation/ proliferation	May be present	Prominent	May be present
Atypical stromal/ epithelial cells	Absent	Present	Absent
Hyperplastic changes	Absent	Absent	Prominent
Thrombi	Present	May be seen	May be seen

IBD, *Inflammatory bowel disease.*

Acute Colitis

Biopsies that show features of activity but without features of chronicity are best categorized as *active colitis*. The term *acute colitis* is reserved for patients who have no history of IBD. It is helpful to separate biopsies with active colitis into those that have an ischemic/hemorrhagic appearance and those that do not. The former may be diagnosed as *acute hemorrhagic colitis*.

TABLE 13.13 Differential Diagnosis of Inflammatory Bowel Disease

Feature	UC before Treatment	UC after Treatment	Crohn's Disease
Diffuse disease	Always	May be present	May be present
Rectal involvement	Always (except children)	May be absent	May be absent
Segmental involvement	Rare (cecal patch, appendix)	May be present	Present
Ileal involvement	Mild	Distal 1-5cm	Mild → severe, >5cm
UGI involvement	Rare	Rare	Usually present
Granulomas	Mucin-related	Mucin-related	Non–mucin-related
Anal disease	Absent	Absent	Usually present

UC, *Ulcerative colitis;* UGI, *upper gastrointestinal tract.*

Acute Hemorrhagic Colitis

The most common causes of an acute ischemic/hemorrhagic colitis pattern of injury are ischemia, infection, radiation injury, certain drug reactions, and some phases of IBD (Fig. 13.33). *Escherichia coli* and *Clostridium difficile* are two of the more common infections that cause acute hemorrhagic colitis. Injury to the bowel mucosa is mediated by toxins released by these organisms that lead to intestinal ischemia, resulting in an ischemic-like acute hemorrhagic colitis. Ultimately, the most useful way to differentiate these two disorders is by analysis of stool for C. *difficile* toxin and special cultures for growth of *E. coli* O157:H7. The discriminating features of these disorders are discussed in more detail in Chapters 4 and 17.

Table 13.14 summarizes some of the characteristics that distinguish primary acute ischemia from infectious colitis (e.g., *E. coli* O157:H7) and acute radiation injury. For example, ischemia often involves watershed areas of the bowel such as the splenic flexure and shows prominent withering crypts and lamina propria hyalinization, whereas infectious colitis more often involves the right colon, shows more prominent edema and hemorrhage and neutrophils, and has less prominent withering crypts. Radiation colitis should be suspected in patients who have had a prior pelvic carcinoma. The changes of acute radiation injury are typically limited to the left colon. Common features of radiation injury include dilated and proliferating lamina propria and submucosal blood vessels and atypical epithelial and/or stromal cells. In some cases, lamina propria fibrosis or hyalinization is prominent, mimicking collagenous colitis (see Chapters 4 and 17).

Acute (Nonhemorrhagic) Colitis

Biopsies that show active (acute) colitis but without a hemorrhagic or ischemic appearance (Fig. 13.34) are most often caused by infection, drugs, or IBD. Acute infectious colitis is often referred to as *self-limited colitis* because the symptoms and signs typically improve without treatment. The most common causes of acute self-limited (infectious) colitis in the colon are *Salmonella*, *Shigella*, *Campylobacter*,

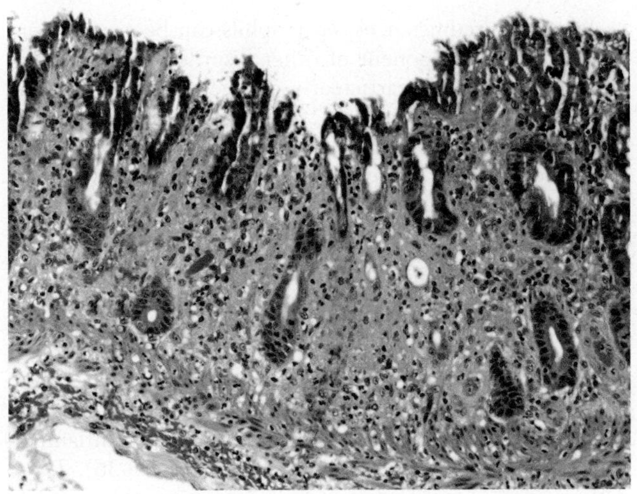

FIGURE 13.33 An acute ischemic/hemorrhagic colitis pattern of injury is characterized by hyalinization of the lamina propria, withering crypts, and regenerative epithelial changes, with or without intravascular fibrin thrombi. This pattern may be associated with ischemia, infection, radiation, or drug-induced mucosal injury.

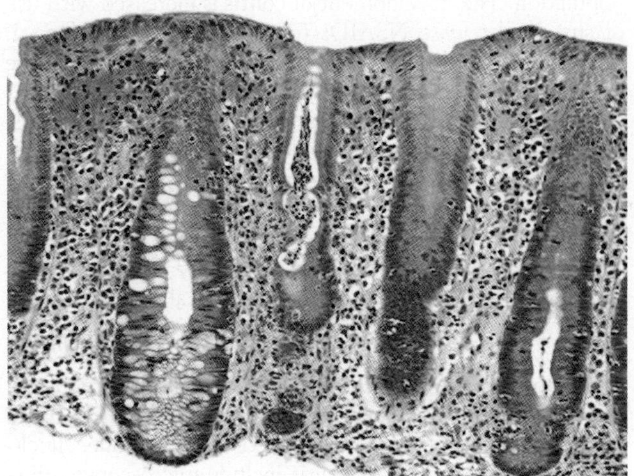

FIGURE 13.34 Acute nonhemorrhagic colitis is most often infectious, drug induced, or a manifestation of early inflammatory bowel disease. The lymphoplasmacytic inflammation is confined to the upper half of the mucosa and is accompanied by an active (neutrophilic) component of variable severity.

TABLE 13.14 Active Colitis, Ischemic/Hemorrhagic Type Pattern of Injury

Feature	Ischemia	Infection (*E. coli*)	Radiation
Anatomic distribution	Watershed	Right > Left	Left > Right
Edema/hemorrhage	Present	Common	Present
Withered crypts	Prominent	May be present	May be present
Fibrin thrombi	May be present	May be present	May be present
Neutrophils	May be present (in early phase)	Prominent	May be present
Atypical epithelial and stromal cells	Absent	Absent	Present
Dilated blood vessels	May be present	Absent	Prominent
LP hyalinization	Prominent	May be present	May be present

LP, *Lamina propria.*

Aeromonas, and *E. coli* (see Chapters 4 and 17). Although there is substantial overlap in histological features among these infectious colitides, some organisms are associated with certain characteristics that help identify them (see Chapter 17). Most infectious colitides are characterized by predominantly neutrophilic inflammation in the lamina propria and crypts, often involving the upper half of the mucosa more significantly than the lower half. Features of chronicity, such as basal plasmacytosis and crypt distortion, are typically absent. Infectious colitides are often segmental or patchy in distribution and may involve the right colon more often than the left. The pattern of involvement may help suggest one type of organism over another. However, the precise diagnosis is ultimately established by stool culture.

In some cases, patients with IBD, particularly if it is mild, show features of infectious colitis (without well-established features of chronicity). Posttreatment biopsies from patients with IBD may show similar features. Finally, many types of drug reactions can mimic infectious colitis (see Chapter 12 for a more detailed discussion of drug-induced colitis). NSAID use is one of the most common causes of colitis in the general population. The development of colitis is increased with use of sustained-release NSAIDs (e.g., fenamates, diclofenac). NSAID-induced colonic injury can mimic almost any type or pattern of colitis, including infectious colitis, IBD, ischemic colitis, microscopic colitis, and even eosinophilic colitis. Therefore a drug reaction should be considered in the differential diagnosis of all inflammatory disorders of the GI tract, including the colon. More notably, anti–PD-1 and anti–PD-L1 agents, which have been approved by the US Food and Drug Administration for a wide variety of cancers (e.g., melanoma, renal cell carcinoma, colorectal cancers), have been associated with an acute colitis pattern of injury. In these instances, it can be difficult to differentiate acute self-limited infectious colitis from immune checkpoint inhibitor–related colitis (see Chapter 17 for additional details). Other known patterns of injury associated with immune checkpoint inhibitor–associated colitis include microscopic colitis and an IBD-like pattern of injury.

Eosinophil-Predominant Colitis

Eosinophils are a common component of inflammatory infiltrates in many different types of disorders of the colon. However, their occurrence as the predominant, or only, type of inflammatory cell elicits a specific differential diagnosis that includes allergic colitis, eosinophilic gastroenteritis, parasitic infection, and certain mast cell disorders. Eosinophilic colitis (known as *allergic colitis*) is mainly a disorder of young infants and neonates and usually involves the rectum (Fig. 13.35). Eosinophilic gastroenteritis is a poorly understood condition that often affects children and young adults. However, this condition involves mainly the esophagus, stomach, and/or small intestine. The colon is rarely involved in isolation from these other organs.

Parasitic infections often elicit a prominent eosinophilic infiltrate, but the eosinophils are usually in the form of microabscesses, and they do not typically involve the epithelium or cause epithelial injury. Mast cell disorders such as systemic mastocytosis can elicit a prominent eosinophilic response in some cases, but these patients usually have a known history of systemic mastocytosis.

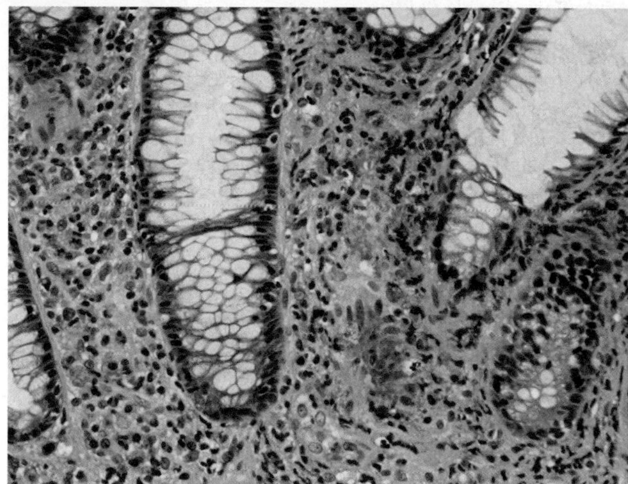

FIGURE 13.35 An eosinophil-predominant pattern of injury is seen more often in pediatric biopsies and is characterized by a marked increase in eosinophils in the lamina propria associated with intraepithelial infiltration and epithelial damage.

In some circumstances, eosinophils can be a prominent inflammatory component of other disorders, such as IBD, microscopic colitis (particularly collagenous colitis), many different types of drug reactions, and vasculitis. These other conditions usually reveal other, more typical histological features and other types of inflammatory cells that are characteristic of the specific disorder that is causing the patient's illness.

Paucicellular Colitis

Colitis associated with a minimal inflammatory component or none at all is a common reaction pattern in many different types of (resolving) inflammatory disorders of the colon. However, certain inflammatory conditions are more typically associated with paucicellular lamina propria inflammation at the peak of the patient's illness (Fig. 13.36). These include drug reactions, certain infections, and systemic disorders that involve the colon (e.g., amyloidosis). A common pattern in this group is apoptotic colopathy, defined as colitis associated with apoptosis as a prominent histological feature of the disorder. Apoptoses may be associated with other types of inflammatory cells, or it may be present in isolation.

The differential diagnosis of apoptotic colopathy is outlined in Box 13.3. Some bowel preparation solutions are associated with the development of prominent apoptoses in the bases of the crypts. The right colon is often affected more severely than the left colon. In this condition, there is usually no evidence of colitis other than the presence of apoptosis. Chemotherapeutic drugs and other immunosuppressants, such as mycophenolate, are associated with prominent apoptosis and apoptotic microabscesses. GVHD, transplant rejection, cord colitis syndrome, certain infections (CMV or HIV), and radiation injury can also cause prominent apoptotic injury to the epithelium. Certain phases of IBD are also associated with prominent apoptosis, but other features of IBD usually provide clues to the correct diagnosis in this condition.

Mycophenolate-induced colitis may mimic GVHD, but the former condition often shows more prominent eosinophils and neutrophils in the inflammatory infiltrate, and only rare endocrine cell aggregates compared with GVHD (see Table 13.14). CMV infection can also be difficult to differentiate from GVHD, and both conditions can be present in the same patient. Considering this differential diagnosis, crypt distortion, hypereosinophilic crypts, and prominent crypt necrosis and dropout are more characteristic of GVHD than CMV infection, particularly in patients who have severe disease. In bone marrow transplant recipients in whom GVHD-like changes in the colon develop and in whom viral inclusions are identified, it is probably best to consider the latter a superimposed infection, particularly if the patient has evidence of GVHD in other organs of the body (e.g., skin, liver, upper GI tract).

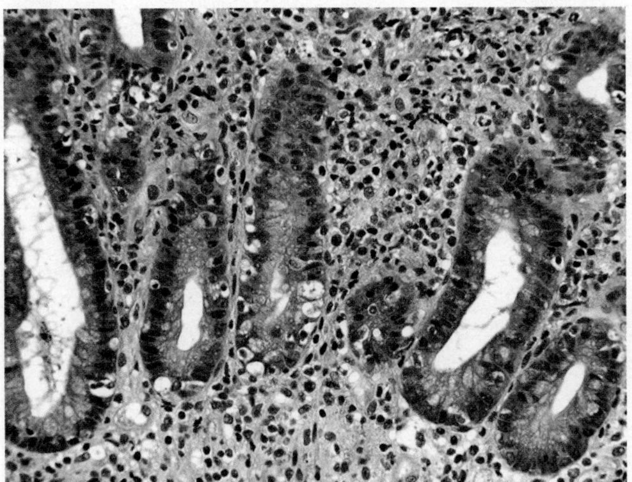

FIGURE 13.36 A paucicellular inflammatory pattern in the colon may be associated with increased apoptosis, as illustrated here. This pattern is typically seen in graft-versus-host disease and its mimics, including mycophenolate-induced mucosal injury and infectious colitis.

BOX 13.3 Differential Diagnosis of Apoptotic Colopathy

Bowel preparation
Drugs (chemotherapy, mycophenolate)
GVHD
Transplant rejection
Infection (CMV, HIV)
IBD
Radiation

CMV, *Cytomegalovirus;* GVHD, *graft-versus-host disease;* HIV, *human immunodeficiency virus;* IBD, *inflammatory bowel disease.*

Lamina Propria Infiltrates

The causes and differential diagnosis of lamina propria infiltrates of the colon are covered extensively in Chapter 6. Fig. 13.37 shows an example of xanthomatous infiltrates. Table 13.15 separates infiltrates into pigmented and

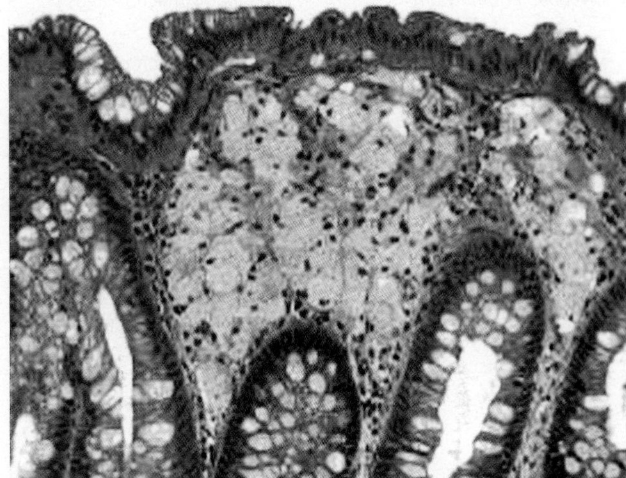

FIGURE 13.37 Histiocytic lamina propria infiltrates in the absence of a significant inflammatory component are seldom of much clinical consequence in the colon. Xanthomatous infiltrates *(shown here)* and melanosis coli are the two most common types of infiltrates seen in colon biopsies.

TABLE 13.14 Differential Diagnosis of Graft Versus Host Disease

Feature	GVHD	Mycophenolate Mofetil–Induced Colitis	CMV	Cord Colitis Syndrome
Crypt architecture	Usually distorted (except in mild cases)	Usually distorted	Usually preserved	Usually distorted
Prominent eosinophils	Absent	Present	Absent	Absent
Lymphoplasmacytic inflammation	Absent	Absent	Absent	Present
Clusters of neuroendocrine cells in lamina propria	Present	Absent	Absent	Absent
Loose aggregate of epithelioid histiocytes	Absent	Absent	Absent	Present; usually related to crypt injury
Hypereosinophilic crypts	Present	May be present	Absent	Absent
Crypt dropout and necrosis	Present; usually in grades 3-4	May be present	Absent	Absent
Viral inclusions	Absent	Absent	Present	Absent

CMV, *Cytomegalovirus;* GVHD, *graft-versus-host disease.*

TABLE 13.15 Lamina Propria Infiltrates

Diagnosis	Histology	Histochemical	Immunohistochemical
Pigmented			
Melanosis	Dark brown, granular macrophages	PAS and acid-fast positive	CD68 positive (must bleach pigment)
Pseudomelanosis	Black, subepithelial macrophages	Iron positive	CD68 positive
Brown bowel syndrome	Brown smooth muscle cells	PAS, acid-fast positive Yellow autofluorescence	N/A
Barium granuloma	Gray, finely granular refractile pigment	PAS negative	N/A
Chronic granulomatous disease	Golden-brown macrophages	Fat stain and PAS positive	N/A
Nonpigmented			
Xanthoma	Clear, foamy macrophages	Fat stain positive on unfixed tissue	α_1-Antitripsin, monocyte chemotactic and activating factors
Muciphages	Clear, foamy macrophages	d-PAS, Alcian blue positive	CD68 lysozyme positive
Mycobacterium avium	Pink, foamy macrophages	Acid-fast or Fite positive d-PAS diffuse positive	CD68 positive
Malakoplakia	Pink, foamy macrophages with nuclear grooves Michaelis-Gutmann bodies (MGB)	d-PAS positive MGB positive for calcium and iron	CD68 positive
Granular cell tumor	Pink, granular histiocytic cells	d-PAS positive	S100 positive
Signet ring cell carcinoma	Clear cytoplasm with displaced nucleus	d-PAS, Alcian blue, and mucin positive globules	Cytokeratin positive
Clear cell carcinoid tumor	Clear cells with foamy cytoplasm	d-PAS and mucin negative	Chromogranin positive
Malignant histiocytosis	Granular Langerhans cells with irregular elongate nuclei and nuclear grooves	d-PAS and mucin negative	S100 and CD1a positive

d-PAS, *Periodic acid–Schiff stain with diastase digestion.*

nonpigmented types and provides a summary of the histological, histochemical, and immunohistochemical methods for separating these two disorders. Most infiltrative disorders do not cause colitis, but cause expansion of the lamina propria and distortion of the crypts by the infiltrate. Therefore, although technically not a form of "colitis," lamina propria infiltrates may cause an endoscopic appearance of colitis and a diarrheal illness.

Neoplasia

Neoplastic conditions of the colon are covered in detail in Chapters 17, 22, and 27. Some neoplastic conditions, such as dysplasia, arise in patients with chronic inflammatory diseases of the colon (e.g., ulcerative colitis, Crohn's disease). Distinguishing regenerative changes from dysplasia in IBD are also covered in Chapter 17.

CHAPTER 14

Inflammatory Disorders of the Esophagus

Margaret H. Collins, Robert D. Odze, Deepa T. Patil

Contents

INTRODUCTION

Inflammatory disorders of the esophagus are extremely common. Among the most common is gastroesophageal reflux disease (GERD), a chronic condition, affecting as many as 40% of people in the Western world.[1] Because of the ease and frequent use of upper endoscopy for diagnosing gastrointestinal (GI) illnesses, biopsy specimens procured from esophageal mucosa to evaluate the presence or absence of inflammatory diseases—particularly GERD and its attendant complication, Barrett's esophagus (BE)—are commonly encountered by surgical pathologists. This chapter focuses on myriad inflammatory conditions that affect the esophagus, beginning with GERD.

GASTROESOPHAGEAL REFLUX DISEASE

Clinical Features

GERD is an extremely common chronic condition, particularly in Western countries.[1] Estimates based on an assumption that reflux-like symptoms are an indicator of the disease suggest a prevalence rate of 20% to 40%.[2,3] GERD is associated with considerable healthcare costs; in the United States in 2015 esophageal disorders accounted for $18.1 billion in health care expenditures, including $12.4 billion for acid-inhibition therapies.[4] Clinically, GERD is often classified as *erosive* or *nonerosive* based on endoscopic or pathological features, and currently includes the concepts of *proven* and *unproven* GERD in clinical decision-making.[1] One recent review defines GERD as "a family of syndromes attributable to, or exacerbated by, gastroesophageal reflux, evident symptomatically, endoscopically, or by physiological testing, which impart morbidity through troublesome symptoms and/or risk."[5] Using this definition, GERD phenotypes emerge including nonerosive reflux disease, GERD hypersensitivity, low- or high-grade esophagitis, Barrett's esophagus, reflux chest pain syndrome, laryngopharyngeal reflux, and regurgitation dominant reflux. Risk factors associated with GERD include advanced age (especially after age 40 years), certain lifestyle habits (e.g., alcohol consumption), body mass index, and tobacco smoking, although the clinically relevant contributions of many of these factors are not entirely clear. Compared to females, males are at increased risk for erosive esophagitis, Barrett's esophagus, and especially esophageal adenocarcinoma.[6] The symptoms most often associated with GERD are heartburn, acid regurgitation, and dysphagia. Reflux symptoms are common in runners.[7] Atypical or supraesophageal symptoms include asthma, chronic cough, chronic sore throat, pharyngitis, laryngitis, a globus sensation, and noncardiac chest pain. The clinical and pathogenetic aspects of GERD are discussed further in the section on BE.

Pathogenesis

In the traditional view, GERD may also be defined as "a condition in which a normal physiological event is affected by an imbalance between aggressive and defensive factors."[4] Aggressive factors include hiatus hernia, found in patients who have moderate to marked GERD; transient relaxation of the lower esophageal sphincter in GERD patients who do not have hiatus hernia; acid; pepsin; bile acids; alcohol; and acidic foods. Defensive factors include lower and upper esophageal sphincters, esophageal peristalsis, and restoration of normal esophageal pH following a reflux episode by salivary bicarbonate secretion, impaired in patients who have xerostomia or Sjogren's syndrome. Expressed as the "burn hypothesis,"[4] reflux esophagitis is caused by reflux of gastric or duodenal fluid into the esophagus, and refluxed gastric acid, bile, pepsin, and duodenal contents cause injury to the esophageal mucosa.[8-10] Esophageal epithelial injury is greater if pepsin is present in addition to acid in refluxate.[4] With ongoing reflux injury, surface esophageal cells die, triggering both an inflammatory response (infiltration of neutrophils) and a proliferative response (basal cell and papillary hyperplasia). The cause of reflux is multifactorial. Contributing factors in addition to those already stated above include delayed gastric emptying, increased gastric acid production, and bile reflux.[2,3,11-13] Although the data have been somewhat conflicting, there is some evidence to support an association among high body mass index, the presence of hiatal hernia, and GERD.[5,14-18] Likewise, there is evidence to suggest that *Helicobacter pylori* infection may actually protect against the development of GERD and its complications.[5,18,19] Specifically, corpus gastritis is associated with decreased acid secretion, and GERD is less common in patients with severe corpus gastritis.[11,20] When acid secretion returns to normal after the eradication of *H. pylori*, there is an increased risk of developing GERD.[21,22]

Recent studies of the pathogenesis of GERD in animal models [20,23,24] and in vitro indicate that exposing esophageal squamous epithelial cells to acids and bile salts alone can cause epithelial cells to secrete inflammatory cytokines (i.e., interleukin 8 [IL8] and IL1β) that cause inflammatory cells (T-lymphocytes and neutrophils) to migrate into the epithelium. This finding has led to the new inflammation hypothesis asserting that the inflammatory response, not the direct effect of acid, is the initial factor responsible for damaging esophageal mucosa.[6] Evidence supporting the role of inflammation in GERD includes antiinflammatory symptoms reduction, reported by many patients affected by GERD, after commencing proton pump inhibitors (PPI) therapy, because PPI recently have been shown to have antiinflammatory effects on esophageal epithelium.[25] Histological examination in animal models has demonstrated that infiltration of the submucosa by lymphocytes is an early manifestation of inflammation. Neutrophils involve the mucosal surface later in the course of disease progression. These findings provide further support for an alternative concept for the development of reflux esophagitis in humans.[20]

The diagnosis of GERD has rested on the clinical impression of symptoms consistent with pathological reflux and the demonstration of excessive acid reflux. However, the association of symptoms with reflux is generally weak, and the use of additional modalities may add to the diagnostic accuracy. A schema to increase diagnostic accuracy for GERD is shown in Table 14.1.[26]

TABLE 14.1 GERD Diagnosis Based on Multiple Modalities

Endoscopy	Ph or Ph-Impedance	High-Resolution Manometry
Conclusive Evidence for Pathological Reflux		
• High-grade (LA grades C and D) esophagitis • Long-segment Barrett's esophagus • Peptic esophageal stricture	• Acid exposure time >6%	
Borderline or Inconclusive Evidence		
• Low-grade (LA grades A and B) esophagitis	• Acid exposure time 4-6% • Reflux episodes 40-80	
Adjunctive or Supportive Evidence*		
• Histopathology (light microscopy or electron microscopy) • Low mucosal impedance	• Symptoms associate with reflux • Reflux episodes >80 • Low mean nocturnal baseline impedance • Low post-reflux swallow-induced peristaltic wave index	• Hypotensive esophagogastric junction • Hiatus hernia • Esophageal hypomotility
Evidence Against Reflux		
	• Acid exposure time <4% • Reflux episodes <40	

**Increases confidence for pathological reflux if other evidence is borderline or inconclusive.*
Data from Gyawali CP, Kahrilas PJ, Savarino E, et al. Modern diagnosis of GERD: the Lyon consensus. Gut 2018;67:1351–1362.

The role of esophageal biopsy in the diagnosis of GERD is debated. In the schema in Table 14.1, for example, histomorphology is considered adjunctive, to be obtained only in cases not confirmed endoscopically or by pH or pH impedance. Other strategies suggest more liberal use of biopsy including to rule out eosinophilic esophagitis (see Eosinophilic Esophagitis section).[27] However, a recent study concluded that in patients who have refractory GERD symptoms but do not have dysphagia, the prevalence of eosinophilic esophagitis is so low that obtaining biopsies may be considered unnecessary.[28]

Pathology

On endoscopic examination, patients with erosive esophagitis exhibit erosions, ulcers, strictures, or some combination of these. However, as many as 50% to 60% of all symptomatic patients with objective evidence of GERD have normal mucosa or only mild hyperemia at endoscopy.[29] Furthermore, histologically inflamed esophageal mucosa (esophagitis) may appear normal endoscopically; and conversely, hyperemia does not necessarily indicate the presence of esophagitis microscopically. Because of these endoscopic/pathological discrepancies, biopsies are always warranted in symptomatic patients to document the presence of tissue injury and to exclude other entities such as infections, eosinophilic esophagitis (EoE) especially in patients who have dysphagia, BE, and other preneoplastic or inflammatory alterations. This approach is particularly important if empiric reflux therapy has failed.

Biopsies of grossly visible lesions in GERD characteristically reveal evidence of "active" esophagitis, a nonspecific injury pattern that can result from a variety of causes. Pinch biopsies obtained through standard endoscopes are often not adequate for evaluation of early histological changes resulting from reflux because they usually do not include the entire thickness of the mucosa and are difficult to orient.[8,29] Endoscopes with a large-caliber biopsy channel and jumbo biopsy forceps should be used to facilitate accurate histological diagnosis. Use of jumbo forceps does not increase the rate of complications related to endoscopy[30]; rather, it greatly improves the quality of the histological specimens.

Histologically, reflux changes are typically distributed over the distal 8 to 10 cm of the esophagus in a patchy fashion, and multiple biopsies are often necessary to consistently demonstrate histological abnormalities.[31] However, changes are typically worse in the distal esophagus and decrease in intensity more proximally. Because biopsy specimens from the lower 1 to 2 cm of the esophagus, even in asymptomatic subjects, often reveal evidence of mild squamous hyperplasia,[31,32] diagnostic biopsy specimens should be obtained usually more than 2.0 cm above the level of the gastroesophageal junction (GEJ) to diagnose esophagitis reliably, and submitted specimens should state the esophageal site from which the biopsies were obtained.[33] Furthermore, because of a high level of discordance between endoscopic and histological findings, it is recommended that all symptomatic patients undergo biopsy, regardless of the presence or absence of endoscopic abnormalities. Esophageal biopsies are considered more useful for establishing a diagnosis of GERD in infants than in adults.[34]

Reflux esophagitis produces a characteristic, although nonspecific, tissue injury pattern. Features of untreated active esophagitis include basal cell hyperplasia, elongation of the lamina propria papillae into more than two thirds of the thickness of the mucosa, epithelial cell necrosis, increased intraepithelial inflammation (including eosinophils, neutrophils, and lymphocytes), lack of surface maturation (nucleated cells at surface of epithelium), distended pale squamous "balloon" cells, intercellular edema (acantholysis), and, in severe cases, surface erosions or ulcerations (Figs. 14.1 to 14.3). Intercellular edema or dilated intercellular spaces reflecting increased paracellular permeability may be a useful marker of early injury in the absence of endoscopic evidence of injury.[35,36] Scoring several histological features of esophageal biopsies (elongated papillae, basal zone hyperplasia, dilated intercellular spaces, intraepithelial inflammatory cells, necrosis, and erosions) may be useful to distinguish nonerosive reflux disease biopsies from reflux hypersensitivity, functional heartburn, and control biopsies.[26,37,38]

Squamous Hyperplasia

For many years, it was believed that the only true diagnostic criterion for esophagitis was the presence of intraepithelial inflammation. However, in 1970, Ismail-Beigi and co-workers found that some patients who had clinical symptoms of GERD but a normal or only minimally abnormal endoscopic appearance showed hyperplasia of the squamous epithelium, a finding that they postulated was an

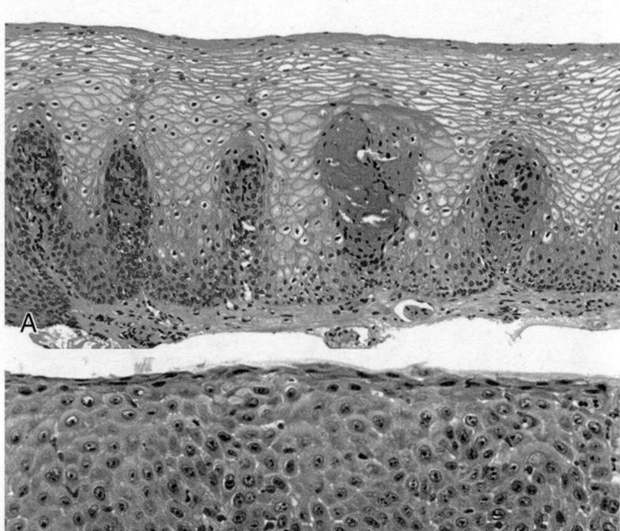

FIGURE 14.1 A, Normal squamous mucosa shows basal and suprabasal cells that involve less than 15% of the thickness of the epithelium. The lamina propria papillae involve approximately 50% of the thickness of the epithelium. **B,** In reflux esophagitis, there is basal and suprabasal cell hyperplasia, elongation of the lamina propria papillae, lack of surface maturation with the presence of nucleated squamous cells at the surface of the epithelium, and increased inflammation in the lamina propria.

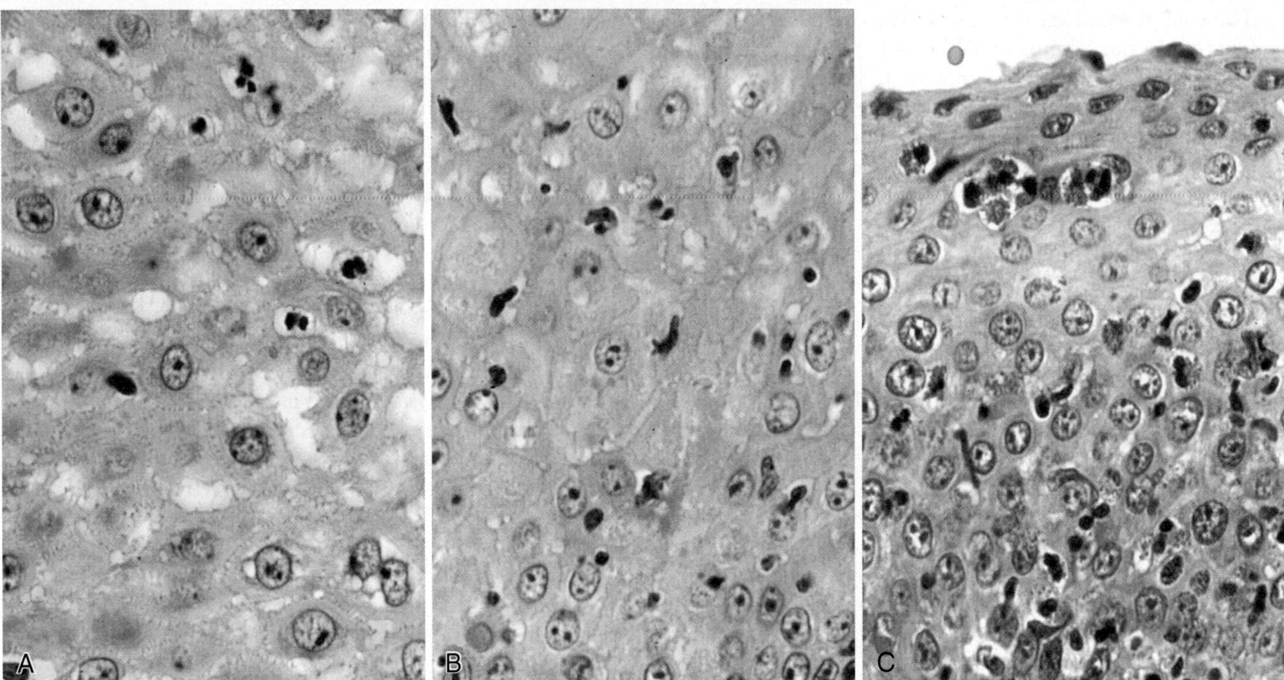

FIGURE 14.2 High-power view of the squamous mucosa in a patient with reflux esophagitis. A, Neutrophils are identified within the squamous epithelium. **B,** There is an increased intraepithelial component of squiggly T lymphocytes. **C,** There is an increased number of eosinophils. In addition, the squamous cells are reactive appearing, with prominent nucleoli. Intercellular edema is evident, particularly in **A.**

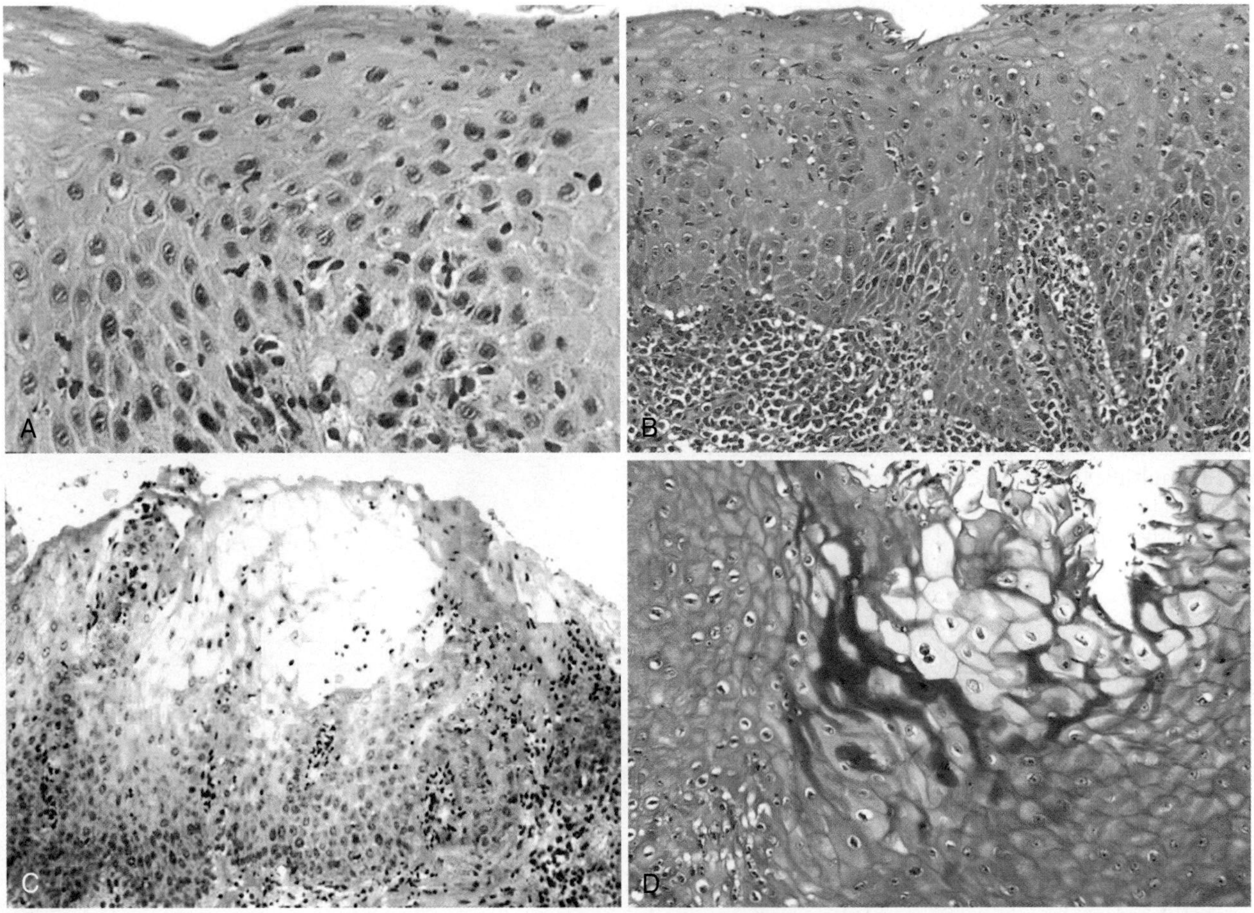

FIGURE 14.3 Reflux esophagitis. A, Mild reflux esophagitis shows reactive squamous cells, increased intraepithelial lymphocytes, and prominent intercellular edema, particularly in the basal and middle portions of the epithelium. **B,** Moderate reflux esophagitis shows an increased number of intraepithelial lymphocytes, scattered eosinophils, and few neutrophils. **C** and **D,** Severe reflux esophagitis. This portion of the squamous mucosa shows increased intraepithelial neutrophils and ballooning degeneration of the squamous cells, particularly in the middle and superficial portions of the epithelium.

early histological manifestation of reflux-induced injury.[39] Squamous hyperplasia was defined by (1) lengthening of the subepithelial lamina propria to more than two thirds of the thickness of the squamous epithelium and (2) expansion of the basal zone of the squamous epithelium to more than 15% of the thickness of the epithelium (see Fig. 14.1). Subsequent studies confirmed these initial observations and also demonstrated a significant positive correlation between the severity of reflux, as measured by 24-hour pH score (a composite quantitative evaluation of acid reflux) and the length of the lamina propria papillae.[40] These histological features also occur in infants with GERD, but with poor correlations between pH score severity and histological severity.[41] Increased mitoses, slight enlargement of basal and suprabasal nuclei, and prominent nucleoli and hyperchromatism are features often associated with true basal cell hyperplasia. True basal cell hyperplasia is best evaluated in well-oriented tissue sections that include at least three consecutive papillae cut longitudinally. Unfortunately, this orientation is rarely achieved in small pinch biopsy samples. Therefore caution should be taken not to overinterpret "mild" changes as evidence in favor of esophagitis.

Inflammation

The principal inflammatory cells in patients with reflux esophagitis include neutrophils, eosinophils, and lymphocytes (see Fig. 14.2).[42] However, depending on the phase of disease and the treatment status, none, one, or all of these inflammatory cells may be present in a single biopsy specimen. Therefore, a diagnosis of (reflux) esophagitis can be established in the absence of inflammation if the basal cell and lamina propria papillae changes are present, particularly in a patient who has begun treatment with antireflux agents.

Neutrophils. Within the esophageal squamous epithelium, intraepithelial neutrophils always indicate a pathological process. However, intraepithelial neutrophils are not a sensitive indicator of reflux esophagitis, because they are present in fewer than 30% of GERD patients with documented reflux. They also are not specific for GERD. Therefore, the presence of a significant number of neutrophils, particularly in association with a surface erosion or ulcer, should prompt the pathologist to search for a viral or fungal (*Candida*) infection.

Eosinophils. Increased numbers of eosinophils often are present in patients with esophagitis.[43] However, because rare, isolated eosinophils may be found in the mucosa of normal adults, particularly in the distal 1 to 2 cm of the esophagus, and of normal children, they are not considered diagnostic of esophagitis if sparse in number and not associated with other features of esophagitis, such as those discussed previously.[44-47] Eosinophils in the lamina propria are considered an even more sensitive indicator of GERD in infants.[34]

Occasionally, large numbers of eosinophils are present in esophageal biopsy specimens of adult patients with putative reflux.[40,48] In this circumstance, causes of esophageal eosinophilia other than reflux, such as primary EoE, drug reaction (including Stevens-Johnson syndrome), pill-induced esophagitis, collagen vascular disease, and, very rarely, parasitic infection,[49] should be excluded. Children with apparent GERD who have prominent eosinophilia may improve clinically when given an elemental diet, which suggests that certain food sensitivities may lead to reflux-like symptoms[50,51] (see Primary Eosinophilic Esophagitis).

Lymphocytes. Lymphocytes are considered a normal intraepithelial component of the esophageal squamous mucosa.[42,52,53] These are largely T lymphocytes and have either a round or an irregular nuclear contour, particularly when deformed by adjacent squamous epithelial cells. Because of their "squiggly" appearance, intraepithelial lymphocytes may resemble granulocytes. These cells have been identified as CD8+ and TIA-1+ T lymphocytes and tend to be more prominent in the peripapillary epithelium.[54] Normal esophageal mucosa contains roughly 10 to 12 lymphocytes per high-power field (HPF).[53,54] Although lymphocytes are present in increased numbers in patients with GERD, this finding in isolation has no independent diagnostic significance, because normal control subjects may also have increased numbers.[53] In addition, other disorders, such as achalasia and Crohn's disease, may be associated with increased numbers of intraepithelial lymphocytes.[55,56]

Other Microscopic Features of GERD

Dilation and congestion of lamina propria capillaries are additional characteristic features of reflux esophagitis,[57] but this finding may also occur in specimens from normal controls, albeit in a mild fashion, possibly as a traumatic biopsy artefact.[58] Other features that may be seen in GERD include ballooning degeneration of squamous cells, intercellular edema (acantholysis) that causes minor separation of individual squamous cells, multinucleation of squamous cells, increased mitoses, and decreased surface maturation. The presence of multinucleated (regenerative) cells may mimic herpetic esophagitis (Fig. 14.4). Multinucleated regenerative squamous cells are distinguished from virally infected cells by the lack of characteristic nuclear inclusions and by their prominence at the base of the mucosa and adjacent to ulcers, rather than in the surface cells, which is characteristic of herpes.[59]

Differential Diagnosis of GERD

The differential diagnosis of GERD includes infectious esophagitis, pill esophagitis, esophagitis caused by ingestion of corrosive agents such as lye, chemotherapy- and radiation-induced esophagitis, primary EoE, trauma, and systemic diseases such as collagen vascular disease, Crohn's disease, Stevens-Johnson syndrome, various bullous diseases, lichen planus, and graft-versus-host disease. Many of these conditions share overlapping morphological features with GERD. Therefore, an accurate diagnosis of "reflux" esophagitis requires correlation with the patient's clinical, endoscopic, manometric, and histological data. In the absence of clinical information, a diagnosis of reflux esophagitis cannot be established on the basis of biopsy findings alone. The histological features are essentially nonspecific. In fact, in this scenario, a "top line" diagnosis of "active esophagitis consistent with reflux" rather than "reflux esophagitis" should be used.

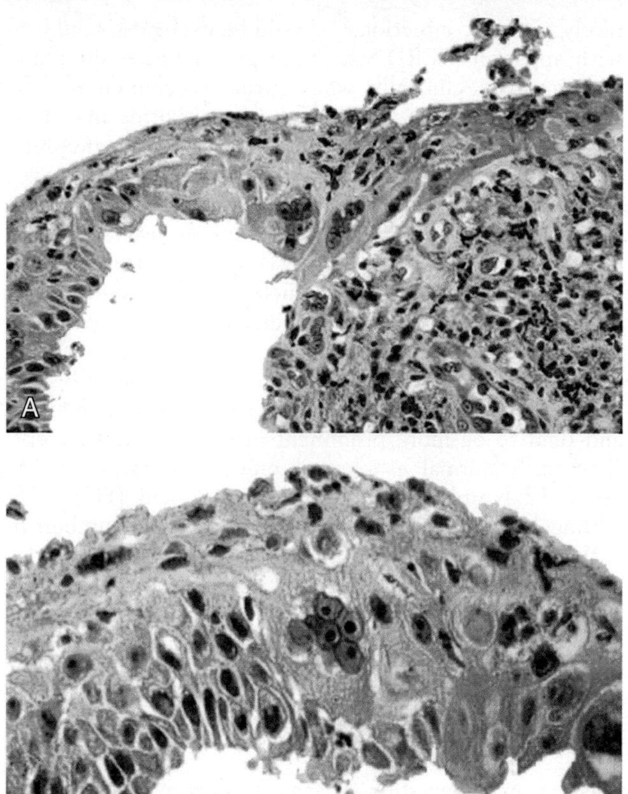

FIGURE 14.4 A and **B,** Multinucleated reactive epithelial cells in a patient with severe reflux esophagitis. The multinucleated reactive squamous epithelial cells are most prominent in the basal layer and in areas of mucosa adjacent to ulceration. The multinucleated cells show a low nucleus-to-cytoplasm ratio and perinuclear cytoplasmic clearing. In addition, there is prominent intercellular edema, epithelial degeneration, increased inflammation, and ulceration.

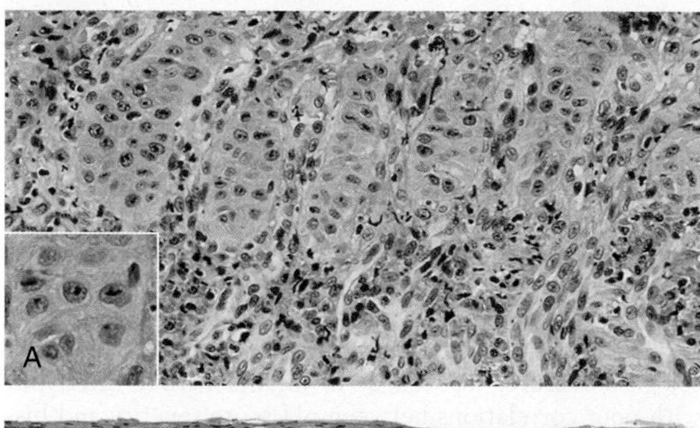

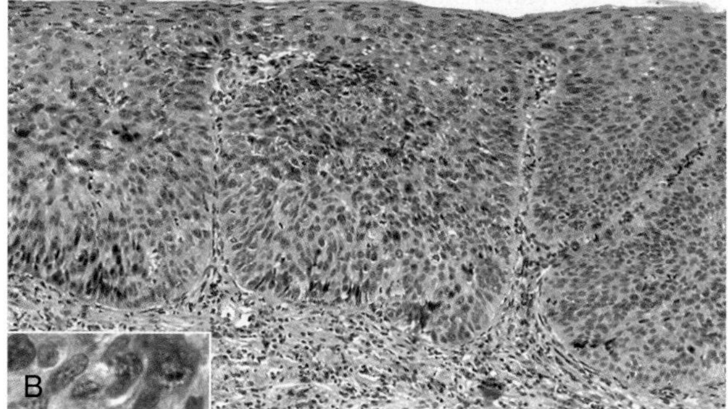

FIGURE 14.5 A, Marked reactive (pseudoepitheliomatous) hyperplasia in a patient with severe reflux esophagitis. Squamous cells are reactive and hyperchromatic and possess prominent nucleoli but do not show significant loss of polarity or nuclear overlap. The papillae are of uniform length and width, and the nuclei, although mildly atypical, are uniform in appearance *(inset)*. **B,** In high-grade squamous dysplasia, the papillae vary in size and shape, and there is considerable nuclear pleomorphism, hyperchromasia, and nuclear overlapping *(inset)*.

Reactive Squamous Hyperplasia versus Dysplasia

On occasion, marked reactive (pseudoepitheliomatous) hyperplasia related to reflux esophagitis may resemble squamous dysplasia histologically (Fig. 14.5). The most helpful distinguishing feature is the presence of *cytoarchitectural uniformity* in cases of hyperplasia, compared with *cytoarchitectural pleomorphism* in cases of dysplasia or carcinoma.

The mucosal architecture in hyperplastic lesions retains its uniformity, showing elongation of papillae that extend to roughly equal depths within the deep lamina propria and are usually of similar width. In contrast, dysplastic squamous epithelium typically displays architectural distortion with absent, sharply angulated, or markedly irregular papillae in terms of their length and width (Table 14.2; see also Chapter 24 for details).

Cytologically, hyperplastic squamous epithelial cells are uniform and do not show loss of polarity or overlapping nuclei. The nuclei may be uniformly enlarged; however, they have smooth nuclear membranes, open chromatin, often prominent nucleoli, and increased mitoses but no atypical mitoses. Dysplastic squamous epithelial cells are typically more pleomorphic in size and shape, are more hyperchromatic, have irregular nuclear contours, and reveal nuclear overlapping and loss of polarity (see Fig. 14.5).

TABLE 14.2 Differential Diagnosis of Reactive Hyperplasia versus Dysplasia of Squamous Epithelium

Feature	Hyperplasia	Dysplasia
Papillae	Regular	Absent or irregular
Nuclear enlargement	++	+→+++
Nuclear pleomorphism	+/–	+→+++
Nuclear overlapping	–	+→+++
Nuclear hyperchromasia	+/–	+→+++
Nuclear membrane	Smooth	Irregular

+, Mild degree; ++, moderate degree; +++, marked degree.

Reactive Changes in Ulcers versus Dysplasia or Carcinoma

Granulation tissue within the base of erosions or ulcers may exhibit large atypical endothelial cells and fibroblasts[60,61] (Fig. 14.6). They are usually distributed in a scattered fashion within otherwise typical granulation tissue. These cells do not form solid clusters of cells and have a normal, or even decreased, nucleus-to-cytoplasm (N:C) ratio. In contrast, carcinoma usually demonstrates groups or sheets of cohesive cells with overlapping nuclei and an increased N:C ratio. In difficult cases, immunohistochemistry for cytokeratins can be helpful in differentiating true carcinoma (positive) from reactive "pseudosarcomatous" alterations of the stromal cells (negative).

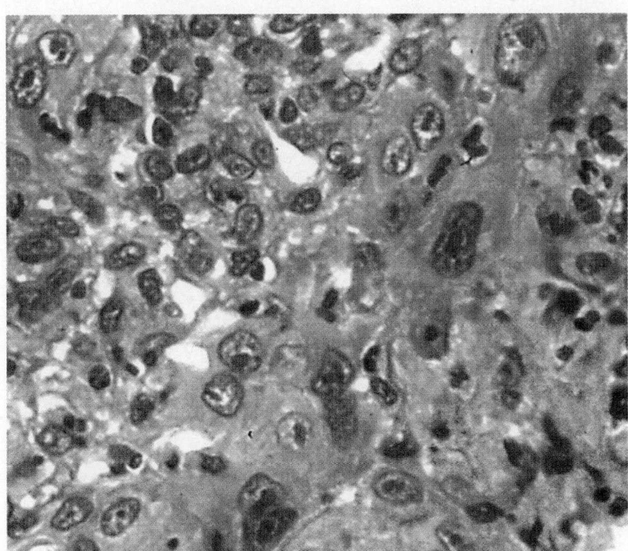

FIGURE 14.6 High-power view of the base of an esophageal ulcer showing increased inflammation and marked, somewhat atypical reactive mesenchymal cells. Although the nuclei are enlarged and irregular in shape, the nucleus-to-cytoplasm ratio of the cells is still maintained. The cells are scattered rather than grouped together, as one would expect in a malignant process.

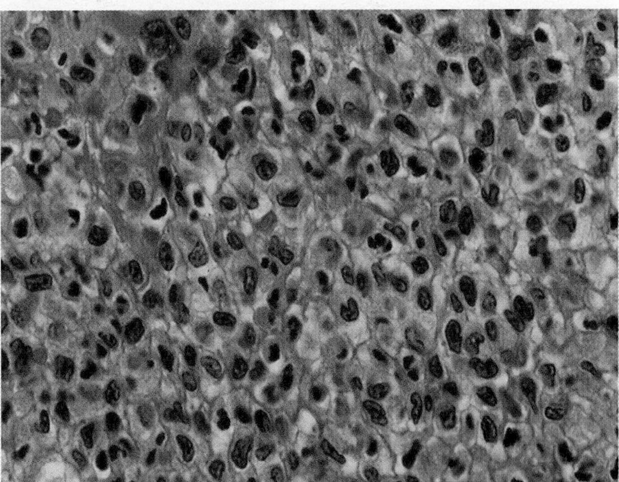

FIGURE 14.7 High-power view of an exudate from a benign ulcer in a patient with reflux esophagitis shows abundant cleaved and activated lymphocytes and macrophages that may simulate a lymphoma histologically. If the lymphocytic infiltrate is limited to the luminal exudate, without infiltration of the underlying tissue, it should be considered benign.

Rarely, the inflammatory exudate within the ulcer or erosion may contain abundant activated and atypical lymphocytes that can simulate lymphoma (Fig. 14.7). In general, these cells are benign when confined to the surface exudate. The infiltrate should raise concern for a lymphoma if it involves the underlying tissue in a dense, confluent, and homogeneous manner.

Natural History and Treatment of GERD

The natural history of GERD in the general population remains uncertain because of the widespread use of acid inhibitors. GERD has multiple phenotypic presentations, and nonerosive reflux disease (NERD), erosive esophagitis, and BE may form a continuum. Most patients with GERD (50% to 70%) have normal mucosa on endoscopy and therefore are diagnosed with NERD.[62-64] Some researchers have proposed that NERD is a discrete entity because of its unique physiologic characteristics, which include a more competent antireflux barrier.[65] However, most authorities believe that GERD is a progressive disease that starts with NERD and progresses with time, to erosive esophagitis or BE or both, in selected high-risk individuals. Some data suggest that progression from NERD to erosive esophagitis occurs in as much as 30% of patients annually,[66-69] but it is unknown whether NERD can progress directly to BE without an erosive phase.[70] Between 1% and 22% of patients with erosive esophagitis progress to a more severe form of disease, whereas regression to a less severe form of disease occurs in 6% to 42% of patients, depending on whether acid inhibitors have been used.[71-73] Erosive esophagitis is a risk factor for BE.[74,75] Barrett's esophagus develops in between 1% to 13% of patients with erosive esophagitis annually.[76] In a recent prospective, follow-up endoscopic study[77] to evaluate the risk of BE in a Swedish general population (the Kalixanda study database),[78] the incidence of BE was 9.9 per 1000 person-years, and the prevalence of BE in this GERD cohort increased from 3% to 8% during a 5-year follow-up period. In fact, progression of GERD to BE in the general population may be higher than previously recognized.[68,79] Interestingly, patients who have GERD have reduced risk of developing microscopic colitis, ulcerative colitis, or Crohn's disease, especially GERD patients who have erosive esophagitis or Barrett's metaplasia.[80]The vast majority of patients with GERD have a recurrent but nonprogressive form of disease that is controlled adequately with acid inhibitor therapy.

Current medical forms of therapy, such as PPI and other acid inhibitors, are highly effective at relieving symptoms and repeat biopsies may show histological improvement or resolution of pre-therapy pathology.[33] However, progressive disease develops in some patients despite ongoing therapy.[81] In one study, as many as 82% of patients who showed healing of their esophagitis with omeprazole relapsed within 6 months after cessation of therapy.[81] In a 10-year follow-up study of 101 patients with reflux esophagitis, significant morbidity related to GERD developed in almost 75%, showing quality of life scores significantly lower than those of a non–GERD control population.[82] Surgical treatment is considered an option for patients with chronic GERD who are not responsive to medical therapy or have a defective LES.[83,84] Esophageal biopsy is indicated for patients who become refractory to therapy or who develop new symptoms to evaluate for emergence of complications such as neoplasms.

Although PPI are the current mainstay for GERD treatment, approximately 30% of GERD patients continue to experience symptoms while receiving once daily label-dose PPI. Use of a bile sequestrant along with a daily label-dose PPI significantly reduced heartburn symptoms compared to a placebo, and regurgitation symptoms were also reduced.[85] A US expert panel of foregut surgeons and therapeutic gastroenterologists recently agreed that surgery was a viable option for GERD patients for whom PPI discontinuation becomes necessary or who want to discontinue PPI therapy.[86] Laparoscopic fundoplication and magnetic sphincter augmentation were considered acceptable options for such patients, and transoral incisionless fundoplication was considered an option for such patients who do not have a hiatal hernia. For PPI-nonresponders, laparoscopic fundoplication was recommended as an appropriate surgical option if a hiatal hernia was present. Magnetic sphincter augmentation was considered appropriate for PPI-nonresponders with regurgitation-predominant disease who had or did not have a hiatal hernia, and transoral incisionless fundoplication was appropriate for PPI-nonresponders who did not have a clinically significant hiatal hernia. Laparoscopic fundoplication and magnetic sphincter augmentation were not considered appropriate surgical options for PPI-nonresponders whose impedance-pH study was negative.

INFECTIOUS ESOPHAGITIS

Infections remain an important cause of esophagitis and can have significant implications in the immunocompromised host. Viruses and fungi cause most forms of acute infectious esophagitis.[87] Bacterial esophagitis occurs in some patients with systemic or upper respiratory infection, but this condition is rarely sampled histologically.

Viral Esophagitis—Herpes

Clinical Features

Herpes esophagitis occurs primarily in immunosuppressed patients. Common causes of immunosuppression include prior chemotherapy, solid organ and bone marrow transplantation, and acquired immunodeficiency syndrome (AIDS). Herpes esophagitis also may occur in otherwise healthy young adults with normal immune function, who usually have a self-limited infection that resolves within 1 to 2 weeks.[88-90] In a recent analysis of 46 patients with herpes esophagitis, 72% were immunocompromised and those with longer symptom duration were more likely to require treatment extension; in addition, 37% of patients had underlying esophageal disease and were more likely to have concomitant *Candida* esophagitis.[91] Symptoms of herpetic esophagitis include odynophagia, dysphagia, epigastric pain, fever, and upper GI bleeding, but some patients are asymptomatic.[92] Coexistent herpes labialis and oropharyngeal ulcers are seen in approximately one fourth of patients.[87,90] Herpetic ulcers in the esophagus may serve as a portal of entry for other pathogens and can be associated with herpetic pneumonitis.[88] Endoscopically, herpetic ulcers are typically shallow, sharply punched-out lesions and are often surrounded by relatively normal-appearing mucosa.

Pathology

Herpes simplex or varicella-zoster virus infects esophageal squamous epithelium. Accordingly, the characteristic inclusion bodies are limited to the squamous epithelial cells, typically accentuated at the superficial lateral margin of ulcers and erosions. In fact, biopsy specimens obtained distant from the immediate edge of the ulcer lesion may not be diagnostic. Microscopic diagnostic criteria include the presence of Cowdry A intranuclear viral inclusion bodies, ground-glass nuclei, nuclear molding, multinucleated giant cells, and ballooning degeneration of infected cells (Fig. 14.8).[88,89] Cowdry A inclusions are eosinophilic to amphophilic round

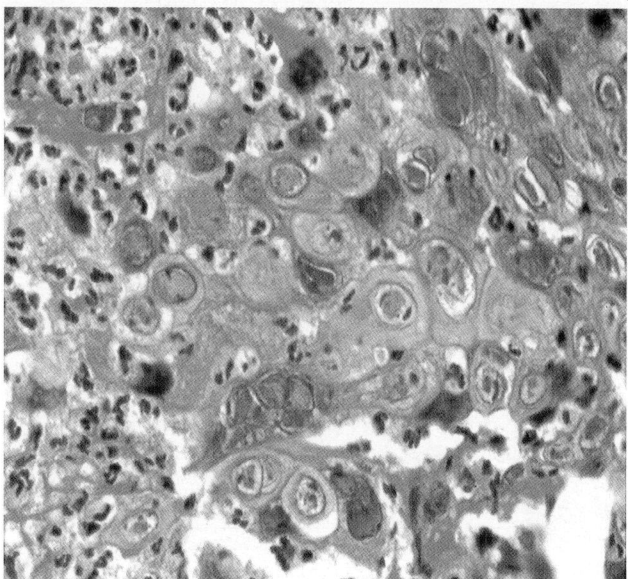

FIGURE 14.8 High-power view of herpes esophagitis showing diagnostic Cowdry A inclusions and multinucleated cells with nuclear molding. These cells are most prominent in the superficial portions of the epithelium and particularly adjacent to areas of ulceration.

bodies separated by a clear zone from a thickened nuclear membrane. Ground-glass nuclei have a smooth, homogeneous chromatin pattern with a pale basophilic quality. Multinucleated giant cell changes in squamous epithelial cells may occur in reflux esophagitis and should not be confused with the cytopathic effects of herpesvirus infection. Reactive cells have prominent nucleoli and perinucleolar clearing, but nuclear inclusion bodies are not present. Large numbers of mononuclear cells, primarily aggregates of macrophages with convoluted nuclei, in the surface exudate adjacent to the infected epithelium have been noted as a characteristic finding in herpetic ulcers and should make the pathologist suspect herpesvirus infection.[93] However, similar cells may be observed in nonherpetic ulcers throughout the GI tract in the absence of herpesvirus infection, so this finding is not specific. Herpes simplex type I is the most common cause of herpetic esophagitis, but on morphological grounds, this type cannot be distinguished from herpes simplex type II or varicella-zoster. Immunohistochemical staining and in situ hybridization, if clinically indicated, can help distinguish these three viral species.

Differential Diagnosis

On occasion, herpetic esophagitis may be difficult to distinguish from squamous dysplasia/carcinoma (Table 14.3). The nuclear inclusions characteristic of herpetic esophagitis may be mistaken for macronucleoli typical of malignant cells. However, in herpes esophagitis, one usually sees a halo located between the nuclear inclusion and the nuclear membrane. In addition, the ground-glass chromatin pattern that is characteristic of virally infected cells shows little structure and is pale, in contrast to the variably granulated and darkly stained chromatin typical of malignant cells. Radiation-induced esophagitis also may be mistaken for herpetic esophagitis, because radiation can result in the formation of enlarged squamous cells with multiple nuclei, nucleoli, and pale chromatin. However, careful attention to

TABLE 14.3 Differential Diagnosis of Viral Esophagitis

Etiology	Endoscopy	Morphology
Herpesvirus	Superficial ulcers	Dense intranuclear eosinophilic inclusions (Cowdry A) Ground-glass chromatin Multinucleated syncytia of squamous cells Detached squamous cells with viral inclusions Macrophages in ulcer base
Cytomegalovirus	Linear ulcers Single deep ulcers	Cytomegaly and nucleomegaly with single large nuclear inclusion or multiple amphophilic cytoplasmic inclusions in endothelial and stromal cells
Radiation esophagitis	Ulcer or stricture	Bizarre epithelial and stromal cells Degenerated and multinucleated squamous cells Preserved nucleus-to-cytoplasm ratio Rare mitotic activity Vascular intimal proliferation Stromal fibrosis and stellate fibroblasts
Squamous dysplasia or carcinoma	Mucosal erythema and friability, erosions, plaques, nodules	Nuclear hyperchromasia Nuclear pleomorphism, increased mitotic rate. Increased nucleus-to-cytoplasm ratio Lack of surface maturation Nuclear overlapping and loss of polarity

the presence or absence of characteristic Cowdry A inclusions and ground-glass nuclei allows their distinction.

Treatment

Empiric treatment for herpetic lesions is often initiated on the basis of clinical suspicion, even in the absence of histological confirmation. Acyclovir (Zovirax) can be administered orally and helps initiate healing of active disease, but it does not prevent recurrences. Other medications, including famciclovir (Famvir) and valacyclovir (Valtrex), have also been shown to be effective therapy for herpes esophagitis. Intravenous medications may be indicated for severe disease.

Viral Esophagitis—Cytomegalovirus

Clinical Features

Cytomegalovirus (CMV) is a member of the human herpesvirus family, with an estimated prevalence rate among adults ranging from 40% to 60% of all cases of infectious esophagitis in resource-rich countries. Like other herpesviruses, CMV is not normally cleared from the body but instead is kept in a state of latency by the immune system. Therefore, chronic CMV infection only rarely causes disease among immunocompetent persons, but it does represent a major cause of morbidity and mortality in immunocompromised patients (especially patients infected with the human immunodeficiency virus [HIV] whose CD4 counts are lower than 50 cells/μL), transplant recipients, patients with malignancies, and patients who have received immunosuppressive therapy.[94]

CMV esophagitis, although less common than herpetic esophagitis, is not infrequently found in patients with AIDS. In one study, CMV infection was found either alone or in combination with *Candida* and herpes in 30% of AIDS patients.[95] Similar to herpes simplex or varicella-zoster esophagitis, CMV esophagitis may also rarely occur in immunocompetent individuals.[96]

Presenting symptoms may include odynophagia, nausea, substernal pain, and fever. Endoscopically, CMV esophagitis has a variable appearance. Most patients with CMV esophagitis have multiple, well-circumscribed ulcers,[97] most often located in the middle to distal esophagus. Deep linear ulcers and shallow ulcers, erythema, diffuse erosive esophagitis, and an inflammatory exudate also may be seen in the setting of CMV esophagitis,[98] but these findings lack diagnostic specificity. However, a recent retrospective study of endoscopic appearances of patients with herpes or CMV esophagitis identified a scoring system with 97% sensitivity and 89% specificity to discriminate CMV from herpes esophagitis.[99] Viral culture is not used routinely because detection of the virus does not confirm active disease.[100]

Pathology

CMV-infected cells typically show marked cytomegaly and nucleomegaly with large ovoid intranuclear inclusions and thick marginated chromatin (Fig. 14.9). The inclusion bodies may be brightly eosinophilic or deeply basophilic and are usually separated from the nuclear membrane by a halo. In addition, small eosinophilic to basophilic granular inclusions may be evident in the cytoplasm of infected cells. Cytoplasmic inclusions typically appear within minute vacuoles. CMV infects mesenchymal and columnar cells, but not squamous cells. Therefore, it is important for endoscopists to biopsy or brush the base of esophageal ulcers to optimize the chance of sampling diagnostic cells.[101] No single technique is 100% sensitive in establishing a diagnosis of CMV esophagitis. A combination of diagnostic modalities is often used.[102] If a careful search of well-prepared, routinely stained tissue sections or cytology preparations fails to reveal CMV inclusions, or at least suspicious cells, then additional ancillary immunohistochemical or in situ hybridization tests may be helpful. Immunohistochemistry may highlight infected cells without typical CMV morphology on routine stained sections and can be more sensitive than light microscopy. As previously mentioned, CMV esophagitis may coexist with herpes and *Candida* infection in both transplant recipients and patients with AIDS.[89]

Treatment

A variety of medications, such as ganciclovir, valganciclovir, foscarnet, and cidofovir, may be effective for the treatment of CMV esophagitis. The specific choice of therapy depends on the site and severity of infection, the level of underlying immunosuppression, the patient's ability to tolerate and adhere to the treatment regimen, and the potential drug interactions.[103]

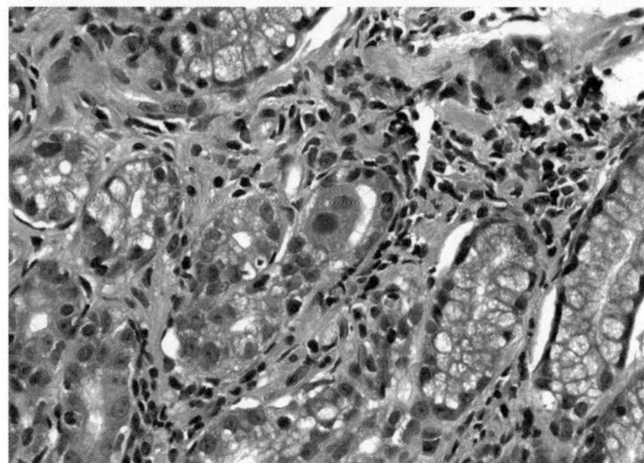

FIGURE 14.9 High-power view of cytomegalovirus esophagitis shows characteristic nuclear and cytoplasmic inclusions in glandular epithelium.

Other Viruses

Symptoms related to esophageal disease are common in AIDS patients.[95] In most, a specific infectious agent such as *Candida*, herpes simplex, varicella-zoster, or CMV can be identified.[95,104] However, in some patients, no apparent cause for the esophagitis or ulcer can be found by standard techniques. Hybridization with specific DNA probes may reveal Epstein-Barr virus in some of these patients.[105] In some HIV-positive patients, however, odynophagia and multiple discrete esophageal ulcers are observed in the absence of an identifiable pathogen. Ultrastructural studies in such patients have revealed the presence of viral particles consistent with retrovirus, which suggests that the esophagus may represent a primary direct target site of acute HIV infection itself.[106,107] Human papilloma virus (HPV) may cause esophageal ulcers, hyperkeratosis and solitary papilloma or papillomatosis.[108] Koilocytosis, perinuclear clearing and giant and multinucleated cells are also features of HPV infection.

Fungal Esophagitis—*Candida*

Clinical Features

Fungal esophagitis is most commonly caused by *Candida albicans* or *Candida tropicalis*. Fungal infection occurs primarily in patients with some type of underlying disease (e.g., AIDS, other immunosuppressive disorders, diabetes) and in patients who have undergone treatment with broad-spectrum antibiotics, acid-suppressive therapy,[109,110] or inhaled [111] or swallowed corticosteroids.[112] It also may be found in otherwise healthy patients.[113] Clinically, the presenting symptoms are dysphagia and odynophagia, but some patients remain asymptomatic, with the infection discovered incidentally at esophagoscopy performed for other reasons, especially in elderly patients.

At endoscopy, esophageal candidiasis typically appears as white plaques of fibrinopurulent exudate, which may be focal or confluent, overlying erythematous mucosa. These plaques can be scraped away to reveal ulceration underneath. This is in contrast to the white patches seen in eosinophilic esophagitis that cannot easily be dislodged from esophageal epithelium (see Eosinophilic Esophagitis).

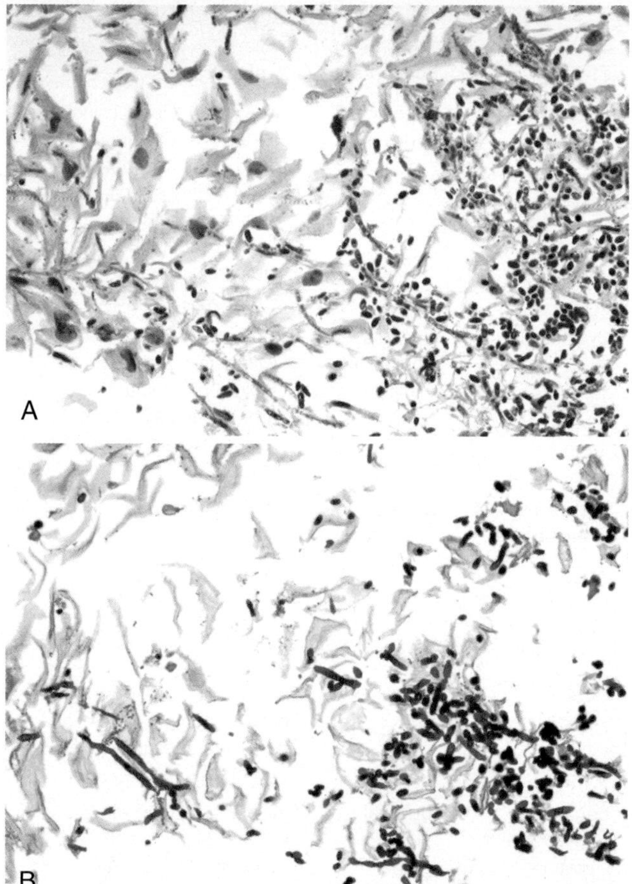

FIGURE 14.10 *Candida* esophagitis shows abundant pseudohyphae and budding yeast forms, readily seen on routine hematoxylin and eosin stain **(A)** and highlighted by periodic acid–Schiff fungus stain **(B).**

Pathology

Morphologically, pseudohyphae and budding yeast forms can be demonstrated in a background of active esophagitis and are easily identified within the ulcer slough and fibrinopurulent exudate (Fig. 14.10). Because *Candida* organisms are part of the normal flora of the GI tract, confirmation of this diagnosis requires more than simply identifying budding yeast forms; pseudohyphae should be detected within tissue to document true infection.[114] Pseudohyphae have a linear or ribbon-like appearance in which small indentations, rather than true septations, are typically noted along the long axis of the organisms. Yeast forms have a slight ovoid contour and frequently manifest budding from the tips.[115] In immunosuppressed patients, who occasionally reveal only minimal inflammation, special stains (silver stain, periodic acid–Schiff [PAS]) should be used to detect small numbers of invasive fungal forms within the tissue. However, special stains cannot be used to speciate the type of *Candida* organisms. C. *tropicalis* is more virulent than C. *albicans* because of its increased potential for tissue invasiveness.[116] *Candida* can colonize preexisting ulcers or any damaged mucosa, and the pathologist should consider the possibility of a dual infection or pathology.[117] C. *auris*, first described in 2009 causing an ear infection, has been isolated from the oral cavity, oropharynx and nares, but has not yet been reported in the esophagus.[118]

Differential Diagnosis

On occasion, the endoscopist may identify small white plaques that, although they resemble *Candida* esophagitis, represent glycogenic acanthosis, ectopic sebaceous glands or inflammatory exudate in EoE. Glycogenic acanthosis occurs as white mucosal plaques that measure 2 to 5 mm.[119] Diffuse esophageal glycogenic acanthosis may occur as a rare manifestation of Cowden syndrome.[120] Biopsy features include distention of squamous epithelial cells with glycogen, which is evident as pale-staining material that is PAS positive and diastase digestible.[121] Ectopic sebaceous glands, which may also appear as small, pale yellow or white, punctate elevations of the mucosa, are rare but are easily recognized in biopsy material by their close resemblance to normal dermal sebaceous glands.[122] White plaques in EoE tend to be smaller than those associated with *Candida* and are composed of exudate containing eosinophils and squamous epithelial cells. EoE plaques are typically more difficult to dislodge than are *Candida*-associated plaques.

Treatment

Fluconazole (Diflucan) is the drug of choice because it is safe and well tolerated, although other drugs, such as itraconazole and ketoconazole, are also effective.[123,124] Amphotericin B is considered a second-line option and is reserved for severe cases and for patients for whom treatment with azole compounds has failed, such as patients who are infected with *glabrata* species of *Candida* which is more commonly azole-resistant than *albicans* species.[108] Echinocandins (e.g., Caspofungin), a new class of antifungal agents that act on fungal cell walls, are being used in randomized trials for patients with *Candida* esophagitis refractory to azole compounds.[125,126] Lack of symptomatic response in patients with *Candida* esophagitis should prompt search for a co-infecting agent such as herpes virus.[127]

Bacterial Esophagitis

Primary bacterial infections of the esophagus are exceedingly rare except in immunocompromised patients; most cases are secondary and occur in areas of ulceration. The most common infecting organisms are normal flora from the mouth and respiratory tract (*Staphylococcus aureus*, *Staphylococcus epidermidis*, *Streptococcus viridans*, and *Bacillus* species). A diagnosis of bacterial esophagitis can be established when sheets of confluent bacteria invade the subepithelial tissue.[87] The number of bacteria appears to be inversely related to the intensity of the inflammatory reaction.[128] Bacterial cultures of biopsy material are not performed routinely but may be helpful to further identify organisms that are detected on routinely stained tissue sections. *Actinomyces* may occur in areas of previous tissue injury; the infection is characterized by the presence of sulfur granules and intertwining thin branching actinomyces filaments within the subepithelial tissue. A distal esophageal microbiome analysis of patients receiving PPI, all of whom had either Barrett's esophagus or GERD without Barrett's esophagus, revealed *Actinomyces* was the only species significantly different in PPI users; it was more abundant in users independent of dose or duration of PPI use.[129] Occasionally, one may encounter *Mycobacterium tuberculosis*, *Mycobacterium avium-intracellulare*, *Histoplasma capsulatum*, or *Toxoplasma gondii* in the esophagus.[130,131]

Parasitic Esophagitis—Chagas Disease

Clinical Features and Pathogenesis

The World Health Organization estimates that approximately 10 million people are infected with *Trypanosoma cruzi* worldwide. Approximately 100 million are at risk of contracting the infection, and these are mostly in Latin America. Humans are accidental hosts for *T. cruzi*. They are usually infected at night via contact with feces of blood-sucking triatomine insects. A second mechanism of transmission, responsible for as much as 10% of cases, is transfusion of whole blood or blood derivatives (except for lyophilized products).[132] A third route of transmission is congenital. The likelihood of congenital transmission in children of chagasic mothers ranges from 1% to 10%.[133] After 2 to 4 months, the acute clinical manifestations (inflammation of the eye, conjunctivitis, palpebral edema, periauricular satellite adenopathy, and generalized infection) disappear and the disease enters a period of clinical latency ("indeterminate" form). Studies performed in endemic areas have provided clinical and radiologic evidence of esophageal disorders in 7% to 10% of people with chronic *T. cruzi* infection, and megaesophagus in 3%.[133-136] Dysphagia of solid and liquid food is the first and most important symptom of digestive disturbance and occurs in 98% of patients.[137] It may begin slowly but leads to malnutrition and severe weight loss.[138-140] Other clinical symptoms include regurgitation, pyrosis, hiccups, cough, and parotid gland hypertrophy. Esophageal pain often appears with deglutition as a consequence of spasmodic contraction of a hypersensitive esophagus.[133] Esophageal involvement is progressive in some patients but not in others, and it evolves independently of heart involvement. The 2018 achalasia guidelines include a statement that there are only minor differences in the clinical presentation of idiopathic achalasia and achalasia caused by Chagas disease.[137]

Pathology

Destruction of neuron plexuses in the esophagus by the inflammatory reaction induced by *T. cruzi* is the main cause of dysperistalsis of the esophagus. In idiopathic achalasia, inhibitory neurons are lost selectively, whereas in Chagas disease both inhibitory and excitatory neurons are lost.[137] This neuronal loss results in gradual narrowing of the distal esophagus with luminal enlargement of the proximal esophagus, sometimes termed *chagasic megaesophagus* (grade I to IV). Microscopically, distal muscular hypertrophy and mononuclear inflammatory infiltrates occur in the muscle layers. The submucosal and myenteric plexuses show an intense mononuclear infiltrate with associated neuronal injury (Fig. 14.11).[49,141] A 2010 report indicates that patients with megaesophagus have a significantly decreased amount of S100-positive and glial fibrillary acidic protein (GFAP)-positive enteroglial cells when compared with seronegative controls and asymptomatic seropositive patients.[134]A 2013 immunohistochemical study identified increased substance P, which has proinflammatory effects, and decreased vasoactive intestinal peptide, which has antiinflammatory effects, in sections of chagasic megaesophagus, suggesting that these

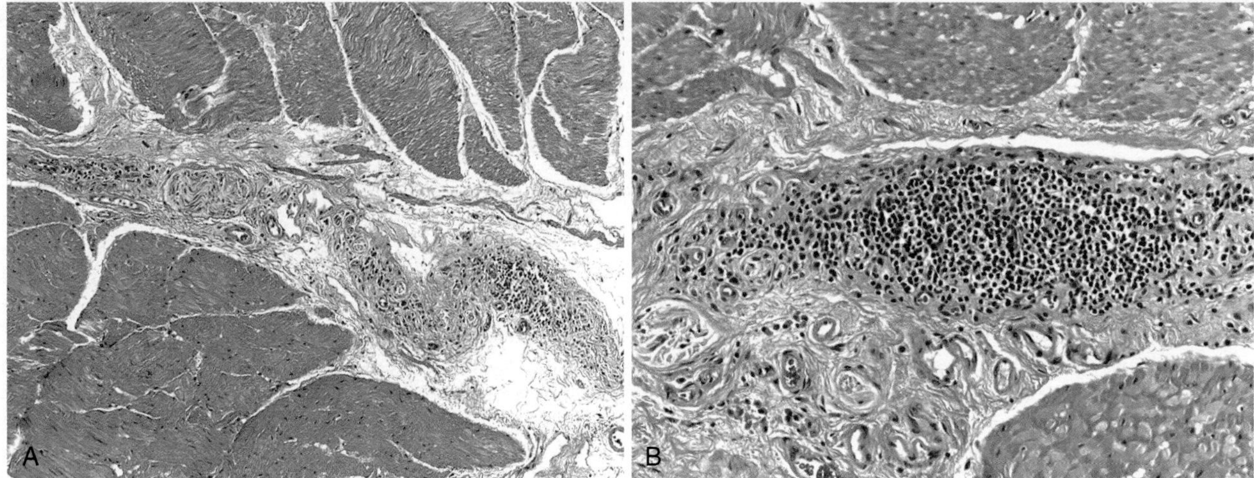

FIGURE 14.11 **A** and **B,** Myenteric plexus in a patient with megaesophagus and Chagas disease. Notice the variable infiltration of the myenteric plexus by mononuclear inflammatory cells and the lack of ganglion cells.

alterations contribute to inflammation that ultimately leads to denervation.[142] With disease progression, there is intense neuronal destruction and denervation of the organ, with loss of function.

Treatment

Only two drugs are effective for the treatment of Chagas disease in the acute and chronic phases: nifurtimox and benznidazole.[143-145] Both are almost 100% effective in curing the disease if treatment is begun soon after infection, at the onset of the acute phase, but their efficacy diminishes with time and duration of infection. Treatment protocols for the chronic phase of disease remain controversial.[145] In the presence of megaesophagus, dilation of the esophagogastric junction may be performed by passing a dilator or air-filled balloon through an endoscope. Repeated dilations may be needed to prevent the development of recurrent strictures. Surgery is indicated in some cases. Cardiotomy is the most frequently performed procedure. Injections of botulin toxin into the esophagus have also been used in some patients but appear to be more effective in idiopathic achalasia than Chagas disease.[134,137,146]

PILL-, DRUG-, AND TOXIN-RELATED ESOPHAGITIS

Pill Esophagitis

Clinical Features

Esophageal injury caused by prolonged direct mucosal contact with ingested, particularly large-sized, tablets or capsules occurs frequently.[147-153] Commonly implicated agents include antibiotics (particularly tetracyclines and clindamycin), nonsteroidal antiinflammatory drugs (NSAIDs), potassium chloride, ascorbic acid, iron supplements, quinidine, and bisphosphonates.[150,151,154] Symptoms include odynophagia, continuous retrosternal pain, and dysphagia. Elderly patients and women are affected most frequently.[154,155] Affected patients often report having ingested a pill with very little or no fluid before nighttime sleep. Most affected individuals do not have an abnormality of esophageal transit. However, in some reports, patients with quinidine-induced or potassium chloride–induced injury had a history of external esophageal compression, such as valvular heart disease with left atrial enlargement, or esophageal entrapment by fixed mediastinal structures and adhesions after thoracic surgery.[149]

Pathology

Pill esophagitis often results in discrete ulcers with normal or only mildly inflamed esophageal mucosa. Ulcers may be shallow or, more commonly, deep with extension into the muscularis mucosae. They are usually located at the junction of the proximal and middle thirds of the esophagus, the area where the aortic arch compresses the esophagus and peristaltic amplitude is relatively low. Patients with left atrial enlargement are especially susceptible to pill-induced esophageal injury.

The histological appearance of pill-induced esophagitis is typically nonspecific. However, prominent eosinophilic infiltration, spongiosis (dilated intercellular spaces), and necrosis of squamous epithelium should always raise the possibility of pill-induced injury, particularly if located in the upper esophagus. Crystalline stainable iron may be identified in cases of ferrous sulfate–induced disease, and polarizable crystalline material may be evident in cases of alendronate-induced injury[151] (Fig. 14.12). Some cases of pill esophagitis are severe and lead to perforation.

Differential Diagnosis

A variety of conditions can cause histological features similar to those found in pill esophagitis. Herpes esophagitis is often a major consideration; a clinical history of immunosuppression and identification of characteristic viral cytopathic inclusions is useful in this differential diagnosis. Other causes of infectious esophagitis, including CMV and *Candida,* may mimic pill esophagitis, both clinically and pathologically. Identification of CMV cytopathic effect or fungal elements is diagnostic. GERD is more common than pill esophagitis; however, it usually is not possible to distinguish these conditions on histological grounds in an isolated esophageal biopsy specimen and in the absence of clinical information. Features potentially helpful in the differential diagnosis are diffusely dilated intercellular spaces that were

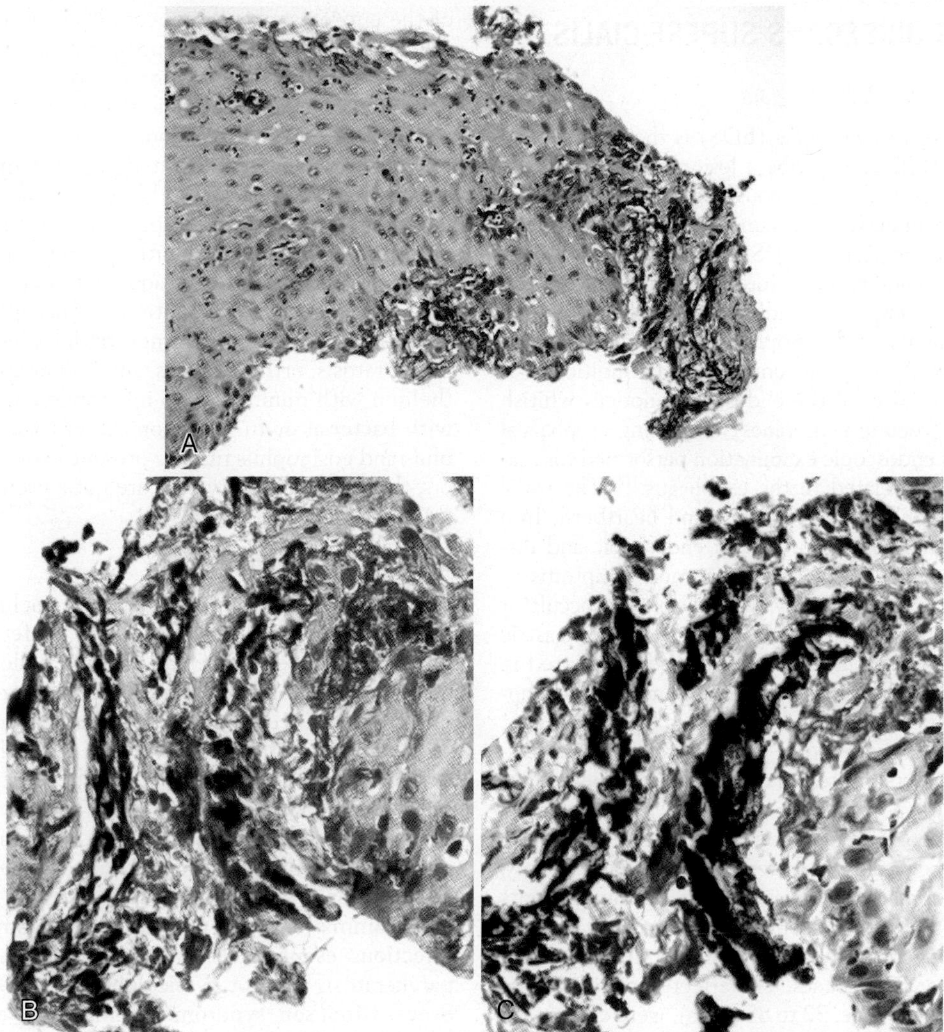

FIGURE 14.12 A, Severe active pill (ferrous sulfate) esophagitis shows marked acute inflammation, ulceration containing pigmented material, and reactive epithelial changes. **B** and **C,** Inflammatory exudate of the base of the esophageal ulcer shows brown crystalline material (**B**), identified as stainable iron by Perls stain (**C**).

found more commonly in a study of 22 cases of pill esophagitis compared to 20 cases of reflux esophagitis, and reactive epithelial changes and papillary elongation that were more common in reflux compared to pill esophagitis.[156]

Corrosive Esophagitis

Clinical Features

Corrosive or caustic esophageal injury occurs in children and adults, most commonly as a result of the ingestion of alkaline (lye) or acid (nitric) substances.[157-159] Gastroduodenal lesions also are common after ingestion of caustic agents. Coughing, crying, and vomiting after ingestion are typical presenting symptoms. Dysphagia, refusal to drink, and mouth or chest pain, with drooling and salivation, may ensue. Airway obstruction and glottic edema can result in respiratory distress and stridor.[160,161]

Pathology

The endoscopic appearance of the esophageal mucosa varies according to the type, physical state, concentration, and volume of the ingested substance. Typically, one encounters mucosal edema, erythema, hemorrhage, and necrosis, sometimes with the formation of circumferential ulcers and mucosal sloughing.

The pathological features are nonspecific and are related to tissue necrosis and subsequent inflammation. Acid injury often produces coagulative necrosis, with the depth of injury limited by the eschar formation. Alkaline injury typically causes liquefactive necrosis with fat and protein digestion. Because a protective eschar does not develop in cases of alkaline injury, the depth of penetration is often greater than with acid injury,[158] and perforation secondary to corrosive esophagitis develops in some patients. Initially, the esophagitis may reveal a dense neutrophilic infiltrate, vessel thrombosis, bacterial invasion, and abundant granulation tissue. Long-term complications include stricture formation, which may require endoscopic or surgical treatment, and, rarely, squamous cell carcinoma.[162] Among 100 children with corrosive esophagitis due primarily to ingestion of an alkaline substance (potash), chromoendoscopy using Lugol's iodine identified unstained (abnormal) areas in the esophagus of 2 of the children, and mild dysphasia was reported in biopsies of their esophagus.[163]

ESOPHAGITIS DISSECANS SUPERFICIALIS

Clinical Features and Pathogenesis

Esophagitis dissecans superficialis (EDS) is the term coined by Rosenberg in 1892 to describe a lesion characterized by extensive dissection of the squamous epithelial lining of the esophagus from its underlying corium in the form of a tubular cast. Dramatic presentations of EDS, with vomiting of esophageal casts, were documented before the endoscopic era.[164] In less dramatic cases, the condition varies from sloughing of large fragments of the esophageal squamous mucosa, which may be coughed up or vomited, to a condition that is not even suspected until the endoscopist notices whitish strips or streaks (pseudomembranes) of peeling esophageal mucosa during an endoscopic examination performed for reasons that may be unrelated to the esophagus.[165] The usual symptoms are dysphagia, odynophagia, and heartburn. In a series of 12 patients with documented endoscopic and histological features of EDS, the most common symptoms or signs leading to upper endoscopy were dysphagia, occult or overt GI bleeding unrelated to EDS, weight loss, epigastric pain, and heartburn.[166] Although EDS has been reported in association with several types of medications (bisphosphonates,[167] NSAIDs,[166] and potassium chloride), hot beverages, chemical irritants, heavy smoking, physical trauma, celiac disease,[168] collagen vascular disorders, and autoimmune bullous dermatoses (pemphigus and pemphigoid),[167,169] the pathogenesis remains poorly understood. A recent report of 31 patients[170] described a similar pattern of injury. In that study, the term *sloughing esophagitis* was used to describe patients whose biopsies showed prominent parakeratosis and superficial sloughing of necrotic squamous epithelium. Endoscopy revealed plaques or membranes. The affected patients were predominantly older (range, 32 to 85 years), were chronically debilitated, and consumed multiple medications. Sloughing esophagitis and EDS are now considered synonymous.[171]

Pathology

Endoscopic features of EDS may include single or multiple white patches of peeling mucosa, extending from the middle to the distal esophagus, or even diffuse sloughing of the entire esophageal mucosa.[166] In addition, long linear mucosal breaks, vertical fissures, and circumferential cracks with peeling mucosa, with or without bleeding, have been described. Three endoscopic diagnostic criteria have been proposed: ≥2cm strips of sloughed mucosa, normal underlying mucosa, and non-ulcerated adjacent mucosa.[171] Histologically, at low power, the biopsy samples consist of long, detached fragments of superficial squamous epithelium with some degree of intraepithelial splitting at varying levels above the basal layer of the squamous epithelium, occasionally associated with separation of the epithelial layers to form bullae.[166] Other common findings include prominent parakeratosis, orthokeratosis, and fragments of necrotic epithelium with minimal or no inflammation, often associated with bacterial or fungal colonization (Fig. 14.13). Neutrophils and eosinophils may be present within the epithelium, but these inflammatory cells are not a prominent feature of this condition.

Differential Diagnosis

The differential diagnosis of EDS includes mechanical trauma related to esophagoscopy, infectious esophagitis (fungal or herpetic), and chronic bullous diseases that involve the esophagus. Repeated attempts to obtain a biopsy, combined with endoscopic trauma, causes layers of squamous epithelium to detach from the mucosa, simulating bullae. Several cases have been reported to occur after traumatic esophagoscopy.[172,173] However, epithelial detachment induced by endoscopic trauma does not reveal necrosis, inflammation, or bacterial colonies on histological examination.

Inflammation and necrosis are common features of infectious esophagitis, but prominent orthokeratosis and parakeratosis are not. Vesiculobullous dermatoses such as Stevens-Johnson syndrome, pemphigus, and pemphigoid may mimic EDS. However, chronic bullous diseases can be excluded by demonstration of an absence of complement and immunoglobulin deposits by direct immunofluorescence (DIF), lack of anti-desmoglein antibodies by enzyme-linked immunosorbent assay (ELISA),[174] and lack of corresponding cutaneous and oropharyngeal lesions. Clinically, patients with EDS show a poor response to steroid therapy.

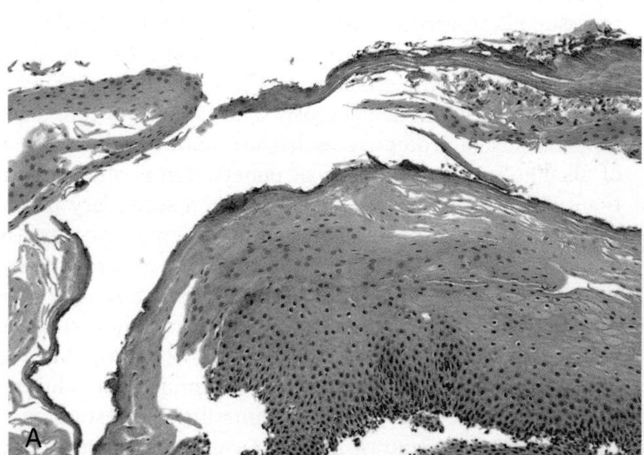

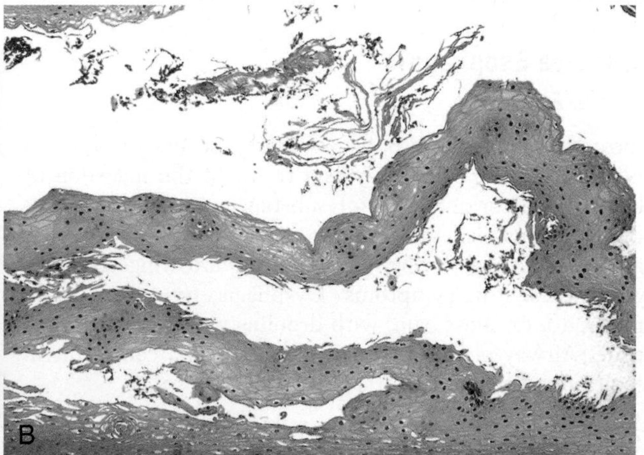

FIGURE 14.13 A, Esophagitis dissecans superficialis characterized by prominent parakeratosis and detached superficial strips of squamous epithelium with parakeratosis, flaking debris, and bacterial colonies in the absence of active inflammation. **B,** Intraepithelial splitting of parakeratotic squamous epithelium with minimal or no inflammation.

Treatment

Despite its sometimes dramatic presentation, EDS in most patients has a positive outcome. A combination of acid suppression, topical analgesics, and discontinuation of any potential precipitating medications results in healing of EDS without sequelae in most cases. Because of the superficial nature of the epithelial injury in this disease, it is presumed that stricture development is rare.

PRIMARY EOSINOPHILIC ESOPHAGITIS (EOE)

Clinical Features

EoE is a chronic, immune-mediated/allergen-driven inflammatory esophageal disorder characterized by symptoms of esophageal dysfunction and eosinophil-rich intraepithelial esophageal inflammation.[175,176] EoE is a clinicopathologic disease with world-wide distribution that was initially recognized at the end of the twentieth century. Since then, both incidence and prevalence have increased; in the U. S., incidence is currently estimated at 23.1/100,000 population and prevalence at 76.6/100,000 population.[177] The annual health expenditure due to EoE in the U. S. is estimated at approximately one billion dollars, and affected patients report significantly reduced quality of life.[178] EoE affects mostly males (male-to-female ratio 3:1), and can affect any age group but typically occurs in young adults who present with food impaction. Signs and symptoms are not sex-based but differ according to age: young patients present with failure to thrive, food refusal, vomiting and abdominal pain, and older children, adolescents and adults complain mostly of dysphagia.[50,179-182] Many EoE patients (28-86% of adults and 42-92% of children) have other allergic diseases including atopic dermatitis and asthma.[183-186] Peripheral blood eosinophilia may occur in primary EoE patients but is usually mild, and noninvasive biomarkers with sufficient specificity and sensitivity to become routinely-used in clinical care have not yet been identified.[187-189]

The relationship between EoE and PPI has evolved. Originally, EoE was distinguished from GERD on the basis of either normal pH-monitoring studies or, more commonly, lack of response to PPI therapy. However, many EoE patients preferred to continue PPI therapy because they reported some symptom relief related to use of PPI. Over time it became apparent that a group of patients who clinically had the characteristics of EoE responded well to PPI and had improved biopsies following PPI therapy. These patients had gene profiles more closely resembling "classic" EoE patients than patients with GERD and they were said to have PPI-responsive esophageal eosinophilia (PPIREE); patients who did not respond to PPI were given the diagnosis of EoE, and those who did were given the diagnosis of PPIREE. Studies of the effects of PPI on cultured esophageal epithelial cells uncovered antiinflammatory activities of PPI, and other basic studies confirmed that PPI could be beneficial to EoE patients, and thus could be used as therapy. A recent statement by an international panel of EoE experts recommends considering PPI as a form of therapy for EoE, rather than a diagnostic test, and removes a trial of PPI therapy from the diagnostic work-up for EoE.[190,191]

Pathogenesis

Among early clinical observations of EoE patients was the recognition that in some families multiple family members were affected, implicating a genetic predisposition.[192] Later studies showed that the risk of developing EoE among first-degree relatives of affected patients was 1.8-2.3% and was higher among males than females. Studies of twins identified a greater contribution of common environment (81%) than genetic heritability (14.5%) to disease development.[193] Subsequent work identified exposures in early life, including antibiotic use and cesarean delivery, as increasing the risk of developing EoE,[194] and showed that environmental factors may modify the risk conferred by genetic susceptibility variants by increasing or decreasing the risk of developing EoE.[195] Increased risk of developing EoE following early antibiotic exposure suggests that the composition of the esophageal microbiome may contribute to disease pathogenesis.

Analysis of esophageal biopsies has shown that gene dysregulation in EoE most commonly affects esophageal epithelium and lymphocytes.[196,197] The first genome-wide microarray analysis of esophageal biopsies from EoE patients identified a transcriptome that differed from controls; the most highly upregulated gene was *CCL26* that encodes the cytokine eotaxin-3 which is secreted by esophageal squamous epithelial cells and attracts and activates eosinophils.[198] IL-13 and IL-5 gene upregulation was also found documenting Th2-involved immune responses; subsequent studies showed that IL-13 induced esophageal epithelial cells to secrete eotaxin-3 and also reduced expression of epithelial differentiation cluster (EDC) genes, specifically filaggrin and involucrin.[199] More recent work has identified additional dysregulated genes at the EDC on chromosome 1q21 including desmoglein 1 (*DSG1*) which is downregulated by IL-13. The strongest chromosomal association with EoE is found at locus 2p23, which encodes the esophagus-specific IL-13-inducible proteolytic enzyme calpain 14 (*CAPN14*). Thymic stromal lymphopoietin (*TSLP*), overexpressed in patients who have atopic diseases including EoE, is released by epithelial cells in EoE and promotes Th2 differentiation as well as activating dendritic and mast cells.[196,197]

Our current understanding is that EoE occurs in patients with predisposing genetic and allergic backgrounds and is triggered by antigens that result in Th2-differentiation and epithelial barrier dysfunction. Dendritic cells are important initiators of the immune cascade and mast cells contribute to symptomatology and to tissue fibrosis and muscle dysfunction. Release of cytotoxic granules by eosinophils likely contributes to the pathology observed in EoE.

Pathology

Gross (Endoscopic) Features

The esophagus in EoE has characteristic, but not pathognomonic, features recognized at endoscopy (Table 14.4; see Fig. 14.4). A classification and grading system useful for both clinical evaluation and for research studies evaluates features with acceptable interobserver agreement among gastroenterologists.[200-202] A memory aid for the features is EREFS which stands for edema, rings, exudates, furrows and strictures. This endoscopic reference scoring system predicts activity in adult[203] and pediatric EoE patients.[204] In some cases, the esophagus appears entirely normal, but more than 90% of affected patients display one or more endoscopic abnormality.[205] Since EoE is a disease characterized by remissions and relapses, patients often undergo numerous endoscopies, which is more concerning in children who require anesthesia. The recent development of a minimally invasive esophageal string test that yields tissue fragments and effluent that correlate with eosinophil counts and biomarkers of disease activity derived from mucosal pinch biopsies may reduce the need for more invasive methods to determine disease status in both children and adults with established EoE diagnoses.[206]

Microscopic Features

Similar to endoscopic features, EoE has characteristic but not pathognomonic microscopic features, with hematoxylin and eosin staining.[207] Histologically, most of the features of EOE overlap with those of GERD, particularly in distal esophageal biopsies. Although biopsies of patients with EOE tend to reveal more numerous intraepithelial eosinophils, typically in the range of 15 or more per high-power field, severe GERD produces pronounced eosinophilia in this range in only a minority of cases. Because intraepithelial eosinophils in both conditions may be patchy in distribution, sampling error can also affect the ability to establish a correct diagnosis.

Histological features of EOE can be divided into major and minor attributes.[208] Major histological features are considered characteristic and necessary to establish a diagnosis, but are not pathognomonic. They include (1) increased intraepithelial eosinophils (≥15/HPF) obtained from the most densely populated areas (peak density), (2) eosinophilic microabscesses (defined as a collection of four or more eosinophils within the epithelium), (3) surface layering of eosinophils (i.e., affiliation of eosinophils to occupy the outer layer of the squamous epithelium), (4) surface sloughing of squamous cells mixed with abundant eosinophils, and (5) extracellular eosinophilic granules (deposition of these proteins, including eosinophil peroxidase and eosinophil derived neurotoxin, indicates degranulation). The distribution of disease is important, because often involves long segments of the esophagus, may be patchy or focal, and typically involves the proximal or middle esophagus and the distal esophagus or GEJ equally. In contrast, patients with GERD typically have higher eosinophil counts in the distal esophagus—an area where reflux affects the esophagus more severely—than in the proximal esophagus (Table 14.5; see Fig. 14.14).[208-210]

Minor histological features are often helpful but are nonspecific and occur in a wider variety of disorders than the major features do. The minor features include (1) marked basal zone hyperplasia (usually >20% of the epithelial thickness), (2) lengthening of the lamina propria papillae (often greater than two thirds of the epithelial thickness), (3) increased lamina propria fibrosis and chronic inflammation, (4) increased intercellular edema, and (5) increased intraepithelial lymphocytes and mast cells.

A histological scoring system (EoEHSS) suitable for clinical work or research evaluates 8 features found in EoE biopsies.[211] (Table 14.6) The EoEHSS is reliable (can be learned by pathologists not involved in its development),[212] and is responsive (scores become more normal in response

TABLE 14.4 Diagnostic Approach to Patients with Suspected Eosinophilic Esophagitis

Clinical	Food impaction/dysphagia in adolescents and adults Feeding intolerance/GERD symptoms in young children Rule out other causes of esophageal eosinophilia
Endoscopic	Edema, rings, exudate, furrows, strictures (EREFS) Obtain multiple biopsies from proximal and distal esophagus Biopsy normal and abnormal areas Biopsy stomach and duodenum if eosinophilic gastritis/duodenitis/gastroenteritis is in the differential diagnosis, or if new symptoms emerge
Pathological	Avoid Bouin fixative Evaluate for eosinophil inflammation, basal zone hyperplasia, eosinophil abscess, eosinophil surface layering, dilated intercellular spaces, surface epithelial alteration, dyskeratotic epithelial cells, lamina propria fibrosis Count eosinophils per HPF in the most dense areas to obtain a peak count

GERD, *Gastroesophageal reflux disease;* HPF, *high-power field.*
Data from references 175, 190, 200, 211.

TABLE 14.5 Differential Diagnosis of Esophageal Eosinophilia

Features	Eosinophilic Esophagitis	GERD	Eosinophilic Gastroenteritis
Esophageal involvement	Proximal and distal	Mainly distal	Proximal and distal
Surface eosinophil layering	+ (prominent)	+/–	+/–
Eosinophil microabscesses	+	–	+
Eosinophil count ≥15/HPF	+	+/–	+/–
Basal zone hyperplasia	+	+/–	+/–
Other GI tract involvement	–	–	+
Peripheral blood eosinophilia	+	–	+
Antireflux therapy response	+	+	–

GERD, *Gastrointestinal reflux disease;* GI, *gastrointestinal;* HPF, *high-power field.*

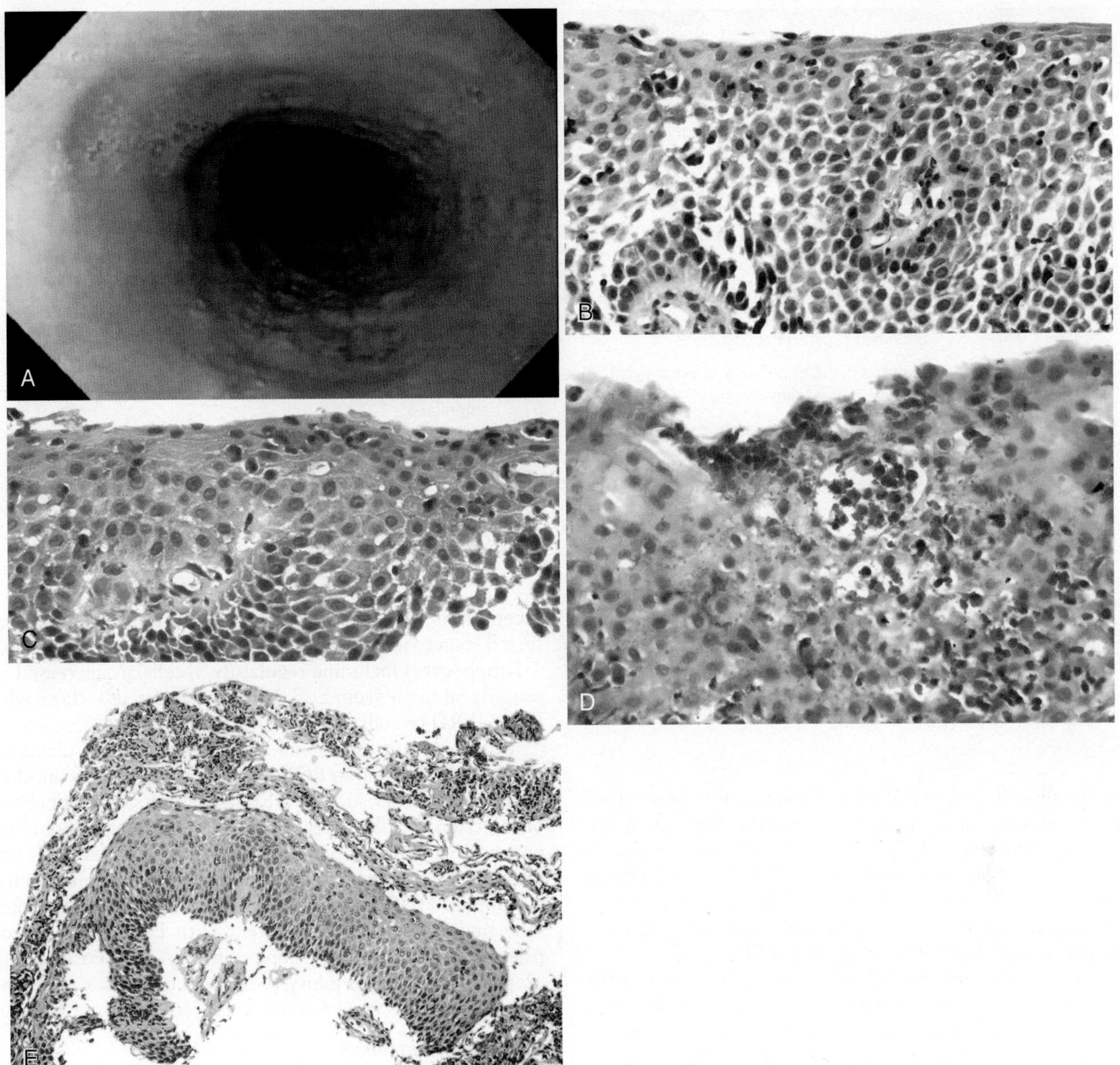

FIGURE 14.14 A, Endoscopic photograph of the esophagus in a patient with primary eosinophilic esophagitis (EOE). The esophageal mucosa shows furrows and concentric rings and is studded with whitish-gray nodular plaques and exudates. The vascular pattern that is seen in normal esophagi is not visible due to edema. Exudates, rings, edema, and furrows, along with strictures not seen in this photograph, are the features evaluated in the eosinophilic esophagitis endoscopic reference score. **B,** Medium-power view of primary EOE shows marked reactive squamous hyperplasia, numerous intraepithelial eosinophils (peak eosinophilic count, >15 per high-power field), and accumulation of eosinophils in the superficial portions of the epithelium. **C,** Medium-power view shows eosinophilic abscesses in the superficial portion of the squamous mucosa. **D,** High-power view of a larger eosinophilic abscess shows aggregation of mainly intact eosinophils in an area of mucosa associated with epithelial cell degeneration. At the epithelial surface, eosinophils are aligned parallel to the esophageal lumen, referred to as eosinophil surface layering. **E,** Accumulation of eosinophils within detached surface epithelial cells forming the exudate that is seen endoscopically.

to therapy known to be efficacious).[201,213] Changes in EoEHSS scores correlate with changes in EREFS scores following therapy.[213] EoEHSS scores correlate with EoE endotypes (pathway classification based on genetic analyses),[214] IgG4 levels (IgG4 deposits may distinguish EoE from GERD),[215] and salivary gland dysbiosis in children with EoE.[216] More importantly, the EoEHSS scores correlate with symptoms.[207,213,217] Although this scoring system has been proposed, many practices still use the peak eosinophil count in their top-line diagnosis.

A vexing clinical problem in EoE is the persistence of symptoms following reduction or eradication of intraepithelial eosinophilic inflammation. Persistent symptoms may signify inflammation and other pathology in the wall of the esophagus that is not usually sampled endoscopically. For example, using biopsies obtained by conventional endoscopy and peroral endoscopic myotomy (POEM) from 10 symptomatic patients, eosinophil infiltrates were found in substantial numbers in muscle layers but few intraepithelial eosinophils were identifed.[218] Symptoms may also persist if

TABLE 14.6 Definitions of Features Evaluated in the Eosinophilic Esophagitis Histology Scoring System

Feature	Definition
Eosinophil inflammation	Based on peak eosinophil count; at least 15 intraepithelial eosinophils in at least one high power field is required for EoE diagnosis
Basal zone hyperplasia	Basal zone that occupies > 15% of total epithelial thickness
Eosinophil abscess	An aggregate of at least 4 eosinophils associated with disruption of the underlying epithelial architecture
Eosinophil surface layering	Eosinophils in the upper third of esophageal epithelium that align parallel to the lumen
Dilated intercellular spaces	Expanded paracellular spaces in which intercellular bridges are seen
Surface epithelial alteration	Surface epithelial cells display pink cytoplasm suggestive of keratinization
Dyskeratotic epithelial cells	Single epithelial cells that display pink cytoplasm and small hyperchromatic nuclei
Lamina propria fibrosis	Thickened lamina propria fibers in which individual fibrils are no longer visible

Data from Collins MH, Martin LJ, Alexander ES, et al. Dis Esophagus. *2017; 30:1-8.*

abnormalities found in endoscopic biopsies are not resolved despite absence of eosinophils. Noting the features of the EoEHSS dichotomously (present or absent), and commenting on severity and amount of tissue that is abnormal affords the clinician the opportunity to prescribe therapy aimed at normalizing those features which could alleviate symptoms in patients who have reduced quality of life.

Special stains are not necessary to recognize eosinophils because of the intense staining of eosinophil granules Only a cell with a nucleus and intensely red cytoplasmic granules should be counted as an eosinophil. Extracellular granules should not be included in a peak eosinophil count. Peak eosinophil count is the current gold standard for the pathology portion of EoE diagnosis and is obtained by counting eosinophils in the area of densest eosinophil inflammation; 15 or more eosinophils in one or more high power fields are required. It is helpful to be able to express the count also as number per unit area because the size of high power fields vary among objectives and reporting counts per unit area overcomes that variability. Mean counts, obtained by averaging the counts from multiple high power fields, are not necessary for clinical work. The presence of extracellular granules does not necessarily indicate that the granules were extruded by an activated eosinophil; several studies have provided evidence that granules may become extracellular because of mechanical forces applied while obtaining biopsies. Antibodies to various eosinophil granule proteins identify their presence in EoE biopsies and correlate with symptoms[219,220] but the antibodies may also demonstrate protein deposition in patients without symptoms.[221] Mast cells may be numerous in EoE biopsies and become less prevalent following EoE therapy.[222] CD117 stains the c-Kit

BOX 14.1 Conditions Associated with Eosinophils in the Esophagus

- Gastroesophageal reflux disease
- Eosinophilic esophagitis
- Eosinophilic gastroenteritis
- Drug hypersensitivity
- Infection
- Hypereosinophilic syndrome
- Gluten-sensitive enteropathy
- Crohn's disease
- Graft-versus-host disease
- Vasculitis
- Connective tissue diseases
- Autoimmune disorders and vasculitides
- Dermatological conditions with esophageal involvement (e.g., pemphigus)
- Achalasia and other disorders of esophageal motility
- Mendelian disorders (Marfan syndrome type II, hyper IgE syndrome, PTEN hamartoma tumor syndrome, etc)

Data from Dellon ES, Liacouras CA, Molina-Infante J, et al. Gastroenterology. *155:1022-1033 2018.*

receptor on the surface of mast cells, but tryptase is the preferred stain to identify mast cells because it is more specific. T lymphocytes including regulatory T cells are increased in esophageal tissue from EoE patients compared to those who have GERD or controls.[223]

Influx of neutrophils and the development of ulcers or erosions are unusual in EOE unless complicated by another unrelated disorder such as GERD, pill-induced esophagitis, or infection.[208] Ultimately, the top-line diagnosis should be nonspecific, and it is helpful to include a note as well. For example: "Active esophagitis with increased intraepithelial eosinophils (>15/HPF)," followed by a note indicating that "the findings could be consistent with EoE in the appropriate clinical and endoscopic setting," or "Eosinophilic esophagitis pattern of injury, see comment" with a comment listing conditions known to cause esophageal eosinophilia.

Differential Diagnosis

Mucosal infiltration by eosinophils is a component of a variety of esophageal inflammatory conditions (Box 14.1), including GERD, EoE, eosinophilic gastroenteritis, Crohn's disease, collagen vascular diseases, infectious esophagitis (secondary to herpes, *Candida*, or parasites), drug-induced esophagitis, and hypereosinophilic syndrome.

The major histological differential diagnosis for EoE is GERD. Histologically, most of the features of EoE overlap with those of GERD, particularly in distal esophageal biopsies. Although biopsies of patients with EoE tend to reveal more numerous intraepithelial eosinophils, typically 15 or more per high-power field, severe GERD may also uncommonly produce pronounced eosinophilia in this range. Because intraepithelial eosinophils in both conditions may be patchy in distribution, sampling error can also affect one's ability to establish a correct diagnosis. The distribution of disease is important, because EoE often involves long segments of the esophagus, may be patchy or focal, and typically involves the proximal or middle esophagus in addition to the distal esophagus or GEJ. In contrast, patients with GERD typically have higher eosinophil counts in the distal esophagus—an area where reflux affects the esophagus more severely—than in the proximal esophagus (Table 14.5; see Fig. 14.14).[208-210]

In parasitic and fungal infections, eosinophils aggregate intensively in areas of infection, even forming abscesses in the lamina propria, and are often associated with neutrophils. The plaques and exudates observed in patients with EoE may suggest *Candida* esophagitis endoscopically, but on microscopy, the plaques in EoE consist of sloughed squamous cells admixed with eosinophils, which are easily distinguished from the fungal elements characteristic of *Candida* esophagitis.

Eosinophilic gastroenteritis is characterized by tissue eosinophilia that is often patchy in distribution and may involve any portion, and any layer, of the GI tract (i.e., mucosa, muscularis propria, and serosa). Mucosal biopsies in patients with eosinophilic gastroenteritis often show numerous eosinophils, and extracellular granules, infiltrating the lamina propria, muscularis mucosae, and epithelium and usually involve one or more anatomic locations such as the esophagus, stomach, and duodenum. Therefore, obtaining biopsy specimens from the stomach and duodenum and correlating the findings with clinical symptoms such as nausea, vomiting, and diarrhea is helpful in establishing a correct diagnosis. Unlike patients with EoE, most of those with eosinophilic gastroenteritis have increased serum total and food-specific immunoglobulin E (IgE) levels. The original description of eosinophilic gastroenteritis was based on examination of both mucosal biopsies and resected bowel specimens, generally removed because of obstructive symptoms. The use of systemic steroids to relieve obstructive symptoms has greatly reduced resections due to eosinophilic gastroenteritis involving the muscularis propria, and endoscopy has become an increasingly safe and common procedure. Eosinophilic gastrointestinal disorders is the current descriptor for eosinophilic GI disease which is based in virtually all cases on examination of mucosal biopsies. In the context of eosinophilic gastrointestinal disorders, eosinophilic gastroenteritis is the descriptor used for eosinophil-rich inflammation in mucosal biopsies from more than one site in the GI tract. Among patients who have multiple sites of eosinophilic inflammation in the GI tract, the esophagus is the most common second site, and the most common combination is esophagus and stomach and small intestine, followed by esophagus and stomach.[224] A recent population-based analysis uncovered increased risk for Crohn's disease or ulcerative colitis in patients who have EoE, and increased risk for EoE in patients who have Crohn's disease or ulcerative colitis.[177] In patients with both EoE and IBD, complications of IBD, but not EoE, were increased. Esophageal involvement by Crohn's disease can reveal nonspecific esophagitis, sometimes associated with increased numbers of eosinophils. The presence of non-necrotizing granulomas is a helpful diagnostic feature, but granulomas are relatively uncommon, observed in only 7% to 9% of patients with esophageal Crohn's disease.[225] Crohn's disease never involves the esophagus in the absence of stomach, small intestine, or colon involvement, and other features such as erosions, sinuses, fistulas, neutrophils, and increased lymphoid tissue are often present in addition to increased eosinophils.

Drug-induced esophagitis can manifest with eosinophilia. It is helpful to establish a temporal clinicopathologic association between use of the drug, onset of symptoms, and tissue eosinophilia in determining that diagnosis. Resolution is often demonstrated when the drug is withdrawn from use.

Vasculitides, including eosinophilic granulomatosis with polyangiitis (EGPA, previously known as Churg-Strauss syndrome) and polyarteritis nodosa, affect the GI tract in approximately 20% to 30% of cases. Eosinophil-rich granulomas, with necrosis, involving medium to small-sized vessels, are typically found in EGPA, whereas arteritis in a background of eosinophilic inflammation is typical of polyarteritis nodosa.[226]

Natural History

There are limited data regarding the natural history of EoE. Currently, it appears to be a chronic disease that is manageable but not curable. EoE often leads to persistent dysphagia if left untreated. In one study of 30 untreated patients who were observed for an average of 7.2 years, dysphagia persisted in 29 patients (97%).[227] Successfully treated patients experience relapse in 25% to 40% of cases. The long-term outcome for patients with EoE who receive treatment, and the proportion of patients who require multiple courses of treatment, are unknown.[228] To date, no malignant potential has been associated with this disease. Few reports have suggested an association with BE,[229,230] but a recent study of a national pathology database suggests that there is a strong inverse relationship between Barrett's metaplasia and eosinophilic infiltrates in the esophageal mucosa. In that study, the observed prevalence rate of the simultaneous occurrence of these two conditions was one third of what would be expected if they occurred independently (odds ratio, 0.29; 95% confidence interval, 0.27 to 0.33; $P < .0001$).[231]

Treatment

Several types of therapeutic modalities are available for patients with EoE. The efficacy of any particular treatment is best evaluated clinically by showing relief of symptoms, or a reduction in the degree of eosinophilic infiltration, or both. Currently, therapy for esophageal inflammation is based on antigen elimination trials, antiinflammatory medications, and physical dilation if strictures are present. Dietary elimination is a treatment modality frequently used in children, but it is often not well tolerated by adults because it is restrictive and compliance is difficult to achieve. Corticosteroids, either systemic or topical, have been effective in the treatment of this disorder in both children and adults.[232] Systemic steroids are used for acute exacerbations, such as severe dysphagia, hospitalization, and weight loss. Topical glucocorticoids are used to provide long-term control. Glucocorticoids show a significant positive effect in reducing esophageal eosinophilia. Before 2007, swallowed fluticasone was primarily used.[233,234] Since then, oral budesonide has also been shown to be effective.[213,235-237] An orodispersible budesonide formulation is approved for treating EoE in Europe but not yet in the United States.[238] Treatment of EoE with cromolyn sodium, leukotriene receptor antagonists, or immunosuppressive agents is not recommended.[176] Humanized antibody therapy directed to block IL5, IL13, or both IL4 and IL13 reduces esophageal eosinophil inflammation with variable effects on symptoms.[201,239-242]

Esophageal dilation is performed for adult patients whose presenting symptoms include symptomatic esophageal narrowing resulting from fixed strictures. However, this procedure usually needs to be repeated regularly and does not reduce the degree of inflammation.[243]

LYMPHOCYTIC ESOPHAGITIS

Lymphocytic esophagitis was first recognized in 2006. In the original description of 20 cases, Rubio and associates[244] emphasized the occurrence of high numbers of CD3+, CD4+, and CD8+ lymphocytes in peripapillary squamous epithelium in the absence of granulocytes (neutrophils and eosinophils). Dilated intercellular spaces were frequently detected. Eleven of the patients were children, seven of whom had Crohn's disease. Purdy and colleagues[245] further characterized this entity in 42 patients with increased intraepithelial lymphocytes in the esophagus. In their study, no significant associations with clinical features were detected. In a report by Haque and coworkers,[246] lymphocytic esophagitis, defined histologically as the presence of increased lymphocytes in the peripapillary esophageal epithelium associated with markedly dilated intercellular spaces in the absence of neutrophils and eosinophils, was detected in approximately 0.1% of an endoscopic population of patients during an 18-month period (Fig. 14.15). Of the 119 study cases, more than two-thirds of patients had symptoms of dysphagia or odynophagia that elicited clinical suspicion for EoE or GERD. Although more than a decade has passed since its recognition, threshold values for increased intraepithelial lymphocytes vary and include 20 lymphocytes/HPF,[247,248] 30/HPF,[249] and at least 40 CD3+ lymphocytes/HPF.[250] Suggested diagnostic criteria for lymphocytic esophagitis include intraepithelial lymphocytosis with evidence of epithelial injury (dilated intercellular spaces and dyskeratosis) involving areas of the esophagus other than the GE junction (where lymphocytosis is common in GERD).[247] Thus defined, most affected patients are female with immune-mediated disorders and disorders elsewhere in the GI tract involving lymphocytosis. Endoscopically, the mucosa may appear normal but findings suggestive of EoE, including rings, furrows, and white plaques, may be seen.[247] Strictures are identified in one-third of patients in one study.[246] Analysis of a large national database yielded data demonstrating a 3.07 odds ratio of patients with microscopic colitis also developing lymphocytic esophagitis, suggesting a common pathogenesis for lymphocytic disorders affecting the upper and lower GI tracts.[249]

Although the clinical significance of lymphocytic esophagitis remains to be defined, evidence suggests that this condition probably represents injury by a variety of potential insults, although an autoimmune etiology has been postulated in some cases. In a number of studies,[244,245,251,252] lymphocytic esophagitis was associated with a multiple clinical conditions, including *H. pylori* gastritis, celiac disease, duodenal lymphocytosis, and Crohn's disease in children and more rarely in adults.[250,253-256] In a study of adults who had lymphocytic esophagitis (defined as 20 peripapillary intraepithelial lymphocytes/HPF without granulocytes, N=94), eosinophilic esophagitis (N=344), and normal biopsies from patients who did not have GERD (N=5202), significant risk factors for developing lymphocytic esophagitis were age over 60 years, use of aspirin or statin drugs, and history of achalasia.[248]

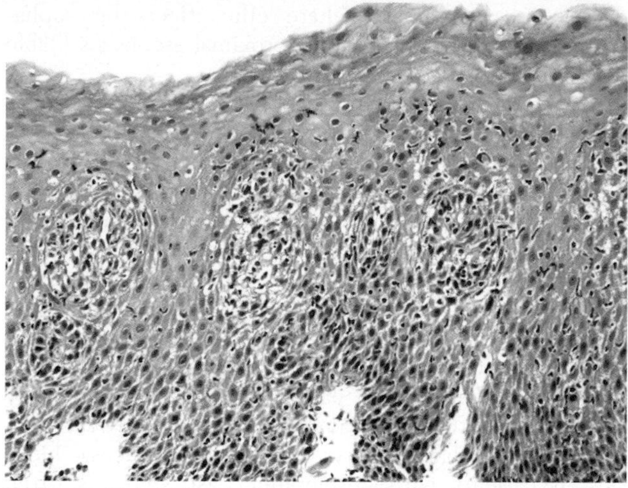

FIGURE 14.15 Lymphocytic esophagitis. The esophageal mucosa shows peripapillary intraepithelial lymphocytosis with basal zone hyperplasia. No significant numbers of eosinophils or neutrophils are identified.

Although the original reports of lymphocytic esophagitis emphasized the lack or paucity of granulocytes, recent studies suggest a relationship between lymphocytic esophagitis and EoE. In a study of 311 patients with symptoms of dysphagia and food impaction predominantly who had increased lymphocytes in their esophageal biopsies, defined as 40 or more CD3+ cells/HPF, 33 (10.6%) had biopsies with lymphocytic esophagitis and EoE, an esophageal phenotype referred to as compound lymphocytic—eosinophilic oesophagitis.[250] In a study of 238 patients with food bolus impaction, EoE and compound lymphocytic—eosinophilic esophagitis (defined at ≥40 lymphocytes/HPF and ≥15 eosinophils/HPF) were significantly more common causes of impaction in patients under 50 years of age, in contrast to GERD that was the most common cause for food bolus impaction in patients over 50 years of age.[256] In a different study, among 69 patients with primary esophageal motility disorder (non-achalasia), lymphocytic esophagitis was strongly associated with the motility disorder (adjusted odds ratio 7.93) compared to 70 patients undergoing fundoplication for GERD.[257]

Successful therapy includes PPI, especially for those who report GERD symptoms which are common in patients with lymphocytic esophagitis, swallowed steroids, and dilation for patients who have strictures.[247] The clinical course appears to be chronic but benign.[247] Compared to patients who have EoE, patients with lymphocytic esophagitis are more likely to respond clinically and to manifest improved biopsies following therapy.[248] A recent review identified a variety of clinicopathologic characteristics reported for lymphocytic esophagitis, and called for consensus criteria for diagnosis of this still somewhat enigmatic disorder.[258]

MECHANICAL CAUSES OF ESOPHAGITIS

Achalasia

Clinical Features

Achalasia is a chronic incurable esophageal motility disorder that is characterized by an inability of the LES to relax after swallowing, which results in periodic esophageal obstruction. It is a rare disease affecting 20,000-40,000 individuals in the United States, men and women equally, who are predominantly 30-60 years of age.[259] The symptoms of achalasia may appear gradually. Patients present initially with a history of dysphagia to solid foods, and later with difficulty swallowing liquids. Often there is a history of weight loss, regurgitation of undigested food, and avoidance of certain solid or bulky foods. Half of the patients complain of chest pain or heartburn[260] and may be initially misdiagnosed as having GERD.[259] Discomfort or fullness under the breastbone and a history of aspiration or aspiration pneumonia may be elicited as well.

High resolution manometry is cited as the test of choice for diagnosis of achalasia.[137,261] As many as 95% of the patients with achalasia have a positive result on esophagography with barium contrast and timed barium esophagram is recommended for both the diagnostic pathway and also to evaluate treatment outcome in recent achalasia guidelines.[137,262] A positive barium study shows characteristic tapering of the distal esophagus and the so-called "bird's beak" sign at the level of the esophageal hiatus. Esophageal endoscopy is typically performed to evaluate for other causes of esophageal obstruction.

Pathogenesis

The pathophysiology of achalasia is linked to destruction of ganglion cells in the esophageal wall and LES, which leads to an impairment of relaxation of the LES. Loss of LES relaxation is believed to be a consequence of loss of the inhibitory activity of vasoactive intestinal peptide and nitric oxide.[259] Destruction of ganglion cells is associated with an inflammatory response, which seems to suggest an autoimmune, viral, or chronic degenerative process.[263] In addition to lymphocytes, mast cells are implicated in the pathophysiology of achalasia because mast cells in LES muscle in patients with achalasia are associated with loss of interstitial cells of Cajal and neuronal degeneration.[264] In a minority of patients with Allgrove syndrome, a mutation on chromosome 12 is implicated in the development of achalasia. Secondary achalasia (or pseudoachalasia) may develop as a result of obstructing lesions, such as GEJ tumors, Chagas disease, or amyloidosis, and closely mimics primary achalasia clinically. In addition, functional obstruction of the LES may be induced by a fundoplication or by gastric banding procedures.

Pathology

The primary histological abnormality in achalasia is a marked reduction, or complete absence, of myenteric ganglion cells (Fig. 14.16).[54,265] Myenteric nerve inflammation, with a predominance of T lymphocytes, and myenteric neural fibrosis are present.[54,266,267] Other alterations include diffuse squamous hyperplasia, florid lymphocytic esophagitis, lymphocytic inflammation of the lamina propria and submucosa, and submucosal glandular atrophy with periductal and glandular inflammation. Mucosal changes in patients with achalasia are variable. In a series of 48 untreated patients, 10 had changes suggestive of GERD,[268] whereas others had normal mucosa.[269] Mucosal/submucosal biopsies from 32 patients with achalasia showed mostly lymphocytic inflammatory cell infiltrates in 87.5% and dilated intercellular spaces in 84.4%, both more common than in controls; muscularis mucosa atrophy (40.6%) and an irregular epithelial surface (28.1%) were found only in achalasia patients.[270] In a study of 72 mucosal specimens from subjects who had and had not undergone myotomy, as well as few resections from subjects with end stage achalasia, mild squamous epithelial inflammation was found with a predominance of CD4-positive T cells and CD4:CD8 ratio on average 2.08:1 in proximal esophagus, 1.83:1 in mid esophagus, and 1.51:1 in distal esophagus. The CD4:CD8 ratio in the myenteric plexus of the resected specimens was 1.40:1. The authors attribute lack of CD8 dominant inflammation in Auerbach's plexus to the lack of neurons, and conclude that the epithelial infiltrates are reactive and cannot be used to identify achalasia.[271] Numerous eosinophils and extracellular protein deposits such as major basic protein, a component of eosinophils granules, have been identified in the muscularis propria of 24/28 subjects undergoing POEM procedures, confirming earlier findings of muscle eosinophilia in (22/42) resected esophagi,[54] with few myenteric ganglion cells, suggesting that eosinophils and their granule proteins may be pathogenic in a subset of subjects who have achalasia.[272] However, some studies identify eosinophils in the muscularis propria of dysmotile esophagi with diagnoses other than achalasia, suggesting that a relationship between tissue eosinophilia and esophageal dysmotility.[273] The principal role of pretherapy biopsies is to rule out all potential causes of pseudoachalasia, including neoplastic alterations or infections.

Treatment

Management of achalasia includes several therapeutic modalities. Pharmacologic management with sublingual nitrates and calcium channel blockers has a high failure rate and is poorly tolerated, and in recent guidelines the use of nitrates, calcium channel blockers or phosdiesterase inhibitors are not recommended as therapy for achalasia.[137,274] Injection of the LES with botulinum toxin is effective for short-term relief of dysphagia but is not recommended for patients under 50 years of age.[137,275,276] Dilation remains a valuable option for nonsurgical candidates. Minimally invasive Heller myotomy has low rates of morbidity and mortality; both it and laparoscopic Heller myotomy with partial fundoplication are durable, safe, and effective treatment options for patients with achalasia.[277-279] POEM is less invasive than laparoscopic Heller myotomy and was recently shown to be noninferior to laparoscopic Heller myotomy to alleviate symptoms of achalasia, but GERD was more common among patients who underwent POEM.[280]

Muscular Dystrophy

Some forms of muscular dystrophy (myotonic form) are associated with esophageal dysmotility and may be associated with a nonspecific esophagitis (see Chapter 7).

Mallory-Weiss Tears and Other Traumatic Esophageal Disorders

Esophageal perforations, either full thickness (Boerhaave syndrome) or partial thickness (Mallory-Weiss tears), and hematomas are manifestations of spontaneous and iatrogenic traumatic esophageal disease.[281]

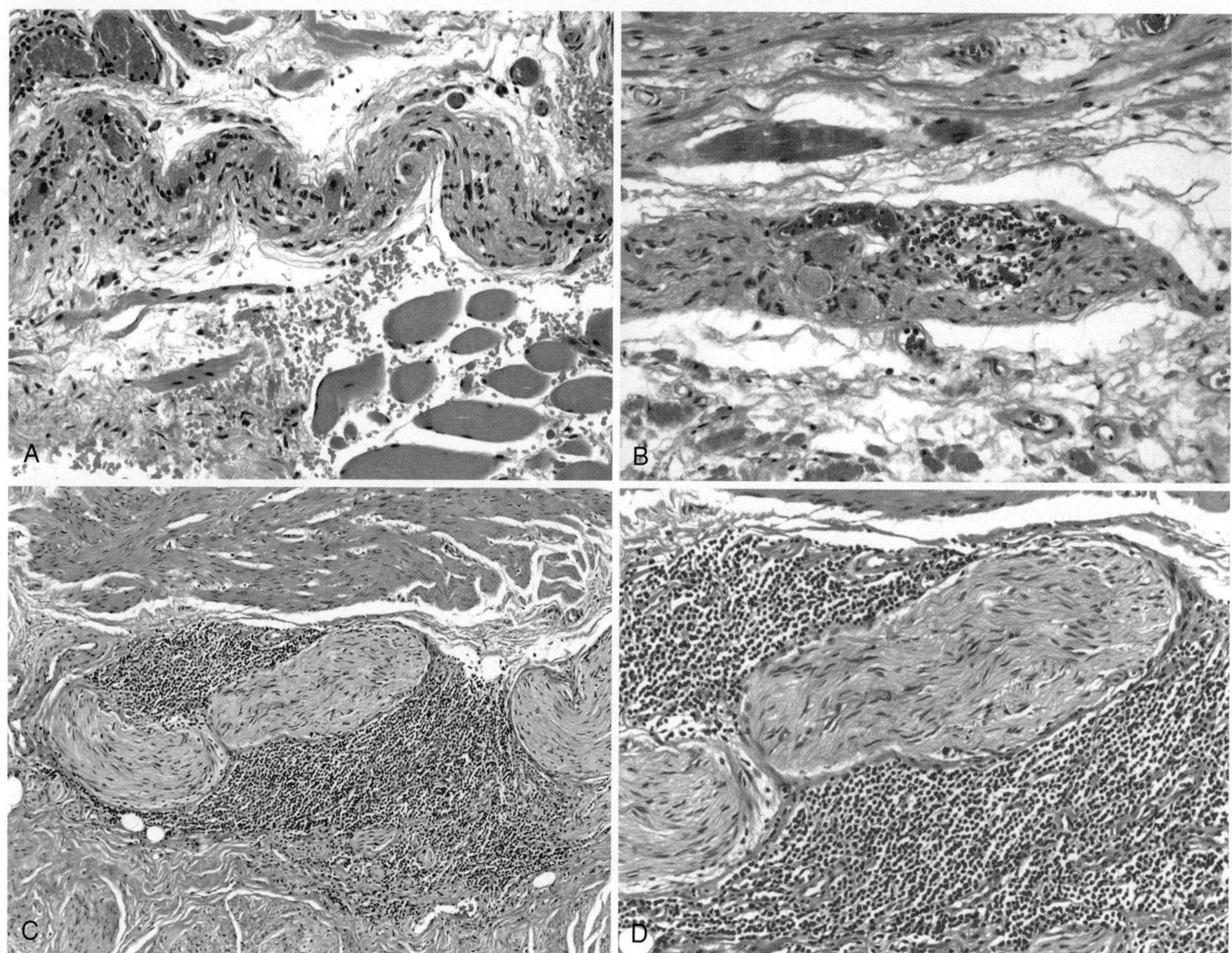

FIGURE 14.16 Histopathology of achalasia. A, Normal myenteric plexus shows multiple ganglion cells and no significant inflammation. **B,** Mild myenteric plexus infiltrate of lymphocytes exhibits few intact ganglion cells. **C** and **D,** Severe inflammation of the myenteric plexus is characterized by a dense infiltrate of mononuclear cells. Ganglion cells are not identified.

Mallory-Weiss tears are mucosal lacerations in the distal esophagus and proximal stomach. Histologically, longitudinal tears of the mucosa extend into the submucosa but do not involve the muscularis propria. These lacerations are accompanied by acute hemorrhage with organizing fibrin, with or without accompanying neutrophilic inflammation. The prevalence of tears among patients with upper GI bleeding is approximately 5%.[282] Precipitating factors include retching, vomiting, straining, coughing, blunt abdominal trauma, and cardiopulmonary resuscitation. Between 40% to 80% of patients have a history of heavy alcohol use leading to vomiting.[282,283] The presence of hiatal hernia is also considered a predisposing factor and is found in 35% to 100% of patients.[284] It has been proposed that, in patients with a hiatus hernia, a higher pressure gradient develops in the hernia sac compared with the rest of the stomach during retching, increasing the potential for mucosal laceration.[281] Others consider a sudden increase in intraabdominal pressure to be the causative factor. The prognosis of Mallory-Weiss tears is generally good. Bleeding from these lesions stops spontaneously in 80% to 90% of cases without therapy. With conservative therapy, the lesions heal within 48 to 72 hours.

Boerhaave syndrome, or postemetic rupture of the esophagus, results from a sudden increase in intraluminal esophageal pressure due to vomiting. In the modern medical context, instrumentation of the esophagus represents the most common cause.[285,286] Clinically, patients experience sudden-onset severe chest pain in the lower thorax and upper abdomen after repeated episodes of retching or vomiting. Often, they have fever or pain after forceful vomiting, esophageal instrumentation, or chest trauma. Typically, acute upper GI bleeding is not seen after esophageal rupture, which helps distinguish it from the more common Mallory-Weiss tears. However, untreated Mallory-Weiss tears may lead to Boerhaave syndrome, and Boerhaave syndrome may be recurrent.[287,288] The most common location of the rupture is at the posterolateral wall of the lower third of the esophagus, 2 to 3 cm proximal to the GEJ.[289,290] Contrast esophagography using a water-soluble agent initially, followed by a barium study if the initial result is negative, represents the most reliable test for documenting the presence and location of the perforation.[291] The initial phase of therapy includes physiologic monitoring, limiting the extent of ongoing mediastinal contamination, cessation of oral intake, and administration of broad-spectrum antibiotics. An overwhelming majority of patients require some type of surgical intervention that depends on the location, extent, and cause of the injury. Boerhaave syndrome may occur in patients who have EoE.[292]

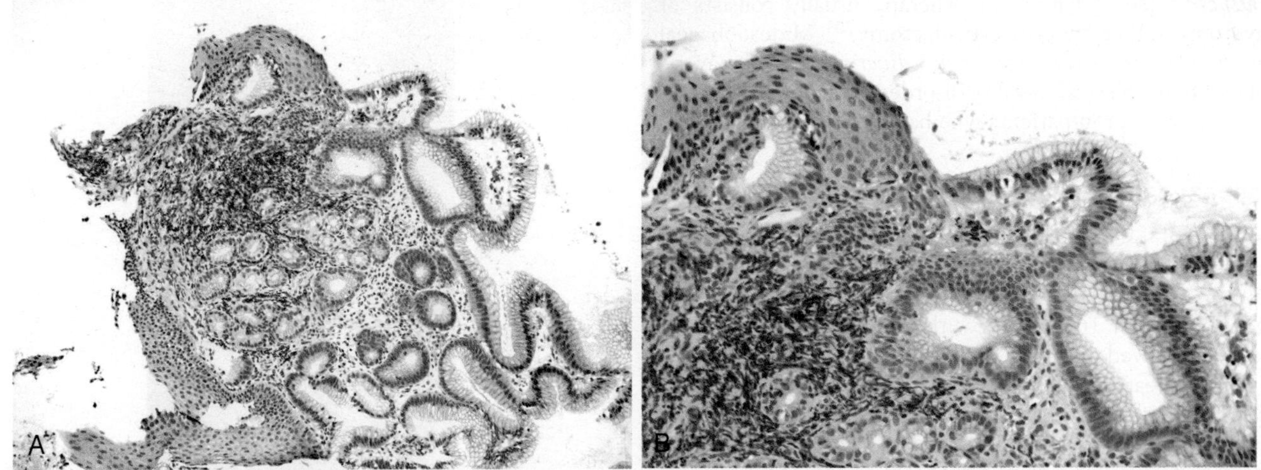

FIGURE 14.17 Histopathology of gastric inlet patch. A, Proximal esophageal biopsy shows gastric mucosa in continuity with esophageal squamous epithelium. **B,** Higher power of the transition between the two types of epithelium shows foveolar epithelium continuous with squamous epithelium.

CONGENITAL AND ACQUIRED DEFORMATIONS

Inlet patch

Gastric inlet patch is a congenital lesion that typically occurs in the proximal esophagus and is recognized as a salmon-colored oval or round area often with heaped margins.[293] The incidence at endoscopy is cited as 0.18-14% and the incidence is greater if chromoendoscopy is used. Rates reported at autopsy are up to 70% suggesting that inlet patches are under-recognized endoscopically. Inlet patches may be asymptomatic or may be found in patients complaining of dyspepsia, reflux, globus, cough, hoarseness, odynophagia or dysphagia. For patients with reflux symptoms who do not respond to PPI use, ablative procedures may be required.[294] Oxyntic type mucosa is most commonly found in inlet patches, but cardiac, antral and antral/oxyntic mucosa has also been reported (Fig. 14.17). Inlet patches often contain H. pylori in patients who have H. pylori in their stomach, but H. pylori may be isolated to an inlet patch. Complications include bleeding, ulcers, strictures, perforations and fistulas. A relationship between inlet patch and malignancy risk is controversial, but proximal esophageal adenocarcinomas have been attributed to inlet patches.[295] Typical inlet patches do not require biopsy for diagnosis, but biopsy may be indicated for atypical appearing mucosa in a typical inlet patch, for patches in unusual areas such as mid or distal esophagus, and lesions with atypical configurations such as polyps. Inlet patches may be associated with rings and webs (see below).

Esophageal Rings and Webs

Structural esophageal abnormalities include esophageal rings and webs. Although many patients are asymptomatic, some experience dysphagia, regurgitation, aspiration, or other symptoms of esophagitis.[296]

An esophageal ring is defined as a concentric, thin (2 to 5 mm) diaphragm of tissue located in the distal esophagus, although rings and strictures may be found associated with circumferential esophageal inlet patches which occur in the proximal esophagus.[297] A Schatzki ring most commonly develops at the squamocolumnar junction (SCJ) at the proximal border of a hiatal hernia, but rings may occur anywhere in the esophagus. The prevalence of esophageal rings is unknown, because most are asymptomatic. Based on data from barium studies, these lesions are present in approximately 6% to 14% of endoscopic examinations.[296] Microscopically, Schatzki rings are composed of both mucosa and submucosa, with basal cell hyperplasia, hyperkeratosis, and, often, eosinophil infiltration. Cases with prominent eosinophils most likely represent a subtype of primary EoE (see earlier discussion).[298,299]

Esophageal webs are defined as eccentric, thin (<2 mm) membranes of tissue in the esophagus, but they are most common in the proximal region. Because most cases are asymptomatic, the prevalence of this condition is unknown. Esophageal webs that occur in association with dysphagia, iron deficiency anemia, glossitis, and koilonychia are referred to as Plummer-Vinson syndrome in the United States and Paterson–Brown Kelly syndrome in the United Kingdom.[300] This condition is most common in thin white women and usually responds to treatment of the patient's underlying iron deficiency state.[296,300] The incidence of Plummer-Vinson syndrome appears to be declining, possibly due to declining incidence of iron deficiency. Webs generally appear histologically as folds of normal mucosa overlying fibrous tissue, but in Plummer-Vinson syndrome that epithelium may be atrophic or hyperplastic with hyperkeratosis, and in some cases contain chronic inflammation.[301] Patients with Plummer-Vinson syndrome are considered at increased risk to develop squamous cell carcinoma of the proximal esophagus.[301] The cause of esophageal webs is unknown, but they are associated with an array of conditions, including cutaneous blistering disorders (e.g., epidermolysis bullosa, cicatricial pemphigoid), Zenker diverticula (see below), esophageal duplication, and cysts. Webs may also occur in association with lymphocytic esophagitis, gastric inlet patch, and Schatzki ring.[299,302,303]

Esophageal Diverticula

Esophageal diverticula occur most commonly in elderly men and consist of full-thickness outpouchings involving all layers of the esophageal wall, usually in the cervical esophagus, where they are termed *Zenker diverticula* or *pharyngeal pouches*[304] (see Chapter 8). Therapy usually consists of myotomy rather than diverticulectomy.[305] Midesophageal diverticula are termed *epiphrenic diverticula* and may be related to esophageal motility disorder.[306] Esophageal diverticula may occur in patients who have Schatzki ring.[299]

Esophageal Pseudodiverticulosis

Esophageal pseudodiverticulosis is an uncommon benign condition that occurs potentially in all age groups but typically in the elderly, with a slight male predominance. A recent study of 16 patients with esophageal pseudodiverticulosis showed mean age of 50.8 years (standard deviation was 17.4 years).[307] The condition usually manifests with dysphagia, which is typically not severe but intermittent or slowly progressive. There is a high incidence of esophageal narrowing, usually in the upper third of the esophagus; in many cases, this may mimic carcinoma. In barium studies, multiple small (1 to 4 mm) flask- or collar stud–shaped outpouchings are present in the esophageal wall. Radiology offers the most sensitive method of diagnosis (Fig. 14.18). Endoscopy is not helpful for diagnosis because the orifices of the pseudodiverticula are difficult to recognize and most often only nonspecific mucosal inflammatory changes are seen. In addition, mucosal biopsies usually are not helpful, because the pseudodiverticula are deep in the submucosa.[308]

Histologically, as the name implies, outpouchings do not represent true diverticula; instead, they consist of dilated and inflamed submucosal esophageal gland ducts. Pseudodiverticula are confined to the submucosa of the esophagus and are lined by cuboidal to stratified squamous epithelium. Often, the squamous epithelium replaces the submucosal glands and duct epithelium entirely, with preservation of the normal round and smooth configuration of the glands. A prominent inflammatory infiltrate composed of lymphocytes, eosinophils, and plasma cells typically surrounds the pseudodiverticula (see Chapter 24). The lack of an infiltrative growth pattern and lack of squamous dysplasia help distinguish pseudodiverticula from invasive squamous cell carcinoma. The cause of this disorder is unclear. Postulated theories of pathogenesis include glandular secretory dysfunction, esophageal dysmotility, and chronic recurrent esophagitis.[296,309] Among 16 patients with esophageal pseudodiverticulosis, 5 had endoscopic/histological evidence of EoE and a clinical diagnosis of EoE.[307] The EoE patients were more likely to have pseudodiverticula in the mid or distal esophagus compared to patients without EoE, and were younger, more likely to have food bolus impactions, and to have other atopic diseases. A causative relationship between EoE and esophageal pseudodiverticulosis has not been established, but the association may be more common than currently realized.

Treatment is directed at relieving esophageal obstruction, if any, and dealing with the underlying inflammatory condition. Long-term follow-up studies indicate that the condition may remain stable for long periods.[310,311]

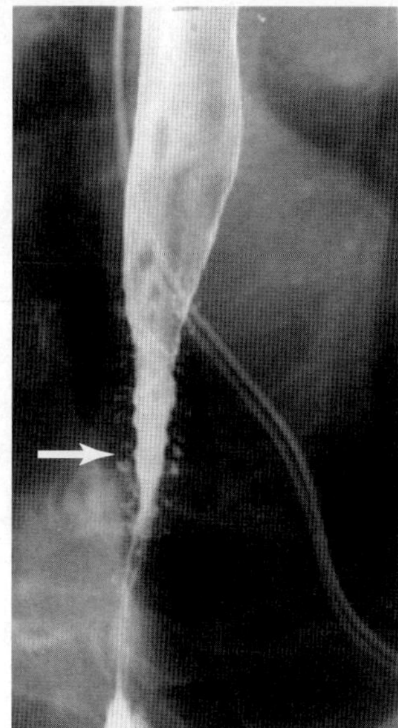

FIGURE 14.18 Esophagography shows multiple esophageal intramural pseudodiverticula as flask-shaped outpouchings (*arrow*) in longitudinal rows parallel to the long axis of the esophagus.

ESOPHAGEAL INVOLVEMENT IN SYSTEMIC DISEASE

Eosinophilic Gastroenteritis

Eosinophilic gastroenteritis (EGE) is a condition that is characterized by patchy or diffuse eosinophilic infiltration in various parts of the bowel wall (mucosa, muscularis propria, and serosa) at one or more sites in the GI tract. The mucosal subtype is the most common (25% to 100%), perhaps because of its accessibility to diagnosis by routine endoscopy and biopsies.[312] The disease selectively involves the stomach (26% to 100%) and small intestine (28% to 100%),[313-316] but involvement of the esophagus has been reported in some cases.[313,314] In a series of 21 patients with eosinophilic gastroenteritis, 9 had histological involvement of the esophagus.[317] Mucosal biopsy specimens from patients with eosinophilic gastroenteritis often show numerous eosinophils, frequently associated with extracellular granules, infiltrating the lamina propria, muscularis mucosae, and epithelium; the lesions usually involve one or more sites of the esophagus, stomach, and duodenum. Pediatric patients who have eosinophilic gastritis may have mucosal eosinophilia in the esophagus contemporaneously, prior to or subsequent to their diagnosis of eosinophilic gastritis.[318,319] Therefore, the onset of new symptoms in EoE patients that may indicate lower GI tract involvement, particularly abdominal pain or protein-losing enteropathy and should prompt endoscopy for re-evaluation of sites in addition to the esophagus.

The diagnosis of EGE is challenging clinically, and also pathologically. EoE is the only eosinophil-rich inflammatory GI disease for which consensus recommendations exist for diagnosis. Therefore, to establish a correct EGE diagnosis, it is helpful to obtain biopsies from the stomach and duodenum and correlate the findings with clinical symptoms of generalized mucosal involvement, such as nausea, vomiting, diarrhea, weight loss, and protein-losing enteropathy. Unlike patients with EoE, many with EGE have increased serum total and food-specific IgE levels and positive skin test responses to a variety of food antigens.[226,312] One or more years before developing definitive signs and symptoms, patients who have eosinophilic granulomatosis with polyangiitis (EGPA, formerly known as Churg-Strauss syndrome) may have gastrointestinal symptoms with biopsies showing excess eosinophils, including in the esophagus, with a resulting diagnosis of eosinophilic gastroenteritis.[320] Therefore when submucosa is present in biopsies consistent with EGE the blood vessels should be specifically examined for evidence of EGPA.

A recent update in terminology addressed the evolution of *eosinophilic gastroenteritis* from a term that applies to small intestine disease to a term that also indicates gastric disease only, or a combination of gastric and small intestinal disease. An international multidisciplinary group recommends that the term *eosinophilic gastroenteritis* be used sparingly and only to refer to disease in both the stomach and the small intestine, and that other forms of eosinophilic gastrointestinal disorders are designated with Eo precursors, such as EoG for *eosinophilic gastritis, EoN* for *eosinophilic enteritis*, and so forth. More specific terminology will hopefully facilitate both clinical care and research efforts.[320a]

Esophageal Involvement in Collagen Vascular Disorders (Including Scleroderma)

Collagen vascular disorders, including progressive systemic sclerosis (scleroderma),[321] systemic lupus erythematosus,[322] rheumatoid arthritis,[323] mixed connective tissue disorders, polymyositis, dermatomyositis,[324] and Sjögren syndrome,[325] may involve the esophagus.[326] Common esophageal manifestations in these conditions include myoneuroenteric dysmotility, esophagitis secondary to reflux, drug-induced esophagitis, and opportunistic infections. Esophageal pathology may be related to the underlying collagen vascular disease, the associated inflammatory conditions, or the side effects of immunosuppressive or other types of drug therapy.

GI complications are found in 90% of scleroderma patients.[327] The esophagus is the mostly commonly affected part of the GI tract followed by the anorectum and small bowel. Symptoms may be absent or mild until severe organ damage occurs. GI involvement portends reduced survival (15% at 9 years). Esophageal symptoms include dysphagia, odynophagia, heartburn, regurgitation, chronic cough or hoarseness.[327] Reflux and dysphagia occur in 34.8% and 4.3% of patients, respectively, and GERD may contribute to the development of interstitial lung disease in affected patients. Scleroderma has been associated with an increased risk of BE and its neoplastic complications.[328] In a series of 63 patients with scleroderma referred for upper GI symptoms, GERD was documented histologically in 53%, strictures in 29%, and BE in 16%.[329] A similar series detected BE in 37% of patients with scleroderma, including two with adenocarcinoma.[330] The mucosal changes are a result of esophageal hypomotility and aperistalsis, with incompetence of the LES.[331] Atrophy and fibrosis predominate in the inner circular layer of the muscularis propria in this condition (Fig. 14.19). Autopsy and functional studies show that smooth muscle atrophy, ,is the most significant alteration in the esophagus.[332] Genes expressed in esophageal biopsies from

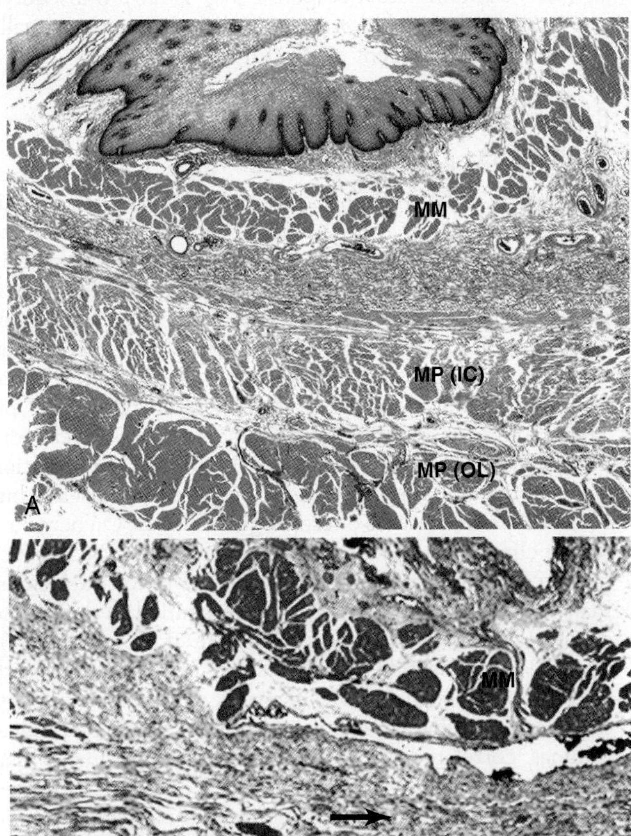

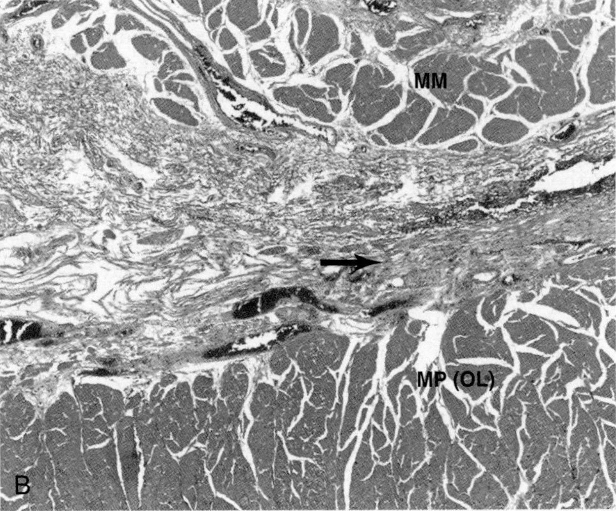

FIGURE 14.19 Histopathology of scleroderma. A, Normal esophagus with intact muscularis mucosae (*MM*) and muscularis propria (*MP*) containing well-defined inner circular (*IC*) and outer longitudinal (*OL*) layers. **B,** In a patient with scleroderma involving the esophagus, marked atrophy of the IC layer of the MP is present (*arrow*), and there is encroachment of the muscle fibers by fibrous tissue. **C,** Trichrome stain confirms the presence of collagen deposition with atrophy and few residual strands of the IC layer (*arrow*).

16 patients with diffuse cutaneous scleroderma compared to controls included upregulated *IL17*, *IFNAR1*, and *PDGFRA*, and downregulated *CCL2* and several human leukocyte antigen genes.[332] One subset of scleroderma patients had an inflammatory gene profile and another subset had a gene profile consistent with cell proliferation. Using basal zone hyperplasia and intraepithelial lymphocytes as markers for GER, differences were not found in those features in biopsies from the lower esophagus of patients with either gene profile, suggesting that the inflammatory gene profile was independent of reflux. Lamina propria collagen deposition (30% of biopsies had lamina propria) was also not different in biopsies from patients with either gene profile.[232] A high incidence of EoE has been identified in patients who have inherited connective tissue disorders.[333]

Esophageal Manifestations of Dermatological Diseases

The esophagus may be affected in many different types of primary dermatological conditions, including drug-induced diseases such as Stevens-Johnson syndrome[334] and bullous diseases such as bullous pemphigoid, benign mucous membrane pemphigoid, epidermolysis bullosa acquisita, pemphigus vulgaris, and lichen planus[335-338] (see Chapter 6). Esophageal disease may develop in the presence or absence of skin lesions.

Pemphigus vulgaris is the most common of the autoimmune mucocutaneous diseases characterized by bulla formation, affecting 0.1 to 0.5 per 100,000 people per year.[338] This condition occurs predominantly in middle-aged to elderly patients of Jewish or Mediterranean descent. Although oral mucosa is most consistently involved, one report suggested that the majority of patients with pemphigus vulgaris who undergo endoscopy with biopsy show evidence of esophageal involvement[339] and esophageal involvement is indeed increasingly recognized.[338] This disorder is caused by loss of integrity of the normal intercellular attachments within the epidermis and mucosal epithelium,[340] which results in the development of flaccid bullae of various sizes. Additional endoscopic abnormalities include erythema, longitudinal red lines, erosions, deep ulcers, exfoliative esophagitis, stenosis, and esophagitis dissecans superficialis.[338] Histologically, intraepithelial blisters are caused by loss of intercellular attachments (acantholysis). For instance, the basal cells may appear separate from one another but remain attached to the basement membrane. Hence, the diagnostic hallmark of pemphigus vulgaris is acantholysis with bulla formation in the suprabasal region combined with a "row of tombstone-like" basal cells.[341] A mild superficial mixed inflammatory infiltrate, which includes eosinophils both within and surrounding the bullae and in the lamina propria, often accompanies blister formation. Desmoglein expression in the esophagus has been shown to be regulated by Th2 cytokines, specifically IL-13.[342] The diagnosis is confirmed by DIF, which shows intercellular IgG, rarely IgA, and complement C3 deposits. ELISA to detect desmoglein 1 and 3 antibodies may be a simpler and more quantifiable method than immunofluorescence.[174] In pemphigus vulgaris patients with mucous membrane involvement only, desmoglein-1 antibodies are detected, and in patients with skin involvement also desmoglein-3 antibodies are also detected.[343]

Bullous pemphigoid is a chronic autoimmune subepidermal bullous disease that affects the skin and sometimes the mucous membranes.[344] IgG autoantibodies bind to the basement membrane, thereby activating complement and inflammatory mediators; this leads to the release of proteases, degradation of hemidesmosomal proteins, and blister formation. Eosinophils are characteristically identified, although their presence is not necessary to establish a definite diagnosis. DIF helps demonstrate the presence of in situ deposition of complement components (typically C3) and linear deposits of IgG at the level of the basement membrane of the esophagus.[344]

The term *epidermolysis bullosa* refers to a group of inherited disorders caused by mutations of genes that encode for structural proteins located at the dermal-epidermal junction. The disorder is characterized by the formation of blisters after minor trauma.[345] Trauma from boluses of food may lead to bullae formation, ulceration, and scarring of the esophageal mucosa with the formation of webs, strictures, and stenoses, most commonly in the proximal esophagus. Esophageal lesions are similar to those in the skin, revealing subepithelial blisters formed by the separation of the esophageal squamous epithelium, with degenerated basal cells from the lamina propria in a clean plane of cleavage without significant inflammatory response (Fig. 14.20). Subsequent ulceration and granulation tissue formation may eventually lead to the development of strictures and webs.

Graft-versus-Host Disease Involving the Esophagus

Esophageal graft-versus-host disease (GVHD) may manifest acutely; it can cause bullous disease and complete sloughing of the esophageal mucosa with the formation of an esophageal cast[346-349] or only nonspecific esophageal ulcers, erythema, and edema. The histological features of esophageal GVHD are similar to those in other parts of the GI tract. Apoptosis and individual cell damage, manifested in squamous mucosa as dyskeratotic keratinocytes, are typically prominent features in combination with a lichenoid interface inflammatory infiltrate (Fig. 14.21). Ulceration and submucosal fibrosis reflect long-standing disease but are not specific features of esophageal GVHD. On occasion, severe clinical disease may show only minor focal changes on mucosal biopsies. Because of the focality of the lesions, many serial tissue sections are recommended to detect the diagnostic features of esophageal GVHD if they are not evident on initial sections.[350] In a study of 51 patients with acute GVHD, vacuolar degeneration, single cell apoptosis, clefts and denuded mucosa were found; those esophageal findings correlated with GVHD involving stomach and duodenum also, as well as clinical signs of GVHD in other organs.[351] In a study of biopsies from 46 patients with and 46 patients without GVHD, duodenal biopsies had the highest sensitivity (89%) among upper tract biopsies.[352] Among 197 patients with clinical suspicion for GVHD, upper tract biopsies to evaluate for GVHD were obtained during 331 endoscopies (Table 14.7)[353] and were evaluated using criteria of McDonald and Sales (grade 0 – normal, grade

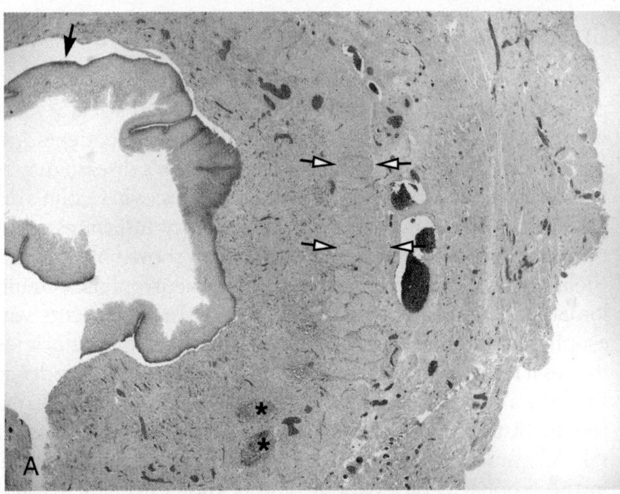

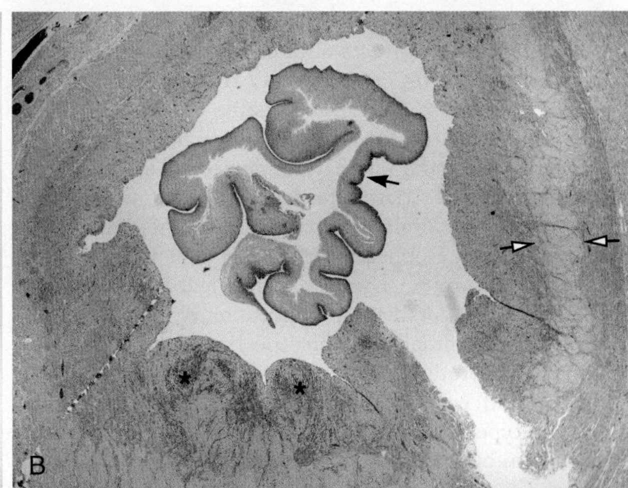

FIGURE 14.20 Histopathology of epidermolysis bullosa esophageal stricture. A, The epithelium is partly detached from the underlying esophageal wall (*black arrow*). The lamina propria is markedly thickened (*white arrows*), and there are multiple lamina propria lymphoid aggregates (*asterisks*). **B,** In a different level of this stricture, the esophageal epithelium is completely detached from the underlying lamina propria (*black arrow* points to basal layer), thickened muscularis mucosa is again seen (*white arrows*), and there is more diffuse chronic inflammation (*asterisks*). (Courtesy Dr. David Einstein, Cleveland Clinic.)

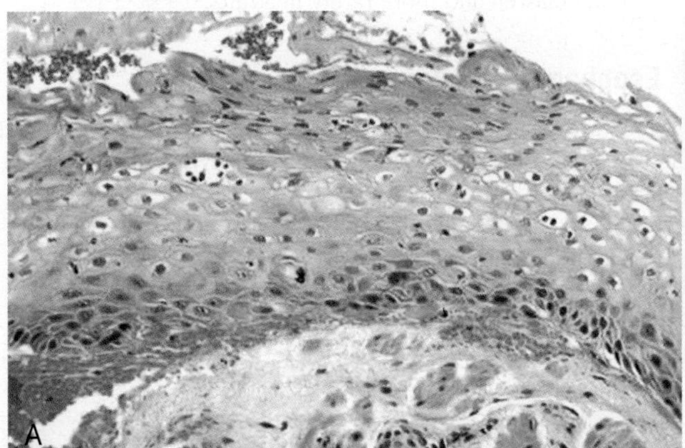

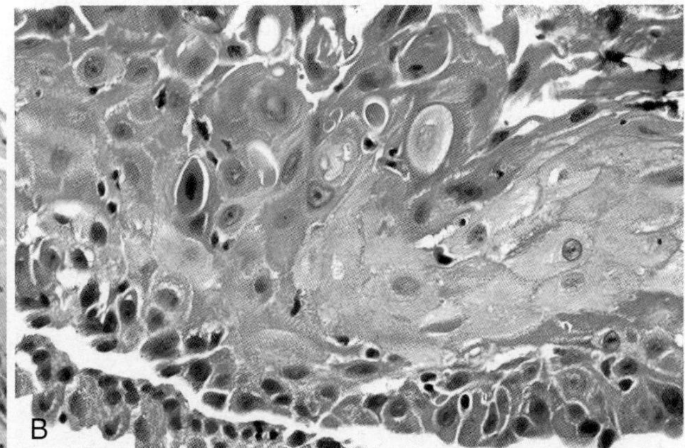

FIGURE 14.21 A, Graft-versus-host disease (GVHD) of the esophagus after bone marrow transplantation. The squamous mucosa is separated from the underlying lamina propria. Lack of surface maturation manifest as the presence of nucleated squamous cells at the surface (ovoid cells), ballooning degeneration of squamous cells, and marked reactive changes are seen. **B,** High-power view of desquamated squamous mucosa in a patient with GVHD shows individual cell necrosis, separation of the epithelium from the underlying lamina propria and marked basal (atypical) reactive changes. The surface squamous cells appear degenerative in nature, and there is marked intercellular edema.

TABLE 14.7 Characteristics of Upper Tract Biopsies to Detect Graft-versus-Host Disease

	Sensitivity (%)	Specificity (%)	Positive Predictive Value (%)	Negative Predictive Value (%)
Esophagus (n=19/331 endoscopies)	33	100	100	41
Stomach (n=324/331 endoscopies)	89	30.6	63.8	67
Duodenum (n=18/331 endoscopies)	80	62.5	57	83.3
Overall	85.6	34.6	64.2	63.7

*Data from Velasco-Guardado A, Lopez-Corral L, Alverez-Delgado A, et al. Endoscopic evaluation and histological al findings in graft-*versus-host *disease. Rev Esp Enferm Dig. 2012;104:310–314*

1 = single cell apoptosis visible at medium power, grade 2 = epithelial damage, grade 3 = crypt/gland dropout, grade 4 = denudation).[354] The data suggest that findings of GVHD in either stomach or duodenum (high sensitivity) coupled with supportive findings in the esophagus (high specificity) are optimum to diagnose GVHD.

Chemotherapy- and Radiation-Induced Esophageal Injury

Esophageal injury is a common side effect of chemotherapy and radiation therapy.[355,356] Esophagitis can occur as a complication of treatment for lung, esophageal, and mediastinal tumors and lymphomas. Acute radiation toxicity typically begins 2 to 3 weeks after therapy. Patients complain of dysphagia, odynophagia, chest pain, or a combination of these symptoms. Late effects of radiation therapy manifest 3 or more months after completion of therapy and include dysphagia, strictures, ulcers, and fistula formation.[357,358] PD1 inhibitors and/or antityrosine kinase inhibitors used concurrently with radiation may accelerate radiation injury, including esophageal stricture formation.[359] Immune checkpoint inhibitors in combination with chemotherapy rarely are associated with esophageal stricture, which may respond to anti-IL-6 therapy.[360] The histological features are similar to those of chemoradiation-induced injury in other parts of the GI tract. Initially (within the first 48 hours), one encounters apoptotic bodies in the mucosal basal zone. Thereafter, and within the first 4 weeks after therapy, a nonspecific type of active esophagitis develops, often with the formation of erosions and ulcers. Bizarre epithelial and stromal cell cytologic atypia may be detected in the chronic phase of disease (Fig. 14.22). Although there are macrocytic changes in epithelial and stromal cells, the N : C ratios are typically well preserved, and mitotic figures are rarely present. Nuclear and cytoplasmic degeneration and multinucleation are common. Chronic radiation-induced cytologic atypia of stromal cells may persist indefinitely. Chronic vascular alterations include the development of sclerosis, intimal foam cell arteriopathy, and obliterative vasculitis. Submucosal fibrosis, mural scarring, and strictures also may complicate deep-seated chemoradiation-induced esophageal ulcers.

Crohn's Disease

Crohn's disease may involve the esophagus with a variable prevalence rate of 0.2% to 11% [361,362] and esophageal involvement should be considered in all Crohn's disease patients with upper tract symptoms.[363] Very rarely, Crohn's disease may be restricted to the esophagus.[363] Mucosal biopsies in Crohn's disease demonstrate nonspecific inflammatory infiltrates which may be predominantly eosinophilic, may show only intraepithelial lymphocytes, or may be mainly neutrophilic. Granulomatous lesions are observed in 7% to 9% of patients with esophageal Crohn's disease.[225] The superficial nature of most mucosal biopsies may account for this relatively low incidence. Usually, a definite diagnosis is established only when characteristic histological features (strictures, deep ulcers, transmural inflammation, granulomas, mural fibrosis) are identified in the esophagus of a patient who is known to have Crohn's disease elsewhere in the GI tract (Fig. 14.23). The mid and distal esophagus are most commonly involved.[363] Upper tract involvement by Crohn's disease correlates with disease progression and recurrence.[363] Some investigators have shown an association between lymphocytic esophagitis and Crohn's disease in children and more rarely in adults.[244,253-255,364]

Esophageal Amyloidosis

The esophagus may be involved in systemic amyloidosis, which, in addition to deposition of amyloid, may result in

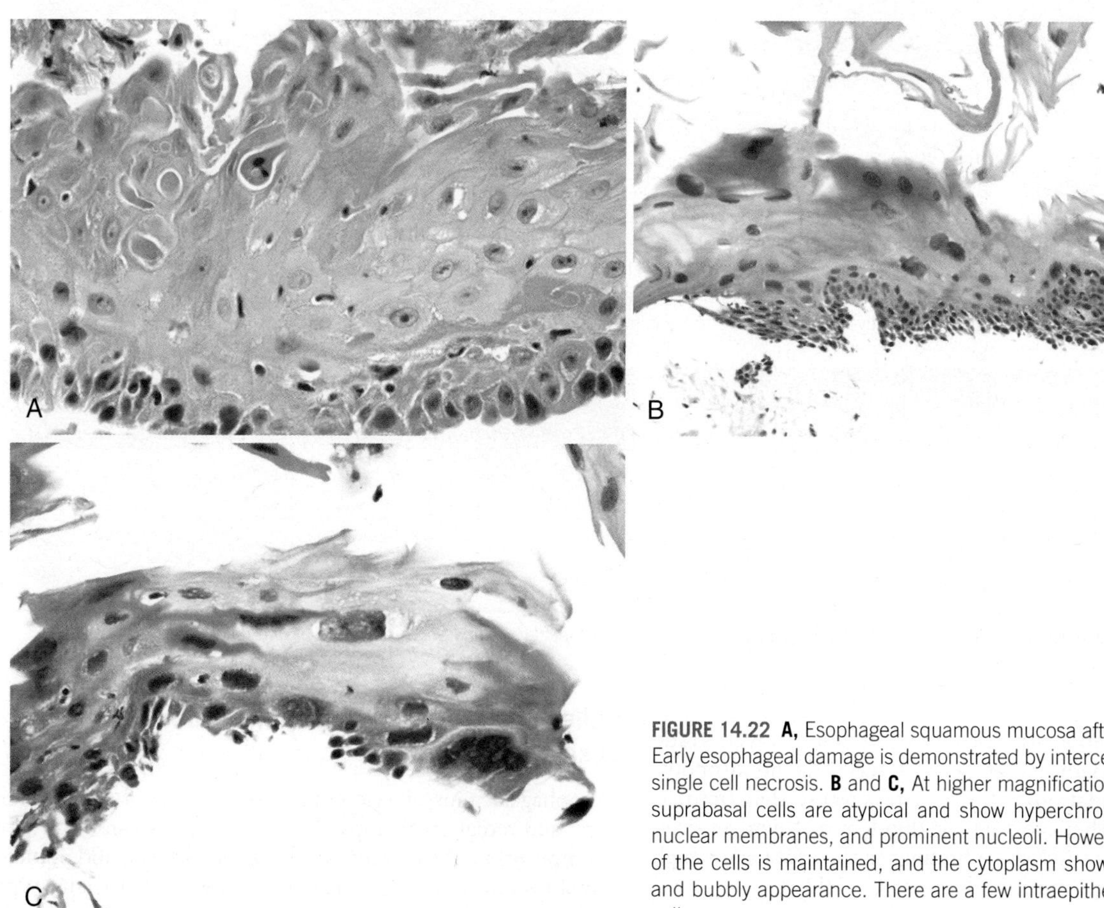

FIGURE 14.22 A, Esophageal squamous mucosa after chemotherapy. Early esophageal damage is demonstrated by intercellular edema and single cell necrosis. **B** and **C,** At higher magnifications, the basal and suprabasal cells are atypical and show hyperchromaticity, irregular nuclear membranes, and prominent nucleoli. However, the N : C ratio of the cells is maintained, and the cytoplasm shows a degenerative and bubbly appearance. There are a few intraepithelial inflammatory cells.

a nonspecific form of esophagitis. In one series, as many as 72% of patients with GI amyloidosis were shown to have esophageal involvement.[365] Amyloid is usually present in the deeper layers of the esophageal wall, and therefore is not usually detectable in superficial biopsy specimens. However, in some cases, the lamina propria and its associated blood vessels may show involvement as well (Fig. 14.24), and vascular compromise may contribute to ulcers found in some patients with esophageal amyloidosis.[366]

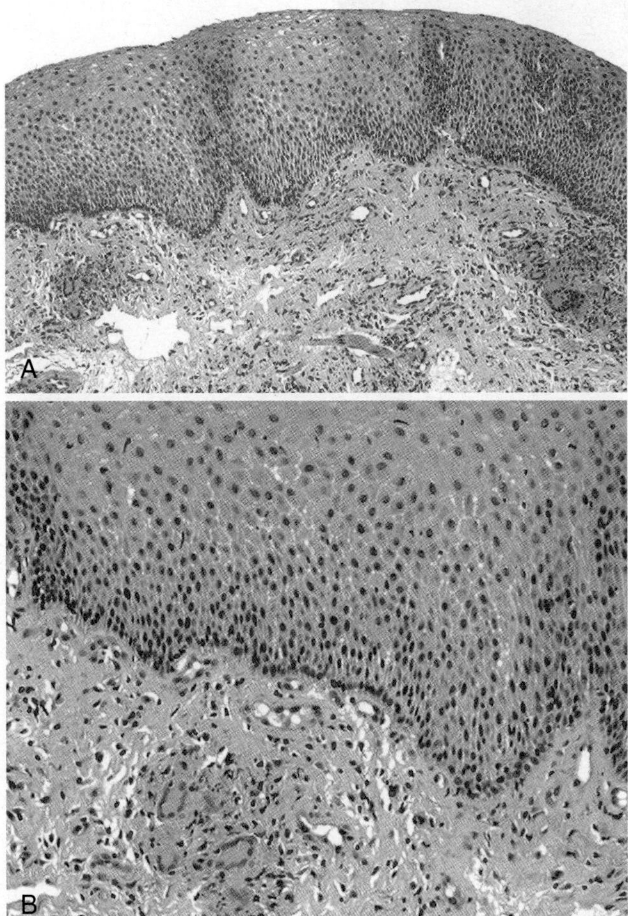

FIGURE 14.23 **A,** Esophageal involvement by Crohn's disease. Basal zone hyperplasia with elongated vascular papillae is identified. The lamina propria contains chronic inflammatory cells and two sarcoid-like granulomas. **B**, High-power magnification shows a well-defined and compact granuloma without central necrosis or evidence of foreign material.

ESOPHAGEAL EPIDERMOID METAPLASIA (ESOPHAGEAL LEUKOPLAKIA)

Esophageal epidermoid metaplasia is a rare condition characterized endoscopically by well-demarcated areas of white, cobblestone-appearing mucosa similar to oral leukoplakia (Fig. 14.25A), which histologically demonstrates an undulating squamous mucosa with flattening of the rete pegs, acanthosis, prominence of the granular layer and varying degrees of hyperorthokeratosis and parakeratosis (Fig.14.25B,C). A study consisting of 25 cases from 18 patients showed that this condition usually affects middle-aged to elderly females who typically present with dysphagia.[367] Mid and distal esophagus is involved more commonly than the proximal esophagus. Risk factors include tobacco smoking and alcohol intake. Similar to its oral counterpart, esophageal epidermoid metaplasia is frequently found adjacent to high-grade squamous dysplasia and squamous cell carcinoma. A subsequent targeted next-generation sequencing study revealed that 67% of esophageal epidermoid metaplasia specimens had alterations in genes often associated with esophageal squamous cell carcinoma. The most frequently mutated genes consisted of *TP53* (n=10), *PIK3CA* (n=2), *EGFR* (n=2), *MYCN* (n=1), *HRAS* (n=1), and the *TERT* promoter (n=1). Sequencing of synchronous and metachronous high-grade squamous dysplasia/esophageal squamous cell carcinomas identified shared genetic alterations with corresponding esophageal epidermoid metaplasia specimens. Additionally, the presence of a *TP53* mutation in esophageal epidermoid metaplasia specimens correlated with concurrent or progression to high-grade squamous dysplasia/esophageal squamous cell carcinoma.[368] In a recent series of 40 patients, 10 (25%) patients had squamous neoplasia before, at, or after a diagnosis of epidermoid metaplasia, with focal findings in 7, and diffuse involvement in 3 patients. Based on these studies, close follow-up or endoscopic treatment is warranted in patients with epidermoid

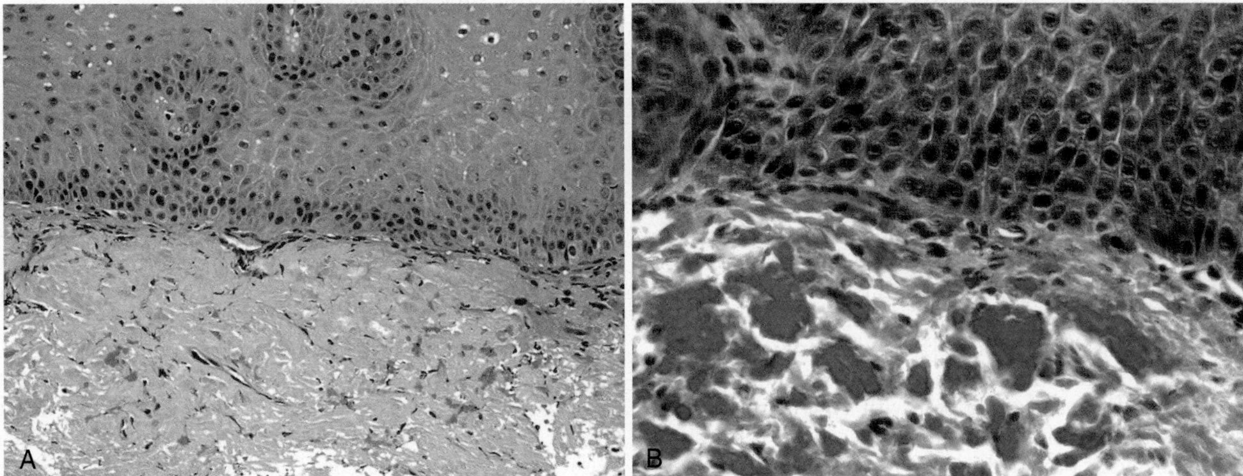

FIGURE 14.24 **A,** Amyloid deposits in the esophagus are usually present in the deeper layers but occasionally may involve the lamina propria in the form of pink, homogeneous, extracellular material. **B,** The same histological section as in **A**, stained with Congo red. The amyloid deposits are congophilic and stain bright orange-red.

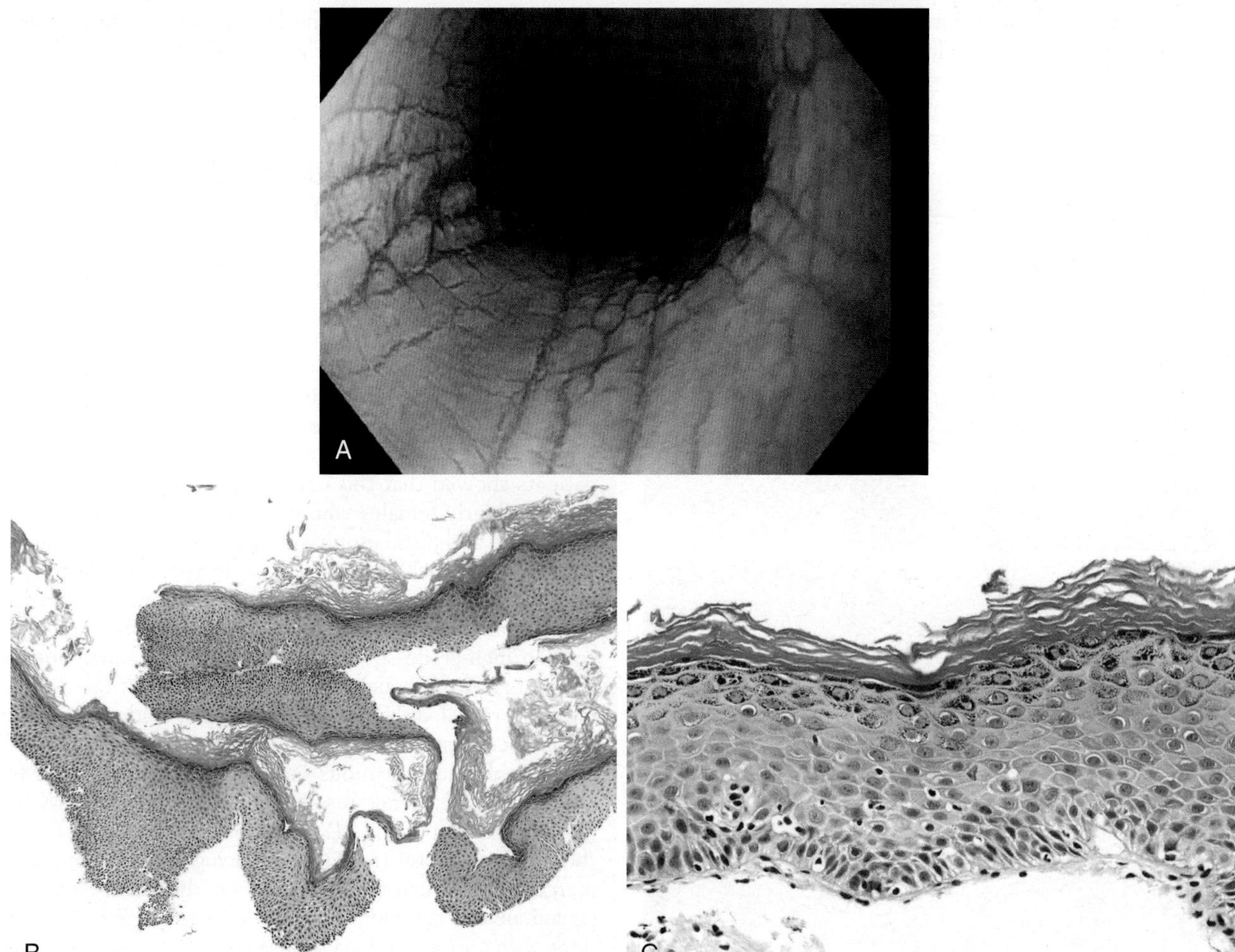

FIGURE 14.25 A, Endoscopic appearance of epidermoid metaplasia (esophageal leukoplakia). The esophageal mucosa shows white, cobblestone appearance involving almost the entire esophagus. **B,** Histologically, epidermoid metaplasia is characterized by an undulating squamous mucosa with varying degrees of hyperorthokeratosis and parakeratosis. **C,** Higher magnification shows flattening of the rete pegs, acanthosis, and a prominent granular layer and hyperorthokeratosis and parakeratosis.

metaplasia without dysplasia. Endoscopic mucosal resection is advocated for easily resectable and/or small dysplastic lesions, and endoscopic ablation therapy such as radiofrequency ablation may be performed for larger lesions with dysplasia.[369]

BARRETT'S ESOPHAGUS

Barrett's esophagus (BE) is characterized by the conversion of normal squamous epithelium of the esophagus into metaplastic columnar epithelium.[370] This disorder is caused by chronic GERD.[371] A very small proportion of cases are congenital in origin, but most are acquired. A familial predisposition for BE and esophageal adenocarcinoma (EAC) has been documented in familial clusters. This has become known as the familial Barrett's esophagus (FBE) phenotype. Chak and colleagues[372,373] found that 20% of relatives in families with this disorder have BE, compared with 10% of relatives of patients with sporadic BE. Sun and colleagues,[374] using segregation analysis, provided epidemiologic evidence in support of one or more rare, autosomally inherited, dominant susceptibility alleles in families with the FBE phenotype. BE is becoming a condition more frequently diagnosed in children, most likely because of the increased performance of upper endoscopy in young patients. A recent report[375] showed that BE may develop in children with reflux symptoms after a mean period of 5.3 years.

The most important clinical aspect of BE is that it predisposes patients to the development of dysplasia and adenocarcinoma.[371,376,377] As a result, it is recommended that patients with BE undergo periodic endoscopic surveillance to detect early neoplastic complications (dysplasia) and prevent the development of cancer.[378,379] Because of recent advances in diagnostic and therapeutic endoscopy (discussed later), there is a growing trend toward recommending esophagectomy only for patients with either extensive high-grade dysplasia (HGD) or invasive adenocarcinoma that invades into and/or beyond submucosa (see section on endoscopic submucosal dissection). As a result, it is now incumbent on the pathologist to be as accurate as possible with regard to distinguishing reactive changes from dysplasia and dysplasia from invasive carcinoma in mucosal biopsy specimens. The discussion here focuses on the current understanding of BE and emphasizes areas in which significant advances may be expected in the near future.

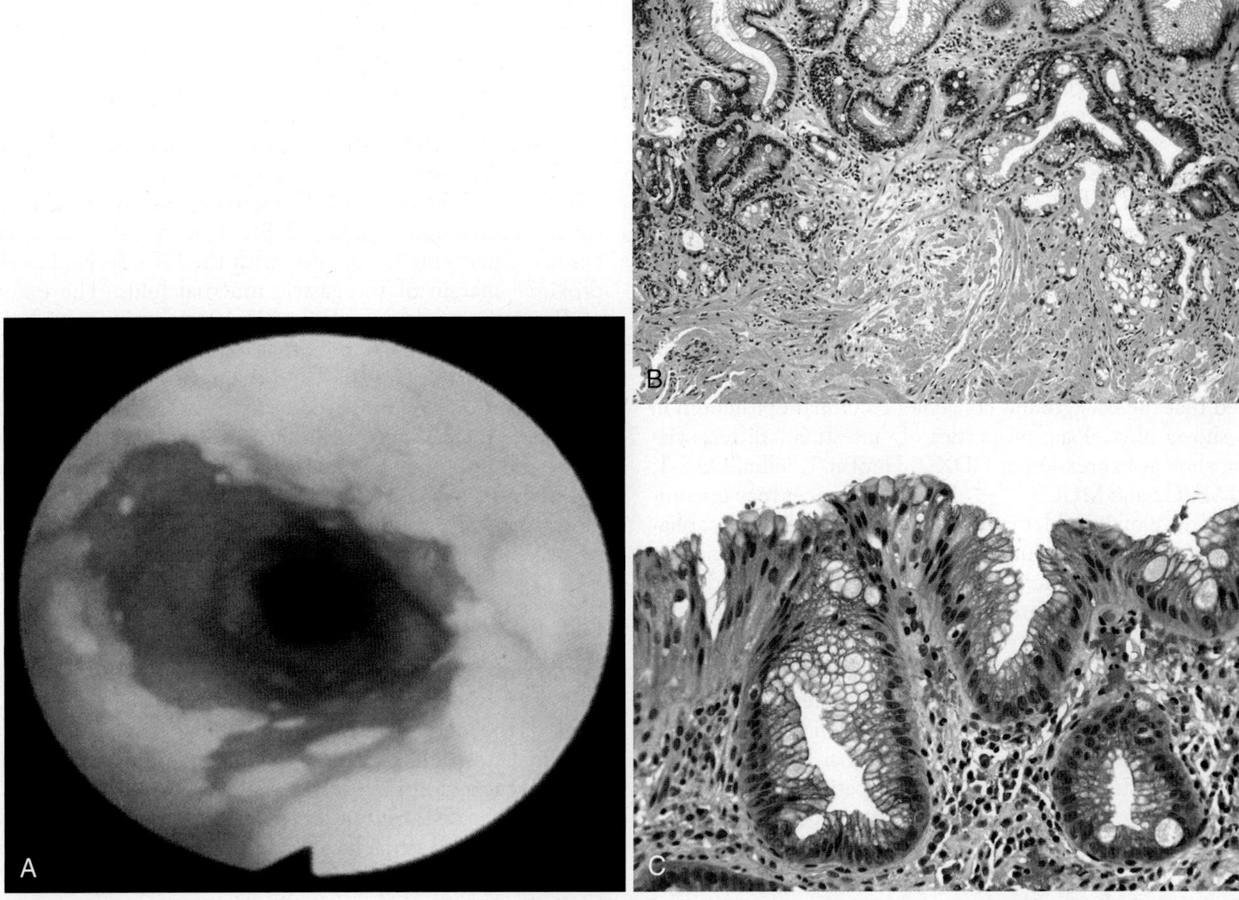

FIGURE 14.26 A, Endoscopic appearance of Barrett's esophagus (BE). Tongues of gastric-appearing columnar mucosa extend proximal to the gastroesophageal junction in an irregular circumferential fashion. Notice the presence of squamous islands within the columnar mucosa. **B,** Histological appearance of BE is characterized by the presence of incomplete intestinal metaplasia, mucous columnar cells, scattered goblet cells, and reactive changes in the bases of the crypts. Notice the presence of splayed fibers of muscularis mucosae at the bottom of the field. Nondysplastic BE shows mildly distorted crypt architecture characterized by increased crowding, branching, and budding. **C,** A high-power view of the surface epithelium shows slight pseudostratification, a serrated (or hyperplastic) luminal contour, and reactive changes characterized by cells with prominent nucleoli. Several pseudogoblet cells are also present in the top portion of the surface epithelium. The lamina propria shows a mild lymphoplasmacytic infiltrate.

Definition

The American College of Gastroenterology (ACG) defines BE as endoscopically recognizable extension of salmon colored mucosa into the tubular esophagus, extending ≥1 cm proximal to the gastroesophageal junction (GEJ), that is confirmed pathologically to contain intestinal metaplasia, the latter defined by the presence of goblet cells.[379] Based on this definition, both the endoscopic and the pathological component must be present to establish a diagnosis of BE (Fig. 14.26). By definition, this disease does not include patients who have intestinal metaplasia (goblet cells) of the gastric cardia or when goblet cells are identified in patients who have a normal Z line or a Z line with <1 cm of variability.[378-380] As much as one third of GERD patients who lack columnar mucosa within the distal esophagus show intestinal metaplasia (goblet cells) in their otherwise anatomically normal GEJ, and these patients do not qualify as having BE based on the ACG definition.[377,381] This position is based on the assumption that the presence of a few intestinalized glands in the GEJ region of patients without endoscopically apparent columnar metaplasia of the distal esophagus does not confer the same increased risk of malignancy as endoscopically visible BE.[376,377,381,382] Similarly, in large cohort studies with long-term follow-up, patients who demonstrate intestinal metaplasia in segments <1cm (referred to as specialized intestinal metaplasia at GEJ) have not shown an increase in development of neoplasia compared to patients with segments of intestinal metaplasia >1 cm.[382]

However, there is no worldwide agreement that intestinal metaplasia (goblet cells) should be required for a diagnosis of BE. The British Society of Gastroenterology does not require intestinal metaplasia to establish this diagnosis.[383] Similarly, in Japan, the GERD Society Study Committee does not require histological confirmation of goblet cells in esophageal columnar epithelium.[384,385] There are data to suggest that most patients with at least 2 cm of columnar-lined esophagus are found to have intestinal metaplasia if enough biopsy samples are obtained from the columnar-lined segment.[386] Therefore, sampling error is a confounding factor. Some patients with significant lengths of columnar-lined esophagus do not have documented intestinal metaplasia despite analysis of many biopsy specimens, but this is exceedingly rare. Several studies have found a similar risk of progression to dysplasia or cancer in patients with and without goblets cells in columnar-lined esophagus.[387,388] Furthermore, some data indicate that the immunohistochemical and molecular characteristics of columnar-lined esophagus with and without goblet cells are similar, so the significance of goblet cells, and their density, are controversial at this time.[389-391]

Defining BE by pathological confirmation of intestinal metaplasia (goblet cells) is problematic for a few other reasons as well. This definition is based primarily on the fact that intestinal-type esophageal epithelium is at highest risk for neoplastic progression. However, it is now well recognized that the background nongoblet columnar epithelium in BE shows physiologic properties of "intestinal" differentiation, such as expression of CDX-2, HepPar-1, villin, DAS-1, and MUC2 and MUC3.[381,392] Moreover, cancer may uncommonly develop in goblet cell–poor or even nongoblet esophageal columnar epithelium. There is also some evidence to suggest that neoplastic progression in BE is associated with loss of goblet cell differentiation. In fact, the true relationship between the *density* of goblet cell metaplasia and cancer risk has never been defined specifically since patients with columnar metaplasia, but without goblet cells, are not enrolled in formal surveillance programs. In a retrospective cohort study of 260 patients with columnar lined esophagus without intestinal metaplasia and 262 patients with intestinal metaplasia, density of goblet cells or percentage of intestinal metaplasia did not correlate with risk of HGD/EAC.[393]

The chance of detecting goblet cells in mucosal biopsy specimens of the esophagus from patients with suspected BE is proportional to the length of BE and the site of the biopsy and, of course, is subject to sampling error.[394-396] In one study, 30.5% of patients with 1 to 2 cm of columnar-lined esophagus had goblet cells in their biopsy specimens, compared with 90% of patients with more than 6 cm of esophageal columnar mucosa.[395] The likelihood of detecting goblet cells increases proportionally with the number of specimens obtained and depends on their location as well. For instance, biopsies obtained from the neo-SCJ show a higher rate of detection of goblet cells than distal biopsies.[394] In one study, goblet cells were detected in 68% of endoscopies in which eight biopsies were obtained, compared with only 35% of those in which four biopsies were analyzed.[396] Based on these data, the current American Gastroenterology Association (AGA) guidelines recommend that in patients with suspected BE, at least eight random biopsies should be obtained to maximize the yield of intestinal metaplasia on histology. In those with shorter segments (1-2 cm), at least four biopsies per cm of circumferential BE, and one biopsy per cm in tongues of BE, should be obtained.[379] Finally, detection of goblet cells has been shown to be dependent on patient age in pediatric studies. Goblet cells are rare in patients younger than 10 years of age but increase in number progressively with age.

Classification

Traditionally, BE has been separated into long-segment, short-segment, and ultrashort-segment types, depending on the length of involved esophageal mucosa (>3 cm, 1 to 3 cm, or <1 cm, respectively). However, the biologic significance of this classification system remains unclear. Several studies have evaluated the risk of dysplasia and cancer in relation to the length of BE.[397-402] A recent multicenter cohort study suggests an 11% increased risk of HGD and EAC for every 1 cm increase in BE length.[402] The increased risk associated with longer lengths of BE has been attributed to a larger surface area at risk for neoplastic progression.[401] The *Prague C & M criteria*[403] were developed to standardize the endoscopic grading of BE. Endoscopic criteria are based on anatomic landmarks, with the GEJ defined as the proximal margin of the gastric mucosal folds. The extent of Barrett's mucosa is then calculated by measuring (in centimeters) the most proximal extent of circumferential columnar mucosa (C value) and the maximal extent of noncircumferential columnar mucosa (M value) above the GEJ. For example, if Barrett's mucosa is circumferential for 2 cm above the GEJ and the maximal extent of noncircumferential Barrett's mucosa is 6 cm above the GEJ, the BE would be graded C2M6. This scoring system has been shown to be reliable in assessing the extent of endoscopic BE (Fig. 14.27).[403,404]

Endoscopic Landmarks

Several landmarks are important for endoscopists to identify when evaluating patients with possible BE.[405] The GEJ, which is the junction between the tubular esophagus and the proximal stomach, is defined in North America as the most proximal aspect of the gastric folds.[405] Endoscopists in Asia often use the distal extent of the palisade vessels, which are fine longitudinal veins located in the lamina propria of the distal esophagus, as their landmark for the GEJ.[406-408] The SCJ, also known as the Z-line, is the junction of squamous and columnar mucosa. It does not necessarily correspond to the location of the GEJ and is irregular in many apparently normal individuals with and without GERD symptoms. The endoscopist should provide the pathologist with knowledge about the relationship of the SCJ to the GEJ (i.e., whether it is located at or above the GEJ) and the precise location of the biopsy relative to these anatomic

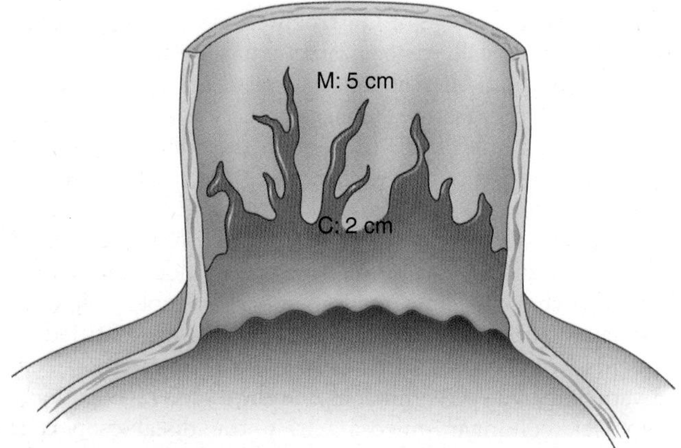

FIGURE 14.27 Prague C & M criteria for grade C2M5 Barrett's esophagus. The circumferential (C) extent of columnar metaplasia is 2 cm above the gastroesophageal junction (GEJ), and the maximal extent is 5 cm (tallest tongue of columnar metaplasia extending above the GEJ). (Courtesy Dr. Michael Huba, Cleveland Clinic.)

landmarks. The distal 2 to 3 cm of the tubular esophagus corresponds to the LES (Fig. 14.28) and is an anatomic region of increased intraluminal pressure. However, there are no anatomic landmarks demarcating the beginning and end of this physiologic sphincter. Therefore, if the SCJ is observed to be proximally displaced relative to the GEJ, biopsies of the GEJ, the SCJ, and the intervening (salmon-pink colored) columnar mucosa should be obtained to help establish a diagnosis of BE.

Clinical Features

As discussed earlier, BE is an acquired condition secondary to GERD, which usually, but not always, manifests clinically as heartburn.[371] It affects both adults and children, but the prevalence of BE among children with GERD is low, between 0.3% to 4.8%.[409-411] A more recent study has suggested that more widespread use of proton pump inhibitors has resulted in an even lower prevalence rate of BE. In a recent retrospective series of 36,041 children who underwent 1 or more upper endoscopic procedures at 2 large volume pediatric facilities over 12 years, the prevalence rate for BE was found to be 0.055%.[412] Esophagitis secondary to GERD is among the most common medical conditions in Western countries.[371] Approximately 25% to 40% of healthy adult Americans experience symptomatic GERD, most commonly manifested clinically as heartburn, at least once per month,[413] and approximately one third of those individuals have endoscopic evidence of esophagitis. BE is found in approximately 5% to 15% of patients who undergo endoscopy for symptoms of GERD,[414-418] compared with 1.3% to 1.6% of the general population.[419,420] One population-based report identified a 28-fold increase in the incidence of BE between 1965 and 1997.[421] BE is the major risk factor for EAC and probably most GEJ adenocarcinomas as well.[422]

Compared with the general population, patients with BE have a 10 to 55-fold increased risk of EAC.[423] Of those with non-dysplastic BE, 0.33% per year show progression to EAC.[424]It is unclear why BE develops in some patients with GERD and not in others. Several sociodemographic and lifestyle risk factors have been identified. For instance, BE is more frequent in men, by a ratio of 3 : 1.[425] The prevalence rate increases with age, with a mean age at diagnosis of 63 years.[425,426] Aside from chronic GERD, other risk factors for the development of BE include hiatal hernia, white ethnicity, the degree of duodenal-gastric reflux, delayed esophageal acid clearance, and decreased resting pressure of the LES.[371] Data are insufficient on the possible roles of dietary intakes of fruits and vegetables, fiber, and fat as risk factors for BE. Obesity, as measured by body mass index and intraabdominal distribution of body fat, has been shown to be a strong risk factor for BE, EAC,[427-432] and GERD.[371,429,433,434] Some authorities propose that high abdominal adiposity has a stronger association for BE than body mass index, which may help explain the male predominance of this condition.[431] Although the use of tobacco and alcohol are well-established risk factors for squamous cell carcinoma of the esophagus, their contribution to the development of BE and EAC remains controversial.[371] There is increasing evidence that cigarette smoking contributes to progression from BE to EAC, rather than conferring an increased risk of BE itself.[435]

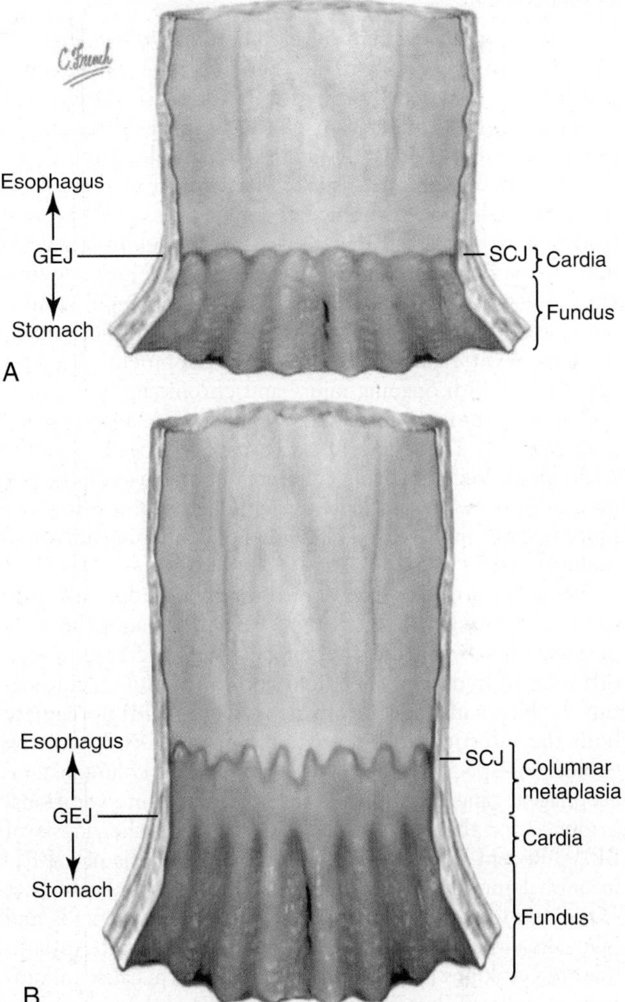

FIGURE 14.28 A, Normal gastroesophageal junction (*GEJ*). The squamocolumnar junction (*SCJ*) lies directly at the GEJ, which is located at the most proximal point of the gastric folds. The cardia represents the most proximal aspect of the gastric mucosa, which is composed of either mucous glands or mixed mucous and oxyntic glands. **B,** Schematic depiction of an ultrashort segment of Barrett's esophagus. A short segment of gastric columnar-appearing mucosa (<1.0 cm in length) extends into the distal esophagus, proximal to the level of the GEJ. In this case, the SCJ is irregular in outline and located proximal to the GEJ.

Although a small proportion of patients with BE are entirely asymptomatic,[378] most exhibit GERD symptoms such as heartburn (e.g., retrosternal burning, tight sensation radiating toward the neck) and acid regurgitation. Less common symptoms include dysphagia and a sensation of a lump in the throat. Heartburn and acid regurgitation often occur after eating, particularly after large meals. BE is rare in children, despite the fact that GERD is common in the pediatric age group.[436,437] The reason for this is unclear. The clinical expression of BE in children is similar to that in adults, except that strictures are more common in the former group, and the endoscopic appearance of the mucosa is not always typical.[436] As mentioned earlier, goblet cells also are less commonly identified in pediatric patients with BE. Therefore, the diagnosis requires careful documentation of the anatomic landmarks and often requires the use of large-sized biopsies. In general, surveillance and treatment of BE are similar in children and adults.

Pathogenesis

The precise mechanism of development and the cell of origin of BE remain unknown, but there has been much recent progress in this area. In any case, chronic GERD leads to inflammation and ulceration of the esophageal squamous mucosa which, if persistent and recurrent, ultimately leads to columnar metaplasia, usually with intestinal metaplasia characterized by the presence of goblet cells.[438-440] Several studies have suggested that squamous epithelium converts initially to columnar epithelium that is morphologically similar to the gastric cardia (i.e., composed of mucinous columnar epithelium with underlying mucous glands or mixed mucous/oxyntic glands) before the development of goblet cells.[441,442] With ongoing injury and chronic inflammation, mucinous columnar epithelium converts to an intestinal phenotype.[381] The length of cardia-type mucosa in patients with short segments of columnar metaplasia increases progressively with age, and longer lengths of cardia-type mucosa show an increased likelihood of containing intestinal metaplasia.[441,443]

Some investigators have shown that bile acids contribute to the development of BE.[438,440,444] Bile acids alter the ionic permeability of mucous membranes, with increased back-diffusion of hydrogen (H^+) ions and intracellular acidification.[444] Bile acids (specifically deoxycholic acid) upregulate both the intestinal differentiation factor, CDX-2, and the goblet cell–specific gene, *MUC2*, in normal columnar and esophageal cancer cell lines, thus providing some additional evidence for the role of bile acids in the pathogenesis of BE.[438] Recent developments in the pathogenesis of GERD in animal models[20,23,24] and in vitro studies indicate that exposing esophageal squamous epithelial cells to acids and bile salts alone can cause epithelial cells to secrete inflammatory cytokines (IL8 and IL1β) that, in turn, cause inflammatory cells (T lymphocytes and neutrophils) to migrate into the epithelium. Given these data, some have proposed that it is the inflammatory response, not the acid directly, that ultimately damages the esophageal mucosa. Using a rat model of reflux esophagitis via surgical esophagojejunostomy, Agoston et al. showed that metaplastic, columnar-lined esophagus develops via a wound healing process, and not via genetic reprogramming of progenitor cells. Re-epithelialization of ulcerated squamous mucosa at the level of the surgical anastomosis was found to occur via proliferation and expansion of immature glands that arose directly from adjacent jejunal crypts, and the neoglandular epithelium was found to harbor an immunoprofile similar to that of the native proliferating jejunal crypt epithelium.[445]

The development of goblet cells appears to represent a multistep process in which many factors lead to stimulation of both mesenchymal and epithelial cells and promote differentiation of the epithelium towards an intestinal phenotype.[438,439] The identity of Barrett's progenitor cells is not fully understood, but a number of potential candidates have been proposed. For instance, GERD may cause mature esophageal squamous cells to transdifferentiate into columnar cells or cause immature esophageal progenitor cells (in the basal layer of the squamous epithelium or in the ducts of esophageal submucosal glands) to undergo columnar rather than squamous differentiation (a process known as transcommitment). In transdifferentiation, the reflux-induced inflammatory environment (mediated by prostaglandin E2 (PGE2), nuclear factor-κB (NF-κB), TNF and other molecules leads to increased sonic hedgehog signaling and decreased Notch signalling.[446]

Since intestinal-type cells that characterize BE are not normally found in the esophagus, stomach, or bone marrow, and reprogramming would be required for any of the progenitor cell candidates to give rise to Barrett's metaplasia.[447] With regard to transcommittment, evidence from mouse models suggests that progenitor cells (marked by expression of stem cell marker LGR5) from the gastric cardia to distal esophagus can occur under the influence of Notch signalling.[448]

Other possible primary sites of origin of stem cells include the basal layer of the esophageal squamous epithelium, mucosal and submucosal glands and their respective ducts.[449] There is also in vitro experimental evidence to support the possibility that stem cells may be derived from undifferentiated mesenchymal cells, either in the lamina propria of the esophagus or in the bone marrow.[450,451] Wang and colleagues[452] studied TP63-deficient mice, which lack squamous epithelium, and found that TP63-null embryos rapidly developed intestine-like metaplasia and gene expression profiles similar to Barrett's metaplasia when exposed to acid reflux. These investigators detected a population of potential embryonic cells at the SCJ.[452]

Regardless of these theories, there is accumulating evidence that the squamous-to-columnar cell metaplastic reaction occurs through an intermediate or transitional phase characterized by the presence of epithelium that shows combined squamous and columnar features. Several types of cells are present in columnar-lined segments that show mixed squamous and columnar differentiation, but they are difficult to recognize without special studies or electron microscopy. One type of epithelium with mixed features is termed *multilayered epithelium (ME)* (see also Chapter 15).[441,453,454] ME expresses a mucin and cytokeratin profile similar to that of fully developed columnar epithelium in BE and shows a high capacity for cell proliferation, differentiation, and expression of intestinal transcription factors.[441] In retrospective and prospective studies, the presence of ME has been strongly associated with GERD-induced inflammation of the GEJ region and has been shown to be almost 100% specific for BE.[454] The significance of ME for pathologists is related to the fact that its identification in a mucosal biopsy specimen from the GEJ region, or most certainly from the distal esophagus, helps define the epithelium in that particular biopsy sample as esophageal and therefore metaplastic in origin. Given the recent change in the definition of BE with regard to the distance from the GEJ (defined as intestinal metaplasia extending for ≥1cm above GEJ), distinction between esophageal versus cardiac origin of columnar epithelium in GEJ junction region biopsies is now less relevant.

Pathological Features

Gross (Endoscopic) Features

Barrett's esophagus is characterized by the presence of salmon-colored mucosa in the tubular esophagus that may show focal areas of surface erosion or ulceration (see Fig. 14.26, *A*).[378] Many patients with BE who are taking high-dose PPIs also exhibit islands of reepithelialized squamous mucosa within a background of salmon-colored mucosa.[455,456] In a high proportion of cases, buried metaplastic epithelium is identified in biopsy specimens from these squamous islands.[455] Squamous islands also develop frequently after endoscopic laser or photoablation therapy of BE[457] and, less commonly, after radiofrequency ablation (RFA) therapy (discussed later). With these latter forms of therapy, as much as 90% of patients may show complete reversal of their Barrett's segment to squamous mucosa.[458] However, with procedures other than RFA, a significant proportion of patients with apparent reversal of their Barrett's segment to squamous mucosa are shown to have buried intestinalized crypts or dysplasia, both of which make continued endoscopic surveillance more difficult.

Barrett's esophagus-related dysplasia is usually subtle and often flat and endoscopically undetectable. However, it may appear as a localized area of surface irregularity, nodularity, polypoid growth, velvety area of mucosa, ulceration, or stricture.[459] With recent advancements in endoscopy techniques (e.g., narrow band imaging), dysplasia detection may improve considerably, particularly in regard to better targeted biopsies.

Microscopic Features

Barrett's esophagus is characterized by both epithelial and mesenchymal changes in the esophagus.[460,461] The crypt and surface epithelium, which may be flat, undulating, or even villiform, is typically lined by mucinous columnar cells with scattered goblet cells, enterocytes, and cells with intermediate or combined intestinal and gastric features (see Fig. 14.26B,C). Scattered endocrine cells and Paneth cells are not uncommon. Depending on the level of associated active inflammation, the epithelium may also show a variable degree of hyperplastic (serrated) and regenerative features. Areas of surface erosion or ulceration may be present as well. In areas of active inflammation or ulceration, the epithelium often shows lack of surface maturation, characterized by mucin depletion, increased size and hyperchromaticity of the cell nuclei, slight nuclear stratification, and increased mitoses. These changes should not be misinterpreted as dysplastic when they are associated with marked active inflammation or ulceration.

The glandular compartment of BE is variable and somewhat dependent on the particular location within the segment of columnar-lined esophagus, the duration and extent of BE, and presence and degree of dysplasia as well. For instance, some studies suggest that there is a positive association between increasing levels of atrophy of the BE gland compartment and advancing grades of BE and dysplasia. In the distal portion of BE, there is usually a higher proportion of oxyntic-type (acid-secreting) glands, or mixed mucous- and oxyntic-type glands, compared with the more proximal regions of BE,[460] where goblet cells are often seen in greater density. Areas of pure mucous-type glands predominate in most individuals with BE, particularly in the more proximal regions of the columnar-lined segment. As mentioned previously, the chance of detecting goblet cells increases with the length of BE. Therefore, more goblet cells are often detected at the region of the neo-SCJ and in the proximal esophagus than in the distal esophagus. Goblet cells may populate the crypts and surface epithelium and may range from focal and few in number to diffuse and numerous. Dystrophic goblet cells are common in BE. They are goblet cells that have lost their polarity and in which the base of the cell is not in direct contact with the basement membrane or the apical mucin vacuole is not in direct contact with the lumen. Pancreatic acinar metaplasia is common in BE, particularly in the region of the distal esophagus and GEJ.[462]

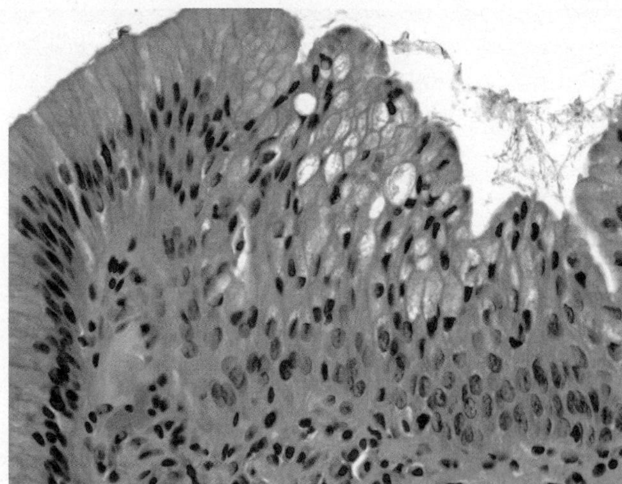

FIGURE 14.29 Surface epithelium in a patient with Barrett's esophagus shows a focus of multilayered epithelium (ME) characterized by basally located squamoid cells and superficial mucinous columnar cells. ME can often be seen to extend from the underlying gland ducts.

A variety of intermediate cell types, such as ciliated mucous cells, cells that show a combination of squamous and mucinous cytoplasmic qualities, and ME, may be seen in as much as 40% of patients with BE (Fig. 14.29).[441,454,460] The chance of detecting ME is greatest in regions near or adjacent to the neo-SCJ and in areas that overlie esophageal glands and ducts.[441] Surface and, less commonly, crypt mucous cells may show barrel-shaped cytoplasmic distention that mimics goblet cells; these cells are termed *pseudogoblet cells*. Differentiation of pseudogoblet cells from true goblet cells is discussed later. ME is composed of epithelium that shows squamoid features in the basal layers and mucinous features in the surface layers of the epithelium, often with scattered pseudogoblet cells. It is much less common to detect true goblet cells in ME. ME may range from 3 to 10 cells in thickness and can often be seen extending up from the submucosal glands and ducts, particularly in areas near the neo-SCJ.

A mild degree of chronic inflammation in the lamina propria, composed of lymphocytes, plasma cells, and scattered eosinophils, is common in BE. In areas of active mucosal injury, chronic inflammation and neutrophilic infiltration in the lamina propria as well as crypt and surface epithelium is common. Areas of active inflammation are typically patchy and are most pronounced in the proximal portion of BE adjacent to the neo-SCJ, where epithelial regenerative changes are often most severe.

Because of ongoing and recurrent inflammation, ulceration, and repair, nondysplastic BE (negative for dysplasia) typically shows mild architectural and cytologic changes that differ from normal intestinal epithelium[463] For instance, the crypts in BE normally show a mild degree of budding, atrophy, branching, increased mitotic activity, dystrophic goblet cells, mucin depletion, nuclear enlargement, nuclear

TABLE 14.8 Histological Features of Dysplasia in Barrett's Esophagus

	Surface Maturation	Architecture	Cytology
Negative	Usually present	Preserved	Smooth nuclear membranes Open chromatin pattern Preserved N : C ratio Nuclear enlargement or stratification limited to crypt bases Variable number of typical mitoses
Low-grade	Usually absent	Absent or only mild abnormalities including irregular crypt shapes, rare crypt budding/ branching, preserved lamina propria between crypts	Nuclear elongation Dense chromatin pattern Increased N : C ratio Nuclear stratification limited to basal half of epithelium or full crypt Increased number of mitoses (typical or atypical) Preserved or mild loss of nuclear polarity
High-grade	Usually absent	Absent or abnormal crypt budding, branching, marked crowding with decreased lamina propria between crypts	Nuclear elongation Dense chromatin pattern Increased N : C ratio Full-thickness stratification Prominent loss of nuclear polarity Increased number of atypical mitoses Mild to marked nuclear pleomorphism

N : C ratio, *Nucleus-to-cytoplasm ratio.*

hyperchromasia, and even mild pseudostratification and a minimal degree of loss of cell polarity, particularly at the bases of the crypts (Table 14.8). Thus, BE typically lacks the presence of evenly spaced, test tube–like crypts that are characteristic of the normal small and large intestine. (Table 14.9). In fact, non-dysplastic mucosa normally shows a spectrum of cytologic "atypia" (referred to as "baseline" or "basal" atypia) within the bases of the crypts (FIGURE. 14.30) which is presumably related to the stage of progression of the underlying BE, although this has not been sufficiently investigated. The degree of (non dysplastic) basal crypt atypia ranges from those with little to no atypia, where the crypts are lined by cells with small normochromatic nuclei and without stratification or mitosis, to mild atypia, where there is more nuclear hyperchromasia and enlargement and rare mitoses, to moderate atypia, where the cells are typically enlarged and elongated, focally stratified, mucin depleted, slightly irregular in shape and often with increased mitoses. This degree of crypt atypia may be associated with p53 positivity, but still falls short of the features characteristic of true crypt dysplasia (see section on dysplasia for more details) (Fig.14.30D,E F). The "baseline" phenotype of BE as described above is likely a reflection of the evolution and proliferation of clones of cells with cumulative genetic errors, and progressive degrees of *genomic instability*.[464,465] The process of clonal evolution begins early in BE, prior to phenotypic expression of dysplasia, when metaplastic epithelial cells acquire mutations that provide them with a selective proliferative advantage relative to genetically normal cells.[464,466]

Clonal molecular aberrations, such as in *CDKN2A* (*p16*), are detected in as much as 90% of BE patients.[467] *CDX2* and *TP53* mutations have been shown to develop at an early phase of columnar metaplasia, before the onset of morphological dysplasia.[370,466,468-470] Furthermore, DNA content abnormalities are not uncommon in patients with nondysplastic BE.[390] Consequently, the epithelium in conventional nondysplastic BE often shows a variable degree of

TABLE 14.9 Reactive Atypia vs Dysplasia in Barrett's Esophagus

Feature	Regeneration/ Reactive Atypia	Dysplasia
Inflammation	Very common	May be present
Ulceration	Common	May be present
Surface epithelial maturation	Present	Absent (except crypt dysplasia which is accompanied by surface maturation)
Pleomorphism	Absent	May be present
Loss of polarity	No	May be present (usually in HGD)
Atypical mitoses	Absent	May be present
Abrupt transition from normal to abnormal epithelium	No	Yes
Surface villiform change	May be present	May be present
Mucin depletion	May be present	Usually present
N:C ratio	Usually maintained	Increased

architectural and cytologic changes that may appear atypical to the untrained eye. (See section Indefinite for Dysplasia for more information on how to differentiate BE from dysplasia.)

There are also characteristic mesenchymal changes that occur in BE.[390] Most, if not all, patients with BE show duplication, thickening, and fraying of the muscularis mucosae. When the muscularis mucosae is duplicated, the new (superficial) layer of muscularis mucosae is in contact with the bases of the BE crypts, and it is often frayed in appearance.[471] The lamina propria may contain an increased number and size of blood vessels, lymphatic spaces, and nerve fibers.[390] A thin, often edematous, lamina propria usually separates the more luminally situated, frayed muscularis mucosae from the deep muscularis mucosae, which represents an extension of the original muscularis mucosae of the squamous-lined esophagus. Some studies have shown increased vascularity in BE segments, particularly in areas of dysplasia.[471]

Ki67 typically stains the lower third of the crypt epithelium in BE.[461,466] However, in areas of active inflammation or ulceration, Ki67 positivity can extend to the upper third of the crypts and even onto the surface epithelium. Weak and heterogeneous p53 positivity is common in the basal portions of the crypts in BE (Fig 14.31), but strong nuclear positivity (overexpression) or complete lack of p53 staining (null pattern) is usually restricted to cases with true underlying *TP53* mutations (missense TP53 mutations in cases with overexpression and deletions or truncating mutations in cases with null pattern of expression) (Fig.14.31B,C),. In any case, the use of Ki67 or p53 is not advocated in routine diagnostic evaluation of patients with BE or in those

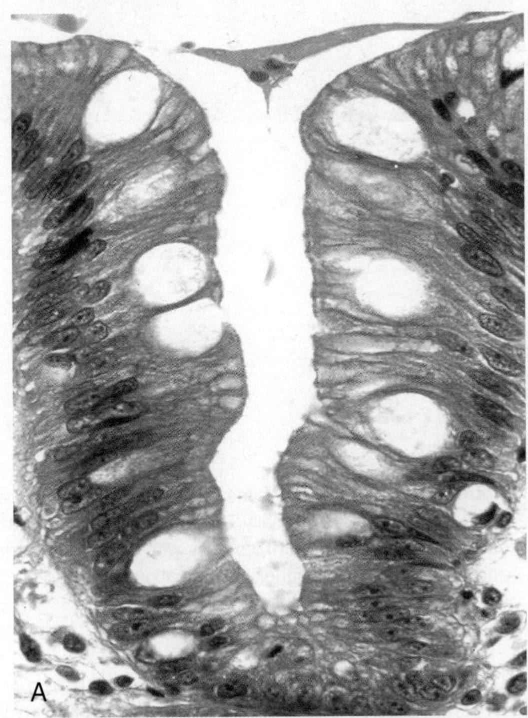

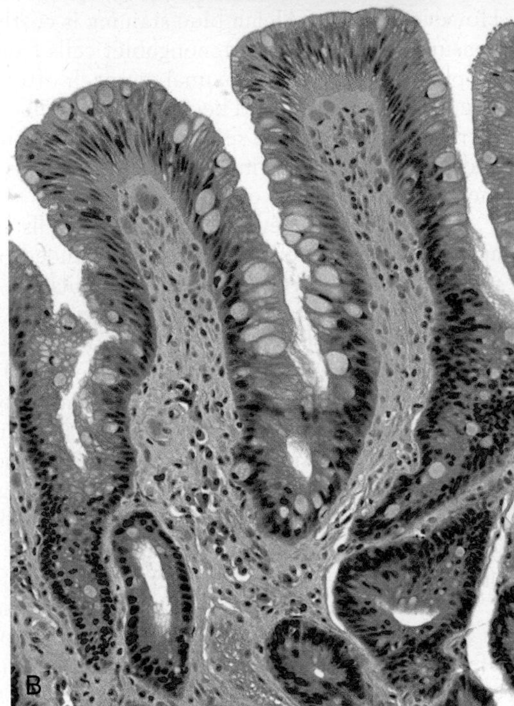

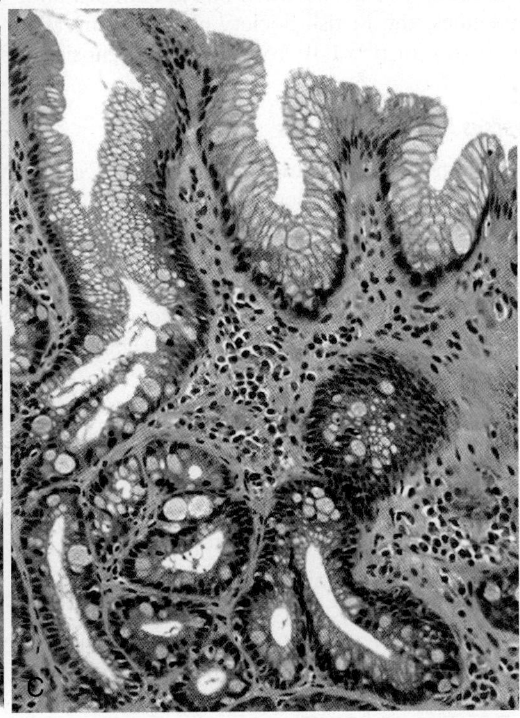

FIGURE 14.30 **A** and **B,** Reactive epithelium in a patient with Barrett's esophagus shows mucinous columnar epithelium, pseudoabsorptive cells with an incomplete brush border, and several goblet cells. The nuclei are slightly enlarged, elongated, and pseudostratified and contain multiple small nucleoli. The retention of cell polarity, absence of atypical mitotic figures, and presence of an orderly basal orientation of the nuclei all denote reactive changes rather than true dysplasia. **C,** Notice that a mild degree of crypt distortion and crowding is a normal component of metaplastic epithelium. In addition, there is maturation of the epithelium toward the surface.

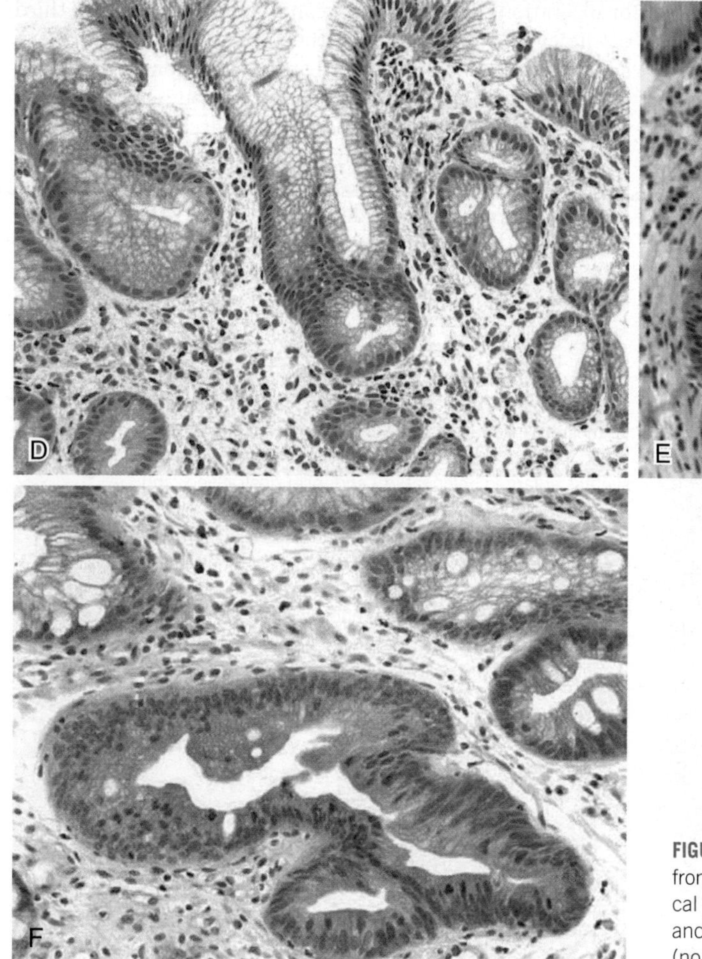

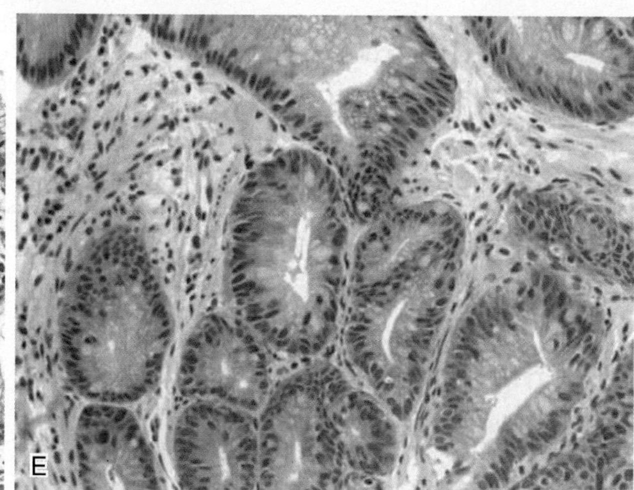

FIGURE 14.30 cont'd. Baseline atypia within crypts can range from bland cells with basally located nuclei with abundant apical mucinous cytoplasm **(D)** to cells with nuclear hyperchromasia and elongation **(E)**. **F,** Higher magnification of baseline crypt atypia (nondysplastic).

with dysplasia or carcinoma. However, in addition to differences in the definition of BE between North America and European guidelines, the British Society of Gastroenterology endorses the use of p53 IHC to support a diagnosis of dysplasia.[472]

Goblet Cells versus Pseudogoblet Cells

Barrett's epithelium (also sometimes referred to as *specialized columnar epithelium*) is histologically and biochemically similar to the incomplete (type II or III) intestinal metaplasia that occurs in the stomach of patients with chronic gastritis (see Chapter 15).[473] Less commonly, BE may show complete (type I) intestinal metaplasia. However, subtyping of intestinal metaplasia has no practical clinical significance in diagnosing or treating BE.

As described earlier, the epithelium in BE has three major cell types: goblet cells and intervening columnar cells that resemble either intestinal-type absorptive cells or gastric-type mucous cells. The brush border of intestinal-type absorptive cells is normally only partially developed. True goblet cells have a rounded "goblet" shape, have clear or slightly blue-tinged cytoplasm, and contain an eccentrically located and sometimes compressed nucleus. Goblet cells are typically distributed randomly in both the crypt and surface epithelium and contain acid mucin that stains intensely blue with Alcian blue at pH 2.5 (Fig. 14.32). The cytoplasmic mucin is composed of a mixture of both sialomucins and sulfomucins, but sialomucins usually predominate.[474,475] However, routine Alcian blue staining is costly and time-consuming and mucinous, nongoblet cells from the distal esophagus, GEJ, and proximal stomach often stain positive. For this reason, and because goblet cells can be readily recognized in tissue sections stained with hematoxylin and eosin (H&E), routine use of Alcian blue is not recommended for diagnosis of BE.

As mentioned previously, mucinous cells in BE often appear barrel-shaped or contain distended cytoplasmic vacuoles that impart an appearance similar to goblet cells (Fig. 14.33, *A*).[475] These pseudogoblet cells represent a potential source of error in the diagnosis of BE, particularly in biopsies from the GEJ region (Table 14.10). Although pseudogoblet cells typically stain less intensely than true goblet cells with Alcian blue at pH 2.5 (see Fig. 14.33B), this difference is usually quite subtle. The distinction is best made on the basis of their H&E-stained cytologic features. On a routine H&E stain, goblet cells typically show a bluish cytoplasm while pseudogoblet cells harbor pale pink mucinous cytoplasm.

In contrast to true goblet cells which are usually present as single cells in a background of columnar epithelium in BE, pseudogoblet cells are typically arranged in the form of linear contiguous stretches of cells on the surface and upper portions of the crypts, without intervening columnar

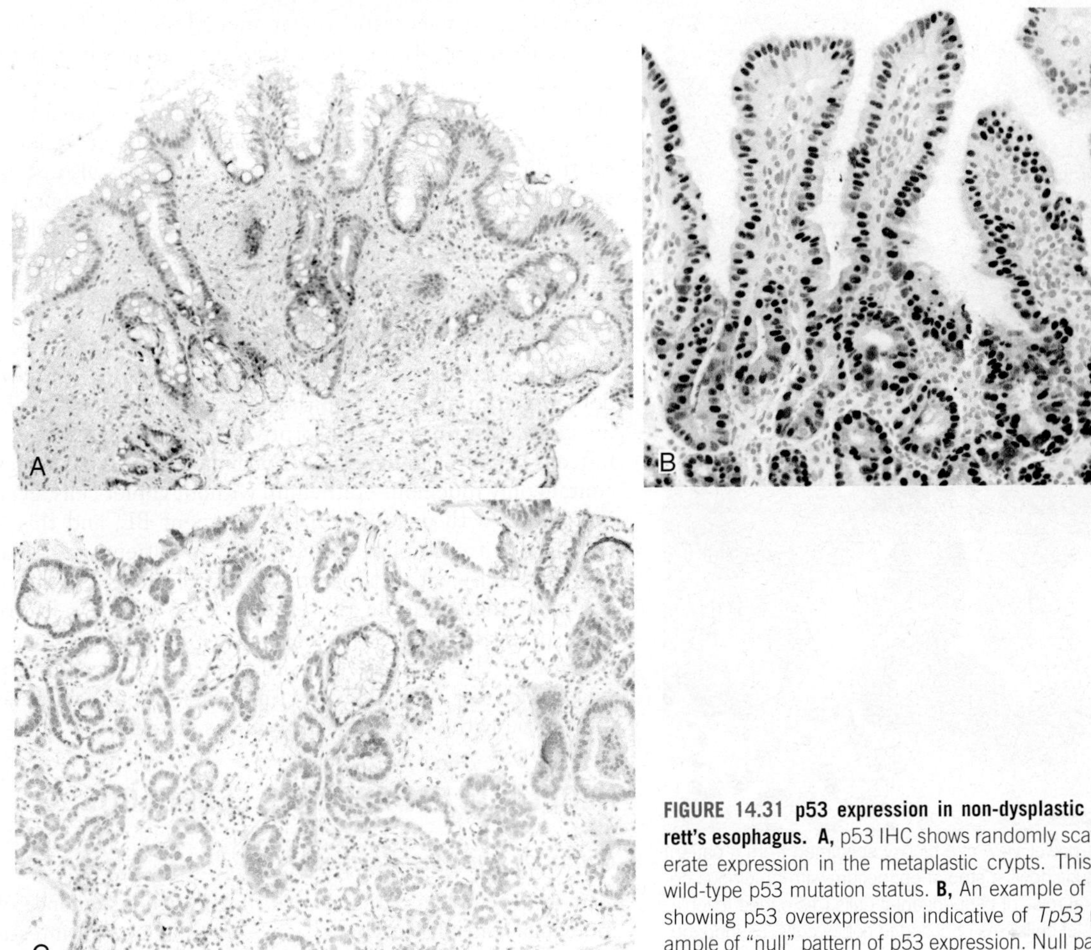

FIGURE 14.31 p53 expression in non-dysplastic and dysplastic Barrett's esophagus. A, p53 IHC shows randomly scattered weak to moderate expression in the metaplastic crypts. This pattern represents wild-type p53 mutation status. **B,** An example of low-grade dysplasia showing p53 overexpression indicative of *Tp53* mutation. **C,** An example of "null" pattern of p53 expression. Null pattern usually results from deletions or truncating mutations in *TP53* gene.

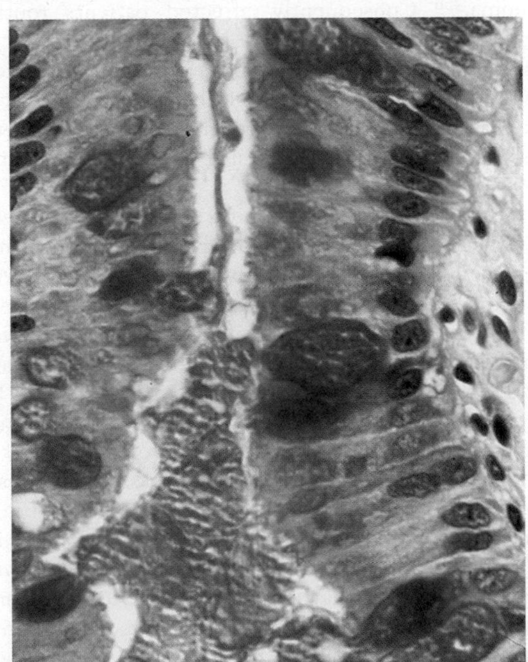

FIGURE 14.32 Biopsy specimen from a patient with Barrett's esophagus, stained with Alcian blue at pH 2.5, shows strong staining of goblet cells. However, this stain is not recommended to diagnose the presence of goblet cells or to distinguish goblet cells from pseudogoblet cells. This distinction is best made on hematoxylin and eosin (H&E)-stained sections, because both types of cells may be positive with Alcian blue.

cells. Pseudogoblet cells are rare in the deeper portions of the crypts and contain a hazy, ground-glass cytoplasmic appearance.

Pseudogoblet cells also reside in the proximal stomach (cardia), particularly in areas of active inflammation and regeneration. Their identification in a biopsy sample by no means implies that the columnar epithelium in the specimen was derived from the anatomic esophagus. Furthermore, even nondistended mucinous foveolar epithelium in the proximal stomach may stain weakly positive with Alcian blue at pH 2.5.[475] Esophageal mucosal and submucosal glands and their corresponding ducts are usually intensely positive with this stain as well. However, differentiation of esophageal glands from true columnar metaplasia usually is not difficult, because the former have a lobular configuration similar to minor salivary glands and are located in the deep mucosa rather than at the surface. The gland ducts may have a mucinous or transitional type of epithelium and may also be Alcian blue positive. Of course, the finding of esophageal glands or ducts helps identify a particular mucosal biopsy specimen as esophageal in origin.[473] Columnar epithelium identified in the same specimen would, by definition, represent metaplastic epithelium.

Differential Diagnosis

On occasion, BE may be confused with congenital islands of ectopic gastric mucosa, termed *inlet patches*. Inlet patches occur in as much as 10% of individuals (see Chapter 19).[476]

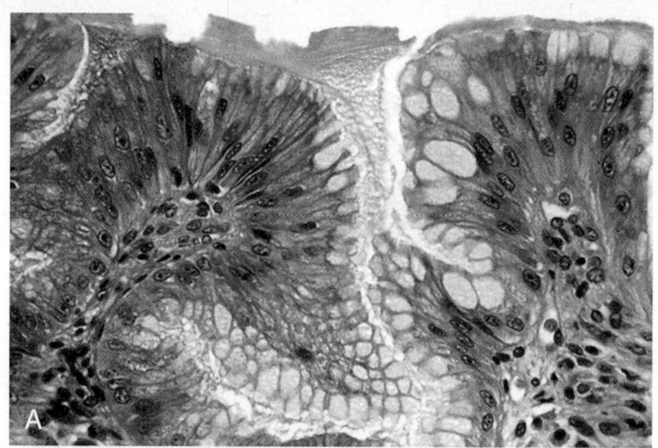

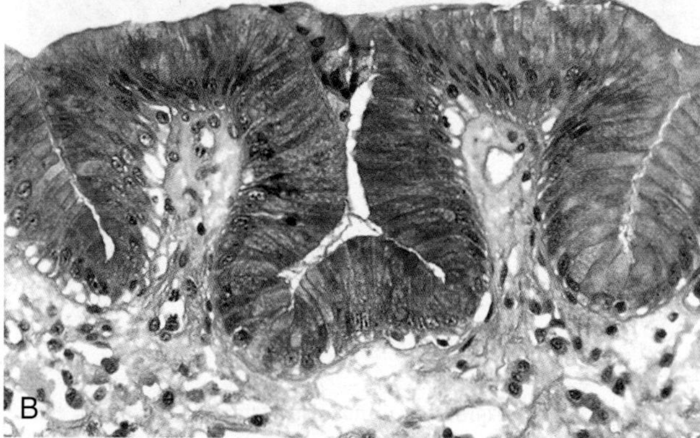

FIGURE 14.33 A, High-power view of a biopsy specimen from a patient with Barrett's esophagus shows a strip of epithelium with mucinous columnar cells and several rows of pseudogoblet cells (distended foveolar cells that resemble goblet cells). As opposed to goblet cells, pseudogoblet cells are typically arranged in linear groups and stain less intensely (but still positively) with Alcian blue at pH 2.5 **(B).** However, because of subjectivity in interpretation of the intensity of an Alcian blue stain and overlap in the intensity of staining between these two cell types, use of Alcian blue at pH 2.5 to distinguish goblet from pseudogoblet cells is not recommended.

TABLE 14.10 Morphological Features of Goblet Cells versus Pseudogoblet Cells

	Goblet Cells	Pseudogoblet Cells
Shape	Rounded "goblet" shape	Elongated, distended cytoplasmic vacuoles
Cytoplasm	Bluish cytoplasm	Pale eosinophilic cytoplasm
Location	Superficial epithelium Crypts	Superficial epithelium Rarely in crypts
Distribution	Random	Linear Nonrandom

In contrast to BE, inlet patches occur predominantly in the upper third of the esophagus and are separated from the stomach by normal squamous epithelium. Inlet patches may contain gastric or intestinal-type mucosa or, rarely, thyroid, parathyroid, or sebaceous gland tissue. Extremely rare cases of cancer in inlet patches have been reported.[476-478]

Biopsy specimens obtained from patients with GERD, or even *H. pylori* gastritis, in the region of the GEJ may reveal foci of pancreatic acinar metaplasia.[462,479] Pancreatic acinar-like cells are characterized by groups or lobules of cells with supranuclear eosinophilic granular cytoplasm and subnuclear basophilic cytoplasm similar to normal pancreatic acini. This type of metaplasia is usually an incidental finding. Foci of pancreatic acinar metaplasia also occur commonly in BE. Regardless of its location, most authorities believe that it represents a metaplastic reaction to injury, although some suggest it is congenital in origin. It has no clinical significance.

Columnar-Lined Esophagus without Goblet Cells

Most, if not all, patients with long-segment BE (>3 cm) demonstrate columnar epithelium with admixed goblet cells, intestinal-type absorptive cells, and gastric-type mucous cells.[480] However, individual biopsy specimens may contain only mucinous epithelium without goblet cells, even in patients with unequivocal long-segment BE, and this is usually due to sampling error. Rarely, in patients (particularly children) with endoscopically visible long lengths of columnar metaplasia in the esophagus no goblet cells are seen, even after inspection of multiple biopsy specimens. Because of the rarity of this situation, the clinical significance and risk of malignancy in long-segment columnar metaplasia without goblet cells remains unknown.[480]

NEOPLASIA IN BARRETT'S ESOPHAGUS

Definition and Classification

Cancer develops in patients with BE through a sequence of molecular and phenotypic changes that begin with intestinal metaplasia (although not always) and then progresses through various grades of dysplasia, ultimately to adenocarcinoma.[466] Consequently, affected patients routinely undergo endoscopic surveillance for early detection of neoplasia. This approach forms the basis of cancer prevention in patients with BE.[377,379] Histological evaluation of dysplasia in esophageal mucosal biopsy specimens is the main method of risk assessment in the surveillance and management of BE.[463]

Dysplasia is defined as unequivocal neoplastic epithelium that remains confined within the basement membrane of the epithelium from which it developed.[481] In most Western countries, including the United States, specimens evaluated for dysplasia in BE are classified as negative, indefinite, or positive (either low-grade or high-grade).[481] The diagnosis and grading of dysplasia is based on evaluation of both cytologic and architectural abnormalities. However, many pathologists, particularly those from Europe and Asia, prefer the more recently proposed Vienna classification system (Table 14.11).[482] The Vienna system is similar to the one outlined earlier except that it uses the terms *noninvasive neoplasia* instead of *dysplasia* and *suspicious for invasive carcinoma* for lesions that show equivocal cytologic or architectural features of tissue invasion. The categories in the Vienna system are as follows: negative for neoplasia, indefinite for neoplasia, noninvasive low-grade neoplasia, noninvasive high-grade neoplasia (including noninvasive carcinoma in situ and suspicion of invasive carcinoma), and invasive neoplasia (intramucosal and submucosal). The Vienna system was developed in an effort to reduce discrepancies in

TABLE 14.11 Revised Vienna Classification and Reid Classification of Neoplastic Precursor Lesions in Barrett's Esophagus

Revised Vienna	Reid
Negative for neoplasia (ND)	Negative for dysplasia
Indefinite for neoplasia (ID)	Indefinite for dysplasia
Mucosal low-grade neoplasia (LGD)	Low-grade dysplasia
Low-grade adenoma	
Low-grade dysplasia	
Mucosal high-grade neoplasia (HGD)	High-grade dysplasia
High-grade adenoma/dysplasia	
Noninvasive carcinoma (carcinoma in situ)	
Suspicious for invasive neoplasia	
Intramucosal carcinoma	Intramucosal adenocarcinoma
Submucosal invasion by carcinoma	Invasive adenocarcinoma

interpretation of dysplasia between Western and Japanese pathologists and to reach a worldwide consensus on the nomenclature of GI neoplasia.

Risk Factors and Pathogenesis

Risk factors for dysplasia in BE (see earlier discussion) are similar to those for the development of adenocarcinoma and are reviewed more extensively in Chapter 24.[371,466] Adenocarcinoma of the esophagus develops mainly in patients who have metaplastic intestinal-type epithelium, although carcinomas may, less commonly, develop in goblet cell–depleted or even goblet cell–absent BE. While some investigators believe that lack of goblet cells in BE-related adenocarcinomas is due to neoplastic glands overgrowing the native intestinalized metaplastic glands, others have shown that clonal expansion, progression and *TP53* mutations can be identified in metaplastic epithelium without goblet cells.[483-485]

Several clinical and endoscopic parameters, such as the presence of a hiatal hernia and longer lengths of BE, are associated with an increased risk of progression to cancer in some studies.[397,398,486] Both GERD and obesity have been shown to be independent risk factors for the development of cancer.[371] Some data suggest that increased dietary fat and tobacco use also increase the risk for neoplastic progression, and that increased dietary intake of fruits, vegetables, and fiber decreases the risk.[371,487-489]

The development of adenocarcinoma in BE follows a metaplasia–dysplasia–carcinoma sequence that is characterized by the accumulation of multiple genetic and epigenetic alterations, many of which occur before the onset of morphological dysplasia.[466] (See Chapter 24 for discussion of molecular pathogenesis.) Many of the molecular events are related to alterations or modifications of the cell cycle, apoptosis, cell signaling, and adhesion pathways.[466,490] The most common genetic alteration in BE is inactivation of the *CDKN2A* (also known as p16, INK4, or p16INK4a) tumor suppressor gene on chromosome 9p21.[491] Inactivation of both alleles of *CDKN2A* is an early event that causes clonal expansion. Loss or mutations of *TP53*, a tumor-suppressive gene located on chromosome 17p13, are also common in BE and are occasionally found in morphologically nondysplastic epithelium.[469,470,492-494] BE shows proliferative abnormalities, reflected by an increased S-phase fraction on flow cytometry and immunohistochemically by overexpression of cell proliferation markers such as proliferating cell nuclear antigen (PCNA) and Ki67.[493] BE and the progression of neoplasia are characterized by widespread genomic abnormalities, losses and gains in chromosome function, and especially DNA instability, which is characterized most often by aneuploidy.[464,465] Aneuploidy is a rather late neoplastic change in BE and has been shown to predict progression to adenocarcinoma.[464,465,470]

Pathology

Endoscopically, dysplasia may be undetectable or may appear as flat, irregular, plaquelike, nodular, polypoid, eroded, or ulcerated mucosa.[461,495] The natural history and risk of malignancy are somewhat dependent on the macroscopic features of the dysplastic lesion.[463] Patients with one or more macroscopic lesions are more likely to develop high-grade dysplasia and cancer than patients without an endoscopically identifiable dysplastic lesion.[496,497] In one study, 60% of patients with dysplastic nodules had cancer, compared with only 23% of patients without endoscopically apparent nodules.[495] In another study by Montgomery and colleagues, a high proportion of BE patients with ulcers had high-grade dysplasia or adenocarcinoma, compared with patients without ulcers, and the presence of an ulcer with high-grade dysplasia increased the likelihood of detecting carcinoma in a subsequent resection specimen.[496]

Rarely, dysplasia in BE may grow as a well-defined, adenoma-like polyp. However, because of the strong association of these lesions with high-grade dysplasia and adenocarcinoma, as well as with adjacent flat, high-grade dysplasia, these lesions should be designated as polypoid dysplasia rather than adenoma, which usually has a benign connotation in rest of the GI tract(see Chapter 24).

Negative for Dysplasia

A diagnosis of "negative for dysplasia" is typically applied to cases of BE that show metaplastic columnar epithelium that is either unremarkable or shows regenerative changes (See section on microscopic features of BE above).[461]

Indefinite for Dysplasia

On occasion, regenerative changes can be marked, particularly in areas of active inflammation or ulceration, and, as such, they may be difficult to distinguish from true dysplasia (Fig. 14.34). In this context, the temporary diagnostic category "indefinite for dysplasia" is often applied until further biopsies can be obtained after the inflammation or ulceration has subsided or healed. This diagnostic category is used most often in situations involving (1) technical issues, (2) atypia related to inflammation and ulceration, and (3) atypical (dysplasia-like) changes present only in the bases of the crypts, but with evidence of surface maturation (see later discussion).[436,461,498,499] Tangential or thick tissue sectioning, poor orientation, suboptimal fixation or staining, denuded surface epithelium, and the presence of marked cautery artifact can make interpretation of dysplasia difficult and can lead to an interim diagnosis of indefinite for dysplasia. In the

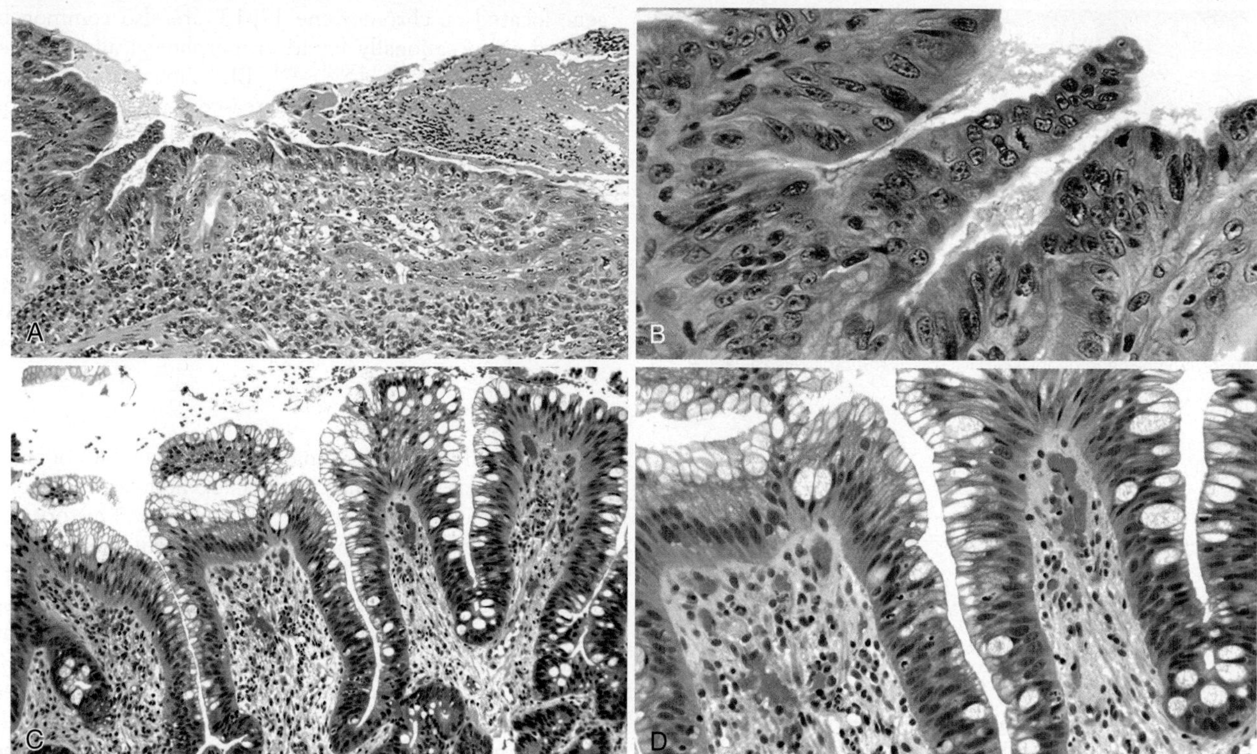

FIGURE 14.34 Barrett's esophagus, indefinite for dysplasia. In **A** and **B,** an area of atypical surface and crypt epithelium is present adjacent to an area of ulceration. At high power **(B)**, the epithelium shows pseudostratification, loss of polarity, and increased mitoses. However, the epithelium is tufted and reveals intraepithelial inflammation as well. On the basis of its location adjacent to an ulcer, this specimen is best qualified as indefinite for dysplasia and would be best reevaluated after the ulcer has been treated. **C** and **D,** Indefinite dysplasia without ulcer. Notice the stratification of the nuclei in the surface epithelium with few intraepithelial neutrophils. While we (the authors) think these changes are likely reactive due to the presence of partial surface epithelial maturation, if unsure it is reasonable to diagnose these examples as indefinite for dysplasia and reevaluate after the inflammation and ulceration has healed and subsided.

presence of ulceration or active (neutrophilic) inflammation, regenerative changes can become extreme, and the crypts may show marked nuclear stratification (particularly at the bases of the crypts), mucin depletion, increased mitoses, and hyperchromaticity. However, even in instances of marked regeneration adjacent to areas of ulceration, some degree of surface maturation is usually evident in nondysplastic BE. Furthermore, the presence of a gradual transition from atypical epithelium to nonatypical epithelium, particularly in association with decreased inflammation, is considered a strong criterion for regeneration rather than dysplasia. Therefore, interpretation of dysplasia, particularly in the setting of active inflammation or ulceration, should be performed with great caution if the atypical changes are low grade and the architecture of the epithelium is well maintained. Crypt-only atypical changes are discussed later in this chapter. Of particular clinical importance is the fact that this diagnostic category should not be considered an intermediate phase between BE with no dysplasia and BE with low-grade dysplasia biologically, but instead it simply represents an interim diagnosis used when a pathologist is unsure if the morphological features truly represent any type or degree of dysplasia or cancer vs non-neoplastic BE.

Positive for Dysplasia

The two most common histological patterns of dysplasia are intestinal (adenoma-like) and nonintestinal (foveolar type). A third type that has serrated architecture (serrated dysplasia) may also show either intestinal or foveolar cytoplasmic features.[380,461,500] Many cases show a mixture of intestinal and foveolar dysplasia, or, rarely, a mixture of all three types. Intestinal dysplasia is far more common; the name denotes the cytologic resemblance of the neoplastic nuclei to sporadic adenomas of the colon. Finally, rare dysplasia cases show no obvious cellular differentiation, and thus have been termed *non-adenomatous* or *null* dysplasia. However, in a recent study, even these cases showed some evidence of gastric (foveolar) differentiation by immunohistochemistry (MUC5AC, and MUC6 positivity [marker of gastric foveolar mucin]).[501]

Intestinal Type Dysplasia. Low-grade (intestinal-type) dysplasia is characterized by crypts with mild (baseline) architectural changes, similar to nondysplastic Barrett's epithelium (Fig. 14.35). The epithelial cell nuclei are typically elongated, crowded, and hyperchromatic; they show an irregular contour and contain dense chromatin, with or without multiple, small, inconspicuous nucleoli.[481,497] Dysplastic cells are usually mucin depleted and show a marked decrease in goblet cell differentiation. In fact, goblet cells may be decreased in number or completely absent from adjacent nondysplastic BE mucosa in biopsy specimens with dysplasia.[497] In low-grade dysplasia, the nuclei are pencil shaped and stratified but for the most part are limited to the basal portion of the cell cytoplasm. Other features include increased mitoses, both typical and atypical, preservation or only mild loss of cell polarity limited to the bases of the crypts, increased N:C ratio, and lack of surface maturation which is characteristic of dysplasia in general. Most notably, dysplastic epithelium often shows an abrupt transition to

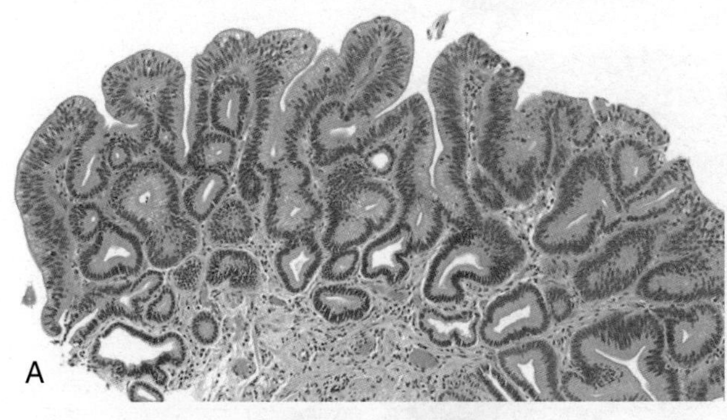

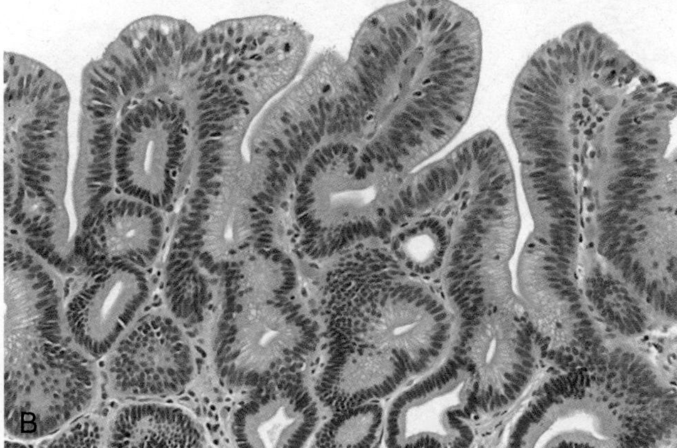

FIGURE 14.35 A, Medium-magnification view of low-grade (intestinal-type) dysplasia in Barrett's esophagus. Overall, there are mild architectural abnormalities. The architecture of the crypts is similar to that seen in nondysplastic Barrett's epithelium. **B,** At higher magnification, the epithelium shows enlarged pencil-shaped nuclei, increased nucleus-to-cytoplasm ratio, stratification of the nuclei limited to the basal half of the cell cytoplasm, slight loss of nuclear polarity, increased mitoses, mucin depletion, and a distinct lack of surface maturation.

nondysplastic epithelium, and this is a helpful feature in distinguishing true dysplasia from regenerating epithelium. The presence of an abrupt transition and of uniform nuclear changes that extend from the bases of the crypts to the mucosal surface in the absence of inflammation is considered diagnostic of low-grade dysplasia.

High-grade (intestinal-type) dysplasia is characterized by epithelium with more severe cytologic changes and is usually accompanied by more significant architectural abnormalities compared with nondysplastic or low-grade dysplastic epithelium (Fig. 14.36).[461,481,497] Architectural abnormalities include villiform change, increased crypt complexity, cribriforming, variability in size and shape of the crypts, crowding, irregularity, and extensive branching. Cytologically, high-grade dysplastic epithelium shows pronounced nuclear stratification (usually reaching the surface of the cells) throughout the full length of the crypts, marked loss of polarity and pleomorphism even at the upper levels of the crypts, prominent enlarged nucleoli, and increased atypical mitotic activity involving the surface epithelium as well. As in low-grade dysplasia, mucin depletion and decrease or complete absence of goblet cell differentiation is typical of high-grade dysplasia. Important features to distinguish high-grade from low-grade dysplasia include full-thickness nuclear stratification, marked loss of cell polarity, particularly at higher levels of the crypt and in the surface epithelium, atypical mitoses in the upper levels of the crypt and in surface epithelium, and considerable architectural distortion (see Table 14.8).

In high-grade dysplasia, the crypts may show intraluminal papillae or bridges. However, prominent intraluminal bridges, intraluminal necrosis, and a back-to-back crypt pattern should raise the possibility of intramucosal adenocarcinoma. Two recent studies[502,503] attempted to ascertain the likelihood of finding adenocarcinoma in the resection specimen using rigorous histological criteria for high-grade dysplasia versus high-grade dysplasia with features suspicious for carcinoma. Another acceptable term for biopsy features suspicious for adenocarcinoma is "high-grade dysplasia with marked glandular architectural distortion; cannot exclude intramucosal adenocarcinoma." The presence of adenocarcinoma in resection specimens was significantly higher in cases with features suspicious for carcinoma. This category included those with solid (back to back glands) or cribriform architecture, ulcers occurring within the high-grade dysplastic mucosa, three or more dilated dysplastic tubules containing necrotic debris, large numbers of neutrophils within high-grade dysplastic epithelium, and dysplastic tubules that were incorporated into the overlying squamous epithelium.[502-504]

Crypt Dysplasia. As discussed earlier, the presence of surface maturation is generally considered a feature of regenerating epithelium rather than dysplasia. However, in some circumstances, dysplasia may also mature to the surface .Lomo and colleagues were the first to describe 15 cases of true dysplasia limited to the crypt bases but without surface involvement (i.e., surface maturation was present)[498] (Fig. 14.37).This is termed "crypt dysplasia". Most cases of crypt dysplasia show features of low-grade dysplasia, but in rare instances, it may consist of high-grade dysplastic cells limited to the crypt bases (Table 14.12; see Fig. 14.37D). Lomo and co-workers provide evidence to suggest that in the early stages of neoplastic progression, dysplasia begins in the crypt bases and may involve only that portion of the epithelium in some circumstances. Eighty-seven percent of their patients with this finding also showed areas of conventional full-crypt dysplasia or adenocarcinoma in other regions of the patient's esophagus. Patients with crypt dysplasia also showed a significantly higher frequency of 17p loss of heterozygosity (LOH) and flow cytometric abnormalities, compared with patients without dysplasia.[498] In another study, the bases of the crypts in foci of crypt dysplasia showed cellular DNA content abnormalities similar to those of basal crypt cells in foci of traditional full-crypt low-grade dysplasia, but the surface epithelium in areas of basal crypt dysplasia was diploid.[499] These findings provide further evidence that dysplasia begins in the crypt bases and progresses, with time, to involve the full lengths of the crypts and surface epithelium.

A study by Coco et al. suggests that crypt dysplasia can be diagnosed reliably, with a moderate level of interobserver agreement.[505] Nevertheless, from a practical point of view, crypt dysplasia is uncommon and should not be diagnosed in mucosal biopsy specimens that also show active inflammation or ulceration, because in these situations, it is often difficult to determine whether the dysplasia-like basal crypt changes are truly dysplastic. Biopsies such as these should be considered indefinite for dysplasia until further specimens

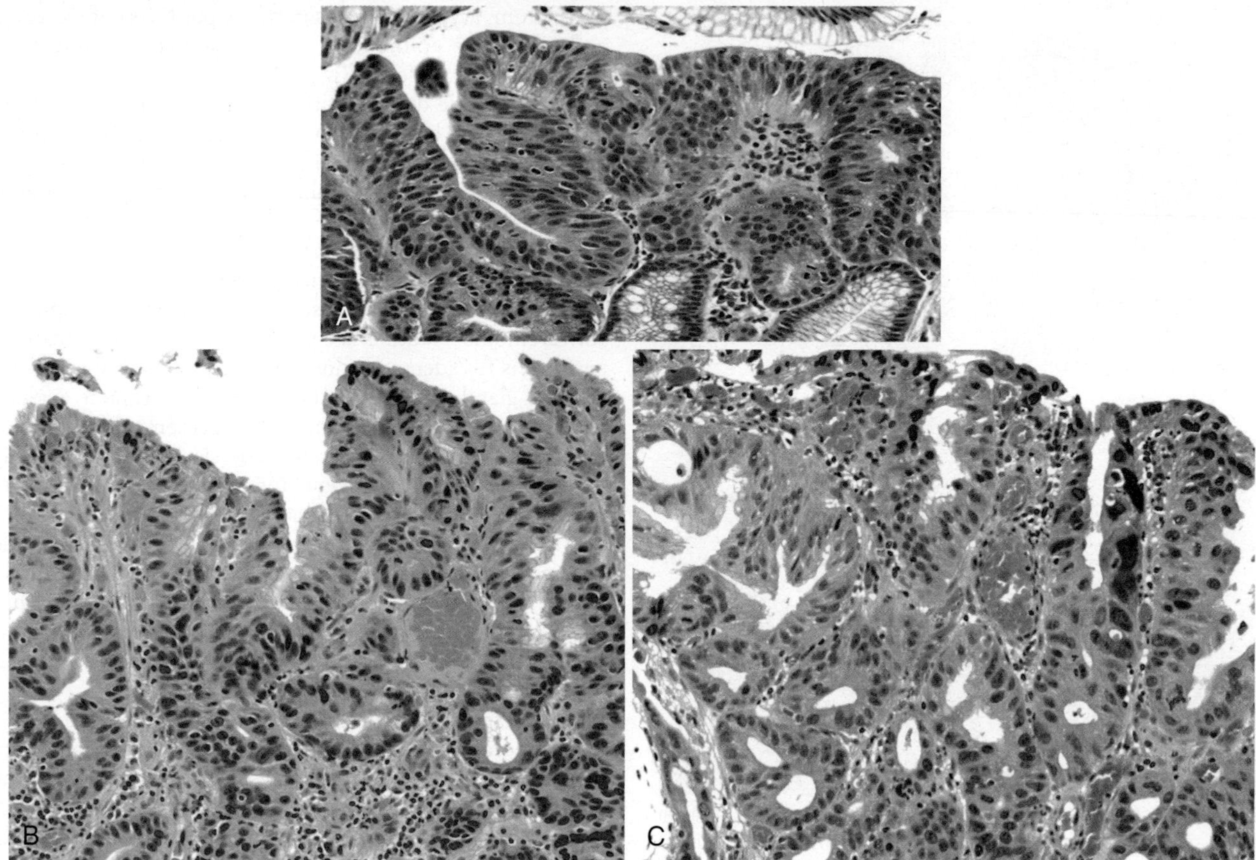

FIGURE 14.36 High-grade dysplasia in Barrett's esophagus. A, In contrast to low-grade dysplasia, high-grade dysplasia shows full-thickness nuclear stratification, increased nucleus-to-cytoplasm (N:C) ratio, increased loss of polarity and pleomorphism, and atypical mitoses. Despite the presence of intraepithelial inflammation, the degree of cytologic and architectural atypia qualifies this lesion as high grade. **B,** Another focus of high-grade dysplasia shows a marked degree of nuclear pleomorphism, loss of polarity, increased N:C ratio, and full-thickness stratification. Even in the absence of architectural distortion, the degree of cytologic atypia warrants a diagnosis of high-grade dysplasia. **C,** High-grade dysplasia with architectural distortion, marked nuclear pleomorphism, atypical mitoses, and increased N:C ratio of the cells.

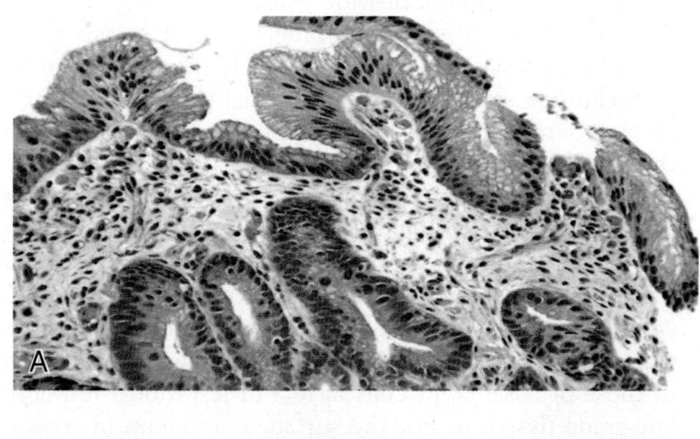

FIGURE 14.37 Crypt dysplasia in Barrett's esophagus (BE). Low-power **(A)** and high- **(B)** power views of a biopsy specimen from a patient with BE show low-grade dysplasia limited to the crypt bases but with evidence of surface maturation. **C,** In this focus, the basal portions of the crypts show dysplastic-appearing cells characterized by nuclear enlargement, stratification, and loss of nuclear polarity.

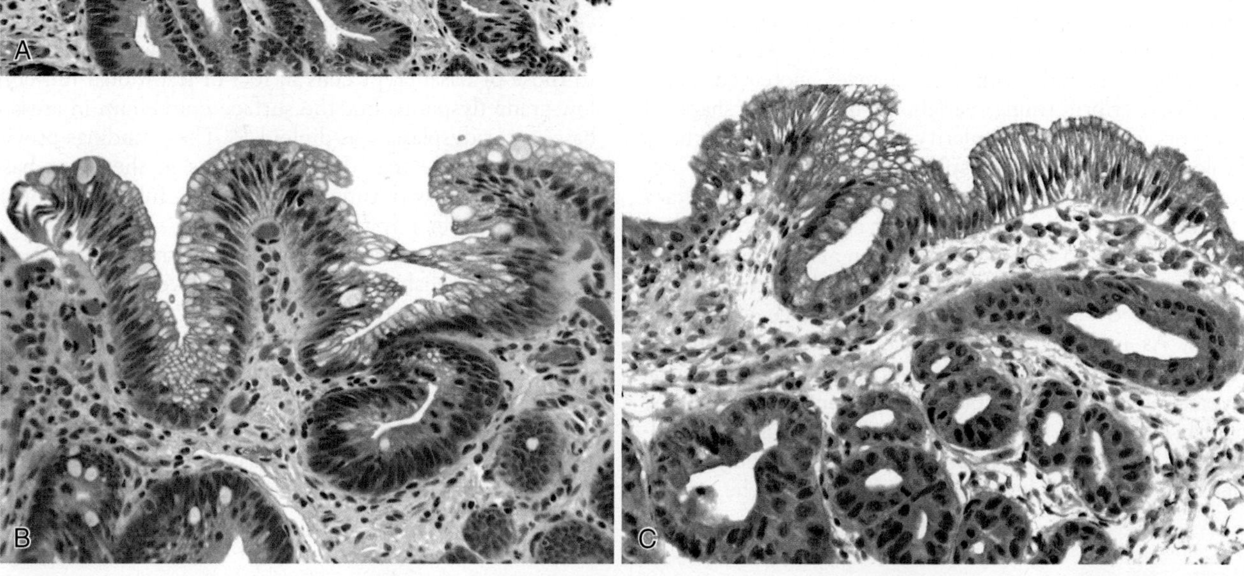

TABLE 14.12 Histological Patterns of Dysplasia in Barrett's Esophagus

Morphological Type of Dysplasia	Low Grade	High Grade
Intestinal dysplasia	Penicillate, elongated nuclei with nuclear stratification Maintenance of nuclear polarity (long axis of nucleus is perpendicular to the basement membrane of the gland) Absent or few goblet cells Mild glandular crowding	Hyperchromatic nuclei with prominent nucleoli Loss of nuclear polarity Crowded glandular architecture with budding and/or cribriform arrangement
Crypt dysplasia	Penicillate, elongated, hyperchromatic nuclei with nuclear stratification in basal crypts with preservation of surface epithelial maturation	Hyperchromatic nuclei with prominent nucleoli Loss of nuclear polarity Crowded glands with budding Surface maturation present
Foveolar dysplasia	Single layer of cuboidal cells with basally oriented round to oval nuclei Nuclear size is two to three times the size of an adjacent lymphocyte or plasma cell nucleus Lack of nuclear stratification	Single layer of cuboidal cells with basally oriented round to oval nuclei Lack of nuclear stratification Increased nuclear size (typically three to four times the size of a lymphocyte or plasma cell nucleus) Variably prominent nucleoli Mild to moderate pleomorphism
Serrated dysplasia	Mild nuclear stratification Small oval-shaped nuclei with an open chromatin pattern Eosinophilic cytoplasm, wispy in appearance	Small oval-shaped nuclei with an open chromatin pattern Prominent nucleoli Eosinophilic cytoplasm, wispy in appearance Hyperchromatic and stratified nuclei and increased mitotic rate

can be obtained after the inflammation has subsided. Nevertheless, if a focus of crypt dysplasia is suspected in a mucosal biopsy, further sectioning of the tissue block and careful analysis of adjacent crypts may help uncover evidence of traditional full-crypt low- or high-grade dysplasia

The natural history of crypt dysplasia has not been fully studied, but there is some preliminary data to suggest that it progresses at a rate much higher than non-dysplastic BE and even approaching that of traditional low-grade dysplasia. For instance, a large series of 4,545 patients who had two sequential samples (separated by ≥12 months) obtained using the WATS3D (wide-area trans-epithelial sampling with 3 dimensional computer-assisted analysis) technology, progression to HGD or adenocarcinoma occurred in patients with baseline non-dysplastic BE at a rate of 0.08%/patient-year. In contrast, the rate of progression was significantly higher (1.42%/patient-year) for patients with baseline crypt dysplasia and 5.79%/patient-year for those with baseline LGD.[506] Furthermore, several studies published in abstract form suggest rates of progression of crypt dysplasia are similar to traditional low grade dysplasia.[507,508] These results indicate that patients with crypt dysplasia likely warrant close follow-up similar to those with LGD, but this needs to be evaluated in further prospective studies.

Foveolar Dysplasia. Based on a series of 200 consecutive BE dysplasia patients, the prevalence of foveolar-type dysplasia was found to be 15% at the patient level, and 20% at the biopsy level.[509] This study also showed that foveolar-type dysplasia is more often high-grade, and occurs mostly in women, in patients who, on average, are a decade older than those with intestinal-type dysplasia. Foveolar dysplasia is more often tubular than villiform.

Criteria for grading foveolar dysplasia have been proposed, but they have not been validated and their reproducibility has not been tested.[509] In general, foveolar dysplasia is characterized by cells that are more cuboidal in shape and have abundant mucinous cytoplasm (see Table 14.12). Although the background non-dysplastic epithelium may show goblet cells, goblet cell differentiation within dysplastic glands is usually either completely absent or sparse when present. Foveolar dysplasia commonly expresses MUC5AC and is generally negative for intestinal markers such as MUC2, CDX2, and villin.[510] Foveolar dysplasia may show a range of cytologic atypia (see Fig. 14.39). Low-grade dysplasia is characterized by cells that have a low N/C ratio (far lower than intestinal type dysplasia) because the cytoplasm contains abundant apical mucin, and the nuclei are not stratified (Fig. 14.38A). Thus, distinguishing reactive atypia from low-grade foveolar dysplasia can be quite challenging. A study by Patil et al. showed that surface nuclear stratification, "top- heavy" atypia, and noncrowded, villiform architecture were highly characteristic of reactive cardiac epithelium in GERD patients (Fig. 14.38B), in comparison to true dysplasia that more often revealed monolayered nuclei within crowded glands that occupied the full thickness of the mucosa.

In contrast, high-grade foveolar dysplasia often shows cells with markedly increased N/C ratio, with nuclei that often measure 3-4 times the size of lymphocytes or plasma cell nuclei. They may show an open chromatin pattern and often contain macronucleoli as well. As mentioned above, this type of dysplasia most characteristically lacks nuclear stratification so typical of intestinal type dysplasia (Fig. 14.38C). Rather, the nuclei in foveolar dysplasia normally maintain a basal and largely monolayer pattern in most circumstances.

With regard to the natural history of foveolar dysplasia, pure foveolar dysplasia is frequently high-grade and associated with a higher risk of neoplastic progression compared to mixed gastric and intestinal-type dysplasia.[509] In one

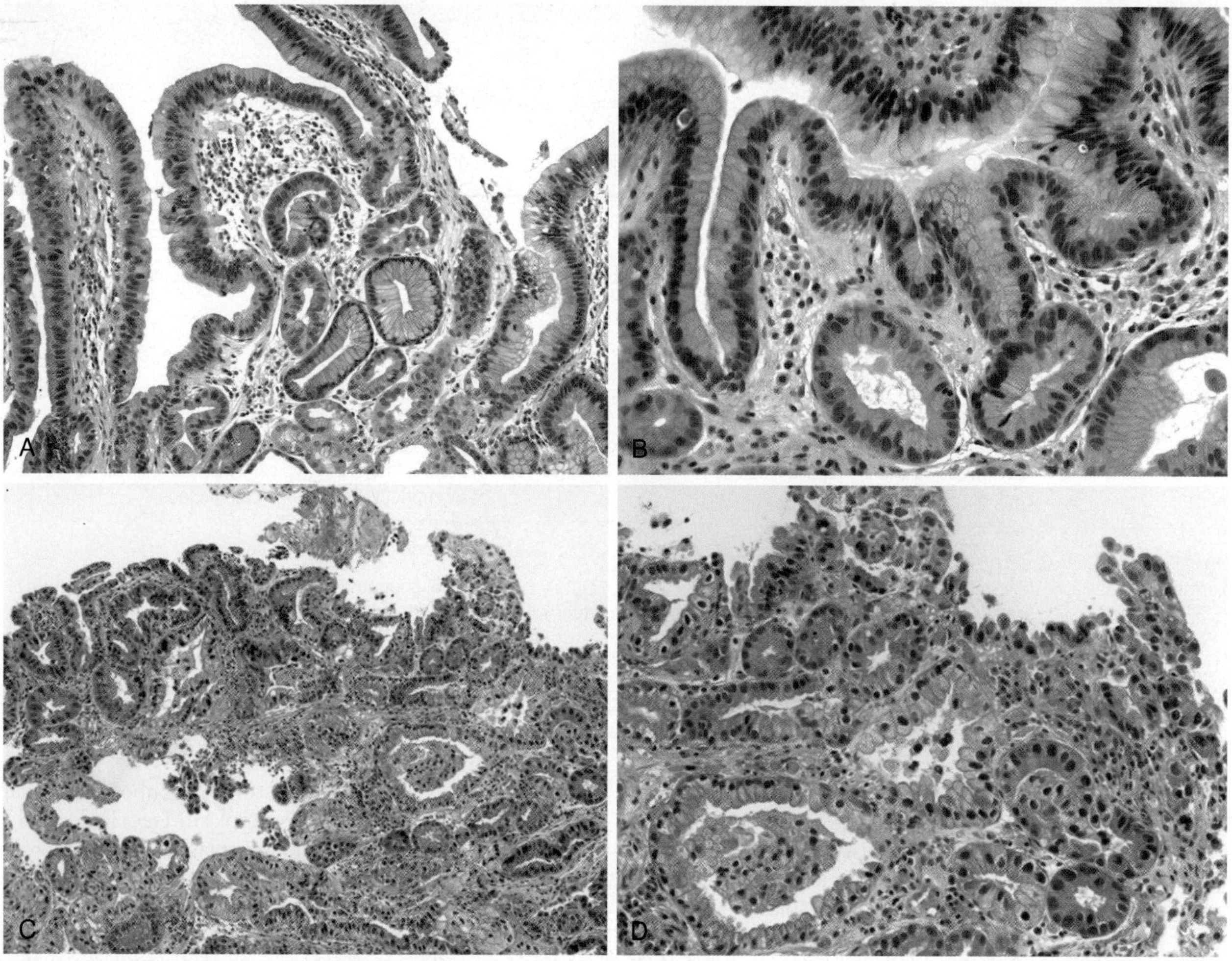

FIGURE 14.38 Foveolar dysplasia in Barrett's esophagus. In contrast to intestinal-type dysplasia, the cells have a more cuboidal or low columnar appearance, the nuclei are round or oval and irregular in shape, there is less nuclear stratification, and there is retention of the apical mucinous cytoplasm with a monolayer arrangement of cells. **A,** Low magnification; **B,** High-magnification. **C,** High-grade foveolar dysplasia is characterized by a back-to-back arrangement of atypical glands lined by cells with prominent nuclear atypia (nuclear size is usually greater than 3-4 times the size of an adjacent lymphocyte or plasma cell nucleus). **D,** On higher magnification the cells show prominent nucleoli and vesicular chromatin pattern.

study of 18 BE patients with non-intestinal ("foveolar") dysplasia from a cohort of 270 high risk BE patients, patients with non-intestinal dysplasia showed a high association with HGD of intestinal type elsewhere in the esophagus, and also showed a significantly higher rate of DNA flow cytometric abnormalities.[500]

Serrated Dysplasia. Serrated dysplasia is the least common type (Fig. 14.39). This type of dysplasia reveals a "hyperplastic" and/or "serrated" phenotype with a saw-toothed configuration of the epithelium and luminal infolding, similar to serrated polyps of the colon. The cells show small, oval-shaped nuclei with an open chromatin pattern, often with prominent nucleoli and less nuclear stratification. The cytoplasm is typically eosinophilic and wispy in appearance, especially at the surface. In high-grade cases, the nuclei are more hyperchromatic and stratified and show an increased mitotic rate. In a study (published in abstract form) consisting of 214 BE patients, the frequency of serrated dysplasia was found to be 2.8% (6/214). Of these 6 patients, 3 progressed to cancer, suggesting a high potential for adenocarcinoma.[511] Additional studies with larger number of patients with long term follow-up are needed to validate these observations.

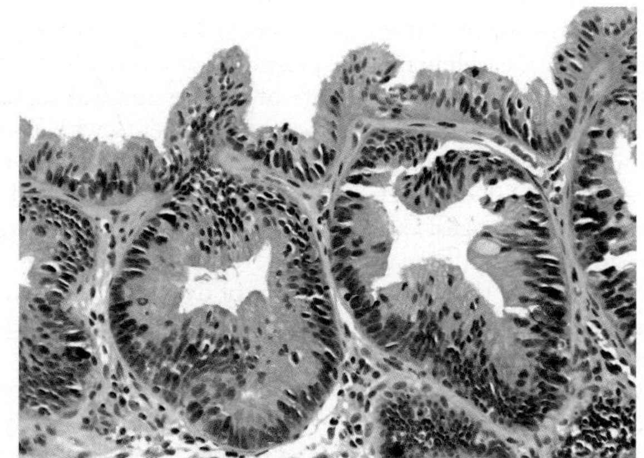

FIGURE 14.39 Serrated dysplasia is characterized by a hyperplastic and serrated phenotype with a saw-toothed configuration of the epithelium and luminal infolding, similar to serrated polyps of the colon.

Mixed Dysplasia. Foveolar and serrated dysplasia may occur in pure form, but in up to 94% of cases, there is

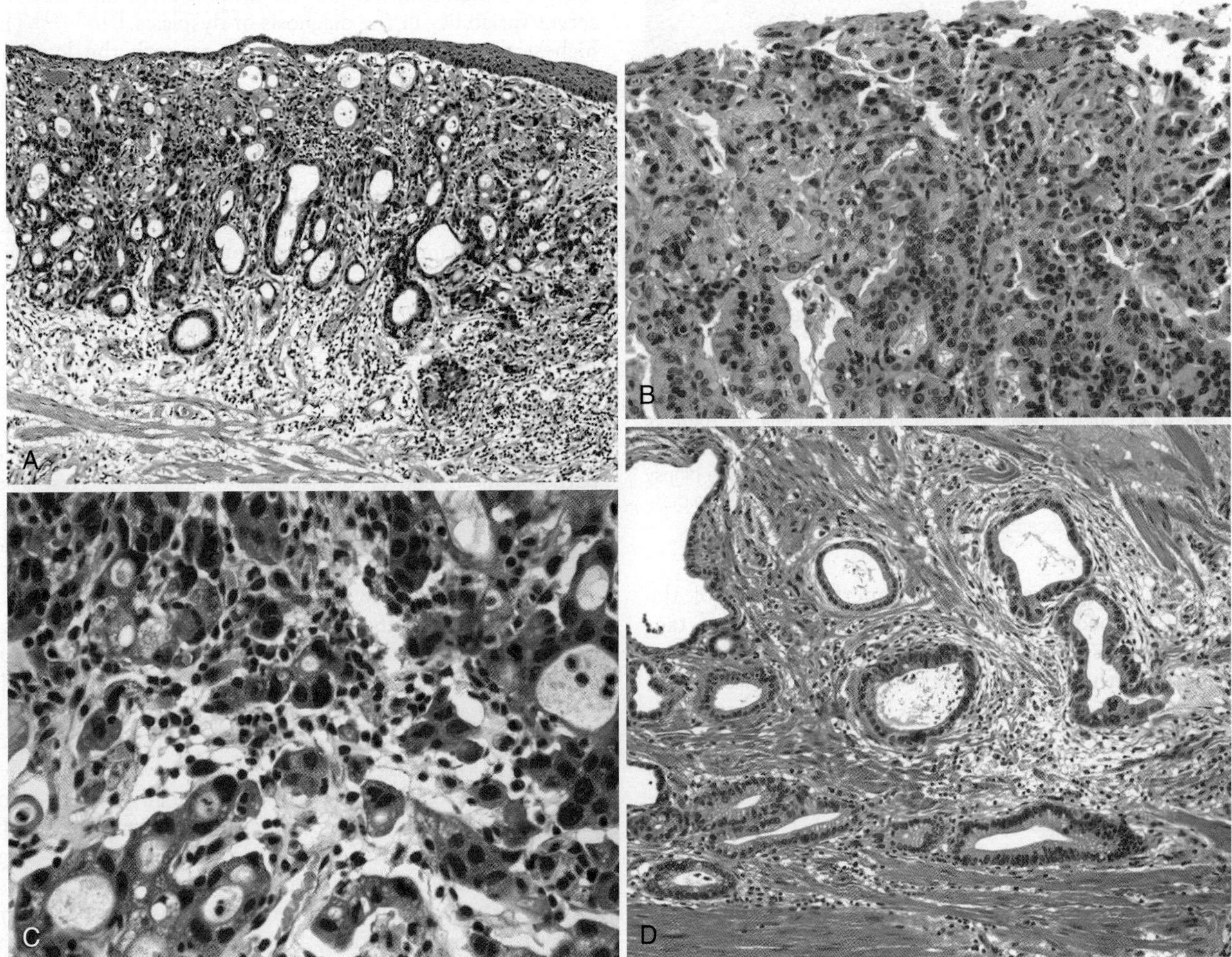

FIGURE 14.40 Intramucosal adenocarcinoma in Barrett's esophagus. A, Intramucosal adenocarcinoma underneath reepithelialized squamous epithelium. It is characterized by a proliferation of small, irregular glands with marked atypia without intervening lamina propria. **B,** Higher magnification shows marked distortion and irregular budding, combined with a back-to-back gland pattern and poor distinction between the basement membrane and the lamina propria. **C,** Individual neoplastic cells are infiltrating the lamina propria in another case of intramucosal adenocarcinoma. **D,** Neoplastic glands are entrapped in the duplicated fibers of muscularis mucosae.

an association with conventional intestinal type dysplasia, either adjacent to or elsewhere in the patient's esophagus.[500] Mixed dysplasia is present when both intestinal and foveolar cells (and/or serrated) reside adjacent to each other,[510] or in rare circumstances, when the dysplastic epithelium itself shows mixed intestinal and foveolar features (which is not uncommon when the cytology is high-grade).

Intramucosal Adenocarcinoma

Intramucosal adenocarcinoma is defined as neoplastic epithelium that has invaded beyond the basement membrane into the surrounding lamina propria or muscularis mucosae but has not extended beyond the deep margin of the original (deep) muscularis mucosae (Fig. 14.40). Because of the presence of lymphatics and blood vessels in the mucosa of the esophagus, intramucosal adenocarcinoma poses a risk of lymph node metastasis in the range of 1% to 2%.[512-515] Well-defined criteria have not been promulgated for this category of neoplasia in BE. In fact, there is a high degree of interobserver variability in the distinction between high-grade dysplasia and intramucosal adenocarcinoma.[504,516] This distinction is relevant when patients with intramucosal adenocarcinoma may be managed differently from those with high-grade dysplasia. However, based on current clinical practice recommendations, most institutions treat high-grade dysplasia similar to intramucosal carcinoma (see later discussion).[517] Recommended criteria for the diagnosis of intramucosal carcinoma include: (1) individual neoplastic cells that invade into the lamina propria and lack a connection to the crypts; (2) sheets of malignant cells without gland formation; (3) markedly angulated, infiltrative-appearing glands that reside in the lamina propria or muscularis mucosae; (4) a complex, anastomosing gland pattern within the lamina propria; and (5) neoplastic glands or cells arranged in a back-to-back or highly irregular architectural pattern that cannot be explained by the presence of preexisting Barrett's epithelium. Intramucosal adenocarcinoma often shows intraluminal necrosis within the neoplastic glands.

Adenocarcinoma with Submucosal Invasion

Adenocarcinoma that shows penetration beyond the original (deep) muscularis mucosae is considered submucosally invasive adenocarcinoma (Fig. 14.41). In superficial biopsies, this diagnosis can be challenging, because entrapped

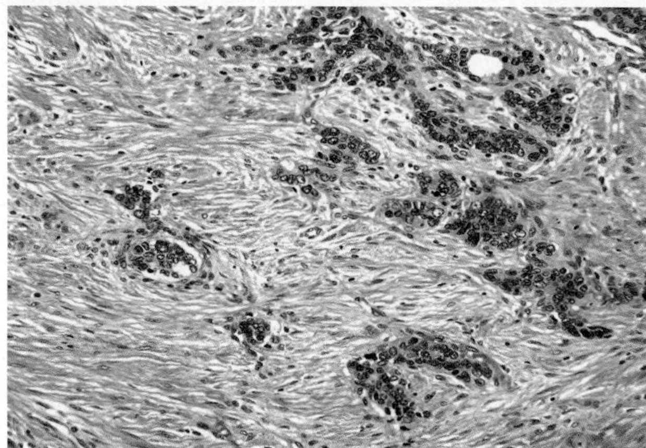

FIGURE 14.41 Submucosally invasive adenocarcinoma in Barrett's esophagus. Irregular malignant glands are present in association with a desmoplastic tissue response. Regardless of the location of the biopsy (i.e., above or below the muscularis mucosae), these features are diagnostic of invasive adenocarcinoma.

dysplastic glands located within superficial fibers of the newly developed muscularis mucosae, particularly in tangentially cut tissue sections, often simulate invasive adenocarcinoma with at least submucosal invasion. However, the presence of a desmoplastic stroma is considered strong evidence in favor of invasive (submucosal) adenocarcinoma. Invasive submucosal adenocarcinoma is best assessed in endoscopic mucosal resection (EMR) or endoscopic submucosal dissection specimens (see Treatment).[518]

Diagnostic Problems Related to Dysplasia

Sampling Error

Dysplasia is often endoscopically undetectable and may vary in amount from focal and minimal to diffuse and extensive, the latter possibly involving the entire segment of BE.[519] The chances of detecting dysplasia are proportional to the number, size, and thoroughness of biopsies obtained at endoscopy. In one study,[386] a minimum of eight biopsies was needed in to provide maximum yield for detection of dysplasia. Four-quadrant, well-oriented, jumbo biopsies obtained at intervals of 1 to 2 cm along the entire segment of BE were shown to have a high degree of sensitivity for detection for dysplasia in one study.[520] However, protocol biopsies of this type are only rarely performed in medical centers in the United States and abroad, being restricted mainly to specialty centers with a high academic or scientific interest in high-risk BE. With the advent of new, more sensitive diagnostic endoscopic techniques such as methylene blue application (chromoendoscopy), confocal endoscopy, and narrow band imaging, the detection rate of dysplasia is expected to increase. The yield of dysplasia is always considerably higher in biopsies from targeted lesions, such as areas of ulceration, nodularity, or mucosal irregularity.

Intraobserver and Interobserver Variability

Given the subtle gradation of changes that occur in the progression of dysplasia in BE, the fact that neoplastic progression occurs on a linear rather than a graded scale, and the wide range of morphological patterns of atypia related to epithelial regeneration and repair, it is not surprising that there is a significant degree of intraobserver and interobserver variability in the diagnosis of dysplasia.[481,497,504] The highest degree of variability occurs at both the low and the high end of the spectrum (i.e., separating regenerative atypia from low-grade dysplasia and separating high-grade dysplasia from adenocarcinoma). As a result, the ACG and the American Gastroenterological Association (AGA) have strongly recommended that all potential dysplasia diagnoses be confirmed by at least one experienced GI pathologist before embarking on a management plan.[378,379] This point was emphasized by several studies showing a strong correlation between the number of pathologists who agree with a dysplasia diagnosis and the rate of neoplastic progression.[521-526] For example, in a study by Skacel and co-workers, when two GI pathologists agreed on a diagnosis of low-grade dysplasia, 41% of patients progressed to high-grade dysplasia or cancer after a mean of 11 months. However, when three GI pathologists agreed on a diagnosis of low-grade dysplasia, 80% of patients progressed.[523] In a study by Srivastava and colleagues in which three GI pathologists agreed on a diagnosis of low-grade dysplasia, 45% of patients progressed to adenocarcinoma during a long follow-up period.[522]

In the general pathology community, there is a tendency to overdiagnose dysplasia. In one study of 485 patients, almost 40% of those who were diagnosed with high-grade dysplasia by a general pathologist had their diagnosis downgraded (11% to no dysplasia, 12% to indefinite dysplasia, and 16% to low-grade dysplasia) after review by three experienced GI pathologists.[521] In fact, a small proportion of patients in that study did not even fulfill the criteria for BE. In another study of 147 cases of low-grade dysplasia diagnosed by community pathologists, an expert GI pathologist agreed with that diagnosis in only 15% of cases, concluding that 0.6% were high-grade, 10% indefinite, and 75% negative for dysplasia.[525] Careful attention to the pathological criteria of high-grade dysplasia, as outlined earlier, and particularly to the presence or absence of significant loss of nuclear polarity (which is common in high-grade dysplasia and absent in low-grade dysplasia), can help avoid this problem of overdiagnosis.

Regenerative atypia versus Dysplasia

Distinguishing regenerative atypia from true dysplasia represents one of the most common challenges in Barrett's pathology (see Table 14.9). Regenerative epithelial changes are always present in areas of neutrophilic inflammation and erosion/ulceration. There is a gradual transition between uninflamed mucosa and inflamed mucosa. The surface epithelium often shows mild nuclear hyperchromasia, slight nuclear elongation, and mucin loss. However, the N:C ratio is usually preserved. In contrast, dysplastic changes often show an abrupt transition between normal and abnormal glands. Nuclear hyperchromasia, elongation, stratification, atypical mitotic activity, and increased N:C ratio, without evidence of surface maturation are features that support a diagnosis of dysplasia.

More recently, Waters et al. proposed using cytologic architecture of the surface columnar epithelium to separate non-dysplastic from dysplastic BE.[527] Based on this system, BE that is negative for dysplasia typically maintains its cellular architecture in the surface columnar epithelium. This architecture has been referred to as the 4-line architecture with line 1 being the gastric type mucin vacuole, line 2 being the base of the mucin vacuole, line 3 being the cytoplasm and line 4 being the nuclei. In contrast, dysplastic epithelium typically does not normally maintain this 4-line architecture and is accompanied by loss of the apical mucin vacuole and nuclear stratification wherein the nuclei are no longer aligned side by side from cell to cell with a line of cytoplasm above them. Using these criteria, the authors noticed a 50% reduction in the proportion of cases diagnosed as indefinite for dysplasia.

Low-Grade Dysplasia versus High-Grade Dysplasia

Because dysplasia progresses to cancer on a continuous (linear) scale, no well-defined cutoff points separate low- from high-grade dysplasia. In general, the overall grade of dysplasia is determined by the most abnormal (highest-grade) epithelium. However, the absolute number or proportion of high-grade dysplastic crypts that is necessary to upgrade a biopsy specimen from low to high grade has never been investigated. Furthermore, not only the presence but also the extent of dysplasia is an important prognostic parameter in patients with BE (see later discussion). Therefore, a practical approach for pathologists to use is to report the highest grade of dysplasia in a particular biopsy specimen and to indicate also, whenever possible, the relative proportion of low- versus high-grade dysplasia within that specimen. For instance, one may sign-out a biopsy as "BE with dysplasia, predominantly low-grade but with focal high-grade." Fortunately, regardless of the proportion of high-grade dysplasia, a patient with a diagnosis of HGD typically undergoes a repeat endoscopy using high-definition white light endoscopy after a period of 6-8 weeks to evaluate for the presence of a visible lesion, which is then removed by EMR.

High-Grade Dysplasia versus Intramucosal Adenocarcinoma

At the high end of the spectrum of neoplasia, the degree of architectural distortion may reach a point at which a diagnosis of intramucosal carcinoma is impossible to exclude with complete certainty (Fig. 14.42),[516] particularly when glands grow in a cribriform or back-to-back pattern or contain intraluminal necrotic debris. In such cases, a diagnosis of "high-grade dysplasia with features suspicious for adenocarcinoma," as advocated by the Vienna classification, may be most appropriate. If the treatment differs for these two diagnoses, further biopsies and an EMR are justified. In a study at the Cleveland Clinic, overall agreement among several GI pathologists for distinguishing high-grade dysplasia from intramucosal adenocarcinoma was only fair (κ = 0.30).[504] These data call into question clinical management decisions that are based solely on a pathologist's ability to differentiate high-grade dysplasia from intramucosal carcinoma in mucosal biopsy specimens. Because many institutions now consider EMR followed by ablative therapy to be the main form of treatment for high-grade dysplasia or intramucosal adenocarcinoma and reserve esophagectomy for treatment of submucosal adenocarcinoma, it becomes less important for pathologists to distinguish these two situations.

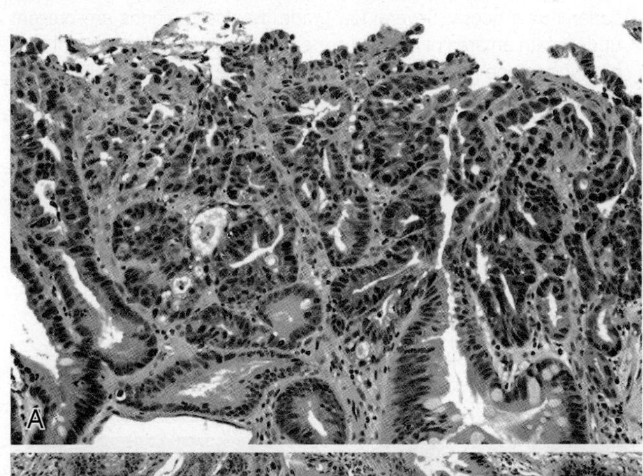

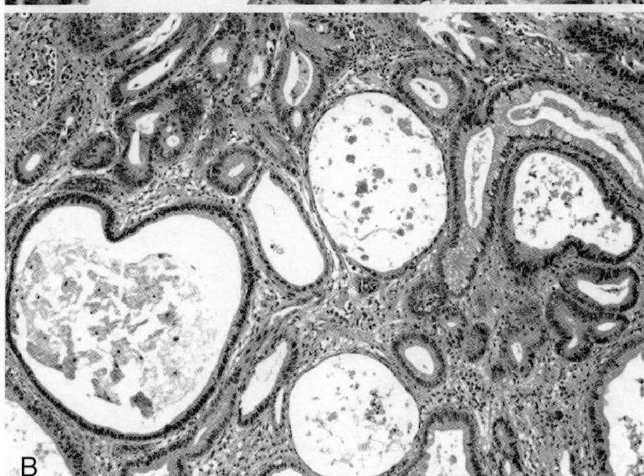

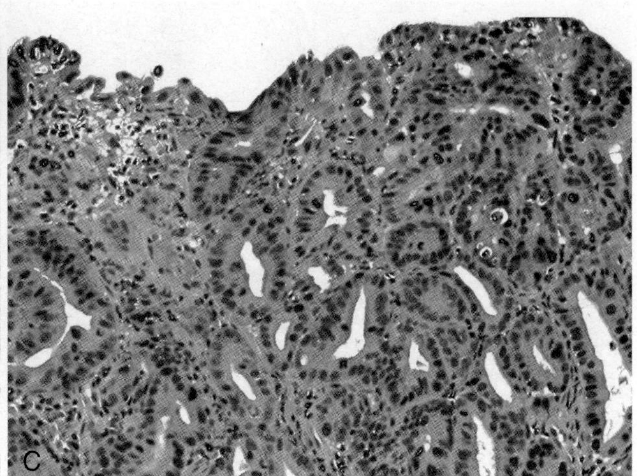

FIGURE 14.42 High-grade dysplasia with foci suspicious for intramucosal adenocarcinoma. A, High-grade dysplastic crypts are bordering an area of crowded crypts suspicious for intramucosal adenocarcinoma. One small crypt, on the left side of the field, also contains intraluminal necrosis. **B,** Diffuse high-grade dysplasia with cystically dilated dysplastic crypts at the base of the mucosa contains luminal necrotic debris suspicious for intramucosal adenocarcinoma. **C,** High-grade dysplastic crypts show a tight back-to-back gland pattern without intervening lamina propria—features quite suspicious for intramucosal adenocarcinoma.

Intramucosal versus Submucosal Adenocarcinoma

Dysplastic glands may be located between frayed fibers of muscularis mucosae, and differentiation of misplaced noninvasive dysplastic epithelium from truly invasive epithelium can be difficult. One must be cautious not to overinterpret entrapped glands as indicative of invasive tumor, particularly if the glands contain cytologically bland or only low-grade dysplastic features. Because tangentially sectioned pieces of tissue may impart a false appearance of invasion into the muscularis mucosae, possible invasion should be considered only in well-oriented, and preferably deep, biopsy specimens. Given that most patients with BE have a duplicated muscularis mucosae, dysplastic glands that invade into, or even through, the new (superficial) muscularis mucosae are still considered "intramucosal" for management purposes.[528] However, in most superficial and even jumbo-forceps–derived mucosal biopsies, the deep (original) muscularis mucosae is not evident. Determination of true submucosal invasion is not possible in that circumstance.

Squamous Overgrowth (Buried Barrett's Esophagus)

As a result of newer, more effective methods of medical (i.e., PPIs) and surgical antireflux therapy and use of ablative forms of endoscopic therapy, squamous reepithelialization of the Barrett's segment (neosquamous epithelium) or islands of squamous mucosa within BE develop in many patients with BE (Fig. 14.43).[529] In patients who have not had endoscopic ablation, buried metaplasia can be found at the SCJ in up to 28% of cases[530] and at squamous islands in as many as 38.5% of cases.[531] In treated patients, buried metaplasia has been found more frequently after photodynamic therapy than after RFA. In 22 reports describing the results of photodynamic therapy for 953 patients with BE, buried metaplasia was found in 135 patients (14.2%) during follow-up intervals that ranged from 4 weeks to more than 5 years. In 18 reports describing the results of RFA for 1004 patents, buried metaplasia was found in only 9 patients (0.9%) during follow-up of 8 weeks to 5 years.[532] Several studies have demonstrated a complete absence of buried metaplasia, or buried dysplasia, in almost 100% of patients after RFA.[533-535] Subsquamous neoplasia has been reported in several patients after RFA of BE.[536]

The neoplastic potential of buried nondysplastic Barrett's epithelium is unknown. Studies suggest that buried Barrett's epithelium, particularly glands that are not in contact with the luminal surface, have significantly lower crypt proliferation rates and increased DNA stability than crypts exposed to the luminal surface.[455,537] Nevertheless, patients who have undergone endoscopic ablation should continue to have surveillance biopsies obtained from the areas of reepithelialized squamous mucosa over the entire original length of the Barrett's segment to exclude buried dysplasia or

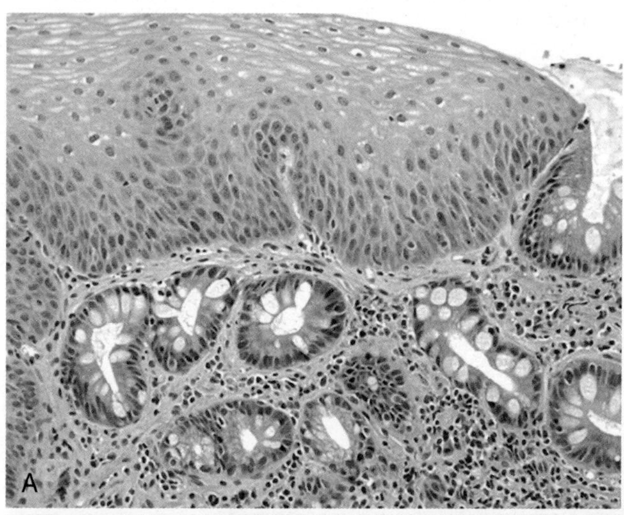

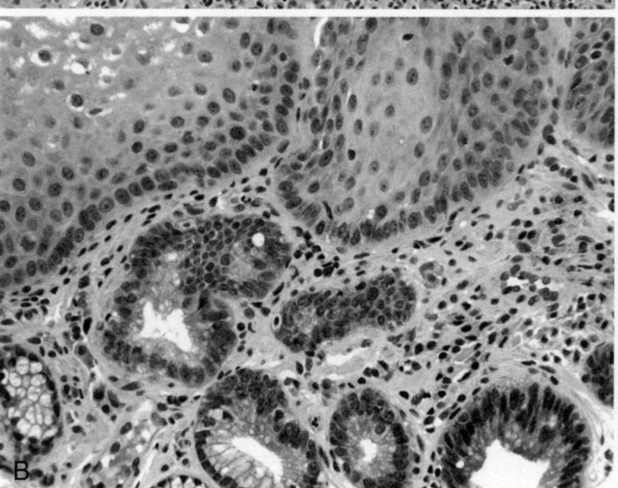

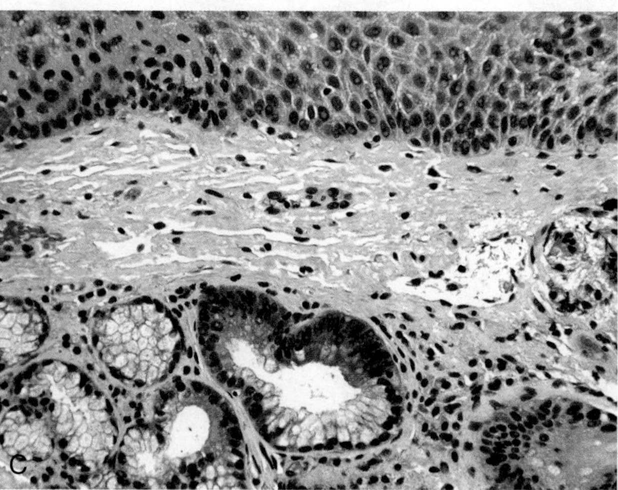

FIGURE 14.43 A, Barrett's esophagus without dysplasia present underneath squamous mucosa, also called buried Barrett's esophagus. **B**, Low-grade dysplasia situated underneath islands of reepithelialized squamous mucosa. Several low-grade dysplastic glands are present underneath an area of reactive squamous epithelium in a patient who had undergone photodynamic therapy. **C,** The dysplastic cells involve the mucosal glands, and there is an abrupt transition between nondysplastic mucinous cells and dysplastic columnar cells.

adenocarcinoma. Buried BE may show marked regenerative changes, such as nuclear hyperchromasia, nuclear stratification, prominent nucleoli, and increased mitotic activity in a background of mild lamina propria inflammation. Pathological evaluation of dysplasia is particularly challenging because the cardinal features used in evaluation of traditional dysplasia, including involvement of the upper crypts and surface epithelium, which help differentiate regenerating epithelium from true dysplasia, are absent. In these cases, the degree of cytologic atypia and architectural complexity that helps distinguish traditional low-grade from high-grade dysplasia should be applied. However, pathologists should be extremely careful not to overdiagnose dysplasia in cases of buried atypical epithelium that shows borderline features between regeneration and dysplasia. In some cases, a diagnosis of indefinite for dysplasia may be appropriate.

Adjunctive Diagnostic Tests of Dysplasia

There are few, if any, reliable adjunctive diagnostic techniques for differentiating nondysplastic from dysplastic epithelium in mucosal biopsy specimens from the esophagus.[463] Markers such as Ki67, PCNA, cyclin D1, TP53, and insulin-like growth factor-II mRNA-binding protein 3 (IGF2BP3, or IMP3)[538] have not been shown to be clinically useful in this regard.[466,539] Although several studies have shown that the extent and distribution of Ki67 staining correlates with increasing grades of dysplasia, regenerating epithelium may also demonstrate increased proliferation, which in some instances can approach the degree seen in high-grade dysplasia.[463,493] Similarly, although the frequency of p53-positive staining has also been shown to be proportional to the grade of dysplasia and may have predictive value in assessing risk of malignancy in patients with BE (discussed later), p53 may also be detected in as many as 10% of biopsy specimens that are histologically negative for dysplasia, and its staining results have high false-positive and false-negative rates (Table 14.13).[463,539] Regardless, in some parts of the world, p53 is used for detection and confirmation of dysplasia. Kastelein et al evaluated p53 immunohistochemical staining patterns in esophageal biopsy samples from 635 patients with BE with clinical follow-up. They found aberrant p53 staining in 11% of biopsy samples without dysplasia, 38% in low-grade dysplasia, 83% in high-grade dysplasia, and in 100% of adenocarcinomas.[469] Kaye et al. found that adding p53 immunostain to histological evaluation decreased interobserver variability with respect to dysplasia classification, and also increased the predictive value of the histological diagnoses.[540] However, in the USA, none of these markers, including p53, are advocated for routine diagnostic use in patients with BE.

One marker of potential diagnostic value is alpha methylacyl-CoA racemase (AMACR), an enzyme involved in β-oxidation of branched-chain fatty acids that has been used as a biomarker in neoplasms from the colorectum, stomach, and prostate gland. In one large study by Dorer and Odze, AMACR staining was negative in all cases of BE considered negative for dysplasia, compared with 38% positivity in low-grade dysplasia cases, 81% in high-grade dysplasia cases, and 72% in adenocarcinomas.[541] Subsequent studies have reported similar findings.[542-544] However, one other study suggests that the sensitivity of this technique is low.[545] Thus, because of the low sensitivity, but high specificity, of AMACR for dysplastic epithelium in BE, a positive result may be helpful to establish a diagnosis of dysplasia in diagnostically difficult cases, but an absence of staining does not necessarily rule out true dysplasia in an atypical focus.

TABLE 14.13 Rate of p53 Expression In Nondysplastic Barrett's Esophagus and Neoplastic Lesions

Diagnostic Category	Rate of p53 Expression
Negative for dysplasia	0 - 11%
Low-grade dysplasia	60 - 95%
High-grade dysplasia/ Adenocarcinoma	83% - 100%

Data from Jones DR et al. Ann Thorac Surg. 1994 Mar;57(3):598-603; Srivastava A et al. Am J Surg Pathol. Volume 41, Number 5, May 2017.

IMP3, also known as K-homologous domain–containing protein (KOC)[546] and L523S, is an oncofetal mRNA-binding protein that regulates transcription of insulin-like growth factor II (IGF-II) and is involved in embryogenesis. In normal tissue, its expression is confined to the placenta. However, it is also present in many neoplastic cells, including carcinoma of the uterine cervix, endometrium (specifically, endometrial serous carcinoma), ovaries, pancreas, kidney, stomach, colon, rectum, lungs, and thyroid.[547-551] In one study, strong cytoplasmic granular expression was reported in 94% of invasive EACs, 93% of metastatic EACs, and 49% of high-grade dysplasia. In contrast, 14% of low-grade dysplasia and 7% of BE without dysplasia were positive.[538]

Biomarkers of Barrett's Esophagus

Many studies have attempted to define various clinical, endoscopic, pathological, immunohistochemical, and molecular markers to help predict the development of cancer in patients with BE.[397,398,486,490] Clinically, as mentioned earlier, the presence of a hiatus hernia and the length of BE have been associated with an increased risk of progression to cancer.[552] In a study from Southern Europe, the annual risk of EAC was 0.57% for patients with long-segment BE but only 0.26% for patients with short-segment disease.[553] In a prospective study of 550 patients by Weston et al, patients with less than 6 cm had a 2.4% risk of progression to cancer, compared with a 6.8% risk in those with more than 6 cm of BE.[486] However, cancer may develop even in patients with short or ultrashort segments of BE.[554,555] There are a number of genetic and epigenetic alterations that occur in BE, and early stage esophageal cancer, that have the potential to be used as predictive biomarkers of BE progression, and some of these are discussed further below.

A number of markers have been studied to risk stratify BE patients with the goal of potentially sparing the "low risk" group from the cost, inconvenience and risks associated with routine endoscopic surveillance. Of these markers, p53 and aneuploidy have been the most extensively studied.[464,491,494] For instance, in a study by Younes and coworkers[539] and another by Weston and coworkers,[556] the frequency and degree of p53 staining (in nondysplastic epithelium) was shown to correlate with an increased risk of progression to high-grade dysplasia or cancer.[539,556] In one of the largest studies to date (n=635 patients), aberrant p53 immunostaining was found to be significantly associated with the risk of neoplastic progression after adjusting for age, gender, BE length, and esophagitis (relative risk [RR] 5.6 [95% CI 3.1–10.3] and RR 14.0 [95% CI 5.3–37.2], respectively). However, only 49% of patients who progressed had aberrant p53 immunostaining, which significantly limits its potential clinical utility.[557,558] Although this assay is not currently advocated for routine diagnostic use due to concerns related to low sensitivity and reproducibility, there is emerging data to suggest that evaluation of p53 abnormalities can contribute to risk prediction in patients with nondysplastic BE.

DNA content abnormalities (as detected by flow cytometry or, more recently, by image cytometry) and genetic alterations in *TP53* and *CDKN2A* appear to be the most promising biomarkers studied to date.[464] DNA aneuploidy, increased 4N fraction, and S-phase fraction all increase in prevalence with histological progression of dysplasia in BE. In one flow cytometry study by Reid and colleagues, none of the patients who were without detectable DNA content abnormalities in their baseline biopsies progressed to adenocarcinoma within 5 years, compared with 28% of BE patients who had either aneuploidy or increased 4N fraction.[494] Moreover, DNA content abnormalities have been shown to have predictive value independent of the histological grade of dysplasia.[559] Data show that a combination of biomarkers is more predictive of cancer risk than single markers. For instance, in one long-term follow-up study of more than 200 patients with BE, 79% of those who had a combination of 17p LOH, DNA content abnormalities, and 9p LOH showed progression to adenocarcinoma within 10 years, compared with only 12% of those who were without any baseline genetic abnormalities.[491] Additional information on nonmorphology-based biomarkers can be found in several articles.[490,550,560,561]

A variety of somatic mutations, aberrantly methylated genes, overexpressed miRNAs, as well as deregulated proteins have also been investigated as tools for BE patients who are at a high-risk of progression to cancer. For instance, loss of 9p encompassing the p16/CDKN2A locus has been found in BE, HGD and EAC cases. Both HGD and EAC can harbor losses on chromosome 5q, 13q and 18q while high-level amplification at ERBB2 on chromosome 17q has been documented in EAC.[562] More recently, a combined panel of methylated *VIM* and methylated C*CNA1* DNAs was recently shown to detect 95% of BE, dysplasia and EAC cases at 91% specificity, including detecting 96% of BE with dysplasia and 96% of EAC.[563]

With regard to morphology, studies have suggested that both the presence and the extent of dysplasia affect the risk that cancer will develop in BE.[495,522,564] In one study of 100 patients with BE and high-grade dysplasia, the risk for adenocarcinoma was greater in those who had "diffuse" high-grade dysplasia (i.e., involving ≥5 crypts in a single biopsy specimen or present in more than one biopsy fragment) than in those with "focal" high-grade dysplasia (involving a single focus or <5 crypts).[495] However, another study failed to confirm these findings and instead showed a lack of correlation between "diffuse" dysplasia and cancer at esophagectomy.[564] Finally, in a comprehensive case-control study that evaluated the relationship between extent of dysplasia and the development of adenocarcinoma, a strong association was observed between the extent of low-grade dysplasia (expressed as the proportion of dysplastic crypts among the total number of crypts per patient) and the development of adenocarcinoma; of 77 patients with BE, 44 eventually developed carcinoma during long-term endoscopic surveillance.[522] Therefore, from a pathologist's perspective, it seems reasonable to attempt to define both the presence and grade of dysplasia and the extent of dysplasia when evaluating biopsy specimens from patients with BE.

Tissue Acquisition Techniques for Biomarker Assessment

Non-endoscopic technologies for sampling BE have also gained significant interest as they are minimally invasive and have the potential for widespread applicability in the primary care setting (Table 14.14). These technologies include Cytosponge, which is an encapsulated sponge tethered to a string, which when swallowed and withdrawn out of the esophagus, collects cells from the esophageal lumen.[565] EsophaCap, a sponge-on-string device that is similar to but slightly smaller than Cytosponge, has been used in combination with methylated DNA biomarkers for diagnosing BE.[566] Another such device is EsoCheck, which uses a swallowable encapsulated balloon device to sample the distal esophagus.[567]

Wide area transepithelial sampling with computer-assisted three-dimensional analysis of disaggregated tissue specimens, termed WATS3D, is an approach that has shown enhanced detection rates of intestinal metaplasia and dysplasia in BE.[568] Compared to forceps biopsies, WATS3D samples a much broader area of mucosa, reducing sampling error. Also, the procedure has been associated with decreased interobserver variability in readings.

Another novel approach is based on assaying volatile organic compounds (VOCs) by detecting conductance changes in the patient's breath. Exhaled VOCs are analyzed to create a BE breath profile, which can then be possibly used as a noninvasive screening tool for identifying BE.[569]

Natural History and Risk of Malignancy

The absolute annual cancer risk of patients with BE without dysplasia is approximately 0.1% to 0.5% per year.[570-573] A recent meta-analysis that included 57 studies demonstrated a pooled annual incidence of cancer in patients with nondysplastic BE was 0.33% (95% CI 0.28- 0.38%), lower than what has been previously reported (Table 14.15).[424] In patients with short segment BE, the annual risk of cancer is 0.19%.

The natural history of low-grade dysplasia in BE is more controversial. Some studies have found that the risk of cancer is no greater than in patients with nondysplastic BE,[403,465,574] whereas others have observed higher rates.[497,522,524] Reported progression rates vary between 1% and 47%.[497,522,523,525,556,575] One reason for this uncertainty is the high degree of interobserver variability in the diagnosis of low-grade dysplasia, even among experienced GI pathologists.[497,524] This theory is supported by the observation that, among patients whose diagnosis of low-grade dysplasia was confirmed by two or more pathologists, the incidence of cancer is substantially higher (5.2 - 9.1%) than among patients whose diagnosis was based on one pathologist's observation.[497,524-526] In a study by Srivastava and

TABLE 14.14 Novel Methods for Screening and Surveillance In Barrett's Esophagus

Method	Sample Obtained and Parameter Assayed	Advantages	Proposed Use
Imaging-Based Techniques			
Narrow band imaging (virtual chromoendoscopy)	Mucosal biopsy, histology	Wide-field imaging, enhances mucosal pit pattern and superficial vasculature of the mucosa	Detection and surveillance
Transnasal endoscopy	Mucosal biopsy, histology	Ultrathin endoscope; better tolerance; no sedation	Detection and surveillance
Capsule endoscopy	No sample obtained	Safe and portable, allows visualization of esophagus without obtaining biopsy	Detection and surveillance
Confocal laser endomicroscopy	Imaging-targeted mucosal biopsy, histology	In vivo histology, probe can be used in any endoscope	Detection and surveillance
Optical coherence tomography	Imaging-targeted mucosal biopsy	In vivo assessment of tissue architecture, no contrast; ability for subsurface imaging	Detection and surveillance
Detection of volatile content in breath (Breath biopsy)	Volatile organic compounds	Create a Barrett's breath profile	Screening
Blood, Stool, or Saliva Biomarker-Based Assays	Blood, stool or saliva, detect methylated DNA, circulating microRNAs, metabolite panels and peptides	Easy access of samples and safety of collection	Screening and/or surveillance
New Esophageal Collection Devices			
Sponge-on-string and encapsulated balloon devices (Cytosponge, EsophaCap, EsoCheck)	Exfoliated cells at the GEJ and from the entire length of the esophagus	Safe, portable, does not require sedation	Screening and surveillance
WATS3D	Brush smear of esophageal lining epithelium	Samples broader area of mucosa, reducing sampling error, uses artificial neural network to create 3-dimensional images of sampled cytology specimens	Screening and surveillance

TABLE 14.15 Risk of Neoplastic Progression in Barrett's Esophagus

Barrett's Esophagus	Risk of Progression to HGD or Cancer (or to Cancer for HGD) per 100 Person-Years	Annualized Rate of Progression
Negative for dysplasia	EAC: 0.33 HGD/EAC: 0.26-0.68	0.2%-0.5% per year
Crypt dysplasia	1.42 per patient-year*	Unknown
LGD	EAC: 0.54-2.51 HGD/EAC: 1.73-5.18	0.4%-13.4% per year
HGD	EAC: 6.6	5%-8% per year

EAC, Esophageal adenocarcinoma; HGD, high-grade dysplasia; LGD, low-grade dysplasia.

**Data based on Shaheen NJ, Smith MS, Odze RD. Gastrointest Endosc. 2021;S0016-51075.*

associates[522] in which three GI pathologists agreed on all diagnoses of low- or high-grade dysplasia in biopsies from 77 patients with BE, 45% of those with a maximum diagnosis of low-grade dysplasia progressed to adenocarcinoma during the follow-up interval. In the same study, it was suggested that the "extent" of low-grade dysplasia, defined as the proportion of crypts that exhibit dysplastic change, was a highly significant risk factor for development of cancer. Other factors, such as variability in the number of biopsies and frequency of surveillance endoscopy, presence or absence of a visible lesion (e.g., polyp, stricture, nodule, ulcer), and lack of distinction between prevalent and incident dysplasia may affect the reported progression rates of low-grade dysplasia.

The progression rate of low- or high-grade dysplasia to cancer is also affected by the growth pattern of the lesion. For instance, high-grade dysplasia associated with a nodule has an association with cancer in 60% of cases, compared with only 23% for high-grade dysplasia without an endoscopic abnormality. In a recent follow up study consisting of 318 patients with non dysplastic BE and 301 with LGD, 7 (1.1%) BE and 21 (3.4%) LGD subjects progressed to HGD/EAC in the follow up period. In this study, BE length [hazards ratio (HR), 1.16; 95% confidence interval (CI), 1.03-1.29], presence of nodularity (HR, 4.98; 95% CI, 1.80-11.7), and baseline LGD (HR, 2.57; 95% CI, 1.13-6.57) were significant predictors of progression on multivariate analysis.[576] Finally, a small proportion of patients may develop adenocarcinoma without seemingly progressing sequentially through all stages of metaplasia and dysplasia.[574] In fact, some reports have revealed patients who developed cancer even though their prior surveillance biopsies showed only metaplasia, but not dysplasia. Of course, this finding may have resulted from a failure to detect dysplasia as a result of sampling error.[574,577]

The risk of cancer in patients with HGD was examined in a meta-analysis of 4 studies and 236 patients. In this study, the weighted annual incidence rate of cancer was found to be 7% (95% CI 5–8).[578] However, the AIM-Dysplasia trial that randomized 127 patients with dysplasia to ablation therapy compared with surveillance reported a much higher yearly progression rate of 19% in the HGD surveillance arm.[458]

The wide range in the incidence rates is partially explained by differences in outcome among patients with "prevalent" versus "incident" dysplasia. *Prevalent* dysplasia is defined as dysplasia that is detected at the initial screening endoscopy or during the first 12 months of surveillance. *Incident* dysplasia is dysplasia that is detected during the course of endoscopic surveillance and, therefore, is presumably less advanced in terms of its natural history. Another possible source of variability in the reported rates of EAC in patients with BE is that patients with intestinal metaplasia of the gastric cardia or GEJ were included in some of the pathology registry-based studies.

Treatment

Most patients with BE (>95%) live relatively normal lives without developing cancer, and their treatment is predominantly aimed at controlling acid reflux and monitoring dysplasia. Although endoscopic surveillance remains controversial because of a lack of randomized trials supporting its value, many retrospective studies indicate that survival is statistically enhanced if cancers are detected earlier by endoscopic surveillance.[579-581] It is recommended that endoscopic surveillance follow the so-called Seattle protocol, which mandates four-quadrant biopsies, with jumbo biopsy forceps, obtained from every 2 cm of Barrett's mucosa and from every 1 cm within previously known dysplastic areas, with targeted biopsies of all grossly apparent mucosal abnormalities (Table 14.16).[519] Cases without dysplasia or with

TABLE 14.16 Recommendations For Surveillance And Management Of Barrett's Esophagus

Society (Year)	Negative for Dysplasia	Indefinite for Dysplasia	Low-Grade Dysplasia	High-Grade Dysplasia
AGA (2011)	• EGD every 3-5 years	• Not specified	• EGD every 6-12 months • Consider endoscopic eradication therapy	• EGD every 3 months • Endoscopic eradication therapy rather than surveillance or surgery
• ASGE (2012)	• EGD every 3-5 years • Consider no surveillance • Consider ablation in select cases	• Repeat EGD with maximal acid suppression	• Repeat EGD in 6 months to confirm LGD • EGD every year • Consider endoscopic therapy	• EGD every 3 months (only patients who are not candidates for endoscopic or surgical treatment) • Consider endoscopic treatment • Consider surgical consultation
• BSG (2014)	• Irregular Z-line: no surveillance • BE <3 cm without IM: no surveillance • BE <3 cm with IM: EGD every 3-5 years • BE ≥3 cm: EGD every 2-3 years • Consider no surveillance on the basis of patient's fitness and risk of progression	• Repeat EGD at 6 months with maximal acid suppression	• Surveillance: EGD every 6 months • Ablation cannot be recommended routinely	• Mucosal irregularity: EMR • Endoscopic therapy is preferred over esophagectomy or surveillance
• ACG (2016)	• EGD every 3-5 years	• Repeat EGD at 3-6 months after optimization of acid suppression • Persistent indefinite for dysplasia: EGD after 1 year	• Endoscopic treatment (patients without life-limiting comorbidity) • EGD every 12 months	• Endoscopic treatment (patients without life-limiting comorbidity)
• ESGE (2017)	• BE <1 cm: no surveillance • BE 1-3 cm: EGD every 5 years • BE 3-10 cm: EGD every 3 years • BE ≥10 cm: referral to BE expert center • Consider discharge for patients with limited life expectancy and advanced age	• Repeat EGD at 6 months with optimization of anti-reflux medication	• Repeat EGD at 6 months • If persistent LGD: endoscopic ablation	• Repeat EGD • Visible irregularity: EMR • Persistent HGD: ablation • No dysplasia: repeat EGD at 3 months

ACG, American College of Gastroenterology; AGA, American Gastroenterological Association; ASGE, American Society of Gastrointestinal Endoscopy; BSG, British Society of Gastroenterology ; EGD, esophagogastroduodenoscopy ; EMR, endoscopic mucosal resection; ESGE, European Society of Gastrointestinal Endoscopy

indefinite or low-grade dysplasia are typically managed by endoscopic surveillance according to guidelines put forth by the ACG and AGA (see Chapter 2).[379,517,582] In brief, the current guidelines recommend a follow-up surveillance interval of 3 years if two consecutive endoscopies with biopsy within 1 year show an absence of dysplasia. Cases diagnosed as indefinite for dysplasia are usually treated more aggressively with antireflux medication to decrease the amount of inflammation, followed by rebiopsy after 3 to 6 months to reevaluate the indefinite focus. However, in some institutions, such cases are managed similarly to low-grade dysplasia. For cases of low-grade dysplasia, a repeat examination within 3–6 months with high-definition white-light endoscopy (HD WLE), and preferably optical chromoendoscopy, should be performed to rule out the presence of a visible lesion, which should prompt endoscopic resection. In a recent meta-analysis (19 studies and 2746 patients), the impact of RFA was evaluated in LGD patients. This analysis showed a significant reduction of progression in the RFA arm compared with the surveillance arm (RR 0.14%; 95% confidence interval [CI], 0.04–0.45; p=0.001) The cumulative rate of progression to high-grade dysplasia/EAC was lower in RFA compared with surveillance (1.7% vs. 12.6%, p <0.001).[583] Thus, after repeating an endoscopic procedure using HD-WLE, if no HGD is found, then both RFA and continued endoscopic surveillance are reasonable options for patients with LGD (Table 14.12).[517]

The management of high-grade dysplasia is more controversial and variable among different institutions. The finding of high-grade dysplasia in flat mucosa should lead to confirmation by an expert GI pathologist and a subsequent endoscopy using high-definition white light endoscopy within 6-8 weeks, with biopsies to rule out visible HGD. Continued surveillance or definitive intervention is typically determined on an individual basis. Patients who have high-grade dysplasia with mucosal irregularity should undergo EMR.[379] Updated AGA guidelines recommend endoscopic ablation (e.g., RFA) after EMR for visible lesions (Table 14.16).[517,584] The updated ACG and AGA guidelines[379,517] recommend that all dysplasia diagnoses should be confirmed by at least one experienced GI pathologist before treatment is instituted.

Endoscopic Ablation

Endoscopic mucosal ablative therapies are categorized into tissue-acquiring (i.e., EMR) and non–tissue-acquiring types. The latter group includes RFA, photodynamic therapy, thermal ablation techniques, argon plasma coagulation, and cryotherapy. Here, the most commonly used techniques and the histopathologic implications for the surgical pathologist are outlined.

RFA is the most common, and most effective, mucosal ablation technique and is rapidly gaining widespread acceptance worldwide. It is a form of ablation that uses high-frequency electrical current to destroy target tissue by thermal heating. It can be applied in a stepwise circumferential fashion or as a focal ablation procedure. Primary circumferential ablation is performed with the use of a balloon-shaped bipolar electrode that has been sized to fit a specific outer diameter. The ablation catheter is inflated, and, on contact with mucosa, radiofrequency energy is delivered to the electrode. Secondary treatment of residual or focal islands of Barrett's mucosa may be performed with an endoscope-mounted bipolar electrode on an articulated platform.[585] Shaheen and colleagues[458] conducted a multicenter, sham-controlled trial in which 127 patients with dysplastic BE were randomly assigned, in a 2:1 ratio, to receive either RFA or a sham procedure (control group). Participants were randomly assigned according to the length of Barrett's mucosa and grade of dysplasia. In the intention-to-treat analyses, among patients with high-grade dysplasia, complete eradication occurred in 81.0% of those in the ablation group but only 19% of those in the control group ($P < .001$) after 12 months of follow-up. Among all patients, complete eradication of all intestinal metaplasia occurred in 77.4% of the treatment group and 2.9% of controls. Progression of high-grade dysplasia to cancer was reported in only 2.4% of the RFA group compared with 19% of controls. The mean number of RFA treatments in the study group was 3.5. Adverse effects included chest discomfort, which usually resolved by 8 days after therapy, and strictures in 6% of patients. Predictors of complete eradication included younger age, shorter Barrett's segment, lower body mass index, and shorter history of dysplasia.[458] After 3 years, dysplasia remained eradicated in more than 85% of patients, and intestinal metaplasia in more than 75%.

RFA has an acceptable safety profile, is durable, and is associated with a low risk of disease progression.[586] One systematic review[587] suggested that success rates with RFA are superior, with approximately 90% of patients showing no high-grade dysplasia after therapy, and this effect seems to be maintained over time.[458,588-591] Despite the success of RFA in eradicating dysplasia, however, its efficacy for eradication of intestinal metaplasia varies widely. Complete response rates range from 46% and 98%.[458,533,590-592] Based on these data, RFA is not considered cost-effective for patients with BE without dysplasia.[593] Factors associated with persistent intestinal metaplasia after RFA therapy include baseline dysplasia, severity of ongoing reflux exposure, hiatal hernia size, and length of Barrett's mucosa.[594,595] The rate of recurrence of intestinal metaplasia following RFA is approximately 8%–10% per patient-year of follow-up, and it may occur more commonly early in follow-up rather than in later years. A recent meta-analysis of 39 prospective and retrospective studies that evaluated the recurrent rates of intestinal metaplasia and dysplasia after complete eradication of BE showed that the pooled incidence of any recurrence (intestinal metaplasia or dysplasia) including patients treated with RFA with or without EMR and stepwise complete EMR was 7.5 (95% CI, 6.1 – 9.0)/100 patient years; pooled incidence of IM recurrence rate was 4.8 (95%CI 3.8 – 5.9)/100 patient years, and dysplasia recurrence rate was 2.0 (95%CI 1.5 – 2.5)/100 patient years. Compared to the complete EMR group, the RFA group had significantly higher overall [8.6 (6.7 – 10.5)/100 patient years vs. 5.1 (3.1 – 7)/100 PY, P = 0.01] and IM recurrence rates [5.8 (4.3 – 7.3)/100 PY vs. 3.1 (1.7 – 4)/100 patient years, P < 0.01] with no difference in recurrence rates of dysplasia. This analysis also highlighted significant heterogeneity in recurrence rates across studies, with most recurrences being amenable to repeat endoscopic eradication therapy.[596] Interestingly, majority of recurrences are detected in the distal 2 cm of the esophagus. Thus, given the not so insignificant rates of recurrences, it is recommended that the entire neosquamous mucosa should be sampled starting immediately above the GEJ.[517]

Photodynamic therapy is based on the ability of chemical agents known as photosensitizers to produce cytotoxicity in the presence of oxygen after stimulation by light at an appropriate wavelength. After intravenous administration, the photosensitizer is retained at higher concentration by the neoplastic tissue. Approximately 48 hours later, photoradiation is performed endoscopically with the use of lasers in conjunction with cylindrical fibers or localizing balloons. The target tissue is destroyed and reepithelializes with squamous mucosa. In a study of 208 patients randomly assigned to photodynamic therapy plus PPI versus PPI alone, photodynamic therapy with porfimer sodium, 630-nm red light, and photoradiating balloons was shown to decrease the risk of carcinoma by 50% after 48 months of follow-up.[597,598] One important drawback of this technique is that the photosensitizers are also taken up by other tissues, so patients are warned to avoid direct sunlight and excessive room light for 4 weeks after treatment. Vomiting, chest pain, and strictures develop in as much as 36% of patients.[597]

Endoscopic Resection

In most major centers, endoscopic mucosal resection (EMR) has become the standard of care as a diagnostic, as well as therapeutic, method of managing patients with BE who have high-grade dysplasia, intramucosal adenocarcinoma, or, in some cases, early invasive adenocarcinoma.[229,599] EMR is particularly recommended for visible neoplastic lesions. In this technique, the endoscopist injects saline into the submucosa to lift the tissue into the lumen and enhance the ability to remove the tissue with clean, deep resection margins. Failure of the lesion to lift with saline injection is considered a poor prognostic sign; it may preclude obtaining adequate deep margins and increases the chance of finding a more advanced (invasive) tumor. Endoscopic submucosal dissection (ESD) is another recent method that is rapidly gaining popularity as a means of en-bloc resection for visible neoplastic lesions.

In the evaluation of EMR or ESD specimens, pathologists should (1) designate and ink (lateral and deep) margins for evaluation of completeness of resection (Fig. 14.44), (2) stretch the specimen gently and mount it on small, premade slabs of wax or other substrates that can be easily removed from fixative containers, (3) photograph the specimen to correlate the histological with the endoscopic findings, (4) obtain serial tissue sections at 2-mm intervals after fixation, and (5) if applicable, obtain radial sections at both ends of the specimen to further evaluate the status of the lateral margins.

The diagnostic value of EMR and ESD specimens resides in the enhanced ability of pathologists to establish an accurate diagnosis and provide an accurate stage of invasion (if any) when compared with evaluation of mucosal biopsies. Interobserver agreement of BE-related neoplasia on EMR specimens is significantly higher than on pre-EMR biopsy specimens. This is probably related to larger tissue sampling and the ability to evaluate mucosal landmarks more easily.[518] Perfect agreement in tumor staging by EMR and esophagectomy was reported in a study[600] in which preoperative EMR findings were compared with those of subsequent histological examination of 25 esophagectomy specimens.

Pathology reports of EMR and ESD specimens (Box 14.2) should include (1) size of the specimen, (2) status of the circumferential/lateral margins and deep margin (it might also be informative to report whether the lateral margins are composed of metaplastic or squamous epithelium), (3) grade of the neoplastic lesion (low-grade, high-grade, intramucosal or invasive adenocarcinoma), (4) degree of differentiation, (5) depth of invasion, and (6) status of vascular invasion. The presence of vascular invasion may dictate further management.

An important aspect in the morphological examination of EMR and ESD specimens is to recognize the presence of a double layer of muscularis mucosae, which is almost always present in BE.[471,538,601,602] The muscularis mucosae layers are often not well delineated. They may appear as wisps of smooth muscle fibers located within the lamina propria (see Fig. 14.44, *B*). The deep layer represents the original muscularis mucosae, and the superficial layer is considered new. The superficial muscularis mucosae separates the lamina propria into two compartments that do not differ substantially

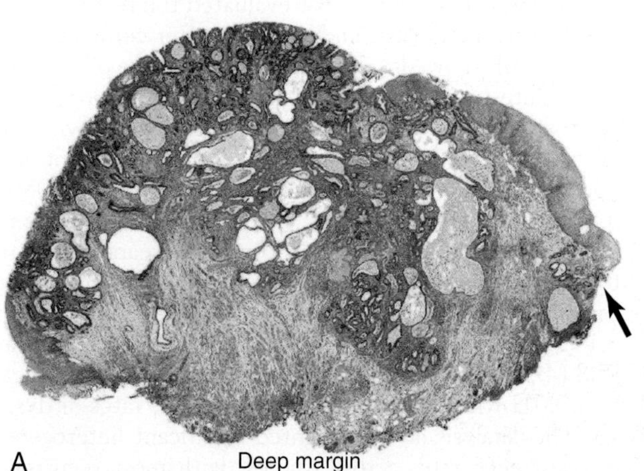

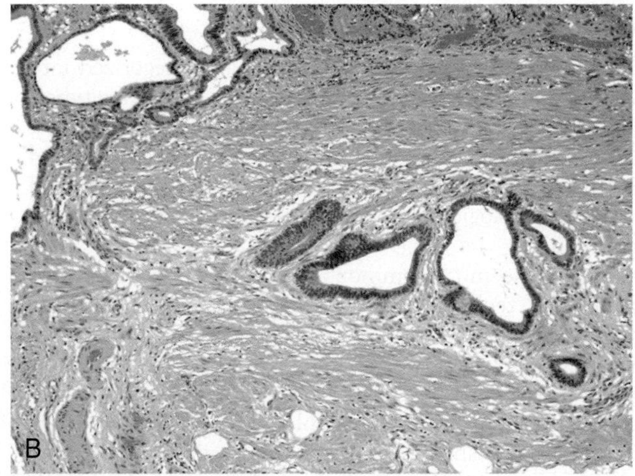

FIGURE 14.44 **A,** Intramucosal adenocarcinoma treated by endoscopic mucosal resection. The neoplastic glands involve the duplicated layers of the muscularis mucosae. There is appropriate inking of the deep and lateral margins. The deep margin and the lateral mucosal margin on the left are uninvolved, but the opposite lateral mucosal margin contains neoplastic glands (*arrow*). **B,** High-power magnification shows neoplastic glands between the original muscularis mucosae fibers and the layers of the superficial duplicated muscularis mucosae.

BOX 14.2 Endoscopic Mucosal Resection and Endoscopic Submucosal Dissection: The Role of the Pathologist

DIAGNOSTIC
- Staging
- Proper gross examination of the specimen including size along with designation of circumferential/lateral margins and deep margin
- Status of the circumferential/lateral margins and deep margin
- Type of epithelium at lateral margins (metaplastic or squamous epithelium)
- Grade of lesion (low-grade, high-grade, intramucosal, or invasive adenocarcinoma)
- Degree of differentiation (if adenocarcinoma)
- Depth of invasion; depth of invasion into submucosa (in microns) for submucosally invasive cancer
- Status of vascular invasion

THERAPEUTIC
- Removal of Barrett's mucosa with and without dysplasia and intramucosal adenocarcinoma
- EMR/ESD is often combined with RFA for ablation of remaining Barrett's mucosa
- Positive deep margin indicates need for further therapy

EMR, *Endoscopic mucosal resection;* RFA, *radiofrequency ablation;* ESD, *endoscopic submucosal dissection.*

in their vascular constituents.[471] Therefore, a diagnosis of submucosal invasive carcinoma (T1b or T1 submucosa) is justified only when the invasive component extends beyond the original (deeper muscle) layer.[603] The risk of lymph node metastasis in patients with intramucosal adenocarcinoma ranges from 0% to 7% of cases.[513-515,604] For patients whose tumors extend into the true submucosa, the frequency of lymph node metastasis often exceeds 20%.[513,514,605]

As mentioned above, assessing depth of submucosal invasion can also pose significant challenges. While dividing the submucosal compartment into three equal thirds (SM1, superficial one-third submucosa; SM2, intermediate one-third of submucosa and SM3, outer one-third of submucosa) is a good approach, it is often difficult to create these divisions due to the lack of muscularis propria in endoscopic resection specimens. As a result, the Paris classification recommends measurement of submucosal invasion in microns.[606] Depth of invasion in the submucosa should be measured from the outermost extent of the outer (deeper) muscularis mucosae. There is recent evidence to suggest that early stage, low-risk adenocarcinomas defined as pT1sm1 cancers with submucosal invasion ≤ 500 μm, without any other histological al risk factors for nodal metastasis may be managed by endoscopic therapy, followed by close endoscopic follow-up.[517]

In addition to its role in staging neoplasms in BE, EMR and ESD are occasionally used to eradicate Barrett's mucosa, high-grade dysplasia, intramucosal adenocarcinoma, and, in some cases, early Barrett's adenocarcinoma (see Box 14.2). Some cohort studies have found that EMR can achieve complete eradication of Barrett's mucosa in 75% to 100% of cases and complete eradication of dysplasia in 86% and 100% of cases.[607-611] However, the usefulness of EMR as a therapeutic procedure is limited by the high reported rates of positive margins, which vary from 62% to 83% in some studies, and by demonstration of metachronous lesions elsewhere in BE on follow-up.[612,613] Therefore, EMR is often combined with RFA for ablation of the remaining Barrett's mucosa. EMR combined with RFA is the best proven ablative therapy for visible high-grade dysplasia and for ablation of BE in patients with high-grade dysplasia.[584]

In many institutions, esophagectomy still remains an important method of treatment of BE with high-grade dysplasia, but it is usually reserved for treatment failures, for high-grade dysplasia not amenable to less aggressive therapy, and, of course, for all patients with submucosally invasive and deep mural adenocarcinomas.

References may be accessed online at Elsevier eBooks for Practicing Clinicians.

CHAPTER 15

Inflammatory Disorders of the Stomach

Bence Kővári, Robert D. Odze, Gregory Y. Lauwers

Contents

HISTORICAL PERSPECTIVE

In 1947, at the dawn of gastroscopy, Rudolf Schindler deemed gastritis "one of the most debated diseases of the human body" and predicted that its significance would be discussed "for some time to come."[1] From the mid-1800s, when Cruveiller exposed the inaccuracies of Broussais's first descriptions of gastritis in autopsy material, to the early 20th century, the concept of gastritis as a disease had been virtually abandoned.[2]

After gastritis was acknowledged as a distinct entity, the search for its cause began. Since 1870, tiny, curved bacteria within gastric mucosa have been described by human and veterinary pathologists, but the organisms were dismissed as irrelevant contaminants.[3] Schindler claimed that the bacteriological cause of chronic gastritis had not been proved convincingly in a single case.[1] Instead, a wide range of etiological theories were proposed, such as improper mastication, a "coarse" or "miserable" diet, alcohol, caffeine, nicotine, condiments and spices, drugs, heavy metals, thermal injury, chronic infections of the tonsils and sinuses, circulatory disturbances, and psychogenic factors. Not surprisingly, researchers were successful in debunking theories put forth by their colleagues but were quite unsuccessful in proving their own.

Subsequently, accurate morphological data were gathered by pathological examination of autopsy material[4] and from endoscopic biopsy specimens. Distinct types and patterns of gastritis were recognized, which led to the conception, presentation, dismissal, and replacement of many classification systems. Some systems were based on solid morphological information and proposed valid clinicopathological associations (e.g., peptic ulcer and gastric cancer), but the lack of therapeutic implications reduced almost all classifications to little more than an academic exercise.

In 1984, when Warren and Marshall proposed that chronic idiopathic gastritis had a bacterial cause (i.e., *Helicobacter pylori*),[5] it was not surprising that their hypothesis was met with skepticism. However, within a few years, the associations of *H. pylori* gastritis, peptic ulcer, and gastric cancer were recognized and, ultimately, accepted.[6] In 1990, guidelines for the classification and grading of gastritis were developed by a group of investigators in Sydney, Australia. The Sydney system correlates topographic, morphological, and etiological information with clinically useful diagnoses.[7]

Four years after its introduction, the Sydney system was updated with the development of a consensus terminology for gastritis, improved guidelines for histological grading, and streamlined diagnostic process.[8] Subsequently, modifications were made to improve the criteria for evaluation of atrophy.[9,10] In 2006, an international consensus was reached on a diagnostic reporting system designed to use the staging of gastritis as a tool for assessing the risk of gastric cancer.[11-15] This chapter provides the terminology and diagnostic approach proposed by the updated Sydney system and its subsequent modifications.

GENERAL PATHOLOGICAL FEATURES OF GASTRITIS

Gastric mucosal injury causes a spectrum of inflammatory responses and epithelial changes that largely depends on the type of noxious events, its intensity, the location, and the duration of injury. Various degrees and types of tissue responses may occur both synchronously and metachronously. A diagnosis of "gastritis" rests on the pathological recognition of patterns of tissue responses, their intensity, and their location. It is essential to understand the normal appearance and inflammatory state of gastric mucosa before determining the type of disorder present (Figs. 15.1 and 15.2; Table 15.1). In the following few sections, a review of the basic pathological tissue reactions of the gastric mucosa to injury is described in detail.

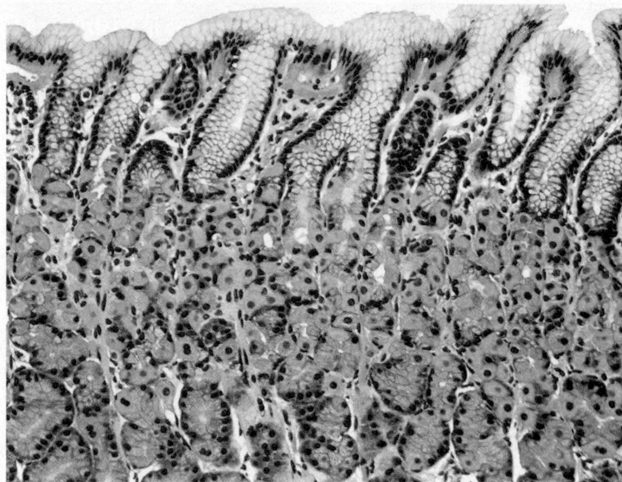

FIGURE 15.1 The normal superficial foveolar (neck) region of the gastric body contains rare or no mononuclear cells and no neutrophils.

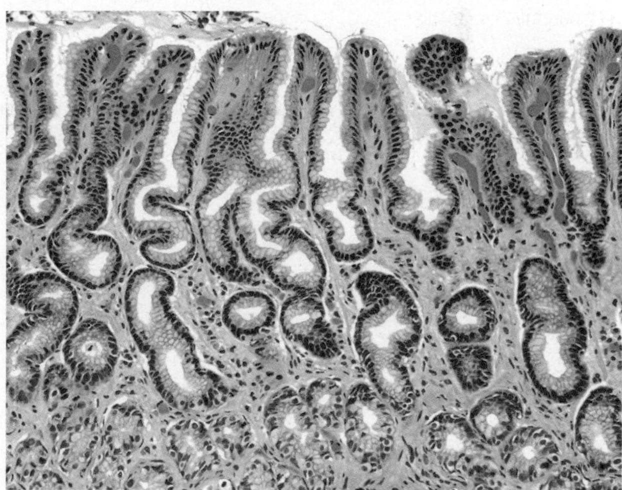

FIGURE 15.2 The normal gastric antrum may contain rare lymphocytes, plasma cells, and eosinophils in the lamina propria, as well as thin strands of smooth muscle. Examination of the distal antrum reveals an extended neck region that results in a mild tortuosity and villous-like configuration of the epithelium.

Neutrophil Infiltration

The lamina propria of normal gastric mucosa may contain rare neutrophils. However, infiltration of the epithelium by neutrophils always represents a pathological response, and when present always constitutes an active component of gastritis. The term *active* is used to indicate an ongoing inflammatory process. In industrialized nations, active inflammation is most commonly caused by *H. pylori* gastritis, but many other infectious and inflammatory conditions (e.g., syphilis,[16] Crohn's disease[17]) may cause neutrophil infiltration as well.

The intensity and location of neutrophil infiltration may help differentiate various types of gastritis. For instance, the acute phase of infectious gastritis (such as phlegmonous gastritis) is likely to present with an abundant neutrophilic infiltrate, while the active phase of *Helicobacter*-induced gastritis may have moderate to severe levels of neutrophils, depending on a variety of factors. For instance, the density

TABLE 15.1 Common Histological Features in Gastritis and Their Significance

Histopathological Component	Normal Setting	Pathological Settings
Neutrophils	Rare in lamina propria Absent in normal epithelium	In active gastritis *(Helicobacter pylori)* Near erosion or ulcer in reactive gastropathy May be present in autoimmune gastritis (almost 50% of cases)
Mononuclear cells	Scattered isolated lymphocytes and plasma cells in lamina propria (antrum > corpus), increase with age None or rare in epithelium	In chronic gastritis (*H. pylori,* autoimmune) and lymphocytic gastritis (if intraepithelial)
Lymphoid aggregates	Rare aggregates, basally located in oxyntic mucosa, without germinal centers	In *H. pylori* infection
Lymphoid follicles	None	In *H. pylori* infection
Eosinophils	Scattered in lamina propria, increase with age Not present in normal epithelium	Moderate increase in *H. pylori* gastritis Autoimmune gastritis Severe with clusters or intraepithelial in eosinophilic gastroenteritis
Edema of the lamina propria	None	In chemical injury, particularly bile reflux
Hyperemia, congestion	None	In any form of active inflammation *(H. pylori),* chemical injury, or vasculopathies (e.g., GAVE)
Surface epithelial degeneration	None Regular, tall cuboidal cells with distinct apical mucin droplet is normal	In *H. pylori* infection, reactive gastropathy
Erosions	None	In chemical injury (flat, not inflamed); *H. pylori* infection (elevated, inflamed)
Foveolar hyperplasia	None	In reactive gastropathy; mucosa adjacent to ulcer; *H. pylori* infection
Intestinal metaplasia	None	Antrum: *H. pylori* infection; chemical injury Corpus and fundus: multifocal atrophic gastritis, autoimmune gastritis, *H. pylori* infection
Atrophy	None Antrum: orderly pits separated by little matrix, no fibrosis Corpus and fundus: parallel, tightly packed oxyntic glands reaching muscularis mucosae	Antrum: *H. pylori* infection (rare without intestinal metaplasia) Corpus and fundus: multifocal atrophic gastritis, autoimmune gastritis, *H. pylori* infection
Endocrine cell hyperplasia	None; no obvious G cells on H&E staining; no clusters or nests	With chronic PPI therapy; atrophy, particularly autoimmune gastritis
Parietal cell alterations	No prominent protruding parietal cells; no lumen or dilations in oxyntic glands	With chronic PPI therapy
Interfoveolar smooth muscle hyperplasia	Scattered fibers between antral foveolae; no bundles	Reactive gastropathy, GAVE

GAVE, *Gastric antral vascular ectasia;* H&E, *hematoxylin and eosin stain;* PPI, *proton pump inhibitor.*

of neutrophils detected in *H. pylori* gastritis usually (but not universally) correlates with the density of *H. pylori* infection.[18-20] Conversely, in cases with rare neutrophils but with features otherwise suggestive of *H. pylori* infection, such as a plasma cell-rich infiltrate, an intense hunt for the bacteria is usually warranted, either with or without ancillary tests.[21] Acute hemorrhagic gastritis resulting from nonsteroidal antiinflammatory drug (NSAID)– or alcohol-induced chemical injury often shows only a minimal neutrophilic infiltrate, unless an erosion is present. In such cases, biopsies are typically devoid of a rich background of plasma cells. Mild and focal neutrophilic infiltration can be seen in some phases of autoimmune gastritis.[22]

Mononuclear Infiltration

Antral mucosa normally contains a few mononuclear cells in the lamina propria (i.e., lymphocytes and plasma cells), whereas normal corpus mucosa contains virtually none. However, the density of "normal" mononuclear cells in the lamina propria of patients without disease varies considerably according to a number of factors, such as their geographic location and ethnicity, their age, and, of course, their diet and medication profile, among others (see Fig. 15.2).[23] It is generally recommended that "gastritis" not be diagnosed unless there are at least several clusters of about five or more mononuclear cells in the lamina propria, or the infiltrate is diffuse and bandlike. In general, if the epithelium is healthy and does not reveal either regenerative or degenerative changes, then it is unlikely that a mononuclear infiltrate in the lamina propria is considered "pathological" or abnormal. In the corpus and fundus, rare single mononuclear cells in the lamina propria are considered a normal finding. Under normal conditions, intraepithelial lymphocytes are not present anywhere in the gastric epithelium.

Mucosal infiltration by plasma cells, lymphocytes, and often some eosinophils and mast cells is characteristic of chronic *H. pylori* gastritis. This infiltrate is typically band-like and located mainly in the superficial portion of the lamina propria. It usually starts in the antrum, but it may progress proximally in the stomach, particularly in patients receiving proton pump inhibitors (PPIs) and without proper antibiotic therapy. In autoimmune gastritis, the corpus and fundus of the stomach are selectively involved, the infiltrate is more diffuse[24] (usually centered around the deep portions of the mucosa), and the infiltrate consists mainly of lymphocytes rather than plasma cells.

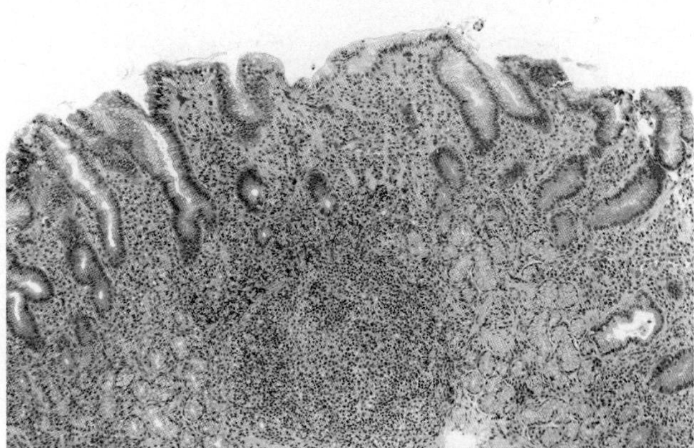

FIGURE 15.3 Antral mucosa with well-developed lymphoid follicle in a patient with *Helicobacter pylori* gastritis. Neither lymphoid aggregates nor follicles are found in the normal antrum.

Lymphoid Aggregates and Follicles

Normal gastric mucosa, particularly the corpus, may contain occasional, small lymphoid aggregates, usually basally located close to the muscularis mucosae. In contrast, lymphoid follicles (i.e., with germinal centers) are rare in normal gastric mucosa of *H. pylori*–negative adults.[25] In studies with extensive biopsy sampling, lymphoid follicles or aggregates have been detected in almost all individuals with *H. pylori* gastritis. Subsequently, detection of lymphoid follicles is highly suggestive of *H. pylori* infection (Fig. 15.3). In *H. pylori*–infected children and young adults, lymphoid follicles may be quite numerous, and it may in fact produce an endoscopic appearance of nodularity that is often referred to as *follicular gastritis*.[26,27]

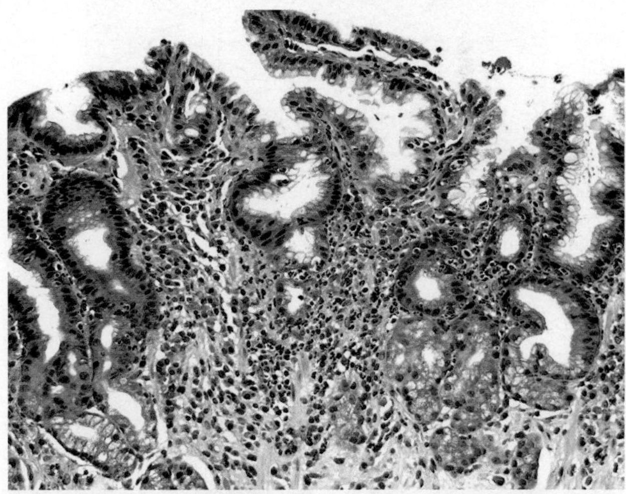

FIGURE 15.4 Eosinophils may compose some portion of the inflammatory infiltrate in *Helicobacter pylori* gastritis.

Eosinophil Infiltration

Rare, scattered eosinophils may be present in the gastric mucosa of normal healthy patients, particularly in individuals who live in a suboptimal public health environment. However, prominent eosinophilic infiltration usually represents a pathological process, such as eosinophilic gastritis or gastroenteritis.[28,29] Eosinophil infiltration may occur in a wide variety of disorders, such as gastric anisakiasis and other granulomatous or parasitic infections of the stomach as well.[30]

In *H. pylori* gastritis, if detected, eosinophil infiltration is usually mild. However, a greater eosinophilic component of the inflammatory infiltrate may manifest in children with *H. pylori* infection (Fig. 15.4).[31] After *H. pylori* eradication, eosinophils may persist for a long time, similar to mononuclear cells.[18] Eosinophils can be a prominent component of the inflammatory infiltrate in autoimmune gastritis as well.[22]

Mucosal Hyperemia

Mucosal hyperemia (congestion) is frequently an indicator of chemical injury. Interestingly, a significant correlation has been reported between the degree of hyperemia and the concentration of bilirubin within gastric fluid.[32] However, congestion may also be detected in many other conditions, such as *H. pylori* gastritis, and may be related to an increased infiltration of mast cells (Fig. 15.5).[33,34]

Surface Epithelium Regeneration and Degeneration

Surface epithelium regeneration and degeneration (or both) represents a nonspecific cellular response to a variety of injuries to the mucosa. For instance, degenerative changes may result in the emergence of cuboidal (rather than columnar) cells and depletion of mucin. Regenerative changes are particularly prominent in a variety of conditions, such as chemical gastropathy (resulting from bile reflux, ethanol, or NSAIDs), vascular gastropathies, and *H. pylori* gastritis as well.[35-37] When prominent, epithelial regeneration in *H. pylori* gastritis may result in the accumulation of tufts and buds of cells at the surface of the mucosa (Fig. 15.6).[38]

Surface Erosion

Surface erosions are the result of severe epithelial injury that leads to necrosis. By definition, erosions are ulcers that

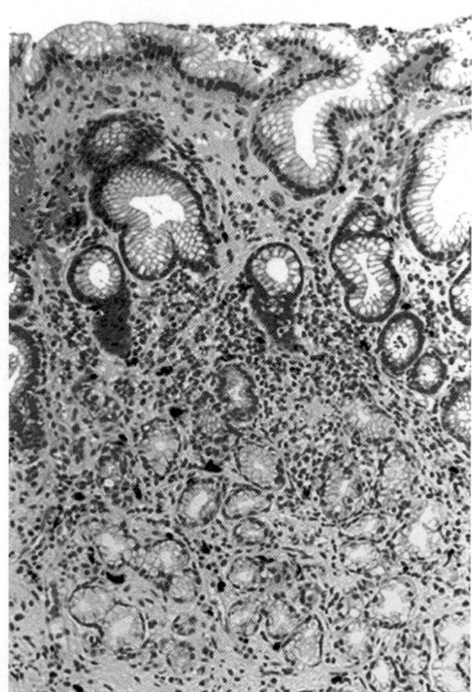

FIGURE 15.5 An increase in the number of mast cells may be seen in many types of gastritis, particularly those caused by *Helicobacter pylori* (tryptase stain).

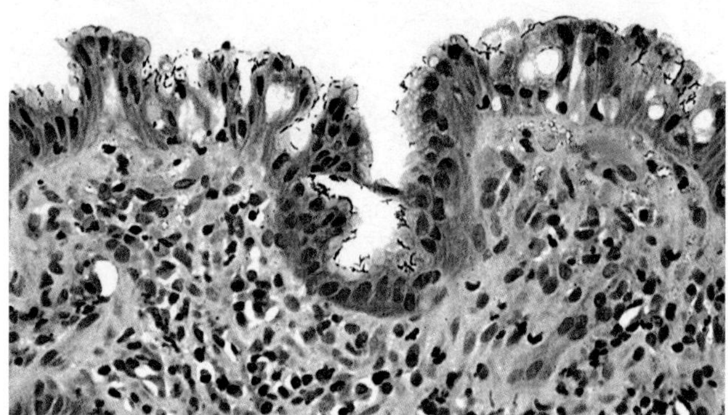

FIGURE 15.6 Surface epithelial degeneration (i.e., mucin-depleted epithelial cells) is typically found in *Helicobacter pylori*–infected stomachs, even in areas where bacteria are rare or absent. Focal loss of cells (i.e., microerosions) is evident. Bacteria occupy the empty spaces created by dropout of individual cells and areas of mucin depletion (silver triple stain).

do not extend beyond the muscularis mucosae. Chemically-induced flat surface erosions are characterized by a relatively paucicellular lamina propria, neutrophilic infiltration, hyalinization of the lamina propria, and a withering pit and gland epithelium, giving the mucosa an ischemic appearance. They often result from the acute effects of drugs, alcohol, bile reflux, or ischemia (Fig. 15.7).[39,40] Elevated surface erosions are typically associated with *H. pylori* gastritis. These erosions are usually characterized by a superficial layer of fibrinopurulent debris (i.e., fibrinoid necrosis, neutrophils, and cellular debris) associated with a plasma cell–rich lamina propria infiltrate and hyperplastic, regenerative-appearing epithelium at the margins (Fig. 15.8).[41]

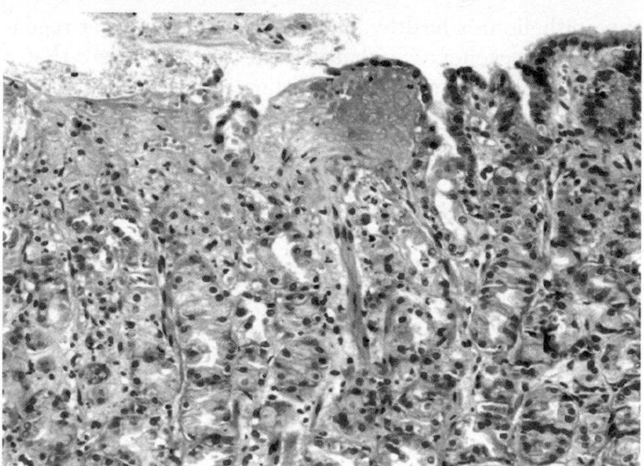

FIGURE 15.7 Typical appearance of a flat surface erosion with homogeneous eosinophilic necrosis resulting from an acute toxic injury, such as nonsteroidal antiinflammatory drugs, alcohol, or bile reflux.

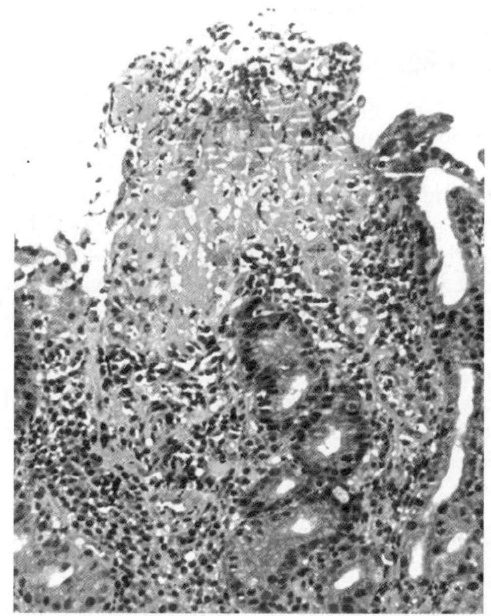

FIGURE 15.8 Superficial erosion in *Helicobacter pylori* gastritis. A superficial layer of nonhomogeneous fibrinoid necrosis that contains granulocytes and cell debris may be found in severe cases of *H. pylori* gastritis.

Foveolar Hyperplasia

Foveolar hyperplasia is defined as proliferation, elongation, and tortuosity of gastric pits that results in a corkscrew configuration to the pits. It is a regenerative phenomenon. It represents a compensatory tissue response to increased exfoliation of the surface epithelium, and it is a visual surrogate for increased cell proliferation and cell turnover (Fig. 15.9). Foveolar hyperplasia may be diagnosed readily when several cross-sections of the same gastric pit are visualized in a single, well-oriented gastric biopsy specimen.[42,43] Other features of foveolar hyperplasia include hyperchromatic nuclei, high nucleus-to-cytoplasm ratio, upper pit mitoses, mucin depletion, and cuboidalization of the epithelial cells.

Foveolar hyperplasia is a characteristic feature of reactive gastropathy, including bile reflux and NSAID gastritis, particularly in long-term users.[32,42,43] The degree of foveolar

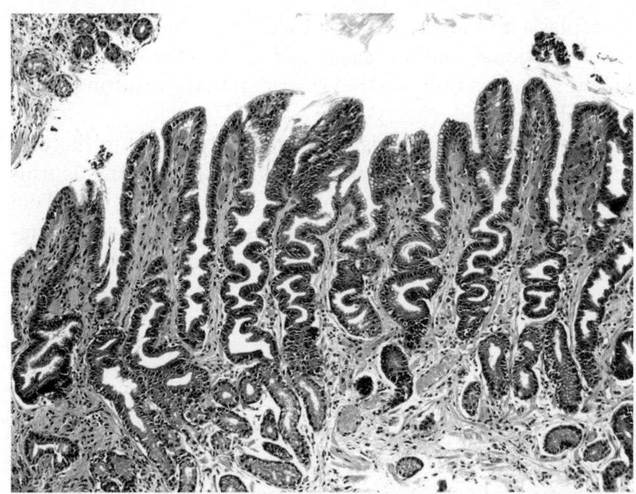

FIGURE 15.9 Reactive (chemical) gastropathy shows marked foveolar hyperplasia (i.e., elongated and coiled gastric pits), vascular congestion, and smooth muscle bundles that extend upward into the superficial lamina propria.

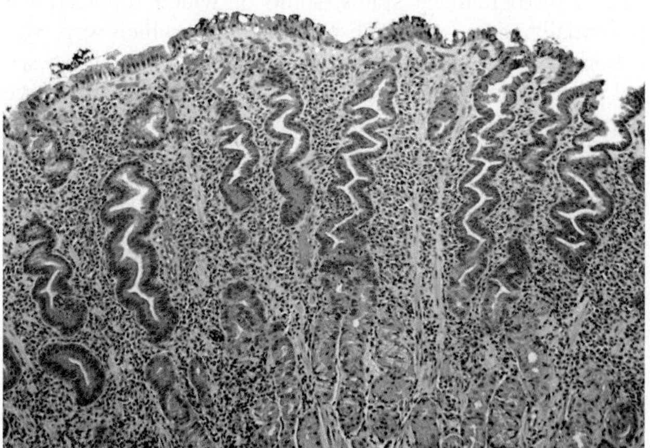

FIGURE 15.10 Foveolar hyperplasia is commonly seen in *Helicobacter pylori* gastritis, but the marked elongation shown herein suggests the possibility of coexistent chemical injury.

hyperplasia (together with smooth muscle hyperplasia and congestion) has been used to score the severity of reactive gastropathy.[44] A mild degree of foveolar hyperplasia is common in patients with *H. pylori* gastritis; however, marked hyperplasia often indicates coexistent chemical injury (Fig. 15.10).[45] Foveolar hyperplasia may also be prominent in autoimmune gastritis, sometimes with the development of hyperplastic polyps. Finally, the use of PPIs can also lead to foveolar hyperplasia.[46]

Intestinal Metaplasia

Intestinal metaplasia is defined as replacement of gastric-type foveolar epithelium with intestinal cells (i.e., goblet cells, enterocytes with brush border, and Paneth cells) (Fig. 15.11).[47] Two types of intestinal metaplasia (I and II) have been described. Metaplastic epithelium that closely resembles normal small intestinal epithelium, containing acid mucin–producing goblet cells and absorptive enterocytes with a brush border, is considered complete metaplasia (type I). Incomplete metaplasia (type II) shows a disorderly mixture of irregularly shaped goblet cells (intestinal and immature intermediate mucous cells) that contain acidic sialomucins and sulfomucins. Although the clinical importance of their distinction has long been debated, a recent meta-analysis reemphasized that incomplete intestinal metaplasia is associated with a higher risk of gastric cancer.[48] Incomplete metaplasia is further subdivided into type IIa and type IIb (also referred to as type III) by the presence of sulfomucins within nongoblet (mucinous) cells in the latter.[49] Although type IIb has been shown to be associated with an even higher increased cancer risk, the practicability of subtyping incomplete intestinal metaplasia is limited in clinical practice. In fact, most patients with intestinal metaplasia have a mixture of the incomplete and complete types when extensive areas of mucosa are sampled,[47] and the degree of incomplete intestinal metaplasia (including type IIb) parallels the extent of intestinal metaplasia in general. Furthermore, one meta-analysis indicated that intestinal metaplasia in the antrum and corpus is associated with a higher cancer risk than when it is limited to the antrum,[48] which underscores a positive correlation between the extent of any type of intestinal metaplasia and risk of progression to carcinoma.

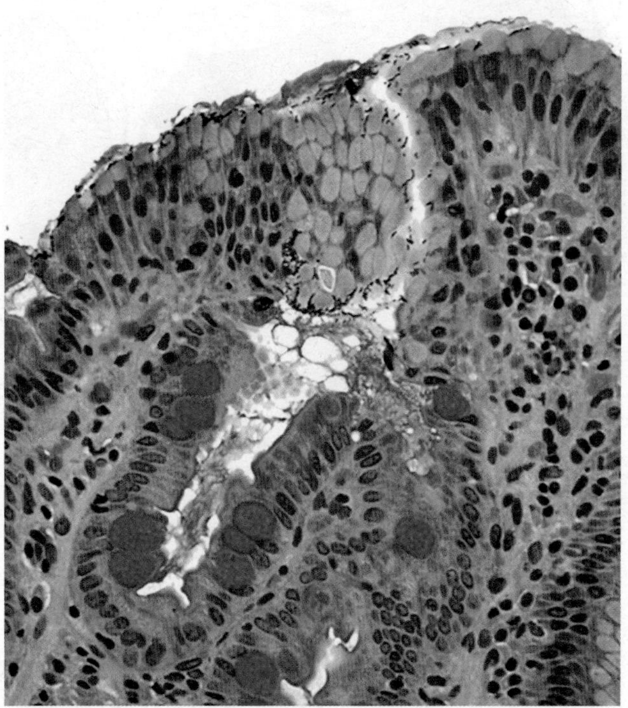

FIGURE 15.11 In the high-power photomicrograph of metaplastic gastric mucosa stained with a triple stain (hematoxylin and eosin, Alcian blue, and a modified Steiner stain), the goblet cells are bright blue. *Helicobacter pylori* organisms adhere only to the nonmetaplastic portions of the epithelium.

Intestinal metaplasia can be identified and its extent evaluated with the use of hematoxylin and eosin (H&E) stain, although specific mucin histochemical stains can be used to highlight metaplastic areas. For instance, the Alcian blue/periodic acid–Schiff (AB/PAS) stain at pH 2.5 is an excellent method for demonstrating the type and extent of intestinal metaplasia, particularly when used in combination with a hematoxylin counterstain (Fig. 15.12).

Mucin histochemical stains, some of which reported are potentially toxic (e.g., high-iron diamine), which were traditionally used to determine the specific type of intestinal metaplasia by helping to detect sulfated mucins, have been largely replaced by immunohistochemical stains that identify proteins associated with particular mucin-encoding genes. Although more than 20 such mucin genes have been identified, only a few (i.e., *MUC1*, *MUC2*, *MUC5AC*, and *MUC6*) are commercially available, and even these are used mainly in the research setting (Table 15.2).

Intestinal metaplasia may develop in a variety of pathological settings, but its presence always indicates an underlying chronic, and often atrophic, gastritis. Intestinal metaplasia occurs frequently in patients with *H. pylori* gastritis.[50,51] Because *H. pylori* organisms do not normally adhere to intestinal-type epithelium (see Fig. 15.11), they commonly disappear in mucosa with extensive intestinal metaplasia and atrophy. Intestinalized epithelium may provide additional defense against *H. pylori* through changes in the composition of the gastric mucus resulting from metaplasia.

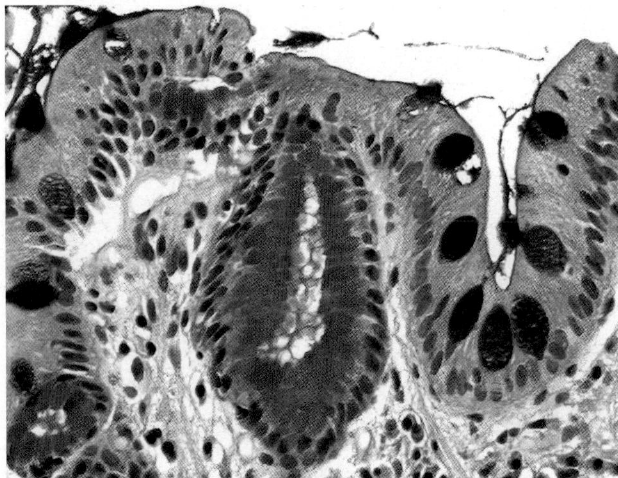

FIGURE 15.12 The Alcian blue stain, periodic acid–Schiff (PAS) stain, and hematoxylin counterstain highlight the acid mucin-producing goblet cells *(purple)* and neutral mucin-containing foveolar cells. The purple color results from a combination of acid mucins *(blue)* and neutral mucins *(red)* within goblet cells.

Intestinal metaplasia is also frequently found in the corpus of patients with autoimmune gastritis, and this is usually associated with pseudopyloric metaplasia as well. Foci of intestinal metaplasia are common in patients with reactive gastropathy after Billroth II surgery.[43] Metaplasia can be detected in individuals with an otherwise completely normal stomach.

Atrophy

Gastric atrophy is defined as loss of gastric glands.[10,52] Atrophy is a histological finding, not a nosological entity. When the gastric mucosa is damaged, regardless of the cause, it may (1) regenerate to normal (restitutio ad integrum) or (2) undergo an adaptive reparative change with replacement of native glands with other types of tissue (i.e., metaplasia) (Fig. 15.13).[53] When injured glands fail to regenerate, the stromal space they previously occupied may be replaced by fibroblasts and extracellular matrix (i.e., fibrosis) (Fig. 15.14). Ultimately, the result of metaplasia and fibrosis is loss of functional epithelium (i.e., atrophy).

Diffuse atrophy of the corpus and fundus typically occurs in autoimmune gastritis as a consequence of immune-mediated destruction of oxyntic epithelium. Less severe and more focal atrophy, which is usually limited to the antrum, may also occur in reactive gastropathy. *H. pylori* gastritis usually triggers multifocal atrophy in the antrum, which spreads to the oxyntic mucosa in the advanced stages of the disease.

The updated Sydney system recognizes multifocal atrophic gastritis (MAG; referred to as *environmental atrophic gastritis* in the pre–*H. pylori* era) as an entity distinct from nonatrophic gastritis and autoimmune atrophic gastritis.[8,54] The distinction between gastritis with focal atrophy and atrophic gastritis has not been well defined (Fig. 15.15). This issue is important because scattered foci of intestinal

TABLE 15.2 Mucin Immunohistochemistry in the Stomach

Mucin Expressed*	Normal Gastric Epithelium	Intestinal Metaplasia Type I		Intestinal Metaplasia Type II		Intestinal Metaplasia Type III	
		G	*C*	*G*	*C*	*G*	*C*
MUC1	++ (foveolar epithelium; chief and parietal cells)	–	–	++	++	+++	+++
MUC2	–	+++	–	++	+	++	±
MUC5AC	+++ (foveolar epithelium; all mucous neck cells)	–	–	++	++	++	++
MUC6	+ (antral glands; mucopeptic cells of neck zone in corpus)	–	–	–	±	±	±

**Expression of the most common mucin proteins in the normal stomach and the three types of intestinal metaplasia is detected by immunohistochemical staining. Because the intensity of the staining and the percentages of cells assessed as positive vary and interpretation is highly subjective, the use of these stains to determine the type of intestinal metaplasia and any inference of cancer risk in individual patients is strongly discouraged.*

C, *Columnar or absorptive cells;* G, *goblet cells.*

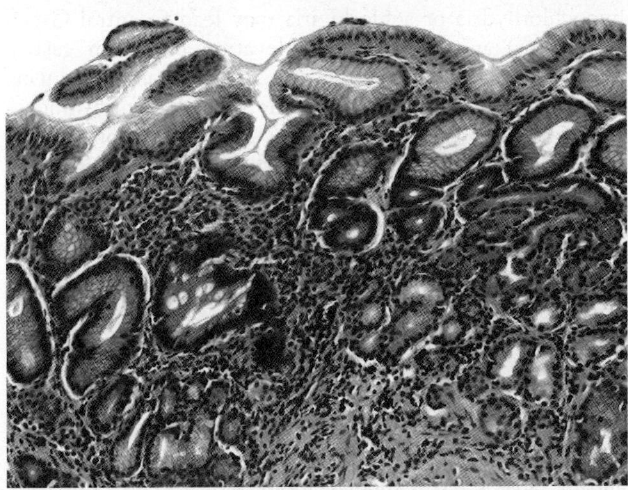

FIGURE 15.13 Atrophic oxyntic mucosa with pyloric or pseudopyloric metaplasia as well as focal intestinal and pancreatic acinar metaplasia as observed in autoimmune gastritis.

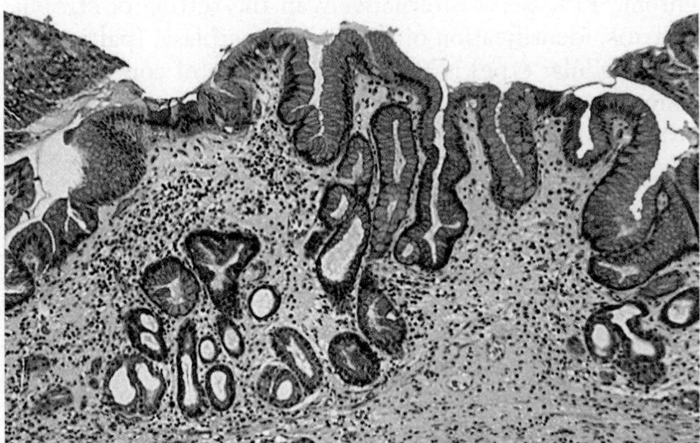

FIGURE 15.14 Nonmetaplastic atrophy in the antrum, which is associated with long-standing *Helicobacter pylori* infection or prolonged chemical injury, is uncommon. However, when associated with *H. pylori* infection and severe atrophic gastritis, the condition can predispose to gastric cancer.

metaplasia are found in the antrum of most patients with *H. pylori* gastritis and in a small percentage of noninfected adults. It is not appropriate to classify these individuals with "atrophic" gastritis, a diagnosis that implies altered gastric function and an increased risk of cancer. In the absence of established guidelines, we suggest that a diagnosis of MAG should be made only when there is evidence of atrophy either with or without intestinal metaplasia in at least 50% of a generously biopsied stomach (i.e., minimum of two samples from the antrum and two from the corpus or fundus).

Several pathology workshops have been devoted to the development of a reproducible method for grading atrophy in mucosal biopies.[9,10] Pathologists have recommended that atrophy be evaluated according to its two subtypes: *nonmetaplastic* or *metaplastic*. The subtype known as *nonmetaplastic atrophy* (see Fig. 15.14) is an area of mucosa with true glandular loss, replaced by stromal elements (usually fibrosis). In *metaplastic atrophy* (i.e., metaplasia equals atrophy), the native glands that are physiological for that site may be replaced by those with a pyloric phenotype (i.e., pyloric or pseudopyloric metaplasia) or an intestinal phenotype (i.e., intestinal metaplasia) comprising goblet cells and absorptive cells (either with or without a brush border) (see Fig. 15.13). Intestinal metaplasia may develop anywhere in the stomach, whereas pyloric (pseudopyloric) metaplasia occurs in the corpus or cardia. In both types of atrophy, the degree of gland loss may be broadly graded as mild, moderate, or severe, which corresponds to a scale of 1 to 3 (Fig. 15.16).

Problems may arise when gastric biopsies are labeled as "stomach" or "antrum-body," in which case it may be difficult to determine whether there is true pyloric metaplasia or the biopsy is simply representative of the antrum or antral-fundic transition. In this instance, immunohistochemical staining for gastrin-positive endocrine cells can help identify mucosa derived from the antrum. However, this method is not fool-proof because gastrin-positive cells may, on occasion, be present in metaplastic and atrophic

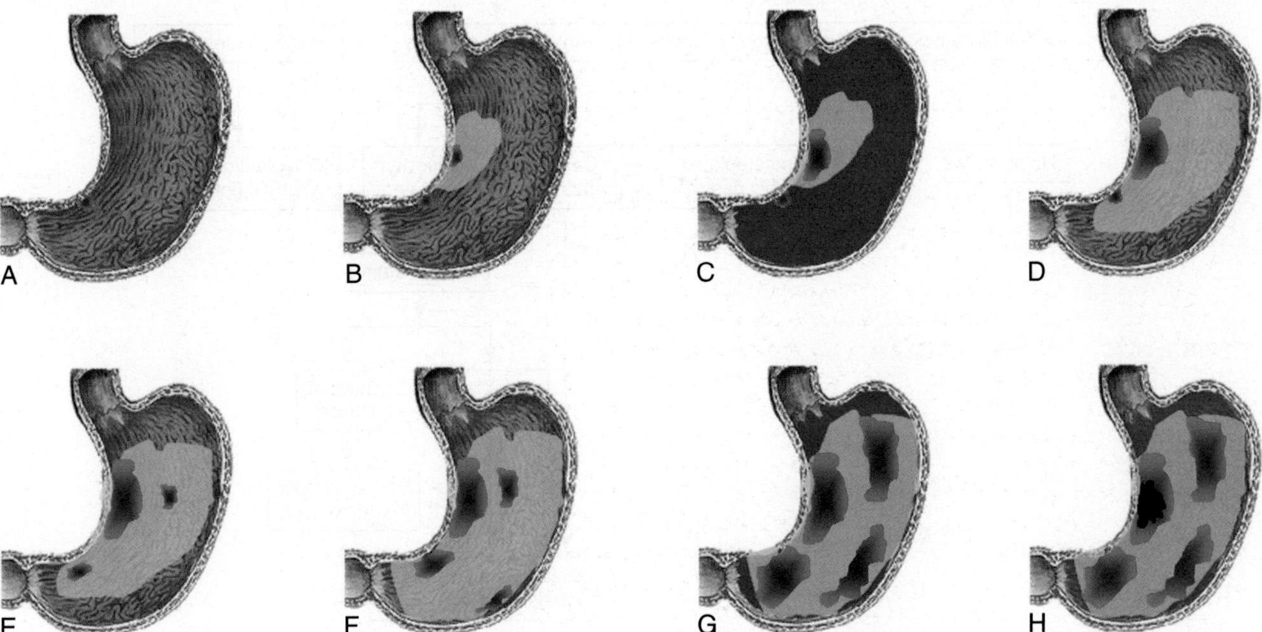

FIGURE 15.15 Spectrum of atrophy *(pink)* and metaplasia *(blue)*. Although it is intuitive that stomach **A** has nonatrophic gastritis and that stomachs **F, G,** and **H** have atrophic metaplastic gastritis, stomachs **B** to **E** are difficult to assign to a particular category, particularly when only limited biopsy samples are available.

areas of the fundus. Thus it is not just the finding of a gastrin-positive cell that should be considered, but also its quantity and location in the epithelium and its association with other mucosal structures. The algorithm depicted in Figure 15.17 summarizes an approach to the evaluation of atrophy in gastric biopsies.

Endocrine Cell Proliferation

Endocrine cell hyperplasia develops as a consequence of functional changes in the stomach and is most prominent in autoimmune atrophic gastritis. In this condition, hypochlorhydria or achlorhydria may lead to antral G-cell hyperplasia and a secondary elevation of serum gastrin levels.[55,56] Hypergastrinemia causes histamine-producing enterochromaffin-like (ECL) cells within oxyntic mucosa to proliferate. Neuroendocrine cell proliferation can be detected in patients with advanced atrophic gastritis and in biopsies of patients who take PPIs.[57] Although antral G-cell hyperplasia can be detected easily on H&E–stained tissue sections (Fig. 15.18), hyperplasia of ECL cells in oxyntic mucosa is best visualized and quantified with specific immunostains (Fig. 15.19).

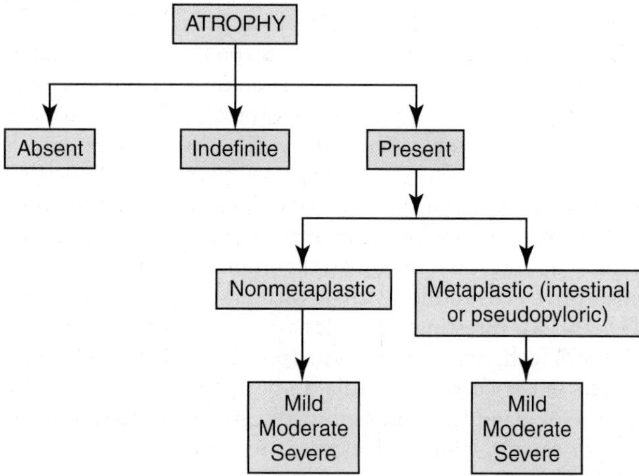

FIGURE 15.16 The types and degrees of atrophy are based on the Atrophy 2000 classification. (*Modified from Rugge M, Correa P, Genta RM, et al. Gastric mucosal atrophy: interobserver consistency using new criteria for classification and grading. Aliment Pharmacol Ther. 2002;16:1249–1259.*)

The most widely used classification system of ECL cell hyperplasia consists of simple or diffuse, linear, micronodular, and adenomatoid hyperplasia; ECL cell dysplasia; and neoplasia (i.e., neuroendocrine tumors). These are reviewed later in this chapter in the Autoimmune Gastritis section and in Table 15.3. A mild to moderate degree of ECL cell hyperplasia may occur in patients who use PPIs for extended periods. However, in these patients, the oxyntic mucosa is not atrophic and commonly displays parietal cell hypertrophy and oxyntic gland dilation, both frequently seen in chronic PPI users. Alternatively, in the setting of atrophic gastritis, identification of ECL cell hyperplasia (particularly micronodular type) is a diagnostic feature of corporal autoimmune atrophic gastritis.

Parietal Cell Alterations

Apocrine-like protrusion and pseudohypertrophy of oxyntic cells are frequently attributed to chronic use of PPIs (Fig. 15.20A).[58,59] However, identical histological changes have been reported in other clinical settings; therefore the findings are not pathognomonic.[60] Use of PPIs may lead to dilation of oxyntic glands, which in extreme cases may produce

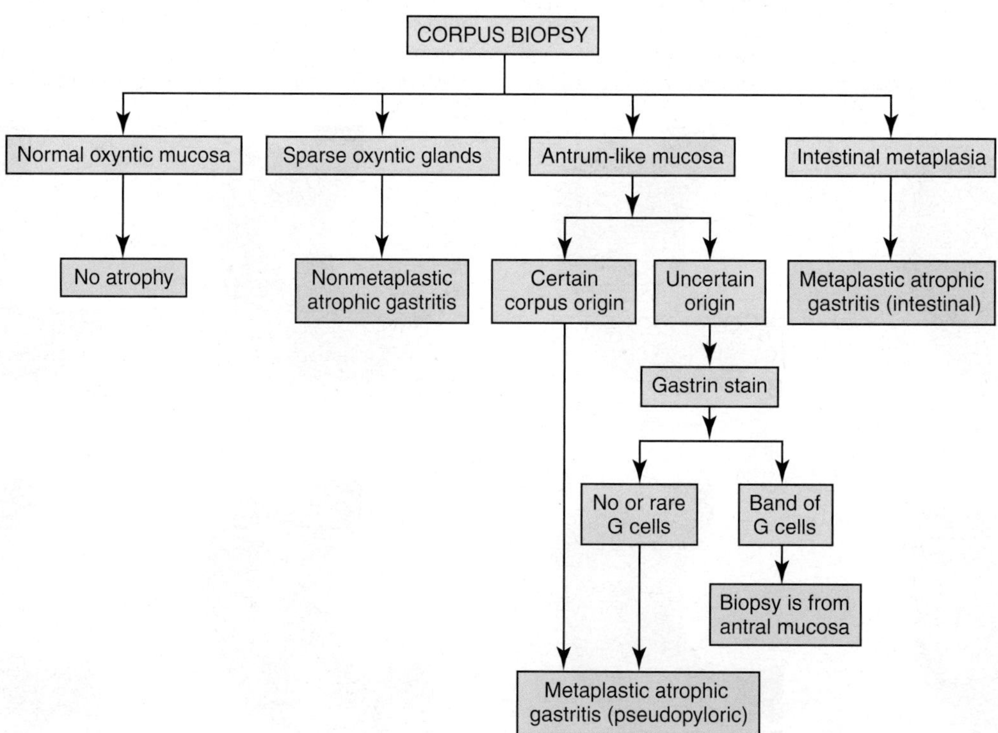

FIGURE 15.17 Algorithm for the diagnosis of atrophy in biopsy specimens obtained from the gastric corpus.

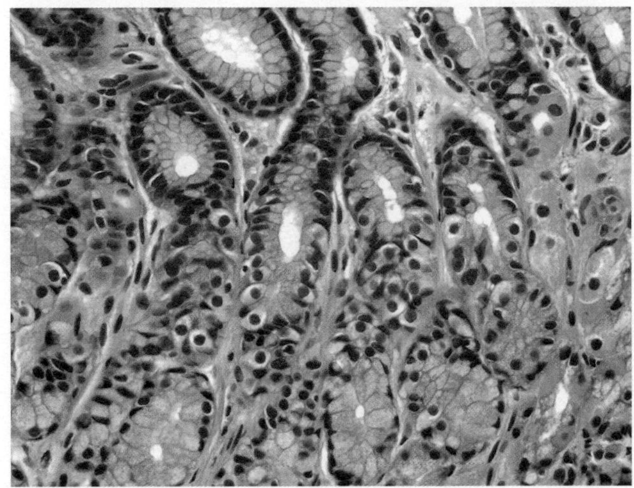

FIGURE 15.18 Gastrin-producing endocrine cell hyperplasia can be suspected on routine staining by the grouping of cells with distinct pale cytoplasm and central dark nuclei (i.e., fried egg appearance). Antigastrin immunohistochemical stain can be used to confirm this finding.

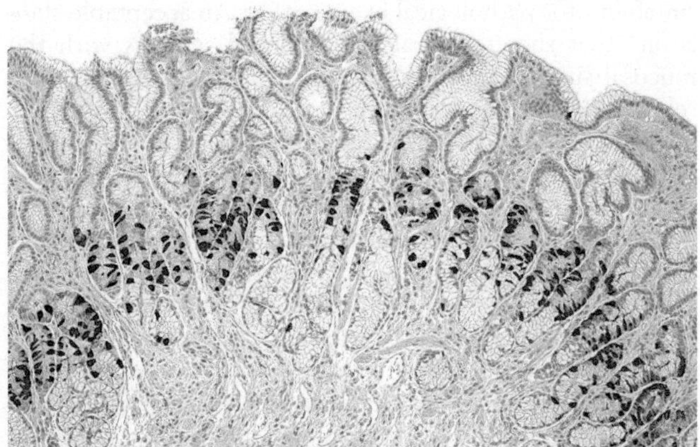

FIGURE 15.19 Example of linear G-cell hyperplasia in the antral mucosa by immunohistochemical staining.

multiple fundic gland–type polyps that impart an appearance of the gastric mucosa that inspired the picturesque description of *gastric acne*.[61,62] Cytoplasmic vacuolation of parietal cells has been reported in patients using PPIs as well as rare cases with pseudo–signet ring cell morphology (Fig. 15.20B). Because most chronic users of NSAIDs also take PPIs to reduce the risk of NSAID-induced ulceration, oxyntic gland alterations are frequently seen in conjunction with reactive (chemical) gastropathy.[43,63,64]

Interfoveolar Smooth Muscle Hyperplasia

In the normal stomach, smooth muscle fibers are generally confined to the muscularis mucosae, where they run parallel to the mucosal surface. Several studies have shown that reactive (chemical) gastropathy is often associated with proliferation of smooth muscle fibers that run perpendicular to the muscularis mucosae within the interfoveolar lamina propria (see Fig. 15.9). The changes may be caused by the pulling effect of prolapsing mucosa, similar to that seen in *solitary rectal ulcer syndrome* and other prolapse-type polyps.[65] Another proposed mechanism is the release of platelet-derived growth factor (PDGF), a known smooth muscle stimulant, as a result of epithelial damage. However, smooth muscle hyperplasia is not specific for NSAID-induced gastritis and may be seen in a variety of other conditions, such as gastric antral vascular ectasia (GAVE), bile reflux gastritis, and even in simple reactive mucosa adjacent to ulcers.[43,64]

UPDATED SYDNEY SYSTEM

The updated Sydney system provides guidelines for generating systematic, uniform diagnostic reports. The goal of the system is to enhance consistency so that pathologists issue clinically relevant and precise diagnoses, and allow clinical studies to be performed and evaluated in an

TABLE 15.3 Classification of Enterochromaffin-Like Cell Proliferations

Diagnosis	Criteria for Increased Endocrine Cells	Common Disorders
Hyperplasias		
Simple or diffuse hyperplasia	>2 × standard deviations (age and gender matched)	ZES, Early AIG, PPI therapy
Linear hyperplasia	Linear groups of five or more cells inside the glandular BM	ZES, Early AIG, PPI therapy
Micronodular hyperplasia	Clusters of five or more cells within epithelium measuring <150 μm in diameter	Autoimmune atrophic gastritis
Adenomatoid hyperplasia	Aggregates of five or more micronodules in lamina propria	Autoimmune atrophic gastritis, MEN-ZES
Dysplasias		Autoimmune atrophic gastritis, MEN-ZES
Enlarged micronodules	>150 μm	
Adenomatous micronodules	Collections of at least five closely adherent micronodules, intervening BM only	
Fused micronodules	Adenomatous micronodules with no intervening BM	
Microinfiltrative lesions	Infiltration of the lamina propria	
Neuroendocrine tumor (type 1)		Autoimmune atrophic gastritis, MEN-ZES
Intramucosal	Expansile or infiltrative nodules > 0.5 mm	
Invasive	Any size tumor within submucosa	

AIG, *autoimmune gastritis;* BM, *basement membrane;* MEN, *multiple endocrine neoplasia;* ZES, *Zollinger-Ellison syndrome.*
Data from Solcia E, Fiocca R, Villani L, et al. Hyperplastic, dysplastic, and neoplastic enterochromaffin-like cell proliferations of the gastric mucosa: classification and histogenesis. Am J Surg Pathol. *1995;19(suppl 1):S1–S7.*

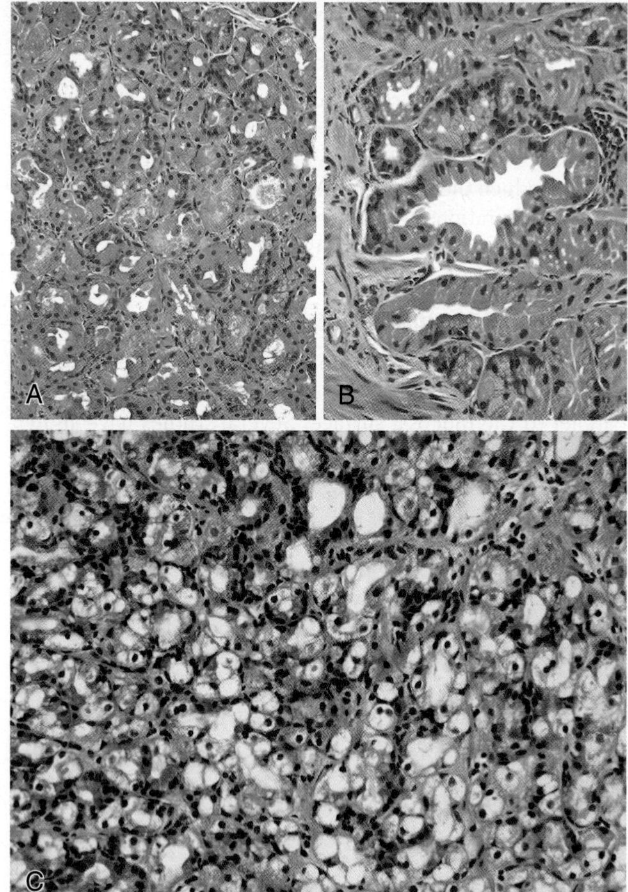

FIGURE 15.20 Proton pump inhibitor therapy–related changes. Mild glandular dilation with parietal cell apocrine-like blebs **(A)** and more pronounced dilation with oxyntic cell hypertrophy **(B)**. **C,** Clear cell changes can also be observed in the glandular component of the transitional mucosa.

unambiguous manner. To create a pathology report suggested by the updated Sydney system, at least five biopsy specimens should be evaluated and the findings synthesized (Fig. 15.21). The system (Table 15.4) classifies chronic gastritis into three broad categories on the basis of topography, morphology, and when possible, on the basis of cause as acute, chronic, or special (distinctive).[8] The latter category includes entities of uncertain pathogenesis and gastropathies. This system also separates chronic gastritis into atrophic and nonatrophic forms (Fig. 15.22).

Biopsy Protocol

The biopsy protocol depicted in Figure 15.21 is recommended to obtain satisfactory mucosal sampling. Specimens from three compartments (i.e., antrum, incisura angularis, and corpus) should be separately designated when submitted to the pathology laboratory. Proper specimen orientation is critical for optimal evaluation and is best accomplished at the time of tissue embedding. Unfortunately, in routine clinical practice, gastroenterologists do not often adhere to such a rigorous sampling and labeling protocol (see Reporting Gastritis in the Absence of a Complete Biopsy Set), and this limitation is not addressed by the Sydney classification.

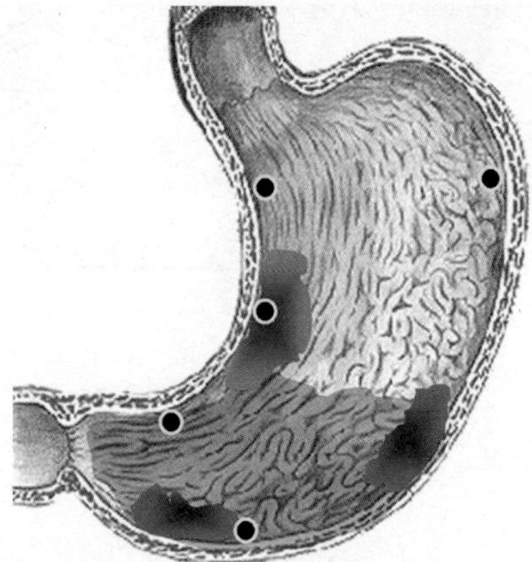

FIGURE 15.21 The five biopsy sites *(circles)* recommended by the updated Sydney system.

Evaluation of Histological Variables

Each mucosal biopsy specimen should be assessed for its suitability for pathological examination. An acceptable slide is one that shows several well-oriented sections with the mucosal surface and the muscularis mucosae visible. Each relevant pathological feature (e.g., density of *H. pylori*, intensity of neutrophilic and mononuclear inflammation, atrophy of the antrum and corpus, intestinal metaplasia) should be graded on a standardized visual analogue scale (Fig. 15.23). Each feature is assigned a numeric or descriptive value: 0 for absent, 1 for mild, 2 for moderate, and 3 for marked or severe. The values of each specimen are determined separately for each anatomic compartment (i.e., antrum and corpus). A minimum of two specimens from the antrum, one from the incisura angularis, and two from the corpus, should be evaluated.

Determination of Gradient of Inflammation

After evaluation of the histological variables, the next step in the Sydney system is to document the degree of inflammation in the two main gastric compartments to determine whether the inflammation is similar in intensity (i.e., pangastritis) or more severe in the antrum (i.e., antrum-predominant gastritis) or the corpus (i.e., corpus-predominant gastritis). To conclude that inflammation in one compartment is predominant, the difference in the inflammatory variables should be at least two grades. This helps minimize the effect of interobserver variability. The degree of atrophy and metaplasia can also be assessed according to the Atrophy 2000 guidelines.[10] The last step in the Sydney classification is to decide whether focal atrophy or diffuse atrophy (metaplastic or nonmetaplastic) is present.

Diagnosis

The final diagnosis according to the Sydney system represents a synthesis of the observations outlined previously, including information regarding possible cause. Examples of diagnostic reports are "*H. pylori* antrum-predominant gastritis" and "corpus-restricted atrophic gastritis without *H. pylori* infection, suggestive of autoimmune gastritis" (Fig. 15.24).

TABLE 15.4 Sydney System Classification of Gastritis

Type of Gastritis	Etiological Factors	Gastritis Synonyms
Nonatrophic	*Helicobacter pylori*	Superficial
	Other factors (?)	Diffuse antral gastritis (DAG)
		Chronic antral gastritis (CAG)
		Interstitial-follicular
		Hypersecretory
		Type B
Atrophic		
Autoimmune	Autoimmunity	Type A
	H. pylori (?)	Diffuse corporal
Multifocal atrophic gastritis (MAG)	*H. pylori*	Pernicious anemia–associated
	Environmental factors	Type B, type AB
		Environmental
		Metaplastic
		Atrophic pangastritis
		Progressive intestinalizing pangastritis
Special forms		
Chemical	Chemical irritation	Reactive
	Bile	Reflux
	NSAIDs	
	Other agents (?)	
Radiation	Radiation injury	
Lymphocytic	Idiopathic (?)	Varioliform
	Autoimmune mechanisms (?)	Celiac disease associated
	Gluten (?)	
	Drugs (e.g., ticlopidine)	
	H. pylori (?)	
Noninfectious granulomatous	Crohn's disease	Isolated granulomatous
	Sarcoidosis	
	Wegener's granulomatosis	
	Foreign substances	
	Idiopathic (?)	
Eosinophilic	Food sensitivity	Allergic
	Other allergies (?)	
Other infectious gastritides	Bacteria (other than *H. pylori*)	Phlegmonous, syphilitic, others
	Viruses	Cytomegalovirus
	Fungi	Anisakiasis
	Parasites	

CAG, *Chronic antral gastritis;* DAG, *diffuse antral gastritis;* MAG, *multifocal atrophic gastritis;* NSAIDs, *nonsteroidal antiinflammatory drugs.*

Reporting Gastritis in the Absence of a Complete Biopsy Set

The Sydney system guidelines can be applied only when a full set of biopsy specimens is available (see Fig. 15.21). In routine practice, pathologists are usually asked to make a diagnosis based on only one or two biopsies and often from unspecified sites. In these cases, an empiric approach is recommended.

Most types of gastritis, including those caused by *H. pylori*, can be diagnosed without extensive tissue sampling. In contrast, assessment of the degree of atrophy requires adequate sampling and knowledge of the site of origin of each specimen to distinguish MAG from autoimmune metaplastic atrophic gastritis. A diagnosis of gastritis based on only a few nonrepresentative or inadequately identified biopsy specimens should not include any statements regarding topographic distribution of disease. If a specimen labeled as "corpus" contains pyloric-appearing glands and lacks parietal and chief cells, suggesting that it may be derived from the antrum, an immunostain for gastrin can help resolve the issue. The finding of numerous gastrin-positive cells, typically in the midgland region, is evidence in favor of the antrum, whereas atrophic pyloric-type glands from metaplastic corpus may contain either rare, scattered, or no gastrin-positive cells at all. In addition, recognition of nodular ECL-cell hyperplasia will raise the possibility of autoimmune gastritis. If uncertainty persists, a less-specific diagnosis (e.g., chronic inactive gastritis with atrophy and intestinal metaplasia) may be used, along with a comment regarding the differential diagnosis, including a suggestion that a more extensive sampling would be helpful to determine an exact etiology. Other information, such as clinical evidence of pernicious anemia, hypergastrinemia, achlorhydria, and the presence or absence of circulating anti–parietal cell antibodies, may help establish a precise diagnosis of autoimmune metaplastic atrophic gastritis.

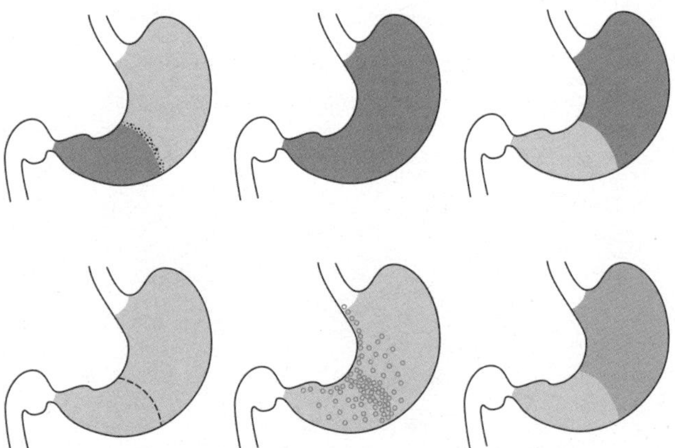

FIGURE 15.22 The Sydney system separates chronic gastritis into atrophic and nonatrophic forms, each representing one of the extremes of the spectrum of gastritis.

OLGA AND OLGIM SYSTEMS

Building on the current knowledge of the natural history of gastritis and its associated cancer risk, the Operative Link for Gastritis Assessment (OLGA) staging system has been proposed.[11,66] The system places the histological phenotypes of gastritis on a scale of progressively increasing gastric cancer risk, from the lowest (stage 0) to the highest (stage IV).

Use of a well-defined biopsy sampling protocol (Sydney system) is considered the minimum requirement for reliable staging of chronic gastritis. The stage of gastritis is determined by a combination of the extent of atrophy (scored histologically) with its topographic location (resulting from the mapping protocol). Consistent with the Sydney recommendations, OLGA staging system reporting includes information about the likely cause of gastritis (e.g., *H. pylori*, autoimmune).

The OLGA system is based on the atrophy score. Atrophy is scored as a percentage of the atrophic glands. Nonmetaplastic and metaplastic subtypes are considered together. At each biopsy sample level (irrespective of the area from which it originates), atrophy is scored by using a four-tiered scale: atrophy absent (0%) = 0, mild (1% to 30%) = 1, moderate (31% to 60%) = 2, and severe (>60%) = 3. The OLGA gastritis stage (I to IV) is determined by combining the overall antrum score with an overall corpus score for atrophy (Table 15.5). Details on how to apply the OLGA scores in clinical practice are provided in a well-illustrated step-by-step tutorial.[13,14]

A subsequent modification of the OLGA staging system that only considers intestinal metaplasia rather than

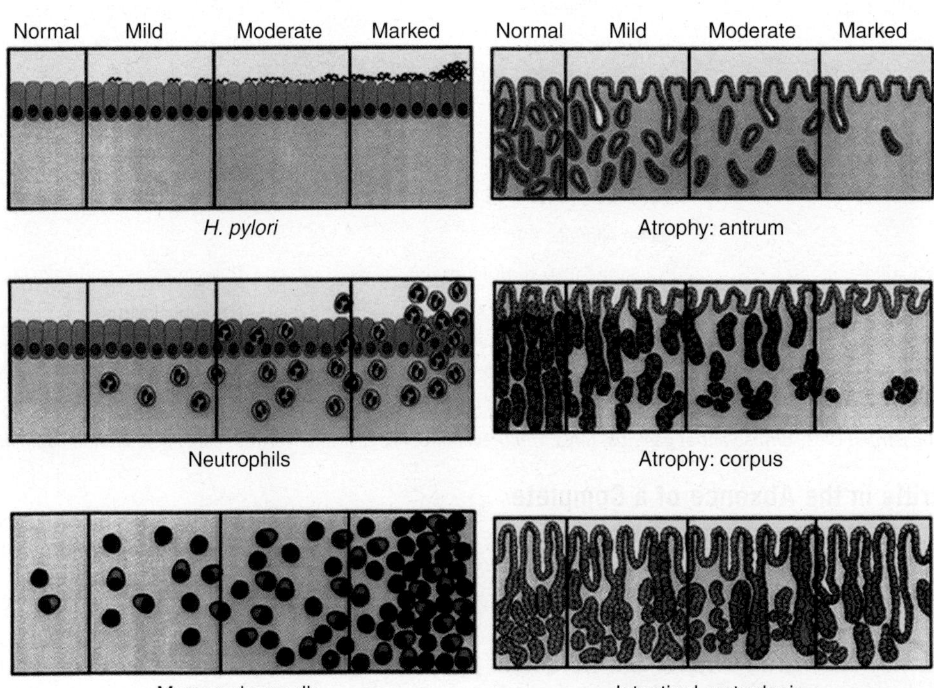

FIGURE 15.23 The visual analogue scale proposed in the updated Sydney system.

atrophy as the main parameter for assessment of gastric cancer risk (i.e., Operative Link for Gastric Intestinal Metaplasia [OLGIM]) has been proposed. This scheme may be less vulnerable to interobserver variability because intestinal metaplasia can be recognized and quantified more reliably than atrophy, especially for general pathologists.[67,68] However, considering that pseudopyloric metaplasia is often the dominant phenotype of atrophy in patients with autoimmune gastritis, a substantial proportion of potentially high-risk individuals can be missed when using the OLGIM system.

A recent meta-analysis has underscored the significant association between advanced OLGA/OLGIM stages (i.e., stages III and IV) and risk of gastric cancer.[69] The conclusion is already reflected in the European guidelines for the management of gastric precancerous lesions, which recommends endoscopic surveillance every 3 years for patients with high-risk OLGA/OLGIM stages.[70]

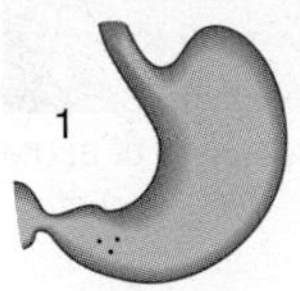

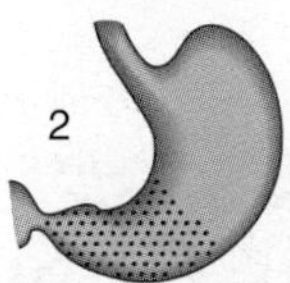

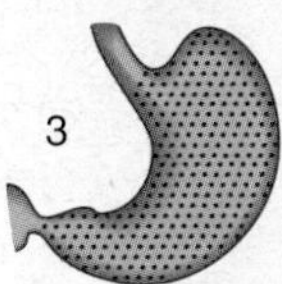

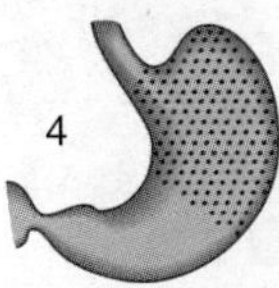

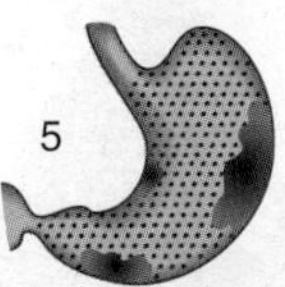

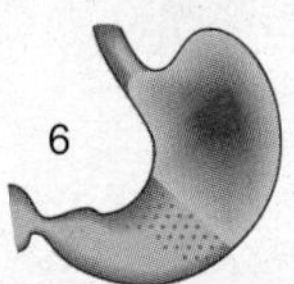

FIGURE 15.24 Examples of diagnoses generated according to the recommendations of the updated Sydney system. Areas of gastritis *(red)*, intestinal metaplasia *(blue)*, and atrophy *(gray)* are indicated.

ACUTE AND SUBACUTE MUCOSAL INJURY (ACUTE GASTRITIS)

This section describes acute conditions that typically present with sudden onset and rapid evolution, and often result from an imbalance between acute mucosal injury and tissue repair. Histologically, *acute gastritis* is defined as any form of gastritis that shows acute ("active") features of epithelial injury and inflammation, but without well-established features of chronicity. For instance, it may represent the initial phase of *H. pylori* infection or of an acute bacterial (suppurative) gastritis, such as phlegmonous gastritis, which is much less common.[71-74] Acute hemorrhagic gastritis is a common form of an acute gastritis that is usually caused by ingestion of large quantities of alcohol or medications including NSAIDs or antibiotics.[75] Corrosive acidic and alkaline substances can cause extensive, severe necrotic lesions that are usually not biopsied. Unless perforation develops, the lesions typically heal, sometimes with scarring and organ deformity. An acute manifestation of autoimmune enteropathy has been reported in the stomach.[76] This condition is briefly discussed in the differential diagnosis section of Autoimmune Gastritis later in this chapter and more extensively in Chapter 11.

Acute Hemorrhagic Gastritis

Clinical Features

Acute hemorrhagic gastritis (also known as acute *hemorrhagic erosive gastropathy*) is defined as acute gastritis associated with hemorrhage and congestion of the mucosa and/or deeper layers of the stomach. It is most often characterized by diffuse mucosal hyperemia associated with bleeding, erosions, and ulcers.

TABLE 15.5 Operative Link for Gastritis Assessment (OLGA) Staging System

	Corpus			
Antrum	**No Atrophy (Score 0)**	**Mild Atrophy (Score 1)**	**Moderate Atrophy (Score 2)**	**Severe Atrophy (Score 3)**
No atrophy (score 0), including incisura angularis	Stage 0	Stage I	Stage II	Stage II
Mild atrophy (score 1), including incisura angularis	Stage I	Stage I	Stage II	Stage III
Moderate atrophy (score 2), including incisura angularis	Stage II	Stage II	Stage III	Stage IV
Severe atrophy (score 3), including incisura angularis	Stage III	Stage III	Stage IV	Stage IV

Ingestion of large doses of toxic chemical substances, including various medications such as aspirin, other types of NSAIDs, iron (ferrous sulfate) pills, and less frequently, a variety of other drugs (e.g., doxycycline), may cause acute mucosal injury ranging from edema and hyperemia to frank erosion and ulceration. These lesions may occur suddenly, without prior pain or discomfort, in both first-time and chronic NSAID users.[63] Similar, but usually less severe, changes may be caused by ingestion of large quantities of alcohol.[77] Because alcohol and aspirin act synergistically to alter mucosal defenses, many cases of hemorrhagic gastritis are caused by alcohol users who consume aspirin to prevent hangover sickness.[78] More specifically, NSAIDs act by interfering with prostaglandin synthesis, whereas alcohol causes direct damage to the gastric mucosa.[39]

Pathological Features

Grossly, acute hemorrhagic gastritis is characterized by hyperemic edematous-appearing mucosa, surface erosions, and active bleeding (Fig. 15.25). The damage is usually centered on the antrum. The clinical history (e.g., shock, burns, ingestion of large doses of NSAIDs) rather than the pathological features helps determine the precise cause. In addition, multiple subepithelial petechiae may develop after large quantities of strong alcoholic beverages are consumed over a short period.[39,79]

Microscopically, acute hemorrhagic gastritis, regardless of its cause, is characterized by dilation and congestion of mucosal capillaries, edema, and interstitial hemorrhage within the lamina propria. Surface erosions are typically usually small and appear ischemic, showing superficially hyalinized lamina propria. Aggregates of fibrin and neutrophils replace eroded epithelium and often project above the mucosal surface to form small, elevated clumps of necrotic debris (Fig. 15.26A). The foveolar epithelium underneath and adjacent to erosions and ulcers show regenerative changes reminiscent of epithelial "withering" observed in ischemia, but also elongation, increased tortuosity, and mucin depletion. Enlarged and hyperchromatic nuclei and increased mitoses are common features and should not be misinterpreted as dysplasia. Recalling the location of the normal regenerative zones in the antrum (i.e., gland base) and corpus (i.e., mucous neck cell region) can help mitigate an overdiagnosis of dysplasia. In the absence of concurrent *H. pylori* infection, unaffected areas of the stomach do not usually show increased chronic inflammation. In the setting of *H. pylori* infection, the pathologist may see chronic active inflammation in the mucosa, which may obscure or worsen the changes caused by NSAIDs or alcohol.

Natural History and Treatment

The prognosis of acute hemorrhagic gastritis depends on the type and amount of noxious chemical agents ingested. Cases without deep ulcers are usually self-limited, although severe damage may lead to perforation or healing with distorting scars in rare cases. In extreme cases, erosion of an underlying large blood vessel may cause catastrophic hemorrhage and death. The mainstay of treatment is cessation of ingestion of the offensive corrosive agent. Suppression of acid secretion with PPIs helps reduce the severity of mucosal damage and facilitates mucosal healing.

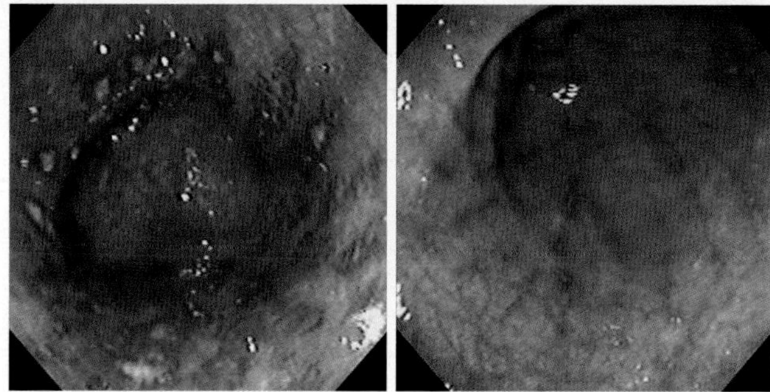

FIGURE 15.25 Two views showing the endoscopic appearance of acute hemorrhagic gastritis. (*Courtesy David Y. Graham, MD, Houston, Texas.*)

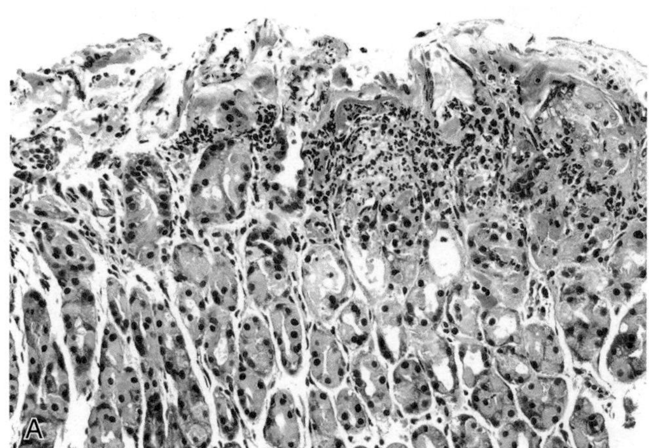

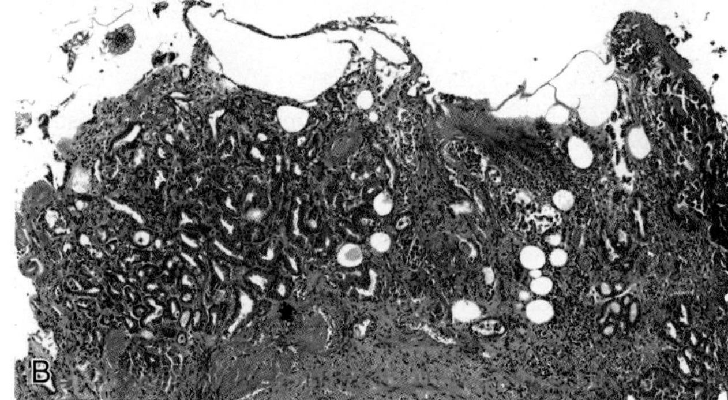

FIGURE 15.26 A, Superficial erosion in the corpus mucosa of a patient with acute hemorrhagic gastritis. **B,** Rare example of emphysematous gastritis with distinct pneumatosis of the lamina propria in addition to active inflammation with focal erosion.

Stress-Induced Gastritis

Clinical Features and Pathogenesis

This subtype of acute gastritis occurs in patients with major physiological distress, such as severe trauma, especially brain injury with increased intracranial pressure; burns; severe hypothermia; shock; sepsis; coagulopathy; severe liver and renal insufficiency; and prolonged mechanical ventilation.[80] Gastric mucosal damage may develop in up to 75% of these patients; however, improvements in critical care have led to a decline in mortality. For instance, the development of clinically important gastrointestinal (GI) bleeding in critical care units has recently decreased from 25% to 0.6% to 4%.[81-83]

Stress-induced gastritis is usually precipitated by a sudden imbalance between injurious agents and protective factors involved in the maintenance of mucosal integrity. The putative pathogenesis is mediated by hypotension–related stasis, the release of vasoconstrictive substances, increased vascular permeability, and reperfusion injury. The luminal acidity is also known to be essential, exerting its noxious effect by inhibiting and causing loss of integrity of mucosal defense mechanisms (e.g., mucus-bicarbonate barrier). The role of concurrent *H. pylori* infection in severe stress-induced mucosal injury has also been postulated.[84]

Pathological Features

Stress-induced gastritis usually affects the oxyntic mucosa with edema, ecchymoses, and multiple superficial erosions. Ulcers are usually more than 0.5 cm in diameter and form well-delineated craters of various depths.[81,85] Stress-induced gastritis is microscopically indistinguishable from acute hemorrhagic gastritis caused by toxic chemicals. The lamina propria shows hemorrhage and congestion without notable inflammatory infiltrate. Regenerative atypia of the epithelium is common and may be severe. Ischemic features with withering pit epithelium are also not uncommon. Erosions are frequently covered by a fibrinopurulent exudate.[75]

Natural History and Treatment

The 90-day mortality rate of intensive care patients with clinically important GI bleeding is up to 55%, significantly exceeding the mortality rate of similar patients without overt GI bleeding (25%).[82] Enteral nutrition, PPIs, and histamine 2 receptor antagonists are recommended as prophylactic measures in critically ill patients.[83,86]

Phlegmonous and Emphysematous Gastritides

Clinical Features

Phlegmonous and emphysematous gastritis are rare types of acute gastritis that commonly affect patients with severe comorbidities and conditions that cause delayed gastric emptying. Rare examples have developed after endoscopic fine-needle aspiration and endoscopic resection of gastric neoplasms.[87,88] Infection by gas-forming microorganisms such as *Escherichia coli*, *Streptococcus*, *Klebsiella*, and *Pseudomonas* species are associated with the phlegmonous variant, whereas emphysematous gastritis is most frequently caused by *Proteus* and *Clostridium* species. CT imaging can be diagnostic by revealing gastric wall thickening and pneumatosis.[89]

Pathological Features

Endoscopic features include hyperemic and swollen edematous gastric folds and multiple erosions or ulcers coated with a purulent-appearing discharge. Microscopic evaluation can show a spectrum of alterations ranging from various degrees of reactive epithelial changes, to erosions and ulcerations association with fibrin deposition, severe and diffuse, sometimes transmural neutrophilic infiltration, abscess formation, and necrosis. In addition, emphysematous gastritis shows characteristic expansion of the mucosa by gas bubbles of various sizes (Fig. 15.26B).[89]

Differential Diagnosis

Phlegmonous gastritis can be differentiated from other forms of gastritis by the presence of severe neutrophilic infiltration of the gastric wall that usually spreads both longitudinally and vertically. The differential diagnosis of emphysematous gastritis includes gastric pneumatosis (on imaging studies) and pseudolipomatosis at the microscopic level resulting from air that becomes trapped in the mucosa through a mucosal defect incurred during gastroscopy.[90] Rarely, the entrapped gas may lead to mucosal elevation suspicious for a neoplastic process.

Natural History and Treatment

Early diagnosis and treatment are essential. Emphysematous gastritis is frequently associated with a fulminant clinical course with a mortality rate up to 60%. Gastric strictures develop in one-fourth of surviving patients. Management of these patients can be either conservative (i.e., antibiotic therapy covering anaerobes and gram-negative bacilli) or surgical (i.e., gastrectomy) in severe cases.[90]

Reactive (Chemical) Gastropathy

General Comments and Definition

The Sydney system defines chemical gastropathy as "the constellation of endoscopic and histological changes caused by chemical injury to the gastric mucosa."[8] Implicit in this definition is the absence of independent specific endoscopic or histological features in patients with a history of endogenous or exogenous chemical damage to the stomach. Nevertheless, compared with chronic gastritis, the lamina propria is devoid of a significant inflammatory infiltrate and shows dominantly regenerative mucosal (both epithelial and stromal) architectural changes. *Bile reflux gastritis* was the first recognized form of reactive gastropathy.[32,91-94] Subsequently, it was determined that NSAID use may cause similar mucosal lesions, and the term *chemical gastritis* was introduced. Additional synonyms include *reactive gastropathy*, *type* C *gastritis*, and *chemical gastritis*. Morphologically identical alterations may occur in mucosa adjacent to ulcers of any kind, mass lesions, and vascular disorders, such as portal hypertensive gastropathy and GAVE. Thus the feature of reactive gastritis must be interpreted in conjunction with the clinical and endoscopic information of the patient.

Clinical Features

Several chemical agents, including numerous medications, are commonly associated with damage to gastric mucosa. Although some agents cause acute destructive and ulcerating lesions, others may induce only subtle and mild changes of reactive gastritis. Before the discovery of *H. pylori* as a cause of gastritis, several types of food items, such as caffeine and hot peppers, were also thought to cause gastritis. However, the role of many of those food items was eventually discounted. Most patients with mild reactive gastritis are asymptomatic. Severe cases may be associated with dyspepsia, loss of appetite, nausea, and vomiting. Upper GI tract bleeding or perforation can develop in cases with deep ulcers.

Etiological Factors and Pathogenesis

Duodenopancreatic (Bile) Reflux

Historically, bile reflux gastritis was initially recognized as a complication of partial (Billroth II) gastrectomy, which was a procedure used for benign conditions such as peptic ulcer disease. With the discovery of *H. pylori* as the principal cause of peptic ulcer disease and with the use of effective medical treatment, Billroth II antrectomies for benign disease have become increasingly uncommon. Subsequently, the prevalence of anastomotic and stomal gastropathy is expected to decline. Some patients have developed polypoid growths at the anastomotic site and gastric outlet obstruction when the lesions attain a large size, prompting endoscopic assessment.

Reflux of bile, or other luminal components of the duodenum, into a normal, nonoperated stomach is difficult to demonstrate in clinical practice, and the relevance of this condition needs further clarification. However, reactive gastritis, in the absence of known NSAID therapy or any other specific cause, is most commonly induced by duodenogastric bile reflux. Some degree of bile reflux is believed to occur in most healthy individuals and particularly those who smoke and have a duodenal ulcer, or those who have chronic respiratory disease, suffer from alcohol abuse, or are postcholecystectomy.[95] Gastric mucosa chronically exposed to bile may undergo pathological changes similar to those that occur in a gastric stump. Patients with bile reflux documented by 24-hour ambulatory monitoring of intragastric bilirubin absorbance and pH values were found to have significantly more active and chronic inflammation, intestinal metaplasia, atrophy, and *H. pylori* infection (particularly in the corpus and incisura) than dyspeptic patients without bile reflux.[96] A high prevalence of *H. pylori* infection was reported for antrectomized patients in Israel.[97,98] These data contrast with previous observations that bile reflux tends to eliminate, or suppress, *H. pylori* infection.[99,100]

Duodenogastric reflux with alkaline pancreatic and duodenal secretions, acids, bile salts, and lysolecithin results in disruption of the mucosal barrier and direct chemical damage to gastric surface epithelium. Loss of this barrier allows back-diffusion of hydrogen ions and secondary injury.[101] This combined injury leads to accelerated exfoliation of surface epithelium and a histamine-mediated vascular response that manifests histologically as edema and hyperemia. Persistent epithelial damage promotes the release of other proinflammatory agents, such as PGDF, which stimulates smooth muscle and fibroblastic proliferation.

Medications

The most commonly used drugs and drug categories that can damage gastric mucosa when consumed at therapeutic doses are listed in Table 15.6. The most common pattern of drug-induced gastric mucosal injury is reactive gastritis (Fig. 15.27), although some drugs induce other patterns of injury. The most common forms of drug-induced gastritis are discussed in more detail in the next dedicated section.

Pathological Features

In patients with duodenogastric bile reflux, the gastric mucosa may exhibit congestion, edema, and surface erosion. In postgastrectomy patients with bile reflux, gross examination of the anastomotic site may also reveal polypoid lesions.[102,103] Nonspecific superficial erosions may occur in the more proximal areas of the gastric stump.

Microscopically, reactive gastritis is characterized by a variable degree of foveolar hyperplasia distinguished by tortuosity of the surface epithelium, regenerative changes including mucin depletion, thinning and loss of the columnar shape of the foveolar epithelium (i.e., cuboidalization), increased mitoses, nuclear hyperchromasia, occasional superficial erosions (see Fig. 15.7), and congestion, edema, and smooth muscle proliferation in the lamina propria.[94,104] Although a diagnosis of chemical gastritis can be suspected when these features are detected, a firm diagnosis necessitates correlation with supportive clinical data (e.g., medication history) and exclusion of *H. pylori* infection.[43] The algorithm in Fig. 15.28 provides a common-sense approach to the evaluation of reactive gastritis. Usually, the features of

TABLE 15.6 Drug-Induced Gastric Injury

Drug or Drug Family	Predominant Morphology of Gastric Injury
NSAIDs, aspirin, alcohol	Erosions, ulcers, reactive gastropathy
Proton pump inhibitors	Parietal cell hypertrophy and hyperplasia, fundic gland cysts and polyps
Iron	Reactive gastropathy and erosions with Fe^{2+} deposits
Doxycycline	Reactive gastropathy and erosions; characteristic eosinophilic necrosis of the wall of superficial capillaries with luminal microthrombi and neutrophils
Sodium polystyrene sulfonate sorbitol (Kayexalate)	Crystal deposition (i.e., rhomboid or triangular, nonpolarizable, basophilic crystals adherent to the surface epithelium or within sloughed inflammatory exudates)
Cholestyramine	Crystal deposition (similar to Kayexalate crystals)
Colchicine or taxane-based chemotherapy	Abundant metaphase mitoses (especially ring mitoses), epithelial pseudostratification, loss of polarity, increased apoptosis in pit epithelium
Chemotherapy	Mucosal sloughing, enlarged gland cells with normal N:C ratio, gland loss
Immune checkpoint inhibitors	Chronic active gastritis with increased intraepithelial lymphocytosis and prominent apoptosis or focally enhanced gastritis
HAIC or SIR-Spheres therapy	Ulceration with nuclear atypia; numerous enlarged, bizarrely shaped nuclei with vesicular chromatin and large, irregular nucleoli
Bisphosphonates (e.g., alendronate)	Ulcerations (rare in the stomach, most common in the esophagus)
Corticosteroids	Possibly increased acid secretion, synergistic ulcerogenic effect with aspirin and NSAIDs

Fe^{2+}, *Ferrous iron ion;* HAIC, *hepatic arterial infusion chemotherapy;* N:C *ratio, nucleus-to-cytoplasm ratio;* NSAIDs, *nonsteroidal antiinflammatory drugs;* SIR-Spheres, *selective internal radiation microspheres.*

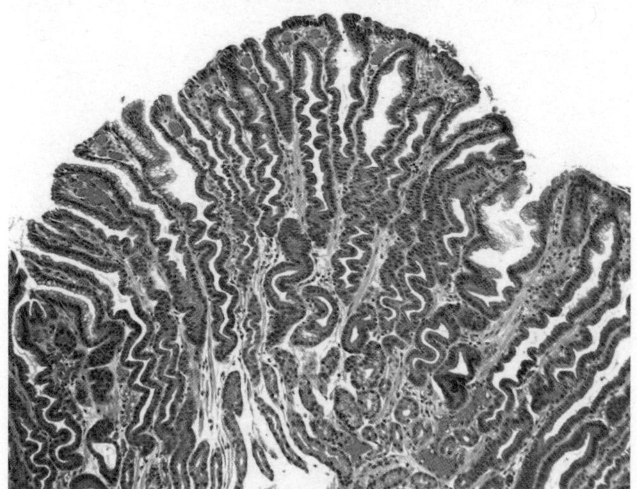

FIGURE 15.27 Stomal gastropathy (after Billroth II chronic gastritis) showing sparse chronic inflammation and marked foveolar hyperplasia, mucin depletion, vascular congestion, edema, and smooth muscle hyperplasia.

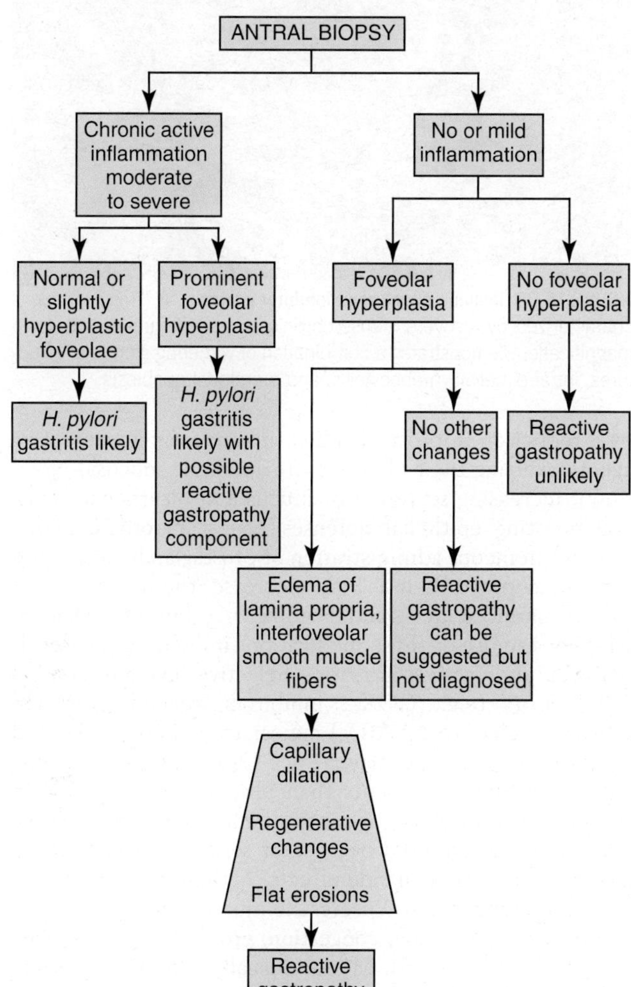

FIGURE 15.28 Diagnostic algorithm for reactive (chemical) gastropathy. (*Modified from Genta RM. Differential diagnosis of reactive gastropathy. Semin Diagn Pathol. 2005;22:273–283.*)

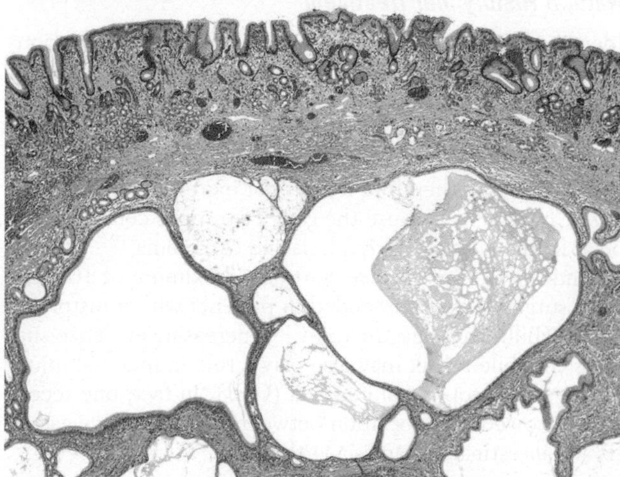

FIGURE 15.29 Gastritis cystica polyposa in a patient with chronic atrophic gastritis. Notice the lobular configuration of the submucosal epithelium and the rim of normal lamina propria.

reactive gastritis (see Fig. 15.27) are limited to the antrum. The corpus of previously nonoperated stomachs only rarely show findings of reactive gastritis. However, corpus mucosal biopsies are usually the only ones available for study from patients who have had Billroth II surgery.

Between 10% and 30% of patients who undergo a partial gastrectomy will develop mucosal lesions adjacent to the anastomosis or stoma site. These cystic lesions are formed from dilated, irregular, and cystic foveolae that frequently show regenerative changes (Fig. 15.29). When the lesion forms a polyp, it is referred to as *gastritis cystica polyposa;* when the lesion is predominantly inverted, forming a prominent submucosal lesion or mass, the term *gastritis cystica profunda* is used[105] (see Chapter 20 for details).

Differential Diagnosis

Differentiating drug-induced reactive gastropathies from other causes is difficult and may be impossible without knowledge of the patient's medication history. One feature that should always raise the possibility of drug-induced mucosal injury is the presence of ischemic-like erosions including the presence of withering pits and hyalinized lamina propria. Unfortunately, chronic inflammation (particularly when it is moderate or severe), either with or without neutrophils, tends to obscure the features of chemical gastritis. Furthermore, *H. pylori* infection may induce some of the features traditionally considered characteristic of chemical gastritis as well (see Fig. 15.9). Although a combination of reactive gastritis with a chronic lymphoplasmacytic infiltrate is not necessarily indicative of multiple etiologies, a combination of their deleterious effects is not uncommon because agents that cause mucosal injury (e.g., NSAID use or *H. pylori* infection) affect a large population of patients. In a large Central European study, more than 5% of patients diagnosed with gastritis showed a combination of different histological patterns of injury.[106]

Finally, as mentioned earlier, changes identical to those of chemical gastritis may occur in the mucosa adjacent to ulcers, mass lesions, and a variety of other disorders, such as portal hypertensive gastropathy and GAVE.

Natural History and Treatment

Identification and discontinuation of the offensive noxious agent(s) usually leads to mucosal healing without further treatment. Focal intestinal metaplasia may develop in reactive gastritis if ingestion is chronic, but this does not normally progress into antrum-restricted atrophic gastritis or to corpus atrophy; therefore it does not increase gastric cancer risk. Conversely, because the gastric stump is considered to be at increased risk for dysplasia and carcinoma,[107,108] regular endoscopic surveillance starting a maximum of 10 years after surgery is recommended in patients with a history of partial (Billroth II) gastrectomy.[109] Increasing evidence suggests that bile reflux may also play a role in mucosal injury of the gastroesophageal junction (GEJ). In fact, one recent study showed an association between antral reactive gastritis and intestinal metaplasia at the GEJ.[110]

Drug-Induced Gastritis and Other Iatrogenic Mucosal Changes

The list of medications known to cause injury to gastric mucosa is ever-increasing. Some of these medications (e.g., NSAIDs) are available over the counter in many countries. In addition to NSAIDs, other agents, such as iron, potassium, gold, and corticosteroids may cause gastric mucosal damage, with some associated with more distinctive histological findings. The most commonly used drugs and drug categories that can damage gastric mucosa when consumed at therapeutic doses are listed in Table 15.6. Although the most common pattern is reactive gastritis (see Fig. 15.27), some drugs induce other patterns of injury as well. For example, immune checkpoint inhibitors most frequently cause active chronic gastritis, or rarely, focally enhanced gastritis.[111] A graft-versus-host disease (GVHD)–like pattern of injury, with increased apoptosis, may be observed in patients treated with mycophenolate, immune checkpoint inhibitors, colchicine, or taxane-based chemotherapy (Fig. 15.30)[111-114]

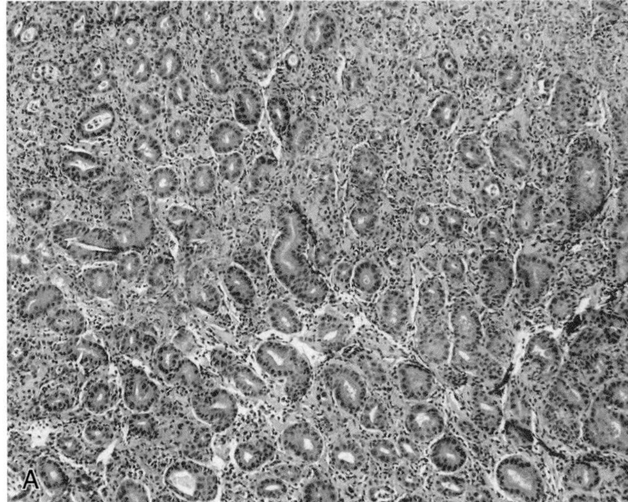

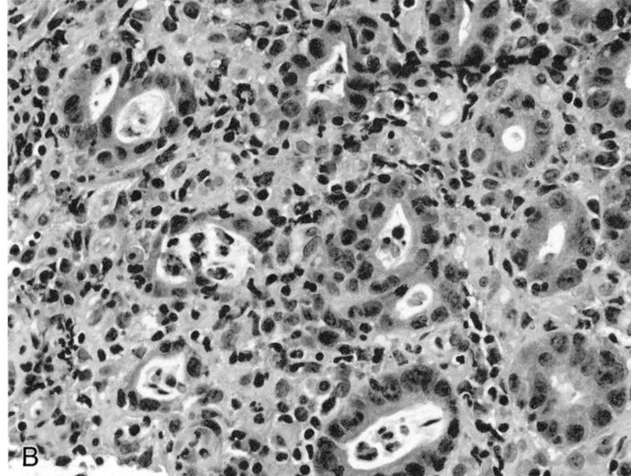

FIGURE 15.30 Immune checkpoint inhibitor gastritis. A, This example is characterized by a severe diffuse chronic active inflammation. **B,** High magnification demonstrates a combination of withering glandular structures, intraepithelial lymphocytosis, and prominent apoptosis.

Confirmation of the etiology of a suspected iatrogenic gastritis may be impossible without knowledge of the patient's medication history. However, some histological feature such as ischemic-like erosions, brisk apoptotic activity, and ring mitoses should prompt a review of the patient's prescribed drugs. In a minority of cases, the specific drug (e.g., Kayexalate resin) itself may be microscopically identified based on its characteristic morphology (Fig. 15.31).[115]

Nonsteroidal Antiinflammatory Drug–Induced Gastritis

Although millions of people ingest NSAIDs daily, severe GI complications such as a bleeding gastric ulcers develop in only approximately 2% per year.[63] These patients may represent a specific subset who have a genetic predisposition to the breakdown of mucosal defense mechanisms in response to these medications. Unfortunately, specific risk factors for severe complications from NSAIDs have not been identified. In routine practice, reactive gastritis is probably one of the most common diagnoses of gastric biopsies in the industrialized world.[64] However, it remains unclear whether gastroenterologists should change or discontinue NSAID use or, at a minimum, add a PPI to the daily medication list for patients with a biopsy-proven diagnosis. Epithelial injury after exposure to NSAIDs appears to be mediated by a reduction in prostaglandins (important cytoprotective agents exerting their effects by maintaining mucosal blood flow), increasing secretion of mucus and bicarbonate ions, and boosting epithelial defenses against cytotoxic injury. The simultaneous administration of prostaglandin analogues (e.g., misoprostol) and PPIs decrease the incidence of NSAID-induced ulcers and bleeding,[63,116] but it is unknown whether the use of these medications influences the development of reactive gastritis. Selective cyclooxygenase-2 inhibitors (e.g., COX-2 inhibitors, second-generation NSAIDs, selective NSAIDs) appear to be better tolerated by gastric mucosa and may reduce GI symptoms, but they still cause more GI events than placebos.[117,118] Although the indications for use of many of these compounds have been drastically limited because of serious concerns about possible cardiovascular side effects,[119] their use persists.

In long-term NSAID users, the mucosa may appear normal or show erythema, congestion, erosions, or ulcers (see Figs. 15.25 and 15.26). Microscopically, NSAIDs typically induce a reactive gastropathy pattern of mucosal injury. Although some histological features are observed more frequently in long-term NSAID users, their specificity and predictive value are uncertain because of the difficulty of

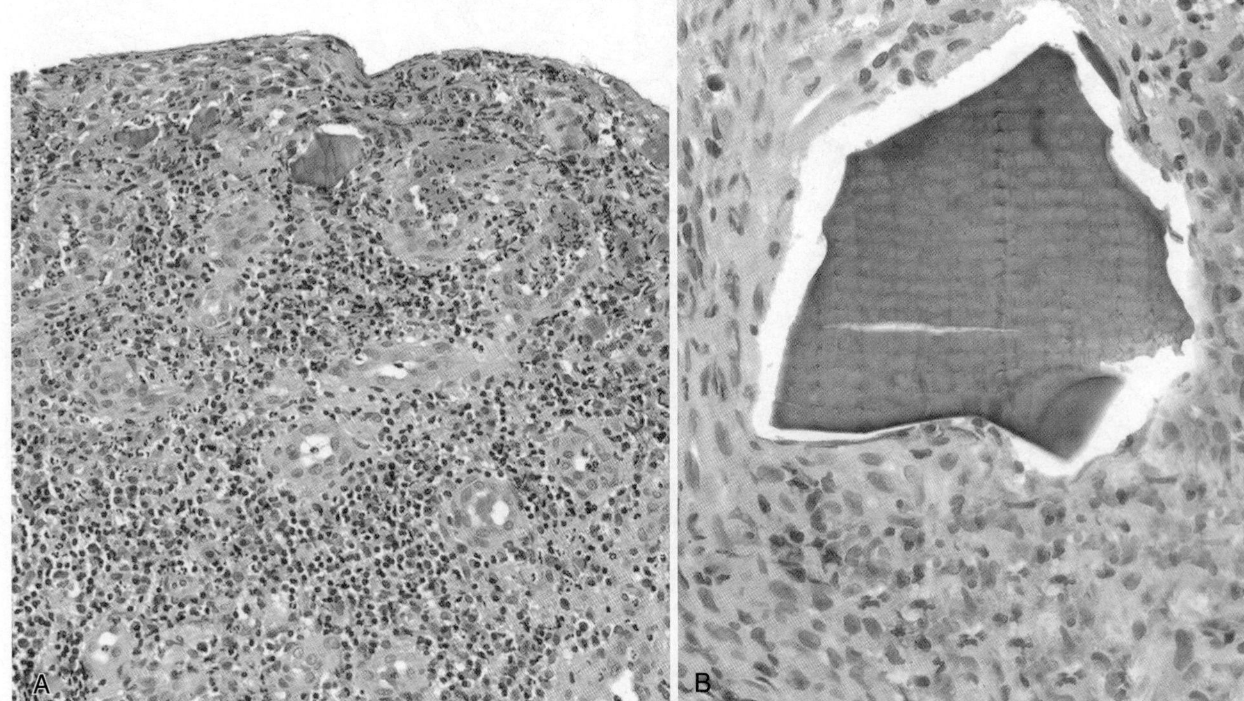

FIGURE 15.31 **A** and **B,** Rhomboid, purple, platelike crystals are characteristic of the side effects of Kayexalate given for the treatment of hyperkalemia in uremic patients.

obtaining normal controls. Further, many patients fail to declare NSAID use, or ingestion of other substances (e.g., alcohol) that may cause mucosal changes similar to those of NSAIDs. Finally, there is always the possibility of clinically silent bile reflux.[45,120] Nevertheless, a possible giveaway of NSAID-induced reactive gastropathy is the presence of erosions/ulcers showing an ischemic-like pattern with withering pits and hyalinized lamina propria. A similar morphology but with additional brown pigment embedded in the necrotic debris and hyalinized material at the base of an erosion is a common feature in ferrous sulfate (iron pill)–induced injuries (Fig. 15.32).[121] Eosinophilic capillary wall degeneration (i.e., fibrinoid necrosis) and luminal microthrombi should raise the possibility of doxycycline related mucosal damage (Fig. 15.33).[122]

Iron

Iron tablets are used widely for the treatment of anemia. A reactive gastritis pattern of injury with mucosal erosions or ulcers develops in some users. The mucosa may show changes reminiscent of ischemic injury, with withering pits and superficially hyalinized lamina propria. Characteristic brown pigment (representing fragments of iron tablets) may be identifiable among granular debris on the mucosal surface within the ulcer exudates or within inflamed tissues.[123,124] The ferrous nature of the pigment can be highlighted by use of a special stain for iron (Fig. 15.32A,B). These findings should not be confused with a glandular siderosis pattern with faint brown pigmentation of the glandular epithelial cells that is usually caused by systemic iron overload (Fig. 15.32C,D), whereas the nonspecific siderosis pattern with hemosiderin-laden macrophages in the lamina propria is usually a consequence of previous mucosal injury and hemorrhage.

Colchicine and Taxane-Based Chemotherapy

Colchicine is an alkaloid widely used for the treatment of gout and a variety of other medical conditions. The effect of colchicine at the cellular level is attributed to its ability to bind tubulin and inhibit its polymerization into microtubules, thereby inhibiting mitosis. Abdominal pain, cramping, and diarrhea are well-known clinical side effects. The pathological features of colchicine toxicity include multiple and sometimes numerous metaphase epithelial mitoses arranged in a distinctive ringlike configuration (Fig. 15.34). Other alterations include epithelial pseudostratification, loss of nuclear polarity, and increased apoptosis, which can mimic dysplasia. These findings may develop anywhere in the GI tract, but they are most prominent in the duodenum and gastric antrum, with relative sparing of the gastric body.[125] Conversely, taxanes inhibit the process of cell division by preventing depolymerization of microtubules and may induce noticeable histological changes at nontoxic therapeutic dosage.[113] The findings are similar to that of colchicine toxicity (Fig. 15.35). However, in addition to mitotic arrest, taxanes may causes coagulative necrosis of the epithelium, a feature not associated with colchicine toxicity.

Kayexalate

Kayexalate (sodium polystyrene sulfonate in sorbitol) is a cation exchange resin used to treat hyperkalemia in uremic patients. GI side effects (resulting from the hyperosmolar sorbitol component that is used to prevent constipation) include erosions, ulcers, and sometimes infarction in the esophagus, stomach, and intestines. Histologically the epithelium may show an ischemic pattern of injury. Biopsies may reveal characteristic purple, polygonal, platelike Kayexalate crystals (see Fig. 15.31).[126]

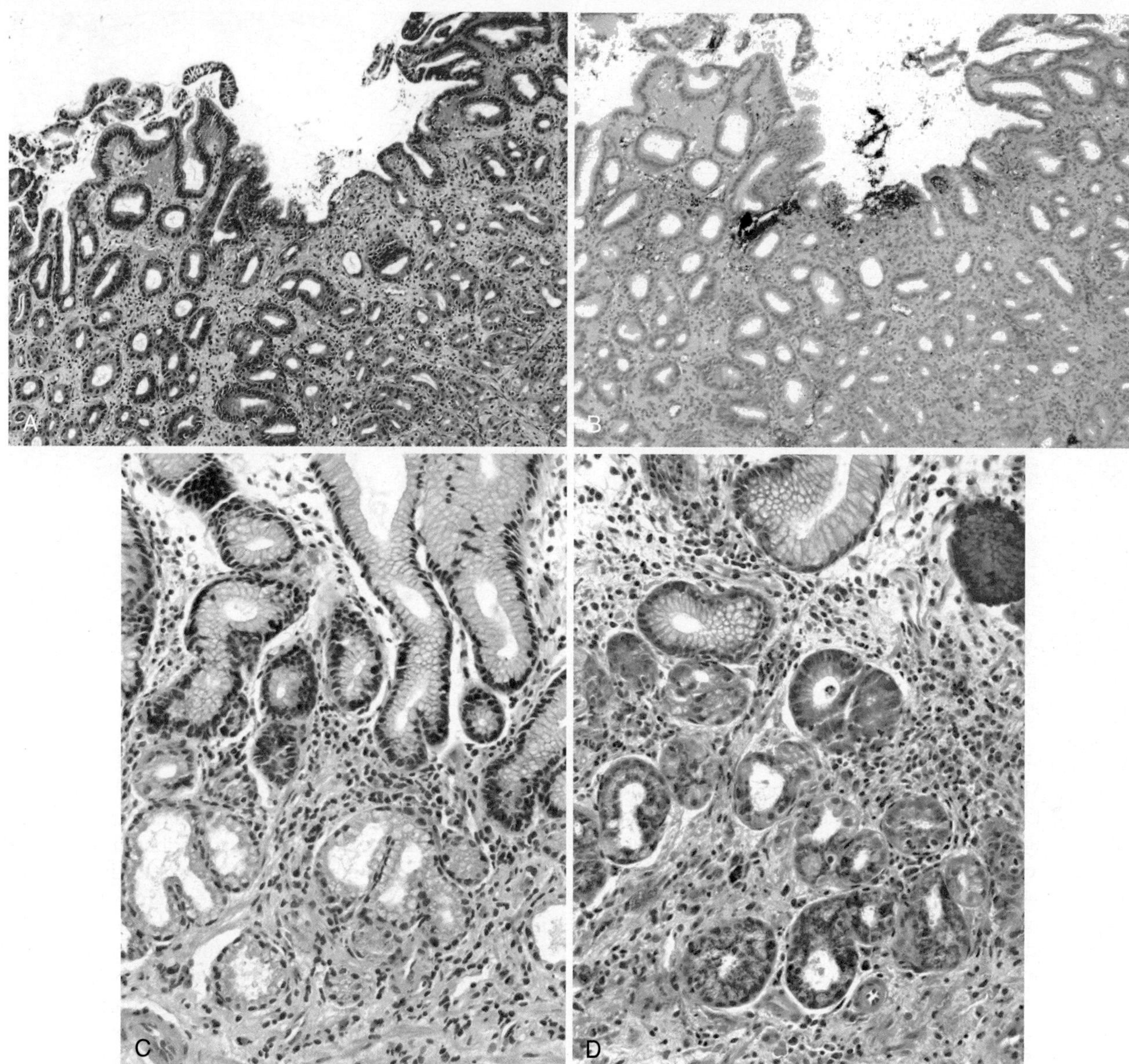

FIGURE 15.32 **A,** Mucosal erosion associated with chronic iron tablet intake. **B,** The ferrous nature of the pigment in the erosion is highlighted by a Prussian blue stain. These changes should not be confused with glandular siderosis, which is most common in systemic iron overload, which is characterized by golden-brown intracytoplasmic pigments **(C)**. **D,** Prussian blue stain shows that the pigment reflects epithelial iron deposition.

Chemotherapy- and Radiation-Induced Gastritis

Mucosal lesions may result from external irradiation of the epigastric region or infusion of selective internal radiation microspheres, as well as chemotherapeutic agents systemically or by intraarterial perfusion. Early (acute) changes consist of apoptosis and necrosis of the epithelium and fundic glands, edema, congestion, and mild mononuclear cell infiltration either with or without erosions or ulcers.

Radiation therapy causes vascular dilation, prominent and sometimes atypical endothelial or stromal cells, and occasional subendothelial collections of histiocytes. With chemotherapy and, to a lesser extent, radiation therapy, epithelial atypical cytological changes (e.g., striking nuclear pleomorphism with irregular and prominent nucleoli) mimicking dysplasia or adenocarcinoma are often noted.[127,128]

Clues that the cytological atypia represents iatrogenic injury includes preservation of the glandular architecture; large, irregular nuclei with a normal or low nucleus-to-cytoplasm ratio (Fig. 15.36); cell-to-cell variations in the degree of atypia; cytoplasmic vesiculation; and an overall gradual transition from cytologically atypical to more normal-appearing epithelium with surface maturation. In addition to being provided with clinical history, one way to determine that the atypia is radiation-induced is to identify the causative agent; such as selective internal radiation microspheres (SIR-Spheres or yttrium-90 microspheres) that can be found in the biopsies often in association with ulceration (Fig. 15.37).[116,129] Chronic changes resulting from radiation therapy include disruption of the mucosal architecture, fibrosis, and abnormalities of blood vessels that can persist indefinitely (Fig. 15.38).[130,131]

Proton Pump Inhibitor Therapy

In addition to the changes in oxyntic mucosa (i.e., parietal cell hyperplasia, hypertrophy, and dilation) described earlier

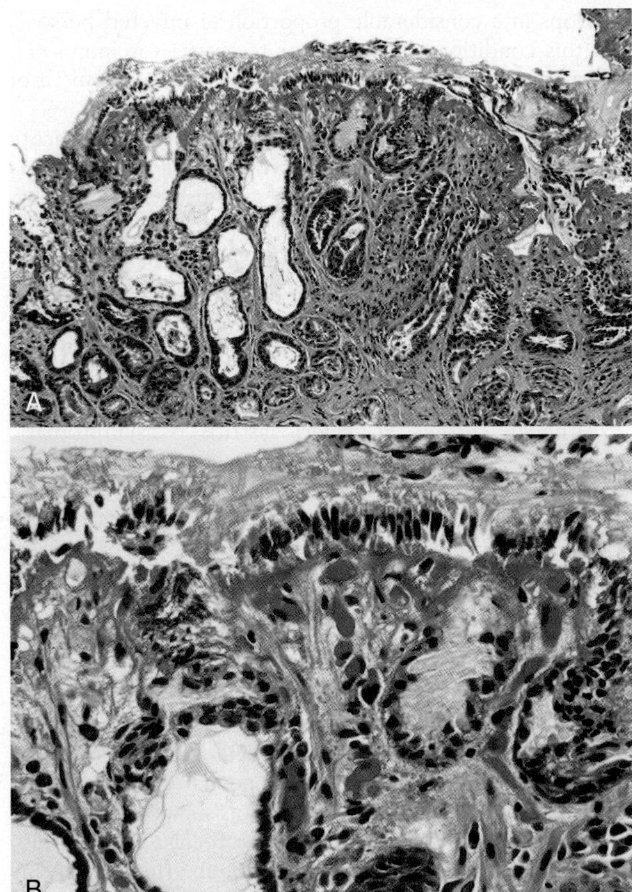

FIGURE 15.33 Doxycycline-induced gastritis. A, Low-power view shows surface erosion and scattered acute inflammation among withering glands with reactive epithelial changes. **B,** Higher-power examination shows the characteristic degenerative fibrinoid necrosis of the subepithelial capillaries with scattered fibrin thrombi. Reactive foveolar epithelium and mucin extrusion can also be seen.

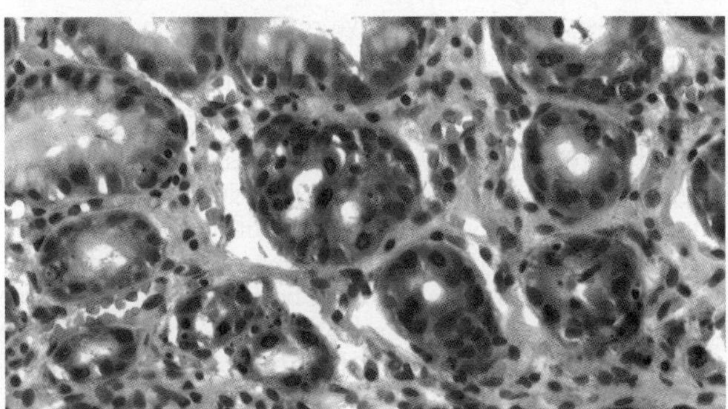

FIGURE 15.34 Colchicine toxicity may be suspected when the gastric epithelium shows prominent metaphase mitoses in a characteristic ringlike configuration. In some cases, epithelial pseudostratification with loss of polarity and apoptosis may mimic epithelial dysplasia.

(see Fig. 15.20), prolonged use of PPIs can lead to the formation of fundic gland polyps.[132,133] These lesions have little or no known association with neoplastic progression and are reversible on discontinuation of therapy.[134]

Patients with *H. pylori* gastritis who receive PPIs for prolonged periods may show changes in the intensity and distribution of gastritis.[135,136] Acid suppression with PPIs tend to cause a reduction in the bacterial and inflammatory burden; after months of therapy, inflammation is often reduced in the antrum and migrated to the corpus (i.e., corpus-predominant gastritis).[137,138] Subsequently, *H. pylori* organisms are frequently undetectable in the antrum and may only be present deep within the oxyntic glands and within the canaliculi of oxyntic cells (Fig. 15.39C,D; Fig. 15.40). The ensuing severity of corpus gastritis can accelerate the development of atrophy in that portion of the stomach,[135,136] with possible increased risk of neoplastic transformation.[48,139] However, to date there is no long-term clinical data to indicate an adverse outcome.

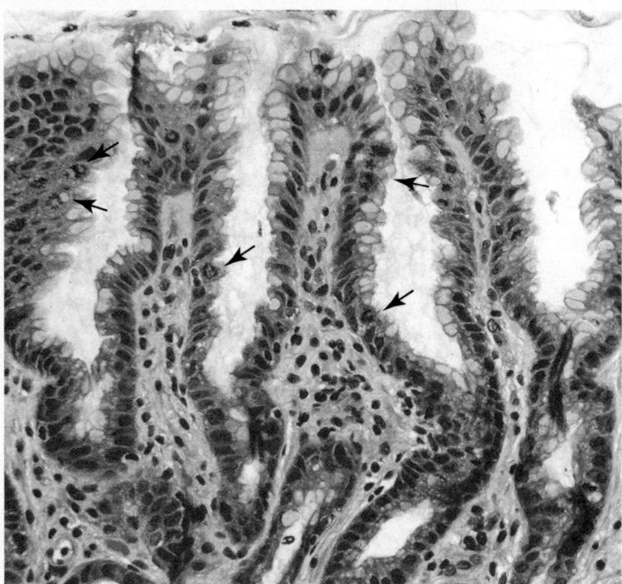

FIGURE 15.35 Example of Taxol-induced toxicity in a treated breast cancer patient. Observe the ringlike mitoses in the superficial foveolar epithelium *(arrows)*.

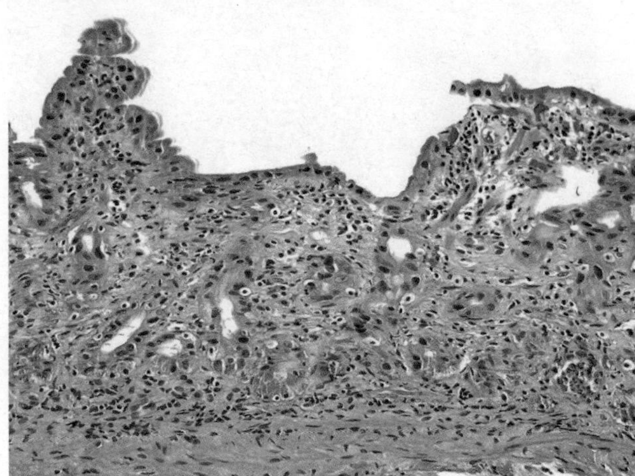

FIGURE 15.36 Chemotherapy-induced gastritis. Distinctive cytonuclear reactive atypia is present in this case. Maintenance of the normal glandular architecture, nuclear variability, and a low nucleus-to-cytoplasm ratio are characteristic features.

The guidelines of the Houston Consensus and the Maastricht Consensus of the European *H. pylori* Group recommend the detection (and treatment) of *H. pylori* before initiating long-term PPI therapy.[140,141]

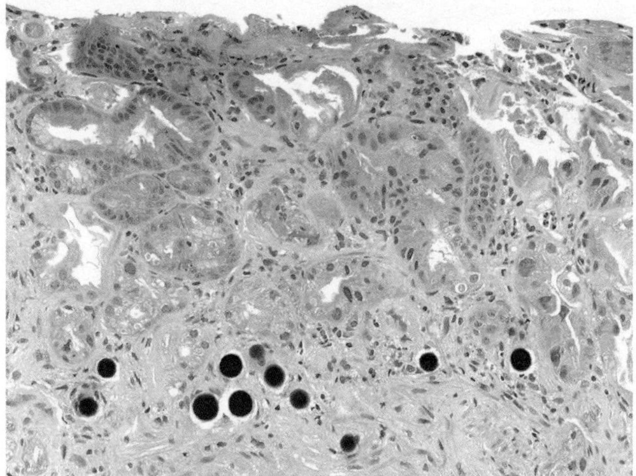

FIGURE 15.37 Radiation-induced cytological atypia can be determined by identifying the causative agent. The microspheres used in selective internal radiation therapy can be found in biopsies of gastric mucosa, often in association with ulceration.

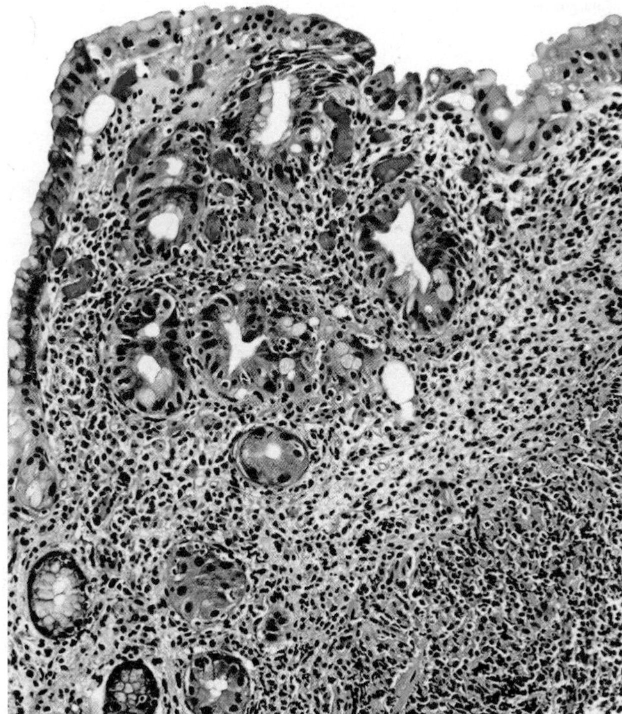

FIGURE 15.38 Radiation gastritis. This example shows fibrotic lamina propria with withering irradiated glandular structures. The inflammation is limited. Scattered residual neuroendocrine cell clusters can be noted.

CHRONIC GASTRITIS

Helicobacter pylori Gastritis

Clinical Features

Chronic *H. pylori* gastritis affects two-thirds of the world's population and is one of the most common chronic inflammatory disorders of humans.[142,143] It is causally related to most non–NSAID-induced duodenal and gastric ulcers, and most gastric mucosa–associated lymphoid tissue (MALT) lymphomas. In certain regions of the world, atrophic gastritis develops in a considerable proportion of infected persons, and this condition is a precursor to gastric carcinoma. *H. pylori* gastritis is a strong risk factor for the development of gastric cancer, particularly the intestinal type.

The early phase of *H. pylori* infection elicits an acute inflammatory response that is asymptomatic or has short-lived clinical manifestations, such as nausea and vomiting. Because most patients with early *H. pylori* gastritis do not undergo endoscopy, information regarding the clinical, endoscopic, and pathological aspects of acute *H. pylori* infection is limited.[142,144-146]

Endoscopically, manifestations of acute *H. pylori* gastritis are typically found in the antrum and characterized by hemorrhagic lesions and multiple erosions or ulcers.

Although chronic *H. pylori* gastritis is asymptomatic in most infected individuals, its impact on human health is profound. *H. pylori* gastritis confers a 15% to 20% lifetime risk for peptic ulcer disease, and 70% of gastric cancers and 85% to 90% of primary gastric MALT-type extranodal marginal zone lymphomas are directly linked to chronic *H. pylori* infection.[147-150]

Current guidelines recommend *H. pylori* eradication in all patients in whom infection is identified.[140]

Although programs for global eradication of *H. pylori* have been advocated with the goal of preventing gastric carcinoma, insufficient supportive evidence has prevented widespread acceptance of the proposals.[151,152] Critics of these programs cite the increasing resistance of *H. pylori* to the antibiotics used in current protocols. There is also much attention to the development of an effective vaccine to prevent *H. pylori* infection.[153]

Epidemiology

According to two recent meta-analyses, the overall global prevalence of *H. pylori* infection among adults is 44.3%, with approximately 4.4 billion infected individuals.[154,155] The rate of *H. pylori* infection approaches 80% to 90% in many developing countries, particularly those in the tropics. Cross-sectional studies have revealed a high prevalence of infection among children, indicating that exposure to the bacterium probably occurs relatively early in life. In industrialized parts of the world (e.g., Western Europe, United States, Canada, Australia), exposure tends to occur later in life, with an average of 20% to 50% of adults being infected.[154,155] The global prevalence of *H. pylori* infection in children (33%) is significantly lower than in adults.[154] Prevalence rates as low as 5% have been reported in Norwegian children between 1 month and 3 years of age,[156] and in China (Guangzhou province), the infection rate for children between 1 and 5 years of age was noted at 19% in 2003.[157]

Concerning the global trends with time, the prevalence of *H. pylori* infection in the 1970–1999 period was compared with those of the 2000–2016 period. *H. pylori* prevalence decreased in Europe (from 49% to 40%), Northern America (from 43% to 27%), and Oceania (from 27% to 19%), whereas prevalence data are stable in Asia and South America.[155] In eastern Asia (e.g., Japan, South Korea), where improved sanitation methods were introduced after World War II, there is a clear trend toward a lower rate of *H. pylori* infection.[154]

Despite declining rates of *H. pylori* infection in industrialized counties, the prevalence of *H. pylori* among patients

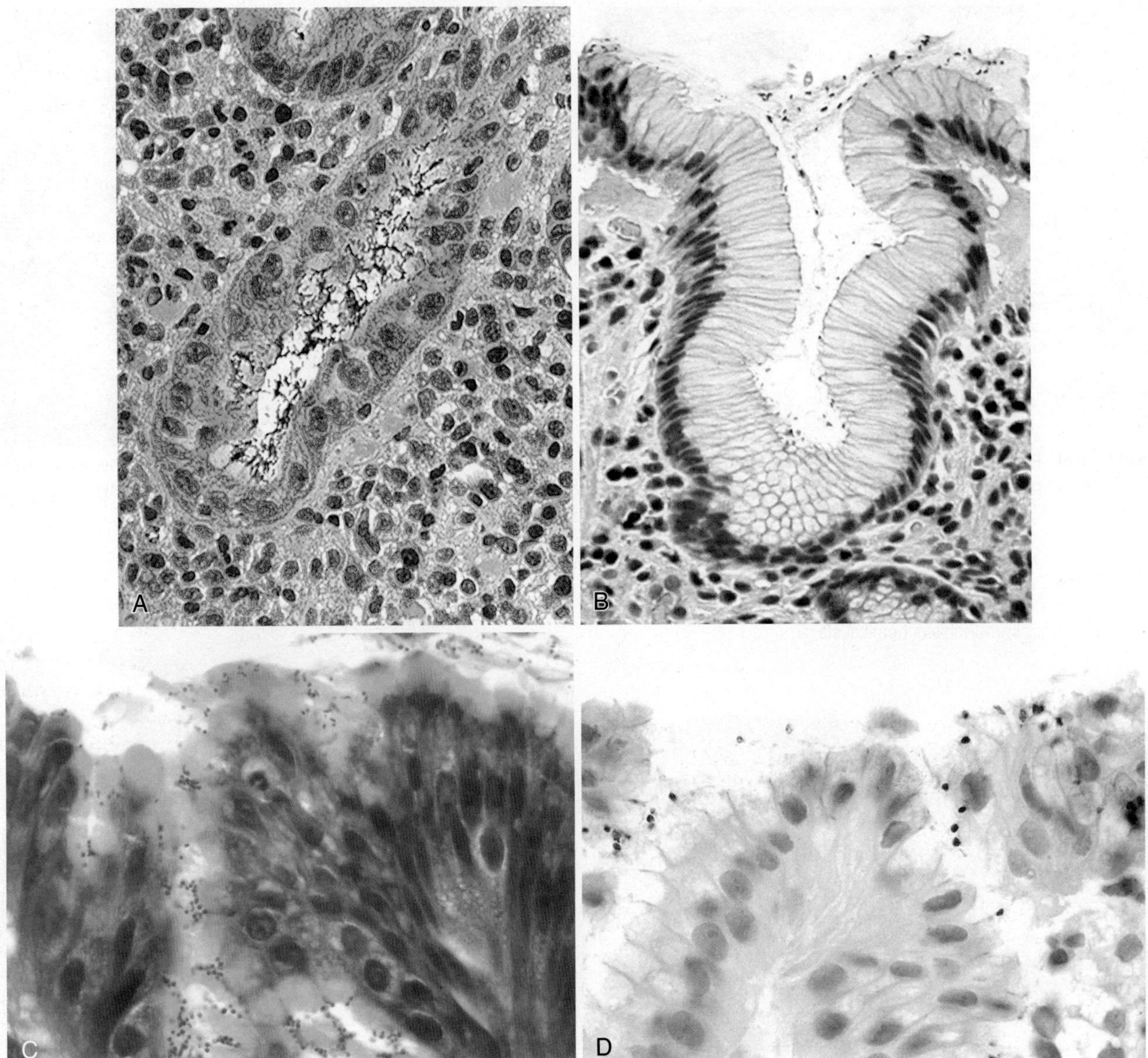

FIGURE 15.39 A, Innumerable *Helicobacter pylori* organisms (triple stain) are seen within the lumen of a pit and in the intercellular spaces of the foveolar cells. **B,** A gastric pit stained with an anti–*H. pylori* immunohistochemical stain. Coccoid forms of *H. pylori* (which usually result from unsuccessful eradication therapy) are stained with the *H. pylori* blue stain **(C)** and with an anti–*H. pylori* immunohistochemical stain **(D).**

who undergo endoscopy remains significant, and *H. pylori* should be considered in all gastric biopsy specimens examined, regardless of the patient's age or history.

Pathological Features

Grossly, there are no distinct endoscopic patterns of chronic *H. pylori* gastritis. Depending on the stage and type of gastritis, hyperemia, erosions, hypertrophy, and atrophy may coexist in various combinations. Unfortunately, none of these endoscopic features has proved useful for predicting the presence or absence of *H. pylori* gastritis. A diagnosis of *H. pylori* gastritis rests on pathological evaluation of gastric mucosal biopsies or detection of urease in mucosal specimens by the *Campylobacter*-like organism (CLO) test or the urea breath test.[158] Polymerase chain reaction (PCR) testing is discussed later.

Microscopically, *H. pylori* infection normally triggers mixed mucosal inflammation consisting of various proportions of active (i.e., neutrophil granulocytic) and chronic (i.e., lymphoplasmacytic) inflammation. Although "activity" has been regarded as the hallmark of *H. pylori* gastritis, inactive *H. pylori* gastritis is increasingly common in the era of widespread PPI use.

Given the increasing number of mildly active or inactive cases, the most characteristic feature of *H. pylori* gastritis is a plasma cell–rich mononuclear infiltrate, in a typically bandlike pattern, located in the superficial part (or neck region) of the lamina propria (Fig. 15.41). Historically, this distribution prompted use of the term *chronic superficial gastritis*, although this term should not be used as a clinical diagnosis.[54] If such a pattern of inflammation is recognized, the specimen should be intensively evaluated for the presence of *H. pylori* organisms, even in the absence of active inflammation. In some cases, a prominent diffuse intraepithelial lymphocytosis can be seen as well.[159-161] Another rare feature may be accumulation

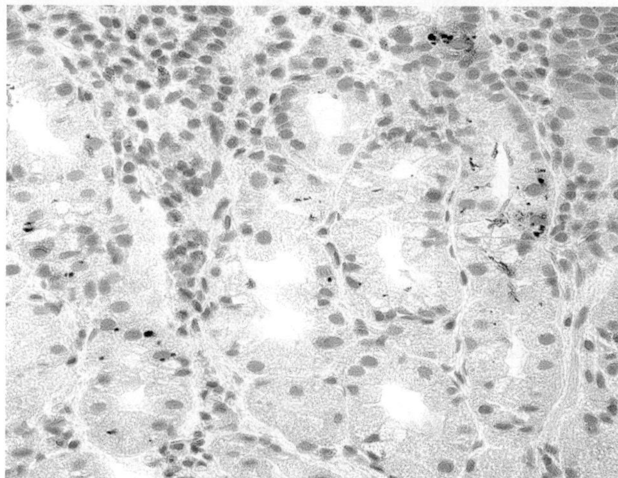

FIGURE 15.40 Patients with *Helicobacter pylori* gastritis may have additional proton pump inhibitor–related changes. These changes include a milder intensity of antral inflammation accompanied by a greater intensity in the corpus, few or no detectable organisms in the antrum, and a peculiar redistribution of *H. pylori* in the deeper portions of the oxyntic glands, even reaching the intracellular canaliculi of the parietal cells, as demonstrated by this section from the corpus stained with an anti-*Helicobacter* immunohistochemical stain.

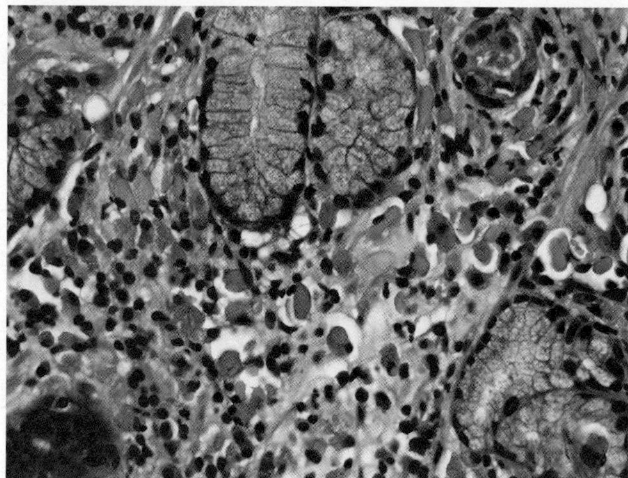

FIGURE 15.42 Russell body gastritis characterized by the accumulation of Mott cells (i.e., plasma cells containing a Russell body).

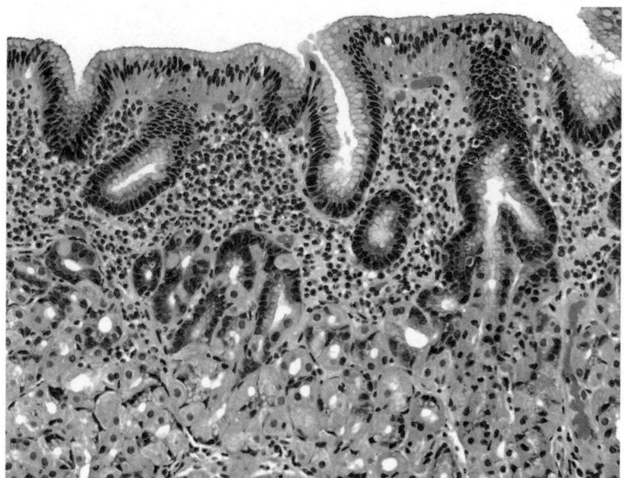

FIGURE 15.41 Chronic superficial gastritis. Lymphocytes and plasma cells form a band that fills the lamina propria of the mucous cell neck region, a common feature in *Helicobacter pylori* gastritis. Although the term *superficial gastritis* accurately describes the distribution of inflammation, the Sydney system refers to it as *mild, chronic, active (H. pylori), nonatrophic gastritis.*

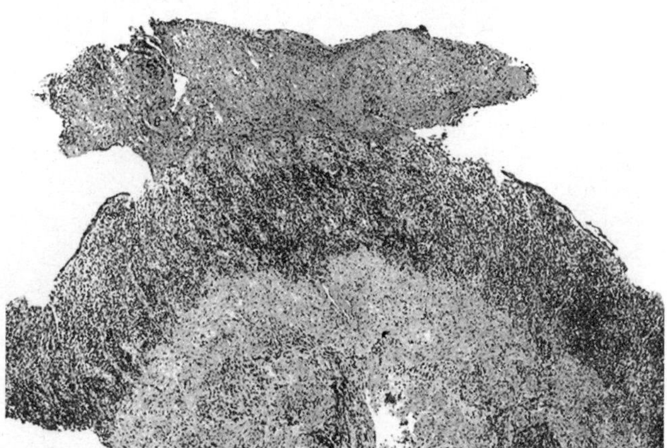

FIGURE 15.43 Acute severe *Helicobacter pylori* infection. Fibrinopurulent material is seen over a superficial erosion. The mucosa is extensively infiltrated by neutrophils.

of Russell bodies (i.e., eosinophilic immunoglobulin-containing inclusions) in plasma cells, and the term *Russell body gastritis* is used by some authors if this feature is prominent (Fig. 15.42). Lymphoid follicles with germinal centers are found in almost all *H. pylori*–infected patients, and their presence is highly specific for *H. pylori* gastritis (see Fig. 15.3).[25,162,163] Occasionally, lymphoid infiltrates may be large and irregular, with lymphoepithelial lesions at the periphery. In such cases, additional evidence of gastric extranodal marginal-zone lymphoma of MALT-type[164-166] should be sought (see Natural History and Complications section). Pathological features that warrant further immunohistochemical and molecular investigation include an expansile monotypic infiltrate, a monocytoid appearance of the lymphocytes, lymphoepithelial lesions associated with glandular destruction, and endoscopic evidence of a mass or nodularity. A diagnosis of atypical lymphoid infiltrate may be rendered when immunohistochemical and molecular tests yield equivocal results. Although the intensity of the neutrophilic infiltrate responds quickly to antibiotic therapy, the density of the mononuclear cell infiltrate typically declines slowly after successful eradication of infection, and the underlying chronic inactive gastritis may persist for several years in as many as 30% of patients. Lymphoid follicles also decline in number and size, although they may persist indefinitely in some patients.

In severe acute infection, grossly visible pseudomembranes and pus adherent to inflamed mucosa have been described (Fig. 15.43).[167] Neutrophils are a common histological feature of *H. pylori* infection. The intensity of neutrophilic infiltration correlates positively with the density of *H. pylori* organisms (see Detection of *Helicobacter*

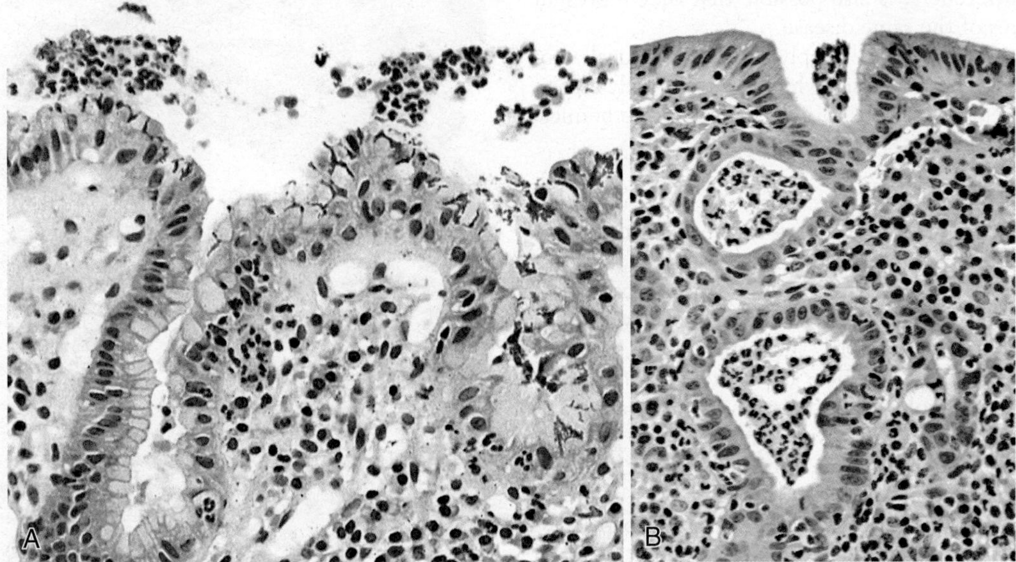

FIGURE 15.44 **A,** In *Helicobacter pylori* infection, neutrophils typically infiltrate the lamina propria and the surface, foveolar, and glandular epithelium. **B,** In severe cases, pit abscesses may be found.

pylori Organisms section). Neutrophils are more abundant in the antrum and cardia than in the corpus, where they may be rare or completely absent despite the presence of organisms in other areas of the stomach. Neutrophils may be seen in the lamina propria and within the surface and foveolar epithelium (Fig. 15.44). In severe infection, neutrophils may fill the lumen of the gastric pits, forming pit microabscesses and a surface exudate. Pediatric *H. pylori* gastritis is more likely to lack severe acute inflammation compared with adult cases.[168] In patients with atrophy, active neutrophilic inflammation only rarely occurs in areas of metaplasia. As previously noted, after successful eradication therapy, neutrophils disappear rapidly, and their continued presence is considered a valuable indicator of therapeutic failure.[18]

Various epithelial alterations can be also detected. In chronic *H. pylori* gastritis, epithelial degeneration is particularly prominent because of intimate contact of the *H. pylori* organisms with the surface cell membrane (see Fig. 15.6).[169]

The epithelial cells often become irregular and cuboidal in shape, have decreased apical mucin content, and occasionally drop out, leaving small gaps in the epithelium that contribute to a ragged, disorderly appearance to the surface. Notably, the density of *H. pylori* organisms may be reduced in areas with reactive, mucin-depleted, foveolar epithelium. The characteristic alterations are caused by bacterial toxins, such as VacA and CagA, urease, ammonia, acetaldehyde, and phospholipases, which have a direct effect on epithelial cells.[170-172]

In addition, *H. pylori* causes mast cells to release platelet-activating factors, which leads to thrombosis.[173] The disturbance of the local microcirculation may result in ischemic loss of epithelial integrity and ultimately in surface erosions and ulcers.[172]

Subtypes of Helicobacter pylori Gastritis

H. pylori infection may show different patterns of gastritis associated with various outcomes and may ultimately be associated with the development of glandular atrophy.

Nonatrophic Antrum-Predominant Gastritis

Nonatrophic antrum-predominant gastritis is the most common pattern of *H. pylori* gastritis (i.e., hypersecretory, diffuse antral, or superficial antral gastritis) in the Western world. It is characterized by moderate to severe inflammation of the antrum, normal or mild inflammation of the corpus, and absence of atrophy. This clinical presentation is associated with normal or increased acid secretion and a 20% estimated lifetime risk of duodenal ulceration.[174-176]

Nonatrophic Corpus-Predominant Gastritis

Nonatrophic corpus-predominant gastritis is restricted mainly to patients who use PPIs chronically. The density of *H. pylori* organisms and the intensity of inflammation are low in the antrum and more pronounced in the corpus. In many cases, even in the corpus, the active inflammation is mild or absent (i.e., inactive gastritis), and the *H. pylori* may only be recognized deep in the lumina of the oxyntic glands. Ancillary studies may be necessary for their detection. Several studies have shown that corpus atrophy proceeds at an accelerated rate in these patients.[177,178]

Nonatrophic Pangastritis

In some individuals chronically infected with *H. pylori*, marked inflammation is evenly distributed throughout the stomach, with little difference between the antrum and corpus. This pattern of gastritis is particularly common in poorly sanitized areas, where *H. pylori* infection is highly endemic. Pangastritis is widely thought to be the background condition in which atrophy develops.[179-181]

Antrum-Restricted Atrophic Gastritis

Biopsies in this condition show extensive patches of intestinal metaplasia and atrophy restricted to the antral mucosa (including the incisura angularis). This is usually associated with moderate to severe inflammation and either a normal, or only mildly inflamed, corpus without atrophy. The relationship between antrum-restricted atrophy and MAG is unknown. Although it is possible that these entities are biologically different, it is also possible that they represent different stages of the same disease.

This terminology does not apply to mild and focal atrophy or to intestinal metaplasia, which are frequently associated with current or previous *H. pylori* infection or chemical gastropathy.

Multifocal Atrophic Gastritis

MAG was formerly referred to as *environmental chronic atrophic gastritis* and, in its most advanced stage, as *atrophic pangastritis*.[7,182] This pattern of gastritis is most prevalent among populations who live or have recently lived in suboptimal sanitary conditions, such as parts of southern and eastern Asia, Latin America, and Europe.[183-186] Exceptions to this epidemiological association include Japan and Korea, where despite high levels of sanitation and personal hygiene, there is one of the world's highest prevalence rates of atrophic gastritis and gastric adenocarcinoma.[187-189] In contrast, in Equatorial Africa, which has a precarious socioeconomic environment, inadequate sanitary conditions, and an *H. pylori* prevalence of almost 90%, there is a surprisingly low prevalence rate of atrophic gastritis and gastric adenocarcinoma.[190-192]

Determination of the *H. pylori* genotype has not proved reliable in predicting the phenotype of gastritis, including atrophy.[193] As a result, other than consideration of the country of origin, it is difficult to predict the risk for atrophic gastritis in an individual patient in industrialized countries.

Atrophic gastritis is a risk factor for gastric ulceration and, more importantly, noninvasive neoplasia (i.e., dysplasia) and intestinal-type adenocarcinoma.[194-197] In biopsy specimens with MAG, foci of atrophy and intestinal metaplasia may be found in antral and corpus mucosa. In contrast with antrum-restricted atrophic gastritis, MAG often displays severe inflammation in the corpus mucosa, and acid secretion may be reduced, suggesting a more advanced state of disease.

Detection of Helicobacter pylori Organisms

The gastric mucosa is covered by a thick layer of mucus that is the primary site of *H. pylori* colonization and often contains large numbers of organisms.[198] When in contact with epithelium, *H. pylori* organisms characteristically attach to but do not penetrate the surface mucous cells (see Fig. 15.39A,B). *H. pylori* naturally infects the antrum, and in advanced cases, the proximal stomach. *H. pylori* organisms rarely colonize intestinal epithelium, and in patients with extensive areas of metaplastic atrophy, organisms are usually confined to the nonmetaplastic, nonatrophic areas of mucosa. A sample that consists primarily or exclusively of intestinalized gastric mucosa is inadequate to evaluate the possibility of *H. pylori* infection. If only an atrophic biopsy specimen is available, it should be documented, and additional samples should be requested. The density of organisms is also reduced overlying mucin depleted regenerative epithelium including the edges of an ulcer, even in a background of severe *H. pylori* gastritis. *H. pylori* organisms rarely colonize necrotic tissue. If specimens from other areas are available, the issue can be easily resolved; unfortunately, frequently only one specimen labeled "gastric ulcer—rule out *H. pylori*" is received. In these cases, the pathologist

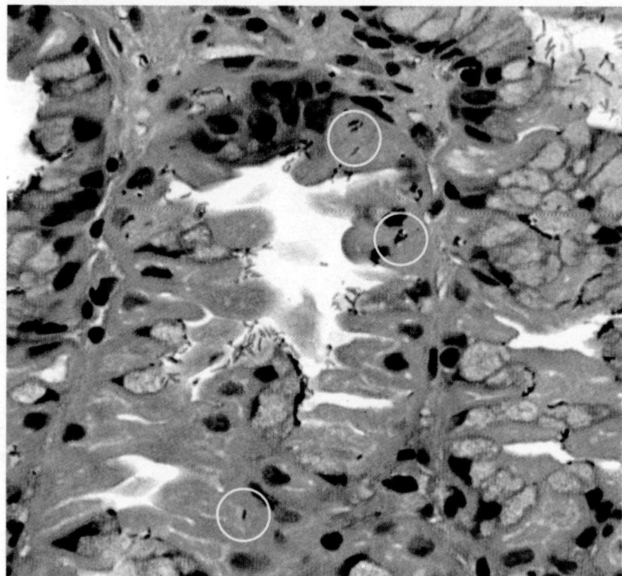

FIGURE 15.45 *Helicobacter pylori* organisms are identified in the deep portion of oxyntic glands and within canaliculi of oxyntic cells *(circles)*. This feature is seen only in patients who use long-term proton pump inhibitors.

should suggest more extensive sampling or the performance of a noninvasive test (e.g., urea breath test).

In patients who use PPIs, the distribution of the *H. pylori* organisms may change. The *H. pylori* organisms tend to be rare or even absent in the antrum, and a corpus predominant disease can develop. In such cases, the bacteria may be difficult to detect even in the corpus, disappearing from the surface mucus, and sometimes they can be recognized only in the lumina of the pyloric or oxyntic glands.[137,199] Patients treated with antibiotics before gastric biopsy may also demonstrate a markedly reduced number of organisms and often have atypical (coccoid) forms (see Fig. 15.39C,D).[199]

Interestingly, without an established clinical significance, intracellular invasion has been observed in surface mucous cells, chief cells, and parietal cells (rare), particularly in patients who have received PPIs (Fig. 15.45).[200-203]

The intensity of neutrophilic infiltration correlates to the density of *H. pylori* organisms.[18-21] As many as 70% of gastric biopsy specimens from *H. pylori*–infected subjects reveal organisms by routine H&E staining. In the remaining 30% of cases, a more sensitive stain is usually needed. Many laboratories routinely stain all gastric biopsies, even those without significant inflammation, for *H. pylori* to ensure identification of organisms. Nevertheless, to avoid unnecessary charges, the use of ancillary studies can be cost-effectively tailored in both adult and pediatric populations, based on the inflammatory pattern seen on the H&E-stained slides[168,204] *H. pylori* infection should always be suspected when chronic gastritis presents with a superficial bandlike lymphoplasmacytic infiltrate,[204] and the organisms can be easily identified on H&E stain in cases with active inflammation. Ancillary techniques are typically only needed in cases of inactive chronic gastritis, and they can be ordered after first screening the H&E slides for *H. pylori* organisms.[21,168,204,205] Conversely, biopsy specimens with noninflamed mucosa (e.g., normal or reactive gastropathy), including those from patients with a positive

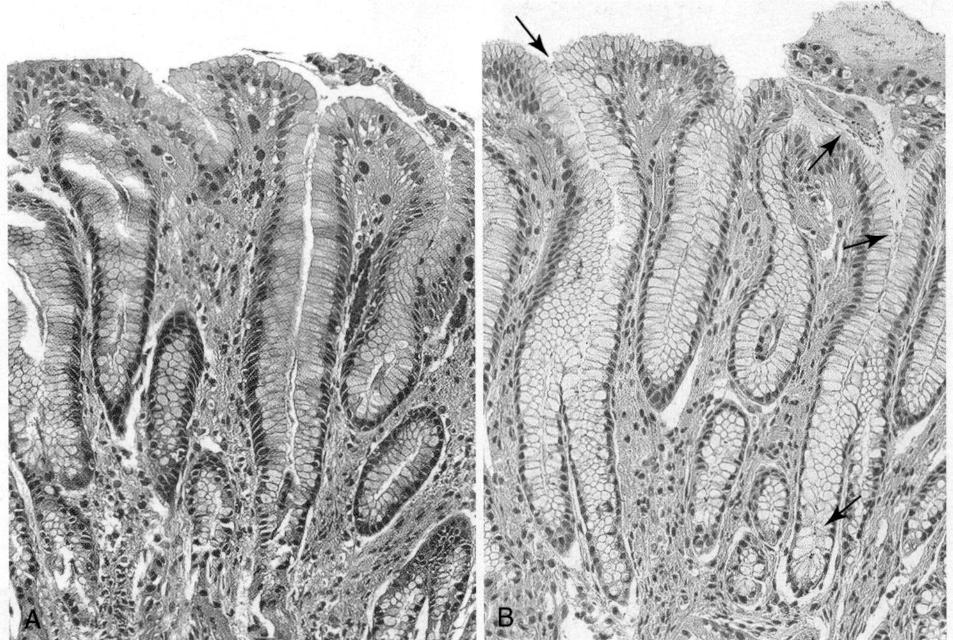

FIGURE 15.46 **A,** Although this is extremely rare, even a normal gastric mucosa can harbor *Helicobacter pylori* infection. **B,** Although the pathologist may not suspect infection in such cases, organisms can be detected by an immunohistochemical stain *(arrows)*.

Campylobacter-like organism test,[206] very rarely contain *H. pylori* organisms (Fig. 15.46). In such cases, ancillary techniques are usually also unable to detect *H. pylori* organisms.[204,205]

Commonly used and relatively inexpensive stains, such as Giemsa and Diff-Quik, are adequate for identification of most cases of *H. pylori* organisms.[207,208] The triple stain simultaneously allows visualization of *H. pylori* organisms (silver-impregnation; see Fig. 15.6, Fig. 15.11, and Fig. 15.39A)[209] and allows inconspicuous foci of intestinal metaplasia (Alcian blue at pH 2.5) to be detected (see Fig. 15.11). Immunohistochemical stains for *H. pylori* increase sensitivity and are particularly useful for detecting coccoid forms of the organism and rare organisms located deep within the glands.[210,211] After *H. pylori* treatment, organisms may be best visualized with an immunohistochemical stain. Immunohistochemistry is recommended as the preferred ancillary technique by at least one GI pathology society (see Fig. 15.39B,D).[212]

The prevalence of *H. pylori* strains resistant to antibiotics is increasing worldwide, especially clarithromycin resistance rates, which have reached 30% to 50% in some countries (e.g., Italy, Turkey, Japan, and China). Susceptibility testing is recommended by some guidelines before the prescription of a clarithromycin-based triple eradication therapy in populations with a high (>15%) clarithromycin resistance rate.[140] This can be performed either by culture and antibiogram or by molecular testing of gastric tissue samples. FISH and PCR used on gastric biopsy specimens have been evaluated for identification of antibiotic sensitivity, which could be a valuable clinical application.[213] Lately next-generation sequencing assays to detect multiple resistance mutations were also developed.[214] Nevertheless, in clinical practice, most patients are still prescribed *H. pylori* eradication treatment without antibiotic susceptibility testing, and clarithromycin triple therapy fails to eradicate the organism 20% of the time.[215,216] The primary culprit appears to be resistance to clarithromycin, which can be significant (about 15% to 20%) in certain populations. Resistance has been related to point mutations in bacterial 23S rRNA, and genotypic (PCR) evaluation of resistance is more sensitive than phenotypic (culture) testing. However, PCR-based testing correlates less well than culture with treatment outcomes and therefore has a low predictive value.[217]

Peptic Ulcer

An *ulcer,* in contrast with *erosion,* is defined as a loss of the entire mucosa, including the muscularis mucosae. Ulcers may extend deep into the submucosa and even muscularis propria. Ulcers typically begin as erosions, but not all erosions progress to ulcers. Gastric ulcers may be acute or chronic. Peptic ulcers are always considered chronic and are most often solitary. They may occur in any portion of the GI tract that is exposed to acid peptic juices. Approximately 98% of peptic ulcers occur in the stomach and duodenum, with an incidence ratio of approximately 1:4. *H. pylori* is detected in the stomach of almost all patients with duodenal peptic ulcer and in more than 90% of gastric ulcer patients who are not NSAID users.[218,219] Zollinger-Ellison syndrome, a rare condition, is characterized by the presence of multiple peptic ulcers induced either by sporadic hypergastrinemia or as part of a multiple endocrine neoplasia type 1 (MEN 1)–related gastrinoma.[220]

Pathological Features

Most peptic ulcers occur on the lesser curvature of the stomach in the antrum close to the incisura angularis.[221,222] They are typically sharply demarcated lesions, which may appear erythematous, edematous, and only slightly elevated above the level of the surrounding mucosa (Fig. 15.47). Peptic ulcers are usually small (0.5 to 2.0 cm in diameter), but some can be more than 3.0 cm in diameter. Large (i.e., giant) ulcers may be misdiagnosed endoscopically as malignant.[223,224]

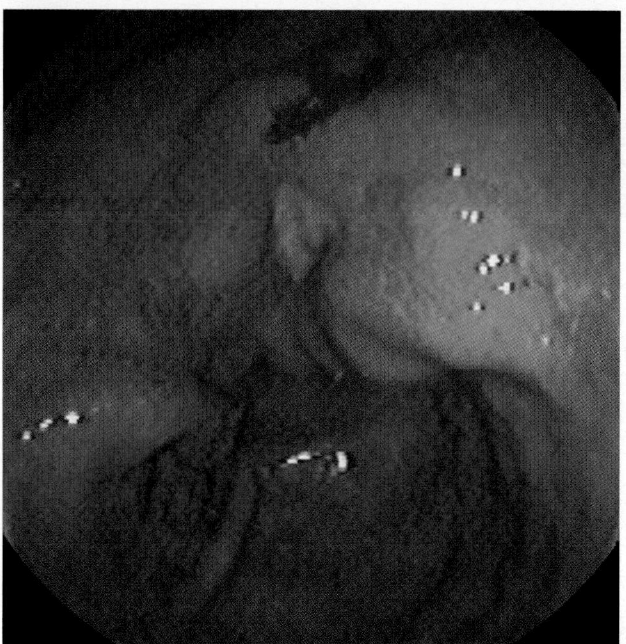

FIGURE 15.47 Endoscopic view of an antral peptic ulcer. Notice the discrete border with adjacent flat, normal-appearing mucosa.

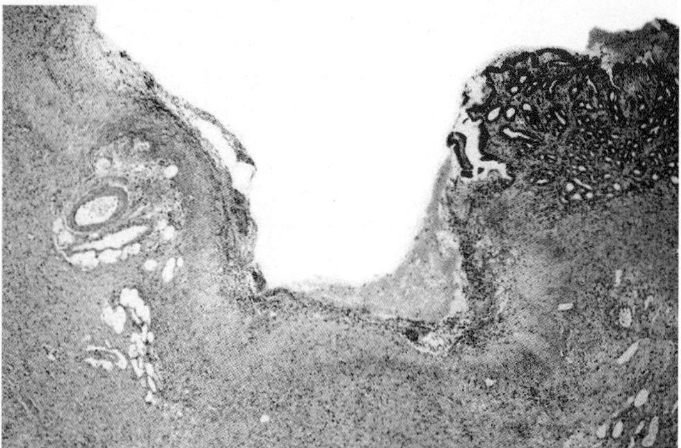

FIGURE 15.48 Low magnification of a gastric peptic ulcer. The ulcer crater contains a small amount of fibrin and necrotic debris with underlying granulation tissue. The mucosa immediately adjacent to the ulcer shows regeneration.

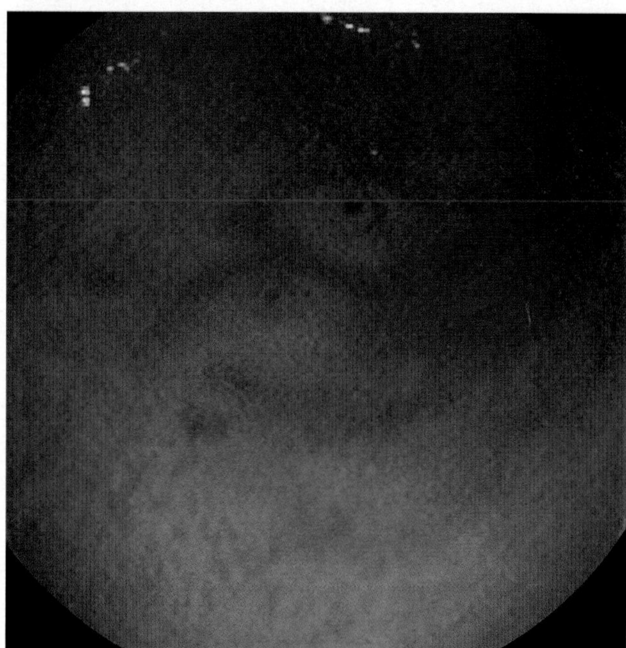

FIGURE 15.49 Stress ulcer with clean borders in the antrum. Some ulcers have evidence of recent hemorrhage.

Perforating ulcers penetrate into adjacent structures, most commonly the pancreas. Endoscopically, peptic ulcers are usually surrounded by flat, normal mucosa or a radiating pattern of rugal folds. In some cases, extensive fibrosis may lead to atypical endoscopic presentations.[225]

Microscopically, the mucosa surrounding peptic ulcers typically shows chronic active inflammation and marked regenerative changes, increased mitoses, mucin depletion, and foveolar hyperplasia—features that can mimic dysplasia (Fig. 15.48). Features that support regeneration include evidence of surface maturation, mitotic activity confined to the deeper foveolar regions, and nuclei without loss of polarity that have even chromatin, thin nuclear membranes, and uniform, central punctate nucleoli. A gradual transition from atypical to normal epithelium favors regeneration.

The base or crater of peptic ulcers consists of necroinflammatory debris, granulation tissue, and fibrosis with chronic inflammation from the luminal surface to the deep portions of the gastric wall. Substantial lymphoid infiltrates arranged in follicles may lie adjacent to ulcers, in some cases mimicking malignant lymphoma.[162] At the ulcer's base, blood vessels proliferate, often showing prominent inflammation and arteritis obliterans. When disrupted, these arteries may bleed profusely. Bizarre stromal cells represent proliferating regenerative mesenchymal cells that may show significant nuclear atypia, and they should not be misinterpreted as a neoplastic process.

Differential Diagnosis

Acute stress ulcers in intensive care patients are usually multiple. They measure more than 0.5 cm in diameter and usually present as well-delineated superficial craters. Fibrinoid material intermixed with acute inflammatory exudate and necrotic debris form the ulcer bed. Because of frequent hemorrhage, blood clots may fill the ulcer crater[81,85] (Fig. 15.49).

Medications including NSAIDs and less frequently iron supplements (i.e., ferrous sulfate) and doxycycline can also induce ulcerative mucosal injury. Gastric ulcers that occur in the greater curvature and in other parts of the proximal stomach are more likely to be related to chronic NSAID use rather than *H. pylori* infection.[221,222]

Other infections including gastric tuberculosis, cytomegalovirus (CMV), and histoplasmosis (rare) may also cause gastric ulceration, especially in immunocompromised patients.[226-228]

Benign and malignant tumors may become ulcerated. Malignant ulcers occur most often with adenocarcinoma and stromal tumors and less commonly with lymphomas, metastases, and direct extension of a surrounding extragastric malignancy. In contrast with the usually flat borders of nonneoplastic ulcers, characteristic endoscopic features of malignant ulcers are heaped-up mucosal borders and irregular rugal folds. Nevertheless, ulcers associated with malignant lymphomas are often flat or only slightly elevated, are frequently multiple, and may reach large sizes (10 to 12 cm in diameter).[225]

Natural History and Complications

The most common complications of peptic ulcer disease, in order of frequency, are hemorrhage, perforation, and obstruction. Clinically, approximately one-third of patients have been reported to experience at least one of these complications during the course of disease. Gastric outlet obstruction may develop as a result of distortion and narrowing of the pyloric area because of fibrosis, edema, and smooth muscle spasm. Surgical treatment may become necessary if endoscopic dilation fails.[229,230] Bleeding occurs when ulcers erode underlying blood vessels. Rarely, ulcers may form a fistula with the small intestine, transverse colon, or gallbladder or may perforate adjacent organs such as the pancreas or liver. They may also result in an inflammatory pseudotumor that clinically mimics a malignant tumor. However, effective antibiotic therapy for *H. pylori* and PPI therapy have changed the frequency of these complications over the past few decades.[231] Eradication of *H. pylori* facilitates healing of peptic ulcers and essentially prevents their recurrence. In contrast, more than 80% of patients treated only with acid inhibition experience recurrence within 1 year.[232]

Helicobacter heilmannii *Infection*

More than 50 species of *Helicobacter* have been described, but only a few non–*H. pylori Helicobacter species* cause gastritis in humans, which are frequently designated as the *Helicobacter heilmannii sensu lato* (*H. heilmannii s. l.*) group. They include *H. bizzozeronii, H. felis, H. salomonis, H. suis, H. fennelliae, H. cinaedi, and H. heilmannii sensu stricto* (formerly known as *Gastrospirillum hominis*). *H. heilmannii s. l.* is responsible for 1% of all human *Helicobacter* infections.[233-235] In some rural areas in eastern Europe and Asia, infection with *H. heilmannii* is more common, supporting the hypothesis that it is acquired by zoonotic transmission.[236] The organisms are 5 to 9 µm long (twice as long as *H. pylori)* and have five to seven spirals.

Although *H. heilmannii s. l.* organisms are easily visualized with any of the common histochemical *H. pylori* stains (Fig. 15.50), their detection may be difficult because they tend to be less numerous and more focally distributed than *H. pylori*. Polyclonal immunohistochemical stains for *H. pylori* also react with *H. heilmannii s. l.*, as do some

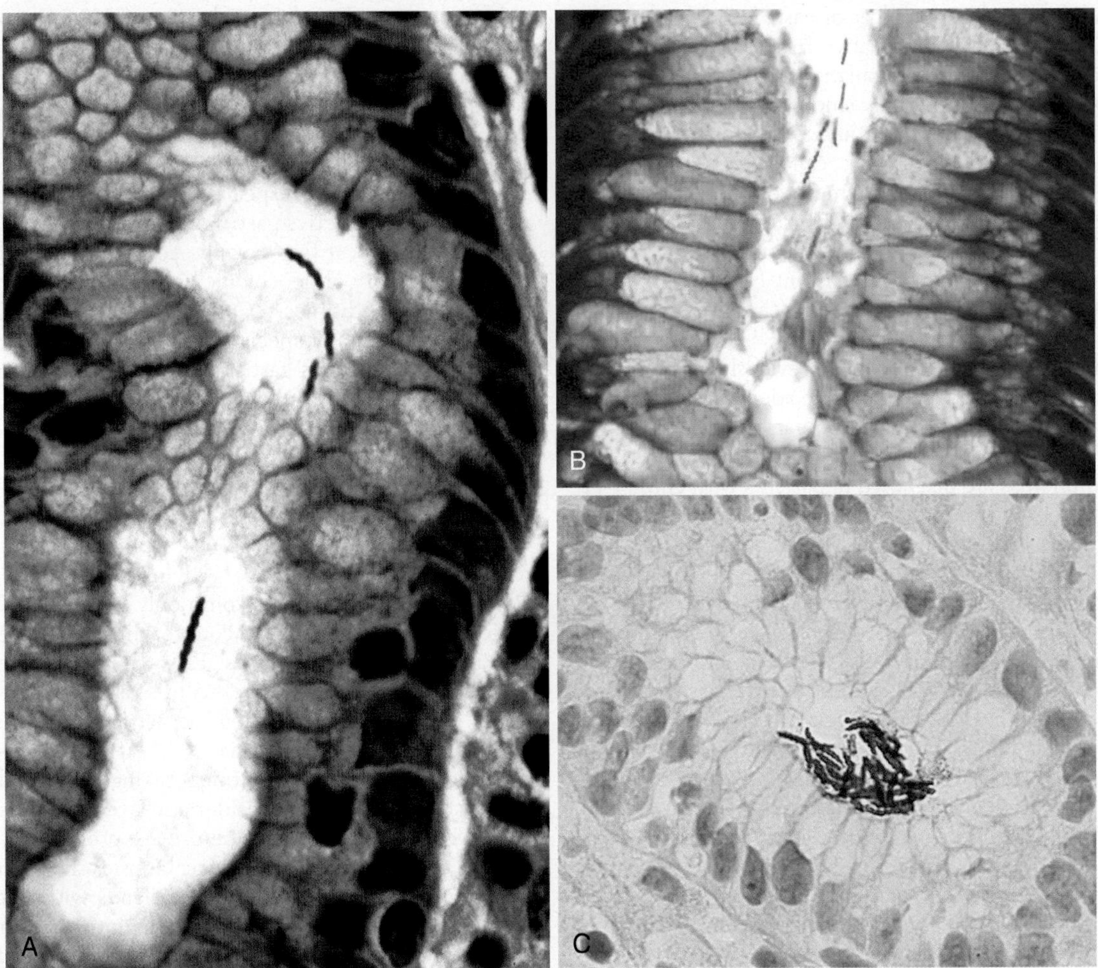

FIGURE 15.50 *Helicobacter heilmannii* organisms are at least twice as long and considerably thicker than *Helicobacter pylori*. Their characteristic tightly spiraled shape is clearly visible at high power with the triple stain **(A)**, the *H. pylori* blue stain **(B)**, and most polyclonal anti-*Helicobacter* immunohistochemical stains **(C)**.

commercially available monoclonal stains. *H. heilmannii s. l.* can be missed by those who rely exclusively on these immunostains for their diagnosis.

Gastritis caused by *H. heilmannii s. l.* differs from *H. pylori* gastritis. It is more common in children and usually milder and patchier in its distribution, with fewer erosions and ulcers. The inflammation tends to be more circumscribed, mainly affecting the antrum, although cases of severe corpus active gastritis may develop as well. The diagnosis rests on morphological recognition of the organisms, although differentiation of the various *H. heilmannii s. l.* species is not possible by light microscopy. These organisms have not been cultured successfully in vitro, and the specific antibiotic susceptibility of *H. heilmannii s. l.* has therefore not been well studied. Clinically, *H. heilmannii s. l.* patients are treated identically to those with *H. pylori* infection, and rates of successful outcomes are similar.[237]

Similar to *H. pylori, H. heilmannii s. l.* infection has been linked to the development of gastric adenocarcinoma[238] and MALT lymphoma. Regression of lymphoma after successful eradication therapy has been reported.[239,240]

Natural History and Complications

H. pylori is a lifelong infection that if left untreated may progress from nonatrophic to atrophic gastritis and, in some cases, gastric and duodenal peptic ulcer disease, gastric carcinoma, and MALT lymphoma. The relative risk of these complications varies among different populations and is related to bacterial, environmental (especially smoking), and host genetic factors.[241] The extent of atrophy and type of intestinal metaplasia are associated with gastric cancer risk. Incomplete intestinal metaplasia and involvement of the corpus have been identified as an increased risk factor for gastric carcinoma compared with complete and antrum-restricted metaplasia/atrophy.[48] Patients with persistent *H. pylori* infection have a higher probability of developing these sequelae than those who were successfully eradicated.[241] In a large North American series of individuals with previously diagnosed *H. pylori* gastritis, the incidence of gastric adenocarcinoma after *H. pylori* diagnosis at 5, 10, and 20 years was 0.37%, 0.5%, and 0.65%, respectively.[242] Although 85% to 90% of gastric MALT lymphomas are diagnosed in patients with chronic *H. pylori* infection, over 75% will regress for extended periods with successful eradication of the infection.[239,243-245]

Polymorphisms in genes coding cytokines (e.g., IL-1β) that modulate the inflammatory response triggered by *H. pylori* organisms, proteins involved in DNA repair, and epigenetic modulations including DNA methylation are host factors that contribute to the susceptibility to gastric adenocarcinoma.[246,247] The different levels of risk for the various aforementioned complications vary worldwide in relation to different *H. pylori* strains. Routine *H. pylori* genotyping with evaluation of virulence factors including vacA+/babA2+/oipA might prove helpful in predicting patients at higher risk of gastric cancer or lymphoma. For example, the presence of the *cagA* gene and subsequently produced serum antibodies were found more prevalent in patients with gastric high-grade B-cell lymphoma compared with MALT lymphoma.[248] Gastric epithelial dysplasia is discussed in detail later in this chapter. Carcinoma and lymphoma are discussed in Chapters 25 and 31, respectively.

Helicobacter pylori–Negative Chronic Gastritis

Although chronic active gastritis has been considered virtually synonymous with *H. pylori* infection, and active gastritis has been regarded as an essential component of *H. pylori* infection, there is a common perception among pathologists practicing in the West that the incidence of chronic active and inactive gastritis in patients without detectable *H. pylori* organisms (i.e., *H. pylori*–negative chronic active gastritis) is increasing.[20,106,249] The rate of mild *H. pylori*–negative chronic gastritis also depends on the threshold that pathologists use for a pathological lamina propria lymphoplasmacytic infiltrate. One commonly used cutoff is >5 plasma cells per high-power field (HPF). *H. pylori*–negative chronic gastritis may represent an *H. pylori* gastritis in which the organisms are undetectable, or it may represent injuries or disease states unrelated to *H. pylori* infection. The presence of *H. pylori* organisms may remain undetected as a result of extensive intestinal metaplasia or regenerative epithelial changes at the edges of an ulcer. Antibiotic therapy administered to treat other infections, the masking effect of PPIs, and inadequate sampling or suboptimal staining techniques may be, likewise, responsible. When anti–*H. pylori* immunohistochemical stains are used for all gastric biopsies with a bandlike superficial lymphoplasmacytic infiltration (see Fig. 15.41), organisms can often be found in cases considered negative based on evaluation of H&E-stained slides.

Regardless of the method used, it is important to consider all the circumstances that can result in chronic active inflammation of gastric mucosa in the absence of visible *H. pylori* organisms. Neutrophilic inflammation may be present in almost 50% of cases of autoimmune gastritis.[22] Inflammatory bowel disease, especially Crohn's disease, is another possible cause of active gastritis, although the inflammation may be more focal (see Focally Active [Enhanced] Gastritis) and a history of ileocolonic disease may help in steering the differential diagnosis. Other infectious (e.g., CMV and syphilitic gastritis) or special types of gastritis (e.g., lymphocytic and collagenous gastritis) as well as iatrogenic injury (e.g., drugs and GVHD) should also be considered, depending on the clinical circumstances.[250]

Causes That May Lead to False-Negative H. pylori Detection

Proton Pump Inhibitor Use

PPIs are one of the most commonly prescribed GI medications available over the counter in the United States and in many other countries. PPIs are highly effective for chronic gastroesophageal reflux disease (GERD), eosinophilic esophagitis, prevention of gastric damage associated with NSAIDs, and dyspepsia.[138,251] After they are recommended, most people continue taking them indefinitely, and gastroenterologists consider any attempt to discontinue the medication for 2 weeks before the procedure futile.

As a consequence, most gastric biopsies show a presumed PPI effect: focally dilated oxyntic glands with flattened or hypertrophic parietal cells protruding into the lumen.[58,252] Many features of *H. pylori* gastritis may also be altered by PPI therapy, including a milder intensity of antral inflammation accompanied by a greater intensity in the corpus, few or no detectable organisms in the antrum, and a redistribution of *H. pylori* organisms in the deeper portions of the oxyntic glands, even reaching the intracellular canaliculi of the parietal cells[135,253-257] (see Fig. 15.40). PPI use can cause false-negative results for urea breath tests. Subsequently, most guidelines recommend discontinuing the medication 2 to 4 weeks before *H. pylori* testing.[140,141]

Recent Antibiotic Treatment

A large swath of the general population receive antibiotic treatment for a variety of confirmed or suspected infections (e.g., ear, throat, and urinary tract infections and after dental procedures). Because these treatments are usually not coordinated with gastroenterologists, endoscopies may be done on patients who recently received or are still taking antibiotics. Some of these antibiotics affect *H. pylori*, but when used outside of a coordinated triple or quadruple therapy, they rarely cure the *H. pylori* infection. They may, however, temporarily decrease the bacterial load and make the infection, which is still active and capable of inducing inflammation, histologically undetectable. Such incidental antibiotic treatments are proposed to be one of the most common causes of *H. pylori*–like chronic active gastritis.

In practice, a urea breath test or monoclonal stool antigen test, performed at least 4 weeks after completion of therapy, is recommended as the best option for confirmation of *H. pylori* eradication.[140,141] Posteradication follow-up biopsies are uncommon, but if performed, are likely to reveal one of two findings. If the therapy was successful (i.e., *H. pylori* infection was eradicated), the mucosa shows various degrees of chronic gastritis, possibly some lymphoid follicles, but no active inflammation.[18,258] If the therapy failed, a recrudescence occurs, and the chronic active gastritis is often more severe than before the unsuccessful therapeutic trial.

Chronic Active Gastritis Unrelated to *Helicobacter* Infection

In some biopsies, the features of reactive gastropathy are accompanied by those of mild chronic gastritis, either with or without foci of active inflammation. Because the features of *H. pylori* gastritis may overlap with those of reactive gastropathy (and the two types may coexist in patients), a careful search for *H. pylori* organisms is imperative. The two causes can usually be discerned. In contrast with *H. pylori* gastritis, the chronic infiltrate of reactive gastropathy is typically loose and less well defined, does not form a subepithelial band (formerly designated *superficial gastritis*), and rarely shows significant numbers of plasma cells. Neutrophils, if present, tend to be confined to the lamina propria, sparing the glandular epithelium, where they are often associated with eosinophils. Intraepithelial neutrophils, aggregates of neutrophils, and regenerative epithelium are usually found only in the vicinity of erosions, which are often revealed by deeper tissue sections.

Although active inflammation is not widely recognized as a common histological feature of autoimmune gastritis, one comprehensive study identified intraepithelial neutrophilic infiltration in at least one gland in 45% of cases, while neutrophilic gland abscess formation was less frequently observed.[22]

Focally Active (Enhanced) Gastritis

The finding of either individual or just a few gastric foveolae, or glands surrounded and infiltrated by lymphocytes, macrophages, plasma cells, or neutrophils, in a background of normal gastric mucosa, is referred to as *focally enhanced gastritis*.[17]

Although focal and often intense gastritis has been described in a high percentage of patients with inflammatory bowel disease (and more specifically Crohn's disease), its positive predictive value (which is approximately 5%) has been contested in adult patients.[259] However, its significance is better established in the pediatric population (positive predictive value approximately 75%).[260] Children are also more likely to be affected by Crohn's disease (55%). However, ulcerative colitis patients may also include patients with focally enhanced gastritis (30%).[261] This type of inflammatory pattern can also develop in patients without inflammatory bowel disease,[262-264] including those with iatrogenic colitis (e.g., immune checkpoint inhibitor therapy[111] or GVHD) (Fig. 15.51A).[259] Of note is the fact that *H. pylori* infection can also be patchy at times, although typically with a less striking contrast between inflamed and adjacent, less inflamed, or even normal-appearing mucosa than in cases related to inflammatory bowel disease. Nevertheless, when focal gastritis is detected, an effort should be made to detect *H. pylori* (Fig. 15.51B).

Other Infections

Other bacteria (e.g., syphilitic gastritis; Fig. 15.52A), fungi, and viruses (e.g., Epstein-Barr virus [EBV] and CMV) may infect the gastric mucosa, but only rarely do they produce a histological appearance of chronic active gastritis. Rather, they typically elicit a more mixed type of inflammatory infiltrate and one that is less superficial (such as CMV gastritis) (Fig. 15.52B,C). Unless specific clinical information is available (e.g., an immunosuppressed patient, disseminated aspergillosis), a search for infectious agents other than *Helicobacter* species in gastric mucosa is likely to be laborious and, ultimately, unrewarding.

Summary

If a biopsy demonstrates a superficial bandlike inflammatory pattern of injury, but no organisms are detected after a meticulous search (including anti–*H. pylori* immunohistochemistry), it is wise to inform the clinician that, despite an inability to identify organisms, the histological appearance is still suspicious for *H. pylori* gastritis. In fact, if the pathologist is able to elicit a clinical history of recent antibiotic treatment, he or she may suggest a plausible explanation for *H. pylori*–negative chronic active gastritis. The pathologist can indicate that the inadequately treated infection may reemerge, and other detection methods (e.g., urea breath; stool antigen test) or even a new set of biopsies after a few weeks, may ultimately reveal the presence of *H. pylori* organisms. Finally, receiving only antral biopsies from patients who may have corpus-predominant pangastritis can be frustrating. A reminder to the clinician regarding the effects of PPIs on *H. pylori* distribution in the stomach may help persuade them to sample both the antrum and corpus.

Autoimmune Gastritis

Clinical Features

Autoimmune gastritis is a type of corpus-restricted, chronic atrophic gastritis associated with serum anti–parietal cell

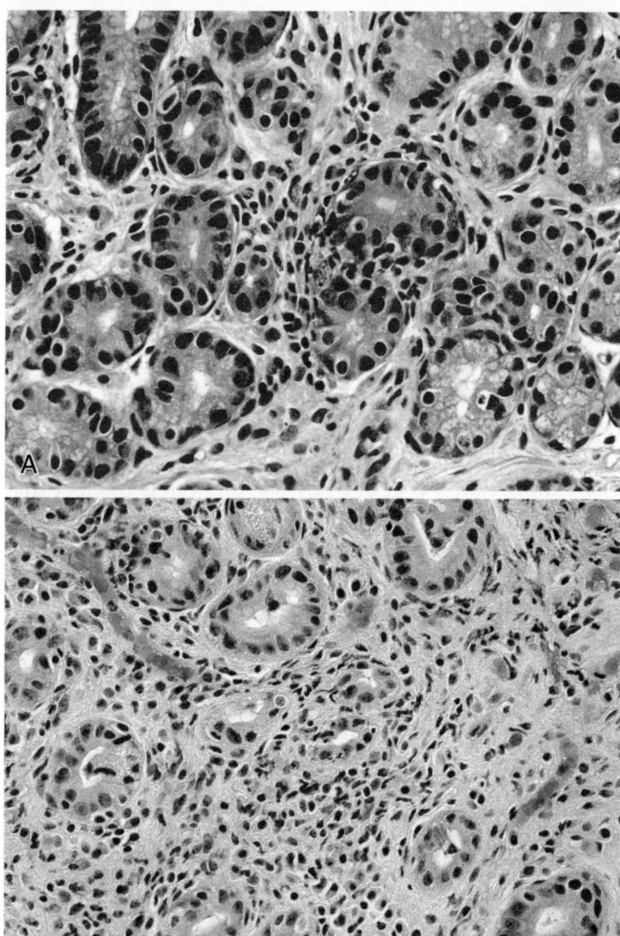

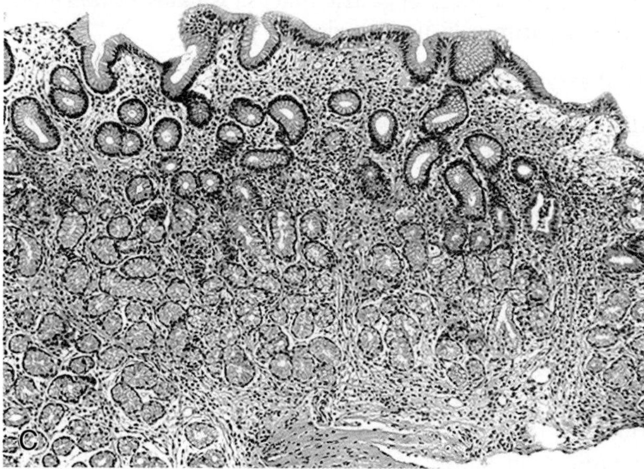

FIGURE 15.51 Focally enhanced (*Helicobacter pylori*–negative) chronic active gastritis. It is characterized by patchy lymphoplasmacytic and neutrophilic infiltrates, sometimes limited to only one or a few glands. This morphology can be observed in the setting of graft-versus-host disease **(A)** or Crohn's disease **(B),** which can also present with more diffuse chronic gastritis **(C).**

and anti–intrinsic factor antibodies. It results in intrinsic factor deficiency either with or without anemia.[265,266] Autoimmune gastritis does not cause specific clinical manifestations until a critical decrease point has occurred in the parietal cell mass, after which anemia develops. Years before the onset of anemia, patients may show various degrees of hypochlorhydria, hypergastrinemia, and loss of pepsin and pepsinogen secretion.

Achlorhydria, which is a direct result of destruction of acid-producing parietal cells, typically occurs in the most advanced stage of disease. However, hypochlorhydria may occur in patients with a large number of preserved parietal cells, which suggests that there may be a possible role for anti–proton pump antibodies or inhibitory lymphokines released by inflammatory cells in the pathogenesis of this disease. Atrophy of the corpus and hypochlorhydria leads to hypergastrinemia that tends to correlate with disease severity.[267,268] Damage to chief cells results in a reduction of pepsin activity in gastric juice and in the level of pepsinogen in serum. The finding of a low pepsinogen I (primarily produced by oxyntic mucosa) level (<20 ng/mL) or a decreased pepsinogen I–to–pepsinogen II (dominantly secreted by the antral mucosa) ratio is a sensitive and specific indicator for corpus atrophy.[267,269]

Iron-deficiency (microcytic) anemia or pernicious (macrocytic) anemia develops in many patients with autoimmune gastritis. Achlorhydria is a major contributor to the pathogenesis of iron-deficiency anemia because acidity is important for absorption of nonheme iron, which supplies at least two-thirds of the nutritional iron supply in most Western diets.[270] Pernicious anemia, which results from loss of intrinsic factor production by parietal cells, is usually an end-stage manifestation and is preceded by corpus-restricted chronic atrophic gastritis and reduced or absent acid secretion of at least 10 years' duration.[271,272] Autoimmune gastritis is a risk factor for gastric hyperplastic and adenomatous polyps, pyloric gland adenomas, carcinomas, and neuroendocrine tumors. Polyps are detected in 20% to 40% of patients with pernicious anemia; they are mostly sessile, less than 2 cm in diameter, and often multiple. Most are hyperplastic, but up to 10% of cases contain foci of dysplasia.[132,273] Gastric adenocarcinomas associated with pernicious anemia are mostly of the intestinal type and arise from intestinal metaplasia, suggesting that they likely develop through a metaplasia-dysplasia-carcinoma pathway.[274]

Epidemiology

Pernicious anemia is an uncommon disease with a reported prevalence rate of approximately 1%, even among older adults and in high-incidence regions of the world. However, autoimmune gastritis is likely underdiagnosed because most patients have microcytic or macrocytic anemia and are treated with iron, folate, and cobalamin without undergoing a thorough investigation of the underlying cause. However, targeted studies suggest an overall prevalence rate of 2%, with a peak of 4% to 5% among elderly women.[275]

Pathogenesis

The cause of autoimmune gastritis is unknown. Most likely there are two different scenarios in which autoimmune gastritis can develop: "de novo" or initiated by *H. pylori* infection.[276] A high prevalence of antibodies with specificity for gastric mucosal antigens has been reported for patients with *H. pylori*–associated gastritis.[277,278] Twenty percent of *H. pylori*–positive individuals have autoantibodies that react with canaliculi of parietal cells, which are a primary antibody target in autoimmune gastritis. Studies

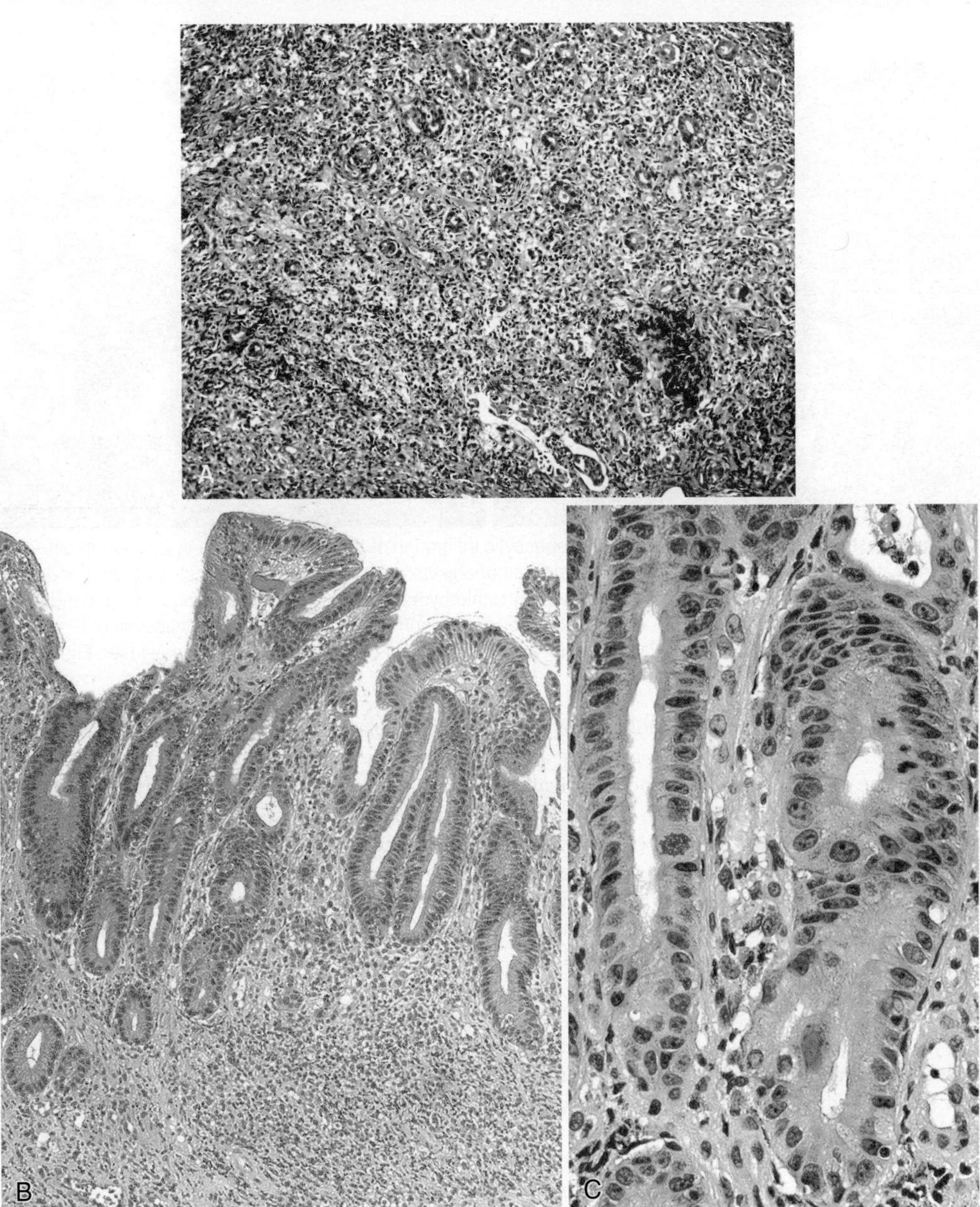

FIGURE 15.52 Chronic active gastritis with no detectable *Helicobacter pylori* organisms. **A,** Syphilitic gastritis showing diffuse infiltration of the mucosa by a mixed inflammatory infiltrate with a predominance of plasma cells. Note the effacement of the glandular architecture. Immunohistochemical staining for *Treponema pallidum* will highlight the spirochetes. **B,** In this second example of *H. pylori*–negative gastritis, the chronic inflammation is located in the lower half of the antral mucosa, and the density of plasma cells is relatively low. **C,** A single cytomegalovirus inclusion is magnified.

with cloned T cells from *H. pylori*–infected patients and patients with autoimmune atrophic gastritis have identified molecular mimicry between *H. pylori* and hydrogen and potassium receptors and ATPase, suggesting that infection may stimulate T cells that target parietal cells.[153] These studies provide support for the concept of a cross-reactive mechanism between *H. pylori* organisms and gastric epithelial antigens that may be responsible for, or at least participate in, the pathogenesis of autoimmune gastritis.[279] The role of genetic susceptibility, such as an association with certain HLA isoforms (HLA-DRB103 and HLA-DRB104), has also been identified.[276] The role of IgG_4 in autoimmune gastritis may be similar to that in autoimmune pancreatitis. One study found IgG_4-immunoreactive plasma cells in gastric biopsies to be 100% specific (albeit not highly sensitive) for autoimmune atrophic gastritis and pernicious anemia.[280]

From the morphological perspective, Pittman et al. investigated the available original prediagnosis samples of biopsy-proven autoimmune gastritis patients in a North American population. The majority of cases (66%) showed diagnostic features of autoimmune gastritis. The second most common pattern (24%) was inactive chronic gastritis, whereas only two cases showed active chronic *H. pylori* gastritis.[281]

Pathological Features

Grossly, the mucosa of the corpus in patients with autoimmune gastritis is usually thinner than normal and shows a reduction or complete absence of rugal folds. Fine submucosal vessels are usually easily recognizable on endoscopic

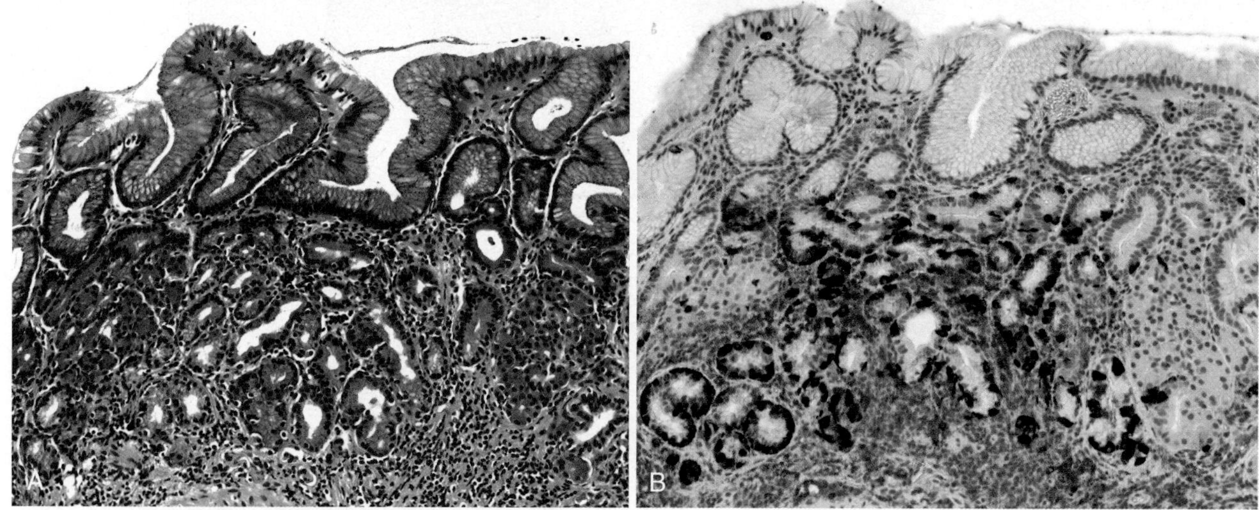

FIGURE 15.53 Autoimmune gastritis. A, Biopsy shows marked lymphocytic infiltration of the corpus mucosa in addition to diffuse pseudopyloric and focal intestinal and pancreatic acinar metaplasia. **B,** Synaptophysin immunohistochemistry highlights distinct linear and nodular enterochromaffin-like cell hyperplasia**.** The atrophy of the oxyntic mucosa and subsequent achlorhydria triggers a feedback mechanism and induces gastrin cell hyperplasia in the gastric antrum (see Fig. 15.18), which can be highlighted by gastrin immunohistochemistry. Identification of G cells can help distinguish corpus biopsies with extensive pseudopyloric metaplasia mimicking antral mucosa (–) from true antral mucosa (+) (see Fig. 15.19).

examination in advanced cases. Hyperplastic polyps are also common in advanced-stage disease. Chronic gastritis and mucosal atrophy may be patchy and may endoscopically mimic polyposis (i.e., pseudopolyposis) with the spared nonatrophic mucosal islands appearing polypoid between the depressed atrophic areas. This may lead to a clinicopathological conundrum with polypoid lesions signed out as "normal" or near-normal gastric mucosa, which underscores the importance of sampling both the nonpolypoid and polypoid mucosa, the former of which yields the correct diagnosis in this situation.[282]

Microscopically, the main pathological features of uncomplicated autoimmune gastritis are diffuse corpus-restricted chronic gastritis with a variable degree of atrophy, metaplasia (Fig. 15.53A), and ECL cell proliferation (Fig. 15.53B). Three phases can be identified during the course of autoimmune gastritis in corpus mucosa, termed *early, florid*, and *end-stage*.

The early phase is characterized by multifocal or diffuse lymphocytic and plasma cell infiltration. In contrast with the superficial bandlike pattern characteristic of *H. pylori* gastritis, the inflammatory infiltrate in autoimmune gastritis is either basal predominant or involves the entire thickness of the lamina propria.[22,281] Some degree of oxyntic gland destruction is frequently observed in this stage,[281] and intraepithelial lymphocytes and apoptotic bodies may be focally detected within the oxyntic glands. Hypertrophic changes of the residual parietal cells may be present and may indicate a high level of compensatory stimulation related to hypergastrinemia.[60,281,283] Patchy pseudopyloric metaplasia is frequently present at this stage as well, but focal intestinal metaplasia may also be visible. Although the histology may suggest the etiology, a positive diagnosis at this stage normally requires demonstration of circulating anti–parietal cell autoantibodies, a test rarely performed in routine clinical practice.[284]

The florid phase of autoimmune gastritis is characterized by marked atrophy of oxyntic glands, diffuse lymphoplasmacytic infiltration of the lamina propria, and normal or reduced thickness of the mucosa with a relative increase in the thickness of the foveolar component. In about 50% of cases, eosinophils are a prominent (>30/HPF) component of the inflammatory infiltrate.[22,281] Pseudopyloric metaplasia is often extensive, whereas intestinal metaplasia is usually limited. The presence of pancreatic acinar metaplasia in a corpus biopsy is considered specific for an autoimmune etiology, thus its presence should always raise the suspicion for autoimmune gastritis (see Fig. 15.53A).[22] At this stage of disease, the pathological features of autoimmune atrophic gastritis are sufficiently distinctive, particularly if the antrum is not inflamed. However, demonstration of antibodies directed against parietal cell and intrinsic factor antigens is still necessary for confirmation.

The end stage of disease is characterized by a near-complete reduction in oxyntic glands (see Fig. 15.53A), foveolar hyperplasia with elongation and microcystic change, hyperplastic polyp formation, and an increasing degree of pseudopyloric, pancreatic acinar, and intestinal metaplasia. The glands may be shorter, with a gap between the base of the glands and the muscularis mucosae, while the muscularis mucosae may be thickened. At this stage, inflammation is usually minimal or absent, although scattered lymphoid aggregates may persist.

During the florid and end stages, hypochlorhydria and achlorhydria cause antral gastrin cell hyperplasia and hypergastrinemia, which stimulates ECL cell proliferation in the corpus (Fig. 15.53B). Although ECL cell proliferation may also occur in patients using PPIs or in those with Zollinger-Ellison syndrome, multiple endocrine neoplasia syndromes, and *H. pylori*–associated MAG, it is usually less prominent, and its degree does not normally reach the "micronodular" pattern. Solcia et al. proposed a rather arbitrary classification of ECL hyperplasia that helps categorize the various stages of ECL cell hyperplasia and neoplastic ECL cell proliferations, although the clinical significance of this classification system remains to be determined (see Table 15.3 and

Chapter 29). For example, a neuroendocrine tumor (NET) is defined by Solcia as an expansile or infiltrative endocrine growth that is more than 0.5 mm in diameter.[285] Although ECL cell NETs may arise during the florid phase, they are found most commonly in patients with end-stage disease.[274] NETs associated with ECL cell hyperplasia occur in 5% to 8% of patients with autoimmune gastritis and severe hypergastrinemia, and they account for 70% to 80% of all gastric NETs. These type 1 NETs are relatively innocuous and are associated with a 5-year survival rate greater than 95%, in sharp contrast with the less common solitary, sporadic type 3 NETs, which are biologically more aggressive (<35% 5-year survival rate).[286] Therefore it is important to convey to clinicians the clinical and pathological context in which a gastric NET is diagnosed.

The antral mucosa in autoimmune gastritis may be completely normal, or it may show mild, chronic inflammation, even with small foci of intestinal metaplasia similar to that observed in an age-matched general population unrelated to autoimmune gastritis. However, in 30% to 50% of the cases, a reactive gastropathy can be detected in the antrum, with foveolar hyperplasia,[22,287] which may also be induced by the trophic effects of hypergastrinemia. In addition, hyperplasia of gastrin cells, caused by achlorhydria, is often present as well (see Fig. 15.53C,D).

Differential Diagnosis

H. pylori gastritis must be differentiated from autoimmune gastritis in some cases. Other than demonstration of *organisms,* the presence of a bandlike distribution of the inflammatory infiltrate is usually more superficial and pronounced, and the neutrophilic infiltration (i.e., activity) is more severe. In addition, the absence of characteristic lesions of autoimmune gastritis, such as the selective atrophy of the oxyntic mucosa and neuroendocrine ECL-cell hyperplasia are helpful.

Another diagnosis to consider is gastric involvement by autoimmune enteropathy. This exceedingly rare panenteric condition, more common in the pediatric population, is related to various complex etiologies and preferentially affects the mid gut. However, it may also involve the hindgut and the foregut, including the stomach. Gastric biopsies commonly show mild to moderate chronic gastritis with expansion of the lamina propria by a lymphoplasmacytic infiltrate. Deep crypt apoptosis and neutrophilic activity have been reported in some cases, as well as a lymphocytic gastritis pattern of disease. Loss of oxyntic glands, pseudopyloric metaplasia, and ECL cell hyperplasia have been reported as well, and this mimics autoimmune gastritis.

SPECIFIC PATTERNS OF GASTRITIS

Lymphocytic Gastritis

Clinical Features

Lymphocytic gastritis is a condition characterized pathologically by large numbers of mature lymphocytes that infiltrate the surface and foveolar epithelium. This pattern of gastritis has been reported in 0.3% to 4% of patients who undergo upper endoscopy. Lymphocytic gastritis is most commonly diagnosed in the fifth decade of life, and it affects women more than men, especially when it is associated with celiac sprue.[288]

Lymphocytic gastritis is, essentially, a pathological reaction pattern without specificity for any particular disease. An allergic or autoimmune pathogenesis has been proposed.[288]

Almost all intraepithelial lymphocytes in this condition are CD8+ T cells, similar to those found in the duodenal mucosa of celiac disease patients. Lymphocytic gastritis is frequently observed in patients with celiac disease, but also less commonly following other conditions, such as *H. pylori* infection. It has also been associated with drug use, including NSAIDs, omeprazole, and checkpoint inhibitor immunotherapy.[111] Other associations include Ménétrier disease,[289,290] lymphocytic or collagenous colitis, Crohn's disease, human immunodeficiency virus infection, chronic variable immunodeficiency, autoimmune enteropathy, lymphoma, and esophageal carcinoma.[291]

Pathological Features

Endoscopically, patients (including those with celiac disease) may present with scattered superficial erosions in the corpus or antrum, or they may have normal-appearing gastric mucosa. Varioliform gastritis, which represents a specific endoscopic appearance of the disease rather than a distinct pathogenetic disorder, is characterized by the presence of multiple small nodules with central depressions (i.e., "octopus sucker gastritis"). This condition most likely represents a peculiar form of *H. pylori* infection.[159,160]

The gastric distribution of the intraepithelial lymphocytosis correlates roughly with the etiology of the disease. Celiac disease–associated cases are typically antral predominant, whereas *H. pylori*–associated lesions are usually body predominant. Drug-induced (e.g., NSAID) cases frequently manifest as pangastritis.[291,292]

Microscopically, lymphocytic gastritis is rather loosely defined by the presence of more than 25 intraepithelial lymphocytes per 100 epithelial cells, although lymphocyte counting is usually unnecessary because the morphological picture in its entirety is often more helpful and indicative of true disease (Fig. 15.54).[211,218] The histological features are easily distinguishable from those of typical *H. pylori* gastritis (see Fig. 15.41) in which only rarely are more than 5 or 6 intraepithelial lymphocytes per 100 epithelial cells present, and the lymphocytes are usually more irregularly distributed as well. The gastric distribution of intraepithelial lymphocytosis may help suggest a specific etiology. Celiac disease–associated cases are typically antrum-predominant, whereas *H. pylori*–associated lesions are usually corpus-predominant.[291,292] The severity of the lamina propria inflammatory changes in lymphocytic gastritis also varies considerably. In mild cases, there is only a minor increase in chronic inflammation, and without neutrophils. At the other extreme, marked chronic inflammation may be seen in the lamina propria that is occasionally associated with surface erosions. The lamina propria infiltrate is typically composed of lymphocytes, with scattered plasma cells, eosinophils, and mast cells. Prominent neutrophils may be an indicator of *H. pylori* infection.[293] Other features of lymphocytic gastritis include a variable degree of degenerative epithelial changes, mucin depletion, foveolar hyperplasia, and increased mitoses. Because *H. pylori* infection is the second most common etiology,[291] but the number of

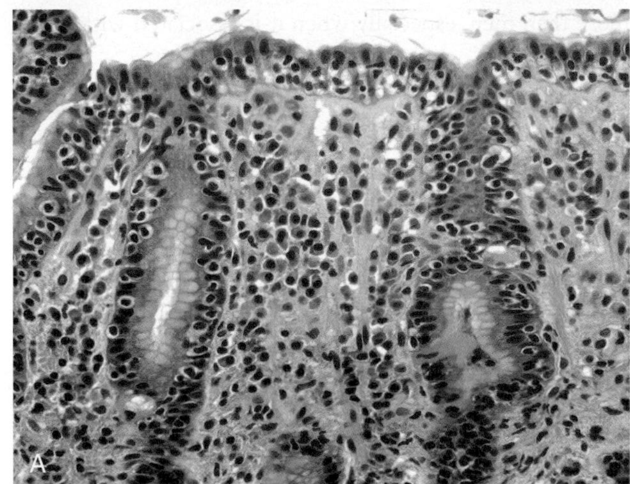

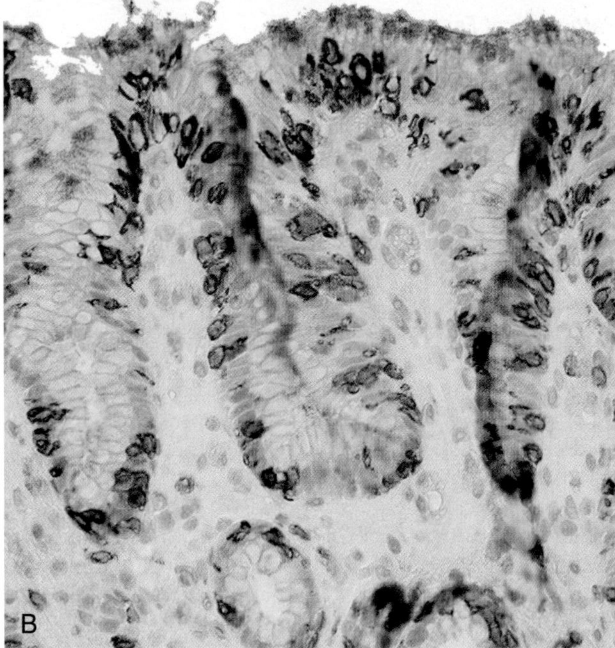

FIGURE 15.54 A, Lymphocytic gastritis with marked intraepithelial lymphocytosis and a marked plasma cell and lymphocytic infiltrate in the lamina propria. **B,** CD3 immunohistochemistry highlights the intraepithelial T cells.

organisms may be low, anti–*H. pylori* immunohistochemistry is recommended for all cases if *H. pylori* is not detected on H&E-stained slides.[212]

Collagenous Gastritis

Collagenous gastritis is a relatively recently described rare entity that is histologically similar to collagenous colitis and is characterized by the presence of a distinct subepithelial collagen band and lamina propria inflammatory infiltrate. The disease may affect both adults and children. In the pediatric setting, there is no gender predilection, whereas a female predominance is observed among adult patients.[294] In contrast with observations in early literature, recent data suggest that pediatric and adult age groups share a similar clinical presentation, characterized by anemia, endoscopically nodular mucosa resembling cobblestones, chronic abdominal pain, and variable watery diarrhea.[294-296] Collagenous gastritis has been associated with celiac disease, collagenous and lymphocytic sprue, as well as collagenous and lymphocytic colitis, especially in adult patients.[294,296-301] In one series, almost half of all adult patients were taking medications known for causing other immune-mediated GI diseases (e.g., olmesartan and antidepressants).[295]

The histological hallmark of collagenous gastritis is the subepithelial collagen band, which is usually >10 μm thick in well-oriented tissue sections, demonstrates a ragged interface with the underlying lamina propria, and may contain entrapped capillaries (Fig. 15.55). However, the collagen band is focal or patchy in about 50% of cases and may be missed by limited tissue sampling. In problematic cases, the subepithelial collagen may be highlighted with tenascin immunohistochemistry.[294] The distribution of the collagen band has been reported to be more frequently corpus-predominant in the pediatric setting, whereas it is usually antrum-predominant in adult patients.[294,302] Focal detachment and degenerative atypia of the surface epithelium has also been noted.[294] The lamina propria often shows a variable lymphoplasmacytic infiltrate. In addition to the characteristic collagen band, biopsies may demonstrate any or all of the following superimposed patterns: (1) eosinophil-rich pattern (>30 eosinophils/HPF in the lamina propria); (2) lymphocytic gastritis-like pattern with intraepithelial lymphocytosis; or (3) an autoimmune gastritis-like corpus-predominant atrophic pattern with reduction of oxyntic glands, pseudopyloric and intestinal metaplasia, splaying of hyperplastic smooth muscle in the lamina propria, and rarely, mild ECL cell hyperplasia.[294,295,303] Neutrophils may be detected, albeit active inflammation is usually only focal and mild. Despite treatment, in the majority of the cases, both the histological features and the clinical symptoms of collagenous gastritis persist after treatment.[295,296,302]

The differential diagnosis includes fibrosis associated with autoimmune gastritis, healed ulcer, or radiation therapy and scleroderma in which the collagen deposition is not specifically subepithelial and may involve deeper levels of the bowel wall.

Eosinophilic Gastritis

Clinical Features and Definition

Eosinophilic gastritis belongs to a group of eosinophilic gastrointestinal disorders (EGIDs) that also includes eosinophil esophagitis, eosinophilic gastroenteritis, and eosinophilic colitis. In a North American study of 317 children and 56 adults with EGID, 41% developed eosinophilia outside of their primary disease location. Eosinophilic gastritis was the most common nonesophageal EGIDs, with 38% of patients showing gastric eosinophilia.[304] Idiopathic (isolated) eosinophilic gastritis is a poorly characterized condition, thus only limited literature is available, other than in sporadic case reports.[304-309] It affects both children and adults without a gender predilection.

Endoscopically the disease may present with erosive/ulcerative or nodular lesions, but near-normal mucosa can also occur. The gene expression patterns of these two endoscopic presentations overlap, implying that they represent only morphological variations of the same disease. [310] Epigastric pain, nausea, and vomiting were the most common

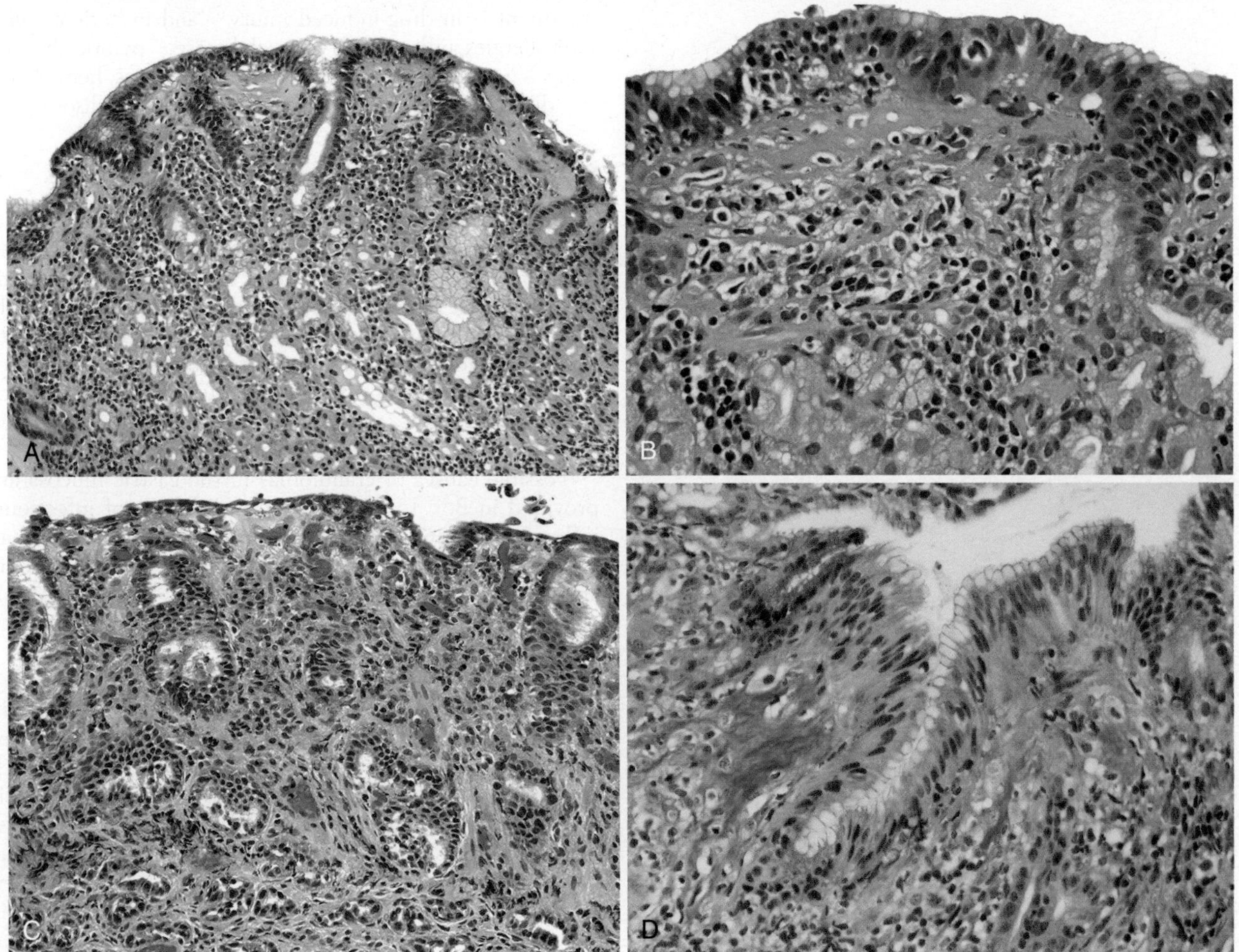

FIGURE 15.55 **A** and **B,** Examples of collagenous gastritis showing a thickened and irregular subepithelial collagen plate on a background of chronic gastritis. **C,** The mucosa may become atrophic with splitting of the muscularis mucosa. **D,** Trichrome stain highlights the subepithelial collagen deposition.

reason for endoscopy in adults and children, followed by reflux disease and dysphagia.[304] The majority of patients have symptomatic, endoscopic, and histological improvements after treatment.[304]

Pathological Features

The normal range of gastric mucosal eosinophils has not been firmly established.[311-314] Although most observers consider the finding of a few eosinophils in the lamina propria common, the updated Sydney system posits that intraepithelial eosinophils in gastric mucosa are abnormal.[315]

In a biopsy series from northern Sweden, a mean lamina propria eosinophil count of 11 eosinophils/5 HPFs in the cardia, body, and antrum of asymptomatic adult volunteers has been reported.[313] In the United States, patients (range 4 to 81 years of age) with no history of relevant GI disease and histologically unremarkable gastric biopsies[29] demonstrated a mean eosinophil count of 4 eosinophils/HPF (±4 standard deviations [SD]), equivalent to 15 eosinophils/mm^2 (± 17 SD; range 0 to 110 eosinophils/mm^2). There were no significant differences in the counts in biopsies from the antrum compared with the corpus, and no significant variation by age or geographic location. DeBrosse et al. reported peak eosinophil counts of 8 eosinophils/HPF in antral biopsies and 11 eosinophils/HPF in oxyntic mucosal biopsies from 19 children from the United States,[312] while a Canadian study demonstrated a mean eosinophil count of 12.3 (±8.7 SD) in the antrum and 7.6 (±6.5 SD)/HPF in the corpus.[316] A recent multicenter study from Greece, Italy, and Spain evaluated biopsies of 111 pediatric patients and found a median eosinophil count ranging from 0 to 3.2 eosinophils/mm^2, with significant differences among the three centers.[317]

We recommend that the term *histological eosinophilic gastritis* be used for the diagnosis of patients who have no known clinical cause of eosinophilia, but their gastric biopsies show at least 30 eosinophils/HPF in at least five separate hot spot HPFs. Eosinophilic degranulation and clustering may be noted.[318] Sheets of eosinophils are seen in over 50% of cases. Eosinophils tend to surround the foveolae (Fig. 15.56A) and infiltrate the epithelium (Fig. 15.56B), but they only rarely form eosinophilic pit abscesses. Involvement of the muscularis mucosae or submucosa may occur. Although reactive epithelial changes similar to those found in chemical gastropathy are common, neither foveolar hyperplasia nor intestinal metaplasia is characteristic.

If *H. pylori* organisms are detected, a diagnosis of eosinophilic gastritis can be established only if the mucosal

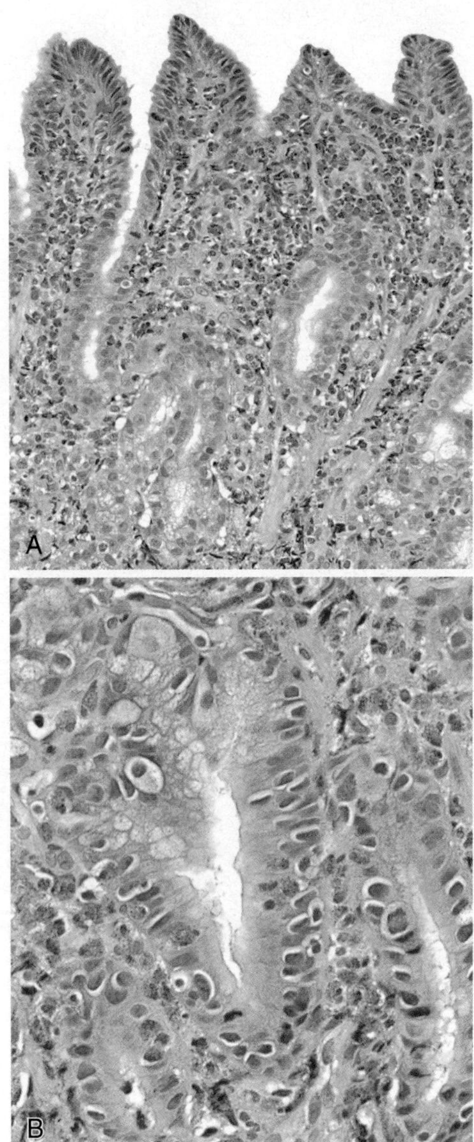

FIGURE 15.56 A, There are innumerable eosinophils in the lamina propria in this example of eosinophilic gastritis. **B,** Eosinophils occur within the muscularis mucosae. Eosinophils tend to surround the foveolae and infiltrate the epithelium, but they only rarely spill into the lumen to form eosinophilic pit abscesses.

eosinophilia persists several months after successful eradication therapy. When regenerative epithelial changes are observed in a gastric biopsy with significant eosinophilic infiltrates that fall below the recommended quantitative threshold, we suggest a diagnosis of "reactive gastropathy with increased eosinophils." The diagnosis should include a comment mentioning the possibility of eosinophilic gastritis among other differential diagnoses deemed appropriate in the context of the patient's specific clinical situation.[29]

Other conditions associated with increased numbers of eosinophils in the lamina propria have been reported. Among those is autoimmune gastritis, in which increased eosinophilia is more common than in *H. pylori* gastritis.[22,319-321] Abnormally elevated eosinophils have also been documented in a variety of conditions, including infection with *Anisakis* spp.[322] or *Strongyloides stercoralis*,[323] after *H. pylori* treatment,[18] in drug-induced injury,[63] and in patients with food allergies, inflammatory bowel disease,[29] pyloric obstruction,[324,325] tumors,[326] connective tissue diseases, hematopoietic disorders, and rare eosinophil-associated GI disorders.[28]

Granulomatous Gastritis

Granulomatous gastritis is a nonspecific histological pattern of disease characterized by the presence of multiple granulomas in gastric mucosa (Fig. 15.57). The morphological appearance of the granulomas does not usually provide useful clues regarding their cause, except when foreign material, acid-fast bacilli, or fungal forms are identified; the latter two entities occasionally cause central necrosis or caseation. In most cases, the cause cannot be determined without specific clinical and laboratory information.

Possible causes of granulomas in the gastric mucosa are provided in Box 15.1, including many types of infectious, inflammatory, and neoplastic diseases; however, they may be seen in otherwise healthy individuals. The endoscopic appearance of the stomach may be normal, or it may exhibit characteristics of the specific disease entity that caused the granulomas to form.

Mycobacterial and Fungal Infections

Worldwide, tuberculosis is the most common cause of granulomatous disease of the GI tract. However, the stomach was only affected in approximately 6% of all GI tuberculosis cases in one large multicenter study of 104 patients.[327] Gastric tuberculosis may manifest in various clinicopathological forms including (1) localized gastric tuberculosis with a primary complex (caseation of celiac lymph nodes), (2) gastric tuberculosis secondary to pulmonary disease, (3) as part of a more extensive GI tuberculosis, or (4) miliary tuberculosis in immunocompromised patients (e.g., HIV positive).[328] Primary gastric tuberculosis has been reported mostly in developing countries with a high prevalence of *Mycobacterium tuberculosis* infection and caused by the ingestion of unpasteurized milk infected with *Mycobacterium bovis*.[329-332] The prepyloric and antral regions, especially in the lesser curvature, are the most frequently affected sites of involvement.[333] Many cases manifest as a large, nonhealing ulcer or may mimic a submucosal neoplasm.[333,334] Microscopic examination may reveal epithelioid granulomas with patches of caseating necrosis (see Fig. 15.57A,B).[333,334] Scrutinizing acid-fast stains for bacteria may prove unrewarding, and PCR analysis for mycobacterial DNA fragments is a more sensitive method of detection.[335]

Fungal infections may also induce granulomatous gastritis, and a few cases of primary gastric infection by *Histoplasma capsulatum*[336-338] as well as *Aspergillus* species have been reported.[339,340] These patients often have signs and symptoms of a large gastric ulcer.[336-338] Microscopically, neutrophilic infiltrate within the granuloma may be noted.[340]

Helicobacter pylori Infection

Unexplained granulomas may be found in less than 10% of patients with *H. pylori* gastritis, and the role of this organism in causing granulomas is unknown and controversial.[341] Because gastric granulomas are not rare and may also be seen in healthy individuals, the discovery of granulomas in

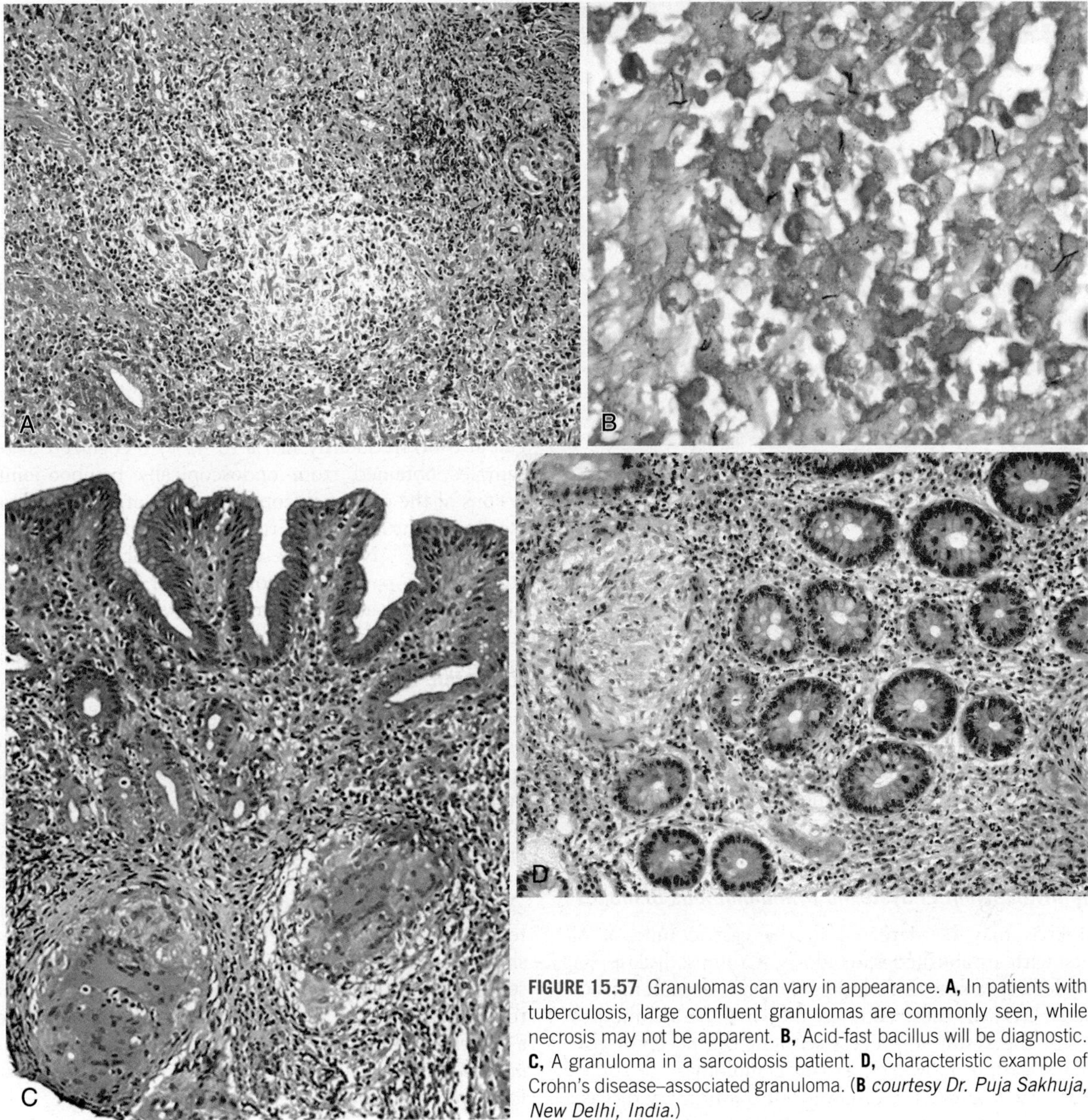

FIGURE 15.57 Granulomas can vary in appearance. **A,** In patients with tuberculosis, large confluent granulomas are commonly seen, while necrosis may not be apparent. **B,** Acid-fast bacillus will be diagnostic. **C,** A granuloma in a sarcoidosis patient. **D,** Characteristic example of Crohn's disease–associated granuloma. (**B** *courtesy Dr. Puja Sakhuja, New Delhi, India.*)

patients with *H. pylori* gastritis may represent a coincidental finding. Alternatively, granulomas in this setting may indicate a second disorder.

Parasites

The nematodes most commonly associated with the formation of gastric granulomas are *Anisakis* spp. Early lesions show interstitial edema accompanied by loose, predominantly eosinophilic inflammation, and late lesions may show overt eosinophilic microabscesses. Well-preserved larvae are often detected. In late lesions, the most common findings are foreign body granulomas, which are sometimes associated with fragments of helminthic cuticles.[30,342] Rarely, fragments of larvae interpreted as *Strongyloides stercoralis* have been observed in gastric granulomas.[343,344] These conditions are discussed further in Chapter 4.

Foreign Bodies

Suture material is a common cause of granulomas in patients who have undergone a partial gastrectomy. Histology may disclose the engulfed foreign material within histiocytes. Examination under polarized light should always be performed in cases of granulomatous gastritis. In patients with gastric ulcer, food particles may become engulfed by the ulcer crater, where they may cause a foreign body reaction. When granulomas are found in biopsies obtained from active ulcers, their origin is readily apparent. However, diagnostic difficulties may arise when granulomas are found in specimens from healed ulcers and the pathologist lacks the appropriate clinical information. In rare cases, ingestion of nonnutritive substances (e.g., onychophagia) has been reported as a cause of granulomatous gastritis.[345]

BOX 15.1 Causes of Gastric Granulomas

INFECTIONS
Bacterial
- Tuberculosis
- Syphilis
- Whipple disease
- *Helicobacter* (?)
- *Actinomycosis*

Fungal
- Histoplasmosis
- *Aspergillosis*

Parasitic
- *Anisakiasis*
- *Strongyloidosis* (?)

FOREIGN BODIES
Sutures
Food

Xanthogranuloma
Tumors
- Carcinoma
- Lymphoma
- Plasma cell granuloma

Granulomatous diseases of unknown origin
- Immune-mediated vasculitis
- Granulomatosis with polyangiitis (Wegener's granulomatosis)
- Inflammatory bowel disease: Crohn's disease
- Sarcoidosis
- Isolated granulomatous gastritis

Immune-related pathology

Tumors

Rarely, adenocarcinomas (particularly mucin-producing lesions) may induce the formation of granulomas in gastric mucosa or in lymph nodes. Granulomas have also been observed in patients with gastric non-MALT lymphomas.[346]

Other Unusual Causes

Granulomatous gastritis is, rarely, part of an immune-mediated vasculitis syndrome, such as Wegener's granulomatosis. Sometimes, it may assume a xanthogranulomatous pattern, akin to that seen in some cases of cholecystitis or pyelonephritis.[347,348]

Gastric Involvement in Systemic Granulomatous Diseases

Granulomas may be detected in the gastric mucosa of patients with established sarcoidosis, Crohn's disease, or immunological diseases including chronic granulomatous disease (CGD). In these settings, they may be assumed to be part of the systemic process without the need for further investigation. However, gastric granulomas are sometimes detected before the discovery of the primary disease in other organs. In these cases, correct interpretation of the biopsy findings may prompt diagnosis of a condition that may otherwise remain obscure for a long time.[349]

Isolated gastric sarcoidosis, or sarcoidosis initially manifesting in the stomach without involvement of other organs, is rare. Sarcoidosis involving the GI tract is occasionally discovered at autopsy, but it is rarely of clinical importance. In one recent study, only 4% of patients with sarcoidosis undergoing gastric biopsy showed epithelioid cell granulomas.[350] Nevertheless, severe disease can produce gastric outlet obstruction or bleeding. Endoscopic findings include nodularity, polyps, erosions, ulcers, and segmental (usually distal) rigidity that may resemble a neoplastic lesion, including linitis plastica.[351-353] There are no pathognomonic histological findings of gastric sarcoidosis, therefore the histology must be interpreted in conjunction with clinical and radiological information. Nevertheless sarcoidosis more frequently shows numerous and well-formed granulomas with Langerhans-type giant cells (see Fig. 15.57C), whereas Crohn's disease is usually associated with ill-formed epithelioid cell clusters and smaller granulomas without giant cells (see Fig. 15.57D). Schaumann and asteroid bodies are not typically seen in gastric sarcoidosis.

Although gastric involvement in Crohn's disease was initially reported to be rare, recent studies conducted after the technological improvement of endoscopy found a higher incidence (30% to 60%) of upper GI manifestations.[262,354-359] Granulomas in gastric Crohn's disease (see Fig. 15.57D) can be accompanied by focally enhanced gastritis, and either active or inactive *H. pylori*–negative chronic gastritis.[17,261,360] The reported detection rate of epithelioid granulomas shows high variability (3.4% to 63%) based on the sampling method (biopsy vs. resection) and location (antropyloric vs. oxyntic) as well as the extent of examination (e.g., number of samples and serial sections examined).[354-358,361] Granulomas are generally more prevalent in the antropyloric region than in oxyntic mucosa. However, granulomas can also be frequently (10% to 45%) recognized in biopsy samples obtained from endoscopically bamboo-joint–like lesions of the proximal stomach, which are characterized by swollen longitudinal folds traversed by erosive fissures or linear furrows.[362] Nevertheless, detection of granulomas in the stomach in a patient with other features of gastric Crohn's disease should always prompt further investigation of the remainder of the GI tract for further evidence of disease.

Idiopathic Granulomatous Gastritis

After all of the previously discussed etiological diagnoses have been excluded and appropriate tests have been performed, a specific etiology of the granulomatous gastritis may still not be identified. However, isolated or idiopathic granulomatous gastritis should not be considered a distinct nosological entity but rather treated as a holding category and applied as a temporary diagnostic term in cases for which the primary cause of the granulomas awaits determination.[363] Support for this approach is derived from several studies that have shown that most unexplained gastric granulomas may represent concurrent or incipient Crohn's disease or another systemic disorder such as sarcoidosis.[349,353,359] For such cases, a descriptive diagnosis such as *nonnecrotizing granulomatous mucosal inflammation* is preferable to use of a term such as *idiopathic granulomatous gastritis*.

VASCULAR GASTROPATHIES

Vascular gastropathies are a heterogeneous group of disorders characterized endoscopically by alterations in the gastric mucosal blood vessels and microscopically by the presence of little or no inflammation. The most characteristic vascular gastropathies are GAVE and portal hypertensive gastropathy.

Gastric Antral Vascular Ectasia

Clinical Features

GAVE, also known as *watermelon stomach*, is a rare condition of unknown origin. It is frequently associated with gastric atrophy and with autoimmune and connective tissue disorders.[364] More than 70% of cases occur in women older than 65 years of age. Occult bleeding (melena) is the presenting sign in up to 90% of cases, with chronic blood loss that causes iron-deficiency anemia. Sixty percent of patients have severe acute bleeding and hematemesis.

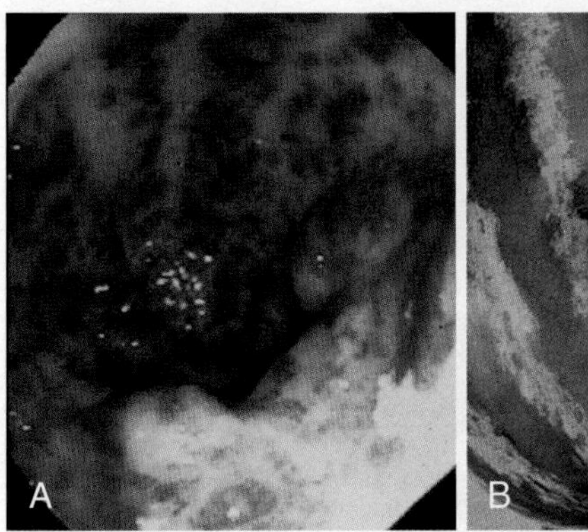

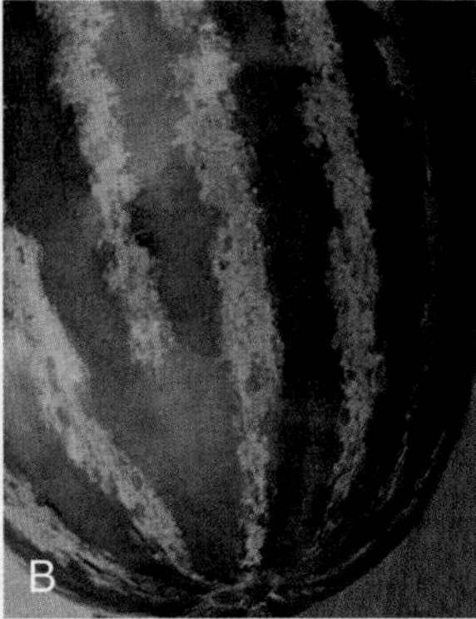

FIGURE 15.58 Watermelon stomach (i.e., gastric antral vascular ectasia). **A,** Endoscopic view of the erythematous lines converging toward the pyloric region of the stomach. **B,** The mucosal appearance resembles stripes of a watermelon.

Pathological Features and Differential Diagnosis

The term *watermelon stomach* is derived from the endoscopically visible ectatic vessels that appear along the longitudinal mucosal folds that converge concentrically from the proximal antrum to the pylorus, resembling the stripes on a watermelon (Fig. 15.58).[365] Various degrees of bleeding and clotting may be seen on the mucosal surface.[364]

Microscopically, GAVE has a characteristic appearance in antral biopsies. The background setting resembles reactive (chemical) gastropathy. The foveolar epithelium shows characteristic elongation, hyperplasia, increased tortuosity, mucin depletion, nuclear hyperchromasia, increased mitoses, and other degenerative changes. The lamina propria, which typically is not inflamed, may contain radiating smooth muscle proliferation oriented perpendicular to the mucosal surface as well as mild fibrosis. Edema may be prominent. The characteristic findings are significantly dilated mucosal capillaries (with a diameter approximating that of adjacent glands).[365] In most cases, fibrin thrombi develop within dilated mucosal capillaries.

Reactive gastropathy, including those caused by bile reflux and drugs (i.e., NSAIDs or iron pill), may mimic the epithelial changes observed in vascular gastropathies. Although not pathognomonic, the presence of fibrin thrombi helps distinguish GAVE from reactive gastropathy (Fig. 15.59) as well as portal hypertensive gastropathy and other causes of mucosal congestion.[366]

Treatment

In contrast with portal hypertensive gastropathy, GAVE does not resolve after lowering portal pressure. The management of GAVE is empiric and involves general measures of acute and chronic GI bleeding treatment. Iron supplements are usually sufficient for patients with minimal bleeding, but therapeutic endoscopy with argon plasma coagulation of the affected area of antral mucosa or antrectomy may be necessary in severe cases.[367-371]

Portal Hypertensive Gastropathy

Clinical Features

Portal hypertensive gastropathy is characterized by dilation and congestion of mucosal blood vessels, which often cause chronic bleeding, and manifests as iron-deficiency anemia and less frequently with acute hemorrhage.[372] It is caused by portal hypertension, which usually results from hepatic cirrhosis.[370,373] For patients with severe portal hypertension, the mucosa is usually diffusely involved, and there is a high risk of acute bleeding. Portal pressure–reducing drugs, bypass surgery, or transjugular intrahepatic portosystemic shunting are the most effective measures for decompressing portal hypertension and reducing the risk of hemorrhage.[372]

Pathological Features and Differential Diagnosis

The endoscopic appearance of portal hypertensive gastropathy has been described as resembling mosaic, snake skin, scarlatina rash, or cherry-red spots (Fig. 15.60).[372,374,375] However, these patterns are nonspecific and do not correlate with the degree of portal hypertension.[376] The mosaic pattern has been found to be the most reliable indicator of mild portal hypertensive gastropathy and a low risk of hemorrhage.[311] Red marks suggest more severe degrees of portal hypertension and a greater risk of mucosal hemorrhage.

The microscopic changes of portal hypertensive gastropathy include foveolar hyperplasia, edema, and a paucity of inflammation, all of which resemble reactive gastropathy (Fig. 15.61). They are usually most prominent in the corpus. The characteristic features are dilation, tortuosity, and occasional thickening of small submucosal arteries and veins. In an appropriate clinical and endoscopic setting, a diagnosis of portal hypertensive gastropathy can be established by recognition of these vascular changes.[377,378]

Although the submucosal blood vessels are most severely affected, the mucosal capillaries are also congested and dilated, giving the appearance of proliferation (see Fig. 15.61). Although in the absence of severe coagulopathy, biopsies are generally considered to be safe, the reluctance to obtain large, deep biopsy samples from patients with an increased risk of bleeding hinders the biopsy diagnosis of portal hypertensive gastropathy. The absence of fibrin thrombi and the predominantly corpus localization of vascular changes are the most important features in the differential diagnosis of GAVE, the importance of which is emphasized by the difference in their clinical management.[372]

Treatment

Current management of portal hypertensive gastropathy aims to reduce portal pressure with somatostatin analogues as the first-line therapy. Because hemorrhage is typically diffuse and its source is often difficult to localize, endoscopic therapy is uncommonly used. Transjugular intrahepatic portosystemic shunting (TIPS) and shunt surgery are last-resort therapy for patients who fail medical treatment.[379]

Dieulafoy Lesion

A Dieulafoy lesion, also known as a *caliber-persistent artery*, refers to a prominent artery that maintains its large caliber while penetrating the submucosa and may protrude into the gut lumen and cause recurrent and sometimes massive hemorrhage when the overlying mucosa becomes ulcerated. These lesions have been described in all parts of the GI tract, but they are most common at the GEJ and in the lesser curve of the stomach. Dieulafoy lesions account for the 0.5% to 14% of patients in whom acute upper GI bleeding develops. Treatment options include endoscopic injection, cautery, ligation, embolization, and surgery.[229,230]

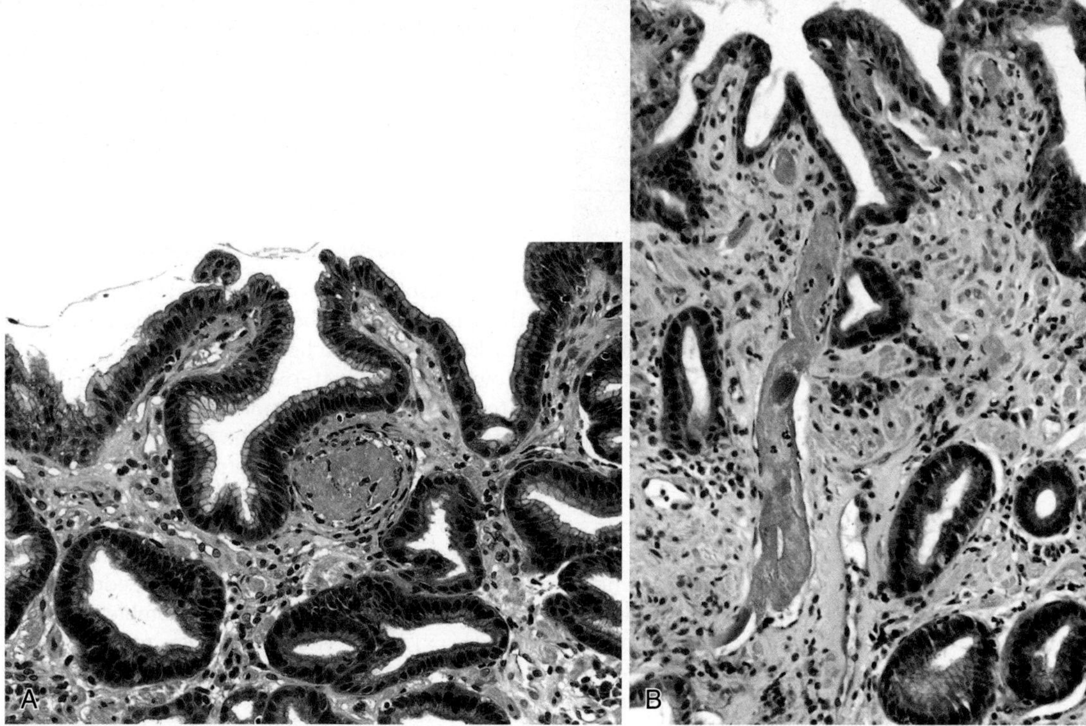

FIGURE 15.59 **A** and **B,** Two examples of gastric antral vascular ectasia show a reactive gastropathy pattern with dilated mucosal blood vessels, some of which contain thrombus material.

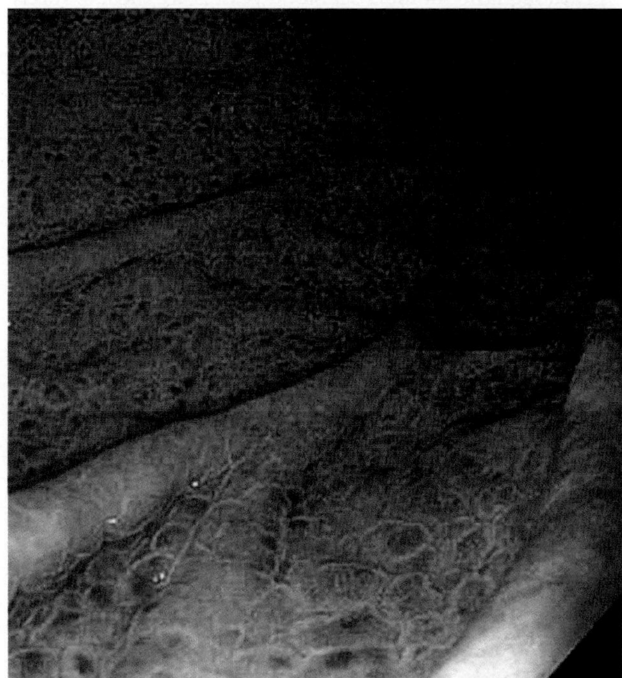

FIGURE 15.60 Characteristic snake skin endoscopic appearance of the antrum in portal hypertensive gastropathy.

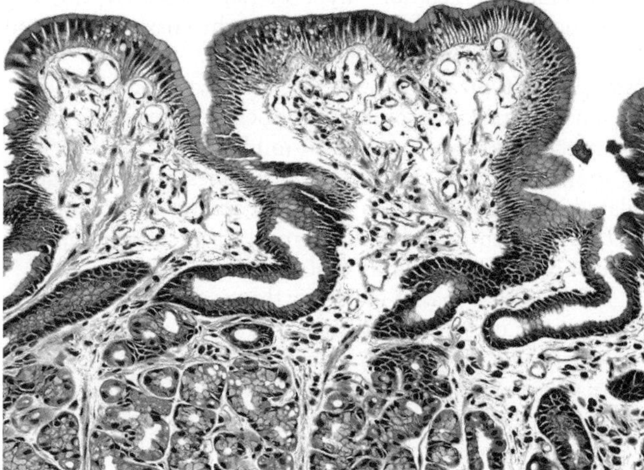

FIGURE 15.61 In portal hypertensive gastropathy, numerous dilated mucosal capillaries impart an edematous appearance to the mucosa.

GASTRIC MUCOSAL DEPOSITIONS

Calcium Deposits

Interstitial calcium deposits in the lamina propria (Fig. 15.62) may, rarely, impart an endoscopic impression of a small, white plaque or sessile polyp. Deposits are typically found in patients with end-stage renal disease, but they may occur in patients with other diseases.[380] The surrounding mucosa is usually unremarkable, but occasionally it may be ulcerated. Some pathologists have proposed that ulceration induces calcium deposits, although direct evidence for this association is lacking.

Siderosis

Gastric mucosal siderosis has been described in association with hemochromatosis as well as in alcoholics and in patients who consume oral iron-containing medications.[381,382] Gastric mucosal hemosiderosis is identified in approximately 2% of gastric biopsies when evaluated by Prussian blue stain.

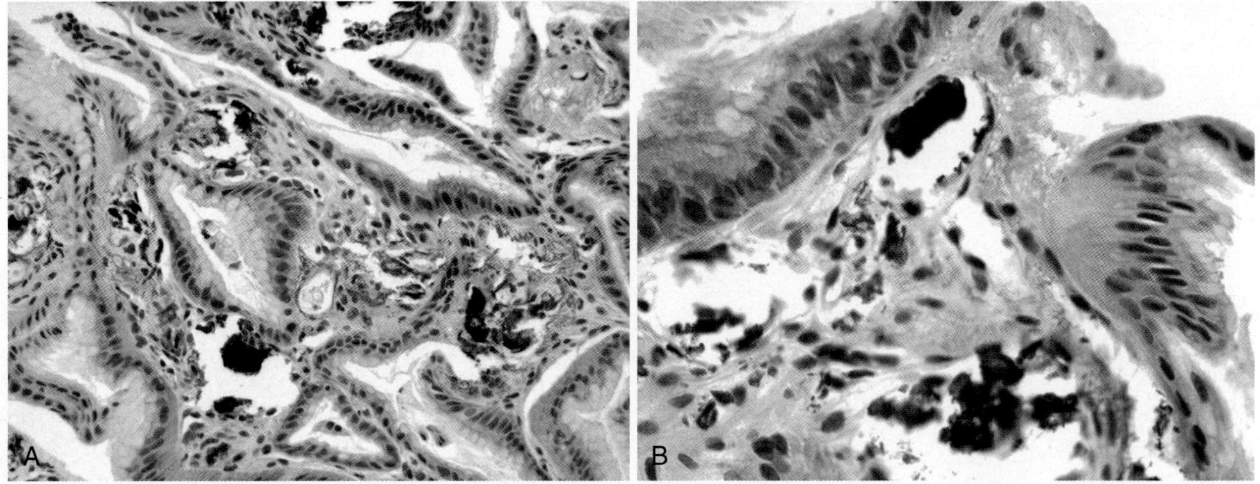

FIGURE 15.62 Stromal calcifications. A and **B,** Microcalcifications within the lamina propria occur in association with chronic renal failure.

One study describes three histological patterns of gastric mucosal siderosis.[383] The first pattern is patchy iron deposition in stromal cells, including macrophages, with only focal epithelial deposition. This type is frequently associated with gastric inflammation, and it may represent iron deposition from prior mucosal hemorrhage. The second pattern is patchy, mostly extracellular iron deposition and focal, mild gastritis or reactive gastropathy–type changes. This type is typically associated with oral iron-containing medications. In these cases, brown crystalline material within the lamina propria may be associated with fibrosis, inflammation, and a foreign body reaction.[382] The third pattern of siderosis is diffuse deposition predominantly in glandular epithelium (see Fig. 15.32C,D). It is often associated with systemic iron overload or hemochromatosis.

GASTRIC CARDIA AND THE GASTROESOPHAGEAL JUNCTION

The GEJ is a poorly defined anatomic area situated between the distal esophagus and the proximal stomach (i.e., gastric "cardia"). GERD and *H. pylori* infection are the major causes of inflammation and intestinal metaplasia of the GEJ region.[384] Other less common causes include reactive gastritis and autoimmune gastritis. In some individuals, multiple etiological agents may act synergistically to cause inflammation.[385-388] Other etiological factors, such as NSAIDs and other drugs, may be responsible for inflammation in the GEJ region in some patients, but these less common causes have not been investigated thoroughly. GERD and *H. pylori* induce chronic inflammation and intestinal metaplasia, which increases the risk of neoplasia.[389]

Until recently, a commonly accepted definition of the *cardia* was "the segment of mucosa that extends for about 1 to 2 cm distal to a normally situated squamocolumnar junction (Z-line) in a patient without columnar metaplasia in the distal esophagus." It consists mainly of mucous-type glands similar to those of the antrum and prepyloric region. However, a mixture of mucous and oxyntic glands is also common. Because no particularly interesting pathological processes were believed to affect this small territory of gastric mucosa that connects two well-characterized segments of the digestive system, the gastric cardia was virtually ignored by gastroenterologists, pathologists, and physiologists for generations. However, during the past several decades, there has been a dramatic rise in the incidence of adenocarcinoma of the cardia/GEJ region.[390] In fact, the increased incidence of GEJ cancer affects the same populations in which the incidence of gastric cancer is decreasing, and the upsurge is presumed to be related to GERD or *H. pylori*, or both.

Histology of the Gastroesophageal Junction Region

The true anatomic GEJ corresponds to the most proximal aspect of the gastric folds, which is an endoscopically apparent transition point in most individuals.[391] The anatomic GEJ usually corresponds to the histological transition point between the esophageal squamous epithelium and the gastric mucinous columnar epithelium in patients without columnar metaplasia of the distal esophagus. The transition point is termed the *Z-line*. However, most adults, particularly those with either physiological or pathological GERD, reveal a slightly proximally displaced ("irregular") Z-line, indicating that the histological squamocolumnar junction is actually located proximal to the anatomic GEJ.[392]

The true gastric cardia is the area of mucosa located distal to the anatomic GEJ and proximal to the portion of stomach composed entirely of oxyntic glands (i.e., corpus and fundus). Inflammation of this anatomic region is termed *carditis,* and it is often caused by *H. pylori* infection, although accumulating evidence suggests that GERD may also cause carditis.[384,389,393,394] However, in GERD cases, it is often difficult to determine whether the inflamed mucosa is esophageal or gastric in origin. It is also important to note that many endoscopists use the term *cardia,* generically, to indicate the location of a mucosal biopsy from the GEJ region, even though the biopsy may have actually been obtained from the distal esophagus.[389,395]

Intestinal metaplasia in the GEJ region may represent at least two different entities: ultrashort-segment Barrett's esophagus (i.e., columnar metaplasia of the distal esophagus with goblet cells less than 1.0 cm long) or chronic carditis with intestinal metaplasia (Table 15.7).[392,396,397]

TABLE 15.7 Differentiation of Esophageal Columnar Metaplasia from Gastric Carditis

Feature	Esophageal Columnar Metaplasia	Gastric Carditis
Clinical Features		
Hiatus hernia	+	−
GERD clinical profile	+	−
Heartburn	+	±
White, male	++	±
Young age	++	±
Alcohol	++	±
Tobacco	++	±
Irregular Z-line or tongues	+	−
Pathological Features		
Squamous overlying intestinalized glands	+	−
Hybrid glands	+	−
Esophageal glands or ducts	+	−
Multilayered epithelium	+	−
Marked atrophy or disarray	+	−
Complete intestinal metaplasia	+	±
Esophagitis (histological)	++	±
Distal gastritis	±	++
Eosinophils	++	±
Neutrophils, lymphocytes, plasma	±	++
Helicobacter pylori	±	++

GERD, *Gastroesophageal reflux disease.*

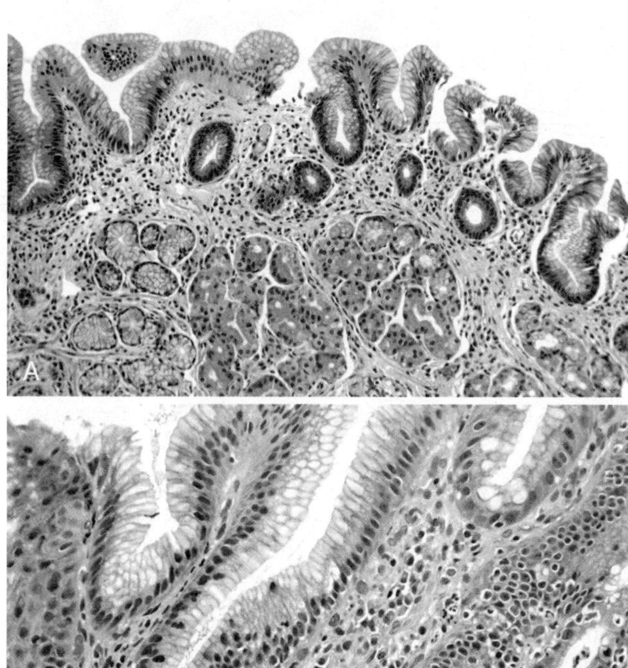

FIGURE 15.63 A, Medium-power view of the true gastric cardia in an adult without symptoms of gastroesophageal reflux disease. The mucosa is composed of a mixture of mucous glands *(left)* and oxyntic-type glands *(right)* with overlying mucinous columnar epithelium. A mild lymphoplasmacytic infiltrate is typical in the cardia of most adults. This biopsy was obtained immediately distal to the most proximal aspect of the gastric folds, the latter of which is defined as the anatomic gastroesophageal junction (GEJ). **B,** Mucosal biopsy from the GEJ shows squamocolumnar junctional mucosa and moderate acute and chronic inflammation of the lamina propria in a patient with *Helicobacter pylori* carditis.

The histological characteristics of short segments of esophageal columnar metaplasia located proximal to the anatomic GEJ are similar to the gastric cardia being composed of pure mucous glands or mixed mucous and oxyntic glands, which leads to difficulty in distinguishing columnar metaplasia of the distal esophagus from the true gastric cardia in biopsies from the GEJ region.[395,398] This distinction is clinically important because columnar metaplasia of the esophagus is caused by GERD, and it may represent an early nonintestinalized precursor of Barrett's esophagus (the latter of which is defined by the presence of intestinal metaplasia and goblet cells).[392,399,400]

There is controversy regarding the origin and histology of the true gastric cardia (see Chapter 1).[384,387,393,401-403] Some authorities believe that the neonatal gastric cardia is composed of surface mucinous columnar epithelium and underlying oxyntic glands identical to the gastric corpus, whereas others maintain that the true anatomic cardia is, ab initio, composed of mucinous columnar epithelium with underlying mucous glands or mixed mucous and oxyntic glands.[392] Proponents of the former theory believe that the mere presence of mucous, or mixed mucous and oxyntic glands, in the mucosa from the GEJ region indicates that it is metaplastic in origin.[386,387,403] However, several studies, including a recent one in heart-beating organ donors, have essentially confirmed that the true gastric cardia in most individuals is composed of either pure mucous or mixed mucous and oxyntic glands underlying mucinous columnar epithelium (Fig. 15.63).[386,393,401,403-405]

The length of the gastric cardia mucosa composed of this morphological appearance normally ranges from 1 to 4 mm.[401] A minority of individuals may reveal pure oxyntic glands in biopsies from the cardia region[387,404-406]; however, this finding is often focal and does not usually involve the entire circumference of the lumen. There is also evidence to suggest that the length of mucosa composed of either pure mucous glands or mixed mucous and oxyntic glands increases with age, and this is presumed to be related to ongoing physiological GERD.[401,403,406-408] Thus the increasing length of cardia-type mucosa with age is believed to result from columnar metaplasia of the distal esophagus (proximal to anatomic GEJ), but in some circumstances (e.g., autoimmune gastritis, *H. pylori* infection), the length of cardia-type mucosa may actually increase as a result of distal extension into the proximal corpus.[409]

Intestinal Metaplasia of the Gastroesophageal Junction

Almost one-third of patients without endoscopic evidence of Barrett's esophagus reveal intestinal metaplasia in the GEJ region in biopsy studies.[384,410] Not surprisingly, the chance of detecting intestinal metaplasia increases proportionally with the number of biopsies obtained.[411] Some evidence suggests that the prevalence of intestinal metaplasia is higher among patients with longer segments of cardia-type mucosa as described earlier, but this finding is more frequently related to GERD than to *H. pylori* infection.[384,387,406] The type of metaplasia may suggest its cause because gastric cardia biopsies from *H. pylori* patients may show a mixture of complete (i.e., containing goblet cells and absorptive-type enterocytes) and incomplete (i.e., goblet cells only) types of intestinal metaplasia more often than GERD, whereas intestinal metaplasia related to GERD-induced "carditis" and to Barrett's esophagus is usually entirely of the incomplete type.[410-412]

The most widely accepted theory regarding the pathogenesis of intestinal metaplasia is that chronic inflammation stimulates its development in the GEJ, regardless of the cause.[389,407,413,414] In GERD patients, chronic reflux leads to inflammation and ulceration of the native squamous epithelium. The damaged mucosa repairs itself via metaplasia to columnar epithelium initially composed of mucinous columnar epithelium with underlying pure mucous, or mixed mucous and oxyntic, glands, and later to epithelium with intestinal metaplasia.[403,412,414]

The cell of origin of metaplastic columnar epithelium in the esophagus is unknown (see Chapter 14 on Barrett's esophagus for more details).[392,410] Possible sites of multipotential stem cells include the basal layer of the native squamous epithelium, esophageal mucosal or submucosal glands and ducts, gastric cardia epithelium, congenital rests of gastric or intestinal epithelium in the esophagus, and even the subepithelial mesenchyme of the esophagus.[392,410,413-415] Studies also suggest that metaplastic and dysplastic epithelium in the stomach may be derived from bone marrow cells, but this theory has not been well investigated in the esophagus.[416] Animal experiments suggest that metaplastic epithelium in the esophagus is derived from cells native to the esophagus rather than the stomach.[413,417] Esophageal mucosal ducts may harbor stem cells that can differentiate into columnar epithelium as well.[410,414]

There is also evidence that indicates that the transition from squamous to columnar cells in the distal esophagus occurs through an intermediate (transitional) phase before intestinalization.[403,410,413,418] In 1993, Shields et al. reported a distinctive type of "multilayered" epithelium that revealed morphological and cytochemical characteristics of both squamous and columnar epithelium (Fig. 15.64).[419] Multilayered epithelium is phenotypically similar to fully developed Barrett's esophagus and has the capacity for cell proliferation and differentiation.[410] One prospective biopsy study found that multilayered epithelium was strongly associated with Barrett's esophagus and GERD-induced inflammation of

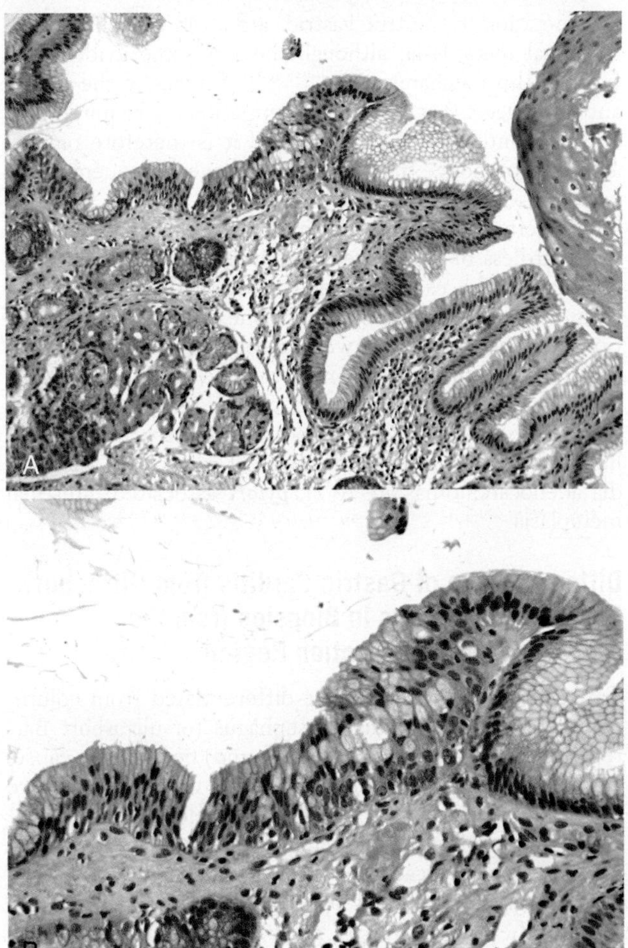

FIGURE 15.64 A, Mucosal biopsy from the gastroesophageal junction (GEJ) region in a patient with reflux symptoms and an irregular Z-line located immediately proximal to the anatomic GEJ. The biopsy shows squamocolumnar junctional mucosa in which there is mild chronic inflammation in the lamina propria, mixed mucous and oxyntic glands in the lamina propria, and overlying mucinous foveolar epithelium with a focus of multilayered epithelium. **B,** High-power magnification of multilayered epithelium shows squamoid cells at the base and mucinous columnar cells at the surface. Overall, the biopsy findings are consistent with columnar metaplasia of the distal esophagus without goblet cells.

the GEJ.[355] Multilayered epithelium is identified in mucosal biopsies from up to 30% of patients with GERD-induced inflammation of the GEJ region.[413,418] Regardless of its putative role in the development of columnar metaplasia in the esophagus, the presence of multilayered epithelium in a biopsy from the GEJ region is considered a surrogate marker for GERD and a likely indicator of GERD as the cause of metaplastic columnar epithelium in the distal esophagus.[357] Multilayered epithelium is usually detected at the level of the squamocolumnar junction, and also often in the vicinity of the openings of the submucosal gland ducts, supporting the theory that the submucosal gland ducts may also contain stem cells that give rise to metaplastic columnar epithelium of the esophagus.[410,418,420]

In contrast, intestinal metaplasia that develops in the true gastric cardia as a result of chronic *H. pylori* infection represents a direct nongoblet-to-goblet cell type of intestinal metaplasia. It is unclear whether GERD-induced inflammation in the true gastric cardia can lead directly to intestinal metaplasia, although there is some evidence in favor of this mechanism.[387,392,406,411] Studies of the gastric antrum suggest that chronic inflammation is a required precursor of intestinal metaplasia, and it is therefore reasonable to hypothesize that the same pathogenic sequence may occur in the gastric cardia of *H. pylori*–infected patients, but objective scientific confirmation is still lacking.[392]

Regardless of the cause, most intestinal-type adenocarcinomas of the esophagus and stomach develop in areas of intestinal metaplasia.[421-424] In one study, 86% of junctional adenocarcinomas were associated with intestinal metaplasia within adjacent mucosa. The cause of intestinal metaplasia may have an impact on the risk of malignancy because distal esophageal adenocarcinomas are more closely linked to GERD-associated intestinal metaplasia than cardia adenocarcinomas are to *H. pylori*–associated intestinal metaplasia.[369,361]

TABLE 15.8 Differentiation of Ultrashort Barrett's Esophagus from Gastric Carditis with Intestinal Metaplasia

Feature	Ultrashort Barrett's Esophagus	Gastric Carditis
Clinical characteristics	Male > female, older	Male = female, younger
Cause	GERD	*Helicobacter pylori*, other
Pathogenesis	Squamous → columnar	Columnar → columnar
Cancer risk	Higher	Lower
Treatment	Acid suppression, surgery, surveillance	Antibiotics, no surveillance

GERD, *Gastroesophageal reflux disease.*

Differentiation of Gastric Carditis from Ultrashort Barrett's Esophagus in Biopsies from the Gastroesophageal Junction Region

True gastric carditis should be differentiated from columnar metaplasia of the distal esophagus (or ultrashort Barrett's esophagus if goblet cells are found) because the cause, pathogenesis, natural history, and risk of malignancy are different for these two conditions (Table 15.8).[389,392,421] Because it is often difficult for endoscopists to know the precise anatomic location of a biopsy obtained from the GEJ region (e.g., whether the biopsy is derived from proximal or distal to the anatomic GEJ), pathologists should attempt to establish the precise location and cause of the inflammatory condition in mucosal biopsies from the GEJ region whenever possible.

Helicobacter pylori

Despite some overlap, the clinical, endoscopic, and pathological features of *H. pylori*–induced carditis are often distinct from those seen in GERD.[392] For example, a young or middle-aged white man who consumes alcohol or tobacco is more likely to have GERD-associated inflammation in biopsies from the GEJ region.[392] *H. pylori* carditis usually affects older patients and is equally common in men and women. Endoscopically, a hiatal hernia, an irregular and proximally located Z-line relative to the anatomic GEJ (either with or without signs of columnar mucosa extending into the distal esophagus), and evidence of esophagitis also support GERD as the cause of inflammation of the GEJ region.

Pathologically, GEJ region biopsies from GERD patients often show only a mild degree of mononuclear inflammation (Fig. 15.65).[387,407] However, active inflammation of the deep or surface epithelium, either with or without surface erosion, may also be seen. Similar to reflux esophagitis, eosinophils are often a prominent component of the inflammatory infiltrate.[407,413] Plasma cell infiltrates and reactive lymphoid follicles are uncommon in GERD, unless there is concurrent *H. pylori* infection.[413]

In patients with *H. pylori* infection, the cardia mucosa appears similar histologically to that seen in *H. pylori* antral gastritis, including increased lymphocytes and plasma cells in the lamina propria, active inflammation, and reactive lymphoid aggregates, with few or no eosinophils.[413] Patients with *H. pylori* carditis, but without GERD, have no inflammation of the esophageal squamous epithelium. When the histology suggests *H. pylori* infection, use of special stains is recommended for detection of organisms not visible on routine stains.[19,425] *H. pylori* organisms do not normally colonize intestinal-type epithelium, and detection may be difficult in biopsies that contain only a limited amount of gastric foveolar-type epithelium.

Identification of certain histological landmarks, such as submucosal or mucosal esophageal glands and squamous-lined ducts, can help prove that a particular biopsy labeled as "GEJ" was derived from the tubular esophagus rather than the gastric cardia. The finding of multilayered epithelium in a biopsy from the GEJ region confirms the esophageal origin of the tissue sample.[392,426] Similarly, origin of tissue from the esophagus can also be inferred from findings of marked glandular atrophy and disarray, incomplete intestinal metaplasia (particularly when it comprises more than 50% of crypts), the presence of squamous epithelium overlying crypts with intestinal metaplasia, and the presence of hybrid glands (i.e., deep glands composed of intestinal metaplasia and mucinous columnar cells)[426] (see Table 15.7 and Fig. 15.65).

Other findings may help in the differential diagnosis as well. For example, most cases of *H. pylori* carditis show evidence of *H. pylori* infection in the corpus and antrum,[425] just as active esophagitis in the squamous epithelium (especially in the setting of a normal antrum or corpus) is strong evidence in favor of GERD as the cause of inflammation in the GEJ region.[413,426]

Basic mucin histochemical stains, such as PAS, Alcian blue, and high-iron diamine, have not proven helpful in distinguishing esophageal-derived metaplastic columnar epithelium from the true gastric cardia.[412,427-429] Both nongoblet and goblet cells may be positive with these stains, regardless of the site of origin. Some investigators have advocated use of Alcian blue at pH 2.5 to distinguish distended foveolar pseudogoblet cells (i.e., light staining) from true goblet cells (i.e., dark staining). Others have documented that both cell types can stain weakly or strongly with this stain, regardless of their site of origin.[412,427-429] Immunohistochemical markers, such as DAS-1, CDX2, HepPar1, and CD10, have been

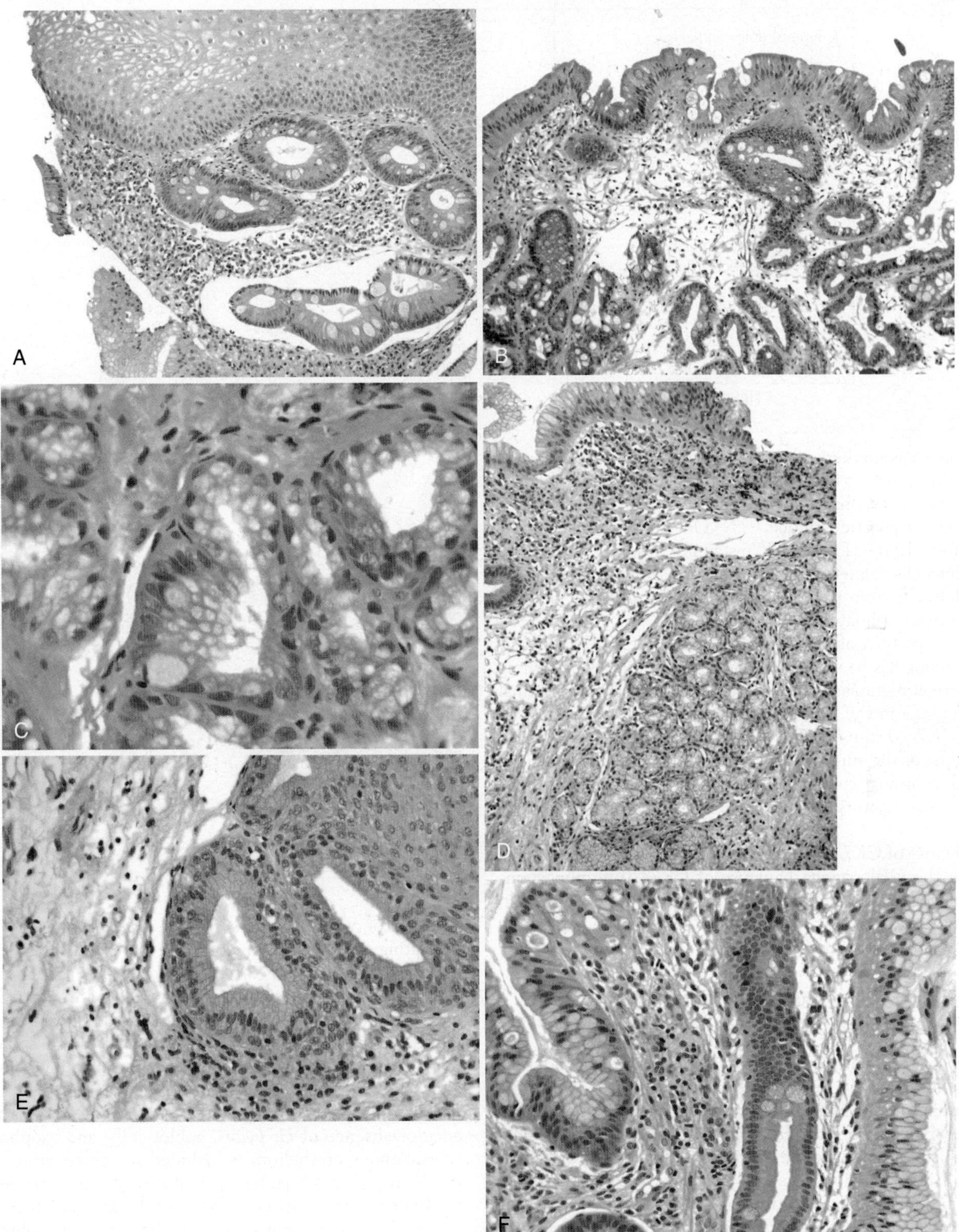

FIGURE 15.65 Mucosal biopsies for the gastroesophageal junction (GEJ) region from patients without endoscopic evidence of Barrett's esophagus but with a slightly irregular Z-line. These patients had no evidence of *Helicobacter pylori* gastritis. **A,** Reepithelialized squamous epithelium overlies glands with intestinal metaplasia. The lamina propria shows a mild degree of chronic inflammation. **B,** The mucosa shows diffuse, incomplete intestinal metaplasia with marked glandular atrophy and replacement of the glands with intestinalized epithelium. There is also irregular branching and horizontal growth of the crypts. **C,** High-power view of the base of the mucosa reveals hybrid glands characterized by incomplete intestinal metaplasia and mucinous columnar epithelium. **D,** Columnar mucosa with a mild chronic inflammatory infiltrate and a well-formed cluster of esophageal mucosal glands in the center of the field. **E,** High-power view of a submucosal gland duct. Any of the features depicted in **A** to **E** seen in a biopsy from the GEJ region indicate columnar metaplasia of the distal esophagus. **F,** Mucosal biopsy from the true gastric cardia in a patient with *Helicobacter pylori* gastritis. There are abundant mucinous foveolar cells, barrel-shaped pseudogoblet cells, and a focus of complete intestinal metaplasia *(center)*. The lamina propria shows a mild degree of lymphoplasmacytic inflammation and scattered neutrophils and eosinophils. This histological picture, particularly the complete intestinal metaplasia, is highly unusual for Barrett's esophagus, and in the presence of *H. pylori* organisms, it is diagnostic of *H. pylori* carditis.

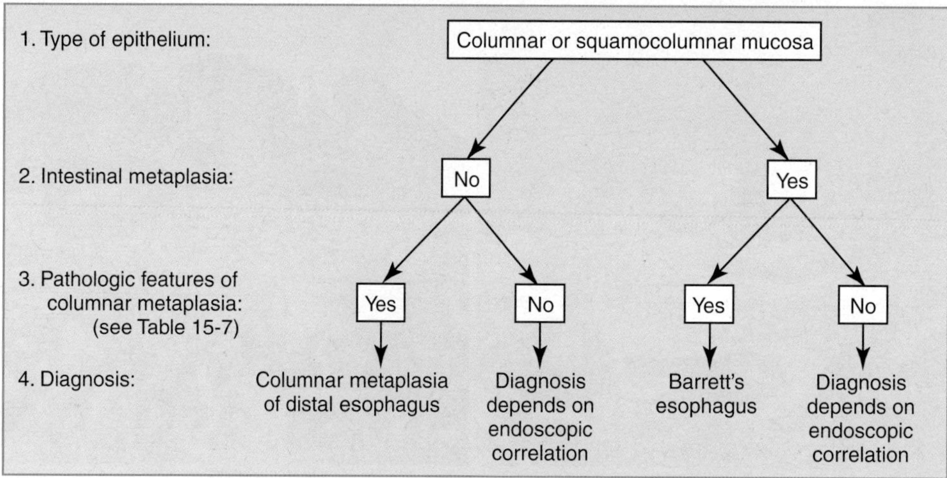

FIGURE 15.66 Strategy for signout of a gastroesophageal junction mucosal biopsy.

proposed as markers of intestinal metaplasia in the esophagus, but none has been shown to be reliably specific for differentiating esophageal from gastric columnar epithelium in routine diagnostic practice.[430-433] One study suggested that combined MUC1 and MUC6 staining was 90% specific for goblet cells related to Barrett's esophagus compared with goblet cells from patients with gastric carditis, but this has never been validated.[434]

The pattern of cytokeratin 7 and 20 (CK7/20) immunostaining has been reported to be helpful in distinguishing intestinal metaplasia in the distal esophagus from intestinal metaplasia in the true gastric cardia.[435] The so-called *Barrett CK7/20 staining pattern* consists of diffuse, strong CK7 staining of the surface and gland epithelium and superficial weak columnar staining with CK20. Unfortunately, several other investigators have not been able to confirm these findings, [395,403,414,425,426,436,437] and there are many limitations to the use of CK7/20 immunostaining in evaluating biopsies from the GEJ region. Thus use of CK7/20 immunostaining is not recommended in daily pathology practice to help distinguish esophageal from gastric intestinal metaplasia in biopsies from the GEJ region.[395]

Strategy for Diagnostic Reporting in Biopsies Obtained from the Gastroesophageal Junction

The strategy outlined in Fig. 15.66 is an easy and reliable method that pathologists can use to help distinguish columnar metaplasia (gastric or intestinal type) of the distal esophagus from the true gastric cardia. When *H. pylori* organisms are detected in cardiac-type mucosa with chronic active inflammation, it is likely that the carditis is part of the patient's concurrent distal *H. pylori* gastritis. It should be emphasized that *H. pylori* carditis is not a distinct entity; rather, it should be viewed as a topographic manifestation of *H. pylori* gastritis.

Many patients without clinically apparent GERD and without *H. pylori* infection have significant inflammation in the cardia and GEJ region. Although it is likely that many of these individuals have asymptomatic GERD, this has yet to be proven. In this setting, the term *carditis* (chronic or chronic active) should be used only if the biopsies are determined by endoscopy to be unequivocally from the

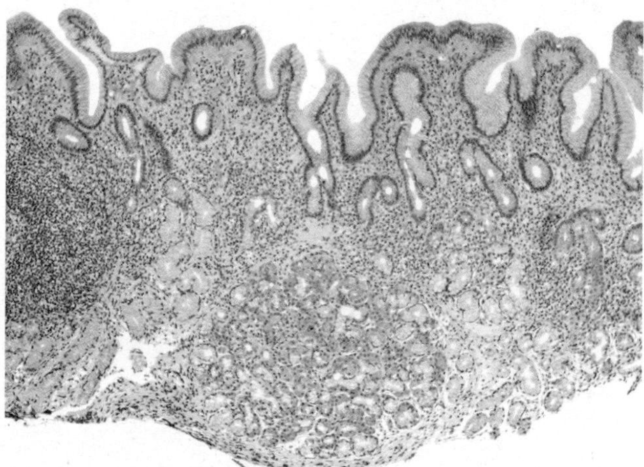

FIGURE 15.67 Pancreatic acinar metaplasia in the cardia of a patient with chronic gastritis.

cardia; otherwise, a brief descriptive diagnosis is preferable, indicating the type of mucosa, the type and intensity of inflammation, and the existence of other relevant features (e.g., erosions). Mild or moderate forms of chronic inflammation in biopsies from the cardia and GEJ region are likely within normal limits, and carditis should be diagnosed only when there is significant activity, epithelial injury, or a dense lymphoplasmacytic infiltrate accompanied by lymphoid follicles. The diagnosis should mention the presence or absence of *H. pylori*, goblet cells, and esophagitis (if squamous epithelium is included in the specimen). If the biopsy shows histological features that are frequently associated with or specific for the tubular esophagus (see Fig. 15.65), a comment should indicate that "the columnar mucosa most likely represents columnar metaplasia of the distal esophagus" (or Barrett's esophagus if goblet cells are found).

Small aggregates of pancreatic-type acinar glands are found in 1% to 5% of biopsy specimens from the GEJ region, usually in deeper portions of the mucosa (Fig. 15.67). Although the origin of these glands (i.e., metaplasia or heterotopia) is unknown and their significance and associations remain elusive, they are usually reported as pancreatic acinar metaplasia,[438] therefore clinicians do not need to alter surveillance or other follow-up protocols based on this finding.

The presence or absence, grade, and extent of dysplasia should be reported for all biopsies from the GEJ region. This is particularly true if the patient has clinical or endoscopic evidence of Barrett's esophagus.[439]

THE STOMACH IN THE YOUNG AND ELDERLY

The constellation of functional and morphological changes that occur in the gastric mucosa of elderly people has been described as "aging" of the stomach.[440] Significant drops in levels of gastric bicarbonate, sodium ion, and parietal fluid secretion affect, to some degree, the gastric mucosa of every aging human, and this results from a decline in the synthesis of prostaglandins.[441,442] Because these products represent the first line of protection against luminal acid-pepsin and exogenous noxious substances, the consequence of a decline is progressive weakening of gastroprotection, which leaves the stomach of elderly people more vulnerable to the noxious effects of endogenous acid and exogenous substances, particularly NSAIDs.

The second set of processes includes pathological conditions that affect various proportions of the elderly, depending on genetic and environmental factors. These alterations may be promoted by the aforementioned decline in physiological gastroprotection. Most complications of chronic gastritis, including intestinal metaplasia and mucosal atrophy, are slowly progressing diseases; therefore they often manifest clinically (as gastric epithelial dysplasia, cancer, and MALT lymphoma) at an advanced age.

Lymphoid Hyperplasia

Nodular gastritis is the endoscopic correlate of a vigorous lymphoid response to *H. pylori* infection.[23,431] Histologically, it is characterized by hyperplasia of lymphoid follicles in the lamina propria; the prominent follicles cause elevations of the mucosa that appear endoscopically as a myriad of granules. Although it may occur in adults, this pattern is more characteristic of children infected with *H. pylori*.[429,430]

Eosinophils

Eosinophils are more common in the gastric mucosa of children than adults. When numerous, eosinophils form microabscesses and infiltrate the muscularis mucosae, a diagnosis of eosinophilic gastritis or gastroenteritis must be entertained and clinical correlation sought. However, an inflammatory infiltrate with an abundance or predominance of eosinophils in the gastric mucosa of an *H. pylori*–infected child (particularly from less industrialized parts of the world) represents a normal response to the infection in most cases.

Atrophy

Atrophy develops in response to years of inflammation-induced injury to the mucosa. Atrophic gastritis is an unusual disorder in young children and adolescents from developed countries. However, in regions where *H. pylori* infection is acquired early in life and environmental factors contribute to a high prevalence of atrophic gastritis in adults (e.g., East Asia, South America), atrophy and intestinal metaplasia may occur in young children.[443-446]

For individuals without *H. pylori* infection or autoimmune gastritis, there is no evidence that atrophic gastritis is more prevalent among older adults compared with children. However, the prevalence of focal intestinal metaplasia, particularly in the distal antrum and pylorus, does increase with age. It is unclear whether this phenomenon is caused by prior *H. pylori* infection, prior episodes of environmental or chemical gastritis, or the cumulative effects of repeated subclinical mucosal injury of any type.

GASTRIC EPITHELIAL DYSPLASIA

Gastric dysplasia is defined as a noninvasive unequivocally neoplastic epithelial process. According to the 2019 edition of the World Health Organization (WHO) Classification of Tumors, gastric intraepithelial neoplasia is an acceptable alternative term for this entity.[447] Gastric dysplasia results from a combination of predisposing environmental conditions combined with various genetic and epigenetic abnormalities.[448] It shares, albeit at a lower frequency, many of the early molecular alterations characteristic of gastric carcinoma. In clinical practice, a diagnosis of gastric dysplasia is an indication for endoscopic therapy and surveillance.[70,449]

Dysplasia Precursor Lesions

Gastric epithelial dysplasia (GED) develops through a well-defined carcinogenic sequence that begins with chronic gastritis and ends with intestinal-type adenocarcinoma.[49,448,450-456] In the United States, *H. pylori* infection is the most common cause of chronic gastritis. It leads to long-standing chronic inflammation in the mucosa and, if left untreated, results in the formation of pseudopyloric and intestinal metaplasia and finally atrophic gastritis.

Intestinal metaplasia is categorized as complete or incomplete (described earlier).[456] Incomplete intestinal metaplasia is associated with a higher gastric cancer risk[48] and occurs in background mucosa in up to 95% of gastric intestinal-type cancers, but in only 0% to 33% of diffuse-type carcinomas.[49,457] The extent and severity of atrophy and intestinal metaplasia is a more important marker of cancer risk. Some studies have reported an 11% risk of adenocarcinoma in patients with atrophy or intestinal metaplasia after a 10-year follow-up period.[51,458] Although mild and focal antral atrophy and intestinal metaplasia do not convey a significantly increased gastric cancer risk, involvement of both the antrum and corpus represent a greater gastric cancer risk than atrophy and intestinal metaplasia limited to the antrum.[48,70,241,449,459,460] Therefore several recent guidelines advise endoscopic surveillance at 1- to 3-year intervals for patients with moderate or severe atrophic gastritis affecting both the antrum and corpus (OLGA/OLGIM stages III/IV).[70,449] Patients with less extensive atrophy, but with a family history of gastric cancer, incomplete intestinal metaplasia, autoimmune gastritis, or persistent *H. pylori* infection indicate a higher gastric cancer risk, therefore surveillance should be offered because they are considered at higher risk for development of cancer.[70]

The neoplastic potential of *pseudopyloric metaplasia of oxyntic epithelium* (see Fig. 15.13) has also been postulated recently. This metaplastic process is observed frequently in the setting of autoimmune gastritis and in the background of some proximal gastric carcinomas. Presenting with an antral morphology and expressing spasmolytic polypeptide, its frequent association with remnant cancers in patients who have had a previous antrectomy implicate it as a probable precursor of gastric adenocarcinoma.[197,461]

Clinical Features and Incidence

In the general population, gastric dysplasia is typically diagnosed in the sixth to seventh decade of life.[462,463] Men are affected more often than women, and the male-to-female ratio is typically between 2.4 and 3.9 to 1.[463,464] Many patients are asymptomatic, but some present with vomiting, weight loss, anemia with iron deficiency, and hematochezia.[465] The lesser curvature of the antrum and the incisura angularis are the most commonly affected regions, although dysplasia may occur anywhere in the stomach.[463,465,466]

The prevalence of dysplasia follows closely the prevalence of gastric cancer, although with marked worldwide variations. This variation likely results from differences in the genetic makeup of different populations and in environmental factors, such as the prevalence of *H. pylori* infection and its different strains. High-risk areas (e.g., parts of Asia and South America) have prevalence rates of 9% to 20%, whereas in Western countries, the prevalence ranges from 0.5% to 4%.[467-469]

The prevalence of dysplasia varies according to the underlying cause. For instance, dysplasia is reported in up to 40% of patients with pernicious anemia,[470-472] but the increased risk for adenocarcinoma is still relatively modest among these patients compared with the general population.[473] Patients with familial adenomatous polyposis (FAP) are at higher risk for flat or, more commonly, polypoid dysplasia (i.e., adenomas). Among FAP patients, the reported rate of dysplasia varies between 2% and 50%, with lesions (often multiple) typically occurring in the antrum.[474-483]

Some studies suggest that patients who have undergone a Billroth II partial gastrectomy and those with Ménétrier disease or Peutz-Jeghers's syndrome are at increased risk for dysplasia and adenocarcinoma.[484-486] In retrospective studies, high-grade dysplasia has been identified in 40% to 100% of early gastric cancers and in 5% to 80% of advanced adenocarcinomas.[487-490]

Dysplasia is also a marker of risk for cancer elsewhere in the gastric mucosa. In one Japanese study, up to 12.5% of patients with dysplasia or an adenoma had concurrent gastric cancer.[487] Fifty-seven percent of gastric cancers discovered during follow-up of patients with dysplasia are considered early forms and are potentially curable, which underscores the importance of endoscopic surveillance.[195,491,492]

Pathological Features

Endoscopically, dysplasia may appear grossly normal or show mucosal irregularity, plaques, nodularity, polypoid growth, erosions or ulcers,[463] mucosal scars, and diffuse inflammatory changes.[462,491] Some studies suggest that most lesions are nonpolypoid (71%),[465] whereas the reverse has been observed by others (27% nonpolypoid).[493]

Dysplasia is characterized by a combination of cytological and architectural atypia. Two major histological subtypes of dysplasia are recognized. *Intestinal-type* ("adenomatous") dysplasia, named for its resemblance to colonic adenomas, is the more common type. Microscopically, intestinal-type dysplasia is characterized by the presence of crowded tubular glands lined by atypical columnar cells with a luminal brush border and overlapping, pencillate, hyperchromatic nuclei with pseudostratification and inconspicuous nucleoli (Fig. 15.68).[494] Various degrees of goblet cell, Paneth cell, and neuroendocrine cell differentiation may be present. The second, less common and less well-recognized histological variant is termed *foveolar (gastric) dysplasia* or type II dysplasia. This type of dysplasia often develops in nonmetaplastic gastric epithelium.[494] Microscopically, foveolar dysplasia is composed of foveolar-type epithelium with cytological and architectural atypia. The foveolae reveal various sizes and shapes, and they occasionally show papillary infoldings and luminal serration. The dysplastic cells are typically cuboidal or low columnar in shape, have clear or eosinophilic cytoplasm containing an apical mucin cap, and contain round to oval vesicular nuclei with nucleoli (Fig. 15.69). Other common cytological features, which are more obvious in intestinal dysplasia, include mucin depletion, crowding, loss of polarity, increased mitoses, nuclear pleomorphism, and lack of surface maturation. Genetic differences between these two histological subtypes of dysplasia support the concept that they likely represent distinct pathways of carcinogensis.[495,496]

Although intestinal-type and foveolar-type dysplasia can be reliably distinguished on the basis of their morphology, in the majority of cases, the two subtypes may also be differentiated using immunohistochemistry. Intestinal-type dysplasia expresses MUC2 and CD10 in most cases, whereas foveolar-type dysplasia most commonly expresses MUC5AC, but not MUC2 or CD10. However, hybrid (mixed) cases do occur. There is currently no established practical use for these stains in routine practice.

Dysplasia may show another form of gastric differentiation in which the cuboidal cells are reminiscent of normal pyloric glands and composed of granular eosinophilic cytoplasm and round nuclei. This type of dysplasia occurs in pyloric gland adenomas (see Chapter 20 for details) and most frequently manifests as a polypoid lesion within oxyntic mucosa. It is frequently found in the setting of autoimmune gastritis and most commonly in elderly women.[497]

As observed in Barrett's esophagus, recent evidence also suggests that dysplasia-like cytological atypia located at the base of the pits but not reaching the surface epithelium likely represents an early stage of dysplasia.[498] This early pattern of dysplasia has been termed *basal gland dysplasia, pit dysplasia,*[499] *pit dysplasia–like atypia,*[500] *intestinal metaplasia with basal gland atypia,*[501] and *immature proliferative lesions*[502] in the published literature (Fig. 15.70).

Most pathologists interpret the presence of surface maturation in an atypical gastric epithelial lesion as a feature of regenerative epithelium. Thus distinction of pit dysplasia from regenerative epithelium may be difficult. Because these lesions normally consist of architecturally regular pits, pathologists should rely mainly on the cytological abnormalities of the epithelium in question (whether they are dysplasia-like), the absence of active inflammation, and the

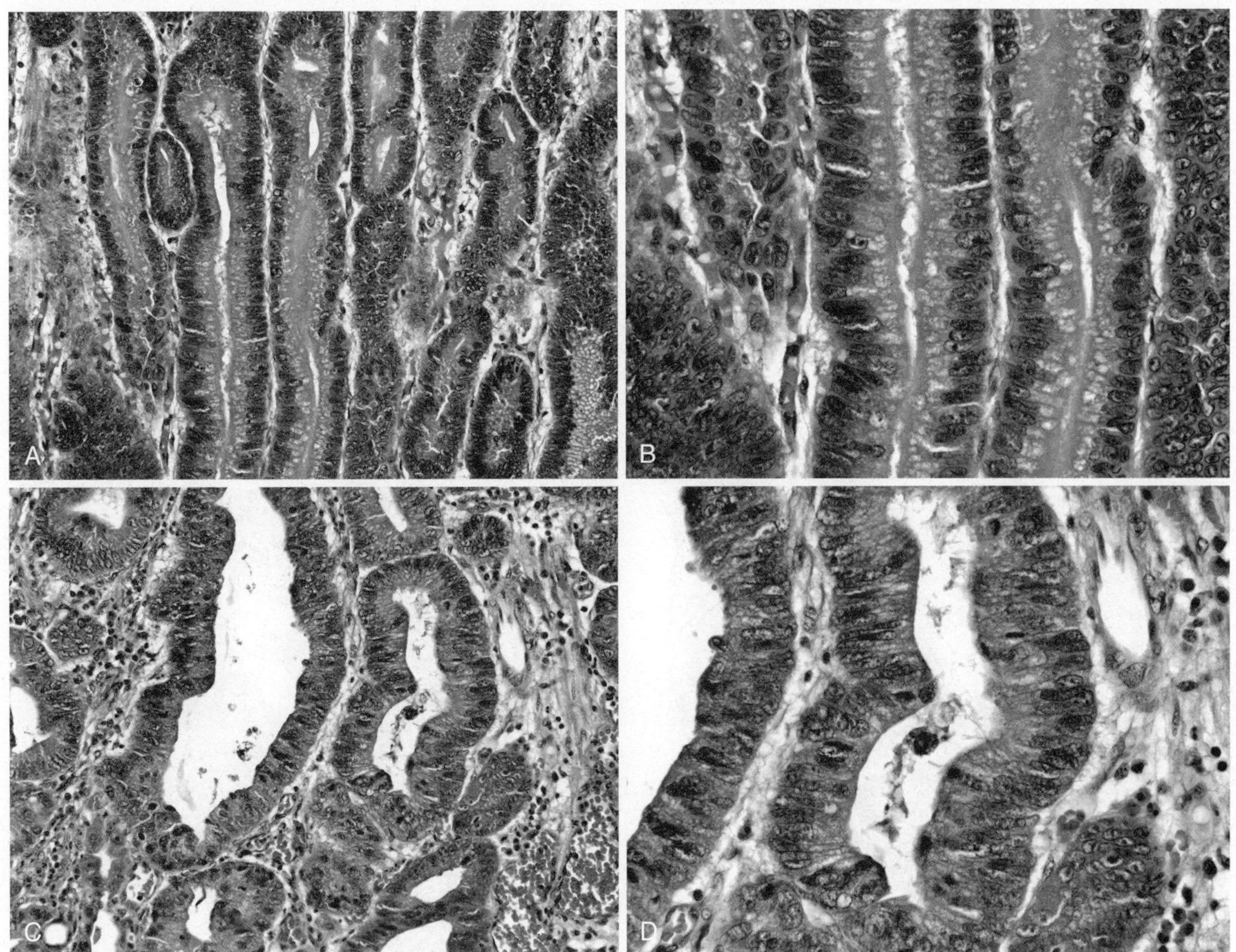

FIGURE 15.68 A, Low-grade, intestinal-type gastric epithelial dysplasia (GED). The lesion is characterized by limited glandular disarray and increased cellularity. **B,** Cytological features of low-grade GED include hyperchromatic, cigar-shaped nuclei confined to the basal half of the cell cytoplasm. Mild nuclear pleomorphism is evident. **C,** High-grade, intestinal-type GED. In contrast with the low-grade type, marked glandular disarray and increased cellularity are observed. **D,** The cytological features of the high-grade type include enlarged, irregularly shaped nuclei extending toward the lumen (upper half of the cell cytoplasm). Clearing of the chromatin is common, and macronucleoli can be observed.

presence of an abrupt transition with adjacent epithelium when diagnosing pit dysplasia. Evaluation of multiple levels may help assess whether there is involvement of the surface epithelium typical of conventional low-grade dysplasia. Referral to an expert GI pathologist is recommended for difficult cases.

In a retrospective study, 38% of cases of pit dysplasia persisted, whereas 25% progressed to conventional low-grade dysplasia in the follow-up period.[438] Furthermore, as additional evidence in favor of its neoplastic nature, pit dysplasia may be identified in adjacent mucosa of 72% of gastric cancers in one study.[499] To date, no management guidelines have been offered for pit dysplasia. Nevertheless, management similar to that for "indefinite for dysplasia" or low-grade dysplasia is considered prudent.[503]

Grading of Gastric Dysplasia

In clinical practice, a two-tier grading system of dysplasia is commonly used: low grade and high grade (Table 15.9; see Figs. 15.68 and 15.69).[462,489,494,504-507] This method of grading has proven to be more reproducible than a three-tier system (i.e., mild, moderate, and severe).[448] It also provides a clinically meaningful method of risk stratification that is used to guide treatment decisions.[508]

Furthermore, there are some differences among pathologists in different parts of the world with regard to the grading of dysplasia. For instance, noninvasive intramucosal neoplastic lesions with high-grade cellular and architectural variations are often referred to as *intramucosal carcinoma* by Japanese pathologists, whereas the same lesions are usually interpreted as *high-grade dysplasia* by Western pathologists. In response to these and other differences in interpretation, a consensus scheme (i.e., Vienna classification) was developed.[509] In the Vienna classification system (Table 15.10), which also considers management implications, high-grade premalignant lesions without invasion of the lamina propria and invasive adenocarcinomas confined to the lamina propria (i.e., intramucosal adenocarcinomas) are considered a single neoplastic group (category 4) because both are usually amenable to endoscopic resection.[510]

Because of their distinct morphological features, there are subtle differences in the grading of intestinal-type and foveolar-type gastric epithelial dysplasia. In both types, the

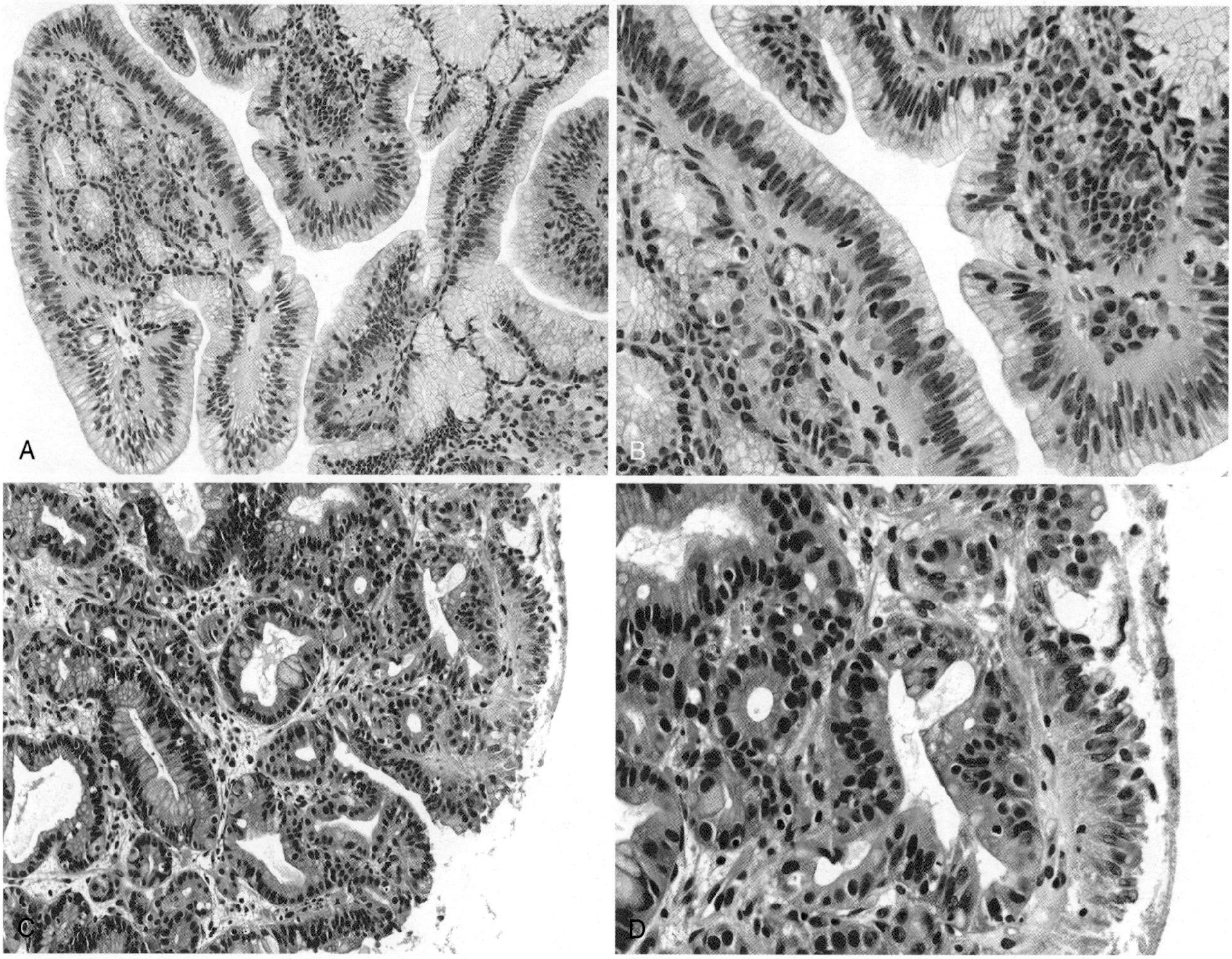

FIGURE 15.69 **A,** Low-grade, foveolar-type gastric epithelial dysplasia (GED) with limited glandular disarray along with increased cellularity and basally located hyperchromatic, cigar-shaped nuclei. **B,** The distinctive feature is the presence of well-formed supranuclear mucin caps. **C,** High-grade, foveolar-type GED, in contrast, shows only minimally altered architectural disarray but is diagnosed on the basis of increased cellularity with severe cytological pleomorphism, including enlarged, irregularly-shaped, overlapping, and stratified nuclei along with increased mitoses **(D).**

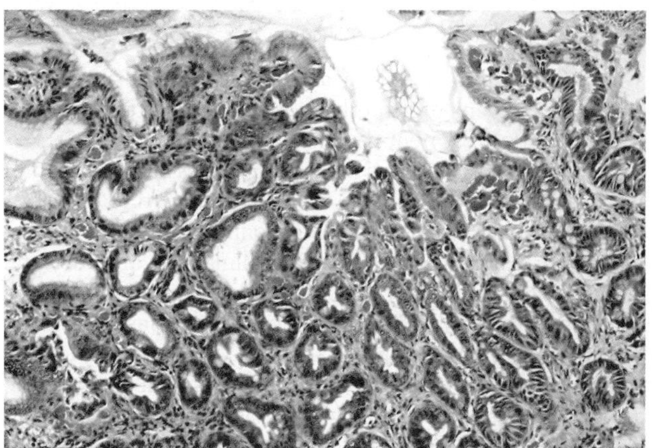

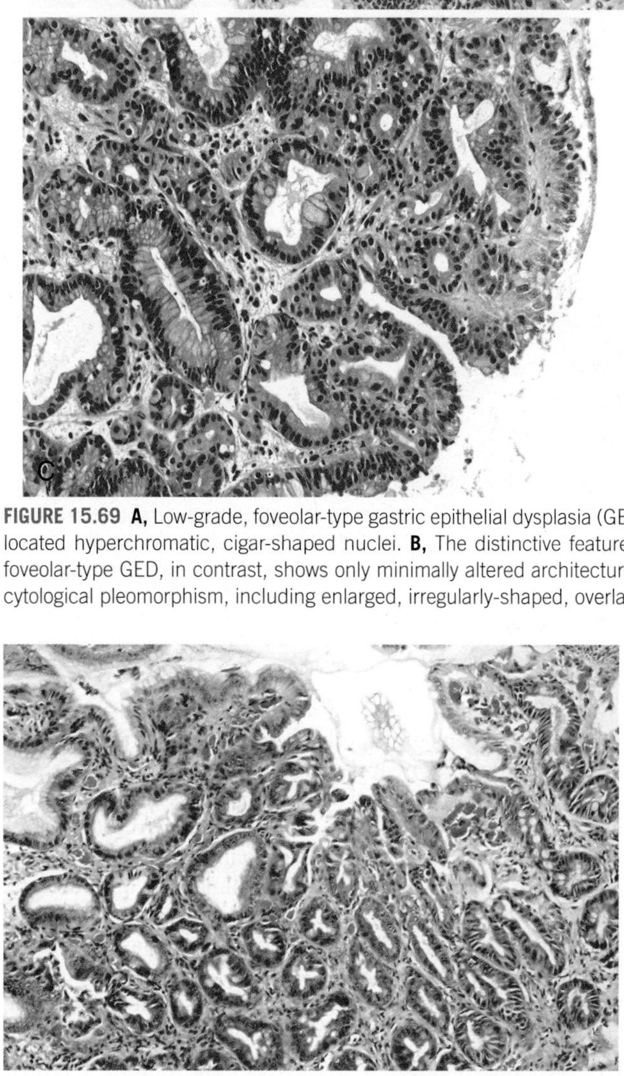

FIGURE 15.70 Hyperproliferative lesion. This biopsy shows immature tubules with scant goblet cells with nuclear hyperchromasia and mucin depletion. Mild architectural disarray is observed. Note the distinct maturation toward the surface.

increasing degree of dysplasia may manifest in both architectural and cytological changes (see Table 15.9; see Figs. 15.68C,D and 15.69C,D). Although both are often present, the finding of either high-grade cytological or high-grade architectural aberrations alone is considered sufficient to establish a diagnosis of high-grade dysplasia.

Intestinal-Type Dysplasia

Low-grade intestinal-type dysplasia is characterized by epithelium with no or only minimal architectural irregularity (i.e., tubular morphology). In contrast with the foveolar counterpart, pseudostratification is common. The cells are closely packed, with retained cellular polarity. Cigar-shaped nuclei are usually confined to the basal half of the cell with a narrow rim of apical cytoplasm with occasional floating mitoses. Nuclear hyperchromasia and irregularity is mild to moderate (see Fig. 15.68A,B).[448,509,511,512]

High-grade intestinal-type dysplasia shows increasing architectural complexity with crowding, back-to-back crypts, complex villous morphology, and marked pseudostratification. The loss of cell polarity and larger-sized round nuclei reaching the apical cell membrane is also a high-grade feature (see Fig. 15.68C,D).

Foveolar-Type Dysplasia

Low-grade foveolar-type dysplasia is characterized by simple, predominantly tubular architecture. The cells are

TABLE 15.9 Histological Features and Differential Diagnosis of Gastric Epithelial Dysplasia Variants

Type of Dysplasia	Histopathological Features: Low-Grade	Histopathological Features: High-Grade	Ancillary Features	Differential Diagnosis
Intestinal	Mucin-depleted (eosinophilic) columnar epithelium Cigar-shaped nuclei Nuclear hyperchromasia Nuclear pseudostratification	Glandular crowding, budding and branching Enlarged and irregular nuclei Loss of polarity with marked stratification Prominent nucleoli	MUC2 [+] CDX2 [+] CD10 [+]	Intestinal metaplasia with reactive changes. Other types of dysplasias (especially foveolar) Very well-differentiated adenocarcinoma
Foveolar	Cuboidal to low columnar foveolar epithelium with pale cytoplasm and apical mucin Hyperchromatic round- to oval-shaped nuclei Minimal to no nuclear stratification	Enlarged ovoid to irregular vesicular nuclei with clumped chromatin Variable stratification Prominent nucleoli	MUC5AC [+] MUC6 [+]	Foveolar hyperplasia with reactive atypia. Other types of dysplasias (especially intestinal-type and pyloric gland adenoma) Adenocarcinoma

TABLE 15.10 Modified Vienna Classification of Gastrointestinal Epithelial Neoplasia

Category	Definition	Common Usage Equivalent
1	No neoplasia	
2	Indefinite for neoplasia	Indefinite for dysplasia
3	Low-grade adenoma or dysplasia	Low-grade dysplasia
4	High-grade neoplasia	High-grade dysplasia
4.1	High-grade adenoma or dysplasia	
4.2	Noninvasive carcinoma (carcinoma in situ)	
4.3	Suspicious for invasive carcinoma	
4.4	Intramucosal carcinoma	Intramucosal carcinoma
5	Submucosal invasive carcinoma	Submucosal adenocarcinoma

cuboidal to low columnar in shape with uniform and basally oriented nuclei that are usually round to ovoid. Nuclear stratification is less common than in the intestinal subtype. Features of foveolar differentiation, such as an apical mucin cap, are well developed (see Fig. 15.69A,B). High-grade foveolar-type dysplasia can show crowded architecture with branching along with budding, although frequently high-grade transformation is represented primarily by abnormal cytological features, such as irregular nuclear contours, a clumped chromatin pattern, and prominent nucleoli. Mitoses are more numerous, and atypical mitoses are more conspicuous compared with low-grade dysplasia. The cells usually become cuboidal rather than columnar and show a higher nucleus-to-cytoplasm ratio. Evaluation of cell polarity is less useful because of the cuboidal shape of the cells with round nuclei (Fig. 15.69C,D).[513]

When architectural complexity is extensive showing irregularly interconnected, fused, and cribriform structures, the lesion should be categorized as *intramucosal adenocarcinoma* because desmoplasia is typically absent when invasion is limited to the lamina propria. Intraluminal necrotic debris and the presence of small haphazardly distributed glands, buds, or isolated cells in the lamina propria also argue in favor of intramucosal adenocarcinoma (Fig. 15.71).

Unusual Variants

Precursor Lesion of Poorly Cohesive Carcinomas

Tubule neck dysplasia, characterized by the presence of enlarged, "globoid," pale, and polygonal neoplastic cells confined to the basement membrane (i.e., in situ signet ring cells), typically occupies the neck region of the gastric glands, sparing the mucosal surface and the deep gastric glands (Fig. 15.72).[514,515] Differentiating tubule neck dysplasia from marked reactive changes can be extremely challenging.[516] Major diagnostic pitfalls include CDH1-associated in situ hereditary diffuse-type gastric cancer (see later) and pseudo–signet ring cell changes noted in association with PPI treatment. The latter most probably represents degenerative vacuolar changes of epithelial cells in the neck region of oxyntic glands. One major difference is the negativity of the vacuoles for mucin stains, including PAS, in pseudo–signet ring cell change, whereas true signet ring cells in tubule neck dysplasia contain mucin.[517] In patients with hereditary diffuse gastric cancer, who most frequently harbor E-cadherin gene *(CDH1)* mutations, in situ diffuse carcinoma and pagetoid spread of signet ring cells have been reported in up to 50% of patients. Morphologically, the latter condition consists of neoplastic signet ring cells that are interspersed with normal foveolar cells and are confined by the basement membrane.[518,519]

Polypoid Dysplasia in Familial Adenomatous Polyposis

Gastric dysplasia develops in 6% to 50% of patients with FAP,[520-522] most commonly in the fourth decade of life.[496] The prevalence rate increases with age, similar to colonic adenomas. Dysplastic lesions are usually small and multiple, and they often are interpreted as *adenomas* when they are polypoid.

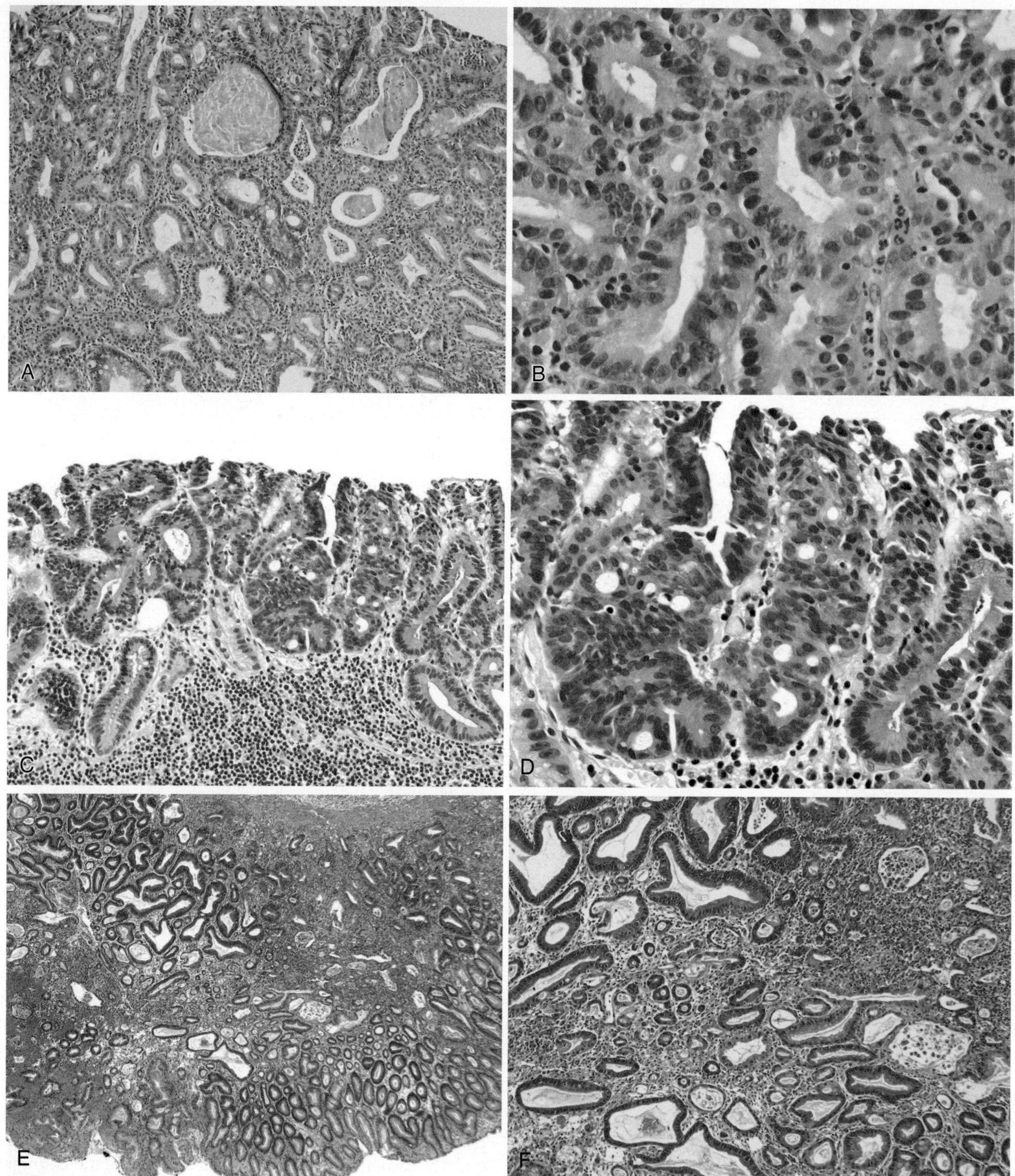

FIGURE 15.71 Examples of intramucosal adenocarcinoma. *Case 1:* In this example the diagnosis is paused on the basis of back-to-back glandular proliferation, the presence of small withering neoplastic glands and intraglandular necrosis (**A**). High-power magnification confirms the fusing of neoplastic glands and high grade nuclear features (**B**). *Case 2:* The focal significant architectural atypia with bridging and intraglandular cribriforming (**C**) along with severe cytologic atypia (**D**) are also diagnostic of intramucosal adenocarcinoma. *Case 3:* This case is characterized by cellular crowding and glandular disarray (**E**). Higher magnification shows disrupted invasive glands and isolated cellular clusters (**F**).

Dysplasia and carcinoma may also develop within fundic gland polyps.[522] Dysplasia occurs in 25% to 62% of FAP-associated fundic gland polyps. It is usually of the foveolar subtype and typically low grade. Despite rare reports of carcinoma arising in fundic gland polyps,[460-462] most gastric cancers that develop in patients with FAP are associated with polypoid areas of dysplasia (i.e., adenomas).[475,524]

Dysplasia may also develop within gastric hyperplastic polyps, particularly those that are larger than 2.5 cm in diameter. Several studies have reported that dysplastic changes occur in 1.8% to 16.4% of hyperplastic polyps.[525-529]

Differential Diagnosis

Dysplasia vs. Regeneration

Differentiating reactive changes from dysplasia can be challenging, particularly in the setting of active inflammation and/or ulceration (Table 15.11).[495,530,531] The cells of regenerative epithelium are usually cuboidal in shape and appear immature based on the finding of basophilic cytoplasm and mucin depletion. Regenerating nuclei are usually large and vesicular and may show mild stratification with pleomorphism and delicate uniform nucleoli, but they do not normally show loss of polarity or marked nuclear membrane irregularity. Mitoses are frequently observed, although not on the surface, and abnormal mitoses are typically absent. Most importantly, regenerating epithelium shows cellular differentiation and maturation near the luminal surface, which is referred to as *surface maturation*. The reactive changes typically blend seamlessly with the adjacent epithelium, whereas in dysplasia there is typically an abrupt transition with nondysplastic epithelium.[532] For cases in which a definite distinction between reactive changes and dysplasia cannot be made with certainty, the term *indefinite for dysplasia* is appropriate (Fig. 15.73A,B).

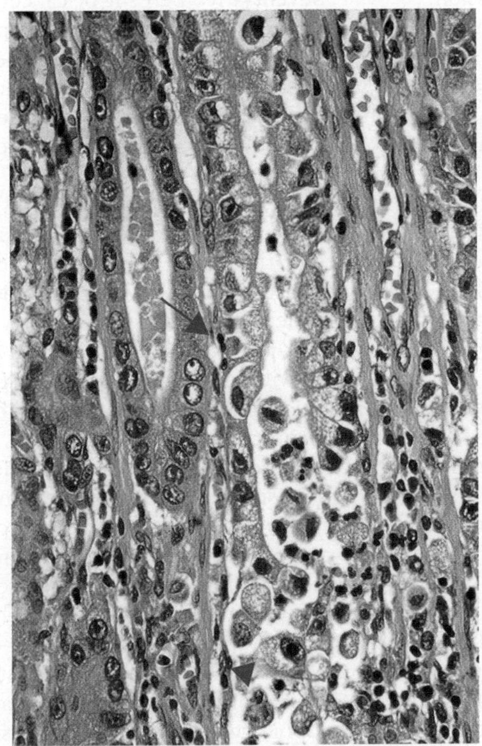

FIGURE 15.72 Tubule neck dysplasia. The tubular epithelial lining contains large globoid cells with clear cytoplasm and atypical vesicular nuclei *(arrow)*. Some cells appear to show early lamina propria invasion *(arrowhead)*.

High-Grade Dysplasia vs. Carcinoma

Differentiating high-grade dysplasia from intramucosal carcinoma can be difficult. Intramucosal adenocarcinoma typically shows overt architectural complexity with irregularly interconnected, fused, and cribriform structures; haphazardly distributed small, budding glands; or single, infiltrating cells within the lamina propria, typically in the absence of desmoplasia[533,534](see Fig. 15.71). With the development of techniques such as endoscopic mucosal resection, distinction of high-grade dysplasia from intramucosal adenocarcinoma has become less important clinically because the lesions are usually treated similarly. This is true, particularly for well-differentiated lesions even up to 2 cm in diameter.[535]

Natural History and Treatment

Gastric dysplasia portends an increased risk of progression to gastric cancer. Unfortunately, the natural history of dysplasia has been poorly studied (Table 15.12).

In some studies, low-grade dysplasia has shown regression in 38% to 75% of cases and persisted in 19% to 50% of

TABLE 15.11 Features of Epithelial Regeneration and Dysplasia

Feature	Regeneration	Dysplasia	Intramucosal Adenocarcinoma
Cellular immaturity	Mild to moderate	Marked	Marked
Vesicular nuclei	None to moderate	None to moderate	Moderate to marked
Mucin depletion	Mild to moderate	Moderate to marked	Marked
Nuclear pleomorphism	Minimal	Moderate to marked	Moderate to marked
Pseudostratification	None to minimal	Mild to marked	Usually marked
Surface maturation	Usually present	Limited to absent	Absent
Transition to adjacent epithelium	Gradual (no border)	Abrupt (distinct border)	Abrupt (distinct border)
Loss of polarity	No or minimal	Yes	Yes
Abnormal mitosis	No	Yes	Yes
Architectural disarray	None or minimal	Mild to moderate	Marked architectural irregularly with interconnected and fused glands Cribriforming Haphazardly distributed, infiltrating small buds, clusters, or single tumor cells

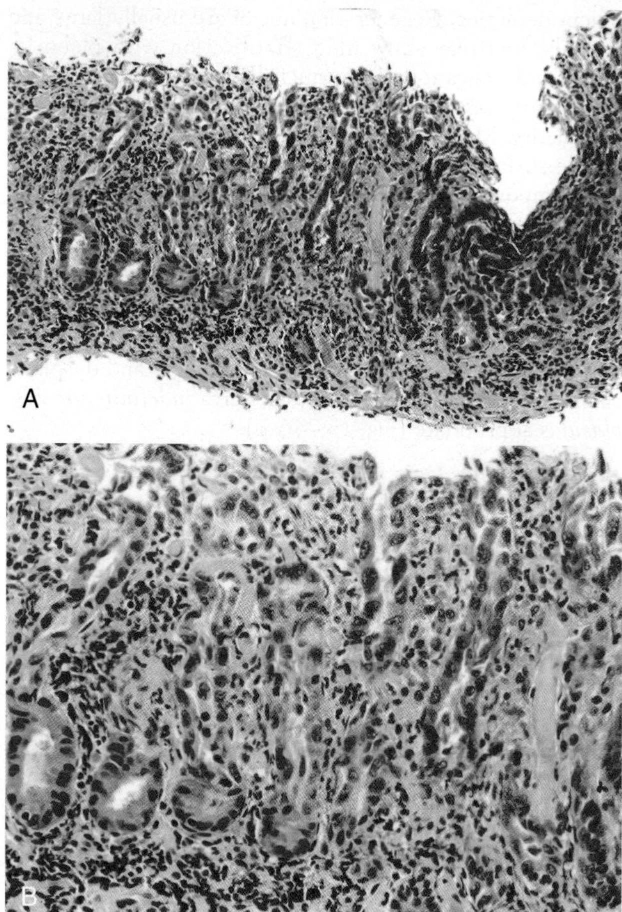

FIGURE 15.73 A, Biopsy at the edge of an ulcer demonstrates considerable glandular cytoarchitectural atypia. **B,** At high magnification, the cuboidal epithelium shows basophilic cytoplasm, mucin depletion, and prominent nucleoli without the loss of polarity. Large, regenerating nuclei show mild, focal pleomorphism. However, nuclear stratification and abnormal mitoses are not seen. Note the marked neutrophilic infiltrate in the stroma.

cases.[462,465,468,536] High-grade dysplasia has shown regression in 0% to 16% of cases, but has persisted in 14% to 58% of cases. In one study, progression to adenocarcinoma occurred in 0% to 23% of cases of low-grade dysplasia in a mean interval of 10 months to 4 years. For high-grade dysplasia, the reported rate of malignant transformation ranges from 4.8% to 100% during a median interval of 4 to 48 months.[462-465,491,537-539] In a large population-based study, 3.5% and 4.3% of patients with low-grade gastric dysplasia were diagnosed with a gastric adenocarcinoma within and after the first year of index endoscopy, respectively.[540] A diagnosis of carcinoma established within 12 months of a diagnosis of dysplasia is very common in cases of high-grade gastric dysplasia and more likely to represent failure to recognize a preexisting cancer rather than true neoplastic progression.[463,465,491] Seventy-five percent of cancers diagnosed after an initial diagnosis of high-grade GED represent missed lesions rather than interval cancers.[465] In the same population-based study, after the first year of follow-up, only 4.5% of high-grade dysplasia progressed to adenocarcinoma, whereas almost 60% developed adenocarcinoma within the first year.[540]

The management of dysplasia has evolved significantly over the past 10 years, and it now takes into account the endoscopic appearance of the lesion, the degree of dysplasia, and the severity of gastric atrophy, which is sometimes indirectly evaluated by the serological pepsinogen level (see Chapter 2).[541,542] Biopsy-proven visible dysplastic lesions should be staged (e.g., with endoscopic ultrasonography) and resected, preferentially using endoscopic techniques, followed by annual endoscopic surveillance.[70,449] Some guidelines recommend endoscopic mucosal resection for lesions less than 1 cm in size and endoscopic submucosal dissection for lesions more than 1 cm in greatest dimension.[449] In patients with nonvisible dysplastic lesions, follow-up endoscopy should be repeated annually in cases with low-grade dysplasia and every 6 months in cases with high-grade dysplasia.[70,449] If no dysplastic lesion is found during follow-up endoscopies (e.g., on three consecutive gastroscopies), three yearly follow-up or further surveillance according to the stage of atrophic gastritis should be considered (see Table 15.12).[70,449]

With recent advanced progress in endoscopic techniques, larger dysplastic lesions and even some adenocarcinomas (i.e., moderately and well-differentiated submucosal cancers invading less than 0.5 mm and without lymphovascular invasion) can be managed conservatively by endoscopic submucosal dissection.[543] Surgical resection remains necessary if an adenocarcinomatous component with adverse prognostic markers is recognized in an endoscopic resection specimen.[544]

The full reference list may be accessed online at *Elsevier eBooks for Practicing Clinicians.*

TABLE 15.12 Guidelines for Management of Gastric Dysplasia and Intramucosal Adenocarcinoma

Lesion	Endoscopic Lesion Type	Grade of Dysplasia	Management	Endoscopic Surveillance	Annual Risk of Progression to Adenocarcinoma/ Development of Metachronous Gastric Cancer
Epithelial dysplasia	Nonvisible	Low-grade	Second endoscopy Extensive sampling to rule out advanced lesion	Annual; Switch to 3 yearly if no dysplasia was found on three consecutive endoscopies	Unknown
		High-grade		Every 6 months	
	Visible	Low-grade	<10 mm: EMR	Annually	0.6%
		High-grade	>10 mm: ESD		6%
Intramucosal adenocarcinoma (tubular-type)	Nonulcerated	Well or moderately differentiated	EMR/ESD	Every 3-6 months for 1-2 years, every 6-12 months for 3-5 years, and annually thereafter	2.5%-3.5%
		Poorly differentiated	<20 mm: EMR/ESD >20 mm: Surgery		
	Ulcerated	Well or moderately differentiated	<30 mm: ESD >30 mm: Surgery		
		Poorly differentiated	<20 mm: Endoscopic resection >20 mm: Surgery		

EMR, endoscopic mucosal resection; *ESD*, endoscopic submucosal dissection.

CHAPTER 16

Inflammatory Disorders of the Small Intestine

Marie E. Robert, Joanna A. Gibson

Chapter Outline

DISORDERS OF MALABSORPTION

Box 16.1 lists intestinal malabsorptive disorders by disease category.

Celiac Disease

Epidemiology and Clinical Features

Celiac disease (also known as gluten-sensitive enteropathy) is an autoimmune disorder that results in damage to the small intestinal mucosa and leads to malabsorption of nutrients. Although this disease was described more than a century ago,[1,2] it is only since 1950 that the role of dietary gluten in its pathogenesis has been recognized.[3] Celiac disease has a worldwide distribution, but is most common in countries with populations of European descent (Europe, North and South America, and Australia), where the prevalence rate is approximately 1%.[4,5] Although historically less common in Asia and Africa, the incidence of celiac disease is rising in these countries due to increased wheat consumption.[4,6,7] A recent change in the gluten reaction landscape is the emergence of nonceliac gluten sensitivity as a separate, poorly understood and possibly immune-mediated (not autoimmune) condition, that along with wheat allergy and celiac disease, form a spectrum of gluten-related disorders.[5,8] This discussion is limited to celiac disease.

Celiac disease may appear at any time in life, from early childhood to late adulthood. Factors governing the timing of clinical disease in genetically at-risk patients are complex and appear to relate to a combination of environmental triggers, including age and amount of gluten in the initial gluten exposure years, usual viral infection exposures, and microbiome alterations.[9-16] Because of the tremendous variability in clinical presentation, patients, especially adults, often have a greater than 10-year lag between symptom onset and diagnosis. Classic symptoms

BOX 16.1 Intestinal Malabsorptive Disorders by Disease Category

- Autoimmunity
  - Celiac disease
  - Autoimmune enteropathy
- Hypersensitivity
  - Protein allergy (milk, soy)
  - Eosinophilic gastroenteritis
- Infection
  - Tropical sprue
  - Bacterial overgrowth/blind loop
  - Other infections
- Nutritional deficiencies
  - B_{12}/folate deficiency
  - Protein-calorie deficiency
  - Zinc deficiency
  - Iron deficiency
- Inherited/metabolic/malformation
  - Microvillous inclusion disease
  - Abetalipoproteinemia
  - Primary intestinal lymphangiectasia
  - Chronic granulomatous disease
  - Disaccharide deficiencies
- Neoplastic/infiltrative disorders
  - Waldenström's macroglobulinemia
  - Amyloidosis
  - Lymphoma
- Immune disorders
  - Graft-versus-host disease
  - Radiation or chemotherapy
  - AIDS enteropathy
- Systemic diseases
  - Lipid storage diseases
  - Histiocytosis X
  - Other
- Nonintestinal diseases
  - Pancreatic insufficiency
  - Bile salt insufficiency
  - Short gut syndrome

include abdominal discomfort, diarrhea, and steatorrhea.[17,18] However, some patients have no gastrointestinal (GI) manifestations, and instead exhibit other signs and symptoms, including short stature, infertility, neurological disorders, recurrent aphthous stomatitis, or dermatitis herpetiformis.[5,13,17-22] In some adults with occult celiac disease, complaints of fatigue often uncover the presence of iron-deficiency anemia, which ultimately leads to the correct diagnosis.[13,23] Further, some patients are entirely asymptomatic and present initially only with histological changes on biopsy analysis. The term *latent celiac disease* has been used to describe patients with this presentation (see later).[24,25] Factors governing the type of clinical presentation and the expression of symptoms are poorly understood. While it was once thought that the development and severity of symptoms were related to the length of intestine involved rather than the severity of mucosal pathology in a single biopsy specimen,[25] additional studies appear to refute that theory.[26,27] At the time of this writing, attention is focused on the action of interleukin (IL)-15 as a promoter of gluten-sensitized T lymphocytes that increase mucosal cytokine levels as a determiner of clinical symptoms, regardless of severity or length of mucosa showing villous blunting.[27-31]

Pathogenesis

Celiac disease is an immunological disorder that occurs in genetically susceptible hosts. Environmental influences are important as well. The familial nature of the disease was originally established in a study of 17 probands, and their families, who underwent small bowel biopsies.[17] This study found an increased incidence of celiac disease in first-degree relatives of symptomatic patients. Studies have documented that 10% to 20% of asymptomatic first-degree relatives have mild histological changes, such as increased intraepithelial lymphocytes without villous blunting, or have mild villous blunting.[17,32,33] In the asymptomatic setting, the decision to institute a gluten-free diet depends on a variety of factors. When symptomatic first-degree relatives are assessed, up to 44% of patients have villous blunting and tissue transglutaminase antibody titers in the diagnostic range.[34]

Genetic studies have established a strong association with major histocompatibility complex (MHC) class II *HLA-DQ2* (majority) and *DQ8*, with up to 95% of patients carrying one of these two genes.[35-39] However, these genetic phenotypes do not explain the pathogenesis entirely, because 30% of the normal population carry the DQ2 haplotype without disease, and not all patients with celiac disease carry this specific phenotype.[35,37] Genome-wide association studies have identified more than 100 non-HLA genes associated with an increased risk of celiac disease, including *CCR3* and *IL2-IL21*.[13,40,41] Some of the identified genes are also common in type 1 diabetes, and rheumatoid arthritis, suggesting that they impart a generalized increased risk of autoimmunity.[29,42-44] Further, evidence linking transcription factors operating across multiple disease loci related to Epstein-Barr virus proteins suggest mechanisms that may be important in numerous autoimmune diseases.[45] The reader is referred to several reviews on the genetics of celiac disease.[13,29,40-42,46-48]

In the proper genetic environment, exposure to gliadins, or the prolamin fraction of gluten found in wheat, rye, and barley, results in both a local and systemic immune response.[18,28,49,50] Additional environmental components may be related to previous infections, for example, with adenovirus 12, reovirus, enterovirus, and perhaps other microbes.[11,12,51-53] The E1b protein of adenovirus has been shown to contain amino acid sequence homology with α-gliadin antibodies, and T cells that recognize these viral proteins cross-react with gliadin.

In 1997, the crucial role of intestinal tissue transglutaminase (tTG), a ubiquitous enzyme in human tissues, in the pathogenesis of celiac disease was uncovered. This enzyme catalyzes cross-link formation between glutamine and lysine residues in substrate proteins.[54] tTG is believed to stabilize extracellular matrix molecules in the setting of mucosal injury and granulation tissue. In their landmark description, Dieterich et al. demonstrated that dietary gliadin, rich in the amino acid glutamine, serves as a substrate for tTG.[54] It is thought that the resulting cross-linked molecules

BOX 16.2 Common Clinical Tests for Celiac Disease

Antitissue transglutaminase antibody
 Always accompanied by serum total IgA assessment
Anti-endomysial antibody
Anti-deamidated gliadin peptide
HLA serotype
 Must be HLA DQ2 or DQ8 positive to be at risk for celiac disease

(gliadin–gliadin or gliadin–tTG) become antigenic epitopes for a subsequent immune response. Of the more than 50 T-cell–stimulating epitopes in gluten proteins, a 33-mer peptide that may be the primary initiator of the inflammatory response in celiac disease has been identified, although it is likely other epitopes also play a role.[55] Gliadin can also cause an immediate, transient increase in tight junction permeability, affecting the barrier function of the gut.[13,56] Investigations into the role of tTG in celiac disease have led to improved[11] diagnostic tests, described further later.[57]

The immune response to dietary gluten involves both the innate and adaptive immune systems in a complex interplay of cytokines, T and B lymphocytes, dendritic cells, and transglutaminase 2.[58-60] Antibody-induced injury may occur via antigen–antibody complex deposition with complement activation and also by the induction of cell-mediated cytotoxicity. Activated mucosal T cells have been shown to cause epithelial injury through the release of cytokines, including interleukin 15.[28,50,61,62]

The clinical diagnosis of celiac disease depends on detecting the appropriate combination of symptoms, laboratory evidence of malabsorption, the presence of serum autoantibodies, and mucosal injury in duodenal biopsies. It is important that pathologists are aware that new algorithms in children allow for the correct diagnosis of celiac disease to be made without endoscopy and biopsy.[63]

Highly accurate serological tests have been added to the "diagnostic tool kit" for celiac disease (Box 16.2).[64] These include the enzyme-linked immunosorbent assay for IgA anti-tTG antibodies, which has a high degree of sensitivity and specificity (77% to 100% and 91% to 100%, respectively). tTG antibody determination has become the serological test of choice for celiac disease and has replaced the antiendomysial antibody test as a first-line approach.[65-67] The antiendomysial antibody (EMA) test remains as sensitive and specific as the anti-tTG test using human recombinant protein, but the immunofluorescence-dependent EMA test is labor intensive and relies on a more subjective interpretation than anti-tTG determinations.[7] Today, EMA antibody testing is often used as a confirmatory test when tTG testing or clinical/biopsy findings are ambiguous. The older anti-gliadin antibody test no longer has a place in celiac disease diagnosis because of its lack of specificity. However, a new generation of antigliadin antibodies, deamidated gliadin peptides (DGPs), are a widely used IgG-based test, with high concordance with both tTG and EMA antibody tests, and possibly greater sensitivity in children and in early disease.[5,64,68-70] This test also has the advantage of detecting celiac disease in IgA-deficient patients. HLA testing to detect susceptible HLA phenotypes (DQ2 and DQ8) is frequently used as a confirmatory test in ambiguous settings or in order to avoid biopsy in children. The absence of DQ2 or DQ8 virtually excludes the diagnosis.[71,72] Finally, transglutaminase-specific IgA deposits can be found in frozen sections of small intestine mucosal biopsies by immunofluorescence in patients with celiac disease, even those with normal to near normal histology.[73-75] However, it is unlikely this technique will become widely used as a diagnostic test.[75] For a more detailed discussion of the current approach to clinical diagnosis and management of celiac disease, several excellent reviews and guidelines are available.[5,64,67,70-72,76-79]

Pathological Features

Background

In Western countries before 1990, celiac disease was a diagnosis that was made with ease and confidence on small bowel biopsies. The pathological diagnosis required severe villous blunting (flat mucosa), usually accompanied by increased intraepithelial lymphocytes (IELs) and lamina propria inflammation in duodenal biopsies obtained distal to the duodenal bulb. A diagnosis of untreated celiac disease was not normally considered when a biopsy did not show significant loss of villous architecture.

Since the early 1990s, several changes in our understanding of celiac disease have altered the diagnostic algorithm for this disease and have eliminated the gold standard status of small bowel biopsies.[5,63,64,80] These changes include (1) recognition that latent or occult (minimally symptomatic) celiac disease in adults represents a large, previously unappreciated disease population[24,25,80,81]; (2) revision of histological criteria to include minimal inflammatory changes with intact, or only mildly abnormal architecture as a part of the histological spectrum of celiac disease[25,80,82,83]; and (3) the discovery that tTG is the target autoantigen of antibodies in patients with celiac disease, and the subsequent development of a highly accurate diagnostic test for anti-tTG antibodies that can now be used in combination with the tests described in the previous section.[54,65,66,84]

These developments have had a great impact on pathologists, who can now correlate minimal histological findings with objective clinical and serological evidence of celiac disease. They have also decreased the need for reliance on small bowel biopsy findings, which can be subject to interpretive challenges due to orientation and nonspecificity of changes. At the time of this writing, the sophisticated pathologist and clinician must understand that evaluating patients for celiac disease may or may not include the need for mucosal biopsy, especially in children (Fig. 16.1).[63,64] In children, small intestinal mucosal biopsies can be obtained to help fulfill diagnostic criteria, or may be reserved for patients in whom serological laboratory results are inconclusive, the caveat being that histological findings in the latter category of patients may also be inconclusive (Box 16.3). Notwithstanding these considerations in children, there is still general consensus worldwide that adults being considered for a diagnosis of celiac disease should undergo small bowel biopsy as part of the diagnostic workup (Box 16.4).

Gross Pathology

In a landmark study, Rubin et al. described the appearance of normal duodenal mucosa on biopsy samples with the use of a hand lens and showed that the mucosa is characterized by

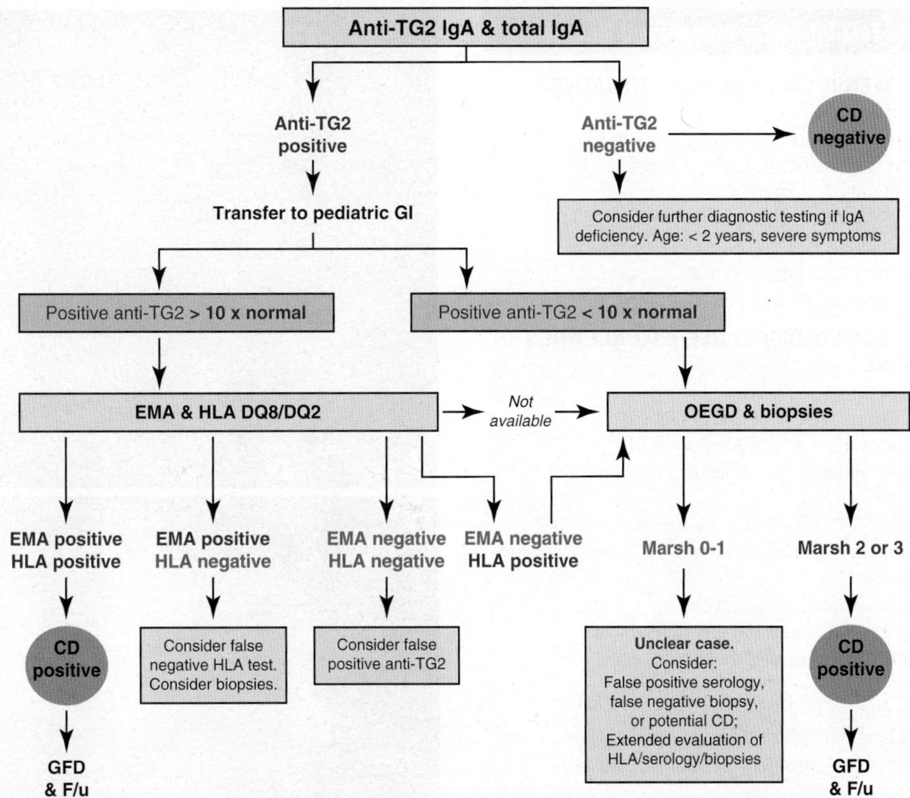

FIGURE 16.1 Approach to diagnosis of celiac disease in children. Note that in some settings a duodenal mucosal biopsy may not be deemed necessary to establish the diagnosis of celiac disease. TG2, IgA anti-tissue transglutaminase 2 antibodies; EMA, IgA anti-endomysial antibodies; CD, Celiac disease; GFD, gluten free diet; OEGD, esophagogastroduodenoscopy. (*Modified from Husby S, Koletzko S, Korponay-Szabó I, et al. European Society Paediatric Gastroenterology, Hepatology and Nutrition Guidelines for Diagnosing Coeliac Disease 2020. J Pediatr Gastroenterol Nutr. Jan, 70(1); 141–156.*)

BOX 16.3 Diagnostic Criteria for Celiac Disease*

Typical symptoms of celiac disease
Positivity of serum celiac disease IgA class autoantibodies at high titer
HLADQ2 or HLA-DQ8 genotype
Celiac enteropathy at the small intestinal biopsy
Response to the gluten-free diet

HLA, *Human leukocyte antigen;* IgA, *immunoglobulin A.*
* *At least four of the five criteria must be met (or three of four if the HLA genotype is not performed).*
Modified from Catassi C, Fasano A. Celiac disease diagnosis: simple rules are better than complicated algorithms. Am J Med. *2010;123:691-693.*

numerous slender villi with a delicate capillary network that floats in formalin like "the tentacles of a sea anemone."[85,86] In contrast, biopsies from patients with celiac disease have a barren, stubby surface, without normal villi, and contain widely spaced irregular capillaries (Fig. 16.2).

Endoscopic findings in patients with celiac disease are subtle and often unreliable.[87,88] A flat, scalloped appearance of the duodenal mucosa, most likely reflecting loss of villi, may be seen.[85,86] One endoscopic study found that a reduction of folds, scalloping, mosaic pattern, and nodular mucosa were sensitive, but not specific, endoscopic findings in celiac disease, as they were also noted in some dyspeptic patients without celiac disease.[89] Likewise, a meta-analysis of studies testing the diagnostic sensitivity and specificity of video capsule endoscopy in celiac disease reports that the images seen can correctly diagnose the condition.[90] However, there are insufficient data on the performance of this instrument in mild histological forms that are recognized today. Of note, at least one capsule endoscopy study reports endoscopic abnormalities (reduction of Kerckring folds, scalloping, and mosaic pattern) limited to the jejunum with normal duodenal appearances in some celiac disease patients, although no confirmatory biopsies were taken.[91] Endoscopic diagnosis appears to be far less reliable in children than in adults.[92,93] Advanced techniques, such as confocal laser microscopy,[94] narrow-band imaging,[95] and immersion technique,[96] may improve diagnostic accuracy, but are as yet not widely tested in clinical practice.

Microscopic Pathology: Biopsy Strategy

As a supplement to the following sections, the reader is referred to the best practices guidelines statement on the use of biopsy as a diagnostic tool for celiac disease, a bulleted summary of which is presented in Box 16.5.[97] Celiac disease is a disease of the proximal small intestine in most patients, with severity usually greatest in the duodenum and proximal jejunum. The ileum may be involved in severe cases, but it is not a reliable site for biopsy diagnosis.[86,98-100] It is now widely recognized that many patients with celiac disease do not have diffusely abnormal small intestinal histology, but instead show mild and patchy involvement in duodenal mucosal biopsies.[101-103] The duodenal bulb, once strictly avoided in the evaluation of celiac disease due to its susceptibility

BOX 16.4 Whom to Test for Celiac Disease and Method

DUODENAL BIOPSY EVEN IF CD SEROLOGY IS NEGATIVE

- Chronic nonbloody diarrhea
- Diarrhea with features of malabsorption (e.g., weight loss)
- Iron-deficiency anemia in absence of other causes
- GI symptoms with a family history of CD
- GI symptoms with autoimmune disease or IgA deficiency
- Failure to thrive in children
- Skin biopsy proven dermatitis herpetiformis
- Video capsule findings suggestive of villous atrophy

CD SEROLOGY IS INDICATED: BIOPSY NEEDED ONLY WHEN SEROLOGY IS POSITIVE

- Irritable bowel syndrome
- Elevated otherwise unexplained liver transaminases
- Chronic GI symptoms without a family history of CD
- Chronic GI symptoms with a personal history of autoimmune disease
- Microscopic colitis
- Hashimoto's thyroiditis and Graves' disease
- Osteopenia/osteoporosis
- Unexplained ataxia or peripheral neuropathy
- Recurrent aphthous ulcerations/dental enamel defects
- Infertility, recurrent miscarriage, later menarche, early menopause
- Chronic fatigue syndrome
- Acute or chronic pancreatitis after excluding other causes
- Epilepsy; headaches; mood disorders; or attention deficit disorders
- Hyposplenism or functional asplenia
- Psoriasis or skin lesions other than dermatitis herpetiformis
- Pulmonary hemosiderosis
- IgA nephropathy

CD, *Celiac disease;* GI, *gastrointestinal.*

Modified from Al-Toma A, Volta U, Auricchio A. European Society for the Study of Coeliac Disease (ESsCD) guideline for coeliac disease and other gluten-related disorders. United European Gastroenterol J, *2019:5:583-613.*

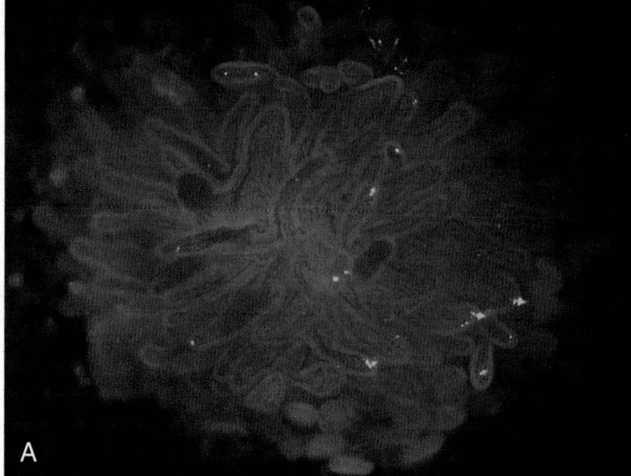

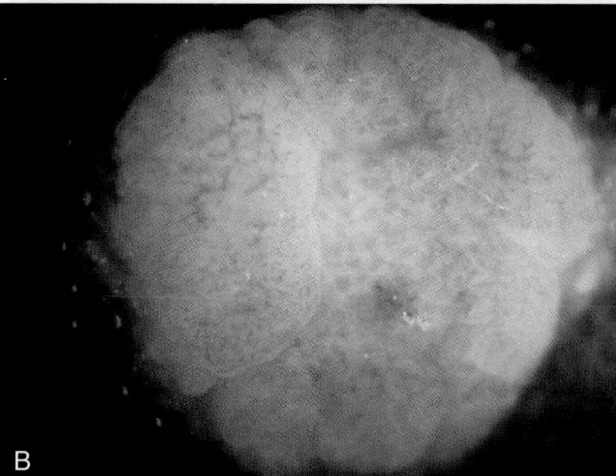

FIGURE 16.2 A, Normal small bowel mucosa viewed with a dissecting microscope (zirconium arc lighting). The villi are slender and translucent, allowing visualization of the underlying delicate capillary network (unstained). **B,** Small bowel mucosa from a patient with celiac disease. The surface is irregular and devoid of villi (unstained). (*From Rubin CE, Brandborg LL, Phelps PC, et al. Studies of celiac disease: I. The apparent identical and specific nature of the duodenal and proximal jejunal lesion in celiac disease and idiopathic sprue. Gastroenterology. 1960;38:28–49.*)

to "peptic" injury and prominent Brunner glands, is now a recommended biopsy site, as it is reliably involved in patients with patchy disease.[102,104-107] In a pediatric study, 16% of children had patchy villous atrophy, but all of these had involvement of the duodenal bulb, and, in four patients, the bulb was the only site of abnormality.[107] Duodenal bulb biopsies may also be more sensitive in patients on a low-gluten diet.[108] Further evidence supporting the validity of duodenal bulb biopsies as a diagnostic site is found in the study by Walker et al. in which paired IEL counts were identical in the duodenal bulb and second portion of the duodenum in celiac disease patients.[109] Based on studies in both adults and children, it appears that the most reliable biopsy protocol to detect all cases of celiac disease is a six biopsy regimen that includes two biopsies from the duodenal bulb and four biopsies from the post-bulb duodenum.[76,97,102,107,110,111]

Once received in the laboratory, accurate evaluation of small bowel biopsy specimens in suspected cases of celiac disease requires proper orientation in tissue blocks to assess mucosal architecture and to avoid overinterpretation of short villi in poorly oriented sections as abnormal. Although biopsies are rarely perfectly oriented, an attempt should be made to find three to four well-oriented villi in a row to assess architecture. This requires the frequent employment of level sections to optimize the number of well-oriented

BOX 16.5 Key Best Practices in Use of Duodenal Biopsy for the Diagnosis of Celiac Disease

Endoscopic findings do not reliably diagnose celiac disease.

Specimen quality is improved by obtaining one biopsy per pass of endoscope.

Practitioners should obtain at least 4 specimens from the distal and 2 from the proximal duodenum (bulb).

Serial sections should be employed routinely in order to achieve well-oriented villi for evaluation.

The evaluation of villous architecture must occur in well-oriented sections; avoid lymphoid aggregates, gastric heterotopia, and regions of prominent Brunner glands.

In biopsies with normal villous architecture, a quantitative assessment of IELs should be performed (see text and Table 16.4).

Assessment of IELs should avoid lymphoglandular complexes.

Pathologists and clinicians must be aware of the differential diagnostic considerations for inflammatory changes seen in duodenal biopsies, especially drugs.

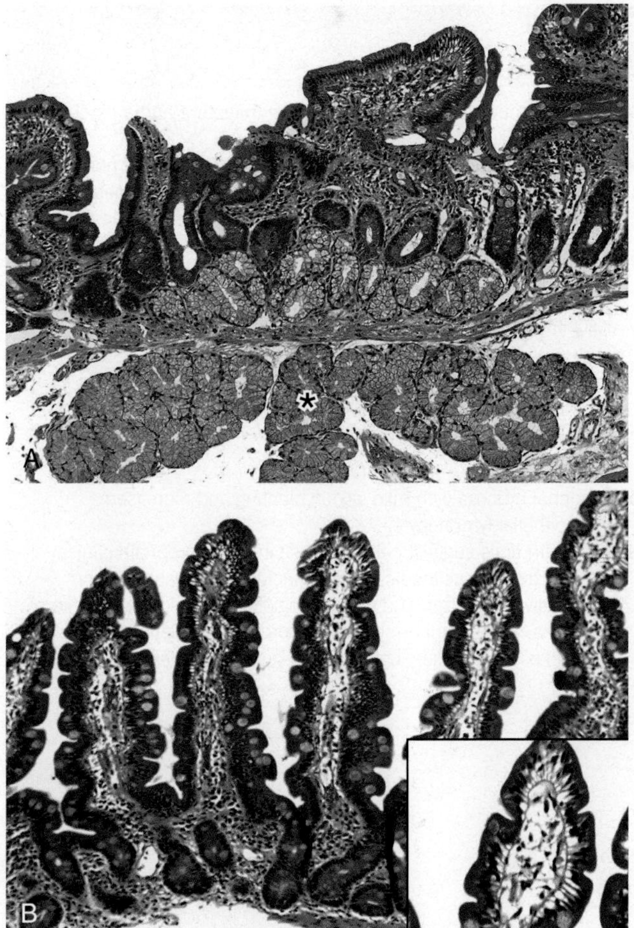

FIGURE 16.3 A, Normal duodenal bulb. The duodenal bulb is a transition zone that is normally subjected to physiological peptic injury. Brunner glands *(asterisk)* and increased mononuclear inflammation are frequently present in the mucosa, resulting in broader and shorter villi. **B,** Normal second duodenum and proximal jejunum. The villous-to-crypt ratio is between 3:1 and 5:1. There are, on average, two intraepithelial lymphocytes per 10 enterocytes *(inset)*.

villi for evaluation.[97,112] Similarly, now that duodenal bulb biopsies are requested in this setting, care must be taken to distinguish commonly observed changes, often referred to as "peptic injury" (neutrophils, gastric surface metaplasia, and surface injury) as well as villous blunting due to mucosal Brunner glands from celiac disease. IEL assessments should be helpful in making this distinction.

Histology of Untreated Disease

Normal small bowel mucosa exhibits a villous height-to-crypt depth ratio of from 3:1 in the proximal duodenum to 5:1 in more distal locations (Fig. 16.3). Epithelial cells lining the villi contain basally located nuclei with abundant mature cytoplasm and a preponderance of absorptive cells admixed with goblet cells. A faint density, representing the microvillous brush border, can be appreciated on hematoxylin and eosin (H&E)-stained tissue sections. Studies have confirmed that there are approximately 20 lymphocytes per 100 epithelial cells in health, with minor variations.[113-117] In health, IELs are most numerous in the base of villi and taper from the base to the villous tip, where they are less numerous.[118] This is in stark contrast to the distribution in untreated celiac disease, in which villous tip IELs are markedly increased. The lamina propria normally contains a mixture of plasma cells, lymphocytes, and occasional eosinophils. Each of the three mucosal components (architecture, epithelium, and lamina propria) should be carefully examined in cases of suspected celiac disease, and, indeed, in the assessment of all small bowel biopsies.

In the following paragraphs, the pathology of celiac disease is described in conjunction with a grading scheme that can be used in pathology reports (Table 16.1). At the time of this writing the Marsh-Oberhuber classification is used regularly in Europe but is far less widely used in the United States in routine pathology reports. Including the Marsh-Oberhuber subtype requires prior knowledge (e.g., by serology) of the patient's having celiac disease, information often not provided in biopsy requisition forms.[80,83] In addition, differences among types 0, 1, and 2 in the Marsh scheme are subtle, so that a high degree of observer variability between pathologists exists. To avoid these issues, it is reasonable to discuss abnormalities in villous architecture with a descriptive modifier (e.g., mild, moderate, or severe; or partial vs. complete), as detailed later, to reflect the degree of villous blunting, adding classification designations as agreed upon by pathologists and clinicians.[97]

Even if not utilized in reports, it is important from both a research and clinical perspective to be aware of the Marsh-Oberhuber classification scheme (Table 16.2).[80,83] This system describes five histological lesions associated with celiac disease, termed preinfiltrative (grade 0), infiltrative (type 1), infiltrative-hyperplastic (grade 2), flat-destructive (grade 3), and atrophic-hypoplastic (grade 4). Two modifications to this scheme have been proposed in an attempt to simplify the diagnosis for pathologists and clinicians.[119,120] Neither has been universally accepted, but both are included for the sake of completeness in Table 16.3.

Biopsies Without Villous Blunting

Preinfiltrative lesions (Marsh-Oberhuber grade 0) refer to normal mucosa seen predominantly in patients with dermatitis herpetiformis but without evidence of malabsorption.

Infiltrative lesions (Marsh-Oberhuber grade 1) refer to finding increases in IELs with preserved villous architecture, whereas infiltrative-hyperplastic lesions (grade 2) show the additional feature of elongated crypts. Both of these patterns of injury are seen in patients with celiac disease (with or without symptoms) as well as in first-degree relatives of patients with celiac disease and in patients with dermatitis herpetiformis. Phenotypic analyses have shown that the increase in IELs is the result of increased numbers of γ/δ T cells.[121-123] Biopsies with these subtle changes are challenging to interpret and require clinical correlation with serology in order to confirm a diagnosis of celiac disease, as similar histology is seen in other conditions. By definition, the villous height and the villous-to-crypt ratio is normal or near normal (Fig. 16.4). The diagnosis relies on the detection of increased IELs, the assessment of which is now a routine part of small bowel biopsy interpretation (see later). The proportion of patients with these minimal histological changes who eventually develop severe histological lesions and symptoms is unknown.[24,25,118] One small study suggested that 4 of 12 people (33%) with mild changes (Marsh-Oberhuber 1–2) on duodenal biopsies

TABLE 16.1 Diagnostic Terminology for Pathology Reports

Histology	Pathology Report*
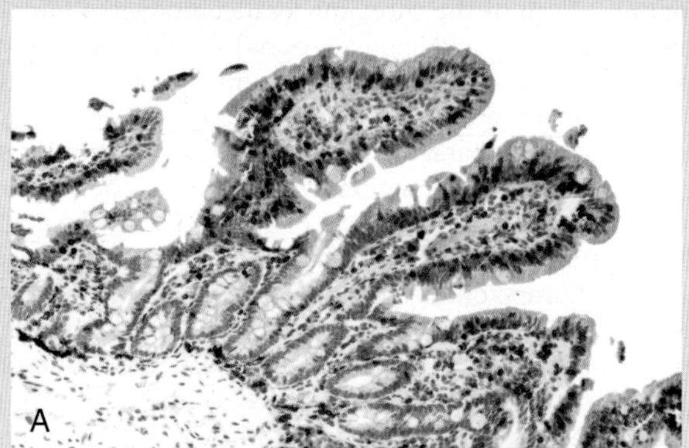	**A,** Duodenal mucosa with normal villous architecture and a patchy/diffuse increase in intraepithelial lymphocytes. **Note:** Increased intraepithelial lymphocytes in the setting of normal villous architecture can be seen in patients with symptomatic or asymptomatic celiac disease. Other associations include *Helicobacter pylori* gastritis, medications (especially NSAIDs and olmesartan and related angiotensin II receptor blockers), infections, and immune-mediated disorders. Correlation with celiac disease–associated serological and/or genetic tests may be considered.
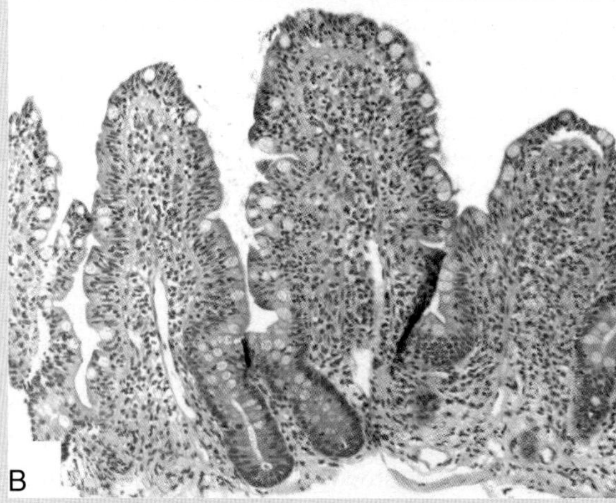	**B,** Duodenal mucosa with mild villous blunting and increased intraepithelial lymphocytes. **Note:** The findings suggest celiac disease in the appropriate clinical setting. Other associated conditions include medication injury (especially olmesartan and related angiotensin II receptor blockers), infections, and immune-mediated disorders. Correlation with celiac disease–associated serological and/or genetic studies is suggested.
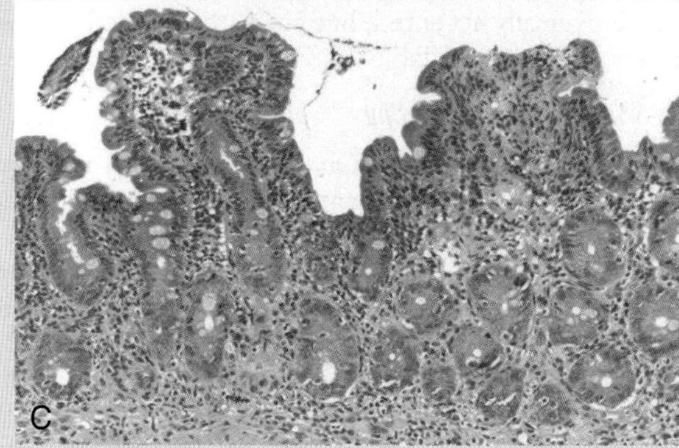	**C,** Duodenal mucosa with moderate villous blunting and increased intraepithelial lymphocytes. **Note:** The findings suggest celiac disease in the appropriate clinical setting. Other associated conditions include medication injury (especially olmesartan and related angiotensin II receptor blockers), infections, and immune-mediated disorders. Correlation with celiac disease–associated serological and/or genetic studies is suggested.
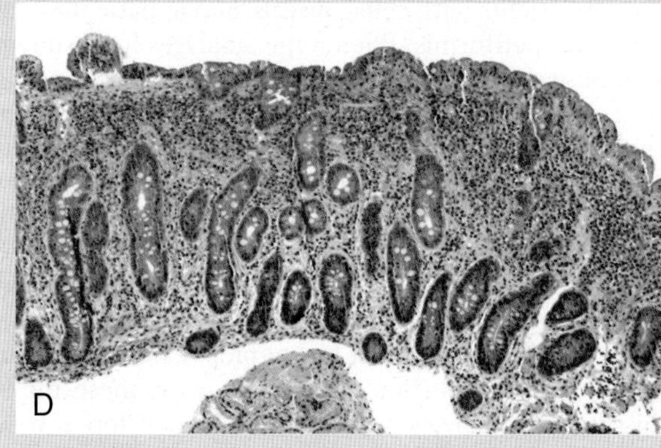	**D,** Duodenal mucosa with severe villous blunting and increased intraepithelial lymphocytes. **Note:** The findings suggest celiac disease in the appropriate clinical setting. Other associated conditions include medication injury (especially olmesartan and related angiotensin II receptor blockers), infections, and immune-mediated disorders. Correlation with celiac disease–associated serological and/or genetic studies is suggested.

**The content of the note will depend on the clinical information provided and findings in gastric and other biopsies. Whenever possible, tailor the report to fit the clinical situation. (Modified from Robert ME, Crowe SE, Burgart L, et al. Statement on best practices in the use of pathology as a diagnostic tool for celiac disease: a guide for clinicians and pathologists.* Am J Surg Pathol. *2018;42:e44-e58.)*

TABLE 16.2 Marsh-Oberhuber Classification of Celiac Disease

Type*	IELs per 100 Epithelial Cells	Crypts	Appearance of Villi
Preinfiltrative type 0	Normal (<40)	Normal	Normal
Infiltrative type 1	>40	Normal	Normal
Hyperplastic type 2	>40	Hypertrophic	Normal
Destructive type 3a	>40	Hypertrophic	Mild blunting
Destructive type 3b	>40	Hypertrophic	Moderate blunting
Destructive type 3c	>40	Hypertrophic	Severe blunting (flat)
Hypoplastic type 4	>40	Atrophic	Severe blunting (flat)

IELs, *Intraepithelial lymphocytes.*

**Types 0 to 2 are rarely seen and occur most frequently in patients with dermatitis herpetiformis, asymptomatic patients, and first-degree relatives of patients with celiac disease. Types 3a to 3c are usually found in patients with celiac disease symptoms. Type 4 is rare and is seen in refractory cases (see text).*

Modified from Oberhuber G, Granditsch G, Vogelsang H. The histopathology of celiac disease: time for a standardized report scheme for pathologists. Eur J Gastroenterol Hepatol. *1999;11:1185-1194.*

TABLE 16.3 Classification Schemes for Pathological Evaluation of Gluten-Sensitive Enteropathy

Marsh, 1992	Oberhuber et al., 1999	Corazza and Vilanaci, 2005	Ensari, 2010
Type 1	Type 1	Grade A	Type 1
Type 2	Type 2	Grade A	Type 1
Type 3	Type 3A	Grade B1	Type 2
	Type 3B	Grade B1	Type 2
	Type 3C	Grade B2	Type 3
Type 4	Type 4	Obsolete	Obsolete

Modified from Ensari A. Gluten-sensitive enteropathy (celiac disease): controversies in diagnosis and classification. Arch Pathol Lab Med. *2010;134:826-836.*

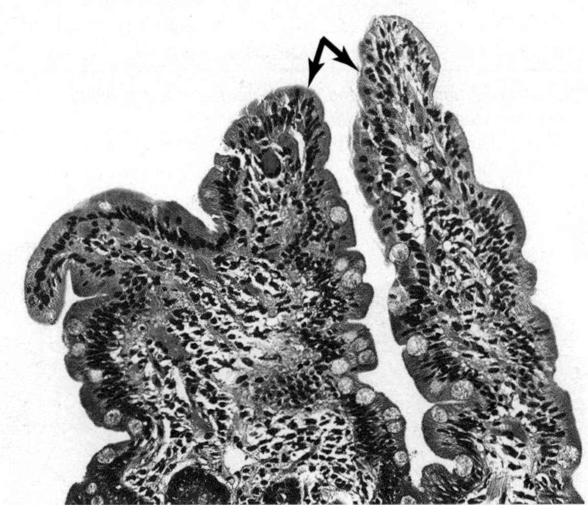

FIGURE 16.4 Untreated celiac disease. This duodenal biopsy was taken from an asymptomatic patient who was discovered to have antitissue transglutaminase antibodies. Normal villi are present, but there is a marked increase in the number of intraepithelial lymphocytes *(arrows)*.

progress to celiac disease with flat mucosa, at follow-up, and a second study found that 3 of 5 (60%) patients with positive tTG antibodies and initial Marsh-Oberhuber 1 lesions progressed to Marsh-Oberhuber 3c at follow-up.[118,124] However, in a larger study with 8 to 25 years of follow-up, only 5 of 236 patients (2.1%) with biopsies showing increased IELs, or a slight reduction in villous-to-crypt ratio, eventually developed celiac disease.[125] These data are complicated by the newer knowledge that patchy histological findings are more common in celiac disease than once appreciated. Sampling error in the above studies cannot be excluded.

Counting Intraepithelial Lymphocytes in Biopsies Without Villous Blunting. Numerous studies have shed light on appropriate methods to count IELs (Table 16.4). Reassessment of the normal range of IELs in the second portion of the duodenum has been performed by several investigators, using H&E-stained sections and sections stained for CD3 antigen, establishing an upper limit of 20 lymphocytes per 100 epithelial cells in normal mucosa in the duodenum.[113-117,126] Careful analysis using CD3 and γ or δ T-cell stains have shown that IEL counts of greater than 25 per 100 epithelial cells (or a ratio of greater than 1:4) merit suspicion for potential celiac disease, whereas counts greater than 29 per 100 epithelial cells provide sound diagnostic evidence for active celiac disease, in serologically positive patients.[114,117,127,128] However, it is entirely impractical to count IELs per 100 enterocytes in busy clinical practices.

A more practical approach, the villous tip counting method, has been validated in at least four studies.[109,114,118,128] Averaging IELs per 20 epithelial cells in five well-oriented villous tips was found to result in a rapid

TABLE 16.4 Methods of Counting IELs in Architecturally Normal Duodenal Biopsies*

Interpretation	Counts	Stain
Diagnosis by Counting IELs per 100 Enterocytes (300-500 Cells Counted)		
Upper limit of normal	20/100 25/100	H&E CD3
Borderline increased	25-29/100	H&E or CD3
Definitely increased	>29/100	H&E or CD3
Diagnosis by Villous Tip Method (5 Villi, 20 Enterocytes per Villous Tip, Mean Count)		
Upper limit of normal	5/20	H&E or CD3
Definitely increased	≥6/20	H&E or CD3

H&E, *Hematoxylin and eosin;* IELs, *intraepithelial lymphocytes. See text for references.*
**Avoid all lymphoglandular complexes. Average the sum of at least five villi.*

and accurate assessment of IEL counts in either H&E- or CD3-stained sections. Using this approach, lymphocyte counts of 6 to 12 IELs per 20 epithelial cells in the tips of villi in architecturally normal mucosa are found in patients with serological or other evidence of celiac disease. The IEL counts are lower than in untreated flat celiac disease biopsies, and higher than in normal controls. Although CD3 stains were used for cell counting in one study,[128] equivalent results were obtained using H&E stains in the other two.[114,118] The counts obtained using the villous tip method correlate well with previously cited studies counting IELs in 100 consecutive enterocytes that found that greater than 29 IELs per 100 epithelial cells is abnormal.[117] A slightly different counting approach was taken in a landmark prospective study comparing IEL counts with serology in a random adult population.[109] IELs were counted in a total of 50 enterocytes (in groups of 10) along the sides and tops of villi. In this study, counts of >25 IEL/100 detected celiac disease, while higher cutoffs missed 50% of cases. Importantly, this study found equally elevated IELs in 3.8% of nonceliac controls, most of whom had *Helicobacter pylori* gastritis. The terms "lymphocytic enteropathy" and "duodenal lymphocytosis" have emerged to describe the spectrum of patients with increased IELs and normal villous architecture. The term "lymphocytic duodenosis" has been proposed to refer to the subset of this group that is proven serologically to not have celiac disease.[109]

Numerous conditions other than celiac disease are associated with increased IELs in architecturally normal duodenal biopsies (Table 16.5). These include *H. pylori* gastritis (Fig. 16.5), viral gastroenteritis (Fig. 16.6), tropical sprue, cow milk protein sensitivity, bacterial overgrowth, some immune conditions, and an ever-expanding list of medications.[109,129-137] Further, the reliability of IEL assessments to detect celiac disease is entirely dependent on active gluten consumption by the patient at the time of endoscopy. Duodenal biopsies from patients already on low- or no-gluten diets will have fewer IELs and less villous blunting.[116]

In summary, the following approach is recommended for biopsies in patients with normal or near-normal villous architecture and a perceived increase in IELs, or with the clinical potential for a diagnosis of celiac disease (i.e., positive tTG serology). First, perform a low- to medium-magnification scan of villi and villous tips, looking for either a diffuse or patchy increase in IELs. Avoid areas of lymphoglandular

TABLE 16.5 Disorders Showing Histological Overlap with Gluten-Sensitive Enteropathy

Conditions Associated with Increased Intraepithelial Lymphocytes*	Conditions Associated with Villous Blunting
Helicobacter pylori gastritis	Common variable immunodeficiency
Viral gastroenteritis	Microvillous inclusion disease
Autoimmune enteropathy	Autoimmune enteropathy
Tropical sprue	Tropical sprue
Refractory sprue	Refractory sprue
Protein intolerance	Protein intolerance
Bacterial overgrowth	Bacterial overgrowth
NSAID injury	Radiation or chemotherapy
Immune checkpoint inhibitors	Nutritional deficiencies
	Eosinophilic gastroenteritis
	Crohn's disease
	Immune checkpoint inhibitors
	ARB injury (Olmesartan and others)
	Idelalisib

**Not all conditions associated with increased intraepithelial lymphocytes also show villous blunting.*
ARB, Angiotensin II receptor blocker; *NSAID*, nonsteroidal antiinflammatory drug.

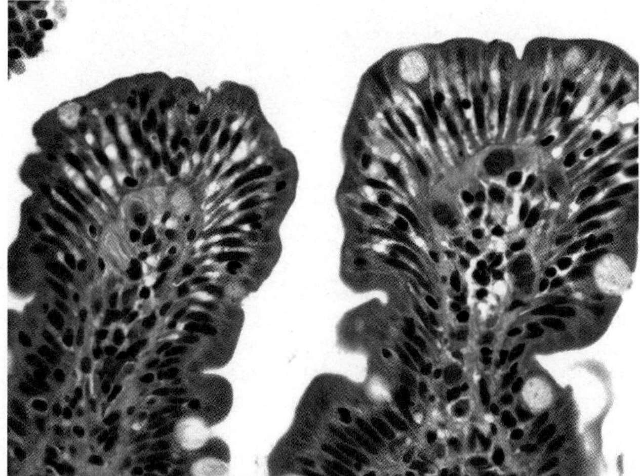

FIGURE 16.5 *Helicobacter pylori*–associated duodenitis. An increase in intraepithelial lymphocytes in the first and second portions of the duodenum is not uncommon in the setting of *H. pylori* gastritis. Gluten-sensitive enteropathy is not suggested in this setting unless clinical evidence supports that diagnosis.

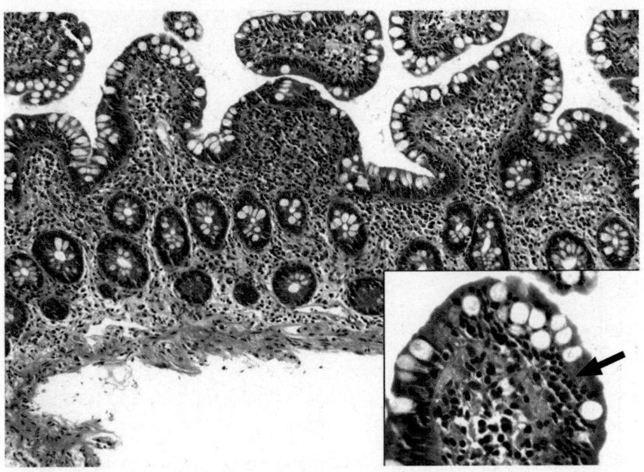

FIGURE 16.6 Viral gastroenteritis. This biopsy specimen from the second duodenum reveals mild villous blunting and a marked increase in the number of intraepithelial lymphocytes *(arrow in inset)*. Viral studies revealed acute infection with rotavirus in this patient, who recovered spontaneously.

complexes, as they lead to falsely elevated IEL counts. If a striking increase in IELs is detected, there is no need to perform an IEL cell count. Evaluation of the number of IELs can be performed with the villous tip method for subtle cases, if desired, without the need for CD3 or γ/δ T-cell immunostains.[97,138,139] If a CD3 stain is employed, care must be taken to not include lymphocytes just beneath the epithelial basement membrane, a region often challenging to distinguish on immunohistochemical stains.

Because correlation with serology is required in all cases, use of excessive time or expense counting IELs in the diagnostic setting is not recommended. Further, reporting exact numbers of IELs in pathology reports is not a standard practice outside of research settings, and is not recommended as a rule. Qualitative comparisons to prior biopsies are useful and should be performed when possible, as this provides important follow-up information to clinicians and patients. Pathology reports should contain a descriptive diagnosis, such as "duodenal mucosa with normal villous architecture and increased intraepithelial lymphocytes," with a note listing the differential diagnosis and a recommendation to correlate with serological evidence of celiac disease (see Table 16.5; Table 16.6). Further, an indication that the IEL increase is patchy or diffuse is appropriate to report. A partial list of causes of increased IELs in the small intestine is provided in Table 16.7.[78,129-131]

Biopsies with Blunted Villi

The flat-destructive pattern (Marsh type 3) is the classic mucosal lesion associated with symptomatic, untreated celiac disease. Duodenal biopsies showing type 3 changes reveal loss of normal small intestinal architecture resulting from a decrease in the height of villi (villous blunting) accompanied by crypt hyperplasia. Type 3 has been further subdivided by Oberhuber into types 3a (mild blunting), 3b (moderate blunting), and 3c (severe blunting).[83] Interobserver variability among pathologists in assessing the degree of villous blunting is recognized, such that a proposed scheme of normal villi, partial blunting, and flat mucosa may be more reproducible than a four-tiered approach.[140,141] This is especially worthy of consideration because studies show a lack of correlation between Marsh score and clinical disease severity.[30,97,142]

In assessing villous architecture in duodenal mucosal biopsies, several well-oriented villi must be visualized, away from lymphoid aggregates, gastric heterotopia, and extensive mucosal Brunner glands. The liberal use of level sections to achieve well-oriented regions should be considered the routine standard of care, not an exceptional practice. The histology of celiac disease with villous blunting is characteristic but variable. Biopsies from the duodenum reveal loss of normal architecture caused by a decrease in the height of villi. In many cases, the mucosa appears completely flat. In others, the villi may be broad and only mildly to moderately shortened, or they may show irregularity. In clinical practice, histological overlap between mild, moderate, and severe blunting is often observed in a single biopsy series[143,144] (Fig. 16.7). Loss of villous height is usually matched by crypt elongation or hyperplasia, such that the overall width of the mucosa usually remains unchanged.[86] The degree of injury observed in surface and crypt epithelia can vary widely and does not always reflect the degree of villous blunting or the severity of symptoms.[86] When the condition is histologically severe, the surface epithelium shows loss of columnar shape, mucin depletion, vacuolization, and enlargement of cell nuclei (see Fig. 16.7A). Cells may show loss of polarity, with stratification, pyknosis, and fragmentation of nuclei. IELs are increased, especially in the tips of villi.[145-147] Surprisingly, the epithelium situated along the sides of blunted villi may appear entirely normal, despite the proximity to severely affected cells at the surface. The cells at the base of hyperplastic crypts often show nuclear enlargement and increased mitoses, reflecting an increase in proliferative activity.[112,144]

The lamina propria in celiac disease typically shows a variable increase in plasma cells. Neutrophils, crypt abscesses, and increased eosinophils are not classic findings but are present in a substantial minority of patients at diagnosis.[144,148,149] However, the finding of diffuse or marked acute inflammation should prompt consideration of other diagnoses, such as drug reactions, "peptic duodenitis," Crohn's disease, and refractory sprue.

It is suggested that pathology reports be accompanied by a note, the content of which depends on the degree of clinical information available at the time of sign-out (see Table 16.1). This is especially needed when clinical information is not provided. If a prior history of celiac disease is known or positive tTG antibodies have been identified, the note could read, "The histological findings support a clinical diagnosis of celiac disease." Comparison to prior biopsies should be included if at all possible. In some specialized celiac centers, synoptic templates are utilized.[112]

Atrophic-hypoplastic lesions (type 4) are rare and are similar to the lesions described in biopsies from patients with refractory, or unclassified, sprue (see later).[21] The finding of atrophic mucosa may correlate with a lack of response to a gluten-free diet.

Histology of Treated Disease (Response to a Gluten-Free Diet)

Patients who respond clinically to a gluten-free diet are not routinely subjected to repeat biopsy. Studies have shown

TABLE 16.6 Differential Diagnosis of Celiac Disease: Distinguishing Clinicopathology

Disease	Increased IEL's	Villous Blunting	Distinguishing Pathological Features	Distinguishing Clinical Features
Helicobacter pylori gastritis	Yes	Rare, if present mild	Fewer IELs than in CD. Blunting almost never present.	May need to do serology to exclude CD
Peptic duodenitis	No	Yes, variable	Neutrophils, erosions, changes usually confined to bulb; gastric surface metaplasia common, but may be physiological	No specific clinical symptoms in peptic duodenitis
NSAID injury	Yes	Patchy	Patchy involvement, erosions, neutrophils	History of NSAID use; lack of typical celiac symptoms/serology
Tropical sprue	Yes	Yes, moderate	Changes extend to ileum. Usually not severe blunting	Patient demographics, and travel history
Bacterial overgrowth	Yes	Sometimes	Most biopsies normal in this setting, but no distinguishing features when abnormal	Condition predisposing to intestinal stasis.
Soy and cow's milk protein intolerance	Sometimes	Yes	Colitis and enteritis, including ileum, prominent eosinophils	Usually children with feeding intolerance
Crohn's disease	Sometimes	If present, not usually diffuse	Patchy involvement, erosions, ulcers, crypt branching, granulomas (rare)	Usually occurring in setting of known Crohn's disease with distal intestine involvement
UC-associated duodenitis	Not usually	Sometimes	Diffuse lamina propria expansion with basal plasmacytosis, IELs not usually increased	Usually discovered in setting of known UC
ARB injury (olmesartan and others)	Yes	Yes	No distinguishing features, may show collagenous sprue	History of ARB use; must have high index of suspicion
Immune modulatory drugs (including checkpoint inhibitors)	Rarely	Yes	Mixed inflammation, with neutrophils, apoptosis, and occasionally crypt branching. Involves upper and lower GI tract	Usually easily distinguished by clinical setting
CVID	Yes	Sometimes	Absence of mucosal plasma cells, giardiasis, BNLH	History of chronic infections.
Autoimmune enteropathy	Not usually	Yes, variable	Neutrophils, crypt apoptosis, decreased goblet and Paneth cells, involves entire small bowel, stomach and colon, usually no increase in IELs	Often infants, syndromic, gut epithelial autoantibodies
Refractory celiac disease	Often	Yes	Thin mucosa, basal plasmacytosis, collagenous sprue; histology may be indistinguishable from untreated responsive celiac disease. In some patients, loss of CD8 and surface CD3 antigens in IELs on IHC.	Refractory clinical course after initial response to GFD or never responded to GFD

ARB, *Angiotensin II receptor blocker;* BNLH, *benign nodular lymphoid hyperplasia;* CD, *celiac disease;* CVID, *common variable immunodeficiency;* GFD, *gluten-free diet;* IEL, *intraepithelial lymphocytes;* IHC, *immunohistochemistry;* NSAID, *nonsteroidal antiinflammatory drugs;* UC, *ulcerative colitis.*

Modified from Robert ME, Crowe SE, Burgart L, et al. Statement on best practices in the use of pathology as a diagnostic tool for celiac disease: a guide for clinicians and pathologists. Am J Surg Pathol. *2018;42:e44-e58.*

TABLE 16.7 Criteria for Refractory Celiac Disease Types I and II

Criteria Pathological/Clinical	RCD Category	
	RCD I	RCD II
Abnormal intraepithelial lymphocyte phenotype by IHC or flow cytometry	No	Yes
Monoclonal γ or δ T-cell receptor gene rearrangement	No	Yes
Clinical response to incremental therapies	No	Variable
Risk of EATL	Rare	Frequent

EATL, *Enteropathy associated T-cell lymphoma;* IHC, *immunohistochemistry;* RCD, *refractory celiac disease.*

Modified from Rubio-Tapia A, Murray, JA. Classification and management of refractory coeliac disease. Gut. *2010;59:547-557.*

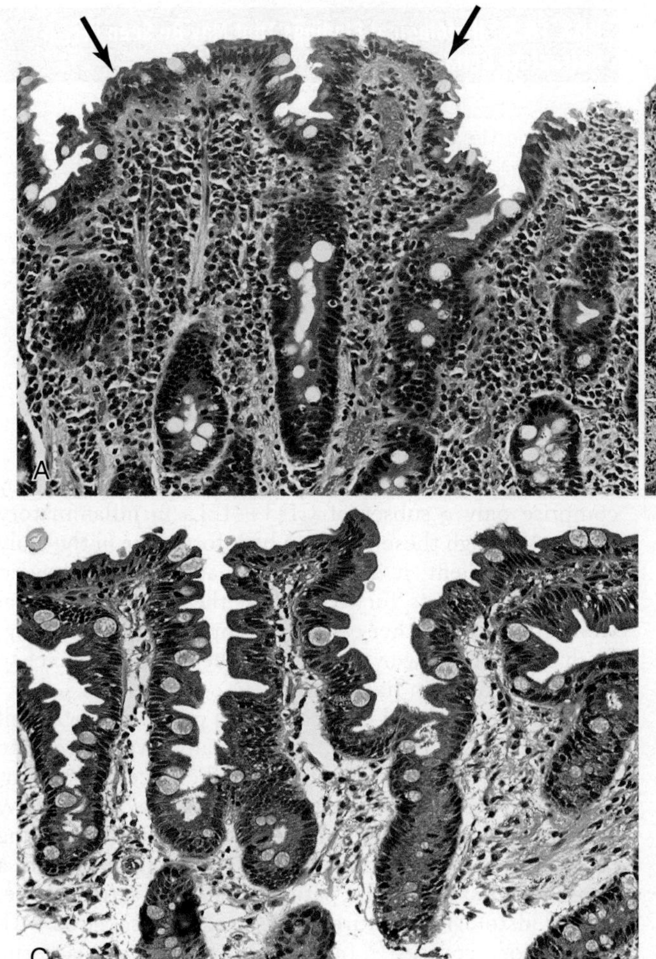

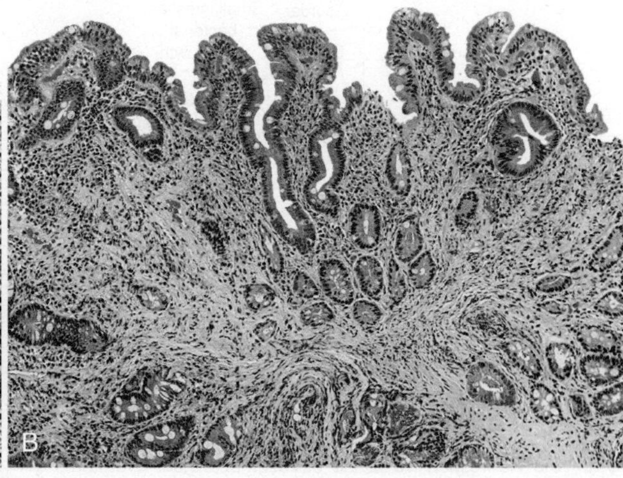

FIGURE 16.7 Celiac disease. A, Severe lesion. The surface epithelium shows loss of its columnar shape and mucin depletion. There is a marked increase in the number of intraepithelial lymphocytes (IELs) *(arrows)*. The elongated crypts show increased mitotic activity and enlarged nuclei. The lamina propria is expanded by plasma cells and lymphocytes. **B,** Moderate lesion. In many cases of untreated celiac disease, only mild to moderate villous blunting is present. In this duodenal biopsy specimen with moderate villous blunting, all the other hallmarks of the disease, including increased number of IELs and crypt hyperplasia, are present. **C,** Treated celiac disease. Duodenal biopsy specimens obtained from patients consuming a gluten-free diet may reveal persistent mild abnormalities. In this example, the villous architecture is almost normal, but a slightly increased number of IELs and mild reactive changes are present.

that mucosal injury, including persistently increased IELs and villous blunting, may persist for up to 1 year after following a strict gluten-free diet.[26,99] However, in many patients, biopsies show a return to normal or near normal within a year or less if diet adherence is achieved (see Fig. 16.7C). Some patients show persistence of moderate or even severe lesions despite marked clinical improvement. Repeat biopsies are indicated when the clinical response is poor and when other disorders, such as refractory sprue, lymphoma, or infection are under consideration.

Refractory Celiac Disease

Approximately 10% of patients with celiac disease have persistent symptoms despite good faith attempts to adhere to a gluten-free diet, so-called nonresponsive celiac disease. Only 10% of those, or approximately 1% of all celiac patients, develop refractory celiac disease (RCD) with a female-to-male ratio of 2:1. RCD is defined as an absent or incomplete clinical response to a strict gluten-free diet, usually in a patient with prior serological or genetic evidence of celiac disease, and is further subdivided into RCD I and RCD II based on clinicopathological criteria (see later).[150-152] When considering reasons for nonresponsive celiac disease, inadvertent gluten ingestion should be ruled out, in addition to other potential causes of diarrhea or malabsorption, such as pancreatic insufficiency, concomitant collagenous colitis, lymphoma, or other rare entities, such as adult-onset autoimmune enteropathy (Fig. 16.8).[145-147] These entities leading to "apparent refractoriness" must be excluded carefully by clinicians before considering the serious and potentially life-threatening condition of RCD.[153] Expert reviews and multicenter studies of this rare condition highlight the salient features of RCD. The prevalence is unknown, with approximately 900 unique patients reported from referral centers as of 2018[150,154-156]; precise definitions vary between centers; the pathogenesis is poorly understood; and therapies are based on anecdotal practices and opinion.[150,157] The following information appears to be supported by numerous studies.

RCD is categorized into two types based on the immunophenotype and clonality of IELs in duodenal tissue, and also based on responses to incremental therapies (see Table 16.7). Patients with RCD I have normal intraepithelial T-cell phenotype by flow cytometry or immunohistochemical analysis (CD3+, CD8+), do not show

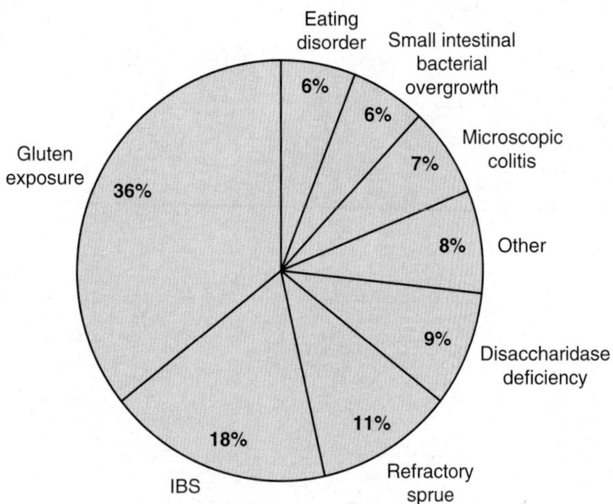

FIGURE 16.8 Nonresponsive celiac disease. Persistent symptoms in patients with celiac disease are most likely due to causes other than refractory celiac disease. *(From Celli R, Hui P, Triscott H, et al. Clinical insignificance of monoclonal T-cell populations and duodenal intraepithelial T-cell phenotypes in celiac and nonceliac patients. Am J Surg Pathol. 2019 Feb;43(2):151–160.)*

clonal rearrangements of the *TCR* gene, often respond to generic immunosuppression regimens, have a low risk of progression to enteropathy-associated T-cell lymphoma, and have a normal life expectancy.[158,159] By definition, patients with RCD II have abnormal intraepithelial T cells (CD3 cytoplasmic +/surface−, CD8−), often have monoclonal *TCR* gene rearrangements, are usually refractory to immunosuppression, and are at increased risk of progression to lymphoma and death.[151,158-165] These findings have led to the theory that a significant proportion of refractory sprue cases represent a form of in situ, or cryptic, T-cell lymphoma. There is no agreement on appropriate therapy, but numerous chemotherapeutic and immunomodulatory regimens have been used.[160,163,166,167] Specific regimens that have been attempted include cladribine,[166] recombinant IL-10,[168] alemtuzumab (an anti-CD52 monoclonal antibody), and most recently, anti-IL-15 antibodies.[169,170] A seven-center study of 232 RCD patients found that an algorithm combining age, albumen levels, and detection of abnormal lymphocyte populations or presence of clonal populations accurately predicted 5-year survival in RCD.[154]

The pathologist's role in considering a diagnosis of RCD is pivotal. While much of the RCD literature states that TCR clonality studies and immunostains for CD3 and CD8 are useful in confirming a diagnosis of RCD and in distinguishing RCDI from RCD II,[150-152,160,161,163,171] newer data have shown monoclonality established using polymerase chain reaction (PCR) in formalin-fixed, paraffin-embedded tissue to be unreliable and nonspecific, especially if common causes of persistent symptoms have not been excluded.[153] Monoclonal *TCR* gene rearrangements are present in new-onset celiac disease, in patients not adhering to a gluten-free diet, in *Helicobacter pylori*–associated duodenitis, and in RCD I.[153] Likewise, by immunohistochemistry, RCD II should be considered only when CD8+ IELs are almost nonexistent, since they comprise only a subset of CD3+ IELs in inflammatory states. Although these tests can be informative in the truly refractory patient, it is important that pathologists avoid embarking on tests for RCD until the extensive clinical workup to detect other causes is complete. In that setting, fresh tissue for flow cytometry may be a useful adjunct to findings in formalin fixed tissues.[172]

BOX 16.6 Histological Findings That May Be Seen in Refractory Celiac Disease (I or II)

- Persistent mucosal inflammation with increased intraepithelial lymphocytes despite strict adherence to a gluten-free diet
- Flat or variable villous architecture over multiple time points
- Subcryptal space with basal lymphoplasmacytosis
- Mucosal atrophy (thin mucosa)
- Collagenous sprue
- Acute inflammation/ulceration
- Enteropathy-associated T-cell lymphoma
  - In refractory celiac disease II patients or de novo
- Rare B-cell intestinal lymphoma

From a histological (not causative) point of view, small bowel biopsies in refractory sprue usually reveal moderate to severe villous flattening despite adherence to a gluten-free diet (Box 16.6). The lesions are typically patchy and variable in distribution, although diffuse flattening of the entire small intestine may occasionally occur. In a longitudinal study of 10 patients with refractory sprue, several histological features were strongly associated with a refractory course.[173] In that study, collagenous sprue developed in five patients. In addition, basal plasmacytosis and mucosal thinning (corresponding to Marsh type 4) were found almost exclusively in biopsies from refractory patients.

Collagenous sprue has since been reported in several series as a pattern of injury seen in the setting of RCD or unclassified sprue.[150,174,175] Like its counterpart in the colon, collagenous sprue is a female-predominate injury pattern characterized by increased deposition of collagen beneath the surface epithelium basement membrane.[176] Rigorous diagnostic criteria, including entrapment of small capillaries and fibroblasts in the collagen layer, should be applied to establish this diagnosis (Fig. 16.9). A trichrome stain to highlight collagen is often helpful. Collagen deposition may be patchy and often appears late in the course of illness. Associated collagenous gastritis and collagenous colitis may occur. Clonal T-cell populations are sometimes found by PCR analysis of fixed tissue, but this may be a prognostically insignificant finding.[174] While early reports suggested dismal clinical outcomes,[173,176] more current literature provides evidence that collagenous sprue represents a histological pattern with a heterogenous clinical outcome. Some patients respond to a gluten-free diet and steroids, others require total parenteral nutrition and chemotherapy, and some die of intractable disease.[150,174,175] In summary, collagenous sprue is a histological injury pattern that usually is seen in patients who fulfill criteria for RCD. Its presence

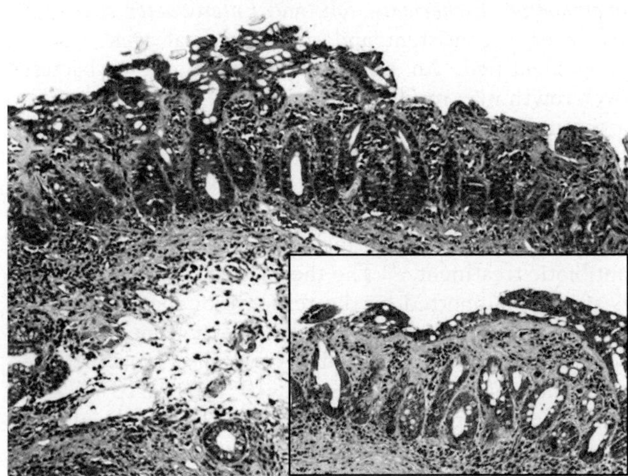

FIGURE 16.9 Collagenous sprue. Cellular elements, including blood vessels and fibroblasts, are entrapped within a thickened collagen layer. Inset highlights subepithelial collagen deposition with trichrome stain.

cannot, by itself, be used to discriminate between RCD I and RCD II.

Malignancy in Celiac Disease

An association between celiac disease and an increased incidence of lymphoma and carcinoma has been reported.[177-179] While some studies suggest a relative risk of approximately 30-fold,[177] recent population-based studies suggest that the increased risk may be lower.[180-184] In two large population-based studies of patients with latent celiac disease, defined as positive serology with normal biopsy, there was no increase in mortality or lymphoma risk on follow-up.[180,183] The role of adherence to a gluten-free diet in decreasing the risk of malignancy in patients with celiac disease is controversial.[177,185,186] A number of studies have confirmed that strict dietary compliance, especially beginning in childhood, probably confers protection from malignant complications.[187-190]

Intestinal lymphoma in celiac disease, first documented in 1937,[191] occurs in 5% to 10% of patients in some series.[192-194] Lymphomas that arise in this setting were originally classified as reticulum cell sarcomas[195] or malignant histiocytosis.[196] In some reports, the term *ulcerative jejunitis* (now understood to be synonymous with lymphoma) was used to describe tumors that develop in the setting of malabsorption.[197] The term *enteropathy-associated T-cell lymphoma* is the current terminology in use, based on their characterization in 1985 by Isaacson et al.[198,199] However, rarely, B-cell lymphomas may develop in association with refractory sprue as well.[173]

Lymphoma may present as solitary or multiple tumors and may involve any portion of the small bowel, either with or without involvement of the mesenteric lymph nodes.[192-194] Clinically, the onset of lymphoma is frequently associated with relapse of malabsorption in previously gluten-free diet–responsive patients.

Studies of the risk of carcinoma in celiac disease patients are inconclusive. While older studies cite an increased frequency of carcinomas, especially those arising in the GI tract, in patients with celiac disease,[192-194,200] recent population studies in Sweden and the United Kingdom suggest no increase in solid tumor incidence in celiac disease, but confirm an increase in lymphoproliferative disorders.[180-183] In a meta-analysis of cancer risk, an increase in overall and small intestinal carcinomas was found, which may decrease on diet adherence.[201] Interestingly, the molecular pathogenesis of celiac disease–associated small bowel carcinoma may differ from that occurring in patients with Crohn's disease.[202]

Other Complications in Celiac Disease

A variety of intestinal and extraintestinal pathological conditions occur in patients with celiac disease. These include lymphocytic gastritis,[203] collagenous gastritis,[204] lymphocytic colitis,[205] collagenous colitis,[145,206,207] dermatitis herpetiformis,[22,208] nonspecific intestinal ulceration, [209,210] and a variety of other associations.[211,212]

Differential Diagnosis

As with mild infiltrative lesions, the villous blunting of type 3 lesions is not specific for celiac disease (see Tables 16.5 and 16.6).[213,214] Flattening of small intestinal villi can be seen in several conditions, such as tropical sprue,[215] bacterial overgrowth,[216,217] unclassified sprue,[173] specific food allergies,[218] common variable hypogammaglobulinemia,[134] and an ever-increasing list of medications (see Box 16.7 and the section Drug Injury of the Small Bowel). Villous blunting is also noted in infants and young children with viral gastroenteritis or cow's milk protein intolerance. Small bowel Crohn's disease and eosinophilic gastroenteritis may rarely result in villous blunting.[219,220] Distinction of these entities from celiac disease rests primarily on clinical, not pathological, data. However, in the rare instance of a flat mucosal biopsy in common variable hypogammaglobulinemia, the lack of lamina propria plasma cells and concurrent infection with *Giardia* are clues to the correct diagnosis. Biopsies in tropical sprue are only rarely completely flat, and a history of residence in tropical climates allows distinction from celiac disease, although this may be a less reliable indicator since the incidence of celiac disease is rising around the world. Above all, serum antibody tests, a careful medication history, and a response to a gluten-free diet are of paramount importance in distinguishing celiac disease from other conditions.

Other Disorders of Protein (Cow's Milk and Soy Protein) Intolerance

The syndromes of cow's or breast milk and soy protein intolerance in infancy and childhood are well documented.[135,218,221-228] Hypersensitivity to other foods has been reported in both children and adults but are not as well understood. Here, the discussion is limited to milk and soy allergy because these disorders are associated with reproducible histological patterns of injury in the GI tract. Clinically, affected infants introduced to either cow's milk or soy-based formulas may develop a variety of symptoms, including acute (frequently bloody) diarrhea, vomiting, abdominal pain, and weight loss. Laboratory abnormalities may be seen, such as hypoalbuminemia, anemia, and metabolic acidosis.[228] Peripheral eosinophilia may or may not be present. Symptoms usually improve rapidly after removal of the inciting agent. However, in some individuals, the symptoms may be prolonged, and steroids may be required.

The pathogenesis of GI protein allergies is diverse, with approximately half related to IgE-mediated hypersensitivity and the other half related to non-IgE T-cell–mediated reactions.[229] Early prospective studies have documented that histological injury in soy protein intolerance develops within 12 hours of ingestion and may resolve within 4 days after dietary exclusion.[218] Recent studies have revealed a prominent T_H2 phenotype to cow's milk–specific lymphocytes and a lack of immunosuppressive cytokines in children with milk-induced GI disease.[230] In some patients, overlap is seen between milk protein intolerance and the more generalized condition of eosinophilic gastroenteritis. Both disorders may be associated with peripheral eosinophilia. Patients with eosinophilic gastroenteritis may initially present with symptoms apparently related to milk protein intolerance. However, their clinical course is more refractory, and they are also more likely to have an atopic phenotype.[223]

The distribution of pathological findings in soy or milk protein intolerance is variable, and includes proctocolitis, food protein–induced enteropathy, and food protein–induced enterocolitis syndrome.[228,229,231] Proctocolitis consists of mild to severe mucosal eosinophilic infiltrates, intraepithelial eosinophils associated with epithelial injury, and edema.[223] In the small bowel the ileum is more affected than the duodenum. Varying degrees of villous blunting may be seen, with mucosal edema, mucin depletion, and increased IELs and eosinophils. When severe, the histological features may resemble untreated celiac disease. However, the finding of increased eosinophils can help distinguish between these two entities. Eosinophils are not always significantly increased in protein intolerance. In such cases, clinical correlation with patient age and dietary history is required to establish the diagnosis. Colorectal changes in allergic disease are discussed in greater detail in Chapter 17.

Tropical Sprue (Environmental Enteropathy)

Epidemiology and Clinical Features

Tropical sprue is a chronic malabsorptive syndrome, often associated with folate and vitamin B_{12} deficiency, that occurs in residents of, or visitors to, the Indian subcontinent and parts of Southeast Asia, Central America, and the Caribbean.[232-237] Notable exceptions are Jamaica and sub-Saharan Africa. In tropical populations, adults are more severely affected than children. The disease occurs in both endemic and epidemic forms. Patients present with chronic nonbloody diarrhea, weight loss, bloating, and abdominal cramps. In severe cases, secondary vitamin deficiencies can lead to complications of nutritional deficiencies (such as subacute combined degeneration of the spinal cord due to vitamin B_{12} deficiency).

The cause of tropical sprue remains unknown, although the preponderance of evidence supports an infectious origin.[236,238-243] The illness probably begins with an acute infection of the small or large intestine that may be bacterial, viral, or parasitic in origin.[238] Subsequently, a chronic infection, with colonization of the small bowel by aerobic enterotoxigenic bacteria, is believed to occur, which probably results in ongoing injury to enterocytes. Bacteria isolated from patients with tropical sprue include *Klebsiella pneumoniae*, *Escherichia coli*, and *Enterobacter cloacae*.[238] However, a consistent and specific causal agent has not been identified. An environment conducive to bacterial overgrowth may result from the release of enteroglucagon, a potent inhibitor of peristalsis, during the acute infectious phase of the disease.[238] A study from India documented contamination of the small bowel with aerobic bacteria, and prolonged orocecal transit time in patients with tropical sprue, with both abnormalities reversing after prolonged antibiotic treatment.[239] The theory of bacterial overgrowth is strongly supported by the response of some patients to broad-spectrum antibiotics, such as tetracycline, along with folic acid. In addition, studies have shown an increased frequency of HLA antigens Aw19 and Aw13 in some patients with tropical sprue. However, the role of HLA antigens in the pathogenesis of this disease remains poorly understood.[244]

The entire small bowel is usually affected in tropical sprue, including the ileum,[233,245] leading to vitamin B_{12} and folate deficiency in most symptomatic patients. Vitamin deficiencies may lead to proliferative injury (e.g., megaloblastic change) to the intestinal crypts and other epithelia.[246] Megaloblastic change, or macrocytosis, refers to the nuclear and cytoplasmic enlargement of epithelial cells that occurs in the setting of interrupted DNA synthesis and cell division (see Chapter 7).

Pathological Features

Asymptomatic native populations susceptible to tropical sprue often harbor pathological changes that include villous shortening and increased inflammation. The degree of abnormality in asymptomatic people is generally minor but is occasionally pronounced.[233,235] Evidence of malabsorption is also frequently found in asymptomatic native residents.

As stated above, the entire small bowel, including the ileum, is usually affected in tropical sprue.[233,245] This is in contrast to celiac disease, in which pathological lesions are present in the duodenum and jejunum and only rarely extend into the ileum. The patterns of distribution of these two diseases are consistent with their pathogenesis. Tropical sprue is caused by colonization of the bowel by bacteria, whereas celiac disease is a response to a dietary antigen that is present in highest concentrations in the proximal gut.

Gross Pathology

Early studies of small bowel mucosa (using a dissecting microscope) revealed that biopsies from symptomatic patients, and from some asymptomatic patients in endemic areas, show an abnormal villous pattern characterized by fusing and broadening of the villi.[233,245,246] The jejunum is usually more severely affected than the ileum, which may appear normal under the dissecting microscope despite being abnormal histologically.[245]

Microscopic Pathology

There is significant overlap in the histological features of tropical sprue and celiac disease. Small bowel biopsies in tropical sprue reveal varying degrees of villous blunting, crypt hyperplasia, and increased mitotic activity (Fig. 16.10).[239,246,247] An increase in lamina propria lymphocytes, plasma cells, and eosinophils, as well as IELs, is also seen. In tropical sprue, IELs are more numerous in the crypts than in the surface

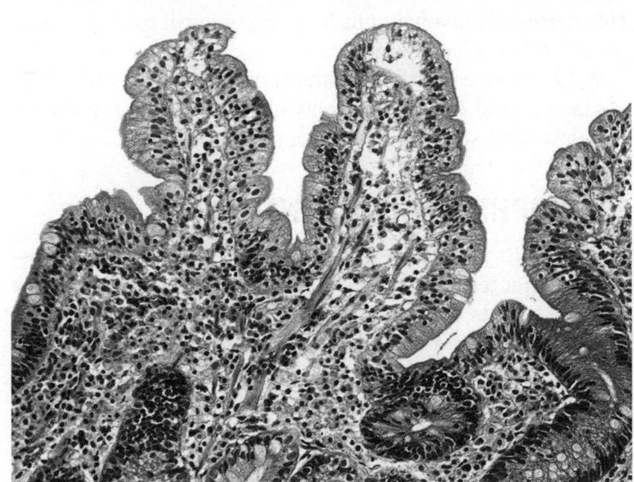

FIGURE 16.10 Tropical sprue. A variable degree of villous blunting is seen in tropical sprue. In this duodenal biopsy specimen, only mild villous blunting is present. A marked increase in the number of intraepithelial lymphocytes, and this is more prevalent in the crypts than in the surface epithelium. The lamina propria is expanded with mononuclear cells. (*Courtesy of Raymond Yesner, MD, Yale University.*)

cells, unlike celiac disease, in which the reverse situation occurs.[248] In severe cases, decreased mitotic activity is combined with a lack of surface epithelial cell maturation. The cells acquire a cuboidal shape, become mucin depleted, and accumulate cytoplasmic fat droplets.[233,235,245,246] As previously mentioned, concomitant folate and vitamin B_{12} deficiency may lead to mucosal atrophy, manifested by crypts lined by cells with markedly enlarged (megaloblastic) nuclei. Completely flat mucosa, common in celiac disease, is almost never seen in tropical sprue.

Electron microscopic studies of small bowel biopsies in tropical sprue have revealed irregularities of microvilli, increased lysosomes, accumulation of fat in surface epithelium, and the presence of dense material beneath the basal lamina.[235]

Differential Diagnosis

The histological changes in tropical sprue are nonspecific and can be seen in a variety of conditions (see Fig. 16.8).[249] Thus a clinical history of residence in, or prolonged visits to, endemic areas is critical in establishing a correct diagnosis. Parasitic and other specific infections must be excluded before a diagnosis of tropical sprue can be made confidently. Biopsies that show completely flat mucosa should arouse suspicion for other diseases such as celiac disease and drug reactions. However, mild to moderate mucosal lesions can be seen in both celiac disease and tropical sprue. Clinical improvement after treatment with broad-spectrum antibiotics further supports a diagnosis of tropical sprue.

Small Intestinal Bacterial Overgrowth (Blind-Loop Syndrome, Stasis Syndrome)

Pathogenesis

Bacterial overgrowth by coliform bacteria in the small intestine occurs in a variety of conditions, all of which predispose the individual to decreased motility and stasis.[216,250,251] These include motor and neural disorders such as scleroderma, diabetes mellitus, pseudo-obstruction, and amyloidosis; structural defects such as diverticulosis and strictures; genetic conditions such as pancreatic deficiency due to cystic fibrosis; and surgical manipulations that lead to isolated bowel segments, such as Billroth II gastrojejunal anastomosis or short bowel syndrome.[252-261] Immune deficiency states, such as AIDS and common variable immune deficiency, may also result in bacterial overgrowth and may contribute to the diarrheal illness that frequently occurs in these conditions.[216,251] Clinically significant bacterial overgrowth also occurs in older adult patients without any other predisposing features, especially among those with disabilities.[262,263] Several studies have documented bacterial overgrowth in patients with irritable bowel syndrome.[264-267] Small intestinal bacterial overgrowth has become a subject of renewed study as the role of the microbiome in general health has come to light.[268]

Clinical Features

Regardless of the underlying cause, this syndrome is characterized by overgrowth of anaerobic bacteria, normally confined to the colon, within the small intestine.[216,250,251] Patients with this condition typically have abdominal pain, bloating, diarrhea, and steatorrhea, although malabsorption of vitamin B_{12}, carbohydrates, and other nutrients can occur as well. Proposed theories of pathogenesis include deconjugation of bile salts by anaerobic bacteria, which leads to fat malabsorption.[158] In addition, certain nutrients, such as vitamin B_{12}, may be depleted by luminal bacteria. Ultrastructural studies of this condition have revealed evidence of damage to surface epithelium and the brush border, with some evidence of defective fat transport and absorption.[269]

Several methods of diagnosis have been used to detect bacterial overgrowth. The traditional gold standard is small intestinal aspirate culture showing growth of at least 10^5 colony-forming units of bacteria per milliliter of small bowel fluid (normal small bowel has fewer than 10^4 colonies per milliliter).[270] Typically, multiple organisms are identified and include species of *Bacteroides*, *Enterococcus*, and *Lactobacillus*. Other diagnostic tests include the ^{14}C-D-xylose or hydrogen breath tests.[271] When bacterial overgrowth is suspected or proven, antibiotic therapy may result in marked improvement.[216,272-274]

Pathological Features

Small bowel biopsies from patients with bacterial overgrowth may be histologically normal despite clinical evidence of malabsorption. When abnormal, biopsies typically reveal mild to moderate villous blunting with increased chronic inflammation in the lamina propria and epithelium, as well as crypt hyperplasia (Fig. 16.11).[216,269,275] Vacuolated epithelial cells, probably containing lipid, may also be seen. One study found that villous blunting, defined as a villous-to-crypt ratio less than 3:1, was the most common abnormality present in small bowel biopsies of patients with bacterial overgrowth versus controls. However, in the same study, more than half of the biopsies from patients with bacterial overgrowth were scored as histologically unremarkable.[276] In contrast to celiac disease, IELs may not be increased in bacterial overgrowth. When present, histological abnormalities tend to be patchy and vary from segment to segment, so that biopsies taken during the same procedure from different sites may show variable changes.

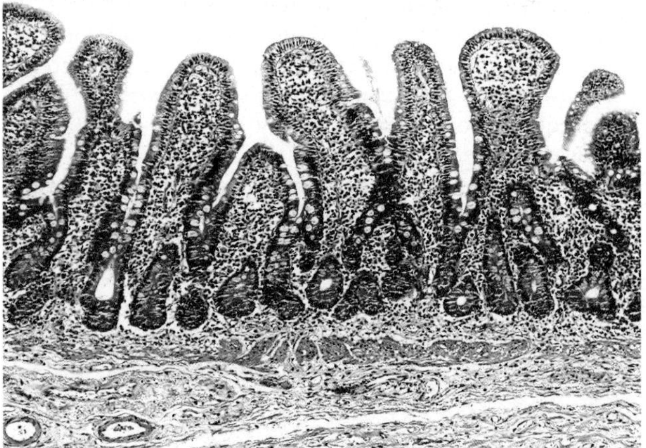

FIGURE 16.11 Bacterial overgrowth. This medium-power image was obtained from a resection specimen of a patient with bacterial overgrowth. The appearance of the mucosa can vary, and this example shows increased numbers of intraepithelial lymphocytes and lamina propria plasma cells. Villous architecture is largely preserved. The histology is nonspecific and shows overlap with many other conditions, as described in the text. (*Courtesy of Joel Greenson, MD, University of Michigan.*)

This pattern of involvement helps distinguish bacterial overgrowth from celiac disease.

As in other conditions characterized by villous blunting, the histological features are entirely nonspecific and do not correlate with severity of clinical symptoms.[269]

EOSINOPHILIC GASTROENTERITIS

Eosinophilic gastroenteritis includes a spectrum of diseases characterized by eosinophilic infiltration of one or more segments of the GI tract, peripheral eosinophilia in some patients, and the frequent coexistence of allergies or asthma.[219,277-282] This rare condition typically appears in children or young adults with symptoms related to the particular segment of GI tract that is involved with disease. The stomach is the most common site of involvement, followed by the duodenum, jejunum, and ileum, which are involved approximately equally. Small bowel disease and gastric disease often occur together.[219] Eosinophilic esophagitis, a related but distinct clinical entity that can occur in isolation or in association with eosinophilic gastroenteritis, is discussed in Chapter 14. Because of the rarity of eosinophilic gastroenteritis, the epidemiology of this disorder is not well understood. Following earlier descriptions, Klein et al. categorized eosinophilic gastroenteritis into three anatomic patterns (mucosal, mural, and serosal), based on the layer of the bowel wall that is primarily infiltrated by eosinophils[278] (Table 16.8). Approximately 50% of patients have mucosal disease, followed by mural

TABLE 16.8 Eosinophilic Gastroenteritis

	Mucosal	Mural	Serosal
Pathology	Mucosal eosinophils with degranulation, crypt eosinophilic microabscesses, eosinophilic clustering, variable villous blunting	Thickened wall, mural and subserosal eosinophilic infiltrates, edema; mucosa may be normal	Eosinophils and edema limited to serosa and subserosa, ascitic fluid with abundant eosinophils
Clinical characteristics	Diarrhea, hemorrhage, protein-losing enteropathy	Abdominal pain, obstruction, nausea, and vomiting	Abdominal pain, obstruction, ascites, nausea, and vomiting
Differential diagnosis	Allergy Infections (parasitic, fungal, *H. pylori*) Drug reaction Crohn's disease Systemic vasculitis Connective tissue disease Neoplasia (carcinoma, lymphoma) Celiac disease Graft-versus-host disease Systemic mastocytosis Pneumatosis intestinalis Idiopathic/primary		
Ancillary laboratory testing	Peripheral eosinophilia Elevated IgE Positive skin test Erythrocyte sedimentation rate Ascites fluid analysis Stool examination Autoantibodies (e.g., ANA, RF)		

Adapted from Klein NC, Hargrove RL, Sleisenger MH, et al. Eosinophilic gastroenteritis. Medicine (Baltimore). *1970;49:299–319; McCarthy AJ, Sheahan K. Classification of eosinophilic disorders of the small and large intestine.* Virchows Arch.*2018;472(1):15-28; Zhang M, Li Y. Eosinophilic gastroenteritis: a state-of-the-art review.* J Gastroenterol Hepatol. *2017;32(1):64-72.*

disease, and, least commonly, serosal disease.[278,283] There appears to be a slight male predominance.

Clinical Features

Symptoms of eosinophilic gastroenteritis vary according to the layer of the bowel wall that is involved. The mucosal form most frequently manifests with GI hemorrhage, nausea, vomiting, and diarrhea. Protein-losing enteropathy and other forms of malabsorption may also occur. Patients with primarily mural disease usually have abdominal pain and symptoms of small bowel obstruction, such as nausea and vomiting.[284] The serosal form often manifests with ascites, as well as abdominal pain, nausea, and vomiting. A rare case of perforated duodenal ulcer in the setting of eosinophilic gastroenteritis has been reported.[285]

Once the condition has been accurately diagnosed, treatment consists of steroids. Surgical resection of obstructed segments of small bowel is frequently performed before diagnosis, because it is difficult to establish a diagnosis by biopsy if the mucosa is not involved (mural disease) or cannot be sampled. Although some diagnostic importance is given to the finding of peripheral eosinophilia, it may be absent in as many as 25% of patients.[269,286] The natural history of eosinophilic gastroenteritis remains largely unknown. In a recent study, three different clinical courses of disease were identified: single flare, recurring disease, and continuous course. In the same study, approximately 40% of patients demonstrated spontaneous remission, while the remainder were treated and showed greater than 95% response to steroids.[287] Recently, the integrin blocker vedolizumab was shown to induce clinical and histological remission in patients with steroid refractory disease.[288]

Pathogenesis

The pathogenesis of eosinophilic gastroenteritis remains unknown but may be different for the three types described (mucosal, mural, and serosal). Familial cases do occur, [289] but no specific genetic abnormalities or inheritance patterns have been identified. In some patients with mucosal disease, eosinophilic gastroenteritis appears to be related to food allergy or other hypersensitivity reactions.[277,279,281,290] IgE is elevated in some patients. Several studies have shown that the degree of tissue injury and the severity of symptoms are related to the degree of eosinophilic infiltration and to eosinophilic activation and degranulation.[176,289,291,292] Extracellular major basic protein and eosinophil cationic protein are present at increased levels in affected mucosa.[293] Experimental models with electron microscopy have demonstrated neuronal damage secondary to eosinophil infiltration and degranulation.[294,295] Eotaxin 1, a highly selective eosinophil chemokine, is important for the migration of eosinophils into the GI tract in health and disease.[296,297] IL-5 may work synergistically with eotaxin 1 in eosinophil migration.[298] The triggers for chemokine activation in eosinophilic gastroenteritis are unknown but are presumably related to altered immune responses to environmental antigens in susceptible hosts. In contrast to mucosal disease, the mural and serosal forms of the disease appear to be unrelated to hypersensitivity. The pathogenesis of this group of disorders is not understood.

Pathological Features

Eosinophils are a normal constituent of the GI lamina propria; they serve a protective role against infections, particularly parasitic infestations. When eosinophil numbers are increased, the diagnosis of eosinophilic gastroenteritis should be considered. The pathological changes in eosinophilic gastroenteritis depend on the anatomic location of disease.[278,292] In mucosal type eosinophilic gastroenteritis, an increase in both intact and degranulated eosinophils is seen in the lamina propria and infiltrating the epithelium (Fig. 16.12). Some specimens may show eosinophilic crypt abscesses, surface erosion, or ulceration. The infiltrate may be severe and diffuse or mild and patchy. Biopsies from multiple sites are often needed to detect the presence of mucosal disease.[160,214,219,222,229] In the small intestine, the mucosal architecture is usually normal, or it may show mild villous blunting. However, severe mucosal lesions (flat mucosa) have also been reported in rare instances.[279] In addition to the lamina propria, eosinophils may accumulate in the muscularis mucosae and the superficial submucosa. The density of eosinophils is often greatest in the deepest portion of the mucosa. Counting of eosinophils in the small intestine is of limited clinical value, as eosinophilic gastroenteritis can be patchy and well-defined criteria and clinically validated cutoffs for this disease are lacking. Numerous studies have shown that there is a broad range of eosinophils throughout the normal small intestine and elsewhere in the GI tract. Cutoffs for an increased number of eosinophils have varied in different case series, between >20 to >70 eosinophils per high-power field, counted in 1 to 5 high-power fields, depending on the anatomic location, patient age, geographic location, and other variables.[282,299-302]

Because mucosal biopsies are frequently normal in the mural and serosal forms of disease, the finding of normal mucosa in biopsy specimens from patients with suspected eosinophilic gastroenteritis does not exclude the diagnosis.

The pathology of the mural form of eosinophilic gastroenteritis is characteristic (Fig. 16.13). Resection specimens show thickening and induration of the intestinal wall on gross examination. Ulceration may be present.[219,303]

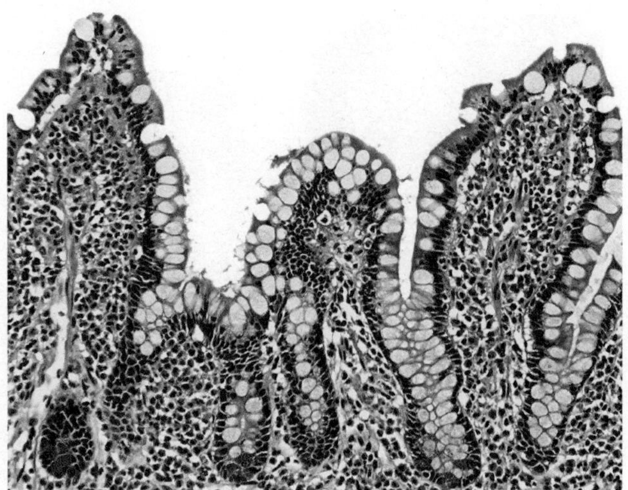

FIGURE 16.12 Eosinophilic gastroenteritis. The epithelium may not show significant injury. In other cases, the epithelium may be infiltrated by eosinophils, with the formation of crypt abscesses and ulceration.

Microscopically, prominent edema and a marked eosinophilic infiltrate are the hallmarks of mural eosinophilic gastroenteritis. Submucosal edema is frequently prominent and may also extend into the muscle layer. As in mucosal biopsies, eosinophilic infiltration is usually of a severe degree, but it can also be patchy. Dense eosinophilic infiltrates may extend into the subserosa.[219,292,303,304] In serosal eosinophilic gastroenteritis, edema and eosinophils are limited to the subserosal layers. In this setting, the diagnosis can usually be made by ascitic fluid cytology.

Differential Diagnosis

Mucosal eosinophils can be increased and prominent in a variety of inflammatory conditions of the small intestine. The differential diagnosis of eosinophilic gastroenteritis includes conditions that lead to elevated tissue eosinophil levels, such as parasitic infections, vasculitis, drug reactions, and Crohn's disease. Parasites must be excluded by having a high index of clinical suspicion, careful examination of tissue sections and by stool examination. In vasculitis, the inflammation tends to be centered in and around blood vessels, and ischemic changes may be present. Although clinical and radiological confusion with Crohn's disease may occur, the distinction from Crohn's disease is relatively simple in histological sections of resection specimens. The differential diagnosis in mucosal biopsies is more difficult, especially if the stomach is not involved and the degree of eosinophilic infiltration is patchy. However, certain features of Crohn's disease, such as focally enhanced neutrophilic exudates and granulomas, are rarely seen in eosinophilic gastroenteritis. Occasionally, duodenal biopsies from patients with celiac disease may show increased mucosal eosinophils.[292] However, clinical correlation with serum autoantibodies and attention to the other characteristic features of celiac disease usually make distinguishing it from eosinophilic gastroenteritis straightforward. The concurrent or subsequent development of celiac disease and dermatitis herpetiformis has been reported in patients with eosinophilic gastroenteritis.[305]

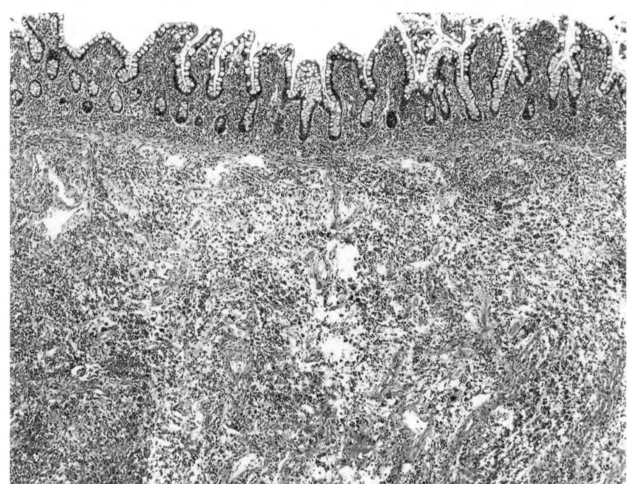

FIGURE 16.13 Eosinophilic gastroenteritis. In the mural form, edema and eosinophils extend into the submucosa and muscularis propria.

NUTRITIONAL DEFICIENCIES

A variety of nutritional deficiencies may lead to characteristic morphological abnormalities in the small intestine. It is important to note that nutritional deficiencies often occur in the setting of other pathological conditions of the small bowel, such as celiac disease, intestinal infections, and Crohn's disease, resulting in a complex pathological picture. Several pathological changes, including those related to vitamin B_{12}, protein, zinc, and iron deficiencies, are described here.

Vitamin B_{12} Deficiency

Absorption of vitamin B_{12}, an essential nutrient required for normal DNA synthesis, occurs primarily in the distal small bowel.[306] Vitamin B_{12} deficiency, such as that resulting from pernicious anemia, is characterized by macrocytosis, a decrease in the number of mitoses, and villous blunting (Fig. 16.14).[307,308] The mechanism by which B_{12}

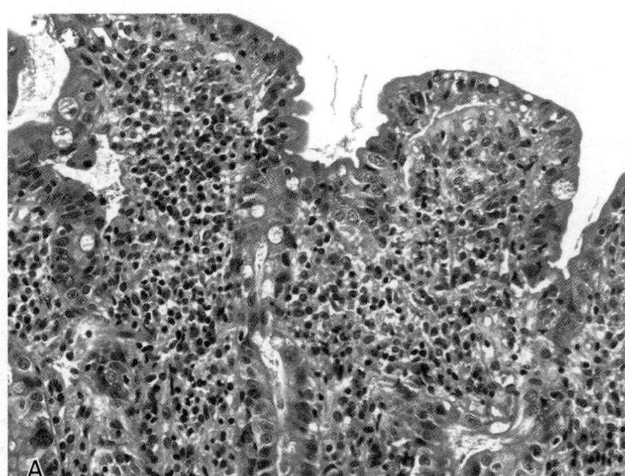

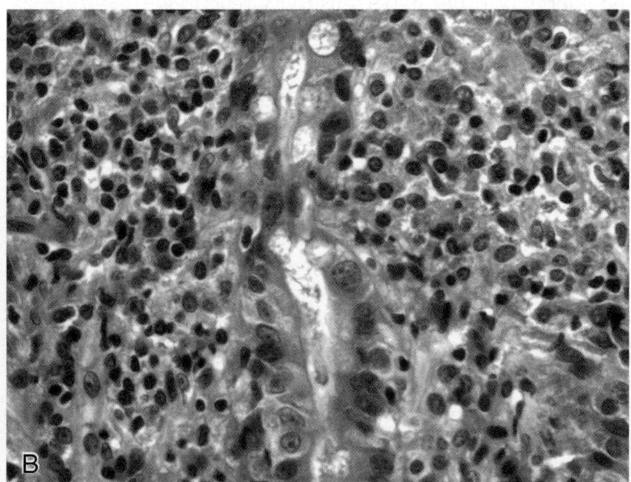

FIGURE 16.14 Duodenal biopsy specimen from a patient with pernicious anemia and vitamin B_{12} deficiency. A, In the low-power view, the villi are blunted, and there is increased inflammation in the lamina propria. The crypt nuclei are enlarged and irregular and show lack of maturation toward the surface. **B,** High-power view of the crypt shows the nuclear enlargement (macrocytosis) that is characteristic of vitamin B_{12} deficiency.

deficiency leads to macrocytosis is thought to be impaired DNA synthesis and inhibition of cell division.[307] These changes are similar to those seen in folate deficiency, chemotherapy, and radiation injury, and are reversed by B_{12} administration. Several patient populations are at risk for B_{12} deficiency, including the elderly, gastric bypass patients, premature infants, and cancer patients with long-term decreased nutritional intake.[309,310] Patients with celiac disease and Crohn's disease are at risk for secondary B_{12} and other nutritional deficiencies secondary to malabsorption.[306,311] Tropical sprue may also result in B_{12} deficiency and may show identical small-intestinal pathology. After treatment, the mitotic rate has been shown to return to normal within several days, whereas the macrocytic and architectural changes take longer (approximately 2 months) to normalize. Of note, B_{12} deficiency secondary to pernicious anemia rarely, if ever, is associated with evidence of malabsorption.

Protein Deficiency

Although rare in Western societies, protein malnutrition remains an important cause of death in infants and children in African and Asian countries. Kwashiorkor is a syndrome associated with low protein intake but normal or high caloric intake, and marasmus is a condition of both low protein and low caloric intake. Most patients also show concurrent parasitic infection or tropical sprue, which complicates the clinical and histological picture.[312-315]

Pathological features in untreated kwashiorkor or marasmus typically include mild to moderate villous blunting, increased mononuclear lymphocytes in the lamina propria, normal or mildly decreased mucosal width, cuboidalization of epithelial cells, and a decrease in the number of mitotic figures.[312-315] In some studies, Paneth cells are also decreased in number, and cytoplasmic lipid droplets are present in epithelial cells.[316] Macrocytosis may be present and may reflect dietary folate deficiency. The overall appearance bears similarity to celiac disease. Changes vary from minimal to severe and correlate with the degree of protein malnutrition, but severe changes are uncommon.

Electron microscopic studies in malnutrition reveal abnormalities in the microvillous brush border, decreased endoplasmic reticulum, dilated cytoplasmic vesicles, and phagocytic vacuoles.[317] Functional studies have revealed a decrease in the activity of mucosal disaccharidase, as well as other enzymes that may contribute to nutrient malabsorption.[312,313] Duodenal biopsy specimens from patients with kwashiorkor had lower levels of heparan sulfate proteoglycan when compared with those from patients with marasmus.[315] The biopsy appearance in marasmus is less pronounced than in kwashiorkor, despite a higher degree of caloric depletion. The mucosa is typically slightly thin, with a marked decrease in mitotic rate. However, a near-normal crypt-to-villous ratio is usually seen.[314]

Little is known about the molecular pathways within the intestinal cell in a protein deprivation environment. In a recent study using human cell lines and mouse models, researchers showed that protein deprivation leads to increased intracellular kinase activity, thereby limiting apoptosis of intestinal cells, providing evidence for a compensatory protective mechanism under nutritional stress.[81] One long-term study found a return to normal histology only after 4 to 10 years of protein supplementation.[313]

Acrodermatitis Enteropathica (Zinc Deficiency)

Acrodermatitis enteropathica is a rare autosomal recessive syndrome characterized by the presence of dermatitis, alopecia, diarrhea, growth retardation, and depressed mental function in early childhood.[318,319] It occurs in all races and affects males and females equally. The discovery, in 1973, that acrodermatitis enteropathica is caused by zinc deficiency has allowed the successful treatment of this once-fatal condition by dietary supplementation with zinc sulfate.[320] The disorder is caused by mutations in the *SLC39A4* gene on chromosome 8q24.3, which encodes a protein that appears to be involved in zinc transportation.[321] In patients with acrodermatitis enteropathica, zinc remains bound to this peptide and is unavailable for absorption.[322] Acquired acrodermatitis enteropathica, affecting adults, occurs as a result of zinc deficiency secondary to either decreased zinc intake or zinc loss, as can occur in malabsorption. Cases of acquired acrodermatitis enteropathica have been reported in patients with total parenteral nutrition[323,324] and present similarly to the autosomal recessive syndrome. In one case report, a 41-year-old female patient presented with acrodermatitis enteropathica due to autoimmune enteropathy.[325]

Small bowel mucosal biopsies in patients with acrodermatitis enteropathica may be entirely normal. However, a number of studies have reported varying degrees of villous blunting, lamina propria inflammation, and edema.[318,326,327] In rare cases, flat lesions similar to those seen in celiac disease have been documented.[327] The degree of abnormality may reflect the severity of zinc deficiency at the time of biopsy. In any case, the histological features are nonspecific. Several electron microscopic studies have revealed peculiar rhomboid and ovoid lysosomes within Paneth cells in patients with acrodermatitis enteropathica.[326,328] These changes may be related to zinc deficiency; at least one study reported their disappearance after zinc replacement.[328]

Iron Deficiency

Iron deficiency is a well-known result of malabsorption such as that due to celiac disease. However, iron deficiency itself may lead to mucosal injury and subsequent steatorrhea and malabsorption. In a study of 14 infants and children with iron-deficiency anemia, in whom celiac disease had been excluded, duodenal biopsies revealed mild to moderate villous blunting and increased lamina propria inflammation in approximately 50% of the patients.[329] The mechanism of injury is unknown but may be related to the role of iron in the normal metabolism of epithelial cells.[330]

Other Rare Metal Deficiencies

Other rare metal deficiencies have been described, frequently in the setting of celiac disease or other causes of malabsorption, including copper deficiency[331] and niacin deficiency.[332]

PEPTIC DUODENITIS AND DUODENAL ULCER

Peptic duodenitis and duodenal ulcer, once considered separate disease entities, are now recognized to represent two ends of the spectrum of peptic injury.[333,334] The proximal duodenum may be viewed as an extension of the gastric antrum, but without the protective coating of mucus and bicarbonate-secreting surface cells. The duodenal bulb, in particular, is physiologically exposed to a higher acid content than the remainder of the small intestine. In fact, some workers object to labeling the mild morphological changes described in this section as "peptic duodenitis," arguing that these findings represent normal physiological alterations. In the setting of increased gastric acid secretion, such as in antral-predominant *H. pylori* gastritis, duodenal inflammation and ulceration may occur. An extreme version of peptic injury is also seen in Zöllinger-Ellison syndrome, in which ulceration and diffuse Brunner gland hyperplasia may also involve the distal duodenum and jejunum.[335]

Current understanding of the pathophysiology of peptic duodenitis is that chronic exposure to acid induces both gastric surface metaplasia and hyperplasia of Brunner glands in the duodenal bulb.[334,336-341] In patients with *H. pylori* gastritis, foci of gastric surface metaplasia may become colonized with bacteria and incite an inflammatory response that can lead to ulceration.[334,340-342] This hypothesis is strongly supported by the finding that 95% to 100% of duodenal ulcers occur in patients with *H. pylori* gastritis and that duodenal ulcers heal faster and recur less frequently after eradication of *H. pylori*.[260,263,264]

Kreuning et al. were among the first to document the presence of duodenitis, which they studied in asymptomatic volunteers.[333,336] Patients with dyspepsia are more likely to have moderate to severe duodenitis or duodenal ulcer.[333] A high proportion of asymptomatic and symptomatic patients (64% and 94%, respectively) have foci of gastric surface metaplasia and prominent mucosal Brunner glands in biopsy specimens from the duodenal bulb.[333,336] Fundic gland (gastric) heterotopia, found less frequently than gastric surface metaplasia in duodenal mucosal specimens, is associated with the development of chronic duodenitis and duodenal ulcer disease.[254,256,265] In one study of more than 28,000 patients with duodenal biopsies, acute duodenitis, but not foveolar metaplasia, was more common in patients with *H. pylori* infection. In addition, gastric heterotopia was associated with fundic gland polyps and the authors suggested that use of proton pump inhibitors may enhance its endoscopic detection.[343]

Pathological Features

Peptic duodenitis is characterized by the presence of three main pathological features, all of which may vary in severity: increased plasma cell infiltration, neutrophils in the lamina propria or epithelium (or both), and reactive epithelial changes, including villous blunting.[333,334,336,339] Gastric surface metaplasia is not always used as an absolute criterion for peptic duodenitis, because it may be found in cases without inflammation and therefore may simply represent an adaptive response to chronic acid exposure.[334] However, most cases of peptic duodenitis show extensive gastric surface metaplasia, which can be highlighted with a periodic acid–Schiff (PAS) stain (Fig. 16.15). The distribution of changes is often patchy and can be missed as a result of sampling error.

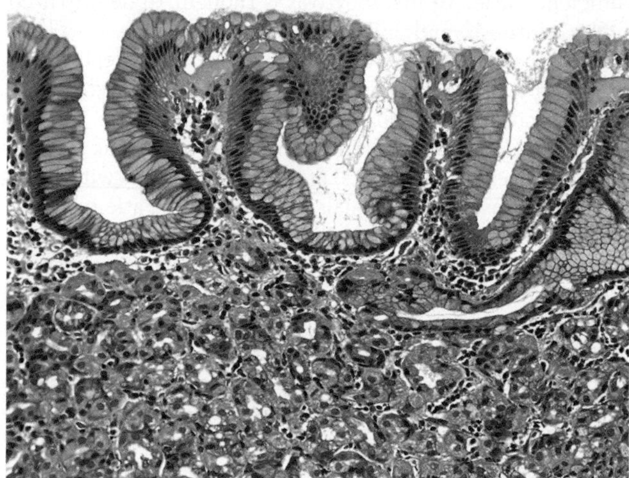

FIGURE 16.15 Peptic duodenitis secondary to heterotopia. Both gastric mucous cells and oxyntic glands are present.

In mild cases, near-normal mucosa can be seen with only a borderline increase in plasma cells and subtle reactive epithelial changes. These changes are not usually associated with symptoms and therefore may be physiological.[333,334,336] In moderately active peptic duodenitis, the epithelium is infiltrated by neutrophils and shows mucin depletion, a syncytial growth pattern, and more marked reactive epithelial changes, such as nuclear hyperchromasia and increased mitoses. Surface cells containing abundant PAS-positive mucin (gastric surface metaplasia) are usually easily identifiable. Brunner glands are hyperplastic and, as a result, may be prominent in the mucosa above the level of the muscularis mucosae. Severe cases show erosion or ulceration. If the ulcer is caused by peptic injury, concomitant *H. pylori* gastritis is frequently present.[340,342] In one prospective study of 731 French patients with peptic ulcer disease, 40% of patients had *H. pylori* infection, 18% had a history of gastrotoxic drug intake, 20% had a history of both, and the remaining 20% had neither *H. pylori* infection nor gastrotoxic drug intake and were classified as having idiopathic peptic ulcer.[344]

Differential Diagnosis

Pathological changes in peptic duodenitis are nonspecific. Nonsteroidal antiinflammatory drug (NSAID) injury, Crohn's disease, celiac disease, and infections may have a similar histological appearance. Clinical correlation and

BOX 16.7 Drugs Causing Small Bowel Injury

- Nonsteroidal antiinflammatory drugs (NSAIDs)
- Immunomodulatory drugs
  - Mycophenolate mofetil
  - Ipilimumab
  - Azathioprine
  - Tocilizumab
  - Methotrexate
- Chemotherapy and radiation
  - Taxanes
  - Irinotecan
  - Yttrium-90 (^{90}Y)-selective internal radiation microspheres
- Miscellaneous
  - Kayexalate
  - Colchicine
  - Benicar
  - Ferrous sulfate
  - Antibiotics
  - Isotretinoin

stains for organisms (including *H. pylori*) should be performed to help differentiate among these conditions. However, the degree of gastric surface metaplasia, combined with prominent Brunner glands, especially in a patient with documented *H. pylori* gastritis, often helps in establishing a diagnosis of peptic duodenitis.

DRUG INJURY OF THE SMALL BOWEL

Small bowel injury caused by drugs, medications, and other pharmaceuticals occurs in numerous clinical settings and is likely underrecognized and underreported (Box 16.7).[345] The patterns of injury are varied and depend on the pharmacological properties of the specific agent. The most common and consistently observed small bowel drug-related injury is caused by NSAIDs, a widely used class of drugs available both over the counter and by prescription. Other frequently encountered medications that cause small bowel injury include antibiotics, Kayexalate (sodium polystyrene sulfonate in sorbitol), sevelamer (an anion-exchange resin), ferrous sulfate, chemotherapeutic agents (e.g., taxanes), and immunosuppressants. With a few exceptions, most of these drugs produce nonspecific histological patterns of injury, and a high index of suspicion by the clinician and pathologist is required to detect them.

Nonsteroidal Antiinflammatory Drug–Induced Enteropathy

Clinical Features

GI toxicity resulting from NSAID use is increasingly common, causing as many as 100,000 hospital admissions annually in the United States and many more worldwide.[346-349] Ulceration of the stomach and proximal duodenum resulting from NSAIDs has long been recognized.[350] However, numerous studies have documented ulceration leading to significant hemorrhage, perforation, or obstruction occurring in the distal small bowel and colon as a result of NSAID use.[351-358] The term *NSAID enteropathy* has been used to describe this condition. Patients may have persistent iron-deficiency anemia despite the absence of gastroduodenal involvement.[351,352,357] The incidence of small bowel inflammation and ulceration has been reported to be as high as 46% to 70% among long-term NSAID users.[353] A more modest increase was found in an autopsy series, wherein 8.4% of patients previously taking NSAIDs had jejunal or ileal ulcers, compared with 0.6% of controls.[351]

Pathogenesis

The cause of NSAID enteropathy is most likely multifactorial, involving a sequence of events.[359] Local topical irritation, enterohepatic recirculation, and increased mucosal permeability secondary to cellular injury and loss of tight junction function, as well as microcirculatory events, all play a role.[352,359,360] These events may allow infiltration by luminal antigens, bile, and bacterial products, which in turn incite an inflammatory response. Newer types of NSAIDs, known as selective cyclooxygenase-2 (COX-2) inhibitors, are associated with a significantly lower incidence of intestinal side effects, but they still carry a risk of ulceration and hemorrhage, especially in long-term users.[274,277] The use of concomitant proton pump inhibitors has led to an overall decrease in gastroduodenal NSAID-related complications, presumably due to a decreased contribution of acid to the injury in the upper part of the small bowel, while NSAID injury in the distal small bowel has risen in number.[349,361]

Pathological Features

A wide spectrum of histological changes may occur in the small bowel as a result of NSAID injury. Mild lesions consist of superficial erosions with nonspecific neutrophilic and plasmacytic infiltrates (Fig. 16.16).[362-364] Erosions are frequently multiple and can progress to form deep ulcers, which may cause severe hemorrhage.[355,365] In one surgical study of 11 patients who underwent emergent small bowel resection for NSAID-induced ulceration, ulcers were observed in the ileum in eight and in the jejunum in four, and they were multiple in 50% of cases.[365] The ability to obtain jejunal biopsies during push enteroscopy has led to the documentation of more subtle changes, including mild villous blunting in some cases.[366] However, severe, diffuse villous blunting has not been reported in NSAID injury.

A rare but more distinctive form of NSAID enteropathy is referred to as *diaphragm disease* (Fig. 16.17).[367-371] This condition involves numerous thin, weblike mucosal septa that project into the lumen and cause significant narrowing and obstruction. The middle small intestine and the ileum are the preferred sites of involvement.[372] The mucosal diaphragms consist of mucosa with reactive epithelial changes, with or without surface erosions, and prominent submucosal fibrosis. The bands of fibrous tissue are characteristically oriented perpendicular to the surface of the mucosa. Mild chronic inflammation is usually present. The fibrosis is thought to result from recurrent ulceration and scarring. These diaphragms are fairly specific for NSAID injury.

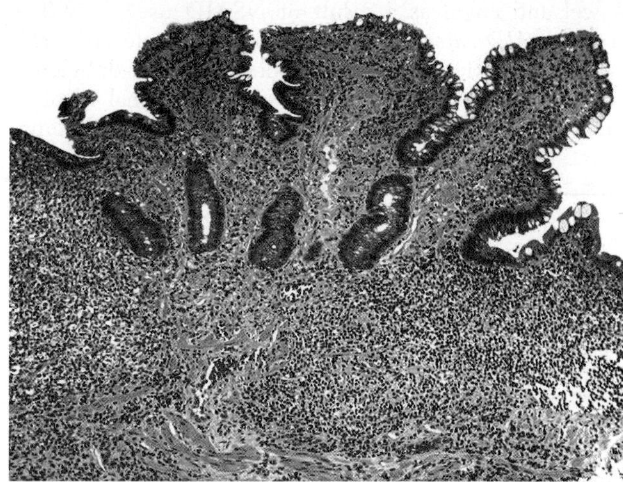

FIGURE 16.16 Nonsteroidal antiinflammatory drug injury. In this biopsy specimen of the terminal ileum, marked expansion of the lamina propria is seen, with cuboidal shape and mucodepletion of surface epithelium. Neutrophils and aphthous lesions are common, but not uniformly present.

Differential Diagnosis

The differential diagnosis of the common ulcerating form of NSAID injury includes peptic and *H. pylori*–induced duodenitis, Crohn's disease, and, rarely, infections such as *Giardia*. The lack of specificity of the histological changes seen in some of the previously discussed entities can cause diagnostic dilemmas, especially in biopsies of the terminal ileum, where the distinction between NSAID injury and Crohn's disease has significant clinical implications. Aphthous lesions may occur in both diseases, but significant plasma cell infiltrates, crypt distortion, and pseudopyloric metaplasia are much less common in NSAID injury. In the upper GI tract, gastric biopsies help distinguish *H. pylori*–related injury from NSAID-induced injury to the proximal duodenum. In addition, peptic duodenitis, which is frequently associated with marked gastric surface metaplasia in the duodenum, is not specifically associated with NSAID injury. Appropriate clinical information is important to differentiate between these disorders. The differential diagnosis for NSAID-induced diaphragm disease includes radiation or chemotherapy injury, chronic ischemia, Crohn's disease, and the rare entity CMUSE (cryptogenic multifocal ulcerating stenosing enteritis; see later discussion).

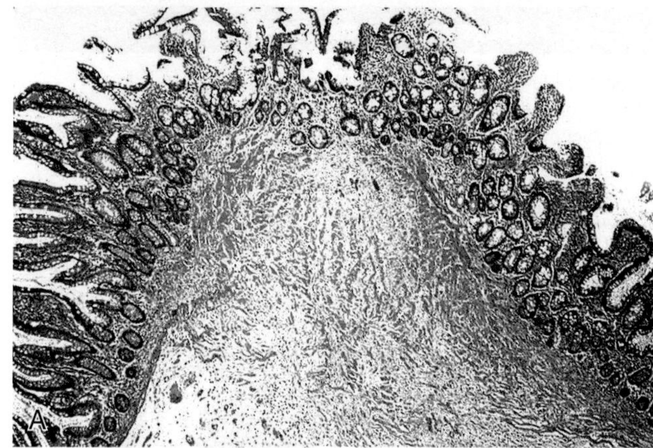

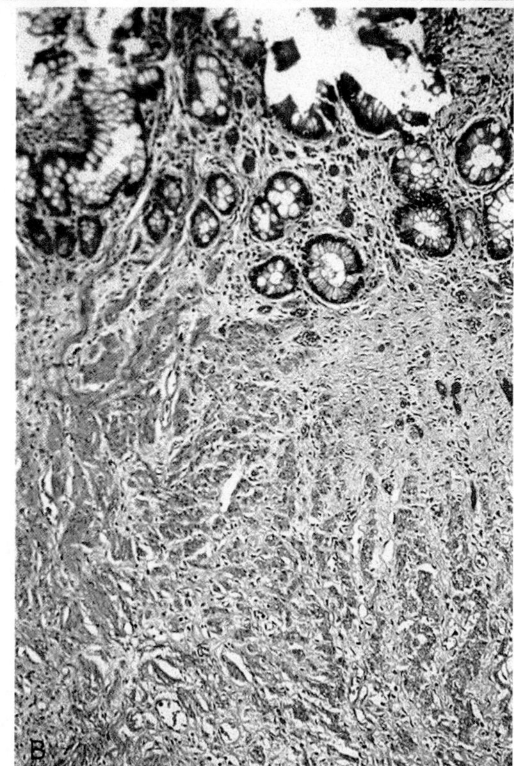

FIGURE 16.17 Nonsteroidal antiinflammatory drug (NSAID) injury. A, Low-power view of NSAID-induced diaphragm disease. This cross section is through one of the thin fibrous septa that form the luminal diaphragm. Submucosal fibrosis is prominent. **B,** High-power view shows a slightly disorganized mucosa with reactive changes and submucosal fibrosis. (*Courtesy of Robert Odze, MD, Brigham and Women's Hospital.*)

Radiation- and Chemotherapy-Induced Enteritis

Radiation Injury

The GI tract is exquisitely sensitive to radiation. The small intestine is the most sensitive portion of the gut, followed by the stomach, colon, and esophagus.[373-376] Radiation injury related to therapy is subdivided into acute and chronic forms.[377]

Acute Radiation Injury

In the acute stage, clinical symptoms related to small-intestinal involvement include diarrhea, abdominal pain, and bloating. The severity of toxicity is related to the radiation dose and to the volume of intestine exposed.[378] This syndrome, frequently called *radiation enteritis*, occurs in 20% to 70% of exposed patients and can appear within hours after exposure.[379,380] However, biopsies are not usually obtained at this stage unless the clinical features suggest that other conditions, such as opportunistic infections, may be present. The earliest histological changes occur in the surface and crypt epithelia, which show mitotic arrest, nuclear enlargement, and hyperchromasia as well as flattening and separation of cells.[381] Increased numbers of apoptotic bodies in the crypts are typical.[382,383] Ultrastructurally, loss of microvilli, vacuolization of endoplasmic reticulum, and other changes have also been reported.[384] In a mouse model of acute radiation-induced intestinal injury, researchers show that mesenchymal stems cells support the growth of endogenous intestinal crypt cells to promote repair of the small intestine within hours following radiation exposure.[385]

After 7 or more days of therapy, the area of the epithelial surface is reduced by approximately 40%,[298,302] and the mucosa is notable for villous blunting, crypt hypoplasia, and a marked decrease in the number of lymphocytes in the lamina propria. Ulceration can occur at this stage and may be widespread if exposure is persistent. In addition to epithelial changes, endothelial cells are similarly damaged, resulting in increased vascular permeability and submucosal edema.[375,376] The acute syndrome is transient; symptoms and histological changes usually resolve within several weeks after cessation of radiation.

The most important differential diagnosis in the setting of acute radiation therapy is opportunistic infection. Special stains and cultures should be used to exclude infections in these, as in all other immunocompromised patients. Acute radiation injury may also mimic the early phase of ischemic injury. In addition, the degree of epithelial atypia often present in acute radiation injury may occasionally be mistaken for dysplasia, particularly if the clinical history is unknown.

A unique and novel form of radiation brachytherapy consists of selective internal radiation therapy using biocompatible resin-based yttrium-90 (^{90}Y)-labeled microspheres that are delivered via arterial catheters to selectively target inoperable tumors, such as metastatic lesions of the liver. If delivery of the spheres is imperfect, the spheres can travel to the GI tract, leading to mucosal damage, including ulcerations, days to months after exposure.[386,387]

Chronic Radiation Injury

Chronic intestinal radiation injury develops years after radiation exposure, regardless of the presence or severity of previous acute radiation injury. The reported incidence of chronic radiation injury after radiotherapy has ranged from 1% to 36%.[388,389] With the use of current radiotherapy regimens and protective measures, the incidence is now reported to range from 5% to 10%.[375,376,390] The incidence and severity of chronic radiation injury has been shown to be related to the overall dosage and to the volume of small bowel irradiated.[390,391]

Clinical symptoms are variable but usually reflect chronic ulceration (pain, hemorrhage), stricture formation (obstruction), or perforation. The symptoms are related to long-term, irreversible pathological changes in mesenchymal tissue that ultimately lead to vascular insufficiency. Most likely, these changes occur secondary to sustained overexpression of inflammatory and fibrogenic cytokines.[391] Although epithelial and villous architectural changes usually return to normal after acute radiation injury, stromal cells, especially fibroblasts, and endothelial cells undergo a variety of persistent changes. Enlargement of fibroblasts, with expansion and vacuolization of their cytoplasm, an increase in nuclear size, and hyperchromasia are common. Although the cells increase in size, the nucleus-to-cytoplasm ratio typically stays within the normal range.[121,392] Submucosal fibrosis and, occasionally, fibrosis of the muscularis propria may be present as well (Fig. 16.18A,B). Intimal proliferation of small and medium-sized arteries, with partial or total occlusion of the vascular lumen, is a frequent finding in surgical specimens removed because of stricture formation (see Fig. 16.18C). Ischemic changes in the overlying mucosa are often present (see Fig. 16.18D).[121,393] Mucosal biopsies obtained from strictured segments may show ulceration, mucosal fibrosis, crypt branching, and inflammation. Although these findings are nonspecific, they are compatible with chronic radiation injury in the proper clinical setting.

Mucosal telangiectasia and vascular proliferations may also develop as a long-term sequela of radiation therapy (see Fig. 16.18E).[392,394] They may be missed on histological examination because thin-walled vessels frequently collapse after biopsy.

Chemotherapy Injury

Cytotoxic chemotherapy agents frequently cause acute enteritis that may be debilitating.[395-398] The pattern of injury occurs in four phases: (1) an influx of inflammatory cells into the lamina propria, demonstrated in animal models[397]; (2) loss of epithelial cells and mucosal structure; (3) disruption of large areas of epithelial lining; and (4) recovery with regrowth of epithelium and a return to normal structure and function.[397] In fact, the histological changes seen in small-intestinal biopsies after chemotherapy are similar to those seen in acute radiation injury. Biopsies obtained shortly after chemotherapy show reactive nuclear and cytological atypia and macrocytosis (Fig. 16.19). These changes reflect an arrest of maturation, which occurs within hours after administration of the drug.[399,400] Mitotic figures are usually decreased in number, and an increase in apoptotic bodies is observed in epithelial crypts, along with villous blunting, which may be severe. Cytotoxic chemotherapy is associated with an increase in a variety of proapoptotic proteins, including TP53, caspase 3, and Bax and Bak in small-intestinal crypt cells.[401] Necrosis of crypt epithelium may follow, with the development of surface erosions. These changes are transient, and the mucosa usually returns to normal within a few weeks after cessation of treatment.

Taxanes, such as paclitaxel or docetaxel, are a common component of many cancer regimens. Taxanes bind microtubules of the mitotic spindle apparatus and prevent depolymerization, resulting in mitotic arrest and the formation of numerous ring mitoses.[402,403] The appearance of ring mitoses occurs early in the course of the disease, which is then followed by apoptosis. The presence of ring mitoses can mimic dysplasia in otherwise normal tissue, and a helpful distinguishing feature is that taxane-induced mitotic arrest is limited to the proliferative zone.[404] Because of the timing of taxane-induced mitotic arrest, this change is most frequently encountered in asymptomatic patients and should not be interpreted as toxicity.[403]

Immunomodulatory and Other Antineoplastic Drugs

Immunomodulatory drugs are a growing class of medications used in a variety of clinical contexts, particularly in the treatment of autoimmune diseases and stem cell or organ transplantation. Mycophenolate mofetil (MMF)

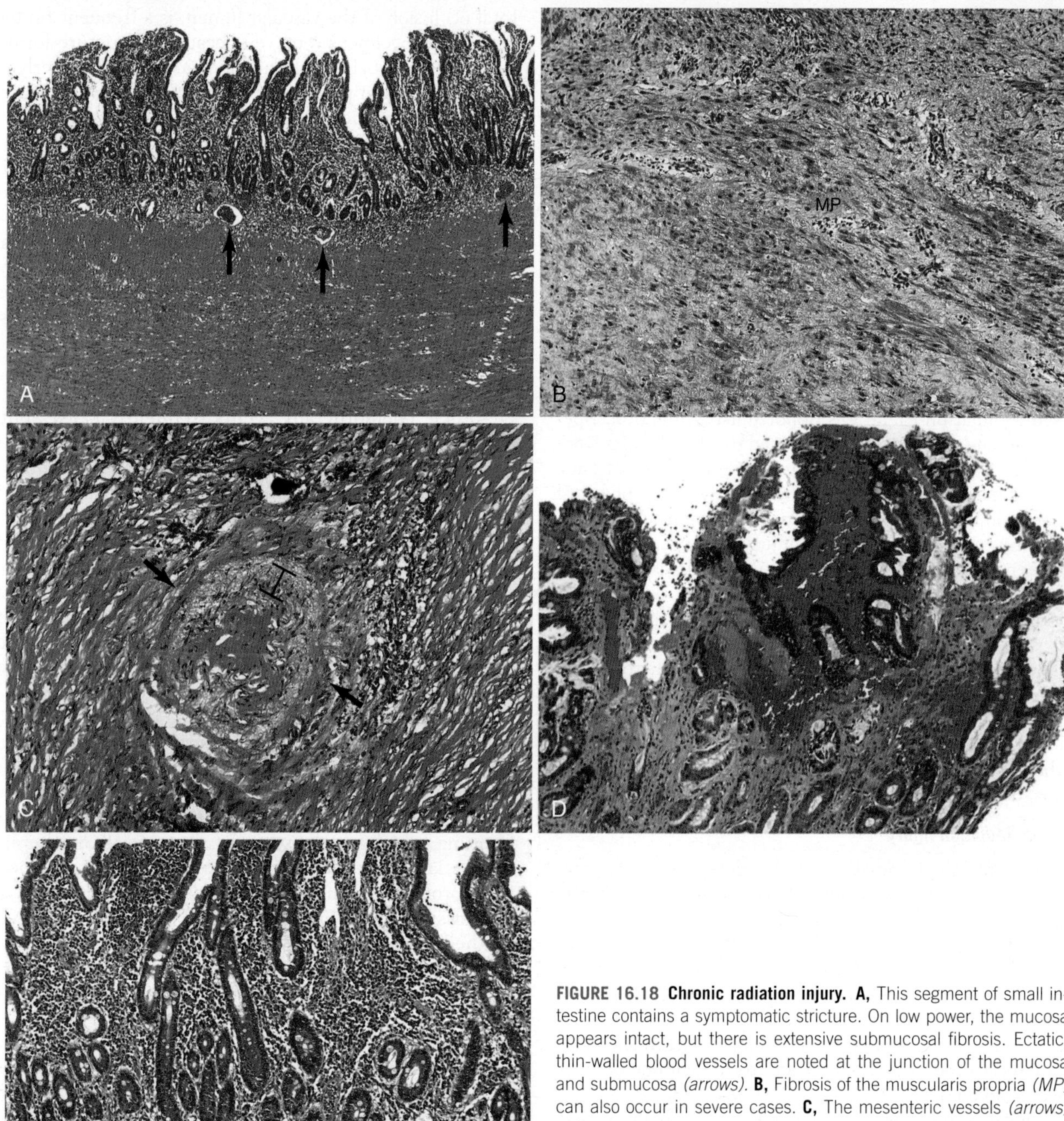

FIGURE 16.18 Chronic radiation injury. A, This segment of small intestine contains a symptomatic stricture. On low power, the mucosa appears intact, but there is extensive submucosal fibrosis. Ectatic, thin-walled blood vessels are noted at the junction of the mucosa and submucosa *(arrows).* **B,** Fibrosis of the muscularis propria *(MP)* can also occur in severe cases. **C,** The mesenteric vessels *(arrows)* within the subserosa frequently show severe intimal proliferation *(bar),* thrombosis, and occlusion of the vessel lumen. **D,** Mucosal biopsies may show ischemic-type surface erosions. **E,** Ectatic vessels are present in the mucosa and submucosa. Radiation-induced telangiectasias are often associated with bleeding. Mild architectural distortion of the crypt epithelium can be seen.

is an immunosuppressant drug that selectively inhibits B- and T-cell proliferation by blocking the de novo pathway of purine synthesis, a pathway on which enterocytes depend. MMF is used to prevent rejection in the setting of solid organ transplantation and to prevent graft-versus-host disease (GVHD) in bone marrow transplantation. It is also used increasingly in the treatment of severe autoimmune disease, such as lupus or psoriasis.

MMF-induced toxicity has been well recognized and is associated most frequently with diarrhea and several histological patterns of enteritis and colitis. Several studies have documented changes resembling GVHD in mucosal biopsy specimens from small and large intestine in patients taking MMF.[405] In such cases, there is increased apoptosis in epithelial crypts with only scant inflammation (Fig. 16.20).[406] A second, Crohn's-like pattern consists of patchy

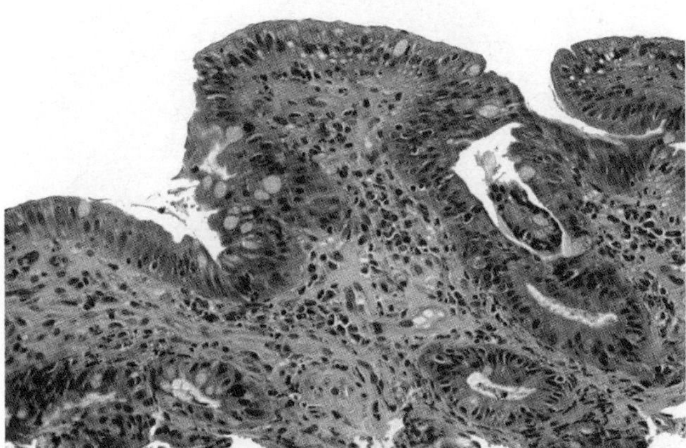

FIGURE 16.19 Chemotherapy injury. Small bowel biopsy specimens obtained shortly after chemotherapy often reveal villous blunting, nuclear enlargement, and cytoplasmic basophilia. A decrease in mitotic activity is seen, caused by an arrest of cell proliferation. No significant inflammation is observed.

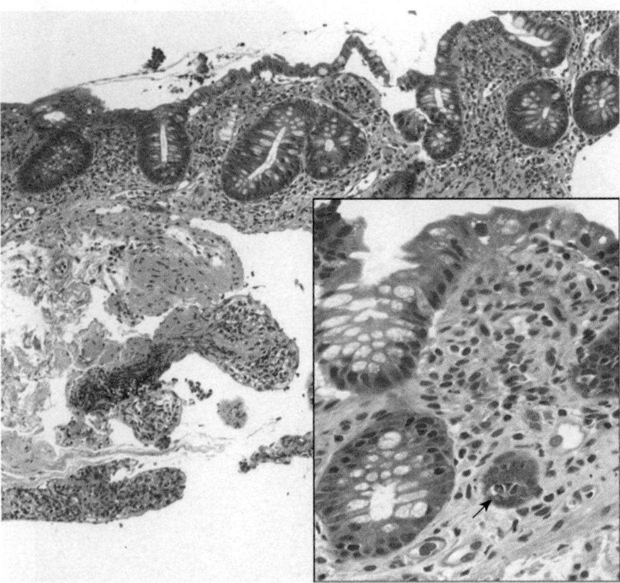

FIGURE 16.20 Injury caused by mycophenolate mofetil (CellCept) in the terminal ileum. Reactive epithelium is present without increased inflammation. Increased epithelial apoptosis is present in crypt cells *(inset, arrow).*

inflammation of the upper and lower GI tract with erosions and architectural distortion.[407,408] In both settings, infections must be carefully excluded before the changes can be attributed to drug toxicity. In addition, rare case reports have described a celiac disease–like enteropathy in renal transplant patients treated with MMF. Biopsies show increased IELs and moderate villous blunting.[409]

Recognition of MMF effect is important, because reduction of dose or discontinuation can lead to symptom improvement. However, many patients with MMF-associated diarrhea have no pathological changes on biopsy. In bone marrow transplant patients, in whom MMF is frequently administered, the distinction from GVHD is particularly important and can be challenging. Both conditions have similar histological features of increased apoptosis and scant inflammation. In a study of 57 patients, researchers found that minor histological features, including increased eosinophils, lack of endocrine cell aggregates, and lack of apoptotic microabscesses favor a diagnosis of MMF-induced colitis over GVHD.[410] In addition, other clinical variables (for example, GVHD affecting other organs, recent medication changes) can be useful to distinguish between these conditions.

Another class of drugs strongly linked to intestinal injury are the immune checkpoint inhibitors (CPIs).[411,412] Despite promising therapeutic anticancer activity, the immune-related adverse events associated with CPIs are increasingly recognized as a cause of significant morbidity in cancer patients undergoing treatment with this class of drugs. An early example of CPI is ipilimumab, a CTLA4-inhibiting antibody,[413] most frequently used for treatment of metastatic melanoma as well as other malignancies. Ipilimumab induces autoimmune syndromes in a variety of organs (thyroiditis, hepatitis, colitis), including GI sites in up to 20% of patients.[414,415] Histologically, mucosal specimens from patients with ipilimumab toxicity can show a variety of inflammatory changes, including mixed acute and chronic lamina propria inflammation, IELs, and apoptosis (Fig. 16.21).[414,416] Perforation can occur. Further, a case report describes the development of celiac disease, responsive to a gluten-free diet, following ipilimumab therapy, raising the possibility that immunomodulatory therapy could serve as a trigger to unmask celiac disease.[417] Anti-PD-1/PDL-1 therapy, another CPI, is becoming common in the treatment of malignancies. GI toxicity due to anti-PD-1/PDL-1 targeted therapy (e.g., pembrolizumab, nivolumab) is also becoming increasingly recognized and shares many clinical and histological features with ipilimumab-induced mucosal injury.[418,419]

Other immunosuppressant drugs, such as methotrexate and azathioprine, have rarely been associated with GI injury and have been reported to cause changes resembling celiac sprue.[420,421] Idelalisib, a kinase inhibitor employed in the therapy of hematological malignancies, induces apoptosis and has been associated with both colitis and enteritis, with villous blunting.[422]

Miscellaneous Drugs

Colchicine

Colchicine is an alkaloid-based medication with antimitotic activity that is used primarily to treat gout. Patients with concurrent renal disease are particularly susceptible to the toxic effects of colchicine.[423] If left untreated, colchicine toxicity can lead to diarrhea, shock, multiorgan failure, and even death. In biopsy specimens, the duodenal epithelium shows multiple metaphase mitoses, particularly with a ringlike formation (Fig. 16.22). Epithelial pseudostratification, increased apoptosis, and loss of polarity are also present and at times are mistaken for changes of dysplasia. These changes are present predominantly in the duodenum and gastric antrum and appear to correlate with clinical signs of colchicine toxicity that are not seen in patients who are taking colchicine without clinical signs of toxicity. The pathological changes appear to resolve after discontinuation of colchicine. As mentioned

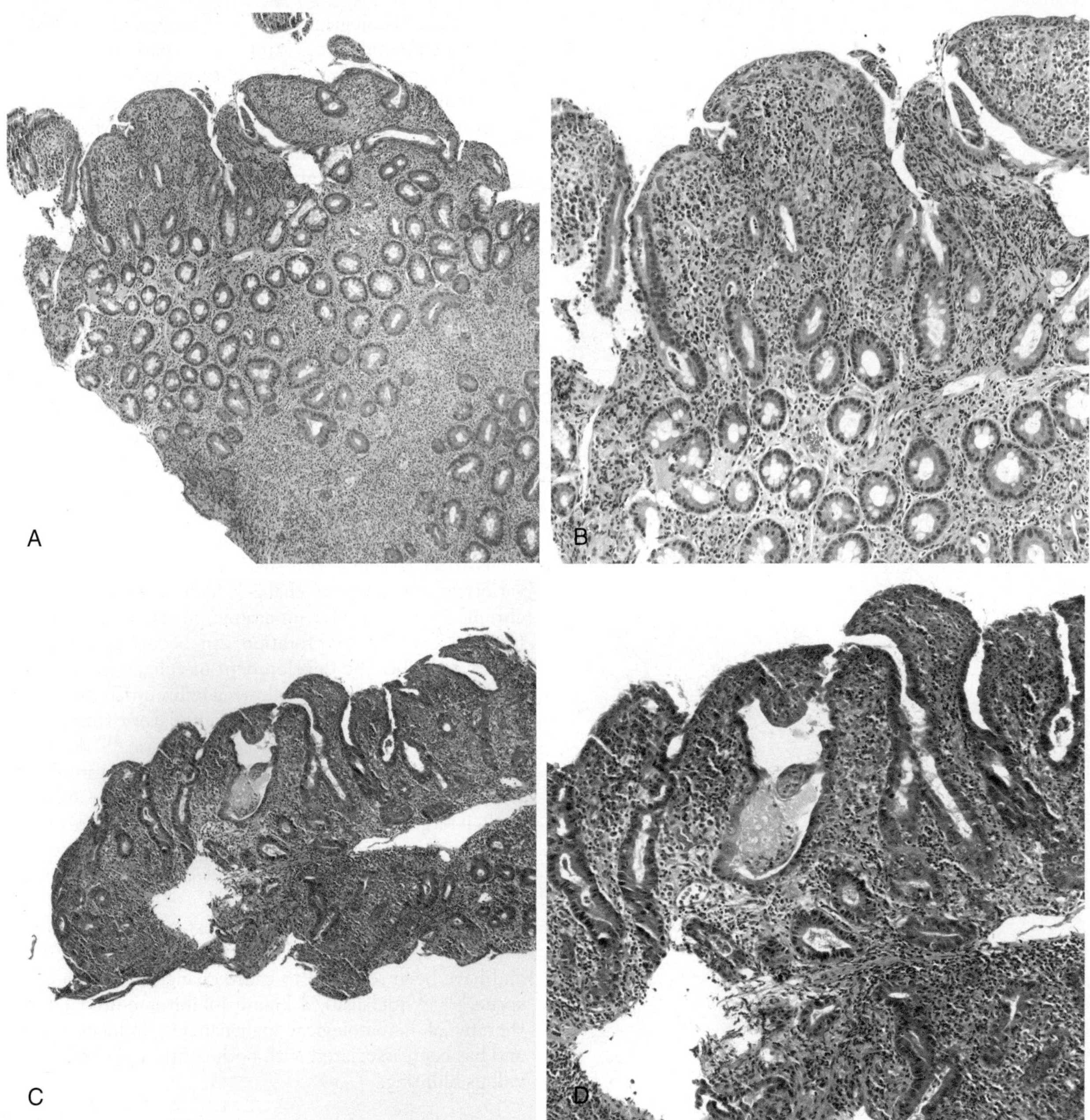

FIGURE 16.21 **A** and **B,** Anti-PD-L1antibody induced duodenitis, showing partial villous blunting, acute inflammation, and lamina propria expanded by chronic inflammation. **C** and **D,** Anti-CTLA4 antibody (ipilimumab)-induced duodenitis, showing partial villous blunting, acute inflammation, and lamina propria expanded by chronic inflammatory cells.

above, similar mitotic arrest changes are seen with other chemotherapeutic agents, such as taxanes. However, in the case of taxanes, the mitotic arrest is not associated with toxicity.[403]

Kayexalate

Kayexalate (sodium polystyrene sulfonate) is a cation-exchange resin used in the treatment of hyperkalemia, particularly in patients with chronic renal disease or renal failure. It can be administered either as an enema or orally, usually in a suspension of hypertonic sorbitol. Kayexalate has been known to cause colonic necrosis. Upper GI tract injury has also been reported.[424] Small bowel biopsy specimens most commonly show mucosal injury characterized by erosive changes and associated lightly basophilic and refractile (but not polarizable) crystals (Fig. 16.23). The crystals have a characteristic regular mosaic pattern that distinguishes them from cholestyramine crystals. Sevelamer is another example of an anion-exchange resin frequently used to treat patients with hyperphosphatemia in the setting of chronic kidney disease. Swanson et al. reported a series of seven patients on sevelamer who had several mucosal abnormalities, including acute inflammation, ulceration, and necrosis, associated with sevelamer crystals.[425] The sevelamer crystals differ from Kayexalate and cholestyramine crystals and can be distinguished by their irregular broad "fish scales" with a variable eosinophilic to brown color on H&E stain.[402]

Sartans

Sartans are a class of angiotensin II receptor agonists used in the treatment of hypertension. Rubio-Tapia et al. published a series of 22 patients who presented with a severe spruelike disorder in the setting of olmesartan administration.[426] In that series, duodenal biopsies demonstrated villous blunting, mononuclear-cell rich inflammation, and marked subepithelial collagen deposition. Celiac disease was excluded due to negative serological studies and lack of response to a gluten-free diet. In 18 patients, there was histological recovery after discontinuation of olmesartan. Since this initial report, additional case reports and case series have published similar findings, including in association with other sartans.[427]

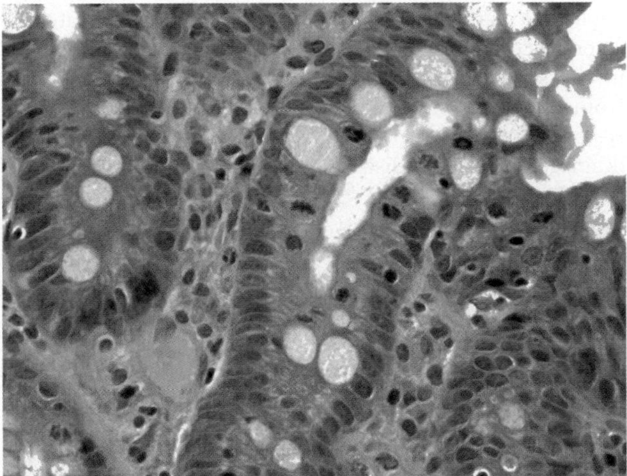

FIGURE 16.22 Colchicine effect. Multiple metaphase mitoses, particularly with a ringlike formation, are seen throughout the epithelium.

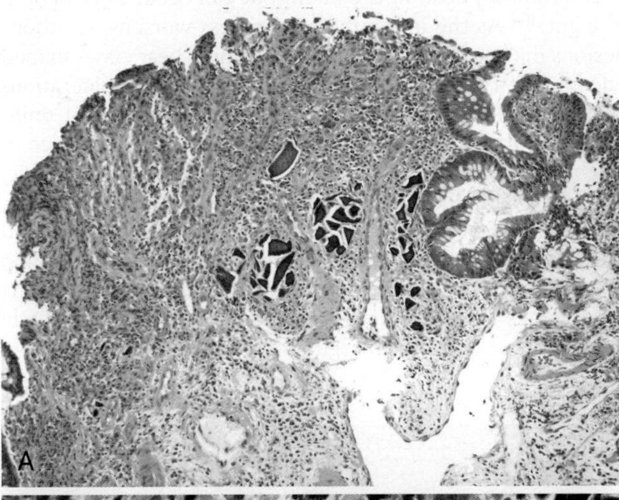

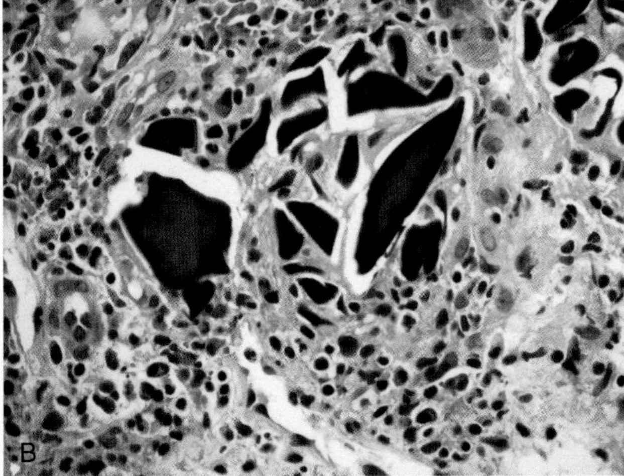

FIGURE 16.23 A and **B,** Kayexalate injury. The ulcer is associated with basophilic, sharp-edged crystals showing a mosaic pattern.

INFLAMMATORY BOWEL DISEASE

Crohn's Disease

Crohn's disease is an idiopathic chronic inflammatory condition. Unlike other inflammatory bowel diseases, it can involve any segment of the GI tract and is characterized by transmural inflammation with frequent stricture and fistula formation, as well as the presence of noncaseating granulomas in approximately 50% of biopsy and resection specimens (see also Chapter 17).

Epidemiology and Pathogenesis

Crohn's disease has a worldwide distribution but continues to be more prevalent in Western countries. The annual incidence in northern Europe and North America has risen sharply in recent years and is now roughly 10 per 100,000 population, with prevalence rates of 200 to 300 per 100,000 population.[428-431]

Genetic susceptibility has been demonstrated in both family and population studies, with a higher incidence in relatives of patients with Crohn's disease, disease concordance between twins, and increased incidence in certain ethnic populations, such as Ashkenazi Jews.[432,433] Most patients present in the second or third decade of life. However, a smaller, second peak occurs in the sixth to seventh decade of life.[434]

Although much remains to be learned, significant advances in our understanding of the biology, environmental factors, and genetic associations of Crohn's disease have occurred in the past 10 years utilizing tools such as genome-wide association studies.[430,431,433,435-438] A detailed discussion of genetics is beyond the scope of this chapter; however, at the time of this writing, at least 37 Crohn's disease genetic susceptibility loci have been identified (some of which are also associated with ulcerative colitis).[433,436] These include the association of Crohn's disease with frameshift mutations in the *CARD15* (*NOD2*) gene on chromosome 16; the *IBD5* locus on chromosome 5; certain variants of the *IL23R* gene on chromosome 1; ATG16L1, LRRK2, IRGM, STAT3, JAK2, and Th17 pathways, as well as other genes that regulate autophagy.[433,435,437-441] Many of these genes regulate the host immune response to microbial organisms, collectively termed the gut microbiota.[442] Current research supports the hypothesis that both Crohn's disease and ulcerative colitis represent responses to alterations in gut microbiota in genetically susceptible hosts. For additional details, the reader is referred to several excellent reviews on the genetic associations of Crohn's disease.[430,431,435,443-445] In this chapter, involvement of the small intestine is considered, with emphasis on the terminal ileum, the most common site of involvement, and the duodenum. A discussion of Crohn's colitis and its distinction from ulcerative colitis can be found in Chapter 17.

Pathological Features

Gross Pathology

On gross examination, Crohn's disease of the small intestine is characterized by thickening of the bowel wall, strictures, fistula formation, and fat wrapping (Fig. 16.24 and Table 16.9).[446-451] The bowel wall is usually firm and stiff due to a combination of fat wrapping, submucosal fibrosis, obliterative muscularization of the submucosa, and hypertrophy of the muscularis propria.[451-454] In addition, nerve and vessel alterations are frequently present in the intestinal wall. *Fat wrapping,* or "creeping fat," is the term used to describe adherence of mesenteric adipose tissue to the intestinal wall, in part or in whole. This finding is usually associated with transmural inflammation in the underlying bowel segment, especially deep lymphoid aggregates.[450] There is convincing evidence to suggest a role of adipocytes in the secretion of proinflammatory mediators.[455-459] Far from a passive phenomenon, adherence of mesenteric fat is now known to be related to abnormalities in lymphatic drainage in Crohn's disease and may have a direct role in initiating mural fibrosis.[460-463] Fat wrapping is frequently found in association with stiff, "hose pipe" strictures of the involved segment of bowel. Bowel loops frequently adhere to one another via mesenteric fat. When this occurs, fistula tracts can extend from one segment to another or from the diseased segment to other abdominal organs. It is especially common to find a diseased segment adhering to a normal segment of bowel. Mesenteric lymph nodes are often enlarged.

The mucosal surface in Crohn's disease shows a variety of changes that may be seen radiologically, endoscopically, and in surgical resections.[446-449] The earliest change consists of aphthous lesions, which are tiny erosions that are commonly seen in the ileum but can occur anywhere in the gut.[464] As the inflammatory process worsens, aphthous lesions may coalesce and deepen, forming bear claw–shaped ulcers. With progression of disease, longitudinal ulcerations and crevices develop, which tend to outline areas of uninvolved mucosa and give rise to a cobblestone appearance of the mucosa, as well as inflammatory pseudopolyps (see Fig. 16.24C). Knifelike fissures that penetrate into, or through, the muscularis propria may develop.[450,453] Intramural and mesenteric abscess cavities and sinus tracts may also develop in severe cases. Skip areas of involvement are characteristic of Crohn's disease. An abrupt transition between grossly involved and uninvolved segments is often seen.

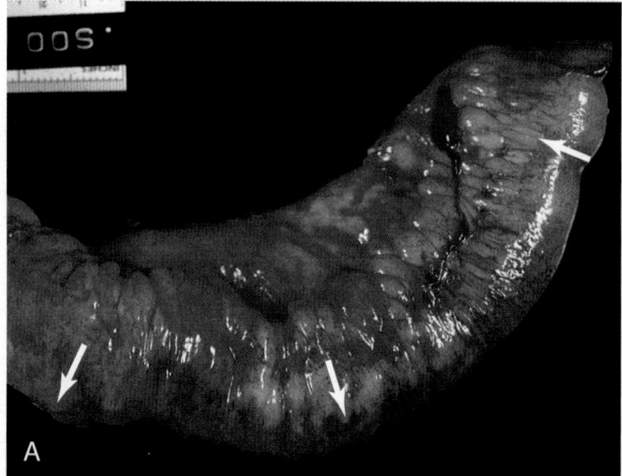

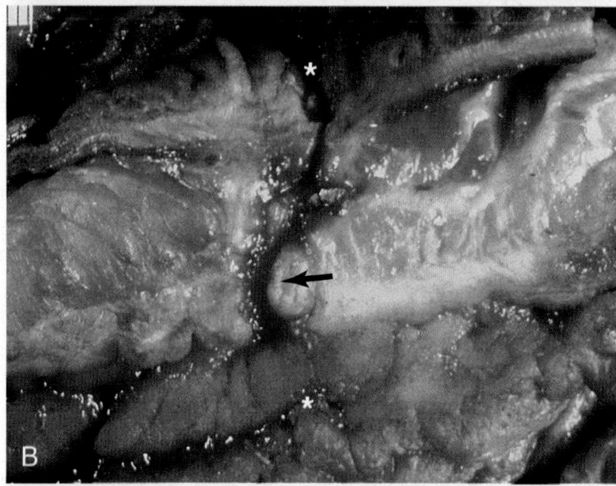

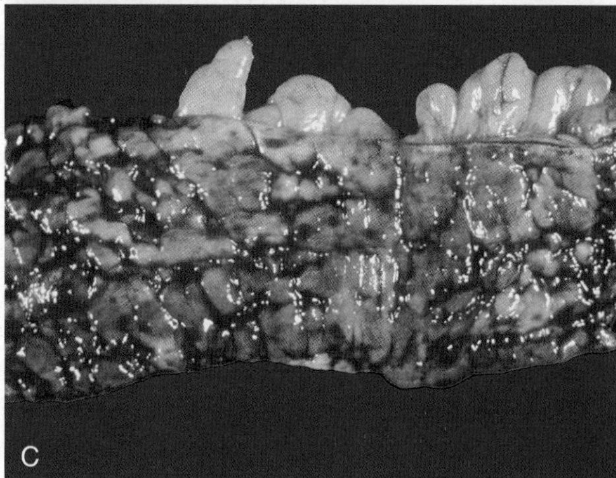

FIGURE 16.24 Crohn's disease. A, Fat wrapping *(arrows)* is prominent in this case. **B,** In this example, two segments of intestine *(asterisks)* are connected by a fistula tract *(arrow)*. **C,** The mucosal surface may exhibit a cobblestone appearance, characterized by the presence of serpiginous, anastomosing ulcers outlining islands of residual intact mucosa.

TABLE 16.9 Characteristic Pathological Features of Crohn's Disease*

Gross Pathology	Microscopic Pathology
Serosal Fat wrapping Wall stiffness Adhesions to other structures Fistulas Strictures	Erosions (aphthous lesions) Crypt architectural distortion Increased lymphocytes and plasma cells Neutrophilic cryptitis, crypt abscesses Pseudopyloric metaplasia Submucosal fibrosis Neuronal and muscular hypertrophy
Mucosal Aphthous lesions Cobblestone appearance Serpiginous and "bear claw" ulcers	Noncaseating granulomas Fissuring ulcers, sinus tracts Transmural lymphoid aggregates Vasculitis

**Segmental involvement is characteristic.*

Microscopic Pathology

Varying degrees of active (neutrophilic) inflammation and chronic inflammatory changes (architectural distortion, chronic inflammation, fibrosis, stromal hypertrophy) are usually present in some, or all, layers of the bowel wall (see Table 16.9).

Aphthous lesions consist of a small surface erosion associated with a neutrophilic infiltrate (Fig. 16.25A).[465,466] They frequently occur in epithelium overlying lymphoid aggregates and are often surrounded by normal mucosa. In the earliest stage, neutrophils infiltrate the base of a single crypt and traverse the epithelial layer into the lumen. Fissuring ulceration, which develops in more advanced cases, begins at the base of aphthous ulcers and extends into the deeper layers of the bowel wall (see Fig. 16.25B,C). In addition to aphthous lesions, the mucosa in Crohn's disease shows other chronic and active changes, such as increased numbers of lymphocytes and plasma cells, crypt architectural irregularity, and neutrophilic infiltrates. Of note, cryptitis and increased neutrophils within the lamina propria are more common than crypt abscesses. Hyperplasia of Paneth cells and pseudopyloric metaplasia (mucous gland metaplasia) within the deep mucosa are also commonly present.[467] The latter refers to a proliferation of small glands lined by cells that contain clear mucin, similar to those seen in the gastric antrum. A marked variation in the degree of morphological changes, even within one involved segment of bowel, is a hallmark of Crohn's disease. When present in resection specimens, the mucosal changes described here are typically patchy.

Mural changes in Crohn's disease, loosely called transmural inflammation, consist of myriad findings. Deep, flask-shaped or knifelike (fissure) ulcers may extend into the submucosa or muscularis propria in a haphazard, irregular fashion and are associated with acute and chronic inflammation, granulation tissue, edema, and fibrosis. Submucosal fibrosis and "obliterative muscularization" of the submucosa are associated with areas of stricturing.[450,451] Neuronal and smooth muscle hypertrophy within the muscularis mucosa, submucosa, and muscularis propria are common. A morphometric study of mural and vascular remodeling in resections of ileal strictures in Crohn's disease revealed a 17-fold expansion of the muscularis mucosae by a combination of smooth muscle hyperplasia and collagen type 5 deposition.[468] In addition, submucosal vessels displayed eccentric smooth muscle and collagen deposition oriented toward the gut luminal aspect of the vessels. There is some evidence to suggest that resections performed after the use of antitumor necrosis factor-α therapy leads to a decrease in granuloma formation and a distinct pattern of hyalinized submucosal fibrosis, in addition to the expected decrease in active mucosal inflammation.[469]

Deep fissuring ulcers are often lined by abundant histiocytes or foreign body giant cells, or both, which should not be mistaken for granulomas. One feature that is characteristic of Crohn's disease is the presence of transmural lymphoid aggregates, with or without germinal centers, that may be present anywhere in the bowel wall, from the mucosa to the subserosa. A frequent observation in resection specimens, referred to as "the string of beads" (or "rosary" sign), consists of a linear distribution of lymphoid aggregates in the submucosa and subserosa (Fig. 16.26).[446-449]

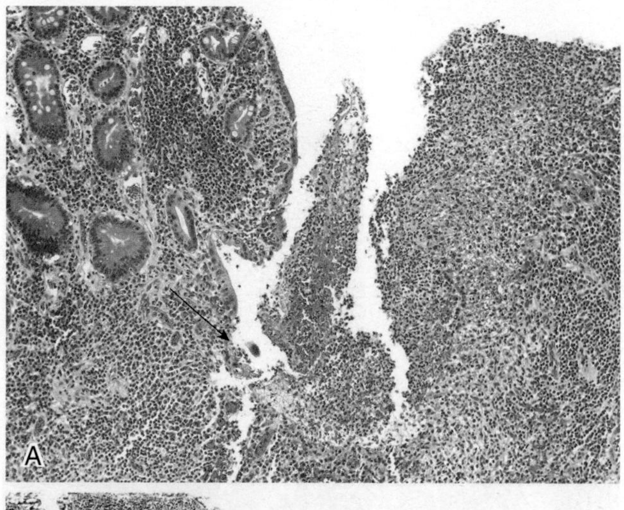

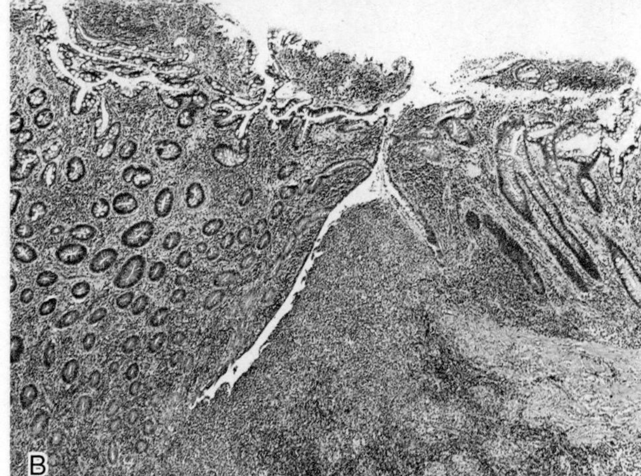

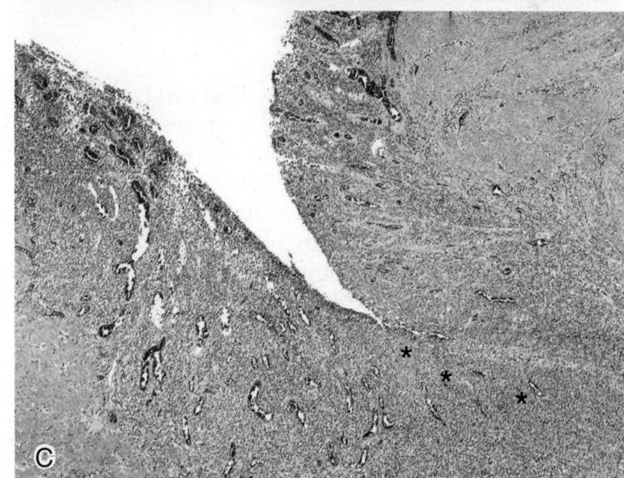

FIGURE 16.25 Crohn's disease and aphthous lesion. A, Aphthous lesions are small erosions that are associated with a neutrophilic infiltrate *(arrow)*. They frequently occur on the surfaces of lymphoglandular complexes. **B,** Early fissures often develop, initially from the base of an aphthous lesion. **C,** An early fissuring ulcer extends into the submucosa.

Nonnecrotizing granulomas are also a characteristic finding in Crohn's disease. Granulomas are found in 50% to 60% of resection specimens [446,470,471] and in approximately 35% of biopsy specimens (Fig. 16.27).[446,471,472] They may be found in any segment of the intestine, including uninvolved areas, and may be located throughout the

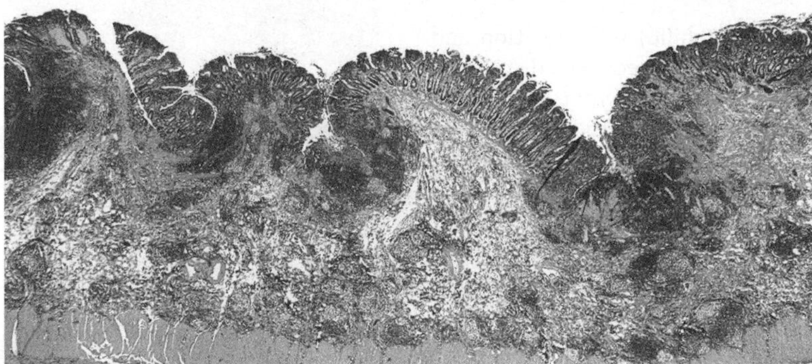

FIGURE 16.26 Crohn's disease. Transmural lymphoid aggregates are a hallmark of Crohn's disease. They frequently have a "string of beads" appearance at the junction of the muscularis propria and the subserosa.

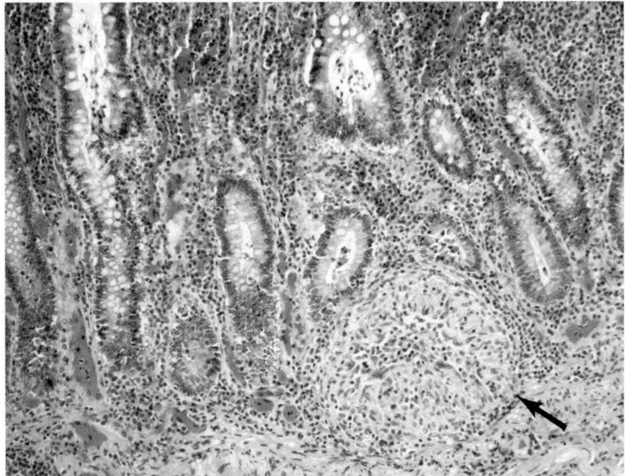

FIGURE 16.27 Crohn's disease. A small collection of epithelioid histiocytes *(arrow)* is seen in this mucosal biopsy.

bowel wall, from mucosa to serosa. Regional lymph nodes contain granulomas in up to 40% of resections.[446,470] Granulomas may vary in size and shape, ranging from small, loose collections of epithelioid cells to large, well-formed granulomas with giant cells. The latter are frequently surrounded by a rim of lymphocytes. Special stains and molecular techniques to identify and exclude infections, especially *Mycobacterium tuberculosis*, should be used in cases with unusual clinical or histological features, or when the granulomas contain evidence of necrosis.[473] Rarely, granulomas in Crohn's disease may show a small amount of central necrosis, and, in that setting, a full infectious workup must be initiated. Care should be taken to not mistake small epithelioid collections associated with damaged crypts as an indication of Crohn's disease. These are essentially foreign body granulomas and may be seen in any crypt injury condition, including in the colon in ulcerative colitis.

Several studies suggest that, in addition to classic granulomas, microaggregates of macrophages within gastric and duodenal mucosa may be a useful marker of Crohn's disease.[474-476] Aggregates of 5 to 10 macrophages not forming recognizable granulomata and identified only by CD68 immunohistochemical stains were present in gastric and duodenal biopsies from patients with Crohn's disease, but not from patients with ulcerative colitis.[476] However, it is unlikely that a definitive diagnosis can be made on the basis of this finding alone.

Vascular changes are common in Crohn's disease. The changes observed in mural vessels include endothelial injury, intimal proliferation, thrombosis, and, rarely, granulomatous or fibrinoid vasculitis.[458,468,477,478] Most of these changes have been observed in arterioles that are located adjacent to or underneath areas of ulceration. Granulomas may also occur in a perivascular distribution. These findings have led some authors to suggest that vasculitis may be an important mechanism of injury in Crohn's disease.[458,477,478]

Risk Factors for Anastomotic Recurrence Following Surgery

Recurrent perianastomotic disease is a significant problem for Crohn's disease patients undergoing resection for strictures and fistulas. While studies have presented conflicting data with respect to the importance of active disease at surgical margins, there appears to be more evidence that the presence of inflammation at either the ileal or colonic margin in ileocolectomy specimens is associated with an increased risk of clinical recurrence.[479,480] The presence of isolated inflammation of nerve plexes (myenteric plexitis) at surgical margins has also received attention as a predictor of recurrence.[481,482] On the other hand, a large study reported that recurrence of Crohn's disease was unaffected by the width of the macroscopic margin of resection or the presence of microscopic disease at margins.[483] Another study found that patients resected for fistulizing disease had an increased risk of early recurrence compared with those resected for strictures.[484] Studies on granulomas reveal conflicting results, with at least one study reporting an association between the presence of granulomas in resections with subsequent recurrent disease.[485] However, a subsequent study correlating the presence of granulomas in resection specimens with outcome found an association with increased extraintestinal manifestations, perianal disease, and younger and female patients, but no correlation between the presence of granulomas and disease progression or recurrence rates.[486] Although the importance of the above factors has not been fully established, pathologists should specifically report the degree of inflammatory changes present at surgical margins in resections performed for Crohn's disease, and also note the presence of granulomas.

TABLE 16.10 Differential Diagnosis of Crohn's Disease in Biopsies of the Small Intestine

	Distinguishing Features
Duodenum	
NSAID injury	Patchy acute inflammation, surface erosion, lack of significant architectural distortion
Peptic duodenitis	Frequently confined to duodenal bulb, often associated with gastric heterotopia, mucous cell metaplasia
Eosinophilic gastroenteritis	Diffuse (not focal) eosinophilic infiltration
Involvement by ulcerative colitis	Diffuse chronic inflammation with architectural distortion, lack of granulomas
Infection	Lack of architectural distortion, lack of features of chronicity
Gluten-sensitive enteropathy	Diffuse increased number of intraepithelial lymphocytosis, villous blunting, absence of acute inflammation
Terminal Ileum	
NSAID injury	Patchy mild acute inflammation, surface erosions, lack of significant architectural distortion, with or without pyloric metaplasia
Backwash ileitis	Patchy mild acute inflammation, distal few centimeters of ileum only, rare ulceration or pyloric metaplasia
Yersinia infection	Associated with lymphadenopathy, suppurative inflammation, necrotizing granulomas
Behçet's disease (rare)	Association with oral and genital ulcers, uveitis, vasculitis, and thrombosis
Vasculitis or ischemia	Mucosal necrosis, "withering" crypts, hyalinization of lamina propria, congestion, hemorrhage, edema; lack of features of chronicity (granulomas, architectural distortion, pyloric metaplasia)

NSAID, *Nonsteroidal antiinflammatory drug.*

Special Considerations for Biopsy Specimens

Terminal Ileum

Although Crohn's disease can usually be specifically diagnosed in resection specimens, evaluation of biopsy specimens from the small intestine may be difficult because of the lack of specificity of the inflammatory changes in small tissue fragments, the lack of deeper portions of bowel wall that would allow assessment of mural inflammation, and the need for close correlation with endoscopic findings, including distribution of gross abnormalities (Table 16.10). The histological features of Crohn's disease in terminal ileal biopsies vary with the severity of disease and the site of biopsy (Fig. 16.28). When cobblestone ulcerations and stricture formation are present, the corresponding biopsies are usually diagnostic or at least consistent with the disease. However, when endoscopic findings are more subtle or consist only of aphthous lesions, the histology may be near normal or entirely nonspecific. In the setting of active disease, characteristic histological features include those of chronicity, such as pseudopyloric metaplasia, crypt and villous architectural changes (atrophy, branching, cystic change), as well as features of activity, including increased acute and chronic inflammation in the lamina propria, neutrophilic cryptitis, crypt abscesses, and surface erosion or ulceration. Granulomas are helpful when present but are found in less than 50% of biopsy specimens. These changes often occur in a patchy or segmental fashion. Distinction from NSAID injury and backwash ileitis in the setting of ulcerative colitis can be challenging (see Differential Diagnosis, later). Detecting fibrosis and other mural changes is not possible in mucosal biopsies.

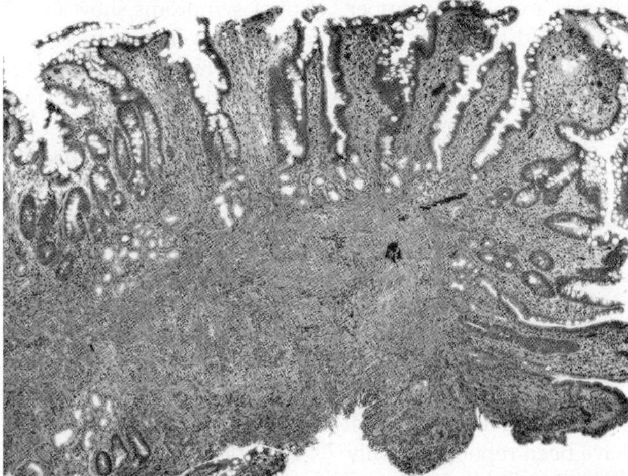

FIGURE 16.28 Crohn's disease. Inflammatory changes in the terminal ileum of a patient with Crohn's disease. Findings include architectural distortion, villous blunting, and increased plasmacellular inflammation. Granulomas are found in only a minority of biopsies.

Duodenal Crohn's Disease

Duodenal involvement in Crohn's disease was previously considered rare (noted in 1% to 7% of cases).[487,488] However, the incidence of involvement is rising, possibly related to the growing use of upper endoscopy as a diagnostic tool. Several studies have highlighted the importance of performing upper endoscopy in patients with suspected inflammatory bowel disease, because of the high incidence of detection of inflammatory changes (up to 81%), even in patients without upper GI symptoms.[489-494] Most patients with involvement of the duodenal bulb also have involvement of the gastric antrum, sometimes in a pattern described as focal active gastritis.[491-493] However, distal duodenal involvement is not always associated with gastric involvement.[478,487,488,495-497] The vast majority of patients with duodenal involvement have distal ileal or colonic disease. Rarely, the duodenum is the only site involved by Crohn's disease.[487,488,497,498] Of interest, inflammatory changes in gastric and duodenal biopsies have also been found in up to 70% of patients with ulcerative colitis (see later).[489,492,494]

The clinical manifestations of proximal small bowel Crohn's disease are similar to those of distal disease. Symptoms are usually related to ulceration and stricture formation and include epigastric pain, hemorrhage, nausea, and vomiting. As mentioned, many patients with Crohn's disease and without upper GI tract symptoms show endoscopic and histological evidence of involvement. In several studies, 24% to 64% of patients with histological involvement of the duodenum or stomach had no upper GI tract symptoms.[488,493,496]

The endoscopic findings of proximal Crohn's disease are variable. Asymptomatic patients frequently have small aphthous lesions or notching of duodenal folds, whereas symptomatic patients may show granularity, a cobblestone mucosal pattern, linear ulcerations, and stricture formation.[488,495,497,499] Scalloping of the duodenal folds, in a manner sometimes found in celiac disease, has also been reported.[500]

Histological findings in the proximal intestine are similar to those with distal disease. Noncaseating granulomas have been reported in only 7% to 15% of duodenal biopsies [488,495,497,501] but in up to 75% of resection specimens from this area.[487] Granulomas may be found in endoscopically normal mucosa as well. Because granulomas are relatively uncommon in proximal small bowel biopsies from patients with Crohn's disease, the diagnosis frequently relies on the presence of other chronic inflammatory changes (Fig. 16.29). These include increased lymphocytes, plasma cells, and eosinophils; basal plasmacytosis; crypt architectural irregularity; and cryptitis and crypt abscesses with or without surface erosions or ulceration. One study of 49 patients reported that acute inflammation within otherwise normal small bowel mucosa was seen only in Crohn's disease, not in *H. pylori*–related gastritis.[501] Diffuse villous blunting is rare, but patchy architectural distortion may be pres ent.[487,488,495-497] The finding of increased IELs with normal villous architecture may also be a manifestation of Crohn's disease.[502,503] However, this finding has numerous associations, including celiac disease, such that a de novo diagnosis of Crohn's disease should not be made on the basis of that finding alone.

To summarize, a diagnosis of duodenal involvement with Crohn's disease relies heavily on the finding of patchy or segmental inflammatory changes, with or without granulomas, in patients without another obvious cause of inflammation (such as peptic injury). Most duodenal biopsies are accompanied by gastric and esophageal biopsies, which allows a more global assessment of inflammatory changes. Finally, it should be remembered that most patients have concomitant distal disease. As a practical guideline, the information gained from upper endoscopy should be correlated with the results of colonoscopy in patients with potential inflammatory bowel disease.

Differential Diagnosis

An increasing number of medications are associated with both small and large intestinal mucosal inflammation and show histological changes that bear similarity to that seen in inflammatory bowel disease (see later section). These include immune checkpoint inhibitors, sartan-related compounds, MMF, and idelalisib.[97,414,417,419,422,426,504]

Because of their widespread use, injury due to NSAIDs is a common concern in the differential diagnosis of ileal Crohn's disease. The pathogenesis of NSAID mucosal injury is multifactorial and includes a direct topical effect, COX inhibition, decreased prostaglandin synthesis, increased cell membrane permeability, and alterations in microbiome.[349]

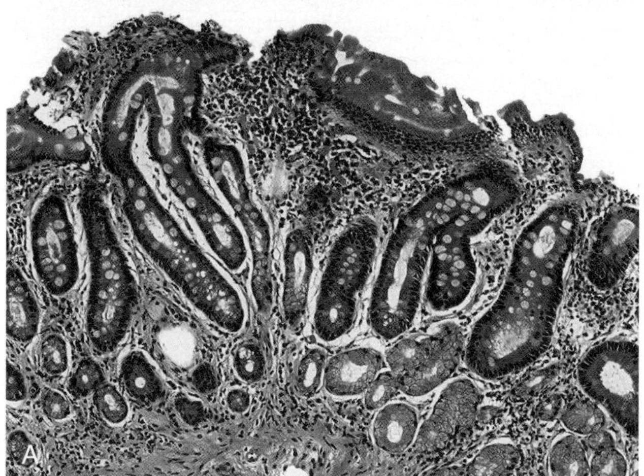

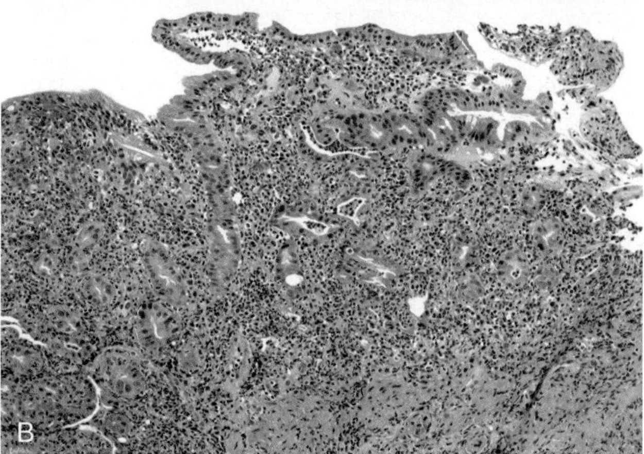

FIGURE 16.29 Crohn's disease. A, Duodenal involvement by Crohn's disease may be difficult to distinguish from peptic or nonsteroidal antiinflammatory drug injury. In this patient with both ileal and gastroduodenal Crohn's disease, mild architectural distortion and increased lamina propria inflammation can be seen. **B,** In this example of duodenal Crohn's disease, active inflammation with marked architectural distortion and crypt abscesses are present.

NSAID-induced injury may resemble Crohn's disease both endoscopically and histologically, as both are associated with aphthous lesions. Severe changes at endoscopy, such as cobblestone mucosa and strictures, and chronic pathological changes such as crypt irregularity and lymphoplasmacytic infiltrates point strongly away from NSAID injury. As a practical guideline, when aphthous lesions are seen as the only endoscopic abnormality in patients taking NSAIDs, it is prudent to recommend a trial of NSAID removal before considering a de novo diagnosis of Crohn's disease (see Table 16.10). Further, aphthous lesions are not infrequently found in asymptomatic patients undergoing screening endoscopy, with or without NSAID use. In a follow-up study of 29 patients with isolated ileitis, including aphthous lesions and even features of chronicity, no patients with asymptomatic ileitis progressed to overt Crohn's disease in a 2-year follow-up period.[505] Continued patient follow-up and close examination of medications in use are needed to determine the clinical significance of this "incidental" finding.

In the ileum, Behçet's disease and vasculitis can mimic Crohn's disease. Behçet's disease of the GI tract is rare in Western countries, occurs primarily in Asians, and is frequently associated with generalized thrombosis and large genital ulcers. This condition can be difficult to distinguish from Crohn's disease on the basis of histological analysis because small erosions and superficial ulcers of the terminal ileum may occur in both diseases. However, strictures and sinus tracts do not occur in Behçet's disease, and clinical information often helps separate these two entities. Other forms of vasculitis can be distinguished from Crohn's disease by the predominantly vascular and perivascular location of the inflammatory response, the presence of ischemic changes, and the clinical history of a generalized vasculitic syndrome. *Yersinia* infection may cause appendicitis and ileocolitis that can resemble Crohn's disease histologically (see Chapter 4).[506,507] Serology, culture, and PCR analysis can be useful to detect *Yersinia* species in suspected patients.

Distal ileitis in patients with ulcerative colitis has received renewed attention that calls into question the theory of "backwash" as the mechanism that leads to ileal inflammation.[508] Original descriptions of backwash ileitis in patients with severe pancolitis may have included patients with Crohn's disease (see also Chapter 17).[509-512] More contemporary studies report ileitis, with both active and chronic mucosal changes, as an occasional finding in ulcerative colitis patients without pancolitis and with only mildly active disease at surveillance colonoscopy.[510,513,514] The term ulcerative colitis–associated ileitis has been proposed to describe the minor inflammatory changes sometimes noted in the ileum at colonoscopy in patients with ulcerative colitis, regardless of the degree of cecal inflammatory activity.[508,513] The concept of extracolonic intestinal involvement in ulcerative colitis is not new, since it is well established that the duodenum and stomach may be affected in this disease (see later). Pathologists and clinicians must evaluate small intestinal inflammation in the context of the entire clinical picture in order to distinguish ulcerative colitis–associated ileitis from Crohn's disease. In general, the endoscopic and histological findings are milder and less extensive in ulcerative colitis-associated ileitis than in Crohn's-related ileitis, with extension beyond 5 cm in length being unusual in the former. Acute inflammation with cryptitis and crypt abscesses is the most common finding in ulcerative colitis–associated ileitis (Fig. 16.30). It was previously believed that crypt distortion and metaplasia precluded a diagnosis of so-called backwash ileitis, but detailed studies of resection specimens have shown that pseudopyloric metaplasia, villous atrophy, and crypt distortion can be seen, rarely, in this setting.[509,510] In a study of 100 newly diagnosed pediatric patients with inflammatory bowel disease with pancolitis and ileitis, detailed histological assessment coupled with clinical data allowed for accurate discrimination between Crohn's disease and ulcerative colitis–associated ileitis.[515] In that study, the presence of crypt distortion, lamina propria expansion, and acute lamina propria inflammation were useful discriminators when combined with clinical data. The clinical significance of ulcerative colitis–associated ileitis is controversial. In one study of 100 consecutive colectomy patients with ulcerative colitis, 22% had ileitis. These patients had a shorter duration of disease, were more likely to have had fulminant colitis, and had a higher frequency of pouchitis.[512] Other studies found no relationship between backwash ileitis and pouchitis.[492,516,517]

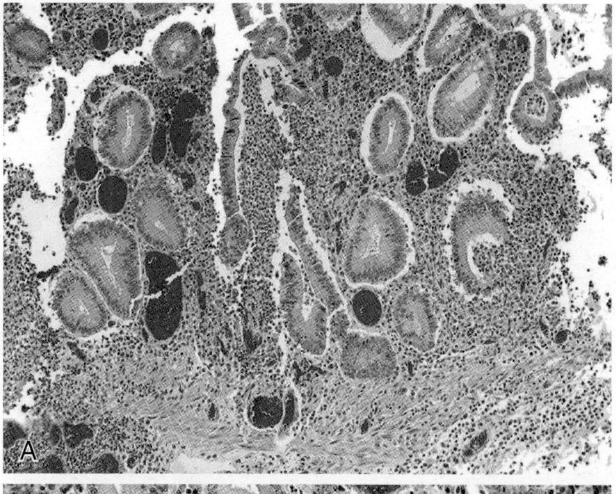

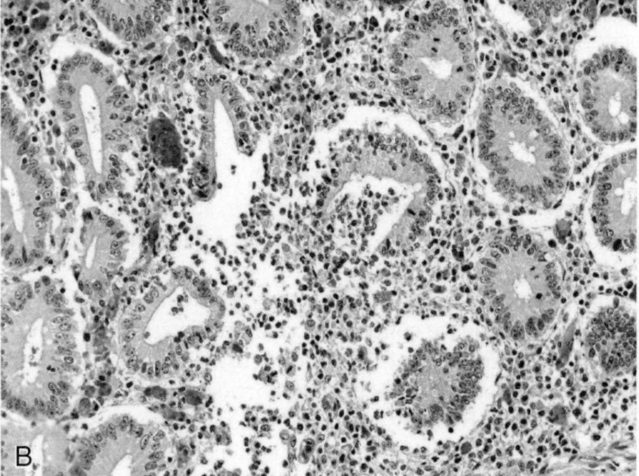

FIGURE 16.30 Ulcerative colitis associated ileitis (backwash ileitis). A, Backwash ileitis consists of a mild influx of neutrophils within the lamina propria or epithelium. The villous architecture is usually normal, although mild distortion has been reported. **B**, High-magnification view illustrating cryptitis and crypt abscesses with reactive epithelial changes.

In the proximal small intestine, mimickers of Crohn's disease include peptic duodenitis, *H. pylori*–associated duodenal inflammation, eosinophilic gastroenteritis, celiac disease, and infectious enteritis (see Table 16.10). NSAID- and other medication-induced injuries are always in the differential diagnosis of duodenal inflammation and ulceration.

Duodenal Involvement by Ulcerative Colitis

Traditionally, ulcerative colitis is viewed as a disease limited to the colon, with only occasional involvement of the contiguous terminal ileum. However, a number of studies have reported the presence of chronic active inflammation in the duodenum and/or stomach in patients with ulcerative col itis.[489,490,503,518-524] These findings were initially reported in pediatric patients, in whom upper GI endoscopy is frequently a routine part of the initial workup for inflammatory bowel disease. Studies have since shown similar upper GI changes in adults as well.[523,525,526] While this finding challenges a basic tenant historically used to distinguish ulcerative colitis from Crohn's disease, upper GI involvement in ulcerative colitis is being increasingly recognized as a unique diagnostic entity with specific clinicopathological

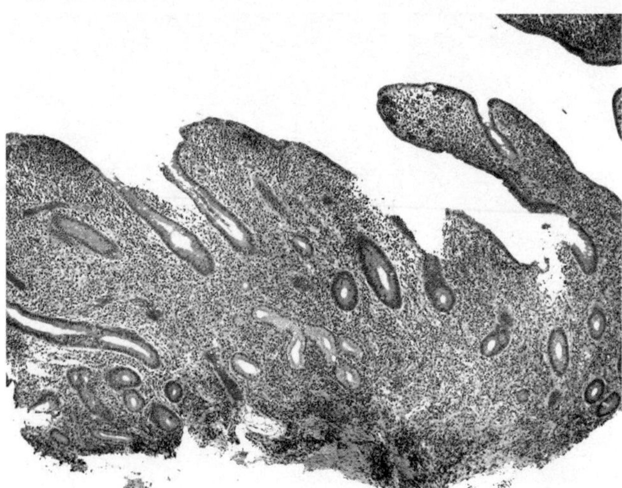

FIGURE 16.31 Diffuse duodenitis in ulcerative colitis. This duodenal biopsy specimen, obtained from a patient with ulcerative colitis, exhibits increased lamina propria plasma cells and an extensive neutrophilic infiltrate. These changes were present diffusely throughout the involved segment. (*Courtesy of Robert Odze, MD, Brigham and Women's Hospital.*)

features. Generally believed to be rare, studies estimate the prevalence of duodenitis in ulcerative colitis patients to be 3% to 7.6%.[492,527,528]

The most distinctive pattern of duodenal injury in the setting of ulcerative colitis, described in several case reports and studies, consists of diffuse mucosal inflammation with crypt and villous architectural distortion, basal plasmacytosis, and crypt abscesses involving the duodenum and, occasionally, the jejunum and ileum (Fig. 16.31; see also Chapter 17).[521,523,526] In one review the term ulcerative colitis–associated enteropathy is proposed to describe these cases.[526] In some patients duodenal inflammation develops only after colectomy and is associated with pouchitis.[523,527,529] One study found duodenitis in 40% of ulcerative colitis patients who had colectomy with subsequent duodenal biopsies.[523] Further, duodenal inflammatory changes were more severe in patients with pancolitis than in patients with only left-sided ulcerative colitis.[530] It has been proposed that patients with ulcerative colitis and diffuse enteritis likely represent a separate category of inflammatory bowel disease that bears more resemblance, overall, to ulcerative colitis than to Crohn's disease.[526]

Ileal–Anal Pouch Inflammation (Pouchitis)

Clinical Features

Pouchitis is a syndrome defined by the presence of inflammation in ileal pouch mucosa, associated with clinical signs and symptoms and endoscopic abnormalities. Many clinicians diagnose pouchitis exclusively on the basis of clinical criteria, reserving endoscopic examination and biopsy for patients with chronic refractory pouchitis or for those with possible Crohn's disease involving the pouch. A common classification scheme based on the duration of symptoms or the response to antibiotics is shown in Table 16.11.[531]

Pouchitis is the most common complication of ileal pouch–anal anastomosis, the procedure of choice for the surgical management of patients with chronic ulcerative colitis.[531-537] Pouchitis occurs almost exclusively in patients with chronic ulcerative colitis and is uncommon in patients who have had an ileal pouch–anal anastomosis procedure for familial adenomatous polyposis.[532,534] Pouchitis has also been reported in Kock's continent ileostomies.

TABLE 16.11 Classification of Idiopathic Pouchitis

Activity	• Active • Inactive
Presentation	• Acute (<4 weeks' duration) • Chronic (>4 weeks' duration)
Clinical pattern	• Single episode • Infrequent (<4 episodes/year) • Relapsing (>4 episodes/year) • Continuous
Response to antibiotics	• Antibiotic responsive: Infrequent episodes (<4/year) responding to a 2-week course of a single antibiotic • Antibiotic dependent: Frequent or persistent episodes requiring long-term, continuous therapy for maintaining remission • Chronic antibiotic refractory: No response to 4-week course of metronidazole or ciprofloxacin. Requires prolonged therapy of at least 4 weeks, consisting of 2 or more antibiotics, oral or topical 5-ASA, corticosteroids, AZA/6-MP, or biologics

5-ASA, 5-aminosalicylates; AZA, *azathioprine;* 6-MP, *6-mercaptopurine.*
Modified from Shah H, Zezos P. Pouchitis: diagnosis and management. Curr Opin Gastroenterol. *2020, 36:41-47.*

Approximately 50% of patients who have had an ileal pouch–anal anastomosis procedure experience at least one episode of pouchitis. The incidence of pouchitis decreases proportionally with the length of follow-up, ranging from 23% to 46% over 10 years.[531] The incidence of pouchitis decreases dramatically after the first 6 months after surgery. In one study, the risk of pouchitis was 80% at 1 year after surgery and 48% at 10 years after surgery.[533] Despite the high incidence of pouchitis, pouch excision is necessary in less than 1% of patients.[535]

Patients with pouchitis usually present with an increased frequency of bowel movements (with or without bloody diarrhea), tenesmus, low-grade fever, malaise, and anorexia. Occasionally, patients develop anal fissures, perianal abscesses, strictures, and fistulas, all of which should raise a strong suspicion for Crohn's disease involving the pouch.

Pathogenesis

A variety of risk factors have been associated with the development of pouchitis.[538,539] Some of these include greater extent and severity of inflammation in the colon, the presence of extraintestinal manifestations, tobacco smoking, serum positivity for antineutrophil cytoplasmic antibodies, and the presence of primary sclerosing cholangitis. Studies also suggest that severe pan-ulcerative colitis and the presence of appendicitis associated with chronic ulcerative colitis may also increase the risk of development of pouchitis after surgery.[539] Whether ulcerative colitis–associated ileitis and gastroduodenitis are associated with the development

BOX 16.8 Classification of Pouchitis

Idiopathic pouchitis
Secondary pouchitis
- Infectious
  - Bacterial: *Clostridium difficile, Campylobacter jejuni, Salmonella typhi, Escherichia coli, Klebsiella* sp., *Pseudomonas*
  - Fungal: *Candida*
  - Viruses: cytomegalovirus
- Ischemic
  - NSAID associated
  - Autoimmune associated
  - Crohn's disease
  - Cuffitis
  - Irritable pouch syndrome

Modified from Shah H, Zezos P. Pouchitis: diagnosis and management. Curr Opin Gastroenterol. *2020;36:41-47.*

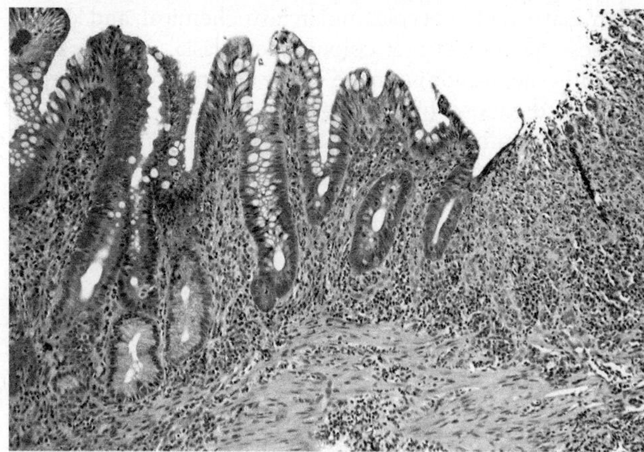

FIGURE 16.32 Chronic idiopathic pouchitis in a patient who underwent an ileal pouch–anal anastomosis procedure for severe pan-ulcerative colitis. The biopsy specimen shows acute and chronic inflammation, villous atrophy, ulceration, and a focus of pseudopyloric metaplasia.

of pouchitis is unsettled. Genetic associations include the *TLR9-1237C* and *CD14-260T* alleles, and polymorphisms in *IL1RN* and *NOD2*.[540-542]

While the etiology of pouchitis is not completely delineated, bacterial dysbiosis (alterations in pouch microbes) has emerged as a leading factor in the pathogenesis of so-called idiopathic pouchitis (Box 16.8).[531,535,543,544] It is thought that changes in the quantity and type of luminal microbiota induce or exacerbate the mucosal immune response in susceptible individuals.[531,545,546] Additional factors include infection with specific pathogens such as C. *difficile* and cytomegalovirus (CMV), ischemic complications, decreased availability of short-chain fatty acids, altered immunity, NSAID use, and Crohn's disease.[531,536,537,547]

Pathological Features

Grossly, the most frequent findings in pouchitis are erythema, edema, granularity and friability, loss of vascular pattern, hemorrhage, and superficial erosions and ulcerations. Rarely, pseudomembranes may develop. The presence of fissures, fistulas, sinus tracts, and deep bear claw ulcers or fissuring ulcers should raise a strong suspicion for Crohn's disease.

Microscopically, pouchitis may be classified as active, chronic, or chronic-active. Typical findings include mixed neutrophilic and lymphocytic infiltrates in the lamina propria and epithelium, with or without erosions or ulcerations.[535,548,549] Mild to moderate villous atrophy is common. However, severe cases may show complete villous atrophy. Chronic changes, such as crypt and villous distortion; pseudopyloric metaplasia; crypt hyperplasia; expansion of the lamina propria by inflammation composed of lymphocytes, eosinophils, plasma cells, and histiocytes; and Paneth cell hyperplasia are common in severe cases and particularly in recurrent cases (Fig. 16.32). Granulomas, either necrotizing or more commonly nonnecrotizing, may be present and do not necessarily indicate a diagnosis of Crohn's disease, since granulomas may be related to mucin, foreign material (e.g., sutures), and infectious agents. Moreover, transmural inflammation in resected pouches is not pathognomonic for Crohn's disease of the pouch. In one study, 30% of patients resected for chronic antibiotic-refractory pouchitis (not Crohn's disease of the pouch) had transmural inflammation in resection specimens.[550] Rarely, dysplasia and even adenocarcinoma may develop in pouch mucosa.[551] A pouchitis disease activity index has been developed that combines information from clinical, endoscopic, and histological findings, but it is not widely used in clinical practice.[552] It has been subsequently shown that histology has a somewhat limited role in grading pouchitis, when compared with endoscopic and clinical scoring.[553] However, biopsies are useful in evaluating the presence of specific pathogens, ischemia, and dysplasia.

In considering a diagnosis of pouchitis, pathologists should be aware that most ileal pouches undergo an early adaptive response to the new luminal environment. This is characterized by mild neutrophilic and eosinophilic inflammatory infiltrates in the lamina propria, partial villous atrophy, Paneth cell hyperplasia, and a partial transition to a colonic mucin phenotype characterized by an increase in sulfomucins.[554] These changes should not be misinterpreted as indicative of pouchitis in the absence of appropriate clinical symptoms or signs.

Differential Diagnosis

The differential diagnosis of pouchitis includes ischemia, infection, and Crohn's disease.[535] Features of ischemia in pouch mucosa are similar to those observed in other portions of the GI tract (see Chapter 11) and usually develop within a short time after surgery. Infections, such as with *Shigella*, *E. coli*, *Salmonella*, or *Clostridium*, can induce histological features similar to those of chronic idiopathic pouchitis, but these infectious agents are usually identified by stool culture. CMV infection may occur if patients are significantly immunocompromised. Crohn's disease involving the pouch should be considered in cases that contain nonnecrotizing granulomas, deep ulcers, sinus tracts, fistulas, or fissures. In these cases, examination of the patient's prior colectomy specimen is essential, in order to search for subtle changes of Crohn's disease. Other less frequent causes of pouch dysfunction should also be considered before definitive treatment. These include pelvic sepsis, inflammation of the retained cuff of rectal mucosa (referred to as cuffitis), and anastomotic strictures. Finally, because most ileal pouches develop early and persistent morphological, inflammatory, phenotypic, mucin histochemical, and kinetic changes characteristic of colonic metaplasia, a diagnosis of pouchitis should not be made in the absence of appropriate clinical and endoscopic findings.

Chronic inflammation of the ileum proximal to the pouch, so called pre-pouch ileitis, has been described in patients who underwent colectomy for chronic ulcerative colitis.[555] In one study, 15 patients with chronic ulcerative colitis, verified by reexamination of colectomy specimens and clinical data, developed contiguous ileal inflammation from 1 to 50 cm proximal to the ileal pouch. Only half had concomitant pouchitis. Other features of Crohn's disease were absent, and patients responded variably to antibiotics. Although the etiology is unknown, pre-pouch ileitis may represent a distinct entity with features more similar to pouchitis than to Crohn's disease. A second study found that pre-pouch ileal ulcers were associated with NSAID use in some patients.[556]

Treatment

The first line of treatment of pouchitis is antibiotics. Anti-inflammatory agents and steroids are typically used for antibiotic-resistant cases. Immunosuppressive agents, such as azathioprine and infliximab, may be used for long-term maintenance therapy. Finally, surgical excision of the pouch should be considered when all available drugs have failed (chronic antibiotic-resistant pouchitis).[536]

ISCHEMIC DISORDERS OF THE SMALL INTESTINE

The intestines are supported by a rich anastomosing network of blood vessels that originate from three main vessels: the celiac artery, the superior mesenteric artery, and the inferior mesenteric artery.[557] The small intestine derives its blood supply almost exclusively from the superior mesenteric artery and its branches, although the first portion of the duodenum is also frequently supplied by a branch of the hepatic artery. Because of the extensive network of communicating vessels, vascular insufficiency of the small intestine does not usually occur until there has been severe compromise in blood flow or the patient has underlying medical conditions that contribute to vascular injury, such as hypotension, sepsis, collagen vascular disease, vasculitis, severe atherosclerosis, or chronic radiation.[558]

Injury in intestinal ischemia occurs via two mechanisms. The first is deprivation of oxygen that is needed for normal cellular metabolism.[559] The second is reperfusion injury that occurs when blood flow is reestablished to a previously anoxic region.[560] This process results in the generation of superoxide radicals that increase the permeability of capillaries and other cell membranes. Implicit in reperfusion injury is a transient loss of blood flow. Hence, reperfusion injury does not account for the changes seen in bowel infarcts after acute vascular occlusion but does lead to additional injury if the patient survives the initial ischemic insult and blood flow is reestablished.

Ischemic injury can result from an array of conditions, and the outcome is variable, depending on its severity, the abruptness of onset of oxygen deprivation, the length of bowel involved, and the length of time of the disruption (Box 16.9) (see Chapter 11 for details).[559-564] Most of the entities listed in Box 16.9 are described in other chapters. In this chapter, three causes of ischemia are discussed: acute mesenteric insufficiency, focal segmental ischemia, and neonatal necrotizing enterocolitis.

BOX 16.9 Causes of Vascular Insufficiency of the Small Intestine

- Occlusive
  - Embolic
    - Superior mesenteric artery
  - Thrombotic
    - Superior mesenteric artery
    - Superior mesenteric vein
- Low flow
  - Low cardiac output
  - Hypotension/shock
- Mechanical
  - Hernia
  - Volvulus (including Meckel diverticulum)
  - Trauma
- Hypercoagulable states
  - Disseminated intravascular coagulation
  - Clotting disorders
- Infections
  - Neonatal necrotizing enterocolitis
  - Bacterial infections (clostridial)
- Collagen vascular diseases
- Vasculitis
- Radiation injury
- Drugs
  - Potassium chloride
  - Digitalis
  - Vasopressor agents
  - Oral contraceptives

Acute Mesenteric Insufficiency

Acute disruption of mesenteric blood flow is a catastrophic condition associated with a high mortality rate secondary to infarction and perforation of the intestines.

Causes

The four main causes of mesenteric insufficiency are embolism, arterial thrombosis, nonocclusive (low-flow) ischemia, and mesenteric vein thrombosis.[559,561,563-568]

Embolism accounts for 25% to 30% of acute intestinal ischemia.[561,563,564] The majority of emboli arise from the heart in the setting of atrial fibrillation. Other sources of emboli include left ventricular thrombi, valve vegetations, and atheromatous plaques in the aorta. The clinical presentation is that of acute abdominal pain, usually in a patient with a history of a cardiac abnormality. Vomiting and bloody diarrhea ensue as tissue injury progresses from reversible ischemia to frank infarction. Peritoneal signs and shock indicate transmural necrosis. Treatment usually consists of emergency embolectomy and resection of the infarcted bowel segment.[569-571]

Arterial thrombosis accounts for 10% to 15% of cases of acute mesenteric ischemia.[561,563,564] This syndrome occurs in the setting of severe atherosclerosis of the superior mesenteric artery, typically at its origin, and may be temporally related to episodes of low blood flow. The clinical presentation is often milder than ischemia resulting from embolism, with intermittent, mild to moderate abdominal pain, or even a complete absence of symptoms, until frank infarction develops.

Nonocclusive mesenteric ischemia occurs in patients with low cardiac output and low mesenteric blood flow.[561,563,564,572] Predisposing factors include congestive heart failure, preexisting peripheral vascular disease, and, potentially, use of cardiac glycosides such as digitalis (because of their vasoconstrictive action). Once again, the severity of symptoms is variable. However, once significant tissue ischemia occurs, the syndrome is identical to that of mesenteric artery occlusion.

Mesenteric vein thrombosis causes fewer than 10% of cases of acute intestinal ischemia.[561,563,564] This condition occurs in a variety of clinical settings, such as trauma, hypercoagulable states, portal vein thrombosis, low-flow states, intraabdominal sepsis, neoplasms, and mechanical bowel obstruction. Symptoms are often subtle and of long duration before frank infarction occurs.

Pathological Features

Gross Pathology

The length of the small intestine affected in acute mesenteric ischemia depends primarily on the point of occlusion of the affected vessel or the severity of loss of cardiac output, and the length of time before embolectomy or thrombectomy is performed.[467,559,573] For example, an embolus lodged at the origin of the superior mesenteric artery will result in infarction of the entire small bowel, from the ligament of Treitz to the splenic flexure of the colon, if not removed expeditiously.

Evidence of ischemia or infarction may be diffuse and confluent, or patchy and multifocal. The serosal aspect often appears congested and blue-black in color (Fig. 16.33). Perforation may be present, but it may not be accompanied by a well-developed fibrinous exudate if the resection occurred shortly after clinical presentation. Pneumatosis intestinalis may be present.[574] In arterial occlusions, the mesentery may appear pale, whereas in venous thrombosis, the mesentery is usually congested and hemorrhagic. There is typically an abrupt demarcation between uninvolved and involved segments of bowel.[561,564] The intestinal lumen is invariably filled with blood. The mucosal surface appears beefy red, boggy, and ulcerated and may contain irregularly protruding islands of mucosa. This mucosal appearance gives rise to the characteristic thumbprinting sign commonly seen on abdominal radiographs of patients with this condition. Pseudomembranes may also be present. Transmural hemorrhage may be seen, and the wall may be friable and thin. In mesenteric vein thrombosis, thrombi may be visible in mesenteric veins on gross examination.[573]

Microscopic Pathology

Microscopically, features of arterial ischemia are similar throughout the GI tract.[575] The earliest changes occur in the mucosa, but occasionally the submucosa is affected first in animal models.[575,576] Characteristically, the mucosa shows loss of epithelium, which occurs progressively from the villous tips to the base of the crypts (sometimes referred to as withering crypts) and is associated with edema and congestion. The lamina propria often reveals deposition of pink proteinaceous material as a result of "leaky" blood vessels. Within hours of the injury, neutrophils flow into the damaged area. Experimental studies have shown that early histological changes in ischemia consist of hemorrhage, congestion, and edema of the submucosa, sometimes associated with preservation of the overlying mucosa. Submucosal changes may then lead to various degrees of mucosal necrosis, with or without ulceration, luminal hemorrhage, and pseudomembrane deposition (Fig. 16.34).[467,575] Depending on the extent and severity of occlusion, mucosal changes may recover to normal if the ischemic insult is halted. However, if recovery occurs after a more persistent or severe episode, tissue healing may result in fibrosis and stricture formation.[575] In the acute setting, there is typically an absence of a chronic inflammatory response, although neutrophils may be seen if enough time has elapsed since the onset of the occlusion.

In resections, infarcted segments reveal coagulative necrosis and hemorrhage. Examination of mesenteric vessels

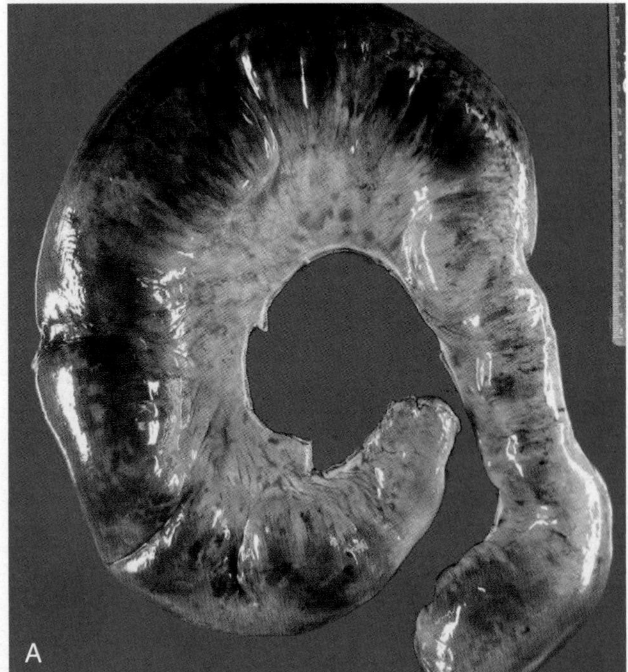

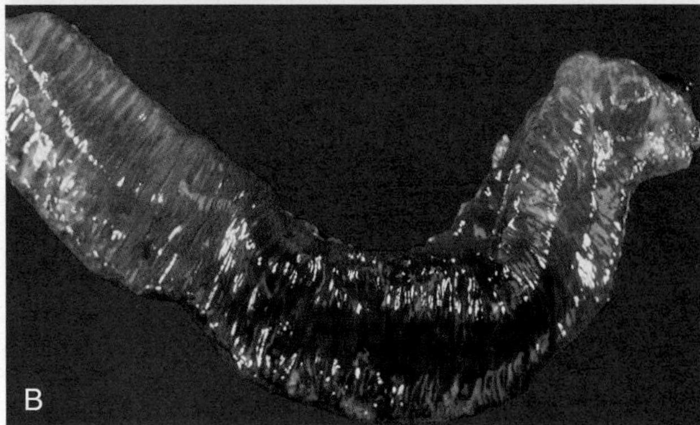

FIGURE 16.33 Ischemia. A, In this example of superior mesenteric artery embolism, a large segment of jejunum is infarcted. The serosal surface is intensely congested and hemorrhagic. **B,** This specimen illustrates focal, segmental infarction, such as might occur with an incarcerated hernia. (**A** *courtesy of Brian West, MD, Yale University.*)

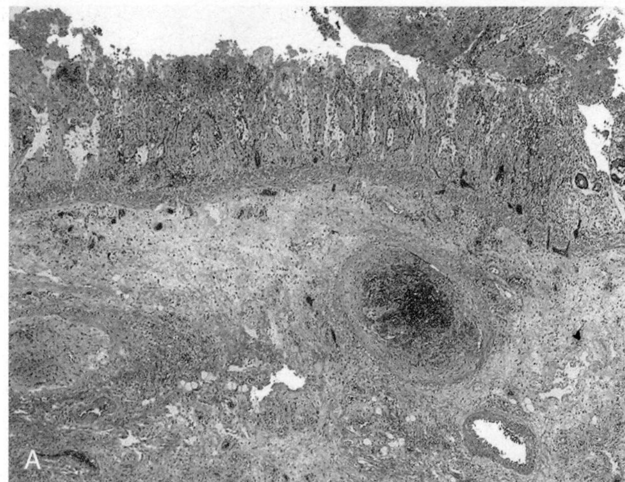

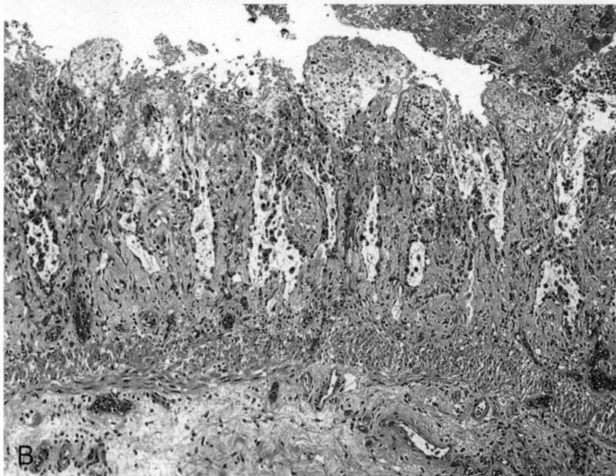

FIGURE 16.34 Ischemia. A, Transmural infarction resulting from ischemia. **B,** High-power view reveals surface epithelial necrosis with focal crypt preservation. There is a fibrinous neutrophilic exudate on the surface.

may be confusing because thrombi may develop acutely as a response to stasis and congestion. Clinically significant thrombi show evidence of organization, which implies their presence over a significant period of time. Fibrin thrombi may be present in small arterioles in areas of necrosis and do not, by themselves, indicate vasculitis or a hypercoagulable state.

Focal Segmental Ischemia

Vascular compromise that involves short segments of intestine is clinically less severe than the global insults just discussed. Focal segmental ischemia may result from atheroemboli lodging in smaller vessel branches, trauma, or mechanical abnormalities, such as bands and adhesions, incarcerated hernias, volvulus, intussusception, neoplasms, and congenital anomalies.[561,565,566,577,578] The gross and microscopic findings of focal segmental ischemia are similar to acute mesenteric insufficiency. The main difference is that in focal segmental ischemia, smaller lengths of intestine are involved and a spectrum of changes may occur, ranging from mild reversible disease to chronic irreversible injury.[577]

Neonatal Necrotizing Enterocolitis

Neonatal necrotizing enterocolitis occurs in premature infants during the first week of life and affects the colon and terminal ileum.[579] The pathogenesis is related to ischemia and subsequent infection of the bowel.[580] The hallmark radiological and pathological findings include pneumatosis intestinalis and ischemic necrosis of the bowel wall. This disorder is discussed in greater detail in Chapters 10 and 17.

CRYPTOGENIC MULTIFOCAL ULCERATING STENOSING ENTERITIS

Cryptogenic multifocal ulcerating stenosing enteritis (CMUSE) is a term used to describe a rare and poorly understood entity of the jejunum and ileum that is characterized by the presence of multiple small intestinal strictures that often require surgical intervention or therapy with steroids (or both).[581-585] The typical presenting symptoms described in case reports and small series are abdominal pain, intermittent obstruction, vomiting, and weight loss.[586,587] A retrospective study of 20 patients with a histopathological diagnosis of CMUSE showed that most patients had characteristic radiological features, including multiple short strictures and shallow ulcers of the small intestine, typically without significant obstruction.[588] CMUSE is also associated with endoscopy capsule retention.[589] There has been no association with any of the other forms of inflammatory bowel disease, and affected patients have not used NSAIDs. Some patients have autoimmune disorders, and one case associated with type I C2 deficiency has been reported.[582] More recently, in one reported series, 3 of 12 patients showed abnormalities of jejunal or ileal arteries on angiography, consisting of stenoses and aneurysms, suggesting a variant of polyarteritis nodosa.[583] The lack of association of this entity with Crohn's disease or ulcerative colitis and its association with only minimal inflammation and occasional vascular abnormalities have led investigators to postulate that CMUSE is an independent entity, possibly a form of vasculitis.[590] A singular association with an X-linked reticulate pigmentary disorder has been reported.[591] In one study of two siblings with CMUSE, genome-wide single-nucleotide polymorphism homozygosity mapping found an association with the *PLA2G4A* gene.[592]

The pathology of CMUSE is characteristic. Resection specimens typically reveal numerous (as many as 25) short stenoses separated by several centimeters of normal intestine. Central ulceration in areas of stenosis is common. On microscopic examination, fibrinous exudates are observed in the mucosa and are associated with a modest infiltrate of mixed acute and chronic inflammatory cells in the mucosa and submucosa (Fig. 16.35). In some patients, eosinophils are also prominent. Inflammation is normally limited to areas of stenosis, which show submucosal fibrosis. The muscularis propria and subserosal layers are typically normal. No definite arteritis has been described in resection specimens. However, several cases with focal phlebitis and thrombosis of small venules have been described.[583]

The main differential diagnosis is diaphragm disease resulting from NSAID use, although in some instances a positive history of NSAID use is the only way to distinguish these two entities.[587]

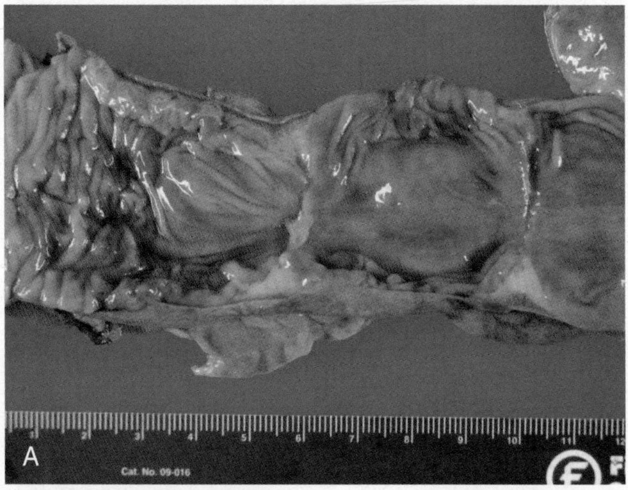

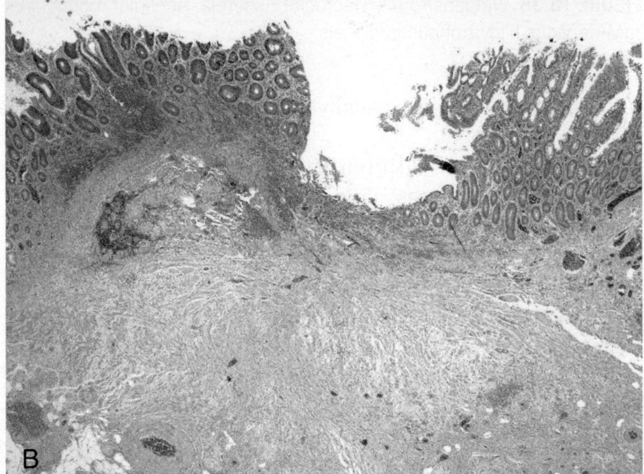

FIGURE 16.35 Cryptogenic multifocal ulcerating and stenosing enteritis (CMUSE). A, Gross photograph of resection specimen shows multiple discrete small bowel strictures. **B,** Low-power view of the small intestine taken from an area of stricture reveals mucosal ulceration with submucosal fibrosis. The muscularis propria *(not shown)* is unaffected.

GRAFT-VERSUS-HOST DISEASE

Acute and chronic GVHD occurs in the setting of stem cell transplantation and, rarely, solid organ transplantation.[593] In this disorder, donor cytotoxic T lymphocytes incite an immunological reaction to certain host cells. The GI tract, along with skin and liver, is a common site of injury.[594] Approximately 10% to 40% of patients who undergo stem cell transplantation develop acute GVHD, and endoscopic biopsies and histological examination are a mainstay in the assessment of patients presenting with digestive symptoms in the post–stem cell transplant period.[595,596] The disease usually involves the colon more severely than the small intestine, and the colon is a reliable area to survey for the presence of disease.[597,598] Nevertheless, when involved, the small intestine demonstrates characteristic findings. Epithelial apoptosis, gland destruction and loss, mild villous blunting, and surface erosions develop and are associated with GI symptoms (Fig. 16.36).[595,599] The histological changes of GVHD are not entirely specific, and disorders such as infection, drug-related injury (in particular mycophenolate mofetil), ischemia, and rarely inflammatory bowel disease

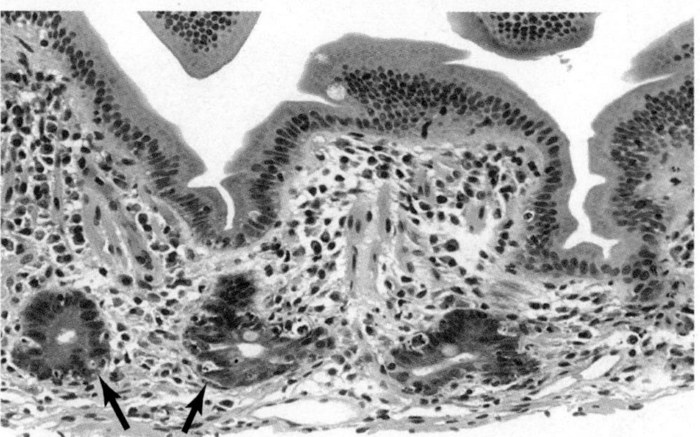

FIGURE 16.36 Graft-versus-host disease (GVHD). This biopsy specimen shows mild GVHD characterized by an increased number of apoptotic epithelial cells in the crypts *(arrows)*. No increase is seen in the amount of inflammation.

are part of the differential diagnosis.[595] This disorder is discussed in more detail in Chapter 5.

INTESTINAL LYMPHANGIECTASIA

Lymphangiectasia can be primary or secondary; the latter condition is more common.

Primary Lymphangiectasia

Primary intestinal lymphangiectasia (Waldmann's disease) is a rare congenital disorder that is characterized by severe protein loss (protein-losing enteropathy), peripheral edema, steatorrhea, chylous effusion, and lymphocytopenia. [600-605] The basis for this disease is a profound structural abnormality of the lymphatic system that consists of dilation and tortuosity of lymphatic channels resulting in lymph stasis in the intestinal tract. The disease onset is variable but primarily affects children and young adults.[606,607] Lymphangiectasia can be diffuse or localized. Endoscopically, the characteristic finding is the presence of punctate white spots. Histologically, the small bowel shows dilated lymphatic channels within the small intestinal mucosa. The etiology of primary intestinal lymphangiectasia remains unknown. Secondary causes of intestinal lymphangiectasia should be excluded. This condition is discussed extensively in Chapter 9.

Secondary Lymphangiectasia

The term *secondary lymphangiectasia* refers to the presence of diffusely dilated lymphatics that is not associated with protein-losing enteropathy but is related to a local inflammatory or neoplastic process. Conditions associated with secondary lymphangiectasia include lymphoma, carcinoma, Crohn's disease, systemic lupus erythematosus, Behçet's syndrome, chronic pancreatitis, radiation therapy, trauma, heart disease, hematological malignancies, and prior liver transplantation.[608-616] Rarely, there is no detectable underlying condition.[609] Clinical correlation with patient age and severity of symptoms allows the distinction between primary and secondary forms, and all causes of the secondary form should be excluded before

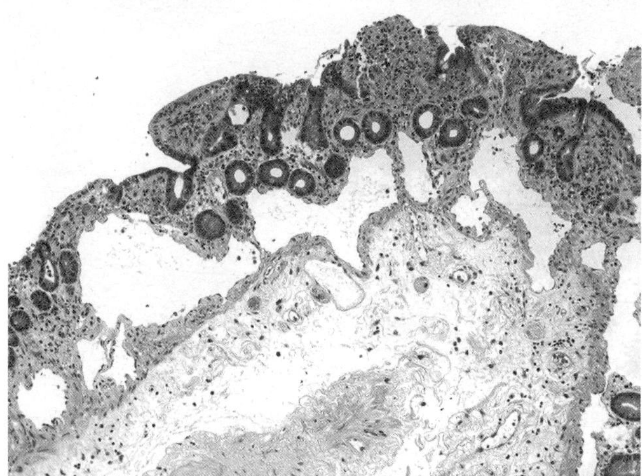

FIGURE 16.37 Secondary lymphangiectasia. Endoscopically, small white nodules may be seen that exude white fluid on biopsy. Dilated lymphatic channels are present in the mucosa and are lined by endothelial cells. Occasional dilated mucosal lymphatics are also a frequent finding in otherwise normal mucosa and are usually of no clinical significance.

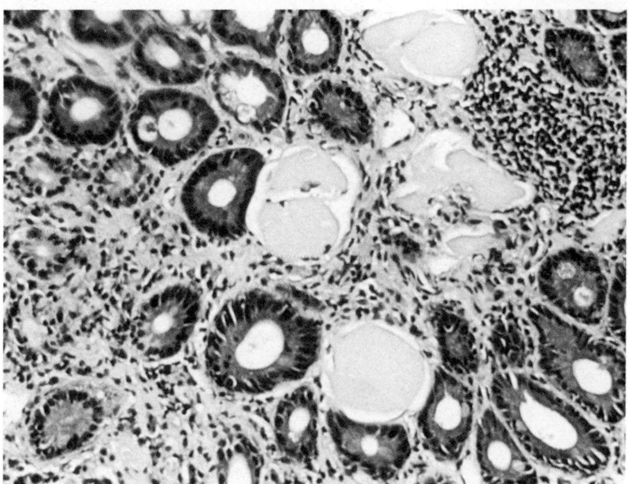

FIGURE 16.38 Waldenström's macroglobulinemia. Acellular monoclonal IgM deposits fill lymphatic channels.

a consideration of primary intestinal lymphangiectasia is established. Although secondary lymphangiectasia is not typically associated with malabsorption, protein-losing enteropathy has been reported in patients with secondary lymphangiectasia in association with heart disease (e.g., constrictive pericarditis) and after liver transplantation.[608,609] The diagnosis of lymphangiectasia is based on endoscopic features and corresponding pathological findings on histological examination of the small bowel, either in a biopsy or resection specimen.

Pathological Features

The endoscopic appearance of secondary lymphangiectasia is variable, and the distribution of lesions depends on the underlying cause.[617] Affected areas may show white dots, corresponding to dilated mucosal lacteals, or larger white nodules or plaques that leak chylous material when biopsied. Diffusely edematous jejunal mucosa with finger-like projections have been noted on capsule endoscopy and at resection.[608,609,613] Cystic mass lesions may be present within the mesentery or wall of the intestine.

Microscopically, dilated lymphatic channels lined by endothelium may be seen in the superficial and deep mucosa and may extend throughout the bowel wall (Fig. 16.37). The dilated structures may appear empty or may contain faintly eosinophilic proteinaceous material. Frequently, no associated inflammatory changes are seen. The major importance of recognizing mucosal lymphangiectasia in small intestinal biopsies is to alert the clinician to the possibility of an underlying malignancy.

Differential Diagnosis

The differential diagnosis of lymphangiectasia includes Waldenström's macroglobulinemia and pneumatosis intestinalis. Immunoglobulin deposits in macroglobulinemia are densely eosinophilic, unlike the proteinaceous material seen in dilated lymphatics. Immunohistochemical stains for IgM can also help distinguish these two entities. The cysts in pneumatosis intestinalis lack a clearly defined endothelial lining and instead are usually lined by foreign body giant cells.

In addition to differentiating lymphangiectasia from other specific diseases, care should be taken not to overinterpret the finding of focally dilated lymphatics, which are often present in mucosal biopsies in the normal population. In addition, tissue artefact may lead to the creation of a space (probably representing trapped air) immediately beneath the epithelial basement membrane of small bowel villi that can be mistaken for a dilated lymphatic. False spaces can be distinguished from true lymphatic vessels by the lack of an endothelial lining in the former.

WALDENSTRÖM'S MACROGLOBULINEMIA

Waldenström's macroglobulinemia is a rare and indolent lymphoproliferative disorder characterized by neoplastic B cells with plasmacytic differentiation and the production and deposition of monoclonal IgM throughout the body, resulting in hyperviscosity syndrome.[618] Lymphoplasmacytic lymphoma is the most common underlying disease, although other IgM-producing lymphomas and plasma cell dyscrasias can lead to this syndrome. Patients develop diarrhea and malabsorption secondary to IgM deposits in mucosal lymphatics.[619,620] Symptoms of intestinal involvement vary from mild to severe and are sometimes the presenting complaint that ultimately leads to the correct diagnosis.

The endoscopic appearance of the small intestine is of numerous gray to white granular mucosal nodules.[621] On microscopy, a variable degree of "clubbing" and blunting of villi is seen, combined with a mildly increased lymphoplasmacellular infiltrate. The most striking histological finding is the deposition of acellular, eosinophilic material within lymphatic channels in the tips of villi and in the base of the mucosa (Fig. 16.38).[621-623] Foamy macrophages are also frequently present in the lamina propria. Occasional atypical lymphocytes may be seen as well.[619,620] Macroglobulinemia may be associated with diffuse lymphangiectasia, which in turn may cause malabsorption and protein-losing enteropathy. The amorphous deposits are PAS positive, diastase resistant, and Congo red negative and may be focally

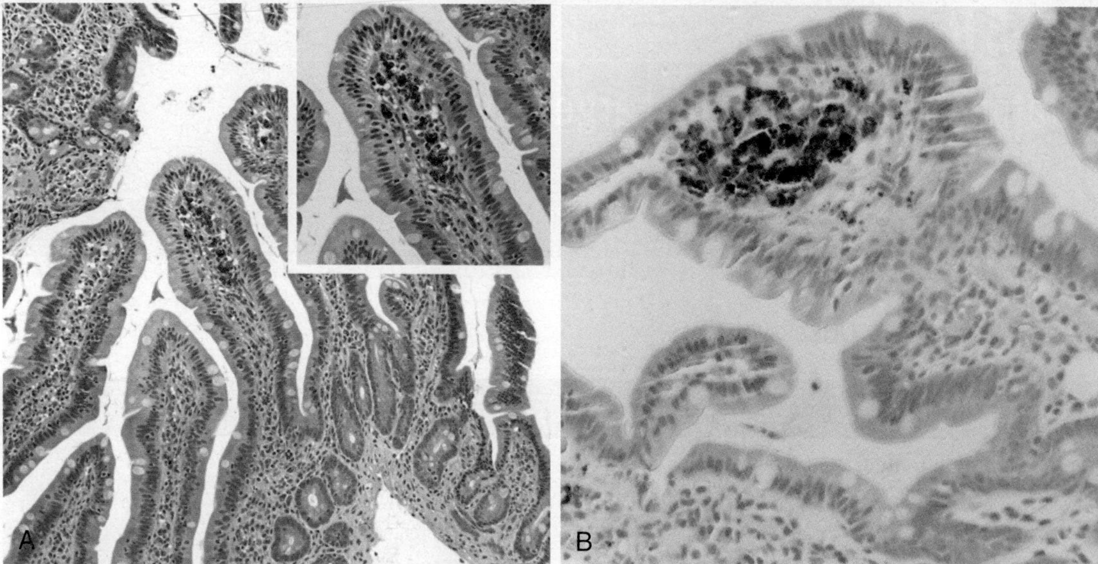

FIGURE 16.39 Pseudomelanosis duodeni. A, Dark brown pigment is seen within the lamina propria of duodenal villi. *Inset* shows detail of pigment. **B,** Iron stain of pseudomelanosis duodeni shows variable positivity.

positive with oil red O. Immunohistochemical stains reveal strong diffuse positivity for IgM, with light-chain restriction.[620] Deposits show a mixture of granular electron-dense material and lipid droplets on electron microscopy.[620] Amyloid and collagen fibrils are not normally present.

The differential diagnosis of Waldenström's macroglobulinemia in mucosal biopsies includes amyloidosis (which tends to accumulate around vessels and can be distinguished by Congo red stains), lymphangiectasia (which lacks the densely eosinophilic material within the lymphatic spaces), Whipple's disease, and *Mycobacterium avium-intracellulare* infection (both of which can be distinguished by stains for organisms, electron microscopy, and PCR), and any other disorder that leads to macrophage accumulation.

PNEUMATOSIS CYSTOIDES INTESTINALIS

The term *pneumatosis cystoides intestinalis* refers to the accumulation of gas-filled cysts within the wall of the intestine. It may occur at any site in the GI tract but is most common in the small intestine.[624,625] The pathogenesis is not well understood, and the clinical relevance varies greatly, from benign pneumatosis to life-threatening complications. It typically occurs in the setting of an underlying intestinal disease, such as inflammatory bowel disease, neonatal necrotizing enterocolitis, infectious colitis or enteritis, or diverticulosis. Recent publications have also reported an association with repeat upper endoscopy procedures, connective tissue diseases or autoimmune diseases, and drugs.[626-631] Additional reports have linked the development of pneumatosis intestinalis to the use of targeted chemotherapeutic agents, such as the antiepidermal growth factor receptor inhibitor osimertinib or the monoclonal antibody bevacizumab.[632,633] It also occurs in association with a variety of systemic diseases (e.g., cystic fibrosis, chronic obstructive lung disease, cirrhosis).[634,635] Pathologically, the entity is characterized by the presence of empty cysts lined by macrophages and giant cells within the submucosa and subserosa.

PSEUDOMELANOSIS DUODENI

Pseudomelanosis of the small intestine, most commonly involving the duodenum, is a rare finding during upper endoscopy.

Clinical Features

Patients with pseudomelanosis duodeni are detected incidentally during endoscopic examination of the upper GI tract.[636-640] The classic endoscopic appearance consists of foci of black or brown pigment peppered throughout the small bowel mucosa.[638,640] Patients with this finding have undergone upper endoscopy for a variety of symptoms thought to be unrelated to the presence of pseudomelanosis. In the majority of reported cases, the patients are 50 years of age or older and there is an association with hypertension, chronic kidney disease, anemia, and diabetes.[636] There are no known or reported long-term consequences to pseudomelanosis duodeni. Microscopically, dark brown-black, granules may be seen within macrophages within the mucosa, especially toward villous tips (Fig 16.39). The granules will stain with Perl's Prussian blue iron stain.

Pathogenesis

The etiology of pigment deposition is unclear. The pigment, initially believed to be melanin, has been found in subsequent studies to be a mixture of substances, including ferrous sulfide, hemosiderin, ceroid, and lipofuscin, among others.[637] Postulated causes of the pigment deposition, include iron deposition (such as in the setting of iron pill ingestion or superficial bleeding), the effects of macrophage metabolism of medications, and charcoal or other substance ingestion. Medications that have been associated with pseudomelanosis duodeni include hydralazine, furosemide, and hydrochlorothiazide.

The full reference list may be accessed online at Elsevier eBooks for Practicing Clinicians.

CHAPTER 17

Inflammatory Disorders of the Large Intestine

Deepa T. Patil, Robert D. Odze

Contents

APPROACH TO EVALUATING COLITIS

Pathologists are asked to evaluate colorectal biopsy specimens for a variety of reasons, but often only a pattern of injury can be identified, at best. This evaluation is performed with the hope that a specific diagnosis can be rendered once appropriate clinical, radiological, and laboratory information is obtained. However, some forms of colitis, such as lymphocytic colitis, collagenous colitis, and ischemic colitis, do have specific histological features, and a diagnosis can be rendered in the absence of clinical information. Many histological features are characteristic of chronic inflammatory bowel disease (IBD). However, it is often difficult or impossible to distinguish ulcerative colitis (UC) from Crohn's disease (CD) on the basis of colorectal biopsy specimens only, particularly after the patient has been treated medically, in which case the features of these two disorders overlap considerably.

Normal vs. Abnormal Colitis

Perhaps the most important aspect of evaluating colorectal biopsy specimens is to differentiate normal from abnormal colitis, which can often be difficult because of the presence of bowel preparation and biopsy procedure artifacts. Artifacts include surface epithelial degeneration, edema, hemorrhage and congestion (Figs. 17.1 and 17.2), aggregation of inflammatory cells, pseudolipomatosis (intramucosal air; Fig. 17.3), mucin depletion, and even neutrophilic cryptitis, among others. Pathologists should not be reluctant to render a diagnosis of *normal colon* if the histological features fall into one or more of the artifact categories, particularly if the patient is asymptomatic. After all, *normal* is the most common diagnosis in the general population. Terms such as *nonspecific (or increased) chronic inflammation, nonspecific colitis,* and *increased acute and chronic inflammation* are inappropriate pathological diagnoses that often cause confusion for clinicians and thus should be avoided.

Pathologists should be aware of several important points when evaluating colorectal biopsy specimens, particularly with regard to histological findings that are considered normal. For example, lymphocytes and plasma cells are always present in the lamina propria of colorectal mucosa, regardless of the anatomic location. However, the density of lamina propria inflammatory cells varies among the different anatomic locations. In general, the cecum and right colon are more cellular than other segments of the colon. A progressive decrease in the cellular constituents of the lamina propria is normal from the right to the left colon (Fig. 17.4). In addition, although the colonic crypts are mostly arranged in a straight and tubular configuration, show an even distribution, and typically extend to the level of the muscularis mucosae, the distal rectum may show some variation in crypt architecture under normal circumstances (Fig. 17.5). Lymphocytes are normally present in the surface epithelium of the colorectal epithelium and number approximately 5 per 100 epithelial cells.[1] Surface intraepithelial lymphocytes are generally more prominent in the cecum and right colon than in the remainder of the distal colon. In addition, intraepithelial lymphocytes are more numerous in areas of mucosa overlying lymphoid follicles (Fig. 17.6).[2,3] Eosinophil counts also vary substantially in different portions of the colon (more in the right colon than in the left), and "normal" numbers depend on other

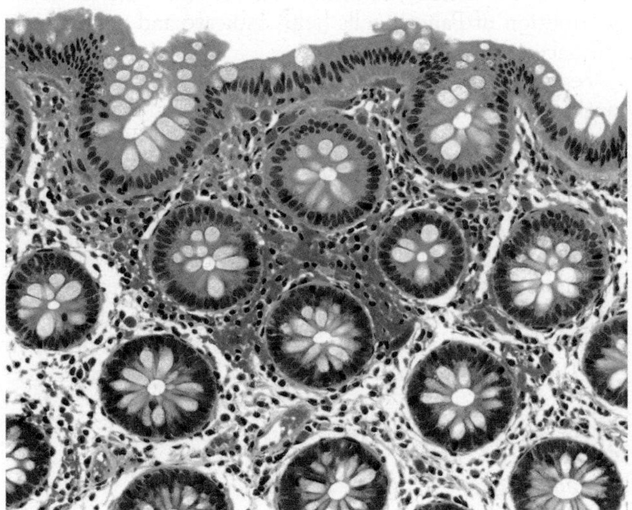

FIGURE 17.1 Colonic biopsy specimen showing biopsy artifact with lamina propria hemorrhage and congestion.

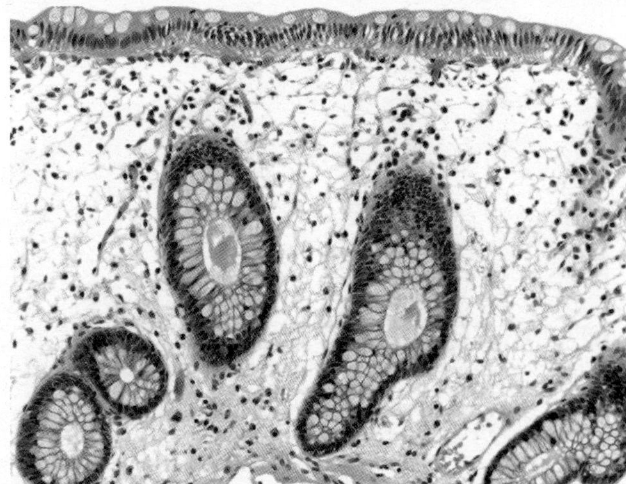

FIGURE 17.2 Colonic biopsy specimen showing lamina propria edema related to bowel preparation.

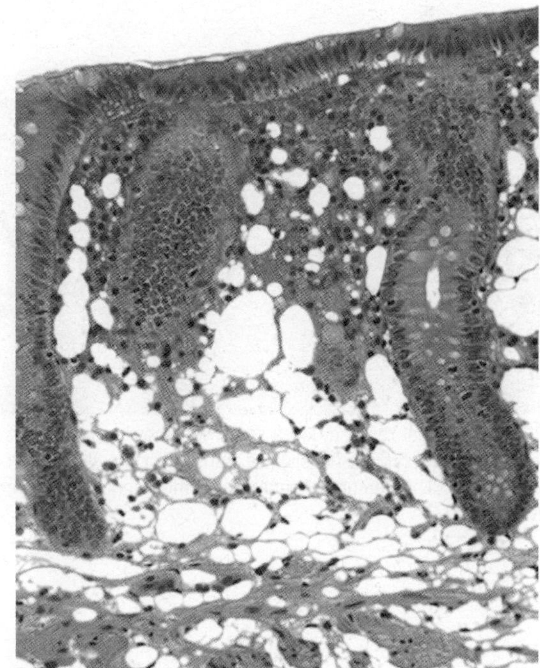

FIGURE 17.3 Colonic pseudolipomatosis composed of intramucosal air resulting from bowel insufflation during endoscopy.

factors, such as the geographic location and the latitude of the patient's principal habitat.[4,5] Individuals who live in the southern states of North America, or closer to the equator, have a higher number of lamina propria eosinophils compared with individuals who live in more northern states.[4] Knowledge of the anatomic location of the colonic biopsy specimens is also important, but this has become increasingly difficult in recent times mainly because gastroenterologists have a tendency to place biopsy specimens from different sites into one specimen container.

Acute vs. Chronic Colitis

Evaluation of patterns of injury in colorectal biopsy specimens is often best performed at low magnification (see Chapter 13).

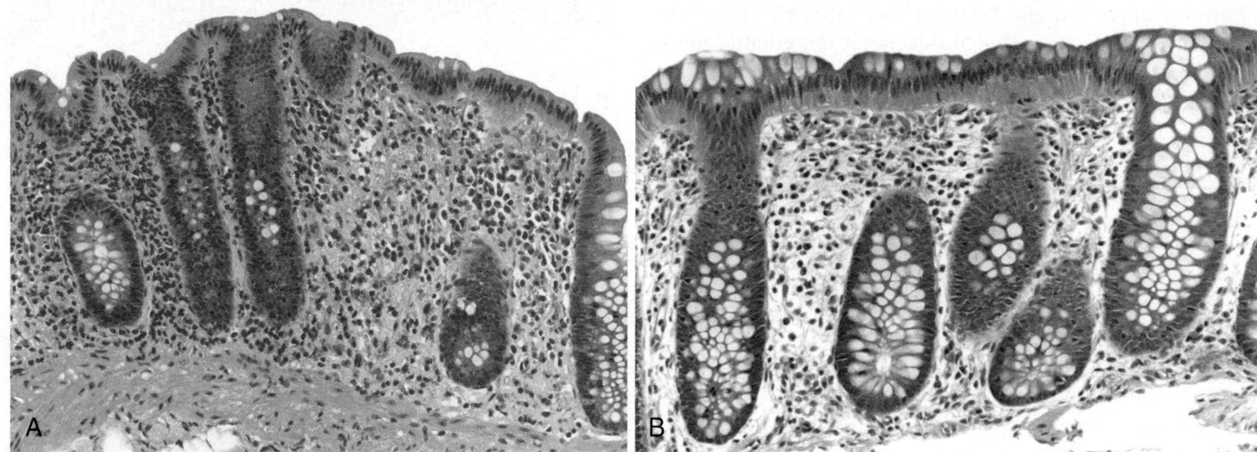

FIGURE 17.4 Biopsies from the right colon **(A)** and left colon **(B)** showing differences in the cellular constituents of the lamina propria. The lamina propria in the right colon is usually more cellular than in the left colon and shows increased numbers of lymphocytes, plasma cells, and eosinophils.

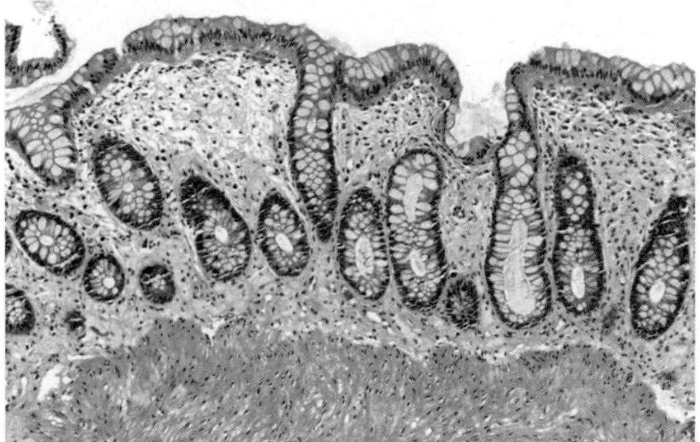

FIGURE 17.5 Normal rectal mucosa specimen showing mild crypt distortion, shortened crypts, and slight expansion of the lamina propria by muciphages. This feature should not be misdiagnosed as chronic inactive colitis.

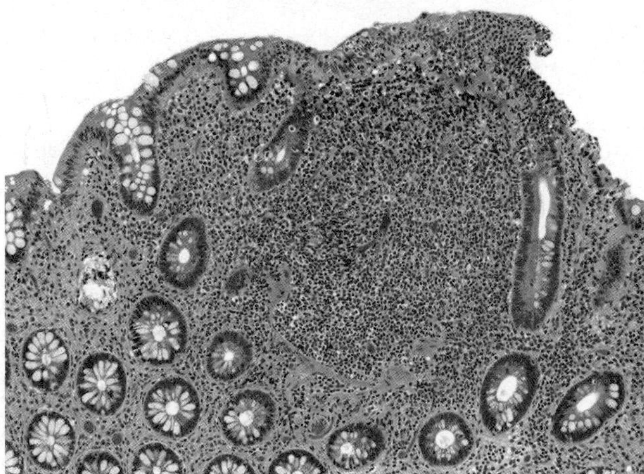

FIGURE 17.6 Colonic mucosa with lymphoid aggregate showing lymphocytes and neutrophils within the surface epithelium. This feature represents trafficking of inflammatory cells as a part of normal mucosal defense.

For example, lamina propria cellularity and crypt architecture are easier to evaluate at low magnification than at high magnification. In addition, it is easier to compare histological changes among different fragments of tissue within the same specimen block under low-power examination.

After a biopsy is determined to be *abnormal,* distinction of acute from chronic changes is important clinically. The most consistent and reliable markers of chronic injury are crypt architectural distortion, basally located lymphoid aggregates, basal plasmacytosis, diffuse mixed inflammation, Paneth cell (or pyloric gland) metaplasia (or hyperplasia in biopsy specimens from the right colon), and lamina propria fibrosis (Table 17.1). Many types of colitides, including acute infectious colitis, may result in expansion of the lamina propria by plasma cells; however, basal plasmacytosis, wherein plasma cells fill the space between the bases of the crypts and the muscularis mucosae, is an excellent histological marker of chronic colitis.[6] This feature is also helpful to differentiate acute infectious colitis from acute-onset IBD in most circumstances. In IBD, features of chronicity are almost always present in the cecum, right colon, and proximal portion of the transverse colon[7]; even in these portions of the colon, an increase in the number and a change in the distribution of Paneth cells helps indicate and confirm the presence of chronic injury.

Features of *active injury* in the colon include, most importantly, regenerative and degenerative epithelial changes, even in the absence of increased inflammatory cells. However, often other inflammatory infiltrates are present. The most common are neutrophil- or eosinophil-mediated injury in the form of cryptitis, crypt abscesses, mucosal erosions, and ulceration. Edema and hemorrhage also may be prominent in some forms of colitis, and there are several other forms of active injury as well (see Chapter 13). These changes may be superimposed on a background of chronic colitis, in which case the diagnostic term *chronic active colitis* is used.

ULCERATIVE COLITIS

Epidemiology

UC is a chronic, episodic inflammatory disease of the colon. It has a propensity to develop in adolescents and young

TABLE 17.1 Microscopic Features of Acute vs. Chronic Colitis

Feature	Acute Colitis	Chronic Colitis
Crypt architecture	Preserved	Often distorted
Expansion of lamina propria	Usually superficial, predominantly neutrophils ± eosinophils	Diffuse (superficial and deep), mixed lymphocytes and plasma cells
Basal lymphoid aggregates	Usually absent	Often present
Basal plasmacytosis	Usually absent	Almost always present
Granulomas	Usually absent	Present in Crohn's disease; related to crypt rupture in ulcerative colitis
Cryptitis and crypt abscesses	Present, superficial	Present, superficial and deep
Pyloric or Paneth cell metaplasia	Absent	Often present
Lamina propria fibrosis	Absent	May be present

adults, although there is a second incidence peak among middle-aged men. The incidence and prevalence rates of UC are highest in North America, England, northern Europe, and Australia. Estimates of the annual incidence of UC in North America and Europe range from 1.5 to 20.3 cases per 100,000 individuals.[8] The incidence of UC appears to have stabilized during the past 25 years and is no longer increasing, unlike that of CD, which seems to be increasing in incidence. It has been estimated that UC will develop in approximately 1% of the U.S. and European population during their lifetime. There is marked ethnic variation in the incidence of UC, with a high incidence in the Jewish population. In the United States, the annual incidence of UC among Jewish individuals is 13 per 100,000 person-years, compared with 3.8 per 100,000 among non-Jewish whites.[9] Recent data indicate a prevalence of 286 cases per 100,000 population in the United States.[10] UC is more common in industrialized countries compared with less-developed countries, and in urban compared with rural populations. The incidence rate of UC among immigrants who have moved to high-risk geographic regions is higher than that of the same ethnic groups in their native countries.

Clinical Features

The clinical symptoms of UC vary depending on the phase and extent of disease. They include urgency, passage of mucus, tenesmus and rectal bleeding in patients with proctitis, and diarrhea (mainly bloody), rectal bleeding, abdominal pain, fever, and weight loss in patients with extensive colitis. Among patients with fulminant colitis, symptoms include fever, generalized abdominal pain, rectal bleeding, and abdominal distention. Patients may also complain of symptoms related to anemia and hypoalbuminemia, such as fatigue, dyspnea, and peripheral edema. In general, the clinical symptoms correlate with the severity of disease. However, on occasion, there may be evidence of histologically or endoscopically active disease in asymptomatic patients. The onset of symptoms is typically slow and insidious. In most cases, patients are symptomatic for weeks or months before seeking medical attention. Some patients with UC present clinically more acutely and thus show symptoms that mimic acute infectious colitis. In fact, in some instances, infection such as with *Salmonella* or *Clostridium difficile* precedes an initial episode of UC (see Acute Self-Limited [Infectious] Colitis).

Extraintestinal manifestations of UC can affect any organ system but are most common in the skin, eyes, mouth, joints, and liver. Cutaneous hypersensitivity, photosensitivity, and urticarial rashes may occur in response to medical therapy (especially sulfasalazine) rather than the underlying disease itself. Erythema nodosum occurs in 2% to 4% of patients with UC. It manifests as single or multiple, tender, erythematous nodules on the extensor surfaces of extremities. Pyoderma gangrenosum is less common, occurring in 1% to 2% of patients with UC. The lesions may be single or multiple and may occur on the trunk, extremities, face, breast, and stoma sites. Less common skin manifestations include Sweet's syndrome and oral aphthous ulcers.

The two most common ocular manifestations of UC are episcleritis and uveitis; these occur in 5% and 8% of patients, respectively. Seronegative arthropathy (type 1, pauciarticular or type 2, polyarticular) occurs in 5% to 20% of individuals with UC and is more common than axial arthropathy; the latter manifests as sacroiliitis and ankylosing spondylitis. In terms of liver involvement, most patients with UC have mild elevations of serum aminotransferase and alkaline phosphatase levels. The most important complication is primary sclerosing cholangitis (PSC), which occurs in almost 3% of patients with UC. Unlike all of the complications listed previously, which typically follow the colonic disease activity, PSC may follow an independent progressive course, even when UC has been stable or inactive for years, and it may appear before onset of UC as well.

Patients with mild or moderately severe disease usually exhibit minimal signs on physical examination. The affected portion of the colon may be tender on abdominal palpation, but abdominal rigidity or guarding is highly unusual. Severe (fulminant) colitis is usually associated with generalized abdominal tenderness, with either normal or hyperactive bowel sounds, which decrease with disease progression. Distention of the abdomen with absent bowel sounds is an ominous sign that suggests peritoneal irritation in cases of fulminant colitis. Other signs that may be associated with UC include aphthous ulceration of oral mucosa, clubbing of fingernails (typically in long-standing UC), peripheral edema, and mild perianal disease. Digital rectal examination is often normal but may occasionally reveal velvety and edematous mucosa. In addition to anemia that results from acute or chronic gastrointestinal (GI) blood loss, patients with UC are predisposed to hypercoagulability and its complications, such as deep vein thrombosis, pulmonary embolism, renal artery thrombosis, cerebrovascular accidents, mesenteric vein thrombosis (and consequent ischemic colitis), and coronary thrombosis.[11]

Laboratory findings in UC depend on disease activity. Anemia, leukocytosis, thrombocytosis, increased erythrocyte sedimentation rate (ESR), elevated C-reactive protein (CRP) level, and hypoalbuminemia are typically associated with active disease. Stool cultures for organisms such as *C. difficile*, *Campylobacter* species, and *Escherichia coli* are usually performed to exclude an infectious cause or complication. Perinuclear antineutrophil cytoplasmic antibodies (pANCA) are positive in 60% to 80% of patients with UC.[12] Immunoglobulin A (IgA) anti–*Saccharomyces cerevisiae* antibody (ASCA) is found in fewer than 1% of patients with UC, whereas IgG ASCA may be seen in as many as 20% of patients (see Ancillary [Serologic] Diagnostic Tests for Inflammatory Bowel Disease).

Radiological studies help provide a general assessment of the extent of disease and complications associated with UC. Plain radiographs are indicated in cases of severe UC to assess for the presence of intraperitoneal air. The finding of marked colonic dilation suggests fulminant colitis. Because the transverse colon is the least dependent part of the colon, a diameter larger than 5 cm is highly suggestive of toxic megacolon. In the earliest stage of UC, a double-contrast barium enema may show a fine granular appearance of the colon. With advanced disease, deep submucosal ulcers result in characteristic "collar-button" ulcers. Diffuse absence of mucosal haustrations, thumbprinting, and narrowing or shortening of the colon are some of the features associated with pancolitis. Computed tomography (CT) is not very helpful in detecting mucosal changes in early disease. However, in advanced UC, the hallmark finding is the presence of mural thickening. In almost 70% of patients with UC, CT with contrast reveals the classic *target* or *double halo sign* caused by inhomogeneous enhancement of the thickened bowel wall. Rectal narrowing and widening of the presacral space are typical findings of long-standing UC.[13]

Assessment of disease activity and prognosis is based on clinical, endoscopic, or histological findings or a combination of these indices. Although it is not standardized, a widely accepted clinical classification is that of Truelove and Witts.[14] Frequency of bowel movements, rectal bleeding, fever, tachycardia, anemia, and elevated ESR are used to classify disease activity as *mild, moderate*, or *severe*. Because this classification does not correlate with disease status in patients with limited colitis, a numerical disease activity score, known as the Sutherland index or Ulcerative Colitis Disease Activity index, is now more commonly used, especially in clinical trials. It combines scores from four components (stool frequency, rectal bleeding, sigmoidoscopic findings, and physician's global assessment).[15]

Risk Factors and Pathogenesis

The exact etiology of UC still remains unknown. However, its pathogenesis is related to a combination of three major elements: genetic susceptibility of the host, immunity, and environmental factors. Although specific agents may incite an inflammatory response in a susceptible host, such agents have not yet been identified. However, studies have shown that luminal microorganisms, their metabolic byproducts, and interactions with normal epithelial structures play key roles in stimulating a host immune response in UC.[16]

Genetic Factors

The observation that 10% to 20% of patients have at least one other affected family member lends support to the role of genetic factors in the development of UC.[17] The strongest evidence of a genetic influence is derived from three European studies wherein 6% to 16% of monozygotic twin pairs had concordant UC, compared with 0% to 5% of dizygotic twin pairs.[18-20] The lifetime risk of developing disease is higher among first-degree relatives of a patient of Jewish descent and among relatives of patients with early-onset disease.[21]

A wide array of genes are responsible for conferring genetic susceptibility, disease specificity, and phenotype in patients with UC.[22] Linkage analyses have demonstrated that chromosomes 1, 2, 3, 5, 6, 7, 10, 12, and 17 harbor susceptibility genes for UC.[23] Specifically, the *IBD2* locus on chromosome 12 has a strong association among families with UC.[24] Additionally, the C3435T polymorphism of the human multidrug resistance 1 *(MDR1)* gene is also linked to susceptibility to UC.[25]

Besides susceptibility genes, human leukocyte antigen (HLA) alleles also influence disease behavior in UC. A significantly increased frequency of HLA-A11 and HLA-A7 has been observed to occur in patients with UC. Specifically, HLA-DR1 *(DRB1*0103)* has been associated with severe colitis.[26] HLA-DR2 *(DRB1*1502)* has been associated with UC in Japanese and Jewish populations.[27,28]

Recent studies in patients with very-early-onset IBD and in those with both a family history of IBD and severe manifestations of the disease have helped identify rare genetic variants that interfere with biochemical cellular pathways that ultimately may lead to increased inflammation. For example, a rare mutation that affects the regulatory function of the X-linked inhibitor of apoptosis *(XIAP)* gene was found to result in early-onset refractory IBD in a 15-month old boy.[29] Furthermore, mutations in the interleukin (IL)-10 receptor *(IL10RA)* gene region, which can ultimately manifest as early-onset IBD, have also been found to be characterized by Mendelian-like inheritance with highly penetrant variants.[30] Nevertheless, these mutational events only account for 10% to 25% of IBD cases, and not all cases have been associated with these types of genetic abnormalities, which suggests that IBD is very likely a complex polygenic disease.[31]

Environmental Factors

It is now widely accepted that continuous antigenic stimulation by commensal bacteria, fungi, or viruses leads to chronic inflammation in individuals who have defects in immunoregulation, mucosal barrier function, and microbial killing. The distal terminal ileum and colon contain the highest concentrations of bacteria (almost 10^{12} organisms per gram of luminal content), and they are a source of constant antigenic stimulus to the host immune system. Animal studies have shown rapid development of colitis when germ-free HLA-B27 transgenic rats[32] and IL-10–deficient mice[33] are populated with normal specific pathogen-free bacteria. Administration of antibiotics effectively prevents and reduces the severity of colitis in these animal models.[34]

There are several postulated mechanisms by which gut flora may initiate or contribute to the development of colitis (see Immune Factors). By virtue of their ability to adhere to or invade the surface epithelium or to produce enterotoxins, microbial organisms stimulate production of inflammatory cytokines. Alteration of the balance between protective and harmful bacteria (e.g., *Bacteroides* species) reduces the concentration of short-chain fatty acids, which provide nourishment to colonocytes. The most frequently observed changes include a decrease of *Firmicutes,* an increase in *Proteobacteria* and *Bacteroidetes,* and an increase in mucolytic bacteria and sulfate-reducing bacteria, such as *Desulfovibrio.*[31] An impaired mucosal barrier and inability to kill microbes because of impaired host defense mechanisms also contribute to hyperresponsiveness and production of high levels of inflammatory cytokines. Abnormal antigen processing, loss of tolerance, autoimmunity, and an abnormally excessive T-cell response are some other mechanisms that influence the severity of inflammation.

A T-cell α-chain receptor knockout mouse model of colitis has demonstrated lack of development of inflammation after appendectomy in animals at 3 to 5 weeks of age.[35] Subsequent case-control studies on humans have also suggested that appendectomy may have a beneficial effect on the disease course.[36-38] However, there have been no prospective studies confirming a possible protective effect.

The best-characterized environmental factor associated with UC is cigarette smoking. UC is more common in nonsmokers than in current smokers.[39] In fact, the second incidence peak in middle-aged men may, in part, be linked to patients who have stopped smoking later in life. A recent prospective study of a cohort of 229,111 women who were followed over a period of 32 years (Nurses Health I and II cohort) showed that the risk of UC is highest during the first 2 to 5 years after cessation of smoking but remains elevated for more than 20 years.[40] The postulated mechanisms for the protective effect of smoking include modulation of cellular and humoral immunity, increased generation of oxygen free radicals, and alteration of cytokine levels.

The use of medications, most notably antibiotics, has also been associated with an increased risk of IBD.[41] This association may result from changes in the intestinal microbiome after use of antibiotics during early stages of life, when the microbiota plays a critical role in shaping immune cell development. Nonsteroidal antiinflammatory drugs (NSAIDs), contraceptives, and statins are medications that have been associated with a nearly twofold increased risk of UC.[42,43]

Immune Factors

Intestinal Barrier and Innate Immunity

The intestinal barrier, consisting of intestinal epithelial cells (IECs) and innate immune cells, maintains the equilibrium between luminal contents and the mucosa. Enterocytes, goblet cells, neuroendocrine cells, Paneth cells, and M cells each appear to play distinct roles in maintaining this equilibrium. Genetic deletion of Muc2 (mucin 2), a major goblet cell-derived secretory mucin, results in spontaneous colitis in murine models.[44] Dendritic cells have been found to accumulate in the mucosa of patients with IBD. Blockage of CD40/CD40L interactions between dendritic cells and effector T-cell populations prevents experimental T-cell–mediated colitis.[45]

Adaptive Immune Response

Both humoral and cell-mediated immunological mechanisms play major roles in the pathogenesis of UC. UC is associated with an increase in the synthesis of IgG, notably the IgG_1 and IgG_3 subclasses. Most patients have circulating antibodies to a variety of dietary, bacterial, and self antigens that are of the IgG_1 subclass, and these are polyclonal in nature. Because serum antibody titers usually do not correlate with disease activity or course, it has been postulated that cross-reactivity between antibodies to bacterial antigens and colonocyte epithelial epitopes may help trigger an immunological response that leads to mucosal inflammation.[46]

UC is associated with several autoimmune diseases such as diabetes mellitus, pernicious anemia, and thyroid disease. The possibility that UC is an autoimmune disease is supported by the fact that patients with UC have serum antibodies directed against lymphocytes, ribonucleic acid, smooth muscle, gastric parietal cells, and thyroid tissue. Patients also have antibodies to epithelial cell–associated components, notably an autoantibody against a 40-kDa epithelial antigen found in normal colonic epithelium. This IgG autoantibody was eluted specifically from colonic mucosa of patients with UC and was not found in patients with CD or other colonic inflammatory conditions.[47] This antigen also shares epitopes with antigens found in the bile ducts, skin, eyes, and joints, sites that are commonly associated with extraintestinal manifestations of UC. The other autoantibody associated with UC is pANCA. It is found in 60% to 80% of UC patients and belongs to the IgG_3 subclass. The exact antigen to which pANCA is directed is unknown. There is some evidence that the antigen is a 50-kDa nuclear envelope protein that is specific to myeloid cells.[48] The pathogenic relevance of pANCA is unclear. It appears to be associated with an aggressive disease course and development of pouchitis.[49]

Bacterial antigens also trigger innate immunity by activation of pattern-recognition receptors, which include Toll-like receptors (TLRs) and nucleotide-binding oligomerization domain (NOD)-like receptors (NLRs). Activation of TLRs and NLRs results in downstream activation of nuclear factor κB (NF-κB), which further stimulates production of various proinflammatory cytokines and chemokines. Defects in any of these pathways can result in abnormal bacterial processing and possibly IBD.[50]

Colonic epithelial cells express class II major histocompatibility complex (MHC) antigens and can initiate an inflammatory response by acting as antigen-presenting cells.[51] Increased turnover of colonic epithelium, reduced metabolism of short-chain fatty acids, abnormal membrane permeability, and altered composition of mucosal layers contribute to the pathogenesis of UC.[52,53] Animal models of colitis produced by disruption of colonic epithelium further support the role of epithelial cells in the pathogenesis of IBD.[54]

Release of various cytokines from the T-cell inflammatory pathways may also lead to increased epithelial cell permeability and alteration of the endothelium, contributing to diarrhea and localized ischemia, respectively.

Pathological Features

Gross Features

In untreated cases, the extent of colonic involvement depends on the clinical severity of disease. UC classically involves the rectum with variable, but continuous, involvement of the colon more proximally (Fig. 17.7). According to the Montreal classification, the extent of UC is divided into *ulcerative proctitis* (involvement limited to the rectum), *left-sided* or *distal* UC (involvement of the rectum and sigmoid but not beyond the splenic flexure), and *extensive* UC or *pancolitis* (involvement of the rest of the colon proximal to the splenic flexure).[55] At the initial onset of disease, pancolitis occurs in approximately 20% of patients, left-sided colitis in 50% to 60%, and proctitis or rectosigmoiditis in approximately 45% of patients.[56] Skip lesions, in the form of appendiceal, periappendiceal, or ascending colon/cecal involvement, have been observed in as many as 80% of patients with subtotal UC (see Unusual Morphological Variants of Ulcerative Colitis).[56] Based on a long-term follow-up study by Farmer and colleagues, pancolitis eventually develops in almost one-half (46%) of patients with proctitis or rectosigmoiditis and in more than 70% of those with left-sided colitis.[57]

In the active phase of disease, the mucosa usually appears diffusely congested, granular, and edematous. Ulcers, when present, are usually small and oriented longitudinally in relation to the teniae coli. They often appear to undermine adjacent areas of mucosa, which leads to the formation of polypoid mucosal folds or inflammatory pseudopolyps. In such cases, the mucosa may have a cobblestone appearance, similar to that observed in CD. Rarely, an exaggerated form of pseudopolyp formation, known as *filiform polyposis*, may be present (Fig. 17.8). It is characterized by the presence of elongated, slender, villiform, wormlike, polypoid mucosal projections and usually spares the rectum. In severe cases, ulcers may be extensive, involve large segments of bowel, and lead to near-total or total mucosal loss.

In cases of toxic megacolon, the bowel wall appears extremely thin, dilated, and congested. The serosal surface usually demonstrates fibrinous or fibrinopurulent exudate. Rarely, there is evidence of perforation. The mucosal surface in these cases is extensively denuded, hemorrhagic, ulcerated, and often covered with purulent exudates.

In the quiescent (inactive) phase of UC, the mucosa may appear completely normal, or it may show diffuse granularity, either with or without inflammatory pseudopolyps. In some cases of long-standing UC, the bowel wall is thickened and contracted ("colonic foreshortening"), and the mucosal surface may appear atrophic.

In treated UC, especially when patients have been given steroid enemas, the rectal mucosa may show minimal or no abnormalities on gross examination. Similarly, in patients who have received medical treatment before surgical resection, there may be focal, diffuse, or even widespread areas of grossly normal-appearing bowel between areas of affected bowel.

Microscopic Findings

Depending on the phase of disease and the degree of inflammatory activity, UC is categorized histologically as *chronic inactive*, *chronic active*, or *active* (without features of chronicity) for the purpose of diagnostic sign-out. Chronic colitis (regardless of "activity") is defined by the presence of histological features of chronicity (Box 17.1), such as crypt architectural distortion, crypt atrophy, diffuse mixed lamina propria inflammation, basal plasmacytosis, basally located lymphoid aggregates, and Paneth cell metaplasia (in the left colon). Other changes of chronicity include lamina propria fibrosis, pyloric gland metaplasia, and Paneth cell hyperplasia in the right colon. Common changes of "activity" include neutrophilic or eosinophilic cryptitis, crypt abscesses, regenerative or degenerative epithelial changes, hemorrhage, necrosis, erosions, and ulceration.

Unfortunately, there is no universally accepted method of grading histological activity in biopsy specimens from patients with UC. At least 18 different histological scoring systems have been proposed to categorize activity, but these are mainly used in research protocols and do not have much relevance to clinicians when deciding how to manage their patients.[58] Scoring systems that have been used in clinical studies range from use of stepwise methods, in which disease activity is divided into rather subjectively assessed grades, to others that prefer use of a

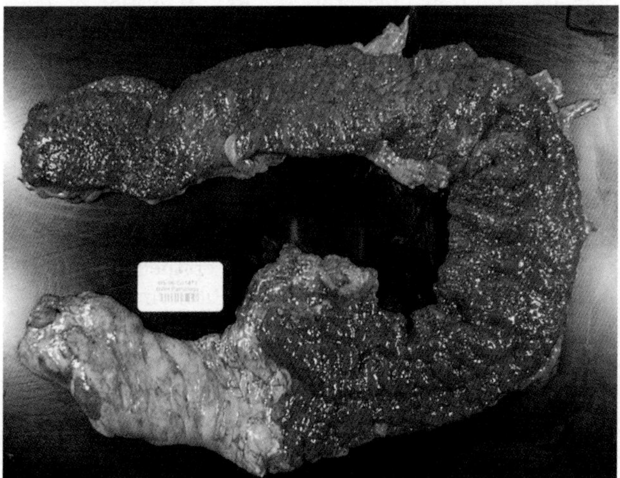

FIGURE 17.7 A gross specimen of subtotal ulcerative colitis showing diffuse continuous disease starting from the distal rectum and continuing up to the midportion of the ascending colon.

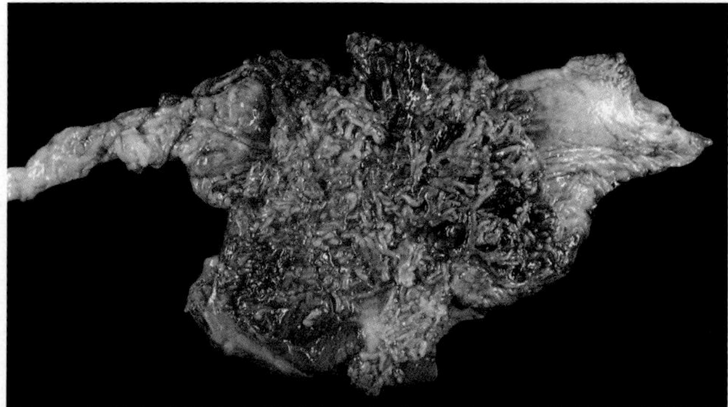

FIGURE 17.8 Gross specimen of ulcerative colitis showing numerous filiform polypoid mucosal projections that represent an exaggerated form of inflammatory pseudopolyp formation (filiform polyposis).

BOX 17.1 Histological Features of Activity and Chronicity in Ulcerative Colitis

FEATURES OF ACTIVITY

Neutrophilic (or eosinophilic) cryptitis
Crypt abscesses
Necrosis
Regenerative and degenerative epithelial changes
Erosions
Ulcers

FEATURES OF CHRONICITY

Crypt architectural distortion
- Crypt atrophy
- Crypt foreshortening
- Irregular spacing of crypts
- Irregular size of crypts
- Crypt branching or budding
- Loss of crypt parallelism
- Villiform surface contour

Basal plasmacytosis
Basal lymphoid aggregates
Diffuse mixed lymphoplasmacytic infiltrate within the lamina propria
Paneth cell metaplasia in the left colon (hyperplasia in the right colon)
Pyloric gland metaplasia
Lamina propria or submucosal fibrosis
Thickening or duplication of the muscularis mucosae

more quantitative methods, by using numerical scores that correspond to specific histological features. For instance, the Riley scoring system[59] uses a four-point score (*none, mild, moderate,* and *severe*) to assess six histological features: presence of an acute inflammatory cell infiltrate (neutrophils in the lamina propria), crypt abscesses, mucin depletion, surface epithelial integrity, chronic inflammatory cell infiltrate (round cells in the lamina propria), and crypt architectural irregularities. This scoring system was applied in a prospective study that was aimed at predicting recurrence in 82 outpatients with asymptomatic UC in endoscopic remission. This scoring system was later modified (Modified Riley score)[60] to rank the degree of inflammation hierarchically, and to exclude crypt architectural changes, which according to the authors, are not responsive to clinically relevant changes in inflammation. This system has never been validated but has been used in multiple randomized control trials.[58]

Geboes et al.[61] developed a scoring system that categorizes histological changes as grade 0 (structural change only), grade 1 (chronic inflammation), grade 2 (2a, lamina propria neutrophils and 2b, lamina propria eosinophils), grade 3 (neutrophils in the epithelium), grade 4 (crypt destruction), and grade 5 (erosions or ulcers). This system generates a score from 0 to 5.4 that increases with disease severity or activity. The Geboes scoring system has been shown to be reproducible to some degree, where the authors found moderate to good interobserver agreement among three pathologists (kappa 0.59 to 0.70).

More recently, two histological scoring methods have been developed and validated: the Nancy index and the Robarts histopathological index (RHI).[62,63] Both of these scoring systems demonstrate mostly a high degree of intraobserver and interobserver agreement. The RHI was developed by scoring biopsies according to the Geboes score and then determining which features were reproducible and correlated best with the pathologists' interpretation of disease severity using a visual analog scale. Four features were found to correlate best with overall disease severity, including lamina propria chronic inflammation, lamina propria neutrophils, neutrophils in the epithelium, and the presence of ulcers and erosions. The Nancy index is a stepwise 5-item method that assesses lamina propria lymphoplasmacytic inflammation, neutrophilic inflammation, and ulcers to arrive at the final grade.[63]

One simple and reproducible type of grading system that is commonly used in clinical practice by the authors of this chapter is as follows. The degree of activity is graded as *mild* if less than 50% of the mucosa shows evidence of activity, and the lamina propria is only mildly expanded by inflammatory cells. It is graded as *moderate* if more than 50% of the mucosa shows activity and/or if the lamina propria inflammatory component is moderately or severely dense, but there are no surface erosions or ulcers. It is graded as severe if surface erosion or ulceration is present, regardless of the density of inflammation in the lamina propria or epithelium. In this simple classification, "activity" includes any of the features outlined earlier in this chapter, and in this manner, it takes into account the fact that patients who are in an active phase of disease clinically may not necessarily show peak neutrophil influx at that point in time (see Figs. 17.10 to 17.12).

Chronic Active Colitis. Histologically, previously untreated UC in adults typically involves the colon in a diffuse and continuous manner, always beginning at the distalmost portion of the rectum and extending proximally to the point at which inflammation stops, which in most cases is rather abrupt (Table 17.2). Typically, specimens from involved regions of the colon have a similar appearance. Usually, each biopsy fragment shows a homogeneous and diffuse pattern of injury, although the severity of inflammation may vary from region to region in the bowel (usually worse distally) or between individual biopsy fragments from one area of the colon, especially posttreatment (see discussion on posttreatment features later in this chapter).

UC characteristically involves the mucosa and sometimes involves the superficial submucosa as well (Fig. 17.9). The histological findings vary depending on the clinical phase of disease. Ultimately, in periods of clinical activity, UC is predominantly a lymphoplasmacytic inflammatory process with superimposed neutrophils, hemorrhage, and epithelial degeneration and regeneration. A dense, homogeneous lymphoplasmacytic infiltrate typically expands the lamina propria (Fig. 17.10).[64-66] The density of plasma cells is usually greatest in the basal region of the lamina propria (termed *basal plasmacytosis*). Basally located lymphoid aggregates (situated between the bases of the crypts and the muscularis mucosae) are also common. They may show germinal centers. Expansion of the lamina propria and the presence of basal lymphoid aggregates contribute to irregular spacing of the crypts.

TABLE 17.2 Features of Untreated Ulcerative Colitis and Crohn's Disease

Untreated Ulcerative Colitis	Crohn's Disease
Diffuse, continuous disease	Segmental disease
Rectal involvement	Variable rectal involvement
Disease worse distally	Disease severity is variable from segment to segment
No fissures (except in fulminant colitis)	Fissures, sinuses, fistulous tracts common
No transmural aggregates	Transmural lymphoid aggregates
Either no or only mild distal ileal involvement (less than 5 cm in general)	Often moderate to severe ileal involvement, either segmental or diffuse and usually more than 5 cm
Upper GI tract involvement (stomach, duodenum) less common	Upper GI tract involvement (esophagus, stomach duodenum, jejunum) much more common
Anal disease less common	Anal tags, fissures and fistulae are more common
Granulomas are less common, and when present are crypt-rupture (mucin) associated	Epithelioid granulomas unrelated to ruptured crypts common
Appendiceal involvement is more common and resembles chronic active colitis seen in the rest of the colon	Appendiceal involvement is less common

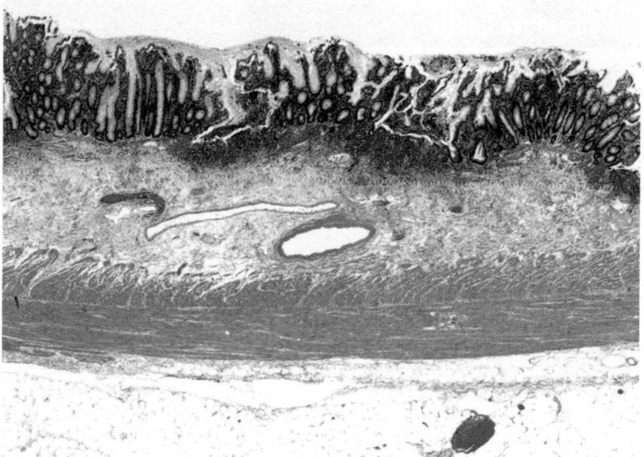

FIGURE 17.9 Resection specimen of ulcerative colitis showing inflammatory changes restricted to the mucosa and superficial submucosa.

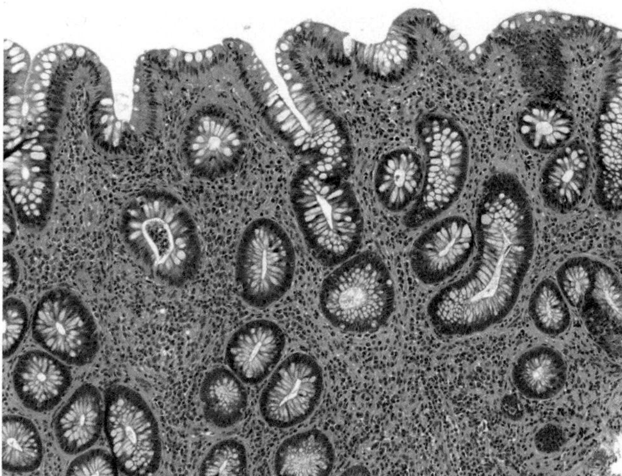

FIGURE 17.10 Distal rectum with mild chronic active ulcerative colitis. The lamina propria is expanded by a lymphoplasmacytic inflammatory infiltrate. Crypt architectural distortion is present with minimal/focal neutrophilic epithelial injury.

One characteristic and frequent morphological feature of UC is crypt architectural distortion, which is characterized by irregularly arranged, branched, dilated, and/or shortened crypts. In some circumstances, branching and shortening of crypts represents morphological manifestations of crypt regeneration. Most patients with new-onset (pretreatment) UC have experienced several weeks to months of subclinical or minimal inflammation, during which time the lamina propria has been inflamed, plasma cells have congregated in the basilar region of the lamina propria, and significant crypt injury with regeneration has occurred. Crypt architectural distortion is considered a hallmark of chronic injury. However, it may develop in any inflammatory disease of the colon that manifests as periods of repeated bouts of injury and repair before full mucosal healing. Thus when the inflamed mucosa is repeatedly exposed to bouts of injury followed by repair, the epithelium does not always heal with perfectly well-formed and aligned crypts. Crypt distortion is therefore not a specific feature of UC (or CD). It occurs in many other types of disorders, such as chronic recurrent ischemia, persistent or recurrent infections (e.g., C. *difficile*), radiation colitis, drug-induced colitis, graft-versus-host disease (GVHD), and even microscopic colitis. Furthermore, not all patients with UC, even in an active phase of disease, reveal crypt distortion in every portion of the colonic mucosa. For this reason, absence of crypt distortion does not necessarily rule out a diagnosis of UC.

Depending on the severity of active disease, a neutrophilic inflammatory cell infiltrate (with or without eosinophils) may be seen within the lamina propria and/or in the surface and crypt epithelium (cryptitis); it may be minimal, focal and patchy, or diffuse and severe. Similarly, aggregates of neutrophils within the crypt lumina (crypt abscesses) may be focal or diffuse (Figs. 17.11 and 17.12). Rupture of crypts caused by inflammation can lead to the development of aggregates of histiocytes, foreign-body giant cells, and even well-developed granulomas as a response to extravasated mucin (Fig. 17.13). These *mucin granulomas* (crypt rupture–associated granulomas) are usually present in the deeper portions of the mucosa, where crypts tend to rupture more often compared with the superficial mucosa. Often, deeper cuts through tissue blocks are necessary to determine whether or not a

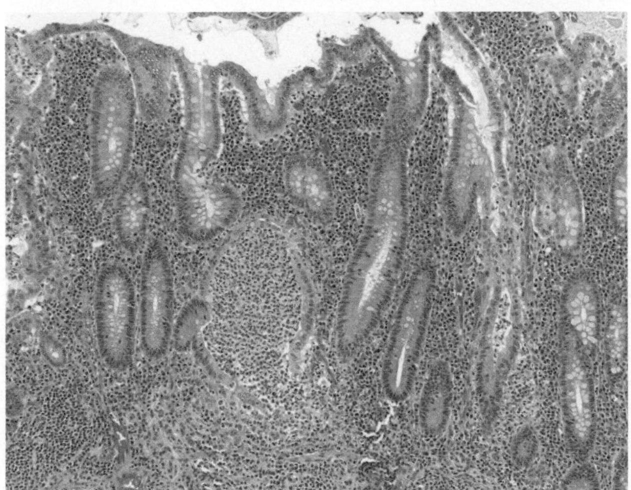

FIGURE 17.11 Moderate chronic active colitis. Greater than 50% of the mucosa shows cryptitis and crypt abscesses. The lamina propria inflammatory component is moderately or severely dense. Slight villiform mucosal architecture is also present in this case.

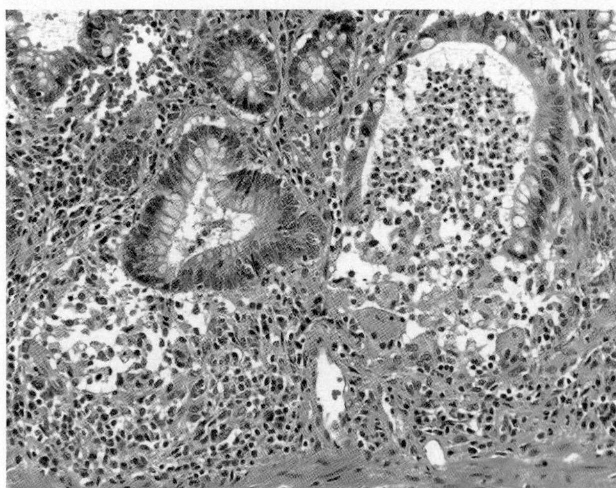

FIGURE 17.13 Ulcerative colitis with crypt rupture–associated granulomas (mucin granulomas). The ruptured crypt abscess is associated with a rim of histiocytes as well as foreign-body giant cells containing engulfed mucin.

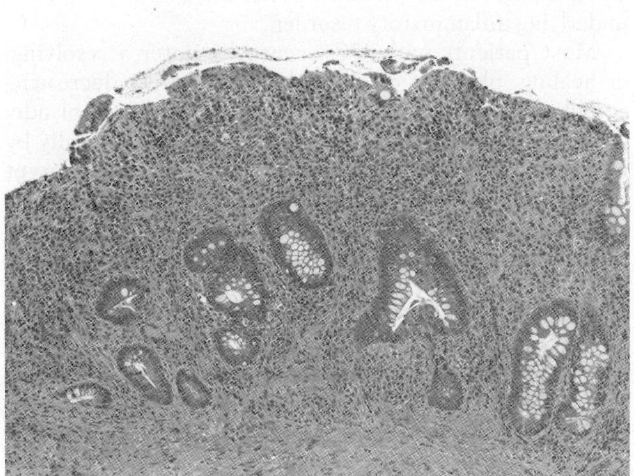

FIGURE 17.12 Severe chronic active ulcerative colitis showing mucosal ulceration with villiform appearance of the adjacent regenerating mucosa and crypt architectural distortion. The lamina propria also shows basal lymphoid aggregates.

granuloma is related to a ruptured crypt. Some patients show a marked foreign-body–type giant cell response or even a fully developed granulomatous response, which can be seen at the base of the mucosa. Distinguishing granulomas in UC from those in CD can be challenging, but the latter are more often randomly located in the mucosa, are more often superficial in location, and are typically unrelated to injured crypts (see Crohn's Colitis). When a mucosal granuloma is identified, serial sections should be evaluated to determine whether it is located immediately adjacent to a ruptured crypt.

In areas of activity, the surface and crypt epithelium always shows regenerative and/or degenerative changes. Features of regenerative changes include loss of mucin, enlarged and variably sized nuclei either with or without nuclear stratification, hyperchromasia, prominent nucleoli, and increased mitotic activity. Features of degenerative changes include cytoplasmic vacuolization and heterogeneity, nuclear fragmentation and pyknosis, and lack of mitotic activity. In addition, the crypts may show increased apoptotic activity. In areas adjacent to erosions and ulcers, degenerative cells may acquire a syncytial appearance, with abundant and prominent eosinophilic cytoplasm (Fig. 17.14). In some instances, the syncytial epithelium overlies stroma that is devoid of crypts and contains actively inflamed granulation tissue. Regenerating surface epithelial cells, which are cuboidal initially and then columnar with maturation, acquire a slightly more basophilic cytoplasm. On occasion, the surface epithelium may be villiform in appearance, resembling small-intestinal mucosa. Regenerative changes may mimic dysplasia (see Dysplasia in Ulcerative Colitis and Crohn's Disease). Mucin reappears slowly, first in cuboidal cells and later in goblet cells. With time, goblet cells may become numerous.

Paneth cell metaplasia in the left colon and pyloric gland metaplasia are reliable histological indicators of chronic injury. In active disease, even the ascending colon, cecum, and transverse colon may show irregularity in the distribution and increased numbers of Paneth cells (Fig. 17.15). Pyloric gland metaplasia is less common in UC than in CD. It is more commonly observed in samples from the proximal colon and is often seen in close proximity to ulcerated mucosa.

Occasionally, the rectum is completely free from inflammatory disease (absolute rectal sparing) or shows less activity than in the proximal colon (relative rectal sparing). This phenomenon is usually caused by the effects of prior medical treatment, either orally or, more commonly, with enemas (e.g., steroid enemas). However, on careful inspection, one often finds one or more subtle features of chronicity, which is evidence of prior inflammation and injury.

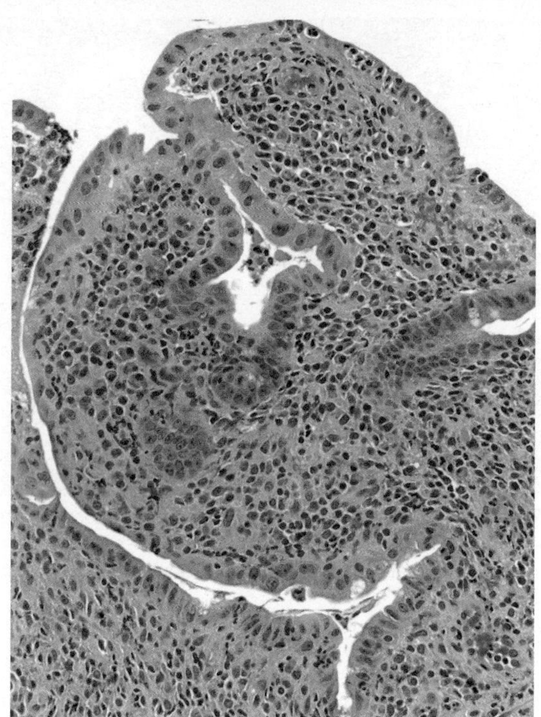

FIGURE 17.14 Active ulcerative colitis with regeneration. The epithelium adjacent to an erosion or ulcer often acquires a syncytial regenerative appearance, containing cells with hypereosinophilic cytoplasm.

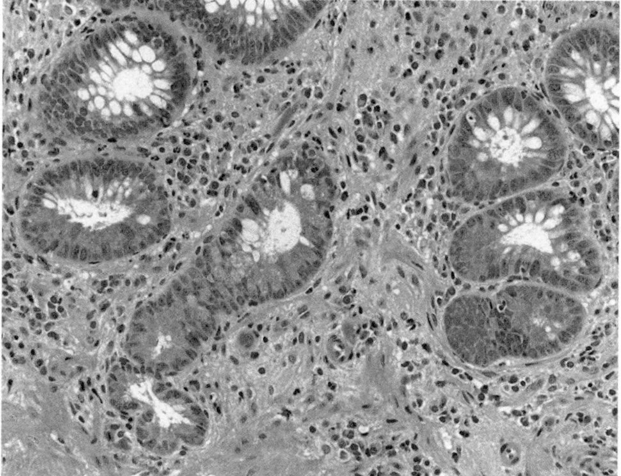

FIGURE 17.15 An ascending colon biopsy specimen from a patient with chronic active ulcerative colitis showing hyperplasia and irregular distribution of Paneth cells.

Grossly normal–appearing colonic mucosa proximal to regions of active colitis may also reveal a spectrum of abnormalities. Most commonly, there is a mild lymphoplasmacytic infiltrate within the lamina propria. However, the crypts are usually more evenly arranged and lack distortion. A few neutrophils may be present in the lamina propria or occasionally within a crypt, but neutrophilic crypt abscesses are rare. Eosinophils may also be increased and may produce small eosinophilic crypt abscesses on occasion. In the context of a patient with classic UC in the more distal colon, these changes in the proximal bowel are a reflection of the underlying inflammatory disorder.

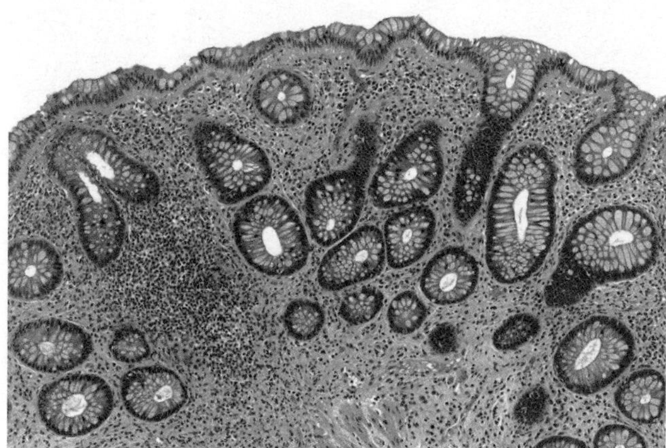

FIGURE 17.16 Resolving phase of ulcerative colitis showing mild crypt architectural distortion with a lymphoid aggregate and patchy lymphoplasmacytic inflammation. This phase of disease is associated with a decrease in the degree of neutrophilic epithelial injury.

Most patients with UC eventually enter a resolving, or healing, phase of disease, characterized by decreasing activity (and symptoms) after an active colitis episode. This phase of disease is characterized morphologically by less activity and less crypt injury, but higher levels of crypt regeneration and remodeling (Fig. 17.16). Injured crypts typically heal from the base of the mucosa progressively upward toward the luminal surface. Neutrophils and other active components of crypt injury decrease first, followed by a reduction in lamina propria lymphocytes and plasma cells. During this initial healing phase, there is often much variability in the type and degree of mucosal inflammatory changes within biopsy fragments from different regions of the colon and even within individual fragments of mucosa from a single site. Neuroendocrine cell hyperplasia occurs in some patients, whereas others develop prominent lymphoid follicles that are more common in the distal colon and rectum (follicular proctitis). Follicular proctitis appears to identify a subgroup of patients who have a less favorable response to medical therapy.[67,68]

Chronic Inactive (Quiescent) Colitis. The resolution period of UC, characterized by decreasing activity and increasing repair, may last for several weeks or months. Thereafter, UC patients may be symptom free for variable but often long periods. This is the "inactive" or "quiescent" period of disease. During this time, the mucosa may be completely normal, or it may show various degrees of chronic inactive disease (mainly crypt distortion), either with or without mild patchy activity (Fig. 17.17). Architecturally distorted crypts represent a" biomarker" of prior bouts of colitis. Alternatively, the colon may heal completely and thus appear normal histologically. The rate at which this occurs is variable among patients. For instance, patients with only mild active colitis of short duration can show complete restitution of architecturally normal mucosa within several months after the initial

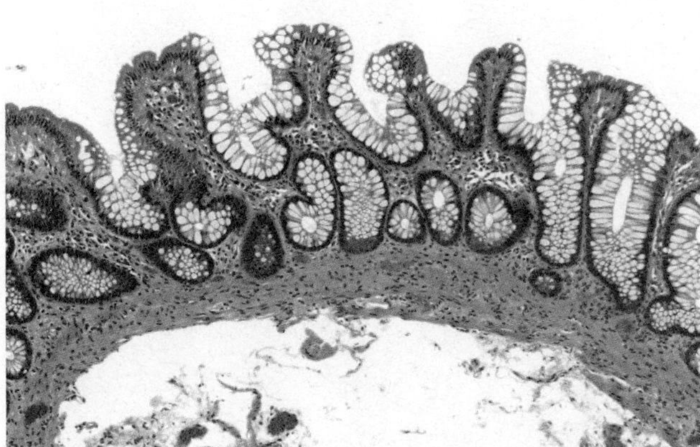

FIGURE 17.17 Chronic inactive ulcerative colitis in a biopsy specimen from the left colon showing crypt architectural distortion, villiform surface contour, and Paneth cell metaplasia.

BOX 17.2 Causes of Unusual (Crohn's-like) Patterns of Disease in Ulcerative Colitis

- Effects of oral or topical therapy
- Low-grade disease in remission
- Cecum or ascending colon inflammation in left-sided colitis
- Appendiceal involvement as a skip lesion
- Pediatric ulcerative colitis (initial presentation)
- Ileitis in ulcerative colitis (backwash ileitis)
- Upper gastrointestinal tract involvement (e.g., duodenitis)
- Crohn's-like aphthous ulcers in ulcerative colitis
- Granulomas (usually related to crypt rupture)
- Fulminant colitis

active episode. The pace of crypt remodeling is usually slow in most patients; such remodeling occurs typically over many weeks to months.

Unusual Morphological Variants of Ulcerative Colitis

A summary of the causes of unusual morphological patterns of disease in UC is provided in Box 17.2. It is important that pathologists recognize these variants so they can avoid falling into diagnostic traps and misdiagnosing UC as CD. This section provides a summary of many of the causes of Crohn's-like changes that may occur in UC as a result of a variety of factors such as treatment effect, age of the patient, systemic manifestations of disease, or simply a result of long-term waxing and waning of inflammatory activity. These include most commonly segmental or patchy involvement of the colon, rectal sparing, skip lesions, ileal or upper GI tract inflammation, aphthous ulceration, and granulomas, among others.

Ascending Colon, Cecum, and Appendiceal Involvement as "Skip Lesions" in Ulcerative Colitis

Some UC patients with either subtotal or limited left-sided colitis may show patchy, mild, chronic, or active inflammation in the cecum or ascending colon that may be falsely interpreted as CD because of the impression of segmental involvement of the colon, which is a classic manifestation of CD in the colon.[69-71] Up to 65% of patients with UC have limited left-sided involvement initially. However, proximal extension occurs in 29% to 58% of such patients.[69,72,73] For instance, in one study by D'Haens and colleagues of 20 patients with established left-sided UC, 6 showed a sharp demarcation between affected and unaffected portions of colon, whereas 14 showed a more gradual transition.[69] The area of transition in such cases may appear somewhat patchy, giving a false impression of skip lesions. Seventy-five percent of this latter group of patients showed an area of inflammation in the cecum, primarily in the periappendiceal mucosa, that was separate from the distal inflamed segment. In a study by Mutinga et al., 14 patients with both left-sided UC and pathologically confirmed patchy right-sided chronic inflammation were compared with 35 control patients who had limited left-sided UC only.[56] The two groups had similar demographic features, extraintestinal manifestations, severity of disease, prevalence of progression to pancolitis, and natural history, which suggests that patchy right-sided inflammation in patients with left-sided colitis has little clinical significance. This phenomenon should be recognized by pathologists so a false diagnosis of CD can be prevented when there is an initial suspicion for segmental disease in the colon.

In a prospective study of 271 patients with UC, including 63 with inactive left-sided or subtotal colitis, periappendiceal cecal mucosal involvement was identified in 32% of patients. Similarly, since the original description by Davison and Dixon in 1990 of "discontinuous involvement" wherein the appendix was found to be inflamed in 21% of 62 cases of patients with only distal colonic UC,[74] several other studies have shown that the appendix may be involved as a "skip lesion" in this disease,[75,76] although at least one other study failed to confirm this finding.[77] In another study by Groisman et al., ulcerative appendicitis was present in 86% and 87% of patients with "nonuniversal" and "universal" UC, respectively.[75] Their study included two cases with limited left-sided involvement combined with appendiceal involvement. Overall, the role of the appendix in UC is poorly understood. Patients with prior appendectomy have been shown to have a lower risk for UC.[78,79] In one study, the severity of appendiceal inflammation (ulceration) in patients with UC was a strong predictor of the development of pouchitis after a total proctocolectomy and ileoanal pouch procedure.[80] In summary, involvement of both the appendix and the cecal or ascending colon can occur in patients with subtotal colitis. This phenomenon should be recognized by pathologists as an acceptable potential skip lesion in UC.

Ulcerative Colitis in Pediatric Patients

Several studies have shown that pediatric patients with untreated UC at initial clinical presentation may show evidence of relative, or even complete, rectal sparing or even patchy colonic disease on biopsy studies.[81-85] Markowitz et al. reported 12 pediatric patients with untreated UC, 5 (42%) of whom showed patchy, mild active inflammation and mild crypt changes in the rectum, but diffuse involvement in the more proximal regions of the colon.[81] In fact, one patient had a completely normal rectal biopsy specimen. A study by Glickman et al. compared the rectal mucosal

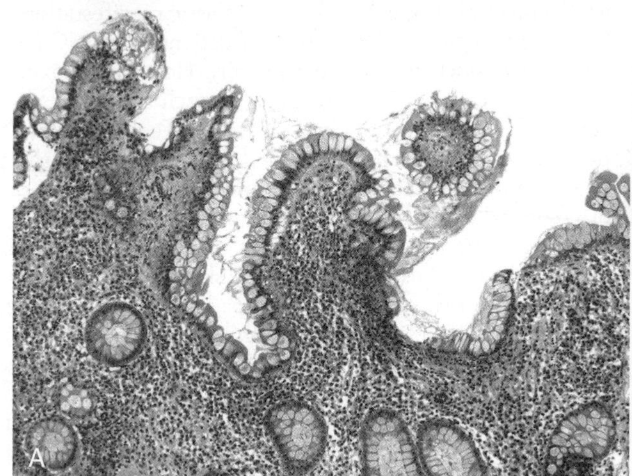

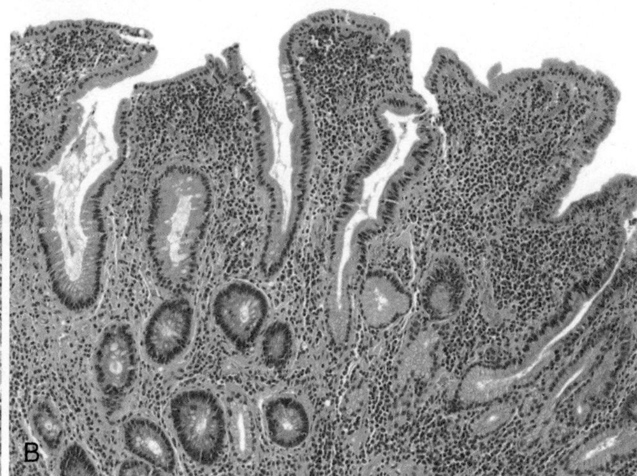

FIGURE 17.18 Ileitis in ulcerative colitis. A, The small-bowel mucosa shows expansion of the lamina propria by neutrophils, eosinophils, and plasma cells. There is mild villous blunting. In some cases, pyloric gland metaplasia **(B)** may be present.

biopsy appearance of 70 pediatric patients who had UC with that of 44 adult patients, all at initial presentation before medical treatment.[82] Compared with adults, the pediatric patients showed significantly fewer cases of chronic active disease and a greater number of patients with microscopic skip areas and relative rectal sparing. In this study, 2 of the 70 pediatric patients had completely normal rectal biopsy specimens at initial clinical presentation, in contrast with none of the adult patients. Thus an absence of features of chronicity or the presence of mild active disease and microscopic skip areas at initial presentation in pediatric patients should not exclude a diagnosis of UC. In adults, relative (but not absolute) rectal sparing (i.e., less severe inflammation in the rectum compared with the proximal colon) may be seen, rarely, at initial presentation before treatment as well.[86,87] In one study, a 31% prevalence rate of relative rectal sparing was noted in a series of 46 adult patients with UC at initial presentation, but even in those cases, histological features of chronicity were almost always present in the rectal mucosa at the time of initial diagnosis.[87]

Ileitis in Ulcerative Colitis

Patients with UC, and particularly those with involvement of the cecum and ileocecal valve, may also show active inflammation in the distal few centimeters of the terminal ileum; a condition that has been historically termed *backwash ileitis* (BWI). The hypothetical mechanism for this phenomenon is that when inflammation of the proximal cecum/ileocecal mucosa is severe enough, it may cause malfunction of the ileocecal junction (ICJ), retrograde flow of colonic contents into the distal terminal ileum, and secondary inflammation of the terminal ileum as a result of a "toxic" reaction to the luminal refluxate.[88,89] This theory was originally proposed in the early 20th century by Crohn and Rosenak[90] in an effort to explain the observation that some patients had a previously undescribed "combined form of ileitis and colitis," a constellation of findings that was unusual in "regional enteritis" or "ulcerative colitis." In a more contemporary study of the ileum in UC patients, Haskell et al. reviewed 200 UC resection specimens and found active ileitis in 17% of cases; in most cases, the inflammation was confined to the distal 1 cm of the ileum.[91] Ninety percent of cases consisted of mild, patchy neutrophilic inflammation in the lamina propria, focal cryptitis or crypt abscesses, and patchy villous atrophy and regenerative changes (Fig. 17.18A). In rare instances, surface ulceration or even pyloric (mucous gland) metaplasia was present as well (see Fig 17.18B). Most interestingly, in their study, a "backwash" mechanism for ileitis in UC was questioned because some patients showed a conspicuous lack of cecal involvement. The authors of that study suggested that ileitis may have developed as a result of drug toxicity (such as NSAIDS) or perhaps as a result of the bowel preparation procedure, rather as a result of backwash. More recently, in a critical evaluation of the literature on BWI by Patil et al., the concept of BWI was discarded in favor of a theory that ileitis in UC patients may more likely be related to primary involvement of the underlying disease, rather than as a result of mechanical backwash of colonic contents into the ileum.[92] The originally proposed backwash theory has never been proven experimentally and, in fact, was postulated during a time when little was known regarding the broad pathological manifestations of CD in the GI tract, including the colon, or the variability of involvement of the upper GI tract in either CD or UC. Regardless, most cases of ileitis in UC, regardless of the precise etiology, show only mild inflammation. Thus when a patient with presumed UC shows more severe ileal findings, such as deep or even fissuring ulceration, abundant submucosal inflammation, non–crypt-rupture related granulomas, or long lengths of ileal involvement (generally >5 cm), a strong suspicion for CD should always be entertained, particularly when the patient does not have inflammation of the proximal cecum and ileocecal valve.

Prognostic Significance of Ileitis in Ulcerative Colitis. In a large case-control study, Arrossi et al. evaluated pouch outcome in patients with UC and in those with IBD of the indeterminate type and reported that the presence of BWI was not a significant risk factor for the development of pouchitis.[93] This has been confirmed in other studies as well.

Previous studies have suggested that the condition referred to as *backwash ileitis* may be associated with an increased risk of colonic adenocarcinoma.[94] For instance, in a study by Heuschen et al., 590 UC patients were classified into those with and without BWI, or limited left-sided colitis and evaluated for the presence of colorectal cancer (CRC) in resection specimens.[95] Twenty-nine percent of 107 BWI patients had CRC compared with 8% and 1.8% of patients without BWI or left-sided colitis, respectively. However, one of the major limitations of this study was that cancer was an indication for proctocolectomy in 25% of their BWI cohort compared with 8% of patients without BWI. Therefore the conclusion regarding the causal association of BWI and CRC cannot be justified based on the data presented in this study. Larger studies performed over the past 20 years[93,96] have shown no significant association between BWI and risk of CRC. In a retrospective case-control study by Navaneethan et al., 178 proctocolectomy specimens with BWI were compared with 537 controls to evaluate the association of BWI and colonic neoplasia.[97] In patients with BWI, colon cancer was seen in 18% of patients in contrast with 12% and 9% in those with extensive colitis without BWI or left-sided colitis, respectively. Within the BWI group with colon cancer, low-grade dysplasia and high-grade dysplasia was noted in 4% and 8% cases, respectively. With dysplasia as the end-point, multivariate analysis revealed that BWI with extensive colitis was associated with an increased risk of any colonic neoplasia (odds ratio [OR] = 3.53; 95% confidence interval [CI] 1.01–12.30, $P = 0.04$). It is important to note that dysplasia/colon cancer was an indication for colectomy in 13% cases with BWI and 10% cases without BWI. Unfortunately, the retrospective nature of this study precludes evaluation of the causal association of BWI and colorectal neoplasia.

Other Causes of Ileitis in Ulcerative Colitis. There are other factors that may lead to the development of active inflammation in the distal ileum ("active ileitis") in patients with UC. These include various infections, drugs (e.g., NSAIDs), and, most commonly, the effects of certain bowel preparation agents.[98-100] For instance, in a prospective study consisting of 50 patients with active UC, 16% had ileal inflammation, but without involvement of the cecum, indicating that backwash was surely not the cause of the ileitis ("non-BWI").[101] These patients revealed higher levels of ileal inflammatory cytokines (IL-6, IL-8, and tumor necrosis factor-α [TNF-α]) and also had extraintestinal manifestations of UC (e.g., arthritis, pyoderma gangrenosum) at the time of clinical presentation. This condition should not be confused with CD of the terminal ileum. In CD, the distal ileum typically shows longer lengths of involvement (often >5 cm) and is associated with histological features of chronicity, such as pyloric gland metaplasia, ulceration, and established radiological abnormalities.[89]

Gastric and Duodenal Involvement in Ulcerative Colitis

Gastric and/or duodenal involvement may rarely occur in patients with clinically and pathologically confirmed UC.[102-108] For instance, Valdez et al. described four patients with chronic active inflammation in the duodenum similar in appearance to the patients' colonic disease.[102] In another study, five patients had chronic active gastritis, and four had chronic active duodenitis; in these cases, the upper GI findings resolved after colectomy.[107] Several similar cases have been reported in the Japanese literature.[109] In a study by Lin and colleagues, esophageal, gastric, and duodenal biopsies from 69 patients with proven UC were compared with those of 97 control subjects.[110] The most common pattern

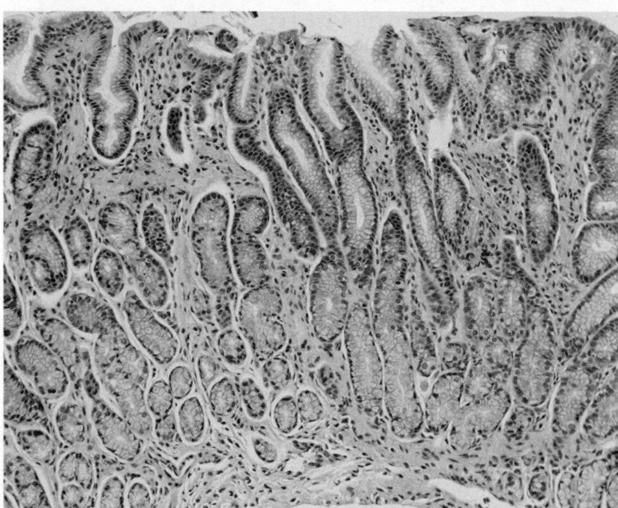

FIGURE 17.19 Gastric involvement in ulcerative colitis. The biopsy shows gastric antral mucosa with expansion of the lamina propria by lymphocytes and plasma cells. The inflammation is localized to superficial lamina propria. The biopsy was negative for *Helicobacter pylori* organisms.

of inflammation in the upper GI tract was "focal gastritis," followed by the presence of mixed inflammation in the basal aspect of gastric mucosa, and superficial plasmacytosis (Fig. 17.19). Diffuse chronic duodenitis was observed in 10% of UC patients, and these changes persisted after colectomy. The authors did not find specific mucosal changes in esophageal biopsy specimens from patients with UC. Until such cases have been followed for longer periods, it is difficult to know with certainty whether the finding of upper GI inflammation in UC represents a primary manifestation of UC or simply an unrelated, coincidental inflammatory disorder. Ultimately, more precise characterization of these types of UC cases will likely require long-term follow-up to help establish specific criteria of upper GI involvement in patients with UC.

Aphthous Ulcers in Ulcerative Colitis

Although aphthous type ulcers are common in CD, they may occur in other types of colitides and even in UC, as well. For instance, they have been reported in infectious colitis, diverticular disease–associated colitis, and diversion colitis, among other conditions.[98] In one study, aphthous-type ulcers were present in 17% of UC resection specimens.[80] In this study, manifestations of CD did not develop in any of the patients, nor was the presence of aphthous ulcers associated with the subsequent development of pouchitis on follow-up.

Granulomas in Ulcerative Colitis

Some cases of active UC, particularly the more severe ones, may develop granulomas in the deep mucosa, and these are most often associated with ruptured crypts (see Fig. 17.13). This finding may be prominent in some UC patients and may, in fact involve several contiguous crypts in the deep mucosa. Granulomas may also develop in UC from degenerated collagen, particulate matter, superimposed infections, or as a result of a drug reaction, therefore not all are related to ruptured crypts.[111-115] In equivocal cases, "mucin granulomas" related to ruptured crypts may be distinguished from primary granulomas in CD by the use of histochemical stains or by evaluation of multiple deep tissue sections to find the ruptured crypts. In general, granulomas located in the superficial aspects of the mucosa (and certainly in the submucosa) are more likely to be CD-related compared with basally located mucosal granulomas, which are more often crypt rupture–related in etiology.

Natural History and Treatment

Medical Therapy

Current therapeutic strategies for UC are separated into those that treat active disease (induction therapy) and those that prevent disease recurrence once remission has been achieved (maintenance therapy). Medical therapy focuses on agents that alter the host's immune response in an effort to decrease mucosal inflammation. First-line therapy consists of oral 5-ASA preparations such as sulfasalazine, Pentasa, Asacol, and balsalazide. Sulfasalazine induces remission in 39% to 62% of patients with mild to moderate UC.[116] Topical 5-ASA enemas can be used to treat disease located as much as 20 cm from the anal verge. Moderate to severe flares of UC are treated with systemic glucocorticosteroids. Azathioprine and 6-mercaptopurine are two purine analogue immunomodulators that interfere with nucleic acid metabolism and exert a cytotoxic effect on lymphocytes. Cyclosporine A, another potent inhibitor of cell-mediated immunity, is primarily indicated in patients with severe steroid-refractory disease.

Several recent advanced biological therapies and small molecules have shown clinical efficacy in patients with moderate to severe colitis who have previously failed to improve with corticosteroids and/or thiopurines. These therapies include anti–TNF agents like infliximab,[117] adalimumab,[118] and golimumab,[119] anti-$\alpha_4\beta_7$-integrin antibody (vedolizumab),[120] anti-IL-12/IL-23p40 antibody (ustekinumab),[121] and small-molecule antibody preferentially targeting JAK1 and JAK3 (tofacitinib).[122]

Evaluation of Medical Therapy

The goal of medical therapy is to achieve clinical remission. In current clinical practice, disease activity is monitored by assessing patients' clinical symptoms and severity of colonic inflammation by colonoscopy. However, there is evidence to suggest that endoscopic findings do not necessarily correlate with histological disease, especially after treatment.[123,124]

Effects of Prior Treatment on the Histology of Ulcerative Colitis

In patients who have received medical therapy (oral or enema), mucosal histological changes can vary considerably. Portions of mucosa may heal completely, whereas others may still be active. Healing occurs in a segmental or patchy fashion. This pattern of healing gives an impression of segmental or patchy disease (skip lesions), which may be mistaken for CD. In this circumstance, exceptions to the classic principles of UC pathology may lead to diagnostic confusion.

Classic teaching emphasizes that UC is characterized morphologically by the presence of diffuse fixed architectural or cellular mucosal changes (or both) that categorize the process as chronic. However, in 1993, Odze and colleagues prospectively evaluated 123 rectal mucosal biopsy specimens from 14 patients with pathologically confirmed UC treated with either 5-aminosalicylic acid (5-ASA) or placebo enemas.[125] During the course of treatment, 29% of rectal biopsies from 64% of patients were histologically normal, showing no evidence of chronic or active disease. Patients treated with 5-ASA showed a significantly higher percentage of normal biopsy specimens (obtained from areas of mucosa previously shown to be involved with chronic active disease) than did the placebo group. This was the first report to demonstrate that "fixed" chronic features in UC may revert to normal in the natural course of the patient's illness and that topical therapy may enhance this phenomenon. Subsequent studies by Kleer and Appelman,[126] Bernstein and colleagues,[127] and Kim and colleagues,[128] all of whom evaluated patchiness of disease and patterns of involvement in UC colorectal biopsy specimens with time, confirmed and expanded the initial findings of Odze's group.

In these studies, 30% to 59% of patients, some of whom were treated with oral sulfasalazine or steroids (or both), showed either patchiness of disease or rectal sparing on follow-up surveillance biopsies. Awareness of these data should prevent misinterpretation of the findings of a normal rectal biopsy specimen or patchiness of disease in medically treated patients with UC as evidence against this diagnosis or as representing skip areas characteristic of CD. In addition, patients with low-grade indolent disease, particularly those in clinical and pathological remission, may show minimal architectural features of chronicity or perhaps even a completely normal-appearing biopsy specimen during the natural waxing and waning course of their illness. However, it must be emphasized that these data relate primarily to biopsy material from treated patients. They do not apply to patients whose UC has not yet been treated or in whom a diagnosis is being considered on the basis of the evaluation of a resection specimen. Evaluation of disease "continuity" by analysis of mucosal biopsies is not useful to distinguish UC from CD of the colon in previously treated IBD patients. In contrast, large portions of mucosa from a resection specimen with a normal histological appearance are an indication of true segmental disease and normally provide reliable evidence in support of an alternative diagnosis such as CD.

Histology of Patients in Clinical Remission

The European Crohn's and Colitis Organization[129] and the International Organization for the Study of Inflammatory Bowel Disease (IOIBD) [130] define *remission* as complete resolution of clinical symptoms and endoscopic mucosal healing. Endoscopic mucosal healing in UC is defined by resolution of visible mucosal inflammation and ulceration, often assessed by using the Mayo endoscopic scoring method.[131] As discussed earlier Chronic Inactive (Quiescent) Colitis, as mucosal healing occurs, there is quite a lot of variability in the type and degree of inflammatory changes such that at any given point of time, mucosal biopsies may show changes ranging from active colitis, chronic active colitis, chronic inactive colitis, or completely normal mucosa on histological examination. In fact, in a prospective observational study of 103 patients with UC in clinical remission, histological inflammation was found in 54% of patients receiving maintenance therapy, and 37% had at least moderate inflammation based on histology scores. Of the 52 patients with endoscopic evidence of left-sided colitis, 34% had histological inflammation in the proximal colon.[132]

Deep remission is a more recent concept in IBD management. It is currently defined as the combination of clinical remission and mucosal healing. In a large retrospective study consisting of 252 IBD patients who were treated with anti–TNF-α therapy for ≥11 months, 122 patients achieved deep remission. The majority of patients in deep remission (81%) had "inactive disease," while 19% had active disease histologically.[133]

Histological Features Predictive of Clinical Outcome and Disease Recurrence

Much emphasis has recently been placed on the importance of mucosal healing as an outcome for therapies in patients with IBD. Few studies in UC have shown that despite endoscopic mucosal healing, active histological disease is associated with poor long-term outcomes.[59,134,135] In two studies by Bitton et al.[134] and Bessissow et al.[124] in which biopsies from UC patients with endoscopically inactive disease (defined as a Mayo endoscopic score of 0) and a follow-up period of 12 months were evaluated, basal plasmacytosis, whether present in a focal or diffuse pattern, was found to be an independent predictor of clinical relapse in UC patients with mucosal healing. In a more recent study of 646 UC patients, 60% had endoscopic mucosal healing, 40% had histological quiescence, and 10% had histological normalization on follow-up colonoscopy. Of the 310 patients who were in clinical remission, histological normalization was independently associated with increased odds of relapse-free survival compared with histological quiescence (hazard ratio [HR], 4.31; 95% CI, 1.48 to 12.46; $P = 0 .007$) and histological activity (HR, 6.69; 95% CI, 2.16 to 20.62; $p = 0.001$). [136] Another study by Zezos and colleagues found increased numbers of lamina propria eosinophils in patients with active UC, and severe eosinophilic infiltration was the most significant predictor of treatment failure in these patients.[137] In a recent study consisting of 281 UC patients, histological features of UC activity were associated with increased rates of systemic corticosteroid use, colectomy, and hospitalization in the entire cohort ($P <0.05$ for all) and with increased rates of systemic corticosteroid use in an analysis limited to patients in endoscopic remission ($p <0 .001$); in patients in endoscopic remission, only histological activity was independently associated with use of systemic corticosteroids (multivariate OR, 6.34; 95% CI, 2.20–18.28; $p <0 .001$). Compared with patients without histological evidence of UC activity, patients with only a small number of mucosal neutrophils still had higher rates of systemic corticosteroid use ($p <0.001$).[138] Interestingly, in contrast with the aforementioned studies, this study did not find any association between basal lymphoplasmacytosis or intramucosal eosinophilia and poor clinical outcome.

Lastly, in a large meta-analysis that included 28 studies contributing 2677 UC patients, histologically active disease was associated with an overall increased risk of relapse (OR 2.41, 95% CI, 1.91 to 3.04), with a similar effect noted in the subgroup with an endoscopic Mayo score of 0 versus 0 or 1. More rigorous Geboes cutoffs demonstrated numerically stronger impact on relapse rates: Geboes <3.1 (OR 2.40, 95% CI 1.57–3.65), Geboes <2.1 (OR 3.91, 95% CI 2.21–6.91), and Geboes 0 (OR 7.40, 95% CI 2.00–18.27). Among individual histological features, basal plasmacytosis (OR 1.94), neutrophilic infiltrations (OR 2.30), mucin depletion (OR 2.05), and crypt architectural irregularities (OR 2.22) predicted relapse.[139]

Histological Inflammation as a Predictor of Colorectal Neoplasia

Persistent histological inflammation has been associated with an increased risk for development of colorectal neoplasia in patients with UC. In a case control study of 204 patients with UC, histological and endoscopic activity predicted the development of neoplasia during the 14-year study period on univariate analysis. However, only histological inflammation was predictive on multivariate analysis (OR, 4.69; 95% CI, 2.10 to 10.48; $p <0.001$).[140] In another cohort study of 418 UC patients, 15 developed advanced neoplasia during a median follow-up period of 6.7 years. In this study, the average histological inflammation score correlated with neoplasia development on multivariate analysis (HR, 3.8; 95% CI, 1.7 to 8.6).[141] In a more recent meta-analysis of 1443 patients, Flores et al. showed that the pooled odds ratio for colorectal neoplasia was 3.5 (95% CI, 2.6 to 4.8; $p <.001$) in those with any mucosal inflammation and 2.6 (95% CI, 1.5 to 4.5; $P = 0.01$) in those with histological inflammation, when compared with those with mucosal healing.[142] These findings could have implications on surveillance for CRC screening in patients with long-standing UC where clinicians may consider adjusting screening intervals in individuals who lack mucosal healing at surveillance colonoscopy.

Surgical Therapy

Surgical therapy is indicated in cases of medically refractory disease, recurrent systemic complications, unacceptable side effects of medical therapy, colonic perforation, colonic dysplasia, or carcinoma. Surgical choices include subtotal colectomy with ileostomy, colectomy with ileorectal anastomosis, and proctocolectomy with ileal pouch–anal anastomosis (IPAA). A variety of configurations of the ileal pouch have been designed, with *J*-pouch, *S*-pouch, and *K*-pouch being the most common. The *J*-pouch procedure is commonly performed in patients with refractory UC or UC-associated neoplasia. In patients with UC-associated dysplasia of the rectum or sigmoid colon, mucosectomy of the rectal cuff is often performed during the pouch construction.

Clinical Course

The typical course of UC consists of periods of remission interrupted by flares of activity. In approximately 5% of patients, the course is complicated by toxic megacolon, defined as acute colonic dilation (with a transverse colon diameter >6 cm radiologically) with loss of haustration in a patient with a severe attack of colitis. It is usually encountered early in the course of disease and in some cases may be the initial presentation of UC. Approximately 50% of patients respond to medical therapy alone. Perforation is the most important predictor of mortality. Surgery is recommended for patients with perforation or clinical deterioration after 48 to 72 hours of medical therapy.

Colonic strictures develop in almost 5% of UC patients. Their presence should always prompt a high index of suspicion for malignancy, especially if the stricture is located proximal to the splenic flexure. In a retrospective study comprising 1156 patients, 24% of strictures were found to be malignant.[143] Most of the malignant strictures were located proximal to the splenic flexure, were clinically symptomatic, and developed late in the course of disease (after 20 years). Cancers associated with strictures tend to be more advanced than those not associated with a stricture.

Patients with UC have an increased risk for CRC, and the primary risk factor is the duration and extent of the disease (see Dysplasia in Ulcerative Colitis and Crohn's Disease).

CROHN'S COLITIS

Clinical Features

CD is a chronic inflammatory condition that can affect any part of the GI tract but has a propensity to involve the distal small and proximal large intestine. Descriptions of CD date back to more than three centuries, when it was termed *terminal ileitis, regional enteritis,* and *granulomatous enterocolitis.* Crohn, Ginzburg, and Oppenheimer are credited with the first modern description of CD in 1932.[144]

The clinical classification of CD, known as the *Montreal classification,* is based on age at disease onset, principal anatomic location, and clinical behavior (Box 17.3). It distinguishes disease of the ileum from that of the colon or both the ileum and colon. Approximately 30% to 40% of patients have small bowel involvement only, and 30% to 40% have ileocolonic involvement; only 10% to 20% have exclusive involvement of the colon (Crohn's colitis). In patients with ileal disease, colonic lesions develop in fewer than 20% of patients during a period of 10 years.[145] Similarly, ileal involvement occurs in 20% of patients with colonic disease.[146] In a retrospective analysis of 84 patients with Crohn's colitis, 52% had right-sided colitis, 40% had left-sided colitis, and 6% had pancolonic involvement. Small bowel involvement was more frequently associated with right-sided disease, whereas proctitis and perianal lesions were more frequent in patients with left-sided disease.[147]

Accurate assessment of the incidence and prevalence of CD worldwide is limited because of inconsistencies in diagnostic criteria, lack of thorough clinical evaluation with the use of modern radiological techniques, and, in some cases, an inability to differentiate UC from CD pathologically. Despite these limitations, reproducible epidemiological trends have been discerned. The age-adjusted annual incidence rate was reported to be 9 per 100,000 persons in Olmsted County, Minnesota. More recently, the prevalence of CD in the United States was estimated at 201 per 100,000 adults or 43 per 100,000 people younger than 20 years of age.[8] There is a higher incidence of CD in northern latitudes (e.g., Denmark, 9/100,000; Nova Scotia, 20/100,000) than in southern Europe (e.g., Spain, 0.9/100,000; Italy, 3.4/100,000). In Asian, South American, and most African countries, the incidence is very low.[8] Although all ethnic groups may be affected, CD is more prevalent among white North Americans, northern Europeans, Ashkenazi Jews, Scandinavians, and the Welsh.

Women are slightly more commonly affected than men (female-to-male ratio, 1.3:1). Most patients with CD are diagnosed during the second to fourth decades of life, although there is a smaller peak between the fifth and seventh decades. There is no relationship between pathological findings and age at onset, but some studies have identified a greater proportion of colonic and distal colonic disease among older patients and a predominance of ileocolonic disease in younger patients.[148,149] In one recent study that evaluated 118 patients with either isolated colonic or ileocolonic CD, those with isolated colonic CD were significantly older at disease onset and had a shorter interval from initial diagnosis to surgery. Compared with patients with ileocolonic disease, those with isolated colonic CD more often had subtotal or total colitis and were more likely to have left-sided colitis.[150]

The clinical presentation of CD varies substantially depending on the principal location of disease, the intensity of inflammation, and the presence or absence of specific intestinal and extraintestinal complications. In some cases, weight loss and fever may be the only presenting features, especially in children. Crohn's colitis often manifests with diarrhea, either with or without blood. Depending on the extent of colonic involvement and the severity of inflammation, patients may have a range of initial findings, ranging from minimally altered bowel habits to fulminant colitis. Intermittent and colicky abdominal pain is a common presenting symptom. Although most patients have either relative or complete sparing of the rectum, proctitis may be the initial or even the only area of involvement at presentation in some cases. Perianal skin tags, anal fissures, or ulcers are often present at the time of diagnosis as well. In a subset of patients (almost 24%), perianal disease preceded intestinal symptoms by a mean period of as long as 4 years.[151]

The clinical pattern of disease is typically divided into aggressive fistulizing, fibrostenosing, and cicatrizing disease. Fistulas are a common finding in CD and may involve different segments of the bowel; more rarely, they may involve adjacent organs as well (coloduodenal, cologastric, or rectovaginal fistula). Symptoms of intestinal obstruction or jaundice, or both, are more common in the fibrostenotic form of disease.

Extraintestinal manifestations of CD occur in 6% to 25% of cases and are more common among patients with colonic involvement.[152,153] They include musculoskeletal disorders such as pauciarticular arthropathy (6%), polyarticular arthropathy (4%), and peripheral arthralgias (16%

BOX 17.3 Montreal Classification of Crohn's Disease

Age at diagnosis
- A1 younger than 16 years
- A2 between 17 and 40 years
- A3 older than 40 years

Location
- L1 ileal
- L2 colonic
- L3 ileocolonic
- L4 isolated upper tract disease

Behavior
- B1 nonstricturing, nonpenetrating
- B2 stricturing
- B3 penetrating

p perianal disease

to 20%). Axial arthropathies, granulomatous vasculitis, periostitis, and amyloidosis are other rare rheumatological complications.[154-156] Mucocutaneous lesions include pyoderma gangrenosum, erythema nodosum, and oral aphthous ulcers. Episcleritis and uveitis tend to occur in association with active intestinal disease and occur in as many as 6% of patients. Among hepatobiliary manifestations, more than 25% of cases manifest with symptomatic cholelithiasis. Although it is more commonly associated with UC, PSC may develop in as many as 4% of patients who have colonic CD.[157] Hyperoxaluria with calcium oxalate stone formation, interstitial nephritis, and cardiomyopathy have associations with CD as well.

Patients with CD have a prothrombic tendency and therefore may present with venous thromboembolism or, less commonly, arterial thrombosis. In more than 50% of patients, a predisposing factor cannot be identified.[158,159]

As in UC, there is no specific clinical or laboratory test that establishes a definite diagnosis of CD. The diagnosis is usually established based on a compilation of clinical findings combined with radiological, endoscopic, and pathological findings. Laboratory tests may be completely normal. In some patients, the white blood cell count is elevated, which suggests a pyogenic complication. The presence of anemia, elevated ESR, and elevated CRP in a patient with abdominal pain is not specific for CD but should always prompt a workup for IBD. Stool studies, including culture, examination for ova and parasites, C. *difficile* toxin assay, and serological testing for *Entamoeba histolytica*, are usually performed to exclude an infectious cause. Serological testing shows elevated ASCA levels in 41% to 76% of patients.[160,161]

Barium studies are a popular method of investigation for patients with suspected CD. They are especially helpful in delineating late transmural complications of CD. Aphthous ulcers, thickened mucosal folds, submucosal edema, fistulas, sinus tracts, and fixed strictures are some of the findings that may be detected by barium studies. Currently, CT or magnetic resonance enterography is preferred over barium studies. Radiological findings that correlate with disease activity include mural enhancement and increased density of pericolonic fat.[162,163]

Common endoscopic findings of CD include aphthous ulcers, edema, cobblestoning, and luminal narrowing. Segmental involvement is characteristically present in early-stage disease. Rectal sparing is often present in untreated cases.

Once a diagnosis of CD has been established, clinical disease activity is usually monitored with the use of a composite scoring system. The Crohn's Disease Activity index is a commonly used scoring system that evaluates eight variables (stool count, abdominal pain, general well-being, features of extraintestinal disease, opiate intake for diarrhea, presence of abdominal mass, hematocrit value, and body weight).[164]

Risk Factors and Pathogenesis

The cause of CD is unknown; similar to UC, it probably involves a combination of environmental factors (e.g., luminal bacteria, infectious agents), abnormalities in immune regulation, and genetic predisposition for development of disease.

Many infectious agents, including *Chlamydia*, *Listeria monocytogenes*, *Pseudomonas* species, paramyxovirus, and *Mycobacterium paratuberculosis*, have been etiologically linked to CD as a cause of granulomatous vasculitis and bowel injury. Molecular techniques have detected *M. paratuberculosis* in tissues of some patients with CD.[165] One study by Lamps and colleagues found *Yersinia* species DNA in 31% of Crohn's resection specimens.[165] There are many histological similarities between these infections and CD, and the possibility that one or more of them triggers the development of CD is an appealing hypothesis. However, thus far, there is no conclusive evidence to implicate any one specific organism in the pathogenesis of CD.

Genetic Factors

The relative risk (RR) for development of IBD among first-degree relatives of patients with CD is 14 to 15 times higher than in the general population.[166] Ethnicity also appears to play a significant role. Eastern European (Ashkenazi) Jews have a two-fold to four-fold higher risk for CD than non-Jews from the same geographic location. Further support for a genetic predisposition is provided by data on monozygotic and dizygotic twins.[20,167] The concordance rate for CD is 67% among monozygotic twins and 8% among dizygotic twins, suggesting a strong genetic influence. Although results are inconsistent and vary with the population being studied, numerous studies have found both positive and negative associations between HLA antigens and the development of CD.[168,169]

Genome-wide association studies and computerized meta-analyses have identified 71 susceptibility loci for CD on 17 chromosomes thus far.[170] Three important pathways have been highlighted by these studies. The first susceptibility locus was identified in 2001 as nucleotide-binding oligodimerization domain 2 *(NOD2)* or caspase-recruitment domain 15 *(CARD15)*.[171-173] A homozygous carrier of disease-specific allelic variants has a 17.1-fold increased risk for CD, whereas the OR for a heterozygous carrier is 2.5.[174] Genetic polymorphisms in *NOD2/CARD15* are present in 20% to 30% of patients with CD, and the abnormalities correlate with younger age at onset, ileal location of disease, and an increased likelihood of stricture formation.[175,176] *NOD2/CARD15* mutations are more common in white patients with CD but are rare in Asians and Africans.[177] The *NOD2/CARD15* gene product binds to muramyl dipeptide, a component of bacterial peptidoglycan found in both gram-positive and gram-negative bacteria.[178,179] NOD2/CARD1 is expressed in Paneth cells[180] that produce endogenous antimicrobial peptides known as defensins. *NOD2/CARD15* gene variants interfere with binding to muramyl peptide, resulting in decreased antibacterial defense.

The second important pathway implicated in CD pathogenesis is related to autophagy, a unique process by which cytoplasmic constituents are isolated within a membrane-bound vesicle and then delivered to lysosomes for elimination. Misfolded or misaggregated proteins are eliminated via this pathway without inciting an inflammatory or autoimmune response. Variants in at least two autophagy-related genes have been associated with CD, namely, the autophagy-related 16-like 1 *(ATG16L1)* gene and the immunity-related guanosine triphosphatase family member M *(IRGM)* gene on chromosome 5.[181-184]

The third pathway associated with CD is related to IL-23.[185] IL-23 is a cytokine produced by dendritic cells and macrophages in response to various antigenic signals. In response to IL-6 and transforming growth factor-β (TGF-β), naïve CD4+ T cells upregulate the IL-23 receptor (IL-23R), which results in autocrine generation of effector T cells that produce IL-17. Although most common single nucleotide polymorphisms (SNPs) in the *IL23R* gene are associated with an increased risk for CD and UC, rare variants appear to be protective against the development of CD.[186,187]

Environmental Factors

The gradually increasing incidence of CD has also been attributed to a variety of environmental factors. Higher socioeconomic status, use of oral contraceptives, NSAID use, increased intake of refined sugars, and decreased intake of dietary fiber have all been implicated as risk factors for CD. Zinc deficiency is associated with immunological dysfunction in patients with CD,[188] and some data suggest that an elemental diet may improve CD by reducing intestinal permeability.[189]

In contrast with UC, CD is more prevalent among smokers. Smoking is an independent risk factor for clinical, surgical, and endoscopic recurrences in CD and also appears to influence disease activity after surgery. Although the pathogenesis is unclear, it is believed that smoking causes alteration of intestinal permeability, induces cytokine production, and promotes production of microvascular thrombi.[190,191]

Immune Factors

Similar to UC, disturbance of the intestinal epithelial barrier and innate immunity also plays a role in the pathogenesis of CD. Analysis of intestinal biopsies from patients with CD shows downregulation of the junctional protein epithelial cadherin, which composes the tight junctions of this physical barrier.[192]

Interaction of effector T cells and antigen-presenting cells is vital to the pathogenesis of CD. Processing of luminal antigens by dendritic cells located within the lamina propria and the subsequent interaction between MHC class II molecules and T-cell receptors leads to activation and differentiation of T cells. The helper T-cell Th1 and Th17 responses that characterize CD are influenced by cytokines IL-23, IL-6, and TGF-β. Within mononuclear cells, NF-κB plays a key role in regulating transcription of IL-1, IL-6, IL-8, TNF, and other peptides that generate an inflammatory response. TNF is not only essential in formation of granulomas, but also causes neutrophil activation and, along with interferon-γ, induces expression of MHC class II molecules on IECs.

TNF and other proinflammatory cytokines also promote expression of adhesion molecules on endothelial cells, which leads to trafficking of inflammatory cells into mucosa. Integrins $\alpha_4\beta_7$ and $\alpha_E\beta_7$ have ligands (mucosal addressin cellular adhesion molecule and E-cadherin, respectively) that are specific to the intestinal environment.[193] Antibodies to the α_4 subunit of integrin have a therapeutic role in the management of CD.[194]

Tissue destruction (especially penetrating ulcers, fistulas, and sinuses) ultimately results when proinflammatory substances such as prostaglandins and matrix metalloproteinases are elaborated by mononuclear cells and granulocytes. Mural fibrosis, another characteristic finding of CD, is a result of TGF-β that is released in the presence of inflammation. It stimulates production of type III collagen, which not only promotes healing of ulcers but also contributes to the formation of strictures.[195] Fat wrapping ("creeping fat") is an indicator of transmural disease that is often identified intraoperatively. It results from upregulation of peroxisome proliferator–activated receptor-γ (PPAR-γ), which regulates homeostasis of adipose tissue.[196] Histologically, the finding of pyloric gland metaplasia in the lower GI tract indicates chronic mucosal injury. Pyloric glands are a form of ulcer-associated cell lineage (UACL); they represent budlike glandular structures that develop from the base of intestinal crypts at sites of chronic ulceration. The UACL expresses a variety of peptides implicated in the repair of damaged GI mucosa, notably epidermal growth factor and members of the trefoil peptide family, which restores epithelium in areas of mucosal ulceration.[197]

The pathophysiology of diarrhea in CD is related to multiple factors. Increased mucosal permeability caused by inflammation and production of prostaglandins, biogenic amines, neuropeptides, and reactive oxygen metabolites results in exudation of proteins and fluids. Bacterial overgrowth and altered colonic mobility in areas of strictured bowel also contribute to diarrhea.

Pathological Features

Gross Features

CD is classically characterized by segmental involvement of the affected areas of bowel, although pancolitis, and even proctitis as the only manifestation of colonic involvement may occur in a small proportion of cases (Fig. 17.20A). The serosal surface often appears congested and may be covered with a fibrinous exudate. Fat wrapping (creeping fat) along the antimesenteric border is a common finding in CD. In contrast with UC, the bowel wall in CD is typically thickened. It does not lie flat on opening. Mucosal aphthous ulcers overlying lymphoid aggregates are an early feature of CD. A zone of hyperemia often surrounds larger ulcers. As the disease progresses, ulcers enlarge to form discontinuous, serpiginous, or bear claw–type longitudinal furrows (see Fig. 17.20B). Areas of edematous, mildly inflamed, or even normal mucosa are located between areas of longitudinal ulcers; this results in the development of a cobblestone appearance of the mucosa. Inflammatory pseudopolyps are most commonly encountered in the transverse colon and splenic flexure. In segments of bowel involved by disease, the wall of the bowel is usually thick and fibrotic. Fissures, sinuses and fistulous tracts, and mural or pericolonic abscesses may be present in complicated cases.

Strictures are more common with long-standing disease. Depending on the degree of obstruction, the bowel wall proximal to the stricture may be secondarily dilated and congested (Fig. 17.21). Perforations are uncommon in CD, occurring only in 1% to 3% of cases.[198,199] They occur as a result of superimposed ischemia or infection or as a complication of fissures, sinus tracts, or fistulas. Fibrous adhesions may seal off sites of perforation, so they may not be visible on gross examination of the bowel.

Microscopic Features

General Comments. Histologically, colonic CD (whether isolated or combined with ileal disease) classically shows

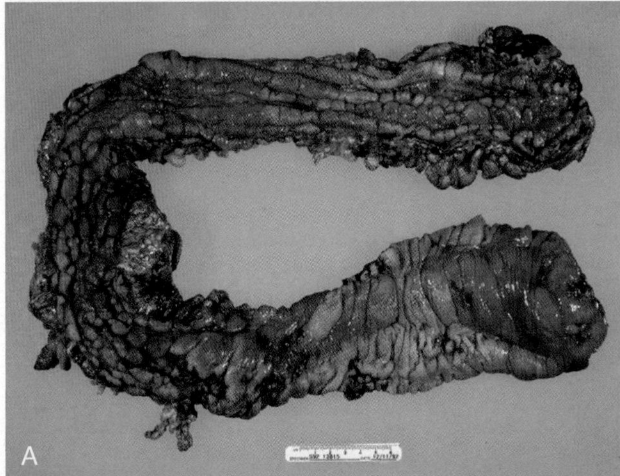

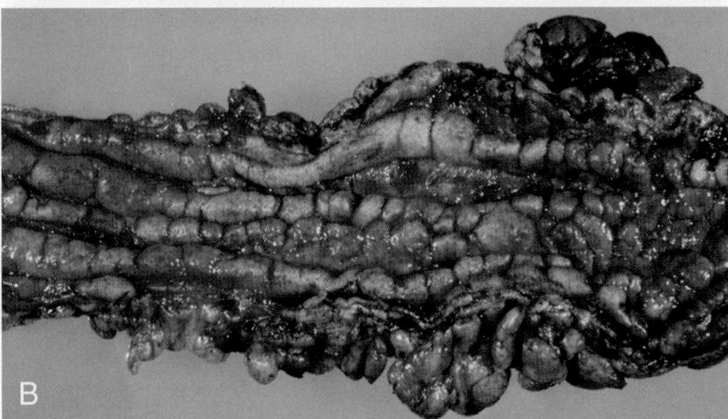

FIGURE 17.20 **A,** Gross specimen of Crohn's colitis showing segmental (patchy) distribution of disease in the right colon. **B,** The affected segment shows deep longitudinal ulcers with a cobblestone appearance of the mucosa.

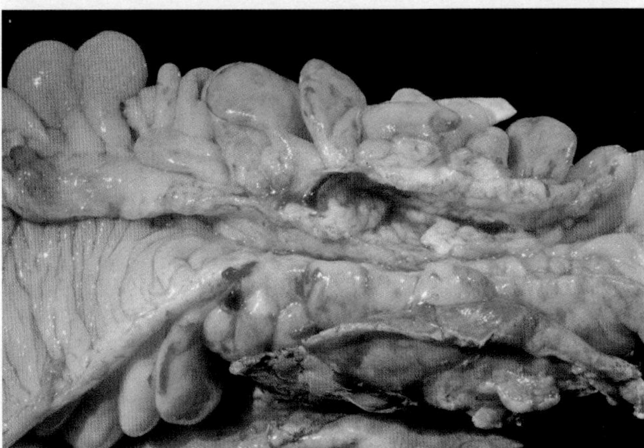

FIGURE 17.21 Gross specimen of Crohn's colitis showing stricture formation with dilation of the proximal colonic segment (*left* aspect of specimen).

skip areas of involvement, both grossly and microscopically. Areas of involvement alternating with areas of normal mucosa are characteristic ("segmental" colitis). However, as mentioned earlier, pancolitis occurs in a small proportion of cases. Overall, CD is characterized by the presence of a wide variety of mucosal and mural changes (Box 17.4). Other major pathological features include aphthous and fissuring ulcers, sinuses and fistulas, transmural lymphoid aggregates, and nonnecrotizing granulomas. All of these features may affect the bowel wall in a patchy and segmental distribution. Other, less characteristic but common features include submucosal fibrosis, neural hypertrophy, muscularis mucosae and muscularis propria hypertrophy, neural plexitis, perivascular lymphoid aggregates, serositis, and pyloric gland metaplasia.

BOX 17.4 Pathological Features of Crohn's Disease

MAJOR PATHOLOGICAL FEATURES

Segmental disease
Creeping fat
Fistulas/sinuses
Skip lesions
Granulomas
Transmural lymphoid aggregates
Aphthous and fissuring ulcers

MINOR OR SECONDARY PATHOLOGICAL FEATURES

Submucosal fibrosis
Neural hypertrophy
Muscularis mucosae hypertrophy
Muscularis propria hypertrophy
Neural plexitis
Perivascular lymphoid aggregates
Serositis
Pyloric gland metaplasia

Mucosal Changes. Similar to UC, and depending on the phase of disease, the mucosa may show a wide spectrum of changes ranging from completely normal to diffuse and severe chronic active inflammation with ulceration. In biopsies, mucosal disease is categorized similar to UC: *chronic inactive, chronic active,* or *active* (see earlier discussion). Histological features of chronicity include crypt architectural distortion, crypt atrophy, diffuse mixed lamina propria inflammation, basal plasmacytosis, basally located lymphoid aggregates, pyloric gland metaplasia, and Paneth cell metaplasia (in the left colon). Other changes of chronicity include lamina propria fibrosis and Paneth cell hyperplasia in the right colon. "Activity" is characterized by the presence of neutrophilic or eosinophilic cryptitis, crypt abscesses, regenerative and/or degenerative epithelial changes, necrosis, erosions, and ulceration. Grading of the degree of inflammation in patients with CD is difficult and has not been standardized. This is also because some areas of the bowel may show severe ulcerating disease, and others adjacent to it may be completely normal. However, in individual biopsies, grading the degree of activity can be done similar to the system proposed by the authors in the Ulcerative Colitis section earlier in this chapter.

In active CD, the disease may be patchy, with foci of injured and inflamed crypts situated adjacent to completely normal crypts. Two types of ulcers are characteristic of active CD: aphthous and fissuring ulcers. Aphthous ulcers arise in focal, mildly active CD. They are well-delineated, small, superficial lesions that overlie lymphoid aggregates. They usually involve a portion of mucosa occupied by about two to four crypts in length. The earliest stage is a mild neutrophilic infiltrate in the superficial half of the lymphoid aggregate. Neutrophils infiltrate the crypts and form small basilar crypt abscesses, producing epithelial necrosis and

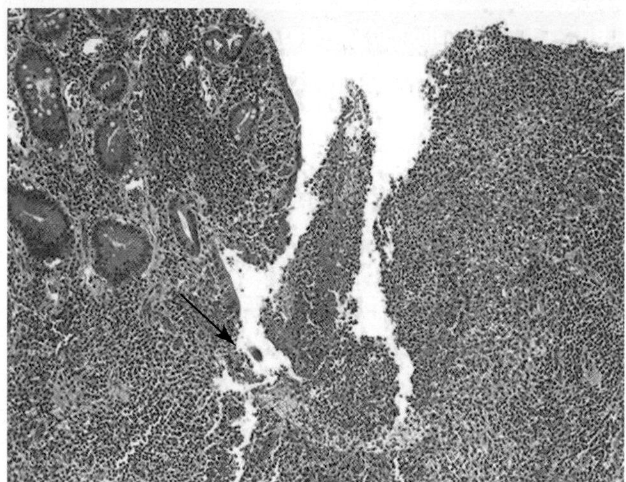

FIGURE 17.22 Aphthous ulcer in Crohn's colitis. Neutrophilic inflammation involves the epithelium overlying lymphoid aggregates, which leads to ulceration *(arrow)*.

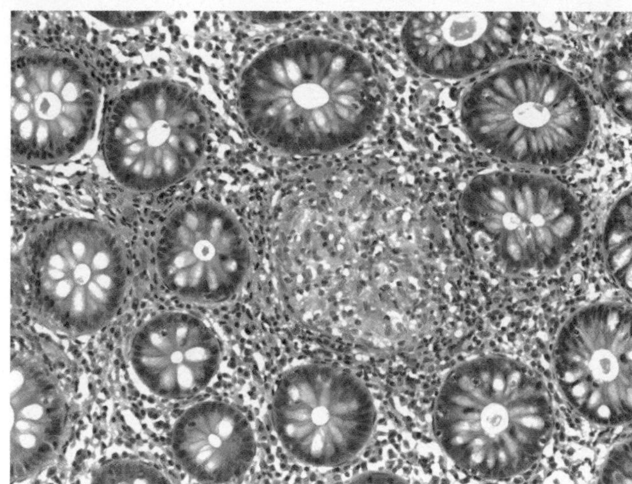

FIGURE 17.24 Crohn's colitis with a well-formed epithelioid granuloma in the lamina propria, not associated with a ruptured crypt.

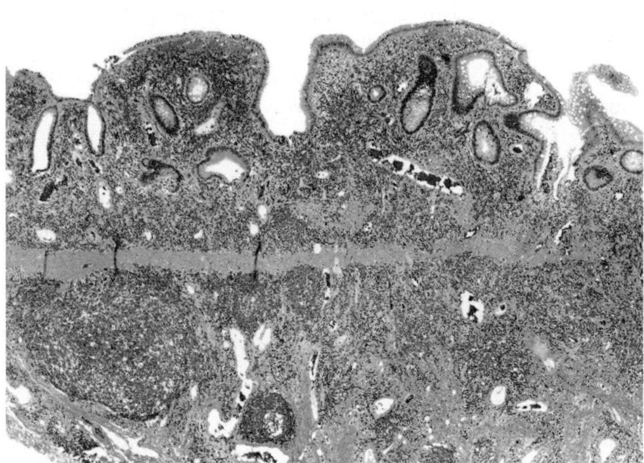

FIGURE 17.23 Active Crohn's colitis with diffuse mixed inflammation, crypt architectural distortion, prominent mucosal and submucosal lymphoid aggregates, thickened muscularis mucosae, fibrosis, and perivascular lymphoid aggregates.

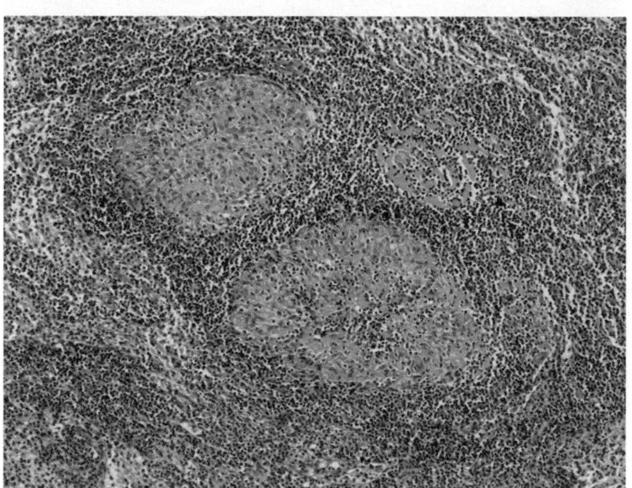

FIGURE 17.25 Crohn's colitis with granulomas within pericolonic lymph nodes.

an intraluminal exudate (Fig. 17.22). Concomitant neutrophilic infiltration and erosion of the superficial epithelium develops into a small microabscess that covers the lymphoid aggregate as the ulcer expands. Irregularly shaped crypts with regenerative epithelial changes are typically found at the edges of older (healing) ulcers. Aphthous ulcers can continue to expand and connect to form serpiginous or longitudinally oriented ulcers.

Crypt disarray is a feature of mucosal involvement in CD, similar to UC. There is significant variation in the size and shape of crypts. Features such as crypt branching and shortening are most easily appreciated at medium or low magnification (Fig. 17.23). Heterogeneity in the density and distribution of lymphoplasmacytic inflammation within the lamina propria is a common finding in CD, as it is in UC. Well-circumscribed, focal collections of lymphocytes that surround several crypts (lymphoid aggregates) simulate normal lymphoid follicles. However, lymphoid aggregates in CD may reveal crypts within their center, whereas in normal lymphoid follicles, the crypts are pushed toward the periphery.

Although nonnecrotizing epithelioid granulomas are characteristic of CD, they are neither specific nor sensitive for this diagnosis.[114,200,201] The prevalence of granulomas in endoscopic biopsy samples ranges from 13% to 50%; in resections, it ranges from 40% to 60%.[202] Granulomas are more frequently encountered early in the course of disease. They are typically sarcoid-like and composed of aggregates of epithelioid histiocytes admixed with lymphocytes and neutrophils (Fig. 17.24). Occasionally, giant cells are present. In some cases, they may be very sparse and poorly formed, consisting only of small, pericryptal collections of closely arranged histiocytes, referred to as *pericryptal microgranulomas*.[203] Serial step sections enhance the likelihood of detecting pericryptal microgranulomas.[204-206] They may be present in involved as well as in uninvolved segments of colon. They may be present in any layer of the bowel wall or within pericolonic lymph nodes (Fig. 17.25).

Granulomas in CD should be distinguished from mucin granulomas that form around ruptured crypts, which is

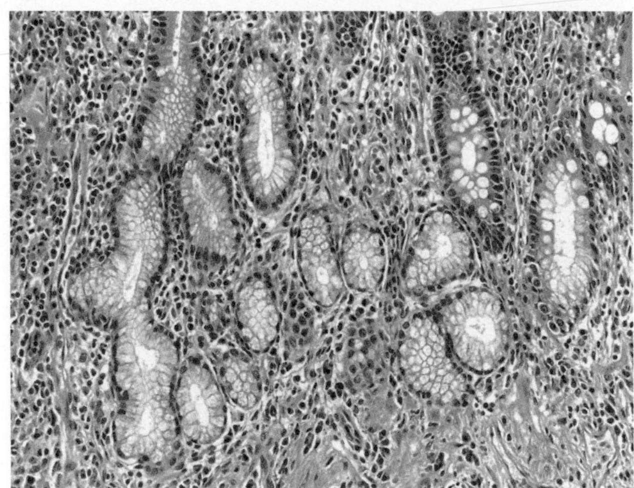

FIGURE 17.26 Chronic Crohn's colitis with pyloric gland metaplasia.

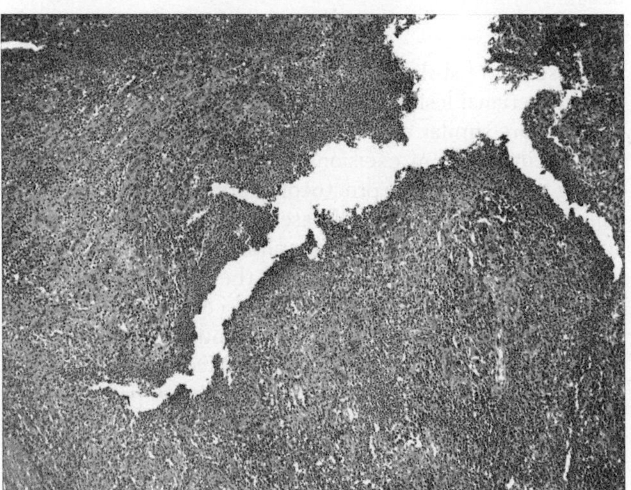

FIGURE 17.27 Crohn's colitis with deep fissuring ulcers.

common in UC (see Pathological Features in the Ulcerative Colitis section earlier in this chapter). Macrophages within mucin granulomas usually have a greater amount of bubbly or clear cytoplasm, which is caused by phagocytosis of mucin and crypt contents. Foreign-body giant cells usually are not a component of CD-related granulomas, but they may be found in mucin granulomas. Mucin stains are not always helpful because a small amount of mucin may also be present in the cytoplasm of macrophages in CD-related granulomas. Thick-walled capillaries, pericryptal fibroblastic sheaths, and tangential sections of germinal centers may mimic the well-formed granulomas of CD. The presence of necrotizing granulomas or a large number of granulomas should prompt a workup for an infectious etiology such as tuberculosis, histoplasmosis, yersiniosis, or sarcoidosis.

Pyloric gland metaplasia is far more common in CD than in UC, and it is frequently present in the small bowel. In colonic CD, pyloric gland metaplasia is more common in the cecum and right colon (Fig. 17.26).

Mural Changes. Among the common mural changes of CD are knifelike fissuring ulcers and sinus tracts, which typically occur at right angles to the longitudinal axis of the bowel.

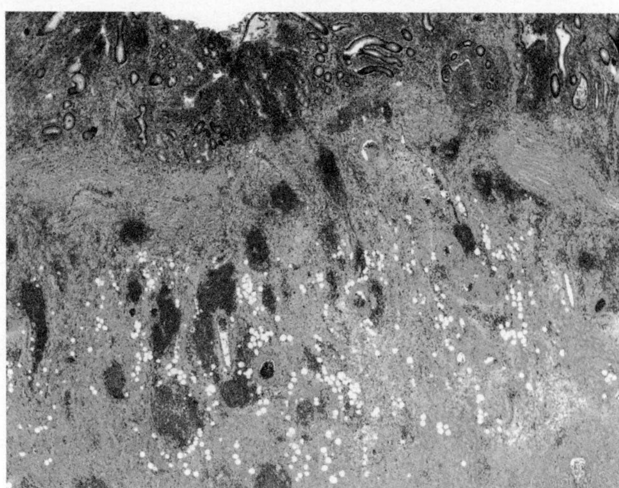

FIGURE 17.28 Chronic active Crohn's colitis associated with abundant transmural lymphoid aggregates.

They may extend through the bowel wall and may develop into a fistula or result in pericolonic abscess formation (Fig. 17.27). They are usually lined by acute inflammatory cells, necrotic and granulation tissue, and loose aggregates of epithelioid histiocytes resembling early granulomas. Multinucleate giant cells may be present as well. Dense lymphoid aggregates, with or without germinal centers, are usually found at the mucosal-submucosal junction. However, transmural lymphoid aggregates that are located in the deeper aspects of the bowel wall, including the subserosal adipose tissue ("Crohn's rosary"), are characteristic of CD (Figs. 17.28 and 17.29). These are defined as collections of predominantly small, mature-appearing lymphocytes of variable size that are distributed throughout the bowel wall. Some cases of CD show prominent perivascular lymphoid aggregates, which may or may not be associated with granulomas, particularly in the submucosa. This feature has led some authorities to postulate that CD may represent a vascular disorder.

Abnormalities in smooth muscle, such as splaying and hypertrophy of the muscularis mucosae and distortion (and hypertrophy) of the muscularis propria, are common in long-standing CD. Proliferation of smooth muscle that obliterates the submucosa ("muscularization of submucosa") occurs more commonly in stricturing CD.[207] CD also affects the neural tissue. There is both hypertrophy of nerve trunks and an increase in the number of ganglion cells.[208,209] Large, abnormal fusiform nerve bundles may be seen throughout the affected bowel wall. Additionally, the myenteric plexuses may show infiltration by lymphocytes *(myenteric plexitis)* (Fig. 17.30). Some studies have shown that myenteric plexitis in the proximal margins of an ileocolonic resection is more likely to be present in resection specimens of patients with a previous surgery for CD and of those with a shorter duration of disease before surgery.[210] The severity of inflammation also appears to correlate with severity of endoscopic recurrence.[211]

Some studies suggest that colonic CD less frequently shows major pathological features than does ileal CD. A study by Soucy and colleagues showed that patients with isolated CD had significantly fewer major pathological

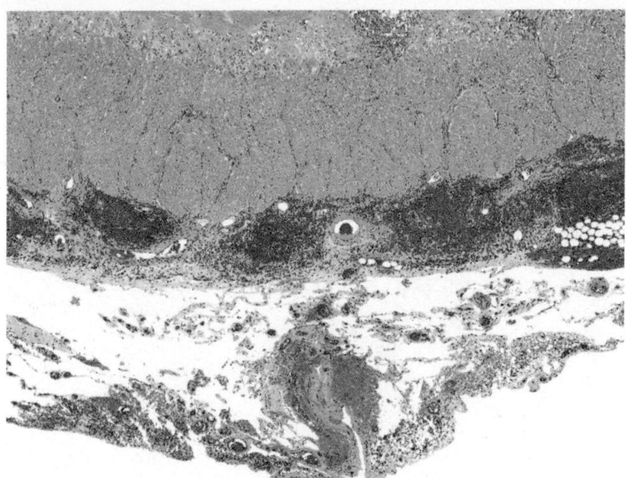

FIGURE 17.29 Crohn's colitis associated with serosal-based lymphoid aggregates. Deep lymphoid aggregates located at the junction of the muscularis propria and subserosal adipose tissue give rise to a characteristic serosal "beading" pattern, also known as *Crohn's rosary.*

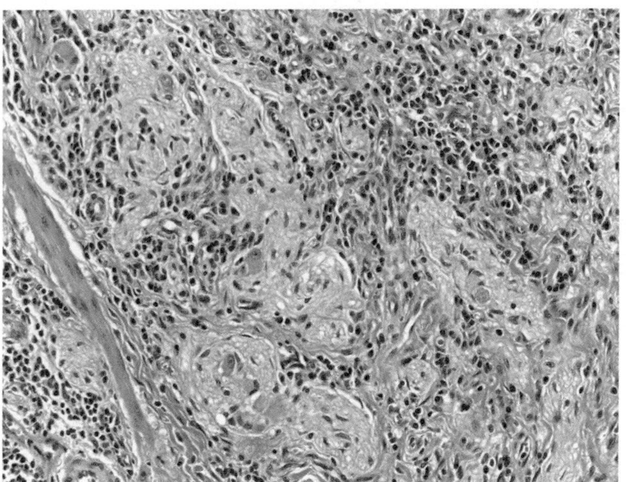

FIGURE 17.30 Crohn's colitis with neural hyperplasia. Lymphocytes and plasma cells also infiltrate the myenteric plexuses (myenteric plexitis).

features of CD, such as strictures/stenosis, pericolonic adhesions, segmental disease, the finding of proximal disease worse than distal disease, perivascular lymphoid aggregates, and pyloric gland metaplasia, compared with those with ileal CD.[150] A small proportion of patients from both groups showed inflammatory changes limited to the mucosa, similar to what is seen in UC (see later discussion).

Perianal Crohn's Disease

Perianal involvement occurs in approximately 74% of CD patients, typically within 10 years of the initial diagnosis, and it generally increases in frequency in patients with more distal colonic disease. In 20% to 36% of patients with CD, the patients' perianal disease actually precedes the intestinal disease.[212] Skin tags or fibroepithelial polyps are the most common type of perianal lesion in CD, being present in 40% to 70% of cases. Histologically, they resemble fibroepithelial polyps that occur in non-CD patients. Other manifestations of anal CD include anal fissures, stenosis, and anorectal abscesses and fistulas, the latter comprising 18% of all CD-related perianal lesions.[213] The histological features of perianal CD are similar to CD elsewhere in the GI tract in that the specimens from excisional biopsies, limited resections during fistula repair, or proctocolectomy for severe or medically refractory perianal disease show mucosal ulceration accompanied by transmural lymphoid aggregates and mural fibrosis. One note of caution is that the fistulae may be associated with a foreign-body–type giant cell reaction, and this should be distinguished from true granulomas when evaluating whether the patient has CD. Medical management remains the main type of therapy for most patients with perianal CD.

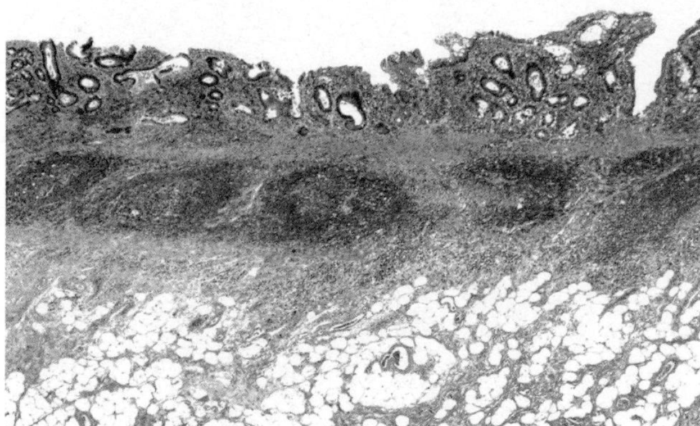

FIGURE 17.31 Superficial (ulcerative colitis–like) Crohn's colitis with inflammatory changes restricted to the mucosa and superficial submucosa. This patient also had involvement of the terminal ileum by Crohn's disease.

Superficial (Ulcerative Colitis–Like) Crohn's Colitis

As mentioned previously, the colon is involved in almost 50% of CD cases, either alone or in combination with the small intestine. However, in some studies, up to 20% of CD patients have disease limited to the colon. Although some cases of Crohn's colitis show classic features of CD (e.g., fissuring ulcers, sinus tracts, transmural lymphoid aggregates, submucosal fibrosis, granulomas), others show few or none of these features and resemble UC, both clinically and, particularly, histologically. These cases have been termed *superficial Crohn's disease* or *UC-like Crohn's disease* because the inflammatory changes are limited to the mucosa and, in some cases, the superficial submucosa, similar to UC (Fig. 17.31).[214-217] In these cases, a diagnosis of CD may be established by noting the presence of typical CD in other regions of the GI tract, such as the distal small intestine or the perianal region, or by showing other cardinal features of CD such as granulomas unrelated to ruptured crypts, segmental involvement of the colon with skip areas unrelated to treatment effect, or absolute rectal sparing from the initial onset of disease. In addition, CD also should be suspected in patients who have UC-like features in the colon and severe anal or perianal disease (e.g., fissures, fistulas). UC-like CD is rare. In one of the earlier studies that evaluated 10 patients with "superficial" CD, the diagnosis of CD was rendered based on the association with classic CD in other segments of the same resection specimens, a previous history of resection for CD, small bowel involvement, segmental or irregular disease distribution, and presence of granulomas.[214]

In a comprehensive case-control study by Soucy et al. comprising 73 patients with isolated colonic CD and 45 patients with ileocolonic CD, all of whom had detailed pathological evaluation of a wide variety of UC and CD features, the incidence of UC-like CD was 14% and 13%, respectively, in the two groups.[150] Patients with UC-like CD were younger than those who had classic CD with mural involvement. In this study, 50% of patients with superficial UC-like CD had only left-sided colitis, whereas 19%, 13%, and 6% showed right-sided, total, and subtotal colitis, respectively. Granulomas were observed in 44% of cases. Of the four UC-like CD patients who underwent an IPAA procedure, none showed an anastomosis breakdown. When the UC-like colonic CD cohort was compared with patients with non–UC-like colonic CD, the mean age at diagnosis was significantly younger in the former group (25 vs. 35 years; $P = 0.02$). However, there were no differences in the pathological (nonmural) features or in overall outcome between these two groups.

In another study consisting of 21 CD patients with UC-like pancolitis at presentation who underwent a pouch procedure, only 14% had pouch complications that necessitated pouch resection.[217] Furthermore, recurrent CD in the small intestine developed in only 5%. Therefore it appears that many patients with UC-like colonic CD have good success after a pouch procedure, and this approach may be a viable option in affected patients who are either resistant to permanent ileostomy or prefer a pouch procedure.

Natural History and Treatment

The natural history of CD is quite variable, and the type of therapy administered also affects the disease course. Two population-based studies that evaluated patient outcome—from Olmsted County, Minnesota (225 patients), and Copenhagen County, Denmark (373 patients)—found that a relapse or exacerbation of disease developed in 10% to 30% of CD patients, respectively, after the first year of diagnosis, 15% to 25% experienced low disease activity, and 50% to 65% were in remission. On long-term follow-up (>10 years), 10% to 13% of patients remained in remission, 67% to 73% experienced a chronic intermittent course, and a chronic course with continuous activity developed in 13% to 20%.[218,219] Penetrating/fistulizing CD, young age at presentation, short duration of disease before first surgery, and ileocolonic disease are high risk factors for CD recurrence after surgery.[219] Based on the outcome data from a detailed clinicopathological study consisting of 118 patients with isolated and ileocolonic CD, colonic recurrence will develop in as many as 28% of patients after surgery, noncolonic recurrence will develop in 10%, and recurrent disease at both sites will develop in 6%, during a mean follow-up interval of more than 5 years.[150] A recent meta-analysis consisting of 21 studies (2481 patients) that assessed positive resection margins, 10 studies (808 patients) that assessed plexitis, and 19 studies (1777 patients) that assessed granulomas in patients undergoing resection for CD showed that positive resection margins increased the risk of clinical recurrence (RR 1.26, 95% CI, 1.06 to 1.49) and surgical recurrence (RR 1.87, 95% CI, 1.14 to 3.08), granulomas increased the risk of clinical recurrence (RR 1.31, 95% CI, 1.05 to 1.64) and endoscopic recurrence (RR 1.37, 95% CI, 1.00 to 1.87), and plexitis increased the risk of endoscopic recurrence (RR 1.31, 95% CI, 1.00 to 1.72).[220]

The goal of therapy is to induce and maintain clinical remission. Aminosalicylates are used in the treatment of mild to moderate CD. Antibiotics, especially metronidazole and ciprofloxacin, are used to treat perianal disease, fistulas, and active luminal CD. Moderately severe CD is treated with tapered doses of prednisone. The thiopurine analogues, azathioprine and 6-mercaptopurine, inhibit cell-mediated immunity and therefore play a role in management of CD. Methotrexate induces remission in patients who do not tolerate thiopurine analogues. Infliximab and adalimumab are monoclonal anti-TNF antibodies that benefit approximately 60% of patients with luminal disease. Forty percent of these patients maintain a good response after 1 year. Among newer therapeutic agents is natalizumab, a humanized monoclonal antibody against α_4-integrin that inhibits leukocyte adhesion and migration into inflamed tissue. It has been found to be an effective induction and maintenance agent for treatment of moderately to severely active CD.[221]

Surgery is most often indicated for patients with intra-abdominal abscess, medically refractory disease, intestinal obstruction, toxic megacolon, hemorrhage, dysplasia, or cancer. Postoperative disease recurrence has been associated with the presence of perianal disease, ileorectal anastomosis, and segmental resection.[222] In a study by Morpurgo and colleagues, patients with either granulomas or segmental colitis at presentation showed a higher recurrence rate when compared with patients without granulomas and patients with pancolitis.[217] In a study by Soucy and colleagues, which specifically evaluated patients with colonic CD at initial presentation, there were no significant differences in the development of adverse outcomes between patients with isolated colonic CD versus those with ileocolonic CD.[150]

Patients with CD are at risk for small-bowel and colorectal adenocarcinoma. The risk is higher in patients with a family history of sporadic CRC, uncontrolled inflammation, shortened colon, or multiple inflammatory pseudopolyps.[223] The range of cumulative prevalence of dysplasia in colonic CD reported in earlier studies was between 2% and 5%.[224,225] More recently, the estimated 25-year risk of dysplasia in colonic CD has ranged from 12% to 25%[226,227] (see Dysplasia in Ulcerative Colitis and Crohn's Disease).

CHRONIC INFLAMMATORY BOWEL DISEASE, TYPE UNKNOWN ("INDETERMINATE" COLITIS)

In a small proportion of IBD cases (1% to 10%, depending on the study), a definite diagnosis of UC or CD cannot be established with absolute certainty after evaluation of the patient's resection specimen. This occurs, most commonly, either because the pathologist has insufficient clinical, radiological, endoscopic, or prior (biopsies) pathological data on the patient and/or because of overlapping pathological features between these two disorders, which occurs most commonly in patients with acute fulminant colitis.[228-232] In these circumstances, the term *indeterminate colitis*

(IC) has been used, but some authorities prefer the term *IBD, unknown type* or *IBD, indeterminate type*. In 1998, Swan and colleagues evaluated 95 patients with "fulminant colitis" with the aim of identifying features that could help separate UC from CD.[233] After all pathological material and clinical follow-up information had been reviewed, microscopic examination correctly diagnosed UC or CD in 91% of cases. Granulomas and transmural lymphoid aggregates located distant from areas of ulceration were the most specific indicators of CD. Overall, the diagnosis of *indeterminate colitis* is a vastly overused term in IBD pathology. Furthermore, in recent years, unfortunately, it has been expanded to use in patients in whom a definite diagnosis of CD or UC cannot be made in endoscopic biopsies. This diagnosis should never be used in biopsies because it is usually not possible to distinguish CD from UC in biopsy studies, especially in IBD patients who have already undergone medical therapy, and in those without CD-like anal disease, clear evidence of CD-like ileal involvement, or multiple granulomas unrelated to ruptured crypts. Furthermore, IC is not a specific disease entity and therefore has no diagnostic criteria. Rather, it represents a provisional term used by pathologists only when a definite diagnosis of UC, CD, or any other cause of chronic colitis cannot be established with complete certainty given the clinical information and pathological tissue available at the time of sign-out of the patient's resection specimen. In as many as 80% of cases, the true nature of the patient's underlying IBD becomes apparent within several years of follow-up or when all of the patient's clinical, endoscopic, and previous pathology material (including all prior mucosal biopsies) is obtained and reviewed in detail.[234]

Historical Perspective

The term *indeterminate colitis* was originally applied to cases of fulminant pancolitis (i.e., severe colitis with systemic toxicity often associated with colonic dilation), a disease in which the classic features of UC may be obscured by the presence of severe, diffuse ulceration with early superficial fissuring ulceration, transmural lymphoid aggregates (in areas of deep ulceration), and relative rectal sparing—features that are normally associated with CD.[233] However, it is now recognized that these "CD-like" features may occur in patients with fulminant UC, so most if not all of the types of specimens originally interpreted as IC can now, more conclusively, be diagnosed as fulminant UC. This is based on data suggesting that with time, patients with fulminant UC who have one or more CD-like features do not develop CD in other portions of the GI tract and have a successful rate of IPAA procedures. For instance, in one study of 21 patients with fulminant pancolitis and superficial fissuring ulcers, the incidence of CD-like complications after total colectomy and IPAA was very low and was statistically similar to that of a control group of patients without fissuring ulcers in their resection specimen.[235] Therefore the presence of these ulcers in patients with fulminant colitis is not considered necessarily indicative of CD and should not be used as evidence to deny the patient an opportunity for an IPAA procedure (Fig. 17.32).

More recently, the term *IC* has been broadened to include any IBD case in which a definite diagnosis cannot be established pathologically in a resection specimen, even in patients who do not necessarily have IBD. There are other potential causes of "IC" other than IBD, such as severe infectious colitis or drug/medication-related colitis requiring surgical treatment. Naturally, the ability to establish a precise diagnosis of either UC or CD is highly dependent on the level of awareness of the pathologist regarding the range of morphological features seen in these disorders and the unusual patterns of injury in each disorder that can mimic the other. In a study by Farmer and associates, 84 IBD colectomy specimens were reviewed by 24 university pathologists, whose diagnostic accuracy was compared with that of a single GI pathologist who had a particular interest in IBD.[231] The GI pathologist rendered a diagnosis that was different from that of the others in 45% of the specimens; in most cases, this decision resulted in a change of diagnosis from UC to CD. Therefore it is highly recommended that pathologists seek the opinion of an expert GI pathologist regarding any case that is ruled indeterminate from their point of view before final sign-out.

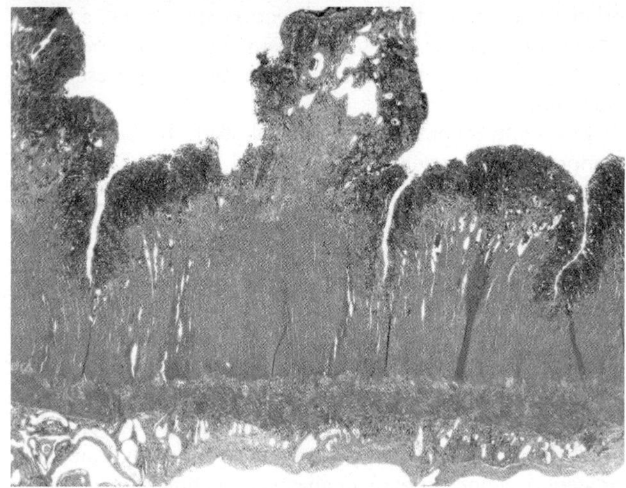

FIGURE 17.32 Fulminant ulcerative colitis. Acute severe (fulminant) ulcerative colitis shows fissuring ulcers that may extend into the muscularis propria. The intervening mucosa often shows inflammatory polyps. Deep or serosal-based lymphoid aggregates are not uncommonly seen in the vicinity of ulcers *(not shown)*. This latter feature may be confused with Crohn's disease.

Pathological Features

The most common (clinical and pathologic) reasons for establishing an interim diagnosis of IC are listed in Box 17.5. In addition to the reasons described in the table, pathologists often diagnose IC when a definite diagnosis of UC or CD cannot be made by evaluation of biopsy specimens. This practice is strongly discouraged because the cardinal features of CD cannot be seen in biopsies, and the pattern of inflammation in both UC and CD becomes altered and more similar after medical treatment (see earlier discussion). Therefore, as mentioned earlier, IC is a diagnosis that should never be made on biopsy material. In many instances, a diagnosis of IC is made because of a lack of awareness of the many types of unusual variants of UC that can mimic CD and the subtypes of CD that mimic UC (i.e., UC-like CD). Finally, in some cases, a diagnosis of IC is made because of the unwillingness of pathologists to accept a particular finding, such as true segmental disease with skip

BOX 17.5 Potential Reasons for a Diagnosis of Indeterminate Colitis

Fulminant colitis
Insufficient clinical, radiological, and pathological information
Interpretation of biopsy specimens
Failure to recognize unusual variants of ulcerative colitis
- Ulcerative colitis with Crohn's-like features
- Discontinuous disease
- Superficial fissuring ulcers
- Aphthous ulcers
- Ileal involvement
- Involvement of the upper gastrointestinal tract
- Granulomas

Crohn's disease with ulcerative colitis–like features
- Pancolitis
- Superficial colitis

Inflammatory bowel disease complicated by infections
- Pseudomembranous colitis
- Cytomegalovirus infection

Chronic recurrent (refractory) pouchitis
Failure to accept hard criteria for Crohn's disease
- Transmural inflammation
- Granulomas
- Deep fissuring ulceration
- Ileal involvement
- Segmental disease

Unusual pathological manifestations of other forms of colitis
- Ischemia
- Radiation

Microscopic colitis with features of inflammatory bowel disease
Diverticular disease–associated chronic colitis
Diversion colitis
Nonsteroidal antiinflammatory drug–induced colitis mimicking inflammatory bowel disease
Acute self-limited colitis
Polyposis disorders that may mimic inflammatory bowel disease
- Solitary rectal ulcer syndrome
- Inflammatory "cap" polyposis
- Juvenile polyposis

lesions in untreated patients, granulomatous inflammation unrelated to ruptured crypts, transmural lymphoid aggregates in patients without fulminant colitis, or deep fissuring ulceration, as a definite diagnostic criterion for CD in colonic resection specimens. In reality, any one of these features should be considered as supportive evidence for a diagnosis of CD in the appropriate clinical setting.

In most studies of IC, the majority of cases diagnosed as IC represent UC; a small proportion (10% to 40%) are, in fact, CD.[229] However, in some circumstances, other pathological mimics of IBD, such as NSAID-related colitis, diverticular disease–associated colitis (DAC), radiation or ischemic colitis, and infectious colitis, may also show histological features in resection specimens that mimic either UC or CD (Box 17.6). These other disorders should always be considered when pathologists are confronted with an IC resection specimen.

Natural History and Treatment

As mentioned earlier, there is a strong clinical need to classify IBD as CD or UC (or some other disorder) because the IPAA ("pouch") procedure is usually contraindicated for patients with CD. In studies of IPAA in CD, there was a

BOX 17.6 Pathological Mimics of Ulcerative Colitis or Crohn's Disease

UNUSUAL PATHOLOGY MANIFESTATIONS OF OTHER FORMS OF COLITIS
Ischemic colitis
Radiation colitis
Microscopic colitis with features of IBD
Diverticular disease–associated chronic colitis
Infectious colitis
- Bacterial infection—*Escherichia coli, Salmonella, Shigellosis,* tuberculosis, syphilis, *Yersinia,* lymphogranuloma venereum
- Protozoan infection—amebiasis

Diversion colitis
Drug-induced colitis (NSAID colitis)
Vasculitis (Behçet's syndrome)
Acute self-limited colitis

POLYPOSIS DISORDERS THAT MAY MIMIC IBD
Solitary rectal ulcer syndrome
Inflammatory "cap" polyposis
Juvenile polyposis

IBD, Inflammatory bowel disease; *NSAID*, nonsteroidal antiinflammatory drug.

high risk for morbidity related to pouchitis, fistulas, incontinence, or anastomotic leaks.[236,237] Many studies have evaluated the pathological features, natural history, and outcome of ileoanal pouches in patients with IC.[230-232,234,238-242] Results vary considerably because most of these studies were retrospective, used varying and poorly defined criteria for IC, and lacked sufficient follow-up information. Nevertheless, in general, approximately 20% of IC patients experienced severe pouch complications, a frequency that is intermediate between that seen in UC (8% to 10%) and in CD (30% to 40%).[232,236,238,240] This finding is not unexpected because in most studies, the IC study group consists of a mixture of true UC and CD patients. In a study by Yu and coworkers of 82 cases of IC and 1437 cases of UC, all of which involved an IPAA operation, patients with IC had higher incidences of pelvic sepsis, pouch fistulas, and pouch failure than patients with UC.[230] However, 15% of the patients with IC ultimately had their diagnosis changed to CD, and when newly diagnosed CD patients were removed from the analysis, the rates of pouch complications in IC and UC patients were statistically similar.

In 1995, McIntyre et al. compared 71 patients with IC and 1232 patients with UC for frequency of bowel movements, incontinence, and prevalence of pouchitis and pouch failure after an IPAA procedure.[238] Although the failure rate in IC was higher than in UC (19% vs. 8%), IC and UC patients had similar overall outcomes, once again suggesting that most patients with IC probably have UC as the cause of the colonic inflammatory disorder. Although a substantial proportion of CD patients who undergo an IPAA operation experience pouch failure (30% to 45%), some studies have suggested that CD patients whose pouches can be retained in situ have acceptable pouch function.[236,243]

Ancillary (Serologic) Diagnostic Tests for Inflammatory Bowel Disease

In certain circumstances, serological testing for ANCAs and ASCAs may be helpful in classifying IC cases as UC or CD.[12,244] In addition to these antibodies, a widely used serological profile by Prometheus Laboratories tests for antibodies against outer membrane porin C (OmpC), a protein belonging to *E. coli* that regulates metabolite and toxin transport, and CBir1, a flagellin that presumably induces colitis through adaptive immune response.[245] A typical profile for CD includes detectable ASCA IgA and anti-CBir1 IgG antibodies and an absence of anti-OmpC IgA and pANCA. Elevated serum pANCA and low levels (below the reference range) of ASCA IgA, anti-OmpC, and anti-CBir1 IgA are usually associated with UC.

ANCAs are detected in the serum of 60% to 70% of patients with UC but in only 10% to 40% of CD patients. Patients with UC who have a high level of pANCA are at an increased risk of pouchitis after IPAA.[246] Of the CD patients who are positive for ANCAs, most have left-sided colitis with clinical, endoscopic, or histological features of UC.[247] ASCAs are present in 50% to 60% of CD patients. As a serum marker for CD, ASCA has a sensitivity of 67% and a specificity of 92%. In a meta-analysis designed to evaluate the diagnostic precision of ANCA and ASCA in IBD, these serological tests were shown to be quite specific but not very sensitive in distinguishing CD from UC. In this study, an ASCA+/ANCA− test result offered the best sensitivity and specificity for CD (55% and 90%, respectively).[12] In fact, these tests showed even higher rates in the pediatric IBD population. In a study consisting of 135 pediatric patients (81 with CD and 54 with UC), an antibody panel consisting of pANCA, ASCA, OmpC, and CBir1 identified 65% of children with CD and 76% of those with UC, with a specificity of 94%.[248] In CD, OmpC has been correlated with increased risk of fibrostenosing disease, internal penetrating disease, and the need for small-bowel surgery.[249] CBir1 has been shown to identify cases of CD not detected with other markers.[245] Approximately 55% of CD patients are positive for anti-CBir1, and this marker independently helps identify a subset of CD patients (particularly those with fibrostenosing disease) who may also be ANCA positive.

Use of serological testing has not been extensively studied for IC. In a prospective European study of 97 patients with a diagnosis of IC, only a small minority showed characteristic serological patterns that helped establish a diagnosis of ASCA+/ANCA− CD or ASCA−/ANCA+ UC. In most patients, there was insufficient information to accurately classify IC patients as having either CD or UC.[250] Therefore the clinical utility of these markers in IC appears limited.

Differential Diagnosis of Ulcerative Colitis vs. Crohn's Disease

Resection Specimens

UC characteristically involves the mucosa in a diffuse and continuous manner. It almost always affects the rectum. The terminal ileum may be affected to a lesser degree and exclusively in patients with pancolitis (i.e., BWI). Infections, drug or medication-related injury (e.g., NSAIDs), and bowel preparation agents can also result in inflammation of the terminal ileum. In contrast, CD shows segmental or patchy involvement of the bowel and often affects longer lengths of terminal ileum, both actively as well as chronically. In a resection specimen, a diagnosis of UC is usually established by the presence of diffuse chronic active colitis or chronic inactive colitis involving the mucosa in the absence of mural changes typical of CD, such as fissuring ulcers, transmural lymphoid aggregates, non–mucin-related granulomas, mural fibrosis, and fistulas or sinus tracts. Neural hyperplasia, hyperplasia of muscularis mucosae, and submucosal fibrosis are also less common in UC than in CD. In addition, involvement of other regions of the GI tract, especially perianal disease, is a sign of CD. Upper GI involvement in UC has been described, but it is unclear whether these changes are specific to UC or represent a nonspecific systemic immune response to a generalized inflammatory condition. A summary of the classic microscopic features of UC and CD is provided in Table 17.2.

Because most resections are performed for medically refractory disease or disease-related complications and therefore have been treated medically, both UC and CD may show patchy, or segmental, histological changes. One may also see a reduction in the amount of transmural inflammation in CD. Granulomas are also far less common after treatment.

Biopsy Specimens—Before Medical (Drug) Treatment

UC and CD demonstrate considerable overlap in morphological features in biopsy samples with chronic and/or active disease. Furthermore, because the characteristic features of CD are typically found deeper in the bowel wall, it is difficult or impossible to distinguish UC from CD based solely on analysis of mucosal biopsy specimens. However, in untreated cases, features in favor of CD are granulomas not associated with crypt rupture, long or multiple segments of small bowel involvement, clear evidence of upper GI involvement (esophagus, stomach, duodenum, jejunum), rectal sparing at disease onset, particularly in adults, fistulas, and CD-like perianal disease, such as recurrent and severe or unremitting fissures, fistulas, anal tags, ulcers, and hemorrhoidal disease. Patchy disease in the same segment before treatment and evidence of deep and prominent submucosal involvement in a patient without fulminant colitis are additional features that favor CD over UC.

Biopsy Specimens: Post–Medical (Drug) Treatment

After medical therapy, either orally, intravenously, or by enema, an uneven pattern of healing caused by the therapeutic effects of drugs used for the disease often cause the histological features of UC to become patchy in distribution, mimicking the pattern of CD in the colon (see Unusual Morphological Variants of Ulcerative Colitis). Thus in the posttreatment setting, pathologists cannot consider "patchiness" of disease or "rectal sparing" as features necessarily indicative of CD. In medically treated patients, unless there is confirmed radiological evidence of CD-like anal or perianal disease, granulomas unrelated to ruptured crypts, or definite CD-like ileal or upper GI involvement, it is almost impossible to distinguish UC from CD in this setting.

DYSPLASIA IN ULCERATIVE COLITIS AND CROHN'S DISEASE

Fewer than 1% of all CRCs in the United States are associated with IBD. Colorectal carcinoma arising in UC was first documented in 1925 by Crohn and Rosenberg.[251] Warren and Sommers were first to document CRC in a patient with CD in 1948.[252] Both UC and CD patients are at increased risk for development of dysplasia and carcinoma. However, estimation of risk is influenced by numerous factors, such as differences in sampling protocols, recognition and classification of disease, treatment regimens, and methods used to detect neoplasia. Evidence from two population-based studies, one from Manitoba, Canada (RR in CD, 2.64; RR in UC, 2.75)[253] and another from Olmstead County, Minnesota (standardized incidence ratio [SIR] in CD 1.9; SIR in UC, 2.4),[254] indicated that the risk of cancer is roughly equivalent in UC and CD in patients with equal lengths of affected colon. In another study, Choi and colleagues found no significant differences in age at diagnosis, duration of IBD, multiplicity and distribution of cancer, presence of dysplasia, or 5-year survival rate in patients with CD-associated versus UC-associated CRC.[255]

Ulcerative Colitis: Incidence and Risk Factors of Dysplasia/Cancer

The overall incidence of CRC after 25 to 35 years of UC ranges from 3% to 43%.[256,257] In two recent population-based cohort studies, UC-associated CRC accounted for only 0.15% to 0.4% of all cases of CRC diagnosed in the general population.[258-260] A meta-analysis of 116 studies estimated the risk of cancer in patients with UC at 2% after 10 years, 8.5% after 20 years, and 17.8% after 30 years of disease.[261] Five years later, data from a 30-year surveillance program at St. Mark's Hospital in the United Kingdom calculated the risk of cancer and dysplasia as 2.5% at 20 years, 7.6% at 30 years, and 10.8% at 40 years.[262] Subsequent population-based studies also suggested that the risk of developing dysplasia/cancer has decreased with time. In a recent study that included 32,911 Danish patients diagnosed with UC, the RR of CRC (1.07; 95% CI, 0.95 to 1.21) was comparable to that of the general population.[263] The change in incidence rate, especially during the first 1 to 10 years after diagnosis, is likely the result of improved surveillance, early use of colectomy for medically refractory disease, and significant improvements in medical therapy.

Features associated with an increased risk of dysplasia and carcinoma in patients with UC include increased duration of disease, increased anatomic extent of disease, associated PSC, a family history of sporadic cancer, young age at onset, and severity of endoscopic and histological disease activity. The RR for dysplasia or cancer significantly increases after 8 to 10 years of disease duration.

Most cases of dysplasia/cancer arise in a background of pancolitis or at least subtotal colitis. Limited left-sided colitis cases carry an intermediate risk, whereas proctitis or proctosigmoiditis carries either little or no risk of cancer at all.[264,265] Compared with RRs of 1.7 and 2.8 for patients with proctitis and left-sided colitis, respectively, patients with pancolitis have an RR of 14.8 for neoplasia.[264]

PSC develops in approximately 2% to 5% of UC patients. In a meta-analysis that included 22 studies, patients with PSC and UC were found to have a fourfold increased risk of dysplasia/cancer.[266] UC patients who have undergone liver transplantation for PSC also have a higher risk of dysplasia/cancer, estimated at 1% per year.[267-269] For these reasons, it is highly recommended that patients undergo annual colonoscopy from the onset of PSC.

A positive family history of sporadic colon cancer is a well-documented predisposing factor for colon cancer, with a more than twofold associated risk.[270] Younger age at onset of colitis has been associated with an 8.6-fold increased risk of dysplasia/cancer.[254,271] However, this estimate must be interpreted with caution because of the lower rates of CRC observed in the general population used for comparison in this age group. Nevertheless, this increased risk likely reflects the high proportion of pediatric IBD patients who have extensive disease.[263,272]

Two previous studies from the United Kingdom demonstrated that the severity of endoscopic and histological inflammation is related to colon cancer risk.[273,274] In a recent meta-analysis, a diagnosis of extensive colitis was associated with a 4.8-fold increased risk of dysplasia/colon cancer.[260]

Crohn's Disease: Incidence and Risk Factors of Dysplasia/Cancer

There is wide variability in the reported risk of dysplasia/CRC in CD, primarily because of inconsistencies in documentation of the duration and location of CD (colonic vs. isolated small-bowel CD).[275,276] In CD, there is also an increased risk for dysplasia and adenocarcinoma in excluded segments of bowel and also in the small intestine.[277]

In a large, population-based survey of 1655 patients with long-standing and extensive CD, the reported RR of CRC was 2.5 (95% CI, 1.3 to 4.3).[278] A meta-analysis of 12 studies showed a higher RR (4.5) for patients with colonic disease.[279] In a recent Danish study, the RR of dysplasia/colon cancer among 14,463 patients diagnosed with CD did not differ significantly from that in the background population, nor did it change over a period of 30 years.[263] This has mostly been attributed to improved medical therapy and surveillance programs.

As in UC, patients with long-standing CD and a family history of sporadic colon cancer are at increased risk for dysplasia/cancer.[270,276,280] There is a convincing association between degree of inflammation and dysplasia/cancer in CD as well.[278] A population-based study from Sweden showed that the RR for colon cancer was 5.6 in CD patients with disease restricted to the colon.[278] The RR was even greater in patients who were younger than 30 years of age at the time of diagnosis. Therefore extent of colitis, duration of disease, family history of sporadic colon cancer, and young age at presentation are risk factors for development of dysplasia and cancer in colonic CD. In contrast with UC, PSC does not seem to increase the risk of colon cancer in patients with colonic CD. This was recently demonstrated in a case-control study consisting of 114 patients with colonic CD.[281]

Pathological Features of Dysplasia in Ulcerative Colitis and Crohn's Disease

Dysplasia is defined as unequivocal neoplastic epithelium confined to the basement membrane. At present, it is the best and most reproducible marker of malignancy risk in patients with IBD.[282] It is present in up to 90% of patients

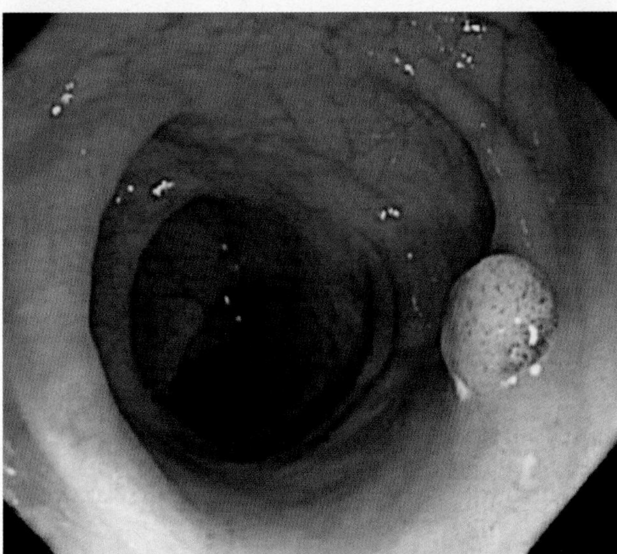

FIGURE 17.33 Endoscopic appearance of an "adenoma-like dysplasia-associated lesion or mass" (DALM) (now termed *visible polypoid dysplasia* based on the SCENIC classification) in a patient with ulcerative colitis. The polypoid lesion (0.8 cm in diameter) is well circumscribed and shows a smooth surface. This lesion was completely resected during endoscopy. The terms "DALM" and "adenoma-like" are no longer used in clinical practice.

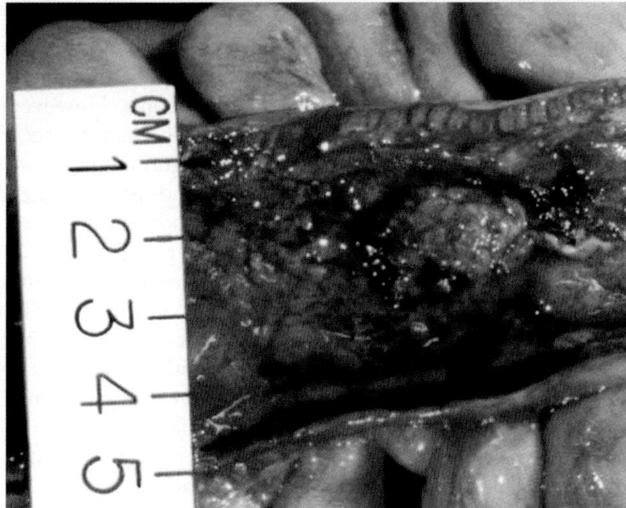

FIGURE 17.34 Colonic resection performed for a "non–adenoma-like DALM" (now *termed visible sessile dysplasia*) in a patient with ulcerative colitis. The lesion measured 2.3 cm in diameter and was broad based with irregular borders. Biopsies showed high-grade dysplasia. However, the resection specimen showed invasive adenocarcinoma. The term "non–adenoma-like" is no longer used in clinical practice.

with UC and up to 87% of patients with CD who have carcinoma. It may occur adjacent to and/or distant from the primary tumor. Dysplasia may occur in any portion of the colon, but it most often parallels the location of cancer; it may occur as an isolated focus, but more often is multifocal. Rarely, it is diffuse.

Terminology and Classification

Before the advent of image-enhancing endoscopic techniques, such as high-definition colonoscopy or chromoendoscopy, dysplasia was classified as either *flat* or *elevated;* the latter types of lesions were termed *dysplasia-associated lesion or mass* (DALM). This classification was considered important because these two types of dysplasia were managed differently.[283-286] There is inconsistency in the literature with regard to the criteria used to define raised, endoscopically visible, dysplastic lesions as DALMs. For instance, the term *flat dysplasia* has been used to describe endoscopically detectable, but slightly raised, lesions in some studies, but not in others.

Raised dysplastic lesions in UC (and CD) were further separated into those that resembled non–IBD-related sporadic adenomas ("adenoma-like") and those that did not resemble adenomas, which were termed *non–adenoma-like.*[286-288] Endoscopically resectable well-circumscribed, smooth or papillary, nonnecrotic, sessile or pedunculated polyps were called *adenoma-like dysplastic lesions* (also known as *adenoma-like polyp, adenoma-like dysplastic polyp, adenoma-like low-grade* or *high-grade dysplasia, polypoid dysplasia,* or *adenoma-like mass*) [284,287] (Fig. 17.33), while velvety patches, plaques, irregular nodules, wartlike thickenings, carpet-like lesions, stricturing lesions, and broad-based masses that could not be resected by endoscopic methods, and therefore required surgery were categorized as non–adenoma-like dysplastic lesions (Fig. 17.34).

Recently, the endoscopic classification system of dysplasia in IBD has changed. The new guidelines have proposed an endoscopic classification system of dysplasia that conceptually aligns with the clinical management of dysplasia. This new classification system is the Surveillance for Colorectal Endoscopic Neoplasia Detection and Management in Inflammatory Bowel Disease Patients: International Consensus Recommendations (SCENIC) (Table 17.3).[289]

This classification is based on the use of high-definition colonoscopy and chromoendoscopy to aid in the visualization of mucosal abnormalities. Based on these recommendations, the terms *DALM, adenoma-like,* and *non–adenoma-like* are no longer used in clinical practice. Instead, dysplasia is now categorized as either *visible* or *invisible* endoscopically. Visible dysplasia is defined as dysplasia identified on targeted biopsies from a lesion visualized at colonoscopy, while invisible dysplasia is identified on random (nontargeted) biopsies of colonic mucosa, without a visible lesion. This classification scheme (modified from the Paris Classification) [290] further divides visible lesions into *polypoid* (pedunculated or sessile) or *nonpolypoid* (superficial elevated, flat or depressed) types (see Table 17.3).

Gross Features

Retrospective studies have shown that most dysplastic lesions in IBD are, in fact, polypoid rather than flat or invisible.[273,291] For instance, in a large retrospective review of 2204 surveillance colonoscopies in UC patients, 77% of the 104 dysplastic lesions found were elevated or polypoid (or both).[273]

Regarding the anatomic distribution of dysplasia in UC, low-grade dysplasia was found in one study to be more commonly localized to the distal colorectum (68%).[292] Similarly, in a pooled analysis, Choi reported that 52% (range, 47% to 62%) of colitis-related CRCs occurred in the rectosigmoid region.[293] Additionally, a 20-year prospective study and a 30-year analysis of surveillance colonoscopy showed

TABLE 17.3 Terminology for Reporting Findings on Colonoscopic Surveillance of Patients with Inflammatory Bowel Disease (SCENIC Guidelines)

Term	Definition
Visible dysplasia	Dysplasia identified on targeted biopsies from a lesion visualized at colonoscopy
Polypoid	Lesion protruding from the mucosa into the lumen >2.5 mm
Pedunculated	Lesion attached to the mucosa by a stalk
Sessile	Lesion not attached to the mucosa by a stalk: entire base is contiguous with the mucosa
Nonpolypoid	Lesion with little (<2.5 mm) or no protrusion above the mucosa
Superficial elevated	Lesion with protrusion but <2.5 mm above the lumen (less than the height of the closed cup of a biopsy forceps)
Flat	Lesion without protrusion above the mucosa
Depressed	Lesion with at least a portion depressed below the level of the mucosa
Invisible dysplasia	Dysplasia identified on random (nontargeted) biopsies of colon mucosa without a visible lesion

that 44% and 58.6% of dysplastic lesions occurred within the rectosigmoid region, respectively.[262,294] A retrospective study of flat dysplasia by Goldstone and colleagues confirmed that in patients undergoing surveillance for long-standing UC, 74.6% of neoplasia (flat low-grade dysplasia, flat high-grade dysplasia, or carcinoma) occurred in the distal colon (64.4% in the rectosigmoid and 10.2% in the descending colon), whereas only 25.4% occurred in the ascending colon, cecum, or transverse colon.[295]

In CD, dysplasia also occurs more often in areas close to, rather than distant from, the primary tumor. Dysplasia distant from cancer has been identified in 38% to 41% of specimens with colonic CD.[277,296] Regardless of the location of the primary tumor, dysplasia/cancer always develops in areas of either prior or current colitis, as in UC. In a study by Sigel and associates, dysplasia was found adjacent to carcinoma in 87% of cases and distant from carcinoma in 41% of cases.[277] In their study of 30 cases of CD-related adenocarcinoma, 27% occurred in the small intestine and 73% occurred in the colon. In a study that evaluated 50 cases of Crohn's colitis-associated dysplasia, 44% of patients were found to have multifocal dysplasia/cancer in segments not affected by colitis.[297]

Microscopic Features

Grading of Dysplasia

According to the grading system proposed by Riddell and colleagues in 1983, dysplastic changes in UC and CD are separated into three distinct categories: *negative for dysplasia, indefinite for dysplasia,* and *positive for dysplasia* (low and high grade).[282] The Vienna grading system, which denotes five diagnostic categories, is used by many pathologists in Japan and Europe.[298] A comparison of the two systems is outlined in Table 17.4. Both visible and invisible dysplastic lesions are graded in the same manner.

TABLE 17.4 Comparison of Vienna and Riddell's Classifications of Dysplasia in Inflammatory Bowel Disease

Vienna	Riddell
1. Negative for neoplasia/dysplasia	Negative for dysplasia
2. Indefinite for neoplasia/dysplasia	Indefinite for dysplasia
3. Noninvasive low-grade neoplasia (low-grade adenoma/dysplasia)	Low-grade dysplasia
4. Noninvasive high-grade neoplasia 4.1 High-grade adenoma/dysplasia 4.2 Noninvasive carcinoma (carcinoma in situ) 4.3 Suspect for invasive carcinoma	High-grade dysplasia
5. Invasive neoplasia 5.1 Intramucosal adenocarcinoma 5.2 Submucosal carcinoma or beyond	Adenocarcinoma* Intramucosal Invasive

*Not described in Riddell paper (see reference 282).

The grade of dysplasia is determined by evaluating a combination of cytological and architectural alterations of the epithelium. A diagnosis of "negative" is reserved for nondysplastic or regenerating epithelium (Fig. 17.35).

Cases are considered "indefinite for dysplasia" when the features of the atypical epithelium resemble dysplasia, but because of other factors such as inflammation, ulceration, or technical artifact, a definite diagnosis cannot be established with complete certainty (Fig. 17.36). Inflammation and ulceration make interpretation of atypical changes difficult (i.e., reactive vs. neoplastic). Regenerating epithelium often shows enlarged and variably sized nuclei, nuclear stratification, prominent nucleoli, and increased mitoses. These changes overlap with those observed in true dysplasia. In some cases, tangential sectioning of the tissue or severe cautery or processing artifact may also render an atypical focus difficult to interpret. In general, the presence of surface maturation is usually (but not always) indicative of a regenerative process. Thus the presence of this feature should always evoke great caution in diagnosing true dysplasia (Table 17.5).

In low-grade dysplasia, the crypts show a tubular and/or villous configuration and may also demonstrate focal or mild crypt budding and crowding. Cytologically, dysplastic crypts are lined by cells that show nuclear enlargement, elongation (often referred to as *pencillate*), increased nucleus-to-cytoplasm (N:C) ratio, hyperchromasia, stratification, a clumped chromatin pattern, single or multiple nucleoli, and hypereosinophilic, mucin-depleted cytoplasm (Fig. 17.37). Dysplastic epithelium normally involves both the crypt and surface epithelium, but early cases may show involvement of the crypts only (*crypt dysplasia;* see later discussion). Mitotic figures are often plentiful, but atypical mitotic figures are less common than in high-grade dysplasia. In low-grade dysplasia, the nuclei are usually limited to the basal half of the cell cytoplasm, and there are no significant architectural abnormalities such as glandular crowding, cribriforming, or a back-to-back gland pattern. Other, less

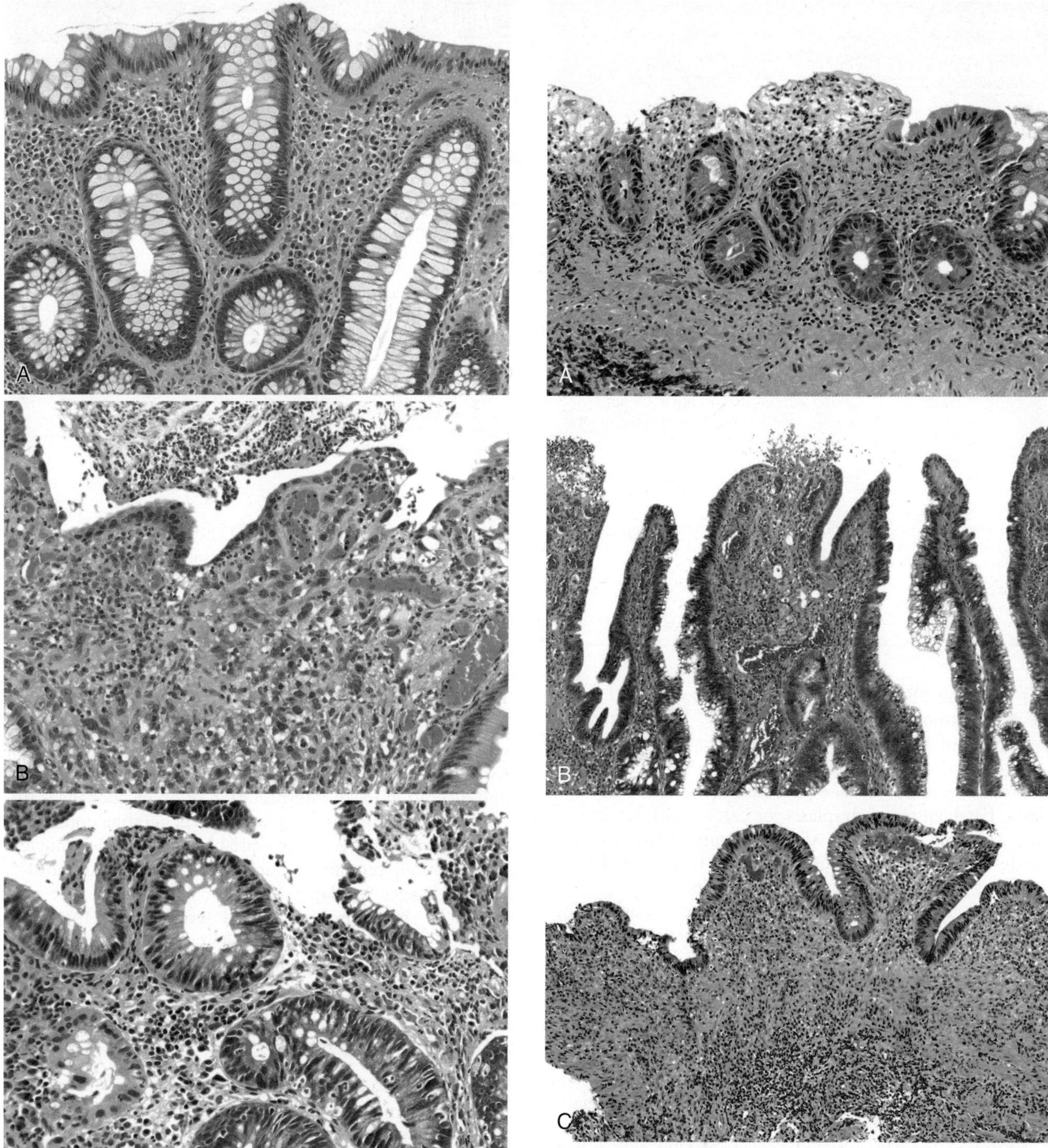

FIGURE 17.35 A, Chronic inactive colitis showing colonic mucosa with complete surface maturation, considered negative for dysplasia. **B,** An area of marked active inflammation with erosion and a monolayer of epithelial cells show regenerative changes. The stromal cells can also show cytological atypia. "Bizarre" (reactive) stromal cells should not be mistaken for sarcoma. **C,** Regenerating epithelium can also show nuclear stratification and hyperchromasia that may be mistaken for dysplasia.

FIGURE 17.36 Ulcerative colitis graded indefinite for dysplasia. A, Colonic biopsy specimen shows crypts lined by cells with enlarged, hyperchromatic nuclei. However, the lack of surface epithelium in this fragment precludes evaluation of surface maturation. Therefore the case is best classified as *indefinite for dysplasia.* **B,** The colonic epithelium in this biopsy specimen shows nuclear hyperchromasia and stratification at the surface. However, these changes are associated with surface erosion on one part of the sample and prominent active inflammation. The latter finding indicates the possibility of reepithelialization of the mucosa, and therefore the case is best categorized as *indefinite for dysplasia.* **C,** Another example of a case considered *indefinite for dysplasia.* Villiform mucosal architecture, stratification, and nuclear hyperchromasia and enlargement are present. However, these changes are adjacent to an erosion, and there is at least partial surface maturation in some of the crypts.

common features of low-grade dysplasia include dystrophic goblet cells and endocrine and Paneth cell metaplasia.

With progression from low- to high-grade dysplasia, the cells acquire more cytological atypia, characterized by even

TABLE 17.5 Regenerative Epithelial Changes vs. Dysplasia

Feature	Regenerative Changes	Dysplasia
Nuclear enlargement	Usually minimal	Always present
Nuclear hyperchromasia	May be present	Always present
Nuclear stratification	May be present near healing ulcers	Present in adenomatous (intestinal)-type dysplasia
Nuclear pleomorphism	Usually minimal	Always present
Irregular nuclear contour	Usually minimal	Always present
Loss of nuclear polarity	Absent	Present (in high-grade dysplasia)
Prominent nucleoli	May be present	Present in high-grade dysplasia
Vesicular chromatin	Usually absent	Present (especially in high-grade dysplasia)
Loss of surface maturation	Absent	Present (except in crypt dysplasia)
Increased mitoses	May be present	Usually present
Atypical miotic figures	Usually absent	Present
Increased nucleus-to-cytoplasm ratio	May be present	Always present
Syncytial appearance of cells with abundant eosinophilic cytoplasm	Present	Usually absent
Villous configuration	May be present	Present
Mucin loss	Present	Present
Epithelial "atypia" overlying inflamed stroma that lacks glands	Present	Usually absent
Intraepithelial neutrophils	Usually present	May be present
Complex glandular architecture	Absent	Present in high-grade dysplasia

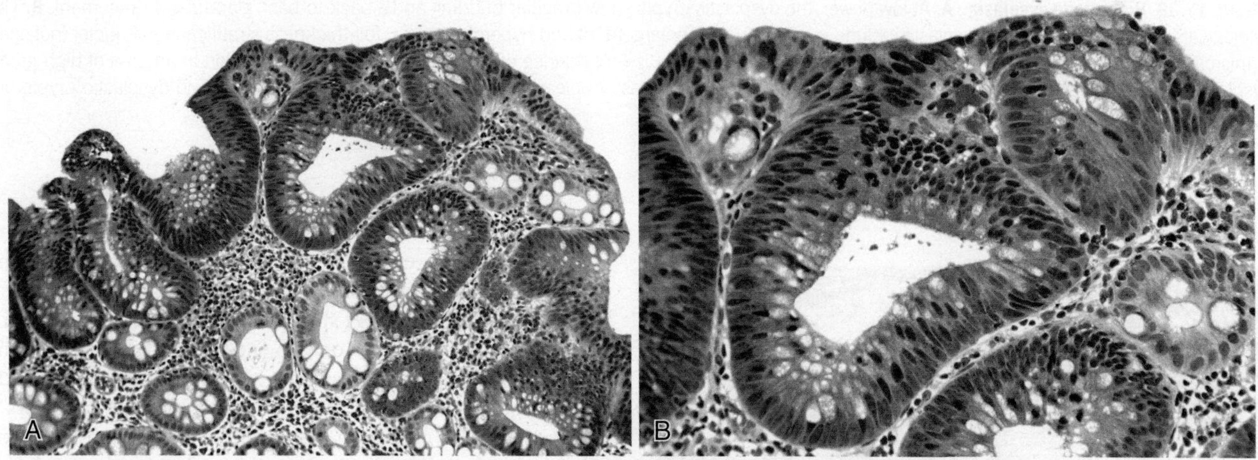

FIGURE 17.37 Low-grade dysplasia (A, low-magnification; B, high-magnification). The crypts are lined by cells that demonstrate nuclear hyperchromasia, stratification, and enlargement. Increased mitoses are observed, and there is a distinct lack of surface maturation.

more pronounced nuclear enlargement, pleomorphism, hyperchromasia and, in particular, loss of nuclear polarity (Fig. 17.38). The nuclei may show a more "open" chromatin pattern and contain prominent and enlarged nucleoli. Full-thickness nuclear stratification is characteristic when the nuclei are pencil shaped. However, many high-grade lesions show enlarged, but irregular, round nuclei rather than pencil-shaped nuclei. In these cases, nuclear stratification may not be present. Architecturally, back-to-back glands or cribriforming may be present, and this is always considered a high-grade feature, especially when it is prominent and even if the nuclei appear more low-grade cytologically. Mitotic figures, both typical and atypical, are more frequent than in low-grade lesions and are usually present in both the upper and lower portions of the crypts and in the surface epithelium. In general, the features of the most atypical portion of dysplastic mucosa determine the overall grade of dysplasia in any particular biopsy sample. However, there

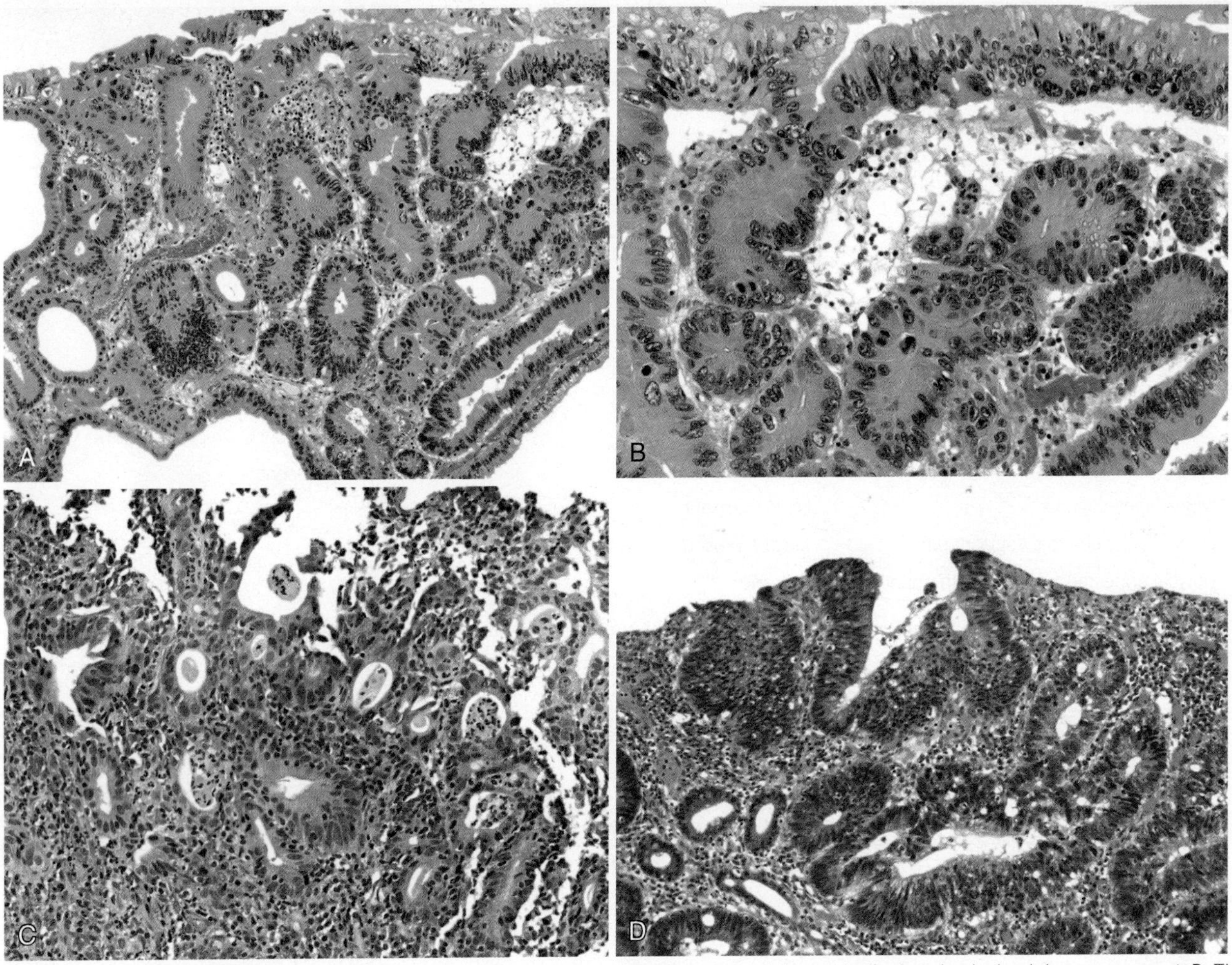

FIGURE 17.38 High-grade dysplasia. A, At low power, the dysplastic crypts show irregular budding and a back-to-back glandular arrangement. **B,** The cytological features of high-grade dysplasia include marked nuclear enlargement and hyperchromasia, full-thickness stratification of nuclei (not seen in this case), increased pleomorphism, and a loss of cell polarity. There is no evidence of surface maturation. **C,** Ulceration in an area of high-grade dysplasia. **D,** Another example of high-grade dysplasia shows full-thickness nuclear stratification with cytological atypia. The dysplastic crypts are crowded and show glandular budding.

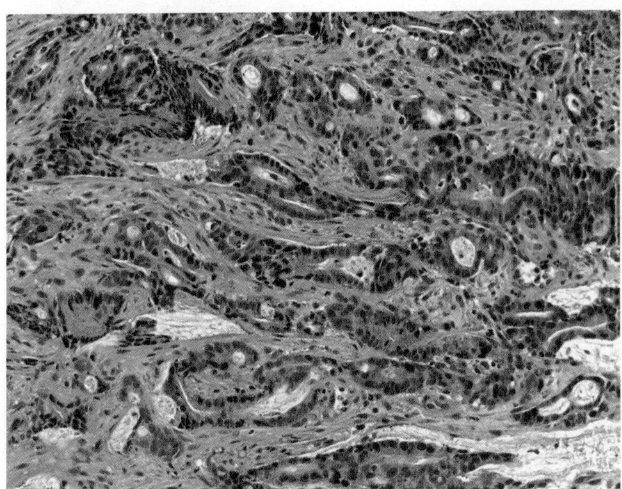

FIGURE 17.39 Invasive adenocarcinoma in a biopsy specimen from a patient with long-standing ulcerative colitis. The infiltrating neoplastic glands are surrounded by desmoplastic stroma.

is no uniform agreement regarding the proportion of high-grade dysplastic crypts that is necessary to upgrade a biopsy from low to high grade. A simple rule of thumb is that there should be more than one or two (i.e., more than rare) high-grade crypts present to designate a biopsy as high-grade, but admittingly, this number varies among expert pathologists.

Intramucosal carcinoma is defined by the presence of cells or glands that have penetrated into, but not beyond, the lamina propria or muscularis mucosae. Common patterns of early invasion include single-cell or small-gland infiltration, glands with irregular jagged contours, and extensive cribriforming with pushing borders. Desmoplasia is absent when the carcinoma is limited to the mucosa. Thus its presence is normally diagnostic of submucosal invasion (Fig. 17.39).

Morphological Types of Dysplasia

Historically, *intestinal* ("adenomatous"), *hypermucinous/villous,* and *serrated* dysplasia were considered the predominant morphological subtypes of dysplasia in IBD. In one study of IBD cancers, 52% of dysplastic lesions were villous, 29% were serrated, 5% were tubular (adenomatous), and 13% showed mixed features.[299] However, more recently, an international group of IBD pathology experts proposed a novel histological classification system of IBD-associated dysplastic lesions that serves to recognize several additional variants that are rare and often difficult to recognize (Table 17.6).[300] This new classification includes four general categories: *intestinal, gastric, mixed intestinal and gastric,* and *unclassifiable.* The intestinal type of dysplasia is further separated into *tubular/villous (adenoma-like), goblet cell–deficient, crypt cell, sessile serrated lesion (SSL)-like, traditional serrated adenoma (TSA)-like,* and *serrated, not otherwise specified (NOS)* subcategories. The tubular/villous (adenoma-like) intestinal-type of dysplasia remains the most common and most well-characterized type, both histologically and clinically, However, there is emerging data with regard to the other subtypes, and this is discussed in more detail later. Unfortunately, much of the prior dysplasia literature either does not specify clearly the type of dysplasia under study or refers specifically to the intestinal type. As a result, the following discussion applies mainly to the tubular/villous intestinal type of dysplasia, unless otherwise specified.

Intestinal Dysplasia

Tubular/Villous "Adenoma-like" Dysplasia. This type of dysplasia is by far the most common type of dysplasia encountered in patients with IBD. Morphologically, it resembles conventional colorectal adenomas. The growth pattern is tubular and/or villous, and the crypts are often crowded. The nuclei are enlarged, elongated, hyperchromatic, and stratified. The density of goblet cells is variable. The intervening columnar cells are enterocyte-like but may contain a small amount of microvesicular mucin. Some lesions contain prominent Paneth cells or endocrine cells. Surface maturation is minimal or absent except near villous tips (see Fig. 17.37).

Goblet Cell–Deficient Dysplasia. This form of dysplasia is characterized by crypts that either lack completely, or show only

TABLE 17.6 Morphological Subtypes of Dysplasia in Inflammatory Bowel Disease

Category of Dysplasia	Description
Intestinal Type	
a. Tubular/villous (adenoma-like)	• Tubular and/or villous architecture with crowded crypts • Nuclei are enlarged, elongated, hyperchromatic, and stratified • Density of goblet cells is variable • Some lesions may contain prominent Paneth cells or endocrine cells
b. Goblet cell–deficient	• Crypts either lack completely or show only rare goblet cells • Nuclei are stratified, hyperchromatic, and elongated
c. Crypt cell dysplasia	• Crypts are usually noncrowded and show a uniform flat tubular growth pattern • Crypts are lined by "terminally differentiated" enterocytes interspersed with goblet cells, basally located Paneth cells, and scattered endocrine cells • Nuclei are round- or oval-shaped, enlarged, hyperchromatic, or vesicular
d. Sessile serrated lesion–like	• Similar to SSLs seen in a sporadic setting • Crypt serrations may involve the basal or superficial crypts, or both • Crypts show dilation, with or without lateral extension, resulting in *L*- or *T*-shaped configurations • Unlike sporadic SSL, the presence of flat bases is not a required feature • Cells have microvesicular cytoplasm with interspersed smaller numbers of goblet cells • Nuclei are round- to oval-shaped or slightly elongated, hyperchromatic, and may contain inconspicuous nucleoli
e. Traditional serrated adenoma–like	• Resembles a sporadic TSA • Villiform epithelial proliferation containing slitlike epithelial serrations • Ectopic crypts or aberrant crypt foci are characteristic • Individual cells show pencillate nuclei with fine chromatin and prominent eosinophilic cytoplasm
f. Serrated NOS	• Serrated crypt architecture that cannot be readily categorized into SSL or TSA-like lesion
Gastric Type	
a. Tubular/villous (mucinous/ hypermucinous)	• Tubular and/or villous architecture • Crypts show either no or only a few rare goblet cells • Cells show small, hyperchromatic, basally oriented nuclei with minimal or no cytological atypia • Abundant mucinous cytoplasm
b. Serrated	• Serrated growth pattern • Nuclei are round and vesicular and show little or no reduction in size near the surface • Abundant mucinous cytoplasm
Mixed Intestinal and Gastric Type	• Combination of two or three morphological types of dysplasia • May include subtypes of the same category (e.g., tubular/villous subtype of intestinal dysplasia and TSA-like dysplasia) or mixture of separate categories (e.g., tubular/villous form of intestinal dysplasia and gastric-type dysplasia)
Unclassifiable	• Lesion that cannot be readily classified into any of the aforementioned categories

NOS, Not otherwise specified; *SSL,* sessile serrated lesion; *TSA,* traditional serrated adenoma.

rare, goblet cells. The cells show nuclear hyperchromasia and stratification and elongation of nuclei, and it involves the crypts as well as the surface epithelium (Fig. 17.40). In the original study that described this morphological variant of dysplasia, it was associated with the highest interobserver agreement (95% agreement) among all GI IBD pathology experts.[300]

Crypt Cell Dysplasia. Crypt cell dysplasia is characterized by a noncrowded, uniform flat tubular growth pattern of the epithelium. The crypts are lined by "terminally differentiated" enterocytes interspersed with goblet cells, basally located Paneth cells, and scattered endocrine cells (Fig. 17.41). The nuclei are typically round or oval-shaped, enlarged, hyperchromatic, or vesicular. As opposed to normal or reactive epithelium, crypt cell dysplasia shows lack of maturation to the surface with the nuclei showing either very little or no reduction in overall size. Paneth and endocrine cells may be sparse or completely absent in some cases. The term *crypt cell dysplasia* is a consensus-based revision of the original term *dysplasia with terminal epithelial differentiation* in the prior study that described the rare morphological subtypes of dysplasia.[300]

Serrated Dysplasia (Sessile Serrated Lesion–like Dysplasia, Traditional Serrated Adenoma–like Dysplasia, and Serrated Dysplasia Not Otherwise Specified). It has been known for quite some time that serrated lesions, both visible and invisible, may develop in IBD patients. In fact, some early studies had suggested that serrated dysplasia is quite common, and in some studies, even more common than the intestinal type. Unfortunately, early studies did not differentiate the various subtypes of serrated dysplasia or recognize that even IBD patients may develop sporadic serrated lesions. Thus the old literature is now difficult to interpret. Serrated lesions may be visible or invisible. Visible lesions are often polypoid, and these range from those that resemble conventional hyperplastic polyps (Fig. 17.42A) at one end of the cytological atypia scale to SSLs and TSAs at the other end of the scale. In some cases, serrated lesions may not quite fit nicely into any of these categories, and in these cases the term *serrated dysplasia NOS* may be used. Invisible (randomly sampled) and nonpolypoid colonic mucosa may also reveal dysplastic lesions with a serrated pattern of growth and even some with cytological and architectural features identical to that of an SSL or TSA.

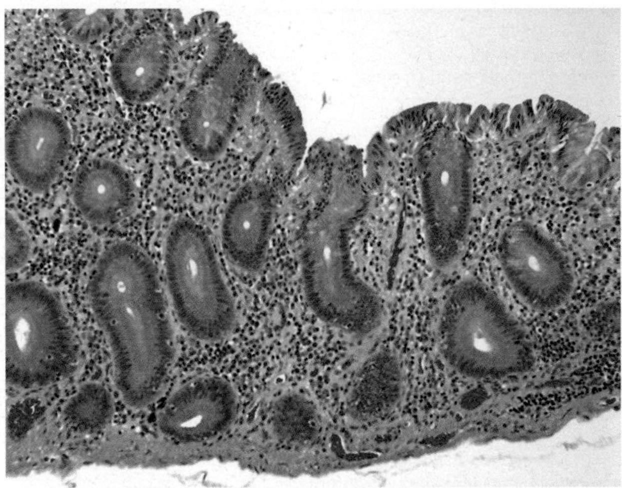

FIGURE 17.40 Goblet cell–deficient dysplasia. The lesion is characterized by crypts that either lack goblet cells completely or show these only rarely. The cells show nuclear hyperchromasia, stratification, and elongation of nuclei, and it involves the crypts and the surface epithelium.

Sessile serrated lesion–like dysplasia is similar to SSLs seen in the sporadic setting and is characterized by crypts with serrated architecture wherein the serrations may involve the basal or superficial crypts, or both. The crypts show dilation, with or without lateral extension, resulting in *L*- or *T*-shaped configurations (see Fig. 17.42B). However, unlike sporadic SSL, flat crypt bases are not a required feature. The cells have microvesicular cytoplasm and are interspersed with smaller numbers of goblet cells. The nuclei are round to oval or slightly elongated, hyperchromatic, and may contain inconspicuous nucleoli. They are basally located and may be slightly stratified at the crypt base, and there may be maturation at the surface. This category excludes lesions that resemble conventional SSLs without cytological dysplasia.

Traditional serrated adenoma-like dysplasia resembles a sporadic TSA in which the lesion is composed of villiform epithelial proliferation containing slitlike epithelial serrations along with ectopic crypts or aberrant crypt foci. The individual cells show pencillate nuclei with fine chromatin and prominent eosinophilic cytoplasm (see Fig. 17.42C). In a recent study that evaluated 52 TSA-like lesions in 30 IBD patients, the prevalence of TSA-like lesions in IBD patients was found to be 0.4%.[301] In this series, 23/27 TSA-like

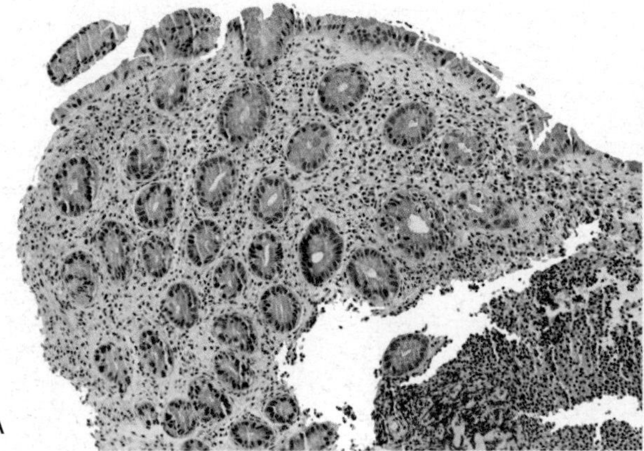

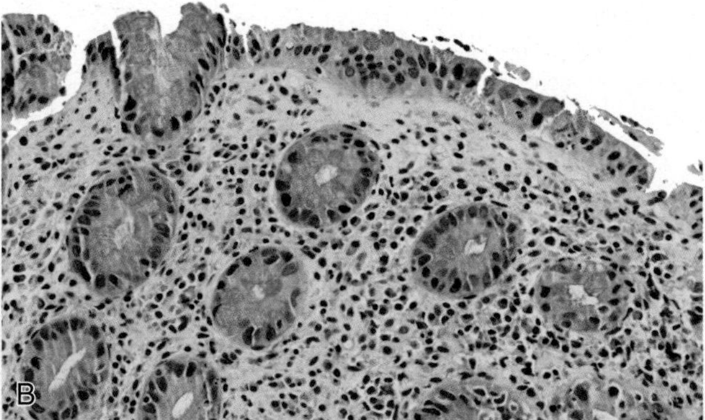

FIGURE 17.41 Crypt cell dysplasia. A, Crypt cell dysplasia characterized by a noncrowded, uniform, flat tubular growth pattern. The crypts are lined by "terminally differentiated" enterocytes interspersed with goblet cells, basally located Paneth cells, and scattered endocrine cells. The nuclei are round or oval, enlarged, and hyperchromatic or vesicular. **B,** There is a lack of surface epithelial maturation.

lesions identified in colectomy specimens presented as ill-defined plaquelike areas of the mucosa with a granular appearance, and low-grade and high-grade serrated dysplasia was found in 15 of 27 and 10 of 27 cases, respectively.

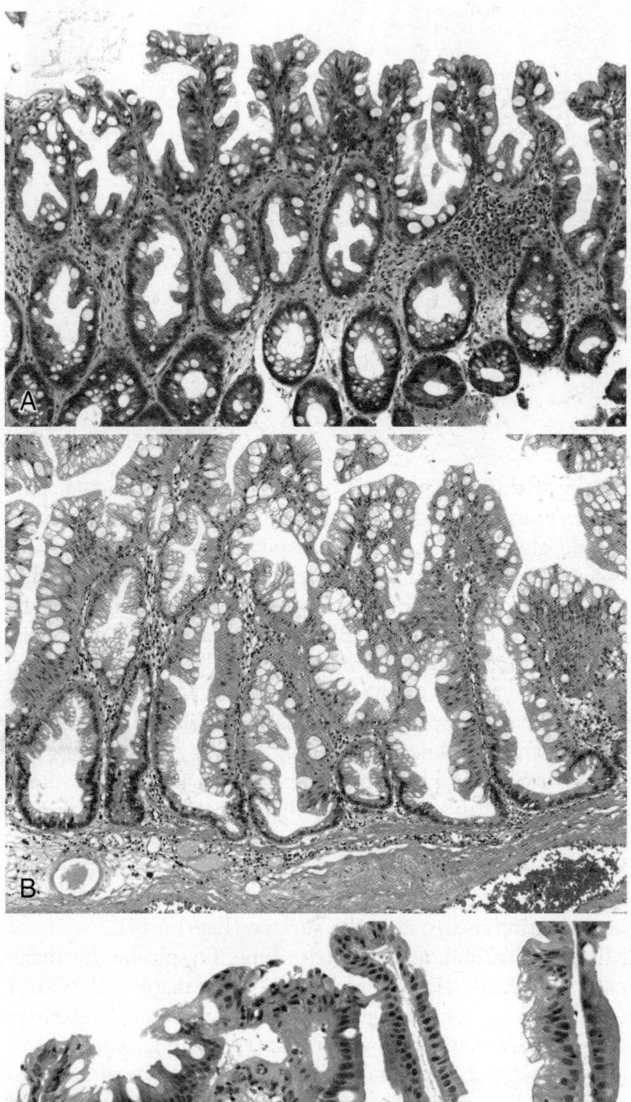

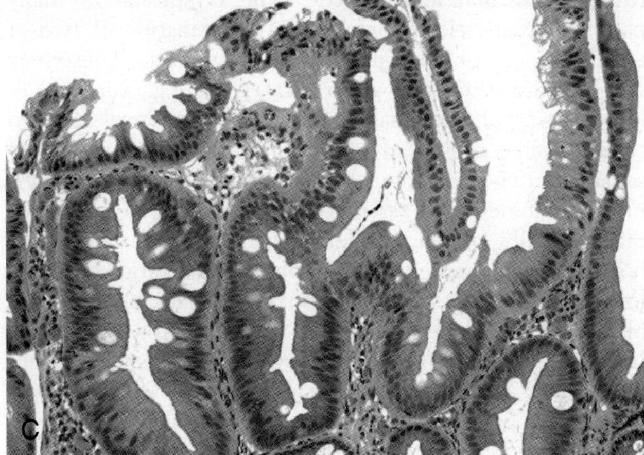

FIGURE 17.42 Serrated dysplasia in IBD. Serrated lesions in IBD may be visible or invisible. **A,** Hyperplastic polyp in a patient with ulcerative colitis. **B,** Sessile serrated lesion-like dysplasia in a patient with ulcerative colitis. The crypts show serrated architecture, basal dilation, and abnormal growth ("boot-" or "anchor-"shaped crypts). They are lined by cells with slight nuclear stratification and hypereosinophilic cytoplasm. **C,** Traditional serrated adenoma-like dysplasia in a patient with ulcerative colitis. The lesion is composed of villiform epithelial proliferation containing slit-like epithelial serrations along with ectopic crypts or aberrant crypt foci. Individual cells show pencillate nuclei with fine chromatin and prominent eosinophilic cytoplasm.

Little is known regarding the biological characteristics and natural history of serrated lesions in IBD. However, there are some data on hyperplastic changes and hyperplastic-type polyps. In a large clinicopathological and outcome study published in abstract form, 188 polyps from 161 IBD patients with at least 1 serrated polyp were analyzed. Most were hyperplastic polyps (97%) that were detected microscopically, not endoscopically. Adenocarcinoma, adenoma, or flat or elevated dysplasia did not develop in any of the patients, but additional hyperplastic or inflammatory polyps developed in 33% of the patients.[302] In a retrospective study consisting of 94 patients with "hyperplastic polyp-like changes" in biopsies of flat mucosa obtained during routine surveillance ("flat serrated change"), the authors found that 12.8% of these patients had subsequent visible dysplasia on follow-up. However, a multivariate analysis did not show a statistically significant difference in the risk between patients with and without these lesions. Based on these results, the authors suggested that there should be no change in routine surveillance protocols for patients with invisible hyperplastic polyp–like serrated change.[303] One study[304] evaluated serrated lesions in 78 IBD patients and classified them as *SSA/P-like* (negative for dysplasia), *TSA-like* (positive for low-grade dysplasia), and *cytologically atypical hyperplasia–like* (indefinite for dysplasia). The authors found that SSA/P-like visible lesions in IBD occurred preferentially in females and in the right colon, similar to sporadic polyps. Nearly 11% of these nondysplastic SSA/Ps were associated with synchronous or metachronous neoplasia over a follow-up period of 103 months. In contrast, TSA-like and cytologically atypical hyperplasia–like polyps were significantly associated with synchronous or metachronous neoplasia (low-grade dysplasia in 17, high-grade dysplasia in 6, and invasive adenocarcinoma in 3).

Serrated Polyposis in Inflammatory Bowel Disease. IBD patients may rarely show numerous hyperplastic and serrated lesions in their colon, reminiscent of the serrated polyposis syndrome. In one study by Srivastava et al., three patients with IBD (UC in 2, CD in 1) developed a wide spectrum of serrated lesions ranging from invisible serrated dysplasia to a broad range of visible lesions such as hyperplastic-like polyps, sessile serrated lesion–like polyps, and TSA-like polyps throughout the colon.[305] The visible lesions contained various grades of dysplasia ranging from little to no cytological atypia up to adenocarcinoma (two patients). In this study, it was not clear whether the study patients had IBD and superimposed serrated polyposis or whether the serrated lesions developed as a direct result of the underlying IBD; however, the latter was favored by the authors of that study.

Thus, in general, in a patient with a visible lesion that resembles a serrated polyp of any kind, it is important to determine whether the lesion has arisen within or outside the segment of bowel affected by IBD. Similar to sporadic adenomas, patients with IBD may develop "sporadic" serrated polyps that are unrelated to IBD. Regardless, until we know more about the clinical behavior of serrated dysplasia that is related to IBD, the clinical management for visible and invisible lesions is similar to that of serrated lesions seen in non-IBD patients.

Gastric Type Dysplasia. Rarely, dysplastic lesions in either UC or CD are composed nearly exclusively of cells with

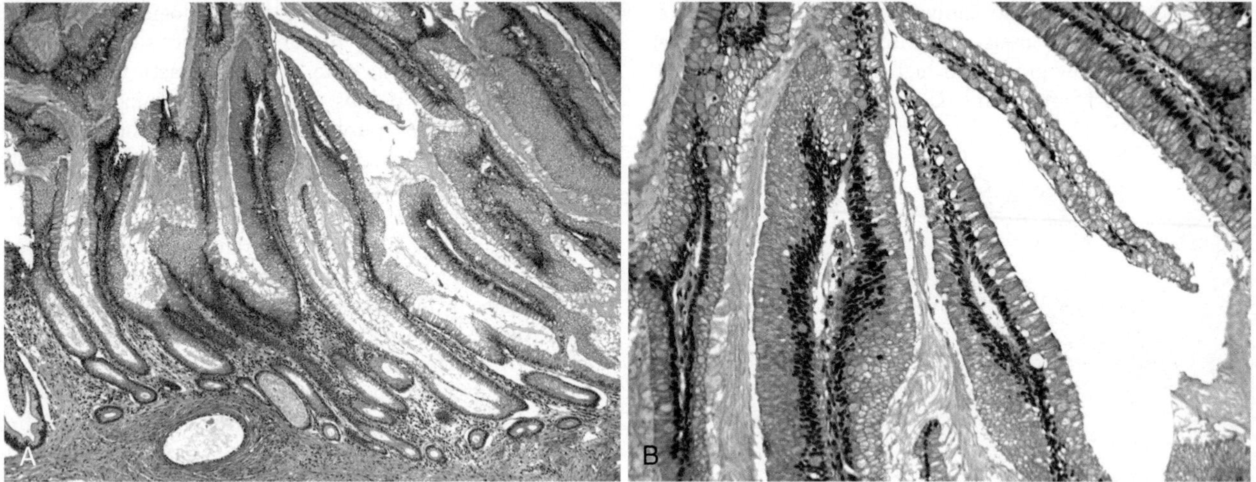

FIGURE 17.43 Mucinous dysplasia. A, The mucosa shows prominent villiform architecture. **B,** Higher magnification shows that the individual cells contain small, hyperchromatic, basally located nuclei with minimal cytological atypia.

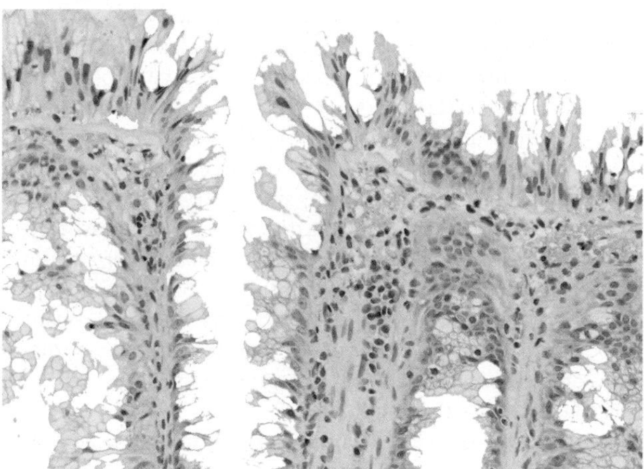

FIGURE 17.44 Serrated dysplasia in inflammatory bowel disease, mixed intestinal/gastric type.

mucinous cytoplasm, similar in appearance to gastric foveolar cells. These cases typically show either no or only a few goblet cells within the dysplastic epithelium. The predominant growth pattern of these lesions may be tubular/villous, completely villous, or even serrated.

Gastric dysplasia has been termed *mucinous, hypermucinous,* or *hypermucinous villous* in prior studies. It is a rare form of dysplasia, and when present, it may show such minimal cytological atypia that it may be difficult to recognize it as unequivocally neoplastic. In general, the dysplastic epithelium shows relatively small, hyperchromatic, basally oriented nuclei with minimal, or in some cases, no cytological atypia.[306,307] (Fig. 17.43). However, more traditional dysplastic changes may be present in higher-grade lesions. These features include a crowded, back-to-back arrangement of glands lined by cells with hyperchromatic and markedly enlarged nuclei. Prominent nucleoli are common. For the most part, the nuclei maintain their basal orientation or are only partially stratified. In general, the colonic epithelium is rather resistant to mucinous metaplasia, with a few exceptions such as pyloric metaplasia, or focally within hyperplastic polyps (in a microvesicular pattern). Thus the finding of gastric-like mucinous metaplasia should always arouse strong suspicion for gastric dysplasia in an IBD patient. In three recent studies (one published in abstract form) that evaluated the different morphological subtypes of dysplasia in IBD, the prevalence of mucinous dysplasia ranged from 6.8% to 14%.[308-310] Given the limited number of cases of mucinous dysplasia reported to date, the natural history and biological characteristics of this variant remain largely unknown.

Gastric serrated dysplasia is similar to tubular/villous adenoma–like dysplasia but is distinguished by a strikingly serrated growth pattern involving both the basal and superficial crypts, sometimes resulting in mucin-filled cystic glands. The nuclei are round and vesicular and show little or no reduction in size near the surface (Fig. 17.44).

Mixed Intestinal and Gastric Type Dysplasia. In many patients, dysplastic lesions show a combination of two or even three morphological subtypes of dysplasia. These may be all within the same general category (e.g., tubular/villous subtype of intestinal dysplasia and traditional serrated adenoma–like dysplasia), or it may occur as a mixture of separate categories (tubular/villous forms of intestinal dysplasia combined with gastric type dysplasia; see Fig. 17.44). Histologically, the various subtypes of dysplasia may occur both within the same foci of dysplasia or as spatially distinct lesions. In a study (published in abstract form) consisting of 50 patients all of whom had a colectomy for dysplasia in IBD (UC = 43, CD = 7), of the 67 foci of dysplasia, there were 16 (24%) foci of mixed dysplasia. The most common mixed pattern was intestinal tubular/villous combined with serrated (*N* = 9/16; 56%). Two of the 16 mixed cases (13%) showed a combination of intestinal (tubular/villous and serrated) and gastric (tubular/villous) dysplasia.[308] In our experience, the mixed form of dysplasia is more likely to be encountered in large-sized visible lesions rather than in small visible lesions.

Early (Crypt) Dysplasia. Although better characterized in patients with Barrett's esophagus, rarely patients with IBD may develop early dysplastic changes limited to the bases of the crypts without involvement of the surface epithelium (i.e., surface maturation is present).[311] The lesions usually have a flat configuration, noncrowded crypts, and cytoplasmic features that simulate the repertoire of normal colonic epithelium. This is also known as *crypt dysplasia* (Fig. 17.45). In our experience, most patients with crypt dysplasia reveal conventional dysplasia (involving both crypt and surface epithelium) elsewhere in the colon at the time of discovery of crypt dysplasia. Because crypt regeneration also shows surface maturation, a diagnosis of crypt dysplasia should not be made in biopsy specimens exhibiting inflammation or ulceration or in those that are not well oriented. At this time, the biological characteristics and natural history of crypt dysplasia in IBD are largely unknown. In a small series of 14 colon biopsies from 7 patients with IBD, aneuploidy was detected in all 14 biopsies with crypt dysplasia in IBD, and 6 patients developed HGD (n = 5) or adenocarcinoma (n = 1) in the same colonic segment where crypt dysplasia was diagnosed within a mean follow-up duration of 27 months.[312]

Natural History and Treatment of Visible Dysplasia

As discussed earlier, the treatment of dysplasia in IBD depends largely on the endoscopic appearance and resectability of the lesion. The SCENIC guidelines define an endoscopically resectable lesion as one that has distinct margins, appears to be completely removed on visual inspection after endoscopic resection, is histologically consistent with complete removal, and the biopsies taken from mucosa immediately adjacent to the resection site are free from dysplasia.

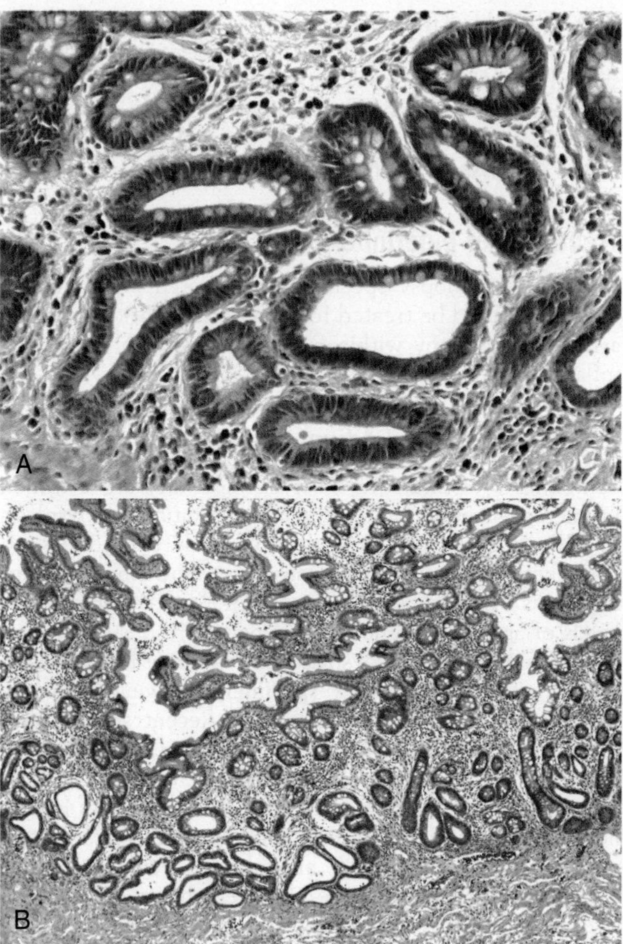

FIGURE 17.45 Crypt dysplasia in a patient with Crohn's colitis. A, Colonic mucosa shows nuclear hyperchromasia, stratification, and enlargement involving the basal crypts. **B,** However, there is no involvement of the surface epithelium (i.e., surface maturation is present).

Historically, distinction between *adenoma-like DALM* (polypoid visible dysplasia in the SCENIC classification) and *sporadic adenoma* was considered important because the former was usually treated by colectomy, whereas the latter was treated by polypectomy.[283] However, more recent data suggest that patients with UC and an "adenoma-like" lesion may be treated adequately by polypectomy and continued surveillance, regardless of the pathogenesis of the lesion.[286-288] In a study consisting of 24 UC patients with an "adenoma-like DALM" within areas of colitis, 10 UC patients with an "adenoma-like DALM" outside areas of colitis, and 49 non-IBD (control) patients with sporadic adenomas,[286] 62.5% patients in the first group developed an additional adenoma-like DALM, only 1 patient (4%) developed a single focus of flat dysplasia, and 1 patient (4%) developed a poorly differentiated adenocarcinoma of the cecum by 7.5 years after polypectomy.[287] Among the patients with adenoma-like DALMs outside areas of colitis, 50% developed additional adenoma-like DALMs proximal to areas of colitis, but none developed invisible dysplasia or carcinoma. This group was not significantly different from the control group, 49% of whom developed further adenomas during the follow-up interval. A subsequent study by Kisiel et al.[313] also showed that of 77 UC patients with polypoid visible dysplasia, 36% developed another polypoid low-grade dysplastic lesion, 5% developed invisible low-grade dysplasia, and only 1 patient (1%) developed carcinoma after a median follow-up interval of 20.1 months.

The presence of high-grade dysplasia within an *adenoma-like DALM* (now referred to as *polypoid visible dysplasia*) is not considered a contraindication to polypectomy. In the study by Blonski et al., invisible dysplasia or carcinoma did not develop in any of 9 UC patients with such lesions during a follow-up period of 76.5 months.[314]

In a recent meta-analysis consisting of 1037 IBD patients undergoing endoscopic resection for a total of 1428 colonic lesions, the pooled risk (rate per 1000 person-years of follow-up) of CRC was 2 (95% CI, 0 to 3), the pooled risk of high-grade dysplasia was 2 (95% CI, 1 to 3), and the pooled risk of any lesion was 43 (95% CI, 30 to 57) after complete resection of the lesion.[315] These data highlight the effectiveness of endoscopic resection and follow-up for patients with visible polypoid dysplastic lesions. Unfortunately, most of the previous studies have not addressed differences in outcome between pedunculated and sessile visible dysplastic lesions.

Biopsy specimens from lesions that are deemed nonresectable via endoscopic techniques (Fig. 17.46) often show only dysplastic epithelium, which usually represents surface sampling of a carcinoma. Several studies have detected a strong association between endoscopically unresectable lesions and cancer at colectomy. Given the high risk of synchronous or metachronous adenocarcinoma, the presence of such lesions is a strong indication for colectomy.[223,316,317]

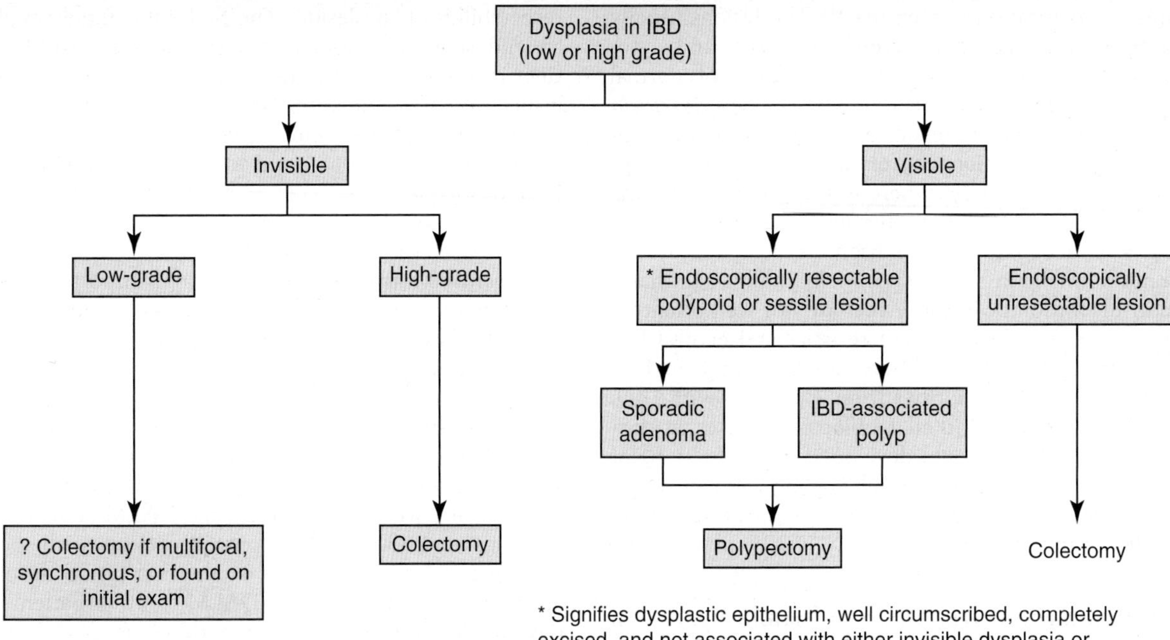

FIGURE 17.46 Algorithmic approach to the treatment of dysplasia in patients with inflammatory bowel disease (IBD).

Natural History and Treatment of Invisible Dysplasia

Most of the data regarding the natural history and treatment of dysplasia in IBD apply mainly to UC. It has been reported that the 5-year rate of development of either high-grade dysplasia or carcinoma in patients with low-grade dysplasia is 54%.[257] As a result, many institutions recommend colectomy for UC patients with invisible low-grade dysplasia, particularly if it is found on initial colonoscopy, is multifocal, or develops in a metachronous fashion.[257,317,318] However, some institutions prefer to place patients with invisible low-grade dysplasia under surveillance (see later discussion). Ullman and colleagues showed that 27% of patients with UC who underwent a colectomy within 6 months after a biopsy diagnosis of invisible low-grade dysplasia had unexpected high-grade dysplasia or cancer in their resection specimen.[319] In contrast, invisible high-grade dysplasia is associated with a higher probability of detecting cancer at colectomy (40% to 67%) and of progression to carcinoma (5-year predictive value, 40% to 90%).[223,257,320] For these reasons, patients with invisible high-grade dysplasia, even if it is unifocal, are referred for colectomy. More recent studies using chromoendoscopy or high-definition white-light endoscopy have reported a 10% incidence rate of invisible dysplasia.[289] Thus random biopsy samples showing invisible dysplasia in older studies may have been obtained from mucosa that may now be recognizable as a distinct mucosal abnormality using modern endoscopic techniques.

In all cases of dysplasia assessment, it is important and highly recommended by the American Gastroenterology Association and the American College of Gastroenterology that the presence or absence of dysplasia be confirmed by at least one pathologist who is skilled in GI pathology or who has broad experience with dysplasia in UC.[223,317]

A study by Kiran and colleagues suggests that instead of segmental colectomy, total proctocolectomy should be strongly considered for CD patients with a preoperative diagnosis of dysplasia because as many as 44% show multifocal dysplasia.[297] Similarly, patients with high-grade dysplasia have a 45% risk of having synchronous cancer.

Treatment of Indefinite Dysplasia

Patients with biopsy specimens considered indefinite for dysplasia should be treated for their inflammation and have a repeat endoscopy within 6 months, preferably after the inflammation has subsided.[223,317]

Sampling Error and Adjunctive Markers

Sampling error and interobserver variability are common problems encountered in the interpretation of dysplasia in IBD.[282] Since the original 1983 study by Riddell and coworkers, several investigations have shown only moderate levels of interobserver agreement.[282,321-323] In general, levels of agreement among pathologists are highest for the category of high-grade dysplasia and negative for dysplasia; they are lowest for biopsy specimens showing low-grade dysplasia or indefinite for dysplasia. Recent studies have focused on finding other, more reproducible, adjunctive methods of assessing malignancy risk in UC. These include a variety of histochemical (e.g., mucins, sialosyl-Tn), immunohistochemical (e.g., proliferation markers, TP53), and molecular (*APC*, *p27*, *p16*, aneuploidy) techniques.[324-329] α-Methylacyl-CoA racemase has been shown to be sensitive and highly specific for dysplasia in IBD.[330] In one study, 90% of low-grade dysplasia, 80% of high-grade dysplasia, and 71% of adenocarcinomas in IBD were positive, in contrast with none of the foci of nondysplastic regenerating epithelium. Several studies have shown increased expression of *TP53* in the progression of neoplasia in IBD,[331,332] but a small proportion of nondysplastic cases may also be positive. Furthermore, TP53 immunostaining is fraught with a high false-positive rate, which makes TP53 less useful for differentiating regeneration and true dysplasia in IBD.

Molecular Features of IBD Neoplasia

Tissue-based studies have demonstrated that IBD-related neoplasia is associated with aberrant methylation in *EYA4*,[333] *ER, CDKN2A, MYOD, CDH1, RUNX3, MINT1,* and *COX-2*.[334-338] A tissue-based study showed that methylation of genes in the WNT signaling pathway is an early event in patients with IBD colitis, and there is a progressive increase in methylation of the WNT signaling genes *APC1A, APC2, SFRP1,* and *SFRP2* during development of IBD-associated neoplasia.[339] In an in-depth analysis of IBD-associated CRCs and sporadic cancers performed using whole-exome sequencing, Robles and colleagues showed a lower rate of *APC* activation and a higher rate of *SOX9* inactivating mutations in the IBD-CRC cohort compared with the sporadic CRC cohort.[340] This study also noted that despite both the cohorts showing similar missense mutations within the DNA-binding domain of p53, the identity and molecular distribution of single substitution mutations were different. In another study, Yaeger and colleagues analyzed genomic alterations in over 300 cancer-related genes in 29 UC and 18 CD-associated cancers using a next-generation sequencing platform. They found 6.2 genomic alterations per tumor, with alterations in *TP53, IDH1,* and *MYC* being more frequent and mutations in APC being less frequent than those reported in sporadic CRCs in The Cancer Genome Atlas database.[341] (See Chapter 23 for more details on the molecular basis of IBD neoplasia.)

Although these markers show some promise as adjunctive biomarkers, additional studies must be performed before any of this knowledge can be translated into clinical management of patients with long-standing IBD.

Surveillance in Inflammatory Bowel Disease

The optimal surveillance strategy for patients with UC remains controversial[342] (see Chapter 2 for more details). Much debate centers on the sensitivity of the detection system, the predictive value of dysplasia for assessing the risk for CRC, and the cost.[343-345] Data supporting the effectiveness of surveillance in patients with UC are not uniform but do suggest a reduction in mortality from carcinoma in those who are willing to undergo prophylactic colectomy should dysplasia be detected. As a result, the overall balance of evidence supports surveillance for dysplasia in UC.

Widespread agreement on appropriate surveillance strategies in patients with UC has not been established.[320,346] The American Gastroenterology Association recommends that surveillance should begin after 8 years of disease in patients with pancolitis and after 15 years in patients with colitis involving the left colon only. Colonoscopy should be repeated every 1 to 2 years.[223,317] Four-quadrant biopsy specimens should be obtained from every 10 cm of mucosa between the cecum to the sigmoid colon and from every 5 cm more distally. In addition, a biopsy should be performed on any suspicious lesions or masses. In a study by Rubin and associates, 33 biopsy specimens were needed to detect dysplasia with 90% probability, and at least 64 biopsy specimens were needed to reach a 95% probability of detecting dysplasia.[324] The finding of dysplasia, when confirmed by an expert pathologist, is usually an indication for colectomy. For patients for whom a colectomy is not feasible or is unacceptable, frequent surveillance (e.g., every 3 to 6 months) is considered an acceptable alternative. At present, surveillance is not indicated for patients with ulcerative proctitis.

In 2% to 16% of CD patients, dysplasia/cancer is detected during the course of the illness. Overall, the survival benefit of endoscopic surveillance in CD is controversial, primarily because of the lack of prospective studies.[278,347,348] However, there is a growing trend toward endoscopic surveillance in patients with long-standing CD.[348] The Crohn's and Colitis Foundation of America consensus conference recommendations for surveillance in patients with colonic CD includes screening colonoscopy for those who have major colonic disease (involving at least one-third of the colon) with a disease duration of at least 8 to 10 years.[223,317] However, surveillance is often difficult to perform because of the presence of strictures that often require the use of a pediatric endoscope. Although most strictures are a manifestation of transmural disease, as many as 12% of CD-related strictures are malignant from the onset.[349]

NON-IBD COLITIS

Acute Self-Limited (Infectious) Colitis

Clinical Features

Acute self-limited colitis (ASLC) is defined as a transient, presumably infectious, acute inflammatory disorder of the colon. Patients typically come to medical attention because of abdominal pain and tenderness, low-grade fever, and in some instances bloody diarrhea as well.[6,350] The inflammatory process usually resolves completely within 2 to 4 weeks. A wide variety of pathogens, most commonly bacterial organisms such as *Campylobacter jejuni, Salmonella, Shigella* species, *E. coli,* and *Yersinia enterocolitica,* result in this pattern of colonic injury. In immunocompromised patients and very rarely in immunocompetent individuals, viral infections such as enteric adenoviruses (serotypes 40 and 41) and infections by parasitic organisms like *Entamoeba histolytica* and *Cryptosporidium* species may also cause a mild, self-limited form of infectious colitis. A detailed description of infectious disorders of the GI tract is provided in Chapter 4. Here, we discuss the clinicopathological features of the most common organisms that cause ASLC in the context of diagnostic biopsy pathology of the colon (Table 17.7).

The clinical presentation of patients with ASLC includes rapid-onset abdominal pain, diarrhea, and fever. Typical laboratory findings include peripheral blood and fecal leukocytosis. In ASLC related to bacterial infection, stool cultures are positive in only 40% to 60% of cases. Therefore a negative result does not entirely exclude an infectious etiology.[6,351] In fact, in most instances, the exact cause of the patient's colitis is never actually determined. Imaging studies may reveal nonspecific thickening of the bowel wall. However, because of the acute onset, they are seldom performed.[350]

TABLE 17.7 Clinicopathological Features of the Most Common Pathogens That Cause Acute Self-Limited Colitis

Organism	Clinical Features	Laboratory Findings	Colonoscopic Findings	Location of Disease	Microscopic Findings	Complications
Campylobacter jejuni	Diarrhea, fever, abdominal pain	Fecal blood and leukocytes, positive stool culture	Erythema, edema, multiple superficial ulcers as large as 1 cm	Any part of the colon may be involved	Neutrophilic cryptitis, histiocyte aggregates	GI hemorrhage, toxic megacolon, pancreatitis, cholecystitis, reactive arthritis, Guillain-Barré syndrome, HUS
Salmonella spp. (*S. enteritidis* and *S. typhimurium*)	Nausea, diarrhea, fever, and bloody diarrhea within 48 hours after exposure	Fecal blood and leukocytes, positive stool culture	Mucosal congestion, granularity, friability, and ulceration	Any part of the colon may be involved	Mucosal edema, congestion, cryptitis, crypt abscesses, thrombi in small venules	Toxic megacolon, bleeding, sepsis
Shigella spp.	Abdominal cramping, fever, and diarrhea	Fecal blood and leukocytes, positive stool culture	Small, ragged ulcers with normal intervening mucosa; severe cases with diffuse mucosal congestion and erosions	Any part of the colon may be involved	Aphthous ulcers, cellular lamina propria with neutrophils, cryptitis, and crypt abscesses	Appendicitis, HUS, myocarditis, pneumonitis, reactive arthritis, toxic megacolon
Escherichia coli (enteroinvasive *E. coli* and enterohemorrhagic *E. coli* [EHEC])	Watery to bloody mucoid diarrhea, tenesmus, fever, abdominal cramps	Fecal blood and leukocytes, positive stool culture (for EHEC)	Segmental involvement with marked mucosal congestion, friability, edema, and diffuse ulcers, rarely pseudomembranes	Right colon is most commonly involved	Neutrophilic cryptitis, crypt abscesses with erosions, ischemic pattern of injury	HUS
Yersinia enterocolitica	Fever, abdominal cramps, diarrhea within 1 to 3 weeks after infection	Fecal blood and leukocytes, stool culture, serology	Focal or diffuse mucosal edema, erythema, and ulcers	Proximal colon more commonly involved than rectosigmoid colon	Mucosal edema, cryptitis, and crypt abscesses (necrotizing granulomas are found only in patients with prolonged disease course)	Septicemia, chronic relapsing fever, appendicitis

GI, Gastrointestinal; *HUS,* hemolytic-uremic syndrome.

Specific Infectious Organisms

Campylobacter jejuni

C. jejuni is one of the most frequently isolated stool pathogens in patients with ASLC. In immunocompromised patients, *Campylobacter fetus* is more frequently isolated. The incidence of *C. jejuni*–related diarrhea is 4% to 11% in the United States. Bacterial transmission usually occurs via contaminated food.[352] In developing countries, the infection is hyperendemic in children younger than 2 years of age. The most common presenting symptoms are diarrhea (90%), fever (90%), and abdominal pain (70%). These may be accompanied by headache, myalgia, and vomiting. Stool examination typically reveals red blood cells and leukocytes. *Campylobacter* DNA may be isolated in as many as 19% of affected patients with acute-onset diarrhea.[353]

Salmonella Species

At least 2000 serotypes of nontyphoid *Salmonella* species have been identified as potential causative agents of gastroenteritis (nontyphoid salmonellosis). Almost 45,000 cases of *Salmonella* gastroenteritis are reported annually.[354] In the United States, *Salmonella enteritidis* and *Salmonella typhimurium* are the most commonly isolated species. Infection is most likely to develop in children younger than 1 year of age. In addition, patients with achlorhydria, hemolytic anemia, immunosuppression, or malignancy (e.g., disseminated carcinoma, hematolymphoid malignancies) are predisposed to *Salmonella* infection. Gastroenteritis develops in 75% of patients infected with this organism. Patients usually present with nausea, vomiting, fever, and bloody diarrhea.

Shigella Species

Shigella infection is the most common cause of bacillary dysentery. The first documentation of shigellosis-related GI illness dates back to the American Civil War period. Currently, the incidence of shigellosis worldwide is reported to be 10% to 20% of infectious diarrhea. Although it is more common in tropical countries and temperate zones, its prevalence in the United States and Europe is increasing. In fact, the incidence of *Shigella sonnei* (which is more common in the United States than *Shigella flexneri*) is 60% to 80% in patients with diarrhea.[355] The infection is common in children 6 months to 5 years of age. Microbiology laboratory workers are also at risk. The clinical presentation consists of lower abdominal pain, rectal burning, bloody diarrhea, and fever.[356] A biphasic illness is characteristic. The initial phase of infection is characterized by fever, abdominal pain, and watery diarrhea, which, after 3 to 5 days, is usually followed by tenesmus and small-volume bloody diarrhea. Very rarely, patients have an acute abdomen secondary to perforation. Presence of red blood cells and leukocytes in stool is a common finding. Stool cultures are often positive during the first few days of infection.

Escherichia coli

Although six major strains of *E. coli* have been implicated in human diarrheal disease, only two specific strains, enteroinvasive *E. coli* (EIEC) and enterohemorrhagic *E. coli* (EHEC), invade colonic tissue and cause ASLC. In the United States, EHEC O157:H7 is the pathogenic strain most commonly isolated from stools of patients with bloody diarrhea.[357] Consumption of infected hamburger meat is a common mode of disease transmission. The disease is most common in Northern climates such as Minnesota, Massachusetts, and the U.S. Pacific Northwest. Clinical symptoms for both EIEC and EHEC begin with watery diarrhea and fever, which is usually followed by 3 to 8 days of bloody diarrhea. Stool examination shows red blood cells and white blood cells. Peripheral blood examination often reveals leukocytosis with an increased number of immature white blood cells. Radiological examination during the first week of illness may reveal a thumbprinting sign, which is the result of subepithelial edema and hemorrhage. Stool cultures are very helpful in establishing a definitive diagnosis. Occasionally, polymerase chain reaction (PCR) and enzyme-linked immunosorbent assay (ELISA) testing for Shiga-like toxins may be necessary to confirm the diagnosis.

Yersinia enterocolitica

Y. enterocolitica causes a spectrum of clinical illnesses that range from mild gastroenteritis to invasive ileitis and colitis.[358] In comparison with the United States, *Y. enterocolitica* gastroenteritis is far more common in Scandinavian and European countries. The serotypes prevalent in these countries also differ. Strain O:8 is more common in the United States, whereas strains O:3 and O:9 are more prevalent in Scandinavian and European countries.[359] Almost two-thirds of infections involve both the small bowel and colon (enterocolitis). Children younger than 5 years of age are commonly affected. Clinical symptoms last for 1 to 3 weeks and include fever, abdominal pain, and bloody diarrhea. As with other causes of ASLC, stool analysis often reveals the presence of blood and leukocytes. Stool culture and serological studies may be helpful to establish a diagnosis. Radiological findings in cases of mild gastroenteritis are nonspecific. In severe cases, the radiological changes may mimic CD.

Pathogenesis

The clinical manifestation of ASLC is mostly related to the ability of microorganisms to invade the mucosa or produce enterotoxins. Although toxigenic organisms usually target the small bowel (and rarely the colon), tissue-invasive organisms typically cause injury to both the terminal ileum and colon.

Tissue-Invasive Organisms

C. jejuni, *Salmonella* and *Shigella* species, *E. coli*, and *Y. enterocolitica* are organisms that invade tissue and cause epithelial injury and death. Tissue invasion also results in the production of inflammatory cytokines that trigger an acute inflammatory reaction. In addition to tissue invasion, *Shigella* species undergo intracellular multiplication that allows for transmission of the infection into adjacent epithelial cells. In cases of *Salmonella* or *Y. enterocolitica* infection, organisms invade the lamina propria and submucosa and disseminate to extraintestinal sites via the bloodstream. Increased intracellular calcium and release of prostaglandin and leukotriene metabolites, serotonin, substance P, and reactive oxygen metabolites contribute to increased fluid output from epithelial cells.

Toxigenic Organisms

Enterotoxins are polypeptides secreted by bacteria that alter the transport of electrolytes and water through colonocytes without causing cellular injury. *Shigella*, enterotoxigenic *E. coli* (ETEC), *Staphylococcus aureus*, *Clostridium perfringens*, and *Vibrio cholera* are most associated with toxin production. Binding of enterotoxins to specific mucosal receptors causes decreased influx of sodium and chloride ions into the cells and active secretion of chloride ions from cells into the intestinal lumen. Thus enterotoxins are responsible for the acute phase of illness. Clinical symptoms are a result of fluid and electrolyte disturbances.[360]

Cytotoxins are polypeptides that cause tissue injury by inhibiting protein synthesis, disrupting actin and tight junction integrity, damaging mitochondria, and depleting adenosine triphosphate (ATP) within cells. Organisms that elaborate cytotoxins include C. *difficile*, enteropathogenic *E. coli* (EPEC), EHEC, and *Shigella*. In addition, EHEC also produces an enterohemolysin that causes endothelial damage. Endothelial injury results in initiation of the coagulation cascade that ultimately leads to an ischemic colitis–pattern of tissue injury.

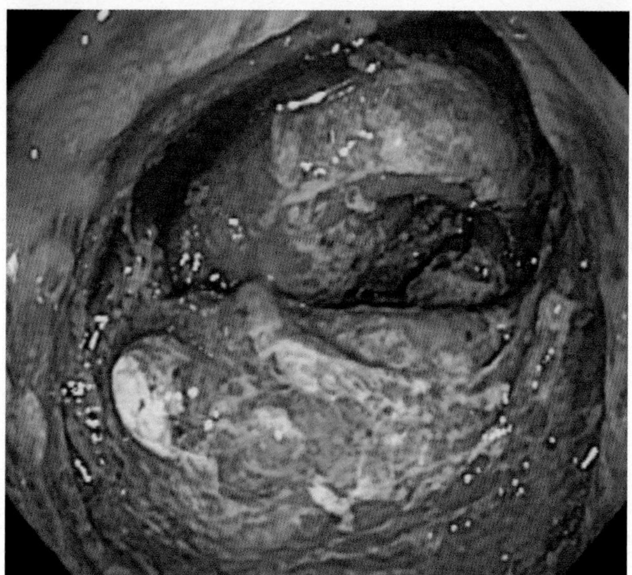

FIGURE 17.47 Endoscopic appearance of colitis secondary to enterohemorrhagic *Escherichia coli* O157:H7 infection. The mucosa shows erythema, edema, and pseudomembrane formation.

Pathological Features

Gross Findings

Grossly, affected colonic mucosa may show minimal changes, such as patchy areas of edema, erythema, loss of the normal vascular pattern, and superficial erosions or ulcers. In severe cases, large segments of colon may be involved and show more severe mucosal friability and ulceration. Some organisms reveal characteristic endoscopic findings. For instance, C. *jejuni* can affect any part of the colon; typically, the mucosa shows numerous, superficial ulcers that range from 2 mm to 1 cm in size. *Salmonella* species may produce hemorrhagic mucosa with granularity, friability, and ulceration; very rarely, toxic megacolon may develop. The colon is the major site of involvement in cases of *Shigella* infection; in most cases, the colonic mucosa shows patchy involvement by small, ragged ulcers with normal intervening mucosa. Aphthous ulcers may also be present. If only the rectosigmoid region is involved, mucosal involvement is usually continuous and consists of diffuse areas of ulceration and granularity. EHEC O157:H7 infection is usually segmental; infection results in friable, erythematous, and edematous mucosa with superficial ulcers. The right colon is more commonly involved than the transverse, or left, colon. Pseudomembranes may develop in severe cases (Fig. 17.47). *Y. enterocolitica* tends to affect the proximal colon more than the distal colon. The mucosa may appear edematous with patchy or diffuse areas of superficial erosions. Pseudomembranes and perforation are uncommon in the early phase of infection.

Microscopic Findings

In the early phase of ASLC, the mucosa typically shows intact crypt architecture, edema, hemorrhage and congestion, and a mild neutrophilic infiltration of the lamina propria, crypt, and/or surface epithelium (Fig. 17.48). More severe cryptitis, crypt abscesses, and even crypt rupture–associated granulomas are not uncommon, but these usually occur a few days after the onset of disease. The epithelium is typically degenerated, and as a result, it may appear flattened, hypereosinophilic, and mucin depleted. Later in the disease, the lamina propria often shows increased lymphocytes, histiocytes, and neutrophils, but usually without prominent plasma cells (Fig. 17.49). Basal plasma cells are not typical of ASLC because this feature develops in patients with long-standing (many weeks to months) and emerging chronic disease.

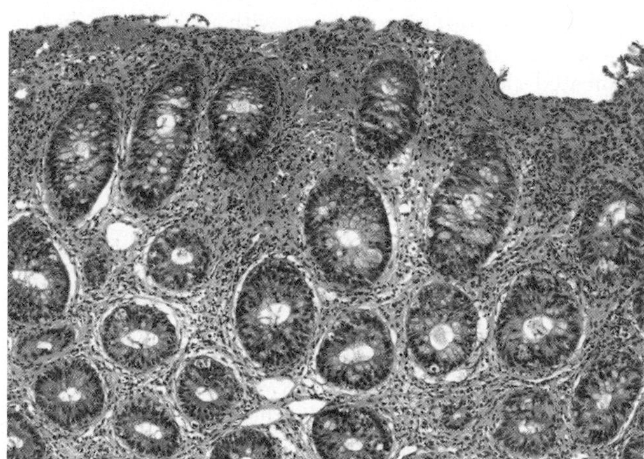

FIGURE 17.48 Low-power view of acute infectious colitis showing intact crypt architecture, one of the key diagnostic features of this entity. There is surface erosion accompanied by hemorrhage, edema, and expansion of the lamina propria by a neutrophil-rich inflammatory infiltrate. Foci of cryptitis and crypt apoptosis are also present.

Unless biopsies are obtained within the first few days of disease, the classic histological phenotype of ASLC, as just described, is uncommon. Biopsies are more commonly obtained several weeks after disease onset, in which case they may show partial histological resolution, characterized by mild or completely absent neutrophilic inflammation, less edema and hemorrhage, increased lymphocytic inflammation, and prominent reactive epithelial changes. After 2 to 3 weeks of infection, the mucosa may, in fact,

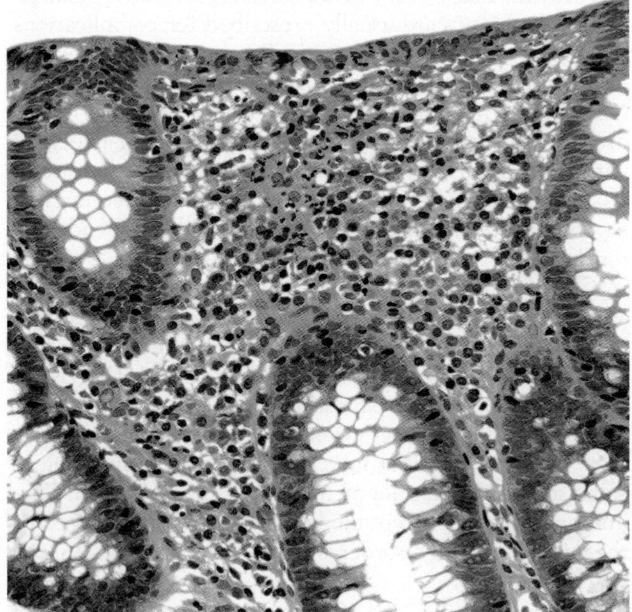

FIGURE 17.49 *Campylobacter jejuni*–associated colitis showing expansion of the lamina propria by neutrophils, eosinophils, plasma cells, lymphocytes, and rare histiocytes.

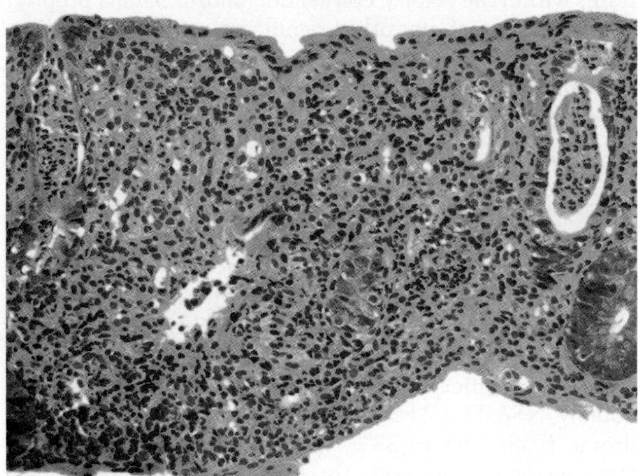

FIGURE 17.50 *Salmonella*-associated colitis showing prominent neutrophilic cryptitis and crypt abscesses.

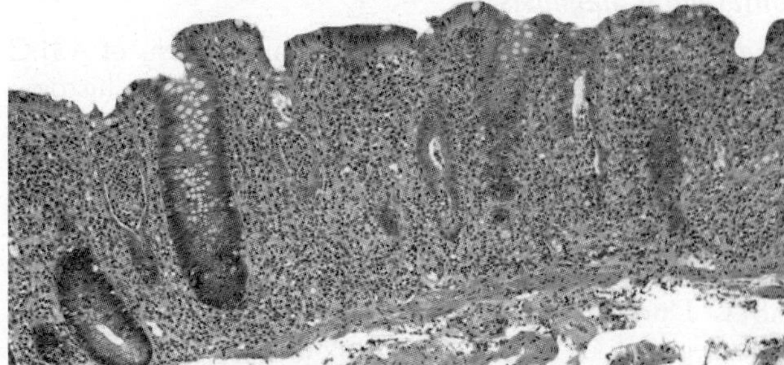

FIGURE 17.51 *Shigella*-associated colitis showing expansion of the lamina propria by a mixed inflammatory infiltrate, cryptitis, and crypt abscesses.

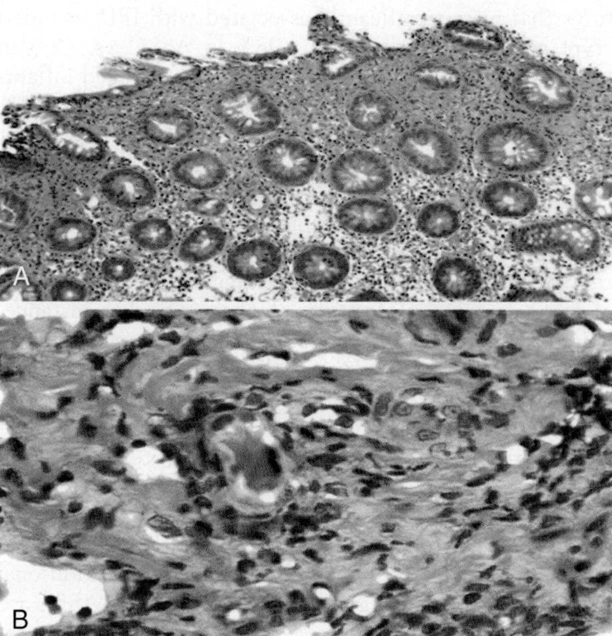

FIGURE 17.52 Enterohemorrhagic *Escherichia coli* O157:H7 infection is often associated with an ischemic pattern of mucosal injury. A, Biopsy specimen shows mucosal erosion with lamina propria hemorrhage and focal hyalinization. The crypt epithelium shows reactive mucin loss. **B,** Capillary thrombus is present within the lamina propria.

be completely normal or may show only residual, patchy, mild inflammation (often referred to *focal active colitis;* see later discussion) and a mildly hypercellular lamina propria. In some cases, resolving ASLC reveals persistent residual surface epithelial damage and increased intraepithelial lymphocytes, reminiscent of lymphocytic colitis, and this may take months to resolve completely.

Some organisms show characteristic microscopic findings. For instance, C. *jejuni* infection may be associated with histiocytic aggregates that resemble granulomas. A Warthin-Starry silver stain performed in the early phase of infection highlights curved rods within crypt and surface epithelium.

Salmonella infection is typically associated with mild and focal changes. Mucosal edema and congestion of capillaries within the lamina propria are usually prominent in mild cases. In severe cases, the mucosa may show numerous crypt abscesses (Fig. 17.50), ulceration, and microthrombi within small venules of the lamina propria.

Early *Shigella* infection is characterized by the presence of aphthous ulcers with patchy foci of cryptitis and reactive epithelial changes in adjacent epithelium. With ongoing injury, the lamina propria typically shows a prominent mixed inflammatory infiltrate composed of neutrophils, lymphocytes, and plasma cells (Fig. 17.51).

EHEC O157:H7 infection may cause marked epithelial and endothelial damage. Neutrophilic cryptitis and occasional crypt abscesses are accompanied by superficial "microerosions" and prominent hemorrhage and edema, hence this disease is designated as a type of *hemorrhagic colitis*. Damage to the endothelium may result in an ischemic pattern of injury characterized by mucosal necrosis, withering crypts, and hyalinization of the lamina propria, either with or without pseudomembrane formation, and even microthrombus formation in mucosal and submucosal blood vessels (Fig. 17.52).

Differential Diagnosis

The most important clinical differential diagnosis of ASLC is IBD. However, several studies have shown that histopathology can help differentiate these two disorders.[6,351,361] In ASLC, endoscopic examination usually shows patchy mucosal involvement. In UC, the mucosal changes are diffuse and continuous. Discrete, serpiginous ulcers are characteristic of CD and are seldom, if ever, encountered in ASLC. During the early phase of illness, the presence of diffuse, regional, or focal active colitis without crypt architectural distortion or other features of chronic mucosal injury (e.g., basal plasmacytosis, Paneth cell metaplasia) and with prominent neutrophilic cryptitis favors a diagnosis of ASLC over IBD.[351,362,363] In a seminal study by Surawicz and colleagues[361] that compared clinicopathological features of 37 cases of ASLC with 14 cases of IBD, the histological features that were significantly associated with IBD included crypt architectural distortion (93% in ASLC vs. 14% in IBD), expansion of the lamina propria by a mixed inflammatory infiltrate (86% vs. 37%), basal plasmacytosis (71% vs. 0%), and basal lymphoid aggregates (43% vs. 0%). Giant cells and even granulomas may be present, but in ASLC they are usually present in the basal half of the mucosa in association with ruptured crypts.

In some infectious cases, the disease is prolonged (typically more than 3 to 4 weeks), leading to the development of some histological features of chronicity. For instance, *Shigella* infection has been associated with crypt distortion mimicking IBD.[362] However, in the "chronic" phase of bacterial infection, lamina propria cellularity typically diminishes with time. In contrast, increased cellularity of the lamina propria, with basal lymphoplasmacytosis, supports a diagnosis of IBD.

During the resolution phase of ASLC, the disease may be patchy and thus mimic Crohn's colitis. Epithelioid granulomas, when present, should raise suspicion of CD. Additional features that help distinguish Crohn's colitis from ASLC are lack of involvement of the rest of the GI tract and clinical resolution of symptoms with supportive therapy.

Natural History and Treatment

Most cases of ASLC resolve within 2 to 3 weeks with supportive therapy. In most bacterial infections, treatment does not provide a significant benefit over conservative management. Antibiotics are usually prescribed for complications, such as sepsis or disseminated infection. Some infections (e.g., C. *jejuni*) may result in the development of pancreatitis, cholecystitis, reactive arthritis, and Guillain-Barré syndrome. Prolonged infection by *Shigella* has been associated with appendicitis, myocarditis, pneumonitis, reactive arthritis, and hemolytic-uremic syndrome. EHEC infection may be complicated by hemolytic-uremic syndrome, end-stage renal disease, seizures, or cerebral edema.

Classic IBD develops in a small percentage of patients after an infectious illness. In one Spanish study, the incidence rate of IBD after an episode of infectious gastroenteritis was 68 per 100,000 person-years.[364] The risk of developing IBD is highest during the first year after an episode of ASLC. The pathogenesis is unknown. One possibility is that the initial infection serves as an initiator, or catalyst, for the development of IBD in a genetically and immunologically susceptible host. However, in some cases, the initial diarrheal disorder is simply misdiagnosed as infectious colitis.

Focal Active Colitis

Focal active colitis is defined as a pattern of colonic injury characterized by the presence of focal neutrophilic infiltrates within the colonic epithelium (and/or lamina propria) in the absence of any other significant microscopic abnormality.[365] The changes may involve a single crypt, a few adjacent crypts, or small regions of mucosa across a series of multiple colorectal biopsy specimens (Fig. 17.53).

Clinical Features

Based on one prospective study[366] and three retrospective studies[365,367,368] that evaluated, in total, 163 adult patients and 31 pediatric patients, a focal active colitis pattern of injury is more common in adult women than in adult men but shows an equal gender distribution in children. The most common causes of focal active colitis in adults are resolving infectious colitis (19% to 55%), drugs (most notably NSAIDs; 24% to 45%), and irritable bowel syndrome (IBS; 14% to 33%) (Table 17.8). Although CD is less common, it accounts for 13% of cases in adults. The presenting symptoms are usually sudden-onset diarrhea,

TABLE 17.8 Prevalence of Conditions Associated with a Focal Active Colitis Pattern of Injury

Diagnosis	Adults[365] (%)	Adults[367] (%)	Adults[366] (%)	Children[368] (%)
Infectious	55	48	19	31
Incidental	40	29	8	26.6
Ischemia	5	10	0	0
Crohn's disease	0	13	11	27.6
Ulcerative colitis	0	0	2.2*	3.45
Drugs	39	0	24	0
Irritable bowel syndrome	14	0	33	0
Allergic	0	0	0	6.9
Hirschsprung's disease	0	0	0	3.45

*Excludes >2 cases of indeterminate colitis.

abdominal tenderness, and fever. C. *jejuni* is the most frequently isolated causative organism. C. *jejuni* DNA is isolated in up to 19% of patients.[353] This pattern of injury may also be observed incidentally (8% to 29%) during colonoscopic assessment for cancer surveillance or in patients with guaiac-positive stools.

In the pediatric population, focal active colitis is most often associated with infectious colitis (31%), CD (28%), allergic colitis (7%), UC (3%), and Hirschsprung's disease (3%). As in adults, this pattern of inflammation is observed as an incidental finding in approximately 28% of cases.[368] Occasionally, bowel preparation agents, especially oral sodium phosphate solutions, cause focal active colitis.

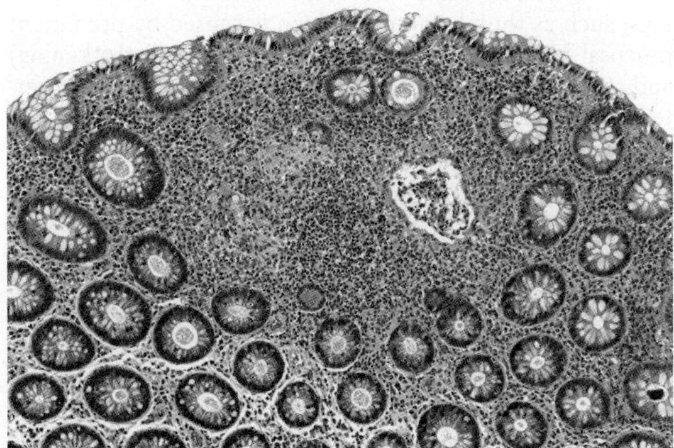

FIGURE 17.53 Focal active colitis. Low-power view of colonic mucosa shows neutrophilic cryptitis and crypt abscesses in a group of two to three crypts. The damaged crypts also show a cuff of mononuclear cells including histiocytes. Notice that the rest of the mucosa is essentially unremarkable.

Pathological Features

Depending on the cause, endoscopic findings range from completely normal to patchy mucosal erythema with scattered aphthous ulcers. Focal active colitis is characterized by the presence of neutrophilic cryptitis that may involve a single crypt or a small collection of crypts (see Fig. 17.53). The lamina propria may be mildly expanded by an inflammatory infiltrate that is rich in neutrophils or eosinophils. The finding of a florid neutrophilic inflammatory infiltrate at the crypt bases associated with prominent crypt apoptosis (so-called *basal focal active colitis*) is often associated with drug therapy, especially NSAIDs, antibiotics, proton pump inhibitors (PPIs), and steroids.[366] Oral sodium phosphate bowel preparations cause cryptitis, often centered on lymphoid follicles (i.e., aphthous lesions), that is identical to that seen in some types of infectious colitis and in CD.[369]

Natural History and Treatment

Between 0% and 16% of adult patients and about 25% of pediatric patients with focal active colitis develop IBD. These patients develop CD more commonly than UC (see Table 17.8).

Ischemic Colitis

Ischemic colitis is the most common form of ischemic injury of the GI tract. The diagnosis is based on a combination of clinical, radiological, endoscopic, and histological findings. Since its original description by Boley[370] and Marston[371] and their colleagues in the 1960s, understanding of the etiology and pathophysiology of this entity has evolved significantly. Ischemic colitis can manifest as an acute transient disorder that is completely reversible on reestablishment of blood flow, as an acute severe and irreversible form of injury, or as a chronic recurrent disorder (Table 17.9).

TABLE 17.9 Patterns of Ischemic Colitis

Pattern	Symptoms and Signs	Pathogenesis/Etiology	Key Histological Features	Outcome
Acute transient (reversible) ischemic colitis	Sudden-onset abdominal cramping, diarrhea, passage of blood within 24 hours after onset of symptoms	Nonocclusive ischemia: low flow state (vascular hypoperfusion, vasospasm associated with medications, infections (see Box 17.7) Sudden embolic event	1-2 hours: mucosal and submucosal edema, hemorrhage, and surface epithelial detachment Reperfusion causes neutrophilic inflammatory infiltrates and cryptitis	Symptoms typically resolve with conservative measures without long-term sequelae
Acute severe (irreversible) ischemic colitis	Early stage: sudden-onset severe abdominal pain, bloody diarrhea Late stage: diffuse and continuous abdominal pain with tenderness	Occlusive ischemia • Arterial and venous thrombosis, vasculitis, small and medium vessel disorders (amyloidosis, diabetes mellitus, radiation) • Hypercoagulable states • Obstruction (colon cancer, strictures, adhesions, volvulus, hernia)Infections: *Escherichia coli*	Early phase: mucosal erosions, ulceration and necrosis, lamina propria hemorrhage, "withered crypts," lamina propria hyalinization Late phase: transmural necrosis, extensive bowel wall edema, serositis	20% of patients require surgical resection Despite surgery, mortality is 60%
Chronic recurrent ischemic colitis	Persistent bloody diarrhea With symptomatic stricture: nausea, vomiting, sepsis	Occlusive ischemia caused by slow-growing atheromatous plaques in mesenteric blood vessels	Mucosal erosions with granulation tissue formation, hemosiderin, and submucosal and/or mural fibrosis	Segmental resection is the choice of therapy; recurrence occurs in 5% of patients

Pathogenesis

Ischemic damage occurs when decreased vascular flow results in deprivation of oxygen uptake by the bowel (typically reduced to less than 50% of normal). Hypoxia initiates a sequence of events that leads to cellular dysfunction, edema, and cell death. The specific pathogenetic mechanisms for the development of ischemia depend on the cause and duration of the ischemic event.

The initial response to ischemia is increased oxygen extraction. This phase of disease is accompanied by transient vasodilation, which allows for compensation of as much as 75% of the reduction in blood flow in some circumstances. This response is normally sustained for a few hours until vasoconstriction and redistribution of blood flow results in the development of mucosal injury. Vasoconstriction persists after the inciting event is resolved. Because the mucosa is most vulnerable to decreased oxygen supply, pathological changes of transient ischemia are usually restricted to the superficial aspects of the mucosa.

Reperfusion of the bowel is required to recover from an episode of ischemia. However, restoration of the flow of oxygenated blood has its own consequences. It results in the generation of oxygen free radicals capable of causing additional structural and functional damage to the epithelial cells. This is referred to as *reperfusion injury*. Parks and Granger demonstrated that the histological changes after 3 hours of ischemia and 1 hour of reperfusion were worse than those after 4 hours of ischemia without reperfusion.[372] Increased microvascular permeability, increased epithelial permeability, and decreased blood flow all contribute to reperfusion injury. During this phase, levels of thromboxane A_2 and leukotriene C_4 (vasoconstrictors) increase by more than 300%, and there is a concurrent decrease in the levels of prostaglandin I_2 (vasodilator).

During an ischemic episode, ATP is metabolized to hypoxanthine. Superoxide ions (oxygen-free radicals) are generated when oxygen combines with hypoxanthine to form xanthine. Oxygen-free radicals cause lipid peroxidation of cell membranes, breakage of DNA strands, and disturbed cellular homeostasis, all of which results in calcium overload and irreversible mitochondrial injury. Oxygen-free radicals are also capable of recruiting neutrophils and activating the complement pathway. Therefore the presence of neutrophils within the mucosa (cryptitis, crypt abscesses) and bowel wall is an indicator of reperfusion injury. Activated neutrophils further release proteases and collagenases, which, in conjunction with complement proteins, result in further tissue damage.

Acute Ischemic Colitis

Clinical Features

Ischemic colitis accounts for 1 of 2000 hospital admissions.[373] The incidence rate in the general population ranges from 4.5 to 44 cases per 100,000 person-years.[374] Ischemic colitis occurs more commonly in women (55% to 64%) but manifests at a significantly younger age in men than in women.[374,375] Patients older than 60 years of age and those with cardiac disease (e.g., cardiac failure, atrial fibrillation, recent myocardial infarction, hypotension) are at a significant risk for ischemic colitis.

Presenting symptoms of acute ischemic colitis usually include sudden-onset crampy abdominal pain, diarrhea, urgency to defecate, and hematochezia within 24 hours. In the nonocclusive form of ischemia (discussed later), pain may be absent in as many as 25% of patients. Physical and radiological examinations in the early phase of acute ischemic colitis often reveal no abnormalities.

There is severe tissue damage in 15% to 20% of cases, and these patients typically complain of diffuse and continuous abdominal pain.[376] If ischemic colitis is complicated by ileus, patients may complain of anorexia, nausea, and vomiting. Physical examination often reveals abdominal distention, a sign that correlates with bowel infarction. Generalized abdominal tenderness is common. Peripheral blood examination often shows leukocytosis. Metabolic acidosis is documented in almost 50% of patients. Radiographs obtained during this phase often reveal nonspecific findings, such as thumbprinting (which is caused by prominent mucosal haustrations as a result of bowel wall thickening) and air-filled loops. Peritoneal free air is an indicator of perforation. Other ominous signs include pneumatosis coli and gas within the mesenteric veins.[377]

Specific Etiological Factors

Bowel ischemia results from a variety of different causes and occurs at various levels, depending on the intensity, rapidity, location, and degree of reduction in blood flow (Box 17.7). Blood flow may be compromised by intrinsic or extrinsic vascular occlusion or by nonocclusive (systemic) disorders.

Thromboembolism in patients with atherosclerotic vascular disease is the most common cause of acute colonic ischemia. Vascular compromise also occurs secondary to mechanical obstruction caused by a tumor, adhesions, volvulus, strangulated hernia, intussusception, or extreme hypovolemia and hypoperfusion after cardiopulmonary bypass surgery. Long-distance running, consumption of oral contraceptives or estrogen compounds, cocaine abuse, or a genetic defect in coagulation factors (e.g., protein C, protein S, factor V Leiden) are some of the etiological factors in young and middle-aged individuals with ischemic colitis. Acute ischemic colitis, when transient and reversible, resolves with restoration of blood flow and is most commonly nonocclusive in nature. It is usually associated with vascular hypoperfusion resulting from decreased cardiac output (e.g., in congestive cardiac failure, myocardial infarction, cardiac arrhythmia), hypovolemia, shock, and excessive physical stress or exercise.

Pathological Features

Gross Findings

The splenic flexure (Griffiths' point) and sigmoid colon (Sudeck's point) are regions where the circulations of the superior mesenteric artery, which supplies the ascending and transverse colon, and the inferior mesenteric artery, which supplies the descending and sigmoid colon, meet. At these anatomic points, there is a very limited collateral vascular network. Therefore these areas of bowel are highly susceptible to ischemic damage and are often referred to as the *watershed* territories of the bowel. The most commonly affected region is the left colon (75% of cases), followed by the splenic flexure (as many as 25%) and right colon

BOX 17.7 Colonic Ischemia: Etiological Factors

IDIOPATHIC (SPONTANEOUS) OCCLUSIVE

MAJOR VASCULAR OCCLUSION

Trauma
Thrombosis or embolization of mesenteric arteries
- Arterial embolus
- Cholesterol embolus
- Aortography
- Colectomy with inferior mesenteric artery ligation
- Midgut ischemia
- Previous abdominal aortic reconstruction

Mesenteric venous thrombosis
- Hypercoagulable states
- Portal hypertension
- Pancreatitis

SMALL AND MEDIUM VESSEL DISEASE

Diabetes mellitus
Rheumatoid arthritis
Amyloidosis
Radiation injury
Systemic vasculitis disorders
- Systemic lupus erythematosus
- Polyarteritis nodosa
- Kawasaki's disease
- Ehlers-Danlos syndrome
- Allergic granulomatosis
- Scleroderma
- Behçet's syndrome
- Takayasu arteritis
- Thromboangiitis obliterans
- Buerger's disease

HEMATOLOGICAL DISORDERS AND HYPERCOAGULABLE STATES

Sickle cell disease
Protein C deficiency
Protein S deficiency
Antithrombin III deficiency

COLONIC OBSTRUCTION

Colon carcinoma
Adhesions
Stricture
Diverticular disease
Rectal prolapse
Fecal impaction
Volvulus
Strangulated hernia
Pseudo-obstruction

NONOCCLUSIVE

VASCULAR HYPOPERFUSION

Cardiac failure
Hypovolemia
Sepsis
Neurogenic insult
Anaphylaxis
Long-distance running or strenuous exercise

DRUGS

Catecholamines
Cocaine
Digitalis preparations
Diuretics
Estrogen compounds
Danazol
Gold
Nonsteroidal antiinflammatory drugs
Neuroleptics
Potassium salts

INFECTIONS

Bacteria (*Escherichia coli* O157:H7)
Parasites (*Ancylostoma ceylanicum, Ascaris*)
Viruses (cytomegalovirus, hepatitis B, hepatitis C)

Data from Gandhi SK, Hanson MM, Vernava AM, et al. Ischemic colitis. *Dis Colon Rectum.* 1996;39:88–100.

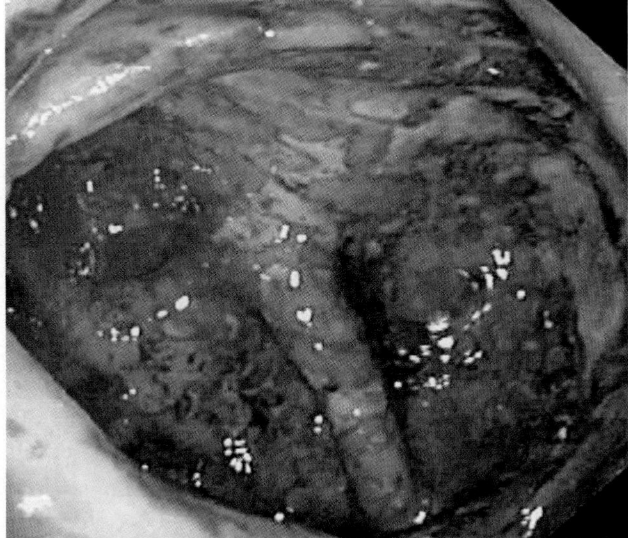

FIGURE 17.54 Endoscopic appearance of ischemic colitis (acute severe irreversible ischemia) showing mucosal erythema, edema, ulcerations, and pseudomembrane formation.

(10%). Because of its dual blood supply from the splanchnic and systemic arterial systems, the rectum is uncommonly affected by ischemia.

In acute reversible colonic ischemia, the mucosa shows minor changes grossly, which mainly consist of mucosal and submucosal edema. With severe and prolonged ischemia, hemorrhage is usually grossly visible. Nodules of hemorrhage correspond to the "thumbprinting" sign seen on radiological studies. Superficial mucosal erosions, petechial hemorrhages, and segmental erythema develop with progressive ischemia. The term *colon single-stripe sign* refers to a single line of erythema with erosion/ulceration oriented along the longitudinal axis of the colon.[378] In cases of irreversible ischemic injury ("gangrenous" ischemia), the bowel appears greenish-gray or black on the serosal surface because of necrosis. The mucosal surface shows ulceration, congestion, and edema. Pseudopolyps and pseudomembranes may also develop (Fig. 17.54).[376] The bowel wall is thin and friable, and perforation may be present. Rarely, ischemia may mimic colon cancer by presenting as a mass lesion. In a recent systematic review of mass-forming ischemic colitis, it was noted that the proximal colon was more likely to

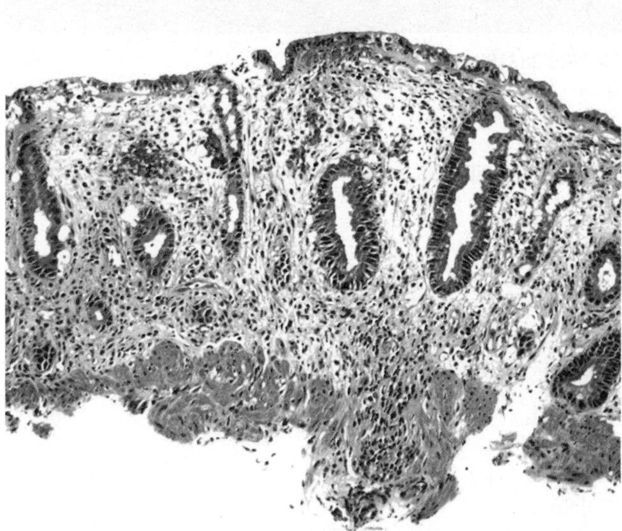

FIGURE 17.55 Early acute reversible ischemic colitis. This biopsy specimen shows mucosal edema, hemorrhage, and detachment of surface epithelial cells. The crypt epithelium shows partial mucin depletion. There is patchy, minimal neutrophilic inflammation.

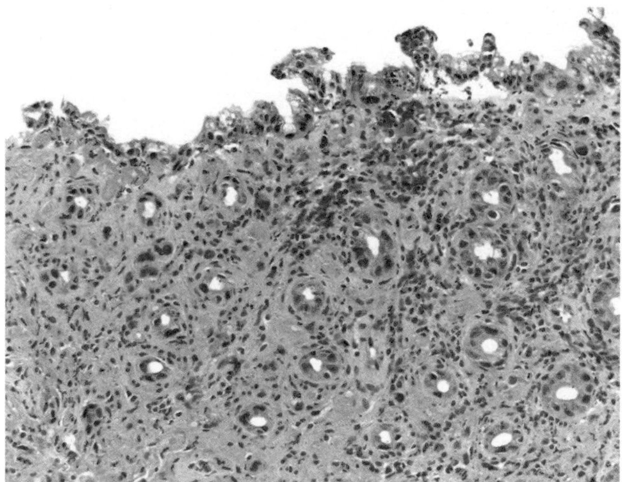

FIGURE 17.56 Ischemic colitis showing superficial mucosal erosion with withered atrophic crypts. The lamina propria has a hyalinized appearance as well as hemorrhage, a finding that is usually associated with ischemic colitis.

be affected.[379] Examination of resection specimens should not only include documentation of the extent of ischemic damage but should also incorporate steps to investigate the cause of ischemia. Therefore sampling of the mesenteric vasculature is critical.

Microscopic Findings

The early phase of acute reversible ischemic colitis is characterized by mucosal edema, hemorrhage, and detachment (and degeneration) of the surface epithelial cells from the underlying basement membrane (Fig. 17.55). With progressive ischemia, there is necrosis of the superficial portion of the mucosa with initial sparing of the deeper crypts, a phenomenon referred to as *withering crypts*[380,381] (Fig. 17.56). Withered crypts are lined by flat, attenuated, and degenerated epithelium. The remaining crypts are typically mucin-depleted and atrophic. Other characteristic findings include hemorrhage, congestion, and hyalinization of the lamina propria.[380] Capillary microthrombi may also be present (Fig. 17.57). Overall, the amount of inflammation is variable and depends on the type, degree, and completeness of blood flow reduction. Complete sudden-onset occlusion results in an infarct with little inflammation if there is no reflow. Neutrophilic infiltrates are characteristic of reperfusion injury. In severe cases, mucosal necrosis may become complete and may show ulceration or pseudomembrane formation, or both. In areas of pseudomembrane formation, sloughed-off surface epithelial cells may assume a signet ring cell–like appearance within the lumen of the degenerated crypts, which mimics signet ring cell adenocarcinoma (Fig. 17.58).

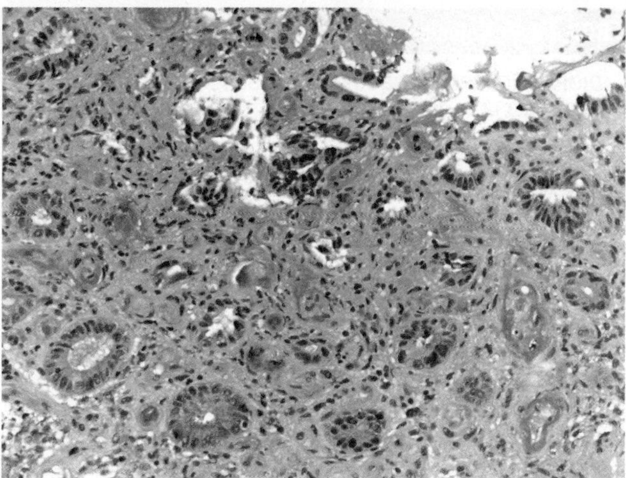

FIGURE 17.57 Ischemic colitis with capillary microthrombi. This biopsy specimen was obtained from a young man with a coagulation disorder.

In cases of irreversible ischemic damage, variably sized but often large segments of the bowel demonstrate transmural ischemic necrosis ("gangrenous" necrosis) often combined with prominent mural edema, congestion, and hemorrhage. A serosal fibroinflammatory response is typically present in areas of perforation. In resection specimens, sampling of the mesenteric vasculature may reveal organizing thrombi, vasculitis, or myointimal hyperplasia, depending on the cause of ischemia. In areas of transmural necrosis, ulceration, and suppurative inflammation, secondary thrombus formation may occur because of development of a localized transient hypercoagulable state within the vascular system (Fig. 17.59). This is caused by localized stasis of blood flow combined with the effects of an inflammatory cytokine-rich microenvironment. Thus the presence of vascular thrombi in regions of bowel distant from necrosis or ulceration is a better indicator of a vascular etiology of the patient's colitis.

During the resolution phase of acute reversible ischemic colitis, the colonic mucosa shows epithelial regeneration and granulation tissue formation. Chronic inflammatory cells gradually replace neutrophils, and mucosal healing occurs within a few days to weeks.

Natural History and Treatment

In transient and reversible forms of ischemic injury, complete resolution of the clinical symptoms usually occurs

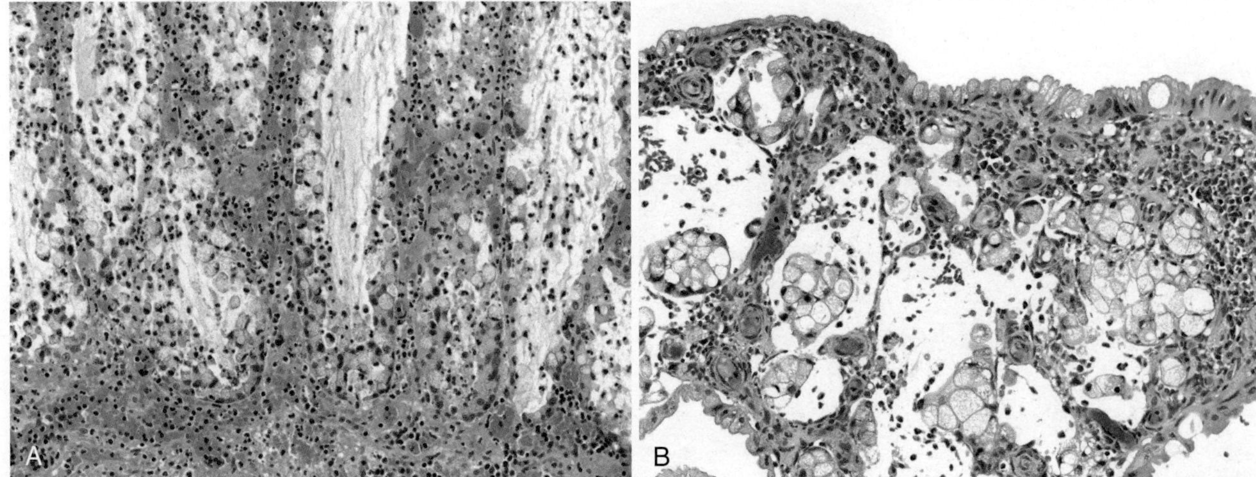

FIGURE 17.58 A, Pseudo–signet ring cells in acute severe ischemic colitis in a patient with history of deep vein thrombosis, infective endocarditis, and septicemia. In areas with prominent mucosal necrosis, the degenerating surface epithelial cells slough off into the crypt lumen and acquire a signet ring cell appearance. **B,** These should not be misdiagnosed as signet ring cell adenocarcinoma, which usually shows clusters as well as single atypical cells infiltrating the lamina propria.

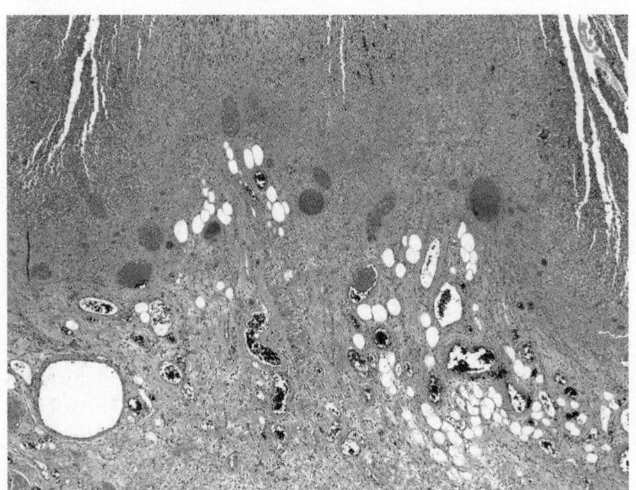

FIGURE 17.59 Secondary thrombus formation in a patient with colonic ulceration and necrosis. The tissue shows vascular thrombi within an area of extensive necrosis and ulceration. Stasis of blood flow and the presence of inflammatory cytokines may result in the development of a localized hypercoagulable state, which leads to thrombus formation.

within a few days. In severe reversible ischemic colitis, patients are treated with medical or surgical therapy. The healing phase may last as long as 6 months. The overall prognosis depends on the severity of ischemia, underlying cause, stage of presentation, and presence of comorbidity. Patients treated medically have a low mortality rate. Stricture formation has been documented in as many as 13% of cases.[382]

Approximately 20% of patients with severe acute ischemic colitis require surgical management.[383] These patients often have evidence of ongoing sepsis refractory to medical treatment, signs of peritoneal irritation, diarrhea and bleeding lasting longer than 10 to 14 days, evidence of pneumoperitoneum, endoscopic evidence of full-thickness ischemia, or protein-losing enteropathy of more than 2 weeks' duration. The mortality rate among those undergoing surgical resection ranges from 18% to 48%, depending on the timing of surgery and the response to initial management.[384]

Chronic Ischemic Colitis

Clinical Features

Chronic ischemic colitis develops in 20% to 25% of patients with ischemic injury.[376] This disorder mainly affects patients older than 60 years of age. Intermittent bloody diarrhea is a common presenting symptom. In cases complicated by stricture formation, patients may have signs and symptoms of intestinal obstruction, sepsis, or both, and it may mimic other disorders such as IBD or diverticular disease, among others. Weight loss and diarrhea may occur as a result of protein-losing colopathy. In patients with chronic ischemia resulting from mesenteric vein thrombosis, signs of portal hypertension and GI bleeding from varices or hemorrhoids may be present. Radiological examination, specifically angiography, is helpful in delineating the source of vascular occlusion.

Specific Etiological Factors

Chronic ischemia most commonly results from longstanding and progressive atherosclerotic disease that involves the celiac axis and superior mesenteric artery. Other causes include ischemia secondary to mechanical obstruction caused by a slow-growing retroperitoneal mass compressing the vasculature, adhesions, volvulus, strangulated hernia, hypercoagulable states, and medications that cause vasospasm, such as selective serotonin receptor agonists (sumatriptan, rizatriptan).

Pathological Features

Gross Findings

In chronic ischemia, the colonoscopic findings are reminiscent of segmental chronic active colitis. The mucosa may show foci of atrophy, granularity, and pseudopolyps. In addition, evidence of ongoing or active ischemic injury in the form of erosions, hemorrhage, and edema may be present. Mural changes in the form of fibrosis and strictures can mimic CD.[381] There may be gross evidence of organizing thrombi within pericolonic blood vessels. The disease

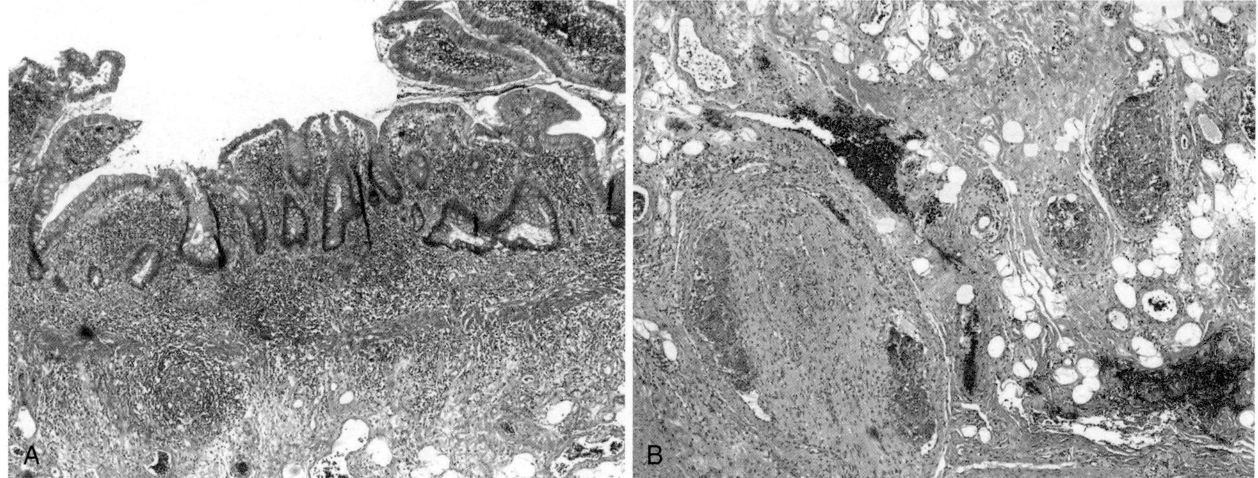

FIGURE 17.60 A, Chronic active ischemic colitis involving the right colon shows changes reminiscent of idiopathic inflammatory bowel disease, with crypt architectural distortion, mixed inflammation, basal lymphoid aggregates, and cryptitis. **B,** Organizing thrombi are present within the pericolonic (serosal) blood vessels.

distribution is similar to that of acute ischemic colitis. The left colon is more commonly affected than the right colon. The rectum is usually spared.

Microscopic Findings

In chronic ischemic colitis, the mucosal changes may be active, showing features of acute ischemic injury, or inactive. In some cases, the histological features mimic chronic active IBD-like colitis (Fig. 17.60A). Mucosal erosions with withering crypts and lamina propria hyalinization may be interspersed with features of chronic mucosal injury that include crypt architectural distortion, Paneth cell metaplasia, increased cellularity of lamina propria (composed of lymphocytes and plasma cells), basal plasmacytosis, basal lymphoid aggregates, and minimal neutrophilic cryptitis and crypt abscesses. The lamina propria may show hemosiderin deposition, granulation tissue, congestion, and hemorrhage. Variable submucosal edema and fibrosis causing fibrotic thickening of the bowel wall is a characteristic finding. In addition, the blood vessels may reveal atherosclerotic changes with myointimal hyperplasia and acute or organizing thrombi (see Fig. 17.60B).

Natural History and Treatment

Mildly symptomatic chronic ischemic colitis frequently responds to supportive management. Colonic strictures may occur during a period of a few months to several years. The treatment of ischemic strictures is endoscopic dilations. However, most patients eventually need surgical resection of the affected segment for symptoms related to obstruction or repeated episodes of diarrhea. Disease may recur in a minority of patients.

Differential Diagnosis

Acute Ischemic Colitis

ASLC can mimic early ischemic colitis by showing expansion of the lamina propria by neutrophil-rich inflammatory infiltrate accompanied by cryptitis and crypt abscess formation. Some organisms such as *E. coli* cause injury through ischemic mechanisms. In these cases, the mucosa may show withered crypts and hyalinization and even mucosal microthrombi.

C. *difficile* colitis can mimic ischemic colitis by showing dense pseudomembranes, edema, hemorrhage, and mucosal necrosis. However, the presence of lamina propria hyalinization suggests ischemic colitis and not C. *difficile* infection.[380] (Table 17.10; see Figs. 17.56 and 17.57.) In addition, in C. *difficile* colitis, pseudomembranes are more diffuse than in ischemic injury, where they are usually patchy in distribution.

Chronic Ischemic Colitis

Chronic ischemic colitis may resemble IBD. There can be an overlap in terms of disease distribution, especially with CD. Almost one-third of patients with CD have isolated involvement of the colon. In CD, total or subtotal involvement of the colon or left-sided colitis is more common.[150] Ischemic colitis also typically involves the left colon more commonly than the right colon and usually spares the rectum. The mucosa in CD as well as chronic ischemic colitis may show evidence of chronic mucosal injury. In areas of ischemic ulcers, lymphoid aggregates within the submucosa and superficial muscularis propria may be present. However, transmural lymphoid aggregates (and epithelioid granulomas) in areas of bowel distant from ulceration or necrosis are not characteristic of ischemic colitis.[381] Patients with IBD are at an increased risk of mesenteric ischemia and ischemic colitis. Although vascular changes such as myointimal hyperplasia and lymphocytic vasculitis have been documented in CD, the finding of organizing thrombi is uncommon; therefore this feature indicates an ischemic etiology or superimposed ischemia in a patient with established IBD.

Radiation Colitis

Clinical Features

Radiation colitis refers to colonic injury caused by exposure to ionizing radiation. Depending on the interval between radiation exposure and onset of symptoms, the injury is

TABLE 17.10 Ischemic Colitis vs. *Clostridium difficile* Colitis

Feature	Ischemic Colitis	*C. difficile* Colitis
Microscopic Findings		
Hyalinized lamina propria	Very common	Absent
Withered or atrophic crypts	Very common	Rare
Lamina propria hemorrhage	Usually present	Rare
Full-thickness mucosal necrosis	Common in severe cases	Rare
Diffuse pseudomembranes	May be present in only severe cases	Present
Endoscopic Findings		
Polyp or mass	May be seen in some cases	Usually absent
Pseudomembranes	May be present	Typically present

From Dignan CR, Greenson JK. Can ischemic colitis be differentiated from *C. difficile* colitis in biopsy specimens? *Am J Surg Pathol.* 1997;21:706–710.

categorized as acute (within 60 days of exposure) or chronic. Radiation colitis occurs most commonly in patients who have received radiation therapy for cervical or prostate cancer. Imaging studies, bone marrow conditioning regimens, and nuclear accidents are other potential sources of radiation exposure. With improved radiation therapy techniques that allow for targeted delivery of high doses of radiation for treatment of pelvic cancers, the incidence of radiation proctitis appears to be decreasing. The cumulative incidence rate of radiation colitis is 10% to 30% for mild disease and 2% to 3% for moderate to severe disease.[385] The incidence of asymptomatic radiation colitis is much higher (almost 80%). Acute radiation colitis occurs within hours to several days after radiation exposure and is caused primarily by damage to the epithelium. Symptoms of bleeding, diarrhea, tenesmus, and abdominal pain usually resolve within 2 to 3 months after cessation of radiation therapy. CT findings of radiation proctitis include regular and symmetric colonic wall thickening, often associated with inflamed perirectal fat.

Chronic radiation colitis occurs in 5% to 15% of patients who receive radiation to the pelvis.[386] It typically occurs over a period of a few months to several years after radiation exposure. Delayed symptoms of chronic radiation colitis include intermittent bleeding and abdominal pain. CT findings in chronic radiation-induced proctitis include the "halo effect," which results from an increase (>1 cm) in the anteroposterior presacral space combined with thickening of the perirectal fascia. Some patients have intermittent constipation and diarrhea because of fibrotic strictures, or, in some cases physiological pseudo-obstruction. Radiation colitis may remain clinically silent for long periods (average range, 6 to 24 months).[386] Once symptoms begin, they often remain for long periods.

Pathogenesis

The degree of damage caused by radiation increases proportionally with the dose and duration of exposure. A dose of 4500 rads is usually required to cause clinically significant complications. A dose of 5000 to 6000 rads causes disease in 25% to 50% of patients.[387] A single whole-body dose of external radiation is more harmful than small, regional doses with appropriate protection. The presence of other concurrent diseases, specifically microvascular injury associated with diabetes, hypertension, severe atherosclerosis, or previous intestinal injury, can further enhance the deleterious effects of radiation.[388]

Radiation selectively damages rapidly dividing cells that are in the G_2/M phase of the cell cycle. Loss of DNA strands leads to irreversible changes and, eventually, to cell death. Because the colonic epithelium regenerates within 5 to 6 days, it is highly susceptible to this form of toxic injury. Free radicals formed as a result of radiation exposure induce microvascular endothelial injury and precipitate cellular apoptosis. Apoptotic cells are usually confined to the crypt bases, which is the zone of highest proliferative activity in normal colonic mucosa.[389,390] TGF-β also plays an important role in the pathogenesis of chronic radiation colitis via its fibrogenic and proinflammatory effects. Increased levels of TGF-β have been found in vascular endothelial cells, fibroblasts, and smooth muscle cells of irradiated tissues.[391] All of these changes result in mucosal ulceration, mural fibrosis, inflammation, and vascular myointimal sclerosis.

In contrast with small bowel injury, which usually manifests with metabolic and nutritional derangements, colonic injury seldom manifests with metabolic abnormalities because of its role in reabsorption of water and as a fecal conduit. Compared with the rest of the colon and because of the proximity to other pelvic organs, the anterior wall of the rectum is the most likely area of the colon to develop radiation injury.

Pathological Features

Gross Findings

In acute radiation colitis, mucosal changes may include pallor, edema, erythema, prominent telangiectasia, and loss of the normal vascular pattern (Fig. 17.61). Occasionally, shallow ulcers may be present.

In chronic radiation colitis, strictures and fistulas are common. The serosal surface may show dense fibrous adhesions. The mucosa may show flattening of the surface with superficial ulcers. If a fistula is present, the subserosal adipose tissue surrounding the fistula tract shows adhesions and organizing fat necrosis.

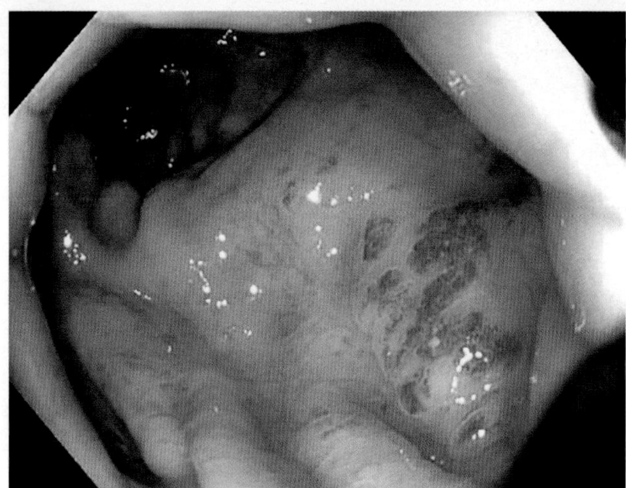

FIGURE 17.61 Endoscopic appearance of radiation proctitis showing mucosal erythema, edema, and telangiectasia.

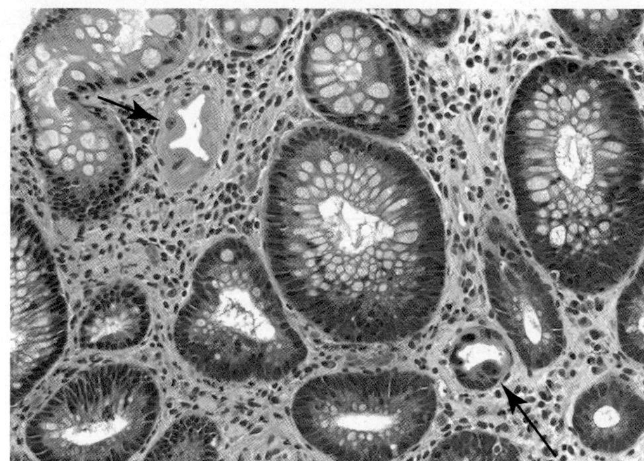

FIGURE 17.63 Radiation atypia mimicking dysplasia. The crypt and surface epithelial cells show cytological atypia. However, the cells *(arrows)* typically show a low nucleus-to-cytoplasm ratio, smudgy nuclear chromatin, and pale eosinophilic or bubbly voluminous cytoplasm.

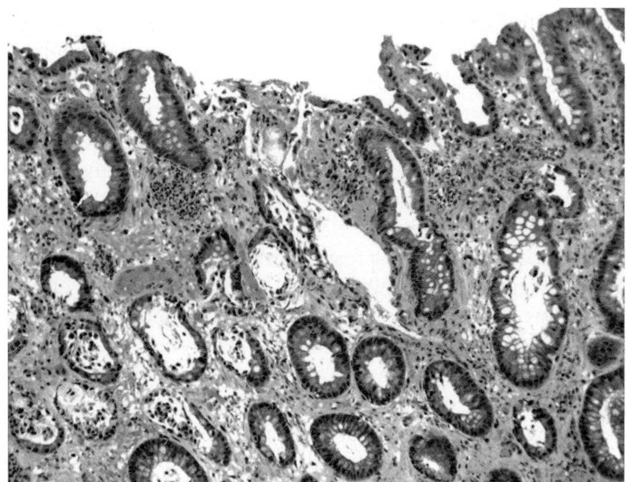

FIGURE 17.62 Acute radiation colitis. The colonic mucosa shows erosion, lamina propria hemorrhage, congestion, edema, and cryptitis. The surface and crypt epithelium also demonstrate mucin depletion.

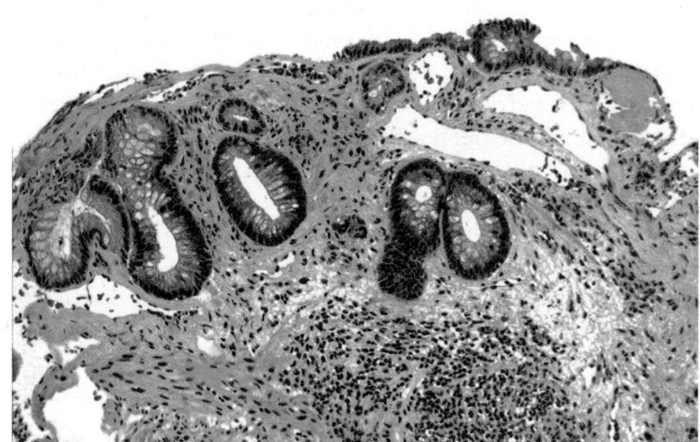

FIGURE 17.64 Chronic radiation colitis in a rectal biopsy specimen shows crypt architectural distortion, hyalinization of the lamina propria, and vascular ectasia.

Microscopic Findings

The histopathological changes of acute radiation colitis develop within several hours of exposure. Loss of integrity of the mucosa typically occurs within 1 to 2 days. The mucosa demonstrates foci of ulceration, edema, and vascular fibrinoid necrosis. Other findings include the presence of crypt abscesses, reduced mitotic activity, neutrophil- and eosinophil-rich lamina propria infiltrate, epithelial flattening and degenerative changes, and mucin loss (Fig. 17.62). Mild crypt architectural distortion and increased crypt apoptosis may also be present. The epithelial cells usually show a low N:C ratio, smudged nuclear chromatin, and a bubbly or wispy voluminous cytoplasm. It is not uncommon to find marked nuclear abnormalities that mimic epithelial dysplasia (Fig. 17.63).

As the acute injury resolves, the inflammatory infiltrate composed of neutrophils and eosinophils is replaced by scattered lymphocytes and plasma cells. The degree of activity (cryptitis and crypt abscesses) also decreases. Some of the biopsy fragments show a variable degree of crypt atrophy and crypt dropout. Regenerating crypts typically demonstrate increased mitotic activity.

Chronic radiation colitis is characterized by the presence of crypt architectural distortion; less commonly, other features of chronic injury, such as Paneth cell metaplasia, crypt atrophy, and reactive epithelial atypia, are present (Fig. 17.64). The typical vascular changes include hyalinized arterioles (Fig. 17.65), foci of healed arterial necrosis, vascular ectasia, and myointimal hyperplasia. Submucosal fibrosis, atypical "radiation fibroblasts" (Fig. 17.66), submucosal neuronal proliferation, and serosal thickening are some of the mural changes encountered in resection specimens. Strictures, fistulas, ulcers, and serosal adhesions may develop during the later stages of radiation-induced injury. However, these are secondary effects of blood vessel narrowing and ischemia. Chronic radiation damage can be subtle in biopsy specimens. The vascular changes such as capillary telangiectasia may be patchy and can be easily overlooked. More importantly, mucosal biopsy specimens

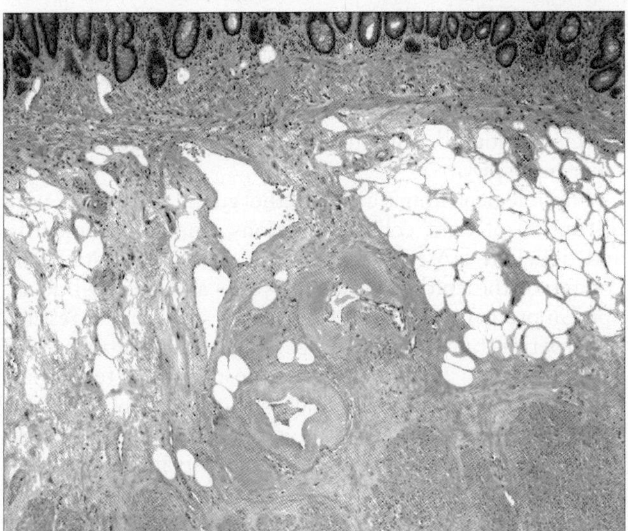

FIGURE 17.65 Chronic radiation colitis with vascular changes characterized by the presence of hyalinized arterioles. This finding should be distinguished from vascular amyloidosis.

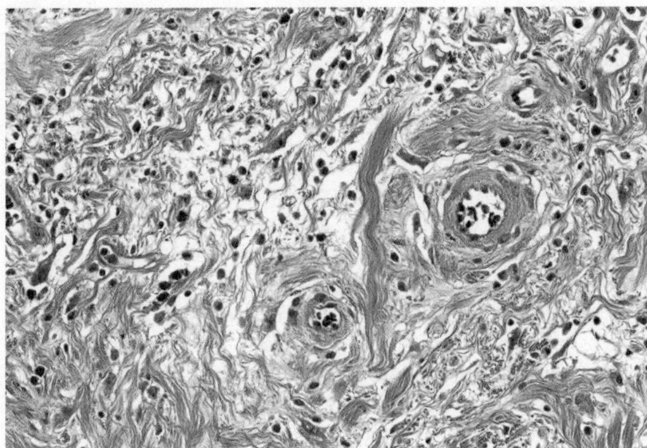

FIGURE 17.66 "Atypical" radiation fibroblasts. The nuclei of stromal cells (fibroblasts) are hyperchromatic and show tapered borders with a smudgy nuclear chromatin pattern. Some fibroblasts may also show prominent nucleoli.

seldom contain submucosal tissue that harbors the vascular changes or radiation fibroblasts characteristic of this entity.

Differential Diagnosis

The differential diagnosis of radiation colitis is broad and includes ischemic colitis, infectious colitis, drug toxicity, allergic or eosinophilic colitis, collagenous colitis, IBD, amyloidosis, and mucosal prolapse, among others.

Distinguishing chronic radiation-induced injury from primary colonic ischemia is often difficult on histological grounds alone. Knowledge of the anatomic location of involvement is helpful because radiation injury has a predilection to involve the rectum, in contrast with ischemia, which more commonly involves the watershed areas of the bowel. The finding of atypical stromal cells, combined with vascular changes characteristic of radiation injury, favors a diagnosis of radiation colitis over primary ischemic colitis.

The early phase and the healing phase of radiation colitis may resemble infectious colitis. However, infectious colitis typically results in expansion of the lamina propria by a neutrophil-rich inflammatory infiltrate. Cryptitis, crypt abscesses, and even crypt rupture–associated granulomas are often present. In contrast, the cytological changes of radiation colitis, such as nucleomegaly with smudged chromatin and bubbly cytoplasm, are not encountered in infectious colitis.

Radiation colitis may, on occasion, demonstrate increased eosinophils within the lamina propria, raising the question of allergic or eosinophilic colitis. Unlike allergic or eosinophilic colitis, the colonic mucosa in radiation colitis does not demonstrate sheets of eosinophils, eosinophilic cryptitis, or crypt abscesses. Peripheral blood eosinophilia and a history of allergies are some of the other factors that help support the diagnosis of eosinophilic colitis.

The histological findings of increased numbers of eosinophils, surface epithelial damage, and lamina propria fibrosis, especially prominent during the healing phase of radiation injury, may mimic collagenous colitis. However, radiation-induced hyalinization does not stain as intensely with trichrome. Furthermore, the hyalinization tends to be random in distribution and may even involve the entire thickness of the mucosa, not necessarily showing the classic subepithelial localization of collagenous colitis.[1] In addition, the lamina propria is typically expanded by an acute inflammatory cell infiltrate rather than a superficial-predominant lymphoplasmacytic infiltrate characteristic of collagenous colitis.

The chronic phase of radiation colitis often shows crypt architectural distortion that mimics IBD. Basal lymphoplasmacytosis, diffuse mixed inflammation of the lamina propria, and nonischemic-type ulcers help distinguish IBD from radiation colitis. The characteristic vascular changes accompanied by stromal atypia and mural fibrosis support a diagnosis of radiation colitis over IBD.

Vascular hyalinization of radiation colitis may also mimic amyloidosis, but this can be excluded by a Congo red stain. Finally, the presence of a fibrotic lamina propria combined with dilated mucosal capillaries may mimic mucosal prolapse. The lack of smooth muscle proliferation and the presence of atypical fibroblasts support a diagnosis of radiation colitis in such cases.

Natural History and Treatment

Most cases of radiation proctitis are self-limited and respond to medical management that includes sucralfate enemas, steroids, and pain control. Patients with severe bleeding are managed by thermal (endoscopic) or chemical (formalin) coagulation.[385] Surgical therapy is indicated in patients with strictures, perforations, or fistulas.

Neonatal Necrotizing Enterocolitis

Clinical Features

Neonatal necrotizing enterocolitis (NEC) is a rapidly progressive, nonocclusive, acute ischemic condition of the bowel that primarily affects premature infants. The condition typically manifests when infants are administered oral food for the first time. NEC affects 2% to 22% of all premature infants, usually during the first 3 months of life. However, its peak incidence is during the first week of life.[392]

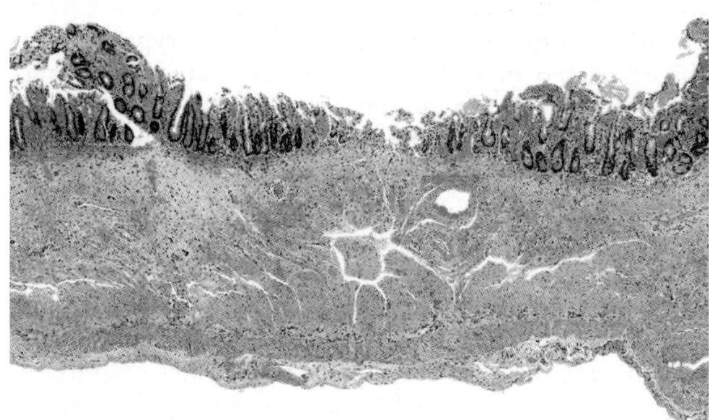

FIGURE 17.67 Necrotizing enterocolitis. The resection specimen shows extensive mucosal ulceration with segmental mucosal necrosis and prominent submucosal edema. There is also a serosal fibroinflammatory reaction.

It affects 1% to 5% of all neonatal intensive care admissions and 5% to 10% of all very-low-birth-weight (<1500 g) infants.[393] NEC is more likely to develop in infants of African descent, particularly males.[394,395]

The disease presentation varies from one that is slow and indolent to one that is progressively severe and results in death. Early signs and symptoms are nonspecific and include bradycardia, lethargy, vomiting, and abdominal distention. In some cases, infants show discoloration of the abdominal wall or a palpable abdominal mass. Metabolic acidosis, thrombocytopenia, and leukocytosis are common laboratory abnormalities. An absolute neutrophil count of less than 1.5×10^9 cells per liter is associated with a poor prognosis.[396] Progressive thrombocytopenia correlates with the presence of severe tissue injury and necrosis. An increase in platelet count after conservative therapy often signals clinical improvement.[397] In as many as 23% of patients, bacterial organisms such as *E. coli*, *Klebsiella*, *Enterococcus*, and coagulase-negative *Staphylococcus* are isolated from blood cultures.[398] Radiological findings are helpful in diagnosing and staging the disease. The hallmark features of NEC include dilated and thickened bowel, pneumatosis intestinalis, and, in severe cases, gas within portal vein branches.[399] A modified Bell staging system, which is based on a combination of systemic signs, laboratory results, and abdominal and radiographic findings, is routinely used to assess the severity of disease and select optimal therapy.[400-402]

Pathogenesis

Although the precise cause of NEC remains unclear, several risk factors related to its pathogenesis have been identified. These are hypoxic-ischemic injury, physiological immaturity of the gut, and alterations in the normal gut flora.

Ischemic injury is believed to be the major inciting factor for development of NEC. It may result from several conditions including but not limited to cardiac anomalies, sepsis, and polycythemia.[403] Reperfusion of the bowel may trigger additional mucosal damage. Ischemia and mucosal inflammation cause an increase in the local concentration of nitric oxide, which results in direct epithelial injury and apoptosis. In addition, overproduction of nitric oxide causes prolonged activation of the inflammatory cascade. Inflammatory cytokines, in turn, upregulate the production of endothelin-1, a potent mediator of vasoconstriction in the neonatal intestinal circulation.[404] This further potentiates intestinal ischemia and injury.

Physiological immaturity of the gut is associated with disruption of tight cellular junctions, impaired peristalsis, and deficient IgA mucosal defense. The composition and volume of the epithelial mucin layer is also not well developed in premature infants. These factors facilitate intestinal hyperpermeability and allow bacterial translocation across the mucosal barrier. Prolonged exposure to bacterial antigens also leads to abnormal microbial colonization.

Altered composition of the endogenous gut flora, with a predominance of pathogenic microorganisms such as *Staphylococcus*, *Enterobacter*, *Enterococcus*, and *Clostridia* species, is observed in premature infants and is believed to contribute to the development of NEC. Feeding practices to reduce its incidence include feeding of human breast milk, a delay in oral feeding, or a switch from formula to breast milk.[399,405]

Pathological Features

Gross Findings

Simultaneous involvement of the small and large bowel is present in as many as 44% of patients, whereas isolated colonic involvement is observed in approximately 26%.[398] The process involves the proximal colon more commonly than the distal colon. In the acute phase of disease, bowel involvement may be patchy, focal, or diffuse. Macroscopic features are similar to those found in severe ischemia.[406,407] The affected segment of colon is dilated, hemorrhagic, and necrotic. The serosal surface typically demonstrates fibrinous exudates and adhesions. One or more perforations are commonly identified during this stage. Pneumatosis intestinalis (numerous air-filled cysts within the bowel wall) is not uncommon. The mucosal surface shows hemorrhage, ulceration, friability, and edema. In the later stages of disease, the bowel wall becomes thickened because of fibrosis. Strictures or stenosis may also be evident at this stage. The left colon is more commonly affected than the right colon in this regard.[408]

Microscopic Findings

In the acute phase of disease, NEC is characterized by coagulative necrosis that may be focal or diffuse in distribution. In most cases, there is diffuse and extensive necrosis with prominent submucosal edema and marked vascular congestion. In less severe cases, necrosis may be limited to the mucosa (Figs. 17.67 and 17.68). The lamina propria is expanded by a mixed inflammatory cell infiltrate composed of eosinophils, neutrophils, lymphocytes, and plasma cells. Crypt abscesses and pseudomembranes are uncommon. The serosal aspect typically shows a prominent fibroinflammatory reaction and adhesions. In areas of perforation, there is organizing fat necrosis, and a foreign-body giant cell reaction to luminal contents may be present. In some cases, submucosal or transmural gas-filled cysts surrounded by a giant cell response may be seen. Vascular thrombi are only rarely identified.

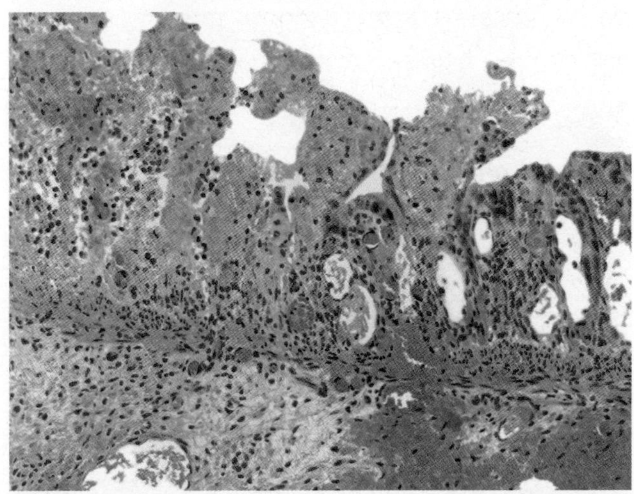

FIGURE 17.68 Necrotizing enterocolitis. Higher magnification shows mucosal necrosis, vascular congestion, hemorrhage, edema, and regenerative changes. Few, if any, neutrophils are present.

In the reparative phase of NEC, regenerating epithelium is accompanied by granulation tissue formation and submucosal fibrosis.

Differential Diagnosis

The main differential diagnosis of NEC includes severe infectious colitis and Hirschsprung disease–associated enterocolitis.

Unlike NEC, infectious colitis is characterized by a neutrophil-predominant inflammatory cell infiltrate with frequent crypt abscesses and lack of transmural ischemic-type necrosis. The profile of pathogenic organisms isolated in NEC includes endogenous bacterial flora such as *E. coli*, *Enterococcus*, and coagulase-negative *Staphylococcus*. In contrast, *Shigella*, *Salmonella*, and *C. jejuni* are the common culprits of infectious colitis.

Hirschsprung disease–associated enterocolitis is a serious and potentially life-threatening complication of Hirschsprung disease (see Chapter 9). It is a clinical syndrome characterized by the presence of diarrhea, abdominal distention, fever, colicky abdominal pain, lethargy, and blood in the stool. This type of enterocolitis affects both the dilated (ganglionic) and the nondilated (aganglionic) portion of bowel.[409] Histological sections usually show prominent neutrophilic cryptitis and crypt abscesses. Crypt architecture is usually preserved. In severe cases, the changes mimic NEC. There may be extensive mucosal ulceration, submucosal edema, and transmural necrosis of the bowel. Lack of ganglion cells in Hirschsprung disease–associated enterocolitis is the key to establishing a correct diagnosis. However, in cases in which segments of colon with ganglion cells are involved, a clinical history of failure to pass meconium, abdominal distention, vomiting (bilious or feculent), and other signs of intestinal obstruction support a diagnosis of Hirschsprung disease–associated enterocolitis.

Natural History and Treatment

Most patients affected by NEC are treated medically. Conservative management includes bowel rest, abdominal decompression with a gastric tube, and administration of broad-spectrum antibiotics. Additional supportive measures include monitoring of fluid and electrolyte balance. Surgery is indicated in cases of bowel perforation or instances of medical therapy failure. Despite significant advances in neonatal care, the incidence of NEC continues to increase, and the mortality rate has remained unchanged. It ranges from 20% to 30% and is even higher in lower-birth-weight infants.[399,405] Segments of the bowel that are injured but not surgically removed may develop strictures (10% to 40%) and become atretic.[407] Approximately 5% of NEC cases recur, either at the original site or elsewhere within the bowel.[410] Recurrence is more common in patients who have an underlying clinical condition, such as congenital heart disease. Another long-term complication of NEC is the development of short bowel syndrome. However, this complication develops only when there has been extensive small-bowel and colon resection.

Eosinophilic Colitides

Unlike in the esophagus, eosinophils are a normal component of the lamina propria of the colon. In fact, eosinophils are an associated component of many disease states such as infections, allergy, IBD, radiation, collagenous colitis, hypereosinophilic syndrome, connective tissue disorders, vasculitis, myeloproliferative neoplasms, and drug hypersensitivity (Box 17.8). However, in some diseases, eosinophils may form the predominant or even the exclusive type of inflammatory cell in the mucosa. When this occurs, the pattern of colitis is usually referred to as *eosinophilic colitis*. The most common causes of eosinophilic colitis include primary eosinophilic (allergic) colitis of infants and young children, parasitic infection, and a variety of drug reactions. In many instances, an underlying cause for mucosal eosinophilia cannot be identified by the pathologist, in which case the term *primary eosinophilic colitis* or *idiopathic eosinophilic colitis* is often used. This is, in fact, a rare phenomenon in the colon specifically (see later). Most of the primary eosinophilic conditions of the GI tract occur in the esophagus, stomach, and small intestine (e.g., eosinophilic esophagitis, eosinophilic gastritis or gastroduodenitis, or eosinophilic enteritis).

Diagnostic Criteria and Approach to Colonic Biopsies with Eosinophilia

As discussed earlier in this chapter, the density of eosinophils is known to be higher in the right colon, particularly the cecum and ascending colon, compared with the left colon. There is also data to suggest that eosinophil density is greater during peak allergy seasons and among individuals living in the southern United States compared with those in the northeastern regions.[4,411] Other studies have also documented a gradient of the eosinophil density from the proximal to the descending colon, such that the proximal colon has three times the number of eosinophils compared with the descending colon.[411-413]

For practical purposes, a general approach to colonic mucosal eosinophilia includes: (1) determining whether the distribution is focal (involving one or two fragments) versus diffuse (involving all biopsy fragments), (2) applying the diagnostic criteria proposed by Turner et al. [414] based on the anatomic location of the biopsy to confirm a diagnosis of eosinophilia (see later), and (3) reviewing medical records

BOX 17.8 Primary and Secondary Causes of Colonic Eosinophilia

Primary
- Eosinophilic colitis

Secondary
- Infections-parasitic (*Strongyloides* and *Schistosoma*) and fungal (*Basidiobolus ranarum*)
- Medications (nonsteroidal antiinflammatory drugs, antiplatelet agents, mycophenolate mofetil, tacrolimus)
- Vasculitis (eosinophilic granulomatosis with polyangiitis—Churg-Strauss syndrome)
- Inflammatory bowel disease
- Radiation colitis
- Neoplasia
- Connective tissue disorders
- Collagenous colitis

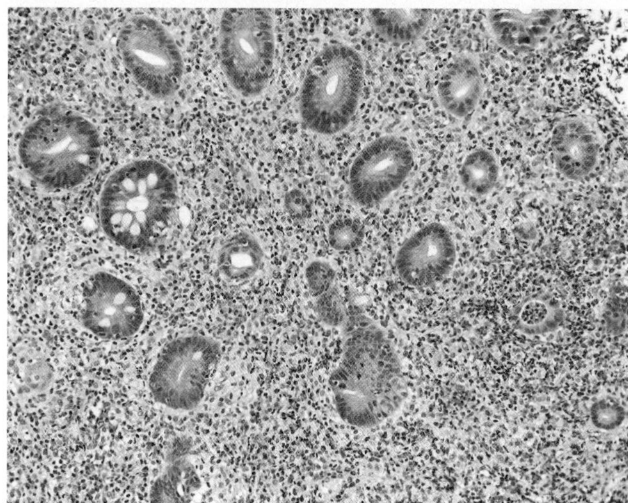

FIGURE 17.69 Eosinophilic colitis.

to determine whether eosinophilia can be explained by any of the aforementioned secondary conditions. Biopsies in which eosinophilia is restricted to one or two fragments are likely to be a result of a parasitic or fungal infection rather than primary eosinophilic colitis. In cases in which a secondary cause can be found, a descriptive diagnosis should be rendered along with a comment indicating the likely etiology. As proposed by Turner, for cases in which no specific cause can be found, a diagnosis of *primary eosinophilic colitis* should be rendered in patients who are clinically symptomatic and/or have mucosal abnormalities detected during endoscopy. In those without any clinical symptoms or endoscopic abnormalities, a biopsy diagnosis of primary colonic eosinophilia is reasonable.[414] Some of the common conditions causing colonic mucosal eosinophilia are described later.

Primary Eosinophilic Colitis

Primary eosinophilic colitis is a clinicopathological entity characterized by the finding of prominent colonic mucosal eosinophilia in tissue samples, but in patients without either a clinically or pathologically apparent cause. It is considered part of the general group of eosinophilic GI disorders, which includes eosinophilic esophagitis, eosinophilic gastritis/duodenitis, and eosinophilic gastroenteritis; albeit it is the least common among this group of disorders.

Clinical Features

As mentioned earlier, the epidemiology of eosinophilic colitis is difficult to study because of the lack of well-defined diagnostic criteria. In most cases, the colon is affected in conjunction with other segments of the GI tract, especially the small bowel and stomach. In a recent series of 43 patients diagnosed with eosinophilic gastroenteritis, the mucosal form of colitis without involvement of the rest of the GI tract was documented in 8% of patients.

Pathogenesis

Eosinophils respond to several stimuli including nonspecific tissue injury, allergens, and infections. Recruitment and activation of eosinophils to sites of inflammation are regulated by cytokines, including IL-5, IL-13, IL-4, and TNF produced by activated Th2 and mast cells. Activated eosinophils produce leukotriene C4, which is then metabolized to LTD4 and LTE4, potent smooth muscle constrictors, and a wide range of cytokines that potentiate the inflammatory response.[415,416] In adults, eosinophilic colitis is more likely a non–IgE-associated disorder that functions through a CD4-positive Th2 lymphocyte–mediated mechanism.

Pathological Features

Most cases show normal-appearing mucosa on endoscopy. Other findings may include patchy mucosal edema, punctate erythema, granularity, and aphthous ulcers, but these are quite uncommon and nonspecific.

Several studies have attempted to establish a diagnostic threshold for *eosinophilic colitis*. As expected, there is a great amount of variability among these studies, in part because of the lack of uniformity in histological criterion used for "increased" intramucosal eosinophils, varying study populations (adults vs. children), and lack of appropriate controls, specifically with regard to anatomic location. For example, it has been stated that the term *eosinophilic colitis* may be used if there are more than 20 eosinophils per high-power field (HPF).[417,418] In a recent retrospective study by Turner and colleagues, the authors established the following thresholds for a diagnosis of *eosinophilic colitis* based on the site in the colon: >50 eosinophils per HPF in the right colon, >35 eosinophils per HPF in the transverse colon, and >25 eosinophils per HPF in the left colon. In this study, the authors selected 194 cases from an adult North American population of approximately 1.2 million patients who had undergone a colonoscopy and mucosal biopsies during a period of 7 years and compared the number of eosinophils per mm^2 with 159 controls.[414] Interestingly, the authors found that about one-third of patients with mucosal eosinophilia but without an underlying disorder were completely asymptomatic.

As discussed earlier, biopsy specimens in eosinophilic colitis typically show sheets or aggregates of eosinophils within the lamina propria and submucosa, often accompanied by degranulation and epithelial injury in the form of cryptitis and crypt abscesses (Fig. 17.69).

Differential Diagnosis

Because primary eosinophilic colitis is, essentially, a diagnosis of exclusion, the differential diagnosis includes all other causes of colonic eosinophilia (see Box 17.8), especially parasitic or fungal infections, vasculitis, connective tissue disorders, IBD, medications (such as NSAIDs, antiplatelet agents, mycophenolate mofetil, tacrolimus), and neoplastic conditions such as systemic mastocytosis and neoplasms such as LCH. Tissue-invasive parasites such as *Strongyloides* and *Schistosoma* are the most common parasites that cause colonic eosinophilia. The eosinophilic reaction is usually present around the eggs or larval forms and may consist of degranulated eosinophils with Charcot-Leyden crystals.[419] Long-standing parasitic infections may result in crypt architectural distortion resulting in a chronic colitis pattern of injury. Among the fungal pathogens, *Basidiobolus ranarum* is a specific pathogen that involves the GI tract and is associated with peripheral eosinophilia and inflammatory masses rich in eosinophils that mimic malignancy. Multiple deeper tissue sections are often required to exclude parasitic and fungal infections as the primary cause of eosinophilia.

Both UC and CD may show prominent eosinophils within the lamina propria. In fact, the presence of severe eosinophilic infiltrate has been associated with treatment failure in patients with active UC.[139] A prior history of IBD is essential to differentiate IBD from eosinophilic colitis.

Vasculitis, particularly eosinophilic granulomatosis with polyangiitis (Churg-Strauss syndrome), is an immune-mediated vasculitis that affects medium- and small-caliber vessels in patients with a history of asthma and/or allergic rhinitis.[420] In addition to small bowel, proximal colon is another commonly affected region within the GI tract.[416] The diagnosis is best established in resection specimens where the blood vessels show fibrinoid necrosis in association with dense eosinophilic infiltrate.

Lastly, neoplastic conditions such as systemic mastocytosis and LCH (see the Mastocytic Disorders section) can show a prominent eosinophilic infiltrate that may mask neoplastic cells. However, epithelial injury as well as sheets or clusters of eosinophils with degranulation are not typically found in these entities. When in doubt, immunohistochemical stains such as CD117 and CD25 for mast cell disorders and CD1a or Langerin stain for LCH can be performed to exclude these possibilities.

Natural History and Treatment

Most patients have just one episode of eosinophilic colitis, without relapse, whereas others are affected by a more relapsing-remitting or chronic form of disease.[421] Corticosteroids are the first line of therapy for eosinophilic colitis. Mesalazine and other immunomodulatory agents such as azathioprine, infliximab, and adalimumab may be administered in severe steroid-refractory cases. Surgical resection is limited to patients who have complications related to bowel obstruction, volvulus, or perforation.

Allergic Proctocolitis

Clinical Features

Allergic proctocolitis (dietary protein–induced proctocolitis) is the most common cause of proctocolitis in infants who are breast-fed or formula fed. Typically, patients will develop blood-streaked stools. It is believed to be caused by an immunological reaction to dietary proteins, such as cow's milk protein (see later). Although allergic proctocolitis is the most common cause of colitis in infancy, the prevalence of this condition is unknown. However, in a prospective series of 22 patients with rectal bleeding, the incidence of allergic proctocolitis was 64%.[422] In a series of children 2 to 14 years of age, the incidence of allergic proctocolitis was 18%.[423] The classic clinical presentation is that of a healthy infant whose parents notice a gradual onset of bloody stools that progressively increase in frequency. Anemia or hypoalbuminemia develops in some infants.[424] Growth delay or poor weight gain is uncommon. Similar to infants, children with allergic proctocolitis may also have rectal bleeding as their major symptom. Other symptoms in this age group include abdominal pain, vomiting, diarrhea, and constipation. By definition, stool cultures should be negative for pathogenic bacteria. Infants with allergic proctocolitis may demonstrate mild peripheral eosinophilia and elevated serum IgE levels and may have a positive family history of atopy.[425-428]

Pathogenesis

Allergic proctocolitis occurs in infants who are fed milk or soy-based formula, but most patients are breast-fed and become sensitized to proteins that are maternally ingested and excreted via breast milk. Cow's milk protein and soy protein are the main culprits in this regard.

Dietary protein–induced proctocolitis is believed to be a non-IgE–associated mechanism. T-cell–mediated immune reaction has been suggested to play a major role in its pathogenesis.[429] In breast-fed infants, the offending maternal dietary protein conjugates with breast milk IgA and is specifically cleaved by microbial IgA proteases present in the rectosigmoid colon.[430] Eosinophils are a major component of the inflammatory cell infiltrate; they have receptors that bind to IgA, leading to degranulation and release of inflammatory cytokines.[430,431]

Pathological Features

Mild and nonspecific endoscopic findings such as focal erythema and friability have been reported in this condition.[426] Microscopically, allergic proctocolitis is characterized by an increase in the number of eosinophils within all compartments of the mucosa (surface and crypt epithelium, lamina propria, and muscularis mucosae) (Fig. 17.70).[426,428,432] The presence of 6 to 20 eosinophils per HPF or more than 60 eosinophils per 10 HPF in the lamina propria has been documented in 90% and 58% of patients with allergic proctocolitis, respectively.[426,432] Eosinophils are usually localized to the lower third of the mucosa, in close proximity to or within the muscularis mucosae. They may also be seen in close association with lymphoid aggregates. Crypt architecture is usually normal. There may be focal areas of surface epithelial degeneration and mucin depletion. Erosions, neutrophilic crypt abscesses, and granulomas are rarely present.[433] Mucosal eosinophilia is usually a focal finding, so the distribution of eosinophils varies within separate biopsy fragments. Therefore biopsies from multiple sites in the colon may be required to establish a diagnosis.[426]

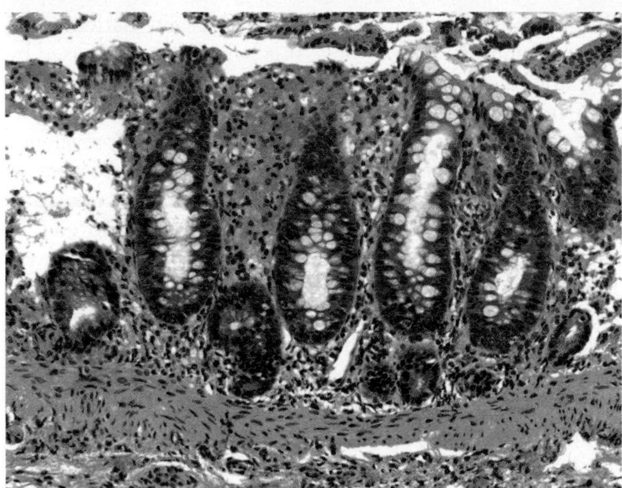

FIGURE 17.70 Allergic colitis in a 7–week-old infant with bloody stools. Notice the increased number of eosinophils, especially in the deep aspect of the lamina propria, some of which are infiltrating the crypt epithelium.

Differential Diagnosis

The differential diagnosis of allergic proctocolitis includes infectious colitis, Hirschsprung disease–associated enterocolitis, and IBD.[432] Infectious colitis usually shows a prominent neutrophilic inflammatory infiltrate within the lamina propria, crypt, and surface epithelium. Eosinophils are typically only a minor component of the inflammatory infiltrate. Positive stool cultures and lack of correlation of symptoms with a specific dietary agent also helps distinguish these two entities.

Hirschsprung disease–associated enterocolitis is a serious complication that may occur before or after resection of the aganglionic colonic segment. Patients have abdominal distention, diarrhea, fever, and bloody stools. Lack of ganglion cells, a prominent neutrophilic inflammatory infiltrate, and, in severe cases, extensive mucosal ulceration and transmural necrosis help distinguish this entity from allergic proctocolitis.[434]

Some cases of CD may show a prominent eosinophilic infiltrate within the lamina propria. However, allergic proctocolitis typically lacks histological features of chronic mucosal injury, such as crypt architectural distortion, basal lymphoplasmacytosis, and Paneth cell metaplasia. Furthermore, neutrophilic crypt abscesses and granulomas are uncommon. The lack of significant endoscopic mucosal abnormalities, the focal nature of the disease, and the lack of disease elsewhere in the GI tract favor a diagnosis of allergic proctocolitis over IBD.

Natural History and Treatment

Treatment of allergic proctocolitis involves dietary manipulation to eliminate the offending agent. In most cases, the bleeding resolves within 72 to 96 hours.[424] However, the endoscopic and histological abnormalities may persist for several weeks.

Microscopic Colitis

Historical Perspective

The term *microscopic colitis* was first coined by Read and colleagues in 1980 for patients with chronic watery diarrhea who had normal sigmoidoscopy and barium enema findings but evidence of mucosal inflammation in their colonic biopsy specimens.[435] After the original histological description of this disease, Kingham and associates noticed increased chronic inflammation within the lamina propria, minimal distortion of the crypts, and reduced numbers of goblet cells in patients with this disorder.[436] A few years before these two studies, the term *collagenous colitis* was introduced for patients with chronic watery diarrhea who demonstrated thickening of the subepithelial collagen table.[437,438]

Use of the term *microscopic colitis* as a pathological diagnosis was challenged by Lazenby and colleagues.[1] They noted that some inflammatory conditions, especially CD, may on occasion be accompanied by normal endoscopic findings combined with histological evidence of colitis. Furthermore, increased chronic inflammation in the lamina propria was believed to be a somewhat confusing observation, given that in the colon, inflammatory cells are a normal constituent of the lamina propria. The true nature of mucosal inflammation in microscopic colitis was further refined by emphasizing the presence of increased surface and crypt lymphocytes, a hallmark feature of both collagenous and lymphocytic colitis. Currently, *microscopic colitis* is considered a clinical term that typically refers to either collagenous or lymphocytic colitis but can include other causes of colitis that result in an absence of endoscopic abnormalities associated with microscopic inflammation.

Collagenous Colitis

Clinical Features

In Sweden and Spain, the annual incidence of collagenous colitis is 0.6 to 5.2 per 100,000 individuals. The incidence in an age- and gender-adjusted population-based study from North America was 3.1 per 100,000 person-years.[439-441] Patients usually are diagnosed in late adulthood (mean age, 63.8 years; range, 29 to 93 years), but young adults and even children may be affected.[442] Women are more commonly affected than men; the female-to-male (F:M) ratio ranges from 3:1 to 9:1.[443] Affected patients have a significant association with concurrent immunological conditions such as autoimmune thyroiditis (21%) and rheumatoid arthritis (7%) as well as other inflammatory disorders such as Raynaud syndrome (3%) and celiac disease (2.9%).[443]

The typical clinical presentation of patients with collagenous colitis is chronic, watery, nonbloody diarrhea that has persisted for an average period of 24 months before diagnosis.[443] Patients may also reveal abdominal pain, fecal incontinence, urgency, and weight loss. Fecal leukocytosis is present in as many as 55% of patients. Autoimmune markers may be positive, including antinuclear antibodies (as many as 50% of patients), pANCA (as many as 14%), rheumatoid factor, and complement C3 and C4.

Pathogenesis

The cause of collagenous colitis remains unknown. In fact, many of the risk factors and putative etiological agents discussed in this section are applicable to both collagenous colitis and lymphocytic colitis.

The most accepted hypothesis is that collagenous colitis develops as a result of an immunological response to intraluminal dietary or bacterial elements. Resolution of symptoms after fecal stream diversion and recurrence of inflammation with restoration of intestinal continuity, especially in cases of collagenous colitis, support this hypothesis.[444] The association of collagenous colitis (and lymphocytic colitis) with celiac disease, a variety of medications, and other autoimmune conditions also suggests a role of luminal antigens in the pathogenesis of this condition.

A number of medications such as NSAIDs, PPIs, HMG-CoA reductase inhibitors (statins), selective serotonin reuptake inhibitors, carbamazepine, ticlopidine, acarbose, flutamide, gold salts, and immune checkpoint inhibitors have been implicated as possible causes of collagenous or lymphocytic colitis.[445,446] Although NSAID consumption has been reported in approximately 30% to 70% of patients, the causal association between this group of medications and collagenous or lymphocytic colitis has not been fully established. One of the proposed mechanisms is that NSAIDs cause mucosal injury, which allows luminal antigens or bacterial organisms to enter the lamina propria and incite an inflammatory response.

Because of their association with a variety of autoimmune conditions, researchers have focused their attention toward investigating HLA haplotypes and serum markers in both collagenous and lymphocytic colitis. Patients with lymphocytic colitis frequently express HLA-A1 antigens (66.6%).[447] Abnormal expression of HLA-DR and HLA-DQ loci has also been documented in both lymphocytic and collagenous colitis.[448,449]

Malabsorption of bile acids has also been suggested as an etiological factor in collagenous colitis and, less commonly, lymphocytic colitis. Isolation of organisms such as C. *jejuni*, Y. *enterocolitica*, and C. *difficile* in some patients with lymphocytic or collagenous colitis suggests a possible infectious etiology.

A genetic predisposition within families (especially among sisters) has been observed in both lymphocytic and collagenous colitis.[450,451]

The pathogenesis of expansion of the subepithelial collagen layer in collagenous colitis is unclear. In normal colon, the collagen band is composed of type IV collagen, whereas in collagenous colitis, it is composed of type VI collagen, tenascin, and a minor amount of types I and III collagen. Tenascin is an extracellular matrix protein that is synthesized by intestinal subepithelial myofibroblasts. Therefore disturbances in the function of subepithelial myofibroblasts may lead to an increased synthesis or decreased degradation of extracellular matrix proteins, either of which could lead to increased collagen deposition.[452]

Diarrhea in collagenous and lymphocytic colitis is of the secretory (nonbloody) type and most likely results from the effects of direct epithelial injury. The severity of inflammation has been correlated with decreased colonic fluid absorption.[448] Increased mast cell activity and bile acid malabsorption are some of the other proposed mechanisms for diarrhea in these disorders.

Pathological Features

Gross Findings

Most patients with collagenous colitis have a normal-appearing colon. Patchy erythema, edema, friability, an abnormal vascular pattern, and even frank ulcerations may occur in a minority of patients. Some cases, in fact, may show pseudomembranes and linear mucosal breaks *(cat-scratch colon)*.[453-455] The latter is thought to be caused by barotrauma as a result of insufflation of air into the colon at the time of endoscopy, combined with the endoscope trauma. The mucosa in collagenous colitis is particularly prone to endoscope trauma and even perforation.

Microscopic Findings

In classic cases, collagenous colitis is characterized by preservation of crypt architecture combined with an increase in inflammatory cells within the lamina propria, especially in the superficial half, and degeneration of the surface epithelium. Inflammatory cells include lymphocytes, plasma cells, and eosinophils (Fig. 17.71A). The pathognomonic finding is the presence of a thickened or irregular subepithelial collagen layer, which is usually thicker than 10 μm (range, 20 to 60 μm). One rapid method of evaluating the thickness of the collagen layer is to count the number of lymphocyte nuclei (which are 5 μm in diameter) that can be accommodated within the collagen layer. Collagen thickening may be continuous or patchy in distribution and is often more pronounced in the right colon compared with the left. Often the collagen layer shows an irregular and ragged appearance at the deep edge, with entrapment of inflammatory cells, stromal cells, and even small-sized capillaries[456] (see Fig. 17.71B). In some cases, the collagen layer is not thickened at all, but instead shows an irregular, jagged, or fibrillary appearance, either with or without entrapped of inflammatory cells (see Fig. 17.71C). Eosinophils are often closely associated with the collagen layer. A trichrome stain may be performed to highlight the collagen layer and irregularity of its basal border (see Fig. 17.71D).

In most cases, the surface epithelium demonstrates infiltration by lymphocytes, which may be focal or diffuse. Epithelial injury, in the form of mucin depletion and nuclear degeneration, is often present as well. Another very characteristic finding is the presence of epithelium that has been stripped away from the underlying collagenous layer (see Fig. 17.71B).

Several studies have documented the distribution and histological abnormalities in collagenous colitis (and lymphocytic colitis). The cecum and transverse colon usually show the most severe changes and the thickest collagen layer[457]; therefore biopsies from these anatomic regions have a higher diagnostic yield (80%) than biopsies from the rectum (30%). However, in 90% of cases, a diagnosis of collagenous colitis can be established by flexible sigmoidoscopy if biopsy specimens are obtained from above the rectosigmoid junction.[458] In a more recent study consisting of 101 patients with collagenous and lymphocytic colitis, it was found that obtaining two samples (one from the ascending colon and one from the descending colon) was sufficient to diagnose microscopic colitis in all patients.[459]

As many as 30% of cases show histological changes similar to those seen in IBD, but these are typically focal and mild. For instance, cryptitis, crypt abscesses, Paneth cell metaplasia, crypt architectural distortion, or surface ulceration may be present in 2.5% to 44% of cases.[460] In one study, Paneth cell metaplasia and crypt distortion were associated with refractory disease.[461] Rarely, collagenous colitis

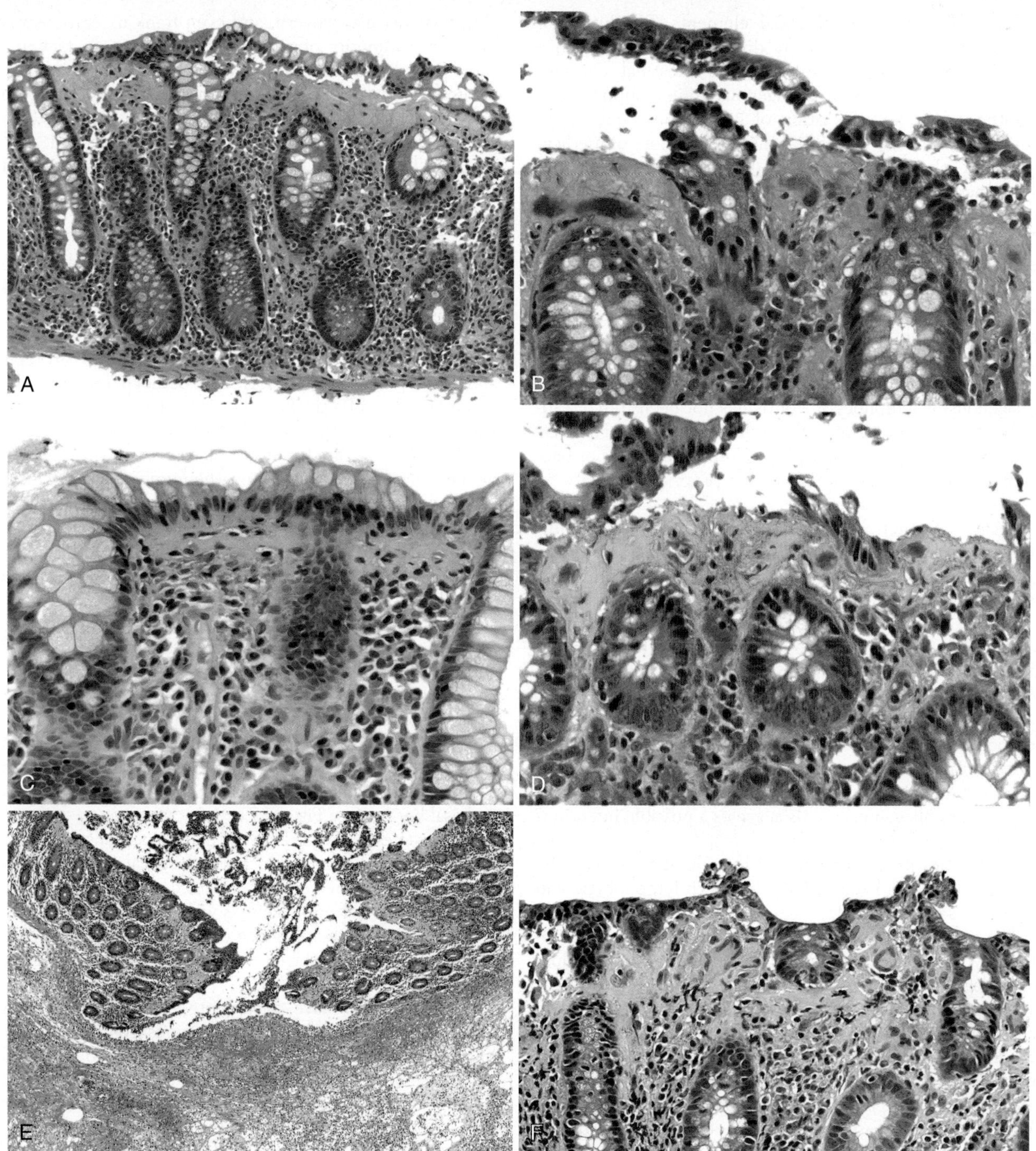

FIGURE 17.71 Collagenous colitis. A, The mucosa shows intact crypt architecture and a thickened subepithelial collagen layer. There is expansion of the lamina propria by lymphocytes, plasma cells, and eosinophils. **B,** Higher magnification shows thickening and irregularity of the collagen layer, which may entrap small capillaries, stromal cells, and inflammatory cells. The surface epithelium shows intraepithelial lymphocytes and degenerative changes. In addition, stripping of the surface epithelium from the underlying collagen layer is present. **C,** Collagenous colitis with minimal thickening of the subepithelial collagen layer. The collagen layer appears irregular, jagged, or fibrillary and shows entrapment of inflammatory cells. **D,** Trichrome-stained section of collagenous colitis highlights the subepithelial collagen layer that entraps stromal and inflammatory cells. Notice the irregular, jagged appearance of the lower border of the collagen layer. **E,** Collagenous colitis with ulceration and perforation. The adjacent mucosa shows changes characteristic of collagenous colitis. **F,** Collagenous colitis with subepithelial giant cells. The figure shows a thickened subepithelial collagen layer with entrapped multinucleate giant cells and epithelioid histiocytes.

may be associated with ulceration and pseudomembranes (see Fig. 17.71E), which may be related to superimposed C. *difficile* infection or ischemia.[453] Similarly, rare cases show subepithelial giant cells and even granulomas as a reaction to the subepithelial collagen (see Fig. 17.71F).[462]

Differential Diagnosis

The differential diagnosis of collagenous colitis includes lymphocytic colitis, IBD, solitary rectal ulcer syndrome (SRUS) or mucosal prolapse, ischemia, radiation colitis, and amyloidosis (Table 17.11).

TABLE 17.11 Differential Diagnosis of Microscopic Colitis

Feature	Collagenous Colitis	Lymphocytic colitis	SRUS/Mucosal Prolapse	Ischemic Colitis	Radiation Colitis	Amyloidosis
Crypt architecture	Usually intact	Usually intact	Distorted with dilated and branching crypts	Usually intact, may be distorted in chronic ischemia	Usually intact, may be distorted in chronic radiation colitis	Usually intact
Expansion of lamina propria by lymphocytes and plasma cells	Common, usually restricted to upper half of lamina propria	Common, usually restricted to upper half of lamina propria	Absent	Absent	Absent	Absent
Prominent eosinophils within lamina propria	Absent	Present, common	Absent	Absent	Present, common	Absent
Thickening of the subepithelial collagen layer	Present	Absent	Rare	Absent	Absent	Absent
Entrapment of inflammatory cells within thickened collagen layer	Common	Absent	Absent	Absent	Absent	Absent
Full-thickness hyalinization of lamina propria	Absent	Absent	Rare	Present, common	Rare	Absent
Withered or atrophic crypts	Absent	Absent	Uncommon	Present, very common	Present, common	Absent
Epithelial "atypia"	Absent	Absent	Present, common, (reactive atypia may mimic dysplasia)	Rare (reactive atypia may mimic dysplasia)	Present common, (reactive atypia may mimic dysplasia)	Absent
Fibromuscular replacement of lamina propria	Absent	Absent	Present	Rare	Absent	Absent
Amyloid deposits within lamina propria and blood vessels	Absent	Absent	Absent	Absent	Absent	Present

SRUS, Solitary rectal ulcer syndrome.

Lymphocytic colitis appears similar to collagenous colitis but lacks the characteristic thickened subepithelial collagen layer. Additionally, the degree of intraepithelial (and lamina propria) lymphocytosis is usually more prominent in lymphocytic colitis than in collagenous colitis, although eosinophils are usually more prominent in collagenous colitis.

Compared with collagenous colitis, UC and CD usually show a greater degree of and a more diffuse crypt architectural distortion and neutrophilic infiltration in the active phase of disease. Basal lymphoplasmacytosis and basal lymphoid aggregates are more common and diffuse and are not associated with significant lymphocytosis. In contrast with IBD, the inflammatory infiltrate in collagenous colitis is usually localized to the upper half of the lamina propria. Classic forms of IBD are not associated with subepithelial collagen layer thickening. In IBD, fibrosis, if present, usually involves deeper aspects of the lamina propria (Table 17.12).

SRUS or mucosal prolapse may mimic collagenous colitis because of the presence of a fibromuscular lamina propria in the former. This finding is typically identified adjacent to the crypts, rather than beneath the surface epithelium, and does not entrap inflammatory cells, stromal capillaries, or fibroblasts. The surface epithelium in mucosal prolapse is often ulcerated, and the crypts do not show intraepithelial lymphocytosis.

Ischemic colitis is associated with hyalinization of the lamina propria that may be mistaken for collagen. However, this reaction is more fibrinous, or hyaline, in quality and typically involves the entire mucosa. Other findings, such as lymphocyte-mediated epithelial injury, are not features of ischemic colitis.

Radiation colitis is associated with hyalinization of the lamina propria, which is often accompanied by the presence of telangiectatic blood vessels and atypical endothelial cells and fibroblasts. Hyaline material does not stain as intensely as collagen with the trichrome stain, and it lacks the other typical findings of collagenous colitis, such as entrapment of inflammatory or stromal cells.

In amyloidosis, the distribution of amorphous, acellular, eosinophilic amyloid deposits occurs along the basement membranes of crypts and blood vessels within the lamina propria and superficial submucosa, as opposed to the

TABLE 17.12 Microscopic Colitis vs. Inflammatory Bowel Disease

Feature	Lymphocytic Colitis	Collagenous Colitis	Inflammatory Bowel Disease
Cryptitis or crypt abscesses	Focal, when present	Focal, when present	Prominent
Crypt distortion	Focal, when present	Focal, when present	Prominent
Basal plasmacytosis	Usually absent	Usually absent	Typically present (except in patients with remission and inactive disease)
Basal lymphoid aggregates	Usually absent	Usually absent	Present
Paneth cell metaplasia	May be seen	May be seen	Usually present
Prominent lymphocytic or plasmacytic inflammation within lamina propria	Usually present, restricted to upper half of the lamina propria	Usually present, restricted to upper half of the lamina propria	Usually present, but restricted to lower half of the lamina propria
Neutrophils in lamina propria	May or may not be seen	May or may not be seen	Often present, especially in active disease
Prominent eosinophils	No	Yes	May or may not be present
Thickened or irregular subepithelial collagen layer	No	Yes	Rare (but with no entrapment of inflammatory cells)
Ulcer or erosion	Rare	Rare	Common

typical superficial distribution of the thickened collagen layer in collagenous colitis. A Congo red stain is useful in this regard.

Natural History and Treatment

The natural history of collagenous colitis is variable. Patients usually reveal episodes of remission and exacerbation. In approximately 25% of patients, collagenous colitis undergoes spontaneous clinical remission, accompanied or followed by histological improvement. Studies have shown complete normalization of the inflammatory infiltrate with budesonide treatment in as many as 69.2% patients and a partial reduction in approximately 30.8% of cases.[463] Another study documented a decrease in the thickness of the subepithelial collagen layer, from 19 µm in the initial biopsies to 14 µm in follow-up biopsies during an average period of 24 months.[464] Patients with shorter duration of disease (<6 months) have an increased chance of spontaneous remission.[465] As mentioned earlier, patients with collagenous colitis may, on rare occasions, experience bowel perforation after colonoscopy or barium enema.[466]

The choice of therapy for collagenous colitis depends on the severity of disease and the adverse effects of medications. Common types of medical therapy include antidiarrheal agents (e.g., loperamide), bismuth subsalicylate (e.g., 5-ASA), cholestyramine, steroids (e.g., budesonide), and immunosuppressive agents (e.g., 6-mercaptopurine, azathioprine, methotrexate). Budesonide induces remission in up to 85.7% of patients, but the disease recurs in at least 60% of cases after discontinuation of the drug.[467] Rarely, surgical intervention is advised for patients who have severe symptoms that are unresponsive to medical therapy. Diversion of the fecal stream by creation of an ileostomy results in improvement of clinical symptoms. However, the disease typically recurs on reestablishment of bowel continuity.

Lymphocytic Colitis

Clinical Features

Lymphocytic colitis was originally described in 1989 when Lazenby and colleagues identified a subset of patients with microscopic colitis who demonstrated prominent intraepithelial lymphocytosis in biopsy specimens of the colon.[1] Compared with European studies that document an incidence rate of 1.1 to 3.1 per 100,000 per year, a study from North America showed that the incidence rate gradually increased to 5.5 per 100,000 between 1985 and 2001.[440,441] The peak incidence is in the sixth or seventh decade of life (mean age, 60.7 years; range, 19 to 98 years).[443] Rare cases of lymphocytic colitis have been reported in children. Similar to collagenous colitis, lymphocytic colitis is more common in women, but with a lower F:M ratio (between 2.4:1 and 2.7:1).

Lymphocytic colitis is associated with other autoimmune diseases, particularly thyroiditis (19%), rheumatoid arthritis (4%), fibromyalgia (5%), celiac disease (3%), and lymphocytic gastritis (1%).[443,468] The prevalence of celiac disease in patients with established lymphocytic colitis ranges from 3.5% to 30% in various studies. In fact, some patients with celiac disease show lymphocytic infiltration of the epithelium in all regions of the GI tract *(lymphocytic gastroenterocolitis)*. This pattern of colitis also occurs in other types of diseases, such as CVID, autoimmune enterocolopathy, and other immune deficiency disorders.

Presenting symptoms include chronic, watery, nonbloody diarrhea, usually with little or no abdominal discomfort, nausea, or vomiting. The diarrhea may be sudden or insidious in onset. The average duration of symptoms ranges from 3 months to 30 months before diagnosis.[469] Patients may also complain of abdominal pain (as many as 70%), urgency (as many as 65%), flatulence (as many as 59%), and weight loss (as many as 48%). Very rarely, constipation is a presenting symptom. In one study, there was seasonal variation in onset of clinical symptoms, which was significantly

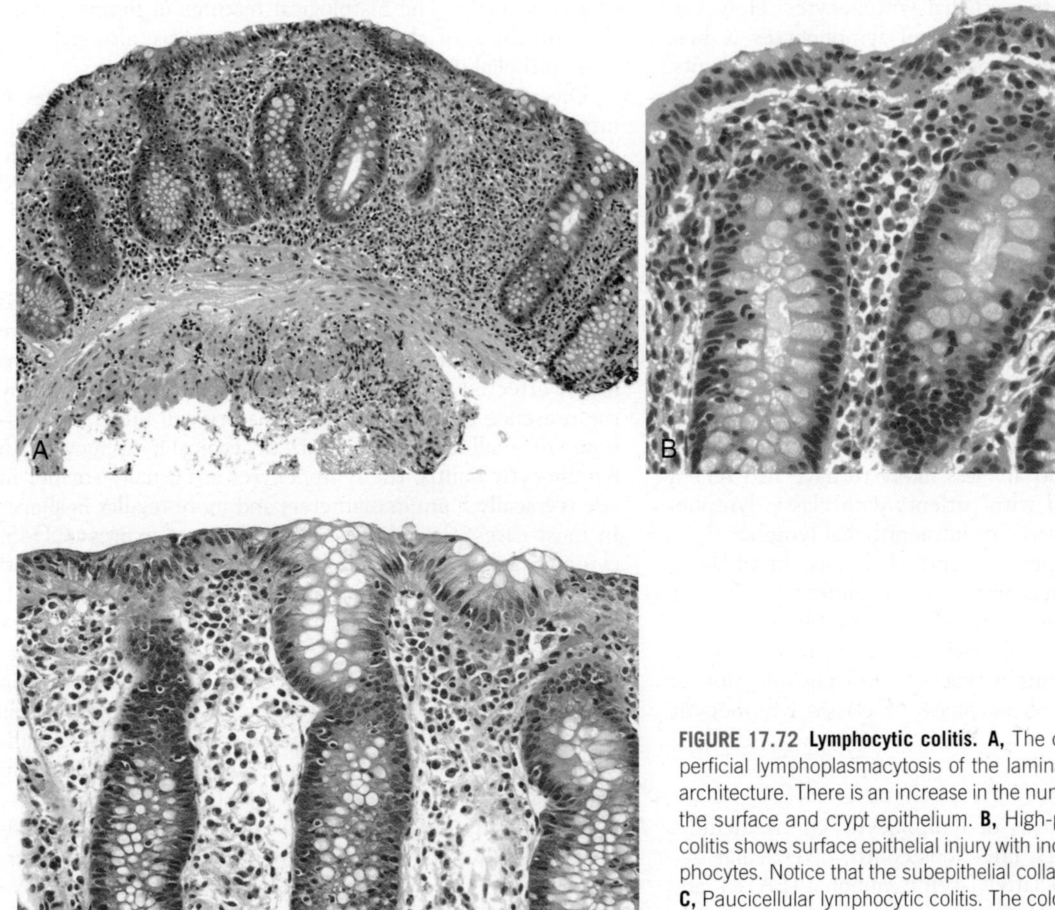

FIGURE 17.72 Lymphocytic colitis. A, The colonic mucosa shows superficial lymphoplasmacytosis of the lamina propria with intact crypt architecture. There is an increase in the number of lymphocytes within the surface and crypt epithelium. **B,** High-power view of lymphocytic colitis shows surface epithelial injury with increased intraepithelial lymphocytes. Notice that the subepithelial collagen layer is not thickened. **C,** Paucicellular lymphocytic colitis. The colon biopsy specimen shows a mild increase in lamina propria inflammatory cells and increased intraepithelial lymphocytes in crypt and surface epithelium.

associated with summer and fall seasons.[470] The results of physical examination and routine laboratory studies are usually normal.

Pathogenesis

The cause of lymphocytic colitis remains unknown. However, as in collagenous colitis, many drugs have been associated with this condition, such as ranitidine ruscus extract (Cyclo 3 Fort),[471] PPIs, β-adrenergic receptor blockers, statins, bisphosphonates, selective serotonin reuptake inhibitors, ipilimumab, and immune checkpoint inhibitors, among others.[445,446,472] Compared with collagenous colitis, an even stronger association has been found between lymphocytic colitis and celiac disease (as many as 30% of patients).[438,471,473] Although this association suggests the possibility of similar pathogenetic mechanisms, patients often do not respond to a gluten-free diet. They also do not possess HLA haplotypes associated with celiac disease (HLA-B8 and HLA-DR3), although an increased incidence of the HLA-A1 haplotype has been observed in patients with lymphocytic colitis.[447] Additional details regarding proposed theories of pathogenesis were discussed earlier in the Collagenous Colitis section.

Pathological Features

Most patients with lymphocytic colitis have normal-appearing colonic mucosa. However, a minority of patients may show mucosal erythema, congestion, and decreased vascular markings at endoscopy. As in collagenous colitis, rare cases show ulceration resulting from superimposed infections or drug reactions.

Lymphocytic colitis may be diffuse or patchy in distribution. Several studies have shown more severe involvement of the right colon versus the left colon. Rectal sparing has been observed in as many as 8% of cases.[440]

Surface epithelial injury (epithelial degeneration, mucin depletion, cytoplasmic hypereosinophilia, epithelial flattening) with increased intraepithelial lymphocytes (typically >20 per 100 surface epithelial cells) is the hallmark histological feature of lymphocytic colitis (Fig. 17.72A–B).[1] Crypt architecture is usually normal or near normal, and the superficial (and sometimes deep) lamina propria is characterized by the presence of a mixed inflammatory infiltrate composed mainly of lymphocytes and plasma cells. In contrast with collagenous colitis, eosinophils are either absent or few in number. In classic cases, the degree of intraepithelial lymphocytosis is marked, and one does not need to enumerate intraepithelial lymphocytes. However, in borderline cases, quantitation of lymphocytes is best performed in the surface epithelium between the crypts. IBD-like features such as cryptitis, crypt abscesses, Paneth cell metaplasia, and crypt architectural irregularity have also been described in lymphocytic colitis, but, as in collagenous colitis, they are usually focal and mild when present.[460]

Some cases of lymphocytic colitis show minimal histological changes, and only a slight increase in intraepithelial lymphocytosis (*atypical, paucicellular,* or *minimal change lymphocytic colitis*). In these mild cases, the disorder is characterized by only a mild increase in lamina propria inflammatory cells, usually limited to the superficial half of the mucosa (see Fig. 17.72C). The findings may be focal and patchy. Some cases are associated with giant cells.[462,474-476] Patients with "paucicellular lymphocytic colitis" are generally younger in age and are less likely to have had recent weight loss, compared with patients with classic lymphocytic colitis.[477] The degree of intraepithelial lymphocytosis ranges from 7 to 20 per 100 epithelial cells. In addition, epithelial flattening, degeneration, detachment, and mucin depletion are less prominent or even completely absent. Currently, it is not entirely clear whether this pattern of lymphocytosis represents a type of resolving infection or simply an early or evolving phase of classic lymphocytic colitis.

Differential Diagnosis

The differential diagnosis of lymphocytic colitis includes collagenous colitis, IBD, infectious colitis, diverticular disease, enteropathy-associated T-cell lymphoma (EATL), and autoimmune enteropathy (especially in pediatric patients).

Collagenous colitis may be confused with lymphocytic colitis, particularly if only rectal biopsies are obtained or if the subepithelial collagen layer in collagenous colitis is patchy or only mildly increased in thickness or only qualitatively abnormal. In collagenous colitis, the degree of intraepithelial lymphocytosis is less than in lymphocytic colitis, and the lamina propria infiltrate reveals more eosinophils.

IBD-like features in lymphocytic colitis are usually focal (see Table 17.12). The presence of significant crypt architectural distortion, basal lymphoplasmacytosis, and marked cryptitis and crypt abscess formation should alert the pathologist to IBD, especially if the patient has bloody diarrhea. Intraepithelial lymphocytosis may be seen in CD as well.[478] In these cases, lack of superficial expansion of the lamina propria by a lymphoplasmacytic infiltrate and the presence of disease elsewhere in the GI tract, especially the small bowel, favor a diagnosis of CD.

Acute infectious colitis is characterized by neutrophilic inflammatory cell cryptitis and crypt abscesses without dense lymphocytes or plasma cells. Therefore prominent and diffuse intraepithelial lymphocytosis supports a diagnosis of lymphocytic colitis over acute infectious colitis. During the resolving phase of infectious colitis, biopsy specimens may show focal intraepithelial lymphocytosis. In these cases, the self-limited nature of the disease, accompanied by residual cryptitis, crypt abscesses, and positive stool cultures, helps separate these two entities. Within the spectrum of infectious colitis is *Brainerd diarrhea.*[479] Bryant and colleagues originally described this entity as an epidemic form of chronic diarrhea linked to the water supply of a cruise ship. The histological features in Brainerd diarrhea are those of classic lymphocytic colitis, although surface epithelial damage is typically less prominent.

Diverticular disease may be associated with focal areas of intraepithelial lymphocytosis that may mimic lymphocytic colitis. Presumably, this is caused by bacterial overgrowth. Knowledge of the location of the biopsy (usually sigmoid colon) and the endoscopic finding of diverticula should alert the pathologist to this disorder.

Marked intraepithelial lymphocytosis and surface epithelial injury is also a hallmark feature of enteropathy-associated T-cell lymphoma (EATL). Most patients with EATL have celiac disease, although some do not. The colon is uncommonly affected by this condition. EATL is characterized by the presence of a diffuse inflammatory cell infiltrate composed of small- and medium-sized, atypical lymphocytes. In lymphocytic colitis, the lymphocytes are usually smaller in size (typically 5 μm in diameter) and more regular in shape. In most cases, the neoplastic lymphocytes express CD45, cytoplasmic CD3, and CD7 and are negative for CD4 and CD8. In addition, they may show T-cell–restricted intracellular antigen 1 (TIA-1), granzyme B, and perforin expression. Molecular genetic studies reveal the presence of clonal rearrangements of the T-cell receptor β-chain and γ-chain genes.[480] The lymphocyte population in lymphocytic colitis is usually CD8 positive and does not express TIA-1, granzyme B, or perforin. Furthermore, clonal rearrangements in lymphocytic colitis are rare.

In children, the differential diagnosis of colonic lymphocytosis includes colonic involvement by autoimmune enteropathy.[481,482] Patients with autoimmune enteropathy have chronic diarrhea with severe protein loss. Colonic biopsies may reveal diffuse mild expansion of the lamina propria by lymphocytes, plasma cells, and eosinophils. In severe cases, goblet cells may be depleted (or completely absent); crypt intraepithelial lymphocytosis, architectural distortion, and occasional crypt abscess formation may be present. However, in autoimmune enteropathy, surface intraepithelial lymphocytes are not prominent. In diagnostically challenging cases, serological testing for antienterocyte and anti–goblet cell antibodies may be helpful.

Natural History and Treatment

Spontaneous resolution of symptoms has been documented in as many as 18% of patients with lymphocytic colitis.[483] Salicylates (mesalazine) and budesonide therapy can cause clinical remission in 86% of patients.[483,484] Medical treatment leads to histological resolution in as many as 73% of patients. Clinical relapse of illness may occur as early as 2 months after an initial response to treatment. Most relapses occur between 14 months and 3 years after treatment, and relapse rates range from 25% to 44%.[483,484]

Other Causes of "Microscopic" Colitis

At different phases of disease, various disorders such as infectious colitis, drug-induced colitis, IBD, allergic colitis, radiation colitis, or even amyloidosis may show completely normal mucosa at endoscopy but reveal evidence of inflammation in mucosal biopsy specimens. Therefore not all clinical cases of "microscopic colitis" necessarily represent either lymphocytic or collagenous colitis. As a result, the term *microscopic colitis* should be avoided in pathology reports in favor of disease-specific diagnoses.

Association Between Microscopic Colitis and Inflammatory Bowel Disease

Although the exact pathophysiology of microscopic colitis and IBD is still largely unknown, recent studies have suggested a possible association between these disorders. For instance, some studies suggest that a microscopic colitis histological pattern can be seen as an attenuated form of IBD, and some of these patients eventually develop either classic UC or CD. A number of studies, including two recent genome-wide association studies, have identified associations between HLA haplotypes, DQ2 and DQ8, and risk of both collagenous and lymphocytic colitis.[485-487] Interestingly, a number of these variants also have been associated with risk of IBD.[488] Similar to IBD, the gut microbiome in microscopic colitis is also associated with marked dysbiosis and decreased diversity.[489,490] Additionally, higher expression of proinflammatory cytokines such as interferon-γ, TNF-α, and IL-17, similar to those seen in IBD, have been demonstrated by investigators who have studied mucosal gene expression and immune response in microscopic colitis.[491]

In a recent prospective nationwide cohort study, Khalili et al. demonstrated that compared with population comparators, microscopic colitis was associated with a 17-fold relative increase in risk of IBD.[492] All of these findings suggest that microscopic colitis may represent a risk factor, particularly for later-onset IBD.

From a pathologist's point of view, it is important to recognize that some patients with well-established UC or CD may develop periods during the natural history of their illness in which biopsies of their colon may resemble lymphocytic colitis or even collagenous colitis, either focally or diffusely. Etiological possibilities for this phenomenon include (1) new-onset microscopic colitis (in a patient with quiescent IBD), (2) recurrent IBD manifesting with microscopic colitis–like histological changes (in which case the findings are usually only focal), or (3) recurrent microscopic colitis in a patient whose original IBD diagnosis was incorrect. When confronted with this situation, it is helpful to reevaluate the patient's prior colonic biopsies for accuracy and correlate the most recent biopsy findings with the clinical and endoscopic features of the patient's current episode to sort through these various diagnostic possibilities. For instance, patients who have IBD that has been reconfirmed both clinically and pathologically but develop nonbloody diarrhea associated with either minimal or no endoscopic abnormalities and show diffuse microscopic colitis-like changes in their biopsies are more likely to represent new-onset microscopic colitis than recurrence of the original IBD. Of note is that focal and mild IBD like changes can also occur in patients with well-established microscopic colitis (see the Lymphocytic Colitis and Collagenous Colitis sections earlier in this chapter for more details).

MASTOCYTIC DISORDERS

Mast cells play an important role in immune defense in the GI tract. Overproduction or overactivation of mast cells can cause GI disorders that are amenable to drugs that target mast cell function specifically. Mast cell disorders include mastocytic enterocolitis and systemic mastocytosis.

Mast cells compose 2% to 5% of mononuclear cells in the lamina propria of the normal GI tract. Their numbers are highly dependent on the location of the biopsy and the immune status of the individual. For demonstration of increased mast cells, immunohistochemical stains for tryptase or CD117, the surface receptor for stem cell factor, are recommended. CD117 highlights all of the mast cells, whether or not they have degranulated, while the presence of tryptase, or lack thereof, indicates the degree of degranulation. In our experience, CD117 tends to have a cleaner background compared with tryptase.

The pathogenesis of the aforementioned mast cell disorders is overproduction or overactivation of mast cells in response to GI tract–specific stimuli. However, the precise stimuli that mediate mast cell activity are unclear. Mast cells are preferentially located adjacent to nerve terminals within the lamina propria. When activated by neuropeptides such as substance P, they release inflammatory mediators such as serotonin, histamine, and other inflammatory cytokines. Release of histamine and prostaglandin D_2 contributes to the development of diarrhea and increased intestinal motility. Degranulation also stimulates visceral motor neurons, causing diarrhea and abdominal pain. In patients with IBS, stress-induced mast cell activation can lead to a similar cascade of physiological events in the GI tract.[493-495]

Mastocytic Enterocolitis

The term *mastocytic enterocolitis* was coined by Jakate and coworkers to describe patients with chronic diarrhea of unknown etiology in whom an increase in mucosal mast cells was observed.[496] It is somewhat controversial whether this entity truly represents a distinct clinicopathological disorder. Patients usually reveal a history of diarrhea of at least 4 weeks' duration. Abdominal pain occurs in as many as 45% of patients. Routine laboratory tests, including stool analysis for ova and parasites, are typically negative. Serum tryptase levels are usually within normal limits. The disorder appears to be slightly more common in women, and the age at diagnosis ranges from 21 to 78 years.[496]

Colonoscopic findings in patients with this disorder are typically normal. Jakate and coworkers found that the concentration of mucosal mast cells in normal colon biopsy specimens in a control population was 13.6 ± 3.1 (mean ± standard deviation). Taking this value into consideration, a cutoff value of ≥20 mast cells per HPF (>2 standard deviations) was considered to represent a significant increase in mast cell density in the patients in their study (Fig. 17.73). In this series, up to 67% of patients who received treatment with antihistamines or sodium cromolyn, or both, showed either cessation of or a significant reduction in diarrhea.[496] Subsequently, Hahn and colleagues evaluated a series of biopsy specimens from patients with IBS but they could not document an increase in mucosal mast cell concentration.[497] In another recent study, the mean number of mast cells was 26 (range, 11 to 55) per HPF in 100 completely asymptomatic patients undergoing routine colonoscopy.[498] Given the substantial overlap in the mucosal mast cell density in patients considered to have mastocytic enterocolitis and those who are completely asymptomatic, the threshold

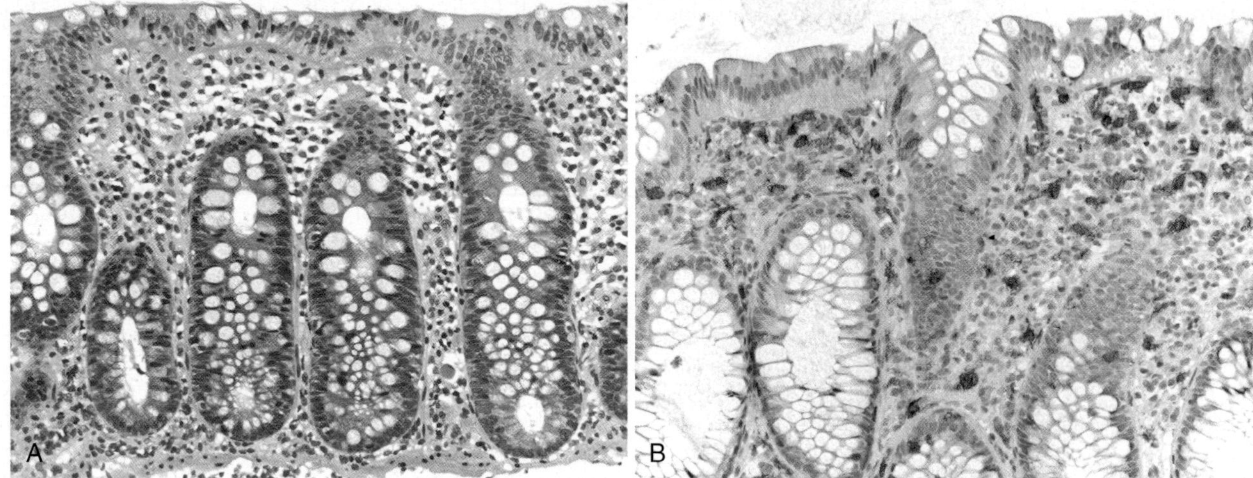

FIGURE 17.73 Mastocytic enterocolitis in a patient with a history of chronic diarrhea. A, Colonic mucosa with normal crypt architecture without epithelial injury or alteration of the lamina propria. **B,** An increase in the number of mucosal mast cells (>20 per HPF) is highlighted by CD117 immunohistochemical stain.

of ≥20 mast cells per HPF raises question about the diagnostic utility of this cutoff and hence, counting mucosal mast cells in patients presenting with chronic diarrhea is not recommended.

Systemic Mastocytosis

Clinical Features

Systemic mastocytosis is defined as a clonal, neoplastic proliferation of mast cells that accumulates in one or more extracutaneous organs, either with or without evidence of skin lesions. A nonneoplastic increase in the number of mucosal mast cells must be differentiated from systemic mastocytosis, wherein 60% to 80% of patients have GI symptoms.[499] Presenting symptoms include abdominal pain, diarrhea, nausea, and vomiting. Some cases are associated with peptic ulcer disease. A diagnosis of systemic mastocytosis normally requires confirmation of one major and one minor criterion, or three minor criteria (Box 17.9). The major criterion is 15 or more mast cells per HPF detected in the bone marrow or in other extracutaneous organs. Minor criteria are spindle-shaped cells composing 25% of the mast cell infiltrate, detection of a D816V *KIT* mutation, expression of CD2 and/or CD25 on CD117-positive mast cells, and a serum tryptase level of 20 ng/mL or greater.[500]

Pathogenesis

More than 90% of patients with systemic mastocytosis have a somatic gain-of-function mutation in the KIT receptor tyrosine kinase, primarily an aspartic acid to valine substitution (D816V) in the second catalytic domain. This point mutation results in enhanced survival and cell autonomous growth of neoplastic mast cells.[501]

Pathological Findings

Endoscopically, the colonic mucosa usually appears edematous and nodular.[499] However, in some instances, the mucosa may look completely normal. Biopsy specimens from patients with GI involvement by systemic mastocytosis may demonstrate an expansion of the lamina propria caused by oval to spindle-shaped cells admixed with numerous eosinophils (Fig. 17.74A–C). Mild crypt architectural distortion, in the form of irregular crypt spacing and crypt foreshortening, may also be present. In a study by Hahn and colleagues of nine cases of systemic mastocytosis with GI involvement, the mean mast cell density was 209 per HPF (range, 110 to 301).[497] In all cases, the mast cells expressed CD25 (see Fig. 17.74D). In a series of 24 patients with systemic mastocytosis, Doyle and colleagues found the mast cell density to be highly variable, ranging from 20 to 278 per HPF (mean, 116).[498]

A recent study has proposed that the finding of an atypical mast cell population (defined as mast cell aggregates with mast cells coexpressing both CD117 and CD25) in mucosal biopsy specimens from patients who are either completely asymptomatic or present with nonspecific symptoms may not necessarily indicate a neoplastic mastocytic disorder. In a series of 16 patients with incidentally discovered abnormal

BOX 17.9 Criteria for Systemic Mastocytosis

MAJOR CRITERION

Multifocal, dense infiltrates of mast cells (≥15 mast cells in aggregates) detected in sections of bone marrow and/or extracutaneous organs.

MINOR CRITERIA

1. In biopsy specimens of bone marrow and/or extracutaneous organs, >25% of the mast cells in the infiltrate are spindle-shaped or have atypical morphology.
2. Detection of activating point mutations at codon 816 of *KIT* in bone marrow, blood, or another extracutaneous organ.
3. Mast cells in bone marrow, blood, or other extracutaneous organs express CD2 and/or CD25 in addition to mast cells markers.
4. Serum total tryptase persistently exceeds 20 ng/mL (unless there is an associated clonal myeloid disorder, in which case this parameter is not valid).

Modified with permission from Horny HP, Metcalfe DD, Bennett JM, et al. Mastocytosis. In: Swerdlow SH, Campo E, Harris NL, et al. *WHO Classification of Tumours of Haematopoietic and Lymphoid Tissues.* Lyon, France: IARC Press; 2017:61–69.

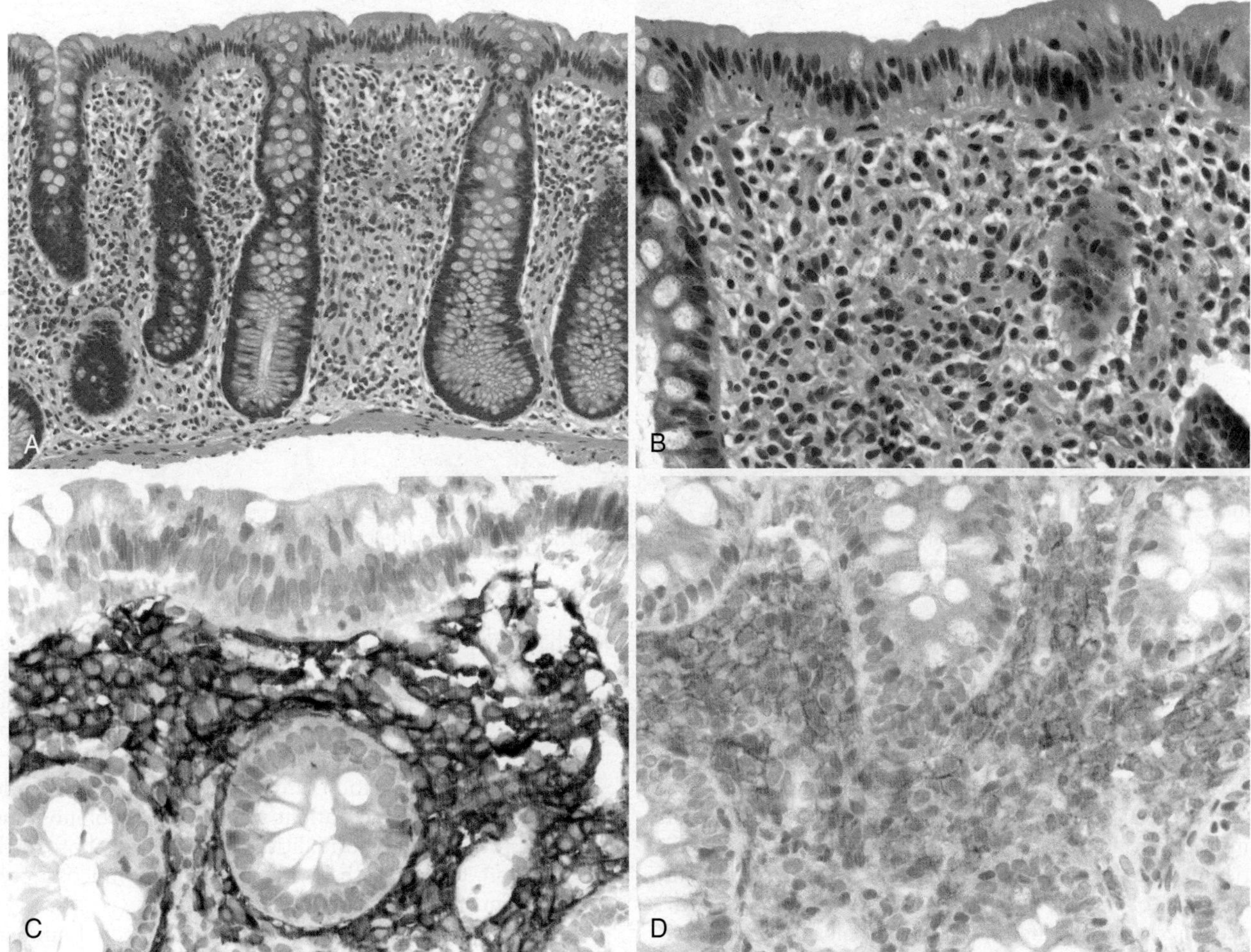

FIGURE 17.74 Systemic mastocytosis involving the colon. A, This colon biopsy specimen shows normal crypt architecture with a subtle increase in cellularity of the lamina propria. **B,** On higher magnification, there is expansion of the lamina propria by bland oval- to spindle-shaped cells with a moderate amount of pale eosinophilic cytoplasm, admixed with eosinophils. The mast cells are diffusely positive for CD117 **(C)** and show aberrant expression of CD25 **(D).**

mast cell aggregates in GI mucosal biopsy samples, none of the patients developed systemic mastocytosis during the follow-up period.[502]

Differential Diagnosis

The differential diagnosis of systemic mastocytosis involving the GI tract includes LCH, a much rarer entity. LCH of the GI tract is a disease that primarily affects male children who are younger than 2 years of age. The presenting symptoms include vomiting, abdominal pain, intractable diarrhea, malabsorption, bloody stool, and protein-losing enteropathy. In a recent series of 12 adult patients with LCH, the majority of patients were found to be women who were asymptomatic on clinical presentation.[503] Biopsies from patients with GI involvement by LCH show expansion of the lamina propria with histiocytic infiltrates arranged in sheets, nests, or clusters. The nuclei are kidney bean–shaped with nuclear grooves, fine chromatin, and a prominent nucleolus (Fig. 17.75). The infiltrate is rich in eosinophils; thus, it mimics systemic mastocytosis histologically. In contrast with systemic mastocytosis, these cells express S-100 protein, CD1a, and Langerin, and they lack CD117 immunoreactivity.

Natural History and Treatment

GI involvement by systemic mastocytosis is usually managed medically by drugs that limit mast cell activation and degranulation, such as H_1 and H_2 histamine receptor antagonists, cromolyn sodium, leukotriene antagonists, and occasionally short-term glucocorticoid therapy. Cytoreductive therapy with interferon or cladribine (nucleoside analogue) is indicated for aggressive disease with organ dysfunction caused by mast cell infiltration. Response to therapy is usually temporary, and repeated treatments are necessary. Specific tyrosine kinase inhibitors such as imatinib can be administered to patients either with or without the D816V *KIT* mutation. Other agents such as dasatinib and protein kinase C (PKC) inhibitors are currently under investigation to improve the symptoms and the mast cell infiltration.[504]

Irritable Bowel Syndrome

IBS is a functional GI disorder characterized by the presence of abdominal discomfort or pain associated with diarrhea, constipation, or a combination of both lasting at least 6 months. The prevalence of IBS in the United States varies from 3% to

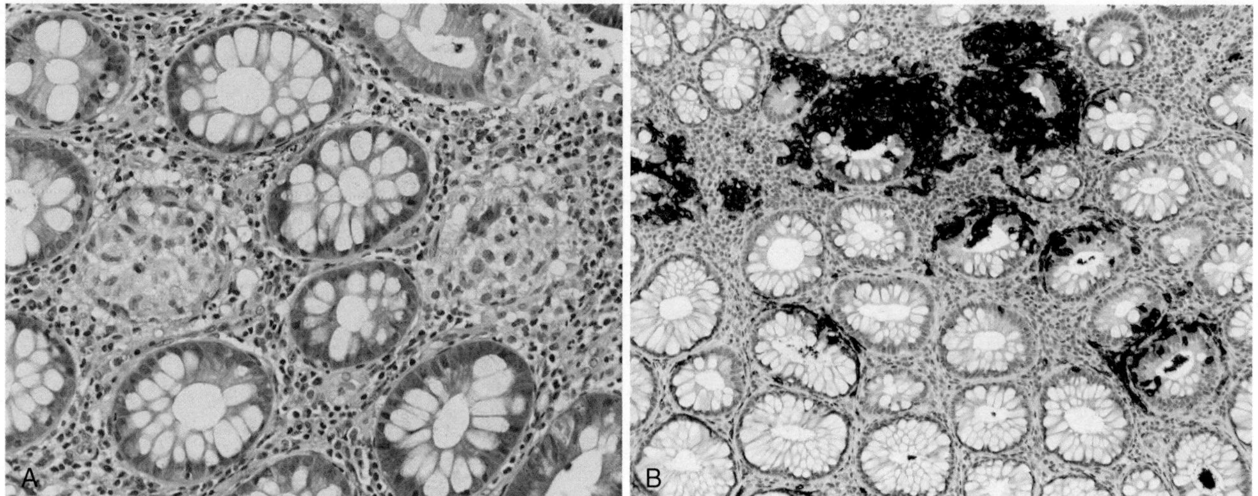

FIGURE 17.75 Langerhans cell histiocytosis involving the colon. A, This colon biopsy shows expansion of the lamina propria with histiocytic infiltrates arranged in sheets, nests, or clusters. The nuclei are kidney bean–shaped, with nuclear grooves, fine chromatin, and a prominent nucleolus. The infiltrate is rich in eosinophils. The neoplastic cells are positive for Langerin **(B).**

20%. Younger individuals, typically between 30 and 50 years of age, have a higher prevalence of IBS.[505] Women are more likely to be affected than men (F:M ratio, 2:1).[506,507]

Abdominal discomfort or pain relieved by defecation is a common symptom. The pain is often localized to the lower abdomen, and its onset may be associated with an increase or decrease in stool frequency. Based on the predominant symptom, the illness is classified as by the Rome IV criteria into diarrhea-predominant, constipation-predominant, mixed bowel habits, and unclassified subgroups.[508] Currently, there is no biochemical, histopathologic, or radiological test for establishing a diagnosis of IBS. IBS is diagnosed clinically by applying symptom-based criteria (Rome IV criteria).

A number of different pathogenic mechanisms have been associated with the development of IBS, including abnormal motility, visceral hypersensitivity, low-grade inflammation, and stress.[509,510] Diarrhea occurs as a result of increased high-amplitude propagated contractions, an enhanced gastrocolic response, and possibly rectal hypersensitivity.[511] In contrast, constipation results from increased segmental (nonpropulsive) contractions, decreased high-amplitude propagated contractions, and reduced rectal sensitivity.[512]

Bacterial gastroenteritis precedes the development of IBS in 7% to 30% of patients. Colonic inflammation causes an increase in the local concentrations of 5-hydroxytryptamine (5-HT), prostaglandins, bradykinins, and adenosine. 5-HT acts on intrinsic afferent neurons to initiate a peristaltic reflex, which leads to diarrhea.[513] The dysbiosis of microbiota in IBS has been recognized as a plausible contributing factor to this condition. IBS symptom severity has been associated with a distinct fecal microbiota signature, and patients with severe IBS have lower microbial richness and exhaled methane as well as a reduced presence of the *Methanobacteriales* and *Prevotella* enterotype, but an increased presence of the *Bacteroides* enterotype.[514]

Stress induces changes in intestinal secretion and permeability responses in healthy subjects. Therefore it is likely that stress plays a role in the onset and persistence of IBS-related symptoms. Depression and fatigue in patients with IBS have been associated with an increase in colonic mast cells. Because mast cells communicate with both the enteric and the central nervous systems, it has been suggested that excess mast cells in the colon may be related to the symptoms of depression and fatigue in patients with IBS.[515]

Endoscopic examination is often performed to exclude an organic cause of the patient's symptoms. Colonoscopy does not reveal any abnormalities. However, in those with constipation, there may be evidence of rectal mucosal erythema or mucosal prolapse.

Increased numbers of mast cells have been found in the cecum, terminal ileum, and jejunum of patients with IBS.[516-518] Jakate and colleagues found that 45% of patients with an increase in the number of mucosal mast cells had a history of abdominal pain and a presumed diagnosis of IBS-D.[496] In two recent studies, the mean number of mast cells was found to be 30 (range, 13 to 59) per HPF in 100 patients with IBS.[498,519]

Management of IBS includes dietary adjustments such as increased fiber intake. Antispasmodics and anticholinergics are indicated for the treatment of abdominal pain. Loperamide, 5-HT antagonists, alosetron, antidepressants, and antibiotics are known to provide symptom relief in most patients. Some patients have spontaneous improvement over time. However, in general, IBS is a relapsing disorder. Prolonged duration of symptoms accompanied by psychological stress portend a poor clinical prognosis. In our experience, clinicians often request that pathologists perform a mast cell stain on biopsies from patients suspected to have IBS. Given that there is no diagnostic cutoff with regard to the density of mucosal mast cells in patients with IBS, it is recommended that pathologists objectively report the highest density of mast cells per HPF found in a biopsy, without offering any clinical interpretation or information regarding the diagnostic threshold.

Apoptotic Colopathy

A variety of disorders of the colon are associated with apoptosis as the prominent, or in some cases, the only significant

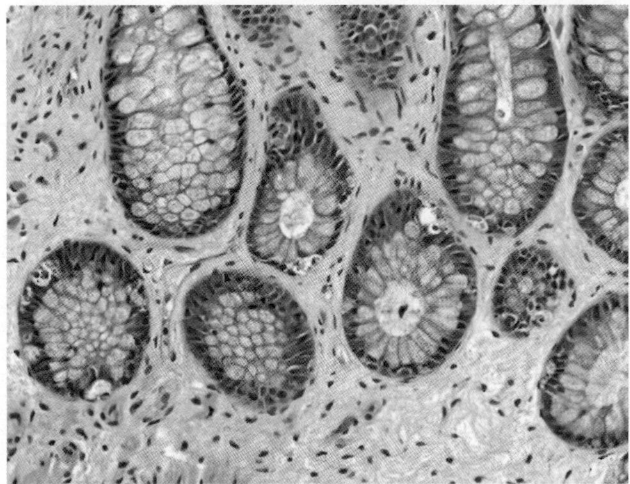

FIGURE 17.76 Apoptotic colopathy. The colonic mucosa shows increased numbers of crypt apoptotic bodies. The remainder of the mucosa did not show any other abnormality.

histological abnormality in tissue. For instance, In disorders such as GVHD, cytomegalovirus (CMV) colitis, autoimmune enteropathy, mycophenolate mofetil (MMF) toxicity, and immune checkpoint inhibitor–related colitis, apoptosis is one of several histopathological manifestations of the disease. Nevertheless, colon biopsies may, on occasion, reveal prominent or increased numbers of apoptotic bodies in the absence of any other significant microscopic abnormalities (Fig. 17.76). Diagnostic possibilities in these cases include bowel preparation injury and drug effect. McKenna and coworkers described a pattern of colopathy characterized by prominent apoptosis in the crypt bases in biopsies of the colon without any other alterations. In their study, 9 of 11 patients had watery diarrhea and abdominal pain at presentation. Patients were mainly women ranging in age from 14 to 68 years. Endoscopic examinations were normal in all cases for which clinical information was available. Mucosal biopsies from these patients demonstrated normal mucosal architecture with a marked increase in crypt epithelial apoptosis at the crypt bases. In 9 of the 11 patients, there was evidence of cryptitis and a mild expansion of the lamina propria by a mixed inflammatory infiltrate composed of lymphocytes, plasma cells, and eosinophils. None of the patients had biopsy changes of lymphocytic or collagenous colitis.[520] This study did not specifically address the cause of the histopathological findings in these patients. Based on the available information, apoptotic colopathy is best considered a pattern of injury that is associated with several colonic disorders that must be differentiated on the basis of a combination of clinical and pathological findings (Box 17.10).

Diverticular Disease

Colonic diverticula are defined as outpouchings of either all or portions of the colonic wall. They are further classified as either true diverticula, when the outpouchings are composed of all the layers of the bowel wall, or false diverticula (pseudodiverticula), when only the mucosa and submucosa protrude into the muscularis propria. True diverticula are usually congenital in origin. False diverticula are the most common type observed in the colon. The term *diverticulosis* refers to the presence of single or multiple diverticula. *Diverticulitis* is defined as inflammation of one or more diverticula, with or without micro or macro perforations.

BOX 17.10 Disorders Resulting in Apoptotic Colopathy

- Graft-versus-host disease
- Cord colitis syndrome
- Cytomegalovirus infection
- Autoimmune enterocolopathy
- Medications
  - Mycophenolate mofetil
  - Immune checkpoint inhibitors

Clinical Features

Most patients with diverticulosis are asymptomatic, making determination of the true incidence of this condition difficult. However, reported prevalence rates range from 12% to 49%, and the rate is known to increase with age.[521] In individuals younger than 40 years of age, the rate is less than 10%, whereas the estimated rate in patients 80 years of age or older is as much as 66%.[522] Worldwide, the United States, Europe, and Australia have the highest prevalence rates, and diverticulosis has been referred to as a "disease of Western civilization." Right-sided colonic diverticula are more common in Asians, whereas more than 90% of patients in Western countries have only left-sided disease. Diverticulosis is equally common among men and women.

Most cases of diverticulosis are discovered incidentally during screening colonoscopy. Others may present with symptoms such as left lower quadrant pain that may worsen on eating or a change in bowel habits. Other symptoms include constipation, diarrhea, bloating, and passage of mucus per rectum. Physical examination may reveal mild tenderness in the left lower quadrant. However, guarding is typically absent unless the patient has diverticulitis and peritonitis.

Studies have shown that the rate of occult bleeding in diverticulosis is similar to that in the healthy adult population. Therefore the presence of a positive occult blood test should not necessarily be attributed to diverticulosis clinically.[523]

Acute diverticulitis is the most common clinical manifestation, affecting 10% to 25% of patients with diverticulosis.[522] Diverticulitis results from inflammation of diverticula, which is considered an uncomplicated form of diverticulitis. Complications such as perforation, abscess formation, fistula, obstruction, or bleeding occur in 5% to 25% of patients with acute diverticulitis. Hemorrhage in patients with acute diverticulitis usually manifests as painless, sudden-onset hematochezia. Some patients pass fresh blood or blood clots per rectum.

Patients with acute diverticulitis typically have left lower quadrant pain at presentation. However, in the presence of a redundant sigmoid colon, the pain may be localized to the suprapubic region or to the right side of the abdomen. Because Asians have a predilection for right-sided diverticulosis, right-sided pain is a predominant symptom in this population. Anorexia, nausea, vomiting, and occasionally dysuria (caused by irritation of the bladder wall) are some of the other symptoms of acute diverticulitis.

Signs of acute diverticulitis include localized tenderness either with or without guarding. Rectal examination may reveal the presence of a mass that corresponds to a localized abscess or phlegmon. Peripheral blood leukocytosis is typically the only major laboratory finding in patients with this disorder. Plain radiographs (erect chest films) are helpful in detecting pneumoperitoneum, which may be seen in up to 11% of patients. Contrast enemas (with a water-soluble agent such as Gastrografin) have a sensitivity of 62% to 94% for detecting acute diverticulitis. CT is the diagnostic procedure of choice, with a sensitivity ranging from 93% to 98%. Another advantage of CT is that it helps distinguish diverticulitis from colonic cancer, especially in patients who present with right-sided disease.

Pathogenesis

The anatomy of the colon predisposes humans to the development of diverticula. Unlike the small bowel or rectum, the colon lacks a concentric outer longitudinal layer of muscularis propria. Instead, the outer longitudinal layer is condensed into three longitudinal bands of tissue, known as *teniae coli*. Teniae coli are arranged along the mesenteric, medial, and lateral aspects of the bowel wall. The blood supply of the mucosa and submucosa arises from mesenteric vessels (vasa recta) that traverse through the subserosa and penetrate the circular layer of muscularis propria at two points between the mesenteric and antimesenteric teniae. The bowel wall is weakest at these locations and provides outward access for mucosal herniations. The colonic vasa recta arise at regular intervals from the main mesenteric arteries, and diverticula tend to follow their distribution. They are usually found in two to four parallel longitudinal rows between the mesenteric and the two antimesenteric teniae.[524]

Diverticular disease is believed to be caused by inherent structural alterations of the colonic wall, motility abnormalities, and low levels of dietary fiber. Early descriptions of specimens alluded to thickening of the colonic wall and shortening of the teniae, which results in accordion-like folds of the colonic wall. This is also referred to as *myochosis* (from the Greek *myo*, "muscle" and *chosis*, "a heaping up"). This may cause the mucosa to be arranged into multiple folds, which are then susceptible to prolapse *(polypoid prolapsing mucosal folds)*.[525] It has been suggested that the thickening of the colonic wall is a result of hypertrophy resulting from an increase in elastin deposition within the muscle cells of the teniae.[526] Increased deposition of elastin has been partly attributed to increased absorption of proline, which is present in significant concentrations in typical Western diets. Additionally, increased synthesis of type III collagen and increased cross-linking of colonic collagen is directly related to age.[527] This theory is further supported by the fact that patients with connective tissue disorders such as Ehlers-Danlos syndrome, Marfan syndrome, and scleroderma have higher rates of diverticulosis.[528]

Early studies demonstrated abnormal motility and increased intraluminal pressures in patients with diverticular disease. However, the exact mechanism for this finding is unclear. Although the myenteric and submucosal plexuses are normal in appearance in affected patients, the numbers of interstitial cells of Cajal are reduced.[529] Imbalances in the excitatory cholinergic signals and inhibitory adrenergic signals may also contribute to abnormal motility of the bowel wall in patients with diverticular disease.[530]

One of the most widely accepted precipitating factors for the development of diverticular disease is a low-fiber diet. There is epidemiological evidence for an association of diverticular disease with the industrial development of refined sugar and milled grains in the 20th century.[531] Because more countries have adopted Western dietary habits, the incidence of diverticular disease has increased worldwide.[532] Low-fiber diets are deficient in cellulose, which binds water and salt and increases the bulk of stools. Low-volume stools have longer transit time, and straining results in higher intraluminal pressures. Based on the law of Laplace, the sigmoid colon, which has the smallest diameter, also has the highest intraluminal pressure, and diverticula occur most commonly in this segment of colon.[533,534]

The pathogenesis of diverticulitis is believed to be similar to that of appendicitis: Fecal material or fecaliths obstruct diverticular sacs, typically at their neck, and cause mucosal erosions and inflammation. Inflammation and edema further obstruct drainage of sac contents, leading to prolonged exposure to bacterial flora. Inflammation also causes diminished venous blood flow, which results in localized ischemia that further exacerbates tissue injury.

Complicated diverticulitis results when the immune response cannot contain the inflammation and the bacterial organisms and accompanying inflammatory contents perforate the muscle and extend through the bowel wall. Fistula formation occurs when perforations extend to adjacent loops of bowel wall or other organs. Diverticular hemorrhage occurs as a result of weakened arteries where they course through the muscle wall. Inflammation further destroys arterial walls and results in abrupt-onset bleeding.

Pathological Features

Gross Findings

Diverticular disease most commonly involves the sigmoid colon (>90%). The cecum and ascending colon are affected in fewer than 5% of patients. Pancolonic involvement occurs in 16% of cases.[535] Characteristic gross findings include thickening and shortening of the bowel wall, with or without abscesses, serosal fat wrapping, and adhesions if there have been previous bouts of diverticulitis. The diverticula usually range in size from 5 to 10 mm and are surrounded by erythema or ulcers (Fig. 17.77A–C). The adjacent mucosa may show prolapse-type inflammatory polyps.[525] Giant diverticula can measure as much as 25 cm in diameter.[536]

Microscopic Findings

Diverticula consist of flask-shaped mucosal outpouchings that may extend deep into the bowel wall, through the muscularis propria into the subserosal adipose tissue (see Fig. 17.77D). The superficial aspect of the outpouchings usually reveals a thin layer of muscularis mucosae. The mucosa within the diverticulum may be normal in appearance or may show features of active or chronic inflammation, such as reactive lymphoid aggregates (see Fig. 17.77E), increased numbers of lymphocytes and plasma cells, cryptitis, crypt abscesses, mild crypt architectural distortion, and Paneth

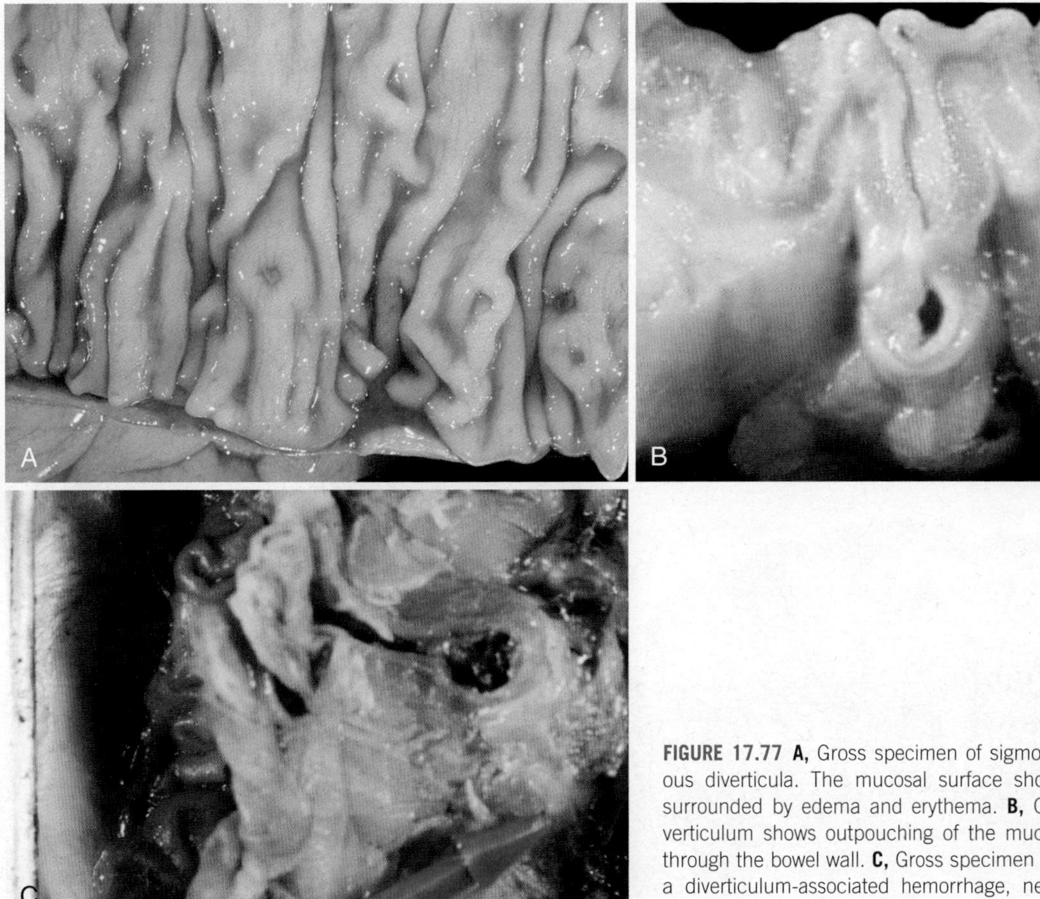

FIGURE 17.77 A, Gross specimen of sigmoid colon with numerous diverticula. The mucosal surface shows diverticular ostia surrounded by edema and erythema. **B,** Cross-section of a diverticulum shows outpouching of the mucosa and submucosa through the bowel wall. **C,** Gross specimen of diverticulitis shows a diverticulum-associated hemorrhage, necrosis, and abscess formation.

Continued

cell metaplasia (see Fig. 17.77F).[537] These changes are usually most prominent in the deep portions of diverticula. Erosions or ulcers may also be present.

Diverticulitis is characterized by suppurative inflammation of the diverticulum and peridiverticular abscess formation (see Fig. 17.77G).[538] Mucosal edema, hemorrhage, foreign-body giant cell reaction to luminal contents, and lymphoid hyperplasia are often present. In the vicinity of infected diverticula, there is fibrosis of the muscularis propria. The arterial walls may exhibit medial hypertrophy and duplication of the internal elastic lamina. Serositis and fat necrosis are usually associated with cases complicated by perforation and fistula formation. Inflammatory masses may form when there is marked peridiverticulitis. These changes grossly mimic a neoplasm.

Crohn's-Like Diverticulitis

In some individuals, diverticulitis is associated with patchy chronic active colitis, serpiginous ulcers, serosal fat wrapping, granulomas, transmural lymphoid aggregates, and mural fibrosis, similar to CD *(Crohn's-like diverticulitis)*. Vascular changes including occlusive arterial fibroplasia and active lymphohistiocytic vasculitis may also be present.[539] The presenting symptoms in patients with these features of Crohn's-like diverticulitis usually include abdominal pain, intermittent constipation, and bleeding. In a series of 29 such patients (mean age, 63 years) who did not have prior or concurrent CD, Goldstein and colleagues found that most had evidence of fistulas at the time of surgery.[539] During a mean follow-up period of 7.6 years that included a series of endoscopic and radiological studies, most of the patients (92%) did not show evidence of Crohn's enteritis or colitis. In two patients (8%), signs and symptoms of perianal and small-bowel CD developed within the first 6 months after surgery. Therefore in their study, the Crohn's-like changes in most patients represented a reaction to diverticulitis rather than coexistent CD in a patient with diverticulitis.

Differential Diagnosis

Coexistent Crohn's Disease and Diverticulitis vs. Crohn's-like Diverticulitis

The differential diagnosis of Crohn's-like diverticulitis includes preexisting CD and, on occasion, new-onset CD in patients with already established diverticulitis. Unlike CD, which usually shows a patchy distribution of disease throughout the colon and even ileal involvement, pathological changes of Crohn's-like diverticulitis are limited only to the segment of bowel involved by diverticular disease. Other features, such as neuronal hyperplasia, pyloric gland metaplasia, and villiform mucosal changes are not as common in Crohn's-like diverticulitis.[539] One key distinguishing

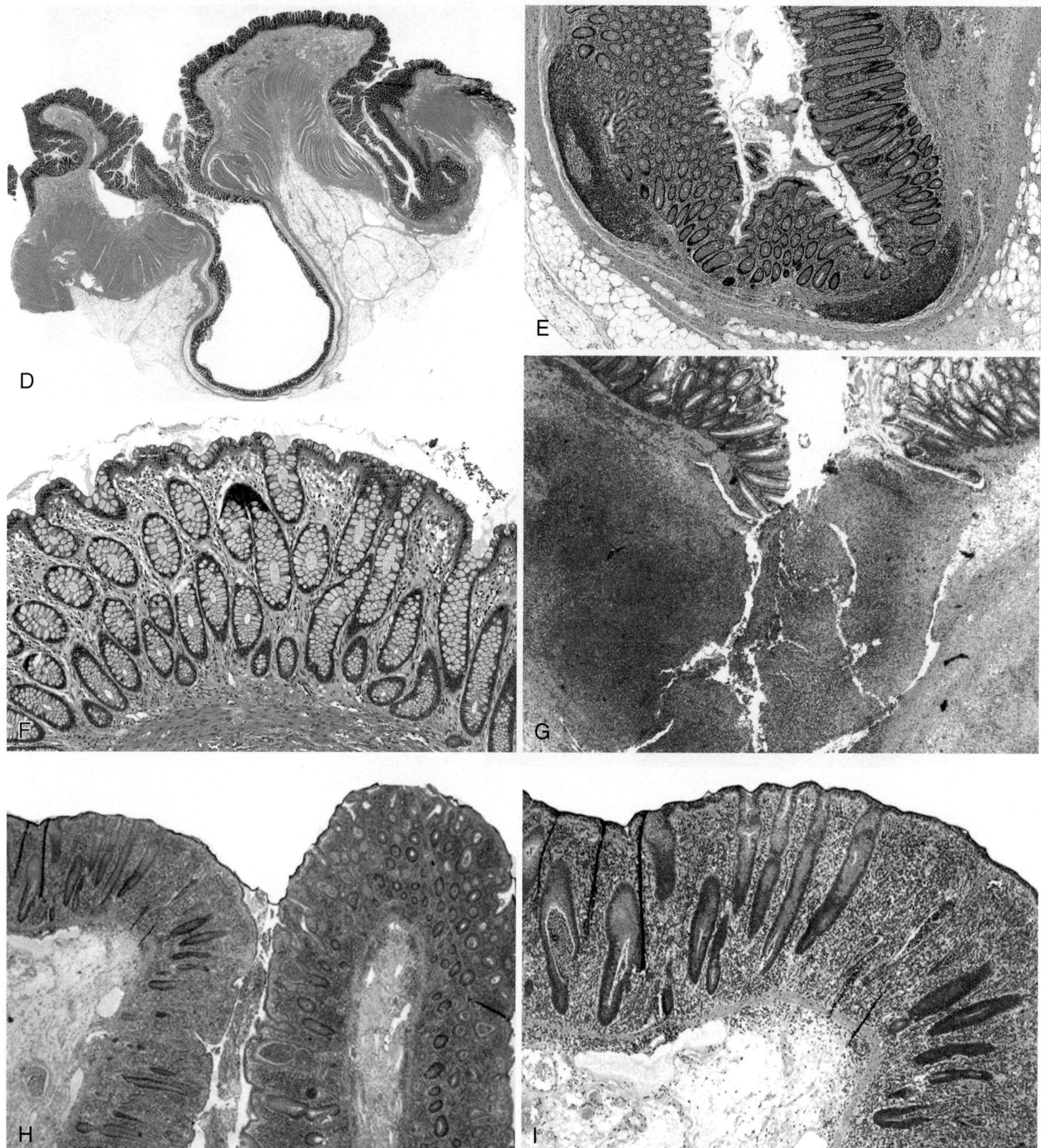

FIGURE 17.77, CONT'D **D,** Histological section through a diverticulum shows flask-shaped mucosal outpouchings that extend deep into the bowel wall, through the muscularis propria into the subserosal adipose tissue. **E,** Diverticulum with prominent submucosal lymphoid aggregates localized to the deep aspect of the diverticulum. **F,** Diverticulosis with focal mild crypt architectural distortion and Paneth cell metaplasia. These mucosal changes are typically restricted to the segment of colon affected by diverticular disease. **G,** Diverticulitis complicated by diverticular abscess formation. **H,** Diverticular disease–associated colitis. Low-power view shows ulcerative colitis–like inflammatory changes in the interdiverticular and diverticular mucosa. **I,** High-power view shows increased mixed inflammation in the lamina propria, crypt abscesses, crypt distortion and atrophy, and basal plasmacytosis, all features reminiscent of chronic active ulcerative colitis.

feature is that the rectum and interdiverticular mucosa in patients with Crohn's-like diverticulitis are typically normal, lacking features of active or chronic IBD-like mucosal injury. Additionally, lack of disease in the remainder of the GI tract (including perianal disease) further supports a diagnosis of Crohn's-like diverticulitis instead of CD. In patients who develop new-onset CD in the setting of preexisting diverticular disease, in addition to potential involvement in other portions of the GI tract in patients with the former, differences may also be found within the interdiverticular mucosa as well. The interdiverticular mucosa in diverticular disease may show features of prolapse-type changes, but not IBD, whereas in patients with CD, the interdiverticular mucosa may show classic IBD features.

Natural History and Treatment

Diverticulosis often remains asymptomatic for many years. Complications related to diverticulitis develop in 10% to 25% of patients. Treatment includes increased dietary fiber, 5-ASA, antibiotics, anticholinergics, and antispasmodics. Surgery is indicated for patients who have had at least two episodes of diverticulitis[540] and for those who demonstrate signs of subclinical diverticulitis, fistula formation, intestinal obstruction, or perforation. Surgery is performed either in a single stage (i.e., resection with primary anastomosis) or as a two-stage procedure (primary resection with Hartmann pouch, followed by reanastomosis). One study from the Mayo Clinic showed that 76% of patients who underwent sigmoid colectomy without prior signs of systemic infection showed histological evidence of active or chronic inflammation with reactive lymphoid aggregates, cryptitis, crypt abscesses, mild crypt architectural distortion, and Paneth cell metaplasia. Within 1 year after surgical resection, complete resolution of pain and other related symptoms occurred in most patients.[541]

Hemorrhage is usually managed endoscopically. Between 7% and 45% of patients experience recurrence of diverticulitis. Almost 50% of the recurrences occur within 1 year after surgical resection.[542] Younger age at presentation and persistence of postoperative symptoms are associated with a higher risk of recurrent diverticulitis after resection.[543]

Diverticular Disease–Associated ("Segmental") Colitis

Clinical Features

Diverticular disease–associated colitis (DAC) is defined as a form of mucosal-based UC-like chronic colitis that is anatomically confined to the colonic segment involved by diverticula in individuals with otherwise uncomplicated diverticular disease. The incidence of DAC is estimated to be 0.3% to 1.3% of all patients with diverticulitis.[544] Most patients are men (F:M ratio, 1:2) and older than 60 years of age (range, 32 to 87 years). Presenting symptoms include left lower quadrant cramping pain, diarrhea, and rectal bleeding. Fever, leukocytosis, and weight loss are uncommon. IBD-like extraintestinal symptoms, such as arthropathy and pyoderma gangrenosum, have also been reported in some cases.[539,545,546]

Pathogenesis

The pathogenesis of DAC remains unclear; however, it is most likely related to a combination of multiple factors, such as mucosal prolapse, fecal stasis, and mucosal ischemia.[467] Some studies suggest that patients with diverticulitis are also at an increased risk for IBD.[547-549] Therefore the association between IBD and diverticulitis is probably not simply a coincidence and raises the possibility that this may represent a form of UC-like immune-mediated disease. In one study, 82% of IBD patients with diverticulosis had segmental sigmoid colitis, compared with only 62% of matched control patients without diverticulosis.[548]

Pathological Features

Gross Findings

Gross findings include UC-like mucosal erythema, edema, friability, or ulceration in the interdiverticular mucosa of the area of bowel involved by diverticular disease. The diverticular orifices are usually normal in appearance. However, in contrast with UC, the rectum is typically spared in DAC, as is the area of colon proximal to the diverticulosis.

Microscopic Findings

DAC resembles UC histologically in the interdiverticular mucosa (see earlier discussion). The disease is typically restricted to the mucosa and, as mentioned earlier, affects the interdiverticular area of the colonic segment that is affected by diverticular disease. The histological changes include diffuse mixed lymphoplasmacytic infiltrate within the lamina propria with crypt architectural distortion, cryptitis, crypt abscesses, lymphoid aggregates, and Paneth cell metaplasia (see Fig. 17.77H–I). Crypt rupture–associated granulomas may develop as well. Superficial erosions and ulcers accompanied by regenerating epithelial changes may also be present. In essence, all of the features of typical UC may be seen in DAC.

Differential Diagnosis

Diverticular Disease–Associated Colitis vs. Ulcerative Colitis

Because of the histological similarities between DAC and UC, distinguishing these two entities can be challenging if one is not aware of the differences regarding the distribution of disease in these two disorders. Knowledge of the location of disease in relationship to areas of diverticulosis is critical. For instance, rectal sparing is extremely unusual in UC, except in patients who have received prior oral or enema treatment, or at initial onset of disease in children. Mucosal inflammation in UC typically extends in a continuous fashion and often involves the proximal colon as well. In contrast, in DAC, the rectum is normal, and the mucosal inflammation is characteristically restricted to the segment of colon involved by diverticular disease.

Natural History and Treatment

Most patients with DAC respond to conservative therapy that includes antiinflammatory drugs such as mesalamine or sulfasalazine. Antibiotics or steroids are prescribed if the patient does not respond to this initial line of therapy. In most patients, resolution of symptoms occurs within 6 months of medical therapy. Rarely, surgery is performed for medically refractory disease or for patients who present with complications related to obstruction or bleeding. Thus far, recurrence of disease after resection has not been documented. Progression to UC has been documented in three studies, in which a minority of patients (9/60) developed endoscopic and pathological evidence of UC.[544,550,551] The onset of UC occurred 4 to 25 months after the initial diagnosis of DAC. In more than one-half of these patients, progression to UC occurred after surgery for DAC.

Diversion Colitis

Clinical Features

Diversion colitis is a clinicopathological syndrome caused by diversion of the fecal stream that, ultimately, results in the development of colitis within diverted segments of bowel. This disorder was first recognized by Morson and Dawson in 1972.[552] However, it was not until 1981 that Glotzer et al. coined the term *diversion colitis* by demonstrating a causal association between fecal diversion and subsequent colonic inflammation.[553]

Surgical diversion of the fecal stream is performed for a variety of reason; however, obstruction of the sigmoid colon or rectum caused by cancer or complicated diverticular disease (Hartmann operation) is the most common reason to divert the fecal stream. Gender reassignment surgeries, Hirschsprung disease, severe IBD, traumatic injury to the bowel, severe infectious colitis, idiopathic constipation, and pseudomembranous colitis are some of the other conditions that may lead to surgical diversion. Diversion colitis occurs more commonly in patients who had surgery for IBD (87%) than in patients with other (noninflammatory) conditions, such as familial adenomatous polyposis (28%).[554] Most patients are clinically asymptomatic. In the others, presenting symptoms include passage of mucus and/or blood per rectum or abdominal pain.[553,555] Disease onset most commonly occurs 3 to 36 months after surgery.

Pathogenesis

The pathogenesis of diversion colitis remains controversial. The most accepted theory is that diversion colitis results from luminal deficiency of short-chain fatty acids (SCFAs), which are usually derived from the fermentation of dietary starches by normal colonic bacterial flora.[556] Once the fecal stream has been diverted, dietary starches are no longer available as a source of fuel for endogenous bacteria. This results in decreased bacterial counts, lower numbers of strict anaerobes, and increased numbers of *Enterobacteriaceae* and nitrate-reducing bacteria. The distal colonic epithelium is more dependent on SCFAs as a metabolic substrate than the proximal colon.[557] In support of this hypothesis, Harig and colleagues demonstrated that a subset of patients who were given enemas containing SCFAs showed endoscopic and histological resolution within a few weeks.[556] However, a prospective, randomized, double-blind trial showed that butyrate enemas neither affected the bacterial population in the diverted colon nor provided resolution of endoscopic or histological parameters in a study of 13 patients.[558]

Recent experimental models of diversion colitis have shown that colonic mucosa devoid of exposure to the fecal stream produces high levels of reactive oxygen species. These molecules cause cellular damage and loss of mucosal integrity that allows translocation of the luminal bacteria and antigens into the submucosal layer, leading to development of colitis.[559] However, this theory has not been confirmed in human subjects.

Another proposed mechanism for development of diversion colitis is ischemia. It has been suggested that SCFAs cause relaxation of the vascular smooth muscle, and thus in a diverted bowel, butyrate deficiency may result in increased vascular resistance in pelvic arteries that eventually leads to ischemia and pathological changes of diversion colitis.[560]

Pathological Features

Gross Findings

Gross features of diversion colitis include mucosal erythema, friability, edema, and nodularity.[553] In severe cases, ulcers and hemorrhage may be present. Pseudopolyps and strictures may develop in chronic cases.

Microscopic Findings

Virtually all segments of bowel that have been diverted from the fecal stream for a minimum of a few weeks ultimately reveal characteristic histological changes in the colon, even in patients without the typical clinical signs and symptoms of diversion colitis.[561] Thus unless patients are symptomatic, the post-diversion morphological changes that occur are considered normal "baseline" changes of the defunctioned bowel and represent an adaptive response to the new luminal microenvironment. Thus a diagnosis of *diversion colitis* is considered a combined clinical and pathological syndrome. In asymptomatic patients and those with established clinically evident diversion colitis, the defunctioned bowel characteristically shows prominent diffuse nodular lymphoid hyperplasia. The lymphoid nodules often show prominent germinal centers (Fig. 17.78A).[562] The prominent lymphoid aggregates result in marked distortion (bending, atrophy) of the crypts (see Fig. 17.78B). The lamina propria shows expansion by an inflammatory cell infiltrate composed of lymphocytes and plasma cells, which tends to be denser in the upper half of the mucosa. Cryptitis, crypt

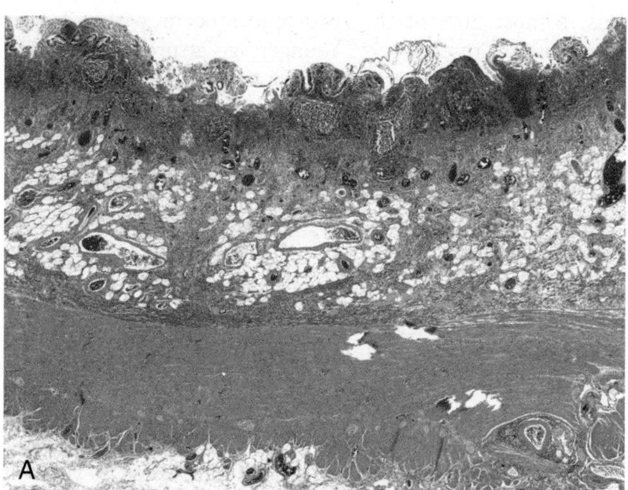

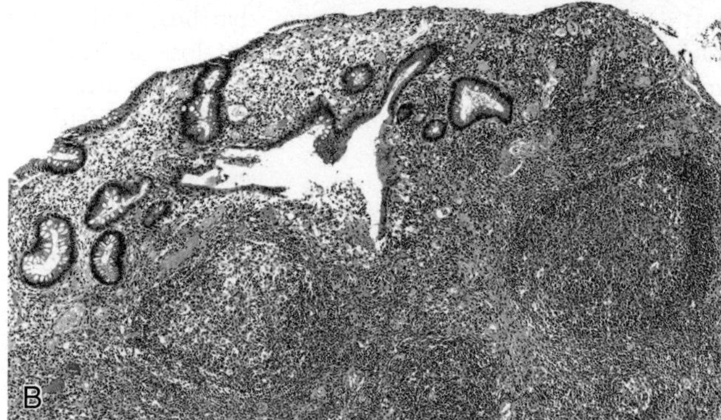

FIGURE 17.78 A, Diversion colitis in a resection specimen from a patient with a Hartmann pouch. Low-power view shows mucosal erosion with enlarged lymphoid aggregates. **B,** High-power view shows mucosal erosion with reactive lymphoid hyperplasia. The reactive follicles often expand the lamina propria and superficial submucosa and cause crypt architectural distortion.

abscesses, villiform surface change, epithelial mucin depletion, Paneth cell metaplasia, and erosions (aphthous ulcers) may also be present. More severe histological changes are more likely to be present in symptomatic patients, but this has never been confirmed scientifically (see Fig. 17.78B). Crypt rupture–associated granulomas and surgery-related changes, such as suture granulomas toward the deep aspect of the bowel wall, are also not uncommon.

Defunctioned segments of bowel in patients with IBD (UC or CD) not uncommonly may also show the effects of diversion of the fecal stream, and these changes may be superimposed on the underlying IBD, depending on the activity level of the latter. In fact, a combination of true diversion colitis and recurrent UC within the same segment of diverted colon may result in the development of a severe form of chronic active colitis that is often accompanied by transmural lymphoid aggregates, fissuring ulcers, and crypt rupture–associated granulomas. These changes can easily be misconstrued as CD.[563] In a long-term follow-up study of patients with IBD and a defunctioned rectum, none of the 22 patients who had a preoperative diagnosis of UC demonstrated granulomas within the diverted segment of bowel.[564]

Differential Diagnosis

Diversion Colitis vs. Recurrent Ulcerative Colitis of a Hartmann Pouch

To differentiate diversion colitis from UC in cases in which a portion of bowel, typically the rectum, is diverted as part of surgical management for the latter condition, it is necessary to know the status of the rectum before surgery to help differentiate residual/recurrent UC from diversion colitis as the principle cause of the patient's new-onset symptoms. Most patients with UC have rectal involvement at disease onset, so it is assumed that the postsurgical (defunctioned) rectum may naturally be susceptible to recurrence of active UC. Diversion colitis is typically associated with prominent follicular lymphoid hyperplasia that is most striking toward the distal aspect of the defunctioned segment of bowel (Table 17.13). In contrast with UC, crypt architectural distortion in diversion colitis is usually minimal and is mainly caused by the presence of enlarged and reactive lymphoid follicles rather than basal lymphoplasmacytosis, which is characteristic of UC. The lymphoplasmacytic inflammatory infiltrate in diversion colitis tends to be restricted to the upper half of the mucosa and is usually minimal or mild in degree. The extent of crypt inflammation is also usually minimal compared with active UC. In some cases, these histological differences are helpful in separating the two processes. However, in most cases, it is difficult, or even impossible, to distinguish recurrent UC in the rectum from active diversion colitis with complete certainty, particularly on the basis of mucosal biopsies only. Furthermore, in some instances, the patient's symptoms may actually reflect a combination of both disease processes occurring at the same time, and this should be taken into consideration when considering the future of management of the patient.

Diversion Colitis vs. Recurrent Crohn's Disease of a Hartmann Pouch

Because new-onset CD specifically limited to a newly created diverted segment of bowel is a highly unlikely event, histological changes reminiscent of diversion colitis in the defunctioned segment of colon must be differentiated from CD only in patients who had CD in the rectum documented before the diversion surgery (see Table 17.13). However, diversion colitis normally shows UC-like, not CD-like features, and the inflammation is usually restricted to the mucosa and upper submucosa. Prominent lymphoid aggregates, basal lymphoplasmacytosis, cryptitis, and Paneth cell metaplasia are common findings as well. Intramucosal crypt rupture–associated granulomas should not be mistaken as definite histological evidence of recurrent CD. Patchy distribution of mucosal and mural changes within the affected segment, presence of deep fissuring ulcers, significant crypt architectural distortion, transmural lymphoid aggregates, and true epithelioid granulomas help support a diagnosis of CD. However, as in mucosal biopsies of the colon in patients without prior surgery, none of the histological features of the mucosa, including the presence or absence of granulomas (unless they are not associated with ruptured crypts), can reliably separate recurrence of CD in the diverted rectum from diversion colitis.

Natural History and Treatment

In most patients, surgical restoration of bowel continuity causes rapid and complete reversal of symptoms and histological abnormalities of diversion colitis within a period of 3 months.[555] If reanastomosis cannot be performed, enemas containing SCFAs are usually administered to reduce

TABLE 17.13 Diversion Colitis vs. Inflammatory Bowel Disease (IBD)

Feature	Ulcerative Colitis	Crohn's Disease	Diversion Colitis
IBD mucosal changes	Present	Present	Present
Crypt atrophy	May be present	May be present	More common
Lymphoid hyperplasia	May be present	Rare	More common
Diffuse disease	May be present	Absent	More common
Previous IBD rectum	Present	Present	Absent
Symptoms decrease on exclusion	Yes	Yes	No
Symptoms decrease on hookup	No	No	Yes
Ulcers	Common	Common	Rare
Focal mild patchy cryptitis	Present	Present	More common

inflammation before restoration of bowel continuity. There is no known risk of cancer in patients with diversion colitis who do not have either UC or CD.

DRUG-INDUCED COLITIS

A wide variety of drugs can result in injury to the colon. In fact, almost every morphological pattern of colitis (e.g., IBD-like, ischemia, microscopic colitis, acute self-limited infectious colitis) can develop as a result of drug toxicity of one kind or another. However, certain specific patterns of injury, such as focal active colitis, apoptotic colitis, isolated erosions or ulcers, strictures, pseudomembranous colitis, and ischemic colitis, in particular, should always arouse suspicion of a drug-induced cause of the patient's colitis. This is why it is vital for pathologists to know the drug history of the patient when evaluating their biopsies or resection specimens before establishing a final diagnosis because there are so many drugs that mimic common types of colonic inflammatory disorders. A more detailed description of drug-induced colitis is provided in Chapter 12. In this chapter, the clinicopathological features of NSAID-related colitis, mycophenolate mofetil (MMF)-associated colitis, immune checkpoint inhibitor–associated colitis, cord blood colitis, fibrosing colonopathy, and the effects of chemotherapy and bowel preparation agents on the colon are discussed in more detail.

Nonsteroidal Antiinflammatory Drug–Associated Colitis

Clinical Features

NSAIDs are used widely for management of acute and chronic pain disorders, and it is not surprising that they are perhaps the most ubiquitous agents associated with drug-related colonic injury. In the United States, almost 20% of the general population uses NSAIDs on a regular basis.[565] Because of the increasing use of nonprescription NSAIDs, the incidence of NSAID-associated colitis is difficult to estimate. NSAID-associated colitis affects older individuals. The clinical presentation varies depending on the severity, location, and duration of injury. Most patients have a history of NSAID consumption for a period of at least 1 month before illness. Some patients become symptomatic within 1 to 2 weeks after high-dose NSAID ingestion.[566] In the acute form of NSAID-related colitis, patients present with bleeding, diarrhea, and iron-deficiency anemia. Stool cultures are usually negative. Rarely, patients have abdominal guarding and tenderness because of bowel perforation at presentation. Prolonged NSAID use is associated with chronic bleeding and, on occasion, intestinal obstruction caused by stricture formation.

Pathogenesis

NSAID-related colitis is believed to be a consequence of increased colonic permeability that occurs after drug ingestion.[567] NSAIDs inhibit cyclooxygenase, a key enzyme that regulates the synthesis of prostaglandin, which plays a major role in maintaining mucosal integrity. Loss of mucosal integrity allows luminal bacteria, bile acids, and food antigens to enter the mucosa and incite an inflammatory response. Thus diarrhea and bleeding associated with acute NSAID-related colitis result from direct mucosal damage.

The laxative-like effect of NSAIDs also contributes to diarrhea. Another possible mechanism for diarrhea is the association of collagenous colitis with NSAID ingestion.[445] It has been postulated that thickening of the subepithelial collagen layer is related to exposure to luminal antigens after loss of mucosal integrity because of NSAID injury.

NSAIDs induce release of vasoconstrictors, such as leukotrienes and proteases, which cause local microvascular endothelial damage.[568,569] In conjunction with inflammatory cytokine–induced vasospasm, NSAID use can also result in an ischemic pattern of mucosal injury that manifests as acute or chronic colitis, the latter often associated with stricture formation.[208]

Pathological Features

Gross Findings

In acute NSAID-related colitis, the colonic mucosa shows patchy erythema, friability, erosions, or ulcers. Ulcers are more common in the right colon than in the left colon. As in the small bowel, chronic NSAID use causes *diaphragm disease* of the colon (Fig. 17.79; see Chapter 12). This is characterized by the presence of multiple, concentric luminal protrusions of fibrotic mucosa and submucosa that occlude the lumen.[570] Some cases are associated with strictures and serosal adhesions.

Microscopic Findings

In acute NSAID-induced colitis, the mucosa may be normal or may show mild crypt architectural distortion and patchy, variable expansion of the lamina propria by mixed inflammatory cells composed of lymphocytes, plasma cells, and eosinophils. Neutrophilic cryptitis, focal erosions, and increased crypt apoptosis are frequent findings (Fig. 17.80).[571] In some cases of NSAID injury, the biopsy reveals

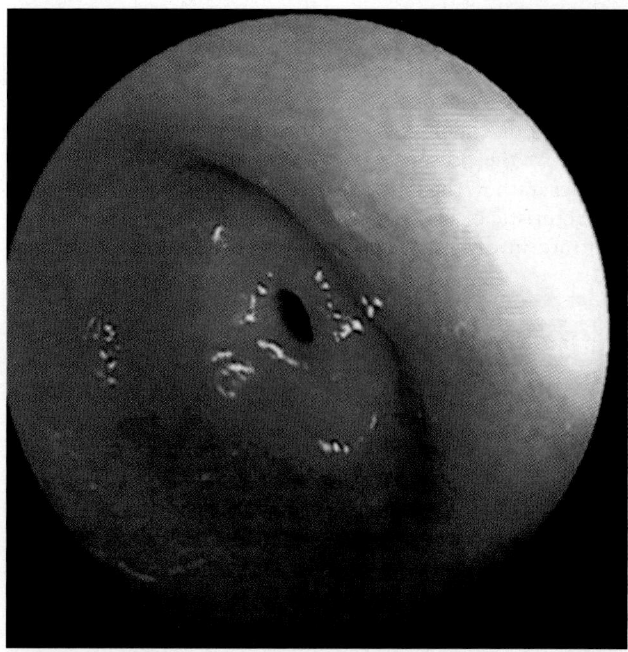

FIGURE 17.79 Endoscopic appearance of colitis related to use of nonsteroidal antiinflammatory drugs (NSAIDs). Concentric, fibrotic thickening of the mucosa and submucosa result in luminal obstruction (diaphragm disease).

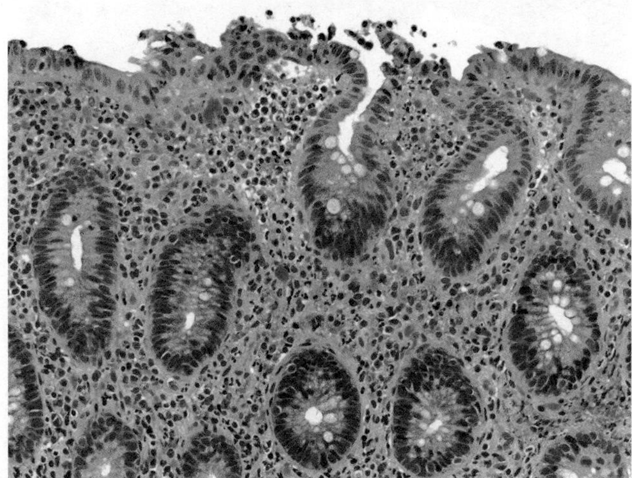

FIGURE 17.80 Acute nonsteroidal antiinflammatory drug colitis. The colonic mucosa shows expansion of the lamina propria by a mixed inflammatory cell infiltrate composed of neutrophils, eosinophils, lymphocytes, and plasma cells. Cases may show a predominance of eosinophils within the lamina propria as well.

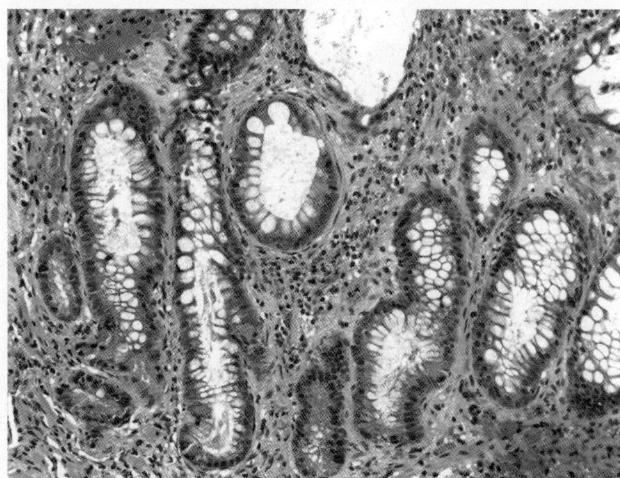

FIGURE 17.81 Chronic nonsteroidal antiinflammatory drug colitis. A biopsy specimen of the descending colon showing crypt architectural distortion, Paneth cell metaplasia, and patchy neutrophilic cryptitis.

an ischemic pattern of injury characterized by lamina propria hyalinization and atrophic crypts. Increased intraepithelial lymphocytes and focal active colitis are some other patterns of mucosal injury associated with NSAIDs (Fig. 17.81). Luminal bands of fibrosis that cause *diaphragm disease* are a rather dramatic and serious chronic complication of NSAID use. These bands are composed of fibrotic mucosa and submucosa that protrude into the lumen of the bowel forming a series of concentric bands that may lead to bowel obstruction. These diaphragms also harbor a variable amount of smooth muscle, nerves, ganglia, and small- to medium-sized blood vessels.

Differential Diagnosis

NSAID-related colitis can mimic many types of colitis, but the most common are ones that mimic acute infectious colitis and IBD. Documentation of NSAID use and exclusion of other causes are key methods to help establish a correct diagnosis. Resolution of symptoms and mucosal changes after cessation of NSAID intake is, ultimately, the only definite way to confirm the diagnosis.

Patients with acute infectious colitis or NSAID-related colitis may have diarrhea and bleeding at presentation. An acute onset of symptoms within hours to days after exposure to a possible infectious agent supports infectious colitis rather than NSAID-related colitis. NSAID-related colitis usually shows a patchier distribution of mucosal injury, fewer neutrophils within the lamina propria, and less prominent neutrophilic cryptitis.

CD may mimic both acute and chronic forms of NSAID-related colitis, and involvement of the small bowel is a common feature of both entities. NSAID-related colitis lacks transmural lymphoid aggregates and epithelioid granulomas that are characteristic of CD, although an isolated case of diclofenac-induced colitis with focal granulomatous inflammation has been reported.[572]

Natural History and Treatment

Therapy for NSAID-related colitis consists of discontinuation of the offending drug, leading to resolution of symptoms and histological abnormalities in most patients. Mucosal ulcers may take months to heal. Because stricture (diaphragm disease) formation is irreversible, endoscopic dilation or surgery is the treatment of choice for patients with this complication.

Mycophenolate Mofetil–Associated Colitis

Clinical Features

MMF is used as an immunosuppressive agent in bone marrow and solid organ transplant recipients as well as in patients with autoimmune disorders such as systemic lupus erythematosus. MMF toxicity produces pathological changes that should be recognized to avoid unnecessary modifications to the patient's immunosuppressive regimen.[573-577]

Almost 50% of patients receiving MMF therapy complain of diarrhea, nausea, vomiting, and abdominal pain. The incidence of bleeding and ulceration ranges from 3% to 8%. Rarely, complications from colonic necrosis or perforation occur.[578] MMF toxicity usually occurs at a dose that ranges between 1000 and 2000 mg per day.

Pathogenesis

In the liver, MMF undergoes conversion to its active metabolite, mycophenolic acid (MPA). MPA inhibits inosine monophosphate dehydrogenase, an enzyme involved in de novo purine synthesis. In addition to its desired inhibitory effect on lymphocyte proliferation, which is highly dependent on purine synthesis, the decreased purine synthesis also affects colonocytes,[578] resulting in decreased crypt epithelial proliferation.[579] MMF effects on the lower GI tract result predominantly from its antimetabolite activity, whereas in the upper GI tract, local mucosal irritation from pill intake also contributes to the epithelial injury.

Pathological Features

In most patients with MMF toxicity, the colonic mucosa shows no endoscopic abnormalities. In a minority of patients, patchy edema, erythema, or aphthous ulcers may be present.

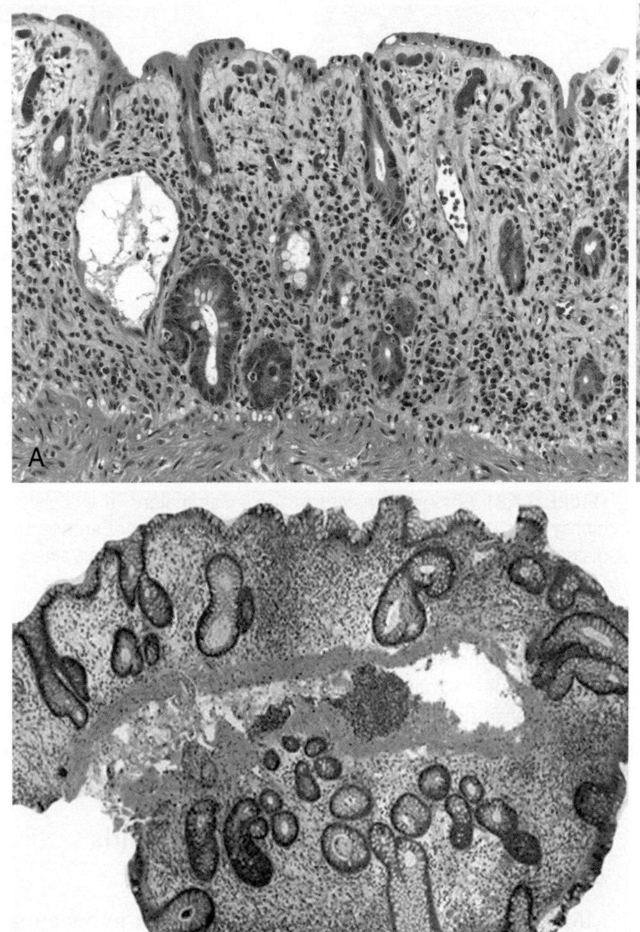
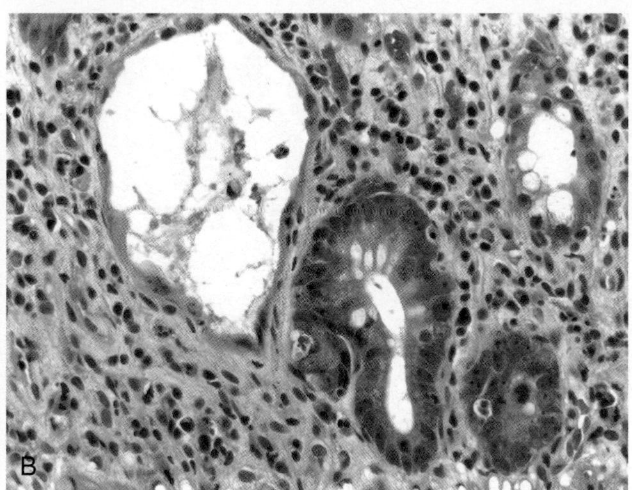

FIGURE 17.82 Mycophenolate mofetil (MMF) colitis. A, The colonic mucosa shows mild crypt architectural distortion, lamina propria edema, and degenerating crypts. The lamina propria usually shows an increase in the number of eosinophils and an increase in the number of crypt apoptotic bodies. **B,** MMF colitis showing degenerated crypts with microcystic change. These crypts contain apoptotic debris and are lined by atrophic epithelium with partial disruption. Notice the crypt apoptotic bodies in adjacent crypts. **C,** Idiopathic inflammatory disease–like pattern of MMF colitis showing crypt architectural distortion, crypt atrophy or loss, and a mild increase in lamina propria chronic inflammatory infiltrate.

Biopsies from patients with MMF toxicity may be completely normal or almost normal (as many as 31%), or they may demonstrate a variety of patterns of injury mimicking IBD, GVHD, acute self-limited colitis, or ischemic colitis.[580] Most commonly, MMF colitis is characterized by the presence of mild crypt architectural distortion, prominent lamina propria edema, increased crypt epithelial apoptosis, mildly increased eosinophils within the lamina propria, and degenerative (hypereosinophilic) crypts (Fig. 17.82A).[581] Degenerated crypts often exhibit microcystic changes and are lined by atrophic epithelium that may show partial disruption and often contain apoptotic cells and apoptotic debris (see Fig. 17.82B). The surface epithelium may reveal regenerative changes as well. Lamina propria edema imparts an empty appearance to the mucosa. Inflammation, when present, is typically composed of patchy neutrophilic infiltrates and prominent eosinophils within the lamina propria, often more than 15 eosinophils per 10 HPFs.[582,583] In some cases of MMF toxicity, there is evidence of crypt architectural distortion, crypt atrophy or loss, Paneth cell metaplasia, and a mild increase in lamina propria chronic inflammatory infiltrate (IBD-like pattern; see Fig 17.82C). Occasionally, the presence of mucosal erosions combined with surface crypt degeneration mimics ischemic colitis.

Differential Diagnosis

In a posttransplantation immunosuppressed patient with a history of diarrhea and consumption of MMF, the main differential diagnosis includes GVHD and infectious colitis, especially CMV-induced colitis. Recurrent episodes of MMF colitis can also mimic IBD.

Differentiation of MMF colitis from GVHD is important because treatment of MMF toxicity requires a reduction in the level of immunosuppression, whereas, depending on the severity of symptoms, GVHD is typically treated with enhanced immunosuppression. MMF colitis is characterized by higher numbers of lamina propria eosinophils, less crypt epithelial apoptosis, less crypt distortion, atrophy, or loss, and an absence of endocrine cell microaggregates in the lamina propria. In one recent study, biopsy specimens from patients with MMF colitis showed fewer lamina propria lymphocytes and crypt apoptotic bodies but significantly more neutrophils and eosinophils than specimens from patients with GVHD. A value of 15 or more eosinophils per 10 HPFs had 100% sensitivity and 67% specificity for a diagnosis of MMF colitis.[582]

CMV colitis is usually associated with prominent crypt epithelial apoptosis and a variable degree of neutrophilic

TABLE 17.14 Common Terminology for Adverse Events: Clinical Grading System for Assessing Severity of Immune Checkpoint Inhibitor–Induced Colitis

Grade	Diarrhea	Colitis
1	Increase of <4 stools/day over baseline	Asymptomatic
2	Increase of >4-6 stools/day over baseline	Abdominal pain, mucous, and blood in the stools
3	Increase of ≥7 stools/day, incontinence, and limiting self-care activities of daily living	Severe pain, fever, peritoneal signs, and ileus
4	Life-threatening consequences (hemodynamic collapse)	Life-threatening consequences (perforation, ischemia, necrosis, bleeding, and toxic megacolon)
5	Death	Death

cryptitis and crypt abscesses. The finding of characteristic intranuclear and intracytoplasmic CMV inclusions is diagnostic of CMV colitis. Immunohistochemistry is a reliable way to confirm CMV infection, especially if viral inclusions are difficult to identify on light microscopy. It is, however, important to note that CMV can develop on a background of MMF (or GVHD) colitis as a superinfection, so the possibility of two simultaneous disorders should always be entertained when confronted with a biopsy specimen containing CMV inclusions.

Unlike IBD, MMF colitis usually lacks significant basal lymphoplasmacytosis, prominent crypt abscesses, and diffuse lymphoplasmacytic infiltrates within the lamina propria. Furthermore, the crypt epithelial changes seen in MMF colitis (dilation with degenerating epithelium and apoptosis) are not typical findings of chronic active IBD.

Natural History and Treatment

Reduction in dosage or discontinuation of the drug is the therapy of choice for MMF colitis. This approach typically leads to reversal of symptoms and tissue injury within a few weeks. In some patients, crypt architectural distortion and atrophy may persist for 12 months.[580]

Immune Checkpoint Inhibitor–Associated Colitis

Clinical Features

Immune checkpoint inhibitors (ICIs) have transformed the treatment landscape in oncology such that they have now become the standard of care for the treatment of numerous types of malignancies. ICIs target immune checkpoints that downregulate cytotoxic T-cell function, thereby promoting their survival and antitumor action. Immune checkpoint proteins cytotoxic T-lymphocyte–associated protein 4 (CTLA-4) and programmed cell death protein 1 (PD-1) are receptors that are expressed on the surface of cytotoxic T cells that interact with their ligands CD80/CD86 (CTLA-4) and programmed death-ligand 1 (PD-L1) for PD-1 on antigen-presenting cells. While enhancing antitumor T-cell activity, ICIs also activate global T-cell responses that induce a variety of immune-related adverse events that include immune-mediated colitis.[584-586] Some of these FDA-approved agents used in clinical oncology include ipilimumab and tremelimumab (anti-CTLA-4); pembrolizumab, nivolumab, and cemiplimab (anti-PD-1); and durvalumab, atezolizumab, and avelumab (anti-PD-L1).

The American Society of Clinical Oncology (ASCO) defines ICI colitis based on clinical symptoms of diarrhea (defined as >3 watery bowel movements a day) and colitis (presence of abdominal pain, rectal bleeding, and mucous in the stools). In 2% to 5% of patients, the symptoms worsen quickly and progress to toxic megacolon, ileus, peritonitis, bowel perforation, and death. Disease severity is graded clinically using the Common Terminology Criteria for Adverse Events (version 5) developed by the National Cancer Institute (Table 17.14).[587] Laboratory blood tests are seldom helpful because the presence of an elevated white blood cell count, increased CRP and ESR levels are nonspecific. In contrast with patient symptoms, which neither correlate with endoscopic findings nor predict response to therapy, endoscopic findings do predict response of enterocolitis to treatment. Therefore endoscopic examination with biopsies is considered the gold standard for diagnosing ICI enterocolitis.[588]

The incidence of ICI is quite variable and depends on the type of drug and dosage. Recent studies describe the incidence of diarrhea as 12.1% to 13.7% for patients treated with anti–PD-1, 30.2% to 35.4% for patients treated with anti–CTLA-4, and 9.4% to 10.6% for those treated with combination therapy.[586,589,590]

Pathogenesis

The pathophysiology of ICI-associated colitis is poorly understood. CTLA-4 plays a critical role in both regulatory T-cell (T_{reg}) function, and in downregulating T-cell responses after activation of naive T cells in the lymph node.[591] This is primarily mediated through binding of CTLA-4 to the costimulatory ligands for CD28, CD80, and CD86. Mouse models have shown that colitis possibly results from inhibition of CTLA-4–dependent T_{reg} function. Interestingly, CTLA-4–associated colitis also shows dose dependency, a finding that is consistent with an incomplete receptor blockade mechanism of action.

PD-1 is a direct inhibitory receptor on T cells, which on binding to its ligands, PD-L1/PD-L2, dephosphorylates multiple signaling proteins downstream of the T-cell receptor and CD28. Experiments in animal models as well as human cancers have shown that the PD-1/PD-L1 pathway downregulates T-cell immunity in the presence of chronic antigen exposure that is either difficult or impossible to clear.[591] In contrast with anti-CTLA4–induced colitis, colitis resulting from PD-(L)1 blockade occurs more variably throughout the treatment course and is more often indolent in nature.

In terms of the type of T-cell infiltrate, anti–PD-1-induced colitis is associated with a higher infiltration of CD8-positive T cells, whereas CD4-positive T cells are more prevalent in patients with CTLA-4–induced colitis. Thus taken together, "hyperactivation" of effector T cells, increased circulating memory T cells, and lymphocytic infiltration of colonic mucosa essentially drive ICI-associated colitis.[592]

Pathological Features

Gross Findings

Although the colon is the most frequently affected site of toxicity, the effects of ICI toxicity can be seen throughout the GI tract as well as the hepatobiliary system.[593] In the majority of patients, the mucosa may show patchy or diffuse erythema, loss of vasculature, edema, friability, exudate, and ulceration. In some cases, cobblestoning either with or without serpiginous ulcers, resembling those in patients with Crohn's colitis, may also be present. In most patients, the entire colon is involved, therefore biopsies from the distal colon and rectum obtained by flexible sigmoidoscopy are usually sufficient for rendering a diagnosis. Nearly 20% to 30% of patients with suspected ICI colitis may show completely unremarkable mucosa. It is recommended that in cases with suspected ICI toxicity, biopsies should be obtained regardless of the endoscopic appearance, especially because ICI colitis can be entirely microscopic.

Microscopic Findings

Histologically, ICI-associated colitis may show a variety of morphological patterns of injury, such as active colitis with prominent apoptosis, microscopic colitis (lymphocytic colitis or collagenous colitis), and an IBD-like chronic active colitis.

Active colitis with prominent apoptosis is the most common histological pattern. It is characterized by expansion of the lamina propria by a mixed inflammatory cell infiltrate composed of neutrophils, eosinophils, lymphocytes, and plasma cells (Fig. 17.83A). Neutrophilic cryptitis and

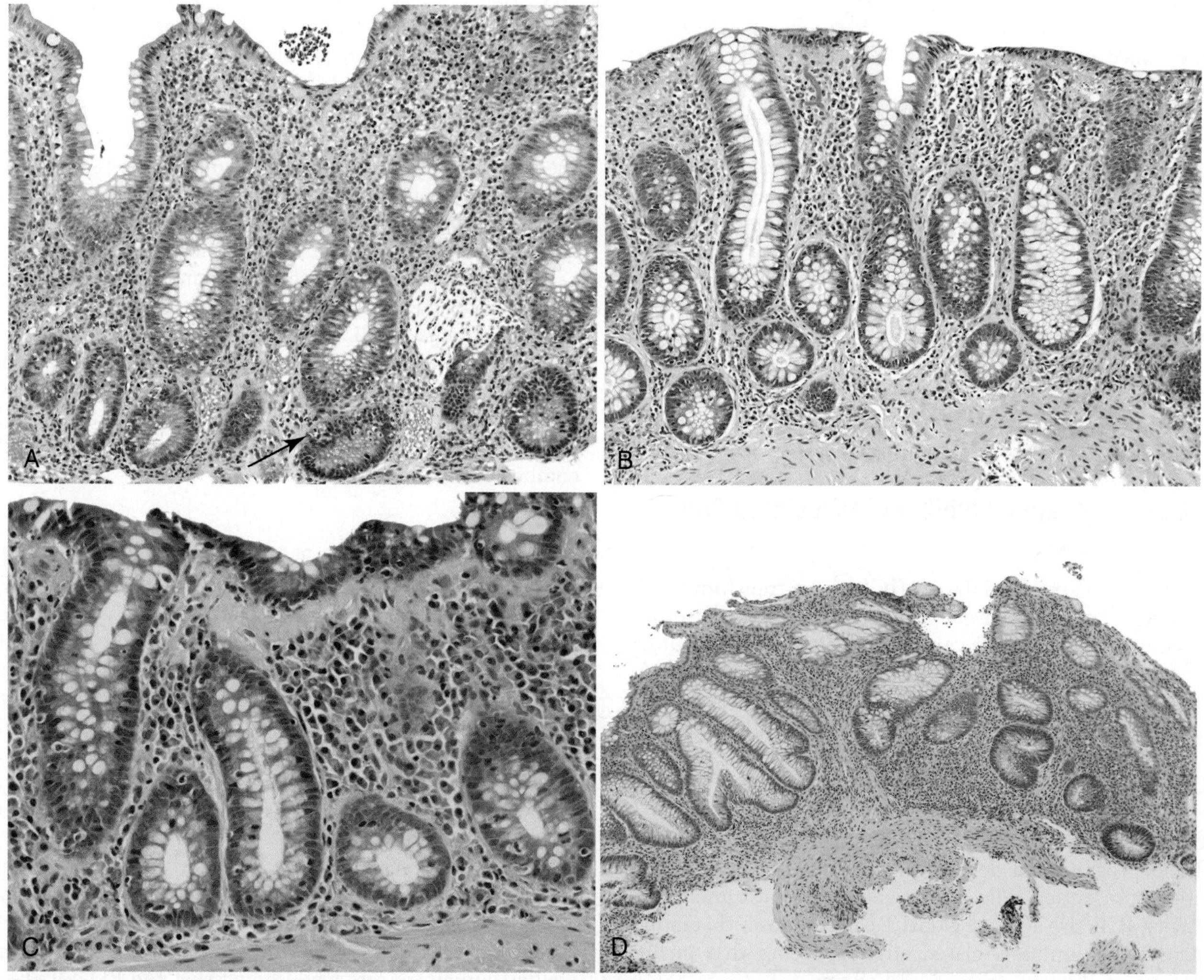

FIGURE 17.83 Immune checkpoint inhibitor–associated colitis. A, Active colitis with prominent apoptosis pattern of immune checkpoint inhibitor (ICI) colitis showing colonic mucosa with erosion, degenerating crypts, crypt abscess formation, and scattered apoptotic activity. Lymphocytic colitis **(B)** and collagenous colitis **(C)** pattern of injury of ICI colitis. This pattern of injury resembles biopsies from patients developing microscopic colitis that is unrelated to ICI therapy. **D,** Idiopathic inflammatory disease–like pattern of ICI colitis showing crypt architectural distortion, crypt atrophy or loss, and increase in lamina propria chronic inflammatory infiltrate that is mostly composed of lymphocytes and plasma cells.

crypt abscesses as well as increased apoptotic activity is common. In this pattern of injury, there may also be a concurrent increase in intraepithelial lymphocytes, both within the crypts as well as within the surface epithelium, but this is only one component of the inflammatory response in contrast with the purer microscopic colitis pattern of injury described later. In more severely injured mucosa, the crypts show attenuated epithelium, often with luminal apoptotic debris. In a recent study consisting of 86 patients with ICI colitis, this "diffuse active colitis" pattern of injury was seen in patients on ipilimumab therapy.[594]

The lymphocytic or collagenous colitis pattern of injury caused by ICI therapy is histologically similar to those that are unrelated to ICI therapy. These patterns of injury have been shown to be more common in patients receiving nivolumab and pembrolizumab.[594] The colonic mucosa shows expansion of the upper half of the lamina propria by a lymphoplasmacytic inflammatory infiltrate. The crypts as well as the surface epithelium show prominent intraepithelial lymphocytosis (see Fig. 17.83B). Thickening of the subepithelial collagen layer with entrapment of inflammatory cells, stromal cells, and capillaries is seen in cases with a collagenous colitis pattern of injury (see Fig. 17.83C). A recent study consisting of 15 patients with ICI-induced microscopic colitis showed that patients who demonstrated a microscopic colitis pattern of injury had an aggressive disease course requiring more steroid therapy and hospitalization compared with cases of microscopic colitis unrelated to ICI therapy.[446]

Finally, the third most common pattern of injury is one that resembles IBD. In this pattern, ICI colitis is characterized by a diffuse expansion of the lamina propria by lymphocytes and plasma cells with crypt architectural distortion and basal plasmacytosis (see Fig. 17.83D). There is usually accompanying neutrophilic cryptitis, either with or without crypt abscesses. Metaplastic changes including Paneth cell metaplasia in the left colon and pyloric gland metaplasia may be present as well.

Much less common patterns of injury include apoptotic colopathy (without active or chronic inflammation) and ischemic colitis. Apoptotic colopathy, resembling GVHD, has been associated with both anti–CTLA-4 and anti–PD-L1 agents, reported in about 20% to 25% of patients with ICI colitis. Rarely, ICI therapy can cause changes similar to those of ischemic colitis. In a series of 17 patients who received anti–PD-1 therapy, an ischemic colitis pattern of injury was observed in 3 patients.[595]

Differential Diagnosis

The differential diagnosis of ICI-associated colitis depends on the predominant pattern of injury. For patients who develop an active colitis pattern of injury, infectious colitis and other concurrent chemotherapy-induced colitides must be considered, especially given that these patients are immunocompromised. In biopsies that show prominent apoptotic activity, CMV colitis and GVHD are also in the differential diagnosis. Microscopic colitis unrelated to ICI therapy is histologically indistinguishable from ICI-related microscopic colitis. Therefore a history of ICI therapy and a temporal association between onset of clinical symptoms and administration of therapy is most helpful in confirming a diagnosis of ICI colitis.

Naturally, the chronic active colitis pattern of injury caused by ICI colitis mimics IBD clinically, endoscopically, and histologically. In fact, there are reports of patients developing IBD following ICI therapy.[596,597] Recent studies have also shown that ICI therapy exacerbates symptoms of colitis in patients with preexisting IBD.[598,599] It is unclear whether ICI colitis causes additional dysregulation in the epithelial barrier function and excessive immune activation in patients who are predisposed to developing IBD. Therefore, ultimately, clinical history is most helpful in distinguishing IBD-like colitis caused by ICI therapy from new-onset or primary IBD.

Natural History and Treatment

Most patients with grade 1 diarrhea are treated symptomatically. For patients with colitis and systemic symptoms, such as fever, tachycardia, and dehydration, the first step is to discontinue the drug. Because anti–CTLA-4 agents are associated with a higher incidence of recurrent colitis, these agents are often permanently discontinued. Systemic corticosteroids followed by a steroid taper are the first-line therapy and have been reported to be effective in nearly 88% of patients.[600] Anti–PD-1/L1 agents are generally resumed as monotherapy once symptoms resolve or improve to grade 1 diarrhea. Some patients develop steroid-refractory disease, in which case, other agents such as infliximab and vedolizumab are added to the treatment regimen.

Cord Colitis Syndrome

Cord colitis syndrome was recently described in a series of 11 patients who underwent cord-blood hematopoietic stem cell transplantation (HSCT) for hematopoietic disorders such as leukemia, myelodysplastic syndrome, non-Hodgkin's lymphoma, Hodgkin's lymphoma, aplastic anemia, and myeloproliferative disorder. It is defined as persistent diarrheal illness (>7 days duration) in a patient who received cord-blood HSCT, that is not caused by acute GVHD, bacterial (including C. *difficile*) or viral infection, posttransplantation lymphoproliferative disease, or any other identifiable etiology on microbiological and histopathological examination.[601] The pathogenesis of this entity is unknown. The prevailing hypothesis is that it is likely bacterial in origin because patients respond well to antibacterial therapy. In a follow-up study by the authors who described this entity, shotgun DNA sequencing on four colon biopsy specimens obtained from two patients with cord colitis revealed 2.5 million sequencing reads that were then computationally assembled into a 7.65-Mb draft genome. This bacterial draft genome was found to have a high degree of homology with genomes of bacteria in the Bradyrhizobium genus, thus indicating that *Bradyrhizobium enterica* (provisional name of the bacterium) may be associated with this syndrome.[602]

In a study consisting of 104 patients who received cord-blood HSCT, 10.6% were diagnosed with this condition. Patients developed watery, nonbloody diarrhea 3 to 12 months after transplantation.[601] There were no associations with demographic factors, the type of primary hematological disease, or the type or dose of conditioning or GVHD treatment regimens. Cord colitis syndrome was more likely to develop in patients with a history of grade 2 (or higher)

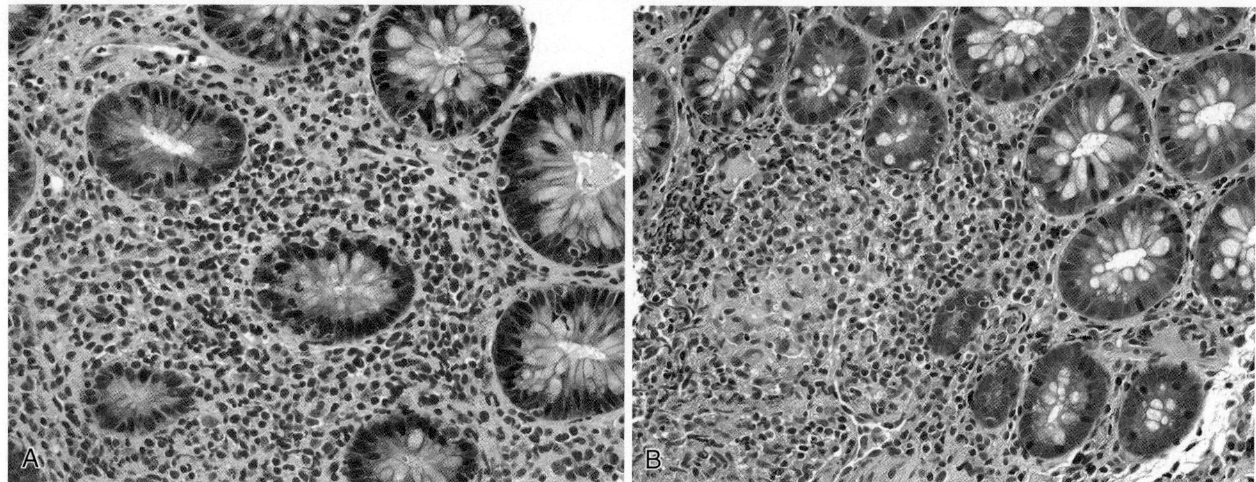

FIGURE 17.84 Cord colitis syndrome. A, The colonic mucosa shows expansion of the lamina propria by a mixed inflammatory infiltrate composed of lymphocytes and plasma cells. Crypt apoptosis is a frequent finding in these cases and may mimic grade 1 graft-versus-host disease. **B,** The biopsy shows loose epithelioid granulomas within the lamina propria. (*Courtesy Dr. Jason Hornick, Brigham and Women's Hospital, Boston, MA.*)

acute GVHD compared with those with grade 1 GVHD, or an absence of GVHD. Radiological imaging showed colonic wall thickening, either diffuse or focal, in most patients.

Grossly, the colon may reveal mucosal erythema, edema, and ulcers. Frank pseudomembrane formation was not present in any of the reported cases. Pathologically, mucosal biopsy specimens show a nonspecific chronic active colitis pattern of injury (i.e., mild crypt architectural distortion, neutrophilic cryptitis, and Paneth cell metaplasia). The lamina propria, in all cases, shows a mixed inflammatory cell infiltrate composed of lymphocytes, plasma cells, and histiocytes. The surface epithelium shows general degenerative changes, including flattening and mucin depletion. A mild increase in crypt epithelial apoptosis, similar to that observed in grade 1 GVHD, is a characteristic finding observed in 73% of reported patients (Fig. 17.84A). Crypt rupture–associated granulomas were more common than well-formed epithelioid granulomas (see Fig. 17.84B).

The main differential diagnosis of cord colitis syndrome is acute GVHD. Unlike cord colitis syndrome, acute GVHD usually does not exhibit increased plasma cells in the lamina propria, prominent neutrophilic crypt injury, Paneth cell metaplasia, or granulomas.[603,604]

Cord colitis syndrome responds well to antibacterial therapy (typically fluoroquinolone and metronidazole). Because discontinuation of therapy may lead to relapse, these patients often require prolonged medical treatment.

Fibrosing Colonopathy

Clinical Features

Fibrosing colonopathy is a distinct clinicopathological entity that was first described in 1994 in patients with cystic fibrosis in whom colonic strictures developed while they were consuming high-strength pancreatic enzymes (typically 24,000 to 50,000 U of lipase per kilogram per day).[605-607]

The condition was initially described in children ranging from 9 months to 15 years of age. Rare cases have since been described in adults.[608] All patients had a history of high-strength pancreatic enzyme therapy for a period of 12 to 18 months before clinical diagnosis. Abdominal pain, nausea, and vomiting related to intestinal obstruction is the typical clinical presentation. Some patients develop diarrhea, ascites, constipation, severe anorexia, and weight loss. Radiological examination (barium enema) in patients with suspected fibrosing colonopathy usually reveals colonic strictures, shortening of the ascending colon, and abnormal haustra.

Pathogenesis

The pathogenesis of fibrosing colonopathy is poorly understood. It has been postulated that impacted viscid fecal material and entrapped enzyme pellets cause pressure necrosis of the mucosa. Direct toxicity from exposure to high concentrations of pancreatic enzymes and altered luminal fatty acids may also contribute to epithelial injury. Proteolytic and lipolytic enzymes are believed to play a role in the development of fibrosis in this condition.

Pathological Features

Gross Findings

The disorder usually affects the right colon initially, followed by the transverse colon. The sigmoid colon and rectum are usually spared, but in rare cases, the condition may affect the entire colon.[609,610] The mucosal surface may demonstrate a cobblestone appearance with patchy surface erosions. Segmental thickening of the colonic wall is characteristic.

Microscopic Findings

Fibrosing colonopathy is characterized by dense fibrosis of the lamina propria and submucosa (Fig. 17.85A). The submucosa often demonstrates keloid-like bands of collagen. Fibrosis extends to the inner circular layer of the muscularis propria. In some cases, both the inner and outer layers of the muscularis propria are completely attenuated and replaced by fibrous tissue.[606] Repeated episodes of mucosal injury cause fraying or complete disintegration of the smooth muscle fibers of the muscularis mucosae. This leads to loss of demarcation of the mucosa and submucosa.

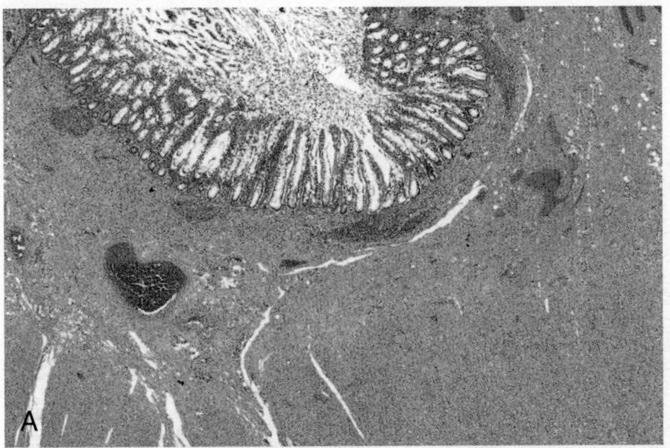

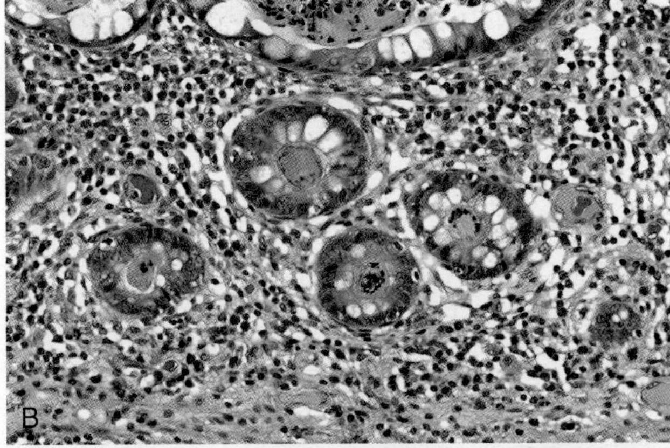

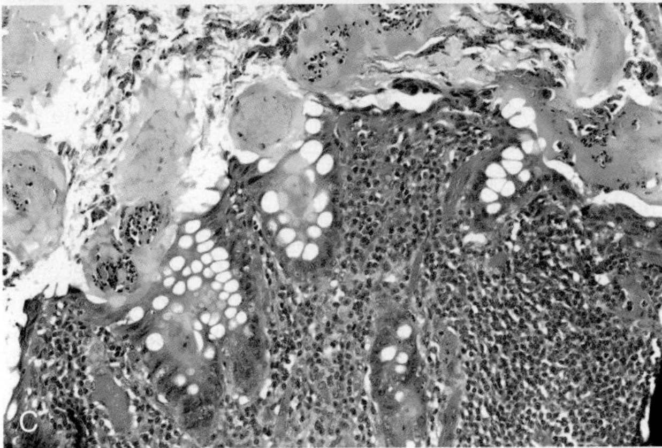

FIGURE 17.85 Fibrosing colonopathy. A, Colon resection specimen shows prominent fibrosis of the lamina propria and submucosa. In some cases, the fibrosis extends into the muscularis propria as well. **B,** Fibrosing colonopathy in a patient with history of cystic fibrosis. Mucosal sample shows colonic crypts with inspissated mucin and neutrophilic injury. **C,** Often, a large amount of mucin is seen overlying the surface epithelium.

The mucosa shows patchy neutrophilic cryptitis and crypt abscesses. Crypt architectural distortion is usually caused by fibrosis of the lamina propria. Some of the crypts may show inspissated mucus within their lumen (see Fig. 17.85B–C). Most cases of fibrosing colonopathy demonstrate a prominent eosinophilic and mast cell infiltrate within all layers of the bowel wall.[606,611] Eosinophil counts range from 26 to 164 per HPF.[606] Additionally, one may find aggregates of morphologically normal ganglion cells toward the basal aspect of the mucosa.

Differential Diagnosis

The young age at presentation, presence of strictures, and preferential involvement of the right colon mimic CD. Although fibrosing colonopathy is associated with mural fibrosis, other pathognomonic features of CD, such as epithelioid granulomas and transmural lymphoid aggregates, are typically absent in this condition.[607]

Fragmentation of muscle fibers and replacement of the submucosa by fibrous tissue mimics colonic involvement by scleroderma. However, scleroderma characteristically demonstrates degenerative changes (cytoplasmic vacuolation, eosinophilia) in the muscle fibers, thickening of the blood vessels, and serosal fibrosis. Clinical information regarding extra-GI manifestations of scleroderma is also helpful.

Hollow visceral myopathy is a muscle disorder that affects both children and adults. Patients usually have chronic intestinal pseudo-obstruction as a presenting symptom. In contrast with fibrosing colonopathy, the bowel wall in hollow visceral myopathy typically shows dilation and thinning. Muscle cell degeneration, muscle cell loss, and fibrosis of the muscularis propria are characteristic changes in hollow visceral myopathy. These changes affect either the circular or the longitudinal layers of muscularis propria, smooth muscle cells of the blood vessels, and the muscularis mucosae. Unlike fibrosing colonopathy, the cytoplasm of myocytes in this condition is vacuolated or rarified, and the boundaries of the smooth muscle cells are often indistinct. Extensive fibrous replacement of both layers of muscularis propria in advanced hollow visceral myopathy can resemble fibrosing colonopathy. At that stage, a clinical history of pancreatic enzyme supplement therapy is the only way to reliably distinguish these two disorders.

The presence of dense hyalinization of the submucosa and muscularis propria in fibrosing colonopathy can mimic amyloidosis. Amyloid deposits characteristically have a homogenous, hyaline quality on hematoxylin and eosin (H&E) stain. They are usually present between muscle fibers and in the walls of blood vessels. A positive reaction with Congo red stain and demonstration of apple-green birefringence on polarization is helpful in distinguishing amyloidosis from fibrosing colonopathy.

Natural History and Treatment

Because this condition is related to high-dose pancreatic enzyme therapy, a U.S. consensus committee recommended that therapeutic doses be restricted to less than 2500 U of lipase/kg/meal to avoid this complication.[612] In patients who develop symptoms of intestinal obstruction, surgical resection remains the main form of therapy.

CHEMOTHERAPY-ASSOCIATED COLONIC INJURY

A multitude of chemotherapeutic agents cause injury to the GI tract. The most common drugs are antimetabolites, such as 5-flurouracil (5-FU), leucovorin, mitomycin, cisplatin, and methotrexate. Within a few hours to several days after exposure to chemotherapeutic agents, patients complain of abdominal pain, nausea, vomiting, and diarrhea. Severe diarrhea occurs in 15% to 20% of patients who receive leucovorin or 5-FU. Methotrexate ingestion can result in severe

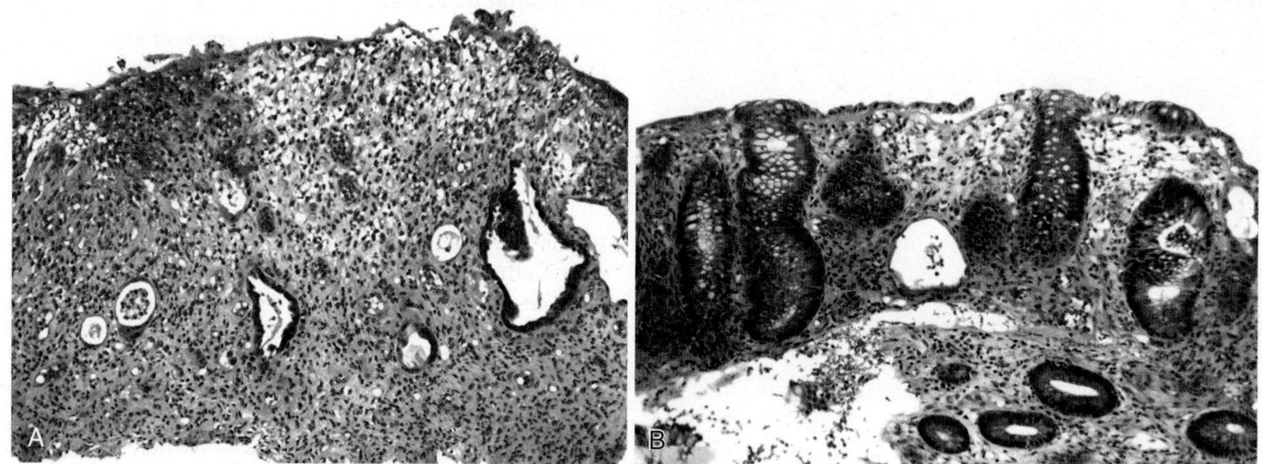

FIGURE 17.86 Colitis secondary to induction chemotherapy in a patient with acute leukemia. A, This biopsy specimen shows almost complete loss of crypts and crypts in different phases of degeneration. The lamina propria shows marked edema and focal hemorrhage but without prominent neutrophils. **B,** Another area of colonic mucosa from the same patient shows patchy crypt destruction, increased apoptosis, and crypt regenerative changes.

complications, such as toxic megacolon. Chemotherapy also predisposes to the development of mucosal infections, neutropenic enterocolitis, and pseudomembranous colitis (caused by C. *difficile* infection). These disorders are discussed in Chapter 4.

Because systemic chemotherapy targets rapidly dividing cells, colonocytes are severely affected (see Chapter 12). The proliferation zone of crypts is the initial target of insult. Specific agents, such as 5-FU, cause an ischemic pattern of injury caused by vasoconstriction resulting from activation of protein kinase C and the coagulation cascade.[613]

Pathologically, colonic mucosa may show mucosal erosions and ulcers acutely. The colon tends to be less severely affected than the remainder of the GI tract. Chemotherapy effects in the colon have been best characterized in patients who have received 5-FU. In this condition, crypt epithelial cells demonstrate loss of nuclear polarity, pyknosis, and apoptosis (Fig. 17.86A). Dilated crypts with intraluminal apoptotic debris are a frequent finding (see Fig. 17.86B). On occasion, the degree of cytological atypia may be severe enough to mimic dysplasia. In these cases, crypt epithelial cells show voluminous, vacuolated cytoplasm and markedly enlarged, hyperchromatic nuclei, but with a normal or low N:C ratio. These changes are often associated with neutrophilic cryptitis and expansion of the lamina propria by lymphocytes, plasma cells, and eosinophils. In fact, in chemotherapy toxicity, it is common to see markedly regenerating crypts located side by side to atrophic and degenerating crypts, and this feature helps distinguish drug effect from other conditions, such as ischemia. Similar to crypt epithelial cells, the stromal cells may also show "bizarre" nuclear changes. During the resolution phase, the crypt epithelium often appears hyperplastic and regenerative.

EFFECTS OF BOWEL PREPARATION AGENTS

Enema solutions containing bisacodyl (Dulcolax), hydrogen peroxide, or hypertonic solutions (e.g., monobasic and dibasic sodium phosphate preparations) are bowel preparation agents that can adversely affect colonic mucosa.[369,614] Soap-containing enemas usually cause diarrhea and rectal bleeding.

Colonic damage presumably occurs by a direct effect of the chemical agent on the mucosa or by its detergent action on epithelial cells. Saline enemas and oral hypertonic solutions generally cause mucosal damage by precipitating withdrawal of water from the mucosal surface.

The mucosal surface characteristically shows erythema and slight friability, often with obliteration of the vascular pattern.[615,616] Occasionally, aphthous ulcers develop. The surface epithelium may show a flattened appearance. Lamina propria edema is common. In some cases, the surface epithelium becomes stripped away from the underlying lamina propria. Extravasated red blood cells may be seen in the lamina propria (see Figs. 17.1 and 17.2). With longer time intervals between enema and endoscopy, the changes may become even more pronounced. If the patient received an enema more than 18 to 24 hours before endoscopy, neutrophils may infiltrate the mucosa as well. Mucosal erosions and even aphthous ulcers, mimicking CD, may be present if the enema contains soap or hydrogen peroxide.[614]

Oral sodium phosphate solutions are specifically associated with surface epithelial vacuolization and detachment of the surface epithelium from the underlying basement membrane, which imparts a "hobnail-like" appearance to the epithelium. Foci of cryptitis and apoptosis may also be present.[369,614] Bisacodyl causes more severe changes, including a pale and vacuolated appearance of both the surface and crypt epithelium.

Bowel preparation artifact may mimic ASLC, CD, or GVHD. In contrast with ASLC, bowel preparation–related changes usually do not cause significant epithelial damage, are often accompanied by prominent lamina propria edema, and demonstrate less neutrophilic epithelial injury.

The presence of aphthous ulcers and cryptitis can mimic CD. However, a clinical history of prolonged diarrhea and bleeding and lack of cytological changes of vacuolation and epithelial detachment in the latter entity are helpful in distinguishing these conditions.

Grade 1 GVHD can be difficult to distinguish from bowel preparation–related changes because oral sodium phosphate preparations are also associated with increased apoptosis.[369] However, apoptotic bodies in GVHD are typically located within the basal compartment of the crypts, whereas apoptotic bodies related to bowel preparation are usually confined to the surface epithelium.[573]

Because colonic epithelium normally regenerates within 5 to 7 days, the changes associated with bowel preparation artifact usually disappear within this time frame. Enemas containing hypertonic solutions have the potential to cause severe water and electrolyte disturbances that can precipitate acute renal failure in patients with other comorbidities[617] (see Chapters 1 and 12 for further details).

EFFECTS OF MUCOSAL PROLAPSE IN THE COLON

Mucosal prolapse syndrome is a distinct clinical and pathological entity that affects any portion of the colon. In the anorectal region, this term is synonymous with *SRUS* (see later). However, localized areas of mucosal prolapse are quite common in the colon, particularly in older patients. For instance, depending on the location and severity of mucosal prolapse, lesions may manifest in the form of polypoid mucosal elevations, either with or without ulceration. These lesions include inflammatory cloacogenic polyps, rectal prolapse, inflammatory cap polyps, inflammatory myoglandular polyps, and even localized colitis or proctitis cystica profunda.[618-620] All of these disorders share similar pathological features because they all develop as a result of chronic mucosal prolapse.

Solitary Rectal Ulcer Syndrome

Clinical Features

The earliest documentation of SRUS dates back to 1830 when Cruveilhier reported four unusual cases of rectal ulcers that were all localized to the anterior wall of the rectum.[621] However, the term *solitary ulcer of the rectum* was first coined by Lloyd-Davis in the 1930s. It was not until 1969 that this condition became well recognized, when Madigan and Morson published a detailed review of 68 cases outlining the histopathological features.[622] Finally, Rutter and Riddle further refined and linked the pathogenesis of this entity to rectal prolapse.[623] SRUS is now considered a distinct clinicopathological entity that occurs as a consequence of compromised blood flow to the rectum leading to localized ischemia and ulceration.

The prevalence of SRUS is quite low (1 to 3.6 per 100,000 per year).[624] Patients with SRUS typically have a long history of chronic constipation and strenuous defecation. Rectal bleeding, mucus discharge, and pain with defecation are common presenting symptoms. The condition has been reported in both adults and children. SRUS is slightly more common in younger adults between 30 and 40 years of age, but almost 25% of patients are older than 60 years of age at clinical presentation.[625]

Pathogenesis

Mucosal prolapse may occur, to some minor degree, in the anorectal region in patients who strain excessively during defecation. However, in patients with SRUS, it is believed that malfunction of the puborectalis muscle specifically leads to excessive straining during defecation, which then manifests as injury to the rectal mucosa.[623] In fact, paradoxical contraction of pelvic floor muscles (puborectalis syndrome or pelvic outlet syndrome) causes increased pressure within the rectum and anal canal, which also contributes to the development of SRUS.[626] In older patients, this is further precipitated by loss of muscle tone, which affects the levator ani muscles. Chronic straining during defecation results in elongation of the muscle attachments from the rectum to the sacrum, which leads to the descending perineum syndrome. Increased mobility of the rectum allows for internal rectal prolapse, which is a form of intussusception. Internal prolapse then causes stretching of the submucosal blood vessels and subsequent ischemia, particularly at points in the mucosa subjected to the most intense pressures. Thus the inflammatory changes, including the development of ulcers, and polyps in SRUS represent the sequela of ischemia, particularly at the most traumatized "lead points" of the internally prolapsed mucosa. Ulcers may also result from direct pressure necrosis caused by fecal impaction within the anal canal. Anatomically, shearing of rectal mucosa most commonly occurs on the anterior rectal wall, typically located 10 to 15 cm above the anal verge, where there is a sharp bend in the rectum as the latter dips into the pelvis. This actually also corresponds to the location of the puborectalis muscle sling, which usually fails to relax in patients with chronic constipation. The chronic and recurrent nature of this illness ultimately leads to repeated bouts of ulceration and repair, eventually resulting in polyp formation and fibromuscular hyperplasia of the mucosa, which is so characteristic of this condition pathologically. When prolapse occurs at the level of the anal verge, an inflammatory cloacogenic polyp may develop, but the latter can certainly occur in patients without the full SRUS.[627] Similar-appearing polypoid lesions may occur in other parts of the colon subjected to mucosal prolapse, such as areas of colon involved by diverticular disease, or surrounding ileostomy or colostomy sites.

Pathological Features

Gross Findings

SRUS is somewhat of a misnomer because, depending on the phase of disease, an ulcer may not necessarily be present, and lesions may, in fact, be multiple. The most common location of pathological changes is the anterior wall of the rectum, anywhere between 4 and 10 cm proximal to the anal verge.[623] Multiple lesions are present in up to 30% of patients.[622] Pathological features consist of polyps (25%), ulcers (21%), or both. In some cases, patchy foci of granular, hyperemic mucosa (18%) may be the only visible abnormality.[628] Ulcers usually range from 0.5 to 4 cm in diameter. In some cases, the base of the ulcer may be indurated, resembling a neoplasm.

Microscopic Findings

The earliest histological changes of SRUS consist of surface ischemic-type erosions or ulcers, often combined with thickening of the subepithelial collagen layer. Characteristic findings in the mucosa include the presence of fibromuscular hyperplasia of the lamina propria, which consists of hyperplastic smooth muscle fibers that extend luminally from the muscularis mucosae, which itself may appear thickened, hypertrophic, and splayed (Fig. 17.87A–B). Vascular congestion, hemorrhage, and edema are also common manifestations of prolapse. The crypts show dilation and elongation, and the epithelium typically reveals regenerative and degenerative changes such as hyperplastic or serrated contour and mucin depletion (see Fig. 17.87C). As mentioned earlier, the superficial mucosa often shows features of ischemia, characterized by necrosis, the presence of atrophic and withered-appearing crypts, and lamina propria hyalinization. The anal squamous mucosa is usually acanthotic and hyperkeratotic.

In long-standing SRUS, repeated mucosal trauma and repair may result in misplacement of the cystically dilated and injured crypts into the superficial submucosa, or sometimes even deeper into the bowel wall. This condition is referred to as *colitis cystica polyposa/profunda*. This phenomenon is most commonly seen in polyps. The misplaced glands show a lobular arrangement and are surrounded by lamina propria elements that may show evidence of trauma in the form of hemosiderin-laden macrophages or extravasated mucin from ruptured glands. The glandular epithelium often shows regenerative epithelial changes in the form of slight nuclear hyperchromasia and mucin loss (see Colitis Cystica Polyposa/Profunda).

Differential Diagnosis

Depending on the morphological appearance of the lesion (ulcer vs. polypoid lesion), the differential diagnosis for SRUS ranges from CD to adenomatous or serrated polyps, Peutz-Jeghers polyps, and even invasive adenocarcinoma (Table 17.15).

Unlike SRUS, ulcerated lesions in CD characteristically lack fibromuscular hyperplasia of the lamina propria and ischemic-type superficial mucosal necrosis. The findings of epithelioid granulomas, Paneth cell metaplasia, and basal lymphoplasmacytosis are helpful in supporting a diagnosis of CD.

On occasion, reactive changes in SRUS can be severe and may resemble dysplasia or the surface of an adenoma. However, because the epithelium is reactive and not neoplastic in SRUS, it shows surface maturation, lack of atypical mitoses, and nonabrupt changes with the surrounding nonatypical epithelium.

Serrated hyperplastic features of crypt epithelium in SRUS may also raise the possibility of a primary serrated

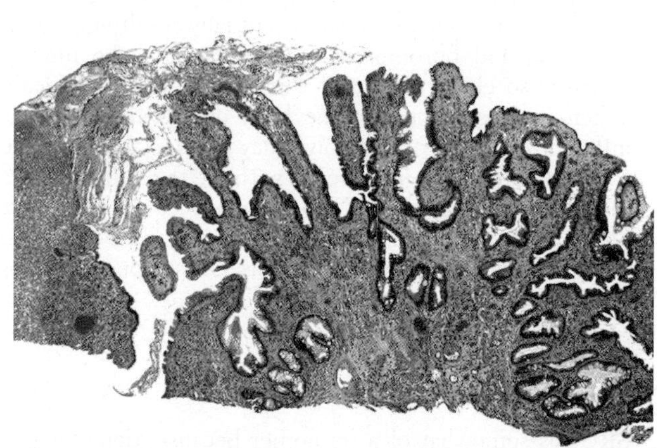

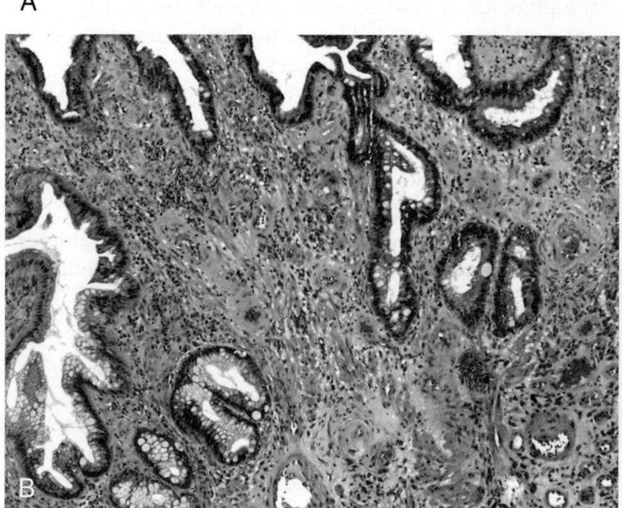

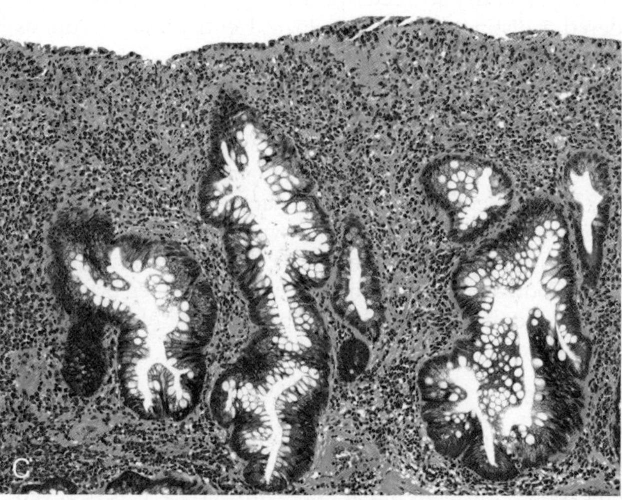

FIGURE 17.87 A, Solitary rectal ulcer syndrome (SRUS), or mucosal prolapse, shows ulcerated mucosa with villiform surface architecture. Crypt dilation, branching, regeneration, and hyperplasia of crypt epithelium are seen. Notice the presence of fibromuscular hyperplasia of the lamina propria. **B,** Higher magnification shows lamina propria edema, actively inflamed granulation tissue, and characteristic fibromuscular proliferation within the lamina propria. **C,** SRUS (mucosal prolapse) shows dilation and elongation of crypts with epithelial changes that range from mucin depletion to a hyperplastic or serrated appearance.

TABLE 17.15 Differential Diagnosis of Solitary Rectal Ulcer Syndrome/Mucosal Prolapse

Feature	SRUS/Mucosal Prolapse	Crohn's Disease	Adenomatous/ Serrated Polyp	Peutz-Jeghers Polyp	Invasive Adenocarcinoma
Crypt architecture	Distorted with dilated and branching crypts; serrations are typically restricted to the upper half of the crypt	Distorted	Crowded crypts with or without branching; when serrated, the serrated changes extend to the basal aspect of the crypts	Distorted with lobular glandular architecture	Distorted with angulated and infiltrative pattern
Expansion of lamina propria by lymphocytes and plasma cells	Absent	Present, typically basal lymphoplasmacytosis	May be present	Absent	Not applicable
Prominent eosinophils within lamina propria	Absent	May be present	May be present	May be present	Not applicable
Fibromuscular replacement of lamina propria with smooth muscle fibers separating individual crypts	Present	Absent	May be present in large lesion	Absent; smooth muscle fibers usually surround groups of glands arranged in a lobular configuration	Not applicable
Ischemic mucosal changes	Common	Absent	Absent	Absent	Absent
Epithelial "atypia"	Present, common, (reactive atypia may mimic dysplasia)	May be present (reactive or dysplasia)	Present	Present (usually reactive atypia)	Present
Stromal desmoplasia	Absent	Absent	Absent	Absent	Present
Transmural lymphoid aggregates, granulomas	Absent	Present	Absent	Absent	Absent

SRUS, Solitary rectal ulcer syndrome.

polyp, such as a hyperplastic polyp or sessile serrated lesion, or even a traditional serrated adenoma. However, the hyperplastic changes in polypoid mucosal prolapse are typically restricted to the upper half of the crypts and are located adjacent to foci of mucosal ulceration. In true serrated polyps, the epithelial changes are uniformly present throughout, and unless the entire hyperplastic polyp has "prolapsed," fibromuscular hyperplasia is extremely unusual.

As many as one-third of hamartomatous polyps in Peutz-Jeghers syndrome arise in the rectum.[629] Sporadic Peutz-Jeghers polyps have also been documented.[630] In contrast with Peutz-Jeghers polyps in the small bowel, those that arise in the colorectum usually show a less well-developed arborizing pattern of smooth muscle fibers. However, unlike in SRUS, in which smooth muscle and fibrous tissue (often with inflammation) separates individual glands or crypts, the muscle fibers in Peutz-Jeghers polyps separate groups of glands, which leads to lobulation of the glandular architecture, and inflammation, ulceration, and reactive ischemia-like changes are not a normal feature of the former. Additionally, a family history of polyps, presence of mucocutaneous pigmentation, and association with other neoplasms (breast, ovarian, cervical) are helpful in excluding Peutz-Jeghers syndrome.

Misplacement of epithelium in SRUS (localized colitis cystica profunda [CCP]) can be difficult to distinguish from invasive adenocarcinoma. The mucin-filled cysts in SRUS are typically arranged in a lobular configuration and are lined by either regenerating or normal colonic epithelium. They are characteristically surrounded by a discrete rim of lamina propria (except in older cysts) along with foci of extravasated mucin, hemorrhage, or hemosiderin. The lining epithelium may appear atypical as a result of reactive mucin loss. Lack of a stromal desmoplastic response and cytological atypia favor a diagnosis of SRUS instead of invasive adenocarcinoma (see Colitis Cystica Polyposa/Profunda). Additionally, invasive adenocarcinoma usually shows an irregular, angulated glandular profile, which is quite distinct from the lobulated growth pattern of misplaced epithelium.

Natural History and Treatment

Surgical excision is the therapy of choice for polypoid lesions related to SRUS. In cases with extensive rectal prolapse, rectopexy is performed. In addition, supportive measures such as increase in the intake of dietary fiber and bowel-training programs provide some benefit. Despite surgical treatment, recurrence of SRUS has been documented in as many as 15% of cases.[614]

Colitis Cystica Polyposa/Profunda

Clinical Features

Colitis cystica polyposa/profunda is a rare pathological reaction pattern characterized by the presence of misplaced epithelium, cysts, or both within the submucosa and in some cases also within the deeper aspects of the bowel wall, including the muscularis propria and even the serosa. CCP was first described by Stark in 1766.[631] In 1863, Virchow reported a patient with submucosal cysts that presented as multiple polypoid lesions and coined the term *colitis cystica polyposa*.[632] However, it was not until 1957 that the term *colitis cystica profunda* was first used to separate this condition from colitis cystica superficialis, a condition characterized by cyst formation restricted to the mucosal layer (as opposed to colitis cystica profunda, where the cysts are located below the muscularis mucosae) in patients with pellagra.[633,634]

CCP develops most commonly in patients with a history of chronic inflammation or trauma, such as UC, CD, radiation injury, SRUS, certain chronic infections (such as *Shigella*), and also surrounding surgical anastomoses and stomas. Rarely, CCP may develop in association with colonic intussusception, diverticulitis,[635] mucosal trauma related to spinal cord injury,[636] or IBS. It may also manifest as a solitary lesion in an apparently completely normal colon, but this is very rare.[637,638] Patients usually report passage of blood or mucus in stools, either with or without abdominal pain and diarrhea. CCP can affect individuals of any age, but patients are commonly between 4 to 68 years of age. The condition is more common in men than in women (F:M ratio as low as 1:7).[633] Radiological evaluation can be misleading because thickening of the bowel wall with filling defects and prominent mucosal folds may be misinterpreted as a neoplastic process.

Pathogenesis

Chronic and often repetitive mucosal damage is a common feature among all conditions that lead to the development of CCP. Originally, CCP was considered to be a congenital malformation.[639] This theory was supported by the fact that CCP is often diagnosed in young adults and children as well as in those with congenital disorders such as Peutz-Jeghers syndrome.

The currently accepted theory is that the condition represents an acquired regenerative phenomenon in response to chronic and repeated mucosal injury. It has been postulated that within areas of mucosal ulceration, failure of the muscularis mucosae to heal completely allows portions of the mucosa to gain access ("herniate") into the submucosa. If the original injury to the bowel wall is deep, then in some instances, mucosa may also become misplaced into the muscularis propria, or even into the serosa. Areas adjacent to lymphoid follicles, at the base of the mucosa, represent weak points within the muscularis mucosae that facilitate mucosal herniation.[640]

Pathological Features

Gross Findings

CCP may be a localized, segmental, or a diffuse process.[641] The localized form can affect any part of the colon, but it is more common in the rectum, where it is often associated with (or caused by) mucosal prolapse (see earlier discussion). CD, diverticulitis, and radiation injury may be associated with the segmental form of CCP.

The diffuse form of CCP is less common. It has been reported in association with UC or radiation injury, especially when the latter involves wide fields of external beam irradiation. Diffuse CCP may also manifest as multiple prominent polypoid mucosal elevations. The polypoid elevations may become confluent to form a masslike lesion. On cut section, the bowel wall may reveal mucin-filled cysts.

Microscopic Findings

The histological hallmark of CCP is the presence of intestinal epithelium, lamina propria, and/or mucin or mucin-filled cysts within the submucosa, muscularis propria, and rarely, the serosa. Mucin cysts may communicate with the lumen of the bowel. They are typically lined by benign colonic epithelium that may show regenerative and/or degenerative changes. Larger cysts may reveal an incomplete or absent epithelial lining (Fig. 17.88A). Mucin extravasation into surrounding tissues is a common finding, and this is often associated with inflammation, presumably as a result of cyst rupture. Misplaced epithelium, whether cystic or not, is usually surrounded by a discrete rim of lamina propria

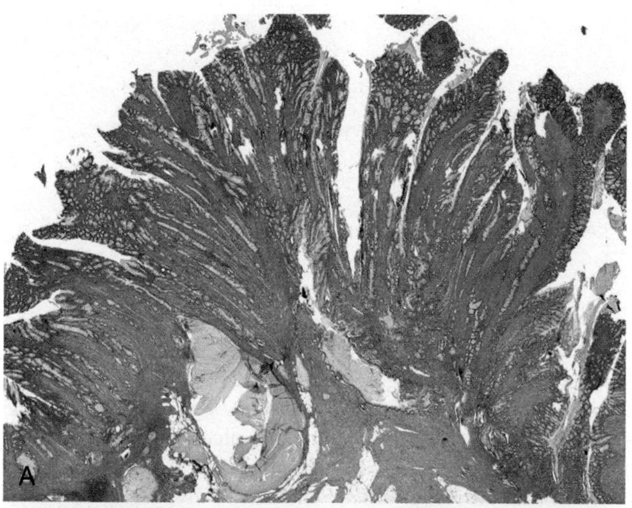

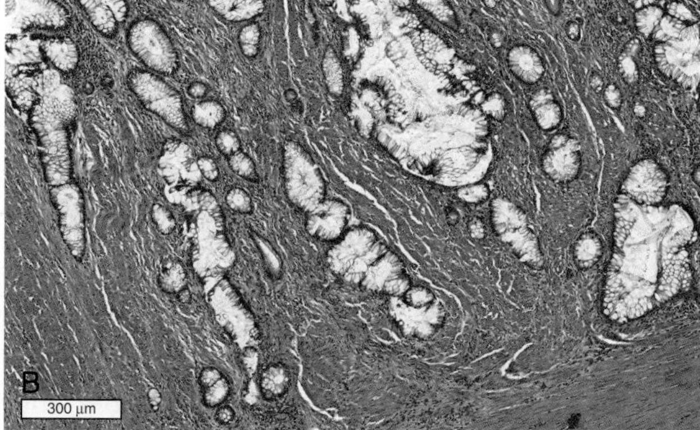

FIGURE 17.88 A, Colitis cystica profunda in a patient with chronic ulcerative colitis. Herniation of mucosa into the superficial submucosa is associated with dilated and distorted crypts, inflammation, and crypt rupture. **B,** At high power, the misplaced crypts show reactive changes and are associated with a rim of lamina propria.

TABLE 17.16 Colitis Cystic Profunda vs. Invasive Adenocarcinoma

Feature	Colitis Cystica Profunda	Invasive Adenocarcinoma
Crypt architecture	Distorted with dilated and branching crypts with lobular/rounded architecture	Distorted with angulated and infiltrative pattern
Extravasation of mucin	Common	May be present
Mucin pools partially lined by epithelial cells	Common; epithelial cells may show reactive atypia that mimics dysplasia	May be present; the lining epithelium is dysplastic
Clusters of free-floating dysplastic epithelial cells within mucin pools	Absent	Present in invasive mucinous adenocarcinoma
Lamina propria elements surrounding the glands	Present	Absent
Epithelial "atypia"	Present, common, (reactive atypia may mimic dysplasia)	Present
Stromal desmoplasia	Absent	Present

(see Fig. 17.88B). However, older cysts may be enveloped by densely fibrotic stroma resulting from involution of lamina propria and subsequent fibrosis. Occasionally, foci of dystrophic calcification or ossification may be present within cysts as well. Because of the secondary mechanism of injury, cases of CCP typically reveal evidence of the initiating inflammatory disease process in the bowel as well as epiphenomenon changes such as hemorrhage, hemosiderin deposition, granulation tissue, and fibrosis.

Differential Diagnosis

CCP should be differentiated from invasive carcinoma (Table 17.16). In some cases, this can be challenging, especially if the cysts are not surrounded by lamina propria or if there is abundant extravasated mucin but with minimal glandular epithelium. It is particularly difficult to differentiate these conditions in biopsies. Thus pathologists should be extra cautious not to overdiagnose cancer in a patient with a stricture, ulcer, nodule, or mass when one of the common precipitating CCP conditions are also known to be present, and especially in patients who have had cancer and were subsequently treated by radiation therapy. Misplaced glands in CCP are usually lobulated, smooth, even, and rounded in contour. They typically lack the angulated and infiltrative pattern of an invasive adenocarcinoma. Lack of significant cytological atypia, stromal desmoplasia, and cells floating within the mucin cysts are additional features that support a diagnosis of CCP. In cases in which there is abundant extravasated mucin, the finding of epithelium at the peripheral edge of mucin pools favors CCP, whereas clusters of free-floating (dysplastic) epithelium within mucin pools usually represents a malignant process.

BEHÇET'S SYNDROME

Clinical Features

Behçet's syndrome is a chronic, inflammatory, vasculitic disorder characterized by the combined presence of oral ulcers, genital ulcers, and iritis. Vasculitis affects large- and small-sized blood vessels of both the venous and the arterial system. Systemic involvement includes the colon, anus, and ileum.[642,643] The disease is more common in Asian and Mediterranean countries than in Western countries. Patients commonly have systemic manifestations in the form of oral and genital ulcers, erythema nodosum, and arthritis. GI tract involvement occurs in 10% to 50% of patients. Although the disease typically occurs in young adults between 20 and 40 years of age, GI involvement may manifest during the fourth to fifth decade of life.[643-645] Men are more frequently affected than women. Clinical symptoms may include anorexia, nausea, abdominal pain, or diarrhea. Rarely, patients have an acute condition in the abdomen and fever as a result of perforation.

Pathogenesis

Patients with Behçet's syndrome are genetically predisposed to the development of this syndrome. Although most cases are sporadic, familial clustering has been reported.[646] Increased risk for Behçet's syndrome has been associated with certain HLA types (e.g., HLA-B51). Genome-wide screening of affected families has identified other, non-HLA genetic alterations that involve the intercellular adhesion molecule-1 *(ICAM1)*, tumor necrosis factor *(TNF)*, vascular endothelial growth factor *(VEGF)*, and familial Mediterranean fever *(MEFV)* genes.[647-649] GI manifestations of Behçet's syndrome are caused by vasculitis-induced ischemia. However, the etiology of the vasculitis is unclear. Multiple factors, including bacterial antigens, environmental chemicals, heavy metal exposure, and infections (CMV, Epstein-Barr virus, parvovirus B19, and herpes simplex virus type 1) have been implicated as triggers of an aberrant immune response in patients with a genetic predisposition to develop the disease.[650,651] Both cellular and humoral immune activation appear to mediate the inflammatory response in Behçet's syndrome. In addition, vascular damage induced by inflammation or intrinsic endothelial dysfunction likely plays a role in thrombogenesis.

Pathological Features

Gross Findings

In the GI tract, Behçet's syndrome manifests as either a localized or a diffuse process. The localized form of disease typically affects the ileocecal region, whereas the diffuse form commonly affects the colon. The mucosal surface typically reveals multiple, discrete, ulcers located along the antimesenteric aspect of the colon. They have a

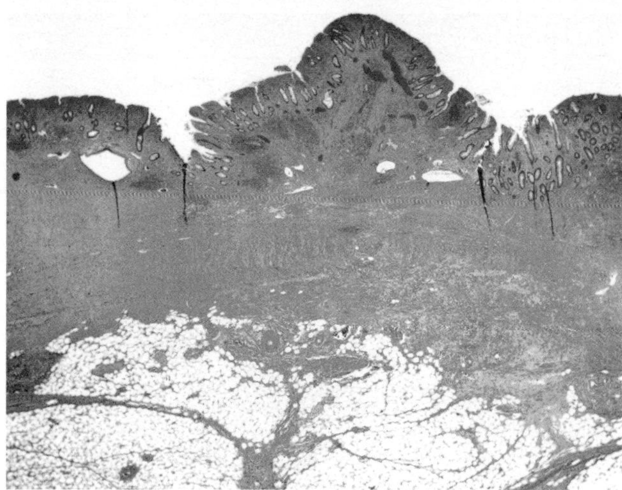

FIGURE 17.89 Behçet's syndrome. This colon resection specimen shows mucosal ulcers with prominent lymphoid aggregates at the base of the ulcers. Mural fibrosis and deep lymphoid aggregates, features that mimic Crohn's disease, are present. (*Courtesy Dr. Elizabeth Montgomery, Johns Hopkins Hospital, Baltimore, MD.*)

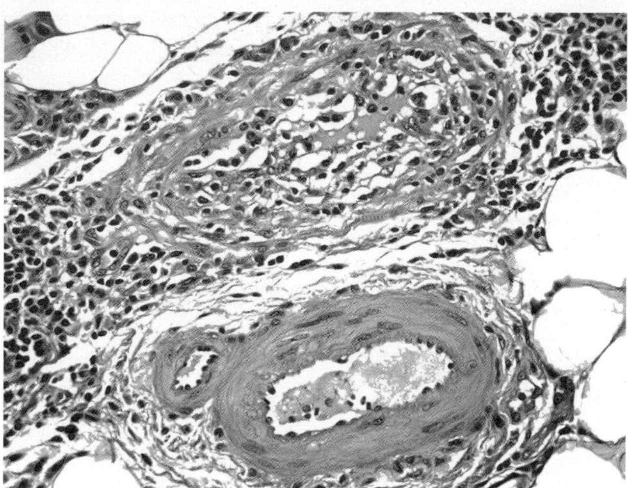

FIGURE 17.90 Behçet's syndrome. The image shows lymphocytic infiltration of the veins with myointimal thickening. The adjacent artery is unaffected by the process. (*Courtesy Dr. Elizabeth Montgomery, Johns Hopkins Hospital, Baltimore, MD.*)

characteristic punched-out appearance and often extend deep into the bowel wall.[642] Cases with perforation reveal marked thinning of the bowel wall and gangrenous changes.

Microscopic Findings

Deep, well-delineated, punched-out ulcers characteristically show prominent lymphoid aggregates at the base of the ulcers (Fig. 17.89). The mucosa between ulcers is usually normal in appearance unless it reveals ischemic changes such as superficial mucosal necrosis, atrophic crypts, and lamina propria hyalinization. Vasculitis affects small venules and arteries. In general, arterial involvement is less common. The inflammatory infiltrate within the vessel wall is predominantly lymphocytic in nature (Fig. 17.90). Vascular changes such as vascular intimal thickening, thrombosis, and fibrinoid necrosis of the vessel wall may be present at different stages of development. In cases complicated by perforation, there is evidence of transmural necrosis and extensive serosal fibroinflammatory reaction. Healed lesions are characterized by submucosal and mural fibrosis.

Differential Diagnosis

Because of its predilection for involvement of the ileocecal region, Behçet's syndrome should be differentiated from CD, especially in young adults. Extraintestinal manifestations are usually not helpful in distinguishing CD from Behçet's syndrome because ocular involvement, genital ulceration, and oral lesions may be seen in CD as well. In fact, oral ulcers in patients with CD are indistinguishable from oral aphthae in Behçet's syndrome. The classic findings of CD, such as granulomas, transmural lymphoid aggregates, thickening of muscularis mucosae, and neural hyperplasia, are typically absent in Behçet's syndrome.[642] Unlike CD, the mucosa adjacent to the ulcers in Behçet's syndrome does not show features of chronic mucosal injury, but it may show ischemic changes. Although the mesenteric vessels in CD may reveal myointimal hyperplasia and thickening of the vessel walls (Crohn's vasculopathy), lymphocytic vasculitis with accompanying fibrinoid necrosis is extremely unusual and should prompt investigation of a primary vascular disorder (see Chapter 10).

Natural History and Treatment

GI involvement in Behçet's syndrome is associated with a poor prognosis. The preferred form of medical therapy is a combination of steroids, NSAIDs, and immunosuppressive agents.[652] Between 5% and 10% of patients require surgical therapy.[653] Surgical resection is usually performed in patients with recurrent abdominal symptoms. Patients who undergo surgical resection often experience recurrence, especially if the initial indication for surgery was intestinal perforation or fistula.[652,654] Recurrence typically occurs within 2 years after surgery and is characterized by the development of ulcers at or in close proximity to the stoma or anastomotic site.

The full reference list may be accessed online at Elsevier eBooks for Practicing Clinicians.

CHAPTER 18

Inflammatory Disorders of the Appendix

Nicole C. Panarelli

Chapter Outline

INTRODUCTION

The appendix is a vestigial organ without proven significant physiological function; however, it is subject to a host of clinically significant inflammatory disorders, some of which involve the appendix exclusively and others that are systemic.

The vermiform appendix arises from the medial aspect of the cecum, inferior and posterior to the ileocecal orifice. It averages 8 cm long (range 2 to 20 cm) and 0.7 cm in diameter.[1] The appendix is most often located behind the cecum and ascending colon, but it may lie behind the ileum and mesentery, along the pericolic gutter, in the subhepatic region, or in the lesser pelvis. The appendix is maintained in its position by a fold of peritoneum that invests mesoappendiceal fat throughout its length. The appendiceal artery is derived from the ileocolic artery, which is derived from the superior mesenteric artery, and it is located at the free edge of the peritoneal fold.

The appendix is composed of the same five layers as the remainder of the large bowel, consisting of mucosa, submucosa, muscularis propria, subserosa, and serosa (Fig. 18.1A). However, in contrast, the mucosa contains abundant, organized lymphoid tissue arranged circumferentially. It closely resembles mucosa from the terminal ileum, particularly in young individuals. The epithelium of the appendix contains goblet cells, absorptive cells, neuroendocrine cells (predominantly Kulchitsky type and basally located), and scattered Paneth cells (Fig. 18.1B).[2] Unlike in the colon, in which crypts are uniformly aligned, appendiceal crypts tend to be more irregularly spaced and can be entirely absent in areas of mucosa adjacent to and overlying lymphoid aggregates. In addition to lymphoid tissue, abundant immunoglobulin A (IgA)–secreting plasma cells are also normally present in the lamina propria.

The muscularis propria consists of an inner circular and outer longitudinal layer of smooth muscle, similar to other parts of the gastrointestinal (GI) tract. The appendix is enveloped by serosa up to the point of attachment of the mesoappendix, where the serosa envelops the mesoappendiceal fat up to the peritoneal fold. Under normal circumstances, neutrophils and eosinophils are absent from the mucosa and wall of the appendix.

CONGENITAL, DEVELOPMENTAL, AND ACQUIRED ANATOMIC ABNORMALITIES

The appendix may exhibit a variety of anatomic abnormalities, such as an atypical location,[3] duplication,[4,5] congenital

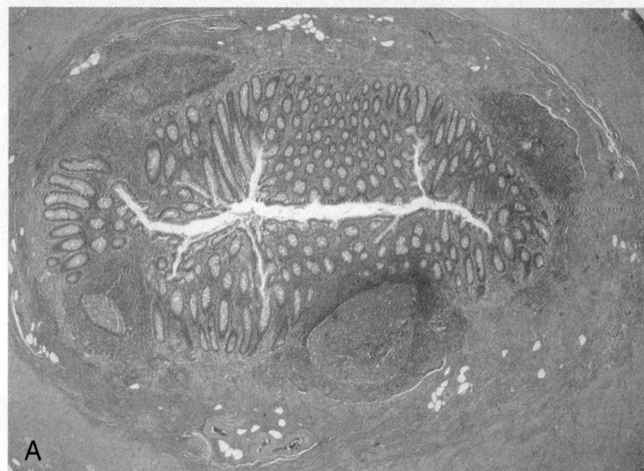

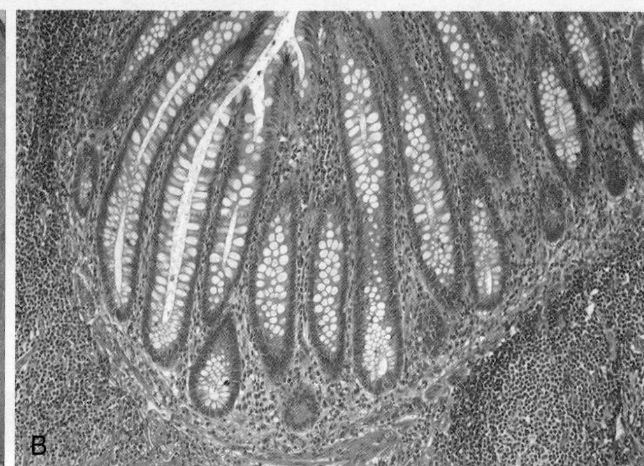

FIGURE 18.1 A, The appendix contains all layers of the intestinal wall including mucosa, submucosa, muscularis propria, subserosa, and serosa. Lymphoid tissue is often prominent. **B,** Epithelial components of the crypts are the same as those in the colon and include, goblet cells, absorptive cells, Paneth cells, and endocrine cells. The crypts are irregularly spaced and may appear distorted around lymphoid aggregates.

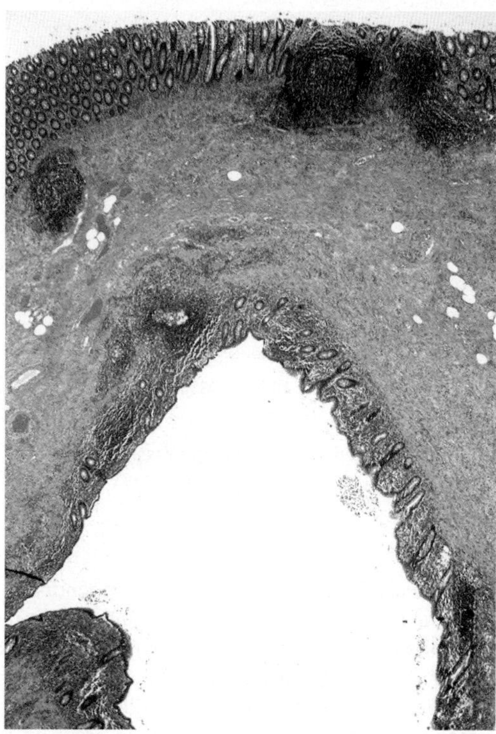

FIGURE 18.2 Complete appendiceal duplication is seen as an extra appendiceal lumen in the wall of the cecum in this case. This finding prompted surgery for suspicion of a cecal mass.

absence,[6] and luminal septal formation.[7] An abnormally long appendix (>7 to 10 cm) has been linked to the development of torsion, although this complication has also been reported for appendices of normal length.[8]

Abnormal Location

The position of the appendix is determined mainly by changes in the position and shape of the cecum that occur during organ development, growth, and rotation. If the cecum does not descend fully, the appendix becomes located retroperitoneally in an ascending retrocecal position, anterior to the right kidney. The frequency of a retrocecal location ranges from 26% to 65%.[9,10] If the appendix lies in a retrocecal position, it may be positioned intraperitoneally in a paracecal pouch of peritoneum, or retroperitoneally either with or without a paracecal fossa formed by the peritoneum.[11]

The clinical manifestations of acute appendicitis depend on the location of the appendix in the abdomen. If the appendix is located retrocecally, it may give rise to an abscess in the pararenal space, or infection may spread along the right paracolic gutter up to the right posterior subhepatic and right subphrenic spaces.[12,13] More than 50% of patients with ascending retrocecal appendicitis have an atypical clinical presentation. They may manifest with right upper quadrant pain or nonlocalizing abdominal pain, instead of the more common presentation consisting of central periumbilical pain followed by localization to the right lower quadrant, signs that are more often seen in cases of classic appendicitis, when the appendix is in its normal anatomic location.[14,15] Because of the atypical clinical presentation, retrocecal appendicitis is more likely to be diagnosed later in its course, resulting in a higher incidence of perforation and more serious complications.[14] However, some studies have not shown an association between retrocecal location and perforation at the time of presentation.[16]

Duplication

Duplication of the vermiform appendix is rare. It is found in approximately 1 of 25,000 patients (0.004%) who have undergone surgery for acute appendicitis.[17] The clinical presentation depends on the location of the appendix in the colon.[17,18] Cave and Wallbridge classified appendiceal duplication into three types.[19,20] Type A shows incomplete duplication; both appendices have a common base. Type B has complete duplication, with the first appendix arising from its usual location at the confluence of the teniae coli, and the second located at various sites along the colon (Fig. 18.2). Type C has complete duplication of the cecum, with each part having its own appendix.[19,20] Duplication of the appendix associated with duplication of the colon has been reported.[21]

Absence and Atresia

Agenesis and atresia of the vermiform appendix are both quite rare, occurring at an estimated frequency of 1 case per 100,000 resected appendices.[6,22] Congenital absence should

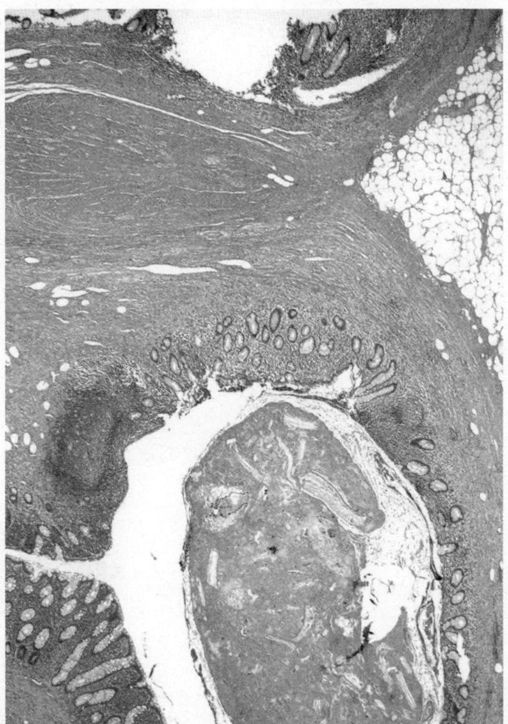

FIGURE 18.3 Acquired appendiceal diverticula are usually found in the distal appendix. They consist of herniations of mucosa and submucosa into the appendiceal wall.

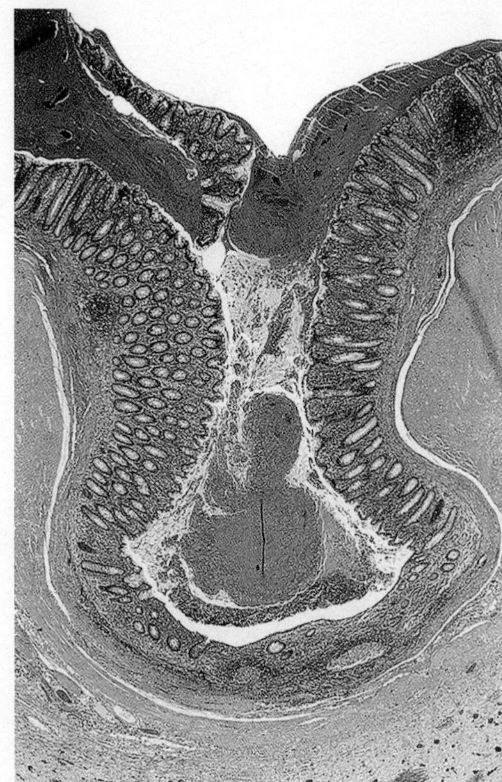

FIGURE 18.4 Acquired appendiceal diverticulum in a patient with cystic fibrosis.

be diagnosed only after thorough examination of the entire ileocecal region to exclude the possibility of an abnormally located appendix. Congenital absence of the appendix has been associated with other congenital malformations, such as congenital diaphragmatic hernia.[23]

Atresia of the appendix may be associated with atresia of the entire ileocecal region[24] or with atresia of other segments of small intestine.[25] Acute appendicitis may occur in an atretic appendix, but the diagnosis of atresia is usually established only after pathological examination of the resection specimen, because radiological findings are often nonspecific and may be obscured by periappendiceal inflammation.[26]

Appendiceal Septa

The appendix can have complete or incomplete septation, a finding that is principally seen in children and young adults, who usually suffer from acute appendicitis at clinical presentation.[7] Possible contributing factors to the formation of septa include congenital abnormality, postinflammatory fusion of mucosal folds, and ischemia caused by thrombosed vessels.

Diverticular Disease of the Appendix

Clinical Features

Diverticular disease of the appendix is rare. It has a reported incidence of 1 case (0.77% to 2%) per 50 to 130 appendectomies, or 1 case (0.004%) per 25,000 for true congenital diverticula.[22,27] Congenital diverticula are outpouchings formed by all mural layers, including mucosa, submucosa, and muscularis propria. Acquired diverticula presumably result from increased intraluminal pressure and subsequent mucosal herniation through a weak area of the muscularis propria, often at the site of a penetrating artery at the tip of the appendix.

Acquired diverticula occur most often in older males. They are located in the distal third of the appendix, (60%) on the mesenteric border, and usually have a diameter of less than 5 mm (Fig. 18.3).[27] Acquired diverticula may be identified in up to 22% of appendectomy specimens from patients with cystic fibrosis who frequently have appendiceal distension by inspissated secretions (Fig. 18.4).[28]

Diverticular disease may be clinically asymptomatic, or manifest with acute or chronic pain, mimicking acute appendicitis.[27,29] Computed tomography (CT) may help visualize inflamed diverticula, which appear as small, cystic outpouchings, but there is a high rate of false positives with this method of imaging.[30] During the acute phase of illness, the incidence of perforation is approximately three times higher than that for patients with classic appendicitis (33% versus 10%).[31] Because acquired diverticula lack a muscular wall, perforation is not surprising. The morbidity and mortality rates are greater than those for patients with classic acute appendicitis.[27]

Pathological Features

Grossly, the appendix may appear edematous, but diverticula may not necessarily be easily appreciated. If perforation has occurred, the serosa may appear dusky and possess a yellow-tan exudate. Histological findings include an outpouching of appendiceal epithelium through the muscularis propria of the appendix, either with or without associated acute, sometimes suppurative, appendicitis. Chronic changes such as muscular hypertrophy and transmural,

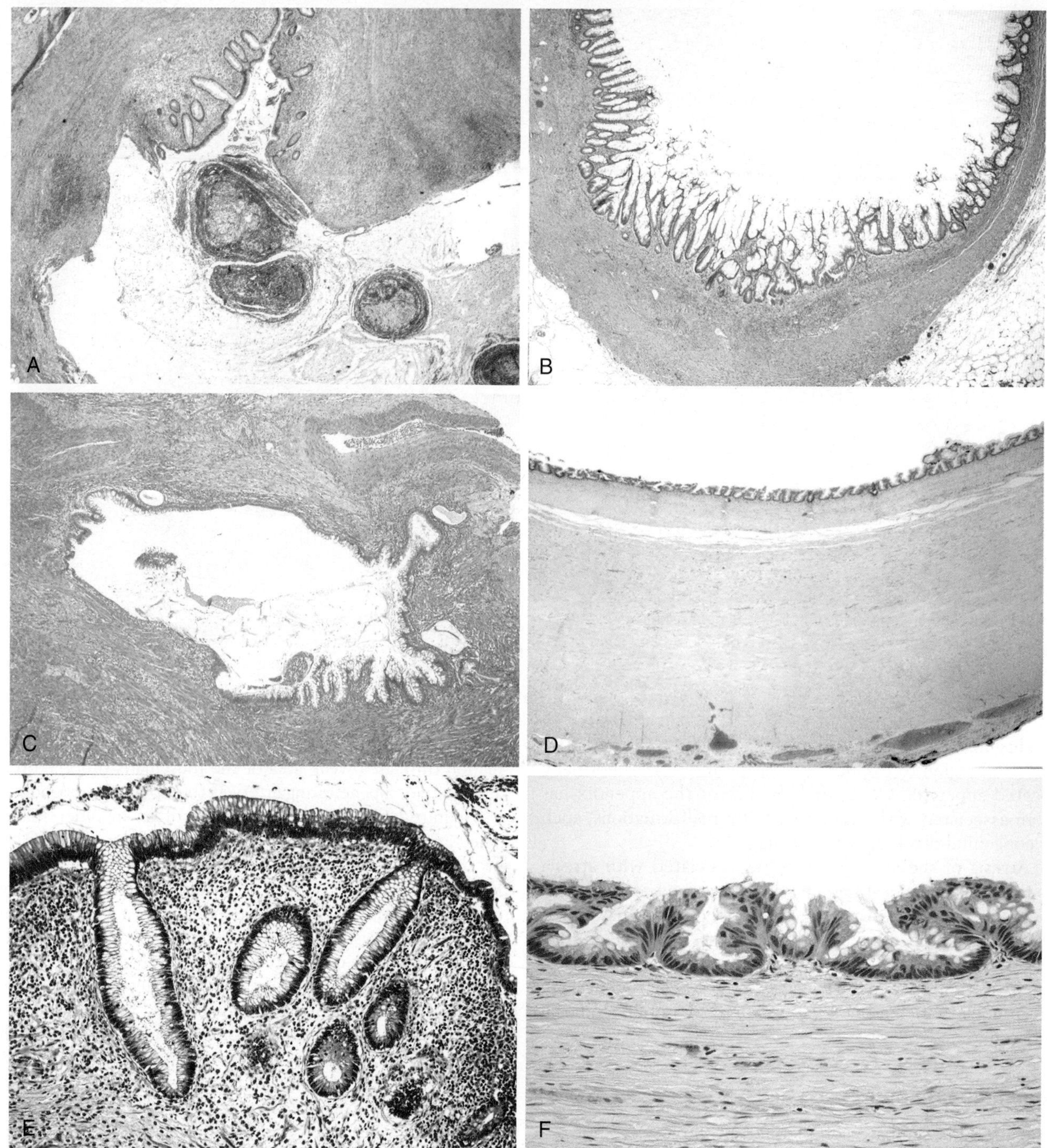

FIGURE 18.5 A, Diverticula may become dilated and contain inspissated mucin, simulating low-grade appendiceal mucinous neoplasm (LAMN). Diverticula are lined by normal-appearing appendiceal mucosa that may be slightly distorted or partially attenuated. **B**, LAMNs are lined by complex, villiform epithelial proliferations with markedly crowded neoplastic crypts. **C**, Diverticula are often associated with muscular hypertrophy, which is not a feature of LAMN. **D**, Increased luminal pressure causes thinning of the appendiceal wall and muscle fibrosis in LAMNs. **E**, The mucosal lining of diverticula contains a mixture of epithelial cells supported by abundant lamina propria. **F**, The epithelial lining of LAMN is monotonous and displays features of low-grade dysplasia. The lamina propria is obliterated.

periappendiceal fibrosis, and lymphoid atrophy, may be present as well.[29,32] In some cases, fibrous obliteration of the lumen may be present. The mucosal lining is essentially that of the normal appendix (see Fig. 18.3), but occasionally, superficial hyperplasia and reactive atypia may simulate a neoplasm, particularly low-grade appendiceal mucinous neoplasm (LAMN), as discussed next.

Differential Diagnosis

The distinction between hyperplastic or regenerative epithelial changes associated with diverticular disease and LAMN is challenging; examination of the entire appendix is recommended, if necessary, to exclude the possibility of LAMN (Fig. 18.5). Mucosal hyperplasia and regeneration, mural distortion, and rupture with spillage of mucin in diverticular

TABLE 18.1 Features Differentiating Diverticular Disease from Low-Grade Mucinous Neoplasms of the Appendix

Feature	Diverticular Disease	Low-Grade Mucinous Appendiceal Neoplasm
Extraappendiceal mucin	May be present Almost always acellular	Frequently present May be cellular or acellular
Crypt architecture	Preserved, slight variations may be present Even spacing maintained	Crowded, villiform, minimal intervening lamina propria
Epithelial morphology	Bland, reactive hyperplastic changes Mixed epithelial cell types including goblet cells, Paneth cells, endocrine cells Maturation normally present	Dysplastic, usually low-grade Lack of maturation Monotonous, nongoblet columnar mucinous cells
Villiform growth pattern	No	Yes
Lamina propria	Present	Usually obliterated by fibrous/hyalinized tissue
Acute inflammation	Usually present	May be present or absent
Mural fibrosis	Usually present	Usually present
Fibrous obliteration	Often present	May be present or absent
Muscular hypertrophy	Usually present	Not usually present
Diffuse pseudomyxoma peritonei	No	May be present or absent

disease all produce striking overlap with mucinous neoplasia. On the other hand, careful study reveals several diagnostically helpful distinguishing features. Mucosal regeneration features superficial gland serration and slight crypt disarray, but overall preservation of the mucosal architecture. The surface displays a smooth contour with evenly spaced crypts, each invested by lamina propria. Some authors note the presence of neuroma-like proliferations in the lamina propria of appendices with diverticulitis. In contrast, LAMNs display a variety of architectural abnormalities. Crowded villous proliferations with filiform projections supported by thin cores of lamina propria are a frequent finding. Areas of LAMN where mucin production causes distention feature completely flat or even extensively denuded epithelial lining with replacement of the lamina propria by fibrosis.[29] Importantly, the epithelial cell composition of reactive hyperplasia is mixed. Although increased goblet cells may be seen in the superficial crypts, hyperplastic proliferations contain a mix of epithelial cell types, including goblet cells, absorptive cells, and Paneth and endocrine cells in the deep crypt regions. The superficial epithelial cells may display reactive atypia, but features of low-grade dysplasia, such as nuclear hyperchromasia, crowding, and elongation are minimal, if present. LAMNs are lined by a monotonous population of columnar epithelial cells with finely vacuolated mucinous cytoplasm, but without discrete mucin vacuoles. Features of low-grade dysplasia are invariably present, although they may be challenging to appreciate in attenuated areas of the neoplasm. Extensive sampling may be necessary to identify the diagnostic findings. The mural changes associated with each of these disorders also overlap. Both produce fibrosis and atrophy of lymphoid tissue. The muscularis propria is often hypertrophic in diverticular disease, whereas LAMN is associated with thinning and fibrous replacement of the muscle. Ruptured diverticula are particularly problematic because they produce changes commonly associated with perforated LAMN. Mucin deposits on the serosa are associated with mixed inflammation, mesothelial hyperplasia, and organizing fibrosis. Detached fragments of diverticular epithelium may be present in the mucin, mimicking localized pseudomyxoma peritonei (Table 18.1). Epithelial cell clusters extruded from ruptured diverticula should display mixed morphology, similar to diverticular lining cells. Efforts should be made to identify diverticula in these challenging cases. Occasionally, they are grossly apparent, but in most cases, they are seen only on microscopic examination. In some instances, communication between the diverticulum and the appendiceal lumen is not seen in the original histological plane of section, but it may become apparent after deeper tissue sectioning.

Intraluminal pressure generated by mucinous secretions in LAMN may, in fact, produce diverticula (Fig. 18.6). In these cases, the diverticular lining appears similar to the tumor cell population in the native lumen.

Fibrous Obliteration of the Appendiceal Lumen

Obliteration of the appendiceal lumen (also known as neuroma or neural hyperplasia) by spindle cells situated within collagenous and myxoid soft tissue is present in approximately one-third of excised appendices. It is usually an incidental finding. The frequency of occurrence increases with patient age.

The tip of the appendix is usually affected, but the whole appendix may be progressively involved. Grossly, the appendix may appear narrow and white in areas of obliteration compared with the adjacent normal appendix. Lesional cells include fibroblasts, Schwann cells, and axons. Admixed mast cells, eosinophils, and scattered endocrine cells may also be present. The infiltrate may be confined to the mucosa, but more commonly, it replaces the entire lumen (Fig. 18.7).

Immunohistochemical staining shows a mixed population of S100 protein–reactive and neuron-specific enolase–reactive spindle cells corresponding to intermingled Schwann cells and axons, respectively. Admixed fibroblasts may be positive for CD34. The finding of lesions with a predominantly neural composition has led to the alternative

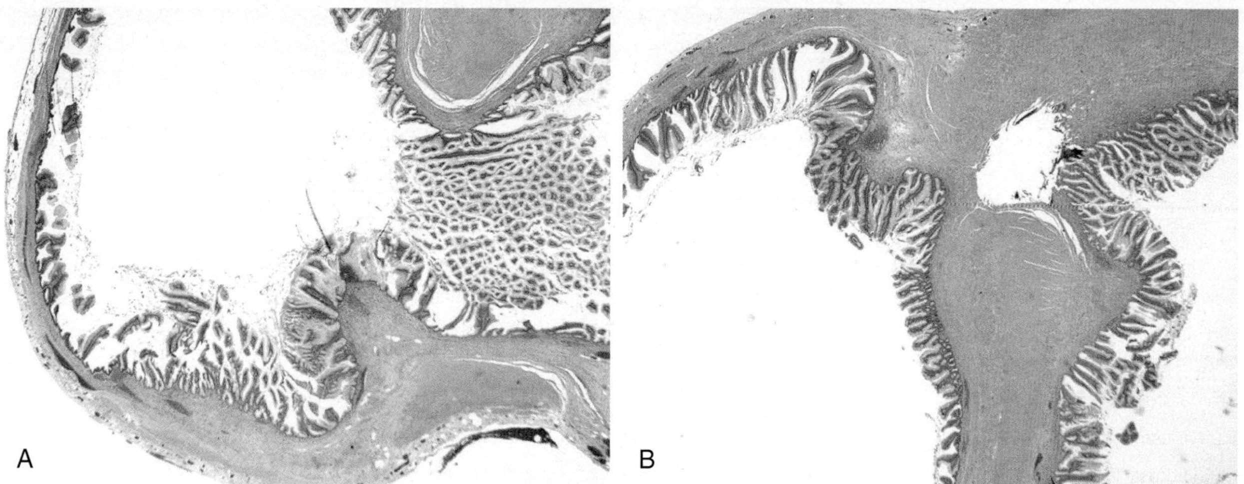

FIGURE 18.6 **A,** A LAMN is seen herniating through the appendiceal muscularis propria to form a diverticulum. **B,** The tumor features exuberant villiform tumor growth, which is appreciable both in the appendiceal lumen *(right)* and in the diverticular lining *(left)*. *(Courtesy Dr. Henry Appelman, The University of Michigan.)*

designation of *appendiceal neuroma*.[33] This phenomenon is thought to be a reactive process, either as a normal part of aging or as a response to prior acute appendicitis, with progressive phases of growth, involution, and fibrosis.[33,34] The common occurrence of fibrous obliteration and neuromatous changes in appendices with ruptured diverticula supports the hypothesis that this phenomenon represents a reactive process.[29]

ACUTE APPENDICITIS AND ASSOCIATED INFLAMMATORY DISORDERS

General Features

Clinical Features

Acute appendicitis is predominantly a disease of children and young adults. It occurs mainly in children and adolescents between 5 and 15 years of age, although no age group is exempt from this condition.[35,36] One crude estimate of the incidence of acute appendicitis in the United States is 11 cases per 10,000 population.[37] Acute appendicitis is more common in Western countries than in Asia or Africa.

The classic symptom triad of acute appendicitis consists of periumbilical pain, which eventually localizes to the right lower quadrant of the abdomen, accompanied by anorexia and nausea. Mild fever, leukocytosis, elevated C-reactive protein level, and right lower quadrant tenderness are usually present. If perforation has occurred, signs of peritonitis may be present. Common clinical mimics of acute appendicitis include mesenteric lymphadenitis (particularly in children), ovarian cysts, appendiceal or colonic diverticulitis, and Meckel's diverticulitis.

Imaging methods, particularly CT, often used to detect acute appendicitis, have improved recently.[38,39] Laparoscopic appendectomy has emerged as a relatively safe operational technique.[40] CT findings suggesting acute appendicitis include distention, wall thickening and enhancement, periappendiceal fat stranding, cecal thickening, and free peritoneal fluid. Approximately 70% of patients suspected of having acute appendicitis by clinical or imaging methods are found to have acute appendicitis at the time of surgery.[41,42]

Some authorities believe that all appendices, even when grossly normal, should be removed when the indication for surgery was suspected acute appendicitis because almost 20% of all grossly normal-appearing appendices may contain acute inflammation on microscopic examination of the tissue.[41,42] One possible exception is for patients who may require urological surgery in the future, because their appendices may prove useful as a potential urinary conduit.[43] Patients with acute appendicitis in the setting of human immunodeficiency virus (HIV) infection have a similar clinical presentation, although sometimes with a less striking elevation in the peripheral white blood cell count. In one surgical series of acute appendicitis in patients with HIV infection, delay before operation increased the likelihood of perforation.[44]

Pathogenesis

The pathogenesis of acute appendicitis is thought by some to reflect an initial insult to the mucosa resulting from luminal obstruction by a fecalith, a fragment of undigested food, lymphoid hyperplasia, or a tumor, followed by bacterial infection that progressively spreads outward from the mucosa and into and through the wall of the organ. However, the evidence for this mechanism is circumstantial at best. Some authorities believe that acute appendicitis represents one manifestation of a range of injuries that include hypersensitivity reactions, infections, and ischemic lesions. The potential causes of acute appendicitis are listed in Box 18.1.

Pathological Features

The appendix may appear grossly normal when inflammation is limited to the mucosa and submucosa. However, when inflammation extends into the muscularis propria, the appendix frequently becomes swollen and erythematous, due in part to dilation of the serosal vessels. When the serosa is affected, the peritoneum is initially dull and gray, but then a purulent exudate may develop. In approximately one-third of cases, a fecalith is identified. Perforation from mural necrosis (i.e., "gangrenous" appendicitis) can follow, which may eventually lead to abscess formation. Sometimes, an appendix resected in the clinical setting of

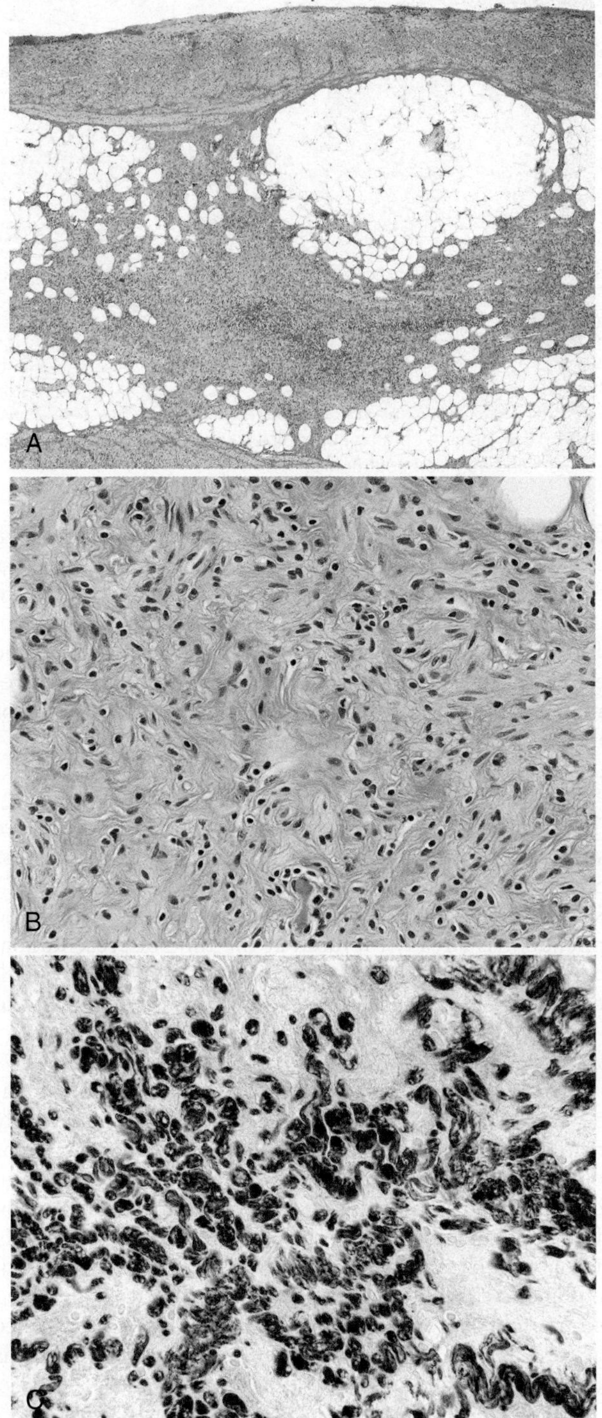

FIGURE 18.7 A, Fibrous obliteration of the appendix usually results in occlusion of the appendiceal lumen. **B,** The lesional cells consist of bland, ovoid to spindle-shaped Schwann cells and scattered mast cells. **C,** S100 protein positivity within the spindle cells confirms their schwannian nature.

acute appendicitis is grossly and histologically normal, even after submission of the complete specimen for histological examination. In these cases, a specific cause is rarely found. Other possible causes are listed in Box 18.2.

On microscopic examination, early changes include mucosal erosions and a neutrophilic infiltrate resulting in cryptitis and crypt abscesses (Fig. 18.8). Later, the inflammation extends into the submucosa and muscularis propria. Collections of neutrophils may be seen in the lumen as well. However, luminal neutrophils alone are not sufficient for a diagnosis of acute appendicitis but raise suspicion of its presence. When inflammation extensively damages the muscularis propria, mural necrosis can lead to perforation. Thrombosed vessels may be present. When the interval between symptom onset and surgery exceeds 72 hours, mural eosinophils may be the predominant inflammatory cell type.[45] When periappendiceal inflammation occurs in the absence of mural involvement, other causes of peritonitis should be sought clinically (see "Periappendicitis"). Anaerobic bacteria are detected in approximately 50% of cases, but they may represent secondary colonization rather than being the primary cause of the acute appendicitis.[46]

BOX 18.1 Causes of Acute Appendicitis

- Obstruction with superimposed bacterial infection
  - Fecalith
  - Lymphoid hyperplasia
  - Polyp or tumor
  - Foreign body
  - Mucin accumulation (e.g., cystic fibrosis)
- Infection
  - Bacterial: *Yersinia, Campylobacter*
  - Parasitic: *Cryptosporidium*, amebiasis
  - Fungal: *Candida*, mucormycosis, aspergillosis
  - Viral: Epstein-Barr virus, cytomegalovirus, varicella-zoster virus, measles virus
- Inflammatory bowel disease
  - Ulcerative colitis
  - Crohn's disease
- Diverticular disease
- Stump appendicitis (after appendectomy)

BOX 18.2 Causes of a Grossly Normal, Histologically Noninflamed Appendix Despite Clinical Symptoms of Acute Appendicitis

- *Yersinia* ileitis or mesenteric adenitis
- Spirochetosis
- Cystic fibrosis
- Other intraabdominal disease (e.g., endometriosis)

Differential Diagnosis

The morphological differential diagnosis, at least for very early appendicitis, includes, among others, infectious gastroenteritis, inflammatory bowel disease (IBD) involving the appendix, and trauma from fecaliths, all of which may result in "mild" superficial neutrophilic inflammation. If inflammation is limited to the mucosa, additional sections may reveal mural inflammation, which would support a diagnosis of primary acute appendicitis. The differential diagnosis with IBD involving the appendix is discussed further below.

Two general and basic patterns of disease progression may occur in patients with acute appendicitis.[47,48] In the first and more common pattern, there is a mixed inflammatory infiltrate ranging from patchy and mild in the early phase, to diffuse and transmural in later phases. In some appendices,

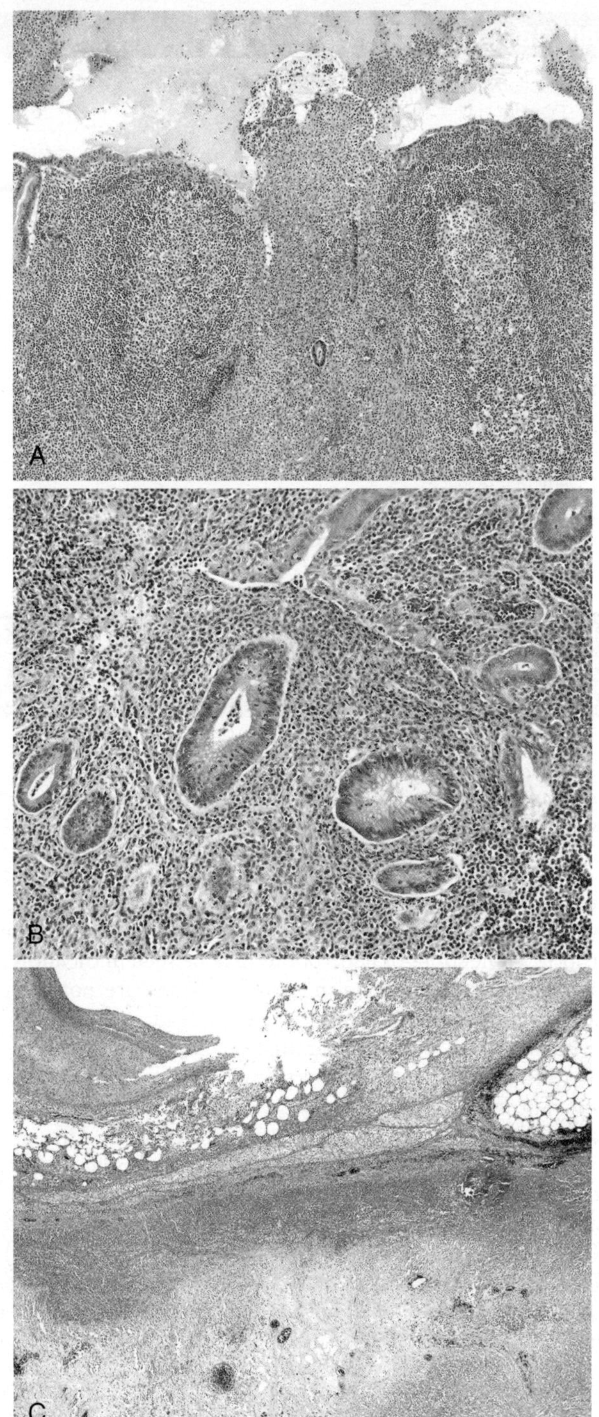

FIGURE 18.8 **A,** Acute suppurative appendicitis consists of a neutrophilic infiltrate that extrudes into the appendiceal lumen from the lamina propria. **B,** Cryptitis and crypt abscesses are invariably present. **C,** Progressive transmural inflammation results in serositis and perforation.

there may be intramural or serosal foreign body–type giant cells surrounded by granulation tissue, suggesting prior rupture. Serositis, fibrous adhesions, and prominent submucosal fibrosis can occur. Mucin extravasation is often present as well. A second, more chronic, pattern, which has been termed *xanthogranulomatous appendicitis*, consists of an infiltrate of foam cells and multinucleate histiocytes, with hemosiderin deposition, luminal obliteration, and sparing of lymphoid follicles (Fig. 18.9). This reaction pattern shares features with Crohn's disease (CD), but lacks epithelioid granulomas, has fewer lymphoid aggregates, and shows less subserosal fibrosis. However, in one study, a patient exhibiting this pattern of inflammation was found to have CD on follow-up, so the features of these two conditions do overlap.[49] Clinical correlation, and determination of disease elsewhere in the small or large bowel, and anus, is important in such cases.

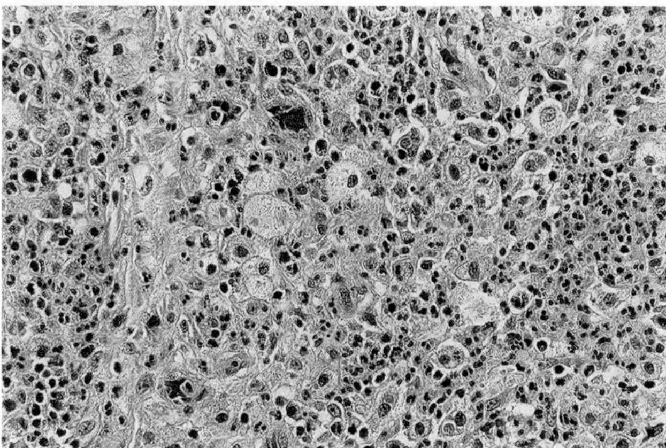

FIGURE 18.9 Healing chronic appendicitis with numerous foamy macrophages and admixed neutrophils.

Natural History and Prognosis

The most common complications of acute appendicitis are perforation, with the development of peritonitis and abscess formation. Young children and elderly adults have the highest risk of perforation. For some patients in whom the appendix has already ruptured at the time of presentation, the surgeon may elect to treat the condition initially with antibiotics and drainage, followed by an appendectomy 4 to 8 weeks later. This approach is termed an *interval appendectomy* (see "Chronic Appendicitis").

Periappendiceal abscesses may result in an inflammatory mass that mimics a neoplasm clinically. If not surgically treated, an abscess may fistulize into the small intestine or colon or onto the skin surface. In women, obstruction of an adjacent fallopian tube may lead to infertility. Inflammation of adjacent blood vessels may result in pylephlebitis. Early diagnosis and surgical intervention (i.e., appendectomy), combined with antibiotic therapy, has drastically reduced the mortality rate associated with acute appendicitis since the early 1900s. The mortality rate for acute appendicitis is now less than 0.5%.[50]

Stump Appendicitis

Clinical Features

Stump appendicitis represents an uncommon late complication of appendectomy. It is defined as residual or progressive acute inflammation in the remaining stump of the appendix after surgery.[51-53] A diagnosis of stump appendicitis is often delayed primarily because of its relatively infrequent occurrence, but a high level of suspicion should be maintained for patients who have signs and symptoms of appendicitis after appendicectomy.[54-56] A history of colicky central abdominal pain that localizes to the right lower quadrant does not often occur in patients with stump appendicitis. Other signs and symptoms include generalized abdominal pain and tenderness, nausea, vomiting, fever, and peritonitis. Abdominal CT findings that reveal a distended appendicular stump, fecalith, pericecal fat stranding, or abscess help to confirm the diagnosis.[51] The consequences of delayed diagnosis include stump necrosis, gangrene, and perforation, which occur in as many as 40% of patients.[51]

Pathological Features

Pathological features of stump appendicitis have not been fully described. However, in most cases, findings are similar to those of classic acute appendicitis, consisting of neutrophils, cryptitis, and some degree of transmural inflammation. Transmural necrosis and perforation can occur in patients with late-stage disease. Granulomatous inflammation has been described in one patient with stump appendicitis.[57]

Natural History and Prognosis

Management usually requires surgical resection of the inflamed residual appendix and antibiotic therapy. It is unclear whether the increasing use of laparoscopic instruments for appendectomy is associated with an increase in the incidence of stump appendicitis.

Periappendicitis

Clinical Features and Pathogenesis

Periappendicitis without mucosal or mural involvement occurs in 1% to 5% of appendices resected for clinically suspected acute appendicitis. Most cases are caused by salpingitis, often in the setting of chlamydia (pelvic inflammatory disease).[58] Other well-described causes include yersiniosis, Meckel's diverticulitis and associated intraperitoneal abscess, urological disorders, colonic neoplasms, infectious colitis, abdominal aortic aneurysm, bacterial peritonitis, and GI perforation.[59,60] The clinical presentation differs somewhat from that of classic acute appendicitis, including longer duration of pain, localization less often in the right lower quadrant, and fewer peritoneal signs.[61]

Pathological Features

Grossly, the serosal surface of the appendix and mesoappendix may appear dull and coated with a fibrinous exudate. Preoperative mechanical manipulation of the appendix may cause mild, diffuse neutrophilic infiltration of the periappendiceal serosa.[58] However, when inflammation in the serosa is accompanied by fibrin deposition or adhesions, it is a potentially significant clinical finding.

Microscopically, a neutrophilic infiltrate is seen within the serosa. The inflammation may extend into the subserosa and rarely into the muscularis propria. Fibrinous adhesions may also be identified. By definition, the mucosa of the appendix is uninvolved. Because the serosal findings are common in patients with acute appendicitis, examination of the entire appendix is recommended to exclude this diagnosis completely. The management of periappendicitis depends on the underlying cause.

CHRONIC APPENDICITIS

The criteria and definition of "chronic appendicitis" as a discrete clinical or pathological disease entity are controversial.

BOX 18.3 Chronic Inflammatory Disorders of the Appendix

Inflammatory bowel disease
- Ulcerative colitis
- Crohn's disease

Interval appendicitis
Diverticular disease
Sarcoidosis
Idiopathic granulomatous appendicitis
Infection
- Bacterial: *Yersinia*, tuberculosis
- Parasitic: schistosomiasis, strongyloidiasis
- Fungal: *Candida, Histoplasma*
- Malakoplakia

Cystic fibrosis

For instance, the term *chronic appendicitis* has been used to describe fibrous replacement of the appendiceal wall after severe or recurrent bouts of acute appendicitis. This process also has been referred to clinically as *subacute appendicitis*. The term has also been used for patients who have had an interval appendectomy, when resection of a perforated appendix was delayed as a result of initial conservative management with antibiotics and drainage. This entity is discussed further later. Thus "chronic appendicitis" is an umbrella diagnosis that encompasses any type of potentially chronic inflammatory condition of the appendix, other than classic acute appendicitis.

Recurrent episodes of acute appendicitis (i.e., subacute appendicitis), ulcerative colitis (UC) and CD of the appendix, granulomatous appendicitis (and its many causes), and cystic fibrosis are also potential causes of chronic appendicitis. The causes of chronic appendicitis are summarized in Box 18.3. Features of disorders classified under this term are detailed next and in Table 18.2.

Ulcerative Colitis Involving the Appendix

Clinical Features

The appendix plays an interesting, but poorly defined, role in patients with UC or CD. For instance, appendectomy is a protective factor in UC. The prevalence of prior appendectomy is lower among patients with UC compared with the general population.[62-64]

Appendicitis, which is usually ulcerating in patients with UC, is typically seen in patients with pancolitis,[64] but it may also occur as a "skip lesion" in patients with subtotal, left-sided, or rectal-only disease. It has an overall incidence of 50% among patients with UC.[65-67]

Pathological Features

Grossly, erythema and ulceration at the appendiceal orifice may be seen endoscopically. Ulcerative appendicitis shows histological features similar to those of the colon in UC (see Chapter 17). Active mucosal inflammation is characterized by cryptitis, crypt abscesses, and suppurative luminal exudate. Chronic changes include lamina propria lymphoplasmacytosis, basal lymphoid aggregates, crypt architectural distortion, and Paneth cell hyperplasia (Fig. 18.10). Early acute appendicitis in non-UC patients exhibits less crypt distortion and plasmacytosis than in UC-associated

TABLE 18.2 Causes of Chronic Appendicitis

Disorder	Clinical Findings	Distribution	Gross Findings	Histological Findings
Ulcerative colitis	Chronic colitis with continuous involvement of the distal colorectum	Appendix may be involved by pancolitis or a "skip lesion"	Mucosal erythema and ulceration	Features of chronic active colitis: cryptitis, crypt abscesses, lymphoplasmacytosis, architectural distortion, Paneth cell hyperplasia
Noninfectious granulomatous appendicitis				
Crohn's disease	Intestinal and extraintestinal manifestations of inflammatory bowel disease	Patchy enterocolitis, not confined to the appendix	Thickening, adhesions, fistulization to adjacent structures	Transmural inflammation, lymphoid hyperplasia nonnecrotic epithelioid granulomata, neural hypertrophy
Interval appendicitis	Mirrors acute appendicitis: adolescents, young adults History of acute appendicitis and delayed appendectomy	Limited to the appendix, localized peritonitis if perforated	Edematous, hyperemic appendix, hemorrhagic contents, fecaliths	Fibrosis, lymphoid hyperplasia, granulomas centered on lymphoid follicles, xanthogranulomatous inflammation
Sarcoidosis	African American patients, 3rd-5th decade Hilar lymphadenopathy, pulmonary and other systemic involvement, elevated serum angiotensin converting enzyme	Systemic disease, affects lung, heart, central nervous system, skin	Fibrosis, may have superimposed acute appendicitis	Nonnecrotic epithelioid granulomata involve all layers of the appendix, may have transmural lymphoid aggregates
Infectious appendicitis with chronic clinical course				
Actinomycosis	Young adults and children	Often confined to appendix, may involve right colon	Markedly enlarged and indurated, adhesions to other intraabdominal structures	Transmural inflammation, lymphoid hyperplasia, granulomas surrounded by neutrophils, "sulfur granules," Splendore-Hoeppli phenomenon, filamentous organisms are gram positive and can be identified with GMS stains
Yersiniosis	Infants, children, young adults, more common in cooler climates	Ileocecal region, appendix, mesenteric lymph nodes	Nodular inflammatory masses, ulcers, perforation	Acute appendicitis with suppurative epithelioid granulomata
Tuberculosis	Immunocompromised, more common in endemic regions and developing countries	Ileocecal, mesenteric lymph nodes	Mural thickening and serosal adhesions	Lymphoid hyperplasia, centrally necrotic confluent granulomas Scarce organism may be seen in AFB stains
Strongyloidiasis	Chronically ill or immunocompromised patients, particularly in tropical climates	Affects multiple organ systems, may be present throughout the GI tract	Edematous and hyperemic appendix	Transmural eosinophil and neutrophil-rich inflammation, larvae in crypts are curved with pointed tails, occasional granulomas
Schistosomiasis	Preferentially affects children, particularly in tropical and developing countries	Affects multiple organ systems, especially the GI and genitourinary tracts	Edematous and hyperemic appendix, may show fibrosis	Transmural eosinophil rich inflammation with granulomatous reaction to ova, ova are ovoid and often calcified

AFB, *acid-fast bacilli;* GI, *gastrointestinal;* GMS, *Grocott's methenamine silver stain.*

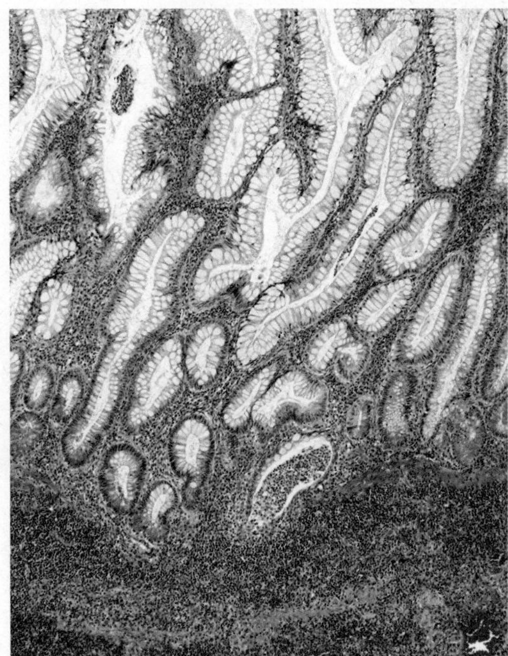

FIGURE 18.10 Ulcerative colitis involving the appendix shows cryptitis, crypt abscesses, architectural distortion, and a basal lymphoplasmacytic infiltrate.

appendicitis. In UC, immunostains may show prominent S100 protein–reactive and MAC387-positive dendritic cells, which are not present in non-UC cases of acute appendicitis.[68] The prognostic implication of appendiceal involvement in UC is dictated by the degree and extent of colonic involvement, but there are little outcome data in this regard.

Crohn's Disease

Unlike for UC, the relationship between appendectomy and CD is not well established. However, one study did find a protective effect of appendectomy on the occurrence of disease after the bias of appendectomy at the time of diagnosis of CD was removed from the analysis.[63] Most appendices removed from patients with CD of the small and large intestine are histologically normal. Patients with appendiceal involvement in CD usually have extensive ileocolonic involvement. Many cases labeled *granulomatous appendicitis* in the past were thought to represent CD. However, more recently this entity has proved to represent a variety of different disorders, all of which feature granulomatous inflammation in the appendix. A crude estimate of the incidence of appendiceal involvement in CD from the recent literature is approximately 20%.[69]

In patients with appendiceal involvement, the histological features are similar to those seen in other sites of the GI tract. Mucosal ulceration, active inflammation with cryptitis and crypt abscesses, granulomas, transmural inflammation, transmural lymphoid aggregates, fissures, and fistulas are characteristic features. Paneth cell hyperplasia may also occur. Scattered nonnecrotizing granulomas are identified in approximately 50% to 80% of cases (Fig. 18.11).[47,70]

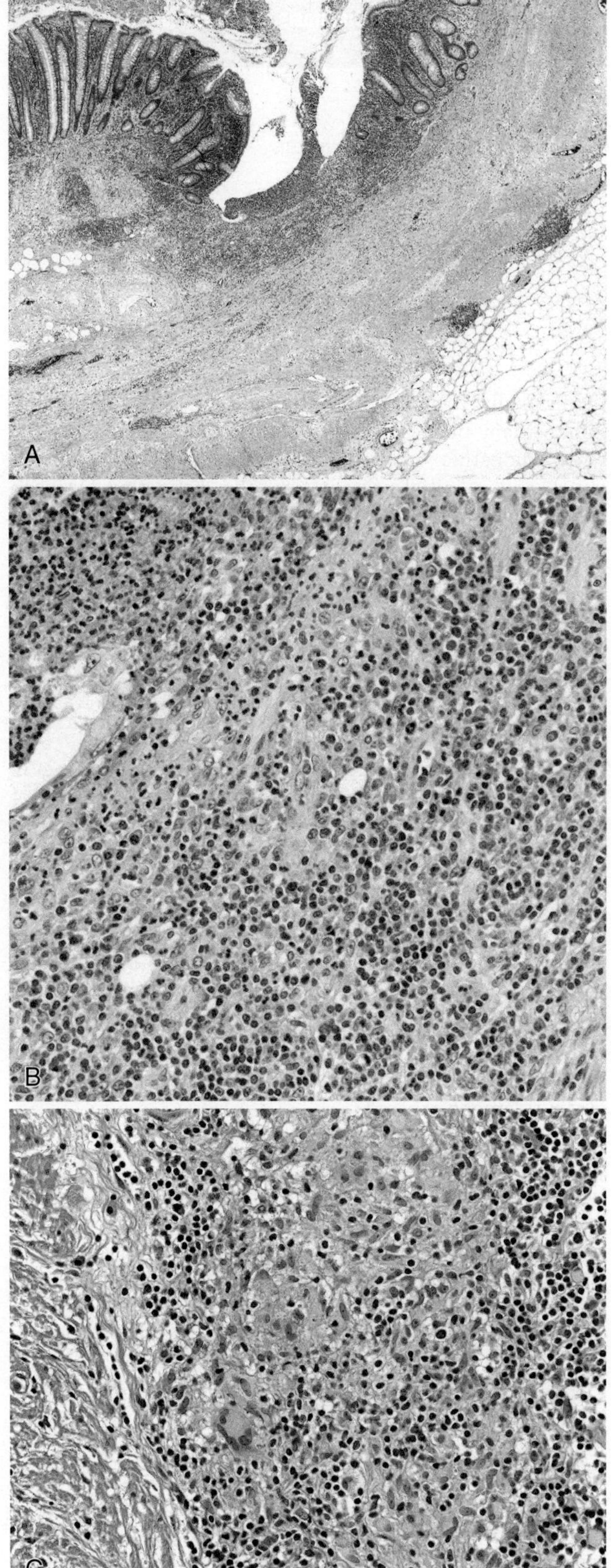

FIGURE 18.11 A, Crohn's disease involving the appendix with transmural lymphoid aggregates and a fissuring ulcer. **B,** Active inflammation of the mucosa. **C,** Scattered nonnecrotizing granulomas.

BOX 18.4 Differential Diagnosis of Granulomatous Appendicitis

Interval appendicitis
Crohn's disease
Idiopathic granulomatous appendicitis
Sarcoidosis
Infection
- Bacterial: *Yersinia*, tuberculosis, actinomycosis
- Parasitic: schistosomiasis, strongyloidiasis
- Fungal: *Candida, Histoplasma*

Foreign body reaction: talc, prior intraabdominal procedures

Occasionally, focal necrosis may be seen within the granulomas. Many of these findings may also be seen in patients with idiopathic granulomatous appendicitis (discussed later), and at initial presentation, the distinction between the two entities may be impossible in the absence of a history of CD elsewhere in the GI tract. Patients with appendiceal CD usually have extensive ileocolic involvement, and the prognosis depends on the degree of extraappendiceal involvement.

Granulomatous Appendicitis

Clinical Features and Pathogenesis

Granulomatous appendicitis is an uncommon finding in appendectomy specimens. It is identified in less than 1% of cases.[71] Historically, most cases of granulomatous appendicitis were thought to result from involvement of the appendix by CD, but more recent data suggest that this is true in only 5% to 10% of cases. Other potential causes of granulomatous appendicitis are summarized in Box 18.4. They include primary (i.e., idiopathic granulomatous appendicitis) and secondary causes such as interval appendicitis, sarcoidosis, foreign body reactions, and infectious disorders (e.g., *Yersinia*, tuberculosis, actinomycosis, schistosomiasis, strongyloidiasis, *Enterobius vermicularis*, *Candida*, *Histoplasma*), among others.[72]

Clinically, patients with granulomatous appendicitis may reveal symptoms that mimic acute suppurative appendicitis or symptoms related to the underlying disease. In some cases, it may be entirely asymptomatic, in which case the finding of granulomatous appendicitis is made in appendectomy specimens that were removed for non–appendix-related disorders.

Pathological Features

Depending on the cause, the size of the appendix may be normal or enlarged. There also may be serosal exudates or fibrous adhesions. Granulomas, which are composed of histiocytes surrounded by a cuff of lymphocytes, may contain multinucleate giant cells, and they may be necrotizing or nonnecrotizing (Fig. 18.12). Necrosis is most commonly seen in infectious disorders, but occasionally granulomas in sarcoidosis and CD may have focal necrosis. Granulomas may involve any layer of the appendiceal wall. The crypt architecture may be distorted. Cryptitis or crypt abscesses may also occur. *Yersinia* and tuberculosis-associated cases are also associated with transmural inflammation and lymphoid hyperplasia and thus mimic CD.

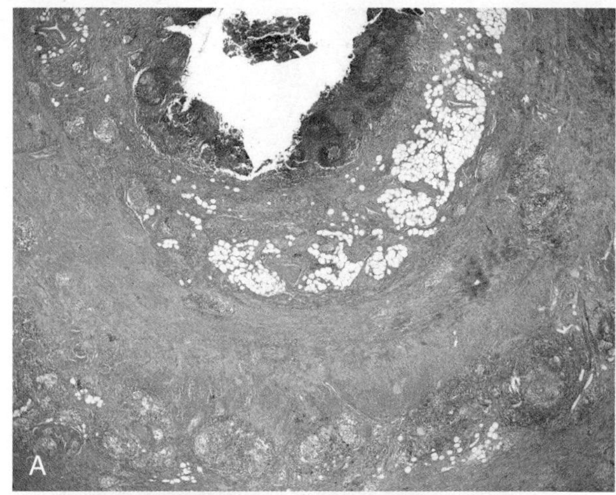

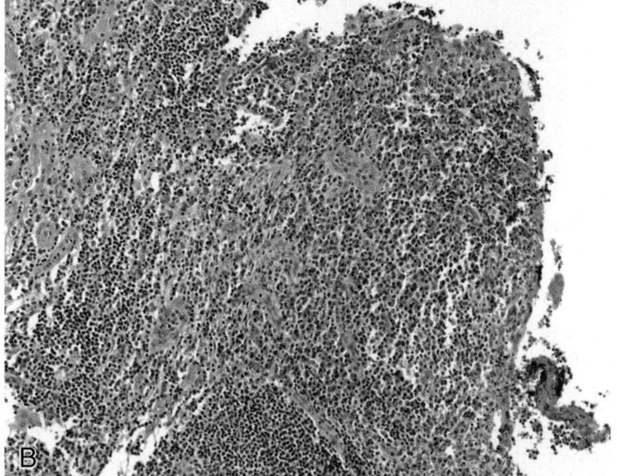

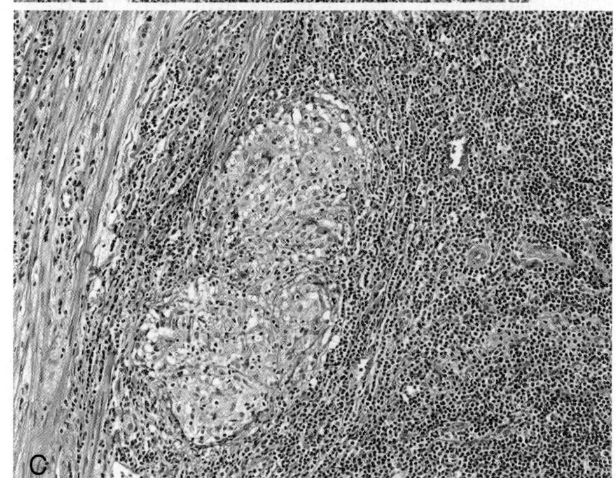

FIGURE 18.12 A, In idiopathic granulomatous appendicitis, multiple granulomas can be seen scattered throughout all layers of the appendiceal wall along with transmural, Crohn's disease–like lymphoid aggregates. **B,** Mild acute appendicitis. **C,** The granulomas are well formed and nonnecrotizing.

Natural History and Prognosis

Management of granulomatous appendicitis depends on the underlying cause. Idiopathic granulomatous appendicitis, sarcoidosis, and infectious causes of granulomatous appendicitis are discussed in later sections. Distinguishing features of the principal causes of granulomatous appendicitis are summarized in Table 18.3.

TABLE 18.3 Distinguishing Features of Granulomatous Appendicitis

Feature	Crohn's Disease	Idiopathic Granulomatous Appendicitis	Interval Appendicitis	Sarcoidosis	Tuberculosis	Yersiniosis
Relevant clinical history	With or without known Crohn's disease	None	Acute appendicitis	With or without known sarcoidosis	Compromised immune system	Young age
Disease distribution	Ileocecal involvement	Limited to the appendix	Limited to the appendix	Systemic, involves mediastinum, liver, central nervous system	Pulmonary and ileocecal involvement	May or may not involve ileocecal region, mesenteric lymphadenopathy
Granulomas	Occasional	Numerous	Occasional (variable)	Numerous	Numerous	Numerous
Distribution of granulomas	Scattered	All layers	Centered on lymphoid follicles	All layers	Concentrated in submucosa	Centered on lymphoid follicles or in the appendiceal wall
Other features of granulomas	Small, epithelioid, lack necrosis	Epithelioid, lack necrosis	Epithelioid, lack necrosis, Xanthogranulomatous inflammation also present	Epithelioid, lack necrosis	Large and confluent with central necrosis	Central necrosis or suppurative inflammation, lymphoid cuff
Active inflammation	Yes	Yes	Variable	Uncommon (mild)	Yes	Variable
Fissures, fistulas	Yes	Occasional	Rarely	No	No	No
Transmural lymphoid aggregates	Yes	Yes	Occasionally	Uncommon	No	No
Fibrosis	Yes	Yes	Yes	Yes	Mild, variable	Mild, variable

Idiopathic Granulomatous Appendicitis

Clinical Features

Idiopathic granulomatous appendicitis is defined as a primary granulomatous inflammatory disorder of the appendix of unknown origin. It shows a predilection for young adults who present with acute or subacute lower abdominal pain, although some are entirely asymptomatic.[70]

Pathogenesis

Most cases historically classified as idiopathic granulomatous appendicitis are probably attributable to infectious causes (e.g., *Yersinia* spp.), interval appendicitis, or other identifiable causes of granulomatous inflammation (e.g., sarcoidosis).[73] True idiopathic granulomatous appendicitis is quite rare, occurring in <0.01% of appendectomy specimens.[74]

Pathological Features

By definition, idiopathic granulomatous appendicitis can only be diagnosed in patients without a history of CD. Also by definition, it is characterized by multiple granulomas, usually nonnecrotizing, involving any, or all, layers of the appendiceal wall. Associated histological findings include a variety of acute changes such as neutrophilic infiltration resulting in cryptitis, crypt abscesses, mucosal erosion, and ulceration. Chronic changes include fissures, transmural lymphoid aggregates, and mural fibrosis.

Differential Diagnosis

Most cases are indistinguishable from CD based solely on evaluation of the appendix. However, idiopathic granulomatous appendicitis is a disorder that is limited to the appendix. Furthermore, most patients who have isolated granulomatous appendiceal disease do not develop CD elsewhere in the GI tract on follow-up.[70,75-78] In contrast, most patients with appendiceal CD have a history of CD or have extensive ileocolonic disease at the time of presentation with appendiceal disease.

Two histological findings may be helpful in distinguishing the two entities pathologically. Fistulization is more common in CD,[70] and the degree of granulomatous inflammation is greater in primary granulomatous appendicitis. Granulomas are not always seen in CD of the appendix; they occur in 50% to 80% of cases. Isolated idiopathic granulomatous appendicitis features approximately 20 granulomas per tissue section, whereas appendicitis associated with CD has fewer than 1 granuloma per section on average.[70] However, one patient reported in a series by Huang et al. who had 21 granulomas per cross section developed CD elsewhere in the gut on follow-up. Thus the number of granulomas

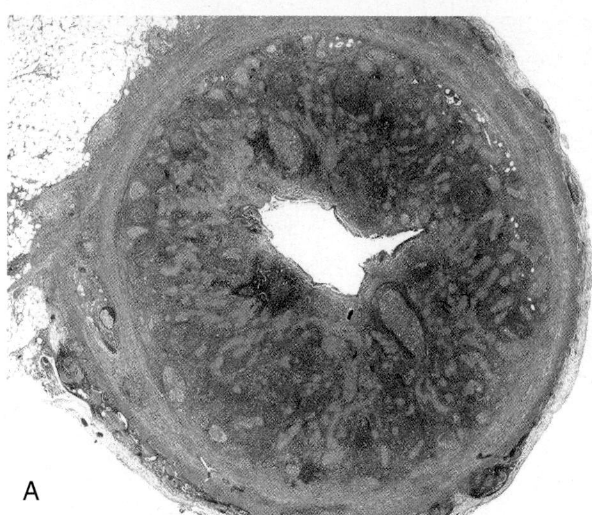

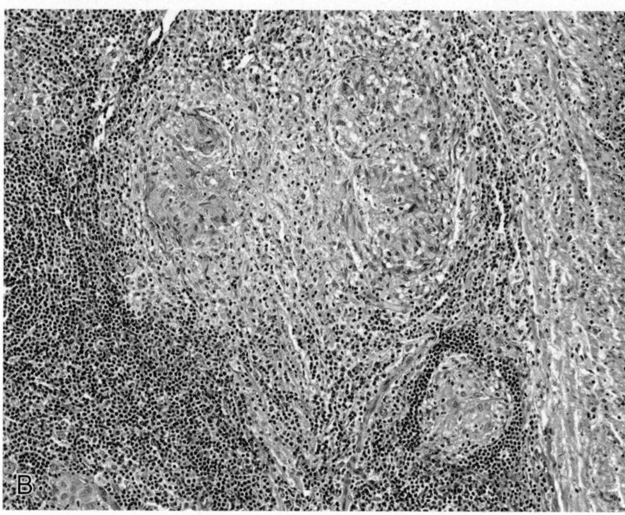

FIGURE 18.13 A, Sarcoidosis of the appendix involves all layers of the appendix and shows well-formed, nonnecrotizing granulomas (**B**).

per cross section is not entirely reliable in separating these entities.[49] In another series, none of nine patients (identified among 1133 consecutive appendectomy specimens) with idiopathic granulomatous appendicitis developed CD within a mean follow-up period of more than 7 years.[78]

Besides CD, other causes of granulomatous appendicitis should be thoroughly investigated before making a diagnosis of idiopathic granulomatous appendicitis. Yersiniosis frequently involves the appendix and ileocecal region but produces suppurative granulomas. The organism may be identified via polymerase chain reaction (PCR). Intestinal tuberculosis also shows a tropism for ileocecal lymphoid tissue. The granulomas are characteristically centrally necrotic and acid-fast stains are helpful in detecting bacilli. Systemic diseases, such as sarcoidosis, are often associated with manifestations in other organ systems. Other features of these disorders are detailed subsequently.

Natural History and Prognosis

Because true cases of idiopathic granulomatous appendicitis are extremely uncommon, the clinical course is not well characterized. However, reports of granulomatous inflammation isolated to the appendix without an identifiable underlying cause describe disease resolution following appendectomy.[79,80]

Sarcoidosis

Clinical Features

Sarcoidosis of the appendix is rare, but its epidemiology parallels that of the systemic disease. Namely, it shows a predilection for young to middle-aged African American patients. Most reports are of patients with known underlying sarcoidosis who present with signs and symptoms of acute appendicitis or chronic nonspecific abdominal pain.[81] Occasional cases wherein appendiceal disease was the initial manifestation of more widespread systemic involvement are also documented.[82] Because appendiceal involvement by sarcoidosis is often asymptomatic, its true incidence is unknown.[71] Although sarcoidosis is posited as one potential explanation for idiopathic granulomatous appendicitis, evidence that true sarcoidosis may be limited to the appendix is lacking.

Pathological Features

The main histological finding is multiple epithelioid granulomas, which are usually nonnecrotizing and involve any, or all, layers of the appendix (Fig. 18.13).[83-85] Features of chronic appendicitis may also be present, including fibrosis, transmural chronic inflammation, and crypt distortion. Patients who present acutely have superimposed features of acute appendicitis, including neutrophilic cryptitis, suppurative inflammation, and acute transmural inflammation. This raises the question of whether sarcoidosis is the cause of appendicitis, in these cases, or an incidental finding in the background of classic acute appendicitis.

Differential Diagnosis

A diagnosis of sarcoidosis is based on exclusion of other causes of granulomatous appendicitis. The differential diagnosis of sarcoidosis is listed in Box 18.4. Absence of central suppuration or necrosis and microorganisms in ancillary studies helps to exclude infection. Ileocecal or other segmental intestinal inflammation is highly suggestive of CD, whereas pulmonary, cardiac, neurological, or dermatological findings favor sarcoidosis.

Natural History and Prognosis

Ultimately, the prognosis of patients with sarcoidosis depends on the extent of involvement of other organs, such as the heart, lungs, and brain. Patients with appendiceal sarcoidosis are at higher risk for perforation, by some reports, but the risk of difficult to assess, given the rarity of the condition.[81]

Interval (Delayed) Appendicitis

Clinical Features

Some patients in whom the appendix has already ruptured at the time of clinical presentation may be treated initially with antibiotics and drainage rather than appendectomy. After a delay of typically 4 to 8 weeks, an appendectomy is usually then performed.[86]

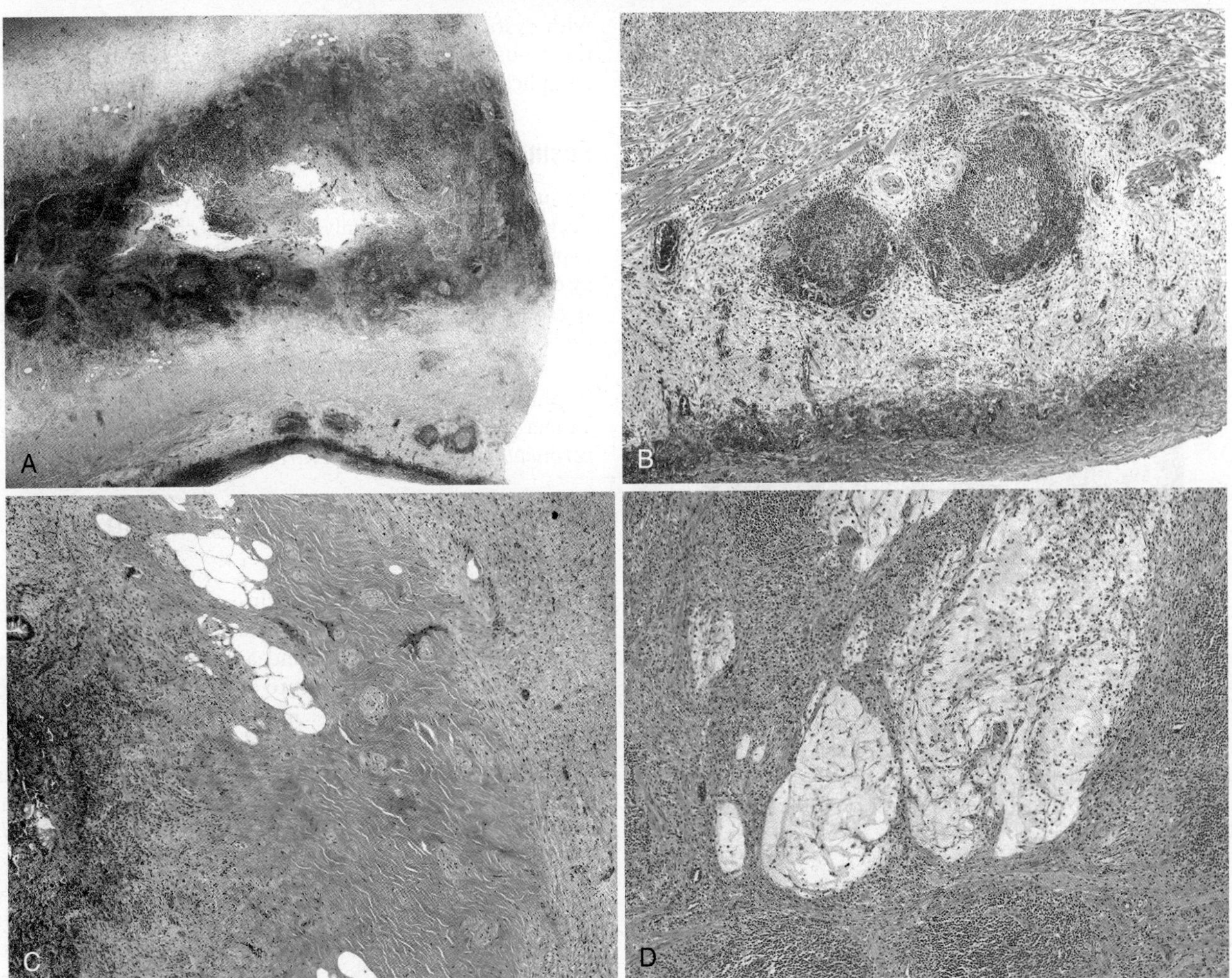

FIGURE 18.14 **A** and **B,** Interval appendicitis frequently shows lymphoid aggregates arranged transmurally in an orderly, string-of-pearls fashion. **C,** Fibrosis of the submucosa and muscularis propria is also common. **D,** Mucin extravasation in interval appendicitis may suggest the differential diagnosis of a mucinous neoplasm.

Pathological Features

The "interval" appendectomy specimen may show a variety of changes, such as cryptitis, crypt abscesses, mucosal crypt distortion, mural fibrosis, and transmural chronic inflammation with lymphoid aggregates, all of which can mimic CD (Fig. 18.14). Interval appendicitis features granulomas and/or multinucleated giant cells in approximately 50% of cases.[48,71] Granulomas often accompany other histological signs and symptoms of a prolonged clinical course, including periappendiceal adhesions and symptom duration >1 week.[86] Xanthogranulomatous inflammation is also frequently present.

Differential Diagnosis

Clinical history is the most important factor for identifying interval appendicitis and distinguishing it from other causes of acute appendicitis. Pathologists should be aware that patients who receive antibiotic therapy for unrelated conditions during an episode of acute appendicitis may have features of interval appendicitis.

Other histological findings of interval appendicitis may mimic CD, including cryptitis, crypt distortion, mural fibrosis, and transmural chronic inflammation with lymphoid aggregates. However, patients do not show clinical signs of CD on follow-up.[48] Other causes of granulomatous appendicitis may be excluded on the bases of special stains (see Table 18.3) and clinical history of concomitant disorders (or lack thereof).

Natural History and Prognosis

Outcomes appear comparable among patients who undergo interval appendectomy compared with those who are treated emergently, and overall complication rates are low. Interval appendectomy may be the preferred approach in settings where more time is required for surgical planning or on the basis of patient and physician preference.[87]

Cystic Fibrosis

Clinical Features

Cystic fibrosis is an inherited, multisystem, autosomal recessive disorder that results in defective chloride transport mechanisms. Mutations occur in the gene that codes for the cystic fibrosis transmembrane conductance protein (CFTR), encoded by a chloride ion channel gene located on chromosome 7q31. Seventy percent of patients have a

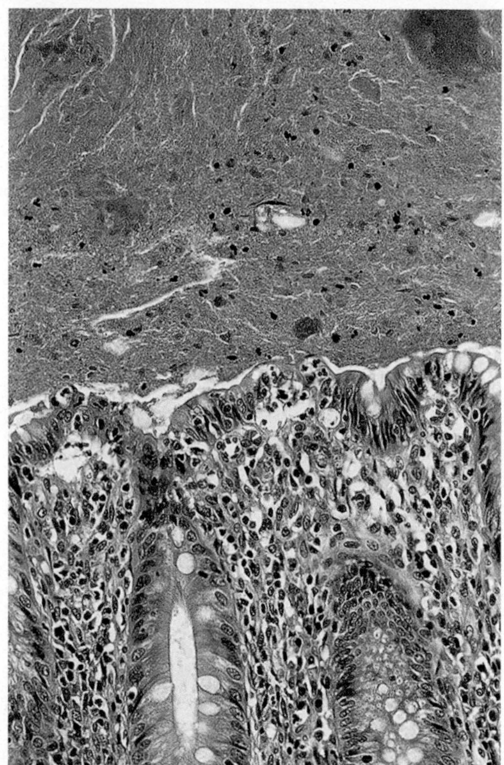

FIGURE 18.15 The appendix in patients with cystic fibrosis shows prominent goblet cells, and the lumen contains thick, inspissated, eosinophilic mucin.

mutation (i.e., deletion of the three-nucleotide codon for phenylalanine) at position ΔF508. Mutations result in defective transcellular salt and water transport and thick mucus secretions. Cystic fibrosis is the most common type of inherited disease among white North Americans and Europeans. It has an incidence of 1 case per 2500 live births.[88]

Pathological Features

The most readily identifiable abnormality is thick, inspissated mucin in the lumen of the appendix (Fig. 18.15). Accumulation of mucin may result in marked expansion and cystic dilatation of the appendix. In some cases, this alone can cause clinical symptoms of appendicitis.[89] The most common histological finding in patients with cystic fibrosis is enlargement and distention of goblet cells, which contain normal-appearing mucin. Inspissated eosinophilic mucin within dilated glands may be seen, but this is a nonspecific finding. Overall, patients with cystic fibrosis have a lower frequency of acute appendicitis (1.5%) compared with the general population (approximately 10%) for unknown reasons.[89] However, the incidence of acquired diverticula is markedly increased (see Fig. 18.4).[28]

Natural History and Prognosis

Treatment of cystic fibrosis includes pancreatic enzyme replacement, ursodeoxycholic acid to stimulate secretion of bile, airway clearance, and organ transplantation. Experimental therapeutic approaches include gene therapy and exogenous administration of nucleoside triphosphate. Insulin-dependent diabetes mellitus develops in approximately 25% of adult patients. The median survival of patients with cystic fibrosis now exceeds 30 years. The most common causes of death include liver disease, cardiorespiratory complications, and complications of organ transplantation.

Eosinophilic Appendicitis

Eosinophilic appendicitis is rare. In a review of 5262 appendectomy specimens, only two cases showed eosinophilic appendicitis.[90] In most cases, eosinophilic appendicitis is associated with parasitic infection, particularly *Strongyloides stercoralis*[91,92] and *Schistosoma japonicum*.[93] Examination of these cases showed an acute suppurative appendicitis with a predominance of eosinophils. Variable numbers of neutrophils may also be present. Increased eosinophils in the lamina propria are rarely found in patients with *Enterobius vermicularis* (formerly *Oxyuris vermicularis*) infection.[94]

INFECTIOUS CAUSES OF ACUTE AND CHRONIC APPENDICITIS

In most patients with classic acute appendicitis, organisms are not identified by histological analysis, although cultures often reveal mixed aerobic and anaerobic bacteria. In one study of 41 children with acute appendicitis, an average of 14 bacterial isolates per specimen was detected.[95] Bacterial isolates are usually composed of normal intestinal flora[95-97] and are thought to play a secondary role after mucosal injury. Bacteria belonging to the *Bacteroides fragilis* group are the most frequently isolated anaerobes, whereas *Escherichia coli* is the most frequently isolated aerobe.[95-97] Bacteria belonging to the *Streptococcus milleri* group are also common aerobes. These organisms may be of greater significance because they have been linked to a higher risk (sevenfold) of abscess formation.[98]

Other types of bacteria, fungi, and parasites cause appendicitis, particularly in immunocompromised and pediatric patients, and in patients from developing parts of the world (Table 18.4). The most commonly identified pathogens in these settings are discussed next.

Bacterial Infections

Yersinia

Clinical Features

Yersinia typically causes acute enteritis in young children and terminal ileitis and mesenteric adenitis in older children and young adults. In a study in which specific cultures were obtained, *Yersinia enterocolitica* was identified in approximately 4% of cases of acute appendicitis.[99]

Pathological Features

In most cases, appendices are grossly normal. Histologically, the characteristic finding is suppurative granulomatous inflammation, but in many cases the appendix may be normal or show only mild superficial acute inflammation (Fig. 18.16).[99] In a study by Lamps and colleagues in 2001, 10 (25%) of 40 patients with granulomatous appendicitis showed evidence of pathogenic *Yersinia* species detected by PCR.[100] Both *Y. enterocolitica* and *Y. pseudotuberculosis* can cause granulomatous inflammation with the formation

TABLE 18.4 Infectious Causes of Appendicitis

Organism	Key Histological Features/Inflammatory Pattern
Bacteria	
Shigella spp.	Acute appendicitis, pseudomembranes, mucosal necrosis
Clostridioides difficile	
Campylobacter spp.	Acute appendicitis, occasional granuloma formation
Yersinia spp.	Suppurative granulomatous inflammation, lymphoid hyperplasia
Actinomyces spp.	Mural and periappendiceal fibrosis, lymphoid hyperplasia, transmural inflammation, nonnecrotic granulomas
Mycobacterium tuberculosis	Large, necrotic, confluent granulomas, transmural inflammation and fibrosis
Viruses	
Adenovirus	Smudgy intranuclear inclusions in epithelial cells, lymphoid hyperplasia
Cytomegalovirus	Active inflammation with ulcers, intranuclear and intracytoplasmic inclusions in enlarged endothelial cells and fibroblasts
Measles	Lymphoid hyperplasia, multinucleated giant cells
Epstein-Barr Virus	Suppurative appendicitis with marked lymphoid hyperplasia
Parasites	
Enterobius vermicularis	Large worms with thick outer cuticle and lateral ala, usually minimal inflammatory response
Schistosomiasis	Eosinophil-rich inflammation, granulomatous reaction to ova
Strongyloidiasis	Eosinophil-rich inflammation, occasional granulomas, curved larvae with pointed tails in crypt lumina

of large, epithelioid, usually nonnecrotizing granulomas surrounded by a prominent lymphoid cuff.[100] In these cases, acute inflammation is common, including central microabscesses within granulomas. Lymphoid hyperplasia is typically present. Regional lymph nodes may also show evidence of granulomatous inflammation with or without suppuration.[100,101] Special stains are not helpful in the identification of *Yersinia*, but the diagnosis can be made via PCR, as mentioned earlier.

Differential Diagnosis

The differential diagnosis of *Yersinia*-associated appendicitis includes other causes of granulomatous appendicitis (see Table 18.3). CD is probably the most important consideration. CD typically features fewer granulomas that lack suppurative inflammation; CD is not limited to the appendix or periappendiceal tissues.

Natural History and Prognosis

Uncomplicated *Yersinia*-related appendicitis usually resolves after surgery. Patients with perforations or immunocompromised patients may require systemic antibiotics.[102]

Mycobacterium tuberculosis

Tuberculosis of the appendix is quite rare, and even most cases of ileocecal tuberculosis spare the appendix. Appendiceal involvement is more likely to occur as a secondary affect of intraabdominal disease, often in patients with pulmonary tuberculosis.[102] Isolated infections of the appendix have been reported.[103,104] The histological findings are identical to those seen elsewhere in the GI tract. They include large, confluent necrotic granulomas associated with transmural inflammation and fibrosis. Acid-fast stain can help to detect bacilli, and PCR analysis can be used to subtype the organism.

Actinomyces

Clinical Features

Actinomyces israelii is an uncommon cause of appendicitis. These gram-positive filamentous bacteria commonly colonize the oral cavity and intestinal tract. Rarely, *A. israelii* can lead to infections of the small intestine, appendix, or colon. Appendicitis presents in adolescence or young adulthood.[105] Patients present with acute abdominal pain, nausea, and fever. Others have a more chronic course with abdominal pain lasting weeks or months before clinical presentation.[106]

Pathological Features

Actinomyces infection produces dense fibrosis that may raise concern for malignancy radiographically and intraoperatively.[107] Associated purulent exudate contains yellow-brown "sulfur granules." Histologically, periappendiceal fibrosis is prominent, as are mucosal lymphoid hyperplasia, transmural lymphoid aggregates, and active mucosal inflammation. Sulfur granules, usually identified in the lumen, contain tangles of long, filamentous organisms staining dark blue on routine hematoxylin and eosin preparations, which are associated with clublike projections of eosinophilic Splendore-Hoeppli material (Fig. 18.17). They can be highlighted by Grocott's methenamine silver (GMS) stains and are gram positive. Nonnecrotic granulomas are often present in all mural layers, and some may be centered on lymphoid follicles. Fistula formation, rupture of the appendix, and abscess formation are common.[108] *Actinomyces turicensis* also has been implicated in causing appendicitis. It is frequently accompanied by aerobic bacterial isolates of the *Streptococcus anginosus* group.[109]

Differential Diagnosis

The main differential diagnoses include other infections causing granulomatous inflammation (see Tables 18.3 and 18.4), CD, and interval appendicitis. In one recent study, *Actinomyces* appendicitis was noted to display a greater degree of periappendiceal fibrosis, lymphoid hyperplasia, and transmural inflammation than CD. *Actinomyces* infection did not feature xanthogranulomatous inflammation, which helps distinguish it from interval appendicitis.[106]

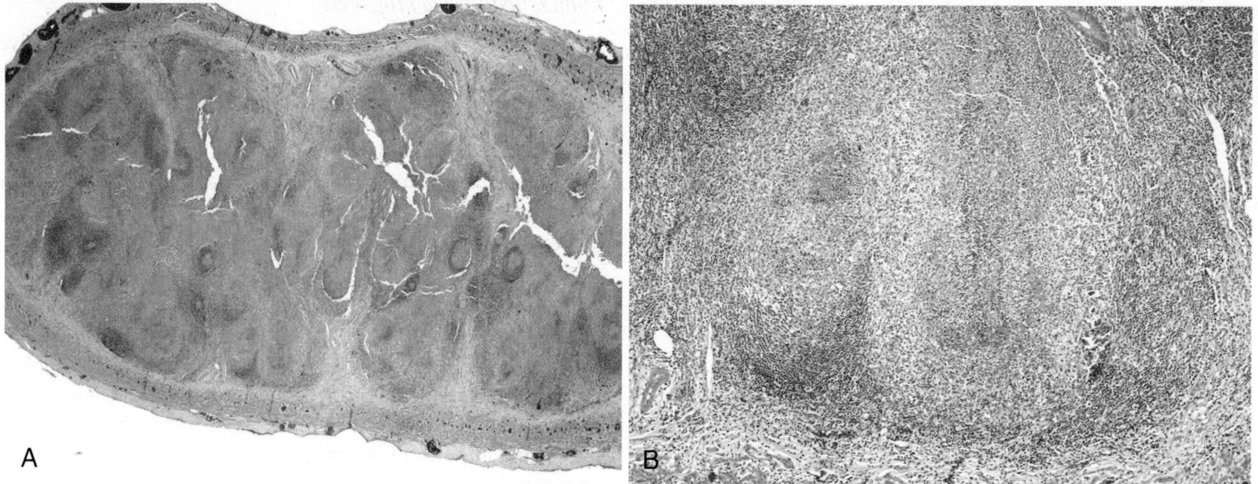

FIGURE 18.16 *Yersinia* appendicitis is characterized by suppurative granulomas and lymphoid aggregates distributed throughout the appendiceal wall as seen at low (**A**) and high (**B**) magnification.

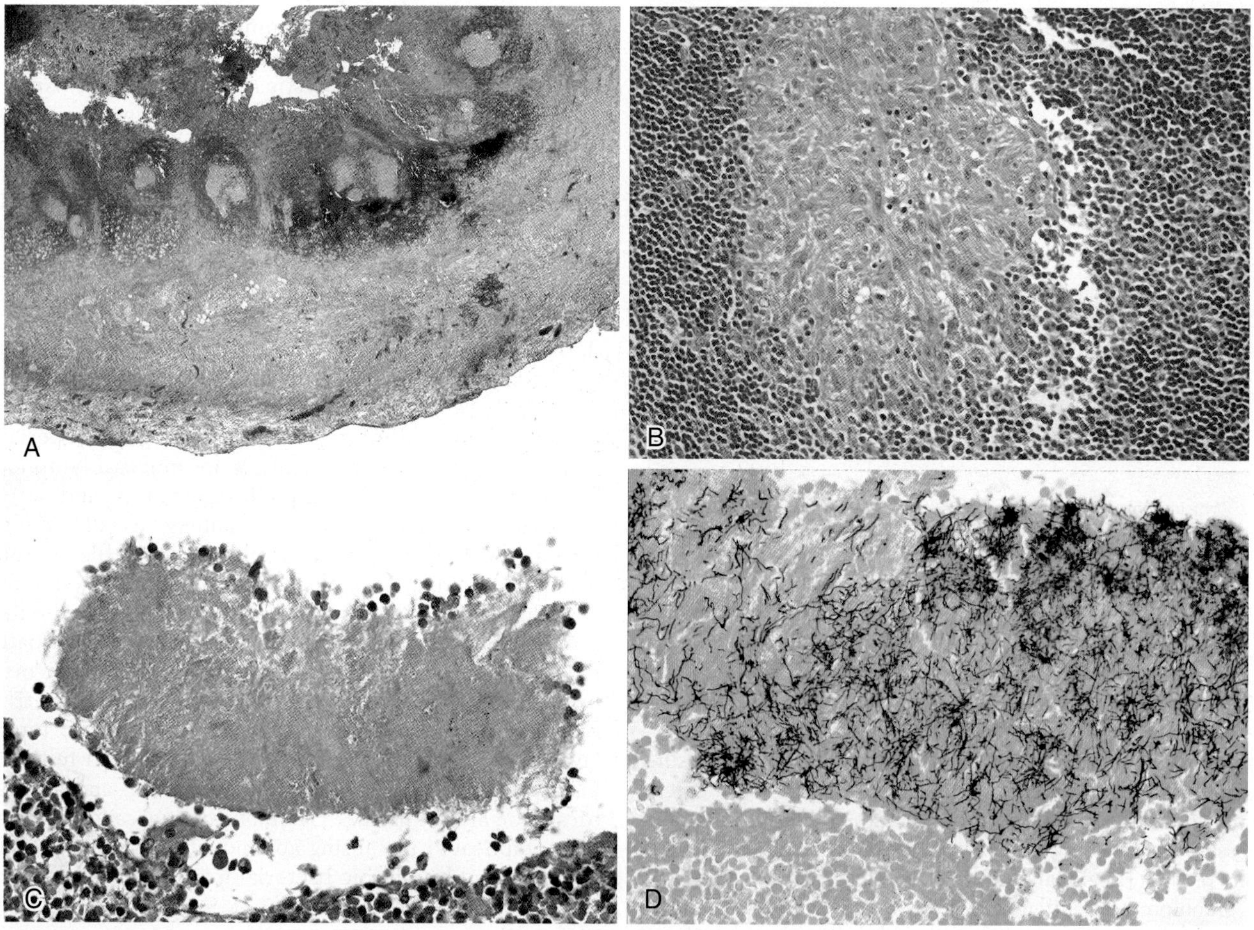

FIGURE 18.17 A, Numerous granulomata are present in the appendiceal mucosa of a patient with *Actinomyces* infection. **B,** The granulomata are epithelioid with a surrounding lymphoid cuff. **C,** "Sulfur granules" contain filamentous blue-staining organisms that are highlighted by a GMS stain **(D)**.

Natural History and Prognosis

In some cases, *Actinomyces* may be an incidental finding rather than the cause of appendicitis. Indeed, some cases wherein the organism was missed in initial review have resulted in no adverse consequences. On the other hand, active infection may result in perforation and intraabdominal actinomycosis, requiring long-term antibiotic therapy.[106]

Campylobacter

Campylobacter jejuni is an uncommon cause of bacterial appendicitis. In one study, *Campylobacter* was detected by immunohistochemical methods in 3 (2.6%) of 116 cases of acute appendicitis.[110] Most patients were young children who had grossly normal appendices. Histologically, active inflammatory changes were limited to the mucosa and consisted

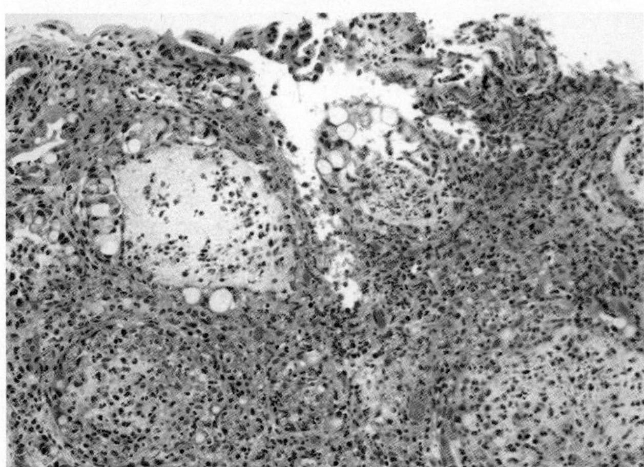

FIGURE 18.18 *Clostridioides difficile* may involve the appendix, particularly in patients with pancolitis. Dilated crypts contain sloughed epithelial cells, inflammatory cells, and mucin. Intercrypt necrosis and inflammation obscure the architecture.

of cryptitis and surface erosions with focal aggregates of histiocytes that occasionally resulted in granuloma formation.[110] One study that used more sensitive PCR techniques found C. *jejuni* DNA in 11 (22%) of 50 cases of acute appendicitis. In that study, all 20 incidental appendectomy specimens (controls) were found to be negative. Whether this organism is a significant cause of acute appendicitis, an innocent bystander, or a cause of superinfection remains unknown.[111]

Clostridium difficile *and* Shigella

Clostridium difficile and *Shigella* infections that involve the appendix are usually associated with generalized colonic disease, although acute appendicitis may rarely represent the initial manifestation. Overall, the histological findings are identical to those seen in the colon. Features include pseudomembrane formation, ulceration, cryptitis, crypt abscesses, and lamina propria hemorrhage (Fig. 18.18).

Malakoplakia

Malakoplakia is most frequently encountered in the urinary tract, but it can also be found in many other organs, including the appendix. In one case report, it was associated with ova of *Taenia* species.[112] Malakoplakia results from an abnormal immune response in which bacteria are incompletely digested and thus accumulate in histiocytes.[113] Typical histological findings include diffuse or nodular thickening of the mucosa resulting from an accumulation of macrophages that contain eosinophilic cytoplasm. Scattered lymphocytes and plasma cells are always present. Michaelis-Gutmann bodies, which are round, laminated structures with a targetoid appearance, are the most characteristic feature (Fig. 18.19). These structures can be highlighted with an iron or calcium stain.

Spirochetosis

Clinical Features

Spirochetosis, most often caused by *Brachyspira aalborgi*, may rarely occur in the appendix. In one study, spirochetosis was detected in 1.9% of incidentally removed appendices, in 0.7% of appendices in patients with histologically proven acute appendicitis, and in 12.3% of patients with clinically suspected acute appendicitis, but histologically normal appendices.[114] These results suggest that spirochetosis may contribute to clinical symptoms in patients with otherwise normal appendices. Spirochetosis of the small intestine and colon is more commonly found in HIV-infected patients than in non–HIV-infected patients. However, little information is available on whether this is also true for the appendix. Overall, adults are more commonly infected than children.[115]

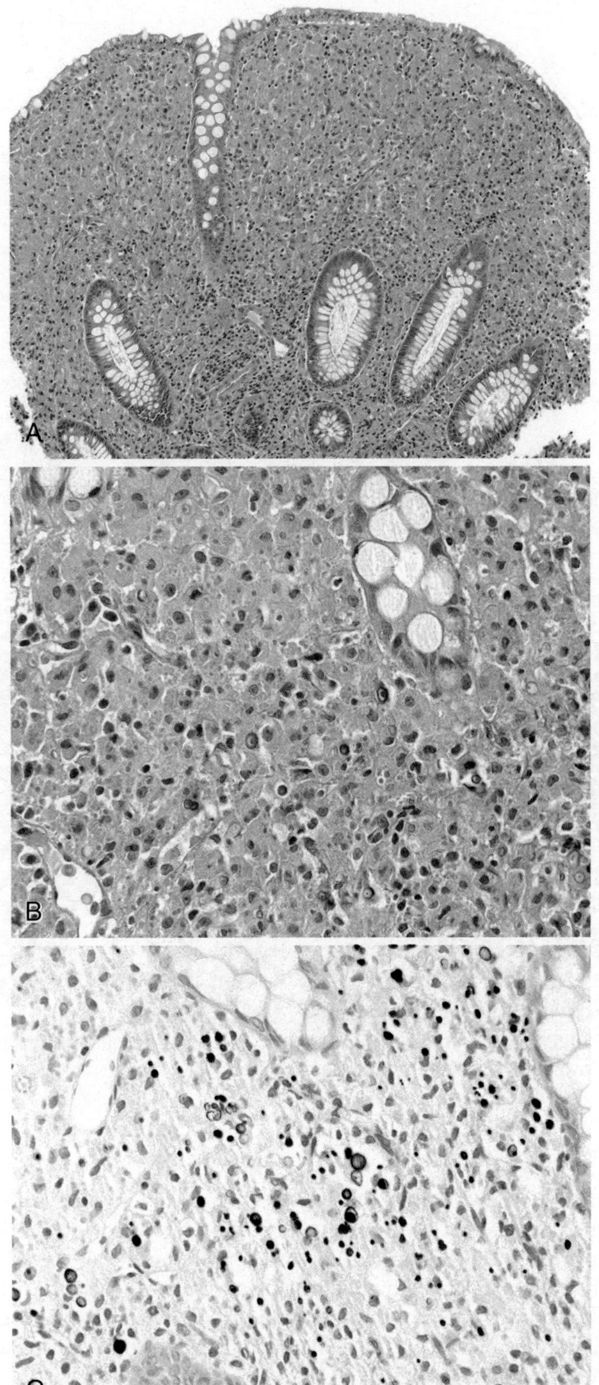

FIGURE 18.19 **A,** Malakoplakia involving appendiceal mucosa is composed of sheets of histiocytes with admixed Michaelis-Gutmann bodies. **B,** They are round, laminated structures with a targetoid appearance. **C,** The Michaelis-Gutmann bodies are highlighted by von Kossa stain.

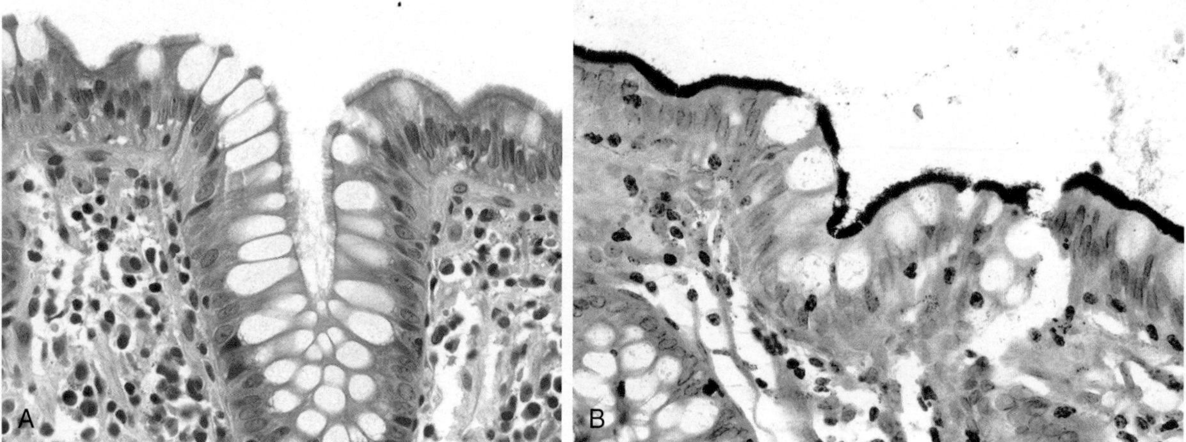

FIGURE 18.20 **A,** Spirochetosis produces a blue "fringe" of adherent organisms without any inflammatory response. **B,** The organisms are highlighted with a Warthin-Starry stain.

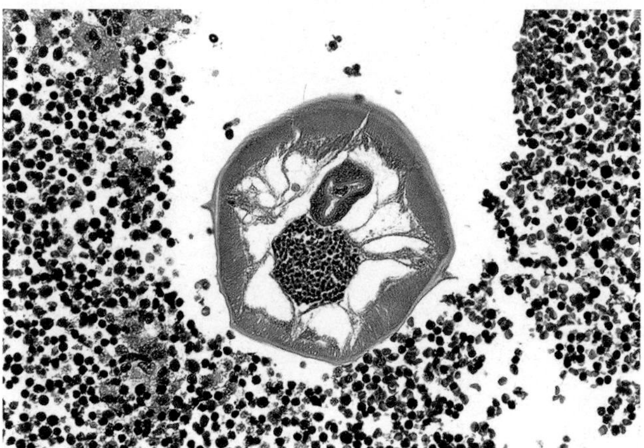

FIGURE 18.21 *Enterobius vermicularis* in the appendiceal lumen. Note the characteristic external cuticle and lateral ala.

Pathological Features

Histologically, spirochetosis is characterized by the presence of a hematoxylin-positive band of organisms, which is approximately 3 μm thick, situated on the surface of the epithelium, and can be highlighted by silver stains (Fig. 18.20). Typically, there is no associated inflammatory response. Electron microscopy reveals organisms within epithelial cells and macrophages.[115]

Helicobacter pylori

Several studies have documented *Helicobacter pylori* organisms in appendices by PCR analysis. Some patients also have acute appendicitis.[116,117] However, a causal relationship between this organism and the development of acute appendicitis has not been confirmed.

Parasitic Infections

Enterobius vermicularis

Clinical Features

Enterobius vermicularis (i.e., pinworm) is one of the most common parasites encountered in the appendix, especially in temperate climates. The overall frequency ranges from 2.4% in Iran[118] to 8.7% in central Europe.[119] At the Johns Hopkins Hospital in Baltimore, Maryland, only 4 (0.25%) of 1584 appendices removed during a 17-year period from patients 15 years of age or younger had proven *Enterobius* infection of the appendix. Another study at Children's Hospital in Columbus, Ohio, showed that 21 (1.4%) of 1549 patients had intraluminal pinworms of the appendix.[120] Children in late childhood and early adolescence (5 to 15 years old) have the highest incidence of infection,[119,121] which is as high as 24% in some studies.

Most patients are asymptomatic. The worm is commonly found in the lumen of the appendix without any significant inflammatory response (Fig. 18.21). However, large worms may obstruct the appendiceal lumen, resulting in development of a mucocele. Eggs and worms in the stool may cause pruritus ani.

Pathological Features

Grossly, the white worms may be visible to the naked eye and usually measure between 2 and 5 mm in greatest diameter. They can also colonize the ileum and proximal colon. Microscopically, the worms have a thick outer cuticle, from which lateral ala project. Internal organs, or eggs, may be visible in the internal aspect of the worm. In one study in which almost 22,000 appendices were evaluated, granulomatous inflammation and increased eosinophils in the lamina propria were rare, occurring in less than 2% of infections.[94] Rarely, worms may invade surrounding tissues, resulting in ulceration and a marked inflammatory response composed of neutrophils and eosinophils. In most cases, there is minimal tissue response to the worm in surrounding tissues. An inverse relationship between active mucosal inflammation and pinworm infection has been observed in several studies.[121-123] Mucosal inflammation has been more strongly linked to the presence of parasite ova.[124] Treatment requires antiparasitic medication such as mebendazole or albendazole.

Strongyloides stercoralis

Strongyloides stercoralis is endemic to tropical and subtropical regions. Eosinophilic appendicitis has been associated with *Strongyloides stercoralis* infection.[91] Morphological features consist of a diffuse infiltrate of eosinophils that is often associated with abscess formation and necrosis. Granulomas may also be present. Larvae are present within crypt lumina; they are basophilic and curved with pointed tails (Fig. 18.22). Identification of the organism in stool specimens is a more sensitive method of detecting infection than analysis of appendiceal tissues.[91,125]

Schistosomiasis

Schistosomiasis is an unusual cause of acute appendicitis; it usually results from *S. haematobium* infection. The disease is endemic in Africa and the Mediterranean and appendiceal involvement is frequent in those areas, although it may be asymptomatic.[126] Symptomatic patients present with symptoms of acute appendicitis or an inflammatory mass. Histological features include transmural eosinophil-rich inflammation with a granulomatous reaction to ova. Eggs are ovoid and calcified; they may be associated with mural fibrosis[102] (Fig. 18.23).

Other Parasitic Infections

Cryptosporidium spp., *Entamoeba histolytica*, *Balantidium coli*, *Toxoplasma* spp., *Trichuris trichiura*, and *Ascaris lumbricoides* rarely infect the appendix.[102,127,128] Parasites in the appendix may be a harbinger of infection elsewhere in the GI tract, so their identification is clinically important.

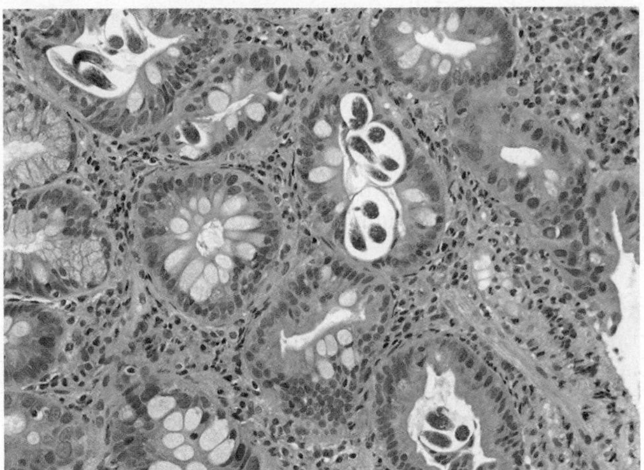

FIGURE 18.22 *Strongyloides* larvae are found in crypt lumina. They are basophilic and curved with pointed tails.

Viral Infections

Viral gastroenteritis does not typically result in appendectomy, although some cases of appendicitis are, no doubt, caused by viral agents. Viral enteritis may lead to surgical excision of the appendix when the infection causes ileocecal intussusception. In such cases, a segment of small intestine, either with or without a segment of the right colon, is also resected. Intussusception is commonly attributed to lymphoid hyperplasia in the terminal ileum, which forms the leading edge of the intussuscepted segment. It classically occurs in infants and young children. Viral agents that are most commonly implicated in this setting are rotavirus, echovirus, and adenovirus.

Adenovirus

Clinical Features

Adenovirus is the most frequently detected virus in the appendix.[129,130] It is an important cause of acute appendicitis and appendiceal intussusception in children. Presumably, viral infection causes lymphoid hyperplasia and consequent appendiceal obstruction. Infection may occur via the enteric route or disseminate hematogenously after upper respiratory infection in immunocompromised hosts. Some evidence indicates that the incidence of adenovirus-associated acute appendicitis is underestimated in adults.[131] This is not surprising, given the subtle nature of histological findings in this infection.

Pathological Features

In appendices infected with adenovirus, lymphoid hyperplasia is prominent, and erosions may be identified. Viral inclusions are typically found in intact mucosal epithelial cells. Zones in which inclusions may be identified are best selected by scanning at low magnification for areas of mucosa that have a ragged appearance to the epithelium. In these areas, the epithelium shows a loss of nuclear polarity and loss of goblet cell mucin, which imparts an eosinophilic appearance to the cells. These zones are frequently

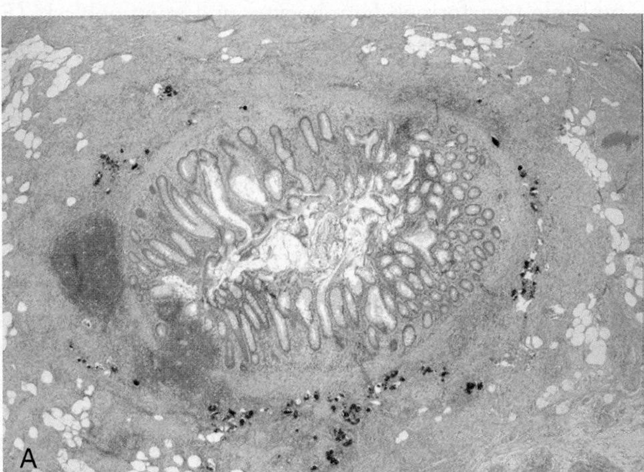

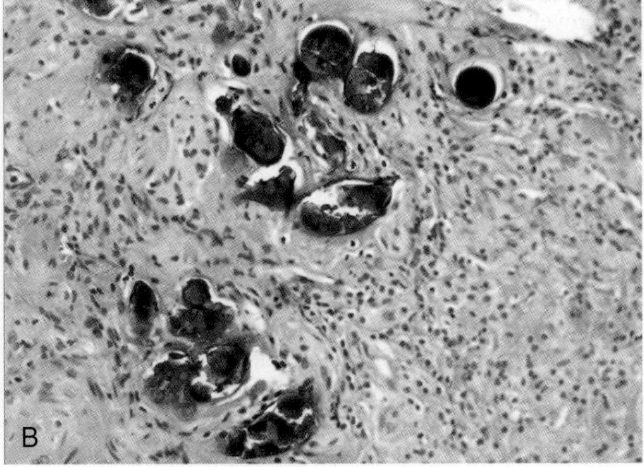

FIGURE 18.23 A, Calcified *Schistosoma* ova are radially arranged in the submucosa. **B,** Calcification, associated fibrosis, and lack of inflammatory reaction reflect remote infection.

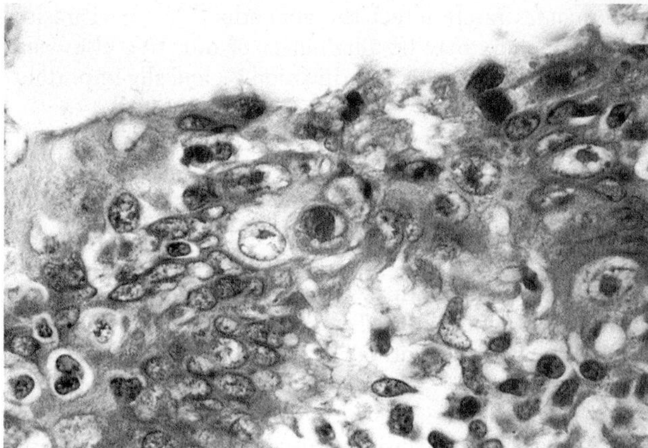

FIGURE 18.24 Adenovirus infection within appendiceal epithelial cells showing Cowdry A and Cowdry B inclusions.

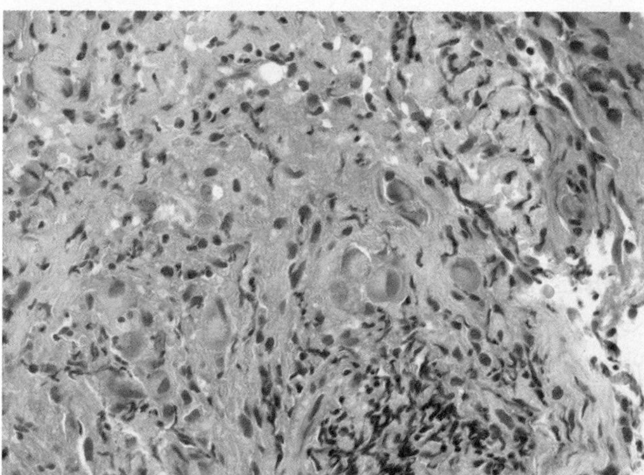

FIGURE 18.25 Cytomegalovirus inclusions are seen in the stromal cells of an ulcer. The nuclear inclusions are eosinophilic and have a lentiform contour. Cytoplasmic inclusions are granular.

associated with reactive lymphoid follicles. Intranuclear adenovirus inclusions are typically Cowdry type B bodies, showing prominent nuclear smudging. Cowdry type A inclusions, which show sharply demarcated intranuclear inclusions surrounded by a clear zone or halo, are found in the minority of cases (Fig. 18.24).

Differential Diagnosis

The main differential diagnosis is cytomegalovirus (CMV). CMV tends to cause appendicitis in immunocompromised hosts. It produces cellular enlargement and intranuclear and intracytoplasmic inclusions that are typically limited to stromal and endothelial cells in the lower GI tract.

Natural History and Prognosis

There is no specific treatment for adenovirus infection. Patients are managed surgically for intussusception and appendicitis and generally experience uncomplicated postoperative courses.[102]

Cytomegalovirus

Clinical Features

Cytomegalovirus (CMV) is an important cause of acute appendicitis in immunocompromised hosts, particularly those with AIDS.[132] The clinical course may be more prolonged than typical acute appendicitis. Patients experience fever, abdominal pain, and diarrhea before developing right lower quadrant pain. The nonspecific early clinical course predisposes to underrecognition and rupture. CMV infection is occasionally responsible for the development of acute appendicitis in immunocompetent patients.[44,133]

Pathological Features

Histological features are similar to those in other infected sites of the GI tract. Viral cytopathic effects are most often detected in endothelial cells, or stromal fibroblasts, rather than in epithelial cells. CMV infection results in granular cytoplasmic inclusions and intranuclear eosinophilic inclusions (Fig. 18.25). Other findings include epithelial cell apoptosis and neutrophilic cryptitis. As in other exuberant inflammatory backgrounds, immunohistochemistry may be necessary to identify viral inclusions.

Differential Diagnosis

Adenovirus inclusions may simulate CMV in the appendix. In contrast to CMV, adenovirus does not produce cellular enlargement, inclusions are exclusively intranuclear, and are smudgy and basophilic.

Natural History and Prognosis

High index of suspicion and thorough pathological examination are necessary to recognize CMV-associated appendicitis. Its identification is important because patients require antiviral therapy, in addition to surgery, and may have systemic infection. The infection responds well to antiviral treatment.[134]

Epstein-Barr Virus

Epstein-Barr virus has been detected in a small subset of individuals with acute appendicitis. It is found in appendices with acute suppurative appendicitis and those with marked lymphoid hyperplasia as the only major histological abnormality.[135-137] In some reports, patients with infectious mononucleosis developed superimposed acute suppurative appendicitis that required surgery.[135] Lymphoid hyperplasia associated with Epstein-Barr virus infection exhibits multiple transformed lymphocytes and immunoblasts (Fig. 18.26). These cells may raise the possibility of lymphoma if the polymorphous nature of the lymphoid proliferation is not appreciated.

Measles Virus

The incidence of measles infection has declined drastically in the past 50 years, mainly because of implementation of vaccination programs. However, small outbreaks still occur. Acute appendicitis may occur in the prodromal or fulminant phases of measles virus infection. In the prodromal phase, the histological appearance is that of marked lymphoid hyperplasia with multinucleate giant cells (i.e., Warthin-Finkeldey cells) either with or without other classic features of acute appendicitis.[138-140] In the late stages of infection, acute suppurative appendicitis may develop, which may be the result of luminal obstruction caused by lymphoid hyperplasia.[141]

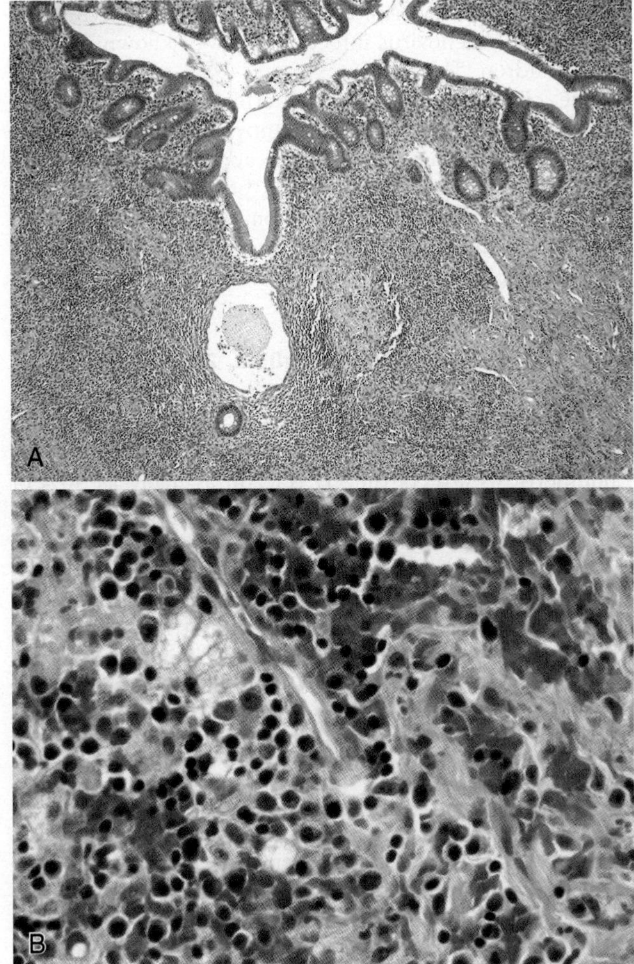

FIGURE 18.26 A, Epstein-Barr virus appendicitis shows mild active inflammation. **B,** A diagnostic pitfall is the presence of prominent activated lymphoid cells that can mimic a high-grade lymphoma.

Varicella-Zoster Virus

Varicella-zoster virus (VZV) associated acute appendicitis has been reported in a 1-year-old boy with active chickenpox. The appendectomy specimen showed an edematous retrocecal appendix with transmural acute inflammation and multiple intranuclear viral inclusions surrounded by a clear halo (i.e., Cowdry type A inclusions). PCR analysis of peripheral blood and appendiceal tissue demonstrated VZV DNA.[142]

Fungal Infections

Fungal infections such as aspergillosis, mucormycosis, histoplasmosis, and candidiasis can involve the appendix,[143,144] but they usually are part of a systemic infection. Patients are typically immunosuppressed because of organ transplantation or chemotherapy. Granulomatous inflammation associated with invasive candidiasis involving the appendix has been reported,[145] but most cases show suppurative inflammation without granulomas. However, because these patients are usually immunosuppressed, the inflammatory infiltrate may be quite mild despite a high volume of organisms. Accompanying epithelial changes, such as denudation and degeneration, are common (Fig. 18.27).

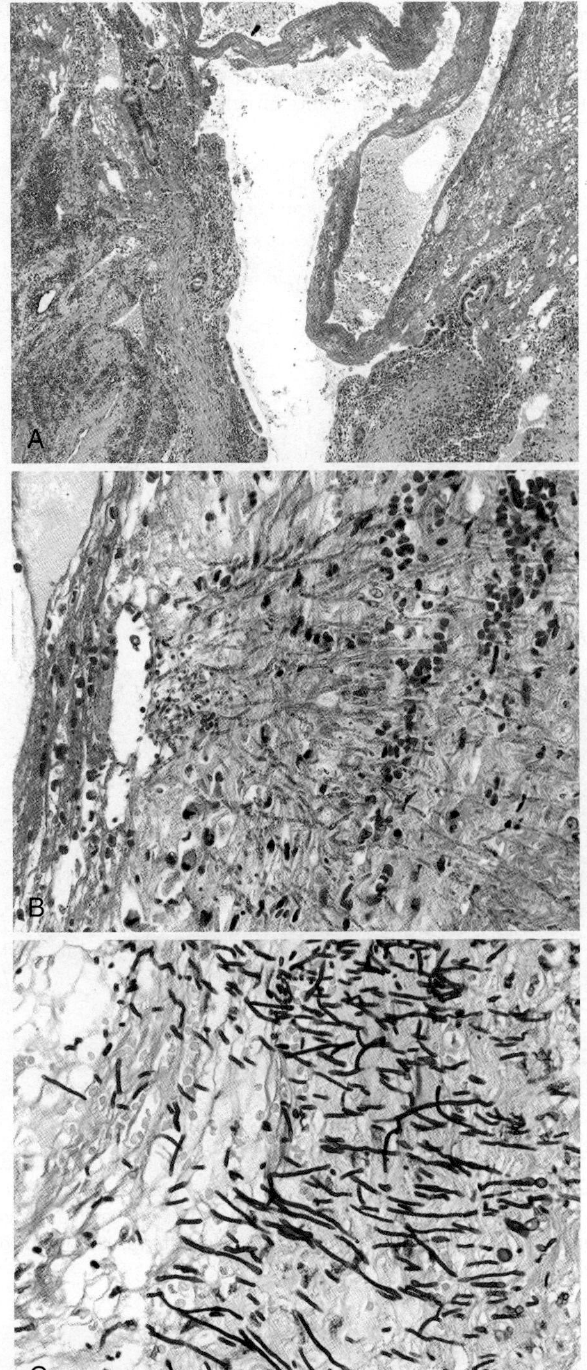

FIGURE 18.27 A, Invasive candidal appendicitis in an immunocompromised patient is evidenced by extensive epithelial denudation and fibrin deposition but a minimal inflammatory infiltrate. **B,** Numerous spores and pseudohyphae are seen on hematoxylin and eosin (H&E) stain. **C,** They are highlighted by periodic acid–Schiff (PAS) stain with diastase digestion.

MISCELLANEOUS DISORDERS OF THE APPENDIX

Intussusception of the Appendix

Intussusception of the appendix is frequently associated with other abnormalities, such as endometriosis or polyps, the latter located mainly in the base of the appendix.[146-148] The causes of appendiceal intussusception include anatomic factors, such as a mobile mesoappendix and wide proximal appendicular lumen, and intrinsic abnormalities, such as polyps, tumors, parasites, endometriosis, and lymphoid hyperplasia. Adenovirus infection is a well-known risk factor in children.[149]

The clinical presentation of affected patients varies. Symptoms include recurrent, crampy right lower quadrant abdominal pain that mimics acute appendicitis. Histologically, affected mucosa may show prolapse-type changes, with crypt architectural distortion, ingrowth of smooth muscle into the lamina propria, and fibrosis. Treatment is usually surgical, consisting of appendectomy, either with or without ileocolic resection.

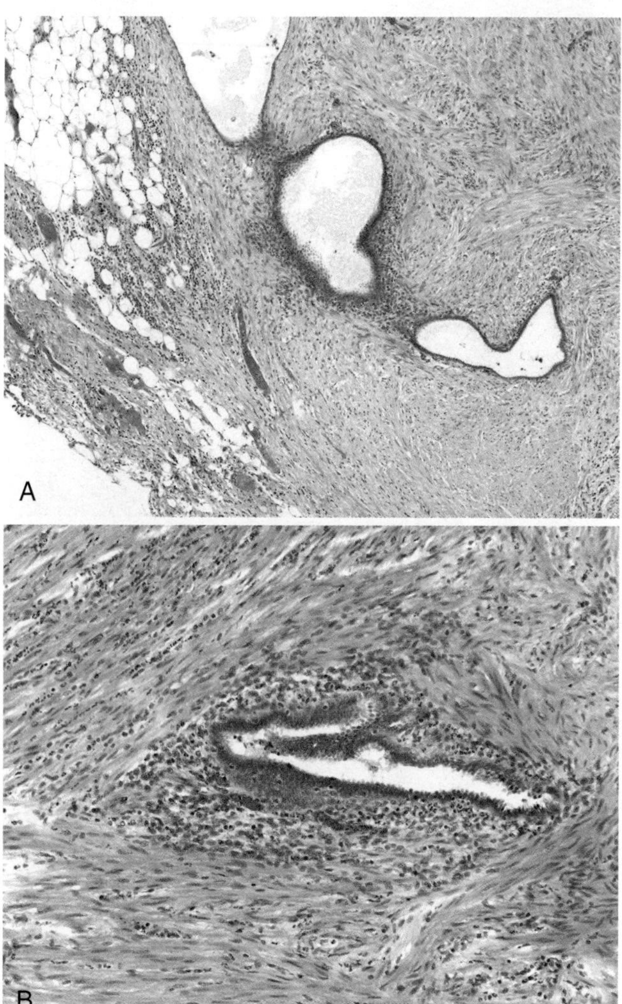

FIGURE 18.28 **A,** Endometriosis, on the serosa of this appendix, acted as a lead point for intussusception. **B,** It comprises endometrial glands surrounded by endometrial stroma that contains extravasation red blood cells.

Endometriosis, Endosalpingiosis, and Deciduosis

Endometriosis

Clinical Features

Endometriosis affects the GI tract in as many as 40% of patients with pelvic endometriosis. The sigmoid colon is the most common site of GI involvement, but the appendix may be involved in up to 15% of cases.[150] The incidence of appendiceal endometriosis is between 0.4% and 2.8%.[151] Although appendiceal endometriosis can masquerade clinically as acute appendicitis,[150,152] patients typically have a nonspecific clinical presentation.[150,152-154] Pain may wax and wane with the menstrual cycle. Occasionally, endometriosis acts as the leading edge for appendiceal intussusception.[147]

Pathological Features

Most cases involve the serosa or muscularis propria and are accompanied by abundant fibrosis and adhesions, although exclusively submucosal cases also occur.[152-154] Cysts filled with hemorrhagic debris may be identified. Histologically, endometriosis of the appendix consists of endometrial-type glands and stroma (Fig. 18.28) associated with hemosiderin deposition and a fibroblastic reaction. The endometrial epithelium undergoes changes in response to the menstrual cycle. For instance, a stromal decidual reaction may be detected in endometriotic foci in pregnant patients (Fig. 18.29).[153] Intestinal metaplasia is well described in endometriosis. It is found admixed with conventional-appearing endometriosis and features goblet-like mucin-containing cells. The mucinous epithelium may appear hyperplastic with tall mucin vacuoles.[155]

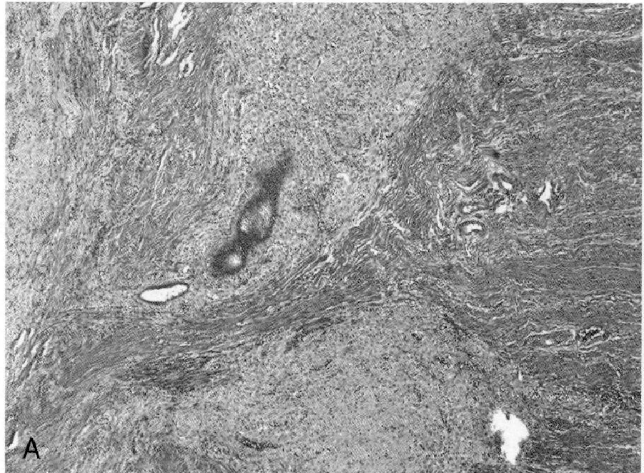

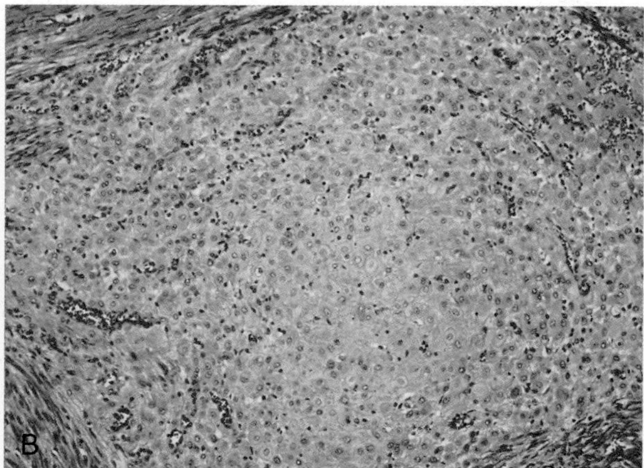

FIGURE 18.29 **A,** Endometrial stroma may become decidualized in pregnant patients. **B,** The stromal cells become polygonal with abundant eosinophilic cytoplasm, and may be mistaken for an epithelial proliferation.

Differential Diagnosis

The diagnosis of endometriosis is usually straightforward, but small endometrial rests may be missed by sampling and lead to an erroneous diagnosis of acute appendicitis, or endometrial glands may not be present in initial sections. Clues to the diagnosis include cellular stromal deposits on the appendiceal serosa, hemorrhage and hemosiderin, and muscular hypertrophy. Step sections may be necessary to identify endometrial glands. Other types of müllerian deposits, namely endosalpingiosis and endocervicosis, may simulate endometriosis. Endosalpingiosis features ciliated epithelium without endometrial stroma. Endocervicosis features mucinous glands that may be admixed with other types of extrauterine müllerian deposits.[156]

Intestinal metaplasia in endometriosis may raise the possibility of dissecting LAMN, particularly when the appendix is distorted and the true lumen is difficult to identify. Immunohistochemistry is helpful in this regard, since endometriotic rests stain for CK7 and ER and are invested by CD10-positive stroma.[155]

Natural History and Prognosis

Most of the morbidity associated with endometriosis results from adhesions, which can lead to infertility, intestinal obstruction, and chronic pain. Management often requires a multimodality approach that includes hormonal therapy and surgical intervention. Rarely, clear cell carcinoma or other primary müllerian carcinomas may arise in endometriotic foci.

Endosalpingiosis

Endosalpingiosis refers to the presence of benign fallopian tube epithelium at extra-müllerian sites, usually the serosal surfaces of the pelvis and peritoneum (Fig. 18.30). Implants may become cystic and clinically simulate acute appendicitis or an appendiceal neoplasm.[157] They comprise ciliated columnar epithelium in glandular formations without endometrial stroma.

Deciduosis

Deciduosis results from the effects of progesterone on extrauterine mesenchymal cells during pregnancy. It is most often seen in ovarian tissues. Deciduosis, in contrast to endometriosis, is more often associated with signs and symptoms of acute appendicitis.[158-160] It usually appears as white plaques or small nodules on the serosa. Deciduosis differs from endometriosis histologically in that it lacks glands. It consists of large polyhedral-shaped cells with abundant granular eosinophilic cytoplasm and small, round nuclei with distinct nucleoli arranged in sheets in the serosa or outer muscularis propria. Rarely, deciduosis occurs in the mucosa of the GI tract.[161] Decidual cells can sometimes be mistaken for malignant (often epithelial) tumors, but immunohistochemical stains for cytokeratins, carcinoembryonic antigen, epithelial membrane antigen, and S100 protein are typically negative. Decidualized cells may show desmin or muscle actin positivity.[158]

Gliomatosis and Other Heterotopias

Gliomatosis peritonei is found in patients with ovarian teratomas and consists of mature glial tissue on the serosal surfaces.[162] Pelvic gliomatosis can affect the serosal aspect of the appendix (Fig. 18.31). It has also been reported as a rare complication of ventricular shunts.[163] Malignant transformation has been recorded.[164,165] Heterotopic gastric and esophageal tissue have also been described in the appendix.[166]

Pigments, Foreign Material, and Processing Artifacts

Melanosis

Melanosis involves the appendix in approximately 7% of individuals older than 40 years. It is histologically identical to that seen in the colon.[167] Pigmented macrophages contain cytoplasmic material (e.g., lipofuscin) that ranges from pale green to dark brown (Fig. 18.32). The pigment lipofuscin accumulates due to ingestion of apoptotic surface epithelial cells by macrophages.[168] The most common cause is laxative use in patients with chronic constipation. Melanosis of the appendix is also relatively common in pediatric patients, and it is thought to represent a response to infection rather than to laxatives.[169]

Barium

Barium can be present in the lumen of the appendix with no associated mucosal response. However, occasionally barium extravasates into the mucosa, where it is phagocytosed by macrophages and induces a granulomatous reaction. Barium is a nonpolarizable, crystalline material that is typically light green (Fig. 18.33).

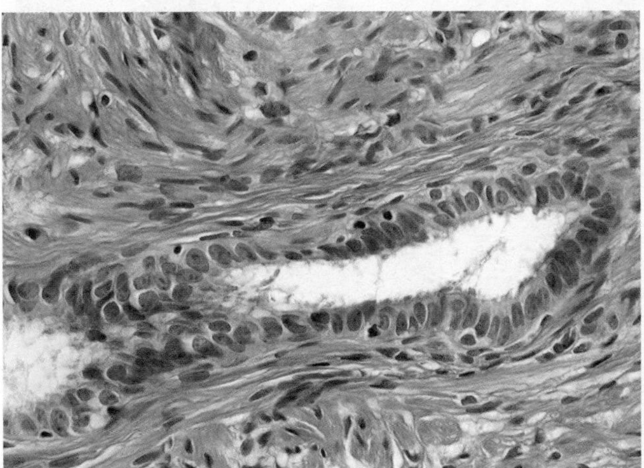

FIGURE 18.30 Fallopian tube epithelium is ciliated and is not invested by stroma in this focus of endosalpingiosis.

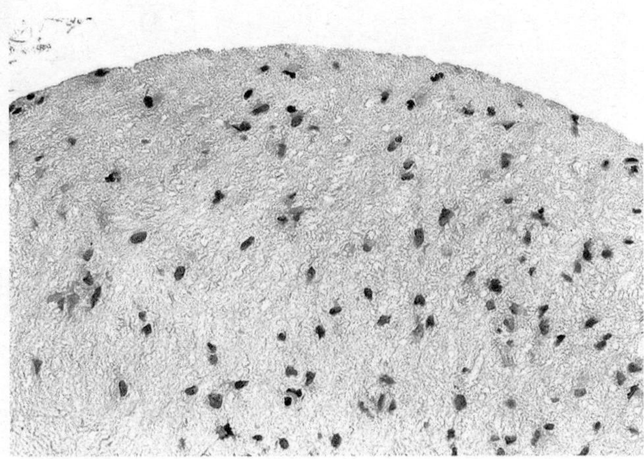

FIGURE 18.31 Gliomatosis consists of nodular glial tissue adherent to the serosa of the appendix.

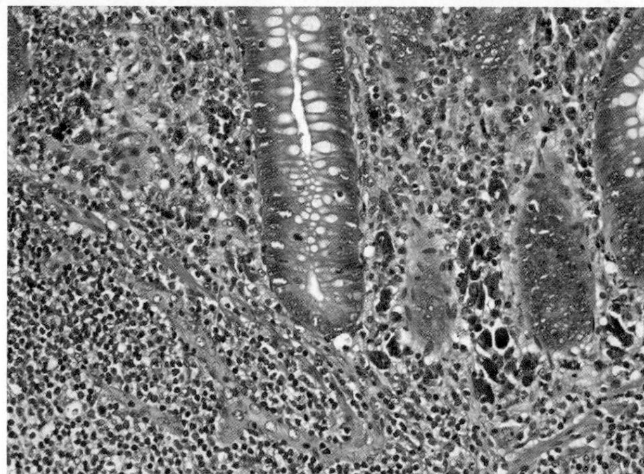

FIGURE 18.32 Melanosis may involve the appendix in patients who take laxatives. Granular brown pigment is present in lamina propria macrophages.

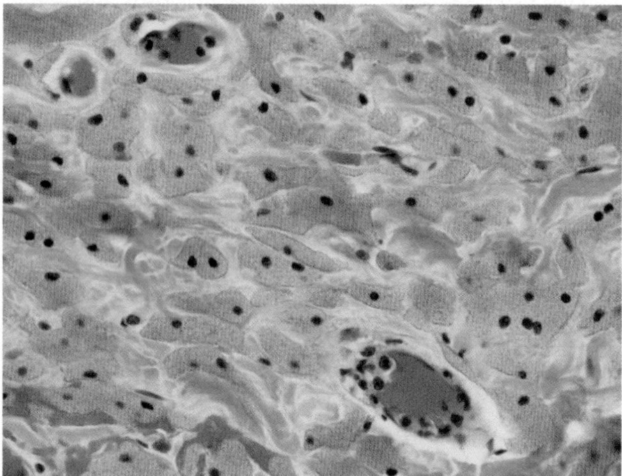

FIGURE 18.33 Barium pigment may be ingested by macrophages. It is grayish green and finely granular. (*Courtesy Dr. Karen Choi, The University of Michigan.*)

Foreign Body Appendicitis

Foreign body appendicitis is rare. However, it has generated considerable interest and has led to a large number of case reports, suggesting it as a potential cause of acute appendicitis. Foreign bodies include dog hair, toothpicks, and lead, among others. A 100-year review of the literature revealed 256 reported cases, with the highest risk associated with stiff or pointed objects.[170] Not all foreign body–associated appendicitis occurs after initial ingestion. Appendicitis may develop years after the offending agent was consumed.[171]

Other foreign materials that can be seen in the appendix include vegetable fragments, which usually do not elicit a mucosal inflammatory response. However, in some cases, vegetable material may obstruct the appendiceal lumen and lead to acute appendicitis. Foreign heterotopic bone formation in the appendix is a rare finding that has been associated with some mucin-producing tumors.[172] Rarely foreign bodies in the peritoneum, such as dialysis catheters, entrap the appendix and lead to acute appendicitis.[173]

Rosai-Dorfman Disease

Rosai-Dorfman disease, also known as *sinus histiocytosis with massive lymphadenopathy,* is a histiocytic, proliferative disorder of unknown origin. It frequently occurs in extranodal locations, but appendiceal involvement is rare with fewer than five reported cases in the literature.[174,175] Patients present with vague abdominal symptoms or a right lower quadrant mass.

The characteristic appearance is sheets of S100 protein–positive histiocytes with abundant, pale cytoplasm that engulf inflammatory cells (i.e., emperipolesis) (Fig. 18.34). Within the GI tract, the proliferation is centered in submucosal tissue, but may be transmural and also focally involve the lamina propria.[174] The background stroma is often collagenous and may contain a scattered, mixed inflammatory infiltrate.

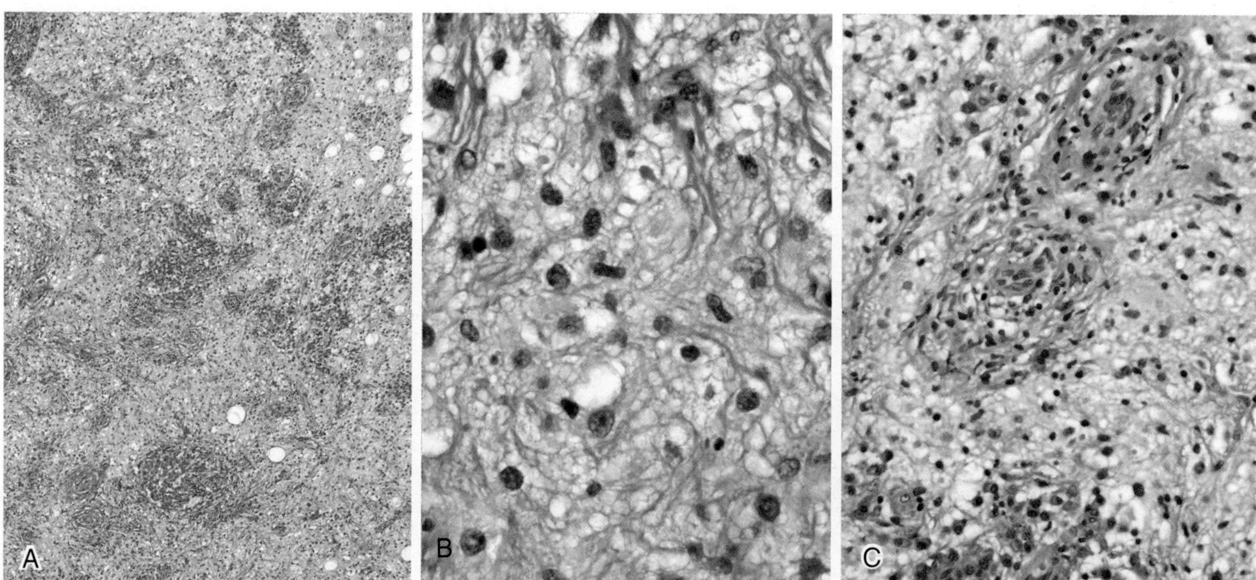

FIGURE 18.34 A, Rosai-Dorfman disease features sheets of histiocytes with scattered lymphoid follicles. **B,** The lesional histiocytes contain abundant rarified cytoplasm. **C,** Vascular inflammation and injury is also a common feature.

The clinical course varies. Although many patients have an indolent clinical course, some die of disease. Chemotherapy has been used with various results.[174,175]

Acute Necrotizing Arteritis of Appendiceal Vessels

Acute necrotizing vasculitis of the arterial vessels of the appendix is rare.[145,176] Vasculitis may be symptomatic, presenting similarly to acute appendicitis, or incidentally detected in a background of other appendiceal pathology. The vascular lesions resemble those of polyarteritis nodosa or microscopic polyangiitis, featuring fibrinoid necrosis of the vessel walls with associated mixed inflammation (Fig. 18.35). Most cases with available follow-up lack clinical signs of systemic disease, indicating that vasculitis may, indeed, be limited to the appendix.[177] In one study, widespread vasculitis in a pattern similar to polyarteritis nodosum developed in as much as one third of patients; thus clinical follow-up is warranted when vasculitis is detected in the appendix.

***The full reference list may be accessed online at** Elsevier eBooks for Practicing Clinicians.*

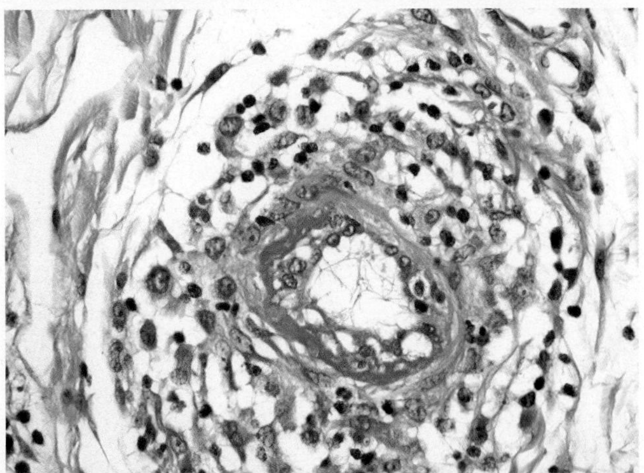

FIGURE 18.35 Necrotizing arteritis is rarely reported in the appendix. It features fibrinoid necrosis of the vessel walls and mixed inflammation.

ACKNOWLEDGMENTS

The author wishes to acknowledge Drs. Leona A. Doyle and Robert D. Odze for their work on previous versions of this chapter.

SECTION III

POLYPS OF THE GASTROINTESTINAL TRACT

CHAPTER 19

Polyps of the Esophagus

Ilyssa O. Gordon

Chapter Outline

INTRODUCTION

Most types of inflammatory lesions of the esophagus do not manifest as endoscopically recognizable polyps. They instead cause only a slight mucosal irregularity or surface erosion. In contrast, most neoplastic processes of the esophagus manifest clinically at an advanced pathological stage. Malignant tumors may form strictures, plaquelike masses, or deeply penetrating or fungating ulcers. Polyps, which are discrete, well-circumscribed luminal protrusions, are uncommon in the esophagus. However, many unusual types of tumors of the esophagus are polypoid.[1] Although esophageal polyps are rare, they often have interesting or unusual pathology.

Esophageal polyps may be divided into epithelial and mesenchymal types. Each type can be further subdivided as benign or malignant. The epithelial nature of an esophageal polyp is usually apparent at endoscopy or on radiographic evaluation because of the formation of a mucosal irregularity. In contrast, most mesenchymal polyps originate within the subepithelial tissues, causing an endoscopically recognizable elevation of the overlying mucosa, but the latter is usually left intact with a smooth contour.

EPITHELIAL POLYPS

Nonneoplastic

Small polyps covered by benign (nonneoplastic) squamous epithelium may develop anywhere in the esophagus (Table 19.1). The pathogenesis and morphological features of these polyps tend to correlate roughly with their site of origin. The two main types of squamous polyps are inflammatory polyps and squamous papillomas.[1]

Inflammatory Polyps

Inflammatory polyps are the most common type of benign, squamous esophageal polyp (Box 19.1). They occur primarily in men at the lower esophageal junction and usually are associated with gastroesophageal reflux disease (GERD).[2-4] Inflammatory polyps represent an exaggerated response to mucosal injury. Some are exuberant, healed ulcer sites. Inflammatory polyps may also develop proximal to the gastroesophageal junction, where they are often associated with mucosal injury caused by embedded pills, infection, or surgical anastomoses.[5]

Histologically, inflammatory polyps often have a smooth, rounded surface and consist of irregular tongues of squamous epithelium that extend deeply within an inflamed lamina propria (Fig. 19.1). Although controversial, some investigators think these polyps represent an endophytic type of squamous papilloma.[6] Human papillomavirus (HPV) was identified in 33% of these polyps by polymerase chain reaction analysis in a study by Odze and colleagues.[6] HPV was postulated to be a promoter of epithelial growth in mucosa that had been damaged by other irritants such as GERD.[6]

Hyperplastic Polyps

At the level of the gastroesophageal junction, hyperplastic polyps composed primarily of gastric hyperplastic foveolar epithelium (Fig. 19.2), with or without hyperplastic and regenerative-appearing squamous epithelium, can develop, presumably as a result of chronic mucosal injury.[5] These gastroesophageal junction polyps have been most often reported in the clinical gastroenterology or radiology literature.[7] Hyperplastic polyps at the gastroesophageal junction may be associated with a short or ultrashort Barrett's

TABLE 19.1 Epithelial Polyps of the Esophagus

Type of Lesion	Pathological Features	Clinical and Pathogenetic Features
Benign		
Inflammatory polyp	Smooth rounded surface; irregular tongues of squamous epithelium; inflamed lamina propria	GEJ, reflux related, represents an exaggerated response to mucosal injury
Hyperplastic polyp	Foveolar hyperplasia, cystic change, regenerative changes, inflammation, ulceration; may also have hyperplastic squamous epithelium	GEJ, associated with chronic mucosal injury usually due to GERD
Squamous papilloma	Finger-like squamous papillae with underlying fibrovascular cores of lamina propria	Exophytic, distal esophagus, most common; also endophytic and spiked Often associated with HPV
Gastric heterotopia	Surface and gland epithelium lamina propria	Proximal esophagus; congenital; also called "inlet patch"
Glycogenic acanthosis	Larger clear squamous cells; endoscopic nodule, PAS+	Increased intracellular glycogen level; if numerous, consider Cowden's syndrome
Precursor Lesions		
Polypoid dysplasia	Resembles colonic adenoma	Setting of Barrett's esophagus
Squamous dysplasia	Nuclear atypia and loss of polarity; mild, moderate, or severe	Precursor to squamous cell carcinoma and spindle cell carcinoma
Malignant		
Spindle cell carcinoma	Biphasic, squamous and spindle cells; keratin+, either component can metastasize	Better prognosis than conventional SCCA as exophytic morphology leads to earlier diagnosis
Squamous cell carcinoma	Usually strictured, ulcerated, or fungating mass	Rarely polypoid
Adenocarcinoma	Usually strictured, ulcerated, or fungating mass	Rarely polypoid

GEJ, *Gastroesophageal junction;* GERD, *gastroesophageal reflux disease;* HPV, *human papillomavirus;* PAS, *periodic acid–Schiff stain;* SCCA, *squamous cell carcinoma.*

BOX 19.1 Key Features of Inflammatory Polyps

- Most common type of benign, squamous esophageal polyp
- Male, gastroesophageal junction, reflux-associated
- Smooth, rounded surface with irregular tongues of squamous epithelium extending deeply within an inflamed lamina propria
- Key differential diagnosis:
  - May resemble endophytic squamous papillomas and may be HPV associated; but these are less frequently diagnosed

HPV, *Human papillomavirus.*

esophagus (33% of cases), and they have less inflammation compared with those arising in a non-Barrett's setting.[8]

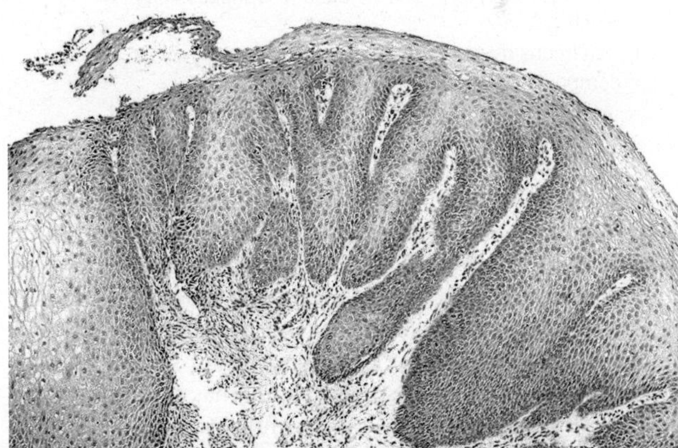

FIGURE 19.1 Squamous-lined inflammatory polyps have an endophytic growth pattern characterized by elongated tongues of benign squamous epithelium extending into the underlying lamina propria. These lesions may represent a subtype of squamous papilloma.

Squamous Papilloma

Squamous papillomas are the other main type of squamous polyp of the esophagus (see Chapter 24) (Box 19.2).[9] They are the most common benign tumor of the esophagus and can occur at any age.[1,6] The reported frequency of squamous papilloma ranges from 0.01% to 0.26% in Europe[10,11] and 0.1% to 0.2% in Asia.[12,13] The presence of multiple polyps (squamous papillomatosis) should raise the possibility of a hereditary syndrome.[14]

Three main histological patterns have been described: *exophytic, endophytic,* and *spiked*.[6] The exophytic type is more common. On endoscopy, these lesions are a few millimeters in size and have a cauliflower-like appearance. Histological examination of the exophytic type reveals finger-like squamous papillae overlying fibrovascular cores of lamina propria (Fig. 19.3). The squamous epithelium may have features of koilocytosis, but it usually lacks the large, hyperchromatic nuclei and binucleation typical of HPV-infected cervical epithelium. Exophytic squamous papillomas occur most frequently in the distal esophagus, but they also occur in the middle and upper esophagus. HPV is associated with as many as 78% of these squamous papillomas,[6,15] although much lower HPV associations have also been reported. For instance, Takeshita et al. reported HPV in 10.5% of squamous papillomas. All of these were located in the middle esophagus of female patients.[13] Recent studies have also found high-risk HPV phenotypes in up to 50% of squamous papillomas.[16,17]

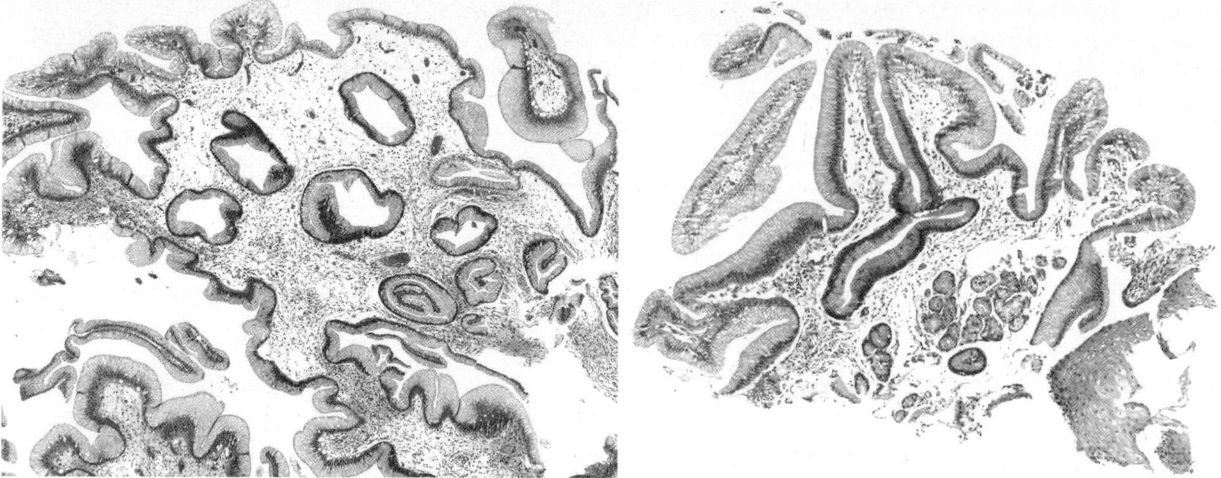

FIGURE 19.2 Gastric foveolar hyperplasia with lamina propria edema and mild inflammation are characteristic of hyperplastic polyps. Squamous mucosa, although not always present in the biopsy, may be hyperplastic or regenerative appearing.

BOX 19.2 Key Features of Squamous Papilloma

- Exophytic is most common histological pattern
  - Finger-like squamous papillae overlying fibrovascular cores of lamina propria
  - May have koilocytic features
  - May be HPV associated
- Endophytic has a smooth, round surface with inverted papilloma appearance
- Spiked are least common, with verrucous appearance, corrugated surface, hyperkeratosis, and prominent granular cell layer
- Benign but small risk for associated malignancy
- Key differential diagnoses:
  - Fibrovascular polyp: usually upper esophagus, larger at presentation
  - Squamous dysplasia and carcinoma: nuclear atypia, invasive component

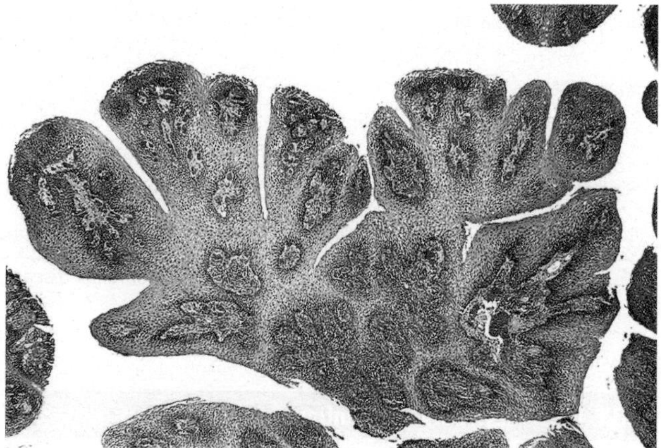

FIGURE 19.3 Squamous papillomas are an exophytic type of squamous polyp that have a finger-like growth pattern. Human papillomavirus infection is strongly associated with these polyps.

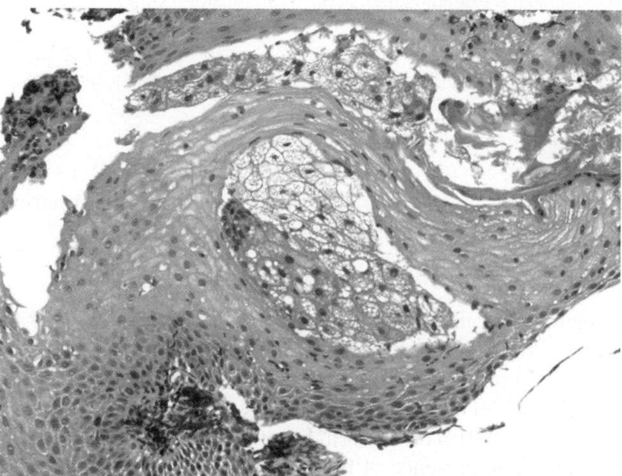

FIGURE 19.4 Examination of this esophageal polyp at high power reveals sebaceous glands embedded within the squamous epithelium.

The endophytic type of papilloma has a round, smooth surface and an inverted papillomatous appearance. Some investigators think they are inflammatory polyps. Spiked squamous papillomas have a verrucous appearance, a corrugated surface, hyperkeratosis, and a prominent granular cell layer. This is the least common form of squamous papilloma. Forty percent of spiked papillomas were shown to harbor HPV in one study.[6] Ratoosh and coworkers described a 60-year-old woman who had a large, verrucous lesion of the distal esophagus and multiple warts on her distal fingertips.[18] HPV-45 DNA sequences were identified in the fingertip and esophageal verrucous lesions, suggesting autoinoculation of the finger wart HPV virus to the esophagus.[18]

Squamous papillomas are benign. Rarely, large squamous papillomas have undergone malignant degeneration.[19] However, whether these lesions represent de novo carcinomas or true malignant degeneration of a squamous papilloma is unknown. Due to the very low risk of malignancy, squamous papillomas should be excised.

Several types of esophageal heterotopias rarely manifest as polypoid lesions on endoscopy (see Chapter 24). Heterotopias occur in 10% of the general population and usually consist of gastric heterotopia, although thyroid, parathyroid, and ectopic sebaceous tissues (Fig. 19.4) have been described.[20] Gastric heterotopias in the esophagus usually contain glands and foveolar epithelium (82% of cases) and are thought to be congenital in origin.[21] Heterotopias are often found in the proximal esophagus and may be called an *inlet patch* on endoscopy. These lesions are distinct from Barrett's esophagus, as described in Table 19.2.

TABLE 19.2 Features Distinguishing Heterotopic Gastric Inlet Patch from Barrett's Esophagus

Feature	Heterotopic gastric inlet patch	Barrett's esophagus
Clinical	Incidental, congenital	Reflux associated
Location	Proximal esophagus	Distal esophagus
Endoscopy	Salmon-colored, velvety patch surrounded entirely by normal gray-white esophageal squamous mucosa	Salmon-colored tongues extending at least 1 cm proximal to, and contiguous with, the GEJ
Histology	Gastric epithelium: glands may be mucinous, oxyntic, or both Typically not inflamed Normally no goblet cells	Goblet cells (intestinal epithelium), may be incomplete: interspersed among gastric-type epithelium

GEJ, *Gastroesophageal junction.*

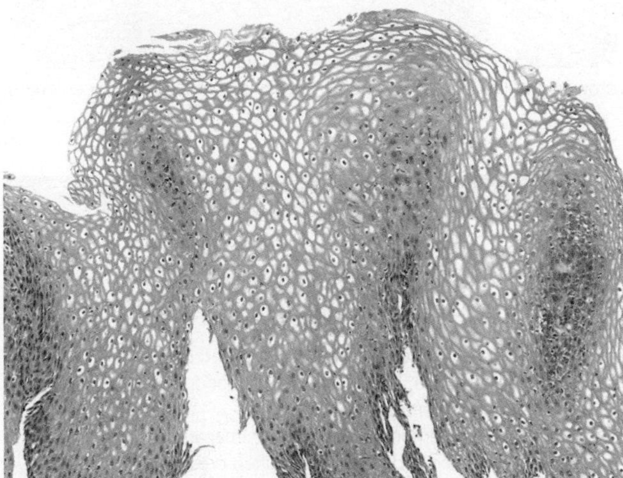

FIGURE 19.5 Thickened squamous mucosa with large clear cytoplasmic accumulation of glycogen is characteristic of glycogenic acanthosis.

Glycogenic Acanthosis

Small, plaquelike or nodule-like lesions can occur in patients with prominent glycogenic acanthosis. They represent focal nodular thickening of the squamous mucosa with cells that contain prominent intracytoplasmic glycogen, seen histologically as clear cytoplasm (Fig. 19.5). Endoscopically, the lesions can resemble squamous papillomas. Patients with Cowden's syndrome or tuberous sclerosis may have numerous polypoid areas of glycogenic acanthosis, and this finding always raises the possibility of one of these diagnoses.[22,23] If making the diagnosis of multifocal glycogenic acanthosis in a patient not known to have already been diagnosed with a syndrome, it is helpful to state in a comment that these clinical syndromes should be considered.

Neoplastic

Polypoid Dysplasia in Barrett's Esophagus

Most so-called adenomas reported in the earlier literature are instead polypoid areas of dysplasia arising in Barrett's esophagus (Fig. 19.6) (see Chapter 24). Endoscopically, lesions are often described as nodules because of their sessile polypoid appearance. Pedunculated polypoid lesions are exceedingly rare.

Histologically, they can resemble colonic adenomas, which led early investigators to label them as adenomas. However, polypoid dysplasia arising in Barrett's esophagus has clinical, pathological, and molecular features similar to those of flat dysplasia and should not be considered benign lesions that can be excised without further follow-up.[24] In one study, all adenoma-like polypoid areas of dysplasia in Barrett's esophagus were associated with carcinoma.[24] Because the term *adenoma* often implies a relatively benign natural history, this term has been replaced with *polypoid dysplasia arising in Barrett's esophagus*.[24-26] The histological features of polypoid dysplasia in Barrett's esophagus are discussed in more detail in Chapter 24.

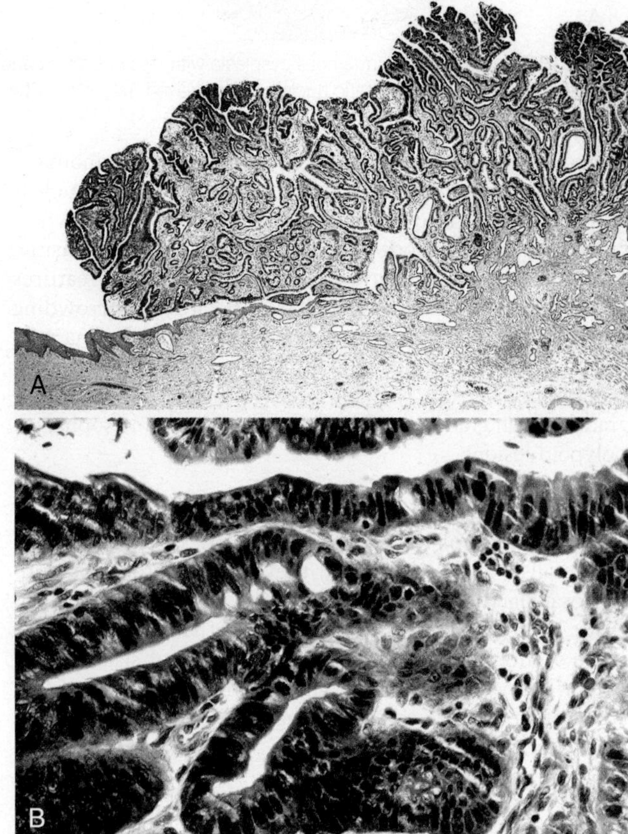

FIGURE 19.6 A, Polypoid dysplasia in Barrett's esophagus. **B,** High-power view reveals high-grade dysplasia.

Squamous Dysplasia

Squamous dysplasia is a precursor lesion to squamous cell carcinoma and to spindle cell carcinoma However, rarely, polypoid squamous dysplasia can present as an incidental finding or in patients with dysphagia or bleeding.[27] As in flat dysplasia, the degree of squamous dysplasia correlates with

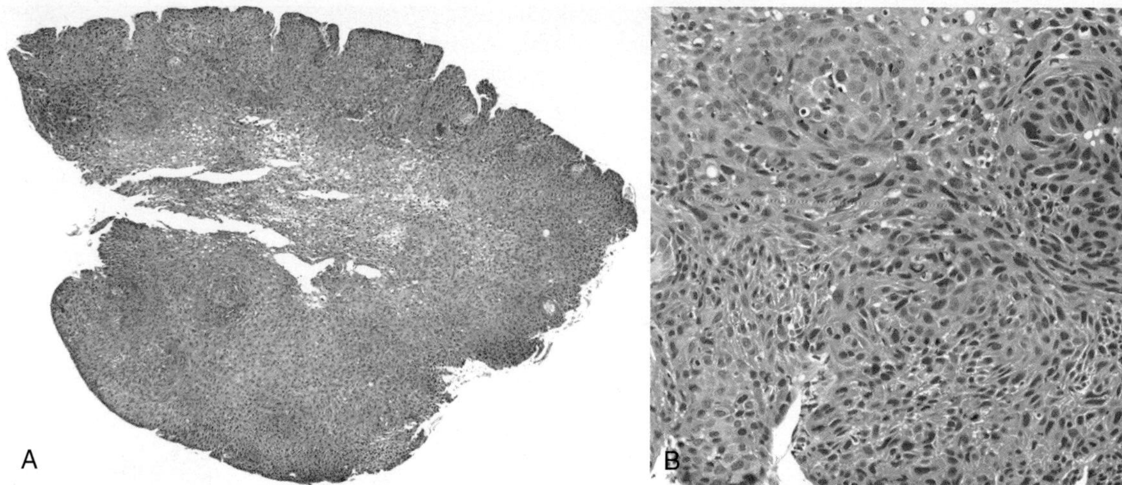

FIGURE 19.7 A, High-grade squamous dysplasia with loss of polarity and cell crowding at low power. **B,** Nuclear atypia is characterized by enlarged, pleomorphic, and hyperchromatic nuclei with increased mitotic activity.

the relative risk of developing squamous cell carcinoma.[28] Cytological features of squamous dysplasia include nuclear atypia, characterized by enlarged, pleomorphic, and hyperchromatic nuclei, along with high nuclear to cytoplasmic ratio and increased mitotic activity.[29] Architectural features of squamous dysplasia include loss of polarity, cell crowding with nuclear overlap, and cell budding into the lamina propria, but without evidence of invasion beyond the basement membrane (Fig. 19.7).[29] Dysplasia is graded as either low grade or high grade,[27] and both can be present in esophageal polypoid lesions.

Adenomas

True adenomas of the esophagus are rare (see Chapter 24 for details). Most commonly, they develop from the submucosal gland or duct system and show a mixture of tubal, cystic, and papillary growth patterns that are similar to those of intraductal papillomas of the breast or sialadenoma papilliferum of the salivary glands. Most of these tumors are benign, but rare cases of malignant transformation have been described.

Spindle Cell Carcinoma

Spindle cell carcinoma (also referred to as carcinosarcoma, pseudosarcoma, polypoid carcinoma, sarcomatoid carcinoma, spindle cell variant of squamous cell carcinoma, and squamous cell carcinoma NOS) is a rare type of malignant tumor that represents 2% of all esophageal carcinomas (see Chapter 24) (Box 19.3).[30,31] Spindle cell carcinomas are bulky, intraluminal masses with exophytic growth that most often develop in the middle portion of the esophagus of middle-aged to elderly men.[32-34] The most common presenting symptom is dysphagia, followed by weight loss and pain.[32]

Typical radiological features include a dilated esophagus expanded by a polypoid, bulky mass with a smooth or scalloped margin. The classic radiological appearance has been referred to as a *cupola sign*.[31,32] Histological examination of these tumors reveals a biphasic growth pattern, showing areas of carcinoma (well, moderately, or poorly differentiated) and areas of malignant, undifferentiated spindle cells.

The epithelial origin of spindle cells has been confirmed by immunohistochemistry, electron micrographic studies, and genetic studies that have shown similar *TP53* mutations in the sarcomatous and carcinomatous components.[1,35,36] The mesenchymal component may show liposarcoma, rhabdomyosarcoma, leiomyosarcoma, chondrosarcoma, or osteosarcoma differentiation. Many previously reported primary soft tissue sarcomas of the esophagus probably instead represent spindle cell carcinomas with a predominant undifferentiated soft tissue sarcoma component. The carcinomatous component is usually squamous, but rarely it can have adenocarcinomatous elements (Fig. 19.8).[37]

Most cases have squamous dysplasia in the overlying or adjacent mucosa, but this finding can be focal and difficult to detect if only a limited number of tissue sections have been obtained. The carcinomatous component may exist only at the base of the polyp and is often overgrown by the more exuberant spindle cell component. Lauwers and colleagues showed that the spindle cell component possessed a greater proliferative index and increased aneuploidy compared with the carcinomatous elements, perhaps providing it with a growth advantage.[38]

Metastases may be composed of either or both of the cellular components. Because these tumors demonstrate prominent exophytic growth with less extension into the esophageal wall, they have been associated with relatively

BOX 19.3 Key Features of Spindle Cell Carcinoma

- Synonyms: carcinosarcoma, pseudosarcoma, polypoid carcinoma, sarcomatoid carcinoma, spindle cell variant of squamous cell carcinoma, and squamous cell carcinoma NOS
- Bulky, exophytic in mid-esophagus
- Mesenchymal component may show liposarcoma, rhabdomyosarcoma, leiomyosarcoma, chondrosarcoma, or osteosarcoma differentiation
- Carcinomatous component can be minimal and may be well, moderately or poorly differentiated, often present at the base of the polyp
- Key differential diagnoses:
  - Sarcoma: complete sampling to exclude a carcinomatous component
  - Benign mesenchymal lesions: lack of malignant features and carcinomatous component

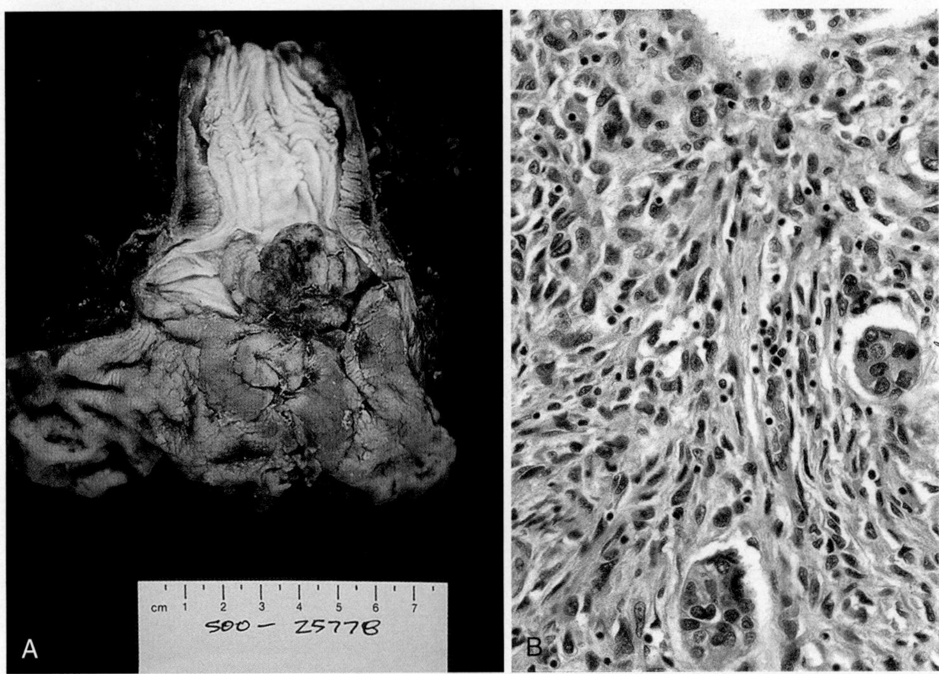

FIGURE 19.8 A, The spindle cell carcinoma is formed by a polypoid intraluminal mass located above the gastroesophageal junction. **B,** Examination of these tumors reveals biphasic histology, typically with a predominance of malignant spindle cells and only focal areas of carcinoma.

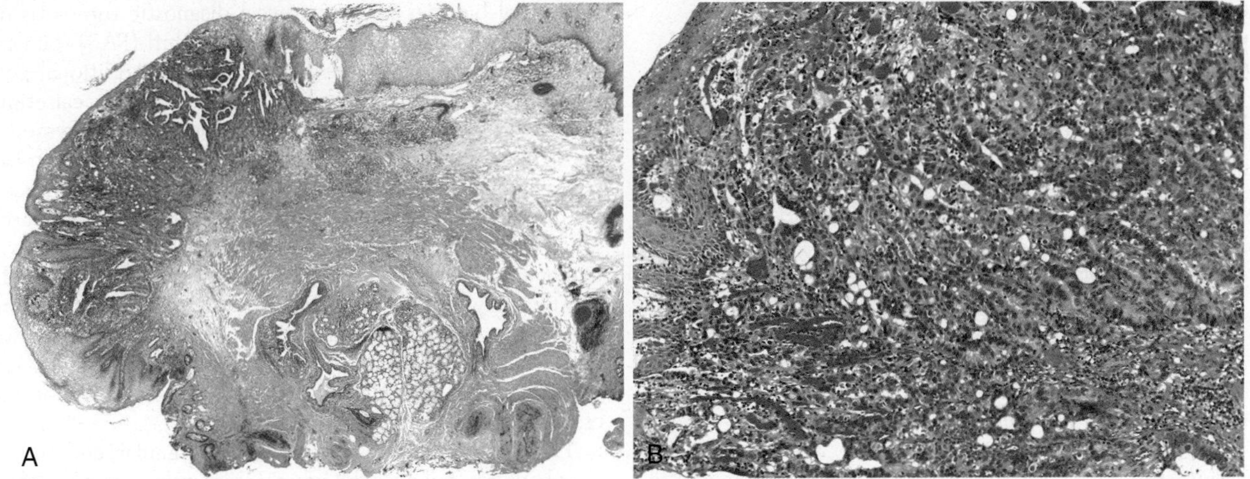

FIGURE 19.9 A, Polypoid intramucosal adenocarcinoma of the esophagus is seen at low power in this endoscopic mucosal resection. **B,** High-power view reveals back-to-back anastomosing gland pattern with scant intervening stroma and nuclear atypia.

good survival rates. In some studies, 50% to 60% of affected patients are alive after 5 years.[1]

Squamous Cell Carcinoma and Adenocarcinoma

In the United States, most squamous cell carcinomas and adenocarcinomas of the esophagus are detected at an advanced stage and grow in the form of strictures, irregular masses, ulcers, or fungating masses. Only approximately 15% of all esophageal malignancies grow in a polypoid fashion, and most of these are spindle cell carcinomas.[33] Intramucosal adenocarcinoma may be polypoid (Fig. 19.9). Conventional squamous cell carcinoma, small cell carcinoma, and adenocarcinoma are only rarely polypoid. Occasionally, early-stage squamous cell carcinomas or high-grade dysplastic lesions may grow as an endoscopically detected polypoid lesion.[39]

Rare Malignant Epithelial Polyps

Malignant epithelial tumors that can rarely present as esophageal polyps or nodules include adenoid cystic carcinoma,[40] adenosquamous and mucoepidermoid carcinomas,[41,42] and neuroendocrine neoplasms.[43,44] See Chapter 24 for details.

MESENCHYMAL POLYPS

Granular Cell Tumors

Granular cell tumors are benign tumors of Schwann cell origin (Table 19.3; Box 19.4). They may develop anywhere in the body but occur most commonly on the skin or the tongue. The gastrointestinal tract is a relatively uncommon site for the development of granular cell tumors, but within that organ system, the esophagus is the most common

TABLE 19.3 Mesenchymal Polyps of the Esophagus

Type of Lesion	Pathological Features	Clinical and Pathogenetic Features
Benign		
Granular cell tumor	Cells with abundant eosinophilic cytoplasm and pyknotic nuclei arranged in sheets or nests, S100+, PAS+	Beware of overlying pseudoepitheliomatous hyperplasia; superficial biopsy may miss the lamina propria lesion; usually asymptomatic in middle-aged adults
Leiomyoma	Spindle cells with abundant eosinophilic cytoplasm, actin+, CD117−, rare mitotic figures	Small, firm, usually in muscularis propria; polypoid more likely when arising in muscularis mucosae
Giant fibrovascular polyp	Large, sausage-shaped polyp with fibrovascular core of loose, myxoid, hyalinized or collagenous fibrous tissue, adipose tissue, edema, and inflammatory cells; enlarged, reactive mesenchymal fibroblasts and myofibroblasts; prominent vessels	Upper esophagus, dysphagia, may flip into airways and cause asphyxiation; may be multiple; consider before diagnosing lipoma or liposarcoma; must prove absence of *MDM2* gene amplification
Cystic and diverticular lesions	Cysts: simple, duplication, bronchogenic Pseudodiverticulosis: flask-shaped outpouchings of dilated submucosal glands	Differentiate by cell lining and wall layer involvement
Malignant		
GIST	Spindled or epithelioid, minimal cytoplasm, CD117+, DOG1+ mitotic figures	Usually larger than gastric GIST, imparting poor prognosis; 50% malignant; KIT may be wild type or mutated

GIST, *Gastrointestinal stromal tumor;* PAS, *periodic acid–Schiff stain.*

BOX 19.4 Key Features of Granular Cell Tumors

- Esophageal location: distal >> mid > proximal
- Size: most are less than 10 mm
- Sheets or nests of cells with abundant eosinophilic granular cytoplasm and small, pyknotic nuclei
- Increased mitotic activity and necrosis may indicate malignancy, which is otherwise defined by metastatic disease (rare)
- Overlying squamous epithelium may have pseudoepitheliomatous hyperplasia, mimicking dysplasia or carcinoma
- Positive for S100, nestin, calretinin, CD68, PAS
- Key differential diagnoses:
  - Squamous dysplasia or carcinoma: look for underlying granular cells
  - Schwann cell hamartoma: lacks granular cytoplasm

PAS, *Periodic acid–Schiff stain.*

location. Granular cell tumors occur primarily in adults (median age, 46 years), are more common in women than in men, and are more common among blacks than whites, particularly in the United States. Patients with granular cell tumors are usually asymptomatic. Most cases are detected incidentally at the time of upper endoscopy.[45-48]

On endoscopy, granular cell tumors appear as yellow or yellow-white firm submucosal lesions (Fig. 19.10A).[49] These tumors are most common in the distal to midesophagus, and they are usually single but can be multiple.[46,47,50] The majority of tumors measure less than 10 mm.[46,47,50] Biopsy or endoscopic resection is typically curative.

Histologically, granular cell tumors are composed of sheets or nests of cells with abundant eosinophilic granular cytoplasm and small, pyknotic nuclei (see Fig. 19.10B). They are most common in the superficial lamina propria. The cytoplasmic granules correspond to autophagic vacuoles filled with myelin-like debris, as documented by electron microscopy, and are lysozyme rich. For unknown reasons, the squamous epithelium overlying granular cell tumors may have marked pseudoepitheliomatous hyperplasia that can mimic dysplasia or carcinoma.[32] Because these tumors are subepithelial, superficial biopsies may not reveal diagnostic tumor tissue. Granular cell tumors are periodic acid–Schiff (PAS) stain and S100 protein positive (see Fig. 19.10C).[46] Additional positive immunohistochemical stains include nestin, calretinin, and CD68, due to the presence of cytoplasmic lysozyme.[27]

Although most granular cell tumors are small and limited to the lamina propria, rare cases may involve the submucosa or muscularis propria.[27,46,51] Deep, infiltrative-appearing growth may prompt concern about malignancy; however, malignant behavior is rare. One patient with a granular cell tumor with an infiltrative growth pattern that was initially diagnosed as malignant with incomplete resection was reported to be alive and well after 22 years of follow-up, suggesting that an infiltrative growth pattern does not necessarily imply malignancy.[52]

Histological features of malignant granular cell tumors have been revised over the years. Ultimately, true malignancy is confirmed by identification of metastasis. However, most malignant tumors show highly atypical features as well as atypical histological features, as reported by Fanburg-Smith et al. include increased nuclear to cytoplasmic ratio, nuclear pleomorphism, vesicular nuclei with large nucleoli, >2 mitotic figures per 10 high-power fields, spindling, and necrosis (Table 19.4). These tumors may be associated with local recurrence but usually not death from disease.[53] Nasser et al. simplified the atypical criteria to include only necrosis and/or mitotic activity (using Ki-67) and renamed these "granular cell tumors of uncertain malignant potential."[54] True malignant esophageal granular cell tumors are exceedingly rare.

Leiomyomas

Leiomyomas are the most common type of mesenchymal tumor of the esophagus (see Chapter 30) (Box 19.5). In autopsy studies, as many as 8% of patients harbored at least one esophageal leiomyoma.[55,56] However,

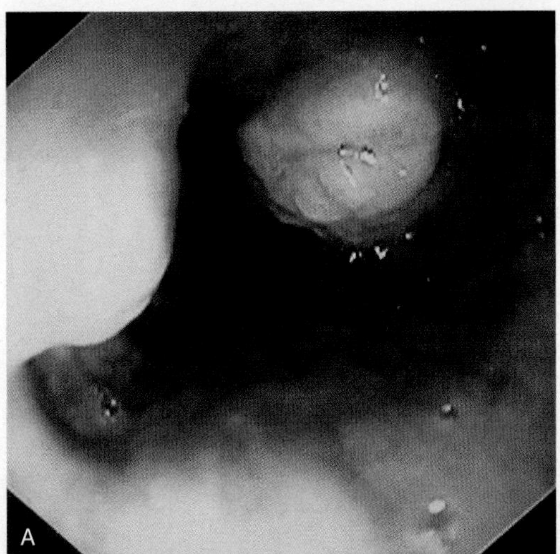

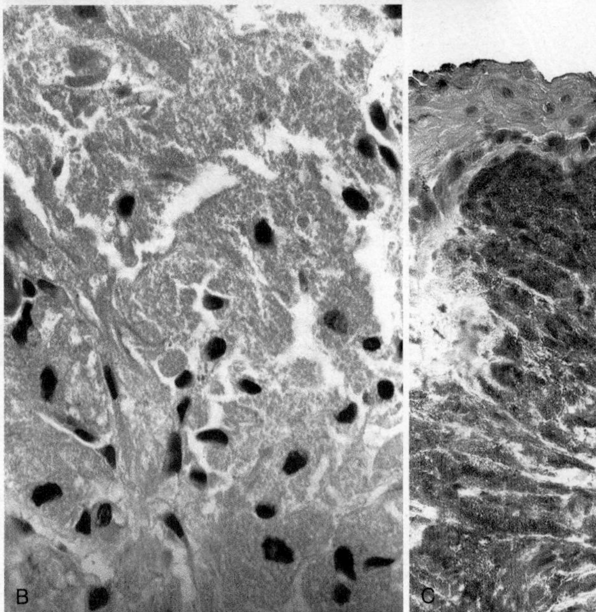

FIGURE 19.10 **A,** Endoscopically, granular cell tumors appear as small, white to yellow, subepithelial nodules. **B,** Histologically, these lesions are composed of large cells with abundant eosinophilic granular cytoplasm and pyknotic nuclei. **C,** A positive immunoperoxidase stain for S100 protein can help to confirm the diagnosis.

TABLE 19.4 Histological Features Distinguishing Benign and Malignant Granular Cell Tumors

Benign Features	Malignant Features
Abundant eosinophilic granular cytoplasm	Increased nuclear to cytoplasmic ratio
Small pyknotic nuclei	Nuclear pleomorphism, vesicular nuclei with large nucleoli
No mitotic figures; negative Ki-67	>2 mitotic figures per 10 high-power fields; positive Ki-67
Plump epithelioid cells	Epithelial and spindle cells
No necrosis	Necrosis

BOX 19.5 Key Features of Leiomyomas

- Most common type of esophageal mesenchymal tumor
- Arise in muscularis propria more often than muscularis mucosae
- Location: distal > mid > proximal
- Bland eosinophilic spindle cells, resembling ordinary smooth muscle, but irregularly arranged, with low mitotic activity
- IHC: positive for SMA, desmin; negative for CD117, DOG1, CD34, S100
- Key differential diagnoses:
    - Gastrointestinal stromal tumor: positive for CD117 and DOG1
    - Schwannoma: positive for S100
    - Inflammatory fibroid polyp: presence of eosinophils, positive for CD34, negative for desmin

IHC, *Immunohistochemistry;* SMA, *smooth muscle actin.*

leiomyomas detected at autopsy are usually minute. In a Japanese study, esophageal leiomyomas had a mean size of 2.5 mm in the greatest dimension and were often multiple. Leiomyomas occur equally in men and women and are usually single, although 24% of patients have multiple lesions. Multiple lesions have been called *seedling leiomyomas*.[56]

Most leiomyomas are located within the inner layer of muscularis propria. However, as many as 18% occur within the muscularis mucosae.[56] Of 48 esophageal leiomyomas collected in one study from the Armed Forces Institute of Pathology and the Haartman Institute in Helsinki, 79% were

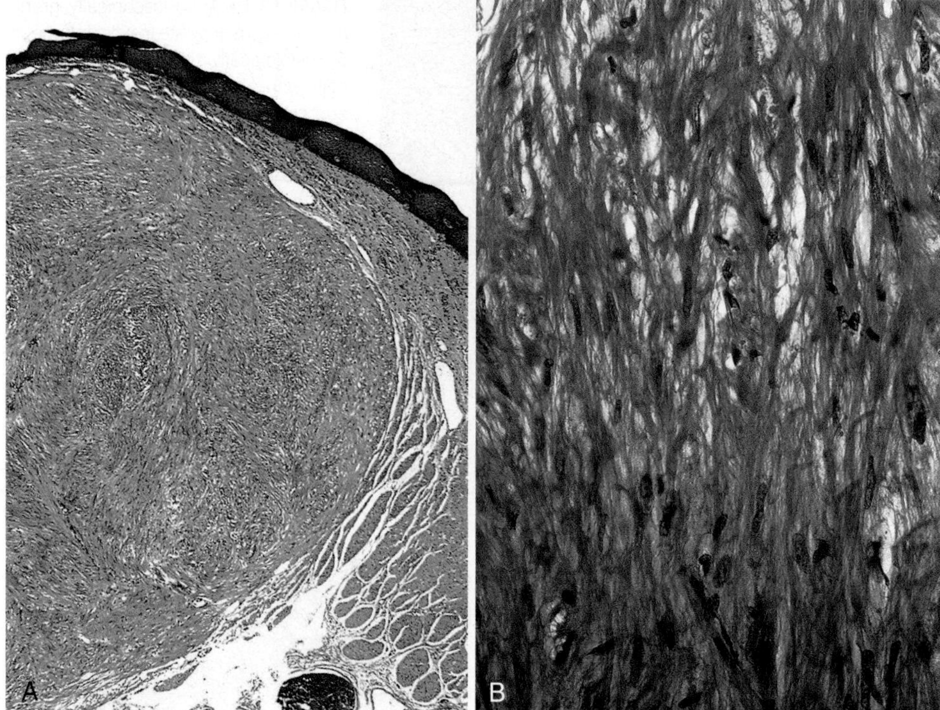

FIGURE 19.11 **A,** The leiomyoma arose from the muscularis mucosae and manifested as an intraluminal nodule. **B,** Histologically, the leiomyoma is paucicellular. The tumor cells are bland and have abundant, fibrillar, brightly eosinophilic cytoplasm without nuclear atypia.

located in the distal esophagus, 18% in the mid esophagus, and 3% in the proximal esophagus.

Multiple, large leiomyomas in the distal esophagus have been called *leiomyomatosis*. Leiomyomas may occasionally grow large, measuring as large as 10 cm in one series.[57] Massive leiomyomas (>1000 g) have rarely been reported.[58] Symptoms related to the tumor, most commonly dysphagia, may develop in patients with large leiomyomas.[57] Most leiomyomas have an intramural location, but in one series, 3% were polypoid.[55] Endoscopic ultrasound is useful for detection and localization of esophageal leiomyomas.[58] Small, pedunculated leiomyomas localized to the muscularis mucosae may be resected endoscopically.[59]

Grossly, esophageal leiomyomas are gray-tan lesions with a firm consistency. Examination usually reveals a cut surface with a whorled appearance similar to that of their uterine counterpart. Histologically, leiomyomas have low cellularity and are formed of bland-appearing eosinophilic spindle cells with bland, slightly oval nuclei and no or minimal mitotic activity (Fig. 19.11). The cells resemble closely the normal fibers of the muscularis, but they are arranged in an irregular fashion and associated with small, thin-walled blood vessels.

Immunohistochemical analysis can confirm the smooth muscle nature of the tumor. These tumors are universally positive for actin, desmin, and high-molecular-weight caldesmon. Immunohistochemical staining for CD117 (KIT) is negative in all cases.[60]

Giant Fibrovascular Polyps

Fibrovascular polyps are rare lesions, but because of their often large size and upper esophageal location, affected patients may have a dramatic clinical presentation (Box 19.6). In one series of 16 cases from the Armed Forces Institute of Pathology, the mean age at presentation was 56 years (range, 32 to 89 years), with men and women being affected equally.[61]

BOX 19.6 Key Features of Giant Fibrovascular Polyps

- Proximal esophagus, large size
- Reactive squamous mucosal surface, may be eroded or ulcerated
- Core consists of:
  - Loose, myxoid, hyalinized or collagenous fibrous tissue with various amounts of adipose tissue, edema, and inflammatory cells
  - Scattered, enlarged, reactive mesenchymal fibroblasts and myofibroblasts
  - Vascular structures
- Negative for *MDM2* gene amplification; recommended to test before making diagnosis
- Key differential diagnoses:
  - Lipoma: bland adipocytes with no fibrous component and fewer vessels
  - Well-differentiated liposarcoma: has *MDM2* gene amplification

These polyps typically occur in the proximal esophagus at the level of the cricopharyngeus muscle.[58] Indolent growth leads to slow onset of symptoms, resulting in their large size at presentation.[59] Large polyps may obstruct the lumen of the distal esophagus or cause asphyxia because of compression of the larynx or regurgitation into the posterior pharynx. Synchronous polyps may be present. Radiologically, the large, sausage-shaped polyps often are easily demonstrated on barium swallow studies.[62] Although most patients have slowly evolving and progressive dysphagia, some have acute respiratory distress or asphyxiation at presentation. Respiratory problems may be caused by obstruction of the upper

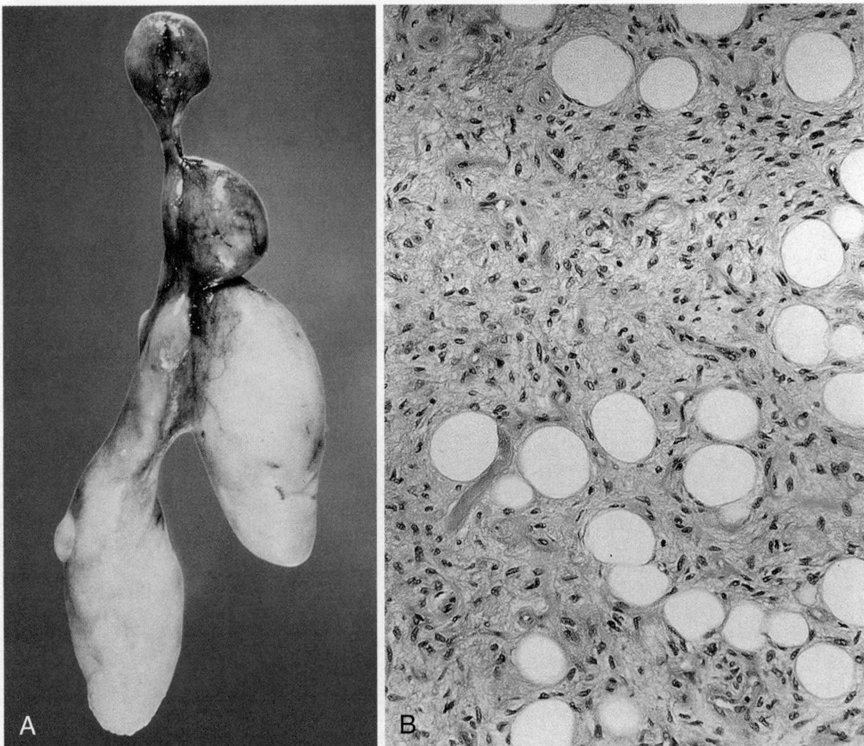

FIGURE 19.12 A, The smooth-surfaced, intraluminal, giant fibrovascular polyp has a long pedicle and is approximately 15 cm long. **B,** The core of the polyp is composed of bland mesenchymal cells, small blood vessels, fat, edema, and scattered inflammatory cells.

airways, particularly when patients vomit, belch, or cough.[63] Endoscopic resection is curative,[49] although recurrence after incomplete resection has been reported.[64]

Pathologically, fibrovascular polyps are elongated tubular structures (up to 15 cm long) covered by benign, often reactive squamous epithelium that may or may not have surface erosion or ulceration (Fig. 19.12A). Histologically, the core of fibrovascular polyps consists of loose, myxoid, hyalinized or collagenous fibrous tissue with various amounts of adipose tissue, edema, and inflammatory cells. Scattered, enlarged, reactive mesenchymal fibroblasts and myofibroblasts are typical. Lesions usually are quite vascular, with a mixture of small- and medium-caliber venous and arterial structures (see Fig. 19.12B).[65] Because of the considerable degree of adipose tissue in some cases, some have been erroneously reported as lipomas or fibrolipomas.[58]

The pathogenesis of fibrovascular polyps is unknown. One theory proposes that they develop as a result of prolapse or redundant folds of mucosa, resulting from excessive swallowing pressure forces. The Laimer triangle, which is located just below the cricopharyngeal muscle, is a region of relative muscular deficiency that has been proposed as the site of origin for these polyps.[66] Graham et al. studied the molecular cytogenetic relationship between lipoma, liposarcoma, and giant fibrovascular polyps, and found that in addition to anatomic and morphological similarities, all five cases originally diagnosed as giant fibrovascular polyp in their study were reclassified as well-differentiated liposarcoma, based on *MDM2* amplification by fluorescent in situ hybiridzation.[67] Multiple case reports of giant fibrovascular polyp histologically mimicking atypical lipomatous tumor/well-differentiated liposarcoma have been reported. Therefore the absence of *MDM2* gene amplification should be confirmed before establishing a diagnosis of giant fibrovascular polyp.

Cystic and Diverticular Lesions

Esophageal cysts and diverticula, which are predominantly mural lesions, may cause a smooth elevation of the overlying mucosa and manifest as polypoid lesions (see Chapter 8 for details). Cysts that arise within the wall of the esophagus are rare. They include simple cysts, duplication cysts, and bronchogenic cysts.[68-70] Simple cysts develop as a result of obstruction and dilation of the esophageal submucosal glands or ducts, or both. They are composed of flattened or atrophic, typically bilayered, cuboidal epithelium in which the lumen is filled with glandular secretions.

Duplication cysts are spherical structures located within the wall of the esophagus. Rarely, the duplicated segment may represent a separate cylindrical tube located parallel to the lumen of the esophagus. Duplication cysts are most frequently located in the distal esophagus and typically include all three layers of tissue (i.e., mucosa, submucosa, and muscularis). By definition, duplication cysts contain both layers of the muscularis propria, but the epithelial lining may be squamous or columnar or a mixture of both. Esophageal duplication cysts may be asymptomatic but can also cause obstructive symptoms, such as dysphagia or respiratory compromise.

Bronchogenic cysts occur in the mediastinum adjacent to the esophagus and often at the same location as esophageal duplication cysts. Bronchogenic cysts are discrete extrapulmonary structures lined by respiratory-type epithelium and contain cartilage remnants and seromucinous glands. The generic term *foregut cyst* may be used for either lesion.[71,72]

Esophageal pseudodiverticulosis is characterized by tiny, flask-shaped outpouchings in the wall of the esophagus. The outpouchings are dilated submucosal gland ducts that may contain inspissated mucin and inflammatory cells (Fig. 19.13). Most cases of pseudodiverticulosis manifest as strictures in the middle and upper esophagus of elderly individuals, and

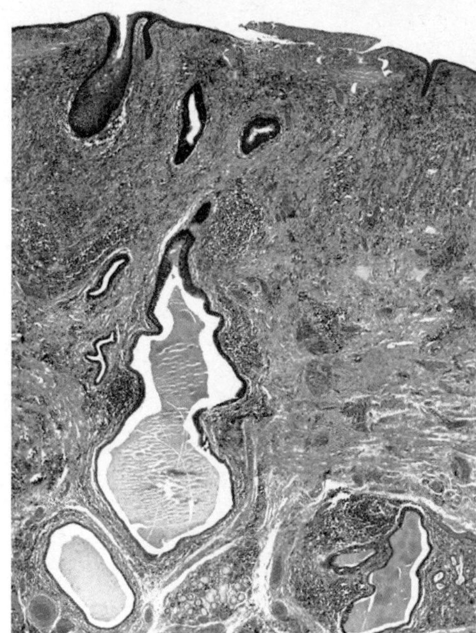

FIGURE 19.13 In pseudodiverticulosis, dilated submucosal gland ducts are filled with mucin and inflammatory cells. The condition usually manifests as a stricture or rarely as an intraluminal mass.

they rarely manifest as intraluminal masses.[73] Mitchell et al. reported a case of a midesophageal diverticulum, associated with a lipoma, which on imaging and endoscopy was initially thought to be a giant fibrovascular polyp.[74]

Rare Benign Mesenchymal Polyps

Rarely, inflammatory fibroid polyps have been reported in the esophagus.[75,76] Other rare benign mesenchymal polyps of the esophagus include lipoma,[77] lymphangioma and lymphangiomatosis,[78,79] schwannoma (Fig. 19.14),[80] hemangioma,[81] pyogenic granuloma,[82] and bacillary angiomatosis.[83]

Gastrointestinal Stromal Tumors

Gastrointestinal stromal tumors (GISTs) are most common in the stomach, followed by the small bowel and the colon, particularly the rectum.[84-86] These tumors rarely arise in the esophagus.[61] In a study by Miettinen and coworkers, esophageal GISTs developed primarily in older patients (median age, 63 years), typically in the lower esophagus, and most patients had dysphagia at presentation.[84] A more recent pooled case series found that esophageal GIST occurred significantly more frequently in men, and presented mainly in patients less than 60 years of age.[85] Larger tumor size, resulting in a high-risk prognostic grouping, has also been found.[85,86] Most esophageal GISTs had an intramural location. However, 17% had an intraluminal polypoid growth pattern. Esophageal GIST has a reported 5-year overall survival ranging from 48.3% to 85.7%, with disease-free survival rates lower than for gastric GIST.[85-87] KIT status may be wild-type or mutated (exon 11).[85,87]

Gross examination of esophageal GISTs reveals a soft, fish-flesh appearance and areas of necrosis. Histologically, most are composed of pure spindle cells, but as many as 25% also have a mixture of epithelioid cells. The appearance of esophageal GISTs ranges from confluent sheets of cells to areas with neuroid-type nuclear palisading to foci with marked myxoid stroma.

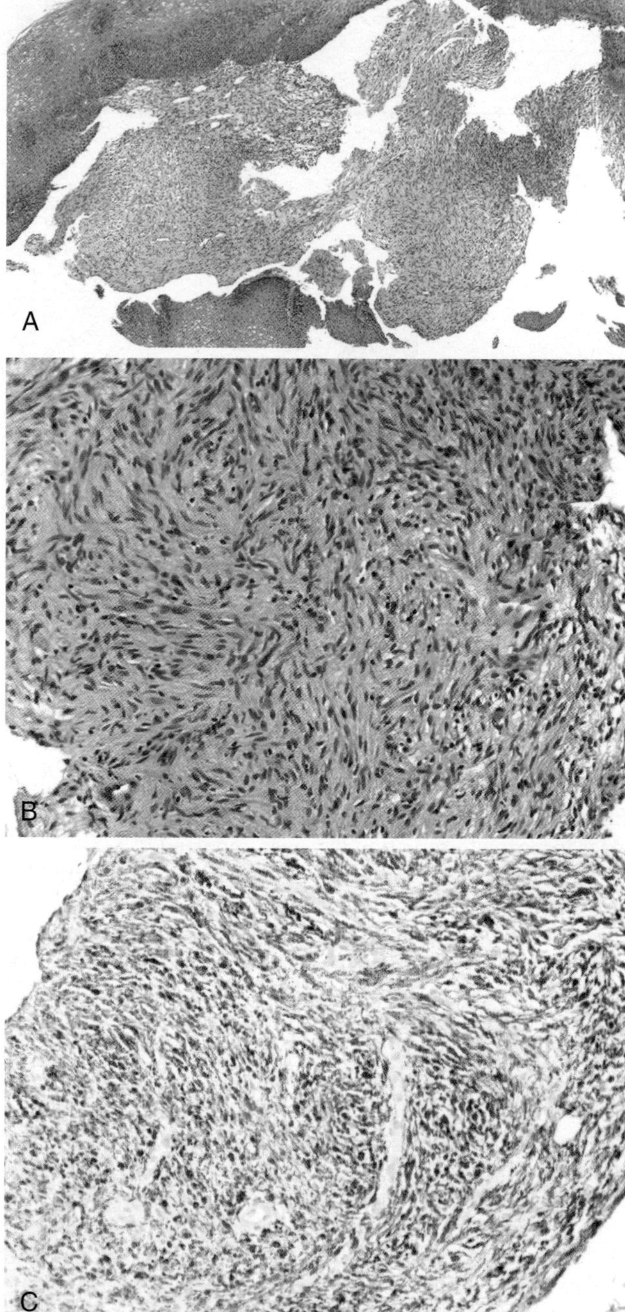

FIGURE 19.14 A, Bland eosinophilic spindle cells are seen under the squamous epithelium at low power. **B,** High-power view shows bland spindle cells with tapered nuclei and eosinophilic cytoplasm, without necrosis and with minimal mitotic activity. **C,** S100 is strongly positive. Immunohistochemical stains are necessary to confirm the diagnosis and exclude mimics.

Unlike most gastric GISTs, more than 50% of esophageal GISTs are malignant. In the study by Miettinen and associates, most malignant GISTs were larger than 5 cm in the largest dimension, contained more than 15 mitotic figures per 50 high-power fields, and had foci of necrosis.[61]

Esophageal GISTs are usually easily differentiated from other mesenchymal neoplasms of the esophagus. Immunohistochemical studies are typically diagnostic, because most

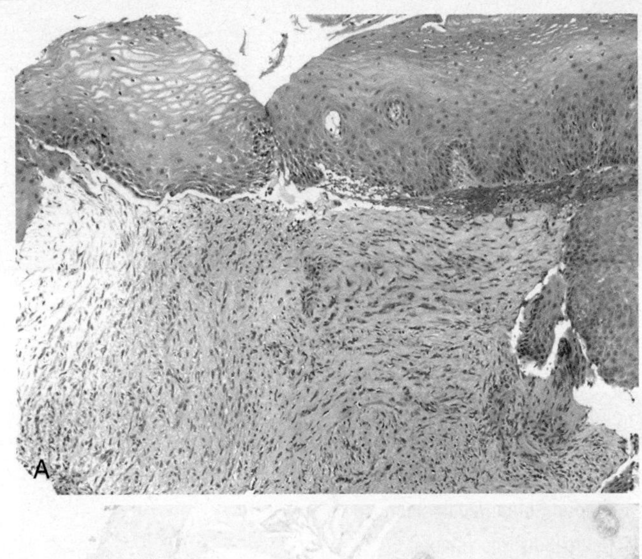

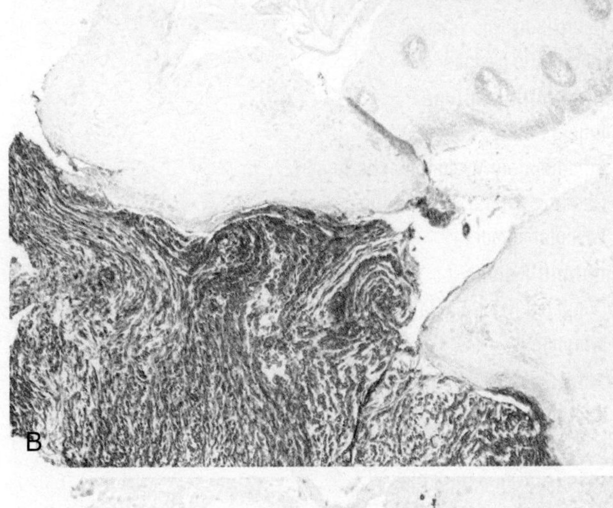

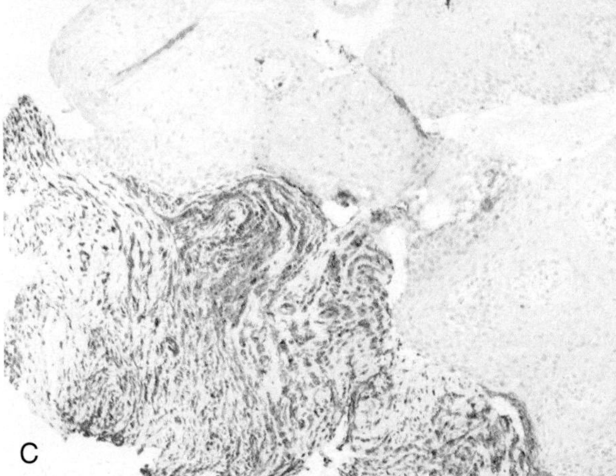

FIGURE 19.15 A, This esophageal gastrointestinal stromal tumor appears as eosinophilic spindle cells that are present beneath the squamous epithelium. Immunohistochemical stains are positive for DOG-1 (**B**) and CD117 (**C**), which confirms the diagnosis.

GISTs are CD117 and DOG1 positive, desmin negative, and usually smooth muscle actin negative (Fig. 19.15).

Rare Malignant Mesenchymal Polyps

Rare mesenchymal polyps of the esophagus that rarely metastasize include inflammatory myofibroblastic tumor,[88,89] solitary fibrous tumor,[90] glomus tumor,[91,92] and Kaposi's sarcoma.[93] Rare malignant mesenchymal polyps include leiomyosarcoma, synovial sarcoma, epithelioid angiosarcoma, and liposarcoma. Leiomyosarcomas occur most commonly in the small bowel and colorectum, followed by stomach and esophagus,[94,95] and are reported much less frequently than before the recognition of gastrointestinal stromal tumors. Cells are spindled in long fascicles with eosinophilic cytoplasm. Nuclei are enlarged and hyperchromatic with prominent atypical nuclei and high mitotic activity. Necrosis may be present. Immunohistochemistry distinguishes leiomyosarcoma from other malignant spindle cell neoplasms, staining positive for smooth muscle actin, negative for GIST markers CD117 and DOG1, and negative for schwannoma marker S100. Leiomyosarcomas can be seen in the sarcomatous component of a spindle cell carcinoma.[96]

Synovial sarcoma more often occurs in the proximal esophagus, but has been reported as a polypoid mass at the gastroesophageal junction, and can be distinguished from carcinosarcoma and gastrointestinal stromal tumor by the characteristic X;18 translocation.[97] Epithelioid angiosarcoma presenting as a large polypoid esophageal lesion with lung metastasis has also been reported.[98] Esophageal liposarcomas are malignancies that can arise in giant fibrovascular polyps of the esophagus, with a favorable prognosis following resection.[99]

BOX 19.7 Key Features of Melanoma Presenting as an Esophageal Polyp

- Polypoid malignant melanoma may be primary or metastatic to esophagus
- Junctional melanocytic activity in esophageal mucosa supports primary site
- Clinical review for melanoma already diagnosed elsewhere supports metastatic site
- Full range of melanoma histology, including spindle and epithelioid patterns
- Pigment may be absent
- Immunostains: S-100+ (most sensitive); also HMB-45+, melan-A/MART-1+
- Many entities are in the differential diagnosis; immunohistochemical stains are most helpful

HMB-45, *Human melanoma black-1;* MART-1, *melanoma antigen recognized by T cells-1.*

OTHER POLYPS

Melanoma

Primary malignant melanomas of the esophagus are rare, but some have been reported to grow as a polypoid mass (Box 19.7).[100,101] These tumors may or may not be pigmented and show a range of histological patterns, including epithelioid and spindle cell elements, often with lentiginous growth pattern.[102,103] Metastatic melanoma may also have a polypoid growth pattern. Differentiation of primary from metastatic melanoma relies on the demonstration of junctional melanocytic activity in the esophageal mucosa[104] and on the absence of melanoma elsewhere in the body.[105] Testing for *BRAF* and *KIT* mutations is important for guiding therapy in these tumors, which generally have a poor overall survival rate.[27,103]

The full reference list may be accessed online at *Elsevier eBooks for Practicing Clinicians.*

CHAPTER 20

Polyps of the Stomach

Till Clauditz, Bence Kővári, Gregory Y. Lauwers

Contents

INTRODUCTION

Gastric polyps are identified in up to 6.3% upper gastrointestinal (GI) endoscopic procedures.[1-7] They may develop as a result of epithelial or stromal cell hyperplasia, inflammation, ectopia, or neoplasia. This chapter classifies gastric polyps according to the predominant cell type (e.g., epithelial, lymphoid, mesenchymal) responsible for polyp growth (Box 20.1). Epithelial polyps can also be categorized according to the epithelial compartment from which they derive. Those that develop from the surface epithelium consist of foveolar or metaplastic intestinal-type epithelium. Other polyp types (e.g., pyloric gland adenomas and oxyntic gland adenomas) arise from the deep glandular component of the mucosa (Fig. 20.1).

The importance of correlation between the clinical signs/symptoms, the endoscopic appearance of the polyp, and the pathological features in the evaluation of gastric polyps cannot be overstated. Anatomic location, number of lesions, and the status of the surrounding non-polypoid mucosa also helps provide essential information for proper classification of gastric polyps. Quality of sampling is also cardinal because incomplete resection has been shown to result in a misdiagnosis in up to 50% of polyps.[8-10]

HYPERPLASTIC POLYPS

Clinical Features and Pathogenesis

Gastric hyperplastic polyps represent an exophytic inflammatory proliferation of foveolar epithelium. Numerous synonyms, including *inflammatory, regenerative,* and *hyperplasiogenous* polyp, have been used to describe these lesions. The prevalence of hyperplastic polyps is predominantly related to the rate of *Helicobacter pylori* infection and to the geographic locale. Although these lesions once accounted for up to 75% of all gastric polyps,[1,11-14] in North America, gastric hyperplastic polyps now represent less than 20% of these lesions.[1]

BOX 20.1 Classification of Gastric Polyps

HYPERPLASTIC POLYPS
Hyperplastic polyp
Polypoid foveolar hyperplasia
(Gastritis cystica polyposa/profunda)

POLYPOID LESIONS IN DISEASES WITH DIFFUSE GASTRIC MUCOSAL HYPERPLASIA
Ménétrier's disease
Cronkhite-Canada syndrome–associated polyp

HAMARTOMATOUS POLYPS
Fundic gland polyp
Peutz-Jeghers polyp
Juvenile polyp
Cowden's syndrome (PTEN hamartoma tumor syndrome)

HETEROTOPIC POLYPS
Heterotopic pancreatic polyp

EPITHELIAL POLYPS
Adenoma
Pyloric gland adenoma
Oxyntic gland adenoma
Neuroendocrine tumor
Polypoid carcinoma
Polypoid metastatic neoplasm

NONEPITHELIAL POLYPS
Inflammatory fibroid polyp
Inflammatory myofibroblastic tumor
Gastrointestinal stromal tumor
Vascular tumor (e.g., Glomus tumor, Kaposi's sarcoma)
Lymphoid hyperplasia
Lymphoma

MISCELLANEOUS POLYPS AND POLYP-LIKE LESIONS
Xanthoma
Langerhans cell histiocytosis
Granuloma
Amyloidosis

Hyperplastic polyps are detected most often in older individuals, with a peak incidence in the sixth and seventh decades of life[1] and with a slight female predominance.[1,15-21] Because they most often appear in the context of chronic gastritis, hyperplastic polyps are usually associated with clinical symptoms related to the underlying chronic gastritis. However, in most cases, patients are asymptomatic. Rarely, large lesions can cause obstructive symptoms if located near the pylorus or the gastroesophageal junction. Anemia and upper GI bleeding may occur if the polyp is eroded. As noted earlier, associated *H. pylori* infection, and to a lesser degree autoimmune gastritis, is common.

More than 85% of hyperplastic polyps occur in patients with chronic gastritis,[13,14,16] and this has led to the hypothesis that these lesions develop as a consequence of an exaggerated mucosal response to tissue injury and inflammation.[1,22,23] It is believed that inflammation initiates the process of injury and that the mucosal healing response results in a stepwise progression through phases of foveolar hyperplasia and polypoid foveolar hyperplasia to, eventually, the formation of a hyperplastic polyp.

Conditions associated with the development of hyperplastic polyps include *H. pylori* gastritis, chronic non–*H. pylori* gastritis including autoimmune gastritis, chemical or reactive gastropathy (including gastritis caused by bile reflux), and gastritis related to Billroth II gastrectomy.[1,17,18,24] The *H. pylori* CagA protein may have a more direct role because expression of CagA in the gastric mucosa of transgenic mice produces hyperplastic polyps.[1,25] The tendency of hyperplastic polyps to occur more proximally in the stomach in patients with autoimmune gastritis compared with other types of gastritis[1] supports the hypothesis that hyperplastic polyps develop as a consequence of chronic mucosal injury.

In one study, 33% of hyperplastic polyps of the gastroesophageal junction were related to Barrett's esophagus, and these presumably developed in the context of reflux.[26]

Finally, another study[23] showed that up to 49% of lesions diagnosed as a hyperplastic polyps presented without a characteristic stromal edema or inflammatory changes, but with cystic glands, thickened and hyperplastic smooth muscle wisps extending toward the mucosal surface, and thick-walled blood vessels—all features similar to anorectal prolapse lesions. These polypoid lesions have been reclassified as *mucosal prolapse polyps*. Notably, these polyps also occurred more commonly in the antrum, or prepyloric region of the stomach, an area of heightened peristalsis.

Rarely, patients may have more than 50 polyps, in which case a diagnosis of gastric hyperplastic polyposis may be considered. However, the specific diagnostic criteria for this syndrome are not well established.[27-29] To date, some 10 cases of hyperplastic polyposis have been reported with and without familiar clustering. Although the pathogenetic background has not been elucidated, an autosomal dominant inheritance pattern was noted in a family with nine cases of hyperplastic polyposis and two cases of poorly cohesive (signet ring cell) carcinoma. Of note, chronic gastritis and *H. pylori* infection was also recognized in most patients.[30] Reported cases with no familiar clustering may represent exuberant sporadic hyperplastic polyps because concurrent *H. pylori* infection, hypergastrinemia, pernicious anemia, proton pump inhibitor therapy, or gastric antral vascular ectasia was documented in most patients.[31] In patients with multiple polyps, other types of polyposis disorders to consider include juvenile polyposis, Peutz-Jeghers syndrome, Cowden's syndrome, and Cronkhite-Canada syndrome (see the "Differential Diagnosis" section).

Pathological Features

Most cases measuring less than 0.5 cm in greatest dimension at the time of endoscopic sampling lack the stromal and epithelial diagnostic features of a classic hyperplastic polyp and, as a result, are reclassified as *polypoid foveolar hyperplasia* (see Differential Diagnosis and Table 20.1).[31] At the other end of the spectrum, true hyperplastic polyps may, rarely, grow up to 12 cm in size.

Hyperplastic polyps occur most commonly in the antrum, but they can develop anywhere in the stomach.[21] They are most often solitary lesions; however, about 20% of cases are multiple, particularly in patients with atrophic gastritis.[1]

Endoscopically, hyperplastic polyps are typically ovoid in shape and show a smooth surface contour, although villiform or pedunculated polyps may develop as well (Fig. 20.2A). Surface erosion often develops as they grow in size.

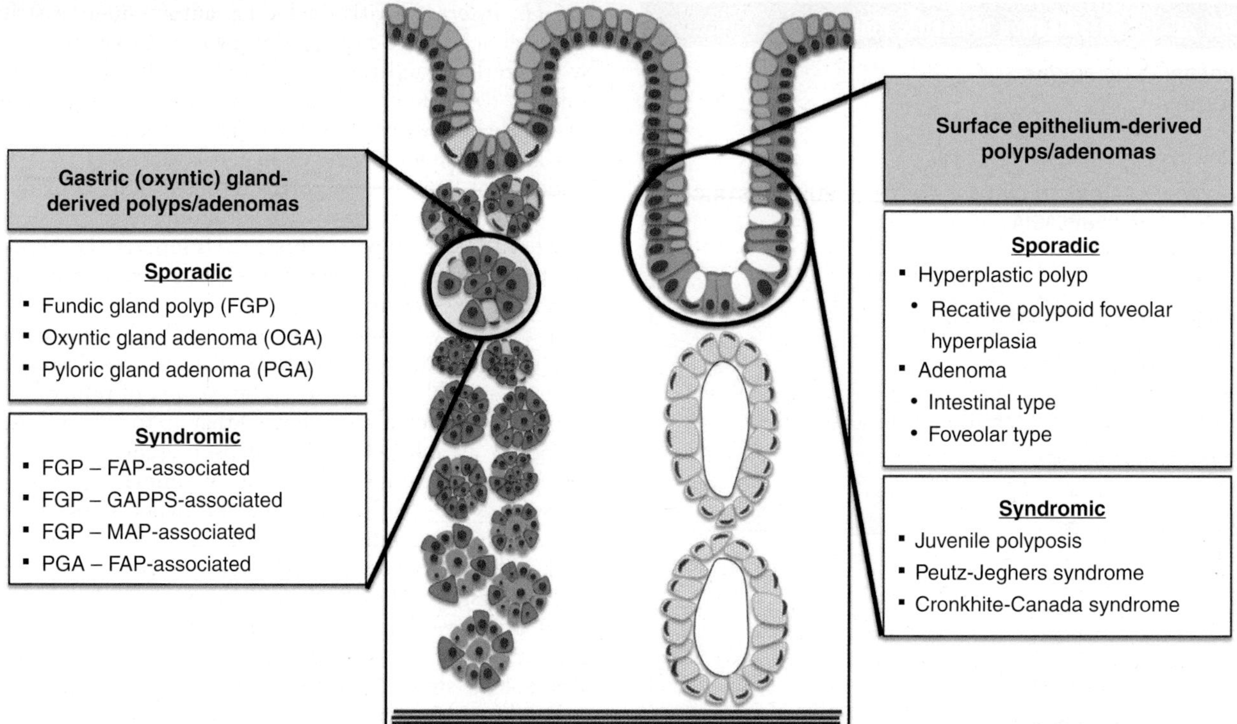

FIGURE 20.1 Histological types of gastric polyps classified according to the epithelial compartment of origin.

Microscopically, hyperplastic polyps are characterized by the presence of architecturally distorted, irregular, cystically dilated, and elongated foveolae (Fig. 20.2B,C). Cellular proliferation and infoldings of the epithelium often impart a corkscrew appearance to the epithelium. Foveolar cells typically have abundant mucinous cytoplasm, but they may be mucin depleted and contain enlarged and hyperchromatic nuclei with prominent nucleoli, which are regenerative features. Mitotic activity may be brisk in areas of active inflammation and surface ulceration.

"Pseudogoblet" or "globoid" mucinous cells are common in hyperplastic polyps. These are hypertrophic foveolar cells that contain an abundance of apically located mucous vacuoles that mimic goblet cells (Fig. 20.2D). Both pseudogoblet and true goblet cells stain blue with Alcian blue histochemistry, however, pseudogoblet cells tend to cluster and form linear segments entirely composed of globoid cells, while true goblet cells are usually intermingled more randomly with columnar cells. These cells should not be mistaken for true intestinal metaplasia. Intestinal metaplasia (i.e., true goblet cells) is identified in less than 25% of hyperplastic polyps and, paradoxically, is more often seen in the surrounding nonpolypoid mucosa than within the polyp itself. Intestinal metaplasia is identified more frequently in polyps located at the gastroesophageal junction because it is presumed that these are associated with Barrett's esophagus.

The lamina propria in hyperplastic polyps is typically edematous and congested, and it usually shows a variable degree of acute and chronic inflammation. Most well-developed hyperplastic polyps also contain bundles of smooth muscle that extend upward from the muscularis mucosae toward the polyp surface. As alluded to previously, some polyps demonstrate broader bands of smooth muscle and thick-walled blood vessels at the base of the polyp, which may indicate prolapse as the pathogenic factor (Fig. 20.2E,F). The inflammatory infiltrate in typical hyperplastic polyps is usually most prominent in the superficial aspects of the polyp and is often associated with surface erosions. Nodular lymphoid aggregates, either with or without germinal centers, may be present as well. Rarely, granulation tissue associated with ulceration may show marked atypical "pseudosarcomatous" reactive stromal fibroblasts and endothelial cells. As noted earlier, *H. pylori* infection is common. These organisms are detected in up to 76% of hyperplastic polyps.[16,32]

Differential Diagnosis

Large polyps may be endoscopically suspicious for a malignant lesion. Furthermore, as they grow in size, they have a tendency to become eroded. Regenerative superficial epithelial changes can be misdiagnosed as a neoplastic process. Thus cautious interpretation of epithelial atypia in the setting of mucosal erosion is advised. Exhaustive sampling of the entire polyp and analysis of multiple levels is often helpful in excluding a true neoplastic transformation.

Another pitfall is the of presence "Pseudogoblet" or "globoid" mucinous cells, as described earlier, which should not be mistaken for signet ring cells if dissociated in an eroded or mechanically damaged polyp.

The differential diagnosis of gastric hyperplastic polyps includes polypoid foveolar hyperplasia; gastritis cystica polyposa or profunda; polyps associated with juvenile polyposis and Peutz-Jeghers syndromes; and polypoid areas in Ménétrier's disease, Cowden's syndrome, and Cronkhite-Canada syndrome. Features helpful in determining the correct diagnosis are summarized in Table 20.1. Polyps in patients with polypoid foveolar hyperplasia and Cronkhite-Canada syndrome are typically smaller in size than hyperplastic polyps

TABLE 20.1 Features of Gastric Polyps

Polyp Type	Prevalence	Site	Architecture	Stroma	Adjacent Mucosa	Malignant Potential	Comments
Hyperplastic polyp	Very common polyp in *Helicobacter pylori* high-prevalence regions	Antrum > body	Elongated, cystic, and distorted foveolar epithelium; often marked regeneration	Inflammation, edema, smooth muscle hyperplasia	Chronic gastritis	<2%	*Helicobacter pylori* or autoimmune gastritis often present; dysplasia in 1%-20%; greatest in polyps >2 cm and in patients >50 years
Polypoid foveolar hyperplasia	Very common	Antrum > body	Elongated foveolar epithelium; no cysts	Normal lamina propria ± edema	Erosion, reactive gastropathy, chronic gastritis, or normal	None	Risk increased with NSAIDs, alcohol, bile reflux, and after Billroth II gastrectomy
Fundic gland polyp	Most common polyp in *H. pylori* low-prevalence regions	Body only	Normal or distorted glands and microcysts lined by parietal and chief cells	Normal ± minimal inflammation	Normal or PPI-associated changes	Rare (except GAPPS)	May be multiple in FAP; dysplasia in as many as 48% of FAP-associated lesions and <1% of sporadic lesions
Adenoma	Common	Antrum > body	Dysplastic intestinal- or gastric-type epithelium; architecture varies with grade	± Inflammation	Chronic gastritis or normal	3%-4% for low-grade adenomas; 5%-30% for high-grade adenomas	Usually solitary
Pyloric gland adenoma	Rare	Body	Tightly packed tubules	Usually scant, uncharacteristic	Chronic atrophic gastritis; normal in syndromic cases	12%-30%	Autoimmune gastritis is a frequent cause; The majority of syndromic cases are FAP-associated
Oxyntic gland adenoma	Rare	Body	Tightly packed tubules	Usually scant, uncharacteristic	Usually normal	Low	The malignant form is named *gastric adenocarcinoma of fundic gland type*
Gastritis cystica polyposa	Rare	Body > antrum	Entrapped, distorted, cystically dilated glands in muscularis; no atypia	Inflammation, edema, smooth muscle hyperplasia	Chronic atrophic gastritis	None	Most common after Billroth II gastrectomy and severe atrophic gastritis
Juvenile polyp	Rare	Body > antrum	Similar to hyperplastic polyp	Inflammation, edema, smooth muscle hyperplasia	Normal	Slight in stomach, greater elsewhere	Clinical history of polyps at other GI sites
Peutz-Jeghers polyp	Very rare	Any site	Normal gastric cell types in arborizing muscle network	Normal lamina propria	Normal	2%-3%	Clinical history of other GI polyps, associated skin changes

Continued

TABLE 20.1 Features of Gastric Polyps—cont'd

Polyp Type	Prevalence	Site	Architecture	Stroma	Adjacent Mucosa	Malignant Potential	Comments
Cowden's syndrome–associated polyp	Very rare	Any site	Irregular or cystic foveolar epithelium	Mildly fibrotic lamina propria	Normal	Low	Frequently associated with esophageal glycogenic acanthosis and various colorectal polyp types including mucosal lipomas and ganglioneuromas
Ménétrier's disease	Very rare	Body only	Foveolar hyperplasia, cysts, atrophy of glands	Normal or increased lymphocytes	Normal antrum Body with diffuse foveolar hyperplasia and oxyntic gland atrophy	Very rare	Diffuse rugal hypertrophy, hypoproteinemia
Cronkhite-Canada syndrome–associated polyp	Very rare	Entire stomach	Foveolar hyperplasia, cysts, atrophy of glands	Edematous, increased eosinophils	Diffuse mucosal foveolar hyperplasia, glandular atrophy, microcystic changes	Very rare	Clinical history of polyps at other GI sites, alopecia, nail atrophy, skin hyperpigmentation, vitiligo

FAP, *Familial adenomatous polyposis;* GAPPS, *gastric adenocarcinoma and proximal polyposis syndrome;* GI, *gastrointestinal;* NSAIDs, *nonsteroidal antiinflammatory drugs;* ±, *with or without.*

and lack cystically dilated, irregular, and tortuous foveolar epithelium. The lamina propria of polypoid foveolar hyperplasia contains less inflammation and lacks smooth muscle hyperplasia.[31]

Gastritis cystica polyposa, or profunda, is closely related to hyperplastic polyps in its pathogenesis and morphology (see Gastritis Cystica Polyposa or Profunda). The surface and intraluminal portions of these lesions may be identical. However, unlike hyperplastic polyps, gastritis cystica polyposa is characterized by cystically dilated, distorted, and irregularly shaped glands or acellular mucin pools located deep to the muscularis mucosae and/or in the submucosa, or even the muscle and serosa in rare circumstances. Polyps related to gastritis cystica polyposa often develop adjacent to anastomotic sites in patients who have had a partial gastrectomy.

Juvenile polyps as well as polypoid areas of gastric mucosa in patients with Ménétrier's disease and Cronkhite-Canada syndrome are histologically very similar to hyperplastic polyps. As a result, these are diagnostically challenging, particularly when evaluating superficial forceps biopsy specimens. However, having appropriate clinical and endoscopic information (i.e., number of polyps and appearance and histology of the non-polypoid mucosa) is essential to helping pathologists establish a correct diagnosis.[33]

Nevertheless, Peutz-Jeghers polyps of the stomach may reveal the characteristic arborizing smooth muscle in the lumina propria, which is typically much more extensive than that of hyperplastic polyps. Unfortunately, most gastric polyps in Peutz-Jeghers syndrome are devoid of this feature, which is usually more prominent in polyps located in the small bowel. Peutz-Jeghers polyps also normally lack significant stromal inflammation and are usually not associated with chronic gastritis unless the latter is a coincidental, synchronous disorder in the patient as a result of other causes.

Natural History and Treatment

The natural history of hyperplastic polyps is poorly understood, but some data suggest that as many as 67% remain stable, 27% may enlarge, and 5% shrink with time.[34,35] Recurrent polyps develop in up to 50% of patients after endoscopic resection.[36,37] Conversely, regression of hyperplastic polyps has been documented in up to 71% of patients with *H. pylori* infection after eradication of the bacteria.[33,38,39] Because of the risk of dysplasia in larger polyps (see Dysplasia and Cancer in Hyperplastic Polyps), resection and a thorough examination is highly recommended for all polyps greater than 1.0 cm in size. In such cases, evaluation of the margins is an important feature if the polyp contains dysplasia or cancer.

Furthermore, because hyperplastic polyps commonly arise on a background of chronic atrophic gastritis, evaluation of the surrounding mucosa is helpful to understand the course of the polyp and the etiology of the patient's gastritis.[40]

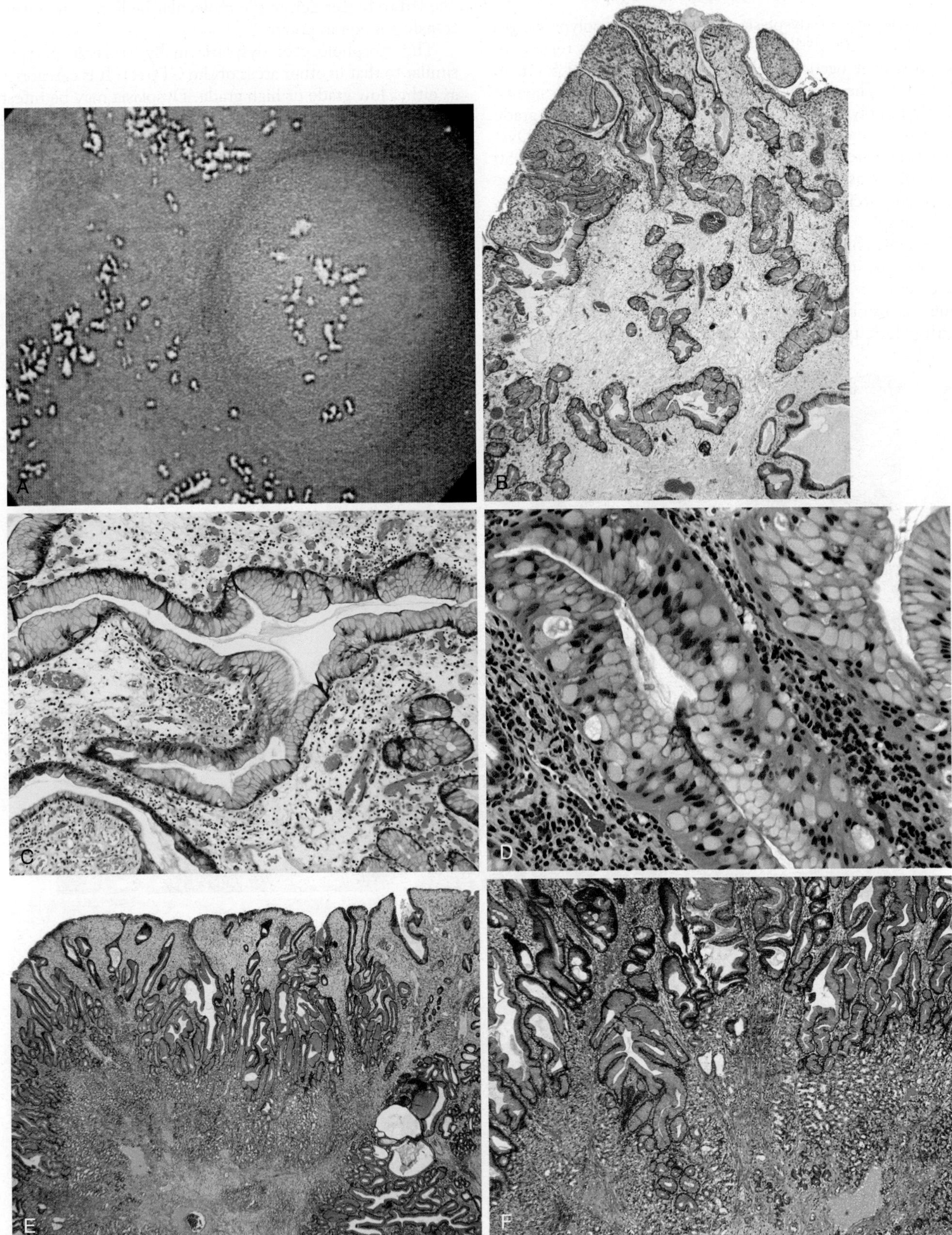

FIGURE 20.2 Gastric hyperplastic polyps. A, This typical sessile hyperplastic polyp is covered by normal-appearing mucosa. **B** and **C,** The polyp is composed of elongated, tortuous, and hyperplastic foveolar epithelium with cystic changes. **D,** The surface epithelium is hyperplastic and can include pseudogoblet cells, which may give a false appearance of intestinal metaplasia or signet ring cell carcinoma in situ. **E** and **F,** Arborizing bundles of muscularis hyperplasia can be seen in the lamina propria. This feature may be suggestive of a mucosal prolapse–associated pathogenesis.

Dysplasia and Cancer in Hyperplastic Polyps

The incidence of dysplasia in hyperplastic polyps ranges from 1% to 20%.[16,41-47] The risk of dysplasia is related to polyp size; it occurs rarely in polyps less than 1.5 cm in diameter. The risk of neoplastic change increases significantly in polyps > 2.5 cm in diameter. In fact, high-grade dysplasia usually occurs in lesions ≥ 5.0 cm in size.[48] Dysplasia and carcinoma tend to occur in patients older than 50 years of age as well.

Adenocarcinoma, when present, is believed to develop from dysplastic epithelium. Some data suggest that *TP53* mutations, chromosomal loss, and chromosomal amplification may be important in the development of dysplasia and carcinoma in gastric hyperplastic polyps. *PIK3CA* mutation has also been identified in a gastric hyperplastic polyp with pyloric type dysplasia.[49] However, further studies are needed to better define the molecular biology of neoplastic transformation in polyps.[50-53]

The morphology of dysplasia in hyperplastic polyps is similar to that in other areas of the GI tract. It is categorized as either low grade or high grade. Dysplasia may be intestinal ("adenomatous"), foveolar, serrated (rarely), or mixed (Fig. 20.3). The spectrum of histological changes of dysplasia are discussed in detail in the Adenoma section later in this chapter. These changes almost always involve the surface epithelium and may involve the deep glands as well.

The principle differential diagnosis of a hyperplastic polyp with dysplasia is a large and eroded polyp with marked regeneration (Table 20.2). The single most useful feature for distinguishing these lesions is the presence of dysplasia-like atypia at the surface of polyps in patients with dysplasia, but an absence of surface atypia in regenerating lesions. Cytological

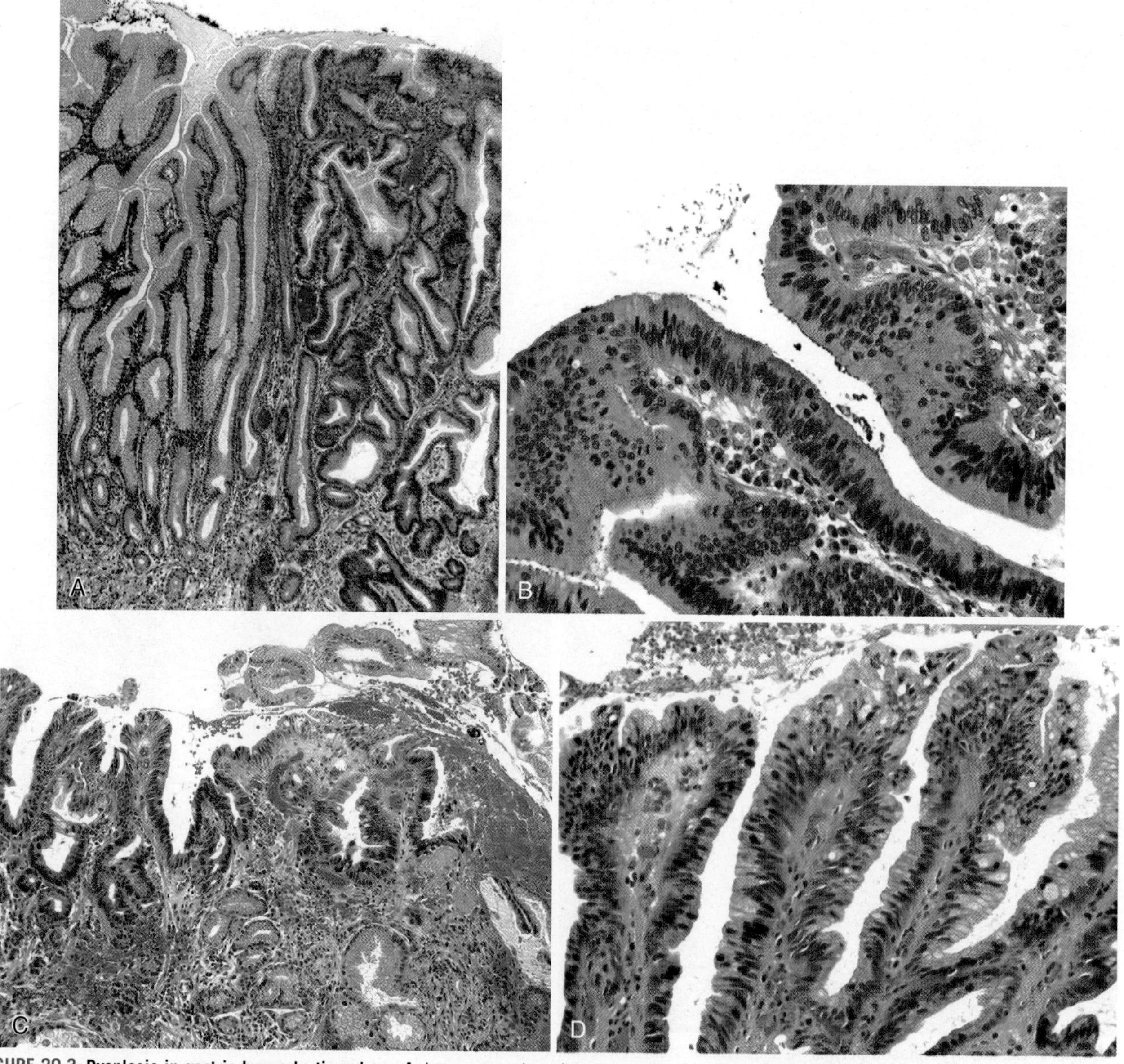

FIGURE 20.3 Dysplasia in gastric hyperplastic polyps. A, Low-power view shows an area of low-grade dysplasia *(right)* adjacent to an area of hyperplastic foveolar epithelium *(left)*. **B,** Higher-power view of low-grade dysplasia with typical intestinal-type cytology. **C,** Dysplasia, which is low grade in this case, is recognizable at low power and usually involves the surface epithelium. **D,** Dysplastic epithelium consists of cells with hyperchromatic, elongated, atypical nuclei and mucin depletion. Surface maturation is absent. This feature can help distinguish dysplasia from regeneration (see Fig. 20.3).

TABLE 20.2 Differentiation of Dysplasia from Regeneration in Gastric Polyps

Feature	Negative for Dysplasia (Regeneration)	Low-Grade Dysplasia	High-Grade Dysplasia
Surface maturation	Present	Absent	Absent
Increased mitoses	Variable	Yes	Yes
Atypical mitoses	No	Few	Increased
Nuclear shape	Ovoid	Elongated	Rounded or irregular
Chromatin pattern	Hyperchromatic	Irregular, hyperchromatic	Irregular, vesicular
Prominent nucleoli	Present	Absent	Present, often multiple
Nuclear stratification	Absent	Mild	Marked in intestinal-type adenomas
Mucin depletion	Variable	Frequent	Frequent
Gland size	Small	Small	Irregular
Budding, branching	Absent	Absent to focal	Prominent
Cribriform profiles	Absent	Absent	Frequent
Inflammation	Often present	Usually absent	Usually absent

atypia limited to the deeper proliferative zones in the polyp with some degree of surface maturation is more often regenerative than dysplastic in nature (Fig. 20.4). However, in the setting of active inflammation and erosion, the degree of atypia in regeneration may be marked, thus a diagnosis of dysplasia should be made with caution. Nuclear pleomorphism and loss of cell polarity, particularly in the absence of prominent nucleoli, also favors a diagnosis of dysplasia. Architectural aberration, such as a cribriform growth pattern, also suggests dysplasia. However, one of the most reliable features is the presence of an abrupt change in the degree of epithelial atypia in the polyp, which strongly favors a diagnosis of dysplasia.

Hyperplastic polyps with dysplasia should also be differentiated from gastric adenomas. Adenomas are characterized by the absence of adjacent or underlying hyperplastic foveolar epithelium, cystic change, and inflammatory stroma, all of which are characteristic of hyperplastic polyps. However, they both may be associated with chronic gastritis in the non-polypoid mucosa.

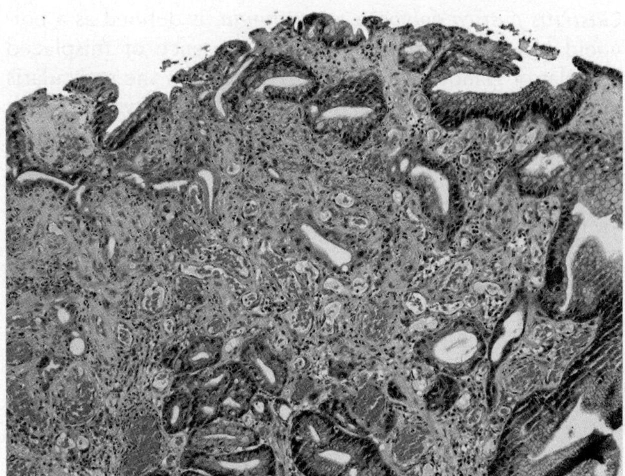

FIGURE 20.4 Regenerative atypia in an eroded gastric hyperplastic polyp. Cytological maturation at the surface is recognizable at low power. In contrast with true dysplasia, surface cells have a decreased nucleus-to-cytoplasm ratio and reduced hyperchromasia relative to deeper epithelium. Proliferating capillaries, which can give the impression of a vascular lesion, can accumulate beneath ulcerated sites.

Morphological Variants

Polypoid Foveolar Hyperplasia

Polypoid foveolar hyperplasia is simply regarded as a precursor of hyperplastic polyps.[23] Similar to hyperplastic polyps, polypoid foveolar hyperplasia is a regenerative lesion associated with chronic gastritis and with other types of acute and chronic mucosal injury.[14] For example, polypoid foveolar hyperplasia often develops at the mucosal edges of surface erosions, ulcers, and carcinomas or adjacent to gastrojejunostomy stomas. It may also be associated with the use of nonsteroidal antiinflammatory drugs, bile reflux, alcohol use, or cytomegalovirus infection.[36,37,54,55] Polypoid foveolar hyperplasia may remain stable in size, regress, or grow. The proportion of these lesions that ultimately progress to hyperplastic polyps is currently unknown.

Grossly, polypoid foveolar hyperplasia usually appears as a sessile lesion 1 to 2 mm in size. These polyps may be single or multiple, and they are most often located in the antrum. Microscopically, polypoid foveolar hyperplasia is characterized by simple hyperplasia of the gastric foveolar epithelium, but without cystic change or significant architectural distortion of the epithelium. The foveolar epithelium is increased in length, and the presence of luminal serration imparts a corkscrew-like pattern to the epithelium (Fig. 20.5). The foveolae are typically crowded and tightly packed, containing little intervening stroma. The quality of the epithelium is variable. In some cases, it is mucin depleted and reactive-appearing with mitotic figures, enlarged nuclei, and prominent nucleoli. In others, cytoplasmic mucin is retained and the epithelium appears mature. Various degrees of intestinal metaplasia may be present as well, but this is much less common than in hyperplastic polyps. The lamina propria may contain a mild lymphoplasmacytic infiltrate, but smooth muscle proliferation is typically absent unless there is associated bile reflux.

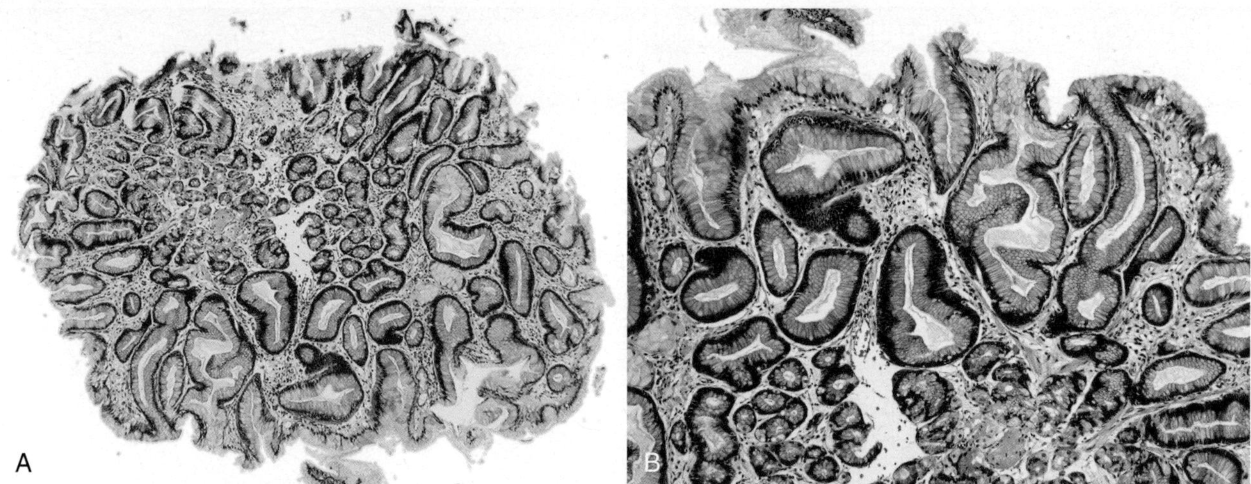

FIGURE 20.5 Polypoid foveolar hyperplasia. A, In contrast with hyperplastic polyps, polypoid foveolar hyperplasia shows elongated, hyperplastic, and tortuous foveolar epithelium without significant cystic change or increased inflammation in the lamina propria. Note also the absence of stromal edematous expansion. **B,** Typical histology of foveolar hyperplasia.

Gastritis Cystica Polyposa or Profunda

Gastritis cystica polyposa, or *profunda,* is defined as a polypoid lesion characterized by the presence of misplaced foveolar or glandular epithelium, or both, in the muscularis mucosae or in deeper portions of the gastric wall, such as the submucosa, muscularis propria, or even the serosa. The lesion is referred to as *polyposa* when an intraluminal polyp is prominent and as *profunda* when the bulk of the lesion is located in the wall of the stomach; both types may result in gastric bleeding.[56-58]

Although these lesions may develop rarely within surgically naive stomachs, they occur more often in patients who have had a partial gastrectomy with subsequent chronic bile reflux, or after surgical or endoscopic manipulation.[58-65] Because of the association of this disease with chronic gastritis and prior gastrectomy, it is presumed that gastritis cystica polyposa/profunda is caused by an exuberant reactive proliferation with trauma- or inflammation/necrosis-induced entrapment of epithelium within the deep portions of the gastric wall. Some authorities have suggested that ischemia and/or mucosal prolapse are critical to the development of this disorder.

Pathologically, polyps associated with gastritis cystica polyposa/profunda are usually located on the gastric side of gastroenteric anastomoses. Rarely, they develop on a background of chronic gastritis. They are grossly indistinguishable from hyperplastic polyps. Polyps may be as large as 3 cm in size and are often associated with enlarged rugal folds. The most characteristic and defining histological feature is the presence of entrapped epithelium and/or glands, either within or beneath the muscularis mucosae of the polyp (Fig. 20.6A–D). Because this is a benign reactive lesion, the epithelial components of the polyp are classically surrounded by lamina propria–like stroma, which is presumably carried along with the epithelium during the process of displacement. The epithelium is often cystic. The cysts are usually entrapped in dense, disorganized bundles of smooth muscle that extend downward from the muscularis mucosae. Marked hyperplasia, reactive changes, and mucin depletion may impart an atrophic appearance to the epithelium, especially when there is associated bile reflux. A mixed neutrophilic and mononuclear infiltrate may be found in the lamina propria in cases with active injury. Superficial erosion and even intestinal metaplasia may be present as well. Dysplasia and even cancer may, extremely rarely, develop in association with gastritis cystica polyposa or profunda.[66] However, it is unclear whether the frequency of occurrence is equal to or greater than that of ordinary hyperplastic polyps.

The principle differential diagnosis is differentiating misplaced epithelium in gastritis cystica polyposa/profunda from a de novo well-differentiated invasive adenocarcinoma, particularly when sampling is limited, such as in biopsies (Fig. 20.6E,F).[67,68] The presence of desmoplasia, cytonuclear pleomorphism, irregularity in the size and shape of the glands, atypical mitoses, and lack of lamina propria surrounding the epithelium in question are all indicative of adenocarcinoma (see Table 20.3 for further details).

MÉNÉTRIER'S DISEASE

Clinical Features

Ménétrier's disease is a rare disorder characterized by the presence of diffuse hyperplasia of the foveolar epithelium of the body and fundus of the stomach combined with hypoproteinemia resulting from protein-losing enteropathy. Other symptoms include weight loss, diarrhea, and peripheral edema. In rare (mostly pediatric) cases, the antrum may be involved as well. In adults, onset typically occurs between 30 and 60 years of age, with a male-to-female ratio of 3 to 1.[69,70]

Although the clinical and pathological features of Ménétrier's disease in children are similar to those in adults, many children have a history of recent respiratory infection, peripheral blood eosinophilia, and cytomegalovirus infection.[71] The disease is usually self-limited in children, lasting only several weeks.[72,73] In contrast, adult Ménétrier's disease is very unlikely to regress.

Pathogenesis

Ménétrier's disease is a form of hyperplastic gastropathy that, in many cases, is driven by excessive secretion of

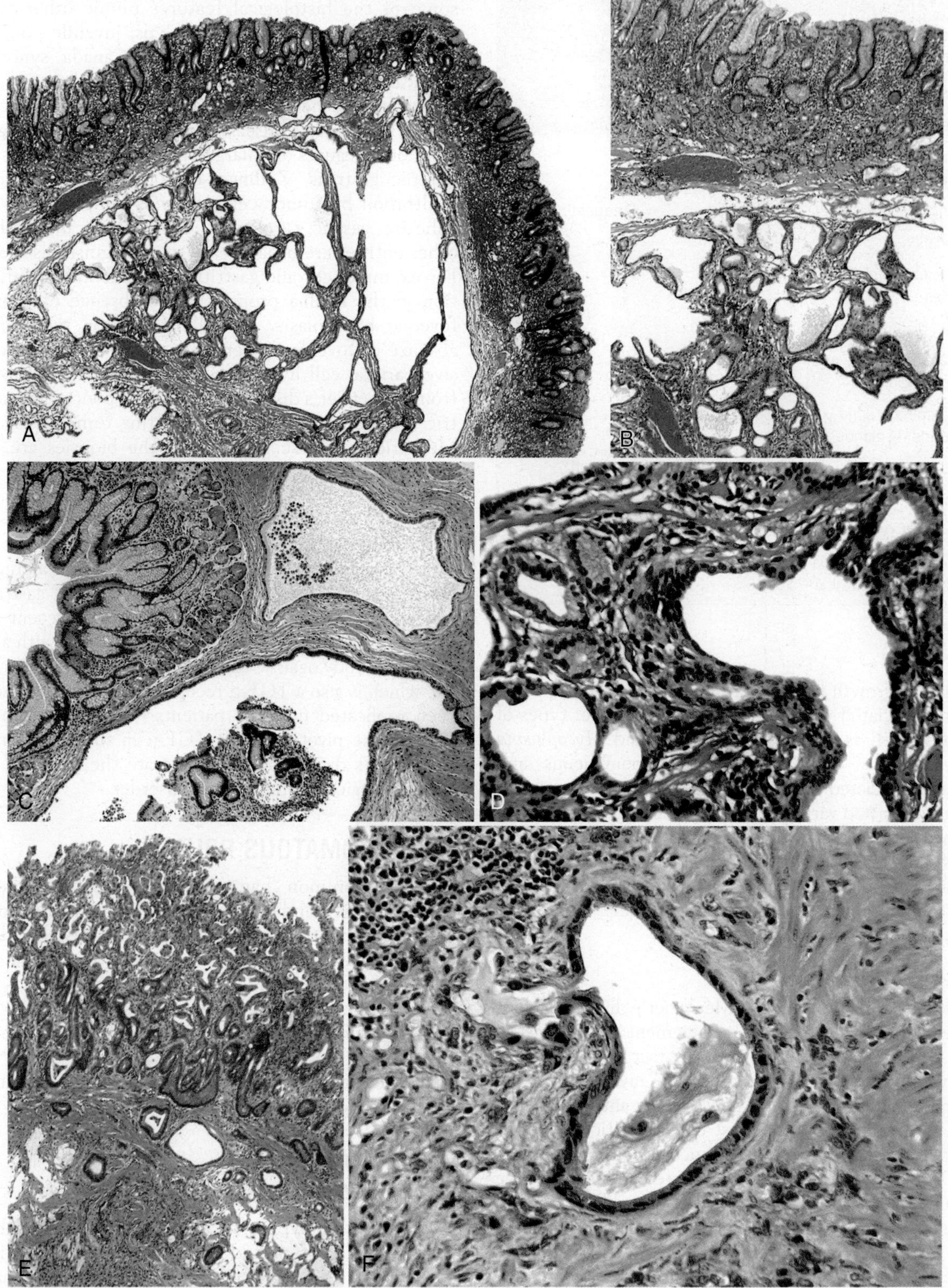

FIGURE 20.6 Gastritis cystica polyposa or profunda. A, The submucosa is replaced by multiple cysts in this case of gastritis cystica profunda. **B,** The mucosa displays features of hyperplastic polyps but also shows a proliferation of cystic glands within the muscularis mucosae and submucosa. **C,** At high power, the misplaced glands show a lobular configuration and are composed of cells with basally located nuclei. A thin rim of lamina propria surrounds the glands. **D,** In some areas, the deep glands can mimic invasive adenocarcinoma. The absence of cytological atypia and lack of desmoplasia are helpful in making this distinction. **E,** Well-differentiated adenocarcinoma associated with chronic gastritis. In contrast with misplaced glands in gastritis cystica polyposa or profunda, carcinomatous glands are highly irregular in size and shape, have jagged edges, and are arranged in a haphazard nonlobular fashion. **F,** At high power, malignant glands show cytological atypia, loss of polarity, and hyperchromasia. Most importantly, in place of a rim of lamina propria, invasive glands are surrounded by desmoplasia.

TABLE 20.3 Differentiation of Gastritis Cystica Polyposa/Profunda from Invasive Adenocarcinoma

Feature	Gastritis Cystica Polyposa or Profunda	Invasive Adenocarcinoma
Overlying hyperplastic polyp	Yes	No
Overlying dysplasia	No	Frequent
Inflammation	Prominent	Absent
Smooth, lobular gland profiles	Yes	No
Irregular, distorted glands	No	Yes
Wide variation in size and shape of glands	No	Yes
Rim of lamina propria surrounding glands	Usually	Never
Mitoses	Rare	Common
Stromal desmoplasia	No	Often
Intraluminal necrosis	No	Occasional
Deep (muscularis propria or serosal) penetration	Rare	Not uncommon

transforming growth factor-α (TGF-α).[74] In children, some cases are associated with cytomegalovirus or other types of infections, such as herpes simplex virus and *Mycoplasma pneumoniae*.[55,71,75-80] In these cases, spontaneous and treatment-associated remissions may occur. Although *H. pylori* infection and various other conditions have been associated with Ménétrier's disease in adults, antibiotics, acid suppression, octreotide, and anticholinergic agents have had only minimal therapeutic benefit in adult patients.[81-83] In contrast, inhibition of TGF-α signaling has been effective in some cases.[84]

Pathological Features

Upon endoscopic examination, Ménétrier's disease is characterized by diffuse, irregular enlargement of the gastric rugae. However, some areas may in fact appear polypoid as well.[85,86] Enlarged rugae typically involve the body and fundus, but they may also involve the antrum in children.[33,87] Histologically, the most characteristic feature of Ménétrier's disease is foveolar (mucous cell) hyperplasia (Fig. 20.7). The foveolae appear elongated and usually have a prominent corkscrew appearance. Cystic dilation of the epithelium is also common. Hyperplastic mucous cells are usually fully differentiated, without regenerative features or mucin depletion. Inflammation is usually only modest or even completely absent, and ulceration is not normally present. Intestinal metaplasia is usually absent. Some cases show marked intraepithelial lymphocytosis, and it may be quite marked in rare instances. Diffuse, or patchy, glandular atrophy and hypoplasia of parietal and chief cells are also characteristic features of Ménétrier's disease.

A diagnosis of Ménétrier's disease may be difficult to establish by evaluation of mucosal biopsies alone because some of the histological features mimic other types of polyps, such as hyperplastic polyps, juvenile polyps, and polyps associated with Cronkhite-Canada syndrome.[33] Clinical information including the endoscopic appearance is essential to help pathologists establish a correct diagnosis. Ménétrier's disease should also be distinguished from other causes of enlarged gastric rugae, such as robust chronic gastritis, Zollinger-Ellison syndrome, and even infiltration by tumor cells, such as lymphoma or poorly cohesive gastric carcinoma. Fortunately, most of these other entities are usually easy to distinguish histologically. For example, chronic gastritis shows abundant inflammation in the lamina propria in the absence of prominent foveolar hyperplasia. In Zollinger-Ellison syndrome, the absence of foveolar hyperplasia and the presence of massive parietal cell hyperplasia helps distinguish this entity from Ménétrier's disease. Lymphoma, poorly cohesive gastric carcinoma, and other infiltrating tumors may mimic Ménétrier's disease grossly, but the biopsies are usually diagnostic.

Treatment

In the past, the treatment of Ménétrier's disease was mainly supportive and provided in the form of serum albumin and nutritional supplementation. In severe cases, gastrectomy was and often still is necessary. However, recent studies have shown remarkable efficacy of treatment with a monoclonal antibody against the epidermal growth factor receptor, which is also a TGF-α receptor.[88] These successes have been replicated in many patients.[84,89-91] These outcomes validate the pivotal role of TGF-α in the pathogenesis of Ménétrier's disease and demonstrate the potential of targeted biological therapy in this disorder.

HAMARTOMATOUS POLYPS

The most common "hamartomatous" lesions of the stomach are fundic gland polyps, although classification of these lesions as *hamartomas* is, in fact, controversial. Other less common hamartomatous polyps are usually associated with distinct polyposis syndromes, such as Peutz-Jeghers syndrome, juvenile polyposis, or rarely, tuberous sclerosis and Cronkhite-Canada syndrome. In most instances, an accurate diagnosis requires correlation of the pathological findings with relevant clinical and endoscopic information.[92]

Fundic Gland Polyps

Clinical Features and Pathogenesis

Fundic gland polyps may be sporadic or familial. They were originally reported as a manifestation of familial adenomatous polyposis (FAP).[93-95] These polyps are now recognized as the most common type of gastric polyp.[1] The apparent increase in incidence reflects the widespread and ever-increasing use of proton pump inhibitors and an overall decreased prevalence rate of *H. pylori* infection, which have been strongly implicated in the genesis of sporadic fundic gland polyp.[96-101] In many series, fundic gland polyps are more common than hyperplastic polyps and, in fact, represent the most common type of gastric polyp

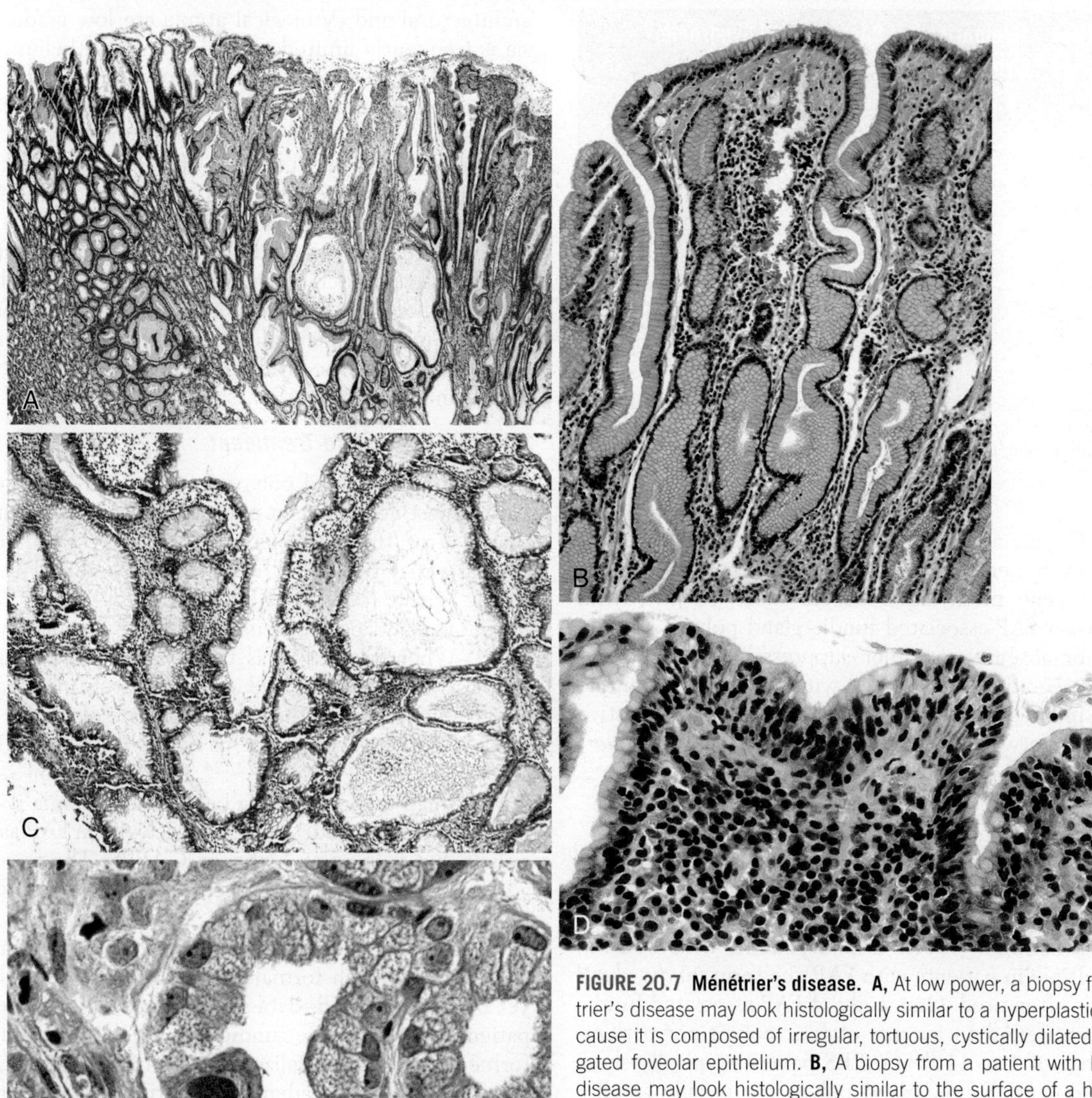

FIGURE 20.7 Ménétrier's disease. A, At low power, a biopsy from Ménétrier's disease may look histologically similar to a hyperplastic polyp because it is composed of irregular, tortuous, cystically dilated, and elongated foveolar epithelium. **B,** A biopsy from a patient with Ménétrier's disease may look histologically similar to the surface of a hyperplastic polyp or foveolar hyperplasia. **C,** In some areas, the mucosa can be replaced by epithelial cysts. The absence of submucosal involvement can differentiate Ménétrier's disease from gastritis cystica polyposa or profunda. **D,** In some cases of Ménétrier's disease, a marked degree of intraepithelial lymphocytosis simulates lymphocytic gastritis. **E,** Although not commonly identified, a cytomegalovirus infection should be considered in pediatric cases of Ménétrier's disease.

(77% of all gastric polyps).[1] However, in some parts of the world, where *H. pylori* gastritis remains prevalent, the hyperplastic polyp remains the dominant type of gastric polyp.

Detection of fundic gland polyps in children should always prompt consideration of FAP. In addition, up to half of fundic gland polyps are associated with symptoms of gastroesophageal reflux.[1] Fundic gland polyps occur more often in women, with an average age of 50 to 60 years at the time of diagnosis.[1,100] Fundic gland polyps may also develop in patients with Zollinger-Ellison syndrome. Up to 90% of patients with FAP have fundic gland polyps within oxyntic mucosa.[93,94,101-105] The same prevalence rate is noted in the recently characterized gastric adenocarcinoma and proximal polyposis syndrome (GAPPS)[106] (see Chapter 25). Less frequently, FGPs may also develop in patients with MUTYH-associated polyposis (MAP).[107]

There are quite distinct natural histories and biological features of sporadic versus FAP-associated fundic gland polyps. In molecular terms, sporadic fundic gland polyps are associated with activating *CTNNB1* mutations in more than 90% of cases, but they show *APC* gene mutations in less than 10% of cases.[103,108,109] Conversely, FAP-associated polyps usually have adenomatous polyposis coli *(APC)* gene mutations[108] and less frequently demonstrate mutations in the gene for β-catenin *(CTNNB1)*, another component of the APC signaling pathway (Table 20.4).[108,110,111] GAPPS and MAP families have point mutations in the promoter 1B

TABLE 20.4 Comparison of Sporadic and Syndromic Fundic Gland Polyps

Feature	Sporadic	Syndromic
Number	Usually solitary (40% multiple)	Typically multiple (90%)
Male-to-female ratio	F > M	M = F
Mean age	52	40
Mutations	*CTNNB1* ≫ *APC*	*APC* > *CTNNB1*
Dysplasia risk	Low (<1%)	High (as much as 48%)
Incidence	0.8%-1.4%	50%-90%

APC, *Gene for adenomatous polyposis coli;* CTNNB1, *gene for β-catenin;* F, *female;* M, *male.*

of the *APC* gene and biallelic mutations in the DNA base excision repair gene, *MUTYH*, respectively.[106,107] Tumor suppressor gene methylation occurs more commonly in sporadic than FAP-associated fundic gland polyps, but the presence or absence of tumor suppressor gene methylation is not specifically associated with the development of dysplasia in these lesions.[90,104,107-111] There is a negative relationship between fundic gland polyps and *H. pylori* infection.[89,112,113]

Pathological Features

Fundic gland polyps are translucent, smooth, sessile, well-circumscribed lesions that occur exclusively within gastric oxyntic mucosa. They may be single or multiple, the latter of which is common in FAP and in patients with GAPPS. When multiple in patients with FAP, the term *fundic gland polyposis* is often used. One study of FAP-associated fundic gland polyps found an average of four polyps per patient, with a range of 1 to 11.[100] GAPPS patients typically show over 100 polyps. Fundic gland polyps are usually smaller than 1.0 cm in diameter, but they may grow to 2 or even 3 cm in size on occasion, especially in polyposis syndromes.

Histologically, fundic gland polyps are composed of cystically dilated and architecturally irregular fundic (oxyntic) glands (Fig. 20.8). In this lesion, the fundic glands assume a microcystic configuration and/or show prominent budding, and they are lined by parietal and chief cells, and occasionally mucinous foveolar cells. Parietal cell hyperplasia is common following PPI therapy and to a lesser degree foveolar cell hyperplasia. Fundic gland polyps in GAPPS tend to be larger in size and also may show inverted foveolar hyperplasia (hyperproliferative aberrant pits) (Fig. 20.8F).[106] Inflammation is typically absent or minimal. The surface and foveolar epithelium in fundic gland polyps is typically atrophic. Regenerative changes are not uncommon, and this is usually restricted to the deep proliferative zones of the polyp, particularly in cases with active inflammation. This should be differentiated from dysplasia that is typically of foveolar type and develops predominantly in patients with syndromic fundic gland polyps. One of the most useful distinguishing features of dysplasia is the sharp transition of atypical and normal adjacent epithelium, whereas regenerative epithelium usually shows a more continuous, seamless transition. In the majority of dysplastic cases, both architectural and cytological atypia are low grade. Dysplasia is frequently limited to the surface epithelium and the neck region. The overall architecture of the oxyntic glands is maintained. Rare cases classified as high-grade dysplasia usually also show low-grade architecture, and only the features of cytological atypia (i.e., loss of polarity, cuboidal rather than columnar cell shape, high nuclear-to-cytoplasm ratio, prominent nucleoli, and atypical mitoses) warrant the high-grade designation. Marked glandular crowding, cribriforming, excessive branching, and budding are usually absent.[119] The morphology of dysplasia in sporadic and syndromic fundic gland polyps is generally similar. The utility of immunohistochemistry in the differential diagnosis is also limited, as β-catenin nuclear positivity is rare in both types.[120]

Natural History and Treatment

Sporadic fundic gland polyps are considered benign lesions with almost no malignant potential. Dysplasia occurs in less than 1% of these lesions.[5,94,103,115,116,121-125] In contrast, dysplasia may be present in 25% to 46% of FAP-associated fundic gland polyps.[5,94,104,113-118,121-124,126,127] Dysplasia in fundic gland polyps is usually of the foveolar type (Fig. 20.9). When present, it is usually low grade. High-grade dysplasia has been reported only very rarely in sporadic fundic gland polyps, but the prevalence rate of high-grade dysplasia in FAP-associated lesions ranges from 0% to 12.5% in several series.[94,115,116,121,122,124] The progression rate from low- to high-grade dysplasia or adenocarcinoma is minimal in sporadic cases, and is approximately 4% in FAP-associated polyps, but it is much higher in GAPPS. The few cases of adenocarcinoma that have been reported have all occurred in syndromic patients.

All dysplastic fundic gland polyps should be completely resected. Although formal surveillance guidelines have not yet been established, data suggest that surveillance of FAP patients for dysplastic fundic gland polyps should be performed on an individualized basis. In FAP patients, surveillance for duodenal adenomas, particularly periampullary lesions and less commonly gastric adenomas, should be carefully performed.

Peutz-Jeghers Polyps

Clinical Features and Pathogenesis

Peutz-Jeghers syndrome is an autosomal dominant syndrome characterized by the presence of mucocutaneous pigmentation and multiple GI hamartomatous polyps.[128,129] The disease occurs equally in men and in women. Patients are usually diagnosed in the second or third decade of life and present with abdominal pain, GI bleeding, or less commonly, obstruction.

Hamartomatous polyps in Peutz-Jeghers syndrome may occur in any portion of the GI tract, but they are most common in the small intestine. Gastric lesions occur in 25% to 50% of patients. Polyps usually develop in the antrum and pylorus, and the median age of onset is 16 years.[130,131] Because of their small size, gastric Peutz-Jeghers polyps are usually asymptomatic. Morphologically identical polyps can occur in McCune-Albright's syndrome, which is caused by somatic activating mutations in the *GNAS* gene.[132]

Most cases (70%) of Peutz-Jeghers syndrome are caused by a germline mutation of the serine-threonine kinase

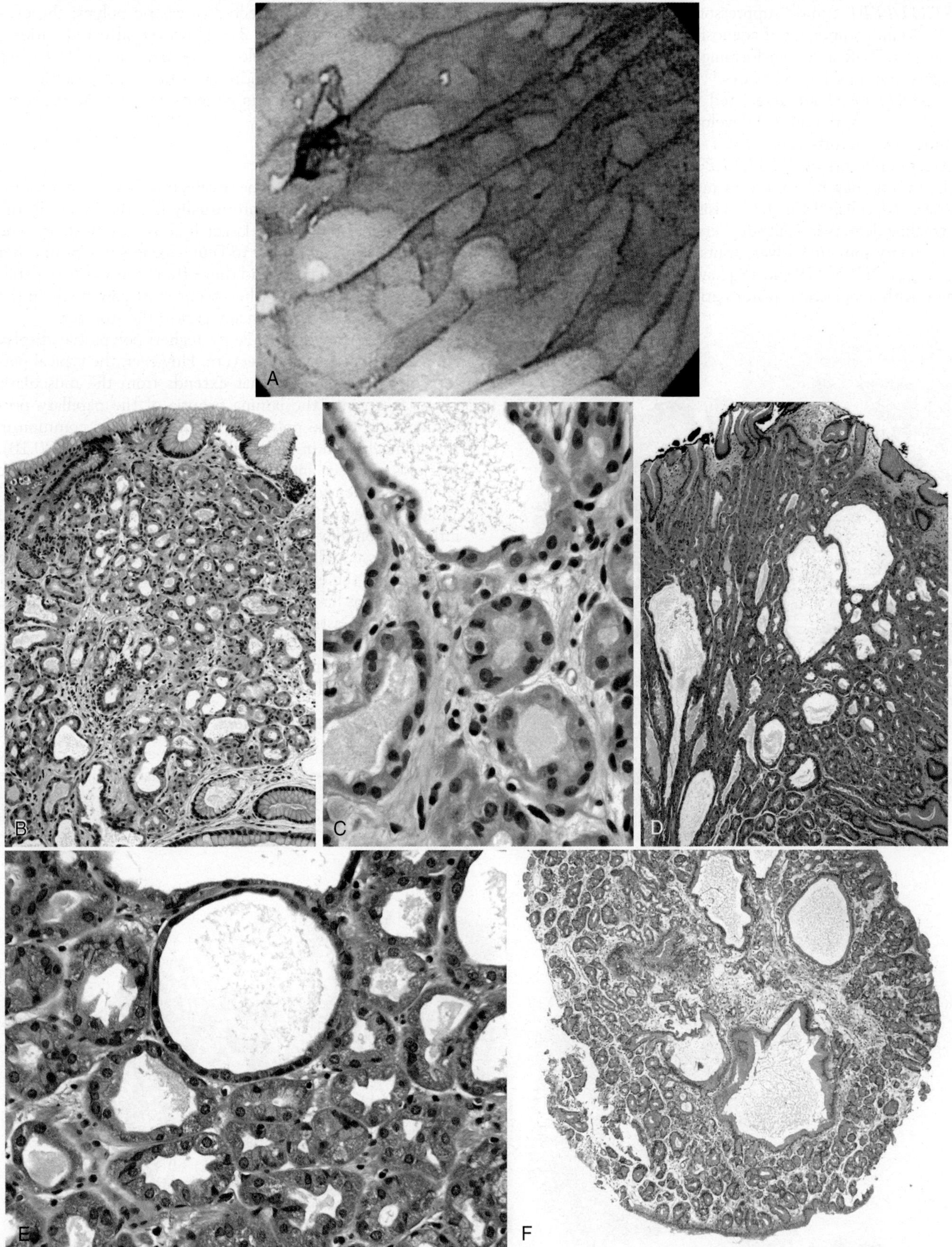

FIGURE 20.8 Fundic gland polyps. A, Endoscopic view shows an unusual case of a patient with numerous fundic gland polyps. The patient was not known to have familial adenomatous polyposis and did not have colonic polyps. **B** and **C,** Microscopic views show that in contrast with hyperplastic polyps, fundic gland polyps have atrophic foveolar epithelium and a marked increase in the number of oxyntic glands, some with irregular budding, and microcystic changes. At high power **(C),** the microcysts are lined by parietal and chief cells, endocrine cells, and variable numbers of mucinous columnar cells. The degree of inflammation in the lamina propria is typically minimal. **D** and **E,** Parietal cell hyperplasia and cysts lined exclusively by parietal cells **(E)** are not typical of fundic gland polyps. The differential diagnosis in this case included Zollinger-Ellison syndrome. **F**, GAPPS-associated syndromic fundic gland polyps are large and are characterized by prominent microcysts lined by inverted foveolar-type epithelium (i.e., hyperproliferative aberrant pits).

STK11/LKB1 tumor suppressor gene,[133-136] which is an important component of adenosine monophosphate (AMP) kinase/mTOR and transforming growth factor-β (TGF-β) signal transduction pathways.[137-140] Truncating mutations of *STK11/LKB1* are associated with an earlier (compared with missense mutations) development of gastric polyps.[130] Tuberous sclerosis genes *TSC1* and *TSC2* are also downstream effectors of *STK11/LKB1*.[139] Some of these signaling events may take place in mesenchymal rather than in epithelial, cells,[141] which is consistent with reports of wnt5a signaling defects in Peutz-Jeghers syndrome.[142-144] Notably, secondary somatic "driver" mutations and loss of heterozygosity (LOH) of 17p and 18q have been detected in association with neoplastic transformation.[133]

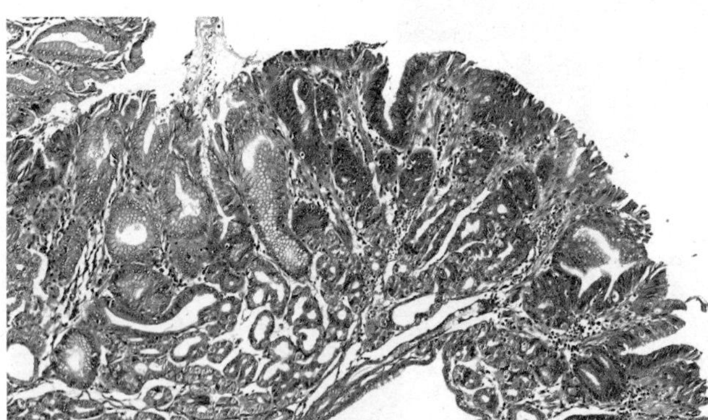

FIGURE 20.9 Dysplasia arising in a fundic gland polyp associated with familial adenomatous polyposis (FAP) typically shows a foveolar phenotype. Hyperchromasia of the surface foveolar epithelium is apparent at low power. The presence of dysplasia is almost pathognomonic for a syndromic (FAP, GAPPS, or MAP-associated) fundic gland polyp. The dysplastic epithelium shows a proliferation of cells containing hyperchromatic, pencil-shaped nuclei with clumped chromatin, pseudostratification, and increased mitoses. Dysplastic epithelium may be seen in the glandular or surface compartment of the polyps.

Dysplasia is rarely detected in gastric polyps; the estimated incidence is 2% to 3%. However, affected patients have a 29% risk of developing gastric cancer.[145] In one series of Peutz-Jeghers syndrome patients with gastric cancer, carcinoma developed in patients with a mean age of 27 years.[146]

Pathological Features

Peutz-Jeghers polyps may be sessile, but they are more commonly pedunculated and are usually less than 1 cm in the largest dimension. Rarely, larger lesions may develop. The gross appearance is similar to Peutz-Jeghers polyps in other portions of the GI tract, and they often have a velvety papillary or villiform surface. They occur most commonly in the antrum but may develop in any part of the stomach.

Microscopically, gastric Peutz-Jeghers polyps may display complex, arborizing architecture. However, the typical pattern of smooth muscle that extends from the muscularis mucosae up into the lamina propria of the papillary projections and to the polyp surface is much less common in the stomach than in the small bowel or colon (Fig. 20.10). Marked surface and foveolar hyperplasia, with cystic change, is often identified. Glandular atrophy is common, and a mild degree of lamina propria edema, congestion, and inflammation may also be apparent. The morphological features are essentially similar to those of gastric hyperplastic polyps, with the exception that some, but not all, hamartomatous polyps have a more fully developed smooth muscle component. Gastric Peutz-Jeghers polyps show defective glandular differentiation.[147] For polyps that occur in the fundic mucosa, this can be recognized by a general depletion of parietal cells.[147]

Natural History and Treatment

Although gastric Peutz-Jeghers polyps are usually clinically silent, large lesions can lead to intussusception. There are also rare examples of patients who have vomited large polyps, presumably as a result of autoamputation.[148] Dysplasia

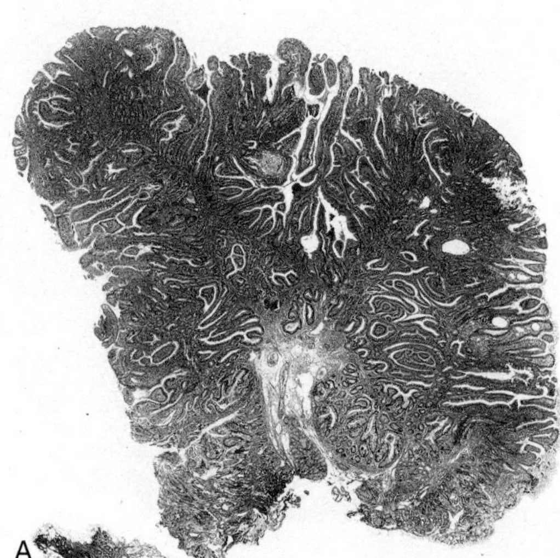

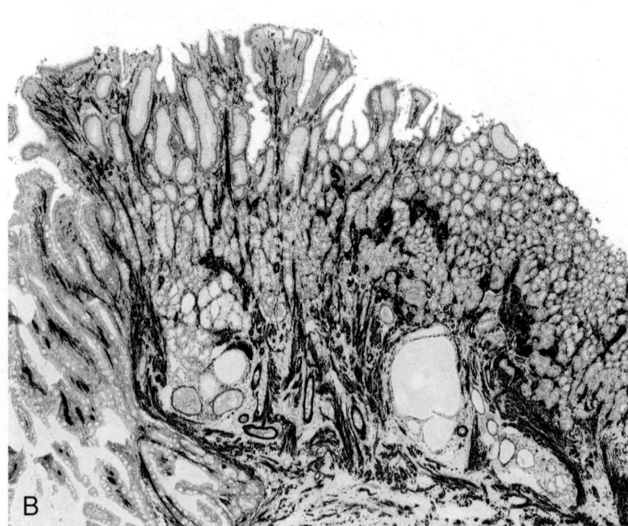

FIGURE 20.10 Gastric Peutz-Jeghers polyp. A, The low-power appearance of a Peutz-Jeghers polyp is similar to that of a hyperplastic polyp. It is composed of an irregular and architecturally distorted proliferation of foveolar epithelium organized in a loose pseudolobular pattern. **B,** Immunohistochemistry (in this case h-caldesmon) may be used to highlight the arborizing smooth muscle bundles and the epithelial nesting pattern, which is frequently inconspicuous on H&E slides.

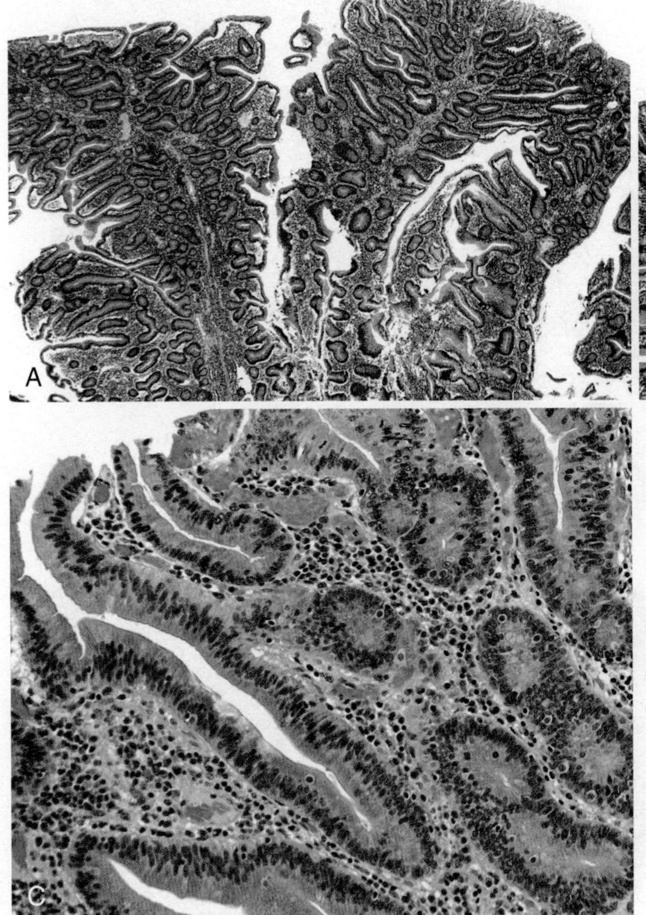

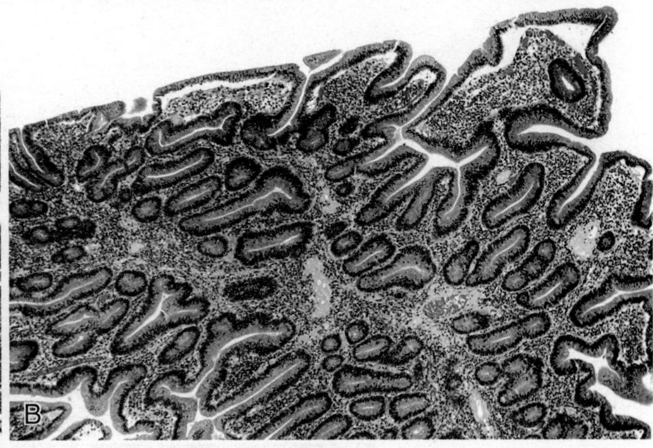

FIGURE 20.11 Dysplasia in Peutz-Jeghers polyps. A, Note the villiform architecture, smooth muscle infiltration, and irregularly shaped glands in this hamartomatous polyp. Even at low power, the absence of epithelial surface maturation is apparent. **B** and **C,** Higher-power views show nuclear elongation, stratification, and hyperchromasia in superficial and deep foveolar cells.

can occur in Peutz-Jeghers polyps (Fig. 20.11), but this is uncommon in gastric lesions. There is no consensus on appropriate surveillance or follow-up of gastric Peutz-Jeghers polyps.[149,150] Novel therapeutic strategies have included the role of mTOR and COX2 inhibitors as well as metformin.[151-153] It has been suggested that surveillance be initiated in the first decade of life, and follow-up endoscopy customized (1- to 3-year interval) based on findings of the first examination.[145]

Juvenile Polyps and Juvenile Polyposis

Clinical Features and Pathogenesis

Sporadic gastric juvenile polyps are rare. They usually occur as part of the generalized juvenile polyposis syndrome, an autosomal dominant syndrome with gastric as well as small and large intestinal manifestations. Other clinicopathological variants of the disease include juvenile polyposis of infancy, isolated colonic polyps, and rarely isolated gastric juvenile polyps (see Table 22.7 in Chapter 22). To establish a diagnosis of juvenile polyposis syndrome, either more than five juvenile polyps of the colon/rectum should be present, or there should be manifestations throughout the entire GI tract, or juvenile polyps occur in association with known family history.[154-156] Gastric polyps are usually detected later in life compared with those that occur in the colorectum (median age 48 vs. 16). Gastric juvenile polyps occur in 15% to 25% of patients with generalized juvenile polyposis coli. Between 20% and 50% of patients with gastric juvenile polyps have a positive family history for juvenile polyposis, which is characterized by a genetic dysregulation of the TGF-β pathway. The mutation most commonly identified involves the *SMAD4/DPC4* gene on Chr 18q21.1 and in BMPR1A on Chr 10q22.23.[157-162] Severe gastric involvement is more common in patients with *SMAD4* mutations than in those with *BMPR1A* alterations. Germline mutations in *PTEN* and possibly *ENG* genes have also been reported.[163]

Pathological Features

The gross and microscopic features of gastric juvenile polyps resemble gastric hyperplastic polyps (Fig. 20.12). The polyps may range from a few millimeters to several centimeters in maximum diameter. The essential microscopic features of juvenile polyps include surface and foveolar hyperplasia, cystic change, edema and inflammation of the lamina propria, and limited smooth muscle hyperplasia. Nevertheless, characteristic features may not be appreciable on superficial biopsies. Intestinal metaplasia may be present as well. Juvenile polyps usually show a less pronounced degree of muscularis hyperplasia and a more prominently inflamed lamina propria, than hyperplastic polyps. However, these features alone are not distinctive. Based on histology alone, it is not possible to

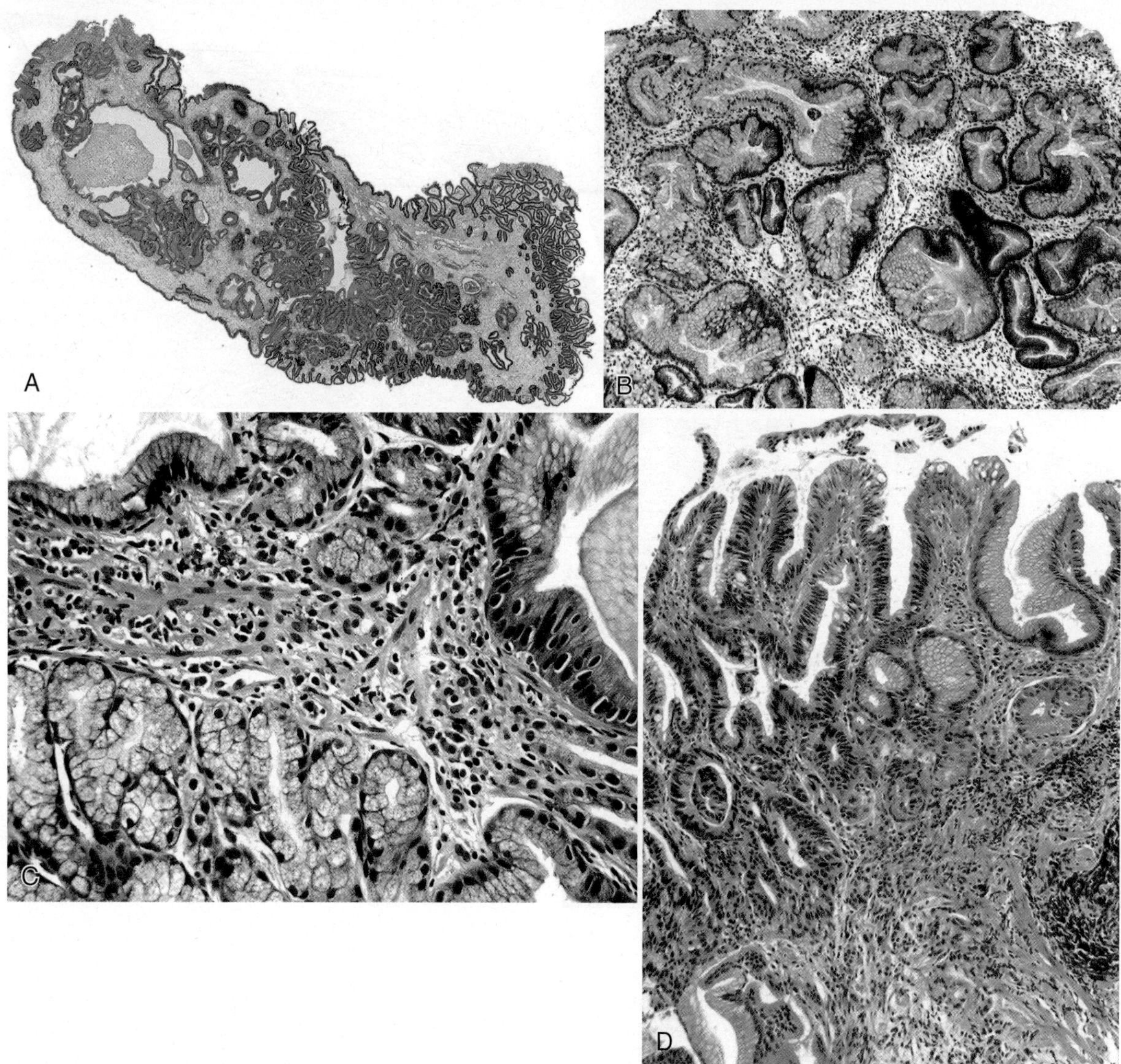

FIGURE 20.12 Gastric juvenile polyposis. A, Similar to hyperplastic polyps, juvenile polyps are composed of irregular, dilated foveolar pits. This polyp occurred in a patient with juvenile polyposis coli. Notice the lobulated organization of epithelial structures in this hamartomatous polyp. **B,** Foveolar epithelium is typical. **C,** The lamina propria is expanded by inflammation. **D,** Low-grade dysplasia *(left)* arises in a gastric juvenile polyp.

reliably distinguish an isolated gastric juvenile polyp from a hyperplastic polyp. Thus knowledge of the clinical context, including the patient's family history, is essential in helping establish a correct diagnosis.[155,164]

Natural History and Treatment

Dysplasia and carcinoma occur with higher frequency in patients with generalized juvenile polyposis coli (Fig. 20.12D). Dysplasia in juvenile polyps appears histologically similar to that in hyperplastic polyps, and it is mostly of the intestinal type. It is characterized by mucin-depleted surface and foveolar epithelium; hyperchromatic, elongated nuclei with clumped chromatin; an increased nucleus-to-cytoplasm ratio; loss of cell polarity; and pseudostratification. Gastric adenocarcinoma has been reported in up to 21% of gastric juvenile polyps,[165] predominantly in patients with a *SMAD4* mutation. Surveillance upper and lower endoscopy are recommended in symptomatic patients from onset of adolescence, with 1- to 3-year intervals.[145] Some guidelines recommend an earlier start in patients with *SMAD4* mutations compared with those with *BMPR1A* alterations.[166]

Cowden's Syndrome/PTEN Hamartoma Tumor Syndrome–Associated Polyps

Clinical Features and Pathogenesis

The spectrum of *PTEN* hamartoma tumor syndromes (PHTSs) encompasses complex disorders usually caused by autosomal dominant germline mutations of the tumor suppressor gene *PTEN*. These include Cowden's disease, Bannayan-Riley-Ruvalcaba syndrome, and Proteus syndrome.[167] Less frequently, other molecular alterations such as *SDHx*, *PIK3CA* and *AKT1* mutations, as well as *KLLN* hypermethylation may be also responsible for the disease. However, *de novo* mutations (without a positive family history) also have been reported.[168-171] The *PTEN* mutation leads to alterations in tissues derived from all three germ layers and results in the development of multiple hamartomas at various anatomic sites. The incidence of Cowden's syndrome is about 1 in 200,000,[172] although this condition is likely underdiagnosed in the community. Newly refined diagnostic criteria for Cowden's syndrome consists of both major and minor criteria (Box 20.2). To reach an operational diagnosis, the suspected patient should present with: (1) >3 major criteria, of which one must be macrocephaly, Lhermitte-Duclos disease (dysplastic gangliocytoma of the cerebellum), or GI hamartomas or (2) two major and three minor criteria. In families with a member who has previously met the clinical diagnostic criteria or has a *PTEN* mutation: (1) any two major criteria or (2) one major and two minor criteria or (3) three minor criteria is enough to establish the diagnosis.[173,174] Regarding GI manifestations, other than gastric polyps, other common GI manifestations include colonic polyps (in 85% to 90% of all cases) and esophageal glycogenic acanthosis (40% to 90%).[175-177] Cowden's syndrome is associated with an increased risk of breast, endometrial, thyroid, and brain cancer as well.[178]

Pathological Features

Almost 50% of Cowden's syndrome patients present with gastric polyps.[176] These are generally sessile and range in size from 0.1 to 2 cm in maximum diameter. Some may closely resemble hyperplastic or juvenile polyps consisting of irregular foveolar epithelium with torturous, cystically dilated, or mucin-filled glands, surrounded by a mildly fibrotic lamina propria with minimal lymphoplasmacytic inflammation.[176,179] Other polyp types, such as ganglioneuromas, fibrolipomas, and intramucosal lipomas (a diagnostic feature that may be unique to Cowden's syndrome) and adenomatous polyps are more common in the colon and show histological features similar to those that occur in the sporadic setting. Recognition of a mixture of polyp types, including some with peculiar mesenchymal component, should always prompt the consideration of Cowden's syndrome.[172,176]

Natural History and Treatment

There are no formal guidelines for surveillance of upper GI manifestations of patients with Cowden's syndrome. However, given that there have been several reported cases of gastric cancer in Cowden's syndrome patients, endoscopic surveillance may be considered on a case-by-case basis.[180] Colonoscopic surveillance is recommended to begin at 35 years of age, with follow-up intervals tailored individually according to symptoms and the presence of polyps at index endoscopy (approximately every 5 years).[181,182]

BOX 20.2 Revised Operational Diagnostic Criteria for PTEN Hamartoma Tumor Syndrome

MAJOR CRITERIA

- Breast carcinoma
- Endometrial carcinoma
- Follicular thyroid carcinoma
- Gastrointestinal hamartomas; ≥3 (excluding hyperplastic polyps)
- Lhermitte-Duclos disease (adult)
- Macrocephaly (≥97th percentile)
- Macular pigmentation of the glans penis
- Multiple mucocutaneous lesions (any of the following):
  - Multiple trichilemmomas (≥3, at least one biopsy proven)
  - Acral keratoses (≥3 palmoplantar keratotic pits and/or acral hyperkeratotic papules)
  - Mucocutaneous neuromas (≥3)
  - Oral papillomas (e.g., on tongue and gingiva), ≥3 *or* biopsy proven *or* dermatologist diagnosed

MINOR CRITERIA

- Autism spectrum disorder
- Colon carcinoma
- Esophageal glycogenic acanthosis
- Lipomas (≥3)
- Mental retardation (i.e., IQ ≤75)
- Renal cell carcinoma
- Testicular lipomatosis
- Papillary thyroid carcinoma (papillary or follicular variant)
- Thyroid lesions (e.g., adenoma, multinodular goiter)
- Vascular anomalies (e.g., intracranial developmental venous anomalies)

From Pilarski R, Eng C. Will the real Cowden syndrome please stand up (again)? Expanding mutational and clinical spectra of the PTEN hamartoma tumour syndrome. J Med Genet. *2004;41(5):323–326.*

Cronkhite-Canada Syndrome–Associated Polyps

Clinical Features

Cronkhite-Canada syndrome is a rare, nonhereditary protein-losing enteropathy that presents as a generalized GI mucosal hyperplasia/polyposis disorder. The condition involves the stomach, small intestine, and colorectum, but spares the esophagus.[183-187] Unlike most syndromic polyposis disorders, Cronkhite-Canada syndrome typically manifests in middle to late adulthood, with a mean age of onset at 59 years. Europeans and Asians are affected most often, with a slight male predominance.[188]

In addition to GI manifestations, patients with this disorder have ectodermal abnormalities including alopecia, nail dystrophy, skin hyperpigmentation, and vitiligo.[189] Common GI complaints include diarrhea, weight loss, abdominal pain, anorexia, weakness, and hematochezia.[183,184,190] Protein-losing enteropathy with hyponatremia, edema, and anemia have also been described.[189] The efficacy of corticosteroids for induction of remission and azathioprine for maintenance (in some patients) and positive immunoglobulin G_4 (IgG_4) staining (in some limited studies of Cronkhite-Canada syndrome polyps, but not in other tissues) have led some authorities to propose an autoimmune basis for this disorder.[191] However, other studies do not support the notion that Cronkhite-Canada syndrome is an IgG_4-related disease[192]; thus the cause of Cronkhite-Canada syndrome remains unknown.

Cronkhite-Canada syndrome is associated with a mortality rate of approximately 50%; most deaths are related to anemia and chronic wasting. Optimal therapy has not been established, but treatment options include nutritional support, antibiotics, corticosteroids, anabolic steroids, histamine receptor antagonists, and surgery, depending on the particular circumstances of the patient.[191-199] Up to 20% of patients with Cronkhite-Canada syndrome develop adenocarcinoma, which may occur in any portion of the GI tract, including the stomach.[200-203] Although cancers may develop within polyps or nonpolypoid mucosa,[204,205] the malignant potential of the polyps themselves remains largely unknown.

Pathological Features

Advanced cases of Cronkhite-Canada syndrome show diffuse, irregular enlargement of the gastric rugae throughout the fundic mucosa and the antrum. Numerous small- to medium-sized sessile polyps that typically measure between 0.5 and 1.5 cm in maximum diameter may be superimposed on a background of enlarged rugae (Fig. 20.13A). In fact, the endoscopic appearance is similar to that of Ménétrier's disease, except that the entire stomach is usually involved. Individual polyps may appear as elongated, papillary, or villiform lesions or, alternatively, as clusters of sessile nodules, which can help in the diagnosis of Cronkhite-Canada syndrome.

Microscopically, changes in the stomach involve both the interpolypoid and polypoid mucosa (Fig. 20.13B). As in Ménétrier's disease, marked surface and foveolar hyperplasia with cystic change and atrophy of the glands are characteristic features. The lamina propria is often edematous and usually shows a mild to moderate degree of inflammation with prominent eosinophils, but intestinal metaplasia is uncommon.[192] The surrounding nonpolypoid mucosa shows alternating areas of atrophy and foveolar hyperplasia with microcystic changes. Unfortunately, a single biopsy from a Cronkhite-Canada syndrome–associated polyp may appear histologically identical to a juvenile polyp, hyperplastic polyp, or Ménétrier's disease.[33,185] However, knowledge of other clinical features of this disorder, particularly when combined with the finding of diffuse enlargement of gastric rugae and multiple polyps in all areas of the stomach, is helpful in establishing a correct diagnosis.

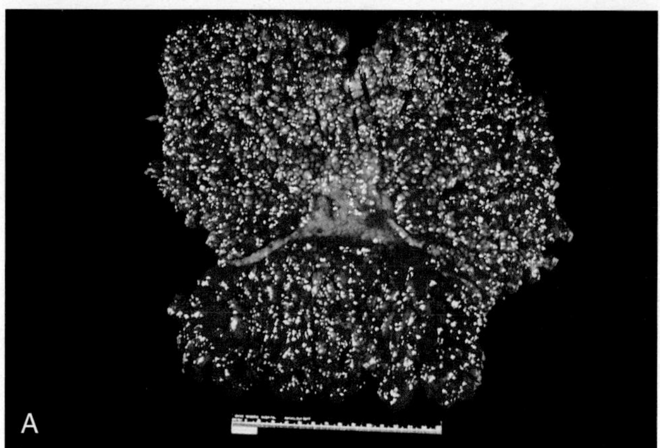

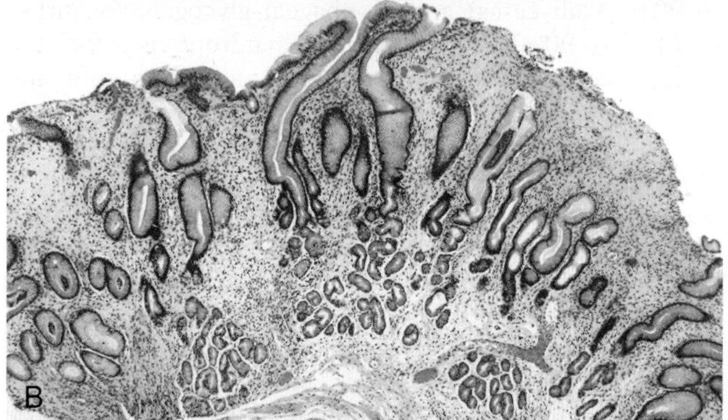

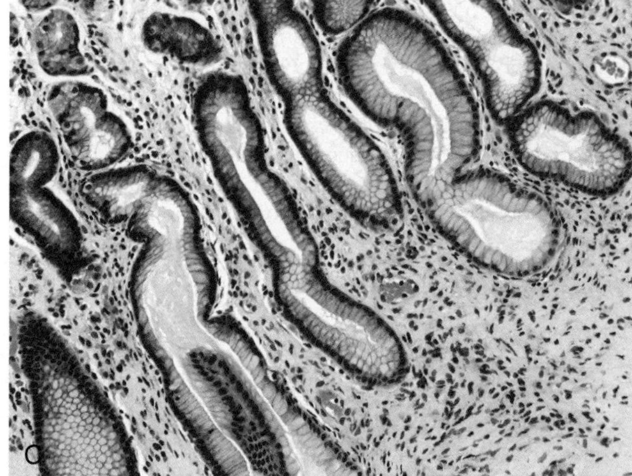

FIGURE 20.13 Cronkhite-Canada syndrome. A, In the resected stomach of a patient with Cronkhite-Canada syndrome, the fundus and the antrum show a carpet-like proliferation of small polyps and enlarged rugae. **B** and **C,** The polypoid and the interpolypoid mucosa show elongated, tortuous, and cystically dilated foveolar epithelium and edema in the lamina propria.

EMBRYONIC RESTS AND HETEROTOPIA

Pancreatic Heterotopia

Clinical Features

Ectopic rests of pancreatic tissue may occur in several parts of the upper GI tract when fragments of pancreas separate during embryonic rotation of the foregut. Foci of ectopic pancreatic tissue are most commonly found in the stomach,[206-208] but they may also occur in the small intestine and colon.[209] Between 0.1% and 4% of all gastric polyps represent pancreatic heterotopia.[210,211] Men and women are affected equally, and the average age at diagnosis is 45 years. However, pediatric patients also may be affected.[212]

Heterotopic pancreatic tissue is susceptible to many of the same disorders that affect the orthotopic pancreas including acute and chronic pancreatitis and cancer.[212-214] Although pancreatic adenocarcinoma in ectopic pancreas is extremely uncommon, such patients usually also have background pancreatic intraepithelial neoplasia in the ectopic focus.[215,216] Some cases may have elevated serum pancreatic enzyme levels.[217]

Pathological Features

Pancreatic heterotopia most commonly occurs in the prepyloric and antral regions of the stomach, but it may rarely occur in the corpus as well.[206,207] Most lesions are less than 3 cm in diameter. Grossly, they consist of small submucosal nodules that protrude through the mucosa, often forming a central dimple or surface erosion, which represents the surface of a draining pancreatic duct. This finding offers an endoscopic clue to the diagnosis.[218] Alternatively, pancreatic heterotopia can form a submucosal mass that can easily be mistaken for other submucosal lesions, such as a gastrointestinal stromal tumor (GIST).[219-221] Ulceration and bleeding are common, although heterotopic pancreas in the stomach is frequently asymptomatic. Clinical symptoms are related to the location and size of the lesion and to the presence or absence of ulceration and/or bleeding.[222,223]

Microscopically, heterotopic pancreatic tissue may be composed of any one or a combination of the three normal components of pancreatic parenchyma (i.e., ducts, acini, and endocrine islets). Most frequently the heterotopic tissue is composed of all these elements. Some have proposed a classification in which type 1 pancreatic heterotopia includes acini, ducts, and islets; type 2 has only two of these elements; and type 3 has only one element, but this classification has no clinical relevance.[209] Cases consisting exclusively of ductal or neuroendocrine elements should not be mistaken for a well-differentiated tubular adenocarcinoma or neuroendocrine tumor. Histologically, each component of a heterotopic pancreas is similar to that which occurs in the orthotopic pancreas (Fig. 20.14). Acini within heterotopic pancreatic tissue typically drains into ducts lined by tall columnar epithelium. However, squamous metaplasia is occasionally identified. Thick, disorganized bundles of hyperplastic smooth muscle are often admixed with acini and ducts. When only smooth muscle and ducts are present, the lesion was previously referred to as an *adenomyoma*.[224] Endocrine elements, representing islets of Langerhans, are found in less than 50% of cases. Acute and chronic inflammation and necrosis, resembling acute and chronic pancreatitis of the orthotopic pancreas, may be present as well. Gastric mucosa overlying heterotopic pancreas often shows reactive changes, including foveolar hyperplasia, as well as various degrees of edema, congestion, and inflammation.

Differential Diagnosis

The differential diagnosis of pancreatic heterotopia includes well-differentiated adenocarcinoma, gastritis cystica polyposa/profunda, and pancreatic acinar metaplasia. Pancreatic acinar metaplasia is far more common than pancreatic heterotopia and does not contain ducts, stroma, smooth muscle, or endocrine cells.[206] Distinguishing well-differentiated adenocarcinoma, gastritis cystica polyposa/profunda, and heterotopic pancreatic tissue, particularly heterotopic foci associated with pancreatic intraepithelial neoplasia, may be difficult if pancreatic acini and endocrine cells are not readily identifiable. However, most examples of pancreatic heterotopia lack architectural and cytological atypia, atypical mitoses, and other features of malignancy that are common in well-differentiated carcinomas. In contrast with carcinoma, the ducts in pancreatic heterotopia normally grow in an organoid or lobular growth pattern. The duct profiles are smooth, rather than irregular or jagged. The smooth muscle hyperplasia often associated with pancreatic heterotopia contrasts sharply with desmoplasia often associated with invasive carcinoma.

Gastritis cystica polyposa/profunda may resemble pancreatic heterotopia, but the former is associated with mucosal hyperplastic changes, inflammation, and erosions. The submucosal epithelium of gastritis cystica polyposa/profunda is composed of mucinous columnar epithelium, either with or without gastric glands, which contrasts with pancreatic duct–type epithelium that is characteristic of pancreatic heterotopia.

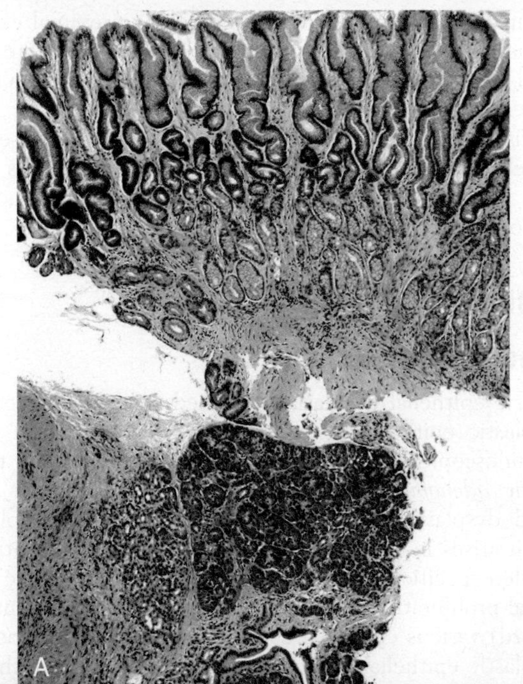

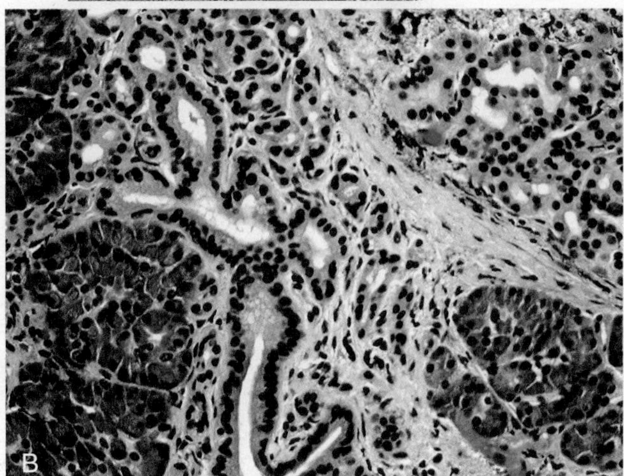

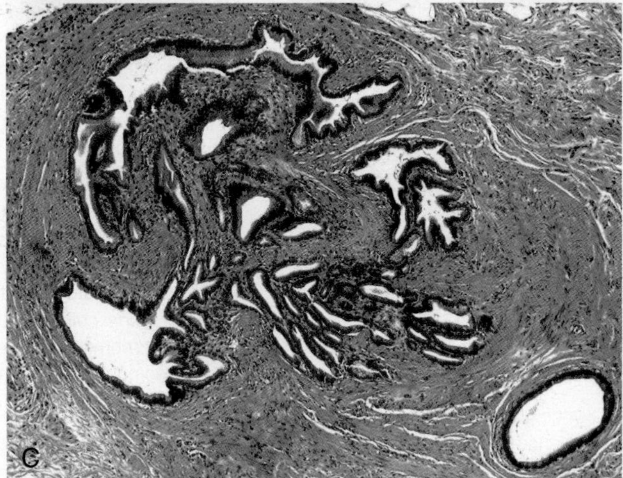

FIGURE 20.14 Pancreatic heterotopia. A, The low-power appearance suggests a nodule of pancreas within the submucosa. **B,** Pancreatic heterotopia can include ducts, acinar glands, and islets. **C,** This adenomyoma is composed only of ducts and smooth muscle.

Brunner's Gland Nodules

In the duodenum, Brunner's gland hyperplasia is usually related to chronic peptic duodenitis. It is unclear whether Brunner's glands in the prepyloric region represent a true hamartomatous process or, more likely, a proximal extension of hyperplastic duodenal Brunner's glands into the distal stomach as a result of hyperchlorhydria, or are a consequence of chronic *H. pylori* gastritis.[225-229]

Histologically, Brunner's gland nodules are composed of densely packed, cytologically benign Brunner's glands that form a prominent submucosal nodule. Pyloric obstruction may occur in rare and extreme cases.[230,231]

NEOPLASTIC EPITHELIAL POLYPS

Nomenclature and Definitions

Gastric epithelial dysplasia is defined as an unequivocally neoplastic epithelial lesion without invasion, which may be endoscopically flat, exophytic, or polypoid. The term *gastric adenoma* specifically refers to exophytic or polypoid dysplastic lesions. Flat gastric epithelial dysplasia, which arises in the setting of chronic atrophic gastritis, is detailed specifically in Chapter 15. Gastric neoplastic epithelial proliferations may be derived from (or differentiate toward) various epithelial compartments. The subtypes of neoplastic epithelial polyps are termed after the epithelial compartment from which they are derived. Foveolar-type and intestinal-type adenomas develop from the surface epithelium. They respectively arise from the foveolar or metaplastic intestinal-type epithelium.

Because the literature tends to differentiate these subtypes according to their morphology despite similar clinical features and management, in this chapter we use the same approach in the following section and discuss surface epithelium–derived adenomas as one entity, but consider the morphological aspects of the individual subtypes separately. Pyloric gland adenomas and oxyntic gland adenomas derived from the gastric glandular epithelium as their respective linages of cellular differentiation are reminiscent of either normal pyloric or oxyntic gland epithelium (see Fig. 20.1). Furthermore, there is also inconsistency in the literature regarding the classification of nonneoplastic polyps (e.g., fundic gland, hyperplastic, or hamartomatous polyps) with dysplasia. In this chapter, if a residual nonneoplastic polyp component is present, we classify the lesion as *dysplastic transformation of the respective entity,* rather than as a *gastric adenoma.*[232] The clinicopathological features of gastric adenoma variants are summarized and compared in Table 20.5.

TABLE 20.5 Clinicopathological Features of Gastric Adenoma Variants

Adenomas	Clinical Association	Histopathological Features	Immunohistochemical Features	Genetic Alterations
Intestinal type	• Chronic atrophic gastritis • *H. pylori* gastritis–related • Autoimmune atrophic gastritis– related • Familial adenomatous polyposis	*Low grade:* Absorptive columnar epithelium with hyperchromatic cigar-shaped nuclei, pseudostratification, and eosinophilic cytoplasm *High grade:* Architectural disarray, crowding, budding, and branching. Enlarged nuclei with nucleoli, irregular contours, and loss of polarity with marked stratification	MUC2 CDX2 CD10	*APC, TP53, KRAS, CTNNB1*
Foveolar type		*Low grade:* Cuboidal to low- columnar shape Gastric surface–type epithelium with pale eosinophilic cytoplasm and apical mucin cap Hyperchromatic round- to oval-shaped nuclei *High grade:* Enlarged ovoid to irregular vesicular nuclei with prominent nucleoli and clumped chromatin Stratification is not as marked intestinal high-grade dysplasia	MUC5AC MUC6	
Pyloric gland adenoma	• Familial adenomatous polyposis • Autoimmune gastritis • Lynch syndrome • Sporadic	*Low grade:* Tightly packed tubules with monolayer of uniform cuboidal to low-columnar shaped cells with pale/eosinophilic cytoplasm Absence of mucin cap Round- to oval- shaped nuclei *High grade:* complex architecture, hyperchromasia, loss of polarity and nuclear pleomorphism with prominent nucleoli	MUC6 MUC5AC	*KRAS* *GNAS* *APC*
Oxyntic gland adenoma	• Sporadic • *Relationship to pyloric gland adenoma under investigation*	Low-grade appearance with tightly packed tubules, cords and clusters of chief cell, parietal cell, or mucous neck cell differentiation Nuclear hyperchromasia, nucleomegaly, and increased nuclear-to-cytoplasm ratio are absent.	Pepsinogen I H+/K+ ATPase MUC6	*GNAS* *CTNNB1* *AXINs* *APC*

Intestinal-type and Foveolar-type ("Surface Epithelial-Differentiated") Adenomas

Clinical Features

Sporadic adenomas, either derived from or differentiating toward the surface epithelium, account for up to 10% of all gastric polyps,[226] but more recent studies suggest that this value may be grossly exaggerated.[1,11] The discrepancy likely reflects the marked variation in the incidence of adenomas and adenocarcinomas in different geographical populations worldwide. For example, gastric adenomas are more common in Asia, where the incidence of gastric adenocarcinoma is high.[3,148,233-235] However, in recent North American studies, gastric adenoma was diagnosed in only 0.1% of patients who underwent an upper endoscopy, and adenomas represented only 0.7% of all gastric polyps.[1,15] In all populations, the incidence of gastric adenomas increases progressively with patient age.[19,20,43,236-238] In Western countries, affected patients are usually in the sixth to seventh decade of life, and the male-to-female ratio is 2 or 3 to 1.[1]

Most adenomas (as well as flat dysplastic lesions) develop on a background of chronic *H. pylori* gastritis with atrophy and intestinal metaplasia or autoimmune atrophic gastritis.[1,239] In contrast, adenomas developing in FAP patients occur more often in the absence of gastritis.

Pathogenesis

The pathogenesis of surface gastric adenomas is unresolved and remains a topic of intense study. Part of the uncertainty lies in the lack of international consensus on the definition and criteria of the conventional (surface-type) adenomas. For instance, in some countries, pure adenomas unrelated to chronic gastritis are rare, whereas in others, it is quite common. Furthermore, some authorities believe that a true adenoma is a lesion that develops in a normal (noninflamed) stomach, whereas others allow the designation of *adenoma* in patients with chronic gastritis, which may actually reflect *polypoid dysplasia* as a result of the underlying inflammatory condition. The molecular features of gastric adenomas are poorly understood. Most adenomas (up to 90%) harbor *APC* or *TP53* mutations, with a tendency to be mutually exclusive.[240] Studies of Japanese patients have found different patterns of genetic changes in high-grade and low-grade adenomas, suggesting that they may arise through different molecular pathways.[241,242] Microsatellite instability is identified in a minority of lesions, but its incidence has been reported to be greater in adenomas that contain carcinoma.[243-248] In contrast, *APC* mutations may occur more commonly in adenomas without carcinoma than in those with carcinoma.[247,249] Furthermore, recent publications proposed that gastric adenomas should be stratified into two groups based on their propensity to progress into malignant tumors. *APC*-mutated adenomas may represent an indolent subtype that rarely progresses to carcinoma, whereas *TP53*-mutated cases are more aggressive and are more frequently associated with invasive adenocarcinoma.[240] In one study, intestinal-type adenomas were more likely than foveolar-type adenomas to have *KRAS*, *APC*, or *CTNNB1* mutations, although no statistically significant differences in any particular genetic alteration were found.[250]

One study of American patients reported that intestinal-type adenomas (adenomas with intestinal-type dysplasia) are more often associated with chronic gastritis, compared with lesions composed exclusively of dysplastic foveolar epithelium. Intestinal-type adenomas were far more likely to contain high-grade cytological features.[251] However, 20% of the patients in this study had a history of FAP, a condition well known for the development of fundic gland polyps, a lesion that characteristically develops foveolar-type dysplasia rather than intestinal-type dysplasia. In our opinion, dysplastic fundic gland polyps represent a unique entity and should not be categorized as adenomas. Other studies of Japanese, Korean, and Portuguese patients found that intestinal markers (i.e., MUC2, CD10, and CDX2) tended to be expressed in "low-grade" adenomas, whereas gastric markers (i.e., MUC5AC and MUC6) were preferentially expressed in adenomas with high-grade dysplasia and intramucosal carcinoma.[252-254] Although further studies are necessary, the different inclusion criteria (e.g., regarding syndromic vs. nonsyndromic patients, polypoid vs. nonpolypoid lesions, and chronic gastritis–associated vs. non–chronic gastritis–associated) and definitions of histological types (H&E vs. immunohistochemistry) and populations of these studies (North American, European, and Asian) may explain the divergent results of "adenoma" worldwide.

Pathological Features

Gross Features

Conventional (surface-type) adenomas occur most commonly in the antrum, but they may develop anywhere in the stomach.[241,251] More than 80% are solitary. Grossly, adenomas are typically well-circumscribed, sessile, or pedunculated lesions that measure less than 2 cm in maximum diameter (Fig. 20.15A). The average size is 1 cm. *Papillary adenomas*, those with a prominent tubulovillous or villous growth pattern, are often larger in size, with an average diameter of 4 cm. Papillary adenomas have a velvety surface contour and a lobulated gross appearance. Most adenomas in the United States develop on a background of chronic gastritis, which frequently shows endoscopically visible atrophic and metaplastic changes. Recently, a "raspberry-like" variant of foveolar adenoma has been proposed as a distinct entity. This subtype appears to develop in non-atrophic, *H. pylori*–negative mucosa. Endoscopically, these lesions have been reported as a small, bright-red protrusion with a raspberry-like fine, granular surface and a papillary or gyrus-like microarchitecture on narrow-band imaging.[255]

Microscopic Features

Histologically, surface epithelium–derived gastric adenomas are divided into intestinal and foveolar subtypes.[250,253,255] However, given the lack of proven clinical relevance, routine histological subtyping is not necessary for clinical management. Intestinal-type adenomas (56% of all cases) are also referred to as *conventional adenomas* by some. Intestinal-type adenomas resemble conventional tubular colonic adenomas histologically. They are composed of intestinal-type columnar epithelium, showing cells with hyperchromatic, cigar-shaped nuclei, pseudostratification, and dense eosinophilic cytoplasm (Fig. 20.16A–B). A distinct brush border is

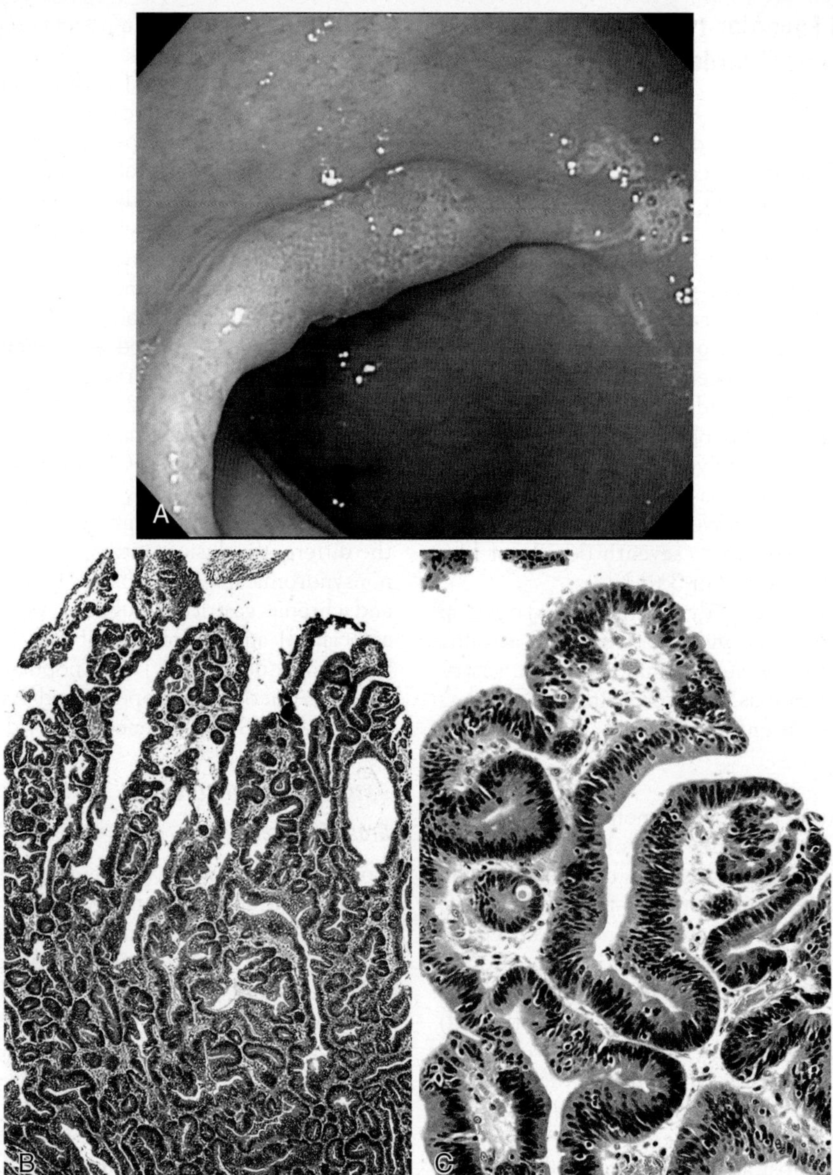

FIGURE 20.15 Gastric adenoma. A, This adenoma presents endoscopically as a thickening of the gastric fold. Note the irregularity of the pit pattern. **B,** Most gastric adenomas appear histologically similar to their colonic counterparts and are composed of cells with stratification, hyperchromatic pencil-shaped nuclei, and mucin depletion. **C,** Higher-power examination shows clear cytological evidence of dysplasia without surface maturation.

often detectable that helps confirm intestinal differentiation in the dysplastic epithelium. Paneth, goblet, and endocrine cell differentiation can be present as well.[250,253,257] These cells are usually arranged as tubules. However, tubulopapillary (tubulovillous) and papillary variants can occur as well, but are less common.[258]

Foveolar-type adenomas represent 41% of cases and are composed of dysplastic mucinous columnar epithelium that resembles the native gastric surface (foveolar) epithelium. The dysplastic cells of these polyps are typically cuboidal to low columnar in shape and contain pale or clear cytoplasm, a characteristic apical neutral mucin cap, and hyperchromatic, round to oval nuclei (Fig. 20.16D,E). Irregular branching of the glands is common. Goblet cell and Paneth cell differentiation is distinctly uncommon. Although gastric adenomas can usually be subtyped into intestinal and foveolar types based on morphology alone, immunohistochemistry can be used to highlight the cellular lines of differentiation in cases that are unclear. Intestinal adenomas are positive for MUC2, CD10, and CDX2, whereas foveolar adenomas characteristically express MUC5AC diffusely and, to a lesser extent, MUC6.[253] A subset of cases show mixed intestinal and foveolar differentiation by morphological and/or immunohistochemical methods.[253] Adenomas with a prominent papillary or villous architecture (i.e., *papillary adenomas*) frequently display marked cellular pleomorphism and brisk mitotic activity, features that are uncommon in nonpapillary adenomas.

Grading of Adenomas

Grading of adenomas is controversial and varies among pathologists in different parts of the world.[259,260] Western pathologists grade dysplasia in adenomas (and flat dysplastic lesions) as either low grade or high grade.[256,257,261] The main advantage of this two-tiered grading system (compared with a three-tiered system [i.e., mild, moderate, or severe]) is that it has a higher degree of interobserver agreement, and it aligns more precisely with clinical management decisions.[256]

Another difference in the evaluation of dysplasia in adenomas (or flat dysplasia) between Western and Eastern (mainly Japanese) pathologists is that the former normally requires unequivocal evidence of lamina propria invasion to establish a definite diagnosis of adenocarcinoma,[261] whereas the latter do not because they place more importance on the cytological features in their assessment of "malignancy." Thus a polyp categorized as an *adenoma with high-grade dysplasia* by Western pathologists may, therefore, be interpreted as an *adenoma with carcinoma* by Japanese pathologists.[261] Recognition of these discrepancies in grading led to the establishment of four international systems for classification of dysplasia (and adenomas) and early cancer in the stomach (Table 20.6).[256,257,260,262] Although it is not essential to formally apply any of these international classifications in routine practice, their use has facilitated international diagnostic consistencies and research.

Intestinal-type low-grade dysplasia shows a predominantly tubular architecture with maintained cell polarity, basally located cigar-shaped nuclei, and apical or "floating" mitoses (see Fig. 20.16). Conversely, high-grade intestinal-type adenomas show architectural complexity with irregular villous architecture, glandular crowding, and back-to-back glands, and they are characterized by marked pseudostratification and loss of cell polarity, with more atypical, round nuclei reaching the apical cell membrane.

Foveolar-type low-grade adenomas typically present with maintained cell polarity, a well-developed mucin cap, and uniform and basally oriented round to ovoid nuclei, which may overlap, but nuclear stratification is less common, even in high-grade lesions (see Fig. 20.16). Similarly to the intestinal counterpart, high-grade foveolar dysplasia may also show increasing architectural complexity. However, in many cases, the high-grade nature is illustrated by cytological changes including markedly increased nuclear-to-cytoplasm ratio, irregular nuclear contours, an open chromatin pattern with prominent nucleoli, increased mitotic rate, and atypical mitoses. In addition, eosinophilic cytoplasmic changes and depletion of mucin cap are common. The evaluation of

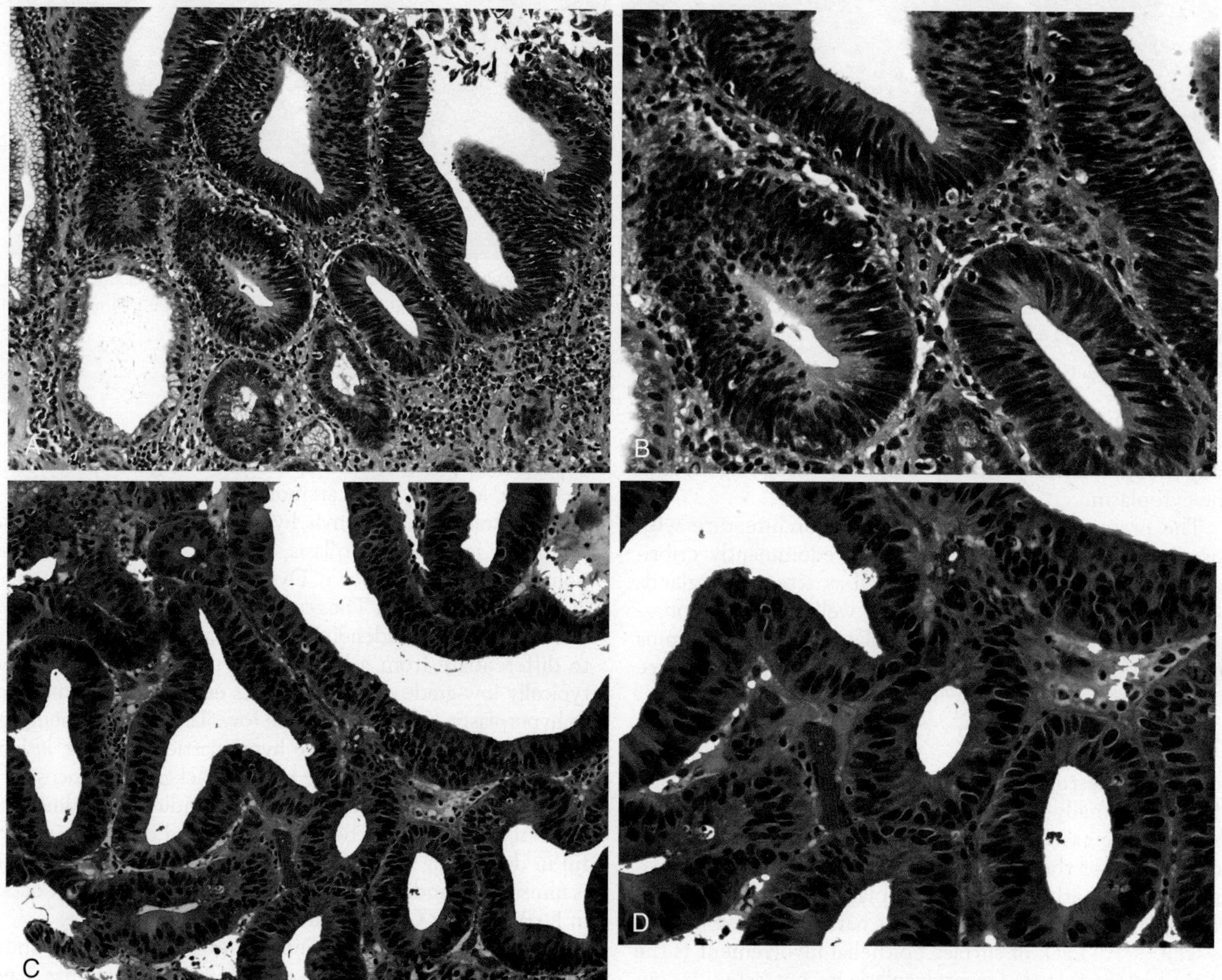

FIGURE 20.16 **A** and **B,** Low-grade adenoma "intestinal type" showing hyperchromatic, cigar-shaped nuclei, limited pseudostratification, and dense eosinophilic cytoplasm. Paneth, goblet, and endocrine cell differentiation and a brush border can be frequently seen in some cases. **C** and **D,** High-grade adenoma "intestinal type" with more complex architectural aberrations and more severe cytological atypia.

continued

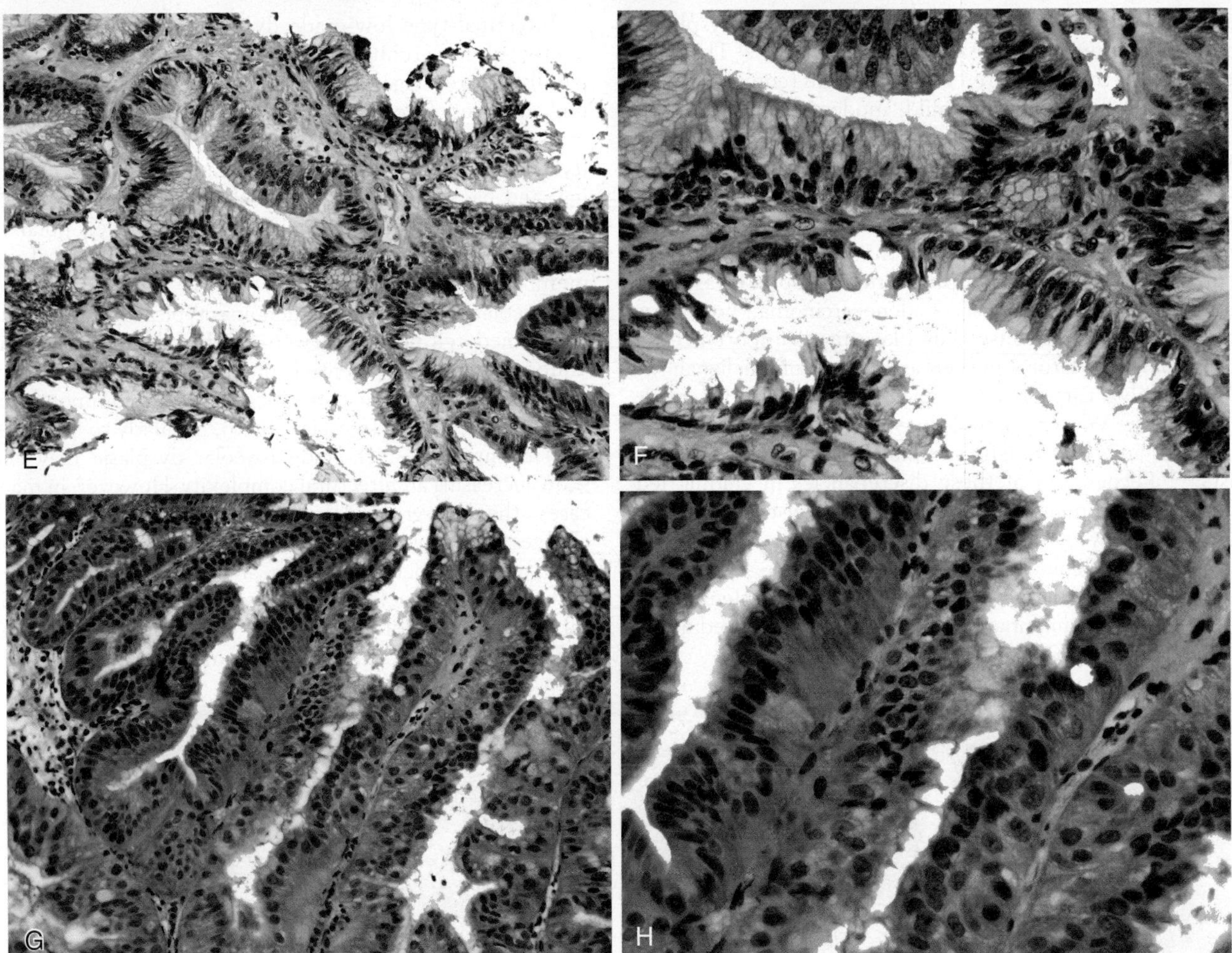

FIGURE 20.16 CONT'D **E** and **F,** Low-grade adenoma "foveolar type" typically showing cuboidal to low columnar cells with pale or clear cytoplasm, a characteristic apical neutral mucin cap, and hyperchromatic, round to oval nuclei. **G** and **H,** High-grade adenoma "foveolar type" with more severe cytological atypia and a loss of polarity.

cell polarity may be challenging as the dysplastic foveolar cells tend to be relatively more cuboidal with physiologically round, relatively larger nuclei easily occupying most of the cytoplasm.

The presence of an overtly crowded architecture with fused, irregularly interconnected or predominantly cribriform and papillary structures as well as attenuated glands with intraluminal necrotic debris as well as small haphazardly distributed glands, buds, or isolated cells in the lamina propria are features of intramucosal adenocarcinoma (see Fig. 20.16).[250,251,253,256,257,263]

Pit Dysplasia

In both intestinal and foveolar adenomas, dysplastic changes normally extend to and involve the mucosal surface. In rare cases, unequivocal dysplasia may be limited to the bases of the pits in the absence of active inflammation.[264] This early pattern of dysplasia is termed *pit dysplasia,*[265] although other synonyms have been used for this as well.[266-268] Lack of surface epithelial involvement is the distinguishing feature for pit dysplasia in contrast with conventional dysplasia. Although our knowledge regarding the behavior of pit dysplasia is limited, 25% of cases progressed to conventional low-grade dysplasia in a recent retrospective study.[266]

Differential Diagnosis

The differential diagnosis of a gastric adenoma includes hyperplastic polyp with dysplasia, fundic gland polyp with dysplasia, and polypoid carcinoma.

In contrast with adenomas, hyperplastic polyps with dysplasia contain foveolar hyperplasia, cystic changes, and inflammation in the underlying polyp. Dysplasia is often focal or patchy in hyperplastic polyps. The recently described "raspberry-like" variant of foveolar adenoma may be particularly challenging to differentiate from a hyperplastic polyp. Because of their typically low-grade dysplasia and its endoscopic resemblance to hyperplastic polyps, low-grade foveolar adenoma should be always considered when large hyperplastic polyp-like lesions are identified in an otherwise healthy background mucosa.[255]

The finding of cystically dilated fundic glands lined by parietal and chief cells beneath the area of dysplasia is helpful in diagnosing a dysplastic fundic gland polyp. Dysplasia is unusual in fundic gland polyps other than those that occur in FAP, MAP, or GAPPS patients.

Both foveolar adenoma and pyloric gland adenoma show gastric differentiation. However, foveolar adenomas have a distinctive PAS-positive luminal mucin cap and characteristically express MUC5AC. Conversely, pyloric gland adenomas lack a mucin cap and are typically predominantly highlighted by MUC6 immunohistochemistry.[253,269]

TABLE 20.6 Classification of Gastric Dysplasia

Western Classification[256,257]	Japanese Classification[261]	Padova Classification[262]	Vienna Classification[260]
Benign reactive	Benign, no atypia (includes intestinal metaplasia, epithelium)	1. Negative 1.0 Normal 1.1 Reactive 1.2 Intestinal metaplasia (IM) 1.2.1 IM, complete type 1.2.2 IM, incomplete type	1. Negative for neoplasia or dysplasia
Indefinite	Benign, with atypia (frequently associated with active inflammation or found within hyperplastic polyp)	2. Indefinite for dysplasia 2.1 Foveolar hyperproliferation 2.2 Hyperproliferative intestinal metaplasia	2. Indefinite for neoplasia or dysplasia
Low-grade dysplasia	Borderline between benign and malignant (dysplastic lesions with architectural and cytological atypia)	3. Noninvasive neoplasia 3.1 Low-grade dysplasia 3.2 High-grade dysplasia 3.2.1 Suspect for carcinoma without invasion 3.2.2 Including carcinoma without invasion	3. Noninvasive neoplasia, low grade (low-grade adenoma or dysplasia)
High-grade dysplasia	Highly suspect for carcinoma (complex architecture)	4. Suspect for invasive carcinoma	4. Noninvasive high- grade neoplasia 4.1 High-grade adenoma or dysplasia 4.2 Noninvasive carcinoma (carcinoma in situ) 4.3 Suspicion of invasive carcinoma
Carcinoma	Invasive carcinoma (stromal invasion)	5. Invasive adenocarcinoma	5. Invasive neoplasia 5.1 Intramucosal carcinoma 5.2 Submucosal carcinoma or beyond

Natural History and Treatment

Gastric adenomas are associated with an increased risk of malignancy. The risk is generally related to the size of the lesion. The risk of intramucosal carcinoma or invasive cancer in gastric adenomas is increased with polyp size greater than 2 cm.[270-272] Depressed-type morphology, red discoloration, and mucosal ulceration have also been associated with an increased risk of carcinoma.[273,274] Overall, carcinoma may be detected synchronously in up to 30% of all gastric adenomas.[38,47,238,275]

In Western populations, 3% to 4% of patients with biopsy-proven low-grade dysplasia progress to adenocarcinoma within 5 years of follow-up, whereas 30% to 60% of polyps with high-grade dysplasia have been reported to progress to adenocarcinoma.[276,277] However, this high rate of progression for high-grade lesions may not represent the natural progression but may represent preoperatively underdiagnosed adenocarcinoma as a result of limitations of endoscopic sampling.[278,279] In the majority of patients with biopsy-proven high-grade dysplasia who are later diagnosed with adenocarcinoma, the upgraded diagnosis is assigned within the first year of follow-up.[276,277] These results suggest that an already existing invasive component may be frequently missed because of undersampling at the initial endoscopy. After the exclusion of the first year of follow-up, only approximately 5% of high-grade dysplastic lesions progress to adenocarcinoma.[276]

Because of recent advances in endoscopic resection techniques, these procedures are currently preferred over surgery. Regardless of size, all adenomas, with any grade of dysplasia, should be resected in their entirety.[40,274,280-282] Whether this requires endoscopic mucosal resection (for adenomas ≤10 mm in size), endoscopic submucosal dissection (for adenomas >10 mm in size), or partial gastrectomy depends on many factors including the size, gross appearance (i.e., flat or polypoid), and location.[40] Endoscopic ultrasound may also be helpful in evaluating polypoid lesions.

Endoscopic suspicion of an adenoma should always prompt a thorough evaluation of the entire stomach, including nonpolypoid mucosa, with biopsies.[210] This evaluation is important because additional biopsies may identify a synchronous dysplasia, or invasive carcinoma, elsewhere in the stomach related to the patient's chronic gastritis. *H. pylori* eradication is also important.[32,210,283]

After resection, a careful follow-up with annual endoscopic surveillance is recommended because a gastric adenoma is also a strong risk factor for metachronous gastric neoplasia in the non-polypoid stomach.[40,248,284,285] Several Korean studies have found a slightly greater incidence of colon adenomas in patients with gastric adenomas.[286-288] These investigators have advocated colonoscopy for all patients with gastric adenomas, which may be justified in Korean populations. Additional studies are needed to determine whether this association holds true in other populations.

Pyloric Gland Adenomas

Clinical Features and Pathogenesis

Pyloric gland adenomas are uncommon lesions. In one frequently cited study, pyloric gland adenomas represented almost 3% of all gastric polyps, but this figure likely overestimated its prevalence because this series did not include fundic gland polyps in the analysis— the most common type of gastric polyp.[258] At clinical presentation, most patients are in their seventh or eighth decades of life. Women account for 60% of the cases.[258,269,289]

Pyloric gland adenomas frequently develop in a background of chronic gastritis with intestinal metaplasia or atrophy, or both (particularly in autoimmune gastritis).[258,289,290] Alternatively, they may also be observed in hereditary cancer predisposition syndromes (e.g., FAP, Lynch syndrome, and juvenile polyposis syndrome).[269,291-293] Molecular analyses of gastric pyloric gland adenomas have identified mutations in *KRAS* (41% to 67%) and GNAS (63% to 83%), which encodes the adenylate cyclase regulatory protein Gαs.[294] The relevance of these mutations to prognosis is unknown. Sporadic and FAP-associated pyloric gland adenomas share common genetic alterations, although the frequency of *APC* mutations is higher in syndromic cases (100% vs. 44%).[295]

Pathological Features

Pyloric gland adenomas are most commonly located in the gastric corpus, but they can be found anywhere in the stomach and may, in fact, be associated with gastric heterotopia in the duodenum, pancreatobiliary ducts, gallbladder, rectum, and uterine cervix.[258,296,297] The median diameter of pyloric gland adenomas is 1.7 cm.

Histologically, low-grade pyloric gland adenomas show tightly packed tubules composed of a monolayer of cuboidal to low-columnar mucus-secreting cells with pale to moderately eosinophilic cytoplasm lacking an apical mucin cap (Fig. 20.17). Reported mainly in the setting of FAP-associated cases, some pyloric gland adenomas can contain scattered parietal cells and cells that express chief cell markers immunohistochemically.[291] The nuclei are typically small, uniform, and round to slightly ovoid, and they contain inconspicuous nucleoli and an open chromatin pattern. High-grade pyloric gland adenomas present with a complex architecture with cribriform structures, a higher nucleus-to-cytoplasm ratio, loss of nuclear polarity, hyperchromasia, and pleomorphism.[289] One study reported high-grade dysplasia in 39% of lesions.[258,289] By immunohistochemistry, pyloric gland adenomas are characteristically positive for MUC6.[258,289,298] MUC5AC, a primarily foveolar marker, is also frequently expressed in pyloric gland adenomas. Recently, based on the expression of these two markers, three subtypes have been described: the most common is the *mixed* type, characterized by a relatively balanced coexpression of both markers, followed by the *pure pyloric* type, which shows diffuse MUC6 labeling and MUC5AC positivity limited to the surface foveolar epithelium, and a rare *predominant foveolar* type that shows diffuse MUC5AC expression and MUC6 positivity restricted to the basalmost part of the glands.[269] MUC2 expression in pyloric gland adenomas is rare, and like CDX2, it occurs only in areas of intestinal metaplasia.[289,298]

Differential Diagnosis

Pyloric gland adenoma should be differentiated from other types of gastric adenomas. Although both foveolar and pyloric gland adenomas reveal cells with pale to eosinophilic cytoplasm, the apical mucin cap that is characteristic of foveolar-type adenomas is absent in pyloric gland adenomas.

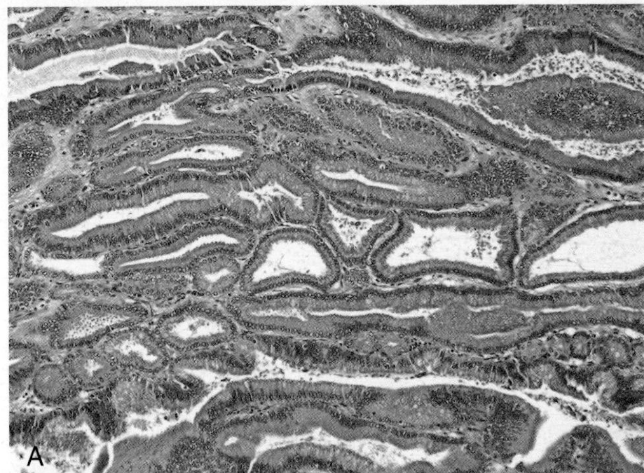

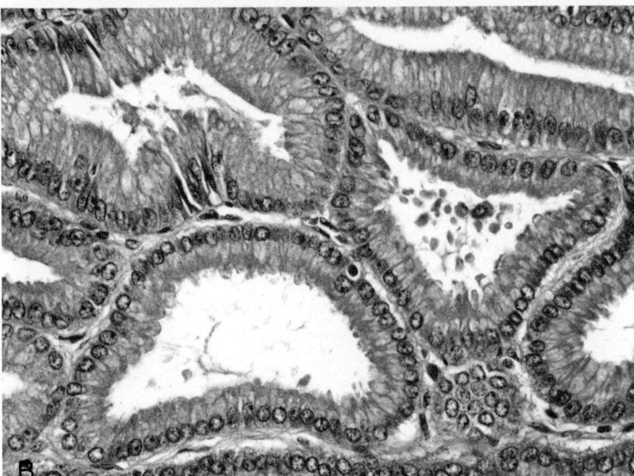

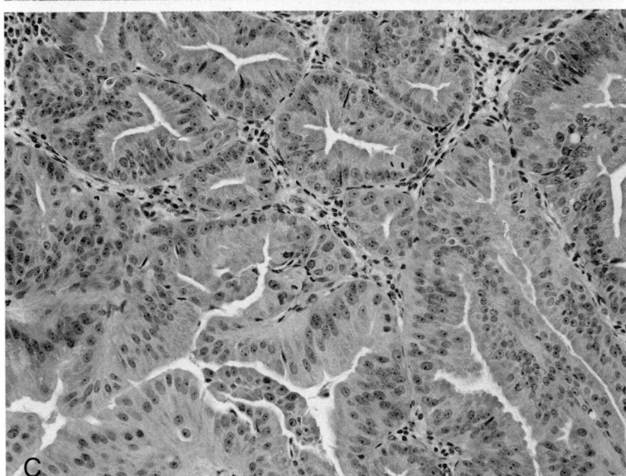

FIGURE 20.17 Pyloric gland adenoma. A, This pyloric gland adenoma features compact tubules and small glands. **B,** These tubules are lined by a monolayer of columnar mucus-secreting cells with pale ground-glass eosinophilic cytoplasm. The uniform round nuclei are also characteristic of pyloric gland adenoma. The absence of an apical mucin cap in pyloric gland adenomas helps differentiate them from foveolar-type adenomas. **C,** High-grade pyloric gland adenoma with more complex architecture and higher nucleus-to-cytoplasm ratio, loss of nuclear polarity, pleomorphism, and more prominent nucleoli.

Concerning ancillary studies, in typical examples, pyloric gland adenomas express MUC6, whereas foveolar adenomas may be highlighted by MUC5ac, although sometimes a mixed expression of these two markers may be detected (see earlier). The presence of goblet cells and Paneth cells, a brush border, and MUC2, CDX2, or CD10 expression are markers of intestinal-type adenomas.

The presence of scattered parietal and chief cells in some pyloric gland adenomas may make differentiation from oxyntic gland neoplasms difficult, especially concerning the subtype with predominantly mucous neck cell differentiation. In fact, both lesions express MUC6 and show overlapping genetic alterations (i.e., *GNAS* mutations) suggesting that these two entities may represent lesions along the same disease spectrum.[291]

Natural History and Treatment

The risk of high-grade dysplasia increases with the size of the lesion, the presence of tubulovillous architecture, a mixed immunophenotype, or a background autoimmune gastritis. A synchronous association with adenocarcinoma (intramucosal or invasive) is reported in 12% to 30% of cases.[258,269,289] In the absence of specific guidelines, the general recommendations established for the management of typical gastric adenomas should be followed. However, based on the accumulated data, complete endoscopic removal should be considered for all pyloric gland adenomas, especially if they are large or show high-grade dysplasia. The local recurrence rate is approximately 10%.[269,299]

Oxyntic Gland Neoplasms

Clinical Features and Pathogenesis

Oxyntic gland neoplasms arise in the gastric corpus and fundus and show chief cell, parietal cell, and mucous neck cell differentiation, thereby closely mirroring the normal cell types of gastric oxyntic glands. Most patients with oxyntic gland adenomas are in their sixth decade of life, and a male predominance has been reported in the largest series to date.[300,301]

These neoplasms were previously referred to as *chief cell hyperplasia*, *oxyntic gland polyp*, or *oxyntic mucosa pseudopolyp*. The term *oxyntic gland neoplasm* is used to emphasize the entire spectrum of tumors that show oxyntic gland differentiation in which *oxyntic gland adenoma* represents the benign variant at one end of the spectrum, and *gastric adenocarcinomas of fundic gland type* represents the most malignant end of the spectrum.[300] However, the vast majority are simple *adenomas*, and these are discussed further in this chapter. Although available data are limited, in half of the genetically studied cases, alterations of several genes involved in the Wnt/b-catenin signaling pathway, including *CTNNB1*, *AXINs*, *APC*, and *GNAS*, have been identified.[302,303]

Pathological Features

Endoscopically, most lesions occur in the gastric corpus. They are usually elevated, although a rare "inverted" form was reported recently. The size ranges from 3 to 40 mm on average.[300]

Microscopically, oxyntic gland adenomas are composed of tightly packed tubules, cords, and clusters of cells with chief cell, parietal cell, or mucous neck cell differentiation (Fig. 20.18). However, most lesions are chief cell–predominant or show an admixture of chief and parietal cells resembling normal oxyntic glands. Less frequently, oxyntic gland adenomas may be composed predominantly of mucous neck cells. This latter pattern is more common in larger-sized lesions and may represent a more aggressive phenotype.[300,304,305] The level of cellular atypia is usually only low grade. Cells show nuclear hyperchromasia, nucleomegaly, anisonucleosis, and an increased nucleus-to-cytoplasm ratio, but with few mitotic figures.[306] High-grade lesions are characterized by a more complex anastomosing glandular or trabecular proliferation, with more pronounced nuclear atypia. Relatively frequently, well-circumscribed clusters of neoplastic tubules extend into the submucosa, but without evidence of desmoplasia. See the Differential Diagnosis (Including Benign vs. Malignant) section that follows.[301]

The diagnosis of oxyntic gland adenoma can usually be reached on H&E-stained slides. However, ancillary studies can be used to highlight the various cellular components. Chief cells are characteristically positive for pepsinogen-I, while parietal cells express H+/K+-ATPase.[307] Similar to pyloric gland adenomas, most tumors are also extensively positive for MUC6.

Electron microscopy reveals cells with enlarged nuclei, irregular nuclear membranes, and disorganization and distortion of the intracellular organelles, such as a rough endoplasmic reticulum and zymogen granules.[300,303]

Differential Diagnosis (Including Benign vs. Malignant)

Fundic gland polyps represent another oxyntic gland–derived lesion that can be excluded based on its less complex architecture and complete lack of cytological atypia. In cases of oxyntic gland adenomas with predominantly mucous neck cell differentiation, pyloric gland adenoma enters the differential diagnosis. Both lesions are formed by pale eosinophilic cells with a ground-glass or foamy cytoplasm and express MUC6. Based on overlapping genetic alterations (i.e., *GNAS* mutations) and the presence of scattered oxyntic cells in some pyloric gland adenomas (reported especially in the setting of FAP-related cases), these entities may represent two morphologically different manifestations of the same disease spectrum.[291] Oxyntic gland adenomas with a predominantly trabecular pattern may be confused with neuroendocrine tumors. The synaptophysin and CD56 expression of oxyntic gland neoplasms may pose a diagnostic pitfall in this regard, but importantly, chromogranin-A positivity was never reported.[308]

The interpretation (benign vs. malignant) of oxyntic gland adenomas that extend into the submucosa is often challenging and is still debated among expert GI pathologists. Lesions with well-circumscribed, expansive borders that involve the muscularis mucosae and expand into the submucosa may represent either prolapse-type changes or true tissue invasion. Considering that the vast majority of patients with submucosal involvement have had neither true recurrence nor progression of disease, the authors of this chapter feel that these lesions should be classified as *benign oxyntic gland adenomas*.[301] However, if the borders of the lesion have an infiltrative appearance and /or reveal desmoplasia, gastric adenocarcinoma of the fundic gland type should be considered.[300]

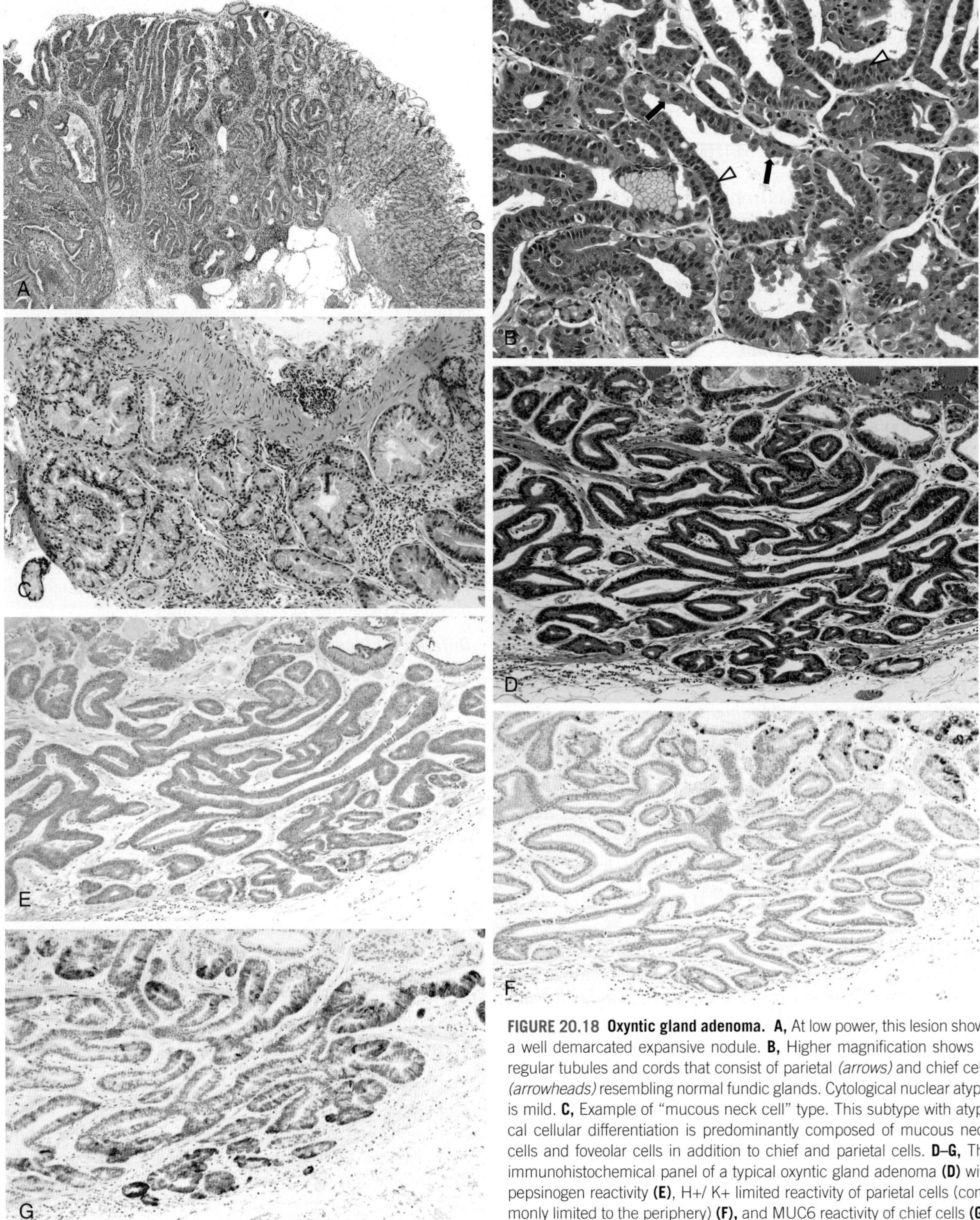

FIGURE 20.18 Oxyntic gland adenoma. A, At low power, this lesion shows a well demarcated expansive nodule. **B,** Higher magnification shows irregular tubules and cords that consist of parietal *(arrows)* and chief cells *(arrowheads)* resembling normal fundic glands. Cytological nuclear atypia is mild. **C,** Example of "mucous neck cell" type. This subtype with atypical cellular differentiation is predominantly composed of mucous neck cells and foveolar cells in addition to chief and parietal cells. **D–G,** The immunohistochemical panel of a typical oxyntic gland adenoma **(D)** with pepsinogen reactivity **(E)**, H+/ K+ limited reactivity of parietal cells (commonly limited to the periphery) **(F),** and MUC6 reactivity of chief cells **(G).**

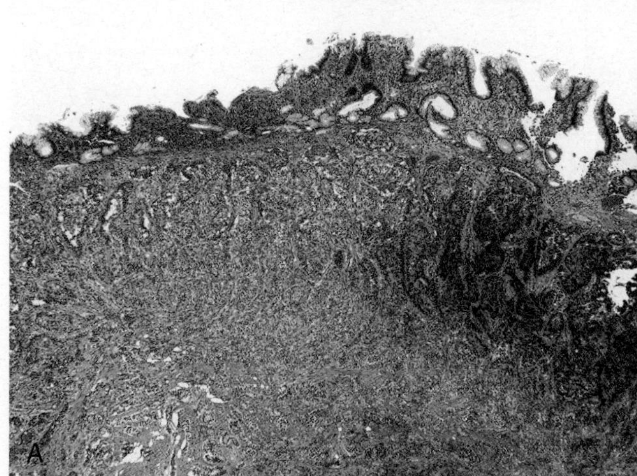

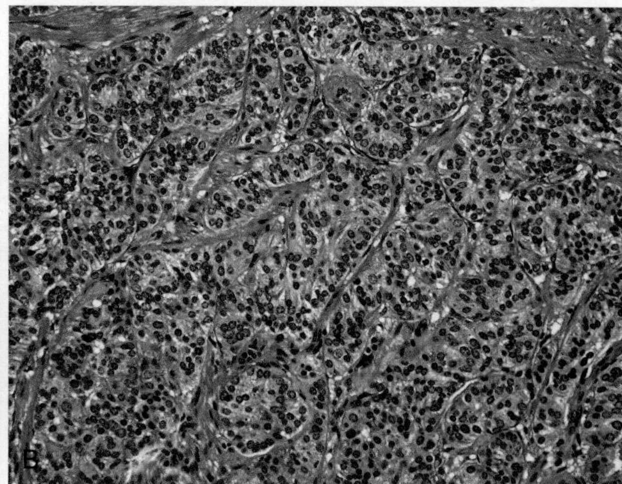

FIGURE 20.19 Neuroendocrine tumor. A and **B,** The intramucosal portion of this well-differentiated neuroendocrine tumor is composed of nests and trabeculae.

Natural History and Treatment

Oxyntic gland adenomas that are limited to the mucosa or those that "herniate" into the submucosa follow a benign course and can be treated endoscopically. In the largest series published to date, no evidence of recurrence or metastasis was reported with a median follow-up of 32 months.[300] Nevertheless, gastric adenocarcinomas of fundic gland type (i.e., with submucosal invasion and desmoplasia) can be associated with lymphovascular invasion.[300] Current guidelines do not offer specific recommendations for the management of oxyntic gland neoplasms. However, the size of the lesion, degree of atypia, and an infiltrative growth pattern should be considered to indicate the need for endoscopic resection or minimally invasive surgery.[300,309]

Neuroendocrine Tumors

Neuroendocrine tumors and other gastric neuroendocrine lesions are discussed more thoroughly in Chapter 29. More than 50% of all gastric neuroendocrine tumors manifest endoscopically as a polypoid lesion (Fig. 20.19A).[1,310] Up to 30% of GI neuroendocrine tumors occur in the stomach, and their incidence is on the rise.[311-314] In North America, 0.06% of all patients who have undergone an upper GI endoscopy are diagnosed with gastric neuroendocrine tumor, which represents 0.6% of all gastric polyps.[1,15] The average age at clinical presentation is 65 years, and there is a female predominance.[1,15]

Gastric neuroendocrine tumors are classified into various clinicopathological subtypes, each of which has a substantially different prognosis. The most common type (80% to 90% of all gastric neuroendocrine tumors) are type 1 neuroendocrine tumors. These occur most commonly in the body and fundus, are often associated with autoimmune gastritis, and have a favorable prognosis (5-year survival is virtually 100%).[239] Type 2 tumors are rare. These arise in patients with multiple endocrine neoplasia type 1 and hypertrophic hypersecretory gastropathy. Type 3 lesions are also less frequent (10% to 15% of gastric neuroendocrine tumors), develop spontaneously without any background mucosal inflammation, and have a more aggressive behavior (5-year survival <50%). Recent studies also propose the possibility of prolonged proton pump inhibitor therapy as a potential cause of indolent gastric neuroendocrine tumors.[315]

Autoimmune gastritis–associated neuroendocrine tumors may be multifocal, and they sometimes manifest as multiple polyposis. Hyperplastic proliferation of scattered enterochromaffin-like neuroendocrine cell nests is a characteristic feature of autoimmune gastritis, and these may progress into a type 1 neuroendocrine tumor if the neuroendocrine cell nests form a nodule that exceeds 500 μm in diameter.[22,316,317] Given the association with autoimmune gastritis, it is not surprising that neuroendocrine tumors are frequently accompanied by gastric hyperplastic polyps and adenomas.[15,318-320]

Recently, an additional variant of mixed neuroendocrine–nonneuroendocrine tumor consisting of an adenoma (noninvasive) and a low-grade neuroendocrine tumor has been recognized. These tumors are termed *mixed adenoma neuroendocrine tumors* (MANETs) and usually present endoscopically as a polypoid lesion.[321]

Treatment of neuroendocrine tumors depends on the type, size, and multiplicity of lesions (see Chapter 29). Endoscopic resection or follow-up is preferred over surgical resection in cases of type 1 tumor.

Metastatic Lesions

According to the largest endoscopic sampling-based study, one-third of all GI metastases show a polypoid endoscopic appearance. A submucosal/intramucosal lesion is the second most common manifestation.[322] In advanced cases, an ulcerated mucosal mass may form. Melanomas are particular prone to bleeding.[323-326] The stomach is the most common target of metastatic spread among the various segments of the tubular GI tract. Thirty-three percent of all GI metastatic tumors occur in the stomach. The majority of lesions are located in the fundus (70% to 80%). One-third of patients have multifocal gastric lesions.[322,327] In contrast with the esophagus, duodenum, colon, and rectum, where secondary tumors usually develop as a result of direct invasion, vascular spread (44%) is the usual rout of dissemination to the stomach.[322]

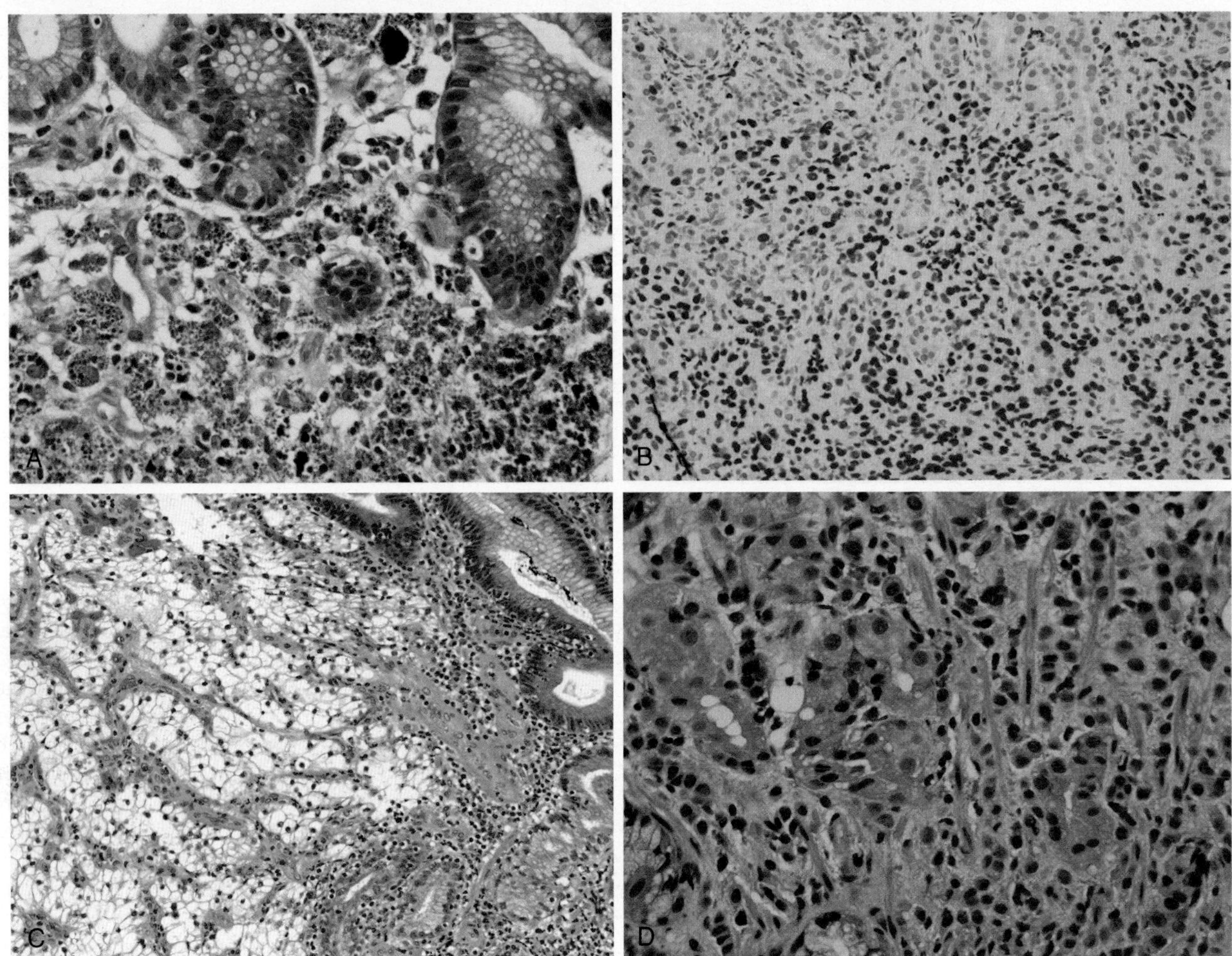

FIGURE 20.20 Metastatic tumors to the stomach. A, Metastatic melanoma with prominent brown pigmentation. **B,** The melanocytic differentiation is highlighted by SOX10 immunohistochemistry. **C,** Metastatic renal clear cell carcinoma. **D,** At low power, metastatic lobular carcinoma of the breast may be mistaken for lymphocytes in association with chronic gastritis. However, at high power, the lobular carcinoma cells appear atypical and show a single-file arrangement of cells, unlike lymphocytes. The malignant cellular infiltrate could easily be mistaken for gastric poorly cohesive carcinoma.

The stomach is most frequently involved by hematogenous metastasis from melanoma (approximately 30% of all gastric metastases), followed by breast carcinoma (12%). Metastases originating from the lung and kidneys as well as direct extension from the esophagus, pancreas, duodenum, and colon are also relatively common (Fig. 20.20).[323-325,327,328] Some tumors may colonize the mucosa and mimic primary gastric adenocarcinoma.[326] Lung carcinomas are one of the most common primary tumors in autopsy series, but they only represent about 5% of all gastric metastases in endoscopic biopsies.[322,324,327] This discrepancy is most likely a result of the dismal prognosis associated with metastatic lung cancer. Metastatic spread of lobular breast carcinoma frequently involves the stomach; however, these cases usually mimic diffuse gastric cancer, with wall thickening rather than distinct polypoid lesions.

In the absence of a clinical history, a panel approach to immunohistochemistry is useful. Notably, metastatic melanomas may be positive for CD117. Conversely, as many as 50% of epithelioid GISTs may express melan-A,[329] but they usually are S100 negative and DOG1 positive.[329] DOG1 positivity can be detected in a plethora of different carcinomas and should not be mistaken for epithelioid GISTs.[330]

NONEPITHELIAL POLYPS

Inflammatory Fibroid Polyps

Clinical Features and Pathogenesis

Inflammatory fibroid polyps are uncommon lesions that can occur anywhere in the GI tract.[331] However, they are most common in the stomach, where they represent up to 3% of all gastric polyps. They frequently arise in the antrum immediately proximal to or overlying the pyloric sphincter.[1,332,333] When large and pedunculated, this location allows intussusception to occur into the duodenum, which is why some inflammatory fibroid polyps can manifest with symptoms and signs of gastric outlet obstruction.[334] However, most are actually small and submucosal lesions that are sometimes associated with overlying mucosal erosion.

Gastric inflammatory fibroid polyps are more common in women,[1,331,335,336] with a mean patient age at clinical presentation of 60 to 75 years.[1,336,337]

The description of one Devonshire family with inflammatory fibroid polyps in three generations of women suggests the possibility of a genetic basis for this lesion. This was referred to as *Devon polyposis*.[338,339] Recent molecular investigations have identified activating mutations of the platelet-derived growth factor receptor-α gene *(PDGFRA)* in up to 70% of gastric and small-intestinal inflammatory fibroid polyps.[331,336,337,340,341] *PDGFRA* is also mutated in some GISTs.[74,342] *PDGFRA* mutations are more often located within exon 12 in small-intestinal polyps, whereas exon 18 *(D842V)* mutations are more common in gastric polyps.[337]

Pathological Features

Inflammatory fibroid polyps are mostly submucosal lesions that frequently extend into the mucosa and are commonly ulcerated. Their median diameter is 1.5 cm. Most lesions are smaller than 3 cm in size. However, polyps as large as 5 cm in diameter have been reported.

Microscopically, inflammatory fibroid polyps often show an abrupt demarcation at the level of the muscularis propria. Unlike small-intestinal lesions, involvement of the muscularis propria is unusual in gastric polyps. Extension of the tumor into the mucosa causes separation of gastric glands, which results in a disordered and atrophic appearance of the mucosa.

Inflammatory fibroid polyps are composed of a loose mixture of spindle-shaped, plump, cytologically bland stromal cells; inflammatory cells; and small, thin-walled blood vessels in an edematous or myxoid background (Fig. 20.21). Stromal cells often proliferate in a concentric fashion surrounding small- and medium-sized blood vessels; this feature can be highlighted by a CD34 immunostain.[333,343]

Mitotic figures are rare, but occasionally they may be found in deeper portions of the lesion. Atypical mitoses are never seen. Eosinophils are typically a prominent inflammatory component and may also be concentrated around blood vessels. In a subset of inflammatory fibroid polyps, only a paucity of eosinophils may be present, and this may be associated with a peculiar type of perivascular hyalinization.[344] Larger lesions may show collagen deposition and smooth muscle proliferation or even giant cell formation.

Immunohistochemically, stromal cells are positive for CD34, vimentin, and fascin.[331,334,343,345,346] In contrast with GISTs, stromal cells in inflammatory fibroid polyps are immunohistochemically negative for CD117 (KIT) and DOG1.[345,347,348] They are also negative for desmin, S100, and anaplastic lymphoma kinase, all of which helps differentiate them from other mesenchymal polyps, such as schwannomas and inflammatory myofibroblastic tumors.

Natural History and Treatment

Inflammatory fibroid polyps are best classified as a benign neoplasm. No reports have described malignant behavior. Nevertheless, recurrence is possible, and thus complete resection is the preferred method of treatment.

Inflammatory Myofibroblastic Tumors

Clinical Features and Pathogenesis

This mesenchymal neoplasm was originally described in the small-intestinal mesentery of preadolescent children.[349] Almost one-third occur in the stomach.[350-353] Tumors may arise in children or adults.[349-351,354] Patients may present with nonspecific symptoms, including fever, abdominal pain, growth retardation, and weight loss.[349,355,356] Elevated leukocyte count, hypergammaglobulinemia, and elevated erythrocyte sedimentation rate are also commonly reported.[357]

The cause of inflammatory myofibroblastic tumors is poorly understood. Approximately 50% of cases display a translocation involving chromosome 2p that rearranges the genes for tropomyosin 3 *(TPM3)* and anaplastic lymphoma kinase *(ALK)* to create a new fusion gene *(TPM3-ALK)*. Other tyrosine kinase receptor genes such as *ROS1* and *NTRK3* can be involved as well.[358-361] Gene rearrangements are more common in patients younger than 10 years of age.[361-363]

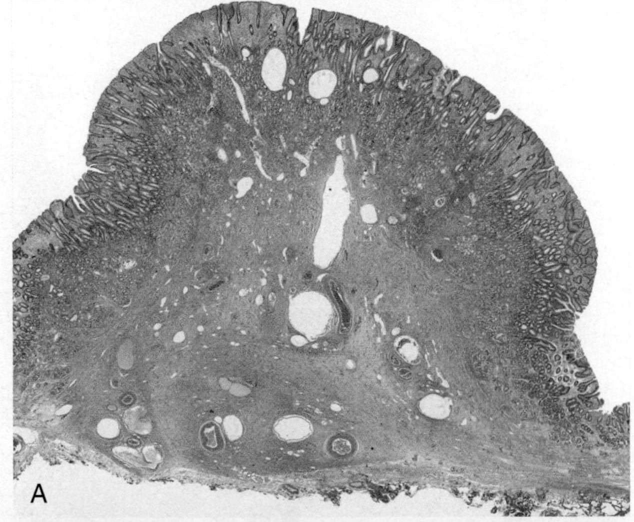

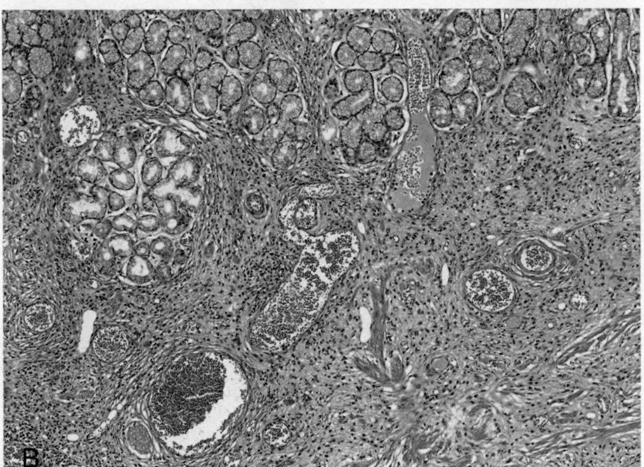

FIGURE 20.21 Gastric inflammatory fibroid polyp. A, At low power, a loose mesenchymal proliferation fills the submucosa and muscularis mucosae and penetrates into the basal portion of the mucosa. **B,** The cytologically bland, spindled mesenchymal cells are accompanied by lymphocytes and eosinophils. The mesenchymal proliferation tends to aggregate in a concentric fashion around blood vessels.

Pathological Features

Inflammatory myofibroblastic tumors may show a wide range (average 8 cm) in size. They typically appear as solid, white lesions with infiltrative borders and with foci of myxoid change. Histologically, they are composed of spindle-shaped cells with vesicular chromatin and small nucleoli, and they show a prominent infiltrate of mature plasma cells and lymphocytes (Fig. 20.22). The plasma cell component is polyclonal.[364] Some lesions are hypocellular, whereas others may show a myxoid stroma.

ALK is expressed in approximately 50% of cases.[365] The spindle cells are also immunohistochemically positive for smooth muscle actin, desmin, vimentin, and cytokeratin.[357,363,366] Tumors may also be focally positive for CD34 and factor XIIIa.[367]

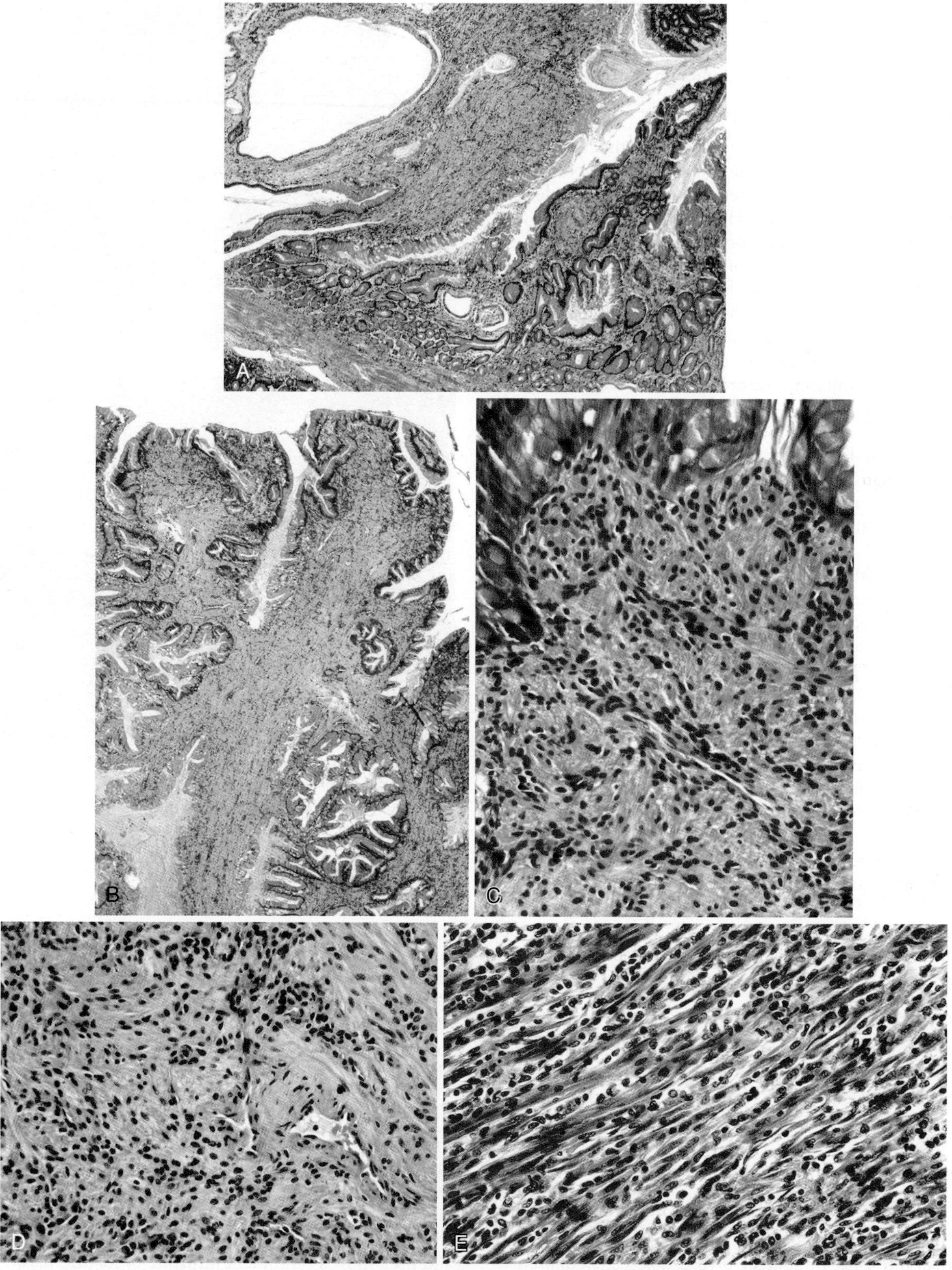

FIGURE 20.22 Inflammatory myofibroblastic tumor. A and **B,** At low power, a dense mesenchymal proliferation fills the submucosa and extends into the muscularis mucosae. **C,** The mesenchymal proliferation extends up to and interfaces with the surface epithelium. **D** and **E,** The mesenchymal cells of an inflammatory myofibroblastic tumor may demonstrate moderate cytological atypia and are embedded in a lymphocyte and plasma cell–rich stroma. This tumor should be differentiated from a gastrointestinal stromal tumor.

Natural History and Treatment

Although inflammatory myofibroblastic tumors are considered lesions of intermediate malignancy, they often recur locally.[352] No specific histological features have been associated with recurrence, but several studies suggest that aneuploidy may help identify particularly aggressive lesions.[352,363] An association between ALK expression and absence of distant metastases has been reported for extra-GI inflammatory myofibroblastic tumors. Anaplastic lymphoma kinase expression may be identified in tumors that recur locally.[354] The risk of local recurrence suggests that complete surgical excision and long-term follow-up are indicated for all patients with inflammatory myofibroblastic tumors.[354]

Gastrointestinal Stromal Tumors

GISTs are discussed in detail in Chapter 30. The stomach is the most common site. When these tumors occur in the stomach, they can manifest as a submucosal polyp (Fig. 20.23).

Vascular Tumors

Benign vascular tumors, such as hemangiomas and glomus tumors, may occur in the stomach and appear as an intraluminal nodule or polyp (Fig. 20.24). These lesions are histologically similar to their counterparts in other areas of the body, such as the skin and elsewhere in the GI tract, and they are uniformly benign. They may be confused with an epithelioid GIST. Kaposi's sarcoma can also involve the stomach and manifest as a cherry-red–colored polyp (Fig. 20.25). Vascular tumors are discussed in detail in Chapters 11 and 30.

LYMPHOID POLYPS

Lymphoid Hyperplasia

Lymphoid hyperplasia with germinal center formation, also known as *follicular hyperplasia* or *chronic follicular gastritis*, is usually a manifestation of chronic gastritis and particularly of *H. pylori* infection.[368,369] Reactive lymphoid nodules are most prevalent in the antrum, but they may occur in the gastric body as well. Nodules are often multiple and usually are smaller than 0.3 cm in the greatest diameter.[370] Eradication of *H. pylori* is associated with a decreased prevalence rate and density of lymphoid follicles.[371]

Lymphoma

Between 4% and 20% of all non-Hodgkin's lymphomas manifest initially in the GI tract.[1,6,7] Most cases involve the stomach. Many lesions initially present as either solitary or multiple polyps. Gastric lymphoma is discussed in more detail in Chapter 31.

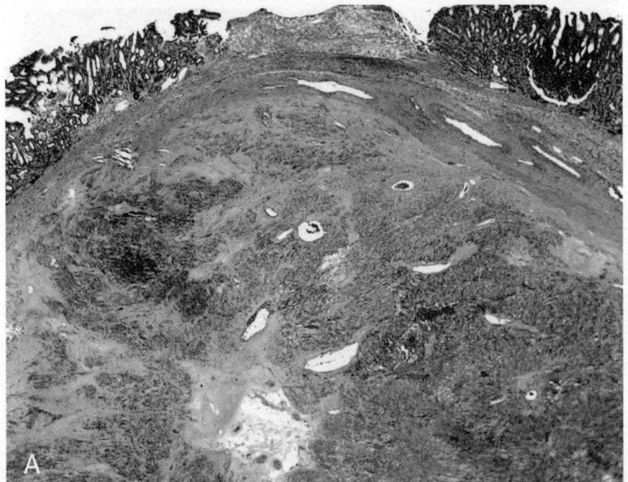

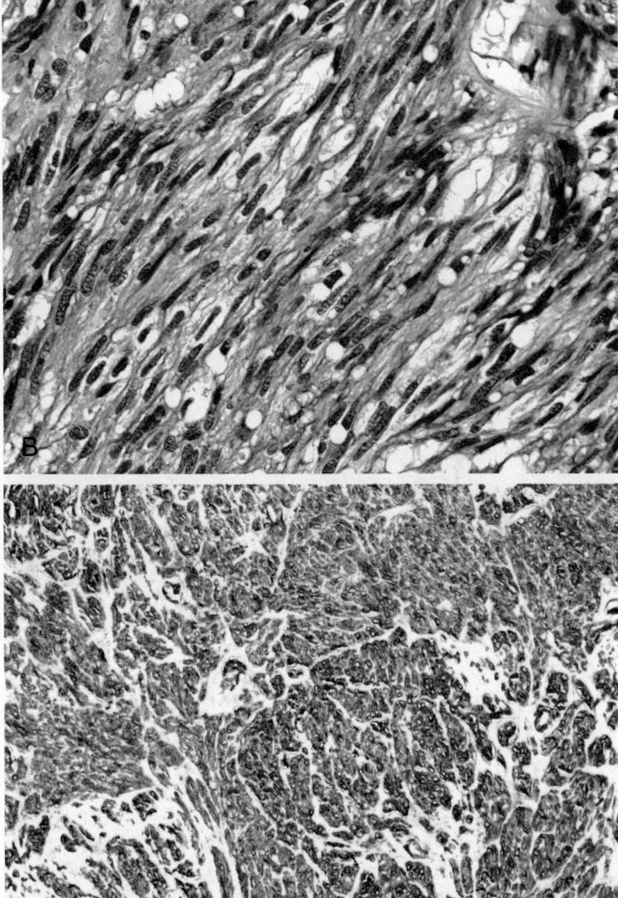

FIGURE 20.23 Gastrointestinal stromal tumor (GIST). A, In contrast with the inflammatory myofibroblastic tumor, GISTs tend to be centered within the muscularis propria. **B,** Characteristic histology of spindle cell GIST. **C,** CD117 immunostaining highlights the spindle cell proliferation.

MISCELLANEOUS RARE POLYPS AND POLYP-LIKE LESIONS

Xanthoma

Xanthomas are small, sessile, yellow-colored mucosal nodules composed of loose aggregates of lipid-laden macrophages in the lamina propria (Fig. 20.26). Xanthomas are most often found in the body and fundus[372,373] of the stomach. Xanthomas are typically multiple and smaller than 3 mm in diameter.

Xanthomas develop most commonly in association with chronic gastritis, especially after partial gastrectomy, and they are thought to form in response to tissue injury. The differential diagnosis of xanthoma includes benign muciphages,

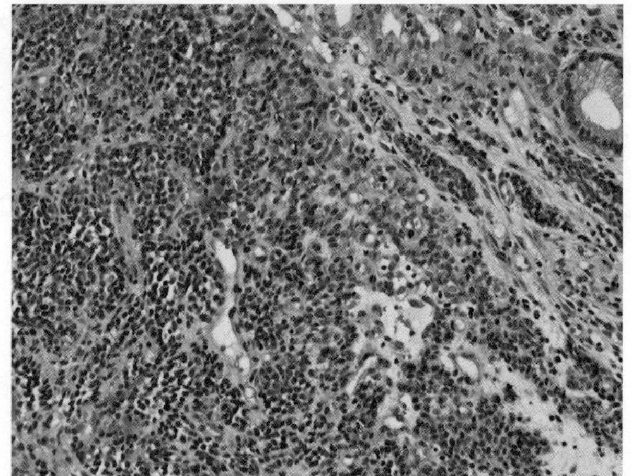

FIGURE 20.24 Glomus tumor. The glomus tumor is composed of nests of a monomorphic infiltrate of round cells with indistinct borders and scant amphophil-to-eosinophil cytoplasm surrounding thin-walled vascular structures.

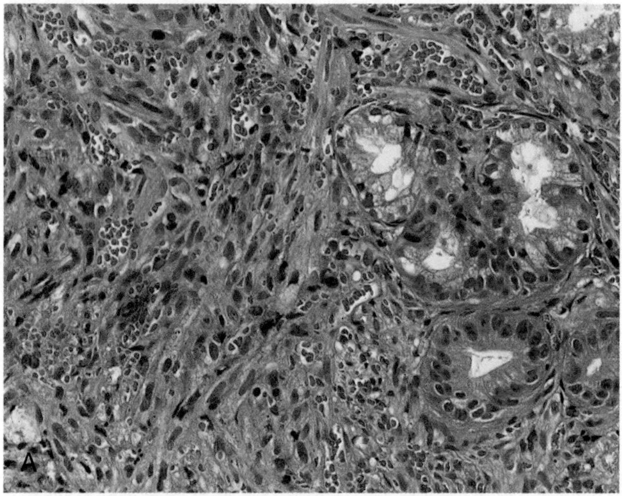

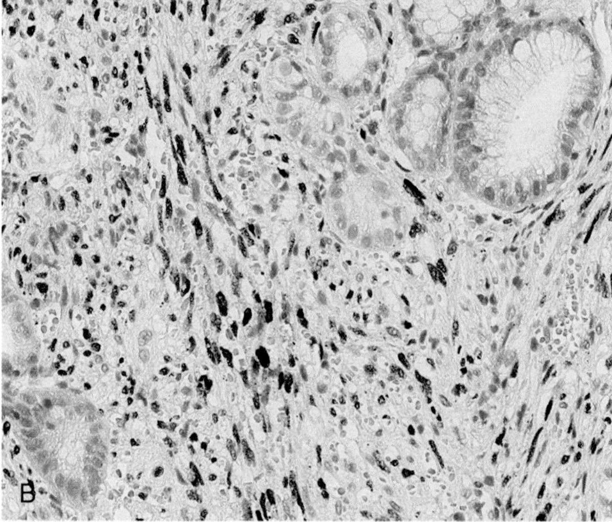

FIGURE 20.25 Kaposi sarcoma. A, Higher-power examination reveals a cytologically bland spindle cell infiltrate that forms slitlike vascular spaces. Hyaline globules can be a clue to the diagnosis. **B**, Positivity for human herpes virus 8 (HHV-8) immunohistochemistry confirms the diagnosis.

granular cell tumor, and signet ring cell carcinoma. Because xanthomas contain intracellular glycolipids that are lost during tissue processing, lesional macrophages are negative for periodic acid–Schiff (PAS) stain, whereas muciphages are strongly positive. The cytoplasmic granules of granular cell tumors stain positively with PAS, but they are also positive for the S100 protein. Signet ring cell carcinomas also contain cytoplasmic mucin, which can be demonstrated with PAS or mucicarmine stain. Signet ring cell carcinomas can be easily differentiated from xanthomas by their overt malignant nuclear cytology and cytokeratin immunoreactivity. *Mycobacterium avium–intracellulare* infection may also lead to the accumulation of foamy macrophages, which are packed with intracellular acid-fast bacilli.

Langerhans Cell Histiocytosis

Langerhans cell histiocytosis, previously known as *histiocytosis X*, is primarily a disease of young children. The guidelines of the Histiocyte Society subclassify this disorder according to the number of organs/organ systems affected, lung manifestation, and the involvement of one of three risk organs (liver, spleen, and bone marrow).[374] Depending on the location of the disease, the terms *eosinophilic granuloma, Hand-Schüller-Christian disease,* and *Letterer-Siwe disease* are also applicable. The single-system, solitary nodular form that may also be denoted as eosinophilic granuloma is occasionally found in the stomach.[375,376]

Histologically, the nodules are composed of tight clusters of coffee bean or kidney-shaped cells with finely granular cytoplasm (Fig. 20.27). Scattered eosinophils may be found in the nodule, but the mucosa is otherwise usually intact. The identity of Langerhans cells is confirmed by positive S100 protein and CD1a immunostaining and by electron microscopy, which shows characteristic tennis racket–shaped intracytoplasmic Birbeck granules. As an isolated gastric nodule, eosinophilic granuloma is typically benign. The granulomas often regress without therapy.

Pseudo–Signet Ring Cells

Rarely, gastric biopsies, particularly those from the fundus, may contain a proliferation of signet ring–like cells located in the deep foveolar and superficial glandular epithelium that produce a small nodule, bump, or polyp. Examination of pseudo–signet ring cells reveals a large, clear cytoplasmic vacuole with an eccentrically compressed nucleus located at the edge of the cell membrane (Fig. 20.28). The cells may occur in isolation or, more commonly, in rows and are not mitotically active. There may be a slight loss of polarity, but pseudo–signet ring cells are almost always confined to the intraepithelial space. Association of pseudo–signet ring cell change with proton pump inhibitor treatment has been reported and is generally regarded as a degenerative phenomenon of parietal and fundic neck cells.[377]

Amyloidosis

Amyloidosis is a heterogeneous group of systemic diseases classified according to the amyloid fibril–forming protein (see Chapter 6). Among the various amyloid types, the kappa amyloid light chain more frequently affects the upper GI tract,

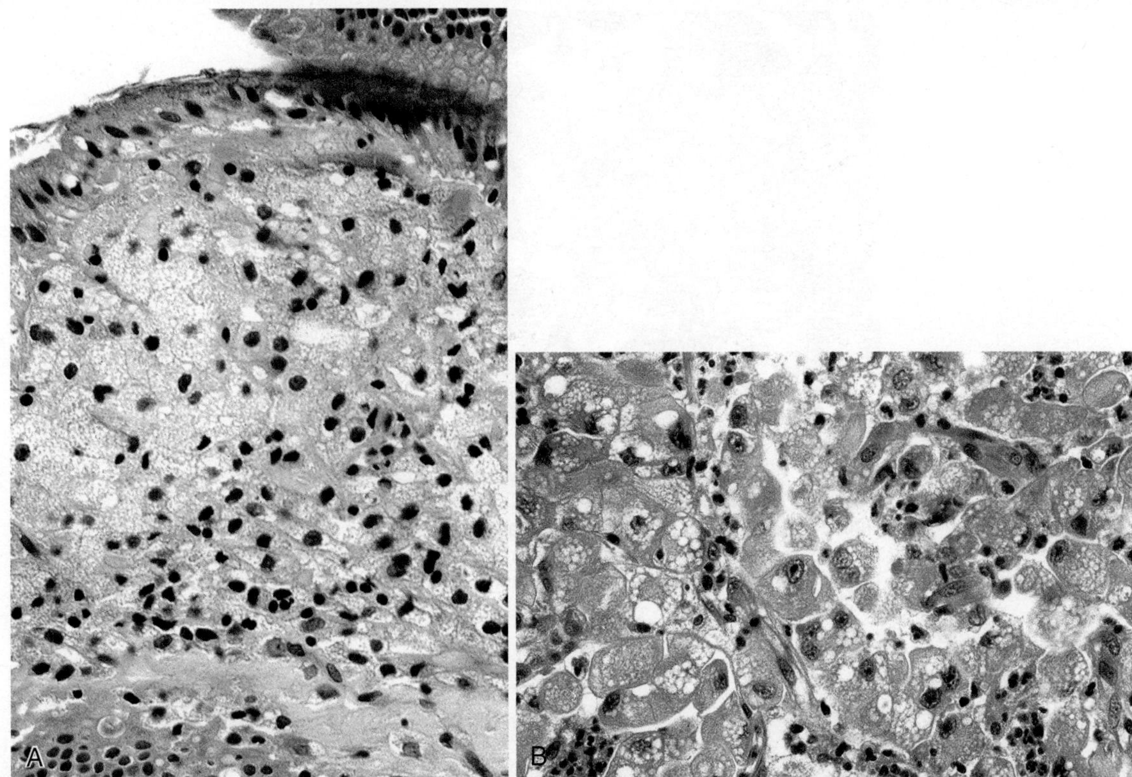

FIGURE 20.26 Gastric xanthoma. A, The mucosa is filled with foamy, lipid-laden macrophages that contain cytologically bland, round to oval nuclei without atypia. As is typical of xanthomas, the result of mucicarmine staining was negative. **B,** Although potentially misinterpreted as a xanthoma, signet ring cell carcinoma cells are pleomorphic with cytological atypia, including nuclear hyperchromasia and increased mitotic activity. Cytoplasmic mucin vacuoles displace eccentrically located nuclei. The result of mucicarmine staining was positive.

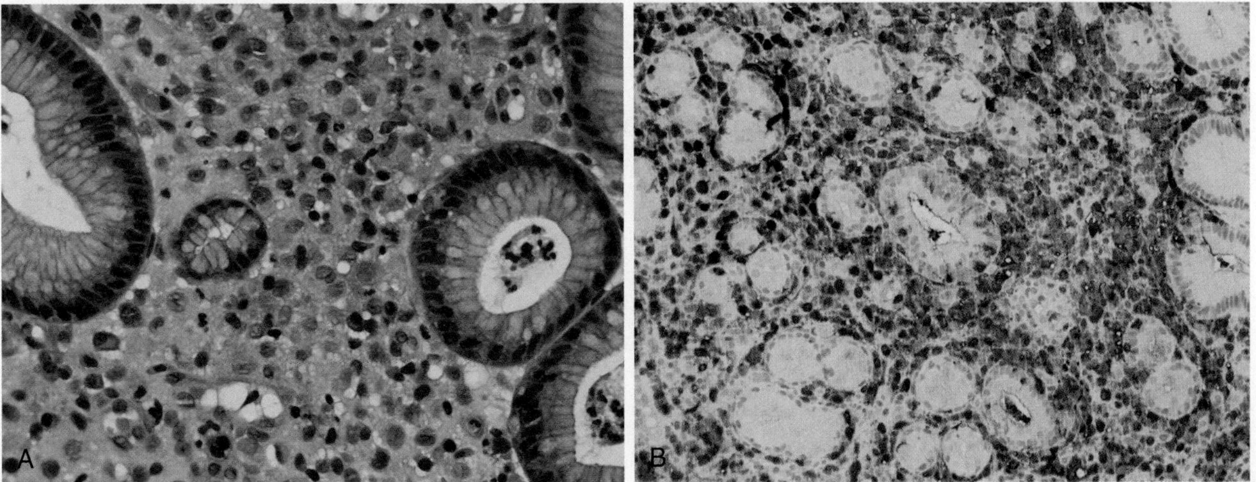

FIGURE 20.27 A, Example of Langerhans cell histiocytosis with expansion of the lamina propria by angulated histiocytic-appearing cells. **B,** The diagnosis is confirmed by CD1a immunohistochemistry.

including the stomach, whereas transthyretin-derived amyloidosis more commonly involves the lower segments of the GI tract. Lambda light chain and amyloid A amyloidoses show no such obvious predilection for specific segments.[378] When it involves the stomach, amyloidosis may cause ulceration or a submucosal nodule or mass. Large-interstitial amyloid deposits may be referred to as *amyloidomas*. Rarely, spontaneous and biopsy-induced submucosal (or mucosal) bleeding caused by rupture of rigid amyloid-laden vessels can also form a polypoid mass. Histologically, amyloid deposits in the stomach are most frequently concentrated in the wall of small- to medium-sized blood vessels.[379] Perineural and interstitial deposits may also develop in the submucosa (Fig. 20.29). The condition may be associated with dysmotility, although this complication occurs frequently in other areas of the GI tract. A diagnosis of amyloidosis can be confirmed by examination of Congo red–stained slides under polarized light.

The full reference list may be accessed online at Elsevier eBooks for Practicing Clinicians

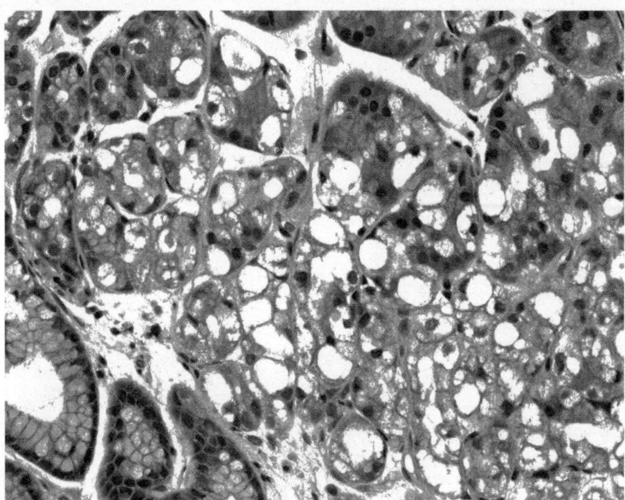

FIGURE 20.28 Pseudo–signet ring cell change. These mitotically inactive cells are predominantly located in the neck region of gastric glands, in isolation or in rows, with clear cytoplasmic vacuoles and eccentric, compressed nuclei.

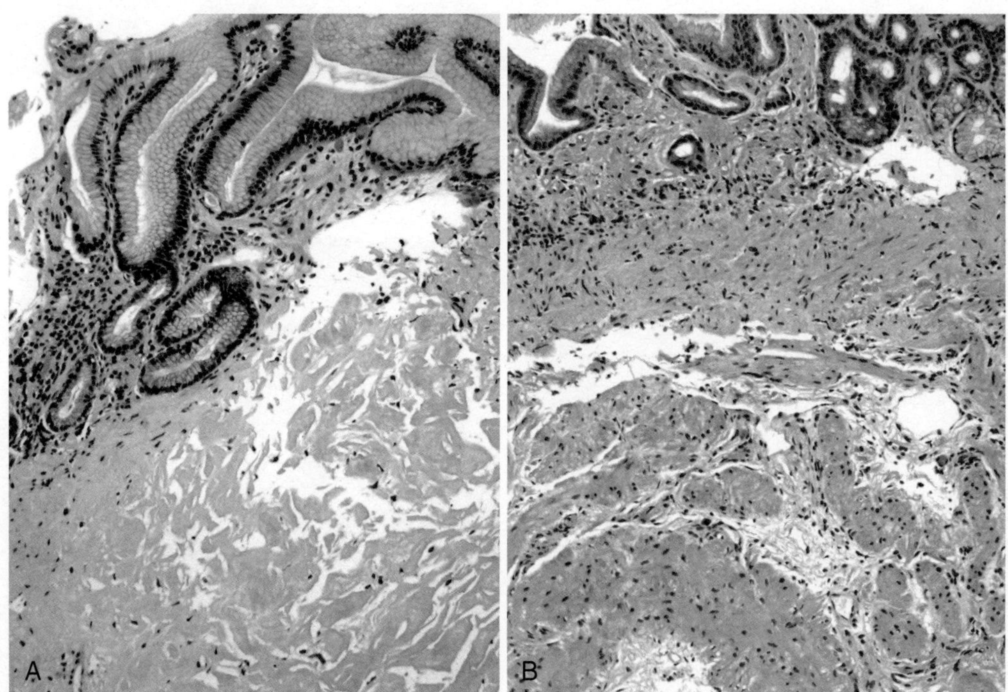

FIGURE 20.29 Amyloidosis. A, Amyloid deposits can form a nodule, or amyloidoma. **B,** In some cases, amyloid deposits within vessel walls can resemble smooth muscle bundles.

CHAPTER 21
Polyps of the Small Intestine

Michael W. Cruise, Erica C. Savage

Contents

INTRODUCTION

Upper gastrointestinal (GI) endoscopy is routinely performed as part of the evaluation of patients with GI symptoms. Newer techniques such as double-balloon enteroscopy and capsule endoscopy also allow for complete visualization of the small intestine. Gastroenterologists may identify and sample a variety of polyps, nodules, excrescences, and subtle abnormalities in the mucosa during the course of the procedure that, before the endoscopic era, would have gone largely unrecognized. Many of these lesions are clinically asymptomatic and occur in the duodenum, which is amenable to upper endoscopic examination. This chapter discusses the clinicopathological features and differential diagnoses of the most common or important lesions that may cause the clinical impression of an intestinal polyp (Box 21.1).

INFLAMMATORY LESIONS

As in other areas of the GI tract, inflammatory lesions of the small intestine may produce polypoid masses. Small polyps are often incidental, whereas larger polyps may be symptomatic as a result of hemorrhage or luminal obstruction.[1] Inflammatory pseudopolyps associated with Crohn's disease are the most common inflammatory polyps of the small intestine; they are commonly encountered in the terminal ileum, where they demonstrate varying degrees of villous architectural distortion, pyloric gland metaplasia, and active inflammation (Fig. 21.1). They can be quite numerous and can even carpet the small bowel with finger-like projections.[1]

Inflammatory-type polyps of the small intestine may arise secondarily from other types of disease. Cytomegalovirus infection can rarely manifest as isolated GI inflammatory polyps, often in immunocompromised hosts (Fig. 21.2).[2,3] Endometriosis of the bowel wall and submucosa may induce inflammatory changes including inflammatory-type polyps. Changes mimicking Crohn's disease have also been reported.[7,8] Endometriosis can also involve the mucosa, resembling dysplasia and even carcinoma (Fig. 21.3). Well-differentiated neuroendocrine tumors (NETs) may also induce an inflammatory reaction in the mucosa away from the main tumor, likely related to mucosal prolapse. These lesions contain numerous ectatic capillaries with admixed smooth muscle bundles and fibrosis.[9]

Xanthomas can also occur in the duodenum, although they are rarer than gastric xanthomas.[4] They are characterized by collections of pale and foamy histiocytes in the lamina propria. Histiocytic differentiation can be documented by immunohistochemical staining with CD163, CD68, or both.

BOX 21.1 Polypoid Lesions of the Small Intestine

Hyperplasias and heterotopias
- Brunner gland hyperplasia/hamartoma
- Gastric heterotopia
- Pancreatic heterotopia

Inflammatory lesions
- Crohn's disease–associated inflammatory "pseudopolyp"
- Inflammatory polyp, CMV associated
- Inflammatory polyp, not otherwise specified
- Xanthoma
- Inflammatory fibroid polyp
- Peutz-Jeghers polyp
- Juvenile polyp (juvenile polyposis syndrome and *PTEN* hamartoma tumor syndrome)
- Polyp of Cronkhite-Canada syndrome

Benign epithelial neoplasms
- Adenoma
- Pyloric gland adenoma
- Hyperplastic polyp

Neuroendocrine neoplasms
- Well-differentiated neuroendocrine neoplasm
- Gangliocytic paraganglioma
- Neuroendocrine carcinoma

Mesenchymal tumors
- Gastrointestinal stromal tumor
- Leiomyoma
- Lipoma
- Hemangioma
- Neurofibroma
- Granular cell tumor
- Ganglioneuroma
- Schwannoma
- Kaposi sarcoma
- Lymphangiectasia

Lymphoid lesions
- Nodular lymphoid hyperplasia
- Diffuse large B-cell lymphoma
- Mantle cell lymphoma (lymphomatous polyposis)
- Low-grade B-cell lymphoma (follicular, MALT-type, Mediterranean fever)
- T-cell lymphoma (gluten sensitivity enteropathy–associated lymphoma)

Metastases

CMV, *Cytomegalovirus;* MALT, *mucosa-associated lymphoid tissue;* PTEN, *phosphatase and tensin homolog.*

Inflammatory fibroid polyps (described in Chapter 30) are also less common in the small bowel compared with the stomach (Fig. 21.4).[5] Similar to their gastric counterparts, they often demonstrate mutations in the *PDGFRA* gene.[6]

HYPERPLASIA AND HETEROTOPIA

Brunner Gland Hyperplasia/Hamartoma

Clinical and Endoscopic Features

Brunner glands are lobular collections of tubular glands within the duodenum, predominantly located in the duodenal submucosa. In the first part of the duodenum, however, Brunner glands commonly transgress the muscularis mucosae and extend into the lamina propria.[10] Brunner glands within the lamina propria are less frequently observed in the middle to distal duodenum.

Occasionally, Brunner glands proliferate, creating small polypoid excrescences or imparting a nodular appearance to the mucosal surface (Fig. 21.5). These Brunner gland proliferative lesions are most commonly encountered in the duodenal bulb, usually as an incidental finding at endoscopy performed for other indications. However, they may be seen as one of a constellation of findings, including villous shortening and gastric foveolar mucous cell metaplasia of the villous epithelium, that are indicative of peptic injury of the duodenum (peptic duodenitis). Proliferative Brunner gland lesions have also been associated with end-stage renal disease and uremia.[11,12]

The nomenclature of Brunner gland proliferative lesions is not well established, and a number of diagnostic terms, including *Brunner gland hyperplasia, Brunner gland adenoma,* and *Brunner gland hamartoma,* have been used. Histologically, it is difficult to distinguish hyperplasia from hamartomas and adenomas, and the distinction between these diagnoses is arbitrary. No well-documented cases of either true glandular dysplasia or carcinoma arising in proliferative Brunner glands have been reported. Careful review of the limited literature reports of Brunner gland adenocarcinoma and dysplasia reveals that the dysplastic glandular epithelium involves the surface epithelium with likely secondary involvement of the underlying hyperplastic Brunner glands.[13-17] In other cases, the adenocarcinomas appear to arise from pyloric gland adenomas and not from hyperplastic Brunner glands.[16,17] Therefore the term *Brunner gland adenoma* is potentially misleading, and we prefer to use the term *Brunner gland hyperplasia* to limit confusion among our clinicians and to highlight the nonneoplastic nature of the entity.

Some authors distinguish between *Brunner gland hyperplasia* and *Brunner gland hamartoma* based on the size of the lesion. However, the size cutoff between these two entities is arbitrary and not well established in the literature.[18] The distinction is of no clinical significance, and a diagnosis of Brunner gland hyperplasia/hamartoma is usually sufficient in large polypoid lesions.

Pathological Features

Brunner glands are composed of neutral, mucin-secreting, cuboidal to columnar cells with basally located nuclei arranged in lobules containing thin, fibrous septa. Brunner glands are histologically indistinguishable from pyloric glands of the distal gastric mucosa. Indeed, biopsies of the gastroduodenal junction may demonstrate a gradual transition of these epithelial types. The predominantly submucosal location of Brunner glands helps identify the biopsy as duodenal in origin.

The diagnostic criteria for Brunner gland hyperplasia are subjective because Brunner glands may be normally seen in the lamina propria of the duodenum, particularly within the duodenal bulb. In addition, proliferation of Brunner glands is commonly observed in peptic-type duodenal injury. We reserve the term *Brunner gland hyperplasia* for those endoscopically visible duodenal nodules that are found to contain lobules of Brunner glands within the mucosa in at least 50% of the length of a biopsy specimen (Fig. 21.6A). Brunner gland hyperplasia may manifest as solitary or multiple nodules that are typically small (<1 cm) and characterized by lobules of glands that are increased in both size and number.

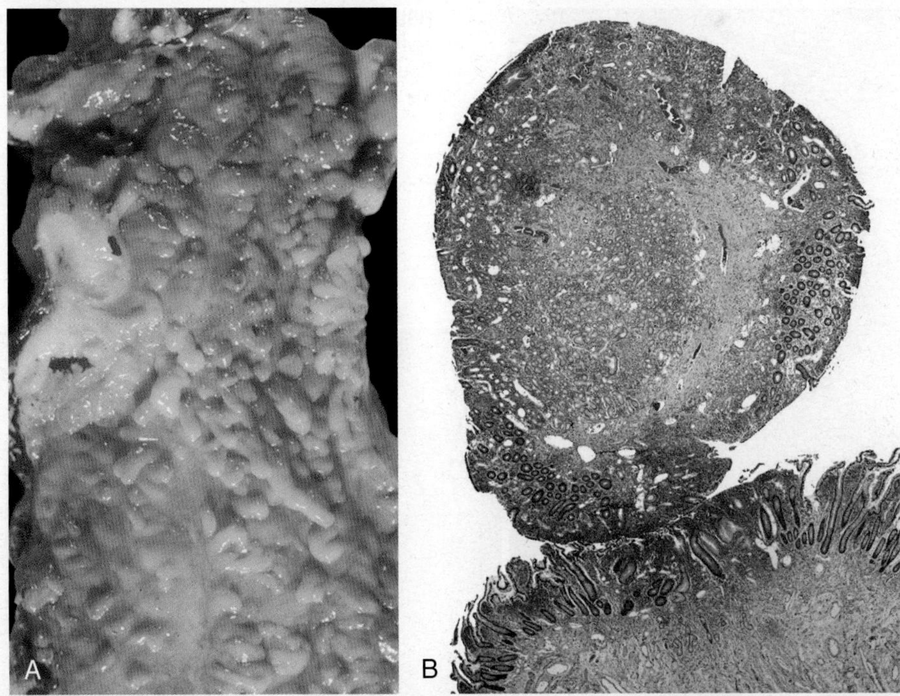

FIGURE 21.1 Crohn's disease–associated "pseudopolyps" of the ileum. A, Much of the ileal mucosa is flattened and atrophic, and residual plaquelike and polypoid areas of mucosa are present. **B,** A polypoid excrescence of mucosa is preserved in an area of the ileum affected by active ileitis.

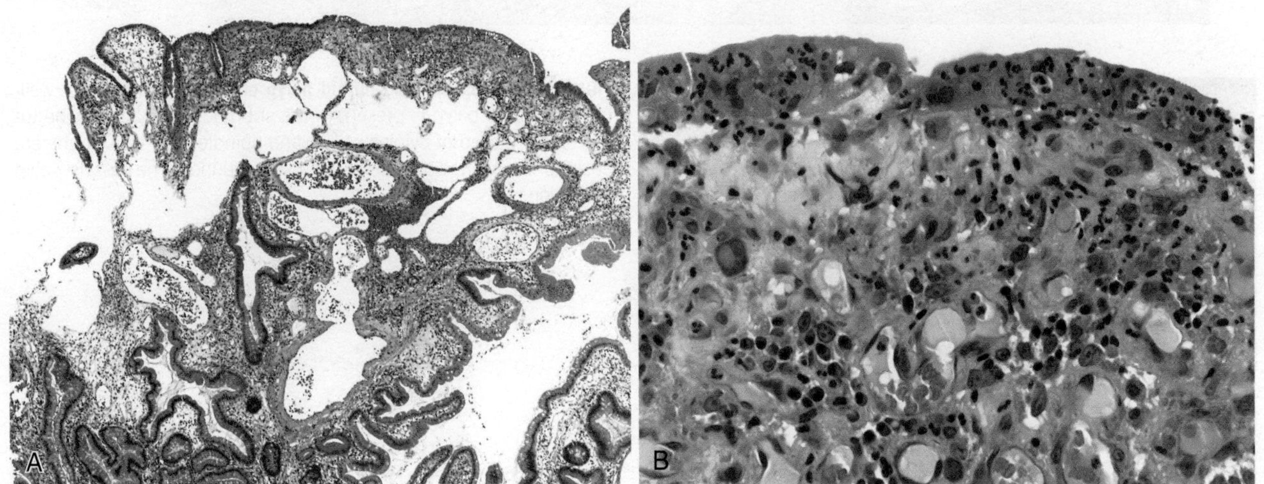

FIGURE 21.2 Cytomegalovirus-associated inflammatory polyp. A, This isolated inflammatory polyp has an expanded and edematous lamina propria with vascular ectasia. **B,** Numerous cytomegaloviral inclusions are identified.

The lobules extend into the mucosa and are separated by delicate fibrous septa. Cystic dilation of Brunner glands may occur, and rare cases of Brunner gland cysts have been reported.[19,20] The cells are cytologically bland with abundant neutral mucin and small, basally located nuclei with minimal to absent mitotic activity.

Large polyps (>2 cm) composed of Brunner glands may produce symptoms of obstruction, intussusception, melena, and anemia requiring endoscopic resection. Such polyps typically display more abundant fibromuscular stroma, likely the result of mucosal prolapse-type changes. Those who advocate for distinction between Brunner gland hyperplasia and hamartoma note that hamartomas consist of Brunner glands admixed with large ducts and bands of smooth muscle, while hyperplastic lesions are composed only of Brunner glands.[21] For such large polyps, however, the diagnosis of *Brunner gland hyperplasia/hamartoma* may be appropriate, as it recognizes the relatively arbitrary distinction between these two diagnoses.

In mucosal biopsy specimens, Brunner glands are commonly crushed, imparting a spindle cell appearance to the epithelial cells (Fig. 21.6B). Crushed Brunner glands may be mistaken for histiocytic collections, raising concern for Whipple disease, particularly given their intense positive reaction on periodic acid–Schiff (PAS) staining. The spindled appearance of crushed Brunner glands may also raise concern for a mesenchymal lesion. Careful histological evaluation with comparison of adjacent partially crushed lobular collections of Brunner glands will allow for identification of this distortion artifact.

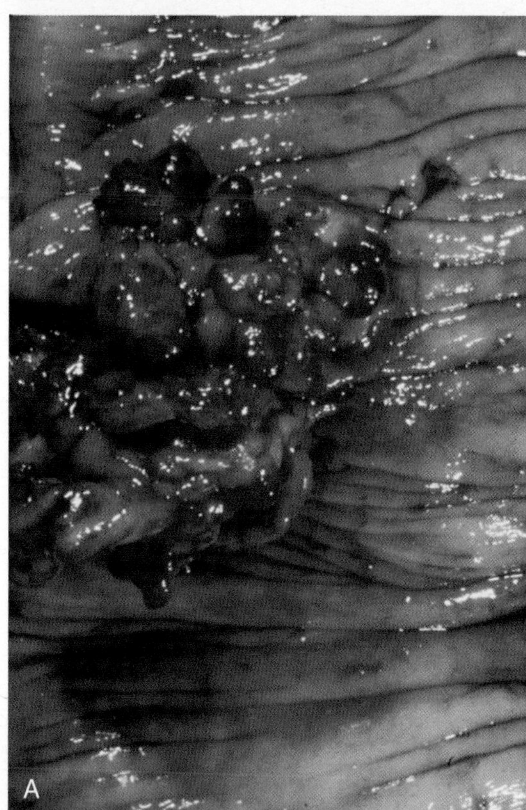

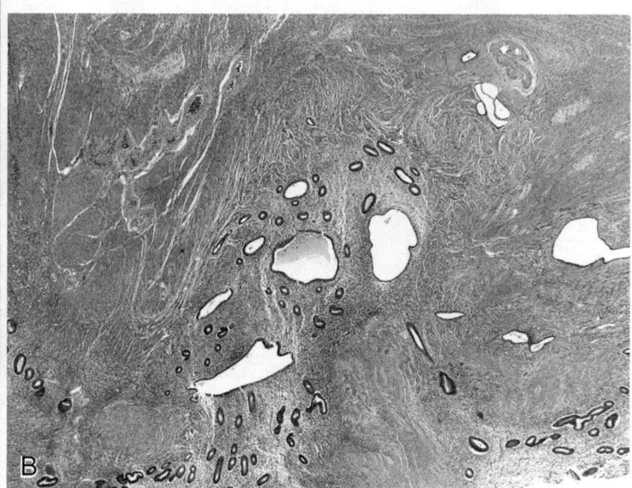

FIGURE 21.3 Endometriosis of the small intestine. A, Multiple erythematous polypoid lesions in an area of endometriosis. **B,** Rounded aggregates of endometrial glands and stroma infiltrate the muscularis propria.

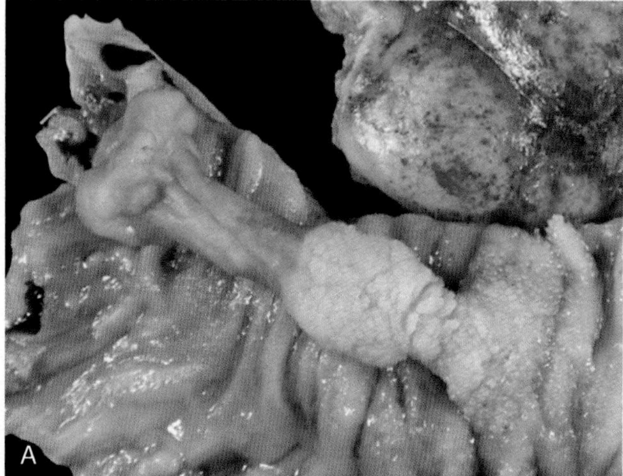

FIGURE 21.4 Inflammatory fibroid polyp of the duodenum. A, A well-circumscribed polyp is present in the submucosa. **B** and **C,** The tumor is composed of cytologically bland spindle cells with prominent eosinophils. A whorling pattern is present around some vessels within the lesion.

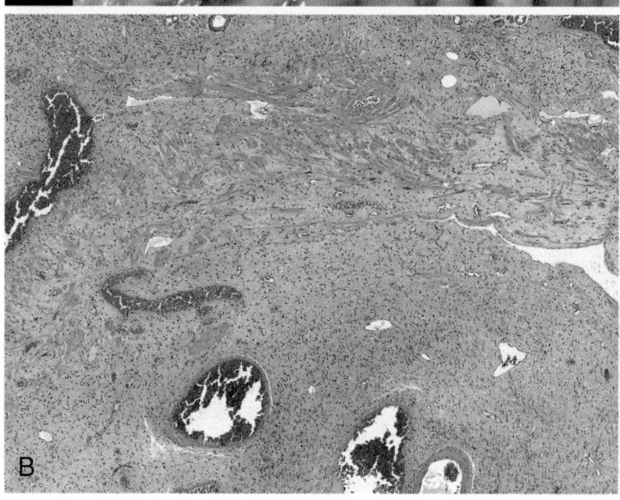

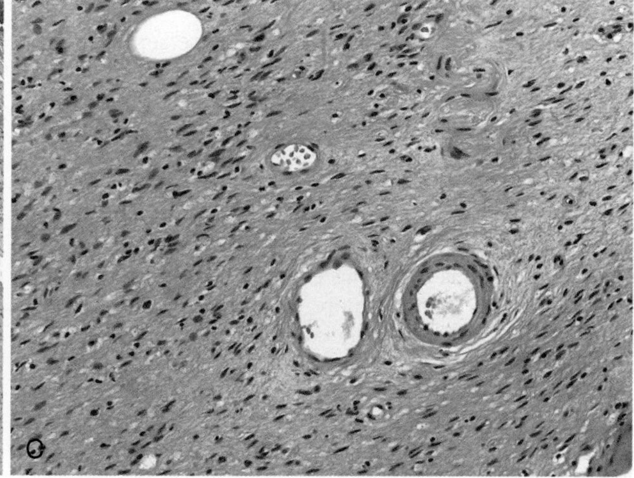

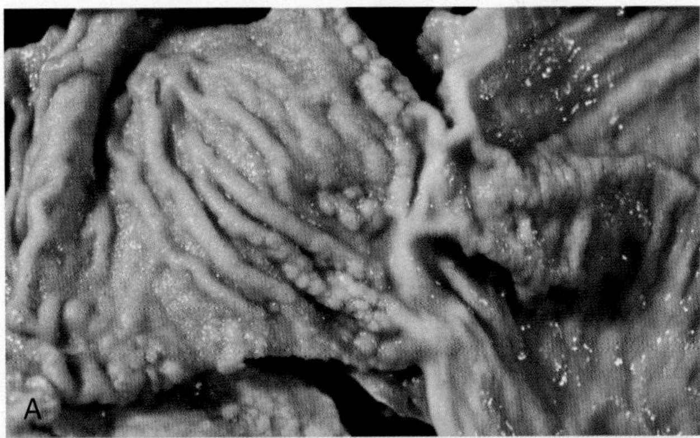

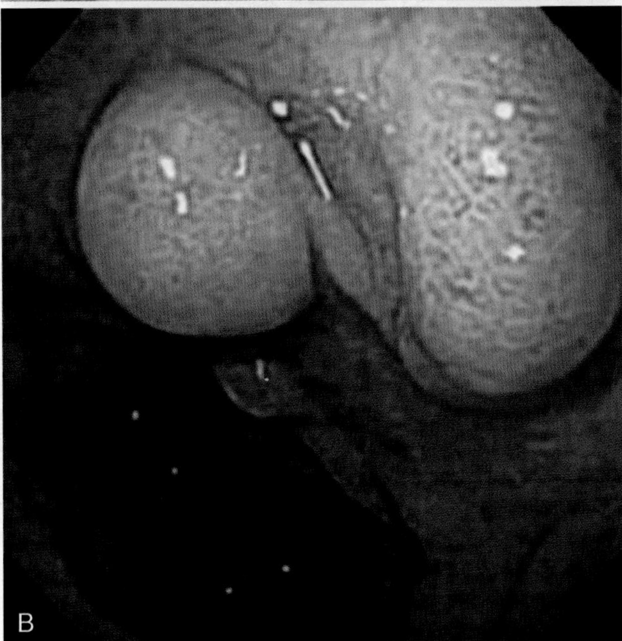

FIGURE 21.5 Brunner gland hyperplasia. Numerous polypoid excrescences are present within the duodenal bulb, imparting a nodular quality to the mucosal surface in a resection specimen **(A),** which may be endoscopically apparent **(B).**

Differential Diagnosis

Histological features of peptic-type injury of the duodenum include any of the following: active inflammation within the lamina propria or epithelium, Brunner gland hyperplasia (Fig. 21.7A), gastric foveolar metaplasia of the surface epithelium (Fig. 21.7B), hemorrhage, and edema. Nodular duodenitis is frequently observed in patients with a history of peptic ulcer disease.[22] In the setting of histological findings indicative of peptic-type duodenal injury, the presence of Brunner gland hyperplasia should be attributed to peptic duodenitis.

Pyloric gland adenoma is a relatively recently described adenoma subtype that can occur in the duodenum and not infrequently evolves into invasive adenocarcinoma. The distinction between *pyloric gland adenoma* and *Brunner gland hyperplasia/hamartoma* is difficult (see later discussion). Both express the mucin core peptide MUC6; however, pyloric gland adenomas usually also demonstrate labeling with MUC5AC, which is not typical of Brunner glands.[23]

Gastric Heterotopia

Clinical and Endoscopic Features

Gastric heterotopias in the duodenum are most commonly identified in the bulb and are usually incidental, small (<1.0 cm) nodules that may be multiple.[24] Patients are typically asymptomatic, but larger polyps may manifest as masses and cause obstruction or intussusception.[25,26] Peptic ulceration resulting from heterotopic oxyntic glands in the proximal duodenum is rare because the acid secretions are quickly diluted by the alkaline duodenal contents derived from the pancreatobiliary system. However, rare cases of massive GI bleeding have been reported, particularly in patients with extensive heterotopias.[25,27] Gastric heterotopia is also associated with concurrent fundic gland polyps of the stomach, suggesting that the increased use of proton pump inhibitors (PPIs) in the general population may enhance its endoscopic detection.[28]

Pathological Features

Biopsies of gastric heterotopias display well-organized oxyntic glands composed of chief and parietal cells (Fig. 21.8A). The overlying surface often exhibits gastric foveolar-type mucinous epithelium with adjacent normal duodenal intestinal villi. Gastric heterotopia in the duodenum may harbor the same pathological processes that affect the stomach, including *Helicobacter pylori* infection (Fig. 21.8B).[28] Large gastric heterotopias may exhibit secondary mucosal prolapse-type changes including prominence of the muscularis mucosae, submucosal fibrosis, cystic dilation of the oxyntic and mucinous glands, and surface epithelial hyperplasia.[29]

Differential Diagnosis

Gastric heterotopia differs from gastric foveolar metaplasia, which is hypothesized to be a response to inflammation caused by peptic injury associated with gastric *H. pylori* infection[30] (Table 21.1). Histologically, peptic-type injury of the duodenum typically results in active inflammation within the lamina propria or epithelium and erosion or ulceration. The metaplastic gastric foveolar epithelium is not associated with the oxyntic glands characteristic of gastric heterotopia.

Pancreatic Heterotopia

Clinical and Endoscopic Features

Pancreatic heterotopia represents the presence of pancreatic tissue outside the normal pancreas without any anatomic or vascular connection to the pancreas. It is synonymous with the terms *pancreatic rest* and *ectopic pancreas*. Pancreatic heterotopia of the small intestine is most commonly located in the proximal duodenum and can be seen either confined to the mucosa or within the muscularis propria. Pancreatic tissue may be normally identified in the region of the minor papilla and does not necessarily qualify as heterotopia.[31] In most cases, pancreatic heterotopia is asymptomatic and only incidentally detected. Mural heterotopias develop most commonly in the periampullary region and are more likely to be symptomatic as a result duodenal obstruction, intussusception, and stricture or stenosis of the ampulla.[32-34]

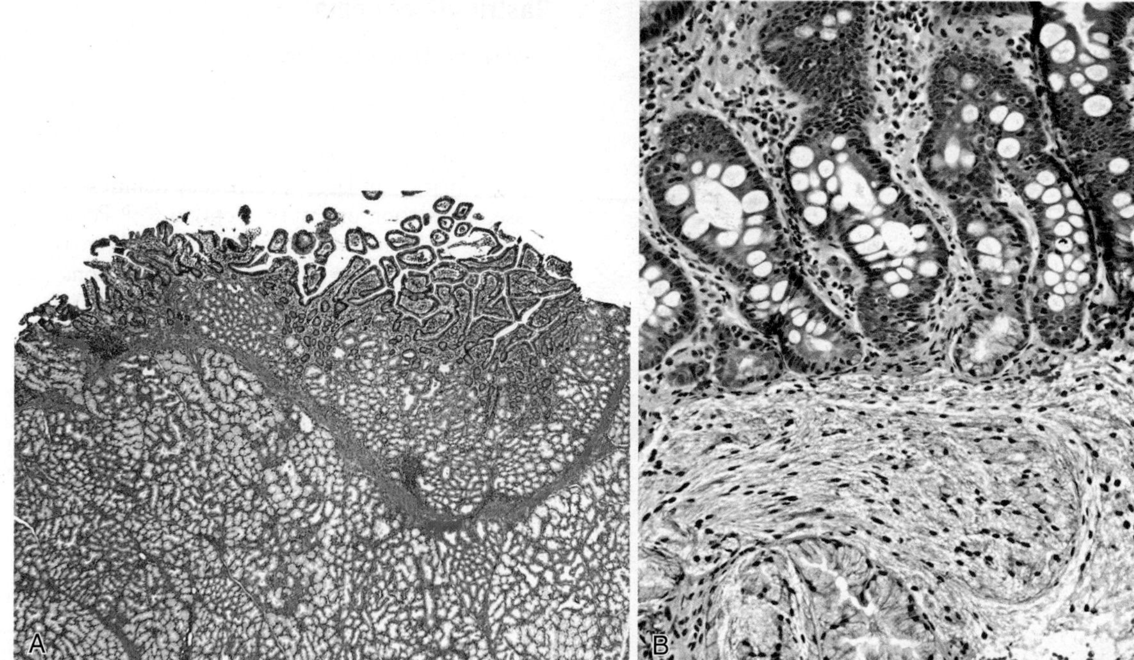

FIGURE 21.6 Brunner gland hyperplasia. A, At low power, lobules of Brunner glands expand the submucosa, extending into and filling the lamina propria. The hyperplastic Brunner glands are separated by delicate fibrous septa. **B,** Brunner glands may become artifactually distorted and contain spindled, compressed epithelial cells.

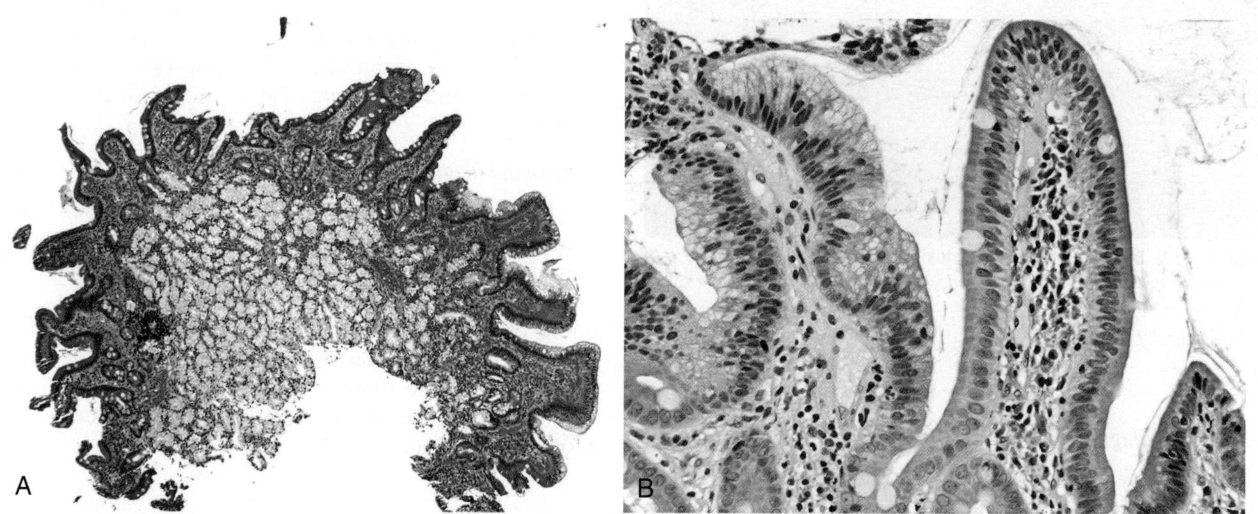

FIGURE 21.7 Nodular peptic-type duodenitis. A, Hyperplastic Brunner glands fill the lamina propria, imparting a nodular appearance to the mucosa. Partial villous shortening and increased lamina propria chronic inflammation are also seen, indicative of duodenitis. **B,** Foveolar-type metaplasia is present on the villous surface of the duodenum. In contrast with the absorptive and goblet cells, the metaplastic cells contain small apical vacuoles, similar to gastric foveolar cells.

Symptomatic mural pancreatic heterotopias often mimic a neoplastic process, leading to surgical resection,[32] and an endoscopic biopsy diagnosis is not possible given the location of the lesion.

Pathological Features

Pancreatic heterotopia may be composed of pancreatic acini, ducts, or islets, either alone or in combination (Fig. 21.9). Most frequently, pancreatic ducts are identified, with a variable number of acinar cells and islets and no relationship between symptoms and the cell type present.[35] Mural lesions are often histologically indistinguishable from normal pancreas. Most mucosal-based lesions are unassociated with inflammation, being present in otherwise normal mucosa of the duodenum. Rarely, ductal adenocarcinoma, mucinous neoplasms, and NETs have been reported to develop in pancreatic heterotopia.[35-39]

Differential Diagnosis

A periampullary duodenal wall cyst (groove pancreatitis) is not often confused with mural pancreatic heterotopias. Although both may contain pancreatic ducts, acini, and islets, a periampullary duodenal wall cyst has characteristic clinicopathological features. Most patients are young to

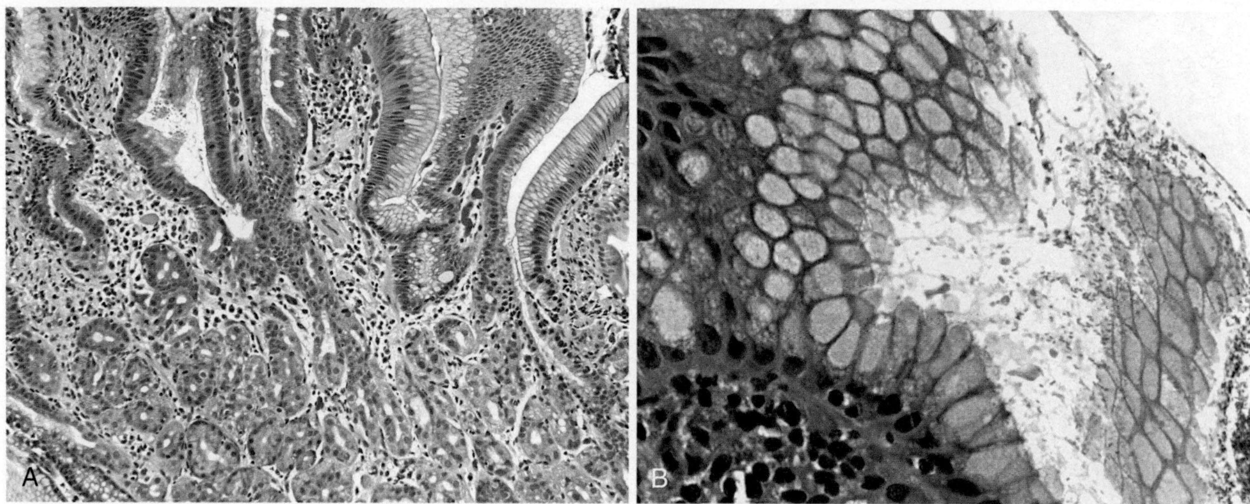

FIGURE 21.8 Gastric heterotopia. A, The duodenal mucosa contains tightly packed aggregates of gastric glands composed of chief and parietal cells. The villous surface of the duodenum also demonstrates gastric foveolar-type metaplasia. **B,** *Helicobacter pylori* organisms can be present with gastric heterotopia, particularly in cases in which gastric foveolar-type cells replace the normal duodenal surface epithelium.

TABLE 21.1 Gastric Heterotopia vs. Gastric Metaplasia

	Gastric Heterotopia	Gastric Metaplasia
Clinical presentation	Usually incidental	Epigastric pain
Endoscopic features	Nodular mucosa	Duodenitis
Histological features	Oxyntic mucosa Normal duodenal mucosa	Gastric foveolar (mucous) cells Villous blunting ± active inflammation Prominent Brunner glands
Clinical implications	None	Peptic injury

middle-aged men who report alcohol use and typically present with pain and vomiting caused by duodenal stenosis.[40-42] Jaundice may also be seen late in the disease course as a result of compression of the common bile duct.[40] The lesion typically involves the area of the minor papilla where pancreatic tissue may normally be identified. Fibrosis and inflammation occur in the "groove" between the superior aspect of the pancreatic head, the common bile duct, and the duodenum. In addition to groove pancreatitis, alternative names include *cystic dystrophy of the duodenal wall* and *paraduodenal pancreatitis*.[31] Most cases are characterized by multiple or solitary cysts varying in size from 1 to 10 cm within the duodenal wall and pancreas (Fig. 21.10). "Solid" types have also been described and are characterized by fibrotic thickening of the duodenal wall with small (<1 cm) cysts.[41] A reactive myofibroblastic spindle cell proliferation is usually present in the duodenal wall, whereas the fibrosis in the groove area is more paucicellular and hyalinized.[43] Cystically dilated ducts partially lined by ductal epithelium and containing inspissated eosinophilic material are characteristic (Fig. 21.11). Squamous metaplasia, granulation tissue, calcium deposition, and giant cell reaction are also frequently encountered.[41,43] It has been speculated that this disorder is a localized form of alcohol-induced pancreatitis occurring in pancreatic tissue present in the area of the minor papilla.[31]

HAMARTOMATOUS POLYPS

By definition, hamartomatous polyps are a haphazard arrangement of normal stromal and epithelial elements. Hamartomatous polyps of the small bowel occur mainly in the setting of polyposis syndromes including Peutz-Jeghers syndrome (PJS), juvenile polyposis syndrome (JPS), and *PTEN* hamartoma tumor syndrome. The latter two syndromes have similar-appearing hamartomatous polyps. Correct classification of these polyps is critical to management because many of these syndromes carry unique risks of GI and extra-GI malignancy (Table 21.2). Rarely, sporadic hamartomatous polyps resembling their syndromic counterparts occur.[44] Other sporadic hamartomatous lesions have been described, including those made predominantly of mesenchymal elements such as adipose tissue, vessels, and nerves. There are numerous reports of neuromuscular and vascular hamartomas in the literature; however, these lesions are not hamartomas but are likely related to injury from nonsteroidal anti-inflammatory drugs (diaphragm disease) (see Chapters 12 and 16).[45,46]

Peutz-Jeghers Polyps

Clinical and Endoscopic Features

PJS is an autosomal dominant hamartomatous polyposis syndrome with a prevalence of 1 in 50,000 to 200,000 births.[47-49] The majority of patients have a positive family history; however, 25% of cases are de novo. A diagnosis of PJS should be considered in patients with any of the following: (1) perioral or buccal mucocutaneous melanin pigmentation, (2) two or more histologically confirmed Peutz-Jeghers polyps, and (3) a family history of PJS.[49] More than 90% of patients with PJS develop small intestinal polyps, most commonly in the jejunum, followed by the ileum and the duodenum. PJS patients are often diagnosed at an early age (approximately 20 years) because these polyps often cause abdominal pain, obstruction resulting from intussusception, and bleeding.[47,50] Surgical intervention often occurs in these

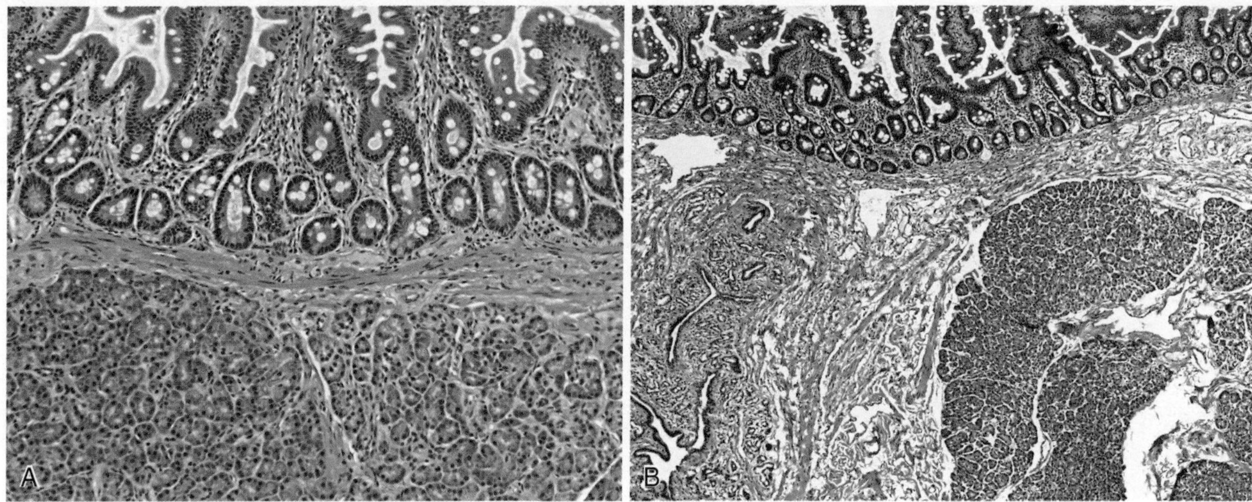

FIGURE 21.9 Pancreatic heterotopia. A, The duodenal submucosa contains rounded aggregates of pancreatic acini. **B,** Lobules of pancreatic acini are associated with ducts and tubules lined by pancreatic ductal epithelium, similar to the parenchyma of the normal pancreas.

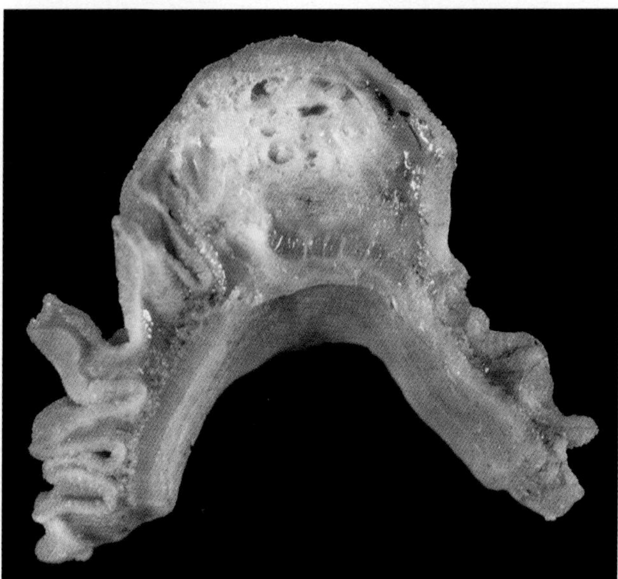

FIGURE 21.10 Paraduodenal pancreatitis (cystic dystrophy of heterotopic pancreas). The cut surface is heterogeneous, with cystic and solid areas that correspond to cysts lined by biliary-type epithelium enmeshed within a stroma rich in smooth muscle.

settings. Indeed, patients are at risk for short gut syndrome resulting from the numerous GI surgeries undertaken to resect these polyps.[51]

Patients with PJS have a significantly increased risk of intestinal adenocarcinoma, particularly of the colon (cumulative risk of 39%) but also of the small bowel (13% cumulative risk).[47,49,52-61] For this reason, patients are enrolled in an endoscopic screening protocol at a very young age.[47] Affected individuals are also at increased risk for other tumors, including breast (24% to 54% cumulative risk), pancreas (11% to 36% cumulative risk), stomach (29% cumulative risk), cervix (10% to 23% cumulative risk for adenoma malignum), ovary (21% cumulative risk for sex cord/stromal tumor with annular tubules and mucinous tumors), lung (7% to 17% cumulative risk), uterus (9% cumulative risk), and testis (9% cumulative risk for large-cell calcifying Sertoli cell tumor).[49,52,59,60,62-64] The cumulative lifetime risk for any cancer approaches 90%.

Given the increased risk of cancer in these patients, an initial colonoscopy, upper GI endoscopy, and video capsule endoscopy is recommended at 8 years of age. If polyps are identified, surveillance colonoscopy, upper GI endoscopy, and video capsule endoscopy is recommended every 3 years. For those without polyps on this initial screen, repeat colonoscopy, upper GI endoscopy, and video capsule endoscopy is recommended at 18 years of age with continued surveillance every 3 years.[49]

Peutz-Jeghers polyps have an irregular, multilobulated endoscopic appearance and lack the velvety texture typical of adenomas (Fig. 21.12). Because they contain prominent smooth muscle, they are tightly anchored to the bowel. Unlike juvenile polyps, they rarely autoamputate.

In 1998, the gene responsible for the majority of sporadic and inherited cases of PJS was identified as *STK11* (also known as *LKB1*), a serine/threonine kinase located on chromosome 19p13.3.[49,50,65-68] *STK11* is a tumor suppressor gene involved in a wide spectrum of cellular functions, including cellular proliferation, cell polarity, and apoptosis.[49,69-71] *STK11* has been shown to interact with other tumor suppressors, including *TP53* and *PTEN*.[69] Approximately one-third of the mutations in PJS patients are caused by large deletions.[49]

There have been case reports of sporadic Peutz-Jeghers polyps, but this is somewhat controversial. In a study at a tertiary care center, three patients with potential sporadic Peutz-Jeghers polyps were identified, but two of them had other features suggestive of PJS, although strict clinical criteria were not met. The authors concluded that if sporadic Peutz-Jeghers polyps do exist, they are extremely rare.[44]

Pathological Features

The hamartomatous polyps of PJS are histologically distinctive and consist of disorganized mucosa with prominent smooth muscle bundles. The smooth muscle fibers of the muscularis mucosae form thick cores and permeate the polyps in an arborizing fashion (Fig. 21.13A). The epithelium lining these polyps is similar to the normal mucosa in that there are goblet cells, absorptive enterocytes, endocrine cells, and Paneth cells (Fig. 21.13B). Rarely, metaplastic bone formation has been reported in these polyps.[72] As

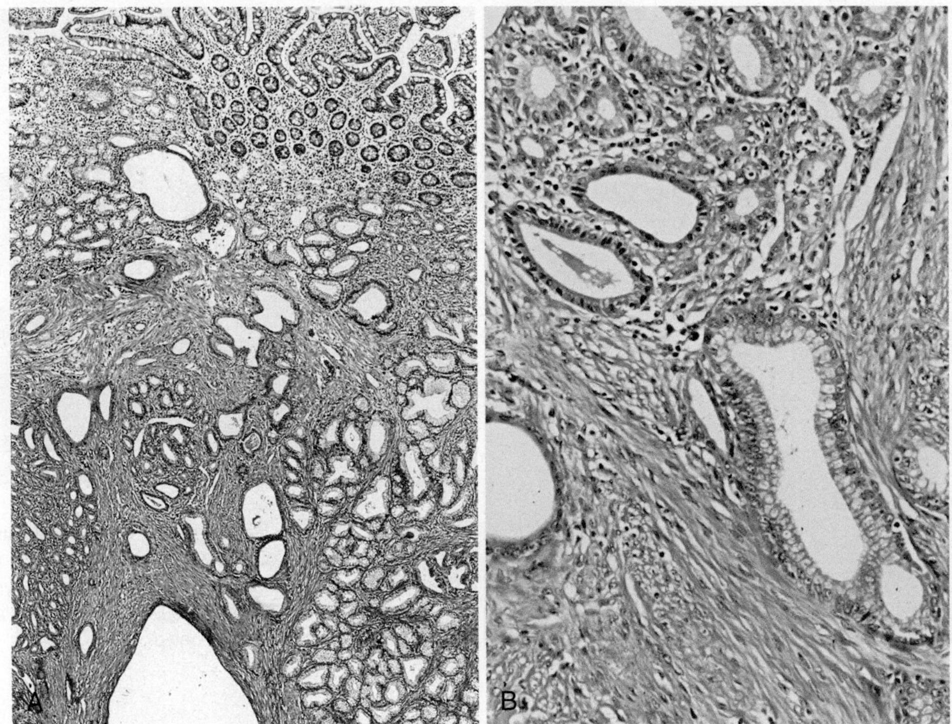

FIGURE 21.11 Paraduodenal pancreatitis. A, Numerous lobules of ductules are present in association with a prominent proliferation of smooth muscle in the submucosa of the duodenum. **B,** The ductules are lined by bland cuboidal and columnar cells containing mucin typical of biliary or pancreatic ductal-type epithelial cells.

TABLE 21.2 Hamartomatous Syndromes Affecting the Small Bowel

Syndrome	Polyp Type	Small Bowel Involvement	Histology	Dysplasia In Polyp*	Gene Mutations	Risk of Small Bowel Adenocarcinoma
Peutz-Jeghers syndrome	Peutz-Jeghers polyp	Frequent (>90%)	Normal mucosal elements with arborizing smooth muscle	Rare; possible increased risk of dysplasia in nonpolypoid mucosa	*STK11/LKB1*	13%
Juvenile polyposis syndrome	Juvenile polyp	Infrequent (<20%)	Inflamed, edematous lamina propria, cystic glands, often ulcerated	Rare	*SMAD4* and *BMPR1A*	~10%
PTEN hamartoma tumor syndrome	Multiple types: juvenile polyps, ganglioneuromas, lipomas, and adenomas	Variable (33%-66%)	Variable	Rare	*PTEN*	Unclear, likely low

**Dysplasia in polyps other than an adenoma.*
PTEN, *Phosphatase and tensin homolog.*

much as 10% of Peutz-Jeghers polyps have foci of misplaced epithelium in which the epithelium is located within the submucosa, the muscularis propria, or both. This phenomenon is encountered more frequently in polyps larger than 3 cm in diameter (Fig. 21.13C).[73]

The development of Peutz-Jeghers polyps is the subject of some controversy. Given the prominent smooth muscle in these polyps and the presence of misplaced epithelium, some authors suggest that patients with PJS are prone to mucosal prolapse.[74] Indeed, the differential diagnosis of Peutz-Jeghers polyps, particularly in the colon, is mucosal prolapse polyps. However, hemorrhage and hemosiderin deposits, commonly seen in prolapse polyps, are not prominent in Peutz-Jeghers polyps.

The sequence of events that results in GI dysplasia and carcinoma is also unclear in relation to Peutz-Jeghers polyps. One occasionally encounters dysplasia and even carcinoma in a Peutz-Jeghers polyp; however, in a study of 2461 Peutz-Jeghers polyps from 63 patients, only 6 polyps contained foci of dysplasia.[75] These results argue that the hamartoma-adenoma-carcinoma hypothesis proposed by some authors rarely occurs.[76] Peutz-Jeghers polyps have also been shown

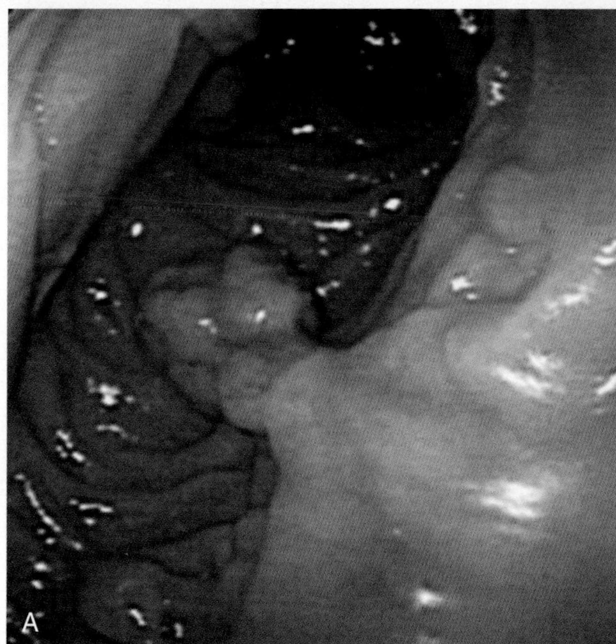

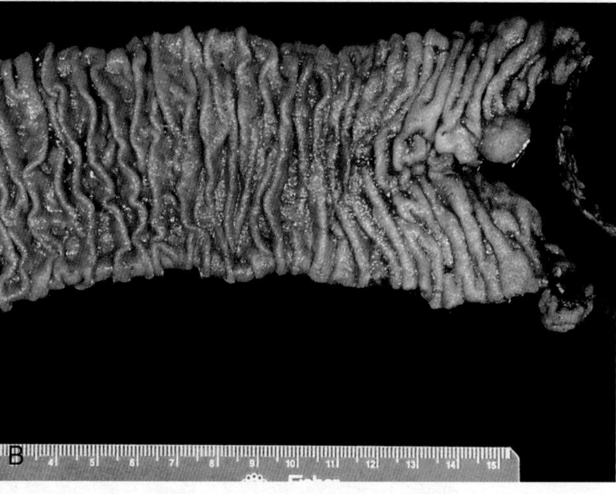

FIGURE 21.12 Peutz-Jeghers polyps of the duodenum. A, The endoscopic appearance of Peutz-Jeghers–type polyps is characteristic. These lesions are variable in size and shape but typically are multinodular and contain a smooth surface and thick stalk. **B,** Gross appearance of a Peutz-Jeghers polyp.

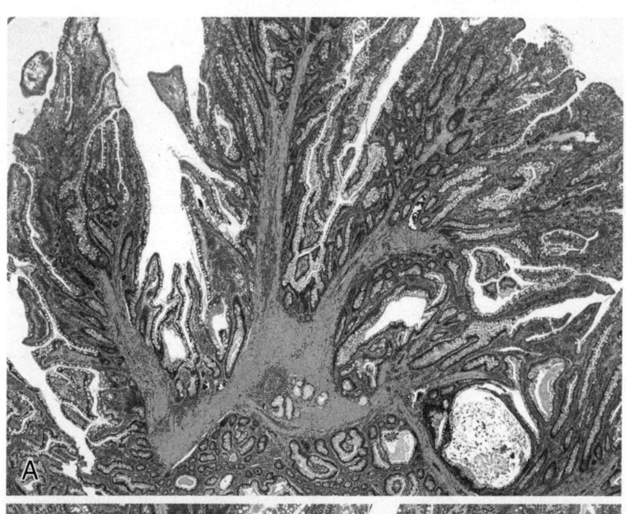

FIGURE 21.13 Peutz-Jeghers polyp of the duodenum. A, The polyp is composed of complex, arborizing fronds lined by absorptive cells, goblet cells, and endocrine cells. **B,** Under higher power, the stroma is seen to be rich in smooth muscle fibers arising from the muscularis mucosae. **C,** Misplacement of the epithelium within the submucosa and muscularis propria is common in Peutz-Jeghers polyps.

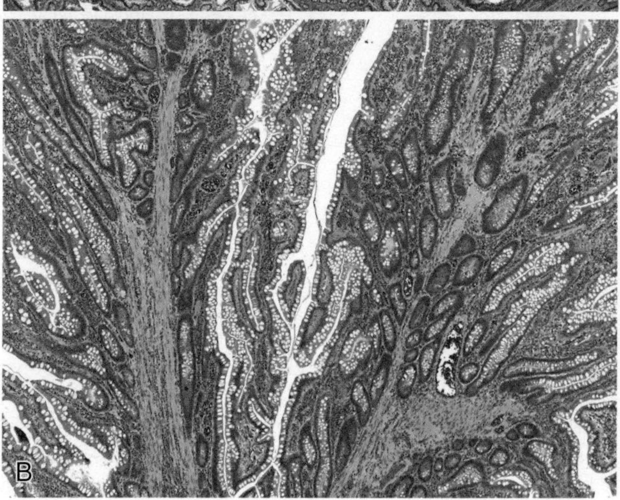

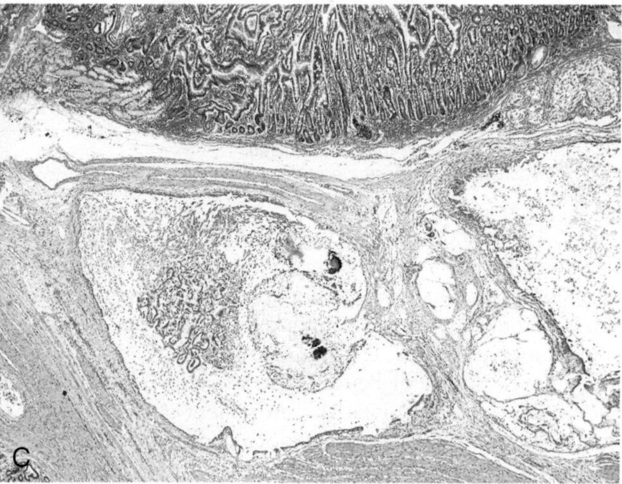

to be polyclonal, arguing against the possibility of malignant potential. Given these results, it is possible that carcinoma develops in surrounding mucosa that may have an accelerated pathway to dysplasia and carcinoma.[59,74]

In any case, when one encounters dysplasia in a Peutz-Jeghers polyp, the dysplasia should be classified according to a two-tier system (i.e., low-grade or high-grade dysplasia). Care must be taken not to interpret misplaced epithelium as invasive adenocarcinoma.[73] The misplaced epithelium should not have desmoplastic stroma or an infiltrative growth pattern. The epithelial cells should have a similar cytology to other parts of the polyps, and the glands should be invested with lamina propria.

Juvenile Polyps

Clinical and Endoscopic Features

Juvenile polyps of the small intestine are rare and occur in two polyposis syndromes: JPS and *PTEN* hamartoma tumor syndrome.[77] Juvenile-type polyps can also be seen in Cronkhite-Canada syndrome, an extremely rare, noninherited disorder associated with diffuse GI polyposis.[78,79] Juvenile polyps tend to be friable and undergo autoamputation. Endoscopically, they appear smooth and often have evidence of hemorrhage. As a result, patients typically present with complaints related to bleeding, such as occult blood loss, hematochezia, fatigue, or anemia.

First described in 1964, JPS is an extremely rare (1 per 100,000 to 160,000 births), autosomal dominant polyposis syndrome with variable penetrance and phenotypic heterogeneity. Diagnostic criteria include (1) at least five colorectal juvenile polyps, (2) any number of extracolonic juvenile polyps, or (3) any number of juvenile polyps in patients with a family history of JPS.[49] Three clinical phenotypes of JPS have been described: *infantile juvenile polyposis*, *juvenile polyposis coli*, and *generalized juvenile polyposis*. Infantile juvenile polyposis syndrome, the most severe type, is characterized by early and diffuse involvement of the entire GI tract. Because these hamartomatous polyps have surface erosion, affected patients usually present with GI bleeding and anemia. JPS is also associated with a significantly increased risk of adenocarcinoma in involved GI sites. The colon is the site most commonly involved by disease, with the risk of colorectal cancer ranging from 17% to 22% by 35 years of age and nearing 68% by 60 years of age.[49] The lifetime risk of developing carcinomas of the stomach, small intestine, or pancreas is approximately 10% to 15%[80]; however, in those with *SMAD4* mutations, the risk of gastric cancer approaches 30%.[49] Prevention of intestinal adenocarcinoma mandates intensive screening, with colonoscopy and upper GI endoscopy every 1 to 3 years, beginning 12 to 15 years of age.[49] Severe GI bleeding may necessitate immediate surgery. Progression to dysplasia in a polyp is not necessarily an indication for surgery, provided that it can be completely removed. Given the increased risk of adenocarcinoma, genetic screening of family members of affected individuals is essential.

Mutations in two genes have been described in patients with JPS: *SMAD4* (also known as *MADH4* or *DPC4*) and *BMPR1A* (also known as *ALK3*).[49,81-86] Approximately 25% of patients with JPS have a negative family history, and their polyps presumably arise from de novo mutations. The proteins encoded by these genes are involved in the transforming growth factor-β (TGF-β) signal transduction pathway. Because the TGF-β signaling pathway mediates growth inhibitory signals, proteins in this pathway function as tumor suppressors. Mutations in *SMAD4* have been shown to be more common in patients with upper GI polyps, whereas patients with *BMPR1A* mutations are more likely to present at a younger age than those with mutations in *SMAD4*.[87]

The term *PTEN hamartoma tumor syndrome* was coined to encompass all hamartoma syndromes that arise through mutations in the tumor suppressor, *PTEN*. This term encompasses Cowden syndrome, Bannayan-Riley-Ruvalcaba syndrome (BRRS), Proteus syndrome, and others.[77,88] Patients with these syndromes have a wide variety of GI, skin, and soft tissue tumors and an increased risk for carcinomas of the colorectum, thyroid, breast, and endometrium.[89]

Cowden syndrome is 50% less common than JPS and is characterized by multiple hamartomatous tumors of endodermal, mesodermal, and ectodermal origin. The most distinctive lesions are mucocutaneous—in particular, trichilemmomas, acral keratosis, subcutaneous lipomas, palmoplantar keratoses, oral cobblestoning, and oral papillomas. Colonic polyps in Cowden syndrome are common and include ganglioneuromas, adenomas, inflammatory-type polyps, juvenile polyps, and less frequently lipomas and leiomyomas.[49] Although rarer, similar polyps can occur in the small intestine and stomach, with frequencies ranging from 37% to 66%.[90,91] Current American College of Gastroenterology (ACG) guidelines recommend surveillance colonoscopy and upper GI endoscopy every 2 years beginning at 15 years of age.[49]

BRRS is also associated with juvenile polyps of the GI tract (mostly limited to the ileum and colon); however, these patients also have neurological findings, including macrocephaly and slowed psychomotor development. Some BRRS patients also develop extraintestinal hamartomatous tumors similar to those seen in patients with Cowden syndrome.[77]

Pathological Features

Juvenile polyps are pedunculated and are histologically characterized by abundant lamina propria, dilated mucin-filled crypts, active inflammation, and surface erosion (Fig. 21.14). The epithelium in these polyps can contain adsorptive cells, goblet cells, endocrine cells, and Paneth cells. Eosinophils are often prominent. Unlike Peutz-Jeghers polyps, juvenile polyps lack prominent smooth muscle bundles. Juvenile polyps in the small bowel are very similar to inflammatory-type polyps. The distinction between these two polyps is mostly based on the clinical context in which they arise. In a patient with a known polyposis syndrome, the diagnosis of a juvenile polyp is appropriate. In cases where multiple inflammatory or juvenile polyps are seen, the possibility of a polyposis syndrome should be considered. If a single juvenile or inflammatory polyp is encountered, one should be cautious in suggesting a polyposis syndrome.

BENIGN EPITHELIAL NEOPLASMS

Adenomas of the Small Intestine

Clinical and Endoscopic Features

Adenomas account for approximately 25% of benign neoplasms of the small intestine and can be divided into

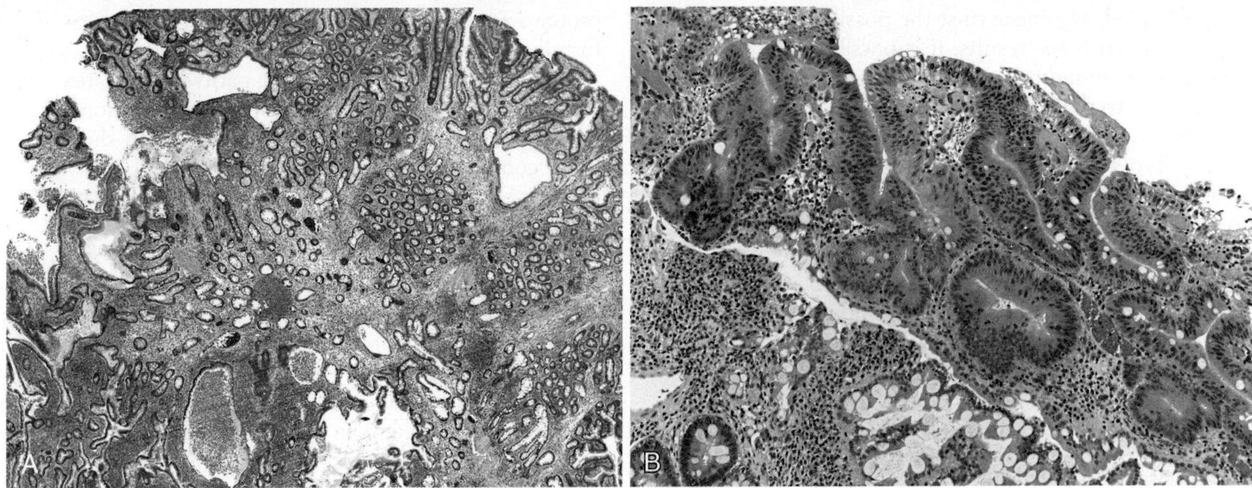

FIGURE 21.14 Juvenile polyp from a patient with juvenile polyposis syndrome. A, The polyp demonstrates an expanded, edematous lamina propria with a mixed inflammatory cell infiltrate. Dilated glands with crypt abscesses are seen. Unlike Peutz-Jeghers polyps, there are no prominent smooth muscle bundles. **B,** Areas of low-grade dysplasia characterized by epithelial cells with pseudostratified, enlarged, and hyperchromatic nuclei are seen focally.

ampullary and nonampullary adenomas, with the majority of nonampullary adenomas occurring in the periampullary duodenum. Several investigators have postulated that the ampulla may be prone to neoplastic transformation because it is chronically irritated by pancreatic juices and bile salts, resulting in long-standing injury to the mucosa and culminating in epithelial cell dysplasia.[92,93] A large proportion of small intestinal adenomas (40%) are sporadic, occurring in older individuals (mean age of duodenal adenomas is 65 years); however, up to 60% occur in patients with adenomatous polyposis syndromes, including familial adenomatous polyposis (FAP) and *MUTYH*-associated polyposis (MAP).[94] Approximately 17% of patients with MAP have duodenal polyposis, and their lifetime risk of duodenal cancer is 4%.[95,96] Small bowel adenomas also occur in Lynch syndrome. Unlike adenomas in MAP and FAP, those in Lynch syndrome may not have such a strong predilection for the proximal small bowel and ampulla. As in MAP, the lifetime risk of small bowel adenocarcinoma in Lynch syndrome is 4%.[97] Given that adenomas may not be amenable to upper endoscopy, capsule endoscopy has been used to identify occult adenomas and carcinomas in Lynch syndrome[98]; however, this is currently not recommended for routine screening.[99]

Although some adenomas located distal to the ampulla produce luminal obstructive symptoms or occult blood loss, most are asymptomatic and clinically silent until complicated by the development of carcinoma. In contrast, ampullary and periampullary adenomas can produce obstructive jaundice before malignant transformation and become symptomatic earlier in their evolution.

Pathological Features

Nonampullary Adenomas. Nonampullary adenomas of the small intestine encompass a variety of histological subtypes, including intestinal-type adenomas, pyloric gland adenomas, and serrated lesions. Serrated and intestinal-type adenomas are endoscopically and histologically similar to those of the colon. Larger adenomas (>1 cm) are more likely to harbor areas of high-grade dysplasia, and approximately 50% have a villous component consisting of long papillary projections lined by columnar, mucin-depleted epithelial cells with enlarged, hyperchromatic nuclei. Paneth cells and endocrine cells are often more numerous in adenomas of the small intestine compared with those of the colon. The criteria for grading dysplasia in adenomas of the small intestine are similar to those for colonic adenomas. *Low-grade dysplasia* is defined as nuclear stratification confined to the lower half of the cells in the absence of complex architectural changes (Fig. 21.15A,B). *High-grade dysplasia* is characterized by architectural complexity (i.e., cribriforming and glandular crowding) in conjunction with high-grade nuclear features (i.e., nuclear enlargement with loss of nuclear polarity, irregular nuclear membranes) (Fig. 21.15C). The terms *severe dysplasia* and *carcinoma in situ* should no longer be used to describe these changes.

Unlike adenomas of the colon, but similar to those of the esophagus and stomach, the lamina propria in adenomas of the small intestine contains a rich lymphatic network. When dysplastic epithelial cells break through the basement membrane and infiltrate the lamina propria, the term *intramucosal adenocarcinoma* is appropriate. Intramucosal adenocarcinoma of the small intestine carries a risk of lymph node metastasis and is staged as pT1a carcinoma, according to the eighth edition of the *Cancer Staging Manual* of the American Joint Committee on Cancer.[99]

Pyloric gland adenomas (PGAs) are composed of tightly packed glands lined by cuboidal epithelium with an even monolayer of round nuclei with abundant mucinous cytoplasm reminiscent of pyloric-type glands (Fig. 21.16A).[23,100] These polyps are likely more common in the stomach, but 46% of pyloric gland adenomas occurred in the duodenum in one study.[23] Given their resemblance to Brunner glands, the distinction between PGA and Brunner gland hamartoma/hyperplasia can be difficult; however, PGAs often do not have overlying intestinalized epithelium when they occur in the duodenum. Furthermore, there is no lobular configuration in these lesions, in contrast with Brunner gland hamartoma/hyperplasia. Immunohistochemically, PGAs express MUC6 and variable MUC5AC.[23]

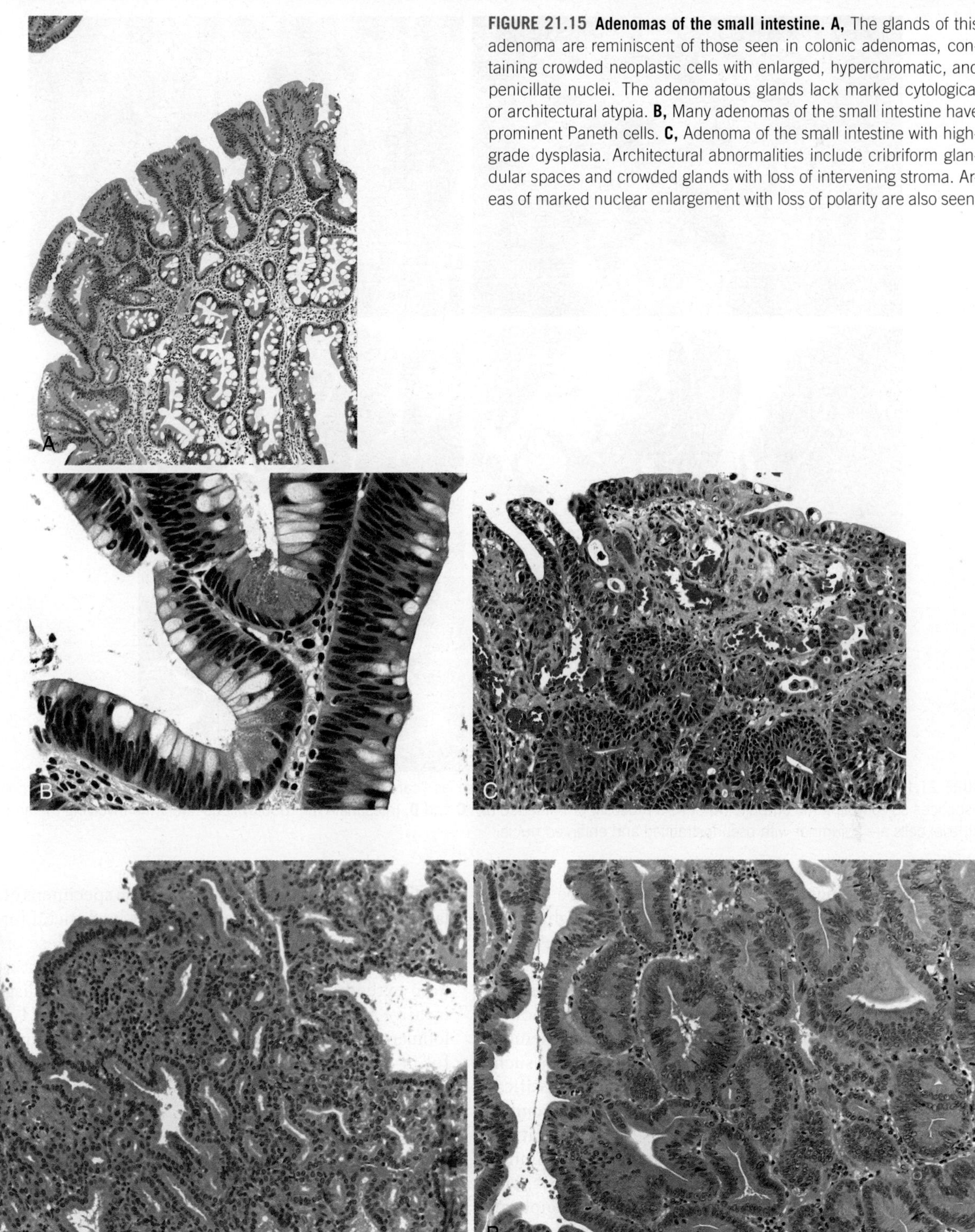

FIGURE 21.15 Adenomas of the small intestine. A, The glands of this adenoma are reminiscent of those seen in colonic adenomas, containing crowded neoplastic cells with enlarged, hyperchromatic, and penicillate nuclei. The adenomatous glands lack marked cytological or architectural atypia. **B,** Many adenomas of the small intestine have prominent Paneth cells. **C,** Adenoma of the small intestine with high-grade dysplasia. Architectural abnormalities include cribriform glandular spaces and crowded glands with loss of intervening stroma. Areas of marked nuclear enlargement with loss of polarity are also seen.

FIGURE 21.16 Pyloric gland adenoma. A, This polyp is composed of tightly packed glands containing epithelial cells with basally located round nuclei. The cells have abundant, slightly eosinophilic to foamy cytoplasm. Occasional dilated glands are seen in this example. No areas of convincing dysplasia are seen in this field. **B,** A pyloric gland adenoma with low-grade dysplasia characterized by nuclear enlargement, stratification, and prominent nucleoli.

By definition, pyloric gland adenomas are neoplastic, with recent genetic studies demonstrating a high frequency of *GNAS* and *KRAS* mutations.[101] Despite being called *adenomas,* some lesions are fairly bland without areas of conventional dysplasia. Nondysplastic pyloric gland adenomas therefore do occur; however, often areas of dysplasia can be identified (classified as either *low-grade* or *high-grade*) (Fig. 21.16B). Between 10% and 30% of pyloric gland adenomas are associated with invasive adenocarcinoma.

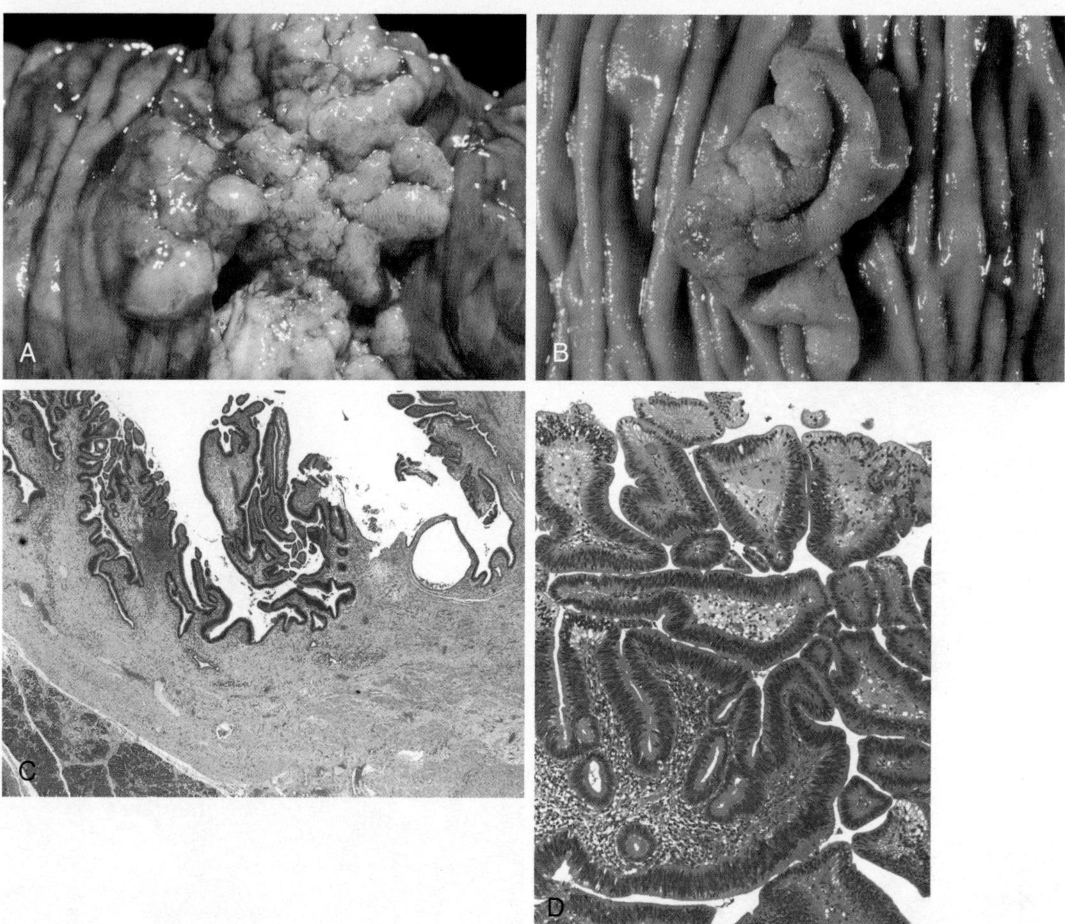

FIGURE 21.17 Villous adenomas of the ampulla. These lesions may appear as "carpet" adenomas composed of velvety papillary and polypoid excrescences surrounding the ampulla **(A)** or as a mucosal prominence **(B)**. **C** and **D,** Intestinal-type tubulovillous adenoma involving the ampulla. The epithelial cells are columnar with pseudostratified and enlarged nuclei.

Ampullary Adenomas. Ampullary adenomas can be divided into *intestinal* and *pancreaticobiliary* types (although mixed lesions also occur). Intestinal-type adenomas are more common (~75%) and resemble colonic and nonampullary intestinal-type adenomas (Fig. 21.17C,D). Pancreaticobiliary-type (or mixed intestinal and pancreaticobiliary) adenomas often have a prominent papillary architecture and resemble intraductal papillary neoplasms of the pancreas. As such, the current World Health Organization (WHO) classification[102] advocates classifying these lesions as *intraampullary papillary-tubular neoplasms* (IAPNs). By definition, IAPNs must be confined to the ampulla with no or minimal involvement of the duodenal papilla, pancreatic duct, and bile duct. The papillary projections are lined by a monolayer of cuboidal epithelial cells with round nuclei and eosinophilic cytoplasm (Fig. 21.18A,B). Varying degrees of dysplasia, both low-grade and high-grade, are common (>80%) in these lesions.[102]

Both intestinal and pancreaticobiliary ampullary adenomas are often associated with adjacent invasive adenocarcinoma. Although most adenocarcinomas of the ampulla arise from adenomas, nonpolypoid (or flat) dysplastic lesions of the ampulla also occur. These dysplastic lesions are almost always associated with an adjacent invasive adenocarcinoma. Some of these lesions have a micropapillary architecture lined by dysplastic cuboidal to columnar cells.

The evaluation of biopsy or resection specimens of ampullary and periampullary adenomas may be difficult for several reasons. Ampullary ducts and glands are in close proximity to bundles of smooth muscle, and when dysplastic epithelium extends into these structures, a mistaken diagnosis of invasive adenocarcinoma may be rendered (Fig. 21.19). The lobular architecture and lack of desmoplasia can be helpful in distinguishing this finding from invasive adenocarcinoma. As with their colonic counterparts, misplacement of the dysplastic epithelium into the submucosa may occur as a consequence of mechanical injury or prolapse in these adenomas. The presence of lamina propria around these dysplastic glands and the presence of hemosiderin deposits and acellular mucin pools are helpful features to differentiate epithelial misplacement from invasive adenocarcinoma. Finally because many patients with ampullary lesions have obstructive jaundice, biliary stents are often placed. Stents cause inflammatory epithelial injury and erosions of the ampullary epithelium with concomitant reactive and regenerative epithelial changes, as well as inflammation of the underlying stroma (Fig. 21.20). This constellation of findings may mimic dysplasia or even invasive cancer. Therefore it is imperative to know the patient's status regarding stenting of the common bile duct to evaluate the specimen properly and avoid overdiagnosing neoplasia. The presence of active inflammation and foveolar metaplasia should

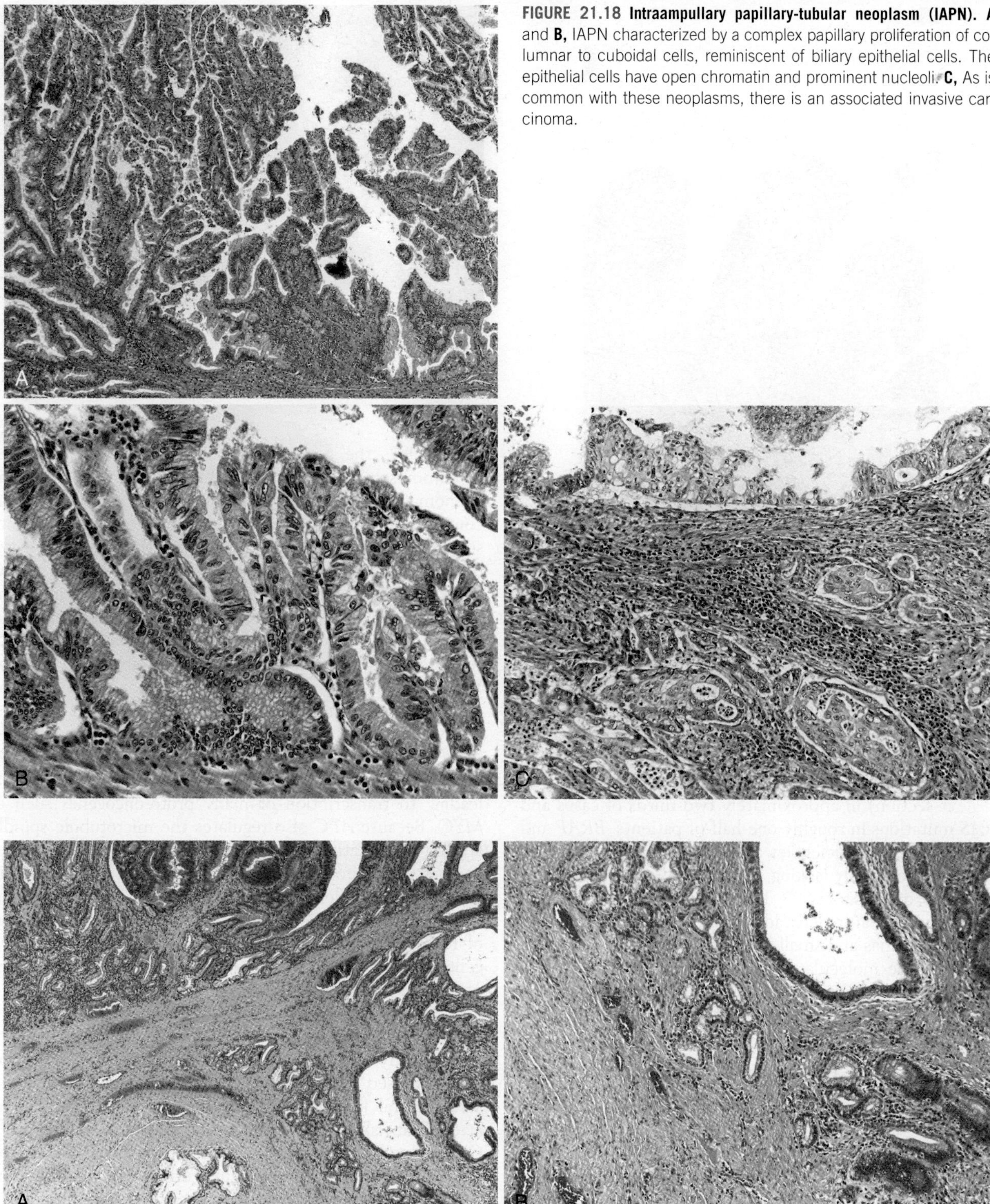

FIGURE 21.18 Intraampullary papillary-tubular neoplasm (IAPN). A and **B,** IAPN characterized by a complex papillary proliferation of columnar to cuboidal cells, reminiscent of biliary epithelial cells. The epithelial cells have open chromatin and prominent nucleoli. **C,** As is common with these neoplasms, there is an associated invasive carcinoma.

FIGURE 21.19 Ampullary adenoma involving periampullary glands. A, Adenomatous epithelium extends into the underlying periampullary glands, which are embedded in smooth muscle. **B,** At higher power, there is an admixture of adenomatous glands and nonneoplastic periampullary glands associated with a rim of lamina propria.

make one cautious in interpreting the epithelial changes as dysplastic.

Immunohistochemical and Molecular Features

Some authors have used immunohistochemistry to differentiate histological subtypes of ampullary and nonampullary adenomas. Intestinal-type adenomas (ampullary and nonampullary), like their colorectal counterparts, express CDX2 and MUC2. Coexpression of CK7 and CK20 is also common.[103] IAPNs with pancreaticobiliary-type epithelium express MUC1, MUC5AC, and MUC6,[104] and PGAs express MUC6 and variable MUC5AC.[23] The considerable

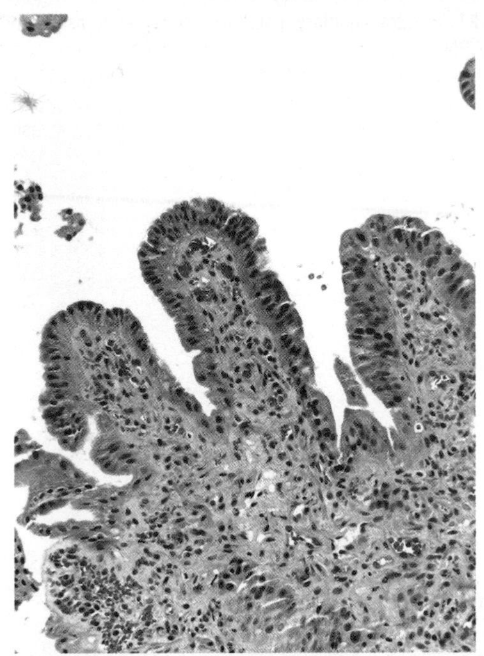

FIGURE 21.20 Regenerative epithelial changes secondary to biliary stenting. In this example, the lamina propria is expanded and inflamed with prominent capillaries suggestive of previous injury. The epithelium demonstrates mucin loss and areas of pseudostratification. However, the nuclei are not markedly enlarged and hyperchromatic. Furthermore, the nucleus-to-cytoplasm ratio is not increased.

overlap in the expression of these proteins among these lesions, however, limits their clinical utility.

Sporadic ampullary and nonampullary adenomas demonstrate molecular abnormalities associated with the WNT signaling pathway, including *APC* mutations (discussed in the next section) in approximately two-thirds of cases and *KRAS* mutations in roughly one-half of patients. *BRAF* and mismatch repair deficiencies are relatively rare, and *TP53* mutations are usually lacking, particularly in the absence of high-grade dysplasia.[89-91,95] Therefore the molecular features of sporadic ampullary adenomas are similar to those of colonic adenomas and small intestinal adenomas associated with FAP. The molecular characteristics of PGAs are less well understood, but recent studies demonstrating a high frequency of *GNAS* and *KRAS* mutations support the neoplastic nature of these lesions.[101]

Familial Adenomatous Polyposis

Clinical and Endoscopic Features

FAP is an autosomal dominant inherited disease occurring in approximately 2 to 3 per 100,000 persons. [49] Clinically, FAP is relatively easy to diagnose, as most affected patients have a strong family history and 100 to 1000 polyps on colonoscopy (classic FAP is defined as the presence of >100 colonic adenomas). An attenuated form of FAP has been described that manifests with significantly fewer colonic polyps, often more than 15 but always less than 100. Small intestinal adenomas occur in approximately 90% of FAP patients (Fig. 21.21). Typically, they are more prominent in the duodenum and ampulla.[105] The incidence of small bowel or ampullary carcinoma was estimated to be 4.5% among those patients enrolled in a screening program.[106,107]

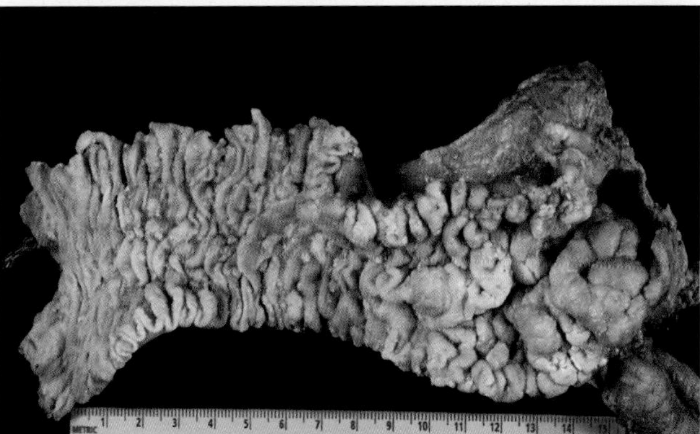

FIGURE 21.21 Duodenojejunal resection specimen from a patient with familial adenomatous polyposis syndrome. Numerous small polyps and exaggerated mucosal folds are present throughout the specimen. In addition, several larger, irregular polyps are seen.

In 1987, the gene responsible for FAP was localized to chromosome 5q21, and in 1991 it was identified as the adenomatous polyposis coli *(APC)* gene.[108] The *APC* gene contains 15 transcribed exons encoding a 312-kDa tumor suppressor. Mutations in *APC* constitute the initial step in the development of colorectal carcinoma in FAP patients. *APC* is involved in a wide variety of cellular functions, including cell adhesion, migration, chromosome segregation, and signal transduction. One of the most important roles of *APC* is to regulate the activity of β-catenin, a protein involved in the Wnt signaling pathway and cellular adhesion. In conjunction with other proteins, *APC* is essential in inducing the phosphorylation and subsequent degradation of β-catenin. Loss of *APC* function through mutation leads to accumulation of β-catenin, which subsequently translocates to the nucleus, leading to transcription of many proto-oncogenes such as *MYC*. Because *APC* also regulates the microtubule spindle apparatus, mutations predispose to aneuploidy and further neoplastic transformation.[109] More than 700 mutations in *APC* have been identified in FAP patients. Interestingly, the location of the mutation has striking effects on the phenotype of FAP. Those occurring in the central portion of the *APC* gene (codons 279 to 1309) correlate with increased numbers of duodenal polyps as well as the size of the adenomas.[110]

Risk of Malignancy

In the early 1990s, Spigelman developed a classification scheme based on the number and size of adenomas, their architectural features, and the degree of dysplasia, in an attempt at risk stratification of FAP patients (Table 21.3).[93] Originally, the dysplasia was classified as *mild, moderate,* or *severe;* however, more recent studies have modified the original Spigelman classification to reflect the division of dysplasia into *high-grade* and *low-grade.*[111] The risk of progression to duodenal or ampullary adenocarcinoma is most likely correlated to the Spigelman stage at initial endoscopy. In a study of 114 patients with FAP, 6 duodenal or ampullary carcinomas were identified. In five cases, the original Spigelman stage was III (one case) or IV (four cases). Only 17% of patients progressed to a higher Spigelman stage during the surveillance program.[112] A more recent study demonstrated a much higher rate of progression in Spigelman stage (40%); however, no patient developed adenocarcinoma.[111] Given that the Spigelman stage depends on villosity and

TABLE 21.3 Modified Spigelman Score*

Factor	1 Point	2 Points	3 Points
Polyp number	1-4	5-20	>20
Polyp size (mm)	1-4	5-10	>10
Architecture	Tubular	Tubulovillous	Villous
Dysplasia	Low-grade	—	High-grade

Stage grouping: stage 0, no polyps; stage I, 1 to 4 points; stage II, 5 to 6 points; stage III, 7 to 8 points; stage IV, 9 to 12 points.

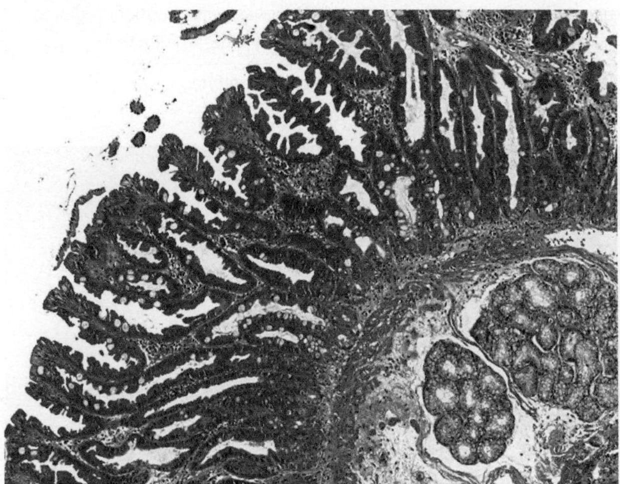

FIGURE 21.22 Duodenal hyperplastic polyp. This polyp is reminiscent of microvesicular hyperplastic polyps of the colon. Prominent epithelial serrations are seen imparting a "sawtooth" luminal outline. This particular polyp demonstrated a V600E *BRAF* mutation that is often seen in colonic hyperplastic polyps. (*Courtesy Dr. Christophe Rosty. University of Queensland, Herston, Queensland, Australia.*)

degree of dysplasia, it is possible that interobserver variability among pathologists could account for these differences. Currently, endoscopic mucosal resection or prophylactic pancreaticoduodenectomy is considered for patients with an advanced Spigelman stage. One recent study, however, reported a significant proportion of duodenal adenocarcinomas occurring in patients without Spigelman stage IV disease. Instead, large duodenal polyp size and high-grade dysplasia were more positively associated with duodenal adenocarcinoma, and the authors propose that revisions to the current Spigelman staging system that prioritize these findings be considered.[113]

Hyperplastic Polyp

Recent reports have described small intestinal polyps with morphological features resembling colonic microvesicular hyperplastic polyps with prominent epithelial serrations and abundant cytoplasm with small mucin droplets (Fig. 21.22).[114,115] In a series of nine polyps, five were found in the second portion of the duodenum. Molecular analysis performed on six of these polyps found a V600E *BRAF* mutation in two polyps and *KRAS* mutations in another two polyps.[115] These polyps also expressed gastric mucins similar to serrated colorectal polyps. Although these findings are suggestive, additional studies need to be performed to further characterize these lesions.

NEUROENDOCRINE NEOPLASMS

The GI tract is a common location for neuroendocrine neoplasms (NENs), in which there is a predilection for the small intestine. Here, we present a brief discussion of small intestinal tract NENs. A more detailed discussion of NENs of the GI tract can be found in Chapter 29.

Small intestinal NENs are most commonly found in the ileum, with only 11% occurring in the jejunum and 2% to 3% occurring in the duodenum.[102,116] NENs of the duodenum and proximal jejunum (i.e., foregut NENs) are frequently associated with characteristic clinical and pathological features distinct from NENs of the distal jejunum and ileum (midgut NENs). Clinically, duodenal NENs can result in hypersecretion of certain hormones and be associated with various clinical syndromes. Immunohistochemical staining for peptide hormones can be performed to confirm the clinical impression of a syndromic NEN; however, routine immunohistochemical staining for peptide hormones is not suggested for clinically nonfunctional NENs and can be potentially confusing. If peptide hormone immunohistochemistry is performed and demonstrates that the majority of the tumor cells exhibit hormone production, then it is acceptable, but not necessary, to supplement the diagnosis of NEN to reflect the corresponding subtype (e.g., gastrin-producing NEN).[102] Specific functional terms such as *gastrinoma* should not be used to describe NENs in the absence of clinical and serological findings indicative of a hormonal syndrome. Although the functional status of a NEN is defined by the clinical and serological findings, it is useful to divide NENs into categories based on their location in the small intestine and the corresponding cell subtype because this allows for discussion of site-related differences among NENs (Table 21.4).

In addition to functional status, a recent study has proposed dividing small intestinal NENs into three molecular subgroups (chromosome 18 loss, no arm-level copy-number variation, and multiple copy-number variation) given different prognostic outcomes. The vast majority (55%) of small intestinal NENs demonstrated chromosome 18 loss and were associated with *CDKN1B* mutations and CpG island methylation phenotype (CIMP) negativity. These tumors occurred in older patients and were associated with a favorable prognosis. No arm-level copy number variation (CNV) (19% of tumors) was associated with CIMP positivity and an indeterminate prognosis. Tumors with multiple CNV (26% of tumors) tended to occur in younger patients and were associated with the poorest prognosis (Table 21.5).[117]

NENs of the small intestine are further classified by using the criteria applicable to all GI and pancreatic NENs published by the WHO in 2019.[102] Well-differentiated NENs demonstrate histomorphological features similar to those of their nonneoplastic counterparts and express immunohistochemical markers of neuroendocrine differentiation (i.e., chromogranin A, synaptophysin, and INSM1). Well-differentiated NENs can be graded based on assessment of mitotic activity and the Ki67 proliferation index (Table 21.6), with the vast majority encompassing grade 1 (<2 mitoses per 10 high-power field [HPF] and/or <3% Ki67 proliferation index) and grade 2 (2 to 20 mitoses per 10 HPF and/or 3% to 20% Ki67 proliferation index) lesions.

Metastatic disease to locoregional lymph nodes and the liver is common in small intestinal NENs (ranging

TABLE 21.4 Clinicopathological Features of Neuroendocrine Neoplasms According to Site and Hormone Production

Tumor Type	Anatomic Site Predilection	Associations	Clinical Course
Gastrin-producing NEN	Duodenum, pancreas, and lymph nodes (primary tumor may be microscopic)	Functional: MEN1 (25%) Nonfunctional: *Helicobacter* infection, long-term PPI?	Functional: frequent regional and distant metastasis Nonfunctional: indolent
Somatostatin-producing NEN	Ampullary/periampullary area and pancreas	NF type 1, adrenal pheochromocytomas	Typically indolent, but larger tumors may metastasize
Gangliocytic paraganglioma	Ampullary/periampullary area	NF type 1	Typically indolent, but larger tumors may metastasize
Serotonin-producing NEN	Distal jejunum and ileum	True carcinoid tumor caused by serotonin production	Malignant with frequent regional and distant metastasis

MEN1, *Multiple endocrine neoplasia type 1;* NEN, *neuroendocrine neoplasm;* NF, *neurofibromatosis;* PPI, *proton pump inhibitor.*

TABLE 21.5 Proposed Molecular Subclassification of Small Intestinal NENs

Molecular Group	Clinical Setting	Associated Abnormalities	Clinical Prognosis
Chromosome 18 loss	55% of small intestinal NENs Older patients	*CDKN1B* mutations CIMP negativity	Favorable
No arm-level CNV	19% of small intestinal NENs	CIMP positivity	Intermediate
Multiple CNV	26% of small intestinal NENs Younger patients	—	Poor

CIMP, *CpG island methylation phenotype;* CNV, *copy-number variation.*

TABLE 21.6 World Health Organization 2010 Classification of Neuroendocrine Neoplasms

WHO Grade	Mitotic Count	Ki67 Index	Terminology
G1	<2 per 10 HPF	<3%	Neuroendocrine neoplasm
G2	2-20 per 10 HPF	3%-20%	Neuroendocrine neoplasm
G3	>20 per 10 HPF	>20%	Neuroendocrine neoplasm

HPF, *High-power field;* WHO, *World Health Organization.*

from 35% to over 60% based on data from either large-population or large referral centers).[118-121] Disease progression is prolonged in most cases, however, with 5-year survival rates of 70% to 100% in those with locoregional disease and 35% to 60% in those with distant metastasis because of the low-proliferation rate of most tumors (grade 1 and grade 2 lesions).[120,122,123]

Neuroendocrine Neoplasms of the Duodenum, Ampulla, and Proximal Jejunum

Gastrin-Producing Neuroendocrine Neoplasms

Clinical Features

Gastrin-producing NENs represent the largest group of duodenal and proximal jejunal NENs, accounting for approximately two-thirds of NENs in the upper GI tract.[124,125] Gastrin-producing NENs can be either nonfunctioning or associated with Zollinger-Ellison syndrome (ZES), which is characterized by hypergastrinemia, gastric hypersecretion, and refractory peptic ulcer disease.[126] The functional status of the NEN is defined by clinical and serological findings and not by the immunohistochemical expression of peptide hormones. Gastrin-producing NENs develop in the pancreaticoduodenal region (gastrinoma triangle); the primary tumor is found with near-equal frequency in the pancreas and in the duodenum. Rarely, a gastrin-producing NEN is identified in a lymph node in the gastrinoma triangle without an apparent duodenal or pancreatic primary tumor, suggesting the possibility of a primary lymph node gastrinoma[127]; however, it is likely that so-called *primary lymph node gastrinomas* represent metastases from microscopic primary tumors that are easily overlooked on routine examination.[128-132]

ZES is found in approximately 40% to 50% of duodenal gastrin-producing NENs.[124,125,133] most of which are sporadic, with approximately 25% associated with multiple endocrine neoplasia type 1 (MEN1). Sporadic ZES NENs most commonly occur in the duodenum (60% to 75%) but can also be found in the pancreas.[130,134] In contrast, most MEN1-associated ZES NENs occur in the duodenum and are often multifocal.[134]

Nonfunctional gastrin-producing NENs typically occur in the duodenal bulb and are localized in the lamina propria and submucosa.[135] Most nonfunctioning gastrin-producing NENs are clinically indolent, small (<1 cm), and asymptomatic; they are often discovered during endoscopy for other reasons or during surgical resection for unrelated causes. Nonfunctioning gastrin-producing NENs of the duodenum have been associated with *H. pylori* infection of the stomach or long-term PPI therapy.[135] It is postulated that *H. pylori* infection and PPI therapy result in G-cell hyperplasia within the duodenum, leading to formation of sporadic nonfunctional gastrin-producing NENs.[135]

Pathological Features

Gastrin-producing NENs resemble NENs elsewhere in the gastroenteropancreatic system and are composed of uniform cells with lightly eosinophilic cytoplasm arranged in trabeculae (most common), anastomosing cords, and tubules (Fig. 21.23A,B). Immunohistochemistry often reveals staining with synaptophysin, chromogranin A, and gastrin (Fig. 21.23C). Other peptides may be detected in a subset of tumor cells.[124,125] Gastrin-producing NENs infrequently label with CDX2[136] but may express PAX8 by immunohistochemistry.[137,138] The nontumorous duodenum can demonstrate gastrin cell proliferation in MEN1-associated gastrinomas and in sporadic nonfunctional gastrin-producing NENs associated with *H. pylori* gastritis and long-term PPI therapy.[135,139] Sporadic ZES NENs typically do not exhibit proliferative gastrin cell changes in the nontumorous mucosa.[139]

Both sporadic and MEN1-associated ZES NENs may be multifocal; however, the pathogenesis varies in these two conditions. Multifocal sporadic ZES NENs from the same patient probably represent metastases because they frequently demonstrate the same somatic *MEN1* gene mutation and similar patterns of X-chromosome inactivation in tumors at different sites within the same patient.[140] Multifocal ZES NENs in patients with MEN1 syndrome have varied genetic abnormalities and probably represent independent primary tumors.[141]

Natural History

Incidentally discovered, nonfunctioning gastrin-producing NENs of the duodenal bulb appear to be indolent tumors without significant risk of aggressive behavior based on early evidence.[135] In contrast, ZES NENs may behave in a clinically malignant fashion with a higher rate of metastasis. Patients with functional gastrin-producing NENs should be evaluated for MEN1 syndrome because patients with this syndrome and their family members are at risk for synchronous or metachronous syndrome-related tumors and would benefit from close surveillance and genetic counseling.

The prognosis of sporadic and MEN1-associated duodenal gastrin-producing NENs is more favorable than that of pancreatic gastrin-producing NENs.[134] Patients who have sporadic ZES NENs with distant metastatic disease typically undergo surgical exploration and resection of the primary tumor and regional lymph nodes.[126,130,132,142] Between 50% and 60% of sporadic duodenal ZES NENs are associated with regional lymph node metastases.[132,142] The management of patients with MEN1 is more complicated because surgery is rarely curative.[143] Nevertheless, recent data suggest that patients with MEN1 syndrome benefit from surgical removal of the NEN, compared with medical management alone.[132,144]

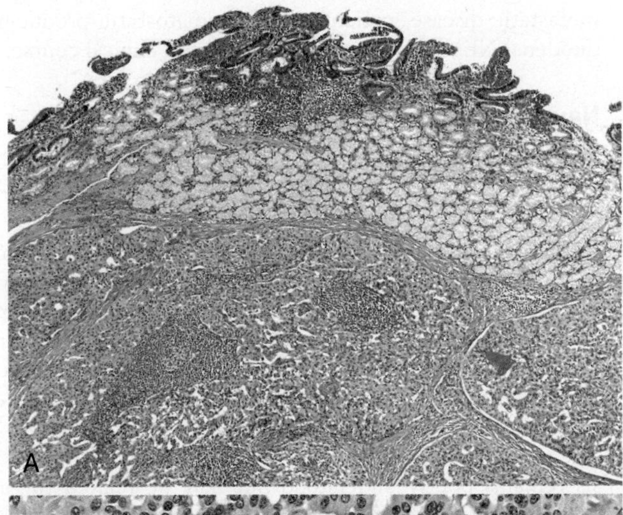
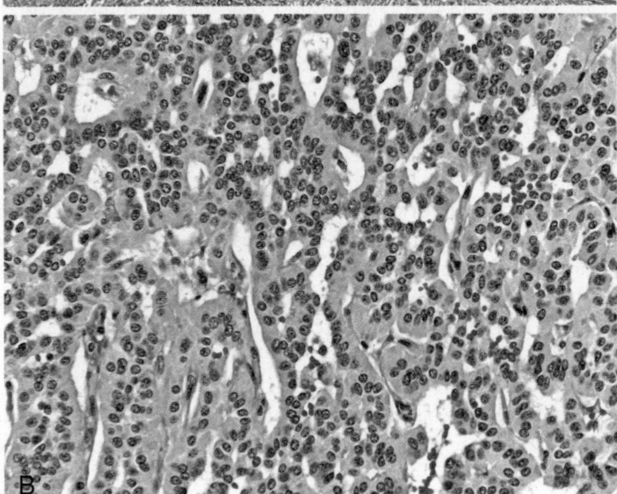
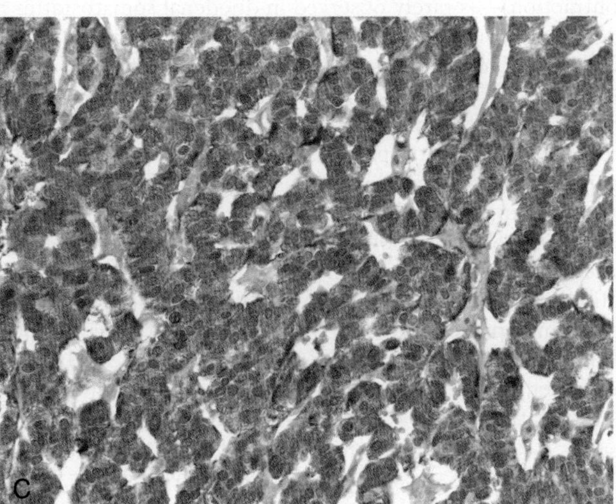

FIGURE 21.23 Duodenal gastrin-producing, well-differentiated neuroendocrine neoplasm. A, The tumor is predominantly located within the duodenal submucosa. **B,** The tumor cells are cytologically bland and are arranged in trabeculae. **C,** The tumor cells display diffuse, strong cytoplasmic staining for gastrin. They also frequently stain for other neuroendocrine markers such as synaptophysin and chromogranin.

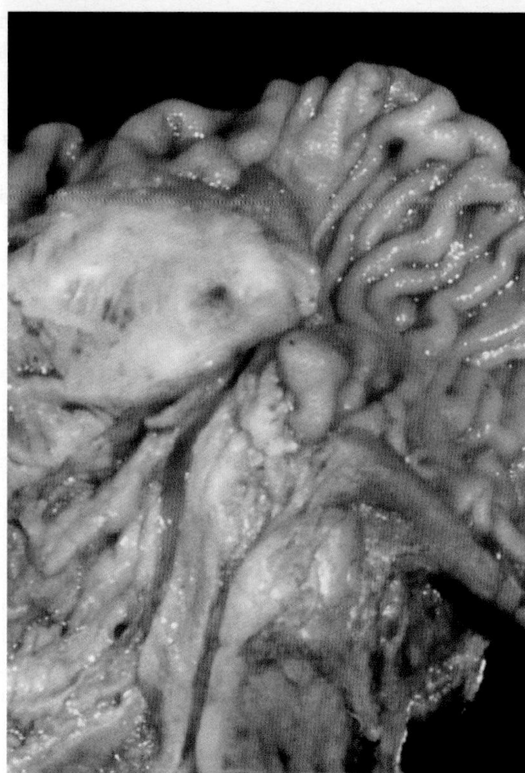

FIGURE 21.24 Ampullary somatostatin-producing, well-differentiated neuroendocrine neoplasm. The tumor is a relatively well-circumscribed, tan-yellow mass within the submucosa of the duodenum at the ampulla.

Somatostatin-Producing Neuroendocrine Neoplasms

Clinical Features

Somatostatin-producing NENs have a predilection for the ampulla and periampullary region (Fig. 21.24).[145-147] Somatostatin inhibits secretion of a number of endocrine and exocrine products and diminishes peristaltic contractions of the gallbladder and stomach.[148] Somatostatinoma syndrome—consisting of diabetes mellitus (caused by inhibition of insulin secretion), steatorrhea (caused by inhibition of pancreatic enzyme secretion), hypohydria or achlorhydria, and cholelithiasis (caused by suppression of cholecystokinin-pancreozymin release and gallbladder contraction)—is rarely observed in duodenal somatostatin-producing NENs.[149-152] In contrast, somatostatin-producing NENs of the pancreas may produce somatostatinoma syndrome.[146,153]

Because of the preferred ampullary and periampullary location, somatostatin-producing NENs of the duodenum typically manifest with symptoms and signs related to bile duct obstruction, abdominal pain, or cholelithiasis.[154,155] Approximately 10% of ampullary/periampullary NENs have been associated with von Recklinghausen disease (neurofibromatosis type 1, or NF1),[156] although the frequency with which patients with NF1 develop these tumors is not clear.[152,157-168] Mutations in *EPAS1* (which encodes HIF2α) have been described in patients with the triad of duodenal somatostatinomas, paragangliomas, and polycythemia.[169] Some patients with ampullary somatostatin-producing NENs also have a pheochromocytoma involving one or both adrenal glands.[159]

Pathological Features

Somatostatin-producing ampullary/periampullary NENs have characteristic morphological features that help distinguish these tumors from other NENs of the duodenum. Approximately 60% of somatostatin-producing NENs display a characteristic mixed pseudoglandular and trabecular architectural arrangement with polarized cells arranged in pseudoglandular structures; the central lumina frequently contain diastase-resistant proteinaceous secretions (Fig. 21.25A).[149,159] Psammoma bodies are seen in approximately 60% of sporadic somatostatin-producing ampullary/periampullary NENs and in almost all NF1-associated somatostatin-producing NENs (Fig. 21.25B).[141,144] In contrast, pancreatic somatostatin-producing NENs less frequently exhibit a pseudoglandular architecture (~20%) or psammoma bodies (~40%).[141] Somatostatin-producing NENs are strongly positive for somatostatin and synaptophysin, whereas chromogranin A may or may not be expressed.[102] A subset of the tumor cells may also express other peptide hormones, including gastrin, calcitonin, and serotonin.[149,170]

Natural History

Both sporadic and NF1-associated somatostatin-producing duodenal NENs may metastasize to regional lymph nodes and to the liver.[141] The risk of metastasis appears to be related to tumor size. Tumors smaller than 2.0 cm have a low metastatic potential, whereas larger lesions are at increased risk of metastatic disease.[161] Even in the setting of metastatic disease, patients with a somatostatin-producing duodenal NEN typically have a protracted clinical course.

Neuroendocrine Neoplasms of the Distal Jejunum and Ileum

Clinical Features

In contrast with duodenal NENs, NENs of the distal jejunum and ileum are derived from serotonin-producing enterochromaffin (EC) cells and may secrete serotonin. Therefore jejunoileal NENs are true carcinoid tumors. These tumors also elicit peritumoral or mesenteric fibrosis that may produce symptoms of recurrent small bowel obstruction, bowel ischemia and infarction, and protracted abdominal pain.[171] The mechanism by which jejunoileal NENs stimulate fibrosis remains poorly understood but may be related to the secretion of serotonin or possibly growth factors by these tumors.[171] A significant percentage (approximately one-third) of jejunoileal NENs are associated with second synchronous or metachronous malignancies, most frequently adenocarcinomas of the GI, genitourinary, and gynecological tracts.[172-175] Gene expression profiling and comparative genomic hybridization analysis of jejunoileal NENs has revealed frequent loss of chromosome 18q with frequent gain of chromosomes 4 and 7 seen in metastases.[176-178] Other genetic analyses have suggested that gain of chromosome 14 predicts poor outcome in ileal NENs.[179]

Pathological Features

Jejunoileal NENs have a variable gross appearance, ranging from the presence of polypoid tan-yellow submucosal nodules to annular masses or strictures secondary to marked fibrosis characteristic of these lesions (Fig. 21.26).

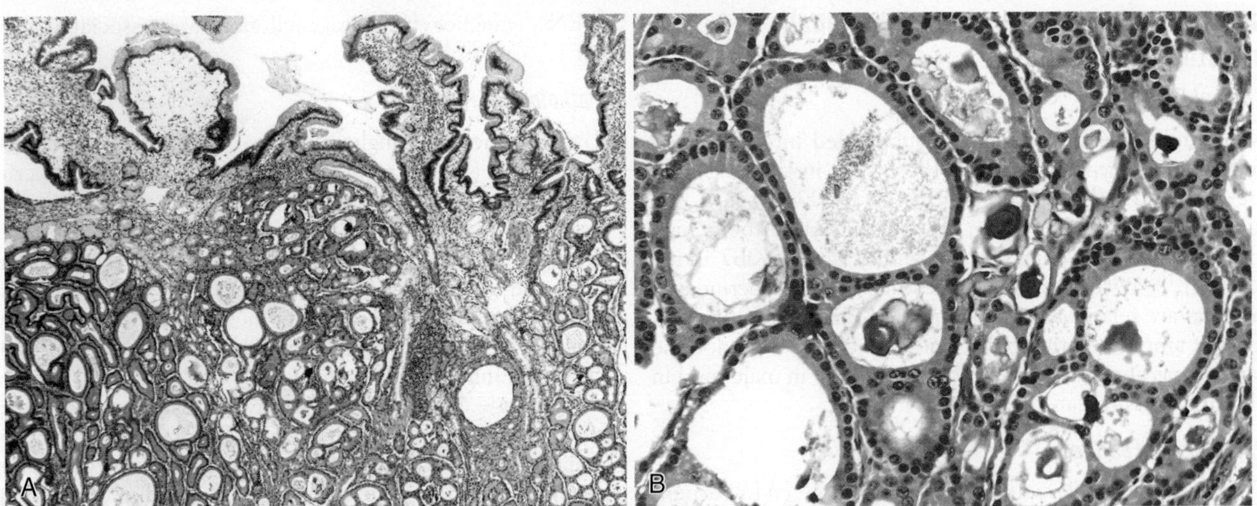

FIGURE 21.25 Ampullary somatostatin-producing, well-differentiated neuroendocrine neoplasm. The tumor is arranged predominantly in glandular structures **(A)**, some of which contain luminal proteinaceous secretions and psammoma bodies **(B)**.

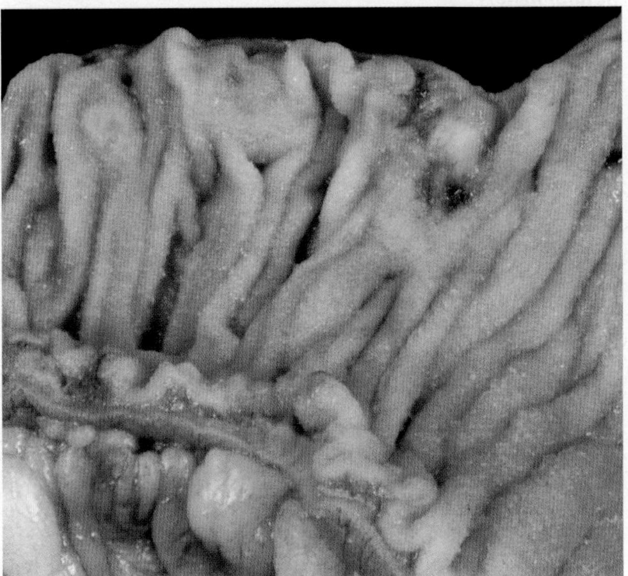

FIGURE 21.26 Multifocal, well-differentiated neuroendocrine neoplasm of the distal ileum has formed small, tan-yellow, sessile, submucosal polypoid masses.

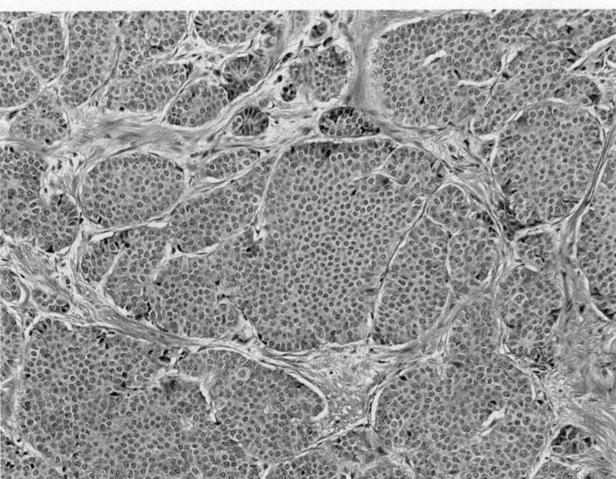

FIGURE 21.27 Well-differentiated neuroendocrine neoplasm of the terminal ileum. The tumor is composed of solid nests of cells enmeshed within a fibrotic stroma. The cells have bland, round nuclei with stippled chromatin and abundant eosinophilic cytoplasm.

Approximately 25% of tumors manifest as multiple mucosa-based polypoid lesions, which is more frequently seen in younger patients.[180] X-chromosome inactivation analysis of multifocal tumors of the small intestine has demonstrated identical X-chromosome inactivation patterns, indicating that multiple tumors represent mucosal metastases in some cases.[181]

Jejunoileal NENs are typically composed of rounded nests of uniform tumor cells with lightly eosinophilic cytoplasm (Fig. 21.27). Anastomosing cords, trabeculae, and cribriform and pseudoglandular structures may also be observed. The tumor cells are associated with densely fibrotic stroma that may compress the tumor cells into a single-file and cordlike arrangement. Most tumors demonstrate perineural and lymphovascular invasion. Jejunoileal NENs are typically strongly positive for synaptophysin and chromogranin and usually display diffuse, strong reactivity for CDX2.[136,182-186] Jejunoileal NENs are negative for PAX8, which may help localize the primary site of a NEN in the setting of metastatic disease to the liver with an unknown primary tumor.[137,138] However, the antibody commonly used for PAX8 may actually recognize another related PAX protein.[187]

Natural History

Because of their relatively small size and submucosal location, jejunoileal NENs are rarely diagnosed until the development of metastatic disease to lymph nodes or distant sites, particularly the liver. In contrast with the more favorable 5-year survival rates for NENs of the duodenum, patients with jejunoileal NENs have a relatively poor 5-year survival rate (55%).[188] Factors associated with aggressive clinical behavior include size (>1 cm), regional lymph node metastases, and metastases to the liver.[189-191] Some groups have found that female sex, age younger than 50 years, multiple mucosal nodules, and the presence of carcinoid syndrome are also associated with a poorer clinical outcome.[180,189]

Neuroendocrine Carcinoma of the Small Intestine and Ampulla

Clinical Features

Neuroendocrine carcinomas are subdivided into small cell and large cell types (similar to those seen in the lung) and are defined by the appropriate high-grade histological features of these tumor types in conjunction with either a high mitotic rate (>20 per 10 HPF) and/or a high Ki67 index (>20%).[102] Within the small intestine, neuroendocrine carcinomas are relatively rare but appear to have a predilection for the ampulla/periampullary area.[192,193] Neuroendocrine carcinomas appear to occur more frequently in males and in older patients (mean age, 68 years).[192,194]

Pathological Features

The distinction between small cell and large cell neuroendocrine carcinoma is based on a variety of cytoarchitectural features. Small cell neuroendocrine carcinoma tumor cells are typically small (less than three times the size of a small lymphocyte) and are arranged in large sheets with areas of necrosis. The nuclei display finely granular chromatin, inconspicuous nucleoli, and prominent nuclear molding.[124,125,193] Large cell neuroendocrine carcinomas usually demonstrate an architectural arrangement similar to that of well-differentiated NENs, often displaying an organoid or trabecular architecture. The tumor cells have larger, more vesicular nuclei, prominent nucleoli, and moderate amounts of cytoplasm.[124,125,193] Both small cell and large cell neuroendocrine carcinomas can be associated with adenomas of the overlying surface epithelium. In addition, adenocarcinoma has been reported to be associated with neuroendocrine carcinomas, particularly of the ampulla.[193-195] If the tumor contains a significant component (>30%) of both tumor types, the term *mixed neuroendocrine–non-neuroendocrine neoplasm (MiNEN)* should be used (this terminology replaces what was previously called *mixed adenoneuroendocrine carcinoma* or *MANEC*).[102,124,125] Rare cases of composite small cell neuroendocrine carcinoma and squamous cell carcinoma of the ampulla have also been reported.[196]

Natural History

Neuroendocrine carcinomas are clinically aggressive, and patients typically present with advanced disease. The mean survival time for patients with metastatic disease is 14.5 months.[192,193]

Gangliocytic Paraganglioma

Clinical Features

Gangliocytic paragangliomas are rare tumors that have a predilection for the ampullary/periampullary region. Gangliocytic paragangliomas occur slightly more frequently in men and usually occur in middle age (mean age, 54 years), but they have been reported to occur in younger patients.[197-199] These lesions manifest as polypoid submucosal nodules ranging in size from 2 to 4 cm. Many patients present with GI bleeding caused by mucosal erosion, but ampullary/periampullary tumors can cause obstructive jaundice.[198,200,201] Similar to somatostatin-producing NENs, gangliocytic paragangliomas are associated with NF1.[156,200,201]

Pathological Features

Gangliocytic paragangliomas are composed of a variable mixture of (1) nests of uniform polygonal neuroendocrine cells that occasionally form tubules, (2) mature ganglion cells, and (3) spindle cells with Schwannian differentiation arranged in broad fascicles or associated with the polygonal cells and ganglion cells (Fig. 21.28).[199,203,204] Psammoma bodies may be identified in the neuroendocrine cell population.[149] The neuroendocrine cells typically stain for both chromogranin A and synaptophysin but can also label for the peptide hormones somatostatin, pancreatic polypeptide, vasoactive intestinal peptide (VIP), and gastrin. The spindle cells show tapered ends, contain faintly eosinophilic cytoplasm, and stain intensely for S100 and neurofilament. The ganglion cells may be dispersed singly, or they may form small clusters and stain for synaptophysin.

Natural History

Gangliocytic paragangliomas usually follow a benign course; however, there are reports of gangliocytic paragangliomas with metastasis to regional lymph nodes, particularly large tumors (>2 cm).[205-209] Most frequently, the metastatic tumor in lymph nodes consists of the neuroendocrine component of the tumor, although cases of metastasis containing all three components have been described.[207] To our knowledge, none of the reported cases of metastatic gangliocytic paraganglioma to regional lymph nodes has resulted in patient death. To date, a review of the literature reveals only one case of malignant gangliocytic paraganglioma in which a patient with regional lymph node metastasis as well as distant metastasis to the liver and pelvis died.[210] Therefore a conservative management approach seems appropriate.

MESENCHYMAL LESIONS

A complete discussion of the clinical and pathological features of mesenchymal tumors is presented in Chapter 30. Most previously reported cases of leiomyomas, schwannomas, and neurofibromas of the small intestine likely represent gastrointestinal stromal tumors (GISTs) because true smooth muscle and nerve sheath tumors are extremely rare in the duodenum, being more likely to occur elsewhere in the GI tract. Lymphatic lesions are commonly encountered; they frequently form endoscopically visible polypoid lesions in the small intestine.

LYMPHATIC LESIONS

Dilated lymphatics are not infrequently encountered during endoscopic evaluation of the small intestine, where they appear as yellow or white plaques or polyps. Abnormalities of the small bowel lymphatics may represent a primary disorder of the small intestine, or they may be associated with numerous secondary processes. However, in one analysis, approximately 13% of patients undergoing endoscopic evaluation of the small bowel harbored incidental yellow or white plaques containing dilated lymphatics that were not associated with any other primary or secondary disorder.[211]

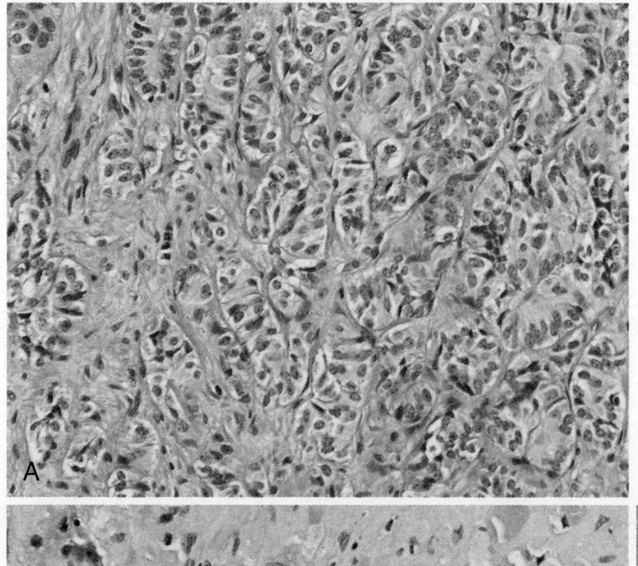

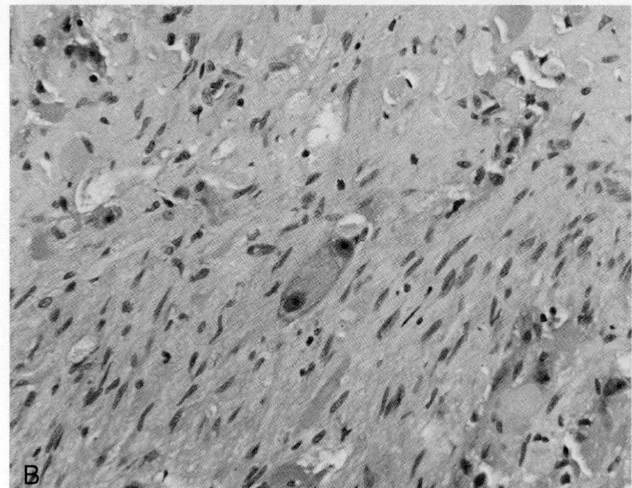

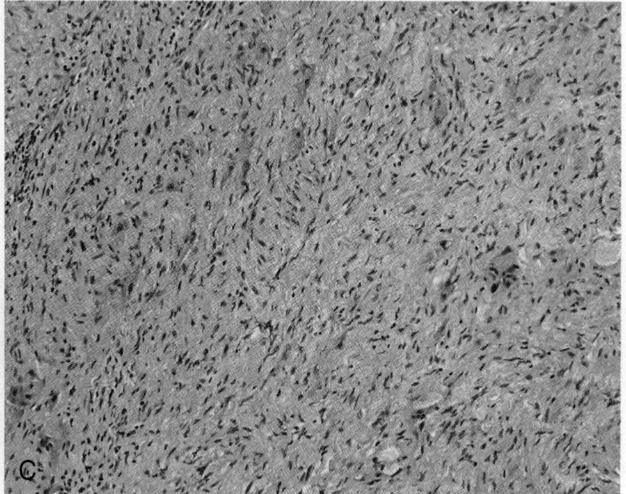

FIGURE 21.28 Gangliocytic paraganglioma. A, The neuroendocrine epithelioid cells are arranged in solid nests and trabeculae. The cells have abundant clear to amphophilic cytoplasm and round, bland nuclei. **B,** Ganglion cells with vesicular round nuclei and prominent nucleoli are characteristically interspersed within the spindle cell population. **C,** The spindle cells are arranged in fascicles that contain abundant eosinophilic cytoplasm and elongated nuclei.

Primary Lymphangiectasia

Primary intestinal lymphangiectasia (PIL), also known as *Waldmann disease,* is a rare protein-losing enteropathy typically seen in children and young adults, although rare cases have been diagnosed in adulthood. The precise etiology remains elusive; however, given the early age of clinical onset, some attention has been given to a possible genetic predisposition. Clinical symptoms vary and include edema (localized or generalized), thickening of the small bowel wall, ascites, pleural effusion, and recurrent diarrhea.[212,213] Computed tomographic imaging is most often used in the diagnosis; it reveals diffuse, nodular thickening of the bowel wall with ascites and hypodense streaks in the small bowel caused by markedly dilated lymphatics.[214,215] Mucosal biopsies are not specific, revealing only multiple dilated lymphatic spaces, but they are often necessary to confirm the presence of dilated lymphatics. Diagnosis of PIL remains challenging, and many patients experience years of symptoms before obtaining a definitive diagnosis. Once diagnosed, treatment consists predominantly of adherence to a protein-rich diet and medium-chain triglyceride (MCT) supplementation. When dietary modifications fail, various medications have been employed (i.e., octreotide and propranolol). Surgical resection remains a treatment of last resort.[213]

Secondary Lymphangiectasia

A number of disorders can give rise to dilated lymphatics in the small intestine. Acute inflammatory disorders including infections frequently display dilated lymphatics. In particular, dilated lymphatics are a common histological finding in Whipple disease, and their presence should prompt a careful evaluation for the characteristic PAS-positive macrophages in the lamina propria. Dilated lymphatics may also be the result of extraluminal compression caused by malignancy elsewhere in the GI tract or regional lymph nodes, malrotation, fibrosis, or lymph node obstruction or infiltration by inflammation, a tumor (Fig. 21.29), or infection.

LYMPHOID LESIONS

Benign Lymphoid Hyperplasia

The lamina propria of the small intestine normally contains a mild chronic inflammatory infiltrate composed predominantly of plasma cells and mature lymphocytes with occasional eosinophils, histiocytes, and mast cells. Lymphoid aggregates, many with germinal centers, are also seen in the small intestine and are found in increasing concentration distally, forming nodular aggregates of lymphocytes in the terminal ileum (Peyer patches). The specialized epithelium

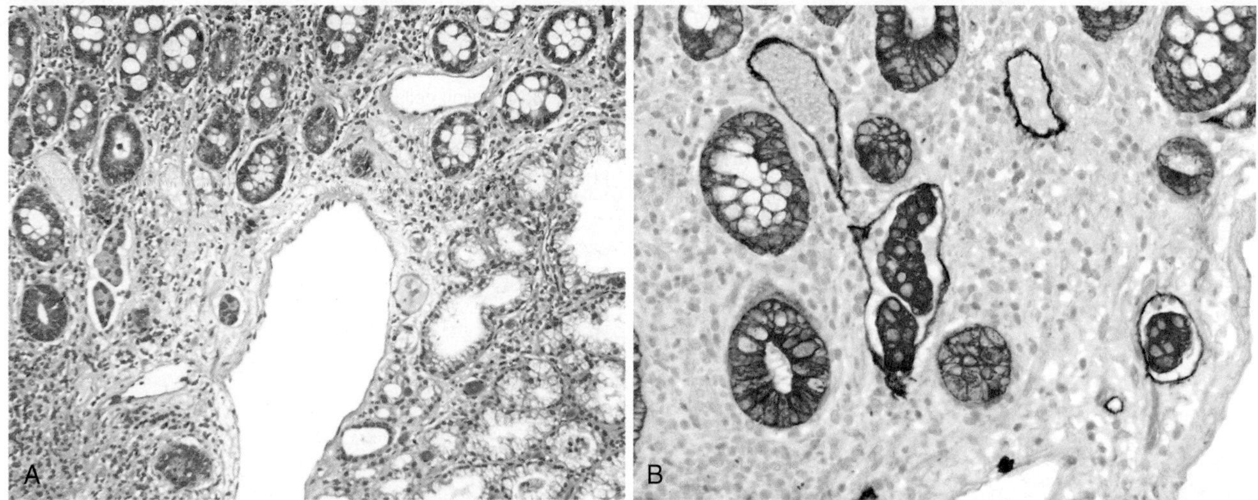

FIGURE 21.29 A, Secondary lymphangiectasia resulting from lymphatic involvement by pancreatic ductal adenocarcinoma. **B,** Cytokeratin/D2-40 double stain demonstrates the malignant cells *(red stain)* within lymphatic spaces *(brown-stained lymphatic endothelium).*

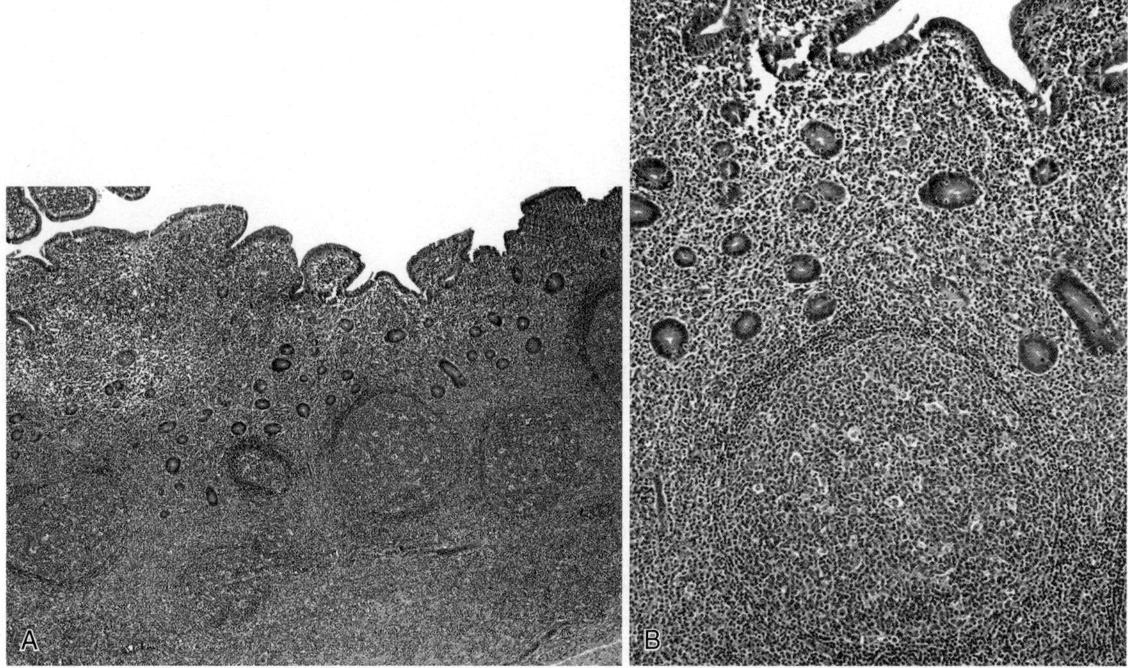

FIGURE 21.30 Nodular lymphoid hyperplasia of the duodenum. A, Confluent lymphoid aggregates are present within the mucosa in an older adult patient. The villi are blunted, and prominent germinal centers are seen **(B).** The patient ultimately proved to have a diffuse large B-cell lymphoma of the ileum.

overlying Peyer patches is distinct from the surrounding mucosa in that it contains fewer goblet cells and is associated with more abundant intraepithelial lymphocytes as well as occasional neutrophils; these findings should not be interpreted as representing enteritis. Reactive lymphoid hyperplasia in the distal ileum may occur in association with a wide variety of inflammatory disorders, including infections (e.g., *Salmonella, Yersinia, Mycobacterium*), as well as idiopathic inflammatory bowel disease.

Nodular lymphoid hyperplasia (NLH), also known as *follicular lymphoid hyperplasia,* is characterized by hyperplastic germinal centers with well-defined lymphocytic mantles located in the mucosa and submucosa (Fig. 21.30).[216] Endoscopically, the nodules may resemble small polyps, prompting biopsy. In children, NLH has been associated with infection and food allergies, and it typically follows a benign course with spontaneous regression.[217,218] In adults, NLH in the duodenum is typically a reactive process caused by a variety of conditions including peptic duodenitis, celiac disease, autoimmune enteritis, and Crohn's disease. A recent report has also linked diffuse duodenal NLH with concurrent *H. pylori*–associated gastritis.[218]

Diffuse NLH of the small intestine, distal to the ampulla, in adults is rare and usually implies the presence of an underlying immune disorder. In adults, NLH is associated most often with common variable immunodeficiency (CVID) and is occasionally seen in patients with selective immunoglobulin A (IgA) deficiency or HIV/AIDS.[217,219,220]

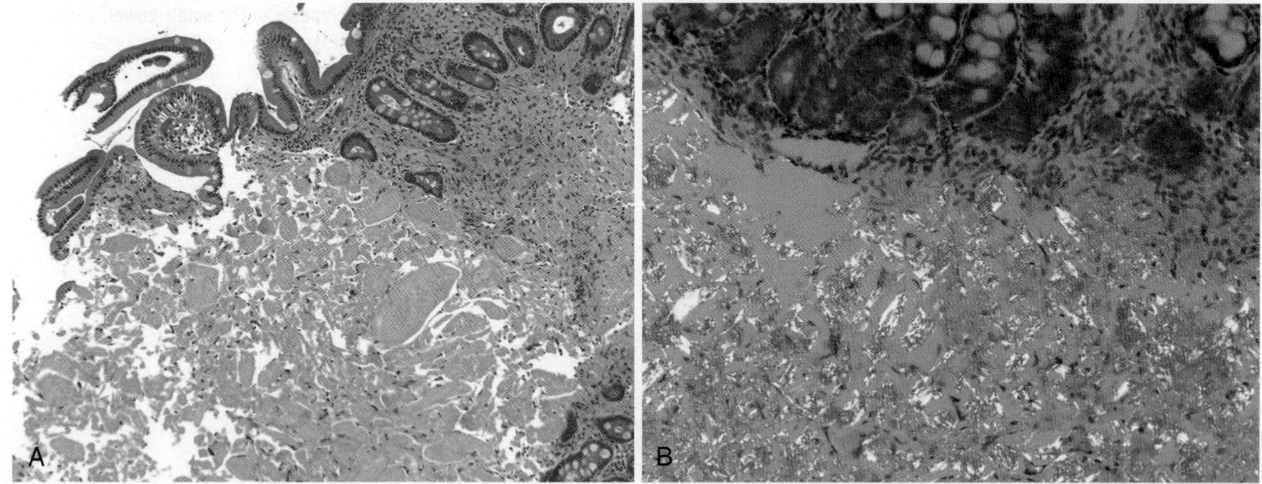

FIGURE 21.31 Polypoid amyloid deposition in a patient with multiple myeloma. A, This polyp contains prominent lamina propria deposits of amorphous eosinophilic material demonstrating characteristic birefringence on a polarized Congo red stain **(B).**

Approximately 50% of adults with CVID have NLH, which can occur diffusely throughout the small intestine.[221] A wide spectrum of histological changes can be observed in CVID. In addition to reactive NLH, prominent mononuclear inflammation in the lamina propria in association with villous blunting and increased intraepithelial lymphocytes may be seen.[221,222] A marked decrease or a complete absence of plasma cells is present in up to two-thirds of patients.[221] Concurrent infection with *Giardia lamblia* is seen in many patients with either IgA deficiency or CVID.[217,221,222] NLH may also be seen with *Giardia* infection in the absence of an identifiable humoral immunodeficiency.[223,224]

Finally, NLH has been reported to be a possible risk factor, or premalignant condition, for the development of lymphoma in the small intestine.[225] Literature reports describe the presence of NLH in the mucosa adjacent to primary small intestinal malignant lymphomas.[220,222,225-227] In such cases, there is often a gradual transition between the hyperplastic and neoplastic lymphoid tissue.[225,226] Although the data linking NLH and the development of malignant lymphoma are limited, the presence of persistent and diffuse NLH should prompt careful evaluation for the possibility of malignant lymphoma.

Malignant Lymphoma

A detailed discussion of hematopoietic malignancies that may affect the small intestine is presented in Chapter 31. With the exception of enteropathy-associated T-cell lymphoma, most lymphomas of the small intestine are B-cell lymphomas, and specific subtypes demonstrate a predilection to affect different regions of the small intestine. Enteropathy-associated T-cell lymphomas usually develop in the jejunum or distal duodenum, reflecting the disease distribution of celiac disease. Most lymphomas of the ileum are diffuse large B-cell lymphomas. Primary follicular lymphoma of the GI tract has a predilection for the duodenum and is typically low-grade with a favorable prognosis.[228-230]

Malignant lymphoid neoplasms can also result in amyloid deposition in any portion of the GI tract including the small bowel (primary amyloidosis). Secondary amyloidosis and inherited amyloidotic disorders can also involve the GI tract.[231,232] The small bowel is most commonly affected. Whereas amyloid deposition within the gut is usually around submucosal vessels, occasionally amyloid deposition can manifest as nodules or polyps (Fig. 21.31).

Multiple Lymphomatous Polyposis

Lymphomatous polyposis is an unusual form of GI involvement by lymphoma that is characterized by innumerable polypoid excrescences (Fig. 21.32). It can affect any portion of the GI tract but frequently produces large polyps in the ileocecal region. Lymphomatous polyposis usually occurs as a manifestation of mantle cell lymphoma, although other lymphoma types, including follicular lymphoma, diffuse large B-cell lymphoma, marginal zone lymphoma, and T-cell lymphoma, can give rise to lymphomatous polyposis.[233-236]

METASTASES

Adenocarcinoma is the most common primary malignancy of the small intestine and is typically identified in the duodenum in the area around the ampulla of Vater, with decreasing incidence in the jejunum and ileum.[237] Virtually any type of malignancy, however, may secondarily involve the small intestine and simulate a primary malignancy, particularly underlying pancreatic adenocarcinomas that invade into the small bowel (Fig. 21.33). When entertaining a diagnosis of primary small intestinal carcinoma, the possibility of metastasis must always be considered because metastatic disease is more common than primary small intestinal adenocarcinoma. Indeed, within the tubal gastrointestinal tract, the small intestine is the most common location for metastasis. Secondary involvement of the small intestine may occur via direct extension from another organ, peritoneal dissemination, or hematogenous or lymphovascular spread. Identifying a metastasis to the small intestine is often straightforward when there is a known history of a primary neoplasm elsewhere. If the initial primary diagnosis is remote or unknown, distinguishing a metastasis from a primary small intestinal adenocarcinoma can be difficult.[238]

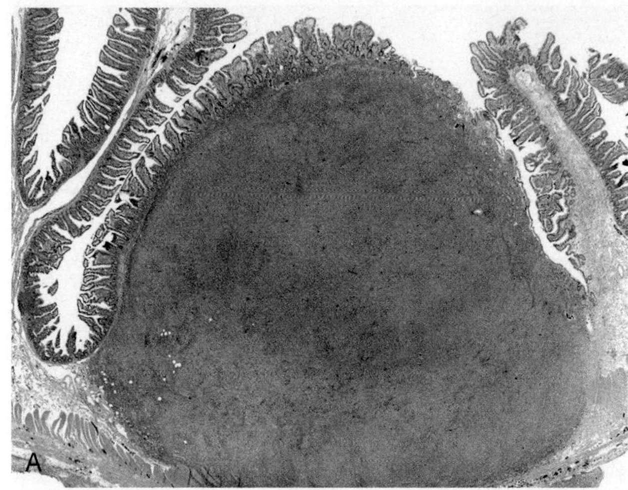

FIGURE 21.32 Lymphomatoid polyposis of the small bowel. Lymphomatoid polyposis caused by diffuse large B-cell lymphoma characterized by polypoid masses **(A)** composed of large neoplastic, CD20-positive lymphocytes **(B). C,** Lymphomatoid polyposis caused by mantle cell lymphoma characterized by an expanded mantle zone surrounding a germinal center.

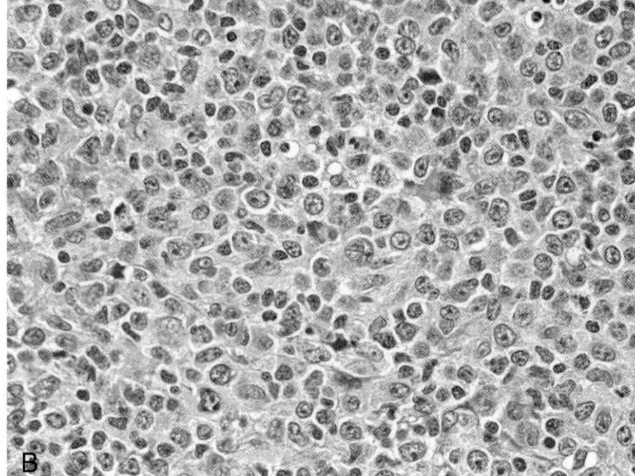

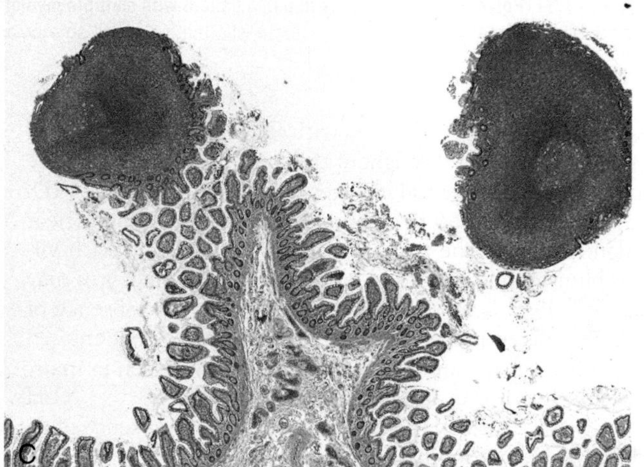

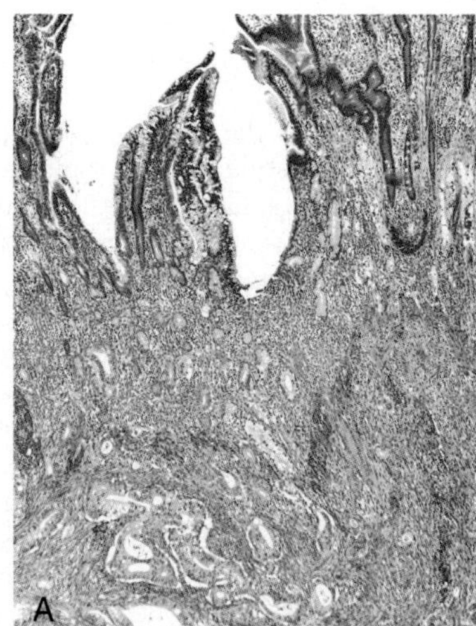

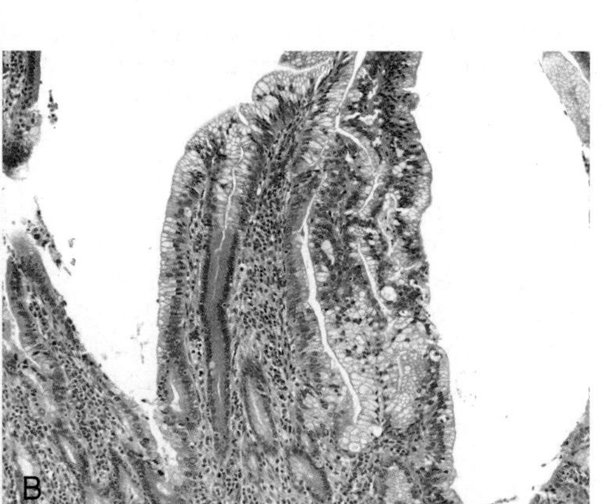

FIGURE 21.33 Secondary involvement of duodenum by pancreatic adenocarcinoma. A, Pancreatic adenocarcinoma invading the duodenum and involving the mucosal surface. Adenocarcinomas that secondarily involve the small intestine may show surface maturation when they transgress the basement membrane. In this case, neoplastic epithelial cells colonize the mucosal surface and mimic an adenoma **(B).**

Although metastases to the small bowel can arise from any number of different primary sites, the most common include the breast (particularly lobular carcinoma), skin (primarily cutaneous melanoma), lung (non–small cell lung carcinomas, particularly adenocarcinoma), gynecological tract (particularly ovarian carcinomas), and other GI tract organs (particularly colorectal adenocarcinoma).[239,240] Metastatic gastrointestinal tract and gynecological tract carcinomas usually involve the small intestine as a result of peritoneal dissemination and typically demonstrate extensive, often multifocal, involvement of the subserosal connective tissue and muscularis propria. Primary carcinomas of the lung, breast, genitourinary tract, and head and neck often secondarily involve the small intestine as a result of hematogenous dissemination, and they may produce solitary lesions limited to the mucosa and submucosa, imitating a primary intestinal carcinoma.[241-243] Breast carcinoma, particularly infiltrating lobular carcinoma, can be challenging and often infiltrates the lamina propria and submucosa without destroying the crypt epithelium (Fig. 21.34).[244]

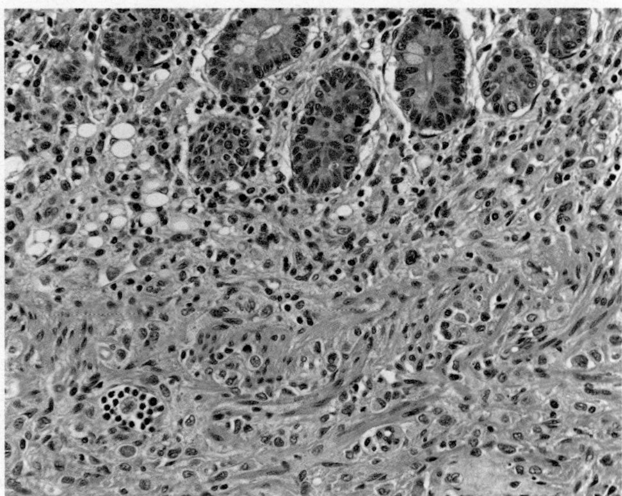

FIGURE 21.34 Metastatic lobular breast carcinoma to small bowel demonstrates subtle involvement of the deep lamina propria and infiltration of the muscularis mucosae between the small intestinal crypts.

Features favoring a diagnosis of metastatic carcinoma include multifocal involvement, extensive mural and serosal disease with minimal mucosal involvement, and extensive lymphovascular invasion. Small intestinal adenocarcinomas are of an intestinal type, and the presence of signet ring cell differentiation or a diffuse-type growth pattern is uncommon in primary carcinomas of the small intestine, especially in areas distal to the ampulla or in tumors unrelated to Crohn's disease.[245] Metastatic adenocarcinoma to the small intestine frequently demonstrates maturation of the neoplastic epithelium as it grows from the serosa toward the bowel lumen; however, it can also reach the mucosal surface of the small intestine and exhibit an in situ growth pattern along intact basement membranes, simulating a "precursor" dysplastic lesion (adenoma). In one analysis, mucosal colonization was observed in 60% of metastatic GI tract adenocarcinomas to the small intestine that involved the mucosa and in 26% of adenocarcinomas from non–GI tract primary sites.[239] Therefore the presence of an apparent in situ dysplastic lesion does not provide evidence for a primary small intestinal carcinoma.

Immunohistochemical stains are particularly helpful when considering metastasis from non–GI tract primary sites, such as the lung or breast, but are not helpful in distinguishing primary small intestinal adenocarcinoma from metastatic GI tract adenocarcinomas. Primary small intestinal adenocarcinomas often demonstrate a CK7-positive/CK20-negative or CK7-positive/CK20-positive immunophenotype. Some authors have suggested that this CK7 and CK20 expression profile may help distinguish primary small intestinal adenocarcinomas from secondary colorectal adenocarcinomas, which typically are CK7-negative and CK20-positive.[246] However, colorectal adenocarcinomas, particularly those with high levels of microsatellite instability, can coexpress CK7 and CK20 or display a CK7-positive/CK20-negative expression profile, limiting the utility of CK7 and CK20 immunohistochemistry in this setting.[247]

Malignant cutaneous melanoma shows a predilection for the GI tract and usually affects the small intestine (Fig. 21.35).[248,249] Metastatic cutaneous melanomas to the GI tract can be either pigmented or amelanotic and may mimic a variety of primary neoplasms, including carcinomas, sarcomas or GISTs, and large cell lymphomas. Immunohistochemical stains (S100 protein, HMB-45, A103 [MART-1], tyrosinase, microphthalmia transcription factor, and SOX10) have been shown to demonstrate high sensitivity and variable specificity for melanoma.[250,251] Importantly, when one is evaluating high-grade spindle cell lesions for which GIST is in the differential diagnosis, one or more melanoma stains should be included in the panel because as much as 50% of malignant melanomas can express CD117.[252-254]

The full reference list may be accessed online at *Elsevier eBooks for Practicing Clinicians.*

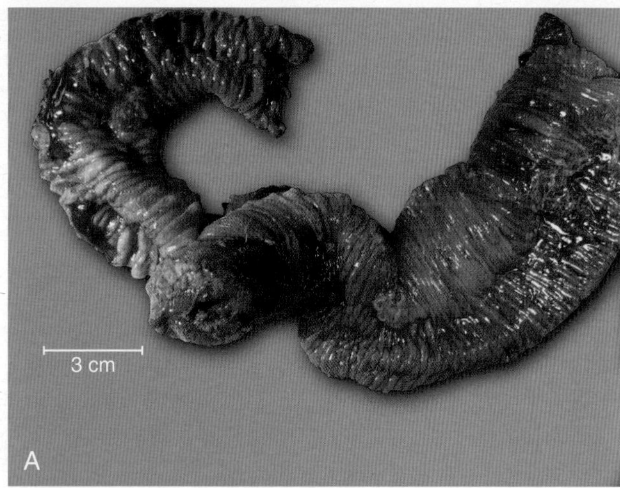

FIGURE 21.35 Metastatic melanoma. **A,** Gross image demonstrates a pigmented lesion involving the small bowel. **B,** Metastatic melanoma diffusely infiltrates the mucosa. The tumor is composed of highly pleomorphic epithelioid cells with prominent nucleoli **(C).**

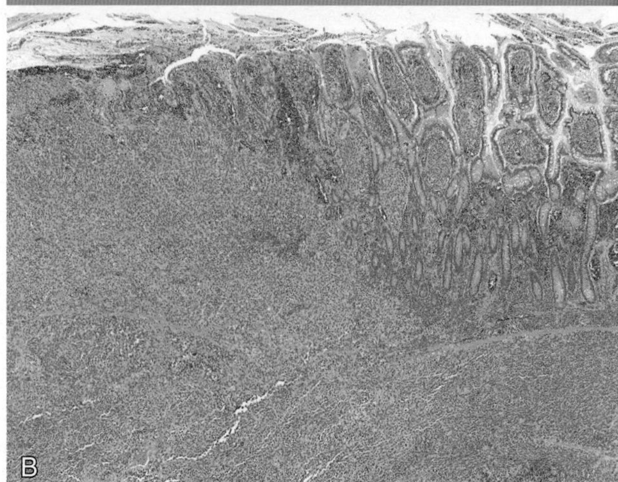

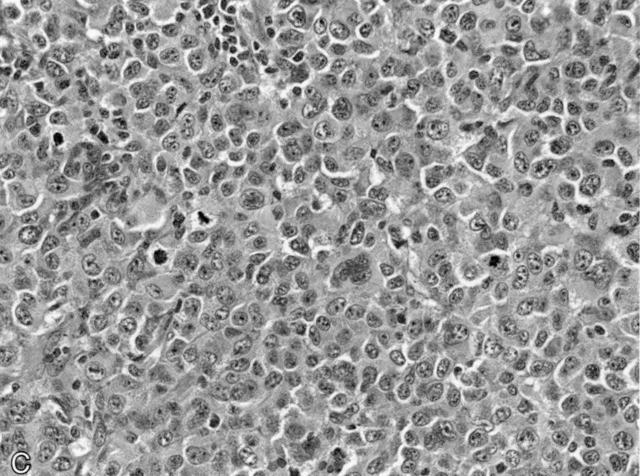

CHAPTER 22

Polyps of the Large Intestine

Rish K. Pai, Jason L. Hornick

Chapter Outline

INTRODUCTION

Large bowel screening programs have been shown to substantially reduce the incidence of colorectal carcinoma by identifying and removing premalignant polyps. Increased use of colonoscopy has led to an increase in the number of polyps encountered in daily pathology practice. Broadly speaking, the term *polyp* refers to any form of lesion that projects above the surrounding colonic mucosa. The vast majority of colorectal polyps are adenomatous, serrated, inflammatory, or hamartomatous. In addition, polyps may develop from mesenchymal proliferations, benign or malignant hematolymphoid tissue, metastatic tumors, and a wide variety of non-neoplastic substances, such as air. The relative proportions of these various types of polyps depends on the type of population undergoing endoscopy (e.g., age, associated risk factors such as inflammatory bowel disease [IBD] or

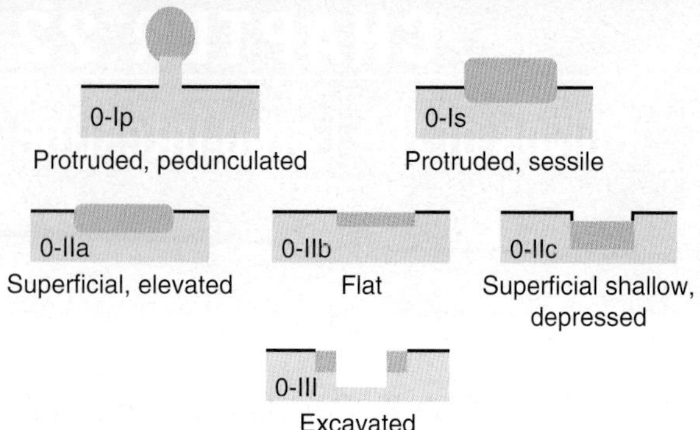

FIGURE 22.1 Paris endoscopic classification for superficial neoplastic lesions. (*Diagram 1 from The Paris Endoscopic Classification of Superficial Neoplastic Lesions: Esophagus, Stomach, and Colon: November 30 to December 1, 2002. Gastrointest Endosc. 2003;58(6 Suppl):S3-S43.*)

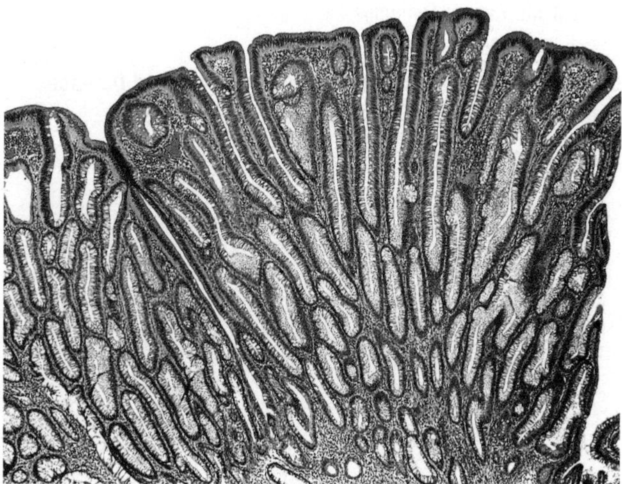

FIGURE 22.2 Tubular adenoma with predominantly tubular architecture. The adenomatous epithelial cells show mild hyperchromasia with enlarged, oval nuclei that occupy the basal half of the cell cytoplasm. Basal polarization of the nuclei is retained, and no significant pleomorphism occurs. Occasional nondysplastic crypts are evident in the deep portion for comparison.

polyposis syndrome) and the method of investigation (e.g., sigmoidoscopy vs. colonoscopy), but serrated and adenomatous polyps are by far the most common polyps in general.

ENDOSCOPIC CLASSIFICATION OF POLYPS

In 2002 an international group of endoscopists, surgeons, and pathologists gathered in Paris, France, to revise and modify a prior Japanese classification of superficial neoplastic lesions. This resulted in the Paris Endoscopic Classification for Superficial Neoplastic Lesions of the colon, and it applies to all polyps and early carcinomas that do not invade deeper than the submucosa (Fig. 22.1).[1] This classification scheme is useful because each subtype of lesion carries a different risk of invasive carcinoma, and it also helps determine the type of endoscopic resection that must be performed.

Subsequently, endoscopists have used narrow-band imaging to classify colorectal lesions as either serrated/hyperplastic, adenomatous, or invasive carcinoma based on the color, the quality of the blood vessels, and the surface mucosal pattern.[2] The Narrow-Band Imaging International Colorectal Endoscopic (NICE) classification system has been shown to have a high degree of sensitivity for predicting the presence of submucosal carcinoma,[3] but it has limited utility in distinguishing adenomatous from serrated polyps in routine clinical practice.[4] The endoscopic pit pattern and granularity have also been used to classify polyps and help predict the risk of submucosal invasive carcinoma.[5-7] Using these various endoscopic features and classification systems, gastroenterologists can determine whether the polyp in question requires an advanced endoscopic technique for removal or it can simply be removed by piecemeal polypectomy.[7]

ADENOMATOUS POLYPS

Conventional Adenoma

Clinical Features

Adenomas are common lesions. They are almost always asymptomatic. However, some patients may develop either overt, or occult, rectal bleeding, and large polyps may lead to iron-deficiency anemia. The clinical importance of adenomas is almost entirely related to their well-established premalignant nature. In general, the prevalence of adenomas increases dramatically with age. By the fifth decade of life, approximately 12% of individuals have adenomas, of which approximately 25% are considered high-risk lesions (see later).[8] After 50 years of age, the prevalence rate of adenomas continues to increase to approximately 50% of the population in high-risk Western countries such as the United States. The likelihood that adenomas will develop is strongly influenced by family history and by a variety of nutritional factors.[9,10]

Pathological Features

Adenomas are defined as in situ dysplastic clonal proliferations of epithelium (Fig. 22.2). Microscopically, adenomas are categorized, architecturally, as either tubular, tubulovillous, or villous (Fig. 22.3). However, precise histological criteria for each of these three categories vary widely. One reasonable rule of thumb is that villous adenomas should contain at least 75% villi, whereas pure tubular lesions should contain less than 25% villi. Thus tubulovillous lesions are those that contain between 25% and 75% villous epithelium. The degree of villous differentiation has been shown to increase with increasing size of the adenoma. Villous lesions are considered "advanced" for the purpose of clinical management (see later discussion).

The lamina propria of adenomas may contain a variable amount of lymphocytes, plasma cells, neutrophils, and eosinophils. Some adenomas, particularly those with high-grade dysplasia, may be ulcerated. Paneth cell or neuroendocrine cell metaplasia is a common finding and may be marked in some cases. Rarely, one may see squamous metaplasia (or squamous morules) in adenomas.[11] Some adenomas, particularly those that are pedunculated, may contain dilated and ruptured crypts with mucin extravasation into the lamina propria. Often, these cases are associated with epithelial displacement into the submucosa. Desmoplasia is not normally seen in benign colonic adenomas. When present, it should raise a very strong suspicion of a submucosal invasive adenocarcinoma.

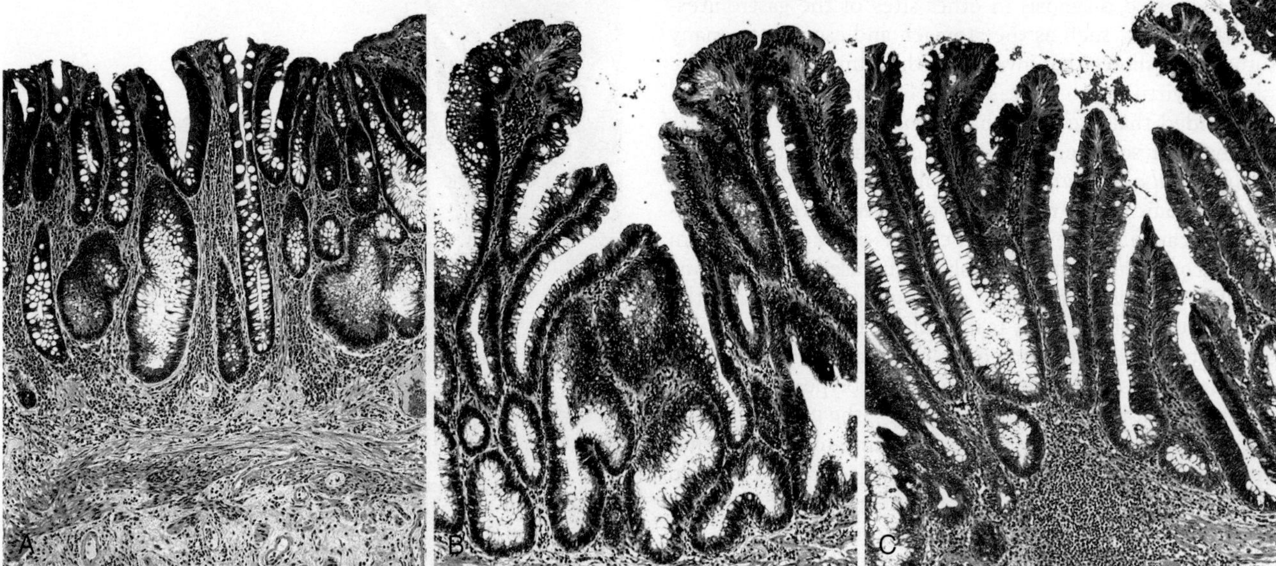

FIGURE 22.3 Each of these three adenomas displays low-grade dysplasia, but the architecture varies from tubular **(A)** to tubulovillous **(B)** to villous **(C)**. The loss of architectural rigidity is a common finding in adenomas.

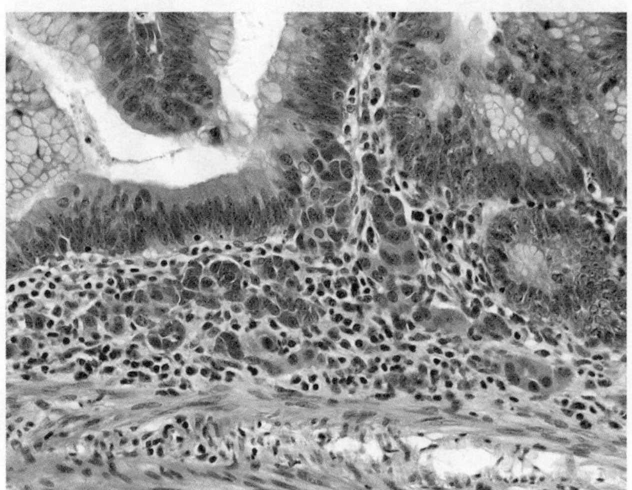

FIGURE 22.4 Composite adenoma-microcarcinoid. Clusters of well-differentiated neuroendocrine cells infiltrate the lamina propria underneath the dysplastic crypts.

Very rarely, adenomas are associated with a minute proliferation of well-differentiated neuroendocrine cells either adjacent to, or underlying, dysplastic crypts in either the mucosa or submucosa.[11-14] These lesions have been referred to as *composite adenoma-microcarcinoid tumors*.[12-14] The neuroendocrine component consists of small clusters and nests of uniform cells with round nuclei and eosinophilic cytoplasm (Fig. 22.4). The vast majority of studies indicate that composite adenoma-microcarcinoid have a benign clinical course, even when the neuroendocrine cells extend into the submucosa; however, care must be taken to exclude a high-grade neuroendocrine carcinoma arising from an adenoma.[12-17]

Grading Dysplasia in Adenomas

Microscopically, by definition, all adenomas contain at least low-grade dysplasia. Dysplasia in adenomas is generally classified as either low grade or high grade based on a combination of cytological and architectural features.[18] This classification system is favored because (1) a decrease in the degree of interobserver variability has been documented regarding interpretation of dysplasia by pathologists; (2) improved clinical pathological relevance is seen with regard to surveillance and treatment options; and (3) the term *carcinoma in situ* is often misinterpreted by clinicians as indicative of malignant behavior, which may lead to an unnecessary colonic resection.

Low-grade dysplasia is defined by the presence of architecturally noncomplex crypts containing nuclei that are pseudostratified, or partially stratified, such that the cell nuclei reach only the lower half of the cell cytoplasm. Mitotic activity may be brisk, but atypical mitoses, significant loss of polarity, and pleomorphism are minimal, if present at all. Apoptosis is usually readily identifiable throughout the adenomatous epithelium. The crypts are arranged in a parallel configuration without significant back-to-back configuration, cribriforming, or complex budding.

High-grade dysplasia is defined by marked pseudostratification, or stratification, of neoplastic nuclei that extend toward the luminal half of the cells and usually contain significant pleomorphism, increased mitotic activity, atypical mitoses, and marked loss of polarity. Architectural changes such as back-to-back gland configuration and cribriforming may also be observed. With progression of neoplasia, glands lose their orderly configuration and become more irregular and complex. In addition, neoplastic nuclei become more "open" in appearance and may contain prominent nucleoli (Fig. 22.5). The N:C ratio of the cells increases, and loss of polarity becomes marked.

The pathological criteria and clinical importance of intramucosal adenocarcinoma in adenomatous polyps is a controversial topic. Intramucosal adenocarcinoma is defined as invasion into the lamina propria, including the muscularis mucosae, but not through the muscularis mucosae into the submucosa (see Fig. 22.5). Although this is a well-recognized diagnosis in other sites of the gastrointestinal (GI) tract, such as the stomach and esophagus, many studies have shown that invasion of the lamina propria of the colon has virtually no increased risk of lymph node metastasis provided that the polyp has been completely excised.[19] This has led some authorities to conclude that the term *intramucosal adenocarcinoma* should not be used in the setting of colonic adenomatous polyps, given the lack of clinical significance. However, other experts argue that the term *intramucosal adenocarcinoma* should be used in any setting in which there is pathological evidence of invasion into the lamina propria, but that it is incumbent on the pathologist, gastroenterologist, and surgeon to understand the biological potential of this phenomenon, and that polypectomy is sufficient to treat these lesions. Ultimately, the goal is to avoid unnecessary surgery for patients with intramucosal adenocarcinoma. However, if one feels compelled to use the term adenoma with intramucosal adenocarcinoma, the diagnostic report should always include a statement regarding the absence of submucosally invasive cancer, the status of the resection margin, and the overall adequacy of resection and need for further therapy, which in most cases is best accomplished with endoscopic polypectomy.

Natural History and Treatment

Screening colonoscopy has played a major role in the steady decline in the incidence of colorectal carcinoma in the United States.[20] The National Polyp Study,[10,21] a large study initiated in 1990, has demonstrated that removal of adenomas by endoscopic polypectomy significantly decreases both the incidence of colorectal adenocarcinoma and colorectal cancer–specific mortality.[22] Patients with colon cancer identified on screening colonoscopy not only have lower-stage disease at presentation, but also have more favorable outcomes independent of their staging.[23] The best predictor for the presence of malignancy within an adenoma at the time of excision is the polyp size. Among adenomas larger than 2 cm, there is a 10% to 20% risk of carcinoma in the polyp at the time of removal. Adenomas measuring between 1 and 2 cm have a 5% risk of harboring cancer, and those smaller than 1 cm have a much lower risk of adenocarcinoma (<1%).[24-26]

The degree of dysplasia also represents an independent risk factor for malignancy in adenomas, regardless of polyp size. Most adenomas harbor only low-grade dysplasia. However, larger lesions have a greater likelihood of harboring high-grade dysplasia.[18,27,28] Nevertheless, high-grade dysplasia within a colorectal adenoma does not increase the risk of carcinoma elsewhere in the patient's colon.[27] Because of the time involved for an adenoma to acquire sufficient molecular changes for it to become invasive, most remain benign. In general, adenomas are slow-growing lesions. The lifetime prevalence rate of adenomas is approximately 50%, whereas the lifetime prevalence of colorectal adenocarcinoma is approximately 6%. Therefore it is evident that only a small minority of polyps ultimately develop adenocarcinoma. Actual longitudinal follow-up data have been difficult to obtain because adenomas are typically removed at the time of endoscopic identification.[24] One cohort of 35 patients, all of whom had an adenoma smaller than 5 mm in maximum diameter, was followed up for 2 years. In 50% of the patients, an increase in size of the adenoma occurred; in the remainder, the lesion remained unchanged or even regressed slightly.[24]

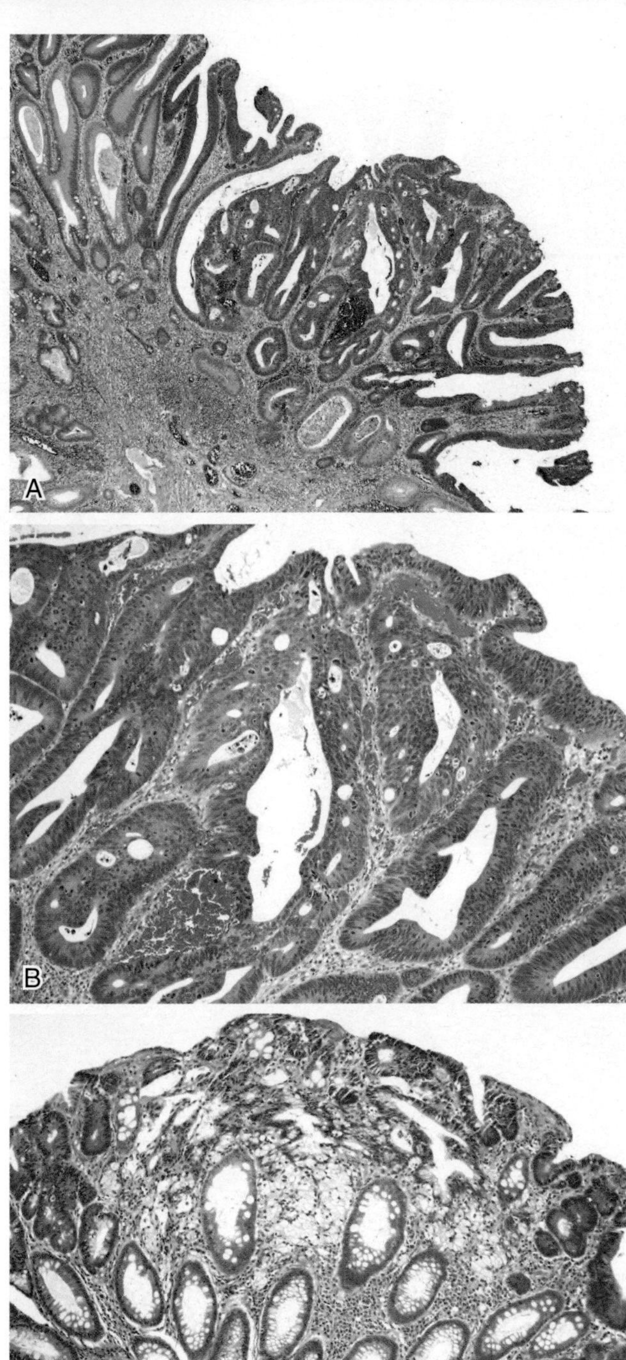

FIGURE 22.5 High-grade dysplasia and intramucosal adenocarcinoma in an adenoma. **A,** This tubulovillous adenoma has a focus of high-grade dysplasia. **B,** This typical focus of high-grade dysplasia shows a marked degree of nuclear hyperchromasia, pseudostratification, and loss of polarity from the base to the surface of the mucosa. The architecture is also complex with areas of cribriform growth. **C,** This adenoma from a patient with known Lynch syndrome has a focus of intramucosal adenocarcinoma with sheetlike growth of signet ring cells within the lamina propria.

BOX 22.1 Guidelines for Adenoma/Carcinoma Surveillance

1. Average risk (no first-degree relative with colon cancer)
Colonoscopy at 50 years of age:
    - If no adenoma or carcinoma, repeat in 10 years
    - If 1 to 2 tubular adenomas <10 mm, repeat in 7 to 10 years
    - If 3 to 4 tubular adenomas <10 mm, repeat in 3 to 5 years
    - If 5 to 10 tubular adenomas <10 mm, repeat in 3 years
    - If adenoma ≥10 mm, repeat in 3 years
    - If adenoma with high-grade dysplasia, tubulovillous or villous architecture, repeat in 3 years
    - If >10 adenomas on single examination, repeat in 1 year (consider genetic testing for these patients and for those with >10 cumulative adenomas)
    - If piecemeal resection of and adenoma ≥20 mm, repeat in 6 months
2. Moderate risk (first-degree relative with colon cancer before 60 years of age or ≥2 first-degree relatives with colon cancer)
Colonoscopy at 40 years of age or 10 years before age of occurrence in relative, whichever comes first: follow guidelines as above
3. High risk (familial adenomatous polyposis [FAP], Lynch syndrome, serrated polyposis)
    - FAP: Colonoscopy every 1 to 2 years beginning at 10 to 12 years of age
    - Lynch syndrome: Colonoscopy every 1 to 2 years beginning at 20 to 25 years of age
    - Serrated polyposis: Colonoscopy every 1 year after diagnosis

The appropriate treatment for all colorectal adenomas, regardless of their size, architectural type, or degree of dysplasia, is complete endoscopic removal with negative margins (Box 22.1).[29,30]

Surveillance Guidelines

Colorectal adenocarcinoma prevention screening recommendations are based on the distribution of adenomas throughout the colon, the age of the patient, and the patient's family history (see Box 22.1). Although most adenomas occur distal to the splenic flexure, up to 40% occur in the proximal colon. At least one-fourth of patients have adenomas that are present only proximal to the splenic flexure.[31-33] For this reason, full colonoscopy is the preferred method for screening in the United States over all other modalities.[34] Yearly fecal immunochemical testing (FIT) is suitable for those who decline colonoscopy. Second-tier tests include CT-colonography every 5 years, FIT-fecal-DNA test every 3 years, and flexible sigmoidoscopy every 5 to 10 years. The current consensus regarding screening guidelines supports the use of colonoscopy starting at 50 years of age, although there have been recent recommendations to reduce the age to 45. Persons with a family history of colorectal carcinoma in a first-degree relative diagnosed before 60 years of age should undergo colonoscopy every 5 years beginning at 40 years of age, or 10 years before the age at which the patient's relative was diagnosed with an adenomatous polyp.[29,35-37] African Americans should undergo initial screening at 45 years of age. Colonoscopy should be repeated every 1 to 10 years, depending on the findings at the initial screening, and the patient's family history. See Chapter 2 for details of screening and surveillance.

Key Reporting Issues for Pathologists

Aside from the diagnosis of an "adenoma," pathologists should also report the architectural pattern (tubular, tubulovillous, or villous), particularly when villous; the presence or absence of high-grade dysplasia; and the status of the polypectomy margins whenever possible. Small, "diminutive" tubular adenomas are usually excised in total, and these are usually removed in such a manner that it is often not possible to evaluate the margins of the specimen. This is normally acceptable from a clinical point of view because the endoscopist is keenly aware of the method used to excise the polyp, and as a result, the possibility of a lack of ability of the pathologist to evaluate margins when removed as such. Similarly, margins cannot normally be evaluated in large adenomas that are removed by piecemeal polypectomy. In this situation, the endoscopist would normally know whether the polyp was removed in total (and as such, determination of the margins by the pathologist is not necessary) and also whether a certain fragment of polyp represented the stalk of the polyp where the deep margin resides. In this case, the pathologist may issue a comment regarding the status of the piece of tissue that was designated as the polyp stalk. For polyps that are removed in piecemeal, it would be expected to find multiple pieces of tissue with cautery effect at the edges of tissue fragments, either with or without dysplasia. These do not normally represent the final margins of the polyp, however. In situations in which the margin cannot be evaluated, it is usually helpful to indicate this in the diagnostic report. In contrast, if a polyp is removed in one piece, then the status of the resection margins should be evaluated and commented on in the pathology report. If possible, the number of each polyp type should be provided; however, this is often difficult when multiple polyps are placed in the same jar. The endoscopic size of the polyp is used for postpolypectomy surveillance guidelines; however, if the endoscopic size is markedly different from the histological size, it is helpful to comment on this finding as well.

A key issue is risk stratification of patients based on the likelihood of developing advanced neoplasia in the future. Patients are divided into those with low risk (defined as 1 to 2 tubular adenomas <10 mm in size), intermediate risk (3 to 4 tubular adenomas <10 mm), and high risk defined as an *advanced adenoma* (adenoma with villous features, high-grade dysplasia, or adenocarcinoma, size ≥10 mm, or five or more adenomas) (see Box 22.1). Advanced adenomas require more aggressive colonoscopic surveillance given the increased risk for further metachronous adenomas and adenocarcinoma.[29] Unfortunately, the degree of interobserver variability is high for determination of the presence and degree of villous architecture and the presence or absence of high-grade dysplasia, even among expert GI pathologists.[37] However, the vast majority of villous adenomas, or adenomas with high-grade dysplasia, are ≥10 mm in size. Thus these polyps are considered "advanced" regardless of the presence or absence of these high-risk features, therefore the lack of interobserver agreement for villosity and/or high-grade dysplasia would not affect surveillance. Importantly, the finding of advanced morphological features should not be considered an indication for colectomy because advanced lesions have no potential for metastasis unless they harbor an invasive cancer.

Adenoma with Epithelial Displacement

Clinical Features and Pathogenesis

Foci of displaced or "misplaced" epithelium or mucin extravasation within the submucosa is a rather common finding in adenomas, particularly in polyps that have a long or pedunculated stalk, and those from the left colon versus the right colon. This may lead to a misdiagnosis of invasive adenocarcinoma.[38-41] This pathological reaction occurs in 2% to 4% of adenomatous polyps; it tends to occur more commonly in the left colon and particularly in the sigmoid colon, where the intraluminal pressures are higher and peristalsis is more vigorous. It occurs in patients of all ages and is slightly more common among males. Displaced epithelium in adenomas is believed to occur secondary to peristalsis-induced twisting and torsion of the polyp stalk, which leads to vascular compromise, inflammation, breakdown of the muscularis mucosae, and eventually herniation of adenomatous epithelium into the submucosa. Thus this reaction occurs much more commonly in polyps that have a long stalk, which are more susceptible to twisting and torsion. Rarely, adenomatous glands can herniate into a submucosal lymphoid aggregate. This results in formation of a "lymphoglandular complex." This phenomenon tends to occur in regions of the mucosa in which the muscularis mucosae is incomplete or shows breaches in its integrity and sites in which blood vessels enter the mucosa from the submucosa.[42] Such adenomas tend to be sessile in structure, in contrast with the more common pedunculated polyp that more often contains epithelial displacement resulting from tissue injury.

Pathological Features and Differential Diagnosis

The intramucosal portion of an adenoma that contains displaced epithelium may have features that range from low- to high-grade dysplasia, and it may be tubular, tubulovillous, or villous. More often than not, foci of displaced epithelium show a similar degree of dysplasia to that in the intramucosal portion of the polyp. The epithelium in the submucosa is usually well-lobulated and composed of well-circumscribed aggregates of crypts in a pattern reminiscent of the mucosal portion of the polyp. Displaced epithelium is usually surrounded by a distinct rim of lamina propria, is often associated with hemorrhage or hemosiderin deposition in the stroma, shows no evidence of desmoplasia, and lacks the cytological and architectural features of invasive carcinoma (Fig. 22.6). Mucin pools, when present in association with displaced epithelium, are usually either acellular or lined by dysplastic epithelium of a grade similar to that in the surface mucosal portion of the polyp. Furthermore, mucin pools are typically smooth and regular, and they are usually associated with extravasated mucin associated with ruptured crypts in the surface of the polyp. In contrast, the presence of irregular, small, jagged mucin pools dissecting through the submucosal stroma or the presence of mucin pools associated with cytologically malignant cells floating in the pools of mucin are features suggestive of adenocarcinoma.

Table 22.1 outlines features of adenomas with displaced epithelium from invasive adenocarcinoma.[40-43] Features suggestive of adenocarcinoma include (1) epithelium that contains a greater degree of cytological and architectural atypia than that of the intramucosal portion of the adenoma; (2) architectural complexity, such as the presence of irregular, tortuous, and jagged crypts; (3) back-to-back and cribriform crypt formation; (4) a nonlobular configuration of crypts; (5) single or small clusters of cells without a surrounding rim of lamina propria; (6) a desmoplastic reaction; and (7) the absence of hemorrhage or hemosiderin deposition in the stroma (Fig. 22.7). Although displaced benign crypts usually demonstrate a communication of the intramucosal portion of the polyp on deeper sectioning, this feature may also occur in cases with adenocarcinoma, but it is more common in the former compared with the latter.

Treatment

Adenomas with epithelial displacement should be excised in total, with confirmation that the mucosal and deep cauterized margins of the polyp are negative, similar to adenomas without epithelial displacement.[44] For management purposes, pools of mucin associated with a rim of dysplastic epithelium at the deep resection margin should be considered "positive" for adenomatous epithelium. The significance of the presence of acellular mucin pools at the cauterized deep resection margin is unclear. As such, this should probably warrant close endoscopic follow-up. Cases in which a definite distinction from invasive adenocarcinoma cannot be made with complete certainty should probably be managed individually according to other clinical health factors (see Malignant Polyps). If invasion cannot be ruled out with certainty, but there are no unfavorable histological features, then polypectomy would be considered adequate treatment regardless. In almost all cases in which uncertainty regarding the presence of a small focus of invasive carcinoma exists, complete polypectomy will usually be sufficient because "unfavorable" histological features are unlikely to be present. However, in cases in which invasion cannot be ruled out with certainty, but the foci of uncertainty involve a deep or lateral resection margin, then surgical resection should be considered if the clinical circumstances support surgery.

Flat or Depressed Adenomas

Flat adenomas are defined as noninvasive dysplastic lesions without an intraluminal polypoid component (Paris 0-IIa, IIb, and IIc).[45-49] They may be slightly raised at the edges, but typically they have a central depression. Some authorities define these as adenomas with a height (thickness) less than two times that of adjacent normal mucosa. Flat adenomas are associated with molecular abnormalities somewhat different from conventional polypoid adenomas.[46,48] The molecular phenotype is thought to be of a more aggressive nature than that of typical adenomas by some authorities, but this is highly controversial. Some reports cite an increased prevalence rate of high-grade dysplasia and a higher rate of progression to adenocarcinoma than conventional adenomas.[47,48] However, one large follow-up study of 474 flat adenomas from the National Polyp Study cohort found neither a higher rate of high-grade dysplasia nor an increased risk of advanced adenomas on follow-up, compared with either conventional sessile or pedunculated adenomatous polyps.[50]

Of practical clinical importance, these lesions may also be more difficult to identify endoscopically. An accurate assessment of the prevalence rate and natural history of these lesions may depend on more extensive studies that utilize chromoendoscopy or high-resolution endoscopy, or both.[45] Lynch et al. described two families with flat adenomatous polyposis.[51-53] The lesions in these patients

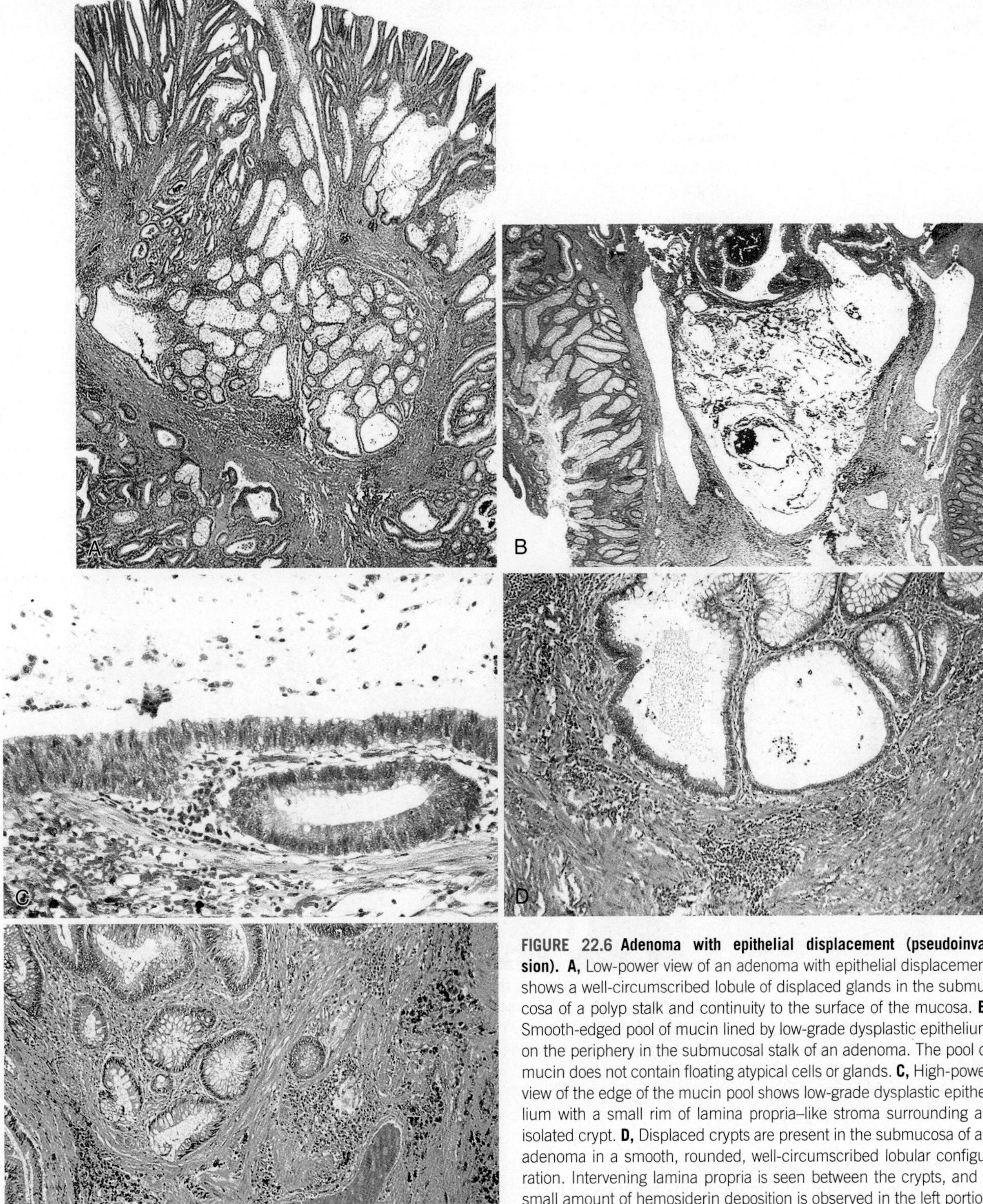

FIGURE 22.6 Adenoma with epithelial displacement (pseudoinvasion). A, Low-power view of an adenoma with epithelial displacement shows a well-circumscribed lobule of displaced glands in the submucosa of a polyp stalk and continuity to the surface of the mucosa. **B,** Smooth-edged pool of mucin lined by low-grade dysplastic epithelium on the periphery in the submucosal stalk of an adenoma. The pool of mucin does not contain floating atypical cells or glands. **C,** High-power view of the edge of the mucin pool shows low-grade dysplastic epithelium with a small rim of lamina propria–like stroma surrounding an isolated crypt. **D,** Displaced crypts are present in the submucosa of an adenoma in a smooth, rounded, well-circumscribed lobular configuration. Intervening lamina propria is seen between the crypts, and a small amount of hemosiderin deposition is observed in the left portion of the photograph. **E,** In another area, the displaced crypts are slightly separated from one another, and marked congestion and hemosiderin deposition are seen around the edges of the displaced epithelium.

TABLE 22.1 Adenomas with Epithelial Displacement vs. Adenocarcinoma

Feature	Displaced Epithelium	Invasive Adenocarcinoma
Pedunculated shape	Usually present	Present or absent
Architecture	Round, smooth, lobular arrangement of crypts	Irregular, variably sized tortuous crypts, single cells, small clusters of cells
Crypts	Noncomplex	Complex, cribriform, budding
Mucin pools	Round, smooth, lined by dysplastic epithelium at periphery	Irregular, floating cells may be present
Hemorrhage/hemosiderin	Usually present	Usually absent
Desmoplasia	Absent	Usually present
Lamina propria around crypts	Usually present	Absent
Communication to surface	Often present	Present or absent
Degree of dysplasia	Similar to polyp surface	Carcinoma-like

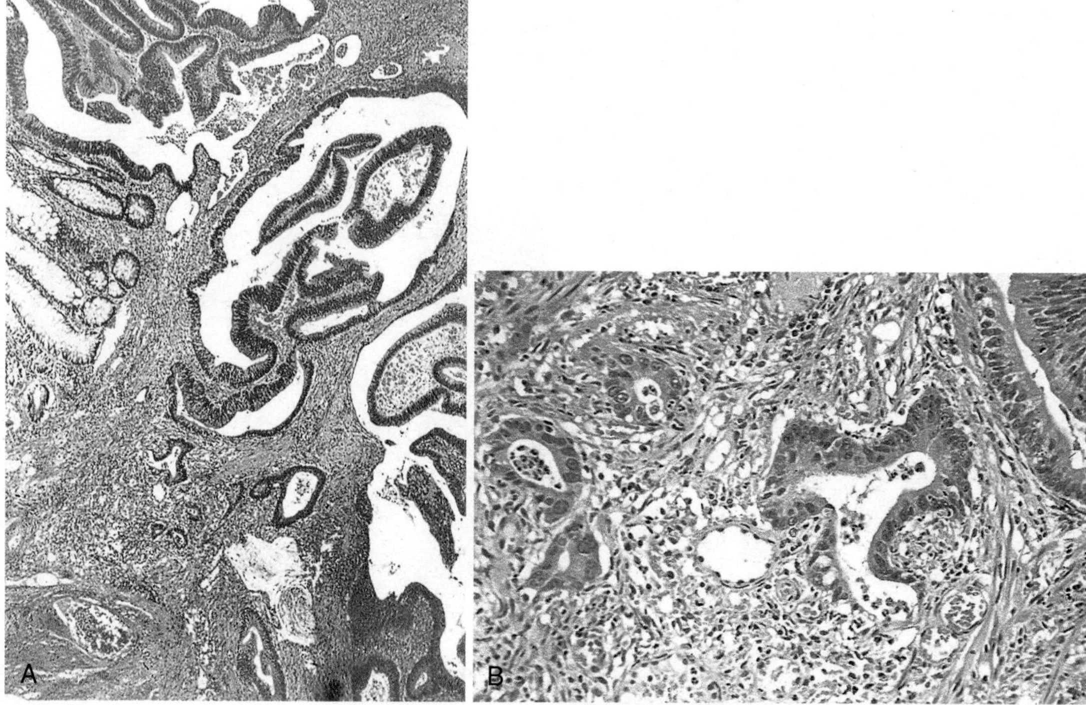

FIGURE 22.7 A, In contrast with adenomas with epithelial displacement, this adenoma contains invasive, well-differentiated adenocarcinoma in the central portion of the polyp stalk. The infiltrating glands are irregular in size and shape and show a lack of lamina propria surrounding the invasive glands; no evidence of hemorrhage or hemosiderin deposition is seen. The infiltrating glands are irregular and jagged in contour and infiltrate in a nonlobular fashion. **B,** High-power view of infiltrating glands shows their irregular profile, surrounding inflammation, and an early desmoplastic reaction.

were predominantly right-sided, but they did not have typical features of familial adenomatous polyposis (FAP) or Lynch syndrome. Subsequent studies showed that patients with so-called *hereditary flat adenoma syndrome* actually have attenuated FAP (see later discussion).[54,55] A flat adenoma may result in the development of flat, or depressed, invasive adenocarcinoma without evidence of residual overlying or adjacent adenomatous epithelium. However, this phenomenon may also occur in large cancers that, upon growth, obliterate the overlying adenomatous epithelium.

Adenomatous Polyposis Syndromes

Familial Adenomatous Polyposis

FAP is an autosomal dominant condition caused by either inheritance of a mutated *APC* gene (located on chromosome 5q) or a new germline mutation in the same gene (up to one-third of cases).[56] Adenomas then develop from loss of the second *APC* allele in colonic epithelial cells.[57] *APC* is a tumor suppressor gene, and its absence allows for additional mutations in other genetic loci, such as in the *KRAS* and *TP53* genes (see Chapters 23 and 27). FAP patients

TABLE 22.2 Adenomatous Polyposis Syndromes

Syndrome	Colorectal Polyps	Extracolonic Lesions	Genetics	Risk of Malignancy
Familial adenomatous polyposis (FAP)	Adenomatous polyps (100s to 1000s)	Duodenal/periampullary adenomas, gastric fundic gland polyps, congenital hypertrophy of the retinal pigment epithelium, osteomas, dental abnormalities, desmoid tumors, brain tumors	Autosomal dominant *APC* mutations	100% risk of colorectal carcinoma (mean age 35-40 years) 3%-5% risk of duodenal/periampullary carcinoma
Attenuated FAP	<100 adenomatous polyps	Similar to conventional FAP	Autosomal dominant *APC* mutations	80% risk of colorectal carcinoma (mean age 50 years)
MUTYH-associated polyposis	Oligopolyposis with adenomas and serrated polyps	Uncertain	Autosomal recessive *MUTYH* mutations	80% risk of colorectal carcinoma
Polymerase proofreading–associated polyposis	>10 adenomas	Uncertain	Autosomal dominant *POLE* and *POLD1* mutations	40%-60% risk of colorectal carcinoma
NTHL1 polyposis	>10 adenomas	Sebaceous skin lesions	Autosomal recessive *NTHL1* mutations	High risk of colorectal carcinoma
MSH3-associated polyposis	>10 adenomas	Duodenal adenomas, gastric cancer, early-onset astrocytoma	Autosomal recessive *MSH3* mutations	High risk of colorectal carcinoma
AXIN2-associated polyposis	>10 adenomas	Ectodermal dysplasia	Autosomal dominant *AXIN2* mutations	High risk of colorectal carcinoma

develop large numbers of colorectal adenomas during late childhood, adolescence, and early adulthood. FAP has been traditionally defined by the presence of more than 100 adenomatous polyps in the colon, although many patients have several hundred or even thousands of polyps. Adenocarcinoma develops in most patients by their mid-30s, but it can occur as early as 17 years of age. FAP accounts for approximately 1% of all colon cancers.

The frequency of FAP is from 1 in 8000 to 1 in 14,000 in the general population, with equal sex representation worldwide.[58] FAP patients may express a variety of extraintestinal phenotypes (see later discussion), but all include the presence of adenomatous polyps of the GI tract. They are predisposed to a high rate of adenocarcinoma. Upper GI tract adenomas and adenocarcinomas may also develop in FAP patients at a high frequency; they are particularly prominent in the first and second portions of the duodenum and in the periampullary region.[59-61] Periampullary adenomas and adenocarcinomas have recently become the most common causes of morbidity and mortality in FAP patients who have undergone prophylactic colectomy. The prevalence of noncolonic adenomas in FAP ranges from 9% to 50% in the stomach and from 50% to 100% in the duodenum. Much less commonly, patients with FAP develop thyroid carcinoma, brain tumors (discussed later), pancreatic carcinoma, and hepatoblastoma.

Cyclooxygenase-2 (COX-2) inhibitors have received considerable attention lately as a method of decreasing polyp burden in FAP patients [62] or reducing or eliminating rectal adenomas in patients who have had a subtotal colectomy.[63] COX-2 inhibitors may also decrease the extent of duodenal polyposis in FAP patients.[64,65] Gardner's syndrome, Turcot's syndrome, and attenuated FAP are considered subtypes of FAP; these are discussed in the following sections (Table 22.2).

For most patients, the treatment of choice is screening during adolescence followed by a postadolescent prophylactic colectomy.

Variants of Familial Adenomatous Polyposis

Desmoid fibromatosis affects 15% of patients with FAP and has been referred to as *Gardner's syndrome,* although use of this term is no longer recommended by the World Health Organization (WHO).[59,66,67] Desmoid tumors in these patients occur most commonly in the small bowel mesentery and abdominal wall. Surgical incisions can also increase the incidence of desmoid fibromatosis. Osteomas (particularly in the mandible, skull, and long bones), epidermoid cysts, dental abnormalities, and congenital hypertrophy of the retinal pigmented epithelium (CHRPE) can also occur. Overall, CHRPE affects 70% to 80% of FAP patients.

Central nervous system tumors can occur in association with both FAP and Lynch syndrome. This is referred to as *Turcot's syndrome,* although this term is also no longer recommended by the WHO as many patients have been found to have constitutional mismatch repair deficiency.[59,68,69] Although medulloblastomas are the most common primary central nervous system tumor in FAP patients,[70] astrocytomas and ependymomas can also occur. In contrast, the most common primary central nervous system tumor in patients with Lynch syndrome and constitutional mismatch repair deficiency is glioblastoma.

Attenuated Familial Adenomatous Polyposis

The term *attenuated FAP* refers to a hereditary colon cancer syndrome with fewer than 100 colonic polyps (usually <30).[54,71] Many such patients, on closer endoscopic examination or with the assistance of methylene blue staining, are found to harbor more than 100 polyps, so these patients may, in fact, have conventional FAP. When patients are seen with a suspicious family history, or mild polyposis, or both, the diagnosis can be further investigated by assaying for mutations in the *APC* gene. In attenuated FAP, as opposed to classic FAP, *APC* mutations tend to occur at the most 5′ or 3′ aspect of the gene.[59,72] Once the mutations are discovered, these patients require close endoscopic screening for removal of polyps and prevention of adenocarcinoma development. In addition to being fewer in number, adenomas and adenocarcinomas develop at a later stage in life compared with classic FAP; the lifetime risk of colorectal carcinoma in attenuated FAP is approximately 80%. These adenomas, and adenocarcinomas, are otherwise of unremarkable morphology, although many of the adenomas in some patients with attenuated FAP are "flat" (see earlier discussion). Upper GI lesions and extraintestinal manifestations develop at a rate similar to that observed in classic FAP.

MUTYH-Associated Polyposis

There is an alternative genetic mechanism for the attenuated FAP phenotype, one that is inherited in an autosomal recessive fashion (unlike the mutations that cause FAP).[59,73] In 2002, Al-Tassan et al. studied a family whose members harbored multiple colorectal adenomas and carcinomas, but lacked *APC* mutations.[74] They discovered that affected patients carried biallelic mutations in the mutY DNA glycosylase gene *(MUTYH)* located on the short arm of chromosome 1, which encodes a base excision repair enzyme responsible for preventing mutations after oxidative DNA damage. Mutations in *MUTYH* results in G→T conversions throughout the genome. Other groups have detected homozygous or compound heterozygous *MUTYH* mutations in 15% to 40% of patients who have between 10 and 100 adenomas.[75,76] The highest frequency of *MUTYH*-associated polyposis is seen in patients with more than 30 adenomatous polyps, but who have no family history of polyposis.[77] Patients with *MUTYH*-associated polyposis can also have multiple serrated polyps, suggesting some overlap with serrated polyposis.[78] Similar to FAP and attenuated FAP, duodenal adenomas and adenocarcinomas occur in these patients. Sebaceous tumors have also been described in affected patients.

Two specific missense mutations (p.Y179C and p.G396D) account for most *MUTYH*-associated polyposis in northern Europeans.[73] Other mutations are more common in southern Europeans (p.E480del), Pakistanis (p.Y104*), and Indians (p.E480*).[79-81] One large population-based study of 2239 cases by Farrington et al. found a 93-fold increased risk of colorectal cancer compared with wild-type controls.[82] The lifetime risk of colorectal carcinoma in affected patients is 80%, and the risk of duodenal carcinoma is 4%.[83] The risk of cancer in heterozygous carriers of an *MUTYH* mutation remains unknown but is probably slightly increased.[82,84,85]

Other Adenomatous Polyposis Syndromes

Recently, germline mutations in the exonuclease domain of *POLE* and *POLD1* have been associated with a clinical phenotype that overlaps with FAP and attenuated FAP.[86,87] Similar to *APC* mutations, mutations in *POLE* and *POLD1* are dominantly inherited. Patients present with oligo adenomatous polyposis and early-onset colorectal and endometrial cancer. The risk of colorectal carcinoma appears higher for *POLD1* mutation carriers compared with *POLE* carriers; however, carriers of both mutations warrant colonoscopic surveillance.[88] The cancers that develop in these patients are characterized by a hypermutated phenotype, and they are amenable to immunotherapy.

NTHL1 is a protein involved in base excision repair similar to MUTYH. Mutations in *NTHL1* result in C→T transitions and predispose to adenomatous polyposis that presents in adulthood, generally by 50 years of age.[89,90] Endometrial carcinoma and sebaceous skin tumors are also seen, which results in overlap with both *MUTYH*-associated polyposis and Lynch syndrome. Other more rare polyposis syndromes include *MSH3*-associated polyposis and *AXIN2*-associated polyposis. *MSH3* encodes the *MMR* gene that is involved in repairing di-, tri-, tetra-, and pentanucleotide repeats.[91] Biallelic mutations in *MSH3* result in multiple adenomas and colorectal carcinoma.[92] Duodenal adenomas, gastric cancer, and early-onset astrocytomas have also been reported. *AXIN2* regulates β-catenin degradation and functions in the same pathway as APC.[93-95] Mutations in this gene result in colonic polyps, colorectal cancer, gastric polyps, and ectodermal dysplasia and is inherited in an autosomal dominant manner.

Lynch Syndrome-Associated Adenomas

Lynch syndrome is an autosomal dominant condition caused by inherited defects in one of the DNA mismatch repair genes *(MLH1, MSH2, MSH6, PMS2)* or *EPCAM* [96,97] that lead to microsatellite instability and a rapid accumulation of somatic mutations in genes that control pathways of tumor progression (see Chapters 23 and 27). Most mutations occur in the *MLH1* and *MSH2* genes and are truncating. Lynch syndrome is the most common form of hereditary colon cancer, accounting for approximately 3% of all colon cancers (see Chapters 23 and 27); universal screening of all colorectal carcinomas is recommended by numerous GI societies. The disorder is characterized by the development of colon cancer, often at an early age, and with predominance of right-sided cancers. Lynch syndrome patients do not usually develop an excess of polyps. However, rarely they can present with multiple adenomas.[98] When adenomas do occur, they carry a significant risk of malignant degeneration. However, individuals with constitutional mismatch repair deficiency caused by biallelic mutations in *MMR* genes develop adenomas at a very young age. Constitutional mismatch repair deficiency also predisposes to a wide variety of other tumors including leukemia, lymphoma, and brain tumors.

The risk of colon cancer in Lynch syndrome varies widely according to the pathogenic MMR gene mutation.[83] The risk is highest in those with *MSH2* mutations (~95%) and lowest in those with *PMS2* mutations (~10%).[99,100]

BOX 22.2 Classification of Serrated Colonic Polyps

1. Nondysplastic serrated polyps
   a. Normal architecture, normal basilar crypt proliferation
      - Microvesicular hyperplastic polyp
      - Goblet cell hyperplastic polyp
   b. Abnormal architecture, abnormal proliferation along the length of the crypts
      - Sessile serrated polyp (or sessile serrated lesion)
2. Dysplastic serrated polyps
   a. Sessile serrated polyp (or sessile serrated lesion) with dysplasia
   b. Traditional serrated adenoma
   c. Serrated adenoma unclassified
3. Unclassifiable serrated polyps (with or without dysplasia)

Immunohistochemical staining of adenomas in patients with Lynch syndrome demonstrates loss of expression of the inherited faulty mismatch repair protein in 50% to 79% of adenomas and is influenced by the adenoma size and the presence of high-grade dysplasia.[101-104] Defective DNA mismatch repair functionality suggests that the progression from adenoma to carcinoma could be quite rapid in these patients. It has also been suggested that Lynch syndrome is associated with a higher proportion of flat adenomas. Patients with Lynch syndrome also have a ~15% lifetime risk of small-intestinal carcinoma; the duodenum and the jejunum are the most common sites.[105,106]

The histological features of colorectal carcinomas in Lynch syndrome are distinctive, similar to those of sporadic microsatellite instability-high (MSI-H) carcinomas (see also Chapters 23 and 27).[107-112] Sixty percent occur in the proximal colon. Compared with microsatellite stable colorectal carcinomas, MSI-H carcinomas more commonly have a mucinous or signet ring cell component, a microglandular or medullary growth pattern, and an expansile ("pushing") margin. These tumors are often poorly differentiated and characteristically show prominent tumor-infiltrating lymphocytes. A peritumoral lymphoid or Crohn's-like response is often seen at the leading edges of the tumors.

SERRATED POLYPS

Recognized by their bland cytological features and classic serrated architecture, serrated polyps were historically considered non-neoplastic and without malignant potential. However, it is now well-recognized that some types of serrated polyps may, in fact, progress to adenocarcinoma.[113,114] Recognition of the potential neoplastic nature of these lesions has led to identification and characterization of the serrated pathway of carcinogenesis,[115-120] which is discussed further in Chapter 27. Box 22.2 describes the classification of serrated polyps. The serrated neoplasia pathway describes a morphological progression that begins in nondysplastic serrated polyps and terminates with the development of carcinomas that have morphological, biological, and clinical characteristics that differ from carcinomas that develop in the conventional adenoma-carcinoma pathway.

Terminology and Classification

Table 22.3[121] outlines the histological and molecular features of serrated colorectal polyps.[121] Two principle morphological subtypes of "hyperplastic polyps" are well-recognized. These are termed *microvesicular polyps* and *goblet cell hyperplastic polyps*. From a clinical point of view, it is not yet considered mandatory or even recommended to distinguish these two variants in diagnostic reports. Rather, it is considered clinically important to recognize and report goblet cell hyperplastic polyps, which can have very subtle serrated features, to distinguish them from normal mucosa and from other types of serrated polyps. They can be difficult to distinguish from normal epithelium if one does not look carefully at the crypts for evidence of numerous goblet cells and a sawtooth surface contour. The microvesicular variant of hyperplastic polyp is the most common. A third type of hyperplastic polyp *(mucin-poor hyperplastic polyp)* was initially described by Torlakovic et al.[114] However, this lesion should not necessarily be regarded as a distinct entity because little is known of its biological nature, and most authorities believe that it likely represents a mucin-depleted variant of a microvesicular hyperplastic polyp, perhaps as a result of tissue injury.

Torlakovic and Snover first recognized an unusual type of serrated polyp that occurred mainly in patients with serrated polyposis.[122] In 2003, Torlakovic et al. provided the first description of serrated polyps in patients without any known polyposis syndrome.[114] Since 2003, this polyp has been termed *sessile serrated adenoma, sessile serrated polyp, sessile serrated adenoma/polyp*, and, more recently, *sessile serrated lesion* (SSL) by the most recent WHO publication.[124] The original argument for including the term *adenoma* in its description was to emphasize clinically that these lesions are in fact valid precursors of colorectal carcinoma. However, over the years, use of the term *adenoma* has resulted in much confusion among clinicians because they have the tendency to associate *adenomas* with *dysplastic epithelium*, which of course most SSLs do not contain. In fact, these polyps have significant differences in their natural history and molecular phenotype compared with conventional adenomas. If dysplasia is present within an SSL, the WHO recommends the term *SSL with dysplasia*. Thus the term *cytological dysplasia* has been dropped in the current edition of the WHO classification of serrated polyps.

Traditional serrated adenoma (TSA) remains the recommended diagnostic term to be used for "serrated adenoma" of the type reported by Longacre and Fenoglio-Preiser in 1990.[182] We have only recently begun to appreciate the wide diversity of molecular and morphological alterations that can occur in these particular lesions (see later). Finally, over the past several years, new and unusual types of dysplastic serrated polyps that do necessarily fulfill the precise diagnostic criteria of a typical TSA or an SSL with dysplasia have been increasingly described. In this setting, the WHO recommends use of the generic term *serrated adenoma unclassified* for unequivocally dysplastic serrated lesions that do not fit neatly into one of the above two discrete diagnostic categories. Another acceptable term for polyps that do not fit into a specific category is *serrated lesion with dysplasia*,

TABLE 22.3 Classification, Histologic, and Molecular Features of Serrated Polyps

Histological Features					Molecular Features		
Type	**Crypt Architecture**	**Proliferation Zone**	**Cytological Features**	**Mucin Type**	***BRAF* Mutation**	***KRAS* Mutation**	**CpG Island Methylation**
Microvesicular hyperplastic polyp	Funnel-shaped crypts with serrations limited to upper two-thirds	Located uniformly in the basal portion of crypts	Small basally located nuclei, no dysplasia	Mixed micro-vesicular and goblet cell	70%-80%	0%	+
Goblet cell hyperplastic polyp	Elongated crypts that resemble enlarged normal crypts; little to no serrations	Located uniformly in the basal portion of crypts	Small basally located nuclei, no dysplasia	Goblet cell only	0%	50%	–
Sessile serrated lesion	Horizontal growth along the muscularis mucosae, dilation (often asymmetric) of the crypt base (basal third of the crypt), and/or serrations extending into the crypt base	Proliferation may be abnormally located away from the crypt base, variable from crypt to crypt	Small basally located nuclei with occasional larger nuclei with inconspicuous nucleoli, no dysplasia	Mixed micro-vesicular and goblet cell	>90%	0%-5%	++
Sessile serrated lesion with dysplasia	As for sessile serrated lesion	As for sessile serrated lesion with more proliferation in dysplastic component	Varied morphological appearance to dysplastic component	Varied type	>90%	0%	+++
Traditional serrated adenoma	Slitlike serrations, often ectopic cryptfoci	Present within ectopic cryptfoci and crypt base	Elongated pencillate nuclei with nuclear stratification and cytoplasmic eosinophilia; may develop overt (conventional or serrated) dysplasia	Occasional scattered goblet cells; rare goblet cell variant has been described	20%-40%	50%-70%	BRAF mutated ++ KRAS mutated +
Serrated adenoma–unclassified	Varied	Varied	Unequivocal dysplasia must be present	Varied	Uncertain	Uncertain	Uncertain

From Pai RK, Bettington M, Srivastava A, Rosty C. An update on the morphology and molecular pathology of serrated colorectal polyps and associated carcinomas. Mod Pathol. *2019;32(10):1390-1415.*

unclassified, although this is not specifically endorsed by the WHO. Regardless, both terms convey the essential feature, which is the presence of a serrated polyp of some kind with dysplasia. Ultimately, knowledge of the presence or absence of dysplasia is important for clinicians to be aware of with regard to assurance of completeness of resection and determination of frequency of future surveillance.

Molecular Alterations in Serrated Polyps

Elucidation of the molecular alterations in serrated polyps has been critical in our understanding the neoplastic progression in the serrated pathway of carcinogenesis (Fig. 22.8).[121] The molecular hallmarks of the serrated pathway include activating mutations involving a component of the RAS-RAF-MAP-kinase signaling pathway as well as methylation of CpG DNA islands. Both microvesicular hyperplastic polyps and SSL commonly demonstrate activating mutations in *BRAF*.[126,127] CpG island DNA methylation is uncommon in hyperplastic polyps but occurs in up to 50% of SSLs.[126,127] Given the histological and molecular overlap between hyperplastic polyps and SSLs, it is likely that SSLs arise from microvesicular hyperplastic polyps, although this still remains a matter of debate. In contrast with SSLs and microvesicular

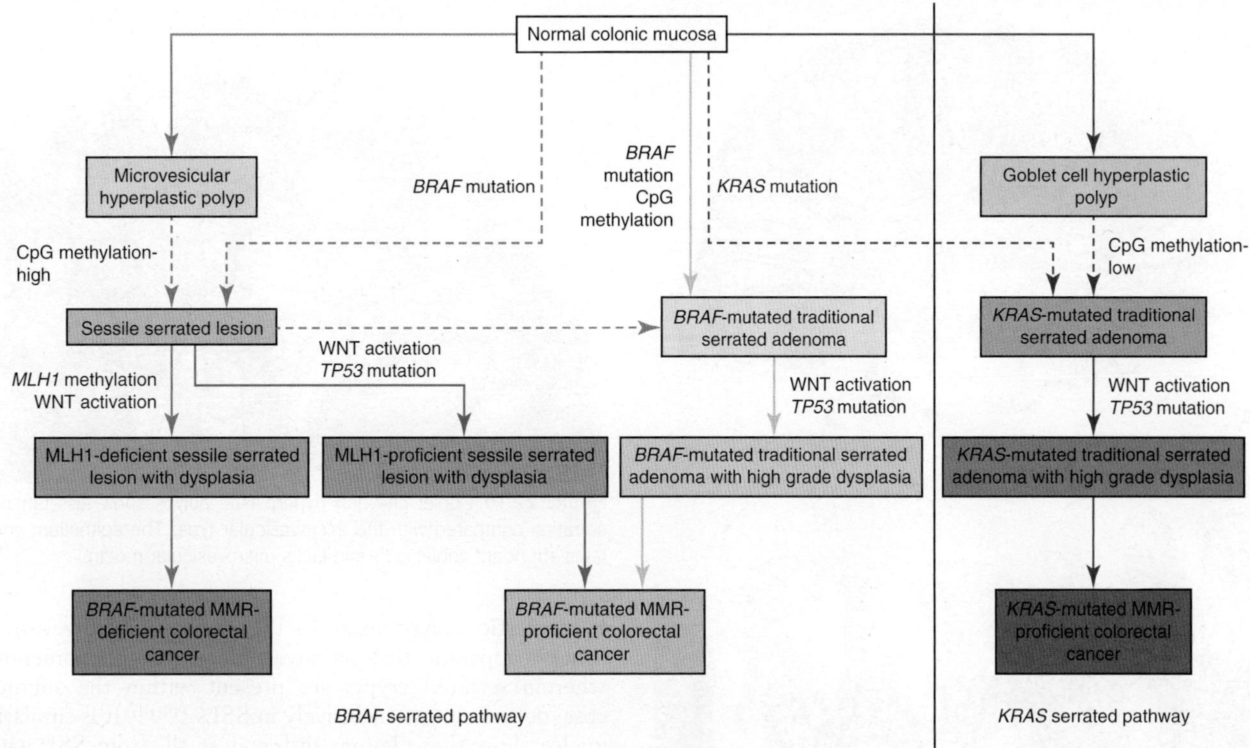

FIGURE 22.8 Serrated neoplasia pathway. (*Pai RK, Bettington M, Srivastava A, Rosty C. An update on the morphology and molecular pathology of serrated colorectal polyps and associated carcinomas. Mod Pathol. 2019;32(10):1390-1415.*)

hyperplastic polyps, goblet cell hyperplastic polyps often demonstrate *KRAS* mutations.[128]

The development of dysplasia in SSLs is frequently accompanied by methylation-induced silencing of the *MLH1* gene. Silencing of *MLH1* results in microsatellite instability and accumulation of mutations in a wide variety of genes, including *CDKN2A* and *TP53*.[129-131] Activation of the WNT pathway also occurs, but this often occurs late in neoplastic progression, in contrast with the conventional adenoma-carcinoma pathway, where aberrant WNT signaling happens early.[132,133]

TSAs have more complex molecular alterations. They are molecularly heterogeneous. Most TSAs also harbor alterations in the RAS-RAF-MAP-kinase signaling pathway. Approximately 50% have a *BRAF* mutation, and 30% have a *KRAS* mutation.[134-136] More extensive CpG island methylation is seen in *BRAF*-mutated TSAs.[135] In addition, many of the *BRAF*-mutated TSAs arise in association with SSL-like and/or microvesicular hyperplastic changes in the surrounding mucosa. The origins of the *KRAS*-mutated cases are less clear, but they also may arise in association with a precursor lesion with features of a goblet cell hyperplastic polyp.[137,138] Additional mutations in TSAs include frequent *RSPO* fusion transcripts in *KRAS*-mutated TSAs and frequent *RNF43* mutations in *BRAF*-mutated TSAs.[139,140] These molecular alterations tend to occur at the transition from precursor polyp to TSA.[141] The development of high-grade dysplasia and invasive carcinoma in TSAs is often accompanied by loss of p16 expression and mutations in *TP53*.[135] In contrast with SSLs with dysplasia, the progression from TSA to invasive carcinoma is never accompanied by *MLH1* inactivation.

Hyperplastic Polyps

Clinical Features

Hyperplastic polyps are considered serrated polyps with normal architecture and normal hierarchical proliferative characteristics. They are small, innocuous lesions that may be found throughout the colon of adults, but they are especially common in the rectum.[142] Up to 90% occur in the left colon. Their prevalence rate increases with age. Up to 35% of asymptomatic individuals older than 50 years of age demonstrate hyperplastic polyps.[142] Specific lifestyle and dietary factors commonly associated with conventional adenomas are also associated with hyperplastic polyps. These include cigarette smoking, alcohol consumption, low folate intake, and obesity.[143,144] These lesions are typically asymptomatic and are often identified as an incidental finding during endoscopic examination of the colon. Endoscopically, hyperplastic polyps are small, sessile, smooth bumps or nodules that appear pale and often flatten on insufflation of air.[145]

Pathological Features

Microvesicular hyperplastic polyps are usually small or diminutive sessile polyps. Endoscopically, they can often have a stellate pit pattern, as described by Kudo et al.[146] Histologically, they are composed of serrated epithelium with funnel-shaped, evenly spaced crypts and with proliferative zones confined to the crypt bases (Fig. 22.9). Nuclear atypia is minimal, but some polyps show a mild degree of nuclear stratification at the base of the polyp, which should not be confused with a conventional adenoma in poorly oriented tissue sections. Dystrophic goblet cells and cells with round vesicular nuclei and prominent nucleoli are rare; if

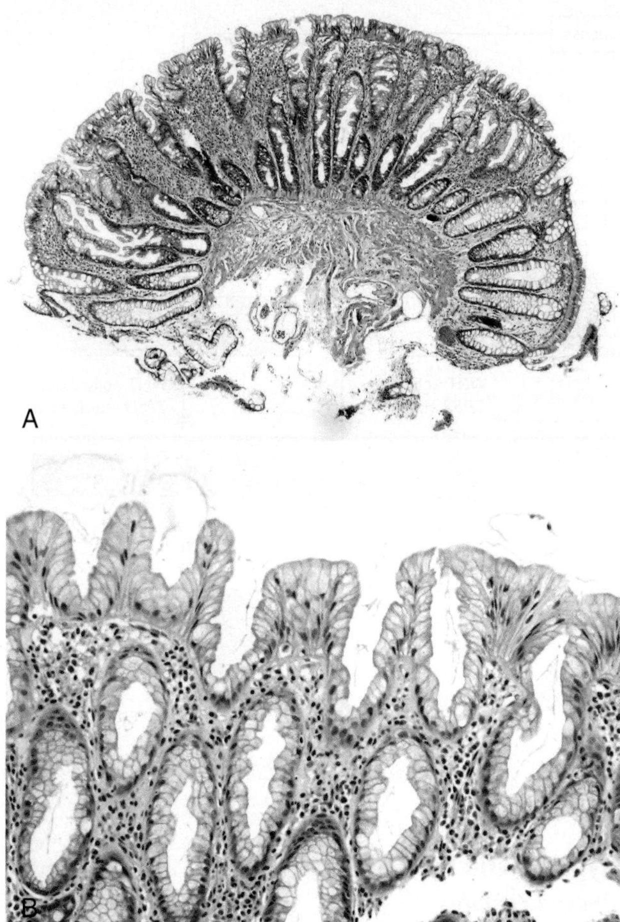

FIGURE 22.9 A, Hyperplastic polyp, microvesicular type, shows marked luminal serration and a mixture of goblet cells and columnar cells with microvesicular mucin. B, These polyps show surface maturation with basally located small nuclei and abundant microvesicular mucinous cytoplasm. Notice the absence of mitoses in the upper crypt and surface epithelium.

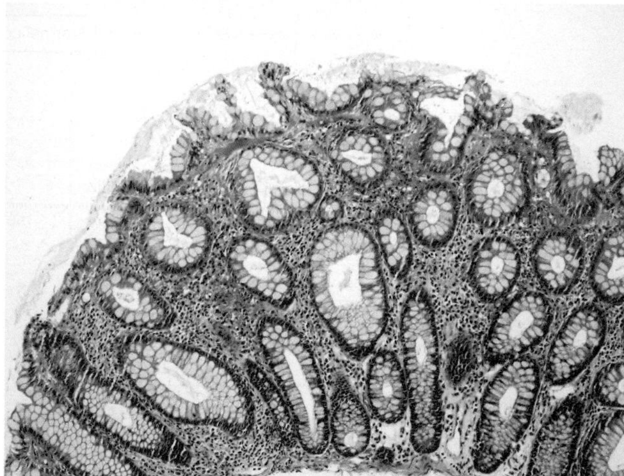

FIGURE 22.10 Goblet cell–rich hyperplastic polyps show less luminal serration compared with the microvesicular type. The epithelium contains abundant goblet cells and lacks microvesicular mucin.

present, they are usually confined to the lower portions of the crypts. Most notably, these lesions show distinct evidence of surface maturation and an absence of cells with eosinophilic cytoplasm characteristic of SSLs and TSAs (see later discussion). The cells lining the crypts consist mainly of goblet cells and cells with abundant fine apical vacuoles containing microvesicular mucin (see Fig. 22.9). The nuclei in the cells in the surface epithelium are basally located and quite small in size. Importantly, the luminal epithelial serrations are usually limited to the upper one-half to two-thirds of the crypt in contrast with SSL (see later).[132] When cut in cross section, the serrated crypts of these polyps have a uniform stellate appearance.

Some polyps also show thickening, and even extension, of the muscularis mucosae into the lamina propria. Occasionally, these prolapse-type changes can be quite striking and result in distortion of the serrated crypts, mimicking an SSL. In addition, larger-sized microvesicular hyperplastic polyps (>0.5 cm) may be slightly distorted and even show mild, often symmetric crypt dilation. In this instance, care should be taken to distinguish these changes from an SSL (see latter discussion). Occasional reports of *inverted* hyperplastic polyps exist in the literature. However, it is now apparent that an inverted growth phenomenon, wherein serrated crypts are present within the submucosa, occurs almost exclusively in SSLs.[114,147] It is similarly unclear how these lesions differ, if at all, from SSL with epithelial displacement.

Goblet cell hyperplastic polyps are the second most common type of hyperplastic polyp. They are typically small (<0.5 cm) sessile lesions and are commonly found in the left colon, but they can certainly be present in the right colon as well. Goblet cell hyperplastic polyps are often overlooked because their morphological alterations are usually quite subtle.[148] These polyps show elongated crypts that are rich in goblet cells without microvesicular mucin (Fig. 22.10). They are normally sessile lesions but demonstrate a far lesser degree of luminal serration than microvesicular hyperplastic polyps. The luminal section is usually limited only to the surface and uppermost portions of the crypts. The crypts may be mildly elongated as well. Nuclear atypia, stratification, and mitoses are not seen in this type of hyperplastic polyp. In these polyps, the crypts are taller and wider than normal. Occasional branching or tortuosity may occur, but this is rare.

Natural History and Treatment

Until recently, small hyperplastic polyps were not believed to require definitive treatment, although they are typically removed in the process of endoscopy with biopsy. However, the biological characteristics and natural history of hyperplastic polyps, particularly the microvesicular type, are now considered controversial. Large lesions, particularly those located in the right colon, should be removed in total.[149,150] Small proximal hyperplastic polyps may carry the same risk of synchronous advanced neoplasia as similarly sized SSLs, although the risk of metachronous neoplasia is unclear.[151] Further studies are needed to determine the natural history and malignant potential of hyperplastic polyps and each of the different subtypes. There is a strong correlation between the occurrence of hyperplastic polyps and conventional adenomas in similar populations worldwide.[152] Although some studies suggest that distally located hyperplastic

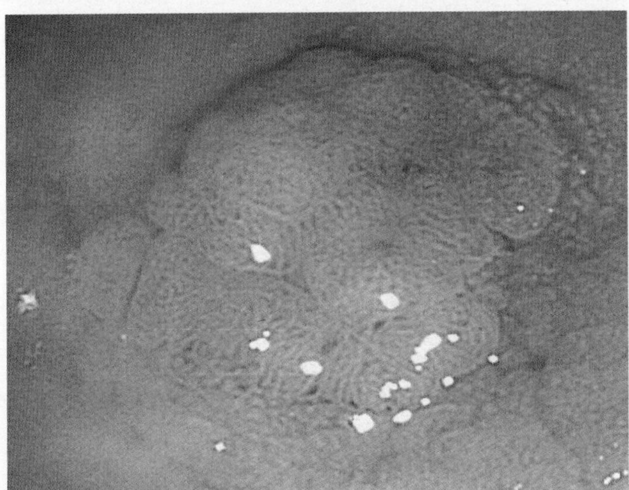

FIGURE 22.11 Endoscopic appearance of a sessile serrated lesion characterized by a superficially elevated lesion with indistinct margins.

polyps predict an increased risk of proximal adenomas or even advanced adenomas, this is controversial.[152-155] Thus at present, the finding of a distal hyperplastic polyp at sigmoidoscopy is not considered to be an absolute indication for full colonoscopy.[142] Furthermore, surveillance for detection of metachronous hyperplastic polyps, or adenomas, after removal of a hyperplastic polyp is not currently recommended.

Sessile Serrated Lesions

Clinical Features

In contrast with hyperplastic polyps, SSLs are usually larger in size (>5 mm) and occur more often in the proximal colon (75%).[156,157] The prevalence of SSLs varies according to endoscopist experience and has been found in up to 20% of individuals undergoing screening colonoscopy by skilled endoscopists.[158] SSLs are associated with female sex, smoking, high body mass index, and alcohol intake.[159,160] SSLs can be difficult to identify at endoscopy. However, awareness and specific training can improve detection. They often appear as ill-defined, sessile, pale lesions with an irregular shape and a "cloudlike" surface (Fig. 22.11).[161,162] These polyps are often covered by adherent mucin, and a rim of bubbles or fecal debris can sometimes collect at the periphery of these lesions.[163] They have a stellate configuration (Kudo pit pattern II) and appear as superficially elevated lesions (Paris classification 0-IIa).[1,146,164] Incomplete resection is common in SSLs given the lack of a sharp demarcation between the SSL and adjacent normal colonic mucosa.

Pathological Features

Morphologically, SSLs show distinctive features, characterized more specifically by the presence of asymmetric crypt dilation, crypt irregularity (horizontally shaped crypts), prominent and often exaggerated lower (and upper) crypt serration, mitoses in the upper levels of the crypts, vesicular nuclei in the upper crypts, reduced amounts of lamina propria between crypts, hypermucinous epithelium, and, occasionally, an inverted (epithelial displacement) growth pattern (Fig. 22.12; see Table 22.3).[114] Rows of cells with eosinophilic ("pink") cytoplasm are not uncommon. These may represent "senescent" cells or possibly early dysplastic cells, but this topic is controversial. The basal portions of the crypts are usually branched and may appear flask- or boot-shaped (similar to an inverted *T*), indicative of horizontal rather than vertical growth. An expert panel of pathologists suggested that the presence of one or more unequivocally architecturally distorted crypts of this kind situated at the base of the lesion is enough evidence to establish a diagnosis of an SSL rather than a hyperplastic polyp in the appropriate clinical and endoscopic setting.[165] This definition has been adopted in the current WHO classification. Mature goblet cells, or mucinous cells, show an irregular distribution by being uncharacteristically located at the bases of the crypts. Some polyps also contain perineurial-like proliferations in the lamina propria.[166]

SSLs may show a variable degree of nuclear atypia. At the low end of the spectrum, lesions show little or no stratification, a low mitotic rate, and clear evidence of surface maturation. SSLs may occasionally show an increased degree of nuclear stratification, consisting of cells with open vesicular chromatin and small nucleoli as well as increased eosinophilia of the cytoplasm. These features approach those of a traditional serrated adenoma, but the cytological changes are often focal and present only in the surface epithelium, not along the entire length of the crypts. This focal eosinophilic change should not be considered indicative of a TSA or an SSL with dysplasia.

It is important to emphasize that the size, location, number, and endoscopic appearance are not part of the pathological diagnosis of a hyperplastic polyp or an SSL. Using these parameters can hamper future efforts to refine the risk profile of patients with serrated polyps, especially in scenarios such as small proximal hyperplastic polyps or large distal hyperplastic polyps. Only a proper morphological classification of serrated polyps will allow for refinement of the risk of metachronous neoplasia in these patients. Results from such analyses can then be used to modify the diagnostic criteria and include other features for the diagnosis if necessary. From a practical perspective, it is extremely rare to encounter a microvesicular hyperplastic polyp >9 mm, and such polyps should be considered advanced serrated polyps for the purpose of subsequent surveillance intervals. The main dilemma occurs when encountering small or diminutive proximal serrated polyps that morphologically are best classified as a microvesicular hyperplastic polyp (see Fig. 22.8). Furthermore, goblet cell hyperplastic polyps are not infrequently seen in the proximal colon. Despite the lack of diagnostic features, there has been a tendency to consider all proximal serrated polyps as SSLs because of the presumption that hyperplastic polyps do not exist in the proximal colon. Such a diagnostic strategy will lead to an increased frequency of colonoscopy for these patients and an increased burden on surveillance programs. In rare cases of polyps with marginal histological features, size and location can be used to tip the diagnosis one way or another.

Sessile Serrated Lesions with Dysplasia

With histological and molecular progression (often characterized by loss of MLH1 immunostaining and microsatellite instability), SSLs may acquire morphological evidence

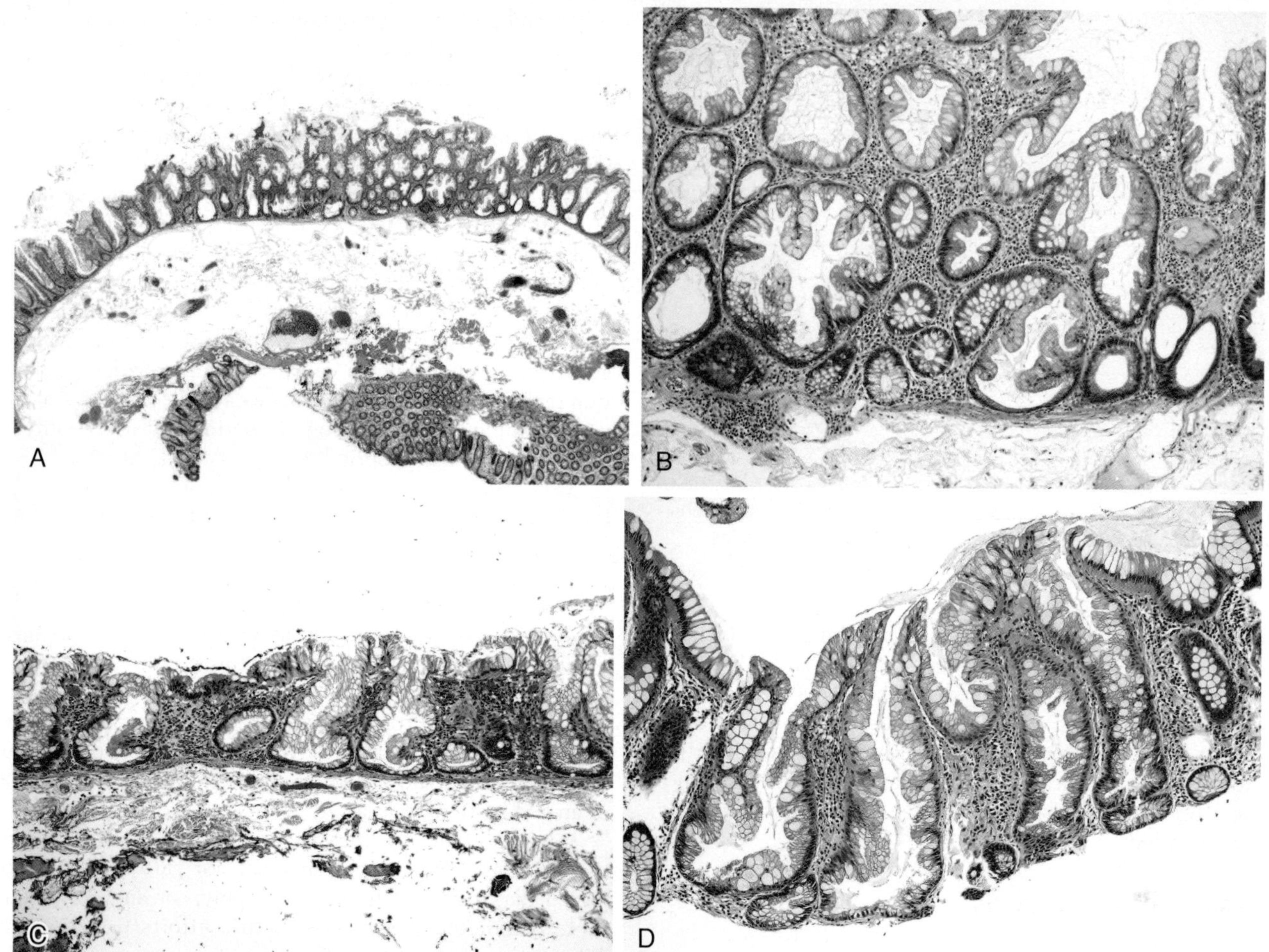

FIGURE 22.12 A, Sessile serrated lesion showing multiple architecturally distorted crypts. **B,** A higher-power view of some serrated crypts from the polyp shown in **A** characterized by deep crypt serrations and asymmetric dilation of the crypt bases. **C,** Multiple crypts in this sessile serrated lesion demonstrate asymmetric growth along the muscularis mucosae. **D,** This small sessile serrated lesion has multiple architecturally distorted serrated crypts.

of dysplasia (see Table 22.3).[119,167,168] SSL with dysplasia represents the most "advanced" type of serrated polyp, and these lesions can progress fairly rapidly to invasive carcinoma (see later discussion). These lesions have been historically referred to as *mixed hyperplastic/adenomatous polyps*. However, it is now well recognized that these polyps do not occur as a result of a coincidental growth of hyperplastic and adenomatous elements, but as a result of dysplastic change within an SSL. Morphologically, these lesions usually show discrete areas of a typical SSL with dysplasia (Fig. 22.13). Occasionally, background SSL-type crypts may not be apparent in polyps that contain a large dysplastic component, and thus have "overgrown" their SSL precursors. In such cases, the presence of any convincing nondysplastic serrated crypts is considered sufficient to diagnose an SSL with dysplasia.

The morphological heterogeneity of dysplasia seen in SSLs has only recently been described.[169] Two general types occur: *serrated dysplasia* and *intestinal-type dysplasia*. However, until more follow-up and natural history data are obtained, it is not necessary to grade or morphologically subclassify the type of dysplasia for clinical purposes. Rather, it is more prudent to recognize the various types of dysplasia seen in these polyps to ensure an accurate diagnosis and for future studies. Most commonly, dysplasia is intestinal and characterized by the presence of elongated, cigar-shaped hyperchromatic nuclei that resemble low-grade dysplasia in conventional adenomas. Architecturally there is often increased complexity characterized by crypt branching, crypt elongation, and a villous and/or cribriform architecture. The dysplasia frequently involves the full thickness of the mucosa and is usually associated with loss of MLH1 expression, although frequencies vary.[169,170] Serrated dysplasia is less common. SSL with serrated dysplasia shows architectural complexity and tightly packed glands composed of epithelial cells with prominent cytoplasmic eosinophilia, luminal serration, enlarged nuclei, and prominent nucleoli (see later; see Fig. 22.13). MLH1 is normally preserved in this type of dysplasia. Polyps composed of a mixture of these two types of dysplasia is also common. Rarely, SSLs can show very subtle cytological and architectural abnormalities, often with glandular crowding, mild nuclear enlargement, a slight change in mucin content, and a slight change in serrations termed *minimal deviation dysplasia*. This is also often associated with loss of MLH1. However, because little is known regarding the biology and natural history of such lesions, more study is needed before this becomes a diagnostic entity. Occasionally dysplasia closely resembles that of a conventional adenoma with typical basophilic cytoplasm, penicillate nuclei, and straight crypts without significant serrations and architectural complexity. The dysplasia is often limited to the surface of the

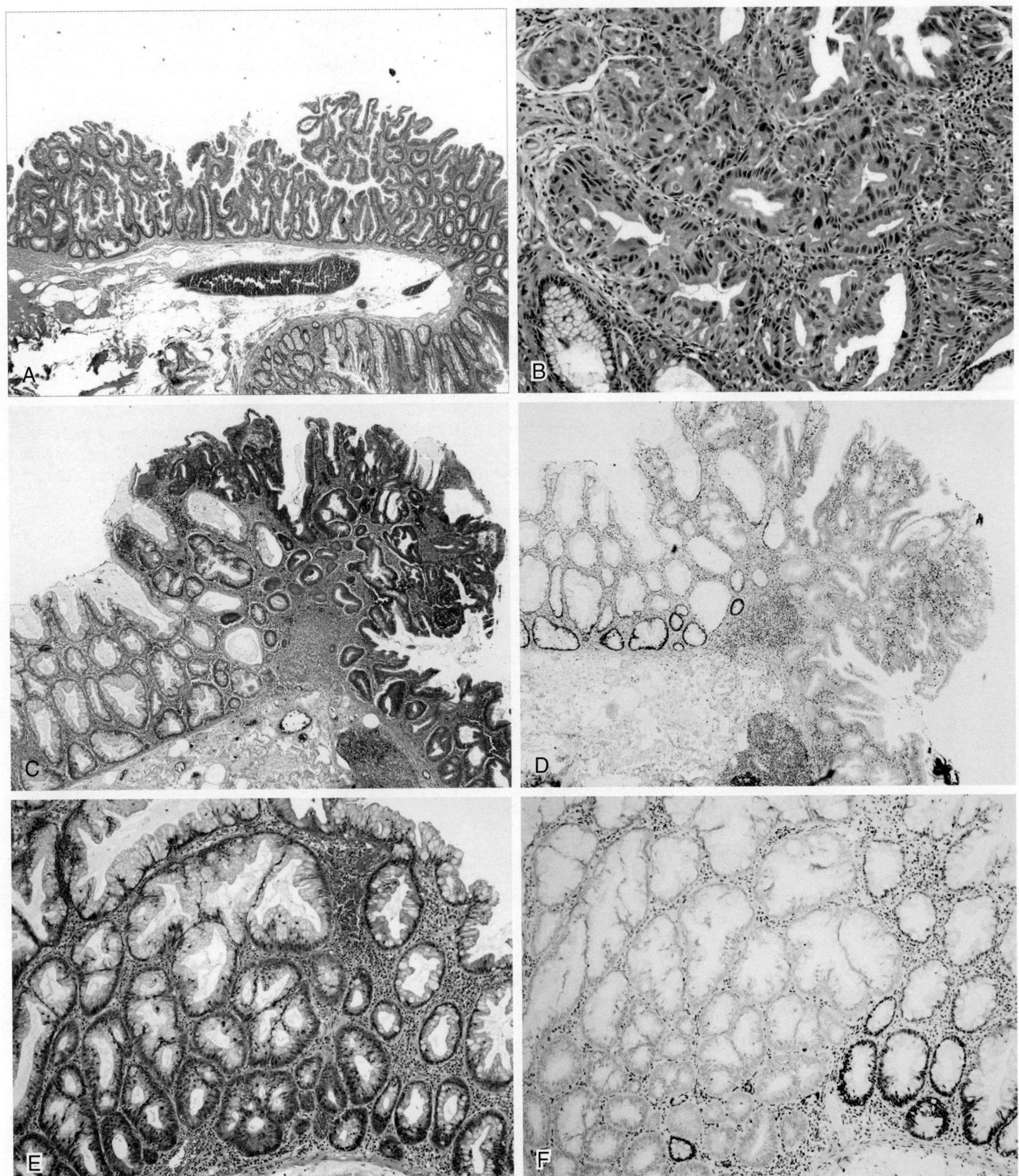

FIGURE 22.13 **A,** Sessile serrated lesion with a typical pattern of dysplasia showing an abrupt transition between nondysplastic serrated crypts and crypts with obvious features of dysplasia. **B,** An area of dysplasia in a sessile serrated lesion characterized by marked glandular crowding, cytoplasmic eosinophilia, and round nuclei with occasional prominent nucleoli. This pattern has been referred to as *serrated dysplasia* by some authors and is often associated with retention of MLH1 by immunohistochemistry. **C,** Another sessile serrated lesion with dysplasia with polypoid growth of the dysplastic focus. **D,** The dysplastic area demonstrates loss of MLH1 by immunohistochemistry. **E,** A focus of dysplasia within a sessile serrated lesion with subtle nuclear enlargement predominantly restricted to the crypt bases with increased architectural complexity. The atypia is predominately restricted to the crypt base. **F,** Loss of MLH1 expression is observed in this focus, supporting the diagnosis of dysplasia. This type of dysplasia has been referred to as *minimal deviation dysplasia* by some authors.

polyp. MLH1 is preserved in this pattern. Recent studies have suggested that such lesions may represent a collision between a conventional adenoma and an SSL given the differences in *BRAF* mutations between the dysplastic component and adjacent SSL.[171]

Natural History

The natural history and risk of progression to malignancy of SSLs are poorly understood but are under intense investigation.[149] The mean age of patients with SSLs with dysplasia is similar to SSLs that harbor invasive carcinoma, suggesting

TABLE 22.4 Surveillance Colonoscopy Recommendations for Serrated Polyps

Organization	Serrated Polyps Only	Serrated Polyps and Adenomas
US Multi-Society Task Force on Colorectal Cancer	10 years for: • ≤ 20 hyperplastic polyps <10 mm 5-10 years for: • 1-2 sessile serrated lesions <10 mm 3-5 years for: • 3-4 sessile serrated lesions <10 mm • Hyperplastic polyp 10 mm 3 years for: • 5-10 sessile serrated lesions <10 mm • Sessile serrated lesion ≥10 mm • Any sessile serrated lesion with dysplasia • Traditional serrated adenoma 6 months for: • Piecemeal resection of sessile serrated lesion ≥20 mm	No specific recommendations because of low quality of evidence (see Box 22.1 for adenoma surveillance recommendations)
British Society of Gastroenterology	3 years: • ≥2 serrated polyps with ≥1 serrated polyp ≥ 10 mm or any with dysplasia • ≥5 serrated polyps (excluding diminutive rectal hyperplastic polyps) • Participation in national bowel cancer screening (fecal immunochemical test) if invited	3 years: • ≥2 adenomas or serrated polyp with ≥1 advanced polyp (serrated polyp ≥10 mm in size or containing any grade of dysplasia, or an adenoma ≥10 mm in size or containing high-grade dysplasia) • ≥5 adenomas or serrated polyps • Participation in national bowel cancer screening (fecal immunochemical test) if invited
Cancer Council of Australia	10 years: • Hyperplastic polyps <10 mm 5 years for: • 1–2 sessile serrated lesions all <10 mm without dysplasia 3 years for: • 3–4 sessile serrated lesions, all <10 mm without dysplasia • 1–2 sessile serrated lesions ≥10 mm or with dysplasia, or hyperplastic polyp ≥10 mm • 1–2 traditional serrated lesions, any size 1 year for: • ≥5 sessile serrated lesions <10 mm without dysplasia • 3–4 sessile serrated lesions, one or more ≥10 mm or with dysplasia • 3–4 traditional serrated adenomas, any size	**Clinically significant serrated polyps and synchronous conventional adenomas** 5 years for: • 2 in total, sessile serrated lesions <10 mm without dysplasia 3 years for: • 3–9 in total, all sessile serrated lesions <10 mm without dysplasia • 2–4 in total, any serrated polyp ≥10 mm and/or dysplasia • 2–4 in total, any traditional serrated adenoma 1 year for: • ≥10 in total, all sessile serrated lesions <10 mm without dysplasia • ≥5 in total, any serrated polyp ≥10 mm and/or dysplasia • ≥5 in total, any traditional serrated adenoma **Synchronous high-risk conventional adenoma (tubulovillous or villous adenoma, with or without HGD and with or without size ≥10 mm)** 3 years for: • 2 in total, sessile serrated lesions any size with or without dysplasia or traditional serrated adenoma 1 year for: • ≥3 total adenomas, sessile serrated lesions any size with or without dysplasia oy any traditional serrated adenoma

that once dysplasia occurs in an SSL, progression to invasive adenocarcinoma occurs fairly rapidly.[129] It is commonly believed that loss of DNA repair ability and subsequent microsatellite instability are mechanisms that drive rapid neoplastic progression.[167] Although SSLs that harbor dysplasia progress rapidly to carcinoma, the acquisition of dysplasia in SSLs takes years to occur.[150,159,172] In one study of 55 patients with SSL who were monitored for a mean of 7 years, colorectal cancer or high-grade dysplasia developed in 15% of patients.[173] In other studies, patients with SSL were found to be at increased risk for synchronous advanced neoplasia and interval adenomas during surveillance.[174] One rational proposal for the management of SSL is based on the fact that most traditional hyperplastic polyps (goblet cell or microvesicular type) are unlikely to progress to carcinoma, and that SSLs without dysplasia are probably slow, but progressive, lesions. Table 22.4 provides a summary of the recommendations from the U.S. Multi-Society Task Force on Colorectal Cancer, British Society of Gastroenterology, and Cancer Council Australia.[175-177]

Treatment

For SSLs without dysplasia, complete endoscopic removal is recommended.[142,149] However, if this is not possible, then repeat endoscopy with biopsies should be performed within 1 year to evaluate for signs of dysplasia, and this should be followed by continued surveillance at shorter intervals until the lesion is completely removed. Surgical excision for large SSLs without dysplasia, particularly those that are recurrent, is also a reasonable alternative, although this is becoming less common with the increased use of advanced endoscopic techniques. In contrast, complete excision is considered mandatory for SSLs with dysplasia based on the likelihood that these lesions have undergone hypermethylation and acquired microsatellite instability and therefore are prone to carcinoma progression. Complete excision should be accomplished by endoscopy or surgical resection. If removed by piecemeal polypectomy, patients usually undergo repeat endoscopy within 6 months to 1 year to ensure that the lesion has been removed in its entirety and that there has been no progression.

Traditional Serrated Adenomas

Due to heterogeneity in the morphology, molecular characteristics, and frequency of association with non-neoplastic serrated or "hyperplastic" precursor polyps, the clinical and epidemiological features of these polyps are poorly understood. Nevertheless, TSAs are relatively uncommon, representing less than 1% to 2% of all colonic polyps in most studies.[178] In one Japanese study, TSAs accounted for only 1.8% of more than 10,000 colonic polyps.[179] Endoscopically, TSAs manifest variable characteristics, but they are more often pedunculated than sessile.[180] In one study, 63% of TSAs were pedunculated, 29% were sessile, and 8% were described as flat or carpetlike.[181] They may occasionally be rather large and filiform in contour. In one study, "filiform" TSAs were exclusively found in the rectum.[180]

Overall, TSAs are more common in females and occur more commonly in the left colon,[180] particularly the sigmoid colon and rectum.[142] Right-sided TSAs, however, do occur, and these may be flat rather than polypoid. The mean age at diagnosis is 60 to 65 years of age, which is typically older than for patients with hyperplastic polyps or SSLs.[182] As mentioned previously, TSAs are molecularly heterogenous: there are *BRAF*-mutated and *KRAS*-mutated types. *BRAF*-mutated TSAs more commonly are associated with a precursor hyperplastic polyp or SSL and occur in the right colon in a higher percentage of cases than the *KRAS*-mutated type. It is based on these observations that some authorities have suggested that these lesions, in particular, may reflect development of TSA-like dysplasia in an SSL, but this topic remains highly controversial. Regardless of the terminology used for these lesions, the treatment ultimately is the same because both are considered, generically, serrated lesions with dysplasia. In fact, it is not currently recommended to diagnose a "TSA arising in an SSL" as diagnostic of an "SSL with TSA-like dysplasia." SSLs with dysplasia are considered advanced lesions that often demonstrate microsatellite instability and CpG island DNA hypermethylation, and they can rapidly progress to carcinoma. In contrast, TSAs typically progress more slowly, have distinctive morphology, and do not normally develop microsatellite instability. Thus future studies are needed to elucidate the true relationship and potential biological continuum between SSLs and TSAs.

The origin of *KRAS*-mutated TSAs is less clear, although goblet cell hyperplastic polyp-like changes can, occasionally, be found at the periphery of these lesions. Of course, this suggests a possible progression pathway of goblet cell hyperplastic polyp to TSA, but further research is needed in this regard.

Pathological Features

Most TSAs are composed of epithelial cells with abundant and intensely eosinophilic cytoplasm and bland oval-shaped palisaded nuclei, usually without significant mitotic activity (Fig. 22.14; see Table 22.3).[135,183,184] The second and probably most typical feature of TSA is the presence of distinctive slitlike serrations, similar to the narrow slits present in normal small-intestinal epithelium.[135,178,180,182,185] The association of both the traditional serrated adenoma cytology and slitlike serrations makes the diagnosis of traditional serrated adenoma straightforward. A third characteristic feature is the presence of ectopic crypt foci. Ectopic crypt foci are small buds of epithelial cells resembling the bases of normal crypts that are not anchored to the muscularis mucosae, but instead are situated perpendicular to the villous projections of the polyp.[186] Ectopic crypt foci are not specific for TSAs. They occur in other polyps, such as conventional adenomas, and as such may simply represent small zones of proliferation in polyps with a villiform growth pattern.[187,188] Interestingly, flat TSA often lack ectopic crypt foci. Some TSAs with typical slitlike serration and at least focal ectopic crypt foci may show a predominance of goblet cells (mucin-rich variant) rather than the characteristic eosinophilic cells with abundant cytoplasm.[189,190]

Architecturally, TSAs are often protuberant and villous, but they can grow as flat, superficially elevated lesions as well. Filiform traditional serrated adenomas show elongated, finger-like villous projections and often show inflammation, ulceration, and dilated lymphatics within the lamina propria. Up to 50% of TSAs reveal an adjacent area of non-dysplastic serrated precursor, either a hyperplastic polyp or SSL. Distal TSAs may show an adjacent "shoulder" area of flat growth at the edge of the protuberant polyp. In a recent study, small (<10 mm) polyps resembling these shoulder areas were shown to be early forms of TSA that can be recognized by subtle superficial serrations and cytoplasmic eosinophilia.[137,138]

Despite being a polyp with malignant potential, most TSAs do not reveal the classic cytological characteristics of "dysplasia" because they lack significant nuclear hyperchromasia and mitotic activity outside of the areas of ectopic crypt foci. It is controversial among experts whether the "baseline atypia" of TSAs represents a very low grade of dysplasia (because molecular aberrations are common in these lesions) versus truly non-dysplastic "senescent epithelium" (based on the absence of significant cytological atypia). Regardless of the term used to describe the cytological features of TSAs without traditional high-grade dysplasia, TSAs are nonetheless considered premalignant polyps because most, if not all, will eventually progress through various stages of overt (conventional) dysplasia to cancer if left untreated. Overt (conventional) dysplasia does develop in TSAs with progression. The dysplasia in TSAs can be either intestinal type, resembling dysplasia seen in conventional adenomas, or serrated type, characterized by tightly

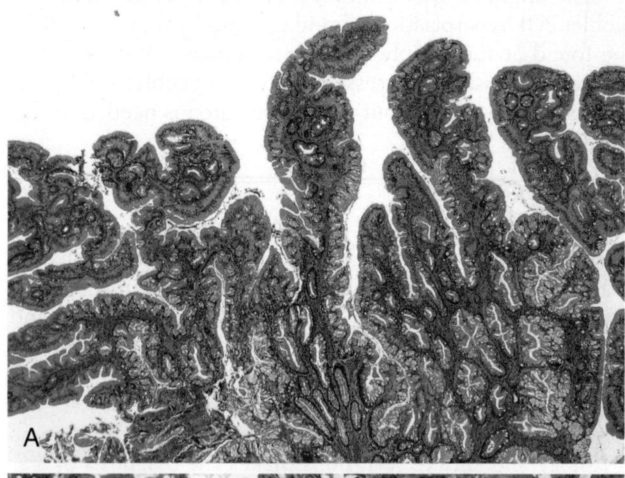

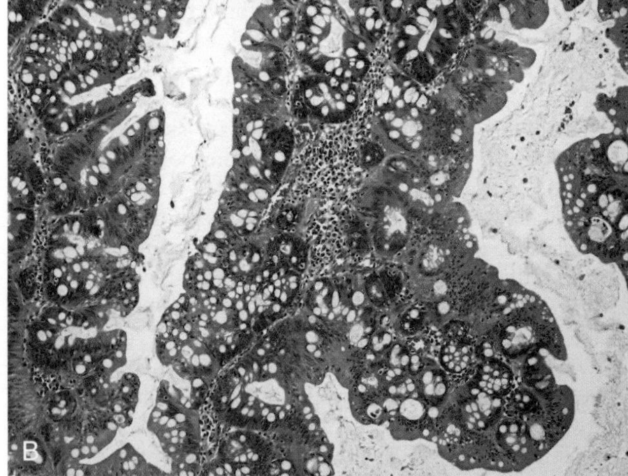

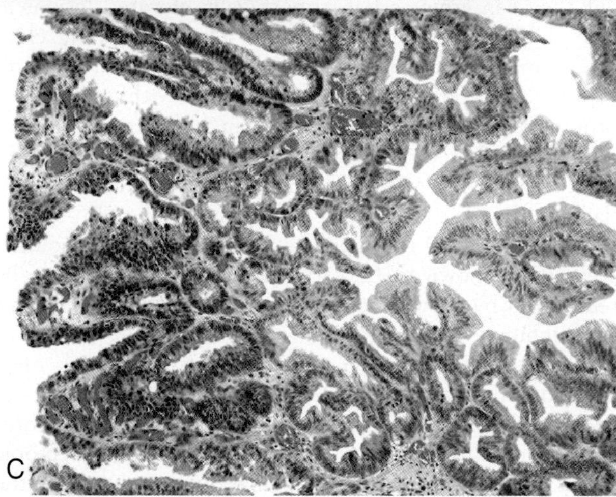

FIGURE 22.14 **A,** The traditional serrated adenoma differs from a sessile serrated lesion by the presence of hypereosinophilic cytoplasm and confluent nuclear stratification. **B,** High-power view shows the characteristic cytological features as well as ectopic crypt foci. **C,** An area of high-grade dysplasia *(left)* within a traditional serrated adenoma.

packed serrated glands composed of epithelial cells with prominent cytoplasmic eosinophilia, enlarged nuclei, and prominent nucleoli (see Fig. 22.14).[135,184] Both high-grade intestinal and serrated dysplasia should be reported when present because this indicates a more advanced stage of the lesion. However, it is also unclear whether "advanced" TSAs, as such, portend any increased risk of further synchronous or metachronous neoplasia or risk of cancer after excision compared with conventional TSAs without high-grade dysplasia. Furthermore, it is similarly unclear whether the risk of progression is affected by the type (intestinal vs. serrated) or extent of dysplasia in the polyp.

Natural History and Treatment

The natural history of TSA and the risk of progression to malignancy are poorly understood given its infrequent occurrence as an isolated polyp.[142,191] Most TSAs occur synchronously with other polyps. An additional complication is the occasional lack of use of consistent terminology, as mentioned earlier. For instance, the terms *TSA with associated SSL* versus *SSL with TSA-like dysplasia* when the lesion occurs on a background of SSL or a hyperplastic polyp. Thus evaluation or progression has been challenging. Nevertheless, progression to high-grade dysplasia was reported in 37% of TSAs in one study.[182] In this study, 11% contained intramucosal adenocarcinoma. In another study of filiform TSAs by Yantiss et al., 22% showed high-grade dysplasia, and another 6% showed invasive adenocarcinoma.[180] Some studies have suggested that the rate of malignant transformation in TSAs is similar to that of conventional adenomas.[179,192] It is likely that the risk of progression is related to the size and location of the lesion.[179] Large TSAs in the proximal colon may progress at a more rapid rate than those in the left colon.

Prior studies suggesting a high risk of concurrent colorectal carcinoma and metachronous adenomas in patients with a baseline TSA were limited by a small number of patients.[193,194] More recently, in a relatively large study of Korean patients with TSAs, the risk of metachronous serrated polyps, conventional adenomas, and high-risk adenomas was higher than a control population with only baseline conventional adenomas.[195] A recent population-based study from Denmark also showed that patients with TSA were nearly five times more likely to develop colorectal carcinoma on follow-up compared with those without TSA.[196] The treatment of TSAs is complete endoscopic removal. The surveillance interval is similar to that for patients with conventional adenomas (i.e., every 3 to 5 years).

Serrated Adenomas Unclassified

Recently, unusual types of dysplastic serrated polyps have been identified that do not fit neatly into a discrete diagnostic category, such as a TSA or SSL with dysplasia. In fact, some tubular, tubulovillous, or villous adenomas may show areas of architectural serration, but these polyps can be distinguished from TSAs most easily by the characteristics of the cytological features of the nuclei (Fig. 22.15).[197] In one study, re-review of 180 distal villous and tubulovillous adenomas resulted in reclassification of 20 polyps as TSA.[187,198] However, some of these so-called *serrated tubulovillous and villous adenomas* also demonstrated molecular features intermediate between a TSA and conventional tubulovillous adenoma. It is unclear why some conventional adenomas acquire a serrated growth pattern, but this may be related to the acquisition of *KRAS* mutations, which has been proposed to add a "serrated" molecular signature to traditional adenomas, and provides evidence of a "fusion" molecular pathway

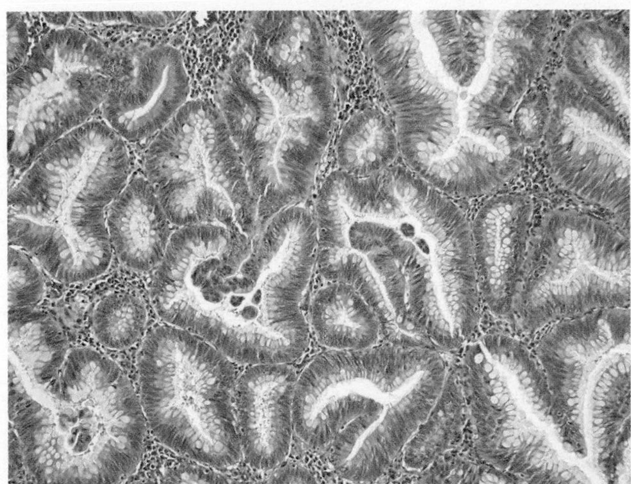

FIGURE 22.15 Conventional adenoma with a serrated architecture. In contrast with traditional serrated adenomas, conventional adenomas with architectural serration harbor cigar-shaped elongated nuclei with clumped chromatin, nuclear stratification, and mucin depletion, similar to traditional tubular or tubulovillous adenomas.

of carcinogenesis in some cases.[168] Some of these polyps may represent TSAs overgrown by conventional intestinal-type dysplasia. Recently, a superficial serrated adenoma has been described that consists predominantly of straight adenomatous glands with only superficial serrations.[137] These polyps lack eosinophilic cytoplasm, slitlike serrations, and ectopic crypt foci of TSA. They have been demonstrated to harbor *KRAS* mutations and *RPSO* fusions similar to TSAs. Some of these likely represent early forms of TSA but lack the features needed to a definitive diagnosis. Finally, some SSLs with small areas of superficial eosinophilic cells can be confusing to classify in some cases. These SSLs have been regarded as having either *low-grade serrated dysplasia, features of TSA,* or *enteric metaplasia* by various authors. These changes can be differentiated from TSA arising from an SSL caused by involvement of the deeper portions of the serrated crypts in TSA compared with SSLs with focal eosinophilic change. However, given the uncertainties in the classification of these unusual serrated lesions, the term *serrated adenoma, unclassified* is proposed by the recent WHO.

Differential Diagnosis of Serrated Polyps

Differentiation between SSL and MVHP can be challenging, and this distinction continues to be problematic, both in the community setting and among GI pathologists.[199-201] In a recent population-based study from Denmark, nearly 25% of all serrated polyps were excluded from the study because of a lack of consensus as to the diagnosis.[196] Regardless, in contrast with hyperplastic polyps, SSLs show dilated crypts, prominent full crypt serration, asymmetric basal crypt dilation with horizontal and branched crypts, increased numbers of dystrophic goblet cells, focal nuclear stratification, and upper crypt mitoses. SSLs also may contain rows of cells with hypereosinophilic "pink" cytoplasm, but these do not occur in hyperplastic polyps. However, some microvesicular polyps, particularly those in the right colon, may show one or more of these features focally. In these instances, correlation with the size, endoscopic appearance, and location of the lesion may be helpful. In general, if the lesion is larger than 0.5 cm in size, is sessile, and is present in the right or transverse colon, it most likely represents an early SSL. It should be emphasized that when making the diagnosis of SSL on a single architecturally abnormal crypt, the changes should be overt, and the polyp should lack features of mucosal prolapse, which can also distort the crypt architecture.[202,203] In equivocal cases, deeper levels may be helpful to identify SSL-type architectural changes.

TSAs are usually easy to differentiate from hyperplastic polyps and SSLs because the former are larger in size, often pedunculated and villiform, and show marked cytoplasmic eosinophilia at all levels of the crypt. TSAs are, for the most part, "dysplastic" lesions; hyperplastic polyps are not. Prolapse-type polyps arising in mucosal prolapse syndrome are frequently inflamed or even ulcerated, and they may show prominent crypt serrations, particularly at the surface of the polyp. They usually have superficial ischemic-type features, contain markedly regenerative epithelium, and show characteristic fibromuscular hyperplasia of the lamina propria. Inflammatory polyps not associated with prolapse may also have focal crypt serrations. However, in inflammatory polyps, the majority of the crypts are not serrated, and the inflamed edematous lamina propria helps differentiate inflammatory polyps from hyperplastic polyps.

Conventional adenomas may show serrated features as well. However, these are diffusely and homogeneously "dysplastic" lesions. They have hyperchromatic, pseudostratified, cigar-shaped (pencillate), atypical nuclei present uniformly throughout the polyp from base to surface. In adenomas with displacement, the crypts also show atypical features, with frequent mitoses and even single-cell necrosis.

Serrated Polyposis Syndrome

Serrated polyposis syndrome is characterized by the development of multiple serrated polyps in the colon, but without involvement of the upper GI tract or extracolonic manifestations. The etiology of this condition is unknown.[204] Up to one-third of serrated polyposis patients have at least one first-degree relative with colorectal carcinoma. A minority (~5%) have a first-degree relative with serrated polyposis.[205,206] To date, no high penetrance causative gene has been identified, although approximately 2% of affected patients have a pathogenic germline variant in *RNF43*, a gene involved in the WNT signaling pathway and mutated in some sporadic serrated polyps.[207-210]

Males and females are equally affected, and most patients are diagnosed in their 50s and 60s.[81,204-206] The diagnostic criteria have been recently revised. It now includes patients with a predominantly distal polyposis phenotype.[165] In addition, one previous criterion (any number of serrated polyps proximal to the sigmoid colon in an individual who had a first-degree relative with serrated polyposis) has been removed from the diagnosis. Thus at present, patients must meet at least one of the following criteria to qualify for a diagnosis of serrated polyposis syndrome.

1. At least five serrated polyps proximal to the rectum, all ≥5 mm, with at least two ≥10 mm.
2. More than 20 serrated polyps of any size, but distributed throughout the large bowel, with at least 5 proximal to the rectum.

Importantly, any histological subtype of serrated polyp may be included in the final count. Also, the diagnosis may be established only after multiple colonoscopies have been performed. Thus polyp count is cumulative over time.

As evident from the two main criteria listed earlier, the phenotype of serrated polyposis is highly heterogeneous. It includes patients with low polyp burden as well as patients with large numbers of polyps. Approximately 45% of patients with serrated polyposis fulfill criterion two, 25% meet criterion one, and 30% meet both criteria.[205,206]

Patients with serrated polyposis have an increased risk of colorectal carcinoma compared with the general population. The prevalence of colorectal carcinoma was reported to be 16% and 29%, respectively, in two recent large serrated polyposis cohorts.[205,206] Often, the diagnosis of colorectal cancer was made either before, or concurrently, with a diagnosis of serrated polyposis. The highest risk of carcinoma is in patients who fulfill both criteria. The presence of multiple SSLs proximal to the splenic flexure, the presence of SSL with dysplasia, and the presence of ≥1 advanced adenoma also increased colon cancer risk in these patients. Cancers occur throughout the colon, with up to 50% occurring in the distal large bowel. Approximately one-half of all colon cancers in serrated polyposis have a molecular phenotype consistent with origination from SSLs, characterized by *BRAF* mutations and CpG island DNA hypermethylation.[211] The remaining patients lack this phenotype, which suggests that many cancers may also develop via the conventional adenoma-carcinoma pathway.

Serrated polyposis is an underdiagnosed entity for a variety of reasons.[212,213] First, pathologists may be unfamiliar with the criteria used to establish the diagnosis. In addition, because the diagnosis is made, in part, based on the cumulative polyp burden, it is impossible to establish a diagnosis if information from all prior colonoscopies is unavailable. For this reason, when a patient has multiple serrated polyps, but the exact location, size, and number are not clear from the colonoscopy report, one should still raise the possibility of serrated polyposis and perform a careful review of all prior colonoscopy data whenever possible.

Once the diagnosis is established, genetic counseling should be performed to exclude rare genetic syndromes that may also present with a serrated polyposis phenotype (*MUTYH*-associated polyposis, hereditary mixed polyposis syndrome, and *PTEN*-hamartoma tumor syndrome).[150,214] The goal of surveillance in these patients is to remove all polyps >3 to 5 mm in size and to enroll patients in a yearly colonoscopy surveillance program to prevent colorectal carcinoma. If the polyp burden is high, and thus it is difficult to be controlled by colonoscopy, surgery should be considered a viable option.[214,215] First-degree relatives should also undergo colonoscopy, given the increased risk of colorectal carcinoma compared with the general population.[81,216]

MALIGNANT POLYPS

Definition

A malignant polyp is defined as a polyp that contains invasive adenocarcinoma.[27,217,218] Invasive carcinoma is defined by the presence of malignant glands that penetrate through the muscularis mucosae into the submucosa. Invasive carcinoma is often recognized by its association with a desmoplastic stromal response, but not all cancers are desmoplastic. Other key features include the presence of neoplastic cells in close association with fat, medium-sized arteries, nerves, ganglia, or large-sized lymphatics. Malignant glands usually reveal irregular, angulated contours and, of course, show cytological features of malignancy. Areas of invasion must be distinguished from areas of displaced epithelium as discussed previously.[38,219] Occasionally, these two phenomenon may occur in the same polyp.

Most submucosally invasive colorectal adenocarcinomas are associated with excellent outcomes, and most patients can be successfully managed conservatively if the lesion can be completely removed endoscopically.[220] However, pathologists play a key role in determining when additional treatment is necessary after endoscopic removal of a polyp with invasive carcinoma has been performed. Previously well-known and research-proven features that are used to determine the need for additional treatment, such as surgical resection, include the grade of the tumor, the presence or absence of lymphatic invasion, and the margin status.[221,222] However, more recently, multiple additional tumor features have been described that may also influence the risk of lymph node metastasis or recurrence, and these are described in more detail later.

Pathological Assessment of Risk in Malignant Polyps

Endoscopic Configuration

Pedunculated adenomas are the easiest to remove endoscopically, and thus much of the older literature has focused on invasive carcinoma that arises within pedunculated lesions. Historically, it was believed that invasive carcinoma arising within a sessile, superficially elevated, flat, or depressed lesion was less amenable to treatment by endoscopic resection because of difficulty removing them in one intact piece. It was also felt that the risk of lymphatic invasion was higher in these lesions. However, when matched for the presence of "high-risk" or "adverse" pathological features, the endoscopic configuration of the polyp itself has not been shown to have an effect on outcome.[223] It is important that gastroenterologists take great care to remove nonpedunculated lesions in one piece so the margin status and depth of invasion can be fully evaluated reliably. Endoscopic mucosal resection, or submucosal dissection, are usually needed for nonpedunculated polyps.

Polyp Size

The risk of invasive carcinoma is tightly linked to the endoscopic appearance, the pit pattern, and endoscopic size of the lesion. However, the size of the polyp is not an independent predictor of an adverse outcome such as lymph node metastasis or recurrence. The size of the invasive carcinoma component does seem to correlate with risk of lymph node metastasis in some studies. For instance, one study measured the area of submucosal invasion using digital analysis and demonstrated that an area >35 mm^2 predicted lymph node metastasis on multivariate analysis.[224] Measurement of the area of invasion is not easy to perform and, as such, is not currently recommended. However, simpler measurement techniques have been proposed by some Japanese investigators.

Margin Status

The presence of carcinoma at the cauterized stalk margin in pedunculated polyps and the presence of mucosal and/or deep margins in nonpedunculated polyps have been shown to be associated with an increased risk of local recurrence in multiple studies. However, what constitutes a "positive" margin has been the subject of debate for many years. Cooper et al. evaluated 140 adenomatous polyps for "unfavorable" histological features and considered the presence of a carcinoma less than 1 mm from the deep cauterized margin as an unfavorable sign.[225] However, Volk et al. considered carcinoma less than 2 mm from the deep margin as "positive" in their study.[226] More recent studies have, indeed, confirmed an increased risk of recurrence when carcinoma is within 1 mm of the deep margin, but others have shown that only carcinoma at the margin confers an adverse outcome.[227,228] Furthermore, although a "positive" margin is associated with an adverse outcome, the presence of a positive margin in any individual patient may not necessarily warrant surgical resection when other adverse pathological risk factors are not present in the polyp. Re-excision of the polypectomy site may be adequate when margin status is the only adverse feature. From a practical point of view, pathologists should report whether carcinoma is present at the cauterized margin of course, but if it is not at the margin, then it is prudent to report the actual distance from the margin in millimeters. This provides clinicians with the precise information they need to help guide the need for further treatment, which often takes into account a variety of variables such as patient age, comorbidities, and location of the tumor, among others.

Tumor Grade and Subtype

Poorly-differentiated ("high-grade") tumors have been associated with an adverse outcome after polypectomy in most studies, although this has not necessarily been a strong predictor of such. According to current American Joint Committee on Cancer and College of American Pathologists guidelines, tumor grade is based on the degree of gland formation, and this suffers from interobserver variability. Furthermore, in several prior studies, the area of the highest tumor grade defined the overall tumor grade for the polyp. However, this usually occurs at the invasive front, in which dedifferentiation and tumor budding may in fact be the principle poor prognostic factors. Regardless, poor tumor differentiation is still regarded as an adverse prognostic feature associated with increased local recurrence and lymph node metastasis and, as such, remains an important component of the pathologist's assessment of malignant polyps.

Poor tumor differentiation occurs commonly in MSI-H carcinomas. However, there are no guidelines available that describe how to incorporate mismatch repair protein expression in the risk stratification of malignant polyps. Signet ring cell, poorly cohesive, and micropapillary carcinomas are considered high risk by definition. Mucinous carcinomas are considered high risk in some studies, although data from other studies do not support this conclusion. Cribriform histology has been associated with increased risk of lymph node metastasis[229,230]; however, additional studies are needed before this feature can be incorporated into risk stratification.

Lymphatic and Venous Invasion

Lymphatic invasion is a well-studied histological feature in malignant polyps and has been shown in multiple studies to be predictive of lymph node metastasis (Fig. 22.16). In one meta-analysis of 1438 polyps, lymphovascular invasion was identified in 17.6% of polyps, and this feature was more common in lymph node–positive versus lymph node–negative cases (35.3% vs. 7.2%).[223] Two more recent studies from Japan have also confirmed the predictive value of lymphatic invasion. For instance, Ishii et al. evaluated 136 patients with submucosal invasive carcinoma who underwent colectomy. Lymph node metastasis was seen in 29% of patients with lymphatic invasion in contrast with 5% of those without lymphatic invasion.[231] Tateishi et al. evaluated 322 patients and demonstrated similar results.[232] Overall, these studies underscore the importance of careful assessment of endoscopically resected polyps with invasive carcinoma for the presence of lymphatic invasion to help guide subsequent therapy.

However, some studies have failed to demonstrate a predictive value of lymphatic invasion in colon polyps.[226] Furthermore, lymphatic invasion may be difficult to identify pathologically. It suffers from only a fair degree of interobserver agreement.[233] Lymphatic invasion is more easily identified, with confidence, if it is present at the leading edge of the carcinoma or outside of the confines of the carcinoma. Immunohistochemistry (D2-40 or CD31) is often helpful in confirming the presence of lymphatic invasion when there is diagnostic uncertainty.

Venous invasion is a well-known poor prognostic factor in colorectal carcinoma, but its significance in adenomas with invasive carcinoma is less clear, given that it is a relatively rare event in this setting. Venous invasion is a relatively rare event in malignant polyps. Venous invasion is defined as the presence of carcinoma within an endothelium-lined space surrounded by a readily identifiable smooth muscle layer or elastic lamina. The use of special stains to identify elastic fibers is usually very helpful. Some studies have shown that venous invasion is associated with lymph node metastasis[232]; however, other studies have not.[234] Regardless, the presence of venous invasion should always be reported if identified histologically so the treating physician can make treatment decisions with all available potentially valuable information.

Tumor Budding

Tumor budding was first described in 1954 by Imai, who identified tumor cells that seemed to be "sprouting" from the invasive tumor front (see Fig. 22.16). Tumor "sprouts" or "buds" are now believed to represent a type of epithelial-mesenchymal transition, and a marker of degree of "invasiveness" of the tumor. Pathologically, this was defined by Ueno et al. in 2002 as a tumor cluster composed of less than five cells.[235] Tumor budding can occur both within the tumor (intratumoral budding) or at the invasive front (peritumoral budding). For instance, in one seminal study of submucosally invasive carcinomas by Ueno et al. in 2004, poor tumor differentiation, lymphovascular invasion, and tumor budding were independently associated with risk of lymph node metastases.[229] Of these three features, tumor budding was the strongest predictor in multivariate analysis. In multiple subsequent studies, peritumoral tumor budding

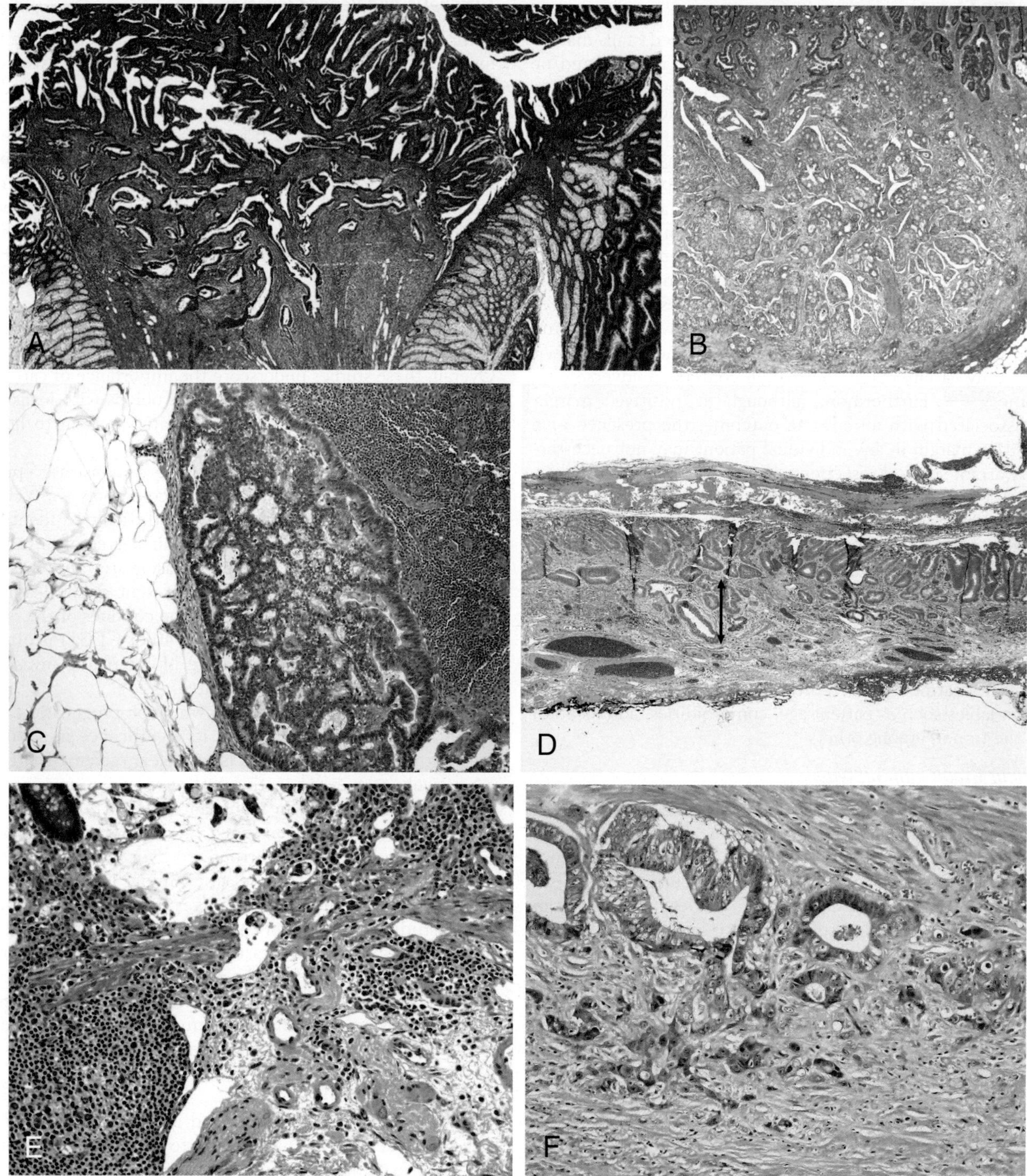

FIGURE 22.16 A, A pedunculated tubulovillous adenoma with a focal invasive well-differentiated adenocarcinoma into the stalk of the polyp. The margin was widely free, and no lymphovascular invasion or grade 2 to 3 tumor budding was identified. **B–C,** The adenocarcinoma arising from this adenoma was poorly differentiated and deeply invasive. No lymphovascular invasion or high tumor budding was identified, but a subsequent colectomy demonstrated two positive lymph nodes **(C)**. **D,** This endoscopic submucosal dissection specimen for a flat adenoma had a small focus of submucosally invasive well-differentiated adenocarcinoma. The depth of submucosal invasion *(double-headed arrow)* was 350 microns. The resection margin was negative for lymphovascular invasion, and high tumor budding was not identified. This polyp is considered to have very low risk of lymph node metastasis. **E,** This poorly differentiated adenocarcinoma arising from a tubular adenoma had a small focus of lymphatic invasion. **F,** In this polyp with invasive carcinoma, there is grade 3 tumor budding, which is an adverse histological feature associated with lymph node metastasis.

has been shown to be an independent prognostic factor associated with lymph node metastases, local recurrence, and cancer-related death.[229,236-240] As a result, the National Comprehensive Cancer Network has recognized the importance of tumor budding in predicting poor behavior in patients with malignant polyps and has recommended incorporation of this feature in therapeutic decision making. In 2017, an international consensus conference was convened, and guidelines were proposed on how to measure tumor budding in malignant polyps.[241] It is recommended that

TABLE 22.5 Evaluation of Polyps Harboring Adenocarcinoma

Favorable Histology	Unfavorable Histology	Reporting Recommendations
Tumor grades 1 and 2	Tumor grades 3 and 4	Essential
No lymphovascular invasion	Lymphovascular invasion	Essential
Grade 1 tumor budding (<5 per 0.785 mm^2)	Grades 2 and 3 tumor budding (≥5 per 0.785 mm^2)	Optional, but recommended
Grade 1 poorly differentiated clusters (<5 per 0.785 mm^2)	Grades 2 and 3 poorly differentiated clusters (≥5 per 0.785 mm^2)	Optional
≤1000 microns depth submucosal invasion (used in some centers) *OR* Kikuchi level sm1 (applicable to sessile polyps with muscularis propria)	>1000 microns submucosal invasion *OR* Kikuchi level sm2 and sm3 (applicable to sessile polyps with muscularis propria)	Optional
Negative margin or ≥1 mm from margin (depending on particular studies)	Positive polypectomy margin or <1 mm from margin (depending on particular studies)	Essential

the invasive front should be scanned at low magnification, and then the area containing the highest number of tumor buds should be identified. The tumor buds should then be counted in a single 20× field in this area. A correction factor should then be applied to determine the number of buds in an area that measures 0.785 mm^2 in dimension. Using this method, a tumor bud count between 0 and 4 is considered "low" (grade 1), 5 to 9 is "intermediate" (grade 2), and ≥10 buds is "high" (grade 3). In the setting of a malignant polyp, a bud count ≥5 (grades 2 to 3) is associated with increased risk of lymph node metastasis.

A similar process termed *poorly differentiated clusters* has also recently been described and has been defined as clusters of five or more cells without gland formation. The presence of poorly differentiated clusters has also been associated with lymph node metastasis and disease-free survival.[242,243] In a recent study, a model combining tumor grade, margin status, lymphovascular invasion, any budding (combining tumor budding and poorly differentiated clusters), and muscular mucosae status (intact muscularis mucosae vs. disrupted muscularis mucosae) was able to predict lymph node metastasis better than a conventional model that included only tumor grade, lymphovascular invasion, and margin status.[243] Future studies are needed to determine whether poorly differentiated clusters should become part of standard reporting in malignant polyps or potentially combined with tumor budding and reported as one feature.

Depth of Submucosal Invasion

The extent of tumor invasion into the submucosa is another feature that has been studied for its potential association with risk of lymph node metastasis. Haggitt et al. in 1985 categorized depth of invasion in pedunculated polyps into four levels.[244] Haggitt levels 1 to 3 correspond to invasion of the head, neck, and stalk, respectively, and have a low risk of lymph node metastasis. Haggitt level 4 corresponds to invasion below the stalk of the polyp and is invariably associated with a positive stalk margin in pedunculated polyps. For this reason, providing Haggitt levels does not provide additional information regarding risk of adverse outcomes. Kikuchi in 1995 divided the submucosa into sm1, sm2, and sm3 representing the inner third, middle third, and outer third, respectively.[245] Only tumors with invasion into the outer two-thirds of the submucosa (≥ sm2) showed a risk of lymph node metastasis. This classification is useful in specimens that contain muscularis propria, such as in transanal excisions. However, this is not normally applied to endoscopic resections.

Measurement of the actual depth of submucosal invasion in millimeters provides an alternative to sm and Haggitt levels. This technique has also been shown to predict lymph node metastasis in multiple studies.[229,232,246-248] For instance, Ueno et al. demonstrated that no tumors with less than 500 μm depth of invasion and only 3.9% of tumors with a depth of 2000 μm of invasion, had lymph node metastasis.[229] More recently, others have demonstrated that tumors with less than 1000 μm depth of invasion have only a low risk of lymph node metastasis. In this study, a cutoff of 1000 μm was recommended to separate low-risk from high-risk polyps. However, in some other studies, depth of submucosal invasion has not been shown in multivariate analysis to be an independent predictor of lymph node metastasis. Given these conflicting data, reporting depth of submucosal invasion is not mandatory at most institutions in the United States.

If one does provide depth of submucosal invasion, the measurement depends on the polyp type. For pedunculated polyps, only invasion into the stalk should be measured. In nonpedunculated polyps, one should measure depth of invasion from the muscularis mucosae (see Fig. 22.16). If the muscularis mucosae cannot be identified, then the depth is measured from the surface of the tumor.

Reporting Malignant Polyps

Key features to include in diagnostic reports of adenomas with invasive carcinoma include histological type, tumor grade, margin status, lymphatic invasion, venous invasion, tumor budding, and depth of submucosal invasion (Table 22.5). If the tumor lacks any of these high-risk features, the risk of lymph node metastasis is extremely low (<1%). Of note, the College of American Pathologists checklist on colorectal carcinoma has tumor budding as an optional element, does not require separating lymphatic from venous invasion, and does not require reporting depth of submucosal invasion. Nevertheless, it is good practice to include these elements in a pathology report on an endoscopic resection of a malignant polyp.

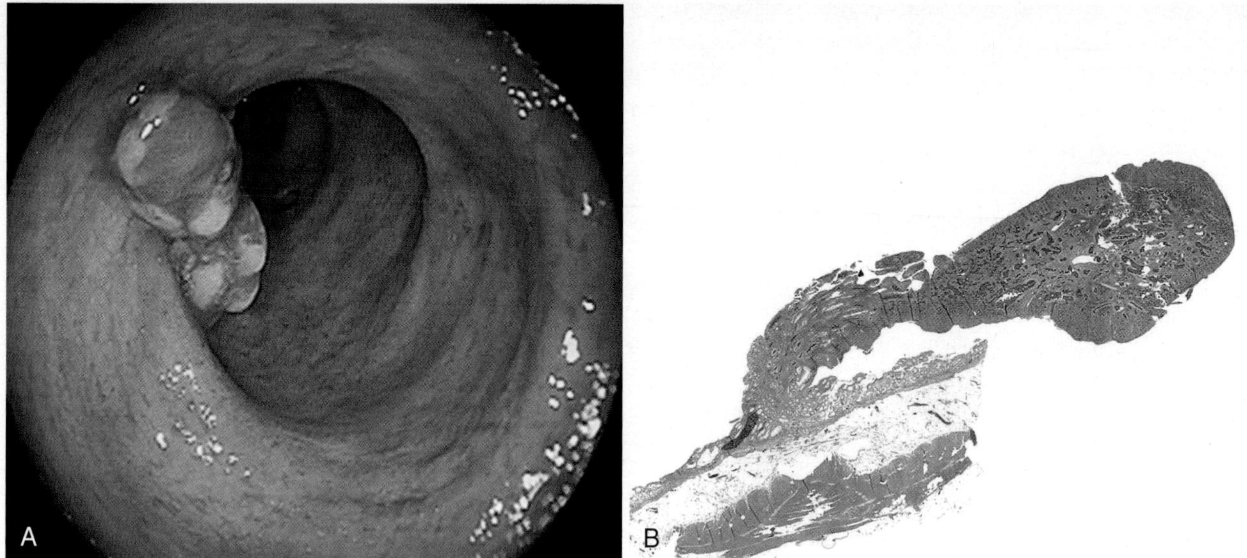

FIGURE 22.17 **A,** Endoscopic appearance of a giant "filiform" inflammatory polyp in a patient with chronic ulcerative colitis. **B,** The inflammatory polyp projects several centimeters above the mucosal surface.

INFLAMMATORY POLYPS

Inflammatory polyps are defined as intraluminal projections of mucosa that are formed of a non-neoplastic mixture of stromal and epithelial components and inflammatory cells. Inflammatory polyps represent areas of inflamed and regenerating mucosa that project above the level of the surrounding mucosa, which is frequently ulcerated. They generally develop as a response to either localized or diffuse inflammatory diseases (e.g., Crohn's disease, ulcerative colitis), but they also occur in association with other disorders, such as ischemic colitis,[249] neonatal necrotizing enterocolitis,[122] and infectious colitis,[123] and they commonly form at the edges of intestinal ulcers and mucosal anastomoses. The pathogenesis is related to ulceration of the mucosa, followed by inflammation and regenerative hyperplasia of the intervening nonulcerated epithelium. In rare cases, the patient may have no apparent underlying inflammatory disorder.

Pathological Features

Grossly, inflammatory polyps may be sessile or pedunculated. They are almost always smaller than 2 cm in size, but so-called *giant inflammatory polyps* may grow to large sizes and cause obstruction.[124,250] *Filiform polyposis* refers to the presence of numerous dense, filamentous polyps that can project several centimeters above the surrounding mucosa (Fig. 22.17).[125] This form of polyposis is usually associated with IBD or, rarely, juvenile polyposis.

Histologically, some polyps, particularly those adjacent to ulcers or anastomotic sites, are formed entirely, or almost entirely, of inflamed granulation tissue. However, most inflammatory polyps (or "pseudopolyps") are composed of a mixture of inflamed lamina propria and distorted colonic epithelium; surface erosions may or may not be present (Fig. 22.18). Colonic crypts are often dilated and branched, and neutrophilic cryptitis and crypt abscesses may be prominent. Some crypts may also have a serrated architecture. In the later stages of development, inflammatory polyps may only consist of many finger-like projections of either completely normal- or near-normal–appearing mucosa, surrounding a core of submucosal tissue. The latter may show fibrosis, chronic inflammation, or other subtle clues as to the origin of the polyp.

Three potential pitfalls may occur in the histological evaluation of inflammatory polyps. First, dysplasia may rarely develop in these lesions, particularly in those associated with IBD. Much more commonly, regenerating epithelium can be extreme, particularly in inflamed or eroded areas, simulating a neoplastic process. Careful attention to surface maturation, which is usually observed in regenerating epithelium and almost never in dysplasia, can help in making this distinction in difficult cases. Second, bizarrely shaped, enlarged, or multinucleated stromal cells that can mimic sarcoma (termed *pseudosarcoma*) may develop in inflammatory pseudopolyps.[251] These cells may be spindled or epithelioid, and they are often located in aggregates at the surface of the polyp, directly underneath the area of ulceration and granulation tissue in a somewhat regular, linear, and organized manner (Fig. 22.19).

Finally, in many instances, the histological appearance of inflammatory polyps may be indistinguishable from that of a juvenile polyp or other hamartomatous polyps. Distinction between these types of lesions is based largely on clinical information, such as the age of the patient (almost all such polyps in young children are juvenile polyps), the presence or absence of a clinical history of a hamartomatous polyposis syndrome (juvenile polyposis, Cowden's syndrome, hereditary mixed polyposis syndrome, and Cronkhite-Canada syndrome can all have juvenile-type polyps),[252] and the presence or absence of an underlying inflammatory disorder.

Natural History and Treatment

Inflammatory polyps tend to persist even after healing of the surrounding mucosa has been achieved. They are frequently found in IBD. Inflammatory polyps have no increased tendency for neoplastic transformation. Treatment is usually directed at the underlying inflammatory condition. Rarely, surgical excision is indicated when large, or numerous, polyps cause symptoms as a result of bleeding or obstruction.[124]

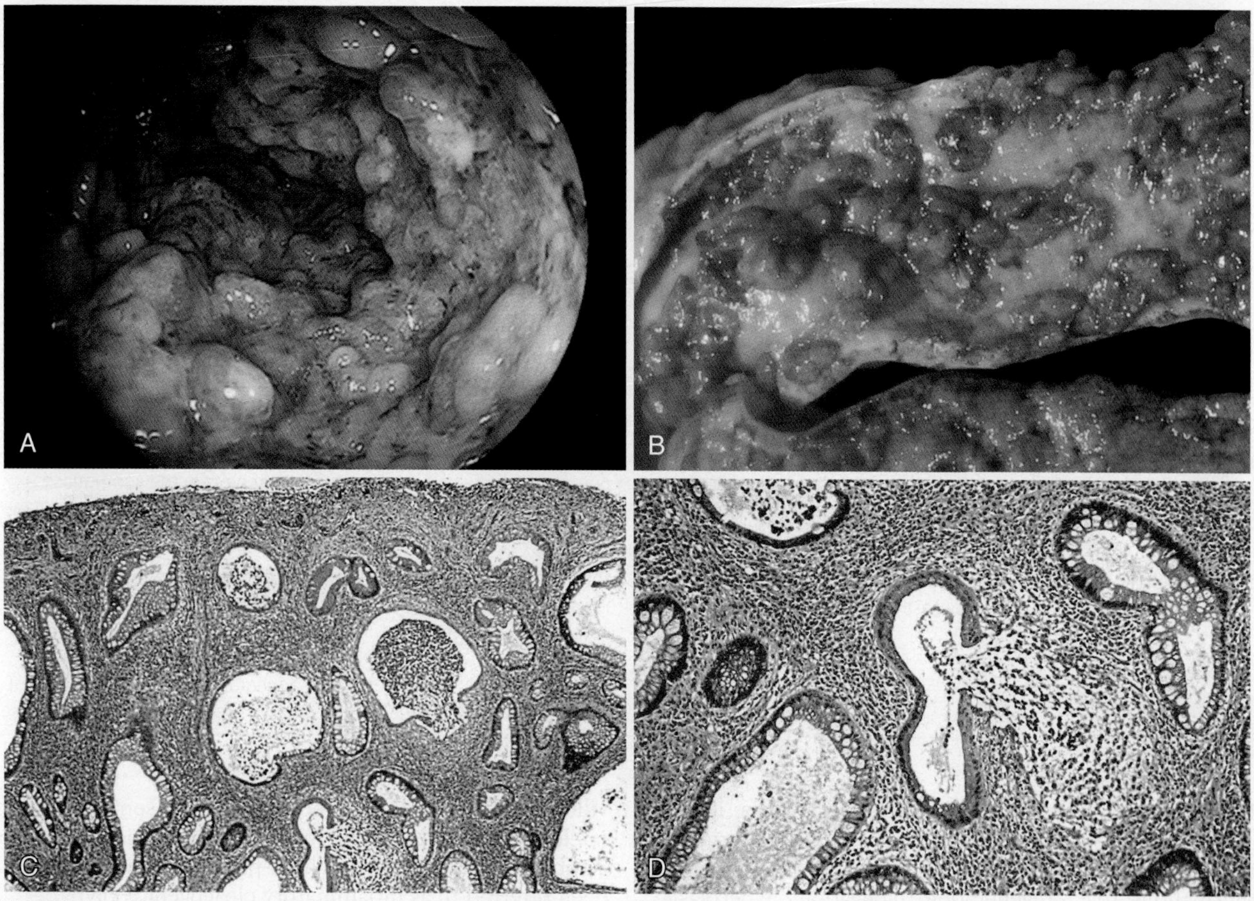

FIGURE 22.18 Inflammatory pseudopolyps. **A,** Endoscopic appearance of diffuse (severe) inflammatory polyposis in a patient with chronic ulcerative colitis. **B,** This colonic resection specimen shows broad, shallow ulcers surrounded by raised, erythematous tags of inflamed mucosa. **C,** Inflammatory pseudopolyps in patients with inflammatory bowel disease are frequently composed of a mixture of acute inflammation, dense mucosal lymphoplasmacytic infiltrate, and distorted dilated crypts with surface erosion, cryptitis, and crypt abscesses. **D,** Crypt abscesses with crypt rupture may be present and may lead to mucin granulomas or mucin extravasation.

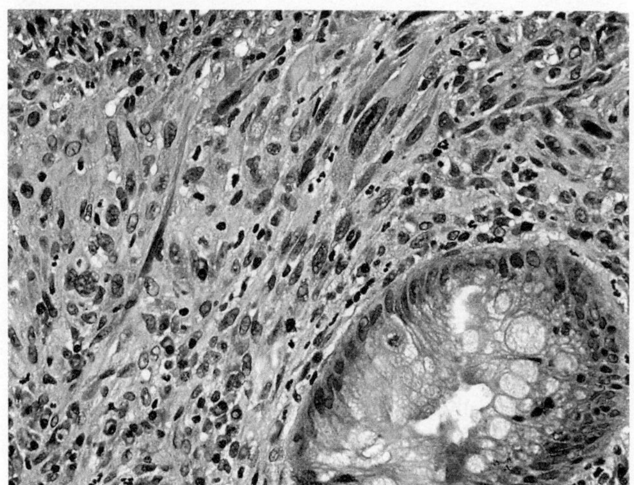

FIGURE 22.19 "Pseudosarcoma" in an inflammatory polyp. Bizarre-shaped, enlarged, atypical stromal cells may occasionally be seen in granulation tissue of an inflammatory pseudopolyp, particularly beneath an area of surface erosion. These cells can be confused with sarcoma, carcinoma, or viral infection (e.g., from cytomegalovirus).

POLYPS ASSOCIATED WITH MUCOSAL PROLAPSE

Prolapse-type polyps develop as a result of localized injury to the mucosa caused by traction, distortion, and twisting of mucosa resulting from peristalsis-induced trauma. This leads to torsion of blood vessels, localized ischemia, tissue damage, and repair in the form of lamina propria fibromuscular hyperplasia. Depending on the anatomic location of the injury and the underlying cause, these lesions may be referred to as *mucosal prolapse syndrome, inflammatory cap polyps, colitis cystica polyposa,* or *diverticular disease–associated polyps* (Table 22.6). All demonstrate some overlapping histological abnormalities that are usually the result of mucosal prolapse, but they all have distinctive clinical or pathological features as well.[253] The majority of polyps encountered in routine sign-out that arise as a result of mucosal prolapse do not have a specific clinical association, and they can simply be signed out as descriptively as *inflammatory polyp with features of mucosal prolapse* or *mucosal prolapse-associated inflammatory polyp.* The classic histological features of prolapse-induced polyps include (1) a

TABLE 22.6 Polyps and Lesions Associated with Mucosal Prolapse

Entity	Clinical Presentation	Endoscopic Features	Pathological Features
Mucosal prolapse syndrome	Rectal bleeding, straining during defecation, sense of incomplete evacuation	Mucosal erythema, ulcers (solitary or multiple), polypoid/ mass lesions	Thickening and disruption of the muscularis mucosae that often runs parallel to the long axis of the crypts, diamond-shaped crypt bases, vascular ectasia, serrated crypt architecture
Inflammatory cap polyps	Diarrhea, mucoid stools, bleeding, pain on defecation	Multiple small, sessile or semipedunculated polyps; most common location is rectum or rectosigmoid	Elongated, dilated, or tortuous hyperplastic colonic crypts with abundant inflammation in the lamina propria and a characteristic "cap" of granulation tissue with adherent fibrin
Colitis cystica profunda/ polyposa	Varied, often accompanies mucosal prolapse syndrome	Polypoid lesions with submucosal component	Multiple cystically dilated, mucin-filled crypts in the submucosa and occasionally in the muscularis propria or serosa
Diverticular disease–associated polyps	Occurs in patients with diverticular disease	Bright red, polypoid, or slightly elevated patches of mucosa in patients with sigmoid diverticulosis	Vascular congestion, hemorrhage, lamina propria fibrosis, and crypt architectural changes. Larger polyps may have a "leaflike" appearance and show changes typically seen in mucosal prolapse

variable degree of fibromuscular hyperplasia of the lamina propria; (2) thickening, splaying, and vertical extension of the muscularis mucosae into the lamina propria; (3) crypt abnormalities (e.g., regeneration, elongation, hyperplasia, architectural distortion, serration); and (4) a variable degree of inflammation, ulceration, and reactive epithelial change (Fig. 22.20).[253,254]

Mucosal Prolapse Syndrome

The term *mucosal prolapse syndrome* was first proposed by du Boulay et al. in 1983 as a unifying term for clinicopathological abnormalities underlying the solitary rectal ulcer syndrome and its related entities.[255] This syndrome affects patients in middle age and presents with rectal bleeding, straining during defecation, and a sense of incomplete evacuation. Endoscopic findings are varied and can range from mucosal erythema, single or multiple ulcers, and polypoid/ mass lesions.[256,257] The etiology of this syndrome is not entirely clear, but paradoxical contraction of the puborectalis muscle during defecation has been observed.[258,259] Given the myriad endoscopic findings, the differential diagnosis is broad and includes IBD, ischemic colitis, neoplasia, and infectious proctitis. There is often a delay in the diagnosis of mucosal prolapse syndrome with an initial incorrect diagnosis occurring in 25%.[260]

Histologically mucosal prolapse syndrome is characterized by thickening and disruption of the muscularis mucosae, diamond-shaped crypt bases, vascular ectasia, erosions and ulceration, and serrated crypt architecture.[261,262] The fibers of the muscularis mucosae often run parallel to the long axis of the crypts. Neutrophilic cryptitis is common, but increased lymphoplasmacytic inflammation of the lamina propria is usually not present. When forming a mass lesion at the anorectal junction, these lesions often have a villous architecture, serrated crypts, and some degree of nuclear enlargement and hyperchromasia, which can mimic a tubulovillous adenoma. These polypoid lesions have also been referred to as inflammatory cloacogenic polyps.

Patients with mucosal prolapse syndrome are often managed conservatively if symptoms are mild or moderate.[256] Avoidance of straining and consumption of a high-fiber diet are recommended. Biofeedback has been shown to be helpful in some patients.[263] Surgery (e.g., rectopexy) may be necessary in patients with severe symptoms or overt rectal prolapse.[256]

Inflammatory Cap Polyp (and Polyposis)

Inflammatory cap polyps were first described in abstract form in 1985 by Williams and coworkers.[264] These rare lesions usually occur in the setting of cap polyposis, a condition in which dozens of these types of polyps develop. There is no sex predilection, and they occur over a wide age range.[265] Clinically, patients with cap polyposis present with diarrhea, mucoid stools, GI bleeding, and/or tenesmus, features that mimic IBD. Occasionally, these symptoms are accompanied by severe hypoproteinemia.[266] The etiology of these polyps is unknown, but abnormal motility is common in affected patients, suggesting that polyps may arise due to repeated trauma from chronic straining during defecation.[267-269]

Endoscopically, most cap polyps are small, sessile, or semipedunculated lesions that range in size from a few millimeters to 2 cm. The most common location is the rectum or rectosigmoid; less commonly, the descending colon is involved.[270-273] Rarely, cap polyps may involve the entire colon and even the stomach.[265,274] Multiple polyps are typically located at the crests of mucosal folds, separated by normal or edematous mucosa.

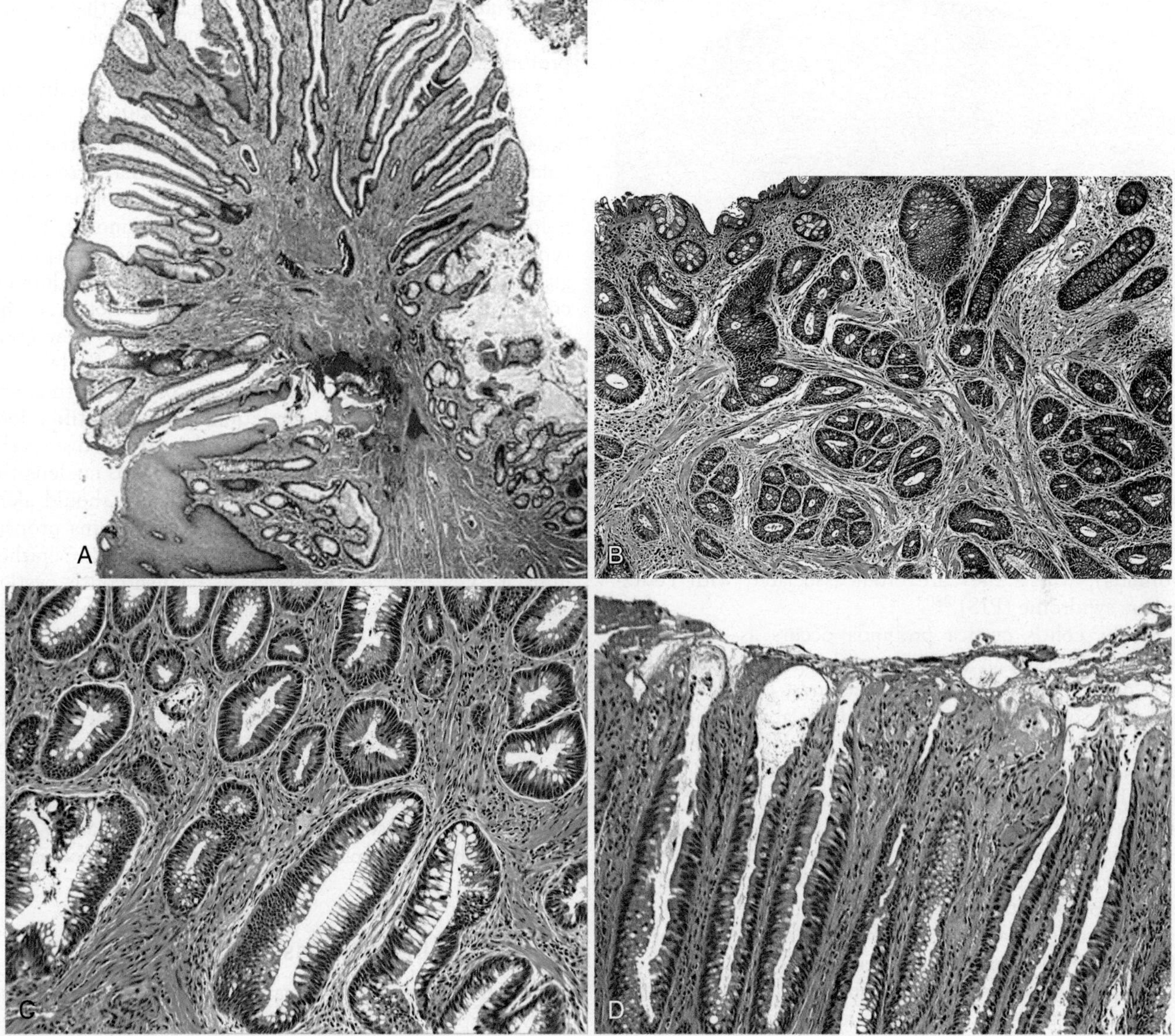

FIGURE 22.20 Mucosal prolapse polyp variants. A, Inflammatory (cloacogenic) polyp of the anorectal transition zone. **B,** Strands of thickened and splayed muscularis mucosae extend around the crypt bases and into the overlying lamina propria. The crypts assume an angulated and distorted appearance. **C,** When embedded tangentially, prolapse polyps show strands of smooth muscle that appear to encircle colonic crypts, which frequently assume a "diamond" shape. **D,** On the surface, mucosal prolapse polyps often contain markedly regenerative, serrated/hyperplastic-appearing epithelium and ischemic-type changes with erosion.

Histologically, cap polyps are non-neoplastic lesions composed of elongated, dilated, or tortuous hyperplastic colonic crypts with abundant inflammation in the lamina propria and a characteristic "cap" of granulation tissue, usually with adherent fibrin (Fig. 22.21). Goblet cells in cap polyps have been shown, by immunohistochemistry, to express nonsulfated mucins.[275] The intervening lamina propria typically contains increased acute and chronic inflammatory cells. Some polyps contain splayed smooth muscle fibers, or fibrosis, suggestive of a mucosal prolapse etiology.[265,271]

Many patients with multiple polyps require surgical resection for resolution of their symptoms,[270,272,273] although some patients improve spontaneously[265] or with therapy to eradicate *Helicobacter pylori* infection.[274] Infliximab may also be effective therapy for cap polypsis.[276] Isolated polyps are treated by simple polypectomy. Cap polyps have no risk of malignancy.

Colitis Cystica Profunda/Polyposa

Clinical Features

Colitis cystica profunda is a rare benign condition characterized by cystic dilation and displacement of mature crypts through the muscularis mucosae into the submucosa, or even into deeper layers of the bowel wall. The term *colitis cystica polyposa* was first used by Virchow in 1863 to describe a case in which multiple polypoid lesions were produced by submucosal cysts.[277] The term *colitis cystica profunda* subsequently came into use in 1957 to encompass cases that show a dominant form of the disease without prominent polyp formation[278]; most affected patients have both submucosal cysts and associated polypoid lesions. Similar lesions are found in the stomach (gastritis cystica profunda), where they most frequently occur after Billroth II gastrectomy,[279] and in the small bowel (enteritis cystica

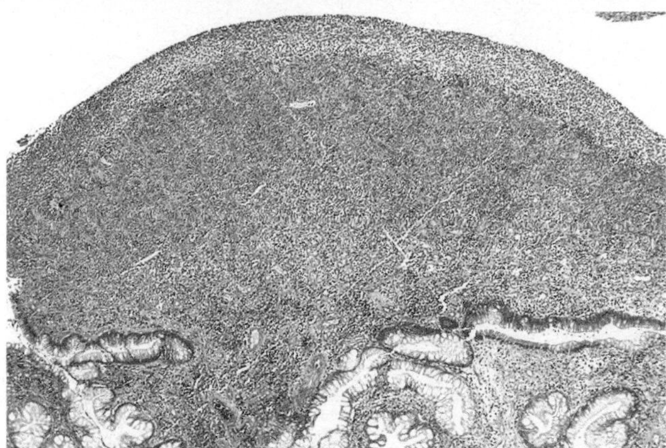

FIGURE 22.21 Inflammatory cap polyp. This type of inflammatory pseudopolyp shows an overlying "cap" of necroinflammatory exudate. These polyps may occur in the setting of cap polyposis, at anastomotic sites, in association with inflammatory bowel disease (as in this case), or in many other conditions that induce mucosal ulceration.

profunda), where they are often associated with Peutz-Jeghers syndrome (PJS).[280]

Rarely, colitis cystica profunda occurs as an isolated lesion (or lesions) in a patient with an otherwise apparently normal colon.[281,282] However, most cases are associated with some form of chronic colonic abnormality, most commonly solitary rectal ulcer syndrome[277,283,284] in which the lesions are located exclusively in the rectosigmoid colon. Distal lesions (sometimes called *proctitis cystica profunda*) have also been reported in paraplegics,[285] in patients with self-inflicted rectal trauma,[286] and in patients with postirradiation colonic strictures.[287,288] Less commonly, a diffuse form of colitis cystica profunda occurs in patients with IBD (including ulcerative colitis, Crohn's disease,[289] and unclassified forms[290]) or infectious dysentery.[277]

The pathogenesis of colitis cystica profunda is believed to be related to prolapse and subsequent torsion with trauma of the mucosa and submucosa that leads to vascular compromise and ischemia.[277] In solitary rectal ulcer syndrome (see Chapter 17), mucosal prolapse results in ischemia and ulceration by virtue of traction exerted on blood vessels at the time of defecation.[277] However, in colitis cystica profunda associated with infectious or idiopathic IBD, the pathological changes probably occur as a result of displacement and entrapment of regenerating glands in the submucosa during the process of reepithelialization and healing of ulcers.

Guest and Reznick[277] reviewed the clinical features of 144 cases of colitis cystica profunda. Patients ranged from 4 to 76 years of age (median, 30 years). Males and females were approximately equally affected. The most common presenting symptoms were blood in the stool (68%), mucoid stools (43%), diarrhea (27%), tenesmus (13%), and abdominal discomfort (12%).[277] Rarely, patients may develop obstruction.[281]

Pathological Features

Grossly, colitis cystica profunda can be a focal, segmental, or diffuse lesion. Focal and segmental lesions can mimic invasive adenocarcinoma. Transrectal ultrasonography and other imaging modalities can aid in making the distinction by demonstrating multiple cysts limited to the submucosa and lack of lymph node involvement in colitis cystica profunda.[291]

Histologically, the condition is characterized by the presence of multiple, usually cystically dilated, mucin-filled crypts in the submucosa and occasionally in the muscularis propria or even the serosa. The stroma surrounding displaced crypts usually consists of lamina propria; this is helpful in distinguishing it from adenocarcinoma, which typically has a desmoplastic stroma. Furthermore, displaced glands in colitis cystica profunda often grow in a lobular configuration without jagged borders and do not show the unusual, irregularly shaped glandular profiles characteristic of adenocarcinoma. Displaced crypts typically show either normal or reactive-appearing colonic epithelium. A mild degree of mucin depletion, pseudostratification, and increased mitotic activity may be observed as well. However, loss of nuclear polarity, an increased nucleus-to-cytoplasm (N:C) ratio, and atypical mitoses should alert one to the possibility of adenocarcinoma. Lamina propria surrounding displaced glands and lack of dysplastic epithelium are key features that help distinguish colitis cystica profunda from invasive adenocarcinoma (see Table 22.1; Fig. 22.22).

Treatment

In many patients with rectal prolapse, treatment of the defecation disorder itself (e.g., education to avoid straining at defecation, a high-fiber diet, bulk laxatives) leads to remission of colitis cystica profunda.[283] Some patients require surgical resection because of obstruction,[281] confusion with carcinoma, severe symptoms, or coexistent IBD.[290]

Diverticular Disease–Associated Polyps

Polyps that occur in association with diverticulosis are of two types: inverted diverticula and polypoid prolapsing mucosal folds. Polyps of the former type have been described in patients with inverted Meckel diverticula of the ileum (wherein they may cause intussusception),[292] isolated inverted colonic diverticula, or inverted sigmoid diverticula in the setting of sigmoid diverticulosis.[293,294] Inverted colonic diverticula usually range from 0.2 to 2 cm in size. They may be sessile or pedunculated, but they characteristically have the same color as the surrounding mucosa.[294] These polyps tend to vanish with gentle pressure from the biopsy forceps or from air insufflation at endoscopy.[294] Bowel perforation may occur as a result of endoscopic polypectomy in cases in which the inverted diverticulum mimics an adenoma.[294]

Polypoid prolapsing mucosal folds are the more common form of diverticular disease–associated polyps. Grossly, these appear as bright red, polypoid, or slightly elevated patches of mucosa in the area of mucosa involved with diverticulosis.[295] Swollen mucosal folds between diverticular ostia may reveal an apical brown discoloration. More advanced lesions characteristically show small, brownish, polypoid protrusions of the mucosal folds. Polyps normally range from 0.5 to 3 cm in size.

Histologically, early lesions show vascular congestion, hemorrhage, and hemosiderin deposition. More advanced

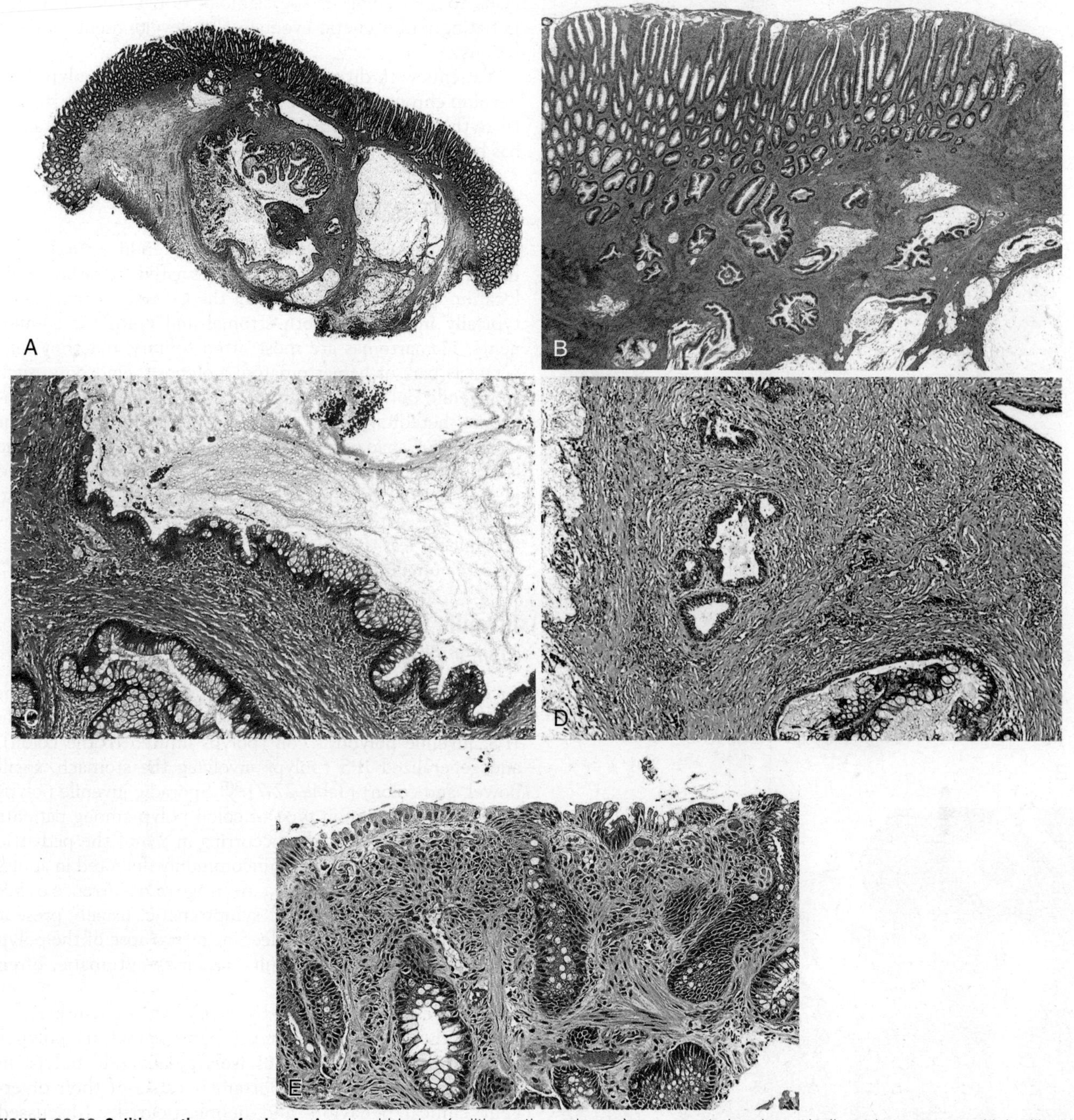

FIGURE 22.22 Colitis cystica profunda. A, A polypoid lesion (colitis cystica polyposa) was resected endoscopically; at low power, multiple dilated, mucin-filled spaces are shown expanding the submucosa. **B,** A case of cystica profunda occurring in association with mucosal prolapse. The thickened muscularis mucosae can be seen *(top),* where it extends around the crypts at the base of the lamina propria. Within the submucosa *(bottom)* is a cystically dilated, mucin-filled crypt. **C,** Keys to recognizing the benign nature of cystica profunda include the lack of cytological atypia in the epithelium of the displaced crypts, which may appear regenerative but maintains the usual low nucleus-to-cytoplasm ratio and basal nuclear polarity. **D,** Hemosiderin deposition in the stroma and the presence of lamina propria surrounding displaced crypts are additional features that separate cystica profunda from infiltrating adenocarcinoma. **E,** One of the most common associations of colitis cystica profunda is with solitary rectal ulcer syndrome (occult rectosigmoid prolapse), in which case the surrounding nonpolypoid mucosa shows characteristic fibromuscular proliferation in the lamina propria.

lesions reveal edema, capillary thrombi, lamina propria fibrosis, and crypt architectural changes, such as dilation and branching. The most advanced, "leaflike" polyps show changes typically seen in mucosal prolapse, such as smooth muscle ingrowth into the lamina propria, crypt hyperplasia, mucin depletion, and serrated hyperplastic changes of the epithelium (Fig. 22.23). Epithelial hyperplasia may be marked and should not be mistaken for an adenoma.[296] Rarely, one may see pseudosarcomatous changes of the stroma, characterized by enlarged and hyperchromatic myofibroblasts that should not be mistaken for sarcoma.[296]

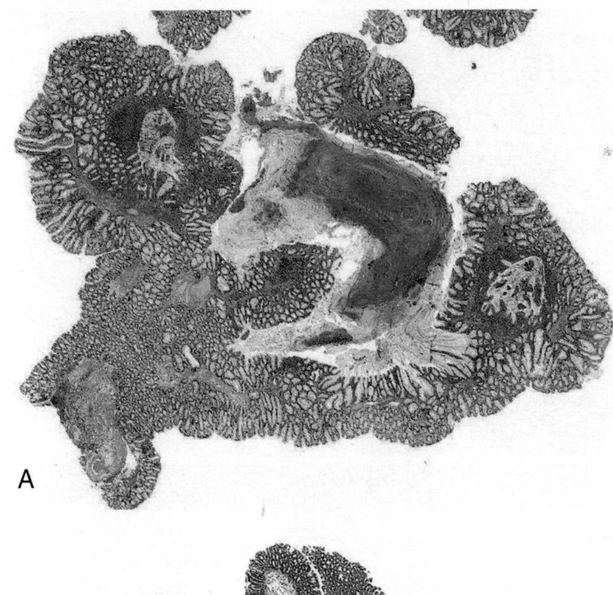

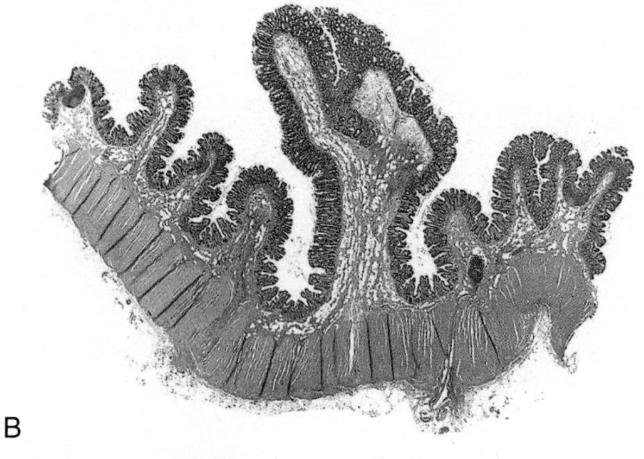

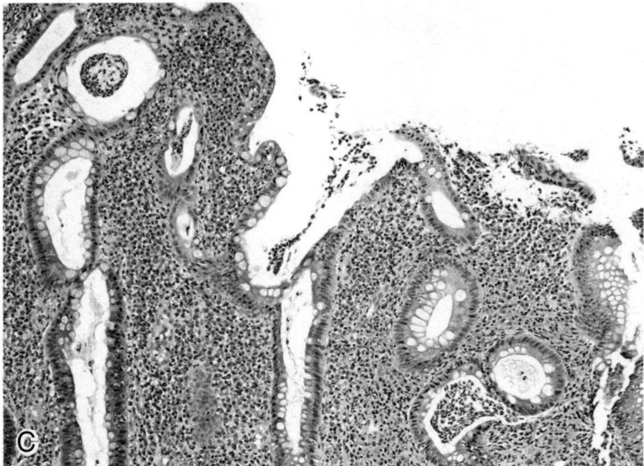

FIGURE 22.23 Diverticular disease–associated polyps. A, Redundant mucosal folds in patients with sigmoid diverticular disease are produced by thickening and shortening of the muscularis propria, as seen in this section. A more prominent redundant fold at the center has the low-power appearance of a pedunculated polyp. **B,** A prominent leaflike polyp located at the mouth of a diverticulum.

Redundant mucosal folds occur in a large majority (90% to 100%) of patients with advanced sigmoid diverticulosis, although only a minority develop grossly polypoid lesions or frank prolapse-like histological alterations of the mucosa (see Fig. 22.23).[297,298] Thickening of the taenia coli, which leads to shortening of the sigmoid, is believed to be the initiating pathogenetic event in the development of these lesions.

Patients with diverticular disease–associated polyps may develop chronic low-grade blood loss.[299] Treatment is similar to that for diverticulosis in general and in many instances has been shown to result in regression of polyps.[299]

HAMARTOMATOUS POLYPS

Hamartomas are defined as irregular or architecturally distorted overgrowths of cells and tissues native to the anatomic location in which they occur. In the GI tract, hamartomas typically incorporate both stromal and epithelial components. Hamartomas are most often solitary, but they may occur as part of hamartomatous polyposis syndrome, such as juvenile polyposis syndrome (JPS), PJS, Cowden's syndrome, hereditary mixed polyposis syndrome (HMPS), or Cronkhite-Canada syndrome. Cronkhite-Canada syndrome is a nonhereditary polyposis syndrome, but it is discussed in this section because of its histological resemblance to JPS. In aggregate, the hamartomatous polyposis syndromes account for less than 1% of the annual incidence of colorectal carcinoma in the United States and Canada.[300]

Juvenile Polyps and Juvenile Polyposis

Clinical Features

Juvenile polyps occur in four distinct settings: sporadic, usually isolated juvenile polyps of the colon, syndromic infantile JPS, juvenile polyposis coli (polyps limited to the colon), and generalized JPS (polyps involving the stomach, small bowel, and colon) (Table 22.7).[301] Sporadic juvenile polyps are the most common type of colon polyp among patients in the first decade of life, occurring in 2% of the pediatric population.[252] They are not uncommonly detected in adults as well. One study reported a mean age of occurrence of 5.9 years of age.[302] Children, if symptomatic, usually present with either painless rectal bleeding or prolapse of the polyp through the rectum.[302] Adults, when symptomatic, often have rectal bleeding.

First described in 1964 by McColl and coworkers,[303] JPS is the most common GI hamartomatous polyposis syndrome. Separation of isolated juvenile polyps in childhood from JPS is important because of their divergent clinical behaviors and neoplastic risks (discussed later).[301] The diagnosis is confirmed when there are (1) ≥5 colonic juvenile polyps, (2) multiple juvenile polyps of the upper and lower GI tract, or (3) any number of juvenile polyps in a patient with a family history of JPS. Hamartomas do not occur outside the GI tract, but congenital birth defects are reported in 15% of JPS patients; these include malrotation of the gut and cardiac and genitourinary defects.[301]

In 1998, linkage analysis in a large Iowa kindred demonstrated that a gene for familial JPS maps to chromosome 18q21.1, a region containing both the *DCC* and the *SMAD4 (DPC4, MADH4)* tumor suppressor genes.[304] Germline truncating mutations in *SMAD4* were shown to be responsible for a subset of JPS patients.[305] In 2001, germline mutations in the gene encoding bone morphogenic protein receptor 1A, *BMPR1A,* were also reported in JPS families

TABLE 22.7 Juvenile Polyps and Polyposis

Association	Diagnostic Criteria	Inheritance	Genetics	Risk of Malignancy
Sporadic	<3 polyps; no family history of juvenile polyposis	None	—	Essentially none
Juvenile polyposis of infancy	Generalized polyposis Often severe symptoms (diarrhea, hemorrhage, malnutrition, intussusception) Often death at a young age Often congenital abnormalities	None	Contiguous *BMPR1A* and/or *PTEN* deletion	Usually fatal before 2 years of age from non-neoplastic complications
Juvenile polyposis coli	Any number of polyps in a patient with family history, *OR* ≥3 polyps* without family history. Polyps are predominantly colonic; small-bowel polyps, if present, are few in number	Autosomal dominant, but family history in only 20%-50%	*BMPR1A* mutation, *SMAD4* mutation, or *ENG* mutation	30%-68% risk of colorectal carcinoma
Generalized juvenile polyposis	Polyps throughout stomach, small bowel, and colorectum, usually numbering from 50 to 200	Autosomal dominant, but family history in only 20%-50%	*SMAD4* mutation > *BMPR1A* mutation	At least 55% risk of gastrointestinal carcinomas, including 20% upper tract (stomach, duodenum) carcinomas

**Some investigators use ≥5 polyps.*

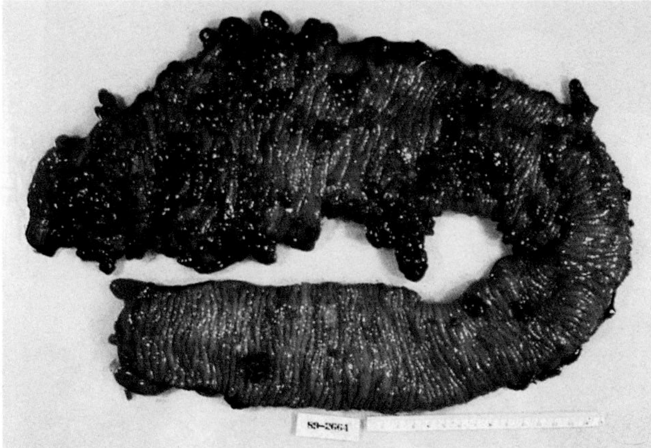

FIGURE 22.24 Juvenile polyposis coli. The resected colon harbors numerous reddish sessile and pedunculated polyps. These polyps are less numerous than those seen in familial adenomatous polyposis and are characteristically grouped in the region of the rectosigmoid. (*Courtesy of Emma E. Furth, MD, University of Pennsylvania, Philadelphia, PA.*)

lacking *SMAD4* mutations.[306] *SMAD4* mutations account for 15% to 20% of patients with JPS, and *BMPR1A* mutations are found in 20% to 25% of JPS patients,[301,307,308] suggesting that there is additional (as yet undefined) genetic heterogeneity in JPS. Patients harboring *SMAD4* mutations have a higher risk of generalized JPS,[301] including massive gastric polyposis, as well as hereditary hemorrhagic telangiectasia.[309-311] Although JPS is transmitted in an autosomal dominant fashion, 25% of newly diagnosed patients have no family history, and thus likely represent de novo mutations.[72]

JPS of infancy (infantile JPS) is a rare disorder with a poor prognosis that typically manifests in the first 2 years of life as generalized polyposis complicated by GI bleeding, diarrhea, rectal prolapse, and/or protein-losing enteropathy.[301] Unlike conventional JPS, no family history is found in patients with JPS of infancy. In 2006, Delnatte et al. reported that four patients with JPS of infancy were heterozygous for a de novo germline deletion of chromosome 10q, including the *PTEN* and *BMPR1A* genes, providing the first evidence of a genetic basis for this disorder.[312]

Pathological Features

Isolated juvenile polyps are most common in the rectosigmoid colon (54%). However, 37% of patients have polyps located proximal to the splenic flexure.[302] In juvenile polyposis coli (polyps limited to the colon), polyps are most common in the rectosigmoid colon and typically number as high as 200 (Fig. 22.24). The classic juvenile polyp (Fig. 22.25), found most frequently in isolated cases, is unilobulated and has a smooth, round surface contour. Histologically, these polyps are characterized by numerous cystic and dilated, often tortuous crypts, some filled with neutrophils and inspissated mucin (which reflects the older term, *mucous-retention polyp*). The intervening lamina propria is usually edematous and expanded by lymphocytes and plasma cells, with occasional neutrophils and eosinophils. A few strands of muscle fibers may be present as well, but this is not usually prominent, if present at all. In ulcerated cases, the epithelium may be markedly regenerative in appearance, simulating dysplasia. In patients with JPS, both classic (typical) and nonclassic (atypical) polyps are usually found. Nonclassic polyps (Fig. 22.26) are often larger in size, multilobulated, and villiform, frequently giving the gross appearance of several polyps attached to a single stalk. Histologically, compared with typical cases, they contain less abundant lamina propria and a greater amount of epithelial

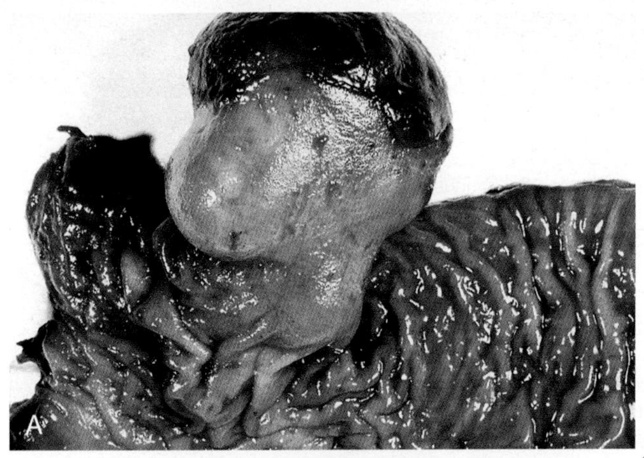

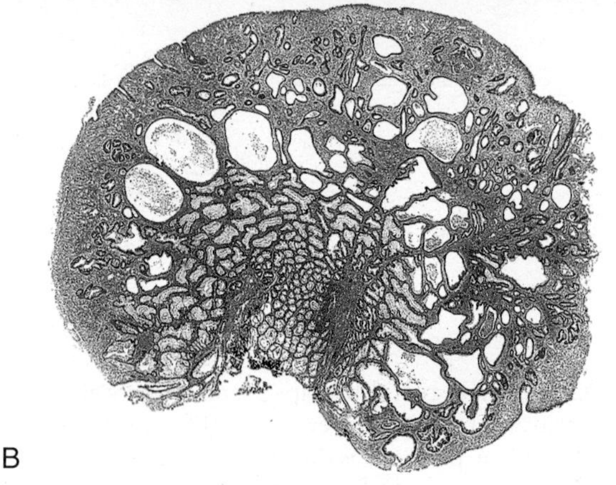

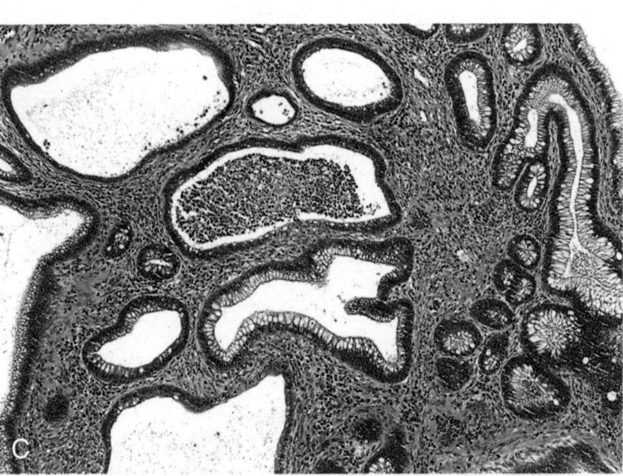

FIGURE 22.25 Classic juvenile polyps. A, These polyps grossly appear rounded, smooth, and unilobular with an erythematous cap of eroded tissue. **B,** Their cut surface reveals multiple dilated, mucin-filled crypts, leading to the term *mucus-retention polyp*. **C,** At higher power, the crypts are dilated and branched. Some contain crypt abscesses, collections of neutrophils, or eosinophils *(center)*. The surrounding stroma is also expanded and contains numerous mixed inflammatory cells. (*A courtesy of Thomas C. Smyrk, MD, Mayo Clinic, Rochester, MN.*)

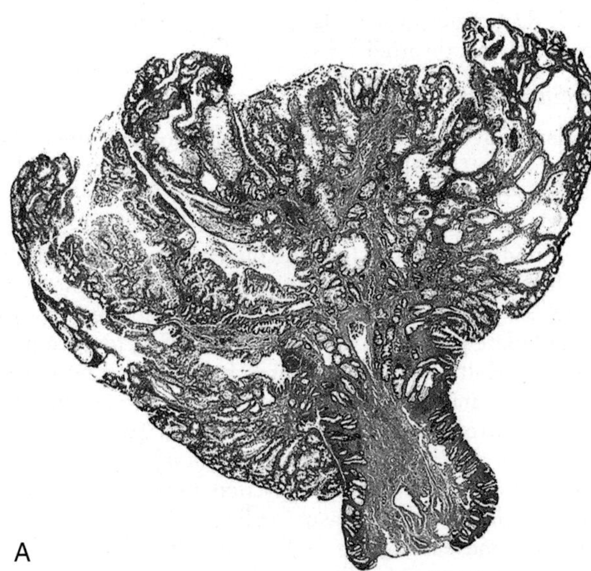

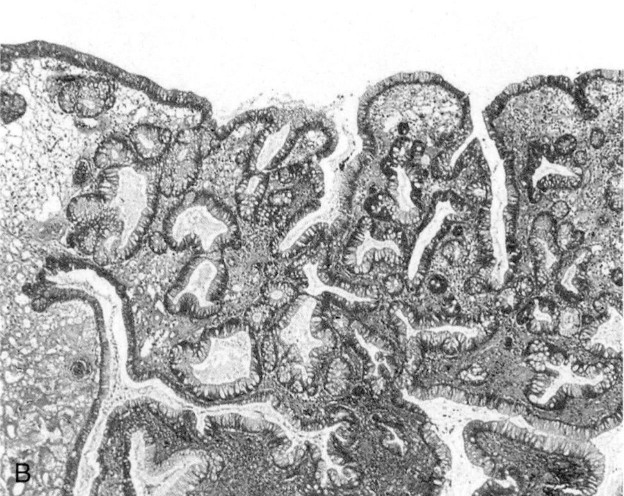

FIGURE 22.26 Atypical juvenile polyp in juvenile polyposis syndrome. A, These polyps have a villiform architecture and frequently give the appearance of several polyps attached to the same stalk. **B,** Atypical polyps exhibit more epithelial overgrowth and less abundant stroma in comparison with classic juvenile polyps. In this case, there is prominent crypt branching and distortion and cytological atypia approaching that of dysplasia.

overgrowth, often containing many elongated, tortuous, and irregularly shaped crypts.[313] The clonal origin of both the epithelium and the fibroblasts in juvenile polyps from *SMAD4* mutation carriers has been shown by fluorescence in situ hybridization.[314] Many patients also have separate adenomas, or polyps with combined features of a juvenile polyp and an adenoma (dysplasia).[315,316] In fact, true dysplasia (Fig. 22.27) has been detected in as many as 30% of polyps of JPS patients.[313,317] Loss of SMAD4 expression by immunohistochemistry can be observed in

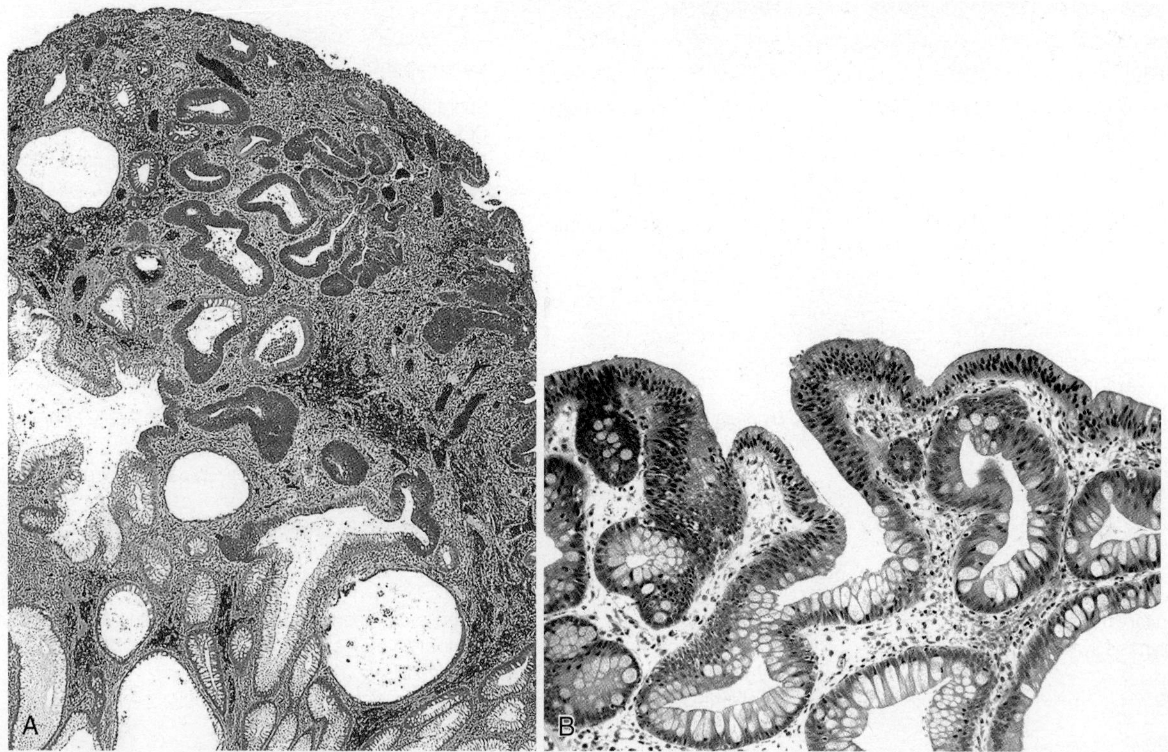

FIGURE 22.27 Dysplasia arising in a juvenile polyp. A, A classic juvenile polyp contains an area of hyperchromatic crypts *(top)*. **B,** At higher power, the involved crypts and surface epithelium, which contain enlarged, hyperchromatic, and crowded nuclei, are cytologically indistinguishable from an adenoma. The crypt at *center* shows a mixture of dysplastic and nondysplastic epithelium.

juvenile polyps from patients with germline mutations, and particularly in polyps with dysplasia.[310] Dysplasia is almost never observed in patients with isolated juvenile polyps. For instance, Gupta et al. reported dysplasia in only 1 of 331 juvenile polyps from 184 nonpolyposis patients.[302]

Natural History and Treatment

Patients with sporadic juvenile polyps have no associated increased risk for malignancy.[318-320] Furthermore, they are not predisposed to the development of new juvenile polyps, and they do not require any particular type of follow-up.[318] In contrast, estimates of the risk of GI carcinoma in JPS have varied widely. In one large kindred, the risk of upper and/or lower GI cancer in affected patients was 55%.[320] In 1995, in a reevaluation of data from the St. Mark's Polyposis Registry, Desai et al. projected that the incidence of colorectal carcinoma through 60 years of age was 68% (Table 22.8).[321] More recent data indicate that the cumulative lifetime risk of developing colorectal carcinoma is approximately 40%, with a median age of onset at 44 years of age. Surveillance recommendations should take into account the risks of both the lower and upper GI tract cancer, including gastric cancer. Upper and lower endoscopy (including visualization of the entire colon) is usually recommended by 15 years of age, and this should be repeated annually. Endoscopic polypectomies followed by histological examination of all removed polyps should be performed until the patient is free from polyps, at which point the surveillance interval may be lengthened to 3 years. Consideration should be given to prophylactic gastrectomy, or colectomy, if diffuse polyposis cannot be controlled by endoscopic polypectomy or if there is a family history of GI carcinoma or dysplasia.[322]

Peutz-Jeghers–Type Hamartomatous Polyps and Peutz-Jeghers Syndrome

Clinical Features

PJS is an autosomal dominant syndrome characterized by mucocutaneous pigmentation; distinctive hamartomatous polyps of the small intestine, colon, and stomach; and an increased risk for both intestinal and extraintestinal malignancies (see Chapters 20 and 21 for details). Estimates of the incidence of PJS vary widely, from 1 in 50,000 to 1 in 200,000 births.[323,324] Significant phenotypic variability can occur within PJS kindreds. Furthermore, patients may not have a family history of PJS. Most patients seek treatment during the second or third decade of life because these polyps often cause abdominal pain, obstruction due to intussusception, and/or bleeding. In one study, the average age at presentation was 18 years of age, with a range of 2 to 62 years.[325] Peutz-Jeghers polyps have also been described in neonates.[326] The main clinical manifestations of PJS include mucocutaneous pigmentation (most characteristically on the vermilion border of the lips), GI polyposis, and an increased risk for GI carcinomas (39% cumulative risk of colorectal carcinoma) and extraintestinal benign and malignant tumors.[327]

In 1997, the PJS locus was mapped to chromosome 19p13.3; this was achieved via use of comparative genomic hybridization of PJS polyps in one patient, followed by targeted linkage analysis in 12 affected families.[328] In

TABLE 22.8 Hamartomatous Polyposis Syndromes

Syndrome	Gene	Polyp Type	Differential Diagnosis	Risk of Malignancy
Juvenile polyposis syndrome	*SMAD4, BMPR1A*	Juvenile/inflammatory polyp	Sporadic inflammatory polyp Cronkite-Canada syndrome Inflammatory bowel disease	~40% risk of colorectal carcinoma ~20% upper tract (stomach, duodenum) carcinomas
Peutz-Jeghers syndrome	*STK11*	Peutz-Jeghers polyp (lobular arrangement of colonic crypts)	Mucosal prolapse polyp	39% risk of colorectal carcinoma 36% risk of pancreatic carcinoma 29% risk of stomach carcinoma 54% risk of breast carcinoma
Cowden's syndrome	*PTEN*	Multiple types: • Juvenile/inflammatory polyp • Ganglioneuroma • Intramucosal lipoma • Lymphoid polyp • Serrated polyps • Conventional adenomas	Juvenile polyposis syndrome Hereditary mixed polyposis	25%-50% risk of breast carcinoma 3%-10% risk of thyroid carcinoma 10%-15% risk of colorectal carcinoma
Hereditary mixed polyposis syndrome	*GREM1*	Multiple types: • Conventional adenomas • Juvenile/inflammatory polyp • Inflammatory serrated polyp • Serrated polyps • Prolapse-type polyps	Juvenile polyposis syndrome Familial adenomatous polyposis Serrated polyposis	Increased risk of colorectal carcinoma uncertain
Cronkite-Canada syndrome	Not hereditary	Juvenile/inflammatory polyp Background mucosa is also abnormal	Juvenile polyposis syndrome	Increased risk of colorectal carcinoma uncertain

1998, two separate reports identified the *STK11* (formerly *LKB1*) gene on 19p13.3 as the main causative gene in PJS.[329,330] Germline mutations in the *STK11* tumor suppressor gene, which encodes a novel serine threonine kinase, disrupt the function of the protein's kinase domain.[330] Overall, however, *STK11* mutations have been found in only approximately 60% of familial and 50% of sporadic cases, suggesting the possibility of genetic heterogeneity in PJS.[331] A definite diagnosis of PJS requires one of the following: (1) detection of ≥3 Peutz-Jeghers polyps, (2) any number of Peutz-Jeghers polyps in a patient with a family history of PJS, (3) mucocutaneous pigmentation in a patient with a positive family history of PJS, and (4) any number of Peutz-Jeghers polyps in a patient with characteristic mucocutaneous pigmentation.[124]

Pathological Features

PJS-associated hamartomatous polyps can occur anywhere in the GI tract, but they are most common in the small bowel (65% to 95%), followed by the colon (60%) and stomach (20% to 50%).[332] Involved segments of bowel may harbor from 1 to 20 polyps, and these may vary in size from 0.5 to 3 cm. Well-developed polyps located in the small intestine and colon tend to be pedunculated in shape.

In the small bowel, the diagnosis is usually straightforward because the hamartomatous polyps of PJS are histologically distinctive. They consist of disorganized and hyperplastic epithelium with a prominent core of smooth muscle arranged in a branching, treelike or arborizing pattern. Colonic polyps also commonly occur in PJS patients. However, in the colon, there is often much more histological overlap with mucosal prolapse polyps. Mucosal prolapse polyps can also have prominent smooth muscle that also involves the lamina propria in between non-neoplastic epithelium. However, prolapse polyps tend to occur in the left colon, whereas PJS polyps usually occur throughout the colon and are multiple. PJS polyps also tend to have a lobular architecture to the epithelium that is not apparent in mucosal prolapse polyps (Fig. 22.28).[333] PJS also does not normally have ischemic features or ulceration. Patient age and location of the polyp can also be helpful in suggesting a PJS polyp in a patient with an isolated colonic polyp. One should exercise extreme caution in suggesting a diagnosis of PJS in older patients based on the morphology of polyps isolated to the left colon. The lamina propria of PJS polyps is usually normal in composition and does not typically demonstrate increased inflammation. The overlying epithelium is composed of all of the normal cells typical of the involved segment of the GI tract. In most colonic Peutz-Jeghers polyps, the epithelium shows epithelial overgrowth and areas of hyperplasia, but the dysplasia is unusual. Nevertheless, nondysplastic epithelium has been shown to be clonal.[329]

Studies of histological and molecular alterations have shown that a subset of polyps may progress through a sequence of hamartoma, dysplasia, and then eventually to carcinoma. Somatic loss of the 19p13.3 allele occurs in a substantial proportion of nondysplastic polyps. This (in

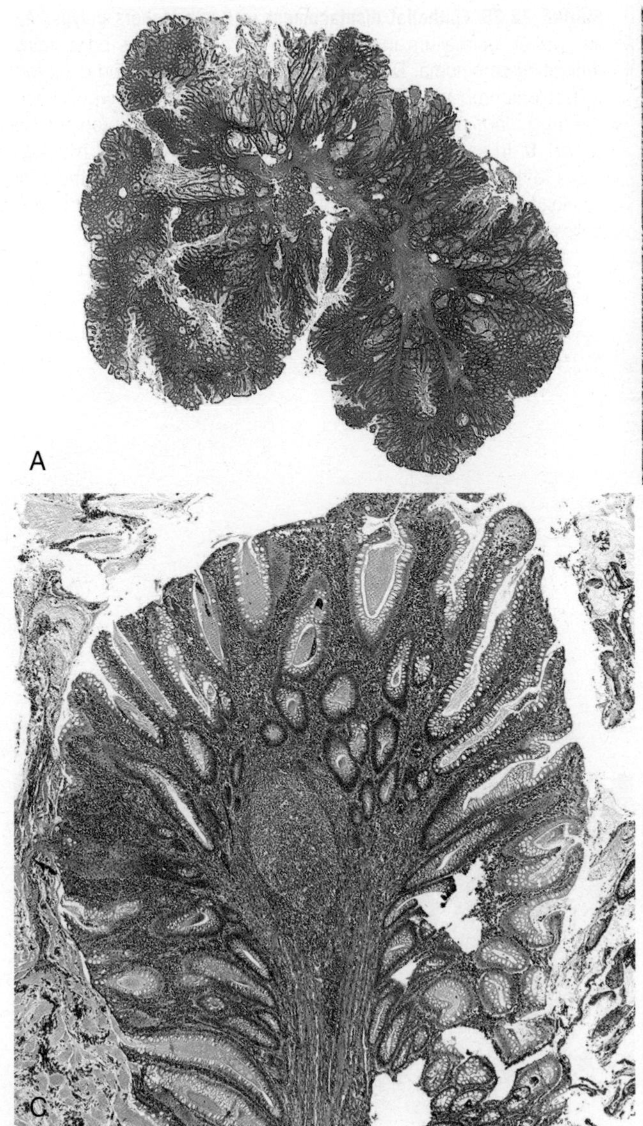

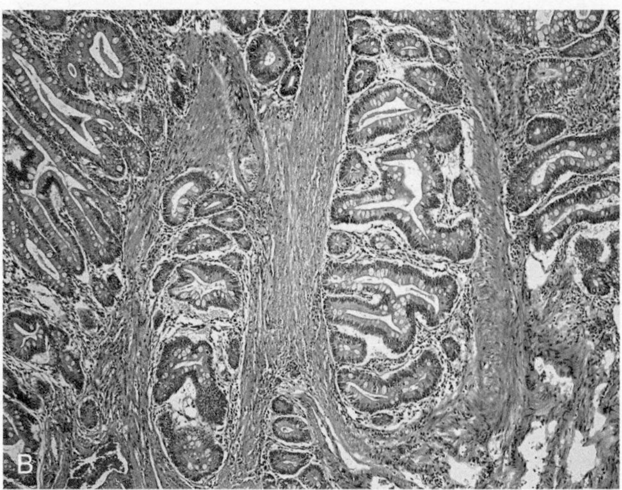

FIGURE 22.28 Peutz-Jeghers polyps. A, Colonic Peutz-Jeghers polyp shows the characteristic overgrowth of epithelium and an arborizing smooth muscle core. **B,** The branching smooth muscle is derived from the muscularis mucosae. **C,** The overlying mucosa is typically nondysplastic and maintains its normal architecture. In contrast with juvenile polyps, the mucosa has a normal ratio of lamina propria to epithelium, and the crypts are not cystically dilated. Cell types normal for that region of the gastrointestinal tract (in this case, goblet cells and absorptive cells) are found within the epithelium.

conjunction with germline mutation at this locus) accounts for hamartoma formation.[334,335] Dysplasia and carcinoma arise in hamartomas via the acquisition of additional genetic alterations at loci such as *TP53* and β-catenin.[335] Hizawa et al. documented "adenomatous" (dysplastic) foci in 12.7% of Peutz-Jeghers hamartomas in the GI tract.[336] In a study of 52 colonic Peutz-Jeghers polyps, Narita et al. found dysplasia in 3 (5.8%).[337] Intramucosal and invasive carcinomas have been documented in Peutz-Jeghers polyps of the stomach, small bowel, and colon. Carcinomas are more likely to arise in patients with familial PJS. Only a single case report has described the occurrence of carcinoma in a nonsyndromic Peutz-Jeghers–type hamartomatous polyp.[338]

Some Peutz-Jeghers polyps show foci of epithelial displacement, pseudoinvasion, or herniation of benign epithelium into the intestinal wall (all synonymous with the phenomenon of enteritis cystica profunda) (Fig. 22.29). Shepherd et al. studied 491 Peutz-Jeghers polyps and reported epithelial displacement in 10% of small-intestinal polyps. However, this phenomenon was not observed in gastric or colonic polyps (see Chapters 20 and 21).[339] Polyps with epithelial displacement are characterized by the presence of intramural mucinous cysts that can involve all layers of the bowel wall, including the serosa. Grossly and histologically, these polyps can simulate invasive adenocarcinoma.[340] Helpful histological discriminators between pseudoinvasion and true carcinoma include the following: lack of cytological atypia in the deep glands, with a normal composition of epithelial cell types; hemosiderin deposition; and the presence of epithelium at the periphery of mucinous cysts. Another potential pitfall is the overdiagnosis of displaced dysplastic epithelium as true invasion.[341] Helpful discriminating features in these cases include the presence of both nondysplastic and dysplastic epithelium within the dilated displaced crypts, the presence of lamina propria around the displaced crypts, and the lack of a desmoplastic response in noninvasive cases.

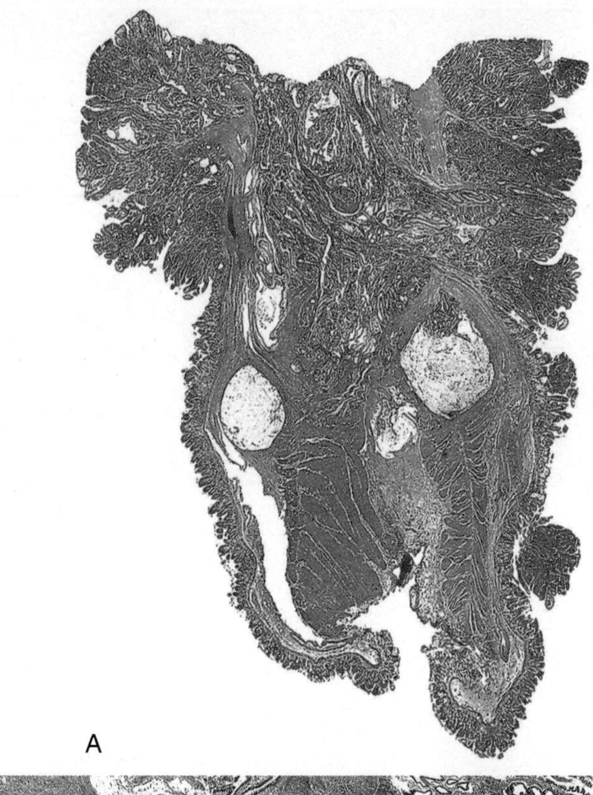

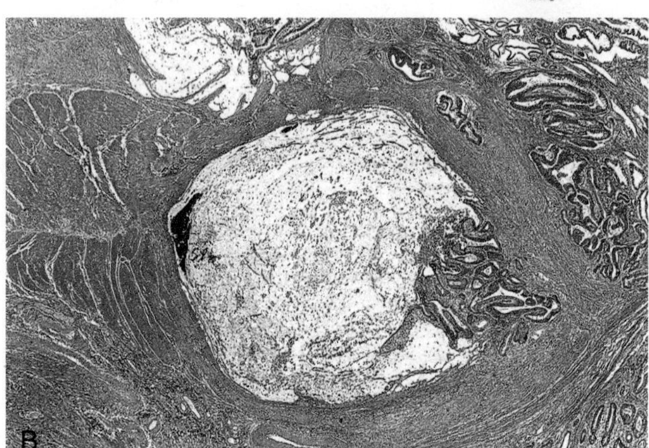

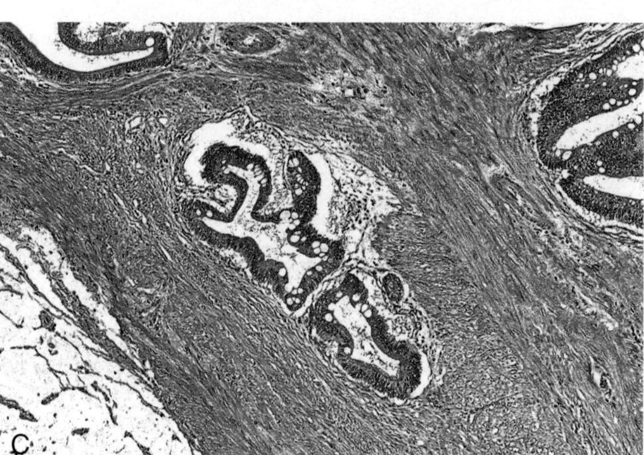

FIGURE 22.29 Epithelial displacement in Peutz-Jeghers polyps. A, At low power, epithelium in the stalk of a Peutz-Jeghers polyp mimics infiltrating carcinoma. Dilated crypts are found within and deep to the muscularis propria *(center).* **B,** A dilated, mucin-filled crypt is seen in the muscularis propria. An epithelial lining with lamina propria is seen *(right).* **C,** In addition to mucin pools and lamina propria, histological clues to the benign nature of the displaced crypts include the benign cytology of the involved crypts, which contain a normal mix of goblet cells and absorptive cells.

Natural History and Treatment

Non-neoplastic GI complications of PJS include GI bleeding and abdominal pain related to intussusception or luminal obstruction by large-size polyps. Intussusception is frequent (occurring in 47% of 222 Japanese PJS patients in a series by Utsunomiya et al.[342]) and is most common in the small intestine, caused in part by the pedunculated nature of the small bowel and colonic polyps. Prolapse of pedunculated PJS polyps through the rectum may also occur.[342]

Neoplastic complications of PJS include an increased frequency of both GI and extraintestinal neoplasms. Numerous early case reports attest to the increased risk of gastric, small-intestinal, and colonic malignancy in PJS, although the absolute risk was initially thought to be relatively low. Subsequent studies suggested a high risk for cancer development. In a retrospective study from the Mayo Clinic spanning 50 years, noncutaneous cancers developed in 18 (53%) of 34 PJS patients, with a mean age of 39.4 years at the time of cancer diagnosis.[343] In particular, the relative risk of GI carcinoma (predominantly colon cancer) in that study was 50.5, and in women with PJS, the relative risk of breast and gynecological cancers was 20.3. In a meta-analysis of cancer risk in PJS, Giardiello et al. calculated a cumulative risk for malignancy of 93% in patients 15 to 64 years of age.[344] In this study, the cumulative risks were as follows: breast cancer, 54%; colon cancer, 39%; pancreatic cancer, 36%; gastric cancer, 29%; ovarian cancer, 21%; and small-intestinal cancer, 13% (see Table 22.8). Furthermore, significantly increased relative risks were found for cancers of the following organs: esophagus (57), stomach (213),

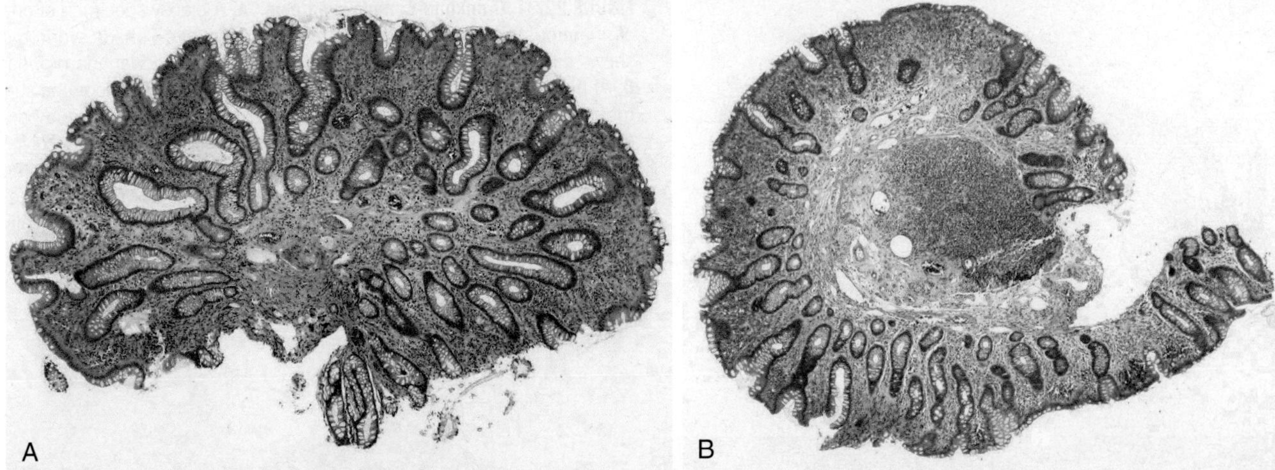

FIGURE 22.30 A, A small hamartomatous polyp from a patient with Cowden's syndrome that is best characterized as an inflammatory polyp. There is mild architectural distortion of the crypts with a hypercellular lamina propria. **B,** Another polyp from the same patient that demonstrates a prominent submucosal lymphoid aggregate.

small intestine (520), colon (84), pancreas (132), lung (17), breast (15.2), uterus (16), and ovary (27). Although a statistically significant increased risk for either testicular cancer or cervical cancer could not be demonstrated in Giardiello's study, distinctive tumors at these sites have been reported in PJS. A study by Lim et al. of 240 PJS patients harboring germline mutations in *LKB1* also reported high cancer risks for these patients.[345] By 60 years of age, the risk of pancreatic carcinoma in PJS patients was 8%, the risk of breast cancer was 32%, and the risk of colorectal cancer was 30%.

Surveillance in PJS is indicated for removal of GI polyps and for the early detection of both GI and extraintestinal neoplasms.[323,327,346] Surveillance recommendations for the GI tract include baseline colonoscopy, and esophagogastroduodenoscopy, at age 8 years to identify those patients with polyps that may cause obstruction in late childhood/adolescence. If polyps are identified, endoscopy is repeated every 3 years. If no polyps are found, then endoscopy is typically repeated again at 18 years of age and every 3 years thereafter. In women, monthly breast self-examinations should begin at 18 years of age, and semiannual clinical breast examinations and annual mammography should begin at 25 years of age. Minimum gynecological surveillance recommendations include annual pelvic examinations and Papanicolaou tests in women and annual testicular examinations in men. Because of the clearly documented increased risk for pancreatic carcinoma, some authors also advocate pancreatic imaging examinations every 1 to 2 years starting at 30 years of age.[300,323,327]

Cowden's Syndrome

Clinical Features

Cowden's syndrome (also known as PTEN-*hamartoma tumor syndrome*) is an autosomal dominant hamartoma/neoplasia syndrome first described by Lloyd and Dennis in 1963.[300] In 1996, the susceptibility locus for this syndrome was mapped to chromosome 10q22-23,[347] and in 1997, germline mutations in the *PTEN* gene (phosphatase and tensin homolog, deleted on chromosome 10) on 10q23 were first reported in families with this syndrome.[348,349] Since that time, mutations of the *PTEN* tumor suppressor gene or its promoter have been identified in 80% to 85% of patients who met the strict operational diagnostic criteria set forth by the International Cowden's Consortium.[350,351]

Hamartomas in Cowden's syndrome affect all three germ cell layers, but most commonly arise from ectodermal and endodermal elements. Almost all patients (90% to 100%) have mucocutaneous lesions such as trichilemmomas, acral keratoses, and oral papillomas.[350] Breast lesions affect the majority of female patients and include fibroadenomas, fibrocystic disease, and adenocarcinomas (25% to 50%).[350] Breast carcinoma has been reported in men as well.[352] Thyroid abnormalities, such as multinodular goiter and follicular adenoma, are found in one-half to two-thirds of patients. Thyroid carcinoma occurs in 3% to 10% of patients.[350] Macrocephaly, cerebellar gangliocytoma, and genitourinary malformations are also frequent components of Cowden's syndrome. An increased risk of endometrial carcinoma and renal cell carcinoma have been added to the operational criteria for this syndrome as well.[351,353]

Pathological Features

GI hamartomas are detected in 50% to 85% of patients with Cowden's syndrome. Hamartomatous polyps may affect the stomach, small bowel, and colon (Fig. 22.30). The most common esophageal manifestation is glycogenic acanthosis. More often, patients affected reveal a striking mixture of polyp types, such as ganglioneuromas, inflammatory polyps, lymphoid follicle polyps, intramucosal lipomas, adenomas, ill-defined "mesenchymal" polyps, and serrated polyps. The frequency of polyp types varies somewhat among the various studies.[354,355] For instance, in a recent study of 43 Cowden's syndrome patients, inflammatory polyps were detected in 21%, polypoid lymphoid follicles in 55%, ganglioneuromas in 52%, adenomas in 48%, serrated polyps in 62%, and lipomatous polyps in 52%.[355] Both submucosal and intramucosal lipomatous polyps develop in these patients.[356] Given that both ganglioneuromas and intramucosal lipomas are rare, it is the presence of these types of polyps that usually triggers consideration of Cowden's syndrome if present in a patient with multiple other types of polyps. Loss

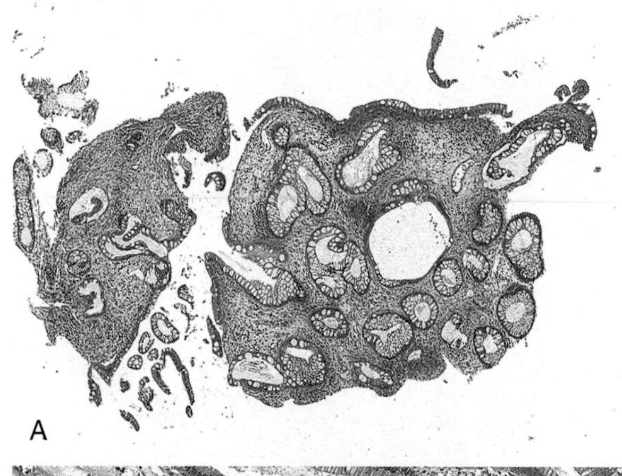

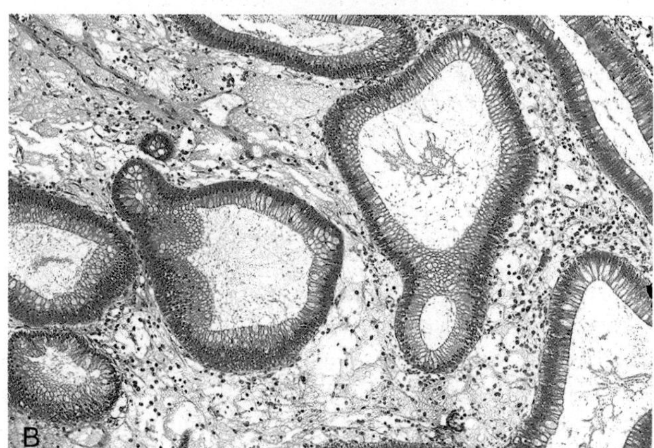

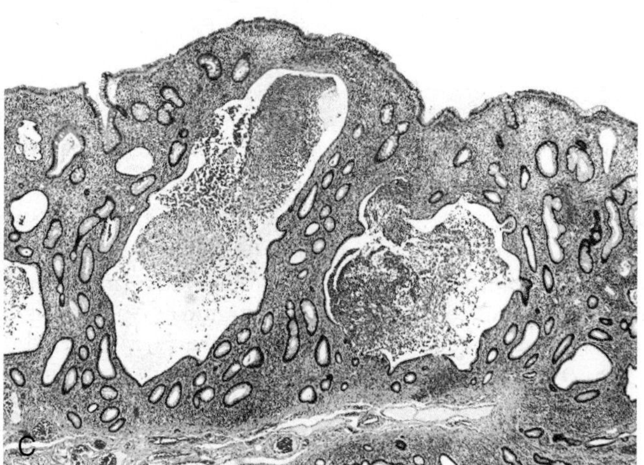

FIGURE 22.31 Cronkhite-Canada syndrome. A, A biopsy specimen of one of numerous colonic polyps in a patient with Cronkhite-Canada syndrome shows dilated and branched crypts within an expanded lamina propria. **B,** At higher power, cystically dilated crypts are filled with mucin; the surrounding lamina propria is edematous and contains increased numbers of mononuclear cells. **C,** Although individual Cronkhite-Canada polyps are histologically indistinguishable from juvenile polyps, biopsy of the intervening nonpolypoid colonic mucosa in a patient with Cronkhite-Canada syndrome shows lamina propria edema and scattered cystically dilated crypts.

of expression of the wild-type *PTEN* allele coupled with the germline *PTEN* mutation was demonstrated in both GI hamartomas and colonic adenomas of several patients with Cowden's syndrome.[357]

Natural History and Treatment

Recent studies have demonstrated that the lifetime risk of colorectal adenocarcinoma in patients with Cowden's syndrome with *PTEN* mutations is 10% to 15%.[358,359] For this reason, endoscopic surveillance of the GI tract has been recommended starting at 15 years of age and then every 2 years thereafter.[327] If the polyp burden is small, the interval period can be lengthened. Perhaps more importantly, screening and surveillance are also directed at breast and thyroid malignancies.[300] Recommendations for women include monthly breast self-examinations, annual clinical breast examinations beginning in late adolescence, and mammography beginning at 25 years of age. Annual clinical examination of the thyroid gland, in both sexes, should begin in late adolescence, either with or without parallel use of thyroid ultrasonography every 1 to 2 years.[300]

Cronkhite-Canada Syndrome

Clinical Features

Cronkhite-Canada syndrome is a nonhereditary polyposis syndrome of unknown etiology (see also Chapter 17). Since the first description of this syndrome by Cronkhite and Canada in 1955,[360] hundreds of cases have been reported. Although it is worldwide in distribution, most cases originate from Japan, Europe, and the United States. Unlike most polyposis syndromes, most patients present to physicians in middle adulthood (mean age, 59 years).[361] Infantile cases of Cronkhite-Canada syndrome have been rarely reported.[362]

Colonic polyps associated with Cronkhite-Canada syndrome occur in association with distinct ectodermal abnormalities such as alopecia of both the scalp and body hair, dystrophy of the nails, and skin hyperpigmentation.[360] Skin lesions are usually manifested by the presence of light to dark brown macules on the extremities, face, neck, palms, and soles.[361] Affected patients often present with a variable combination of diarrhea, weight loss, nausea and vomiting, anorexia, and GI bleeding. In some cases, diarrhea may result in severe electrolyte abnormalities and the development of seizures or tetany.[361]

Pathological Features

Polyps in Cronkhite-Canada syndrome occur throughout the GI tract but spare the esophagus. Histologically, in the colon, they closely resemble juvenile and inflammatory polyps, consisting of cystically dilated, tortuous crypts usually containing inspissated mucin (Fig. 22.31). The intervening lamina propria is typically edematous and contains increased numbers of mononuclear cells and eosinophils.[363] Burke and Sobin compared the histology

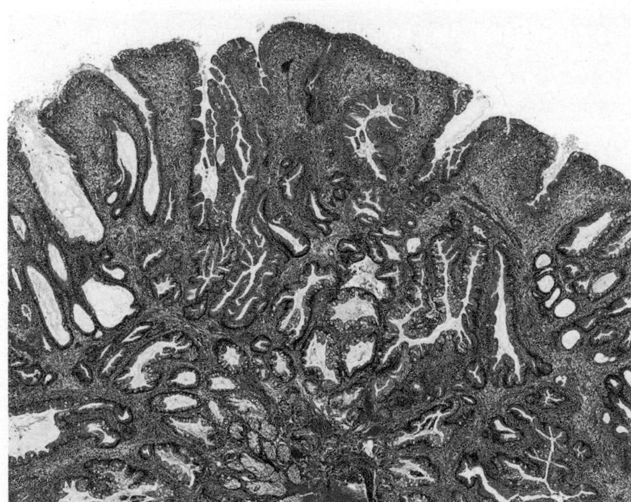

FIGURE 22.32 A characteristic polyp seen in patients with hereditary mixed polyposis syndrome that has features of both an inflammatory polyp and serrated polyp. (*Courtesy of Thomas Plesec, MD, Cleveland Clinic, Cleveland, OH*).

of Cronkhite-Canada polyps with juvenile polyps.[364] In this study, the histological features of each type of polyp were microscopically indistinguishable, although colonic juvenile polyps were more frequently pedunculated.[364] However, in patients with Cronkhite-Canada syndrome, the intervening nonpolypoid intestinal mucosa also shows pathological changes, such as edema, cystically dilated and distorted epithelium, and increased inflammatory cells (see Fig. 22.31), whereas the intervening mucosa in JPS is normal.

Natural History and Treatment

The malignant potential of colonic Cronkhite-Canada polyps is controversial. There have been multiple reports of affected patients who have also had adenoma,[365-367] colorectal carcinoma,[366-368] or gastric cancer.[368] Although dysplastic changes may occur within polyps,[366,368,369] it is not clear whether this represents a coincidental incidental sporadic adenoma or dysplasia within the polyp itself. The mortality rate in Cronkhite-Canada syndrome is high (50% to 60%). Death usually results from malnutrition, GI bleeding, or infection. Treatment includes aggressive nutritional support, antibiotics, immune suppression, and surgical resection of symptomatic segments of the GI tract.[361]

Hereditary Mixed Polyposis Syndrome

Hereditary mixed polyposis syndrome (HMPS) is a recently described attenuated polyposis syndrome that tends to occur in patients of Ashkenazi Jewish descent.[370] These patients have predominantly colonic polyps, including adenomas, serrated polyps, and inflammatory/juvenile-type polyps. The mean age of onset in individuals with known HMPS is 20 years of age, but polyps have been found in affected individuals as young as 10 years of age. A distinctive polyp type has also been described in this syndrome that shows a mixture of inflammatory and serrated polyp features (Fig. 22.32).[371] This, in fact, was the most common polyp type in one kindred with HMPS. HMPS is associated with a high-risk of colorectal cancer. Extracolonic tumors have been reported, but no clear pattern of involvement has been identified. Occasionally, there is considerable overlap with familial adenomatous polyposis; some patients show many colonic polyps.[370] One other family presented with clinical features that raised a suspicion for Lynch syndrome. The diagnosis of HMPS is confirmed by identification of mutations (usually duplications) in the *GREM1* gene on chromosome 15. In affected individuals, colonoscopies should begin at 25 to 35 years of age and repeated at 1- to 2-year intervals if polyps are detected.

VISIBLE DYSPLASTIC LESIONS IN INFLAMMATORY BOWEL DISEASE

Not uncommonly, endoscopically visible lesions that are well-circumscribed occur in patients with ulcerative colitis or Crohn's disease.[372-374] Some of these may represents sporadic adenomas, and others may represent dysplasia resulting from underlying IBD.[374] The distinction between these two types of lesions was formerly considered clinically important because sporadic adenomas are generally treated by polypectomy and continued surveillance, whereas dysplastic lesions associated with an underlying IBD have been regarded as an indication for colectomy in medically fit patients.[372-376] However, the results of three important follow-up studies have suggested that IBD patients with well-circumscribed endoscopically visible dysplastic lesions, regardless of whether they represent sporadic or IBD-related lesions, may be treated adequately by endoscopic removal and continued surveillance if there is no evidence of invisible dysplasia (either low grade or high grade) in the remainder of the colon.[377-380]

In one study by Engelsgjerd et al.[377] and another by Odze et al.[378] representing the long-term follow-up data of the Engelsgjerd study, the clinical outcomes of 24 patients with ulcerative colitis who had an adenoma-like polypoid dysplastic lesion were compared with those of 10 ulcerative colitis patients with a coincidental sporadic adenoma (based on the fact that the lesions were located proximal to areas of histologically confirmed colitis) and 49 nonulcerative colitis patients with a sporadic adenoma. After more than 6 years of follow-up, 59% of the ulcerative colitis patients with an adenoma-like lesion had developed further adenoma-like polyps; this was statistically similar to the findings in the other groups (i.e., ulcerative colitis patients with a sporadic adenoma and non–ulcerative colitis patients with a sporadic adenoma who developed further adenomas). Only one patient with ulcerative colitis and an adenoma-like polyp developed an isolated focus of low-grade dysplasia, and one patient (with primary sclerosing cholangitis) developed adenocarcinoma. Rubin et al. found similar results in a study of 38 ulcerative colitis patients and 18 Crohn's disease patients with 70 "dysplastic" polyps, all of whom were treated with polypectomy and followed for a mean of 4.1 years.[379] In this study, most patients (52%) did not develop any additional polyps, and none developed either flat dysplasia or adenocarcinoma. In a recent meta-analysis of 10 studies comprising 376 patients, the risk of developing colorectal carcinoma was very low after complete endoscopic removal of a

TABLE 22.9 Summary of Features Differentiating Sporadic Adenoma and Inflammatory Bowel Disease–Associated Polypoid Dysplasia

Feature	Sporadic Adenoma	IBD-Associated Visible Dysplasia
Patient age	Older (>60 years)	Younger (<60 years)
Extent of disease	Usually subtotal	Usually total
Disease activity	Usually inactive	Usually activc
Disease duration	Shorter (<10 years)	Longer (>10 years)
Polyp location	Usually nondiseased area (right colon)	Diseased area (left colon)
Associated flat dysplasia	Never	Occasionally
Increased lamina propria and crypt inflammation	Usually absent	Usually present
Villous architecture	Usually absent	Occasionally present
Mixture of benign and dysplastic crypts at surface of polyp	Usually absent	Usually present
Top-down dysplasia	Usually present	Usually absent
Bottom-up dysplasia	Usually absent	Usually present
p53 immunostaining	Usually absent	Usually present
Nuclear β-catenin immunostaining	Usually prominent	Usually absent
LOH of 3p	Uncommon	Common
LOH of *CDKN2A*	Rare	Common

IBD, *Inflammatory bowel disease;* LOH, *loss of heterozygosity.*

polypoid dysplastic lesion in IBD.[381] Based on these studies, the recent SCENIC Consensus guidelines recommend surveillance for these patients rather than colectomy.[380]

Pathological Features and Differential Diagnosis

Grossly, adenomas associated with IBD are endoscopically and histologically identical to those that occur outside that setting (see the Conventional Adenoma section earlier in this chapter).[378,382-385] Lesions that occur proximal to histologically confirmed areas of colitis (e.g., right-sided lesions in a patient with left-sided ulcerative colitis) can be diagnosed reliably as sporadic adenomas because it is well known that dysplasia related to IBD develops only in areas involved with chronic inflammation.[386,387] However, lesions that occur within areas of colitis may be impossible or difficult to distinguish from true adenoma-like polypoid dysplastic lesions related to the underlying colitis. Several clinical, endoscopic, pathologic, and molecular features may help in distinguishing a sporadic adenoma from an IBD-associated polypoid dysplastic lesion, and these are summarized in Table 22.9, although such distinction is no longer essential. Clinically, patients with sporadic adenomas, in contrast with those with IBD-associated adenoma-like polypoid dysplasia, are typically older (>60 years of age) and have less extensive inflammatory disease, less disease activity, and a shorter duration of disease (usually <10 years).[374] Endoscopically, the lesions may be indistinguishable.[388]

Histologically, IBD-associated polypoid dysplastic lesions often show an increased degree of acute and chronic inflammation in the lamina propria, cryptitis and crypt abscesses involving dysplastic crypts, and a mixture of benign and dysplastic crypts at the surface of the polyp—features that are not usually seen in sporadic adenomas (Fig. 22.33).[374] In addition, flat or invisible dysplasia may be detected in the base of the stalk or in the mucosa surrounding the polyp. Stalk dysplasia, if present, should alert the pathologist that dysplasia may be present in the adjacent mucosa and that this is likely to be an IBD-associated lesion rather than a sporadic adenoma. Features such as polyp size, architectural type (tubular, tubulovillous, or villous), degree of dysplasia, and nuclear cytological features are not helpful in distinguishing these two groups of lesions.[374]

By immunohistochemistry, IBD-associated adenoma-like polypoid dysplastic lesions have a higher degree of TP53 and a lower degree of nuclear β-catenin staining, in contrast with sporadic adenomas.[389-391] Furthermore, their molecular characteristics are different.[387,392-396] IBD-associated lesions show a higher prevalence of 3p and *CDKN2A* mutations, indicating different timing and frequency of molecular defects compared with sporadic adenomas. See Figure 22.34[397] for an algorithmic approach to IBD patients with dysplastic lesions.

MESENCHYMAL POLYPS

Although the vast majority of colonic polyps are epithelial in origin (or include an admixture of both colonic epithelium and stroma, as in many hamartomatous polyps and inflammatory polyps), some represent primary stromal cell proliferations. These include both benign and malignant tumors of adipose tissue (lipomas, liposarcomas, and lipomatous hypertrophy of the ileocecal valve), smooth muscle tissue (leiomyomas and leiomyosarcomas), vascular tissue (glomus tumors, vascular malformations, lymphangiomas, and angiosarcomas), and neural tissue (ganglioneuromas, neurofibromas, perineuriomas, granular cell tumors, and mucosal Schwann cell hamartomas), as well as gastrointestinal stromal tumors (GISTs). In addition, mesenchymal polyps of unknown origin, such as inflammatory fibroid polyps, may occur in the colon as well. Some of the more common lesions are described in this section (Table 22.10).

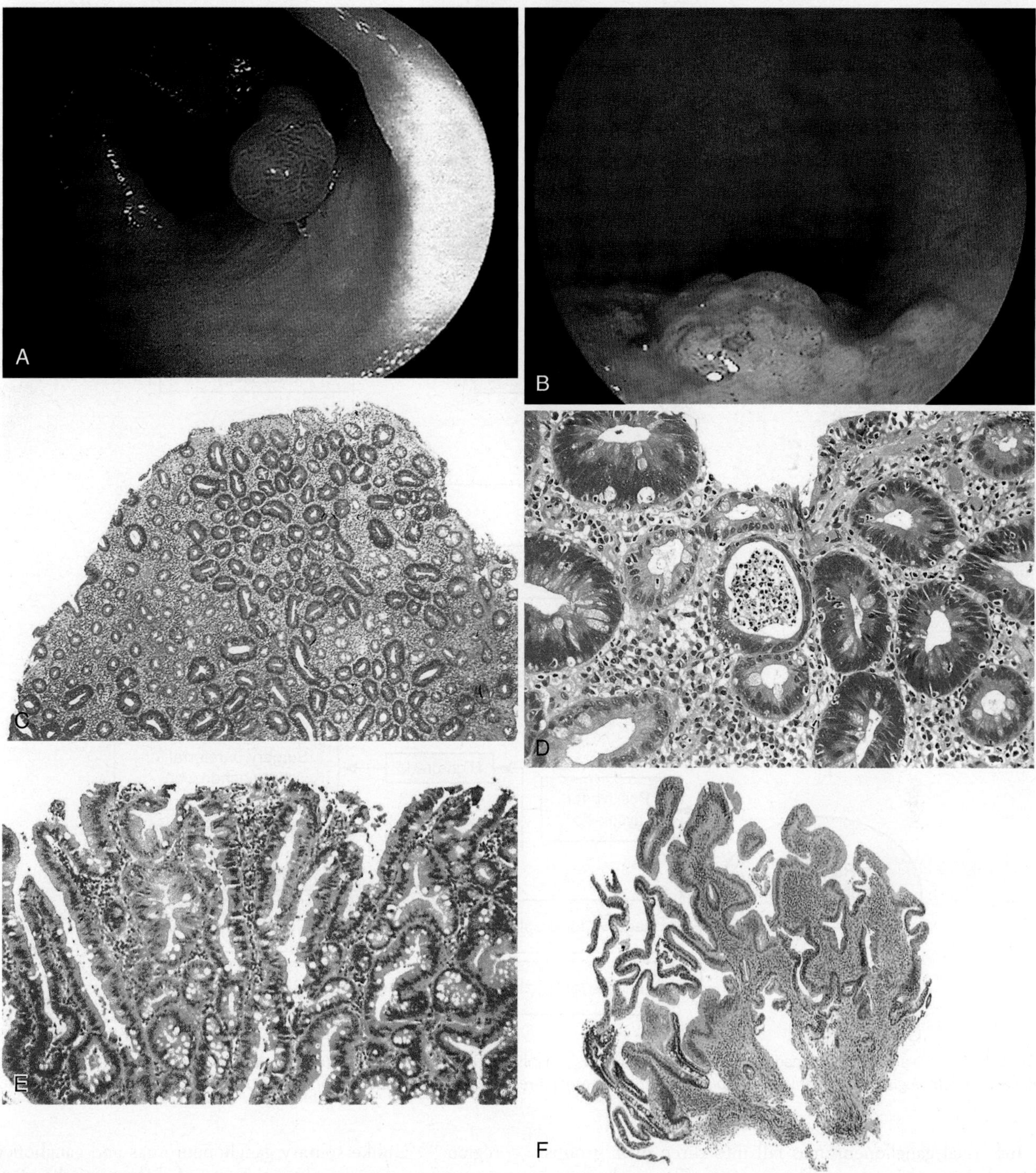

FIGURE 22.33 A, Endoscopic appearance of a well-circumscribed polypoid dysplastic lesion in ulcerative colitis. The lesion is grossly identical to a sporadic adenoma. **B,** In contrast with **A,** this is an irregular visible lesion with indistinct borders. **C,** Low-power view of the polypoid dysplastic lesion seen in **A**. A mixture of low-grade dysplastic and nondysplastic crypts is found in the central portion of the polyp and at the surface of the polyp. **D,** High-power view of one portion of the same polyp as in **C**. Dysplastic crypts are mixed with nondysplastic crypts. One dysplastic crypt in the central portion of the figure shows a crypt abscess. **E,** Another visible lesion in a patient with ulcerative colitis. The histological distinction between a sporadic adenoma and an ulcerative colitis–associated polypoid dysplastic lesion is not possible on morphological grounds alone. **F,** This visible dysplastic lesion in ulcerative colitis shows an irregular distorted villous architecture, irregular crypt budding, and prominent lamina propria lymphoplasmacytic inflammation.

Ganglioneuroma

Clinical Features

Ganglioneuromas are benign tumors composed of a proliferation of nerve fibers, Schwann cells, and ganglion cells. They most commonly arise in the posterior mediastinum and the retroperitoneum. Ganglioneuromas of the intestinal tract are considerably less common. GI ganglioneuromas can occur at any level, from the stomach to the anus, including the gallbladder. They are most common in the colon and rectum.

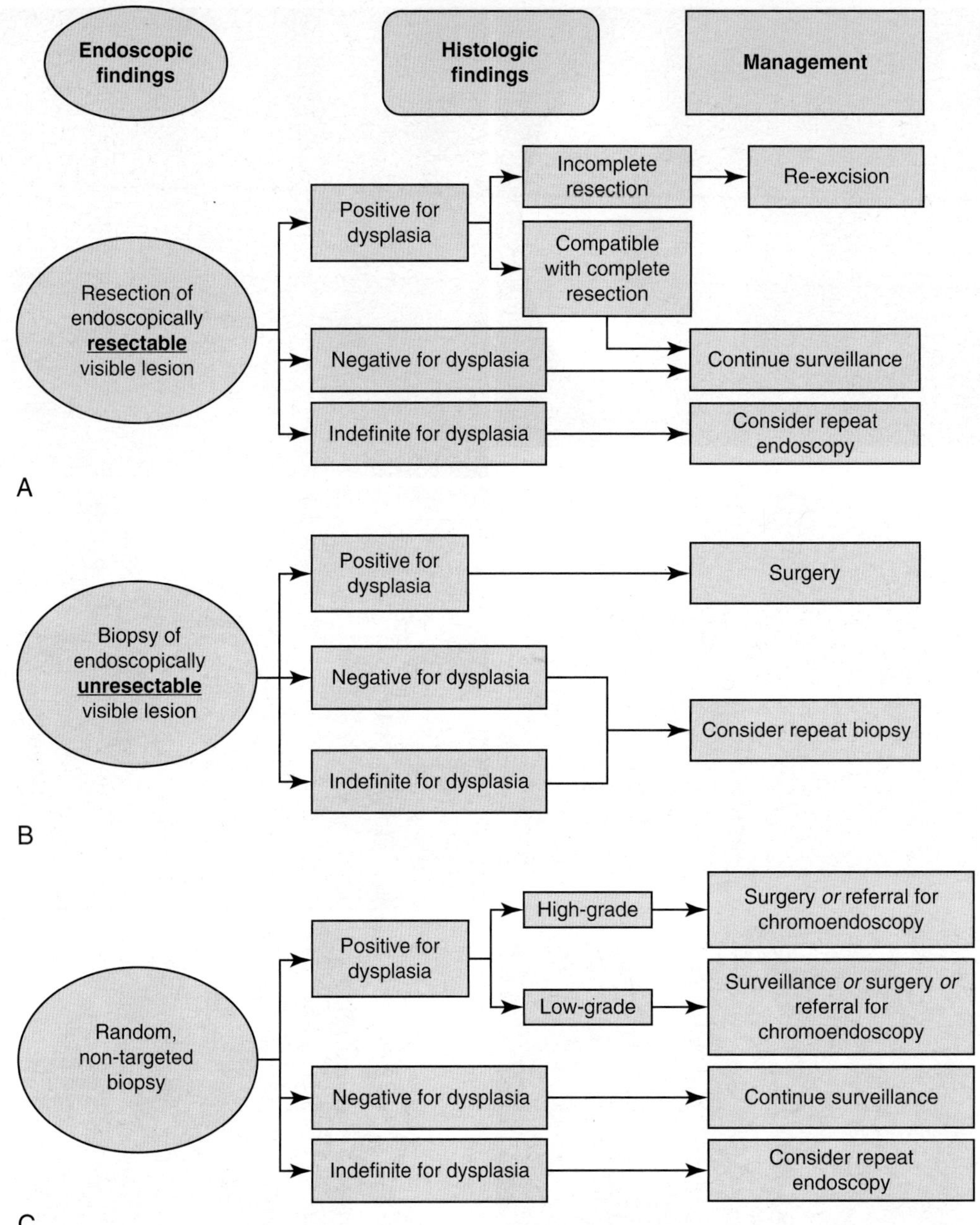

FIGURE 22.34 This algorithm summarizes the treatment of dysplasia in inflammatory bowel disease. *(Chiu K, Riddell RH, Schaeffer DF. DALM, rest in peace: a pathologist's perspective on dysplasia in inflammatory bowel disease in the post-DALM era. Mod Pathol. 2018;31(8):1180-1190.)*

Intestinal ganglioneuromas fall into three main groups: (1) solitary polypoid ganglioneuromas, (2) ganglioneuromatous polyposis, and (3) diffuse (transmural) ganglioneuromatosis. Isolated polypoid ganglioneuromas are most common.[398] These are small sessile or pedunculated polyps that often measure just a few millimeters in size and are endoscopically indistinguishable from adenomas or hyperplastic polyps. No sex predilection has been noted. They do not produce symptoms and are usually detected as an incidental finding at the time of colonoscopy. In ganglioneuromatous polyposis, multiple (dozens to innumerable) polyps occur in the colon. In some patients, polyps are scattered throughout the colorectum, whereas in others, multiple polyps aggregate in only one particular segment of the bowel, such as the rectosigmoid or the terminal ileum/right colon region.[398] Unlike solitary ganglioneuromas and ganglioneuromatous polyposis, the epicenter of diffuse ganglioneuromatosis lies within the submucosa or muscularis propria, which results in mural thickening and sometimes stricture formation. Affected regions of bowel range from 1 to 17 cm in length.[398] However, irregular nodular lesions on the mucosal aspect of the bowel can also be detected in some cases with transmural involvement.

These categories have different clinical implications. Solitary polypoid ganglioneuromas are not associated with systemic manifestations and do not require long-term follow-up.[398] Ganglioneuromatous polyposis is strongly associated with Cowden's syndrome[399-401] and type 1 neurofibromatosis (NF1, also called *von Recklinghausen disease*).[400] Diffuse ganglioneuromatosis occurs in

TABLE 22.10 Differential Diagnosis of Colorectal Mesenchymal Polyps

Type of Polyp	Architectural Features	Cytological Features	Associated Hyperplastic Epithelium	Immunohistochemistry
Polypoid ganglioneuroma	Poorly circumscribed, entraps crypts	Spindle cells with tapered nuclei; occasional ganglion cells; coarse collagenous stroma	No	S100+ (spindle cells) NSE+ (ganglion cells)
Mucosal perineurioma	Poorly circumscribed, entraps and whorls around crypts	Short spindle cells with ovoid nuclei and pale indistinct cytoplasm; fine stroma	Yes (80%)	EMA+ Claudin-1+ (60%)
Mucosal Schwann cell hamartoma	Poorly circumscribed, entraps crypts	Spindle cells with elongated, wavy nuclei and dense eosinophilic cytoplasm	No	S100+
Leiomyoma of muscularis mucosae	Well circumscribed, arises from muscularis mucosae	Spindle cells with blunt-ended nuclei, bright eosinophilic cytoplasm, well-defined cell borders	No	SMA+ Desmin+
Prolapse-type inflammatory polyp	Thickening, splaying of muscularis mucosae; haphazard growth pattern	Spindle cells with ovoid to elongated nuclei; inflammatory cells	Yes	SMA+ Desmin ±
Inflammatory fibroid polyp	Infiltrative, often ulcerated surface	Stellate to spindled cells, concentric perivascular orientation; prominent vascularity; prominent inflammatory cells (especially eosinophils)	No	CD34+ PDGFRA+

EMA, *Epithelial membrane antigen;* NSE, *neuron-specific enolase;* SMA, *smooth muscle actin.*

patients with multiple endocrine neoplasia (MEN) type IIb, NF1, or multiple intestinal neurofibromas.[398,400] Of these, the association between diffuse ganglioneuromatosis and MEN IIb is particularly strong. Carney et al. found that all of their patients with MEN IIb had intestinal ganglioneuromatosis; GI symptomatology (constipation, megacolon, pain, diarrhea) was preceded by endocrine disease in 87%.[402] Smith and coworkers also found diffuse ganglioneuromatosis in all three of their pediatric patients with MEN IIb who presented with pseudo-obstruction mimicking Hirschsprung's disease.[403] Intestinal manifestations preceded the development of medullary thyroid carcinoma in all three cases.

Pathological Features

Biopsies of ganglioneuromatous polyps reveal a hypercellular and expanded stroma that displaces and distorts the adjacent or overlying colonic crypts. The stroma itself is composed of spindle-shaped cells, which are mainly S100-positive Schwann cells admixed with variable numbers of ganglion cells that are neuron-specific enolase (NSE)-positive (Fig. 22.35). In the normal colon, ganglion cells are only rarely present in the lamina propria. Therefore their presence in mucosal biopsies, particularly when there is more than one, should alert the pathologist to the possibility of a ganglioneuroma. Occasionally, ectopic ganglion cells migrate into the lamina propria in response to mucosal injury, such as in Crohn's disease, but these cases lack the characteristic spindle cell proliferation of ganglioneuromas. In some ganglioneuromas, the ganglion cell component is readily identifiable, whereas in others it is rare. Diffuse ganglioneuromatosis (Fig. 22.36) is centered within the myenteric plexus, but it may also affect all layers of the bowel wall.

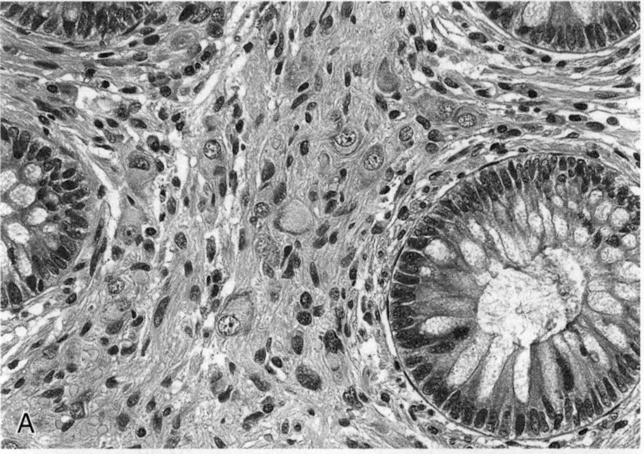

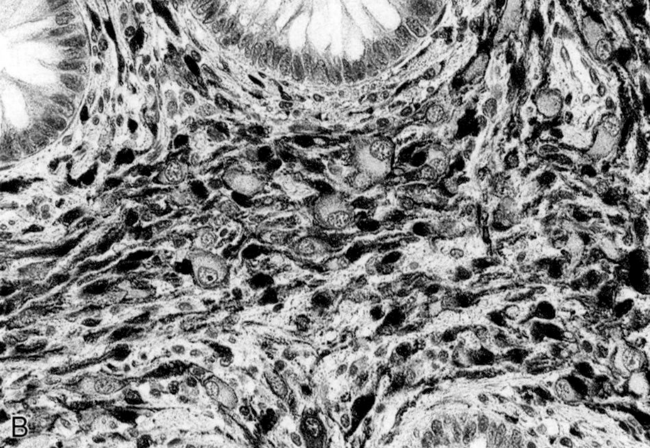

FIGURE 22.35 Mucosal ganglioneuroma (ganglioneuromatous polyp). **A,** At high power, the stromal proliferation is composed of spindle cells and ganglion cells that appear either in clusters (as in this case) or as single isolated cells. **B,** S100 immunostain labels the spindled Schwann cells but not the ganglion cells.

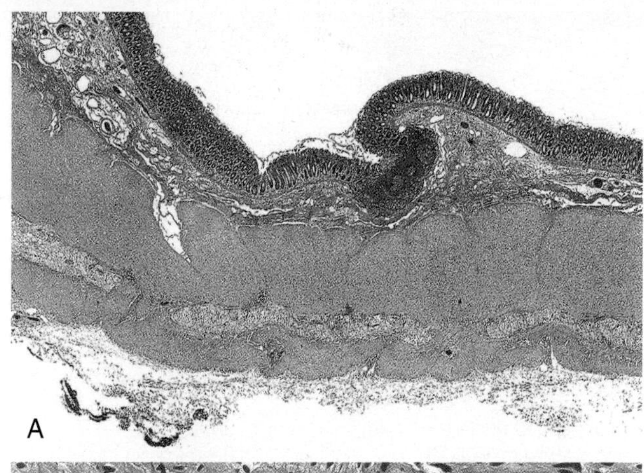

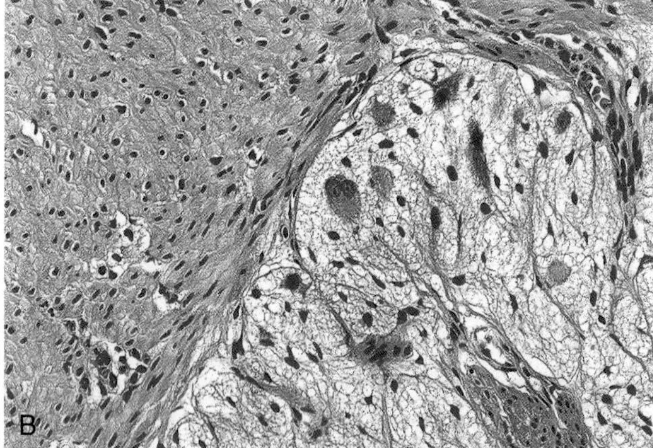

FIGURE 22.36 Diffuse ganglioneuromatosis. A, At low power, the myenteric plexus is diffusely expanded in this patient with multiple endocrine neoplasia (MEN) type IIb syndrome. **B,** A cytologically abnormal, binucleated ganglion cell within the expanded myenteric plexus attests to the neoplastic nature of the lesion.

Neurofibroma

Clinical Features

Neurofibromas may occur as isolated lesions or as part of NF1. Isolated GI neurofibromas outside the setting of NF1 are exceedingly rare. NF1 is one of the most common genetic diseases, affecting at least 1 in 3000 births. The other form of neurofibromatosis—neurofibromatosis type 2 (NF2)—does not involve the GI tract. Patients with NF1 have germline mutations of the *NF1* tumor suppressor gene on chromosome 17q11.2. Although the syndrome is inherited in an autosomal dominant manner, only approximately 50% of patients are members of NF1 families (the other half represent sporadic germline mutations).

Diagnostic criteria for NF1 include the presence of at least two of the following features: (1) more than six café au lait spots; (2) more than two neurofibromas of any type or more than one plexiform neurofibroma; (3) axillary or groin region freckling; (4) optic glioma; (5) more than two Lisch nodules; (6) a distinctive bony lesion, including dysplasia of the sphenoid bone or dysplasia or thinning of the long bone cortex; and (7) a first-degree relative with NF1.[404] In addition to dysplastic lesions and the benign and malignant tumors that may arise in NF1, these patients also tend to have a stature that is smaller than average. Forty percent to 60% of patients suffer from learning disabilities.[404]

GI involvement occurs in as many as 25% of patients with NF1. Severe GI complications are rare in childhood because neurofibromas typically develop after puberty.[405] GI complaints in both children and adults are most frequently related to the presence of a mass lesion, but severe abdominal pain in the absence of a radiologically identified anatomic lesion has also been described.[405] Mass lesions, or polypoid lesions, in NF1 are of variable types. There is an increased incidence of GISTs,[406-409] diffuse and polypoid ganglioneuromatosis (described earlier), GI neuroendocrine tumors (most frequent in the duodenum or periampullary region, often somatostatin-producing lesions),[410] and GI neurofibromas. In addition, an association between NF1 and duodenal gangliocytic paraganglioma has also been described.[411] Finally, there may also be an increased risk for small-intestinal adenocarcinoma in NF1.[412]

Symptomatic GI neurofibromas in NF1 are unusual. They are less commonly reported than GISTs, GI ganglioneuromatosis, or duodenal neuroendocrine tumors.[413-415] Zöller et al. studied benign and malignant tumors arising over a long-term follow-up period in 70 Swedish adults with NF1 and found that GI neurofibroma was suspected in only one patient; this was based on radiological evidence of a prepyloric mass and was not confirmed microscopically.[409] Likewise, GI neurofibromas were identified by abdominal ultrasound screening in only 4 of 62 asymptomatic adults with NF1 in a study by Wolkenstein et al.[416] Neurofibromas involve (in descending order) the jejunum, stomach, and other small-intestinal sites such as the ileum and duodenum, colon, and mesentery.[417]

Pathological Features

Neurofibromas are often plexiform and may involve any layer of the bowel wall. Those that arise in the submucosa often extend into the lamina propria and appear polypoid. Their microscopic appearance is similar to that of other extraintestinal neurofibromas (Fig. 22.37). They consist of proliferating bundles of spindle cells with wavy dark nuclei, strands of collagen, varying amounts of myxoid matrix material, and scattered neurites. Both Schwann cells and fibroblasts are present, but S100 usually labels fewer cells than in ganglioneuromas. Submucosal lesions that extend into the muscularis mucosae may separate the overlying crypts and give the appearance of a juvenile polyp when viewed at low power.

Granular Cell Tumor

Granular cell tumors usually arise in the tongue or dermis but can occur in virtually any anatomic location (see Chapters 19 and 30). Within the GI tract, granular cell tumors are most common in the esophagus. The colon is the second most common GI primary site, followed in descending order by the perianal region, stomach, appendix, and small bowel.[418-420] Colonic granular cell tumors have a predilection for the right colon.[420] In most cases, the granular cell tumor is an incidental finding at the time of colonoscopy or surgical resection, although fecal occult blood or rectal bleeding may have precipitated a colonoscopic examination, particularly if the lesion is within the rectum or anus. Endoscopically, granular cell tumors typically appear as smooth, sessile, submucosal polyps, ranging in size from a

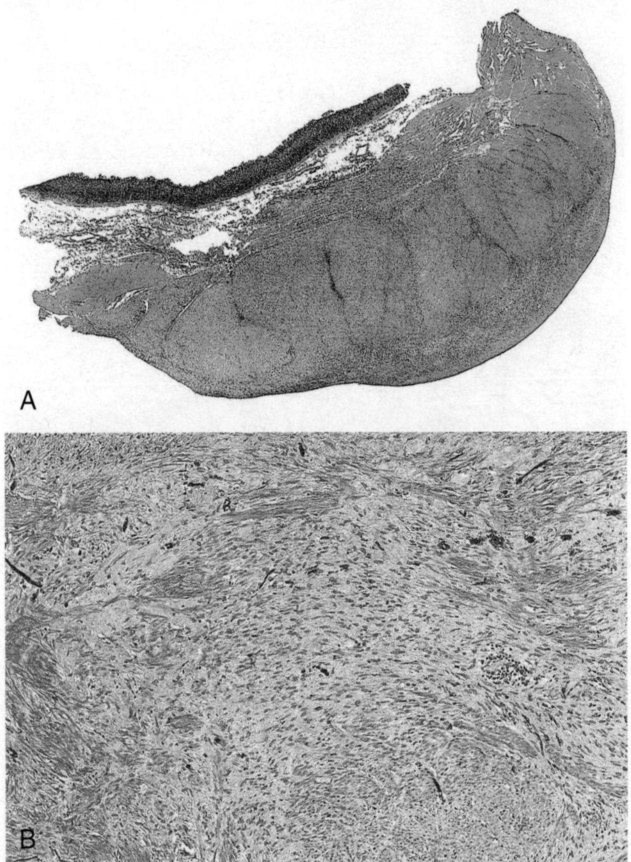

FIGURE 22.37 **Neurofibroma. A,** A fusiform enlargement of the muscularis propria is seen in this diffuse neurofibroma. **B,** At higher power, smooth muscle fibers of the muscularis propria are splayed apart by a proliferation of wavy spindle cells in a fibrotic stroma.

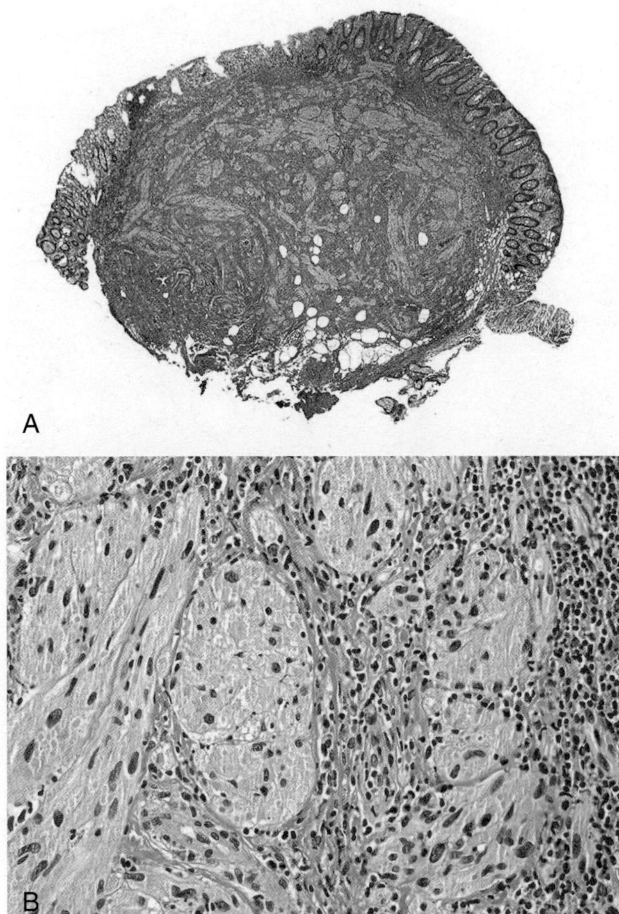

FIGURE 22.38 **Granular cell tumor. A,** This unencapsulated lesion expands the submucosa of the rectum. **B,** The lesional cells are plump, spindle shaped, and rounded with abundant granular cytoplasm.

few millimeters to 2 to 3 cm; they are usually covered by intact colonic mucosa. In 5% of patients, multiple granular cell tumors are present, either in different portions of the GI tract or in GI and extraintestinal sites.[418,421]

Histologically (Fig. 22.38), colonic granular cell tumors resemble those in other portions of the GI tract. They are poorly circumscribed, unencapsulated tumors composed of plump, rounded, or polygonal-shaped cells with uniform small nuclei and abundant granular eosinophilic cytoplasm.[420] They are weakly positive with periodic acid–Schiff (PAS) staining both before and after diastase, and they uniformly label with both NSE and S100. The immunohistochemical profile and ultrastructural appearance of granular cell tumors support Schwann cell differentiation. The term *granular cell tumor* thus contrasts with the previous designation of *granular cell myoblastoma,* an appellation that reflects the earlier concept of a muscle origin. Granular cell tumors harbor inactivating somatic mutations in the endosomal pH regulators *ATP6AP1* or *ATP6AP2,* which explains the accumulation of intracytoplasmic granules in this tumor type.[422]

Endoscopic polypectomy is the treatment of choice. Only very rare granular cell tumors that arise at extraintestinal sites behave in a malignant fashion.[423] In addition to large size and the presence of necrosis, the following histological features have been found to correlate with malignant behavior in extraintestinal granular cell tumors: spindling of tumor cells, vesicular nuclei with large nucleoli, pleomorphism, and increased mitotic activity (>2 mitoses/10 high-power fields).[423] In the largest published series of GI granular cell tumors, none of 75 tumors recurred or metastasized.[418]

Mucosal Perineurioma

Perineuriomas are uncommon, benign peripheral nerve sheath tumors that include soft tissue, intraneural, and sclerosing variants.[424-426] They may arise in the colon and usually manifest as polypoid lesions discovered incidentally at the time of screening colonoscopy or, rarely, as submucosal masses.[427] They are typically found in middle-aged adults, with a female predominance of 3.2:1. Endoscopically, mucosal perineuriomas are small, sessile polyps indistinguishable from hyperplastic polyps or adenomas. Most arise in the rectosigmoid colon and typically measure several millimeters in size.[427,428] In the past, mucosal perineuriomas were referred to as *fibroblastic polyps.*[429-431]

Histologically, mucosal perineuriomas are composed of uniform, short spindle cells with ovoid to tapered nuclei and pale indistinct eosinophilic cytoplasm within a fine collagenous stroma (Fig. 22.39). They usually show irregular borders with the adjacent lamina propria and tend to

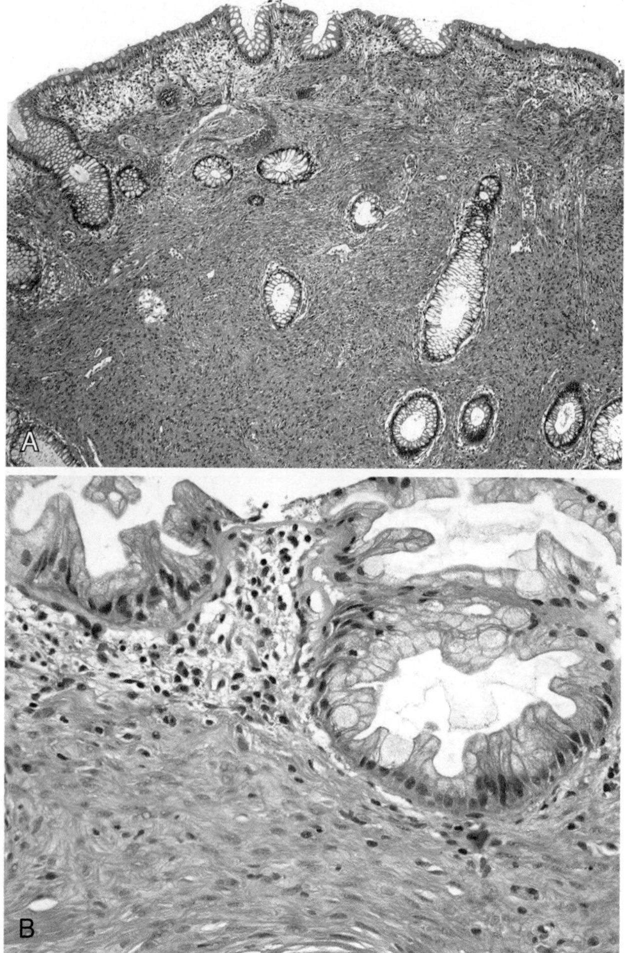

FIGURE 22.39 Perineurioma. A, Mucosal perineuriomas show irregular borders and surround and entrap colonic crypts. **B,** The tumor cells are uniform in appearance and contain bland ovoid to elongated nuclei and pale indistinct eosinophilic cytoplasm within a fine collagenous stroma. These lesions are often associated with hyperplastic polyps.

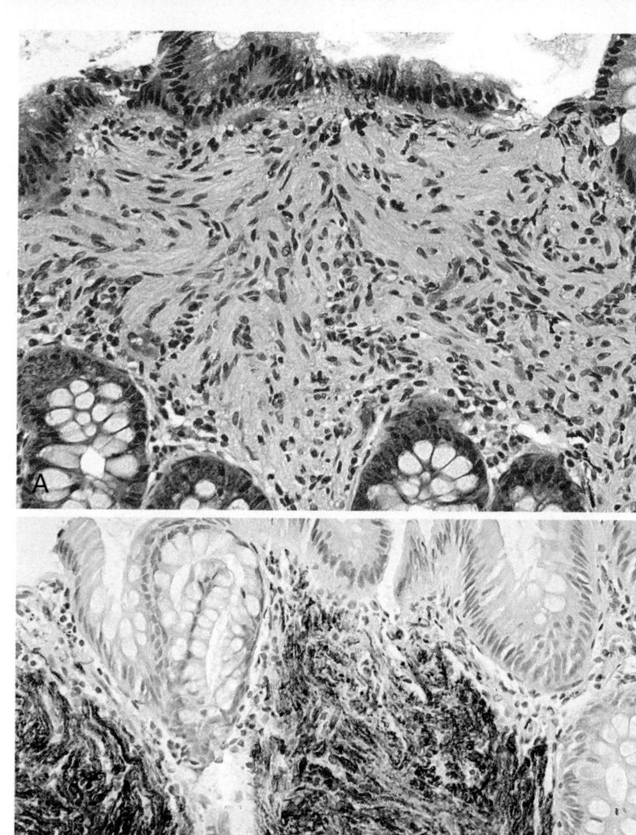

FIGURE 22.40 Mucosal Schwann cell hamartoma. A, The lamina propria contains uniform spindle cells with tapering nuclei and dense, eosinophilic cytoplasm. **B,** S100 protein is strongly positive. In contrast with mucosal perineurioma, epithelial membrane antigen is negative *(not shown)*.

show entrapment and whorling around colonic crypts.[427] The spindle cells lack mitotic activity, nuclear atypia, and pleomorphism. Eighty percent of mucosal perineuriomas are associated with serrated epithelial polyps, usually hyperplastic polyps (see Fig. 22.39), but sometimes SSLs as well.[427-429] In fact, otherwise typical hyperplastic polyps may occasionally contain minute perineurial proliferations within the lamina propria. These findings suggest that perineuriomas associated with serrated polyps may represent a reactive proliferation rather than a true neoplastic growth.[166]

By immunohistochemistry, mucosal perineuriomas are positive for epithelial membrane antigen (EMA), and 60% are positive for the tight junction–associated protein, claudin-1. Of note, EMA expression may be relatively weak (compared with the epithelium), requiring examination under high magnification to confirm immunoreactivity.[427,430] Perineuriomas are negative for S100, which distinguishes them from other morphologically similar nerve sheath proliferations composed of Schwann cells. Studies have identified *BRAF* V600E mutations in both the hyperplastic (or serrated) polyp component, similar to conventional serrated polyps without a perineurial component.[428,432]

Mucosal perineuriomas are not associated with NF1. They are benign tumors that require no clinical follow-up after polypectomy.

Mucosal Schwann Cell Hamartoma

A mucosal Schwann cell hamartoma is usually detected at screening colonoscopy as a small (1 to 6 mm), sessile lesion that is endoscopically similar to a hyperplastic polyp.[433] They are typically found in middle-aged to elderly adults, with a female predominance. The sigmoid colon and rectum are most often involved.

Histologically, mucosal Schwann cell hamartomas are composed of uniform, bland spindle cells with elongated, wavy nuclei, fine chromatin, and indistinct nucleoli; abundant, dense eosinophilic cytoplasm; and ill-defined cell borders with minimal intervening stroma (Fig. 22.40).[433] The spindle cells entrap crypts and show irregular margins with the adjacent lamina propria. Unlike mucosal perineurioma, there is an absence of whorling around crypts, and there is no associated hyperplastic polyp. By immunohistochemistry, lesional cells show strong staining for S100 protein (see Fig. 22.40B). Mucosal Schwann cell hamartomas are negative for EMA, which distinguishes them from mucosal

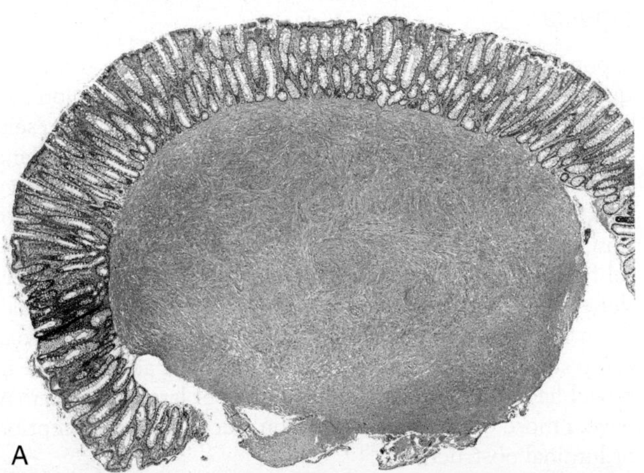

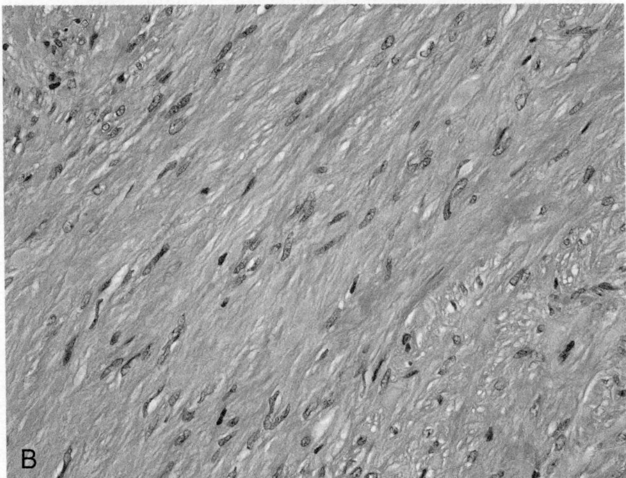

FIGURE 22.41 Leiomyoma. A, The polyp is composed of a nodular expansion of the muscularis mucosae, which is sharply demarcated from the overlying, slightly attenuated colonic mucosa. **B,** The smooth muscle cells contain abundant brightly eosinophilic cytoplasm and are arranged in fascicles.

perineuriomas. They are distinguished from ganglioneuromas by a lack of ganglion cells.

Mucosal Schwann cell hamartomas are not associated with an inherited syndrome. They are benign and require no follow-up after polypectomy.

Leiomyoma of the Muscularis Mucosae

Leiomyomas of the colorectum are benign smooth muscle tumors that arise from the muscularis mucosae (see Chapter 30). They constitute the most common type of mesenchymal tumor of the colon and are almost always discovered as an incidental polyp in patients undergoing screening colonoscopy or in surgical resection specimens removed for carcinoma.[434] In the largest series of 88 such lesions, Miettinen et al. documented a male predominance of 2.4:1 and a median age of 62 years.[435]

Endoscopically, leiomyomas are small, sessile protrusions that appear submucosal in origin. Occasionally, they are pedunculated.[435] Their predominant location is in the rectosigmoid region. Grossly, they are white, firm, well-circumscribed polyps that typically measure several millimeters in size. However, lesions as large as 2.2 cm have also been reported.[435]

Histologically (Fig. 22.41), they are composed of bundles of mature smooth muscle cells that form a sharply demarcated, nodular expansion of the muscularis mucosae. The cells are more haphazardly arranged than the normal muscularis mucosae and contain more abundant cytoplasm; they merge at the periphery of the leiomyoma with the adjoining muscularis mucosae. In Miettinen's series, only 2 of 88 lesions showed significant cytological atypia of the smooth muscle cells, akin to "symplastic" leiomyomas of the uterus, but in only one lesion was there an isolated mitotic figure.[435] The overlying colonic mucosa is usually normal or may be attenuated. In the sigmoid colon (their most common location), leiomyomas outnumber GISTs, but in the rectum they are either as common as or less common than GISTs.[435] In contrast with GISTs, leiomyomas label strongly and diffusely with smooth muscle actin (SMA) and desmin and are negative for CD34, KIT (CD117), and S100.

Endoscopic polypectomy is sufficient treatment for leiomyomas, which are uniformly clinically benign. Even tumors with cytological atypia or mitotic activity need only the assurance of complete endoscopic removal.

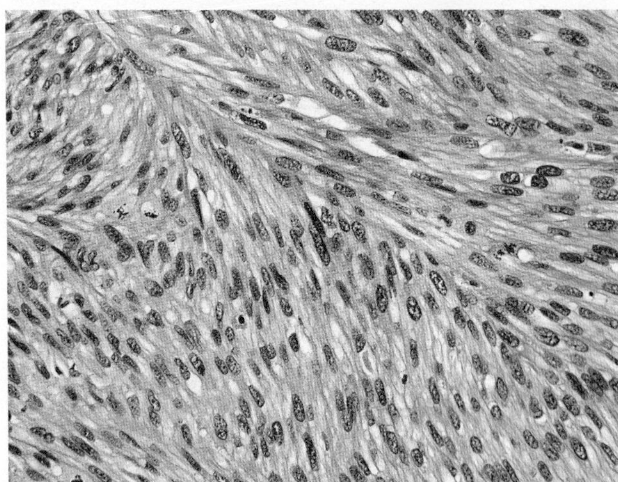

FIGURE 22.42 Leiomyosarcoma. These are more cellular than leiomyomas and contain frequent mitotic figures.

Leiomyosarcoma

True leiomyosarcomas of the colorectum are rare (see Chapter 30 for details); most previously reported cases represent malignant GISTs. Unlike GISTs, true leiomyosarcomas frequently manifest endoscopically as intraluminal polypoid tumors.[434] In a series of seven cases by Miettinen et al., the sex distribution and age range were similar to those of leiomyomas, with a male-to-female ratio of 2.5:1 and a median age of 61 years.[436] Colonic leiomyosarcomas are much less common than either leiomyomas or GISTs, and they differ from both of these lesions in their more frequent location in the right colon. In contrast with leiomyomas, leiomyosarcomas are of a much larger size (mean, 6.0 cm), frequently infiltrate into the overlying colonic mucosa, are often associated with mucosal ulceration, and may show coagulative necrosis.[436]

Leiomyosarcomas are predominantly of high-grade histology. They are composed of mitotically active spindle cells that resemble smooth muscle cells, with cigar-shaped nuclei and eosinophilic cytoplasm. In Miettinen's series, six of seven cases contained more than 100 mitoses/50 high-power fields.[436] Similar to leiomyomas, leiomyosarcomas express SMA (and often, desmin) and are negative for CD34, KIT, and S100 protein (Fig. 22.42). They are not related to GISTs.

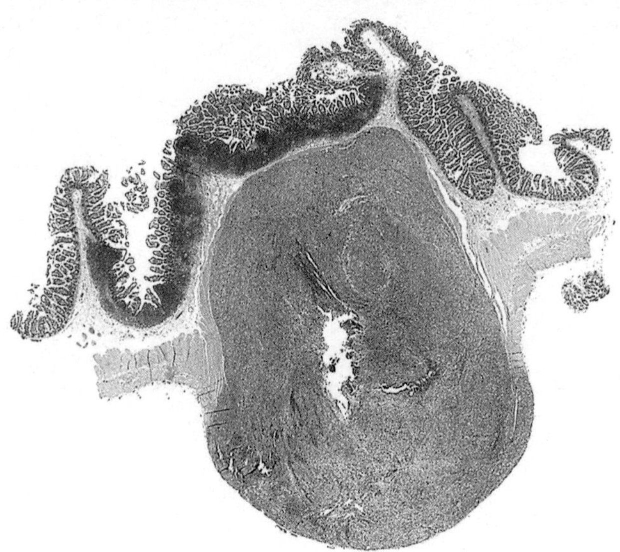

FIGURE 22.43 Gastrointestinal stromal tumor (GIST). Unlike leiomyomas that arise from the muscularis mucosae, the epicenter of GISTs usually lies within the muscularis propria.

Most patients die of their disease within 6 months to 3 years, but long-term survival may occur, even among patients whose tumors have a high rate of mitotic activity.[436] Because of their rarity, no minimal criteria for malignancy have been established for colonic smooth muscle tumors. However, a large, mural smooth muscle tumor at this anatomic site that exhibits any degree of nuclear atypia or more than a rare mitotic figure should probably be regarded as malignant.

Smooth muscle neoplasms classified variably as leiomyosarcomas, leiomyomas, and smooth muscle tumors of uncertain malignant potential also occur in association with human immunodeficiency virus (HIV) infection or with other immunodeficiency states, including solid organ transplantation and congenital immunodeficiencies. The pathogenesis of these tumors is related, in part, to Epstein-Barr virus (EBV) infection and subsequent clonal expansion of smooth muscle cells; in situ hybridization for EBV sequences is positive in these tumors, as are markers of smooth muscle differentiation such as desmin and SMA.[437,438] EBV-associated smooth muscle neoplasms frequently manifest as GI tumors,[437] but they also occur in diverse extraintestinal sites such as the lungs, liver, brain, heart, kidneys, and thyroid gland, among others.[437,439-441] In the GI tract, the lesions typically are single or multiple endoscopically submucosal nodules with central ulceration that measure from less than 1 to 4 cm in size.[442]

Gastrointestinal Stromal Tumor

GISTs are uncommon tumors of the colorectum, where they account for only 5% of all GISTs (see Chapter 30 for details).[443] KIT expression is found in 76% and CD34 expression in only 59% of colonic tumors,[436] but rectal tumors are characteristically (90%) positive for CD34.[435] Unlike leiomyomas and leiomyosarcomas, colorectal GISTs rarely manifest as mucosal polyps because their epicenters are usually within the muscularis propria (Fig. 22.43).[435,436]

Lipoma

Lipomas occur throughout the GI tract but are most frequent in the colon, particularly in the ascending colon and cecum (see Chapter 30).[444] In the colon, they represent the most common submucosal mesenchymal tumor [444] and have a predilection for elderly women.[445] Their incidence varies from 0.56% in autopsy studies [446] to 0.15% in colonoscopy studies.[447] Although many lipomas are an incidental finding, their tendency to produce symptoms is strongly dependent on their size. Patients with lipomas smaller than 2 cm in size are rarely symptomatic, whereas larger lesions can result in rectal bleeding, abdominal pain, and a change in bowel habits.[448] A significant minority of large lipomas may have a more dramatic presentation, such as intussusception or luminal obstruction.[449,450]

Endoscopically, small lipomas are usually soft, sessile polyps that have an intact, smooth overlying mucosa. The mucosa over larger lipomas can be ulcerated and irregular as a result of mechanical trauma or intussusception.[451] Biopsy forceps that reach through the mucosa can expose endoscopically recognizable, yellow adipose tissue in the submucosa. Most lipomas are solitary. In 25% to 30% of patients, multiple lipomas occur.[446] Rarely, lipomatous polyposis has been reported. In one case, hundreds of lipomas studded the colon of a 51-year-old male patient, who underwent colectomy because the polyps mimicked FAP.[452] Endoscopic polypectomy or surgical resection is usually indicated for lesions that are symptomatic or larger than 2.5 cm.[453]

Histologically (Fig. 22.44), most lipomas are discrete but not encapsulated lesions that are localized to the submucosa. In rare cases, the lipoma involves the muscularis propria or arises in the subserosal fat.[444] The overlying colonic mucosa can be normal, atrophic, hyperplastic, or ulcerated. Occasionally lipomas can be predominantly intramucosal. When associated with other hamartomatous polyps, Cowden's syndrome should be considered.[356] It is not unusual to find changes of a hyperplastic polyp or SSL overlying submucosal lipomas. Most lipomas are composed of a uniform population of mature adipocytes. In cases with surface ulceration, one may observe atypical hyperchromatic adipocyte nuclei, mitotic activity, and fibrosis—changes that are interpreted as reactive.[454]

Lipomatous Ileocecal Valve

True lipomas of the ileocecal valve are well-circumscribed lesions that affect only one of the ileocecal valve lips.[455] More commonly, there is a diffuse increase in submucosal adipose tissue that causes the ileocecal valve to appear similar to a set of protruding lips. This has been referred to as *lipohyperplasia, lipomatosis,* and *lipomatous hypertrophy of the ileocecal valve.*

Histologically, deep forceps biopsies show mature adipose tissue within the submucosa, identical to a true lipoma. In the past, barium enema examinations sometimes confused these lesions with malignancy.[455] In current practice, lipomatous ileocecal valves are rarely sampled because their appearance at colonoscopy is characteristic, thus they are rarely confused with neoplasms. Most patients do not experience symptoms, but lipomatous hyperplasia may lead to recurrent intussusception or even appendicitis in rare

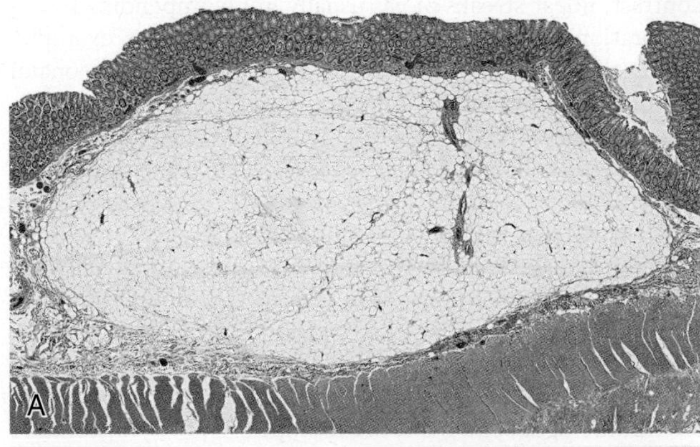

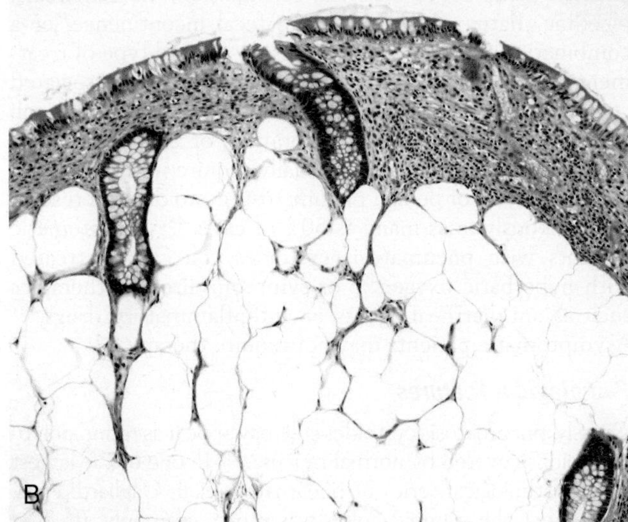

FIGURE 22.44 Lipoma. A, A discrete nodule of adipose tissue is localized to the submucosa consistent with a submucosal lipoma. **B,** An intramucosal lipoma with adipocytes present in the lamina propria.

cases.[456,457] The ileocolonic mucosa overlying the protruding valve can also show nonspecific ulceration related to mechanical trauma.

In one autopsy study, 80.4% of patients had some degree of lipomatous hypertrophy of the ileocecal valve, and it was judged to be marked in 13.7%.[458] The degree of lipohyperplasia correlated with greater body weight and with fatty infiltration in the right ventricle and pancreas.[458]

Inflammatory Fibroid Polyp

Inflammatory fibroid polyps are histologically and clinically benign lesions that occur throughout the GI tract (see Chapters 20 and 21). They are most common in the gastric antrum and terminal ileum, but they have been reported in many locations, including the esophagus, duodenum, and ileoanal pouch.[459,460] Inflammatory fibroid polyps may occur in the colorectum.[461-466] In one study, only 4 (12%) of 33 lesions arose in the colon.[467] Patients of all ages can be affected, and there is no significant sex predilection. Although occasional inflammatory fibroid polyps have been reported in patients with Cowden's syndrome,[468] in chronic IBD including ulcerative colitis[460] and Crohn's disease,[469] and in a familial setting spanning three generations,[470] there

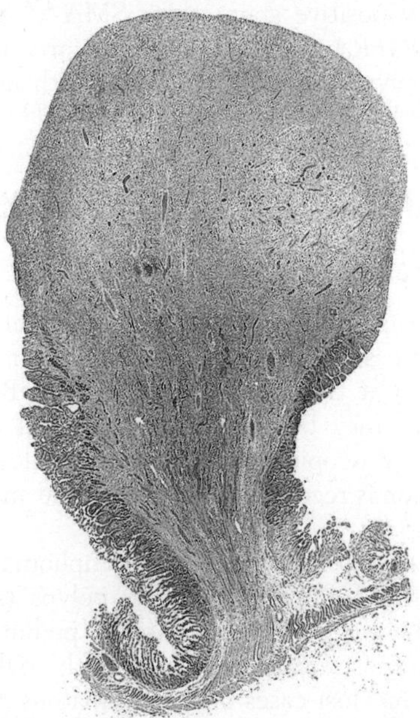

FIGURE 22.45 Inflammatory fibroid polyp. This pedunculated inflammatory fibroid polyp has its epicenter within the submucosa.

is no specific association between inflammatory fibroid polyps and any particular type of underlying GI disease. Intestinal lesions most commonly manifest with symptoms (in decreasing order) of abdominal pain, bloody stools, weight loss, or diarrhea[461]; those on the ileocecal valve can cause obstruction.[471] A single patient was reported to have colocolic intussusception related to an inflammatory fibroid polyp of the cecum,[461] but this complication is, by far, more common with small-bowel lesions.

Endoscopically, colonic inflammatory fibroid polyps are usually solitary, sessile polyps that appear submucosal and range from 1.5 to 7 cm in size.[461] In most cases, the overlying colonic mucosa is ulcerated. Histologically (Fig. 22.45), inflammatory fibroid polyps are similar in appearance to those that occur in the small intestine. The epicenter of the tumor is usually in the submucosa, but it can infiltrate into the overlying mucosa and the muscularis propria or serosa. Some cases are localized entirely within the mucosa. The lesion shows highly vascularized, fibromyxoid stroma that contains abundant inflammatory cells. The vascular network ranges from capillaries to larger, thick- and thin-walled blood vessels, which may be occluded.

The inflammatory infiltrate is usually dominated by eosinophils. Some cases show a short fascicular growth pattern and only a few eosinophils, whereas others show prominent hyalinization.[463] Lymphocytic aggregates lacking germinal centers may also be present, and plasma cells, histiocytes, and neutrophils may be seen as well. A characteristic cell type is the stellate or spindle-shaped, bland stromal cell that tends to be arranged in an onion-skin pattern around blood vessels and crypts when there is mucosal involvement. Cytological atypia of the stromal cells is only infrequently present and is, at most, mild. The stromal cells are reactive for vimentin,[472] CD34 (82% to 100% of cases),[473,474] fascin,[474] calponin,[474] and CD35 (typically staining a small subset of lesional cells)[474]; however, in contrast with GISTs, they are negative for KIT. One-fourth of cases show positive staining for SMA.[474] Studies have identified *PDGFRA* mutations in the majority of inflammatory fibroid polyps and positive staining with anti-PDGFRA antibodies.[475-477] Local excision is curative.[461]

MISCELLANEOUS POLYPOID LESIONS

Lymphoid Polyp

Prominent lymphoid follicles in the colorectal lamina propria, which are a normal finding, may appear as a minute mucosal polyp at the time of colonoscopy. Because lymphoid follicles may be the only histological finding in a biopsy of an endoscopically apparent polyp, deeper sectioning of the lesion is recommended to exclude an adenoma or serrated polyp.

Lymphomatous polyposis refers to lymphoma in the colon that grows in the form of multiple polyps (see Chapter 31).[478,479] These are typically smooth, pedunculated polyps. They are most commonly found in the right colon and terminal ileum. Most cases of lymphomatous polyposis are mantle cell lymphomas. Morphological and immunophenotypic assessment is needed to accurately subtype these tumors because a minority are low-grade follicular lymphoma or low-grade B-cell lymphoma.[480,481]

Pneumatosis Coli

Clinical Features

The hallmark of pneumatosis is the presence of gas within the bowel wall. Radiologically, the gas may appear as linear streaks or cysts adjacent to the muscularis propria. When it is predominantly cystic, the designation *pneumatosis cystoides intestinalis* is usually applied. The term *pneumatosis coli* refers to either linear or cystic forms that are limited to the wall of the colon. Although frequently cited as a rare diagnosis, pneumatosis is often asymptomatic and is likely underreported.[482] Pneumatosis itself is not a single disease entity but rather represents the common end point of multiple pathogenic conditions. It is primary (idiopathic) in only 15% of cases.[483] The other 85% of cases occur secondary to diverse predisposing conditions that include trauma from endoscopy or endoscopic polypectomy,[484,485] blunt abdominal trauma,[486] sigmoid volvulus,[487] collagen vascular disease,[488] appendicitis,[489] neonatal necrotizing enterocolitis, adult ischemic bowel disease, infectious colitis (e.g., *Clostridium difficile* colitis),[490] AIDS,[483] idiopathic IBD, pyloric stenosis, and various pulmonary conditions such as asthma, cystic fibrosis, and emphysema.[491]

Three main (and, in some cases, interrelated) mechanisms have been proposed for gas accumulation: (1) in patients with pulmonary disease, air from ruptured pulmonary blebs may pass through the retroperitoneum, along the loose adventitia of mesenteric blood vessels, and into the subserosa of the bowel wall; (2) increased intraabdominal pressure may force gas through minute defects of the intestinal epithelium, where it accumulates in the loose connective tissue of the submucosa and subserosa; and (3) intestinal necrosis may allow gas-forming anaerobic organisms to proliferate within the intestinal wall. Depending on the associated condition, or lack thereof, pneumatosis can be clinically benign or can represent a surgical emergency. The cystic form is often an incidental finding in adults who have clinically benign disease. In contrast, linear streaks of gas usually imply impending bowel perforation resulting from epithelial necrosis. For example, this is the form of pneumatosis typically seen in neonatal necrotizing enterocolitis. One paradoxical exception occurs in patients with AIDS, in whom linear pneumatosis has been reported to follow a benign course, even when associated with infectious colitis.[483]

Of particular relevance to this chapter is the cystic form of pneumatosis coli, which can result in endoscopically (or grossly) polypoid lesions. Whereas in the older literature, small-intestinal pneumatosis predominated, pneumatosis cystoides coli is now the more common form in adults and usually follows a benign course.[491,492] Most affected patients are middle-aged, and many are asymptomatic. Symptomatic patients complain of diarrhea, constipation, mucoid stools, bleeding, flatus, abdominal pain, fecal incontinence, or a combination thereof.[492] The necessity for and type of treatment depends on the patient's symptoms and any associated colonic pathological process. Rare cases of pneumatosis coli associated with ischemia, perforation, or anaerobic infection are life threatening and usually require immediate surgery. The cysts of benign pneumatosis cystoides coli resolve spontaneously in as many as 50% of cases.[482] Symptomatic patients with pneumatosis cystoides coli can be treated with hyperbaric oxygen[493] or symptom-directed therapies such as antidiarrheal agents or antiinflammatory drugs.[491] Asymptomatic patients may not require therapy.[494]

Pathological Features

Grossly, pneumatosis cystoides coli may appear as round polypoid lesions covered by normal mucosa.[493] In one of the largest clinicopathological series of pneumatosis coli, Gagliardi et al. found that the sigmoid colon was most commonly affected (40%), followed in decreasing order by the rectum, descending colon, transverse and ascending colon, and cecum.[491] Grossly, cystic collections of gas can be found in any layer of the bowel wall, but they predominate in the loose fibrofatty tissues of the submucosa, and less prominently in the subserosa. In severe cases, the affected segment may have a spongy appearance caused by the presence of closely packed gas cysts.[489]

Microscopically (Fig. 22.46), the cysts appear as empty spaces lined by epithelioid macrophages and multinucleated giant cells that represent a foreign body–type reaction; rarely, foamy macrophages predominate.[491] The macrophage lining cells may be attenuated but can be highlighted by immunohistochemistry for macrophage markers (e.g., CD68, CD163), if necessary. The overlying mucosa may also contain small cystic spaces and epithelioid macrophages or giant cells within the lamina propria. In Gagliardi's series, associated mucosal abnormalities were detected in all cases, including mild atrophy or mild crypt distortion in almost all, chronic inflammation in three-fourths, and active inflammation in almost one-half of the patients.[491]

Mucosal Pseudolipomatosis

Pseudolipomatosis is a minor procedural complication of endoscopy that results from air insufflation, mild mucosal trauma, and penetration of gas into the lamina propria.[495-497] Most cases involve middle-aged to older adults who undergo colonoscopic screening for rectal bleeding.[498,499] Endoscopically, lesions may be solitary or multiple, raised, white to

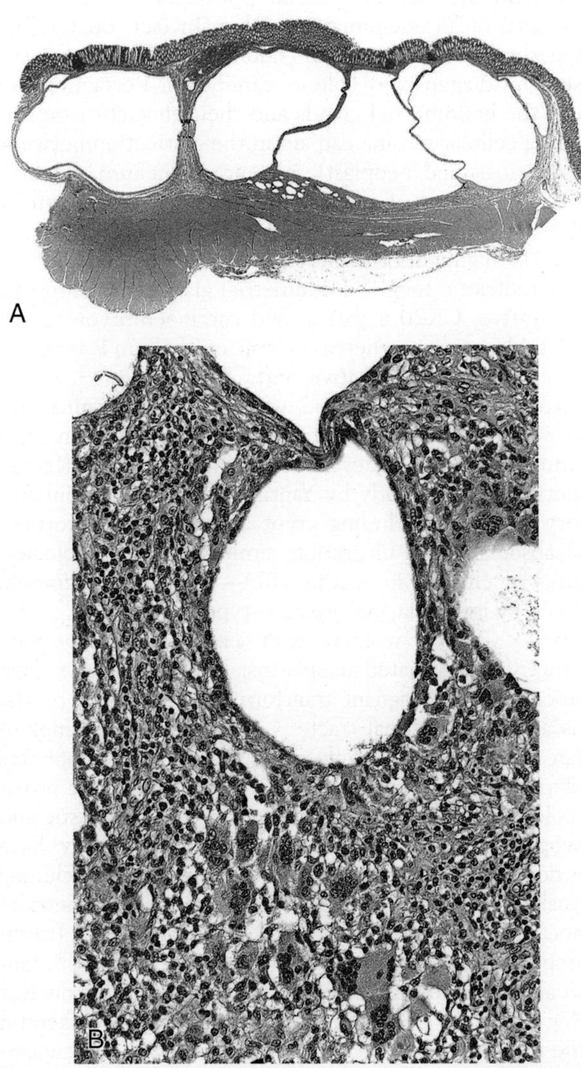

FIGURE 22.46 Pneumatosis coli. A, Large cysts characteristically predominate in the submucosa. **B,** Biopsy specimens may contain cystic spaces in both the mucosa and the submucosa; these gas-filled cysts appear "empty" and are lined focally or diffusely by histiocytes and foreign body–type giant cells. Histiocytes lining the gas-filled cysts may be flattened and attenuated. Often, other chronic inflammatory cells, including lymphocytes and plasma cells, are admixed with the submucosal macrophages.

yellow plaques measuring from 1 to 3 cm in size.[499] Histologically, numerous vacuolated spaces within the lamina propria, measuring from 20 to 240 μm, can be identified (Fig. 22.47).[498] The clear spaces have no epithelial lining, but on ultrastructural examination are bounded by collagen and ground substance.[500] In 1985, Snover et al. proposed the term *mucosal pseudolipomatosis* for these lesions, based on histochemical and ultrastructural evidence that the vacuoles are composed of trapped gas rather than adipocytes, as was previously believed.[501] Many cases resolve within weeks.[497]

Endometriosis

Clinical Features

Endometriosis is estimated to affect as many as 15% of menstruating women.[502] Pelvic involvement is most common,

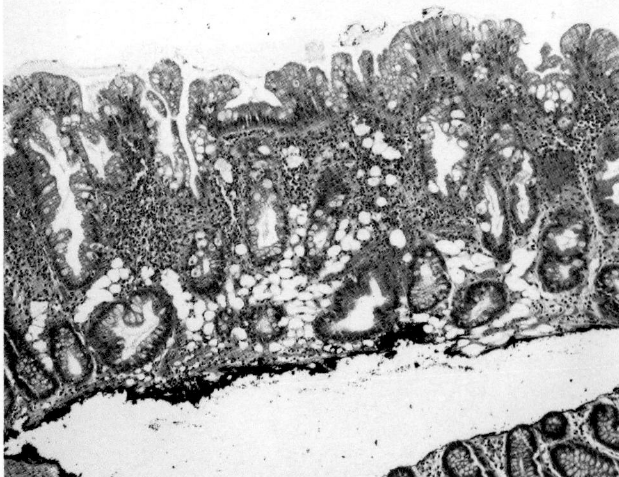

FIGURE 22.47 Mucosal pseudolipomatous. In this sessile serrated lesion, numerous vacuolated spaces within the lamina propria are identified. The clear spaces have no associated epithelial lining and are not associated with an adipocyte nucleus.

but diverse extrapelvic sites can be affected irrespective of the presence or absence of pelvic disease. The intestinal tract is involved by endometriosis in 15% to 37% of patients with pelvic endometriosis.[503] The most commonly affected site is the rectosigmoid colon, followed by the rectovaginal septum. Any site in the large or small bowel may be affected, but gastric or esophageal involvement does not appear to occur.[503] Although most patients are in their childbearing years, symptomatic sigmoid endometriosis has been documented to occur even in older postmenopausal women who have not received hormone replacement therapy.[504]

An unknown number of patients with intestinal endometriosis are asymptomatic, but those who come to medical attention suffer from abdominal pain, mass effect, bowel obstruction, rectal bleeding, infertility, diarrhea, or urinary frequency, in decreasing order.[503] Numerous case reports have described patients whose endometriosis clinically and surgically mimicked a primary colonic carcinoma.[505] More commonly, intestinal endometriosis simulates inflammatory diseases such as diverticulitis, appendicitis, or Crohn's disease.[503] Treatment is similar to that for pelvic endometriosis, including pain medication and hormonal therapy; patients with complications such as obstruction, perforation, or a mass lesion that simulates carcinoma may require surgery.

Pathological Features

The gross features of resected bowel specimens depend on the site of involvement of the bowel wall and the size of the implants. Subserosal endometriotic foci typically elicit a fibrotic response and serosal adhesions. Those in the muscularis propria can elicit smooth muscle hypertrophy akin to that seen in uterine adenomyosis, with irregular mural thickening, strictures, or mass lesions that grossly simulate a stromal tumor. More germane to the topic of colonic polyps are the lesions produced by either submucosal or mucosal involvement. In one of the largest systematic studies of intestinal endometriosis, Yantiss et al. found that 66% of affected patients had endometriotic foci in either the submucosa or the mucosa, including involvement of the lamina

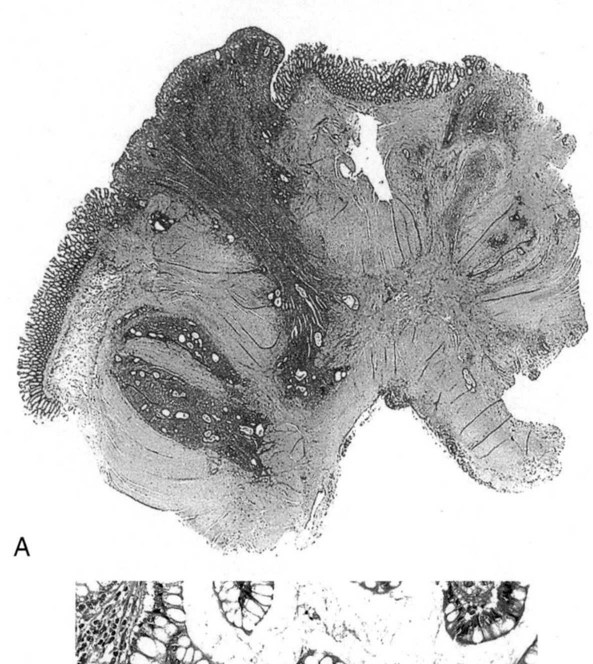

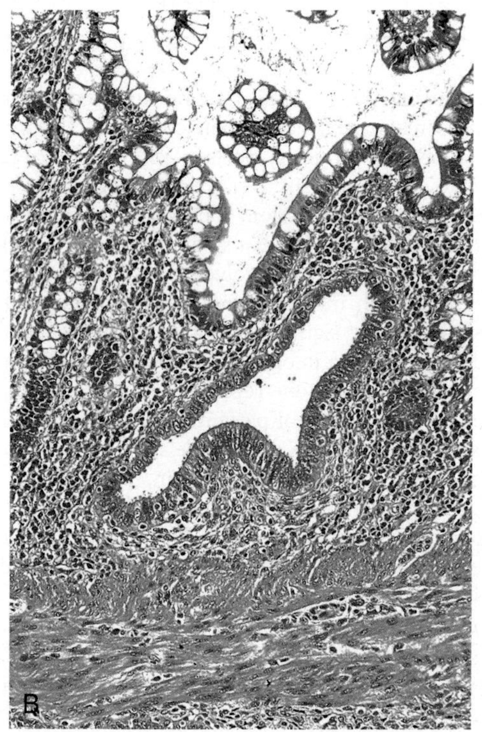

FIGURE 22.48 Endometriosis. A, A polypoid lesion projects above the surrounding colonic mucosa *(center)*. In addition, several endometriotic foci can be seen in the muscularis propria, which is characteristically markedly thickened. **B,** Endometriotic glands contain more hyperchromatic nuclei and appear mucin depleted relative to the normal colonic epithelium. They can merge with colonic crypts, giving the appearance of adenoma or dysplasia. Recognition of endometrial stromal cells adjacent to the hyperchromatic glands is key to the correct diagnosis.

propria in almost 30%.[503] Grossly, these lesions are likely to mimic either primary colon cancer, with production of ischemic mucosal ulceration over a submucosal mass, or an adenomatous polyp.

Histologically (Fig. 22.48), the hallmark of endometriosis is the presence of ectopic endometrial glands and stroma. In the lamina propria, the hyperchromatic columnar nuclei and mucin-depleted cells of endometriotic glands can merge with the adjacent colonic epithelium, creating the appearance of an adenomatous polyp. In fact, dilated and irregularly shaped submucosal endometrial glands can easily cause a misdiagnosis of colonic carcinoma. Recognition of cilia in the endometrial glands and their characteristic surrounding cellular stroma can aid in the distinction between endometriosis and neoplastic colonic epithelium. In difficult cases, a panel of immunohistochemical stains can be useful. Estrogen and progesterone receptors are positive,[502] and CD10 highlights the endometrial stromal cells in 88% of endometriotic foci.[506] Endometrial glands are uniformly CK7-positive, CK20-negative, and carcinoembryonic antigen (CEA)-negative, whereas colonic epithelium is typically CK7-negative, CK20-positive, and CEA positive.[502]

Ectopic endometrial tissue, whether in the lamina propria or in deeper layers of the bowel wall, results in reactive mucosal abnormalities in more than one-half of affected patients.[503] In the study by Yantiss, active chronic inflammatory changes—including crypt architectural distortion, crypt abscesses, and ulceration, similar to the pathological features of chronic idiopathic IBD—were most common, followed by ischemia and prolapse-type changes.[503]

Up to 1% of women with endometriosis develop endometriosis-associated neoplasms; the ovary is the most common site of malignant transformation, followed by the pelvis and the intestinal tract.[507] Akin to the frequency of benign endometriotic involvement, most such neoplasms develop in the rectosigmoid colon, with fewer in the proximal colon or ileum.[507,508] The entire range of neoplastic and preneoplastic changes of primary uterine pathology have been documented to occur within intestinal sites, including atypical hyperplasia, adenocarcinoma in situ, endometrioid adenocarcinomas, malignant mixed Müllerian tumors (carcinosarcomas), and endometrial stromal sarcomas.[507,508] Yantiss et al. suggested that "dirty necrosis," higher-grade nuclear cytology, and a CK7-negative/CK20-positive cytokeratin profile were most helpful in distinguishing colonic adenocarcinoma from endometrioid adenocarcinoma.[508] Prolonged unopposed estrogen therapy may be a predisposing factor.

Heterotopias

The colon is an unusual site for heterotopic tissue. Pancreatic and gastric heterotopia has been reported.[509,510] Gastric heterotopia of the large bowel more commonly occurs in the rectum and often presents as a polypoid lesion or a raised erythematous area. Histologically, oxyntic mucosa predominates (Fig. 22.49). In one study, pyloric gland adenoma and even invasive carcinoma have been reported, suggesting rare neoplastic transformation.[510] Pancreatic heterotopia occurs much more commonly in the stomach, followed by the duodenum and jejunum. Only case reports of colorectal pancreatic heterotopia exist.[509] These can rarely harbor pancreatic ductal adenocarcinoma.

Benign Infiltrative Processes

Muciphages

Scattered, isolated histiocytes are present in the lamina propria in most colonic biopsy specimens, but they do not tend to form aggregates, and therefore usually remain inconspicuous (see Chapter 7). However, biopsy specimens obtained

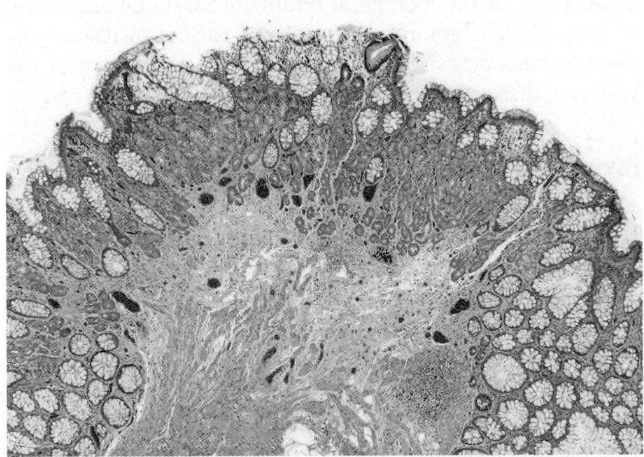

FIGURE 22.49 A rectal polyp characterized by gastric heterotopia. The gastric mucosa is composed predominately of oxyntic glands.

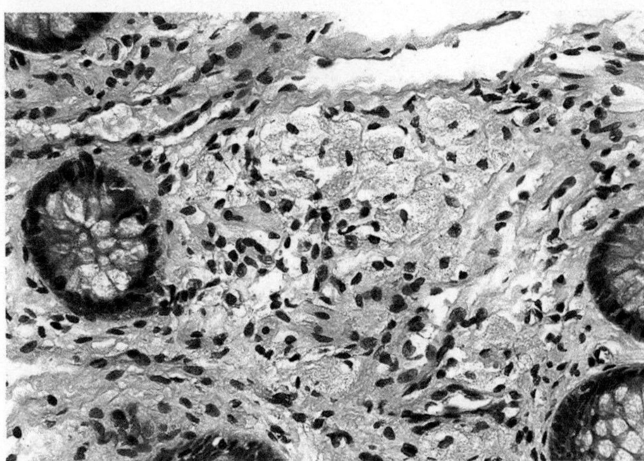

FIGURE 22.50 Muciphages. A cluster of lightly basophilic, foamy macrophages is present in the lamina propria of this rectal biopsy specimen.

from the rectosigmoid region may show prominent histiocytic aggregates that may impart a nodular or polypoid appearance to the mucosa. In a series of 100 consecutive rectal biopsy specimens, Bejarano et al. found foamy histiocytes in 40%; aggregates of large foamy histiocytes were moderate to intense in 23%.[511] In most cases, infiltrates are present in the superficial aspect of the lamina propria, but they can also involve the muscularis mucosae. Immunohistochemical stains reveal these cells to be CD68-positive and cytokeratin-negative macrophages. This immunoprofile and the lack of nuclear enlargement or atypia help distinguish them from signet ring cell carcinomas. In 20% of patients, histiocytic aggregates were the only histological finding to account for the endoscopic impression of a small nodule or polyp.[511]

In most cases, the foamy histiocytes represent muciphages that contain neutral and acidic mucins, mainly sialomucins.[511] Common histological abnormalities of the associated rectal mucosa include mild to moderate fibrosis of the lamina propria, mild crypt atrophy, and mild chronic inflammation, suggesting that muciphages are the residua of previous mild mucosal injury (Fig. 22.50).[511]

Xanthomas and Xanthogranulomas

In a minority of cases, histiocyte aggregates represent true xanthomas, or localized collections of lipid-containing histiocytes. These cases are not distinguishable from muciphages based on their appearance with hematoxylin and eosin (H&E) stain. The nature of these histiocytes is revealed by negative mucin histochemical stains, including PAS with diastase, Alcian blue at pH 2.5 and pH 1.0, and mucicarmine. In addition, lipid-containing histiocytes have a characteristic granular, dotlike cytoplasmic labeling for CD68 that contrasts with the usual, more clumped cytoplasmic CD68 labeling of muciphages.[511] In contrast with muciphages, true xanthomas are unusual. The most common GI site of involvement is the stomach. Colorectal xanthomas are almost all located in the sigmoid colon or rectum, where they are seen endoscopically as cream-colored to yellow papules or polyps that typically measure from 1 to 4 mm in size.[511-514] They are almost always found incidentally at colonoscopy and may be solitary or multiple. Xanthoma cells are histologically similar to muciphages and can involve both the lamina propria and the muscularis mucosae (or even the submucosa if the biopsy is deep enough), but most cases are limited to the lamina propria. Most reported patients with xanthomas are middle-aged, and no clear sex predilection has been observed. Most patients have neither hyperlipidemia nor associated skin lesions.[513]

More extensive xanthomatous or xanthogranulomatous inflammation that involves the deeper layers of the bowel wall, including the muscularis propria, is a rare cause of intestinal obstruction. These lesions have been reported in the ileocecal valve [515] and the rectosigmoid colon.[516,517]

Differential Diagnosis of Histiocytic Infiltrates

The finding of histiocytes in the lamina propria may raise a differential diagnosis with lipid storage disease or infection (fungal organisms, acid-fast bacilli, and the Whipple bacillus, among others). In addition, signet ring carcinoma cells may, on occasion, be confused with histiocytes. Histiocytes are usually readily distinguished from signet ring cell carcinoma by their lack of nuclear enlargement and atypia on routine H&E staining. In questionable cases, immunohistochemical stains for CD68 and cytokeratin can be performed; histochemical stains for mucin are of no utility in this differential diagnosis because both muciphages and carcinoma cells contain cytoplasmic mucin. Stains for infectious organisms are not usually performed unless the patient is immunosuppressed, the histiocytic aggregates are located proximal to the rectosigmoid colon, or another clinical indication requires it. Mucosal infiltrates and their differential diagnosis are explained in detail in Chapter 7.

Systemic Mastocytosis

Patients with systemic mastocytosis are seen with diarrhea or abdominal pain, usually secondary to the release of mast cell mediators into the circulation.[518] Intractable diarrhea or malabsorption is more often seen in patients with direct infiltration of mast cells into the colonic mucosa.[518] Endoscopically, colonic involvement by systemic mastocytosis may have a polypoid or nodular appearance, although in other cases the mucosa may be flat, erythematous, or entirely unremarkable.[519,520]

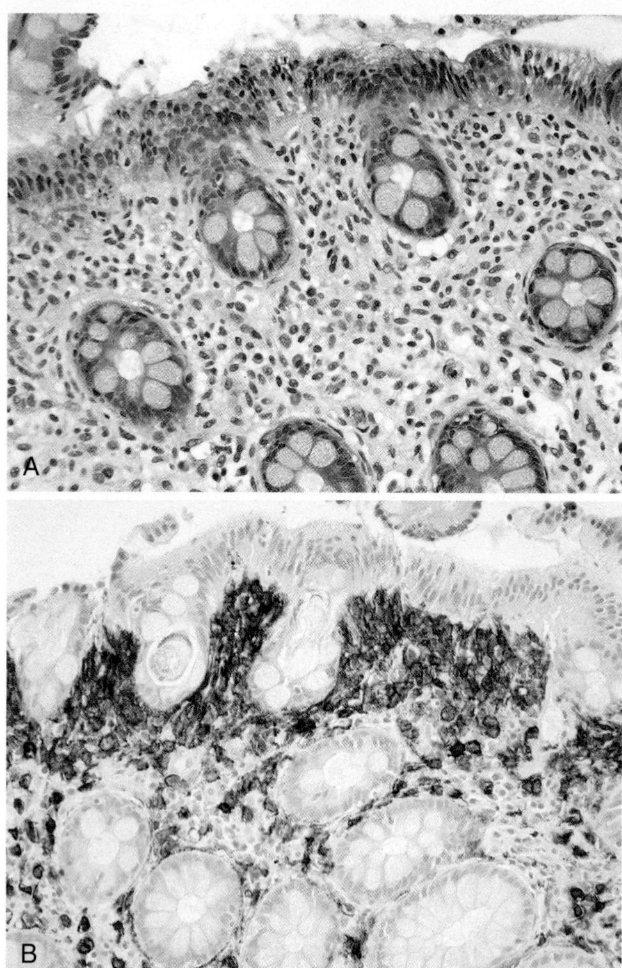

FIGURE 22.51 **Systemic mastocytosis. A,** The mucosa contains an infiltrate of mononuclear cells with pale cytoplasm. **B,** An immunostain for KIT (CD117) is positive, confirming that the mononuclear cells are mast cells and highlighting the sheetlike growth pattern in the superficial lamina propria.

Histologically, the lamina propria may contain small clusters, larger aggregates, or confluent sheets of mononuclear cells with abundant pale cytoplasm (Fig. 22.51).[519,520] A bandlike subepithelial infiltrate is a typical finding. In contrast with the round nuclei in normal mast cells, neoplastic mast cells usually contain ovoid or spindle-shaped nuclei.[519] Prominent admixed eosinophils are common, and this can be a helpful clue to the diagnosis of mastocytosis, although it may also lead to a misdiagnosis of eosinophilic colitis.[518-520] Mastocytosis involving colonic mucosa can be quite subtle and therefore easily mistaken for normal histiocytes. By immunohistochemistry, neoplastic mast cells are strongly positive for KIT (CD117) (see Fig. 22.51B) and tryptase and show aberrant staining for CD25, whereas CD25 is negative in mast cells in both normal mucosa and inflammatory conditions.[518] KIT immunostain highlights the abnormal distribution of mast cells and is very useful to help establish a diagnosis of systemic mastocytosis. One recent study has suggested that the incidental finding of mast cell aggregates or sheets in the colorectal mucosa in patients without suspected mastocytosis may not indicate the presence of the systemic disease.[521]

Inverted Appendix

Appendiceal intussusception is a rare condition. It was found in only 0.01% of 71,000 appendectomies studied during a 40-year period in one large series.[522] All ages, from infants to the elderly, can be affected, but it is more common in the first decade of life and among males.[523] Anatomically, there are several main types of appendiceal intussusception, which have been reviewed in detail by Langsam et al.[524] Briefly, either the distal or proximal appendix can intussuscept and give rise to either a completely or partially inverted appendix that protrudes into the cecum. An inverted appendix should therefore be considered in the radiological and histological differential diagnosis of polypoid cecal lesions.[525,526]

Most patients with an inverted appendix are symptomatic; their abdominal complaints are nonspecific but can include abdominal pain, nausea and vomiting, and blood in the stool.[527-529] Predisposing conditions include abnormal peristalsis (either of the intestine or the appendix itself), anatomic abnormalities such as a mobile mesoappendix or a wide appendicular lumen, and mass lesions that form a focal point for intussusception.[523] In the last category, inverted appendices have been reported in patients with appendiceal mucocele,[528] appendiceal adenoma,[525,526] juvenile polyp,[527] endometriosis,[525] and PJS,[531] among other conditions. In some cases, the appendix has no apparent abnormality.[529]

Pathologically, the inverted appendix with a mass lesion, such as an adenoma, can appear as a pedunculated polyp in which the inverted appendix forms the "stalk."[530] Histologically, the layers of the appendiceal wall are reversed. The mucosa forms the external layer, and the submucosa and muscularis propria form the internal layer. The mucosa may show increased acute and chronic inflammation, and the submucosa may show fibrosis.[523,529] In some cases, it is histologically normal.[529] Ischemic changes secondary to inversion can also occur.

Mucosal Tag

Small excrescences of histologically normal mucosa are a frequent incidental finding at colonoscopy. Termed *mucosal polyps* by some authors, they represent benign elevations of colonic mucosa. They are most often sampled to exclude an adenoma or hyperplastic polyp. In one autopsy study of 502 Cretan patients (median age, 65 years), incidental colorectal polyps were identified in 21.1% of cases, and 6.9% of these were mucosal tags.[531] Even higher frequencies are documented when only diminutive (<5 mm) polyps are considered. Weston and Campbell reported that 17.9% of diminutive polyps represented either mucosal tags or lymphoid follicles,[532] and in a study by Hoff et al., 23% of diminutive polyps were mucosal tags.[24] Mucosal tags may diminish in size with time when monitored endoscopically.[24]

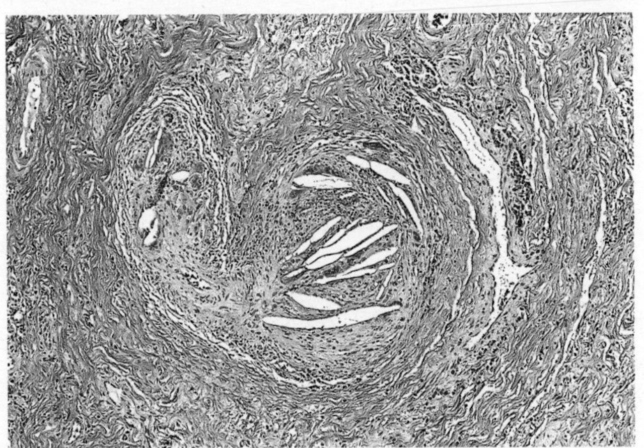

FIGURE 22.52 Atheroemboli-associated polyp. Within the underlying submucosa, an arterial lumen is occluded by atheroembolic material that contains cholesterol clefts.

Atheroembolus-Associated Polyps

Some cases of localized colonic ischemia produce the endoscopic appearance of a mass or a polyp. In a study of the histological features distinguishing ischemia from C. *difficile* colitis, for example, Dignan et al. reported that the endoscopic impression was that of a mass lesion or polyp in 7 of 24 patients with ischemic colitis.[533] Atheroemboli can rarely cause polyp formation through an ischemic mechanism (Fig. 22.52).[534,535] Submucosal edema that develops in ischemic colitis contributes to this appearance by elevating the overlying ischemic mucosa.[536] Rarely, atheroemboli are discovered as an incidental finding on biopsies of adenomatous polyps.[536]

The full reference list may be accessed online at Elsevier eBooks for Practicing Clinicians.

SECTION IV

EPITHELIAL NEOPLASMS OF THE GASTROINTESTINAL TRACT

CHAPTER 23

Molecular Diagnostics of Tubal Gut Neoplasms

Nancy M. Joseph

Contents

INTRODUCTION

The genomic revolution is inexorably changing our understanding of nearly all medical conditions, and it is changing our clinical practices in the fields of diagnostic pathology and oncology. Indeed, genomic biomarkers have dramatically improved clinical algorithms for diagnosis, prognosis, treatment, and disease monitoring of cancer. It is now well recognized that all clonal neoplasms result from accumulating alterations in the genome that are usually acquired or "somatic" in nature.[1,2] Occasionally, there are inherited or "germline" genetic alterations that increase an individual's chances of acquiring sufficient mutations in order to form a neoplasm. The genomic landscape of the most common cancer types have now been largely described by large sequencing efforts including The Cancer Genome Atlas (TCGA) program and the International Cancer Genome Consortium (ICGC). The development of a genome atlas for all cancer types has been accompanied by the development of targeted therapies.

This chapter will highlight the most common molecular alterations of tubal gastrointestinal (GI) tract neoplasms (Fig. 23.1) and will discuss the clinically relevant alterations and methodologies most commonly used for molecular testing in clinical practice (Table 23.1). Although this chapter does not provide a comprehensive reference of all genetic alterations in all tubal gut neoplasms or an exhaustive treatise on the specific intricacies of all molecular diagnostic techniques, it outlines the molecular techniques routinely used in diagnostic laboratories, with a specific focus on the advantages and limitations for each methodology. The goal of this chapter is to help practicing GI pathologists select the best method of testing for each type of cancer specimen that will achieve the best molecularly integrated diagnosis and fulfill the standard of care of molecular testing for optimal clinical management.

TYPES OF GENETIC ALTERATIONS IN CANCER

Cancer arises from accumulations of genetic alterations in the genome.[1,2] Genetic alterations are defined as changes in the DNA sequence and/or DNA content resulting from single nucleotide point mutations; small or large insertions or deletions (indels); copy number changes including large-scale chromosomal gains and losses as well as focal amplifications or deep deletions; and structural rearrangements/translocations. In addition to changes in the DNA sequence/content, epigenetic changes can also occur that modify gene expression or function. One of the most common forms of epigenetic alterations is methylation of CpG islands in the genome, which are enriched in promoter regions and generally lead to decreased gene expression. CpG island methylation cannot be detected with standard DNA sequencing without bisulfite treatment of the DNA. It is thus important to understand what types of genetic alterations can be detected by each molecular method.

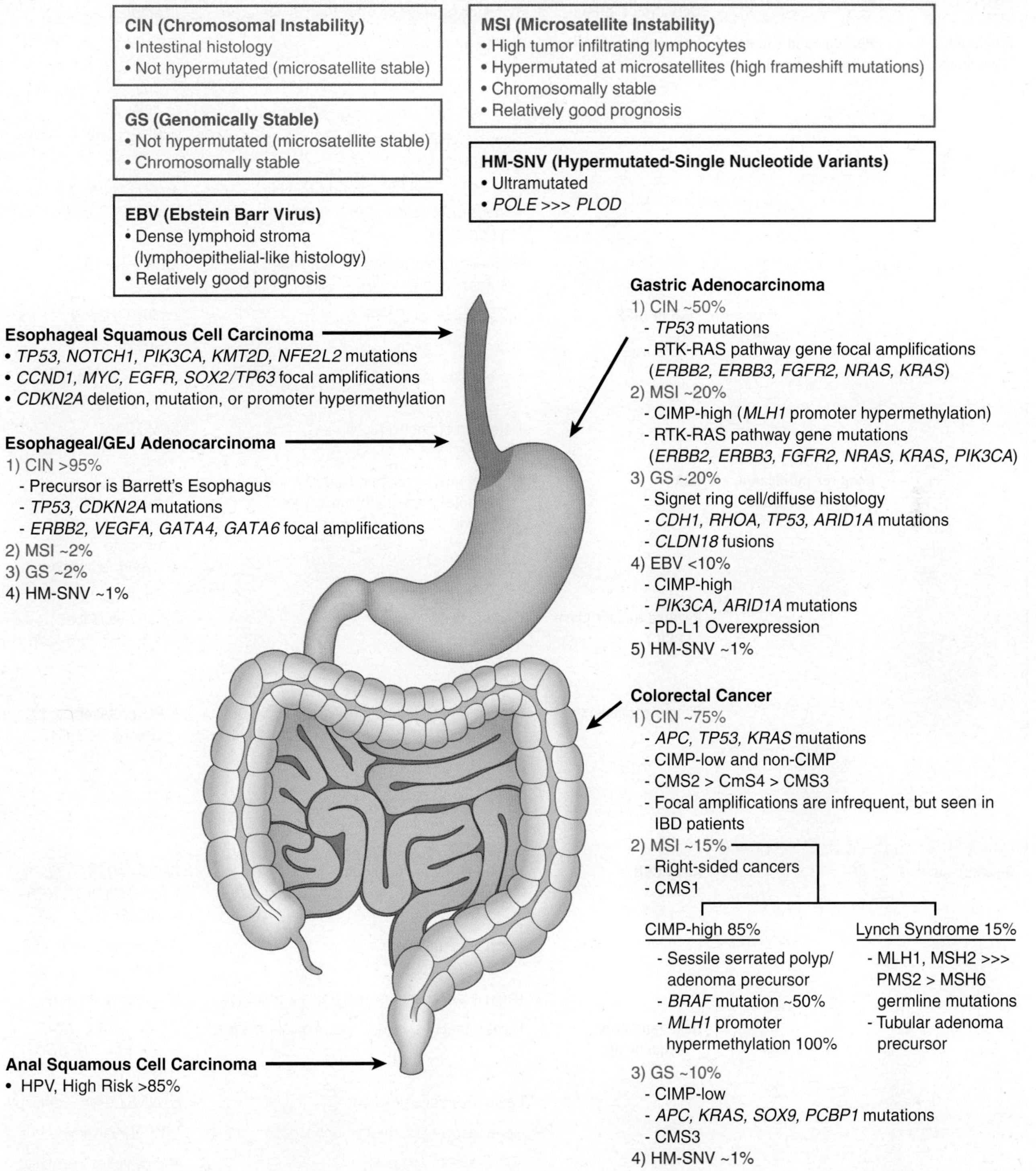

CIN (Chromosomal Instability)
- Intestinal histology
- Not hypermutated (microsatellite stable)

GS (Genomically Stable)
- Not hypermutated (microsatellite stable)
- Chromosomally stable

EBV (Ebstein Barr Virus)
- Dense lymphoid stroma (lymphoepithelial-like histology)
- Relatively good prognosis

MSI (Microsatellite Instability)
- High tumor infiltrating lymphocytes
- Hypermutated at microsatellites (high frameshift mutations)
- Chromosomally stable
- Relatively good prognosis

HM-SNV (Hypermutated-Single Nucleotide Variants)
- Ultramutated
- *POLE* >>> *PLOD*

Esophageal Squamous Cell Carcinoma
- *TP53, NOTCH1, PIK3CA, KMT2D, NFE2L2* mutations
- *CCND1, MYC, EGFR, SOX2/TP63* focal amplifications
- *CDKN2A* deletion, mutation, or promoter hypermethylation

Esophageal/GEJ Adenocarcinoma
1) CIN >95%
- Precursor is Barrett's Esophagus
- *TP53, CDKN2A* mutations
- *ERBB2, VEGFA, GATA4, GATA6* focal amplifications
2) MSI ~2%
3) GS ~2%
4) HM-SNV ~1%

Anal Squamous Cell Carcinoma
- HPV, High Risk >85%

Gastric Adenocarcinoma
1) CIN ~50%
- *TP53* mutations
- RTK-RAS pathway gene focal amplifications (*ERBB2, ERBB3, FGFR2, NRAS, KRAS*)
2) MSI ~20%
- CIMP-high (*MLH1* promoter hypermethylation)
- RTK-RAS pathway gene mutations (*ERBB2, ERBB3, FGFR2, NRAS, KRAS, PIK3CA*)
3) GS ~20%
- Signet ring cell/diffuse histology
- *CDH1, RHOA, TP53, ARID1A* mutations
- *CLDN18* fusions
4) EBV <10%
- CIMP-high
- *PIK3CA, ARID1A* mutations
- PD-L1 Overexpression
5) HM-SNV ~1%

Colorectal Cancer
1) CIN ~75%
- *APC, TP53, KRAS* mutations
- CIMP-low and non-CIMP
- CMS2 > CmS4 > CMS3
- Focal amplifications are infrequent, but seen in IBD patients
2) MSI ~15%
- Right-sided cancers
- CMS1

CIMP-high 85%
- Sessile serrated polyp/adenoma precursor
- *BRAF* mutation ~50%
- *MLH1* promoter hypermethylation 100%

Lynch Syndrome 15%
- MLH1, MSH2 >>> PMS2 > MSH6 germline mutations
- Tubular adenoma precursor

3) GS ~10%
- CIMP-low
- *APC, KRAS, SOX9, PCBP1* mutations
- CMS3
4) HM-SNV ~1%

FIGURE 23.1 The genetic landscape of tubal gut carcinomas. The molecular subtypes and most frequent genetic alterations seen in the most common carcinomas of the gastrointestinal tract. *CIMP,* CPG island methylator phenotype; *CMS,* consensus molecular subtype; *GEJ,* gastroesophageal junction; *HPV,* human papilloma virus; *RTK,* receptor tyrosine kinase. (Drawing courtesy Sarah Bowman.)

Detection of single nucleotide changes along with small insertions and deletions in an unknown nucleic acid sample is the most common assay performed in molecular diagnostics. These assays are performed to identify hereditary germline disease–associated mutations and somatic or acquired mutations in tumor cells. Although sequencing is the "gold standard" method, it was not always the most practical approach before next-generation sequencing (NGS) because of the size of the target gene that must be analyzed, the limited DNA sample that may be available, or the rarity of the variant sequence in the nucleic acid population to be analyzed. Many different approaches to screening for mutations have evolved in the past 20 years in response to improved technologies. The most common methods used today include Sanger sequencing, polymerase chain reaction (PCR), and NGS,

TABLE 23.1 Methods for Detection of Genetic Alterations*

		Detection Method	Types of Alterations That Can Be Detected	Examples
Single-gene methods	**Performed in situ on a tissue section**	**Immunohistochemistry**	Point mutations	*BRAF* p.V600E, *IDH1* p. R132H, *TP53* dominant-negative hotspots
			Gene amplification or gene expression caused by fusion event	*ERBB2 (HER2), NTRK, STAT6*
			Loss-of-function mutation (frameshift, nonsense, splicing) or deletion of tumor suppressor	*MLH1, MSH2, MSH6, PMS2, SDHB, TP53*
			Promoter hypermethylation causing loss of tumor suppressor expression	*MLH1, SDHB*
		FISH or CISH	Amplification of a gene	*ERBB2 (HER2)*
			Deletion of a gene	*CDKN2A, PTEN*
			Gene rearrangements/fusions	*EWSR1, PRKACA* rearrangement
			Detection of oncogenic viruses	*EBV, HPV*
	Requires purification of nucleic acids	**PCR**	Hotspot mutations, microsatellite instability, promoter hypermethylation (needs bisulfite treatment)	*BRAF* V600E, microsatellite instability, *MLH1* promoter hypermethylation
		Reverse transcriptase PCR	Gene fusions	*EWSR1-FLI1* fusion, *DNAJB1-PRKACA* fusion
		Sanger sequencing	Point mutations, small insertions or deletions	*KRAS* mutations in codons G12, G13, G61, G146
Genomic methods		**Array CGH**	Focal gene amplifications	*ERBB2 (HER2), EGFR, MYC, CCND1, KRAS, BRAF*
			Focal gene deletions	*APC, PTEN, RB1, TP53, CDKN2A*
			Large-scale chromosomal gains and losses	Monosomy, trisomy
		Next-generation sequencing	Point mutations, small insertions or deletions	*KRAS, NRAS, BRAF, PIK3CA, KIT, PDGFRA, CTNNB1*
			Large insertions/deletions	*CTNNB1* exon 3 deletion
			Gene rearrangements/fusions	*EWSR1* rearrangement
			Microsatellite instability	Microsatellite instability
			Tumor mutation burden (TMB)	Hypermutation
			Focal gene amplifications	*ERBB2 (HER2)*
			Focal gene deletions	*APC, PTEN, RB1, CDKN2A*
			Large-scale chromosomal gains and losses	Monosomy, trisomy
		DNA methylation profiling (by array or NGS of bisulfite-converted DNA)	Epigenetic subgroups	CIMP-high, CIMP-low, non-CIMP subtypes

**Methods performed on nucleic acids usually require at least 30% to 40% tumor content, and microdissection of unstained FFPE slides is often required to enrich for tumor content before DNA extraction.*

CGH, Comparative genomic hybridization; *CISH*, chromogenic in situ hybridization; *EBV*, Epstein-Barr virus; *FISH*, fluorescence in situ hybridization; *HPV*, human papillomavirus; *PCR*, polymerase chain reaction.

TABLE 23.1 Methods for Detection of Genetic Alterations*—Cont'd

Tissue Requirement	Tumor Fraction Requirement	Advantages	Disadvantages
Single unstained section per antibody	Tumor fraction can be low because analysis occurs in situ	Widely available, rapid turnaround time, inexpensive, limited tissue and tumor content requirement	A negative result does not exclude mutations in the gene as only one amino acid change is detected. For example, *IDH1* p. R132C would not be detected Staining result could be equivocal. Example: 2+ Her2 staining Loss of staining can be difficult to interpret Antibodies are not widely available for most molecular alterations
Single unstained section per probe set	Tumor fraction can be low because analysis occurs in situ	Widely available, rapid turnaround time, relatively inexpensive, limited tissue and tumor content requirement	Can only assay a single gene per test Break-apart probes can capture any rearrangement involving EWSR1, but cannot tell you the fusion partner
5-10 unstained slides for extraction of tumor DNA	≥40% tumor fraction required for MSI, MLH1 promoter methylation*	Fast and inexpensive	MSI does not inform as to which of the four mismatch repair proteins is mutated or hypermethylated
5-10 unstained slides for extraction of tumor RNA and generation of cDNA	Can be low because sensitivity is high	Easy to generate primers for any gene fusion of interest, can determine the fusion partner	RNA in FFPE samples can be degraded; may require multiple primer pairs to detect fusion transcripts with different breakpoints
5-10 unstained slides for extraction of tumor DNA	≥40% tumor fraction required*	Easy to generate primers for any gene exon of interest	Have to amplify and sequence every exon of interest; labor intensive and expensive. (e.g., activating *KIT* mutations occur in exons 9, 11, 13, 14, 17, and 18; inactivating mutations in tumor suppressor genes like *TP53* can occur in any of numerous exons)
10 unstained slides for extraction of tumor DNA	≥30% tumor fraction required*	High-resolution copy number data	No data for mutations or rearrangements
5-10 unstained slides for extraction of tumor DNA or tumor RNA	Sensitivity for mutation detection is high, but sensitivity for copy number changes and fusion detection usually requires ≥30% tumor fraction*	Can detect all types of alterations in many genes in a single assay	Requires resources for bioinformatic data processing and storage, 1- to 2-week turnaround time
5-10 unstained slides for extraction of tumor DNA	>40% tumor fraction required*	Outperforms conventional histologic-based methods for tumor classification and prognostic stratification	Not yet clinically validated or reimbursable for tubal gut neoplasms

each of which is discussed briefly in the following sections with an emphasis on the advantages and limitations of each method.

Chromosomal copy number changes and structural variations are a hallmark of cancer and include abnormal chromosomal number (i.e., trisomies, monosomies, aneuploidy), translocations, focal amplifications, and subchromosomal deletions.[3] Although deletions and abnormalities in chromosome number are among the most common changes, particularly in solid tumors, translocations and focal amplifications have garnered the most interest because of their association with oncogenic activations that may be susceptible to targeted inhibition. The most common methods used in the characterization of chromosomal copy number changes and structural variations include fluorescence in situ hybridization (FISH), comparative genomic hybridization (CGH) array methods, reverse transcriptase PCR (RT-PCR), and NGS.

METHODOLOGIES FOR DETECTION OF GENETIC ALTERATIONS

Sample Collection and Processing

Clinical tumor samples are most frequently formalin-fixed paraffin-embedded (FFPE) samples, so most molecular methodologies used for tumor samples are optimized for FFPE tissues. Most germline genetic testing, on the other hand, is performed on high-molecular-weight genomic DNA or RNA extracted from white blood cells in whole-blood samples. Improved methods use more limited samples, such as blood spots and buccal smears. A thorough discussion of all methods is beyond the scope of this chapter, so we will focus on testing of surgical pathology samples and other samples that may harbor neoplastic cells, including cytopathology samples and cell-free DNA that may be used for molecular screening and diagnosis.

Detection of Genetic Variants in Tissue Sections

Immunohistochemistry

Immunohistochemical staining on FFPE sections is a routine method in all surgical pathology practices, and there are an increasing number of antibodies that can help detect genetic alterations. For example, there are numerous antibodies against tumor suppressor proteins that are commonly lost in cancer as a result of deletion, truncating mutations, or promoter methylation. Also available are antibodies against proteins that are overexpressed in tumor samples as a result of amplification or translocation; antibodies against oncoproteins that aberrantly localize to the nucleus based on genetic alterations; antibodies against proteins that serve as surrogate markers of defining genetic alterations in tumors; and most recently, mutant-specific antibodies that recognize hotspot mutations in oncoproteins. Examples relevant to GI neoplasms are provided in Table 23.1. Advantages of immunohistochemistry include rapid turnaround time, minimal tissue requirement (single 5-micron section per stain), and in situ visualization of the results, which allows for accurate interpretation in samples with low tumor content. The major limitation is that only a small fraction of clinically relevant mutations currently have a mutant-specific antibody available, and it is unlikely that there will ever be antibodies available for all clinically relevant molecular alterations.

Fluorescence in Situ Hybridization and Chromogenic in Situ Hybridization

FISH and chromogenic in situ hybridization (CISH) are widely used methods that can be applied to detection of DNA and RNA variants. Metaphase FISH is a cytogenetic technique that requires culture of live cells, and this allows detection of much smaller abnormalities than are detected by conventional karyotyping. Interphase FISH does not require culture of live cells, and it is therefore a practical method that is commonly used to study routinely fixed tumors.

For interphase FISH analyses, DNA probes in the 60- to 200-kb range are covalently attached to a fluorescent molecule, hybridized to a complementary target sequence in cellular DNA, and visualized under a fluorescent microscope as a point of fluorescent light in the nucleus of the cell. Probes are designed with specificity to any region of interest within the genome and are widely available for centromeric regions (i.e., CEN probes) and telomeres. Multiple probes may be hybridized simultaneously and analyzed separately by using different colors of fluorescent dyes.

Known, recurrent oncogenic translocations are commonly detected by FISH by using dual-fusion probes or break-apart probes. Dual-fusion probes contain two probes, each labeled with a different fluorescent dye and designed to bind regions spanning the breakpoint of each translocation partner. In the absence of a translocation, two distinct nuclear signals are observed for each colored probe. In the presence of a translocation, there is a single distinct signal for each color from the nontranslocated chromosomes, and the other two signals then combine, or fuse, together both colors for the translocation. Dual-color, break-apart probes are particularly useful in detecting translocations in which one gene can recombine with multiple partners, like *EWSR1*. This approach consists of two probes that bind to the intact gene flanking the breakpoint. In the setting of a translocation, the two probes break apart from each other and yield two distinct signals rather than a single hybrid signal.

Copy number aberrations are also well suited for detection by FISH. Centromeric probes give an accurate count of chromosome number and are useful in the detection of aneuploidy. When centromeric probes are used in combination with probes that target specific genes or hotspot chromosomal regions, they also allow a readout of regions of genomic deletion or amplification. Diploid tumor cells have two distinct centromeric probe signals and only one chromosomal arm signal in the setting of a deletion, but more than two in the case of amplification. Multiple cells are typically scored, and a signal ratio is calculated and compared with validated positive and negative control ratios.

Detection of Genetic Variants in Purified Nucleic Acids

Microdissection to Enrich for Tumor Purity

Tumor samples are a complex mixture of neoplastic cells, stromal cells, inflammatory cells, and background (normal) tissues. Some carcinomas, like those of the pancreas and biliary tree, are characterized by scattered, small neoplastic glands embedded within abundant desmoplastic stroma. Other cancers may be infiltrated by a dense lymphocytic response. As a result, unenriched tumor samples may vary in neoplastic cellularity from a high of approximately 80% to a low of only 5% to 10% tumor cell fraction. The success of many molecular diagnostic assays depends on a neoplastic cellularity or tumor cell fraction of at least 40%, and microdissection is usually required to enrich the sample for neoplastic cells. Manual microdissection often involves scraping specified regions of unstained FFPE sections under direct guidance of an adjacent and aligned hematoxylin and eosin (H&E)-stained section.[4] These approaches can produce marked improvements in neoplastic cellularity.

Laser microdissection methods may be used to dramatically enrich neoplastic populations, although the yield of tissue is significantly reduced by these labor-intensive methods. Assay requirements must be tailored to the tissue parameters to determine which enrichment methods are needed. In liquid-phase enrichment, cells are digested to release them in a suspension and then purified by bead-tagged antibodies that target cell surface antigens. These approaches are common in research applications, but are used much less frequently in clinical practice.

In addition to tissue samples obtained from sections cut from paraffin blocks, cytopathology samples may also be used in molecular diagnostic assays. The number of cells and quantity of DNA available for testing from cytology preparations have recently been shown to be consistently adequate for a variety of methodologies, including NGS.[5-8] The use of cytological specimens in molecular assays must be closely supervised by a pathologist who can ensure that an adequate specimen is collected during the biopsy procedure, and because the process may consume the permanent diagnostic record.

Liquid Biopsies and Circulating DNA

Small amounts of detectable cell-free DNA circulate in the plasma and serum of healthy individuals, and in those with a variety of disease states. In patients with cancer, this includes DNA and RNA from tumor cells. Detection of a variety of tumor mutations, microsatellite alterations, methylation abnormalities, and chromosomal alterations has laid the foundation for development of assays for use in cancer screening, diagnosis, and therapeutic monitoring.[9] In a similar manner, DNA from other biofluids (e.g., effusions, fecal samples, biliary aspirations, luminal washings) may be used in molecular diagnostic assays. These technologies are an extremely active area of research and hold promise for the development of a variety of novel assays. One significant obstacle with cell-free DNA is the low fraction of tumor-derived DNA, which means alterations will all have low mutant allele frequencies, and both the sensitivity and specificity of variant detection is markedly decreased. Thus cell-free DNA is a commonly used method of monitoring disease burden, rather than making an initial diagnosis.

Nucleic Acid Extraction and Purification

Historically, extraction of high-quality DNA and RNA has required fresh or frozen tissue samples. If processed very quickly after surgical removal, these samples provide excellent nucleic acids for subsequent investigations. However, degradation of nucleic acids may occur. Degradation depends on several factors: tissue necrosis, duration of acute surgical ischemia, the time from resection to tissue harvesting, DNase and RNase activity during extraction, and improper storage. Attempts to use formalin-fixed, paraffin-embedded tissue samples create unique challenges and are usually less successful because of DNA fragmentation, DNA cross-linking, and contaminants. However, these samples are much more widely available, and improvements in nucleic acid recovery and subsequent testing have greatly increased the utility of these samples.

Traditional extraction of good-quality high-molecular-weight DNA requires a three-step extraction procedure. First, cell and tissue lysis use detergents, proteinase K, and RNase. Second, proteins are removed, avoiding RNA and chemical contamination. Third, DNA is purified. Conventional manual extraction techniques use phenol-chloroform purification and precipitation by using ethanol or isopropanol. Newer, kit-based approaches use a variety of bead-based elution technologies to purify DNA.[10] Some methods yield DNA of lesser purity and lower molecular weight, although this result is acceptable for many applications. The methods used must appropriately balance ease of use, expense, quality, and downstream assay requirements.

RNA is extracted by two predominant methods: phenol-based extraction (e.g., TRIzol reagent) and silica matrix or glass fiber filter-based binding. TRIzol methods retain small RNAs, including microRNA (miRNA) and small interfering RNA (siRNA). TRIzol reagent also includes guanidine isothiocyanate to maintain the integrity of RNA while disrupting cells and dissolving cell components.

After extraction, nucleic acids must be accurately quantified to assess the success of the extraction and to determine the correct quantity of template for subsequent applications. Quantification is typically performed by using either ultraviolet spectrophotometry or fluorometric quantification with a known control or standard.

Sanger Sequencing

Sanger sequencing is currently known as *first-generation sequencing*. Sanger sequencing was described by Frederick Sanger in the 1970s[11] and is based on electrophoretic separation of randomly terminated linear sequence extensions. Modern day automated Sanger sequencing uses fluorescent chemistry (different fluorescent dyes label the four dideoxynucleotide chain terminators: ddATP, ddCTP, ddGTP, ddTTP) and capillary electrophoresis.[12] It has served as the primary machine for single-gene diagnostics in molecular diagnostics laboratories and as the workhorse for the first generation of the human genome sequencing project that was completed in 2003.[13] Sanger sequencing is accurate, has well-defined chemistry, and is best suited for reading 300-base pair (bp) to 1-kilobase (kb) DNA fragments in a single reaction.

Sanger sequencing has technical limitations, particularly throughput (i.e., number of bases per second that can be read). Electrophoretic separation is the predominant rate-limiting step that severely limits the speed and cost of assays. For example, it has been estimated that one automated sequencer would require several decades and tens of millions of dollars to sequence a single genome today.[14] Another limitation is sensitivity. The lower limit of detection is 20% mutant allele frequency, which means a sample would need to contain at least 40% tumor content to reliably detect a heterozygous mutation.

Polymerase Chain Reaction

PCR is a fast and inexpensive technique used to amplify, or copy, small segments of DNA of interest. The amplified PCR products can then be used in numerous molecular and genetic analyses, including modern day Sanger sequencing, DNA fingerprinting or specimen identity analysis, microsatellite instability (MSI) analysis, and melting curve analysis.

For simplicity, sequence variant detection methods may be divided into PCR-based technologies and sequencing technologies. Methodological approaches may be tailored to the range of expected results. For instance, the approaches used to detect a common known sequence variant at a set codon (e.g., *BRAF* V600E mutation in thyroid cancer) are very different from mutation screens applied to an entire exon, multiple exons, entire genes, or a panel of genes. PCR-based approaches use a variety of different techniques. Common approaches include PCR primers that are designed to amplify specific recurrent mutations and real-time PCR melting curve analysis. However, as sequencing technologies have improved and reactions have become simpler and cheaper to perform and analyze, sequencing approaches have become the first choice for sequence variant detection. PCR is still commonly used for detection of MSI and MLH1 promoter hypermethylation, although MSI is becoming more routinely performed as part of NGS panels.

Methylation-specific PCR starts with bisulfite treatment of the DNA. Methylated DNA is characterized by the conversion of cytosine to 5-methylcytosine, which results in suppression of gene transcription when it occurs in the regulatory promoter region. During bisulfite treatment, unmethylated cytosine residues are deaminated, which converts them to uracil, whereas 5-methyl cytosines are unchanged. Possible methylation of key DNA sequences may then be evaluated by methylation-specific PCR, which uses sets of primers that are complementary to T residues for unmethylated cytosines or C residues for methylated cytosines.

Reverse Transcriptase Polymerase Chain Reaction

Known, recurrent translocations are readily detectable by RT-PCR or PCR performed on cDNA that is reverse transcribed from purified RNA. Different methods use the same general principles; several primer pairs and sets of primer pairs are designed to detect all possible known breakpoints for a given translocation. Each primer pair consists of a forward primer that flanks the fusion junction on one side and a reverse primer that flanks the fusion junction on the other side. Multiple primers are needed because of the limitation in the size of PCR products and the large genomic variability in known breakpoints for some translocations. This RT-PCR reaction can be performed either quantitatively to measure amplicon production in real time or can be followed by gel electrophoresis of the reaction product to determine whether an amplicon was produced, which indicates that the specific fusion transcript being assayed is present. The RT-PCR product can also be sequenced by Sanger sequencing to confirm and visualize the fusion transcript.

Comparative Genomic Hybridization Array

Array-based hybridization is a technology that uses a large number of targets that are densely arrayed on a small, readable substrate, allowing multiple, simultaneous hybridizations. Array targets are immobilized on glass slides or other materials and may consist of DNA, cDNA, PCR products, oligonucleotides, RNA, or proteins. Array-based hybridizations were originally developed on nitrocellulose and nylon membranes and were moved to treated glass slides in 1987. The development of technology to deposit small spots of target on glass substrates led to a rapid increase in the miniaturization of spots and the array density of spots. High-density oligonucleotide arrays with oligonucleotides covering the entire human genome have been developed and are commercially available for research or clinical use including from Affymetrix (CytoScan HD Array and OncoScan FFPE Assay), Illumina (HumanCytoSNP BeadChip and Infinium CytoSNP-850K BeadChip), Agilent (SurePrint G3 Human CGH Array), and others.

CGH arrays are designed to test DNA. Specific genomic DNA sequences are spotted onto an array corresponding to loci known to be amplified or deleted in human tumors or possibly encompassing a much more comprehensive representation of the human genome.[15] Genomic DNA from the test sample is purified, fragmented, fluorescently labeled, and hybridized, typically in a competitive two-color hybridization with a known normal or control sample. To facilitate application to limited tissue samples, several methods have been developed to globally amplify test DNA before CGH analysis. Competitive hybridization allows a readout of the relative genomic copy number across all assayed genomic loci.

Expression arrays are designed to determine the relative expression level of a vast number of genes in a single sample. Typical experiments use labeled mRNA in a competitive, two-color fluorescent hybridization with a known control sample.[16] These tests simultaneously measure the transcript level of thousands of genes compared with a control or normal specimen. This transcriptional profiling (i.e., transcriptome analysis) is commonly applied to human neoplasms in the research setting.

Next-Generation Sequencing

Also known as *second-generation sequencing* and *massively parallel sequencing,* NGS technologies are capable of sequencing large numbers of different DNA or cDNA sequences in parallel (i.e., in a single reaction).[14] NGS technologies were developed in part from focused investment by the National Human Genome Research Institute (NHGRI) in an effort to markedly reduce the expense of large-scale sequencing and thereby rapidly advance the realization of personalized medicine. As opposed to the pre-NGS era, when it cost roughly $10 million to sequence a single human genome (3 billion bases), the 2021 cost to sequence one human genome is now below $1000, making it possible to perform whole-genome sequencing on an individual basis. Whole-genome sequencing does not yet have routine validated clinical applications, though it has been used with great success in selected cases[17] and research studies. Whole-exome sequencing refers to large-scale sequencing of all the coding exons in the whole genome, which compose only approximately 2% of the genome. Exome sequencing may be directed at the whole exome of approximately 30,000 genes, or it may target the approximate 3000 genes or smaller subsets known to be involved in human disease.

Despite the explosion of research studies using whole-genome and whole-exome sequencing unveiling the genetic basis of countless human diseases and cancers, validated clinical applications remain limited and are predominantly targeted at smaller subsets of disease-associated genes. The drastic sequencing cost reduction makes it actually cheaper to sequence all of the exons of several hundred cancer genes (~1 to 3 megabases [Mb]) of an individual cancer patient's tumor using NGS than it is to sequence a few exons of a few genes (~1 to 3 kb) using Sanger sequencing. Furthermore, by sequencing a larger footprint of the genome, NGS allows for detection of multiple types of genetic alterations (mutations, indels, copy number alterations, and structural variants) in a single test, which is one of the biggest advantages of NGS testing.

Template Generation

The general starting point for all NGS assays is double-stranded DNA (dsDNA). It is obtained from a variety of sources, including genomic DNA and reverse-transcribed RNA (i.e., complementary DNA [cDNA]). All starting dsDNA must be converted into a sequencing library wherein fragmentation, size selection, and adapter ligation are used to generate an unbiased representation of the DNA population to be sequenced. Limitations in the detection sensitivity require that sequencing reactions be amplified before sequencing, which may introduce bias (e.g., loss of representation of rare sequences) and errors, which are particularly problematic in clinical applications. The latest technological platforms can sequence from single-molecule templates, which represents such a significant improvement that some authorities refer to them as *third-generation platforms.*[14]

For NGS, hundreds of thousands of template molecules are immobilized and spatially arrayed on solid surfaces (i.e., flow cell) or beads, thus allowing for massively parallel sequencing reactions. Although the various platforms of NGS use the same four basic steps (i.e., sample collection, template generation, sequencing reaction, and detection), they use substantially different methods of template generation and sequence interrogation. Because NGS represents the most important technological development in molecular diagnostics, it is considered in more detail in the following sections.

Sequencing Reaction

NGS platforms use a series of repeating chemical reactions that apply DNA polymerase or ligase to add and detect nucleotides on a repetitive nucleotide-by-nucleotide basis. This process, referred to as *sequence by synthesis*, represents a dramatic improvement to Sanger sequencing, which requires discrete separation and detection of fragments that differ in length by 1 bp. The simultaneous analysis of massive numbers of reactions by NGS is largely responsible for the more than 100,000-fold decrease in per base sequence cost during the past decade.

Data Analysis

Compared with Sanger sequencing (which typically reads 500 bp to 1 kb in a single reaction), most NGS platforms offer shorter average read lengths (50 to 400 bp). Because NGS reactions generate millions of these short reads, data analysis is a much more difficult task, making heavy demands on data acquisition, storage, tracking, quality control, analysis, and interpretation.[14] NGS data generation can vastly outpace analytic and interpretation resources.

Typically, the first phase of analysis is base calling, which is usually performed by the proprietary software associated with the sequencing platform. Base calling is followed by sequence alignment and assembly, an area of extremely active computational research.[18] The last phase of analysis requires interpretation of the final sequence data. Third-generation platforms may offer longer reads, which could vastly reduce the challenges of data analysis, but these underdeveloped platforms are not widely available.

Sequencing Coverage

All NGS platforms have inherent errors in base calling. The rate of error varies with each specific platform and chemistry. To counter qualitative errors, each base pair is sequenced multiple times in separate, parallel sequencing reactions. The degree to which each nucleotide is quantitatively resequenced is referred to as the *coverage* or *coverage depth of sequencing.*

Because there may be biases in coverage depth during any NGS experiment, evolving standards suggest a need for 50 to 100 times coverage to ensure 100% accuracy in detection of single-nucleotide sequence variants. Clinical sequencing for germline variants, which are expected to be present at a mutant allele frequency of 50%, usually requires less depth of coverage than clinical tumor sequencing. Tumor samples are never pure, and variants can be either clonal or subclonal, so deeper sequencing with high coverage (500 to 1000×) is often performed. The higher the coverage, the higher the sensitivity of the assay, allowing for detection of subclonal variants or rare variants present at low mutant allele frequencies. The occurrence of errors and the need for coverage contribute to the plateau in the cost reduction of whole-genome sequencing. This plateau may be overcome by the increased fidelity associated with third-generation technologies that use single-copy DNA.

Targeted Sequencing

Targeted sequencing with NGS technology requires enriching DNA regions of interest before sequencing. Enrichment strategies include hybrid capture or multiplex PCR enrichment. Hybrid capture generally allows for more accurate quantification of variant allele frequencies and copy number alterations because PCR duplicates can be removed during data processing. Using targeted panels of genes to capture relevant mutations or alterations for specific disease types allows for deeper sequencing while maintaining a low cost. NGS becomes cost-effective compared with Sanger sequencing when multiple genes must be sequenced. Examples include panels of genes for the diagnosis of genetic diseases and for the detection of oncogenic driver mutations in cancer.

Some of the first multigene targeted oncogenic assays have been established for lung cancer, for metastatic disease that has failed other therapeutic options, and for a variety of research studies, and they have offered significant advantages to traditional molecular diagnostic approaches.[19,20]

Other early panels, including those developed for screening known genes associated with colorectal polyposis and Lynch syndrome, have been powerful and cost-effective tools that eliminate the traditional stepwise approach to genetic characterization.[21,22]

PRINCIPLES OF TARGETED THERAPY

The heterogeneity of tumors is a challenge for traditional cytotoxic forms of cancer therapy. Cancer cells are characterized by the genetic instability that accompanies uncontrolled cell division, increasing the likelihood of multiple mutations and replication errors. In addition, dynamic variations in the tumor microenvironment influences cancer cell behavior in a manner that involves direct communication with cancer cells.

Conventional cytoreductive chemotherapy generally exploits toxic compounds that affect all proliferating cells. Thus successful therapy relies on finding drug combinations and dosage limits that allow selective killing of neoplastic cells without targeting nonneoplastic cells. Although the past 50 years of cytotoxic therapy have seen major strides in cancer management, these approaches do not take advantage of the exceptional biological understanding that now broadly exists for most human cancers and can be routinely achieved on a personalized level. Targeted therapies attempt to exploit the identification and inhibition of target genes that are thought to be essential for tumorigenesis. Targeted therapies are individualized to the genetic aberrations in a specific tumor and have transformed trial-driven oncology into one of the leading frontiers of personalized therapy.[23] Because targeted therapies are based on specific gene aberrations in a given tumor, these approaches have transformed diagnostic pathology and prompted development of a wide range of companion tests that support the application of tailored therapeutic options.[24,25] Here, we discuss some of the principles and therapies that are most relevant to tubal gut neoplasms.

Driver Mutations and Oncogene Addiction

Targeted therapies are successful, in large part, because they focus on the genetic mechanisms that underlie the development and progression of human tumors. Human neoplasia is a genetic disease driven by acquisition of clonal genetic alterations that confer a growth advantage. Some of these mutations are major drivers of the transformation process.[26] Driver mutations have diverse effects in cells alone or in combination, and they may drive either inhibitory or stimulatory pathways. In some cases, the long-term proliferative effect of driver mutations may be associated with a decrease in activity of other normal cellular growth regulatory pathways. The cellular tolerance of subsequent downstream mutations may depend entirely on the ongoing effects of these driver mutations.

The net result of these processes is that cancer cells become dependent on driver mutations. In some cases, shutting off the drivers results in a sudden increase in inhibitory signals, an absence of compensatory stimulatory signals, and unopposed activities of other genes that become detrimental to the cell.[27] Shutting drivers off may result in more striking antiproliferative and apoptotic effects than otherwise predicted. This concept, known as *oncogene addiction*, has been demonstrated in cell culture and animal models of human neoplasms.[27,28]

Early targeted therapies exhibited dramatic effects in different liquid and solid tumors. The tyrosine kinase inhibitor (TKI) imatinib was effective in chronic myeloid leukemia (CML) with *BCR-ABL* translocations, which exhibit constitutively active ABL tyrosine kinase activity, as well as in GI stromal tumors (GISTs) with activating *KIT* mutations.[29] The epidermal growth factor receptor *(EGFR)* inhibitor gefitinib was potent in lung cancers with activating EGFR mutations.[30] These early successes of targeting and shutting down key oncogenic driver mutations in human cancer formed the cornerstone of modern developmental cancer therapeutics with small molecules and monoclonal antibodies.

Small Molecule Signal Transduction Inhibitors

Cancer cells are generally characterized by hyperactivated signaling pathways leading to uncontrolled cell growth, which are often driven by mutated, overexpressed, or amplified oncogenes. Blocking these pathways can lead to apoptosis or growth arrest.

The nature of these signaling cascades has made protein kinases attractive targets for the development of therapeutic compounds. Both receptor and nonreceptor tyrosine kinases initiate signaling pathways crucial to cell growth and transformation. Thus small molecule TKIs can be effective antineoplastic agents. These are designed to compete with ATP or substrate binding, or bind in an allosteric fashion and alter activity because of a conformational change of the protein.

The first TKIs (tyrphostins) were identified in 1988, designed to specifically inhibit the activity of EGFR but not other receptor or nonreceptor tyrosine kinases.[31] This early work paved the way for the development of a series of TKIs, including imatinib, an inhibitor of ABL, the oncogenic target of BCR-ABL translocations in CML.[32] The therapeutic efficacy of imatinib in CML and later in GIST has been a major driving factor in the development of new TKIs throughout the pharmaceutical industry. However, long-term use of imatinib in some late-stage GIST or CML patients can cause drug resistance. This typifies an issue with signal transduction inhibitors; dynamically complex oncogenic signaling networks lead to an escape from oncogene addiction as further mutations occur. Luckily, the next generation of ABL TKIs have proven to be effective for imatinib-resistant patients. A steady flow of new inhibitors is moving into early clinical trials, with many more in the development pipeline.

Many tumors are driven by mutation, amplification, or epigenetic upregulation of the EGFR family of tyrosine kinases that includes EGFR (HER1), ERBB2 (HER2), ERRB3 (HER3), and ERBB4 (HER4). Binding of EGF or its homologs to these receptors induces receptor homo- or hetero-dimerization and subsequent tyrosine transphosphorylation, leading to activation of downstream signaling pathways including phospholipase C, Ras/MAP kinase, PI-3 kinase, mTOR, and others (Fig. 23.2). The expression or activity of these receptors is increased in many cancers (colon cancer, breast carcinomas, gliomas, and non–small cell lung carcinomas) leading to cell proliferation. Two

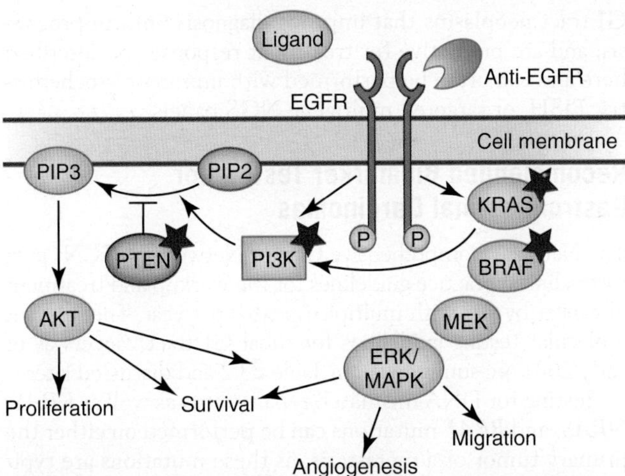

FIGURE 23.2 Epidermal growth factor receptor (EGFR) signaling pathway. Ligand binding results in dimerization of EGFR, autophosphorylation, and activation of downstream signaling cascades. *Stars* mark proteins that are activated (KRAS, BRAF, and PI3K) or inactivated (PTEN) in colorectal cancer, potentially causing resistance to anti-EGFR therapy. *AKT,* A serine/threonine-specific protein kinase, also called protein *kinase B (PKB)*; *ERK,* extracellular signal–regulated kinase (now called *MAPK*); *MEK,* a tyrosine/threonine kinase (also known as *MAPKK*); *P,* phosphate; *PI3K,* phosphatidylinositide 3-kinase; *PIP2,* phosphatidylinositol (4,5)-bisphosphate; *PIP3,* phosphatidylinositol (3,4,5)-trisphosphate.

selective EGFR TKIs, gefitinib and erlotinib, were approved by the U.S. Food and Drug Administration (FDA) and are indicated as first-line therapy in patients with *EGFR*-mutated lung cancer.

In addition to tyrosine kinases, small molecule inhibitors have been investigated for downstream targets, including small G proteins such as oncogenic Ras and its target RalA; protein serine/threonine kinases such as B-Raf, MEK, mTOR, and Akt; and lipid kinases such as different isoforms of PI-3 kinase.[33] Although many of these efforts remain under investigation, Raf and MEK inhibitors have been widely used in cancer therapy. Ras, Raf, and MEK reside in a linear pathway that is key to cellular growth control, and numerous mutations have been found in Ras, Raf, and even MEK in most cancer types, especially colorectal and pancreatic carcinomas and melanomas. Although there are Ras inhibitors in late-stage investigation, both Raf inhibitors (sorafenib, vemurafenib) and MEK inhibitors (trametinib, cobimetinib, binimetinib) have been approved for use alone and in combination in different settings.

Monoclonal Antibody Therapies

The search to produce therapeutic antibodies has been ongoing for more than 100 years. Early therapeutic efforts focused on nonhuman monoclonal antibodies, but they are highly immunogenic and therefore associated with a short half-life. The first successful therapeutic antibody was the chimeric mouse/human anti-CD20 drug rituximab (Rituxan).[34] Chimeric antibodies are approximately 65% human, resulting in decreased immunogenicity and a much longer serum half-life. Cetuximab (anti-EGFR) is also a chimeric antibody.

Second-generation therapeutic monoclonals, referred to as *humanized monoclonals,* are 95% human, resulting in an even greater reduction in immunogenicity. Trastuzumab (anti-HER2) and bevacizumab (anti-VEGF) are examples of humanized antibodies.

Later methods allowed the development of fully human monoclonal antibodies, including panitumumab (anti-EGFR) and ipilimumab (anti-CTLA4).[35] The fully human monoclonals have an extended half-life and improved pharmacokinetics, resulting in increased dosage intervals for these expensive therapies. Monoclonal antibody therapies are particularly useful for targeting cell surface receptors. They have been among the most successful targeted therapies during the past 10 years and include the checkpoint inhibitors targeting CTLA4, PD-1, and PD-L1. Additionally, numerous studies are underway to conjugate monoclonal antibodies with cytotoxic drugs to improve cancer therapy, and some of these antibody drug conjugates (ADCs) are already approved.

Tumor Heterogeneity and Acquired Resistance to Targeted Therapy

Despite good initial tumor responses, acquired resistance often develops, even after relatively short intervals of response. The resistant tumor clones typically are characterized by two types of genetic alteration not found in the original tumor analysis. First, mutations in the target gene block the drug binding site or confer new activity that is no longer responsive to the targeted therapeutic agent.[36] Second, alterations bypass the targeted signaling blockade by activation of downstream or parallel pathways.[37]

Although the term *acquired resistance* implies that the tumor has evolved during the course of treatment, mathematical models suggest that the resistant clones may exist at the outset of therapy as very small subpopulations within the original tumor.[38] The course of therapy eliminates the bulk of sensitive cells, but the resistant subclones are unaffected and continue to grow in the same location, resulting in the emergence of recurrent tumors. The significant degree of heterogeneity in most human tumors has been the subject of numerous investigations.[39]

These concepts about tumor heterogeneity are shifting the way we think about the diagnosis and management of cancer. Rather than administering targeted therapeutic agents consecutively, it may be advantageous to use two or even three targeted agents simultaneously.[38] It may become important for the molecular diagnostics laboratory to characterize the dominant genetic aberrations and the subclones that may harbor mutations important for the development of resistant tumors.[39] The need for more comprehensive genomic profiling may drive the development of assays that are better able to survey the entire tumor, such as those based on circulating tumor cells or DNA.

GASTROINTESTINAL CARCINOMAS

The Landscape of Genetic Alterations in Gastrointestinal Carcinomas

The preceding discussions on sequencing and array technologies provide insight into the depth of genomic and gene expression data that can be harvested from analyses of a pathology specimen. The Cancer Genome Atlas (TCGA)

Project, the International Cancer Genome Consortium (ICGC), and others have recently detailed the genetic and epigenetic aberrations of large cohorts of colorectal, gastric, and esophageal carcinomas assayed by multiple technological platforms including whole-genome and whole-exome DNA and RNA NGS as well as genome-wide methylation profiling.[40-46] Major highlights from these and other studies are summarized in Figure 23.1, with a focus on the five molecular subtypes of GI tract adenocarcinomas outlined by the TCGA. Four of the five subtypes (chromosomal instability [CIN], microsatellite instability [MIS], genomically stable [GS], and hypermutated single nucleotide variants [HM-SNVs]) are found in both upper and lower GI tract locations, but the Epstein-Barr virus (EBV) subtype is only found in the stomach. The four consensus molecular subtypes (CMS1, msi-immune; CMS2, canonical; CMS3, metabolic; and CMS4, mesenchymal) of colorectal adenocarcinoma based on transcriptomic analyses of primary colorectal cancers[47] are also integrated in Figure 23.1. More rare epithelial cancers of the tubal GI tract including small bowel adenocarcinomas, appendiceal adenocarcinomas, and neuroendocrine carcinomas have been genomically profiled in smaller cohorts by multiple independent research groups, often using targeted NGS assays rather than whole-genome and whole-transcriptome assays.

Although Figure 23.1 highlights the most common genetic alterations in the most common epithelial GI tract cancers, most cancer patients do not yet clinically need whole-genome, whole-exome, whole-transcriptome, or genome-wide methylation profiling as only smaller subsets of genes have been clinically validated to be actionable. However, the use of targeted multigene NGS assays is becoming more and more routine in clinical practice, with the expansion of targeted therapies. Clinically useful molecular testing in GI tract neoplasms that improve diagnosis, inform prognosis, and are predictive for treatment response are described here and can often be performed with immunohistochemistry, FISH, or targeted multigene NGS panels.

Recommended Biomarker Testing for Gastrointestinal Carcinomas

The National Comprehensive Cancer Network (NCCN) puts forth clinical practice guidelines for the workup and treatment of cancer by site with multiple updates per year. The relevant molecular testing guidelines for tubal GI tract cancers as of early 2021 are summarized in Table 23.2 and discussed later.

Testing for DNA mismatch repair status as well as *KRAS*, *NRAS*, and *BRAF* mutations can be performed on either the primary tumor or a metastasis, as these mutations are typically early events in GI cancers. These mutations would be expected to be clonal within colorectal cancers because they typically occur as an early event during the development of an adenoma or sessile serrated lesion and are therefore present in all subsequent generations of evolving malignant and metastatic clones.

DNA Mismatch Repair Status in Gastrointestinal Carcinomas

Evaluation of the DNA mismatch repair protein complex is now recommended for all GI tract adenocarcinomas and has two major clinical utilities: (1) to screen for Lynch syndrome in colorectal cancer and (2) to identify all locally advanced or metastatic tumors with deficient mismatch repair (dMMR)/MSI because prognosis and treatment algorithms differ for these tumors. MSI occurs in approximately 15% of colorectal adenocarcinomas, 20% of

TABLE 23.2 NCCN Biomarker Testing Guidelines for Locally Advanced, Unresectable, or Metastatic Gastrointestinal Tract Carcinomas

	Biomarker Testing					
Cancer Type	**MMR or MSI**	***HER2* Overexpression**	***KRAS, NRAS* Mutation**	***BRAF* Mutation**	***PD-L1* Expression**	**TMB**
Esophageal squamous cell carcinoma					X	X
GEJ adenocarcinoma	X	X			X	X
Gastric adenocarcinoma	X	X			X	X
Small-bowel adenocarcinoma	X	X			X	
Colorectal adenocarcinoma	X	Only if Ras and Raf wild type	X	X		
Clinical utility	Predicts response to immune checkpoint inhibition; good prognosis	Predicts response to anti-HER2 therapy	Predicts resistance to anti-EGFR therapy	No benefit from anti-EGFR therapy unless combined with a BRAF inhibitor; BRAF-positive, microsatellite stable cancers have poor prognosis	Predicts response to immune checkpoint inhibition	High TMB predicts response to immune checkpoint inhibition

GEJ, Gastroesophageal junction; *HER2*, human epidermal growth factor receptor 2; *MMR*, mismatch repair; *MSI*, microsatellite instability; *PD-L1*, programed death ligand 1; *TMB*, tumor mutation burden.

small-intestinal adenocarcinomas, and 20% of gastric adenocarcinomas and is seen at lower frequencies in esophageal/gastroesophageal junction (GEJ) adenocarcinomas (see Fig. 23.1). DNA mismatch repair deficiency is associated with a dramatic decrease in the fidelity of postreplicative DNA repair, particularly at microsatellites, which are short, repetitive DNA sequences scattered throughout the genome in both coding and noncoding regions. Thus tumors with DNA mismatch repair deficiency exhibit a high mutation burden with widespread mutations at microsatellites, labeled as MSI. Because high mutation burden increases the likelihood for expression of neoantigens, dMMR tumors have increased immunogenicity and typically demonstrate many tumor infiltrating lymphocytes. Indeed, dMMR tumors are exquisitely sensitive to checkpoint inhibitor therapy,[48-50] leading to FDA approval of pembrolizumab in 2017 for all unresectable or metastatic tumors with dMMR/MSI. Thus screening for mismatch repair deficiency is the standard of care for all locally advanced unresectable or metastatic GI adenocarcinomas. Mismatch repair status may be assayed by immunohistochemistry or MSI testing, which both have approximately 90% to 95% sensitivity, though immunohistochemistry offers several advantages.

Mismatch Repair Immunohistochemistry

The DNA mismatch repair protein complex is composed of four mismatch repair proteins (MLH1, PMS2, MSH2, and MSH6) and is expressed in all proliferating cells, including normal crypt base epithelium and most cancers. The majority of inactivating mismatch repair gene defects result in total loss of mismatch repair protein expression, which is readily identifiable by immunohistochemistry.[51] Immunohistochemistry for mismatch repair proteins is commonly used as the initial screening test because it offers several advantages. It is rapid and inexpensive, does not require tissue microdissection or DNA extraction, can be readily preformed on any tissue sample including small biopsies with low-tumor content, and can be used to guide subsequent genetic testing to identify Lynch syndrome in the case of an abnormality (see Universal Screening for Lynch Syndrome). The interpretation of mismatch repair protein immunohistochemistry is discussed in more detail in Chapter 27.

Microsatellite Instability Testing

MSI was first described in a subset of predominantly right-sided colorectal cancers in 1993.[52-55] Multiplex PCR tests that amplify a panel of DNA microsatellites (in both tumor and normal DNA from the same patient for comparison) were developed and validated several years later.[56] Later panels demonstrated that the use of relatively monomorphic mononucleotide repeats allows MSI testing to be performed on tumor DNA samples without accompanying normal DNA.[57] After PCR amplification of the microsatellites, the amplified products are typically resolved using capillary gel electrophoresis that can resolve 1- and 2-bp shifts in microsatellite sizes (see Fig. 27.52). A positive MSI test result has extremely high specificity for an underlying DNA mismatch repair deficiency, but does not inform as to which of the four DNA mismatch repair proteins is defective. MSI can also be readily identified as part of a multigene NGS assay.

Colorectal Cancer: Biomarker Testing for Anti-EGFR Therapy

In addition to universal dMMR/MSI testing of all newly diagnosed colorectal cancers, several authorities including American Society for Clinic al Oncology (ASCO), American Society for Clinical Pathology (ASCP), College of American Pathologists (CAP), and Association for Molecular Pathology (AMP), and the NCCN[58,59] also recommend extended RAS testing for all advanced or metastatic colorectal cancers to guide anti-EGFR therapy. The epidermal growth factor receptor gene *EGFR* (also known as *HER1* or *ERBB1*) encodes a transmembrane glycoprotein with intrinsic protein tyrosine kinase activity. EGFR is expressed constitutively throughout the body, including in many epithelial tissues, and it is a key activator of the RAS-RAF-MAPK signaling pathway (see Fig. 23.2).[60] EGFR is upregulated in a wide variety of cancers, is overexpressed in 60% to 80% of colorectal cancers, and has been associated with an increased risk of metastasis and poor survival.[61,62] Whereas activating *EGFR* mutations are common in some cancers like lung cancer and *EGFR* amplification is common in others like brain cancer, epigenetic upregulation appears to be the predominant mechanism of activation in colorectal cancer.[63] *EGFR* amplification occurs in only approximately 15% of colorectal cancers,[64] and point mutations in *EGFR* have rarely been described.[65]

Effective inhibition of EGFR is one of the major breakthroughs of personalized medicine in the past 15 years. Small molecule inhibitors (i.e., erlotinib and gefitinib) are highly effective in some cancers, including lung cancer, which have activating mutations in exons 18 to 21 of the *EGFR* gene, but they have not been effective in colorectal cancer, likely because of the absence of activating point mutations. However, anti-EGFR monoclonal antibodies (i.e., cetuximab and panitumumab) have been very effective in colorectal cancer and have come into routine use in patients with advanced disease.[58]

Monoclonal anti-EGFR antibodies bind to the extracellular domain and impede ligand binding, which inhibits downstream EGFR signaling through the RAS-RAF-MAPK pathway and thus prevents tumor cell growth, angiogenesis, invasion, and metastasis, and also induces apoptosis.[63] Although several potential predictors of resistance to anti-EGFR therapy have been suggested, only *KRAS*, *NRAS*, and *BRAF* mutations are strongly supported by all lines of evidence for use in patient stratification. Patients with activating mutations in exons 2, 3, or 4 of the *KRAS* or *NRAS* genes should not be treated with the anti-EGFR inhibitors cetuximab or panitumumab.[66-79] A *BRAF* p.V600E mutation makes response to cetuximab and panitumumab very unlikely unless given with a BRAF inhibitor.[66-71,75,78-81]

KRAS and *NRAS* Mutation

Hotspot mutations in *KRAS* or *NRAS* result in oncogenic constitutive activation of the RAS-RAF-MEK-MAPK signaling pathway (see Fig. 23.2). *KRAS* is one of the most frequently mutated oncogenes in human cancer, and mutations occur in 40% to 50% of colorectal cancers.[40,82] *NRAS* mutations occur in approximately 3% to 10% of colorectal cancers and are mutually exclusive with *KRAS* mutations.[40,82] Because KRAS and NRAS sit downstream of EGFR, activation of KRAS or NRAS can bypass the inhibitory effect of anti-EGFR therapy. Indeed, numerous studies have now demonstrated resistance to the anti-EGFR inhibitors cetuximab and panitumumab in patients whose colorectal cancers harbor activating *KRAS* or *NRAS* mutations in exon 2 (codons 12 and 13), 3 (codon 61), and 4 (codon 146) of either gene.[66-77,79] Thus *KRAS* and *NRAS* exon 2, 3, and 4 mutation testing is a requirement of standardized chemotherapeutic protocols before cetuximab or panitumumab therapy is considered.[58] The requirement for testing all six exons makes multigene NGS sequencing a more attractive and increasingly more common approach for testing than PCR or Sanger sequencing.

Of note, two early retrospective studies suggested that cetuximab therapy may have some efficacy in patients whose colorectal cancers harbored the *KRAS* p.G13D mutation.[76,83] However, later studies demonstrated that tumors with a *KRAS* p.G13D mutation were no more likely to respond to EGFR inhibitors than tumors with other *KRAS* mutations.[84-87] Thus all hotspot *KRAS* and *NRAS* mutations are a contraindication to treatment with cetuximab or panitumumab.

BRAF Mutation

BRAF is a key member of the RAS-RAF-MEK-MAPK signaling pathway (see Fig. 23.2) and is mutated in approximately 5% to 10% of colorectal cancers.[40,82] A *BRAF* mutation is seen in approximately 50% of dMMR/MSI colorectal cancers and only 3% to 9% of microsatellite-stable (MSS) colorectal cancer, with the higher frequencies in metastatic MSS cancers, as a *BRAF* mutation in MSS cancers confers a poor prognosis.[40,88,89] BRAF lies downstream of KRAS in the EGFR signaling pathway, and like KRAS, mutations that constitutively activate BRAF can bypass the therapeutic effect of anti-EGFR therapy. Several studies suggested that patients with *BRAF*-mutated metastatic colorectal cancers may receive some benefit from anti-EGFR therapy[79,88] and that BRAF was not predicative of response to anti-EGFR therapy.[70] However, numerous other studies, including two large meta-analyses, demonstrated no added benefit or even a detrimental effect of anti-EGFR therapies in *BRAF*-mutated tumors.[80,81,90-95] However, later studies using combination therapies that include a BRAF inhibitor with an EGFR inhibitor, either with or without a MEK inhibitor, have demonstrated promising overall response rates, leading the NCCN to recommend treatment of metastatic *BRAF*-mutant colorectal cancers with a combination of the BRAF inhibitor encorafenib and an EGFR-inhibitor, although not yet in the first line.[58,96-98] Thus a *BRAF* p.V600E mutation makes response to cetuximab and panitumumab very unlikely unless given with a BRAF inhibitor.

HER2 Amplification

Metastatic colorectal cancers that are wild type for *KRAS*, *NRAS*, and *BRAF* do not all respond to anti-EGFR therapy. An example is *HER2*-amplified colorectal cancers. Although *HER2* amplification is infrequent in colon cancer (~3% overall), the frequency is slightly higher in the *KRAS*, *NRAS*, *BRAF* wild type subset (5% to 14%). *HER2* signaling can bypass the therapeutic effect of anti-EGFR therapy by activating a parallel signaling pathway. The possible role of HER2 amplification in anti-EGFR resistance was first described in the setting of acquired resistance.[99] Other studies have found that *HER2* amplification may predict initial resistance to anti-EGFR therapy.[100,101] Furthermore, other studies have demonstrated promising results using anti-HER2 therapy in HER2-positive colorectal cancer.[102]

Acquired Resistance to Anti-EGFR Therapy

As with many other targeted therapies used in cancer patients, despite a favorable initial response to anti-EGFR therapy, acquired resistance eventually develops.[68,69] Although the discovery of several mechanisms of acquired resistance represents an exciting advance in the development of tailored colorectal cancer therapy, ongoing studies continue to explore therapeutic options. Resistance mechanisms include amplification of HER2, which has been observed in some colorectal cancer patients with acquired resistance to cetuximab therapy.[99] Early studies combining cetuximab and trastuzumab suggested that the combined toxicity of these agents outweighs the benefit,[103] but a later study demonstrated promising results using dual therapy with trastuzumab and lapatinib.[102] Ongoing studies are exploring these therapeutic options.

Acquired *EGFR* mutations have also been observed in some colorectal cancer patients with acquired resistance to cetuximab therapy. These mutations result in a conformational change to the extracellular domain of EGFR that prevents cetuximab binding.[104] This conformational change does not appear to effect panitumumab binding, raising the possibility that these tumors may remain sensitive to panitumumab. Although preliminary evidence indicates that switching to panitumumab may have clinical benefit in this setting, additional clinical studies are required to further characterize this application.[105,106]

HER2 Testing in Gastroesophageal and Gastric Adenocarcinoma

The human epidermal growth factor receptor 2 gene (*ERRB2*, also known as *HER2* or *HER2/NEU*) is a member of the EGFR receptor tyrosine kinase family that activates a downstream signaling cascade, including RAS, RAF, MAPK, PI3K, and mTOR. The *HER2* gene is amplified and the protein overexpressed in several human cancers, most notably breast cancer, and promotes tumorigenesis through important biological effects on cell growth, differentiation, survival, and migration.[107] HER2 activation is a driver mutation in breast cancer, which led to the development of a highly efficacious targeted monoclonal antibody therapy called trastuzumab (Herceptin, Genentech), which binds to the extracellular domain of HER2, thereby blocking HER2 activation and silencing downstream signaling.[108]

HER2 gene amplification or protein overexpression is known to occur in subsets of both gastroesophageal junction (GEJ) and gastric adenocarcinoma. The reported frequency of *HER2* amplification or protein overexpression varies widely in different studies.[109] The recent TCGA publications on esophageal, gastroesophageal, gastric, colorectal, and GI carcinomas[40-43] demonstrate *ERBB2* amplification in approximately 30% of gastroesophageal adenocarcinomas and 20% of gastric adenocarcinomas, with most cases occurring in the chromosomal instability CIN subtype of GEJ and gastric cancer, with fewer cases seen in the EBV and GS subtypes of gastric cancer. About 5% of colorectal adenocarcinomas and 3% of esophageal squamous cell carcinomas also show *ERRB2* amplification.

In 2010, results of the international phase III randomized controlled ToGA (trastuzumab for gastric cancer) trial demonstrated that trastuzumab plus chemotherapy significantly prolonged overall survival compared with chemotherapy alone in patients with HER2-positive advanced gastric and GEJ adenocarcinoma.[110] This study led to FDA approval of trastuzumab with chemotherapy for first-line use in patients with HER2-positive advanced GEJ or gastric cancer in 2010. Thus assessment of *HER2* status is a routine component of management of advanced gastric and gastroesophageal cancers, with many experts recommending initial testing of all newly diagnosed patients as an important component of therapeutic planning.[111]

Several authorities, including CAP, ASCP, ASCO, and NCCN put forth guidelines recommending HER2 testing for all patients with inoperable locally advanced, recurrent, or metastatic adenocarcinoma of the GEJ or stomach for whom HER2-targeted therapy is being considered.[112-114] Furthermore, the guidelines recommend an algorithmic approach that starts with HER2 immunohistochemistry (IHC), followed by HER2 FISH (or ISH) only for cases with an IHC score of 2+ (equivocal), as outlined in Figure 23.3.

Immunohistochemistry for HER2 should be accurate, reproducible, and validated in an accredited laboratory.[112] Scoring HER2 expression by IHC in gastric and GEJ cancer should use the Ruschoff/Hofmann scoring method, which was used in the ToGA trial and many other studies demonstrating excellent correlation between IHC and gene amplification methods.[110-112,115] The degree of lateral or basolateral membranous positivity is scored on a scale from 0 to 3+, as outlined in Table 23.3 and illustrated in Figure 23.4. Cases with positive (3+) or negative (0 or 1+) HER2 IHC results do not require further testing, but those with equivocal (2+) results require *HER2* FISH or ISH.

Dual-color, FDA-approved commercial probe kits for *HER2* FISH typically include a chromosome 17 centromeric probe (CEP17) and a 17q12 *HER2* probe. Results are enumerated by counting at least 20 tumor cell nuclei. A *HER2*:CEP17 ratio of ≥ 2 is considered positive for amplification (Fig. 23.5). For FISH or ISH assays without a centromeric reference probe, an average *HER2* copy number of ≥ 6 signals per cell is considered positive for amplification. FISH results may be scored manually or by using validated automated image analysis systems.

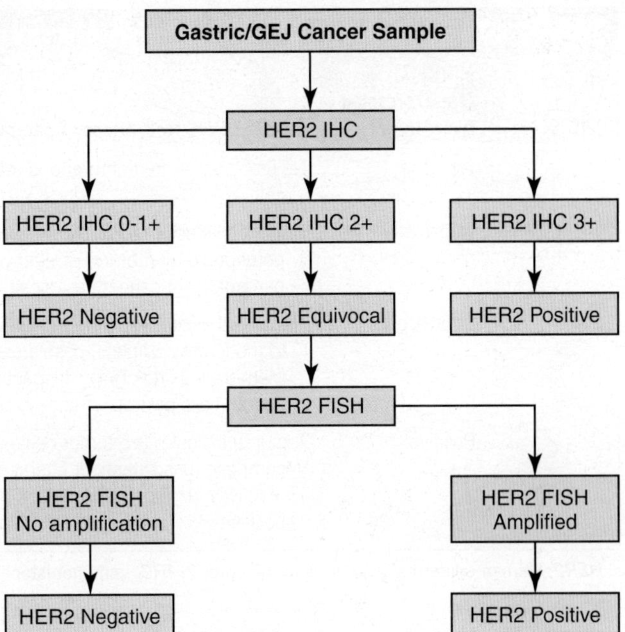

FIGURE 23.3 Algorithm for HER2 testing in gastroesophageal adenocarcinoma. HER2 cases that are scored 2+ by immunohistochemistry (IHC) are considered equivocal and are subjected to fluorescence in situ hybridization (FISH) for further analysis. *GEJ*, Gastroesophageal junction.

Tumor Mutation Burden and PD-L1 for Immune Checkpoint Therapies

In addition to tumors that show dMMR, immune checkpoint therapies have demonstrated robust responses in tumors with high tumor mutation burden (TMB) and with expression of PD-L1. Like dMMR tumors that show hypermutation specifically at microsatellites called MSI, cancers can display other types of hypermutation including hypermutation caused by *POLE* mutation leading to defective exonuclease proofreading activity during DNA replication, or hypermutation caused by UV-related mutagenesis in skin cancer or smoking-related mutagenesis in lung cancer. All hypermutated tumors are thought to have an increased neoantigen load, leading to immune cell infiltration. One mechanism that tumors use to evade the immune system is upregulation of the checkpoint protein programmed death ligand 1 (PD-L1). PD-L1 on tumor cells binds to PD-1 on infiltrating T cells, and this binding prevents the T cells from killing tumor cells. Tumors without hypermutation, like EBV-driven gastric cancer, can also upregulate PD-L1 as an immune evasion mechanism. Numerous ongoing studies continue to evaluate both TMB and PD-L1 expression as predictors of response to immune checkpoint inhibitor therapies in each cancer type, and testing for these is becoming more and more routine. TMB testing requires a multigene NGS assay, and PD-L1 testing is performed by immunohistochemistry and uses specific antibodies and scoring criteria for each cancer type.

GASTROINTESTINAL STROMAL TUMORS

GISTs are the most common sarcoma of the GI tract and one of the most common sarcomas overall. Derived from interstitial cells of Cajal, GISTs share almost universal expression of the tyrosine kinase receptor KIT, which is a common immunohistochemical marker used in the diagnosis of GIST. GISTs are resistant to conventional chemotherapies, so abundant interest was generated when activating *KIT* mutations were first described in GISTs in 1998.[116] This finding raised the possibility that targeting by a TKI could prove to be an effective management strategy and eventually led to the discovery that imatinib mesylate (Gleevec, Novartis) produced dramatic therapeutic responses in these tumors.[117-122] GISTs have subsequently become one of the premier models for personalized therapy in cancer management. Imatinib was approved by the FDA for use in GISTs in 2002, and it has become the first-line therapy for most metastatic or unresectable GISTs. Approximately 80% of patients respond to initial imatinib therapy; however, the development of resistance is common, and progressive disease develops in more than one-half of patients within 2 years. Numerous

TABLE 23.3 Interpretation of HER2 Immunohistochemistry in Gastroesophageal Adenocarcinoma

IHC Score	HER2 Overexpression Assessment	Staining Pattern in Biopsy Specimen	Staining Pattern in Surgical Specimen
0	Negative	No reactivity or no membranous reactivity in any tumor cell	No reactivity or membranous reactivity in <10% of tumor cells
1+	Negative	Tumor cell cluster (≥5 tumor cells) with a faint or barely perceptible membranous reactivity irrespective of percentage of cancer cells positive	Faint or barely perceptible membranous reactivity in ≥10% of cancer cells; cells are reactive only in part of their membrane
2+	Equivocal	Tumor cell cluster (≥5 tumor cells) with a weak to moderate complete, basolateral, or lateral membranous reactivity irrespective of percentage of cancer cells positive	Weak to moderate complete, basolateral, or lateral membranous reactivity in ≥10% of cancer cells
3+	Positive	Tumor cell cluster (≥5 tumor cells) with a strong complete, basolateral, or lateral membranous reactivity irrespective of percentage of cancer cells positive	Strong complete, basolateral, or lateral membranous reactivity in ≥10% of cancer cells

HER2, Human epidermal growth factor receptor 2; *IHC,* immunohistochemistry.

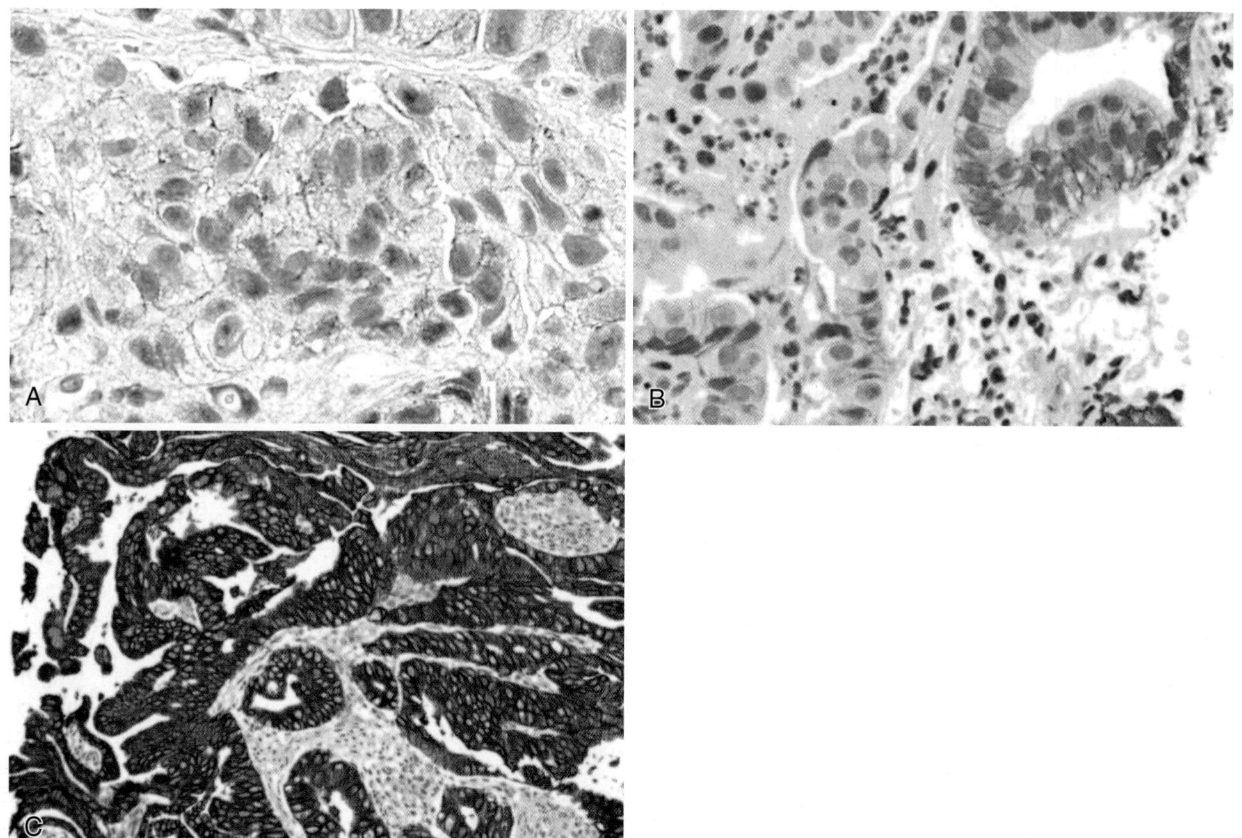

FIGURE 23.4 HER2 immunohistochemical analysis in gastric cancer. A, HER2 case that is scored 1+ has faint, barely perceptible membranous reactivity that requires a 40× objective to visualize. **B,** HER2 case with a 2+ score has moderate, complete basolateral membranous reactivity. **C,** HER2 case with a 3+ score has strong, complete membranous reactivity, which is readily identified with a 10× objective.

studies have tested additional TKIs to treat imatinib-resistant GIST, leading to FDA approval of sunitinib, regorafenib, and repritinib in 2006, 2012, and 2020 for second-, third-, and fourth-line use, respectively. Additionally in 2020, avapritinib was FDA approved for first-line used in a subset of patients with primary resistance to imatinib (Table 23.4).

Landscape of Genetic Alterations in Gastrointestinal Stromal Tumors

Activating mutations in the *KIT* gene are present in 75% to 80% of GISTs, and activating mutations in platelet-derived growth factor receptor-α *(PDGFRA)*, a member of the same type III receptor tyrosine kinase family as KIT,

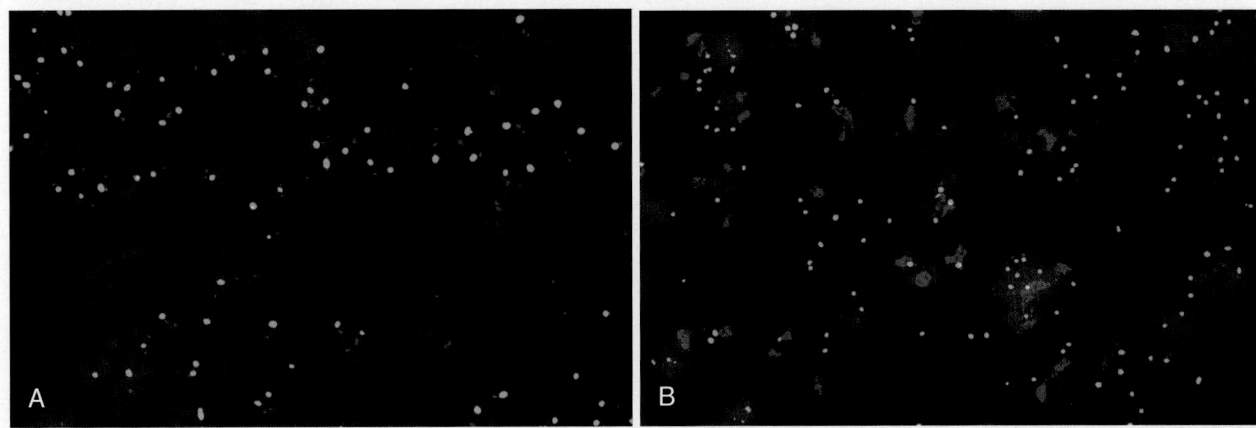

FIGURE 23.5 HER2 fluorescence in situ hybridization analysis in gastric cancer. Gastric cancer samples were hybridized with a chromosome 17 centromeric (17 CEN) probe *(green)* and a locus-specific HER2 probe *(red)*. **A,** Cancer with no *HER2* amplification has a HER2 : 17 CEN probe signal ratio of less than 1.8 to 1. **B,** Cancer with *HER2* amplification has a HER2 : 17 CEN probe signal ratio of 15.4 to 1. Nonneoplastic cells without HER2 amplification can be seen to the right of the field.

are seen in 5% to 10% of GISTs.[123-127] *KIT* and *PDGFRA* mutations result in constitutive activation of the MAPK and PI3K pathways. The majority of *KIT* mutations occur in the juxtamembrane domain encoded by exon 11, and mutations in the extracellular domain encoded by exon 9 are the second most common.[128,129] On the other hand, most *PDGFRA* mutations occur in exon 18, which encodes the tyrosine kinase 2 domain.[130]

Approximately 10% to 15% of GISTs are wild type for *KIT* and *PDGFRA*. Anywhere from 42% to 88% of GISTs lacking mutations in *KIT* and *PDGFRA* have been shown to have deficiency of one of the succinate dehydrogenase complex subunits (SDHA, SDHB, SDHC, and SDHD), either caused by mutation in one of the four *SDH* genes or promoter hypermethylation of *SDHC*.[131-136] Importantly, all GISTs with mutations or promoter methylation of any of the *SDH* genes demonstrate loss of SDHB staining by immunohistochemistry, which can be used to screen for SDH-deficient GISTs.[131] SDH-deficient GISTs resulting from mutation in one of the *SDH* genes are almost always found to be germline (>80%), thus patients with SDH-deficient GISTs should be referred to a genetics clinic. SDH-deficient GISTs characteristically occur in the stomach, show epithelioid morphology, display multinodular architecture, and are usually seen in younger patients, so cases with these characteristics or cases known to be wild type for *KIT* and *PDGFRA* should be evaluated with an SDHB immunostain.

GISTs that are wild type for *KIT* and *PDGFRA* and retain intact SDHB expression by immunohistochemistry have been shown to harbor mutations in *NF1*, *BRAF*, or *RAS*, and rare cases have also been shown to harbor oncogenic fusions involving *BRAF*, *NTRK3*, or *FGFR1*.[136-139] Thus testing for mutations in GIST has evolved from *KIT* mutation testing to multigene panel testing by NGS. The 2020 NCCN guidelines for GIST recommend *KIT* and *PDGFRA* mutation testing for all advanced or high-risk GISTs in which targeted therapy is being considered.[140] GIST that are wild type for *KIT* and *PDGFRA* should be evaluated for loss of SDHB staining and those with intact SDHB should have multigene NGS testing.

Targeted Therapy in Gastrointestinal Stromal Tumors

TKI therapy is the primary therapeutic modality for unresectable or metastatic GISTs and is also used in the adjuvant setting for high-risk GISTs. Imatinib is used in the first-line setting for most GISTs and has shown durable responses in numerous studies.[119,121,122,141,142] Imatinib is an oral, small molecule receptor TKI that works by blocking the adenosine triphosphate (ATP) binding site of the constitutively activated mutant KIT or PDGFRA protein.[143] Binding effectively shuts down signaling.

The type of mutation in *KIT* or *PDGFRA* is the best predictor of response to initial imatinib therapy (summarized in Table 23.5).[143,144] Mutations in *KIT* exon 11, which encodes the intracellular juxtamembrane domain, are the most common *KIT* mutations and are associated with the most favorable response to imatinib. Mutations in *KIT* exon 9, which encodes the extracellular domain, are the second most common, and they are less responsive to imatinib therapy and require higher dosing.[145-147] Mutations in *KIT* exon 13 (encoding the ATP-binding pocket) and KIT exon 17 (encoding the activation loop) are rare and are resistant to imatinib. Approximately 60% of *PDGFRA*-mutant GISTs harbor the D842V mutation in exon 18, which encodes the tyrosine kinase 2 domain and is structurally analogous to *KIT* exon 17. The *PDGFRA* D842V mutation is resistant to imatinib.

Overall, approximately 10% to 15% of patients have primary resistance to imatinib therapy. Most of these patients have imatinib-resistant mutations in exon 9 of KIT or exon 18 of *PDGFRA* or are wild type for *KIT* and *PDGFRA*.[143,144] Furthermore, secondary resistance develops in patients whose tumors are initially sensitive to imatinib, typically at a median of 18 to 24 months. Secondary mutations are a common mechanism of secondary resistance, and these mutations are most common in exons 13, 14, or 17 of *KIT* or exon 18 of *PDGFRA*.[143,144,148,149] Because secondary mutations are a common mechanism of resistance to imatinib, switching to a different TKI with activity against the secondary mutation is a common strategy for management of imatinib-resistant disease.

TABLE 23.4 Mutations in Gastrointestinal Stromal Tumors and Sensitivity to Tyrosine Kinase Inhibitor Therapy

							FDA-Approved Tyrosine Kinase Inhibitors for GIST (year of approval)				
Gene	Protein Domain	Exon	Common Amino Acid Changes	Primary Mutation Frequency	Clinicopathological Correlates	Secondary Mutation Frequency	Imatinib (2002), First-Line	Sunitinib (2006), Second-Line	Regorafenib (2012), Third-Line	Repritinib (2020), Fourth-Line	Avapritinib (2020), First-Line for D842V
KIT	Extracellular domain	9	A502_ Y503Dup	10%-20%	80% occur in the small intestine	0%	+*	+	+		
	Juxtamembrane domain	11	Inframe indels involving W557_K558	60%-70%		0%	+	+	+		
	Tyrosine kinase domain 1 (ATP binding pocket)	13	K642E, V654A	1%-3%		50%-60%	–	+	–	+	
		14	T670I				–	+	+	+	
	Tyrosine kinase domain 2 (activation loop)	17	D816V	1%		40%-50%	–	–	–	–	
			Non-D816V (e.g., D820, N822)				–	–	+	+	
		18	A829				–	–	+	+	
PDGFRA	Juxtamembrane domain	12	V561D	1%	Most occur in the stomach, decreased c-Kit expression by IHC, often epithelioid morphology		+	+	+	+	+
	Tyrosine kinase domain 1 (ATP binding pocket)	14	N659K	<0.5%			+				
	Tyrosine kinase domain 2 (activation loop)	18	D842V	5%-6%		10%-15%	–	–	–	–	+
			Non-D842V	2%-3%			+	+	+	+	+
SDHA, SDHB, SDHC, SDHD	Any	Any	No hotspots	4%-6%	Younger patients, most occur in the stomach, multinodular architecture, epithelioid morphology, metastases common but indolent course, all can be detected by loss of SDHB staining		–		+		
SDHC promoter hypermethylation	No mutations			2%-3%							

Drug sensitivity is indicated with a + symbol, and resistance with a – symbol.
*Exon 9 KIT mutations are sensitive to higher doses of imatinib.

TABLE 23.5 Molecular Genetic Diagnosis of Polyposis and Other Hereditary GI Cancer Syndromes

Entity	Gene	Proportion of Cases Attributable to Gene
Polyposis Syndromes		
Familial adenomatous polyposis (FAP)	*APC*	>95%
Attenuated adenomatous polyposis (AFAP)	*APC*	20%-30%*
	MUTYH (MYH)†	20%-50%
Gastric adenocarcinoma and proximal polyposis of the stomach (GAPPS)	APC promoter region (exon 1B)	>95%
Peutz-Jeghers syndrome (PJS)	*STK11 (LKB1)*	Familial 100%; simplex 90%
Juvenile polyposis syndrome (JPS)	*SMAD4*	20%
	BMPR1A	20%
Cowden syndrome (PTEN hamartoma tumor syndrome)	*PTEN*‡	85%
Bannayan-Riley-Ruvalcaba syndrome (BRRS)	*PTEN*‡	65%
Proteus or proteus-like syndrome	*PTEN*‡	20%-50%
Hereditary mixed polyposis syndrome	*SCG5, GREM1*	
Serrated polyposis syndrome	Unknown	
Hereditary Nonpolyposis Colorectal Cancer (HNPCC)		
Lynch syndrome	*MLH1*	50%
	MSH2	40%
	MSH6	7%-10%
	PMS2	5%
	EPCAM (TACSTD1)§	1%-3%
Familial colorectal cancer type X	Unknown	
Lynch-like syndrome	Unknown	
Others		
Hereditary diffuse gastric cancer	*CDH1*	30%-50%
Syndromic GIST (can occur in Carney-Stratakis syndrome or Neurofibromatosis type 1)	*SDHA, SDHB, SDHC, SDHD*	>95%
	NF1	
	KIT	
	PDGFRA	
Familial Barrett's esophagus	Unknown	

*The proportion of cases with *APC* mutations increases with increasing numbers of adenomas.
†AFAP caused by *MUTYH* mutations is also known as *MUTYH-associated polyposis* (MAP). Some *MUTYH* mutation carriers have more than 100 polyps at presentation, and these cases are differentiated from FAP by the absence of an autosomal dominant family history and patient age older than 35 years.
‡The term *PTEN hamartoma tumor syndrome* (PHTS) is used to describe cases with *PTEN* mutations.
§Hereditary *EPCAM* mutations cause Lynch syndrome by inducing MSH2 methylation and gene silencing in colonic epithelial cells.

Sunitinib is an oral multikinase inhibitor that is active against KIT, PDGFRA, and other receptor tyrosine kinases. Like imatinib, sunitinib binds the ATP-binding pocket, but has a smaller molecular profile than imatinib, allowing greater activity against exon 13 and 14 *KIT* mutations and a broader range of exon 9 *KIT* mutations and wild type *KIT*. After demonstration of effectiveness in clinical trials,[150] sunitinib was approved by the FDA in 2006 for use in patients with an advanced GIST that is resistant to imatinib therapy and for those who cannot tolerate imatinib. Overall, approximately 50% of patients with imatinib-resistant disease can benefit from sunitinib therapy, although the median progression-free survival is only 6 months.[143] Exon 17 *KIT* mutations and exon 18 *PDGFRA* mutations remain resistant to sunitinib.

Regorafenib, a TKI with broad activity against KIT, PDGFRA, and VEGFR, was shown to be effective in advanced GISTs that failed treatment with imatinib or sunitinib[151] and was FDA approved for third-line therapy in 2012. Newer compounds including repritinib and avapritinib are TKIs that have more potent activity against mutations in the activation loop and have demonstrated success in recent clinical trials, leading to FDA approval of both compounds in 2020, with repritinib approved as a fourth-line therapy and avapritinib approved as a first-line therapy in patients with the *PDGFRA* D842V mutation.[152,153] Many other receptor tyrosine kinase agents continue to be evaluated in a variety of clinical trials.[143,144] Targeting of downstream signaling has also been considered, including mTOR inhibitors, PI3K inhibitors, and MEK inhibitors, and immunotherapies are also being trialed.

Tumor heterogeneity, with different mutations identified in different lesions or within a single metastasis, is also seen. Surgical resection or ablation is recommended in patients who are initially responsive but in whom limited progression occurs. By removing the imatinib-resistant clone, therapy may be continued in otherwise responsive disease.

Finally, monitoring for the emergence of resistant mutations plays an important role in therapeutic monitoring and decision making regarding second-, third-, and fourth-line therapies. Unfortunately, the location and multiplicity of resistant disease makes biopsy sampling impractical, especially knowing that different metastases may have different resistant mutations. Emerging technologies that can detect mutations in cell-free fluid samples such as serum and plasma offer significant gains in clinical utility in this setting as mutations from any of multiple metastases could all be detected in a single liquid biopsy.

MOLECULAR DIAGNOSTICS OF HEREDITARY GASTROINTESTINAL CANCER

Molecular diagnostics were applied to hereditary GI cancer syndromes, with germline testing for familial adenomatous polyposis and Lynch syndrome beginning in the early and mid-1990s, respectively.[82] In the past 20 years, hereditary cancer testing has expanded to include all of the polyposis syndromes, familial gastric cancer, and syndromic GISTs (see Table 23.3).

With the exception of Lynch syndrome and syndromic SDH-deficient GISTs, hereditary GI cancer molecular testing does not involve anatomical pathology specimens. Germline testing for hereditary cancer mutations is performed on genomic DNA extracted from white cells obtained from peripheral blood. Single-gene mutational testing is typically performed by Sanger sequencing; however, with the advent of NGS, most germline mutation testing is now being combined into panels of genes, allowing significant reductions in cost and turnaround time.[21,22] In addition to the sequence variants identified by sequencing, some inherited defects in the hereditary cancer genes consist of much larger genomic deletions or duplications that are not routinely detected by sequencing. They are particularly common in familial adenomatous polyposis, accounting for approximately 10% of cases or families.[154] If sequencing fails to identify a pathogenic variant, comprehensive adenomatous polyposis coli *(APC)* gene testing programs include assays to detect larger aberrations, including Southern blot, quantitative PCR, and CGH arrays.

Surgical pathologists should be aware that testing is available for most of the hereditary GI cancer syndromes. Because pathologists may be the first clinicians to recognize that a patient is affected by one of these syndromes, they can play a key role in suggesting referral to a genetics counselor for assessment and testing. Here, we discuss Lynch syndrome in more detail because surgical pathologists play a key role in universal screening of all colorectal cancers for Lynch syndrome.

Universal Screening for Lynch Syndrome

Individuals with Lynch syndrome have a hereditary predisposition for colorectal cancer, endometrial cancer, and other GI tract cancers. Lynch syndrome is caused by germline mutations in one of the DNA mismatch repair genes (*MLH1*, *MSH2*, *MSH6*, or *PMS2*) or the *EPCAM* gene, which induces methylation silencing of *MSH2*. Lynch syndrome causes approximately 2% to 4% of all colorectal cancers.[51,155] Originally described as Lynch syndrome I (site-specific colorectal cancer), Lynch syndrome II (colorectal and extracolonic cancer), and Muir-Torre syndrome (skin tumors and visceral malignancies), it is now understood that all three syndromes share the same basic underlying molecular pathogenesis. The genetic basis for differences in the tumor spectrum between individuals and families most likely reflects genotype-phenotype relationships of different mutations or the effects of other modifier genes or environmental influences that are not yet fully understood.

Many Lynch syndrome patients have family histories with strong autosomal dominant patterns and, therefore, meet Amsterdam I or II family history criteria for hereditary nonpolyposis colorectal cancer (HNPCC). The HNPCC criteria describe a family history of colorectal cancer predisposition, therefore not all HNPCC patients have Lynch syndrome.[51] As many as 50% of HNPCCs (e.g., familial colorectal cancer type X) may be caused by unknown genes. Additional clinical, pathological, and pathogenetic aspects of Lynch syndrome are discussed in Chapter 27.

Despite the identification of germline mismatch repair gene mutations as the cause of Lynch syndrome more than 20 years ago, identification and genetic testing of possible Lynch syndrome patients has been slow to catch on in clinical practice.[51] Although some of this disparity was related to failure of the clinical community to rigorously screen all newly diagnosed colorectal cancer patients for a family history of cancer, many Lynch syndrome patients do not meet the traditional family history criteria. Approximately 40% of Lynch syndrome patients do not meet Amsterdam I or II criteria, including approximately 25% who do not meet the much less stringent Bethesda criteria.[156]

Because effective screening tests are readily available, and the morbidity and mortality associated with Lynch syndrome are greatly reduced with intensive colonoscopic screening, several authorities, including the Evaluation of Genomic Applications in Practice and Prevention (EGAPP), United States Multi-Society Task Force on Colorectal Cancer, ASCP, CAP, AMP, ASCO, American Gastroenterological Association, and the NCCN all recommend universal screening of newly diagnosed colorectal cancer cases by using either MSI PCR testing or mismatch repair immunohi stochemistry.[58,59,157-162] Both tests have approximately 90% to 95% sensitivity for detection of a mismatch repair defect; in the setting of a strong family history, a second test is recommended if the initial screening test result is negative.

Many centers use immunohistochemistry as the initial screening test because it offers the important advantage of determining which of the four mismatch repair proteins is deficient. Approximately 15% of all colorectal cancers will show deficient mismatch repair, but only 15% to 20% of those are caused by Lynch syndrome, while the remaining cases are caused by somatic promoter hypermethylation of *MLH1*. Thus any case with intact MLH1 by IHC (loss of MSH2 and MSH6 or isolated loss of MSH6 or PMS2) represents a case that most likely represents Lynch syndrome and should be referred to a genetics clinic for follow-up germline genetic testing. Cases that show loss of MLH1 (which is accompanied by loss of PMS2), on the other hand, need further workup to differentiate between sporadic versus hereditary cases.

Characterization of MLH1-Deficient Colorectal Cancers

Most MLH1-deficient colorectal cancers are caused by promoter hypermethylation of *MLH1*, which occurs in approximately 12% to 15% of colorectal cancers. However, loss of *MLH1* can also occur if the patient has Lynch syndrome with a germline mutation in the *MLH1* gene and the tumor loses the second copy of *MLH1*. To discriminate between these possibilities, additional testing for either *BRAF* or *MLH1* promoter methylation testing can be performed.

Although *BRAF* mutations occur in only 5% to 10% of colorectal cancers, they are enriched in cases with sporadic MLH1 promoter hypermethylation, occurring in approximately 50% of hypermethylated cases (see Figure 23.1, colorectal cancer). Furthermore, *BRAF* mutations are almost never identified in Lynch syndrome–associated colorectal cancers. Thus identification of a *BRAF* mutation in an MLH1-deficient colorectal cancer excludes the need for further evaluation for Lynch syndrome.[163] In colorectal cancer, *BRAF* mutations usually are limited to the V600E variant, which is readily evaluated in paraffin-embedded tissue by sequencing or *BRAF* V600E mutation–specific immunohistochemistry. If the MLH1-deficient colorectal cancer is also wild type for *BRAF*, the case has a 50/50 chance of being hereditary, and either referral to genetics for germline testing or *MLH1* promoter methylation testing can be performed if available.

If available, testing for *MLH1* promoter methylation is a more direct approach to definitively determine whether the MLH1 loss is caused by promoter methylation or by Lynch syndrome. In fact, *BRAF* testing is not necessary if *MLH1* promoter methylation testing is readily available. *MLH1* methylation analysis is usually performed by methylation-specific PCR or sequencing; both are performed after bisulfite treatment of template DNA.

Germline Testing for Lynch syndrome

Putative Lynch syndrome patients should be sent for genetic evaluation and counseling before germline testing, which is usually only undertaken in patients whose tumors are shown to have deficient MMR or MSI. Furthermore, this group of patients can be narrowed down to those with MLH1-deficient tumors that are *BRAF* wild type or show unmethylated *MLH1* promoter, as well as those with loss of MSH2 and/or MSH6, or isolated loss of PMS2. Rarely, tumors from Lynch syndrome patients have no detectable abnormalities by MSI testing and mismatch repair immunohistochemistry and some with normal screening results but a strong family history may still be referred for germline testing. Germline testing is performed by sequencing of genomic DNA obtained from white blood cells from peripheral blood. In addition to germline sequence variants and genomic deletions, rare families have heritable methylation silencing of MLH1 and MSH2 expression.[163,164]

The full reference list may be accessed online at *Elsevier eBooks for Practicing Clinicians.*

CHAPTER 24

Epithelial Neoplasms of the Esophagus

Jonathan N. Glickman, Robert D. Odze

Chapter Outline

INTRODUCTION

Most benign and malignant neoplasms of the esophagus are epithelial in origin (Box 24.1). Overall, an estimated 17,650 new diagnoses of esophageal carcinoma, and 16,000 deaths, occurred in the United States in 2019.[1] The incidence of esophageal carcinoma has increased in the United States and Europe in the past 30 years, principally because of a marked rise in Barrett's esophagus (BE)–associated adenocarcinoma.[2]

BENIGN NEOPLASMS AND TUMOR-LIKE LESIONS

Squamous Papilloma

Clinical Features

Esophageal squamous papilloma is the most common benign type of epithelial tumor of the esophagus.[3,4] The prevalence rate is estimated to be 0.1% to 0.5%, with some suggesting a recent increase in incidence in some patient populations.[5] These lesions may affect patients of all ages and both sexes. Most are asymptomatic, but large lesions may cause epigastric pain, dysphagia, or symptoms related to luminal obstruction. Key features are summarized in Box 24.2.

Pathogenesis

The pathogenesis of esophageal squamous papilloma is controversial. Many studies have shown an association (10% to 50%) with human papillomavirus (HPV) infection.[3-5] When detected, both low-risk and high-risk subtypes (e.g., types 6/11 and 16, respectively) have been reported. However, the prevalence of HPV is variable among studies, likely resulting from differences in the techniques used to detect viral antigens or DNA and the possibility that as yet unidentified subtypes of HPV may be involved. Others have proposed that at least a subset of these lesions develop as a result of chronic mucosal irritation, perhaps secondary to gastroesophageal reflux disease (GERD).

Pathological Features

Grossly, esophageal squamous papillomas are usually small, discrete, sessile, soft, tan lesions that are most commonly 0.3 to 0.5 cm in size but may be larger. They occur most commonly in the distal or middle esophagus but may develop anywhere in the esophagus (Fig. 24.1). As many as 20% of cases are multiple, and rare cases of diffuse papillomatosis have also been reported.[6,7] Microscopically, three distinct histopathological types have been recognized: exophytic, endophytic, and spiked (verrucoid) (Fig. 24.2).[3] The exophytic type, which is the most common, is composed of finger-like papillary fronds. The endophytic type shows a smooth, round surface contour and an inverted papillomatous proliferation. Least common is the spiked or verrucoid type, which has a spiked surface contour, a prominent granular cell layer, and marked hyperkeratosis.

All types are characterized by the presence of a branched fibrovascular core of lamina propria with a variable degree of acute and chronic inflammation and vascular congestion. The overlying squamous epithelium in all types is

BOX 24.1 Epithelial Tumors of the Esophagus (Including WHO Classification of Digestive System Tumors, 5th ed.)

BENIGN NEOPLASMS

Squamous papilloma
Adenoma (gland/duct)
Barrett's esophagus–associated polypoid dysplasia
Squamous dysplasia

MALIGNANT NEOPLASMS

Squamous cell carcinoma NOS
Squamous cell carcinoma variants
- Basaloid carcinoma
- Spindle cell carcinoma
- Verrucous carcinoma
- Esophageal carcinoma cuniculatum

Adenocarcinoma NOS
- Barrett's esophagus–associated
- Non–Barrett's-associated
  - Heterotopia-associated
  - Esophageal gland duct associated
  - Adenoid cystic carcinoma

Mixed squamous and glandular tumors
- Adenosquamous carcinoma
- Mucoepidermoid carcinoma

Neuroendocrine neoplasms
- Neuroendocrine tumor (grades 1, 2, 3)
- Neuroendocrine carcinoma (grade 3)
  - Large cell neuroendocrine carcinoma
  - Small cell neuroendocrine carcinoma
- Mixed neuroendocrine–nonneuroendocrine carcinoma
  - Mixed adenocarcinoma–neuroendocrine carcinoma
  - Mixed squamous cell carcinoma–neuroendocrine carcinoma

Undifferentiated carcinoma
- Lymphoepithelioma-like carcinoma

Choriocarcinoma
Pleomorphic giant cell carcinoma
Metastases

Adapted from WHO Classification Editorial Board. Tumours of the Esophagus. In Digestive System Tumors. *5th ed. Lyon: IARC Press; 2019, 23-58.*

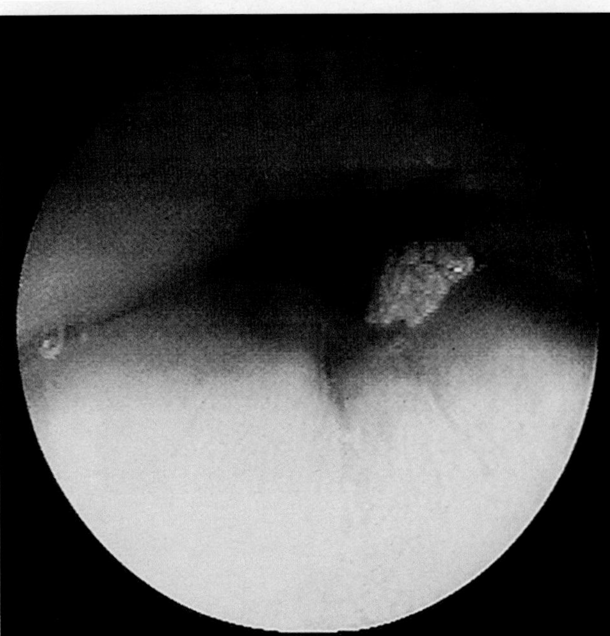

FIGURE 24.1 Endoscopic photograph of an exophytic squamous papilloma of the esophagus showing a well-circumscribed, broad-based nodule with a verrucoid irregular surface.

BOX 24.2 Esophageal Squamous Papilloma: Key Features

Clinical/endoscopic
- M = F, wide age range
- Asymptomatic, usually incidental finding
- Solitary whitish polypoid lesion (up to 5 mm), rarely multiple
- Benign

Histological
- Mature squamous epithelium and fibrovascular cores
- Subtypes: exophytic (most common), spiked/verrucous, endophytic

Special/immunohistochemical stains: none

Molecular
- HPV (low risk or high risk) in 10% to 50% of patients

Differential diagnosis
- Pseudoepitheliomatous hyperplasia (associated with esophagitis)
- Verrucous carcinoma (large plaquelike lesion)

Prognostic factors
- (Rare: Multiple papillomas or papillomatosis may require resection)

acanthotic, often reactive, showing a prominent basal cell zone and complete surface maturation, with occasional parakeratosis or dyskeratosis (see Fig. 24.2E). Up to 50% of lesions show histological features of HPV infection, such as koilocytosis or bi- or multinucleation. Mitoses may be present in the basal and suprabasal epithelial layers, particularly in cases with active inflammation.

Differential Diagnosis

A papilloma that is large, is oriented poorly, or shows marked reactive changes may, on occasion, be difficult to distinguish from a well-differentiated squamous cell carcinoma or a verrucous carcinoma. However, esophageal squamous papillomas lack cytological atypia, mitoses in the middle and upper levels of the squamous epithelium, atypical mitoses, and an infiltrative growth pattern characteristic of carcinoma. Furthermore, their gross (endoscopic) appearance is distinctive. In contrast to carcinoma, papillomas are well localized and well demarcated, smooth, discrete polyps without necrosis, stricture formation, or heaped-up borders. They lack the central keratinous crater characteristic of verrucous carcinoma (Table 24.1).

Papillomas may also be confused with pseudoepitheliomatous hyperplasia occurring adjacent to a healing ulcer or overlying a granular cell tumor. However, the latter type of lesion lacks a fibrovascular core and other features of HPV infection such as koilocytosis. Unlike esophageal squamous papillomas, pseudoepitheliomatous hyperplasia often shows abundant inflammation and surface erosion.

Prognosis

Squamous cell papillomas are benign lesions with little or no malignant potential.[3,8] However, rare cases associated with squamous dysplasia, or even squamous cell carcinoma, have been reported, often in association with extensive esophageal papillomatosis, and may warrant ablation or resection.[7]

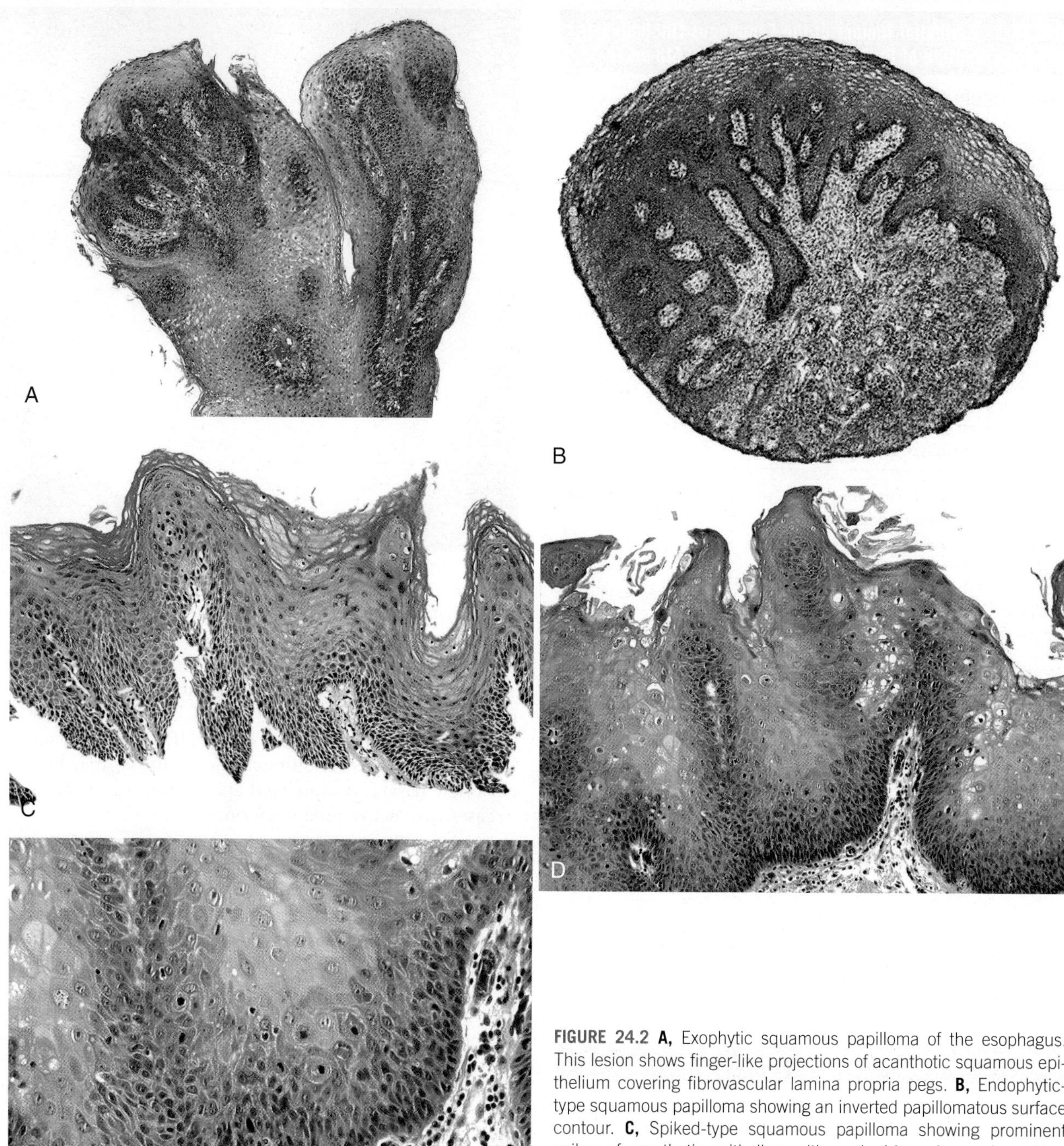

FIGURE 24.2 A, Exophytic squamous papilloma of the esophagus. This lesion shows finger-like projections of acanthotic squamous epithelium covering fibrovascular lamina propria pegs. **B,** Endophytic-type squamous papilloma showing an inverted papillomatous surface contour. **C,** Spiked-type squamous papilloma showing prominent spikes of acanthotic epithelium with marked hyperkeratosis and hypergranulosis. **D,** Medium-power photomicrograph of a case of diffuse papillomatosis. Notice the superficial keratinocytes with koilocytosis. **E,** The deep portion of the same papilloma as in **D** shows basal zone hyperplasia.

Adenoma

Adenomas of the esophagus are defined as benign epithelial proliferations located within the esophagus. True adenomas develop from neoplastic transformation of the submucosal gland or duct system. Polypoid dysplastic lesions arising in BE, which have been referred to in the past as adenomas, are not true adenomas and are better regarded as a neoplastic complication of the underlying metaplastic disorder.

Submucosal Gland or Duct Adenoma

Adenomas that develop from the submucosal glands or gland ducts are rare. They are most often histologically similar to those that arise from the minor salivary glands. This is not surprising because, embryologically, the esophageal submucosal glands are considered a continuation of the minor salivary glands of the oropharynx. They are usually submucosal and develop as well-circumscribed

TABLE 24.1 Esophageal Squamous Papilloma: Differential Diagnosis

Feature	Reactive Hyperplasia	Papilloma	Verrucous Carcinoma
Clinical			
Frequency	Common	Common	Rare
Age	All ages	All ages	50-70
Sex	M = F	M = F	M > F (80%)
Location	Distal > mid	Mid = distal	Mid
Pathological			
Size	Grossly inapparent	<3 cm	>3 cm
Polyp	–	++	–
Ulceration	+	–	+/–
Mucosal inflammation	+	–	–
Stricture	–	–	+/–
Circumferential involvement	–	–	+/–
Growth pattern	Endophytic	Exophytic > endophytic > spiked	Exophytic
Fibrovascular core	–	++	–
Pushing margin	–	–	+
Extension into submucosa	–	–	+
Lymph node metastases	–	–	+/–
Cytological atypia	–	–	+
Koilocytosis	–	+/–	–
Outcome/treatment			
Clinical behavior	Benign	Benign	Aggressive
Therapy	None	None/excision	Surgical resection

+, Consistently present; ++, key feature; –, not present; +/–, sometimes present.

lesions that resemble pleomorphic adenomas,[9] Warthin tumors (Fig. 24.3B), or, more rarely, pancreatic or ovary-like serous cystadenomas.[10]

Other examples exhibit tubal, cystic, and papillary growth patterns similar to intraductal papillomas of the breast or sialadenoma papilliferum of the salivary glands.[11] The epithelium typically contains two cell layers (similar to the normal submucosal gland ducts) with only mild to moderate cytological atypia and infrequent mitoses (see Fig. 24.3A). The immunophenotype of the tumor cells is also similar to that of the normal esophageal gland ducts.[12] A mixed inflammatory infiltrate may be present as well. In all instances, adenomas should be distinguished from non-neoplastic cystic dilatation of esophageal glands or ducts, which can occur secondary to duct obstruction. Most of these tumors behave in a benign fashion,[13] although rare carcinomas have been reported.[14]

Polypoid Dysplasia in Barrett's Esophagus

Polypoid dysplastic lesions resembling adenomas may develop in BE (see Chapter 14). Endoscopically, these lesions usually appear as well-defined sessile or pedunculated polyps that range in size from 0.5 to 1.5 cm and usually occur in the middle or distal esophagus within areas of BE (Fig. 24.4). Histologically, these polyps are composed of a tubular or tubulovillous proliferation of low- or high-grade dysplastic epithelium. Similar to the surrounding flat nonpolypoid BE, the epithelium is most commonly of the intestinal type, but it may also show a gastric (foveolar) phenotype or mixed features of both.[15]

In one study, these lesions showed proliferative and molecular abnormalities (loss of heterozygosity of *APC* and *TP53*) similar to those of flat BE-associated dysplasia.[16] Polypoid or nodular mucosal abnormalities in BE are associated with an increased risk of underlying adenocarcinoma or subsequent progression. In fact, in one study of 10 cases, 9 were associated with adenocarcinoma.[16] Patients with nodular or polypoid dysplastic foci in the BE segment should be treated according to accepted protocols for Barrett's dysplasia, with a preference for endoscopic mucosal resection to adequately stage the lesion and guide further therapy.[17]

Tumor-Like Lesions

Developmental Cysts and Duplications

Congenital cystic lesions and duplications may occur in the esophagus and mimic a malignant tumor because of their mass effect. These lesions, which are discussed more thoroughly in Chapter 8, are categorized into two principal groups: duplications and neurenteric (dorsal enteric) remnants. They may occur anywhere in the esophagus but are most common in the upper third. Clinically, they may be asymptomatic, or they may cause dysphagia or pain secondary to compression of nearby respiratory or alimentary tract structures.

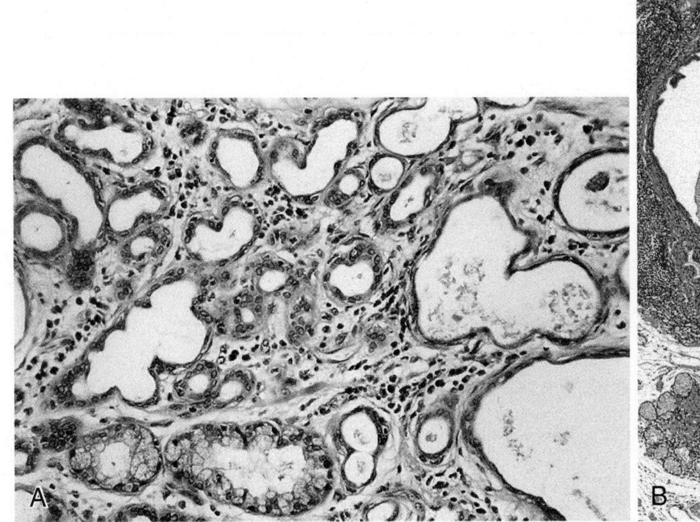

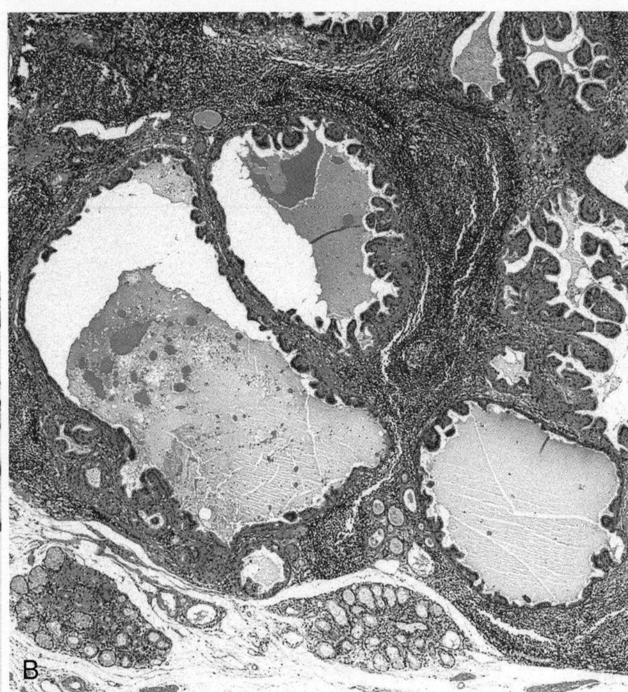

FIGURE 24.3 Benign gland/duct adenoma of the esophagus. A, This lesion is composed of a proliferation of irregular glands lined by flattened, cuboidal to low columnar epithelium focally showing two cell layers. No mitosis or significant atypia is noted. **B,** Another gland- or duct-associated lesion has the morphology of a Warthin tumor, with eosinophilic cuboidal epithelium and a lymphoid stroma. A normal esophageal submucosal gland is visible at the lower left.

Duplications most likely develop as a result of abnormal recanalization of the esophageal lumen during embryogenesis, and often present during childhood but may also be noted in adults.[18,19] They may be extramural or intramural, and may become cystic if there is no communication with the esophageal lumen. They are usually isolated but may also be associated with other congenital foregut lesions such as pulmonary cystic malformations.[20] Histologically, these unilocular cysts may be lined by respiratory, gastric, oxyntic, squamous, or simple cuboidal epithelium, and usually contain all layers of the gastrointestinal (GI) tract (muscularis propria, enteric nerve plexuses) in the cyst wall. A lymphoepithelial cyst, lined by squamous or cuboidal epithelium and surrounded by a dense mononuclear inflammatory infiltrate, has also been reported in the cervical esophagus.[21]

Tracheobronchial duplications (also known as bronchogenic cysts) are a duplication subtype resulting from anomalous budding of bronchial structures derived from the embryonic foregut. They are typically unilocular and located in the mediastinum or in the wall of the esophagus.[22] Microscopically, they are lined by ciliated columnar epithelium and frequently contain cartilage, smooth muscle, and mucous glands in the surrounding cyst-lining tissue (Fig. 24.5).

Neurenteric remnants (also termed *dorsal enteric cysts*) occur primarily in the posterior mediastinum of infants and are thought to arise from incomplete closure of the notochordal remnant.[23] These cysts may be associated with additional congenital defects, including spina bifida and vertebral anomalies. Microscopically, they are lined by gastric, intestinal, squamous, or respiratory epithelium and are usually surrounded by all the normal tissue layers of the bowel wall.

Developmental cysts and duplications are benign. However, they may become infected as a result of rupture, or may produce symptoms due to mass effect.[24] Extremely rarely, adenocarcinoma or squamous cell carcinoma may develop from these lesions.[25,26]

Among acquired cystic lesions, mucoceles are not uncommon. They may develop in excluded segments of esophagus created after surgery for esophageal atresia or perforation.[27] In large or chronic cases, the cystic lining may not be apparent microscopically, revealing only inflammation and fibrous tissue.

Heterotopias

Gastric, thyroid, parathyroid, pancreatic, or even sebaceous tissue may be present as heterotopias in the esophagus. These deposits are presumed to be congenital in origin, although, as discussed later, some possible relationships with clinical conditions such as GERD and BE have been proposed.

Gastric heterotopia ("inlet patch") is by far the most common type, being present in an estimated 2% to 14% of the general population.[28-30] These lesions are usually located in the upper third of the esophagus. Although they are often asymptomatic, they may give rise to symptoms that result from complications of acid secretion, such as heartburn, dysphagia, active esophagitis, ulceration, bleeding, stricture, and perforation. Patients with *Helicobacter pylori* gastritis frequently show concurrent colonization of the heterotopic mucosa.[31] Although heterotopias are often identified endoscopically, the diagnosis is confirmed by finding gastric glandular (usually oxyntic type) and surface epithelium in the esophagus in patients without intervening BE (Fig. 24.6A). Some investigators have found

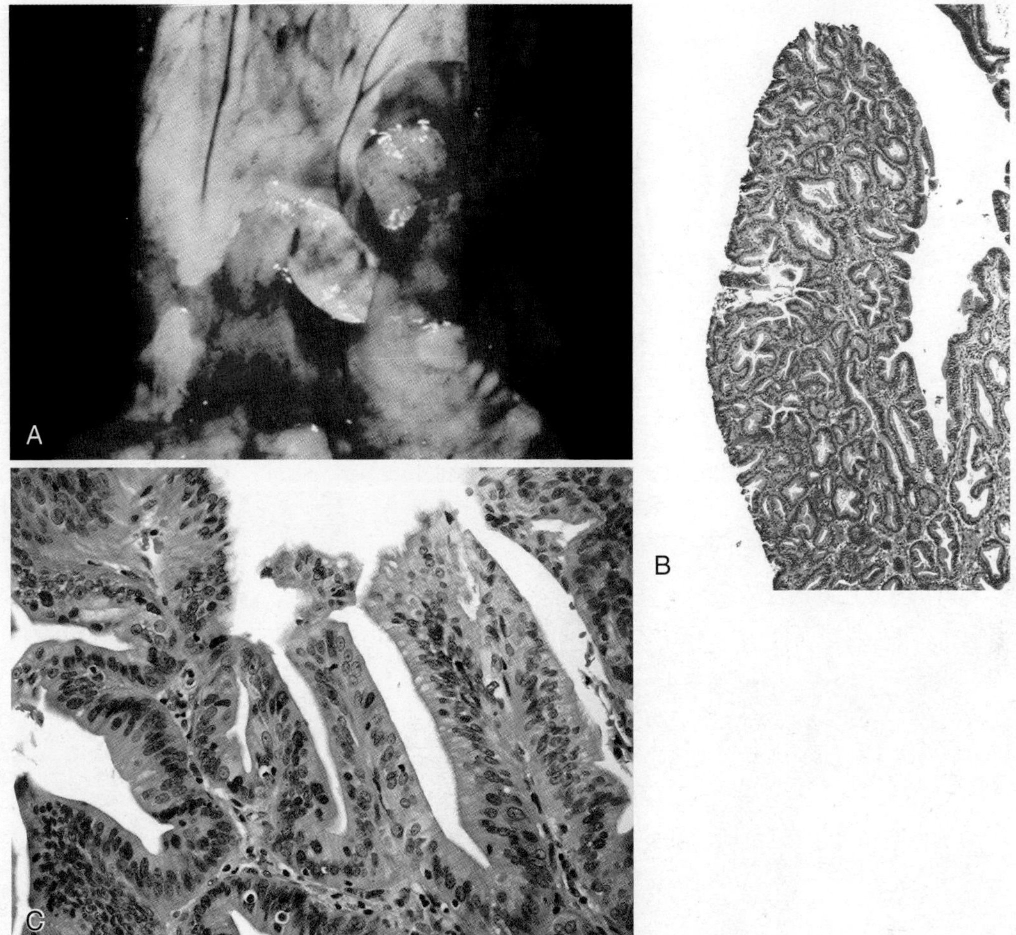

FIGURE 24.4 Polypoid dysplasia in Barrett's esophagus. A, Gross image of two well-circumscribed pedunculated polyps situated just above the gastroesophageal junction and arising on a background of Barrett's mucosa. The squamous mucosa of the normal esophagus is seen just above the polyps. **B,** Low-power photomicrograph of the circumscribed polypoid area of dysplasia in another example. Notice that the polyp is formed of tightly packed, convoluted, dysplastic glands and is arising from columnar mucosa with intestinal metaplasia. **C,** The polyp is composed of high-grade dysplastic columnar epithelium.

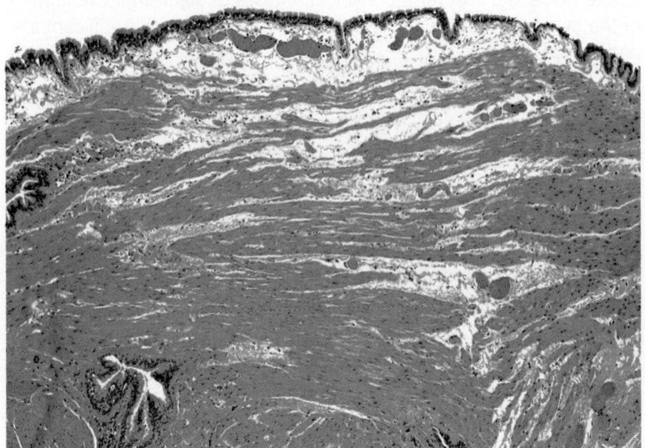

FIGURE 24.5 Bronchogenic cyst. The epithelial lining consists of ciliated columnar epithelium overlying a wall of fibromuscular tissue.

a positive correlation with the presence of BE, although the basis for this association, if any, is unknown.[28,29] No therapy is required in most patients, although large inlet patches, or those causing symptoms, may be ablated. Rarely, adenocarcinoma may develop in gastric heterotopia (see Fig. 24.6B),[32,33] and an intraductal papillary mucinous neoplasm arising from a pancreatic heterotopia has been reported.[34]

Heterotopic sebaceous glands are the second most common form of heterotopia in the esophagus. They may occur at any level of the esophagus, are frequently multiple, and usually appear as slightly elevated, yellowish lesions, 1 to 2 mm in diameter.[35] Microscopically, these lesions show sebaceous cells within the epithelium or in the lamina propria (Fig. 24.7). Sebaceous cells are microvesicular and contain vacuolated cytoplasm filled with lipid substances. An excretory duct, with or without a connection to the surface epithelium, may be present as well. Although it has been suggested that sebaceous glands may represent a metaplastic process in the setting of GERD, no clear relationship to symptoms or other pathological findings has been established in large population-based studies of asymptomatic individuals.[36]

Pseudoepitheliomatous Hyperplasia

Pseudoepitheliomatous hyperplasia is a morphological pattern of reactive squamous epithelium that most commonly occurs adjacent to healing ulcers. It is characterized by

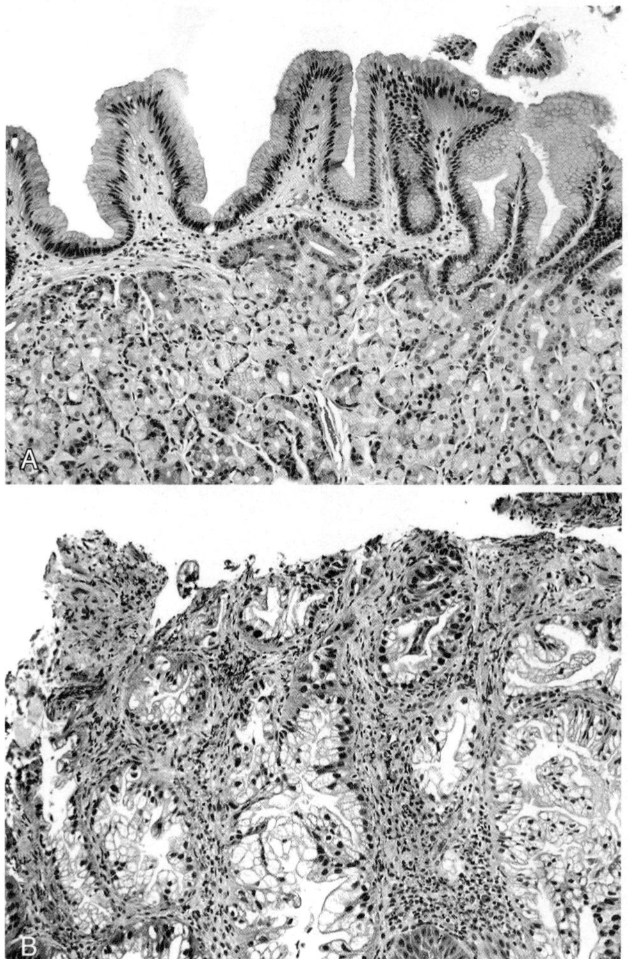

FIGURE 24.6 Gastric heterotopia. **A,** Gastric surface epithelium and oxyntic glands from a heterotopia in the upper esophagus. **B,** Poorly differentiated adenocarcinoma *(bottom)* is arising in a focus of gastric heterotopia.

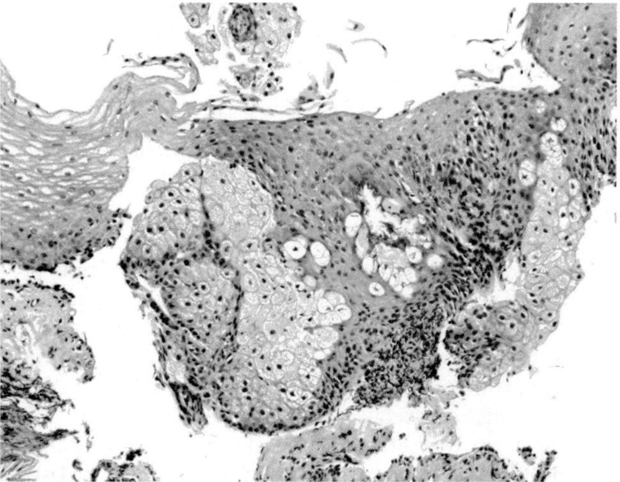

FIGURE 24.7 Sebaceous heterotopia of the esophagus. Associated with the squamous epithelium is a proliferation of vacuolated sebaceous cells mixed with keratin debris.

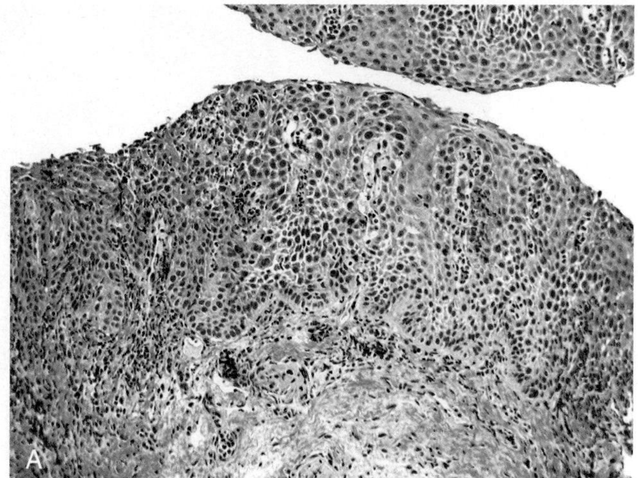

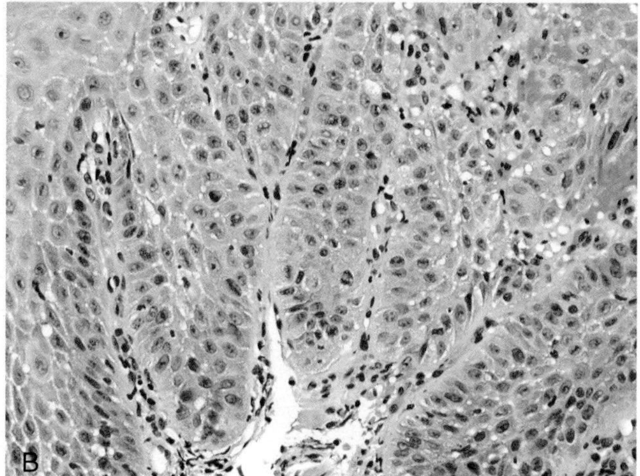

FIGURE 24.8 Pseudoepitheliomatous hyperplasia of the esophagus. **A,** This marked reactive change is characterized by a proliferation of irregular pegs of squamous epithelium that extend into the underlying lamina propria with a moderate amount of chronic inflammation. **B,** High-power view shows that the epithelium is composed of hyperchromatic cells with a slightly increased nucleus-to-cytoplasm ratio and visible nucleoli. However, no atypical mitoses or significant overlapping of the cells and their nuclei is observed. In addition, no significant loss of polarity is seen.

parallel, elongated, and typically evenly spaced and uniform columns (pegs) of highly reactive squamous cells with prominent nucleoli and mitoses, which may extend deep into the lamina propria (Fig. 24.8). Inflammation, both acute and chronic, is usually present, and this assists in recognizing the reactive nature of the cell proliferation. Lack of surface maturation (nucleated cells at surface) and parakeratosis may be present as well. Its appearance may simulate invasive squamous cell carcinoma, although the lack of either cytological atypia or deeply infiltrative growth supports its benign nature.[37] Furthermore, the squamous cells in reactive hyperplasia usually retain their polarity with respect to each other (absence of overlapping nuclei) and with respect to the basement membrane. Nevertheless, if the columns (pegs) of squamous epithelium are irregular and nonuniform, particularly in areas immediately adjacent to ulcers, and this feature is present in abundance, suspicion for a malignant process should be higher.

On occasion, this pseudoepitheliomatous reaction may be endoscopically visible and polypoid; some authors refer to these lesions as "hyperplastic" or "inflammatory" polyps.[38] In addition, polypoid foci of pseudoepitheliomatous hyperplasia may be confused with the endophytic type of squamous papilloma. However, the latter lesions usually lack the significant inflammation and epithelial damage associated with hyperplasia. Finally, pseudoepitheliomatous hyperplasia may be encountered in squamous mucosa overlying subepithelial granular cell tumors.[39]

MALIGNANT NEOPLASMS

Squamous Dysplasia

Clinical Features

Esophageal squamous cell carcinoma, similar to its counterparts in the skin or cervix, is believed to develop through a progression of premalignant or dysplastic precursor lesions. Dysplasia is defined as the presence of unequivocal neoplastic cells confined to the epithelium. The terms dysplasia and intraepithelial neoplasia (IEN) are synonymous, the former being used in the United States and the latter being preferred in Europe and Asia. Squamous dysplasia is more common in patients at high risk for squamous cell carcinoma and is adjacent to squamous cell carcinomas in 60% to 90% of cases.[51] In addition, dysplasia is frequently multifocal, and carcinomas associated with dysplasia are more likely to be multifocal in origin.[41] Dysplasia is currently classified as low-grade or high-grade, based on the degree of cytological atypia and the proportion of the epithelial thickness involved by dysplasia. In this two-tiered system, *low-grade squamous dysplasia* roughly corresponds to the previously used terms mild and moderate dysplasia, and *high-grade squamous dysplasia* includes severe dysplasia and carcinoma in situ (see later discussion).

Pathological Features

Gross Pathology

Dysplastic epithelium appears erythematous, friable, and irregular in more than 80% of cases.[42,51] Erosions, plaques, and nodules may also be present. However, dysplasia may appear completely normal endoscopically. When available, enhanced endoscopic visualization techniques such as narrow-band imaging are also helpful in highlighting dysplastic mucosa that is otherwise grossly nondescript.[52] Mucosal staining with Lugol iodine may also be helpful to highlight dysplastic mucosa, but this technique has proven inferior to narrow band imaging in comparative studies.[52] Dysplastic cells may also be harvested by exfoliative balloon cytology, a technique that is often used for screening in high-risk areas such as China (see Chapter 3).[53]

Microscopic Pathology

Dysplastic squamous epithelium is characterized by a combination of architectural and cytological abnormalities that vary in extent and severity, and this is reflected in the grade (Fig. 24.9). The epithelium is usually hypertrophic but may be atrophic in rare circumstances. In 20% of cases, dysplastic epithelium spreads into esophageal mucosal gland ducts and simulates stromal invasion.[54] Low-grade dysplasia reveals involvement of the basal (lower) half of the squamous epithelium with neoplastic cells with mild cytological atypia, whereas high-grade lesions involve more than half of the epithelial thickness. High-grade dysplasia is diagnosed when severe cytological atypia (markedly increased nucleus-to-cytoplasm [N:C] ratio, significant nuclear pleomorphism and hyperchromasia) is present regardless of the extent of epithelial involvement (see later). In addition, dysplastic cells may occasionally grow as isolated cells in a horizontal pagetoid fashion, although this pattern must be distinguished from the more common pagetoid involvement of the squamous epithelium by adenocarcinoma.[55,56]

Cytological changes of low-grade lesions include nuclear enlargement, varying degrees of nuclear hyperchromasia, mildly increased N:C ratio, and increased mitotic rate. High grade lesions show markedly increased N:C ratio, coarsened chromatin, greater degrees of nuclear hyperchromasia, pleomorphism, and irregularity. Nucleoli may be present but are not a consistent feature and are not specific because they are also frequently present in reactive squamous epithelium (discussed later). When present, nucleoli may be unusually large in size and irregular in shape. Architecturally, dysplastic cells display disorganization, loss of polarity, overlapping nuclei, and lack of surface maturation, which are key features in helping to distinguish true dysplasia from nonneoplastic (reactive) processes (see Fig. 24.9C). Mitotic figures are usually increased in number and may be found at any level of the epithelium (base, midepithelium, or surface). Abnormal (tripolar or disorganized) mitotic figures may be present as well, particularly in high-grade lesions.

Rarely, precursor dysplastic lesions may reveal a proliferation of disorganized large cells (with a normal or even low N:C ratio) with open irregular nuclei, prominent enlarged and irregular single or multiple nucleoli, peripheral condensation of chromatin, and multinucleation (see Fig. 24.9D,E). In these cases, the border between the epithelium and the lamina propria is often highly irregular, showing sharp, budding, or bulbous expansions of epithelium protruding deep into the lamina propria. This type of dysplastic epithelium is often associated with inflammation and surface maturation, although the latter to a much lesser degree than in either normal or reactive squamous epithelium. In these cases, distinguishing dysplastic epithelium from either markedly reactive squamous epithelium or very well-differentiated squamous cell carcinoma may be extremely difficult. Often, repeat biopsies from deeper portions of the lesion and close correlation with the gross endoscopic appearance are necessary to help establish a final diagnosis. In these cases, invasion should not be diagnosed unless there is unequivocal evidence of irregular clusters of neoplastic cells within the deep lamina propria that are clearly disconnected from the overlying surface epithelium (on deeper levels of tissue sectioning) and associated with a peritumoral stromal desmoplastic response.

Differential Diagnosis (Reactive versus Neoplastic)

Squamous dysplasia must be distinguished from reactive epithelial changes associated with esophagitis. Although regenerating squamous cells may show mild nuclear enlargement, hyperchromasia, and expansion of the basal cell layers, they lack significant nuclear pleomorphism, overlapping nuclei, and nuclear crowding and do not display abnormal mitoses (see Fig. 24.9). Unlike in dysplasia, the chromatin is typically fine and homogeneous, and nucleoli, when present, are small and regular in shape. Architecturally, reactive squamous epithelium often displays some degree of surface maturation.

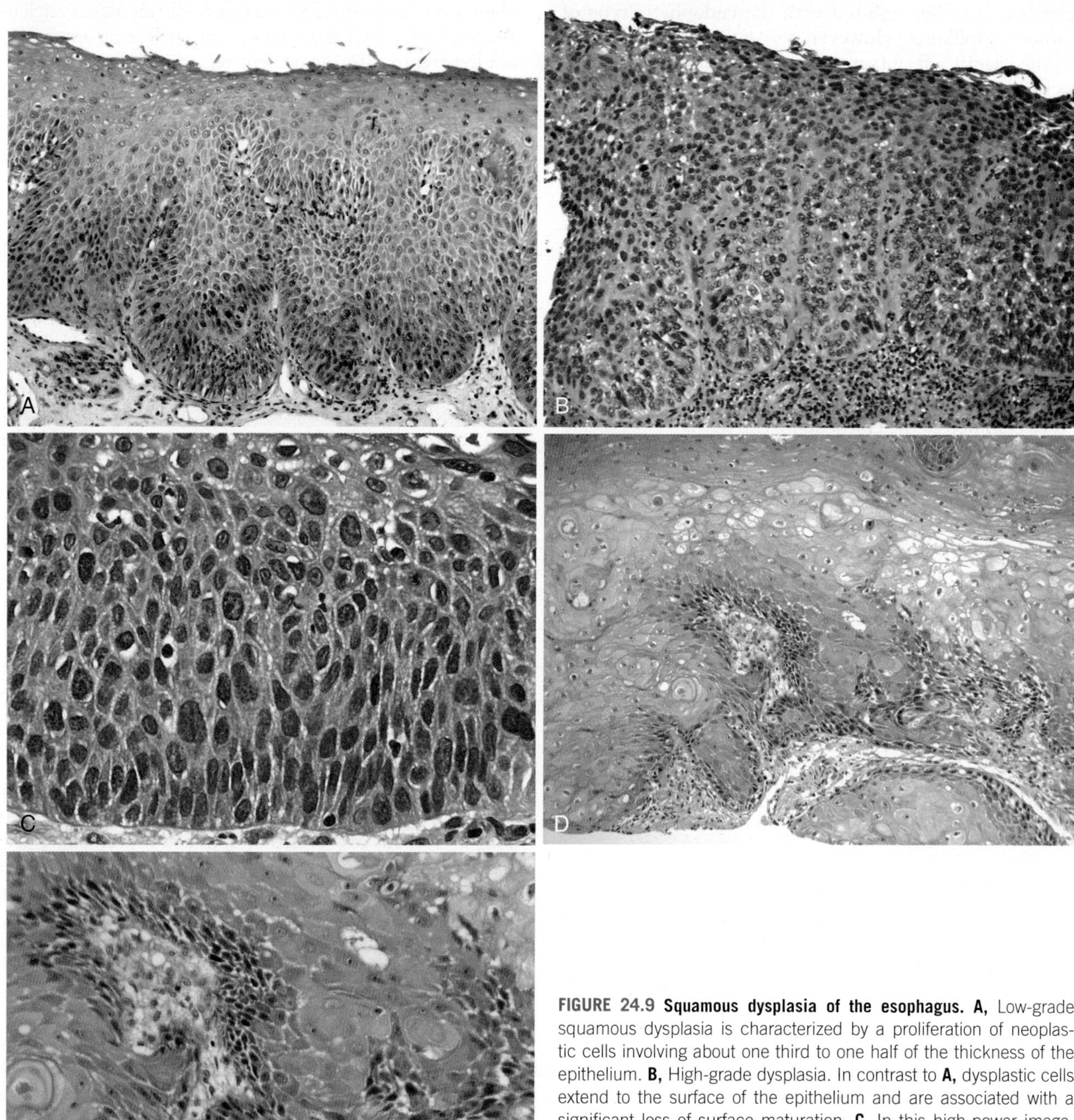

FIGURE 24.9 Squamous dysplasia of the esophagus. A, Low-grade squamous dysplasia is characterized by a proliferation of neoplastic cells involving about one third to one half of the thickness of the epithelium. **B,** High-grade dysplasia. In contrast to **A,** dysplastic cells extend to the surface of the epithelium and are associated with a significant loss of surface maturation. **C,** In this high-power image, dysplastic cells are shown to have an increased nucleus-to-cytoplasm ratio, marked hyperchromatic nuclei, significant loss of polarity, and overlapping of the cells and their nuclei. **D,** This unusual morphological appearance of squamous dysplasia is characterized by disorganized large cells with open nuclei. **E,** High-power photomicrograph of the dysplastic cells seen in **D**.

Essential to the benign, nonneoplastic diagnosis is the fact that the basal and suprabasal layers maintain their polarity and orderly spacing in reactive lesions. Mucosal inflammation frequently accompanies reactive squamous epithelium, and in the presence of inflammation, a diagnosis of dysplasia should be rendered with caution. In biopsy specimens in which the epithelial changes appear sufficiently marked to suggest dysplasia but a reactive process cannot be excluded because of inflammation, a diagnosis of "indefinite for dysplasia" is appropriate. In such cases, follow-up biopsies after treatment of the underlying esophagitis frequently help resolve the diagnostic uncertainty. The results of ancillary stains, such as strong nuclear staining for TP53 (indicative of inactivating mutations) and extensive, suprabasal cell proliferation highlighted by the proliferation marker Ki-67, may also support a diagnosis of dysplasia in problematic cases.[57] Histological features useful in the differential diagnosis of squamous dysplasia are summarized in Table 24.2.

TABLE 24.2 Reactive Hyperplasia versus Dysplastic Squamous Epithelium

Feature	Reactive	Low-Grade Dysplasia	High-Grade Dysplasia
Clinical/Endoscopic			
Esophageal SCC risk factors	+/–	+	+
Normal appearance	+/–	+/–	+/–
Erythema	+/–	+/–	+/–
Irregular/nodular	–	+/–	+/–
Abnormal Lugol/ chromoendoscopy	–	+	+
Pathological			
Nuclear pleomorphism	–	+/–	++
Increased N:C ratio	+/–	+	++
Nuclear hyperchromasia	+/–	+	++
Increased mitotic rate	+/–	+	++
Abnormal mitoses	–	+	++
Nuclear crowding, disarray	–	+	++
Surface maturation	+	+	–*
Inflammation	+	+/–	+/-
Immunohistochemical/Molecular			
TP53 mutation/abnormal p53 staining	–	+	+
Full-thickness Ki-67 staining	–	–	+
DNA aneuploidy	–	+	+

N:C ratio, *Nucleus-to-cytoplasm ratio;* SCC, *squamous cell carcinoma; +, consistently present; ++, key feature; +, consistently present; –, not present; +/–, sometimes present.*

**Some examples of high-grade dysplasia show surface maturation, with high-grade dysplastic epithelial cells limited to the lower half of the epithelium.*

In biopsy specimens from patients who have received chemotherapy or radiotherapy, the squamous epithelium may contain markedly atypical cells with enlarged hyperchromatic nuclei that raise the possibility of dysplasia. However, in contrast to dysplasia, these cells do not have an increased N:C ratio and often contain distinctive vacuolization in their cytoplasm. Furthermore, unlike in dysplasia, mesenchymal cells showing similar changes may also be present in the lamina propria, as well as other characteristic stromal changes of chemotherapy or radiotherapy (Fig. 24.10A). Therefore awareness of the patient's clinical history is critical.

Biopsy specimens from patients with esophagitis caused by GERD or other causes such as drug effects occasionally contain multinucleated epithelial giant cells, raising the possibility of dysplasia (see Fig. 24.10B,C).[58] In these cases, no other cytological or architectural features of dysplasia are present, and results of special studies for viral inclusions are negative. In inflammation-induced multinucleation, the nucleated squamous cells are typically basal or suprabasal in location and may be increased in number adjacent to areas of ulceration. In contrast, multinucleated virally infected cells (e.g., herpes simplex) are common in the surface epithelium and adjacent to sloughing epithelium.

Prognosis and Treatment

Squamous dysplasia frequently occurs adjacent to invasive carcinoma. For example, 30% of patients with a biopsy diagnosis of high-grade dysplasia show invasive squamous cell carcinoma in subsequent endoscopic resections.[42] In addition, patients with squamous dysplasia are at increased risk for squamous cell carcinoma on follow-up. In a 13-year follow-up study of patients from China, 106 with low-grade dysplasia and 23 with high-grade dysplasia, those with low-grade dysplasia had a 3- to 8-fold increased risk, and patients with high-grade dysplasia had a 28- to 34-fold increased risk for invasive carcinoma.[51] In another study, 15% of patients with low-grade dysplasia progressed to high-grade dysplasia, whereas invasive carcinoma developed in 30% of patients with high-grade dysplasia during an 8-year follow-up period.[59] However, dysplasia may also regress or disappear, although sampling error certainly may account for a normal finding on follow-up biopsy in a patient with dysplasia in a prior biopsy specimen. Therefore patients with a diagnosis of squamous dysplasia require thorough endoscopic examination with biopsies, first to exclude synchronous invasive squamous cell carcinoma (particularly if associated with a visible mass lesion or ulceration) and second to detect the development of early invasive tumor on follow-up. Low-grade dysplasia without a mass or associated carcinoma may be managed with repeated biopsies and continued surveillance in most patients. Mucosal ablation is an option in patients with flat dysplasia, and this technique provided durable remission in 86% of patients over a period of 5 years in one study.[60] A patient with any grade of squamous dysplasia associated with a mass lesion should be

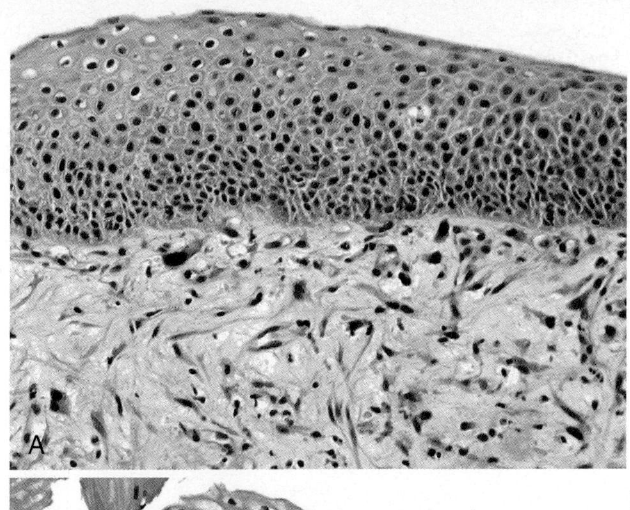

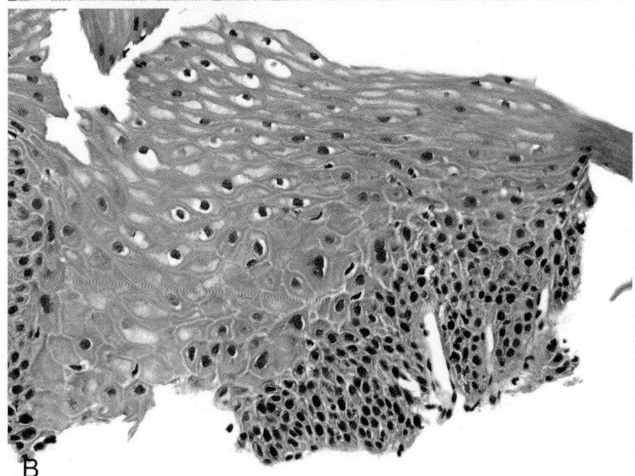

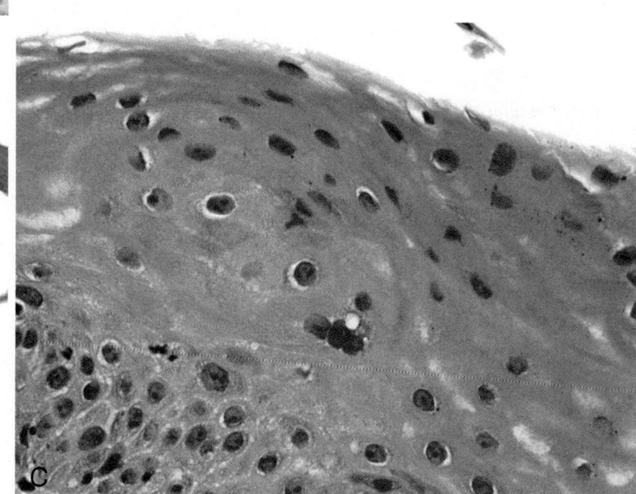

FIGURE 24.10 **A,** Reactive squamous epithelium with nuclear atypia from a patient who received chemoradiotherapy. Nuclear changes are present in both epithelial and stromal cells. **B,** Reactive epithelial giant cell changes are seen in the basal portion of the epithelium adjacent to a healing ulcer. **C,** High-power image of another multinucleated epithelial giant cell shows increased nuclear size and prominent nucleoli but a low nucleus-to-cytoplasm ratio. These cells are usually located in the basal portion of the epithelium, as shown here.

considered as having carcinoma until proven otherwise, and managed accordingly. Some endoscopically subtle invasive carcinomas have been reported that apparently arose from low-grade dysplasia, further emphasizing the need for careful endoscopic scrutiny and adequate sampling in patients with any grade of squamous dysplasia.[61]

Endoscopic mucosal resection or endoscopic submucosal dissection, which permits removal of dysplastic lesions or even early superficial cancers, aids in the diagnosis and staging of early invasive tumors and is performed increasingly in specialized centers. Use of both methods have been associated with complete resection rates of greater than 90%, though endoscopic submucosal dissection may be preferable for larger (>15 mm) lesions.[62]

Squamous Cell Carcinoma

Clinical Features

Squamous cell carcinoma is the most common malignant tumor of the esophagus worldwide. However, in the United States and western Europe, the incidence of this type of esophageal cancer has been declining over the past 20 years, both in absolute terms and relative to esophageal adenocarcinoma (see later discussion). In 2012–2016, the overall incidence of squamous cell carcinoma in the United States was approximately 1.3 per 100,000 person-years, accounting for approximately 31% of all esophageal cancers.[1,2] It affects predominantly men (two to three times more often than women) with a peak incidence in the seventh decade of life. There is a marked geographical and ethnic variation in incidence: the highest rates (as many as 161 per 100,000) occur in China, Iran, South America, and South Africa.[40] In the United States, the disease is approximately four times more common in black men than in white men.[1] Common presenting symptoms include dysphagia and weight loss. As many as 14% of patients with head and neck squamous cell carcinoma have synchronous or metachronous esophageal squamous cell carcinoma.[41]

Pathogenesis

The pathogenesis of squamous cell carcinoma is multifactorial and varies significantly among different regions of the world.[42,43] Many cases develop without an identifiable cause or predisposing condition. Known risk factors in high-prevalence areas such as China and Iran include consumption of food or water rich in nitrates and nitrosamines, which results in the development of chronic esophagitis. Additional risk factors, common to both Western and developing countries, include tobacco smoke, alcohol, and various vitamin deficiencies. Other predisposing conditions include achalasia,[44] Plummer-Vinson syndrome, strictures resulting from acid or lye ingestion, and the rare autosomal dominant condition tylosis (keratoderma palmaris et plantaris).[45] Individuals related to affected family members are also at increased risk for esophageal carcinoma.

HPV infection has been implicated in tumorigenesis in many squamous epithelia. However, its precise role in esophageal carcinoma is controversial. HPV DNA has been isolated from esophageal tumors at prevalence rates of 0% to 66%.[40,43] Viral types most commonly identified include HPV types 16 and 18. Varying rates of HPV positivity among studies may be attributed to differences in the techniques used to detect HPV and to different populations of patients studied. Importantly, evidence of active HPV infection, such as HPV seropositivity, viral DNA integration, or p16^{INK4a} activation, is lacking from the vast majority of squamous cell carcinomas,[46] indicating that HPV is most likely a causative factor in only a small fraction of tumors.

Molecular Features

At the molecular level, the most common alterations are overexpression of cell cycle regulatory proteins (e.g., amplification of cyclin D1 in 50% of tumors) and inactivation or loss of tumor suppressor proteins (e.g., p16 [CDKN2A] in as many as 80% of cases).[47] Environmental risk factors such as tobacco, alcohol, and diet appear to produce mutations through the production of reactive oxygen species and DNA adducts. Polymorphisms in the *ALDH2* and *ALDH1B1* genes, which encode enzymes involved in alcohol metabolism, and in CYP1A1, a detoxification enzyme for xenobiotics, are associated with elevated risk for squamous cell carcinoma.[43] Most of these tumors also express high levels of the epidermal growth factor receptor (EGFR), seen in 19% to 68% of the cases in some studies.[48] Some of these alterations, such as inactivating mutations of *TP53* and *CDKN2A* and increased cell proliferation, appear to occur early in neoplastic progression and are frequently detectable in squamous dysplastic precursor lesions as well.[49] Epigenetic silencing of gene promoter hypermethylation, such as the transcription factor SOX2 in a subset of aggressive squamous cell carcinomas, also has been observed.[50] For more information on molecular features, refer to Chapter 23.

Pathological Features

Gross Pathology

Squamous cell carcinomas may be separated into early (superficial) and late (advanced) types. Superficial squamous cell carcinomas are defined as tumors that invade the lamina propria and submucosa but do not penetrate the muscularis propria. These tumors constitute approximately 15% to 20% of all invasive squamous cell carcinomas, with higher prevalence rates in populations that routinely undergo endoscopic surveillance.[51,59,62] The key features are summarized in Box 24.3.

Squamous cell carcinomas occur in the middle third of the esophagus in 50% to 60% of cases, the distal third in 30%, and the proximal third in 10% to 20%.[40,63] Superficial tumors most commonly appear as mucosal plaques or slightly elevated flat lesions but may also be ulcerated, polypoid, or even grossly inconspicuous. Superficially invasive tumors are more commonly multicentric (as much as 20% of cases) when compared with advanced tumors. This finding may reflect either the presence of synchronous primary tumors occurring in a background of dysplasia or the presence of satellite tumor nodules resulting from intramural metastasis.[41,51,64]

The gross appearance of advanced tumors may be classified as exophytic (protruding) (type 1 in the Japan Esophageal Society classification; 60% of cases), ulcerative (types 2 and 3; 25% of cases), or infiltrative (type 4; 15% of cases) (Fig. 24.11).[40] However, this feature is not a significant prognostic factor. In patients treated with preoperative irradiation or chemotherapy, the tumor may be invisible or perhaps replaced by a shallow surface erosion.

BOX 24.3 Esophageal Squamous Cell Carcinoma: Key Features

- Clinical/endoscopic
  - Male > female, 6th to 7th decade
  - Middle third of esophagus > distal third > proximal third
  - Fungating (most common), ulcerative, or infiltrative mass
  - Aggressive, poor prognosis (overall 5-year survival, 10%)
- Histological
  - Pushing border, or infiltrating nests of tumor cells
  - Well differentiated: sheetlike growth, ample keratinization, squamous pearls, intercellular bridges; few basaloid cells
  - Moderately differentiated (most common): variable keratinization: significant proportion of basaloid cells
  - Poorly differentiated: small or large nests; predominantly basaloid cells, or marked pleomorphism
  - Subtypes: basaloid, spindle cell, verrucous
- Special/immunohistochemical stains
  - p63/p40 positive
  - CK5/6, CK7, CK14 positive
  - Neuroendocrine markers negative or focal
- Molecular
  - TP53 mutation
  - Cyclin D1 overexpression
  - Epidermal growth factor receptor overexpression
- Differential diagnosis
  - Pseudoepitheliomatous hyperplasia
  - High-grade squamous dysplasia
  - Neuroendocrine carcinoma (small cell or large cell)
- Prognostic factors/features to report
  - Tumor stage (Tumor–Node–Metastasis classification)
  - Tumor grade/differentiation
  - Lymphovascular, perineural invasion
  - Residual tumor after neoadjuvant therapy
  - Deep/adventitial margin

Microscopic Pathology

Superficially invasive tumors consist of irregular, elongated projections of dysplastic epithelium that extend into the lamina propria, muscularis mucosae, or submucosa as isolated cells or clusters of cells with a minimal desmoplastic response. Invasion of mucosal and submucosal lymphatics is not uncommon and is likely to account for the occasional instances of intramural metastasis. Advanced carcinomas spread through the esophageal wall, either with an infiltrative pattern composed of individual small nests of tumor cells or with an expansile (pushing) growth pattern composed of a solid mass of tumor cells with a smooth advancing edge. A prominent lymphocytic infiltrate occasionally surrounds the tumor.[65-68]

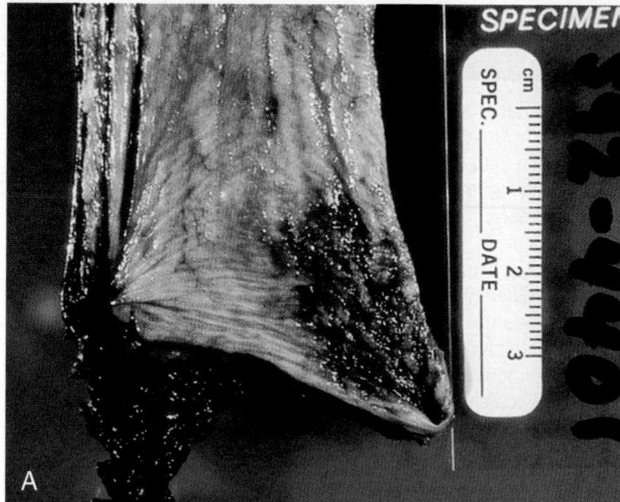

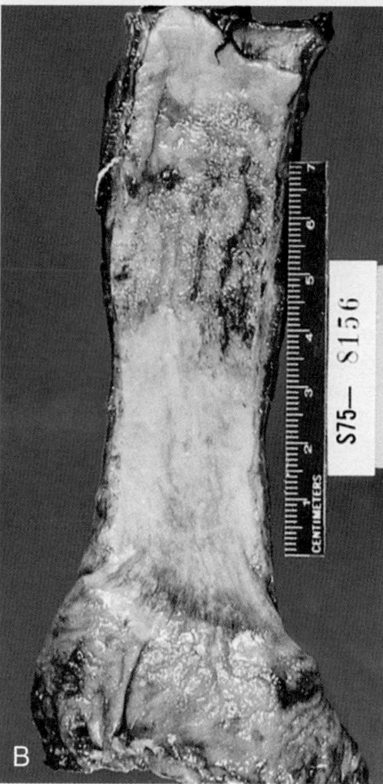

FIGURE 24.11 A, Gross appearance of a superficial squamous cell carcinoma of the esophagus *(right lower corner)*. **B,** Exophytic and ulcerating advanced squamous cell carcinoma of the esophagus is seen in the midportion of the organ.

Squamous cell carcinomas show a range of differentiation from well to poor (Fig. 24.12). Well-differentiated tumors show variably sized nests of polygonal epithelioid cells with ample eosinophilic cytoplasm, easily recognizable intercellular bridges, and abundant keratinization (squamous pearls), with relatively few compact basaloid cells. Moderately differentiated tumors account for approximately two thirds of squamous cell carcinomas. They contain a higher proportion of primitive basaloid cells than well-differentiated tumors, and they are typically arranged in irregular nests and trabeculae with only focal keratinization. Poorly differentiated or undifferentiated tumors show no evidence of keratinization, grow in solid sheets or as single cells, and may contain large, bizarre pleomorphic cells. Since squamous cell carcinomas commonly show varying degrees of differentiation within a single tumor, even a small squamous component should be searched for in an otherwise undifferentiated carcinoma. Focal mucinous differentiation occurs in as many as 20% of cases.[69,70] If the tumor contains an admixture of distinct components of adenocarcinoma and squamous cell carcinoma, it may qualify as an adenosquamous carcinoma (see Carcinoma with Mixed Squamous and Glandular Elements).[40] Focal neuroendocrine or small cell differentiation has also been reported.[71]

Special studies are rarely required to establish a diagnosis of conventional squamous cell carcinoma but may be useful in small biopsy specimens or when rare tumor cells are present, such as for patients who have received neoadjuvant chemoradiotherapy. By immunohistochemistry, squamous cell carcinoma cells are positive for broad-spectrum keratins and for keratins 13, 14, 18, and 19.[72,73] CK7 reactivity is present in as much as 29% of cases, but most cases are negative for both CK7 and CK20.[74] In addition, most tumors express p63, p40, and CK5/6, similar to squamous cell carcinomas that arise in other sites, as well as SOX2.[73,75] Mucin stains may show focal positivity in a high proportion of cases, but this finding alone should not imply that the tumor is an adenosquamous carcinoma. Focal positivity for neuroendocrine markers, such as chromogranin and synaptophysin, also does not exclude a diagnosis of squamous cell carcinoma if it is present in a minority of the tumor cells and if the tumor is otherwise morphologically typical of a squamous cell carcinoma and does not show areas of small cell or large cell neuroendocrine carcinoma.[71,76] Up to 45% of tumors show expression of the immune checkpoint molecule PD-L1, which is the target of immunotherapy in appropriately selected patients.[77]

Differential Diagnosis

In small, poorly oriented biopsy specimens, distinguishing between in situ neoplasia (dysplasia) and invasive squamous cell carcinoma may be difficult. Squamous dysplasia, unlike invasive carcinoma, displays smooth-edged papillations with a continuous basement membrane and a connection to the surface epithelium and lacks single-cell infiltration, the presence of irregular discontinuous nests of cells, and desmoplastic stroma. However, the diagnostic criteria for squamous cell carcinoma differ between Western and Japanese pathologists, and many lesions that would be considered "high-grade dysplasia" by Western pathologists are diagnosed as "carcinoma" by Japanese pathologists solely on the basis of nuclear features.[78]

Invasive squamous cell carcinoma must also be distinguished from nonneoplastic lesions such as pseudoepitheliomatous hyperplasia and pseudodiverticulosis. Pseudoepitheliomatous hyperplasia, similar to other reactive squamous proliferations, does not show significant nuclear pleomorphism, loss of polarity, or overlapping of nuclei and always reveals a connection to the surface epithelium (see Fig. 24.8). Reactive lesions do not show desmoplasia. Pseudodiverticulosis is a rare condition that produces numerous islands of reactive squamous epithelium in the mucosa and submucosa, some of which may be irregular in shape, simulating a carcinoma (Fig. 24.13).[79] This condition is caused by extensive squamous metaplasia of the esophageal ducts and glands, which may occur in association with strictures or motility disturbances. On radiological examination,

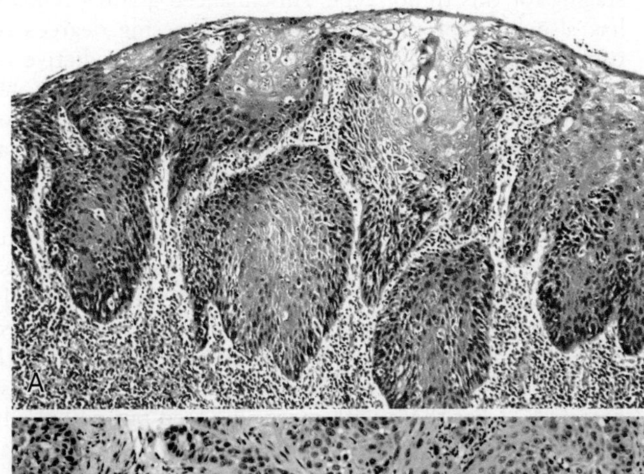

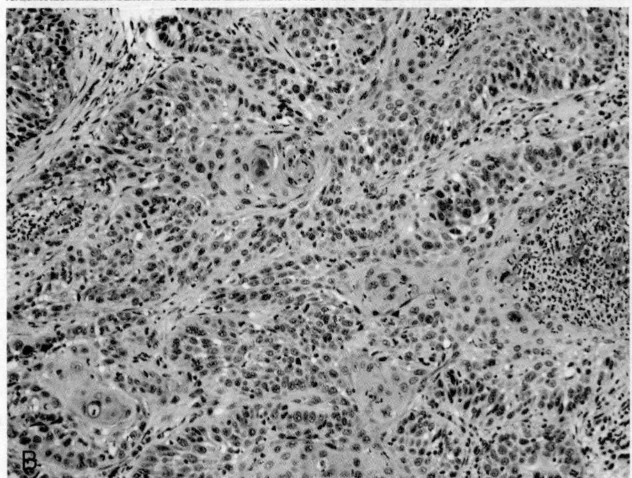

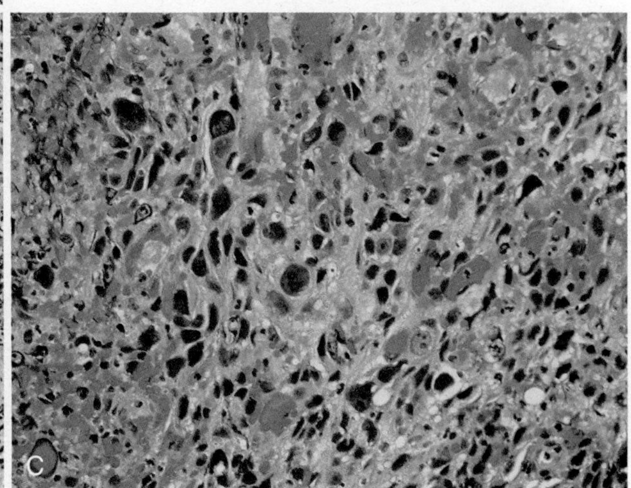

FIGURE 24.12 A, Well-differentiated squamous cell carcinoma characterized by a proliferation of atypical squamous epithelium forming irregular pegs that extend into the underlying lamina propria. This is associated with a mild desmoplastic reaction and chronic inflammation. **B,** Moderately differentiated squamous cell carcinoma. In this image, the tumor shows a mixture of keratinizing and basaloid epithelial elements. **C,** Poorly differentiated squamous cell carcinoma characterized by marked nuclear pleomorphism. However, focal areas of cellular keratinization are present.

pseudodiverticulosis may mimic carcinoma by showing irregular stricture formation. Identifying characteristic diverticula with a barium swallow procedure helps separate this condition from carcinoma radiologically. Pathologically, these lesions are distinguished from invasive carcinoma by the lack of an infiltrative growth pattern, absence of dysplastic squamous epithelium, and the presence of smooth, often rounded, islands of reactive squamous epithelium associated with, or replacing, the submucosal glands and ducts with a prominent inflammatory infiltrate.

Biopsy or resection specimens from patients who have been treated with neoadjuvant chemoradiotherapy may contain only scattered atypical cells, which can occasionally make it difficult to distinguish residual carcinoma from reactive mesenchymal cells. Carcinoma cells may be identified by positive immunostaining for keratins and an increased N:C ratio; reactive mesenchymal cells are typically keratin negative and have expanded, often bubbly or "wispy" cytoplasm. Typically, the N:C ratio of these cells is maintained.

Poorly differentiated tumors may be difficult to recognize as squamous in phenotype, and neuroendocrine carcinoma, melanoma, or even lymphoma may be suspected on morphological grounds. Positivity for keratins, lack of widespread expression of neuroendocrine markers, and negativity for melanocytic and lymphoid markers may help eliminate these alternative diagnoses. In some patients, pulmonary squamous cell carcinoma involves the esophageal wall by metastasis or direct extension (see later discussion) and may be confused with a primary esophageal tumor. Adjacent squamous dysplasia provides strong evidence for an esophageal origin of the tumor. In addition, approximately 10% to 20% of lung squamous cell carcinomas show nuclear immunostaining for thyroid transcription factor 1 (TTF-1), which is not expressed in esophageal epithelium or in tumors derived from it.[80]

Prognosis and Treatment

Squamous cell carcinomas may spread horizontally, but more typically they invade vertically through the esophageal wall and in this manner spread to involve contiguous organs such as the trachea, aorta, and pericardium. Intramural metastasis was detected in as much as 6% of resection specimens in one study, and is a sign of aggressive behavior and a risk factor for postoperative recurrence.[81] Regional lymph node metastasis is present in approximately 60% of patients at the time of diagnosis, and the lymph node positivity rate correlates with depth of invasion (<5% for intramucosal carcinomas and as much as 45% for submucosal carcinomas).[62,82] Carcinomas originating in the upper thoracic esophagus are more likely to metastasize to cervical or upper mediastinal nodes, whereas tumors from the middle and lower thirds of the esophagus metastasize to lower mediastinal or perigastric nodes.[40,63] However, skip nodal metastases are not uncommon in esophageal cancers. Distant metastasis, which most frequently involves the lung or liver, is present in as much as 60% of patients at autopsy.[83]

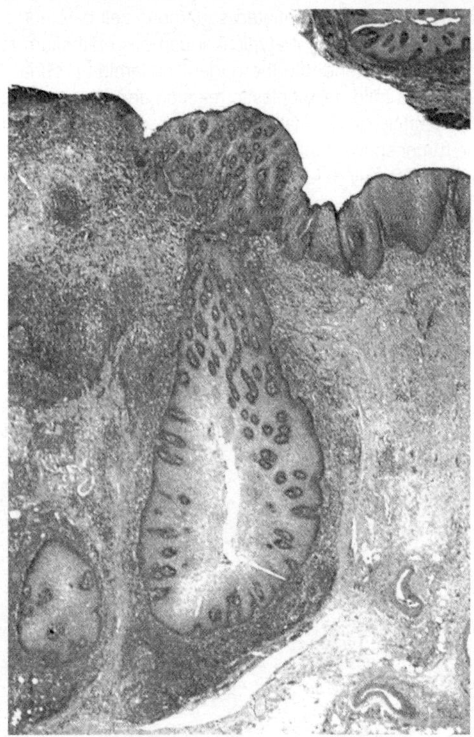

FIGURE 24.13 Pseudodiverticulosis of the esophagus. Low-power image shows a reactive proliferation of squamous epithelium extending into the submucosal gland ducts and associated with a marked chronic inflammatory infiltrate. In contrast to carcinoma, the borders of the squamous proliferation are smooth and do not show atypia or other features of malignancy, such as desmoplasia.

Overall, the 5-year survival rate for patients with squamous cell carcinoma is approximately 15% to 20%, but it approaches 30% to 40% for patients treated with esophagectomy.[1,40,84,85] The most significant prognostic factor is tumor stage, which is based on the American Joint Committee on Cancer (AJCC) tumor–node–metastasis (TNM) classification.[85,86] Patients with tumors that penetrate into the submucosa have 5-year survival rates in the range of 60% to 75%, compared with 40% to 60% and 25% to 30% for patients with tumors that extend into the muscularis propria and the adventitia, respectively.[85]

The presence of lymph node metastasis and a greater number of positive lymph nodes are also correlated with worse prognosis.[82] Patients who have higher numbers of lymph nodes harvested have improved survival, which may reflect either more accurate staging or the therapeutic effect of lymphadenectomy.[87] Therefore, although the minimal number of lymph nodes needed for adequate staging has not been determined,[86] all lymph node candidates in resection specimens should be submitted for microscopic examination in order to maximize lymph node yield.

In patients who have received neoadjuvant chemoradiotherapy, the presence of residual tumor is correlated with reduced survival. In one study of 175 patients, 55 (31%) had complete histological tumor response; their median survival time was 125 months, compared with 21 months for those who had residual tumor.[88] Some authors have also found that poor tumor differentiation is an independent prognostic factor,[84,89] and tumor differentiation as well as tumor location are now incorporated into the AJCC staging for this tumor type. An enhanced grading scheme has also been proposed, in which increasing degrees of tumor budding and small cell nest size are predictive of worse patient outcomes.[90] Intramural metastases[81] and lymphovascular invasion[91] have also been found to be predictive of regional lymph node metastasis and poor survival in some studies, but these findings need to be tested in a prospective manner.

The mainstay of treatment for esophageal squamous cell carcinoma is surgical resection, most commonly transthoracic esophagectomy.[92] As mentioned previously, early (intramucosal or submucosal) carcinomas in selected patients have been managed with endoscopic resection, with low rates of tumor recurrence or metastasis in specialized centers.[42,62] For those with more advanced but potentially resectable (stage II and III) tumors, neoadjuvant chemoradiotherapy followed by surgery induces tumor regression and improves survival in a subset of patients.[88,92]

Basaloid Squamous Cell Carcinoma

Clinical Features

Basaloid (squamous) carcinoma is an unusual variant of squamous cell carcinoma that also occurs in the upper aerodigestive tract (e.g., hypopharynx, base of tongue). The true incidence of esophageal basaloid squamous carcinoma is difficult to determine, but it has been estimated to be from 1% to 3% of squamous cell carcinomas.[93-95] These tumors, like conventional squamous cell carcinomas, characteristically occur in older men with presenting symptoms of dysphagia and weight loss.

Pathological Features

Grossly, basaloid squamous carcinomas are large, bulky, fungating tumors that frequently ulcerate and form strictures. They most commonly arise in the middle and distal esophagus.

Microscopically, the basaloid component comprises anywhere from 5% to 90% of the tumor and shows a variety of morphologies such as solid, cribriform, trabecular, and ductal growth patterns.[93] The characteristic basaloid tumor cells are oval to round, large, and somewhat pleomorphic with an open pale chromatin pattern, small nucleoli, and scant cytoplasm; cells are arranged in solid or cribriform lobules, often showing central necrosis and peripheral palisading (Fig. 24.14). Mitoses are usually easily identifiable. An in situ or invasive squamous cell carcinoma component is often present, at least focally. In addition, other lines of differentiation, including adenocarcinoma, small cell carcinoma, or even spindle cell carcinoma may coexist with the basaloid component.[93,94] On the basis of these findings, basaloid carcinoma has been proposed to arise from a multipotential stem cell, or basal cell, in the native squamous epithelium.

Special Studies

A mucoid matrix that stains positive for periodic acid–Schiff (PAS) and Alcian blue may be present in the cribriform spaces of some tumor cell nests. By immunohistochemistry, basaloid carcinomas typically show weak staining for broad-spectrum keratins (in a membrane-type pattern) and for p63 or p40 with an absence of staining for neuroendocrine markers. The basal cells stain strongly for CK14 and CK19.[93-96]

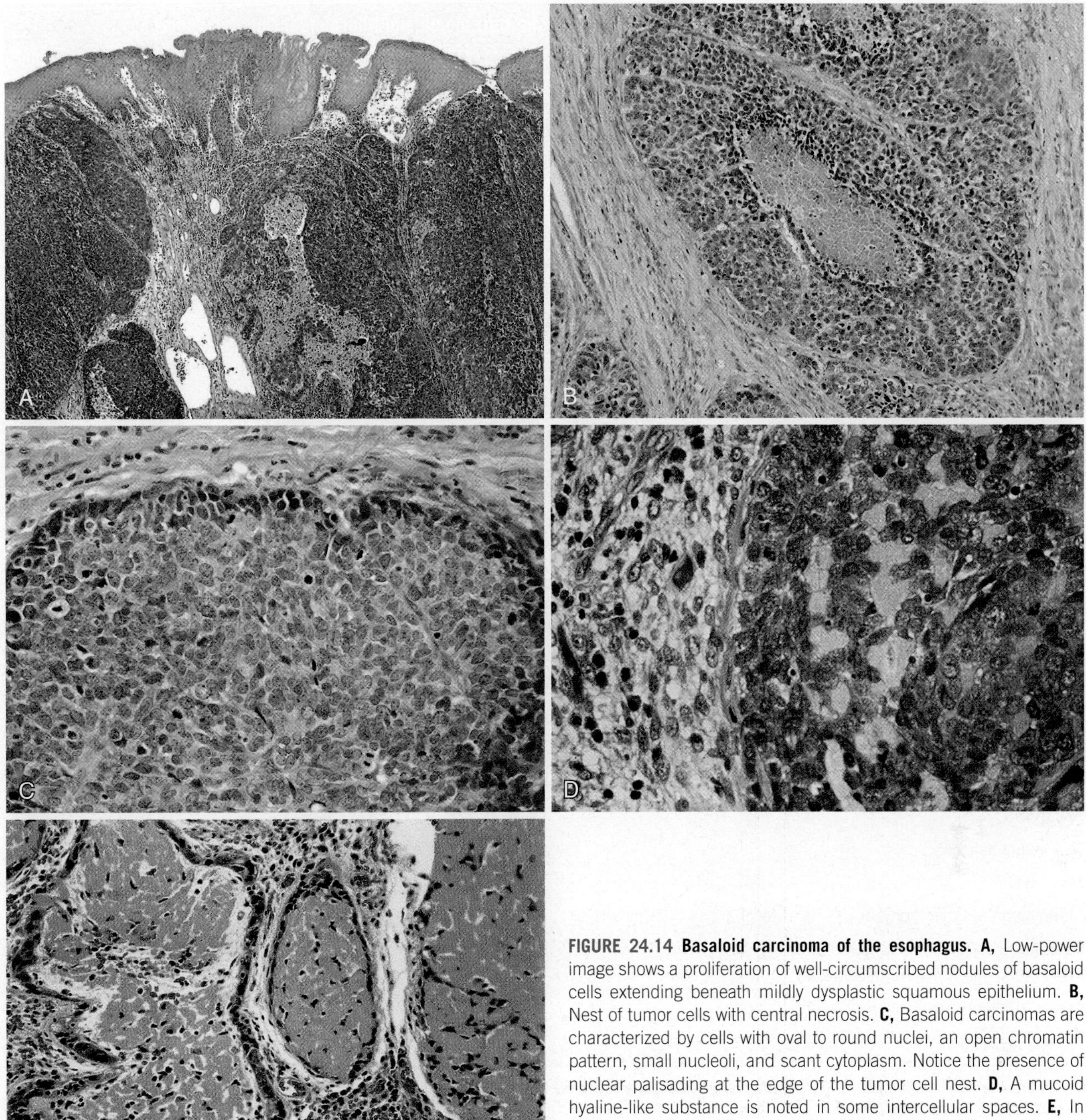

FIGURE 24.14 Basaloid carcinoma of the esophagus. A, Low-power image shows a proliferation of well-circumscribed nodules of basaloid cells extending beneath mildly dysplastic squamous epithelium. **B,** Nest of tumor cells with central necrosis. **C,** Basaloid carcinomas are characterized by cells with oval to round nuclei, an open chromatin pattern, small nucleoli, and scant cytoplasm. Notice the presence of nuclear palisading at the edge of the tumor cell nest. **D,** A mucoid hyaline-like substance is noted in some intercellular spaces. **E,** In some cases, basaloid carcinomas show marked intratumoral necrosis, which gives the false appearance of gland formation and an adenoid cystic carcinoma–like quality to the tumor nodules.

Some tumors show focal actin and vimentin positivity in the basaloid cells and carcinoembryonic antigen (CEA) positivity in the pseudoglandular spaces. At the molecular level, basaloid carcinomas are similar to conventional squamous cell carcinomas, particularly with regard to the frequency of alterations of cyclin D1, and the *TP53* and retinoblastoma *(RB)* tumor suppressor genes.[95,96] However, these tumors are consistently negative for HPV.[95]

Differential Diagnosis

The differential diagnosis of basaloid carcinoma includes conventional (pure) squamous cell carcinoma, adenoid cystic carcinoma, and neuroendocrine carcinoma (NEC). Cases with a prominent basaloid mucoid matrix (Alcian blue positive, PAS positive) or extensive necrosis can adopt a pseudoacinar or cribriform pattern that may be mistaken for adenoid cystic carcinoma (see Fig. 24.14D,E). This is an important distinction, because true adenoid cystic carcinomas of the esophagus are less aggressive than basaloid carcinomas (see Adenoid Cystic Carcinoma). Unlike basaloid carcinomas, adenoid cystic carcinomas form true epithelial lumina do not coexist with conventional squamous cell carcinoma or squamous dysplasia, and lack significant pleomorphism, mitoses, and necrosis (see Fig. 24.25). The basal (myoepithelial) cells of adenoid cystic carcinoma are smaller and more hyperchromatic and

TABLE 24.3 Basaloid Squamous Carcinoma versus Adenoid Cystic Carcinoma and Neuroendocrine Carcinoma

Feature	Basaloid Carcinoma	Adenoid Cystic Carcinoma	Neuroendocrine Carcinoma
Clinical			
Age (years)	>60	40-60	40-80
Sex	M > F	F > M	M > F
Smoking history	+/–	–	+/–
Location middle third	+	+	+/–
Gross appearance	Exophytic	Submucosal nodule	Fungating, ulcerative
Aggressive clinical course	++	+/–	++
Pathological			
Squamous dysplasia	+	–	+/–*
Invasive squamous carcinoma	+/–	–	+/–*
Invasive adenocarcinoma	–	–	+/–†
Ductal and basaloid cells	–	++	–
True epithelial lumina	–	++	–
Pleomorphism	++	–	+
Increased mitoses	++	–	++
Nuclei			
Open chromatin	+/–	–	–
Dense compact chromatin	–	++	+/–*
Nucleoli	+	–	+/–†
Large nuclei	++	–	+/–†
Immunohistochemistry			
S100 protein, actin in basal (myoepithelial) cells	–	+	–
p63, p40	+	+	–
CEA in luminal cells	+	+	–
c-kit/CD117	–	+	–
Chromogranin, synaptophysin	+/– (focal)	–	++
Molecular			
TP53 mutation	+	–	+
Cyclin D1 overexpression	+	–	ND
EGFR amplification	+/–	–	ND

CEA, *Carcinoembryonic antigen;* EGFR, *epidermal growth factor receptor;* ND, *not determined; +, consistently present; ++, key feature; –, not present; +/–, sometimes present.*
**Small cell neuroendocrine carcinoma.*
†Large cell neuroendocrine carcinoma.

regular in size compared with basaloid carcinoma, and they stain strongly for S100 and actin, whereas the basal cells of basaloid carcinoma are typically positive for CK14 and CK19.[96,97] In conventional squamous cell carcinomas, a significant proportion of tumor cells have eosinophilic cytoplasm, grow in irregular infiltrative clusters rather than in rounded nests, and show focal keratinization. However, the distinction between basaloid and conventional squamous carcinoma may be arbitrary and of little prognostic value. The differential diagnosis of basaloid carcinoma, adenoid cystic carcinoma, and NEC is summarized in Table 24.3.

Differentiation of basaloid carcinoma from NEC is usually easily and best performed by immunohistochemical staining with chromogranin, synaptophysin, or CD56. Basaloid carcinomas may show focal and rare weak staining with endocrine markers, but this contrasts greatly with diffuse strong staining in most NECs. Although small cell carcinoma may show only weak or focal staining, these tumors are characterized by the presence of small hyperchromatic cells without nucleoli and with prominent nuclear molding. This contrasts with basaloid carcinomas, which have larger nuclei, lack molding, and have prominent nucleoli.

Prognosis

Basaloid squamous carcinoma is a highly aggressive tumor that carries a prognosis similar to that of pure squamous cell carcinoma. Most studies show no difference in overall survival between these two tumor types,[98] although one study of early (T1) basaloid squamous cell carcinomas showed a lower incidence of lymph node metastases compared with conventional squamous cell carcinoma.[99]

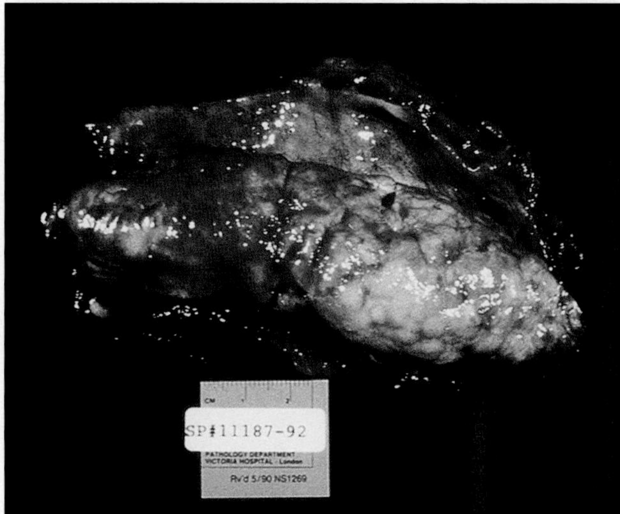

FIGURE 24.15 Gross image of a polypoid spindle cell squamous carcinoma of the distal esophagus. The lesion protrudes into the lumen of the esophagus and is associated with a gray hemorrhagic and necrotic surface.

Spindle Cell Squamous Carcinoma

Clinical Features

Spindle cell squamous carcinoma, also known as carcinosarcoma, polypoid carcinoma, and sarcomatoid carcinoma, was first described by Virchow in 1865; it represents approximately 2% of esophageal carcinomas. Similar to squamous cell carcinoma, it predominantly affects men (80%) in middle to late adult life (40 to 90 years).[100] Because of the typical exophytic intraluminal growth pattern of these tumors, presenting symptoms are commonly related to esophageal obstruction.

Pathological Features

Grossly, these tumors may grow to large sizes (1 to 25 cm) and show a predilection for the middle and distal segments of the esophagus. Eighty percent of lesions are polypoid and have an exophytic growth pattern (Fig. 24.15), whereas only 10% of cases show an infiltrative growth pattern.

Microscopically, the tumor is characterized by a combination of epithelial and spindle cell (or other mesenchymal) elements (Fig. 24.16). The epithelial element is typically moderately to well-differentiated squamous cell carcinoma. In some cases, only in situ carcinoma is present.[100] In fact, some cases show only a small amount of the epithelial component, and this is usually either at the base of the polyp or at the periphery of the invasive tumor. The sarcomatous component is commonly a high-grade spindle cell sarcoma.

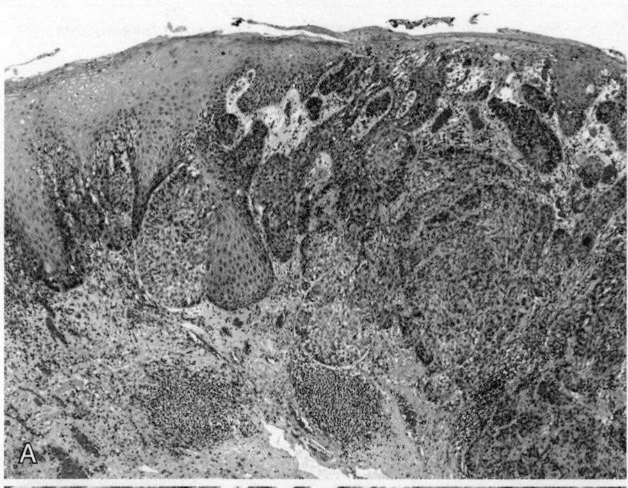

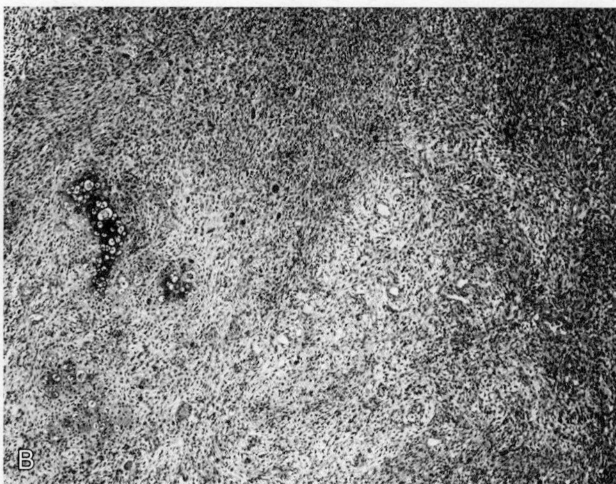

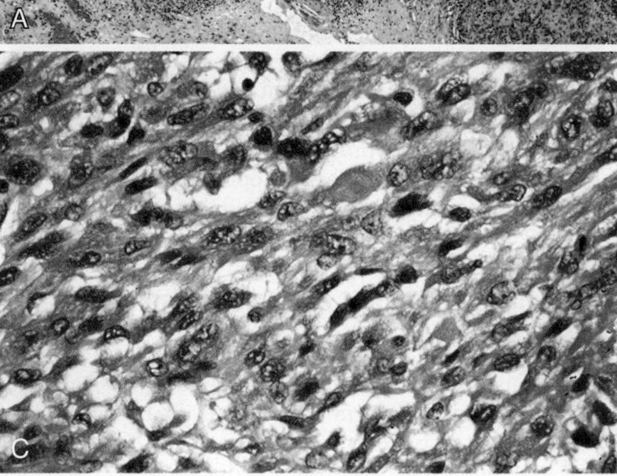

FIGURE 24.16 **A,** Microscopic appearance of spindle cell squamous carcinoma. The superficial portion of this tumor comprises a proliferation of epithelioid malignant squamous cells. **B,** The sarcomatous component of this tumor shows focal chondroid differentiation *(left),* as well as areas of undifferentiated spindle cell sarcoma *(right).* **C,** High-power view of undifferentiated sarcomatous area shows spindle cells with hyperchromatic, elongated nuclei.

TABLE 24.4 Esophageal Spindle Cell Squamous Carcinoma versus Primary Sarcoma and Mesothelioma

Feature	Spindle Cell Carcinoma	Primary Sarcoma	Mesothelioma (from Pleura)
Clinical			
Age (yr)	40-90	Broad	>60
Sex	M > F	M = F	M > F
Location middle third	+	+/–	–
Gross appearance	Exophytic, polypoid	Expansile nodule, polypoid	Infiltrative, extrinsic
Aggressive clinical course	++	++	+
Histological			
Squamous dysplasia	+	–	–
Invasive squamous carcinoma	+/–	–	–
Spindle cells	++	++	+/–
Mesenchymal elements	+/–	+/–	–
Epithelioid elements	–	–	+/–
Immunohistochemistry			
Broad-spectrum keratins	+/–	–	+
Vimentin	+	+	–
Calretinin	–	–	+
WT-1	–	–	+
Molecular			
TP53 mutation	+	–	–
Cyclin D1 overexpression	+	–	ND
EGFR amplification	+	–	ND

EGFR, *Epidermal growth factor receptor;* ND, *not determined; +, consistently present; ++, key feature; –, not present; +/–, sometimes present.*

However, osteosarcomatous, rhabdomyosarcomatous, or chondrosarcomatous differentiation may be present as well.

Immunohistochemically, the epithelial component is typically keratin positive, whereas the sarcomatous component usually stains with vimentin. However, keratin or vimentin may be seen occasionally in either component of the tumor.

By electron microscopy, a mixture of cell types has been identified, ranging from pure epithelial cells, to cells that show a combination of epithelial and sarcomatous features, to cells with pure sarcomatous differentiation.[101] It is these ultrastructural findings, combined with the histological finding in most cases of areas of transition between epithelial and sarcomatous differentiation, that have led to the prevailing theory that these tumors are derived from diverse differentiation (metaplasia) of the carcinomatous element. In addition, molecular studies have found shared chromosome losses and mutations in both the carcinomatous and sarcomatous elements, with additional changes found only in the sarcomatous areas, further supporting this theory of histogenesis.[102]

Differential Diagnosis

Esophageal spindle cell carcinomas must be differentiated from pure sarcomas (e.g., liposarcoma, leiomyosarcoma), including those primary to the esophagus and those involving the esophagus by direct spread or metastasis. Recognition of the distinctive gross features and pattern of esophageal involvement, as well as the presence of malignant or premalignant epithelial elements, strongly favors a diagnosis of spindle cell carcinoma (Table 24.4). Extensive sampling of the tumor and keratin immunostains are often necessary. On occasion, biphasic malignant mesotheliomas may spread from the pleura to involve the esophagus, but these are distinguished by the appropriate clinical history and by the distinctive immunophenotype of mesothelioma (positive for D2-40, WT-1, and calretinin; negative for CEA, MOC31, Ber-EP4).[103]

Prognosis

Spindle cell carcinomas are potentially aggressive tumors, with roughly 50% of cases having lymph node metastasis at the time of diagnosis. Nevertheless, the overall survival rate for this tumor type in recent series has approached 60% (better than conventional squamous cell carcinoma), in part reflecting the larger proportion of tumors detected at an early stage because of their exophytic growth.[100,104] The sarcomatous component usually exhibits a more aggressive biologic behavior and a higher propensity to metastasize.

Verrucous Squamous Cell Carcinoma

Clinical Features

Verrucous carcinoma is a rare low-grade malignant neoplasm, first described in the oral cavity by Ackerman in 1948. Affected patients range from 36 to 76 years of age, and the disease has a male predilection. These tumors may grow very large before the onset of symptoms, with a

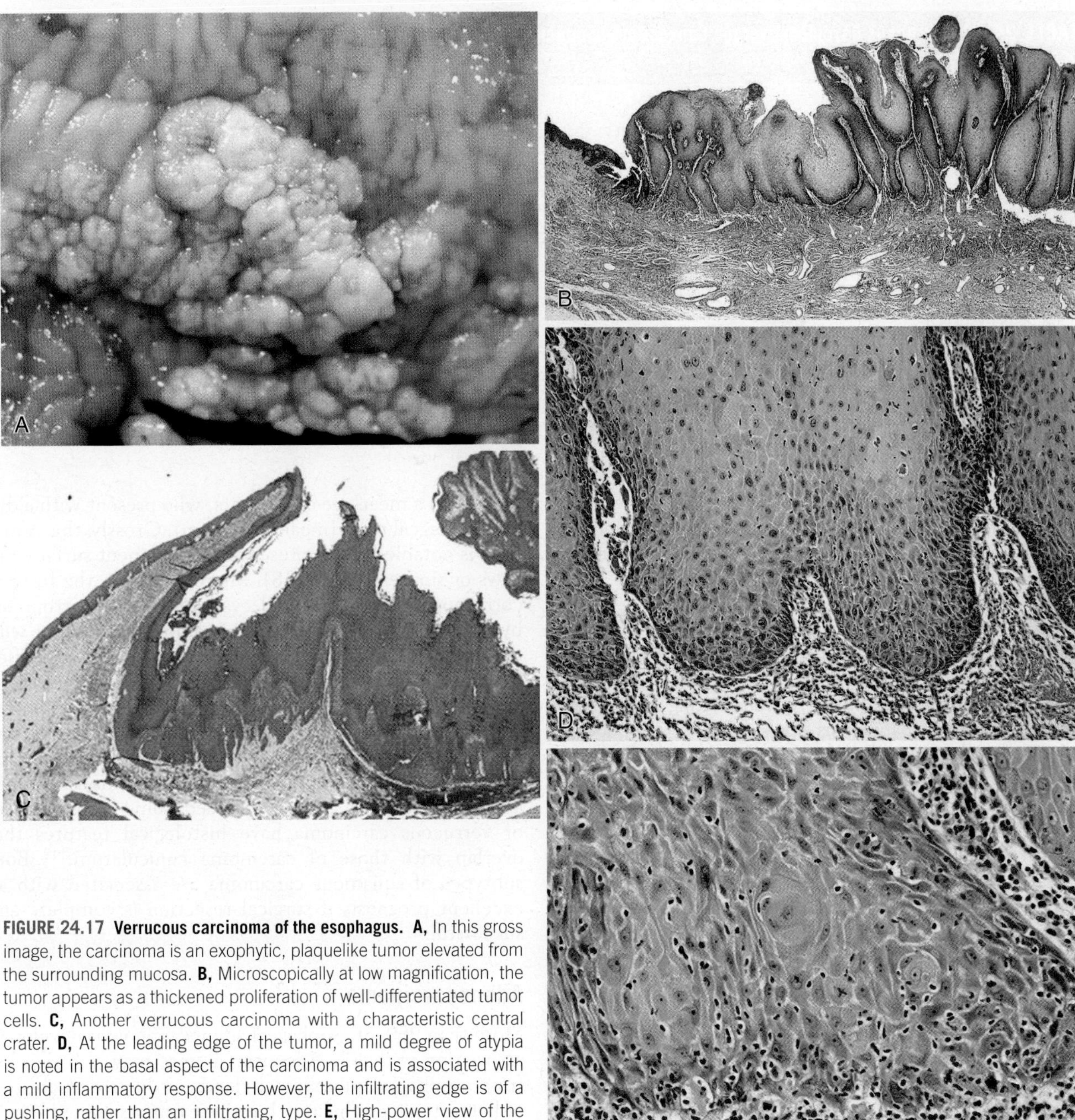

FIGURE 24.17 Verrucous carcinoma of the esophagus. A, In this gross image, the carcinoma is an exophytic, plaquelike tumor elevated from the surrounding mucosa. **B,** Microscopically at low magnification, the tumor appears as a thickened proliferation of well-differentiated tumor cells. **C,** Another verrucous carcinoma with a characteristic central crater. **D,** At the leading edge of the tumor, a mild degree of atypia is noted in the basal aspect of the carcinoma and is associated with a mild inflammatory response. However, the infiltrating edge is of a pushing, rather than an infiltrating, type. **E,** High-power view of the basal aspect of the tumor shows enlarged irregular nuclei, prominent nucleoli, and slight loss of polarity of the tumor cells.

resultant long delay in diagnosis. Presenting complaints are usually dysphagia, weight loss, coughing, and hematemesis. The pathogenesis has been related to various causes of chronic mucosal irritation such as caustic injury (lye), achalasia, lichen planus, diverticular disease, and GERD.[105,106] No definite link with HPV infection has been established.[107]

Pathological Features

Pathologically, verrucous carcinomas have an exophytic papillary growth pattern and often occupy most, or even the entire, circumference of the esophageal lumen. These tumors show characteristic luminal stricturing and erosion, with necrotic and keratinaceous surface debris. Microscopically, the characteristic features are those of a very well-differentiated verrucoid, or papillomatous, proliferation of squamous cells with mild cytological atypia, prominent acanthosis, hyperkeratosis, swollen rete pegs, and inflammation (Fig. 24.17). Invasion is usually difficult to assess because it is typically in the form of broad pushing margins. Classic tumors show a central "crater" of keratin with heaped up edges due to acanthotic squamous epithelium. Mitoses may be limited to the basal layers of the tumor or, rarely, scattered in the mid layers as well. Although the degree of cytological atypia is considered "mild," often the cells are larger in size than their benign counterparts and show enlarged nuclei with irregular nuclear contours, prominent nucleoli, and slight pleomorphism with loss of polarity. These features may extend several layers above the basal

TABLE 24.5 Verrucous Carcinoma versus Conventional Squamous Cell Carcinoma versus Reactive Squamous Epithelium

Feature	Verrucous Carcinoma	Conventional SCC	Reactive Squamous
Clinical			
Risk factors	Chronic mucosal irritation	Alcohol, tobacco	Esophagitis
Sex	M > F	M >> F	M = F
Age range	4th-8th decade	7th decade and older	Wide
Behavior	Locally aggressive	Aggressive, metastases	Benign
Pathological			
Gross appearance	Plaquelike	Exophytic, ulcerative, or infiltrative	Esophagitis
Squamous dysplasia	+/–	+	–
Nuclear pleomorphism	–	+	–
Infiltrative border	–	+	+

SCC, *Squamous cell carcinoma. +, consistently present; ++, key feature; –, not present; +/–, sometimes present.*

layer of the squamous epithelium. Furthermore, some areas of these tumors may show lack of surface maturation. A mild inflammatory response at the tumor–stroma interface is common.

Differential Diagnosis

The key entity in the differential diagnosis is benign squamous papilloma (see Table 24.1). Clinical and endoscopic findings are usually helpful in differentiating these two tumors. Squamous papillomas are small (<3 cm), localized, discrete lesions, whereas verrucous carcinomas more commonly show extensive or circumferential involvement of the esophageal wall. Microscopically, papillomas may display koilocytosis and do not show a pushing deep margin, submucosal extension, or the mild but definite cytological atypia of verrucous carcinomas. Accordingly, pathologists should be cautious about making a diagnosis of verrucous carcinoma based on a biopsy specimen because the superficial aspects of both lesions may be indistinguishable, and both may even be mistaken for regenerative epithelium if the endoscopic findings are unknown. However, reactive squamous epithelium is usually associated with esophagitis and not with a mass lesion, and the normal mucosal architecture of rete ridges will be maintained. Finally, the diagnosis of verrucous carcinoma should be reserved for tumors with the characteristic pushing lower border and should not be used for well-differentiated squamous cell carcinomas that show an infiltrative growth pattern and higher cytological grade in even a portion of the tumor (Table 24.5).

Prognosis

Lymph node metastasis may be present rarely, but no cases with distant metastasis have ever been reported.[108,109] However, these are locally aggressive tumors that often form fistulous tracts with surrounding organs and, as a result, may cause significant morbidity and mortality.[110]

Esophageal Carcinoma Cuniculatum

Carcinoma cuniculatum is an unusual, extremely well-differentiated variant of squamous cell carcinoma that has been reported in approximately nine patients.[111] The tumor is more common in men (male-to-female ratio, 7:2), with a mean age of 57 years, who present with a distal esophageal mass (mean size, 4 cm). Grossly, this tumor type is notable for the presence of prominent surface furrows or sinuses (Fig. 24.18). Microscopically, the furrows correspond to keratin-filled cysts or cavities surrounded by acanthotic, hyperkeratotic squamous epithelium with only mild atypia. Squamous dysplasia was not identified in the surrounding mucosa in any of the published cases, and studies for HPV were consistently negative. None of the reported patients showed lymph node metastasis, and none died of disease after surgical resection. Distinction of this tumor type from verrucous carcinoma is difficult and may, in fact, be arbitrary. Indeed, some reported cases of verrucous carcinoma have histological features that overlap with those of carcinoma cuniculatum.[112] Both subtypes of squamous carcinoma are associated with an excellent prognosis if surgical resection is complete and successful.

Adenocarcinoma

More than 95% of esophageal adenocarcinomas develop in association with BE. Adenocarcinomas may also develop from esophageal submucosal glands or ducts or from foci of heterotopic epithelium, but these tumors are extremely rare (see Non–Barrett's-Associated Adenocarcinoma). Adenocarcinomas that arise in the gastric cardia are discussed further in Chapter 25. Key features are summarized in Box 24.4.

Clinical Features

The incidence of adenocarcinoma of the esophagus has increased dramatically in the past 2 to 3 decades. This tumor now constitutes more than 50% of all esophageal carcinomas diagnosed in the United States, and it is the most common tumor in the distal esophagus.[1,2,40] In 2016, the overall incidence of esophageal adenocarcinoma in the United States was estimated at 3.0 per 100,000 population.[1,2]

The demographic characteristics of patients with adenocarcinoma are similar to those of patients with BE. BE-associated adenocarcinoma affects predominantly older men (mean age, 60 years; male-to-female ratio, 3:1 to 7:1), and more than 80% of patients are white.[2,40] Depending

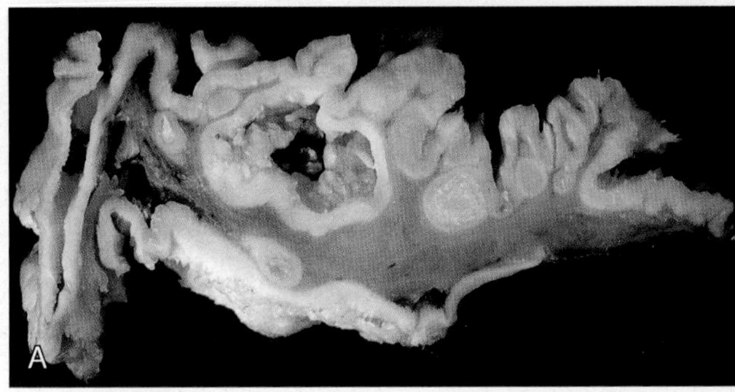

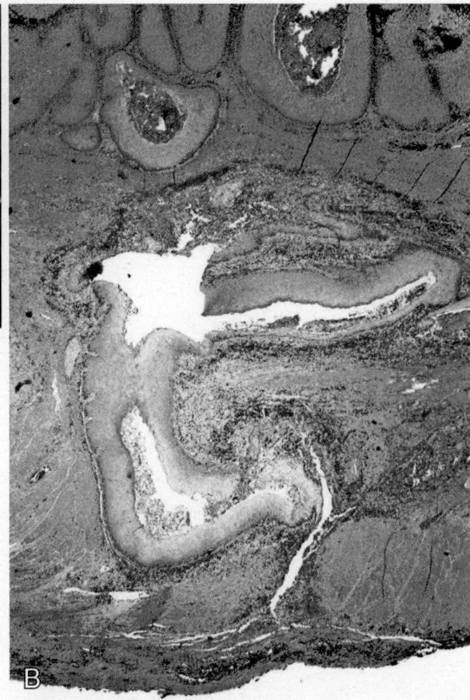

FIGURE 24.18 Esophageal carcinoma cuniculatum. A, Gross photograph of the tumor, showing prominent surface furrows and sinuses. **B,** Low-power photomicrograph of the same tumor shown in **A** demonstrates nests of well-differentiated squamous epithelium and central cavitation. (*Courtesy Dr. Xiuli Liu, MD, Cleveland Clinic, Cleveland, Ohio.*)

BOX 24.4 Esophageal Adenocarcinoma: Key Features

Clinical/endoscopic
- Mean age, 60 years; M > F, 80% white
- Dysphagia, odynophagia, or obstruction; weight loss.
- Majority lower third of esophagus or gastroesophageal junction
- Infiltrative > fungating > flat > polypoid (protruding)
- Aggressive, poor prognosis

Histological
- Grade 1: >95% of tumor composed of glands
- Grade 2: 50% to 95% of tumor composed of glands
- Grade 3: <49% of tumor composed of glands
- Subtypes: mucinous, signet ring, hepatoid

Special/immunohistochemical stains
- Alcian blue, mucicarmine positive
- CK7+/CK20–
- CDX2+

Molecular
- P53, cyclin D1
- HER2 amplification in 15% to 25%

Differential diagnosis
- High-grade dysplasia in Barrett's esophagus
- Gastric adenocarcinoma (tumor location >2 cm distal to esophagogastric junction)
- Metastatic adenocarcinoma

Prognostic factors/features to report
- Tumor stage (Tumor–Node–Metastasis classification)
- Tumor grade/differentiation
- Lymphovascular, perineural invasion
- Residual tumor after neoadjuvant therapy
- Deep/adventitial margin

on the size and location of the tumor, patients may present with dysphagia, odynophagia, or obstruction. Progressive dysphagia and weight loss are ominous signs that are usually associated with advanced disease.

Pathogenesis and Risk Factors

The most significant risk factor for adenocarcinoma is BE, currently defined in the United States by the presence of columnar epithelium (with goblet cells) anywhere in the tubular esophagus; BE develops in approximately 6% to 12% of patients with GERD[113,114] (Table 24.6). Obesity, most likely through its association with GERD and BE, is associated with an increased risk of developing adenocarcinoma compared with a normal body mass index, although the precise magnitude of risk and influence of weight loss on risk modification are uncertain.[115] Tobacco use confers an elevated risk for developing adenocarcinoma both in the general population and in BE patients, although the magnitude of risk (approximately two- to threefold) does not approach the levels observed for esophageal squamous cell carcinoma. No consistent association between alcohol use and adenocarcinoma has been found in recent epidemiological studies. Other environmental factors implicated in increased risk include reduced fruit and vegetable consumption, increased dietary fat, and decreased physical activity. An inverse association with NSAID and statin use has been reported.[115]

The overall prevalence of adenocarcinoma in patients with BE was estimated to be between 5% and 28% in early studies.[116] However, many of the early studies of adenocarcinoma in patients with BE were retrospective and overestimated

TABLE 24.6 Risk Factors for the Development of Barrett's Esophagus and Barrett's Esophagus–Associated Adenocarcinoma

Factor	BE	BE-Associated Dysplasia, Adenocarcinoma
Risk Factors		
Chronic GERD	++	–
Age >50 years	+	+
Male sex	+	–
Central obesity	+	+
Caucasian race	+	–
Tobacco use	+	+
Hiatus hernia	+	+
First-degree relative with BE	+	–
Length of BE	+	+
Alcohol use	–	–
Protective factors		
NSAIDs	–	+
PPI	–	+
Statin	–	+
Helicobacter pylori infection	+	+

Adapted from Odze RD, Montgomery EA, Wang HH, et al. eds. Tumors of the Esophagus and Stomach. *AFIP Atlas of Tumor Pathology, Fourth Series, Fascicle 28. Arlington VA: American Registry of Pathology; 2019, 51-91.*

BE, *Barrett's esophagus;* GERD, *gastroesophageal reflux disease;* NSAIDs, *nonsteroidal antiinflammatory drugs;* PPI, *proton pump inhibitors. +, consistently present; ++, key feature; –, not present.*

the magnitude of risk.[117] More recent studies suggest that patients with BE have an approximately 11-fold increased risk for the development of adenocarcinoma compared with the general population.[118] Indeed, only a small percentage of patients with BE (1% to 5%, or 0.1% to 0.5% per year) develop adenocarcinoma when followed prospectively.[118-123] Factors that increase the risk for adenocarcinoma include the presence, grade, and extent of dysplasia in BE[119,124-126]; the presence of DNA aneuploidy in BE[127]; greater lengths of BE[124,125,127]; and the presence of a hiatal hernia.[113,119,125] As noted earlier, tobacco use also contributes to the risk of malignant progression in BE patients.[114]

It should be noted that although metaplastic epithelium is found adjacent to most carcinomas, the majority (up to 88%) of esophageal adenocarcinomas are identified in patients who have not been previously diagnosed with BE.[123] This observation has led some investigators to hypothesize that distinct patient populations with rapid and slow progression of BE to adenocarcinoma may exist, although the basis for such a distinction has not been identified.[128]

Goblet Cell versus Nongoblet Columnar Metaplasia

One current area of controversy concerns the magnitude of risk for adenocarcinoma in patients with metaplastic esophageal columnar mucosa without intestinal metaplasia (goblet cells). Although intestinal (goblet cell) metaplasia has traditionally been used to define BE,[17] some clinical guidelines, such as in the UK, require only the endoscopic finding of columnar lined esophagus, regardless of whether intestinal metaplasia is present, to establish a diagnosis of BE.[129] Biopsy specimens from columnar-lined esophageal segments may contain large areas devoid of goblet cells. However, these nongoblet areas have been found to express markers of intestinal differentiation such as CDX-2, MUC2, and TFF3,[113] and to harbor genetic alterations associated with neoplastic progression.[130,131] A retrospective study of 712 BE patients found that the risk for adenocarcinoma was similar whether the index esophageal biopsy samples had glandular mucosa with intestinal metaplasia or nonintestinalized glandular mucosa (4.5% and 3.6%, respectively, after a 12-year follow-up period).[132] Furthermore, in several series of BE-associated "early" adenocarcinomas, 34% to 57% occurred within nongoblet columnar mucosa.[133,134] Although additional population-based and preferably prospective studies are needed to more precisely define the relative importance of nonintestinal mucosa as a precursor to adenocarcinoma, current evidence suggests that this pathway accounts for a definite, albeit small, percentage of malignant esophageal tumors.

Molecular Features

The molecular genetic alterations that underlie the development of BE-associated adenocarcinoma have been the subject of extensive study.[47,113,128,135] Similar to most epithelial malignancies, esophageal adenocarcinomas show multiple changes, which are acquired in a stepwise fashion during the progression of dysplasia to carcinoma. Widespread genomic instability is the molecular hallmark of progression to malignancy, and it is believed to be the cause, not the consequence, of carcinogenesis in BE. Most, if not all, chromosomes are affected in this process, either by increased number or by alteration of content (e.g., additions, deletions). In fact, alterations in DNA content (aneuploidy) in nondysplastic BE is a strong predictor of progression to high-grade dysplasia and adenocarcinoma.[113,128] By contrast, DNA mismatch repair defects resulting in microsatellite instability occur infrequently (5% to 10%) in BE-associated adenocarcinomas.[136] Abnormalities in DNA content can be measured in a variety of ways, including fluorescence in situ hybridization (FISH), chromosomal karyotyping, comparative genomic hybridization, flow cytometry, and, more recently, image cytometry.

Among the most common single marker alterations are inactivation (through mutation or transcriptional silencing) of the tumor suppressor proteins p16, p27, and p53 and of the adenomatous polyposis coli *(APC)* gene (75% to 92% of tumors) and overexpression or amplification of cyclin D1 (22% to 64% of cases).[128,137] Amplification of the genes for the growth factor receptor EGFR (13% to 30%), ERBB2/HER2 (15% to 25%), and MET (2%), although present in only a minority of adenocarcinomas, have significant therapeutic implications.[138-140] Many of these abnormalities occur even before the onset of morphological dysplasia. For example, p53 alterations were found in nondysplastic mucosa of up to 69% of BE patients who subsequently progressed to high-grade dysplasia or adenocarcinoma.[141] In another study, methylation, loss of heterozygosity (LOH), or mutations in p16 were observed in as much as 80% of BE patients before the onset of dysplasia or carcinoma.[137]

Some of these techniques are currently being proposed as potentially providing prognostic information in BE patients.[113,119,128] However, at present, no specific biomarkers or biomarker panel has been recommended for routine clinical use to help manage BE by potentially altering the frequency of surveillance endoscopies.[17]

Pathological Features

Gross Pathology

BE-associated adenocarcinomas are located almost exclusively in the distal third of the esophagus in areas of involvement with BE. Distal tumors frequently show extension into the proximal stomach. They may be classified as polypoid (protruding) (5% to 10%), flat (10% to 15%), fungating (20% to 25%), or infiltrative (40% to 50%) (Fig. 24.19A,B).[40,142] Early carcinomas may be undetectable or may appear only as slightly irregular, depressed or elevated lesions.[143] Diffusely infiltrative tumors are uncommon. Large tumors may obliterate the underlying or adjacent Barrett's mucosa, particularly those that arise in the distal esophagus at or near the level of the esophagogastric junction (EGJ). In such instances, it may occasionally be difficult to determine whether an adenocarcinoma located near or at the EGJ is, in fact, esophageal (BE-related) or gastric in origin. Careful attention to the location of the epicenter and proximal and distal extent of the tumor with respect to anatomic landmarks, and sampling of tumor and adjacent mucosa, can aid in this distinction. Patients who have been treated with preoperative chemotherapy or radiation therapy may have little or no gross residual tumor left in their resection specimen. In fact, as much as 50% of patients treated with neoadjuvant therapy show either no, or only minimal, microscopic residual tumor after surgery.[144,145]

Microscopic Pathology

These tumors, like squamous cell carcinomas, typically spread vertically through the esophageal wall and metastasize to regional lymph nodes. Adenocarcinomas are graded as well, moderately, or poorly differentiated. The AJCC grading system classifies tumors by the proportion of tumor that is composed of glands.[85] However, most tumors are moderately or well differentiated.[40,142] Some tumors show variations in grade within the same tumor, and the highest grade is usually recorded for prognostic purposes.

Well-differentiated (grade 1) carcinomas (i.e., >95% of tumor composed of glands) are made almost entirely of irregularly shaped or cystic glandular and tubular profiles that infiltrate the mucosa, submucosa, and muscularis (see Fig. 24.19C). The tumor cells are cuboidal to columnar in shape and contain irregular nuclei with coarse or vesicular chromatin, prominent nucleoli, and a variable amount of eosinophilic or clear cytoplasm. In moderately differentiated (grade 2) carcinomas (50% to 95% of tumor composed of glands), tumor cells are arranged in solid nests and irregular clusters as well as glands (see Fig. 24.19D). In these tumors, the cells within the glandular profiles may adopt a cribriform pattern and show considerable stratification. Poorly differentiated (grade 3) carcinomas (5% to 49% of tumor composed of glands) often infiltrate the esophageal wall in a diffuse manner and usually with a prominent desmoplastic stroma. The tumor cells are arranged in sheets and in poorly formed glandular lumina; signet ring cells and bizarre pleomorphic tumor cells may be present. Interestingly, a subset of poorly differentiated adenocarcinomas involve the surface squamous epithelium in the form of single cells that grow in a pagetoid fashion.[56] Other intestinal cell types, such as Paneth cells and endocrine cells,[146] are present focally in as many as 20% of adenocarcinomas.

Approximately 5% to 10% of adenocarcinomas contain areas of mucinous (colloid) histology, characterized by tumor cell clusters floating in pools of mucin.[147] Another 5% contain areas of infiltrating signet ring cells (see Fig. 24.19E), and occasional cases show clear cell morphology (see Fig. 24.19F). Rare tumors may show multidirectional differentiation, with coincident areas of glandular, squamous, or neuroendocrine differentiation (see later discussion).

In patients treated with preoperative chemoradiotherapy, residual tumor cells may be present merely as individual cells or as small, isolated clusters of cells, in association with ulceration, dense fibrosis, or pools of mucin.[144,145] These cells are frequently pleomorphic, showing extreme nuclear irregularity and enlargement; on occasion, they may be difficult to distinguish from reactive mesenchymal cells. Immunohistochemistry for keratins often helps in this situation, being generally positive in the tumor cells and negative in the mesenchymal cells. Clusters of residual keratin-positive endocrine cells may be present in the deep lamina propria of treated areas, but these should not be mistaken for residual carcinoma.[148] Sometimes, the only sign of a treated tumor is acellular pools of mucin dissecting through the layers of the esophageal wall (Fig. 24.20). However, acellular mucin pools do not result in an increased risk of recurrence or metastasis.[144,145] Complete examination of the tumor bed is necessary to exclude the possibility of residual tumor and provide accurate prognostic information.[149] The degree of response to neoadjuvant therapy is scored using a standardized scoring system (Table 24.7).

Special Studies

Special studies are not usually necessary to establish a diagnosis of esophageal adenocarcinoma, but they can occasionally be useful in characterizing poorly differentiated lesions, identifying resections with little or no residual tumor after neoadjuvant therapy, or distinguishing primary esophageal tumors from metastases. Tumor cells are positive for mucin by histochemical stains including mucicarmine, PAS-diastase, and Alcian blue, although positive cells may be rare or nonexistent in poorly differentiated tumors. Adenocarcinomas stain positively for broad-spectrum keratins and are positive for CK7 and negative for CK20 in approximately 70% to 90% of cases.[150] Reactivity for the intestine-specific transcription factor CDX2 is present in 34% to 92% of cases.[151] While in our experience these tumors do not show extensive expression for the lung/thyroid epithelial marker TTF-1, focal expression is present in a proportion of esophageal tumors, and this marker should be interpreted in clinical context and in combination with other stains.[152] Focal positivity for neuroendocrine markers, such as chromogranin, can be found in 20% to 50% of cases.[146,153]

Assessment of HER2 status is recommended for all cancer patients who are candidates for adjuvant chemotherapy.[139] The easiest initial method is by immunohistochemistry, with staining scored 0+ to 3+ using recently

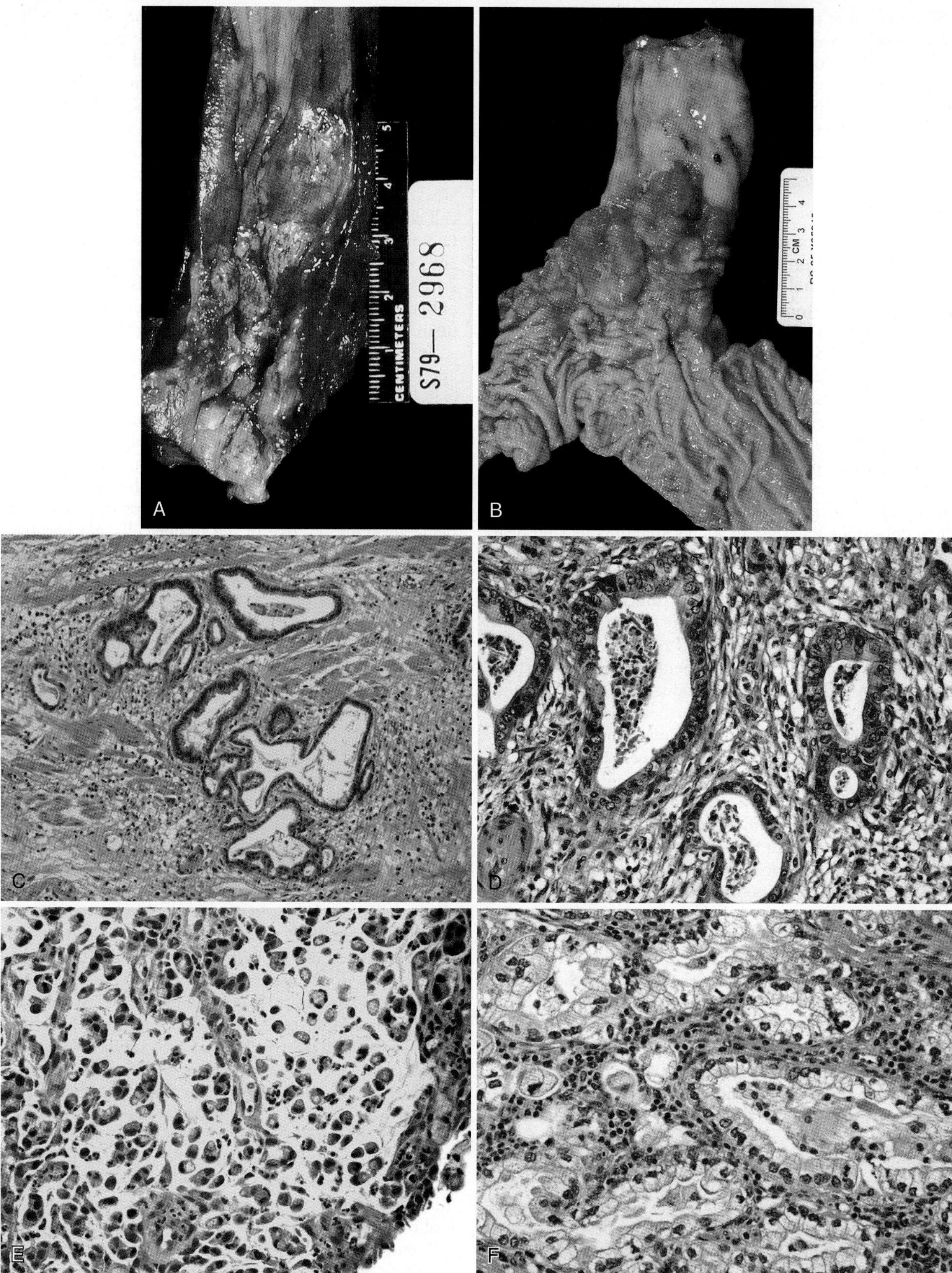

FIGURE 24.19 Barrett's esophagus (BE)-associated adenocarcinoma. A, An irregular, ulcerating, constricting tumor is present just above the level of the esophagogastric junction (EGJ) in association with tongues of BE. **B,** Gross photograph of a tumor arising at the EGJ. Although no Barrett's mucosa is grossly evident, it was discovered on sections taken from the proximal edge of the tumor. **C,** Well-differentiated adenocarcinoma, composed entirely of infiltrating tubular glands. **D,** Microscopic appearance of a moderately differentiated adenocarcinoma characterized by gland formation and more marked nuclear pleomorphism. **E,** A poorly differentiated tumor composed of signet ring cells floating in pools of mucin. **F,** Clear cell–type adenocarcinoma. Notice the tumor cell cytoplasm.

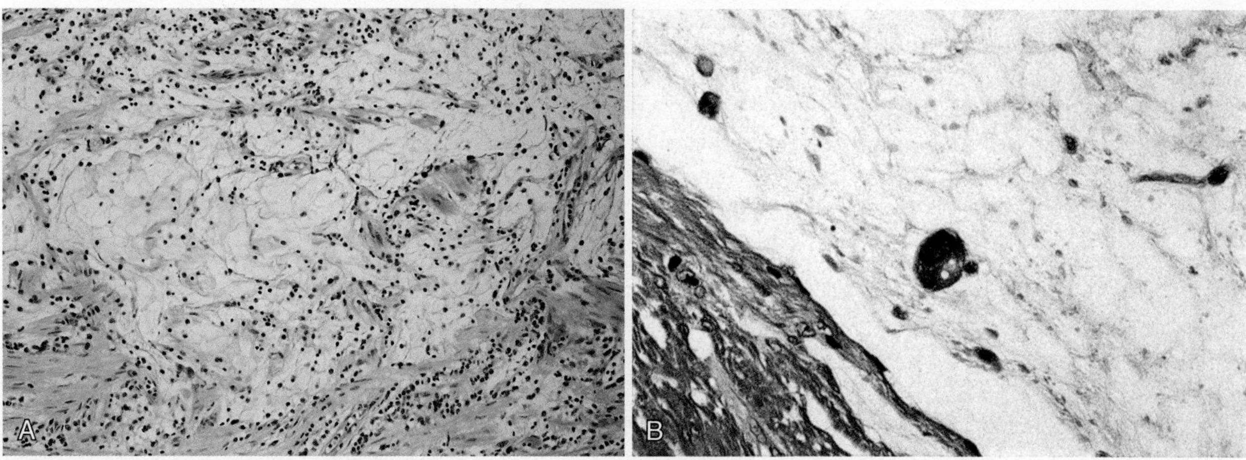

FIGURE 24.20 A, Acellular pools of mucin in the wall of the esophagus in a patient who had neoadjuvant chemoradiotherapy for esophageal adenocarcinoma. No malignant cells are present. **B,** Another case shows rare, highly atypical, enlarged, treated tumor cells floating within a pool of mucin.

TABLE 24.7 Tumor Regression Score for Esophageal Carcinomas

Description	Tumor Regression Score
No viable cancer cells (complete response)	0
Single cells or rare small groups of cancer cells (near complete response)	1
Residual cancer with evident tumor regression, but more than single cells or rare small groups of cancer cells (partial response)	2
Extensive residual cancer with no evident tumor regression (poor or no response)	3

Adapted from Shi C, Berlin J, Branton P, et al. Protocol for the examination of specimens from patients with carcinoma of the esophagus. College of American Pathologists; 2017. https://documents.cap.org/protocols/cp-esophagus-17protocol-4000.pdf. Accessed June 1, 2019.

published criteria (Table 24.8). Patients with 3+ staining have been found to respond to anti-HER2 agents such as trastuzumab. Patients with 2+ immunohistochemical staining are heterogeneous with respect to the amplification of the HER2 locus, which in these patients is assessed by FISH. Because expression and amplification of HER2 may be heterogeneous within gastric and esophageal carcinomas, the region with the highest staining should be used for scoring. Up to 45% of adenocarcinomas express the immune checkpoint protein PD-L1, making these patients potentially eligible for immunotherapy with pembrolizumab or other immune-checkpoint inhibitors.[154]

Differential Diagnosis

Most of the difficulties related to diagnosing adenocarcinomas occur in the evaluation of endoscopic biopsy specimens, in which the distinction between high-grade dysplasia and intramucosal or invasive carcinoma may be uncertain. Architectural features such as single cell infiltration of the lamina propria, sharply angulated glands, small glands in a back-to-back pattern, confluent glands or a sheetlike growth pattern, and glandular intraluminal necrosis support a diagnosis of adenocarcinoma (Fig. 24.21).[155] It is not uncommon for dysplastic glands to be situated within the fibers of the muscularis mucosae, which in BE is often duplicated and fragmented. This finding should not be overinterpreted as representing submucosally invasive tumor unless other features mentioned earlier are also present.

For patients treated with preoperative chemoradiotherapy, keratin immunostaining may be necessary to distinguish rare residual tumor cells from mesenchymal cells with treatment effect. In some patients, it may be necessary to exclude the possibility of metastasis or spread to the esophagus from another primary site such as the stomach, lung, or breast. The presence of BE and dysplastic epithelium adjacent to the carcinoma is normally considered convincing evidence that the tumor has arisen from the esophagus. In addition, primary esophageal adenocarcinomas are negative or only focally positive for TTF-1[152] or estrogen receptor,[156] markers of lung and breast tumors, respectively.

Distinguishing an esophageal adenocarcinoma from a proximal gastric tumor can be difficult, particularly if the tumor has obliterated adjacent or underlying Barrett's epithelium (Table 24.9). Distal gastric adenocarcinomas often arise in a background of intestinal metaplasia of the gastric mucosa and are positive for CK20 in as many as 90% of cases, compared with esophageal adenocarcinomas, which less commonly stain for this antigen.[150,156,157] However, esophageal and gastric cardia adenocarcinomas have very similar CK7 and CK20 staining patterns in most studies, which makes distinction of these tumors difficult on the basis of immunohistochemistry alone.[158,159] In some investigators' views, differentiation between esophageal and EGJ or cardia adenocarcinomas has no epidemiological or biological basis, and all tumors that arise in this region should be considered "esophageal" adenocarcinomas secondary to GERD.[159] In fact, under current AJCC and WHO guidelines, cancers of the esophagus and esophagogastric junction (if the epicenter of the tumor is located within 2 cm of the EGJ) are considered together for staging and management purposes.[40,85,86,92] As stated above, evidence indicates that a subset of EGJ carcinomas

TABLE 24.8 HER2 Immunohistochemistry of Esophageal and Gastroesophageal Junction Carcinoma

Surgical Specimen: Staining Pattern	Biopsy Specimen: Staining Pattern	Score	HER2 Expression Assessment
No reactivity or membranous reactivity in<10% of tumor cells	No reactivity or no membranous reactivity in any tumor cell	0	Negative
Faint/barely perceptible membranous reactivity in≥10% of tumor cells; cells are reactive only in part of their membrane	Tumor cell cluster* with a faint/barely perceptible membranous reactivity irrespective of percentage of tumor cells stained	1+	Negative
Weak to moderate, complete, basolateral or lateral membranous reactivity in≥10% of tumor cells	Tumor cell cluster* with a weak to moderate, complete, basolateral or lateral membranous reactivity irrespective of percentage of tumor cells stained	2+	Equivocal
Strong, complete, basolateral or lateral membranous Reactivity in≥10% of tumor cells	Tumor cell cluster* with a strong, complete, basolateral or lateral membranous reactivity irrespective of percentage of tumor cells stained	3+	Positive

**Tumor cell cluster (>5 neoplastic cells).*

Adapted from Bartley AN, Washington MK, Ventura CB et al. HER2 testing and clinical decision making in gastroesophageal adenocarcinoma: guideline from the College of American Pathologists, American Society for Clinical Pathology, and American Society of Clinical Oncology. Am J Clin Pathol. *2016 Dec; 146(6): 647-669.*

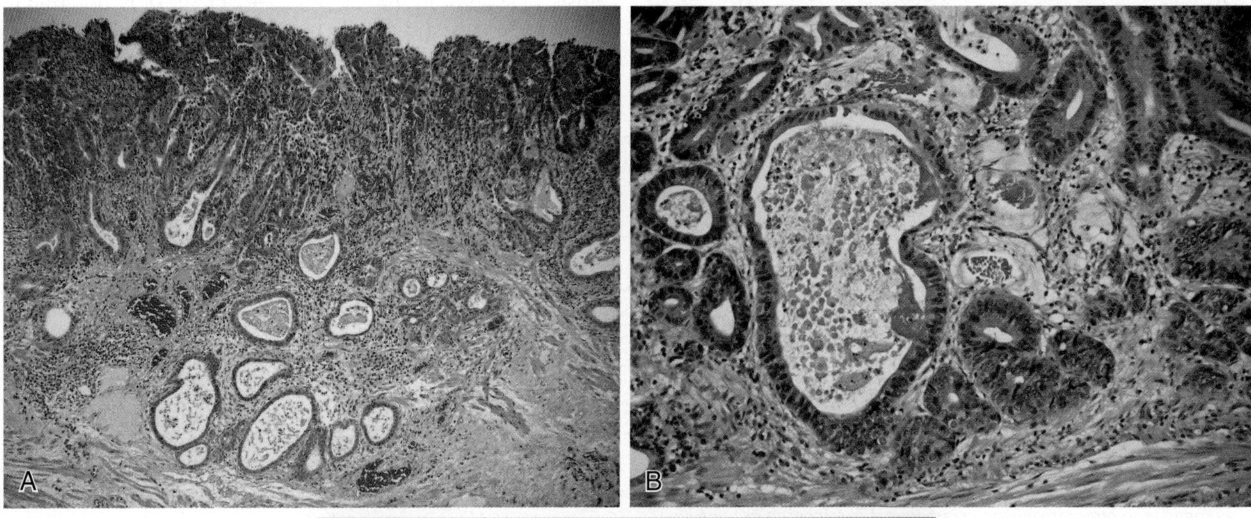

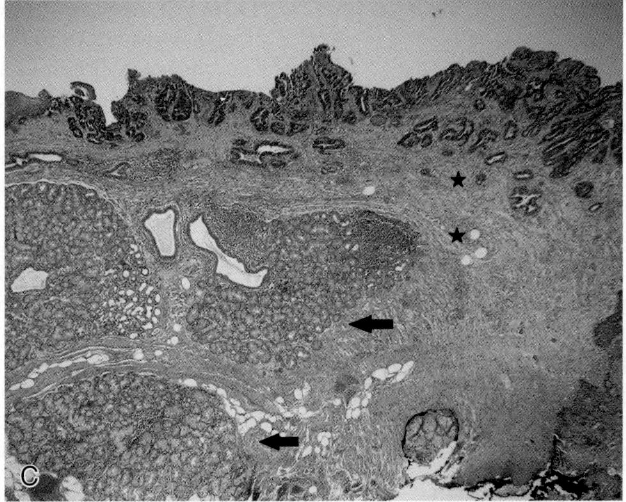

FIGURE 24.21 A, Intramucosal adenocarcinoma of the esophagus associated with high-grade dysplastic Barrett's esophagus. The lamina propria shows a proliferation of glands infiltrating the lamina propria above the level of the muscularis mucosae *(bottom)*. **B,** High magnification of intramucosal adenocarcinoma, showing luminal necrosis, poorly formed "back-to-back" glands, single cells, and clusters of cells. **C,** Low magnification image of endoscopic mucosal resection for Barrett's esophagus–associated intramucosal adenocarcinoma. Note the thickened and duplicated muscularis mucosae *(stars)* and submucosal glands *(arrows)*.

TABLE 24.9 Barrett's Esophagus (BE)–Associated Adenocarcinoma versus Proximal Gastric Adenocarcinoma

Feature	BE-Associated Adenocarcinoma	Proximal Gastric Adenocarcinoma
Clinical		
Age (yr)	>60	40-60
Sex	M >> F	F = M
GERD risk factor	++	+/–
Helicobacter pylori risk factor	–	+/–
Autoimmune gastritis	+/–	++
Midpoint of tumor	Proximal or at EGJ	Distal to EGJ (epicenter >2 cm)
Gross appearance	Exophytic, ulcerative	Fungating
Pathological		
Adjacent BE	+	–
Adjacent gastric intestinal metaplasia	–	+
Tubular type	+	+
Mucinous type	+/– (10%-15%)	+/–
Signet ring cell type	+/–	+/–
Immunohistochemistry		
CK7+/CK20–	++	+/–
CDX2	+	+
Chromogranin, synaptophysin	+/– (focal)	+/– (focal)
Molecular		
TP53 mutation	+	+
HER2 amplification	+/–	+/–
EGFR amplification	+/–	+/–

EGFR, *Epidermal growth factor receptor;* EGJ, *gastroesophageal junction;* GERD, *gastroesophageal reflux disease; +, consistently present; ++; key feature; –, not present; +/–, sometimes present.*

arise in a background of nonintestinalized gastric mucosa and may reflect a different carcinogenesis pathway that is less highly associated with GERD.[133,134,160,161] Additional study is needed to determine whether EGJ carcinomas of this type should be regarded as a separate biological entity with a natural history distinct from BE-associated adenocarcinomas.

Prognosis and Treatment

The most important prognostic factor in esophageal adenocarcinomas is the AJCC TNM pathological stage. Patients with tumors limited to the mucosa or submucosa have an 80% to 100% 5-year survival rate, compared with 10% to 20% for patients with tumors that extend into or through the muscularis.[85,92,142,143] Lymph node metastasis and a higher number of positive lymph nodes are also associated with reduced survival.[162,163] Lymph node micrometastases, consisting of single tumor cells or small clusters of cells, are present in as many as 30% of patients when sought by keratin immunohistochemistry. Although some studies have found that micrometastases confer a worse prognosis in patients who are otherwise node negative, these data are controversial.[164-166]

The majority of esophageal adenocarcinomas show spread into or through the muscularis propria at the time of clinical presentation. Advanced tumors may spread directly into the mediastinum, aorta, or stomach, and distant metastases to the liver, lungs, and other portions of the gastrointestinal tract are not uncommon. Metastasis to regional (periesophageal and perigastric) lymph nodes is present in approximately 50% to 60% of patients.[142,143,162,167] The likelihood of lymph node metastasis is related to tumor depth.[168,169] In one study of 120 submucosal (T1b) adenocarcinomas, 7.5% of tumors limited to the superficial submucosa had lymph node metastases, compared with 45% of tumors that penetrated into the deep submucosa.[168] In contrast, intramucosal adenocarcinomas have only a 1% to 2% risk of lymph node metastasis, according to a recent meta-analysis.[169] It is important to recognize that up to 90% of patients with BE develop duplication of the muscularis mucosae and separation of the original lamina propria into superficial (new) and deep (original) compartments. However, preliminary studies suggest that lymphatics and blood vessels are present in both lamina propria compartments, but that larger vessels are limited to the original (deep) lamina propria.[170] Indeed, tumors that penetrate through the superficial muscularis mucosae but not the deep (original) muscularis mucosae have rates of lymph node metastasis and survival similar to those of intramucosal carcinomas and should be classified as such with regard to T stage.[171]

With regard to tumor type, mucinous histology is associated with a trend toward poorer overall survival after resection in both univariate and multivariate analyses.[172] In addition, for patients who have undergone preoperative chemoradiotherapy, a complete pathological response (indicating absence of residual tumor) has been found to be an excellent prognostic factor, with rates of survival between 90% and 100%.[144,145,173] Higher tumor grade has been found to be prognostically useful in early-stage tumors and has been incorporated into the most recent AJCC stage groupings. Other histological parameters, such as lymphovascular invasion and circumferential margin involvement, are also adverse predictors of survival.[174] Finally, some molecular alterations, such as loss of p27, and amplification of ERBB2/HER2, MET, or EGFR have been shown to correlate with aggressive tumor behavior and poorer patient survival and form the basis for targeted chemotherapy in selected patients.[138-140]

Adenocarcinomas that have not metastasized to distant sites are treated with esophagectomy. Neoadjuvant chemotherapy or radiotherapy has been advocated as a means of improving resectability and has shown some survival benefit compared with surgery alone in some randomized clinical trials.[88] In patients who have early (intramucosal) adenocarcinomas or in whom the presence of invasion is uncertain, endoscopic mucosal resection may be performed to remove the neoplastic lesion and to more accurately stage the carcinoma as an aid to therapeutic decision making.[175] In a medically unfit patient who is not a candidate for esophagectomy and has an early lesion, esophageal adenocarcinoma may be managed conservatively with a variety of ablative techniques (e.g., photodynamic therapy, which has shown tumor eradication in as many as 90% of patients in some studies).[175,176]

In BE patients with high-grade dysplasia and even intramucosal adenocarcinoma, radiofrequency ablation has resulted in eradication of neoplasia in 80% to 90% of patients, and eradication of metaplastic epithelium in 55% to 75%, in several studies.[17,176] However, dysplasia and carcinoma may persist in such cases, particularly in patients with extensive dysplasia, and may even become buried underneath squamous epithelium, making detection and surveillance still more difficult.[177] With the discovery that nonsteroidal antiinflammatory drugs may reduce the risk of adenocarcinoma, the role of these drugs or other agents in chemoprevention and surveillance is an area of active interest and investigation.[178]

Endoscopic Mucosal Resections for Barrett's-Associated Dysplasia and Carcinoma

Endoscopic resection techniques (endoscopic mucosal resection and endoscopic submucosal dissection) have become accepted and increasingly widely used techniques in the management of Barrett's-associated neoplasia.[175] Handling of these specimens requires proper orientation of resection fragments, with identification and inking of lateral (mucosal) and deep margins, sectioning and embedding perpendicular to the mucosal surface.[179] Parameters reported in addition to the diagnosis (grade of dysplasia or adenocarcinoma) include depth of invasion, differentiation state, presence of lymphovascular invasion, and status of margins with respect to dysplasia and adenocarcinoma (Box 24.5). As mentioned earlier, recognition of a thickened or duplicated muscularis mucosae, and identification of definitive submucosal landmarks such as mucous glands and thick-walled vessels, are helpful in accurately assessing depth of invasion (see Fig. 24.21).

BOX 24.5 Endoscopic Mucosal Resections for Barrett's-Associated Dysplasia and Adenocarcinoma

Gross examination and handling
- Ink lateral (mucosal) and deep margins
- Note orientation if present
- Serially section

Histological parameters to report
- Diagnosis (low-grade dysplasia, high-grade dysplasia, adenocarcinoma)
- Depth of invasion (intramucosal, submucosal)
- Differentiation state
- Lymphovascular invasion
- Margin status (adenocarcinoma and dysplasia)

Dysplasia in Barrett's Esophagus

There is compelling evidence that most, if not all, esophageal adenocarcinomas arise through progression of premalignant or dysplastic lesions in patients with BE. Dysplasia in BE is defined as unequivocal neoplastic change within the columnar epithelium without invasion of the lamina propria. Types of dysplasia include intestinal (most common), foveolar (gastric), serrated, and mixed. Some types show no obvious cytoplasmic differentiation and have been termed nonintestinal or "null." Dysplastic BE shows a range of cytological and architectural abnormalities and is classified as either low-grade or high-grade on the basis of the severity of these features (Fig. 24.22 and Table 24.10).[113] The architecture of dysplastic epithelium may be normal or may show villiform or papillary change, crowding, or irregular glands. Additional distorted architectural features include back-to-back gland formation, increased budding, branching or tortuosity of the crypts, and cribriform change. Cytological features include decreased mucin production, nuclear hyperchromasia and pleomorphism, loss of nuclear polarity, increased N:C ratio, increased mitotic rate with abnormal mitotic figures, and nuclear stratification. Dysplasia in Barrett's esophagus is covered in detail in Chapter 14.

In most cases of dysplasia, the neoplastic epithelium involves the full length of the crypts and surface epithelium. This feature helps distinguish it from reactive epithelium, which usually shows evidence of surface maturation. However, it has been recognized that dysplasia originates in the crypt bases; in early cases, it may involve only the basal portion of the crypts, without evidence of surface involvement.[180] In one study, patients with "basal crypt dysplasia" also had a high rate of molecular aberrations in adjacent Barrett's epithelium and a high association with traditional "full-crypt" dysplasia in other parts of the esophagus. Crypt dysplasia is most often composed of low-grade intestinal-type dysplasia, but high-grade changes may occur less commonly (see Fig. 24.22F).

Variants of Adenocarcinoma

Hepatoid Adenocarcinoma

Rarely, BE-associated adenocarcinomas may show areas of hepatoid morphology, composed of polygonal shaped tumor cells with eosinophilic cytoplasm, arranged in trabeculae or solid sheets resembling hepatocellular carcinoma[181] (Fig. 24.23). Similar to hepatoid adenocarcinomas

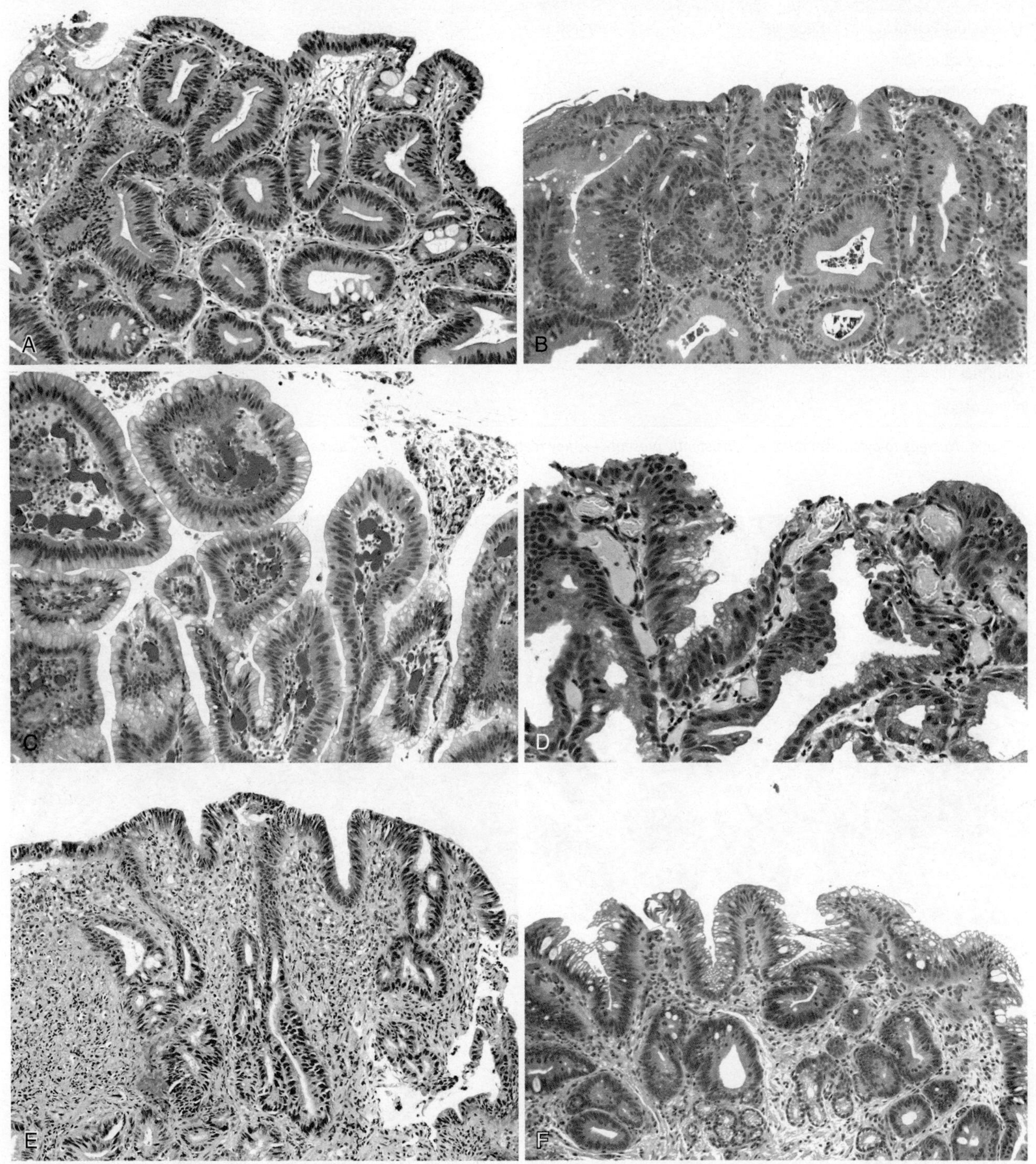

FIGURE 24.22 Dysplasia in Barrett's esophagus (BE). A, Typical appearance of low-grade dysplasia characterized by epithelium containing a proliferation of hyperchromatic pencil-shaped nuclei and a distinct lack of surface maturation. In low-grade dysplasia, the dysplastic nuclei occupy predominantly the basal portion of the cell cytoplasm. **B,** High-grade dysplasia shows a more tightly compact arrangement of highly atypical glands with marked hyperchromaticity, pseudostratification, nuclear pleomorphism, and loss of nuclear polarity. Lack of surface maturation is also apparent in this lesion. **C,** Foveolar variant of dysplasia shows mucinous columnar cells resembling gastric surface epithelium, with enlarged, hyperchromatic, basally located nuclei. Notice the absence of goblet cells. **D,** Serrated-type dysplasia. In this example of dysplasia, the dysplastic cells assume a grooved or serrated apical border. **E,** Low-power image of a biopsy specimen from a patient with BE shows columnar atypia considered indefinite for dysplasia. Although the epithelium demonstrates mild nuclear pseudostratification and hyperchromaticity, a slight degree of surface maturation is seen focally, and the lesion is associated with a significant degree of acute and chronic inflammation and lamina fibrosis suggestive of healing erosion. **F,** Crypt dysplasia. The dysplastic epithelium, which shows significant nuclear pleomorphism and loss of polarity, is found only in the deep portion of the epithelium. The surface epithelium present in the section exhibits nuclear hyperchromasia but is categorized as reactive.

TABLE 24.10 Differential Diagnosis of Dysplasia in Barrett's Esophagus

Histological Feature	Reactive	Indefinite	Low-Grade	High-Grade
Surface maturation	+	+	+/–	+/–
Villiform architecture	–	+/–	+/–	+/–
Mucin depletion	+/–	+	+	++
Irregular glands	–	+/–	+	++
Glandular crowding	–	+/–	+	++
Cribriform glands	–	–	–	+
Increased N:C ratio	+/–	+	++	++
Nuclear stratification	–	+	+ (Basal only)	++ (Full thickness)
Nuclear pleomorphism	–	+/–	+	++
Increased mitotic rate	+	+	+	++
Abnormal mitoses	–	+/–	+	++
Inflammation	++	+	+/–	+/–

N:C ratio, *Nucleus-to-cytoplasm ratio; +, consistently present; ++, key feature; –, not present; +/–, sometimes present.*

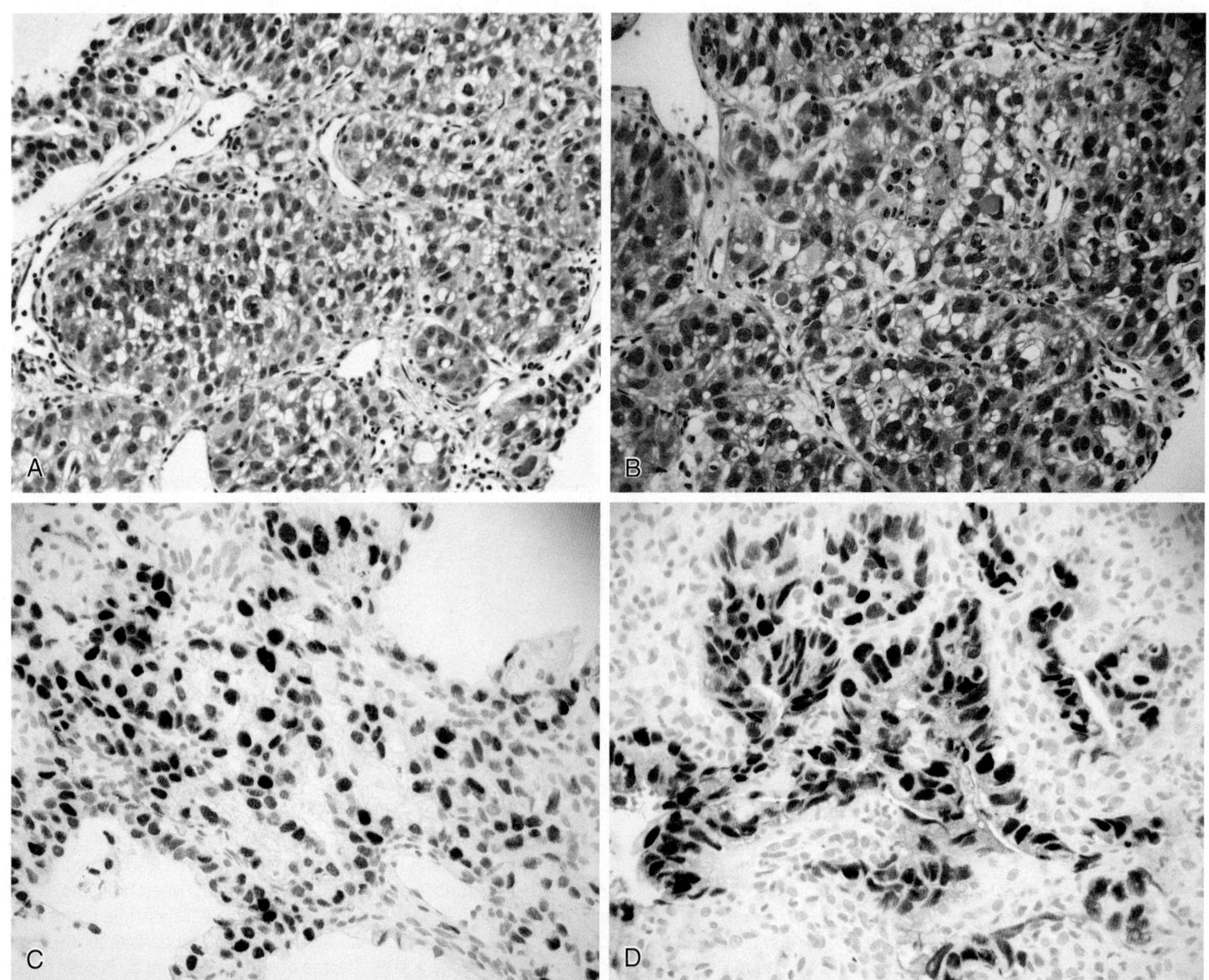

FIGURE 24.23 Hepatoid adenocarcinoma. A, The tumor is comprised of cells with abundant eosinophilic cytoplasm, arranged in trabeculae or solid sheets resembling hepatocellular carcinoma. **B,** Another area of the tumor cells with clear cytoplasm, arranged in nests and trabeculae. **C,** This example expressed the stem cell marker SALL4. **D,** The tumor cells were also positive for the intestinal marker CDX2.

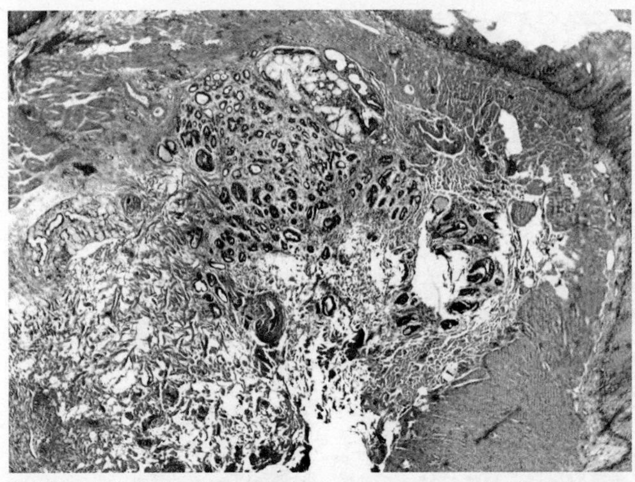

FIGURE 24.24 Well-differentiated adenocarcinoma arising from the submucosal gland or duct system. Residual benign gland is present just superficial to the neoplastic lesion, which is composed of infiltrating tubules. (*Courtesy Dr. Hong-Zen Yeh, Taichung Veterans General Hospital, Taichung, Taiwan.*)

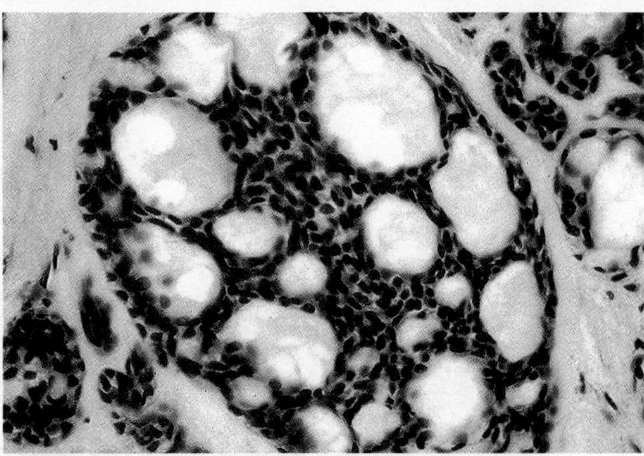

FIGURE 24.25 True adenoid cystic carcinoma of the esophagus. In contrast to basaloid carcinomas, adenoid cystic carcinomas show a proliferation of small hyperchromatic cells with less variation of nuclear size, infrequent mitoses, and no necrosis. The glandular lumina contain a basement membrane–like extracellular material.

arising in the stomach and other organs, these tumors express markers characteristic of hepatocellular carcinoma, such as α-fetoprotein and glypican 3, as well as stem cell markers such as SALL4.[182,183] Recognition of the origin of a hepatoid adenocarcinoma can prove challenging when evaluating biopsies of metastatic lesions. Attention to clinical history (e.g., lack of risk factors for cirrhosis or hepatocellular carcinoma) and radiological findings, and the presence of areas of more typical glandular morphology, are useful in distinguishing these lesions from primary or metastatic hepatocellular carcinoma. Hepatoid adenocarcinomas appear to show an aggressive course with frequent metastases.

Non–Barrett's-Associated Adenocarcinoma

Esophageal adenocarcinomas unrelated to BE are extremely rare and arise either from foci of gastric heterotopia[32,33] or from the submucosal gland/duct system.[14,184] Clinically, patients with heterotopia-associated adenocarcinomas are middle-aged and are seen with symptoms related to dysphagia. Morphologically, adenocarcinomas that arise in ectopic gastric mucosa show a range of differentiation and have also been reported to show a papillary growth pattern (see Fig. 24.6B). Adjacent gastric oxyntic-type mucosa is usually present. Intestinal metaplasia and dysplasia have been reported adjacent to these adenocarcinomas as well. Although these tumors morphologically resemble Barrett's-associated adenocarcinoma, that diagnosis is ruled out by the proximal location of the tumor and the absence of Barrett's epithelium between the tumor and the true EGJ.

Tumors reported to have arisen within the submucosal gland/duct system are typically tubular adenocarcinomas consisting of flat or cuboidal cells with eosinophilic cytoplasm, similar to the native esophageal gland ducts (Fig. 24.24).[184] Another reported example showed a biphasic tumor comprised primarily of a tubular adenocarcinoma with a bilayered structure mimicking gland ducts and a minor element of admixed squamous cell carcinoma.[185] Because of their rarity, little is known about their biological behavior.

Adenoid Cystic Carcinoma

True adenoid cystic carcinomas of the esophagus are extremely rare.[186,187] They are histologically and immunophenotypically identical to the salivary gland type of adenoid cystic carcinoma. Most of the cases previously termed "adenoid cystic carcinoma" were most likely basaloid squamous carcinomas with adenoid cystic carcinoma–like features.[97] True adenoid cystic carcinomas are more common in men, are typically present in the seventh decade, and show no histological association with squamous cell carcinoma or squamous dysplasia (i.e., are derived from the submucosal glands).

Grossly, early tumors form well-circumscribed, solid nodules in the submucosa, but at more advanced stages are ulcerative or protruding. Adenoid cystic carcinoma is composed of two distinct populations of cells: luminal epithelial and myoepithelial cells. The myoepithelial cells are small and hyperchromatic, and show no or only minimal pleomorphism (Fig. 24.25). The luminal cells form solid nests or cribriform spaces, often associated with abundant basement membrane material, which may appear basophilic or undergo hyalinization. The overlying squamous epithelium does not exhibit dysplasia in most instances. Immunohistochemically, adenoid cystic carcinomas show strong keratin, CEA, and c-kit/CD117 staining in the luminal epithelium and weak keratin plus strong p63, S100 protein, and smooth muscle actin positivity in the myoepithelial cells.[97,188] The principal diagnostic challenge is to differentiate adenoid cystic carcinoma from basaloid squamous carcinoma, as discussed earlier (see Table 24.3).

So few true adenoid cystic carcinomas have been reported that clinical follow-up data are scarce. However, these tumors seem to have a better prognosis than typical squamous or basaloid carcinomas. The majority are slow-growing tumors that rarely metastasize and therefore are associated with excellent overall survival, although some aggressive examples have been reported.[114,187]

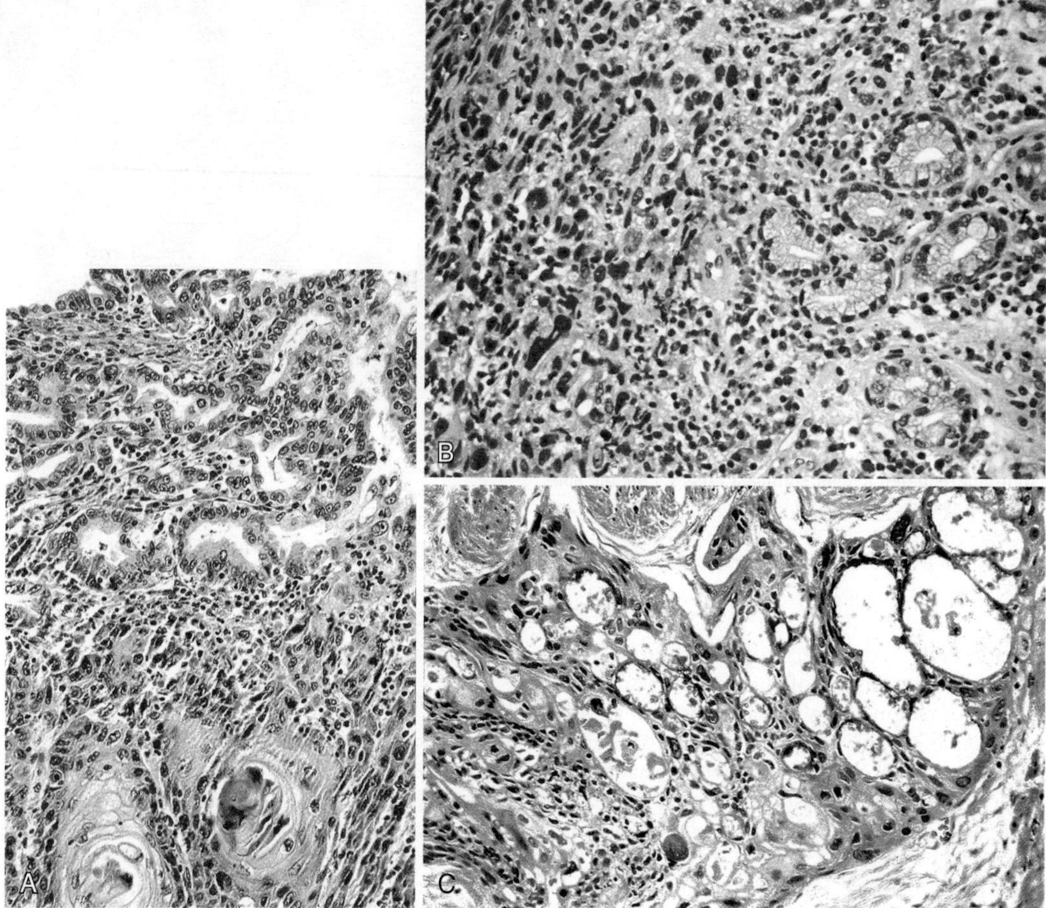

FIGURE 24.26 **A,** Adenosquamous carcinoma of the esophagus characterized by a proliferation of malignant glands *(top)* adjacent to malignant squamous epithelium *(bottom)*. **B**, In another example of adenosquamous carcinoma, the squamous component *(left side)* is poorly differentiated and the glandular component *(right side)* is well differentiated. **C,** This mucoepidermoid carcinoma is characterized by large aggregates of cells that have features of malignant squamous cells toward the periphery of the cellular units intimately mixed with centrally located cells that contain mucin.

Carcinoma with Mixed Squamous and Glandular Elements

Esophageal carcinomas (squamous carcinomas and adenocarcinomas) show a high propensity to exhibit divergent differentiation. In one study,[189] ultrastructural examination of 43 esophageal carcinomas (15 squamous cell carcinomas, 22 adenocarcinomas, 5 small cell carcinomas, 1 adenosquamous carcinoma) showed evidence of multidirectional differentiation in 25% of cases. Tumor cell heterogeneity may also occur in Barrett's-associated adenocarcinomas.[190] In a study by Lam and colleagues,[191] 496 cases of primary esophageal tumor were reviewed. Of these, 11 (2.2%) showed evidence of both squamous cell carcinoma and a mucin-secreting component. The age, sex, and site distribution of these tumors were similar to those of pure squamous cell carcinomas. Histologically, most tumors showed poorly differentiated squamous cell carcinoma with varying amounts of mucin or glandular differentiation.

Tumors composed of both squamous and glandular (mucinous) differentiation have been variously termed *composite tumors, adenoacanthomas, mucoepidermoid carcinoma*, or *adenosquamous carcinoma* (Fig. 24.26).[192,193] The literature is inconsistent regarding nomenclature, primarily because strict diagnostic criteria have not been defined. The WHO classification currently defines an *adenosquamous carcinoma* as a tumor that has admixed but separate malignant squamous and glandular components[40] (Table 24.11). While the proportions of the various components sufficient for this diagnosis have not been set, some investigators have suggested that at least 20% of each component should be present, otherwise the tumor should be classified according to the predominant component. In *mucoepidermoid carcinomas*, malignant squamous elements are admixed with mucin-producing and intermediate cells, similar to the salivary gland neoplasm of the same name. Tumors meeting the latter criteria appear to be extremely rare. The most widely accepted pathogenetic mechanism for tumors of mixed glandular and squamous morphology is the neoplastic transformation of a multipotent epithelial progenitor cell, possibly located in the esophageal submucosal gland or gland duct, which undergoes heterogeneous differentiation. The results of direct molecular assessment of clonality in one case of adenosquamous carcinoma support this hypothesis.[194]

The prognosis for patients with these mixed tumors is uncertain because of their relative rarity. In addition, the reported clinical behavior for patients with mucoepidermoid carcinoma may be misleading, since older patient series likely included a mixture of patients with variants of squamous cell

TABLE 24.11 Adenosquamous Carcinoma versus Mucoepidermoid Carcinoma

Feature	Adenosquamous Carcinoma	Mucoepidermoid Carcinoma
Clinical		
Age (yr)	40-80	40-70
Sex	M > F	M > F
Squamous carcinoma risk factors	+/–	–
Adenocarcinoma risk factors	+/–	–
Location of tumor in esophagus	Middle third, lower third	Middle third
Gross appearance	Ulcerative, infiltrative	Infiltrative
Median 5-year survival	20%	25%-40%
Pathological		
Associated with squamous dysplasia	+/–	–
Associated with Barrett's esophagus	+/–	–
Malignant squamous elements	++	++
Malignant glandular elements	++	++
Relationship of squamous and glandular elements	Admixed but separate	Intimately admixed
Intermediate cells	–	++

++; key feature; –, not present; +/–, sometimes present.

carcinoma as well as true mucoepidermoid carcinomas. Some studies of adenosquamous carcinoma have reported a wide range of survival data (19% to 65% at 5 years), most likely a result of small cohort sizes and variations in the tumor size, stage, and inclusion criteria.[192,195] Despite this uncertainty, tumors with mixed squamous and glandular differentiation are probably best regarded as biologically similar to, and should be staged similarly to pure squamous cell carcinoma, regardless of the terminology used to describe the tumor.[85,86]

Neuroendocrine Neoplasms

As in other locations in the gastrointestinal tract, neuroendocrine neoplasms of the esophagus, by definition, are epithelial neoplasms with neuroendocrine differentiation, usually documented by immunohistochemistry (Table 24.12). Based on this definition, they are quite uncommon. As at other anatomic sites, grading is based on determination of mitotic rate (grade 1: <2 per 10 high-power fields [HPFs], or per 2 mm^2; grade 2: 2 to 20 per 10 HPFs, or per 2 mm^2; grade 3: >20 per 10 HPFs, or per 2 mm^2), Ki-67 proliferation index (grade 1: <3%; grade 2: 3% to 20%; grade 3: >20%), or both,[40,85,86] which correlate well with clinical aggressiveness.[196] Esophageal neuroendocrine neoplasms likely arise from a multipotential cell in the squamous epithelium. However, another theory is that these tumors arise from neuroendocrine (or Merkel) cells in the squamous epithelium, which are present in a high proportion of the general population[197] (Box 24.6).

Neuroendocrine Tumor (Grades 1, 2, 3)

Neuroendocrine tumors (previously termed *carcinoid tumors*) of the esophagus are the least common type of esophageal neuroendocrine neoplasm, comprising 10% or fewer of the total. They have been reported either as isolated polypoid tumors or as incidental findings in esophagectomies for adenocarcinoma.[198,199] However, some tumors referred to in prior case reports as "atypical carcinoids" were not graded using modern approaches and probably represent poorly differentiated NECs.[200] They are histologically similar to those that occur in other parts of the gastrointestinal tract, and are comprised of uniform well-differentiated tumor cells with round to oval nuclei, finely granular chromatin, and moderate amounts of cytoplasm.

Although they have not been well studied because of their rarity, all reported examples appear to have behaved in a relatively benign fashion (see Chapter 29 for additional discussion).

Neuroendocrine Carcinoma (Grade 3)

Large Cell Neuroendocrine Carcinoma

Overall, esophageal NECs are more common than low-grade neuroendocrine tumors, but they still account for only approximately 1% of all esophageal malignant neoplasms.[40] Approximately 70% of NECs are of the large cell type. These tumors arise most commonly in the distal esophagus of elderly patients (mean age, 61 years), with a strong (8:1) male predilection.[76,201] Patients are seen with symptoms of dysphagia or obstruction. The tumor comprises cells with a moderate amount of cytoplasm, conspicuous nucleoli, and coarse chromatin, growing in nests and acinar structures with focal necrosis (Fig 24.27A–C). They may be confused with poorly differentiated squamous cell carcinoma or adenocarcinoma. However, these two latter tumor types should be negative, or show only focal immunoreactivity, for neuroendocrine immunohistochemical markers such as chromogranin, synaptophysin, or CD56.

Small Cell Neuroendocrine Carcinoma

NECs of the small cell type are more frequently encountered in Asian patients and are most common in middle-aged to older adults (median age, 60 years; range, 40 to 90

TABLE 24.12 Neuroendocrine Neoplasms of the Esophagus

	Neuroendocrine Tumor		Neuroendocrine Carcinoma		Mixed Neuroendocrine–Nonneuroendocrine Carcinoma
Feature	**Grade 1**	**Grades 2, 3**	**Large Cell (Grade 3)**	**Small Cell (Grade 3)**	
Clinical					
Age (yr; range)	61 (48-82)	ND	60 (50-80)	60 (40-90)	60 (50-80)
Sex	M = F	ND	M >> F	M > F	M >> F
Location	Middle, distal	ND	Distal	Middle, distal	Middle, distal
Gross appearance	Nodule	Ulcerating	Infiltrative, fungating	Ulcerating	Infiltrative, fungating
Pathological					
Mitotic activity (per 10 HPFs , or per 2 mm^2)	<2	2-20 (gr 2); >20 gr 3)	>20	>20	>20
Necrosis	–	+/–	++	++	+
Nuclear pleomorphism	–	–	++	+	+
Nuclear molding	–	–	–	++	+/–
Nucleoli	–	–/+	++	–	++
Cytoplasm	+	+	+	–	+
Admixed SCC or adenocarcinoma	–	–	+/– (<30%)	+/– (<30%)	++ (>30%)
Immunohistochemical					
Chromogranin/ synaptophysin	++	++	++	++	++
Ki-67 proliferative index (%)	<3	3-20 (gr 2); >20 (gr. 3)	>20	>20	>20
p63	–	–	+/–*	+/–*	++ *
CEA	–	–	+/–†	+/–†	++†
TTF-1	–	–	–	+/–	+/–
Prognosis					
Aggressiveness	–	+	++	++	++

CEA, *carcinoembryonic antigen;* HPF, *high-power field;* ND, *not determined;* NET, *neuroendocrine tumor;* SCC, *squamous cell carcinoma;* TTF-1, *thyroid transcription factor-1; +, consistently present; ++, key feature; –, not present; +/–, sometimes present.*
**In foci of squamous cell carcinoma.*
†In foci of adenocarcinoma.

years), with a slight (2:1) male predilection.[201,202] Grossly, the tumors usually form large exophytic or polypoid masses and arise in the middle or distal third of the esophagus. Similar to the large cell type, they are high-grade tumors, with a high proliferative rate (>20% Ki-67 labeling index) and/or a high mitotic rate (>20 per 10 HPFs).[40,85,86] In small cell carcinomas, the tumor cells are small to intermediate in size, with scant cytoplasm, irregular hyperchromatic nuclei with molding, absent nucleoli, and frequent single-cell necrosis (see Fig. 24.27D). Reactivity for neuroendocrine markers, such as chromogranin or synaptophysin, is usually present. Approximately 10% to 20% of reported cases of small cell carcinoma reveal admixed areas of squamous cell carcinoma or, less commonly, adenocarcinoma, but these tumors should not be classified as mixed unless 30% of each component is present (see later). The differential diagnosis includes poorly differentiated squamous cell carcinoma particularly, the basaloid type, which should be negative for neuroendocrine and positive for squamous immunohistochemical markers (see Table 24.3). The possibility of metastasis or spread of tumor from other anatomic sites (e.g., lung) should also be considered and correlated with clinical history and imaging studies. Unfortunately, immunostains are of limited utility in this distinction, because TTF-1 (a marker of pulmonary epithelial differentiation) is positive in as much as 71% of esophageal small cell carcinomas.[201]

Mixed Neuroendocrine–Nonneuroendocrine Carcinoma (Grade 3)

As discussed earlier, some esophageal malignancies reveal multiple cell lineages. For instance, in one study of 40 esophageal NECs, 15 tumors (12 large cell, 3 small cell) also contained distinct areas of glandular differentiation.[76,190] A mixed neuroendocrine–nonneuroendocrine carcinoma is defined as a tumor that contains at least 30% of each cellular component.[40,114] Because of the occurrence of mixed tumors, a finding of NEC in an esophageal biopsy does not necessarily exclude the possibility of another malignant cell

BOX 24.6 Esophageal Neuroendocrine Neoplasms: Key Features

Clinical/endoscopic
- Male > female, 7th decade
- Bulky, ulcerated or fungating tumors

Histologic
- Neuroendocrine tumor (grades 1, 2, 3)
- Large cell neuroendocrine carcinoma (grade 3)
- Small cell neuroendocrine carcinoma (grade 3)
- Mixed neuroendocrine–nonneuroendocrine carcinoma (>30% each component) (grade 3)

Special/immunohistochemical stains
- Diffuse positivity for at least one neuroendocrine marker (chromogranin, synaptophysin) in neuroendocrine component.
- p63/p40+ in squamous foci, CEA+ in glandular foci
- Ki-67 proliferation index: <3% (grade 1); 3% to 20% (grade 2); >20% (grade 3)

Differential diagnosis
- Metastatic neuroendocrine carcinoma
- Poorly differentiated squamous cell carcinoma (including basaloid type)

Prognostic factors
- Tumor grade
- Tumor stage (tumor–node–metastasis classification)

lineage, which may be diagnosed only on further sampling or after analysis of a resection. Mixed adenocarcinoma–neuroendocrine carcinoma (MANEC) appears to be much more common than the squamous cell-neuroendocrine carcinoma combination, at least based on studies in Western patient populations[114] (Fig. 24.28). Most reported examples of mixed adenocarcinoma-neuroendocrine carcinoma arise in the seventh decade with a strong male preponderance and are associated with Barrett's esophagus.[203] They are staged similar to adenocarcinomas.

Overall, esophageal NECs are highly aggressive neoplasms. Median survival time is typically 12 to 24 months and is slightly less for patients with pure NECs compared with those with an admixed nonneuroendocrine component.[76,199,201]

Choriocarcinoma

Choriocarcinoma of the esophagus is extremely rare and affects adults of both sexes. Of the eight cases reported, three were associated with BE-associated adenocarcinoma and three others with squamous cell carcinoma.[204,205] Grossly, these are large, exophytic tumors with extensive necrosis, usually located in the distal third of the esophagus. Microscopically, a mixture of cytotrophoblastic and syncytiotrophoblastic giant cells is present. Immunohistochemical stain for human chorionic gonadotropin is positive in the trophoblastic cells. The principal differential diagnoses are spread of a mediastinal germ cell tumor and squamous cell carcinoma containing pleomorphic giant cells. The prognosis in all reported cases is exceedingly poor; most patients show widespread metastases at presentation and survival of only a few months' duration.

Undifferentiated Carcinoma

Undifferentiated carcinomas, comprised of tumor cells without apparent squamous, glandular or neuroendocrine differentiation, arise predominantly (9:1 ratio) in male patients in the seventh decade. A proportion of the reported examples appear to be associated with Barrett's esophagus, suggesting they represent an extremely high-grade adenocarcinoma.[206] Nevertheless, these tumors should be extensively sampled to identify foci of glandular or squamous differentiation before the diagnosis of undifferentiated carcinoma is rendered. Tumor cells may show a combination of spindled, rhabdoid, syncytial, or giant cell morphology with large pleomorphic nuclei (Fig. 24.29A,B). Positive staining for keratins confirms the epithelial nature of the neoplasm, and a large proportion of cases are also positive for SALL4. A proportion of these tumors are characterized by loss of expression of the chromatin remodeling genes SMARCA2 or SMARCA4 in the undifferentiated areas. [207] Undifferentiated carcinomas are aggressive neoplasms with a median survival of 10 months. The AJCC staging system for esophageal squamous cell carcinomas is used.

A subset of undifferentiated esophageal carcinomas are associated with a prominent lymphoid infiltrate, and are referred to as *lymphoepithelioma-like carcinomas*.[40] Most cases have been reported from Japan and have clinically resembled conventional squamous cell carcinomas.[65,66] These tumors are histologically similar to their counterpart in the nasopharynx, showing syncytia of primitive-appearing epithelioid cells surrounded by a dense inflammatory infiltrate including lymphocytes and plasma cells (Fig. 24.29C,D). By analogy with the tumors in these other organs, Epstein-Barr virus has been suggested as an etiological agent. However, the virus has been detected in only a minority of esophageal tumors by various methods, including in situ hybridization, immunohistochemistry, and DNA amplification.[67,68] Although the clinical behavior of these tumors is incompletely understood because of their rarity, some authors have suggested that they have a slightly better prognosis than ordinary squamous cell carcinomas.[66]

Pleomorphic Giant Cell Carcinoma

Other rare tumors of the esophagus have been reported, including a pleomorphic giant cell carcinoma arising in a 52-year-old man. This tumor was focally positive for keratins by immunohistochemistry but was also extensively positive for the histiocytic marker CD68 and for neuroendocrine markers such as chromogranin and synaptophysin.[208]

Melanoma

Malignant melanoma, strictly speaking, is not an epithelial tumor, but it deserves mention as a primary esophageal neoplasm, because the squamous epithelium contains resident melanocytes, and melanoma may enter into the differential diagnosis of poorly differentiated esophageal neoplasms. Esophageal melanomas are uncommon; only approximately 300 examples have been reported in the literature. These tumors typically arise in older adults and show a predilection for the middle and distal esophagus. A precursor

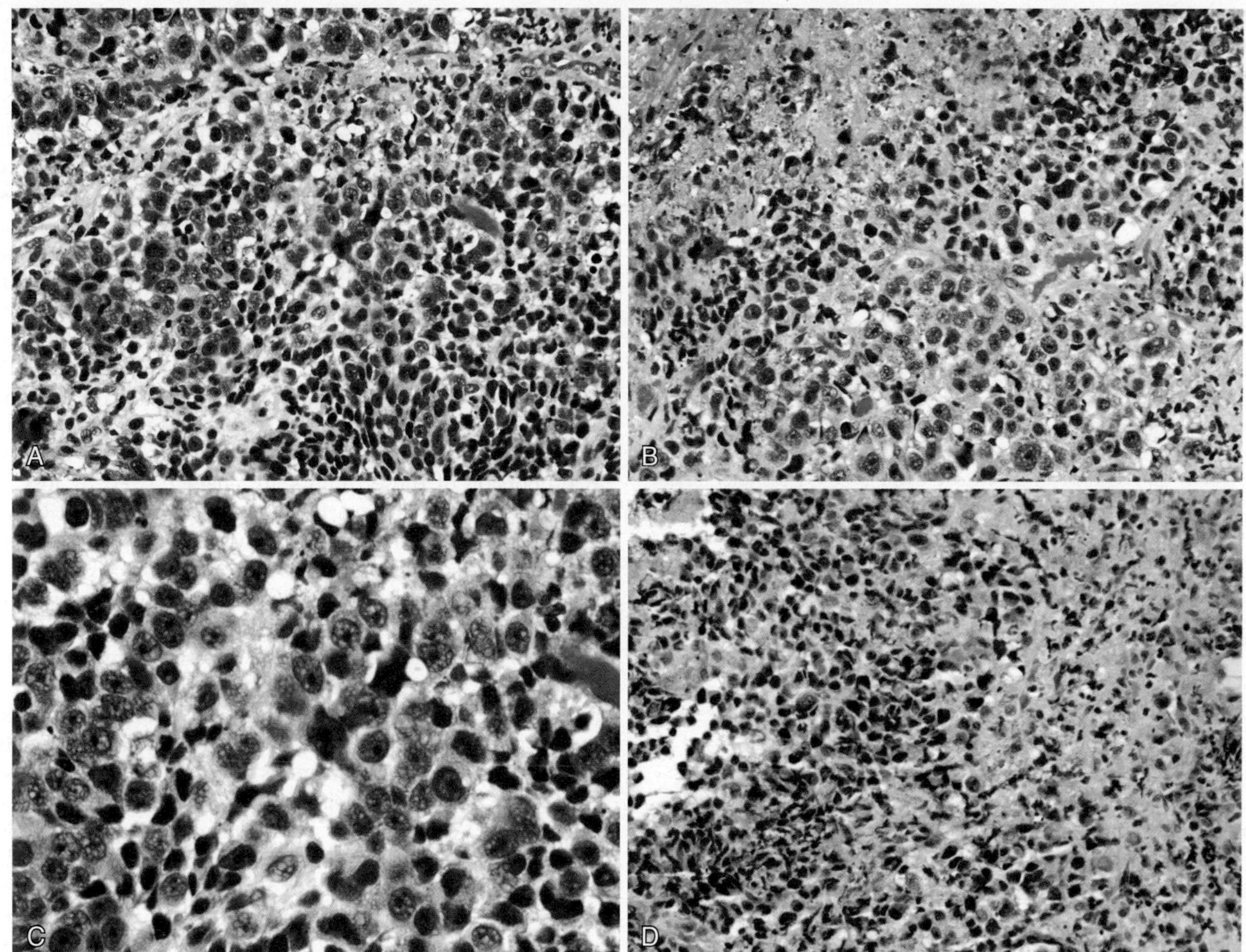

FIGURE 24.27 Esophageal neuroendocrine carcinoma (NEC). A, Large cell NEC. The tumor cells grow in solid sheets and large nests. **B,** Another view of large cell NEC illustrates the frequent finding of tumor necrosis *(top left)*. **C,** At high magnification, the tumor cells contain a moderate amount of cytoplasm, conspicuous nucleoli, and coarse chromatin. **D,** Typical appearance of a small cell carcinoma of the esophagus, which is histologically identical to small cell carcinomas that occur in the lung. This tumor is characterized by a proliferation of small "blue" cells with marked nuclear hyperchromaticity, lack of nucleoli, nuclear molding, and individual cell necrosis.

melanocytic lesion is present in the squamous epithelium in most cases, confirming that these are primary tumors rather than metastases. The tumor cells show a wide variety of morphological appearances (epithelioid, spindle cell, small cell, and signet ring cell) and are almost always positive for markers, such as S100 protein, SOX10, and HMB-45, and negative for keratins (Fig. 24.30). These tumors are highly aggressive, with a mean survival time of 10 to 15 months after surgical resection.[209,210]

Metastases

Metastases to the esophagus are not rare and originate mostly from carcinomas of the lung, breast, and stomach (Fig. 24.31).[211,212] However, almost any type of tumor can metastasize to this location, including renal cell carcinoma. Metastatic lesions typically form nodules in the submucosa but may also produce large, symptomatic, obstructive tumors. Attention to the clinical history, the distribution of the lesion, and the absence of premalignant squamous or glandular epithelium is usually sufficient to distinguish these tumors from primary esophageal carcinomas. In difficult cases, the use of immunostains for CK7 and CK20[74,150,156] or organ-specific markers such as TTF-1 (lung),[80,152] GATA-3 and estrogen receptor (breast),[156] or CDX2 (gastrointestinal tract)[151] may be helpful in suggesting a likely primary site.

The full reference list may be accessed online at Elsevier eBooks for Practicing Clinicians.

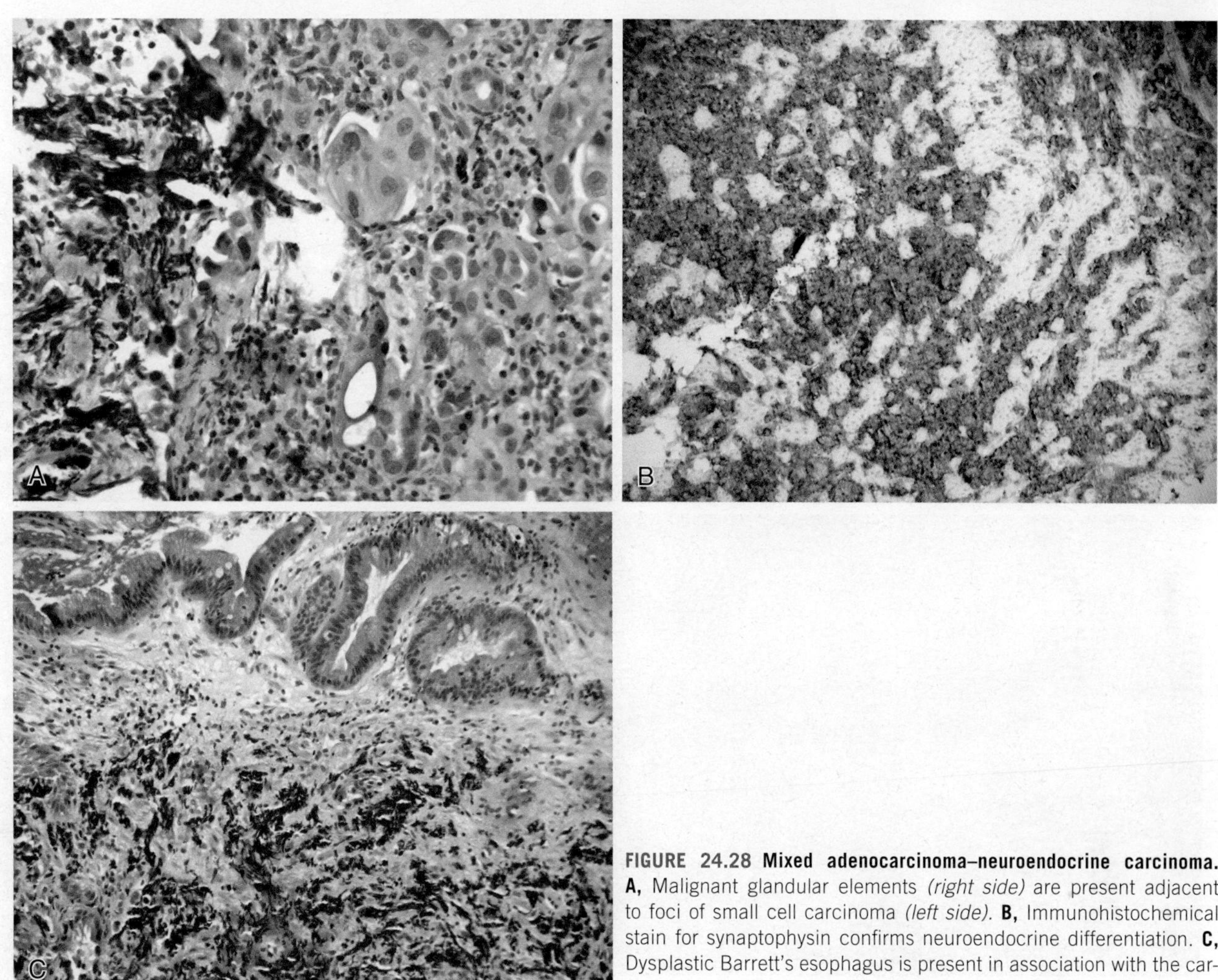

FIGURE 24.28 Mixed adenocarcinoma–neuroendocrine carcinoma. A, Malignant glandular elements *(right side)* are present adjacent to foci of small cell carcinoma *(left side)*. **B,** Immunohistochemical stain for synaptophysin confirms neuroendocrine differentiation. **C,** Dysplastic Barrett's esophagus is present in association with the carcinoma, as is the case for the majority of mixed carcinomas.

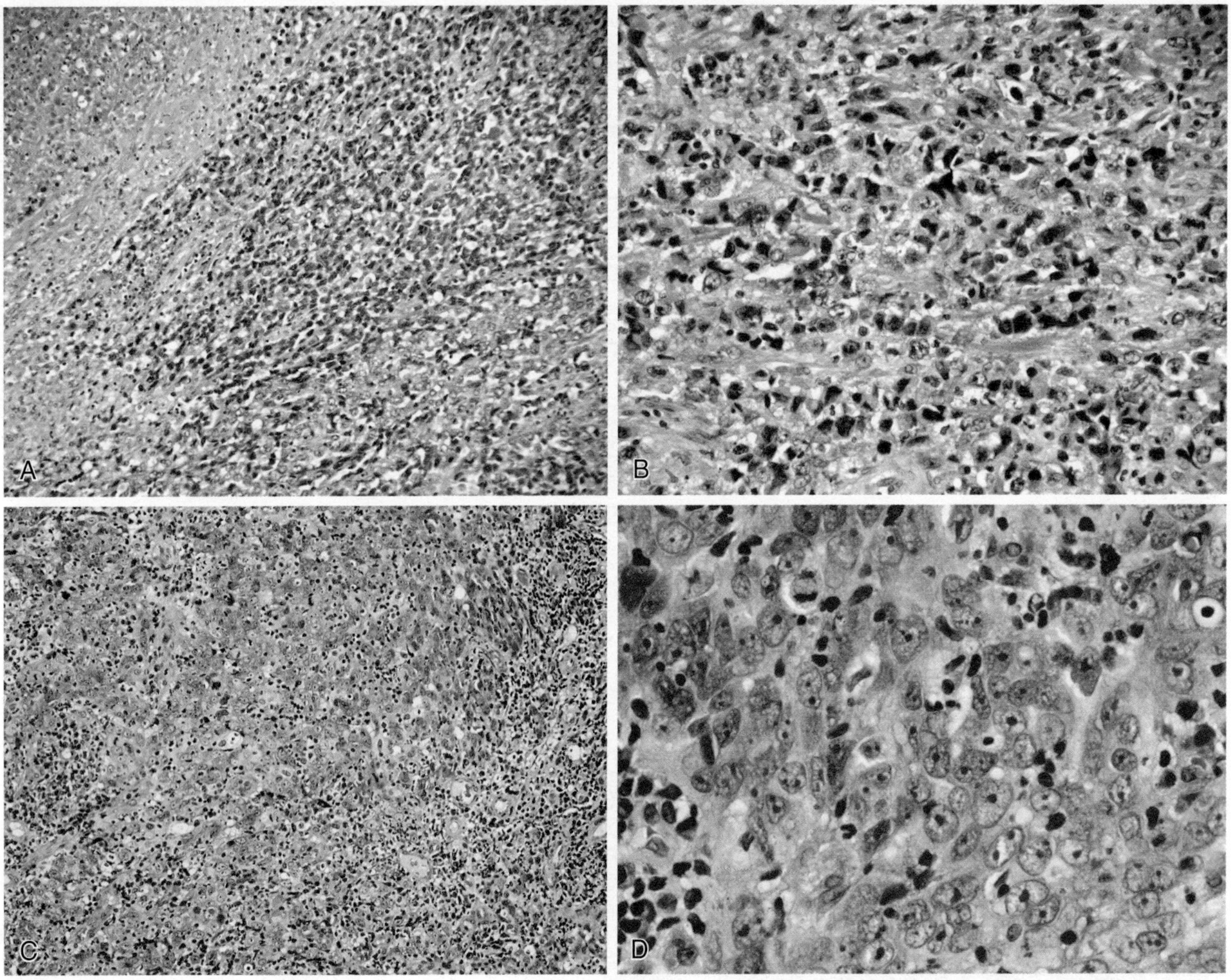

FIGURE 24.29 A, Esophageal undifferentiated carcinoma, comprised of cells without squamous or glandular differentiation, with associated necrosis *(to left).* The tumor was focally positive for cytokeratins by immunohistochemistry. **B,** High magnification view of tumor in **A**. Note the abundant mitoses, nuclear pleomorphism, and coarsened chromatin. **C,** Lymphoepithelioma-like carcinoma subtype. Low-magnification image shows a sheetlike proliferation of undifferentiated epithelioid cells. Notice the abundant lymphoid infiltrate adjacent to and among the tumor cells. **D,** High-power view of tumor cells illustrates the syncytial growth pattern, marked nuclear pleomorphism, and brisk mitotic activity.

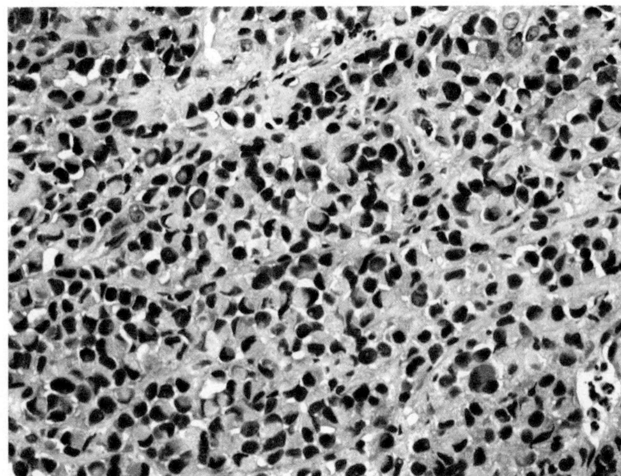

FIGURE 24.30 Esophageal melanoma. This example is characterized by signet ring tumor cell morphology. The tumor cells are positive for melanocytic immunohistochemical markers (S100 protein, HMB45) and negative for keratins. (*Courtesy Dr. Xiuli Liu, Cleveland Clinic, Cleveland, Ohio.*)

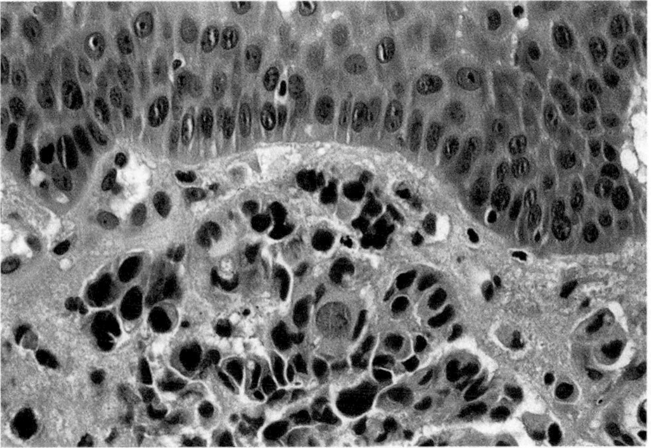

FIGURE 24.31 Metastatic, poorly differentiated carcinoma of the breast to the esophagus. A proliferation of highly atypical cells, some in a single-cell file arrangement, is seen just beneath the epithelium in the upper portion of the lamina propria. The tumor stained positively for estrogen receptor protein, progesterone receptor protein, and gross cystic disease fluid protein.

CHAPTER 25

Epithelial Neoplasms of the Stomach

Fátima Carneiro, Gregory Y. Lauwers

Contents

INTRODUCTION

Gastric cancer remains an important cancer worldwide and is responsible for over 1 million new cases in 2020, and an estimated 769,000 deaths (equating to 1 in 13 deaths globally), ranking fifth for incidence and fourth for mortality globally.[1,2] Over the past 50 years, the incidence and mortality rates of distal gastric cancer have been uniformly decreasing in North America, Europe, and, more recently, in many Asian and Latin American countries.[3,4] However, the absolute number of gastric cancer cases remains stable or may even increase as a result of the predicted growth of the world population and increasing longevity.[5,6]

There is wide variation in incidence on different continents, with the highest rates in Asia, central and Eastern Europe, and South America. Incidence rates are markedly elevated in Eastern Asia (e.g., in Mongolia, Japan, and the Republic of Korea), whereas the rates in Northern America and Northern Europe are generally low and are equivalent to those seen across the African regions.[1,2]

The topographic distribution of gastric cancer has also changed in recent years. In regions of high incidence, about 80% of cases are distal (occurring in the gastric body, antrum, and/or pylorus), with a relative predominance of antral-pyloric location, and *Helicobacter pylori* is the most important risk factor. In countries with low incidence (e.g., North America and Europe), 50% to 60% of gastric cancers are localized in the proximal stomach and the esophagogastric junction (EGJ), and they are associated with gastroesophageal reflux disease.[7] *H. pylori* infection is also a risk factor for proximal gastric carcinoma if esophageal and junctional adenocarcinoma has been properly excluded.[8]

Changes in clinical practice have also led to diagnosis of a higher percentage of early-stage cancers. The widespread increased use of upper gastrointestinal (GI) endoscopy has led to more frequent detection of early superficial cancers, currently treated endoscopically. This trend has had a dramatic impact on the mortality rate (and therapy related morbidity) to the point that gastric cancer is now considered potentially curable if it is detected at an early stage. In the United States, the survival rates of surgically resected gastric cardia cancer patients had a significant improvement between 1988 to 1997 and 2008 to 2015, which may relate to early diagnosis and chemoradiotherapy.[9]

Recent notable findings concern an increase in the incidence of stomach cancer among young adults (<50 years of age) in both low-risk and high-risk countries, including the United States, Canada, the United Kingdom, Chile, and Belarus.[10,11] Because the prevalence rate of *H. pylori* has decreased,[12] autoimmune gastritis may represent an alternative cause of the increasing incidence of gastric cancer in females younger than 50 years of age.[13]

PATHOGENESIS

The pathogenesis of sporadic gastric dysplasia and gastric carcinoma is a multifactorial process in which both environmental and host-related factors play a major role.[14] At least 89% of all noncardia gastric cancers are caused by *H. pylori*.[15,16] In most cases, it is associated with a stepwise carcinogenic process that involves progression from chronic gastritis to atrophy with hypochlorhydria or achlorhydria, intestinal metaplasia, dysplasia, and, ultimately, adenocarcinoma.[17-19] In this sequence, intestinal metaplasia and, subsequently, dysplasia and early adenocarcinoma develop initially in the neck region of the antral or fundic glands, supporting the hypothesis that precursor cells are located in this region.[20] However, the so-called *Correa model* does not explain all carcinogenic steps because a proportion of adenocarcinomas arise in nonintestinalized mucosa and retain a gastric phenotype.[21,22]

The well-known geographic variations in incidence data obtained from studies of changes in dietary and sanitary conditions among immigrants have underscored the role of environmental influences in the development of the intestinal type of sporadic gastric carcinoma, which is the most common type.[23-25] Furthermore, the worldwide decrease in the incidence of intestinal-type gastric cancer has paralleled the decline in *H. pylori* infection, which confirms this bacterium as a major environmental cause of this type of cancer. Long-standing *H. pylori* infection induces chronic gastritis by promoting proinflammatory cytokine release that gradually results in atrophy, achlorhydria, and intestinal metaplasia.[26,27] There is a four-fold to nine-fold increased risk of gastric lesions among patients with *H. pylori* infection, particularly if infection began in early childhood.[28-30] Chronic acid suppression also increases the risk for development of atrophy in patients with *H. pylori* gastritis.[31]

Certain strains of *H. pylori* are more virulent and have been associated with risk of gastric cancer. For instance, strains that produce oncoproteins such as cytotoxin-associated gene A (CagA) and vacuolating cytotoxin A (vac A) lead to upregulation of oncogenes, silencing of tumor suppressors genes, and increased levels of reactive oxygen and nitrogen species.[32] Infection with CagA-positive *H. pylori* strains is the strongest risk factor for the development of gastric carcinoma.[33] Although infection with the most virulent vacA s1, m1, and i1 strains is associated with an increased risk of gastric adenocarcinoma, the predictive value of vacA virulent genotypes observed in the United States and Colombia, was not confirmed in some studies from eastern and southeastern Asia. [33,34] Genetic susceptibility is also involved, such as single-nucleotide polymorphisms (SNPs) of inflammation-associated genes (*IL1B*, *TNF*).[35-37] Interestingly, a distinct genomic profile was identified in *H. pylori*–associated gastric cancer.[38]

However, gastric cancer does not develop in most individuals who are infected by *H. pylori* (<5% of infected hosts will develop cancer), likely because of differences in bacterial genetics, host genetics, age of infection acquisition, and environmental factors.[1] Conversely, about 20% of patients in whom gastric cancer develops are *H. pylori* seronegative.

Chronic *H. pylori* infection leads to reduced acid secretion, which may allow the growth of a different gastric bacterial community. Detailed analysis of the gastric microbiota revealed that patients with gastric carcinoma exhibit a dysbiotic microbial community with genotoxic potential, which is distinct from that of patients with chronic gastritis and may increase aggression to the gastric mucosa and contribute to malignancy.[39-41]

Other environmental and host factors play an important role in the pathogenesis of this disease.[17,42] Diets that are rich in salt (e.g., dried and salted fish and meats, soy sauce, smoked fish, pickled foods) and contain low levels of micronutrients, vitamins, and antioxidants[25] favor intraluminal formation of genotoxic agents, such as specific *N*-nitroso compounds (formed by nitrosation of ingested nitrates) and have been associated with the development of gastric cancer.[17,43,44] In contrast, diets rich in fresh vegetables, citrus fruits, and ascorbic acid are inversely associated with risk of gastric cancer.[45,46] The analysis of multiple studies calculated a potential 50% higher risk of gastric cancer associated with intake of pickled vegetables in East Asia.[47] In contrast, adherence to a Mediterranean diet has been shown to be associated with reduction in gastric cancer.[48] Further, a positive association was found between dietary inflammatory index and gastric cancer risk.[49,50]

Bile reflux has been associated with the development of adenocarcinoma in surgical stumps.[51] With regard to host factors, polymorphisms of the interleukin-1 *(IL-1)* gene have been associated with an increased risk of gastric cancer in *H. pylori*–infected individuals. Furthermore, the presence of a proinflammatory *IL-1* genotype, which plays a role in hypochlorhydria and atrophy, is clearly associated with an increased risk of the intestinal type, but not the diffuse type, of gastric cancer.[52]

Epstein-Barr virus (EBV) infection is another risk factor for the development of gastric cancer.[53-55] The virus can cause aberrant DNA methylation, which results in the inactivation of tumor suppressor genes in the early carcinogenic sequence. Further, EBV can exacerbate gastric cancer formation in the setting of chronic *H. pylori* infection in part by downregulating host defenses that antagonize CagA.[14]

In contrast with the intestinal type of gastric cancer, the diffuse type is more common in younger individuals, with equal incidence in both high- and low-risk geographic regions. Its development is more regulated by genetic factors than is intestinal-type gastric cancer.[25,56] The importance of genetic factors is also underscored by the existence of familial clustering [57] and by the increased incidence of atrophic gastritis in relatives of patients with gastric cancer (see Hereditary Gastric Cancer Syndromes).

Finally, an increased risk of gastric adenocarcinoma in patients with pernicious anemia and autoimmune gastritis has been recognized.[13] However, the magnitude of the risk is debated; it is reported to be around three times that of the general population,[58-62] while a large U.S. population–based cohort study found an incidence of gastric cancer of only 1.2%, similar to that of the general population.[63] Importantly, risk appears to be associated with high-risk gastritis stages (OLGA III–IV).[64]

TABLE 25.1 Intestinal Metaplasia: From Microscopy to Immunohistochemical Profiles

Type	Microscopy	PAS and HID	Immunohistochemical Profiles
Type I (complete)	Columnar cells (nonsecreting, mature, absorptive enterocytes) Goblet cells Paneth Cells	Neutral (PAS+) Sialomucins	CD10 on enterocytes MUC2 in goblet cells
Type II (incomplete)	Columnar cells (secreting, immature, nonabsorptive) Goblet cells	Neutral (PAS+) Sialomucins Sialomucins	CD10 is not expressed MUC5 and MUC6 in columnar cells MUC1 and MUC2 in goblet cells
Type III (incomplete)	Columnar cells (secreting, immature, nonabsorptive) Goblet cells	Sulfomucins Sialomucins and sulfomucins	CD10 is not expressed MUC5 and (MUC6) in columnar cells MUC2 in goblet cells

TABLE 25.2 Staging Systems for Operative Link for Gastritis Assessment (OLGA) and Intestinal Metaplasia (OLGIM)

	CORPUS	No Atrophy No IM	Mild Atrophy Mild IM	Moderate Atrophy Moderate IM	Severe Atrophy Severe IM
ANTRUM	***SCORE***	***0***	***1***	***2***	***3***
No atrophy No IM	0	Stage 0	Stage I	Stage II	Stage II
Mild atrophy Mild IM	1	Stage I	Stage I	Stage II	Stage III
Moderate atrophy Moderate IM	2	Stage II	Stage II	Stage III	Stage IV
Severe atrophy Severe IM	3	Stage III	Stage III	Stage IV	Stage IV

IM, Intestinal metaplasia.

HISTOLOGICAL PRECURSORS OF GASTRIC CARCINOMA

In most instances, the development of gastric adenocarcinoma represents the culmination of an inflammation-metaplasia-dysplasia-carcinoma sequence, known as the *Correa cascade of multistep gastric carcinogenesis*.[19] Mucosal atrophy and intestinal metaplasia confer a high risk for the development of gastric cancer; however, gastric epithelial dysplasia (or *adenoma*, if it is a polypoid lesion) represents a direct neoplastic precursor lesion[19,65] (see Chapters 15 and 20 for more details).

The two main types of intestinal metaplasia are classified as *complete* (type I), and *incomplete* (types IIA/II and IIB/III)[66,67] based on the detection of sialomucin and sulphomucin). Type III, the most closely associated with intestinal gastric cancer, is characterized by the presence of sulphomucin secreting columnar mucous cells.[18,68] Using expanded criteria and novel immunohistochemical stains, incomplete intestinal metaplasia displays goblet and columnar nonabsorptive cells without brush border and coexpression of gastric mucins and MUC2. Complete-type intestinal metaplasia displays well-spaced goblet cells and enterocytes and shows decreased/absent expression of gastric mucins (MUC1, MUC5AC, and MUC6) and expression of MUC2 (an intestinal mucin) (Table 25.1).[69] Factors associated with the progression of gastric intestinal metaplasia include family history, smoking, and genetic susceptibility factors.[70-72]

Another metaplastic lesion, spasmolytic polypeptide-expressing metaplasia (SPEM), develops characteristically in the oxyntic mucosa and is associated with chronic *H. pylori* infection or any other chronic injury. The lesion expresses a metaplastic mucous cell lineage with phenotypic characteristics of deep antral/pyloric gland cells, including strong expression of Trefoil Factor 2 (TFF2; previously designated as spasmolytic polypeptide), as well as MUC6. One marker that is present uniquely in SPEM is the protease inhibitor HE4 (*WFDC2*).[73] Pyloric-type metaplasias in the stomach are initially reparative; their maintenance in the setting of chronic inflammation can lead to deleterious neoplastic scenarios in animal models.[73-77] The role as a direct precursor of cancer in humans is debated.[78]

Proposed in 2005, the OLGA Staging System is another classification of gastritis taking into account the natural history of gastric atrophy[23] and the risk of cancer.[79,80] The scheme stratified the pattern of gastritis based on increasing mucosal atrophy using a four-scale system. The risk of developing gastric cancer is extremely low with stages 0, I, and II but high with stages III and IV, characterized by extensive atrophy of both antral and oxyntic mucosa. An alternative staging method proposed as a modification of the OLGA System is OLGIM, which evaluates exclusively the extension of IM, as assessed in both antral and oxyntic biopsy samples (Table 25.2).[81] However, these two systems have little value in general practice when limited mucosal sampling and follow-up endoscopic strategy is not developed.

Finally, gastric epithelial dysplasia (or *adenoma,* if it is a polypoid lesion) represents a direct neoplastic precursor lesion.[19,65] The neoplastic cells composing gastric dysplasia can follow various lines of differentiation. Most gastric epithelial dysplasias (or adenomas) have an "intestinal" phenotype (type I), resembling colonic adenomas. [82] However, various subtypes have recognized such as foveolar type (type II),[83] serrated type, and gastric pit/crypt dysplasia.[84-89] Finally, the exceedingly rare tubule neck dysplasia is believed to be a precursor of diffuse-type gastric carcinoma.[90] Of those, foveolar type (type II) has been the best characterized, representing less than 30% of the cases and possibly a more biologically aggressive type[21,83] (see Chapter 20 for a more extensive review of the subject). Guidelines for the management of epithelial precancerous conditions and lesions in the stomach are regularly updated.[70] Other putative precancerous conditions include autoimmunity, pyloric metaplasia, gastric ulcers, gastric hyperplastic polyps, previous gastric surgery, and Menetrier's disease.

EARLY GASTRIC CARCINOMA

Clinical Features

An invasive adenocarcinoma confined to the mucosa or submucosa, regardless of the presence of lymph node metastasis, is defined as early gastric carcinoma (EGC) (Fig. 25.1). EGC represents an early stage in development, before invasion of the muscularis.[91] Because of an increased number of upper endoscopies performed worldwide, detection rates for this lesion are on the rise. In Western series, EGC represents 15% to 24% of all newly diagnosed gastric cancers, whereas in Japan it accounts for more than 50% of cases.[92-95] In a large-scale study undertaken in 2017 by the International Gastric Cancer Association (IGCA), the proportion of EGC was found to be significantly higher in Japan (58%) and Korea (48%) than in the West (28%) and other Asian countries (18%).[96] A higher prevalence of gastric cancer, more liberal use of upper endoscopy and chromoendoscopy, and differences in diagnostic criteria help explain the differences between Western and East Asian studies.

Similar to dysplasia, most EGCs are diagnosed in men older than 50 years of age; this is a younger age than for advanced adenocarcinoma, reflecting the amount of time required for progression from early to advanced disease.[95,97] Most patients are asymptomatic, but some complain of symptoms that mimic peptic ulcer disease.[95,98] Epigastric pain and dyspepsia are the most frequently reported symptoms. They usually occur only within the last few months before diagnosis.[99] Most EGCs are small, between 2 and 5 cm, and they are typically localized on the lesser curvature around the angularis region.[99,100] In 3% to 13% of patients, multiple primary sites are present, and this has been shown to be associated with a poorer prognosis.[101]

Pathological Features

Gross/Endoscopic Features

EGCs are divided based on their endoscopic appearance (Fig. 25.2): protruding (type I), flat/superficial (type II), and excavating (type III) (Table 25.3).[102,103] Type II is further subdivided into IIa (elevated) (Fig. 25.3), IIb (flat), and IIc (depressed). Superficial EGCs (type II) account for the highest proportion of cases (80%), with type IIc being most common.[104] Type IIb accounts for 58% of tumors that are smaller than 5 mm.[105] The endoscopic appearance of EGCs has been shown to be a good indicator of the rate of lymph node metastasis, with the lowest rates reported in type I or IIa EGCs.[99] Type IIa, which is defined as a lesion that is twice as thick as normal mucosa, and type IIc, which mimics benign ulcers, are difficult to detect endoscopically

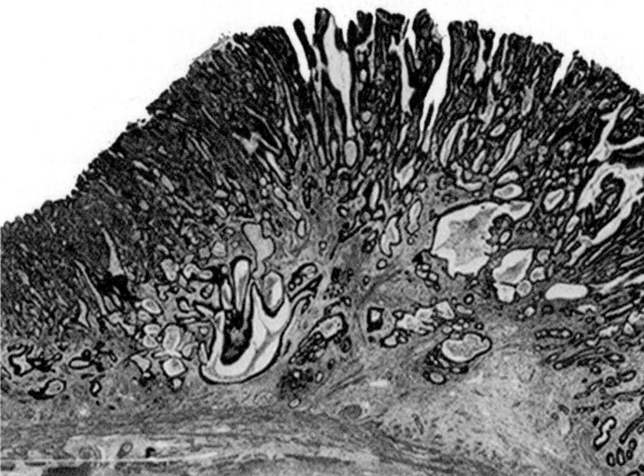

FIGURE 25.1 Early gastric cancer. Scanning view shows involvement of the mucosa.

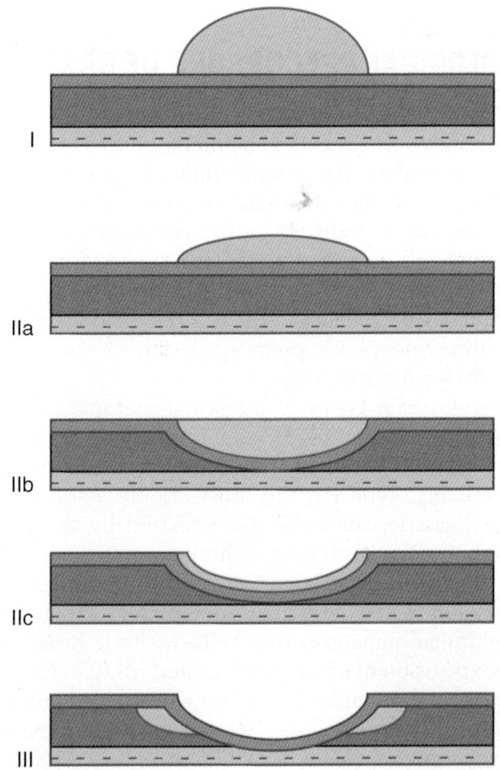

FIGURE 25.2 Endoscopic classification of early gastric cancer (Paris classification).

because of subtle features such as ease of bleeding and an irregular interface with surrounding mucosa.[106] In such cases, obtaining multiple biopsies is advisable to secure a diagnosis.

Microscopic Features

Microscopic variants of EGCs have been reported. Minute EGCs measure less than 5 mm in diameter, and although most are limited to the mucosa, submucosal extension is detected in as many as 15% of cases.[107,108] Superficial spreading EGCs are characterized by the presence of large, serpiginous ulcerations with neoplastic cells that spread laterally over a large area of mucosa.

The majority of EGCs are well-differentiated glandular carcinomas. Tubular and papillary variants represent 52% and 37% of cases, respectively, and may be difficult to differentiate from dysplasia because of the lack of obvious tissue invasion. Signet ring cell (SRC)/diffuse carcinoma (Fig. 25.4) and poorly differentiated carcinoma represent 26% and 14% of cases, respectively, and are usually depressed or ulcerated (types IIc and III).[92,109] Diffuse-type (poorly cohesive) EGCs tend to show greater depths of invasion.[99] The morphological classification of EGC is important

TABLE 25.3 Endoscopic PARIS Classification

Category	Description	Subcategory
0-I	Protruding lesions	0-Ip pedunculated
		0-Is sessile
		0-Isp semipedunculated
0-II	Flat	0-IIa flat elevation
		0-IIb flat mucosal change
		0-IIc mucosal depression
0-III	Ulcerative	Excavated ulcer

because, in addition to the size and the endoscopic appearance (i.e., presence of erosion or not), patients may be treated conservatively via endoscopic resection rather than surgery.[102]

Differential Diagnosis

The differential diagnosis of EGC includes (polypoid and flat) high-grade dysplasia. However, the distinction is subjective and fraught by significant interobserver variation. In contrast with high-grade dysplasia, which shows only limited architectural atypia, EGC is composed of fused or branching tubular structures in some cases. Cribriforming and/or small withering glands can be seen in other examples. In most cases limited to the mucosa, fibroblastic desmoplastic response is absent, or only myxoid transformation of the lamina propria is observed.

Natural History and Treatment

In a series of patients with EGC followed conservatively without surgery, 63% of EGCs progressed to advanced carcinoma during a 6- to 88-month period.[110] With resection, the prognosis of EGC is excellent, with 5-year survival rates greater than 90% reported in most series.[17,92,98,111,112] Size of the tumor and depth of invasion are the two major prognostic indicators, and larger tumors have a greater risk of submucosal infiltration.[93,113-115] However, the risk of invasion should not be overlooked, even in very small tumors. In one series, 15.5% of tumors that measured 3 to 5 mm in diameter showed invasion into the submucosa.[108] Lymph node metastases have been reported in 0% to 7% of intramucosal EGCs and are associated with a 5-year survival rate of almost 100%.[92,114,115] The rate of lymph node metastases for EGCs that extend into the submucosa varies between 8% and 25%, and the 5-year survival rate for these tumors is 80% to 90%.[92,115]

Endoscopic resection has now become the first-line therapy for early gastric cancer, with very low risk of node metastasis. Important characteristics considered in the decision making include the size of the lesion, whether it is ulcerated, the morphological subtype, and the differentiation.[116-120]

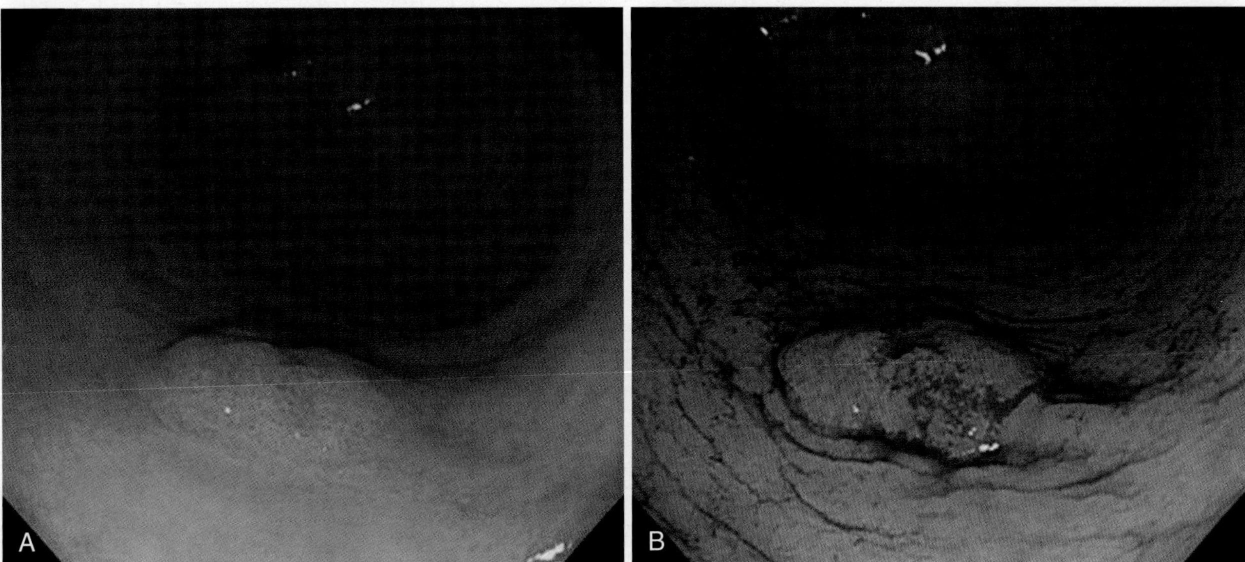

FIGURE 25.3 Endoscopic features of early gastric cancer. A, Endoscopic view of type IIa (elevated) early gastric cancer. **B,** Methylene blue dye (chromoendoscopy) improves detection of carcinoma.

The risk of nodal metastasis is extremely low in a completely resected EGC that is devoid of vascular invasion and has no other unfavorable criteria (i.e., size and ulceration), and the procedure is deemed curative.[120,121] Because of the limitations of endoscopic mucosal resection (EMR) (limited to small lesions, frequent fragmentation, limitation in evaluating lateral margins), the vast majority of all early gastric cancers in East Asia (and a few centers in the West) are now treated by endoscopic submucosal dissection (ESD). Both, EMR and ESD techniques have distinct advantages and disadvantages. The selection of one technique over the other depends greatly on the location and characteristics of lesions (Table 25.4) as well as the expertise of the gastroenterologist.[122] EMR uses a snare and additional ancillary techniques (Cap EMR, band EMR) and frequently results in piecemeal resection. Consequently, EMR is associated with a higher risk of positive microscopic margins and local recurrence. ESD with a submucosal plan of resection provides a larger specimen with en-bloc removal. ESD is technically more challenging and is associated with a higher risk of perforation.[122] A systematic approach for handling and assessing ER specimens is recommended to evaluate the key prognostic features appropriately. Correct handling starts with pinning the specimen before fixation, meticulous macroscopic assessment with orientation of appropriate margins, systematic sectioning, and microscopic assessment of the entire specimen.[122]

Whether eradication of *H. pylori* improves prognosis is unclear. However, the eradication of *H. pylori* decreased significantly the risk of metachronous gastric cancer.[123] In a study of 132 patients with EGC who underwent endoscopic mucosal resection, no new cases of gastric cancer were observed after eradication, while in contrast new early-stage intestinal-type gastric cancer developed in 13.5% of untreated patients.[124]

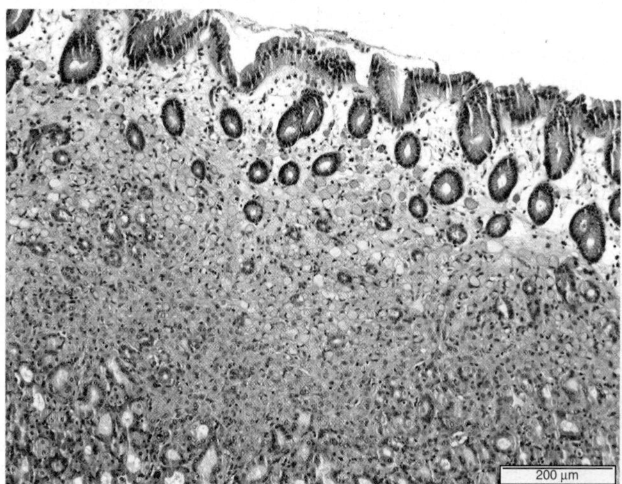

FIGURE 25.4 Early gastric cancer, signet ring cell/diffuse type. Cancer is limited to the upper half of the mucosa, with preservation of the deep glands.

ADVANCED GASTRIC CARCINOMA

Clinical Features

Advanced adenocarcinoma is defined as a tumor that invades the gastric wall beyond the submucosa. Most patients are men (male-to-female ratio of 2:1) in their fifth to seventh decades of life. Clinically, symptoms commonly include epigastric pain, dyspepsia, anemia, weight loss, hematemesis, and symptoms of gastric outlet obstruction.[125] Some patients, particularly younger ones, have intraabdominal dissemination at presentation. Metastatic ovarian lesions (Krukenberg tumors) composed of diffuse-type/poorly cohesive cancer cells may develop in female patients. Advanced-stage gastric cancer (which cannot be surgically treated) has a median survival of approximately 9 to 10 months.[14]

Pathological Features

Gross Features

Advanced gastric carcinomas may display several different gross appearances, such as *exophytic, ulcerated, infiltrative,* and *combined*. These growth patterns form the Borrmann classification, which remains the most widely used system, albeit with limited therapeutic value. It divides gastric carcinomas into four distinct types[126] (Fig. 25.5): polypoid (type I) (Fig. 25.6A), excavating with sharply demarcated and raised margins (type II) (Fig. 25.6B), ulcerated without definite limits, infiltrating into the surrounding wall (type III) (Fig. 25.6C), and diffusely infiltrating (type IV) (Fig. 25.6D). The latter is also referred to as *linitis plastica* when it involves the majority of the stomach. Type III represents the most frequent type, followed by types II, IV, and I.[127,128]

Microscopic Features

Gastric adenocarcinomas display marked heterogeneity at both the cytological and the architectural level. Cytologically, a combination of gastric foveolar, intestinal, and endocrine cell types usually constitutes at least a portion of all tumors.[129] Ciliated tumor cells may also be observed.[130] Mucin histochemical and immunohistochemical stains (MUC1, MUC2, MUC5AC, MUC6, and CD10) may be useful in highlighting the different cellular components.[22,129,131,132] In fact, based on mucin immunohistochemistry (IHC), a phenotypic classification of gastric cancer encompasses four phenotypes: G (gastric; MUC5AC+ and/

TABLE 25.4 Indications for Endoscopic Submucosal Dissection of Early Gastric Cancer

	Intramucosal (T1a) Carcinoma				Submucosal Carcinoma	
	Not Ulcerated		*Ulcerated*		*SM1*	*SM2*
	≤20 mm	>20 mm	≤30 mm	>30 mm	≤30 mm	Any size
Well differentiated						
Poorly differentiated and poorly cohesive						

Classic indications | Indications for surgery | Extended criteria for ESD

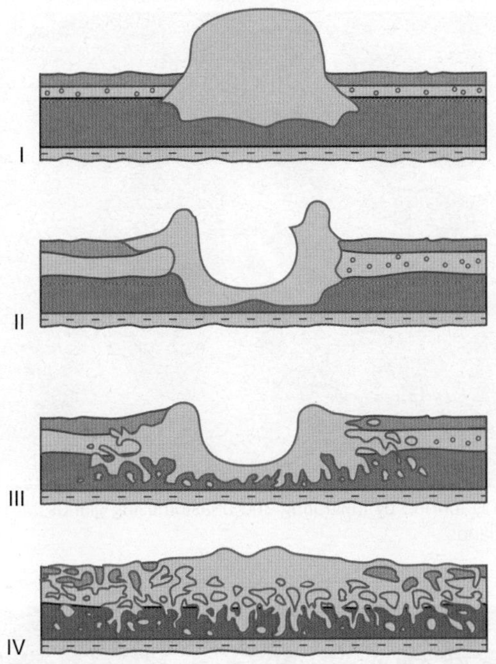

FIGURE 25.5 Borrmann four-stage macroscopic classification of advanced gastric carcinoma.

or MUC6+; MUC2− and CD10−), I (intestinal; MUC2+ and/or CD10+; MUC5AC− and MUC6−), GI (gastric and intestinal); and N (null).[131,133,134] Type I (intestinal) is more common in differentiated gastric cancers than in undifferentiated ones. The loss of MUC5AC expression was identified as an independent, poor prognostic factor in EGC, regardless of the histological type.[133] At variance, other studies showed that the foveolar phenotype (characterized by MUC5AC expression) was associated with poor prognosis in differentiated early gastric cancers.[135] Moreover, epithelial nonpolypoid dysplasia of the stomach with gastric immunophenotype was shown to display features of biological aggressiveness and may represent the putative precursor lesion in a pathway of gastric carcinogenesis originated de novo from the native gastric mucosa, leading to gastric-type adenocarcinoma.[21] For each histological subtype, a shift from the gastric to the intestinal phenotype is commonly observed with tumor progression.

Natural History

The 5-year survival of patients with advanced gastric cancer is estimated to be approximately 20%, and only surgery, including lymphadenectomy, can offer cure.[135a,135b]

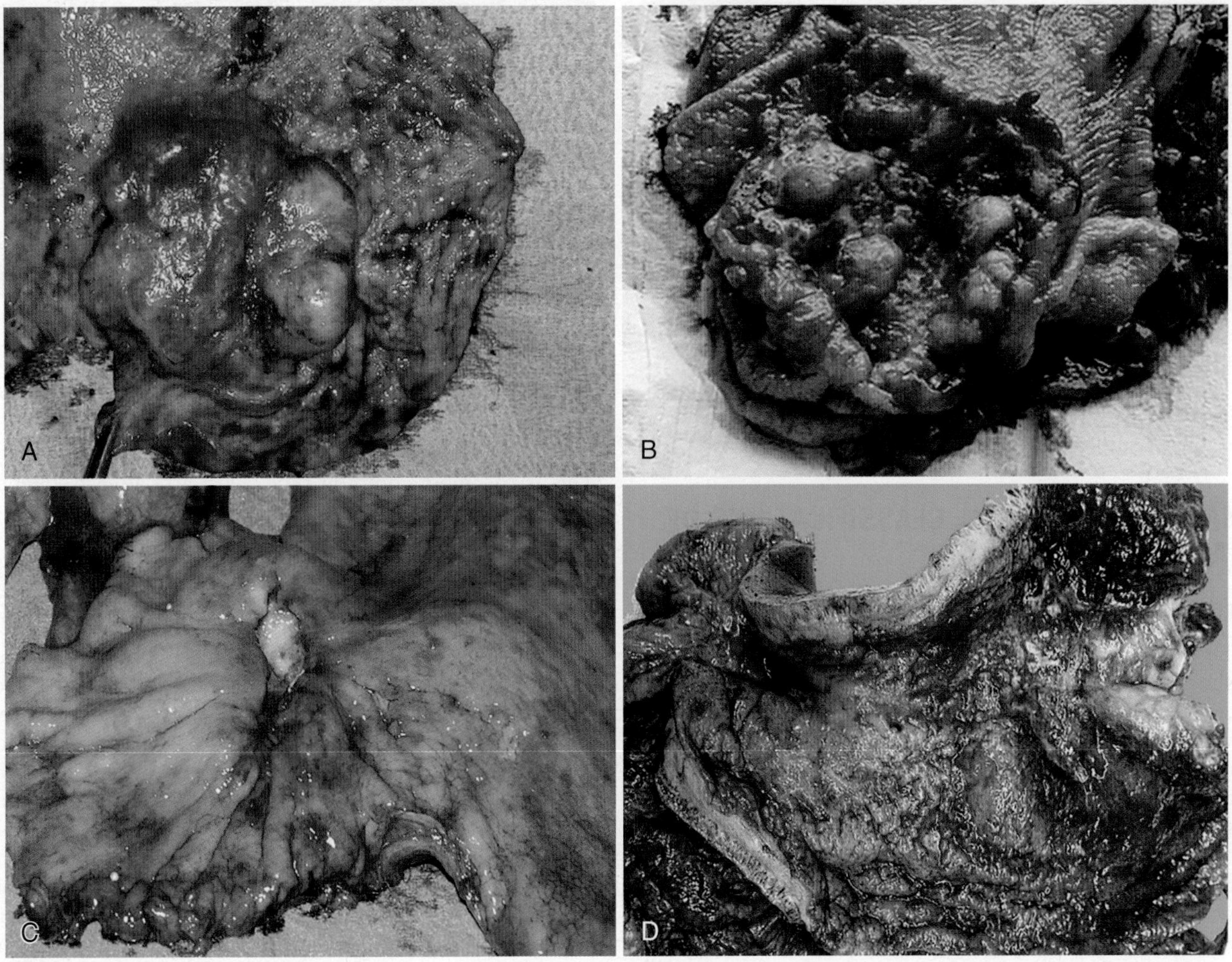

FIGURE 25.6 Growth patterns of gastric carcinoma. A, Polypoid (type I). **B,** Excavating with sharply demarcated and raised margins (type II). **C,** Ulcerated without definite limits, infiltrating into the surrounding wall (type III). **D,** Diffusely infiltrative (type IV).

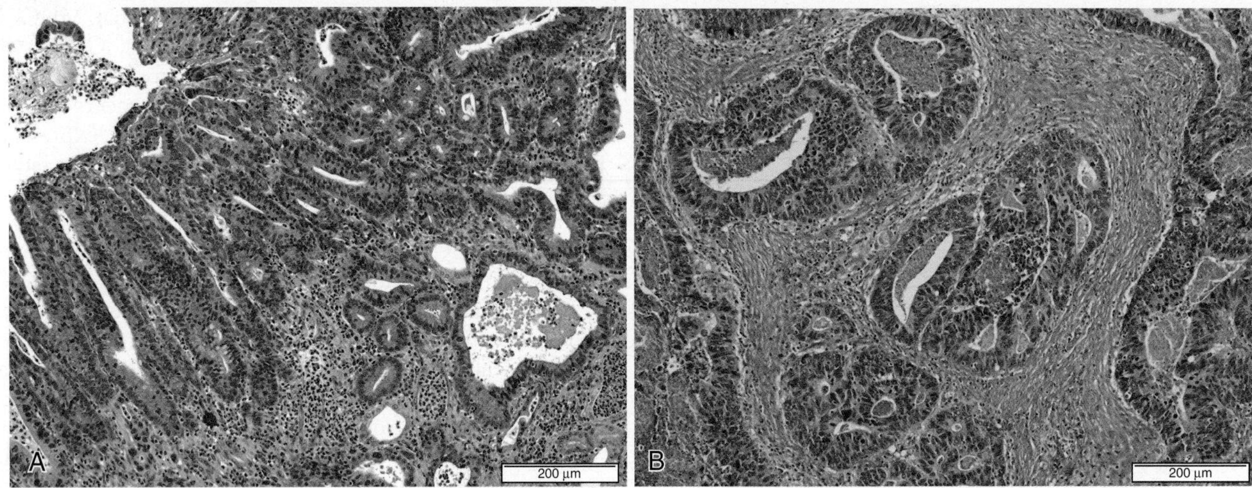

FIGURE 25.7 Tubular (WHO), intestinal (Laurén) adenocarcinoma. A, The neoplasm is formed by infiltrating and anastomosing glands with various degrees of differentiation. **B,** Intraluminal mucin or cell debris is observed in some glands.

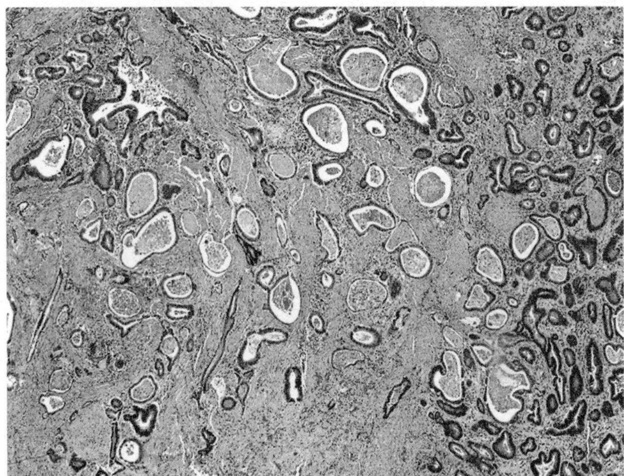

FIGURE 25.8 Tubular (WHO), intestinal (Laurén) adenocarcinoma. The neoplasm is composed of well-formed tubules, some of which are cystically dilated.

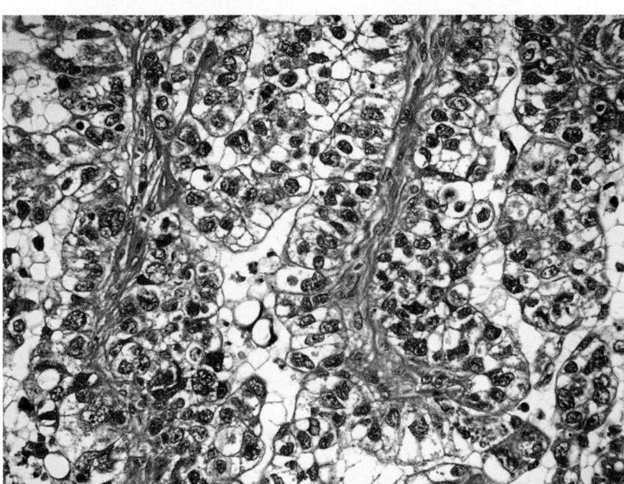

FIGURE 25.9 Tubular (WHO), intestinal (Laurén) adenocarcinoma, clear cell variant. *(Courtesy Professor Ushiku, Tokyo, Japan.)*

However, early detection and new anticancer drugs have prolonged survival.[135c,135d]

MAJOR HISTOLOGICAL CLASSIFICATIONS OF GASTRIC CARCINOMA

World Health Organization Classification

The *WHO Classification of Tumours,* 5th edition, published by the World Health Organization in 2019, is the classification that should be favored in reporting because it will bring uniformity worldwide. The classification recognizes five major types of gastric adenocarcinoma (tubular, papillary, mucinous, poorly cohesive, and mixed) as well as other rarer subtypes (gastric (adeno)carcinoma with lymphoid stroma, hepatoid adenocarcinoma and related entities, micropapillary adenocarcinoma, and gastric adenocarcinoma of fundic gland type). Other histological types of gastric malignant epithelial tumors encompass squamous cell carcinoma, adenosquamous carcinoma, and undifferentiated carcinoma.

Tubular Adenocarcinoma

This is the most common type, with a relative frequency ranging from 45% in Europe to 64% in Japan, and even higher in elderly patients.[136] Tubular structures, branching glands, or acinar structures compose it (Fig. 25.7A). The neoplastic cells can be columnar, cuboidal, or flattened by intraglandular luminal mucin or cell debris (Fig. 25.7B), and the glands can display cystic dilation (Fig. 25.8). A clear cell variant has been described (Fig. 25.9), with a predilection for the esophagogastric region. A poorly differentiated component may coexist, composed of compact sheets of tumor cells (Fig. 25.10). At the other end of the spectrum, (extremely) well-differentiated gastric adenocarcinoma has been described (Fig. 25.11),[137] either with gastric or intestinal differentiation,[138,139] some mimicking complete-type intestinal metaplasia in the stomach.[140] Tubular adenocarcinoma is usually diagnosed in older patients (commonly in the antrum or body), tends to form polypoid or fungating masses, and is strongly linked to chronic *H. pylori* infection, atrophic gastritis, and intestinal metaplasia.

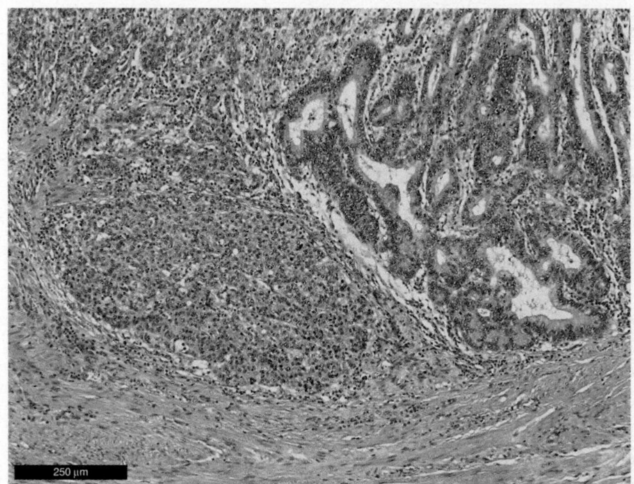

FIGURE 25.10 Tubular (WHO), intestinal (Laurén) adenocarcinoma, with a poorly differentiated component, composed of compact sheets of tumor cells.

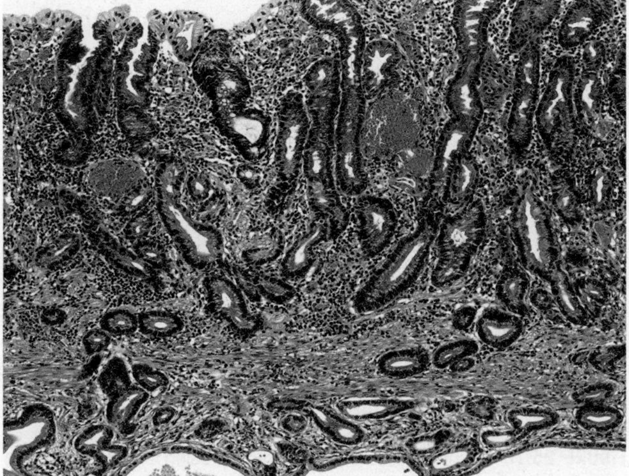

FIGURE 25.11 Very well differentiated tubular (WHO), intestinal (Laurén) adenocarcinoma. *(Courtesy Professor Ushiku, Tokyo, Japan.)*

Papillary Adenocarcinoma

This type is characterized by long epithelial projections scaffolded by central fibrovascular cores (Fig. 25.12) and usually shows an exophytic growth pattern. It accounts for 6% to 11% of all gastric carcinomas, affects older patients, occurs mainly in the proximal stomach, and is frequently associated with liver metastases. A higher rate of lymph node metastases has been reported for papillary adenocarcinoma compared with tubular adenocarcinoma. Combined tubulopapillary variants are also common.

Poorly Cohesive Carcinomas, Including Signet Ring Cell Carcinoma and Other Subtypes

Poorly cohesive tumors were previously included in a general category of SRC carcinoma, even in cases in which SRCs were not identified. The current WHO classification recognizes that a general category of poorly cohesive tumors better reflects the wide diversity of tumors composed of neoplastic cells that are isolated or arranged in small aggregates and may display various morphologies. The SRC type is composed predominantly or exclusively of signet ring cells characterized by a central, optically clear or eosinophilic, globoid droplet of cytoplasmic mucin with eccentrically placed nuclei with crescent shapes (Fig. 25.13A–B). Gland formation is not a normal component of this tumor. Signet ring cells may form a lacelike glandular or delicate microtrabecular pattern, especially in the mucosa (Fig. 25.14).

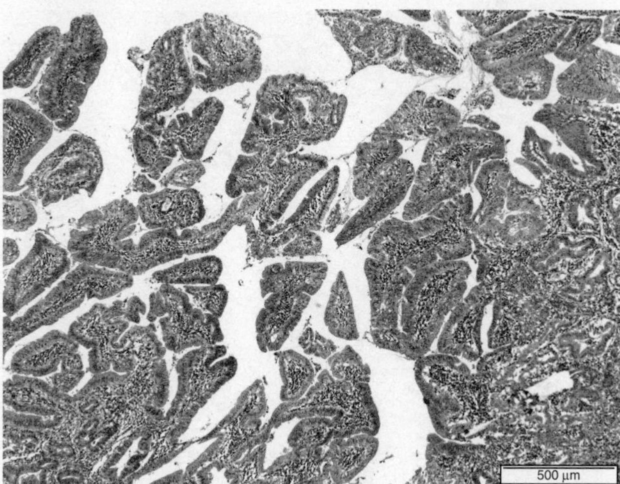

FIGURE 25.12 Papillary (WHO), intestinal (Laurén) adenocarcinoma. The papillary projections are lined by neoplastic cells.

Other variants of *poorly cohesive carcinomas* (non-SRC type) have also been observed, such as tumors that contain cells resembling histiocytes, deeply eosinophilic cells with neutral mucin, and anaplastic cells with little or no intracellular mucin (Fig. 25.15). The latter display bizarre/pleomorphic cells and are related to poor prognosis.

When poorly cohesive carcinomas invade to deeper levels of the gastric wall, they commonly initiate a marked desmoplastic reaction with loss of the morphological features of SRCs (Fig. 25.16). PAS stain may be useful to identify the neoplastic cells (Fig. 25.17A–B).

Poorly cohesive carcinomas are found most commonly in the gastric body and in younger patients, and they account for 20% to 50% of gastric adenocarcinomas, with higher frequencies in Japan.[141-143]

Although associated with *H. pylori* infection, the carcinogenetic sequence of the poorly cohesive gastric cancer is not well characterized.[17,144]

Mucinous Adenocarcinoma

This type of gastric adenocarcinoma is characterized by pools of extracellular mucin that compose at least 50% of the tumor volume; it accounts for 2% to 10% of all gastric carcinomas.[87,145] The cellular component may be formed of glands (Fig. 25.18A) or of irregular clusters of cells, including SRCs that float freely in the extracellular mucin (Fig. 25.18B). Cases with abundant mucin that compose less than 50% of the tumor volume can be referred to *adenocarcinoma with mucinous differentiation.*

Mixed Adenocarcinoma

This type is characterized by a mixture of two or more distinct histological components: glandular (tubular and/

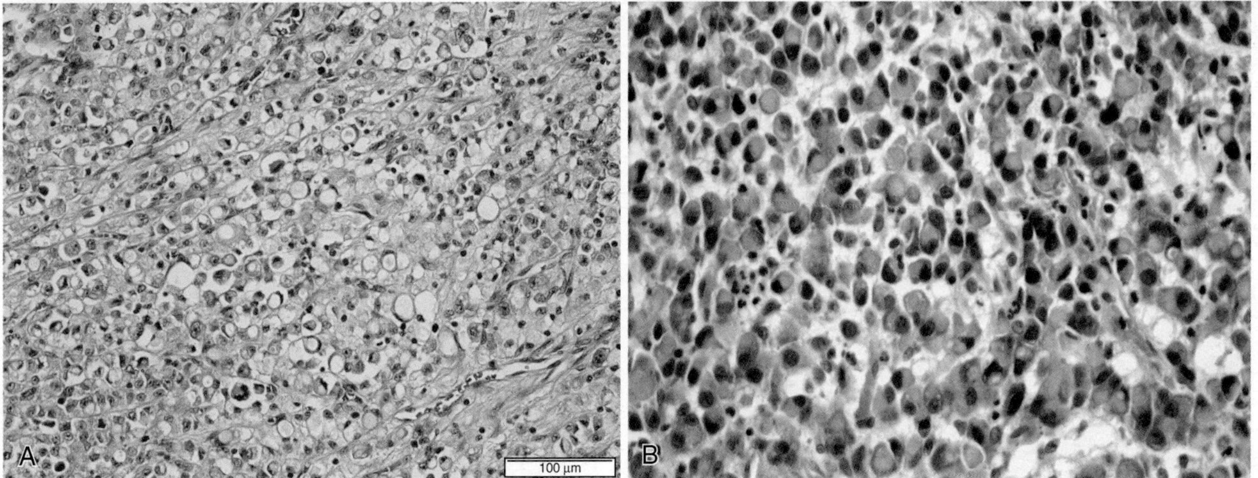

FIGURE 25.13 Signet ring cell (WHO), diffuse (Laurén) carcinoma. This type of carcinoma is characterized by the presence of a prominent intracytoplasmic mucin droplet with an enlarged, eccentrically located, flattened nucleus. **A,** Clear cell cytoplasm. **B,** Eosinophilic cytoplasm.

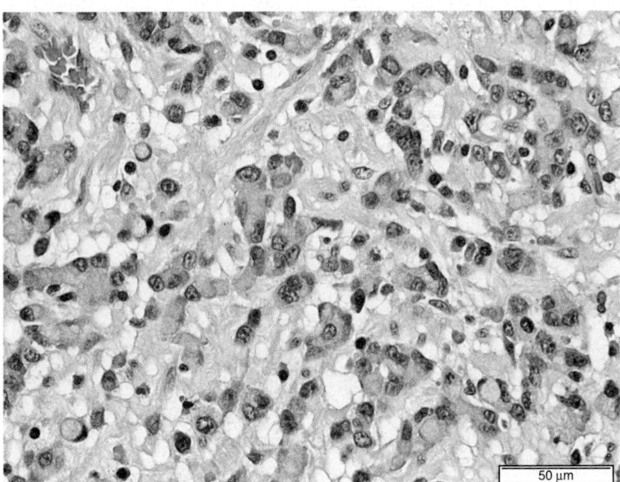

FIGURE 25.14 Signet ring cell (WHO), diffuse (Laurén) carcinoma. The cytoplasm of the neoplastic cells is eosinophilic and the cells display a lacelike glandular or delicate microtrabecular pattern.

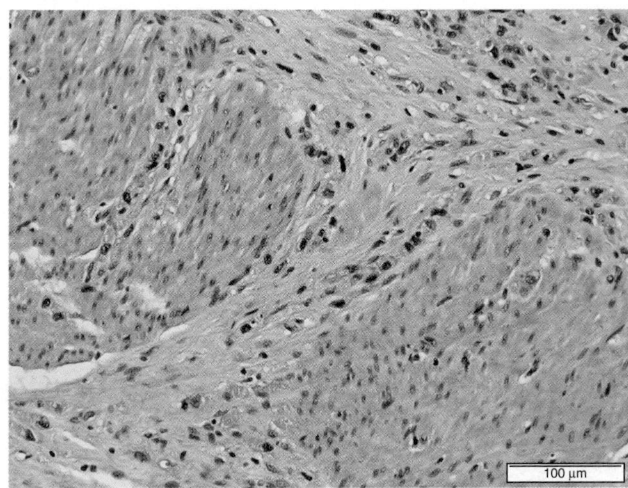

FIGURE 25.16 Poorly cohesive carcinoma. Invasion to deep levels of the gastric wall is accompanied by desmoplasia, with loss of the morphological features of signet ring cells.

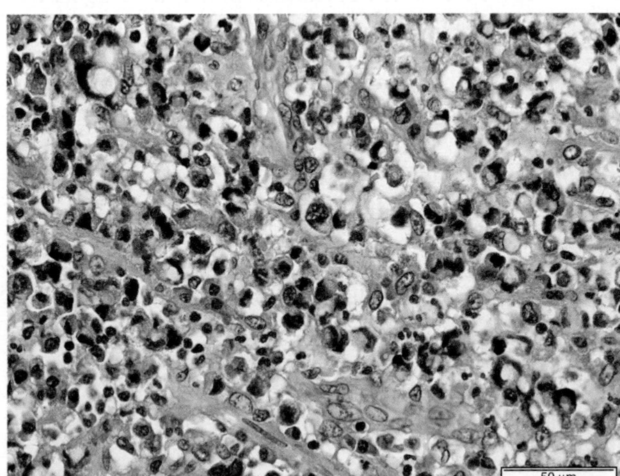

FIGURE 25.15 Poorly cohesive carcinoma, non–signet ring cell type. The neoplastic are bizarre/pleomorphic. Very few signet ring cells can be identified.

or papillary) and SRC/poorly cohesive (Fig. 25.19A–B). The distinct components can be separate or intermingled (Fig. 25.20). It is traditional to report the distinct histological components to gain insights into these tumors. The reported relative frequency is 6% to 22%.[141,142,146] Mixed adenocarcinomas are more aggressive than those with only one histological component.[146-148] The mixed histotype was shown to be an independent risk factor for nodal metastases in submucosal gastric cancers.[149] Mixed adenocarcinomas have been shown to be clonal,[146,150] and the phenotypic divergence has been attributed to a somatic mutation in the E-cadherin gene *(CDH1)*, restricted to the poorly cohesive component.[151] Enhanced promoter CpG island hypermethylation also has been implicated in the histogenesis of mixed carcinoma.[152]

Gastric Carcinoma with Lymphoid Stroma

The morphological subtype defined as *gastric carcinoma with lymphoid stroma* (GCLS), also known as *medullary*

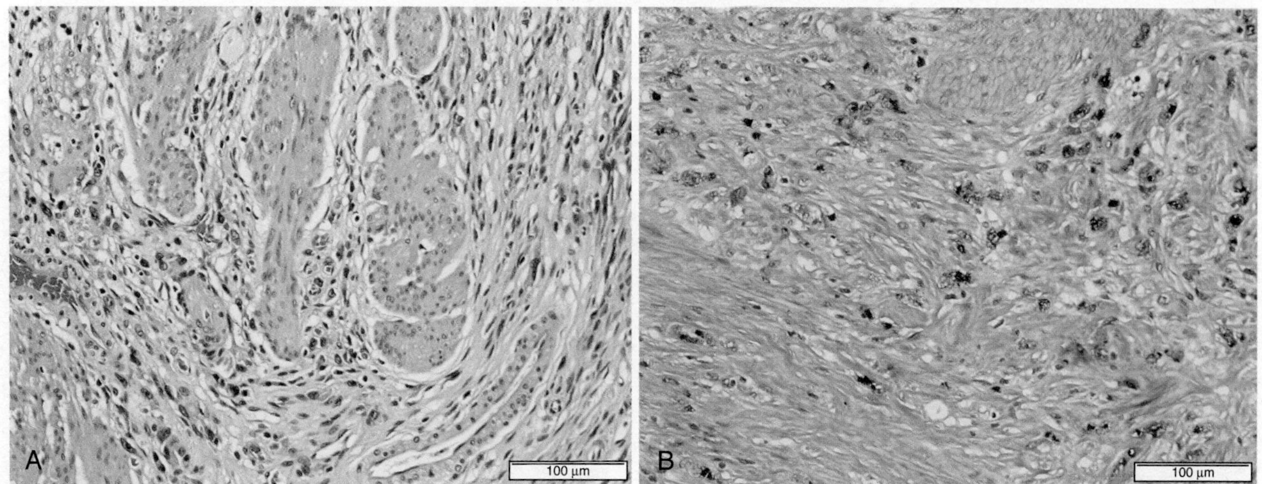

FIGURE 25.17 Poorly cohesive carcinoma. A, Invasion of the muscle layer. **B,** PAS staining may be helpful for the identification of the neoplastic cells.

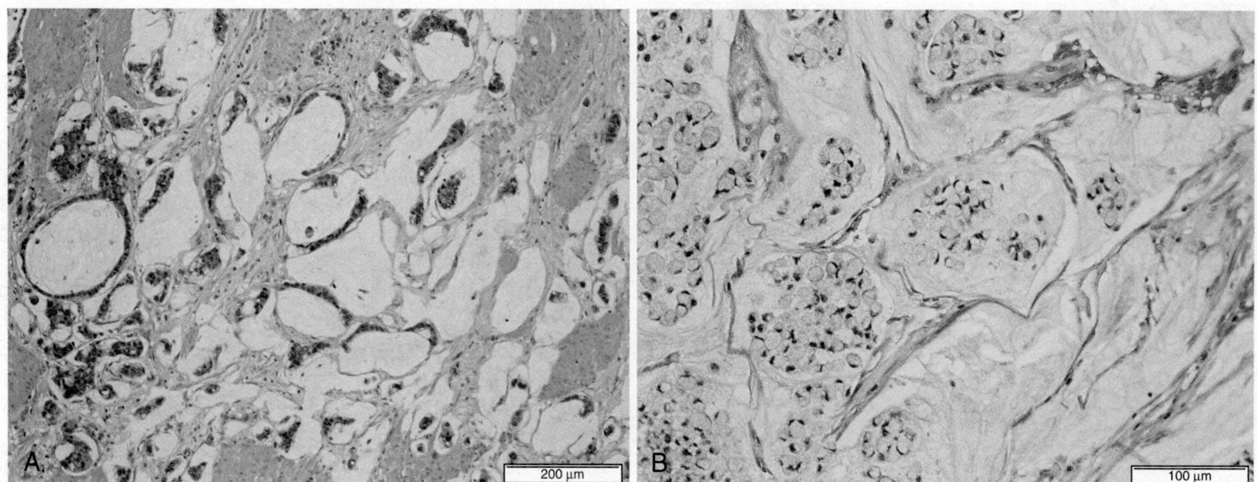

FIGURE 25.18 Mucinous carcinoma. The neoplasia is characterized by pools of extracellular mucin that compose at least 50% of the tumor volume. **A,** The neoplastic cells display a glandular arrangement. **B,** The neoplastic cells (signet ring cells) float in the extracellular mucin.

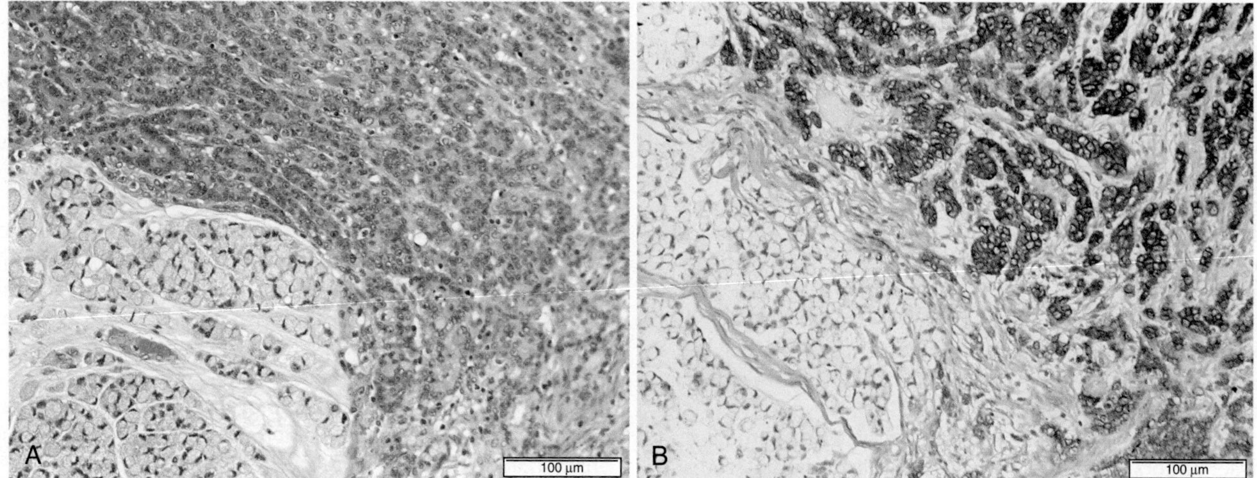

FIGURE 25.19 Mixed carcinoma. A, The neoplasia is composed of two distinct components: one is tubular *(top right),* and the other is constituted by signet ring cells *(bottom left).* **B,** E-cadherin is expressed in the tubular component and is absent in the signet ring cell component.

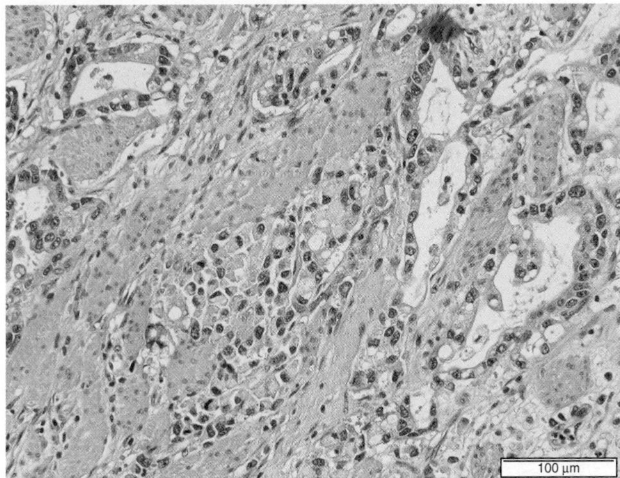

FIGURE 25.20 Mixed carcinoma. The neoplasia is composed of two intermingled components, tubular and poorly cohesive carcinoma (non-SRC type).

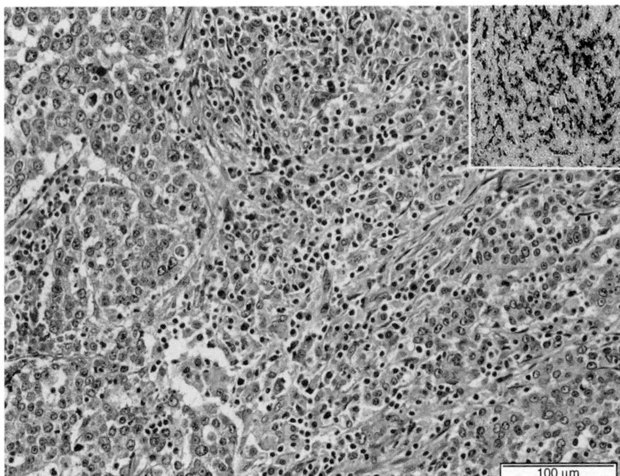

FIGURE 25.21 Gastric adenocarcinoma with lymphoid stroma (GCLS). This type of carcinoma is composed of irregular sheets of polygonal-shaped cells and numerous intratumoral lymphocytes. *Inset:* Intranuclear expression of EBV-encoded small RNA (EBER) by in situ hybridization.

carcinoma,[153] *undifferentiated gastric carcinoma with intense lymphocytic infiltrate,*[154] or *lymphoepithelioma-like carcinoma,*[155] is characterized by the presence of prominent lymphoid infiltration of the stroma. This subtype has been reported to account for 1% to 8% of all gastric carcinomas.[156,157] However, within GCLS, the reported rates of EBV infection vary from 22.5% to 100%,[155,157,158] and the highest frequencies (>80%) are detected by EBV-encoded small RNA (EBER) in situ hybridization.[159-163] A subset of gastric adenocarcinomas with microsatellite instability (MSI) and/or mismatch repair deficiency (MMRd) has a similar histological phenotype but a different transcriptomic profile.[164]

GCLS affects men more frequently than women, and these tumors are more common in the proximal stomach and in the remnant stomach in patients who have had a subtotal gastrectomy.[165]

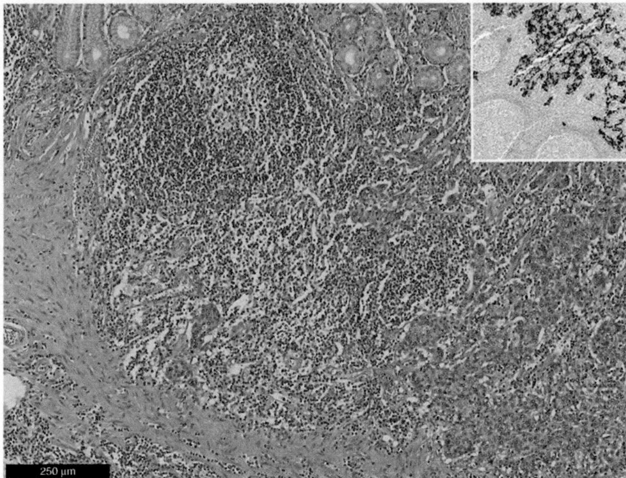

FIGURE 25.22 Epstein-Barr virus–associated gastric carcinoma (EBVaGC) with Crohn's disease–like lymphoid reaction. This carcinoma is composed of tubules and cords surrounded by prominent lymphoid follicles with germinal centers. *Inset:* Intranuclear expression of EBV-encoded small RNA (EBER) by in situ hybridization. *(Courtesy Professor Irene Gullo, Porto, Portugal.)*

GCLS usually shows a pushing tumor border and is typically composed of sheets, trabeculae, ill-defined tubules, or syncytia of polygonal cells surrounded by prominent lymphocytic infiltrate, with occasional lymphoid follicles (Fig. 25.21).[161,166,167] In its early stage, GCLS shows a characteristic "lacelike" pattern with anatomizing or branching glandular structures.[55,168,169]

Rarely, giant cells may be observed[170] CD8+ T lymphocytes are the predominant type of inflammatory cell, although B lymphocytes and plasma cells are usually present as well. Intranuclear expression of EBV-encoded small RNA (EBER) can be demonstrated by in situ hybridization (Fig. 25.21).

Two other histological variants of gastric EBV-associated gastric carcinomas (EBVaGCs) have been reported. Tubular carcinomas with limited desmoplasia, a smaller number of lymphocytes than tumor cells, and prominent lymphoid follicles with active germinal centers are termed *carcinoma with Crohn's disease–like lymphoid reaction* (Fig. 25.22).[169] The other is *conventional-type adenocarcinomas,* such as tubular carcinomas, with scant lymphocytic infiltrate (Fig. 25.23).[169]

The prognosis of patients with these tumors is more favorable than for typical gastric cancers.[153,155,163,171-175] Patients with GCLS have the best overall and disease-free survival rates, followed by those with Crohn's disease–like reaction and, finally, conventional-type adenocarcinoma.[176]

There is some debate about the role played by EBV infection in gastric carcinogenesis, either a direct role or simply a secondary effect.[177] Infection likely occurs early in the carcinogenesis because EBV can be found in adjacent dysplasia,[178] although it has not been observed in normal gastric mucosa or intestinal metaplasia.[179] In GCLS and other EBVaGCs, there is a monoclonal proliferation of carcinoma cells with EBV infection, as demonstrated by polymerase chain reaction (PCR) and EBER in situ hybridization.[180] These tumors are characterized by a stable genome, without p53 expression or *TP53* mutations, and generally are

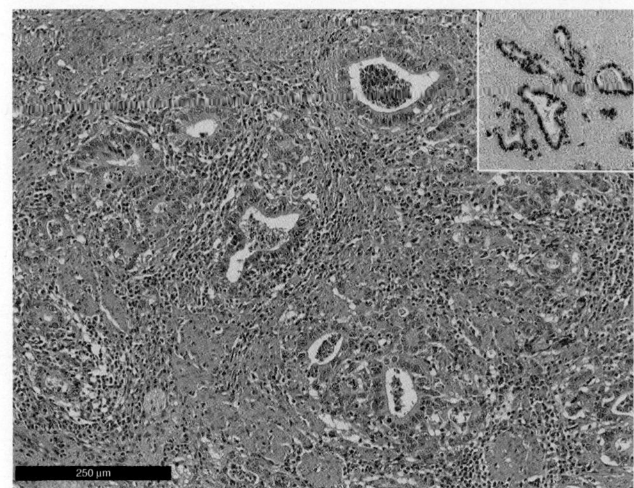

FIGURE 25.23 EBV-associated gastric carcinoma (EBVaGC) of conventional type. This is a tubular carcinoma with less lymphoid stroma than GCLS. *Inset:* Intranuclear expression of EBV-encoded small RNA (EBER) by in situ hybridization. *(Courtesy Professor Irene Gullo, Porto, Portugal.)*

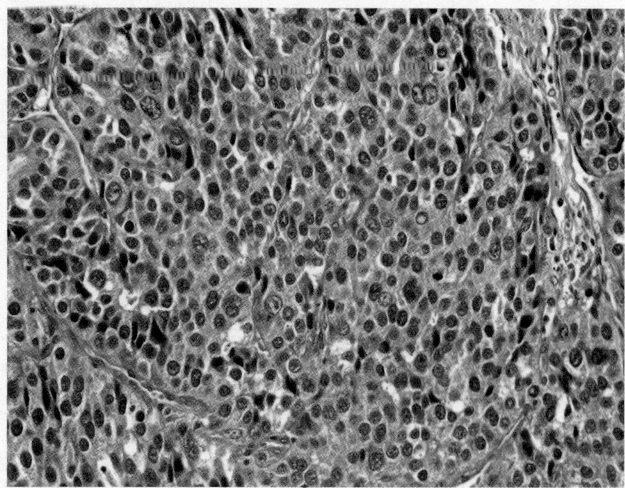

FIGURE 25.24 Hepatoid adenocarcinoma. The neoplastic cells are large, polygonal cells with eosinophilic cytoplasm disposed in trabeculae, resembling hepatocellular carcinoma. *(Courtesy Professor Ushiku, Tokyo, Japan.)*

not associated with *H. pylori* infection. In rare instances of co-infection (*H. pylori* and EBV), EBV potentiates the oncogenic effects of *H. pylori* in the stomach.[181,182] EBV-positive GCLS tumors commonly possess a CpG island methylator phenotype, with frequent aberrant methylation of multiple genes.[183] Because of the overexpression/amplification of *PD-L1/L2* in 30% to 50% of cases, EBVaGCs are good candidates for therapy with immune checkpoint inhibitors.[184-186]

Hepatoid Adenocarcinoma and Related Entities

Hepatoid adenocarcinoma and other gastric adenocarcinomas characterized by the production of α-fetoprotein (AFP) are herein described. The reported frequencies of hepatoid carcinoma and AFP-producing carcinomas are 0.3% to 2%[187,188] and 2.6% to 5.4%[187,189] of all gastric carcinomas, respectively.

Hepatoid adenocarcinomas are composed of large, polygonal cells with prominent eosinophilic cytoplasm disposed in trabeculae or acinar structures—features that resemble hepatocellular carcinoma (Fig. 25.24).[190,191] Hepatoid areas are frequently interspersed with areas of more typical adenocarcinoma, often showing a papillary pattern and less-differentiated areas containing bizarre giant cells and spindle cells.[191,192] Molecular evidence supports the clonal origin of hepatoid adenocarcinoma and coexistent adenocarcinoma.[193] AFP can be detected by IHC in tumor cells and in the serum. Bile and periodic acid–Schiff (PAS)-positive, diastase-resistant intracytoplasmic hyaline globules can be observed (Fig. 25.25A–B).[191,192] Based on the immunohistochemical expression of several differentiation markers, it was suggested that these tumors arise from carcinomas with an intestinal phenotype.[194] Clinically, hepatoid adenocarcinoma is characterized by extensive venous and lymphatic invasion, reflected in the high incidence of hepatic and nodal metastases and a poorer prognosis compared with conventional adenocarcinomas.[191,195-199]

The diagnosis is usually straightforward in terms of the primary tumor, but it can be more challenging when one is evaluating liver metastases. In such cases, negativity for Hep-Par 1 and positivity for cytokeratin 19 and 20 are helpful in excluding a primary hepatocellular carcinoma.[200] AFP (80%) and glypican 3 are detected in 80% to 92% and 56% to 100% of the cases, respectively. PLUNC (palate, lung, and nasal epithelium carcinoma–associated protein) is a marker for gastric hepatoid adenocarcinoma.[201,202] Spalt-like transcription factor 4 (SALL4), a marker of fetal gut differentiation and claudin-6 IHC, may also be useful in distinguishing hepatoid adenocarcinoma from hepatocellular carcinoma.[203] In 2010, Ushiku et al. evaluated a large series of AFP-producing gastric carcinoma and reported diffuse SALL4 expression in most hepatoid (89%) neoplasms and to lesser degree in glandular (57%) and clear cell (39%) neoplasms and none of HCCs controls.[203] Similarly, claudin-6 appears as a reliable marker of AFP-producing gastric adenocarcinomas, detected in 90% of the cases.[204]

Other AFP-producing gastric carcinomas include well-differentiated papillary or tubular adenocarcinomas with clear cytoplasm[205,206] (Fig. 25.26), gastric adenocarcinoma with enteroblastic differentiation (GAED),[207] and yolk-sac tumor–like carcinoma.[208-211] A combination of these histological types may be seen in some cases.

GAED is a tumor showing tubule-papillary architecture and is composed of columnar neoplastic cells with clear cytoplasm. GAED may represent an example of "primitive enterocyte phenotype" cancer because of its morphological resemblance to early fetal gut epithelium (Fig. 25.27); frequent upregulation of oncofetal proteins such as AFP and glypican 3 (GPC3); and several embryonic stem cell marker genes, including *SALL4*, *LIN28*, and claudin-6 *(CLDN6)*.[187,188,204] These tumors are associated with a very aggressive biological behavior.[187,207] However, the survival of patients with GAED is more favorable than that of patients with hepatoid adenocarcinoma.[212] Molecular characteristics include frequent *TP53* mutations and weak association with EBV and MSI. In terms of TCGA molecular subclassification, this group comprises a distinct subset of tumors with chromosomal instability (CIN).

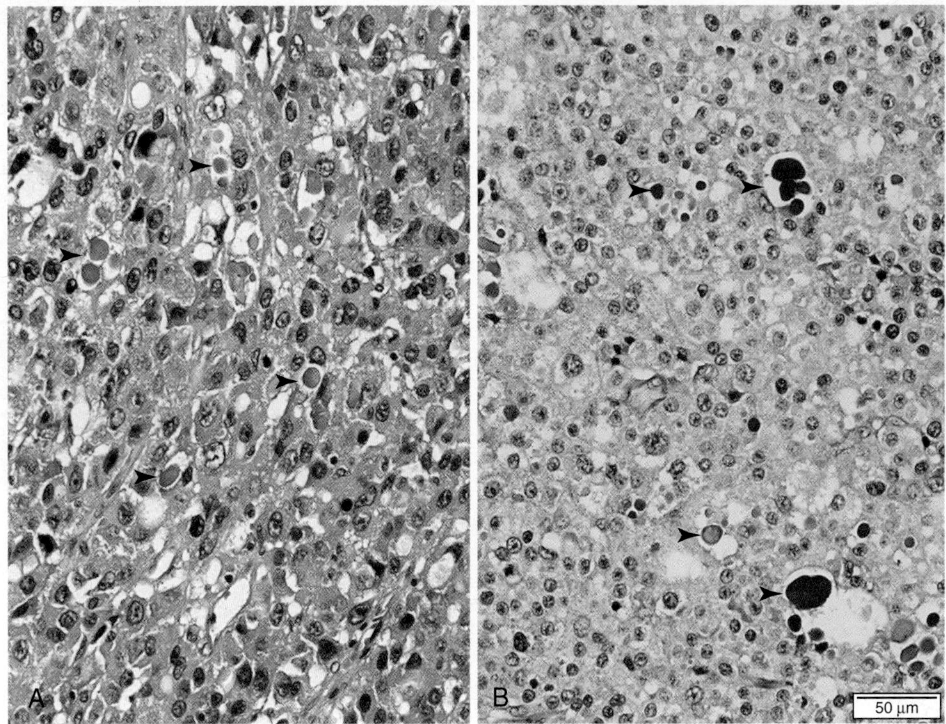

FIGURE 25.25 Hepatoid adenocarcinoma. A, Intracytoplasmic hyaline globules can be observed *(arrowheads).* **B,** These globules can be highlighted with PAS staining *(arrowheads).*

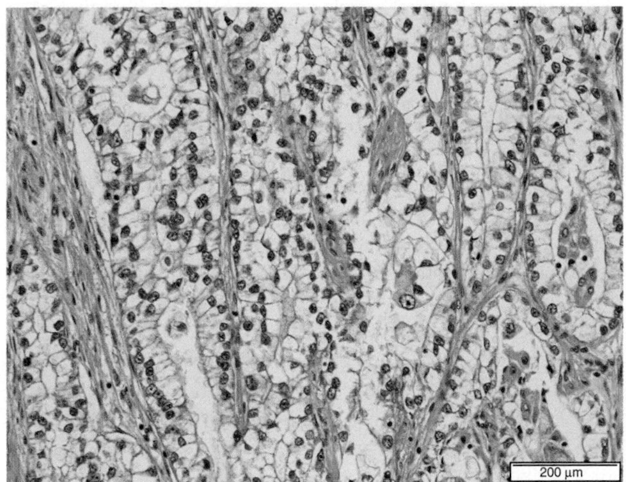

FIGURE 25.26 Clear cell adenocarcinoma. The neoplastic cells are arranged in tubules and display clear cytoplasm. This is a type of α-fetoprotein (AFP)-producing gastric adenocarcinoma.

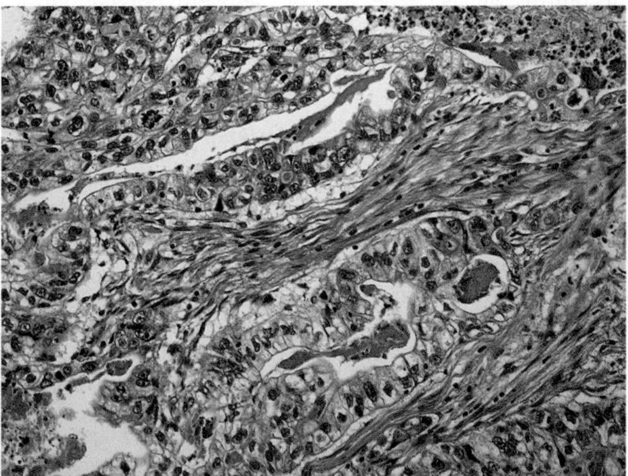

FIGURE 25.27 Gastric adenocarcinoma with enteroblastic differentiation (GAED). The tumor shows tubular architecture and displays columnar neoplastic cells with clear cytoplasm, resembling early fetal gut epithelium. This is a type of α-fetoprotein (AFP)-producing gastric adenocarcinoma.

Micropapillary Adenocarcinoma

This subtype is characterized by the presence of small clusters of tumor cells without fibrovascular cores protruding into clear spaces (Fig. 25.28). This component ranges between 10% and 90% of the entire tumor and is accompanied by tubular or papillary components.[87,213] Micropapillary adenocarcinoma has an unfavorable prognosis, and patients often present with lymph node metastasis.[213-215]

Gastric Adenocarcinoma of Fundic-Gland Type

This subtype is a well-differentiated neoplasm of oxyntic mucosa, assumed to develop from oxyntic gland adenoma.[216] It accounts for 1% of early gastric adenocarcinomas treated by endoscopic submucosal dissection.[217] The characteristic oxyntic gland differentiation can be divided into three subcategories on the basis of the tumor's composition: chief cell–predominant (~99% of reported cases) (Fig. 25.29), parietal cell–predominant, and mixed phenotype.[216] One case is reported in the literature of gastric adenocarcinoma of fundic gland type coexisting with a SRC carcinoma.[218] Submucosal invasion is observed in 60% of cases.[216] IHC demonstrates positivity of both pepsinogen I and MUC6.[219] Some cells also show

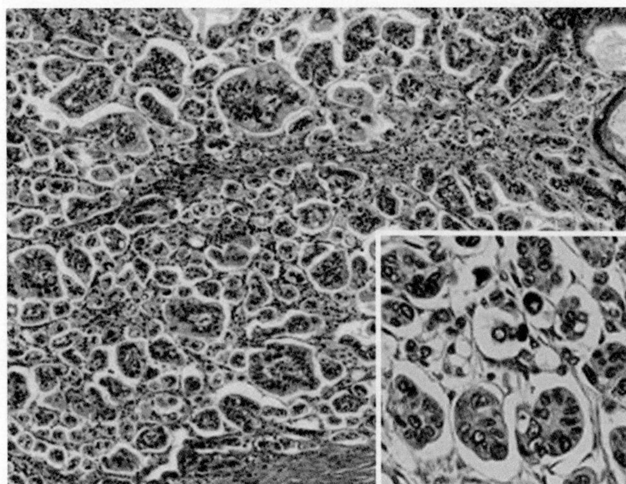

FIGURE 25.28 Micropapillary adenocarcinoma. The neoplastic cells are surrounded by clear spaces resembling lymphatic tumor emboli. *Inset:* Higher magnification of the small clusters of tumor cells without fibrovascular cores protruding into clear spaces.

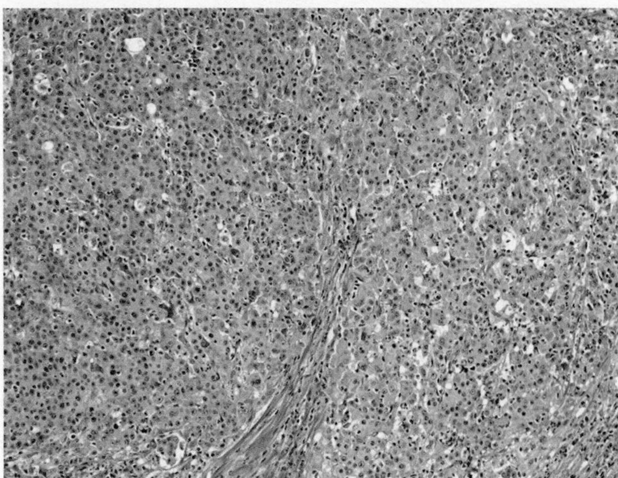

FIGURE 25.30 Undifferentiated carcinoma. The neoplasm is composed of anaplastic cells showing no specific cytological or architectural type of differentiation.

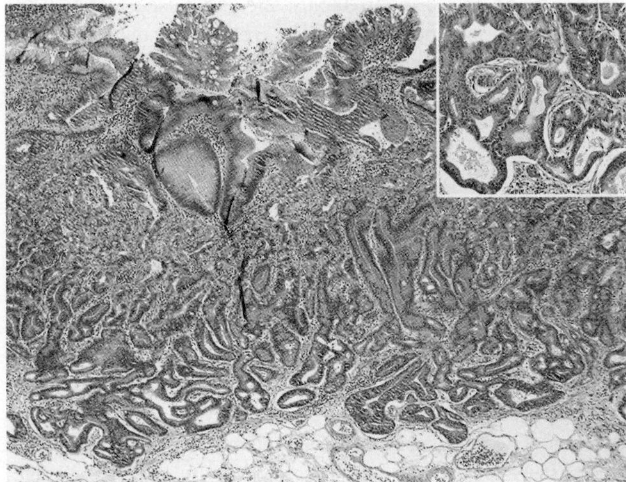

FIGURE 25.29 Gastric adenocarcinoma of fundic-gland type. The neoplasm displays irregularly anatomizing glands and is covered with nonneoplastic epithelium. There is focal invasion of the submucosa. *Inset:* Detail of the neoplastic glands, lined predominantly by chief cells.

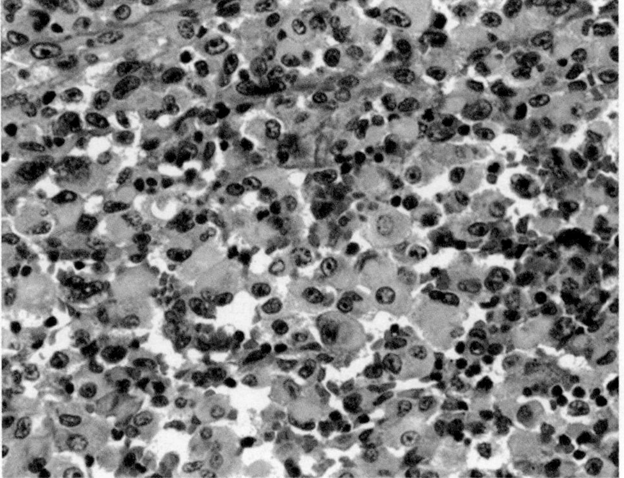

FIGURE 25.31 Malignant rhabdoid tumor. The neoplasm is composed of large cells with characteristic eccentric eosinophilic cytoplasm, large nuclei, and prominent nucleoli.

differentiation toward parietal cells (H+/K+ ATPase–positive).[220] This subtype is slow-growing, and lymph node metastasis is extremely rare.

Undifferentiated Carcinoma

This subtype is a primary carcinoma composed of anaplastic cells showing no specific cytological or architectural type of differentiation (Fig. 25.30). It may resemble lymphomas, metastatic melanoma, germ cell neoplasms, or sarcomas. Variants of undifferentiated carcinoma are rhabdoid carcinoma (Fig. 25.31),[221-223] sarcomatoid carcinoma, carcinoma with osteoclastic–like giant cells (Fig. 25.32),[224,225] and pleomorphic giant cell carcinoma.[87] Immunohistochemical analysis (positive cytokeratin immunolabeling) is often necessary to confirm their epithelial phenotype. EMA immunostaining may be useful in cases with low expression of cytokeratins. Vimentin is consistently expressed, frequently with a perinuclear dot pattern.[226,227] Areas of a glandular component may be found, suggesting an origin of undifferentiated carcinoma via dedifferentiation. In some cases, the undifferentiated phenotype is driven by components of the SWI/SNF chromatin remodeling complex, namely loss of SMARCB1 (INI 1), SMARCA4, and ARID1A.[226,227]

Adenosquamous and Squamous Cell Carcinoma

Adenosquamous carcinomas, which account for 0.25% to 0.4% of all gastric cancers, are tumors in which the neoplastic squamous component composes at least 25% of the tumor volume.[87,228] These tumors are usually deeply penetrating and associated with lymphovascular invasion, and they carry a relatively poor prognosis.[228] However, a few cases limited to only the mucosa and submucosa have been reported, as well as some cases exhibiting a positive response to aggressive chemotherapy.[108,229] A case of adenosquamous carcinoma with EBV infection has been

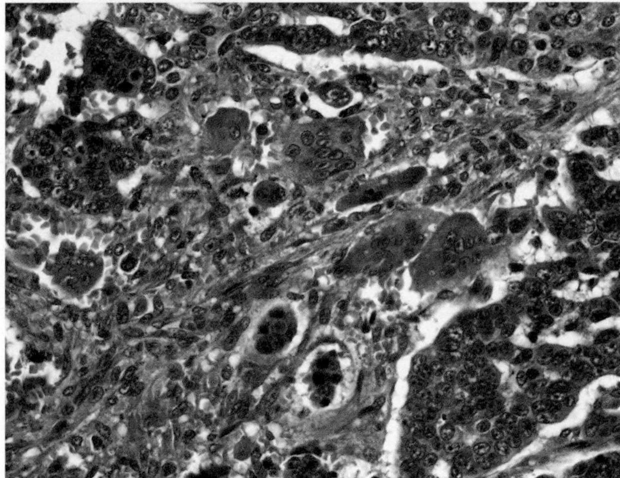

FIGURE 25.32 Carcinoma with osteoclastic–like giant cells. *(Courtesy Professor Ushiku, Tokyo, Japan).*

reported.[229] The pathogenesis of this tumor is unknown. The squamous component may arise from squamous metaplasia of adenocarcinoma cells, from a focus of heterotopic squamous epithelium, or from multipotential stem cells that show bidirectional differentiation.[229-232]

Pure squamous cell carcinomas represent from 0.04% to 0.07%[230] of all gastric carcinomas and affect men five times more often than women.[233] The degree of differentiation varies from moderately differentiated with keratin pearl formation (Fig. 25.33) to poorly differentiated. For tumors of the cardia region, caudal extension of a primary esophageal squamous cell carcinoma should be excluded. Gastric squamous cell carcinomas are often diagnosed at a late stage, and their prognosis is generally poor despite a positive response to chemotherapy.[234]

Laurén Classification

The Laurén classification[235] distinguishes two major types, *intestinal gastric cancer* (IGC) and *diffuse gastric cancer* (DGC). The former is constituted by tubular or papillary structures, while the latter is characterized by poorly cohesive and infiltrative tumor cells that may or may not have SRC morphology. Tumors that present both intestinal and diffuse components are termed *mixed carcinomas*. Other carcinomas that do not fit in one of these subtypes are placed in the *indeterminate* category. Despite dating back to 1965, the Laurén classification is still widely accepted and used, as it distinguishes subtypes with distinct epidemiological settings, clinicopathological profiles, and biological behaviors. These subtypes also correspond to distinct tumor-spreading patterns: IGC tends to metastasize hematogenously to the liver, and DGC usually disseminates through peritoneal surfaces. Mixed gastric cancer shows a poorer prognosis compared with IGC or DGC types[146,236] and a dual metastatic pattern (hematogenous metastases and peritoneal dissemination with lymph node metastases),[148,237] probably because of the cumulative adverse effect of the two components within a single tumor. The relative frequencies of the different subtypes vary a lot in Asian and non-Asian countries.[238-240]

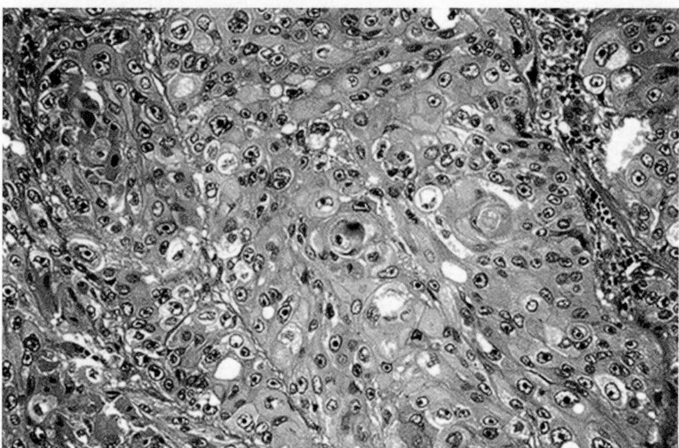

FIGURE 25.33 Gastric squamous cell carcinoma showing a moderate degree of differentiation.

Other Classifications of Gastric Cancer

The Laurén and WHO classifications are most commonly used outside of Japan. In Japan, the Japanese Gastric Cancer Association, updated in 2017, recommends a histological typing system that is similar but not 100% identical to the WHO classification (Table 25.5).[241,242] *Other classification systems* have been proposed, some of which have attempted to correlate certain pathological features of the tumor with its prognosis. The Nakamura classification,[243] extensively used in Japan, divides gastric cancer into two groups: *differentiated* and *undifferentiated*. The former encompasses tubular and papillary adenocarcinomas, and the latter includes poorly differentiated adenocarcinoma and SRC carcinoma. The classification by Mulligan[244] is based on cell differentiation and recognizes a pyloro-cardiac gland type that often shows striking vacuolization or clear cell changes, and occurs predominantly in the "cardia" or pylorus. The classification proposed by Ming[245] is based on the pattern of growth and invasion at the advancing edge, dividing tumors into an expanding (67%) and infiltrative type (33%). Expanding adenocarcinomas correspond to the intestinal type of tumors in the Laurén classification and have a more favorable prognosis than infiltrative carcinomas, which correspond to Laurén diffuse-type adenocarcinomas. The Goseki classification[246] is a four-grade classification based on tubular differentiation and intracellular mucin production: group I consists of well-differentiated tubules with poor intracellular mucin production, group II consists of well-differentiated tubules and plentiful intracellular mucin, group III has poorly differentiated tubules and poor intracellular mucin, and group IV tumors are composed of poorly differentiated tubules and plentiful intracellular mucin. Prognostic value has been attributed to this classification system.[246,247] Italian authors proposed a three-tiered prognostic classification based on histologic, clinicopathologic, and molecular parameters.[248,249]

OTHER TYPES OF GASTRIC CANCER

Choriocarcinoma

Pure gastric choriocarcinomas are rare. Most cases demonstrate a combination of syncytiotrophoblastic and

TABLE 25.5 Comparison of the Different Classification Systems for Gastric Cancer[a]

Laurén (1965)	JGCA[b] (2017)	WHO (2019)
Intestinal	Papillary: pap Tubular 1, well-differentiated: tub1 Tubular 2, moderately-differentiated: tub2	Papillary Tubular, well-differentiated Tubular, moderately differentiated
Indeterminate	Poorly 1 (solid type): por 1	Tubular, poorly differentiated (solid)
Diffuse	Signet ring cell carcinoma (SRC): sig Poorly 2 (nonsolid type): por2	Poorly cohesive, SRC phenotype Poorly cohesive, other cell types
Intestinal/diffuse/ indeterminate	Mucinous	Mucinous
Mixed	Description according to the proportion (e.g., por2 > sig > tub2)	Mixed
Not defined	**Main subtypes[c]:** Adenosquamous carcinoma Squamous cell carcinoma Undifferentiated carcinoma Carcinoma with lymphoid stroma Hepatoid adenocarcinoma Adenocarcinoma with enteroblastic differentiation Adenocarcinoma of fundic gland type Rare subtypes[d]	**Main subtypes[c]:** Adenosquamous carcinoma Squamous cell carcinoma Undifferentiated carcinoma Carcinoma with lymphoid stroma Hepatoid carcinoma Adenocarcinoma with enteroblastic differentiation Adenocarcinoma of fundic gland type Micropapillary adenocarcinoma Rare subtypes[e]

[a]Table prepared in collaboration with Professor Ryoji Kushima, Japan.
[b]JGCA, Japanese Gastric Cancer Association.
[c]Neuroendocrine neoplasms are not included.
[d]Rare subtypes (JGCA): carcinosarcoma, choriocarcinoma, invasive micropapillary carcinoma, yolk sac tumor–like carcinoma.
[e]Rare subtypes (WHO) encompass mucoepidermoid carcinoma, Paneth cell carcinoma, and parietal cell carcinoma.

cytotrophoblastic elements within an otherwise variably differentiated adenocarcinoma (Fig. 25.34).[250-252] Yolk sac and hepatoid carcinoma components may be seen as well.[253] However, some cases of pure gastric yolk sac tumor have been reported.[254,255] Gastric choriocarcinomas are usually exophytic and characterized by prominent necrosis and hemorrhage at both the macroscopic and the microscopic level.[256] Human chorionic gonadotropin can be detected by IHC, and serum levels of this hormone can also be used as a marker of prognosis and serve postoperatively as a marker of tumor recurrence.[257] The commonly accepted pathogenetic explanation is that these tumors represent choriocarcinomatous differentiation or transformation of a typical adenocarcinoma.[258] Hematogenous and lymphatic dissemination are common, with approximately 30% of patients presenting with metastatic disease at diagnosis. The prognosis of affected patients is poor.

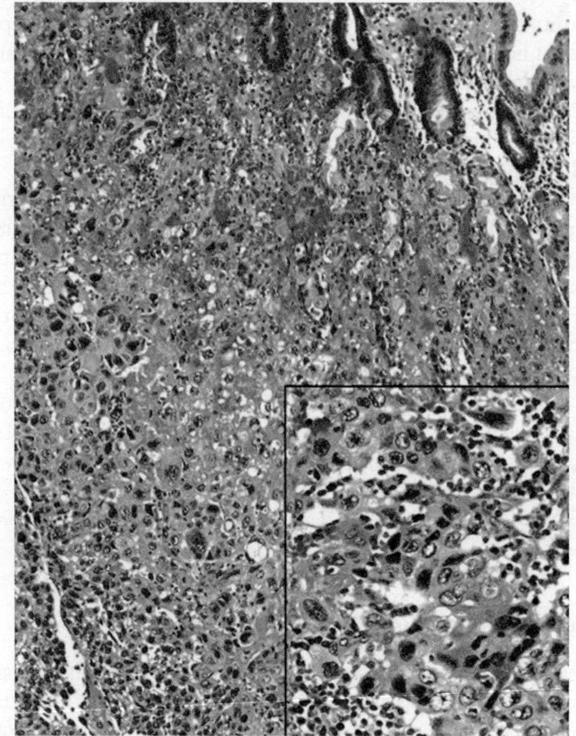

FIGURE 25.34 Gastric choriocarcinoma. The neoplasm is hemorrhagic and shows many multinucleated syncytiotrophoblasts.

Paneth Cell Carcinoma

Paneth cell carcinomas are characterized by tumors with a predominance of cells with Paneth cell differentiation, characteristically showing eosinophilic cytoplasmic granules that are positive for lysozyme and defensin-5 by IHC.[259-261] These tumors are exceedingly rare. Paneth cells can be identified dispersed among typical gastric adenocarcinomas.[262]

Parietal Cell Carcinoma and Oncocytic Carcinoma

Rare examples of parietal cell carcinoma have been reported. These tumors are composed of solid sheets of polygonal cells with abundant, finely granular, eosinophilic cytoplasm that stains with phosphotungstic acid–hematoxylin (PTAH).[263,264] Immunohistochemically, the tumor cells are positive for parietal cell–specific antibodies to H^+,K^+-adenosine triphosphatase and human milk fat globule 2. Ultrastructurally, the tumor cells are characterized by abundant mitochondria, tubulovesicles, intracellular canaliculi, and intercellular lamina filled with undulated microvilli.[263] Some cases of oncocytic gastric carcinomas negative for anti–parietal cell antibodies have been reported.[265] Focal parietal cell differentiation has been reported in a well-differentiated (gland-forming) EGC.[266] It has been suggested that patients with parietal cell carcinoma have a more favorable prognosis than those with usual gastric carcinomas.[267]

Parietal cell and oncocytic carcinomas were originally described before the recognition of gastric adenocarcinomas of fundic-gland type. Despite some similarities, it is worth noting that adenocarcinoma of fundic-gland type, in which parietal cells can be predominant, are commonly small and well-differentiated, and they fail to demonstrate solid sheets of polygonal-shaped cells, as reported with parietal cell carcinomas.

Gastroblastoma

Gastroblastoma is a rare, distinctive epithelial and mesenchymal biphasic tumor that arises in the stomach of children and young adults,[268-272] most commonly in the antrum. These tumors are characterized by mixed spindle and epithelial cellular elements (Fig. 25.35). The epithelial cells have scant pale cytoplasm, round nuclei, and inconspicuous nucleoli. The spindle cell component is monotonous, and the cells are long and slender, often in a myxoid background. Mitoses are rare in most cases, with exceptions, but mitotic counts seem unrelated to outcome.[268,270] Neither the epithelial nor the mesenchymal components display significant atypia or pleomorphism.[268]

Gastroblastoma is characterized by a *MALAT1-GLI1* fusion, and it has been proposed that this fusion gene drives GLI1 oncogenic properties and hedgehog activation.[273,274] By IHC, the mesenchymal component of gastroblastoma expresses CD10, CD56, and vimentin. The epithelial component expresses cytokeratin (AE1/AE3 and CAM 5.2) and may show focal labeling for CD56 and CD10. KIT may be rarely expressed.[274,275] Both components show strong and diffuse staining for GLI1[274] and are negative for DOG1, SMA, calretinin, CD34, desmin, and S100.[268,269,275]

Gastroblastoma rarely recurs following partial or subtotal gastrectomy. Regional and distant lymph node metastases may occur, and liver metastases were reported in two patients at presentation.[275] Local recurrence is rare.[276] Deaths attributable to gastroblastoma have not been documented.[269]

Gastric Neuroendocrine Neoplasms

Neuroendocrine neoplasms (NENs) of the stomach are gastric epithelial neoplasms with neuroendocrine differentiation, including well-differentiated neuroendocrine tumors (NETs), poorly differentiated neuroendocrine carcinomas (NECs), and mixed neuroendocrine–nonneuroendocrine neoplasms (MiNENs)—an umbrella category including mixed adeno-neuroendocrine carcinoma (MANEC).[87]

Metastatic Carcinoma

Metastases to the stomach are uncommon.[277] Among primary tumor entities spreading to the stomach, a high

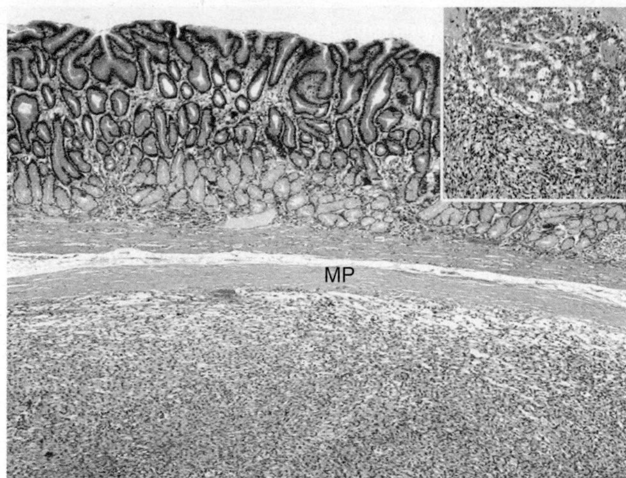

FIGURE 25.35 Gastroblastoma. The tumor develops in the gastric wall. *Inset:* The tumor is biphasic, characterized by mixed spindle and epithelial cellular elements. *MP*, muscularis propria.

prevalence of breast cancer (27%), lung cancer (23%), renal cell cancer (7.6%), and malignant melanoma (7%) has been reported.[278] Furthermore, infiltrations of lymphoma and leukemia in the stomach may occur.[278] In 50% of cases, concomitant metastases are observed in other organs.

In patients with metastasis, infiltration of the deep layers of the gastric wall, combined with a reactive hyperplasia of the overlying mucosa, may mimic hypertrophic gastritis. Metastatic lobular breast carcinoma deserves special attention because its typical single-file growth pattern can resemble diffuse-type carcinoma, SRC carcinoma, or linitis plastica. Breast-associated immune markers are ER, GATA3, BRST-2, and mammaglobin. CDX2, CK20, and HNF4A positivity are suggestive of gastric cancer.[279-281] A combination of GATA3 and SOX10 is useful for the diagnosis of metastatic triple-negative breast cancer.[282]

GASTRIC CARCINOMA IN SPECIAL CLINICAL CIRCUMSTANCES

Gastric Stump Carcinoma

Gastric surgery is associated with an increased risk for the development of gastric cancer, usually after a 15- to 30-year period.[283-286] The incidence of gastric stump carcinoma is estimated as 1% to 2%.[287,288]

Stump carcinomas are more commonly associated with Billroth II surgical reconstruction than with Billroth I and, in the latter, the interval between primary surgery and the diagnosis of stump carcinoma is significantly longer than in the former.[289-293] However, it should be highlighted that the risk of gastric stump is related to the cause of the original gastrectomy. In one study it was shown that patients with original cancer disease developed stump carcinoma in a significantly shorter time interval than those with original benign diseases, mostly peptic ulcers. Specifically, it was shown that the time trend of the reported number of stump carcinomas was quite different in manner between the patients with original cancer diseases and those with benign conditions.[294] Namely, it was the highest at 10 to 15 years followed by a gradual decrease in number thereafter for patients with original cancer diseases, whereas it was the lowest at 10 to 15 years after surgery for patients with original benign diseases, followed by a steady increase thereafter.[294] These data seem to suggest that carcinogenesis in the remnant stomach may occur based on quite different mechanisms. For example, one may come from mucosa with higher risk in the remnant stomach after gastrectomy for cancer diseases, and another may come from some already reported mechanisms developed after gastrectomy for original benign diseases.[294] Animal models suggest that reduction in the serum gastrin level enterogastric reflux of bile and pancreatic secretions may play an important role in the pathogenesis of these tumors.[295,296]

Most carcinomas are diagnosed in the distal residual stomach and preferentially involve the gastric stoma, particularly for patients treated with Billroth II reconstruction, in contrast with nonanastomotic sites in patients treated with Billroth I reconstruction.[284,289-293,297]

Histological lesions of the remnant stomach that predate the development of cancer include intestinal metaplasia, atrophy, foveolar hyperplasia, cystic dilation of the glands, and dysplasia.[297-299] However, the extent of intestinal metaplasia and the incidence of *H. pylori* infection in uninvolved mucosa are significantly less than in usual gastric adenocarcinomas.[297] EBV infection, in association with marked chronic inflammation, is observed in 0% to 12.5% of patients treated with Billroth I reconstruction and in 30.4% to 58.3% among patients treated with Billroth II reconstruction.[300,301]

Interestingly, a higher frequency of MSI is reported in stump carcinomas compared with primary proximal third gastric carcinoma. There is also a significantly higher level of MSI in patients treated with Billroth II reconstruction compared with those treated with Billroth I reconstruction.[302,303]

The pattern of lymph node metastases differs from that of primary gastric cancer, showing an increased risk of hematogenous and liver metastases,[304] possibly related to changes in lymphatic or vascular flow resulting from the patient's original Billroth surgery.

Gastric Carcinoma in Young Patients

Between 2% and 10% of all gastric carcinomas are diagnosed in patients younger than 40 years of age.[305] At variance with a decrease in incidence of gastric cancer overall, the incidence of early-onset gastric cancer is paradoxically increasing.[306,307] The presenting symptoms are usually similar to those in older patients. Female predominance has been reported in young patients with gastric carcinoma.[306-308]

Most cases are of the diffuse type and are not associated with gastric atrophy and intestinal metaplasia.[306,309] *H. pylori* infection (particularly with CagA-positive strains) is thought to be a risk factor in some patients.[71,310,311] Approximately 10% to 25% of young patients with gastric cancer have a positive family history, suggesting that genetic factors are of etiological importance. A different genomic profile has been demonstrated in younger versus older patients with gastric cancer.[312,313] In the former group, alterations of chromosomal regions 11q23.3 and 19p13.3 were common, which likely reflects different pathogenetic mechanisms than those in older patients.[312] In light of the TCGA classification (see Molecular Pathology of Gastric Cancer), adenocarcinomas in young patients are more likely to be genomically stable and of the EBV subtype.[306] Finally, gastric carcinomas in young patients frequently present at a late stage and are associated with a poor prognosis.[309]

MOLECULAR PATHOLOGY OF GASTRIC CANCER

Gastric carcinoma is the result of accumulated genomic, transcriptomic, proteomic, and epigenomic alterations[314] affecting cellular functions. These include self-sufficiency in growth signals, escape from antigrowth signals, apoptosis resistance, sustained replicative potential, angiogenesis induction, and invasive or metastatic potential, but also deregulation of cell energy, escape from immune destruction, tumor-promoting inflammation, genomic instability, deregulation of cell energy, and escape from immune destruction, the so called *hallmarks* of cancer.[315] Recently, four additional hallmarks have been proposed: dedifferentiation and transdifferentiation, epigenetic dysregulation, altered microbioma, and altered neuronal signaling.[316]

Many genes are differentially expressed in different histological types of gastric cancer, including abnormalities in oncogenes, tumor suppressor genes, growth factors, receptor tyrosine kinases, DNA repair genes, matrix degradation enzymes, cell-cycle regulators, and cell adhesion molecules. Furthermore, DNA methylation, histone modification, chromatin remodeling, and regulation by noncoding RNAs are important epigenetic alterations in gastric cancer development.[314,317-320]

Driver Mutations in Gastric Carcinogenesis

Major driver mutations of gastric cancer encompass the following:

1. Mutations in *TP53*, which is the most predominantly mutated driver gene in gastric cancer. Mutations are most frequent in intestinal-type gastric cancer, especially the subtype with CIN (50% to 70%). [321] The mutation rate is slightly lower in diffuse-type gastric cancer and is distinctly uncommon in gastric cancer associated with EBV infection and in gastric cancer with MSI.
2. Mutations in *ARID1A*, which are found mostly in EBV-positive and MSI cancers (70% to 80%).
3. Mutations of *RHOA*, which are found in diffuse gastric cancer (14% to 25%) but not in the intestinal type.[321,322]
4. Mutations in Wnt signaling pathway genes, including a new driver mutation of *RNF43*, occur in gastric cancer with MSI (33% to 60%).[321,323] The mutational incidence of the *APC* gene is more common in the intestinal type (10%) versus the diffuse type (2%). Mutations of beta-catenin occur in around 4% of microsatellite stable (MSS) gastric cancers.[321,323]
5. Mutations in *MUC6*, which encodes a gastric-specific mucin expressed in foveolar neck cells, as well as antral glands, are observed in about 20% of MSI gastric cancers.
6. Mutations in the *KRAS/PIK3CA/PTEN* pathway; mutations in the *PIK3CA* gene have been reported to be frequent in MSI (40%) and EBV-positive gastric cancers (over 60%).[323] Mutations in *KRAS* and *PTEN* are more commonly observed in in gastric cancer with MSI 20% to 30% and 13% to 30%, respectively
7. Mutations in the *CDH1* gene, which are observed mainly in diffuse gastric cancers (25%).
8. Mutations in the *TGFB* signaling pathway, including

frameshift mutations affecting mononucleotide tracts of the *TGFBR2* (90%) and *ACVR2A* (70%), are very frequent in MSI cancers. Overall, 100% of MSI cancers show derangement of the TGFB signaling pathway.[321] Germline mutations in *SMAD4* are responsible for juvenile polyposis syndrome, with florid hyperplastic polyp development in the stomach and a propensity for progression to carcinoma, supporting the important role of *SMAD4* in growth suppression in the gastric epithelium.

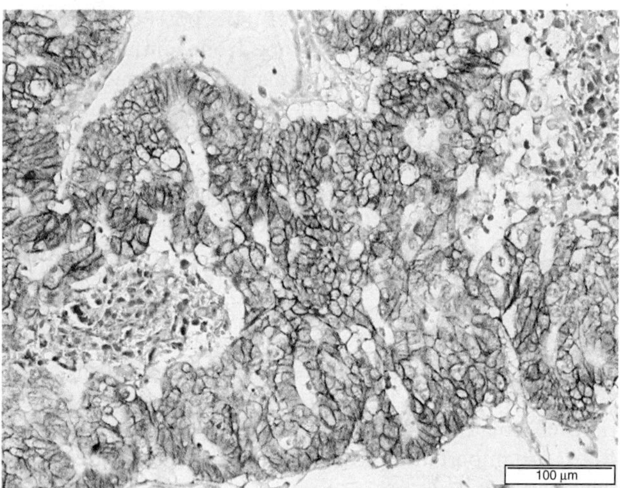

FIGURE 25.36 HER2 expression. The immunohistochemical expression of HER2 is strong and complete at the basolateral membrane of the neoplastic cells (IHC 3+).

9. Other putative driver mutations, most of which affect important cell signaling pathways, encompass hedgehog *(GLI3, ZIC4)*, ERBB (*ERBB2, ERBB3, ERBB4,* and *NRG1*), stem cell *(DCLK1)*, and cell adhesion *(CTNNA2)*.

ERBB2/HER2 alterations are mainly observed in intestinal-type gastric cancer.[14,145,324] *HER2* overexpression and/or amplification are present in up to 20% of gastric cancers.[325,326] IHC expression and in situ hybridization detection of HER2 in gastric cancer are scored as 0, 1+, 2+, or 3+. There is evidence that tumors with HER2 overexpression/amplification may respond to therapy with the humanized monoclonal antibody trastuzumab (Herceptin), as shown in the ToGA trial.[326] Compared with breast carcinoma, HER2 positivity in gastric cancer is frequently heterogeneous, and there is a less stringent correlation between *ERBB2* amplification and protein overexpression (Fig. 25.36).[325] A guideline published from the College of American Pathologists, American Society for Clinical Pathology, and American Society of Clinical Oncology[327] establishes an evidence-based guideline for HER2 testing in patients with gastric cancer. It formalizes the algorithms for methods to improve the accuracy of HER2 testing and provides several recommendations (Fig. 25.37). Given the issue of intratumoral heterogeneity in gastroesophageal adenocarcinoma specimens (Fig. 25.38), testing of multiple biopsy fragments (from a primary or metastatic site) or from the resected primary tumor is recommended. For biopsy specimens, current recommendations state that when possible, a minimum of five biopsy specimens[328] and optimally six to eight should be obtained to account for intratumoral heterogeneity and

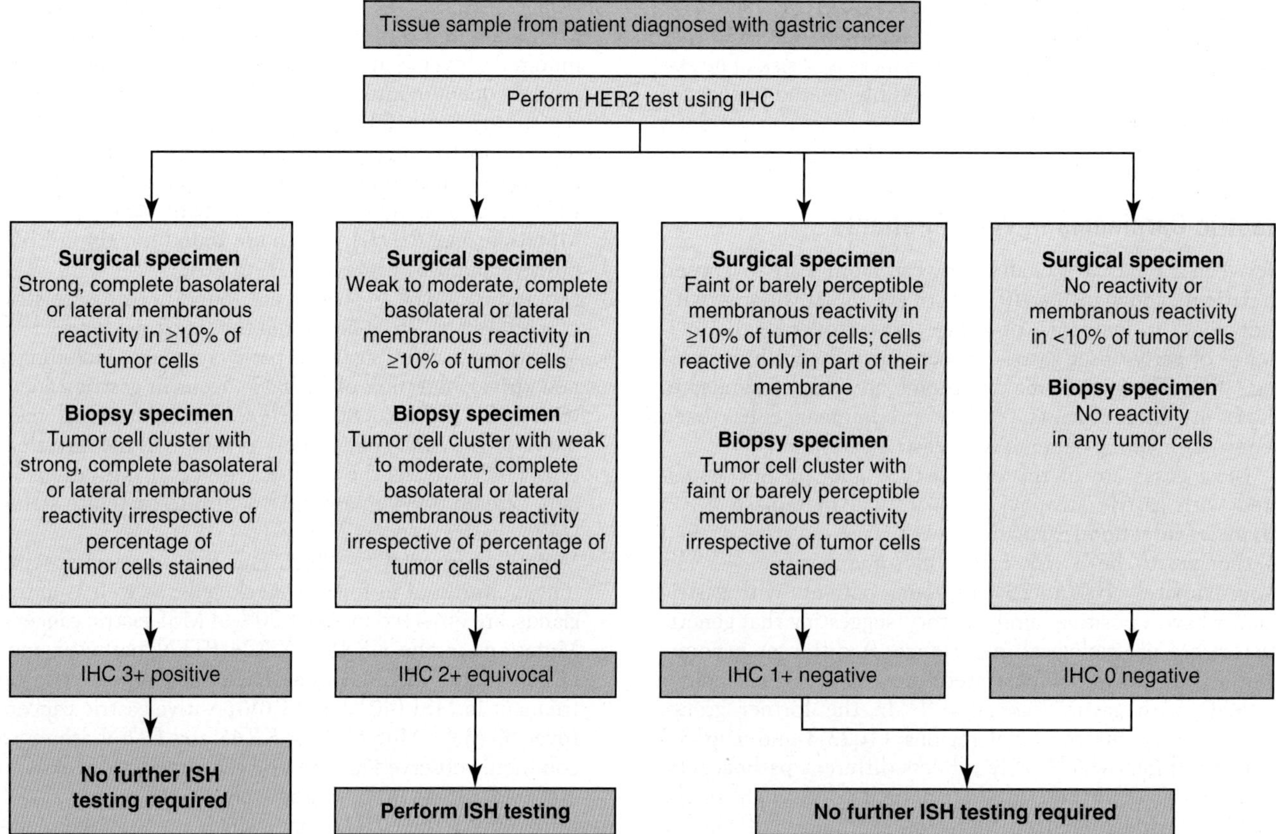

FIGURE 25.37 Evidence-based guideline for HER2 testing in patients with gastric cancer.

to provide sufficient tumor specimens for diagnosis and biomarker testing.[328,329]

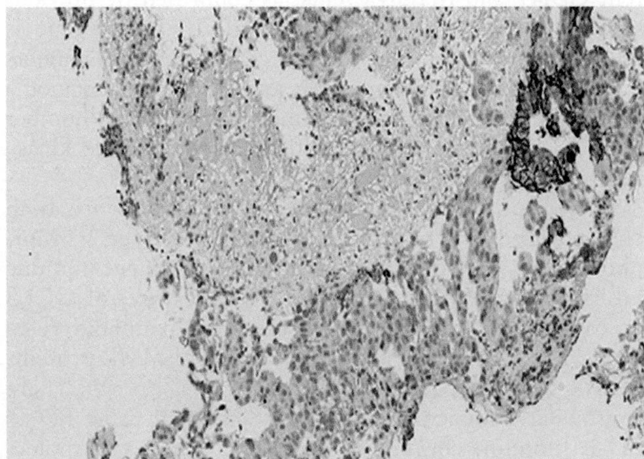

FIGURE 25.38 Heterogeneous HER2 expression in a gastric biopsy. The sample comprises necrotic tissue covering a fragment of gastric carcinoma displaying a small, focal area positive for HER2.

Molecular Classifications of Gastric Cancer

Next-generation sequencing (NGS), whole-genome sequencing (WGS), whole-exome sequencing (WES), RNA sequencing, and targeted sequencing have expanded the knowledge base of molecular pathogenesis of gastric cancer. Several studies analyzed molecular alterations present at high resolution, using various high-throughput platforms, and attempted to achieve integrated molecular classifications of gastric cancer.[323,330-333] These studies attempted to achieve integrated molecular classification schemes, clustering the comprehensive molecular data obtained into subgroups with different molecular signatures and clinical phenotypes.

Deng et al.[334] performed a comprehensive survey of genomic alterations in gastric cancer and found systematic patterns of molecular exclusivity of genes related to receptor tyrosine kinase (RTK)/RAS signaling: *FGFR2* (9%), *KRAS* (9%), *EGFR* (8%), *ERBB2* (7%), and *MET* (4%). These genes were frequently amplified in gastric cancer in a mutually exclusive manner.[334] However, these results were not confirmed in recent studies from Korea, using IHC and in situ hybridization.[324,335] In one of these studies,[335]

TABLE 25.6 Molecular Classifications of Gastric Cancer

Tan et al., 2011 (*n* = 270)			**G-DIF** (44%)	**G-INT** (56%)	
			Cell proliferation **Diffuse GC**	Cell adhesion **Intestinal GC**	
Bass et al., 2014 ("Comprehensive molecular characterization of gastric adenocarcinoma," 2014) (*n* = 295)—TCGA cohort	**EBV** (9%)	**MSI** (22%)	**GS** (20%)	**CIN** (50%)	
	EBV-CIMP *CDKN2A* silencing *PIK3CA* mutations *PD-L1/2* amplification *JAK2* amplification	Gastric-CIMP *MLH1* silencing *PIK3CA* mutations *HER2/3* mutations *EGFR* mutations **Intestinal GC**	*CDH1* mutations *RHOA* mutations *CLDN18-ARHGAP* fusion (RhoA-GTPase) **Diffuse GC**	High *TP53* mutations *TKR-RAS* amplification Amplification of cell-cycle mediators **Intestinal GC**	
Cristescu et al., 2015 (*n* = 300)—ACRG cohort	EBV+ cases included in MSS/TP53+	**MSI** (23%)	**MSS/EMT** (15%)	**MSS/TP53-** (36%)	**MSS/TP53+** (26%)
		MLH1 loss Hypermutation (*KRAS, ARID1A, PIK3CA*) **Intestinal GC**	*CDH1* loss **Diffuse GC**	High *TP53* mutations Genomic instability Oncogene amplification **Intestinal GC**	**Intestinal GC**
Practical algorithm strategy for molecular subtyping	Positive ↑ EBER ISH → (−) →	dMMR/MSI-H ↑ MMRD/MSI IHC/PCR → (−) →	Aberrant ↑ E-cadherin IHC → (−) →	Aberrant ↑ p53 IHC	"wild-type" ↑ p53 IHC

ACRG, Asian Cancer Research Group; *CIMP*, CpG island methylation phenotype; *CIN*, chromosomal instability; *EBV*, Epstein-Barr virus; *EBER ISH*, EBV-encoded small RNA in situ hybridization; *EMT*, epithelial-to-mesenchymal transition; *GC*, gastric cancer; *GS*, genomically stable; *MSI*, microsatellite instability; *MSS*, microsatellite stable; *TCGA*, The Cancer Genome Atlas; TKR tyrosine kinase receptors.

Data courtesy of Professor Irene Gulo, Porto, Portugal, and from references 323, 330, 332.

EGFR was most commonly overexpressed (40%), followed by HER2 (14%) and MET (12%). Furthermore, 2.5% and 11% of cases had simultaneous overexpression of three and two RTKs, respectively. [335] In one study, RTK-amplified gastric cancers (RA-GCs) were observed in 10.5% of 993 consecutive advanced gastric cancer (AGC) patients who underwent radical gastrectomy, not previously submitted to neoadjuvant chemotherapy. It was observed that the RA-GC status correlated significantly with older age, differentiated histology, intestinal or mixed type by Laurén classification, lymphovascular invasion, and mutant pattern of *TP53*. Altogether, these studies suggest that a proportion of gastric cancer patients may be potentially treatable by RTK/RAS-directed therapies.[334,335]

The Cancer Genome Atlas (TCGA) Research Network[323] proposed a four-tiered molecular classification (Table 25.6). The four subtypes are (1) EBV-positive gastric cancer characterized by EBV positivity, stable genome, lack of *TP53* mutations, prevalent *ARID1A* mutation, recurrent *PIK3CA* mutations, frequent *JAK2* and *PD-L1* amplification, and a high level of DNA hypermethylation, as previously reported[336]; (2) gastric carcinoma with MSI (MSI-high), characterized by DNA hypermethylation, *MLH1* silencing, and mutation in druggable target genes such as *RNF43* and *ERBB2*; (3) genomically stable gastric carcinoma, associated with a diffuse histotype and recurrent *CDH1* and *RHOA* events, as confirmed by previous studies[321,322,337]; the *CLDN18-ARHGAP* fusion gene is one of the most frequent somatic genomic rearrangements in this type of gastric cancer[338]; and (4) gastric carcinoma with CIN, exhibiting intestinal morphology, a high number of *TP53* mutations, and amplifications of tyrosine kinase receptors (TKRs).

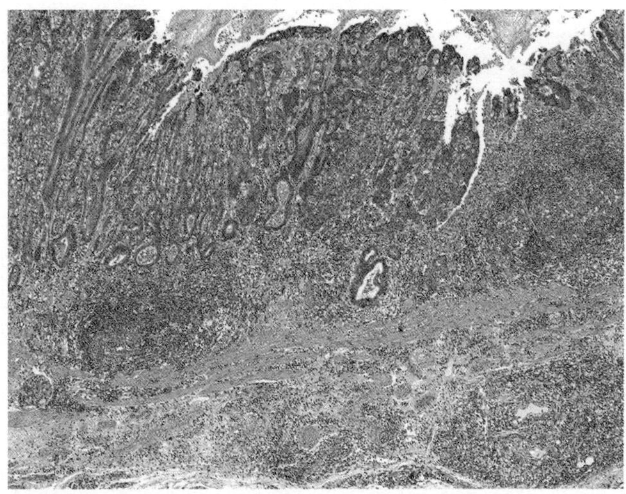

FIGURE 25.39 Tubular carcinoma with Crohn's disease–like lymphoid reaction.

EBV-positive and MSI-high gastric cancers are both characterized by a high-methylation epigenotype.[339] Morphologically, they are characterized by prominent immune infiltrate[248] and frequently display the features of GCLS or carcinoma with Crohn's disease–like lymphoid reaction (Fig. 25.39), with loss of expression of MMR proteins (MMR deficient) (Fig. 25.40A–B).[155,163,172,340-342] There is growing evidence about the possibility of using PD-1/PD-L1 immune checkpoint inhibitors in these two molecular subtypes of gastric cancer.[343,344] In gastric cancer, as in other tumor models, PD-L1 overexpression is associated with high densities of CD3+ and CD8+ tumor-infiltrating lymphocytes,[143,345,346] GCLS morphology,[347] and either EBV+ or MSI-high status.[143,184,185,348,349] Table 25.7 summarizes the key molecular alterations according to TCGA classification.

The Asian Cancer Research Group (ACRG) described four molecular subtypes with distinct prognostic implications (see Table 25.6).[332] These subtypes encompass: MSI-high tumors with intestinal morphology and the most favorable prognosis as previously described[335]; epithelial-to-mesenchymal transition (MSS/EMT) gastric cancer with diffuse morphology and the poorest prognosis; and MSS adenocarcinomas with no EMT signature, either TP53 active (MSS/TP53+) or inactive (MSS/TP53–), and with intermediate prognosis. The MSS/TP53– (inactive) subtype (roughly corresponds to the proliferative 331 and CIN subtypes) is prevalent (36% to 50% of gastric cancers) and harbors genomic amplification of TKR and/or RAS, which are in-use or potential therapeutic targets. Furthermore, some correlation studies of morphological classification and molecular profiles have been carried out.[350,351] Other

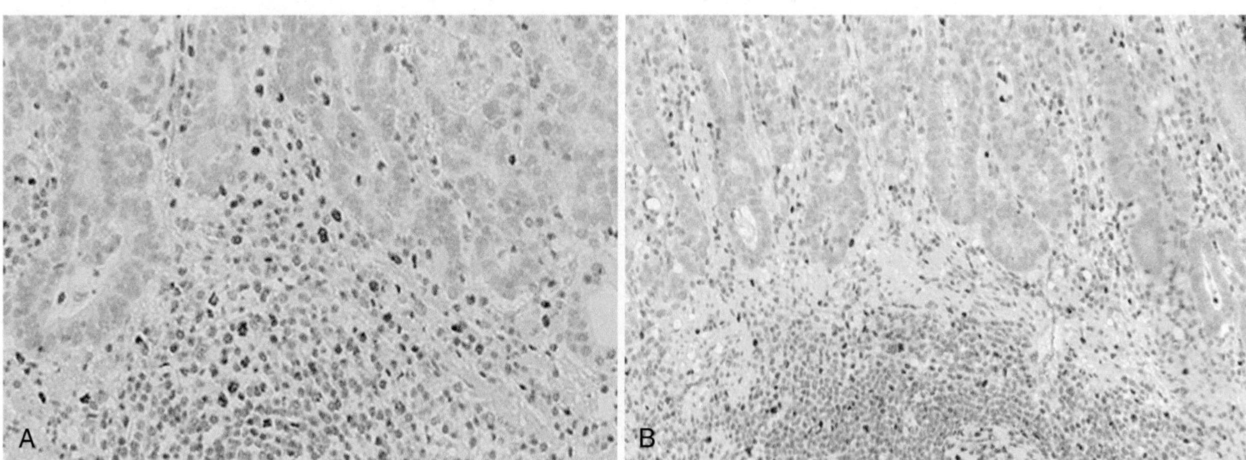

FIGURE 25.40 Mismatch repair deficiency (MMRd). A, Loss of expression of MLH1. **B,** Loss of expression of PMS2.

TABLE 25.7 Key Molecular Alterations According to the Cancer Genome Atlas

Molecular Classification of Gastric Cancer	EBV-positive	MSI	Genomic Stable	Chromosomal Unstable
Relative frequency	9%	22%	20%	50%
Representative histology	**Gastric carcinoma with lymphoid stroma**	**Prominent immune infiltrate**	**Diffuse type***	**Intestinal type***
Methylation				
CpG island	**CIMP**	**CIMP**	Rare	Rare
MSI-high	Absent	All	Absent	Absent
CDKN2A	**All**	**Frequent**	Rare	Rare
MLH1	Absent	**Frequent**	Rare	Rare
Copy number aberrations	Rare	Rare	Rare	**Frequent**
Genomic mutations/alterations	Rare	**Frequent**	Rare	Rare
TP53	Rare	Present	Rare	**Frequent**
CDH1	Absent	Rare	**Present**	Rare
PIK3CA	**Frequent**	**Present**	Rare	Rare
RHOA	Rare	Rare	**Present**	Rare
CLDN18-ARHGAP fusion	Absent	Rare	**Present**	Rare
ARID1A	**Frequent**	**Present**	Rare	Rare
RTK amplification	Rare	Rare	Rare	**Frequent**
RTK mutation	Rare	**Frequent**	Rare	Rare
CD274 (PD-L1) and *PDCD1LG2 (PD-L2)* amplification	**Frequent**	Rare	Rare	Rare

*The Laurén histological classification; see Table 25.5 for the corresponding 2017 Japanese Gastric Cancer Association (JGCA) and 2019 WHO classifications. Modified from Carneiro F, Fukayama M, Grabsch H, Yasui W. Gastric adenocarcinoma. In *WHO Classification of Tumours. Digestive System Tumours.* 5th ed. Lyon, France: International Agency for Research on Cancer; 2019, pp. 85–95.
CIMP, CpG island methylator phenotype; *MSI*, microsatellite instability; *RTK*, receptor tyrosine kinase.

studies from Korea,[324,335] using also IHC and in situ hybridization assay, identified a molecular spectrum of distinct gastric cancer subtypes.

In an attempt to refine the molecular classification of gastric cancer and to identify prognostic/predictive mutational signatures, Li et al.[352] analyzed the mutation burden of the tumors that were classified into regular (86.8%) and hypermutated (13.2%) subtypes. Yamazawa et al.[187] assessed also the expression a panel of primitive phenotypic markers, including embryonic stem cell markers (OCT4, NANOG, SALL4, CLDN6, and LIN28) and known oncofetal proteins (AFP and GPC3), using tissue microarray on 386 gastric carcinomas. These authors observed that gastric carcinoma with primitive enterocyte phenotypes (GAED) is an aggressive subgroup of intestinal type with CIN and suggested that therapeutic strategies targeting primitive markers, such as GPC3, CLDN6, and SALL4, might be considered.[187]

Cost-Effective Strategies for Molecular Classification

Given the complexity and high cost of the experimental approaches needed to stratify gastric cancer according to TCGA and ACRG classifications, which is not always available in daily practice, several studies proposed less costly approaches to reach similar endpoints.[353-363]

On this note, Setia et al.[358] proposed a practical algorithm based on IHC and in situ hybridization techniques currently available in routine diagnostic practice (see Table 25.6). In this study, the authors translated different molecular subgroups into specific immunophenotypes with prognostic and predictive significance. The study of Setia et al. conducted in a Western population[358] was validated in a large-scale Asian cohort.[357]

Pinto et al. used a similar approach to apply the IHC/ISH molecular algorithm to a cohort of gastric cancer patients from Chile.[363] In this study, the authors used targeted NGS sequencing to characterize the four molecular subtypes, identifying *FGFR2* and *KRAS* gene amplification as potential actionable targets in the EMT-like subgroup.[363] Wang et al. studied a gastric cancer Chinese cohort to conclude that it would be possible to reproduce the TCGA and ACRG molecular classifications by using only IHC.[354] In the two most recent cost-effective strategies for gastric cancer molecular classification, Zhao et al.[353] and Tsai et al.[356] used alternative surrogate biomarkers to define MSS/TP53 subgroups and CIN subtype on the basis, respectively, of p21 protein expression and DNA content assessed by DNA flow cytometry.

SPREAD AND METASTASES

Gastric adenocarcinomas can spread by direct extension, metastasis, or peritoneal dissemination. According to the primary site, penetration of the serosa may result in direct spread to the pancreas, liver, spleen, transverse colon, and greater omentum, and this often leads to early transperitoneal dissemination. Diffuse carcinomas have a high propensity to invade the duodenum via submucosal or subserosal routes or via the submucosal lymphatics. Consequently, frozen section examination of margins is desirable, particularly when the clearance is less than 4 cm, to ensure completeness of resection. Lymphovascular invasion should be systematically assessed; it is an indicator of biological aggressiveness and may be a prognostic factor for lymph node–negative gastric cancer.[364,365] Well-differentiated tumors with an intestinal phenotype preferentially disseminate hematogenously and show a high rate of hepatic metastasis. Diffuse carcinomas are more likely to spread to the peritoneum (peritoneal seeding).[237,366] Carcinomas that exhibit both intestinal and diffuse components (mixed carcinomas) possess the metastatic capabilities of each of these tumors and, as a result, have a poorer prognosis.[148] Secondary tumor deposits are common in the omentum, peritoneum, and mesentery but are rare in the spleen. Secondary ovarian deposits are one form of Krukenberg tumor for which bloodstream spread is as likely as transperitoneal spread. Pulmonary lymphangitic carcinomatosis and pulmonary tumor thrombotic microangiopathy may rarely develop in patients with gastric cancer.[367]

PROGNOSIS

The pathological stage (pTNM) remains the strongest independent prognostic indicator in patients with gastric cancer, followed by patient age and comorbidities.[368] The 5-year survival rates for carcinomas that extend into the muscularis propria are 60% to 80%, but they decrease to 50% in cases with serosal involvement. Thorough gross and microscopic examination and, ultimately, accurate staging are important in the pathological examination of gastrectomy specimens. The "N" classification is a cardinal feature of gastric carcinoma evaluation and a minimum of 15 lymph nodes is required for appropriate pathological staging.[369] For every clinical stage group, the detection of nodal disease is an indicator of poorer prognosis, even for superficial neoplasms. For example, clinical stage group I (T1/T2, N0) has a 90% 5-year survival versus 75% for clinical stage IIA (T1/T2, N+).[370,371]

Lymphovascular invasion should be systematically assessed; it is an indicator of biological aggressiveness and may be a prognostic factor for lymph node–negative gastric cancer.

Although the prognosis of advanced gastric adenocarcinoma is poor in general, particularly in the West, some series have shown either stable or slight increase in overall survival.[368,372] The 10-year relative survival rate is approximately 10%. It is worth underscoring that despite increased 5-year survival for operated Western patients (at all stages), the figures do not compare with Eastern Asian series. In Korea, the overall 5-year survival rate for patients with advanced gastric cancer who are surgically treated increased from 43% to 74% between the two calendar periods of 1993 to 1995 and 2010 to 2014.[373]

Whether distal adenocarcinomas have a more favorable prognosis compared with proximal carcinomas is a matter of debate.[374] A historic series of Saito and colleagues reported a 5-year survival rate of 61.6% for patients with carcinoma of the cardia, compared with 82.6% for those with carcinoma of the lower third of the stomach.[375] A recent large Japanese analysis continues to show a somewhat lower 5-year survival for gastric cancer of the upper third of the stomach.[376] Aside from location, the depth of invasion is critical; for example in Japanese centers, survival at 5 years for T1, T2, and T3 carcinomas is >95%, 89.4%, and 69.8%, respectively.[376] However, lymph node status is the single best indicator of prognosis: For positive N1 (pN1) tumors, the 5-year survival rate is 68%, dropping to 43.2% for pN2 tumors and 22% for pN3 tumors.[376] In addition, variation in tumor location, higher frequency of early-stage carcinoma, more accurate staging, and surgical expertise, may help explain improved patient survival rates in Asian compared with Western medical centers.[374] After curative resection, recurrence is locoregional in 40% and systemic in 60% of cases. The former includes the surgical resection margins, the resection bed, and regional lymph nodes.[377] The predominant sites of systemic recurrence are the liver and peritoneum.

MANAGEMENT AND TREATMENT

The various strategies available for the treatment of gastric adenocarcinoma are primarily directed by the stage of the disease. New additional key deciding factors include the detection of biomarkers and the biology of the tumor. Surgery is a mandatory step for early-stage disease. The type of operation is variable, depending on the location of the tumor and the depth of the invasion. Endoscopic resection is now more commonly preferred for early gastric cancers (see earlier) and subtotal or total gastrectomy for more advanced cases. Distal tumors are usually adequately treated by subtotal gastrectomy, whereas proximal tumors can be approached with either a total gastrectomy or a proximal subtotal gastrectomy. Many surgeons consider linitis plastica to be a contraindication to potentially curative resection. To this day, the optimal extent of lymph node dissection remains controversial. East Asian surgeons routinely perform an extended lymphadenectomy, a practice that may account for more favorable survival rates in Asian series compared with Western series.[374] D1 lymphadenectomy refers to a limited dissection of the perigastric lymph nodes, whereas a D2 lymphadenectomy involves removal of lymph nodes along the hepatic, left gastric, celiac, and splenic arteries, as well as those in the splenic hilum. A D3 dissection includes lymph nodes within the porta hepatis and periaortic regions. Arguments in favor of an extended lymphadenectomy include the fact that a larger number of lymph nodes results in more accurate pathological staging and that failure to remove these lymph nodes leaves tumor behind in as many as one-third of patients. However, Western series have failed to show consistent benefit with extended lymphadenectomy.[14] In patients diagnosed as stage pN0, occult tumor cells may be identified in lymph nodes if carefully searched for, which can negatively affect the prognosis.[378] Recent studies point to the putative role of deep-learning models to assist pathologists in detecting lymph nodes with metastases.[379]

Operative success and perioperative mortality rates are also highly dependent on the surgeon's experience.[380] Although surgery remains the only strategy with curative intent, chemotherapy has been shown to offer survival benefit. Perioperative chemotherapy or postoperative chemotherapy plus chemoradiation are the preferred approaches for localized gastric cancer. The therapeutic protocols are numerous, based on stage, toxicity tolerance, and performance status. These variably include platinum compounds plus fluoropyrimidines. Perioperative (preoperative and postoperative) chemotherapy with FLOT (5-fluorouracil/leucovorin, oxaliplatin, docetaxel) is currently recommended for patients with ≥ Stage IB resectable gastric and gastroesophageal junction cancers.[381,382] For patients who are refractory to first-line therapy, options include docetaxel, or irinotecan monotherapy in combination with paclitaxel. Trastuzumab is commonly added to chemotherapy for HER2-overexpressing metastatic adenocarcinoma[383,384] (NCCN Gastric Cancer Guidelines, 2021, Version 2.201). More recently, VEGFR-2 monoclonal antibody has also been used in progressive disease. Finally, PD-L1 monoclonal antibody now plays a major role in the treatment paradigm of gastric cancer, not only for MSI gastric cancers, but also for MSS neoplasms failing other lines of therapy if the tumor is expressing PD-L1 (NCCN Gastric Cancer Guidelines, 2021, Version 2.201).[384,385] The assessment of

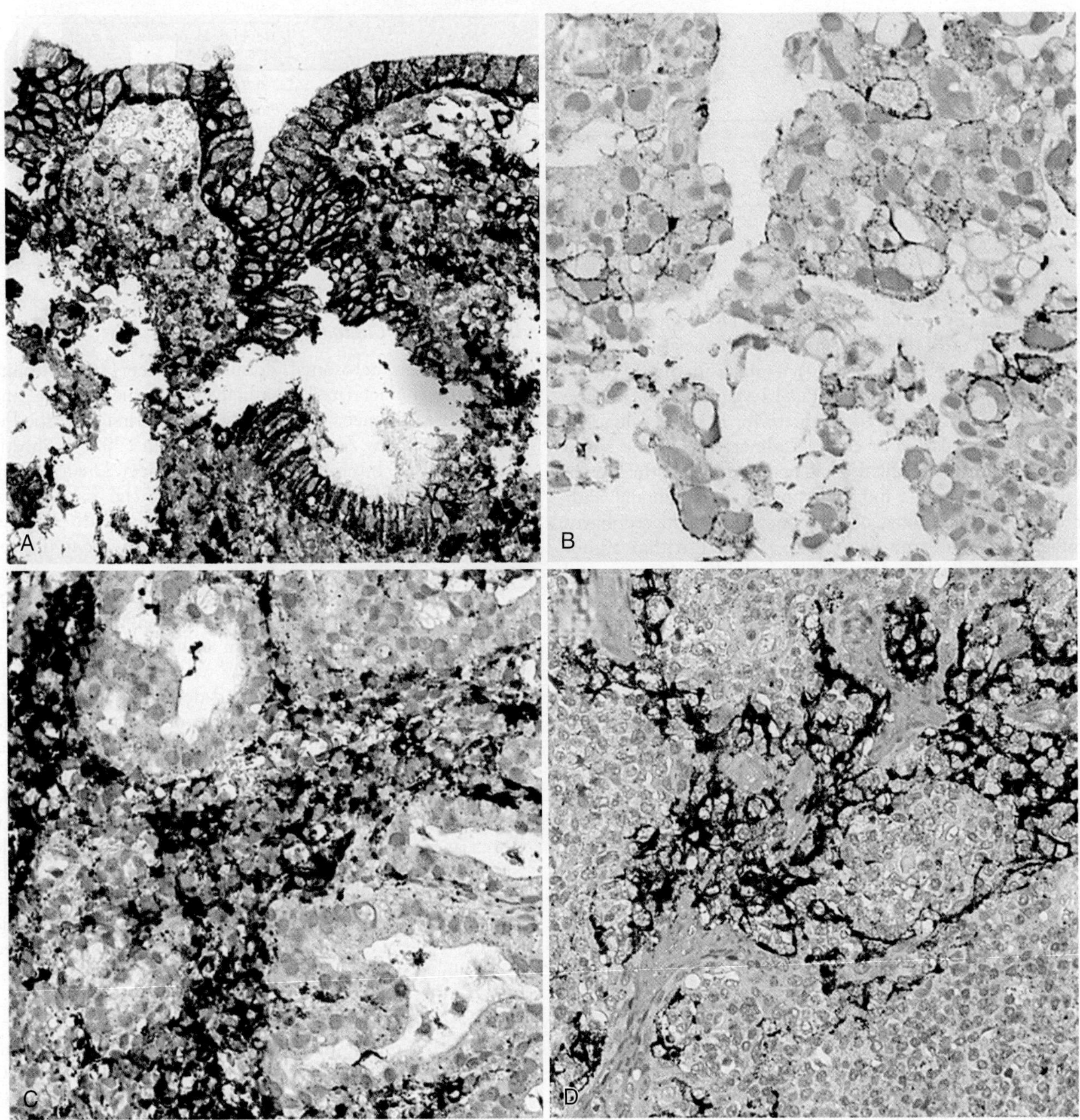

FIGURE 25.41 Patterns of expression of PD-L1 in gastric cancer. A, Strong membranous linear staining of neoplastic cells. **B,** Mild membranous granular staining of neoplastic cells. **C,** Staining restricted to inflammatory cells (lymphocytes and macrophages). **D,** Normal positive control in crypt epithelium (tonsils). One or several of these patterns (A to C) can be present in the same tumor.

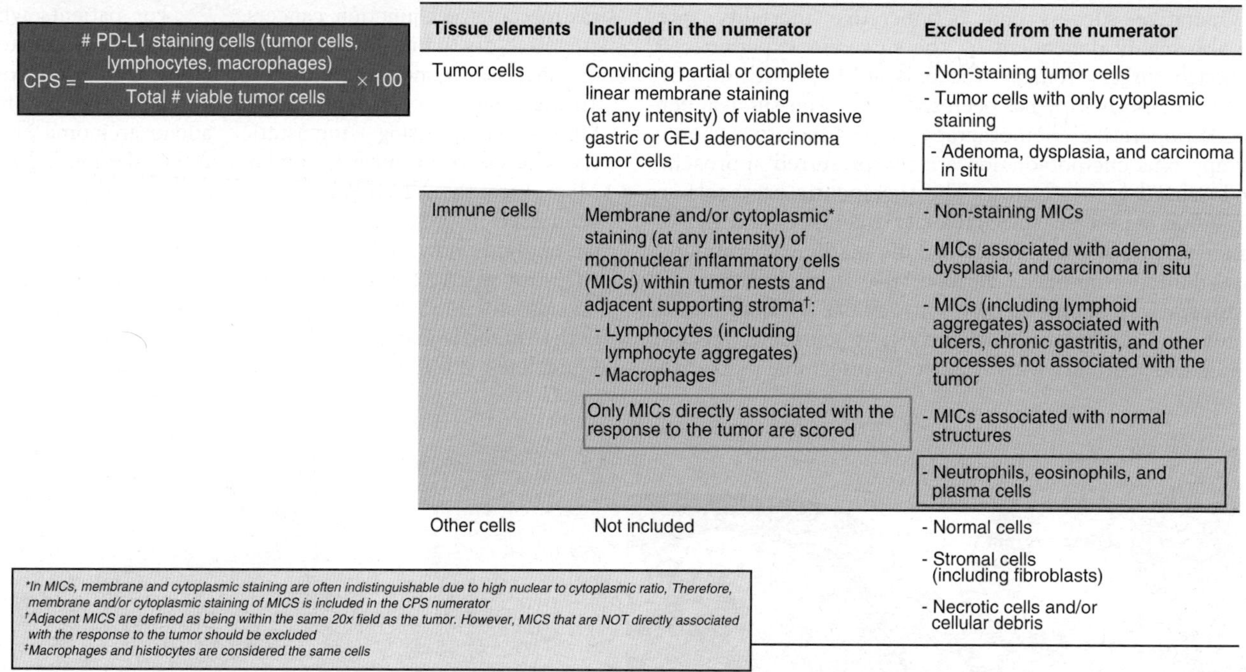

$$CPS = \frac{\text{\# PD-L1 staining cells (tumor cells, lymphocytes, macrophages)}}{\text{Total \# viable tumor cells}} \times 100$$

Tissue elements	Included in the numerator	Excluded from the numerator
Tumor cells	Convincing partial or complete linear membrane staining (at any intensity) of viable invasive gastric or GEJ adenocarcinoma tumor cells	- Non-staining tumor cells - Tumor cells with only cytoplasmic staining - Adenoma, dysplasia, and carcinoma in situ
Immune cells	Membrane and/or cytoplasmic* staining (at any intensity) of mononuclear inflammatory cells (MICs) within tumor nests and adjacent supporting stroma†: - Lymphocytes (including lymphocyte aggregates) - Macrophages Only MICs directly associated with the response to the tumor are scored	- Non-staining MICs - MICs associated with adenoma, dysplasia, and carcinoma in situ - MICs (including lymphoid aggregates) associated with ulcers, chronic gastritis, and other processes not associated with the tumor - MICs associated with normal structures - Neutrophils, eosinophils, and plasma cells
Other cells	Not included	- Normal cells - Stromal cells (including fibroblasts) - Necrotic cells and/or cellular debris

*In MICs, membrane and cytoplasmic staining are often indistinguishable due to high nuclear to cytoplasmic ratio, Therefore, membrane and/or cytoplasmic staining of MICS is included in the CPS numerator
†Adjacent MICS are defined as being within the same 20x field as the tumor. However, MICS that are NOT directly associated with the response to the tumor should be excluded
‡Macrophages and histiocytes are considered the same cells

FIGURE 25.42 Algorithm of analysis of PD-L1 in gastric cancer (see text for details), according to the Interpretation Manual – Gastric or gastroesophageal Junction Adenocarcinoma for the antibody 22C3.

PD-L1 protein expression in gastric cancer is made by an immunohistochemical assay using anti-PD-L1 antibodies for the detection of PD-L1 protein in FFPE tissues from gastric adenocarcinoma (Fig. 25.41A–D): a minimum of 100 tumor cells must be present in the PD-L1-stained slide for the specimen to be considered adequate for PD-L1 evaluation, any convincing partial or complete linear membrane staining of viable tumor cells that is perceived as distinct from cytoplasmic staining, and any convincing membrane and/or cytoplasmic staining of lymphocytes and macrophages (mononuclear inflammatory cells [MICs]) within tumor nests and/or adjacent supporting stroma (directly associated with the response against the tumor). A specimen is considered to have PD-L1 expression if the Combined Positive Score (CPS) ≥1. CPS is the number of PD-L1 membrane-stained cells at any intensity (i.e., tumor cells, lymphocytes, macrophages) divided by the total number of viable tumor cells, multiplied by 100.[386] In Figure 25.42, it is displayed as an algorithm for the analysis of PD-L1 in gastric cancer, according to the interpretation Manual – Gastric or gastroesophageal Junction Adenocarcinoma for the antibody 22C3 (DAKO).

Novel targets that are under investigation in gastric cancer include Claudin 18.2 (more frequently expressed in diffuse gastric cancer).[387]

HEREDITARY GASTRIC CANCER SYNDROMES

Familial clustering is observed in about 10% of the cases of gastric cancer, and 1% to 3% are hereditary, encompassing hereditary diffuse gastric cancer (HDGC)[388] and familial intestinal gastric cancer (FIGC).[389] The stomach is also affected by gastric adenocarcinoma and proximal polyposis of the stomach (GAPPS) syndrome, which was recently recognized as a rare variant of FAP.[390]

Hereditary Diffuse Gastric Cancer

Definition and Clinical Features

HDGC is an autosomal dominant cancer susceptibility syndrome characterized by a high prevalence of DGC and lobular breast cancer (LBC). HDGC was first described in an extended New Zealand Māori family in 1998.[391] Shortly afterward, the International Gastric Cancer Linkage Consortium (IGCLC) was constituted, and the first clinical criteria for early diagnosis of HDGC and identification of *CDH1* carriers was published in 1999[392] and updated three times over 20 years.[388,393,394]

According to the most recent guidelines, HDGC is currently defined by the presence of a pathogenic germline *CDH1* or *CTNNA1* variant in either an isolated individual with DGC or in a family with one or more DGC cases in a first-degree or second-degree relative.[388] The current criteria for genetic testing encompass family and individual criteria (Table 25.8). Individuals who meet the criteria for HDGC genetic testing should first have *CDH1* analyzed. If no variant is identified, these patients should be considered for *CTNNA1* analysis. In Japan and South Korea, it is also recommended that patients with multiple SRC carcinoma lesions, either identified endoscopically or in the gastrectomy specimen, are offered *CDH1* and *CTNNA1* genetic testing.[388] Families that fulfill genetic testing criteria (see Table 25.8) but have no identified pathogenic *CDH1* or *CTNNA1* variant(s) are classified as HDGC-like.

Penetrance of DGC in proven *CDH1* carriers is incomplete, and the time course for the development of clinically significant DGC is unpredictable. The age of DGC presentation is extremely variable, ranging from 14 to 85 years, even within the same family.[388] At the time of clinical presentation, affected individuals present with advanced disease in >90% of cases.[394]

TABLE 25.8 Genetic Testing Criteria for Hereditary Diffuse Gastric Cancer

Family Criteria*
1. ≥2 cases of gastric cancer in family regardless of age, with at least one diffuse gastric cancer (DGC)
2. ≥1 case of DGC at any age, and ≥1 case of lobular breast cancer at age <70 years, in different family members
3. ≥2 cases of lobular breast cancer in family members <50 years of age
Individual Criteria*
4. DGC at age <50 years
5. DGC at any age in individuals of Māori ethnicity
6. DGC at any age in individuals with a personal or family history (first-degree relative) of cleft lip or cleft palate
7. History of DGC and lobular breast cancer, both diagnosed at age <70 years
8. Bilateral lobular breast cancer, diagnosed at age <70 years
9. Gastric in situ signet ring cells or pagetoid spread of signet ring cells in individuals <50 years of age

Data from Blair VR, McLeod M, Carneiro F, Coit DG, D'Addario JL, van Dieren JM, et al. Hereditary diffuse gastric cancer: updated clinical practice guidelines. *Lancet Oncol.* 2020;21(8):e386-e397.

**CDH1* testing is recommended when one of the above criteria has been met and cancer diagnoses have been confirmed. When a criterion involves two or more cancers, at least one cancer should have confirmed histology. Histologically confirmed intestinal-type gastric cancer and nonlobular breast cancer cases should not be used to fulfill testing criteria because these cancers are not part of HDGC. Individuals who are found to be negative for a *CDH1* variant should subsequently be considered for *CTNNA1* analysis.

Pathogenesis

CDH1 (located on chromosome 16q22.1), is a tumor suppressor gene that encodes E-cadherin, a transmembrane protein that is localized to the *adherens* junctions in epithelial tissues and has functions in cell-to-cell adhesion, tension sensing, and signal transduction.[395] *CDH1* germline alterations encompass small frameshift insertions and deletions; splice-site, missense, and nonsense mutations; large rearrangements; and, very rarely, germline promoter methylation. According to the two-hit hypothesis, a second-hit somatic event, leading to bi-allelic inactivation, is necessary for E-cadherin disruption and development of DGC/LBC. *CDH1* second-hit mechanisms include somatic promoter methylation, *CDH1*-large deletions, loss of heterozygosity, or a second (somatic) mutation.[396-398]

Mutations in *CTNNA1*, encoding catenin α-1, another *adherens* junction protein, are also found in a small minority of HDGC cases.[399,400] It was shown that tumors from individuals with *CTNNA1* germline variants lose catenin α-1 protein expression, which suggests that a second-hit event occurs somatically at the *CTNNA1* locus.[400,401] IHC for catenin α-1 may be useful when analyzing tumors from patients with suspected HDGC as catenin α-1 loss seems to be rare in sporadic gastric cancer, while absent or weak expression may suggest genetic susceptibility associated with CTNNA1 germline variants.

Multiplexed panel and WES have been used to identify new candidate genes. So far, there are insufficient data to support that additional genes, other than *CDH1* and *CTNNA1*, predispose specifically to DGC.[388]

Pathology

Macroscopic features differ in stomachs from asymptomatic *CDH1* mutation carriers submitted to prophylactic/risk-reducing gastrectomy and index cases with HDGC. The former generally lack macroscopic alteration.[402] Most index patients present with cancers that are indistinguishable from sporadic DGC, often with linitis plastica, which can involve all topographical regions within the stomach.

The predominant lesions in HDGC are tiny foci of typical SRCs, usually confined to the superficial lamina propria (Fig. 25.43). Larger foci may involve superficial and deep portions of the gastric mucosa and have a characteristic layered structure, with large SRCs in the upper mucosa, small neoplastic cells at the isthmus zone, and deeper mucosa levels displaying a more "immature" phenotype, with small amounts of mucin, vesicular nuclei, and distinct nucleoli.[403]

Two pre-invasive or precursor lesions of SRC carcinoma have been recognized exclusively in *CDH1* pathogenic variant carriers and are important clues to the diagnosis of HDGC. The first is in situ SRC carcinoma corresponding to the presence of SRCs with hyperchromatic and depolarized nuclei within the basal membrane of a gland, replacing the normal cells of the gland (Fig. 25.44), and the second is pagetoid spread of a row of SRCs below the preserved epithelium of glands and foveolae, also within the basal membrane cells (Fig, 25.45).[388,404,405] E-cadherin expression may be abnormal in precursor lesions such as pagetoid spread of SRCs (Fig. 25.46).

Heterogeneous E-cadherin staining patterns have been described in HDGC, including complete loss of expression (Fig. 25.47A), reduced membranous immunoreactivity (Fig. 25.47B), and "dotted" or cytoplasmic staining.[403] However, HDGC may show retained E-cadherin expression and weak membranous immunoreactivity, and sporadic DGC often shows loss of expression. As a consequence, E-cadherin staining should not be used as a pre-screening method for selecting patients eligible for germline *CDH1* variant analysis.

Endoscopic biopsy specimens from *CDH1* pathogenic variant carriers can also have features of non-SRC poorly cohesive (diffuse) gastric cancer with a so-called *aggressive* phenotype, represented by pleomorphic, diffusely infiltrative cells (Fig. 25.48). These features are highly suggestive of disease progression and should be described in the pathology report to prompt staging and clinical intervention.[406]

The histological features of advanced HDGC are similar to advanced sporadic DGC and predominantly present as linitis plastica, with infiltration of the gastric wall by atypical cells with diffuse growth, and cords, microglands, and small mucin lakes.

The morphological features as well as the molecular alterations of early and advanced HDGC are distinct. Intramucosal aberrations, in addition to *CDH1* inactivation, are required for HDGC to gain aggressive features, including aberrant p53 expression,[406,407] p16 overexpression,[408] and activation of cSrc kinase and downstream targets, as the molecular mechanisms supporting epithelial-mesenchymal transition.[409] Concomitant molecular *CDH1* and *TP53* aberrations contribute to the development of aggressive HDGC phenotypes and may play a central role in the cascade of molecular events important for HDGC progression.[403]

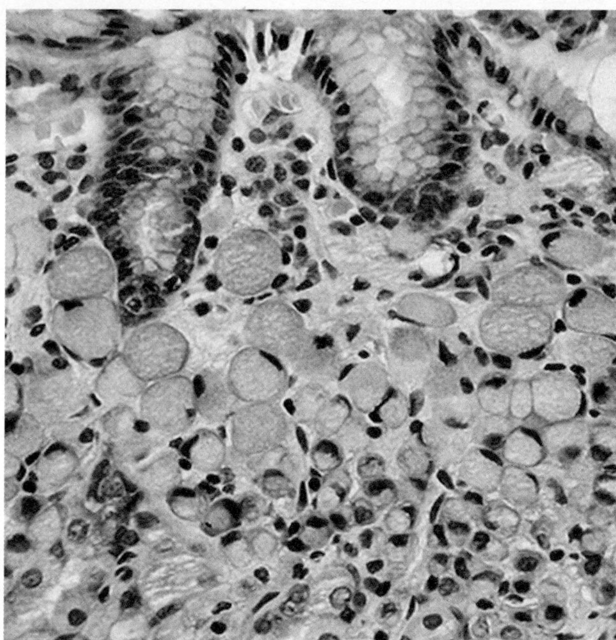

FIGURE 25.43 Hereditary diffuse gastric cancer. Panoramic view of SRC/diffuse carcinoma, restricted to the mucosa. The neoplastic cells display the typical features of signet ring cells (SRCs).

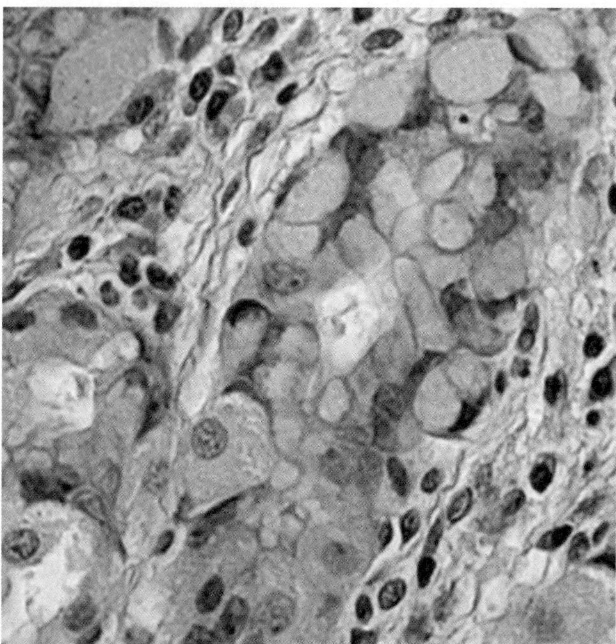

FIGURE 25.44 Hereditary diffuse gastric cancer. In situ signet ring cell carcinoma, characterized by the presence of signet ring cells within the basal membrane substituting the normal epithelial cells.

Histopathological analysis of total (prophylactic) gastrectomies from *CTNNA1* carriers showed foci of SRC carcinoma in the mucosa, resembling the appearance of prophylactic gastrectomies from *CDH1* carriers.[400,410]

When a total-embedding protocol (assessment of the totality of gastric mucosa) is applied for the study of prophylactic gastrectomy specimens performed in asymptomatic

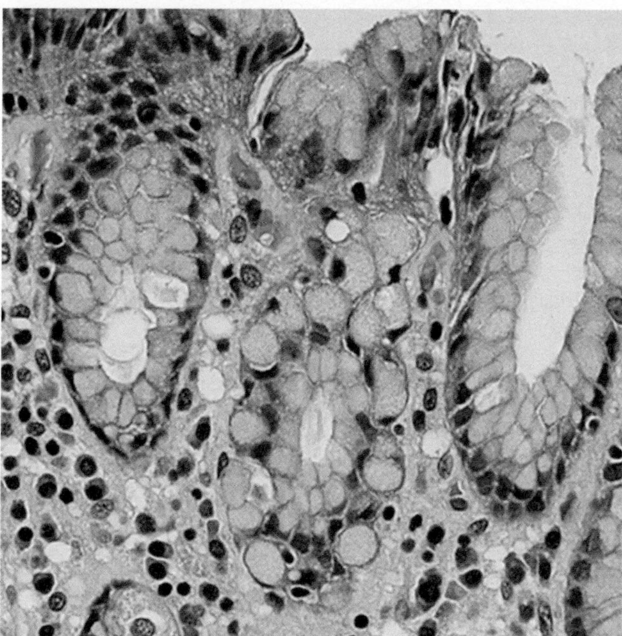

FIGURE 25.45 Hereditary diffuse gastric cancer. Pagetoid spread of signet ring cells (SRCs) that spread below the preserved epithelium of glands and foveolae, within the basal membrane.

carriers of *CDH1* mutations, microscopic cancer foci were detected in 95.3%; when the entire gastric mucosa is not examined, HDGC is found in only 62.5% of total gastrectomy specimens.[402] Total embedding protocol and thorough histopathological examination of the entire gastric mucosa are considered to constitute the gold standard practice for the evaluation of total gastrectomy specimens from *CDH1*/*CTNNA1* carriers. However, for routine histopathology laboratories with constrained resources, total examination of the gastric mucosa may not be feasible. Accordingly, the 2020 updated clinical practice guidelines for the management of HDGC provide different options for pathological examination, depending on the availability of resources.[388]

Prognosis and Management

Early HDGC is considered to have an indolent nature, with a latency period of possibly many years before further progression. On the contrary, advanced HDGC is a very aggressive disease. The neoplastic cells infiltrate diffusely into the gastric wall, spreading eventually into the peritoneal cavity and distant sites.

For asymptomatic carriers of pathogenic *CDH1* mutation, prophylactic/risk-reduction total gastrectomy in early adulthood (20 to 30 years of age) is the treatment of choice. In women, breast magnetic resonance imaging is advised, starting at 30 years of age.[388,394] For carriers of *CDH1* variants of unknown significance (VUS) and individuals from families that are HDGC-like (negative for *CDH1* and *CTTNA1* germline alterations), annual gastric surveillance for at least 2 years is recommended, and prophylactic total gastrectomy is not advised.[388] LBC risk should be managed with either yearly surveillance or bilateral risk-reducing mastectomy.[388]

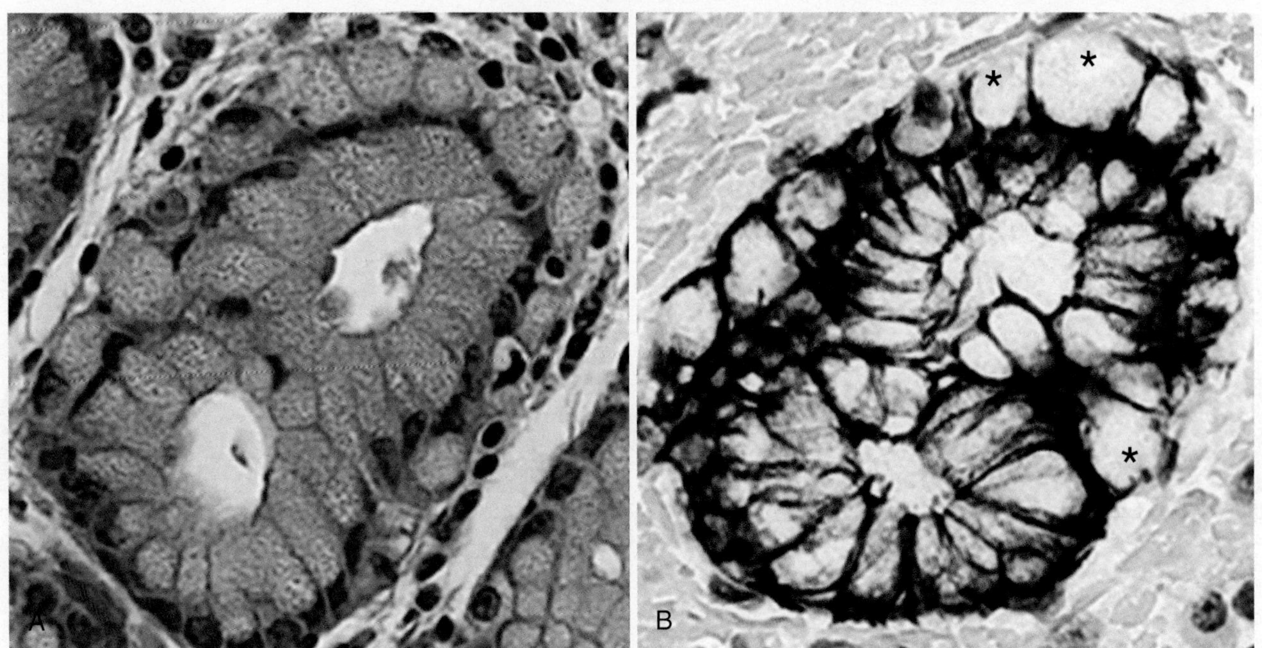

FIGURE 25.46 Pagetoid spread lesion. A, Signet ring cells spread below the preserved epithelium. **B,** In several signet ring cells, there is loss of expression of E-cadherin.

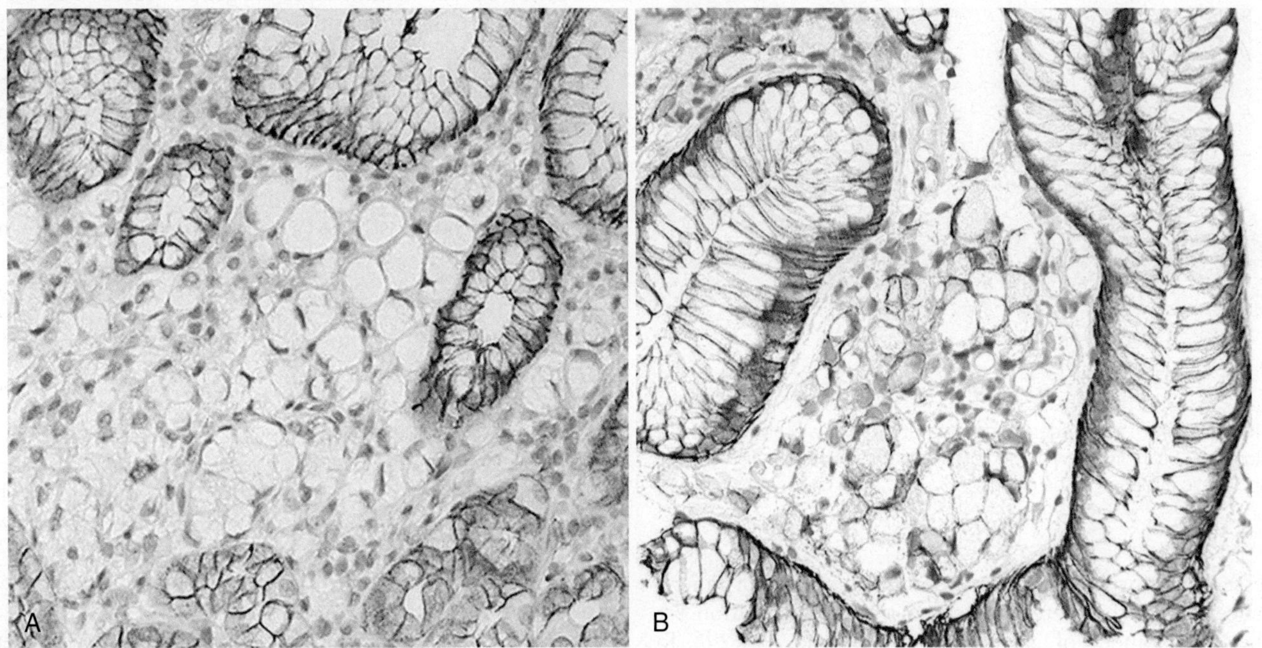

FIGURE 25.47 Heterogeneous E-cadherin staining patterns in hereditary diffuse gastric cancer. A, Complete loss of expression. **B,** Reduced membranous expression.

Carriers of *CTNNA1* pathogenic variants are recommended to undergo yearly endoscopic surveillance at an expert center, with prophylactic total gastrectomy being considered, depending on the results of the biopsies and the penetrance of DGC in the family history.[388]

The prognosis is dismal in individuals with advanced gastric cancer as in patients with advanced sporadic diffuse gastric cancer.

Gastric Adenocarcinoma and Proximal Polyposis of the Stomach

Definition and Clinical Features

GAPPS is an autosomal dominant hereditary gastric cancer syndrome that was identified in 2012.[411,412] It is characterized by extensive involvement of the fundus and body of the stomach, with fundic gland polyps sparing the antrum and

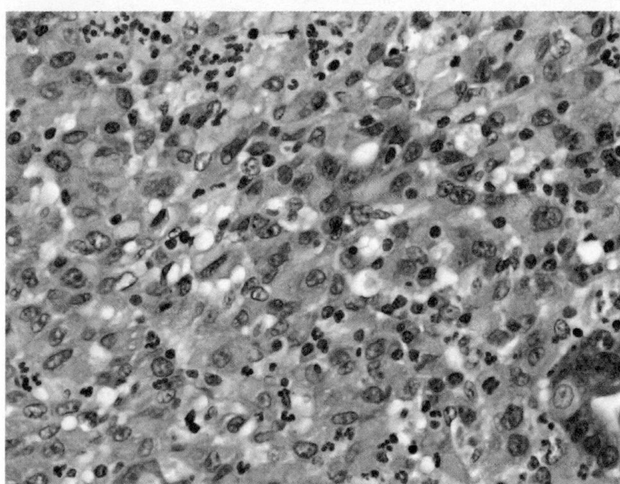

FIGURE 25.48 Endoscopic biopsy from a carrier of *CDH1* pathogenic variant showing features of non–signet cell poorly cohesive (diffuse) gastric cancer with an aggressive phenotype, represented by pleomorphic, diffusely infiltrative cells. Some polymorphs are seen among the neoplastic cells as a result of ulceration *(not shown)*. A preserved gastric gland is seen *(bottom, right corner)*.

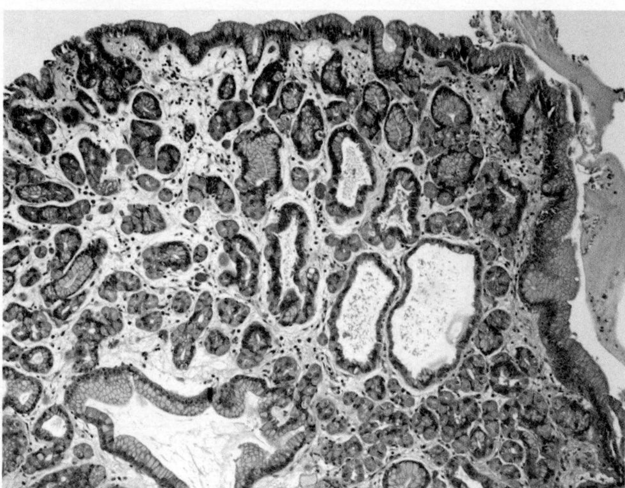

FIGURE 25.50 Gastric adenocarcinoma and proximal polyposis of the stomach. A fundic gland polyp is shown with shortened gastric pits and cystic lesions, lined by mucous, parietal, and chief cells. Some hyperproliferative aberrant pits are seen *(top, left corner)*.

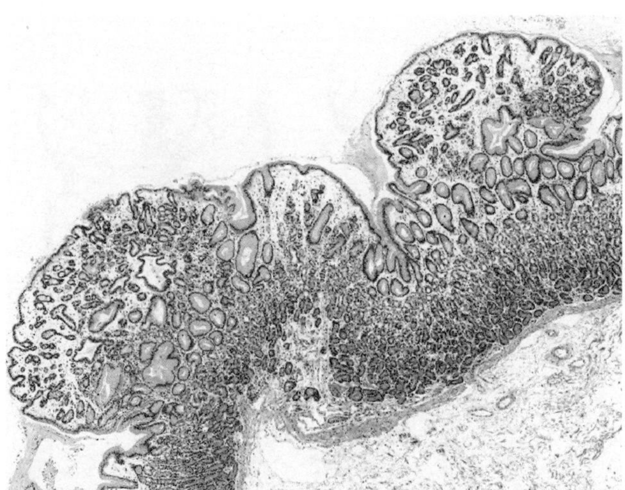

FIGURE 25.49 Gastric adenocarcinoma and proximal polyposis of the stomach. Scanning view of fundic gland polyps, with roundish surface and cystic dilatation of the glands.

lesser curvature; an autosomal dominant pattern of inheritance with incomplete penetrance; and predisposition for the development of gastric adenocarcinoma.[411,413,414] To consider a diagnosis of GAPPS, the presence of polyposis elsewhere in the GI tract should be ruled out to exclude the possibility of (attenuated) FAP.[415]

GAPPS families have been identified in Australia, North America, Europe, and Japan.[411-413,416-421]

Patients can present with nonspecific GI symptoms including abdominal pain, dyspepsia, and melena. Asymptomatic family members present for screening endoscopy because they belong to a known GAPPS family.

The age of onset of gastric cancer is variable, ranging from 23 to 75 years. Fundic gland polyposis with multifocal dysplasia has been detected as early as 10 years of age.[411,416]

Pathogenesis

APC promotor 1B mutations (c.-191T>C, c.-192A>G, and c.-195A>C) were identified as the genetic cause of GAPPS syndrome.[390] All are positioned within the YY1 binding motif of the *APC* gene, reducing the transcriptional level of APC. A second APC hit occurs in most fundic gland polyps in GAPPS by loss of wild-type allele or truncating mutations in the *APC* gene, but this appears to be a late event, occurring in only a subset of the polyp's epithelial cells.[414]

Currently, GAPPS is considered a variant of familial adenomatous polyposis (FAP) with exclusive/predominant involvement of the stomach.[390]

Pathology

GAPPS is characterized by proximal (body and fundus) gastric polyposis with antral sparing, without evidence of colorectal or duodenal polyposis. An arbitrary number of >100 polyps was proposed as a diagnostic criterion, although fewer polyps may be observed in some family members.[411,412] Polyps are predominantly <10 mm in size and are sessile with a smooth surface (Fig. 25.49),[411,421] although in some cases, polyps as large as 40 mm may be present.[416,421]

A range of microscopic features have been described in the literature, including fundic gland polyps (FGPs) (Fig. 25.50), fundic gland–like polyps, hyperproliferative aberrant pits, hyperplastic polyps, gastric-type adenomas (Fig. 25.51), and adenocarcinomas (tubular/intestinal and mixed with a poorly cohesive component).[421] Some lesions show a mixture of the aforementioned features. The larger, dominant fundic gland polyps tend to show foci of dysplasia at the surface (Fig. 25.52) or may be adenomas (foveolar adenomas).[416,421] The main differential diagnosis is fundic gland polyposis in the setting of FAP (mainly attenuated forms). The unique sparing of the antrum and the absence of a colonic polyposis phenotype in patients with GAPPS is an important clinical feature

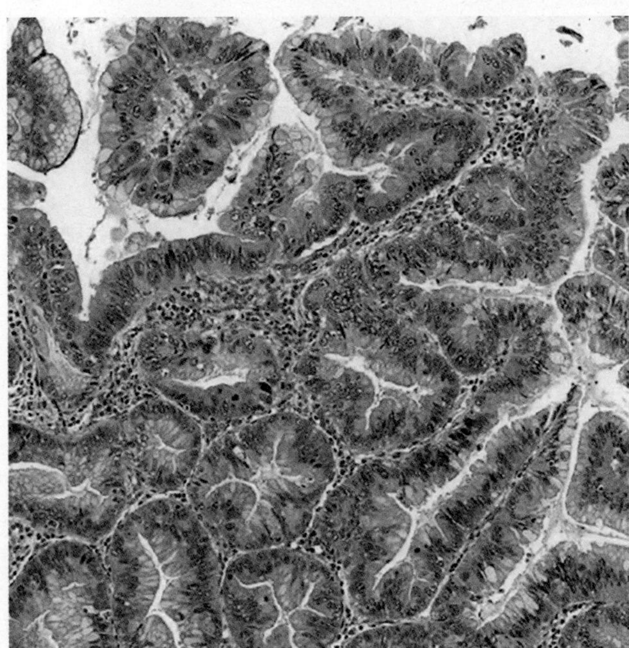

FIGURE 25.51 Gastric adenocarcinoma and proximal polyposis of the stomach. A gastric type polyp is observed. Neoplastic cells display a mucin cap at the apical pole, a feature of foveolar differentiation.

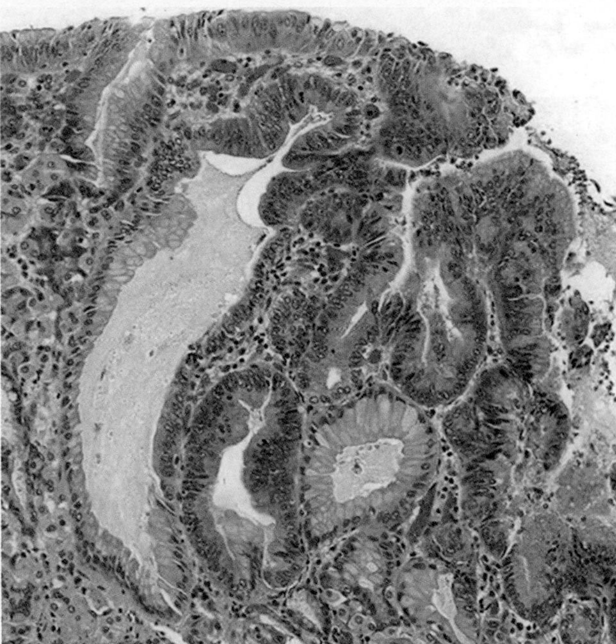

FIGURE 25.52 Gastric adenocarcinoma and proximal polyposis of the stomach. Low-grade dysplasia is observed in the surface of a fundic gland polyp (the dysplastic glands are tortuous, lined by columnar cells with oval nuclei).

that distinguishes GAPPS from (attenuated) FAP.[414] Prolonged use of proton-pump inhibitors may be the cause of FGPs/polyposis without dysplasia and should be considered in the differential diagnosis, mainly on the basis of clinical setting and presence of dysplasia in fundic gland polyps in the GAPPS syndrome.

Gastric adenocarcinomas have been detected in 13% of GAPPS patients and include intestinal-type or mixed-type gastric adenocarcinomas.[411,416]

By IHC, fundic gland polyps and gastric cancers display increased expression of nuclear β-catenin, Ki67, and p53.[422]

Prognosis and Management

Prognosis is often poor in patients with gastric adenocarcinoma. All first-degree relatives of affected patients should be advised to undergo esophagogastroduodenoscopy and colonoscopy.[390,422] Eventually, prophylactic total gastrectomy may be offered because endoscopy may fail to sample polyps with malignant transformation.[413] Because of the limited data available and the heterogeneity of GAPPS patients, recommendations on the management of GAPPS families should be decided on a case-by-case basis.[423]

Familial Intestinal Gastric Cancer

Definition and Clinical Features

Familial intestinal gastric cancer (FIGC) is an autosomal dominant cancer syndrome that is associated with an increased risk of intestinal-type gastric cancer.[389,392] Gastric cancers developed in the setting of gastric polyposis are excluded. Criteria for the diagnosis of FIGC (Table 25.9) were established in 1999 by the International Gastric Cancer Linkage Consortium (IGCLC) and are defined according to gastric cancer incidence.[392]

The mean age at gastric cancer diagnosis is about 10 years earlier than that for patients with sporadic intestinal-type gastric cancers. The disease spectrum is broad, encompassing 18 cancer types. The most frequent is intestinal-type gastric carcinoma, followed by colorectal and breast carcinomas.[389]

Pathogenesis

The genetic cause underlying the disease remains to be fully elucidated. In a previous study of a Dutch family with clustering of intestinal-type gastric cancer, heterozygous mutations were found in the immune response–related gene *IL12RB1*.[424]

In a recent study, NGS approaches were used to test multiple genes implicated in upper GI tract cancer and in cancer susceptibility syndromes across 50 probands with familial aggregation of intestinal-type gastric cancer and no clinical criteria for other GI cancer–associated syndromes. Putative susceptibility genes for FIGC include *SMAD4, PMS1, PRSS1*, and *TP53*. This study supported FIGC as a genetically determined, likely polygenic, gastric cancer–predisposing disease, with earlier onset and distinct from patients with sporadic intestinal gastric cancer (SIGC) at the germline and somatic levels. According to the findings of this study, FIGC is a genetically determined, likely polygenic, gastric cancer–predisposing disease, with earlier onset and distinct from SIGC at the germline and somatic levels.[389]

Pathology

FIGC shows macroscopic and histopathological features that are indistinguishable from those of sporadic intestinal-type gastric cancer.[389]

Prognosis and Management

The prognosis depends on the tumor spectrum and staging. A few recommendations have been suggested for the

TABLE 25.9 Heritable Cancer Syndromes

Heritable Cancer Syndrome	Genetic Testing Criteria	Inheritance Pattern	*Gene(s)*	GC risk (%)	GC Histopathological Subtype
HDGC (Blair et al., 2020)	**Family criteria** (first and second relatives): • At least two cases of GC in family regardless of age, with at least one diffuse GC • At least one case of diffuse GC at any age and one or more cases of LBC at age <70 years in different family members • At least two cases of LBC in family members age <50 years **Individual criteria:** • Diffuse GC at age <50 years • Diffuse GC at any age in individuals of Māori ethnicity • Diffuse GC at any age in individuals with a personal or family history (first degree) of cleft lip/cleft palate • History of diffuse GC and LBC, both diagnosed at age <70 years • Bilateral LBC, diagnosed at age <70 years • Gastric in situ signet ring cells and/or pagetoid spread of signet ring cells in individuals age <50 years	AD	*CDH1* *CTNNA1*	Clinical criteria 2010 56% (F) to 70% (M) (Fitzgerald et al., 2010) Clinical criteria 2015 33% (F) to 42% (M) (van der Post et al., 2015)	Diffuse GC (poorly cohesive, including signet ring cell)
GAPPS (Carneiro et al., 2019)	**Essential criteria:** • Phenotypic features: proximal polyposis with antral sparing; no evidence of colorectal or duodenal polyposis; >100 polyps carpeting the proximal stomach in the index patient or >30 polyps in a first-degree relative of another patient; predominantly FGPs and/or fundic gland-like polyps • Proband or relative with either dysplastic FGPs or GC • Mutation in the 1B promoter of *APC* (YY1 binding motif) **Supportive criteria:** • Autosomal dominant pattern of inheritance • Spectrum of other histological features, including hyperproliferative aberrant pits, hyperplastic polyps, and gastric-type adenomas	AD	Promoter 1B of *APC*	13% (Worthley et al., 2012)	Intestinal and mixed GC arising in the context of fundic gland polyposis of the proximal stomach
FIGC (Caldas et al., 1999)	**IGCLC criteria in high-incidence countries:** • Intestinal GC in three or more relatives; and • One being a first-degree relative of the other two; and • Two or more successive generations affected; and • Intestinal GC at age <50 years in one or more patients; and • Exclusion of gastric polyposis **IGCLC criteria in low-incidence countries:** • Intestinal GC in two or more first-degree relatives • Intestinal GC in second-degree relatives, one diagnosed at age <50 years • Intestinal GC in three or more relatives at any age **Proposal of new criteria (Carvalho et al., 2021)** • GC in two or more relatives at any age; and • At least one intestinal GC	AD	Probable polygenic cause	66% (Carvalho et al., 2021)	Intestinal GC

TABLE 25.9 Heritable Cancer Syndromes—cont'd

Heritable Cancer Syndrome	Genetic Testing Criteria	Inheritance Pattern	*Gene(s)*	GC risk (%)	GC Histopathological Subtype
FAP (Syngal et al., 2015)	**ACG guidelines:** • At least 10 cumulative colorectal adenomas • History of adenomas and FAP-type extracolonic manifestations* • Family history of one of the adenomatous polyposis syndromes	AD	*APC*	4%-7% Asian population (Shibata et al., 2013) Not increased in Western countries	Intestinal GC arising from intestinal-type and pyloric gland adenomas
Lynch syndrome	**Revised Bethesda criteria**: (Umar et al., 2004): • CRC at age <50 years • Synchronous, metachronous colorectal or other Lynch-associated tumor regardless of age • CRC with MSI histology at age <60 years • CRC in one or more first-degree relatives with a Lynch syndrome–related tumor, with one of the cancers diagnosed at age <50 years • CRC in two or more first- or second-degree relatives with Lynch syndrome–related tumors, regardless of age Universal screening for all CRCs and endometrial cancers (Gupta et al., 2019)	AD	*MLH1* *MSH2* *MSH6* *PMS2* *EPCAM*	9% (Møller et al., 2018) 10% (Møller et al., 2018) 7% (Møller et al., 2018) 0% (Møller et al., 2018) 0% (Kim et al., 2020; Latham et al., 2019; Rumilla et al., 2011)	Most cases are intestinal (tubular/ papillary) GC. Poorly cohesive and mucinous GCs have also been described
Peutz-Jeghers syndrome	**WHO criteria**: • ≥3 hamartomatous polyps • ≥1 hamartomatous polyp and positive family history • Mucocutaneous melanosis and positive family history • Mucocutaneous melanosis and ≥1 hamartomatous polyp	AD	*STK11*	29%	Intestinal GC
Juvenile polyposis	**WHO criteria**: • > 3-5 juvenile polyps of the colorectum • Juvenile polyps throughout the GI tract • Any number of juvenile polyps with a family history of juvenile polyposis Exclusion of other syndromes involving hamartomatous gastrointestinal polyps	AD	*SMAD4* *BMPR1A*	10%-30% (Syngal et al., 2015)	Intestinal or diffuse GC arising from juvenile polyps with dysplasia
LFS (Bougeard et al., 2015)	**Revised Chompret criteria:** • Familial presentation (a proband with a LFS tumor at age <46 years and at least one first-degree or second-degree relative with LFS tumor# at age <56 years or with multiple tumors) • Multiple primary tumors (two of which belong to the narrow LFS spectrum, the first being developed before 46 years) • Rare cancers (adrenocortical carcinoma or choroid plexus carcinoma) irrespective of family history	AD	*TP53*	2%-5% (Masciari et al., 2011)	Intestinal or diffuse GC
MAP	Patient with adenomatous polyposis in whom FAP and Lynch syndrome have been excluded by searching for germline mutations in *APC, MLH1, MSH2, MSH6,* and *PMS2*	AR	*MUTYH*	2% (F) to 5% (M) (Win et al., 2016)	Intestinal GC

*Duodenal/ampullary adenomas, desmoid tumors (abdominal > peripheral), papillary thyroid carcinoma, congenital hypertrophy of the retinal pigment epithelium, epidermal cysts, and osteomas.

#Soft tissue sarcoma, osteosarcoma, brain tumor, premenopausal breast cancer, adrenocortical carcinoma, leukemia, and lung bronchoalveolar cancer.

ACG, American College of Gastroenterologists; *AD,* autosomal dominant; *AR,* autosomal recessive; *CRC,* colorectal cancer; *F,* female; *FAP,* familial adenomatous polyposis; *FGP,* fundic gland polyp; *FIGC,* familial intestinal gastric cancer; *GAPPS,* gastric adenocarcinoma and proximal polyposis of the stomach; *HDGC,* hereditary diffuse gastric cancer; *IGCLC,* International Gastric Cancer Linkage Consortium; *LBC,* lobular breast cancer; *LFS,* Li-Fraumeni syndrome; *MAP,* MUTYH-associated polyposis; *M,* male; *WHO,* World Health Organization.

Modified from Gullo I, van der Post RS, Carneiro F. Recent advances in the pathology of heritable gastric cancer syndromes. *Histopathology.* 2021;78(1):125-147.

Data from references 388-390, 393, 394, 411, 414, 428, 429, 431-435, 441-443.

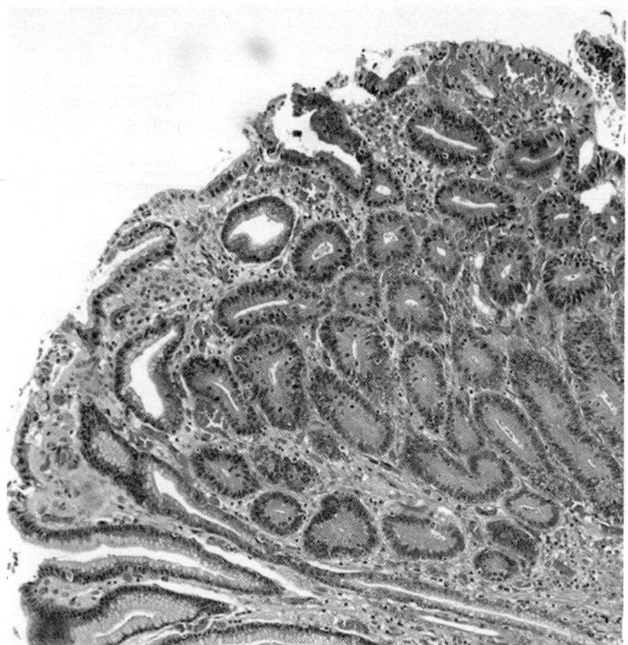

FIGURE 25.53 Familial adenomatous polyposis. Histological view of a gastric adenomatous polyp (adenoma), characterized by intestinal-type glands with low-grade dysplasia *(Courtesy Professor Irene Gulo, Porto, Portugal.)*

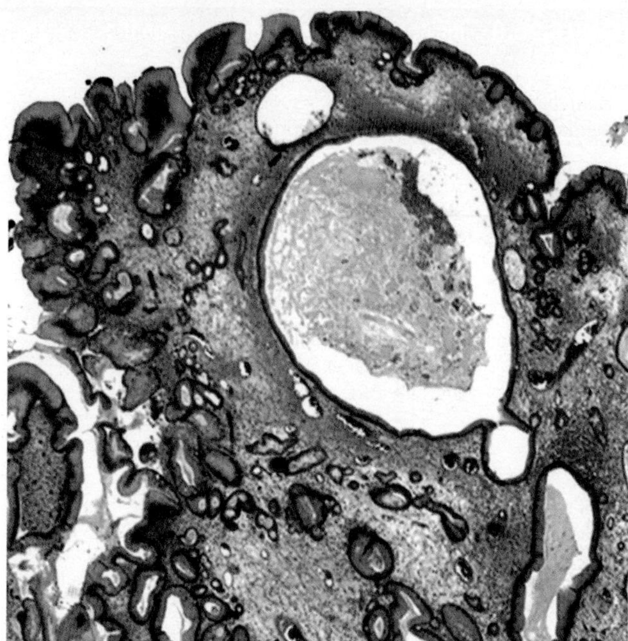

FIGURE 25.55 Juvenile polyposis. Histological view of a gastric polyp displaying dilated glands filled with mucin and prominent edematous stroma.

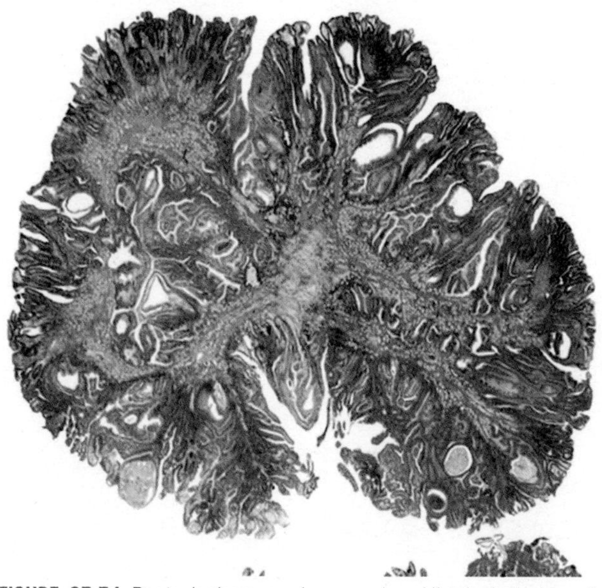

FIGURE 25.54 Peutz-Jeghers syndrome polyp. Histological view of a gastric polyp displaying the typical arborizing muscular framework.

management of patients at risk of developing FIGC, including regular endoscopic surveillance, *H. pylori* eradication, and modification of dietary habits.[389,425]

Gastric Cancer in the Setting of Other Hereditary Cancer Syndromes

Gastric cancer can develop in the setting of other hereditary cancer syndromes (see Table 25.9), such as FAP,[426-429] Lynch syndrome,[428,430-436] Peutz-Jeghers syndrome,[437,438] juvenile polyposis,[439] Li-Fraumeni syndrome,[440-442] *MUTYH*-associated polyposis,[443] and hereditary breast/ovarian cancer syndrome.[444] The lifetime risk of gastric cancer in these syndromes varies substantially among populations studied but is generally low.[445] Figures 25.53 to 25.55 display gastric polyps in the setting of FAP, Peutz-Jeghers syndrome, and juvenile polyposis.

***The full reference list may be accessed online at** Elsevier eBooks for Practicing Clinicians.*

CHAPTER 26

Epithelial Neoplasms of the Small Intestine

Amy E. Noffsinger

Chapter Outline

INTRODUCTION

Epithelial neoplasms develop far less frequently in the small intestine than in the colon, despite the fact that the small intestine has a larger epithelial surface area and a higher rate of cellular turnover. Overall, only 2% of all malignant neoplasms of the gastrointestinal (GI) tract occur in the small intestine.[1] In contrast, 57% of neoplasms arise in the colon. A number of hypotheses have been proposed to explain the relative rarity of small-bowel adenomas and carcinomas.[2] First, the transit time of substances through the small intestine is relatively short compared with the colon, resulting in brief contact time between the mucosa and the luminal contents. Second, unlike the colon, the small intestine does not contain a large quantity of bacteria. Bacteria are known to convert bile salts into potential carcinogens. Third, the luminal contents are more liquid in the small intestine than in the colon. As a result, potentially carcinogenic luminal substances are diluted, and the risk of mechanical trauma is reduced. Fourth, the small intestine is rich in lymphoid tissue, which provides a potentially high level of immunosurveillance against neoplastic cells. Finally, the small intestine is equipped with many microsomal enzymes, some of which may help detoxify potentially carcinogenic substances in the luminal contents.[2]

Epithelial tumors in the small intestine are most commonly located in the duodenum, usually in the vicinity of the ampulla of Vater.[3-5] This finding suggests that biliary or pancreatic secretions play a role in their development, possibly as a result of the carcinogenic effect of bile. Alternatively, constant influx of alkaline bile or acidic pancreatic juice may cause cell damage. Epithelial neoplasms also occur in the jejunum and in the ileum, but much less commonly.[6]

A number of diseases predispose individual patients to the development of small-intestinal adenomas and carcinomas, including familial adenomatous polyposis (FAP), *MUTYH*-associated polyposis (MAP), Lynch syndrome

(LS), Crohn's disease (CD),[7] and celiac disease.[8,9] The risk for small-intestinal carcinomas may also be increased in individuals with hamartomatous polyposis syndromes such as Peutz-Jeghers syndrome (PJS)[10,11] or juvenile polyposis syndrome[12,13] and in patients with long-standing ileostomies.[14,15]

Small-intestinal epithelial tumors are most commonly glandular, although other forms of neoplasia are also seen. Tumors arising in the ampulla of Vater are separately classified from those arising elsewhere in the small intestine because significant treatment and prognostic differences exist for this group of tumors. Box 26.1 summarizes the histological classification of epithelial tumors of the small intestine by the World Health Organization (WHO).[16]

BOX 26.1 World Health Organization Classification of Epithelial Tumors of the Small Intestine (Excluding Neuroendocrine Neoplasms)

BENIGN EPITHELIAL TUMORS AND PRECURSORS

- Adenomatous polyp, low-grade dysplasia
- Adenomatous polyp, high-grade dysplasia
  - Intestinal type, low-grade adenoma
  - Intestinal type, high-grade adenoma
  - Serrated low-grade dysplasia
  - Serrated high-grade dysplasia
  - Noninvasive pancreatobiliary papillary neoplasm with low-grade dysplasia
  - Noninvasive pancreatobiliary papillary neoplasm with high-grade dysplasia
  - Intraampullary papillary-tubular neoplasm

MALIGNANT EPITHELIAL TUMORS

- Adenocarcinoma, NOS
  - Mucinous adenocarcinoma
  - Signet ring cell carcinoma
  - Medullary carcinoma
  - Adenocarcinoma, intestinal type
  - Pancreatobiliary type carcinoma
  - Tubular adenocarcinoma

SMALL-INTESTINAL NEOPLASIA IN POLYPOSIS AND HEREDITARY CANCER SYNDROMES

Familial Adenomatous Polyposis

FAP is associated with adenomatous polyps of the intestinal tract and fundic gland polyps of the stomach. In the small intestine, most FAP-associated lesions arise in the duodenum and tend to cluster around the ampulla of Vater.[17-19] Small-intestinal adenomas are usually multiple and may be numerous (>20 to 50) in some patients.[20] Adenomas are often small, sessile, and tubular, usually measuring less than 1 cm in diameter.[19] Jejunal and ileal adenomas also occur in patients with FAP, especially in those with extensive duodenal polyposis.[21-23]

The prevalence of duodenal adenomas in FAP patients is 50% to 90%, with a 5% lifetime risk for developing small-bowel adenocarcinoma.[24] Patients with FAP who have multiple duodenal adenomas have a 100- to 300-fold increased lifetime risk for duodenal or periampullary cancer compared with the general population.[24,25] In fact, periampullary adenocarcinoma is the most common extracolonic malignant neoplasm in FAP. As a result, patients with known FAP undergo endoscopic surveillance with biopsy examination of grossly normal duodenal and ampullary mucosa to identify potential early precancerous lesions. Duodenal polyposis may be classified with Spigelman staging (Table 26.1).[26] The risk of developing duodenal adenocarcinoma increases with increasing Spigelman stage, and it is reported to be <5% in stages 0 to III and increases to 50% in stage IV.[27-29] Patients should undergo surveillance based on their Spigelman stage.[30]

MUTYH-Associated Polyposis

MAP is inherited as an autosomal recessive disorder. Affected patients carry biallelic missense mutations in the human DNA glycosylase base-excision repair gene *MUTYH*, located on chromosome 1.[31-34] Affected individuals present clinically with features similar to patients with FAP, including multiple adenomatous polyps and early-onset

TABLE 26.1 Spigelman Staging for Duodenal Polyposis in Familial Adenomatous Polyposis

Criterion	1 point	2 points	3 points
Polyp number	1-4	5-20	>20
Polyp size, mm	1-4	5-10	>10
Histology	Tubular	Tubulovillous	Villous
Dysplasia	Mild	Moderate	Severe
Stage	**Spigelman Score**	**Surveillance**	
0	0	Repeat endoscopy every 4 years	
I	1-4	Repeat endoscopy every 2-3 years	
II	5-6	Repeat endoscopy every 1-3 years	
III	7-8	Repeat endoscopy every 6-12 months	
IV	9-12	Surgical evaluation Expert surveillance every 3-6 months Complete mucosectomy or duodenectomy or Whipple procedure if ampulla is involved	

colonic adenocarcinoma and upper GI neoplasms.[32,35-37] Patients with MAP are also at increased risk for colonic serrated adenomas and sessile serrated polyps (sessile serrated lesions) as well as ovarian, bladder, breast, and endometrial neoplasms.[32,33,38,39] Duodenal adenomas and adenocarcinomas also occur commonly in affected patients.[40] In one study,[41] duodenal adenomas were identified in 34% of MAP patients at a median of 50 years of age. Most patients (84%) had only a few small polyps without high-grade dysplasia or villous architecture (Spigelman stages I or II). The lifetime risk for duodenal cancer is estimated to be approximately 4%.[37,41,42] Current surveillance recommendations for MAP patients are the same as for those with FAP.

Lynch Syndrome

LS (also called *hereditary nonpolyposis colorectal cancer [HNPCC] syndrome*) is an autosomal dominant genetic disorder that confers a high risk for both colorectal and endometrial tumors. It occurs as a result of a germline mutation in one of four major DNA mismatch repair genes: *MLH1*, *MSH2*, *MSH6*, or *PMS2*. *MLH1* or *MSH2* mutations make up 90% of LS patients. *MSH6* mutations make up an additional 7% to 10%, and *PMS2* mutations affect <5% of patients. Germline mutations in *EPCAM* (epithelial cell adhesion molecule) may result in inactivation of *MSH2* in a small percentage of patients.[43] Affected individuals have an increased risk for colorectal and endometrial cancer. These patients also exhibit a risk for tumors in other sites, albeit at a lower rate than for colorectal and endometrial cancers. These include urothelial cancers, biliary tumors, and gastric and small-intestinal adenocarcinomas.[44-46]

LS accounts for approximately 3% to 5% of all colorectal carcinomas.[47] The average age at which colonic malignancy develops in the setting of LS is 44 years, compared with an average age of 64 years in sporadic colorectal carcinoma.[43,48] The risk for small-bowel adenocarcinoma in LS patients increases with age. The lifetime risk for small-intestinal adenocarcinoma among these patients is 1% to 4%, approximately 100-fold that of the general population[49-51]; in one-fourth of cases, the small-bowel tumor is the presenting neoplasm of the syndrome.[44,52-54] Unlike patients with FAP, adenomas or adenocarcinomas at any location throughout the small bowel may develop in patients with LS, although a duodenojejunal predominance has been reported.[54] Screening for gastric and duodenal cancer can be considered in individuals at risk for or affected with LS by baseline esophagogastroduodenoscopy (EGD) with gastric biopsy at 30 to 35 years of age. Data for ongoing regular surveillance are limited, but ongoing surveillance every 3 to 5 years may be considered if there is a family history of gastric or duodenal cancer.[30]

Peutz-Jeghers Syndrome

PJS is an autosomal dominant inherited syndrome characterized by mucocutaneous pigmentation and GI polyposis. The disorder has been linked to germline mutations in the serine/threonine kinase gene *STK11* (also called *LKB1*) located on chromosome 19p13.3.[55,56] The most common cancers in this group of patients are gastrointestinal in origin, arising from gastroesophageal, small-intestinal, colonic, and pancreatic sites.[57] The risk for small-intestinal adenocarcinoma among patients with PJS is estimated to be as much as 400 times that of the general population.[58] The lifetime risk for small-bowel adenocarcinoma is 1.7% to 13%, and the risk increases rapidly with advancing age.[59,60]

Surveillance guidelines for PJS are empirical and based on the risk for GI complications and cancer. A consortium review group has recommended that upper GI endoscopy and video capsule endoscopy be performed first at 8 years of age.[61] If polyps are found, the examination should be repeated every 3 years. If none are identified on the initial examination, a second baseline examination should be done at 18 years of age and then every 3 years thereafter.[30]

Juvenile Polyposis Syndrome

Juvenile polyposis syndrome is an autosomal dominant hamartomatous polyposis syndrome caused by defects in either the *SMAD4/DPC4* or *BMPR1A* gene. The polyps arising in association with juvenile polyposis are not limited to the colon and may also occur in the small intestine and stomach.[62,63] These patients exhibit an increased risk for carcinomas of the colon, small intestine, stomach, and pancreas.[12,13,62,63] The exact risk for small-intestinal adenocarcinoma is unknown given the rarity of the syndrome. However, upper endoscopy is recommended every 1 to 3 years beginning at 12 years of age (or earlier for symptoms) and should be repeated every 1 to 3 years, depending on severity, with removal of polyps ≥5 mm. The small bowel past the duodenum should be periodically surveilled, depending on initial polyp findings, by enteroscopy, capsule endoscopy, and/or computed tomographic (CT) enterography if duodenal polyposis is present or if there is unexplained anemia, protein-losing enteropathy, or other small-bowel symptoms.[30]

BENIGN EPITHELIAL TUMORS AND PRECURSORS

The WHO classification for small-intestinal epithelial neoplasms is summarized in Box 26.1.[16] This new classification includes several important changes to the taxonomy of small-bowel neoplasia. As for the current nomenclature used for pancreatobiliary neoplasms, the term *intraampullary papillary-tubular neoplasm* is now used for preinvasive lesions that arise almost exclusively within the ampulla. These lesions represent intraampullary versions of the intraductal papillary and tubulopapillary lesions of the pancreas and bile ducts. Intestinal-type adenomas that arise predominantly on the duodenal surface of the ampulla remain classified as *adenomas*.

Adenomatous Polyps

Small-bowel intestinal-type adenomas are rare,[64] accounting for fewer than 0.05% of all intestinal adenomas. Adenomas peak in incidence in the seventh decade of life but may occur at any age. Most adenomas are asymptomatic. They are usually discovered incidentally in individuals who have undergone endoscopic examination for other reasons. Adenomas that are symptomatic typically involve the region of the ampulla of Vater and manifest with biliary colic and

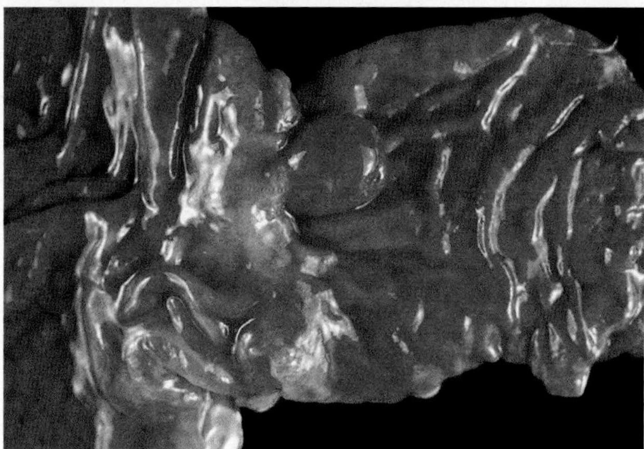

FIGURE 26.1 Duodenal adenoma. Gross photograph shows a pedunculated polypoid lesion projecting into the duodenal lumen. The head of the polyp is smooth and has a somewhat more erythematous appearance than the surrounding non-neoplastic mucosa.

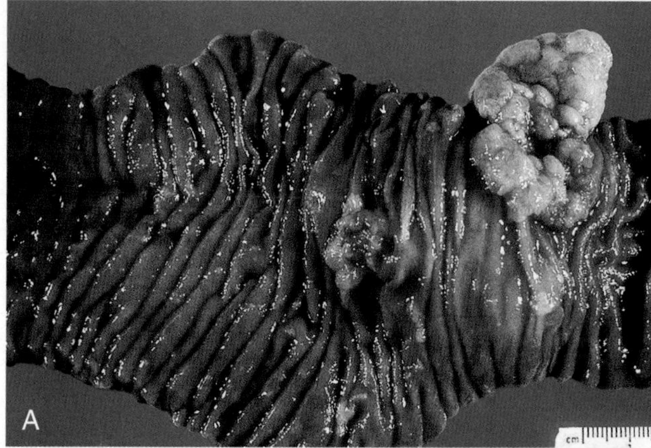

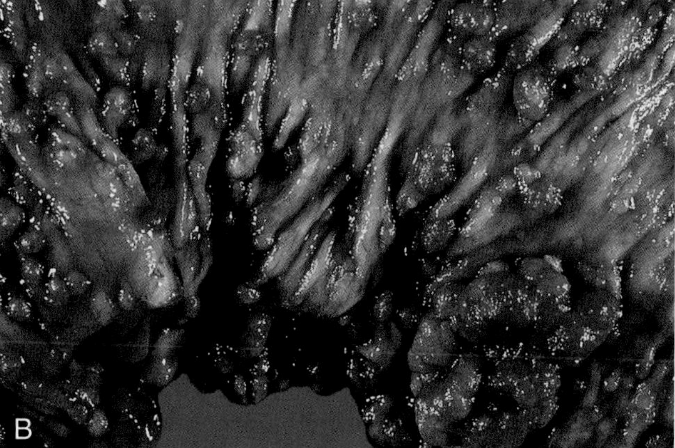

FIGURE 26.2 A, Duodenal resection specimen from a patient with familial adenomatous polyposis. Multiple pedunculated and sessile polyps (adenomas) are present. The largest polypoid lesion represents an adenoma with invasive adenocarcinoma. **B,** The colon from the same patient shows multiple adenomatous polyps as well as an invasive adenocarcinoma *(bottom right).*

obstruction, acute cholangitis, or pancreatitis.[64] Intestinal obstruction, bleeding, nausea, vomiting, anorexia, weight loss, pain, or intussusception may also develop, depending on the size and location of the lesion.[65] Small-intestinal adenomas resemble those that arise in the colon in gross and microscopic characteristics (Fig. 26.1). They are usually lobulated and soft, and they may be sessile, pedunculated, villous, or tubular. A higher proportion of small-intestinal lesions tend to be villous compared with adenomas of the colon; this is most likely a reflection of the underlying villous architecture of the small bowel. Tubular adenomas tend to be small, ranging from 0.5 to 3 cm in maximum diameter. Villous adenomas are often larger, sometimes reaching 8 cm or larger. Intestinal-type adenomas are usually single[65] but can be multiple. The finding of multiple adenomas in the small intestine is rare in patients without a hereditary polyposis syndrome. As a result, identification of multiple lesions should raise suspicion of FAP (Fig. 26.2).

Histologically, intestinal-type adenomas may demonstrate tubular, tubulovillous, or villous growth patterns. They are composed of tall, columnar epithelial cells with elongated, crowded, hyperchromatic nuclei arranged in a "picket fence" pattern. Immature goblet cells may be present. In addition, endocrine cells, squamous cells, and particularly Paneth cells may be numerous (Fig. 26.3). Mitoses, normally seen only in the base of the crypts, may occur at all levels of the adenomatous crypts and villi. A normal-appearing lamina propria is usually present between the neoplastic crypts.

Intestinal-type adenomas can display varying degrees of dysplasia, ranging from low grade to high grade, and they may show intramucosal or associated invasive carcinoma. Although the degree of dysplasia increases, one also tends to see an increased ratio of nucleus to cytoplasm in the cells, loss of cell polarity, and an increased mitotic rate. Prominent crypt budding, nuclear stratification, and loss of mucinous differentiation may herald progression to malignancy.

It is important to distinguish regenerative atypia associated with surface erosion from an adenoma (Fig. 26.4). Regenerating cells tend to mature toward the surface, whereas adenomas do not. The presence of Paneth or endocrine cells in the superficial portions of the lesion is almost always associated with a neoplastic alteration. Prominent acute inflammation with congested capillaries and fibrin deposition, especially when superficial, should alert the examiner to the possibility of regenerative atypia.

Adenomas arising in the small bowel may also be of the pyloric gland type. These lesions typically arise in the proximal duodenum and resemble pyloric gland adenomas arising elsewhere in the GI tract (Fig. 26.5).

Noninvasive Ampullary Neoplasia

Most preinvasive neoplasms in the region of the ampulla of Vater represent intestinal-type adenomas, and approximately 80% of all small-intestinal adenomas arise at this site.[64] Ampullary adenomas resemble their nonampullary counterparts, as described earlier.

Pancreaticobiliary-type ampullary adenocarcinomas are thought to arise from noninvasive papillary and flat intraductal neoplasia reminiscent of that seen in the bile duct and pancreas (Fig. 26.6). The current WHO terminology for these lesions is *intraampullary papillary-tubular neoplasm* (IAPN).[16] An IAPN is defined as a dysplastic, compact, exophytic lesion that is localized almost exclusively within the ampulla and grows predominantly within the ampullary channel, with minimal or no involvement of the

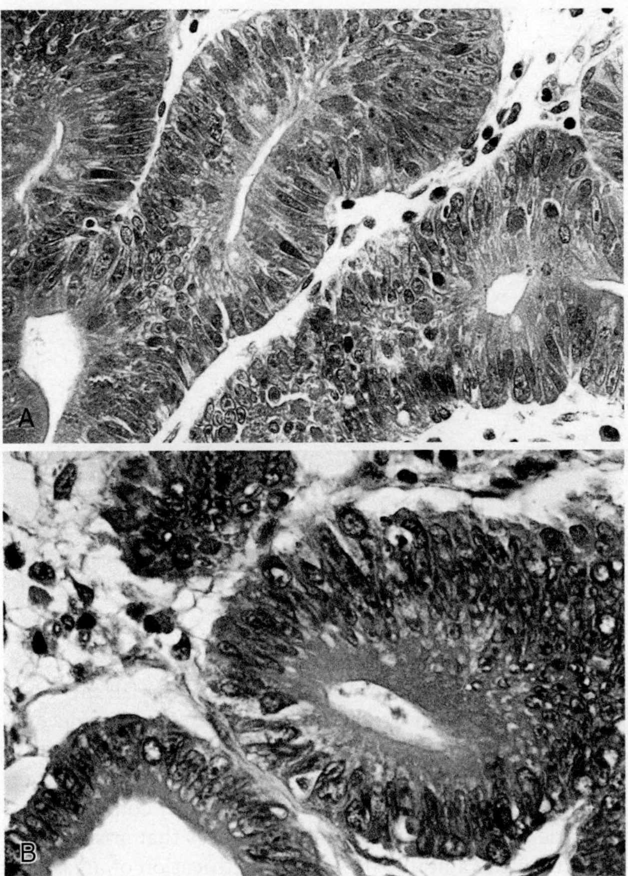

FIGURE 26.3 A, Paneth cells in a duodenal adenoma. Adenomatous crypts contain cells with coarse, eosinophilic, apical vacuoles characteristic of Paneth cells. **B,** This adenoma demonstrates the presence of large numbers of endocrine cells in the glands. These cells have finely granular, eosinophilic cytoplasm. In contrast to Paneth cells, the cytoplasmic granules of endocrine cells are less coarse and are present in a basal location.

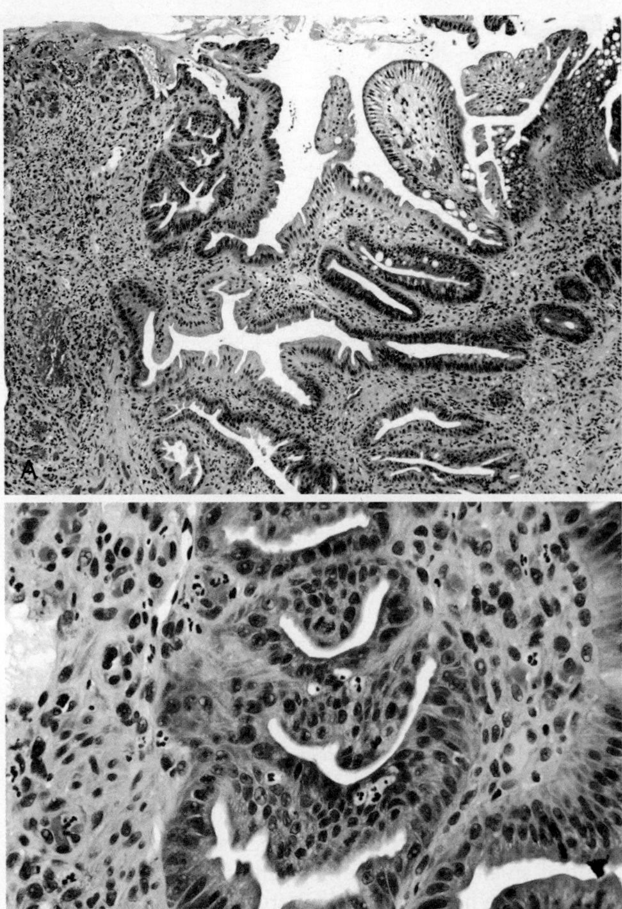

FIGURE 26.4 Regenerative atypia in an ampullary biopsy. A, Low-power view shows distortion of the normal small bowel architecture as a result of chronic inflammation. The deep portion of some crypts appears hyperchromatic, and the nuclei are enlarged. **B,** Higher-power view demonstrates epithelial cells with enlarged nuclei and prominent nucleoli. A large mitotic figure is identifiable in the upper portion of the gland. Active inflammation is clearly present, with neutrophils infiltrating the glands and the lamina propria.

bile duct, pancreatic duct, or duodenal papilla. These preinvasive lesions are encountered infrequently and are usually associated with a coexisting invasive carcinoma.

Histologically, these neoplasms consist of complex, arborizing papillary structures lined by variably atypical epithelial cells. Almost all pancreaticobiliary noninvasive papillary neoplasms have focal high-grade dysplasia, and many have an associated invasive carcinoma.[66-68] The invasive component most commonly has a tubular growth pattern and is the pancreaticobiliary type, although intestinal-type adenocarcinomas may occasionally arise from these papillary precursors.

Serrated Adenoma

Duodenal serrated adenomas are rare lesions, with approximately 35 reported cases in the literature.[69-73] Histologically, they resemble their large-intestinal counterparts. These adenomas have serrated lumens lined by eosinophilic-appearing cells that contain pseudostratified nuclei with prominent nucleoli. Goblet cells are typically not well developed in these lesions. In one study of 13 serrated duodenal lesions, almost one-half demonstrated high-grade dysplasia or progressed to adenocarcinoma.[69]

SMALL-INTESTINAL ADENOCARCINOMA

Clinical Features and Associations

More than one-half of all small-intestinal carcinomas arise in the duodenum, even though this organ constitutes only 4% of the entire length of the small intestine.[5,74,75] The incidence of duodenal adenocarcinoma has increased in recent years, most likely because of the increased use of upper endoscopy[76] and the development of newer techniques such as video capsule endoscopy, double-balloon enteroscopy, and CT enterography.[77,78] In the United States, the incidence of small-intestinal adenocarcinoma is estimated at 0.7 per 100,000 population.[79] Most small-intestinal carcinomas arise in the region of the ampulla of Vater. A smaller percentage of tumors arise in the jejunum, particularly in the first 30 cm distal to the ligament of Treitz. Ileal carcinomas are the least common, except in patients with CD. Small-intestinal carcinomas occur more frequently in men than in women and affect Blacks more often than whites.[3,76]

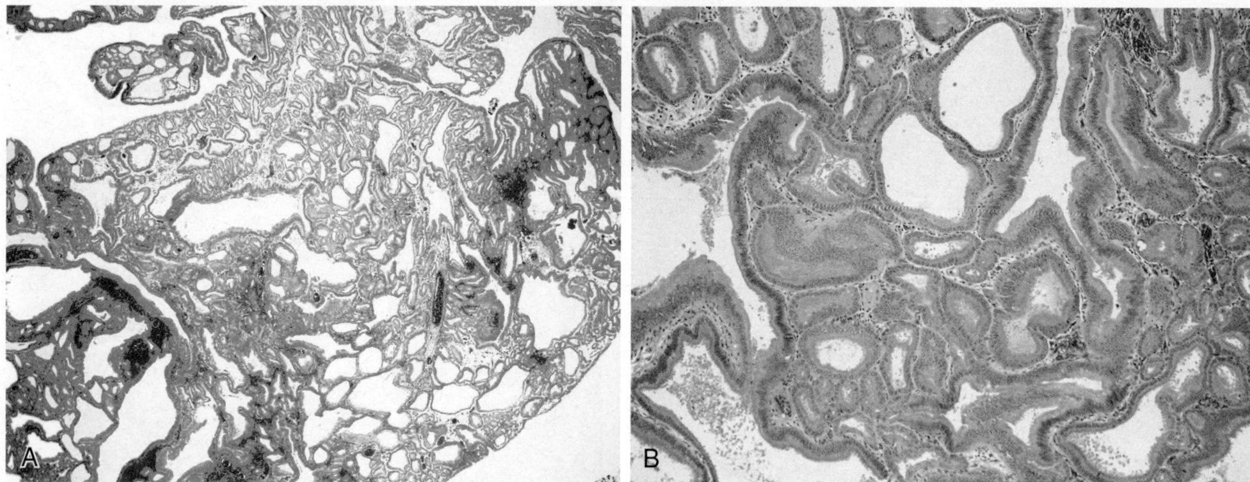

FIGURE 26.5 Pyloric gland adenoma arising in the duodenum. A, Low-power photomicrograph demonstrates a vaguely lobulated polyp composed of tightly packed pyloric gland–type tubules. **B,** Higher-power view demonstrates tubules lined by a single layer of cuboidal epithelial cells with pale to slightly eosinophilic cytoplasm resembling pyloric gland–type cells. The nuclei are round and contain small nucleoli. No dysplastic changes are present in this polyp.

Some diseases (e.g., FAP) are associated with an increased incidence of small-intestinal carcinomas (Box 26.2). Cancers that arise in the upper GI tract, and especially in the periampullary region, represent a major cause of death in these patients. As discussed previously, patients with hereditary polyposis and familial cancer syndromes including FAP, LS, and PJS are at increased risk for development of small-intestinal tumors. In addition, patients with celiac disease have an 80-fold increased incidence of small-intestinal adenocarcinomas compared with the general population.[8] In one study of 175 patients with adenocarcinoma of the small bowel, 13% had celiac disease.[9] The diagnosis of celiac disease preceded that of adenocarcinoma in 63% of these patients. Tumors in these patients often arise in the jejunum.[78]

Ileal adenocarcinomas develop with increased frequency in individuals with long-standing CD (see later discussion). However, in these patients, adenocarcinomas typically arise in the setting of dysplasia (flat or polypoid) rather than in preexisting adenomas.[80]

Most small-intestinal carcinomas manifest in patients between 60 and 70 years of age.[81,82] However, tumors that arise in the setting of a hereditary cancer syndrome are seen in younger individuals. Patients may have presenting symptoms of intestinal obstruction, bleeding, intussusception, or perforation. Ampullary carcinomas often manifest with bile duct obstruction, pancreatitis, and jaundice. Pancreatitis may also develop secondary to pancreatic outflow obstruction.

Pathological Features

Small-intestinal carcinomas may have a flat, stenotic, ulcerative, infiltrative, or polypoid gross appearance (Fig. 26.7). Tumors typically range from 1 to 15 cm in diameter. Larger lesions tend to be found in the more distal portions of the small bowel because lesions in this area often fail to produce symptoms until they are advanced.

Small-intestinal adenocarcinomas are classified by the WHO into six types (see Box 26.1). In general, they are histologically similar to adenocarcinomas that develop elsewhere in the GI tract. However, because small-intestinal cancers usually arise from preexisting adenomas, one may see residual adenomatous changes in the adjacent or overlying epithelium, particularly in smaller lesions. More often, the cancer has overgrown the adenomatous component at the time of diagnosis, especially in tumors that arise in sites other than the ampulla of Vater. Identification of an associated preinvasive lesion allows one to be relatively certain that the tumor is primary to that location. However, some metastatic carcinomas induce significant cytological atypia in adjacent nonneoplastic small-intestinal epithelium that can resemble adenomatous change (Fig. 26.8).

Nonampullary adenocarcinomas are characterized by cellular and nuclear pleomorphism, loss of epithelial polarity, gland-in-gland architecture, and invasion into adjacent tissues. Most small-intestinal adenocarcinomas are moderately differentiated and demonstrate variable degrees of mucin production. Approximately 20% of tumors are poorly differentiated and contain signet ring cells. Other tumors display a prominent extracellular mucinous component. Neoplasms in which more than 50% of the tumor is mucinous should be designated as *mucinous adenocarcinomas* because these tumors tend to have a poorer prognosis than typical gland-forming lesions. Neoplastic endocrine cells and Paneth cells are often present. Squamous cells may also be identified but are less common. The presence of endocrine, Paneth, or squamous cells in a carcinoma has no prognostic significance.

Rarely, small-intestinal carcinomas are of the medullary type. These tumors demonstrate a syncytial pattern of growth with prominent infiltrating lymphocytes. This histological type of small-intestinal carcinoma arises most commonly in elderly females and almost invariably demonstrates a high level of microsatellite instability.[83]

Immunohistochemical Features

Nonampullary small-intestinal adenocarcinomas show more variable expression of cytokeratin 7 (CK7) than do

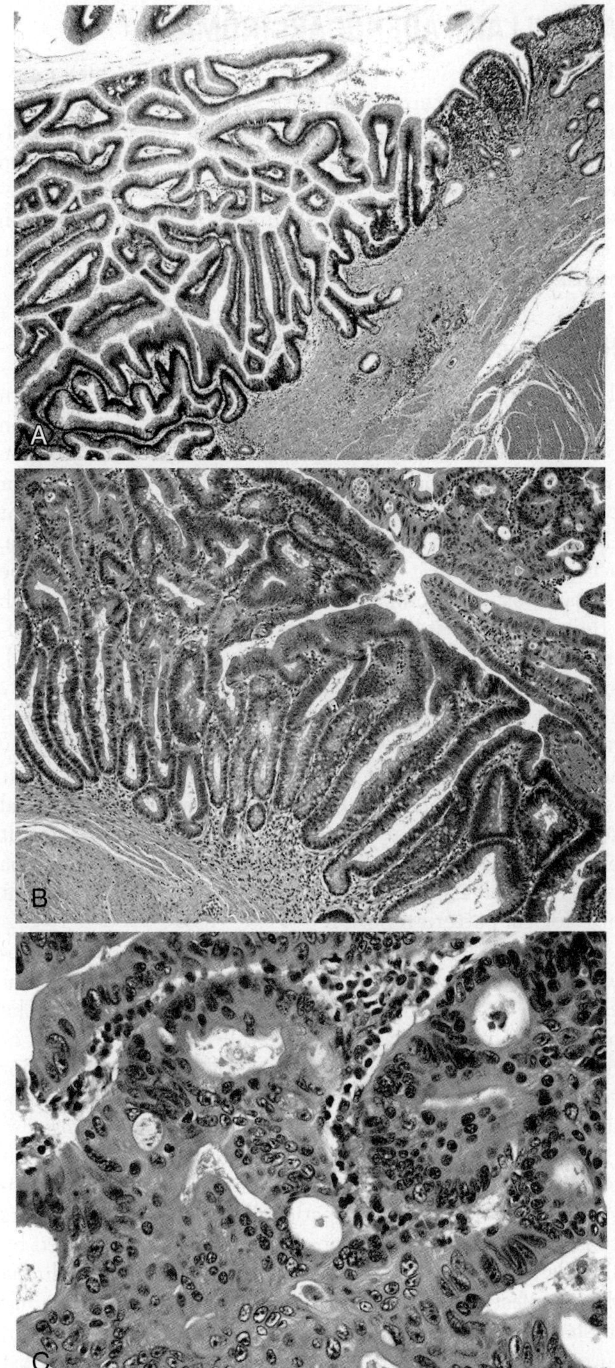

FIGURE 26.6 Intraductal papillary neoplasm involving the ampulla of Vater. A, Low-power photomicrograph demonstrates a papillary intraductal mucinous neoplasm resembling those that arise in the pancreas. **B,** Another in situ ampullary neoplasm more closely resembles an intestinal-type adenoma. **C,** Higher-power view demonstrates a focus of high-grade dysplasia within the noninvasive lesion shown in **B**.

colorectal carcinomas. In one study, diffuse positive CK7 immunoreactivity was identified in 54% of cases, and focal positivity was present in the remaining 46%.[84] In the same study, 67% of cases expressed CK20. Expression of MUC1, MUC2, and MUC5AC occurs in approximately 50%, 36% to 57%, and 40% to 50% of nonampullary adenocarcinomas,

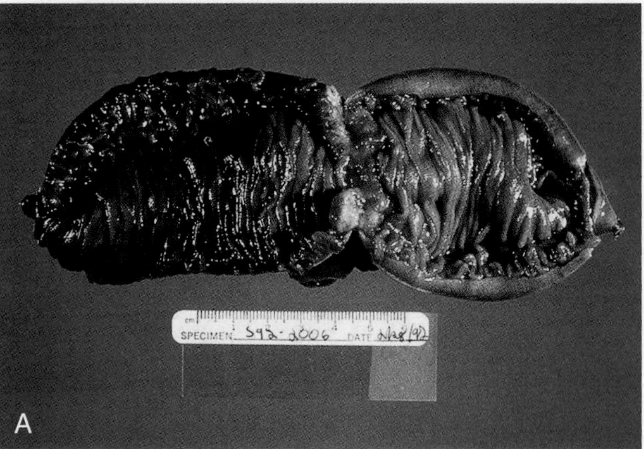

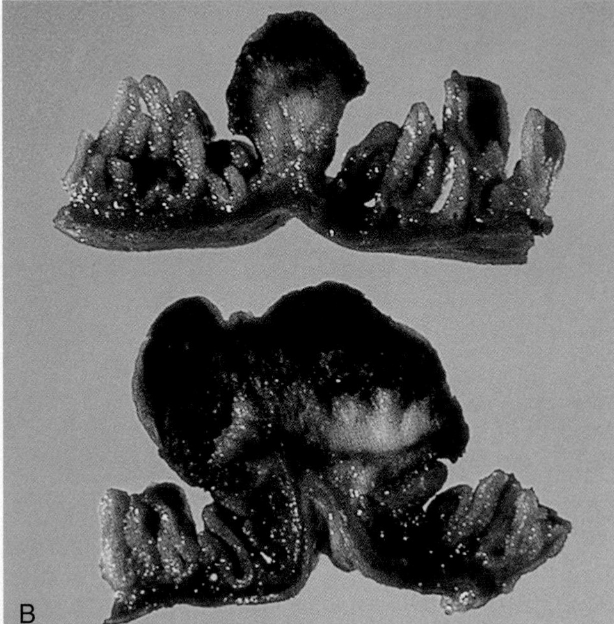

FIGURE 26.7 Gross appearance of intestinal adenocarcinoma. **A,** Jejunal resection specimen demonstrates a circumferential adenocarcinoma constricting the lumen of the small intestine. **B,** Small-intestinal adenocarcinoma demonstrates a polypoid growth pattern. The bulk of the tumor in this case is intraluminal.

BOX 26.2 Conditions Associated with an Increased Risk for Small-Intestinal Carcinoma

Sporadic adenomatous polyps
Congenital anomalies
Long-standing ileostomy
Crohn's disease
Celiac disease
Alpha chain disease
Familial adenomatous polyposis
Gardner's syndrome
MUTYH-associated polyposis syndrome
Peutz-Jeghers syndrome
Lynch syndrome
Juvenile polyposis syndrome

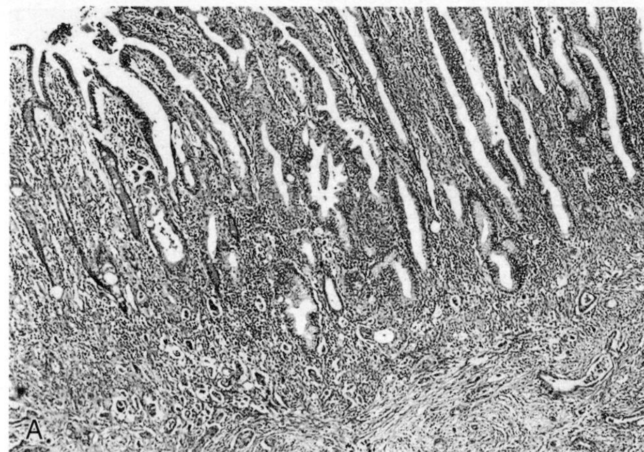

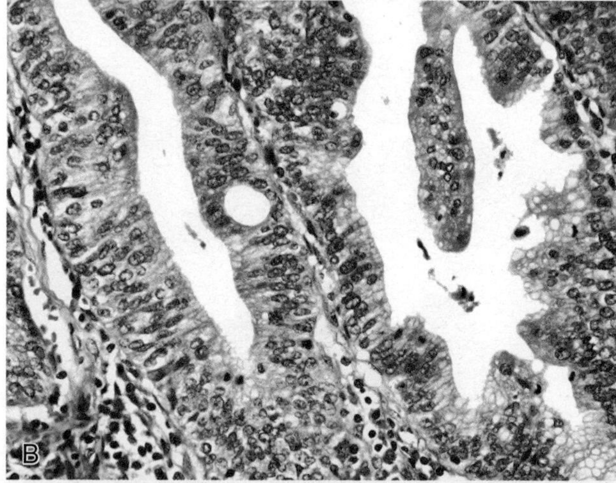

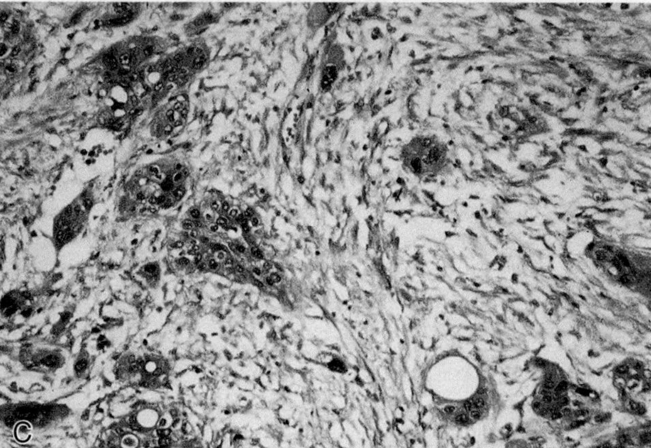

FIGURE 26.8 Metastatic pancreatic carcinoma in the small intestine. A, Low-power photomicrograph demonstrates infiltrating nests of cells within the muscularis mucosae and the submucosa. The epithelium in the overlying mucosa appears complex and irregular. **B,** High-power view of mucosa overlying metastatic pancreatic carcinoma. The epithelium is lined by crowded, mucin-depleted cells with hyperchromatic, somewhat stratified nuclei. The histological appearance is reminiscent of an adenomatous polyp. **C,** High-power view of metastatic pancreatic adenocarcinoma. Infiltrating clusters of highly atypical cells are present within the wall of the small intestine.

respectively.[85,86] Expression of villin is observed in 67% of cases, but the staining is often focal. CDX2 staining is identified in 60% of small-intestinal adenocarcinomas, and the pattern of staining is usually diffuse, similar to colorectal carcinomas.[86]

AMPULLARY ADENOCARCINOMAS

The ampulla of Vater represents the site in the small intestine where most carcinomas arise. The incidence of cancers at this site has increased in the past four decades. Ampullary adenocarcinomas are more common in men than in women.[87] Patients most often have painless jaundice at presentation. Because even small tumors in this location can result in biliary obstruction, many tumors arising in this site are diagnosed at a relatively early stage.

Histological Features

The ampulla is an area in which two types of epithelium converge, that of the duodenum and that of the common bile duct. As a result, carcinomas that arise in this region have historically been classified as either the intestinal or pancreaticobiliary type. Intestinal-type cancers represent the most common histological type of ampullary carcinoma, accounting for 85% of cases.[88] The pancreaticobiliary type is the most common of the remaining tumors, although other unusual histological tumor types may occur, including mucinous, signet ring cell, adenosquamous, clear cell, and neuroendocrine carcinomas. Up to 40% of ampullary adenocarcinomas, however, represent mixed or hybrid phenotypes.[89,90] Nevertheless, classification of an ampullary adenocarcinoma into one of the two major histological types is generally possible with the use of immunohistochemical stains. In cases that remain difficult to classify as a result of hybrid features, a diagnosis of tubular adenocarcinoma with mixed features should be made and the predominant histological pattern reported.[16]

Intestinal-type ampullary adenocarcinomas are histologically indistinguishable from adenocarcinomas that occur elsewhere in the small intestine or colon (Fig. 26.9). The histological pattern varies, from well-formed glandular or tubular structures to cribriform areas or solid nests of tumor cells. As in their colonic counterparts, the glands often contain necrotic or apoptotic debris, so-called *dirty necrosis*.

Pancreaticobiliary ampullary carcinomas closely resemble pancreatic ductal adenocarcinomas or primary adenocarcinomas of the extrahepatic bile ducts. These tumors consist of small, simple, or branched glands surrounded by abundant desmoplastic stroma (Fig. 26.10). The cells lining the neoplastic glands are usually cuboidal to low columnar in shape, and they are typically arranged in a single layer. Intraluminal necrotic debris is infrequently present. Most tumors demonstrate well-formed glandular structures, although less differentiated tumors may contain small clusters and solid nests of tumor cells.

Immunohistochemical Features

Some authors have advocated the use of a variety of immunohistochemical classification systems for evaluation of ampullary carcinomas,[90,91] but exactly which panel of stains should be used remains controversial. The immunoprofile of ampullary adenocarcinoma varies depending on whether the tumor is of the intestinal or the pancreaticobiliary histological type. Intestinal-type ampullary adenocarcinomas are usually CK20 positive (80% to 91%) and CK7 negative (73% to 82%).[91-95] In addition, most of these tumors are

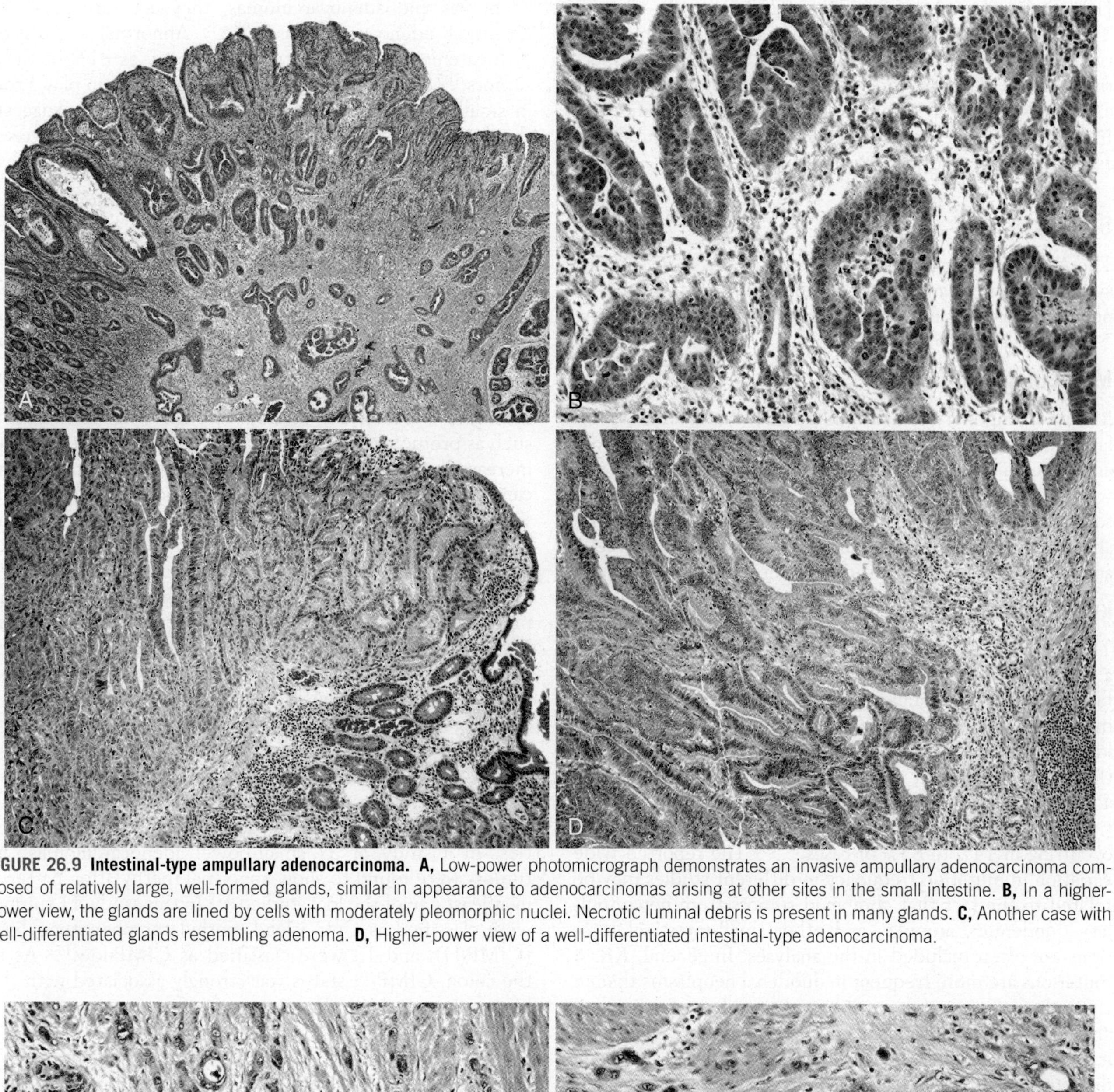

FIGURE 26.9 Intestinal-type ampullary adenocarcinoma. A, Low-power photomicrograph demonstrates an invasive ampullary adenocarcinoma composed of relatively large, well-formed glands, similar in appearance to adenocarcinomas arising at other sites in the small intestine. **B,** In a higher-power view, the glands are lined by cells with moderately pleomorphic nuclei. Necrotic luminal debris is present in many glands. **C,** Another case with well-differentiated glands resembling adenoma. **D,** Higher-power view of a well-differentiated intestinal-type adenocarcinoma.

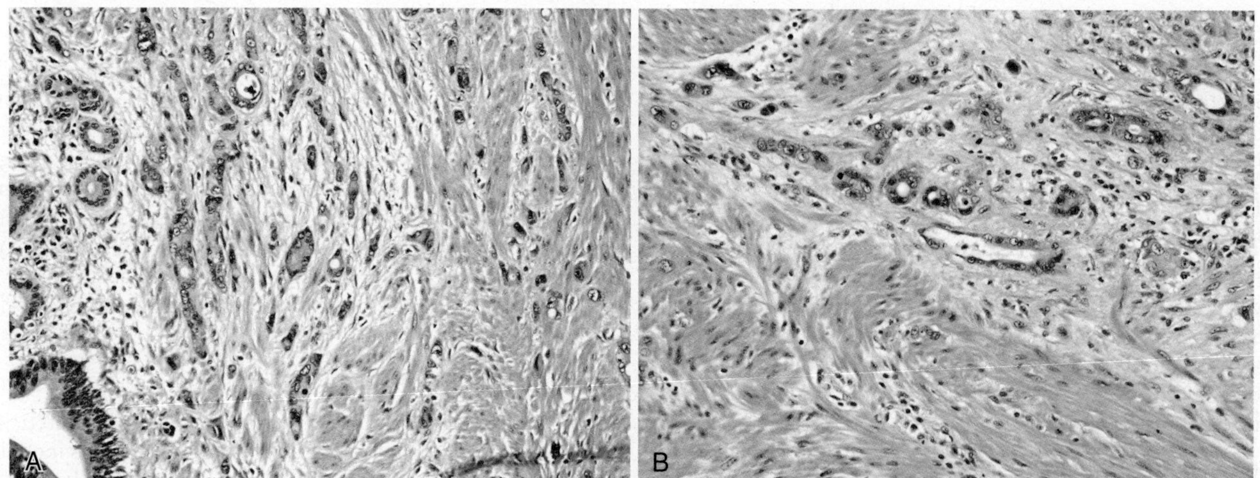

FIGURE 26.10 Pancreaticobiliary-type ampullary adenocarcinoma. A, Infiltrating small, angulated glands resembling those of a pancreatic ductal adenocarcinoma are present in the muscularis propria of the ampulla. **B,** Higher-power view of some of the infiltrating glands. Moderate cytological atypia is present.

positive for CDX2.[91,92,96] They variably express MUC1 (18% to 60%) and MUC2 (47% to 82%).[91,92,95,96]

In contrast, pancreaticobiliary-type ampullary tumors are typically CK20 and CDX2 negative (92% and 83%, respectively) and CK7 positive (96%), and they more commonly express MUC1 (83%) and MUC2 (100%) proteins.[91-96] In some studies, expression of MUC5AC was significantly associated with prognosis.[90]

Staging

The American Joint Committee on Cancer (AJCC) staging system for ampullary adenocarcinomas differs from that of nonampullary carcinomas of the small intestine.

Molecular Features

Most nonampullary and ampullary adenocarcinomas, similar to colonic adenocarcinomas, are believed to arise from an adenoma-carcinoma or dysplasia-carcinoma sequence in which genetic alterations progressively accumulate, leading to cancer development. Small-intestinal adenocarcinomas share many common molecular alterations with colorectal adenocarcinomas, but significant differences also exist.

KRAS *Mutations*

The *KRAS* oncogene encodes a binding protein that plays a key role in transmitting signals from extracellular growth factors to the cell nucleus. *KRAS* mutations occur commonly in colorectal carcinomas and are also frequently identified in colorectal adenomas. Therefore mutations in this gene are thought to represent an early change in the adenoma–carcinoma sequence in the colon. *KRAS* mutations are also found in small-intestinal adenocarcinomas, occurring in 14% to 83% of cases.[97-103] The reported wide variation in mutation frequency in different studies may be related to the fact that combined tumors from nonampullary duodenum, ampulla, and other small-intestinal locations are often included in the analyses. In general, *KRAS* mutations are more frequent in duodenal neoplasms than in those that arise in other small-bowel sites. In a recent meta-analysis, *KRAS* mutations were identified in 45% of ampullary adenocarcinomas.[104] *KRAS* mutations have also been detected in small-intestinal adenomas,[97] suggesting that *KRAS* may play a similar role in both the small-intestinal and the colorectal adenoma-carcinoma sequence.

TP53 *Alterations*

TP53 is the gene most commonly mutated in human cancers. Its function is to facilitate DNA repair before cell replication or, if DNA damage is severe, to initiate apoptosis in the affected cell. As in the colon, *TP53* mutation is a late event in the neoplastic progression of small-intestinal adenocarcinomas.[97,102] Overexpression or mutation of *TP53* is identified in 20% to 53% of cases.[86,97,101,105,106]

APC *and β-Catenin Mutations*

Both the *APC* gene product and β-catenin (encoded by the *CTNNB1* gene) represent important proteins in the WNT signaling pathway. APC binds β-catenin, which leads to its degradation and prevents it from interacting with nuclear transcription factors that initiate cell proliferation. Although *APC* mutations are frequent in both colorectal adenomas and adenocarcinomas, they are rare in small-intestinal adenocarcinomas.[96,97,105] Abnormal expression of β-catenin, however, occurs in as many as 81% of these tumors,[105] suggesting that mutations in β-catenin play a role in small-intestinal adenocarcinoma.[106] One study suggests that loss of β-catenin expression in ampullary carcinomas is associated with poor prognosis and is a predictor of disease recurrence.[107]

Mismatch Repair Genes

Defects in DNA mismatch repair result in high-frequency microsatellite instability (MSI) in colorectal and other cancers and are a characteristic alteration identified in tumors from patients with HNPCC. *MLH1* and *MSH2* are the genes most commonly mutated in patients with HNPCC. These genes are also inactivated in a proportion of sporadic colorectal carcinomas, usually through epigenetic events such as promoter hypermethylation. The overall result is an increased mutation frequency in affected cells. Small-bowel cancers occur with increased frequency among patients with HNPCC,[108-111] suggesting that mismatch repair gene defects likely play a role in sporadic small-intestinal adenocarcinomas as well. MSI has been reported in 18% to 35% of small-bowel carcinomas.[112,113] The frequency of MSI and methylation abnormalities is even higher in small-intestinal adenocarcinomas that arise in the setting of celiac disease.[103,114] The rate of MSI in ampullary adenocarcinomas may be lower, with high-frequency MSI occurring in up to 10% of tumors.[115-117]

Epigenetic Alterations

As with adenocarcinomas of the colon, a subset of small-intestinal adenocarcinomas show methylation abnormalities. In a study of 37 small-bowel adenocarcinomas, 24 tumors were found to show abnormal methylation patterns in at least one of the loci studied.[112] In this study, 11 tumors were classified as CpG island methylator phenotype–high (CIMP-H), and 13 were classified as CIMP-low.[112] As in the colon, CIMP-H status was strongly associated with the high-frequency MSI phenotype.

SMAD4 *Mutations*

The *SMAD4 (DPC4)* gene product was first identified as an important tumor suppressor protein in pancreatic adenocarcinomas. It is part of the transforming growth factor-β signaling pathway, where it plays a role in growth suppression. Deletion or loss of *SMAD4* expression occurs in approximately 50% of pancreatic cancers and in 3% to 50% of colorectal cancers.[118-120] *SMAD4* alterations occur in 24% of nonampullary small-intestinal adenocarcinomas and 34% of ampullary carcinomas.[121,122]

PD1 Pathway Alterations

The programmed death (PD1) pathway is upregulated in the immune microenvironment of many tumor types including melanoma, lung cancers, and renal cancers.[123] It is also upregulated in the MSI-high subset of colorectal cancers.[124] One study[125] found that PD-1 and PD-L1 are additionally highly expressed in both immune cells and tumor cells in most small-intestinal adenocarcinomas. As for colon cancer, PD-L1 expression was most common in MSI-high tumors.

Prognosis

The prognosis of small-intestinal carcinomas is poor. The 5-year survival rate ranges from 14% to 45%, with overall survival ranging from 14 to 40 months.[126] The primary reason for the poor prognosis is that patients are often asymptomatic until late in the course of the disease, and metastases are often present at the time of diagnosis. In general, ampulla of Vater tumors have a more favorable prognosis than distal tumors,[127,128] presumably because they become symptomatic early and therefore tend to be removed at a less advanced stage of growth. Other prognostic factors include tumor size, surgical resectability of the tumor,[129,130] presence of lymphatic or vascular invasion, nodal involvement, depth of invasion into the bowel wall, and presence or absence of invasion into adjacent structures.

CROHN'S DISEASE–ASSOCIATED ADENOCARCINOMA

Clinical Features

Patients with CD are at increased risk for carcinoma of the colon and small intestine.[131-133] The incidence of small-intestinal carcinoma in CD is 20 to 30 times greater than that observed in the general population.[134,135] The cancer risk correlates positively with disease duration and the anatomic extent of the inflammatory process. Risk factors for development of small-intestinal carcinoma in individuals with CD include surgically excluded loops of small bowel, chronic fistulous disease, and male sex. In one study, adenocarcinoma risk was found to be lower in CD patients who had undergone small-bowel resection or who had used salicylates for longer than 2 years.[136] The mortality rate in CD-associated carcinoma is approximately 80%.

Unlike sporadic small-intestinal carcinomas that commonly involve the duodenum, small-intestinal carcinomas that develop in CD arise in areas involved by inflammatory disease. Thirty percent of these tumors arise in the jejunum, and 70% arise in the ileum.

Pathological Features of Dysplasia

It is accepted that dysplasia precedes cancer development in CD, as in ulcerative colitis.[137-139] The diagnosis of dysplasia is sometimes difficult because of recurrent and persistent inflammatory changes associated with the underlying inflammatory bowel disease. Grossly, dysplasia may appear flat or elevated (polypoid). Loss of the normal pattern of mucosal folds may be the only gross manifestation of dysplasia, although a granular or pebbly appearance is not uncommon. On occasion, plaques, nodules, and other irregular polypoid lesions may be identified. Histologically, the diagnosis of dysplasia is based on identification of a combination of architectural and cytological features.[140] Architectural alterations may result in a configuration that resembles adenoma. Cytological abnormalities consist primarily of cellular and nuclear pleomorphism, nuclear hyperchromasia, loss of polarity, and nuclear stratification.

Dysplasia is generally classified as low grade or high grade (including carcinoma in situ). Although invasive carcinoma is more commonly observed in individuals with high-grade dysplasia, it may also be associated with lesser degrees of dysplasia. Low-grade dysplasia is characterized by the presence of tall epithelial cells with elongated, hyperchromatic, pseudostratified nuclei that fail to differentiate into normal goblet or absorptive cells at the mucosal surface (Fig. 26.11). Dystrophic goblet cells may also be present. In low-grade dysplasia, normal basal polarity of the nuclei is maintained. In contrast, high-grade dysplasia demonstrates true nuclear stratification and a greater degree of cytological atypia (see Fig. 26.11B). In high-grade dysplasia, the nuclei lose their polarity; instead of being elongated with the long axis of the nucleus oriented perpendicular to the basement membrane, they are often round and contain prominent nucleoli.

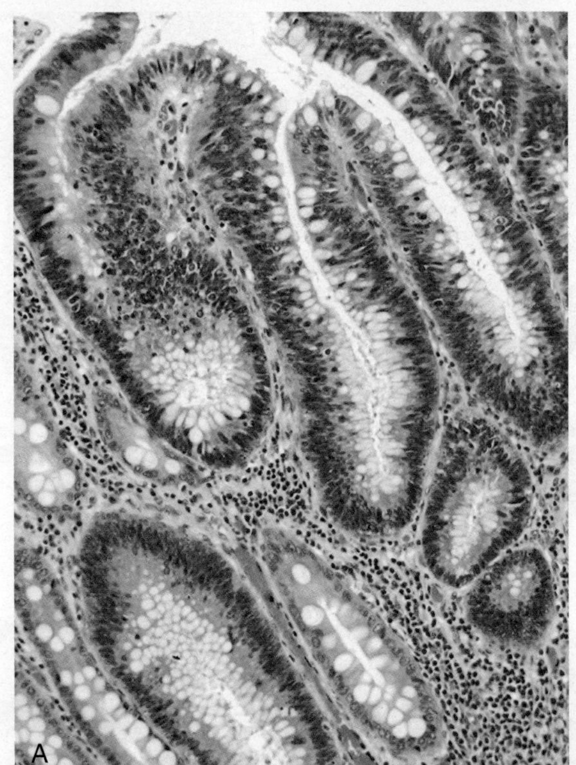

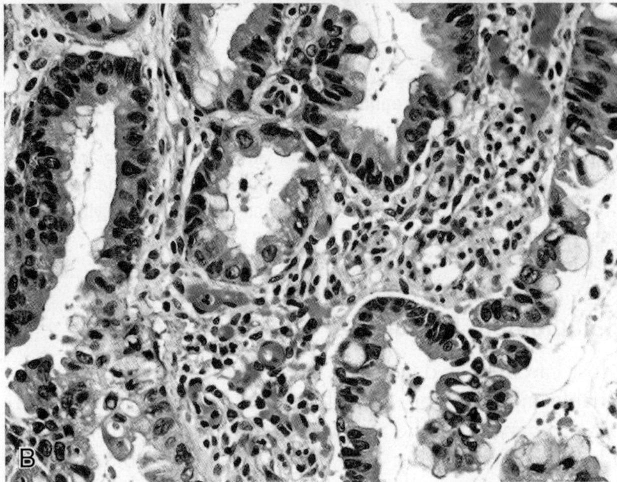

FIGURE 26.11 Dysplasia in Crohn's disease. A, Low-grade dysplasia is characterized by nuclear crowding, elongation, and pseudostratification. The epithelium appears similar to that found in adenomatous polyps. **B,** High-grade dysplasia shows more pronounced crowding, hyperchromasia, and loss of polarity along with true stratification of the nuclei.

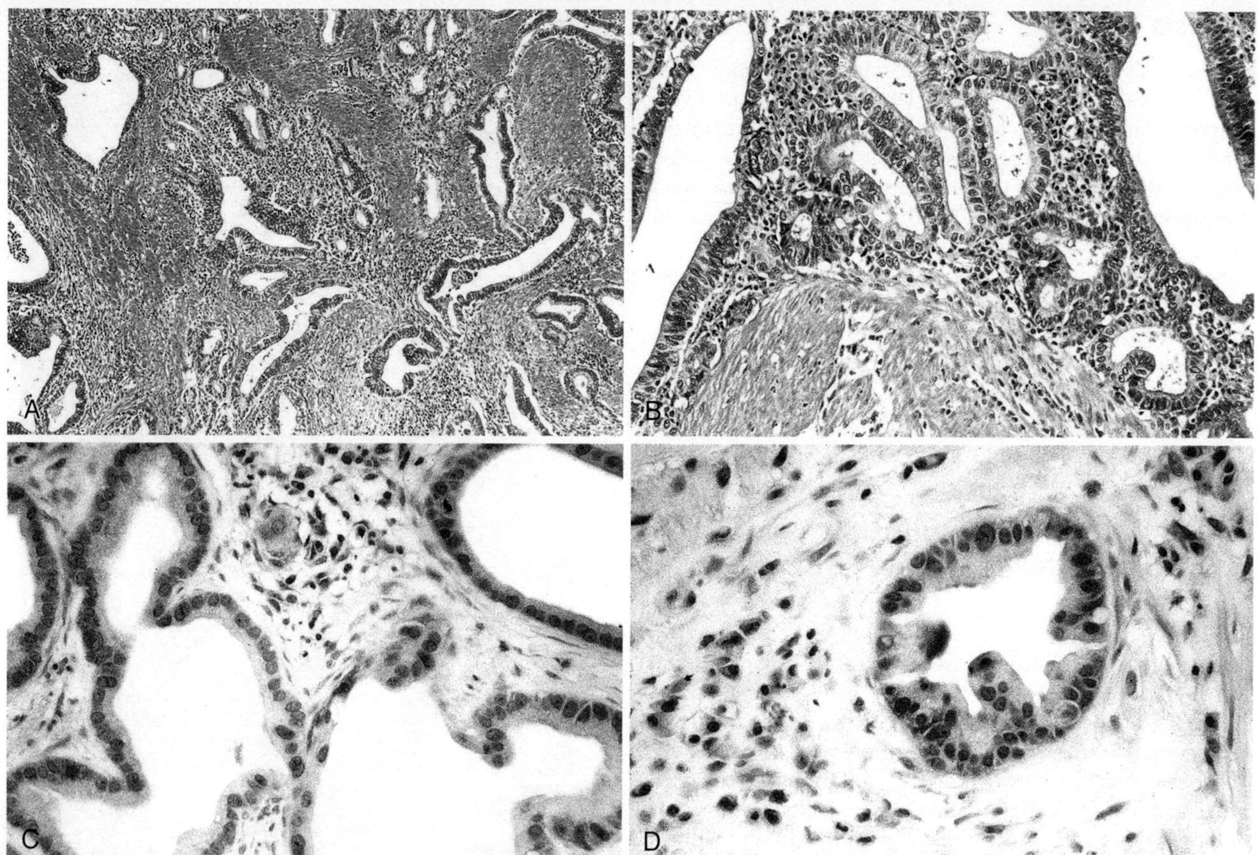

FIGURE 26.12 Misplaced epithelium (pseudoinvasion) versus adenocarcinoma in Crohn's disease. A, Low-power view of an area of epithelial misplacement in a patient with Crohn's disease. Irregular-appearing glands are present in the submucosa but are surrounded by a rim of lamina propria. No desmoplasia is observed. **B,** High-power view of misplaced glands surrounded by lamina propria. The glandular epithelium does not appear dysplastic. **C,** A focus of well-differentiated invasive adenocarcinoma from the same patient as in **A** and **B**. The glands are not surrounded by lamina propria but instead are embedded in a desmoplastic stroma. Mild cytological atypia is seen. **D,** Higher-power view shows a neoplastic gland surrounded by desmoplastic stroma.

Pathological Features of Adenocarcinoma

Most carcinomas develop in areas of macroscopically identifiable inflammatory bowel disease. Grossly, they resemble ordinary, sporadic intestinal carcinomas. Histologically, adenocarcinomas that arise in CD also resemble sporadic tumors. They may show any degree of differentiation, but in patients with CD, there is a higher proportion of poorly differentiated and mucinous tumors compared with the sporadic type.

Differential Diagnosis

In some cases, CD-associated adenocarcinoma is difficult to distinguish from pseudoinvasion, which entails misplacement of epithelium in the submucosa or muscularis that develops as a result of recurrent injury, ulceration, and repair.[141] This represents a form of ileitis cystica profunda. Histologically, epithelial misplacement (pseudoinvasion) is characterized by mucus-filled cysts in the submucosa, muscularis propria, or serosa (Fig. 26.12). The cysts are lined by cuboidal to columnar epithelium–containing goblet cells, enterocytes, and Paneth cells and are normally associated with a rim of lamina propria. On occasion, the cyst lining may regress from pressure atrophy. Features that help rule out malignancy include the absence of desmoplasia and the presence of a rim of lamina propria surrounding misplaced epithelium. Marked cytological atypia, desmoplasia, and angular, irregularly shaped glands are characteristics of invasive adenocarcinoma.

In diagnostically difficult cases, careful sampling and evaluation of the surface epithelium may help resolve the diagnostic dilemma, particularly if dysplastic epithelium is present.

CELIAC DISEASE–ASSOCIATED ADENOCARCINOMA

The rate of development of small-bowel malignant neoplasms among patients with celiac disease is increased as much as 80-fold compared with the general population.[8,99] Adenocarcinoma of the duodenum and proximal jejunum is the most common nonlymphomatous type of malignancy associated with celiac disease, accounting for more than 20% of all small-bowel malignant neoplasms in patients with this disorder[142] (Fig. 26.13). The risk of cancer is highest after 2 years of disease; the tumors may be multifocal.[142-144] Dysplasia similar to that seen in patients with CD[145] may be observed in celiac disease–associated adenocarcinomas as well (see Fig. 26.13D).

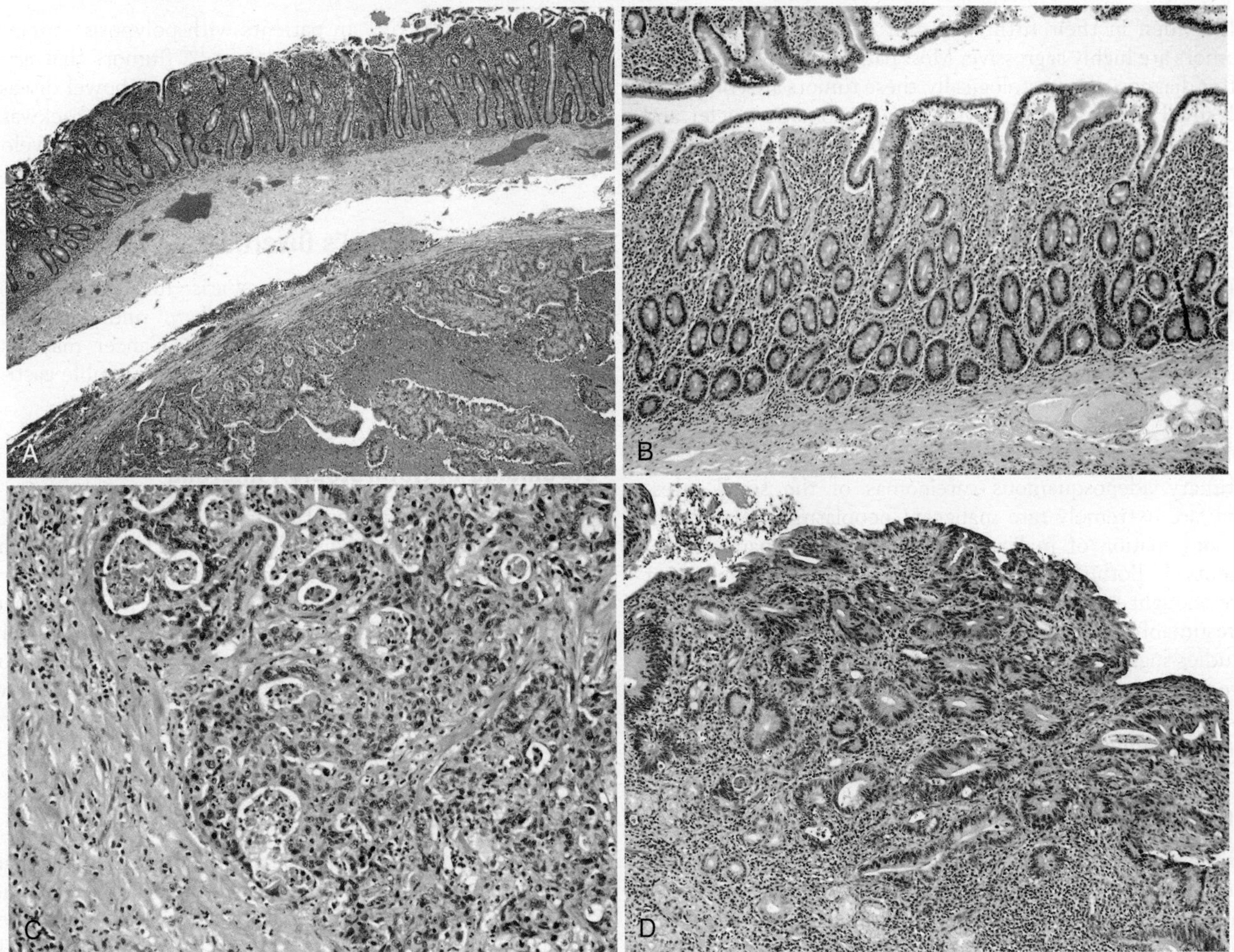

FIGURE 26.13 Intestinal adenocarcinoma arising in association with celiac disease. A, Low-power photomicrograph demonstrates a submucosal tumor and overlying small-intestinal mucosa with prominent villous blunting. **B,** On higher magnification, the overlying mucosa shows moderate villous blunting and a marked increase in intraepithelial lymphocytes typical of celiac disease. **C,** Higher-power view of the invasive adenocarcinoma shows gland formation and intraluminal apoptotic and inflammatory debris. **D,** An area of high-grade dysplasia overlying the invasive adenocarcinoma. The dysplasia appears similar to that seen in association with Crohn's disease.

OTHER TYPES OF CARCINOMA

Hepatoid Carcinoma

Rarely, ampullary cancers may display unusual histological patterns or produce unusual proteins, such as α-fetoprotein (AFP). These tumors are usually moderately to poorly differentiated and resemble gastric AFP-producing hepatoid tumors.[146,147] Histologically, they demonstrate solid, papillary, and tubular growth patterns. Clear cell areas may also be present. α_1-Antitrypsin-immunoreactive hyaline droplets and bile are found in some cases.[146] In addition to hepatoid areas, one usually sees other areas of mucin production and other features of "adenocarcinoma," such as carcinoembryonic antigen (CEA) positivity. Immunohistochemical analysis for antibodies against α-chymotrypsin, prealbumin, transferrin, and AFP is positive, at least focally, in most cases.[147] Elevated AFP may also be detectable in the serum of affected patients.

Choriocarcinoma

Primary choriocarcinomas have been reported in the small intestine but are extremely rare.[148,149] Grossly, these tumors often appear hemorrhagic and partially necrotic. Histologically, they are composed of aggregates of relatively uniform eosinophilic cells with basophilic vesicular nuclei. Multinucleated syncytial cells with irregular cytoplasmic margins and bizarre, anaplastic nuclei are scattered among more uniform smaller cells. Cytotrophoblastic cells are also seen among the syncytial cells. Vascular invasion is often present. Small-intestinal choriocarcinomas produce human chorionic gonadotropin and human placental lactogen, both of which can be documented by immunohistochemistry. Most of the reported cases of choriocarcinoma have been associated with an adenocarcinoma or anaplastic large cell carcinoma, suggesting that these tumors may arise from multipotential stem cells. Before a diagnosis of primary intestinal choriocarcinoma is established, ectopic pregnancy, teratoma, and metastatic disease from an unrecognized primary tumor must be excluded.

Small Cell Carcinoma

Rarely, small cell neuroendocrine carcinomas, similar to those in the lung or large intestine, can arise in the small intestine.[150-152] Patients with small cell carcinoma are often older men in their fifth to eighth decades of life. These tumors are highly aggressive. Most patients die within 1 year after diagnosis.[151] Histologically, these tumors are composed of small anaplastic cells with hyperchromatic nuclei and scant cytoplasm. The cells form broad sheets, solid nests, and ribbon-like strands. They may resemble lymphoma, a tumor that statistically is much more common in the small intestine than small cell carcinoma. Immunohistochemistry and special stains can usually help resolve this differential diagnosis. Small cell carcinomas display immunoreactivity for neuron-specific enolase (NSE), Leu-7, chromogranin A, neurofilament protein, synaptophysin, and low-molecular-weight cytokeratin CAM 5.2.

Adenosquamous Carcinoma

Primary adenosquamous carcinomas of the small intestine are extremely rare malignant neoplasms composed of a combination of malignant glandular and squamous elements.[152] Both the glandular and the squamous component are thought to arise from a single multipotential stem cell, presumably located at the base of the crypts.[153,154] Some studies suggest that adenosquamous carcinomas in the colon are more aggressive than pure adenocarcinomas.[153,155] It is not known whether this fact is also true of small-intestinal adenosquamous carcinomas.

Squamous Cell Carcinoma

Primary squamous cell carcinoma involving the small intestine is extremely rare[156] and usually develops in congenital anomalies such as intestinal duplications or Meckel's diverticula.[157] Squamous cell carcinomas more commonly represent metastases from other sites, such as the cervix or lung.

Sarcomatoid Carcinoma

Sarcomatoid carcinoma of the small bowel is rare, with less than 25 cases reported to date. These neoplasms primarily affect patients in their sixth decade of life, although younger patients may be affected. Small-intestinal sarcomatoid carcinomas have primarily been reported in the distal small intestine.[158-164] They may appear grossly polypoid or endophytic with central ulceration, and they are commonly large (average, 7 cm) at the time of diagnosis. Histologically, these neoplasms may appear biphasic, with admixed epithelioid and mesenchymal elements, or monophasic, composed solely of mesenchymal-type spindle cells. Some tumors demonstrate areas containing anaplastic, bizarre tumor giant cells. Immunohistochemically, both epithelioid and spindle cell components of these tumors show positivity for cytokeratin. Usually, both components also show positivity for vimentin. Focal immunoreactivity for neuroendocrine markers may also be observed.[161] These tumors are negative for CD117 and DOG-1.

Carcinoma in Ileostomies

Adenocarcinomas may arise in ileostomy sites in patients who have undergone bowel resection for FAP or inflammatory bowel disease.[14,165,166] In patients with polyposis, carcinomas develop in adenomatous polyps.[167] Tumors that arise in ileostomies of patients with inflammatory bowel disease occur in those who have had either antecedent backwash ileitis or dysplasia.[14,168] In most cases, the cancers develop many years after creation of the ileostomy.[169]

Carcinoma in Meckel's Diverticula

Tumors with varying histology may arise in Meckel's diverticula. Medullary, mucinous, papillary, and anaplastic carcinomas have all been described.[170] Cancer may also develop in heterotopic gastric mucosa and resemble gastric adenocarcinoma.[171,172]

Carcinoma in Heterotopic Pancreas

Pancreatic heterotopia is the most common congenital abnormality to involve the small intestine. Heterotopic pancreas usually remains asymptomatic, although secondary changes can lead to symptom production. A rare complication is the development of adenocarcinoma, which usually arises from the ductular component of the lesion. Histologically, carcinomas that arise in heterotopic pancreas show the full range of histological changes that occur in ordinary pancreatic carcinomas.[173,174]

Metastatic Carcinoma

Metastatic tumors are significantly more common than primary neoplasms in the small intestine.[175,176] Metastatic carcinomas from many sites may affect the small intestine, although melanoma and lung, breast, colon, and renal cell carcinomas are the most common. Tumors from the mesentery, pancreas, stomach, or colon may spread to the small intestine directly. Metastases from carcinomas of the testes, adrenal glands, ovary, stomach, uterus, cervix, and liver have also been reported. Of these, ovarian tumors are most likely to cause widespread serosal implants.

Secondary adenocarcinomas may closely mimic primary small-intestinal carcinomas both grossly and microscopically. Grossly, secondary tumors often manifest as intramural masses; they may form submucosal nodules or plaques or even produce a polypoid structure or sessile mucosal lesion. Presenting symptoms may include obstruction, intussusception, or perforation. Napkin ring–like circumferential stenotic lesions may also develop and can lead to localized serosal retraction and intestinal kinks. Metastatic lesions may have an infiltrative growth pattern, in which case they may simulate CD or an ischemic stricture.

Differentiation of metastatic from primary carcinomas of the small intestine is sometimes difficult. If the majority of the neoplastic cells are deep within the wall of the small bowel and there is little involvement of the mucosa, the lesion is most likely metastatic (Fig. 26.14). Adenomatous or dysplastic change in the epithelium overlying or adjacent to the invasive tumor strongly favors a small-intestinal primary. However, secondary adenocarcinomas, especially pancreatic carcinoma, can rarely induce marked epithelial atypia simulating adenomatous change in epithelium adjacent to the

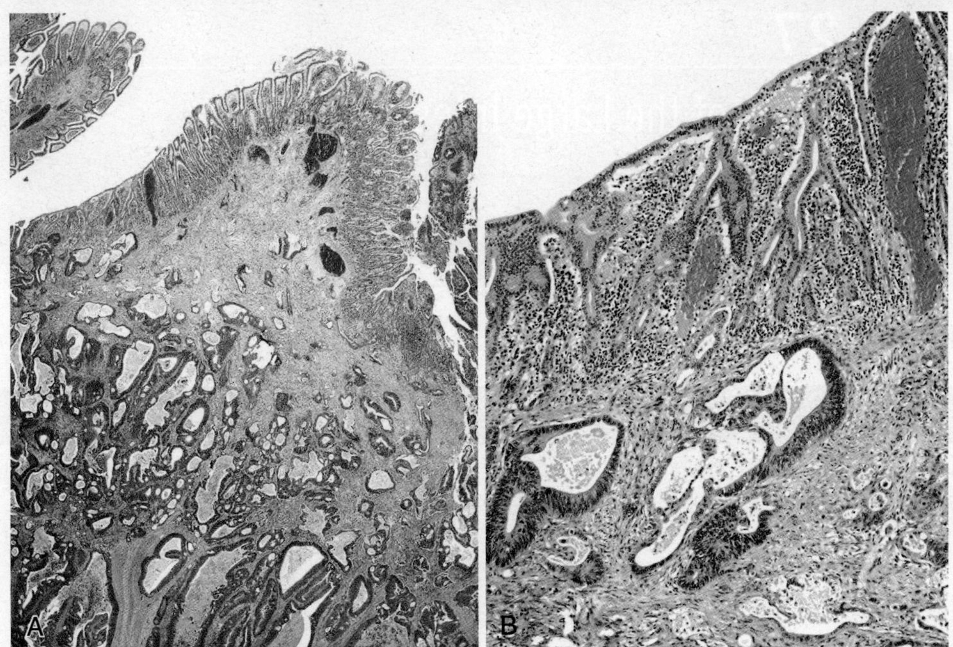

FIGURE 26.14 Metastatic adenocarcinoma in the small intestine. A, The bulk of the tumor is present in the muscularis propria and the submucosa. **B,** The overlying mucosa is inflamed but shows no evidence of precancerous change.

carcinoma (see Fig. 26.7). The cells demonstrate cytological features of malignancy and often appear more disorderly than adenomatous epithelium. However, the pseudostratification of nuclei, typical of adenomatous epithelium, is usually absent. It is unclear whether this epithelial atypia represents neoplastic transformation of the native intestinal epithelium or pagetoid spread of neoplastic cells.

The full reference list may be accessed online at Elsevier eBooks for Practicing Clinicians.

CHAPTER 27

Epithelial Neoplasms of the Large Intestine

Ian S. Brown

Contents

INTRODUCTION

The most common neoplasms of the large intestine are adenomas, conventional or serrated in type (see Chapter 22). Adenomas are the precursor of most primary malignant epithelial neoplasms of the large intestine. Although abundant clinical, morphological, and genetic evidence suggests that primary epithelial malignant neoplasms are a heterogeneous group of tumors, most clinicians consider these neoplasms together to be *colorectal carcinoma.*[1,2] Much of the discussion in this chapter refers to *colorectal carcinoma* (CRC) as a generic single disease, with the recognition that this is an oversimplification. In practice, approximately 85% of CRCs are typical adenocarcinomas; relatively distinct histological subtypes form the remainder (Box 27.1). Recent advances in genetic testing for hereditary colorectal cancer syndromes and for sensitivity to targeted therapies also highlight the clinical relevance of emerging molecular classification systems.

BOX 27.1 World Health Organization Classification of Malignant Epithelial Neoplasms of the Large Intestine

Adenocarcinoma NOS
Serrated adenocarcinoma
Adenoma-like adenocarcinoma
Micropapillary adenocarcinoma
Mucinous adenocarcinoma
Poorly cohesive carcinoma
Signet ring cell carcinoma
Medullary adenocarcinoma
Adenosquamous carcinoma
Carcinoma, undifferentiated, NOS
Carcinoma with sarcomatoid component
Neuroendocrine tumor, NOS
Neuroendocrine carcinoma NOS
Mixed neuroendocrine–nonneuroendocrine neoplasm (MiNEN)

CLINICAL FEATURES

Early-stage CRC is typically diagnosed at the time of screening or during colonoscopy performed for another indication, and it does not usually manifest with symptoms, signs, or other laboratory findings. Advanced cancers are more likely to result in clinical symptoms, such as a change in bowel habits, constipation, abdominal distention, hematochezia, or tenesmus (rectosigmoid lesions). It is important to appreciate that these "colorectal-type" symptoms and signs apply predominantly to left-sided cancers; right-sided cancers often manifest insidiously with nonspecific systemic symptoms and signs such as fatigue, weight loss, and anemia. Only approximately 40% of patients have localized disease at presentation. Approximately 40% have regional metastases, and approximately 20% have distant metastases.[3] Endoscopy with biopsy is the standard diagnostic approach. Computed tomography (CT) and magnetic resonance imaging (MRI) are used to assess depth of invasion, regional spread, and distant metastases; rectal MRI is the "gold standard" used to assess the extent of local spread in rectal cancers, with transrectal ultrasound as an alternative for early lesions.

A variety of screening recommendations have been proposed and endorsed by the American Gastroenterological Association, American Medical Association, and American Cancer Society (Table 27.1).[4-7] Standard guidelines are modified in individuals with a personal or family history of colorectal adenoma or carcinoma.[8] Screening is clinically effective and cost-effective.[8] Screening colonoscopy provides the added benefit of polyp removal, and it is well established that polypectomy can prevent CRC.[9] An estimated risk reduction of at least 20% to 30% for CRC deaths could potentially be achieved by implementing a combination of (1) strategies aimed at improved screening, polyp management, and early diagnosis of CRC, (2) lifestyle modifications, including dietary change and increased exercise, and (3) chemoprevention.[10-12]

TABLE 27.1 Guidelines for Early Detection of Adenomas and Colorectal Cancer in Average-Risk Individuals

Method	Interval*
Tests That Detect Adenomatous Polyps and Cancer†	
Flexible sigmoidoscopy	Every 5 years
Colonoscopy	Every 10 years
Computed tomography colonography	Every 5 years
Tests That Primarily Detect Cancer	
Guaiac-based fecal occult blood test	Annual
Fecal immunochemical test	Annual
Stool DNA test	Every 3 years

Beginning at 50 years of age. The American Cancer Society has proposed that screening should commence at 45 years of age. Discontinuation of screening is recommended at 85 years of age.
†These tests should be encouraged if resources are available and the patient is willing to undergo an invasive procedure.
From Wolf AMD, Fontham ETH, Church TR, et al. Colorectal cancer screening for average-risk adults: 2018 guideline update from the American Cancer Society. CA Cancer J Clin. *2018;68(4):250-281.*

INCIDENCE

Worldwide, malignant epithelial tumors of the colon and rectum are the second most common type of cancer in women (after breast and ahead of uterine cervix) and the third most common cancer in men (after lung and prostate), accounting for 10.2% of all cancers in 2018, with more than 1 million new cases diagnosed each year.[13] There is marked variation in the age-standardized incidence, with a 25-fold difference between high-risk regions (affluent countries including Australia, New Zealand, Europe, the Americas, and Japan) and low-risk regions (developing countries including Africa, India, and other parts of southeast Asia) (Fig. 27.1).[10,12,13] The likely role of environmental and lifestyle influences, particularly diet, alcohol intake, and physical activity, in the genesis of these differences is supported by abundant data. There are also significant global differences in the age at onset of CRC, with a mean age of only 50 years in developing countries.

In the United States, there were an estimated 135,430 new cases of colorectal cancer (71,420 in men and 64,010 in women) in 2017.[3] Seventy percent of these cancers developed in the colon, and 30% developed in the rectum.[3] CRC is the third most common cancer in both men and women

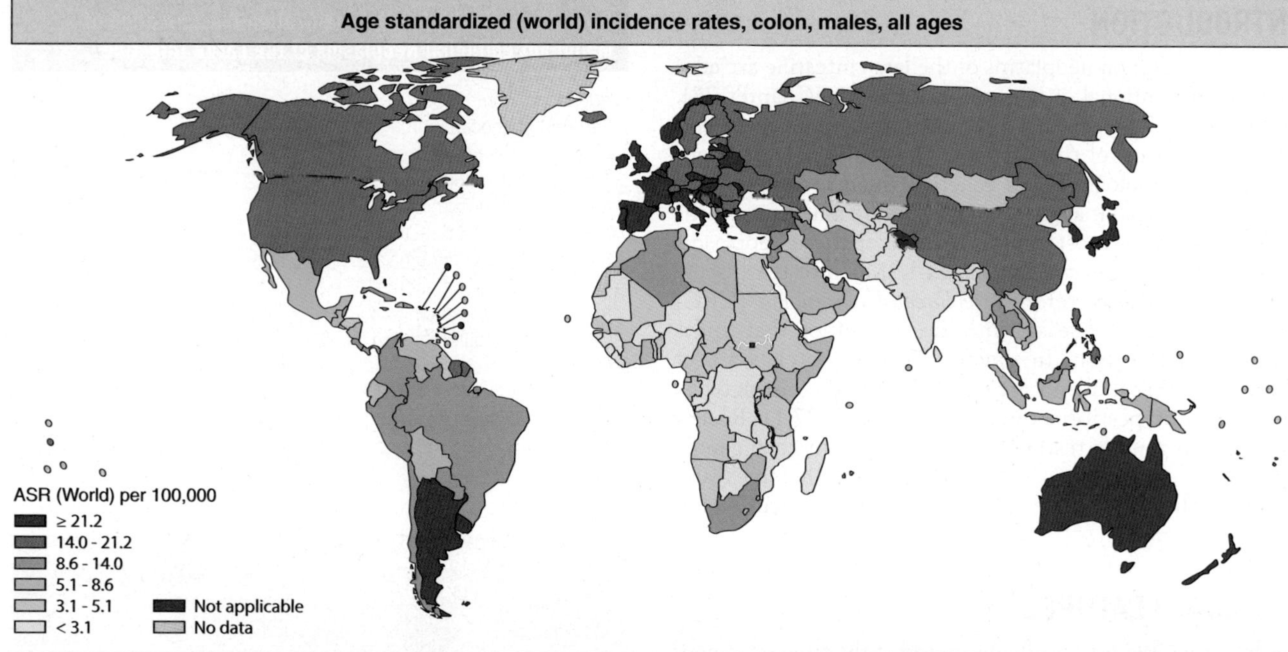

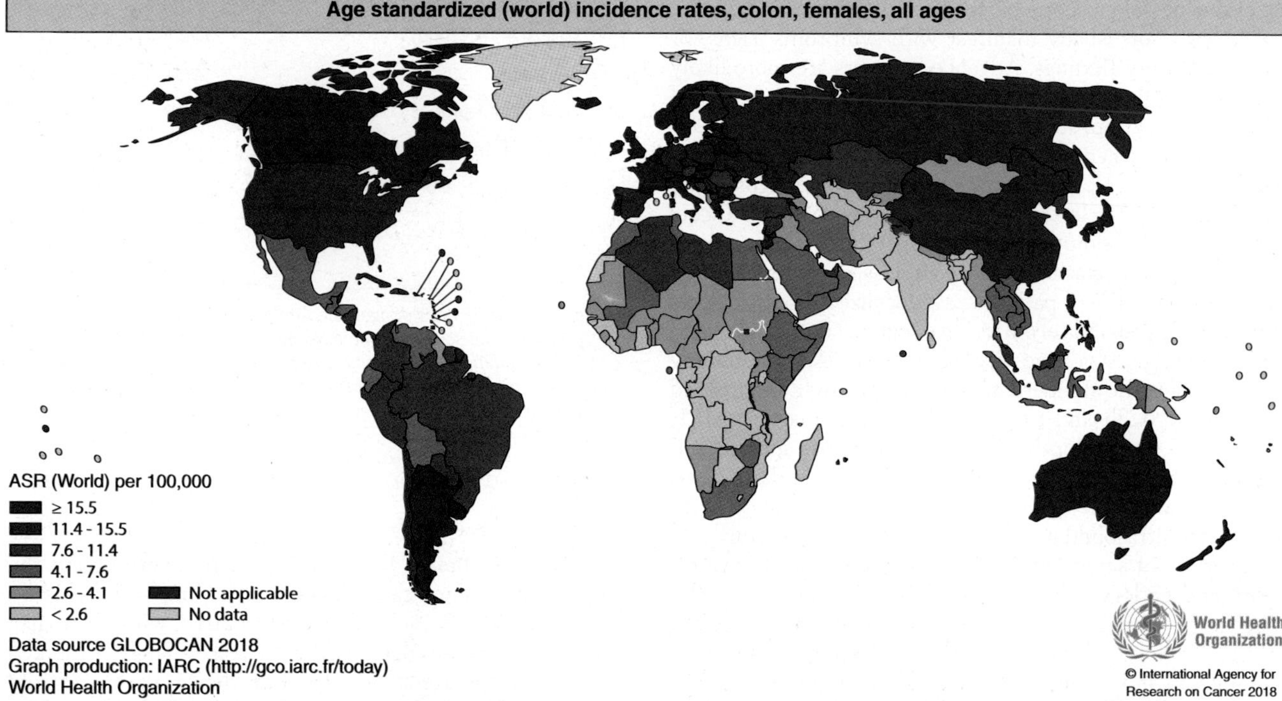

FIGURE 27.1 Colorectal cancer incidence and mortality worldwide in 2018. The estimated age-standardized rates per 100,000 are shown for both males and females. (From Globocan 2018. International Agency for Research on Cancer [IARC]. (*From* https://gco.iarc.fr/today/fact-sheets-cancers.)

and is the fourth most common cancer overall.[6] Overall, it is the second leading cause of cancer death behind only lung cancer, and it is the leading cause of cancer death among nonsmokers.[3] The lifetime risk for development of CRC is estimated at about 5%.[14,15] North American Association of Central Cancer Registries statistics reveal an incidence of 27.6 per 100,000 for colon carcinoma and 11.2 per 100,000 for rectal carcinoma in 2019.[3] CRC is significantly more common in men (combined age-adjusted incidence, 46.9 per 100,000 vs. 35.6 per 100,000 in women); this difference is more striking for rectal cancer than for colonic cancer,[3] and the increased incidence in men is apparent only after 50 years of age. Despite the higher incidence in men, women live longer, so there are a similar number of total cases and cancer deaths in men and women.[3] Fortunately, the incidence and mortality rates have been in decline for several decades as a result of reduction in risk factors (e.g., decreased smoking and red meat consumption, increased use of aspirin, more widespread use of screening tests, and improvements in treatment).[3] The incidence increases with age, with approximately 10% of cases occurring before 50 years of age and only approximately 1% before 35 years of age.[3]

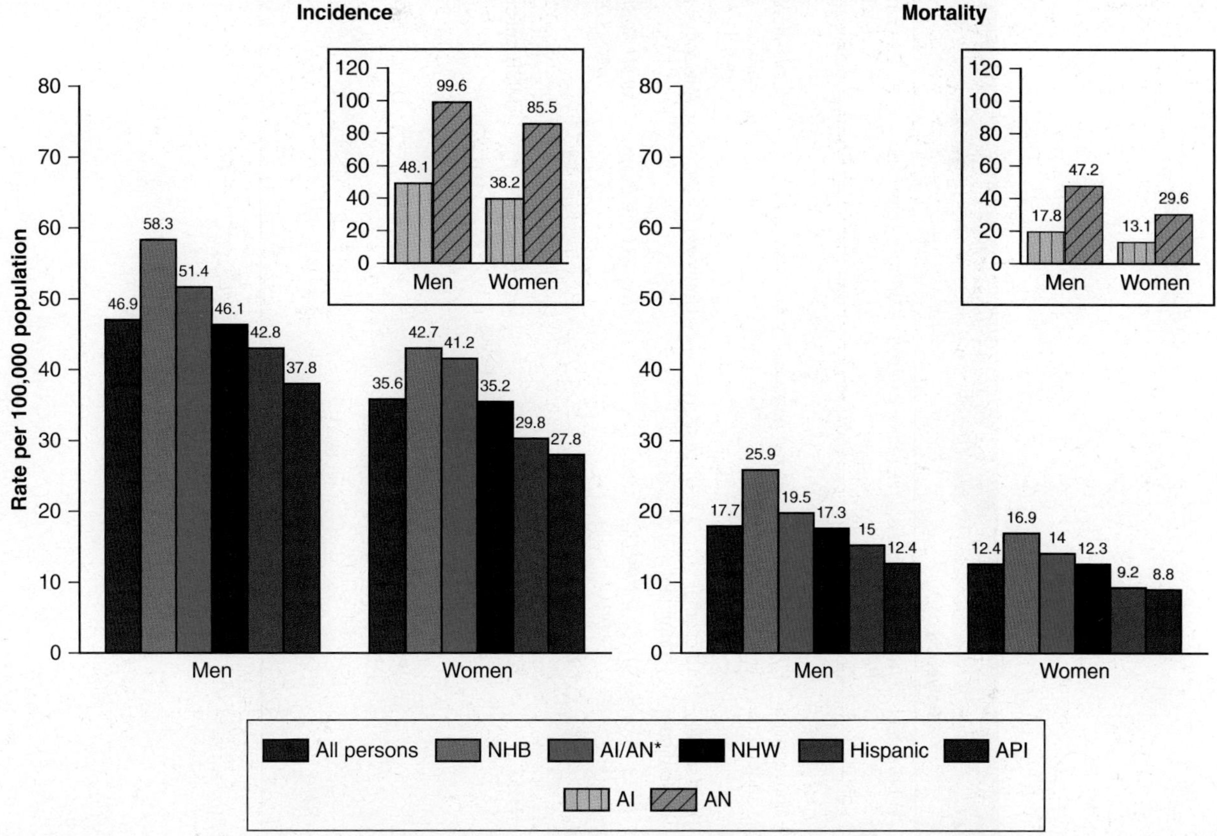

FIGURE 27.2 Incidence (2009 to 2013) and mortality rates (2010 to 2014) of colorectal cancer by Race and Ethnicity, United States. (*From Siegel RL, Miller KD, Fedewa SA, Ahnen DJ, Meester RGS, Barzi A, et al. Colorectal cancer statistics, 2017. CA Cancer J Clin. 2017;67[3]:177-193.*)

TABLE 27.2 Risk Factors for Colorectal Cancer*

Factor	Relative Risk
Family history (first-degree relative)	1.8
Physical inactivity (<3 hours/week)	1.7
Inflammatory bowel disease (physician-diagnosed Crohn's disease, ulcerative colitis, or pancolitis)	1.5
Obesity	1.5
Red meat	1.5
Smoking	1.5
Alcohol (>1 drink/day)	1.4
High vegetable consumption (≥5 servings/day)	0.7
Oral contraceptive use (≥5 years)	0.7
Estrogen replacement (≥5 years)	0.8
Multivitamins containing folic acid	0.5

Modifiable factors are in* ***bold text.*

From American Cancer Society. Cancer Facts and Figures 2002. Atlanta: American Cancer Society; 2002:20.

Data from Colditz GA, Atwood KA, Emmons K, et al. Harvard report on cancer prevention volume 4: Harvard Cancer Risk Index. Risk Index Working Group, Harvard Center for Cancer Prevention. Cancer Causes Control. 2000;11(6):477-488.

In addition to the global variation in CRC incidence, there are significant regional and ethnic differences in incidence within the United States. The incidence varies by approximately 1.5-fold between high-risk regions (predominantly the northeast Atlantic coast) and low-risk regions (predominantly the South and Midwest).[3] Figure 27.2 presents the differences related to racial and ethnic backgrounds. The incidence is highest in non-Hispanic blacks and lowest in Asian Americans/Pacific Islanders.[3]

EPIDEMIOLOGY

The risk of CRC is influenced by both endogenous (constitutional) and exogenous (environmental) factors (Table 27.2).[12,16] For the practicing surgical pathologist, genetic predisposition and long-standing inflammatory bowel disease (IBD) have the most direct clinical impact, and these topics are discussed later. Age, as discussed previously, is the most powerful risk factor. CRC is predominantly a disease of late middle-aged and elderly individuals.[3] The increased risk in males is thought to be related to the protective effect of estrogen.[7,17]

Remaining risk factors are largely related to lifestyle and, importantly, are modifiable, suggesting the potential for interventions aimed at significantly reducing the incidence of CRC.[7,18] The five most convincingly implicated lifestyle factors are obesity, physical activity, and ingestion of red meat, processed meat, and alcohol.[7,12,18] Of these modifiable risk factors, diet has been the most extensively studied, and although there is little doubt that elevated risk is consistently associated with a Western type of diet, it has been difficult to determine which components are most important. Diets with a high calorie intake and those rich in meat, particularly animal fat, have been implicated in many studies.[19-21] Possible mechanisms for this effect include the production of heterocyclic amines, stimulation of higher

TABLE 27.3 Classification of Genetic Syndromes that Predispose to Colorectal Cancer

Phenotype	Nonpolyposis		Polyposis								
Syndrome names	Lynch syndrome	Familial colon cancer type X	FAP	Polymerase proofreading–associated polyposis	*MUTYH* *NTLHL1* Biallelic *MSH3*	AXIN2-associated polyposis	Li-Fraumeni	Juvenile polyposis, Peutz-Jeghers, Cowden's	Hereditary mixed polyposis syndrome	Serrated polyposis	Constitutional mismatch repair deficiency
Description	MMR-deficient CRC	MMR-preserved CRC	Conventional adenomas	Conventional adenomas	Conventional adenomas	Conventional adenomas	Conventional adenomas	Hamartomas	Mixed polyposis	Serrated polyps	Conventional adenomas, MMR-deficient CRCs
Inheritance	Autosomal dominant	Autosomal dominant	Autosomal dominant	Autosomal dominant	Autosomal recessive	Autosomal dominant	Autosomal dominant	Autosomal dominant	Uncertain	Unknown	Autosomal recessive
Genes involved	*MLH1, MSH2, MSH6, PMS2, EPCAM*	*RPS20, EMA4A, HNRNPAO, WIF1*	*APC*	*POLE, POLD*	Base excision repair	Wnt-related genes	*TP53*	*STK11,BMPR1A, SMAD4, PTEN*	*Grem1*	*RNF43* (rare cases)	*MLH1, MSH2, MSH6, PMS2*
Cancer pathway	MMR deficiency		Wnt	DNA proofreading			*TP53*	*TGF mTOR, P13K/AKT*	Bone morphogenetic protein pathway	Wnt (possible)	MMR deficiency
CRC cancer risk	Up to 90%	?	100%	30%-70%	60%-70%	?	?	JPS: 70% PJS: 40% Cowden's:10%	?	?	Up to 50%
Attributable risk	3%	<0.5%	<1%	Rare	0.3%-0.8%	Rare	Rare	Rare	Rare	<0.5%	Rare

FAP, *Familial adenomatous polyposis;* JPS, *juvenile polyposis syndrome;* PJS, *Peutz-Jeghers syndrome.*

levels of fecal bile acids, production of reactive oxygen species, and elevated insulin levels.[20,22] An important role for modification of the normal gut microbiota allowing for an increased susceptibility of the gut epithelium to carcinogens has been proposed.[22] In addition to high-risk factors, there are inverse associations with vegetable and fiber consumption.[20] This effect could be related to anticarcinogens, antioxidants, folate, induction of detoxifying enzymes, binding of luminal carcinogens, fiber fermentation to produce volatile fatty acids, or reduced contact time with epithelium because of faster transit.[19-22] Several studies, including a large pooled multivariate analysis, have found that high folate intake is associated with a decreased risk of CRC, providing some of the most direct evidence of dietary risk factor relationships.[19,20] Finally, alcohol intake has been associated with an increased risk of CRC.[23]

There is an inverse association between use of nonsteroidal antiinflammatory drugs and CRC risk.[11,18,24] Smoking exposure is associated with CRC, although the relative risk is less than for many other tobacco-related malignancies.[18,25] Sedentary lifestyle,[18,26] long-standing IBD[27] (see Colitis-Associated Neoplasia), pelvic irradiation,[28] and ureterosigmoidostomy are also associated with an increased risk of CRC.

Finally, there is evidence that there are important differences in the epidemiological risk factors associated with different subtypes of CRC. There has been a trend in recent years toward the development of more proximal cancers,[29] which may relate to changes in epidemiological risk factors. Furthermore, there are molecular biological differences between right- and left-sided CRCs that would support different epidemiological associations.[30,31] More recently, research has focused on the complex interactions of hormones, energy balance, intestinal flora, and inflammation.[15,18]

Genetic polyposis syndromes account for less than 0.5% of all incident CRCs. Nonpolyposis forms of hereditary CRC have a much higher overall contribution to the causation of CRC and are discussed in detail later in this chapter. The most common genetic syndromes that predispose to CRC are summarized in (Table 27.3).

PATHOGENESIS

Progression from Adenoma to Carcinoma

Most if not all CRCs arise from adenomas, either conventional adenomas, sessile serrated lesions (SSLs), or traditional serrated adenomas (TSAs) (in decreasing order of frequency).[32,33] Residual adenoma is identified in approximately 10% to 30% of CRCs; in the remainder, the adenomas are presumably overgrown by cancer.[34] There are distinct associations between the histological type of precursor lesion and the CRC. These indicate that there are two broad pathways involved in neoplastic progression in the colorectum: the conventional adenoma pathway and the serrated adenoma/lesion pathway.

The conventional adenoma pathway accounts for approximately 70% to 80% of all CRCs and is more prevalent in the left colon and rectum than in the right colon. Conventional adenomas typically precede cancer by approximately 15 years.[35] The prevalence of conventional adenomas in the U.S. population is approximately 25% by 50 years of age and 50% by 70 years of age, and these adenomas have a high lifetime risk of progression if not removed.[36] Exact risks of progression are not known; one study estimated a 10% to 15% chance of progression during 10 years for a 1-cm conventional adenoma,[37] whereas another review puts the risk of developing cancer at 3% to 5%.[38] Endoscopic removal of conventional adenomas decreases the incidence of subsequent CRC.[9,39] The cumulative incidence of new adenomas within 3 years after normal endoscopy averages 27% at follow-up colonoscopy.[40]

The serrated pathway has been increasingly recognized in the past 15 years, and it is estimated to account for approximately 20% to 30% of all CRCs.[41-44] Most CRCs arising in the serrated pathway develop from SSLs, particularly those located in the right colon. The exact progression risk of SSL to CRC is unknown; however, it is unlikely to be higher than for a similar-sized conventional adenoma, and progression is likely to take at least 15 years on average.[45] CRC is typically preceded by the development of dysplasia within these polyps, which marks a rapid acceleration in carcinogenesis.[41,46-49] Historically, conventional endoscopic screening programs have been less effective at reducing right-sided CRC, in large part because the risk of progression of serrated polyps, almost all of which were previously diagnosed as hyperplastic polyps, was not recognized.[50] The progression risk of these polyps is sufficient to warrant their complete endoscopic removal.[48,51] Challenges remain for endoscopic surveillance programs because serrated polyps are difficult to recognize and completely remove endoscopically,[52,53] and the underlying genetic events that drive these lesions allow for development of CRCs in relatively small polyps (see later discussion). Furthermore, SSLs are overrepresented as the precursor lesion of interval cancers (cancers identified between screening intervals).[54,55] TSAs also precede CRC, with typically aggressive features; however, these lesions are much less common.[56] Conventional hyperplastic polyps, particularly those in the left colon, rarely, if ever, progress to cancer.

Aberrant crypt foci represent the earliest stages of colorectal neoplasms and are present before the development of grossly apparent adenomatous polyps.[35,57] Aberrant crypt foci are microscopic lesions most readily identified by examination of methylene blue–stained, stripped mucosal sheets under a dissecting microscope. They are characterized by a localized collection of crypts that show an increase in crypt diameter and an increased number of lining epithelial cells, which imparts a serrated or slitlike appearance. Histological sections of aberrant crypt foci reveal a range of findings, such as normal or only mildly hyperplastic epithelium, features more typical of serrated polyps, or, rarely, true dysplasia (the latter being similar to microscopic adenomas incidentally identified in patients with familial adenomatous polyposis).[57] Aberrant crypt foci may also be visualized endoscopically, although the technical challenges of these methods have prohibited routine clinical applications.[58,59]

Reports of very small (<1 cm) carcinomas that lack any evidence of residual adenoma have raised the possibility that some cancers may arise de novo.[60] However, this is a theory that has lost credibility in recent years. These cancers represent less than 5% of all CRCs. Some studies suggest that they are more likely to be of higher grade than ex-adenoma carcinomas, with a higher risk of lymphatic and blood vessel invasion.[60,61] However, other studies do not support

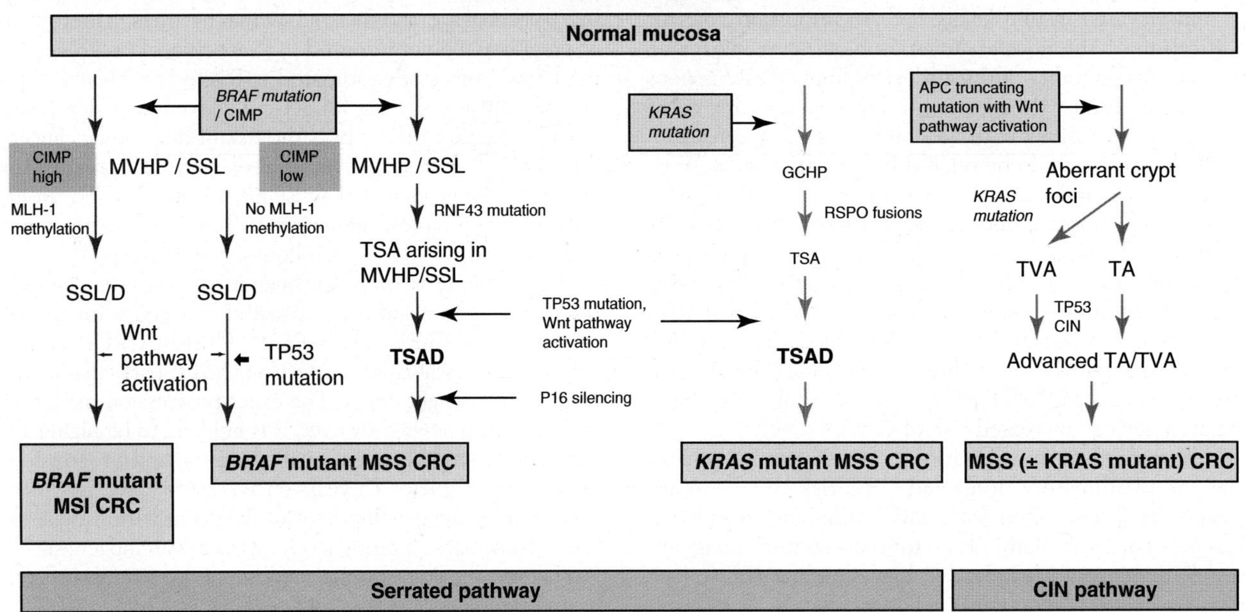

FIGURE 27.3 Molecular pathways to colorectal carcinoma. The pathway for Lynch syndrome–associated colorectal cancers is considered later.

this hypothesis. Hornick and colleagues reported that small carcinomas without a dysplastic component shared clinical and molecular characteristics with small carcinomas that contained a minimal dysplastic component, and with larger carcinomas.[62] It is also possible that some of these lesions represent rapid progression from a small adenoma to cancer because of the early acquisition of high-grade genetic alterations (e.g., aneuploidy, *TP53* mutations).[60]

Molecular Basis of Colorectal Cancer Progression

Human cancers are characterized by an accumulation of a variety of genetic alterations, including mutations that either activate oncogenes or inactivate tumor suppressor genes.[63-65] Accumulation of genetic alterations is critical in the progression from adenoma to carcinoma and likely begins in aberrant crypt foci and other precursor cells that may not manifest morphological features of a neoplasm.[66-68] To accumulate the array of genetic alterations typical of most CRCs, tumor cells must acquire mutations and epigenetic alterations at an increased rate compared with normal crypt epithelial cells.[69,70] Increased acquisition and tolerance of mutations is a hallmark of CRC development and is referred to as *genome instability*.[71,72] Genes involved in the maintenance of the genome have been likened to "caretakers" of the genome.[73] There are three main patterns of genome instability important to the development of colorectal neoplasia: chromosomal instability (CIN), DNA mismatch repair (MMR) defects that result in microsatellite instability (MSI), and CpG island methylator phenotype (CIMP).[73] Additional mechanisms of genome instability result from base excision repair defects and mutations in DNA polymerase proofreading function (POLE and POLD1).[74] Genome instability is in most cases the result of somatic mutations and is important to the two major morphological pathways to CRC evident to histopathologists, the conventional adenoma to carcinoma (CIN predominant) and the serrated pathway (CIMP, DNA MMR–deficiency predominant) (Fig. 27.3).

Chromosomal Instability

CIN is characterized by a persistently increased rate of gains and losses of chromosomal material; it is present in 85% of CRCs.[74-76] The acquisition of abnormalities involving whole chromosomes results in aneuploidy. In addition to whole-chromosome abnormalities, CRCs have other forms of somatic copy number alterations (SCNAs), including abnormalities of whole chromosomal arms as well as focal gains and losses. The underlying genetic basis of aneuploidy in human cancers is poorly understood, although most studies have focused on genes involved in regulation of mitotic spindle assembly and segregation. CIN is a major underlying genetic aberration in the conventional adenoma-carcinoma progression pathway and is, therefore, the predominant form of genomic instability in left-sided CRCs.[75,76]

DNA Mismatch Repair Defects

MSI is characterized by widespread alterations in the size of repetitive DNA sequences. It is present in approximately 15% of CRCs.[76,77] MSI is caused by defective DNA MMR (Fig. 27.4) (see Lynch Syndrome and Other Causes of Hereditary Nonpolyposis Colorectal Cancer). In addition to alterations in the size of repetitive DNA sequences, MSI results in a markedly increased rate of mutations of coding sequences (somatic hypermutation). In general, CRCs with MSI do not harbor abnormalities in chromosomal number or the focal regions of subchromosomal gains or losses that typify cancers with CIN. In most CRCs with MSI, the underlying defect in MMR function is caused by epigenetic CpG island hypermethylation–induced silencing of the *MLH1* gene. This is a characteristic feature of many CRCs that arise in the serrated neoplastic pathway, and most of these cancers are high-frequency CIMP (see later discussion).[41,49,77] MSI is also the mechanism that underlies the

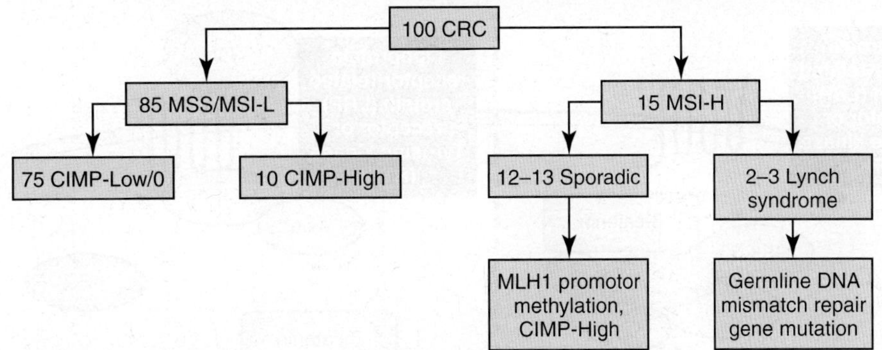

FIGURE 27.4 Breakdown of the molecular pathogenesis of an unselected population of colorectal cancers *(CRCs)*. The numbers are an approximation based on current knowledge. *CIMP,* CpG island methylator phenotype; *MSI-H,* high-frequency microsatellite instability; *MSI-L,* low-frequency microsatellite instability; *MSS,* microsatellite stable.

progression of Lynch syndrome cancers, which are caused by inherited defects in DNA MMR (see later discussion). In Lynch syndrome, MSI develops in conventional adenomas and drives rapid progression to cancer.

CpG Island Methylator Phenotype

CIMP is the acquisition of widespread methylation of CpG dinucleotides in the promoter regions of genes.[78,79] Referred to as an *epigenetic alteration* (because it does not change the DNA sequence), this is a major mechanism of inactivation of tumor suppressor genes such as *CDKN2A* (which codes for p16), *CDHI* (which codes for E-cadherin), and *MLH1*. Widespread CpG island methylation in a single cancer stands in stark contrast with the very limited methylation silencing that occurs in most CRCs and is known as *high-frequency CIMP* (CIMP-H).[79-81] CIMP-H is a characteristic feature of CRC that arises from SSLs and is present in 20% to 30% of CRCs, including almost all cancers that also have *MLH1* hypermethylation silencing. There is a marked difference in frequency depending on the site, with 30% to 40% of sporadic proximal-site colon cancers being CIMP-H (high) compared with 3% to 12% of distal colon and rectal cancers.[81] The underlying genetic basis of the CIMP-H phenotype is poorly understood, but there is evidence that genetic factors and environmental exposures (e.g., smoking, low folate diet, and estrogen withdrawal) may be associated with the development of carcinomas from SSLs.[81,82] A working hypothesis is evolving wherein genetic and epidemiological factors contribute to abnormal methylation events in SSLs of the right colon, which predisposes them to methylation induced silencing of *MLH1*, *MGMT,* and other important genes. This methylation in SSLs has been recently shown to increase progressively with age.[83] An interesting positive interplay appears to exist between *BRAF* mutation and progressive CpG island methylation driving evolution from normal mucosa to SSL to SSL with dysplasia (rarely TSA with dysplasia) and eventually to adenocarcinoma.[45,84,85] The subsequent carcinomas that develop are referred to as *serrated adenocarcinomas* by some authorities (see later discussion), and they are often found to have *BRAF* mutation and MSI-H or CIMP-H, or both, on molecular phenotyping.[41,49]

Implications of Progression Pathways for Screening and Prevention

Screening colonoscopy is more effective for the prevention of left-sided than right-sided CRC, and this difference is thought to be caused by the predominance of the conventional adenoma-carcinoma pathway in the left colon compared with the serrated pathway in the right colon.[50,86] The failure of screening to prevent right-sided colon cancer to the same degree as left-sided colon cancer appears to be related to the particular molecular characteristics of SSLs and difficulties in their endoscopic identification.[54] SSLs are more difficult to completely excise, which could directly lead to colonoscopic screening failures.[87] SSLs are also at greater risk of undergoing rapid progression in a relatively small lesion, secondary to the acquisition of DNA MMR deficiency and MSI.[41] Indeed, studies of interval cancers have found that they are much more likely to exhibit MSI and CIMP-H, both features of CRCs arising in the serrated pathway.[88,89]

Molecular Signaling Pathways Involved in Colorectal Cancer

The preceding text described the major mechanisms by which genomic instability develops in colorectal cancer cells. Molecular events at various points in this development of progressive genomic instability are associated with activation of various cell proliferation–associated signaling pathways. The signaling pathways provide a potential target for personalized therapy (see later discussion).

Wingless and Int-1 Signaling Pathway

The Wingless and Int-1 (Wnt) signaling pathway (also known as the *Wnt/β-catenin signaling pathway*) is an evolutionarily conserved signaling cascade that is critical to embryonic development and intestinal epithelial renewal.[90-93] Two main mechanisms of Wnt pathway activation are encountered in colorectal cancer. By far the most common is biallelic inactivation of the *APC* gene.[68] The *APC* gene was first identified as the gene mutated in most individuals with familial adenomatous polyposis.[94] In this syndrome, affected individuals inherit one mutant copy of *APC* that is functionally inactive. In tumorigenesis, the second allelic copy of the *APC* gene is also inactivated, which fulfills Knudson's paradigm for tumor suppressor gene inactivation. *APC* mutations are also present in 70% to 80% of sporadic CRCs, developing at an early stage during neoplastic development, and they are found in dysplastic aberrant crypt foci.[65,73,94] In normal cells, APC forms a complex with glycogen synthase kinase-3β (GSK3β) and Axin, which degrades β-catenin. *APC* mutations result in inability of the APC complex to

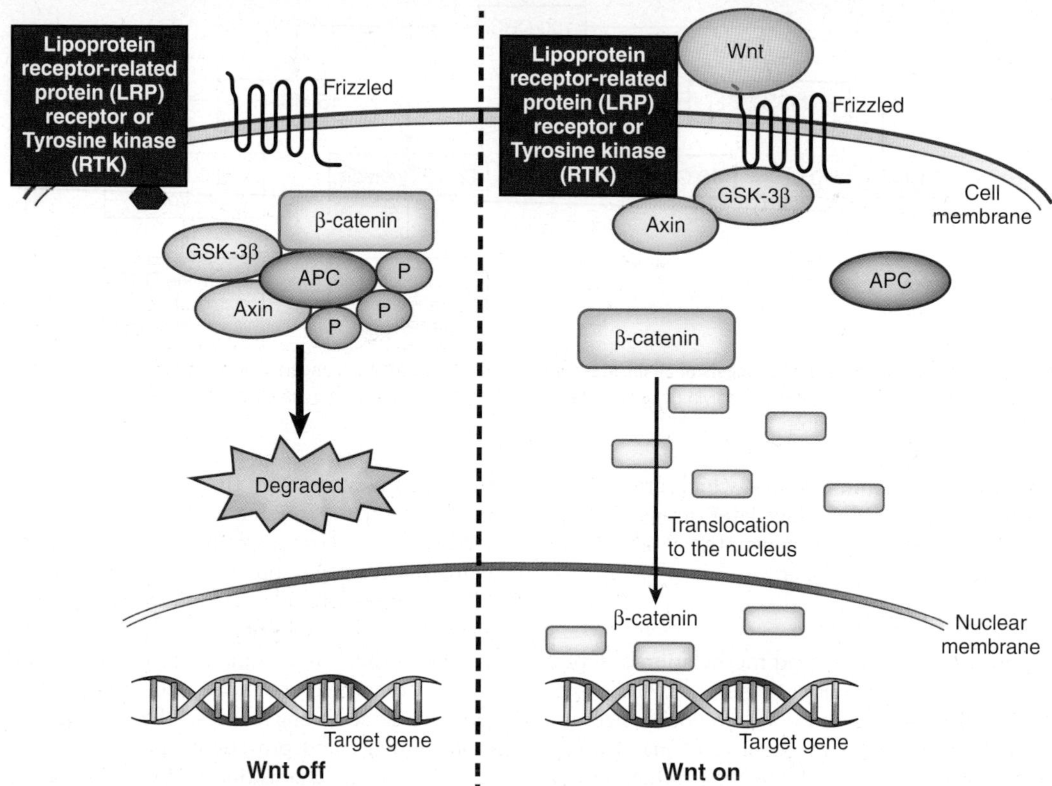

FIGURE 27.5 Canonical Wnt signaling pathway.

bind β-catenin, thereby releasing β-catenin and allowing it to accumulate in the nucleus, where it becomes involved in activating the transcription of a number of other downstream targets, such as cyclin D and Myc. The apparent necessity of *APC* inactivation for the development of early adenomas has resulted in its designation as a "gatekeeper" gene of colorectal neoplasia.[73]

The other main mechanism of Wnt pathway activation is gain-of-function mutations of the gene encoding β-catenin *(CTNNB1)*[68,95] In contrast with the inactivating *APC* mutations, *CTNNB1* mutations target amino acid residues integral to phosphorylation, resulting in persistent activation of Wnt signaling.[65] Finally, mutations have been rarely identified in other Wnt-signaling pathway genes which may result in Wnt pathway activation in CRCs with wild-type *APC*. These mutations involve genes encoding for AXIN1, AXIN2, and TCF4[65] (Fig. 27.5).

Mitogen-Activated Protein Kinase Pathway Activation

The mitogen-activated protein kinase (MAPK) pathway is the major mechanism by which extracellular proliferation factors (mitogens) promote cell growth and proliferation. This is accomplished by binding of the mitogen to a cell surface receptor (e.g., epidermal growth factor receptor [EGFR]), which triggers a phosphorylation cascade that incorporates the upstream transducer protein KRAS and downstream transducer proteins BRAF and ERK. ERK activation regulates nuclear targets such as cyclin D1 and CDK4[96,97] (Fig. 27.6). Mutations in components of the pathway are important to tumor growth, dissemination, and resistance to drug therapy in many human cancers.[96] *KRAS* mutation is present in 30% to 40% of CRCs, while *BRAF* mutation is identified in 10% to 20%.[85,96,98] Importantly, MAPK pathway activation is a critical feature of the serrated pathway to CRC.[41] *KRAS* mutation is also commonly found in the CIN pathway, where it occurs late in adenoma development and results in constitutive activation of the gene and hence the MAPK signaling pathway.[65]

Phosphatidylinositol 3-Kinase (PI3K)/Akt/mTOR Pathway

The PI3K/Akt/mTOR pathway (see Fig. 27.6) is an important pathway involved in cell proliferation, migration, and survival.[99] Constitutive activation of this signaling pathway leads to dysregulated cell proliferation. Somatic mutations in PI3K are identified in 10% to 33% of CRCs, more often in tumors arising in the right colon. There is evidence that these mutations may affect the responsiveness of metastatic CRC to anti-EGFR therapy.[98,100]

TP53

TP53 is important in the DNA damage response and in the cell cycle–arrest pathway, functioning as a tumor suppressor gene. Mutational silencing of TP53 is a common and key step in the genetic progression to CRC and occurs in 34% of right colon tumors and in 45% of left colon and rectal tumors.[98,101] Mutation in TP53 develops earlier in carcinogenesis and with much higher frequency (60% to 90%) in colitis-associated carcinomas.[1] Inactivation of TP53 is seen in both the CIN and serrated pathways, with the prevalence being higher in the former. In both pathways, *TP53* mutation appears to be an important event in the progression from an advanced adenoma to invasive carcinoma.[98] *TP53* mutations in CRC have been associated with increased propensity to vascular invasion, and CRCs with mutant *TP53*

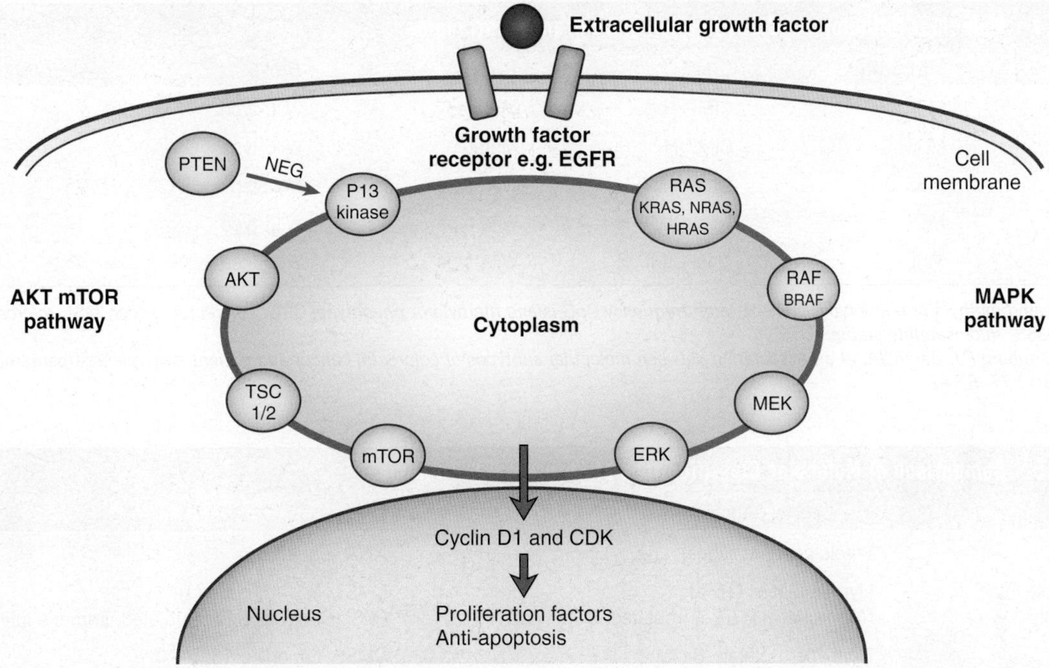

FIGURE 27.6 MAPK and PI3K/Akt/mTOR signaling pathways.

appear to be more chemoresistant and have poorer prognosis than those with wild-type *TP53*.[101]

Other Pathways

Approximately 3% to 7% of CRCs have an *HER2* somatic mutation or gene amplification.[68] This offers a potential target for personalized therapy. The family of transforming growth factor (TGF)-β cytokines represents at least 30 proteins that signal via serine/threonine kinase transmembrane receptors that activate the SMAD family of proteins to regulate proliferation, differentiation, adhesion, migration, and other functions.[102] Surface receptors include TGFBR2, TGFBR1, BMPR2, BMPR1A/1B, ACVR2A/2B, and ACVR1A/1B[102] (Fig. 27.7) Inactivation of the signaling pathway allows for unregulated proliferation. In the setting of colorectal carcinogenesis, this inactivation is important for the transition from low-grade dysplasia to high-grade dysplasia in an adenoma.[98] Common causes for inactivation include germline mutations in *SMAD4* and *BMPR1A* in the setting of juvenile polyposis, and somatic mutations in TGF-β receptor and SMAD family proteins.[98,102] Inactivating mutations in TGF-β receptors often occur in a background of MSI, and more than 50% of colon cancers with MSI contain mutations in *ACVR2A* and *TGFBR2*.[102]

Molecular Classification of Colorectal Cancer

A molecular-pathological classification of CRC has been proposed that is based on microsatellite status (MSI vs. microsatellite stable [MSS]), CIMP status (CIMP-H vs. non-CIMP-H), and the presence of a *BRAF* or *KRAS* mutation (Table 27.4).[100,103,104] This classification results in five subtypes of CRC that have shown to have different prognostic significance.[103] In addition, several of the subtypes have distinct morphology (e.g., MSI-high, see later discussion) and different therapeutic implications in the evolving era

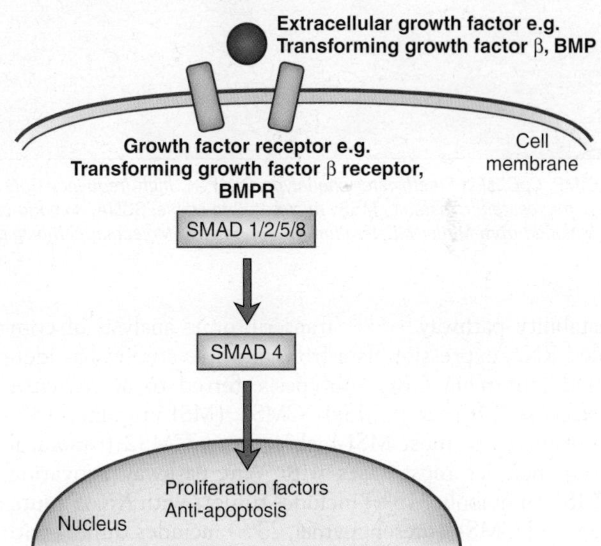

FIGURE 27.7 Transforming growth factor β family signaling pathway.

of personalized therapy (e.g., presence of a *KRAS* or *BRAF* mutation or MSI-high status).

More recently, pure molecular classifications have been developed based on whole-genome sequencing (The Cancer Genome Atlas [TCGA])[105] and RNA sequencing (transcriptomic profiling; the Colorectal Cancer Subtyping Consortium [CRCSC])[106] of a large number of CRCs (Table 27.5). The TCGA classification divides tumors into two broad categories: *hypermutated* or *ultramutated* (15%) and *non-hypermutated* (85%). The hypermutated subgroup shows mostly MSI. In 2% to 3% of cases, the degree of mutation is extreme and is the result of failure of the DNA polymerase proofreading proteins POLE or POLD1.[1,74,105,106] The non-hypermutated cases are MSS with low levels of mutations, and they correspond mostly to tumors of the chromosome

TABLE 27.4 Molecular Pathological Classification of Colorectal Carcinoma

Type	MSI Status	CIMP	*BRAF*	*KRAS*	% of CRCs*
1	MSI	CIMP-H	Mutated	Wild-type	7
2	MSS	CIMP-H	Mutated	Wild-type	4
3	MSS	Non–CIMP-H	Wild-type	Mutated	26
4	MSS	Non–CIMP-H	Wild-type	Wild-type	47
5	MSI	Non–CIMP-H	Wild-type	Wild-type	4

CIMP, *CpG island methylator phenotype;* CIMP-H, *high-frequency CpG island methylator phenotype;* CRC, *colorectal cancer;* MSI, *microsatellite instable;* MSS, *microsatellite stable.*
**Phipps AI, Limburg PJ, Baron JA, et al. Association between molecular subtypes of colorectal cancer and patient survival.* Gastroenterology. *2015;148(1):77–87.e2.*

TABLE 27.5 Comparison of Molecular Classifications of Colorectal Carcinoma

	The Cancer Genome Atlas	CMS
Method	Whole-genome sequencing	RNA sequencing
Subtypes/molecular abnormality	Hypermutated (16%) (MSI, CIMP-H, *BRAF*-mutated, SCNA low)	CMS1: MSI-immune (14%) (MSI, CIMP-H, *BRAF*-mutated, immune infiltration)
	Nonhypermutated (84%) (MSS, SCNA high, Wnt pathway activation)	CMS2: Canonical (37%) (MSS, SCNA high, Wnt pathway activation)
		CMS3: Metabolic (13%) (non–CIMP-H, *KRAS*-mutated, SCNA low, MSS)
		CMS4: Mesenchymal (23%) (MSS, SNCA high, epithelial-to-mesenchymal transition, stromal alteration)
		Mixed features (13%)

CIMP, *CpG island methylator phenotype;* CIMP-H, *high-frequency CpG island methylator phenotype;* CMS, *consensus molecular subtypes;* MSI, *microsatellite instable;* MSS, *microsatellite stable;* SCNA, *somatic copy number alteration.*
Modified from Muller MF, Ibrahim AE, Arends MJ. Molecular pathological classification of colorectal cancer. Virchows Arch. *2016;469(2):125-134.*

instability pathway.[1,74,105] Transcriptomic analysis of compiled RNA expression data from multiple studies has identified four main CRC subtypes referred to as *consensus molecular subtypes* (CMSs): CMS1 (MSI-immune, 14%) corresponds to most MSI-high cancers, CMS2 (canonical, 37%) includes most cases with Wnt pathway activation, CMS3 (metabolic, 13%) includes tumors with *KRAS* mutation, and CMS4 (mesenchymal, 23%) includes tumors with TGF-β pathway activation.[74,105] A further 13% of tumors show mixed RNA expression that does not clearly fit any of the preceding four subtypes. It is said that the CMS classification has the potential to provide for personalized medicine because it better reflects the innate biology of the tumor.[74] However, at present, the molecular classifications for CRC remain a research tool. It remains to be seen what role they will play, if any, in the diagnostic or therapeutic approach to CRC in clinical practice.

GROSS FEATURES AND SPECIMEN HANDLING

The principles for handling, evaluating, and processing CRC resection specimens for pathological examination have been well described and are an essential part of the College of American Pathologists' protocol.[107] The fundamental principles of gross examination are similar for both colonic and rectal resection specimens, but key differences should be observed when dealing with rectal specimens, particularly total mesorectal excision (TME).

With large resection specimens that include multiple subsegments of the colon or rectum, lymph nodes should be designated as either *regional* or *nonregional,* definitions of which are available in the eighth edition of the *AJCC Cancer Staging Manual* of the American Joint Committee on Cancer.[2] Metastases to nonregional lymph nodes are considered to be stage M1.[2]

For carcinomas of the colon, the distance of the tumor from the proximal and distal margins should be measured in the fresh state if possible. All colonic cancer resections have a radial resection margin; in areas of the colon not completely invested by peritoneum (i.e., some cecal tumors, all ascending and descending colon tumors), the radial resection margin is the posterior bare area, which should be inked and sampled for histological examination. In other segments of the colon (e.g., transverse and sigmoid colon), the radial margin is represented by the vascular ties on the so-called "mesocolic" or "mesenteric" margin. In addition to radial margins, it is imperative to assess whether there is tumor extending through the serosal surface. Suspicious areas of serosa are roughened, granular, or hypervascular; such areas should be thoroughly sampled for histological examination. The angle of reflection of the serosa from the mesentery onto the antimesenteric surface of the colon is particularly

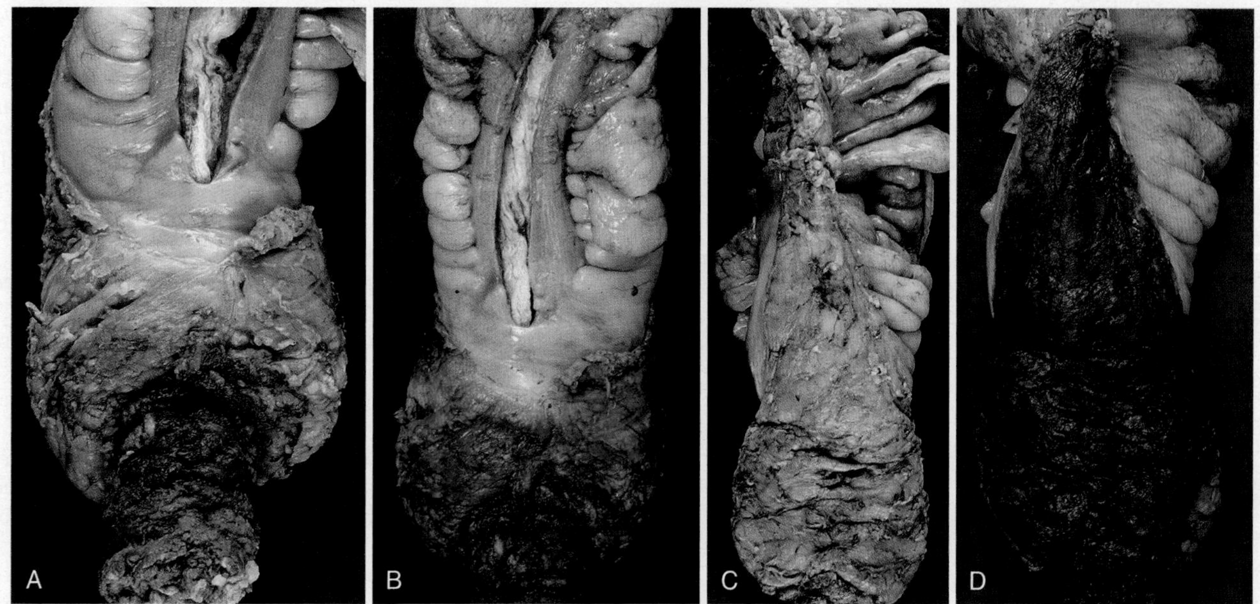

FIGURE 27.8 Example of a total mesorectal excision specimen. Anterior aspect before **(A)** and after **(B)** inking. Posterior aspect before **(C)** and after **(D)** inking.

TABLE 27.6 Parameters Used to Assess the Quality of Mesorectal Excision Surgery for Rectal Carcinoma

Grade	Mesorectal Surface and Bulk	Defects in Mesorectum	Coning	Radial Margin
Complete	Good bulk, smooth surface	No deeper than 5 mm	None	Smooth
Nearly complete	Moderate bulk, irregular surface	Deeper than 5 mm but no visible muscularis propria (except where levator muscles insert)	Moderate	Moderately irregular
Incomplete	Little bulk, irregular surface	Down to muscularis propria	Moderate to marked	Irregular

prone to serosal invasion by carcinoma. All lymph nodes must be found; this is best achieved by removing the fat close to the bowel wall and then using inspection, palpation, and fine slicing. It is important to examine the fat that remains adherent to the bowel wall because this is often a location for small, potentially positive nodes, especially in the immediate vicinity of the tumor (see Special Studies for a discussion of methods to enhance lymph node dissection).

Distinguishing colonic from rectal cancers can be problematic; tumors in the nonperitonealized portion of the left colon are considered rectal in origin, and all tumors located within 15 cm of the anal verge are also considered rectal. Tumors more proximally located for which the exact location is unclear are designated *rectosigmoid*. The point at which the peritoneum no longer surrounds the bowel completely is considered the true rectosigmoid junction; the teniae coli terminate at the junction with the rectum.

For carcinomas of the rectum excised via a TME procedure (Fig. 27.8), the quality and completeness of the mesorectal excision should be assessed before inking and sectioning and graded as either *complete*, *nearly complete*, or *incomplete* (Table 27.6).[108] Macroscopic photographs of the external aspect are useful as a permanent documentation of the appearance. This procedure is best done in the fresh state. The mesorectum is the fatty soft tissue envelope containing lymph nodes, blood vessels, and nerves that surrounds the rectum and is, in turn, surrounded by fascia. The quality of the mesorectal excision procedure and the distance of the tumor from the radial margin are related to the local recurrence rate and overall prognosis in rectal cancer patients, and the procedure for gross examination of these specimens is aimed at optimizing these assessments.[108-111] To assess the quality of the mesorectal surgery, four parameters are evaluated: the bulk of the mesorectum, the presence and depth of any defects in the mesorectum, the presence or absence of coning, and the appearance of the nonperitonealized margin. A complete TME is defined by the presence of an intact mesorectum with only minor irregularities of an otherwise smooth surface, no defects deeper than 5 mm, no coning (progressive narrowing of the mesorectum) toward the distal margin, and a smooth circumferential margin on transverse slicing. A nearly complete TME has moderate bulk to the mesorectum, some irregularity to the surface, and moderate coning, with some defects greater than 5 mm but no visible muscularis propria, except at the insertion of the levator muscles. An incomplete TME has only a little bulk to the mesorectum, defects that extend to the muscularis propria, a greater degree of coning, and an irregular circumferential margin.

The nonperitonealized (radial) margins lie distal to the peritoneal reflections (low on the anterior aspect but high on the posterior aspect), and it is good practice to report the distance of a rectal tumor to the peritoneal reflections. Some rectal tumors also have a serosal surface that requires careful assessment, as in colonic tumors. Tumors in the upper (proximal) rectum have a serosal covering anteriorly

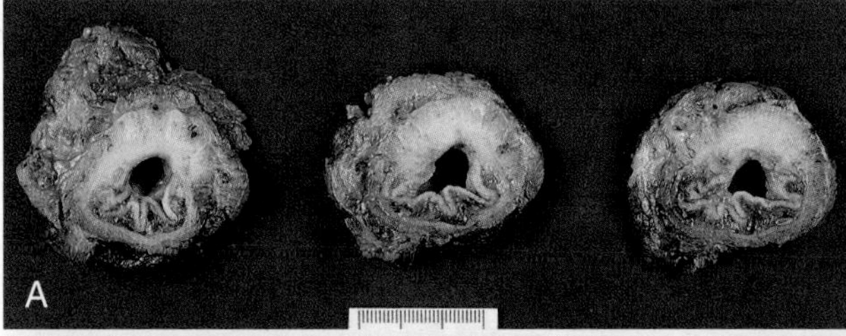

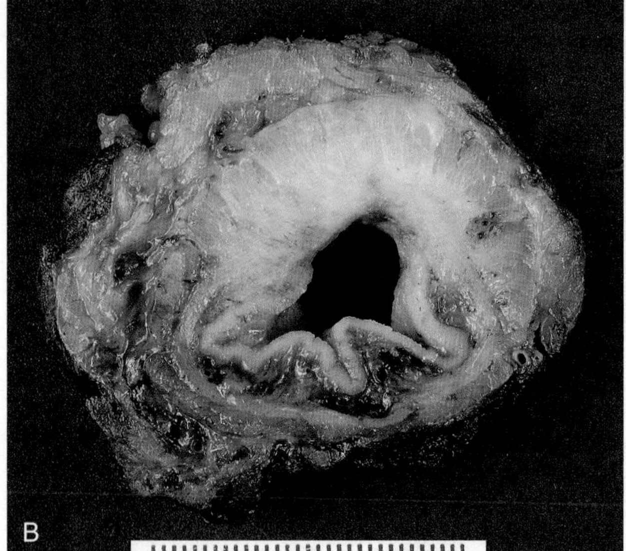

FIGURE 27.9 A, Cross sections of total mesorectal excision specimen. Tumor is visible extending through the muscularis propria and abutting the inked radial margin. **B,** Closer view of one cross-section.

and a radial margin posteriorly, whereas middle to low (distal) rectal tumors have a circumferential radial resection margin.

Ideally these specimens should not be opened through the tumor before fixation; rather, they should be left intact so that the specimen can be transversely sectioned when thoroughly fixed. This is done to optimize assessment of the distance of the tumor to the radial margin. The distance of tumor from the proximal and distal margins should be assessed in the fresh state if possible, and the specimen should be opened along the anterior aspect from proximal and distal, leaving the bowel intact in the immediate vicinity of the tumor. A loose gauze wick, soaked in formalin, is then placed into the unopened segment of bowel. Transverse section is best accomplished after the specimen has been fixed for at least 48 hours (preferably 72 to 96 hours) in an adequate volume of clean formalin. Once fixed, the unopened bowel is sliced at 3- to 5-mm intervals, and the slices are laid out and inspected for (1) appearance of the circumferential radial margin (i.e., smooth, regular, or irregular), (2) extent of tumor invasion, (3) closest distance of tumor to the circumferential radial margin, and (4) any obviously positive nodes and their distance from the circumferential radial margin (Fig. 27.9). Fat away from the tumor is also examined for lymph nodes, taking care not to double-count nodes that are present in multiple slices. At least 12 lymph nodes should be identified; however, all lymph nodes, regardless of how numerous, must be blocked. There are usually fewer lymph nodes in patients who have received neoadjuvant therapy. In one large study, patients who had undergone neoadjuvant therapy had a mean of 5 fewer nodes, and 63% of these patients had fewer than 12 nodes retrieved; the smaller number of nodes retrieved was not associated with poorer disease-specific survival.[112] In another study, mean lymph node harvest was 10.1 (range, 1 to 38). Only 28% had ≥12 lymph nodes, and 32% had <6 lymph nodes.[113] Techniques to facilitate lymph node sampling are discussed later. The concept of lymph node ratio (discussed later) may overcome the issue of low lymph node counts.[114]

The macroscopic appearance of CRCs can be categorized into four general types (Fig. 27.10):

1. **Bulky, exophytic, and polypoid tumors:** These are most common in the cecum, rarely result in obstruction, and often grow large before clinical presentation.
2. **Infiltrative and ulcerating tumors:** These cancers are raised, with irregular edges and a central, excavated ulcerated area that often extends to deep layers of the bowel wall.
3. **Annular and constricting tumors:** These tumors produce the characteristic "apple-core" lesion on barium studies.
4. **Diffuse tumors:** These are analogous to linitis plastica of the stomach and show diffuse flattening and thickening of the colon, initially involving the mucosa, but later involving the entire bowel wall.

There is much overlap among these four patterns of growth, and there is no evidence that gross configuration is a relevant prognostic indicator independent of the histological subtype of the tumor.[115] It is usually not possible to assess accurately the gross appearance of a rectal tumor, given that the specimens are sliced transversely. The importance of properly assessing the radial margin vastly outweighs the importance of determining the macroscopic tumor appearance. In all of these tumor types, the cut surface of the tumor is usually homogeneous in appearance but may show areas of necrosis. There may be dilation of the bowel proximal to the tumor (secondary to obstruction) and alteration of the serosal surface if the tumor extends close to the serosa.

Techniques to Facilitate Lymph Node Detection

Several techniques have been developed to increase the yield of lymph nodes found during tissue dissection. Essentially, these techniques serve two purposes, to make the lymph nodes more visible within the fat or to dissolve the fat around the nodes. Visualization methods are cheaper and simpler. One such technique is the use of GEWF solution, a mixture of glacial acetic acid, absolute ethanol, distilled water, and formaldehyde, all of which are found in most pathology laboratories. GEWF is a lymph node–highlighting solution resulting in lymph nodes becoming more readily identified as chalky-white nodules in fat after immersion in the solution for at least 24 hours. Studies that have evaluated the use of GEWF in CRC specimens have shown mixed results, with some demonstrating increased lymph node yields[116,117] and others showing no benefit related to this technique.[118,119] Another visualization method involves injection of methylene blue into the arterial supply of the fresh specimen before fixation. After fixation, the lymph nodes are highlighted by the blue dye. Again, the literature is divided as to whether there is any benefit in lymph node

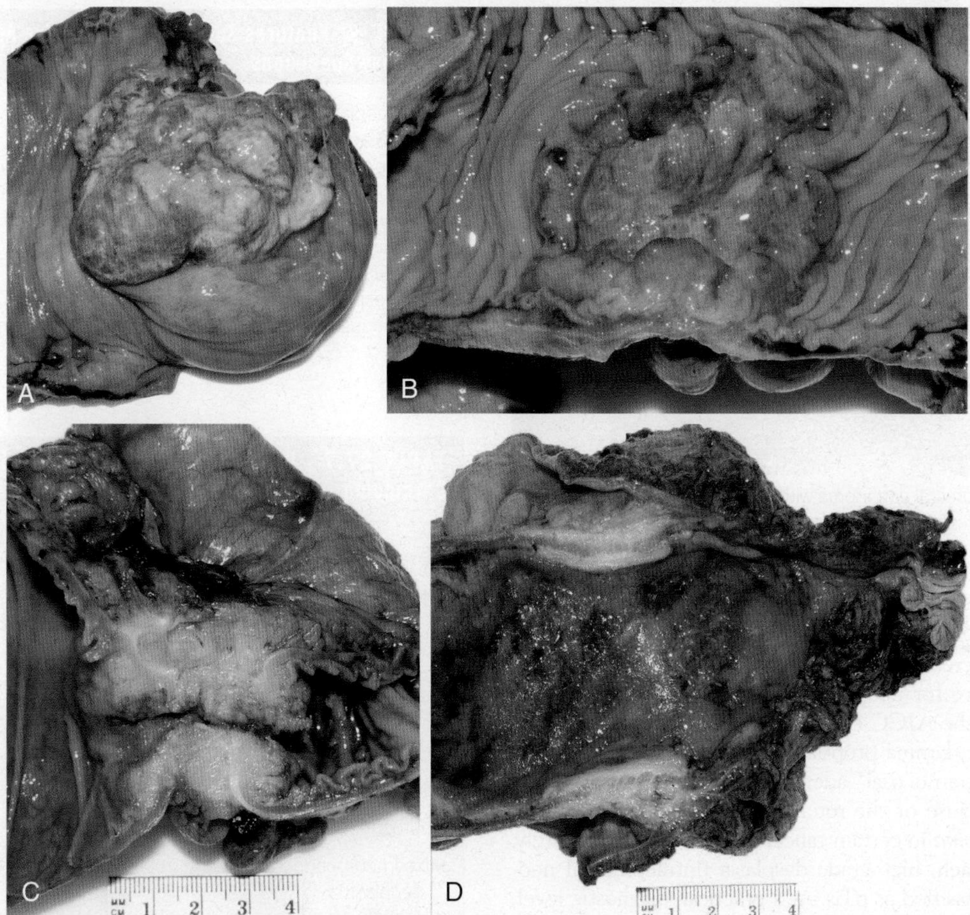

FIGURE 27.10 Colorectal carcinoma. A, Polypoid type. **B,** Infiltrative and ulcerating type. **C,** Annular and constricting type. **D,** Diffuse type.

procurement via this procedure,[120-122] and the dye may create unwanted staining should it inadvertently escape from the vessels on injection.

Fat-clearing techniques involve immersion of the specimen in graded alcohol solutions, followed by xylene to dissolve the fat. Although such methods do increase the yield of lymph nodes,[123] they are time-consuming and expensive (as a result of reagent costs), and there is also the potential of exposure to noxious solvents.

Sentinel Lymph Nodes

The development of distant metastases in 20% to 30% of patients who have a primary tumor confined to the bowel wall is often cited as evidence of undetected metastasis at the time of surgical resection and pathological evaluation. Meticulous pathological evaluation of sentinel lymph nodes (lymph nodes that have the most direct drainage from the tumor) has been investigated in numerous studies. At least three procedures have been used to identify the sentinel node in patients with CRC: injection of methylene blue dye, intraoperative near-infrared fluorescence (NIR) imaging with indocyanine green (ICG), or injection of radiotracer material near the primary tumor.[124,125] The first one to four lymph nodes that change color or exhibit the highest radiation emission are considered the sentinel lymph nodes. Techniques used to evaluate sentinel lymph nodes include intraoperative frozen section, or thin slicing, submission in total, multiple tissue levels, and immunohistochemical analysis of paraffin-embedded material. Unlike the more common situation with breast carcinoma and melanoma in which knowledge of the sentinel node status aims to reduce the extent of surgery, sentinel node status in colorectal cancer is used only to direct more extensive resection. There are some data to suggest sentinel node sampling could also guide a decision toward formal resection in T1 colorectal cancers, which typically have a low likelihood of lymph node metastases; however, at present the data are inconclusive on the benefit of this procedure in early invasive tumors. [126] A meta-analysis of the sentinel lymph node procedure for CRC showed a low sensitivity for sentinel lymph node detection, regardless of T stage, localization, or pathological technique used.[127] Hence, many questions remain regarding the practical utility of the sentinel lymph node biopsy procedure in the management of CRC, and as a result, it remains infrequently performed.

PATHOLOGICAL FEATURES

Criteria for Malignancy and Biopsy Diagnosis

Tumors in which there is invasion confined to the lamina propria and muscularis mucosae (termed *intramucosal adenocarcinoma*) are almost never associated with lymph node metastases. This observation is usually attributed to the paucity of lymphatics in the colorectal mucosa. Therefore colorectal tumors are considered to be "malignant" only if they have invaded through the muscularis mucosae into the submucosa (stage pT1).[2] Although this may be sensible for the management

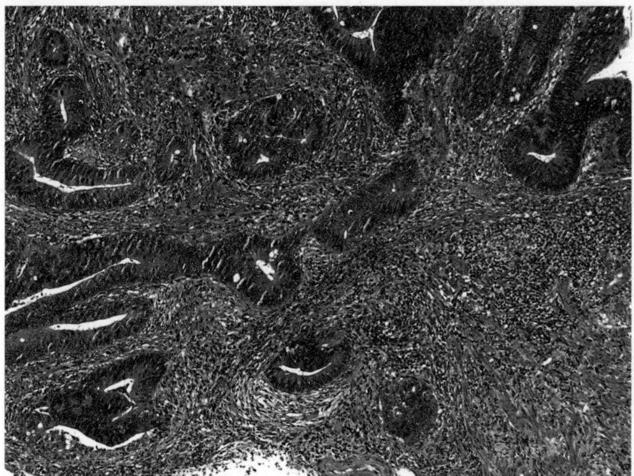

FIGURE 27.11 Colorectal carcinoma with features of early invasion. The tumor cells dissect and disrupt the muscularis mucosae. Sharp angulation is visible in some glands. A desmoplastic stroma is evident around the glands.

of CRC, it has created some controversy about the appropriate nomenclature for neoplasms that do not invade into the submucosa. In the AJCC classification,[2] invasion confined to the mucosa (i.e., lamina propria invasion without submucosal invasion, or "intramucosal" adenocarcinoma) is still classified as stage Tis because of the retention of the term *intramucosal adenocarcinoma* in certain cancer registries. Unfortunately, with this approach, high-grade dysplasia (intraepithelial neoplasia) is also classified as pTis. At a practical, diagnostic level, because of the lack of malignant potential of lamina propria invasion, use of the diagnostic term *intramucosal carcinoma* is not recommended, and the term *carcinoma* should be used only in the context of *invasive adenocarcinoma,* which refers to tumors that have infiltrated into or beyond the submucosa.

Biopsy specimens of sessile or flat lesions are usually superficial, are often poorly oriented, and may be ulcerated. The most important aspect of pathological examination is to determine whether invasion is present. Although the presence of single infiltrating cells or small, markedly irregular glands readily establishes a diagnosis of "invasion," some better-differentiated cancers may not show this pattern of growth. In the absence of definitive pathological features of invasion, a diagnosis of invasion relies heavily on identification of desmoplasia, which is usually present with invasive adenocarcinoma and almost never present in intramucosal cancers. However, differentiation between malignancy-associated desmoplasia and the stromal reaction in an ulcerated adenoma can be difficult. The stroma of an ulcerated adenoma is often more cellular, with more abundant microvasculature, inflammatory cells, and plump fibroblasts. If the muscularis mucosae can be identified, it is helpful to note whether invasion penetrates this layer, but in many biopsy fragments, the muscularis mucosae is difficult to identify clearly. Furthermore, the suspicious tissue may be too small, or the orientation of the suspicious area too inadequate to allow certainty that invasion beyond the mucosa exists. In these cases, the presence of desmoplasia is a helpful indicator that the tumor has penetrated into the submucosa, in which case the carcinoma is at least pT1 (Fig. 27.11). Desmoplasia is rarely, if ever, associated with lamina propria invasion alone. Box 27.2 provides a list of additional features that are suggestive of invasive adenocarcinoma.

BOX 27.2 Features Suggestive of Invasive Adenocarcinoma in Biopsy Specimens

- Desmoplastic stromal reaction
- Irregular gland outlines
- Sharp angulations that appear to dissect through the stroma
- Neoplastic glands situated within fragments of muscularis
- Neoplastic glands adjacent to vessels with a well-developed media layer
- Single neoplastic cells or tumor buds
- Necrosis within glands
- Mucinous morphology with tumor cells floating in mucin pools

TABLE 27.7 Histological Classification of Colorectal Carcinoma

Histological Type	Approximate Frequency (%)
Adenocarcinoma NOS	75-80
Mucinous adenocarcinoma	10
Serrated adenocarcinoma	10
Medullary carcinoma	2-4
Signet ring cell carcinoma	1
Adenoma-like adenocarcinoma	1
Neuroendocrine carcinoma	1
Mixed neuroendocrine–nonneuroendocrine neoplasm	<1.0
Micropapillary carcinoma	<1.0*
Adenosquamous carcinoma	<1.0
Squamous cell carcinoma	<0.1
Other	
Choriocarcinoma	<0.1
Clear cell carcinoma	<0.1
Microglandular goblet cell carcinoma	<0.1
Carcinomas with melanin production	<0.1
Carcinoma with sarcomatoid components	<0.1
Carcinoma with rhabdoid features	<0.1

NOS, *Not otherwise specified.*
**As a pure pattern.*

If one or more of these features is present in an equivocal case, the pathology report should convey that the appearance is suspicious for invasive adenocarcinoma. For those cancers that arise within a polyp, the requirement for surgical resection as opposed to polypectomy is determined on the basis of completeness of excision and the presence of high-risk factors for lymph node metastases (see later).

CLASSIFICATION OF HISTOLOGICAL SUBTYPES

Most CRCs are adenocarcinomas; by definition, they are considered to be of "usual" morphology and are thus designated as *adenocarcinoma, not otherwise specified (NOS)* (Table 27.7). Histological variations may result from the

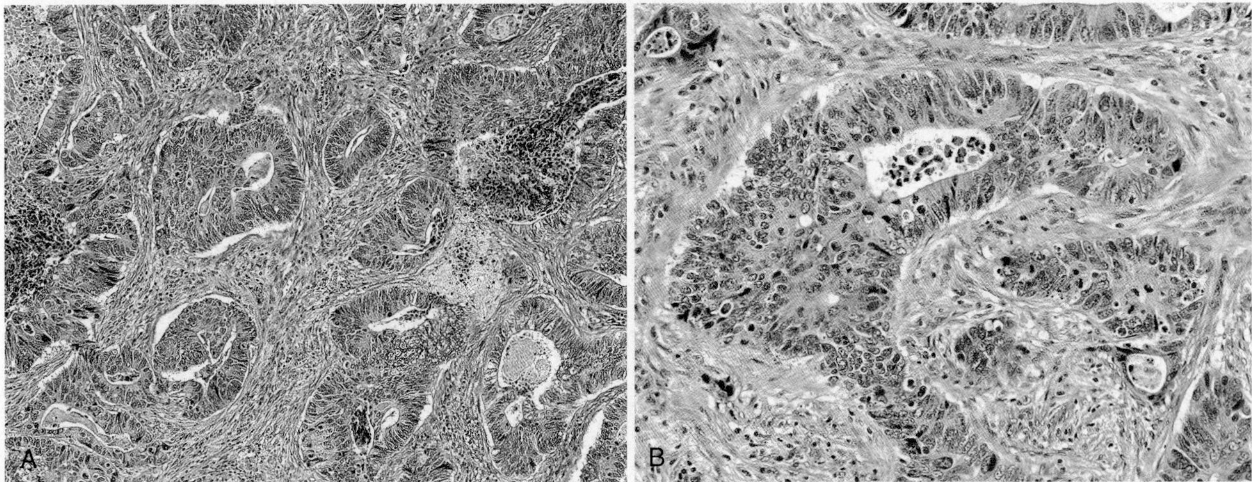

FIGURE 27.12 **A** and **B**, Typical colorectal adenocarcinoma showing irregular glands, some with luminal debris infiltrating a desmoplastic stroma.

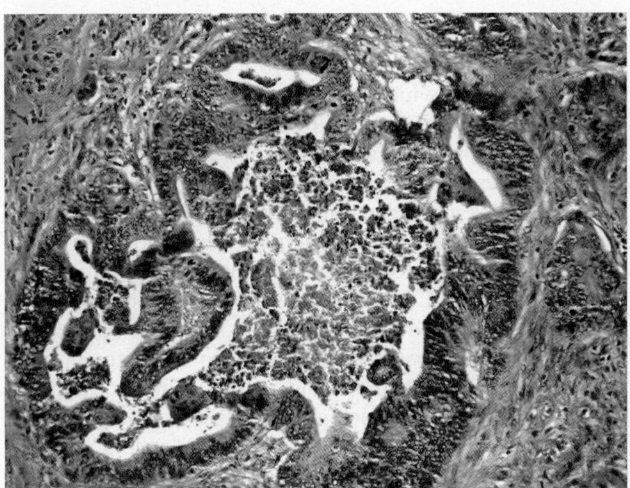

FIGURE 27.13 Typical colorectal adenocarcinoma. There is a proliferation of complex glandular structures, with infolding and bridging of the epithelium. The cells have cylindrical to ovoid nuclei. The lumen contains abundant eosinophilic material and nuclear debris ("dirty" necrosis). This pattern of necrosis is characteristic of colorectal adenocarcinoma.

presence of small components of other histological patterns in an otherwise typical adenocarcinoma. The criteria used to define the various subtypes of colon cancer, such as *mucinous* adenocarcinoma, are described in the following sections. For colon cancer cases in which a second subtype is present but the proportion is not sufficient to meet the specific diagnostic criteria, it is recommended that the presence and percentage of all histological components be commented on in the pathology report (e.g., "moderately differentiated adenocarcinoma with 10% extracellular mucinous component").

Adenocarcinoma, NOS

Most of these adenocarcinomas are moderately to well differentiated (low grade). Typically, there are medium- to large-sized glands, with moderate variability in gland size and configuration and a moderate amount of stroma (Fig. 27.12). In well-differentiated tumors, the epithelial cells are usually tall and columnar and become increasingly cuboidal or polygonal, with decreasing degrees of differentiation. Mitotic figures and apoptosis are usually abundant. Glandular lumina are usually filled with inspissated eosinophilic material as well as nuclear and cellular debris, so-called "dirty necrosis" (Fig. 27.13). When dirty necrosis is present in a metastasis of unknown primary origin, this feature is frequently used to infer a colorectal primary tumor. In general, there tends to be little difference between the superficial and deeper portions of the tumor, although the leading edge is often associated with gland rupture and more frequent foci of small, irregular, and infiltrative-appearing glands. Some tumors have a prominent papillary component, particularly at the surface. Desmoplasia can be prominent, as in cancers of the pancreas and biliary tract. In some instances, the stromal reaction is more collagenous and may show keloidal areas. The nature of the stromal reaction may be of prognostic significance, with myxoid desmoplastic stroma being associated with poorer survival than a collagen-rich stroma.[128,129] In addition to glandular cells, a variable number of Paneth cells, neuroendocrine cells, squamous cells, melanocytes, and trophoblasts can be found in adenocarcinoma NOS.[130-134] Typically, the presence of these other cell types has no prognostic significance. Osseous metaplasia may also be present, possibly related to expression of bone morphogenetic protein by the carcinoma cells.[135]

Mucinous Adenocarcinoma

The World Health Organization (WHO) defines mucinous tumors by the amount of extracellular mucin (i.e., arbitrarily defined as tumor composed of >50% mucin).[1] The terms *adenocarcinoma with mucinous features* or *adenocarcinoma with mucinous differentiation* are often used to describe tumors that have a significant mucinous component (>10% but <50%). Most mucinous adenocarcinomas contain free-floating strips of neoplastic epithelium, or individual tumor cells, in the mucin (Fig. 27.14). A variable number of signet ring cells also may be seen (Fig. 27.15). If more than 50% of the tumor cells have a signet ring cell morphology, the

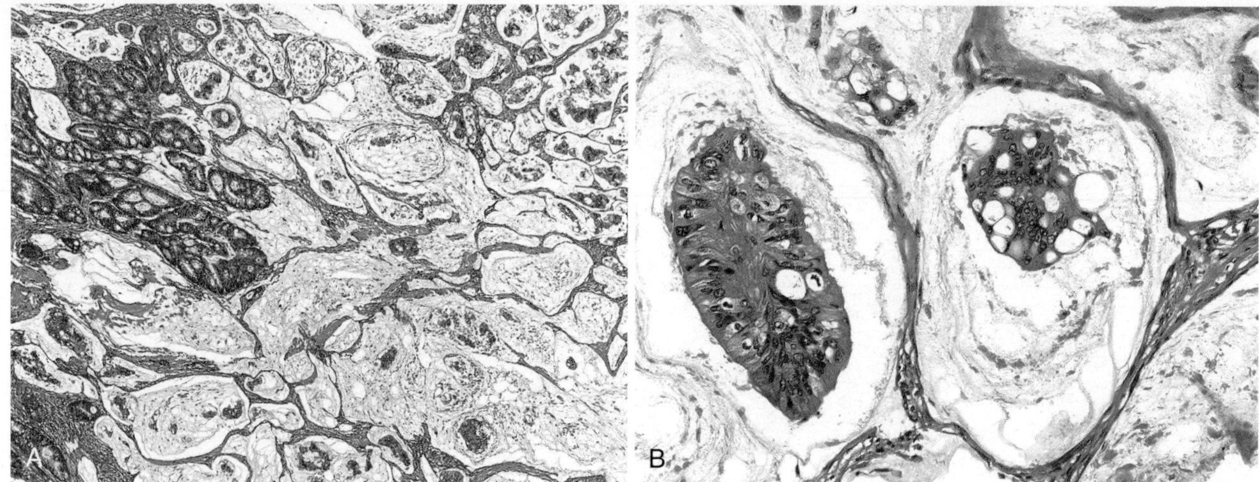

FIGURE 27.14 Mucinous adenocarcinoma. A, The tumor consists of pools of mucin and tumor cells with a cribriform growth pattern. **B,** Most of the mucin pools contain islands of free-floating tumor cells.

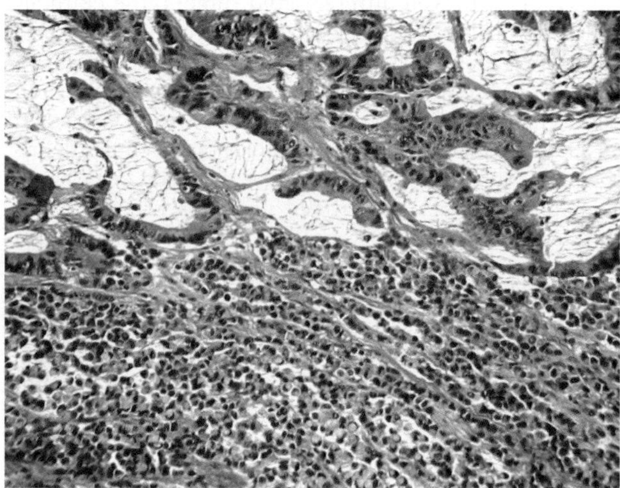

FIGURE 27.15 Mucinous adenocarcinoma with signet ring cell features. This tumor contains a mixture of "mucinous" and signet ring cell carcinoma. Because the signet ring cell areas constitute less than 50% of the tumor volume, this is best classified as a *mucinous adenocarcinoma.* The presence of signet ring cells in mucinous carcinomas is quite common.

tumor is best classified as a *signet ring cell carcinoma,* even if more than 50% of the tumor is composed of extracellular mucin.

Mucinous adenocarcinomas represent approximately 10% of all CRCs.[136] They are more common in patients with Lynch syndrome and with IBD, but are less common in Asian populations.[137] Mucinous adenocarcinoma is more likely to be diagnosed at an advanced stage.[138] The type of genetic alterations identified in these tumors suggests that the molecular pathogenesis is different from that of adenocarcinoma NOS. Higher rates of mutation are found in genes of the MAPK and PI3K/Akt/mTOR pathways. Mucinous colorectal adenocarcinoma is also more likely to demonstrate CIMP-H and to have higher rates of MSI.[138,139] MSI-H mucinous tumors are found more often in younger individuals and are more likely to be exophytic and have an expanding growth pattern compared with non–MSI-H mucinous cancers.[140] Immunohistochemical staining for *TP53* is less frequently positive (30% vs. >50% in adenocarcinoma NOS), which suggests that mucinous carcinomas are less likely to have a stabilizing point mutation in *TP53*. Expression of HATH1, a transcription factor that activates MUC2 expression in intestinal epithelium, is maintained in both mucinous and signet ring cell carcinomas, but is suppressed in nonmucinous carcinomas, which indicates a possible biological basis for mucinous neoplasms.[141] Expression of MUC2 and MUC5AC mucin proteins are both increased; however, there is reduced expression of MUC1 (EMA).[142]

Mucinous adenocarcinoma makes up a greater proportion of right colon tumors and is also more common in females.[143] The cut surface is typically soft and gelatinous with little fibrous tissue, which imparts a "colloid" appearance to the tumor. The tumor is often composed of small nodules of mucin.

On microscopic examination, mucinous adenocarcinomas contain glandular structures or individual tumor cells embedded in pools of mucin; the mucin can be highlighted if necessary, with periodic acid–Schiff or Alcian blue stains. The margins of the tumor can be smooth and expansile or dissecting and infiltrative. In one series of 132 mucinous carcinomas, adjacent precursor adenomas were identified in 31%, a figure similar to that found in adenocarcinoma NOS.[144]

The association between mucinous subtype and survival has been controversial historically. Compared with adenocarcinoma NOS, mucinous adenocarcinoma typically presents at a higher stage at the time of diagnosis,[136,138] is more likely to have peritoneal implants[145,146] and invade adjacent viscera,[147] and is less likely to be cured by surgical resection.[145] Mucinous adenocarcinoma is also more likely to show lymph node involvement beyond the pericolonic region.[147] Two recent meta-analyses of the prognostic significance of mucinous adenocarcinoma concluded that when adjusted for stage, mucinous carcinomas do not manifest an overall poorer prognosis than usual-type adenocarcinoma.[143,148] Furthermore, it does not appear that MSI-H status in mucinous adenocarcinoma is of any prognostic value versus MSI-L or MSS status.[149] Hence, the latest WHO guidelines recommend grading mucinous

BOX 27.3 Mucinous Adenocarcinoma: Key Features

- Greater than 50% extracellular mucin
- Graded on the degree of gland formation
- More likely MSI, *BRAF* mutation or *KRAS* mutation
- More likely to present at a higher stage at diagnosis
- Prognosis similar to adenocarcinoma NOS of the same stage

adenocarcinoma on the degree of glandular differentiation without regard for MSI status.[1] However, there is some evidence that mucinous adenocarcinoma occurring in patients younger than 40 years of age or those developing in the rectum do represent a poorer prognostic group when compared with usual-type CRCs.[150,151] The adverse outcome of rectal location appears to relate to the poorer response of rectal mucinous carcinomas to neoadjuvant therapies, such as chemoradiotherapy, and to the high rates of incomplete resection that have been reported.[142,152] At present, mucinous differentiation is not viewed as a factor in treatment decisions for colorectal cancer.[153] Immunotherapy and therapies directed against increased MUC2 protein expression hold promise for future treatment of this CRC subtype (Box 27.3).[142]

Signet Ring Cell Carcinoma

Signet ring cell carcinoma (SRCC) is defined as a tumor that is composed of at least 50% signet ring cells.[1] For classification purposes, this feature supersedes the presence and amount of extracellular mucin. These tumors represent approximately 0.5% to 1.0% of all CRCs.[154-156] They are slightly more common in men (male-to-female ratio, 1.3:1) and occur at a younger age (mean 63.5 years) than adenocarcinoma NOS.[156] In some studies, more than 50% of signet ring cell adenocarcinomas were detected in individuals younger than 40 years of age.[157] SRCC is also more common in ulcerative colitis, with up to one-third of all signet ring cell carcinomas occurring in patients who have this form of IBD.[158-161] There is also a strong association with Lynch syndrome and more broadly with MSI.[162,163] They frequently exhibit CIMP-H (48%), and *BRAF* mutations are identified in 30% to 33% of cases.[164,165]

Although some reports suggest right-sided predominance, the overall literature is not consistent as to the site of predilection.[154,156,166] Synchronous tumors are found in 14% of patients.[154] SRCCs are usually ulcerating, and approximately two-thirds have an infiltrative gross appearance.[154,156] A linitis plastica growth pattern occurs in up to 20% of cases.[156]

Histologically, tumor cells show a characteristic mucin vacuole that pushes the nucleus to the periphery of the cell (Fig. 27.16). A subset of signet ring cells are round and contain centrally located nuclei without an apparent mucin vacuole. Compared with gastric signet ring cell carcinomas, those in the colorectum are more likely to be associated with abundant extracellular mucin and less commonly result in diffuse infiltration of the tissues. It can be difficult to differentiate colorectal signet ring cell carcinoma from metastatic gastric signet ring carcinoma on morphological grounds, and immunohistochemistry is not helpful because tumors from

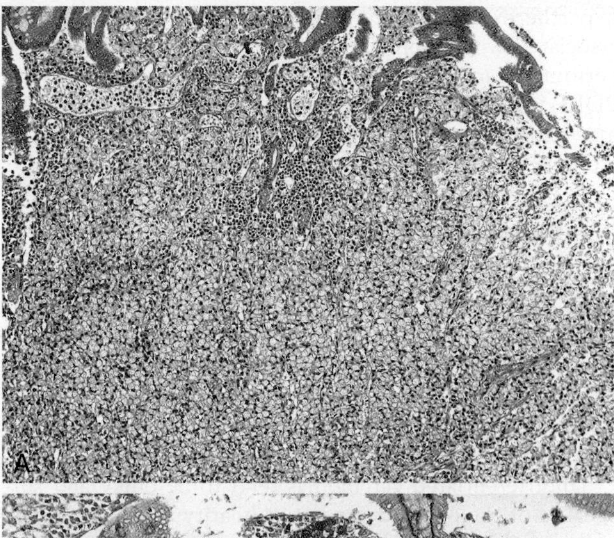

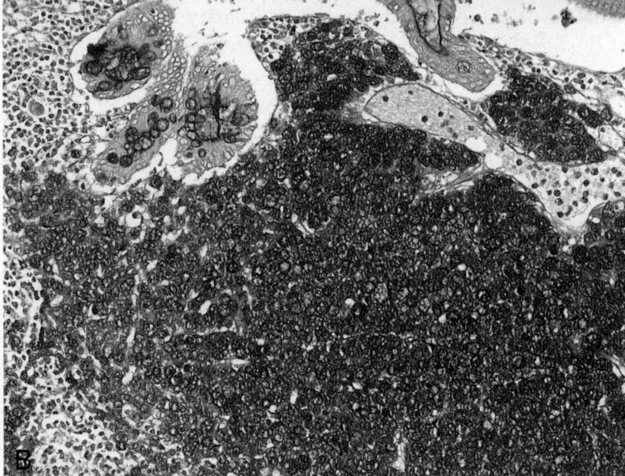

FIGURE 27.16 Signet ring cell carcinoma. A, Sheets of signet ring cells are shown. **B,** Signet ring cells infiltrating through the mucosa and submucosa are highlighted by periodic acid–Schiff stain with diastase digestion.

both sites usually are negative for MUC1 and thyroid transcription factor 1 (TTF1) and positive for MUC2.[167] CDX2 may not be expressed as well. However, the tumor cells are usually reactive for SATB2.[168] In common with most gastric signet ring cell carcinomas, there is loss of E-cadherin expression in most cases.[169]

Similar to mucinous adenocarcinomas, signet ring cell carcinomas are more likely to be diagnosed at an advanced stage.[151,170] Stage III or IV disease is found at the time of diagnosis in approximately 80% of patients.[151,171] Full-thickness penetration of the muscularis propria, vascular invasion, perineural invasion, and peritoneal seeding are more common than in adenocarcinoma NOS.[154-156,162] Some studies have reported distant metastases, often in atypical sites, in as many as 60% of patients at the time of diagnosis.[136,146,172] As a result, surgical resection is less likely to be curative.[157] SRCCs that are MSI-L/MSS are particularly aggressive,[162,173] with 5-year survival rates less than 10% reported.[155,156] Mucin-rich cases may have a more favorable prognosis than mucin-poor cases. [162] Peritoneal carcinomatosis is present in virtually all patients who die of their disease, although liver metastases are present in less than 50% of cases.[154] Cytoreductive surgery with hyperthermic intraperitoneal chemotherapy (HIPEC) is not associated with improvement in prognosis in patients with peritoneal carcinomatosis.[174] The frequent association with PDL1 positivity raises the prospect that immunotherapy may become more important in the treatment of this subgroup in the near future (Box 27.4).[165]

Undifferentiated Carcinoma

The term *undifferentiated carcinoma* is, essentially, restricted to cancers that contain evidence of epithelial differentiation but no obvious gland formation, although most undifferentiated tumors probably represent extremely poorly differentiated adenocarcinoma NOS. For instance, some authors accept this designation for tumors with a very small component (<5%) of gland formation.[1]

Undifferentiated carcinomas tend to be bulky and soft because of their high degree of cellularity and relative lack of desmoplasia, and there is often extensive necrosis. There are typically sheets of cells, cords, or trabecular structures, frequently with an infiltrative growth pattern (Fig. 27.17). The degree of pleomorphism is variable; some tumors show relatively uniform cytological features, whereas others show marked nuclear variability. The distinction between undifferentiated carcinoma and medullary carcinoma can be problematic. Differences from medullary carcinoma include the presence of a more infiltrative border, absence of a syncytial growth pattern, and absence of a heavy lymphocytic infiltrate within undifferentiated carcinomas.[1]

Although pure undifferentiated carcinomas are rare, many adenocarcinomas NOS contain an undifferentiated component (Box 27.5). These tumors are best classified as *adenocarcinoma* but would be considered high-grade in the WHO grading system based on the undifferentiated component. The presence of any undifferentiated component increases the probability that the tumor contains a DNA MMR deficiency, particularly if it is associated with tumor-infiltrating lymphocytes (see Carcinomas with DNA Mismatch Repair Deficiency).

BOX 27.4 Signet Ring Cell Carcinoma: Key Features

- Greater than 50% tumor cells with signet ring morphology
- High grade by definition
- Often associated with extracellular mucin
- More likely MSI and *BRAF* mutation
- Usually present at a high tumor stage, peritoneal carcinomatosis is common
- Poor prognosis

Medullary Adenocarcinoma

This tumor is more often and simply called *medullary carcinoma*, and the WHO classification uses both terms. There is wide variation in the incidence of medullary carcinoma in the literature, which is a reflection of the different diagnostic thresholds used by the reporting pathologists.[175] Overall, between 2% and 4% of CRCs are considered to be the medullary type.[1,176] These tumors are more common in women and typically occur in the cecum or proximal colon.[176,177] Medullary carcinoma has also been referred to as *large cell minimally differentiated carcinoma.*[178]

Most medullary carcinomas are associated with a characteristic genomic profile. These tumors are less likely than usual CRCs to show *KRAS* and *TP53* mutations, and they are more likely to harbor defects in DNA MMR and have *BRAF* mutation[176,178] (see Carcinomas with DNA Mismatch Repair Deficiency). Even when it is present as a small subcomponent of the tumor, a medullary pattern is often predictive of an underlying DNA MMR deficiency.[179] Some authors consider demonstration of MSI to be a requirement for the diagnosis of medullary carcinoma[180]; however, this is not an absolute requirement in the fifth edition WHO classification.[1] Medullary carcinomas are overrepresented in patients with Lynch syndrome.[181]

Macroscopically, medullary carcinomas often present as large, bulky tumors.[181] Histologically, they are characterized by sheets of polygonal-shaped cells with vesicular nuclei, prominent nucleoli, and abundant cytoplasm, and they are associated with numerous tumor-infiltrating lymphocytes[138,182] (Fig. 27.18). Tumor cells may have an organoid or a trabecular architecture, and focal mucin production may also be present. An important diagnostic feature is

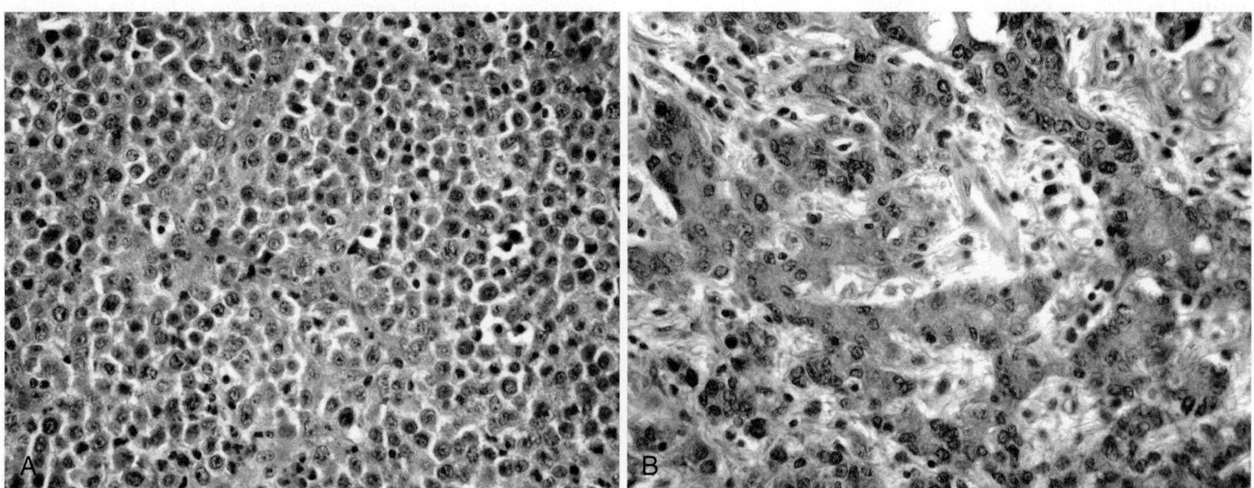

FIGURE 27.17 Undifferentiated carcinoma. A, Sheets of tumor cells without gland formation are shown. The cells were positive for cytokeratin 20 and negative for neuroendocrine markers. **B,** This area illustrates a trabecular growth pattern with possible gland formation focally.

the presence of a pushing border rather than an infiltrative margin, where the latter is better designated as an undifferentiated carcinoma. Immunophenotypically, these tumors are frequently CK20–, are occasionally CK7+, and often show reduced CDX2 expression.[178,183] Differentiation from other nonglandular carcinomas is important because medullary carcinomas have a more favorable outcome.[176] Use of immunohistochemistry for calretinin may be helpful in this regard; in one study, calretinin was positive in 73% of medullary carcinomas but in only 12% of poorly differentiated adenocarcinomas.[183] Also, SATB2 expression is usually retained.[184] Neuroendocrine stains are typically negative.[183,185] PD-L1 expression is more frequent in medullary carcinomas, particularly in tumors that reveal MSI.[186]

Overall, medullary carcinoma has a more favorable prognosis than adenocarcinoma NOS,[176] even though it is more likely to be diagnosed at a higher T stage and have a higher frequency of vascular invasion (Box 27.6).[181]

Serrated Adenocarcinoma

The term *serrated adenocarcinoma* has been used in two main settings: in the first setting, it is used to describe CRCs that arise from serrated precursor lesions, including both SSLs and TSAs; in the second, it is used to describe CRCs that have a distinctive serrated morphology.[104] Consistent with their origin in the serrated pathway, serrated adenocarcinomas are more often proximal than adenocarcinomas NOS in location. Using these definitions, up to 12% of all colorectal adenocarcinomas and up to 17% of all proximal adenocarcinomas can be considered to be of the serrated type.[138,187] Morphologically, these tumors are characterized by a variety of features as well. Architecturally, the tumor has epithelial serrations, and some degree of mucin production is common. In mucinous areas, tumor cells are often present in the form of aggregated balls and pseudopapillary rods that project into mucin. Trabecular areas are common in poorly differentiated cases. Tumor cells have abundant clear or eosinophilic cytoplasm, and the nuclei are vesicular with peripheral condensation of chromatin (Fig. 27.19). Necrosis is uncommon or sometimes focal.[187]

Studies of the molecular pathogenesis of serrated carcinomas have revealed significant heterogeneity, although most of these tumors are associated with a high degree of methylation (CIMP).[104,188] There are at least two major subtypes of serrated carcinomas: proximal MSI cancers that arise from SSL and distal MSS cancers that arise from TSAs.[188] In one study,[189] only 16.1% of all serrated carcinomas were MSI, but 8.2% of the nonserrated adenocarcinomas were also MSI. Therefore most proximal MSI cancers do not show histologically identifiable serrated features, even though they are believed to arise from serrated precursor lesions. In another study of more than 900 CRCs, 9.1% were classified as serrated adenocarcinomas, and about one-half of these had an identifiable serrated polyp precursor lesion.[187] In this series, there was a trend toward decreased 5-year survival, particularly for left-sided cancers. Although the presence of a serrated precursor lesion should always be reported, the fifth edition WHO classification reserves the term *serrated adenocarcinoma* for tumors that show serrated features in the malignant component of the tumor (Box 27.7).[1]

BOX 27.5 Undifferentiated Carcinoma: Key Features

- Less than 5% gland formation
- Variable, sometimes marked, cytological pleomorphism
- Absence of a syncytial growth pattern
- No significant lymphocytic infiltrate
- May be MSI

Carcinoma with Squamous Metaplasia (Adenoacanthoma)

Adenoacanthomas are rare.[134] In one report, they were defined by the presence of adenocarcinoma elements with abundant admixed areas of benign-appearing squamous metaplasia (Fig. 27.20). The natural history and treatment are similar to those of pure adenocarcinomas.

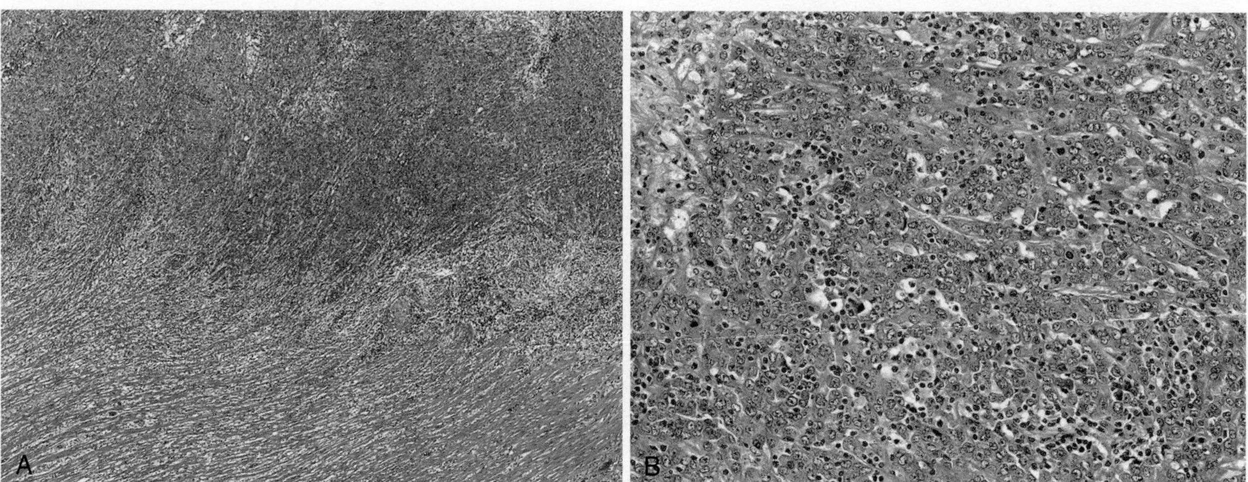

FIGURE 27.18 Medullary carcinoma. A, Low magnification reveals a solid tumor with a well-circumscribed margin at which abundant peritumoral lymphocytes are present. **B,** Tumor cells have large vesicular nuclei, prominent nucleoli, and amphophilic cytoplasm. Numerous tumor-infiltrating lymphocytes are shown.

Adenosquamous Carcinoma

Adenosquamous carcinomas are rare neoplasms, accounting for about 0.06% of all CRCs in Surveillance, Epidemiology, and End Results (SEER) data, although they were reported to be three times more common than pure squamous cell carcinomas in one series.[134,190,191] An association with paraneoplastic hypercalcemia and parathyroid hormone–related protein has been reported with sufficient frequency that a colorectal adenosquamous primary tumor should be considered in the differential diagnosis of patients with this clinical presentation.[134,192,193] This tumor type has also been seen in patients with chronic ulcerative colitis.[191,194] There is an even distribution between the right and left colon.[134] Morphologically, the tumor is composed of both malignant squamous and glandular elements, either as separate components or admixed (Fig. 27.21).

These cancers generally have a higher stage at presentation than adenocarcinomas NOS; in one study, 50% had metastases at the time of diagnosis (Box 27.8).[134] Although the overall survival rate in stage I/II disease is the same as comparably staged adenocarcinoma NOS, the survival rate for stage III/IV disease is significantly lower.[134,190] The overall 5-year survival rate for all adenosquamous carcinomas is 31%.[190]

Squamous Cell Carcinoma

Primary squamous cell carcinomas of the colorectum are exceedingly rare.[195] The etiology and histogenesis are unknown. Most authorities favor an origin from pluripotent stem cells capable of multidirectional differentiation.[196] Some authors have suggested derivation from foci of squamous metaplasia associated with chronic mucosal irritation. Supporting this hypothesis are reported associations with ulcerative colitis and schistosomiasis.[197] In two separate studies, all 31 cases were negative for human papillomavirus (HPV).[134,198] However, there is some limited evidence that HPV may play an etiological role in squamous cell carcinoma of the rectum.[199,200] Most primary squamous cell carcinomas manifest clinically at an advanced pathological stage. The initial presentation is often in elderly patients.

The pathological features are similar to those of squamous cell carcinomas in other organs (Fig. 27.22). Diagnosis of primary squamous cell carcinoma requires (1) exclusion of metastasis from other sites (particularly lung), (2) exclusion of an associated squamous-lined fistula tract (which, if present, is likely the site of origin), and (3) differentiation from carcinomas of the anus that extend proximally into the lower rectum.[196,201] The 5-year survival rate for lymph node–negative squamous cell carcinomas is reported to be 85%. However, squamous cell carcinomas have been reported to have a poorer prognosis than stage-matched adenocarcinoma NOS (Box 27.9).[134,195,196]

BOX 27.6 Medullary Carcinoma: Key Features

- Syncytial growth pattern, uniform cytology, pushing margin, prominent lymphocytic infiltrate
- Frequently MSI, *BRAF* mutation
- Favorable prognosis

Carcinoma with Sarcomatoid Components (Sarcomatoid Carcinoma, Spindle Cell Carcinoma, Carcinosarcoma)

Sarcomatoid carcinomas, also termed *carcinosarcomas* or *spindle cell carcinomas*, are more common in elderly patients, are often bulky or fleshy, and show abundant hemorrhage. Microscopically, these tumors reveal a biphasic growth pattern that combines both epithelial and mesenchymal elements (Fig. 27.23). Histological areas of transition may be observed in some cases.[202] The spindle cell component may be entirely undifferentiated, or it may show osseous, cartilaginous, or smooth muscle differentiation.[203]

Similar to sarcomatoid carcinomas in other anatomic locations, these tumors usually express keratins and epithelial membrane antigen (EMA) in both the carcinoma and the spindle cell components.[203] Carcinoembryonic antigen (CEA) positivity is usually limited to the adenocarcinoma element.[204] Focal S100 and myoglobin positivity has also

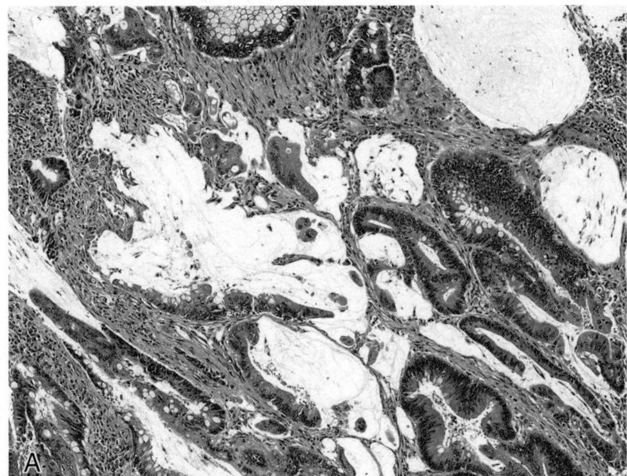

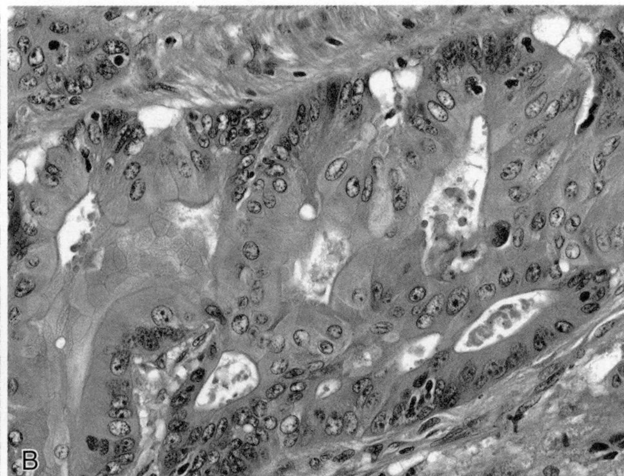

FIGURE 27.19 Serrated adenocarcinoma. A, The glands in this adenocarcinoma show infoldings, and there is a prominent mucinous component. Within some mucin pools, there are "balls" of tumor cells and rod-shaped tumor cell clusters. **B,** Tumor cells have abundant eosinophilic cytoplasm with vesicular nuclei and small nucleoli.

been described in some of these tumors.[205] Metastases may show either one or both of these cellular components. There is evidence in favor of a common progenitor cell origin as a result of the finding of shared *TP53* mutations in both the epithelial and sarcomatoid components.[206] Further subtyping into sarcomatoid carcinomas (which are keratin positive throughout the tumor) and carcinosarcomas (which are keratin negative in the mesenchymal component) has no apparent clinical or prognostic utility.[207] These neoplasms are typically fast-growing and aggressive, with a mean survival of approximately 6 months (Box 27.10).[202]

Carcinoma with Rhabdoid Features

These tumors are considered a variant of carcinomas with sarcomatoid components in the fifth edition of the WHO classification.[1] Most of these tumors occur in the right colon in patients in their seventh decade of life. This carcinoma is characterized by cells with abundant intracytoplasmic eosinophilic inclusions ("rhabdoid cells") (Fig. 27.24). The characteristic tumor cells may be a component of an otherwise typical adenocarcinoma NOS ("composite") or represent a "pure" process. The tumor cells are arranged in diffuse sheets within a variable myxoid background. Spindle and pleomorphic tumor cells may also be encountered, and abortive glandular elements may be present as well.[208] Keratin and vimentin are both expressed in the rhabdoid cells. A diagnostically useful feature is the loss of nuclear expression of SMARCB1 (INI1), a core subunit of the SWI/SNF chromatin remodeling complex.[209] However, INI1 loss is not entirely specific because it may be seen in up to 11% of adenocarcinoma NOS patients. [138] Abnormalities in centrosome structure (ciliary rootlet coiled coil [CROCC]) have also been described.[210] Most colorectal rhabdoid carcinomas display a CIMP-H, *BRAF*-mutated, MSI molecular phenotype.[209,210] Carcinomas with rhabdoid features are highly aggressive, with an overall survival rate of 7.9 months (Box 27.11).[138]

BOX 27.7 Serrated Adenocarcinoma: Key Features

- Origin from either a sessile serrated lesion or a traditional serrated adenoma
- Gland serration, cytoplasmic eosinophilia, often focal mucinous areas
- *BRAF* mutation or *KRAS* mutation (MAPK pathway)

Adenoma-Like Adenocarcinoma (Villous Adenocarcinoma, Invasive Papillary Adenocarcinoma)

Adenoma-like adenocarcinoma is a rare subtype of tumor characterized by ≥50% of the invasive component having an adenoma-like appearance with low-grade villous architecture[211] (Fig. 27.25). This subtype accounted for 8.6% of all CRCs in one series[211]; however, lower incidence rates in the order of 1% to 3% are more generally reported.[1,138] Fewer than one-half of the tumors have severe cytological atypia, and differentiation from a benign adenoma is difficult, either with or without prolapse changes, particularly on biopsy or limited resection material.[212] The distinction is based on the presence of the neoplastic epithelium associated with a desmoplastic stromal response, which is present in almost all malignant cases.[211,212] The invasive margin is typically pushing rather than infiltrating in appearance. *KRAS* mutation is frequently present (58% in one study), and the prognosis is favorable (Box 27.12).[212]

Micropapillary Adenocarcinoma

Micropapillary adenocarcinoma is characterized histologically by small nested clusters of tumor cells that are characteristically retracted from the surrounding stroma[1] (Fig. 27.26). The incidence of this morphological pattern varies from 5% to 20%.[213-215] Although not required to establish a diagnosis, micropapillary adenocarcinoma has a characteristic immunohistochemical finding referred to as an *"inside-out" pattern of reaction* for epithelial membrane antigen EMA (MUC1) whereby expression is on

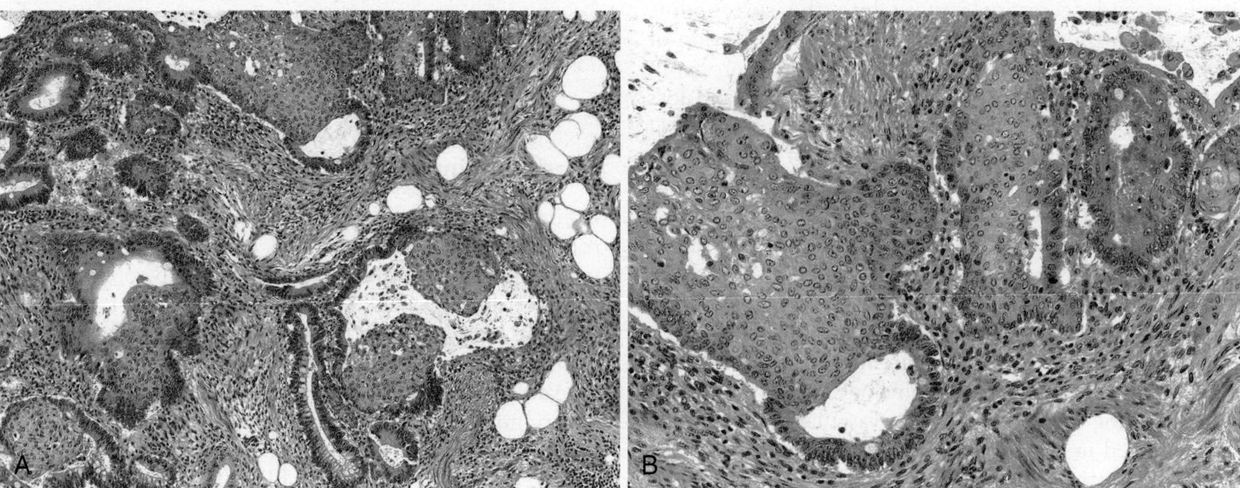

FIGURE 27.20 Carcinoma with squamous metaplasia. A, Typical adenocarcinoma with nests of squamous epithelium. **B,** Malignant glands merge with benign-appearing squamous epithelium.

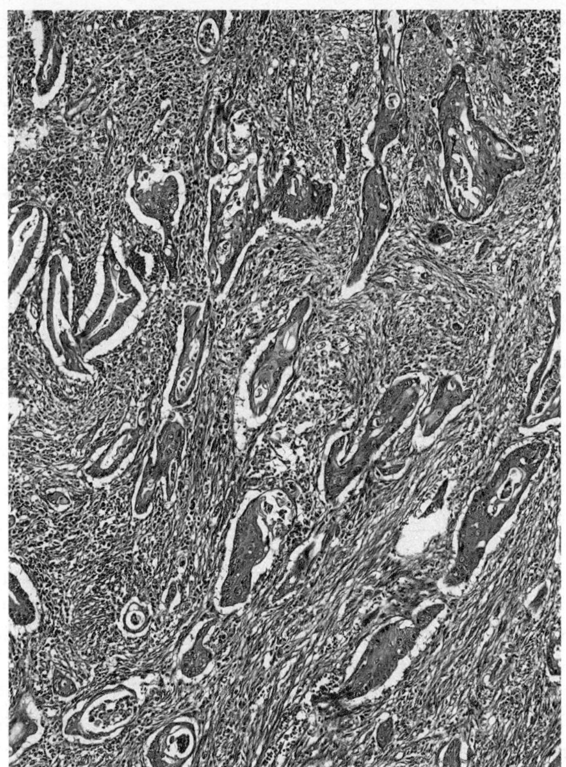

FIGURE 27.21 Adenosquamous carcinoma. Malignant glands merging with a malignant squamous component. This patient had a history of ulcerative colitis.

BOX 27.8 Adenosquamous Carcinoma: Key Features

- Exhibits both malignant squamous and glandular differentiation
- May be associated with hypercalcemia
- Poor prognosis

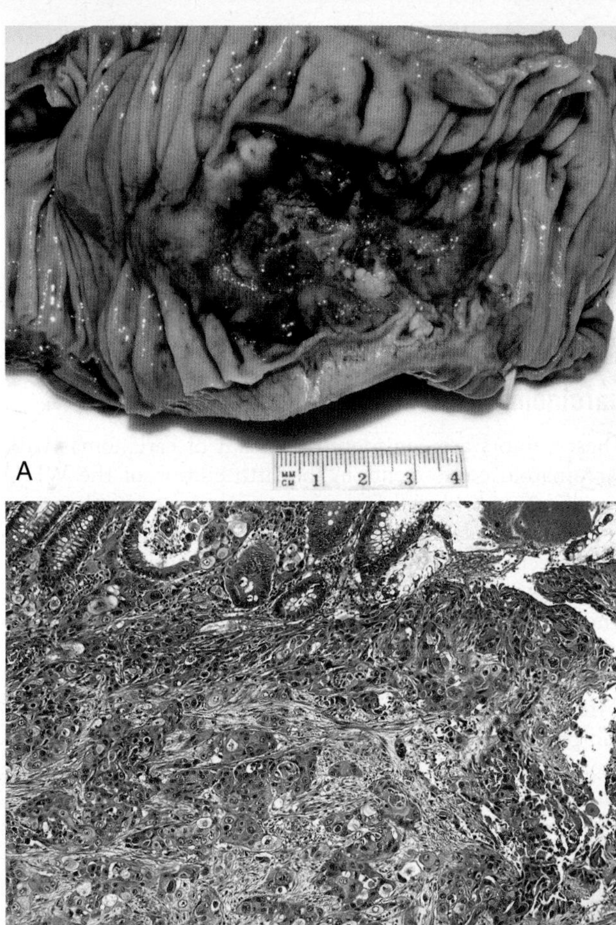

FIGURE 27.22 Squamous cell carcinoma. A, Bulky, ulcerated tumor in the descending colon with macroscopic appearance suggesting a primary carcinoma. **B,** Histologically the tumor comprises pure squamous cell carcinoma. No other primary site of origin was identified.

the external aspect of the epithelial nests rather than on the luminal aspect, as typically seen with adenocarcinoma NOS.[216] This corresponds to the finding on electron microscopy of microvilli on the outer surface of the epithelium and secretory activity into the surrounding stroma, which presumably accounts for the separation of tumor nests from the surrounding stroma.[138] Micropapillary adenocarcinoma also exhibits loss of MUC2 and loss or reduced E-cadherin staining. Tumor cell expression of vimentin and nuclear expression of SMAD4 is also present, which suggests that this morphological pattern represents a form of epithelial-to-mesenchymal transition.[138] Micropapillary adenocarcinoma frequently shows mutation of *TP53*, *KRAS*, or *BRAF*, but they are MSS. Stem cell markers are often expressed.[215] Adenocarcinomas containing a ≥5% component of micropapillary pattern are more aggressive than adenocarcinomas NOS,[217] with an increased proportion of lymph node positivity (up to 80%), reflecting the higher levels of vascular invasion typically identified in this tumor type.[217] In view of this, the WHO classification designates any adenocarcinoma with a ≥ 5% micropapillary component as a *micropapillary adenocarcinoma* (Box 27.13).

BOX 27.9 Squamous Cell Carcinoma: Key Features

- Squamous differentiation without evidence of glandular differentiation
- Must exclude metastasis or extension from the anal canal
- Associated with a history of chronic inflammation/irritation of the mucosa
- Poor prognosis

Choriocarcinoma

Primary choriocarcinoma of the colorectum is rare.[218] In reported cases, patients have been younger than those with adenocarcinoma NOS, with nearly one-half being younger than 50 years of age.[138] These cancers may manifest with massive bleeding from the gastrointestinal tract or from liver metastases.[219,220] Microscopically, the tumor reveals a variable admixture of choriocarcinoma and adenocarcinoma elements. The choriocarcinoma component stains with SALL 4, human chorionic gonadotropin (β-hCG), and α-fetoprotein (AFP).[221] On occasion, choriocarcinoma elements predominate in metastases when the primary tumor was only focally β-hCG+.[222] Increased

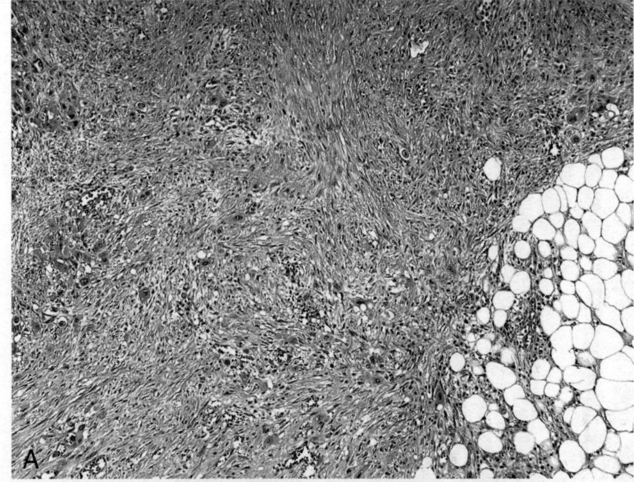

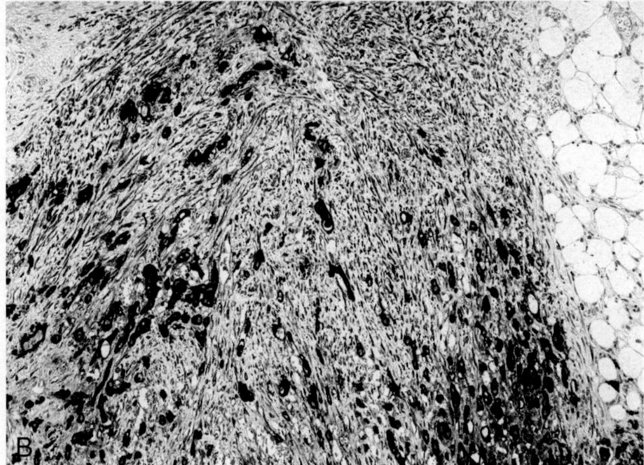

FIGURE 27.23 Carcinoma with a sarcomatoid component. A, High-grade carcinoma with single epithelioid cells merging into spindle-shaped forms and a prominent background collagenous stroma. **B,** AE1/AE3 keratin staining demonstrating keratin expression in the sarcomatoid component.

serum levels of β-hCG [223] and α-fetoprotein[220] have also been reported and serve as useful biomarkers of treatment response. Several theories exist to explain the choriocarcinoma component. The favored theory is dedifferentiation of the concomitant adenocarcinoma.[138] These cancers generally show metastasis to the liver at the time of clinical presentation and follow an aggressive clinical course despite the availability of germ cell tumor–directed chemotherapy (Box 27.14).

Tumors with Neuroendocrine Differentiation

Neuroendocrine Carcinoma

Both small cell and, less frequently, large cell neuroendocrine carcinomas can occur as primary tumors of the colorectum. They arise within adenomas in at least 30% of cases, suggesting a common histogenetic origin with adenocarcinomas.[224,225] These tumors typically manifest in younger patients (mean age, 57 years) compared with adenocarcinomas NOS. At least one-third arise in the rectum.[226,227] They account for approximately 1% of all colorectal tumors, but the incidence appears to be increasing, and they are also possibly underrecognized.[227] The morphological features of these neoplasms are identical to those of neuroendocrine carcinomas in the lung (Fig. 27.27). A minor nonneuroendocrine component may be identified in some cases.[1] Immunohistochemistry usually demonstrates positivity for chromogranin or synaptophysin, although these may be focal. Colorectal neuroendocrine carcinomas generally exhibit reactivity for CDX2 and SATB2, which helps exclude metastatic neuroendocrine carcinoma (e.g., from the lung) to the large intestine. Of these two markers, SATB2 has been shown to be a more sensitive stain.[228]

Neuroendocrine carcinomas of the colorectum are aggressive tumors. Approximately 70% of patients have distant metastatic (stage IV) disease at presentation.[229,230] The median survival time is 10.4 months, and the 3-year survival rate is 13%.[229] In one study, colorectal neuroendocrine carcinomas with a Ki67 index <55% had an increased

BOX 27.10 Carcinoma with Sarcomatoid Components: Key Features

- Exhibit evidence of both epithelial and mesenchymal differentiation
- Mesenchymal differentiation may include osseous, cartilaginous, or muscle differentiation
- Rapid growth
- Poor prognosis

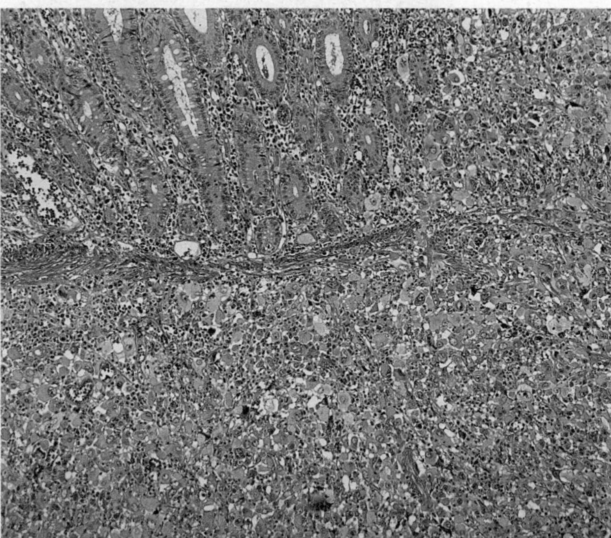

FIGURE 27.24 Carcinoma with rhabdoid features characterized by sheets of tumor cells with abundant intracytoplasmic eosinophilic inclusions. There was loss of INI1 expression in this carcinoma.

BOX 27.11 Carcinoma with Rhabdoid Features: Key Features

- Rhabdoid cells: large epithelioid cells with abundant intracytoplasmic eosinophilic inclusions
- Often admixed spindle and pleomorphic cells
- May be pure or admixed with another adenocarcinoma subtype
- Loss of INI1 expression
- Poor prognosis

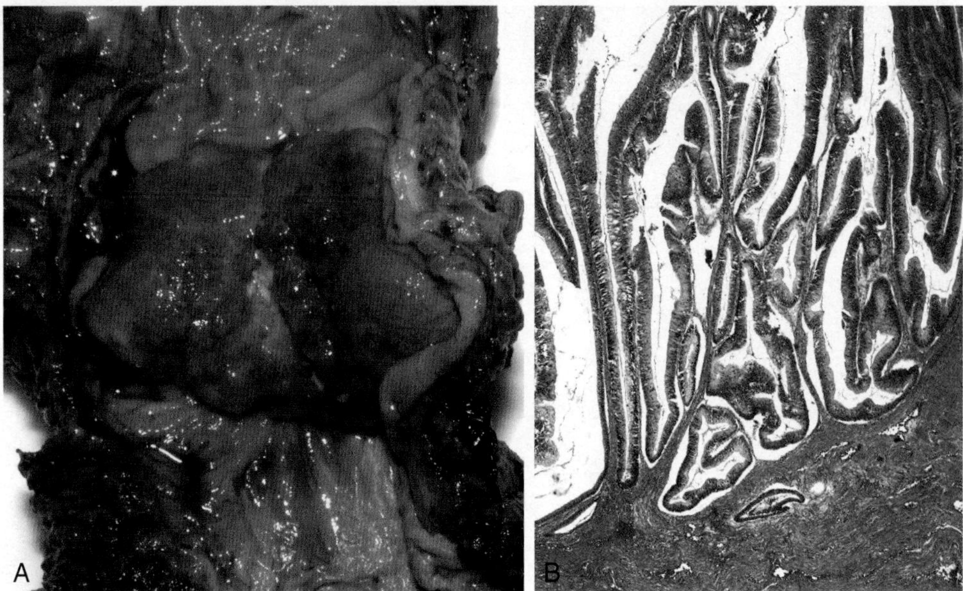

FIGURE 27.25 Adenoma-like adenocarcinoma. A, Macroscopic appearance of an adenoma-like adenocarcinoma occurring in the rectum. **B,** Characteristic low-grade villiform architecture and pushing lower margin.

BOX 27.12 Adenoma-like Adenocarcinoma: Key Features

- Minimal cytological atypia
- Villiform architecture
- Pushing margin with surrounding desmoplasia
- High *KRAS* mutation rate
- Favorable prognosis

median overall survival time (25.4 months) compared with tumors with a proliferation index >55% (5.3 months) (Box 27.15).[231]

Mixed Neuroendocrine–Nonneuroendocrine Neoplasm

In some tumors that show evidence of dual differentiation, distinct separation of pure glandular from pure neuroendocrine tumors is blurred. At one end of the spectrum are adenocarcinomas that contain scattered endocrine cells (detected in up to 20% of all CRCs) [232] and at the other end are neuroendocrine tumors that contain scattered nonneuroendocrine mucinous tumor cells. These features are common and do not affect either tumor behavior or management; they do not warrant classification as distinct entities.

However, the WHO classification refers to tumors that show a significant admixture of adenocarcinoma and neuroendocrine elements (>30% of each component) as *mixed neuroendocrine–nonneuroendocrine neoplasms* (MiNENs).[1] In these composite tumors, the adenocarcinoma and neuroendocrine components are, by definition, intimately mixed. Metastases may show both cellular components or only one. There are no sufficient studies of mixed tumors to make any reasonable conclusion on their clinical behavior.[233]

In contrast with mixed tumors, neoplasms that exhibit both neuroendocrine and glandular differentiation in individual cells are termed *amphicrine neoplasms*. On

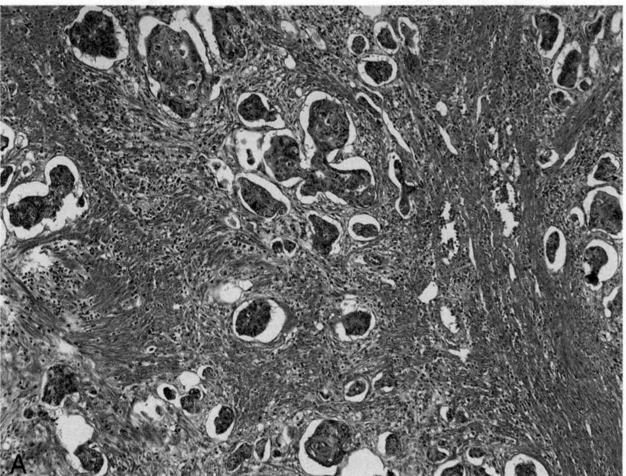

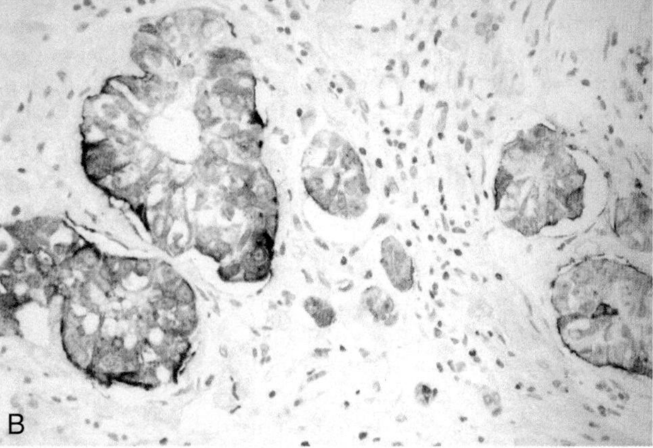

FIGURE 27.26 Micropapillary adenocarcinoma. A, Nested clusters of tumor cells with characteristic retraction from the surrounding stroma. **B,** EMA immunohistochemical stain demonstrating expression on the outside of the nests rather than the lumina aspect.

ultrastructural examination, these tumors show dense-core granules and mucin droplets within the same cells. One variant in the colon has similar characteristics to appendiceal goblet cell carcinoid tumor (goblet cell adenocarcinoma).[234-236] Some contain cells with multiple cellular phenotypes, such as goblet, endocrine, and Paneth cell differentiation (Fig. 27.28). Because these tumors seem to recapitulate the characteristics of normal intestinal crypts, the term *crypt cell carcinoma* has been proposed.[234,235] The malignant potential of these lesions has been well documented, and death is usually the result of intraabdominal rather than disseminated disease (Box 27.16).[234,235]

Other Rare Subtypes of Colorectal Carcinoma

Diffuse carcinoma is a non–signet ring cell carcinoma in the colorectum that exhibits a diffuse pattern of growth similar to those that occur in the stomach. In one study, 15 (0.6%) of 2369 CRCs were "diffuse"; only 7 were signet ring cell type, whereas 8 were "lymphangiosis" type.[237] The lymphangiosis type of diffuse cancer is an adenocarcinoma, often of moderate differentiation, with extensive lymphatic and vascular spread.[237,238] As expected, the prognosis of this type of cancer is extremely poor.[237]

Melanotic adenocarcinoma of the anorectal junction has been reported as a rare primary tumor, although evidence supports phagocytosis of anal melanocytes rather than true melanocytic differentiation in the pathogenesis of these tumors.[239,240]

Clear cell carcinomas have been described in the colon; these tumors have clear cytoplasm, but lack cytoplasmic mucin, lipid, or glycogen[241] (Fig. 27.29). Strong CEA, CK20, and CDX2 expression and an absence of PAX8 and CK7 expression help distinguish this tumor from a metastatic renal cell carcinoma or a carcinoma of Müllerian origin.[241-243] Most cases occurred in the rectum or sigmoid colon, and *KRAS* mutation was found in 80%.[138]

Hepatoid adenocarcinoma is a rare tumor that histologically mimics hepatocellular carcinoma.[244-246] It belongs to a broader group of carcinomas of the gastrointestinal tract that show enteroblastic differentiation, a primitive phenotype reminiscent of the fetal foregut.[245] Patients are often young males. Hepatoid adenocarcinoma is characterized by sheets of large polygonal cells with abundant eosinophilic cytoplasm and central nuclei with prominent nucleoli. Other enteroblastic carcinomas may show characteristic cytoplasmic vacuolation, sometimes with eosinophilic PAS+ globules that represent α-fetoprotein (Fig. 27.30).[245] Hepatoid adenocarcinoma expresses hepatoid markers such as α-fetoprotein, Hep Par 1, and glypican 3.[138] SALL4 is expressed in less differentiated tumors. [245] Overall, the prognosis of hepatoid adenocarcinoma and enteroblastic tumors in general is poorer than for adenocarcinomas NOS.[138,245]

Low-grade tubuloglandular adenocarcinoma is a well-differentiated carcinoma composed of invasive tubular

BOX 27.13 Micropapillary Adenocarcinoma: Key Features

- Greater than or equal to 5% component of small nested clusters of tumor cells that are characteristically retracted from the surrounding stroma
- EMA expression on the outside (periphery) of tumor nests
- Higher rates of *BRAF* or *KRAS* mutation; MSS
- Biologically aggressive with frequent lymph node metastases

BOX 27.14 Choriocarcinoma: Key Features

- Younger patients
- Propensity for hemorrhage
- Choriocarcinoma components
- Immunohistochemical expression of SALL 4, human chorionic gonadotropin (β-hCG) and α-fetoprotein
- Aggressive clinical course

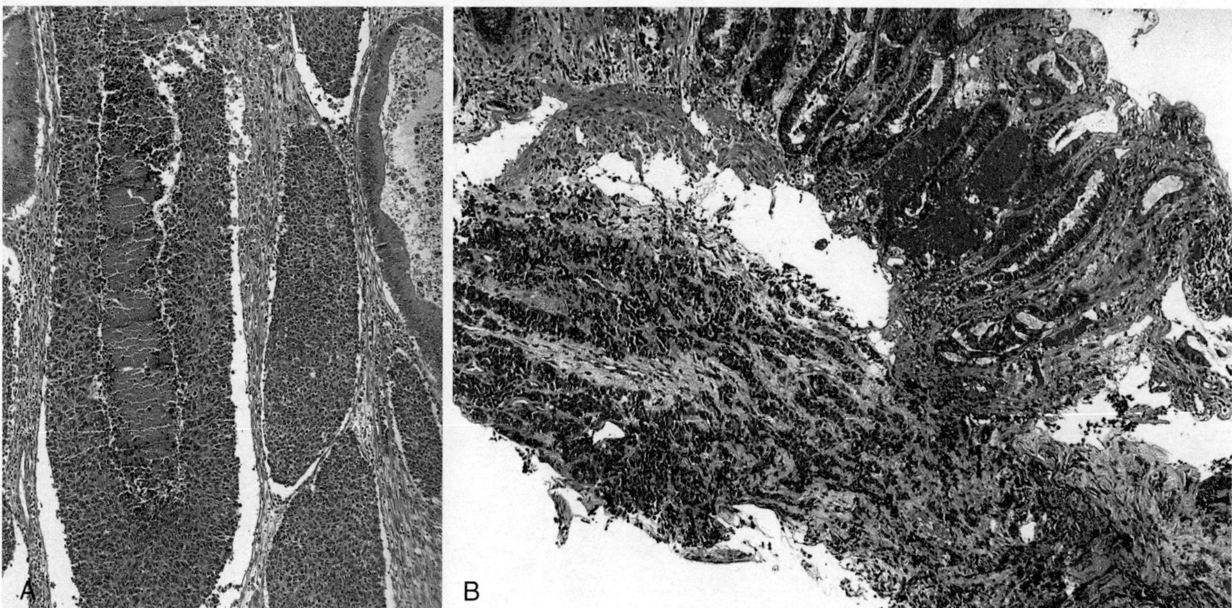

FIGURE 27.27 Neuroendocrine carcinoma. A, Large cell neuroendocrine pattern with islands of larger cells and central necrosis. **B,** Small cell neuroendocrine carcinoma identified in a biopsy specimen. Such cases often receive primary chemotherapy because of associated metastatic disease.

glands lined by minimally atypical neoplastic cells. It is a characteristic appearance of approximately 10% of adenocarcinomas that arise in a setting of IBD[138] (see later discussion). Approximately two-thirds of cases show coexpression of both CK7 and CK20, and approximately one-half show loss of MLH1 expression. There is limited information regarding the prognosis of this subtype; however, it is generally viewed as a favorable subtype of CRC.

Gut-associated lymphoid tissue (GALT)-associated carcinomas (also referred to as *dome-type adenocarcinomas*) are believed to arise from the M cells of the epithelium of lymphoglandular complexes in the colorectum. Macroscopically, they display a plaquelike or "dome"-like appearance. Histologically, they are typically localized to the submucosa and are surrounded by a prominent lymphoid infiltrate with germinal center formation. Desmoplasia is absent. The lining epithelium is cytologically bland, with a sometimes-prominent cytoplasmic eosinophilia and absence of goblet cells. Eosinophilic secretions are present in characteristically dilated lumina; however, the dirty necrosis typical of conventional CRC is not present (Fig. 27.31). The low-power morphological appearance bears some resemblance to Warthin's tumor of the salivary glands.[247,248] By immunohistochemistry, the tumor cells lack expression of MUC2, supporting an M-cell origin. Lymphocytes within the neoplastic epithelium are of B-cell rather than T-cell type.[247] MMR markers are usually retained. Other situations in which neoplastic glandular mucosa is surrounded by a prominent lymphoid stroma occur when inclusion of glandular elements of an adenoma into a lymphoglandular complex occurs (Fig. 27.32), there is prominent peritumoral lymphoid stroma in MSI-H CRC, or a conventional adenocarcinoma NOS invades a lymphoid aggregate. The distinction among these lesions may be difficult.[249] Table 27.8 provides a summary of the features that aid in separation of these entities. The prognosis for GALT-associated carcinoma is overwhelmingly favorable, with no reports of lymph node metastasis.[248] GALT-associated carcinoma is reported to be more common in patients with ulcerative colitis.[250]

BOX 27.15 Neuroendocrine Carcinoma: Key Features

- Mostly small cell in type
- One-third arise in the rectum
- May arise from a preexisting adenoma
- Poor prognosis

Carcinomas with DNA Mismatch Repair Deficiency

Inactivation of DNA MMR plays an important role in the pathogenesis of 15% of CRCs. Although some of these cases

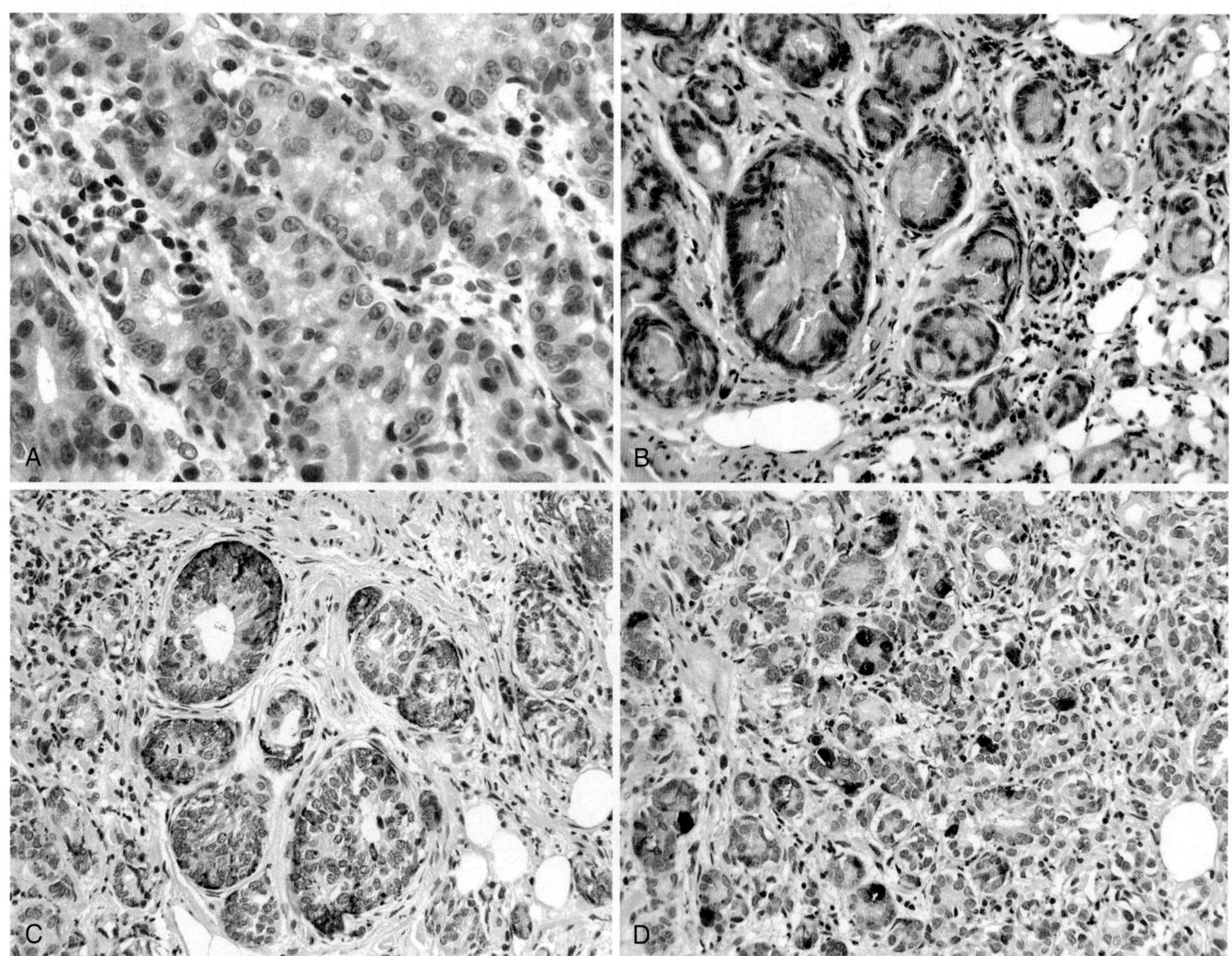

FIGURE 27.28 Mixed crypt cell carcinoma. A, Mixed crypt cell carcinoma shows relatively uniform glands with a mixed cellular population. **B,** Mucin stain highlights goblet cell differentiation. **C,** Chromogranin stain is positive in many tumor cells. **D,** Paneth cell stain highlights neoplastic Paneth cells.

BOX 27.16 Mixed Neuroendocrine–Nonneuroendocrine Neoplasm: Key Features

- Intimate admixture of adenocarcinoma and neuroendocrine elements (>30% of each component)
- Metastases may show only one element

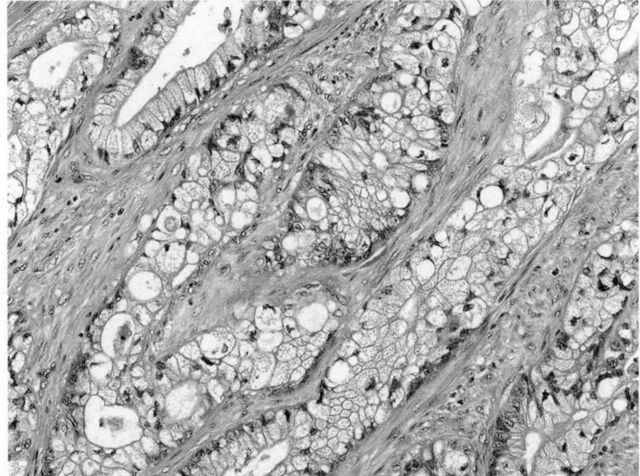

FIGURE 27.29 Clear cell carcinoma. Infiltrating glands contain cells with prominent cytoplasmic clearing. This is typically a result of glycogen accumulation and not mucin.

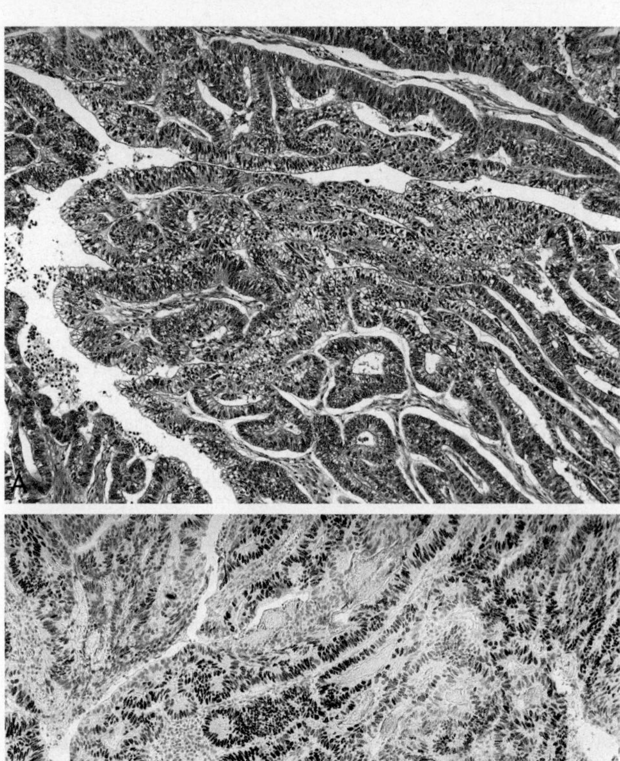

FIGURE 27.30 Enteroblastic pattern. A, Histological appearance with characteristic cytoplasmic vacuolization. **B,** SALL4 expression in this region.

are the result of hereditary alterations in one or more of the MMR genes (see Lynch Syndrome), approximately 80% are sporadic, resulting primarily from promoter hypermethylation and silencing of *MLH1* transcription. In addition to MSI, these cancers contain a variety of specific clinical and pathological associations of importance to surgical pathologists (see Lynch Syndrome for a discussion of immunohistochemical and molecular diagnostics).[77,251]

Sporadic MMR-deficient MSI CRCs with methylation-induced *MLH1* silencing show a marked female predominance (about 4:1), show increased prevalence with age, and are particularly common in women older than 70 years of age.[252] Approximately 90% of sporadic MLH1-deficient MSI CRCs are located in the right colon, where they constitute approximately 50% of all right-sided cancers in women older than 70 years of age.[179] The propensity for right colon involvement mostly underlies the often quoted clinical differences between right-sided and left-sided CRCs.[31] Higher numbers of synchronous and metachronous tumors are found as well.[253] Precursor lesions often reveal characteristics of SSLs in sporadic cases, and conventional adenomas in hereditary cases (e.g., Lynch syndrome).[254] A number of specific pathological associations have also been described in MSI CRCs, which are shared by both sporadic and inherited tumors[179,253,255-259] (Table 27.9). MSI cancers are also more likely to be multiple, have a polypoid or exophytic growth pattern, and show sharply circumscribed, pushing margins and marked grossly visible necrosis. Furthermore, MSI tumors are more likely to show mucinous or signet ring cell features. The association between these histological features and DNA MMR deficiency is high, even when less than 50% of the tumor reveals these features. Therefore the sensitivity and specificity of these histological features for the diagnosis of MSI cancer vary according to the specific criteria used. The presence of a component of any one of the associated histological variants (mucinous, signet ring cell, or undifferentiated) or of a prominent tumor-infiltrating lymphocytic response provides a relatively sensitive guide to identify possible MSI cancers.[260,261]

The character of the host lymphoid response is another feature that shows a striking difference between MSI and MSS cancers. The presence of tumor-infiltrating lymphocytes (Fig. 27.33) is highly predictive of MSI cancer, particularly when present in combination with an undifferentiated tumor (which may or may not be of the classic medullary subtype). In one study, the presence of at least 5 tumor-infiltrating lymphocytes per 10 high-power fields (HPFs) had a sensitivity of 93% and a specificity of 62% for the detection of MSI-H CRC.[262] A number of complex algorithms have been proposed in an attempt to achieve a high degree of specificity for the presence of MSI in any single colon carcinoma. However, in one study, the pathologist's "opinion" (based on an overall evaluation of the features described previously and his or her prior experience with known MSI cancers) was the best predictive factor.[140] Overall, compared with MSI-H Lynch syndrome–associated

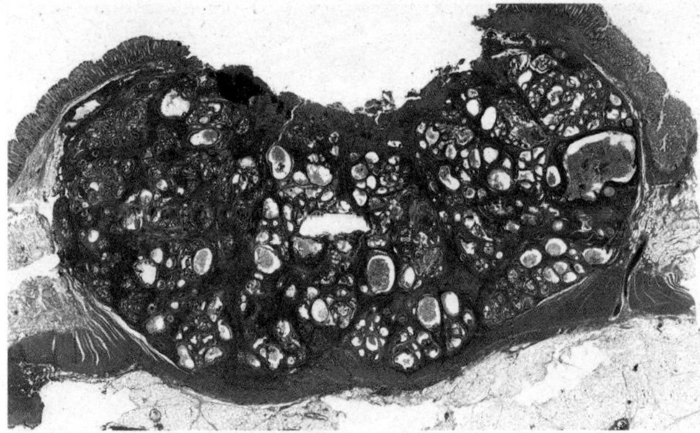

FIGURE 27.31 GALT-associated carcinoma. Dilated glands lined by cells with eosinophilic cytoplasm and a heavy background lymphoid stroma are shown. The lymphocytes are mainly B cells and are found focally within the epithelium. The tumor was microsatellite stable.

colon cancer, sporadic MSI cancers are more frequently heterogeneous, poorly differentiated, mucinous, proximally located, and, as mentioned earlier, associated with a prominent tumor-infiltrating lymphocyte reaction.[263]

Clinically, patients with MSI CRCs are more likely to have an advanced T stage at presentation, but they are less likely to show regional lymph node metastases. In fact, most T4 N0 M0 CRCs are deficient in DNA MMR.[264] When controlled for stage and other standard prognostic parameters, most studies have shown that MSI CRCs are associated with better overall survival compared with MSS colon cancers (see Molecular Genetic Prognostic and Predictive Markers).[264,265]

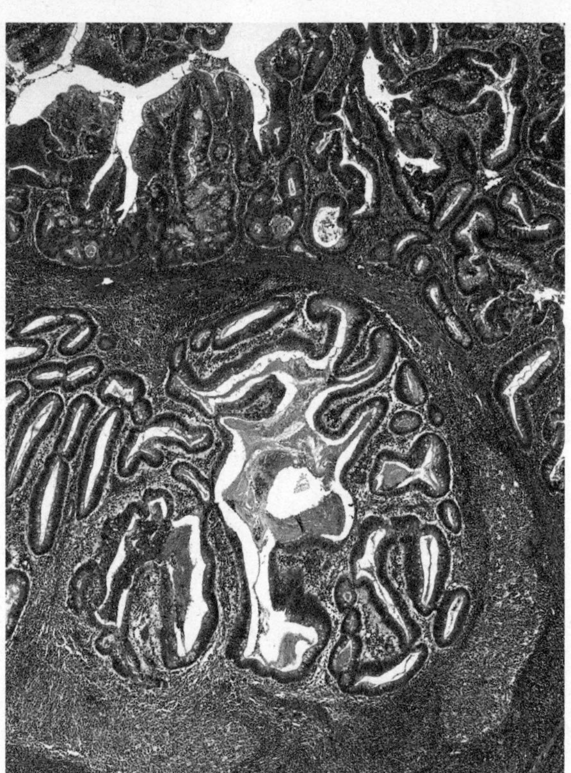

FIGURE 27.32 Adenoma involving a lymphoglandular complex. The surface high-grade tubulovillous adenoma extended into a lymphoglandular complex in the submucosa. Features that indicate the noninvasive nature of this process are the confinement within the surrounding lymphoid tissue, the presence of lamina propria, and the absence of a desmoplastic stroma reaction.

SPECIAL STUDIES

Immunophenotype

Aside from MMR immunohistochemistry, routine examination of CRC specimens does not usually require immunohistochemical studies. However, these studies are often required for characterization of distinctive subtypes (e.g., neuroendocrine carcinoma) or for investigation of primary versus metastatic tumors. The following markers may be helpful in the examination of CRCs:

Keratins

- CRC tumor cells express low-molecular-weight cytokeratins. Most tumors (80% to 100%) are positive for CK20, and the majority (at least 85%) are negative for CK7.[266] MSI adenocarcinomas often show decreased expression of CK20. BRAF-mutated MSS CRCs often display reduced CDX2 and increased CK7 expression.[267] A summary of the frequency of specific keratin profiles in colorectal adenocarcinoma is presented in Table 27.10.

Villin

- Villin is a microfilament-associated actin-binding protein that shows diffuse cytoplasmic expression with brush border accentuation in more than 90% of colorectal adenocarcinomas. Expression may be lost in poorly differentiated tumors.[269] It is also positive in nongastrointestinal tumors that show intestinal differentiation (e.g., lung, bladder).[270,271]

CDX2

- The nuclear transcription factor CDX2 is expressed in more than 90% of all colorectal adenocarcinomas.[272,273] Exceptions include medullary carcinomas and some nonmedullary MMR-deficient carcinomas, which are often negative for CDX2 and CK20 and positive for CK7.[178] Expression is related to differentiation, with high-grade tumors positive in only approximately 50% of cases.[274] There also appears to be an inverse correlation of CDX2 expression with tumor stage.[274] CDX2 is expressed in 10% to 30% of other gastrointestinal malignancies, particularly those with intestinal-type differentiation; in 20% to 65% of mucinous ovarian tumors; and in 50% to 100% of urinary bladder adenocarcinomas.[270,271,274] CDX2 expression is rare in breast, lung, thyroid, kidney, and endometrial adenocarcinomas, although nonbronchioloalveolar mucinous carcinomas of the lung are frequently positive. Several studies have also postulated a role for CDX2 in neoplastic progression, with loss of expression correlating with more advanced/aggressive disease.[275]

SATB2

- SATB2 is a protein selectively expressed in the hind gut epithelium and is therefore a useful marker of a colorectal or appendiceal site of origin.[276] It is found in both epithelial and neuroendocrine cells and in their associated neoplasms of these sites.[228,276] It has greater sensitivity than CDX2 in CRCs, with high levels of

TABLE 27.8 Distinction Between Adenoma Inclusion into a Lymphoglandular Complex, Conventional Adenocarcinoma Invading Superficially into a Lymphoid Aggregate, MSI-High Colorectal Carcinoma, and GALT-Associated Carcinoma

	Adenoma Inclusion into a Lymphoglandular Complex	Conventional Adenocarcinoma Invading a Lymphoid Aggregate	MSI-High Colorectal Carcinoma	GALT-Associated Carcinoma
Size	Any size	Usually ≤20 mm	Usually ≥20 mm	Usually ≥20 mm
Presence of lamina propria	Present	Absent	Absent	Absent
Connection to surface	Surface adenoma with herniation through a gap in the muscularis mucosae	Always	Always; sessile serrated lesion may be present	Minimal or absent
Confinement to surrounding lymphoid tissue	Always	Often invades beyond confines of lymphoid tissue	Always	Always
Desmoplasia	Absent	Present	Present	Absent
Glands	Rounded	Small, fused with necrosis	Often sheetlike growth	Dilated with bright eosinophilic secretions
Lining epithelium	Low-grade cytology	High-grade cytology	High-grade cytology	Cytoplasmic eosinophilia
Lymphocytes within epithelium	Absent	Absent	Present (T lymphocytes)	Present (B lymphocytes)
Lymphovascular invasion	None	Sometimes	Sometimes	None
Immunohistochemistry	Unhelpful	Unhelpful	MMR-deficient	Absence of MUC2 expression

GALT, *Gut-associated lymphoid tissue;* MSI, *microsatellite instability;* MMR, *mismatch repair.*

TABLE 27.9 Pathological Features of High-Frequency Microsatellite Instability Colorectal Carcinomas

Pathological Feature	MSI (%)	MSS (%)	Positive Predictive Value (%)*
Location in right colon	90	34	32
Exophytic/polypoid	82	54	21
Signet ring cell component	13	5	31
Mucinous subtype (>50% extracellular mucin)	15	5	35
Mucinous component (>10% extracellular mucin)	22	7	36
Cribriform pattern	13	28	8
Poor differentiation	38	13	34
Medullary type	14	0.4	71
Medullary component (>10%)	25	3	59
Lymphocytosis	21	3	55
Pushing margin	15	8	25 (NS)
Crohn's-like reaction	49	36	19 (NS)
"MSI" by pathologist	49	11	44

MSI, *Microsatellite instability;* MSS, *microsatellite stable;* NS, *not significant.*
**Assuming a prevalence of MSI-high of 15%.*
From Alexander J, Watanabe T, Wu TT, et al. Histopathological identification of colon cancer with microsatellite instability. Am J Pathol. *2001;158(2):527-535; Kim H, Jen J, Vogelstein B, Hamilton SR. Clinical and pathological characteristics of sporadic colorectal carcinomas with DNA replication errors in microsatellite sequences.* Am J Pathol. *1994;145(1):148-156.*

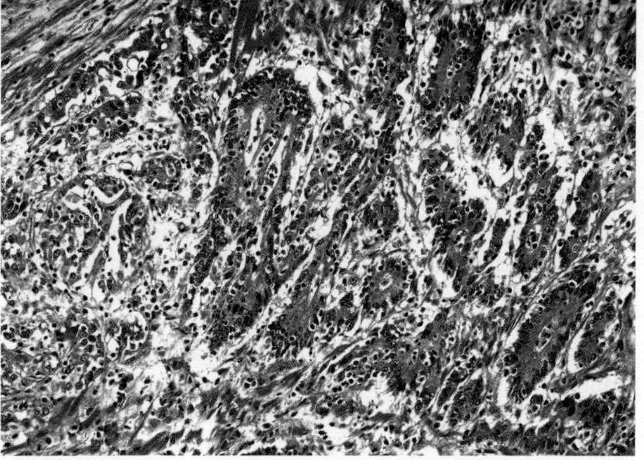

FIGURE 27.33 Adenocarcinoma with numerous tumor-infiltrating lymphocytes in a 75-year-old man. Such carcinomas are show microsatellite instability, and this adenocarcinoma displayed a loss of MSH2 and MSH6 expression indicative of an origin in Lynch syndrome.

methylation, making it a more useful stain in mucinous, signet ring cell, medullary, and undifferentiated CRCs.[168,184,277,278] Recently it has been reported that SATB2 expression is often lost in colitis-associated dysplasia and carcinoma.[279,280] However, expression of SATB2 has been reported in up to 3.6% of extraintestinal carcinomas.[281]

Mucins

- MUC2 is expressed in most CRCs; MUC1 (EMA) expression may be present, but expression of MUC5AC is less common, except in mucinous adenocarcinomas.[142,266]

TABLE 27.10 CK7/CK20 Profile of Colorectal Cancer [268]

CK7	CK20	Prevalence in Colorectal Cancer (%)	Differential
Overall Results			
+		5-15	
	+	85-100	
Profiles			
+	+	5-10	Pancreas, bile duct, urothelial
+	–	0-5	Lung, breast, ovary, endometrial
–	+	75-95	Colorectal, gastric
–	–	0-15	Prostate, adrenal, hepatocellular, renal, carcinoid

CK, *Cytokeratin.*
From Chu P, Wu E, Weiss LM. Cytokeratin 7 and cytokeratin 20 expression in epithelial neoplasms: a survey of 435 cases. Mod Pathol. *2000;13(9):962-972.*

DIFFERENTIAL DIAGNOSIS

Metastasis versus Primary Carcinoma

Metastases to the large intestine are usually readily separated from primary malignancy on the basis of morphology that is unusual for a colorectal primary tumor, a history of primary malignancy at another site, and immunohistochemical findings showing no evidence of colorectal differentiation. Some metastatic lesions remain difficult, such as ovarian and endometrioid carcinoma (discussed later); gastrointestinal tract carcinomas from outside the large intestine, particularly when exhibiting intestinal or mucinous differentiation; and when there is spread of CRC from another site. A useful clue to a primary carcinoma is the presence of an adjacent precursor lesion (adenoma or serrated polyp). However, this is not infallible because metastases to the large intestine can show paradoxical maturation toward the mucosal surface or may involve the mucosa by spread along an intact basement membrane (Fig. 27.34). This finding is most commonly described in metastases to the small intestine; however, an identical process is encountered in the colon and can result in a pseudoadenomatous pattern in the mucosa.[282,283] Additionally, a precursor adenoma is identified adjacent to a colorectal adenocarcinoma in less than one-third of cases.[284] Pathologists should also be aware that hyperplastic "transitional" mucosa adjacent to a carcinoma may simulate a serrated lesion. This is characterized by crypt elongation, superficial crypt widening, and sometimes crypt branching (Fig. 27.35).[285,286] The presence of surface epithelial maturation and the absence of epithelial atypia, deep crypt apoptosis, and irregular glandular architecture are helpful in correctly identifying this as a reactive change. Metastasis is also favored when there is no mucosal involvement, if the bulk of the tumor is deep in the wall with broad serosal involvement, or if there is extensive lymphatic involvement.

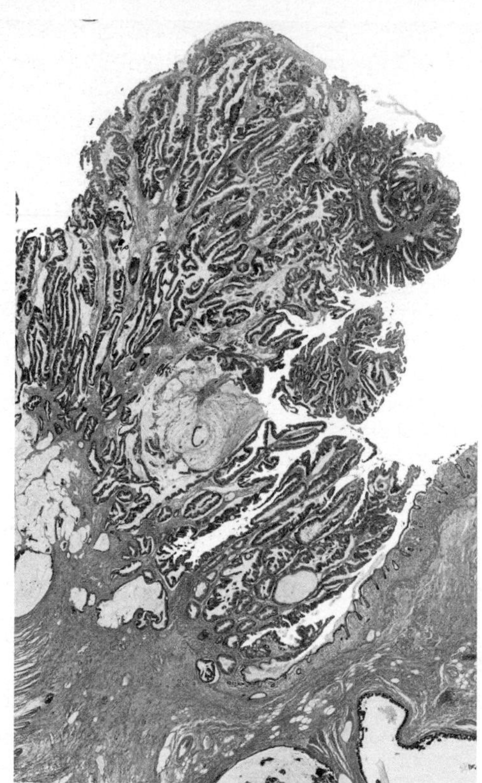

FIGURE 27.34 Metastatic rectal adenocarcinoma not otherwise specified with disseminated peritoneal involvement, invading the right colon and demonstrating paradoxical maturation in the mucosa with a pseudoadenomatous pattern.

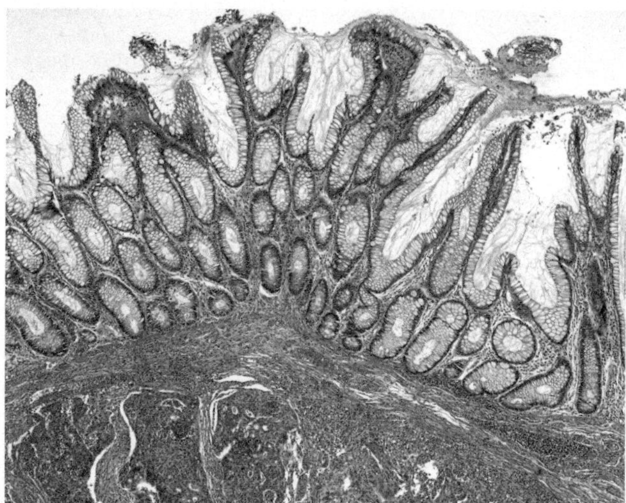

FIGURE 27.35 Transitional mucosa adjacent to a colorectal adenocarcinoma. The crypt hyperplasia and dilation can be mistaken for a precursor serrated lesion at the edge.

A small subset of patients with CRC have multiple colonic tumors. These may represent synchronous primary CRCs or metastases from one tumor to other areas of the colorectum. The presence of multiple tumors that exhibit similar morphology to one another favors metastasis from a single primary tumor, whereas the presence of morphologically dissimilar patterns, at least one of which is of an unusual subtype, favors multiple synchronous tumors rather than metastasis. An underlying condition predisposing to CRC, such as polyposis syndrome or IBD, also favor multiple tumors of colorectal origin. Differences in immunophenotype or molecular marker status may also be helpful in diagnosing multiple synchronous primary tumors, although the latter is rarely used in practice.

Recurrent or Metastatic Carcinoma versus Metachronous Carcinoma

Patients with CRC are at a significantly increased risk for development of additional carcinomas. In these patients, it may be difficult to differentiate tumor recurrence from a distinct metachronous cancer. If a precursor lesion is identified, a diagnosis of a new primary tumor can usually be established easily. However, a metastasis should be favored if there is an absence of mucosal involvement or if there is extensive submucosal-mucosal lymphatic spread in association with multiple tumor nodules, particularly when it is also present at the site of the original tumor. In the remainder of cases, it is often difficult to be definitive. In the absence of a precursor lesion, a diagnosis of tumor recurrence is always favored when a tumor develops at a surgical anastomosis line, even if there are no other supporting features.

Colorectal Adenocarcinoma versus Endometrial or Ovarian Adenocarcinoma

The morphological appearance of some endometrial and endometrioid ovarian carcinomas may show significant overlap with primary CRC. As a result, it may be difficult to firmly establish the correct site of origin of tumors that extensively involve the colorectum and other pelvic organs. The presence of a precursor lesion or the absence of mucosal involvement is helpful in diagnosing a primary colorectal tumor or a noncolorectal tumor, respectively. Endometrioid carcinoma arising from colorectal deposits of endometriosis can be particularly difficult. Although not always present, a high index of suspicion is required when there is background endometriosis near an adenocarcinoma in the large bowel. Some ovarian metastases from a colonic primary tumor may show only unilateral disease and may contain foci suggestive of a primary ovarian tumor of benign nature or low malignant potential.[287] Immunohistochemistry may be useful in this differential diagnosis: CRCs are typically CK7−/CK20+/SATB2+, whereas most endometrial and ovarian cancers are CK7+/CK20−/SATB2−.[288] Furthermore, nuclear expression of WT1 and PAX-8 are often positive in ovarian cancers but negative in CRCs.[289,290]

Colorectal Adenocarcinoma versus Primary Small-Intestinal Adenocarcinoma

Not uncommonly, CRC may directly invade the small intestine or seed the small intestine by intraabdominal spread, which raises the possibility of a primary small-intestinal adenocarcinoma, particularly when there is small-intestinal mucosal involvement. The presence of a precursor lesion generally provides evidence of the original site of origin of the tumor; however, as noted earlier, colonization of the small-intestinal mucosa by CRC can produce a pseudoadenomatous appearance.[282] Immunohistochemistry may be helpful because primary small-intestinal adenocarcinomas are often CK7+ and CK20+, and up to one-third of small-intestinal adenocarcinomas are CK7+ and CK20−.[291] Villin and CDX2 are positive in approximately 60% of small-intestinal carcinomas, compared with 90% of CRCs. A potentially more useful marker is SATB2, which is expressed in most CRCs but less than one-half of small-intestinal adenocarcinomas. Furthermore, unlike the strong and diffuse staining pattern found in CRC, expression of SATB2 identified in small-intestinal adenocarcinoma is typically weak.[292]

NATURAL HISTORY

The overall survival rates for CRC at 1, 5, and 10 years are 83%, 64%, and 58%, respectively.[3] As with most solid tumors, survival correlates with the presence of locoregional disease and distant metastasis. For instance, the 5-year survival rate is 90% for patients with localized disease, 71% for those with regional metastases, and 14% for patients with distant metastasis.[3] However, only 39% of new cases are diagnosed with localized disease alone.[3] Pathological staging in colon cancer (AJCC system) is based on depth of invasion into the bowel wall and surrounding structures, spread to regional lymph nodes, and distant metastasis. With progression, tumors may penetrate the peritoneal lining, resulting in intraabdominal spread or invasion into other abdominal and pelvic structures. Spread through lymphatics or blood vessels may occur at any time (or stage) during the evolution of disease. With further progression, cancer may invade the portal vein tributaries, leading to liver metastases, or the vena cava, leading to lung and bone marrow metastases as well as other distant metastases.

TREATMENT

Surgical Therapy

Patients with colon and rectal cancer are usually managed by surgical resection of the primary tumor, either with or without chemotherapy, depending on the stage of the tumor. Surgical resection is undertaken in all patients unless the tumor is deemed locally unresectable or there is a medical contraindication to surgery. In patients with nonobstructing tumors, a segmental colectomy with en bloc removal of regional lymph nodes is performed. Patients with obstructing tumors may undergo a similar one-stage procedure, a resection with diversion, or a diversion and stent procedure followed by resection. Laparoscopic resection has been shown in several meta-analyses to be as effective as open surgical resection and is associated with shorter hospitalization.[293,294] There are also data to suggest that robotic-assisted surgery may reduce the need for abdominoperineal resection in some low rectal tumors.[295] It is recommended that rectal cancers demonstrating spread beyond the muscularis propria (stage T3), as determined by MRI, are best treated with neoadjuvant chemoradiation before resection.[296]

Surgical resection of liver and pulmonary metastatic disease is also considered if the following criteria are met: the primary tumor was (or will be) resected for cure,[1] complete resection of metastatic disease is feasible either initially or following adjuvant therapy,[2] and maintenance of adequate organ function can be preserved.[3] Ablative therapies and re-resection may be considered in selected patients. Reevaluation for conversion of previously unresectable disease to resectable disease is typically performed every 2 months after initiation of chemotherapy.

Cytotoxic Chemotherapy

Since the 1950s, fluoropyrimidines have been the mainstay of CRC chemotherapy (intravenous 5-fluorouracil [5-FU] plus leucovorin [folinic acid], or oral capecitabine, which is the oral premetabolite of fluorouracil and has comparable efficacy to intravenous 5-FU).[12,297] Subsequently, two new cytotoxic agents—irinotecan, a topoisomerase inhibitor, and oxaliplatin, a third-generation platinum compound—have shown benefit in patients with advanced disease. These chemotherapeutic agents are now widely used in various treatment protocols in the adjuvant and advanced disease settings, typically in combination with 5-FU (e.g., the FOLFOX protocol consists of FOLinic acid + 5-Fluorouracil + Oxaliplatin; the FOLFIRI protocol consists of FOLinic acid + 5-Fluorouracil +IRInotecan; and FOLFOXIRI contains all four drugs). These protocols have been shown to result in increased disease-free survival and overall survival[153,297]; however, the benefit is best in patients younger than 65 or 70 years of age and those with good performance status because of the systemic toxicities associated with these additional agents.[12,297]

Biological and Targeted Therapy

The addition of several different targeted therapeutic agents has shown efficacy in patients with resistant or progressive metastatic disease. Cetuximab and panitumumab are humanized anti–EGFR antibodies that inhibit downstream signaling of cell growth and proliferation, as well as apoptotic pathways that have been shown to be important in the progression of neoplasia. Both are highly effective in advanced CRCs that do not harbor *KRAS* mutations.[153,297] *KRAS* mutation analysis is therefore required in the primary tumor or the metastasis before anti-EGFR therapy is initiated (see Molecular Genetic Prognostic and Predictive Markers).[153] Regorafenib is a small-molecule multikinase inhibitor that has been shown to be effective in metastatic disease that is resistant to other therapies, including *KRAS*-mutant tumors.[153,298] Trifluridine/tipiracil is an orally active antimetabolite agent composed of trifluridine, a thymidine-based nucleoside analogue, and tipiracil, a potent thymidine phosphorylase inhibitor. This drug is useful in refractory metastatic disease or when first-line chemotherapy or biological agents are contraindicated.[299,300] Regorafenib or trifluridine/tipiracil are generally the last-line therapies administered.[153] Bevacizumab is a humanized anti–vascular endothelial growth factor (VEGF) antibody that inhibits soluble protein and results in an antiangiogenic effect in tumors. Aflibercept is another recently developed VEGF inhibitor that has been approved for use in the United States for treatment of metastatic CRC that has failed other modalities.[301,302] Recently immunotherapy with checkpoint inhibitors (nivolumab and pembrolizumab that inhibit PD1 and ipilimumab that inhibits CTLA-4) have shown a favorable clinical response in patients with MSI CRC.[297] Both single-agent nivolumab and pembrolizumab are now FDA approved for metastatic MSI CRC (approximately 4% of all metastatic CRCs), and oxaliplatin- and irinotecan-based regimens are progressing.[303] Whether the benefits of these agents can be transferred to the larger group of metastatic MSS CRCs is currently under investigation.[303]

Investigational Agents

In addition to the aforementioned agents, a number of other chemotherapeutic and biological compounds are under investigation and development (Table 27.11). Several of these agents have proven successful in treating other malignancies. Approximately 5% to 10% of metastatic CRCs harbor the *BRAF* mutation involving V600E. *BRAF* inhibition with vemurafenib or dabrafenib has not been shown to be beneficial as a single-agent therapy; however, there are early promising results when either agent forms part of combination therapy.[303] Up to 7% of CRCs show amplification of HER2. Unfortunately, single therapy with HER2 receptor agonists trastuzumab or lapatinib has not proved to be effective in HER2-amplified xenografts; however, combination therapy using both agents does appear useful in early clinical trials.[304] Fusions in the genes encoding for tropomyosin receptor kinase (TRK) proteins occur in 0.2% to 2.4% of metastatic CRCs and are therefore potential targets for agents such as larotrectinib.[303] One study with small numbers of TRK fusion–positive metastatic CRC has demonstrated apparent benefit.[305] The current status of treatment approaches and ongoing clinical trials are summarized in Table 27.11.

Role of Stage and Pathological Factors in Management

Colon Cancer

Stage I disease (T1/T2 N0 M0) is managed by resection alone, and these patients are not usually offered adjuvant chemotherapy. The management of the commonly encountered situation of invasive malignancy found to be arising in an endoscopically removed polyp is discussed later.

The use of adjuvant therapy in stage II disease is variable and has been the subject of some controversy.[12,307,308] In general, chemotherapy is not offered to patients with low-risk stage II disease (T3 N0 M0 and absence of high-risk features). Adjuvant therapy is typically offered to patients with high-risk stage II disease, which is defined by the presence of poor differentiation (after exclusion of MSI), lymphatic or vascular invasion, bowel obstruction, fewer than 12 lymph nodes examined, perineural invasion, localized perforation, close, indeterminate, or positive margins, or any T4 disease.[153,308,309]

In stage III disease (lymph node positive), adjuvant chemotherapy is widely used.[308] In this setting, regimens containing 5-FU result in a reduction of recurrence rate by 17% and a 13% to 15% increase in overall survival.[310] Capecitabine has a similar efficacy.[12] Many large studies have found that disease-free survival and overall survival are improved when oxaliplatin is added to a fluoropyrimidine in the adjuvant setting. However, as discussed earlier, this is probably only true in patients younger than 70 years of age.[311-313] This combination of drugs is now considered the standard choice for patients who do not participate in new cancer trials and in whom they can be tolerated. In large randomized trials, no benefit has been identified for the addition of anti-EGFR or anti-VEGF therapies in controlled clinical trials in the adjuvant setting.[314,315]

In patients with stage IV disease (Dukes stage D, distant metastases), the added benefit of chemotherapy is firmly established.[153,316] At present, most patients are offered a combination of 5-FU, oxaliplatin, and either anti-VEGF therapy (bevacizumab), an anti-EGFR agent (cetuximab or panitumumab), or a checkpoint inhibitor (nivolumab or pembrolizumab), with the choice depending on MMR status and *KRAS* mutation status (see previous discussion).[153,308]

TABLE 27.11 Therapeutic Approaches in the Treatment of Metastatic Colorectal Carcinoma Currently Under Investigation [306]

Treatment Approach	Nature of Agent	Example
Immunotherapy	Checkpoint inhibitors	Atezolizumab
	Viruses and vaccines (prevention and therapy)	Vaccines against CEA and MUC1 both delivered via an adenovirus
	Immunomodulators	CAR-T cell therapy directed against CEA, HER2 receptor, EGFR, or CRC-associated *KRAS* mutation Tumor microenvironment modulators including CD73, adenosine, TLR9, CCR2, and CCR5
Targeted therapies	Tyrosine kinase inhibitors	MEK1/2 inhibitors (e.g., binimetinib) MAPK inhibitors (e.g., cobimetinib) RAF inhibitors (e.g., donafenib, encorafenib) Multikinase inhibitors (e.g., famitinib)
	Receptor modulators (upregulate or downregulate targeted receptors)	NOTCH transcription complex (e.g., CB-103) EP4 prostaglandin receptor blocker (e.g., grapiprant) Wnt signaling pathway inhibitor (e.g., PORCN)
	Epigenetic modulators (regulation of gene expression via DNA methylation, histone modification, chromatin remodeling, and noncoding RNAs)	DNA methyltransferase inhibition (e.g., guadecitabine); causes genome-wide hypermethylation and is useful in MSS, CIMP-H, and CRC
	Monoclonal antibodies	New agents targeting EGFR and HER2. Many of these represent antibody-drug conjugates to better deliver cytotoxic agents. New VEGFR inhibitors

**This table is meant to represent the array of targets and compounds currently being tested in phase II and phase III trials in colorectal cancer and is not meant to be a comprehensive listing of investigational new agents.*

CAR-T cell therapy, *Chimeric-antigen receptor T-cell therapy;* CEA, *carcinoembryonic antigen;* CIMP-H, *high-frequency CpG island methylator phenotype;* CRC, *colorectal cancer;* EGFR, *epidermal growth factor receptor;* MSS, *microsatellite stable;* VEGFR, *epidermal growth factor receptor.*

Rectal Cancer

The treatment approach to rectal cancer has significant differences with the treatment of colon cancer. Stage II/III disease is now often managed by a combination of preoperative chemoradiation, TME, and postoperative fluoropyrimidines. Although trials are ongoing, current data do not support the addition of other types of agents to this treatment regimen.[317-319] Transanal endoscopic microsurgery (TEM) and transanal minimally invasive surgery (TAMIS) are appropriate for localized superficially invasive rectal carcinomas (T1 N0) in which complete local resection can be obtained.[320] Local resection is only appropriate for T1 N0 early-stage cancers that are small (<3 cm), well-differentiated to moderately differentiated tumors, within 8 cm of the anal verge and limited to <30% of the rectal circumference, in which there is no evidence of nodal involvement.[319]

T1 Colorectal Carcinoma (Malignant Colorectal Polyp)

Most stage I colon cancer presents when an endoscopically resected polyp is found to contain submucosal invasive carcinoma. In most cases, the polyp also contains a preexisting adenoma; however, occasionally no residual precursor lesion is identified (polypoidal carcinoma). Because of the low risk of lymph node metastases, overall approximately 5% to 10%, localized resection (polypectomy) is curative therapy in most cases. Several pathological features have been consistently shown to predict a significantly higher risk for regional lymph node metastases or local recurrence in the wall of the large intestine that warrants surgical resection. These high-risk features include large tumor size/invasive tumor depth, poor differentiation, tumor budding, margin involvement, lymphatic invasion (LI), or venous invasion (VI).[321-327] The more adverse features that are present, the higher the risk for metastatic disease.[325,328] Invasive tumor size has been mostly studied in terms of depth of submucosal invasion. For sessile polyps, Kikuchi levels, representing an approximately equal division of the submucosa into thirds; superficial (200 to 300 μm), mid, and deep levels sm1, sm2, and sm3, respectively, were initially applied.[329] In one well-designed study, the rate of lymph node metastases was 3% when carcinoma was confined to level sm1, 8% for level sm2, and 23% for level sm3.[330] For pedunculated polyps with a clearly evident stalk, Haggitt levels were initially used, with level 1 representing invasion confined to the head of the polyp, level 2 representing invasion to the junction between the head and stalk ("neck of polyp"), level 3 representing invasion into the stalk, and level 4 representing invasion into the native submucosa. Cases with level 3 and level 4 invasion were identified as being at risk for metastatic spread.[331] Use of Kikuchi levels and Haggitt levels have undergone refinement over time, and the approach of direct measurement of depth of invasion is now more widely studied and used. For sessile polyps, a depth of invasion of < 1 mm (<1000 μm), corresponding to Kikuchi levels sm1 and sm2 invasion, represent low-risk lesions, while depth of invasion ≥2 mm, corresponding to sm3 invasion, is associated with an acceptably high risk for metastatic spread.[323,332,333] In assessing depth of invasion, only the extent of submucosal invasion is relevant, so measurements are made from the lowest edge of the muscularis mucosae, unless the muscularis mucosae

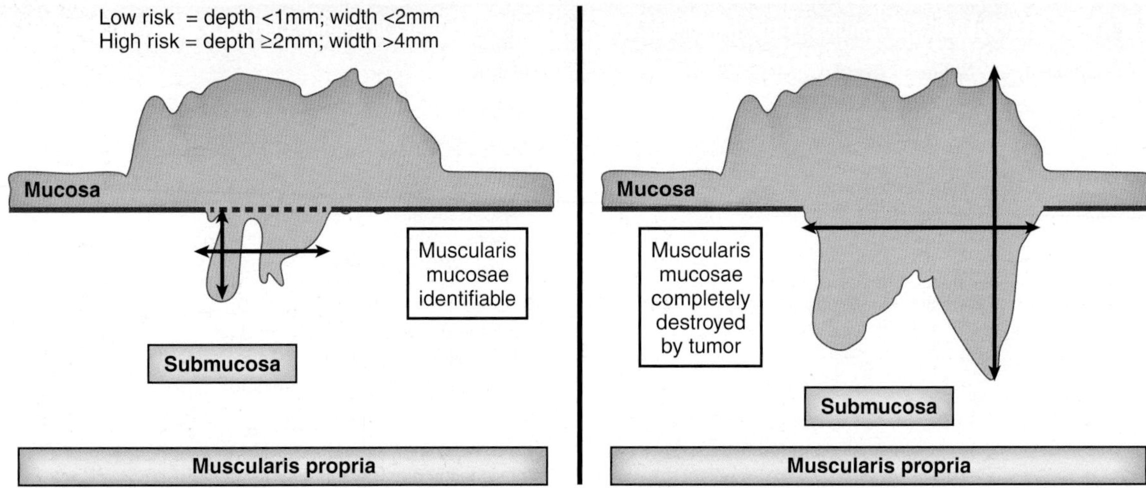

FIGURE 27.36 Method for measuring tumor width and depth in a sessile polyp containing invasive malignancy.

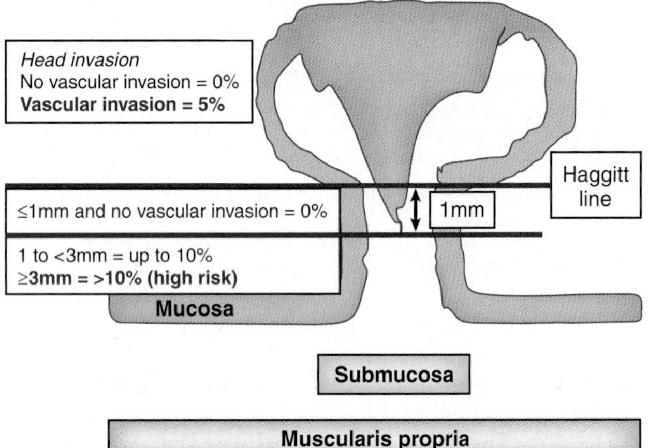

FIGURE 27.37 Method for measuring tumor depth in a pedunculated polyp containing invasive malignancy and the risk for lymph node metastases.

has been entirely destroyed by the invasive tumor, in which case the tumor thickness from surface to greatest point of invasion is measured (Fig. 27.36). For pedunculated polyps, invasion into the head of the polyp has no risk for metastases except when accompanied by vascular invasion.[333] Invasion into the stalk or beyond the stalk, corresponding to Haggitt levels 3 and 4, respectively, for >3 mm (≥3000 μm), represents a point at which the risk of metastases is unacceptably high, and surgical resection is recommended (Fig. 27.37).[333] Invasion into the stalk of a pedunculated polyp for <1 mm has negligible metastatic risk unless vascular invasion is identified, when the risk for lymph node metastases increases to approximately 5%.[333] Invasive tumor width also appears to be an important predictor of lymph node metastasis risk. Width <2 mm is rarely associated with metastatic disease, while width of ≥4 mm represents a high-risk feature.[325,332] Vascular invasion is identified in approximately 20% of malignant polyps, and several meta-analyses have identified this feature as the most important risk factor predicting disease spread and therefore the most significant factor in terms of determining the need for further treatment.[324,334] Poor tumor differentiation is present in approximately 10% of malignant polyps, and the presence of any poorly differentiated area is predictive for adverse behavior.[327] Certain tumor types are automatically considered high grade, such as signet ring cell carcinoma and neuroendocrine carcinoma. The latter is particularly likely to be associated with lymph node metastasis.[325] Patterns of dedifferentiation also represent a high-risk feature. The best studied of these is tumor budding, which is identified in approximately 10% to 20% of early CRCs and has been identified as a significant risk factor in multiple studies.[327,335] The risk is confined to International Tumor Budding Consensus Conference (ITBCC) grades BD2 and BD3.[326] Although less studied, the presence of poorly differentiated clusters probably serves as a similar high-risk marker.[336] Involvement of the polypectomy margin is associated with both recurrence at the local site and an increased risk for metastatic disease.[324,337] However, when the carcinoma does not directly involve the resection margin, there is no significant risk for metastatic disease in the absence of other adverse factors. Although some studies have concluded that the risk for local recurrence only exists when the margin or zone of diathermy artefact is directly involved by carcinoma,[328] others have shown a significant risk for residual disease at the polypectomy site when clearance is <1 mm.[338] There is general agreement that a polypectomy margin of ≥2 mm is not associated with local recurrence risk at the resection site.[322] Other factors that may influence the risk for a malignant polyp include polyp morphology, with sessile polyps being more commonly associated with risk for local recurrence and metastatic spread than pedunculated polyps.[324] Location of the malignant polyp in the distal one-third of the rectum has been identified in several studies as an adverse factor, although the reason for this is unclear.[330,338] Unfortunately, at this site the decision is often a balance between the high risk for metastasis and the higher-risk surgery that is required. Per-anal full-thickness excision followed by adjuvant chemoradiation may be an alternative at this site.[339] Histopathology clearly plays a critical role in triaging patients into those whose polyp has been adequately treated by endoscopic resection alone and those whose adenocarcinoma exhibits features with a significant risk for local recurrence at the site or spread to regional lymph nodes that would be better served by oncological resection. Box 27.17 summarizes

BOX 27.17 Pathological Features to Report in a Colorectal Polyp Containing Invasive Malignancy

Tumor site

Tumor type

Differentiation

Depth of invasion*

Haggitt level (in pedunculated polyps)

Width of invasion

Tumor budding

Vascular invasion

Margin status (millimeters from the margin or "indeterminate" if it is a piecemeal resection)

Mismatch repair immunohistochemistry†

* *Depth below muscularis mucosae in sessile polyps. Depth into the stalk of pedunculated polyps.*

† *Detection of Lynch syndrome may affect the decision for surgery and the extent of resection.*

the features that should be included in the histopathology report, and Table 27.12 provides data on the approximate risk of each factor for regional lymph node spread.

PROGNOSTIC FACTORS

Prognostic factors in CRC may be considered under the following general categories (Table 27.13):

1. Factors related to the patient, such as age, socioeconomic class, and comorbidities
2. Factors related to the appropriate medical diagnosis and treatment of CRC, for instance, the quality of surgery in rectal carcinoma and the detection of sufficient lymph nodes at the time of pathological dissection
3. Factors that are identified by the pathologist, such as extent of tumor invasion, vascular space invasion, and presence of lymph node metastases
4. The presence of molecular changes within the tumor cells that influence the biological aggressiveness of the tumor and its potential response to treatment. Identification of these molecular changes and characterization of the associated risk and potential for

TABLE 27.12 Features Associated with an Increased Risk of Lymph Node Metastases in Stage T1 Colorectal Carcinoma

Feature	Prevalence of Feature	Rate of Lymph Node Metastasis*	Relative Risk for Lymph Node Metastasis	Odds Ratio for Lymph Node Metastasis
Sessile polyp depth ≥2 mm	~60%	~5%	2.5×	3×
Pedunculated polyp with stalk invasion ≥3 mm	Insufficient data	~10%	Insufficient data	Insufficient data
Vascular invasion	~20%	~10%	5×	5×
Poor differentiation	~5-10%	~10%	5×	5×
Tumor budding (BD2/3)	~10–20%	~5%	5×	7×
Resection margin involvement+	~30%	~5%	Insufficient data	Insufficient data
≥1 of: margin involvement/vascular invasion and/or poor differentiation	~40%	~10%		2.5×

**Overall rate observed in studies with this feature reported. Does not account for the concurrent presence of other risk factors.*

+Margin directly involved or undefined.

Data from Brockmoeller SF, West NP. Predicting systemic spread in early colorectal cancer: Can we do better? World J Gastroenterol. *2019;25(23):2887-2897; Beaton C, Twine CP, Williams GL, Radcliffe AG. Systematic review and meta-analysis of histopathological factors influencing the risk of lymph node metastasis in early colorectal cancer.* Colorectal Dis. *2013;15(7):788-797; Hassan C, Zullo A, Risio M, Rossini FP, Morini S. Histologic risk factors and clinical outcome in colorectal malignant polyp: a pooled-data analysis.* Dis Colon Rectum. *2005;48(8):1588-1596; Hashiguchi Y, Muro K, Saito Y, et al. Japanese Society for Cancer of the Colon and Rectum (JSCCR) guidelines 2019 for the treatment of colorectal cancer.* Int J Clin Oncol. *2020;25(1):1-42; Bosch SL, Teerenstra S, de Wilt JH, Cunningham C, Nagtegaal ID. Predicting lymph node metastasis in pT1 colorectal cancer: a systematic review of risk factors providing rationale for therapy decisions.* Endoscopy. *2013;45(10):827-834.*

TABLE 27.13 Overview of Prognostic Factors in Colorectal Carcinoma

Patient Factors	Treatment Factors	Pathological Factors	Molecular Factors	Immunological Factors
Age Sex Socioeconomic status Comorbidity	Surgical Oncological	TNM stage Venous invasion Perineural invasion Tumor subtype	MSI status CMS *KRAS, BRAF, NRAS* mutations Chromosomal abnormality, microRNA	Immunoscore PD-L1 status

response to therapy has become an important part of the pathologist's role in colorectal cancer management;

5. A more recent development is the impact of the immune environment in which the tumor resides.[340] Patient and treatment-related factors are beyond the scope of this textbook and will not be discussed further.

Pathological Prognostic Factors

Pathological Staging

The anatomic extent of tumor spread (pathological tumor stage) is the most important predictor of tumor behavior and outcome for patients with CRC. The TNM staging system, which has replaced the Dukes system and associated modification,[341] is the most widely used system in North America and is outlined in detail in the following sections.[2]

Depth of Tumor Invasion and Peritoneal Involvement

The prognosis of patients with CRC is directly proportional to the depth of invasion and is defined in the T classification of the TNM staging system. As noted previously, the TNM staging of CRC includes *Tis,* a staging term used both for high-grade dysplasia and for intramucosal (lamina propria) invasion including invasion into but not through the muscularis mucosae. In practice, these lesions are best reported as *high-grade dysplasia* to distinguish them from *invasive adenocarcinoma,* which refers to tumors with submucosal invasion (pT1). Tumors that invade into the muscularis propria are stage pT2, and those that invade through the muscularis propria into subserosal adipose tissue or the nonperitonealized pericolic or perirectal soft tissue are stage T3. The extent of tumor invasion beyond the muscularis propria strongly influences prognosis. Substratification of pT3 according to the distance of tumor invasion beyond the outer border of the muscularis propria (pT3a, <1 mm; pT3b, 1 to 5 mm; pT3c, 5 to 15 mm; and pT3d, >15 mm) is significantly related to prognosis; however, it does not currently form part of the TNM staging system.[2]

When tumors invade beyond the muscularis propria, they may penetrate the visceral peritoneum (pT4a) or invade or adhere to adjacent structures (pT4b). Penetration of the visceral peritoneum (serosal involvement) is associated with a significant risk of peritoneal carcinomatosis, and this is an important adverse prognostic factor in patients with CRC.[342-344] Some studies have shown that the presence of localized peritoneal involvement in apparently curative surgical resections independently predicts pelvic recurrence and diminished survival.[344,345] As such, peritoneal involvement is considered an indication for adjuvant therapy in stage II disease, and it must be explicitly reported as positive or negative. However, interpretation of the status of invasion of the peritoneum can be difficult.[346,347] Sections should be taken to show the closest distance of tumor to the serosa, particularly targeting those areas of serosa that appear firm, irregular, or roughened or show prominent vascularity (Fig. 27.38A). The point of reflection of the serosa from the antimesenteric onto the mesenteric aspect of the colon is particularly vulnerable to penetration by tumor. A variety of histological definitions for peritoneal penetration have been used, and this has led to increased interobserver variability.[347,348] Additionally, there is evidence that carcinoma within 1 mm of the serosal surface is associated with a higher rate of peritoneal recurrence.[349] Currently to diagnose peritoneal penetration (pT4a), the tumor should be seen at the serosal surface with associated findings that may include inflammation, mesothelial hyperplasia, erosion, or ulceration (see Fig. 27.38B). [347,348] The use of elastic tissue stains to highlight the peritoneal elastic lamina has been investigated as a potential diagnostic aid. In some of these studies, pT3 tumors demonstrating invasion through the peritoneal elastic lamina were associated with a significantly poorer survival.[350] Unfortunately, the peritoneal elastic lamina is in part an incomplete layer or is thin and difficult to appreciate in elastic tissue stains. This is particularly true for the right side of the colon and effectively precludes any benefit from routine application of these stains.[351] From a practical perspective, carcinoma found invading <1 mm from the serosa should be extensively sampled (at least 5 blocks)[348] and multiple levels cut if the tumor lies immediately beneath, but is not clearly breaching the mesothelial layer in the initial section.

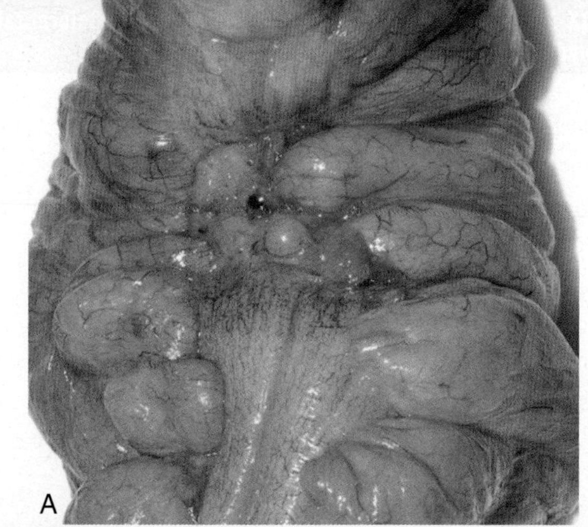

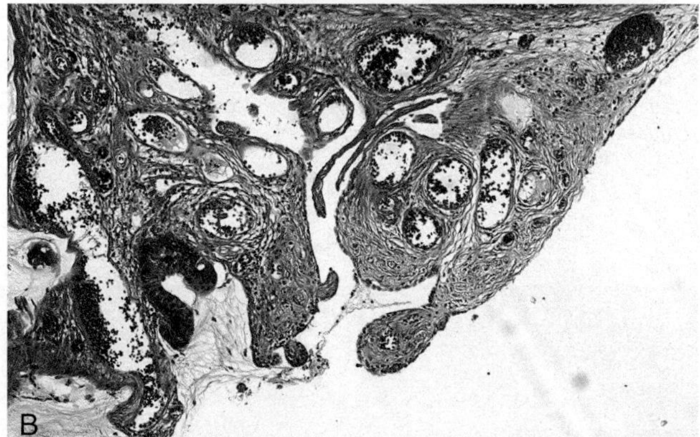

FIGURE 27.38 Serosal invasion. A, Surgical specimen showing roughening, hyperemia, and nodularity on the anterior serosal surface. **B,** Corresponding histological appearance with carcinoma invading beyond the mesothelial layer of the serosa and tumor epithelium identified on the surface.

The T4b substage is also subject to issues in interpretation. Largely, this arises when the site of tumor becomes adherent to an adjacent organ via an inflammatory perforation of a

TABLE 27.14 Features Required for Staging of Colorectal Carcinoma That Is Close to or Involves the Serosa

Stage	Feature
pT4a	• Gross perforation through tumor • Tumor cells on the serosal surface • Tumor cells at the serosal surface with associated mesothelial ulceration and/or inflammatory reaction
High-risk stage pT3	• Tumor ≤1 mm from the serosal surface accompanied by mesothelial hyperplasia, granulation tissue, and fibrin • Tumor-related destruction of the peritoneal elastic lamina deep to the tumor
pT4b	• Tumor within the fibrosis adhering an organ to the colorectal site of tumor • Tumor directly invading into the wall or the parenchyma of an adjacent organ or structure • Tumor invading beyond the sphincteric muscles in the low rectum

peritumoral abscess. At the time of surgery, this appearance will be considered cT4b. Histologically, it may be difficult to determine how deep the tumor invades and whether it, in fact, breached the serosa at the site of origin. However, if tumor is found within fibrosis adhering two organs, it is currently considered to be a pT4b carcinoma, irrespective of whether the fibrosis is a reaction to the tumor invasion itself or purely a response to a peritumoral abscess. Since the latter situation is associated with a prognosis more similar to stage pT3, some suggest that only histologically confirmed invasion of tumor into the muscle wall or parenchyma of an adjacent organ or tissue should be considered stage pT4b.[352]

Lymph Node Involvement

The status of regional lymph nodes in CRC resection specimens is an important parameter used for both prognostication and management. Staging criteria are listed in Table 27.14. The eighth edition of the *AJCC Cancer Staging Manual* states that it is important to obtain at least 12 lymph nodes in colon and rectal cancer resection specimens that have not been subject to neoadjuvant therapy.[2] Although this has become a widely used indicator for assessing the quality of resection specimens, it has also become clear that there should be no upper limit to the number of lymph nodes found in a given resection specimen.[353,354] Furthermore, there is evidence that CRC patients who have more lymph nodes identified do better than those in whom it is difficult to identify lymph nodes.[355,356] The reason for this is uncertain, but it may relate to factors such as quality of surgery, mechanical blockage of tumor spread by lymph nodes, or a higher lymph node count reflecting a more intense immune reaction to the carcinoma.[350] Reasons for a low lymph node count may include the skill of the prosector and factors related to patients themselves. For instance, fewer lymph nodes are found in obese and elderly patients[357] and in those who have received neoadjuvant therapy,[358] whereas more lymph nodes are found in MSI tumors[359,360] and in female patients.[361]

The ratio of involved nodes to the total number of nodes has emerged as a potential prognostic factor. Lymph node ratio is defined as the ratio of the number of positive nodes to the total number of harvested nodes. It is a significant prognostic feature in stage III CRC, when a high ratio predicts both poor overall survival and disease-free survival. The predictive value of this factor appears to be higher than the nodal stage alone.[362-364]

In some studies, lymph node metastases distant from the primary tumor are associated with a poorer outcome. For the TNM classification, the definition of *regional lymph nodes* varies according to the location of the primary tumor, although external iliac and common iliac lymph node metastases are always classified as M1.[2]

A *micrometastasis* is defined as a lymph node tumor deposit that measures >0.2 mm but ≤2 mm in size. These are classified as pN1(mic) or as pM1(mic) when the lymph nodes are nonregional.[2] A recent meta-analysis has confirmed the prognostic significance of micrometastases.[365] *Isolated tumor cells* are defined as single tumor cells, or small clusters of tumor cells, that measure ≤0.2 mm. At present, the clinical significance of this finding is uncertain, and the current recommendation is that they be recorded as N0.[2]

Acellular mucin deposits are not infrequently found in lymph nodes draining rectal carcinoma that has been treated by preoperative neoadjuvant therapy. In the absence of viable neoplastic cells, this finding is regarded as representing tumor regression and does not register in the T or N stage.[366-368] Rarely a situation is encountered in which acellular mucin is found in a lymph node draining a treatment-naive CRC. There is some evidence to regard this finding as an involved lymph node.[369] Certainly, multiple sections are required in this situation to exclude the presence of a small amount of neoplastic epithelium.

Extension of metastatic tumor beyond the lymph node capsule is referred to as *extracapsular spread*. This finding is associated with a significantly increased all-cause mortality and recurrence of disease and should be recorded in the histopathology report.[370]

Tumor Deposits

Interpretation and classification of tumor deposits in the adventitia of the colon that lack identifiable residual lymph node tissue has been problematic, and various definitions have been used in various editions of the *AJCC Cancer Staging Manual* (Fig. 27.39). The seventh edition created a new subcategory, *pN1c*, for tumors without lymph node metastases, but with at least one tumor deposit present. They were defined as irregular, discrete deposits of tumor in the pericolic or perirectal fat, away from the leading edge of the tumor, without evidence of residual lymph node tissue and within the regional lymphatic drainage of the tumor. The definition was further refined in the eighth edition by excluding tumor deposits associated with an identifiable vessel wall or nerve, which are now considered as vascular invasion or perineural invasion, respectively.[2] Demonstration of an associated vascular structure often requires special stains. Unfortunately, concordance between pathologists as to what constitutes a tumor deposit is poor.[371] Because the finding of tumor deposits is associated with poorer prognosis,[372-374] their presence is recorded in the N category as N1c, and the total number of deposits should be recorded in the

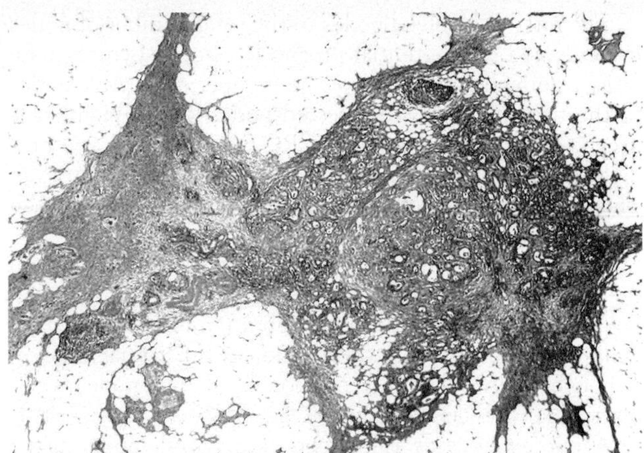

FIGURE 27.39 Pericolonic deposit consistent with venous invasion. The deposit is irregular in shape, showing tumor that extends along connective tissue septa. In addition, residual smooth muscle is shown within the deposit, consistent with the wall of a vein.

TABLE 27.15 Clues That Aid in Separation of Tumor Deposits into Either Lymph Node Metastasis, Perineural or Venous Invasion, or Tumor Deposit

Nature of Deposit	Diagnostic Clue
Lymph node metastasis	Thick capsule Subcapsular sinus Lymphoid tissue present (sometimes a rim of lymphocytes) Round shape
Perineural invasion	Presence in association with neurovascular bundle Nerve demonstrable
Venous invasion	Accompanying artery Vessel wall in continuity (may require deeper levels) Special stains reveal vessel wall (e.g., elastic stains)
Tumor deposit (N1c)	Round outline with no features of the above

pathology report. Five or more tumor deposits have been associated with particularly poor survival.[375] The N1c categorization is used only when there are no identifiable concurrent lymph node deposits. Histological features that aid the separation of tumor deposits into either lymph node metastases or venous and/or perineural invasion are summarized in Table 27.15. There is some debate as to the distance from the invasive edge of the carcinoma that isolated tumor collections must reside before they can be considered a tumor deposit.[375] This issue remains unresolved, but for practical purposes no minimum distance from the invasive edge is required.[2]

Histological Grade

The importance of histological grading as a prognostic factor is supported by the consistent finding of independent statistical significance in studies with multivariate analyses.[113,330] Grading is one of the most widely used pathological variables, but it is also one of the most difficult to define accurately. Use of a two-tiered system of low grade and high grade is recommended and endorsed by the WHO and AJCC.[1,2] This system replaces the traditional classification of well-differentiated, moderately differentiated, and poorly differentiated tumors. It is more reproducible because well-differentiated and moderately differentiated carcinomas behave similarly. Furthermore, well-differentiated tumors make up only a small fraction of tumors in most series. Grading is based on the proportion of tumor composed of glands relative to areas that are solid or composed of nests or cords of cells, and tumors should be classified as either low grade (well or moderately differentiated; >50% gland formation) or high grade (poorly differentiated; <50% gland formation). The WHO classification has added a further nuance by stating that grading is to be performed on the least differentiated component of the carcinoma away from the invasive edge.[1] Grading of biopsy specimens often is inaccurate and fails to reflect the final grade of the tumor in the resection specimen.

Grading of CRCs does not apply to all carcinomas. By definition, signet ring cell carcinomas, undifferentiated carcinomas, and small cell carcinomas are all highgrade. The grading of mucinous carcinomas is based on the degree of gland formation and cytological features, and it is not dependent on MMR status.[1] Tumors that show no or only minimal gland (<5%) formation are classified as *undifferentiated* and likely represent very poorly differentiated adenocarcinomas in most cases. Most importantly, medullary carcinomas should not be classified as either *poorly differentiated* or *undifferentiated* because they are associated with a more favorable overall outcome than these other tumors; medullary carcinomas should probably not be graded at all by the usual methods.[376]

A significant issue with tumor grading based on the extent of gland formation is poor concordance among pathologists.[377,378] In an attempt to produce better concordance and to better refine the prognostic relevance of tumor grade, additional or alternative morphological features have been and continue to be investigated. These factors can be broadly classified into cytological features, presence of tumor dedifferentiation, and molecular markers. The degree of cytological abnormality forms part of the grading system of adenocarcinomas of other sites, for instance, in breast carcinoma. To date, there has been little published data on the role of cytological abnormality in CRC. In one study, the finding of marked nuclear pleomorphism and anaplasia were used to upgrade conventional gland formation–based grading. This combination approach was shown to be better able to predict tumor prognosis.[379] By far, the most interest in morphological features predictive of outcome, and therefore potentially useful in any modified morphological grading system, has been in identifying tumor dedifferentiation. The best studied of these is tumor budding, which is discussed in detail later. Poorly differentiated clusters represent another form of dedifferentiation and frequently coexist with tumor budding. They are defined as clusters of ≥5 tumor cells that lack evidence of gland formation (Fig. 27.40). Poorly differentiated clusters have been shown to predict adverse outcome in all stages of CRC.[380] Because poorly differentiated clusters may be

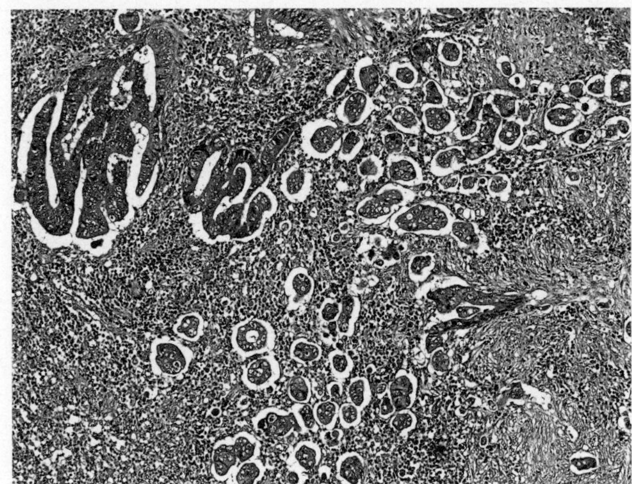

FIGURE 27.40 Poorly differentiated clusters. Clusters of five or more tumor cells that lack evidence of gland formation.

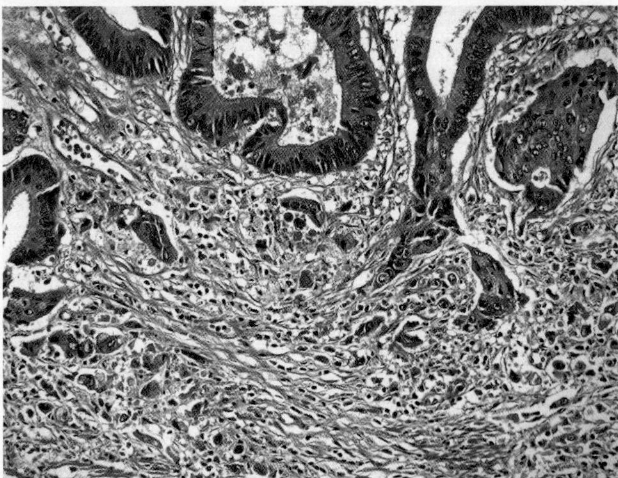

FIGURE 27.41 Tumor budding. Tiny cords and small aggregates of neoplastic epithelium (four cells or less) that detach from tumor glands at the invasive front.

associated with otherwise low-grade adenocarcinoma, their prognostic significance is lost in conventional grading. Ueno et al. proposed a modified grading system based on counting the number of poorly differentiated clusters under a ×20 objective lens in the field containing the highest number of clusters. Tumors with <5, 5 to 9, and ≥10 clusters are classified as grade 1, grade 2, and grade 3, respectively.[381] This system provides better prognostic stratification than the current AJCC grading system and has been shown to have good interobserver reproducibility.[381,382] Conceptually, poorly differentiated clusters lie intermediate in size between tumor budding and micropapillary carcinoma, with all three demonstrating a morphological continuum of tumor dedifferentiation that represents a transition in tumor cells from a cohesive epithelial phenotype to a mesenchymal phenotype possessing the capability of individual cell invasion. Indeed, poorly differentiated clusters display the same reversed polarity pattern by MUC1 immunohistochemistry as seen in micropapillary carcinoma.[383] Another feature of epithelial-to-mesenchymal transition in colorectal cancer is a distinctive peritumoral stromal response resulting from the activation of stromal fibroblasts and the extracellular matrix produced. Several studies have identified a prognostic significance and a potential benefit of a grading system in documenting the presence of this immature stromal reaction that results in keloid collagen and/or abundant myxoid matrix.[129,384,385] The potential role for molecular markers in assigning a clinically relevant tumor grade is discussed earlier in this chapter. At present, the expense and widespread lack of access to molecular testing preclude their use. It seems likely that any further refinement to the grading of CRC may involve a weighted addition of features in addition to extent of gland formation. This is a similar approach to a previous system for rectal cancer devised by Jass and colleagues in the 1980s that used three parameters: lymphocytic infiltration, tubule configuration, and pattern of growth— infiltrative versus expansive.[386]

Tumor Budding

Tumor budding is defined as the presence of tiny cords and small aggregates of neoplastic epithelium (four cells or less) that detach from tumor glands at the invasive front and appear to migrate into adjacent desmoplastic stroma[387] (Fig. 27.41). Tumor budding is present in 20% to 40% of all CRCs.[388] It appears to represent a manifestation of an epithelial-to-mesenchymal transition in the malignant cells.[389,390] The mesenchymal phenotype is characterized by increased migratory capacity, invasiveness, increased resistance to apoptosis, and increased production of extracellular matrix (ECM) components.[388] Pseudopodic extensions from the cytoplasm of the cells within tumor buds have been demonstrated in ultrastructural studies, adding evidence to the mechanism of tumor cell migration. Most recently, transcriptome profiling studies have linked the finding of prominent tumor budding to the mesenchymal subtype (CMS-4) of CRC.[389,391] Tumor budding is now a well-established independent poor prognostic feature in CRC.[387,392-394]

The clinical usefulness of this prognostic feature resides in two settings. The first is in pT1 tumors arising in polyps ("malignant polyps"). In this setting, tumor budding has been associated with increased risk of lymph node metastasis in multiple studies and hence is an important factor to consider in the decision for further surgical treatment.[323,328,395-397] The second situation is in stage II colorectal cancer (pT3/pT4 pN0). In this setting, the presence of tumor budding has been found to predict for a similar prognostic outcome to stage III CRC.[335,398-402] As such, patients with stage II CRC and high-grade tumor budding may benefit from adjuvant chemotherapy.

However, an important issue has been the lack of a standardized method of assessing the degree of tumor budding. To address this, an international consensus has recently proposed uniform reporting guidelines (Box 27.18).[387] It remains to be determined whether standardized reporting will improve interobserver variability in assessing tumor budding, which has ranged from only moderate up to very good, depending on the study.[212] It has been suggested that using cytokeratin immunohistochemistry may improve interobserver variability in tumor budding counts; however, this requires further assessment and is not widely practiced at the present time.[398,403]

BOX 27.18 Recommendations for Reporting Tumor in Budding in Colorectal Carcinoma Based on the 2016 International Tumor Budding Consensus Conference

METHOD FOR ASSESSING TUMOR BUDDING

- Identify the presence of tumor budding at scanning power.
- Scan up to 10 fields at 10× to identify the field with the highest budding density "hot spot."
- Count the number of tumor buds in a 20× field (area 0.785 mm^2) of the hot spot; if the 20× field area is not 0.785 mm^2, the bud count is normalized to this area.
- Grade the tumor budding.
    - 0-4 = low-level budding Bd1
    - 5-9 = intermediate-level budding Bd2
    - ≥10 = high-level budding Bd3

From Lugli A, Kirsch R, Ajioka Y, et al. Recommendations for reporting tumor budding in colorectal cancer based on the International Tumor Budding Consensus Conference (ITBCC) 2016. Mod Pathol. *2017;30(9):1299-1311.*

Histological Subtype

It is now clear from many studies that certain histological subtypes of CRC behave differently from adenocarcinoma NOS. Tumors that behave in a more aggressive fashion include signet ring cell carcinoma, micropapillary adenocarcinoma, carcinomas with a rhabdoid or sarcomatoid component, high-grade neuroendocrine carcinoma, and undifferentiated carcinoma. Tumors with more indolent behavior include medullary carcinoma, adenoma-like carcinoma, and most MSI carcinomas.

Proximal and Distal Resection Margins

The existence of positive resection margins implies the presence of residual tumor in the patient. This situation has led to the residual tumor classification system, whereby R0 indicates no residual tumor, R1 indicates microscopic residual tumor (tumor at the margin or < 1 mm from the margin), and R2 indicates macroscopic residual tumor.[107]

Radial Resection Margin and Total Mesorectal Excision

In recent years, much attention has been paid to proper pathological documentation of the radial (circumferential) margin status in rectal carcinoma, but proper assessment of the radial margin is also important in colonic carcinomas. As described earlier, all colonic cancer resections have a radial resection margin, and, depending on the anatomic location, this may be represented by a posterior bare area or by vascular ties on the mesocolon or mesentery. The radial margin in right colon cancer resections is positive in as many as 10% of cases, and failure to adequately assess these margins may explain tumor recurrence in some of these patients.[404,405]

Awareness of the importance of the circumferential radial margin in CRC has altered both the management and pathological assessment of rectal cancer resection specimens (see Gross Features and Specimen Handling). In 1986, Quirke and coworkers[406] first described the importance of lateral spread and the role of involvement of the radial margin in predicting recurrence of rectal cancer. After slicing the unopened rectal resection specimens serially and analyzing whole-mount sections, positive radial resection margins were found in 14 (27%), and recurrent tumors developed in 12 of these 14 patients.[406] These results were confirmed in larger studies in which positive radial margins predicted not only local recurrence but survival.[407,408] These findings have importance not only for accurate pathological assessment but for surgical management. For instance, Heald and coworkers[409] have long been proponents of surgery that includes TME, which involves a sharp dissection of the entire mesorectum along the finely delimited fascial plane. This procedure removes 2 to 3 cm of perirectal soft tissue (the mesorectal envelope), preserves the pelvic fascia and autonomic plexuses, and represents a significant departure from the usual type of blunt dissection formerly performed by most general surgeons. The clinical effectiveness of TME has been well established.[410-412] It has also been realized that the effectiveness of TME is not simply the result of prevention of positive margins but of the removal of unrecognized tumor deposits that are often located deep within the perirectal adipose tissue.[413]

TABLE 27.16 Relationship Between Outcome and Distance of Tumor to the Radial Margin in Rectal Cancer

Distance to Radial Margin (cm)	Local Recurrence (%)	Distant Recurrence (%)	2-Year Survival (%)
<0.10	16.4	37.6	69.7
0.11-0.20	14.9	21.0	84.8
0.21-0.50	10.3	17.2	87.0
0.51-1.0	6.0	8.2	91.2
>1.0	2.4	10.9	92.8

Data from Nagtegaal ID, van der Velde CJH, van der Worp E, et al. Macroscopic evaluation of rectal cancer resection specimen: clinical significance of the pathologist in quality control. J Clin Oncol. *2002;20(7):1729-1734.*

Results from the Dutch TME trial showed that even when the radial margin is negative, the distance (in millimeters) from the deepest point of tumor penetration to the margin is predictive of local and distant recurrence[414] (Table 27.16). Based on these data, it is recommended that pathologists provide an exact measurement of the distance of the tumor to the radial margin in pathology reports. The Dutch studies have also helped outline specific criteria for assessing completeness of TME specimens (see Gross Features and Specimen Handling).[109,110] In the Dutch series, approximately 55% of TMEs were complete, 20% were nearly complete, and 25% were incomplete. For cases in which the radial margin is negative, this type of gross assessment is predictive of tumor recurrence.

Invasion of Endothelium-Lined Spaces

Invasion of tumor into lymphatics and thick-walled veins should be carefully sought and reported as either present or absent. VI has been defined as a rounded mass of tumor in an endothelium-lined space either surrounded by a rim of smooth muscle or containing red blood cells.[415] Extramural VI (invasion of large veins beyond the muscularis propria)

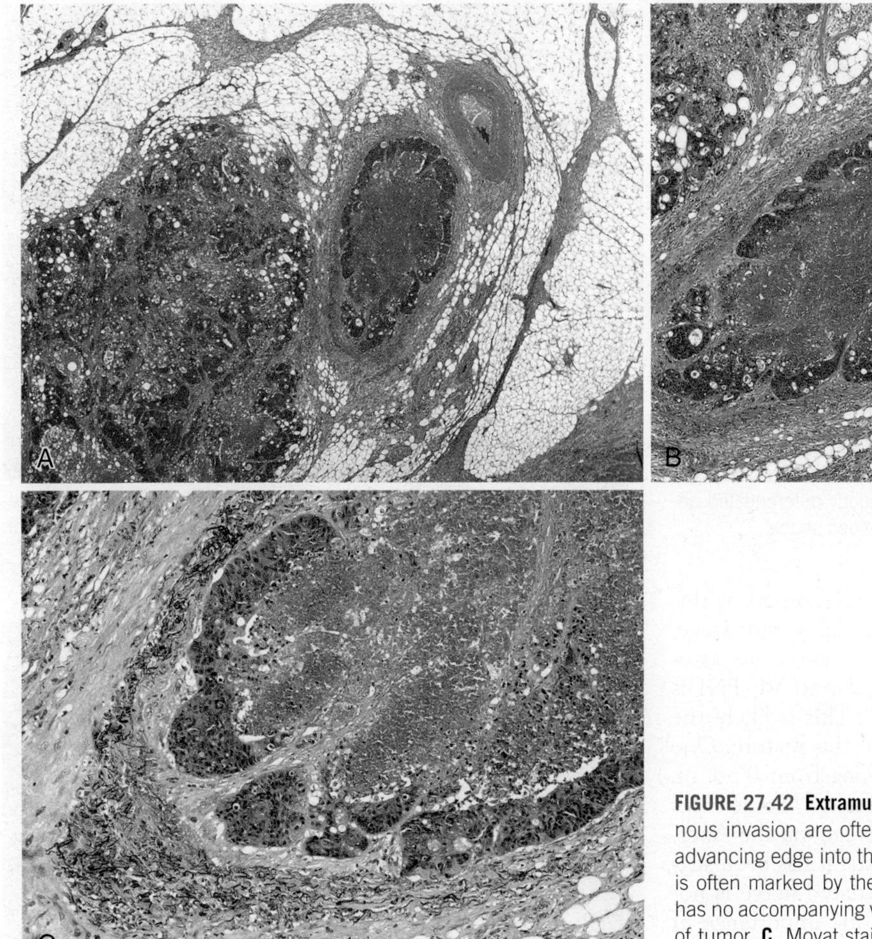
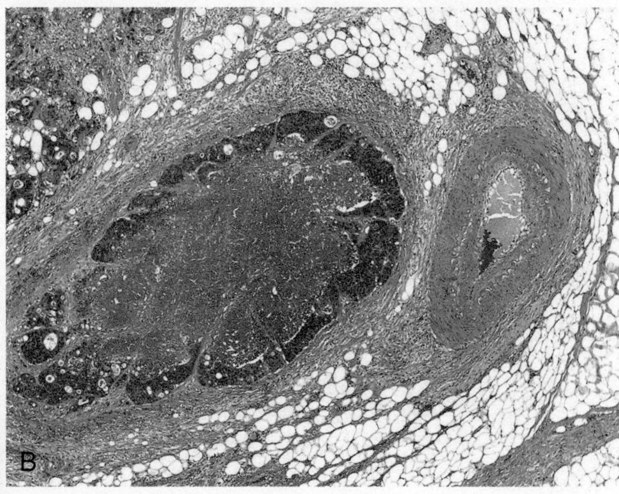

FIGURE 27.42 Extramural venous invasion. A, Foci of extramural venous invasion are often present in tongues that dip down from the advancing edge into the adjacent adipose tissue. **B,** Venous invasion is often marked by the "orphan artery" sign, wherein a large artery has no accompanying vein but instead is adjacent to a rounded focus of tumor. **C,** Movat stain highlights the elastic tissue in the vein wall surrounding the tumor.

is an independent prognostic indicator of disease recurrence and survival in CRC as demonstrated in numerous studies.[416-419] Intramural VI has also been shown to be of prognostic significance in a recent meta-analysis.[420]

Two key histopathological clues to the presence of extramural VI are the "orphan (or unaccompanied) arteriole/artery" sign and the "protruding tongue" sign (Fig. 27.42). The former is defined as a well-circumscribed tumor nodule adjacent to a thick-walled artery, without the presence of an identifiable vein; the latter is a smooth-bordered protrusion of tumor into the pericolic fat, usually adjacent to an artery. The protruding tongue sign often correlates grossly with linear spiculation at the advancing edge of the tumor, and such areas should be sought at gross examination. When these clues are present, an elastin stain is useful to confirm the presence of elastic fibers within the adventitia of the residual vein wall. In one study, use of an elastin stain confirmed the presence of VI in 76% of cases originally deemed equivocal on hematoxylin and eosin (H&E)-stained sections.[421] Several studies have demonstrated the utility of elastic stains in detecting VI when compared with a standard H&E stain.[422,423] Liberal use of elastic stains in the assessment of CRC is encouraged, particularly in cases equivocal for VI, and has been shown to double the detection rate of VI.[423]

Because of its strong predictive value for the development of distant metastases, pathologists should report VI separately from LI or small-vessel invasion. The colorectal dataset from the Royal College of Pathologists, United Kingdom, recommends that extramural VI should be detected in at least 30% of all resected specimens and that this figure should be the audit standard against which individual units compare their reporting outcomes.[424]

Differentiating lymphatics from small, thin-walled postcapillary venules is not always possible, hence there is a need for ambiguous terminology such as *lymphovascular invasion* (LVI) (Fig. 27.43). In some studies, LI has independent prognostic significance, particularly in patients with lymph node–negative disease.[323,397,425,426] The relationship between LI and outcome in individuals with lymph node metastases has not been as clearly ascertained, and attempts to further stratify the prognostic significance according to the location of the lymphatics in the bowel wall have also met with variable success.

Perineural Invasion

Tumor spread along nerves occurs most easily in the perineural space, but occasionally spread may occur in the epineurium or endoneurium of a nerve. All patterns of spread are generally considered together under the designation of *perineural invasion* (PNI).[427,428] Overall, this feature is found in approximately 20% of colorectal cancer resections, although

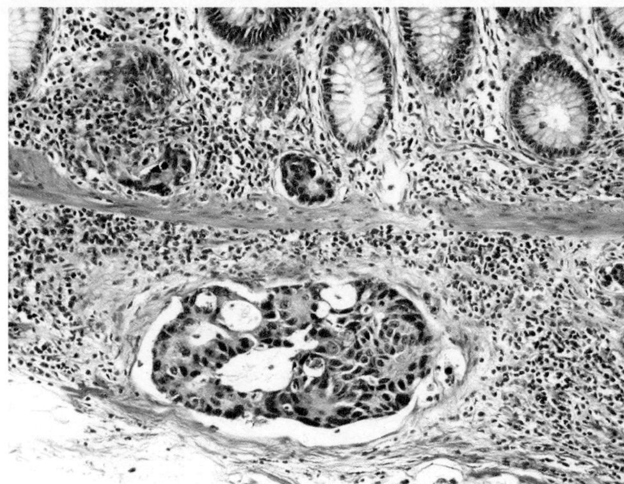

FIGURE 27.43 Lymphovascular invasion. This poorly differentiated adenocarcinoma is present within an endothelium-lined space.

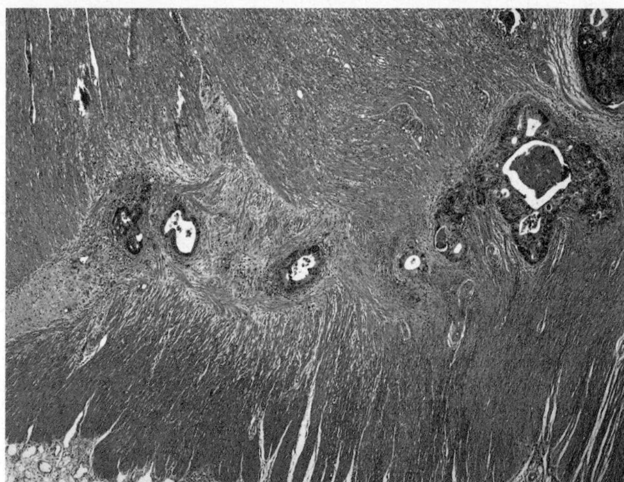

FIGURE 27.44 Perineural invasion. There is a nested pattern of intramural spread via the Auerbach plexus zone with perineural invasion seen at the edge of the photograph.

there is wide variation in prevalence in studies reporting this feature. There is general agreement that high tumor stage, poor tumor differentiation, and rectal location are associated with higher rates of PNI.[429] Similar to VI, PNI is widely underreported by pathologists.[350] This is likely the result of a lack of diligence in looking for this feature. One study has shown detection rates increasing from 0.5% on initial review to 22% following expert review.[350] Some cases show a distinct pattern of intramural spread via the Auerbach plexus zone, which is so characteristic it has been suggested that the identification of an associated nerve is not required[332,430] (Fig. 27.44). The prognostic importance of PNI has been examined in two meta-analyses of published literature, both confirming the importance of PNI for both local recurrence and survival in CRC.[429,431] It is now clear that the prognostic value of PNI is similar to that of other well-established prognostic factors in CRC, arguing that it should be a routinely reported feature.

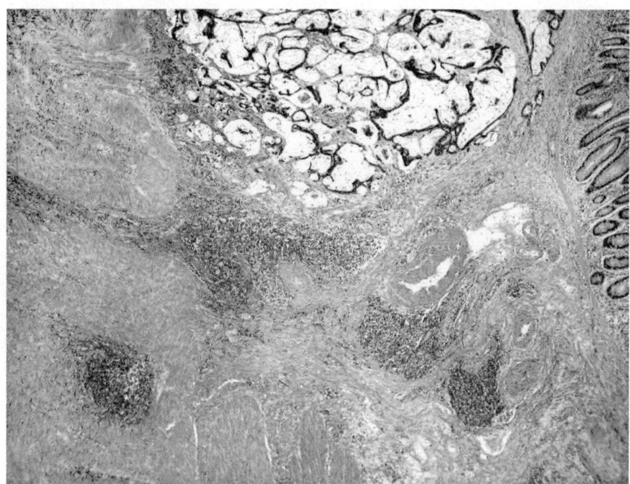

FIGURE 27.45 Peritumoral lymphoid reaction. Prominent lymphoid aggregates are located at the periphery of the tumor; some contain germinal centers.

Host Immune Response

Multiple types of inflammatory and immune reactions occur in response to CRC. In general, the presence of an intense inflammatory response of any type is associated with improved outcome.[432-434] The best studied in terms of prognostic significance are neutrophil infiltration, eosinophil infiltration, and lymphocyte infiltration. The importance of neutrophil infiltration into CRC has been the most controversial of the inflammatory patterns. Recent studies suggest that tumor-associated neutrophils can exhibit either an antitumorigenic or tumor-promoting phenotype, depending on chemical signals from surrounding tissues.[435] Tumor-promoting properties act by way of cytokines that lead to tissue destruction and angiogenesis.[435] Antitumorigenic properties are potentially mediated by several mechanisms. One example is the role of tumor-associated neutrophils in enhancing CD8+ T-cell activation and antitumor immunity.[436] Eosinophil infiltration has been shown to be an independent prognostic marker of favorable progression-free and cancer-specific survival independent of the intensity of overall inflammatory cell reaction.[437,438] The mechanism underlying this is not fully elucidated. Lymphocytic immune reactions have been the most extensively studied and are divided into several patterns: tumor-infiltrating lymphocytes, peritumoral lymphocyte infiltration, and peritumoral lymphoid aggregates (with or without germinal centers), and reactive change in regional lymph nodes (particularly paracortical hyperplasia). Historically, much attention has focused on the development of criteria that can be used to grade the degree of peritumoral lymphocytic response. Graham and Appelman[439] developed the most commonly used criteria for assessing peritumoral lymphoid reaction, which they termed *Crohn's-like lymphoid reaction*. They separated this reaction into three grades: (1) none, (2) mild, defined by the presence of occasional aggregates and scattered lymphocytes, and (3) marked, characterized by the presence of abundant lymphoid aggregates, some with germinal centers, and a prominent peritumoral band of lymphocytes (Fig. 27.45). Defined in this manner, a Crohn's disease–like lymphoid reaction has been found to have independent prognostic significance in several studies.[440-442]

Tumor-infiltrating lymphocytes have gained attention because of their association with MMR-deficient CRCs.[255] This type of immune response is characterized by the presence of lymphocytes that interdigitate between individual malignant cells. Several grading systems have been proposed; one categorizes this reaction as not present, mild, or marked (similar to the grading system used for Crohn's disease–like lymphoid reaction). Other studies have quantified lymphocytes and attempted to develop cutoff points that may be predictive of DNA MMR deficiency.[179,443] For instance, a cutoff of 5 intraepithelial lymphocytes per HPF has a sensitivity of 72% and a specificity of 82% for identification of MSI cancers.[444]

More recently, there has been an explosion of research into the role of immune-mediated responses to CRC and its relationship to molecular subtypes and, in particular, the evolving role of immunotherapy as treatment.[445,446] Tumor-infiltrating lymphocytes have also been associated with decreased likelihood of VI as well as other features of aggressive behavior, and they have been shown to be independently predictive of improved prognosis.[447-449] It is widely believed that the tumor-infiltrating lymphocytic response characteristically seen in MMR-deficient cancers may be directly responsible for the improved outcome of these tumors. Some studies have directly related the immune response to the presence of frameshift peptides in these cancers.[450,451] Others have examined scoring systems that take into account all facets of the immune response (tumor-infiltrating lymphocytes, peritumoral lymphocytes, and intratumoral stromal lymphocytes) in an attempt to provide more robust grading systems.[452] The most prominent scoring system in clinical use is the Immunoscore assay (Integrative Cancer Immunology, Paris, France), which assesses the densities of two lymphocyte populations (CD3+/CD8+) in both the center and at the edge of the tumor.[453,454] A low score on the Immunoscore assay is significantly correlated with poor overall survival.[455] Expression profiles that yield distinctive signatures of immune responses have been examined and are incorporated into the CMS classification of colon cancer, highlighting the link between molecular alteration in the tumor and the host immune reaction.[445,456] Finally, many studies have attempted to quantify T-lymphocyte subsets in the immune reaction.[457] The unifying theme of all of these investigations is a very clear correlation between immune response and prognosis, with all measures of an increased immune response predicting improved outcome.[449,454]

Invasive Margin (Leading Edge) of Tumor

As in other types of human cancer, there is histological variability in the characteristics of the leading edge of CRCs. Smooth, rounded tumors that appear to push into adjacent tissue are at one end of the spectrum, and irregular, infiltrative tumors that aggressively dissect between normal tissue planes are at the other. In the mid-1980s, the characteristics of the leading edge of tumor were found to predict prognosis.[441,458] Proposed grading criteria consisted of a two-tiered system that included both naked-eye and microscopic examination of the tissue.[441] On naked-eye examination, "infiltrating" tumors show ill-defined limits to the invasive border or loss of the host–tumor tissue interface. On microscopic examination, these tumors show "streaming dissection" of the muscularis propria, dissection of the perimuscular adipose tissue by small glands or irregular clusters of cells, or perineural invasion. "Expanding" tumors show none of these features (Fig. 27.46). With these criteria, an infiltrating margin was found to be an independent negative prognostic factor.[459] Other classifications also use a "mixed" category in which the tumoral edge is not purely pushing or purely infiltrative. This category has added utility because tumors that are predominantly pushing or expanding have also been associated with MSI phenotype.[179,255]

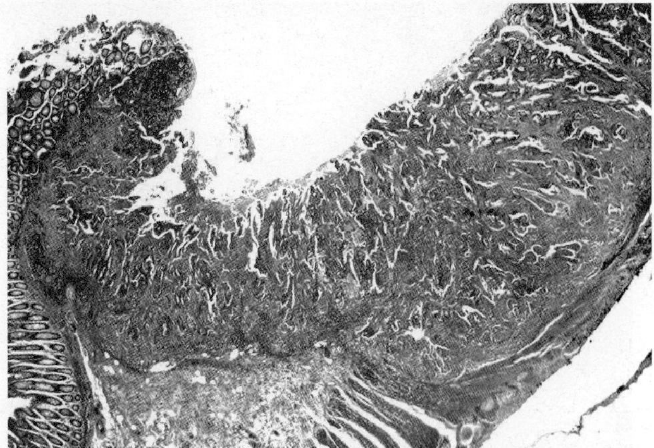

FIGURE 27.46 Pushing or expanding margin of invasion. The invasive tumor edge is smooth and round and is well demarcated from the surrounding tissue. Numerous inflammatory cells are located at the edge of the tumor.

Liver Metastases

Approximately 15% to 25% of patients with CRC have liver metastases at the time of presentation, and in another 20% metastases develop after treatment of their primary tumor.[460] Without treatment, the median survival time after detection of liver metastases is approximately 9 months.[461] There have been significant advances in surgical approaches to liver metastases, and resection of liver metastases has improved outcome in selected patients, with a 35% to 55% overall 5-year survival rate and 25% of patients surviving beyond 10 years. [462,463] However, only 10% to 20% of patients with liver metastases are considered surgical candidates.[462]

In the pathological assessment of resected liver metastases, the resection margin status is considered the most important factor.[464] A margin of less than 1 cm of the tumor was associated with significantly reduced 5-year survival rates compared with margins farther than 1 cm from the tumor.[465] A molecular analysis of tissue samples taken at varying distances from the edge of metastatic tumors showed that no tumor DNA could be detected beyond 4 mm from the tumor edge, suggesting that this extent of clearance may be adequate.[466] Other important pathological factors adversely affecting survival in resectable liver metastases include the presence of portal vein invasion, presence of perineural invasion, presence of micrometastases (small tumor clusters discrete from the main mass), and a thin (<10 layers of collagen) or absent fibrous pseudocapsule.[467] The histological response of colorectal liver metastases to

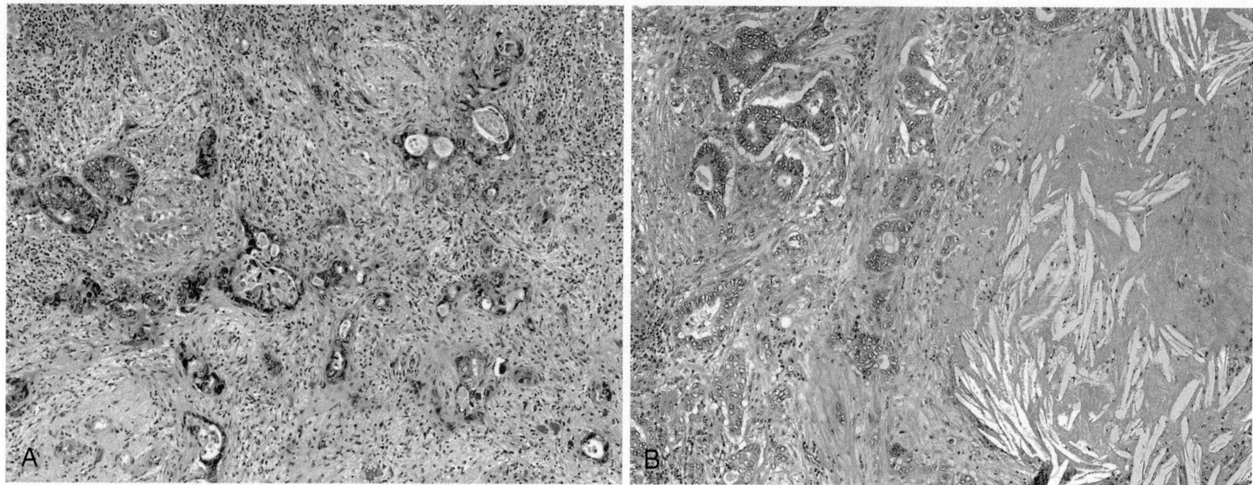

FIGURE 27.47 Metastatic colonic adenocarcinoma in the liver. A, Adenocarcinoma with dirty necrosis. **B,** Adenocarcinoma with infarct-like necrosis.

BOX 27.19 Important Factors to Include in the Histopathology Report for Metastatic Colorectal Carcinoma in the Liver

Number and size of metastases
Distance from resection margin
Presence of lymphatic or venous or perineural invasion
Biliary invasion
Presence of tumor pseudocapsule
Response to neoadjuvant chemotherapy

preoperative chemotherapy has also been shown to have prognostic value, although various methods of assessment of response have been used in each study.[467] One study showed that two different patterns of necrosis can be identified: usual neutrophil and apoptotic material-rich "dirty" necrosis and infarct-like necrosis, characterized by hyalinization, minimal inflammation, and cholesterol clefts. Infarct-like necrosis was associated with improved disease-free survival and may represent a form of therapeutic tumor response to chemotherapy (Fig. 27.47).[468]

It has been proposed that the following pathological features should be recorded in the pathology report of a resected liver metastasis (Box 27.19): number and size of liver metastases, margin distance, presence of lymphatic, venous, perineural, and biliary invasion, mucinous pattern, tumor growth pattern, presence of a tumor pseudocapsule, and pathological response to neoadjuvant chemotherapy.[469]

Peritoneal Metastases

After the liver, the peritoneum is the second most common site of nonnodal metastatic CRC. Peritoneal metastases are present at the time of diagnosis of CRC in up to 10% of patients, and the peritoneum is the site of recurrence of disease in 10% to 35%. The peritoneum is the only site of disease spread in 25% to 35% of metastatic CRCs.[470,471] Colorectal peritoneal carcinomatosis has a poor prognosis, with a median survival of only 6 months if left untreated.[472] Cytoreductive surgery combined with hyperthermic intraperitoneal chemotherapy (CRS–HIPEC) is the only potentially curative treatment option, however, approximately one-half of patients develop recurrent disease within 15 months. In a large multicenter study from the Netherlands examining the outcome of CRS-HIPEC for colorectal peritoneal carcinomatosis, 3- and 5-year survival rates were 46% and 31%, respectively, and overall median survival was 33 months.[473]

Several histological factors have been associated with a high-risk for peritoneal carcinomatosis. These include pT4 disease, pT3 mucinous or signet ring cell carcinoma, involved lymph nodes near the apical tie margin, perforation or fistula formation, and positive resection margin.[474] Recently, it has been reported that CMS4 subgroup tumors, characterized by epithelial-to-mesenchymal transition, are overrepresented in cases of colorectal peritoneal carcinomatosis, representing 70% of cases in this series.[475]

Treatment-Related Factors

Neoadjuvant Therapy for Rectal Carcinoma

In the early 1990s, studies demonstrated that combined-modality preoperative therapy (radiation and 5-FU plus leucovorin) resulted in downstaging and improved local control of rectal cancer after surgical resection.[476,477] Neoadjuvant therapy has become the treatment of choice for T3, T4, and node-positive rectal cancers; it is used in either short-course protocols (more popular in Northern Europe) or long-course protocols (more popular in North America).[319,478] Long-course protocols are preferred when the aim is downsizing of the tumor as they are associated with lower rates of involved circumferential margin at surgery. Long-course protocols are also preferred in larger tumors and distal rectal carcinomas.[12] Because these protocols are stagespecific, accurate radiological preoperative staging is important. Neoadjuvant therapy is associated with a relative risk reduction of local recurrence of 50%.[479]

The role of the pathologist in examining specimens from patients who have had preoperative chemoradiation therapy for rectal cancer is to carefully evaluate for the presence of residual primary tumor and the presence or absence of lymph node metastases. A complete pathological response (i.e., no residual tumor on pathological examination) is seen in approximately

20% of patients.[480] In one study, only 25% of complete clinical responders had a complete pathological response, and an equal proportion of complete pathological responses were found in patients who had a clinical suggestion of residual tumor (usually because of persistent fibrosis or ulceration).[481]

Posttreatment pathological staging is clinically important because downstaging (compared with preoperative clinical stage) is associated with improved rates of overall and disease-free survival at 5 years.[482] Pathological examination of the resection specimen after chemoradiation therapy often reveals fibrosis, mucin pools, hemosiderin-laden and foamy macrophages, ulceration or erosion, residual neuroendocrine cell collections, and epithelial changes such as cytoplasmic eosinophilia (Fig. 27.48).[483] The adjacent mucosa often shows ulceration, architectural irregularity, and reactive epithelial atypia that may be mistaken for dysplasia.[484] Residual tumor, if present, may be located anywhere in the rectal wall or perirectal tissues. The pathological stage is marked with the prescript *y* to indicate that the evaluation was done after treatment (ypTNM). Only residual viable tumor cells are counted in this evaluation, and although it is not always possible to assess the viability of all tumor cells, frankly necrotic tumor should not be included in staging.[2] Nonviable cells are characterized by nuclear hyperchromasia, pyknosis, nuclear fragmentation, and cytoplasmic eosinophilia.[484] A number of validated systems for grading pathological tumor regression have been developed. The relevant features of the most commonly used systems are summarized in Table 27.17.[485]

Careful attention must also be paid to lymph nodes because a complete pathological response may be associated with residual viable lymph node metastases. Note should also be made of the presence or absence of treatment changes and their location in the wall and regional lymph nodes because this information provides a correlate to the original preoperative stage.

Colloid response refers to a tumor response that is predominantly colloid change with or without scattered residual tumor cells. In 15% to 27% of cases, it is the pattern of pathological complete response.[368,486] The 5-year disease-free survival rate is intermediate for these cases, at 64%, compared with 80% for downstaging and 54% for no response.[482] The rate of local recurrence for colloid response is similar to that for tumors with downstaging, whereas distant metastases have a rate of recurrence similar to that in cases with no response.[367] With regard to the finding of acellular mucin pools, these are not considered to represent residual tumor.

Pathological Reporting of Colorectal Carcinoma

The important elements to be included in the pathology report for colorectal carcinoma are listed in Box 27.20.

Molecular Genetic Prognostic and Predictive Markers

Molecular genetic studies have the potential to help predict the outcome of CRC in two main ways. First, they may identify forms of CRC associated with either a favorable or unfavorable prognosis (prognostic markers). Second, they may predict the response to specific therapies (predictive markers).[487] A number of molecular and genetic alterations in CRC have been touted as possible markers of biological behavior and outcome. However, many of these studies have not had the statistical power to determine whether the prognostic implications of these alterations are independent of other known clinical and pathological variables in multivariate analyses. Furthermore, although prognostic information may be of clinical interest, it does not have high clinical utility unless it drives a therapeutic decision tree. Therefore, at the current time, the clinical value of prognostic markers appears to be their usefulness in the identification of subsets of CRC whose outcome is so favorable that there is limited potential benefit from adjuvant chemotherapy.[487,488] Markers that have been validated or that hold the greatest likelihood of independence are listed in Table 27.18.[391,487-489]

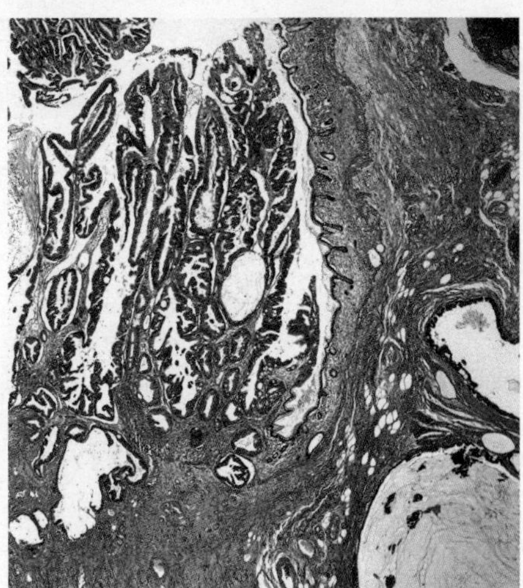

FIGURE 27.48 Rectal adenocarcinoma after neoadjuvant treatment. Mucin pools without malignant cells are present within the muscularis propria, indicative of a complete response to treatment.

Of the molecular alterations that have been most extensively studied, MSI (and other measures of loss of MMR function, particularly immunohistochemical analysis) has emerged as the marker that has the greatest potential utility and has most consistently been shown to have prognostic significance. Many studies have found that MMR deficiency is predictive of a favorable outcome, independent of other standard variables.[391,487-489] This has the greatest clinical relevance for stage II disease, and current management guidelines include incorporation of MMR status with other clinical and pathological factors to identify subgroups of patients with a very favorable outcome and thus no potential benefit from adjuvant chemotherapy.[153] In addition, there is evidence that MMR-deficient cancers may not benefit from fluorouracil-based chemotherapy; in fact, it may have a negative effect on outcome (see later discussion). This evidence provides further impetus to avoid standard fluorouracil-based chemotherapy in stage II disease.

Among the remaining markers, allelic imbalance of chromosome 18 characterized by 18q loss of heterozygosity (LOH) involves loss of the *DCC*, *BCL2*, and *SMAD* genes, including *SMAD4*.[488] Many studies have found that 18q LOH or *DCC* loss is predictive of poor outcome, independent of other standard variables.[490-494] These results are not entirely consistent, however, and some studies found no association between these markers and outcome.[495] In some studies, case ascertainment and molecular methodologies

TABLE 27.17 Pathological Tumor Regression Grading Systems

Descriptive Appearance	AJCC	Mandard	Becker	Dworak
No residual tumor	0 (no residual tumor cells)	1 (no residual cancer cells)	1a (complete regression, 0% tumor)	4 (no vital tumor cells detected)
Near-complete tumor regression	1 (single cell or small groups of cells)	2 (rare cancer cells)	1b (<10% residual tumor)	3 (scattered tumor cells; difficult to find)
Partial tumor regression	2 (residual cancer with desmoplastic response)	3 (fibrosis outgrowing residual cancer)	2 (10%-50% residual tumor)	2 (scattered tumor cells; easy to find)
No tumor regression	3 (extensive residual cancer)	4 (residual cancer outgrowing fibrosis)	3 (>50% residual tumor)	1 (predominantly tumor with significant fibrosis and/or vasculopathy)
		5 (cancer with no changes of regression)		0 (no regression)

AJCC, *American Joint Committee on Cancer.*

BOX 27.20 Important Features to Include in the Pathology Report for Resection Specimens of Colorectal Carcinoma

MACROSCOPIC

Tumor site
Tumor diameter
TME quality (if rectal)
Proximal margin clearance
Distal margin clearance
Circumferential nonperitonealized margin clearance

MICROSCOPIC

Histological subtype
Histological grade
Growth pattern (infiltrating vs. expansile)
Peritumoral inflammatory/immune response
Maximum extent of invasion
Lymphatic invasion
Venous invasion (intramural/extramural)
Perineural invasion
Tumor budding
Tumor regression grade (post–neoadjuvant therapy)
Lymph node status
Total found
Positive nodes
Isolated extramural tumor deposits
Other pathology (e.g., polyps, inflammatory bowel disease)
Mismatch repair protein status
Results of molecular investigations (e.g., extended *RAS* mutation testing, *BRAF* mutation status, *MLH1* methylation status, microsatellite status)

may have had a significant confounding effect on the statistical analysis. Other features that may be independently associated with prognosis, although with less convincing evidence, include DNA ploidy (and S-phase fraction), *TP53* mutation or 17p LOH (loss of chromosomal region 17p, where *TP53* is located), and *CDKN1B (p27)* expression. Studies that have investigated *TP53* have been hampered, in part, by methodological differences between mutation detection and immunohistochemical analysis of TP53 expression.[496,497] Although studies of TP53 immunoexpression have been conflicting, studies of *TP53* mutation have shown an association with poor outcome.[101,498] Poor outcome has been associated with decreased *CDKN1B (p27)* expression.[499,500] The results concerning *KRAS* mutations have been variable, but the consensus of recent studies is that *KRAS* mutations are associated with increased tumor recurrence and death, although this is dependent on the specific mutation[501]; mutations in codons 12 and 61 are associated with poor prognosis, while mutations affecting codon 146 are associated with a more favorable outcome.[502] Currently there are conflicting results as to the prognostic and predictive value of *PTEN* loss,[503,504] *PIK3CA* mutation,[487] *EGFR* overexpression,[340] and *HER2* overexpression.[489]

In recent years, there has been growth in the development of prognostic assays that use multiple genomic and gene expression markers, particularly in the commercial setting. The main aim has been to identify markers that help define the subset of stage II and III colon cancer patients expected to derive benefit from adjuvant chemotherapy, especially in those with borderline indications.[505] The Oncotype DX colon cancer assay (Genomic Health, Redwood City, CA) is predictive of outcome in stage II and III CRC and is available for use in the United States.[506-508] The ColoPrint assay (Agendia, Inc., Irvine CA) is used in combination with pathological factors and MMR status and is predictive of outcome in approximately 70% of stage II CRCs that lack high-risk pathological factors (e.g., pT4 status) and are MMR-proficient.[508-510] At present, it remains unclear whether these commercial multigene assays offer significant improvement to MMR status in the evaluation of stage II and III CRCs.

Improvements in molecular techniques are allowing the detection and analysis of tumor DNA circulating in the bloodstream. This is found in two forms, plasma cell free DNA (cf DNA) and circulating tumor DNA (ct DNA). There are several potential and evolving prognostic and predictive benefits in analyzing circulating DNA. This "liquid biopsy" may allow detection of early-stage CRC before clinical metastases are apparent and hence could become an indication for chemotherapy in stage II CRC.[511] It has also been shown to predict for increased likelihood of tumor relapse following adjuvant therapy.[512] Changes in mutations found in circulating tumor DNA may provide a way of monitoring for disease resistance in patients with metastatic disease undergoing personalized therapy.[513] At present, limitations with this technology include limited sensitivity, which is likely to rapidly improve over time.

TABLE 27.18 Molecular Markers with Prognostic and Predictive Significance In Colorectal Carcinoma

Marker	Prognostic Significance	Predictive Significance
Established Biomarkers		
CIN	Poorer prognosis	Nil
MSI	Favorable prognosis	Poor response to fluorouracil-based chemotherapy Positive response to immunotherapy MMR deficiency predicts a favorable response to irinotecan
KRAS mutation	Poorer prognosis (codon 12, 61) More favorable prognosis (codon 146)	Resistance to anti-EGFR therapy (except G13D)
BRAF mutation	Poorer prognosis if MSS	Probable resistance to anti-EGFR therapy *BRAF* inhibition therapy (investigational)
Emerging Biomarkers		
PIK3CA mutation	Possibly a more favorable prognosis (if taking aspirin)	Limited evidence suggesting resistance to anti-EGFR therapy
HER2 amplification	Uncertain	Potential role for HER2-directed therapy
Molecular profiling studies	CMS classification	Likely differences
Others		
Chromosome 18 allelic imbalance	Possibly a poorer prognosis in stage II and stage III CRC	Nil
TP53	Poorer prognosis	Reduced response to standard treatment
PTEN	Conflicting results	Limited evidence suggesting resistance to anti-EGFR therapy
CDKN1B (p27) expression	Poorer prognosis with decreased expression	Nil
Oncotype DX colon cancer assay	Prognostic information in T3, MMR-proficient, stage II colon cancer	Used to determine benefit of adding oxaliplatin in stage III colon cancer
ColoPrint assay	Prognostic information in T3, MMR-proficient, stage II colon cancer	Predicts increased recurrence risk in stage II colon cancer
Circulating tumor DNA ("liquid biopsy")		Prediction of treatment response or resistance (e.g., *KRAS* mutation). Prediction of shorter disease-free survival
Noncoding RNAs	Potential prognostic information dependent on the effect of the particular noncoding RNA on gene expression	

CIN, *Chromosomal instability;* CRC, *colorectal cancer;* EGFR, *epidermal growth factor receptor;* MSI, *microsatellite instability;* MSS, *microsatellite stable.*

Noncoding RNAs represent several forms of RNA that are not transcribed into protein. It is now clear that these noncoding RNAs serve an important role in regulation of gene expression, which may be to either upregulate or downregulate targeted genes. Most attention has focused on the micro-RNA subtypes of noncoding RNA, and in particular their effect on proto-oncogenes and tumor-suppressor genes such as *MYC*, Wnt signaling pathway genes, and *TP53*. The potential exists to examine panels of micro-RNAs for their expression in CRC that may provide both prognostic information and potential targets for molecular therapy.[514,515] Moreover, circulating micro-RNAs with a signature panel matched to CRCs may function as a biomarker for detection in the bloodstream.[516]

Predictive Factors for Treatment Response

In the adjuvant setting, the use of chemotherapeutic regimes containing 5-FU result in a 15% to 33% improvement in overall survival and reduce the recurrence rate by approximately 15%.[311,517] Although this merits clinical use, most patients with colorectal cancer do not benefit from this type of therapy. Whereas a prognostic marker predicts outcome independent of treatment, a predictive marker is defined by its ability to predict benefit of or response to specific chemotherapeutic agents. Predictive markers have enormous relevance to clinical practice because they allow stratification and tailoring of specific treatment regimens.

Pathological Predictive Factors

In studies that have assessed variables predictive of outcome and benefit from chemotherapy, pathological stage is the most powerful variable. There are two specific scenarios in which additional pathological features are used to predict benefit and thus guide additional treatment.

For patients with stage II disease, the benefit of chemotherapy is either small or unproven in many studies and therefore remains controversial. However, evidence from several studies and expert panels, including the American Society for Clinical Oncology (ASCO), suggests that it

TABLE 27.19 Molecular Genetic Treatment Predictive Markers in Colorectal Cancer

Clinical Predictive Goal	Molecular Genetic Marker
Benefit from chemotherapy in high-risk stage II disease	MSS
Response to fluorouracil	High thymidylate synthase expression
	MSS
	Low levels of dihydropyrimidine dehydrogenase
Response to irinotecan	MSI
	CIMP-H
	High concentrations of topoisomerase I
Response to cetuximab	*EGFR* amplification
	No *KRAS or NRAS* mutation (except *KRAS G13D*)
	No *BRAF* mutation
	Normal functioning of MET and HER2
	Amphiregulin expression present
	Epiregulin expression present
Response to preoperative chemotherapy and radiation therapy	No *TP53* mutation
Response to oxaliplatin	None known
Response to bevacizumab	None known

CIMP-H, *High-frequency CpG island methylator phenotype;* EGFR, *epidermal growth factor receptor;* MSI, *microsatellite instability;* MSS, *microsatellite stable.*

could be offered to patients with high-risk disease, defined by the presence of the following disease-recurrence predictive factors: poor or undifferentiated histology, fewer than 12 lymph nodes evaluated, VI, perineural invasion, positive resection margins, pT4 tumor stage, bowel perforation, or clinical bowel obstruction.[518-520] The use of molecular genetic predictive factors of favorable outcome (and therefore diminished benefit from chemotherapy) is discussed in the previous section.

Molecular Genetic Predictive Markers

There are two broad categories of molecular predictive factors: (1) markers that predict response based on host factors (in particular, germline polymorphisms) that determine bioavailability and activity of the agent (pharmacogenomics), and (2) markers that predict response based on characteristics of the tumor tissue itself. Only the latter are considered in detail here. The clinically validated and most promising tissue markers are listed in Table 27.19.

Predictors of Response to Fluorouracil

Fluorouracil has been the mainstay of CRC chemotherapy for more than three decades, and it has been the subject of numerous studies to identify biomarkers of chemosensitivity and resistance. Of these, the most validated marker is MMR status, assayed by either MSI testing or MMR protein immunohistochemistry.[489] During the past 10 years, multiple studies have found that MMR status is associated with response to 5-FU in the adjuvant setting.[521,522] In fact, there is some evidence that 5-FU may have an adverse effect on outcome in the setting of MSI.[521] The mechanism of this effect is not known. Although the studies have not been consistent on this result, the predominance of evidence supports the use of MMR status in therapeutic decision making. In combination with the favorable prognosis associated with MMR deficiency (see Prognostic Factors), the use of MMR status to identify patients who are not likely to benefit from chemotherapy is rapidly becoming the standard of care for management of stage II and III CRC.[153]

The next most promising line of research in predicting response to 5-FU has been from studies investigating the expression levels of proteins involved in 5-FU metabolism and inhibition of DNA synthesis. One major mechanism of 5-FU activity is believed to be inhibition of thymidylate synthase, an important step in the synthesis of deoxythymidine triphosphate (dTTP), which is one of the building blocks of DNA. Expression levels of thymidylate synthase are related to 5-FU effectiveness, and low levels in tumor tissue samples are associated with a more favorable response.[523] However, the results have not been consistent, and they are complicated by the use of different assay methods (mRNA or immunohistochemistry). To date, thymidylate synthase expression has not been validated sufficiently to predict fluorouracil responsiveness.[524,525] Constitutive genetic factors also play a role in determining response to fluoropyrimidines, and a common polymorphism in the promoter region of thymidylate synthase has been associated with constitutive thymidylate synthase levels. Although this may allow a more reliable prediction of treatment response, further validation studies are required.[526] Enzymes involved in catabolism are also important in predicting 5-FU efficacy. For instance, low levels of dihydropyrimidine dehydrogenase, the major enzyme involved in 5-FU breakdown, predict not only a favorable response to 5-FU but increased toxicity.[526,527] Although research results in the area of pharmacogenomics are promising, these assays have not yet come into widespread clinical use.[527,528]

Predictors of Response to Irinotecan

MMR deficiency has been associated with improved response to irinotecan in several studies and is recommended to be included in the treatment protocol in this situation.[529] Additionally, CIMP-H status is even more strongly associated with response to irinotecan than MMR status.[530] Irinotecan is a semisynthetic camptothecin derivative that selectively inhibits topoisomerase I. The higher the concentration of topoisomerase I, the more sensitive the tumor cells become to irinotecan. High immunohistochemical expression of topoisomerase 1 in tumor cells has been correlated with clinical response to irinotecan.[531]

Other Predictors of Response to Chemotherapy

Much attention has also focused on apoptotic abnormalities and how they may affect patient response to chemotherapy. Studies have shown that *TP53* mutations may be associated

BOX 27.21 *RAS* Mutation Testing in Colorectal Carcinoma

***RAS* MUTATIONS IN COLORECTAL CARCINOMA**

- Mutations in either *KRAS* (~45%) or *NRAS* (~5%) genes occur in approximately 50%.
- Mutations predict for both adverse outcome and poor response to anti-EGFR therapy.

Extended *RAS* testing should be performed in all cases of metastatic colorectal carcinoma (codons 12, 13, 59, 61, 117, and 146).

Modified from Saeed O, Lopez-Beltran A, Fisher KW, et al. RAS genes in colorectal carcinoma: pathogenesis, testing guidelines and treatment implications. J Clin Pathol. *2019;72(2):135-139.*

with resistance to a variety of chemotherapeutic agents, and there are ongoing efforts to find agents capable of restoring the *TP53* function in cancer cells.[101,532,533]

Predictors of Response to Anti–Epidermal Growth Factor Receptor Therapy

The availability of targeted chemotherapeutic agents provides a theoretical possibility of clinically useful predictive assays that can measure the level of the target molecule. Initial trials of cetuximab required immunohistochemical demonstration of EGFR expression in tumor cells for eligibility. However, it is now evident that some patients respond well, even in the absence of detectable EGFR expression, suggesting that this antibody may have an effect on undetectable levels of EGFR expression or on other signaling proteins. Furthermore, the activating mutations that make *EGFR* mutation testing in lung carcinoma helpful are quite rare in CRC.[487] *KRAS* and *NRAS* mutations have been associated with resistance to cetuximab because of activation of signaling downstream of EGFR.[502] Testing for *KRAS* and *NRAS* mutations (a so-called "extended RAS panel") is now routinely performed in all patients eligible for cetuximab therapy, and the presence of a *KRAS* or *NRAS* mutation is a contraindication to therapy (Box 27.21).[487,502,534] It is also important to note that this testing should include specific details of the type of mutation, if present, because several studies suggest that tumors with *KRAS* G13D mutations may still respond to cetuximab.[535,536]

BRAF encodes one of the main downstream cellular effectors of *KRAS* and is mutated in 10% of CRCs. In a manner analogous to *KRAS* activation, *BRAF* mutations could be expected to result in constitutive signaling downstream of EGFR and therefore predict resistance to cetuximab. The data have not been consistent as to whether this is, in fact, the situation; however, a recent meta-analysis supports the view that *BRAF* mutation is associated with resistance to anti-EGFR molecules.[537] Knowledge of *BRAF* mutation status is increasingly being incorporated into the treatment decision process for metastatic CRC.[487,538] Currently, consensus-based guidelines from both the National Comprehensive Cancer Network (NCCN) and European Society for Medical Oncology (ESMO) recommend avoiding the use of cetuximab or panitumumab for patients with *BRAF*-mutated cancers.

Two other downstream targets of EGFR signaling, *PIK3CA* and *PTEN*, function in a signaling pathway that is parallel to *KRAS/BRAF* activation, raising the possibility that aberrations in these genes could also confer resistance to anti-EGFR therapies. *PIK3CA* encodes a lipid kinase that counteracts PTEN and results in Akt phosphorylation and activation. *PIK3CA* is mutated in 15% to 18% of CRCs, providing an alternative method of constitutional signaling, even in the presence of targeted EGFR blockade. Some studies have found that *PIK3CA* mutations are associated with resistance to anti-EGFR therapy.[539,540] Other clinical trials have not supported this result,[541] however, and current evidence suggests that only exon 20 mutations are associated with resistance to anti-EGFR therapy.[542] Similarly, loss of PTEN expression has been associated with poor response to cetuximab therapy, although the results also have not been consistent.[540,543,544] At present, the overall results do not support the use of *PIK3CA* mutation or loss of PTEN as a contraindication to anti-EGFR therapy, and *PIK3CA* mutation testing and PTEN evaluation are not recommended as part of the workup before therapy.[545] It has been recently proposed to consider a *quadruple negative* profile for CRC based on an absence of mutation in *KRAS* exon 2, *BRAF* V600E, *PI3K*-exon 9, and *PTEN* as tumor markers of the highest sensitivity to anti-EGFR treatment.[546]

Although initial anti-EGFR therapy is often very successful, resistance to cetuximab typically emerges in *KRAS* wild-type tumors. Several reasons for this have been identified. One mechanism is the acquisition of *EGFR* mutations resulting in a conformation change that prevents cetuximab binding.[547] These mutations may not block panitumumab binding, suggesting that these tumors may still be sensitive to panitumumab.[547] Several studies have assessed ct DNA in the blood of metastatic CRC patients during anti-EGFR therapy and found that undetectable low-frequency *KRAS*-mutant clones may be selected by anti-EGFR treatment, resulting in a progressive resistance to cetuximab.[548-550] Activation of the PI3K/Akt/mTOR signaling pathway has also been implicated as an important mechanism in the resistance to EGFR inhibitors.[540] Genetic aberrations of the receptor tyrosine kinases MET and HER2 are identified as the bypass mechanisms for acquired resistance to anti-EGFR therapies.[551,552]

Studies have also been conducted to determine whether specific activation of EGFR signaling is associated with improved response to anti-EGFR therapy. EGFR amplification may confer an increased sensitivity to cetuximab, but EGFR testing is not considered a requirement for use of this agent. High expression of amphiregulin and epiregulin, the ligands for EGFR, has also been associated with a favorable response to cetuximab.[553,554] Additional studies are required before these markers are considered for routine clinical use.

Predictors of Response to Anti–Vascular Endothelial Growth Factor Therapy

At present, there are no known molecular genetic markers that predict response to bevacizumab or related anti-VEGF agents.

HEREDITARY COLORECTAL CARCINOMA

Between 2% and 5% of all CRCs are caused by inherited syndromes that have a clearly defined mendelian genetic basis. These genetic syndromes may or may not be associated with

BOX 27.22 Causes of Hereditary Nonpolyposis Colorectal Cancer

- Lynch syndrome
- Constitutional mismatch repair deficiency (non–polyposis-associated cases)
- Lynch-like syndrome
- Familial colorectal cancer syndrome X

BOX 27.23 Amsterdam Criteria for Hereditary Nonpolyposis Colorectal Cancer

AMSTERDAM CRITERIA I

There should be at least three relatives with colorectal cancer; all of the following criteria should be present.

- One should be a first-degree relative of the other two.
- At least two successive generations should be affected.
- At least one colorectal cancer should be diagnosed before 50 years of age.
- Familial adenomatous polyposis should be excluded.
- Tumors should be verified by pathological examination.

AMSTERDAM CRITERIA II

There should be at least three relatives with an HNPCC-associated cancer (colorectal cancer, cancer of the endometrium, small bowel, ureter, or renal pelvis).

- One should be a first-degree relative of the other two.
- At least two successive generations should be affected.
- At least one should be diagnosed before 50 years of age.
- Familial adenomatous polyposis should be excluded in colorectal cancer case(s), if any.
- Tumors should be verified by pathological examination.

Data from Vasen HF, Mecklin JP, Khan PM, Lynch HT. The International Collaborative Group on Hereditary Non-Polyposis Colorectal Cancer (ICG-HNPCC). Dis Colon Rectum. *1991;34(5):424-425; Vasen HF, Watson P, Mecklin JP, Lynch HT. New clinical criteria for hereditary nonpolyposis colorectal cancer (HNPCC, Lynch syndrome) proposed by the International Collaborative Group on HNPCC.* Gastroenterology. *1999;116(6):1453-1456.*

a polyposis (discussed in Chapter 22), and this is a clinically relevant distinction that can direct the genetic search for an underlying cause as well as potentially influence subsequent surveillance. There is a larger group of CRCs, perhaps as many as 35% of all cases, that appear to have an inherited predisposition; however, no causative mutation can be found. It is believed that this group may result from a heterogeneous set of gene mutations that occur at such low allele frequency that they are not identified in genome-wide association studies (GWAS), and their penetrance is too low to have been identified in traditional family linkage studies.[555] In the future, gene sequencing technology offers the potential to identify these low-penetrance mutations, although separating deleterious mutations from nonconsequential abnormalities (variants of uncertain significance) will likely remain a major challenge for some time. The clinical and pathological features of inherited CRC syndromes are summarized in Table 27.3.

Lynch Syndrome and Other Causes of Hereditary Nonpolyposis Colorectal Cancer

Hereditary nonpolyposis colorectal cancer (HNPCC) is a clinical syndrome characterized by hereditary colorectal and other cancers. The term was previously used interchangeably with *Lynch syndrome* but more correctly refers to a broader spectrum of familial CRCs that fulfill the Amsterdam criteria (see later). Hence, this includes other disorders that can mimic the clinical features of Lynch syndrome but lack evidence of germline mutations in MMR genes that characterize Lynch syndrome. Colorectal adenomas may be found in HNPCC; however, they are typically few in number (<10) and therefore do not qualify as a *polyposis*. Several causes for HNPCC are currently known (Box 27.22), of which Lynch syndrome is overwhelmingly the most common.

Historically, the diagnosis of HNPCC was based on clinical criteria, the Amsterdam I or Amsterdam II criteria, the features of which are provided in Box 27.23. Subsequently these clinical criteria were supplemented in the revised Bethesda criteria by a requirement for the pathological documentation of MSI (see Box 27.24).

A major problem for both the Amsterdam and Bethesda criteria has been their low sensitivity in identifying patients with Lynch syndrome. Up to one-half of all patients with a germline mutation diagnostic of Lynch syndrome fail to meet Amsterdam II criteria.[559] Similarly, the Bethesda guidelines have been shown to miss 6% to 25% of patients with Lynch syndrome, although the greater issue is the lack of specificity of the criteria.[559] This led to the development of a number of computer-based clinical models predictive of Lynch syndrome. Examples of these include PREMM5, MMRpredict, and MMRpro.[560,561] Formal genetic testing is recommended when threshold scores are reached via these predictive models, and there is good evidence to support their role in clinical care algorithms.[562] However, as with the Amsterdam and Bethesda criteria before them, these predictive models are now superseded by universal screening of CRC for MMR deficiency and/or MSI (see later discussion).

Lynch Syndrome

Lynch syndrome is the most common inherited cause of CRC. It results from germline alterations affecting the functioning of MMR genes and is inherited in an autosomal dominant fashion. Approximately 3% of all CRCs occur in patients who have Lynch syndrome.[563,564] It is estimated that approximately 0.35% (1 in 279) of the general population has Lynch syndrome,[565] with some geographical variation, depending on the degree of founder effect in some regions.[564,566] There is well-documented variation in the prevalence of mutations in the individual MMR genes in the general population. In one large multi-institutional study, mutations in *PMS2* (1:714) were most commonly encountered followed by *MSH6* (1:758), *MLH1* (1:1946), and finally *MSH2* (1:2841).[565] The difference in pathogenicity of the MMR gene mutations accounts for the finding that loss of MLH1 or MSH2 protein expression are more commonly encountered in CRC than loss of expression of the more commonly mutated genes *MSH6* and *PMS2*.[567]

The cardinal features of Lynch syndrome are summarized in Boxes 27.24 and 27.25, and Table 27.20.[568] It has now become clear that the observed clinical features depend on

BOX 27.24 Revised Bethesda Guidelines for Hereditary Nonpolyposis Colorectal Cancer (Lynch Syndrome)

1. Colorectal cancer diagnosed in a patient who is younger than 50 years of age
2. Presence of synchronous, metachronous colorectal, or other HNPCC-associated tumors,* regardless of age
3. Colorectal cancer with MSI-H† histology‡ diagnosed in a patient who is younger than 60 years of age§
4. Colorectal cancer diagnosed in one or more first-degree relatives with an HNPCC-related tumor, with one of the cancers being diagnosed before 50 years of age
5. Colorectal cancer diagnosed in two or more first- or second-degree relatives with HNPCC-related tumors, regardless of age

* *Hereditary nonpolyposis colorectal cancer (HNPCC)-related tumors include colorectal, endometrial, stomach, ovarian, pancreas, ureter and renal pelvis, biliary tract, and brain (usually glioblastoma as seen in Turcot syndrome) tumors, sebaceous gland adenomas and keratoacanthomas in Muir–Torre syndrome, and carcinoma of the small bowel.*

† *MSI-H = microsatellite instability–high in tumors refers to changes in two or more of the five National Cancer Institute-recommended panels of microsatellite markers.*

‡ *Presence of tumor-infiltrating lymphocytes, Crohn's-like lymphocytic reaction, mucinous/signet ring differentiation, or medullary growth pattern. Five microsatellite loci are originally tested.*

§ *There was no consensus among the Workshop participants on whether to include the age criteria in guideline 3 above; participants voted to keep less than 60 years of age in the guidelines.*

HNPCC, *Hereditary nonpolyposis colorectal cancer.*

From Umar A, Boland CR, Terdiman JP, et al. Revised Bethesda Guidelines for hereditary nonpolyposis colorectal cancer (Lynch syndrome) and microsatellite instability. J Natl Cancer Inst. *2004;96(4):261-268.*

the specific MMR gene that is mutated, the patient's age, and the patient's sex. In general, patients carrying *MLH1* and *MSH2* mutations develop CRC more often and at an earlier age than those with *MSH6* and *PMS2* mutations. Similar findings are noted with Lynch syndrome–associated carcinomas that develop outside of the colorectum. It is worth noting that patients with Lynch syndrome may develop neoplasms that are not related to MMR deficiency.

Pathogenesis

Lynch syndrome is defined by an inherited loss of MMR gene function. For each MMR gene, the two alleles act in a codominant mechanism, so loss of both alleles is required to produce a clinical syndrome. In patients with Lynch syndrome, one abnormal allele is inherited. The remaining normal allele is sufficient to maintain normal expression and functioning of the relevant MMR protein. The clinical syndrome only develops when the second normal allele becomes defective (a "second hit") via a somatic mutation, and the now two abnormal alleles are unable to produce a functional MMR protein. In a small number of cases, MMR gene function is silenced by a mutation in a gene adjacent and downstream to an MMR gene that prevents transcription of the MMR protein. The most common example is mutation in the *EPCAM* gene, which is immediately upstream of the *MSH2* gene and prevents transcription of the *MSH2* gene. Similarly, transcription of the *MLH1* gene is silenced by mutation in the adjacent *LRRFIP2* gene.

BOX 27.25 Key Clinicopathological Features of Lynch Syndrome

- Autosomal dominant inheritance
- Pathogenic mutations in MMR genes *MLH1, MSH2, MSH6,* and *PMS2* or epigenetic mutations with gene silencing *EPCAM* affecting *MSH2, LRRFIP2* affecting *MLH1*
- Earlier average age of CRC onset than in the general population (45 years vs. 69 years), particularly with *MLH1* or *MSH2* mutations
- Right-sided CRC predominance (~70%)
- Accelerated carcinogenesis, with adenoma to carcinoma within 2-3 years in Lynch syndrome vs. 8-10 years in the general population
- High risk of metachronous CRCs
- Increased risk for malignancy at certain extracolonic sites
    - Endometrium (40%-60% lifetime risk for female mutation carriers)
    - Ovary (12%-15% lifetime risk for female mutation carriers)
    - Stomach (higher risk in Asian populations)
    - Small bowel
    - Biliary tree
    - Pancreas
    - Upper urinary tract (transitional cell carcinoma of the ureter and renal pelvis), especially in *MSH2* type
    - Brain (in the Turcot's syndrome variant of Lynch syndrome)
    - Sebaceous adenomas, sebaceous carcinomas, and keratoacanthomas in the Muir-Torre syndrome variant of Lynch syndrome
    - Prostate
- Pathology of CRC
    - More often poorly differentiated, mucinous, and signet-cell ring cell types
    - Crohn's-like reaction, tumor-infiltrating lymphocytes within the tumor
- Prognostic implication
    - Favorable overall
    - Reduced response to conventional chemotherapy
    - Favorable response to checkpoint inhibitor immunotherapy

CRC, *Colorectal cancer.*

Modified from Lynch HT, Lynch PM, Lanspa SJ, et al. Review of the Lynch syndrome: history, molecular genetics, screening, differential diagnosis, and medicolegal ramifications. Clin Genet. *2009;76(1):1-18.*

When both MMR gene alleles are dysfunctional, the DNA mismatches that develop during DNA replication are not adequately repaired. This results in point mutations that affect all aspects of the genome, but particularly the short repetitive triplet base repeats called *microsatellites*. The accumulation of point mutations leads to unstable microsatellite regions (MSIs), which is therefore a good indicator of MMR deficiency. The accumulating point mutations are not limited to microsatellites and affect protein-coding genes.

The mechanism by which the accumulating genomic instability resulting from MMR deficiency results in the development of CRC is not fully established. Recent evidence suggests that there are several pathways (Fig. 27.49). One pathway that is well established is that a significant proportion of Lynch syndrome–associated CRCs develop from a preexisting conventional adenoma. In this pathway, the neoplastic cells in a sporadic, conventional adenoma acquire a second-hit mutation, accelerating the development toward CRC. In this scenario, the MMR deficiency is not the initiating event

TABLE 27.20 Cumulative Cancer Risk in Lynch Syndrome up to Age 75 Years Stratified by MMR Gene Mutation and Sex

Mismatch Repair Gene	Sex	Cumulative Risk of All Cancers (%)	Cumulative Risk of Colorectal Carcinoma (%)	Mean Age of Diagnosis Of CRC (Years)	Cumulative Risk of Endometrial Carcinoma	Cumulative Risk of Ovarian Carcinoma
MLH1	Male	71.4	57.1	43		
	Female	81.0	48.3	43	35.2	11.0
MSH2	Male	75.2	51.4	44		
	Female	84.3	46.6	44	48.9	17.4
MSH6	Male	41.7	18.2	55		
	Female	61.8	20.3	57	41.1	10.8
PMS2	Male	34.1	10.4	59		
	Female				12.8	3.0

From Dominguez-Valentin M, Sampson JR, Seppala TT, et al. Cancer risks by gene, age, and gender in 6350 carriers of pathogenic mismatch repair variants: findings from the Prospective Lynch Syndrome Database. Genet Med. *2020;22(1):15-25; Jang E, Chung DC. Hereditary colon cancer: Lynch syndrome.* Gut Liver. *2010;4(2):151-160.*

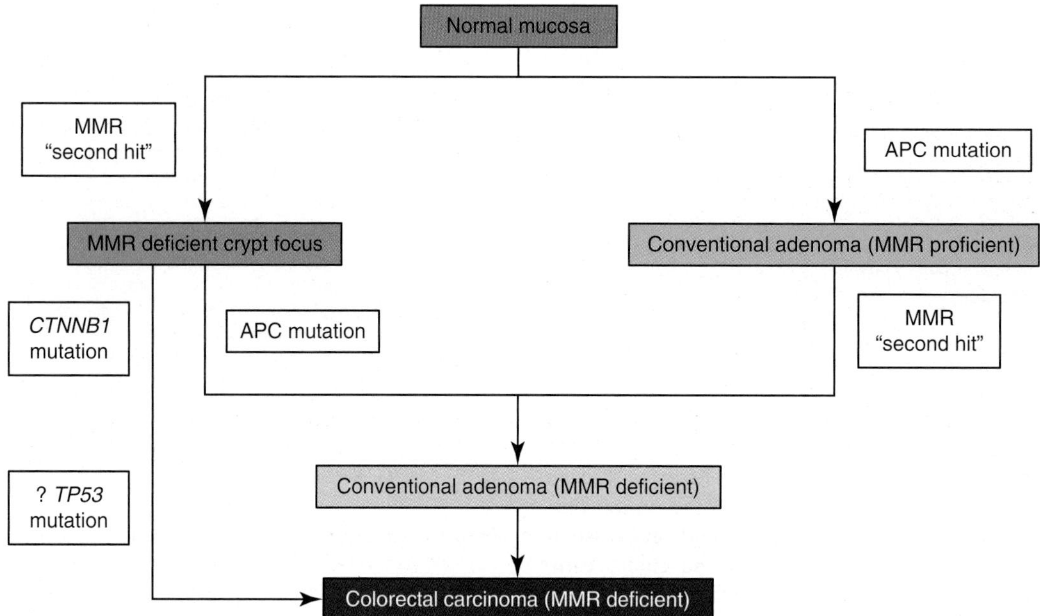

FIGURE 27.49 Pathways to colorectal carcinogenesis in Lynch syndrome.

but occurs later in the growth of the adenoma. Evidence in support of this phenomenon is the heterogeneous/partial loss of MMR expression in some Lynch syndrome–associated adenomas and the propensity for loss of MMR expression to occur only in more advanced adenomas (i.e., larger size, high-grade dysplasia, or villous morphology).[571,572] It is also recognized that Lynch syndrome patients may harbor small (often <5 mm in diameter) conventional adenomas that exhibit high-grade dysplasia, suggesting a second pathway probably exists whereby MMR deficiency develops early during the development of the adenoma or even precedes the development of a visible adenoma.[573] Supporting this proposed pathway is the identification of loss of MMR protein expression in nonneoplastic colorectal crypts in patients with Lynch syndrome, estimated at approximately 1 crypt with MMR protein loss/10,000 crypts (1 cm^2).[574] The term *MMR-deficient crypt foci* has been applied to this finding in a sense that is analogous to the aberrant crypt foci of familial adenomatous polyposis. In one study, nonneoplastic colonic crypts exhibiting loss of expression of MMR protein were identified in 35% of Lynch syndrome patients who had CRC.[575] The molecular mechanism responsible for further progression of MMR-deficient crypts may be a mutation in *CTNNB1*, which encodes for β-catenin and is associated with activation of the Wnt pathway. A secondary acquisition of APC mutations may also provide an alternate mechanism of Wnt pathway activation.[573,576] Interestingly, *CTNNB1* mutations are very rare in the rectum, suggesting a different mechanism is at play in the site.[577,578] MMR-deficient crypt foci may develop into CRC via development of a conventional adenoma with a *CTNNB1/APC* mutation, possibly without ever producing a neoplastic polypoid precursor. Mutations in *TP53*, which are generally rare in MSI CRC, may be important in the latter pathway.[573]

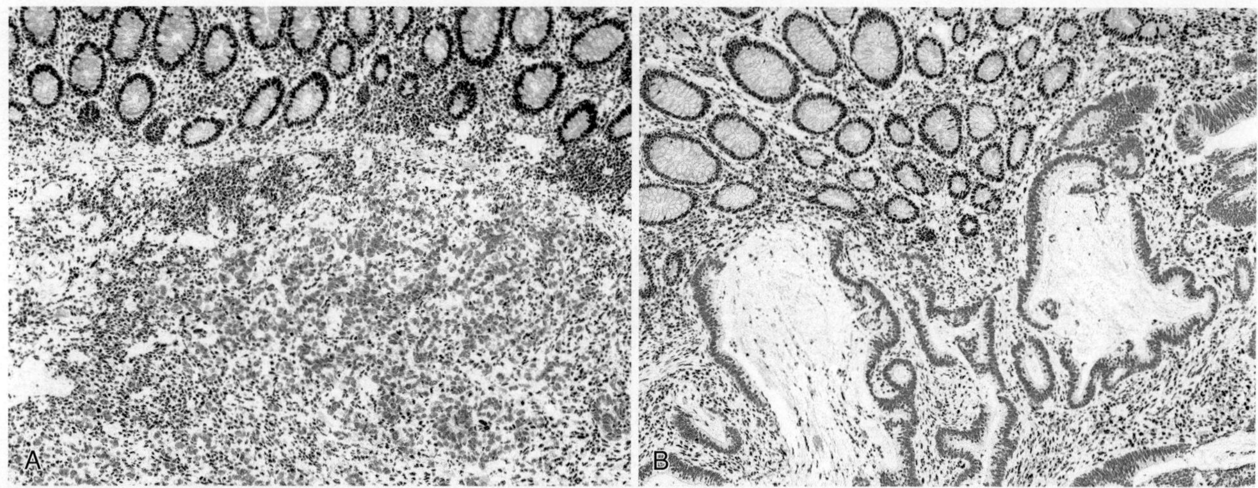

FIGURE 27.50 MLH1 immunohistochemistry. A, There is loss of MLH1 expression in the poorly differentiated tumor cells, whereas normal crypt epithelial cells and lymphocytes maintain expression. **B,** This better-differentiated tumor also shows loss of MLH1 expression in tumor cells with maintenance of expression in normal crypt epithelial cells.

Pathological Features

The gross and microscopic features of MMR-deficient CRCs have been described in detail. Several studies have attempted to define the clinical and pathological features that distinguish sporadic from hereditary MMR-deficient cancers. Compared with sporadic MMR-deficient CRC, Lynch syndrome–associated CRC is more likely to occur in men, to manifest at a younger age (usually <60 years), to be associated with prior CRCs or a characteristic extracolonic tumor, and to be located in the left colon or rectum (approximately one-third overall). As a practical point, all treatment-naive MMR-deficient cancers arising in the rectum should be considered to have a high likelihood to represent Lynch syndrome.[579] Lynch syndrome cancers may be associated with a residual conventional adenoma precursor, whereas sporadic MMR-deficient CRCs are associated with SSLs. When histological features are considered, one study also found that lymphocytic infiltration and tumor budding are more common in Lynch syndrome–associated CRCs, whereas mucin secretion, poor differentiation, tumor heterogeneity, and glandular serration were more common in MLH1 methylated cancers.[254]

One study attempted to determine optimal pathological features that could be used to help identify likely Lynch syndrome–associated CRC in patients younger than 60 years of age. With factors such as patient age, anatomic site, and four pathological features (histological type, grade, Crohn's-like lymphoid reaction, and tumor-infiltrating lymphocytes), they generated the Microsatellite Path (MSI by pathology) score that can be used, on a sliding scale, to help predict the probability that a particular cancer is MSI-H.[444] This morphological approach has been superseded by universal MMR testing of all CRCs.

Ancillary Studies Used by Pathologists for Lynch Syndrome Evaluation

Five separate tests are used to varying degrees in the workup and characterization of Lynch syndrome.

Mismatch Repair Immunohistochemistry. The DNA MMR proteins are ubiquitously expressed in normal human tissues, particularly in proliferating cells, and nuclear expression in crypt epithelium and lymphocytes serves as an internal positive control. In the setting of Lynch syndrome, most hereditary and second-hit mutations in the tumor are inactivating, chain-terminating mutations. As a result of instability of the truncated mRNA transcript or the protein product, these mutations are associated with complete loss of immunohistochemically detectable MMR protein (Fig. 27.50).[261]

Immunohistochemical testing is performed using antibodies to the four genes that harbor the most common known HNPCC mutations: *MLH1*, *MSH2*, *MSH6*, and *PMS2*. During normal DNA MMR activation, MLH1 recruits its binding partner PMS2 to the site of DNA repair. If *MLH1* is mutated (as in Lynch syndrome) and lost from the DNA MMR complex, then PMS2 will also be absent from the repair protein complex. Therefore mutation and loss of MLH1 protein are almost always accompanied by loss of PMS2 expression. The same holds true for MSH2 and the binding partner it recruits during active DNA MMR, MSH6. In contrast, germline mutations in either *PMS2* or *MSH6* are usually associated with the loss of the respective protein alone, as MLH1 and MSH2 can recruit alternative binding partners in this setting.

The sensitivity of MMR immunohistochemistry for identifying loss of protein expression in patients with Lynch syndrome with known mutations is at least 90%, and it has nearly perfect specificity in predicting an underlying MMR defect. Immunohistochemistry has the advantage of identifying which gene is most likely to be affected.[580] However, immunohistochemical staining may be intact in tumors from patients with functionally pathogenic point mutations. In these cases, when point mutations are present in either *MLH1* or *MSH2*, there may be associated abnormalities in expression of PMS2 and MSH6, respectively.

Two pitfalls in the interpretation of MMR immunohistochemistry are staining heterogeneity and unusual combinations of expression patterns. Staining heterogeneity is usually caused by fixation issues or tissue hypoxia and results in false absence staining of one or more MMR proteins. Lack

TABLE 27.21 Interpretation of DNA Mismatch Repair Immunohistochemistry

Pattern of IHC expression (+ = retained; – = absent)					
MLH1	MSH2	MSH6	PMS2	Probability of Lynch Syndrome	Significance/Further Testing
+	+	+	+	Very unlikely	Normal pattern. No further testing unless a strong clinical suspicion of Lynch syndrome exists
–	+	+	–	Sporadic or Lynch syndrome	*BRAF* mutation testing (PCR or immunohistochemistry) or MLH1 methylation If *BRAF* mutation or MLH1 methylation is present, sporadic colorectal cancer. Otherwise investigate for Lynch syndrome by *MLH1*, followed by *PMS2* germline testing.
+	–	–	+	Likely	*MSH2*, followed by *MSH6* germline testing required
+	+	–‡	+	Likely, unless chemotherapy/radiotherapy has been given	*MSH6*, followed by *MSH2* germline testing required. No testing required if postchemoradiotherapy
+	+	+	–	Likely	*PMS2*, followed by *MLH1* germline testing. This can also represent *MLH1* mutation producing protein that is detectable on immunohistochemistry but nonetheless results in PMS2 loss
–	+	–*	–	Unlikely	*MLH1* methylation with a secondary acquired mutation in a mononucleotide microsatellite of *MSH6* gene
–	–	–	–	Possible	Germline loss of *MSH2* and hypermethylation of *MLH1* or hypermethylation silencing of both *MLH1* and *MSH2*
+†	+	+	-	unlikely	*MLH1* promoter hypermethylation

**Partial or complete.*
†Punctate pattern of staining.
‡Can have a nucleolar pattern of staining in post chemotherapy/radiotherapy setting.

of internal control staining is a good indicator of this issue. The absence of staining is often partial, and convincing reactivity elsewhere in the tumor, involving at least 10% of the total area of the tumor, can be reported as retained staining overall.[581] Two other situations may produce focal or extensive loss of MMR protein expression. It is well-recognized that MSH6 may be lost in rectal carcinomas that have had neoadjuvant therapy. Weak expression of the other MMR proteins may also be noted.[582] Clonal loss of MSH6 may accompany MLH1/PMS2 deficiency as a result of acquired instability of a mononucleotide microsatellite within the coding sequence of this gene.[583] Variations in the extent of *MLH1* methylation may be expressed at a protein level as zonal heterogeneity in MLH1/PMS2 expression.[584] Finally, it is important not to overinterpret weak punctate nuclear staining of MLH1 as representing normal expression. This may lead to false assumption of isolated PMS2 loss, indicative of Lynch syndrome, when the primary pathology is methylation-related silencing of MLH1 with secondary loss of PMS2.[585] The more common patterns of MMR expression and their interpretation are summarized in Table 27.21.

Universal Testing for Lynch Syndrome. There is general agreement that identification of patients with Lynch syndrome is an important goal that leads to improved management and decreased mortality among patients and their family members.[586,587] Nevertheless, some Lynch syndrome patients continue to go unrecognized in the United States. At least two major problems lead to suboptimal detection of Lynch syndrome in clinical practice. First, none of the clinical criteria achieve better than 75% sensitivity for detecting Lynch syndrome.[563] Second, implementation of any of the criteria is laborintensive and falls short in clinical practice. As a result, many experts have recommended universal screening for Lynch syndrome in all newly diagnosed CRC patients by using either MMR immunohistochemistry or MSI testing.[588-591] The addition of *BRAF* mutation and MLH1 methylation testing allows definitive classification of MLH1-deficient cancers, thereby providing very practical and effective screening protocols (Fig. 27.51). Some centers use age cutoffs, performing MMR screening only in patients with newly diagnosed CRC who are younger than 60, 65, or 70 years of age; however, this may still miss the significant proportion of Lynch syndrome cases who present beyond these ages.[1,592,593] In particular, mutations in *MSH6* and *PMS2* have an older median age of presentation that is not adequately covered by age-based screening cutoffs.[594] Increasingly, testing all CRCs for MMR status is required to provide clinically important information beyond Lynch syndrome assessment, notably the predictive value of MMR deficiency for response to chemotherapy and checkpoint inhibitor immunotherapy. The decision as to whether the MMR testing is performed on the initial biopsy or the surgical resection specimen depends on the individual laboratory. Advantages for testing initial biopsies are that there are fewer issues with tissue fixation and associated staining artefacts, and identification of Lynch syndrome at the time of biopsy may allow for a different surgical approach. Although in theory, testing only two MMR proteins (MSH6 and PMS2, followed by MLH1 and/or MSH2 if required) should detect all combinations of protein loss, there is an

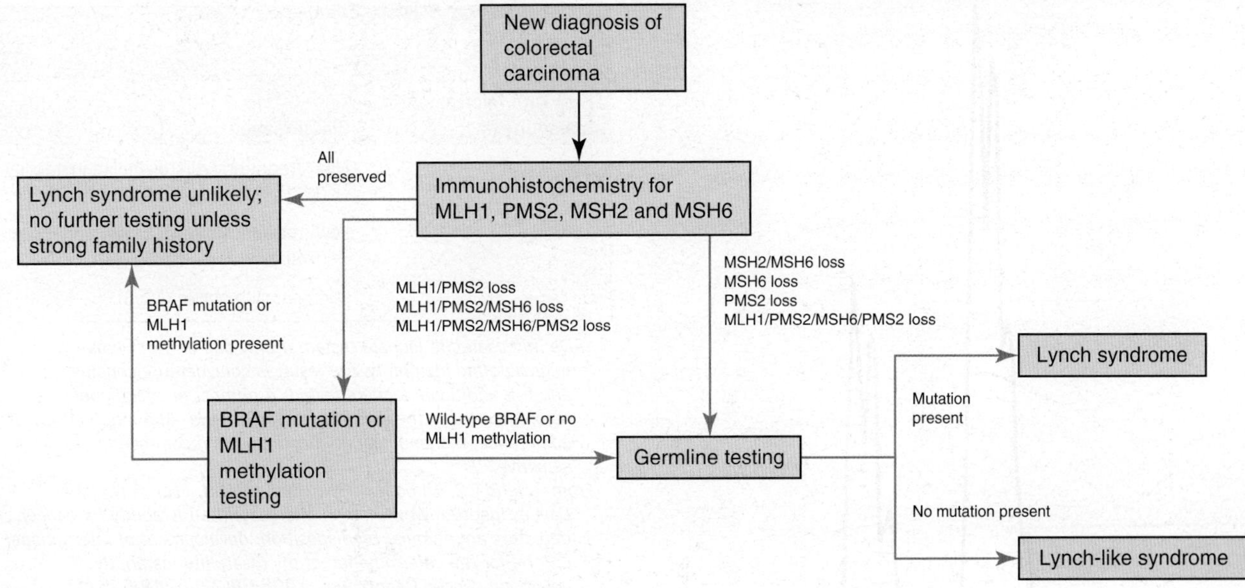

FIGURE 27.51 Suggested screening pathways for Lynch syndrome.

increasing recognition of variant patterns and incomplete loss that may lead to erroneous assessment if all four markers are not evaluated. Furthermore, staining for all four proteins up front prevents a second round of testing in the 15% to 20% of CRCs that lose PMS2 secondary to MLH1 methylation.

***BRAF* Mutation Testing.** *BRAF* mutations are identified in 15% to 20% of CRCs and are mutually exclusive to *KRAS* mutations.[595] Almost all *BRAF* mutations in colorectal neoplasms are V600E point mutations that are readily determined by a variety of polymerase chain reactions (PCRs) and other molecular methodologies.[85] An immunohistochemical stain specific to BRAF V600E (VE1 clone) is also available and has high correlation with underlying *BRAF* mutation,[596] although its usefulness appears to be practice dependent, and molecular methodologies remain the gold standard. *BRAF* mutations are present almost exclusively in serrated pathway neoplasms and are rare (only about 1%) in Lynch syndrome–associated CRC.[597,598] Because of this specificity for the serrated colorectal molecular pathway, *BRAF* mutation testing can be used in a testing algorithm as a means to differentiate sporadic MLH1-deficient (methylated) CRC from Lynch syndrome–associated CRC.[588,599] In MLH1-deficient cancers, *BRAF* mutation testing has a sensitivity of 50% to 70% and a specificity of nearly 100%.[598,600]

***MLH1* Methylation Testing.** Most CRCs with MLH1 deficiency show methylation of the promoter region of the *MLH1* gene, resulting in transcriptional silencing. This abnormality is typically associated with widespread aberrations in DNA methylation (i.e., CIMP), which is present in approximately 25% of CRCs.[79]

These sporadic MLH1-deficient CRCs may be differentiated from Lynch syndrome by *MLH1* methylation testing with molecular PCR assays.[600] This is more efficient than *BRAF* mutation testing for Lynch syndrome because only 65% to 75% of CRCs showing MLH1 methylation have a *BRAF* mutation.[588] An expanded assay of multiple potential sites of methylation, referred to as *CIMP testing*, can also be performed. Although there is no international consensus on the optimal choice of markers for CIMP testing, several loci have begun to emerge as the most sensitive and specific for this type of application.[601]

Microsatellite Instability Testing. Frameshift mutations in microsatellites can be identified by extraction of DNA from both normal and tumor tissue (usually paraffin-embedded tissue), amplification of selected microsatellites by polymerase chain reaction (PCR), followed by analysis of fragment size by gel electrophoresis or an automated sequencer (Fig. 27.52). Criteria have been developed to standardize the molecular classification of MSI (Table 27.22) by using either a Bethesda consensus–defined panel of microsatellites or a revised panel that uses more mononucleotide markers.[558,602] The sensitivity of MSI testing for confirming Lynch syndrome depends on the MMR gene affected and is 80% to 91% for *MLH1 or MSH2* mutations and 55% to 77% for *MSH6 or PMS2* mutations; the specificity of MSI testing is 90%.[589] Only occasional tumors from patients with known pathogenic MMR gene mutations are MSS.[558] The absence of mutations in as many as 20% of Lynch syndrome families with MSI tumors could be caused by the inability of current technology to identify the causative mutation, or it may represent a combination of a somatic mutation of one MMR allele and loss of heterozygosity at the other allele (see Lynch-like Syndrome).[603,604] At present, MSI testing is used primarily in a research setting and does not form part of routine screening algorithms for Lynch syndrome, except in specific next-generation sequencing (NGS) panel testing (see later discussion).

Germline Testing. Genetic workup of Lynch syndrome families aims to identify the underlying germline mutation. Confirmation of the germline mutation allows for the most accurate treatment and follow-up recommendations for the patient and allows predictive testing to be undertaken in interested family members. The initial approach by most laboratories is to analyze the complete coding sequence of the relevant gene or genes (depending on immunohistochemistry results) as well as a portion of the intronic regions important to exon splicing. Some laboratories use a variety

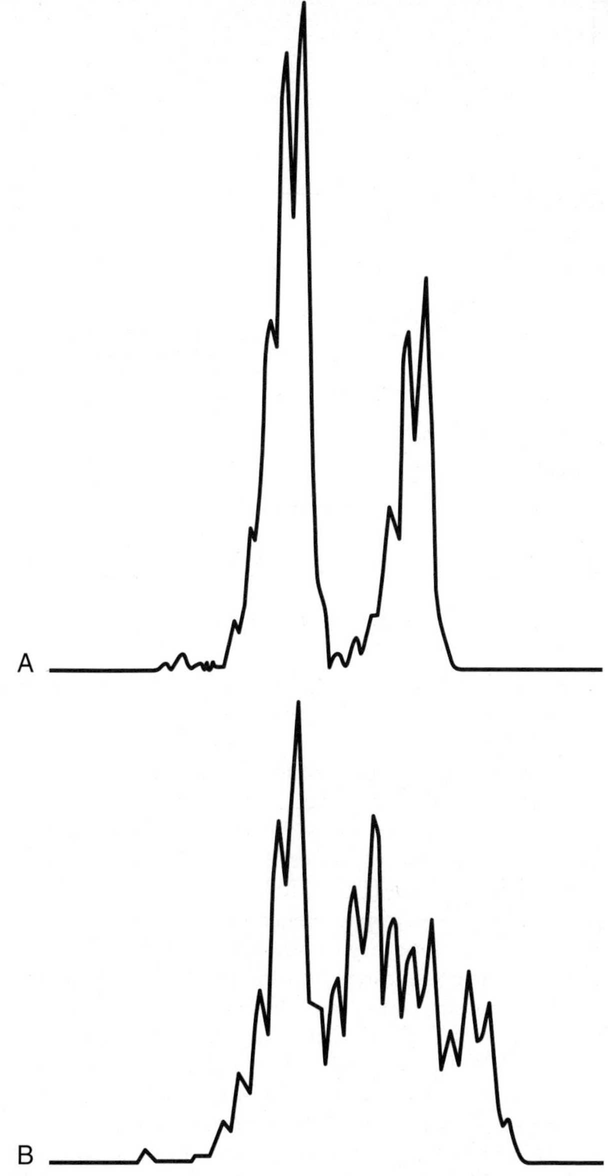

FIGURE 27.52 Molecular analysis for microsatellite instability. Separate DNA samples from normal and tumor tissue have been amplified by polymerase chain reaction and subjected to fragment size analysis in an automated sequencer. **A,** DNA from normal tissue has two distinct peaks indicating that the sample is heterozygous for this allele. **B,** DNA from the tumor reveals multiple additional peaks between the two residual normal alleles, indicative of microsatellite shifts.

of rapid screening approaches to find mutations, whereas others undertake a complete sequence analysis. In certain specific geographic or ethnic settings, screening may begin with testing of founder mutations common to some populations (e.g., the American founder mutation in *MSH2*).[605] If mutations are not detected, testing for mRNA splicing abnormalities and large genomic deletions is indicated, but this may not always be available. The biggest challenge in germline testing relates to the interpretation of point mutations. Criteria for likely pathogenicity have been proposed. An increasing number of functionally insignificant variants is being compiled, but a large number of variants of unknown significance (VUS) remains.[606] In extremely rare families, heritable methylation silencing of *MLH1* and *MSH2* has been reported.[607,608] Germline testing should be undertaken only after informed consent is obtained from the patient and in association with appropriate genetic counseling.

TABLE 27.22 Bethesda Criteria for Microsatellite Instability*

Loci with Microsatellite Instability (%)	Classification
≥40	High-frequency microsatellite instability (MSI-H)
10-30	Low-frequency microsatellite instability (MSI-L)
0	Microsatellite stable (MSS)

Five microsatellite loci are tested; if only one of the five has microsatellite instability, the result is considered inconclusive, and five additional loci are tested. A number of specific loci are recommended in the definition of the criteria. At a later consensus conference, mononucleotide markers were recommended as more sensitive.[558]

From Boland CR, Thibodeau SN, Hamilton SR, et al. A National Cancer Institute Workshop on Microsatellite Instability for cancer detection and familial predisposition: development of international criteria for the determination of microsatellite instability in colorectal cancer. Cancer Res. *1998;58(22):5248-5257.*

Emerging Role of Next-Generation Sequencing. As will be evident from the preceding discussion, the current pathways for detection of Lynch syndrome involve a multistep process. The emerging technology of NGS provides a one-step process for determining the presence of MSI and identifying specific pathogenic variants that can be targeted when subsequent germline sequencing is performed, and it can provide information on predictive and diagnostic biomarkers including BRAF and KRAS. It has been shown that NGS can improve the diagnosis of Lynch syndrome beyond current methodologies and has a diagnostic sensitivity between 96% and 100% and a specificity between 97% and 100%.[559,609]

NGS has become the methodology of choice for germline confirmation of Lynch syndrome. This is generally performed as part of multigene panels that examine the multiple genes defects with known inherited CRC risk. These panels are constantly updated as new pathogenic mutations are identified. It is not uncommon in genetic cancer services for patient samples to be continually retested as new panels become available if pathogenic mutations had not been detected previously despite a strong clinical suspicion of hereditary CRC. Table 27.23 lists the current genes recommended for inclusion by the NCCN in multigene panels for investigation of potential hereditary CRC.

Differential Diagnosis of Lynch Syndrome

In general, the absence of polyposis in Lynch syndrome enables ready differentiation from inherited CRC syndromes that are associated with polyposis syndromes such as familial adenomatous polyposis, attenuated familial adenomatous polyposis syndrome, and MUTYH-associated polyposis. In the past, family and personal history of CRC or other Lynch syndrome– associated cancers raised the possibility of Lynch syndrome clinically. The advent of universal testing of MMR proteins now means that the differential

TABLE 27.23 Comparison of Sporadic Colorectal Cancer and Colitis-Associated Carcinoma

	Risk Factors	Initiating Factors (Normal/Low-Grade Dysplasia)	Progressing Factors (High-Grade Dysplasia/Carcinoma)	Morphology
Sporadic CRC	Environmental Genetic/inherited	*APC* mutation Hypermethylation/*BRAF* mutation Β-catenin accumulation	*KRAS* mutation *TP53* mutation (late) MMR deficiency	Adenocarcinoma NOS
Colitis-associated CRC	Duration, severity, and extent of disease Primary sclerosing cholangitis Family history of CRC	Proinflammatory cytokines (e.g., NF-κB, TNF-α, TGF-β, IL-10, IL-6, and so on) *TP53* mutation Reactive oxygen species Epigenetic changes (e.g., DNA methylation, micro-RNAs)	Noncanonical Wnt pathway Infrequent *KRAS* mutation MMR preserved	Mucinous Signet ring cell Low-grade tubuloglandular More likely synchronous

CRC, *Colorectal carcinoma;* MMR, *mismatch repair;* NOS, *not otherwise specified*

diagnosis for Lynch syndrome mostly exists with tumors showing some form of MMR deficiency in the setting of a possible or probable familial history and/or extracolonic tumors that fit the general spectrum of those associated with Lynch syndrome.

Lynch-Like Syndrome

This is a term given to cases clinically suspected to represent Lynch syndrome on the basis of MSI and deficiency of immunohistochemical staining for an MMR protein; however a germline mutation has not been identified. Other features suggestive of Lynch syndrome may also exist, such as young age at onset, family history, or other Lynch syndrome–associated tumor types. It is widely believed that at least some such cases represent true Lynch syndrome whereby the mutational event that led to silencing of the MMR gene (either in the gene itself or an associated gene) has not been defined at the present time. There also exists the possible explanation that as yet, unidentified mechanisms exist that can silence MMR gene function but are not the result of a genetically inherited syndrome. The most common mechanism that has been demonstrated involves a combination of a somatic mutation of one MMR allele and loss of heterozygosity at the other allele.[603] This results in somatic biallelic loss of an MMR gene, which will be demonstrable by both MSI and deficiency of immunohistochemical staining for an MMR protein. No matter the mechanism, the risk for Lynch syndrome–associated carcinomas in family members is increased compared with the general population but is less than that seen in confirmed Lynch syndrome cases. At present, patients with Lynch-like syndrome are followed up clinically in the same way as those with genetically established Lynch syndrome (Box 27.26).[611]

BOX 27.26 Lynch-like Syndrome

- Microsatellite instability and/or deficiency of immunohistochemical staining for a mismatch repair protein without a detectable germline mutation in a mismatch repair gene
- Potential causes include biallelic somatic inactivation of mismatch repair function or an undetectable germline abnormality

Follow up as per Lynch syndrome

BOX 27.27 Constitutional Mismatch Repair Deficiency Syndrome

- Present in childhood
- Autosomal recessive
- Colorectal carcinoma in one-third; extracolonic malignancy is common
- Café au lait spots
- Loss of mismatch repair protein in both neoplastic and nonneoplastic cells

Constitutional Mismatch Repair Deficiency Syndrome

Constitutional mismatch repair deficiency syndrome (CMMRDS), also referred to as *hereditary biallelic mismatch repair deficiency,* results from inherited biallelic germline mutations in MMR genes, usually either *PMS2 or MSH6.* The biallelic mutations are generally the result of consanguinity, and an autosomal recessive pattern of inheritance is observed. Affected patients present in childhood with a characteristic cluster of tumors including brain (usually glioblastomas), colorectal and small intestinal carcinomas, and hematological malignancies (leukemias and lymphomas). A variety of other epithelial malignancies, including endometrial carcinoma, and rare sarcomas have also been reported.[612] Colorectal adenomatous polyposis has also been described in one-third of patients.[613] Nearly all patients demonstrate café au lait spots, so CMMRDS is often mistaken for neurofibromatosis type I clinically (Box 27.27). Overall, approximately one-third of patients develop CRC,[612] which shows histological features similar to Lynch syndrome–associated CRC. Tumor tissue displays loss of the affected MMR protein by immunohistochemistry, however unlike Lynch syndrome, protein expression is also absent in surrounding nonneoplastic tissue. The unaffected MMR proteins remain preserved.

Polymerase Proofreading–Associated Polyposis Syndrome

Polymerase proofreading–associated polyposis (PPAP) syndrome is an autosomal dominant syndrome resulting from a germline mutation in the exonuclease domain of *POLE* (encoding DNA polymerase epsilon) or *POLD1* (encoding DNA polymerase delta 1). The prevalence is currently unknown, although it is likely to be rare. The clinical phenotype comprises a colorectal polyposis with generally small numbers of adenomas that develop through adulthood and are first evidenced by 20 years of age. The fully developed phenotype is established by 50 years of age. PPAP syndrome accounts for as many as 10% of patients with a phenotype of familial adenomatous polyposis.[614] In contrast with Lynch syndrome, there are no distinctive morphological features allowing histological distinction from sporadic CRC. The development of CRC is earlier than in conventional CRC, with one study finding the risk of CRC up to the age of 70 years for males and females, respectively, to be 28% and 21% for *POLE* mutation carriers and 90% and 82% for *POLD1* mutation carriers. [614] PPAP-associated CRCs demonstrate a hypermutated state, making them good candidates for checkpoint inhibitor treatment. Some cases acquire mutations in MMR genes, resulting in MSI and producing a Lynch-like syndrome.[615]

Familial Colorectal Cancer Type X Syndrome

Familial colorectal cancer type X syndrome is a term used for patients who meet Amsterdam criteria for Lynch syndrome; however, in contrast, the CRCs present at an older age, predominantly in the distal colon or rectum (70%), are more likely to be associated with background polyposis, and do not show histological or molecular evidence of MSI or loss of MMR protein expression.[616] Furthermore, extracolonic tumors typical of Lynch syndrome are not encountered. It is likely that this condition is heterogeneous with many common and uncommon mutations identified in patients meeting clinical criteria for this diagnosis. Some of the described mutations include *BRCA2, SEMA4, NTS, RASSF9, GALNT12, KRAS, BRAF, APC, BMPR1A*, and *RPS20*.[617]

Overlap with Other Hereditary Cancer Syndromes: Hereditary Breast and Ovarian Cancer Syndrome

Because CRC is common, it may develop independently in patients who have an inherited predisposition to non-CRCs. When some of these carcinomas are also associated with Lynch syndrome, such as the pancreas and ovary in the setting of *BRCA1 and BRCA2*, then the clinical scenario may mimic Lynch syndrome. Germline mutation testing will normally clarify the diagnosis. Recently, mutations in the *BRIP1* gene (*BRCA1* interacting protein C-terminal helicase 1) have been linked to early-onset colorectal cancer.[618]

Natural History and Treatment

The lifetime risk of CRC in a patient carrying MMR gene mutations has been estimated at 75%.[619] In men, the lifetime risk of CRC has been estimated at 80%, whereas in women the estimated lifetime risk of endometrial cancer (60%) has been found to be higher than the risk for CRC (50%).[619,620] Many of the studies used to generate these lifetime risks were likely skewed by ascertainment bias; that is, they were based on the most highly penetrant families seen at high-risk genetics clinics. As testing programs have expanded, a broader cross section of families has been included in the risk estimates, which have been significantly reduced.

The most recent estimates for the lifetime cumulative risk of CRC to 70 years of age in carriers of *MLH1, MSH2*, and *MSH6* mutations are 52.8%, 53.1%, and 11.0%, respectively, for men and 47.5%, 52.9%, and 23.9%, respectively, for women.[1,621] *PMS2* mutation is associated with an attenuated phenotype, and the cumulative risk of CRC to 80 years of age is 13% for males and 12% for females.[622] The cumulative risk of metachronous CRC has been reported as 16% at 10 years, 41% at 20 years, and 62% at 30 years after segmental colectomy.[623] The risk of metachronous CRC is reduced by 31% for every 10 cm of extra bowel removed at initial surgery.[623] Metachronous cancers occurred more frequently after subtotal colectomy than after total colectomy (23.5% vs. 6.8%).[624] Even with intensive colonoscopic screening, the risk of a second CRC is 16% at 10 years.[556] These data tend to support extensive surgery at initial CRC resection, although the clinical setting must be taken into consideration. The mean age at diagnosis of first cancer is 40 years in families from high-risk clinics and 56 years in mutation carriers identified in population-based studies.[625]

Based on available evidence regarding risk and outcome, MMR gene mutation carriers or at-risk individuals should be offered colonoscopy every 1 to 2 years beginning at 20 to 25 years of age (or 30 years for *MSH6* and PMS2 mutations).[589,591,610] There is insufficient evidence regarding the benefits of endometrial screening to make clear recommendations, but endometrial ultrasound examination and sampling every year beginning at 30 to 35 years of age should be considered, especially in the setting of a clinical trial.[556] Prophylactic hysterectomy and salpingo-oophorectomy should also be considered, particularly if the patient is undergoing abdominal surgery for any other indication.[556] Additional screening measures that are under investigation include annual urinalysis with cytology, periodic upper gastrointestinal endoscopy, and periodic upper abdominal imaging. There is evidence that nonsteroidal antiinflammatory drugs can reduce the cancer risk in Lynch syndrome; however, this is not sufficiently robust to form part of standard treatment approaches.[589,626] Prophylactic subtotal colectomy has clearly been shown to reduce the risk of metachronous CRC and is the preferred treatment choice in surgical candidates.[589]

COLORECTAL CANCER IN SERRATED POLYPOSIS

Serrated polyposis (SP) is a poorly defined disorder, or group of disorders, characterized by the presence of multiple serrated polyps, which may be hyperplastic polyps, SSLs, TSAs or unclassified serrated adenomas, and an increased risk of CRC. The latest WHO classification has revised the previous diagnostic criteria and simplified these into either of two diagnostic requirements: (1) five or more serrated polyps proximal to the rectum, with two or more being larger than 10 mm in diameter and all being at least 5 mm in size or (2) more than 20 serrated polyps of any size distributed throughout the large bowel, with at least 5 being proximal to the rectum (Box 27.28).[1] When thus defined, 25% of cases meet criterion one, 45%

BOX 27.28 WHO Criteria for Serrated Polyposis Syndrome

1. Five or more serrated polyps proximal to the rectum, with two or more being larger than 10 mm in diameter and all being at least 5 mm in size
2. More than 20 serrated polyps of any size distributed throughout the large bowel, with at least 5 being proximal to the rectum

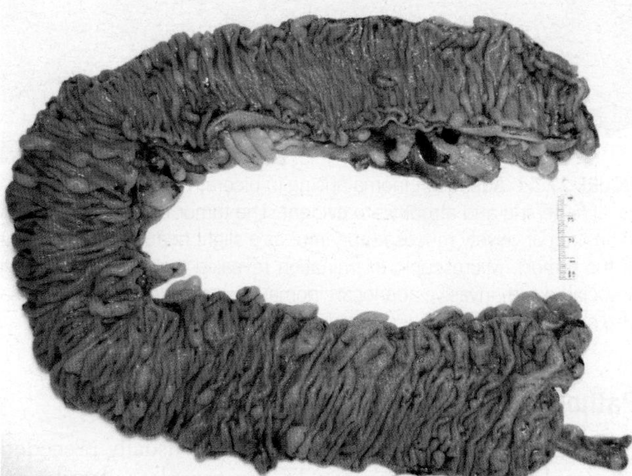

FIGURE 27.53 Colectomy for serrated polyposis. Multiple sessile lesions throughout the colon are shown. Most reside on the ridges of the mucosal folds, which is a typical pattern in this condition.

meet criterion two, and 30% meet both criteria.[627] It is important to note that polyp counts used in the criteria are cumulative counts over time, and SP patients will often not reach clinical criteria for the diagnosis at initial presentation. Furthermore, even when diagnostic criteria are satisfied, the diagnosis is often not appreciated outside of specialized centers.[628] The clinical phenotype is very heterogeneous, with some patients only just reaching the threshold for clinical diagnosis and others demonstrating innumerable polyps (Fig. 27.53). The median cumulative polyp count in serrated polyposis patients is 30 to 40. Serrated polyposis is reported to have a prevalence of 0.1% in primary screening colonoscopies increasing to nearly 1% with cumulative counts in follow-up colonoscopies.[627] SP has an equal sex distribution and a wide age range at presentation, with a median around 50 years. It is associated with an approximately five times increased risk of CRC compared with the normal population. CRC is diagnosed in 16% to 29% of patients with SP, mostly before recognition of the syndrome.[627,629] In patients with known SP undergoing surveillance, 5% of SP patients develop CRC.[630] Specialized centers that deal with large numbers of SP patients have noted an association with lymphoma.[631] In one study of 101 survivors of Hodgkin's lymphoma in the Netherlands, SP was found in 6% of Hodgkin's lymphoma survivors but was absent in controls. Furthermore, the prevalence of advanced serrated lesions was 12% versus 4% in the general population control group.[632]

Serrated polyposis may occur sporadically or with familial clustering, and in some cases it meets the Bethesda criteria for familial CRC.[633,634] Criteria for serrated polyposis may also occasionally be met in other genetic polyposis syndromes, in particular MUTYH polyposis and hereditary mixed polyposis syndrome.[635,636] Approximately one-third of patients with serrated polyposis have a first-degree relative with a history of CRC, and the relative risk of CRC among first-degree relatives of SP patients is 5.4.[627,637] The genetic basis of this syndrome is unknown; an inherited predisposition to abnormal methylation regulation in colonic epithelium and serrated precursors has been hypothesized.[638] A study looking at germline mutations for common polyposis genes was unable to identify any associations with serrated polyposis.[639] In rare cases, a mutation in *RNF-43*, a gene involved in the Wnt signaling pathway, has been documented, but this finding has not been confirmed by others.[640,641] At this time, the condition appears more likely to be the result of complex genetic inheritance rather than a monogenic disorder, and environmental factors such as hormonal milieu and tobacco smoking appear to play a role. Serrated polyps in SP most commonly harbor *BRAF* mutations (73%) followed by *KRAS* mutations (8%),[642] whereas in CRC, the rate of *BRAF* mutations is 50% and *KRAS* mutations is 5%.[643] MLH1 loss is seen in approximately 40% of carcinomas arising in serrated polyposis.[643] Hence, it appears that only about one-half of the carcinomas arise via the serrated pathway.[642] The remaining CRC presumably arise via the conventional adenoma carcinoma pathway. Therefore the presence of conventional adenomas in patients with serrated polyposis is an important feature to record. The most common polyps found in serrated polyposis are hyperplastic polyps and SSLs. Approximately 7% of the SSLs show dysplasia. TSA accounts for approximately 4% of all polyps. Conventional adenomas account for nearly 20% of all polyps.[644] Recommendations for management and follow-up are evolving and depend on the number and size of polyps and the number of concurrent conventional adenomas, but colonoscopy should generally be performed at least every 1 to 3 years.[502]

COLITIS-ASSOCIATED NEOPLASIA

Numerous studies have demonstrated an association between IBD and carcinoma.[27,645] In patients with Crohn's disease, the cancer risk is similar to that for patients with ulcerative colitis, with an equal extent of bowel involvement and disease severity. The risk of colonic cancer is increased with early age of onset of IBD; increased duration, severity, and extent of disease in the colon (pancolitis has the greatest risk); the presence of primary sclerosing cholangitis; and the presence of a family history of colon cancer.[646-649] The risk of neoplasia increases significantly after 8 to 10 years of disease, and this risk was quantified in older studies at approximately 0.5% to 1% per year, plateauing between a 15% to 20% prevalence of CRC by 30 years, which is approximately 20-fold higher than in the general population.[27] More recent studies found that the risk for developing carcinoma is decreasing, presumably as a result of better treatment and surveillance.[650] An updated meta-analysis of population-based cohort studies has quantified the incidence of CRC among IBD patients to be 1%, 2%, and 5% after 10, 20, and >20 years of disease duration, respectively.[651] Cancers occur at a mean patient age of 50 years, which is significantly younger than in the general population.[652] Cancer in IBD is typically preceded by dysplasia, either flat or polypoid, which allows a mechanism for identification and management of patients at a curable stage of their disease. CRC accounts for 15% of all deaths in patients with IBD.

Pathogenesis

Several lines of evidence suggest that the molecular pathogenesis of colitis-associated cancer is distinct from that of sporadic colorectal neoplasia.[653-655] There appears to be four key elements to the pathogenesis.[656] (Table 27.23) First, cytokines released as part of the chronic inflammatory process activate proinflammatory mediators, including nuclear factor kappa B (NF-κB), tumor necrosis factor (TNF)-α, TGF-β, interleukin (IL)-10, IL-6, STAT3, cyclooxygenase-2 (COX-2), PGE2, and IL-23, that promote tumorigenesis by upregulating expression of antiapoptotic genes and stimulating cell proliferation and stromal angiogenesis.[657-659] Second, there is increasing evidence that the microbial dysbiosis found in IBD patients may induce various cell signaling pathways via interaction with metabolites in the feces (e.g., indole, bile acids, retinoic acid) and via expression of noncoding RNAs (e.g., micro-RNAs), leading to dysregulation of normal colonocyte function, perpetuating inflammation, and inducing tumorigenesis.[660-662] Third, there is development of genomic instability via CIN, MSI, telomere shortening, and CIMP pathways. These are similar in mechanism to sporadic CRCs but occur at a different frequency and with key molecular events developing at different points in the progression from dysplasia to carcinoma. Compared with unselected, apparently sporadic cancers, mutations in *APC* and *KRAS*, LOH of chromosome 18q, *BCL2* upregulation, and β-catenin stabilization are all less frequent in colitis-associated cancer. β-catenin signaling may be enhanced by the inflammatory environment. In contrast, *CDKN1A (p21)* downregulation, *CDKN1B (p27)* downregulation, and *CDKN2A (p16)* hypermethylation are all more frequent in colitis-associated cancer. Although there have been some reports that MMR deficiency may play a role in colitis-associated neoplasia, this finding has not been confirmed. There are also significant differences in the timing of genetic events between IBD-associated and sporadic cancers. Of great interest, *TP53* mutations, loss of chromosome 9p (site of the gene encoding *CDKN2A*), and aneuploidy are more likely to be present in colitis-associated dysplasia than in sporadic adenomas.[654,656,663-665] The fourth pathogenic mechanism is via epigenetic changes including DNA methylation, histone modifications, chromatin remodeling, and changes in the regulation of small noncoding micro-RNAs. The disturbance of the regulatory role, usually downregulation of nuclear factors, of micro-RNAs in active ulcerative colitis has received considerable recent attention. In one study that investigated a panel of five target micro-RNAs, MIR1, MIR9, MIR124, MIR137, and MIR34B/C, chosen on the basis of previous publications, methylation of each of the micro-RNAs was significantly higher in nonneoplastic mucosa with colitis-associated carcinoma compared with that in nonneoplastic mucosa from control patients, potentially providing a mechanism for screening patients most at risk of neoplasia.[666]

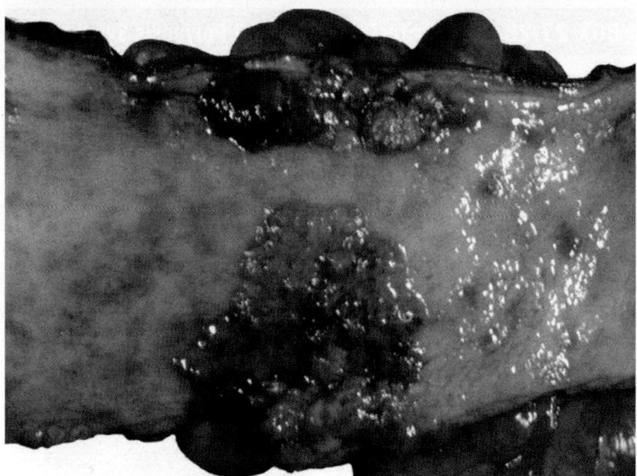

FIGURE 27.54 Adenocarcinoma arising in ulcerative colitis. Severe mucosal flattening and atrophy are evident. The tumor is irregular and lies in an area of velvety mucosa (apparent as a slight nodularity to the right of the tumor). Microscopic examination revealed high-grade dysplasia associated with invasive adenocarcinoma. The surrounding flat mucosa also showed extensive low-grade dysplasia.

Pathological Features

In patients with ulcerative colitis, CRC is usually preceded by dysplasia[667] (see Chapter 17 for complete details). A number of features distinguish colitis-associated from sporadic CRCs[668-670] (Fig. 27.54). Colitis-associated cancers may be difficult to recognize grossly, and they are more likely to grow in a linitis plastica pattern. In one report, up to one-third of cases of high-grade dysplasia or adenocarcinoma were not detected macroscopically.[671] However, the finding of unsuspected carcinoma is generally reported at a lower rate. For instance, in another study, there was only a 3% rate of undetected carcinoma in patients with a preoperative diagnosis of dysplasia.[672] The presence of strictures is a concerning feature that is associated with a finding of low-grade dysplasia in 2%, high-grade dysplasia in 2%, and cancer in 5% of patients with ulcerative colitis and a finding of low-grade dysplasia in 1%, high-grade dysplasia in 0.4%, and cancer in 0.8% of patients with Crohn's disease.[673] In another study, the prevalence of dysplasia in strictures was 3.22% in ulcerative colitis and 2.08% in Crohn's disease.[674] Multiple synchronous cancers are also significantly more frequent in colitis-associated neoplasia; two primary tumors occur in about 20% of patients, and three or more occur in about 10%, compared with 2% in sporadic CRCs.[652,675]

Some studies have suggested that, compared with sporadic cancers, colitis-associated cancers are more evenly distributed throughout the colon and more likely to manifest at an advanced stage, particularly when they are detected outside of a screening or surveillance program.[668] One study suggested that these cancers are much more likely than their sporadic counterparts to arise in the left colon.[652] Signet ring cell carcinomas are significantly more frequent in ulcerative colitis. As many as one-third of all signet ring carcinomas occur in patients with chronic colitis.[159,160] Mucinous adenocarcinomas are also more frequent in ulcerative colitis, averaging between 15% and 20% of all carcinoma patients, with a similar rate also observed in Crohn's disease.[158,676] Approximately 10% of colitis-associated

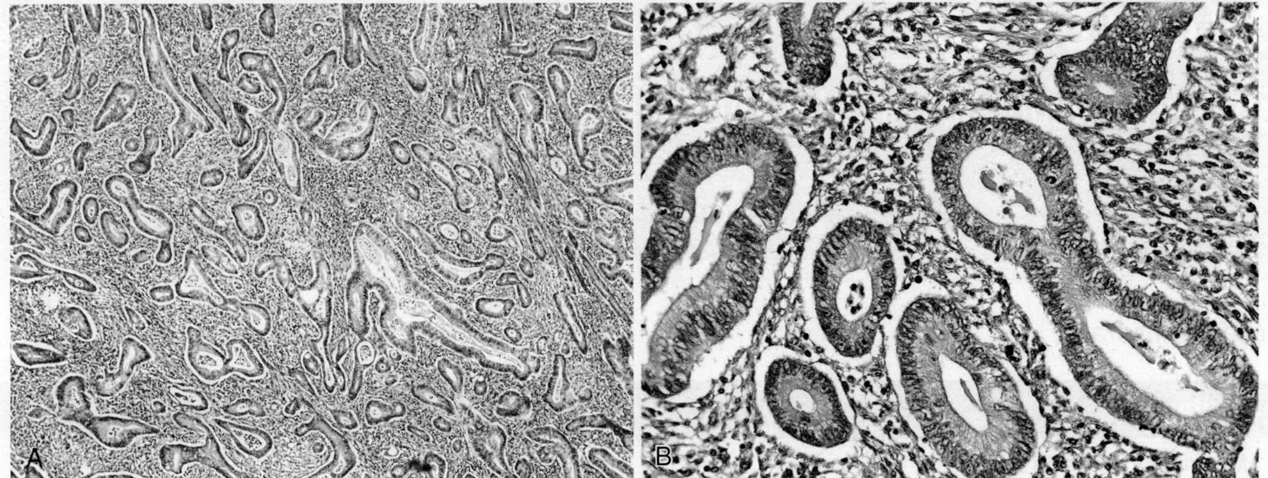

FIGURE 27.55 Low-grade tubuloglandular adenocarcinoma in a patient with ulcerative colitis. A, Proliferation of small to medium-sized neoplastic glands, some with round or tubular profiles, and others with branching. The nuclei show slight stratification. There is no evidence of desmoplasia. **B,** At high power, the low-grade nature of the nuclei is better appreciated.

tumors are composed of very well-differentiated, small- to medium-sized glands with round or tubular profiles, low-grade nuclei, and minimal desmoplasia. These tumors have been termed *low-grade tubuloglandular adenocarcinomas,* and they have been shown to develop directly from low-grade dysplasia, reinforcing the recent trend toward performing colectomy in patients with ulcerative colitis who have only low-grade dysplasia (Fig. 27.55).[677] In general, the degree of tumoral heterogeneity has been found to be greater in colitis-associated carcinomas.[652]

Compared with cancer in patients with ulcerative colitis, cancer in patients with Crohn's disease develops at a slightly older age (but still younger than in the non-IBD general population) and is more likely to be located in the anal or perianal region.[678] Squamous cell carcinoma may develop in this region as a result of long-standing fissures or fistulas.[679] Cancers develop in regions of previous inflammation but also in segments of intestine without endoscopic or pathological evidence of ongoing disease. This is believed to be related to the immunosuppressive effect of treatment on the affected segment rather than the development of carcinoma in non-diseased areas of colon.[668] Surgically excluded segments of the bowel are at particularly high risk for cancer, although procedures that create these segments are performed only infrequently in current practice.[678] Most recent studies suggest that Crohn's disease–associated cancer shows an equal distribution throughout the colon, similar to ulcerative colitis–associated cancer.

Survival of patients with colitis-associated cancer is roughly similar to that of patients with sporadic cancer when controlled for stage and histological subtype.[680,681] As in sporadic cancer, the most important prognostic factors are tumor grade and pathological stage.[682]

The full reference list may be accessed online *at Elsevier eBooks for Practicing Clinicians.*

CHAPTER 28

Epithelial Neoplasms of the Appendix

Joseph Misdraji

Contents

MUCINOUS EPITHELIAL TUMORS

The classification of appendiceal epithelial tumors is shown in Box 28.1. The classification, nomenclature, and histological criteria of mucinous epithelial tumors in the appendix have been the source of considerable controversy. In particular, mucinous epithelial tumors that penetrate deeply into or through the appendiceal wall and disseminate to the peritoneal cavity, resulting in pseudomyxoma peritonei, were the source of much of this controversy. For example, the exact nature of their biological potential (benign vs. malignant, invasive vs. noninvasive) has been a matter of intense debate and has led to nosological confusion. Historically, they were classified as either *ruptured adenomas with dissemination of adenomatous epithelium*[1-6] or as *adenocarcinomas*.[7-11] In 2003, the term *low-grade appendiceal mucinous neoplasm* (LAMN) was introduced[12] for a subset of these tumors, and this term is now universally adopted for tumors that show "pushing" or "broad-front" invasion combined with low-grade cytological features. In contrast, tumors with pushing invasion and high-grade cytological features are termed *high-grade appendiceal mucinous neoplasm* (HAMN). In contemporary classification systems, a diagnosis of adenocarcinoma in the appendix still requires invasion of an infiltrative, not pushing, nature.[13,14]

The nomenclature of goblet cell tumors has also undergone significant recent revision. This enigmatic tumor shows both endocrine and mucinous differentiation and thus has been difficult to classify historically. The classification of these tumors is particularly complicated when they demonstrate high-grade cytological features. For instance, some proposed names for this tumor have included *goblet cell carcinoid, crypt cell carcinoma, mixed adenocarcinoma carcinoid*, and *adenocarcinoma ex goblet cell carcinoid*.[15-17] Recently, these tumors were reclassified as *goblet cell adenocarcinoma*[18] because they typically show glandular or mucinous differentiation, they are staged similarly to adenocarcinomas, and chemotherapy regimens similar to those used for colorectal adenocarcinoma are used in patients with disseminated tumors.

Adenoma

Nomenclature

Historically, the finding of a dilated appendix lined by clearly neoplastic epithelium was often referred to as a *mucinous cystadenoma*, but this term engendered controversy over whether this same tumor, when it spreads to the peritoneum or ovaries, should be termed a *ruptured cystadenoma* or a *cystadenocarcinoma*. However, since the introduction of the term *LAMN* for tumors with similar histological features, the term *mucinous cystadenoma* has been discontinued. *LAMN* is now the accepted term for low-grade epithelial neoplasms that demonstrate pushing invasion and also show spread to the peritoneal cavity.

Whether any tumors should still be classified as *appendiceal adenoma* is unclear and controversial. Some authorities believe that mucinous neoplasms that are confined to the mucosa of the appendix and also show preserved muscularis mucosae should still be recognized as an *adenoma* because of their uniform benign outcome once excised. However, other authorities believe that all mucinous neoplasms should be termed *LAMN*, even if they are restricted to the appendiceal mucosa and without pushing invasion. The Peritoneal Surface Oncology Group International consensus document maintains the designation of *adenoma* only for lesions that resemble their colorectal counterparts; namely, dysplastic lesions that are tubular,

BOX 28.1 World Health Organization Classification of Appendiceal Epithelial Tumors

Appendiceal mucinous neoplasm
- Low-grade appendiceal mucinous neoplasm (LAMN)
- High-grade appendiceal mucinous neoplasm (HAMN)

Serrated lesion and polyp
- Hyperplastic polyp
- Serrated lesion without dysplasia
- Serrated lesion with dysplasia

Adenocarcinoma
- Adenocarcinoma NOS
- Mucinous adenocarcinoma
- Signet ring cell carcinoma
- Undifferentiated carcinoma, NOS

Neuroendocrine neoplasm
- Neuroendocrine tumour (NET)
- Neuroendocrine carcinoma (NEC)
- Mixed neuroendocrine/nonneuroendocrine neoplasm (MiNEN)

Goblet cell adenocarcinoma

tubulovillous, or villous and show features of intestinal-type dysplasia with elongate, hyperchromatic, and pseudostratified nuclei.[13] However, the World Health Organization (WHO) no longer specifically includes the term *adenoma* in its classification of appendiceal tumors. Nevertheless, in this chapter, the term *adenoma* is reserved for dysplastic appendiceal epithelial proliferations that have intestinal-type epithelium, lack hypermucinous features characteristic of LAMN, are tubular, tubulovillous, or villous (and not a flat single layer), and do not show mucin in the wall of the appendix.

Clinical Features

Localized tubular adenomas of the type that occur in the colon are, in fact, rare in the appendix.[5,19-22] However, they may occur in patients with familial adenomatous polyposis.[7,23] Most are incidentally found in appendices removed for other clinical reasons. Large villous adenomas may present with abdominal pain.[24] Tumors in the base of the appendix may represent an extension of a cecal tumor into the appendix, so pathologists should always be aware of this differential diagnosis. The pathogenesis of appendiceal adenomas has never been studied because most of the literature on this topic predates the introduction of the term *LAMN*. They presumably have a similar pathogenesis to colorectal adenomas, but this remains to be tested.

Pathology

Grossly, adenomas of the appendix may show a polypoid or semi-sessile polypoid appearance.[5] By definition, the appendix is not dilated or filled with mucin, as is typical of LAMNs.

The histological appearance of tubular adenomas of the appendix is identical to those that occur in the colon. They may be low grade or high grade. Low-grade tumors show glands lined by cells with elongate, pseudostratified nuclei, with occasional mitotic figures and nuclear debris (Fig. 28.1). High-grade tumors show more architectural complexity, and the glands often show cribriform architecture, micropapillary infoldings, or full thickness stratification. The glands are lined by cells showing high-grade nuclear features, including enlarged nuclei, prominent nucleoli, increased mitotic figures, increased nuclear-to-cytoplasmic (N/C) ratio, loss of polarity, and occasionally pleomorphism.

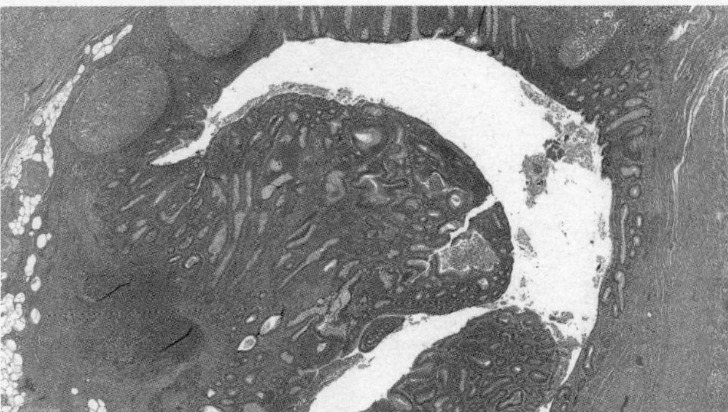

FIGURE 28.1 Tubular adenoma of the appendix. Low-power view shows a polyp projecting into the lumen of the appendix. The polyp shows disordered hyperchromatic glands typical of colorectal tubular adenomas.

Villous adenomas resemble colorectal villous adenomas and are lined by intestinal-type epithelium with hyperchromatic, elongate, and pseudostratified nuclei similar to those that occur in the colon. They can also be low- or high-grade, similar to tubular adenomas.

Differential Diagnosis

The main differential diagnosis is with LAMNs. However, as mentioned earlier, the term *appendiceal adenoma* is reserved for lesions that resemble colorectal-type adenomas and without prominent mucin production. All cystically dilated tumors lined by a single layer of dysplastic epithelium are classified as *LAMN*. Similarly, villous tumors in which the villi are lined by hypermucinous epithelium are more appropriately classified as *LAMN*, even if they are confined to the mucosa.

Natural History and Treatment

Appendiceal adenomas are benign lesions. They are cured by appendectomy. However, if left untreated, they represent a precursor to invasive appendiceal adenocarcinoma.[4] Appendectomy is sufficient treatment for benign appendiceal adenomas.

Low-Grade Appendiceal Mucinous Neoplasm

Nomenclature

LAMNs are mucinous neoplasms with low-grade cytological features that are either confined to the mucosa or show pushing invasion into or through the appendix wall, and, when the appendix ruptures, they may spread to the peritoneal cavity as pseudomyxoma peritonei. Historically, most low-grade mucinous tumors of the appendix were classified as *mucinous cystadenoma*. However, when these tumors spread beyond the appendix, terms such as *ruptured mucinous cystadenoma* or *mucinous adenocarcinoma* have been used, which has created confusion. Because the criteria for tissue invasion in these tumors was believed to

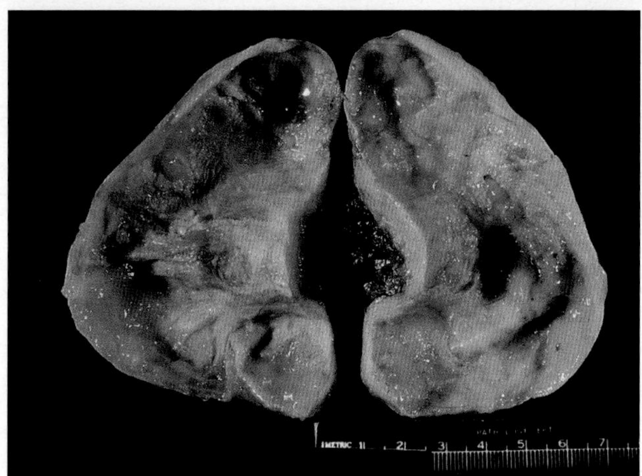

FIGURE 28.2 Gross specimen of a low-grade appendiceal mucinous neoplasm showing cystic transformation of the appendix with marked thickening of the wall. (*From Misdraji J. Epithelial neoplasms and other epithelial lesions of the appendix (excluding carcinoid tumours). Curr Diagn Pathol. 2005;11[1]:60-71.*)

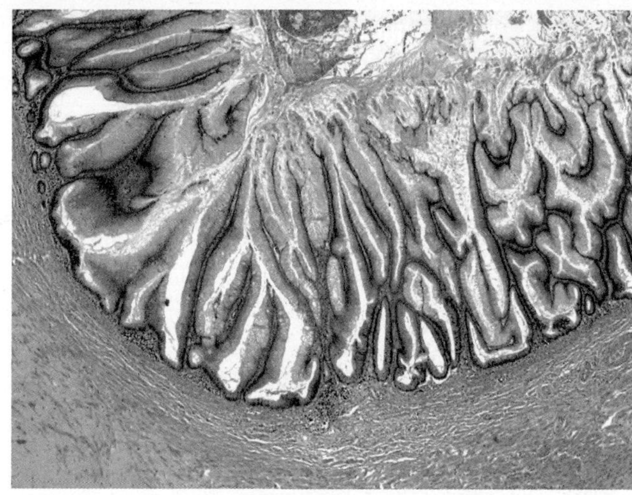

FIGURE 28.3 Low-grade appendiceal mucinous neoplasm. Low-power view shows replacement of the normal mucosa by a villous epithelial proliferation that in this section is confined to the appendiceal mucosa. Note that the villi taper to a filiform appearance and are lined by hypermucinous epithelium, features that are typical of LAMNs.

be poorly defined, other terms that were applied included *mucinous tumor of uncertain malignant potential*[23] or *borderline tumor*. In 2003, the term *LAMN* was introduced[12] for these tumors to circumnavigate the controversy over whether they are benign or malignant and to allow them to be classified regardless of whether they had spread to the peritoneum. This term has gained widespread acceptance and has enabled progress to be made on the clinical, pathological, and molecular aspects of these tumors. However, it should be recognized that in much of the prior literature, so-called *appendiceal adenomas* were in fact LAMNs.

Clinical Features

LAMNs usually present in the sixth decade of life, although the age range at presentation is quite broad (18 to 89 years).[1,5,8,12,25] There is a predilection for fem ales.[1,5,8,26] Patients may present with abdominal pain, a palpable abdominal mass, or even with ovarian metastasis.[1,5,8,12,25] In fact, ovarian metastasis may predate discovery of the primary appendiceal tumor. Other clinical presentations include intussusception of the appendix[27,28] or the finding of mucin within a hernia sac.[29-31] A retrocecal LAMN can present as a retroperitoneal mass or as pseudomyxoma extraperitonei.[32-37] Approximately 15% to 20% of LAMNs are discovered incidentally in patients who have undergone surgery for an unrelated condition.[5,12,26] In some studies, there is an association between LAMNs and other types of colonic neoplasms and polyps.[5]

Pathogenesis

LAMNs show frequent *KRAS* mutations.[38-44] Also, about 50% of LAMNs have *GNAS* mutations.[38,42-44] Activating *GNAS* mutations cause constitutive activation of adenylate cyclase and elevated cAMP levels. In cell lines, this is associated with increased expression of MUC2 and MUC5AC,[38] raising the intriguing possibility that *GNAS* mutations play a role in mucin production, which is a hallmark of LAMNs and its associated complication pseudomyxoma peritonei (see later). LAMNs have not been shown to demonstrate microsatellite instability or other features of the mutator pathway, such as loss of expression of DNA mismatch repair proteins or *BRAF* mutations.[41,42,45] Other mutations occur but are rare, such as *TP53*, *RB1*, *APC*, *MET*, *RNF43*, and *PIK3CA*.[43,44]

Nuclear expression of β-catenin has been observed in LAMNs, but *CTNNB1* mutations are infrequent.[42] Bibi et al. showed that N-cadherin expression is increased in appendiceal mucinous tumors and associated pseudomyxoma peritonei, whereas E-cadherin expression is reduced relative to normal epithelium.[46] They also showed vimentin expression in these tumors. These authors suggested that a shift in cadherin phenotype and vimentin expression may reflect an epithelial-mesenchymal transition in which epithelial cells switch to a mesenchymal phenotype, a process that presumably promotes metastasis.

Pathology

Appendices with LAMNs may appear grossly unremarkable, or they may be cystically dilated and filled with abundant tenacious mucin.[8,12,25,47] The wall may be thin or fibrotic, hyalinized, and calcified (Fig. 28.2).[8,12] Rupture of the tumors with the presence of mucin on the serosal surface or within the peritoneal cavity may be grossly evident.[1,8,12,25] Infrequently, the appendix may be completely encased in mucin or even fused to the right ovary.[12,25,47] The appendix lining may be smooth, granular, or corrugated with intervening smooth areas.[8] Focal outpouchings of the lumen, filled with mucin, have also been described.[25]

On microscopic examination, LAMNs show either villous or flat neoplastic mucinous epithelium, but either way they are often associated with atrophy of lymphoid tissue.[1,12,23] In villous tumors, the villi are typically filiform in appearance and contain scant lamina propria (Fig. 28.3).

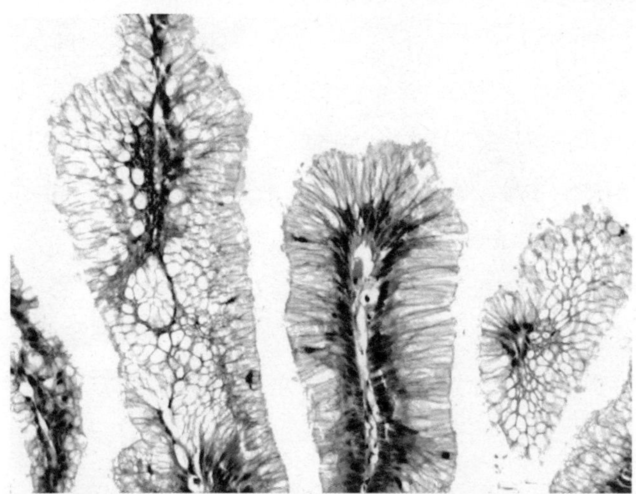

FIGURE 28.4 Low-grade appendiceal mucinous neoplasm. High-power view of the villi shows that they are lined by mucinous epithelial cells with abundant intracytoplasmic mucin. The nuclei show mild nuclear hyperchromasia and pseudostratification, consistent with low-grade dysplasia.

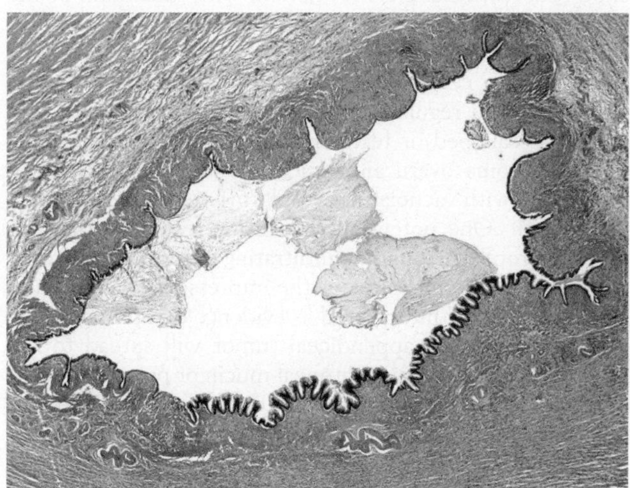

FIGURE 28.5 Low-grade appendiceal mucinous neoplasm. The appendix is dilated with mucin in the lumen, and the mucosal-based tumor is partly flattened and partly scalloped. The term *cystadenoma* is no longer recommended for this lesion.

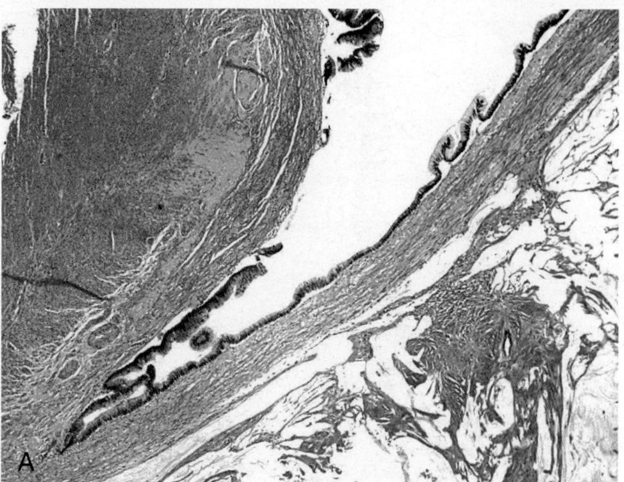

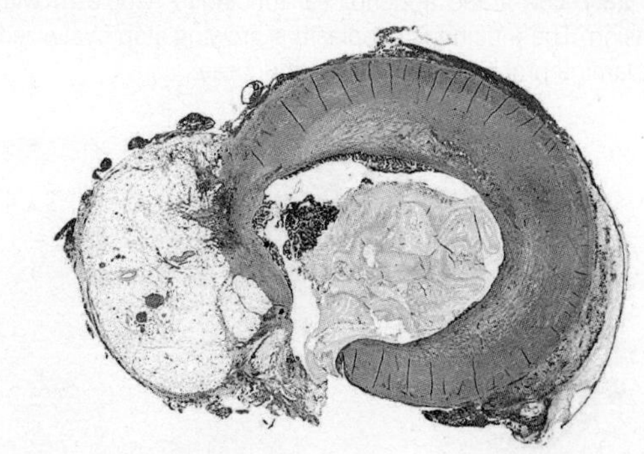

FIGURE 28.6 Examples of pushing invasion in low-grade appendiceal mucinous neoplasm. A, The tumor dissects through the muscularis propria *(upper left)* and merges with dissecting mucin and fibrosis on the appendiceal surface *(lower right).* **B,** Whole-mount view of a LAMN that has perforated the appendix.

The epithelium contains abundant cytoplasmic mucin that may compress the cell nuclei. Cells with small compressed nuclei may appear deceptively benign or even nonneoplastic (Fig. 28.4).[1] The villi are usually straight, but occasionally they show a variable degree of luminal serration. In fact, in some circumstances, these tumors may resemble a hyperplastic polyp or a serrated neoplasm (see later). Alternatively, the epithelium may be flat, scalloped, or undulating in appearance (Fig. 28.5). Denudation of the epithelium is common in these tumors,[1] particularly in those with attenuated epithelium, and in this circumstance, distinction from a benign nonneoplastic retention cyst may be difficult (see later). In some cases, nearly the entire appendiceal mucosa may be denuded of epithelium. In these cases, extensive sampling may be needed to identify the foci of neoplastic epithelium.[7,8] LAMNs are composed of columnar cells that are rich in mucin and typically display low-grade nuclear atypia. Common features include nuclear elongation, hyperchromasia, pseudostratification, inconspicuous nucleoli, infrequent mitoses, and apoptotic nuclear debris.[8,12,48] Bordering areas of neoplastic mucosa may be hyperplastic-appearing epithelium with prominent crypt serration,[22,49] but the significance of this finding is uncertain.

One distinctive feature of LAMNs is that they do not normally invade the appendiceal wall in a conventional manner; they do not show infiltrative and irregular glands or a desmoplastic stroma. Instead, they "invade" by showing broad areas of pushing invasion. Neoplastic epithelium, mucin, or a combination of both may appear to dissect into or through the wall of the appendix and may even cause perforation. Tumor involvement of the appendiceal wall may simulate involvement of a preexisting diverticula. However, in contrast with diverticular involvement by a LAMN, true tumor involvement of the wall of the appendix lacks lamina propria (Fig. 28.6). Fibrosis of the appendiceal wall, which is common in LAMN, may result in the appearance of neoplastic epithelium in direct contact with fibrotic or hyalinized stroma, rather than situated above the muscularis mucosae with surrounding lamina propria (Fig. 28.7). In fact, the appendiceal wall in LAMNs may show alterations

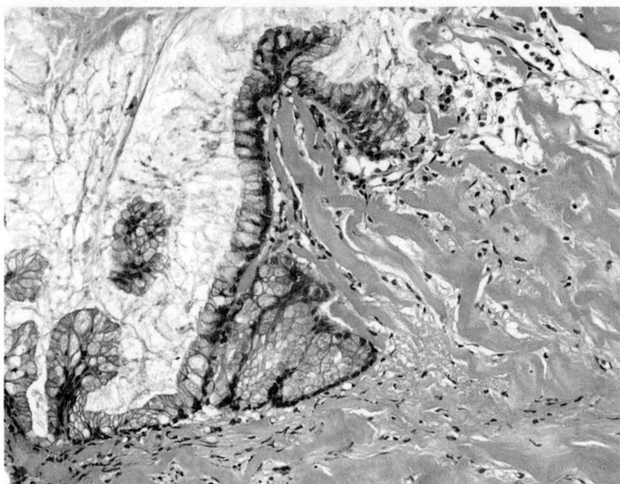

FIGURE 28.7 Low-grade appendiceal mucinous neoplasm with pushing invasion. The mucinous neoplasm is growing atop hyalinized tissue, without lamina propria or muscularis mucosae.

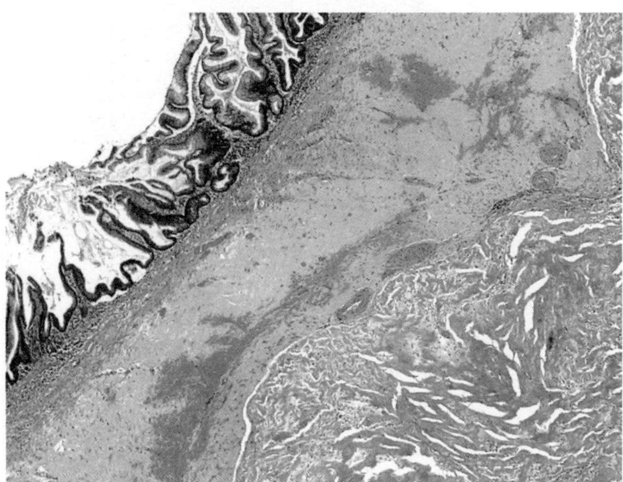

FIGURE 28.8 Low-grade appendiceal mucinous neoplasm demonstrating submucosal fibrosis and marked mural hyalinization with a nodular hyalinized scar *(lower right)*.

of the muscularis mucosae and even total effacement of normal appendiceal landmarks in some cases. Fibrosis and hyalinization of the appendiceal wall may be nodular on occasion (Fig. 28.8), which may represent evidence of prior episodes of mucin leakage and subsequent tissue repair.[12] Dystrophic calcification is common, particularly in areas with prominent mucin.[1,47] Alteration of the wall of the appendix presents pathologists with challenges with regard to pathological staging. For instance, cases in which there is extension into or through the muscularis propria may be difficult to recognize when there is replacement of the muscle layers by fibrous or hyalinized tissue. However, distinction between muscularis propria and fibrotic tissue has little practical importance in patient management for patients in whom the serosa is intact (uninvolved) (see "Natural History").

Tumors that have spread to the ovary often reveal characteristic features that allow distinction from a primary mucinous tumor of the ovary. Most often, the right ovary is the one involved.[25] Involvement of the ovary often

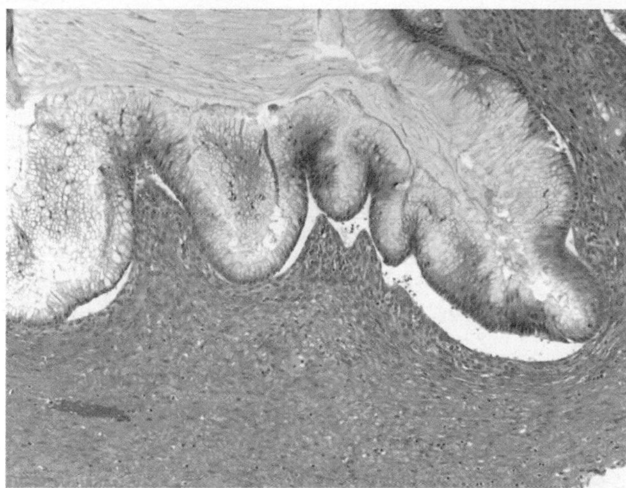

FIGURE 28.9 Ovarian involvement by a low-grade appendiceal mucinous neoplasm. The mucinous tumor typically forms festooning or scalloped glands with a subepithelial cleft. Condensation of the stroma under the neoplastic epithelium resembles a cambium layer, mimicking a primary ovarian neoplasm.

shows subepithelial cleft formation, with separation of the tumor epithelium from the underlying stroma (Fig. 28.9). The characteristic features are elongated glands lined by tall mucinous cells, with pale mucin dissecting the ovarian stroma and regularly spaced shallow invaginations that impart a scalloped or festooned appearance to the glands. Pseudomyxoma ovarii and mucin granulomas (clusters of histiocytes with vacuolated cytoplasm) are frequently present as well. One potentially confusing feature is that the ovarian stroma surrounding infiltrating glands may be more closely packed, which creates the impression of a cambium layer that may be interpreted as evidence of a primary neoplasm.[50] Rarely, an appendiceal tumor will spread to the ovary in the absence of peritoneal mucin or pseudomyxoma peritonei. This situation may cause consideration of a second ovarian primary tumor. One study showed that subepithelial cleft formations are, perhaps, the single best histological feature in the ovary that helps to identify a tumor as a metastatic LAMN, rather than a primary ovarian tumor, but ultimately, a combination of multiple features may be necessary to support an unequivocal origin in the appendix.[51] In isolated cases, molecular studies, such as evaluation of *KRAS* and *GNAS* mutations, may be performed to help determine the true origin of an ovarian tumor.[52]

Appendiceal mucinous neoplasms and their peritoneal metastases usually express keratin 20, and about 25% to 40% coexpress keratin 7.[46,53] CDX-2 and MUC-2 are expressed in nearly 100% of appendiceal mucinous tumors and pseudomyxoma peritonei.[46,53-56] SATB2 is expressed in 80% to 100% of appendiceal mucinous neoplasms, and this marker may be particularly useful to distinguish an appendiceal primary tumor from an ovarian primary tumor.[57,58]

Differential Diagnosis

Appendiceal Adenoma

As per the definition of this tumor discussed earlier in this chapter, appendiceal adenomas represent a tumor that morphologically resembles a colorectal adenoma, with

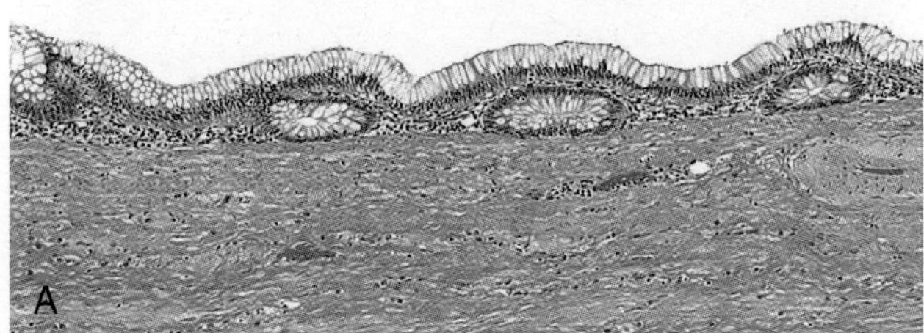

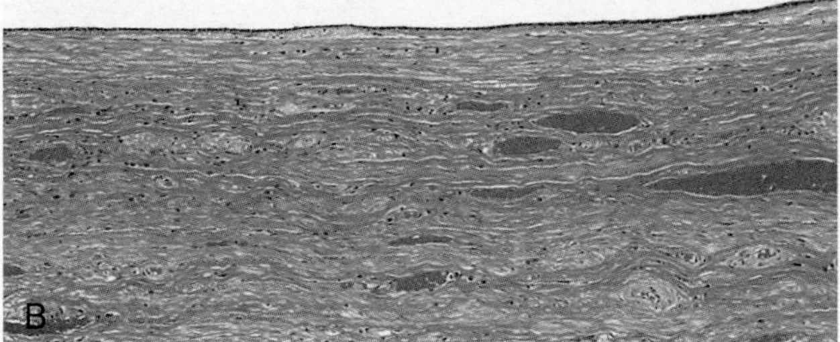

FIGURE 28.10 Retention cyst of the appendix with dilatation of the appendiceal lumen. A, The mucosa is atrophic, but mucosal architecture is still evident in the form of short, flattened crypts within the lamina propria. **B,** In other areas, the cyst lining is composed of an attenuated layer of epithelial cells.

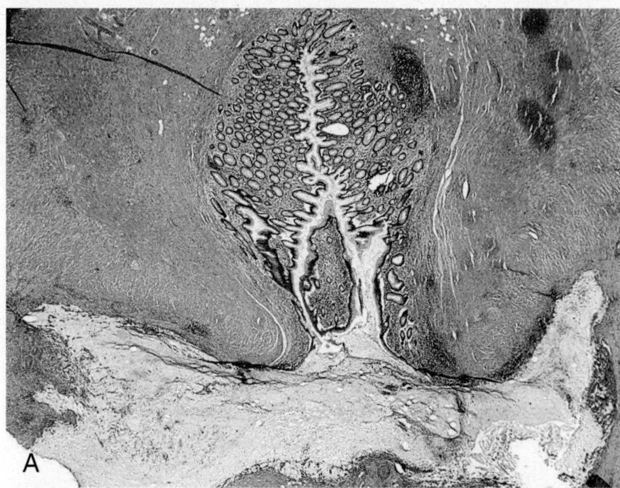

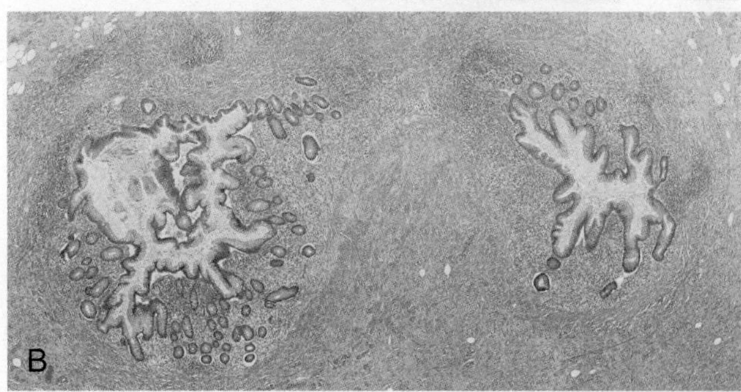

FIGURE 28.11 Appendiceal diverticular disease mimicking a low-grade appendiceal mucinous neoplasm. A, A ruptured diverticulum shows appendiceal mucosa herniating through the muscularis propria, with extravasation of mucin outside the appendix. The mucosa shows architectural disarray, compatible with reactive changes. **B,** Medium-power view of the mucosa in a case of appendiceal diverticular disease shows the typical crypt disarray and hyperplastic changes that are frequently mistaken for evidence of a low-grade appendiceal mucinous neoplasm.

intestinal-type dysplastic epithelium, in either a tubular adenoma or villous configuration, but without excess mucin production. Cystic tumors lined by a single layer of flat, scalloped, or undulating epithelium are, by definition, LAMNs, not adenomas. The villi typical in villous adenomas are lined by intestinal-type epithelium, with a reduced amount of lamina propria, whereas the villi in LAMNs are typically lined by hypermucinous epithelium with virtually no appreciable lamina propria ("filiform" villi). Any tumor that shows a pushing front into the submucosa or muscular wall, perforates the appendix, or is associated with mucin or neoplastic mucinous epithelial cells on the appendiceal serosa or any extraappendiceal site should not be classified as an adenoma.

Retention Cyst

Retention cysts are nonneoplastic benign lesions that develop as a result of obstruction of the appendiceal lumen,[5] although the cause of the obstruction may not necessarily be apparent. Retention cysts are relatively uncommon. They only rarely attain a size larger than 2 cm in greatest diameter.[7] Retention cysts may be fibrotic and chronically inflamed, and they may show extensive epithelial denudation similar to a LAMN. The mucosa may be atrophic with short or flattened crypts, or it may be composed of a single layer of attenuated cuboidal epithelium, mimicking a LAMN (Fig. 28.10).[3,23] Continuity of the attenuated areas with areas of relatively preserved mucosal architecture is an important clue to the diagnosis of a retention cyst.[59] Conversely, the presence of slender filiform villi, even if only a focal finding, is more indicative of a true neoplasm. Retention cysts may also rupture and result in the presence of mucin within the peritoneal cavity.[23] However, unlike pseudomyxoma peritonei that develops due to a neoplasm, the mucin in the peritoneal cavity as a result of a ruptured retention cyst is usually confined to the area of rupture and does not normally accumulate further after appendectomy.

Microscopic examination of the mucin from a ruptured retention cyst may demonstrate varying degrees of tissue reaction and organization (showing granulation tissue in various degrees of development) and mesothelial hyperplasia. Epithelial cells are not present within the mucin in ruptured retention cysts. Thus their presence should exclude this diagnosis unless contamination of the mucin with epithelium may have occurred as a technical complication of specimen prosection.

Ruptured Appendiceal Diverticulum

The presence of diverticula in the appendix should always alert the pathologist to search for a neoplasm that may have caused appendiceal obstruction.[60,61] However, not uncommonly, appendiceal diverticula may rupture and result in extrusion of mucin into the wall of the appendix and on the serosa, which may raise concern for a mucinous neoplasm (Fig. 28.11).[59,62] In addition, the presence of hyperplastic and reactive changes of the epithelium within the diverticula may also be mistaken for a neoplastic process. Some appendices with diverticula are dilated, similar to retention cysts, and reveal an attenuated epithelial lining in continuity with otherwise relatively preserved mucosa.[59] The presence of an everted diverticulum or the presence of fragments of diverticular epithelium at the rupture site on the serosa

BOX 28.2 Features of Ruptured Diverticular Disease of the Appendix That Assist in Distinguishing Diverticular Disease from Low-Grade Appendiceal Mucinous Neoplasm

- Multiple diverticula, many of which are intact, may be present
- Dilatation of the appendiceal lumen, lined by a flat single layer of cuboidalized epithelium segueing into atrophic mucosa with retained crypt architecture
- Mucosal hyperplastic changes with disarrayed but preserved crypts separated by lamina propria
- Absence of slender filiform villi or tightly scalloped mucosal architecture
- Mucosal Schwann cell proliferation
- Chronic inflammation and fibrosis
- A history consistent with interval appendectomy

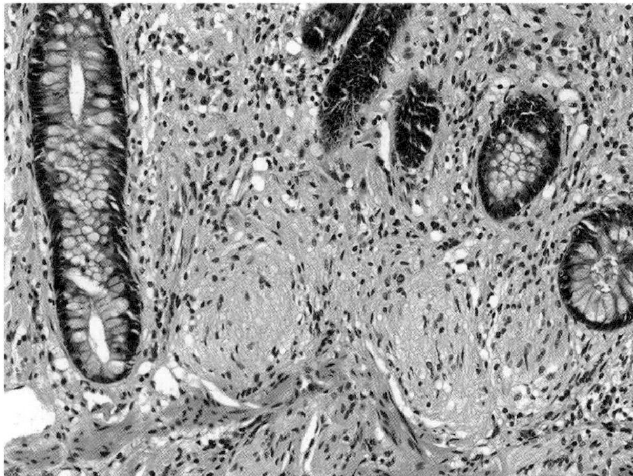

FIGURE 28.12 Mucosal Schwann cell proliferation in appendiceal diverticular disease. The laminar propria contains a vaguely nodular neural proliferation.

may also be confused with localized pseudomyxoma peritonei. There are some features that pathologists can use to differentiate a ruptured diverticulum from a true mucinous neoplasm (Box 28.2). For instance, in some cases of appendiceal diverticula, the appendix may contain several diverticula, which helps alert the pathologist to the correct diagnosis. Hyperplastic epithelium often shows crypt serration, crypt disarray, and hyperplastic changes with abundant mucin-producing cells, which is typically more pronounced in the upper half of the mucosa. Further, nonneoplastic crypts are normally separated by lamina propria, and they show little or no crowding.[59] In contrast, typical LAMNs show back-to-back crypts with scant lamina propria as well as elongated slender villi that protrude into the lumen of the appendix. One other helpful feature is that appendices with diverticula often show Schwann cell transformation of the lamina propria (Fig. 28.12).[62,63] This may be caused by the effects of obstruction.

Endometriosis with Intestinal Metaplasia

Endometriosis of the appendix can cause obstruction with the secondary formation of a retention mucocele, diverticulum, or perforation.[64] In the appendix or cecum, endometriosis may also show intestinal metaplasia of the epithelium,

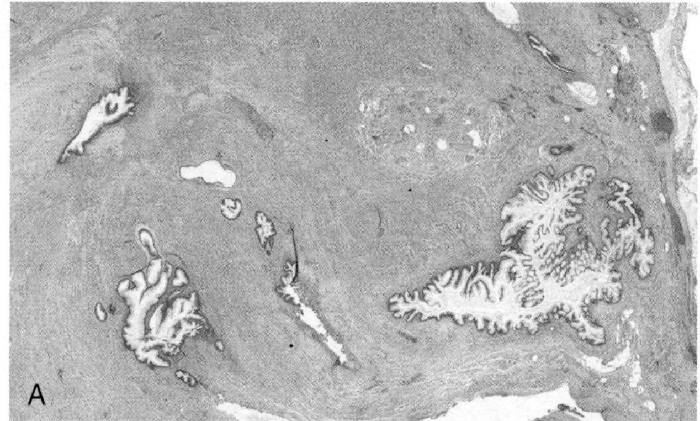

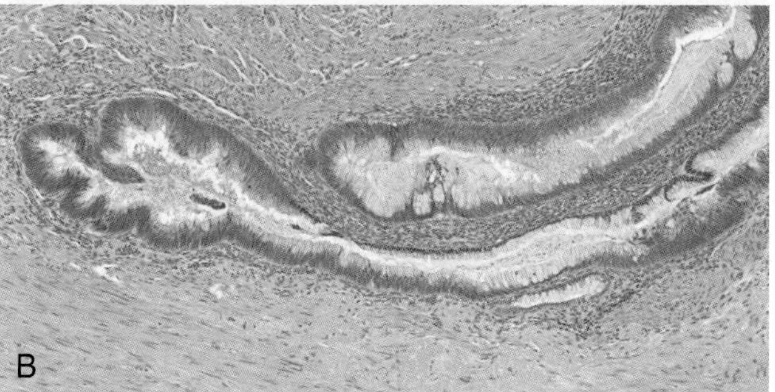

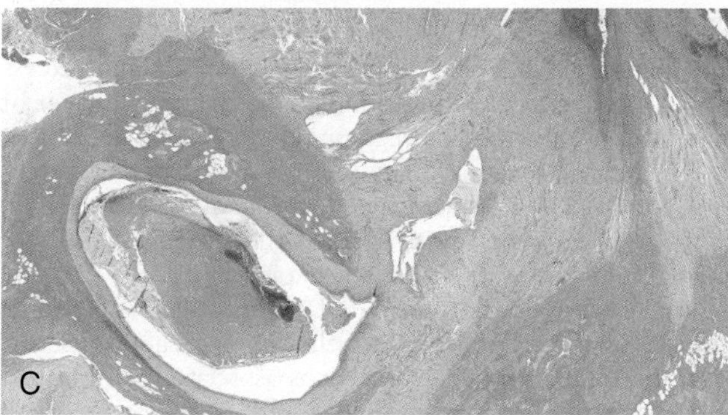

FIGURE 28.13 Appendiceal endometriosis with intestinal metaplasia mimicking low-grade appendiceal mucinous neoplasm. A, Low-power view shows a buckshot pattern of scattered mucinous glands, suggesting an infiltrative mucinous neoplasm. The condensation of the stroma is only slightly visible at this magnification. **B,** Higher magnification confirms that the glands are lined by intestinal-type epithelium but show ovarian-type stroma surrounding them. **C,** In this example of endometriosis with intestinal metaplasia in a pregnant patient, the epithelium lining the glands is the intestinal type, and the stroma is dramatically decidualized.

which can mimic LAMN or a mucinous adenocarcinoma.[65-69] Deposits of endometriosis may reveal the presence of glands lined by mucinous cells, which are occasionally in continuity with endometrial-type glands, and surrounded by a cuff of endometrial-type stroma (Fig. 28.13).[65,67] Stromal decidualization may be present, particularly in pregnant patients.[67] Occasionally, some of the intestinal glands may be cystically dilated with mucin and endometrial stroma. This makes it difficult to distinguish endometriosis from dissecting glands of a LAMN; immunohistochemical stains for estrogen receptor, progesterone receptor, and CD10 may help demonstrate endometrial stroma.[65] Rarely, dysplasia has been reported within endometriotic intestinal glands,[70,71] although reactive changes often mimic dysplasia in this setting, so this feature should be evaluated carefully.

TABLE 28.1 Primary Tumor Staging System for Low-Grade vs. High-Grade Appendiceal Mucinous Neoplasm

T Stage	LAMN	HAMN
Primary tumor cannot be assessed	Tx	Tx
No evidence of primary tumor	T0	T0
Carcinoma in situ (invasion of the lamina propria or invasion into but not through the muscularis mucosae)	Tis(LAMN)	Tis
Tumor or acellular mucin extends into the submucosa		T1
Tumor or acellular mucin extends into the muscularis propria		T2
Tumor or acellular mucin extends into the subserosa or mesoappendix	T3	T3
Tumor or acellular mucin involves the appendiceal serosa	T4a	T4a

HAMN, *High-grade appendiceal mucinous neoplasm;* LAMN, *low-grade appendiceal mucinous neoplasm.*

Natural History

The prognosis of LAMN is highly dependent on stage of the tumor, or, more precisely, the presence or absence of neoplastic epithelium located outside of the appendix, and/or within the peritoneal cavity.[8,12,26] The eighth edition of the *AJCC* includes a new staging system for LAMNs (Table 28.1) in which Tis(LAMN) was specifically created for tumors in which the epithelium, or acellular mucin, pushes into but not through the muscularis propria, and, as a result, there is no T1 or T2 stages in this new system. Cases in which either mucinous epithelium or acellular mucin extends into the subserosa, or mesoappendix, are staged as T3. Tumors that perforate the serosa with either acellular or cellular mucin are classified as T4a. However, it is important to note that the prognosis of LAMN does not necessarily align well with the T stages. Thus a complete and accurate description of the location and extent of mucin and the mucinous epithelial cells should always be described in pathology reports of patients with these tumors.

LAMNs that are confined to the appendix, without extraappendiceal mucin, are almost always cured by an appendectomy.[72,73] This includes tumors that meet the definition of Tis(LAMN) or T3. Although tumors that perforate the serosa, either with or without mucinous epithelial cells on the serosa, are staged as T4a, there is a marked difference in prognosis depending on whether the serosa is involved by acellular mucin only or by epithelial cells. LAMNs associated with acellular mucin on the appendiceal serosa carry a low risk of recurrence or progression to pseudomyxoma peritonei, whereas those with epithelial cells on the serosa or within the peritoneal cavity carry a high risk of recurrence. In one multiinstitutional study,[74] the authors collected 65 patients with ruptured appendiceal mucinous tumors, all of whom had at least 6 months of follow-up. Fifty of these patients had acellular mucin located within the right lower quadrant, and only 2 (4%) of them had local recurrence after 56 and 92 months of follow-up. In contrast, 15 tumors were associated with clusters of low-grade neoplastic epithelium within the extraappendiceal mucin. Five of these cases (33%) recurred in the form of diffuse pseudomyxoma peritonei within 24 to 87 months, and one patient died of disease at 60 months. Pai et al. studied 116 patients with mucinous tumors and came to similar conclusions.[26] They described follow-up for 14 patients with acellular mucin limited to the right lower quadrant. One patient (7%) had a recurrence on follow-up. Three of four patients (75%) with extraappendiceal mucin containing neoplastic epithelium limited to the right lower quadrant also had a recurrence. One recent study reported that five patients with acellular mucin on the serosa did not experience recurrence after a mean follow-up of 45 months.[72]

Acellular mucin located within the peritoneal cavity (beyond the appendiceal serosa) has been shown to confer a low risk of recurrence as pseudomyxoma peritonei. In one recent study,[75] the authors found that patients with acellular mucin located beyond the right lower quadrant had a longer progression-free survival and overall survival compared with patients with cellular mucin deposits. In patients with remote mucinous deposits, the absence of visible disease on CT scan correlated with the presence of acellular mucin. However, one caveat is that sampling error may affect this finding because 5 of 29 patients in this study who were initially classified as having only acellular mucin within the peritoneal cavity were subsequently upstaged to cellular mucinous deposits after complete resection and evaluation of their peritoneal tumor. One series of LAMNs at various stages included eight patients with acellular mucin within the peritoneum, none of whom had a recurrence.[72] In other reports, patients with only acellular mucin after cytoreductive surgery showed a more favorable prognosis than patients with cellular mucin deposits.[76,77]

From these various studies,[26,73-76] it is evident that patients with acellular mucin within the peritoneal cavity have a much more favorable prognosis than patients with cellular peritoneal mucinous tumor deposits, regardless of whether or not the mucin is confined to the right lower quadrant. Thus evaluation for extraappendiceal mucin and neoplastic epithelium should always be performed diligently. Because the presence of acellular mucin on the surface of the appendix may have prognostic significance, it is also important to distinguish mucin carryover as a result of poor specimen handling from true mucin on the serosa. True mucin on the serosa is usually associated with mesothelial hyperplasia and/or neovascularization.[73] Another important issue is determination of the extent of sampling that is necessary in patients with large-volume mucinous ascites to confirm the absence of epithelium. One study demonstrated that of 12 cases that initially revealed acellular mucin within the peritoneal cavity that had been well sampled, an additional 30 blocks of peritoneal mucin found epithelial cells in 2 of the cases.[78] Ultimately, in cases with abundant mucin within the peritoneal cavity, pathologists should sample the mucin thoroughly, beginning with a reasonable number of blocks; if no mucinous epithelium is identified in these initial sections, additional sampling of perhaps another 20 or 30 blocks may be prudent.

In contrast, LAMNs with diffuse (nonlocalized) peritoneal seeding of neoplastic epithelium and mucin typically have a progressive clinical course that frequently results in death of the patient unless managed aggressively (see "Pseudomyxoma Peritonei").

Treatment

Simple appendectomy is considered sufficient treatment for LAMNs that are confined to the appendix. In some cases, the margin of resection reveals the presence of intraluminal mucin, or it may show residual dysplasia. Although some authorities advise additional surgery for patients with a positive margin (defined as either mural dissecting mucin or luminal neoplastic epithelium in a section of the appendiceal margin),[5,79] there are some data to suggest that cases with a positive margin, as defined earlier, are unlikely to show residual neoplasia in a subsequent colectomy specimen or to be associated with an adverse outcome.[26,72,80] However, rare examples of residual tumor, presumably within the remnant of the appendix, have been reported.[81] Thus we feel that the precise status of the appendectomy margin should be reported (describing dissecting mucin, neoplastic epithelium, or other) to help the treating physician make a decision regarding cecectomy versus radiological surveillance in the management of a patient with a "positive" margin.

Given the possibility of peritoneal recurrence in patients with a ruptured LAMN, those with acellular mucin on the periappendiceal serosa should be followed closely to ensure that either localized or diffuse pseudomyxoma peritonei does not develop. Radiographic imaging of the abdomen and pelvis is usually considered the preferred method of surveillance. Tumors that spread to the right lower quadrant reveal a higher risk of recurrence, but appropriate management for these patients remains controversial. For instance, radiological surveillance may be appropriate for some patients.[82,83] Right hemicolectomy offers no additional benefit over appendectomy alone for patients with LAMN, even in patients that contain extraappendiceal mucin and neoplastic epithelium.[84,85] Tumors that have disseminated into the peritoneal cavity are treated either by multiple peritonectomies and heated intraperitoneal chemotherapy (see "Pseudomyxoma Peritonei") or, if the patient is not a candidate for these aggressive approaches, by tumor debulking.

High-Grade Appendiceal Mucinous Neoplasm

Definition

HAMN is a recently introduced term[13,14] proposed for tumors that show architectural features of a LAMN (e.g., pushing-type invasion), but with high-grade cytological features.

Clinical Features

Patients with HAMN present clinically similar to those with LAMN, with abdominal pain and symptoms referable to a mass lesion. However, bulky peritoneal disease may be more frequent in patients with HAMN compared with those with LAMN.[12,86]

Pathogenesis

Similar to LAMNs, HAMNs show frequent *KRAS* mutations, and about 50% also show *GNAS* mutations.[43,86] In addition, HAMNs may show mutations in *TP53, ATM, RNF43*, or *APC*.[42,43,86] They may show p53 overexpression by immunohistochemistry as well.[42]

Pathology

The gross features of HAMN are identical to those for LAMN. Histologically, HAMNs reveal similar architecture to LAMNs (flat, scalloped, undulating, or villous growth of epithelial cells). However, at least focally, and in some cases diffusely, the degree of epithelial atypia is high-grade. High-grade features include marked nuclear enlargement, anisonucleosis, hyperchromasia, prominent nucleoli, and numerous mitoses. In high-grade areas, the epithelium may also show areas of complexity, such as the presence of full-thickness nuclear stratification and the formation of micropapillary or cribriform architecture (Fig. 28.14). The neoplastic cells may also show less mucinous differentiation and appear more columnar, similar to colonic adenomas.

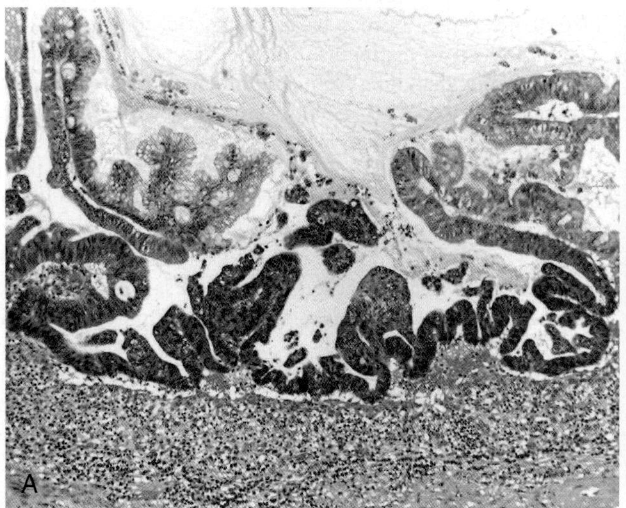

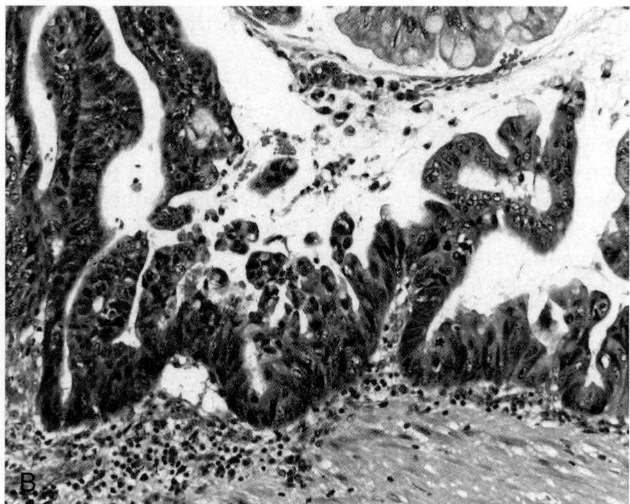

FIGURE 28.14 High-grade appendiceal mucinous neoplasm. A, Medium-power view shows a noninvasive villous tumor within the appendiceal lumen. The villi focally show micropapillary buds. **B,** High-power view shows unequivocal high-grade nuclear cytology with enlarged hyperchromatic nuclei, prominent nucleoli, and increased mitotic figures.

TABLE 28.2 Staging System for Peritoneal Mucin or Mucinous Tumors in the Peritoneal Cavity

Extent of Mucinous Tumor	Stage	Comment
Acellular mucin on peritoneal surfaces other than the appendiceal serosa	pM1a	Requires adequate sampling to exclude mucinous epithelium
Cellular peritoneal mucinous tumor deposits on peritoneal surfaces other than the appendiceal serosa	pM1b	Peritoneal mucinous tumor that pushes into the underlying organ or ovarian involvement are pM1b
Mucinous tumor deposits to sites other than the peritoneal cavity	pM1c	Examples include pleural mucinous tumor deposits or pulmonary metastases

HAMNs may be confined to the mucosa or show pushing invasion, with stromal changes such as fibrosis of the lamina propria, loss of the lymphoid tissue compartment, or fibrosis, elastosis, or calcification of the wall of the appendix. These tumors may rupture, and there can be mucin extrusion either with or without neoplastic mucinous epithelial cells within the extraappendiceal mucin. In contrast with LAMNs, HAMNs are staged according to the T stages used for invasive adenocarcinomas (Table 28.2). Thus a HAMN that pushes into the muscularis propria is classified as T2, not Tis(HAMN). The difference in grading between LAMN and HAMN was initially proposed because of the concern that HAMNs have a higher risk of recurrence (as pseudomyxoma peritonei) compared with LAMNs. However, there is currently no data to substantiate more aggressive staging of HAMNs. For instance, HAMNs that have not perforated the serosa show a low risk of dissemination, similar to LAMNs.[87]

Differential Diagnosis

Low-Grade Appendiceal Mucinous Neoplasm

By definition, LAMNs have low-grade cytological atypia. A diagnosis of HAMN should be reserved for tumors that show high-grade cytological atypia, even if focal.

Appendiceal Adenoma with High-Grade Dysplasia

As mentioned earlier, for a tumor to qualify as an appendiceal adenoma, a tumor should resemble its colonic counterpart (colorectal tubular, tubulovillous, or villous adenoma). It also must be confined to the appendiceal mucosa, without pushing invasion or extraappendiceal spread. A tumor with muscularis mucosae fibrosis, mucin extrusion, mural fibrosis, or extraappendiceal involvement should not be classified as an adenoma. Distinguishing architectural features of a HAMN include a single flat, or undulating, or scalloped layer of epithelial cells, rather than a polypoid growth pattern.

Mucinous Adenocarcinoma

Mucinous adenocarcinomas can show high-grade cytological features, but in contrast with HAMNs, they show infiltrative-type invasion. The presence of crowded mucin pools with floating strips or buds of tumor cells, or the presence of angular glands with desmoplasia, are incompatible with HAMN.

Natural History

HAMNs that have not ruptured more than likely have a negligible risk of progression to pseudomyxoma peritonei.[87] The prognosis of tumors that have spread to the peritoneum depends on the grade and extent of pseudomyxoma peritonei (see "Pseudomyxoma Peritonei"). However, currently no studies have evaluated the outcome of HAMN based on various types of potential treatment, so this will need further investigation before specific recommendations can be made.

Adenocarcinoma

Clinical Features

Adenocarcinomas of the appendix are uncommon. Collins et al. found an incidence of 0.082% among 50,000 appendectomy specimens.[88] There is an increased incidence among men in some series,[4,89-96] but not in others.[97-101] Patients are usually in their fifth to seventh decade of life at clinical presentation[89,91-93,95-98,100,101] and usually present with symptoms of acute appendicitis. Other less common modes of presentation include a palpable mass, obstruction, gastrointestinal (GI) bleeding, or symptoms related to metastases.[3,4,91-94,96-99,102-104] The stage at presentation may be related to the histological type. Mucinous and signet ring cell adenocarcinomas are more likely to present as stage IV disease compared with nonmucinous adenocarcinomas.[105]

Pathogenesis

Several studies have found a high incidence of *KRAS* mutations.[38,41,45,86,106,107] In one study, low-grade adenocarcinomas were far more likely to have *KRAS* mutations than high-grade ones.[107] One study did not find *GNAS* mutations in 3 mucinous adenocarcinomas, and another study found only 1 of 10 tumors with a *GNAS* mutation, suggesting that adenocarcinomas may not necessarily arise from LAMNs or HAMNs.[38,86] *TP53* mutations have been detected in 40% to 75% of tumors.[53,108] With regard to p53 expression by immunohistochemistry, some studies report absent p53 expression,[41,106] whereas others report p53 overexpression in most adenocarcinomas.[45,53] Other mutations that are occasionally observed in adenocarcinomas include *SMAD4*, *APC*, *ARID1A*, *RNF43*, *PI3K*, and *PIK3CA*.[86,107-109] Mutations in β-catenin were not found in one series of 28 appendiceal adenocarcinomas.[109]

Although mucinous carcinomas in the right colon are frequently associated with defective DNA mismatch repair and microsatellite instability,[110-112] most appendiceal adenocarcinomas are, in fact, microsatellite stable.[41,106,107,113] MSI-high tumors usually reveal MSH2/MSH6 loss, and in cases with MLH1 loss, gene-promoter hypermethylation studies and *BRAF* mutation testing are usually negative.[107,113,114] However, even in these patients, testing for Lynch syndrome is often negative.[113] These data indicate that the sporadic pathway of defective DNA mismatch repair is not as biologically relevant in the appendix as it is in the colon, and the immunohistochemical markers for DNA mismatch repair protein expression may not be as specific to detect Lynch syndrome in appendiceal adenocarcinoma as they are in the colon.

Pathology

Grossly, appendiceal carcinomas may be polypoid, ulcerating, or infiltrative.[94,95,104] Obstruction of the lumen may result in cystic dilatation of the appendix. The proximal one-third of the appendix is involved more often than the distal portions.[90,98,102]

Appendiceal adenocarcinomas are classified as *adenocarcinoma not otherwise specified (NOS)*, *mucinous adenocarcinoma*, *signet ring cell adenocarcinoma*, and *undifferentiated carcinoma*.[115] Mucinous adenocarcinomas account for approximately 40% of all appendiceal adenocarcinomas.[92] The histology of invasive mucinous adenocarcinoma of the appendix is similar to those that occur elsewhere in the colon and they are graded similarly. These tumors show irregular pools of mucin of various sizes and shapes that infiltrate the wall of the appendix and are associated with cytologically malignant glandular epithelium, the latter usually arranged as strips, clusters, or complex glandular structures (Fig. 28.15). Mucinous adenocarcinomas may rupture and metastasize transcoelomically to the peritoneum or ovaries,[99,103] but also, less commonly, via a hematogenous route.[3,84,93,106] Histologically, peritoneal metastases resemble those that occur in LAMNs, except that the mucin may be more cellular, and the neoplastic epithelium shows a greater degree of architectural complexity and higher-grade cytological atypia, or it may have signet ring cells, warranting designation as either a grade 2 or grade 3 pseudomyxoma (see the section Pseudomyxoma Peritonei). Other organs, such as the small or large bowel, liver, or ovary, may be affected as well.[6,116]

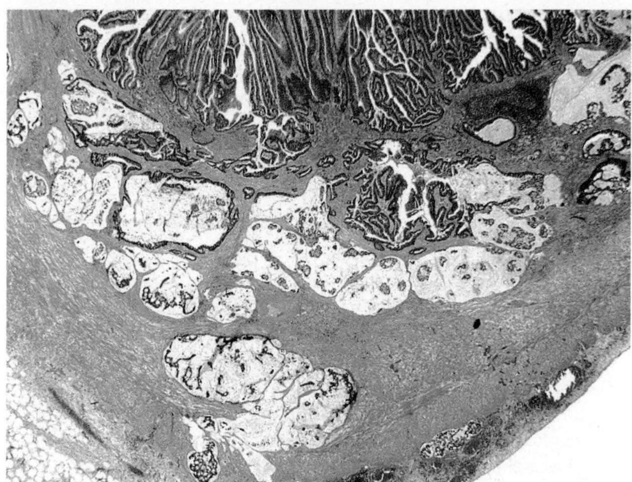

FIGURE 28.15 Invasive mucinous adenocarcinoma of the appendix. Pools of mucin harboring complex atypical epithelial groups dissect into and through the appendiceal wall.

Nonmucinous appendiceal carcinomas show a range of morphological features of the invasive component. For instance, the tumors may resemble colonic adenocarcinomas by revealing malignant glands lined by neoplastic columnar epithelium with dirty necrosis. However, many tumors are composed of well-differentiated tubular glands lined by columnar cells without dirty necrosis and with scant to moderate amounts of extracellular mucin (Fig. 28.16). Rare tumors have glands lined by columnar cells with foamy cytoplasm, reminiscent of pancreaticobiliary adenocarcinomas (Fig. 28.17). Grading is similar to adenocarcinomas of the intestines in general.

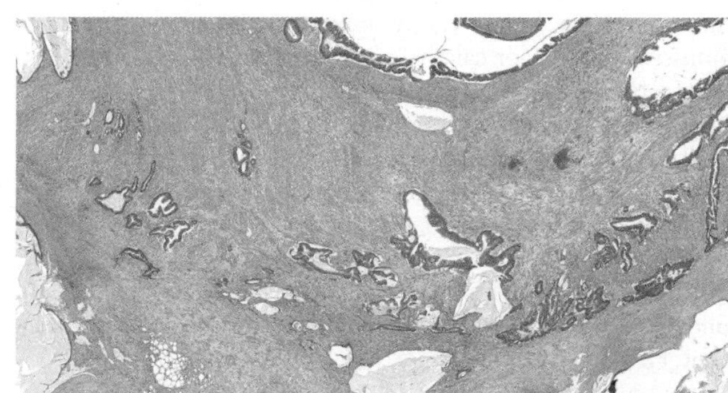

FIGURE 28.16 Invasive adenocarcinoma of the appendix. Typical appearance of an invasive appendiceal adenocarcinoma with intestinal-type malignant glands invading the appendix and a modest amount of extracellular mucin.

Signet ring cell adenocarcinomas are associated with a poor prognosis because of rapid dissemination within the peritoneal cavity.[117,118] The histology is similar to signet ring cell adenocarcinoma at other sites in the GI tract (Fig. 28.18). They are composed of single cells, clusters, and/or sheets of signet ring cells; some tumors have extracellular mucin. Some tumors show areas reminiscent of goblet cell adenocarcinoma, suggesting that the adenocarcinoma may be a high-grade goblet cell adenocarcinoma (see "Goblet Cell Adenocarcinoma").[7]

There is virtually no data regarding potential precursor lesions of adenocarcinoma of the appendix. Adenomas and serrated lesions (see later) may occasionally be seen in the lumen of the appendix in cases of invasive adenocarcinoma. Some adenocarcinomas appear to arise in a pre-existing LAMN or HAMN in that a large cystic tumor with pushing invasion has focal areas of infiltrative-type invasion. In this setting, the identification of unequivocal infiltrative-type invasion, even if focal, qualifies the tumor as an adenocarcinoma.

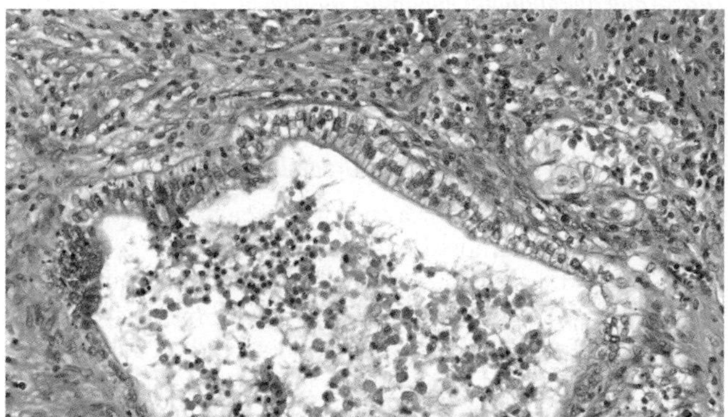

FIGURE 28.17 Invasive adenocarcinoma of the appendix. Rare examples of appendiceal adenocarcinoma have focal or widespread areas in which the malignant glands are lined by columnar cells with foamy or clear cytoplasm, resembling pancreaticobiliary adenocarcinomas.

Differential Diagnosis

Appendiceal Mucinous Neoplasm

Distinguishing an appendiceal mucinous neoplasm (either LAMN or HAMN) from a mucinous adenocarcinoma is based primarily on evaluation of the type of tissue invasion that is present. Appendiceal mucinous neoplasms show pushing-type invasion, with diverticula-like protrusions, fibrosis or hyalinization of the appendix wall, or perforation. Adenocarcinomas show an infiltrative pattern of invasion. Rarely, adenocarcinomas show an infiltrative type of

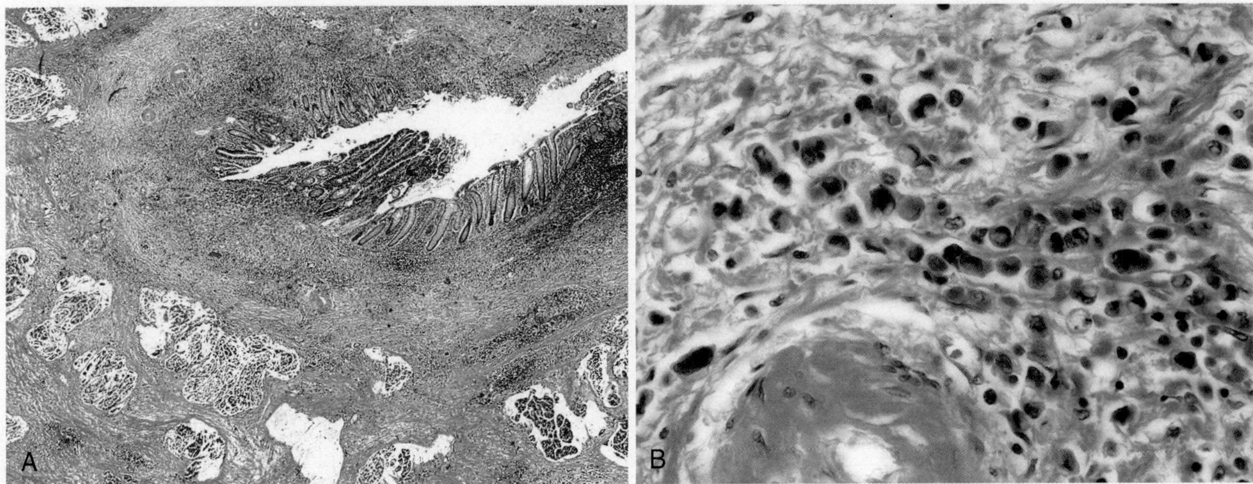

FIGURE 28.18 Appendiceal signet ring cell carcinoma. A, Low-power view shows a cellular neoplasm in the submucosa and muscularis with areas of extracellular mucin production and a predominance of single cells. **B,** High-power view shows that the tumor is composed of single cells, many with an eccentric mucin vacuole.

invasion only focally within a cystic tumor that otherwise would be classified as a LAMN or HAMN. The existence of these types of cases emphasizes the need to submit the entire appendix for tissue sectioning when confronted with a cystic tumor in which an invasive adenocarcinoma is not identified in the initial sections.

Natural History

Numerous studies have shown that the prognosis of appendiceal adenocarcinoma depends primarily on the tumor subtype, histological grade, and stage.[4,89,97,98,102,103,119-121] Patients with mucinous adenocarcinomas reportedly have a more favorable prognosis than those with nonmucinous adenocarcinomas.[97,98,103,105] Population-based survey data show that for patients with stage I to III appendiceal adenocarcinoma, those with mucinous adenocarcinoma have a 5-year survival that ranges from 51.1% to 82%, depending on tumor grade, and those with nonmucinous adenocarcinoma have a 5-year survival between 39.8% and 68.9%, depending on tumor grade. For patients with stage IV disease, those with mucinous adenocarcinoma have a 5-year survival of 11.3% to 56.7%, depending on grade, whereas patients with nonmucinous adenocarcinoma have a 5-year survival of 6% to 29.7%, depending on grade.

Treatment

Invasive adenocarcinoma of the appendix warrants treatment by right hemicolectomy with lymph node dissection to properly stage the tumor and potentially achieve a cure.[97,99,103,120] Most studies have shown that right hemicolectomy offers improved 5-year survival rates compared with appendectomy alone.[48,91,97,99,120,121] However, others have demonstrated no significant advantage to right hemicolectomy in patients with mucinous adenocarcinoma of the appendix.[122] Treatment of patients with peritoneal spread depends on the resectability of the tumor. Patients whose tumors are resectable should be treated aggressively with peritonectomy and postoperative intraperitoneal chemotherapy.[84,123,124] Some authorities advocate oophorectomy in women, both for staging purposes and to remove a frequent site of metastasis.[97,103]

Pseudomyxoma Peritonei

Pseudomyxoma peritonei refers to the accumulation of mucinous tumor deposits within the peritoneal cavity secondary to a mucinous neoplasm.

Nomenclature

Historically, *pseudomyxoma peritonei* was a term reserved for the clinical syndrome in which abundant mucin was present in the peritoneal cavity, and it was recommended not to be used as a pathological diagnosis. Instead, several histological terms were used to denote the finding of mucin, fibrous tissue, and epithelial cells situated within the peritoneum. Over the past three decades, there has been considerable debate regarding the precise nomenclature of, specifically, low-grade pseudomyxoma, which has been termed *disseminated peritoneal adenomucinosis* (DPAM) by some groups[116] and *mucinous carcinoma peritonei* by others.[125] The crux of the controversy is whether low-grade pseudomyxoma is equivalent to peritoneal carcinomatosis. Many authorities objected to terms such as *DPAM* that suggested that low-grade pseudomyxoma peritonei was not a malignant condition. In a recent consensus statement, the authors suggested that the term *mucinous carcinoma peritonei* be used for pseudomyxoma peritonei.[13] Regardless, in the most recent WHO classification of peritoneal mucinous tumors, the term *pseudomyxoma peritonei* (grade 1, 2, or 3) was, in fact, resurrected specifically for peritoneal tumors composed of abundant mucin.[126] This term is most relevant in the context of a primary appendiceal mucinous tumor and is the one recommended by the author of this chapter. However, either *pseudomyxoma peritonei* or *mucinous carcinoma peritonei* are acceptable terms for this condition, depending on specific institutional practices.

With the introduction of the term *pseudomyxoma peritonei* into the lexicon of peritoneal mucinous neoplasia, one point is worth clarifying. In some of the older literature, *pseudomyxoma peritonei* was used to describe the presence of mucin within the peritoneal cavity, even if the mucin was the result of spillage from a nonneoplastic process, such as a ruptured retention cyst, and it was acellular. Today, the term *pseudomyxoma peritonei* is reserved exclusively for the

TABLE 28.3 Nomenclature and Criteria for Grading Peritoneal Mucinous Neoplasms

Peritoneal Mucinous Tumor Nomenclature and Grade	Acceptable Alternative Terminology	Criteria
Acellular mucin (grade not applicable)		Mucin in the peritoneal cavity without mucinous epithelial cells
Pseudomyxoma peritonei, grade 1	Mucinous carcinoma peritonei, grade 1	• Hypocellular peritoneal mucinous tumor as judged at 20× • Low-grade cytological features
Pseudomyxoma peritonei, grade 2	Mucinous carcinoma peritonei, grade 2	• Hypercellular peritoneal mucinous tumor as judged at 20× • High-grade cytological features involving >10% of the tumor • Infiltrative-type invasion with angular or complex glands, desmoplastic stroma, or a pattern of small mucin pools with numerous clusters of tumor cells
Pseudomyxoma peritonei, grade 3	Mucinous carcinoma peritonei, grade 3	Peritoneal mucinous tumor with signet ring cells* or sheets of tumor cells

**The precise percentage of the tumor that must be signet ring cells to qualify for grade 3 has not been defined. Even focal signet ring cell morphology qualifies; however, if the signet ring cells are focal, they must be distinguished from* pseudo signet ring cells, *which are degenerated tumor cells floating in mucin in an otherwise lower-grade tumor. The presence of signet ring cells infiltrating tissue may be more prognostically important than when they are floating in mucin.*

presence of cellular mucinous deposits associated with a mucin-producing tumor, and it is most relevant when dealing with an appendiceal primary. Acellular mucin within the peritoneal cavity should not be referred to as *pseudomyxoma peritonei,* even when it is abundant, but rather simply as *acellular mucin.* If the acellular mucin is the result of a mucinous neoplasm in the appendix or elsewhere, it is then classified as *M1a disease in the peritoneum.* The disease is further staged by whether mucinous tumor deposits are present on peritoneal surfaces other than the appendiceal serosa or are located outside the peritoneal cavity (see Table 28.2).

Clinical Features

Pseudomyxoma peritonei occurs most often in association with a mucinous neoplasm from the appendix, but it has been described with mucinous tumors from other sites, including the ovary (ovarian teratomas), urachus, colon, and pancreas. Approximately 20% of patients with a mucinous tumor of the appendix develop pseudomyxoma peritonei.[127] Patients with pseudomyxoma peritonei typically present in the sixth to seventh decade of life, and women predominate over men in some series.[127-129] Peritoneal mucinous deposits tend to accumulate in particular areas, such as the greater omentum, the undersurface of the right hemidiaphragm, pelvis, right retrohepatic space, left abdominal gutter, and ligament of Treitz.[130] This so-called *redistribution* phenomenon occurs because tumor accumulates in anatomic locations where ascitic fluid is resorbed from the abdomen and in areas most subjected to pooling in the abdomen.[7] Along with the peritoneal cavity, the ovaries are commonly involved with tumor as well.[25,127,129]

Pathogenesis

Molecular studies on pseudomyxoma peritonei have largely examined tumors from appendiceal primary tumors, therefore many of the molecular changes in pseudomyxoma are similar to those in appendiceal mucinous tumors. Pseudomyxoma peritonei very frequently shows *KRAS* mutations.[131-137] *GNAS* mutations are also common, occurring more often in low-grade than in high-grade pseudomyxoma.[131-138] Occasionally, mutations are found in other genes, including those of the transforming growth factor (TGF)β pathway *(SMAD2, SMAD3, SMAD4, TGFBR1, TGFBR1)*, the Hippo pathway *(FAT4, FAT3,* and *DSCH1)*, the WNT pathway (*CTNNβ1*, *WNT7A*, and *WNT10A*), the NOTCH pathway (*NOTCH1* and *NOTCH4*), and the PI3K/AKT pathway (*AKT* and *PIK3CA*).[131,132,134-137] Mutations in genes related to the defective mismatch repair pathway such as *BRAF* or *MLH1* genes are rare.[132] Tumors are almost universally microsatellite stable.[132]

In general, high-grade tumors have a higher mutation rate than low-grade tumors.[134] *TP53* mutations and *MYC* amplification are more frequent in high-grade tumors.[133-135] Other mutations found more often in high-grade pseudomyxoma peritonei include mutations in *PIK3CA, AKT1,* and *PDGFRA*.[133] A subset of high-grade pseudomyxoma peritonei shows overexpression of p53 by immunohistochemistry[132,133,139] and absent SMAD4 expression.[140]

Pathology

Pseudomyxoma peritonei has, as its defining feature, the presence of abundant mucin situated within fibrotic stroma. Currently, pseudomyxoma peritonei is graded according to a three-tier system (Table 28.3).[126,141] Grade 1 pseudomyxoma peritonei is more frequently seen in patients with LAMNs. It demonstrates the presence of abundant mucin, hyalinized or fibrotic stroma, and a variable quantity of low-grade mucinous epithelium (Fig. 28.19). The epithelium is typically arranged as cohesive strips with minimal complexity. This is the appearance of classical pseudomyxoma peritonei. Grade 2 pseudomyxoma peritonei shows complex patterns of epithelium, cribriform glands or angular glands, desmoplastic stroma, or a pattern of small mucin pools with numerous tumor clusters (Fig. 28.20).[12,116] Other criteria for grade 2 pseudomyxoma are high cytological grade affecting greater than 10% of the tumor or high tumor cellularity as judged on a 20× field. The peritoneal tumor may show cells with enlarged nuclei, anisonucleosis, irregular nuclei, or frequent mitoses.

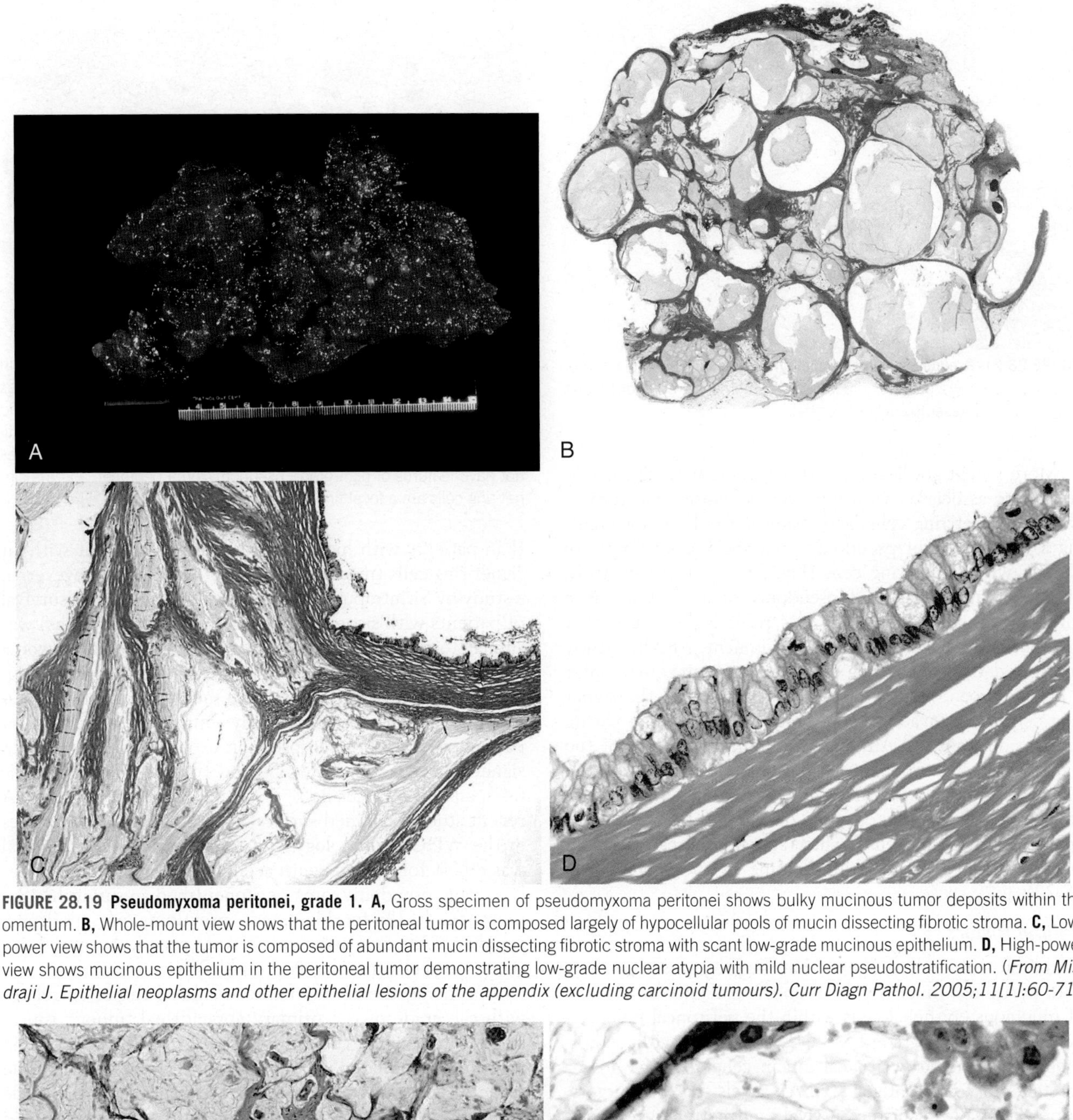

FIGURE 28.19 Pseudomyxoma peritonei, grade 1. A, Gross specimen of pseudomyxoma peritonei shows bulky mucinous tumor deposits within the omentum. **B,** Whole-mount view shows that the peritoneal tumor is composed largely of hypocellular pools of mucin dissecting fibrotic stroma. **C,** Low-power view shows that the tumor is composed of abundant mucin dissecting fibrotic stroma with scant low-grade mucinous epithelium. **D,** High-power view shows mucinous epithelium in the peritoneal tumor demonstrating low-grade nuclear atypia with mild nuclear pseudostratification. (*From Misdraji J. Epithelial neoplasms and other epithelial lesions of the appendix (excluding carcinoid tumours). Curr Diagn Pathol. 2005;11[1]:60-71.*)

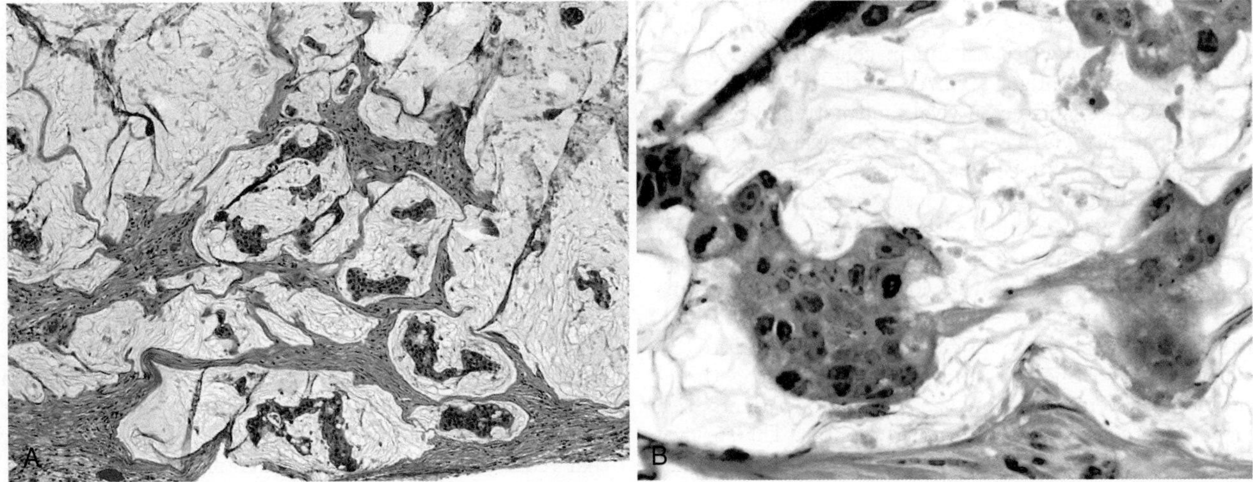

FIGURE 28.20 Pseudomyxoma peritonei, grade 2. A, The peritoneal tumor is composed of crowded pools of mucin harboring many clusters of mucinous epithelium. **B,** High-power view of an epithelial group shows high-grade nuclear atypia, with large nuclei, nuclear hyperchromasia, and nucleoli.

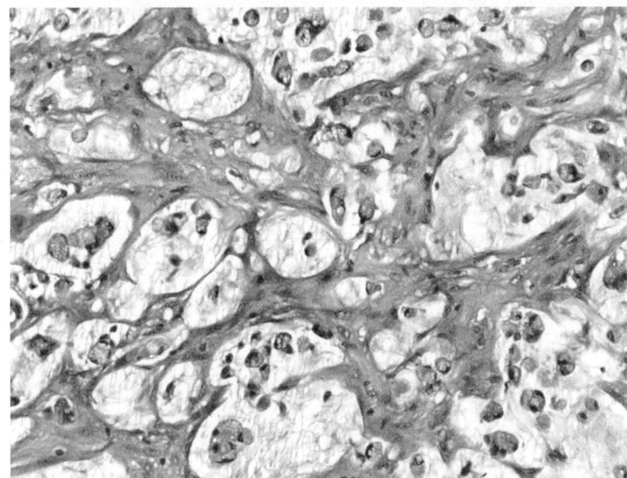

FIGURE 28.21 Pseudomyxoma peritonei, grade 3. The peritoneal tumor in this case shows pools of mucin with numerous small groups and single cells that resemble signet ring cells.

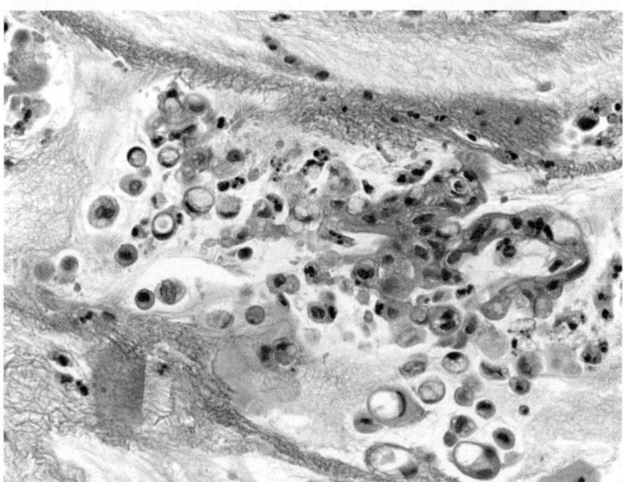

FIGURE 28.22 Pseudosignet ring cells in pseudomyxoma peritonei. In this example of pseudomyxoma peritonei, the peritoneal tumor was hypocellular and showed degenerative changes, including in this field where detached tumor cells floating in the mucin resemble signet ring cells. Pseudosignet ring cells should be suspected when the tumor does not have features of high-grade pseudomyxoma peritonei, and the signet ring cells are a focal finding.

More recent studies noted that tumors with signet ring cells were associated with a poorer prognosis than tumors without signet ring cells, and this was the basis for creating a third grade of pseudomyxoma specifically for those tumors with signet ring cells (Fig. 28.21). In their study, Shetty et al.[142] classified pseudomyxoma peritonei into three grades; the third grade was reserved for cases that demonstrated a signet ring cell component. Another study confirmed that signet ring cells in pseudomyxoma confer a poorer prognosis, but only in cases in which the signet ring cells were invading tissue, rather than floating within mucin pools only.[143] Although a minimum amount of the signet ring cell component has not been defined as yet, the presence of only focal signet ring cells floating within mucin should always raise the question of whether they represent "pseudo–signet ring cells," which actually represent degenerated sloughed tumor cells floating in the mucin (Fig. 28.22).

Natural History

Numerous studies have shown that the prognosis in patients with peritoneal mucin depends on the presence or absence of mucinous epithelial cells within the peritoneal mucin as well as the tumor grade.[125,141,144-147] Patients without epithelial cells in the peritoneal mucin generally have lower carcinoembryonic antigen (CEA) levels before surgery, improved recurrence-free survival, and better overall survival than patients who have cellular peritoneal mucin.[146,147]

Among patients with cellular peritoneal mucinous deposits, patients with low-grade pseudomyxoma have a more favorable outcome than patients with high-grade tumors[148-152] In studies that used a two-tier grading system, the median overall survival for patients with low-grade pseudomyxoma was 100 to 170 months, whereas the median survival for patients with high-grade pseudomyxoma was 32 to 36 months.[152,153] In Shetty's study that introduced a three-tier grading system,[142] the median survival for patients with a signet ring cell component was 40 months. The survival for patients with less than 50% signet ring cells was similar to those with more than 50% signet ring cells (56 vs. 35 months, respectively). Their survival was significantly poorer than patients with high-grade pseudomyxoma but without signet ring cells (median survival 100 months). However, in a study by Sirintrapun and associates,[143] the median survival of patients with signet ring cells in mucin (2.4 months) was similar to that in patients with high-grade pseudomyxoma without signet ring cells (2.9 months), but patients with signet ring cells invading tissue had a median survival of only 6 months. Similarly, a recent study comparing the survival of patients with high-grade pseudomyxoma without and with signet ring cells found a 3-, 5-, and 10-year survival of 84%, 64%, and 38% versus 38%, 25%, and 0%, respectively.[154] A recent study examined survival according to recent changes in the WHO terminology, and found that 10-year survival was 89.6% for patients with acellular mucin only, 63.2% for low-grade pseudomyxoma peritonei (median survival 148.7 months), 40.1% for high-grade pseudomyxoma peritonei (median 63.6 months), and 0% for pseudomyxoma with signet ring cells (median 9.5 months).[82]

In general, the grade of the peritoneal tumor correlates with the grade of the primary appendiceal tumor[6]; thus a single tumor grade can be assigned for both the appendix and the disseminated peritoneal tumor. However, when the grade of the primary tumor in the appendix and the grade of the peritoneal tumor are discordant, both grades should be recorded separately in the pathology report because it is the grade of the peritoneal tumor that ultimately will drive the patient's prognosis. Progression from low-grade pseudomyxoma to high-grade pseudomyxoma has been described in patients who had failure with cytoreduction and chemotherapy treatment.[155,156]

Treatment

Historically, surgical tumor debulking was the mainstay of therapy for pseudomyxoma peritonei, but the majority of patients treated in this manner had disease recurrence that required repeated surgical debulking procedures until adhesions eventually precluded additional surgery, and the patient succumbed to the tumor.[157,158] Survival rates for patients who underwent debulking has been reported to be 86%, 53% to 67%, and 32% at 2, 5, and 10 years, respectively.[157,159] Sugarbaker and colleagues[84,123,124,151] pioneered an aggressive treatment approach that involves peritonectomies and multiple organ resections to achieve complete cytoreduction, hyperthermic intraoperative peritoneal chemotherapy (HIPEC), and additional supplemental cycles of early postoperative intraperitoneal chemotherapy (EPIC). Using this aggressive approach, they achieved 5- and 10-year survival rates of 71.9% and 54.5%, respectively.[84] Other groups have reported similar survival rates using cytoreduction surgery and HIPEC/EPIC.[150,152] In particular, long-term 10-year survival is noted to be better in some studies.[148,149,160]

One of the most important factors associated with success in the management of pseudomyxoma peritonei is the need to achieve complete cytoreduction, which is accomplished in 40% to 91% of cases.[152,160,161] In one study, patients who had complete cytoreduction had 5- and 10-year survival rates of 87% and 74%, respectively, whereas those in whom complete cytoreduction could not be achieved and thus underwent only debulking had 5- and 10-year survival rates of 34% and 23%, respectively.[160] In this regard, the experience of the surgeon may play a role, with specialized centers achieving better survival statistics.[148,149] Patients who experience recurrent disease after their first cytoreduction can undergo repeat cytoreduction, and complete cytoreduction can be achieved in a majority of these patients.[162] The extent of involvement of the peritoneum before cytoreduction affects prognosis,[150,152] perhaps because extensive involvement of the small bowel or mesentery may adversely affect the ability to achieve complete cytoreduction.

Serrated Lesions and Polyps of the Appendix

Serrated lesions and polyps of the colorectum are well-known precursors in the serrated pathway of colorectal tumorigenesis.[163] The terminology for colorectal serrated lesions can also be used in the appendix, but as discussed later, there are some molecular differences between serrated lesions of the colon and the appendix. Because molecular characteristics of colorectal serrated lesions are not entirely shared by appendiceal serrated lesions, it remains unclear whether appendiceal serrated lesions and colorectal serrated lesions are related entities. Also, appendiceal serrated lesions are more morphologically heterogeneous than colorectal ones, which creates challenges when trying to diagnose them according to the classification system used in the colon. The current WHO classification system classifies appendiceal serrated lesions into three broad categories: hyperplastic polyp, serrated lesion without dysplasia, and serrated lesion with dysplasia.[45,164]

Clinical Features

Hyperplastic and serrated lesions of the appendix are most often detected as an incidental finding or in patients who present with acute appendicitis.[7,8,49,165-167] They also occur in patients who have serrated polyposis syndrome.[166] They often affect older adults and are found in men and women equally.[45,167,168] They may be seen in appendices with invasive cancer, and thus probably represent a precursor lesion for invasive adenocarcinoma of the appendix.[45,168,169] However, when an appendix with a serrated lesion ruptures, the serrated lesion does not appear to have the ability to spread as pseudomyxoma peritonei in the same manner as a LAMN.[45,168] Studies have been inconsistent regarding whether or not there is an association between serrated neoplasia of the appendix and synchronous or metachronous colorectal neoplasms.[45,166,170]

Pathogenesis

Mucosal hyperplasia is occasionally seen in appendices that have been inflamed, obstructed, or ulcerated, which is presumably a reaction to inflammation. Thus hyperplastic-appearing serrated proliferations in this clinical/pathological setting may not necessarily be "neoplastic," although *KRAS* mutations have been detected in appendiceal lesions that resemble colorectal hyperplastic polyps.[168] Unlike serrated polyps in the colorectum, molecular features of the colorectal serrated pathway are actually uncommon in appendiceal serrated lesions. Although one study found *BRAF* mutations in 7 of 9 serrated polyps in the appendix,[43] most studies found that *BRAF* mutations are less common in appendiceal serrated lesions compared with colorectal serrated polyps, whereas *KRAS* mutations are relatively common, particularly in appendiceal serrated polyps with dysplasia.[45,166,168,171] Although CIMP-low is occasionally present, CIMP-high is rare, and methylation of the *MLH1* or *MGMT* promoters is generally absent, even in patients with serrated polyposis syndrome.[166] In one study of serrated polyps of the appendix, Yantiss and coauthors[45] found reduced hMLH-1 and MGMT expression across the entire spectrum of serrated lesions, although loss of MLH-1 immunoreactivity was not accompanied by MSI-H.

Abnormal nuclear localization of β-catenin is a reflection of loss of *APC* function, part of the canonical adenoma-carcinoma sequence in the colorectum. To date, studies have failed to demonstrate abnormal nuclear localization of β-catenin in serrated lesions in the appendix.[45,172]

Pathology

Appendiceal serrated lesions may be localized and polypoid, in which case they are usually located at the appendiceal tip, or they may involve broad segments of the appendix and may even involve the entire circumference of the lumen in some cases.[167,168] Grossly, an appendix with a serrated lesion is usually unremarkable, but the lumen may be slightly dilated with mucin, and the mucosa may appear grossly thickened, with minute papillary areas.[8,168]

Hyperplastic Polyp/Mucosal Hyperplasia

A *hyperplastic polyp* of the appendix refers to a discrete polypoid, serrated lesion that morphologically resembles a colorectal hyperplastic polyp. *Mucosal hyperplasia* refers to a more diffuse, segmental or circumferential, serrated mucosal proliferation (with some features of a hyperplastic polyp), particularly one that is associated with a reactive/regenerative process in a postinflammatory setting. Mucosal hyperplasia is particularly common in cases of diverticular disease of the appendix, which also may result from a postinflammatory weak point in the wall of the appendix. Histologically, both hyperplastic polyps and mucosal hyperplasia show elongation of crypts with glandular infolding, producing a serrated luminal

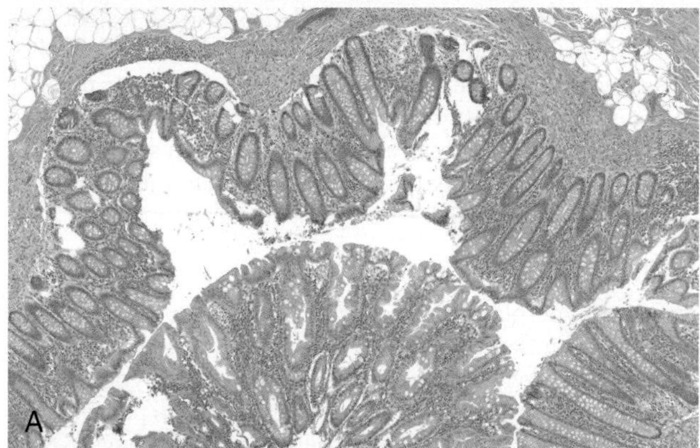

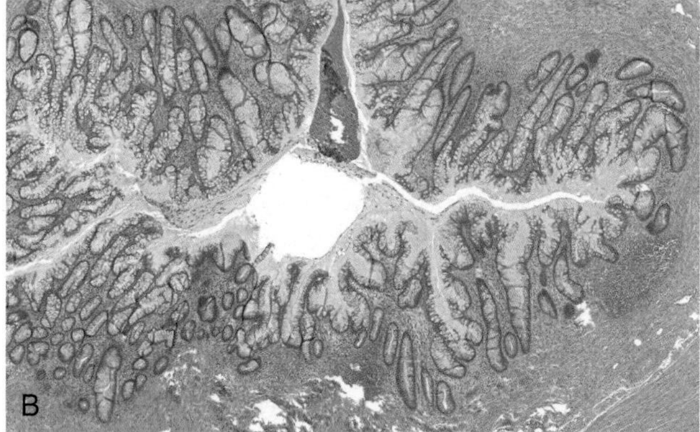

FIGURE 28.23 A, Hyperplastic polyp of the appendix. The appendix shows a polypoid protrusion *(lower half)* in which the crypts show serration of the superficial aspect, similar to hyperplastic polyps in the colon. **B,** Mucosal hyperplasia of the appendix in an example of appendiceal diverticular disease. The mucosa shows serration limited to the superficial aspects of the crypt. The crypt bases are small and round and lack the dilated, inverted T shapes of serrated lesions.

contour that generally involves the superficial portion of the crypts more than the basilar crypts (Fig. 28.23).[8,165] The glands are lined by mucinous cells that differentiate progressively toward the surface, with columnar cells that have apical mucin vacuoles alternating with classic goblet cells.[8,45,165,169] Most crypts taper down to a preserved proliferative zone that contains cells with small, round nuclei.[169] In postinflammatory appendices and in ones with diverticular disease, some degree of crypt disarray may be present, but mitoses are largely restricted to the basal area, and the muscularis mucosae remains intact.[7,8,165]

Serrated Lesion Without Dysplasia

In comparison with discrete hyperplastic polyps or more generalized mucosal hyperplasia, serrated lesions without dysplasia generally show a more florid mucosal proliferation with a more extensive serrated crypt architecture that is not simply limited to the superficial portions of the crypts. The basal portion of the crypts are typically serrated and reveal boot-shaped or inverted T-shaped crypts as well (Fig. 28.24).[45] Other features include prominent serration and dilatation of the crypts, particularly at the bases of the mucosa; fewer neuroendocrine cells; dystrophic goblet cells; increased mitotic figures; and mild nuclear atypia.[45] Essentially, these lesions are morphologically similar to

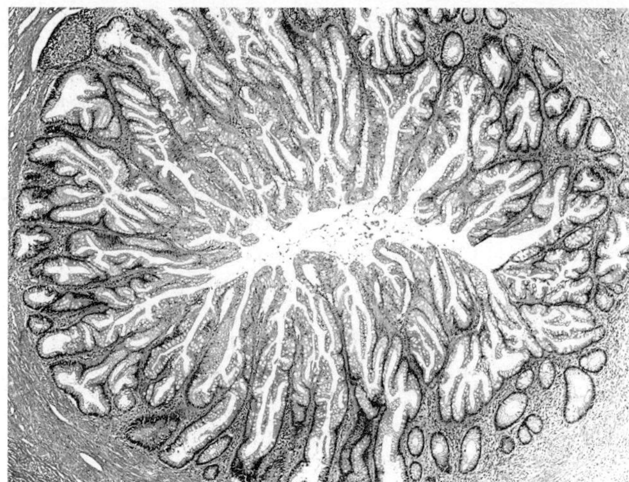

FIGURE 28.24 Serrated lesion without dysplasia. The appendix mucosa is replaced by a mucinous proliferation that shows complex serration of the crypts and an absence of villous architecture. The crypt bases show serration as well. The features are similar to those of sessile serrated lesions in the colon.

sessile serrated lesions (formerly known as *sessile serrated adenoma/polyps*) that occur in the colon.

Serrated Lesion with Dysplasia

Similar to the colon, serrated lesions may develop dysplasia, which can be of the conventional type (adenomatous, intestinal) or the serrated type. In either case, dysplastic epithelium is characterized by cells with enlarged elongated or ovoid nuclei, increased N/C ratio, hyperchromaticity, nuclear debris, infrequent mitoses, and pseudostratification.[45] Rarely, serrated lesions with dysplasia may show a villous growth pattern associated with more complex serration and may show epithelial cells with abundant eosinophilic cytoplasm and elongated nuclei, but with little or no proliferative activity (Fig. 28.25). High-grade dysplasia is characterized by the presence of more severe cytological atypia and/or more complex crypt architecture, such as micropapillary epithelial infolding or cribriform changes with increased nuclear size and irregularity, prominent often enlarged nucleoli, increased hyperchromasia and loss of nuclear polarity, anisonucleosis, and increased mitoses at all levels of the crypts (Fig. 28.26).[45]

One report of 10 serrated lesions with dysplasia in the appendix (referred to as *serrated adenoma* and defined by the presence of serrated fronds in more than 50% of dysplastic structures) showed invasive carcinoma in 4 lesions.[169] In a series by Pai et al., 3 of 7 serrated lesions that were classified as *traditional serrated adenomas* also showed invasive carcinoma,[168] suggesting that lesions that appear similar to traditional serrated adenomas of the colon may rarely occur in the appendix, but they may be more aggressive than those that occur in the colon. However, in one large series by Yantiss et al.,[45] an association between appendiceal *traditional serrated adenomas* and adenocarcinomas was not detected. Clearly, further studies examining many more cases and with long-term follow-up are needed to determine the true biological potential of appendiceal lesions that resemble traditional serrated adenomas of the colon.

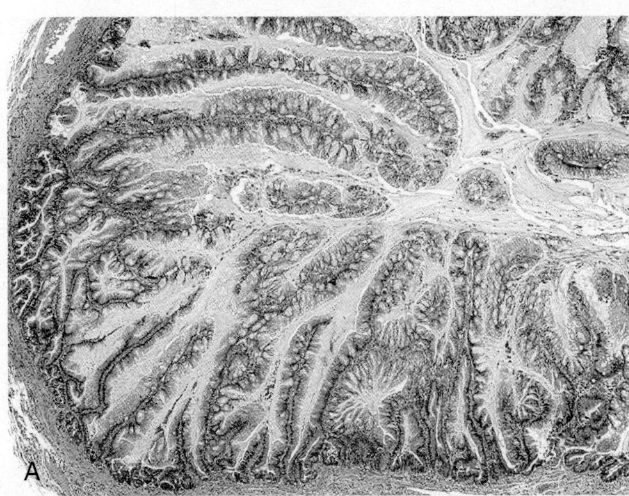

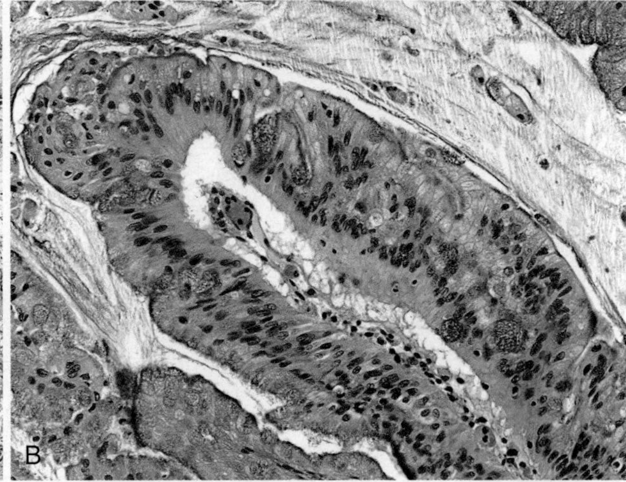

FIGURE 28.25 Serrated lesion with dysplasia resembling a colonic traditional serrated adenoma. A, The appendiceal tumor is composed of villi with complex serration and eosinophilic cytoplasm. **B,** High-power view of the villi shows that they are lined by columnar epithelial cells with cytoplasmic eosinophilia and mild nuclear atypicality with slight nuclear enlargement, grooves, and nuclear pseudostratification.

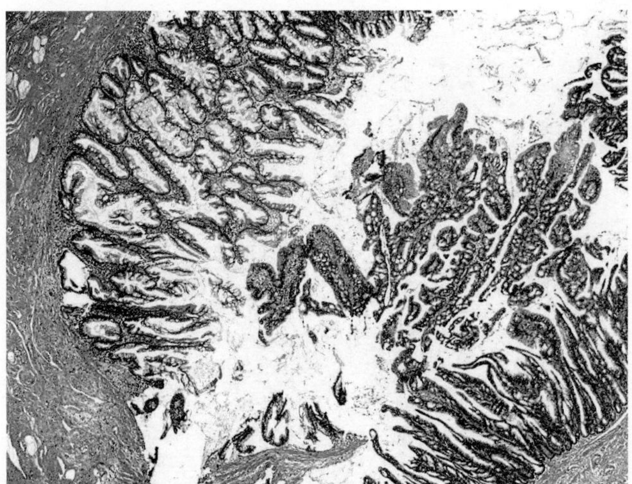

FIGURE 28.26 Serrated lesion with dysplasia. On the *left* side of the image, the neoplasm is a serrated lesion without dysplasia, but on the *right*, the proliferation becomes hyperchromatic with complex serration and cribriforming.

Differential Diagnosis

Low-Grade Appendiceal Mucinous Neoplasm

On occasion, it is difficult to distinguish hyperplastic and serrated lesions of the appendix from LAMNs that show serrated crypt architecture, either focally or diffusely. In contrast with adenomas and LAMNs, which often show slender villi and scant lamina propria, most primary serrated lesions show crypts separated by lamina propria and lack villous architecture (although traditional serrated adenomas can be villous as well). Complex serration favors a serrated lesion rather than a LAMN. Tumors with pushing invasion or those that are associated with pseudomyxoma peritonei are, by definition, considered LAMNs. A particularly challenging situation is the distinction between a LAMN with perforation versus a serrated lesion (whether hyperplastic or neoplastic) in a patient with perforated appendicitis. In these cases, careful attention to the presence of true crypts with lamina propria can help characterize the lesion as a serrated lesion rather than a LAMN. One final area of uncertainty relates to the possibility that LAMNs may arise from a serrated precursor lesion. Currently, no studies have been performed in this regard; however, anecdotal observations indicate that this may be relevant for some LAMNs.

NEUROENDOCRINE NEOPLASMS

Well-Differentiated Neuroendocrine Tumors

Clinical Features

Well-differentiated neuroendocrine tumors (NETs; historically known as *carcinoid tumors*) are found in approximately 0.32% to 0.6% of surgically removed appendices.[173,174] They occur with greatest frequency in the fourth to fifth decade of life,[173-177] although they can occur at any age, including childhood.[178-183] Females are affected more often than males, even after accounting for the increased rate of appendectomy among women.[173-177,181,184] Most cases are found incidentally,[176,185] although these tumors occasionally present clinically with appendicitis or recurrent abdominal pain,[173,184] particularly in children.[178-181,183] In some cases, the tumor may contribute to the development of appendicitis, particularly those that arise at the base of the appendix, by occluding the lumen.[173,185] Clinical presentation with carcinoid syndrome is rather exceptional in patients with neuroendocrine tumors of the appendix.[178,186]

Pathogenesis

There is some evidence to suggest that appendiceal NETs may arise from subepithelial neuroendocrine cells.[187,188] Argentaffin cells within the lamina propria were initially described by Masson in 1928.[189] These cells are associated with S-100–positive, unmyelinated nerve fibers in the periglandular plexus.[190] The number of subepithelial neuroendocrine cells peaks in the third or fourth decade of life and also increases in number in the tip of the appendix.[177,191,192] An increased number of argentaffin cells in the crypts of appendices that harbor NETs has also been reported[193] but has not been confirmed in other studies.[187] The authors of one study found gastrin-releasing peptide and its receptor

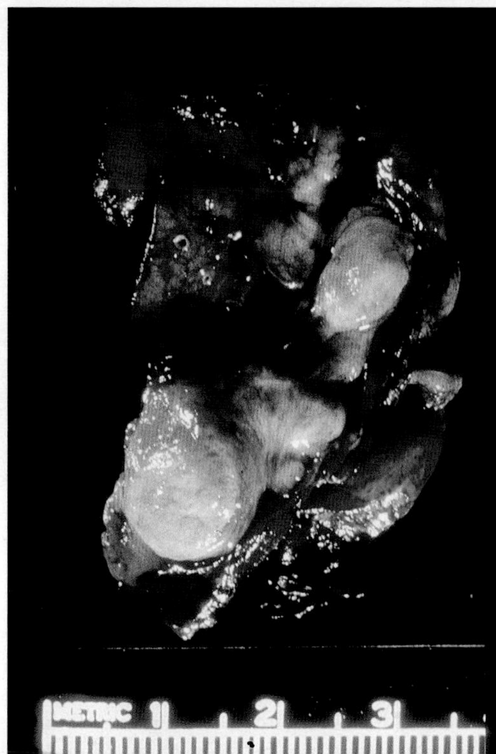

FIGURE 28.27 Gross specimen of appendiceal well-differentiated neuroendocrine tumor (carcinoid tumor) shows a yellow tan nodule in the appendix. (*From Misdraji J. Neuroendocrine tumours of the appendix. Curr Diagn Pathol. 2005;11[3]:180-193.*)

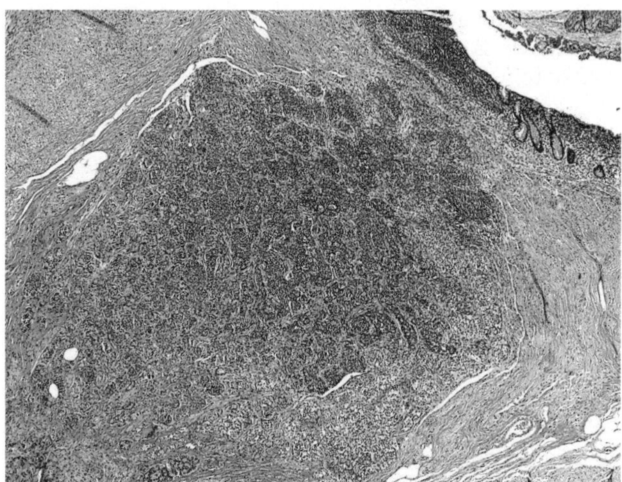

FIGURE 28.28 Well-differentiated neuroendocrine tumor of the appendix (carcinoid tumor) with insular (type A) pattern. A nested tumor is present beneath the mucosa in the appendiceal tip.

coexpression in some NETs, and they suggested a paracrine or autocrine pathway of tumorigenesis.[194]

Pathology

Appendiceal NETs are typically yellow-tan in color with a firm consistency (Fig. 28.27). They are most commonly located at the appendiceal tip (70% of cases), followed by the body and base of the appendix.[173,174,176,185] Approximately 75% are less than 1 cm in diameter and therefore may be hard to detect at gross examination. Approximately 5% are larger than 2 cm in size.[173,174,176,195] Microscopically, most are enterochromaffin cell tumors (ECs) that demonstrate an insular pattern of growth and peripheral palisading of tumor cells (Fig. 28.28).[173] L-cell tumors are less common. They demonstrate more prominent trabecular architecture (Fig. 28.29). Some L-cell tumors demonstrate a pattern of discrete tubules lined by bland, cuboidal-shaped epithelial cells with a small amount of luminal mucin (Fig. 28.30).[16,196] These tumors have been referred to as *tubular neuroendocrine tumors*. The tubules appear compressed within a fibrotic stroma, which may render them difficult to recognize on routinely stained slides.[16,196,197]

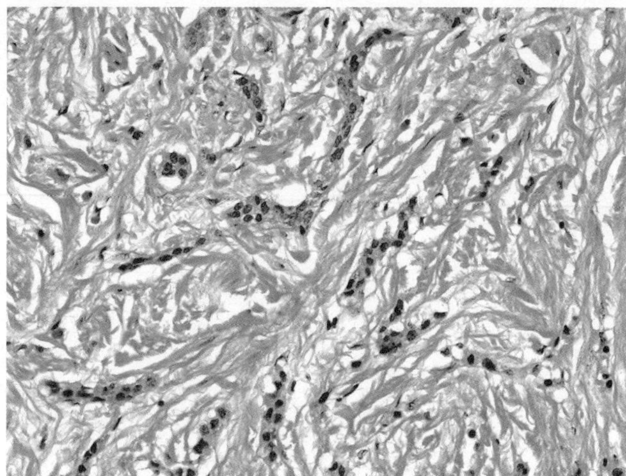

FIGURE 28.29 Well-differentiated neuroendocrine tumor of the appendix demonstrating a trabecular or ribbon-like architecture. These are known as *L-cell neuroendocrine tumors.*

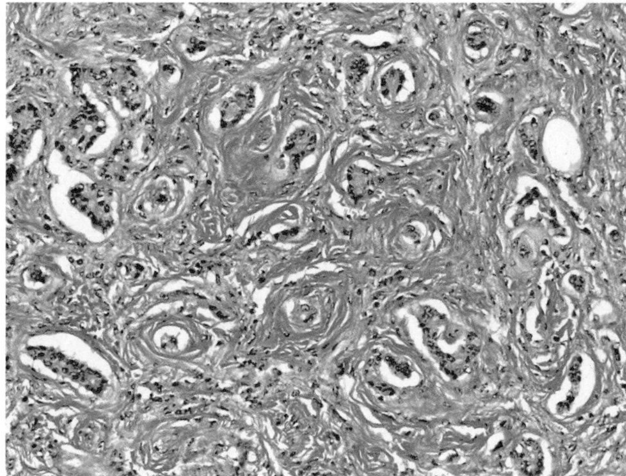

FIGURE 28.30 **Well-differentiated neuroendocrine tumor, tubular L-cell type.** The tumor is composed of uniform small tubules lined by small, bland cells within a fibrotic stroma.

The tumor cells in most neuroendocrine tumors are uniform in size and shape and contain a modest amount of eosinophilic and sometimes finely granular cytoplasm. Tumor cell nuclei show the classic "salt-and-pepper" chromatin pattern of NETs in the GI tract (Fig. 28.31).[173] The intervening stroma may be variably fibrotic and may also

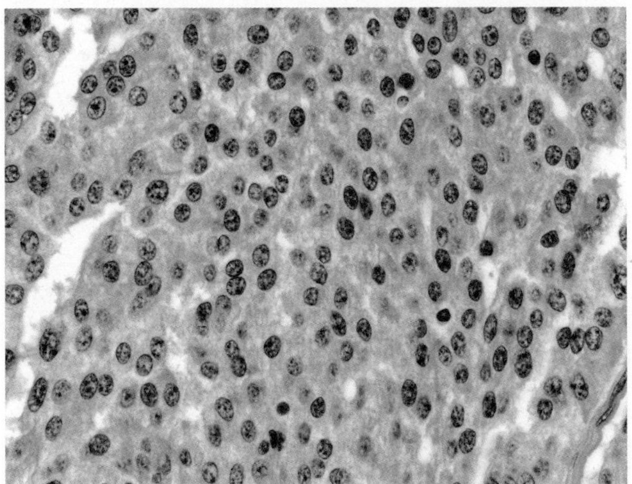

FIGURE 28.31 Well-differentiated neuroendocrine tumor. High-power view shows the characteristic neuroendocrine nuclei, with uniform nuclei and granular "salt-and-pepper" chromatin. *(From Misdraji J. Neuroendocrine tumours of the appendix. Curr Diagn Pathol. 2005;11[3]:180-193.)*

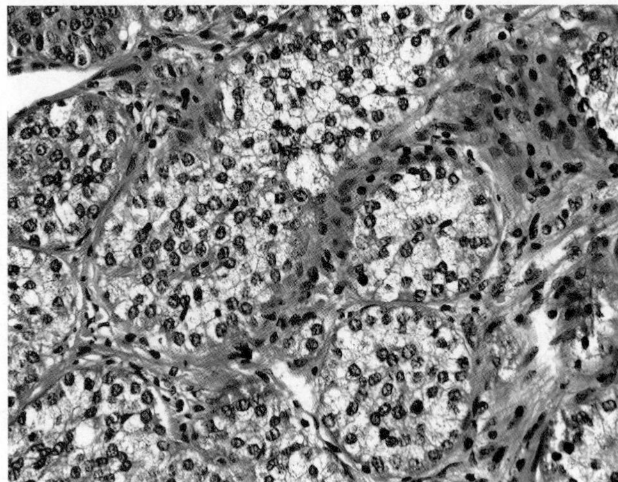

FIGURE 28.32 Well-differentiated neuroendocrine tumor of the appendix with marked cytoplasmic clearing. These so-called *balloon cell neuroendocrine tumors* are otherwise similar to conventional neuroendocrine tumors.

contain a reactive neural proliferation. In some cases, the stroma is densely fibrotic and shows entrapment of tumor cells (scirrhous pattern).[173,174] The overlying mucosa is usually unremarkable, although the tumor may appear to arise from the deep compartment of the mucosa. NETs extend deeply into the wall and even to the peritoneal surface in 33% to 66% of cases.[173,195] Lymphatic invasion is quite common,[173,195] but differentiation of retraction artifact from lymphatic invasion can be difficult.[184,198,199] Perineural invasion is also common, reported in approximately 35% of tumors.[174] Infiltration of the mesoappendix occurs in 7.5% to 27% of cases,[174,184,195] and this feature is generally related to tumor size. Syracuse et al. found invasion of the mesoappendix in 26% of grossly evident tumors, but in only 4% of tumors discovered only on microscopic examination.[185]

Rare NETs demonstrate either clear or foamy cytoplasm as a result of lipid accumulation. This histological change is usually focal, but it may be diffuse on occasion. These tumors are termed *lipid-rich, clear cell,* or *balloon cell NETs*, and they are considered a morphological variant, with a similar immunohistochemical profile and clinical behavior to classical EC NETs (Fig. 28.32).[200,201] Some lipid droplets coalesce to form larger-sized droplets.[201] Tumors with cells containing prominent lipid droplets should be distinguished from goblet cell adenocarcinoma. However, the latter tumor shows large-sized mucin vacuoles and an eccentrically located nucleus. Rare NETs show spindle cell morphology.[202]

Grading of appendiceal NETs is based on mitotic counts or Ki-67 index, similar to NETs in other portions of the GI tract. Tumors with less than 2 mitoses per 2 mm^2 and less than 3% Ki-67 index are graded as G1. Tumors with 2 to 20 mitoses per 2 mm^2 or 3% to 20% Ki-67 index are graded as G2. Tumors with greater than 20 mitoses per 2 mm^2 or greater than 20% Ki-67 index are graded as G3.[203]

Immunohistochemically, EC tumors stain positively with conventional neuroendocrine markers, including chromogranin, synaptophysin, and neuron-specific enolase (NSE). They also express serotonin and substance P.[204,205] S-100–positive cells may be identified surrounding tumor islands, analogous to sustentacular cells.[187,190,197] EC tumors are negative for CEA.[197] p53 is typically negative in appendiceal NET.[206] L-cell neuroendocrine tumors, including so-called *tubular neuroendocrine tumors*, stain for glucagon (Fig. 28.33), pancreatic polypeptide (PP/PYY), and CEA.[204,205,207] These tumors stain with synaptophysin but less consistently with chromogranin.[196,197,207,208]

Differential Diagnosis

Goblet Cell Adenocarcinoma

Clear cell NETs or NETs with a prominent glandular pattern can mimic goblet cell adenocarcinoma (termed *goblet cell carcinoid* before the fifth edition of the WHO classification). Goblet cell adenocarcinomas are generally composed of smaller nests of cells with goblet-like or signet ring–like features, interspersed with eosinophilic granular cells similar in appearance to Paneth cells. The vacuoles in goblet cell adenocarcinomas are typically single in number and larger in size compared with clear cell NETs, which contain foamy, microvesicular, or rarified cytoplasm. Also, goblet cell adenocarcinomas usually infiltrate the appendix in a circumferential manner, unlike typical NETs, which tend to form a discrete mass lesion.

Metastatic Carcinoma

Occasionally, an appendiceal NET (particularly the L-cell variant) can be mistaken for a metastatic carcinoma, such as metastatic breast carcinoma. Attention to the nuclear chromatin pattern, bland nuclear features, and low mitotic activity in NETs helps avoid this diagnostic pitfall.

Natural History

Patients with appendiceal NETs normally have an excellent prognosis. Lymph node metastases are uncommon, and liver metastases are rare.[173,174,176,209] The reported frequency of metastasis ranges from 1.4 to 8.8%,[174,210] but this is highly dependent on tumor size: 0% for tumors less than 1 cm, 3%

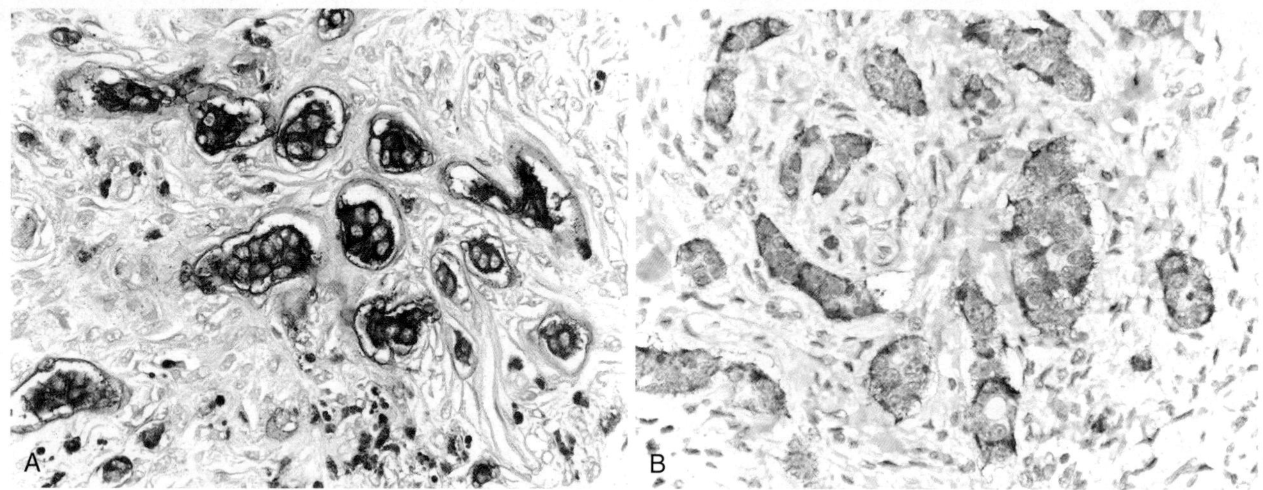

FIGURE 28.33 Well-differentiated neuroendocrine tumor, tubular pattern. A, immunohistochemical stain for carcinoembryonic antigen (CEA) shows strong staining of the tumor. **B,** Immunohistochemical stain for glucagon shows cytoplasmic staining of many tumor cells.

TABLE 28.4 Comparison of UICC/AJCC and ENETS Classifications for Primary Tumor Stage for Appendiceal Neuroendocrine Tumors

Primary Tumor Stage	UICC/AJCC Stage	ENETS Guidelines
X	Primary tumor cannot be assessed	
0	No evidence of primary tumor	
1	Tumor <2 cm	Tumor <1 cm with infiltration of the submucosa and muscularis propria
2	Tumor >2 cm but <4 cm	Tumor <2 cm with infiltration of the submucosa, muscularis propria, and/or minimal (<3 mm) infiltration of the subserosa or mesoappendix
3	Tumor >4 cm or with subserosal invasion or involvement of the mesoappendix	Tumor >2 cm and/or extensive (>3 mm) infiltration of the subserosa and/or mesoappendix
4	Tumor perforates the peritoneum or directly invades other organs or structures (excluding direct invasion into contiguous bowel segments)	Tumor with infiltration of the peritoneum and/or other neighboring organs

AJCC, *American Joint Committee on Cancer;* ENETS, *European Neuroendocrine Tumor Society;* UICC, *Union for International Cancer Control.*

to 6.7% for tumors 1 to 2 cm, and 21% to 30% for tumors greater than 2 cm in maximum dimension.[205,211] Patients with local disease have a 5-year survival rate of 92% to 100%, but this rate decreases for patients with regional metastasis (81%) and those with distant metastasis (31%).[175,176,212]

Several studies have examined prognostic features of appendiceal NETs. The only consistent finding in these studies is that tumors less than 2 cm in size metastasize infrequently, and those less than 1 cm are essentially always benign.[173,174,213] Other factors that have been evaluated but dismissed as prognostic factors include depth of invasion, location of the tumor along the length of the appendix, perineural invasion, lymphatic invasion, and serosal involvement.[174,176,195,213] However, one study found that among tumors less than 2 cm in size, the presence of small-vessel invasion predicted lymph node metastases (60% vs. 0% in tumors without small-vessel invasion), whereas serosal penetration and margin status did not.[214] Studies that have examined the significance of mesoappendix involvement have yielded conflicting results. Some authors reported an increased likelihood of metastatic disease independent of tumor size,[185,215] whereas others showed that mesoappendiceal invasion has no effect on prognosis for tumors smaller than 2 cm in size.[174,198] Still, most authorities feel that the presence of mesoappendiceal involvement and its extent (limited vs. extensive) should be documented in the pathology report.[216] A consensus statement by the European Neuroendocrine Tumor Society (ENETS) notes that neuroendocrine tumors that are less than 1 cm in size with invasion into the subserosa or with mesoappendiceal invasion up to 3 mm in depth and with negative margins pose no risk of recurrence after appendectomy.[217] Tumors that occur at the base of the appendix, are greater than 1 cm, invade deeply into the mesoappendix, or involve the margin have a small risk of recurrence; therefore additional surgery is indicated but not proven to be of benefit.[217] In the ENETS guidelines, mesoappendiceal invasion less than or greater than 3 mm in depth is an important parameter used to stage tumors (Table 28.4).[217]

Treatment

Simple appendectomy is considered curative for NETs less than 1 cm in size if the margin of resection is negative for tumor. According to some authors, the presence of tumor at the margin of resection should prompt consideration of ileocolectomy.[184,185] Tumors greater than 2 cm in diameter have an increased risk of metastatic disease,

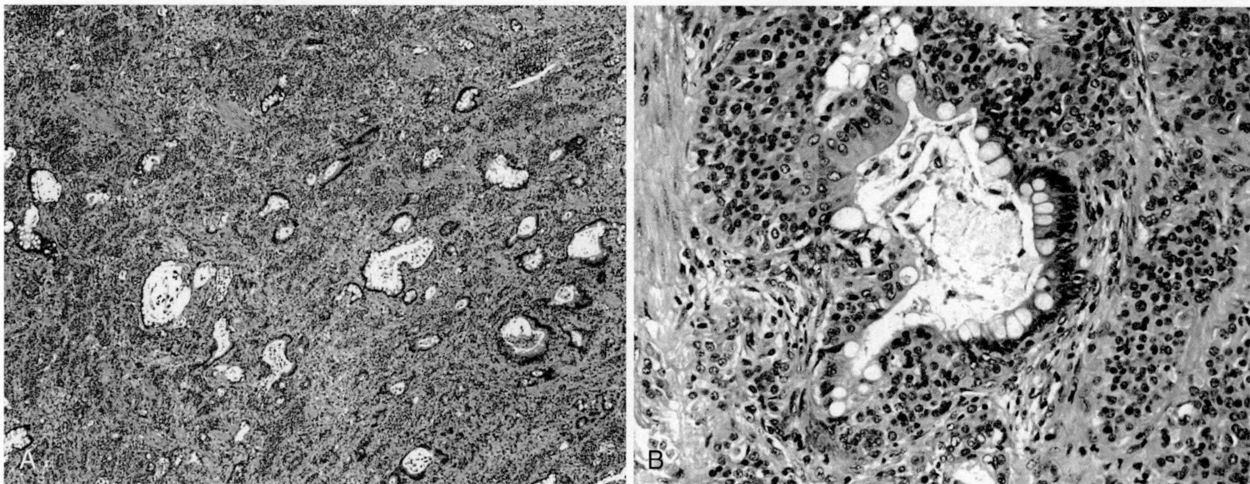

FIGURE 28.34 **Mixed neuroendocrine/nonneuroendocrine tumor. A,** Low-power view shows an insular pattern well-differentiated neuroendocrine tumor with scattered mucinous glands. **B,** High-power view shows merging of intestinal-type glands with nests of well-differentiated neuroendocrine tumor cells.

thus right hemicolectomy is recommended, particularly if there is mesoappendix involvement or vascular invasion.[213] Regardless, less than 20% of hemicolectomy specimens show residual tumor or lymph node metastases.[176,195,209] The management of tumors that measure between 1 and 2 cm in size has not been standardized. Other factors should be considered in the decision process, such as tumor grade, mesoappendiceal and serosal involvement, angiolymphatic invasion, gross evidence of regional lymph node metastases at the time of appendectomy, patient age, and comorbidities.[176,209,211,217] Given that these tumors have a low risk of metastatic disease and an indolent clinical course even when metastatic, conservative management is advised for older adult patients.[176,211,213] Appendiceal NETs in children without metastasis at presentation are often clinically benign.[178] Several authors recommend right hemicolectomy in patients of this age group only for tumors that demonstrate regional lymph node metastases or incomplete resection or in other unusual circumstances.[180-182] However, one study found that tumor size greater than 1.5 cm in children and adolescents was predictive of lymph node involvement, with a sensitivity of 77.8% and a specificity of 66.7%, and recommended right hemicolectomy for these cases.[218]

Neuroendocrine Carcinoma

Overall, neuroendocrine carcinomas are rare in the appendix.[219] Similar to elsewhere in the GI tract, they are poorly differentiated tumors that frequently demonstrate neuroendocrine differentiation when evaluated immunohistochemically and carry a poor prognosis. They are classified as either small cell type or large cell type. Tumor cells in large cell neuroendocrine carcinoma have more abundant cytoplasm, vesicular nuclei, and prominent nucleoli.[219]

Mixed Neuroendocrine/Nonneuroendocrine Neoplasms

Rare tumors in the appendix are composed of histologically distinct components of adenocarcinoma and neuroendocrine tumor. Usually these are high-grade tumors, but rarely the various components are low grade. Examples include composite classical neuroendocrine tumor and adenocarcinoma[220,221] (Fig. 28.34) and mixed adenocarcinoma and high-grade neuroendocrine carcinoma (Fig. 28.35).[222,223] Of note is the fact that the category of mixed neuroendocrine/nonneuroendocrine neoplasms does not include goblet cell adenocarcinomas, which are neoplasms composed of tumor cell clusters with both mucinous and neuroendocrine differentiation, rather than as discrete and separate histological components of each.

GOBLET CELL ADENOCARCINOMA

Nomenclature

Distinctive appendiceal tumors composed of clusters of goblet-like mucinous cells, endocrine cells, and even a variable number of Paneth-like cells have historically been termed *goblet cell carcinoid tumor, mucinous carcinoid tumor,*[224] *adenocarcinoid,*[225] *crypt cell carcinoma,*[15] and *microglandular carcinoma.*[4] Because of the presence of a variable degree of neuroendocrine cells in these tumors as well as their growth characteristics, many authorities have traditionally considered them a variant of neuroendocrine tumor of the appendix. In this context, they were termed *goblet cell carcinoids*. However, use of the term *carcinoid* to describe this tumor type has occasionally led oncologists to manage patients as though they had a neuroendocrine tumor and also to pathologists incorrectly applying neuroendocrine grading and staging systems to this tumor type.[226] In reality, recent data strongly suggest that these tumors behave more similarly to appendiceal adenocarcinomas. Furthermore, they frequently contain extracellular mucin and almost always contain glandular differentiation and intracellular mucin; they are staged similar to adenocarcinomas, and treatments that target adenocarcinoma are appropriate for these tumors when they disseminate. Thus the current WHO classification of appendiceal neoplasms has reclassified these tumors as *goblet cell adenocarcinomas*.[18]

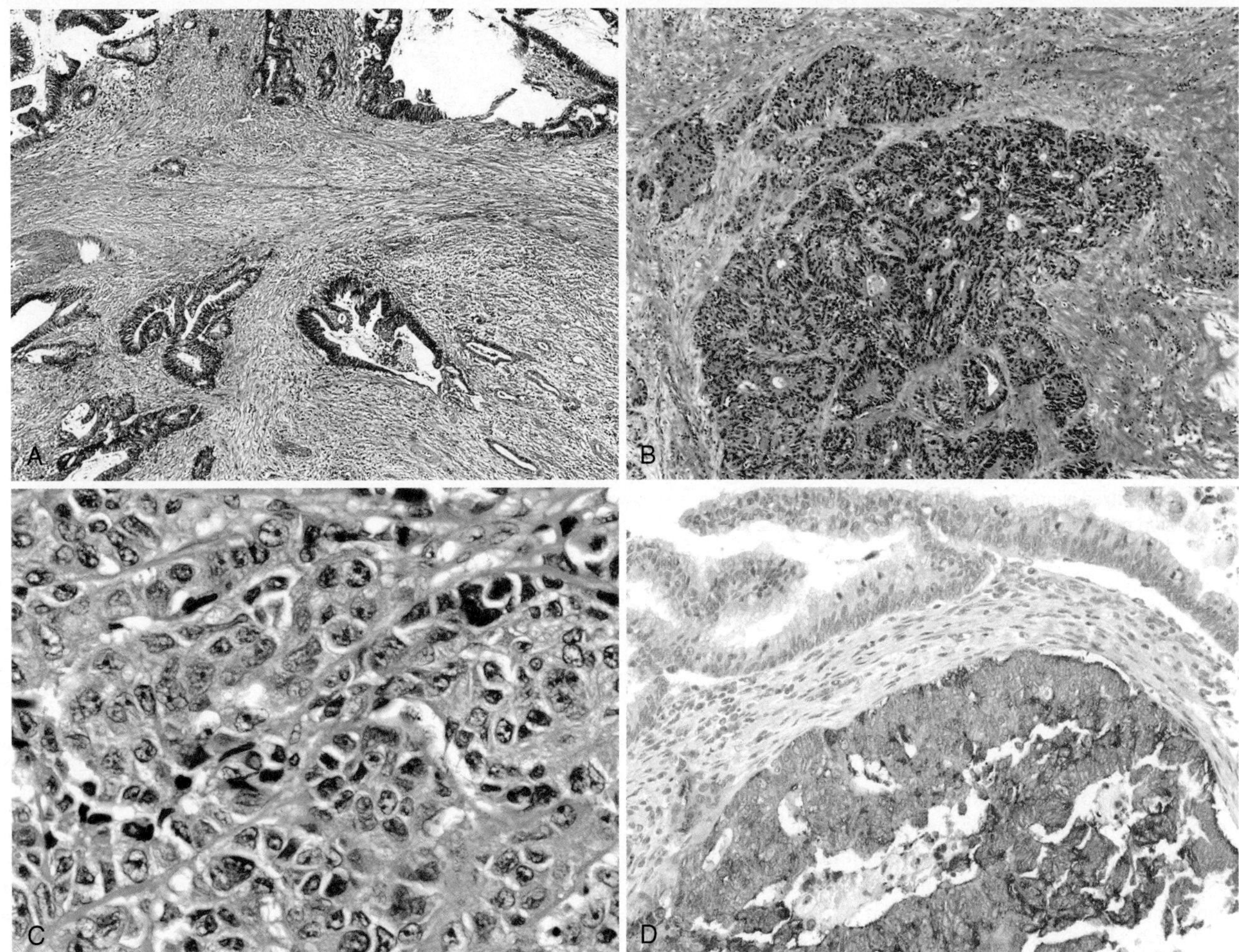

FIGURE 28.35 Mixed adenocarcinoma and large cell neuroendocrine carcinoma. A, Conventional invasive adenocarcinoma. **B** and **C,** Elsewhere, the tumor demonstrates a cribriform/rosetted pattern (**B**) and solid pattern (**C**). **C,** High-power view of the solid areas demonstrates tumor cells with vesicular nuclei, prominent nucleoli, and a moderate amount of cytoplasm. **D,** Synaptophysin stain shows strong staining of the solid and rosetted area *(bottom)* and absent staining of the mucinous neoplasm within the lumen *(top).*

Clinical Features

Goblet cell adenocarcinomas most often affect patients in their fifth decade of life, and they show an equal sex distribution.[227] Tumors may cause symptoms of appendicitis or abdominal pain, but these tumors can also be found incidentally.[228-230] Patients can present when the tumor has metastasized to the peritoneum or, in females, the ovaries.[230-237]

Pathogenesis

In 1981, Isaacson et al. demonstrated that many goblet cell adenocarcinomas are positive for IgA, secretory component, and lysozyme, all of which are features of intestinal crypt cells, and as a result, he proposed the term *crypt cell carcinoma.*[15] Others have also noted the similarities of the tumor nests with normal intestinal crypts. These observations have raised theories regarding the derivation of these tumors and whether they represent proliferation of pluripotential crypt cells or are simply neoplasms that retain the capacity to differentiate into adherent cryptlike units.[15,16,225]

Ultrastructural and molecular studies have shown that the pathogenesis of goblet cell adenocarcinoma shares features with both conventional NET and with adenocarcinoma. Electron microscopic studies have shown evidence of both mucin production and neuroendocrine differentiation (electron-dense granules) within the same cells.[200,238-241] van Eeden and colleagues showed absent staining for p53 and nuclear β-catenin expression, normal DPC4 expression, and rare *KRAS* mutations in 16 goblet cell adenocarcinomas, similar to conventional carcinoid tumors.[242] However, they also found expression of CEA and cytokeratin 7, similar to adenocarcinomas but unlike conventional neuroendocrine tumors. Goblet cell adenocarcinomas also marked with an antibody against the transcription factor Math1, which is involved in the differentiation of intestinal stem cells toward progenitor cells with a secretory phenotype.

Earlier, more limited molecular studies demonstrated shared molecular features between goblet cell adenocarcinomas and conventional neuroendocrine tumors. Stancu and colleagues[227] found allelic loss of chromosomes 11q, 16q, and 18q as frequently in goblet cell adenocarcinomas as in ileal neuroendocrine tumors. They also found absent *KRAS*, *β-catenin*, or *DPC-4* mutations and no p53 overexpression by immunohistochemistry. Ramnani and associates were unable to detect *KRAS* mutations in 22 goblet cell

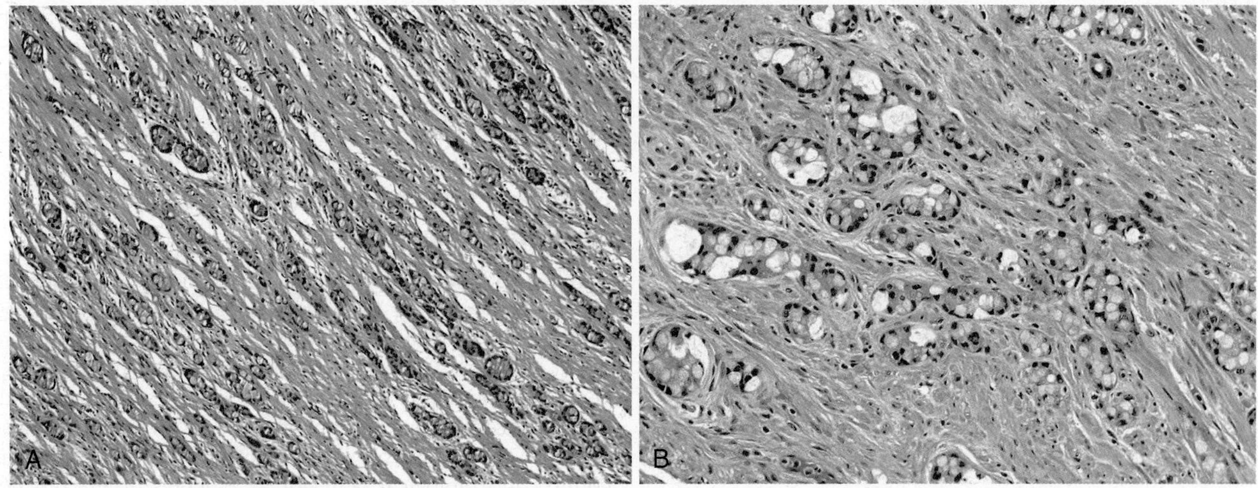

FIGURE 28.36 Goblet cell adenocarcinoma, low-grade pattern. A, Low-power view shows relatively uniform cohesive clusters of tumor cells infiltrating the appendiceal wall without eliciting a stromal reaction. **B,** Medium-power view shows that the cohesive and orderly tumor clusters comprise uniform cells with mucin vacuoles resembling goblet cells.

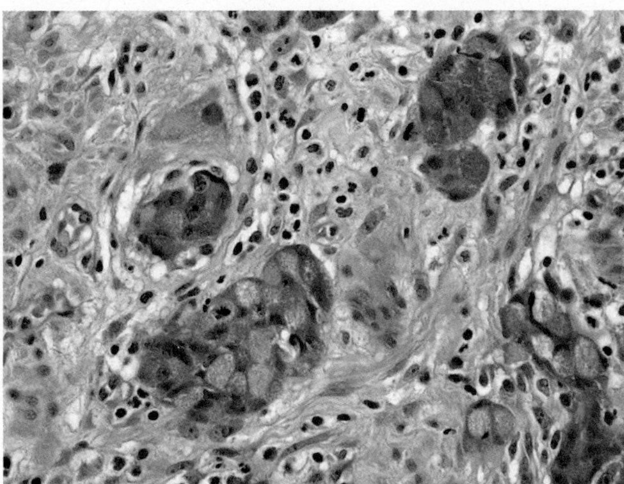

FIGURE 28.37 Goblet cell adenocarcinoma, low-grade pattern. The cohesive tumor clusters include goblet-like or signet ring–like cells and cells with coarse eosinophilic granules analogous to Paneth cells.

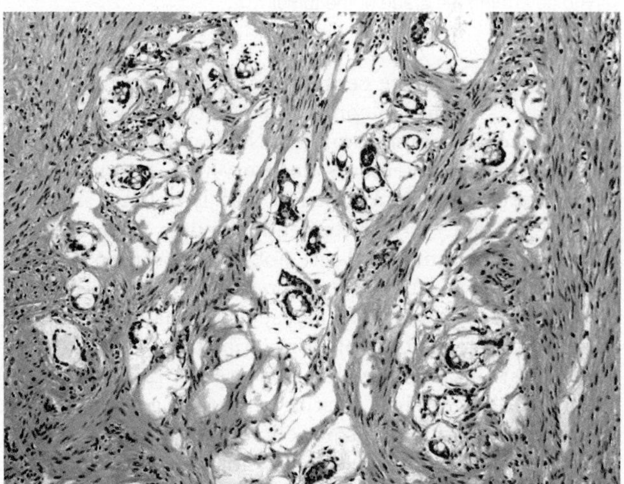

FIGURE 28.38 Goblet cell adenocarcinoma, low-grade pattern. Extracellular mucin pools are a common component of goblet cell adenocarcinomas. The tumor clusters appear as cohesive groups, often with central lumens, resembling floating crypts.

adenocarcinomas.[243] They found *TP53* mutations in 25% of goblet cell adenocarcinomas and 44% of classical neuroendocrine tumors of the appendix. However, although these findings are similar to the molecular features of conventional neuroendocrine tumors, they do not confirm that they are biologically related.

More recently, molecular studies have shown that goblet cell adenocarcinomas commonly have mutations in chromatin remodeling genes, including mutations in *ARID2; ARID1A;* members of the lysine methyltransferase 2 *(KMT2)* family including *KMT2A, KMT2b,* and *KMT2D; DKM6A;* and *NCOR1*.[244,245] Mutations in genes that are observed in gastric signet ring cell carcinoma and lobular breast carcinoma have also been observed, including mutations in *RHOA* and *CDH1*.[244,245] Other reported mutations include those in *GNAS, RHPN2, ATRX,* and *SOX9*. High-grade goblet cell adenocarcinomas have similar mutations, but they acquire additional mutations that are more often seen in colorectal adenocarcinoma, such as *SMAD4, TP53, KRAS, GNAS, BRAF, PI3KCA, APC, ATM,* and *NRAS*.[44,244] Goblet cell adenocarcinomas show retained expression of DNA mismatch repair proteins, and they are microsatellite stable.[246]

Pathology

These tumors usually appear as an area of circumferential thickening of the appendix and thus may be recognized only on microscopic examination of the specimen. The average tumor size is 2 cm.[227] Microscopically, goblet cell adenocarcinomas show circumferential infiltration of the appendix by discrete nests of mucinous cells that resemble goblet cells or, in cases in which the mucin compresses the nucleus to the edge of the cell, signet ring cells (Fig. 28.36).[224] The mucin within goblet-like cells is usually periodic acid–Schiff (PAS) and Alcian blue positive.[224] Often admixed with goblet-like or signet ring–like cells are cells with eosinophilic cytoplasm and, occasionally, Paneth cells (Fig. 28.37).[15,16,225,247,248] Most tumor cell clusters lack a clearly identifiable central lumina.[224,248] Cell clusters

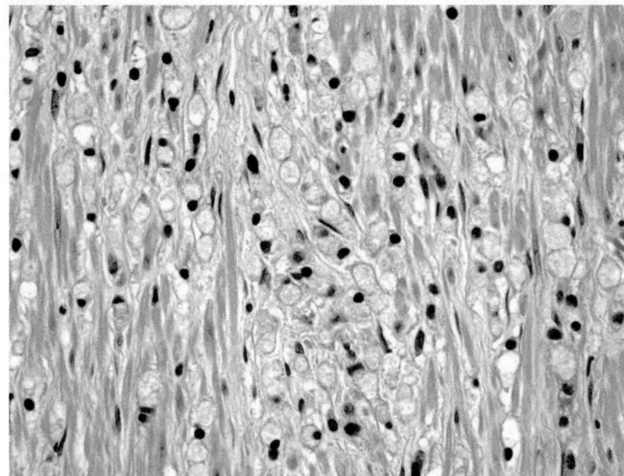

FIGURE 28.39 Goblet cell adenocarcinoma with single cells. Single-cell growth is a high-grade pattern in goblet cell adenocarcinoma, but areas with single cells are commonly present in these tumors, and assessment of the proportion of the tumor demonstrating single-cell growth is necessary to determine the grade of the tumor.

that contain a discrete central lumina resemble intestinal crypts.[16,225] Nuclear pleomorphism is typically mild, and mitoses are infrequent; however, high-grade tumors may show nuclear enlargement, pleomorphism, and more frequent mitoses.[249-251] Perineural and lymphatic invasion may be present.[224,230] Extracellular mucin pools harboring clusters of tumor cells are not an uncommon finding, but unlike pure mucinous adenocarcinomas, the epithelium within pools of mucin usually remains clustered, without the formation of large cribriform-shaped units or linear strips. Some cell clusters reveal preserved central lumina resembling "floating" crypts (Fig. 28.38).[16,248] The tumor typically does not elicit a stromal reaction. In most cases, a precursor lesion is not identified, and the tumor appears to arise without a clear point of origin, or it may seem to arise from the crypts of the appendiceal mucosa.[248] Rare tumors are associated with either a coexisting mucinous neoplasm[252-254] or a component of conventional neuroendocrine neoplasm.[255] Immunohistochemically, goblet cell adenocarcinomas are cytokeratin and CEA positive.[16,239,247] They also express Cam 5.2, cytokeratin 7, cytokeratin 20, CDX2, SATB2, and E-cadherin.[242,256,257] Immunohistochemistry for chromogranin and synaptophysin show variable numbers of neuroendocrine cells, from rare to many.[17,242,258] In some cases, small numbers of cells may be positive for glucagon, particularly in areas that resemble tubular neuroendocrine tumors.[16]

Goblet cell adenocarcinomas that are higher grade demonstrate a variety of more aggressive appearing growth patterns. These patterns vary across different tumors, although some are quite characteristic of high-grade goblet cell adenocarcinomas. The presence of dyshesive mucinous cells among cohesive tubules is a high-grade feature that can occur only focally in otherwise low-grade tumors (Fig. 28.39), but in a more widespread fashion in high-grade tumors. Other high-grade patterns include ribbons and cords of atypical cells, cribriforming or anastomosing tumor clusters, sheets of tumor cells, mucin pools with floating single cells or disorganized clusters, and areas that resemble ordinary intestinal-type adenocarcinomas (Fig. 28.40). A desmoplastic stromal response may be noted in atypical areas. Collectively, these patterns form the basis for grading of these tumors (see the next section on grading).[16,249-251,259]

Grading of Goblet Cell Adenocarcinoma

Historical Perspective

Before 1990, no clear grading systems existed for goblet cell adenocarcinoma. For instance, in one study of 39 tumors, Warkel et al. concluded that extension beyond the appendix at the time of initial surgery, foci of "dedifferentiation," and a mitotic count of 2 or more per 10 high-power fields characterized an aggressive phenotype.[225] Other studies also noted a correlation between cytological grade or mitotic counts, and biological behavior,[260] whereas others did not find Ki-67 proliferation fraction predictive of outcome in goblet cell adenocarcinoma.[261] Thus the overall grading system was controversial and quite uncertain at that time.

The first clinically useful grading system for goblet cell adenocarcinomas was published in 1990 by Burke et al.[16] In this study, the authors defined two grades of goblet cell adenocarcinoma based on the amount of "carcinomatous" growth patterns, the latter of which included the presence of fused or cribriform glands, single-file structures, diffusely infiltrating signet ring cells, or sheets of solid cells. In this study, tumors with less than 25% carcinomatous growth were found to be confined to the appendix and showed a favorable outcome. As a result, they were classified as *goblet cell carcinoid*. However, tumors with greater than 50% carcinomatous growth were found to be more likely high stage at the time of diagnosis and to have aggressive biological behavior. The latter tumors were thus classified as *mixed carcinoid-adenocarcinoma*.

In 2008, Tang et al. proposed a three-tier grading system that promoted the concept that some goblet cell "carcinoids" progress to adenocarcinomas.[17] In this study, tumors with features of goblet cell carcinoid as described by Burke et al. were designated Group A, and two forms of adenocarcinoma associated with this tumor (termed *adenocarcinoma ex goblet cell carcinoid tumor*) were described, an intermediate signet ring cell type (Type B), and a poorly differentiated carcinoma type (Type C). Group B tumors had partial or nearly complete loss of goblet cell clusters, with tumor cells arranged as single cells, disorganized growth, irregular cell clusters with jagged contours, and desmoplasia. In contrast, Group C tumors showed at least 1 low-power field or 1 mm^2 focus in which the tumor was indistinguishable from poorly differentiated or undifferentiated carcinoma. In their study, tumors in group C showed positive staining for p53 and MUC1, but absent MUC2 expression, suggesting progression of the goblet cell adenocarcinoma.

In 2015, Taggart et al. applied both Burke's and Tang's grading systems to a new set of 74 tumors.[250] They found that Burke's method of assessing the percentage of tumor composed of adenocarcinomatous elements predicted outcome, but that Tang's method of classifying the histological subtype of adenocarcinoma (as signet ring cell type or poorly differentiated type) did not. Concurrently, Lee et al. validated Tang's system in a different set of 78 tumors, but these authors proposed a simple two-tier grading system based on scoring

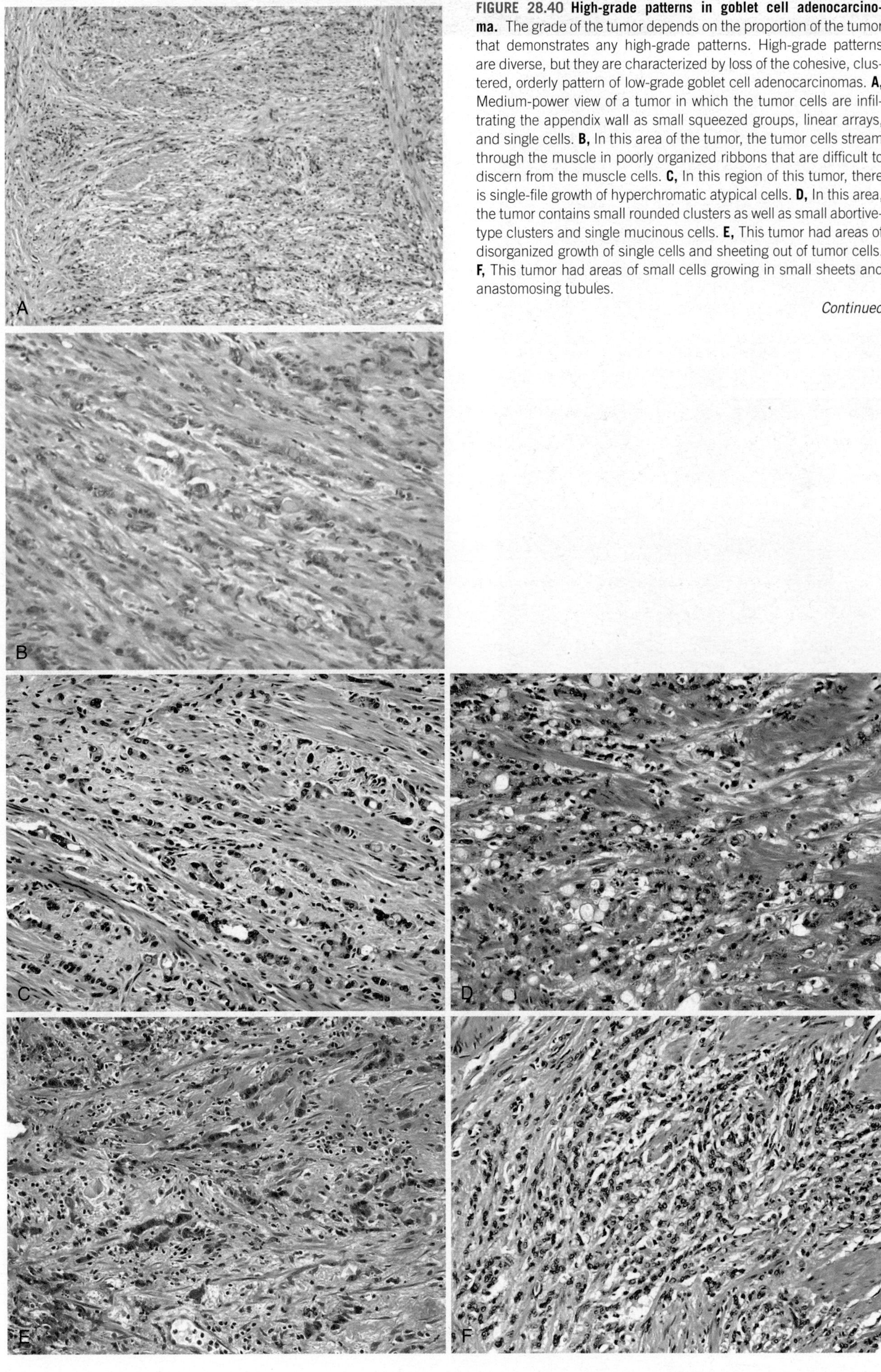

FIGURE 28.40 High-grade patterns in goblet cell adenocarcinoma. The grade of the tumor depends on the proportion of the tumor that demonstrates any high-grade patterns. High-grade patterns are diverse, but they are characterized by loss of the cohesive, clustered, orderly pattern of low-grade goblet cell adenocarcinomas. **A,** Medium-power view of a tumor in which the tumor cells are infiltrating the appendix wall as small squeezed groups, linear arrays, and single cells. **B,** In this area of the tumor, the tumor cells stream through the muscle in poorly organized ribbons that are difficult to discern from the muscle cells. **C,** In this region of this tumor, there is single-file growth of hyperchromatic atypical cells. **D,** In this area, the tumor contains small rounded clusters as well as small abortive-type clusters and single mucinous cells. **E,** This tumor had areas of disorganized growth of single cells and sheeting out of tumor cells. **F,** This tumor had areas of small cells growing in small sheets and anastomosing tubules.

Continued

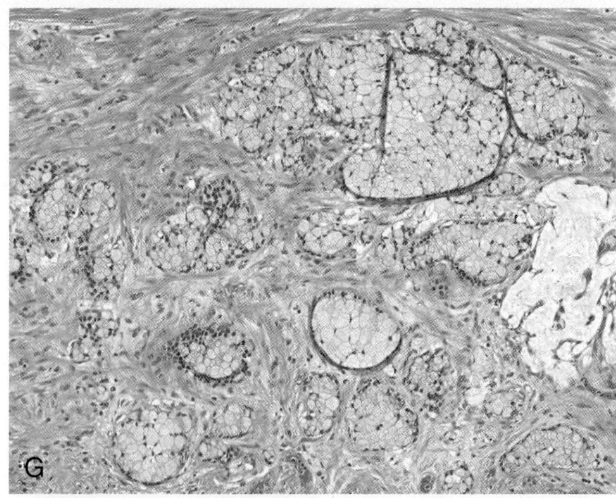

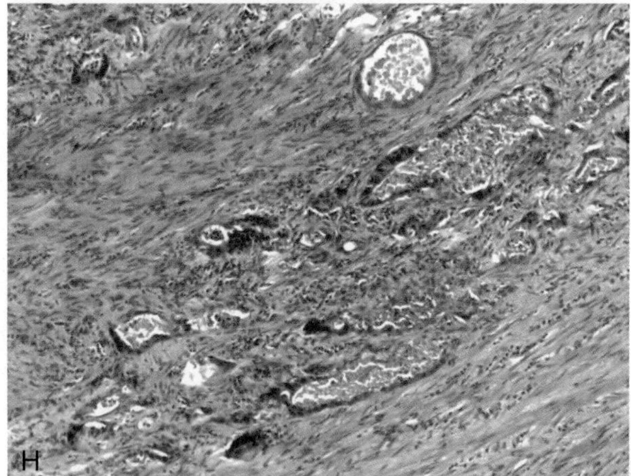

FIGURE 28.40, CONT'D G, The tumor shows large expansile masses of cells rather than the uniform small, cohesive tubules. **H,** In goblet cell adenocarcinoma, there can be areas that resemble conventional adenocarcinoma, such as in this example, with glands lined by atypical columnar cells with necrosis.

the presence of three variables within the tumors: cytological atypia, stromal desmoplasia, and solid growth pattern.[262] Low-grade tumors had, at most, one of these variables, whereas high-grade tumors had two or three of these variables.

Unfortunately, studies on interobserver variability showed only moderate agreement among pathologists when attempting to grade goblet cell adenocarcinomas using either a two- or three-tier system.[263] Each grading system suffers from use of pathological criteria that are open to subjective interpretation, such as the significance of "single cells" or "large tumor clusters," "solid growth," or "desmoplasia" in the setting of appendicitis. For instance, in one study of 77 disseminated tumors by Reid et al., the authors found it difficult to grade the tumors according to either Tang's or Taggart's approach.[249]

Current World Health Organization Grading System

In recent large series of goblet cell adenocarcinomas, the percentage of high-grade histological patterns in the tumor was shown to correlate negatively with survival.[251,259] For instance, Nonaka et al.[251] assessed low- versus high-grade patterns in 105 tumors and found that patients could be separated into four distinct prognostic groups: those with less than 5% high-grade patterns, those with 5% to 39% high-grade patterns, those with 40% to 89% high-grade

TABLE 28.5 Criteria for Grading Goblet Cell Adenocarcinoma

Tumor Grade	Tubular or Clustered Growth (Low-Grade Pattern)	Loss of Tubular or Clustered Growth (Any Combination of High-Grade Patterns)
1	>75%	<25%
2	50%-75%	25%-50%
3	<50%	>50%

patterns, and those with greater than 90% high-grade patterns. Although this conforms, in principle, to Burke's and Taggart's methods of grading, they did not detect a difference in survival between patients with 0% to 25% high-grade patterns and 25% to 50% high-grade patterns. In contrast, Yozu et al. found that these cutoff values were prognostically useful.[259] Yozu and colleagues proposed a clinically useful grading system based on the percentage of well-differentiated tubular, glandular, or clustered growth, using the cutoff values already established by Burke's group and Taggart's group. In this system, a low-grade pattern in goblet cell adenocarcinomas is defined by tumor groups that are largely cohesive with orderly tubules or tumor cell clusters, either with or without extracellular mucin accumulation. Grade 1 tumors are those that contain more than 75% *well-differentiated* tubular or clustered growth. Tumors with 50% to 75% tubular or clustered growth are categorized as grade 2 *(moderately differentiated)*, whereas tumors with less than 50% tubular/clustered growth are categorized as grade 3 *(poorly differentiated)*. High-grade (grade 3) tumors are usually more varied in their appearance. They often show a mixture of microglandular, fused, or cribriform glands, single-cell infiltration or linear arrays of tumor cells, aggregates of disorganized cells within mucin pools, or even areas of conventional adenocarcinoma with larger glands composed of columnar cells with high N/C ratio and stratification similar to conventional colonic adenocarcinoma (Table 28.5). Some specific high-grade patterns are, in general, more frequent in grade 3 tumors, such as single cells or single-file growth, but they all share a general loss of orderly tubular or clustered growth characteristic of low-grade (grade 1) tumors. In summary, the current grading system more closely approximates the approach used for conventional colonic adenocarcinomas by classifying tumor grades according to their overall percentage of well-differentiated glands, which in the appendix are more tubular and clustered than in typical colonic adenocarcinomas. This more simplified approach to grading appendiceal goblet cell adenocarcinomas was adopted in the most recent edition of the WHO.[18]

Differential Diagnosis

Signet-Ring Cell Adenocarcinoma

Goblet cell adenocarcinoma (high grade) may be confused with pure signet ring cell carcinoma (defined as a tumor without a background of a lower-grade goblet cell adenocarcinoma). Signet ring cell carcinomas are more disorganized in their growth pattern and usually more atypical cytologically (increased mitoses, necrosis, pleomorphism) than high-grade goblet cell adenocarcinomas. Regardless, if any portion of an appendiceal tumor shows low-grade goblet cell adenocarcinoma characteristics, even focally, then the tumor is best classified as *goblet cell adenocarcinoma* and graded accordingly.

Metastatic Adenocarcinoma

Some metastatic adenocarcinomas to the appendix can assume a nested appearance, mimicking goblet cell adenocarcinomas. For instance, metastatic breast carcinoma, prostatic adenocarcinoma, pancreatic acinar cell carcinoma, and other tumors can reveal this morphological appearance. However metastatic tumors generally show a much higher degree of cytological atypia and more frequent mitoses. Furthermore, goblet cell adenocarcinomas may have other intestinal-type cells present, such as Paneth-like cells, which is not typical of metastatic adenocarcinomas.

Natural History of Goblet Cell Adenocarcinoma

Similar to conventional carcinomas of the colon, the outcome of goblet cell adenocarcinoma is highly dependent on tumor stage.[16,250,251,259,262,264] Overall survival is 109 to 136 months for stage 2 tumors, 48 to 62 months for stage 3 tumors, and 22 to 37 months for stage 4 tumors.[250,259,264] The 5-year survival is 43% to 87% for stage 2 tumors, 36% to 40% for stage 3 tumors, and 4% to 18% for stage 4 tumors.[230,259,264] Histological grade also affects prognosis,[16,17,251,262] with a median survival of 84 to 204 months, 60 to 86 months, and 29 to 45 months for low-grade (grade 1), intermediate grade (grade 2), and high-grade (grade 3) tumors, respectively.[250,259] A recent study found that among patients with peritoneal metastases of goblet cell adenocarcinoma, WHO grade of the peritoneal metastatic tumor correlated with prognosis.[264] Patients with grade 1/2 peritoneal metastases had a median survival of 98 months and a 5-year survival of 54%, whereas patients with grade 3 peritoneal metastasis had a median survival of 33 months and a 5-year survival of 23%.[264]

Tumors that present with appendicitis and those that perforate are more often diagnosed at an earlier stage, possibly resulting in improved prognosis.[230] Other factors may also play a role in the prognosis of goblet cell adenocarcinomas, such as tumor size, mitotic activity, lymphatic vessel invasion, patient history of a right hemicolectomy, and chemotherapy, although most of these factors have not yet proven to be significant in large series of patients that subjected these variables to multivariate analyses.[230,251,259,262,265]

Treatment

The treatment of goblet cell adenocarcinoma naturally depends on tumor stage and grade. However, determination of whether all patients with goblet cell adenocarcinoma require a right colectomy still remains uncertain. Some, but not all, authorities advocate this approach for all patients.[200,228] ENETS recommends a right hemicolectomy for all patients with appendiceal goblet cell adenocarcinomas,[266] although its benefits are uncertain.[230,265] Oophorectomy should be considered for women with tumors that demonstrate high-grade histology or high stage.[17,265] Tumors that show extension beyond the appendix are usually treated with right hemicolectomy, multi-organ resection, cytoreductive surgery, HIPEC, and postoperative systemic chemotherapy.[230,265,267-269]

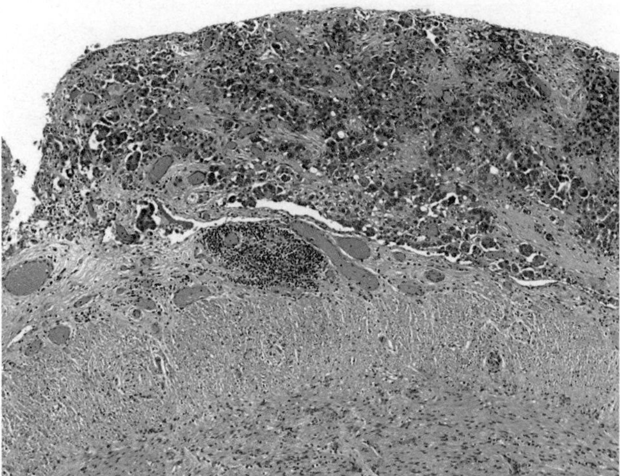

FIGURE 28.41 Papillary serous carcinoma on the appendiceal serosa. A deposit of tumor with papillary features consistent with serous carcinoma is present on the appendiceal serosa.

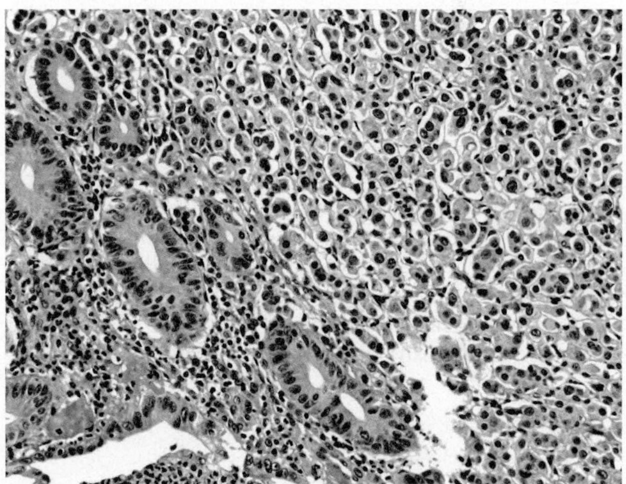

FIGURE 28.42 Metastatic breast carcinoma to the appendix. The mucosa is undermined and infiltrated by a tumor composed of small clusters and single cells with relatively uniform nuclear features. The resemblance of this tumor to goblet cell adenocarcinoma may lead to diagnostic confusion.

SECONDARY TUMORS (OTHER THAN LYMPHOMA)

In females, the most common secondary tumor is metastatic ovarian carcinoma, particularly serous adenocarcinoma, and peritoneal serous carcinoma (Fig. 28.41). The usual scenario is involvement of the appendix with advanced-stage ovarian carcinoma.[270-273] Up to 80% of females with advanced ovarian cancer have appendiceal metastases.[270] However, patients with early disease may rarely be found to have appendiceal serosal involvement on microscopic examination. Therefore some authors advocate appendectomy as part of the primary staging procedure for all patients with ovarian carcinoma.[231,274]

Rarely, gastric carcinoma, breast carcinoma (Fig. 28.42),[275,276] bronchogenic adenocarcinoma and pulmonary small cell carcinoma,[277-281] endometrial carcinoma,[282,283] cervical carcinoma,[284] nasopharyngeal carcinoma,[285]

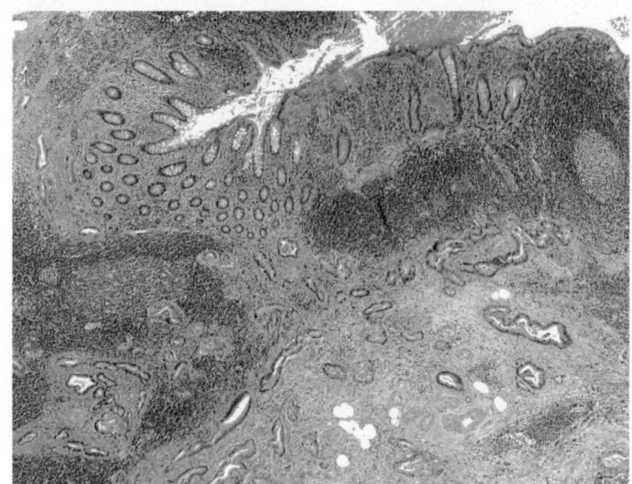

FIGURE 28.43 Metastatic cholangiocarcinoma to the appendix. The appendix shows infiltration of the submucosa and mucosa with irregular glands from a metastatic biliary adenocarcinoma that mimic primary appendiceal adenocarcinoma.

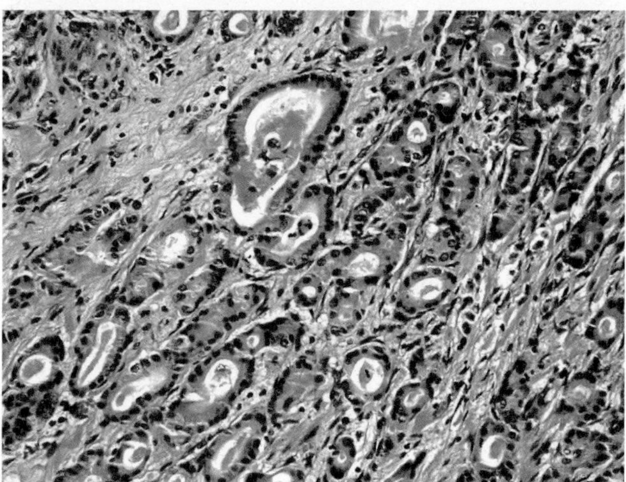

FIGURE 28.44 Metastatic pancreatic acinar cell carcinoma mimicking an appendiceal neuroendocrine tumor. In this case, the glandular differentiation and eosinophilic granular cytoplasm created an appearance reminiscent of a neuroendocrine tumor, and the tubular appearance mimics goblet cell adenocarcinoma.

cholangiocarcinoma (Fig. 28.43),[286] mediastinal choriocarcinoma,[287] transitional cell carcinoma,[288] and prostatic adenocarcinoma metastasize to the appendix.[288,289] Metastatic tumors may obstruct the appendiceal lumen, resulting in the development of acute appendicitis. In some cases, this is the initial manifestation of the malignant neoplasm. Occasionally, it is difficult to determine the location of the primary tumor, particularly in cases with bulky disease. In these instances, determining the location of the greatest bulk of disease can be helpful. For example, Krükenberg tumors with extensive involvement of the appendix, but also of the stomach, are more likely to be primary in the stomach because pure signet ring cell carcinomas are statistically more common in that organ compared with the appendix. Metastatic tumors may also mimic a primary appendiceal tumor, particularly mucinous adenocarcinoma, goblet cell adenocarcinoma, and neuroendocrine tumor (Fig. 28.44).[289]

The full reference list may be accessed online at *Elsevier eBooks for Practicing Clinicians*.

CHAPTER 29

Neuroendocrine Tumors of the Gastrointestinal and Pancreatobiliary Tracts

N. Volkan Adsay, Olca Basturk, David S. Klimstra

Contents

NEUROENDOCRINE CELL SYSTEM OF THE GASTROINTESTINAL TRACT

Neuroendocrine cells in the gastrointestinal (GI) tract altogether constitute the largest endocrine system in the body.[1] In addition to functioning as endocrine cells they have distinctive properties; they also show autocrine, paracrine, and local neuromodulatory effects. They contain neurosecretory granules at the ultrastructural level, and some exhibit neuron-like cell processes. Thus they exhibit features of both conventional endocrine cells and neural cells, also reflected in the neoplasms derived from these cells. Therefore the term *neuroendocrine* (NE) is preferred to distinguish them from other endocrine cells, such as those of the thyroid, adrenal, or pituitary glands.

The NE system of the GI and pancreatobiliary tract is heterogeneous.[1] There are at least 14 different cell types that are responsible for the production of more than 30 peptide hormones and bioamines. Enterochromaffin cells, the most abundant and the presumed origin for most neuroendocrine tumors (NETs), communicate with the crypt/gland lumen, and it is presumed that their tumorigenesis may be partly facilitated by the luminal milieu. At the same time, they are also oriented to secrete their products basally toward the vessels, and NETs of these cells often lead to secretory syndromes, such as carcinoid syndrome (see later). In contrast, enterochromaffin-*like* (ECL) cells occurring in the stomach[2] do not communicate with the lumen, but instead respond to circulating or local hormones. The neoplasms of NE system in the GI tract have traditionally been divided into *foregut*, *midgut*, and *hindgut* categories; however, this is not of much practical use today in surgical pathology because of the elucidation of more organ-specific characteristics of NETs, as discussed later.

Tumors of the NE system are often designated by the hormone they secrete as functional NETs (e.g., gastrinoma, insulinoma). However, this is not based on immunohistochemical expression, but rather serological activity and consequent clinical manifestations. For example, strong immunohistochemical expression of gastrin in a NET is not considered sufficient to diagnose gastrinoma unless it is also clinically functional. One exception is ampullary and duodenal *somatostatinomas* in which there are no measurable circulating levels of somatostatin. Additionally, tumors can secrete different hormones during the course of the disease, further complicating hormone-based classification. Along the same lines, although the specific type of a functional NET can have some loose association with specific histological patterns, these associations are not very consistent, are rather nonspecific, and have no proven significant value in today's practice, with a few exceptions discussed later.

Terminology and Concepts

The terminology for NE neoplasms has always been somewhat problematic. For well-differentiated tumors of the GI-tract, the term *carcinoid tumor* has been widely employed for more than a century,[3-11] although even then some authors were advocating restriction of the term *carcinoid* to serotonin-producing NETs. The term *carcinoid* is now abandoned and replaced with *well-differentiated neuroendocrine tumor*.[3,10,11] Similarly, pancreatic tumors were previously designated as *islet cell tumors* or *pancreatic "endocrine" neoplasms*.[12] Currently, the preferred term,[3] also endorsed by the World Health Organization (WHO; 2017, 2019, and 2021)[10,11,13] is *(well-differentiated) neuroendocrine tumor,* which must be morphologically distinguished from poorly differentiated NE carcinomas such as small cell carcinoma and large cell NE carcinoma. The designation as a well-differentiated neuroendocrine tumor (WDNET) is independent of the stage of the neoplasm, which represents a change from the WHO 2000 and WHO 2004 classifications, which had advocated the *term well-differentiated neuroendocrine carcinoma* for WDNETs with metastases. The term *carcinoma* is now reserved only for poorly differentiated (high-grade) cancers with an overt NE pattern. Accordingly, even in metastatic sites, the neoplasms that were previously called *carcinoid* or *islet cell tumors* are designated as *metastatic neuroendocrine tumors,* not *carcinomas,* although technically speaking they are malignant neoplasms of epithelial nature (i.e., carcinomas).

It is now widely agreed upon that, other than the incipient neoplasms (tumorlet-type lesions) discussed separately later in this chapter, all WDNETs are best considered malignant neoplasms. Low-grade and early-stage neoplasms often follow a protracted or even benevolent clinical course if completely resected. Until recently, some authors had classified these low-grade, early-stage examples as benign *(adenoma)*.[14] In contrast, other investigators have maintained that even the rare occurrence of metastasis is an adequate sign of malignant potential, and they have proposed to classify the entire spectrum of NETs as *carcinoma*.[15-17] It should be noted here that the fact that resected small (low-stage) and low-grade WDNETs are often cured by surgical removal does not necessarily mean they will behave as benign if they are not resected. As the experience with the long-term behavior of these tumors improved in the past few years, it has become clearer that WDNETs may be even more aggressive than previously thought once the hyperplastic precursor type lesions are excluded. Regardless, they remain clinically, pathologically, and genetically distinct from poorly differentiated NE carcinomas.

The identity and definition of poorly differentiated neuroendocrine carcinomas (PDNECs) had remained controversial until recently. Because they are relatively rare, in the past they have been largely included in the grade 3 (Ki67, ≥20%) tumor classification, along with the proliferatively active examples of otherwise morphologically well-differentiated NE neoplasms, or they were analyzed among adenocarcinomas with which they are often admixed. In the WHO 2017 Classification of Tumours of Endocrine Organs[10] and the WHO 2019 Classification of Tumours of the Digestive System,[11] this issue is now clarified, and the poorly differentiated NE carcinomas as defined in the lung are now regarded as a separate category. This distinction is based on morphological grounds alone; however, naturally Ki67 proliferation index and mitotic activity show parallels, with the vast majority of WDNETs showing relatively low Ki67 (median of about 5%, and more than 95% showing <40%), whereas most PDNECs exhibit much higher indices, with virtually all above 40% and most above the 60% range. These two groups also have distinct molecular pathways, with the PDNECs being much closer to (and often admixed with) adenocarcinomas.[18-21] Although WDNETs and PDNECs are now widely accepted to be separate categories, there are cases that are morphologically ambiguous and difficult to classify, and furthermore, there are rare transitions that occur from a WDNET to a PDNEC. However, these latter cases are clearly the exception rather than the rule, and the current approach of classifying these as entirely different entities is warranted until these rare gray zones and overlap cases are better characterized. With advances in treatment, some PDNECs are also downgraded to appearing like a WDNET by morphology or Ki67 index.[22]

The most widely used staging systems for GI and pancreatobiliary NETs are from the College of American Pathologists/American Joint Committee on Cancer (CAP/AJCC)[23,24] and the European Neuroendocrine Tumor Society (ENETS).[25-28] The prognostic value of these staging systems is still being verified. In reporting NETs, it is important to specify which staging system is being employed.

Overview: Gastrointestinal Tract Neoplasms with Neuroendocrine Differentiation

NE differentiation may manifest with various facets in the GI and pancreatobiliary tracts (Box 29.1).

In the ensuing text, general characteristics of these lesions as they relate to each other will be discussed. More detailed discussions and site-specific characteristics can be found in other chapters of this text.

INCIPIENT NEOPLASIA (PROLIFERATIONS, DYSPLASIA/TIS)

Early NE cell proliferations can be seen throughout the GI tract. This phenomenon is best recognized in the stomach, where a spectrum of ECL cell proliferations occur in the setting of hypergastrinemia (usually compensatory to atrophic gastritis-related hypochlorhydria). In this condition, the trophic effects of gastrin lead to a spectrum of ECL cell proliferations ranging from hyperplasia, which can be diffuse, linear, or nodular (Fig. 29.1), to dysplasia, also termed *Tis ("in-situ" neoplasm)*, and finally to full-blown WDNETs.[2] It is difficult to draw sharp lines among these

BOX 29.1 Neuroendocrine Differentiation in Gastrointestinal and Pancreatobiliary Tracts

- **I.** Incipient neoplasia ("dysplasia/Tis"; tumorlets)
- **II.** True neuroendocrine neoplasms
  - **IIa.** Well-differentiated neuroendocrine tumor (WDNET)
  - **IIb.** Poorly differentiated neuroendocrine carcinoma (PDNEC)
- **III.** Mixed tumors
  - **IIIa.** Mixed neuroendocrine and nonneuroendocrine neoplasms
  - **IIIb.** Duodenal gangliocytic paraganglioma
- **IV.** Chimeric tumors (neoplasms with incomplete neuroendocrine differentiation)
- **V.** Goblet cell adenocarcinoma
- **VI.** Non epithelial-origin tumors with NE differentiation
  - **VIa.** Small blue cell tumors
  - **VIb.** Paraganglioma
- **VII.** Induced neuroendocrine differentiation
- **VIII.** Aberrant-focal neuroendocrine differentiation in other tumors
- **IX.** Secondary (metastatic) neuroendocrine neoplasms
- **X.** Mimickers

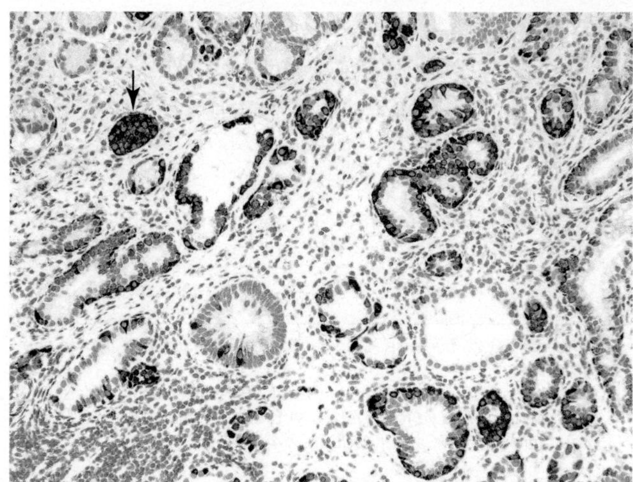

FIGURE 29.1 Incipient neuroendocrine tumor in the setting of autoimmune gastritis. Enterochromaffin-*like* (ECL) cell hyperplasia, linear and micronodular *(arrow),* highlighted by chromogranin immunohistochemical stain in this figure, is common in the setting of secondary hypergastrinemia caused by autoimmune gastritis. These are regarded as precursors of type 1 (or A) gastric neuroendocrine tumors.

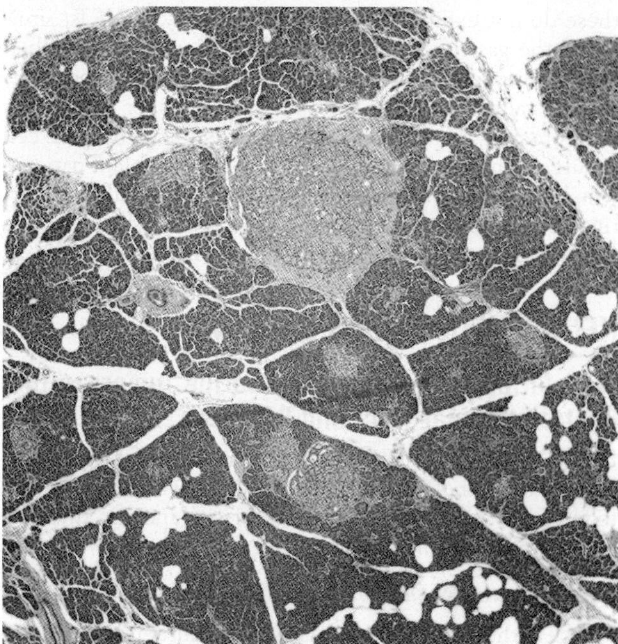

FIGURE 29.2 Incipient neuroendocrine tumor (NET) in a patient with MEN-1 syndrome. Micro-NET (so called *microadenoma*) of the pancreas, characterized by a circumscribed nodule separated from the surrounding parenchyma by a thin band of fibrous tissue. Most examples of this phenomenon have a nesting or trabecular growth pattern and a clonal appearance, which can be highlighted by hormone immunostains.

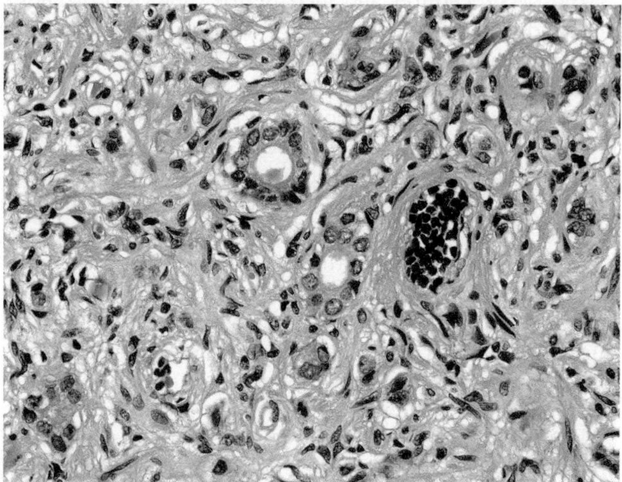

FIGURE 29.3 Microscopic incidental neuroendocrine cell proliferations are not uncommon in the wall of the appendix and are generally of no clinical consequence. This is an example of a tubular variant, which can be mistaken for an adenocarcinoma.

processes, but criteria (albeit arbitrary) have been proposed. For microscopic proliferations, if there is nodular growth of ECL cells >150 microns or if there is a conglomeration of nodules, signs of "microinfiltration," and/or new stroma, then the lesion has been proposed to be classified as *dysplasia or Tis.* These proliferations can be designated as *ECL cell proliferation with micronodule formation,* with further characteristics, including the size, detailed in a comment. It is essential to look for signs of atrophy in the background and investigate the clinical setting to determine the biological significance of the lesion. It is also important to keep in mind that the type 1 and 2 WDNETs that arise in this setting appear to be biologically different and more indolent than sporadic WDNETs.

Another example of incipient NET occurs in the pancreas, multiply in patients with multiple endocrine neoplasia type 1 (MEN-1), vHL, Mahvash disease, and similar "adenomatosis" entities.[1] These patients often develop numerous microscopic nodules that appear to be precursor lesions. Larger ones (<0.5 cm) are referred to as *microadenomas* or *micro-NETs* (Fig. 29.2). Often these can be distinguished by their different morphology from background islets, a fibrous band surrounding them, and often clonal labeling with one of the pancreatic hormones, as opposed to normal islets, which typically show the presence of multiple hormones in an established distribution by immunohistochemistry. As in the gastric ECL cell proliferations, it is often difficult to appreciate where "hyperplasia" ends and true autonomous proliferation of neoplasm begins.

Incidental minute foci of NE cell clusters encountered in the wall of the appendix are also probably examples of the same phenomenon (Fig. 29.3). There are no established guidelines for the terminology or classification of such lesions, and there are no known underlying medical or genetic conditions that predispose to such proliferations. Patchy small clusters that measure less than 1 mm are typically reported as *incidental neuroendocrine cell proliferation,* and a comment regarding their presumed benign nature should be provided. These can be distinguished from true NETs by the small number of cells in each cluster, lack of coalescence of the clusters, and absence of micronodule formation.

Another set of lesions that are increasingly recognized are those associated with adenomas of the GI tract. These occur as small clusters or cords typically forming a thin band at the base of the adenoma. Often the adenoma component is rich in NE cells within the glands in the very same area, leading to speculation that these NE cell proliferations are induced by the local milieu of the adenoma.[29-31] Typically, these do not exhibit the features to qualify as NETs; similar to the gastric and appendiceal proliferations described earlier, they do not form a recognizable tumor and characteristically are composed of a small number of clusters and cords, each composed of a few cells. Incidental NE cell proliferations seen in mucosal biopsies of transplant patients who have undergone drug treatments as well as those occurring in injured mucosa of inflammatory bowel disease are probably representative of the same phenomenon.[32-34]

NEUROENDOCRINE NEOPLASMS

Well-Differentiated Neuroendocrine Tumors of the Gastrointestinal Tract and Pancreas

In the following section, the general characteristics of WDNETs of the GI tract and pancreas will be reviewed, followed by a separate discussion of site-specific findings, with emphasis on how they diverge.

Clinical Features and Epidemiology

Unlike in the lungs, the vast majority of neuroendocrine neoplasms (NENs) in GI/pancreatobiliary tracts are WDNETs. Compared with glandular neoplasms, these are rare, with an estimated annual incidence of 1 to 2 per 100,000. They represent 2% of all tumors of the GI tract. Gastroenteropancreatic neuroendocrine tumors (GEP-NETs) account for 75% of the total proportion of NETs in the body. The increase in incidence of NETs is attributed to the improved diagnostic procedures and increased pathological diagnosis of less differentiated tumors.[35-39] If the minute ECL cell proliferations in the stomach are disregarded, the ileum and appendix are the most common sites for established NETs, but they can occur in any portion of the GI tract. However, NETs are very uncommon in the esophagus (Table 29.1).

Being slow-growing and less infiltrative than ordinary carcinomas (and thus often allowing adaptive processes to take place), NETs are less likely than adenocarcinomas of the corresponding site to present with local symptoms. Instead, they often present with symptoms caused by the hormones they secrete, or they are detected incidentally during workup for other conditions. Some come to attention at an advanced stage with metastasis. Thus the clinical presentation of WDNETs is highly dependent on the site and the cell type. For example, appendiceal primary tumors are often detected incidentally during appendectomy, either as clinically silent small tumors or as the cause of the appendicitis. In contrast, ileal tumors are often not detected until they are metastatic, presumably because they do not lead to local symptoms and remain undetected by routine endoscopy. They are associated with serotonin secretion, and when they metastasize, decreased hepatic metabolism may lead to classical carcinoid syndrome (flushing, diarrhea, asthma, tricuspid regurgitation, and other symptoms). Different functional NETs typically present at different clinical stages. For example, most pancreatic insulinomas manifest early with a set of symptoms and signs called the *Whipple triad*[40]; thus the majority of pancreatic insulinomas are smaller than 2 cm at the time of diagnosis. In contrast, most pancreatic glucagonomas only become symptomatic when the tumor is already fairly large. The severity of the disease and clinical course (and thus prognosis) are also significantly

TABLE 29.1 Staging of Gastrointestinal Neuroendocrine Tumors

Site	Localized %	Regional %	Distant %
Stomach	68	3	7
Small intestine	36	36	22
Appendix	55	29	10
Colon	39	27	25
Rectum	81	2	2

Total is not 100% because some cases are not designated by site and stage.
Based on the SEER database analysis of 13,715 carcinoids; data from Modlin IM, Lye KD, Kidd M. A 5-decade analysis of 13,715 carcinoid tumors. Cancer. *2003:97(4):934-959.*

influenced by the type of hormone produced. For example, the diarrhea caused by VIP-producing tumors (watery diarrhea, hypokalemia, and achlorhydria [WDHA syndrome]) can be debilitating and difficult to control and may even lead to death.

Some WDNETs come to clinical attention at another site based on the effects of their secreted hormone. For example, gastrinomas may lead to peptic ulcers of the duodenum or stomach (Zollinger-Ellison syndrome), or the gastrin they produce may exert a trophic effect on gastric ECL cells and lead to gastric WDNETs.

Gastrinomas also warrant a special note when they arise in the duodenum as an example of an "occult" primary tumor. There, they often present with very small primary tumors that lead to metastases and gastrinoma syndrome, in which the primary is often undetectable, not only clinically but also grossly, composing a minute focus in the duodenal wall[41] or within the "gastrinoma triangle."[42] In fact, in some cases, they present with a large peripancreatic lymph node tumor (presumed to be a metastasis), and no primary tumor can be documented by extensive sampling of the tissues from the triangle, which has led to the question of whether there are true "primary nodal gastrinomas."

Other characteristic clinical presentations should bring the possibility of WDNETs to mind. For example, if there is a large mass in the root of the mesentery without an obvious primary tumor elsewhere, then a GI WDNET, especially of ileal origin, must be considered. Similarly, a WDNET may be the culprit if a very large solitary mass in the liver is encountered without an overt primary tumor, and the patient's liver and general condition are relatively good.

WDNETs may not only lead to syndromes by secreting hormones, but they themselves may be a manifestation of a genetic syndrome. Eighty percent of MEN-1 patients develop pancreatic neuroendocrine tumors (PanNETs), often in the background of multifocal proliferative changes in the islets. Neurofibromatosis may also lead to WDNETs, including the rare but distinctive ampullary somatostatinomas (glandular psammomatous WDNET of the ampullary region). Twenty-five percent of patients with ampullary somatostatinomas prove to have neurofibromatosis.[43,44] In patients with synchronous NETs and GISTs or neurofibromas, neurofibromatosis should be a strong consideration. In vHL syndrome, PanNETs often exhibit clear cytoplasm, presumably as a result of the well-known predilection of

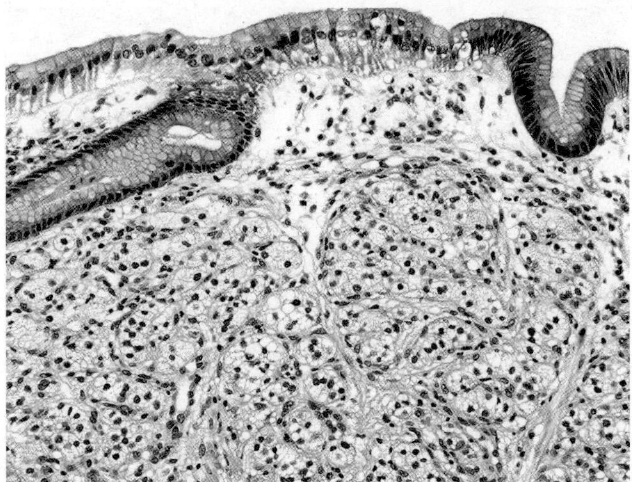

FIGURE 29.4 Clear cell change in a well-differentiated neuroendocrine tumor, which is more common in patients with vHL syndrome, is characterized by cells that have abundant cytoplasm filled with numerous clear vesicles.

vHL patients to develop clear cell tumors with accompanying alterations in glycogen metabolism (Fig. 29.4). WDNETs have also been reported in association with inflammatory bowel disease.

In the clinical diagnosis of WDNETs, PET scans targeting somatostatin receptors have changed the landscape greatly in the past decade. Targeting the type 2 somatostatin receptors that are widely expressed in most WDNETs, this scintigraphic scan has high specificity and sensitivity in detecting these tumors and their metastases. This is typically lacking in the PDNECs, which can be helpful diagnostically.

Pathology

Gross Features

WDNETs are generally well-demarcated and grow with pushing borders. In fact, PanNETs, especially early-stage and indolent ones, may even have capsule-like fibrous tissue surrounding the tumor. WDNETs are typically cellular, stroma-poor tumors, and accordingly, cut sections show a fleshy, homogenous appearance (Fig. 29.5). Having said that, some subsets show substantial sclerosis. The vascularity may lead to darker colors and hemorrhagic foci, especially if the tumor has been manipulated. In formalin-fixed specimens, they become yellow to white. Necrosis and mucosal ulceration can be seen in more advanced cases and are typically signs of aggressive behavior.

In the GI tract, WDNETs often form mucosa-covered, broad-based polypoid lesions, with the bulk of the lesion in the submucosa and muscularis. PanNETs often protrude into the peripancreatic soft tissues, although rare examples may arise from the pancreatic duct wall and appear as sclerotic lesions constricting the duct, causing secondary dilatation of upstream ducts, thus mimicking intraductal papillary mucinous neoplasms (IPMNs).[45,46]

WDNETs are typically solid tumors. However, in the pancreas, some examples (up to 10%) present as a cystic mass as a result of central degeneration, leaving a variably-sized cuff of histologically conventional NET clinging to the cyst wall.

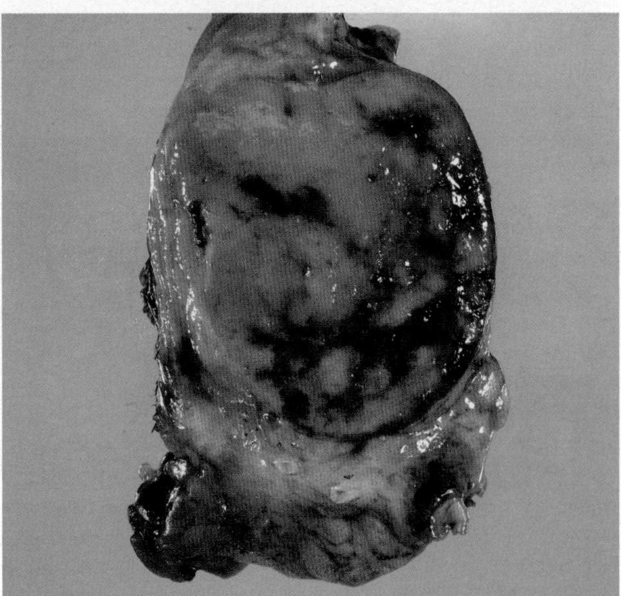

FIGURE 29.5 Gross appearance of a pancreatic well-differentiated neuroendocrine tumor. A solid and well-circumscribed tumor with a soft and fleshy consistency and foci of hemorrhage is shown.

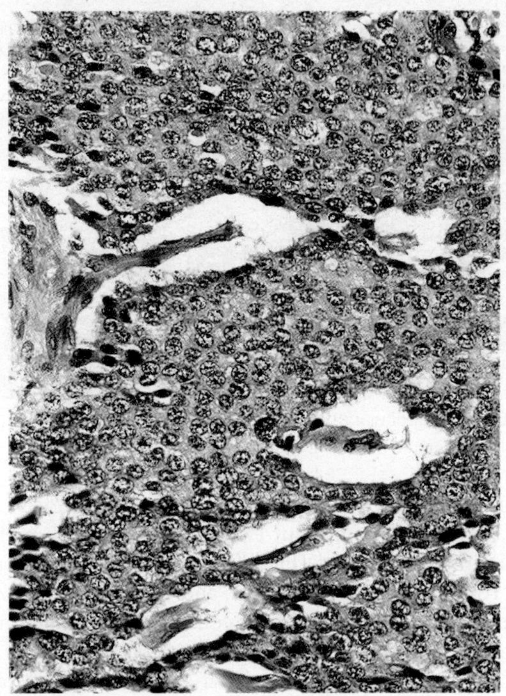

FIGURE 29.6 Well-differentiated neuroendocrine tumors are characterized by monotonous cells with round uniform nuclei and a distinctive chromatin pattern referred as *salt-and-pepper.*

As discussed previously, NETs arising in the background of genetic or medical disorders may be multifocal. In fact, in the pancreas, a multifocal solid tumor often proves to be a NET.

Microscopic Features

Typically, WDNETs are composed of uniform, round cells, with a moderate amount of cytoplasm and coarsely granular, "salt-and-pepper" chromatin (Fig. 29.6). The latter finding is probably the most specific diagnostic feature of these

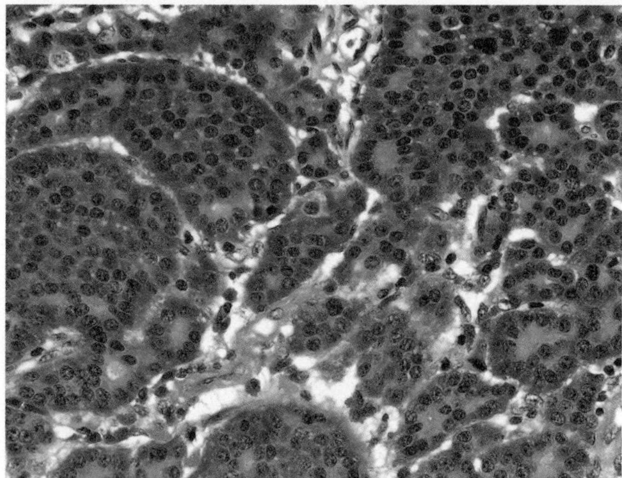

FIGURE 29.7 Although not specific, prominent intracytoplasmic granules at the periphery of the nests, combined with the peripheral rosette-like formations, are more characteristic of well-differentiated neuroendocrine tumors of midgut origin.

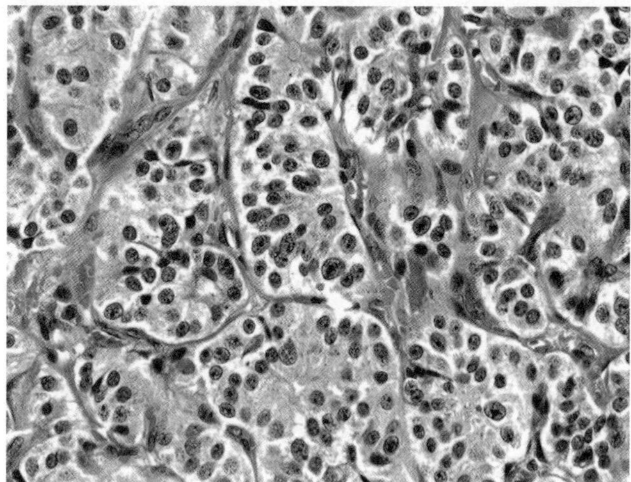

FIGURE 29.9 Most well-differentiated neuroendocrine tumors exhibit nests separated by delicate vasculature. Nucleoli may be evident in some cases, as shown in this example.

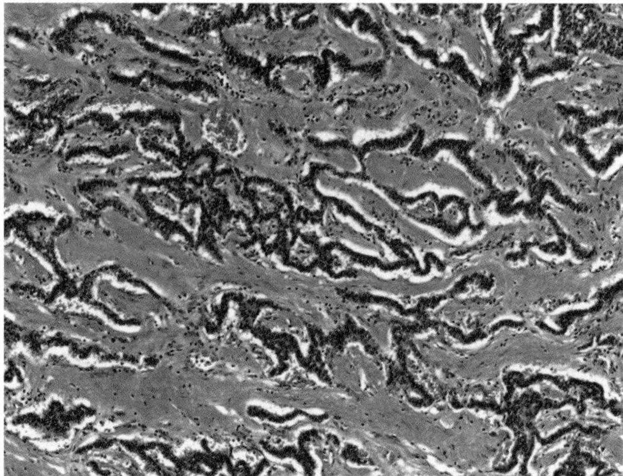

FIGURE 29.8 Trabecular and festoon patterns are characteristics of well-differentiated neuroendocrine tumors.

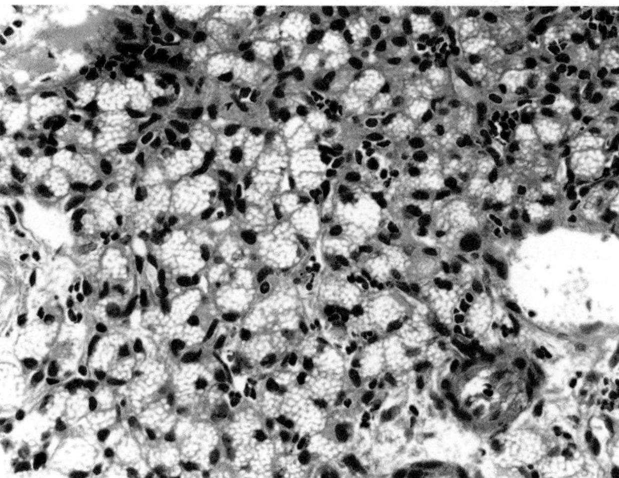

FIGURE 29.10 Lipid-rich neuroendocrine tumors are characterized by abundant microvesicular cytoplasm. Their nuclei can be either round with finely granular chromatin and inconspicuous nucleoli, or they can be relatively small, pyknotic, and partially obscured or even scalloped by the intracytoplasmic vesicles.

tumors. Cytoplasmic granules may be evident and are especially prominent in mid-gut examples, along with melanin/lipofuscin type pigment (Fig. 29.7). The cells grow in nests, acini, rosettes, ribbons, festoons, and trabeculae (Fig. 29.8). Gland formation by the tumor cells is also not uncommon. Delicate vasculature is another hallmark, especially in cases with a prominent nested pattern (Fig. 29.9). Artifactual clefting around the nests is common, particularly in the intestinal examples.

Morphological Variants

There are numerous morphological variants in WDNETs.[47] In most of these, at least one of the three classic NE morphological characteristics (cellular monotony, cytoplasmic abundance, and salt-and-pepper chromatin) is retained. These variants may be important to recognize because some create substantial diagnostic challenges.[47] There is emerging evidence that some may also have clinical significance. In a recent study in the pancreas,[47] these variants were found to cluster in three groups, as described in the following paragraphs.

WDNET variants that have abundant cytoplasm often with prominent nucleoli in a manner seen in metabolically productive cells such as adrenocortical tumors ("lipid rich variant)[48] (Fig. 29.10) or in hepatocytes ("hepatoid variant")[47] and oncocytic cells ("oncocytic variant")[47,49,50] were found to show a tendency to be larger and show more aggressive behavior in the pancreas. They also tend to show a more diffuse growth pattern or broad bands rather than small nests and trabeculae characteristic of more ordinary NETs. Some have dyscohesive growth and resemble solid-pseudopapillary neoplasms. Among these, the lipid-rich variant sometimes lacks the nuclear features characteristic of NETs, potentially leading to misdiagnosis.[51] In other NETs, the cytosolic contents, mostly intermediate filaments,[52] may push the nucleus to the periphery and create a rhabdoid or plasmacytoid[47,52,53] appearance (Fig. 29.11), also mimicking signet-ring cells. Intracellular mucin is lacking, however. Other NETs, especially in the pancreas but also

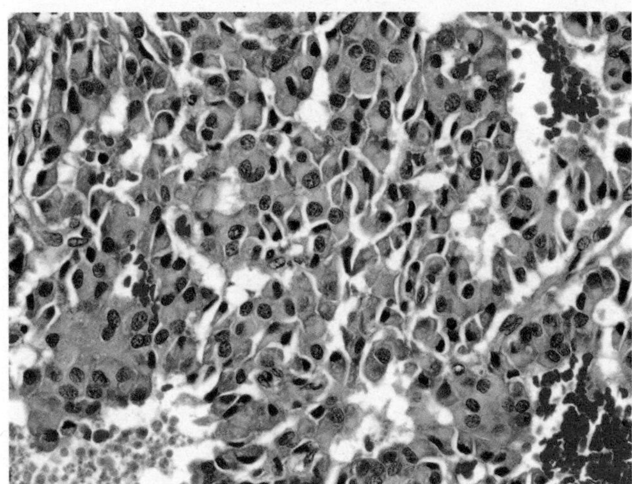

FIGURE 29.11 Rhabdoid morphology in pancreatic neuroendocrine tumors is characterized by peripherally located nuclei resulting from dense cytoplasmic collections composed of whorls of cytokeratin intermediate filaments. This pattern is often associated with dyscohesiveness of the cells and may partly be a product of an artifact.

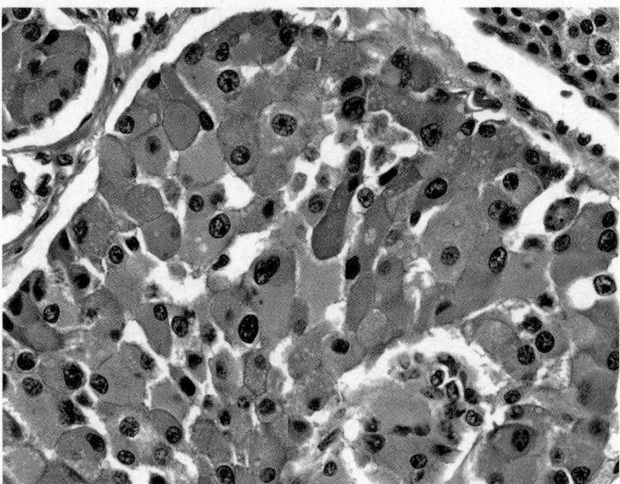

FIGURE 29.12 An oncocytic variant of neuroendocrine tumor with abundant granular eosinophilic cytoplasm and a single prominent nucleolus is depicted. These can resemble hepatocytes and may present a challenge when metastatic to the liver.

occasionally in the stomach or rectum, have oncocytic features characterized by abundant acidophilic granular cytoplasm and single prominent, eccentric nucleoli (Fig. 29.12). A variation in this theme is the hepatoid variant, which may show not only the characteristic histomorphological features of hepatocytes, but may even express reliable hepatocytic markers including arginase and HepPar1.[47] When metastatic to the liver, these oncocytic and hepatoid NETs may easily be mistaken for hepatocellular carcinomas. Some NETs have high nucleus-to-cytoplasm ratio that imparts a "small blue cell" appearance. These cases also often have a more diffuse growth pattern, which further accentuates the concern of a high-grade neoplasm, especially based on small biopsies. Ki67 labeling index is helpful in establishing the well-differentiated nature of such examples. As mentioned previously, these NET variants that resemble metabolic cells and/or show more diffuse growth pattern have been found to be more aggressive in some studies[47,49] and thus may warrant closer attention.

In contrast, the variants that exhibit degenerative changes and more mature elements or organoid patterns appear to be more benevolent. "Endocrine atypia" characteristic of normal endocrine organs may also be seen in WDNETs, represented as large, bizarre, pleomorphic nuclei with smudgy chromatin (Fig. 29.13).[54] This is akin to the degenerative atypia seen in "ancient" schwannomas or "symplastic" leiomyomas. This kind of pleomorphism in NETs can lead to misdiagnosis as more aggressive neoplasms, but some studies have shown that they tend to be smaller and lower grade, and limited data indicate that they may be less aggressive.[47,54] Similarly, NETs that have prominent mature ducts often raise concern for mixed adenocarcinoma, although the tumors displaying these findings are often small and less aggressive. In the pancreas, where these are mostly encountered, they have been also termed *ductulo-insular PanNETs*.[47,55,56] The nature of the ducts is debatable; however, they are often so prominent that they give the impression that they are beyond mere entrapment of normal ductal glandular units of the background tissue.

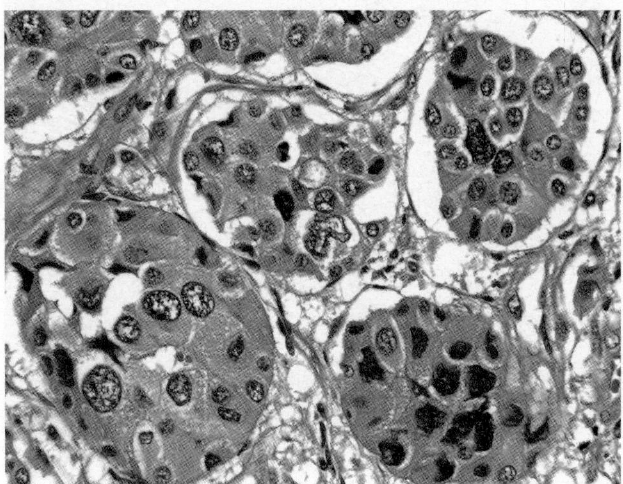

FIGURE 29.13 Symplastic change composed of bizarre degenerative nuclei (neoplastic version of "endocrine atypia") is not uncommon in pancreatic neuroendocrine tumors. However, these nuclei are often accompanied by abundant cytoplasm (cytomegaly), and despite their worrisome appearance, they do not indicate more aggressive biology.

They also are mature, and they do respect the boundaries of the lesion, often stopping at the margins of the NET confined within the NET itself, which help distinguish them from an adenocarcinoma. Another variant that appears to have more benevolent characteristics is the paraganglioma-like variant.[47,57] These can be indistinguishable from a paraganglioma, including the focal presence of sustentacular-like cells in some, but the tumor expresses keratin.

Stromal alterations may also add variety to the morphological spectrum of WDNETs. In some cases, these already hypervascular tumors become massively congested, or hemorrhagic, creating a peliotic appearance. In others, particularly in the stomach, the stroma can exhibit myxoid features (Fig. 29.14). Although most WDNETs are fundamentally stroma-poor tumors, they can exhibit intense stromal sclerosis, especially ileal NETs and PanNETs, which secrete serotonin (Fig. 29.15).[58] In some cases, amidst the sclerotic

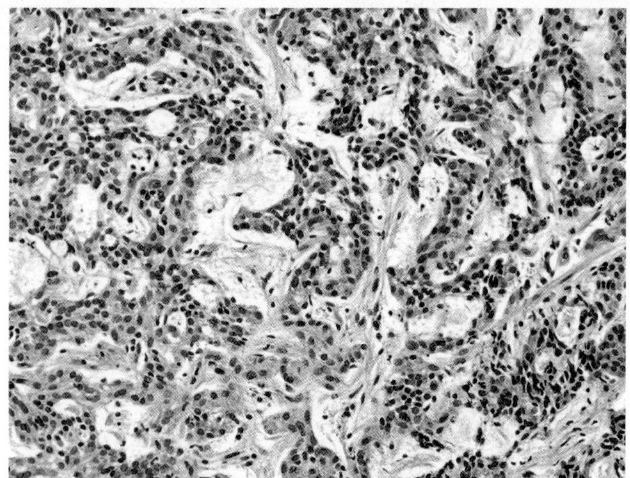

FIGURE 29.14 In rare examples of neuroendocrine tumors, the stroma may appear myxoid.

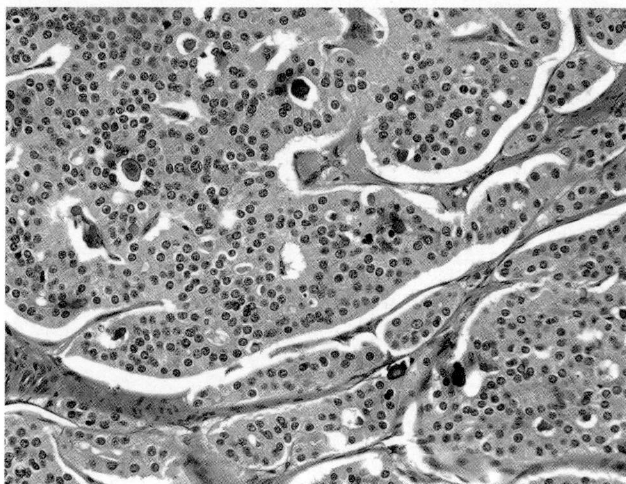

FIGURE 29.16 Ampullary somatostatinomas are characterized by tubule formation and psammomatous calcifications, thus also referred to as *glandular psammomatous neuroendocrine tumor of duodenum.*

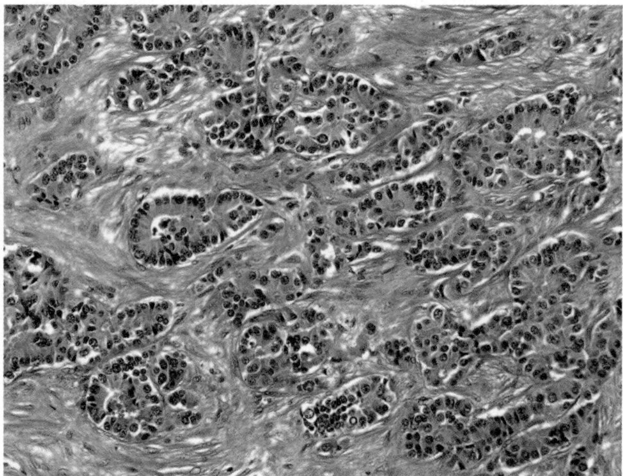

FIGURE 29.15 Although most neuroendocrine tumors have cellular stroma-poor pattern, some cases, as shown in this example, may exhibit sclerotic stroma and mimic adenocarcinoma.

changes, the cellular infiltrates of NET may acquire a cord-like pattern that can be very similar to mammary tubulolobular carcinoma.[47]

Rosette or glandular formations can be prominent in some WDNETs. In fact, in ampullary somatostatinomas, gland formation is so characteristic that the name *glandular psammomatous NET of duodenum* has been applied (Fig. 29.16).[41,44,59,60] They also often entrap the ampullary ductules, which, along with the glands formed by the tumor, can be mistaken for an adenocarcinoma. A variant of WDNETs in the appendix ("tubular carcinoid") is also characterized by gland formation, and considering that NE marker expression may be more limited in this variant, it can be difficult to distinguish from an adenocarcinoma. Ileal WDNETs also tend to have glands, which are often prominent in the superficial/mucosal component of the tumor and are often located at the periphery of the individual nests.

Unlike pulmonary WDNETs (carcinoids), spindle cell morphology is very uncommon in GI and pancreatic NETs. Occasionally, gastric WDNETs may have vague spindle cell morphology. In the ampullary region, trabeculae with prominent elongated cells should raise the question of gangliocytic paraganglioma in which the NE component often exhibits this morphology.

Appendiceal tumors characterized by the presence of goblet cells form a distinct category now termed *goblet cell adenocarcinoma* and are discussed separately later in this chapter.

Immunohistochemistry

WDNETs are defined by the presence of NE granules, which in most (but not all) cases can be highlighted by the widely available NE markers, chromogranin, synaptophysin, and CD56. Among these, chromogranin is the most specific, but its sensitivity is lower. Rectal and a subset of appendiceal NETs (tubular examples) can be devoid of chromogranin A, which is the target of most available chromogranin antibodies. Synaptophysin, on the other hand, is very sensitive but less specific, with a variety of mimickers showing potential expression of this marker. CD56 is even less specific. For the diagnosis of WDNETs, these markers may not be needed, considering the morphology is often distinctive enough. They may, however, become necessary in some of the morphological variants described earlier and of course for the diagnosis of poorly differentiated NE carcinomas (discussed later). INSM1 has attracted attention recently as a marker of NE differentiation with moderate sensitivity and high specificity.[61]

NETs also show epithelial differentiation, and as such they express keratins in the vast majority of cases; however, the type and degree of keratin positivity may vary. Although wide-spectrum keratins are commonly positive, both CK7 and CK20 expression is relatively infrequent. CK19 can occasionally be expressed in PanNETs and has been used as an adverse prognostic marker.[62]

Recently, nuclear transcription factors involved in the embryonic development of site-specific NE cells have been employed in determining the primary site of a WDNET,[63] but they are not entirely specific. For example, CDX2 is commonly expressed in the NETs of GI tract origin (Fig. 29.17A). Islet-1 (isl1) is expressed commonly in PanNETs

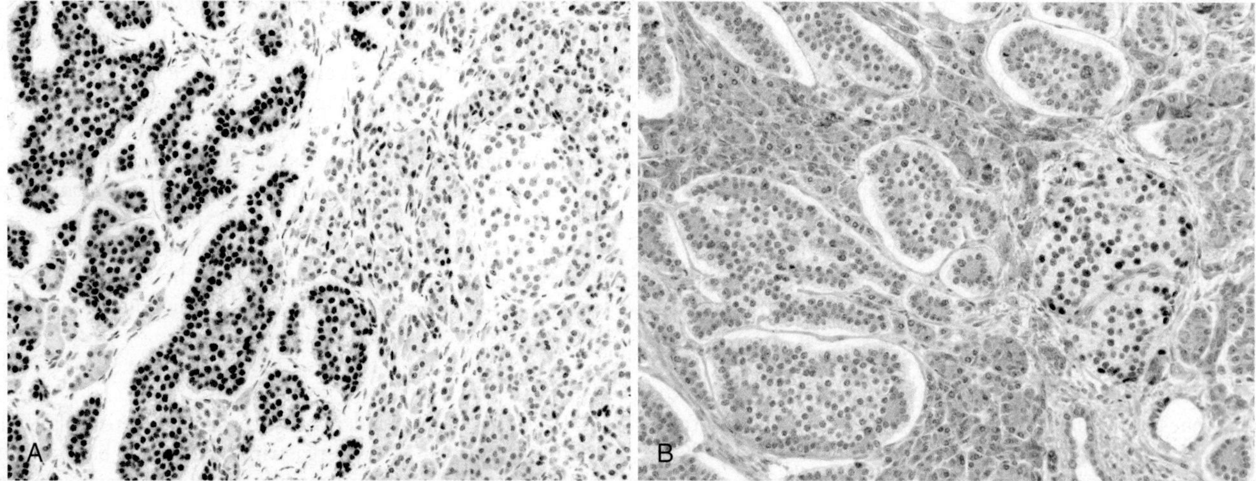

FIGURE 29.17 Midgut well-differentiated neuroendocrine tumors are often positive for CDX2 and negative for Isl-1, as shown in this example metastatic to pancreas. **A,** CDX2 showing diffuse strong labeling in the metastatic neuroendocrine tumor of midgut origin, while the pancreatic tissue on the right is negative, including a negative islet. **B,** Conversely, Isl-1 is positive in the islet but negative in the midgut neuroendocrine tumor.

but is also commonly present in rectal WDNETs (Fig. 29.17B).[64,65] Pancreatic duodenal homeobox 1 (PDX-1) has been shown to be a marker of pancreatic NETs both in primary and metastatic sites,[66] but the specificity of this marker is not known. TTF1 expression is generally uncommon in both pancreatic and GI WDNETs, but its sensitivity for pulmonary carcinoid tumors is quite limited. It should be kept in mind that TTF1 is expressed in small cell carcinomas of any organ. Pax8 is commonly expressed in pancreatic and rectal NETs but is typically absent in ileal NETs. As is true for the pancreatic islet cells, which express progesterone receptors and CD99 presumably due to cross reactivity,[67] PanNETs can also express these markers. Recently, NKX2.2 has been found to be of some value in determining the origin of a metastatic NET.[68]

The molecular pathways commonly abnormal in the adenocarcinomas of respective organs are typically unaltered in WDNETs, whereas they are often also deranged in PDNECs. For example, p53 overexpression and loss of SMAD4 (DPC4, which is commonly altered in pancreatic adenocarcinomas) can be observed in PDNECs but are extremely rare in WDNETs.[21,69-74] Similar observations have been noted for loss of retinoblastoma protein. In contrast, ATRX/DAXX pathway alterations, represented as loss of nuclear expression, which are common in NETs, are seldom detected in PDNECs.

Somatostatin receptor scintigraphy is widely used in the clinical setting and has proven extremely valuable in the clinical diagnosis of WDNETs, follow-up for progression and metastasis, as well as their distinction from other tumors including PDNECs, which typically lack this marker.[69] As the immunohistochemical antibody for SSTR2 is becoming more widely available for daily practice, its potential value in surgical pathology is being evaluated and appears quite promising.[1,14,75]

There are other immunohistochemical caveats to consider. Ileal and rectal WDNETs can express prostate-specific acid phosphatase. In fact, occasionally this may help in determining the origin of a metastatic NET. CEA is expressed in 60% of WDNETs, and CA19-9 positivity may also be seen. S100 can be positive, both nuclear and cytoplasmic, in some WDNETs, especially in the appendix and some ampullary somatostatinomas.

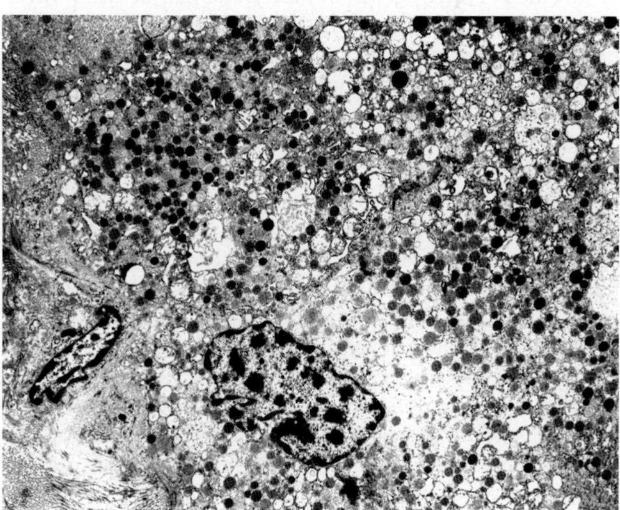

FIGURE 29.18 Electron microscopic examination of well-differentiated neuroendocrine tumors typically shows numerous randomly oriented neurosecretory granules varying in size and electron density.

The value of immunohistochemical analysis of hormone production is not clear. Correlation with functional activity is highly imperfect. Additionally, many tumors have multihormonal activity and may even alter the predominant secretion over time. Therapy may also influence the type of hormone produced by the cells.

Electron Microscopy

Ultrastructural detection of neurosecretory granules represented as membrane-bound dense core granules is helpful in establishing the diagnosis of WDNETs. The pattern of the granules may be helpful in determining the specific cell type (Fig. 29.18). However, electron microscopy is seldom used in modern surgical pathology because of technical impracticalities and the utility of immunohistochemistry. Electron microscopy can be helpful in demonstrating NE differentiation in unusual settings such as poorly differentiated or amphicrine tumors.

Molecular Findings

NETs that arise as a result of familial syndromes (MEN-1, vHL, tuberous sclerosis, or neurofibromatosis type 1) reveal the molecular alterations characteristic of the corresponding syndrome; sporadic tumors may also show these alterations. For example, either somatic mutations or loss of heterozygosity of the *MEN1* gene (11q13) and its protein product menin can be seen in gastric and pancreatic WDNETs, and loss of NF-1 (17q11; neurofibromin) may be found in somatostatinomas. It should be noted here that WDNETs of different sites have different genetic background. For example, ileal NETs are not associated with MEN-1 and vHL syndromes.

As discussed earlier, alterations of genes involved in the pathogenesis of adenocarcinomas of the GI and pancreatobiliary tracts such as *p53*, *Her2*, *CDKN2A*, and *DPC4* are much less common in WDNETs. In contrast, recently, NETs have been found to show mutually exclusive inactivating somatic mutations of *DAXX* (death-domain associated protein) and *ATRX* (alpha thalassemia/mental retardation syndrome X-linked) genes in nearly one-half of cases; these genes are involved in a chromatin remodeling complex, believed to be critical in telomere maintenance. A subset of NETs shows somatic mutation of the genes that encode for proteins in the mammalian target of rapamycin (mTOR) cell signaling pathway and includes somatic mutations of *PIK3CA*, *PTEN*, and *TSC2*. Other molecules that are under investigation and seem to be abnormal in a smaller subset of cases include X-chromosome, Hsp90, IGF1R, and EGFR, among others. There are also more recently described and less well-known genetic alterations implicated in the pancreas characterized by *adenomatosis* (i.e., multiple variably sized NETs in the background of multiple incipient neoplasia). The prototypical example is Mahvash disease,[76-78] which is a rare autosomal recessive disease with inactivating mutations in the glucagon receptor. There are other similar entities such as insulinomatosis of which molecular mechanisms have yet to be characterized.[79,80]

Differential Diagnosis

There is fair amount of fidelity regarding the morphology of these tumors, thus their diagnosis is relatively straightforward in most cases. There are, however, a few situations that lead to diagnostic problems. Limited biopsies or the presence of preservation artifact sometimes leads to misdiagnoses, especially considering that they can be located at the base of the mucosa and thus may be underrepresented in the biopsy. Rosettes and tubules can be mistaken as adenocarcinoma. In crushed specimens, WDNETs may also mimic lymphoid tissue. More problematic are the rare and underrecognized variants as discussed previously. *Clear cell* or *lipid-rich* variants (see Fig. 29.10) are often misdiagnosed as carcinomas from the kidney, adrenal gland, or liver. WDNETs with hepatoid and oncocytic features can be mistaken for a primary hepatocellular carcinoma in the liver (see Fig. 29.12). A *pleomorphic variant* can be mistaken as a high-grade carcinoma (see Fig. 29.13). Tubule-forming examples (such as ampullary somatostatinomas) or ductulo-insular PanNETs often raise concern for an adenocarcinoma. Please see the corresponding organs for the more site-specific discussion of differential diagnosis.

Clinical Outcome and Pathological Prognosticators

GI and pancreatic NETs are now widely recognized as malignant neoplasms, albeit low-grade and even curable when discovered at low stage and low grade. It is the norm that WDNETs have a more favorable prognosis than the conventional adenocarcinomas of the corresponding sites. However, as more data accumulate on the long-term prognosis of these tumors (i.e., 10 years), it is clear that a significant proportion eventually recurs and metastasizes. The preferred sites of distant metastasis are the liver, lung, peritoneum, and bone. Even cases with distant metastasis may have a protracted clinical course.

Clinical Setting

This is best exemplified in the stomach, where WDNETs arising as a result of hypergastrinemia in the background of autoimmune gastritis typically follow a benign clinical course, whereas the sporadic WDNETs of the very same organ are often aggressive.

Primary Location

As the NETs of different sites are increasingly being studied separately from each other, site-specific differences in their behavior are coming to light. For example, appendiceal and rectal NETs are often small and localized when detected, whereas ileal ones usually have metastases. See the Site-Specific Features section later in this chapter for discussion about possible explanations.

Stage

Although part of explanation for the more "benign behavior" of NETs of some sites is in the biology of the cells and anatomy/milieu of these regions, the behavior is also related to the stage at which these tumors are detected. For example, while most appendiceal and rectal WDNETs are small at diagnosis and thus benign behaving, those >2 cm clearly have malignant potential. In fact, just as in any other malignancy, stage is proving to be the most powerful predictor of outcome.[81] There are different staging schemes proposed. In the United States, the TNM system put forth by American Joint Committee on Cancer/Union for International Cancer Control (AJCC/UICC) and endorsed by the CAP is in wider use, although the different TNM staging system proposed by the ENETS may prove to have more validity.[28] In staging these tumors, general principles employed for other cancers are applicable. For example, as a part of the recent paradigm shift,[82,83] an intestinal WDNET should be classified as T4a if the surrogate serosal changes are indicative of clear-cut tumor involvement, even if the tumor cells are not immediately at the serosal surface. One scenario that is challenging for staging is the presence of multiple separate tumors (typically in ileal NETs), considering that the verdict is still out whether these are synchronous primary tumors or metastases. The presence of multicentricity should be noted regardless, considering that these NETs are clearly more aggressive.[84] For staging of PanNETs, the ENETS proposal, which is based on the size of the tumor rather than ambiguous parameters like "peripancreatic soft tissue" involvement used in CAP/AJCC/TNM, may prove to be more applicable and relevant. Recently, in the surgery field, for PanNETs that are smaller than 2 cm, a "watchful waiting" approach has been strongly advocated.[85-89] However, this approach is based on studies that have relatively short follow-up, and they are also mostly based on cases that had already been treated by curative surgery. Even in these studies, about 10% of the cases have metastasis at the time of diagnosis, and another 5% to 10% develop metastasis during follow-up. More importantly, recent studies are making it clear that with longer follow-up, these relatively small NETs often also have malignant behavior if left untreated.

Cell Type

Hormonal activity (cell type) correlates with behavior, but this seems to be a mostly indirect result of the stage at which they present. For example, clinically functioning insulinomas pursue an indolent clinical course in 90% of cases and have even been classified as *benign*, but this favorable outcome is caused, at least in part, by the relatively small size at which these tumors are typically detected. In contrast, other syndromic PanNETs result in recurrence or metastases in 50% to 70% of cases. Duodenal gastrinomas often result in metastases, even when the primary tumor measures less than 1 cm. Therefore both the cell biology and the stage seem to be factors. The cell type determination must be based on the clinical finding of a functional syndrome.

Grade

There is now wide consensus that NETs should be graded and staged separately. The grading system put forth by ENETS and now endorsed by the consensus group[3] and the WHO[10,11,13] classifies NETs into three categories (Table 29.2) based on mitotic activity (per 10 high-power fields [HPF]) and Ki67 proliferation index (percent of cells). This system is applied regardless of the primary location. Naturally, as any other semiquantitative analysis in surgical pathology, this grading system is subject to challenges created by heterogeneity, false positivity by extrinsic factors, methodologies, instruments, operators, and others.[90] Image analysis systems for measuring the Ki67 index,[91] which is not readily available in all centers, is also user dependent. For Ki67 counting, eyeballing, which was considered acceptable until recently, has now been shown to be unreliable for the distinction of grade 1 versus grade 2.[90,92] The preferable approach is the manual or digital counting of captured image of the proliferation hotspots.[93,94] Grading is employed also for metastatic tumors; there are multiple studies showing the value of grading metastases.[95] If the Ki67 count is performed accurately, it often proves to be higher than the mitotic count, perhaps negating the need for the more tedious and even less reproducible mitotic count. Of note, studies are showing that Ki67 may also be valuable in limited cytological specimens (cell blocks).[96,97] For mitotic counting, it is imperative to correct for the microscope's field area, which can vary greatly. Some studies are attempting to reassess the mitotic cut points of the original proposal,[98,99] and variations in optimal cut points may exist among anatomic sites. Some authors advocate changing the cutoff for grade 1 versus grade 2 from 3 to 5; however, emerging evidence fails to support this impression.[100] More data are needed before modifications to the current grading scheme can be implemented. Previously, poorly differentiated NE carcinomas had been mostly included in the grade 3 (Ki67 >20%) WDNET classification. However, this was clarified in the WHO 2017 Classification of Tumours of Endocrine Organs, and PDNECs are now regarded as an entirely separate category.[101] This was based on several studies showing that NE neoplasms with a Ki67 above the 50% range are much more aggressive[102,103] than those with a Ki67 of 20% to 50% with which they were previously classified. It should be noted that this distinction of WDNET and PDNEC is based on morphology.

TABLE 29.2 Grade (Subclassification) of Neuroendocrine Tumors

	Mitotic Rate (per 10 HPFs)*	Ki67 Proliferation Index (%)**
NET, G1	<2	<3
NET, G2	2-20	3-20
NET, G3	>20	>20

HPF, *High-power field;* NET, *neuroendocrine tumor.*
**Mitotic rates are expressed as the number of mitoses per 2 mm² (equaling 10 HPFs at 40x magnification), as determined by counting in 50 fields of 0.2 mm² (i.e., in a total area of 10 mm²).*
***The Ki67 proliferation index value is determined by counting at least 500 tumor cells in the regions of highest labeling (hot spots).*
Data from Klimstra DS, Klöppel G, La Rosa S, Rindi G. Classification of neuroendocrine neoplasms of the digestive system. In: WHO Classification of Tumours Editorial Board editors. WHO classification of tumours, *5th ed. Digestive system tumours. Lyon: IARC;2019:16-19.*

TABLE 29.3 A Pathology Report Example of Primary Neuroendocrine Tumor

Diagnosis

Terminal ileum; resection: Well-differentiated neuroendocrine tumor

- Grade: 1 of 3 in the WHO 2019 Classification of Digestive System Tumours
- Size: 2.5 cm
- Depth of invasion: Muscularis propria
- Lymphovascular invasion: Not identified
- Perineural invasion: Not identified
- Margins: Free of tumor
- Lymph node metastasis: 0/14
- AJCC stage: T2N0; ENETS stage: T2N0

Comment

- Mitotic rate: 1/10 HPF
- Ki67 proliferation index (static image count of hot spot): 2.4%

AJCC, *American Joint Committee on Cancer;* ENETS, *European Neuroendocrine Tumor Society;* HPF, *high-power field.*

Additional Prognosticators

In addition to grade and stage, other histological findings may have prognostic significance in WDNETs and generally should be included in pathology reports (Tables 29.3 and 29.4).

Perineural Invasion. Although subjective, perineural invasion is believed to confer a poorer prognosis. Also, the guidelines are not clear as to whether a nerve entrapped within the lesion is to be regarded as invasion. It is important to recognize that nonneoplastic NE cells can be found

TABLE 29.4 A Pathology Report Example of Metastatic Neuroendocrine Tumor

Diagnosis

Metastatic well-differentiated neuroendocrine tumor
Grade: 2 of 3 in the WHO 2019 Classification of Digestive System Tumours

Comment

This tumor is a WDNET (it is *NOT* a poorly differentiated neuroendocrine carcinoma).
Mitotic rate is 3/10 HPF; Ki67 proliferation index is 13%.
Cytomorphology is suggestive of midgut origin, and CDX2 positivity and Isl1 negativity are supportive of this impression; however, none of these are entirely specific as to the primary of this lesion.

HPF, *High-power field;* WDNET, *well-differentiated neuroendocrine tumor.*

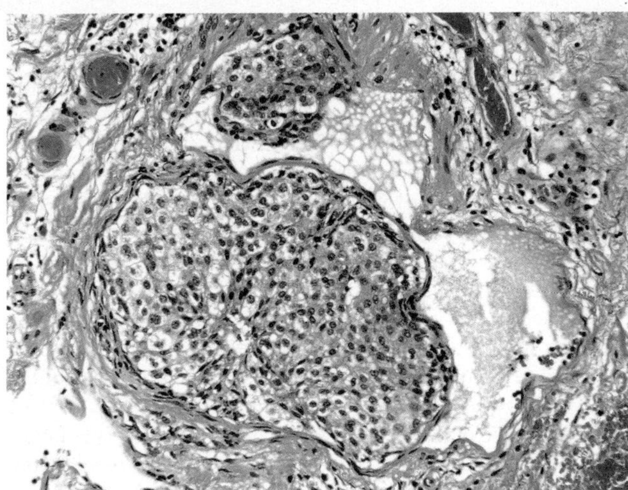

FIGURE 29.19 Vascular invasion of a well-differentiated neuroendocrine tumor.

in a perineural location, particularly in the setting of chronic pancreatitis. Furthermore, in the appendix, NE cell proliferations are intimately admixed with nerves.

Vascular Invasion. Similarly, vascular invasion is a sign of aggressiveness and can occur either as small vessel/lymphatic invasion or in the form of direct extension into larger veins. WDNETs are highly vascularized tumors; therefore vascular invasion can be difficult to recognize within the tumor itself. Moreover, in the small intestine, the characteristic artifactual clefting may also lead to the erroneous impression of vascular invasion (Fig. 29.19). That is why it may not be surprising that the literature on the correlation of vascular invasion with prognosis has shown mixed results. Nevertheless, in some sites like the appendix, it is viewed as an "adverse prognostic factor" and utilized for hemicolectomy indication, although the evidence in support of this is limited at best.[104-106]

Necrosis. In pulmonary NETs, necrosis is used as one of the main criteria in identification of the intermediate grade (atypical carcinoid) group. The meaning of necrosis is less clear for GI and pancreatobiliary tumors. In some studies, it was found to be a strong prognosticator. Clearly it is an important feature of PDNECs, and it has also been found to identify more aggressive versions of ordinary WDNETs, at least in the pancreas.[107] Thus necrosis should be noted in reports of WDNETs.

Ulceration. Mucosal ulceration is also often a sign of aggressive behavior in GI WDNETs.

Morphological Characteristics

As discussed previously, some morphological patterns appear to be associated with more aggressive behavior. For example, some studies have found that cases with more abundant cytoplasm and prominent nuclei (oncocytic, hepatoid, plasmacytoid) or those with a more diffuse growth pattern tend to have a higher rate of progression.[47,50] In contrast, cases with symplastic degenerative changes (pleomorphic variant) or organoid patterns (such as ductulo-insular or paraganglioid PanNETs) appear to be less aggressive, although paradoxically they raise more concern for malignancy by their atypical morphological findings (the presence of bizarre cells in the former, and concern of adenocarcinoma in the latter).

Infiltration Pattern

Although the tumor-host interface is one of the most reliable predictors of behavior in endocrine neoplasia to an extent that, in the thyroid gland, the decision of benign versus malignant is established by it, for NE neoplasia, this issue has not been fully investigated. In a recent study, perhaps not surprisingly, this was found to be an independent prognostic factor, with encapsulated tumors behaving much better than those with high infiltration and a scirrhous pattern.[108,109]

Systemic Markers

As in many other tumors, the markers of systemic inflammation have been found to have some correlation with behavior for some WDNETs.[110]

Tumor Molecular Markers

In addition to the proliferation index, various immunohistochemical and molecular prognostic markers are under investigation. As molecular mechanisms of PanNETs are better elucidated, their potential role as prognosticators is also being recognized. For example, in some studies, WDNETs driven by *MEN1/ATRX/DAXX* have been found to behave differently; however, this could not be confirmed in other studies.[1,18,111] There is also evidence from multiple studies that CK19 expression may have some adverse prognostic significance in PanNETs. C-kit (CD117) has also been advocated as an independent adverse prognosticator.[112] However, none of the markers under investigation has been routinely used in clinical practice.

Margins

As in any malignant neoplasm, it is important to document the margin status for resections of WDNETs. If possible, in polypectomies and mucosal resections, the distance from the deepest tumor to the margin should be reported. It should be noted here that PanNETs often protrude into the peripancreatic soft tissues but are separated from the inked free surfaces by a thin rim of fibrous tissue. These should be documented separately from parenchymal resection margins.

"Clinical Malignancy"

The major morbidity for some functional WDNETs is not the direct effect of the tumor but rather the impact of the hormonal syndrome. For example, VIPomas (WDNETs secreting vasoactive intestinal polypeptide) may be lethal due to massive diarrhea, and serotonin-producing WDNETs may cause serious valvular heart disease.

Given the multiple parameters affecting the outcome of patients, decision support tools like nomograms are being developed to stratify patients.[113]

Treatment

WDNETs are low-grade malignancies. Surgical removal can be curative in early-stage tumors in a significant proportion of cases. Resection or ablation (by radio- or chemoembolization) of metastatic tumors is increasingly being employed, but the specific indications for these procedures are still being debated.[94] If clinically feasible, an oncological operation is preferred, rather than an enucleation or limited excision. On the other hand, management differs by site and stage of the tumor, as discussed later. Although ileal examples warrant resection regardless of tumor size, small appendiceal and rectal examples can be managed by more limited or local removal, appendectomy (if <2 cm) or polypectomy (if <0.5 cm), respectively.

Not surprisingly, being relatively low proliferative lesions, the response of WDNETs to cytotoxic agents is minimal, if any. Therefore this approach is typically reserved for more aggressively spreading tumors.[114,115] Somatostatin analogues (octreotide) have shown some efficacy, but mostly leading to tumor stabilization, rather than remission. Similar experience has been recorded for interferons. Among the targeted therapies, everolimus and sunitinib are now widely employed for WDNETs,[114,115] and many new agents are being investigated,[94] with Hsp90, IGF1R, EGFR, and mTOR pathways as potential targets.[116] Peptide receptor radionuclide therapy including lutetium (77Lu-Dotatate, 90-Y) and octreotide have also been used highly successfully in keeping tumors under long-term control, although they are seldom curative.[117,118]

Site-Specific Features

Although WDNETs show some common characteristics regardless of where they arise, there are also substantial differences based on their origin. These site-specific characteristics of WDNETs are discussed in the respective chapters of this book but are also briefly discussed here.

Esophagus

WDNETs are uncommon in the esophagus; in fact, it is the rarest site among GI NETs, which may be related to the fact that the esophagus does not have a significant NE cell population (although the mucosal glands in the distal esophagus have scattered NE cells). The reported cases occur at an average age in the 60s, with a male predominance. Most cases are distal, especially near the gastroesophageal junction. In one study, 50% of cases were metastatic at the time of diagnosis. There does not seem to be any specific association or histopathological or molecular findings that distinguish esophageal WDNETs. PDNECs, often admixed with adenocarcinomas, are far more common in this site.

Stomach

Gastric NETs represent 6% of all GI NETs. Their incidence appears to be on the rise, attributed partly to the increase in detection as a result of widespread use of endoscopy.[38,119,120]

Although several different GI NE cell types are located in the stomach, 70% of tumors are derived from a single cell type (enterochromaffin-*like* cells) and, less commonly, from G cells or EC cells.

Gastric WDNETs arise in at least three distinct clinical settings, which also affect the biology and management of the tumors (Table 29.5): The first two types, also called *hypergastrinemic types*, are types 1 and 2 (or A and B) arising in the fundic mucosa in the background of hypergastrinemia: type 1, with secondary (compensatory) hypergastrinemia usually caused by the hypochlorhydria of autoimmune gastritis (and indirectly also pernicious anemia) and type 2, as primary hypergastrinemia (gastrin-secreting tumors in Zollinger-Ellison or MEN-1 syndrome). The fundamental process in these tumors is the trophic effect of excessive gastrin on ECL cells, which leads to a spectrum of proliferations of this cell type. Those cases associated with parietal

TABLE 29.5 Clinical Features of Gastric Neuroendocrine Tumors

	Clinical Course	Genetics	Clinical Features	Serum Gastrin Levels	Pathogenetic Mechanism	Number of Tumors
Type 1	Regress spontaneously, endoscopic removal often adequate	May have MEN mutation	Mucosa-covered polyps, superficial, rarely invasive	Secondary hypergastrinemia (caused by achlorhydria)	Autoimmune gastritis	Multifocal
Type 2	Somatostatin analogues effective	Associated with MEN	Mucosa-covered polyps, superficial, rarely invasive	Primary hypergastrinemia (as a result of ectopic gastrin secretion)	Zollinger-Ellison, MEN-1	Multifocal
Type 3		Sporadic	Deep advanced lesions, metastatic	No hypergastrinemia	–	Unifocal

MEN, *Multiple endocrine neoplasia;* MEN-1, *multiple endocrine neoplasia type 1.*

cell hypertrophy or proton pump inhibitor effects have been proposed to be grouped as type 4 and type 5.[1,121-123] Recently, similar cases have been described in Japan in association with *H. pylori*, which may lead to suppression of D cells and secondary hypergastrinemia, but this group is not yet well characterized. Proton pump inhibitor use may also be the cause of NE cell hyperplasia, mimicking the type 1 and 2 pathogenesis mechanism.[124] Type 3 is the sporadic type and can arise anywhere in the stomach.

Types 1 and 2 gastric WDNETs often occur in the background of or evolve from ECL cell proliferations (see Fig. 29.1). It has been proposed[125,126] to classify these as *hyperplasia* (patchy, linear, and micronodular) if they are not forming nodules larger than 150 microns; as *dysplasia* if there are nodules >150 microns (0.15 mm) or fused units or infiltrative nodules; and as *micro-NETs* (micro-carcinoids) if <500 microns (0.5 mm). Recently, the same group of authors attempted to provide a more detailed definition of what qualifies as *hyperplasia*, but this needs to be validated.[2] In daily practice, we typically report these as *enterochromaffin-like cell proliferation* and provide the details regarding their extent and associations. For staging purposes, dysplasias and micro-NETs (micro-carcinoids) can be regarded as *Tis*, although many of them typically exhibit patchy involvement of the muscularis mucosa. Nodules >0.5 mm are regarded as full-blown WDNETs (carcinoids), but the behavior of these is distinctly better than the sporadic type (type 3), the latter with a metastasis rate of about 15%. Thus it is important to recognize the background changes (autoimmune and/or precursor lesions) and clinical correlation. Although type 1 lesions are often benign-behaving and may even regress spontaneously or following the management of hypergastrinemia by administration of somatostatin analogues,[127] some patients continue generating these lesions incessantly and may require antrectomy to eliminate the source of the excess gastrin.

For the diagnosis of the early forms of this proliferation, immunohistochemistry can be very helpful and, in fact, may be necessary, especially if the specific site of the biopsy is not verifiable by histological examination alone because atrophic changes can create substantial mimicry. NE markers (chromogranin and synaptophysin) highlight the NE cell proliferation and distinguish it from other cell populations, and gastrin immunostaining helps establish that the suspect cells are not the native G cells. Evidence of autoimmune and atrophic gastritis in the background is also important to note. Sometimes ECL cell proliferations can be difficult to distinguish from lymphoplasmacytic infiltrates, which are their common companions. Occasionally, type 1 and 2 NETs can have glandular elements entrapped within the established tumor.

Although most type 1 and 2 cases present as mucosa-covered polyps, are often multifocal, and are superficial at the time of diagnosis, type 3 (sporadic) WDNETs are often advanced and involve the stomach transmurally. They also exhibit more aggressive behavior, with lymph node metastases in 60% and liver metastases in 50% of cases. Some examples overlap with the poorly differentiated NE carcinomas, discussed separately in the following sections.

Duodenum

WDNETs of the ampulla and duodenum have different presentation patterns.[60] Ampullary region cases often present with obstructive jaundice. The cell-type based delineation of WDNETs (with the corresponding clinical and pathological characteristics) appears to be most striking in the duodenum. A significant proportion of the gastrin-producing WDNETs occurs in the duodenum, in the so-called *gastrinoma triangle*.[128] One-third of these are associated with Zollinger-Ellison syndrome, and these patients are typically younger and have tumors with more indolent behavior. One-third of the duodenal gastrinomas have lymph node metastasis, despite being small or even occult. Some syndromic gastrinomas appear as primary tumors within peripancreatic lymph nodes, although undetected minute duodenal primary tumors with large nodal metastases likely account for some cases.

Ampullary somatostatinomas[44,59,60,129-132] (glandular psammomatous NET of duodenum) are a distinctive type of WDNET (see Fig. 29.16) that appears to be fairly specific to the ampullary region, and it is discussed in more detail in Chapter 41. A higher percentage is reported in African Americans. These are not called *somatostatinomas* because the patients have somatostatin-related symptoms, but because they typically stain with somatostatin immunohistochemically and are fairly distinctive morphologically with tubular/rosette-like arrangements, intraluminal psammoma bodies (also referred as *psammomatous glandular NETs*), often with abundant acidophilic granular cytoplasm. One-fourth of these patients are documented to have neurofibromatosis,[131] and this close association with NF has been established at the molecular level as well.[133] Some have concomitant GI stromal tumors or GI neurofibromas. Almost one-half have lymph node metastases at presentation, but they appear to be indolent, nevertheless.

Serotonin-producing WDNETs can also occur in the duodenum and appear to be similar to their more common counterparts in the distal small intestine.

Ampullary/duodenal gangliocytic paragangliomas are also a type of NET that occurs almost exclusively in this region and has distinctive characteristics, which are discussed in detail in the respective sections.

Jejunum/Ileum

The distal small bowel is the most common site of clinically relevant WDNETs. These often present with nonspecific findings and may be misdiagnosed as *irritable bowel syndrome* because of the inaccessibility of the site to endoscopic examination. Occasional patients present with intussusception. Small bowel WDNETs have been reported in association with a variety of conditions ranging from celiac disease, Crohn disease, duplications, and Meckel diverticulum, but it is not clear if these are coincidental associations. Most cases appear to be sporadic. Most are serotonin producing (EC cell type), and most of the attributes of the "carcinoids" and carcinoid syndrome in fact refer to this group; however, a variety of hormones can be detected both in the tumor and the serum of these patients. About 5% present with carcinoid syndrome, typically seen in cases with distant metastases that allow the serotonin secreted to bypass liver metabolism. About one-fourth of patients present with multiple mucosal polyps, and it is debated whether these represent true synchronous neoplasms or intramucosal metastases from a single lesion; recent studies and their aggressive behavior favor the latter.[134] Small bowel

WDNETs are also notorious for presenting with mesenteric metastatic disease leading to "buckling" or tethering of the bowel. In fact, in a patient with a large mesenteric mass, the possibility of an ileal/jejunal WDNET should be considered in addition to alternative diagnoses, such as mesenchymal and lymphoid neoplasms. Fibrosis, presumably related to factors secreted by the tumor, can be striking and is believed to contribute to the obstructive symptoms. Some examples have Crohn-like hypervascular polyps adjacent to the tumor, which are attributed to transforming growth factor and largely believed to be secondary.

These are typically mucosa-covered polyps that are firm and homogenous on sections. The muscularis propria may be thickened, attributed to trophic factors. Microscopically, peripheral cytoplasmic granularity, subtle lipofuscin/melanin type pigment formation (see Fig. 29.7), rosettes especially at the periphery of the nests, and the monotony of the polygonal cells appear to be more common or more striking than other sites. Chromatin is also fairly distinctive, even among a salt-and-pepper pattern of NETs showing multiple numerous chromatin clumps. Retraction artifact accentuates the nested pattern. Microproliferations (that can be regarded as hyperplastic) may be seen in the adjacent mucosa. Perineural invasion is common. Lymphatics, especially those immediately adjacent to the mucosa, are often involved and may cause linear spread, which may be responsible for the multifocal mucosal growth in some cases. Medium-size mesenteric arteries may exhibit a peculiar elastotic change, presumably akin to the cardiac changes seen in some patients with carcinoid syndrome. Alterations in chromosome 18 are a common finding in these tumors.

Appendix

If all the small NE cell proliferations discovered in the appendix in autopsies or incidentally in appendectomies are also dignified as NETs, then appendiceal NETs become one of the more common tumors in the body. These proliferations are reported in 0.7% to 2% of all appendices when sampled extensively. About two-thirds are located at the tip of the appendix and therefore are not believed to be the culprits for the appendicitis that brings them to clinical attention. Those located in the tip can lead to the so-called *bell-clapper* configuration. Patients tend to be relatively young, with a mean age of 49 years (approximately 2 decades younger than for other NETs). Whether this is a reflection of the mean age of appendectomy or the peak density of subepithelial NE cells known to occur in the same age group, or both, is an issue of debate. Appendiceal WDNETs are more commonly reported in women, but this may be related to incidental appendectomies performed during gynecological operations. Along these lines, more than 95% of appendiceal WDNETs are ≤2 cm. The incidence of metastasis is very low in these patients. For this reason, appendectomy is considered sufficient treatment for such cases. In contrast, in cases with tumors >2 cm, nodal or distant metastases are noted in one-third. Most authors agree on the need for right hemicolectomy for this group. Whether this operation truly improves survival, however, has yet to be proven. Interestingly, the prognostic role of meso-appendix involvement or perineural invasion has not yet been fully established. The natural occurrence of NE cells and paraganglial cells in association with nerves in this region complicates defining the role of true perineural invasion.

As mentioned previously, appendiceal WDNETs that are presumably L-cell derived can be extensively or exclusively of tubular architecture. This, combined with the paucity or total negativity of chromogranin A staining and the variable CK7/CK20 profile,[135] make tubular WDNETs difficult to distinguish from adenocarcinomas.

The so-called *goblet cell carcinoid of appendix,* now regarded as *goblet cell adenocarcinoma,*[11,136,137] is discussed separately in the following sections.

Colon (Other Than the Rectum)

WDNETs are uncommon in the large intestine. Almost one-half are located in the cecum.[138] They are more common in women, tend to be fairly large at the time of diagnosis, and appear to be more aggressive, with a 5-year survival rate of about 70% for localized tumors and 40% for those with regional spread. For tumors ≤2 cm, reported metastasis rate is about 15%, whereas for those >2 cm, it is 75%. Some produce serotonin; carcinoid syndrome is reported in 5%.

Rectum

Rectal WDNETs are relatively more common, representing 17% of all GI NETs. They are typically diagnosed in the sixth decade. Approximately 50% are asymptomatic and found during routine endoscopy.[138] Additionally, more than two-thirds are smaller than 0.5 cm at the time of diagnosis.[139] The explanation for this does not seem to be merely early diagnosis, but it is at least partly attributable to the biology of the tumors arising in this region from L cells of hindgut. Regardless, the overall metastasis rate is fairly low (14%); <5% of tumors measuring <1 cm are metastatic. Those >2 cm, however, are often metastatic. Some cases are reported in inflammatory bowel disease, and they can be multicentric and atypical.[140,141] Carcinoid syndrome is exceedingly uncommon. Although most rectal WDNETs are straightforward diagnostically, there are a few pitfalls that must be remembered: CEA positivity is common, and the widely available chromogranin A marker is negative in more than 50%, although they do produce neurosecretory granules. In such cases, synaptophysin staining and characteristic morphology together are often conclusive, although synaptophysin may also be negative on occasion, making the morphological evaluation the main decider. Another immunohistochemical pitfall (which can also be used as an advantage in the right setting with combination panels) is the common positivity of prostate-specific acid phosphatase. The rectum is not the only site for positivity of this enzyme in NETs, but it is perhaps the most problematic because of the spread pattern of prostate cancer. However, PSA is typically negative in WDNETs.

Most rectal NETs are initially diagnosed in polypectomy specimens, and if not properly processed, the assessment of the margins can become a problem. If present, ulceration and invasion into muscularis propria are regarded as signs of aggressiveness and are used as additional indications for a radical operation, especially if the tumor is between 1 and 2 cm. Those that are >2 cm are typically treated with low anterior resection or abdominoperineal resection. The fact that the vast majority of rectal NETs are small and cured by polypectomy leads to a bias in which, for example, a metastatic NET in the liver is labeled as *unknown primary tumor* by clinicians, although the patient had a small rectal NET that had been removed years earlier.

Pancreas

PanNETs constitute <5% of pancreatic tumors. Almost one-half are functional, showing serological activity attributable to one of the six hormones that are produced by the islet cells (insulin, glucagon, gastrin, somatostatin, VIP, or pancreatic polypeptide). Most *insulinomas* follow a benign clinical course, likely because they typically are highly symptomatic, even when they are small, which leads to their early detection. Glucagonomas on the other hand tend to be large at diagnosis and have a more aggressive course. PanNETs associated with MEN-1 or other syndromes like vHL and Mahvash and related syndromes (glucagonomatosis and insulinomatosis) tend to be multifocal and less aggressive; these cases also have numerous small nodules termed *microadenomas* (defined as <0.5 cm). More than one-half of PanNET patients have recurrence or metastasis after resection, and many patients come to attention only after the development of metastatic disease that precludes resection.

Microscopically, PanNETs appear to have more morphological versatility than GI WDNETs with the morphological variants discussed earlier (see Figs. 29.10 to 29.13), altogether constituting about one-third of PanNET cases. Among these variants, those with abundant cytoplasm and prominent nucleoli resembling metabolically active cells (hepatoid, oncocytic, and plasmacytoid variants), which also often show a more broad-nested or diffuse pattern or dyscohesive cells resembling solid-pseudopapillary neoplasms, typically present with higher-stage and higher-grade tumors and appear to be more aggressive.[47,49] In contrast, those exhibiting signs of maturation (paraganglioid variant) or with organoid arrangements (ductulo-insular) or with degenerative/symplastic changes (pleomorphic) often have low-grade and low-stage tumors and appear to be more benign (see Fig. 29.13).[47,54] The morphological diversion that characterizes these variants also often extends to include the corresponding immunohistochemical phenotype. For example, hepatoid examples can show arginase and HepPar1, and even bilelike pigment, but they are also often diffusely positive for chromogranin and synaptophysin, and more importantly, they can have more conventional NET components in the same tumor.[47] Similarly, the paraganglioma-like group may show sustentacular-like cells but are positive for keratins as well. The ducts in the so-called *ductulo-insular* variant have a very different keratin profile (Fig. 29.20) than the NET clusters within the same tumor and also show ductal differentiation markers. Some PanNETs show prominent "peliotic" changes with abundant blood and ectasia of vessels. Cystic degeneration is noted in about 10% of cases.

Gallbladder and Biliary Tract

WDNETs are very uncommon in the gallbladder and biliary tract. Some are associated with MEN1 or vHL. They are more common in the bile ducts than in the gallbladder. In fact, in the gallbladder, poorly differentiated NE carcinomas appear to be significantly more common than WDNETs, including some that are associated with conventional adenocarcinomas. In the SEER (surveillance epidemiology and end results database of the NCI), the 5-year survival of WDNETs of the gallbladder is reportedly 40%.

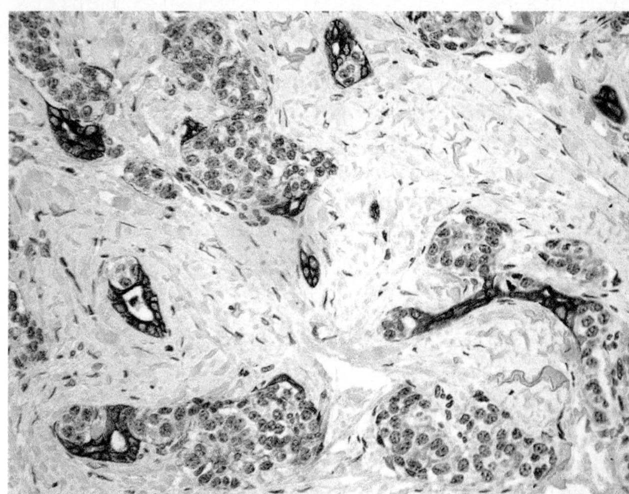

FIGURE 29.20 Pancreatic well differentiated neuroendocrine tumors with significant numbers of small entrapped, nonneoplastic glands (highlighted by CK19 immunohistochemical stain) have been designated as a *ductulo-insular variant.*

Poorly Differentiated Neuroendocrine Carcinomas

The data on poorly differentiated NE carcinomas (PDNECs) of the GI tract are less robust.[103,142-145] These carcinomas occur in essentially every component of the GI tract from the esophagus to the anus. Ampullary carcinomas seem to be more prone to have NE components. In the esophagus and gallbladder, they are more common than the WDNETs of the respective sites. In contrast, in the pancreas, ileum, and appendix, they are far less common than WDNETs.

As in other organs, although some PDNECs are almost identical to pulmonary small cell carcinomas (Fig. 29.21), others are more akin to large cell NECs. Regardless, they are characterized (and also defined) by high mitotic activity (>20 per 10 HPFs, and usually >40 to 50 per 10 HPFs), necrosis, and Ki67 typically over the 50% to 60% range, in addition to their distinctive morphology and high-grade cytology. Immunoexpression of chromogranin and synaptophysin is usually present (and is required for the diagnosis of large cell NE carcinoma), but the intensity and extent of staining are usually less than in WDNETs. In fact, in small cell type PDNECs, the immature cells that characterize this tumor type typically have minimal cytoplasm; therefore the immunohistochemical labeling can also be sparse. They are usually bulky or ulcerated tumors. PDNECs with the morphology as defined in the lung are very uncommon in the pancreas. In fact, pancreatic tumors suspected to be PDNECs often prove to be acinar cell carcinomas[146] (see Chapter 40).

In the current WHO classifications,[101,147-149] PDNECs are now classified as a category distinct from WDNETs, which is in contrast with previous editions in which they were also regarded as a part of grade 3 NETs. In one study, a Ki67 index >55% was found to more appropriately define PDNECs, identifying the group with rapidly progressive behavior and sensitivity to platinum-based chemotherapy.[103]

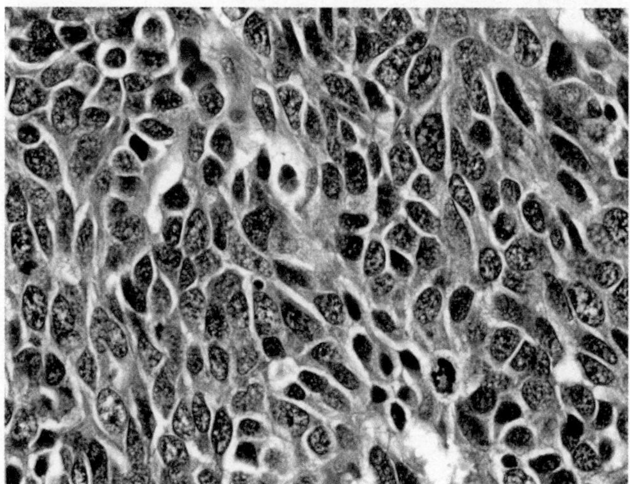

FIGURE 29.21 Poorly differentiated neuroendocrine carcinoma of small cell type in the gallbladder.

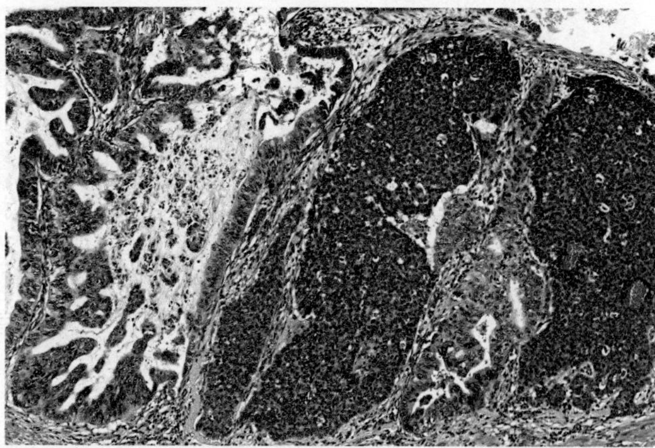

FIGURE 29.22 A neoplasm with morphologically recognizable adenocarcinoma and neuroendocrine carcinoma phenotypes is defined as *mixed adenocarcinoma-neuroendocrine carcinoma* (MANEC).

Of note, it is exceedingly uncommon to see a PDNEC arising in association with a WDNET. Having said that, innocuous WDNETs can acquire more aggressive behavior in time, also manifested as higher proliferation index, but these typically maintain their WDNET morphology. Recent studies have shown that there also appear to be transitional/ambiguous cases, but these are very rare and thus are the exception to the rule. It has also been shown that treatment can attack the more proliferative cells of a PDNEC and decrease the Ki67 index, creating the erroneous impression of a grade 3 WDNET instead of a treated PDNEC.[22] With all of these exceptional situations aside, PDNECs are regarded as a distinct cancer type rather than an advanced version (or a continuum) of WDNETs. In fact, it is clear that PDNECs represent a NE version of adenocarcinoma pathways of the respective organs, whereas WDNETs recapitulate the NE cells, unrelated to adenocarcinomas.

Almost one-half of the PDNECs of the GI tract are associated with conventional adenomas and/or ordinary carcinomas and may thus belong to the conceptual category of so-called *MINENs* (mixed neuroendocrine–nonneuroendocrine neoplasms, see later).[150,151] The amount of PDNEC component can vary from case to case. Based on limited evidence (but also extrapolating from other organs), it appears that even a small PDNEC component must be acknowledged, considering that it may drive the overall tumor behavior and may warrant a different chemotherapy protocol.[103] For this reason, we advocate reporting these carcinomas as *PDNEC with a mixed adenocarcinoma component* and providing the relative proportions in the tumor in a comment.

PDNECs should be distinguished from other high-grade malignancies, and this can be a challenge at times. Poorly differentiated carcinomas NOS or medullary types, as well as melanomas, lymphomas, and metastatic tumors can display nesting growth and monotonous cytology similar to PDNECs. In such cases, nuclear chromatin pattern and immunohistochemical support with chromogranin, synaptophysin, and CD56 is necessary. It should be kept in mind that focal NE cells are often present in other malignancies. Loss of nuclear retinoblastoma labeling, if demonstrated unequivocally, favors a PDNEC but lacks specificity. It should also be noted that PDNECs, especially the small cell carcinomas, are commonly positive for TTF1, regardless of their primary location, and this should not be used as evidence for pulmonary origin. In fact, in select cases, this can be used to favor a PDNEC over another malignancy type. Additionally, akin to their pulmonary counterparts, PDNECs of GI and pancreatobiliary tract origin often show alterations in *TP53*.

PDNECs are highly aggressive tumors that disseminate rapidly. Median survival is between 1 and 2 years, if not less. Current evidence favors treatment with "small cell carcinoma protocols" (platinum based), although additional studies are needed in this regard.

MIXED TUMORS

Mixed Neuroendocrine–Nonneuroendocrine Neoplasms

As discussed previously, in the GI tract, PDNECs are often encountered admixed with an adenocarcinoma, also often with an adenoma component as well.[142] Small cell carcinomas, which in their most classical form preferentially arise in the esophagus or anus, can include squamous cell carcinoma components. Traditionally, terms like *composite*, *collision*, and *amphicrine* have been used for such tumors based on the pattern of association between (and distribution of) the two components; *collision* for those lying side by side, *composite* for those in which the components are intimately intermingled, and *amphicrine* for those with dual differentiation within the same cells. However, all of these most likely represent different facets of the same phenomenon in which the cells in these neoplasms show divergent differentiation, and these patterns are also often seen in a mixture (Fig. 29.22). It should be kept in mind that the term *MINEN* was mostly chosen to designate this umbrella category, more as a conceptual term. For a given case, our approach is to designate the case as *PDNEC admixed with adenocarcinoma* and document the different characteristics of the two components including their individual size and proportion separately, rather than using *MINEN* as a diagnostic term.

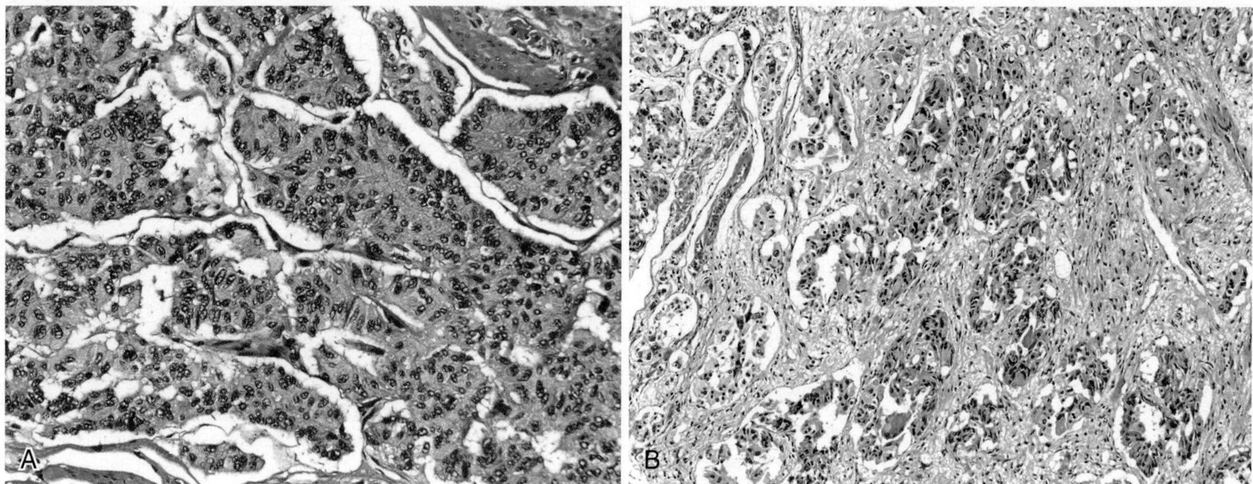

FIGURE 29.23 Duodenal gangliocytic paraganglioma has three components in variable proportions: (1) neuroendocrine cells in compact nests and trabeculae, (2) schwannian-type spindle cells **(A)**, and (3) ganglion-*like* cells **(B)**.

In the GI tract, it is extremely uncommon to see a WDNET in a mixture with adenocarcinoma; in most cases that qualify as MINEN, the NE component proves to be a PDNEC. In the pancreas, however, a distinct WDNET component is often present along with an acinar cell carcinoma, in addition to the common occurrence of scattered individual cells and small clusters[152,153] (see Chapter 40 for details). Current evidence suggests that this may be a sign of maturation because these tumors behave slightly better than ordinary acinar carcinomas. However, it should also be kept in mind that substantial NE differentiation in the form of chromogranin and synaptophysin positivity is a common finding in bona-fide acinar carcinomas. It is important to acknowledge these as acinar carcinomas as it appears to be the main determinant of biological behavior. In the pancreas, the occurrence of a mixture of ductal adenocarcinoma with a well-differentiated PanNET is exceedingly unusual.

In the pancreas, pancreatoblastoma is another tumor type in which NE differentiation can be prominent, along with acinar and ductal components. As in mixed acinar-NE carcinomas, the amount and distribution of NE cells can be highly variable in pancreatoblastomas.

Duodenal Gangliocytic Paraganglioma

Duodenal gangliocytic paraganglioma may also be considered as a "mixed" tumor, in the sense that there is a WDNET component admixed with two other seemingly independent cell types: a mesenchymal component that resembles Schwann cells, and the "ganglion-like" cells (Fig. 29.23).

Incidental Neuroendocrine Cell Proliferations in Other Epithelial Tumors

Occasionally, small NE cell clusters are identified incidentally in the vicinity of glandular epithelial tumors such as adenomas. In the past, this has been dignified with the term *adenoma-carcinoid*[29,154,155] (Fig. 29.24). These have been reported in the colon, but we have also seen examples in the duodenum and ampulla. The WDNET ("carcinoid") component of these lesions is typically small and composed of small cords and minute nests that form a band at the base (adenoma-stroma interface) and typically do not form micronodules that may qualify them as full-blown "tumors." In this regard, they may be similar to the enterochromaffin-like cell proliferations seen in the stomach in the hypergastrinemic conditions discussed earlier. In other words, they may represent proliferations induced by local factors and the tumorous milieu, but they themselves may not necessarily be full-blown WDNETs. More work is needed to determine their nature and clinical significance, if any.

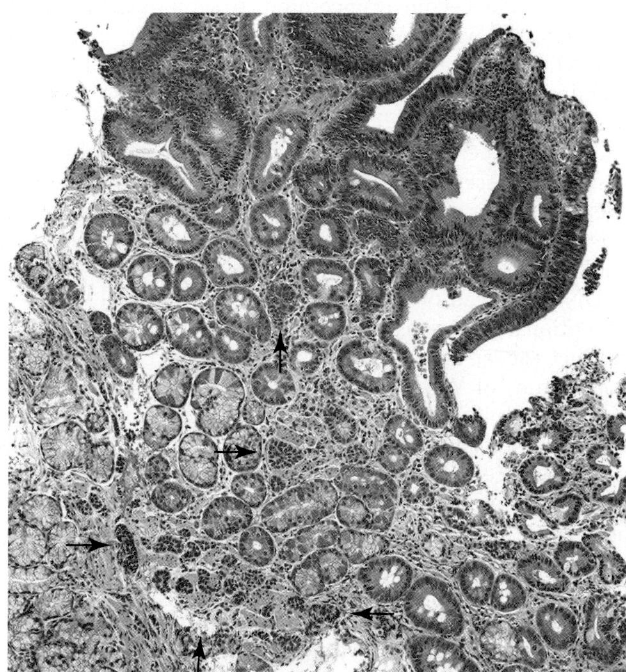

FIGURE 29.24 Small clusters of neuroendocrine cells *(middle; arrows)* may occasionally be seen in the vicinity of an adenoma *(top)*. Although these have been termed *adenoma-carcinoid*, the neuroendocrine cell clusters are typically dispersed and seldom form sizable nodules to warrant concern of a full-blown well-differentiated neuroendocrine tumor.

Goblet Cell Adenocarcinoma (Previously, Goblet Cell Carcinoid and Adenocarcinoma Ex Goblet Cell Carcinoid)

The entity widely known as *goblet cell carcinoid* has been a hotly debated issue since its inception.[136,137,156-161] It is a tumor typically composed of small glandular units with goblet cells (Fig. 29.25) that, for all practical purposes, resemble colonic crypts. Over the years, it has been regarded under various names including *adenocarcinoid* and *crypt cell carcinoma*, but the term most commonly used was *goblet cell carcinoid*.[162-165] The reasons it was regarded in the *carcinoid* family were partly because some showed chromogranin and synaptophysin positivity, albeit often focal and weak. Furthermore, initially they were thought to be more indolent than would be expected from an ordinary adenocarcinoma, and it was believed that they behaved more like a carcinoid. However, later it became clear that this was based on relatively short-term follow-up of cases discovered in appendectomy specimens,[136,158] whereas, with the more advanced cases that had been often mistaken for gynecological malignancies (because of their involvement of gynecological organs and spread to peritoneal surfaces),[136,157] it became clear that these are highly aggressive malignancies. Moreover, they are composed of glandular units of intestinal differentiation (see Fig. 29.25), and they often show mucinous differentiation and spread along the peritoneal surfaces akin to appendiceal mucinous adenocarcinomas. Furthermore, recent studies indicate that the expression of NE markers are often weak and focal or totally absent.[166] Accordingly, in the WHO 2019 Classification of Tumours of the Digestive System, this category was renamed *goblet cell adenocarcinoma*.[11]

Typically, in addition to a conventional goblet cell carcinoid pattern, these tumors show some areas with high-grade cytological features and/or mixed patterns including cordlike infiltration, signet ring cells in cords or as individual cells, a nonmucinous microglandular pattern, an ordinary intestinal pattern, or extravasated mucin (Fig. 29.26). Once disseminated, such tumors exhibit highly aggressive behavior with a median survival less than 3 years. The presence of small round clusters of large goblet-type cells or a rosette-like microglandular pattern are fairly characteristic of these tumors and allow them to be recognized as being derived from the appendix, even at metastatic sites.[136] The most common route of metastasis is through transcoelomic and intraperitoneal invasion in addition to lymph nodes, whereas hematogenous metastasis to the liver or other distant organs is relatively rare. The ovary is the most common site of metastasis followed by abdominal carcinomatosis.

Nonepithelial Origin Tumors with Neuroendocrine Differentiation

Small blue cell tumors with NE type differentiation can occur in the GI and pancreatobiliary tract. Ewing sarcoma and desmoplastic small round cell tumors often show NE differentiation to variable degrees. The latter also often shows evidence of epithelial differentiation. The characteristic molecular and histomorphological patterns of these tumors are beyond the scope of this text, but they should be kept in mind in the differential diagnosis with PDNECs.

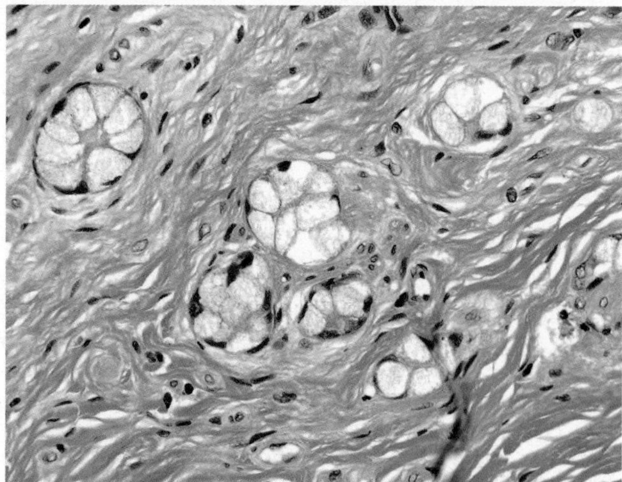

FIGURE 29.25 Distinctive morphology of low-grade goblet cell adenocarcinomas (so-called *goblet cell carcinoid*).Goblet-type tumor cells forming small, round, rosette-like glandular structures closely resembling colonic crypts. Their nuclei are pushed aside as a result of abundant intracytoplasmic mucin within which some neuroendocrine granules are also present and can be highlighted by immunohistochemical stains.

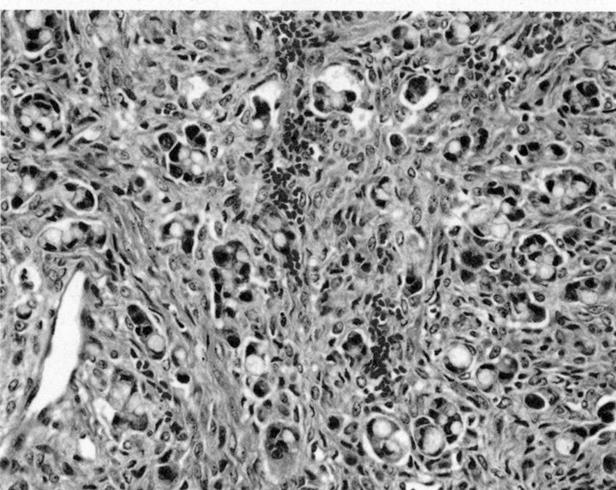

FIGURE 29.26 All high-grade goblet cell adenocarcinomas reveal at least some foci of the so-called *goblet cell carcinoid* pattern, but they also display high-grade features and/or mixed patterns, as illustrated in this example with marked cytological atypia, irregularity of glandlike structures, and few cordlike and individual cells.

Paragangliomas are tumors characterized by NE differentiation and can present as a primary tumor in the vicinity of the GI/pancreatobiliary tract. These tumors are typically keratin negative. Recent evidence suggests a strong familial/genetic background in these cases and may warrant immunohistochemical (for succinate dehydrogenase variants) and genetic testing accordingly. As previously discussed, a variant of WDNET shows a pattern highly reminiscent of paraganglioma but typically is keratin positive.

INDUCED NEUROENDOCRINE DIFFERENTIATION

One peculiar phenomenon that also should be noted here is the emergence of NE features subsequent to therapy in conventional adenocarcinomas. After neo-adjuvant therapy, in some rectal and esophageal adenocarcinomas, the only elements observed in the treatment bed are small clusters of NE cells. The bland appearance of these clusters often raises the question of whether they may be a secondary nonmalignant population within the tumor that survived therapy or should be regarded as *residual tumor.*[167] The current practice, until their nature is better clarified, is to classify and stage these as *persistence of a peculiar clone of neoplastic cells with neuroendocrine transdifferentiation.* It is not clear whether this represents clonal selection/evolution or induction by therapy.

Along the same lines, in the setting of graft-versus-host disease or similar patterns of injury such as mycophenolate-induced injury that leads to disappearance of glands, the remaining epithelium is often rich in NE cells. In some cases, these residual NE cells form cords and minute nests that can mimic a tumor.

FOCAL NEUROENDOCRINE DIFFERENTIATION IN OTHER TUMORS

Scattered NE cells (chromogranin-positive cells) are not uncommon in adenocarcinomas and poorly differentiated carcinomas of the GI and pancreatobiliary tracts. In contrast with the more diffuse (if weak) immunoexpression for chromogranin or synaptophysin found in poorly differentiated NE carcinomas, scattered NE cells in conventional adenocarcinomas usually appear as individual cells with strong immunolabeling in a carcinoma that is otherwise negative for these markers. There are no established guidelines (with proven clinical relevance) as to when these rare NE cells have significance, but most studies suggest they are not prognostically important. Therefore, unless these cells form a zone with a recognizable NE morphology, the convention is to disregard them in terms of clinical management.

SECONDARY (METASTATIC) TUMORS OF NEUROENDOCRINE ORIGIN

Occasionally, NETs from other organs can metastasize to the GI and pancreatobiliary tracts. The small intestine is notorious for being the recipient of metastatic carcinomas, especially from the lung. Additionally, pulmonary PDNECs metastasize to virtually any site in the abdomen, including the pancreas.[168] Because TTF1 is present in PDNECs of any organ, this is not helpful in the differential diagnosis. In the evaluation of such cases, careful clinical analysis is crucial. Features that favor a primary tumor are the presence of an adenoma or adenocarcinoma component or involvement of multiple local lymph nodes without significant lymph node involvement elsewhere. Mucosa-centric distribution is also in favor of a primary tumor, although it can occasionally be seen in metastatic tumors as well.

Of note, Merkel cell carcinoma is another NET type that may present with GI/pancreatobiliary tract metastasis. It is important to recognize this tumor and distinguish it from other PDNECs because its behavior is more indolent, even after metastasis. The distinctive overlapping of round nuclei with washed-off even chromatin, substantiated by the dotlike positivity of CK20 are helpful clues to the diagnosis.

MIMICKERS

WDNETs usually have a distinctive morphology and are easy to recognize. However, certain tumor types are especially prone to mimic NETs at any location. For example, glomus tumors, which can occur in the stomach, often exhibit a nesting pattern and monotony that can closely mimic NETs. Metastasis from the cribriform variant of prostate carcinoma and the nested/alveolar variant of mammary lobular carcinoma are also highly prone to be mistaken as WDNETs. The mimicry of hepatocellular carcinoma and NETs is also well documented,[47] to an extent that many authors advocate the use of NE markers liberally in needle core biopsies of liver mass. Mesenchymal neoplasms with epithelioid histology, particularly the ones with gene fusions involving the *EWSR1* gene or with an SWI/SNF complex deficiency, may also mimic NETs.[169] Additionally, we have seen several examples of epithelioid GISTs that have been mistaken as WDNETs, both in the pancreas and the GI tract.

As discussed earlier, the differential diagnosis of PDNECs from other high-grade malignancies with a nested pattern and monotonous cytology requires careful morphological and immunohistochemical evaluation.

ACKNOWLEDGMENT

The authors are indebted to Dr. Hulya Sahin Ozkan, Dr. Kerem Ozcan, and Ms. Rhonda Everett for their extensive contributions in the preparation of this chapter.

The full reference list may be accessed online at Elsevier eBooks for Practicing Clinicians.

SECTION V

NONEPITHELIAL NEOPLASMS OF THE GASTROINTESTINAL TRACT

CHAPTER 30

Mesenchymal Tumors of the Gastrointestinal Tract

Jason L. Hornick

Chapter Outline

INTRODUCTION

Although epithelial neoplasms predominate in the tubal gut, a variety of mesenchymal neoplasms may originate from or secondarily involve the gastrointestinal (GI) tract. Given the rarity of these lesions and the fact that many have overlapping histological features, accurate classification can be challenging, especially in the setting of limited endoscopic biopsy material. That said, knowledge of a few key details can help narrow an often wide differential diagnosis. For example, mesenchymal neoplasms have favored anatomic locations within the tubal gut as well as characteristic layers of involvement within the wall (mucosa, submucosa, muscularis, or serosa), as described in Table 30.1. An important consideration when faced with an apparent spindle cell lesion involving the tubal gut is to exclude the possibility of a sarcomatoid (spindle cell) carcinoma. In this instance, a panel of broad-spectrum keratin stains can usually correctly identify the lesion as a carcinoma. It is also important to remember that gastrointestinal stromal tumors (GISTs) account for as many as 90% of clinically significant mesenchymal neoplasms within the GI tract; for that reason, GISTs will receive major emphasis within this chapter.

GASTROINTESTINAL STROMAL TUMORS

Although GISTs were once believed to represent smooth muscle neoplasms,[1-3] it has now been established through ultrastructural and immunophenotypic studies and animal models that they arise from either the interstitial cells of Cajal (ICC) or the precursors to those cells.[4-10] ICC are present throughout the wall of the GI tract. They function to coordinate peristalsis by generating and propagating electrical slow waves of depolarization.[7-9,11,12] Although the location and density of ICC vary, in most portions of the GI tract, the largest density occurs around the circumference of the myenteric plexus with extension between the inner and outer layers of the muscularis propria (Fig. 30.1).[13]

KIT (CD117) is a tyrosine kinase receptor that plays a central role in the development and maintenance of ICC[6,14]: the binding of KIT ligand leads to phosphorylation of signal transduction proteins that modulate cell proliferation and inhibit apoptosis.[15,16] Mice that are deficient in Kit or in stem cell factor (Kit ligand) do not have ICC and show evidence of intestinal dysmotility.[17] Activating mutations in *KIT* or in platelet-derived growth factor receptor-α (*PDGFRA*) have been identified in as many as 80% and 10%

TABLE 30.1 Favored Anatomic Locations and Layers of Involvement by Mesenchymal Neoplasms of the Gastrointestinal Tract

Neoplasm	Most Common Anatomic Location	Most Common Layers Involved
Gastrointestinal stromal tumor	Stomach (60%), jejunum and ileum (30%)	Muscularis propria and submucosa
Schwannoma	Stomach	Muscularis propria and submucosa
Gangliocytic paraganglioma	Duodenum	Submucosa
Polypoid ganglioneuroma	Colon	Mucosa
Mucosal perineurioma	Colon	Mucosa
Mucosal Schwann cell hamartoma	Colon	Mucosa
Granular cell tumor	Esophagus	Submucosa
Leiomyoma	Colon and rectum Esophagus	Muscularis mucosae Muscularis propria
Lipoma	Colon	Submucosa
Glomus tumor	Stomach	Muscularis propria
Inflammatory myofibroblastic tumor	Intraabdominal	Mesentery and omentum
Plexiform fibromyxoma	Stomach	Muscularis propria
Perivascular epithelioid cell tumor (PEComa)	Colon and rectum	Variable; mucosa and submucosa or entire thickness of bowel wall
Clear cell sarcoma–like tumor (malignant gastrointestinal neuroectodermal tumor)	Small bowel	Entire thickness of the bowel wall

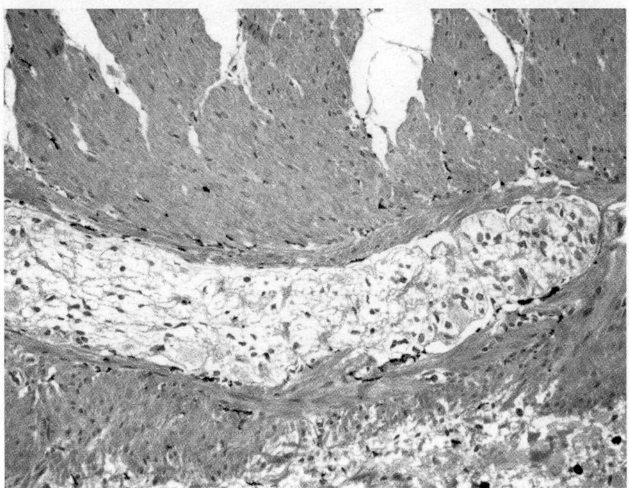

FIGURE 30.1 KIT immunohistochemistry highlights the normal distribution of interstitial cells of Cajal in the myenteric plexus and adjacent muscularis propria.

of GISTs, respectively; these mutually exclusive gain-of-function mutations play a fundamental role in GIST development by leading to constitutive activation.[18-23]

Clinical Features

Approximately 4500 to 6000 GISTs are diagnosed annually in the United States.[18,19] GISTs can arise at almost any age, including childhood, but are most common in middle-aged and elderly adults, with approximately 75% diagnosed in patients older than 50 years.[20-22] They may arise anywhere in the GI tract but are most common in the stomach (60%), followed by the jejunum and ileum (30%), the duodenum (5%), and the colorectum (<5%).[23] Very few cases have been described in the esophagus or appendix.[24,25] GISTs may also occur as primary tumors outside the GI tract, in the retroperitoneum or abdomen (e.g., omentum or mesentery); such tumors are referred to as extra-GISTs (EGISTs).[26,27]

The presenting manifestations of GIST depend on the site of involvement in the GI tract, the size of the tumor, and the portion of the gut wall in which the tumor is located. A significant number of tumors are asymptomatic and are found incidentally at surgery performed for other reasons.[28,29] In fact, studies in which gastrectomy specimens were extensively or entirely examined microscopically have shown that incidental, subcentimeter gastric GISTs (micro-GISTs) can be identified in up to 35% of adults.[30] The most common symptoms are GI bleeding with subsequent anemia, abdominal pain, nausea, vomiting, and weight loss.[31] Signs and symptoms may lead to endoscopy and biopsy. In some cases, a histological diagnosis of GIST can be made if a deep endoscopic biopsy is obtained or if the neoplasm infiltrates the overlying mucosa. Radiographic imaging studies, including use of barium contrast, computed tomography, and endoscopic ultrasound, are commonly used for evaluation and diagnosis of these neoplasms.[32] In addition, GISTs can be diagnosed by fine-needle aspiration cytology.[33]

The behavior of GISTs ranges from benign to malignant. In adults, GIST behavior can be predicted by anatomic site, tumor size, and mitotic activity.[18,20,23,34,35] Metastases usually develop within 2 years of diagnosis, and the expected pattern of metastatic spread is to the liver and peritoneum.[20] Rare cases of metastatic disease outside the abdominal cavity have been seen, most commonly in the lungs, bone, soft tissue, and, very rarely in advanced cases, the brain or skin.[20,36-38] Historically, lymph node metastases in GISTs were thought to be extremely uncommon (<1% of cases). However, more recent studies show that succinate dehydrogenase (SDH)-deficient GISTs (described later) have a propensity for nodal metastases.[39-41]

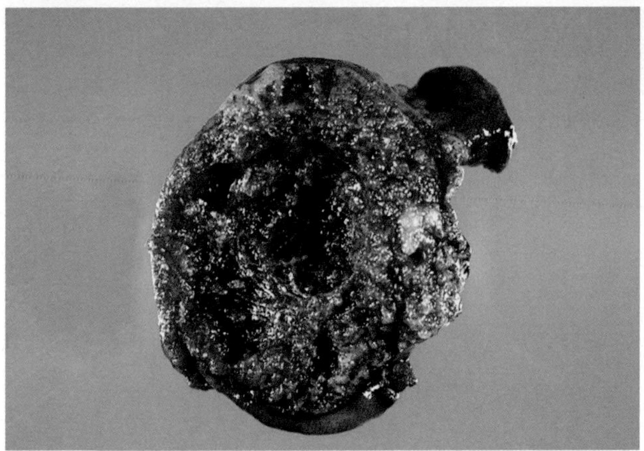

FIGURE 30.2 Gross appearance of gastrointestinal stromal tumor in the stomach. The cut surface is granular and shows foci of hemorrhage. This gross appearance is quite distinct from that of typical smooth muscle tumors, which have a cut surface that is firm and uniform.

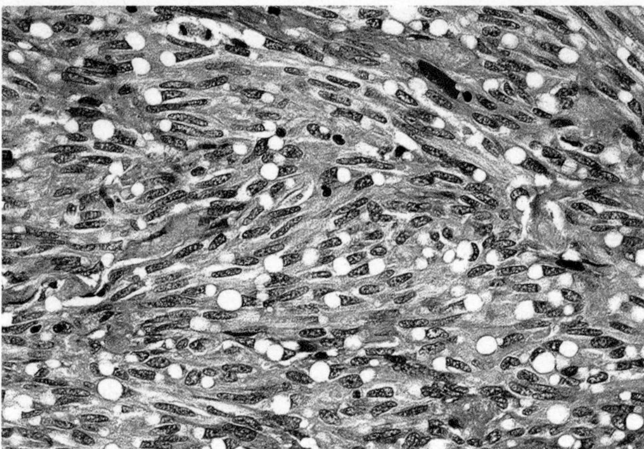

FIGURE 30.4 High-magnification view of a gastric gastrointestinal stromal tumor, spindle cell type, shows the typical prominent paranuclear vacuoles.

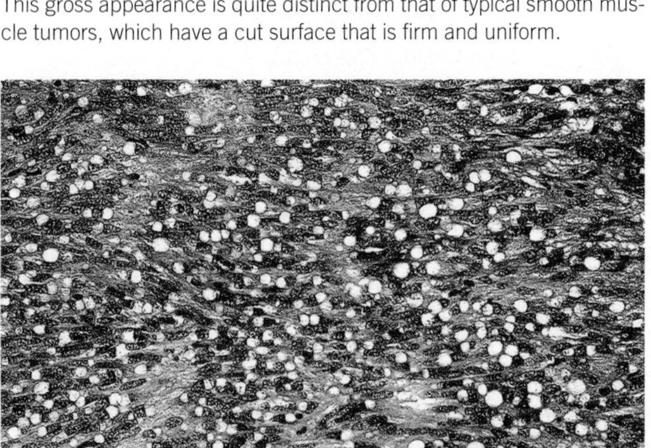

FIGURE 30.3 Gastrointestinal stromal tumor, spindle cell type, composed of uniform cells with modest amounts of pale eosinophilic fibrillary cytoplasm.

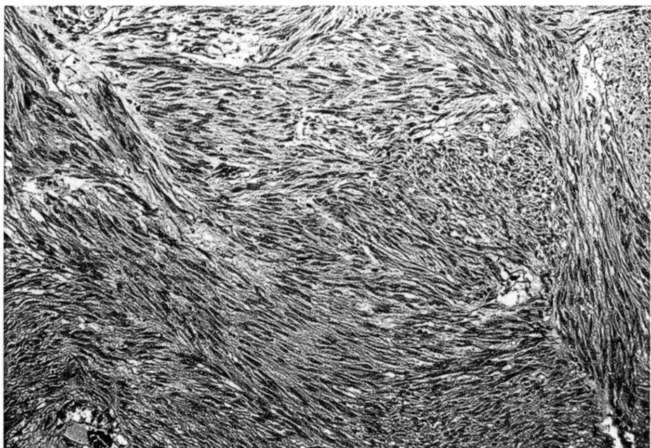

FIGURE 30.5 Gastric gastrointestinal stromal tumor, spindle cell type, arranged in intersecting tight fascicles.

Pathological Features

Gross and Microscopic Features

Most GISTs are uninodular and centered on the bowel wall; however, multinodular or multifocal growth may be observed, especially in the pediatric population and in GIST syndromes. The tumor may ulcerate the overlying mucosa or grow exophytically and protrude from the serosa. Some GISTs are predominantly extramural and may be attached to the serosa of the tubal gut by only a thin stalk of tissue. On cut section, lesions may show areas of hemorrhage, necrosis, or cystic change—features that are not indicative of malignancy in GISTs (Fig. 30.2). The histomorphology varies greatly and includes pure spindle cell, pure epithelioid, and mixed spindle cell and epithelioid types.[18] Epithelioid and mixed cell type GISTs are most commonly encountered in the stomach. [42,43]

Spindle cell GISTs are composed of uniform, elongated cells that are consistent in size and shape. The cells have nuclei with evenly dispersed chromatin, inconspicuous nucleoli, and moderate amounts of pale eosinophilic or basophilic fibrillary cytoplasm (Fig. 30.3). Particular to gastric GISTs is the frequent presence of paranuclear vacuoles that indent the nucleus at one pole (Fig. 30.4). The architecture is that of intersecting short fascicles (Fig. 30.5). The vasculature can range from inconspicuous to hemangiopericytoma-like, whereas the stromal component may be inconspicuous or may exhibit prominent myxoid change, hyalinization, or dystrophic calcification (Fig. 30.6). Prominent collagen fibrils, so-called "skeinoid" fibers, may be observed in small bowel GISTs (Fig. 30.7).[44,45]

Epithelioid GISTs are composed predominantly of cells with either abundant eosinophilic or clear cytoplasm, typically arranged in nests and sheets. The nuclei are round with vesicular chromatin and variable nucleoli (Fig. 30.8). Scattered binucleated cells, multinucleated giant cells, or cells with bizarre nuclei may be present (Fig. 30.9). The stromal alterations may include hyalinization or myxoid change (Fig. 30.10). Confusion with other epithelioid malignant neoplasms can be problematic on endoscopic biopsies, especially when an epithelioid GIST involves the mucosa (Fig. 30.11).

Immunohistochemical Features

KIT (CD117), the product of the *KIT* gene, is a sensitive marker for GIST, irrespective of site; it is expressed in as many as 95% of GISTs.[46] The pattern of immunoreactivity

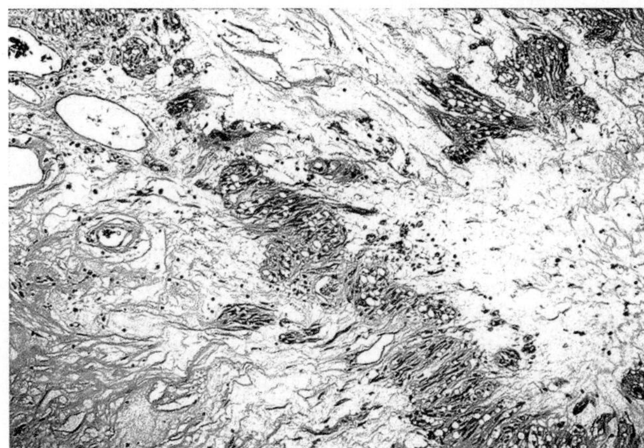

FIGURE 30.6 Gastrointestinal stromal tumor, spindle cell type, showing prominent stromal edema and hyalinization.

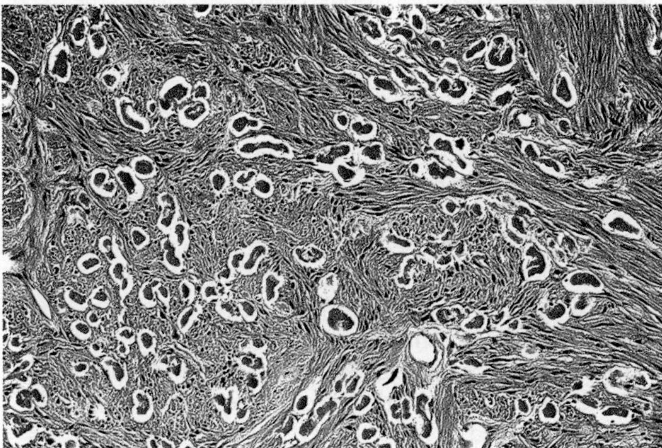

FIGURE 30.7 Small bowel gastrointestinal stromal tumor, spindle cell type, showing numerous eosinophilic collagen globules, so-called "skeinoid" fibers.

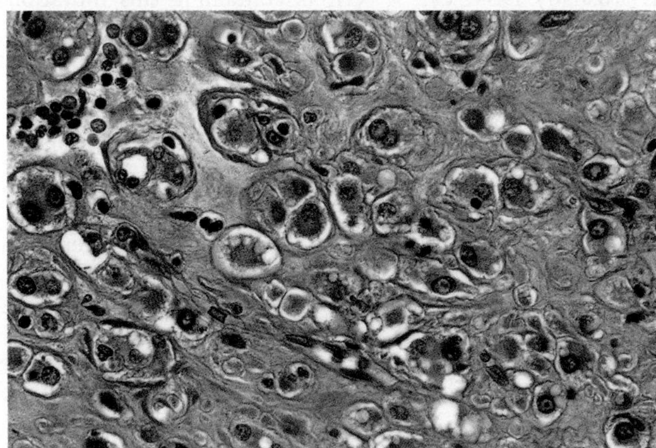

FIGURE 30.8 Gastrointestinal stromal tumor, epithelioid type, composed of cells with rounded nuclei and ample eosinophilic cytoplasm.

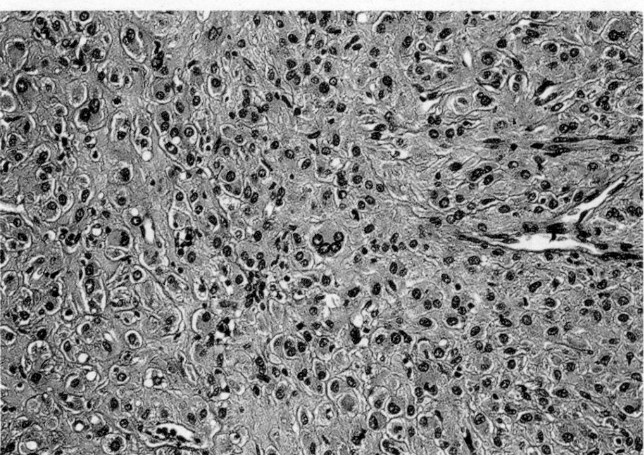

FIGURE 30.9 Gastrointestinal stromal tumor, epithelioid type, in which the cells are arranged in broad sheets with occasional multinucleated cells.

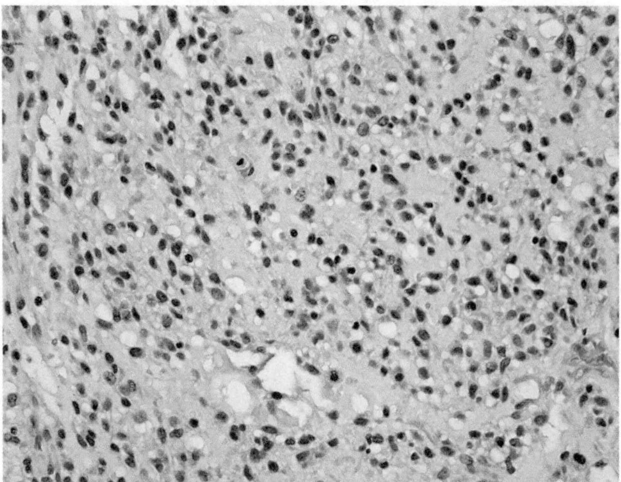

FIGURE 30.10 Gastrointestinal stromal tumor, epithelioid type, showing prominent myxoid stromal change.

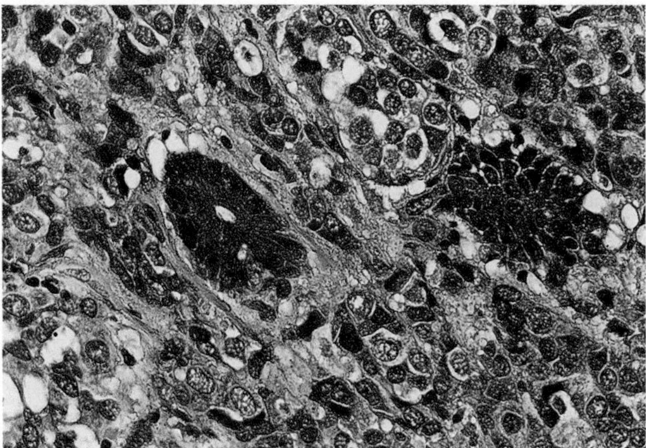

FIGURE 30.11 Small bowel gastrointestinal stromal tumor, epithelioid type, involving the lamina propria.

is typically diffuse and pancytoplasmic (Fig. 30.12), although membranous staining and a paranuclear dotlike pattern may be seen (Fig. 30.13). Approximately 5% of GISTs do not react with antibodies to KIT[47,48]; most KIT-negative tumors are located in the stomach, have epithelioid morphology, and harbor *PDGFRA* mutations.[49] CD34, a hematopoietic stem cell marker, is expressed in roughly 70% of GISTs.[50] Approximately 20% to 30% of GISTs are positive for smooth muscle actin, 5% express S100 protein (usually limited in extent), and 1% to 2% are positive for desmin or keratins.[5,18,46]

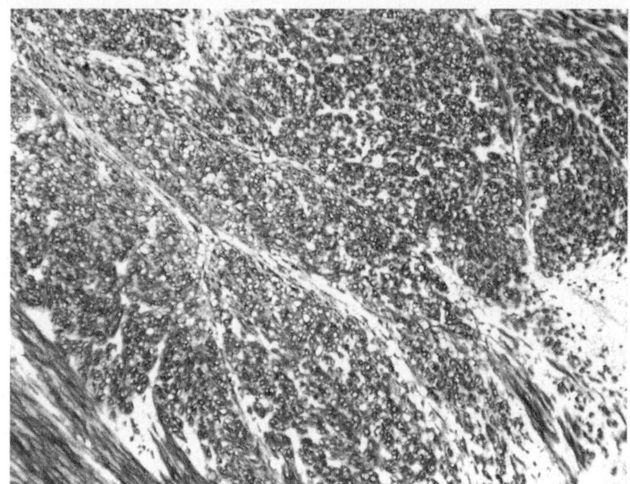

FIGURE 30.12 Pancytoplasmic KIT immunoreactivity is observed in a gastrointestinal stromal tumor, spindle cell type.

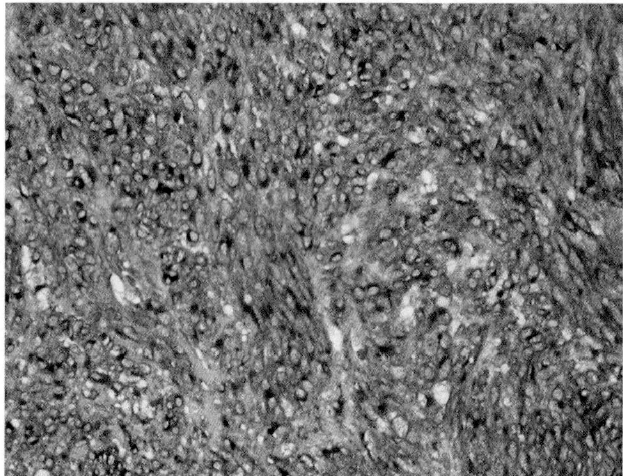

FIGURE 30.13 Paranuclear dotlike accentuation of KIT is observed in some gastrointestinal stromal tumors.

Gene expression profiling studies of GISTs have identified two additional immunostains that are diagnostically useful. *Discovered on GIST 1 (DOG1)*,[51] also known as *anoctamin 1 (ANO1)*, encodes a calcium-regulated chloride channel protein.[52,53] Antibodies directed against ANO1 (DOG1) are immunoreactive with GISTs regardless of their *KIT/PDGFRA* mutational status[54,55] and have sensitivity similar to that of KIT (approximately 95%). However, DOG1 positivity has also been identified in several other mesenchymal tumor types, including a small subset of leiomyomas and synovial sarcomas.[56] Gene expression studies have also shown protein kinase C-theta to be consistently overexpressed in GISTs[57]; immunohistochemical studies have shown that expression of this protein is sensitive and specific for GIST, although few laboratories use this marker clinically.[58] *PDGFRA*-mutant GISTs typically show strong and diffuse expression of PDGFRA, which can also be detected by immunohistochemistry.[59]

Molecular Findings

KIT and *PDGFRA* encode homologous transmembrane glycoproteins[60,61] that contain an extracellular ligand-binding domain with five immunoglobulin-like loops that function in ligand binding and dimerization. The corresponding cytoplasmic domain is composed of a juxtamembrane domain and a tyrosine kinase domain; the juxtamembrane domain regulates KIT tyrosine kinase activity by inhibiting activity in the absence of KIT ligand.[62] As mentioned previously, mutually exclusive mutations in *KIT* or *PDGFRA* are common in GISTs (as many as 80% and 10%, respectively).[18-22] The identification of these mutations in small, incidentally identified GISTs confirms their role as drivers of early tumorigenesis.[28,63] Although most of these mutations are somatic, germline mutations have been identified in rare families (see GIST Syndromes and Succinate Dehydrogenase–Deficient GISTs).[64-68]

Approximately 70% of the mutations involving *KIT* are identified at the juxtamembrane domain in exon 11, resulting in ligand-independent activation of tyrosine kinase activity and ultimately promoting proliferation and cell survival.[62,69-71] The mutations cluster at either the 3′ or the 5′ end of the exon, with the mutation type frequently determining the clinical course. For example, internal tandem duplication mutations have been identified at the 3′ end of exon 11, predominantly in gastric GISTs that follow an indolent course.[72] In comparison, an aggressive clinical course with a higher risk of recurrence and shorter survival time has been observed in GISTs harboring deletions involving exon 11.[73-75] The second most common *KIT* mutation site, seen in approximately 10% of GISTs, is within exon 9 (distal extracellular domain). Patients whose GISTs harbor this mutation commonly have small bowel involvement and a more clinically aggressive neoplasm.[72] Mutations in exons 13 and 17 affect the tyrosine kinase domain of *KIT* and are identified in fewer than 2% of sporadic GISTS.[76,77] The corresponding morphology is typically spindle cell with frequent involvement of the small bowel.[78]

The subset of GISTs that harbor a mutation in *PDGFRA* most commonly have a missense mutation in exon 18 (usually D842V).[79,80] GISTs containing this mutation almost always involve the stomach and have epithelioid morphology.[79-81] Less commonly, *PDGFRA* exon 14 and exon 12 mutations are seen; exon 14 mutations are also associated with epithelioid morphology, location within the stomach, and a favorable clinical course.[79] In general, *PDGFRA* mutations are found within GISTs of the stomach and omentum.[81-83] A primary *BRAF* V600E mutation has been identified in a small subset of GISTs that lack either *KIT* or *PDGFRA* mutations.[84-86] Very rarely, GISTs harbor gene fusions (involving *NTRK3* or *FGFR1*).[87,88]

Differential Diagnosis

GISTs with spindle cell morphology must be distinguished from other spindle cell neoplasms of the GI tract, including smooth muscle neoplasms, nerve sheath tumors, inflammatory fibroid polyp, inflammatory myofibroblastic tumor (IMT), and intraabdominal (desmoid) fibromatosis (Table 30.2).

Although smooth muscle tumors of the GI tract are much less common than GISTs, location is important; leiomyomas are more common than GISTs in the colon, rectum, and esophagus. Esophageal leiomyomas are typically mural tumors, whereas colorectal leiomyomas arise from the muscularis mucosae and present as small polyps. GI

TABLE 30.2 Comparison of Immunophenotype of Spindle Cell Tumors of the Gastrointestinal Tract

Tumor	KIT	CD34	SMA	Desmin	S100
Gastrointestinal stromal tumor	+ (95%)	+ (70%)	+ (30%-40%)	2%	5%
Schwannoma	–	–	–	–	+
Desmoid fibromatosis	–	–	+	Rare	–
Smooth muscle neoplasms	–	10%-15%	+	+	–
Inflammatory myofibroblastic tumor	–	–	+	+	–

SMA, *Smooth muscle actin; –, absent; +, present.*

leiomyomas are composed of spindle cells with cigar-shaped nuclei and bright eosinophilic cytoplasm arranged in fascicles. Leiomyosarcomas of the GI tract are exceptionally rare and show marked nuclear atypia and pleomorphism, features that are uncommonly seen in GISTs. The cells are strongly and diffusely immunoreactive for smooth muscle actin and often for desmin, but there is no expression of KIT.[36,44]

Nerve sheath tumors are also a consideration, including neurofibromas, schwannomas, and malignant peripheral nerve sheath tumors. GI schwannomas, the most common of these nerve sheath tumors, usually occur in the stomach. They are composed of bundles of spindle cells with focal atypia, often arranged in a microtrabecular growth pattern with intercellular collagen, and they are associated with a dense peripheral lymphoid infiltrate. They stain strongly for S100 protein, glial fibrillary acidic protein (GFAP), and SOX10, and are negative for KIT and DOG1. Malignant peripheral nerve sheath tumors rarely arise within the GI tract; they resemble their counterparts in the peripheral soft tissues. In contrast to GISTs, these lesions do not express KIT or DOG1, are variably immunoreactive for S100 protein and SOX10, and often show loss of H3K27me3 (histone H3 with lysine 27 trimethylation).

Less commonly, inflammatory fibroid polyps enter the differential diagnosis. They may arise throughout the GI tract,[89] but they have a predilection for the stomach and terminal ileum, where they form a polyp or intramural mass. These lesions are composed of randomly distributed, spindle and stellate cells associated with numerous rounded blood vessels and inflammatory cells, especially eosinophils, plasma cells, lymphocytes, and mast cells. Frequently, there is concentric perivascular fibrosis with an onion-skin pattern. KIT highlights the scattered mast cells, whereas the spindle cells are negative for KIT. The spindle and stellate cells are immunoreactive for CD34, posing potential confusion with GISTs.[90] Inflammatory fibroid polyps harbor gain-of-function mutations in *PDGFRA* within the same genomic hot spots as those identified within GISTs that lack an activating *KIT* mutation; these mutations lead to high-level expression of PDGFRA, which can be detected by immunohistochemistry.[59,91] Despite having similar activating mutations, inflammatory fibroid polyps behave in a benign fashion and are not related to GIST.

IMTs are most common in children and young adults and can arise as an intraabdominal mass involving the GI tract. The constituent cells have the light microscopic and immunohistochemical features of myofibroblasts, intermingled with inflammatory cells (especially lymphocytes and plasma cells) and collagen. The cells are KIT negative and frequently express anaplastic lymphoma kinase (ALK), caused by rearrangements of the *ALK* gene on 2p23.[92]

Intraabdominal (desmoid) fibromatosis is the most common primary tumor of the mesentery; it often originates from the gastrocolic ligament and omentum. Mesenteric desmoid fibromatosis is arranged in long, sweeping fascicles that have finger-like projections extending into the surrounding soft tissue. Scattered keloid-type collagen fibers may be present, as are dilated thin-walled vessels. The lesional spindle or stellate cells are cytologically bland and monotonous and are distributed evenly within a collagenous or myxoid stroma. By immunohistochemistry, the lesional cells are positive for smooth muscle actin, and they show aberrant nuclear β-catenin immunoreactivity in 80% of cases.[93] These lesions are consistently KIT and DOG1 negative.

GISTs with epithelioid features raise a broad differential diagnosis that includes melanoma, neuroendocrine tumors, and carcinoma; judicious use of immunohistochemical stains is warranted in this setting given the histological overlap (Table 30.3). Because expression of KIT has been identified within a subset of melanomas,[94-96] excluding the possibility of melanoma by performing a panel of melanocytic markers including S100 protein, SOX10, HMB-45, or melan A is warranted. Rare examples of epithelioid GIST show focal keratin immunoreactivity, so the coexpression of CD34 and DOG1 with KIT (or without KIT in epithelioid GISTs containing *PDGFRA* mutations) is essential to avoid misdiagnosis of such cases as carcinoma. Of note, a small subset of gastric adenocarcinomas expresses DOG1.

Overall, nuclear pleomorphism is unusual in GISTs; the finding of marked pleomorphism could suggest other sarcomas (especially leiomyosarcoma and dedifferentiated liposarcoma), sarcomatoid carcinoma, or the very rare dedifferentiated GIST. This dedifferentiation is akin to dedifferentiation in other sarcomas, wherein a transition from a morphologically recognizable conventional tumor to an anaplastic or pleomorphic morphology is appreciated (Fig. 30.14). In the setting of GIST with dedifferentiation, the morphology changes, and the immunophenotype undergoes a transition as well, with loss of KIT and DOG1 immunoreactivity within the anaplastic cells, sometimes with the acquisition of smooth muscle actin or keratins.[97] Dedifferentiation has been described both as a de novo event and after treatment with the selective tyrosine kinase inhibitor imatinib mesylate (Gleevec; Novartis Pharmaceuticals, East Hanover, NJ).[97]

Prognosis and Treatment

Tyrosine kinase inhibitors have played a pivotal role in the management of GISTs, and the U.S. Food and Drug Administration (FDA) has approved four targeted therapies. Imatinib mesylate is a selective tyrosine kinase inhibitor that targets KIT and PDGFRA. Sunitinib malate (Sutent; Pfizer, New York, NY) targets several receptors including those for KIT, PDGFRA, and vascular endothelial growth factor[98-100]; regorafenib (Stivarga; Bayer, Whippany, NJ) is another multikinase inhibitor.[101] Avapritinib (Ayvakit; Blueprint Medicines, Cambridge, MA) targets PDGFRA with exon 18 mutations. The original indication for imatinib was for the treatment of metastatic or unresectable GISTs, with patients showing clinical responses in as many as 80% of cases[102]; current FDA-approved labeling also includes use in the adjuvant setting after complete gross resection of GISTs.[103] Sunitinib is approved for patients who do not tolerate imatinib or who have tumor progression on imatinib therapy. Regorafenib is administered in turn as third-line therapy for patients who fail both other therapeutic agents. Tumor genotype has been shown to correlate with response to these drugs. For example, tumors with an exon 11 *KIT* mutation have shown the best imatinib response rates, whereas tumors without a *KIT* mutation and those with a *PDGFRA* D842V mutation are less likely to have a favorable or a sustained response to imatinib.[49,104] Other studies suggest that patients with an exon 9 *KIT* mutation benefit from a higher dose of this drug.[105,106] Avapritinib was recently approved for patients with advanced *PDGFRA* exon 18-mutant GISTs. Approximately 50% of GIST patients treated with imatinib will acquire a secondary mutation that confers tumor resistance to imatinib,[107-110] and in such cases, sunitinib is approved as a second-line therapy. The most common secondary *KIT* mutations that escape imatinib are *KIT* V654A and *KIT* T670I, both of which are sensitive to sunitinib.

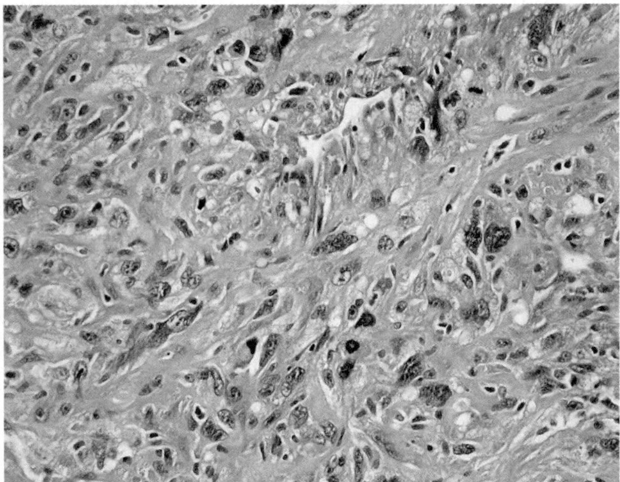

FIGURE 30.14 Dedifferentiated GIST is characterized by areas of marked nuclear pleomorphism that lack immunoreactivity for KIT. In most cases, a recognizable "low-grade" area of conventional GIST is identified.

GISTs are risk stratified based on mitotic rate, size, and anatomic location; these features define the Miettinen criteria for risk stratification (Table 30.4),[23] which establish a risk of progressive disease, defined as either metastatic disease or tumor-related death. The criteria are based on large studies from the Armed Forces Institute of Pathology (AFIP) that evaluated how the clinicopathological features of GISTs within different sites (gastric, small intestinal, duodenal, and rectal locations) affected prognosis in the preimatinib era.[38,42,44,45] To assign an accurate risk of progressive disease, a precise gross tumor measurement with a thorough mitotic count should be performed, evaluating a total area of 5 mm^2. For modern wide-field microscopes, the mitotic count correlating with the total area of 5 mm^2 is obtained from approximately 20 high-power fields (HPFs).

Other factors that have been reported to be associated with poor outcome include tumor necrosis, mucosal invasion, and ulceration.[42,111,112] Tumor rupture, either spontaneous or at the time of surgery, increases the risk of recurrence with intraabdominal seeding.[113,114] Patients

TABLE 30.3 Comparison of Immunophenotype of Gastrointestinal Stromal Tumor with Other Epithelioid Tumors of the Gastrointestinal Tract

Tumor	KIT	SMA	Keratins	S100	HMB-45 or melan A	Chromo	Synapto
Gastrointestinal stromal tumor	+ (95%)	+ (30%-40%)	Rare	5%	–	–	–
Metastatic melanoma	+ (20%-40%)	–	Rare	+	+	–	–
Perivascular epithelioid cell tumor (PEComa)	–	+	–	10%-15%	+	–	–
Glomus tumor	–	+	–	–	–	–	10% (focal)
Neuroendocrine tumor	–	–	+	Rare	–	+	+

Chromo, *Chromogranin;* SMA, *smooth muscle actin;* synapto, *synaptophysin; –, absent; +, present.*

TABLE 30.4 Risk Stratification of Primary Gastrointestinal Stromal Tumor by Mitotic Index, Size, and Anatomic Site

Tumor Parameters		Risk of Progressive Disease* (%)			
Mitotic Index	**Size**	**Gastric**	**Duodenum**	**Jejunum/Ileum**	**Rectum**
≤5 per 5 mm²	≤2 cm	None (0%)	None (0%)	None (0%)	None (0%)
	>2 to ≤5 cm	Very low (1.9%)	Low (8.3%)	Low (4.3%)	Low (8.5%)
	>5 to ≤10 cm	Low (3.6%)	Insufficient data	Moderate (24%)	Insufficient data
	>10 cm	Moderate (10%)	High (34%)	High (52%)	High (57%)
>5 per 5 mm²	≤2 cm	None†	Insufficient data	High†	High (54%)
	>2 to ≤5 cm	Moderate (16%)	High (50%)	High (73%)	High (52%)
	>5 to ≤10 cm	High (55%)	Insufficient data	High (85%)	Insufficient data
	>10 cm	High (86%)	High (86%)	High (90%)	High (71%)

Data from Miettinen M, Lasota J. Semin Diagn Pathol. *2006;23:70-83; Miettinen M, Furlong M, Sarlomo-Rikala M, et al.* Am J Surg Pathol. *2001;25:1121-1133; Miettinen M, Sobin LH, Lasota J.* Am J Surg Pathol. *2005;29:52-68; Miettinen M, Kopczynski J, Makhlouf HR, et al.* Am J Surg Pathol. *2003;27:625-641; and Miettinen M, Makhlouf H, Sobin LH, Lasota J.* Am J Surg Pathol. *2006;30:477-489.*

**Based on long-term follow-up of 1055 gastric, 629 small intestinal, 144 duodenal, and 111 rectal GISTs. Progression is defined as metastasis or tumor-related death.*

†Denotes small numbers of cases.

whose complete resection is complicated by tumor rupture have a significantly shortened survival time, compared with patients with complete resection without tumor rupture.[114-116]

GIST Syndromes and Succinate Dehydrogenase–Deficient GISTs

Although most GISTs are sporadic, almost 5% are associated with a tumor syndrome, including familial GIST syndrome, neurofibromatosis type 1 (NF1), the Carney triad, and Carney-Stratakis syndrome.

Familial GISTs arise from germline mutations in exons 8, 11, and 13 of *KIT* and in exon 12 of *PDGFRA*, identical to the mutations identified in sporadic GISTs.[65,66,117-122] GISTs will develop in almost all patients who harbor these germline mutations, typically within the stomach and small bowel. These lesions most commonly develop in middle-aged patients, but they have been documented in patients as young as 18 years. Other clinical manifestations of *KIT* activation, such as cutaneous mastocytosis and hyperpigmented macules on the skin of the perineum, axilla, hands, and face, may also be found in these patients, as well as a background of diffuse ICC hyperplasia in the bowel wall.[65,68] This latter finding raises the possibility of a hyperplasia to neoplasia sequence, with additional clonal genetic alterations needed to progress from ICC hyperplasia to GIST.[123]

GISTs arising in patients with NF1 have been recognized for some time and are likely the most common GI tract tumor associated with NF1. As estimated from a series of duodenal GISTs reported by the AFIP, patients with NF1 have an increased risk for GIST as high as 180-fold compared with the general population.[44] Most NF1-associated tumors arise in the small bowel, often in a multifocal fashion.[124,125] Distinguishing patients with NF1 and multiple GISTs from patients with sporadic GISTs and multiple metastatic nodules is of major clinical significance. Most NF1-associated GISTs are relatively small, are mitotically inactive, and follow an indolent course. Therefore the index of suspicion for NF1 should be high when one encounters multiple small GISTs, particularly in the small bowel. ICC hyperplasia is sometimes seen in the myenteric plexus adjacent to these tumors. The pathogenesis of NF1-associated GISTs is different from that of sporadic GISTs, as the former tumors rarely harbor *KIT* or *PDGFRA* mutations.[124,126-129]

The identification of GIST arising in the setting of a germline mutation in the SDH complex[130] has led to the recognition of a distinctive group of SDH-deficient GISTs that are found in the stomach and share histological, immunohistochemical, and clinical similarities. These GISTs arise in the setting of Carney-Stratakis syndrome, Carney triad, pediatric GIST, or "pediatric-type" GISTs in adults.[131-133] They have a multinodular or plexiform growth with lobules of tumor separated by bands of smooth muscle, are hypercellular, and have predominantly epithelioid cytomorphology (Figs. 30.15 and 30.16).[131-134] Similar to conventional *KIT*-mutant GISTs, SDH-deficient GISTs express KIT, DOG1, and CD34. However, in contrast to conventional GISTs, which show granular cytoplasmic (mitochondrial) staining for succinate dehydrogenase subunit B (SDHB), GISTs arising in these settings show loss of staining for SDHB (Fig. 30.17).[132] Clinically, these tumors metastasize to lymph nodes and are insensitive to imatinib mesylate; however, despite frequent recurrences and distant metastases, they typically follow a more indolent clinical course.[131,134,135] The clinical behavior of SDH-deficient GISTs cannot be predicted by the Miettinen risk stratification criteria.[136]

Carney-Stratakis syndrome is characterized by paraganglioma and gastric GISTs.[134] This syndrome results from a germline mutation in one of the SDH complex subunit genes and is inherited in an autosomal dominant

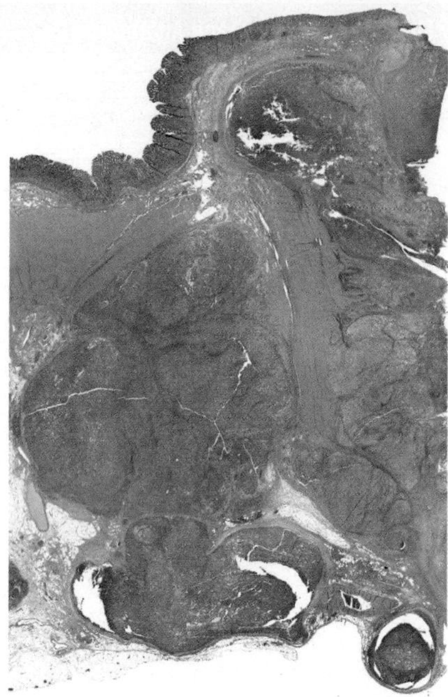

FIGURE 30.15 Succinate dehydrogenase-deficient GIST showing the characteristic multinodular growth pattern through the wall of the stomach.

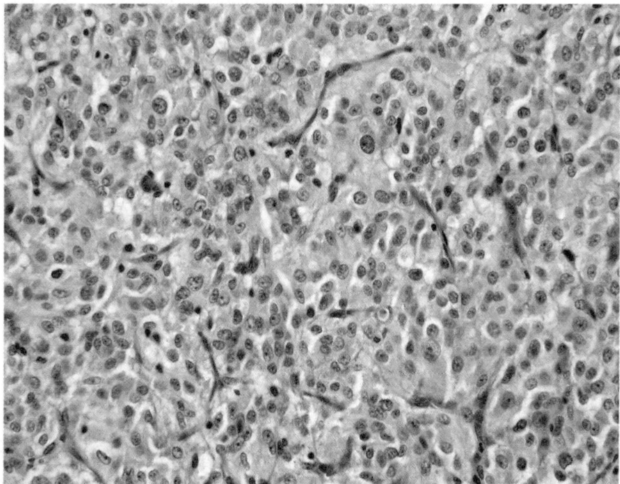

FIGURE 30.16 Succinate dehydrogenase-deficient GIST composed of sheets of epithelioid cells.

manner.[130,137,138] GISTs arising in this setting lack *KIT* and *PDGFRA* mutations.[138]

The nonfamilial Carney triad includes gastric GISTs, paraganglioma, and pulmonary chondroma; GISTs in this syndrome occur exclusively in the stomach and usually arise in much younger patients with a striking female predilection (approximately 85%).[134,139] The SDH-deficient tumors from patients with Carney triad typically show hypermethylation of the *SDHC* promoter.[140]

GISTs may arise in children, albeit rarely, accounting for fewer than 1% of all GISTs.[40] In the pediatric population, GISTs predominate in girls, are usually located in the stomach, and are frequently multifocal with epithelioid or mixed morphology.[141] These lesions often metastasize to lymph nodes, and they often lack mutations in *KIT* and *PDGFRA*; approximately 50% harbor mutations in SDH complex subunit genes, and the remainder show *SDHC* promoter hypermethylation.[142-144] Nearly 5% of GISTs in adults overall are SDH-deficient (formerly referred to as *pediatric-type*); this subtype accounts for roughly 8% of gastric GISTs in adults. Despite the fact that many such tumors appear sporadic clinically, affected patients often harbor *SDHA* germline mutations; *SDHA*-mutant GISTs show loss of both SDHB and SDHA expression by immunohistochemistry.[144,145] These tumors have histomorphology identical to that seen in pediatric patients, Carney triad, and Carney-Stratakis syndrome and a similar clinical course, with nodal metastases, imatinib resistance, and an overall indolent course.[141,146]

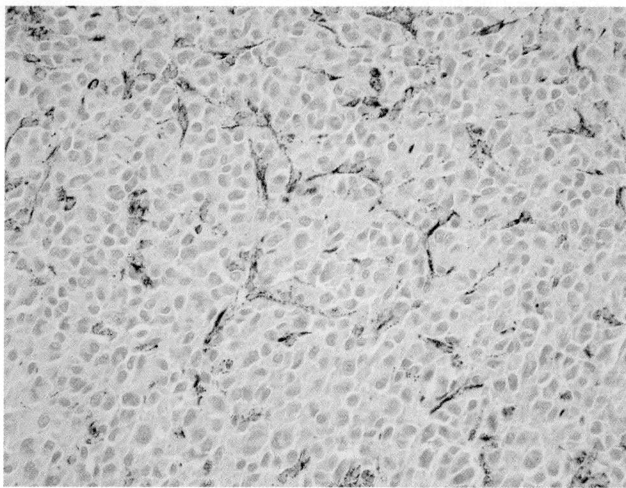

FIGURE 30.17 Immunohistochemistry for SDHB in a succinate dehydrogenase–deficient GIST showing loss of cytoplasmic staining in the tumor cells.

NEURAL TUMORS

Schwannoma

Clinical Features

Schwannomas are most commonly encountered in the stomach,[147] followed by the colon and rectum.[148] These lesions have been rarely described in the esophagus and small intestine.[149-152] Schwannomas have been documented in patients as young as 18 years,[148] but they arise most commonly during middle to late adulthood, with a peak in the sixth decade.[148-153] The largest series evaluating gastric schwannomas documented a female predominance, with a 1:4 male-to-female ratio.[153] Schwannomas typically involve the muscularis propria and submucosa, with frequent ulceration of the overlying mucosa. Those arising in the stomach are usually a mural mass, whereas schwannomas in the colon and rectum often manifest as ulcerated polypoid lesions.[148] The presenting clinical symptoms are typically specific to site. Schwannomas arising in the colon and rectum frequently present with rectal bleeding, abdominal pain, and colonic obstruction,[148] whereas those arising in the stomach present with gastric discomfort and bleeding.[153] It is not unusual for gastric schwannomas to be identified incidentally during other procedures.[153]

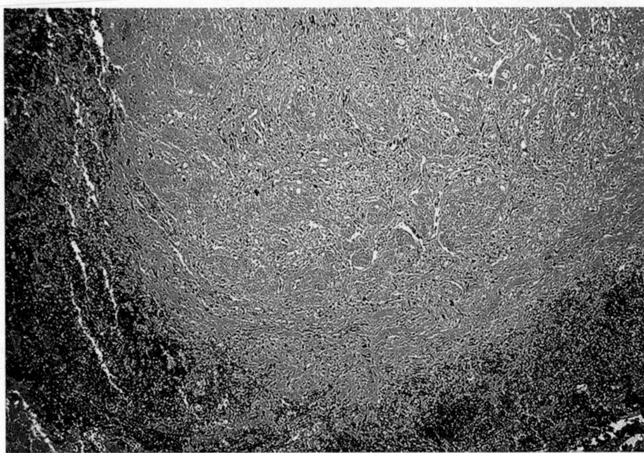

FIGURE 30.18 Gastric schwannoma showing the characteristic lymphoid cuff that surrounds the periphery of the tumor.

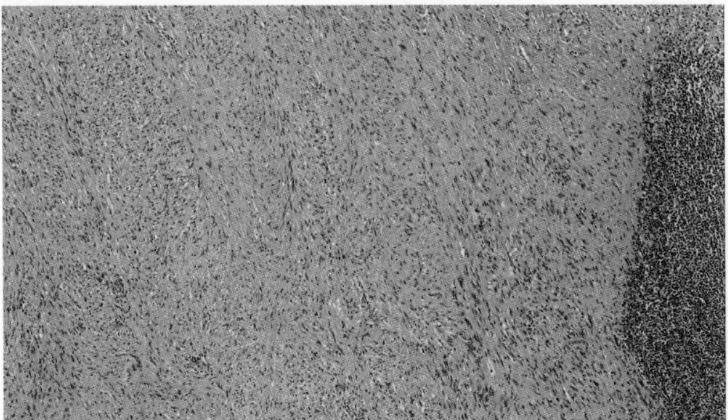

FIGURE 30.19 Gastric schwannoma composed of bland spindle cells arranged in vague fascicles.

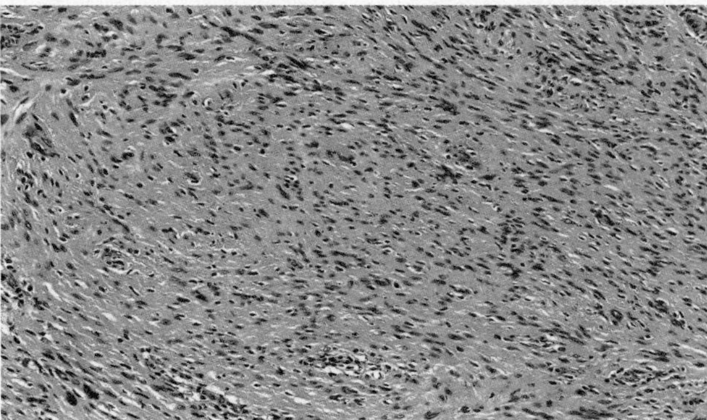

FIGURE 30.20 Gastric schwannoma composed of spindle cells with hyperchromatic nuclei with tapering ends and inconspicuous nucleoli.

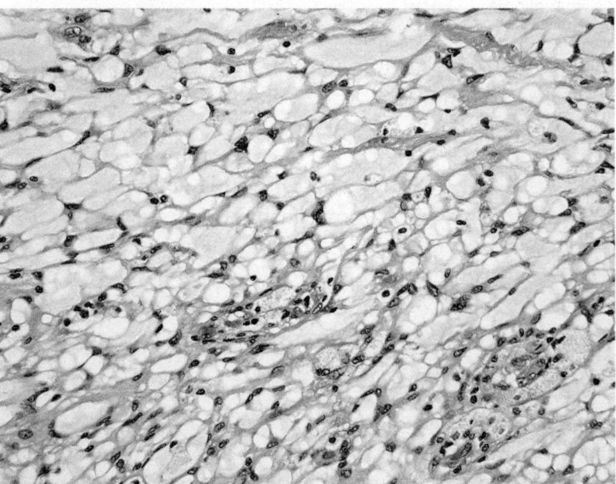

FIGURE 30.21 Microcystic/reticular schwannoma of the stomach composed of an anastomosing network of spindle cells with eosinophilic cytoplasm.

Pathological Features

Gross and Microscopic Findings

Schwannomas are grossly well circumscribed, round or ovoid mural lesions that are devoid of a capsule. Grossly, the lesions are homogeneous and firm with a tan to yellow cut surface without areas of cystic change or necrosis. Histologically, GI schwannomas are quite different from schwannomas of the central nervous system and peripheral soft tissue. The nuclear palisading, Verocay bodies, and hyalinized vessels typically seen in peripheral schwannomas are essentially absent in GI schwannomas. Also, unlike their soft tissue counterparts, GI schwannomas have a discontinuous cuff of lymphoid cells, often with germinal center formation, at the periphery of the lesion (Fig. 30.18). The cellularity of these lesions varies in different portions of the tumor because of the amount of collagenous or myxoid stroma present. Some areas may be highly cellular and contain abortive fascicles or whorls (Fig. 30.19); other, less cellular areas may have a prominent hyalinized or myxoid stroma imparting a microtrabecular pattern. Scattered lymphocytes and plasma cells are often found within the tumor. The spindle cells composing the lesions have elongated, hyperchromatic nuclei with tapering ends, occasional intranuclear inclusions, and inconspicuous nucleoli (Fig. 30.20). Scattered cells with nuclear atypia may be present, but mitotic activity is usually low; rarely, mitotic activity can be greater than 10 per 50 HPFs.[154] Although the lesion is generally circumscribed, it can infiltrate the muscularis mucosae and entrap epithelium.

Although GI schwannomas are predominantly spindled, rare cases of epithelioid schwannoma have been described with the cells arranged in cords, sheets, and even a pseudoglandular pattern.[148] Another rare histological variant of schwannoma described within the GI tract is the microcystic/reticular schwannoma.[154] This variant is different from conventional GI schwannomas in that the usual peripheral lymphoid cuff is lacking and the lesions are composed of anastomosing strands of tumor cells with either round, oval, or tapering nuclei and eosinophilic cytoplasm set within a myxoid, fibrillary, or collagenous stroma (Fig. 30.21).[154]

Immunohistochemistry and Molecular Findings

Similar to their soft tissue counterparts, GI schwannomas are strongly and diffusely immunoreactive for S100 protein, SOX10, and GFAP, and they can show focal CD34 staining. These lesions are consistently negative for KIT, keratins, and muscle markers.

Not only are GI schwannomas histologically different from their conventional soft tissue counterparts, but they are also different molecularly. The somatic *NF2* gene mutations that are common in sporadic soft tissue schwannomas are unusual events in GI schwannomas.[155] GI schwannomas lack an association with neurofibromatosis, with only one reported instance of identification of a gastric schwannoma in a patient with NF1.[127,149,156] In contrast to GIST, which

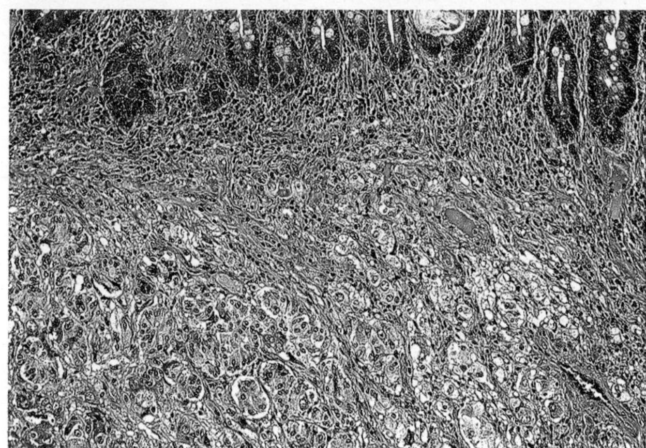

FIGURE 30.22 Low-magnification image of a duodenal gangliocytic paraganglioma.

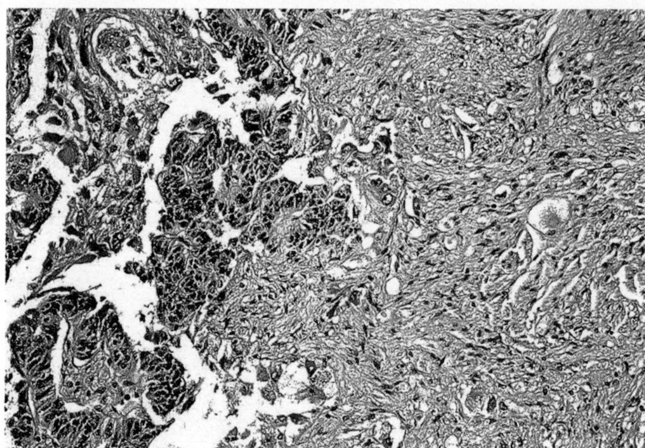

FIGURE 30.23 Gangliocytic paraganglioma composed of an admixture of epithelioid neuroendocrine cells *(left half of image)* and ganglioneuroma-like areas *(right half of image)*.

falls in the differential diagnosis, GI schwannomas lack *KIT* and *PDGFRA* mutations.

Treatment and Prognosis

Studies of GI schwannoma with follow-up have shown benign behavior with no malignant variants or evidence of metastasis identified.[147-153] Complete excision is the preferred management of this lesion.

Gangliocytic Paraganglioma

Clinical Features

The term *gangliocytic paraganglioma* was coined by Kepes and Zacharias in 1971 when they recognized features of both paraganglioma and ganglioneuroma within the same lesion.[157] Gangliocytic paraganglioma is a rare tumor that most commonly arises in the second portion of the duodenum.[158] However, examples have been described in a wide range of anatomic sites.[159] Common presenting symptoms include GI bleeding, abdominal pain, and obstruction.[160,161] Rarely, cases have been identified incidentally at endoscopy or autopsy.[162]

Pathological Features

Gross and Microscopic Findings

Gangliocytic paraganglioma is typically a circumscribed lesion centered in the submucosa and may extend into the muscularis propria. The lesion is a triphasic tumor composed of nests of epithelioid neuroendocrine cells resembling a paraganglioma, ganglion cells or ganglion-like cells, and spindle-shaped Schwann cells in a neuromatous stroma. The components are haphazardly arranged, and one component may predominate. The neuroendocrine component has a ribbon-like or trabecular growth pattern (Figs. 30.22 and 30.23), whereas the ganglion cells have variable degrees of differentiation (Fig. 30.24). The Schwann cell and neuromatous component may have a fascicular architecture.

Immunohistochemistry and Molecular Findings

By immunohistochemistry, a variety of antigens, including CK8 (CAM5.2), neuron-specific enolase (NSE), insulin, glucagon, somatostatin, serotonin, synaptophysin, and

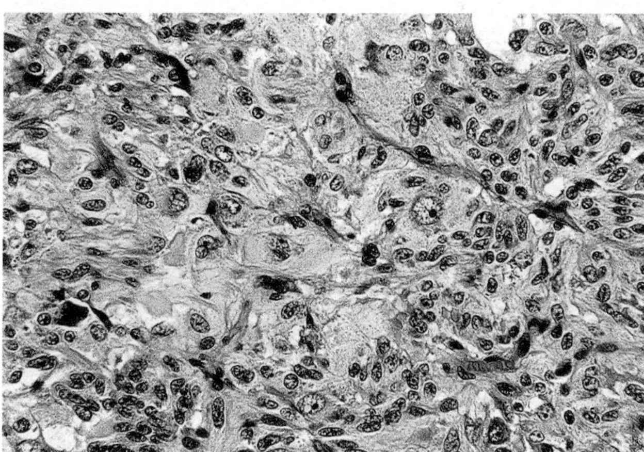

FIGURE 30.24 Gangliocytic paraganglioma containing ganglion cells in various stages of differentiation.

sometimes chromogranin, may be expressed in the neuroendocrine component. The ganglion cells express NSE, synaptophysin, neurofilament protein, and variable chromogranin. The Schwann cells and neuromatous stroma are positive for S100 protein, neurofilament protein, and NSE. S100 protein highlights a sustentacular network surrounding the neuroendocrine cell nests (Fig. 30.25). A recent study has reported *HIF2A* mutations in a subset of gangliocytic paragangliomas.[163]

Treatment and Prognosis

Most gangliocytic paragangliomas behave in a benign fashion, and local resection typically provides adequate treatment. However, rare cases with regional nodal or distant metastases have been reported.[164-168] It has been suggested that prominent nuclear pleomorphism, mitotic activity, and an infiltrative margin raise concern for aggressive behavior,[169] although many of the cases described in the literature with nodal involvement or more distant disease lacked these features. More importantly, the involvement of lymph nodes is not necessarily predictive of an adverse outcome, because patients with nodal disease were alive and well as long as 91 months after surgical resection.[160]

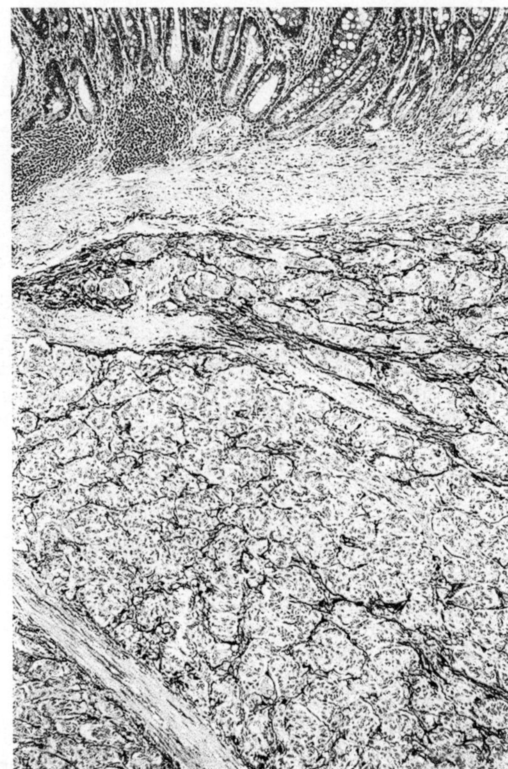

FIGURE 30.25 Gangliocytic paraganglioma showing strong S100 protein reactivity in the sustentacular network.

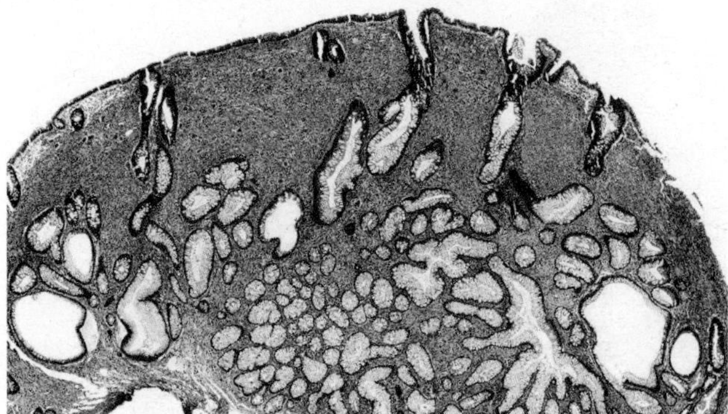

FIGURE 30.26 In this polypoid ganglioneuroma, the lamina propria is hypercellular due to a proliferation of cytologically bland, spindle-shaped cells with schwannian features that distort the adjacent crypt architecture.

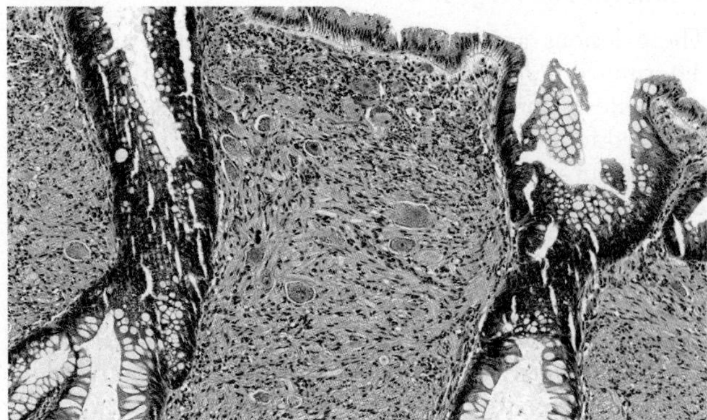

FIGURE 30.27 High-power image of a polypoid ganglioneuroma highlighting the admixture of Schwann cells and ganglion cells.

Ganglioneuroma and Ganglioneuromatosis

Clinical Features

Ganglioneuromas are benign Schwann cell and ganglion cell proliferative lesions that may occur within the GI tract. These lesions may manifest as mucosa-based polyps that arise as sporadic solitary polypoid ganglioneuromas,[170] as ganglioneuromatous polyposis with multiple polyps involving the lower and upper GI tract (in the setting of *PTEN* hamartoma tumor syndrome [Cowden syndrome]),[171-174] or as diffuse ganglioneuromatosis that may involve the deeper aspects of the bowel wall (in multiple endocrine neoplasia type IIb [MEN IIb] and NF1).[175-180] Solitary polypoid ganglioneuroma is usually identified incidentally at the time of colonoscopy; accordingly, it is seen most often in the middle-aged to older adult population who are undergoing screening. In the setting of Cowden syndrome, multiple polypoid ganglioneuromas are seen in addition to a range of other polyp types, including hamartomatous polyps, hyperplastic polyps, adenomas, inflammatory polyps, and lymphoid polyps.[171,173,181] Diffuse ganglioneuromatosis may occur across a wide age range, typically with vague symptoms including abdominal pain, constipation, or diarrhea.[175] Given the multiple cancer risks associated with Cowden syndrome, MEN IIb and NF1, it is prudent to mention the association of these syndromes when diagnosing ganglioneuromatous polyposis or ganglioneuromatosis, so that appropriate genetic testing may be initiated if clinically warranted.

Pathological Features

Gross and Microscopic Findings

Solitary polypoid ganglioneuromas are usually sessile polyps measuring less than 2 cm.[178] Ganglioneuromatous polyposis has a varied extent of involvement; in some cases, polyps are few and small, whereas other examples have shown extensive mucosal involvement. The sporadic and syndromic polypoid ganglioneuromas are histologically similar and contain a hypercellular lamina propria composed of cytologically bland, spindle-shaped cells with schwannian features (Fig. 30.26). Ganglion cells may be arranged in clusters but are often isolated and can be difficult to identify (Fig. 30.27). The glandular epithelium is often splayed apart by the expanded lamina propria, resulting in a distorted appearance at low magnification.

Diffuse ganglioneuromatosis may manifest as bowel wall thickening or a more discrete mass.[175,176,178] Histologically, the submucosal or myenteric plexus may be involved and may show a nodular expansion by Schwann cells and ganglion cells that typically extend into the adjacent submucosa or muscularis propria. Involvement of the mucosa is seen more commonly in NF1.[179]

Immunohistochemistry and Molecular Findings

The ganglion cells are immunoreactive for NSE, and neurofilament protein highlights their processes; the Schwann cells are immunoreactive for S100 protein.

As mentioned earlier, these lesions raise the possibility of MEN IIb, NF1, or Cowden syndrome with germline mutations in *RET*, *NF1*, or *PTEN*, respectively. To date, no recurrent molecular alteration has been identified in sporadic polypoid ganglioneuromas.

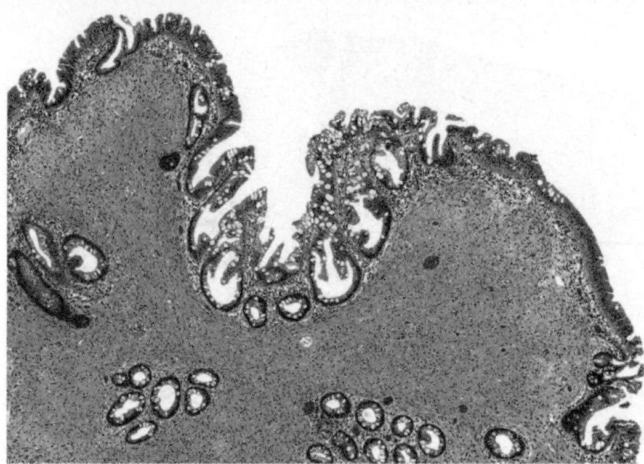

FIGURE 30.28 Mucosal perineurioma composed of bland spindle cells expanding the lamina propria and surrounding colonic crypts. The adjacent colonic mucosa contains a sessile serrated polyp.

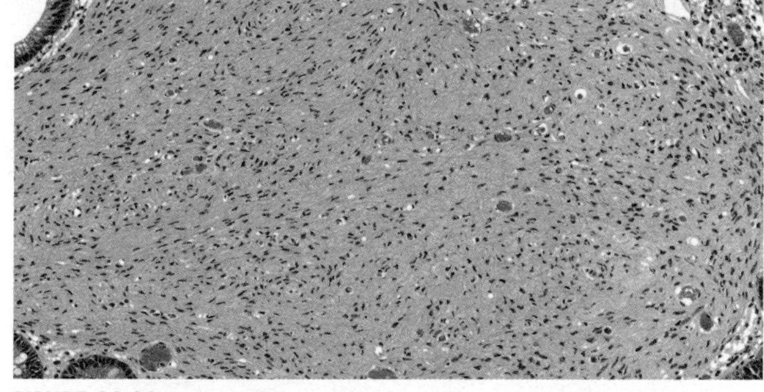

FIGURE 30.29 High-power image of a mucosal perineurioma reveals a haphazard arrangement of bland spindle cells expanding the lamina propria.

Treatment and Prognosis

These lesions are benign, and management is ultimately determined based on whether a germline mutation is identified. Resection of the affected segment of bowel may be required for symptom management in patients with diffuse ganglioneuromatosis.

Mucosal Perineurioma

Clinical Features and Background

The mucosal polypoid lesion that is now referred to as a *mucosal perineurioma* represents what was described in the earlier literature as a "benign fibroblastic polyp."[182-186] Mucosal perineuriomas are benign lesions composed of perineurial cells and are often identified incidentally at colonoscopy.[183] These small, sessile lesions are more commonly identified in women and have a predilection for the rectosigmoid.[182,183,186]

Pathological Features

Gross and Microscopic Findings

Mucosal perineuriomas average 4 mm in diameter and are predominantly solitary lesions composed of bland, ovoid, or elongated spindle cells that expand the lamina propria and splay the crypts, often with a whorled growth pattern around crypts. The proliferation is centered in the mucosa but may extend into the superficial submucosa. The spindle cells contain ovoid or slender nuclei with fine chromatin and pale eosinophilic cytoplasm. In most cases, mucosal perineuriomas are associated with hyperplastic polyps or sessile serrated polyps (Figs. 30.28 and 30.29).[182,184,185]

Immunohistochemistry and Molecular Findings

Mucosal perineuriomas express perineurial markers, including epithelial membrane antigen (EMA), GLUT1, and claudin-1, although EMA staining may be very weak. Mucosal perineuriomas are negative for KIT, S100 protein, smooth muscle actin, and desmin.

The associated serrated epithelium in these lesions has been shown to harbor the V600E *BRAF* mutation typical of sessile serrated polyps and hyperplastic polyps.[184,187] Based on this molecular finding and the frequent association of perineuriomatous stroma within serrated polyps, the perineurial proliferation in hybrid lesions may represent a reactive phenomenon driven by the serrated epithelium.

Treatment and Prognosis

Mucosal perineuriomas are benign, and recurrences have not been documented.

Mucosal Schwann Cell Hamartoma

Clinical Features

Mucosal Schwann cell hamartomas are sporadic polypoid lesions that are found in the colon.[188] They are asymptomatic and are usually identified on screening colonoscopy, predominantly within the sigmoid and rectum.[188] They are most commonly detected in middle-aged to elderly adults, the same group that tends to undergo colonoscopy. There is a female predominance.[188-190]

Pathological Features

Gross and Microscopic Findings

Mucosal Schwann cell hamartomas have a mean size of 2.5 mm and typically are described as small sessile polyps.[188] Histologically, the polyps are composed of a proliferation of spindle cells within the lamina propria that entrap colonic crypts and have an irregular border with the adjacent uninvolved lamina propria (Fig. 30.30). The lesion is composed of uniform, bland spindle cells with elongated or wavy nuclei with fine chromatin, inconspicuous nucleoli, eosinophilic cytoplasm, and indistinct cell borders (Fig. 30.31). Cytological atypia and mitotic activity have not been described.

Immunohistochemistry

By immunohistochemistry, the lesional cells show strong and diffuse reactivity for S100 protein (Fig. 30.32). Other markers that are typically negative include GFAP, EMA, CD34, smooth muscle actin, and KIT.[188]

Treatment and Prognosis

Mucosal Schwann cell hamartoma was first described in 2009 by Gibson and Hornick[188]; limited studies with clinical outcome are available in the literature. However, the

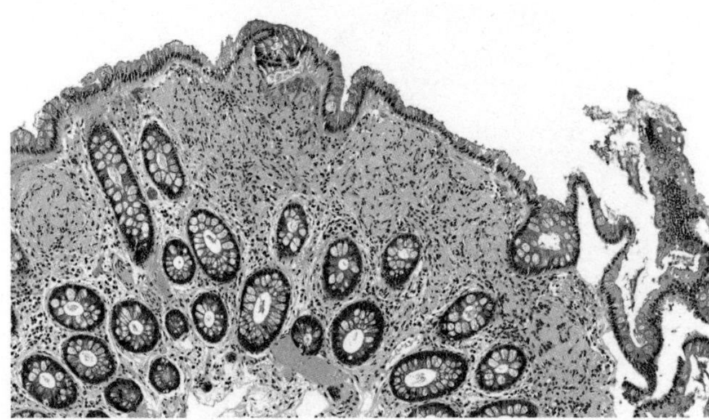

FIGURE 30.30 Mucosal Schwann cell hamartoma composed of a proliferation of elongated spindle cells within the lamina propria that has an irregular border with the adjacent uninvolved lamina propria.

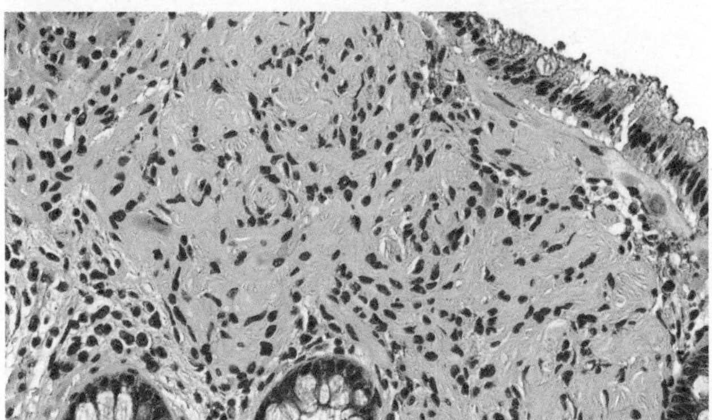

FIGURE 30.31 Mucosal Schwann cell hamartoma at high power shows the uniform, bland spindle cells with elongated nuclei, fine chromatin, inconspicuous nucleoli, and eosinophilic cytoplasm. Notice the absence of ganglion cells.

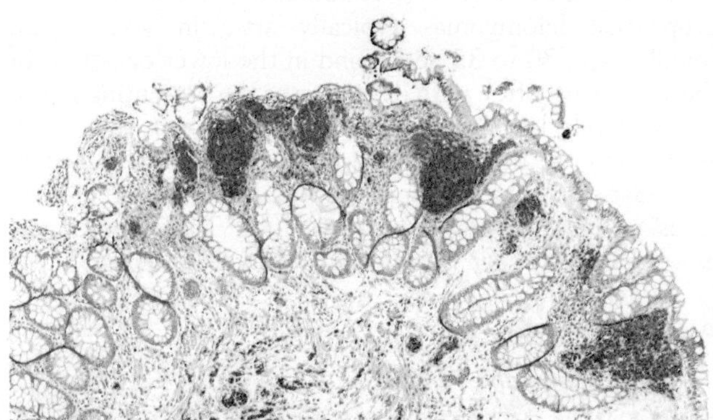

FIGURE 30.32 S100 protein immunoreactivity within the lesional cells of a mucosal Schwann cell hamartoma.

lesion is benign; recurrences have not been documented. To date, these lesions have not been associated with specific inherited syndromes (NF1, MEN IIb, or *PTEN* hamartoma tumor syndrome).

Granular Cell Tumor

Clinical Features

Most granular cell tumors of the gut arise within the esophagus, but they may arise anywhere throughout the GI tract.[191] Occasionally, one encounters multiple lesions

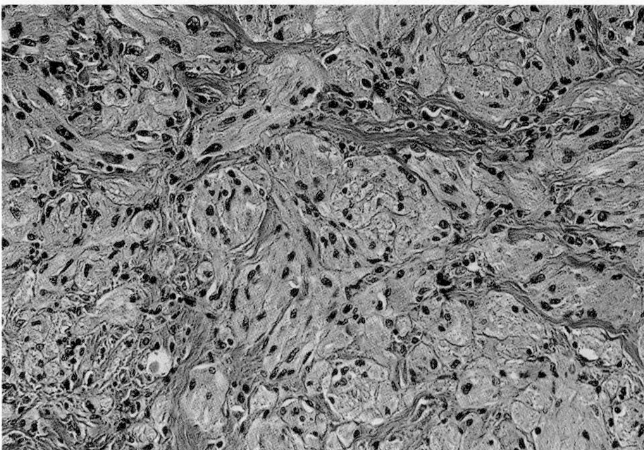

FIGURE 30.33 Granular cell tumor composed of epithelioid or spindled cells with abundant eosinophilic granular cytoplasm. The nuclei are uniform with fine chromatin.

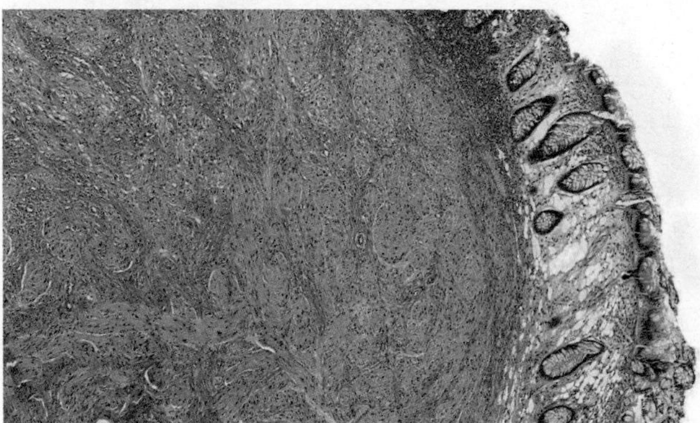

FIGURE 30.34 Granular cell tumor showing neoplastic cells arranged in nests with intervening fibrous tissue or broad sheets.

arising in different portions of the GI tract, either metachronously or synchronously.

Pathological Features

Gross and Microscopic Findings

Granular cell tumors are predominantly located in the submucosa but may involve the muscularis propria, the muscularis mucosae, and the mucosa. The lesional cells are either plump and epithelioid or spindled with abundant eosinophilic granular cytoplasm (Fig. 30.33) containing numerous periodic acid–Schiff (PAS)-positive, diastase-resistant lysosomes. The nuclei may be small and hyperchromatic or large with open chromatin. The cells are typically arranged in nests with intervening fibrous tissue or broad sheets (Fig. 30.34).

Immunohistochemistry and Molecular Findings

Granular cell tumors are uniformly immunoreactive for S100 protein (Fig. 30.35), SOX10, and NSE. Because of the presence of numerous lysosomes, the panmacrophage marker CD68 is typically immunoreactive.[192,193] Granular cell tumors harbor inactivating mutations in the endosomal pH regulators *ATP6AP1* or *ATP6AP2*.[194]

Treatment and Prognosis

GI granular cell tumors nearly always behave in a clinically benign fashion and rarely recur locally, even after incomplete

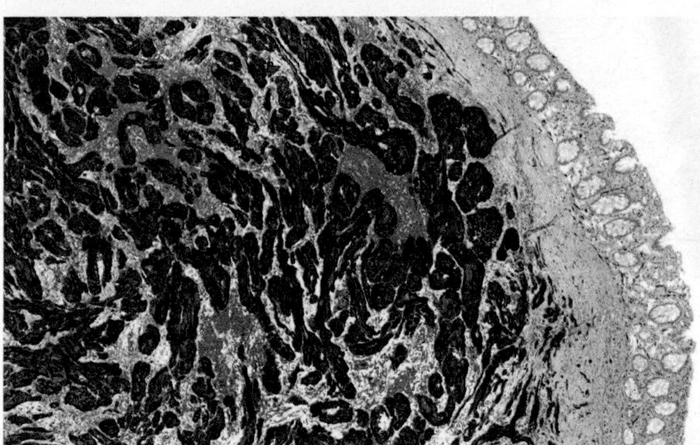

FIGURE 30.35 The typical strong and diffuse S100 protein immunoreactivity is seen within a granular cell tumor.

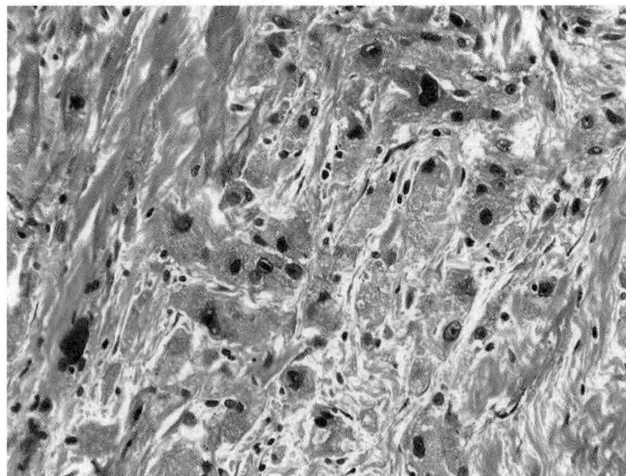

FIGURE 30.36 Rare example of a malignant granular cell tumor of the gastrointestinal tract.

excision. However, rare examples of malignant granular cell tumor have been described in the esophagus (Fig. 30.36). Minimal criteria for malignancy have not been established for GI granular cell tumors.

SMOOTH MUSCLE TUMORS

Smooth muscle tumors of the GI tract arise from the muscularis mucosae or the muscularis propria. They are characterized by positive staining for a variety of muscle markers, including smooth muscle actin and desmin, and a lack of immunoreactivity for KIT.

Leiomyoma

Clinical Features

Leiomyomas that come to clinical attention occur predominantly in the colon, rectum, and esophagus, and are rare in the stomach and small intestine.[36,44] Most are discovered incidentally during evaluations for other processes.[195] Approximately 80% of GI leiomyomas are identified in the colon and rectum as small (<1 cm) nodules that arise from the muscularis mucosae, most commonly in middle-aged to elderly men.[196] Some are attached to the external rectal wall and resemble uterine leiomyomas; estrogen and progesterone receptors may be positive in this subgroup of leiomyomas.[196]

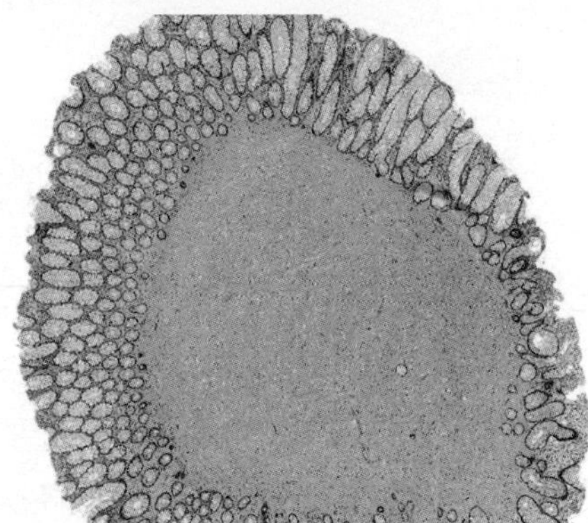

FIGURE 30.37 Colonic leiomyoma of the muscularis mucosae consisting of a low-cellularity spindle-cell lesion arranged in a fascicular pattern.

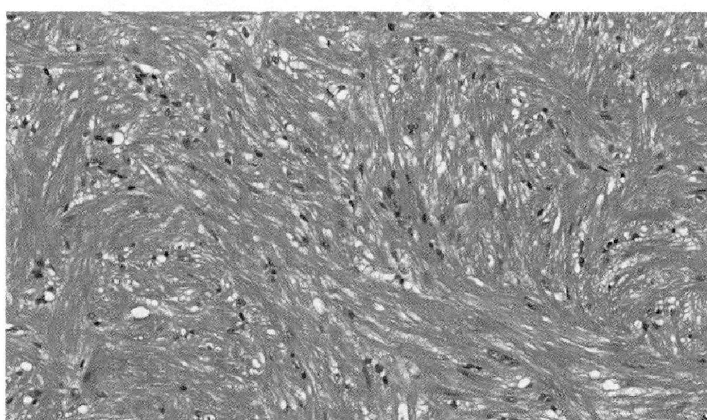

FIGURE 30.38 Colonic leiomyoma at high power showing characteristic bland, spindle-shaped cells with elongated, cigar-shaped nuclei and bright eosinophilic cytoplasm.

Approximately 10% of GI leiomyomas arise in the esophagus, developing from the muscularis propria and forming intramural masses or, less commonly, polypoid masses.[24] Esophageal leiomyomas typically arise in young men (median age, 30 to 35 years) and in the lower one-third of the esophagus, often with dysphagia as the presenting symptom.[24] Rarely, leiomyomas are found throughout the esophagus, where the muscularis propria is essentially replaced by a nodular smooth muscle proliferation, a condition referred to as esophageal leiomyomatosis.[197,198] This condition is most commonly seen in children and adolescents.

Pathological Features

Gross and Microscopic Findings

Colorectal leiomyomas are small polyps, typically with a gross or endoscopically pedunculated appearance.[196] Esophageal leiomyomas are larger lesions given their mural location, with a median size of 5 cm.[24] Histologically, GI leiomyomas, regardless of their site of origin, are characterized by a proliferation of bland, spindle-shaped cells with elongated, cigar-shaped nuclei and bright eosinophilic cytoplasm. The lesions are of low or moderate cellularity and have a fascicular architecture (Figs. 30.37 and 30.38). Mitotic activity is minimal (0 to 1 per 50 HPFs).

Immunohistochemistry and Molecular Findings

Leiomyomas are uniformly positive for smooth muscle actin, desmin, and caldesmon.[24,196] They do not express S100 or the GIST markers CD34, KIT, and DOG1.

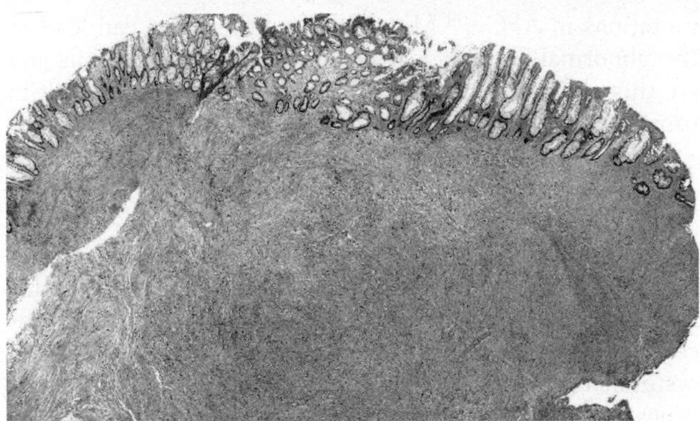

FIGURE 30.39 Leiomyosarcoma of the gastrointestinal tract. Similar to leiomyosarcoma at other sites, the tumor is a moderately cellular to hypercellular spindle cell neoplasm arranged in fascicles with an overall eosinophilic appearance.

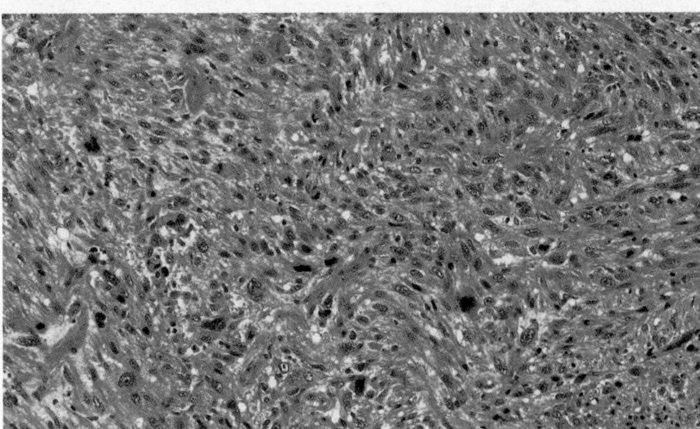

FIGURE 30.40 Leiomyosarcoma of the gastrointestinal tract showing prominent atypia with enlarged, hyperchromatic, and pleomorphic nuclei along with mitotic activity.

Treatment and Prognosis

Leiomyomas have a benign behavior, and those in the colon and rectum are usually excised easily by endoscopic polypectomy.[196] Rarely, they develop as intramural masses in the rectum and require more invasive treatment. For esophageal leiomyomas, resection via enucleation is recommended for symptomatic patients, and asymptomatic patients may be observed.

Leiomyosarcoma

Clinical Features

Leiomyosarcomas of the GI tract are rare and have not been well studied. It is now known that the lesions described as "leiomyosarcomas of the gastrointestinal tract" in previously published studies were in fact predominantly GISTs. Similar to GISTs, these tumors typically occur in older patients.[199] Although they may occur anywhere within the GI tract, they are most commonly found in the small intestine and colon.[195,199] Depending on tumor location, patients may have symptoms ranging from dysphagia, to GI bleeding with anemia, to obstruction.

Pathological Features

Gross and Microscopic Findings

GI leiomyosarcomas have a variable gross presentation as either large lesions that involve the full thickness of the bowel wall or ulcerated polypoid masses that project into the luminal aspect of the GI tract.[36,44] Leiomyosarcomas of the GI tract are indistinguishable histologically from leiomyosarcomas of other sites. They are composed of spindle cells with elongated nuclei and bright eosinophilic fibrillary cytoplasm arranged in fascicles (Fig. 30.39). Marked cytological atypia with enlarged, hyperchromatic and pleomorphic nuclei is typically seen, with brisk mitotic activity (Fig. 30.40). Areas of necrosis are common.

Immunohistochemistry and Molecular Findings

Immunohistochemistry allows for the recognition of leiomyosarcomas as true smooth muscle tumors: these lesions are strongly immunoreactive for smooth muscle actin, with variable expression of caldesmon and desmin. Focal immunoreactivity for CD34, keratins, and EMA is not uncommon.[24] S100 protein, DOG1, and KIT are consistently negative.

Treatment and Prognosis

Based on the limited data that exist, GI leiomyosarcomas are aggressive; they metastasize frequently to intraabdominal surfaces and the liver, and rarely to lymph nodes.[200] Given the rarity of these lesions, minimal criteria for malignancy have not been established. However, malignant features extrapolated from retroperitoneal and abdominal lesions considered to be leiomyosarcomas include a minimum mitotic rate of 1 to 4 per 10 HPFs, some degree of nuclear atypia, and coagulative necrosis.[201,202]

Smooth Muscle Tumor of Uncertain Malignant Potential

As stated previously, identification of atypia within a smooth muscle tumor should raise concern for malignancy. However, some cases that have been well sampled and contain only focal atypia without the presence of mitotic activity are not easily classifiable as leiomyosarcoma. In such instances, the designation "smooth muscle tumor of uncertain malignant potential" may be most appropriate.

FIBROBLASTIC/MYOFIBROBLASTIC TUMORS

Desmoid Fibromatosis

Clinical Features

Intraabdominal desmoid fibromatosis frequently involves the GI tract. Desmoid fibromatosis may arise in the pelvis and mesentery, including those associated with familial adenomatous polyposis (FAP). Desmoid fibromatosis is the most common primary tumor of the mesentery; such examples account for approximately 8% of all desmoid tumors. Most commonly, these tumors arise in the small bowel mesentery, but some originate from the ileocolic mesentery, gastrocolic ligament, retroperitoneum, or omentum. Identifying a mesenteric desmoid fibromatosis in a child should heighten clinical concern for the possibility of FAP.[203,204] Most patients have an asymptomatic abdominal mass at presentation, but some have GI bleeding or an acute abdomen secondary to bowel obstruction or perforation.

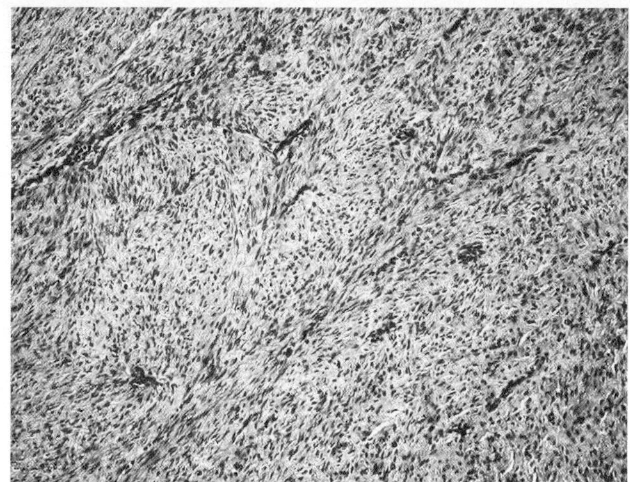

FIGURE 30.41 Low-magnification view showing a mesenteric desmoid fibromatosis composed of bland spindle cells arranged in long fascicles within a collagenous and myxoid stroma.

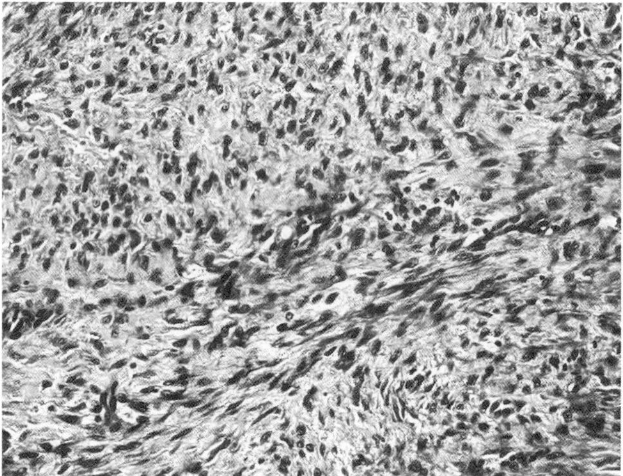

FIGURE 30.42 High-magnification view of a mesenteric desmoid fibromatosis showing bland cells with open chromatin and small nucleoli within a collagenous and myxoid stroma.

Pathological Features

Gross and Microscopic Findings

Most cases of mesenteric desmoid fibromatosis are large (10 cm or larger) at the time of excision. Although grossly circumscribed, these lesions typically infiltrate into the surrounding soft tissues, including the bowel wall. Histologically, desmoid fibromatosis is composed of cytologically bland, spindle or stellate cells that are arranged in long, sweeping fascicles in a collagenous or sometimes myxoid stroma. Scattered keloid-type collagen fibers are often present, as are dilated, thin-walled vessels, sometimes with perivascular edema (Figs. 30.41 and 30.42).

Immunohistochemistry and Molecular Findings

By immunohistochemistry, desmoid fibromatosis frequently shows aberrant nuclear and cytoplasmic β-catenin, as well as smooth muscle actin, whereas KIT, DOG1, and desmin are negative.[54,56] The lesions that arise in the setting of FAP are caused by germline mutations in *APC*, whereas nearly all sporadic cases contain somatic mutations in *CTNNB1* (which encodes β-catenin)[205-208] or, rarely, somatic mutations in *APC*.[209] Mutations in either gene can lead to the abnormal intranuclear accumulation of β-catenin and are thought to activate the downstream genes that result in tumor formation.

Treatment and Prognosis

Similar to desmoid fibromatosis elsewhere, intraabdominal examples are associated with high rates of local recurrence, often seemingly unrelated to margin status. Radiotherapy is part of the National Comprehensive Cancer Network (NCCN) treatment algorithms, as are varied systemic therapies including nonsteroidal antiinflammatory drugs, tamoxifen, methotrexate, and doxorubicin-based chemotherapy.

Inflammatory Myofibroblastic Tumor

Clinical Features

IMT is a distinctive mesenchymal neoplasm that often arises in an intraabdominal location in children and young adults, with an intermediate biological potential. Although IMTs have been reported in virtually every anatomic location, the most common extrapulmonary sites are the mesentery, omentum, and retroperitoneum.[210] The median patient age at diagnosis is 43 years, although IMT has been identified in patients as young as 9 months.[211] These lesions have been described throughout the GI tract, with the stomach, small intestine, and colon most commonly involved.[211] Patients with intraabdominal IMTs often have abdominal pain or an abdominal mass, occasionally with signs and symptoms of GI tract obstruction. Some patients also have prominent systemic manifestations, including fever, night sweats, weight loss, and malaise. A rare aggressive variant of IMT known as epithelioid inflammatory myofibroblastic sarcoma most often presents as multiple intraabdominal (mesenteric or omental) masses in young to middle-aged adults, with a marked male predominance.[212]

Pathological Features

Gross and Microscopic Findings

Grossly, most IMTs are lobular or multinodular with a rubbery cut surface; sometimes the presence of calcifications provides a gritty sensation when the lesion is cut. Although most are solitary lesions, multiple nodules restricted to the same anatomic location are found in as many as one-third of cases.[210] Histologically, a variety of patterns may be seen, either in the same tumor or in different tumors. Some are composed of cytologically bland, spindle or stellate cells arranged in a variably collagenous or myxoid stroma with scattered inflammatory cells, closely resembling nodular fasciitis. Others are composed of a compact proliferation of spindle cells arranged in a fascicular growth pattern (Figs. 30.43 and 30.44). Other foci may be sparsely cellular, with cytologically bland cells deposited in a sclerotic stroma. A lymphoplasmacytic infiltrate is often conspicuous, and small areas of calcification or metaplastic bone may also be observed. Epithelioid inflammatory myofibroblastic sarcoma is composed of sheets of large epithelioid cells with vesicular chromatin, prominent nucleoli, and moderate amounts of amphophilic or eosinophilic cytoplasm, typically embedded in an abundant myxoid stroma with prominent neutrophils (Fig. 30.45).

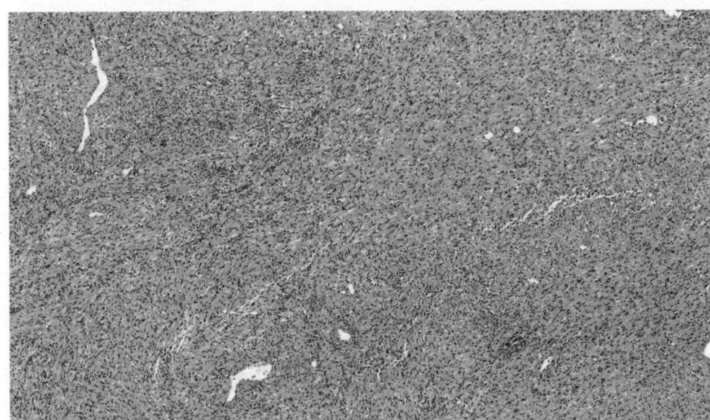

FIGURE 30.43 Inflammatory myofibroblastic tumor composed of spindle cells arranged in vague fascicles with a collagenous stroma.

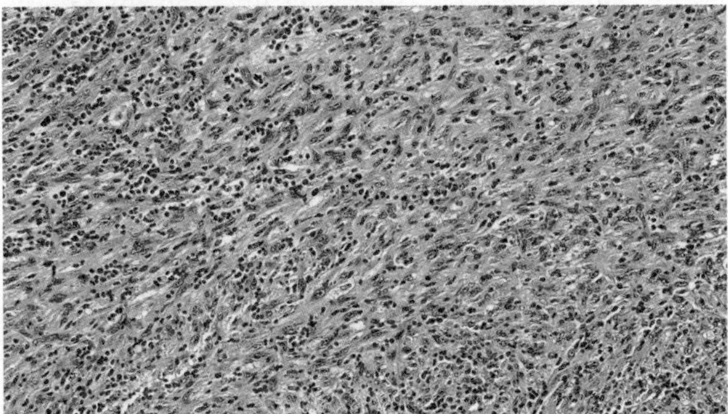

FIGURE 30.44 High-magnification view of an inflammatory myofibroblastic tumor showing bland spindle cells with discernible nucleoli and a prominent lymphoplasmacytic infiltrate.

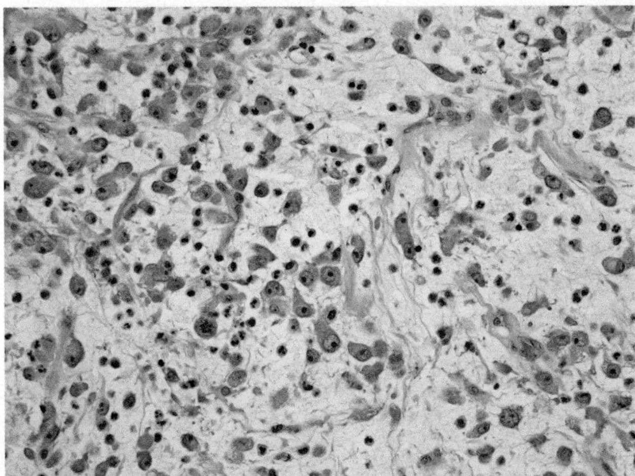

FIGURE 30.45 Epithelioid inflammatory myofibroblastic sarcoma composed of epithelioid cells with prominent nucleoli in a myxoid stroma with scattered neutrophils.

Immunohistochemistry and Molecular Findings

By immunohistochemistry, the neoplastic cells are usually positive for smooth muscle actin and often for desmin.[213] Focal keratin immunoreactivity may be found in up to one-third of cases. Around 60% of IMTs stain for ALK, secondary to clonal cytogenetic aberrations of the *ALK* gene, located on 2p23.[214] A small subset of IMTs is positive for ROS1 (correlating with *ROS1* rearrangements); rare examples harbor other tyrosine kinase receptor gene fusions.[215-218]

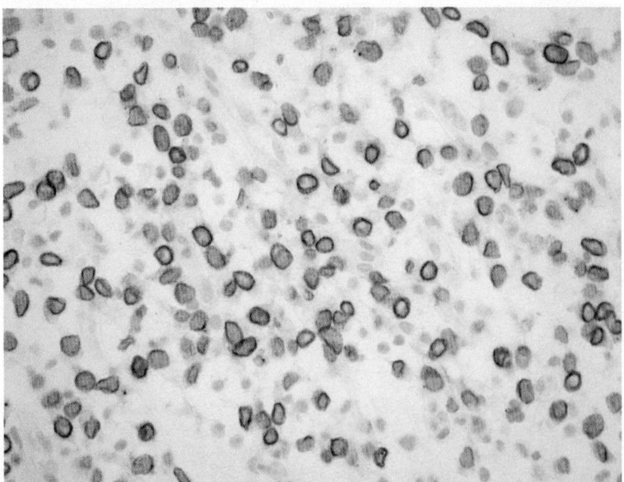

FIGURE 30.46 The characteristic nuclear membrane pattern of ALK immunostaining in an epithelioid inflammatory myofibroblastic sarcoma.

Epithelioid inflammatory myofibroblastic sarcoma is positive for desmin and usually shows a nuclear membrane pattern of ALK staining (Fig. 30.46), less often cytoplasmic staining with paranuclear accentuation; these patterns correlate with particular *ALK* gene rearrangements.[212,219] IMTs can be confused with inflammatory fibroid polyps, benign lesions that most often occur in the stomach and ileum as solitary submucosal polyps.

Treatment and Prognosis

Although most IMTs act in a clinically benign fashion, some tumors in this location have a propensity for more aggressive behavior than their extraabdominal counterparts, with recurrence rates of 23% to 37%.[210,213] A small minority of patients with conventional IMT develop metastatic disease, usually to the lungs and brain.[213] Epithelioid inflammatory myofibroblastic sarcoma pursues an aggressive clinical course with rapid local recurrences and sometimes distant metastases.[212] Patients with aggressive IMTs benefit from treatment with ALK inhibitors such as crizotinib.[220]

VASCULAR AND PERIVASCULAR TUMORS

Hemangiomas and Other Benign Vascular Proliferations

Hemangiomas, lymphangiomas, and vascular malformations are relatively common throughout the GI tract and resemble their counterparts in the peripheral soft tissues. Some are composed of large, cavernous vascular channels, and others contain lobules of small, capillary-sized vessels. These vascular proliferations, particularly lymphangiomas and vascular malformations (the latter referred to as *angiodysplasia* at this site), may sometimes involve large segments of the GI tract. The latter can be associated with life-threatening hemorrhage.

Glomus Tumor

Clinical Features

Glomus tumors are composed of modified smooth muscle cells that are a counterpart of the perivascular glomus

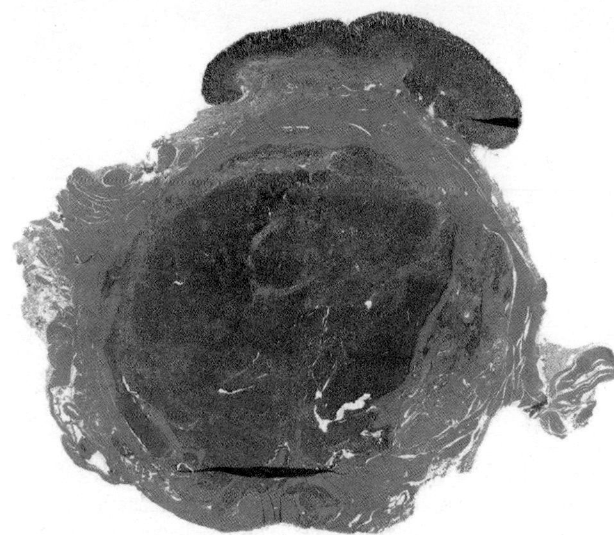

FIGURE 30.47 Low-magnification view showing a gastric glomus tumor involving the muscularis propria as a rounded nodule.

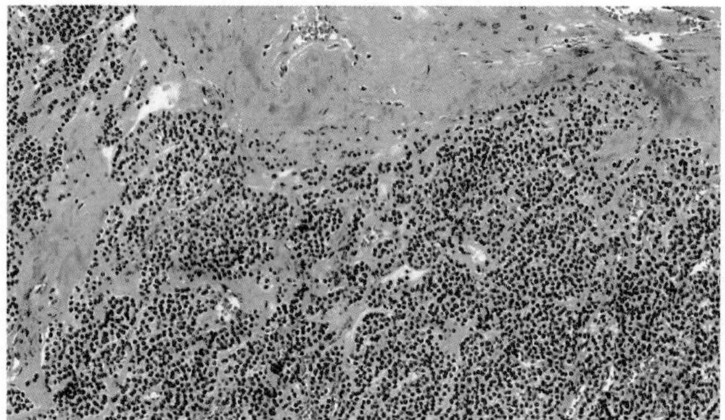

FIGURE 30.48 Gastric glomus tumor composed of uniform cells with an organoid architecture and minimal intervening stroma.

body. These tumors occur most commonly in the peripheral soft tissues, especially the distal extremities. Rare cases have been identified within the GI tract, most commonly within the stomach.[221] In a study of GI glomus tumors by Miettinen et al.,[222] all but 1 of 32 glomus tumors were located in the stomach; the only exception was a cecal tumor. These tumors are found more frequently in women. The median age at diagnosis is 55 years, and the presenting signs and symptoms include GI bleeding or ulcer-like symptoms.

Pathological Features

Gross and Microscopic Findings

GI glomus tumors typically involve the muscularis propria (Fig. 30.47) and are histologically similar to their peripheral soft tissue counterparts. The distinctive glomus cell has a round uniform shape and a discrete round nucleus surrounded by pale to eosinophilic cytoplasm, with characteristic sharply defined cell borders. The cells are arranged in sheets and nests surrounding thin-walled, dilated, and hemangiopericytoma-like vascular spaces in a hyalinized and occasionally myxoid stroma (Figs. 30.48 and 30.49). Mitotic activity is typically low (<5 per 50 HPFs). Focal atypia and vascular invasion have been observed in rare cases.

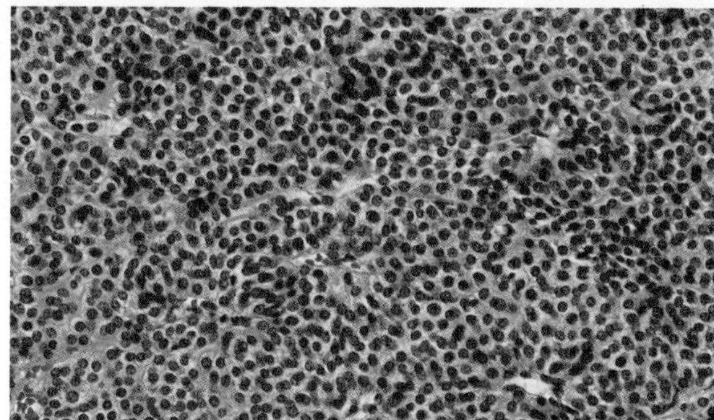

FIGURE 30.49 High-magnification view showing a gastric glomus tumor composed of uniform round cells with round nuclei and pale cytoplasm.

Immunohistochemistry and Molecular Findings

The neoplastic cells are strongly immunoreactive for smooth muscle actin and often for caldesmon, whereas staining for desmin, S100 protein, and KIT is absent. Weak staining for synaptophysin is sometimes observed; this finding may lead to misdiagnosis as a well-differentiated neuroendocrine tumor. Miettinen et al. also report an elaborate network of pericellular collagen type IV and laminin immunoreactivity in these tumors, although these markers are rarely used in clinical practice.[222] Glomus tumors harbor rearrangements involving *NOTCH* genes.[223]

Treatment and Prognosis

Most gastric glomus tumors behave in a clinically benign fashion. In the study by Miettinen et al., follow-up of 32 GI glomus tumors revealed development of metastatic disease in only one patient.[222] In this case, the primary tumor had cytological atypia with focal areas of spindle cell morphology, a low mitotic count, and vascular invasion. In long-term follow-up (median 219 months), the remaining patients all remained disease free.[222]

Angiosarcoma and Kaposi Sarcoma

Clinical Features

Angiosarcoma of the GI tract is exceptionally rare, described in case reports and small series.[224] Involvement of the GI tract by angiosarcoma has been reported mainly in the setting of metastatic disease.[225] Kaposi sarcoma (KS) is seen in the setting of immunosuppression; in the United States, it is most commonly described after transplantation or as an AIDS-related complication. KS is the most common GI tumor in the setting of AIDS.[226] That said, the use of highly active antiretroviral therapy (HAART) has dramatically reduced but not eliminated the incidence of KS. Patients with either angiosarcoma or KS may be asymptomatic, or they may experience weight loss, nausea, vomiting, GI bleeding, or diarrhea.[227] Endoscopic appearances range from multiple flat or slightly elevated purple lesions to larger nodular and polypoid tumors.[228,229]

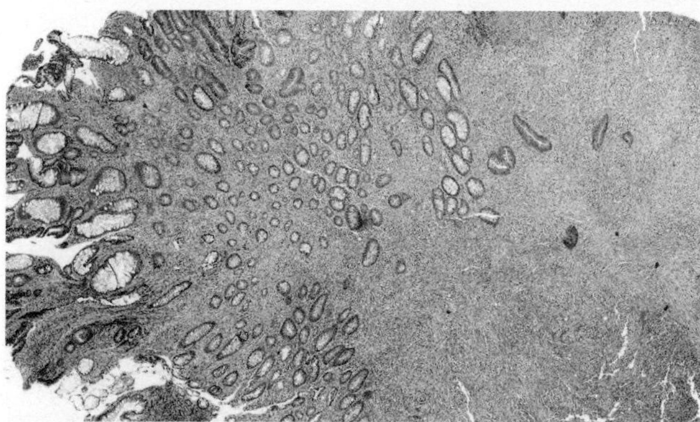

FIGURE 30.50 Low-magnification view of an epithelioid angiosarcoma that manifested as a polyp discovered during colonoscopy for evaluation of gastrointestinal bleeding. Note the expansion of the lamina propria by atypical epithelioid cells splaying apart the colonic crypts.

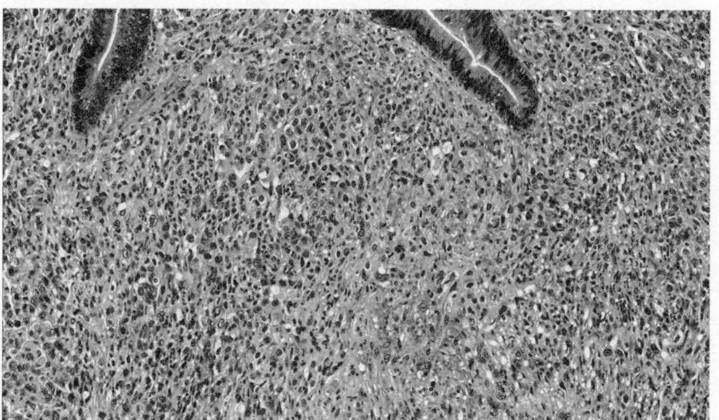

FIGURE 30.51 Colonic epithelioid angiosarcoma composed of sheets of epithelioid cells with large nuclei, prominent nucleoli, and eosinophilic cytoplasm. Extravasated red blood cells are present within the background.

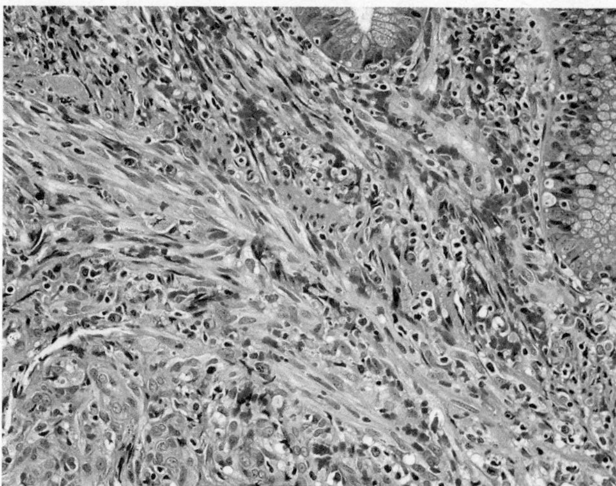

FIGURE 30.52 Kaposi sarcoma of the colon composed of fascicles of uniform and bland spindle cells infiltrating the lamina propria.

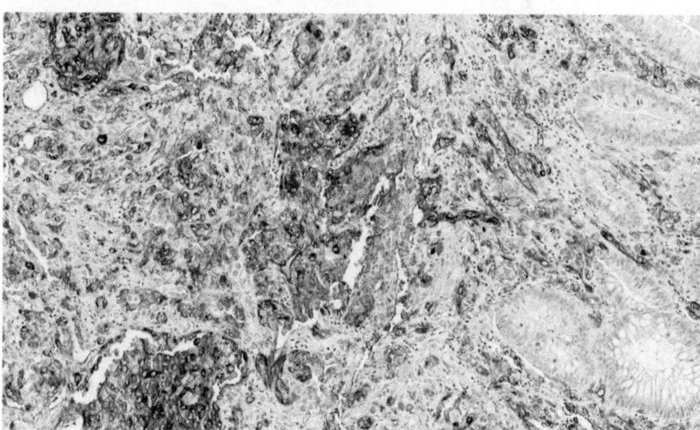

FIGURE 30.53 CD34 immunoreactivity within an epithelioid angiosarcoma.

Pathological Features

Gross and Microscopic Findings

Grossly, both tumor types can have a varied appearance as polypoid mucosal nodules, mucosal ulcerations, or mural and serosal masses with prominent hemorrhage. Angiosarcoma is typified by the presence of spindled or epithelioid cells that form primitive vascular channels that dissect through the tissue. In the GI tract, epithelioid morphology is common and may mimic a poorly differentiated carcinoma (Figs. 30.50 and 30.51).[224] The presence of only rudimentary lumen formation or rare intracytoplasmic vacuoles can also confound the diagnosis. Histologically, KS is composed of monomorphic spindle cells that are separated by slitlike vessels and are arranged in vague fascicles (Fig. 30.52).

Immunohistochemistry and Molecular Findings

In both angiosarcoma and KS, the vascular endothelial markers CD31, CD34, and ERG are typically expressed (Fig. 30.53). The more poorly differentiated the histology, the greater the likelihood that expression of CD34 will be diminished or absent. It is important to bear in mind that the epithelioid variant of angiosarcoma may show keratin immunoreactivity that may be diffuse, mimicking carcinoma.[224]

Human herpesvirus 8 (HHV-8) has been identified as the causative agent of KS.[230] Antibodies to latent nuclear antigen 1 (LNA-1), a protein encoded by HHV-8, have shown excellent sensitivity and specificity in identifying KS (Fig. 30.54).[231,232]

Treatment and Prognosis

Given the rarity of angiosarcoma involving the GI tract, treatment experience is limited. However, localized disease is typically treated with surgical resection, chemotherapy, and radiation therapy. As with angiosarcoma in other sites, the course of disease is rapidly progressive despite aggressive therapy.

The behavior of KS depends on several factors including the immune status of the host, the presence of opportunistic infections, and the stage of the disease. Surgery, other than for tissue diagnosis, is not a mainstay of treatment; rather, chemotherapy and/or radiation therapy are the preferred treatment modalities.

ADIPOCYTIC TUMORS

Lipomas and Liposarcomas

Clinical Features

Lipomas are relatively common tumors in the GI tract. They are most often seen in the right colon as small, submucosal polypoid lesions.[233,234] Although many of these lesions are identified incidentally, large lesions may be ulcerated, with some coming to attention secondary to hemorrhage.[235,236]

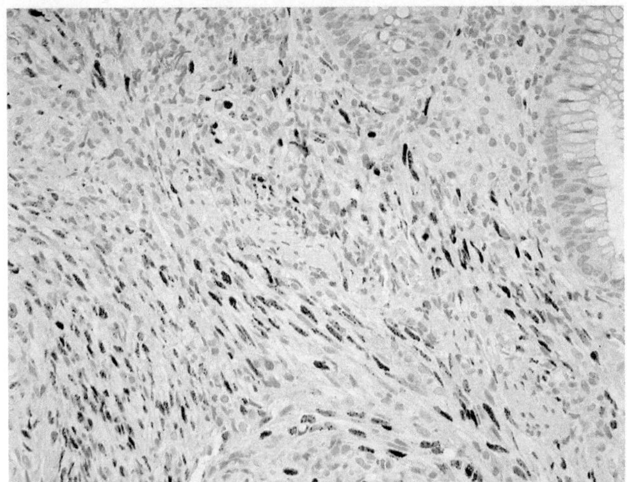

FIGURE 30.54 HHV-8 immunoreactivity in a colonic Kaposi sarcoma.

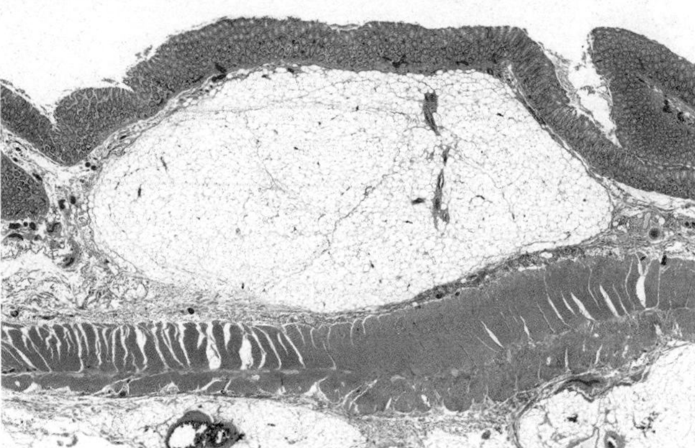

FIGURE 30.55 Colonic lipoma composed of a circumscribed submucosal proliferation of uniform, mature adipocytes without fibrous septa.

Liposarcomas (LPS) involving the GI tract are exceptionally rare. Most are retroperitoneal well-differentiated LPS or dedifferentiated LPS that secondarily involve the gut. Rarely, well-differentiated LPS presents as a large esophageal polyp; such tumors were formerly known as *giant fibrovascular polyp* of the esophagus.[237,238]

Pathological Features

Gross and Microscopic Findings

Lipomas are usually centered in the submucosa and often compress the overlying muscularis mucosae; if large enough, they can cause prolapse-type changes within the adjacent mucosa (Fig. 30.55). Histologically, these tumors are similar to their peripheral counterparts and are composed of mature adipocytes of uniform size. Lipomas lack fibrous septa, nuclear hyperchromasia, or cytological atypia.

As mentioned previously, LPS involving the GI tract represent secondary involvement from tumors arising in the retroperitoneum. Grossly, these lesions are large and typically encase multiple organs, necessitating a large resection. Well-differentiated LPS are composed of adipocytes of variable size with scattered enlarged hyperchromatic nuclei that are frequently best appreciated within the fibrous septa that course throughout the lesion. Well-differentiated LPS may progress to a dedifferentiated LPS that most commonly resembles an undifferentiated pleomorphic sarcoma or a nondescript spindle cell sarcoma; however, most dedifferentiated LPS arise de novo. Polypoid well-differentiated LPS of the esophagus are long tubular structures covered by squamous mucosa; in addition to the features described earlier, such lesions often contain superficial granulation tissue and chronic inflammation, mimicking an inflammatory polyp.

Immunohistochemistry and Molecular Findings

Lipoma is a histological diagnosis rendered on hematoxylin and eosin–stained slides. Difficulty in establishing a diagnosis of well-differentiated LPS can be challenging, especially with small biopsy specimens. That said, the usual clinical scenario is that of a large retroperitoneal mass, which can help guide appropriate ancillary testing when one is faced with a lipomatous lesion. Well-differentiated LPS and dedifferentiated LPS are typified by giant marker and ring chromosomes[239,240] that contain amplified sequences of 12q13–15, resulting in amplification of the *MDM2* gene (12q14) as well as other nearby genes. In cases of potential well-differentiated LPS that lack diagnostic cytological atypia, immunohistochemistry or fluorescence in situ hybridization (FISH) to identify the presence of MDM2 protein overexpression or *MDM2* gene amplification can be useful.[241]

Treatment and Prognosis

Lipomas are benign lesions that only require treatment if symptomatic. Many cases are not excised when recognized by the gastroenterologist at colonoscopy. LPS of the retroperitoneum that involve adjacent organs are often treated by complex multivisceral resection sometimes followed by adjuvant radiation.

MISCELLANEOUS RARE TUMORS

Perivascular Epithelioid Cell Tumor

Clinical Features

The umbrella term *perivascular epithelioid cell tumor (PEComa)* encompasses several mesenchymal lesions that are characterized by mixed smooth muscle and melanocytic differentiation and are composed of so-called "perivascular epithelioid" cells.[242-244] The PEComa family of tumors includes angiomyolipoma, lymphangioleiomyomatosis, and rare PEComas of other diverse anatomic sites.[244] The GI tract is one of the most common anatomic locations for PEComas. Renal angiomyolipoma and pulmonary lymphangioleiomyomatosis are seen frequently in tuberous sclerosis complex, whereas other PEComas are usually sporadic.

GI PEComas occur over a wide age range, with almost one third of cases arising in the pediatric population. These tumors are most frequently identified in the colon and rectum; however, involvement of the small bowel, stomach, and gallbladder has been described.[245,246] Lesions that are large may cause anemia, abdominal pain, or obstruction, but some examples have been identified incidentally during screening colonoscopy.[246]

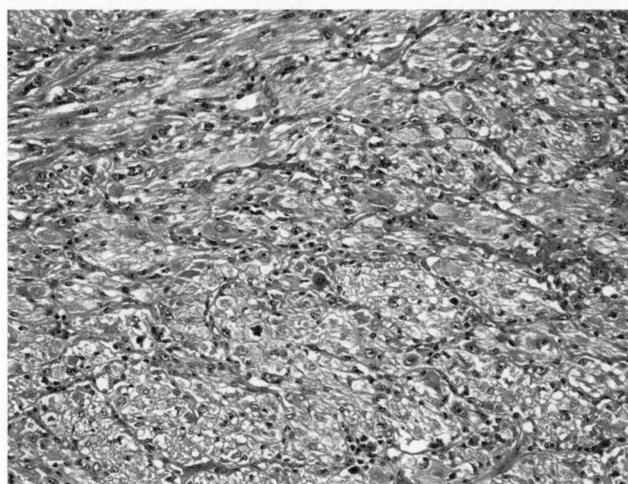

FIGURE 30.56 Gastrointestinal perivascular epithelioid cell tumor (PEComa) composed of epithelioid cells with a nested architecture.

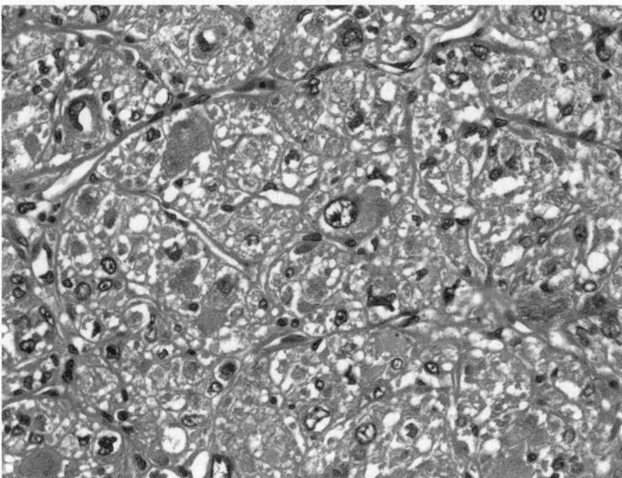

FIGURE 30.57 High-power image of a gastrointestinal perivascular epithelioid cell tumor (PEComa) highlighting the cytological features, including variable nucleoli and granular eosinophilic cytoplasm. This malignant example has prominent cytological atypia.

Pathological Features

Gross and Microscopic Findings

Grossly, the lesions may be either small and centered in the mucosa and submucosa or larger (>5 cm) and involve the full thickness of the bowel wall.[246] Histologically, most PEComas have a nested or trabecular architecture and are composed of epithelioid cells with round to oval nuclei, variable nucleoli, and clear or granular eosinophilic cytoplasm; the nests are surrounded by a delicate capillary vasculature (Figs. 30.56 and 30.57). Often, the lesional cells condense around blood vessels. Rarely, a spindle cell component is identifiable.

Immunohistochemistry and Molecular Findings

PEComas variably express the melanocytic markers HMB-45 and melan A, as well as the smooth muscle markers SMA and desmin.[246] Argani et al. identified a subset of lesions classified as PEComas that harbor *TFE3* gene translocations

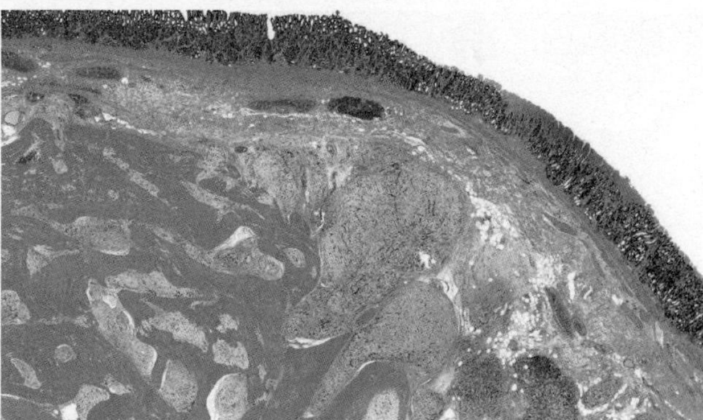

FIGURE 30.58 Plexiform fibromyxoma seen at low magnification as multiple discontinuous myxoid nodules interspersed within the muscularis propria.

(and show nuclear staining for TFE3 by immunohistochemistry).[247] Most other PEComas have *TSC2* mutations.[248]

Treatment and Prognosis

Some PEComas behave in a benign fashion, whereas others follow an aggressive clinical course; currently, there is uncertainty as to which pathological features best predict a poor outcome. It is believed that non-GI PEComas with malignant behavior commonly contain areas of coagulative necrosis, a high mitotic index, and marked cytological atypia.[244,246,249] Doyle et al. have published a series of 35 GI tract PEComas with outcome; the histological features in this series that were significantly associated with metastatic disease included marked nuclear atypia, diffuse pleomorphism, and ≥2 mitoses per 10 HPFs.[246] Resection is the mainstay of treatment; in patients with metastatic disease, mTOR inhibitors have demonstrated some benefit for patients with aggressive malignant PEComas.[250]

Plexiform Fibromyxoma

Clinical Features

Plexiform fibromyxoma is a distinct entity that was previously reported in the literature under the terms *plexiform angiomyxoid myofibroblastic tumor* and *myxoma*.[251-255] The mean patient age is 43 years, with a range from 7 to 75 years; thus far, the male-to-female ratio has been approximately 1:1. Most of these tumors have involved the antrum and pyloric region, with presenting symptoms including anemia, gastric ulcer, nausea, and pyloric obstruction. One case was identified incidentally during cholecystectomy.[252] On endoscopy, the lesions have been described as submucosal masses, frequently with overlying mucosal ulceration.

Pathological Features

Gross and Microscopic Findings

The lesions have a mean size of 6.3 cm (range, 1.9 to 15 cm), and they arise in the antrum, with one third of cases extending into the duodenum.[251-255] Grossly, the lesions are unencapsulated and lobulated masses that may be submucosal or transmural with serosal extragastric components that may form submesothelial nodules; on cut section, a

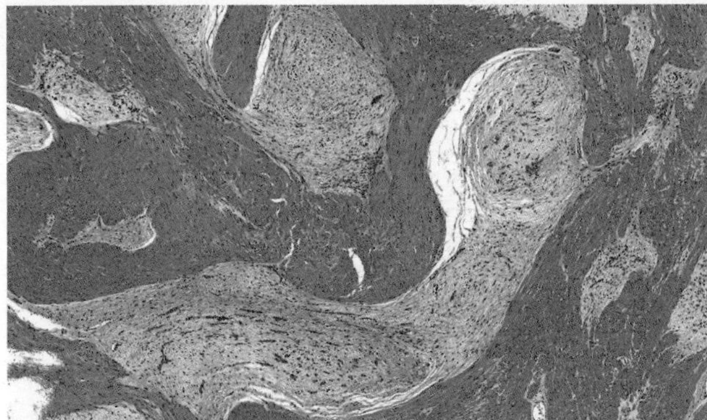

FIGURE 30.59 Plexiform fibromyxoma containing hypocellular myxoid nodules composed of spindle cells that are bland with eosinophilic cytoplasm and inconspicuous nucleoli.

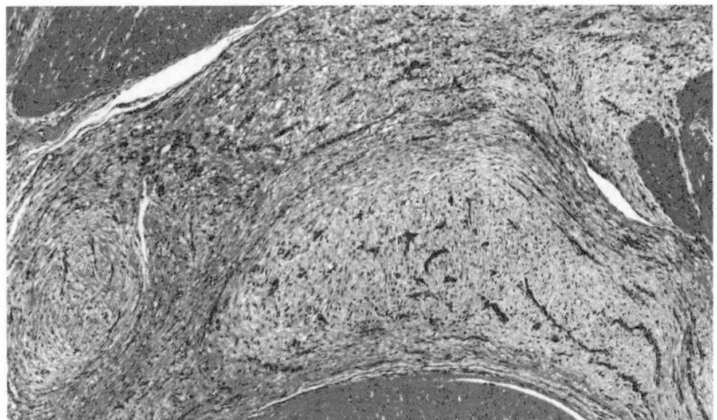

FIGURE 30.60 High-power image of a plexiform fibromyxoma showing a prominent arborizing capillary network within the stroma.

typical gelatinous or mucoid appearance is appreciated.[254] Histologically, these lesions have a multinodular appearance at low power, with discontinuous myxoid nodules typically interspersed within the muscularis propria (Fig. 30.58). The myxoid nodules are relatively hypocellular; myxoid or fibromyxoid matrix separates the component spindle cells, which are bland with eosinophilic cytoplasm and inconspicuous nucleoli (Fig. 30.59). Frequently, a rich arborizing capillary network is appreciated within the stroma (Fig. 30.60). Mitotic figures are scarce; the maximum number reported has been 4 per 50 HPFs.

Immunohistochemistry and Molecular Findings

Most of these lesions have shown immunoreactivity within the spindle cells for smooth muscle actin and muscle-specific actin (HHF35), with variable expression of desmin; none of the lesions has shown expression of KIT, CD34, DOG1, ALK, S100 protein, EMA, or keratins.[254] A subset of plexiform fibromyxomas harbors *MALAT1-GLI1* gene fusions.[256]

Treatment and Prognosis

Plexiform fibromyxoma is benign; neither recurrences nor metastatic disease have been reported after surgical resection. Miettinen et al. reviewed the largest series with long-term follow-up after excision and found that histological features typically worrisome for aggressive behavior (e.g., ulceration, mucosal invasion, vascular invasion) were not indicative of an adverse outcome.[254]

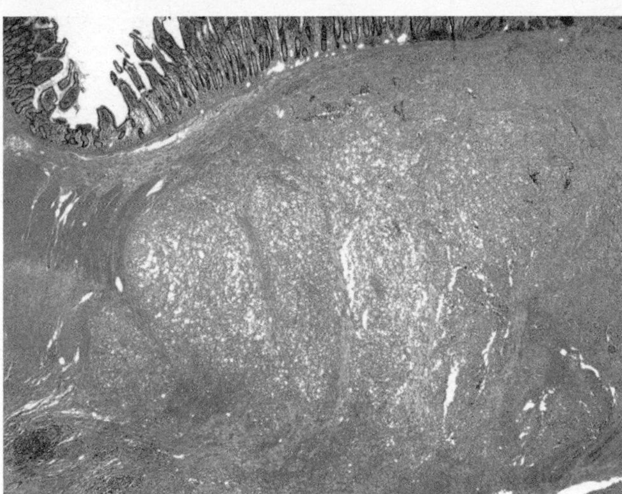

FIGURE 30.61 Gastrointestinal clear cell sarcoma–like tumor in the small bowel showing ulceration of the mucosa and involvement of the entire thickness of the bowel wall.

Gastrointestinal Clear Cell Sarcoma–Like Tumor (Malignant Gastrointestinal Neuroectodermal Tumor)

Clinical Features

A distinctive aggressive sarcoma that somewhat resembles clear cell sarcoma (CCS) of tendons and aponeuroses arises in the GI tract; such tumors have been referred to as *GI CCS-like tumor* and *malignant gastrointestinal neuroectodermal tumor (GNET)*.[257-263] These lesions have been observed in both children and adults and are most frequently identified in the small bowel.[257-263] Depending on the site of involvement, patients may experience obstruction or have nonspecific complaints of abdominal pain, nausea, or diarrhea.

Pathological Features

Gross and Microscopic Findings

These lesions typically involve the full thickness of the bowel wall, with ulceration of the overlying mucosa (Fig. 30.61). GI CCS-like tumors typically have variable growth patterns, including sheetlike, nested, and alveolar or pseudopapillary architecture. The neoplastic cells have eosinophilic to clear cytoplasm and may be round, oval, or spindled. The nuclei have an overall uniform appearance, with vesicular chromatin and small nucleoli; mitotic activity is variable (Fig. 30.62). GI CCS-like tumors often have prominent osteoclast-like giant cells (Fig. 30.63), in contrast to the occasional wreath-like tumor giant cells of conventional soft tissue CCS.[259]

Immunohistochemistry and Molecular Findings

GI CCS-like tumors are strongly positive for SOX10 and S100 protein; in contrast to conventional CCS, most GI tract tumors are negative for melanocytic markers.[263-265] However, rare primary GI tumors that are histologically identical to soft tissue CCS express melan A and HMB-45; such tumors represent conventional CCS arising in the GI tract.[264,266] NSE, synaptophysin, and CD56 may be focally positive in GI CCS-like tumors, whereas KIT, smooth muscle markers, and keratins are negative.[265]

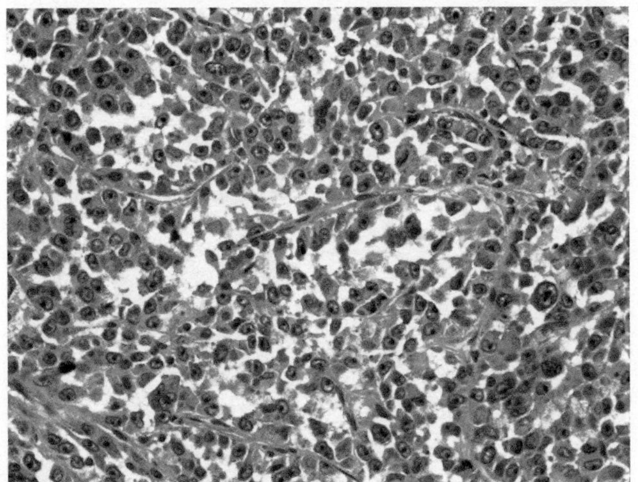

FIGURE 30.62 Gastrointestinal clear cell sarcoma–like tumor showing a nested architecture and delicate fibrovascular septa. The neoplastic cells have uniform, large nuclei with prominent nucleoli and eosinophilic cytoplasm.

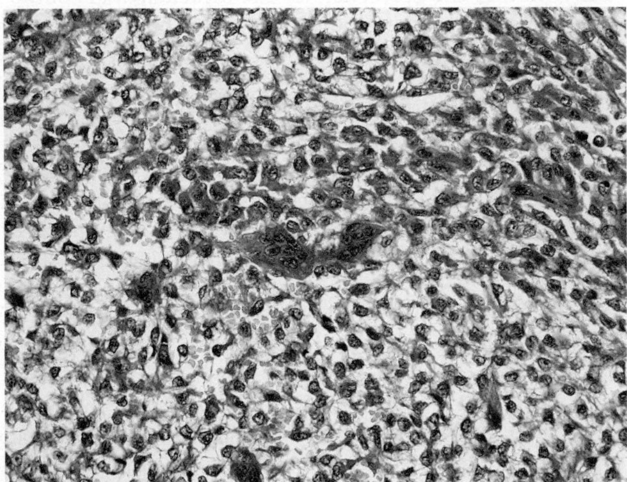

FIGURE 30.63 Multinucleated osteoclast-like giant cells may be seen within a gastrointestinal clear cell sarcoma–like tumor.

GI CCS-like tumor shares cytogenetic features with conventional CCS; both lesions harbor alterations of *EWSR1* (22q12). Most soft tissue CCS have a t(12;22)(q13;q12) translocation that results in an *EWSR1-ATF1* rearrangement,[266,267] whereas GI CCS-like tumors harbor either the *EWSR1-ATF1* or an *EWSR1-CREB1* fusion.[263,265]

Treatment and Prognosis

GI CCS-like tumor shows highly aggressive behavior, with frequent regional lymph node and liver metastases.[265] No effective systemic therapy for this sarcoma type has been identified.

Synovial Sarcoma

Clinical Features

Synovial sarcoma most commonly occurs in the extremities and harbors a characteristic t(X;18)(p11;q11) translocation that results in *SS18-SSX1* or *SS18-SSX2* rearrangements. Rare primary cases of synovial sarcoma have been documented within the GI tract, most commonly in the stomach,

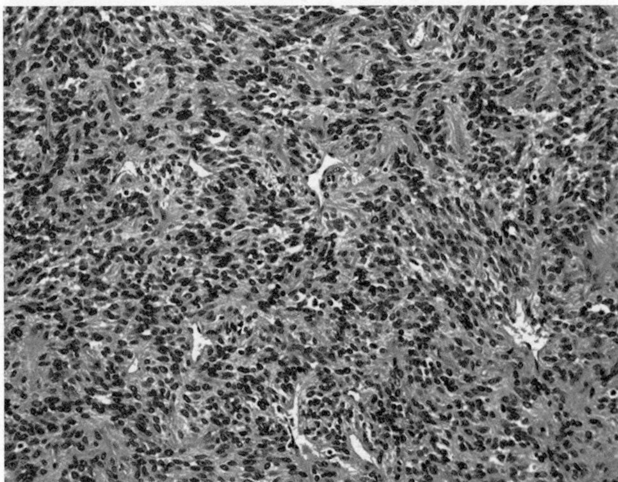

FIGURE 30.64 Monophasic synovial sarcoma composed of uniform spindle cells with a hemangiopericytoma-like vasculature.

with rare reports of synovial sarcoma at other GI sites.[268-275] GI synovial sarcomas usually affect young to middle-aged adults and appear to be somewhat more common in men.

Pathological Features

Gross and Microscopic Findings

The most common finding is that of a submucosal polypoid mass that has a luminal component. Although monophasic, biphasic, and poorly differentiated morphologies have been described in GI tract examples, the monophasic pattern predominates at this site (Fig. 30.64). Monophasic synovial sarcoma is composed of uniform spindle cells with fine chromatin, tapering nuclei, and limited cytoplasm arranged in a tight fascicular growth pattern. A variably collagenous background may be present.

Immunohistochemistry and Molecular Findings

As in their peripheral counterparts, focal keratin and EMA expression is often seen, but there is no expression of CD34 or KIT. Strong nuclear TLE1 is a typical finding. Identifying either *SS18-SSX* fusion transcripts or the presence of an *SS18* rearrangement by FISH is important to establish this diagnosis.

Treatment and Prognosis

The prognosis of these lesions is variable and appears to be dependent on tumor size and histological grade, with larger tumors and those with poorly differentiated histology exhibiting more aggressive behavior.[271]

Gastroblastoma and Duodenoblastoma

Clinical Features

Most biphasic tumors in the GI tract with epithelial and mesenchymal components represent high-grade sarcomatoid carcinomas ("carcinosarcomas") that typically arise in the older adult population and follow an aggressive clinical course.[276-280] However, in 2009, Miettinen et al. published a small series of a novel epitheliomesenchymal biphasic tumor of the stomach that occurred in a younger patient group and was typified by bland epithelial and mesenchymal components without overt nuclear pleomorphism—so-called "gastroblastoma."[281] Since that time, small numbers

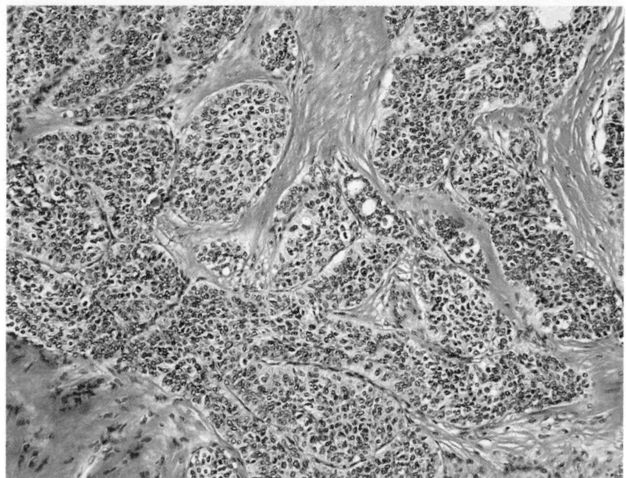

FIGURE 30.65 Gastroblastoma showing an infiltrative growth pattern through the muscularis propria. Note the focus of epithelial differentiation with a tubular architecture in the center of the field.

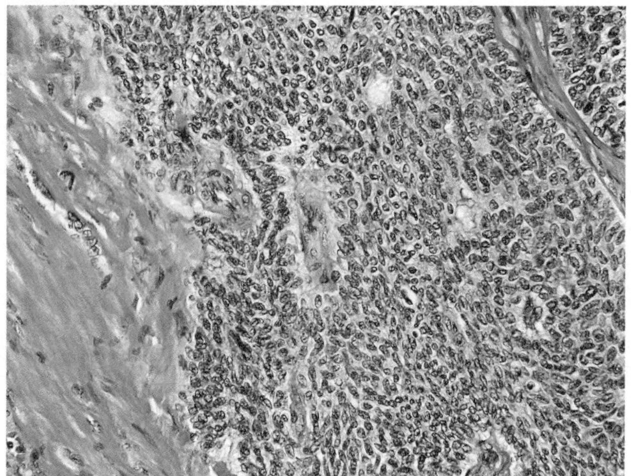

FIGURE 30.66 The mesenchymal component in a gastroblastoma composed of uniform and bland short spindle cells.

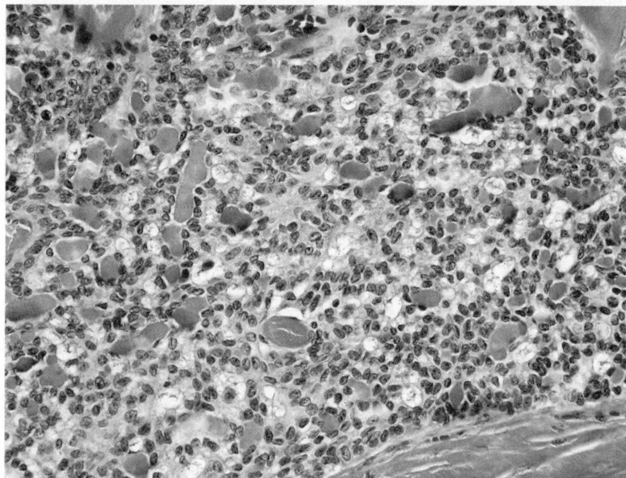

FIGURE 30.67 The epithelial component in a gastroblastoma showing tubular differentiation and luminal eosinophilic secretions.

of additional case reports of this tumor type have been published,[282,283] and a single case report described a similar lesion within the duodenum ("duodenoblastoma").[284] These tumors mostly occur in young adults but show a wide age distribution and appear to be more common in males.

Pathological Features

Gross and Microscopic Findings

The reported tumors have ranged in size from 3.8 to 15 cm and were described as multinodular with cystic areas. They have shown variable involvement of the gastric wall and may be transmural or limited to the muscularis propria or serosa. Microscopically, they contain varying proportions of epithelial and mesenchymal elements with an overall infiltrative growth pattern (Fig. 30.65). The mesenchymal component consists of a uniform population of mildly atypical, spindled to ovoid cells (Fig. 30.66).[281] The epithelial component is variable, with primitive epithelioid clusters merging with the spindled component; more well-developed tubules with open lumina containing eosinophilic inspissated secretions are also seen (Fig. 30.67).[281]

The mitotic rate is highly variable but often low. Importantly, neither the epithelial nor the mesenchymal components have shown the requisite atypia to be diagnostic of carcinoma or sarcoma.

Immunohistochemistry and Molecular Findings

The epithelial components have uniformly been found to express keratins AE1/AE3 and low-molecular-weight keratins, whereas expression of high-molecular-weight keratins has been negative and EMA has been variable. With respect to the spindle cell component, immunoreactivity for CD10 has been identified, but no expression of CD34, KIT, smooth muscle actin, desmin, or CD99 has been reported.[281] The duodenoblastoma described had similar keratin staining of the epithelial component, but the spindle cell component showed immunoreactivity for desmin, focal smooth muscle actin, and CD99.[284] Importantly, none of these lesions had evidence of an *SS18* gene rearrangement, distinguishing them from synovial sarcoma, which would fall into the differential diagnosis given the biphasic nature of the lesion. A recent study has identified a recurrent *MALAT1-GLI1* rearrangement in gastroblastoma, remarkably the same gene fusion found in some plexiform fibromyxomas.[285]

Treatment and Prognosis

Given the varied morphology, accurate diagnosis of this lesion on endoscopic biopsy is unlikely, and thorough evaluation of the resection specimen would be required. In the series by Miettinen et al., no recurrent or metastatic disease was observed in their three patients with follow-up at 3.5 years, 5 years, and 14 years. Because of the limited number of cases, the authors suggested that the prognosis of gastroblastoma is uncertain, and this lesion is best considered a low-grade malignancy.[281] Wey et al. described a gastroblastoma with evidence of histologically confirmed regional lymph node metastasis as well as clinically evident metastatic disease to the liver and pelvis with peritoneal studding, confirming that some gastroblastomas have malignant potential.[283] After surgical resection of the duodenoblastoma, there was no evidence of recurrence or disease progression at 16 months of follow-up.[284]

The full reference list may be accessed online at Elsevier eBooks for Practicing Clinicians.

CHAPTER 31

Hematolymphoid Tumors of the Gastrointestinal Tract, Hepatobiliary Tract, and Pancreas

Judith A. Ferry

Contents

INTRODUCTION

In 55% to 75% of gastrointestinal (GI) lymphomas, the stomach is the primary site. Lymphoma accounts for 1% to 7% of all gastric malignancies.[1,2] Diffuse large B-cell lymphoma and extranodal marginal-zone lymphoma of mucosa-associated lymphoid tissue (MALT lymphoma) are the most common types, with some series having more of the former, and others more of the latter. Other types of lymphoma are quite uncommon, but occasional cases of follicular lymphoma, Burkitt's lymphoma, mantle cell lymphoma, and peripheral T-cell lymphoma may arise in the stomach (Table 31.1). The proportion of gastric T-cell lymphomas appears to be higher in Asian countries than in Western countries, although diffuse large B-cell lymphoma is still more common than T-cell lymphomas.[3]

In 15% to 35% of GI lymphomas, the small intestine or the ileocecal region is the presenting site.[1,2,4] Within the intestines the ileocecal region is the most common site for lymphoma, accounting for about 40% of cases.[5-7] Lymphoma accounts for approximately 25% of small intestinal neoplasms.[1] The proportions of different types of lymphomas vary from one series to another, depending on the age and ethnic background of patients studied, and the part of the world in which the study was performed. The most common type is diffuse large B-cell lymphoma, followed by extranodal marginal-zone lymphoma of mucosa-associated lymphoid tissue (MALT lymphoma, including immunoproliferative small intestinal disease), Burkitt's lymphoma, T-cell lymphomas, mantle cell lymphoma, and follicular lymphoma.[1,4,7-10] The ileum is more commonly affected than the duodenum or jejunum.

TABLE 31.1 Lymphomas of the Digestive Tract

Stomach	Small Intestine	Colon	Anus	Appendix	Liver	Gallbladder	Pancreas
MZL	DLBCL*	DLBCL	DLBCL	DLBCL	DLBCL	DLBCL	DLBCL
DLBCL	MZL (including IPSID)	MZL		Burkitt	Burkitt	MZL	Burkitt
Burkitt	Burkitt	Mantle cell		Follicular	MZL	Follicular	ALCL
Mantle cell	Mantle cell	Follicular		MZL	HSTCL		MZL
Follicular	Follicular	Burkitt					
PTCLs	EATL	MEITL					
	MEITL	Other PTCLs					
	Other PTCLs						
	Extranodal NK/T-cell, nasal type						

Note: The types of lymphoma are listed according to frequency, with the most common at the top.
ALCL, *Anaplastic large cell lymphoma;* DLBCL, *diffuse large B-cell lymphoma;* EATL, *enteropathy-associated T-cell lymphoma;* HSTCL, *hepatosplenic T-cell lymphoma;* IPSID, *immunoproliferative small intestinal disease; MEITL, monomorphic epitheliotropic intestinal T-cell lymphoma;* MZL, *marginal-zone lymphoma;* PTCL, *peripheral T-cell lymphoma.*
**Including subtypes and variants.*

Lymphomas that arise in the ileocecal region are mostly diffuse high-grade B-cell lymphomas (diffuse large B-cell lymphoma or Burkitt's lymphoma) (see Table 31.1).[3,5,11]

The large intestine is the primary site in 3% to 20% of GI lymphomas[2,12,13] and in 21%[5] to 35%[6] of all intestinal lymphomas. Lymphoma accounts for only about 0.5% of malignant neoplasms of this site.[1,14] The most common type of lymphoma is diffuse large B-cell lymphoma, followed by extranodal marginal-zone lymphoma, mantle cell lymphoma, and rare cases of follicular lymphoma, Burkitt's lymphoma, and peripheral T-cell lymphoma. The cecum is the most common site of involvement in the large intestine, followed by the rectum; other portions of the colon are only rarely affected.[1,11,15] Anal lymphomas are very rare; they are usually diffuse large B-cell lymphomas (see Table 31.1).[16]

A variety of lymphomas may present with multifocal GI involvement, including mantle cell lymphoma, follicular lymphoma, enteropathy-associated T-cell lymphoma, marginal-zone lymphoma, and diffuse large B-cell lymphoma.[11]

The most common presenting findings associated with GI lymphomas are abdominal pain, anorexia or weight loss, obstruction, palpable mass, diarrhea, nausea or vomiting, fever, perforation, and bleeding. Intussusception may be seen with bulky lymphomas in the ileocecal region. In a few cases, the lymphoma may be discovered as an incidental finding.[2,4-6,8,9,14,17-19] Symptoms distinctive for different types of lymphoma are noted in the corresponding sections. The more common types of lymphoma, based on pathological subclassification, will be discussed individually. Lymphoma of the appendix is also discussed separately.

GASTRIC MARGINAL-ZONE LYMPHOMA OF MUCOSA-ASSOCIATED LYMPHOID TISSUE (MALT LYMPHOMA)

Clinical Features

The stomach is the most common site for the development of extranodal marginal-zone lymphoma, accounting for about one-third of all cases.[20,21] Gastric marginal-zone lymphoma (extranodal marginal-zone lymphoma of mucosa-associated lymphoid tissue [MALT lymphoma]) affects similar numbers of men and women, with a slight male preponderance in some series. Most patients are older adults, with a median age in the sixth or seventh decade. Infrequently, young adults and even adolescents are affected.[22-28] Patients present with epigastric pain or dyspepsia; nausea and vomiting, bleeding, and weight loss may occur but are unusual.[29] The symptoms often suggest gastritis or peptic ulcer disease rather than lymphoma.[30]

Pathological Features

On endoscopy, or on gross examination of a gastrectomy specimen, this type of lymphoma often consists of erosions, shallow ulcers, mucosal granularity, or thickened mucosal folds, or it appears as a diffusely infiltrative, ill-defined lesion. The appearance may mimic gastritis.[24,30,31] Lymphomas usually involve one portion of the stomach, but tumors may be multifocal and widespread.[24,30-32] Multifocal, widespread, or ill-defined lymphomas may be associated with positive resection margins in gastrectomy specimens.[10,27] Superficial lesions are more common than large masses. A discrete, localized, polypoid tumor,[10] or an exophytic lesion mimicking carcinoma[33] may be found, but this is much less common. Most lymphomas are confined to the mucosa or submucosa. Lymph node involvement is unusual with superficially invasive lymphomas, but it is common when there is invasion into the muscularis propria.[27]

Microscopic examination reveals a diffuse or vaguely nodular infiltrate of marginal-zone cells, small- or medium-sized cells with oval to slightly irregular nuclei, and a distinct rim of clear cytoplasm. In about a third of cases, there is prominent plasmacytic differentiation, often in the form of a bandlike infiltrate of plasma cells in the most superficial portion of the lymphoma. The plasma cells may have the appearance of normal, mature plasma cells or may have cytoplasm with crystalline inclusions, or nuclei with Dutcher bodies. Small clusters of neoplastic cells often infiltrate and disrupt gastric glands to form lymphoepithelial lesions. It is

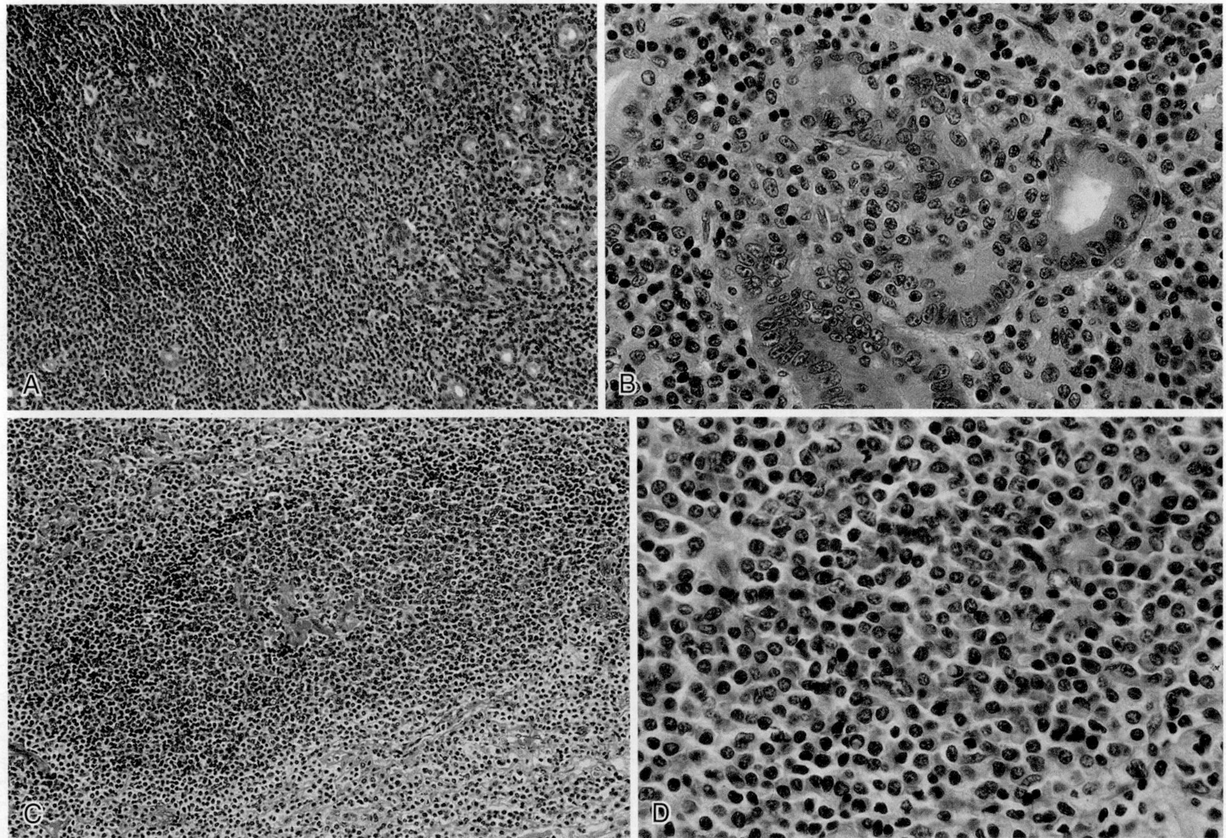

FIGURE 31.1 Gastric marginal-zone lymphoma. A, Low-power view shows a diffuse infiltrate of marginal-zone B cells with a reactive follicle *(upper left).* **B,** Marginal-zone cells infiltrate and disrupt gastric glands, forming lymphoepithelial lesions. **C,** A follicle has been replaced by neoplastic cells ("follicular colonization"). **D,** High-power view shows that the "colonizing" cells are plasma cells, some with Dutcher bodies.

usually possible to identify reactive lymphoid follicles in the lymphoma, often with infiltration and replacement by neoplastic cells (follicular colonization). The cells that colonize the follicles are most commonly marginal-zone–type cells, but plasma cells or large lymphoid cells may also be found. Even when follicles cannot be seen on routinely stained sections, evidence of preexisting follicles can generally be found using antibodies to follicular dendritic cells, such as CD21 or CD23. A few large cells can often be found scattered among the marginal-zone cells (Fig. 31.1).[10,30]

Biopsies of the gastric mucosa also frequently show evidence of infection with *Helicobacter pylori*, detectable on routinely stained sections in some cases, or with special stains such as the thiazine or Steiner stain, or by immunohistochemistry. Alternatively, evidence of *H. pylori* infection can be detected using the rapid urease test (CLO test), stool antigen test, or serology. The likelihood of finding *H. pylori* is greater with lymphomas that are superficial (confined to the mucosa or submucosa) and those that are entirely low grade (rather than having areas of progression to diffuse large B-cell lymphoma).[34] In addition, the frequency of *H. pylori* positivity varies among studies. Although some series report that 80% to 100% of patients harbor *H. pylori*,[28,36] in other studies it is only a minority.[32]

After therapy to eradicate *H. pylori*, complete histological regression of lymphoma is characterized by a lamina propria with a distinctive empty appearance, basal aggregates of small lymphocytes, and scattered plasma cells (Fig. 31.2). Partial regression shows areas of empty lamina propria with foci of atypical lymphoid cells or lymphoepithelial lesions, or both.[35]

Early involvement of lymph nodes often takes the form of bands of marginal-zone cells along sinuses, sometimes with parafollicular aggregates with a marginal-zone pattern, progressing to confluent sheets of marginal-zone cells either with or without monocytoid B cells and follicular colonization.[30,36] The appearance is indistinguishable from that of nodal marginal-zone lymphoma (Fig. 31.3).

Immunohistochemistry

Immunophenotyping shows CD20+, CD5−, CD10−, BCL6−, cyclin D1−, and monotypic surface immunoglobulin (sIg)+ B cells, with plasma cells expressing polytypic or monotypic cytoplasmic immunoglobulin (cIg). The immunoglobulin expressed by neoplastic cells is most often IgM, but in some cases it is IgA or IgG. The neoplastic cells are BCL2+, although BCL2 may be lost in colonized follicles. CD43 is coexpressed in up to one-third of cases. An immunostain for cytokeratin can be helpful for highlighting lymphoepithelial lesions. The proliferation fraction, as measured with Ki67, is low, although it is characteristically high in residual reactive germinal centers.[27,30,31,37]

Molecular Genetic Features

Molecular genetic studies show clonally rearranged immunoglobulin heavy- and light-chain genes. Analysis of

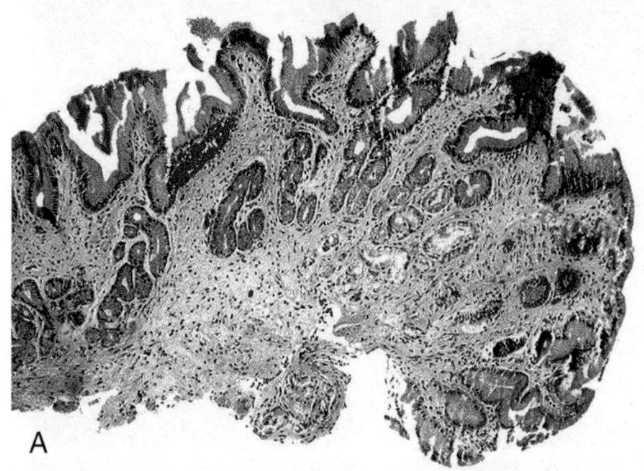

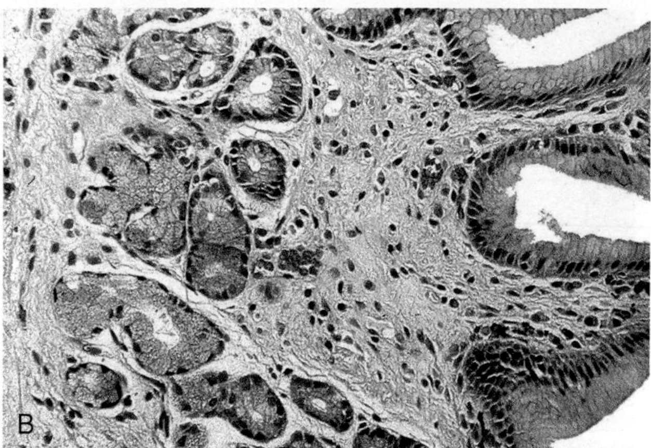

FIGURE 31.2 Gastric mucosa after regression of marginal-zone lymphoma. A, Low-power view shows a pale hypocellular lamina propria. **B,** The lamina propria contains loose connective tissue, fibroblasts, and rare lymphocytes.

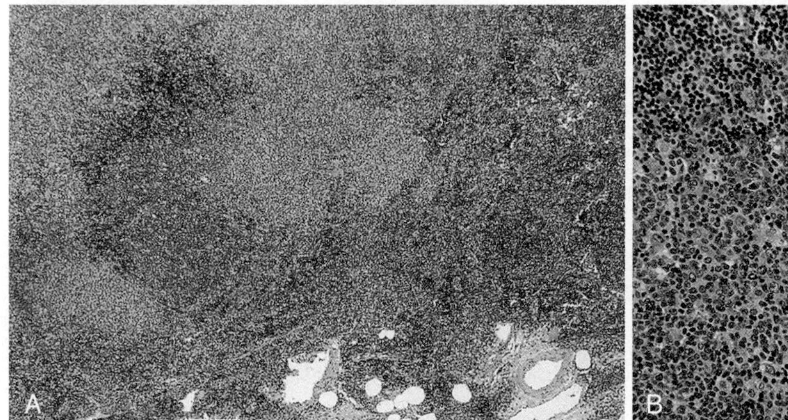

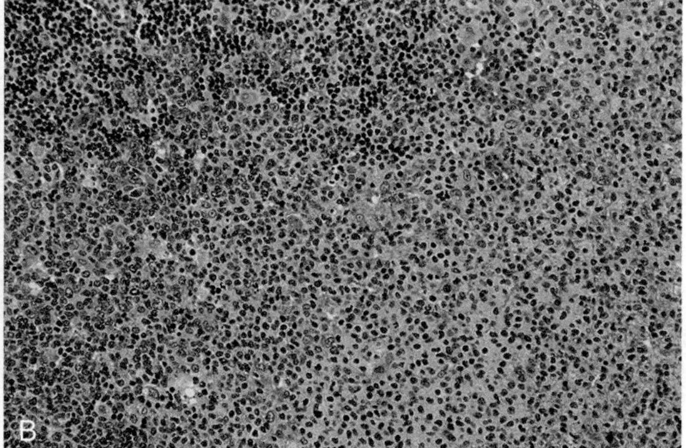

FIGURE 31.3 Perigastric lymph node involved by marginal-zone lymphoma. A, Large aggregates of neoplastic cells replace much of the lymph node, surrounding and invading a reactive follicle. **B,** Monocytoid B cells with abundant pale cytoplasm encroach on a germinal center.

heavy-chain genes shows somatic hypermutation, consistent with neoplastic cells at a postgerminal center stage of development. MALT lymphomas often show biased usage of certain IGHV segments; together with the presence of ongoing somatic mutation, these findings suggest the proliferation of clonal lymphoid cells could be antigen driven.[38] Translocation t(11;18)(q21;q21) is the most common cytogenetic abnormality in gastric marginal-zone lymphoma,[39] although its frequency varies widely,[39-41] from 5% to 50% of cases in different series. This translocation involves *BIRC3* on chromosome 11 and *MALT1* on chromosome 18; it results in a chimeric transcript that can be detected by reverse transcriptase polymerase chain reaction (RT-PCR). The fusion is believed to confer a survival advantage to the neoplastic cells via activation of nuclear factor–kappa B (NFκB). This translocation is found nearly exclusively in extranodal marginal-zone lymphoma.[42] The t(11;18) is associated with a number of clinical and pathological correlates. Marginal-zone lymphomas that fail to regress with *H. pylori* therapy may harbor the t(11;18), whereas t(11;18) is consistently absent in cases that do regress with such therapy. This translocation tends to be associated with higher-stage disease.[43,44] A higher proportion of *H. pylori*–negative gastric marginal-zone lymphomas is also associated with t(11;18)(q21;q21); this could be because of a different pathogenesis[44] or related to the tendency of lymphomas with this translocation to present at an advanced stage, when the lymphoma is able to grow independent of the presence of the bacteria. The t(11;18) is only very rarely found in cases of diffuse large B-cell lymphoma, suggesting that marginal-zone lymphomas with this translocation are very unlikely to undergo large-cell transformation. In general, the proportion of European gastric marginal-zone lymphomas that are positive for t(11;18) has been higher than the proportion of Asian or North American cases. The reason for this variation is uncertain, but possibilities include host factors related to genetic makeup; prevalence of different strains of *H. pylori*; study of resection specimens as opposed to biopsies, because larger, more deeply invasive tumors more often harbor the t(11;18); inclusion of marginal-zone lymphomas in some series secondarily involving stomach; and possibly techniques used (RT-PCR vs. fluorescence in situ hybridization) (Table 31.2).

Another cytogenetic abnormality associated with gastric marginal-zone lymphoma, although less commonly, is t(1;14) (p22;q32), involving the genes for *BCL10* and immunoglobulin heavy chain (IGH). This change results in deregulation of the *BCL10* gene, with resultant loss of its normal proapoptotic activity and acquisition of oncogenic potential.[43] The t(1;14) is also associated with failure of

TABLE 31.2 GI Lymphomas: Pathological Features

Type of Lymphoma	Composition	Usual Immunophenotype	Genetic Features
B-Cell Lymphomas			
Extranodal marginal-zone lymphoma, MALT type	Small lymphocytes, marginal-zone B cells, plasma cells, reactive follicles, lymphoepithelial lesions	Monotypic sIg+, cIg+/– (IgM > IgG or IgA), CD20+, CD5–, CD10–, BCL6–, BCL2+, CD43–/+, cyclin D1–	IGH clonally rearranged; t(11;18) (*BIRC3-MALT1*) in some gastric and intestinal cases; trisomy 18 or trisomy 3 in some cases; t(14;18) (IGH-*MALT1*) in some hepatic cases
Diffuse large B-cell lymphoma	Large centrocytes, centroblasts, immunoblasts and/or anaplastic large B cells	Monotypic sIg+, CD20+, BCL6+/–, CD10–/+, BCL2+/–, MUM1+/–, CD43+/–; can be GCB or non-GCB type	IGH clonally rearranged; *BCL6* abnormalities (translocations or amplifications) are common; t(8;14) (*MYC*-IGH) sometimes found; t(14;18) (IGH-*BCL2*) uncommon
Burkitt's lymphoma	Medium-sized atypical lymphoid cells with round nuclei, basophilic cytoplasm, tingible body macrophages	Monotypic sIgM+, CD20+, CD10+, BCL6+, BCL2–, cMYC+, Ki67 ~100%	IGH clonally rearranged; t(8;14), t(2;8) or (8;22) (*MYC*); rearrangements of *BCL2* and *BCL6* are absent; ~all endemic cases and minority of sporadic and immunodeficiency-associated cases are EBV+
Mantle cell lymphoma	Small to medium-sized, slightly irregular cells with scant cytoplasm	Monotypic sIgMD+, CD20+, CD5+, CD10–, CD43+/–, cyclin D1+, usually SOX11+	IGH clonally rearranged; t(11;14) (*CCND1*-IGH)
Follicular lymphoma	Mixture of centrocytes and centroblasts, follicular dendritic cells	Monotypic sIg+, CD20+, CD10+, BCL6+, BCL2+, CD5–, CD43–, cyclin D1–; hollow FDC meshworks (CD21+, CD23+)	IGH clonally rearranged, t(14;18) (IGH-*BCL2*)
Plasmablastic lymphoma	Plasmablasts, sometimes with more mature plasmacytoid cells, high mitotic rate	CD20–, MUM1+, CD79a–/+, CD138+/–, cIg+/–, Ki67 high, HHV8–	IGH clonally rearranged; *MYC* commonly rearranged or amplified; EBV+, most cases
T/NK Cell Lymphomas			
Enteropathy-associated T-cell lymphoma	Medium-sized and/ or large, sometimes bizarre cells, many admixed reactive cells	CD3+, CD5–; CD4–/CD8– >CD8+; granzyme B+, perforin+, CD56–, CD30+/–, SYK–, Alk1–, CD103+; TCRab–/TCRgd–> TCRab+> TCRgd+	T-cell receptor genes clonally rearranged; EBV–; gains of 9q34 (*NOTCH1, ABL,* and *VAV2*) OR deletions of 16q are common; gains of 5q *(APC)* are common; mutations of JAK-STAT pathway genes and of chromatin modifiers such as *SETD2* are common
Monomorphic epitheliotropic intestinal T-cell lymphoma	Small- to medium-sized cells with pale cytoplasm; admixed reactive cells are sparse	CD3+, CD5–, CD4–, CD8+, CD56+, CD30–, granzyme+, perforin+; MATK+, TCRgd+ > TCRab+	T-cell receptor genes clonally rearranged; EBV–; gains of 9q34 (*NOTCH1, ABL,* and *VAV2*) OR deletions of 16q are common; mutations of JAK-STAT pathway genes and of chromatin modifiers such as *SETD2, MYC* amplification and upregulated MAPK signaling are common
Extranodal NK/T-cell lymphoma, nasal type	Small, medium-sized, and/or large atypical lymphoid cells, necrosis, vascular damage	cCD3+, CD2+, CD4–, CD8–, CD5–, CD56+, granzyme+, perforin+	T-cell receptor genes germline; EBV+; mutations of JAK-STAT pathway genes are common
Hepatosplenic T-cell lymphoma	Medium-sized cells with oval nuclei, fine to condensed chromatin, small to absent nucleoli, pale cytoplasm; can become larger and more atypical over time	CD2+, CD3+, CD5–/+, CD4–, CD8–/+, CD7+/–, CD16+/–, CD56+/–, CD57–/+, TIA1+, granzyme B–, perforin–, TCRgd+ > TCRab+	T-cell receptor genes clonally rearranged; mutations of JAK-STAT pathway genes and of chromatin modifiers such as *SETD2* are common; isochromosome 7q and other changes of chromosome 7 are common

cIg, *Cytoplasmic immunoglobulin;* EBV, *Epstein-Barr virus;* FDC, *follicular dendritic cell; IGH, immunoglobulin heavy-chain gene;* sIg, *surface immunoglobulin.*

lymphoma to regress with antibiotics. The t(1;14) is associated with strong nuclear expression of BCL10 protein; the t(11;18) is associated with moderate nuclear expression of BCL10. Some cases lacking both translocations demonstrate moderate BCL10 expression, so that the protein expression is not specific for a certain cytogenetic change.[45] Rare cases show a t(14;18) involving the genes IGH and *MALT1*.[39,41] The three translocations—t(11;18), t(1;14), and t(14;18)—are mutually exclusive. All three are believed to contribute to lymphomagenesis via activation of NFκB.[45-49] Trisomy 3 and trisomy 18 are found in a subset of cases.[40,41,50] The *BCL1* (cyclin D1) and *BCL2* genes are germline.[10,30]

Genetic features of *H. pylori* may also have an impact on lymphomagenesis. In patients with *H. pylori* infection, t(11;18) shows a tendency to be more frequent when the *H. pylori* strain is positive for cytotoxin-associated gene A (*cagA*). CagA+ strains are associated with a more prominent neutrophilic infiltrate and thus with more reactive oxygen species capable of causing DNA damage, predisposing to the acquisition of translocations.[45] In one study *H. pylori* with multiple HopQ (*H. pylori* outer membrane Q) types, truncated *cagPAI* (pathogenicity activity island) with increased expression of cagT, LEF1 (left end of cagA gene 1), and vacAs1 alleles were more often associated with B-cell lymphoma (MALT lymphoma or diffuse large B-cell lymphoma) than nonneoplastic gastric mucosa.[51]

Staging, Treatment, and Outcome

Staging reveals disease confined to the stomach in an estimated 63% to 88% of cases[26,31,32,52]; regional lymph nodes are involved in the remaining cases, and in a few, there is more widespread disease.[26,31,52] Patients with widespread disease may have involvement of another MALT site, especially the small intestine or colon, but also the lung, kidney, salivary gland, thyroid, ocular adnexa, and others; a few have bone marrow involvement.[2,10,31,32,39] The lymphoma is indolent and may remain localized for years, even without specific therapy.[10]

In 1993, Wotherspoon and colleagues described the remarkable observation of regression of gastric marginal-zone lymphoma after eradication of *H. pylori* with antibiotics.[53] Since then, many other medical centers have reported the same phenomenon, with response rates typically ranging from 60% to 90%.[22,23,35,38] The interval to histological regression may be prolonged, with a range of 1 to 35 months and a median of 3 to 10 months.[25,28,31,35] Features associated with failure of regression include invasion beyond the submucosa, spread beyond the stomach, absence of *H. pylori*, and presence of certain chromosomal abnormalities: t(11;18) and t(1;14).[10,28,31,33,43] A component of diffuse large B-cell lymphoma also decreases the chance of regression. Remarkably, however, complete regression of some cases of diffuse large B-cell lymphoma arising in association with marginal-zone lymphoma confined to the stomach with antibiotic therapy alone has been described[54-58]; regression appears more likely to occur when the lymphoma is superficial (confined to the mucosa or submucosa) on endoscopic ultrasound.[54,56-58]

A minority of patients experience relapse of lymphoma; in some cases this is precipitated by *H. pylori* reinfection.[23] In patients who are histologically negative for lymphoma after *H. pylori* eradication, clonal B cells can be detected by polymerase chain reaction (PCR) for months to years later.[10,22,31,35] Microdissection studies suggest that the clonal cells reside in basal lymphoid aggregates.[35] Clonal B cells can be detected by PCR at presentation in endoscopically normal mucosa in a subset of cases; this finding may predict a longer time to achieve histological remission.[25]

When the lymphoma does not respond, or relapses, after *H. pylori* eradication, other modalities (e.g., surgery, radiation, chemotherapy) may be used,[20,28,31-33,35,38] and cure can usually be obtained. The 5-year survival rate of patients with gastric marginal-zone lymphoma is at least 90%,[10,26,28,52] and the 10-year survival rate is between 80% and 90%.[33] Gastric marginal-zone lymphoma patients have better progression-free survival than extranodal marginal-zone lymphomas arising in most other sites.[21] Of note patients with *H. pylori* infection with or without MALT lymphoma appear to be at increased risk for gastric carcinoma. Follow-up of patients with MALT lymphoma reveals development of gastric carcinoma in occasional cases. The carcinomas may occur in a background of atrophy with intestinal metaplasia, in the same site previously involved by lymphoma.[28]

Pathogenesis

The majority of gastric marginal-zone lymphomas are believed to arise from a background of gastritis with a component of acquired MALT induced by *H. pylori* infection. Persistent infection with chronic antigenic stimulation leads to the appearance of a clonal population of B cells. Surprisingly, the B cells do not have specificity for *H. pylori*; instead, they produce antibodies that may be reactive with a variety of autoantigens. It is the T cells in the infiltrate that have strain-specific reactivity for *H. pylori*. In the early phase of the disease, the B cells require *H. pylori* and the T cells to proliferate. Accordingly, in this phase, the lymphoma remains localized and may respond to antibiotic therapy directed against *H. pylori*. With time, the clonal B cells acquire genetic abnormalities associated with autonomous growth, leading to a low-grade lymphoma that does not regress with *H. pylori* eradication and that may spread beyond the stomach. Additional genetic abnormalities, such as *TP53* inactivation and allelic loss,[10] *CDKN2A* (gene for p16^{Ink4A}) deletion,[59] and *MYC* translocation[30,59,60] may occur and lead to large-cell transformation.

Important pathogenetic questions remain. Only a small proportion of individuals with *H. pylori* gastritis develop marginal-zone lymphoma. It is possible that host factors and environmental factors play a role in the pathogenesis of this type of lymphoma. One study suggests that certain polymorphisms in the T-cell regulatory gene *CTLA4* (cytotoxic T-lymphocyte antigen 4) may be associated with an increased or decreased risk for marginal-zone lymphoma.[61] Others describe an increased risk of gastric marginal-zone lymphoma with certain polymorphisms of genes involved in inflammatory response and antioxidative capacity, with those individuals with a stronger inflammatory response to *H. pylori* and diminished antioxidative capacity more likely to develop gastric marginal-zone lymphoma.[62] Also, in some cases, there is no evidence of *H. pylori* infection,[32] even in patients studied by histology, immunohistochemistry, urease test, serology, or a combination of these methods.[44] In such cases, it is not clear whether infection was present previously and resolved at a stage after the lymphoma attained autonomous growth, or whether there are other, as yet unrecognized, etiological agents for gastric marginal-zone lymphoma.

Factors other than *H. pylori* infection occasionally contribute to lymphomagenesis. A few *H. pylori*–negative marginal-zone lymphomas (as well as a small proportion of cases of chronic gastritis) may be caused by non–*H. pylori* species, such as *Helicobacter heilmannii*. *H. heilmannii* is detectable on histological examination as long, thin, spiral bacilli adjacent to the surface epithelium.[63,64] A case of an Epstein-Barr virus (EBV)+ gastric marginal-zone lymphoma has been reported in a severely immunosuppressed allogeneic stem cell recipient, thus representing an EBV+ posttransplant lymphoproliferative disorder.[65]

Differential Diagnosis

Gastric marginal-zone lymphoma versus gastritis: In favor of a diagnosis of lymphoma, on routinely stained sections are the presence of an expansile, destructive infiltrate with loss of glands, cytological atypia of the infiltrating cells (having the appearance of marginal-zone rather than normal small lymphocytes), frequent lymphoepithelial lesions, and Dutcher bodies. Immunohistochemical studies are often of assistance. Demonstration of monotypic Ig light-chain expression (detectable mainly in cases with plasmacytic differentiation) confirms a diagnosis of lymphoma. A diffuse infiltrate of B cells, and coexpression of CD43 by B cells, both favor a diagnosis of lymphoma. In selected cases, gene rearrangement studies to detect clonal B-cell populations can be useful to distinguish marked chronic gastritis from early involvement by marginal-zone lymphoma.[66]

Gastric marginal-zone lymphoma versus other low-grade lymphomas: In the stomach, marginal-zone lymphoma is much more common than either follicular lymphoma or mantle cell lymphoma. However, either of these may involve the stomach and mimic marginal-zone lymphoma. Marginal-zone lymphoma is composed of CD5−, CD10− B cells with relatively abundant clear cytoplasm, and may show plasmacytic differentiation and an admixture of a few large cells. Mantle cell lymphoma typically is composed of a monotonous population of small- to medium-sized CD5+, cyclin D1+ B cells with scant cytoplasm, without a large-cell or plasmacytic component. However, in a small proportion of mantle cell lymphomas the neoplastic cells may have pale cytoplasm and resemble marginal-zone cells,[67] so that relying on morphology alone may occasionally be misleading. Follicular lymphoma generally has a more distinct follicular architecture and is typically composed of CD10+, BCL6+ B cells with nuclei that are usually more irregular, and cytoplasm that is usually more scant, than marginal-zone cells (see Table 31.2).

Histological progression to diffuse large B-cell lymphoma versus gastric marginal-zone lymphoma: When there are sheets or confluent clusters of large, transformed cells found outside of follicles in a background of marginal-zone lymphoma, a diagnosis of diffuse large B-cell lymphoma, arising in association with marginal-zone lymphoma should be made. "High-grade MALT lymphoma" is not the preferred nomenclature and should not be used.[68] Before diagnosing focal large-cell transformation, it is important to exclude the possibility that the large cells are residual reactive germinal center cells, or neoplastic large cells colonizing follicles. Immunohistochemical stains to demonstrate a follicular dendritic network can be helpful in resolving these uncertainties. The diffuse large B-cell lymphomas that arise in association with gastric marginal-zone lymphomas are often positive for BCL6, and immunostaining for BCL6 may be helpful in highlighting possible areas of large-cell transformation.[69] However, reactive germinal centers are also positive for BCL6, so, as noted earlier, stains for follicular dendritic cells can be performed to investigate this as a possibility.

Poorly preserved high-grade lymphoma versus gastric marginal-zone lymphoma: In a small biopsy with artifactual degenerative change in diffuse large B-cell lymphoma, or Burkitt's lymphoma, there may be cellular shrinkage and distortion leading to a false impression of low-grade lymphoma. The presence of apoptotic debris or mitotic figures suggests a higher-grade tumor. Staining with the proliferation marker Ki67 can be quite helpful in distinguishing low-grade from high-grade lymphomas. Clinical information, such as the endoscopic appearance of the tumor, can also provide a clue to the correct diagnosis.[10]

Plasmacytoma versus marginal-zone lymphoma: Convincing cases of GI plasmacytoma are rare. Most reported cases are more likely marginal-zone lymphomas with prominent plasmacytic differentiation. In favor of a diagnosis of lymphoma are the presence of a component of B lymphocytes, lymphoepithelial lesions, and IgM+ neoplastic cells (marginal-zone lymphomas may express other heavy chains, but IgM expression by a plasma cell neoplasm would be very rare).

INTESTINAL MARGINAL-ZONE LYMPHOMA OF MUCOSA-ASSOCIATED LYMPHOID TISSUE (MALT LYMPHOMA)

Clinical Features

Intestinal marginal-zone lymphoma is the second most common type of lymphoma to arise in the intestines (after diffuse large B-cell lymphoma), accounting for approximately 10%[53] to 18%[64] of all primary intestinal lymphomas. Almost all patients are middle-aged or older adults. Both men and women are affected.[9,41,70,71] Patients occasionally have concurrent gastric marginal-zone lymphoma. Rare patients have inflammatory bowel disease (IBD) or are status post solid organ transplantation,[71] suggesting a role for an immunological abnormality in lymphomagenesis.[71] Many patients are asymptomatic, and the lymphomas may be detected during screening colonoscopy.[71] This type of lymphoma may be located in any portion of the small or large intestine, but a disproportionately large number arise in the rectum,[53,11,41,70,71] with the cecal area next most often affected.[71] In the majority of cases, disease is localized to the bowel, either with or without regional lymph node involvement.[17,30,70] A few patients have serum M components.[9]

The prognosis is favorable. Intestinal marginal-zone lymphoma has a better prognosis than any other type of intestinal lymphoma.[43,57,17] In one study, 80% of patients with marginal-zone lymphoma were alive and well at last follow-up.[9] The 5-year overall survival for intestinal marginal-zone lymphoma in one large series was 88%.[53] In another, 5-year progression-free survival, overall survival, and disease-specific survival were 92%, 94%, and 98% respectively.[71]

Rare patients with intestinal marginal-zone lymphoma respond to antibiotic therapy,[17,72-74] suggesting that *H. pylori*,[74] or some other organism,[75] plays a role in the pathogenesis of a subset of these lymphomas.

Pathological Features

On gross examination, these lymphomas form raised or polypoid masses, sometimes with ulceration, [9,17,18,72] or infrequently they have the appearance of multiple, small, slightly raised lesions with erosion and erythema,[74,75] akin to early gastric marginal-zone lymphoma. Most are single lesions, but occasionally they are multiple.[18,70] The lymphomas can be superficially[17,70] or transmurally invasive.[9,18] In a few cases, the lymphoma may have the appearance of multiple lymphomatous polyposis (see Mantle Cell Lymphoma, later).[76] In one series, the lesions were subclassified into subepithelial tumor type (most common), polyposis type, epithelial mass type, and ileitis type (least common).[71]

The histological, immunophenotypic, and genetic features of marginal-zone lymphoma of the intestine are similar to those seen in the stomach.[47,9,30] Rarely there is associated amyloid deposition, without evidence of systemic amyloidosis. The t(11;18) resulting in the *BIRC-MALT1* fusion is found in 12% to 42% of cases in different series.[40,41,70,77] In one series, the presence of t(11;18) was associated with marginal-zone lymphomas that were larger and higher stage, and they more often affected men.[70] As for gastric marginal-zone lymphoma, trisomy 3 and trisomy 18 are relatively common, and t(1;14) (involving the *BCL10* and IGH genes) and t(14;18) (involving the IGH and *MALT1* genes) are rare or absent (see Table 31.2).[40,41]

A substantial number of marginal-zone lymphomas involving the intestine are secondary; in these cases, the stomach is the most common primary site. Secondary intestinal marginal-zone lymphomas have an even higher proportion of cases with t(11;18), correlating with the tendency of this translocation to be associated with higher-stage disease.[41]

Immunoproliferative Small Intestinal Disease

The frequency of small intestinal lymphoma is higher in the Middle East than in Western countries. The small intestine is the most common primary site for extranodal lymphoma, accounting for 50% of such cases, and for 75% of GI lymphomas in adults in the Middle East. Approximately half of these small intestinal lymphomas have been of the distinctive immunoproliferative small intestinal disease (IPSID) type. Over the past several decades, however, the incidence of IPSID appears to have declined. Although IPSID is found mainly in the Middle East and in countries around the Mediterranean Sea, occasional cases have been described in South Africa, the Far East, Europe, and the United States. Because of its geographic distribution, IPSID has also been called Mediterranean lymphoma.[78-80] IPSID is now considered to be a distinct subtype of extranodal marginal-zone lymphoma. In an association similar to that between *H. pylori* and gastric marginal-zone lymphoma, *Campylobacter jejuni* is hypothesized to be an important factor in the development of IPSID.[81,82] A unique case of IPSID that developed in a Pacific Islander with multiple enteric infections (*C. jejuni*, *Vibrio fluvialis*, whipworm) as well as *Escherichia coli* lymphadenitis and *H. pylori* gastritis has been reported.[83]

Clinical Features

Most patients are young adults (median age, 25 years), ranging from adolescence to middle age. Males and females are equally affected. IPSID tends to be associated with lower socioeconomic status. Patients present with abdominal pain, malabsorption, diarrhea, and weight loss of months' to years' duration. Many patients also have digital clubbing.[78,79,84] Obstruction, bleeding, and perforation are uncommon, in contrast to other types of small intestinal lymphoma.[79] At laparotomy, patients may have one or more recognizable intestinal masses, diffuse mural thickening and/or luminal dilation, or normal-appearing bowel. The abnormalities involve the proximal small intestine, the entire small intestine, or, rarely, just the ileum, or the small intestine in combination with either the stomach or colon.[79] Mesenteric lymph nodes are often enlarged.[30,79,80,84] As with gastric marginal-zone lymphoma, in the early phase of the disease the lymphoma may respond to broad-spectrum antibiotics. Nonresponders may be treated with chemotherapy. Later in the course of disease, when muscle invasion or transformation to a high-grade lymphoma occurs, the lymphoma behaves in an aggressive manner.[10] For resectable stage Ie or IIe1 disease, the 5-year survival rate is 40% to 47%. For higher-stage, unresectable disease, the 5-year survival rate has been reported to be from 0% to 25%.[1] However, patients treated with anthracycline-containing combination chemotherapy have a better outlook, with a complete remission rate of approximately 60%.[78,84]

In about half of cases, there is a highly characteristic laboratory abnormality: the serum contains free α heavy chains without associated light chains. Free α heavy chain may also be found in body fluids, such as intestinal fluid, urine, and saliva. Secreted α heavy chain is more likely to be found in early stages of IPSID. Cases with this abnormality have been called α heavy-chain disease. Closer analysis of this paraprotein reveals that it is a truncated α_1 heavy chain lacking the variable region and the first constant region, and unable to bind light chain. The corresponding mRNA shows an internal deletion of V_H and C_H1. It has been suggested that IPSID develops in patients with recurrent, or persistent, intestinal infections, leading to chronic antigenic stimulation of IgA-secreting lymphoid tissue in this site, with a resultant clonal population that acquires mutations, leading to the production of α heavy chain with the internal deletion noted earlier.[84]

Pathological Features

IPSID is typically characterized by a dense, continuous, bandlike mucosal lymphoid or lymphoplasmacytic infiltrate that is uninterrupted along the length of the small intestine.[79] The mucosa also shows broad villi, although the intestinal epithelial cells usually remain intact.[80,84] The extent of the infiltrate explains the pathogenesis of the malabsorption that affected patients experience. The histological features are similar to those of marginal-zone lymphomas in other extranodal sites, except that in IPSID there consistently is

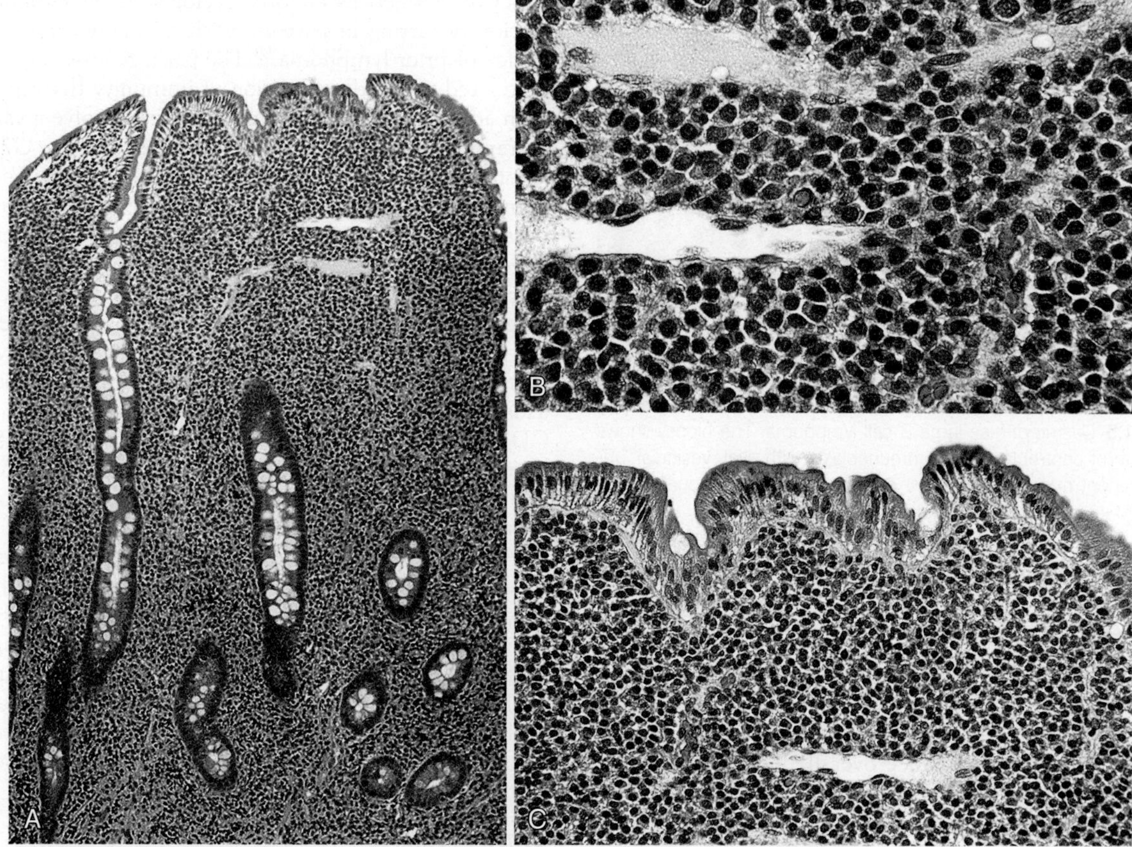

FIGURE 31.4 Immunoproliferative small intestinal disease (IPSID), stage A. A, The lamina propria is filled and expanded by a dense cellular infiltrate. **B,** Higher power view shows numerous plasma cells, one with a Dutcher body, and scattered small lymphoid cells. **C,** Despite the intensity of the cellular infiltrate, the surface epithelium is well preserved.

marked plasmacytic differentiation. The following staging system has been proposed to subclassify the infiltrate in IPSID.

Stage A: Lymphoma is confined to the small intestinal mucosa and mesenteric lymph nodes. The infiltrate consists predominantly of plasma cells, with smaller numbers of marginal-zone cells. The B cells may be inconspicuous, and an immunostain for CD20 can help with recognition of B cells and also of lymphoepithelial lesions.[30] There is variable villous atrophy (Fig. 31.4).

Stage B: In addition to the findings characteristic of stage A, the infiltrate has areas of nodularity that correspond to reactive lymphoid follicles colonized by neoplastic B cells. There are also occasional atypical, immunoblast-like cells. The infiltrate invades beyond the muscularis mucosae.

Stage C: Stage C is characterized by high-grade B-cell lymphoma, typically diffuse large B-cell lymphoma, with formation of one or more large masses. The lymphoma is composed of large cells, sometimes with the appearance of immunoblasts or plasmacytoid immunoblasts. In other cases, the neoplastic cells are pleomorphic and bizarre. The high-grade lymphoma is almost always in the bowel, but in one case, the high-grade lymphoma presented with tonsillar involvement.[83]

Immunohistochemical analysis usually shows expression of α heavy chain without light chain, correlating with the serum paraprotein. In a minority of cases, monotypic light chain is expressed. Molecular genetic analysis has shown clonal rearrangement of Ig heavy and light chains, even in early cases responsive to antibiotic therapy. Previously, early phases of IPSID were thought to be inflammatory, but this information indicates that the infiltrate is neoplastic despite response to antibiotics.[30,78]

Differential Diagnosis

IPSID and celiac sprue are both characterized by lymphoplasmacytic infiltrates and villous atrophy. Patient demographic data should provide a strong clue to the diagnosis, because patients with celiac disease are predominantly of northwestern European descent and they improve on a gluten-free diet, in contrast to IPSID patients. Histological features in favor of a diagnosis of celiac disease include total villous atrophy (in contrast to the villous broadening seen in early-stage IPSID), hyperplastic, elongated crypts, intraepithelial lymphocytosis, and surface epithelial damage.[84] High-grade lymphomas may be found in association with either, but the lymphoma that complicates celiac disease is a T-cell lymphoma prone to cause multifocal perforation.

It may be difficult to distinguish nonspecific chronic inflammation from early-stage IPSID, particularly on a small biopsy sample. In favor of a diagnosis of IPSID is a dense, predominantly plasmacytic infiltrate distorting the mucosal architecture in a patient with clinical features compatible with IPSID. Immunohistochemical stains showing plasma cells expressing only α heavy chain help establish the diagnosis.

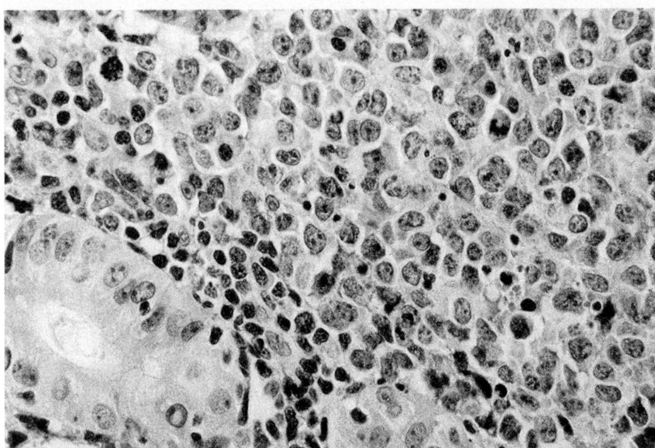

FIGURE 31.5 Gastric diffuse large B-cell lymphoma. The biopsy shows an infiltrate of centroblasts and immunoblasts with oval, vesicular nuclei, prominent nucleoli, and scant cytoplasm, with occasional mitotic figures and interspersed cellular debris.

GASTRIC DIFFUSE LARGE B-CELL LYMPHOMA

Clinical Features

Gastric diffuse large B-cell lymphoma (DLBCL) is mainly a disease of older adults, with a median age in the seventh decade; younger adults are affected only occasionally. There is a slight male preponderance overall.[24,26,27,85,86] Patients may have a palpable mass on physical examination.[10] Some arise in association with marginal-zone lymphoma, consistent with large-cell transformation of the low-grade lymphoma, whereas other large B-cell lymphomas appear to arise de novo; the proportion of cases in the two categories varies among series.[2,24,26,52,86,87] Anemia is common, likely related to bleeding from the lesion.[88] Constitutional symptoms are uncommon. Most patients have normal lactate dehydrogenase (LDH).[88,89]

Pathological Features

On gross examination, the lymphomas are usually single, but occasionally, one may encounter multiple large ulcerated or exophytic lesions. The DLBCLs are usually transmurally invasive and may invade adjacent viscera.[10,24] The corpus and antrum are affected more often than the fundus or cardia.[88] Microscopic examination reveals a diffuse proliferation of large cells with round, oval, irregular, or lobated nuclei, distinct nucleoli, and a narrow but distinct rim of cytoplasm (Fig. 31.5). Immunophenotyping reveals CD20+ B cells coexpressing CD43 in about half of cases. In some cases, expression of monotypic immunoglobulin is demonstrable.[52] The large-cell lymphomas that arise from extranodal marginal-zone lymphoma are CD5−, CD10− (nearly all), BCL6+/−, MUM1−/+, BCL2−/+, with a high proliferation index.[90] Gastric DLBCL includes both germinal center B-cell (GCB, CD10+ or CD10−, BCL6+, MUM1−), and nongerminal center B-cell (non-GCB, CD10−, BCL6+, MUM1+, or CD10−, BCL6−) types (see Table 31.2). A minority are MYC+.[6,87,89,91,92]

Most DLBCLs arising in the GI tract would be subclassified as DLBCL, not otherwise specified (NOS) according to the World Health Organization (WHO) Classification. The WHO has defined a number of other types of lymphomas of large B cells, some of which may involve the GI tract. One of these is EBV+ diffuse large B-cell lymphoma, NOS, which is defined as an EBV+ clonal B-cell lymphoproliferation occurring in patients with no known immunodeficiency or prior lymphoma.[93] The pathogenesis is thought to be related to the deterioration of immunity that may occur with advancing age. This lymphoma can involve a variety of extranodal sites (as well as lymph nodes), but the GI tract is among the more common. The composition may be monomorphous, with a predominance of large, atypical lymphoid cells, which may have the appearance of immunoblasts or Reed-Sternberg–like cells and variants. In some cases, the composition may be more polymorphous, with B cells of a range of stages of maturation including large atypical cells and also reactive cells, including histiocytes, small lymphocytes, and plasma cells. Necrosis is common. Tumor cells usually express pan B-cell antigens (CD20, Pax5, and/or CD79a), often CD30, and occasionally express CD15. They have a non-GCB phenotype, with expression of MUM1. CD10 and frequently BCL6 are negative. By definition, EBV is present in tumor cells.[93-95]

Anaplastic lymphoma kinase (ALK) + DLBCL is a rare type of large B-cell lymphoma (Fig. 31.6); a case of this type of lymphoma arising in the stomach of a 21-year-old man has been reported.[96] Other lymphomas of large B cells are plasmablastic lymphoma and HHV8+ large B-cell lymphoma. Both of these rare types of lymphoma may be encountered in the GI tract, but as they occur most often in HIV+ individuals, they are discussed below, under GI Lymphoproliferative Disorders in Abnormal Immune States.

Genetic Features

Immunoglobulin heavy and light chains are clonally rearranged. Complex cytogenetic abnormalities are common.[97] In contrast to nodal large B-cell lymphomas, *BCL2* rearrangement is rare and *MYC* rearrangement is common.[98] Abnormalities of the *BCL6* gene are more common in gastric than nodal diffuse large B-cell lymphoma. *BCL6* abnormalities include both translocation and somatic hypermutation.[87] One study documented frequent (42% of cases) loss of heterozygosity (LOH) on chromosome 6q in sites of putative tumor suppressor genes, as well as a smaller number of cases with LOH of tumor suppressor genes, including *TP53* and *APC*. Amplification of genomic material in the *BCL6* locus, the *KMT2A* (formerly MLL/mixed-lineage leukemia) gene, and others were also found.[97] Homozygous deletion of *CDKN2A*, encoding $p16^{Ink4A}$, has also been described in high-grade gastric lymphoma.

Activation of the NFκB pathway is important in the pathogenesis of lymphomas of a variety of types. Recently mutations in *A20*, *CARD11*, and *ABIN-1* and *ABIN-2* (A20 binding inhibitor of NFκB) likely to contribute to activation of the NFκB pathway have been documented in DLBCL of the GI tract.[99] Mutations of *A20* were associated more often with DLBCLs with the non-GCB phenotype (according to the Hans algorithm, earlier) and with significantly worse overall survival and event-free survival.[99] A small minority (14% in one series[89]) harbor the *MYD88* L265P mutation.[89]

Unless a component of low-grade lymphoma is identified, it may not be possible to distinguish between de novo DLBCL and DLBCL arising from histological progression of marginal-zone lymphoma (or other low-grade lymphoma). Genetic and cytogenetic features may be helpful. Despite the high frequency of t(11;18) and trisomy 3 in gastric marginal-zone B-cell lymphoma, they are uncommon in

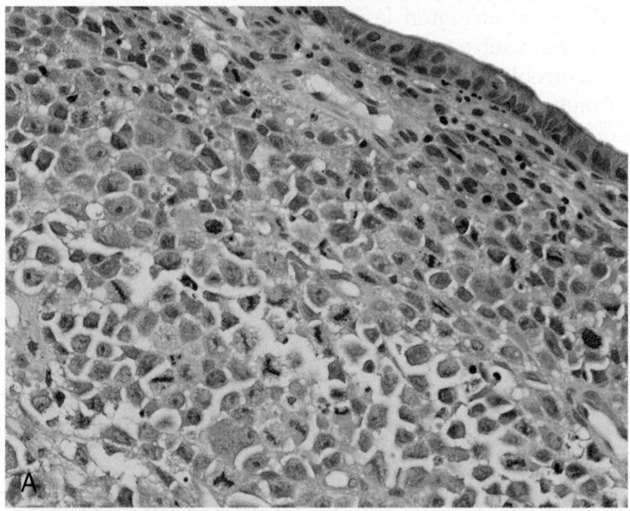

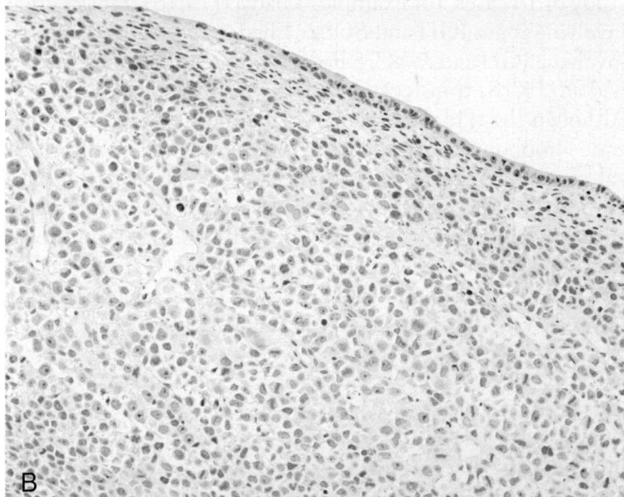

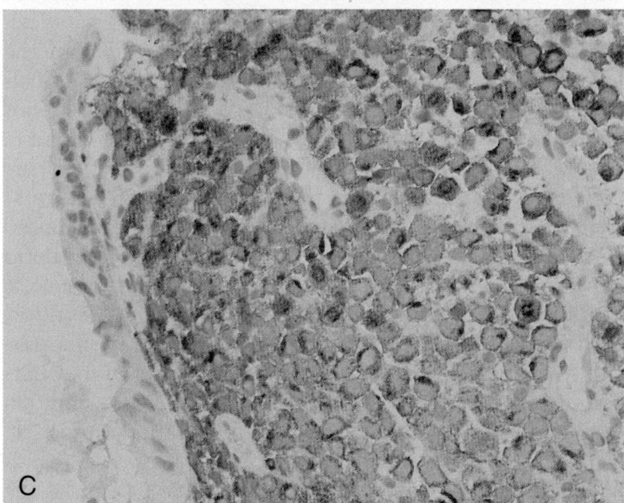

FIGURE 31.6 ALK+ diffuse large B-cell lymphoma, gastric relapse of lymph nodal primary. A, The lamina propria of this gastric biopsy is replaced by a diffuse proliferation of large lymphoid cells with round nuclei and prominent nucleoli. **B,** The lymphoma is negative for CD20. **C,** The lymphoma shows granular cytoplasmic staining for ALK. (**B** and **C** immunoperoxidase stains on paraffin sections.)

gastric DLBCL, suggesting they are not important in transformation of marginal-zone lymphoma to large B-cell lymphoma.[50,59] One report suggests that trisomies (most often involving chromosomes 12 and 18) are more common in large-cell lymphomas that have arisen through transformation of marginal-zone lymphoma than in de novo large B-cell lymphomas.[50]

A variety of mechanisms may lead to transformation of MALT lymphoma to DLBCL, including *TP53* mutation, alterations in *BCL6*, aberrant DNA hypermethylation, and others.[69,100] Translocations involving *BCL6*[87] and *MYC*[98] may play a role in progression of gastric marginal-zone lymphoma to DLBCL, although these alterations may be involved in the pathogenesis of de novo DLBCL as well. Recently, overexpression of Myc was shown to alter microRNA signature in gastric lymphomas. In the setting of Myc-repressed miRNAs normally showing tumor suppressive activity, FoxP1 was overexpressed, theoretically promoting lymphomagenesis and large-cell transformation.[100] Accordingly, MALT lymphomas are typically negative for Myc and FoxP1 by immunohistochemistry while DLBCLs are often positive.[100]

Staging and Outcome

In the majority of cases, patients present with stage I or II disease.[26,52,86,88,101] Patients may be treated with surgery, radiation, chemotherapy, or a combination of these modalities. In a study of patients treated with R-CHOP +/− radiation or surgery, 5-year overall and event-free survival were 85.8% and 89.6%, respectively.[88] Some studies have documented pathological features that have an impact on prognosis. In one study, large B-cell lymphoma associated with a component of marginal-zone lymphoma, or with lymphoepithelial lesions formed by small cells, had a 5-year cause-specific survival rate of 84%, compared with 64% for de novo large B-cell lymphoma. Lymphoepithelial lesions formed by large cells were not associated with a favorable prognosis.[86] In one study using immunophenotyping to subclassify gastric diffuse large B-cell lymphoma as germinal center or non–germinal center type, patients with germinal center type had a significantly better outcome.[87]

Stage is also prognostically important. Patients with stage Ie or IIe1 have a better outcome than those with IIe2 or higher.[26,52] Older age, male sex, Black race, high LDH, and ascites have been associated with a poor outcome.[85,101] Other factors reported to have an impact on prognosis are International Prognostic Index (IPI) score, B symptoms, and Eastern Cooperative Oncology Group (ECOG) performance score.[88]

Differential Diagnosis

Poorly differentiated carcinoma may be composed of discohesive-appearing cells that form few or no glands, and thus may be difficult to distinguish from diffuse large B-cell lymphoma. Lymphoid cells may show artifactual vacuolar change and mimic signet ring cells, but mucin stains and immunohistochemical stains are helpful in distinguishing between lymphoma and carcinoma.

INTESTINAL DIFFUSE LARGE B-CELL LYMPHOMA

Clinical Features

Diffuse large B-cell lymphoma (DLBCL) is the most common type of intestinal lymphoma, accounting for up to two-thirds of cases.[53] Most patients with intestinal DLBCL are middle-aged to older adults. Few cases occur in younger adults or children. There is a slight male preponderance

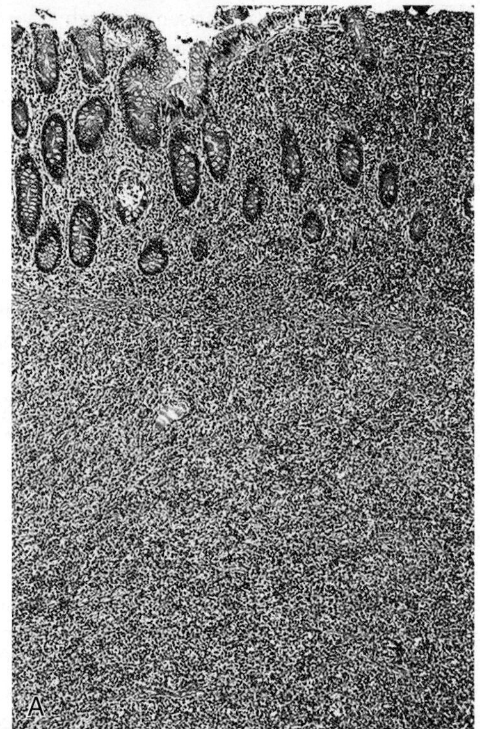

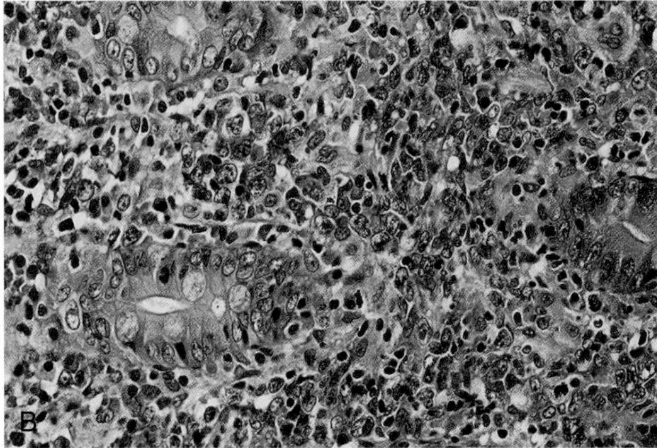

FIGURE 31.7 Diffuse large B-cell lymphoma, arising in the cecum of an HIV+ patient. A, A diffuse infiltrate of lymphoid cells obliterates much of the bowel wall. **B,** The tumor cells are large atypical lymphoid cells with oval or irregular nuclei and prominent nucleoli. Their appearance is consistent with that of centroblasts.

among adults, whereas affected children are almost exclusively male. DLBCL in children is virtually found only in the ileocecal area.[9,14,15,18,70] In the majority of cases, the lymphoma is confined to the bowel except for regional lymph node involvement.[9,14,70] In the remainder, disease is more widespread.[70,89] Anemia is common but constitutional symptoms are usually absent.[89]

This type of lymphoma is relatively aggressive but potentially curable.[10,15,30,70] In one report, de novo DLBCL had a less favorable outcome than DLBCL that arose in association with marginal-zone lymphoma.[17]

Pathological Features

On gross examination, the tumors are similar to, or larger than, low-grade lymphomas.[17,18] They are elevated or infiltrative, ulcerated lesions that are usually transmurally invasive. A subset shows perforation.[4,70] Most are composed of centroblasts, often with an admixture of immunoblasts, or multilobated large lymphoid cells, whereas a minority are composed almost exclusively of immunoblasts (Fig. 31.7).[4,9] A case of intravascular large B-cell lymphoma involving the colon and mimicking ulcerative colitis has been reported.[102]

In some cases, a component of marginal-zone lymphoma is found, which is consistent with large-cell transformation of a low-grade lymphoma. The proportion of cases with an underlying low-grade lymphoma varies greatly in different series, from 10% to more than 50% of large B-cell lymphomas.[4,9,17,70] The immunophenotypic features overlap with those found in gastric DLBCL. De novo intestinal DLBCLs can have a germinal center or a non–germinal center B-cell immunophenotype.[89,92]

Intestinal DLBCL is genetically heterogeneous. In one study of 14 cases, for example, 3 had a t(14;18) translocation involving genes IGH and *BCL2*, 1 had a t(8;14) translocation involving IGH and *MYC*, 5 had a *BCL6* rearrangement, and 1 had a t(11;18) translocation involving *BIRC3* and *MALT1*.[77] Although the t(11;18) characteristic of a subset of marginal-zone lymphomas is generally considered to prevent histological progression to DLBCL, rare cases of intestinal DLBCL harbor t(11;18), which suggests large-cell transformation of an underlying marginal-zone lymphoma with this translocation may occur (see Table 31.2).[70,77] The *MYD88* L265P mutation, which is common in DLBCLs arising in certain other extranodal sites, is rare in the GI tract.[89]

Differential Diagnosis

The differential diagnosis for intestinal DLBCL is similar to that for gastric DLBCL. In addition, floridly reactive lymphoid tissue in the intestine occasionally raises the question of lymphoma. The bowel normally harbors hyperplastic lymphoid tissue in the terminal ileum (Peyer's patches), but hyperplastic lymphoid tissue in other portions of the intestine, when prominent, may suggest lymphoma. This problem may arise with lymphoid polyps, polypoid lesions composed of reactive lymphoid tissue that may be found in the colon. Large collections of hyperplastic lymphoid tissue may develop in the rectum; these have been referred to as *rectal tonsils*, which are large, discrete nodules of organized lymphoid tissue with reactive follicles, often showing florid hyperplasia, located in the lamina propria or submucosa. Rectal tonsils may be accompanied by overlying cryptitis, mild architectural distortion, intraepithelial lymphocytes, and lymphoepithelial lesions, typically without crypt obliteration.[103] In lymphoid follicular proctitis, a condition characterized by congested, nodular mucosa and often associated with rectal bleeding, reactive lymphoid tissue, including lymphoid follicles, is found in the distal portion of the GI tract.[104] Familiarity with these entities and appreciation of the follicular architecture, with enlarged B cells mostly confined to follicles, can avoid overdiagnosis as lymphoma.

MANTLE CELL LYMPHOMA

Clinical Features

Mantle cell lymphoma affects middle-aged or older adults with a male preponderance. Almost all patients are 50

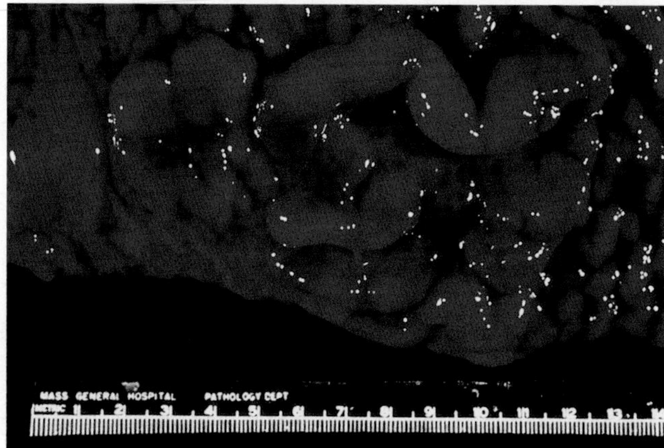

FIGURE 31.8 Multiple lymphomatous polyposis. Gross examination reveals marked expansion of mucosal folds, producing multiple serpiginous and polypoid masses. Microscopic examination showed mantle-cell lymphoma.

years of age or older.[18,30,76,105,106] Mantle cell lymphoma usually presents with widespread disease with involvement of lymph nodes and a variety of extranodal sites; GI involvement is common. Patients may present initially with GI tract involvement. Any portion of the GI tract may be affected,[17,30] and frequently the lymphoma affects multiple sites (stomach, small intestine, colon, and, on occasion, the esophagus).[76,106] GI tract involvement can result in abdominal pain, diarrhea, bloody stool, and weight loss. Mantle cell lymphoma often takes the form of innumerable polyps and then is termed multiple lymphomatous polyposis[76]; this pattern is particularly prevalent in the intestines.[106] The ileocecal region tends to contain the largest polyps.[17,30] In some cases, particularly when mantle cell lymphoma involves the stomach, it takes the form of a smaller number of protruded, ulcerated or fold-thickening lesions.[106] Mesenteric lymph nodes are usually involved by lymphoma.[30] Staging frequently reveals widespread disease away from the GI tract. Although there is usually a good response to chemotherapy, relapses are common and survival is usually only 3 to 5 years. Predisposing factors for the development of mantle cell lymphoma are unknown.

Pathological Features

On gross examination, multiple lymphomatous polyposis has the appearance of multiple fleshy white nodules, 0.5 to 2 cm in greatest dimension, involving the mucosa, but sometimes with superficial submucosal involvement (Fig. 31.8). Less commonly, mantle cell lymphoma takes the form of a discrete mass or an ulcerated lesion.[10]

Microscopic examination shows a bandlike infiltrate, or multiple ill-defined nodules, of atypical, monotonous lymphoid cells that are slightly larger and more irregular than normal lymphocytes, with scant cytoplasm and without conspicuous nucleoli. Single epithelioid histiocytes may be scattered among the neoplastic cells. Remnants of reactive follicle centers may be identified in some nodules. The lymphoma tends to displace and obliterate intestinal glands, but formation of true lymphoepithelial lesions is not a feature (Fig. 31.9).[30,67,105]

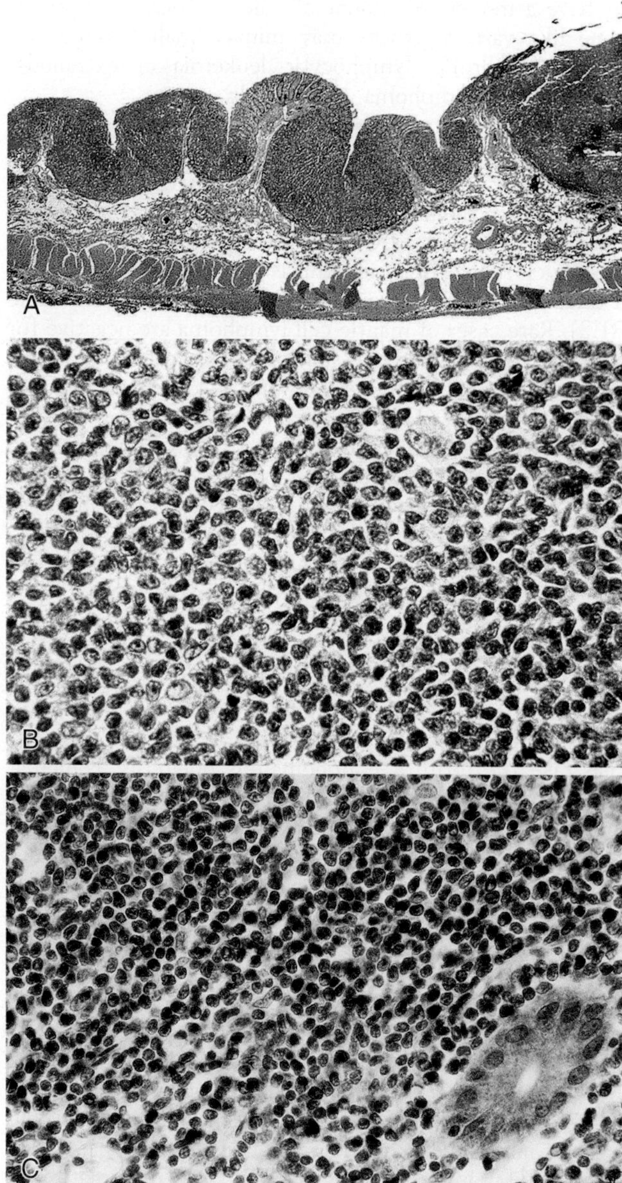

FIGURE 31.9 Multiple lymphomatous polyposis. A, Low-power view. **B,** High-power view shows small, slightly irregular lymphoid cells with scant cytoplasm and few interspersed single epithelioid histiocytes. **C,** With antibody to cyclin D1 there is staining of the nuclei of many of the atypical cells, confirming a diagnosis of mantle cell lymphoma.

A minority of cases of mantle cell lymphoma are characterized by histological features suggesting more aggressive behavior; these "aggressive variants" include blastoid and pleomorphic variants. In the blastoid variant, neoplastic cells have finely dispersed chromatin, and the mitotic rate is high (usually >20 mitoses/10 high-power fields [hpf]) so that the appearance is reminiscent of lymphoblastic lymphoma. In the pleomorphic variant, neoplastic cells are larger and more pleomorphic than in the usual mantle cell lymphoma, and in contrast to typical mantle cell lymphoma, nucleoli are often prominent in at least some of the neoplastic cells. The appearance may mimic diffuse large B-cell lymphoma.[67] Occasional cases of mantle cell lymphoma are composed of small, uniform, dark cells (small cell variant), or have a moderate amount of pale cytoplasm (marginal-zone–like variant); these may mimic small lymphocytic lymphoma/chronic lymphocytic leukemia or extranodal marginal-zone lymphoma, respectively.

Immunophenotyping typically shows CD20+, CD5+, CD43+, CD10−, CD23−, cyclin D1+ B cells expressing monotypic immunoglobulin, IgMD type, with λ being more frequent than the κ light chain. With antibodies to follicular dendritic cells such as CD21, a loose, expanded dendritic network is seen. This lymphoma is associated with t(11;14), a translocation that involves *CCND1* and IGH (see Table 31.2). Rare cases of mantle cell lymphoma are negative for cyclin D1. Nuclear expression of SOX11 has been demonstrated in >90% of cases of mantle cell lymphoma[107]; expression of SOX11 can be helpful in identifying the rare cyclin D1− cases. Of note, however, nonnodal mantle cell lymphoma, which often behaves in a more indolent manner than typical mantle cell lymphoma involving lymph nodes +/− extranodal sites, is often negative for SOX11. Expression of α4β7, the mucosal homing receptor, by mantle cell lymphoma is highly associated with GI involvement.[30,76,108]

Differential Diagnosis

On occasion, other types of lymphoma have the endoscopic or gross appearance of multiple lymphomatous polyposis. In addition, as noted earlier, not all mantle cell lymphomas take the form of lymphomatous polyposis. Follicular lymphoma,[10,17,76] extranodal marginal-zone lymphoma,[76] and even T-cell lymphomas[109] can have the appearance of lymphomatous polyposis. Mantle cell lymphoma without the classic polyposis appearance may be mistaken for other small B-cell lymphomas, particularly if the cytomorphology of the neoplastic cells is that of the small cell or marginal-zone–like variant. Small lymphocytic lymphoma/chronic lymphocytic leukemia (SLL/CLL), another CD5+ B-cell neoplasm, can secondarily involve the GI tract; the case of a patient with severe diarrhea due to SLL/CLL infiltrating the bowel has been reported.[110] SLL/CLL and marginal-zone lymphoma are negative for cyclin D1 and SOX11, in contrast to mantle cell lymphoma. A diagnosis can be readily established in most cases with careful study of hematoxylin and eosin (H&E)-stained slides augmented by immunohistochemistry. The distinction is important, because mantle cell lymphomas have a poor outlook compared with other low-grade B-cell lymphomas.

In cases of the blastoid variant of mantle cell lymphoma, occurrence in an older adult is a clue that lymphoblastic lymphoma is unlikely, and the immunophenotype (CD20+, CD5+, cyclin D1+, monotypic surface immunoglobulin+) confirms a diagnosis of mantle cell lymphoma and excludes lymphoblastic lymphoma. In cases of the pleomorphic variant, even though there are many large pleomorphic neoplastic cells, there is often an admixture of medium-sized cells more closely resembling those more typically seen in mantle cell lymphoma. Cyclin D1 expression by neoplastic cells confirms a diagnosis of mantle cell lymphoma.

DUODENAL-TYPE FOLLICULAR LYMPHOMA

Follicular lymphoma of the GI tract is rare, accounting for less than 4% of all primary GI lymphomas.[13] The 2017 WHO Classification recognizes a distinct variant of follicular lymphoma arising in the GI tract, designated "duodenal-type follicular lymphoma."[111] Affected patients are mostly middle-aged adults with a mean or median age in the 50s.[112-115] There is a slight to moderate female preponderance in some series[112,114,116] while others report men and women equally affected.[117,118] Precise evaluation of distribution of disease is evolving with the availability of techniques allowing more complete evaluation of the small bowel, including double balloon enteroscopy and capsule endoscopy. The duodenum is the site most often involved, most commonly the second portion.[113,114,116,118] Duodenal involvement is frequently accompanied by jejunal or ileal involvement.[115,118] The stomach and colorectum are affected less often. Only 3% of gastric B-cell lymphomas were follicular lymphomas in one large series.[24] Esophageal involvement is rare.[115,117] Patients present with a variety of symptoms, but abdominal pain is the most common. Others have mild or vague GI symptoms. A few have diarrhea, nausea, vomiting, or bleeding. Bleeding is more common with colorectal lesions. In centers with active screening for GI cancers, it is common for the lymphoma to be an incidental finding.[114,115,117,118] Elevated LDH is distinctly unusual, and the Follicular Lymphoma International Prognostic Index (FLIPI) is typically low.[118]

On endoscopy, nodularity of the mucosa is most common, sometimes with the picture of multiple lymphomatous polyposis, which may involve part or all of the GI tract.[76,114,117] The nodules are typically 1 to 2 mm, white or yellow-white, and scattered or confluent. The presence of multiple small nodules is more common with follicular lymphomas that involve the duodenal second portion.[118] GI follicular lymphoma may also take the form of a large, discrete, polypoid or ulcerated mass,[114,117] although such cases may not represent "duodenal-type" follicular lymphoma. The finding of single lesions, or of small numbers of lesions, may be more common in the stomach[117] and colorectum.[114] The lymphomas may be confined to the bowel wall or show regional nodal involvement. More distant spread suggests origin outside the GI tract.

The lymphomas consist of follicles, usually lacking mantles, that are composed of a monotonous population of centrocytes with few to scattered centroblasts distorting the normal glandular architecture. Very often there are increased numbers of lymphoid cells outside follicles, including the stroma of small intestinal villi. Lymphoepithelial lesions are not characteristic. The vast majority are low-grade (grade 1 to 2 of 3), with only rare grade 3 follicular lymphomas.[114,117]

GI follicular lymphomas typically have an immunophenotype similar to that found in nodal follicular lymphomas (CD20+, CD10+, BCL2+, BCL6+) (Fig. 31.10).[13,112-114,116,117,119] Often some of the lymphoid cells outside follicles are B cells with a similar immunophenotype, although CD10 and BCL6 may be more dimly expressed. Proliferation index with Ki67 is low. Follicular dendritic meshworks are hollow rather than intact.[120]

Molecular genetic and cytogenetic studies show clonally rearranged Ig heavy- and light-chain genes and *BCL2* rearrangement,[119,121] although rare cases negative for BCL2 protein and for *BCL2* rearrangement have been reported.[76] The pathological features of GI follicular lymphoma are

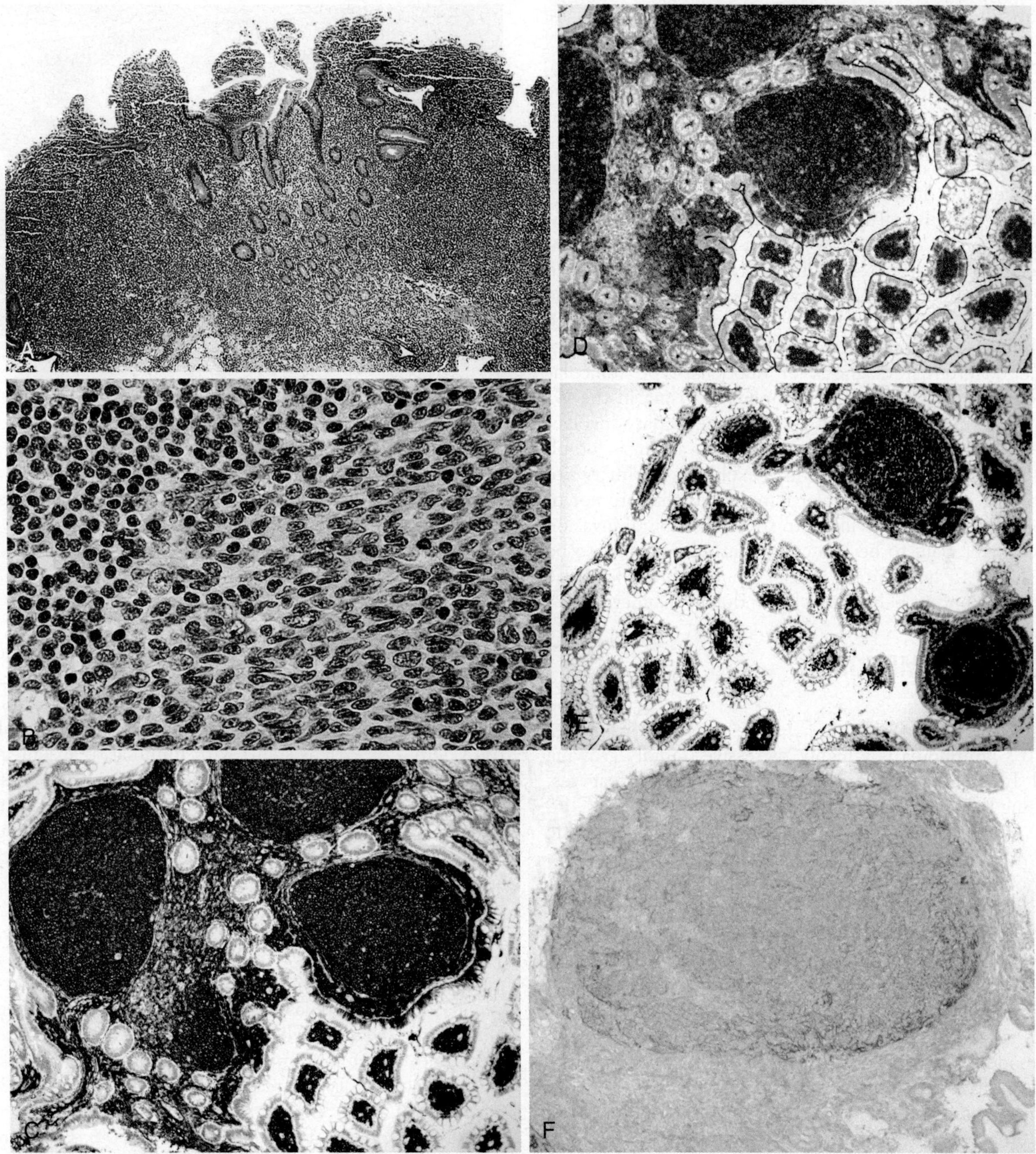

FIGURE 31.10 Follicular lymphoma, grade 1 of 3, duodenal type. A, The duodenal mucosa contains several large, poorly circumscribed lymphoid follicles. **B,** The lymphoid cells in this follicle are a monomorphous population of centrocytes with only a few large cells. The centrocytes are larger than the small lymphocytes in the adjacent mantle. Immunostains on another case show multiple follicles, as well as B cells in stroma of villi outside follicles, coexpressing CD20 **(C)**, CD10 **(D)**, and BCL2 **(E)**. **F**, CD21 highlights a follicle with dendritic staining concentrated around the follicle's periphery while staining is attenuated in the center of the follicle. (**C–F,** immunoperoxidase stains on paraffin sections.)

thus similar to lymph nodal follicular lymphoma. In contrast to follicular lymphoma arising in lymph nodes, however, expression of α4β7 integrin, a mucosal homing receptor, by GI follicular lymphomas is described.[122] Investigators have noted ongoing somatic hypermutation in the absence of activation-induced cytidine deaminase expression and restricted usage of variable regions of the immunoglobulin heavy chain gene, which together with the hollow dendritic meshworks, are features reminiscent of extranodal marginal-zone lymphoma that suggest response to antigen is important in the pathogenesis of these lymphomas.[123] Gene expression profiling studies have shown that duodenal-type follicular lymphoma has features more in common with gastric marginal-zone lymphoma than with nodal follicular lymphoma.[120]

Treatment has varied widely, and the best therapy has yet to be determined. Watchful waiting may be appropriate in many cases.[78] Patients generally do well, although some have persistent lymphoma, and some experience relapse. Relapses may involve the GI tract, lymph nodes, or other sites. Rare instances of response to antibiotics are reported,[117] although in general antibiotics are ineffective.[114] Some authorities recommend a "watch and wait" approach, with careful monitoring of disease for asymptomatic patients with low tumor burden.[115] A superior progression-free survival has been associated with female gender, lack of symptoms at diagnosis, and involvement of the second portion of the duodenum.[118] Histological transformation to diffuse large B-cell lymphoma has been described, but is uncommon. In one case the patient progressed on watch-and-wait surveillance from follicular lymphoma, grade 1 to follicular lymphoma, grade 3A at 5.5 years, to diffuse large B-cell lymphoma at 6 years of follow-up.[124] Death due to lymphoma is very uncommon.[76,112-114,116,118]

The differential diagnosis of duodenal-type follicular lymphoma includes follicular lymphoma arising in the GI tract that is not of duodenal type, and secondary involvement of the GI tract by follicular lymphoma arising in lymph nodes. Staging studies are helpful in excluding a primary site outside the GI tract. Follicular lymphomas that are not of duodenal type are more likely to show transmural invasion of the bowel wall, to be less consistently low grade, to be more likely to have intact (rather than hollow) dendritic meshworks, and to behave in a less indolent manner.[111,125]

BURKITT'S LYMPHOMA

Clinical Features

Burkitt's lymphoma is a highly aggressive, rapidly growing B-cell lymphoma with distinctive pathological features, including the presence of a translocation involving *MYC*.[126] In the WHO classification of tumors of the hematopoietic and lymphoid tissues,[126] three clinical variants of Burkitt's lymphoma are described: endemic, sporadic, and immunodeficiency associated. Endemic Burkitt's lymphoma occurs mainly in young children in sub-Saharan Africa. A complex interplay of environmental and host-related factors—climate, malaria, EBV, age and developmental stage of the patient—appear to play a role in the development of this subset of Burkitt's lymphoma. Most patients with immunodeficiency-associated Burkitt's lymphoma are HIV+, and a few have an underlying iatrogenic[127] or congenital immunodeficiency.[128] Patients with sporadic Burkitt's lymphoma are those who are neither immunodeficient nor fit the epidemiology for endemic Burkitt's lymphoma. Sporadic Burkitt's lymphoma is rare, although among children who develop lymphoma, it accounts for 30% to 50% of all cases of lymphoma.[126]

Burkitt's lymphoma accounts for about 5% of all intestinal lymphomas.[53] Involvement of the ileocecal region is the most common manifestation of sporadic Burkitt's lymphoma. Ileocecal disease is occasionally seen with endemic and immunodeficiency-associated Burkitt's lymphoma, although presentation with disease outside of the GI tract is more common. Infrequently, sites in the GI tract other than the ileocecal area, including the stomach and more distal portions of the colon, are involved.[47,15,24] Only 1% of gastric B-cell lymphomas were Burkitt's lymphomas in one large series.[24] GI Burkitt's lymphoma affects children and young adults, with a marked male preponderance.[47,15] In some cases, staging reveals disease beyond the GI tract.

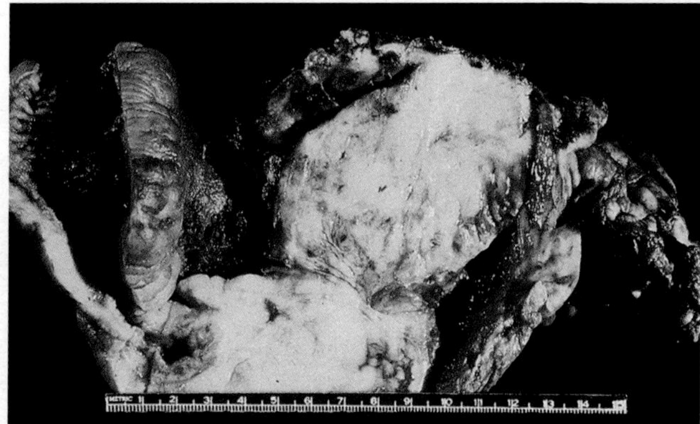

FIGURE 31.11 Burkitt's lymphoma. A large fleshy tumor arises in the ileocecal region.

Immunocompetent patients with Burkitt's lymphoma who are treated with aggressive, high-intensity, short-duration chemotherapy have an excellent prognosis.[129]

Pathological Features

On gross inspection, the GI tumors are usually bulky exophytic lesions, sometimes with ulceration (Figs. 31.11 and 31.12A).[17] Microscopic examination typically reveals a diffuse infiltrate of densely packed, uniform, medium-sized cells with round nuclei, granular chromatin, 3 to 4 small nucleoli, and a distinct rim of deeply basophilic cytoplasm (on Giemsa or Wright stain) with minimal to absent intervening stromal elements. There are typically numerous tingible body macrophages that produce a "starry sky" pattern. The mitotic rate is usually very high. Occasionally the nuclei of neoplastic cells show greater pleomorphism, and nucleoli are fewer in number but tend to be more prominent (see Fig. 31.12B–D). If the immunophenotype and genetic features are typical of Burkitt's lymphoma, such cases are still acceptable as Burkitt's lymphoma. In some instances neoplastic cells have plasmacytoid differentiation, with eccentric basophilic cytoplasm and a single central nucleolus. Nuclei may be somewhat pleomorphic. This tends to be found most often in immunodeficient patients.

Immunophenotyping reveals monotypic IgM+, CD20+, CD10+, BCL6+, CD5−, BCL2−,MYC+,TdT− B cells with a proliferation fraction of nearly 100%. Cytogenetic analysis reveals t(8;14), t(2;8), or t(8;22), corresponding to translocations involving *MYC* gene and either the IGH or, less often, the κ or λ light-chain gene. Translocations involving *BCL2* or *BCL6* are absent. Other than the translocation involving *MYC*, cytogenetic abnormalities are few or absent. EBV is found in about one-third of sporadic and immunodeficiency-associated Burkitt's lymphomas and is typically present in all endemic Burkitt's lymphoma (see Table 31.2).[126] The B-cell receptor (BCR) signaling pathway appears to be important in the pathogenesis of Burkitt's lymphoma. Next-generation sequencing analysis has disclosed mutations of the transcription factor *TCF3* (also known as *E2A*) or its negative regulator *ID3* in about 70% of sporadic cases of Burkitt's lymphoma. These mutations activate BCR signaling, which sustains survival of neoplastic cells via the PI3K pathway.[126] Other recurrent mutations, each of which may be encountered in a minority of cases

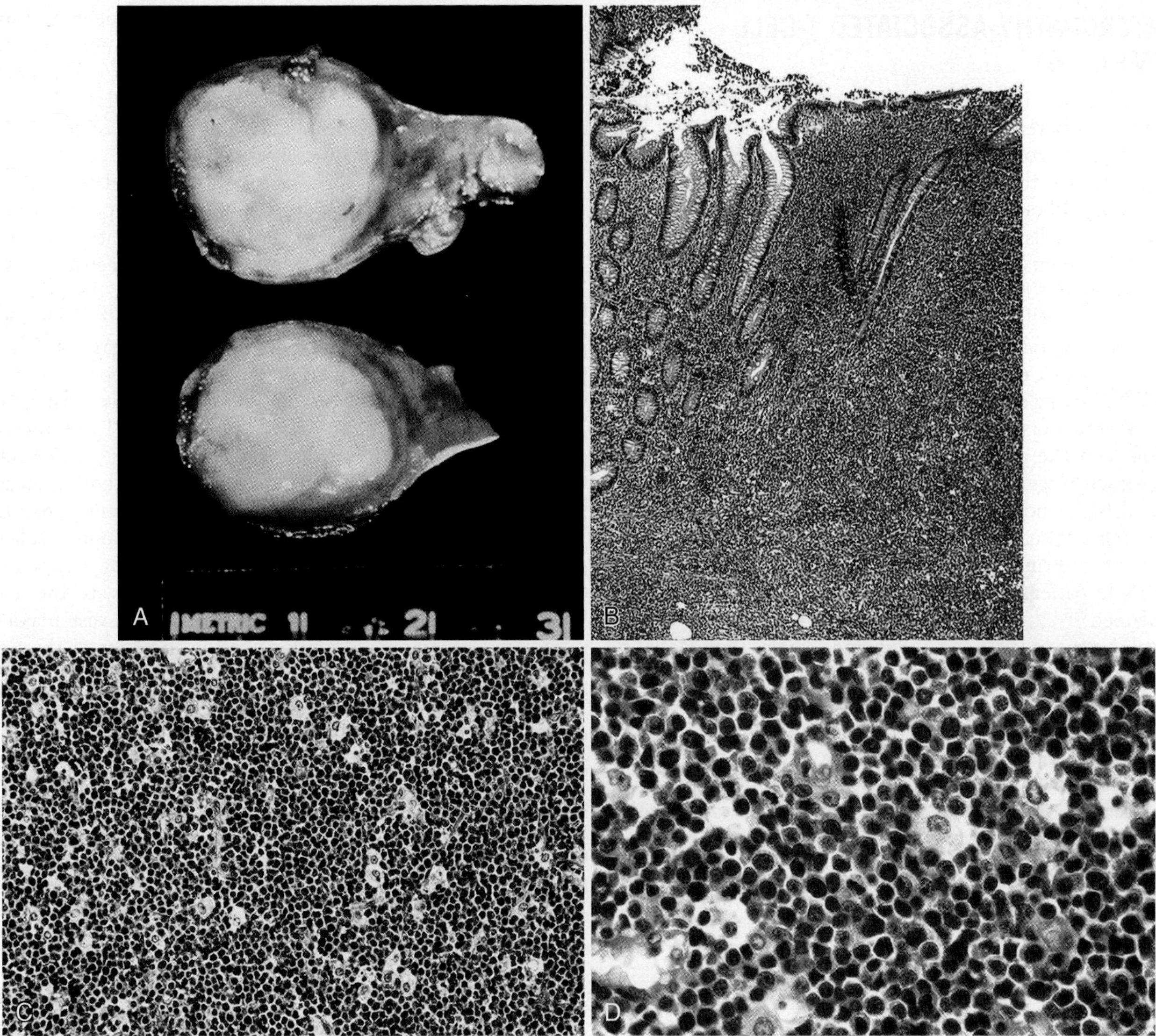

FIGURE 31.12 Burkitt's lymphoma. A, The appendix has been cross-sectioned to reveal that it is replaced by homogeneous white tumor. **B,** A dense, diffuse infiltrate of lymphoid cells involves the appendiceal wall. **C,** A "starry sky" pattern is prominent in many areas. **D,** Neoplastic cells are slightly pleomorphic, medium-sized cells with one or more nucleoli and a scant to moderate quantity of cytoplasm.

of Burkitt's lymphoma include *CCND3*, *TP53*, *RHOA*, *SMARCA4*, and *ARID1A*. Both the number of mutations overall and the proportion of cases with mutations in *TCF3* or *ID3* are fewer in endemic than sporadic Burkitt's lymphoma. An inverse correlation between EBV infection and the number of mutations is reported, suggesting that these mutations may serve in place of the virus for the activation of the BCR signaling.[126]

Differential Diagnosis

The differential diagnosis of Burkitt's lymphoma mainly includes other high-grade B-cell lymphomas, such as diffuse large B-cell lymphoma and high-grade B-cell lymphoma (NOS, and high-grade B-cell lymphoma with *MYC* and *BCL2* and/or *BCL6* rearrangements ["double-hit" lymphoma]).[130] The high-grade B-cell lymphomas have histological features that can mimic Burkitt's lymphoma. A clue to the diagnosis is that, in contrast to Burkitt's lymphoma, these double-hit lymphomas often express BCL2 protein, particularly if there is a *BCL2* rearrangement.[131] They also often have a lower proliferation index than Burkitt's lymphoma, do not have an association with immunodeficiency or EBV, and do not affect children or young adults. Careful attention to clinical, histological, and immunophenotypic features, supplemented by cytogenetic analysis will help to avoid misdiagnosis.

Of note, on a small biopsy, a floridly hyperplastic germinal center could mimic Burkitt's lymphoma. Reactive germinal center cells, like Burkitt's lymphoma, are CD20+, CD10+, BCL6+, BCL2−, with Ki67+ in nearly 100% of cells. A lymphoid follicle should be associated with a follicular dendritic meshwork, so that immunostains for CD21 or CD23 can be helpful, while such meshworks are typically absent in Burkitt's lymphoma. Clinical information regarding presence or absence of a large mass is helpful as well.

ENTEROPATHY-ASSOCIATED T-CELL LYMPHOMA

An association between malabsorption and intestinal lymphoma was noted early in the 20th century. Analysis of lymphomas that arose in association with celiac disease initially suggested that they were a distinctive type of malignant histiocytosis, although later studies showed that the neoplastic cells were T cells consistent with an unusual type of peripheral T-cell lymphoma,[132,133] termed enteropathy-associated T-cell lymphoma (EATL), and previously designated enteropathy-associated T-cell lymphoma, type I. According to the WHO classification, EATL is defined as a neoplasm of intraepithelial T cells that occurs in individuals with celiac disease and exhibits varying degrees of cellular pleomorphism, often with an inflammatory background, typically with enteropathic changes in the adjacent mucosa.[134] EATL with no history of refractory celiac disease (see later) is referred to as de novo EATL, and EATL in patients with a history of refractory celiac disease is designated secondary EATL.[135] Rare cases of intestinal T-cell lymphoma with features of EATL arising in patients with autoimmune enteropathy have been described[136,137]; the full complement of risk factors for the development of GI T-cell lymphoma remains to be defined.

Recent data suggest that the intraepithelial lymphocytes (IELs) that represent the cell of origin of EATL (and of refractory celiac disease II, see below) are innate IELs (NK/T-cell precursors) rather than postthymic T cells.[138]

EATL is uncommon, although it is the most common type of T-cell lymphoma to arise in the intestine. In areas with a high prevalence of celiac disease, such as Europe, there are an estimated 0.05 to 0.14 cases per 100,000 population and it accounts for about 1% of all non-Hodgkin lymphoma.[139] It accounts for approximately 5.4% of all peripheral T-cell or NK-cell lymphomas, although with substantial geographic variation: EATL represents 9.1% of this group in Europe and 5.8% in North America.[140] EATL is rare in Asia. Although an increased risk for lymphoma among celiac disease patients is greatest for primary GI lymphomas of T lineage, a large population-based study revealed an increased risk for B-cell lymphoma, and for lymphoma arising outside of the GI tract as well.[141]

Clinical Features

Enteropathy-associated T-cell lymphoma (EATL) occurs in adults over a wide age range (20 to > 90 years, with a mean or median age in the 50s or 60s), with a male preponderance in some series[135,139,140,142-144] and similar numbers of males and females in a few others.[145] The development of this type of lymphoma is closely linked to celiac disease. It is almost exclusively a disease of Caucasians and is more prevalent among individuals of European descent and, in particular, among those from the United Kingdom, especially Ireland and Wales.[143,145] Patients often have a history of celiac disease, which may be of long or short duration.[143,146,147] Strict adherence to a gluten-free diet reportedly diminishes, but does not eliminate, the risk of development of lymphoma while poor compliance with a gluten-free diet is associated with an increased risk for development of lymphoma.[146,148] In one large study of 1757 individuals with celiac disease, followed for a mean of 18 years after the diagnosis of celiac disease, approximately 0.5% developed EATL.[146] A subset of patients with EATL have no prior history of celiac disease; in some of these cases, there is histological evidence of enteropathy, suggesting that the patients had subclinical celiac disease. Even when enteropathy is not found, the presence of antibodies to gliadin or endomysium, or the human leukocyte antigen (HLA) class II haplotypes HLA-DQ2 or DQ8, or HLA genotype (*HLA DQA1*0501, DQB1*0201*) characteristic of celiac disease may be found.[149]

Patients with EATL present with abdominal pain, weight loss, diarrhea, vomiting, symptoms related to perforation or obstruction, fever, night sweats, or a combination of these findings. Among patients with a history of celiac disease, symptoms may suggest worsening of the celiac disease, with loss of response to a gluten-free diet.[47,135,139,143,145] Only a small minority present with a palpable mass on physical examination, and peripheral lymphadenopathy is very uncommon.[143] Rarely, patients present initially with symptoms related to distant spread of disease.[150] Lymphoma is often confined to the small intestine at the time of presentation.[135] EATL affects the jejunum or ileum or both in nearly all cases. The jejunum is affected more frequently than the ileum. The stomach and the colon are uncommonly involved. Mesenteric lymph nodes may be involved by lymphoma. Staging reveals spread, in a minority of cases, to the liver, and rarely to the bone marrow.[139,143] In the vast majority of cases, lymphoma is confined to the abdomen at the time of presentation.[143] In one series of patients with EATL, the Ann Arbor stage was I in 19% of cases, II in 58%, and IV in 23%.[143] Similar results were found in another series: 75% of patients had stage I or II disease.[144]

EATL has a poor prognosis. Patients treated with anthracycline-based chemotherapy have a slightly better prognosis than those treated with surgical resection alone. Treatment is complicated by the severe malnutrition that characterizes many of these patients. Some patients do not complete their planned chemotherapeutic regimens because of toxicity or disease progression.[135,139,143,144] Chemotherapy may be complicated by perforation, GI bleeding, or sepsis.[143] The majority of patients (84% in one series)[143] die of lymphoma or of complications of therapy.[143,146] Median survival ranges from 3 to 10 months.[139,140,144,145] However, a few patients treated with chemotherapy achieve remission and become long-term survivors, suggesting that chemotherapy is effective in a small subset of cases.[143,144]

In an attempt to improve outcome, newer agents or high-dose chemotherapy followed by stem cell transplant have been tested. In a few studies outcome appears to be improved, leading to 5-year survival on the order of 50% to 60%.[135,139] The perforation associated with intestinal involvement is the most common cause of death, but in some cases, dissemination of disease to lymph nodes and a wide variety of extranodal sites, such as liver, spleen, brain, heart, bone marrow, lungs, kidney, and thyroid, and toxicity due to therapy, contribute to mortality.[133,143]

Patients with secondary EATL have a slightly worse outcome than those with de novo EATL in some series.[135]

Pathological Features

EATL most commonly involves the jejunum or the ileum. Presentation with disease outside the small intestine is rare. Lesions may be single or multiple. They take the form of plaques, nodules, or strictures, with circumferential ulceration and often with perforation. Large masses are less common (Fig. 31.13).[47,134,143]

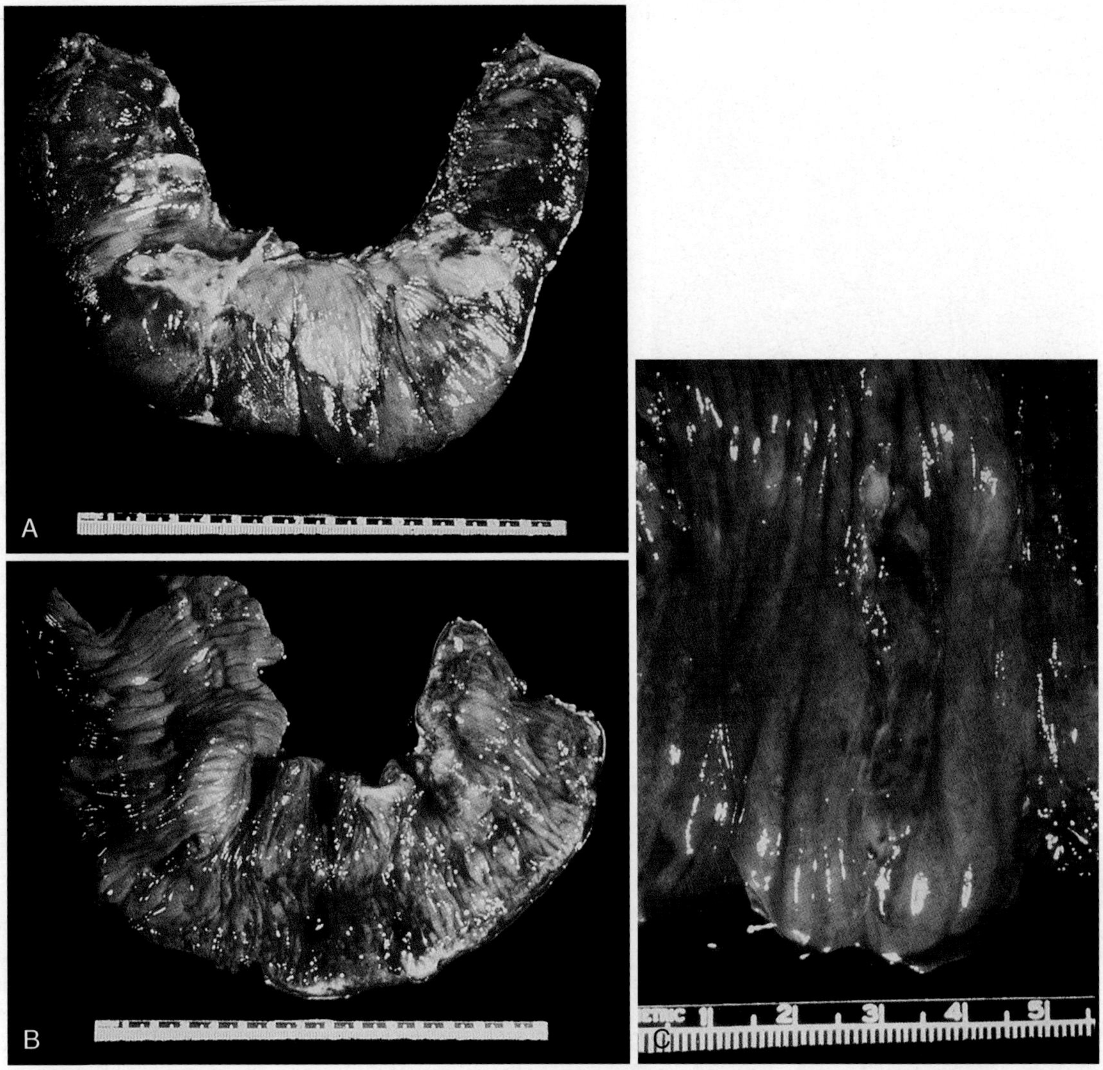

FIGURE 31.13 Enteropathy-associated T-cell lymphoma. A, The small intestine is dilated and its serosal surface is covered by a fibrinopurulent exudate resulting from perforation. **B,** The bowel is opened to reveal multiple small ulcerated lesions, but no large, discrete mass. **C,** Higher power view of one of the circumferentially oriented linear ulcers. (*From case records of the Massachusetts General Hospital. Weekly clinicopathological exercises. Case 53-1987. A 55-year-old woman with one year of malabsorption and the recent development of abdominal pain. N Engl J Med. 317:1715-1728, 1987 Copyright © 1988 Massachusetts Medical Society. All rights reserved.*)

Microscopic examination reveals a dense, diffuse infiltrate of atypical lymphoid cells associated with ulceration and a variable admixture of inflammatory cells. The neoplastic population usually consists of medium-sized and/or large atypical lymphoid cells with round or irregular nuclei, prominent nucleoli and scant to moderate quantity of pale cytoplasm. Tumor cells may occasionally have the appearance of immunoblasts or may be large and bizarre, with an anaplastic appearance. There is often an admixture of histiocytes, eosinophils, small lymphocytes, and plasma cells, which can occasionally obscure the neoplastic population.[84,133,140,143] Careful examination commonly reveals intravascular clusters of tumor cells. Changes of celiac disease are often seen in the mucosa away from the lymphoma, including increased numbers of IELs, villous atrophy, crypt hyperplasia, and a lymphoplasmacytic infiltrate in the lamina propria (Figs. 31.14 and 31.15).[84,133,134,140,143]

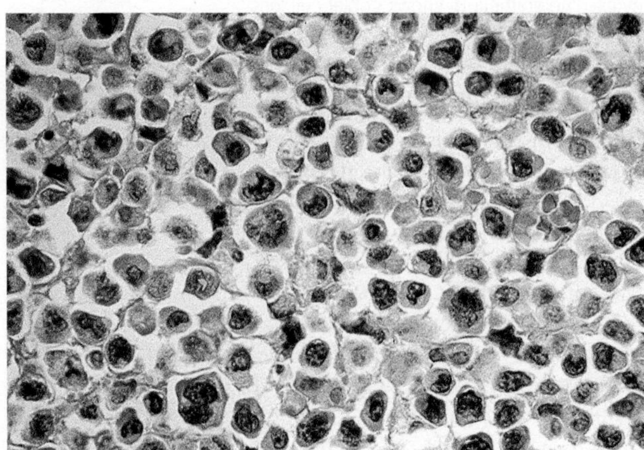

FIGURE 31.14 Enteropathy-associated T-cell lymphoma. High-power view shows large, bizarre pleomorphic cells. They were positive for CD30 (not shown).

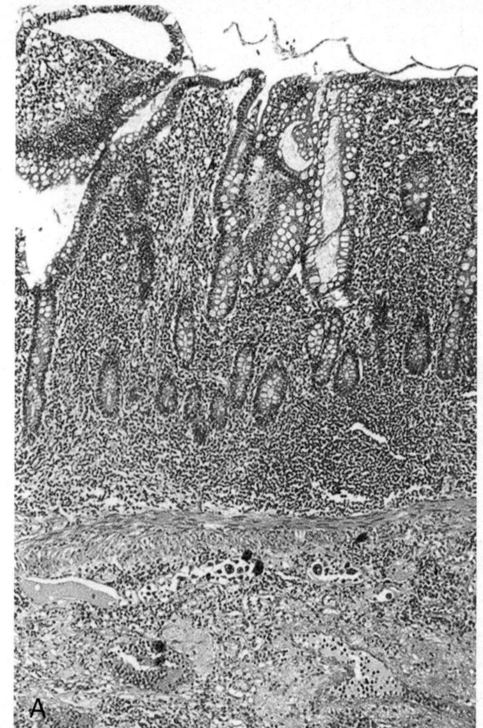

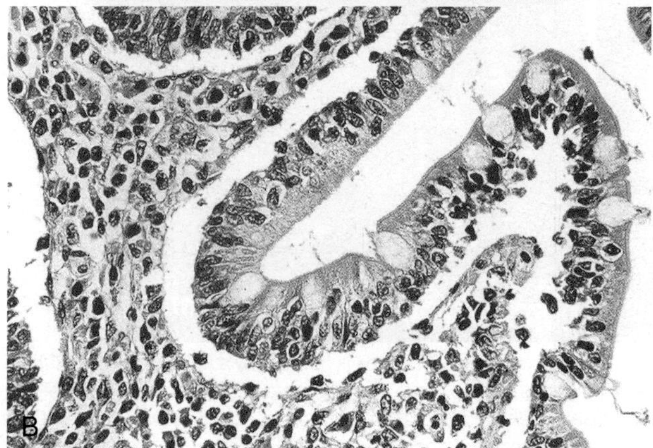

FIGURE 31.15 Enteropathy-associated T-cell lymphoma, changes in surrounding mucosa. **A,** The mucosa shows villous blunting. Tumor cells are seen in the lumen of a small vessel just deep to the muscularis mucosae. **B,** There are increased numbers of intraepithelial lymphocytes. The epithelium shows goblet cell loss.

Immunohistochemical Features

Immunohistochemistry shows that neoplastic cells usually express leukocyte common antigen (CD45), cytoplasmic CD3, and CD7 and consistently lack CD1a, TdT, and CD57. CD4, CD5, and CD56 are usually negative. CD8 is absent in most cases but can be expressed. Many cases are negative for both αβ T-cell receptor (TCRαβ) and for TCRγδ. A minority of cases expresses TCRαβ or less often TCRγδ, or rarely, both.[134,145,147] Neoplastic cells are SYK−.[147] CD30 is expressed by some cases of EATL, especially those with anaplastic morphology; Alk1 is not expressed. The neoplastic cells have a cytotoxic phenotype: they express cytotoxic granule proteins (T-cell intracellular antigen-1 [TIA-1], granzyme B, and perforin).[133,142] The cytotoxic nature of the neoplastic cells, and of the IELs from which they arise, could be responsible for tissue damage, including the villous atrophy, ulceration, and necrosis seen with celiac disease and EATL. In most cases, CD103, the human mucosal lymphocyte antigen (HML-1), is expressed. CD103 is expressed by intestinal IELs and by a subset of lamina propria lymphocytes. Its expression is characteristic of EATL.[151] CD103 is also expressed in hairy cell leukemia, some cases of monomorphic epitheliotropic intestinal T-cell lymphoma (MEITL) (see later), and a subset of cases of HTLV1+ adult T-cell leukemia/lymphoma.[152]

Lymph Node Changes

Mesenteric lymph nodes are almost always enlarged, although they are not always involved by lymphoma. In partially involved lymph nodes, the lymphoma may be found in sinuses or in the paracortex.[30] Enlarged nodes free of tumor may show nonspecific reactive changes, edema, or mesenteric lymph node cavitation. In the latter condition, lymph nodes may be markedly enlarged (up to 8 cm) and show cystic change, so that the lymph node consists of a thickened capsule and a thin rim of lymphoid tissue surrounding clear or turbid fluid that most likely represents lymph.[153] Mesenteric lymph node cavitation is not specific for EATL; it may be seen in celiac disease without lymphoma, and in refractory sprue. The condition may be related to severe malnutrition. When malnutrition is corrected, the lymph node changes may regress.[150]

MONOMORPHIC EPITHELIOTROPIC INTESTINAL T-CELL LYMPHOMA

Clinical Features

Monomorphic epitheliotropic intestinal T-cell lymphoma (MEITL), previously designated EATL type II, has clinical and pathological features that distinguish it from EATL.[144] In contrast to EATL, it does not appear to be associated with celiac disease or with an increased frequency of HLA types associated with celiac disease.[142] Almost all cases of MEITL affect Caucasians, Asians, or Hispanics.[145,154] When MEITL and EATL are considered together, MEITL is less common, accounting for approximately 20% of cases among Caucasians[140,144,155] Most patients are middle-aged and older adults with a median age in the 50s or 60s, and a male:female ratio that ranges from approximately 1:1 to 3:1 in different series.[145,147,155-157]

Patients present with abdominal pain, perforation, and/or obstruction typically without a history of malabsorpt ion.[145,155,157-160] The lymphoma often involves the small bowel, with the jejunum being the segment most often involved. There may be concurrent involvement of the colon or stomach. In contrast to EATL, occasional cases of MEITL are reported to involve the colon without small intestinal involvement.[8,140,157,161,162] The lymphoma is usually localized (stage I or II) but occasionally it may also involve other intraabdominal structures, omentum, mesentery, and less often more distant sites, including bone marrow, inguinal lymph nodes, and brain.[155,157,159,160] The clinical course and response to therapy are similar to EATL, and the prognosis is equally poor.[145,155-157,159]

Pathological Features

On endoscopy or gross examination, lymphomas take the form of diffuse mucosal thickening, sometimes with granularity, nodularity, hyperemia or edema, or of unifocal or multifocal lesions, usually accompanied by ulceration and often by perforation.

Microscopic examination reveals sheets of monotonous lymphoid cells, often with transmural invasion. Neoplastic cells are relatively monotonous small- or medium-sized, occasionally medium-sized to large lymphoid cells with dark to stippled chromatin, small to absent nucleoli and scant to moderate quantity of pale cytoplasm without a conspicuous component of admixed reactive cells such as histiocytes and eosinophils and without conspicuous fibrosis. Most lymphomas show surface ulceration, but away from sites of ulceration and perforation, necrosis is typically absent. At the periphery of the lymphoma, tumor cells often involve the mucosa with less involvement of deeper portions of the wall of the bowel. Examination of mucosa away from the lymphoma usually shows a marked increase in IELs. Villous blunting and crypt hyperplasia are often absent, and if present, are usually mild. The areas with increased IELs may be adjacent to, or at a distance from the lymphoma (Fig. 31.16).[155-157,161-164]

The most common immunophenotype of the neoplastic cells is CD3+, CD5−, CD4−, CD8+, CD56+, CD30−, MATK (megakaryocyte-associated tyrosine kinase)+, TIA1+, although there is deviation from this classic immunophenotype with respect to one or more of these markers in some cases.[142,155,157,160,162,163] In a few cases, aberrant coexpression of CD20, and rarely of CD79a, has been reported, although other B-cell markers are not expressed.[155,159,165,166] The majority of cases express TCRγδ, and thus appear to be of γδ T-cell origin, although βF1+ cases of αβT-cell origin are also described.[155,157] In one study, 55% were TCRγδ+ and 30% were TCRαβ+, while a TCR silent phenotype was uncommon.[147] There is aberrant overexpression of SYK (spleen tyrosine kinase) in nearly all cases, likely related to *SYK* promoter hypomethylation.[147] EBV is absent.[155,159] The immunophenotype of the IELs is similar, or identical to that of the neoplastic cells in the lymphoma.[155] When the immunophenotype of the IELs deviates from that of the lymphoma, the most common differences involve expression of CD8 or CD56.[155,159]

Compared with EATL, MEITL is composed of a more monomorphic population of smaller cells more often expressing CD8 and CD56, less often expressing CD30, with fewer admixed inflammatory cells, less necrosis, less fibrosis and less often with typical changes of celiac disease (prominent villous blunting, crypt hyperplasia) in the surrounding mucosa (see Table 31.2).[144,155,167]

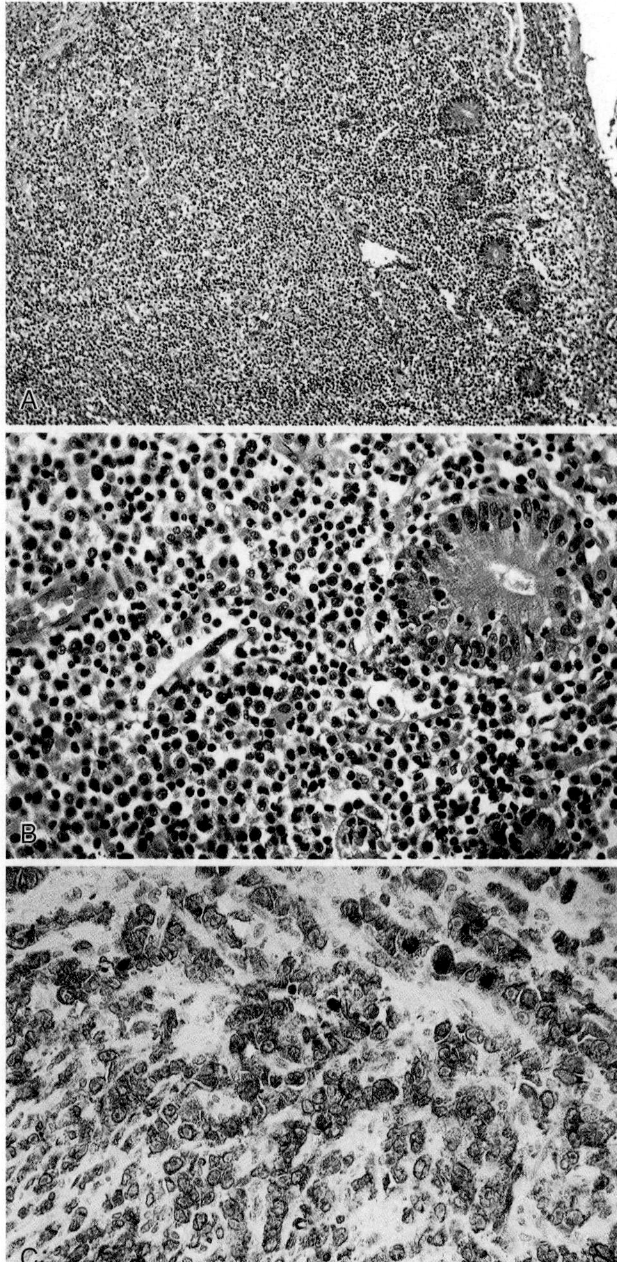

FIGURE 31.16 Monomorphic epitheliotropic intestinal T-cell lymphoma. A, A diffuse infiltrate of lymphoid cells occupies the bowel wall. **B,** Higher power view shows small and medium-sized atypical lymphoid cells. **C,** Neoplastic cells expressed CD3 (immunoperoxidase technique on paraffin section).

Molecular Genetic Features of EATL and MEITL

EATL and MEITL show overlapping genetic abnormalities; these are discussed together in this section. Molecular genetic studies have shown clonal rearrangement of the TCR β- and γ-chain genes.[144,156,167,168] EATL usually shows monoallelic rearrangement of the TCRγ chain gene, while MEITL usually show biallelic TCRγ rearrangement[169] In situ hybridization using probes for EBV encoded RNA (EBER) to detect EBV is typically negative; the presence of EBV should suggest a diagnosis of extranodal natural killer (NK)/T-cell lymphoma (see Differential Diagnosis, later).

EATL and MEITL both show a high frequency of genetic imbalances affecting multiple loci. Both EATL and MEITL often show either gains of the 9q34 region (location of protooncogenes *NOTCH1*, *ABL1*, and *VAV2*) or show deletions of 16q. Gains of chromosomes 1q and 5q (*APC* locus) are common in EATL, and are typically described as rare in MEITL,[134,142,154,169,170] although in one study, all 7 cases of MEITL evaluated showed a gain of 1q21.[163]

Both EATL and MEITL are characterized by mutations in chromatin modifiers, especially *SETD2* (32% of cases), and less often *TET2* and *YLPM1*. JAK-STAT is the most commonly mutated signaling pathway, with mutations in *STAT5B*, *JAK1*, *JAK3*, and *STAT3*, and also in the negative regulator of the pathway *SOCS1*. Occasional cases have mutations in RAS family genes *(NRAS, KRAS)*. *SOCS1* is more often mutated in EATL, while *KRAS* and *STAT5B* are more often mutated in MEITL.[145] Activation of the G-protein–coupled receptor (GPCR) signaling pathway is also described in cases of MEITL.[158,164] DNA repair gene *TP53* is also mutated in some cases of EATL and MEITL,[145] and there may be loss of 17p in the area of *TP53*. LOH at chromosome 9p21 (location of the cell-cycle inhibitor *CDKN2A/B*), is also relatively frequent; this abnormality is more common in EATL than in MEITL but has been described in both.[169,171] Cases with loss of genetic material in this area show loss of p16 protein expression, which suggests that this genetic change is functionally significant.[171]

In MEITL, gains in the area of the *MYC* locus on 8q, leading to *MYC* amplification, are common, but are rare in EATL.[142,156] Gains of Xp and Xq appear to be common in Asian cases of MEITL.[156] MEITL shows upregulation of MAPK signaling, correlating with strong expression of MAPK protein.[145]

COMPLICATED CELIAC DISEASE: REFRACTORY SPRUE AND ULCERATIVE JEJUNITIS

Refractory sprue and ulcerative jejunitis are serious, potentially fatal, manifestations of celiac disease. Refractory sprue is characterized by persistent or worsening malabsorption despite strict adherence to a gluten-free diet for >12 months, after other possible etiologies have been excluded. Approximately 2% to 5% of celiac disease patients have refractory celiac disease.[135,172] Biopsies typically show changes consistent with untreated celiac disease. Ulcerative jejunitis, or ulcerative jejunoileitis, consists of histologically benign mucosal ulcers occurring in patients with celiac disease. Patients with refractory sprue often have ulcerative jejunitis, and vice versa. Patients with refractory sprue or ulcerative jejunitis may develop EATL, and patients with EATL often have, or have had, refractory sprue or ulcerative jejunitis. When EATL follows refractory sprue or ulcerative jejunitis, the same clone is found in the lymphoma as in the histologically benign disorders.[168,173] The same clonal rearrangement is also found in EATL and in surrounding mucosa.[167]Activating mutations of the JAK-STAT pathway are described in RCD II, as in EATL,[138] underscoring their close relationship. These observations suggest a relationship between EATL and complicated celiac disease.[132,150] Refractory celiac disease is discussed in greater detail in Chapter 16.

Differential Diagnosis

EATL often does not form a large mass, and numerous inflammatory cells may be admixed, obscuring the neoplastic population. MEITL is characterized by relatively bland cytology, and in some cases, there is no conspicuous discrete mass. These features may result in misinterpretation as an inflammatory process such as ulcerative colitis or lymphocytic colitis.[174] Careful examination of routine sections for atypical cells, augmented by immunohistochemistry and, if necessary, molecular genetic studies, should help lead to the correct diagnosis. Any ulcerated lesion occurring in a patient with clinical or histological evidence of celiac disease should be approached with suspicion.

The differential diagnosis includes other types of neoplasms as well. The most important of these is diffuse large B-cell lymphoma; the appearance of the neoplastic cells may not be helpful in distinguishing B-cell from T-cell lymphoma. However, in contrast to EATL, diffuse large B-cell lymphoma tends to be found distally, in the ileum, and to be multifocal less often than EATL. Diffuse large B-cell lymphomas produce larger, exophytic or annular masses.[47,175] Unless the diffuse large B-cell lymphoma has arisen on a background of IPSID (see Immunoproliferative Small Intestinal Disease, earlier), the villi are typically normal. Immunohistochemical studies help to confirm the diagnosis. The uniform small-to-medium–sized cells of MEITL could potentially mimic MALT lymphoma; immunostains readily distinguish these two entities.

Extranodal NK/T-cell lymphoma, nasal-type, arising in the upper aerodigestive tract occasionally spreads to the GI tract,[176] and may even rarely arise in the GI tract. The histological and immunophenotypic features of EATL and MEITL show overlap with extranodal NK/T-cell lymphoma, nasal type. Features that favor NK/T-cell lymphoma over EATL include CD56 expression, presence of EBV in tumor cells, absence of histological and serological evidence of celiac disease, and the presence of angiocentric growth. Absence of clonal T cells also provides support for extranodal NK/T-cell lymphoma, as most lymphomas in this category are of NK cell origin and do not show rearrangement of their TCR genes. MEITL shares CD56 expression and lack of an association with celiac disease with extranodal NK/T-cell lymphoma, but MEITL often has a prominent increase in intraepithelial T cells, shows clonal TCR gene rearrangement, and is negative for EBV. (See also Extranodal NK/T--Cell Lymphoma, Nasal Type, later.)

The finding of a T-cell lymphoma in the absence of clinical or histological evidence of enteropathy, antigliadin or antiendomysial antibodies, or celiac disease–associated HLA type tends to exclude EATL, and raises the question of a diagnosis of peripheral T-cell lymphoma, NOS. The specimen should be evaluated carefully to exclude other specific types of T-cell lymphoma as well as unusual reactive processes. Primary intestinal peripheral T-cell lymphoma, NOS is reported to be less often multifocal, less often associated with perforation, and to have a somewhat better prognosis than EATL.[157]

NK-cell enteropathy is a rare atypical NK-cell lymphoproliferative lesion of unknown etiology, characterized by an atypical lymphoid infiltrate involving the GI tract, but in which the clinical course is much more indolent than that of extranodal NK/T-cell lymphoma or T-cell lymphoma.[177,178] The term *lymphomatoid gastropathy* has been used to describe cases of what appears to be the same disorder involving the stomach.[179] Patients are adults without celiac disease who have multiple small, superficial ulcerated lesions involving one or more portions of the GI tract (stomach, small intestine, colon). Biopsies show an interstitial or diffuse infiltrate of medium-sized to large atypical lymphoid cells with acute inflammation. Glandular destruction is found in more advanced cases, but lymphoepithelial lesions and epitheliotropism are not features of this disorder. The infiltrate involves the mucosa and sometimes the muscularis mucosa, but typically does not invade more deeply. The immunophenotype is consistent with NK lineage: cCD3+,

CD5−, CD7+, CD4−, CD8−, CD56+, TIA1 and/or granzyme B+. In one case, mutations of AXL and JAK3 were identified,[180] suggesting that NK-cell enteropathy may be a neoplastic, rather than an unusual reactive disorder. In contrast to extranodal NK/T-cell lymphoma the atypical cells are negative for EBV. In contrast to T-cell lymphoma clonal rearrangement of TCR genes is absent. Follow-up in most cases has been short; although the mucosal lesions may persist or recur, the patients have otherwise been well.[178]

The differential diagnosis with adult T-cell leukemia/lymphoma is discussed later, under Other GI T-Cell Lymphomas. Other poorly differentiated malignant tumors, such as metastatic melanoma and anaplastic carcinoma, may also be considered in the differential diagnosis.[175] Pertinent clinical history and immunophenotyping usually establishes a correct diagnosis in these cases.

EXTRANODAL NK/T-CELL LYMPHOMA, NASAL TYPE

Extranodal NK/T-cell lymphoma, nasal type, rarely arises in the intestine. It appears to be more common in Asians than in other racial groups, although even in series from East Asia, GI extranodal NK/T-cell lymphoma is uncommon. It accounted for only about 3% of all intestinal lymphomas in a series from Korea.[53] In a large series of extranodal NK/T-cell lymphomas from any site, 7% of cases arose in the small or large bowel.[181] Patients are mostly young to middle-aged adults, with men more often affected than women. They usually present with fever, abdominal pain and GI bleeding. This type of lymphoma appears to affect the small intestine and colon more than the stomach, although rare cases primary in the stomach[176,182] and even the esophagus[182] are reported. Disease is often multifocal within the GI tract and associated with perforation. On staging, disease may be localized or may be associated with distant spread at the time of diagnosis.[157,182,183] Patients presenting with an extranodal NK/T-cell lymphoma apparently arising in the GI tract should have careful evaluation to exclude an occult primary in the upper aerodigestive tract. The lesions are ulcerated but often do not form a bulky exophytic mass.[182]

Microscopic examination reveals neoplastic cells with morphology that varies from case to case. In most, tumor cells consist of medium-sized, or a mixture of medium-sized and large, atypical lymphoid cells with dark, often irregular, pleomorphic nuclei and scant to moderately abundant pale cytoplasm. The usual immunophenotype of the tumor cells is cytoplasmic CD3+, CD5−, CD4−, CD8−, CD56+, with expression of cytotoxic granule proteins, and presence of EBV, best demonstrated by in situ hybridization, in essentially all neoplastic cells (Fig. 31.17). Most extranodal NK/T-cell lymphomas are of NK-cell origin and do not rearrange their TCR genes, while a few cases are of T-cell origin and show clonal TCR rearrangement.[184] Genetic sequencing studies (not restricted to GI cases) have shown mutations in JAK-STAT pathway genes including *JAK3*, *STAT3*, and *STAT5B*, leading to constitutive activation of JAK-STAT signaling; mutations in RNA helicase genes DDX3X (20% of cases); and mutations in epigenetic modifiers (MLL2, ARID1A, EP300, ASXL3), reviewed in Chan and Lim.[158]

The prognosis is very poor. Most patients die of lymphoma, with a median survival that has usually been less than a year.[5,157,181,182] Improvements in therapy in recent years, including chemoradiation with L-asparaginase- or platinum-based chemotherapy, and novel, targeted therapies, have led to a less dismal prognosis.

OTHER GI T-CELL LYMPHOMAS

Infrequently, T-cell lymphomas other than EATL or MEITL, or other specific types of T-cell lymphoma, arise in the GI tract. These T-cell lymphomas have been designated intestinal T-cell lymphoma, NOS.[185] They are aggressive lymphomas that can be unifocal or multifocal in the GI tract. In many cases there is widespread disease at presentation. Neoplastic cells are medium-sized to large, epitheliotropism is not conspicuous, and most cases are CD4+ or CD4−/CD8−. The prognosis is unfavorable, but it is typically better than that of EATL or MEITL. Intestinal T-cell lymphoma, NOS is a somewhat heterogeneous entity, and may not represent a single distinct type of lymphoma.

Adult T-cell leukemia/lymphoma (ATLL) is a peripheral T-cell neoplasm caused by the retrovirus human T-cell leukemia virus type 1 (HTLV1).[186] Patients are mostly from Japan or from the Caribbean, in accordance with the distribution of individuals who are HTLV1+. Among patients with ATLL, GI involvement in the setting of widespread disease is fairly common while primary GI ATLL is rare.[187,188] In some instances, patients present initially with disease related to GI tract involvement, although staging usually reveals more extensive disease.[109,189,190] The stomach is the portion of the GI tract most commonly involved, followed by colon and the small intestine.[191] The most common endoscopic finding is multifocal ulceration; other manifestations include giant folds, polypoid lesions, submucosal tumors, and diffuse erosion.[192] In the GI tract, neoplastic cells often infiltrate epithelium to form small nests, and there is often an increase in reactive IELs in areas uninvolved by lymphoma. Neoplastic cells typically have highly irregular or multilobated nuclei; leukemic involvement of peripheral blood is common, where the appearance of the nuclei has given the neoplastic cells the designation of "flower cells." CD103 expression is common. The tendency for epitheliotropism by T cells that may express CD103 may result in misdiagnosis as MEITL or EATL. ATLL expresses T-cell antigens and is typically CD4+, CD7−, in contrast to MEITL and EATL.[152] Immunophenotyping, and evaluation for underlying HTLV1 infection and celiac disease can help to avoid misdiagnosis. In general, ATLL is an aggressive disease associated with a poor prognosis.

Rare cases of primary GI anaplastic large-cell lymphoma (ALCL) are also reported, including both ALK− and fewer ALK+ ALCL (Fig. 31.18).[2,64,11,193] Patients are affected over a wide age range; the median age of those with ALK+ ALCL is slightly younger than those with ALK- ALCL. Men are more often affected than women. The small intestine and the stomach are the portions of the GI tract most often involved.[193] Histological and immunophenotypic features (CD30+; variable, usually limited expression of T-cell antigens; B-cell antigens−; MUM1+; EBER−; ALK+ or ALK−) are overall similar to ALCL arising outside the GI tract, although compared with systemic ALK− ALCL, GI

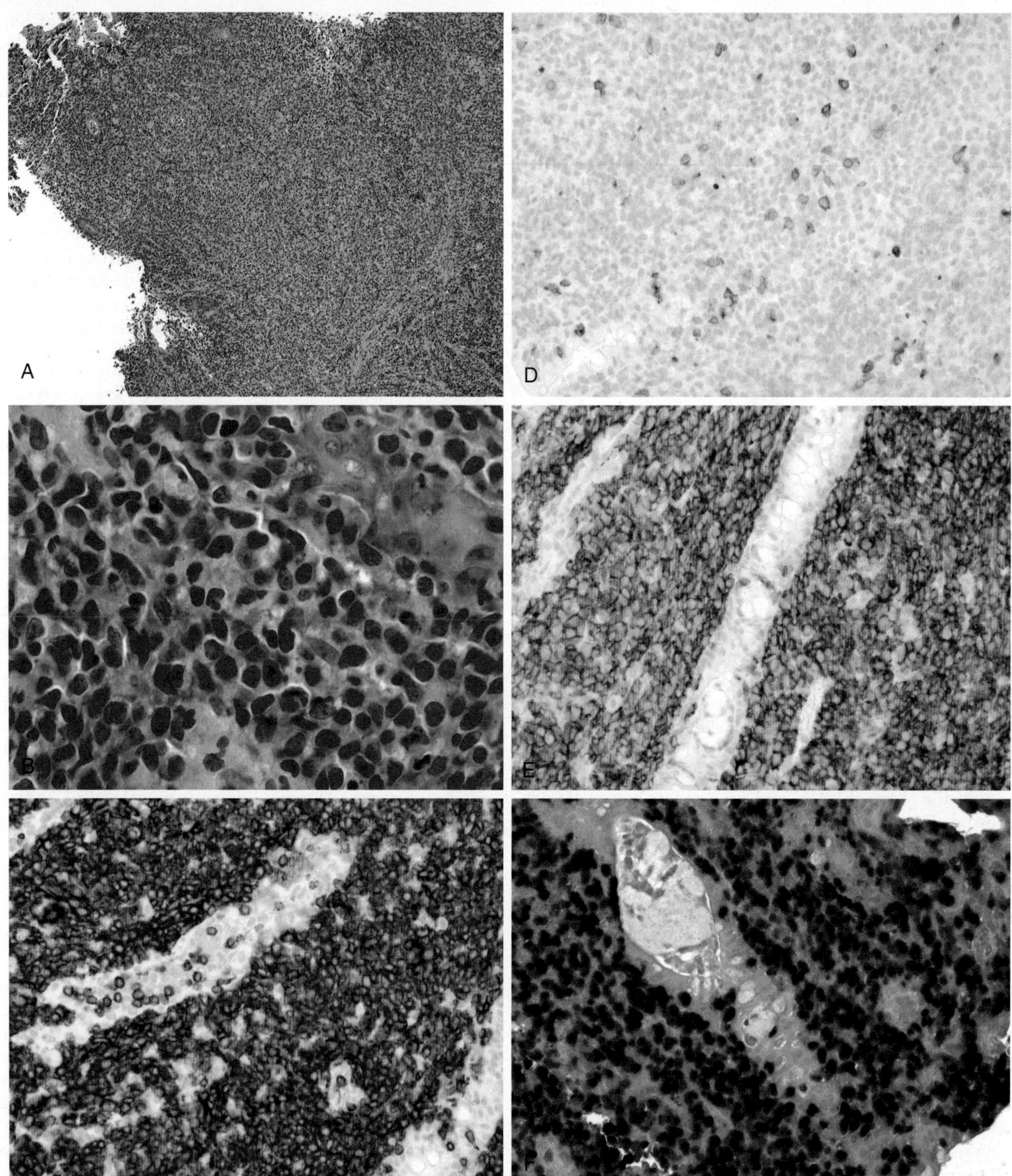

FIGURE 31.17 Extranodal NK/T-cell lymphoma involving descending colon and rectum. A, Low-power view shows a dense, diffuse lymphoid infiltrate. **B,** High power shows medium-sized to large atypical lymphoid cells with dark, irregular nuclei. Neoplastic cells are CD3+ **(C)**, CD5– **(D)**, CD56+ **(E)**, and EBER+ **(F)**. (**C–E,** immunoperoxidase stains on paraffin sections; **F,** in situ hybridization on paraffin sections.)

ALK− ALCL is more often EMA+ and granzyme B+, and less often TCRβF1+.[193] HHV8+ large B-cell lymphomas can mimic ALCL; for completeness, a stain for HHV8 should be performed to exclude this possibility. The prognosis of ALK+ ALCL is favorable, with 5 of 6 patients in one review alive and well at last follow-up. The prognosis of ALK− ALCL is poor.[193]

INDOLENT T-CELL LYMPHOPROLIFERATIVE DISORDER OF THE GI TRACT

Indolent T-cell lymphoproliferative disorder (LPD) is a clonal T-cell lymphoid proliferation that can involve the mucosa in any portion of the GI tract but most commonly involves the small intestine and colon.[194] Affected individuals are adults with a male preponderance. Some patients

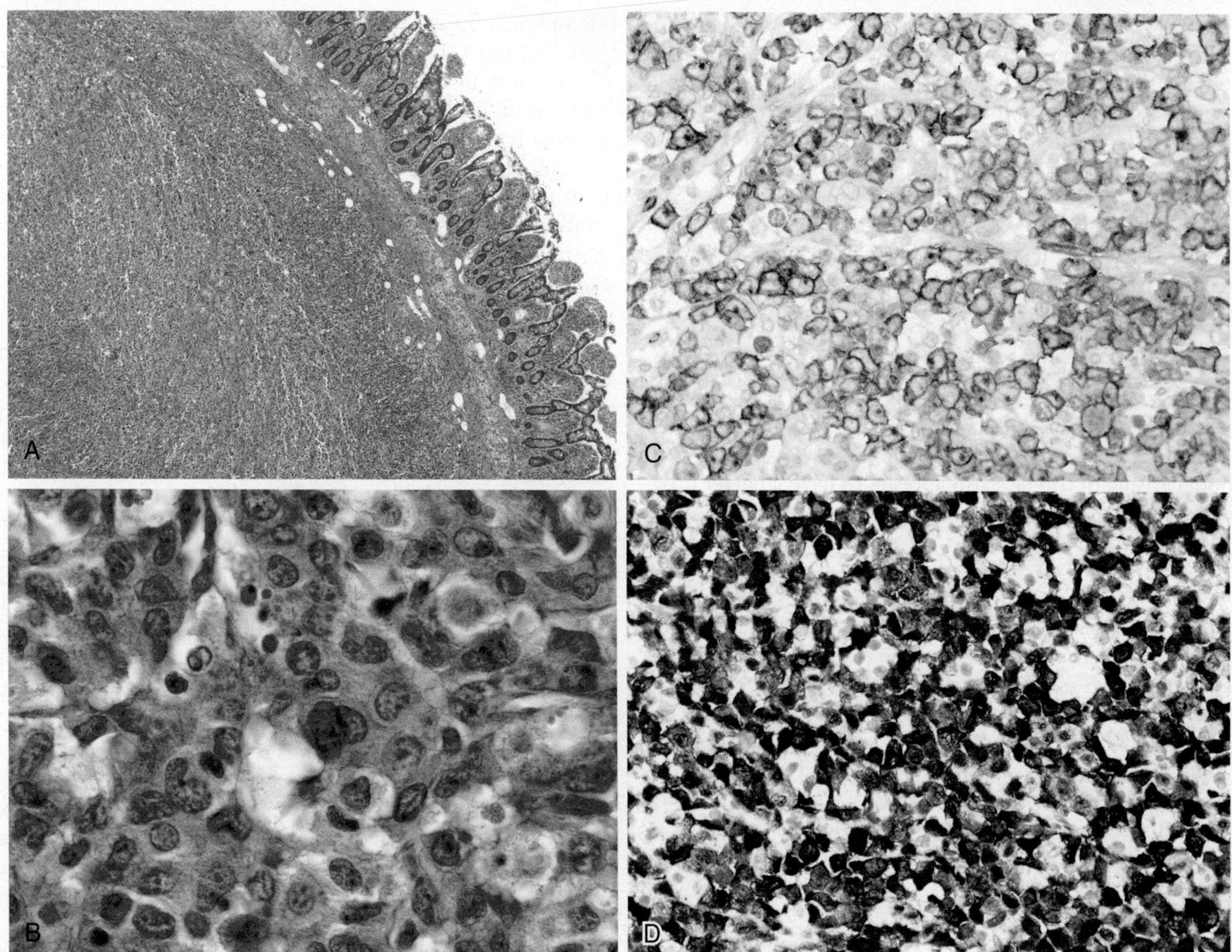

FIGURE 31.18 ALK+ anaplastic large cell lymphoma, arising in small bowel in an adolescent male. A, A dense, diffuse infiltrate of neoplastic cells invades deep into the wall of the bowel. **B,** High-power view shows pleomorphic tumor cells. Note the "hallmark" cells with indented, bean-shaped nuclei. **C,** Neoplastic cells are diffusely positive for CD30, and for ALK **(D)** in a nuclear and cytoplasmic pattern. (**C** and **D,** immunoperoxidase stains on paraffin sections.)

are reported to have prior Crohn's disease, although it is possible that the changes thought to represent Crohn's disease were actually indolent T-cell LPD. Patients present with abdominal pain, weight loss, vomiting, and diarrhea. The LPD often involves multiple sites in the GI tract. The mucosa is thickened, sometimes with small nodules, polyps, or prominent folds, sometimes with superficial erosions.

Microscopic examination reveals a dense, nondestructive infiltrate of the lamina propria, sometimes also extending to involve the muscularis mucosa and submucosa, by small monotonous lymphoid cells. Epitheliotropism is not conspicuous. In some cases, there are also epithelioid granulomas. The infiltrate is composed of mature T cells (typically CD3+, CD2+, CD5+, CD7 variable, TCRαβ+), with proliferation index of <10%. Most cases are CD4+ or CD8+, rarely CD4+, CD8+ or CD4-, CD8-. CD8+ cases are TIA1+, granzyme B-. EBV is absent. Cytogenetic analysis of CD4+ cases often shows a t(9;17) translocation corresponding to *STAT3-JAK2* fusion. On staging, some patients have mesenteric lymphadenopathy, but peripheral lymphadenopathy is absent. Response to chemotherapy has not been shown. The course is chronic, relapsing, and indolent overall, but rarely there is progression to disseminated disease, or transformation to a high-grade lymphoma.[194,195] In one report, a patient with indolent T-cell LPD later developed diffuse large B-cell lymphoma involving the GI tract.[196]

APPENDICEAL LYMPHOMA

Clinical Features

Appendiceal lymphoma is discussed separately because of its distinctive clinical features. The appendix is a rare primary site for lymphoma. Only 1 lymphoma was found in each of two large series, 1 of 1060 appendectomies[197] and another of 1970 appendectomies.[198] In a pediatric series of 209 appendiceal tumors, 12% were lymphomas.[199] In one series, only 2 of 117 GI lymphomas were found to have appendiceal involvement.[19] In a series of 39 small and large intestinal lymphomas, only 1 was appendiceal.[9] Other series have had no appendiceal lymphomas.

Lymphoma of the appendix affects mainly children and young to middle-aged adults,[15,197,200-205] although older adults may be affected as well.[206] Males are affected more often than females.[204-206] Appendiceal lymphoma has been reported in association with HIV infection,[206] but most patients are well before developing lymphoma. Almost all patients present with right lower quadrant abdominal pain that may mimic acute appendicitis.[197,204,206,207] GI bleeding may occur.[206] Some have a palpable mass.

The most common type of appendiceal lymphoma is diffuse large B-cell lymphoma, followed by Burkitt's lymphoma, follicular lymphoma, and MALT lymphoma, with rare cases of T-cell lymphoma and B lymphoblastic lymphoma also reported.[205] Most cases have had Ann Arbor stage I or II disease,[203,204] but localized disease is important for the cases to be convincing examples of primary appendiceal lymphoma. Patients with low-grade lymphomas are often treated with resection alone, and patients with higher-grade tumors have usually been treated with resection combined with radiation or chemotherapy.[201,203,204] The prognosis is good overall[197,204,205,207] and is excellent in children.[199] It is possible that a favorable outcome is related to the limited nature of the disease in most cases, but lymphoma arising in this site still appears to have a better prognosis than most other types of GI lymphomas.

Pathological Features

On macroscopic examination, the tumors may appear as swollen or nodular masses, sometimes described as fleshy and whitish gray, that usually expand the appendix circumferentially, sometimes invading adjacent fat.[197,206] Lymphoma may be confined to the distal appendix or may protrude into the cecum.[201,203,204,207] The most common type is diffuse large B-cell lymphoma, followed by Burkitt's lymphoma (see Fig. 31.11).[9,15,203,206] Rare cases of extranodal marginal-zone lymphoma of mucosa-associated lymphoid tissue (MALT lymphoma) have been reported as well.[197,200,203,207] One case of peripheral T-cell lymphoma has also been described.[201] Mantle cell lymphoma, involving the appendix in the form of multiple lymphomatous polyposis, has been described.[206]

Differential Diagnosis

The differential diagnosis is the same as that for the same types of lymphoma in other sites. Another entity that enters the differential diagnosis of appendiceal marginal-zone lymphoma is atypical marginal-zone hyperplasia of mucosa-associated lymphoid tissue, an uncommon condition described in the tonsils and appendices of children.[208] It is characterized by expansion of the marginal zone with follicular colonization. The expanded marginal zones are composed of CD20+, CD43+ B cells expressing monotypic lambda light chain+, and coexpressing μ and δ heavy chains. These features make these proliferations highly suspicious for marginal-zone lymphoma. In contrast to lymphoma these cases have not shown clonal immunoglobulin gene rearrangement, and patients have been alive and well with no evidence of lymphoma, although follow-up has not been long. The authors describing these cases suggest that they represent preferential expansion of λ light chain+ B cells, the etiology of which is uncertain.[208] This entity is somewhat controversial; others have described similar changes involving lymph nodes and extranodal sites in children and have interpreted them as marginal-zone lymphoma.[209]

HODGKIN LYMPHOMA OF THE GI TRACT

The GI tract is rarely the primary site for Hodgkin lymphoma. All reported cases have been classic Hodgkin lymphoma. Fewer than 0.5% of cases of Hodgkin lymphoma arise in the GI tract.[210] Because of the rarity of Hodgkin lymphoma in this location, strict criteria for its diagnosis should be used, including absence of peripheral and mediastinal lymphadenopathy; absence of substantial hepatic or splenic involvement; predominant GI lesion, with or without involvement of adjacent lymph nodes; and histological and immunohistological features characteristic of Hodgkin lymphoma.

Clinical Features

Only a small number of cases of primary GI Hodgkin lymphoma have been reported, and only a handful of them have been well documented, making precise evaluation of this entity difficult. With this limitation in mind, the disease appears to affect adults over a broad age range, with a male preponderance. In the general population, the sites involved, in descending order, are stomach, small intestine, and colon. Some patients reported to have GI Hodgkin lymphoma have had IBD, almost always Crohn's disease, often for many years, treated with immunosuppressive therapy.[210-212] The Hodgkin lymphoma affects the small intestine, colon, or both in cases associated with IBD. Patients with intestinal tumors have hematochezia, pain, nausea, vomiting, diarrhea, or symptoms related to perforation. In patients with Crohn's disease, the symptoms may resemble exacerbation of the original disease.[210,211]

Although by convention, the bulk of the tumor is in the GI tract at presentation, staging often reveals regional nodal involvement[211,213] and sometimes reveals foci of distant spread.[210] Patients have a favorable prognosis, with good response to therapy in many cases.[210-214]

A case of classic Hodgkin lymphoma presenting with anal pain and perianal fistula in a patient with Crohn's disease has been reported. Evaluation revealed Hodgkin lymphoma involving lymph nodes, anal mucosa and perianal fistula.[215] Given the extreme rarity of Hodgkin lymphoma arising in the GI tract, the lymphoma most likely arose in lymph nodes and secondarily involved the anus.

Pathological Features

The tumor tends to involve the full thickness of the bowel wall multifocally, usually resulting in ulceration.[210,212,213] In patients with Crohn's disease, there is preferential involvement of areas with fissures and preexisting severe inflammation.[210,212] Classic Hodgkin lymphoma of mixed cellularity and nodular sclerosis subtypes have been reported. Immunophenotyping shows that Reed-Sternberg cells and variants, are CD15+, CD30+, focally CD20+ or CD20−, CD3−,[210-212,214,216] CD79a−, and CD45−,[210] typical of Hodgkin lymphoma. Neoplastic cells have shown consistent positivity for EBV using in situ hybridization[210,212,217] and immunohistochemistry for latent membrane protein in the small number of cases that have been tested.[210]

The tendency for Hodgkin lymphoma to occur in areas of inflamed bowel suggests that the tumor is pathogenetically related to the chronic inflammatory process. The history of azathioprine or prednisone therapy in most cases associated with IBD and the presence of EBV suggest that immunosuppression plays a role in the genesis of Hodgkin lymphoma in this site.[210]

Differential Diagnosis

EBV+ mucocutaneous ulcer must be considered in the differential diagnosis of GI Hodgkin lymphoma. The two entities have overlapping histological and immunophenotypic features, and it is possible that some cases previously reported as GI Hodgkin lymphoma represent EBV+ mucocutaneous ulcer (see separate section later). The differential diagnosis of GI Hodgkin lymphoma also includes non-Hodgkin lymphoma and anaplastic carcinoma. It may be possible to distinguish these tumors on routine sections, but if immunohistochemistry is used, it should be noted that, as for Reed-Sternberg cells, carcinoma is CD45−and may be CD15+. An immunohistochemical panel that includes cytokeratin often helps establish a correct diagnosis.

GI LYMPHOPROLIFERATIVE DISORDERS IN ABNORMAL IMMUNE STATES

Human Immunodeficiency Virus Infection

Lymphoma is the second most common malignancy in HIV-infected patients, following Kaposi's sarcoma. In the years before the availability of highly active antiretroviral therapy (HAART), the risk of lymphoma was 50 to 60 times greater for HIV+ patients than for individuals without HIV infection.[218,219] HAART has been associated with a decrease in the frequency of Kaposi's sarcoma and of some types of lymphoma. The proportion of extranodal lymphomas among HIV+ patients is higher than in the general population, and the GI tract is the extranodal site most often affected, with about one-third of all HIV-associated non-Hodgkin lymphomas arising in this site.[219]

Patients are almost all young or middle-aged homosexual men.[219,220] The frequency of lymphoma in different parts of the GI tract is the opposite of that seen in HIV− patients: the colon and anorectal area are most often affected, followed by the small intestine, with the stomach being the least involved.[219] It has been suggested that a high proportion of anorectal lymphomas may result from repeated trauma and chronic inflammation, with uncontrolled proliferation of EBV+ B cells.[220] Grossly, the lymphomas have the appearance of ulcers, masses, or fistulas; the appearance may mimic that of inflammatory or infectious conditions. They are usually confined to the GI tract.[219] The lymphomas are almost all high-grade B-cell lymphomas; diffuse large B-cell lymphoma, often of the immunoblastic type, is most common, followed by Burkitt's lymphoma and polymorphous high-grade B-cell lymphoma (see Fig. 31.6). Almost all anorectal cases tested have been EBV+ by in situ hybridization.[220]

Plasmablastic lymphoma is a distinctive type of diffuse large B-cell lymphoma, often associated with immunodeficiency. Plasmablastic lymphoma has been described in the GI tract, most often in the anorectal area,[221] but also in the intestines[222] and rarely in the esophagus.[223] Most plasmablastic lymphoma patients are HIV+, but plasmablastic lymphoma has been reported in a Crohn's disease patient who had received multiple therapies, including infliximab.[222] GI involvement by plasmablastic lymphoma has also been reported in patients without known immunodeficiency.[223] Patients present with a mass, pain, or bleeding. Plasmablastic lymphomas are composed of a diffuse infiltrate of large atypical lymphoid cells with the appearance of plasmablasts and immunoblasts. Diagnosis may be difficult because plasmablastic lymphomas lack CD20 expression; they often express markers found in later stages of B-cell differentiation, such as CD79a, CD138, and MUM1. As they are plasmacytoid, they may also express monotypic cytoplasmic immunoglobulin. Cellular proliferation, as measured by Ki67, is high, and in most cases tumor cells harbor EBV. Rearrangements involving *MYC* are a common underlying genetic event in plasmablastic lymphoma, and neoplastic cells are often MYC+.[224] The prognosis is poor.

Primary effusion lymphoma is a rare type of HHV8+ large B-cell lymphoma that presents as an effusion, without a solid tumor mass; it occurs most often in HIV+ patients. A few cases of extracavitary primary effusion lymphoma (HHV8+), with features similar to those seen in primary effusion lymphoma except for presentation as a solid mass or masses rather than as an effusion, have presented with gastric or intestinal involvement in HIV+ patients. Rarely patients have endoscopic findings of multiple lymphomatous polyposis.[225] In some cases, patients also developed lymphomatous effusions.[226-228] The lymphomas are composed of large atypical cells with immunoblastic, plasmablastic, or bizarre, anaplastic morphology. Mitotic figures and apoptotic debris are often abundant. Nuclei of neoplastic cells are positive with an immunostain for HHV8. Tumor cells are typically CD45+, and are often positive for CD30, CD138, and EBV, but are mostly negative for B- and T-cell -specific markers. There may be aberrant expression of T-lineage markers, leading to a misdiagnosis of T-cell lymphoma.[229] Clonal rearrangement of immunoglobulin heavy and/or light chain genes is usually demonstrable, without clonally rearranged TCR genes, confirming B lineage.[228] The lymphomas can be treated with surgery and chemotherapy, but the prognosis is poor, with many patients succumbing to lymphoma or other complications of HIV infection.[218,219] Patients receiving HAART may be better able to tolerate therapy, and they appear to have a better outcome.[227]

Several cases of Hodgkin lymphoma in HIV+ patients have been described (see Hodgkin Lymphoma of the GI Tract, earlier).[217]

In summary, GI lymphoma in HIV+ patients affects younger patients with a higher proportion of male patients, shows preferential involvement of distal GI tract, and is more often high grade and more often EBV+ than lymphoma in the general population.[219,220]

Lymphomas Associated with Iatrogenic Immunosuppression in Transplant Recipients

Allograft recipients have an increased risk of lymphoproliferative disorders compared with the general population.[127,230] The posttransplantation lymphoproliferative disorders (PTLDs) have features that differ from lymphoma in the nonimmunosuppressed population. PTLDs are characterized by heterogeneous pathological features, a strong association with EBV, a variable response to therapy, and an often unpredictable clinical course. The median interval from transplantation to PTLD is typically short, often within 6 months in cyclosporine-treated patients. However, PTLD may occur at any time, sometimes many years after transplant. Patients may respond to decreased levels of immunosuppression, or they may require surgical resection, chemotherapy, or radiation. The prognosis is guarded; many patients succumb to PTLD. The risk of PTLD is higher among nonrenal allograft recipients, patients receiving higher levels of immunosuppressive therapy, and patients seronegative for EBV before transplant. Many cases arise in extranodal locations; among patients receiving cyclosporine, the proportion of PTLDs arising in the GI tract is particularly high. Up to approximately one-third of PTLDs in the setting of cyclosporine-based immunosuppression appear with involvement of the GI tract. The small intestine is affected more often than the stomach or colon.[231]

PTLDs are classified according to the criteria of the WHO classification as (1) nondestructive PTLDs (including infectious mononucleosis, florid follicular hyperplasia, and plasmacytic hyperplasia), (2) polymorphic PTLDs, (3) monomorphic PTLDs, both B-cell neoplasms (including diffuse large B-cell lymphoma, Burkitt's lymphoma, plasma cell myeloma, and plasmacytoma) and T-cell neoplasms, and (4) classic Hodgkin lymphoma PTLD.[127,230] Nondestructive lesions usually involve Waldeyer's ring or lymph nodes rather than the GI tract. The lesions show at least some architectural preservation. Infectious mononucleosis PTLD resembles lymphoid infiltrates seen in infectious mononucleosis in the general population, florid follicular hyperplasia PTLD shows follicular hyperplasia, and plasmacytic hyperplasia PTLD shows mainly a proliferation of plasma cells with a few immunoblasts. They are usually polyclonal, EBV+ B-cell proliferations. Polymorphic PTLDs produce destructive mass lesions and show the full range of B-cell differentiation, with lymphocytes, plasma cells, immunoblasts, plasmablasts, and cells resembling follicle center cells (Fig. 31.19). Immunophenotyping reveals B cells that express either polytypic or monotypic Ig, but genetic studies almost always show clonal B cells infected with EBV. Most cases of monomorphic PTLD have morphological, immunophenotypic, and genetic features of diffuse large B-cell lymphoma (Fig. 31.20). Occasional cases are Burkitt's lymphoma. Monomorphic PTLDs of B lineage are usually EBV+. Plasma cell myeloma, plasmacytoma, and classic Hodgkin lymphoma PTLDs are rare. The polymorphic and monomorphic PTLDs of B lineage are those most likely to be encountered in the GI tract.[231-233] There are rare EBV+ GI marginal-zone lymphomas in transplant recipients, which are considered PTLDs[65]; however, in general, EBV− low-grade lymphomas, despite their occurrence after transplant, are not considered to be PTLDs.[127] A few cases of GI peripheral T-cell lymphoma have arisen after solid organ transplant, usually many years after transplantation, and usually involving the small intestine. Some are EBV+. Most of these patients died of their PTLD.[234] Hepatosplenic T-cell lymphoma can occur in transplant recipients (see Hepatic Lymphoma, later).[127,230]

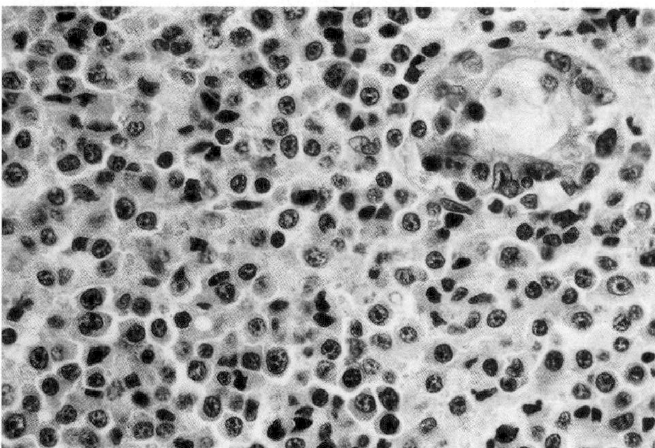

FIGURE 31.19 Posttransplantation lymphoproliferative disorder, polymorphic (nomenclature change). This intestinal tumor is composed of a mixture of small and large lymphoid cells, many with plasmacytoid features.

Inflammatory Bowel Disease–Associated Lymphoma

Non-Hodgkin lymphoma rarely arises in patients with IBD. Whether or not there is an increased incidence of lymphoma in patients with IBD compared with the general population is controversial.[235] In one recent population-based study, an increased risk of borderline statistical significance for the development of lymphoproliferative disorders among those treated with immunosuppressants was identified for IBD overall.[236] Increased numbers of lymphoproliferative disorders were found among patients with Crohn's disease and also ulcerative colitis. However, lymphoma in this setting does have characteristic features. For patients with either ulcerative colitis or Crohn's disease, lymphoma is almost

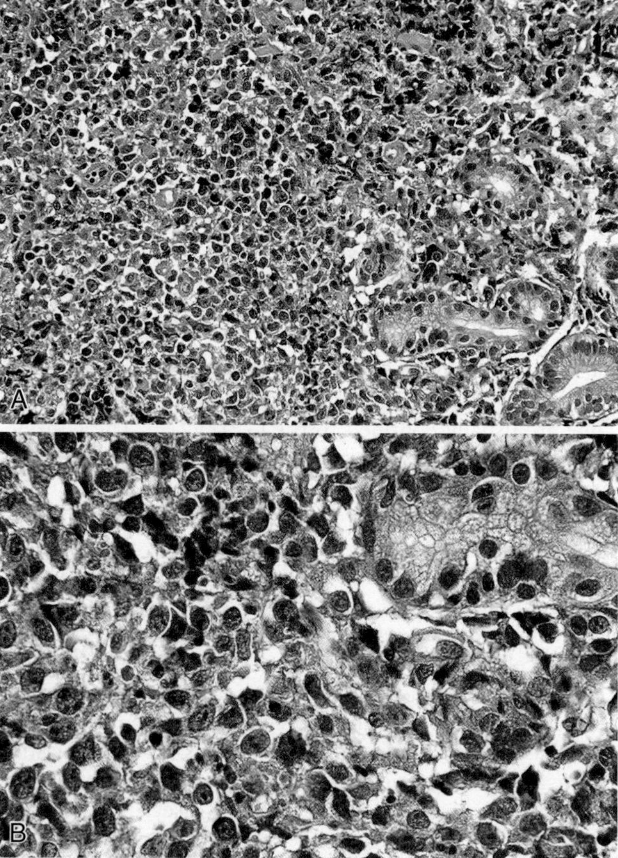

FIGURE 31.20 Posttransplantation lymphoproliferative disorder, monomorphic, involving the stomach. At low **(A)** and high power **(B)**, the histological features are indistinguishable from those of sporadic gastric diffuse large B-cell lymphoma.

never suspected preoperatively, and in rare instances, a diagnosis of lymphoma is only established at autopsy. Patients typically present with symptoms that suggest worsening of IBD. Some have perforation, presence of a mass, hemorrhage, or symptoms thought to represent IBD intractable to treatment, prompting surgical resection.[237]

In one series of 117 GI lymphomas, one arose in a patient with ulcerative colitis.[19] In other series of colorectal lymphoma, from 3% to 15% of cases were in patients with ulcerative colitis.[14,18,202] Compared with other colonic lymphomas, the lymphomas in patients with ulcerative colitis are more often multiple (38% compared with 10% in the general population) and more often distally located in the colon, in contrast to the preferential involvement of the cecum seen in patients without ulcerative colitis.[202,238] The lymphomas are almost always found in sites of active inflammation in patients with long-standing ulcerative colitis (median interval, 8 to 12 years, with wide variation).[237-239] In one report, the incidence of lymphoma appeared to be increased, and the interval to lymphoma appeared decreased (3.1 years) in patients with ulcerative colitis treated with immunosuppressive therapy, compared with cases in older reports.[240] This suggests that immunosuppressive therapy may accelerate the development of lymphoma in potentially susceptible patients. The lymphomas are usually described as high grade, but a minority are low grade; most have been diffuse large B-cell lymphomas.[237,239,240] Others have been low- or high-grade polymorphic B-cell lymphomas[241] with rare cases of extranodal marginal-zone lymphoma.[238,239] The lymphomas that have been tested often harbor EBV, supporting the idea that these lymphomas have arisen in the setting of an abnormal immune state, with iatrogenic immunosuppression contributing to the immune dysregulation.[237,239] Most of the lymphomas are confined to the intestine; in a few patients, disease is widespread. Behavior tends to depend on the grade of the lymphoma.

Approximately 42 cases of lymphoma (two gastric, 19 colonic, 21 small intestinal [most often in the terminal ileum]) arising in association with Crohn's disease have been reported.[237,239,242] Men are affected much more often than women. Patients are typically adults with a wide age range. Most have long-standing Crohn's disease before development of lymphoma. The lymphoma usually arises in areas affected by Crohn's disease. A minority are classified as Hodgkin lymphomas (see Hodgkin Lymphoma of the GI Tract, earlier). The remainder are non-Hodgkin lymphoma; diffuse large B-cell lymphoma is the most common type.[239,240,242] Rare marginal-zone lymphomas (MALT lymphomas) and mantle cell lymphomas occurring in areas of the GI tract uninvolved by Crohn's disease are reported; these may represent sporadic lymphomas unrelated to IBD.[237] Approximately half of patients are alive and free of lymphoma at last follow-up, and the others died, sometimes of lymphoma, sometimes in the postoperative period, and sometimes of other causes.[242] In a study of GI lymphoma arising in 5 patients with ulcerative colitis and 10 patients with Crohn's disease, disease-specific survival was 78% at 1 year and 63% at 5 years. A better prognosis was associated with stage I lymphomas.[237]

A few cases of hepatosplenic T-cell lymphoma have been described in patients with IBD treated with a combination of infliximab, a tumor necrosis factor α blocking agent, and other immunosuppressive medication[243] (see Hepatic Lymphoma, later).

X-Linked Lymphoproliferative Disorder

X-linked lymphoproliferative disorder is a rare, X-linked recessive disorder affecting young boys and characterized by a selective immunodeficiency for EBV. On exposure to EBV, these children develop severe, often fatal, infectious mononucleosis or malignant lymphoma. Lymphomas affect the GI tract in 76% of cases; the ileocecal area is most often involved. They are B-lineage lymphomas that can be classified as Burkitt's lymphoma or diffuse large B-cell lymphoma. When tested, EBV is usually present.[244,245]

Common Variable Immunodeficiency

Common variable immunodeficiency is typically an adult-onset immunodeficiency syndrome characterized by decreased levels of one or more classes of immunoglobulin and susceptibility to a variety of infections including *Giardia*. These patients have an increased risk of neoplasia, the most common of which is non-Hodgkin lymphoma. Rare cases of small intestinal lymphoma, usually classified as diffuse large B-cell lymphoma, have been reported in patients with common variable immunodeficiency, in a background of nodular lymphoid hyperplasia.[246,247]

Wiskott-Aldrich Syndrome

Wiskott-Aldrich syndrome is a rare disorder with X-linked inheritance characterized thrombocytopenia (with small platelets), eczema, and recurrent infections. The disorder is caused by mutations in *WAS*. Individuals with Wiskott-Aldrich syndrome have an increased risk of lymphoma that approaches 100% by 30 years of age. The small intestine is the second most commonly involved site, after the central nervous system.[128]

EBV+ Mucocutaneous Ulcer

EBV+ mucocutaneous ulcer (MCU) is a lymphoproliferative disorder occurring in patients with underlying immunosuppression of various causes including advanced age and iatrogenic immunosuppression.[248-250] Patients have sharply circumscribed ulcerated lesions of skin or mucosal sites, the most common of which is the oral cavity, without formation of a large mass. Other sites include the GI tract and tonsils. EBV+ MCU is characterized by localized but sometimes locally aggressive lesions. Clinical course is overall indolent, sometimes with spontaneous regression. Constitutional symptoms are rare. The lesions may arise in association with local trauma or inflammation, for example, IBD.

Reported cases of EBV-MCU involving the GI tract have affected adults over a broad age range, with a median age of 64 years and a M:F ratio of 1.5.[250] Most patients were iatrogenically immunosuppressed; underlying conditions included prior organ transplantation, IBD, and rheumatoid arthritis. One patient had hypogammaglobulinemia. Most commonly involved is the colorectum, followed by small intestine, esophagus, anus, and stomach. Most patients experienced complete remission with decreased immunosuppression alone, or decreased immunosuppression combined with rituximab. One patient with Crohn's disease who had been treated with infliximab and methotrexate had multifocal EBV-MCU that persisted for 18 months, then progressed locally, with the development of large lesions with transmural involvement and active hemorrhage, and with spread to lymph nodes and to the liver, with multiple hepatic lesions. The patient was treated as for classic Hodgkin lymphoma, and achieved remission.[251] Thus rare cases of EBV-MCU can behave in an aggressive manner, and careful follow-up of patients with EBV-MCU is required.

The EBV+ lesional cells include atypical immunoblasts and Reed-Sternberg–like cells and have an immunophenotype that overlaps with that of Hodgkin lymphoma (CD30+, CD15+ or −, CD20 heterogeneous, Pax5+, CD79a+/−, CD10−, BCL6−, OCT2+, BOB1 variable, MUM1/IRF4+), with a polymorphous background of lymphocytes (including medium-sized cells with irregular nuclei), histiocytes, plasma cells, and eosinophils. EBER in situ hybridization stains the large atypical cells as well as some smaller cells. LMP1 is also often positive. CD8+ T cells are a conspicuous part of the infiltrate. A dense band of T cells forms the deep aspect of the lesion. Apoptotic debris, angioinvasion, and necrosis may be seen. Clonal rearrangement of IGH is detected in <50% of cases. Identification of a clonal or oligoclonal T-cell population is common; clonal CD8+ T cells with decreased functionality may play a role in the pathogenesis of EBV-MCU. Isolated regional lymphadenopathy may be seen, and may show reactive lymphoid hyperplasia, but histologically documented involvement by an infiltrate as described earlier would be strong evidence against EBV-MCU. Systemic lymphadenopathy, hepatosplenomegaly, and involvement of bone marrow are so rare as to also be strongly against a diagnosis of EBV+ MCU.[249,252] However, as noted earlier, rare cases of EBV-MCU can apparently relapse or spread to distant sites.[251]

This disorder can potentially mimic either classic Hodgkin lymphoma, diffuse large B-cell lymphoma, or, in transplant recipients, a polymorphous posttransplant lymphoproliferative disorder. If B-cell antigen expression is prominent on these atypical cells, the possibility of diffuse large B-cell lymphoma may be considered. However, EBV+ mucocutaneous ulcer is characterized by well-circumscribed superficial lesions with a conspicuous rim of T cells at the base of the lesions, which would be unusual for both Hodgkin lymphoma and diffuse large B-cell lymphoma. Classic Hodgkin lymphoma typically shows Reed-Sternberg cells and variants in a background of small lymphocytes, histiocytes, eosinophils, and/or plasma cells, without medium-sized atypical cells or immunoblasts. In addition, Hodgkin lymphoma is so uncommon in the GI tract that the diagnosis should be viewed with suspicion unless the pathological features are truly convincing. The cellular composition of EBV+ MCU is more polymorphous than typically seen in diffuse large B-cell lymphoma. EBV+ MCU usually behaves in an indolent manner, without progression to disseminated disease, with some spontaneous remissions, making the distinction from an aggressive lymphoma important. Hodgkin lymphoma presenting as a cutaneous or mucosal lesion is very rare and establishing a primary diagnosis of Hodgkin lymphoma in skin or mucosa should be performed with extreme caution.[249]

HEPATIC LYMPHOMA

Primary Hepatic Lymphoma

Clinical Features

Primary hepatic lymphoma—that is, lymphoma arising in and confined to (or nearly entirely confined to) the liver—is very uncommon, but it is a well-documented entity often associated with an underlying immunological abnormality. Some authors have suggested that this type of lymphoma has been increasing in frequency recently,[253,254] although it is also possible that more cases of primary hepatic lymphoma are being recognized. Indeed, in many earlier reports, the diagnosis was made only at autopsy.[253] Most cases occur in middle-aged and older adults, but occasional cases arise in young adults, and rare cases in children, have been reported. Patients' ages have ranged from 2 to 87, with a median in the sixth decade. The male-to-female ratio is 2:1 to 3:1. Patients present with right upper quadrant or epigastric pain, nausea, vomiting, anorexia, and/or weakness. On physical examination, patients often have hepatomegaly or a palpable mass. In up to about half of cases, they have B symptoms (fever, night sweats, or weight loss), but only a minority develop jaundice.[255-259]

Hepatic marginal-zone lymphoma (MALT lymphoma) has arisen in adults from 30 to 80 years of age (mean, 62), with a M:F ratio of approximately 1.4:1.[260] LDH is frequently elevated, and hepatic transaminases may also be elevated; however, α-fetoprotein and carcinoembryonic antigen levels are generally normal or only slightly elevated.[255,259,261,262] In a few cases of extranodal marginal-zone lymphoma, the lesion was an incidental finding during abdominal surgery or radiographic evaluation performed for other reasons.[263,264] In one case classified as lymphoplasmacytic lymphoma, and in one case of marginal-zone lymphoma, patients had monoclonal serum proteins that disappeared postoperatively.[263,265]

Associated Disorders

In approximately 40% of cases, patients have some other significant disease, often in the form of an immunodeficiency or chronic stimulation of the immune system.[253,261,266] The disorders include HIV infection; hepatitis B or hepatitis C virus infection, sometimes associated with chronic active hepatitis, cirrhosis, or hepatocellular carcinoma; iatrogenic immunosuppression in transplant recipients; systemic lupus erythematosus; Felty's syndrome (rheumatoid arthritis, neutropenia, and splenomegaly); autoimmune hemolytic anemia; immune thrombocytopenic purpura; primary biliary cirrhosis; prior Hodgkin lymphoma; active tuberculosis; and others.[253,254,256,257,261,264,266-275] Patients who have HIV infection are younger, and are almost exclusively males, in contrast to patients who are HIV−.[267] Primary hepatic lymphoma among children also appears to have a strong male preponderance.[259]

The relationship between lymphoma and hepatitis C virus (HCV) is controversial. Findings in various studies differ, but some show a significantly increased prevalence of HCV infection in patients with primary hepatic lymphoma, suggesting that HCV may play a role in lymphomagenesis.[257] HCV may contribute to lymphomagenesis by chronic antigenic stimulation, or by a "hit and run" mechanism in which there is a transient viral infection that causes permanent genetic changes in host lymphocytes, predisposing them to neoplastic transformation.[276,277] Successful treatment of HCV is reported to be associated with a superior overall survival in patients with marginal-zone lymphoma and also with diffuse large B-cell lymphoma.[276] In a study performed in a HCV-endemic area, HCV has been reported in half of all patients with primary hepatic lymphoma and in a majority of patients with primary hepatic DLBCL.[274] Lymphomas in HCV+ patients in general are usually low-grade B-cell lymphomas; however, most primary hepatic lymphomas in HCV+ patients are DLBCL.[258] Evidence of HCV infection is more common in primary hepatic DLBCL than in primary hepatic marginal-zone lymphoma or in lymphomas involving the liver secondarily.[274] Examined from the opposite point of view, in a study of HCV-infected patients with lymphoma, the liver was the second most frequently involved extranodal site (after the spleen).[278] Interestingly, hepatic involvement by lymphoma was more frequent when HCV+ patients had cirrhosis or hepatitis.[278] In addition to cases of hepatic marginal-zone lymphoma associated with HCV,[264,274] hepatic marginal-zone lymphoma has also arisen in patients with hepatitis B, primary biliary cirrhosis, hepatocellular carcinoma,[260] *H. pylori* infection, and in one case, with nonalcoholic steatohepatitis and metabolic syndrome.[279]

Pathological Features

In most cases, the lymphoma forms a solitary mass which can be small or large[266,274,279]; in occasional cases the lymphoma takes the form of multiple nodules.[266] In about 5% of cases, there is diffuse hepatic enlargement without a discrete mass.[253,255,259,261] Most are DLBCL. The remainder are mostly extranodal marginal-zone lymphoma (MALT lymphoma); rare cases of follicular lymphoma, Burkitt's lymphoma, and peripheral T-cell lymphoma, NOS; and anaplastic large-cell lymphoma are reported.[253-257,262,264-266,268,270,272,274] Most of the HCV-associated lymphomas that arise in liver are DLBCL, as noted earlier,[257] a subset of which arise via transformation of prior low-grade B-cell lymphomas, mostly extranodal marginal-zone lymphoma. Almost all lymphomas in HIV+ patients are DLBCL or Burkitt's lymphoma.[267] The few cases reported in children have been Burkitt's lymphoma or DLBCL.[259] The DLBCLs are often extensively necrotic.[253,255,256] Sclerosis is infrequent. Lymphomas with diffuse hepatic enlargement may show prominent sinusoidal involvement (Fig. 31.21).[255] A case of hepatic DLBCL that arose in a patient with successfully treated HCV had an extra copy of 14q23, and lacked rearrangement of MYC, BCL2, and BCL6.[277] Posttransplantation lymphoproliferative disorders may involve the liver in cases in which the liver is the allograft or when another organ has been transplanted. They are usually monomorphic B-lineage posttransplantation lymphoproliferative disorders with features of DLBCL.[275] Marginal-zone lymphoma arising in a hepatic allograft has been reported.[273]

The extranodal marginal-zone lymphomas have ranged in size from <1 cm to 9 cm (mean, 3.5 cm). Lesions are single or occasionally multiple.[260] Histological features similar to those seen in other sites, include the presence of marginal-zone cells, monocytoid B cells, reactive follicles, and lymphoepithelial lesions formed with bile duct epithelium. The marginal-zone B cells markedly expand the portal tracts, form intersecting broad serpiginous bands entrapping nodules of hepatocytes, and, in some areas, form a diffuse, confluent infiltrate.[263,271,273]

Immunohistochemical features of hepatic lymphomas are similar to those seen at other anatomic sites. The DLBCLs express CD45 and CD20, and in a subset of cases, CD10, BCL6 and/or BCL2.[274] A case of primary hepatic plasmablastic lymphoma (CD20−, CD3−, BCL6–, MUM1/IRF4+, CD138+, EBER+, with Ki67 > 95%) in an HIV+ male has been reported.[280] The extranodal marginal-zone

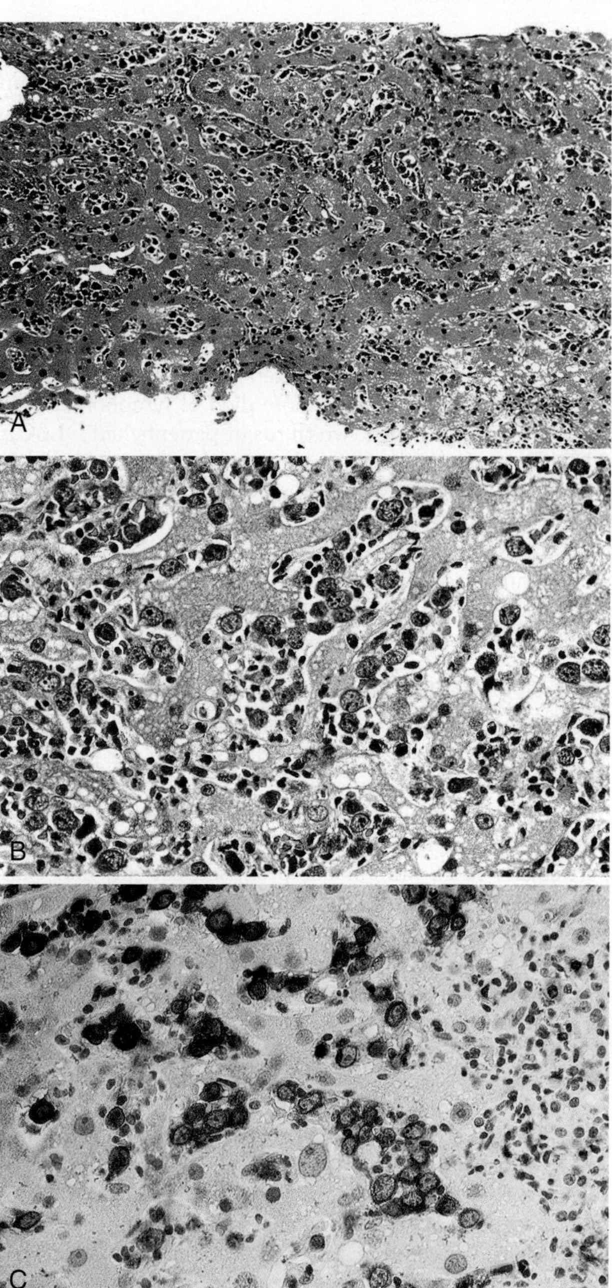

FIGURE 31.21 Hepatic large B-cell lymphoma, involving sinusoids. A, A core biopsy of liver shows markedly increased numbers of cells in hepatic sinusoids. **B,** The cells are large atypical lymphoid cells with round nuclei and prominent nucleoli. **C,** Neoplastic cells expressed B-cell antigens (CD79a is shown) (immunoperoxidase technique on paraffin section).

lymphomas express CD20 but not CD5 or CD10 and often have a component of plasma cells expressing monotypic cytoplasmic immunoglobulin.

Cytogenetic evaluation reveals that the t(14;18), resulting in IGH–*MALT1* fusion, is common in hepatic marginal-zone lymphoma.[39] The t(11;18)(q21;q21) common in marginal-zone lymphomas in certain sites is very unusual in the liver.[45] Next generation sequencing in a case of primary hepatic marginal-zone lymphoma showed mutated *TNFAIP3* and *CREBBP*.[279] These genetic changes suggest that NFκB activation was important in lymphomagenesis, at least in these cases.

Prognosis

Most patients with hepatic marginal-zone lymphoma survive disease free after resection with or without adjuvant therapy, while others die of unrelated causes. A few patients develop relapse of marginal-zone lymphoma in another extranodal site.[263-265,271,274] Death due to hepatic marginal-zone lymphoma is rare.[260] Among patients with intermediate- and high-grade lymphoma, the prognosis is relatively good, with mortality sometimes related to complications of surgery or therapy, as well as to persistent or progressive disease. In one review of primary hepatic lymphoma, the 2-year survival rate was estimated to be 66%. No patient who survived for 2 years or more died of lymphoma.[261] In another series, in which two thirds of patients had DLBCL, 70% of patients had sustained a complete remission.[257] In another study, patients with primary hepatic DLBCL treated with chemotherapy plus rituximab had a better outcome than those treated with chemotherapy without rituximab who in turn had a better outcome than those who did not receive chemotherapy.[274] Among children treated optimally in recent years, survival has been excellent.[259]

Differential Diagnosis

The finding of one or more hepatic lesions raises the question of primary or metastatic carcinoma, and the possibility of lymphoma often is not considered before obtaining tissue for pathological evaluation. The combination of a high LDH and normal carcinoembryonic antigen and α-fetoprotein, particularly in an immunocompromised patient, may raise the question of lymphoma, but histological examination is required to establish a diagnosis.[256,257,261] In some cases, the differential diagnosis based on histological features includes poorly differentiated carcinoma,[255] but careful examination of routine sections and judicious use of immunohistochemical studies are generally sufficient to establish a correct diagnosis.

A rare, nonneoplastic lesion that may enter the differential diagnosis of hepatic marginal-zone lymphoma is hepatic pseudolymphoma, also known as nodular lymphoid hyperplasia.[281] Patients typically have one, occasionally more than one, lesion within hepatic parenchyma. Some of them have other forms of underlying liver disease related to disorders such as hepatitis B infection or primary biliary cirrhosis. On microscopic examination the lesions are composed of organized lymphoid tissue containing lymphoid follicles with reactive germinal centers and an interfollicular area with small lymphocytes, occasional immunoblasts and sometimes, epithelioid histiocytes in clusters or multinucleated histiocytic giant cells. Lymphoepithelial lesions are not seen. The lymphoid infiltrate may extend beyond the main lesion into surrounding portal tracts. Immunohistochemistry shows B cells in follicles and predominantly T cells outside follicles. Any plasma cells present are polytypic. PCR is negative for a clonal B-cell population. Features helpful in distinguishing hepatic pseudolymphoma from marginal-zone lymphoma include absence of a component of B cells with the appearance of marginal-zone cells outside lymphoid follicles, absence of lymphoepithelial lesions, and absence of clonal IGH in hepatic pseudolymphoma.

Hepatosplenic T-Cell Lymphoma

Clinical Features

Hepatosplenic T-cell lymphoma (HSTCL) is a rare peripheral T-cell lymphoma that accounts for 1% to 2% of all peripheral T-cell lymphomas.[282] Hepatosplenic T-cell lymphoma typically involves liver, spleen, and bone marrow. The M:F ratio ranges from 2:1 to 4:1 in different series.[283] Most patients are adolescent or young adult males, with a median age of 35 years.[282] Some patients (up to approximately 20%) are chronically immunosuppressed. HSTCL has been reported in transplant recipients,[284] typically as a late-onset posttransplant lymphoproliferative disorder. Most transplant patients are renal allograft recipients, although occurrence in liver allograft recipients has also been described.[285] Some cases of HSTCL have been described in patients with IBD, all of whom received immunosuppressive therapy, which was most often infliximab, a tumor necrosis factor α blocking agent, in combination with other immunosuppressive agents such as azathioprine or steroids.[243] Rare patients with psoriasis or rheumatoid arthritis being treated with tumor necrosis factor inhibitors and immunomodulators have developed HSTCL.[282]

Cases initially described were of γδT-cell origin (TCRγδ+, TCRαβ−; hepatosplenic γδT-cell lymphoma) but subsequently TCRαβ+cases of HSTCL were identified. The αβ variant appears to affect patients over a wider age range, including children and older adults, with a slightly older median age and a higher proportion of females,[286] but otherwise the γδ and αβ variants are similar clinically.

Patients present with abdominal pain and often have fever, night sweats, or weight loss. Elevated LDH and bilirubin, and abnormal liver function tests are common. The spleen and sometimes the liver are diffusely, often strikingly, enlarged. Involvement of other extranodal sites and peripheral lymphadenopathy are against a diagnosis of HSTCL. Patients may have peripheral blood cytopenias, especially thrombocytopenia, which may be severe. Circulating tumor cells may be found at presentation, but a lymphocytosis is uncommon. In some cases, patients develop an overt leukemic picture late in the course of the disease. Response to anthracycline-based chemotherapy is poor, with a median survival of less than a year.[283,286-289] Treatment with other types of chemotherapy, allogeneic stem cell transplant and targeted therapy may prove useful in improving the prognosis of HSTCL patients.[283]

Pathological Features

Neoplastic cells preferentially involve hepatic sinusoids and splenic red pulp. Pathological features are similar for αβ and γδ variants, except that in a minority of cases, hepatic involvement in αβ cases is periportal in addition to sinusoidal.[286] Neoplastic cells in the marrow are often confined to vascular sinuses, and they may be inconspicuous on routinely stained sections. The sinuses are often expanded by tumor cells. HSTCL rarely forms nodular aggregates or shows diffuse involvement. Immunostains for T cells may be helpful in highlighting abnormal cells in an apparently normal marrow. Neoplastic cells are typically medium sized with oval nuclei with fine to condensed chromatin, small or inconspicuous nucleoli, and a rim of pale cytoplasm (Fig. 31.22A,B).[282,286-289] With disease progression neoplastic cells may become larger and more overtly atypical.[282] The normal counterpart of the neoplastic cell appears to be a mature, nonactivated cytotoxic T cell of the innate immune system.[282]

Immunohistochemical analysis typically shows CD2+, CD3+, CD5−/+, CD4−, CD8−/+, CD7+/−, CD16+/−, CD56+/−, CD57−/+, TCRγδ+(majority), or TCRαβ+ T cells that express the cytotoxic granule–associated protein TIA-1 (Fig. 31.22C). Other cytotoxic molecules (granzyme B and perforin) are negative in most cases. Rare cases with aberrant coexpression of CD19 are described.[290] Molecular genetic analysis shows clonal TCR gene rearrangement. The T cells in the γδ variant are of the Vδ1 subset.[284] Mutational analysis commonly shows mutations of JAK-STAT pathway genes (*STAT5B* or *STAT3*), or of chromatin modifiers such as *SETD2*[283]; these changes may initiate neoplastic transformation of T cells. Isochromosome 7q, with duplication of 7q and loss of 7p, is detected in the majority of cases. Other common changes include trisomy 8 and additional abnormalities affecting chromosome 7 (such as ring chromosome 7),[290] particularly with disease progression.[284,291] EBV is typically absent (see Table 31.2).[282]

The differential diagnosis of HSTCL includes other peripheral T-cell neoplasms, in particular, T-large granular lymphocytic leukemia. HSTCL and T-large granular lymphocytic leukemia show overlapping features, and a minority of cases of T-large granular lymphocytic leukemia has a γδ phenotype, but distinguishing them is important, because in contrast to HSTCL, T-large granular lymphocytic leukemia is characterized by an indolent course and a good prognosis. Compared with T-large granular lymphocytic leukemia of γδ lineage, HSTCL is characterized by more frequent B symptoms (80% vs. 29%), massive splenomegaly (76% vs. 0%), neoplastic cells expanding bone marrow sinuses (100% vs. 0%), lymphocytes lacking azurophilic granules (93% vs. 0%), and a CD3+, CD5−, CD4−, CD8−, CD56+, TIA1+, granzyme B−, TCR γδ+phenotype (71% vs. 14%, allowing one discrepant marker). [292] T-large granular lymphocytic leukemia is more likely to have a peripheral lymphocytosis (29% vs. 7%).[292]

For those uncommon cases of HSTCL with a leukemic phase and blastic neoplastic cells with prominent nucleoli, the possibility of acute leukemia may enter the differential diagnosis. Information on immunophenotype, clinical setting, anatomic distribution of disease, and pattern of marrow involvement (preferentially intravascular in HSTCL) will help establish a diagnosis.[283]

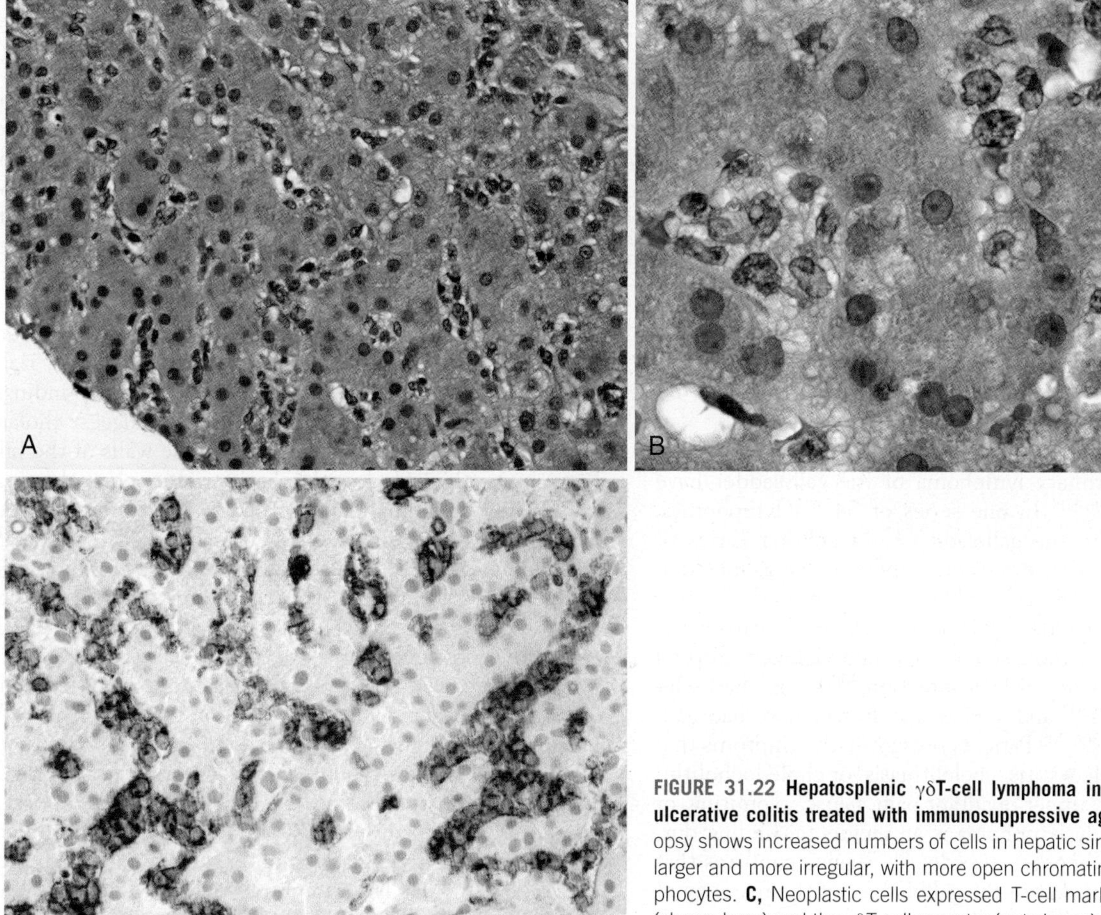

FIGURE 31.22 Hepatosplenic γδT-cell lymphoma in a young man with ulcerative colitis treated with immunosuppressive agents. A, A liver biopsy shows increased numbers of cells in hepatic sinusoids. **B,** They are larger and more irregular, with more open chromatin, than normal lymphocytes. **C,** Neoplastic cells expressed T-cell markers including CD2 (shown here) and the γδT-cell receptor (not shown). (**C,** immunoperoxidase technique on paraffin section.)

Hepatic Involvement in Widespread Lymphoma

In cases of widespread lymphoma, hepatic involvement is common.[258,293] Involvement by non-Hodgkin lymphoma is more common than by Hodgkin lymphoma.[258,274] The lymphomas are of a wide variety of types. Some types of lymphoma have characteristic patterns of hepatic involvement, even though they are not confined to the liver at presentation. Diffuse large B-cell lymphoma, for example, most often involves the liver in the form of tumor nodules obliterating normal parenchyma, but it may also predominantly involve the portal tracts with or without sinusoidal infiltration.

T-cell/histiocyte–rich large B-cell lymphoma (THRBCL), a subtype of diffuse large B-cell lymphoma, often involves the liver, as well as the spleen, at presentation. In the liver, THRBCL has a characteristic appearance, with irregular expansion of the portal tracts by an infiltrate of many small lymphocytes, histiocytes, and occasional neoplastic large atypical lymphoid cells, with little or no spread into sinusoids. Other findings include loss of bile ducts in the infiltrate, necrosis or steatosis of hepatocytes adjacent to the lymphoma, bile stasis, and sinusoidal dilation. Neoplastic cells may be inconspicuous, and the reactive lymphohistiocytic component may damage adjacent parenchyma in a pattern reminiscent of piecemeal necrosis, so that THRBCL may be mistaken for chronic active hepatitis. The combination of large tumor cells in a mixed reactive background may suggest Hodgkin lymphoma. Immunophenotyping is helpful in establishing a diagnosis by demonstrating CD20+ large atypical B cells in a background of T cells and histiocytes.[294,295] Intravascular large B-cell lymphoma is rare but when it occurs, it often involves the liver and shows preferential sinusoidal involvement.[274] Follicular lymphomas show predominantly portal involvement. Hodgkin lymphoma tends to predominantly involve the portal tracts, but it can also form solid nodules of tumor.[293,294] Burkitt's lymphoma almost always takes the form of tumor nodules. Chronic lymphocytic leukemia and mantle cell lymphoma both preferentially involve portal tracts but can occasionally form nodules or involve sinuses.[293]

LYMPHOMAS OF THE GALLBLADDER

Clinical Features

Rare cases of primary lymphoma of the gallbladder have been reported.[296-307] In one series of 54 GI lymphomas, only one arose in the gallbladder.[12] In another series of 56,000 autopsies that evaluated tumors of the gallbladder, no lymphomas of the gallbladder were identified.[302] Most patients have been older adults (mean age of 63 years in one review),[308] with a modest female preponderance. Several patients had a history of HIV infection,[308,309] one had sclerosing cholangitis[307] and approximately half have had gallstones.[297,301,303,306-308] Patients present with symptoms that often mimic cholecystitis, cholelithiasis, or choledocholithiasis, such as right upper quadrant pain, nausea, vomiting, or jaundice.[296] Rarely lymphoma is an incidental finding during evaluation of another disorder.[307] Staging confirms that lymphoma is confined to the gallbladder in the majority of cases.[298-300,302-304,307,308] Patients with extranodal marginal-zone lymphoma and follicular lymphoma have usually done well,[300,301,303,304,308] but patients with diffuse large B-cell lymphoma have often had relatively aggressive disease.[308]

The etiology of lymphoma of the gallbladder is not known, but it has been suggested that lymphomas of extranodal marginal-zone type may be related to bacterial infection and could arise from a background of cholecystitis, analogous to the pathogenesis of gastric marginal-zone lymphoma.[297,301,304]

Pathological Features

Gross examination of the gallbladder usually shows mural thickening or one or more discrete nodules.[297,298,300,307,310] The lymphomas have most often been extranodal marginal-zone type (MALT lymphoma),[296,297,300,301,305,306,310] followed by diffuse large B-cell lymphoma.[308] Several cases of follicular lymphoma have been described.[303,307,308] Other lymphomas primary in the gallbladder that have been encountered include rare cases of lymphoblastic lymphoma, mantle cell lymphoma, extracavitary primary effusion lymphoma, and plasmablastic lymphoma, the latter two in HIV+ men.[308] The marginal-zone lymphomas exhibit a striking female preponderance; their histological and immunohistological features are similar to those of marginal-zone lymphomas in other sites.[300,301,303,304] In one case fluorescence in situ hybridization (FISH) demonstrated t(11;18)(q21;q21) resulting in an *BIRC3-MALT1* fusion,[310] an abnormality that is common in gastric MALT lymphomas, as noted above.

LYMPHOMAS OF THE EXTRAHEPATIC BILE DUCTS

Lymphoma may, on occasion, involve lymph nodes in the porta hepatis and compress the extrahepatic biliary tree, resulting in jaundice. Lymphoma arising primarily from the extrahepatic biliary tree is a very rare phenomenon, however, with only approximately 20 cases reported. Patients with lymphoma of the biliary tree have all been adults over a broad age range, with a mean of 47 years in one review.[308] There is a possible slight female preponderance. Several patients were HIV+. They present most often with obstructive jaundice, but some also have fever, weight loss, right upper quadrant pain, or a combination of these findings. The clinical and radiographic features often suggest cholangiocarcinoma or sclerosing cholangitis. The walls of the bile ducts appear thickened, with biliary stricture on cholangiography. The lymphoma may also take the form of a discrete mass; lesions measuring 3 cm[311] to 8 cm are described.[312] Lymphoma may infiltrate the adjacent liver.[313] In a minority of cases in which lymphoma presents primarily with involvement of the extrahepatic bile ducts, staging reveals regional lymphadenopathy.[308,311,314]

Diffuse large B-cell lymphoma is more common than any other type of lymphoma to arise in this location.[311-317] Follicular lymphoma appears to be next most common, although only a handful of cases are reported.[308,313,318] MALT lymphoma is rare but has been described.[314] MALT lymphoma may form lymphoepithelial lesions with biliary epithelium. The follicular lymphomas have included both low-grade follicular lymphoma positive for CD20, CD10, BCL6, and BCL2,[318] as well as high-grade (grade 3) follicular lymphomas negative for BCL2.[308,313] In one BCL2− case

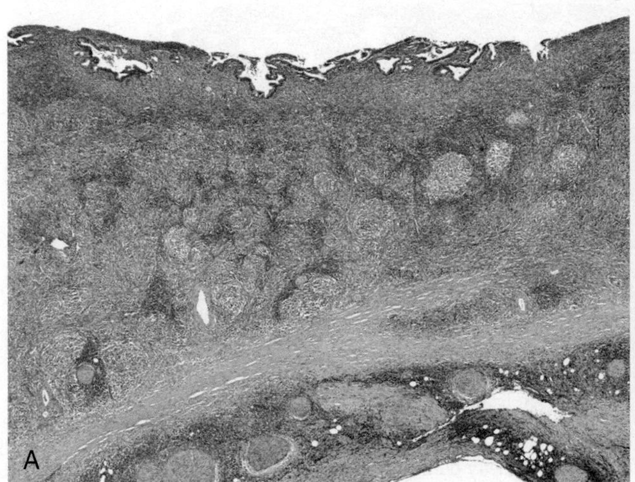

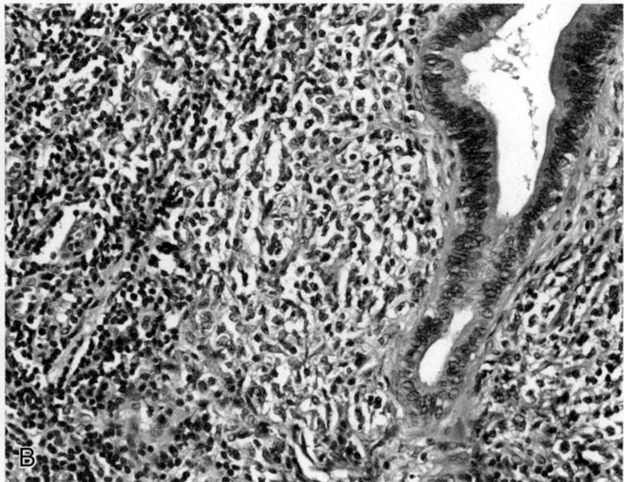

FIGURE 31.23 Follicular lymphoma, common bile duct. A, Low-power view shows mural thickening resulting from a proliferation of ill-defined follicles with associated sclerosis. **B,** Higher power view shows atypical lymphoid cells with irregular nuclei, consistent with centrocytes.

molecular studies showed clonal IGH but FISH was negative for translocations involving *BCL2, BCL6,* and IGH.[313] (Fig. 31.23). Patients diagnosed in recent years and treated optimally have often had an uneventful follow-up.[311-314]

In contrast to lymphomas arising in the gallbladder, lymphomas arising in the extrahepatic bile ducts tend to affect patients who are somewhat younger, less often with associated cholelithiasis, less often with involvement of regional lymph nodes and with a much lower proportion of extranodal marginal-zone lymphoma.[308]

PANCREATIC LYMPHOMA

Clinical Features

Primary pancreatic lymphoma is a rare disorder, comprising less than 0.2% of all pancreatic malignancies,[319] and less than 0.7% of non-Hodgkin lymphomas.[320] Secondary involvement of the pancreas by lymphomas arising in other sites is much more common than primary pancreatic lymphoma.[321] Pancreatic lymphomas often invade or surround and encase adjacent structures such as the duodenum, retroperitoneal soft tissue, mesentery, or large blood vessels. Some show peripancreatic lymph nodal involvement.[322,323] In some cases, origin from the pancreas can be inferred only because the bulk of the tumor involves the pancreas. Only a handful of cases are confined to the pancreas.[322]

Almost all patients are adults, with ages ranging from the first to the ninth decade, and with a male-to-female ratio of greater than 2:1.[321,322,324-333] Rare patients are HIV+[333] and one lymphoma arose in a pancreatic allograft,[334] but with these exceptions, patients have not had conditions predisposing to the development of lymphoma. They present with complaints of abdominal pain, anorexia, nausea, vomiting, weight loss, or malaise, or a combination of these findings.[321,322,325,327,328,330] Invasion into the duodenum may lead to GI hemorrhage.[326] Rare cases have been associated with diabetes mellitus and pancreatic exocrine insufficiency.[329]

On physical examination, patients are often jaundiced, and occasionally they have a palpable mass.[322,323,325,327,328,331] Because signs and symptoms are so similar to those of the much more common pancreatic adenocarcinoma, patients have often undergone laparotomy and resection of tumor, although others have had an open biopsy, and in some cases CT-guided percutaneous biopsy has provided diagnostic material. The prognosis is difficult to assess, as most of the information is in individual case reports, and patients have not been treated uniformly. Although many patients have succumbed to their lymphomas, those treated in recent years may have a better prognosis.[333]

Pathological Features

The tumors take the form of large masses (often >6 cm) involving the head, body, or tail of the pancreas, or the entire pancreas. The lesions are sometimes described as being cystic, or having central necrosis. Invasion into adjacent structures and involvement of abdominal lymph nodes are common.[321-328,330-333]

The lymphomas have almost always been B-lineage tumors,[330-333] although T-cell lymphomas have been reported.[330] Diffuse large B-cell lymphoma is the most common type (Fig. 31.24),[330,333] with rare reports of Burkitt's lymphoma,[329,331] follicular lymphoma,[323,330,332] and extranodal marginal-zone lymphoma.[324] Several anaplastic large-cell lymphomas (ALCLs, 2 ALK+) have been described.[325-327,330] In contrast to most other pancreatic lymphomas, ALCL is of T lineage, and mostly affects younger patients (second to third decade).

Differential Diagnosis

Pancreatic lymphoma may mimic pancreatic adenocarcinoma clinically. Clues that may provide a hint to a diagnosis of lymphoma include its large size compared with most carcinomas.[321] On endoscopic retrograde cholangiopancreatography, lymphoma may compress or distort ductal structures, but generally it does not invade their walls, in contrast to carcinoma.[322] Establishing a diagnosis requires obtaining tissue for pathological examination.

On occasion chronic pancreatitis, in particular IgG4-related pancreatitis, can be associated with a prominent lymphoplasmacytic infiltrate that could raise the question of a

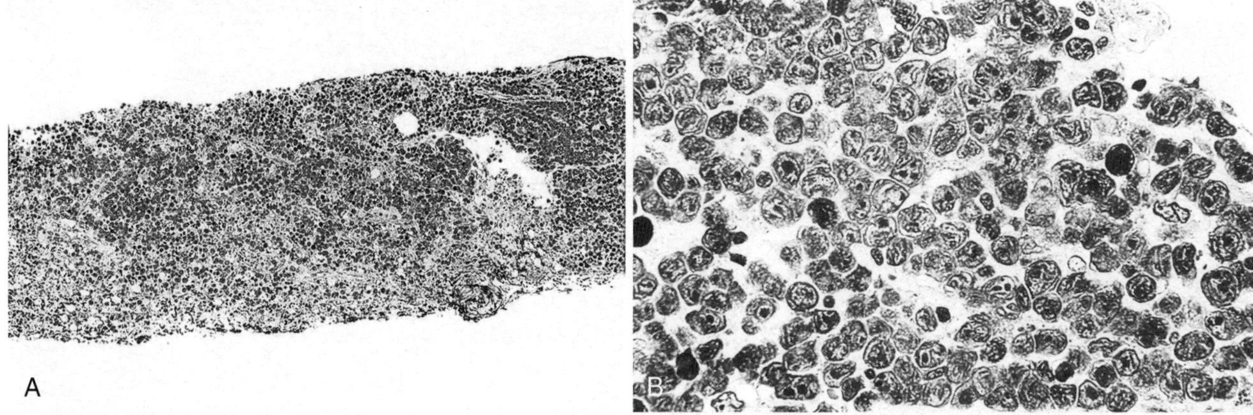

FIGURE 31.24 Pancreatic large B-cell lymphoma. A, A needle core biopsy of a pancreatic mass shows a diffuse infiltrate of lymphoid cells. **B,** Higher power view shows a monotonous population of large lymphoid cells. Immunohistochemistry demonstrated their B-cell nature, and flow cytometric analysis confirmed the presence of a monotypic population of B cells (data not shown). (**A** and **B,** Giemsa stain.)

low-grade lymphoma on a small biopsy. The absence of cytological atypia among lymphoid cells, and presence of a mix of B and T cells, without antigen loss or abnormal antigen coexpression, accompanied by polytypic plasma cells tend to support a reactive process. In IgG4-related pancreatitis there is in addition an increased proportion of IgG4+ plasma cells.

PROLIFERATIONS OF HISTIOCYTES AND DENDRITIC CELLS IN THE GI TRACT AND LIVER

A variety of proliferations of myelomonocytic cells, histiocytes, and antigen-presenting cells can affect the GI tract and liver. In the text that follows are discussed those with distinctive features in these sites. Whipple's disease is characterized by a histiocytic proliferation that often involves the GI tract, but it is discussed separately (see Chapter 4).

Hemophagocytic Lymphohistiocytosis

Hemophagocytic lymphohistiocytosis (HLH, also called *hemophagocytic syndrome*) is a potentially fatal systemic illness related to immune dysregulation that may affect individuals of any age but mainly affects young children. It is characterized by clinical and laboratory findings that may include fever, splenomegaly, cytopenias, markedly elevated ferritin, and decreased NK cell activity. Microscopic examination of bone marrow, liver, spleen, or lymph nodes may disclose hemophagocytic histiocytes, although they are not required, nor are they sufficient by themselves, for the diagnosis of HLH; the appropriate clinical and laboratory findings must be present to establish a diagnosis. HLH may be caused by a mutation in the gene for perforin, a cytotoxic granule protein, or by abnormalities of genes related to cytotoxic activity. In the absence of one of these mutations HLH may also be precipitated in susceptible individuals by severe infections, rheumatological disorders, and some malignancies.[335,336] Among malignancies, lymphomas, particularly those that are EBV+ such as extranodal NK/T-cell lymphoma, may be associated with the development of HLH.[336,337]

The hemophagocytic histiocytes are present in variable numbers and may not be seen in every biopsy performed to search for them. In other instances they are numerous, replacing zones of bone marrow or expanding splenic red pulp or hepatic sinusoids. The histiocytes contain red cells and leukocytes at various stages of degeneration. Over time, the contents of red blood cells may disappear while their membranes remain, so that the histiocytes may take on the appearance of sacks of pale vacuoles, with each vacuole representing a degenerated red cell. On pathological evaluation distinction of HLH from lymphoma is typically straightforward. Although a number of lymphomas can have a sinusoidal pattern in the liver, as described above, in HLH phagocytic macrophages typically predominate, and the lymphocytes present show no significant cytological atypia or immunophenotypic abnormality (Fig. 31.25). If the patient has a lymphoma-associated hemophagocytic syndrome, the lymphoma and the hemophagocytic histiocytes do not necessarily involve the same anatomic sites.

Rosai-Dorfman Disease of the GI Tract and Liver

Rosai-Dorfman disease, also called sinus histiocytosis with massive lymphadenopathy when it involves lymph nodes, is a proliferative disorder of histiocytes with distinctive characteristics. Rosai-Dorfman disease can involve any of numerous extranodal sites in addition to lymph nodes; GI tract and liver are among the most rarely involved of these sites.[338]

Patients are children or young to middle-aged, occasionally older, adults, with both males and females affected. The GI tract or hepatic involvement may occur in a patient already known to have Rosai-Dorfman disease in other sites, or it may represent the initial presentation of Rosai-Dorfman disease. Clinically appreciable manifestations that may develop include vague abdominal discomfort, hematochezia and hepatomegaly; occasionally GI tract or hepatic involvement by Rosai-Dorfman disease is an incidental finding in a patient with disease in other sites.[338,339] In the GI tract the lesions have been identified in the small and large bowel and in the appendix. They are typically submucosal but may extend to involve the lamina propria[338] or muscularis propria.[339] Rare cases of Rosai-Dorfman disease clinically and radiographically mimicking cholangiocarcinoma[340,341] and a case involving stomach and sigmoid colon[342] have been reported, both with involvement of adjacent lymph nodes. Rare cases with pancreatic involvement are also described.[338,341] In nearly all cases digestive tract involvement is present in the setting of Rosai-Dorfman disease that also involves lymph nodes and one or more extranodal sites. Isolated colonic disease has been documented rarely.[338,339]

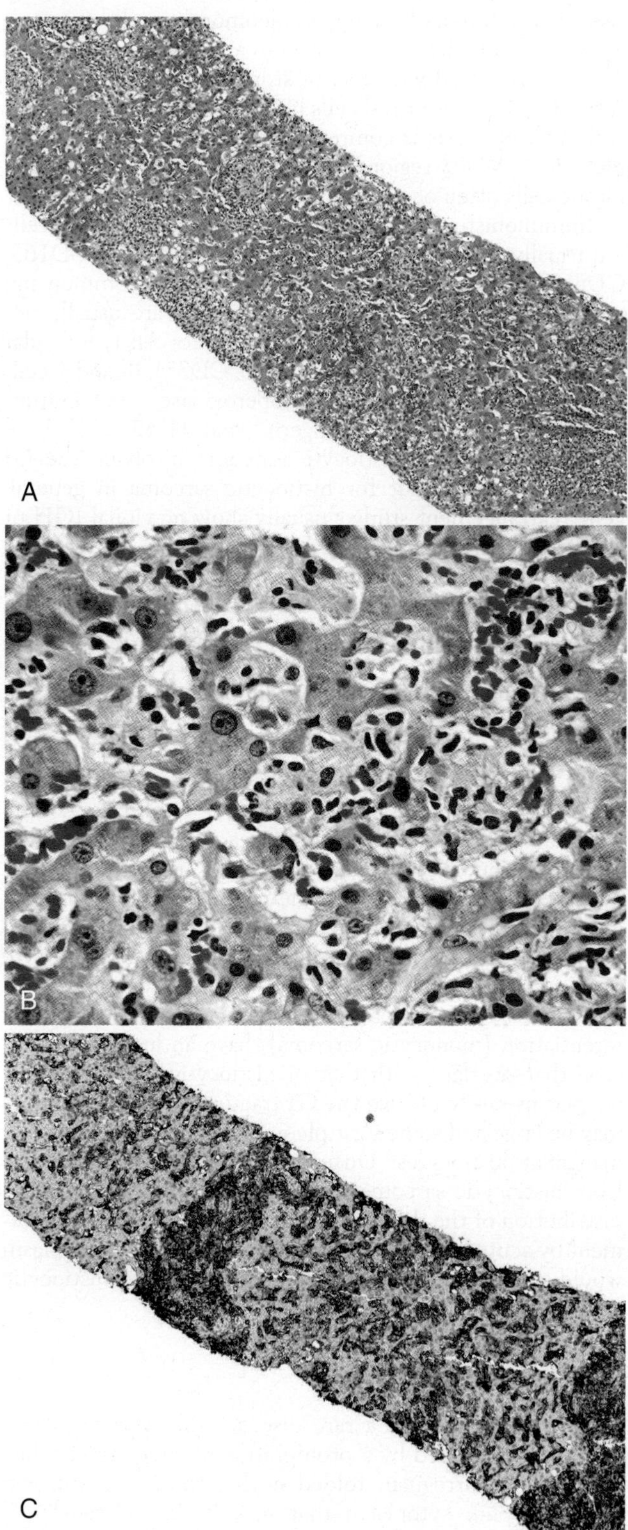

FIGURE 31.25 Hemophagocytic lymphohistiocytosis, hepatic involvement. A, Low-power view shows a core of hepatic parenchyma with increased numbers of lymphocytes and histiocytes in aggregates and within sinusoids. **B,** High-power view shows numerous histiocytes, including hemophagocytic forms, within sinusoids. **C,** An immunostain for CD163 highlights the dramatic increase in histiocytes, predominantly in hepatic sinusoids.

The lesions are composed of large histiocytes with large oval or slightly irregular nuclei, vesicular to finely dispersed chromatin, distinct nucleoli and abundant finely granular eosinophilic, occasionally vacuolated cytoplasm. The most distinctive feature of the histiocytes is the presence of intact leukocytes within their cytoplasm (emperipolesis); emperipolesis may be present in only a fraction of the histiocytes. There is typically an admixture of small lymphocytes and plasma cells (Fig. 31.26). Granulocytes are usually inconspicuous. The collections of histiocytes may mimic granulomas. The histiocytes express S100 but not CD1a or langerin. The S100 immunostain may help to highlight histiocytes with emperipolesis. Hepatic involvement may be subtle and not detected unless specifically sought in a patient known to have Rosai-Dorfman disease in other sites.[338]

Rosai-Dorfman disease in the form of localized lymphadenopathy has an excellent prognosis, with disease often regressing spontaneously. When Rosai-Dorfman disease involves multiple extranodal sites, which is the usual situation in patients with GI tract or hepatic involvement, the prognosis is not as favorable. Patients may have persistent or relapsing disease for years and may eventually succumb to the disease.[338] One patient with disease confined to the colon was well 15 months after surgical resection.[339] One

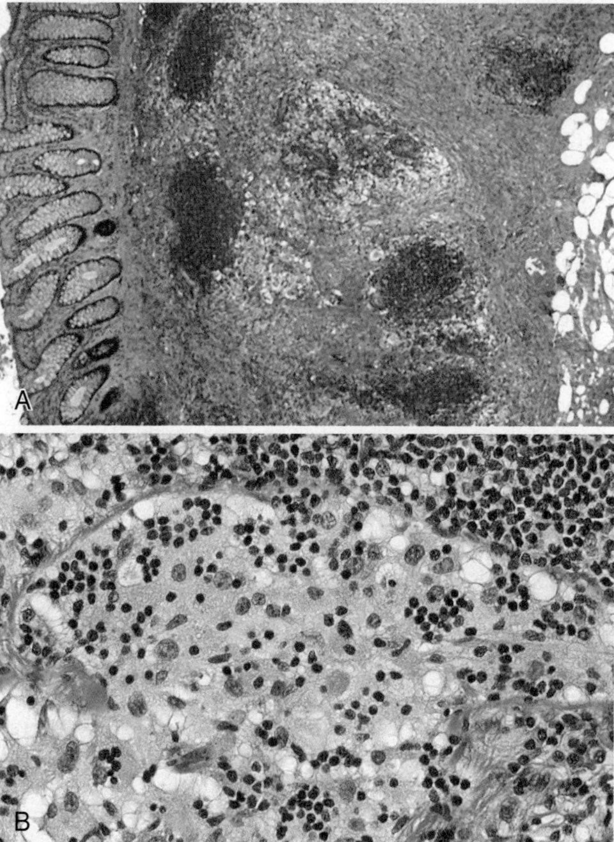

FIGURE 31.26 Rosai-Dorfman disease of the GI tract. A, The wall of the bowel shows a patchy lymphohistiocytic infiltrate. **B,** High-power view shows many histiocytes with large oval nuclei, distinct nucleoli and abundant pale, delicately vacuolated cytoplasm with emperipolesis of small lymphocytes. (*Courtesy of Dr. Gregory Lauwers, Massachusetts General Hospital.*) (**A** *and* **B** *from Lauwers GY, Perez-Atayde A, Dorfman RF, Rosai J. The digestive system manifestations of Rosai-Dorfman disease (sinus histiocytosis with massive lymphadenopathy): review of 11 cases. Hum Pathol. 2000;31:380-385.*)

patient with widespread follicular lymphoma developed Rosai-Dorfman disease that was apparently confined to the liver; when the lymphoma was treated and the patient achieved a remission, and the Rosai-Dorfman disease also resolved.[343]

Differential Diagnosis

The differential diagnosis of Rosai-Dorfman disease is broad and includes reactive and neoplastic processes. The enlarged nuclei of the characteristic histiocytes are atypical and may suggest a malignant neoplasm. The abundant cytoplasm, and thus the low N:C ratio suggests caution in rendering a diagnosis of malignancy. The histiocytic nature of the cells may be appreciated but unless the distinctive cytomorphology with emperipolesis is noted, the differential diagnosis will include other types of reactive and neoplastic histiocytic proliferations.

Histiocytic Sarcoma of the GI Tract

Histiocytic sarcoma is a malignant neoplasm composed of cells with the morphological and immunophenotypic features of mature histiocytes.[344] Before the availability of immunohistochemical and molecular techniques to establish a diagnosis of lymphoma, many cases of what are now recognizable as anaplastic large-cell lymphoma and diffuse large B-cell lymphoma were interpreted as histiocytic sarcoma.[345,346] Enteropathy-associated T-cell lymphoma was previously thought to represent malignant histiocytosis of the intestine associated with celiac disease.[133]

Convincing cases of histiocytic sarcoma (previously sometimes designated true histiocytic lymphoma) are rare. However, they do represent a distinct type of tumor with characteristic clinical and pathological features. Histiocytic sarcomas arise in lymph nodes and extranodal sites. Among extranodal sites, the skin/soft tissue and the GI tract are those most commonly involved. Histiocytic sarcoma arising in the GI tract mainly affects adults over a broad age range, with men and women affected in similar numbers. They present with abdominal pain, weight loss and hematochezia. Obstruction is common among tumors affecting the small intestine.[345,347] In addition to small intestinal involvement, histiocytic sarcoma may arise in the colon, with cases documented in the sigmoid colon and rectum, and rarely in the stomach and anus. Rarely more than one discontinuous portion of the GI tract is affected.[345,347,348] Involvement of regional lymph nodes is common. Hepatic involvement by GI tract histiocytic sarcoma has been documented.[345] A case of bile duct involvement by histiocytic sarcoma mimicking choledocholithiasis has been reported.[348]

Patients with GI tract involvement typically undergo resection of the lesion. Postoperative treatment is variable, as is the outcome. Some patients remain free of disease while others succumb to their disease. Relapses involving bone and lymph nodes have been documented.[345,347]

The neoplasms usually form bulky exophytic lesions that may be polypoid or annular. On microscopic examination they are infiltrative tumors that invade the overlying mucosa, resulting in ulceration. The neoplastic cells grow diffusely and may appear cohesive or discohesive, usually with interspersed inflammatory cells, including lymphocytes, neutrophils, and/or eosinophils and occasionally plasma cells. Tumor cells are large, with large oval to irregular nuclei with vesicular chromatin, often with prominent nucleoli, with abundant pink, granular, sometimes focally clear or vacuolated, cytoplasm, and sharp cell borders. Binucleated and multinucleated tumor cells are commonly seen. Some tumors have highly pleomorphic cells or tumor giant cells. Spindle cells are seen in a minority of cases and may be associated with foci of storiform growth. Phagocytosis of leukocytes or red cells has been described but is not common. Necrosis is common. The mitotic rate is usually high.[345,347] When regional lymph nodes are involved, neoplastic cells often occupy sinuses.[345]

Immunohistochemical analysis shows that neoplastic cells are usually positive for CD45, CD45RO, CD68, CD163, CD4, and lysozyme. Staining for S100 is fairly common and may be focal or diffuse. CD30 and EMA are usually not expressed. Neoplastic cells are negative for Alk1, follicular dendritic cell markers (CD21, CD23, CD35), B- and T-cell-specific markers, CD34, myeloperoxidase, cytokeratins, CD117, desmin, CD1a, langerin, and HMB45.[344,345,347] Genetic studies on histiocytic sarcoma involving the GI tract are limited, but for histiocytic sarcoma in general, gene rearrangement studies usually show no clonal IGH or TCR gene rearrangement.[347] A subset of cases has a history of B-cell lymphoma; in these patients, clonal IGH may be found, likely representing a transdifferentiation phenomenon.[344] The BRAF V600E mutation has been identified in a subset of cases of histiocytic sarcoma (5 of 8 in one series),[349] likely representing an important change in the pathogenesis of this neoplasm.

Differential Diagnosis

Certain neoplasms, in particular B- and T-cell lymphomas, may have a large component of reactive histiocytes that may raise the question of a histiocytic neoplasm. Histiocytic neoplasms are rare and meticulous care in examining immunostains is required to ensure that cytologically malignant cells, and not reactive histiocytes, express histiocyte markers before rendering a diagnosis of histiocytic sarcoma. Myeloid sarcoma, in particular those with monocytic differentiation (monocytic sarcoma), have an immunophenotype that overlaps with that of histiocytic sarcoma; these neoplasms rarely involve the GI tract and liver. Monoblasts may be large and somewhat pleomorphic and may resemble malignant histiocytes. Differentiating monocytic sarcoma from histiocytic sarcoma may depend on investigating the distribution of the disease, as marrow and/or blood involvement by acute myeloid leukemia or other myeloid neoplasm would strongly support monocytic sarcoma over histiocytic sarcoma.

ALK+ Histiocytosis

ALK+ histiocytosis is a rare disorder that affects infants and is characterized by a proliferation of large atypical histiocytes with irregular, folded nuclei, small nucleoli, and abundant pink cytoplasm that may be vacuolated.[350,351] The histiocytes may be erythrophagocytic, and may show emperipolesis, imparting an appearance that mimics Rosai-Dorfman disease. The patients (typically 3 months or younger) present with anemia, thrombocytopenia, and prominent hepatosplenomegaly. In the liver, histiocytes mainly occupy hepatic sinusoids, although involvement of portal tracts has been described. The atypical histiocytes may also infiltrate the bone marrow, although involvement may be subtle on routinely stained sections and immunostains may be required to identify the atypical cells.[350] Renal involvement has been described.[351]

The histiocytes express histiocyte-associated markers (CD68, CD163, lysozyme), S100, and fascin but not CD1a, langerin, CD30, or B- or T-cell-specific markers. They are positive for ALK, in a membranous and cytoplasmic pattern.[350,351] FISH analysis can be used to demonstrate the presence of an ALK translocation.[351] In one case a gene fusion involving TPM3 and ALK was documented using RT-PCR.[350] Patients have either received chemotherapy or have been followed without specific therapy. In the very small number of cases reported, the disorder has slowly resolved over a period of years, and patients have done well.

A variety of disorders can be considered in the differential diagnosis, but the very young age of the patients and the expression of ALK set this disorder apart from other reactive and neoplastic histiocytic proliferations. ALK expression is characteristic of only three other known neoplasms: ALK+ anaplastic large-cell lymphoma, ALK+ large B-cell lymphoma, and ALK+ inflammatory myofibroblastic tumor, but their manners of presentation, histological features, and immunophenotype apart from ALK expression distinguish them from ALK+ histiocytosis.

Follicular Dendritic Cell Sarcoma

Follicular dendritic cell (FDC) sarcoma is a rare neoplasm with morphological and immunophenotypic features of follicular dendritic cells, which are the dendritic cells that provide the framework for the formation of lymphoid follicles. The majority of FDC sarcomas arise in lymph nodes and a minority arises in any of a number of extranodal sites including the GI tract.[352] A case of FDC sarcoma that presented with pancreatic involvement has been reported.[353] A variant of FDC sarcoma with distinctive features, EBV+ inflammatory FDC sarcoma, also called inflammatory pseudotumor–like FDC sarcoma, arises almost exclusively in the liver or the spleen.[354-356]

Clinical Features

FDC sarcoma affects patients over a wide age range. Nearly all are adults and most are young or middle-aged adults, with men and women roughly equally affected. Most patients present with a painless mass, usually without constitutional symptoms. The tumor usually behaves in a relatively indolent manner. Local recurrences are common. Metastases eventually occur in approximately 25% of cases but these may not develop until many years following initial diagnosis. The outcome appears less favorable in cases with a large mass (>6 cm), marked cytological atypia, extensive coagulative necrosis, frequent mitoses (≥5 per 10 hpf), and high proliferation index.[352,355]

The EBV+ inflammatory FDC sarcoma shows a female preponderance and may be more common among Asians. These patients typically present with abdominal pain and often have systemic symptoms such as fever, malaise, or weight loss. Although their tumors are intraabdominal and may achieve a large size before patients come to medical attention, the outcome does not appear to be significantly different from that of other FDC sarcomas.[354,356]

Pathological Features

FDC sarcoma forms a solitary mass lesion that varies widely in size, from <1 cm to >20 cm, and that is usually described as well circumscribed. Larger lesions may be associated with hemorrhage or necrosis. Microscopic examination typically reveals a proliferation of spindle-shaped to ovoid cells with oval to elongate nuclei, vesicular or stippled chromatin, small but distinct nucleoli, and moderate quantity of eosinophilic cytoplasm with indistinct cell membranes forming whorls, fascicles, or ill-defined nodules. Tumor cells may take on storiform pattern of growth or may form sheets. Nuclear membranes are generally more delicate than those of large lymphoid cells. Bi- and multinucleated cells are common. Although in most cases tumor cells are relatively bland, cytological atypia is pronounced in occasional cases. Small lymphocytes are usually scattered among tumor cells. In addition, lymphocytes may collect in greater numbers in a perivascular distribution. Rarely, this tumor arises in association with hyaline-vascular Castleman's disease,[352,355,357] in which there are follicles with involuted germinal centers that may contain abnormal FDCs.

Immunohistochemistry shows staining of tumor cells for CD21, CD23, or CD35, and usually for more than one of these FDC-associated markers. Tumor cells usually express desmoplakin, vimentin, and fascin and are variably positive for S100, EMA, and CD68. Clusterin is often strongly expressed. Tumor cells are negative for CD1a, lysozyme, CD30, CD3, myeloperoxidase, CD34, Alk1, and CD79a. The proliferation index is variable, with Ki67 staining ranging from 1% to 25% of cells. Admixed lymphocytes may be predominantly B cells, predominantly T cells, or a mixture of B and T cells.[352,355,357] Neoplastic cells are negative for EBV in FDC sarcoma of the conventional type.[357]

EBV+ inflammatory FDC sarcoma usually takes the form of a solitary fleshy tumor, commonly with hemorrhage and necrosis. In addition to the cytological and immunophenotypic features described earlier for FDC sarcoma of the conventional type, this variant of FDC sarcoma harbors a prominent lymphoplasmacytic infiltrate. Tumor cells are thus often scattered singly among the inflammatory cells, although focally they may form fascicles. Nuclear atypia is variable, and occasional bizarre cells or Reed-Sternberg–like cells may be seen. The tumor cells consistently harbor EBV, which is present in clonal, episomal form (Fig. 31.27).[354-356]

Evaluation of cases of FDC sarcoma (mostly involving sites other than the digestive tract) shows that a minority harbor the BRAF V600E mutation; the mutation has been identified in both the conventional type and the inflammatory pseudotumor–like type of FDC sarcoma.[349]

Differential Diagnosis

The differential diagnosis of FDC sarcoma includes other spindle cell sarcomas that may involve the GI tract, including GIST and smooth muscle neoplasms. Careful attention to the histological features and judicious use of immunohistochemistry should allow a diagnosis to be established. Inflammatory pseudotumor–like FDC sarcoma raises a different set of differential diagnostic considerations. If neoplastic cells are bland and inconspicuous they may be

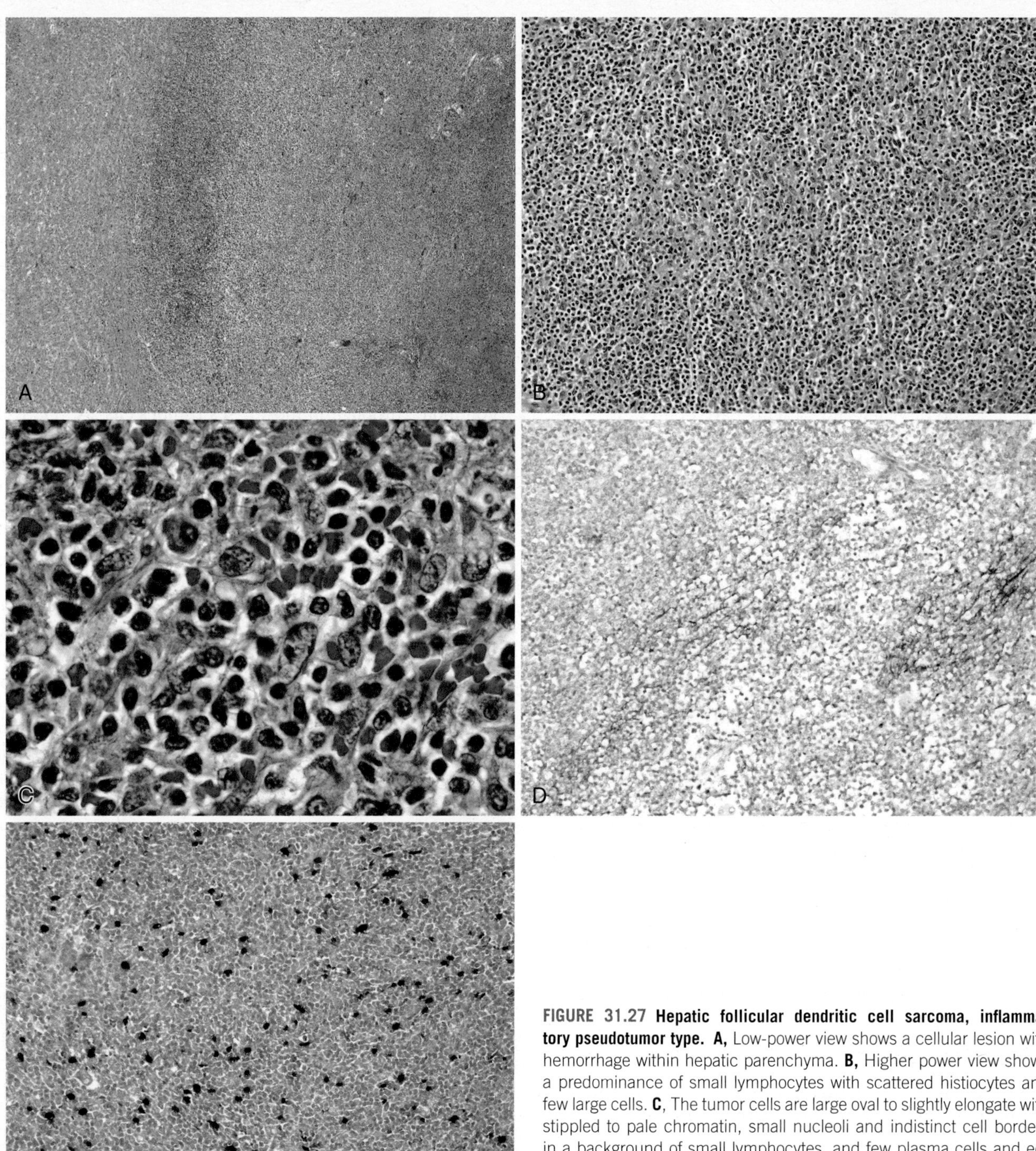

FIGURE 31.27 Hepatic follicular dendritic cell sarcoma, inflammatory pseudotumor type. A, Low-power view shows a cellular lesion with hemorrhage within hepatic parenchyma. **B,** Higher power view shows a predominance of small lymphocytes with scattered histiocytes and few large cells. **C**, The tumor cells are large oval to slightly elongate with stippled to pale chromatin, small nucleoli and indistinct cell borders in a background of small lymphocytes, and few plasma cells and eosinophils (oil immersion). **D,** There is patchy CD35+ dendritic staining (immunoperoxidase stain on a paraffin section). **E,** Tumor cells contain EBV (in situ hybridization for EBER on a paraffin section).

overlooked, and the dense lymphoplasmacytic infiltrate may suggest a low-grade B-cell lymphoma. If neoplastic cells are bizarre and Reed-Sternberg–like, their presence in a reactive background may suggest Hodgkin lymphoma. The presence of EBV in neoplastic cells may heighten the resemblance to Hodgkin lymphoma, as about 40% of all cases of classic Hodgkin lymphoma are EBV+. However, the neoplastic follicular dendritic cells are negative for CD30, which should prompt consideration of other diagnostic possibilities.

Langerhans Cell Histiocytosis of the GI Tract and Liver

Langerhans cell histiocytosis (LCH) typically occurs in one of three clinical scenarios: (1) as unifocal disease (previously known as solitary eosinophilic granuloma), (2) as multifocal, unisystem disease (formerly known as Hand-Schüller-Christian disease), or (3) as multifocal, multisystem disease (formerly known as Letterer-Siwe disease).

Multisystem disease can be subdivided into cases with low risk, involving skin, bone, lymph nodes, or pituitary and those with high risk, with disease involving spleen, liver, bone marrow, or lung.[358,359] The prognosis for LCH has improved over time, and overall survival is now very good; however, survival for pediatric patients with multisystem disease with high-risk organ involvement remains poor.[359] Hepatic involvement by LCH affects adults less often than children. An adult male with hepatic LCH who also had osseous LCH has been described; the LCH invaded bile ducts, mimicking sclerosing cholangitis, and was successfully treated with liver transplantation.[360]

LCH of the GI tract is rare; it manifests differently in children compared with adults. GI tract involvement by LCH among children often occurs in the setting of high risk, widespread disease, and is associated with a poor prognosis. The peak incidence is before age 2 years, and patients are predominantly male. They are symptomatic, presenting with failure to thrive, bloody diarrhea, anemia, hypoalbuminemia, or a combination of these findings. The lesions of LCH may be multiple, affecting more than one portion of the GI tract.[358]

In contrast, LCH among adults more often affects women than men, and it is usually an incidental finding on screening colonoscopy, or on investigation performed to evaluate unrelated symptoms.[358,361] The most common finding is a single polypoid lesion in the colorectum; gastric, small intestinal, and anal involvement is also described. Occasionally patients have multiple lesions in the GI tract.[358,361] Adults with LCH involving the GI tract typically have localized disease and are free of disease on follow-up. A minority of patients develop involvement of other sites on follow-up. Cutaneous involvement has been described in this setting.[358] Based on evaluation of very limited numbers of patients, there is a suggestion of greater risk of relapse when GI tract lesions are multiple rather than single.[358]

In children and adults LCH takes the form of one or more lesions that are sometimes ulcerated and which are usually <1 cm in size. On microscopic examination LCH in the GI tract has an appearance similar to that seen in other sites. The lesions may be well delineated or infiltrative. They are composed of sheets, nests, or clusters of large Langerhans cells with large, pale, oval, folded, or indented nuclei with longitudinal nuclear grooves, inconspicuous nucleoli, and moderate quantity of eosinophilic, sometimes finely granular cytoplasm with indistinct cell borders. There is typically an admixture of eosinophils, small lymphocytes, plasma cells, and neutrophils in numbers which vary from one case to another. The overlying mucosa may show reactive changes. Mitoses are typically not identified among the Langerhans cells. Uncommon findings include the presence of multinucleated giant cells, Langerhans cells with prominent nucleoli, or focal necrosis. Immunostains show that neoplastic cells express S100, CD1a, and CD207 (langerin), and are negative for keratin, HMB45, and CD117.[358] Evaluation of cases of LCH (mostly involving sites other than the digestive tract) shows that many cases harbor mutations leading to MAPK pathway activation, most often BRAF V600E mutation,[349] followed by mutations of MAP2K1.[362]

Differential Diagnosis

The differential diagnosis includes other types of histiocytic proliferations that may involve the GI tract, including Rosai-Dorfman disease and histiocytic sarcoma (discussed earlier), and also systemic mastocytosis (discussed in the section that follows). Of note, Langerhans cells are antigen-presenting cells commonly identifiable in a variety of inflammatory and other neoplastic disorders. In LCH they typically form solid aggregates, while in other disorders they are scattered singly among other reactive cells or among neoplastic cells and do not form the bulk of the lesion.

Mastocytosis: Manifestations in the GI Tract and Liver

Mastocytosis, a neoplastic proliferation of mast cells, occurs in a number of different forms, each with distinctive clinical and pathological features. These include cutaneous mastocytosis, systemic mastocytosis (including indolent and aggressive systemic mastocytosis and systemic mastocytosis with an associated hematological neoplasm), and mast cell sarcoma.[363] The majority of patients with systemic mastocytosis, even in the absence of documented GI tract involvement, have symptoms related to the GI tract, commonly including abdominal pain, diarrhea, and nausea and vomiting. Occasionally patients have GI bleeding. Some studies describe an increase in peptic ulcer disease. The symptoms represent a major cause of morbidity.[364-366] GI tract involvement is rare. When it occurs, it is almost always by systemic mastocytosis, although a case of GI tract involvement by mast cell sarcoma, an extremely rare neoplasm, has been reported.[367] When systemic mastocytosis involves the GI tract, the colon is most often involved, while small intestinal involvement, or involvement of both small and large bowel is uncommon.[368]

The abnormalities in the GI tract, like symptoms related to the GI tract, are diverse, and morphological findings do not necessarily correlate with symptoms, as mast cells outside the GI tract can release the contents of their granules and cause symptoms away from anatomic location of mast cell infiltrates. Thus lack of mast cell infiltrates on endoscopic biopsies does not exclude a diagnosis of mastocytosis.[365] The stomach can show peptic ulcer disease, thickened folds, small nodules consistent with urticarial lesions, and increased lamina propria inflammatory cells, sometimes including mast cells. [364] The small bowel may show dilatation; thickened, edematous nodules and folds; villi that may be blunted or partially or entirely atrophic; infiltration by eosinophils; and/or infiltration by mast cells (less common). The colon may show urticarial lesions, and occasionally shows increased numbers of mast cells in the lamina propria.[364] There may be associated erosions and evidence of chronic mucosal injury. Eosinophils may be present in increased numbers in the lamina propria.[366,368] Plasma cells are often sparse.[368]

To make a diagnosis of systemic mastocytosis involving the GI tract there should be at least one dense aggregate of at least 15 mast cells within GI tract mucosa, although the mast cells may form larger aggregates or take the form of a more diffuse, extensive infiltrate in the lamina propria. The mast cell infiltrate may take the form of a polypoid lesion, a confluent subepithelial band of mast cells, or multifocal aggregates of mast cells.[368] The neoplastic mast cells are small to medium-sized with oval, irregular or elongate nuclei, smooth chromatin, inconspicuous nucleoli, and moderate quantity of pale cytoplasm, distorting the normal glandular architecture (Fig. 31.28).[363,366] In the absence of dense aggregates of mast cells, so that mast cells are scattered in increased numbers in the mucosa without formation of compact clusters, it is possible to render a diagnosis

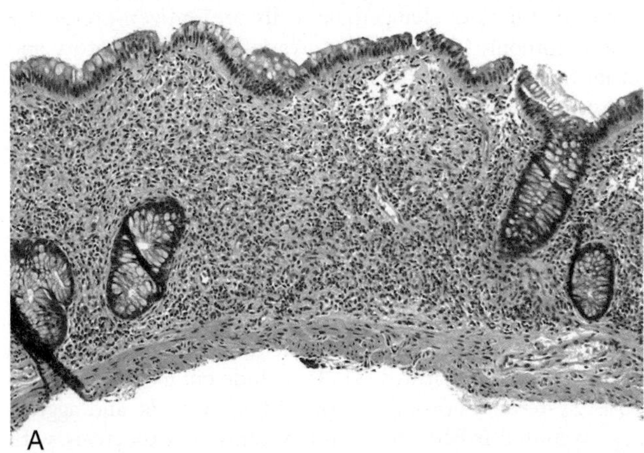

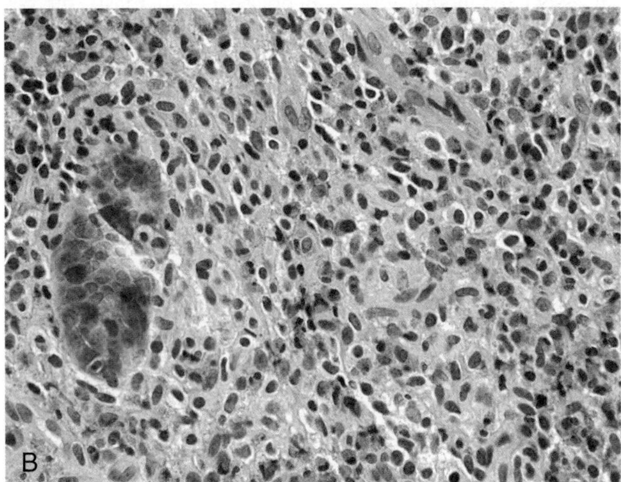

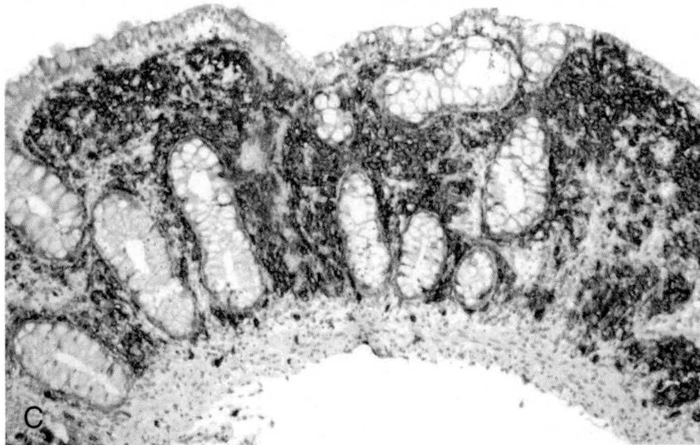

FIGURE 31.28 Colonic involvement by systemic mastocytosis. A, The normal architecture is distorted, with prominent gland loss, by a cellular infiltrate in the lamina propria. **B,** The infiltrate is composed of many cytologically bland mast cells with slightly elongate nuclei and pale cytoplasm, with scattered admixed eosinophils. **C,** The mast cells are strongly positive for CD117 (immunoperoxidase stain on a paraffin section); they also expressed mast cell tryptase and CD25 (not shown).

of systemic mastocytosis if the mast cells have an abnormal immunophenotype, or demonstrate an activating point mutation of KIT.[363] Mast cell sarcoma takes the form of a diffuse proliferation of large, often epithelioid cells, with abundant pink or pale cytoplasm. There are often admixed eosinophils that may provide a clue to diagnosis.[367] The neoplastic cells do not resemble normal mast cells, but their staining with Giemsa and with immunohistochemical stains is similar to that in other types of mast cell neoplasms.

Normal and neoplastic mast cells have purplish granules on Giemsa stain; neoplastic mast cells may have only sparse granulation. On immunohistochemical evaluation mast cells are positive for CD117 (Fig. 31.28C) and for mast cell tryptase, although tryptase staining, which tends to correlate with the degree of granularity, may be weakly expressed.[368] Abnormal mast cells may coexpress CD2 and/or CD25; this finding is consistent with neoplastic mast cells.[365]

Systemic mastocytosis may be associated with hepatomegaly. Microscopic examination commonly reveals portal infiltrates of mast cells and other inflammatory cells, fibrosis (usually without cirrhosis), and extramedullary hematopoiesis. Some patients have portal hypertension, which may be accompanied by ascites.[364]

The prognosis is variable, with some cases of indolent systemic mastocytosis behaving in an indolent manner and aggressive systemic mastocytosis, systemic mastocytosis with an associated hematological neoplasm, and mast cell sarcoma behaving more aggressively. Treatment typically includes two different aspects. The first is treatment to limit the symptomatic impact of systemic mastocytosis by attempting to prevent mast cell degranulation. The second is to control and/or decrease the extent of mast cell infiltration in tissue.[365] Activating mutations of KIT are present in most cases, raising hope that specific tyrosine kinase inhibitors will prove effective in controlling disease.

Differential Diagnosis

Making a diagnosis of systemic mastocytosis in the digestive tract can be challenging, particularly if the patient does not have a previously established diagnosis of mastocytosis. The clinical manifestations related to the GI tract can be striking, but they are nonspecific. On microscopic examination, the mast cell infiltrates are often subtle, and can easily be mistaken for nonspecific chronic inflammation.[368] In one reported case, GI tract involvement by systemic mastocytosis was misinterpreted as IBD.[366] Careful examination of routinely stained slides will reveal the mast cells, and immunostains will readily confirm their identity and help to determine whether they are neoplastic. The histological features of mast cell sarcoma are somewhat nonspecific, but the presence of an epithelioid malignant neoplasm with interspersed eosinophils should raise the question of mast cell sarcoma.

The full reference list may be accessed online at *Elsevier eBooks for Practicing Clinicians*.

SECTION VI

ANAL PATHOLOGY

CHAPTER 32

Inflammatory and Neoplastic Disorders of the Anal Canal

Kelsey E. McHugh, Thomas P. Plesec

Contents

EMBRYOLOGY AND ANATOMY OF THE ANUS AND ANAL CANAL

The anal canal forms during the fourth to seventh weeks of gestation after partitioning of the cloaca into the ventral urogenital membrane and dorsal membrane.[1] The epithelium of the superior two-thirds of the primitive anal canal is derived from the endodermal hindgut; the inferior one-third develops from the ectodermal proctodeum. The dentate line, also known as the *pectinate line,* is located at the inferior limit of the anal valves and delineates where these two epithelial derivatives fuse. The dentate line also indicates the approximate former site of the anal membrane that ruptures in the eighth week of gestation. The outer layers of the wall of the anal canal are derived from the surrounding splanchnic mesenchyme.

The anal canal is defined surgically by the borders of the internal anal sphincter (Fig. 32.1) and varies from 3 to 4 cm in length.[2,3] The surgical anal canal begins at the apex of the anal sphincter complex. This is a palpable landmark (anal rectal ring) and is located approximately 1 to 2 cm proximal to the dentate line. It ends where the nonkeratinizing squamous mucosa terminates at the perianal skin.[4] The internal sphincter is the most distal portion of the internal circular layer of the muscularis propria and is continuous with the muscularis propria of the colorectum. The surface of the anal canal is lined by vertical mucosal folds termed *anal columns (columns of Morgagni)* and is separated by anal sinuses *(sinuses of Morgagni)*. The columns connect at the most distal end by a horizontal row of mucosal folds known as the *anal valves*. Anal valves are typically most evident in children, but they may become more prominent with advancing age.

The location of the anal valves corresponds to the dentate line, which is located approximately at the midpoint of the surgically defined anal canal. The dentate line corresponds, generally, to the squamocolumnar junction. This is not an abrupt transition, but an actual transition zone that extends from several millimeters to just over 1 cm in length. Microscopically, the epithelium lining the anal transition zone varies from a type that resembles the lower genitourinary tract to stratified squamous, columnar, or cuboidal, with islands of colorectal-type epithelium also frequently present[1] (Fig. 32.2). Despite its resemblance to bladder epithelium, the anal transition zone expresses cytokeratins (CKs) CK7 and CK19, but not CK20.[5,6] Immunohistochemical studies for HMB45 and S100 protein have also demonstrated the presence of melanocytes in the anal transitional epithelium, although these are usually more prominent in the anal squamous zone.[7] Microscopically, the mucosal lining superior to the transition zone is columnar,

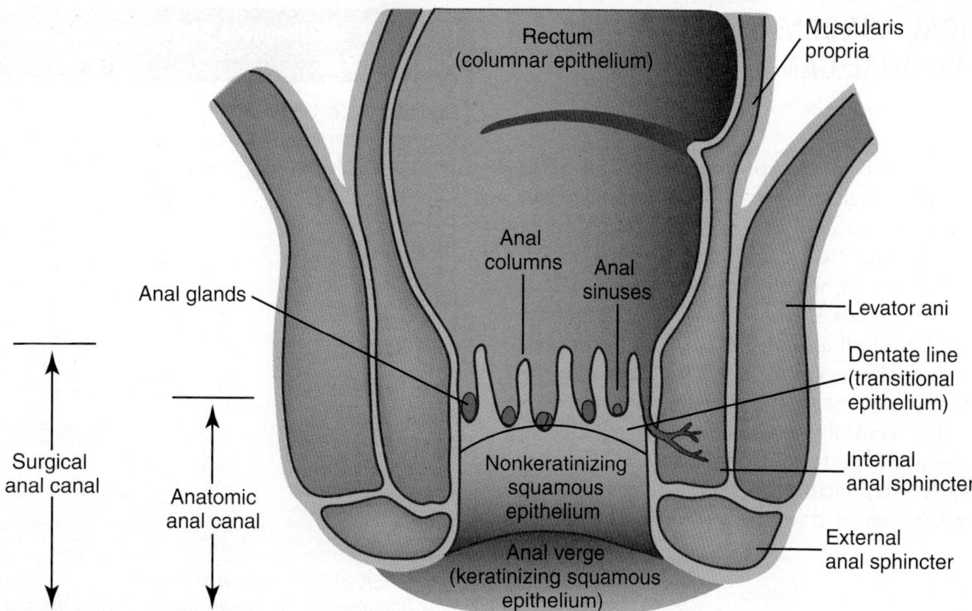

FIGURE 32.1 Anatomical features of the anal canal.

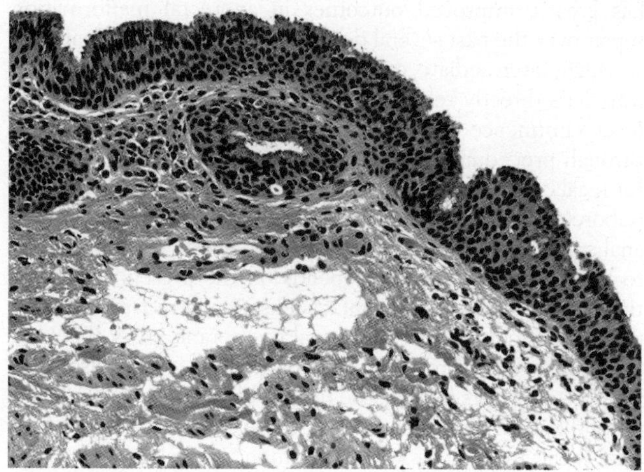

FIGURE 32.2 Normal histological appearance of the anal transition zone. The cells are cuboidal and stratified similar to transitional epithelium of the urinary tract. The photomicrograph also contains an anal duct lined by anal transitional epithelium.

whereas the mucosa inferior to the transition zone is stratified squamous. The squamous mucous membrane is devoid of hair and other cutaneous appendages and does not keratinize. The anal canal ends at the anal verge, where the anal squamous mucosa merges with the true anal skin and one can detect hair follicles, sweat glands, and apocrine glands.

The anal ducts are long, tubular structures that closely approach or penetrate the internal sphincter muscle and may even undermine the rectal mucosa. These ducts are lined by transitional epithelium and mucus-producing cells, which are most common at the terminal portion of the ducts before their opening into the anal crypts. Nodules of lymphoid tissue are often seen surrounding these ducts. The epithelium lining the ducts shows a similar immunohistochemical profile to that of the overlying transitional mucosa (CK7+ and CK20–).[5,8]

The dual embryological origin of the anal canal results in a dual blood supply, venous and lymphatic drainage, and nerve supply.[9-11] The superior two-thirds of the anal canal is supplied by the superior rectal artery, a continuation of the inferior mesenteric artery; the venous drainage of the superior anal canal flows into the superior rectal veins, tributaries of the inferior mesenteric vein. The lymphatic drainage of the superior two-thirds of the anal canal is to the inferior mesenteric lymph nodes. In contrast, the inferior third of the anal canal is supplied primarily by the inferior rectal arteries, which are branches of the internal pudendal arteries. The venous drainage of this portion of the anal canal is to the inferior rectal veins, which are tributaries of the internal pudendal veins and, ultimately, the internal iliac veins. Lymphatic drainage is to the superficial inguinal lymph nodes. The nerve supply of the superior two-thirds of the anal canal is through the autonomic nervous system; the inferior third is supplied by the inferior rectal nerve through the sacral plexus.

These aforementioned differences in embryology, blood supply, drainage, and nervous innervation are clinically relevant, particularly when evaluating congenital malformations of the anal canal and predicting patterns of spread of neoplasms. In surgical pathology practice, it may be difficult to determine whether a tumor has arisen within the distal rectum, the anal canal, or the anal margin/perianal skin because these anatomical zones overlap. Furthermore, bulky tumors often obliterate the normal anatomy. The eighth edition of the *American Joint Committee on Cancer Staging Manual* states that adenocarcinoma proximal to the dentate line/anorectal ring should be staged as rectal cancers and squamous cell carcinomas distal to the dentate line/anorectal ring should be staged as anal canal cancers. Identification of skin appendages helps delineate perianal skin carcinomas from true anal canal cancers. Perianal cancers are also defined by the presence of a tumor that is located within a 5-cm radius of the anus and is completely visualized after gentle traction is placed on the buttocks. An anal canal tumor should not be completely visualized after gentle traction.[12] Perianal cancers are staged as anus/anal canal carcinomas.

EMBRYOLOGICAL ABNORMALITIES OF THE ANUS AND ANAL CANAL

Clinical Features

Anorectal malformations occur in approximately 1 in 5000 live births[13,14] and affect males slightly more commonly than females.[15] They range from minor anal anomalies to complex cloacal malformations. The most common congenital anomaly of the anus is anal atresia, which accounts for up to 75% of all anorectal malformations.[16] Anorectal agenesis accounts for approximately 10% of all anal atresias. Up to two-thirds of congenital anal anomalies occur in association with anomalies in other organ systems, most often the genitourinary system, but also the central nervous system, skeleton, cardiovascular system, and gastrointestinal tract.[16-18] Patients usually present early after birth with failure to pass meconium or with meconium that extrudes from a fistulous opening.[19]

Pathogenesis

The cause of anorectal malformations is multifactorial. Given that about 5% to 10% of malformations arise in children with a chromosomal abnormality, most commonly trisomy 21, and that a number of monogenetic syndromes reveal anorectal malformations as one of their features,[18] genetics are considered an important component of their pathogenesis. Furthermore, anorectal malformations are more common in siblings of patients with anorectal malformations.[20] Ninety-five percent of patients with trisomy 21 and anorectal malformations have an imperforate anus without a fistula, compared with only 5% of all patients with anorectal malformations. Lastly, an association with congenital abnormalities, including anorectal malformations, has been found in infants conceived by assisted reproduction methods.[21]

Pathology

Anorectal malformations are recognized by their gross (anatomical) features. The "Wingspread" classification of anorectal malformation is subdivided into high, intermediate, and low atresia based on the level of termination of the anorectum in relation to the levator ani muscle.[22,23] This classification does not help guide surgery or help predict outcome, however.[15] Fistula formation is a common finding in anorectal malformations, particularly in high and intermediate forms of anal atresia, and it may be rectovesical, rectoprostatic, rectourethral (most common type in males), or anocutaneous in males and rectovaginal, rectovestibular (most common type in females), or anoperineal in females. More recently, the classification of anorectal malformations has been revised into the Krickenbeck scheme (Box 32.1), which adds emphasis on the type of fistula associated with the malformation. The type of fistula helps determine the location of the blind pouch and also helps guide the surgeon's expectations regarding the length of the atretic segment to be resected at the surgical pull-through procedure.[24] In patients with a cloacal disorder, a single perineal orifice is found where the urinary tract, vagina, and rectum all converge into a common channel.

BOX 32.1 Krickenbeck Classification of Anorectal Malformations

CLINICAL GROUPS
Perineal (cutaneous) fistula
Rectourethral fistula
Prostatic
Bulbar
Rectovesical fistula
Vestibular fistula
Cloaca
No fistula
Anal stenosis

RARE VARIANTS
Pouch colon
Rectal atresia/stenosis
Rectovaginal fistula
H fistula
Other

From Holschneider A, Hutson J, Peña A, et al. Preliminary report on the International Conference for the Development of Standards for the Treatment of Anorectal Malformations. J Pediatr Surg. *2005;40(10):1521-1526.*

Prognosis and Treatment

A posterior sagittal approach is considered the gold standard for defining and repairing anorectal anomalies.[20] This approach has greatly improved outcomes in anorectal malformation repair over the past several decades.[24,25] The level of anal atresia (high, intermediate, or low) in relationship to the levator ani muscle is directly related to functional prognosis and rates of fecal continence or constipation following a surgical pull-through procedure.[22] Anorectal agenesis has a poor prognosis for fecal continence because affected patients lack a functional puborectalis sling mechanism as well as internal and external anal sphincters. The prognosis for anal atresia located inferior to the levator ani muscle depends on the presence of functional sphincters as well as intact sensation; atresias isolated to the anus, such as imperforate anal membrane, carry the most favorable surgical prognosis. In patients with cloacal disorders, prognostic factors include the quality of the sacrum, the quality of the muscles, and the length of the common channel. Surgical repair for patients with a common channel less than 3 cm in length is feasible for most pediatric surgeons, whereas surgical repair for patients with a common channel greater than 3 cm in length should be performed at a specialized center by an experienced surgeon.[20] In the first 24 to 48 hours after birth of an infant with an anorectal malformation, the major issues relate to identification of life-threatening anomalies and whether to repair the defect immediately or to perform a protective colostomy with repair at a later date. These decisions are based on the infant's physical examination, the extent of the malformation, and any significant changes that occur in the first 24 hours of life. Once this critical period passes and the features of the infant's malformation are recognized, the surgeon can proceed to repair the defect.

BENIGN TUMOR–LIKE LESIONS OF THE ANUS AND ANAL CANAL

Hemorrhoids

Clinical Features

About one-third of patients undergoing screening colonoscopy are found to have hemorrhoids, but precise prevalence data are not available.[26] Men and women are likely equally affected, and the peak age at diagnosis is between 45 and 65 years of age. Whites are affected more often than African Americans.[27] Painless bleeding is the most common sign of hemorrhoids; pain may occur if the hemorrhoids become thrombosed or strangulated. Hemorrhoids rarely lead to anemia; thus, if a patient presents with anemia, other potential causes should be investigated. With age, the hemorrhoidal tissue may gradually engorge and extend further up into the anal canal, where it becomes susceptible to the effects of straining at defecation. Internal hemorrhoids usually become symptomatic only when they prolapse, become ulcerated, bleed, or thrombose. External hemorrhoids may be asymptomatic or associated with discomfort, acute pain, or bleeding from thrombosis or ulceration.

Pathogenesis

Current evidence indicates that hemorrhoids actually represent cushions of fibrovascular and connective tissue normally present in the anal submucosa and consist of direct arteriovenous communications, mainly between the terminal branches of the superior rectal and superior hemorrhoidal arteries. These cushions serve a protective role during defecation and help maintain continence.[11,26,28] Hemorrhoidal tissues are thought to arise from abnormal dilation of the internal hemorrhoid venous plexus, distention of the arteriovenous anastomoses, prolapse of these cushions, or elevations of anal sphincter pressure with resultant vascular congestion; however, this theory has not been rigorously tested. Thus any cause of elevated intraabdominal pressure, such as straining at defection, inadequate fiber intake, prolonged lavatory sitting, constipation, diarrhea, and conditions such as pregnancy, ascites, and pelvic space-occupying lesions, have all been implicated in hemorrhoid development, but not necessarily proven.[26,27] Portal hypertension, in itself, is not associated with hemorrhoid formation. Rather, hemorrhoidal bleeding in the presence of portal hypertension may be related to the presence of a coagulopathic disorder, rather than simply venous engorgement.

Pathology

Hemorrhoidal tissue is located on the left lateral, right anterior, and right posterior aspects of the anal canal. Internal hemorrhoids are classified according to their site of origin; the dentate line serves as an anatomic/histological border for classification and grading. External hemorrhoids originate distal to the dentate line, arising from the inferior hemorrhoidal plexus, and are lined by modified squamous epithelium. Internal hemorrhoids originate proximal to the dentate line, arising from the superior hemorrhoidal plexus, and are covered with rectal or transitional mucosa. Microscopically, excised specimens show evidence of dilated thick-walled submucosal vessels and sinusoidal spaces, often with thrombosis and hemorrhage into the surrounding connective tissues (Fig. 32.3). Internal hemorrhoids are graded from I to IV based on degree of prolapse and their ability to be reduced (Table 32.1).

All tissues excised as clinical hemorrhoids should be examined histologically because the differential diagnosis of an anal mass and anal bleeding includes entities such as colorectal or anal carcinoma, anal melanoma, inflammatory bowel disease, and infection.[29] Furthermore, hemorrhoidectomy may be complicated by subsequent anal incontinence.

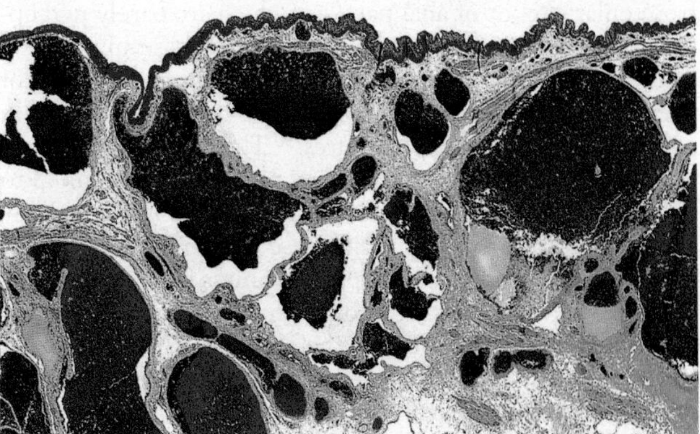

FIGURE 32.3 Low-power view of a hemorrhoid showing vascular dilation and thrombosis. Chronic inflammation of the intervening stroma is also present.

TABLE 32.1 Classification of Internal Hemorrhoids

Grade	Clinical Feature
I	No prolapse during Valsalva maneuver
II	Prolapse during Valsalva maneuver, but spontaneously reduce
III	Prolapse during Valsalva maneuver and need manual reduction
IV	Cannot be reduced

From Cengiz TB, Gorgun E. Hemorrhoids: A range of treatments. Cleveland Clin J Med. *2019;86(9):612-620.*

While anal sphincter injury secondary to hemorrhoidectomy is typically assessed via endoscopic ultrasonography, documenting the histological presence or absence and quantity of smooth muscle and skeletal muscle bundles may be helpful to guide physicians as to the potential cause of the patient's incontinence. Anal fibroepithelial polyps, discussed in the next section, are often confused clinically with hemorrhoids because of their similar gross appearance.

Prognosis and Treatment

Nonoperative measures, such as Sitz baths, analgesics, topical anesthetics, increased dietary fiber, and stool softeners, can be offered to patients with mild symptoms or minimally symptomatic hemorrhoids. If these methods fail, sclerotherapy, rubber band ligation, cryotherapy, or surgical therapy should be considered. Surgical treatment should be individually tailored to each patient according to the degree of symptoms, coexisting anorectal diseases, and the degree of external anorectal component. Complications of hemorrhoidal disease are mostly related to treatment. Mild complications include pain, urinary retention, and constipation. Severe complications include fistula formation, rectal prolapse, and incontinence.

Hypertrophied Anal Papillae/Fibroepithelial Polyps

Clinical Features and Pathogenesis

Hypertrophied anal papillae, also known as *anal fibroepithelial polyps*, are benign polypoid projections of anal squamous epithelium and subepithelial connective tissue. They result from enlargement of anal papillae, which are barely perceptible triangular protrusions located at the base of the anal columns (columns of Morgagni). They are present in 45% of patients who undergo proctoscopic examination and are believed to be acquired structures.[30] They are twice as common in men as in women, and they range in size from 0.3 to 1.9 cm, with a mean diameter of approximately 1 cm. They may be asymptomatic, in which case they are usually found in isolation as a solitary firm, palpable mass on digital examination, or develop in association with an irritation, infection, or chronic fistula or fissure in the anal canal.[30-32] They may also coexist with hemorrhoids and, not surprisingly, are confused with hemorrhoids clinically.[33]

Pathology

Hypertrophied anal papillae/fibroepithelial polyps may have the clinical appearance of a hemorrhoid and are often submitted to the pathologist with this designation.[32] Unlike hemorrhoids, fibroepithelial polyps usually do not contain microscopic evidence of dilated or thick-walled vessels, recent or remote hemorrhage, or organizing thrombi. The mucosa covering the polyp is typically squamous, and the submucosal tissue is composed of loose fibrovascular connective tissue characteristic of this region (Fig. 32.4). Some polyps may contain large, multinucleated, or stellate CD34+ stromal cells or hyalinization of stromal vessels, all thought to result from a reactive process of the stroma.[34,35] Some authors prefer to reserve the diagnosis of *hypertrophied anal papillae* for cases in which the stroma is composed of loose fibrovascular tissue and use *anal fibroepithelial polyp* when the stroma shows predominantly fibrous changes.[31] In essence, hypertrophied anal papillae and anal fibroepithelial polyps are identical to fibroepithelial polyps (acrochordons) of the cutaneous skin.

The clinical differential diagnosis of a polypoid mass in the anal canal includes hemorrhoids, infection/abscess, or other more serious disorders such as anal carcinoma or anal melanoma. Routine histological examination is usually adequate to determine the underlying pathological process. On occasion, the squamous epithelium of a fibroepithelial polyp will contain unsuspected intraepithelial neoplasia.

Prognosis and Therapy

Hypertrophic anal papillae tend to enlarge over time and may convert from an asymptomatic to a symptomatic mass associated with pruritus, anal discharge, and discomfort. Surgical resection in symptomatic cases often results in relief of symptoms. When anal papillae accompany an underlying chronic process, treatment is often aimed at correcting the primary etiology in association with removal of the hypertrophied papillae.[31]

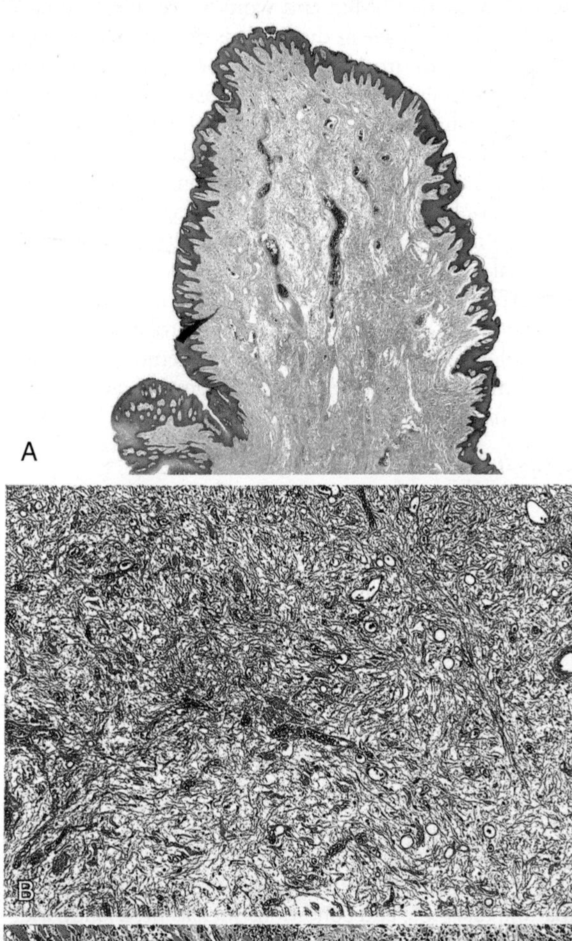

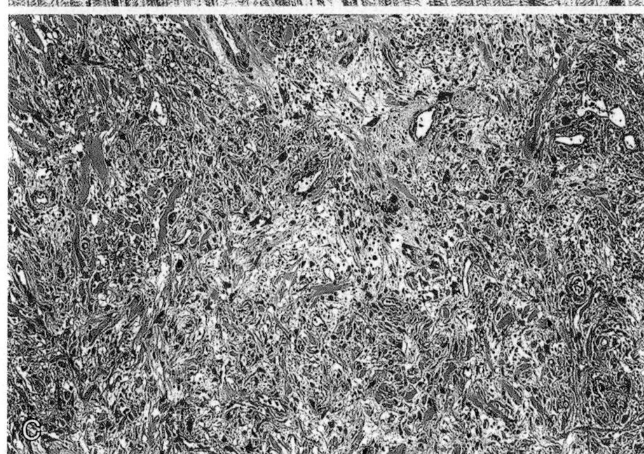

FIGURE 32.4 A, Low-power view of hypertrophic anal papillae (fibroepithelial polyp). In this example, the "tag" is lined by squamous epithelium and composed of fibrovascular connective tissue. **B,** High-power view of the fibroepithelial polyp stroma. **C,** In some anal tags, the stroma may contain numerous stellate fibroblasts with bizarre-shaped and multiple nuclei. These changes are reactive in nature and should not be confused with a stromal malignancy.

Inflammatory Cloacogenic Polyps and Mucosal Prolapse

Clinical Features

Inflammatory cloacogenic polyps (ICPs) occur predominantly in middle-aged patients, although they have also been described in children.[36] Men and women are equally affected. The most common presentation is rectal bleeding or mucous discharge. Patients who report straining at defecation are at increased risk for development of an ICP. ICPs represent one aspect of mucosal prolapse disorders of the gastrointestinal tract, which include inflammatory cap polyps, inflammatory myoglandular polyps, polypoid prolapsing folds of diverticular disease, colitis cystic profunda, and polyps associated with solitary rectal ulcer syndrome, among others. Furthermore, any type of mucosal polyp may undergo secondary prolapse changes, with resultant misplacement of mucosal elements into the submucosa or deeper layers.

The pathogenesis of ICP is believed to be similar to that of other mucosal prolapse disorders.[37] It is likely related to chronic mucosal prolapse that occurs in long-term disorders with constipation and defecation with secondary associated ischemic, inflammatory, and reactive changes of the overlying mucosa.[38-40]

Pathology

These polyps are located in the anterior anal canal, may be single or multiple, and are typically sessile (see Chapter 22 for details and figures). They are variable in size, but usually range from 1 to 2 cm grossly. Histological features include fibrosis of the lamina propria, thickening of the muscularis mucosae, hyperplasia of the mucosal glands (often with a villous-like configuration) leading to a serrated contour of the epithelium, and telangiectasia of surface vasculature, either with or without fibrin thrombi (Fig. 32.5). The muscularis mucosae is typically thickened and irregular, with frequent extension of fibromuscular strands into the lamina propria that results in the formation of "diamond-shaped" crypts and deposition of mucosal elastin. The presence of elastin is particularly distinctive because it is otherwise not seen in the normal rectum (Fig. 32.5C). The surface epithelium is characteristically composed of a mixture of colorectal, transitional, and squamous mucosa. Ischemic-type erosion of the surface epithelium is a common finding, which may contribute to regenerative or hyperplastic (serrated) epithelial changes.

Differential Diagnosis

A variety of entities enter into the differential diagnosis of an ICP.[41] Because of their location in the anal canal and low-power appearance, ICPs may resemble a tubulovillous adenoma or a traditional serrated adenoma of the distal rectum. Recognition of the regenerative (nonneoplastic) epithelial cytology and eroded surface in ICPs and an absence of cytological dysplasia helps distinguish ICP from an adenoma. In addition, ICPs typically contain both transitional and squamous epithelium. The fact that adenomas are somewhat uncommon in the age group in which ICPs are often diagnosed is also useful. In some ICPs, prominent misplacement of the reactive epithelium into the underlying fibrous stroma combined with hyperplastic musculature, also known as *proctitis cystica profunda*, may simulate an invasive mucinous carcinoma (Fig. 32.6; see Chapter 22 for details). Although prolapse changes may also be found in invasive carcinomas, they are more prominent in ICPs, and the "misplaced" epithelium is usually accompanied by lamina propria tissue. In addition, nonneoplastic epithelium surrounding mucin pools may be found in cases of benign proctitis cystica profunda, whereas neoplastic epithelium is often found floating within mucin pools in cases of invasive mucinous adenocarcinoma. In some cases, features of prolapse may be the only finding in the mucosa overlying a malignancy; thus an underlying malignancy should always be considered when biopsy findings of a "mass lesion" reveal prolapse changes, but without neoplasm.[42]

The presence of inflammation and a granulation tissue cap may cause diagnostic confusion with a juvenile/hamartomatous polyp or an inflammatory polyp (related to

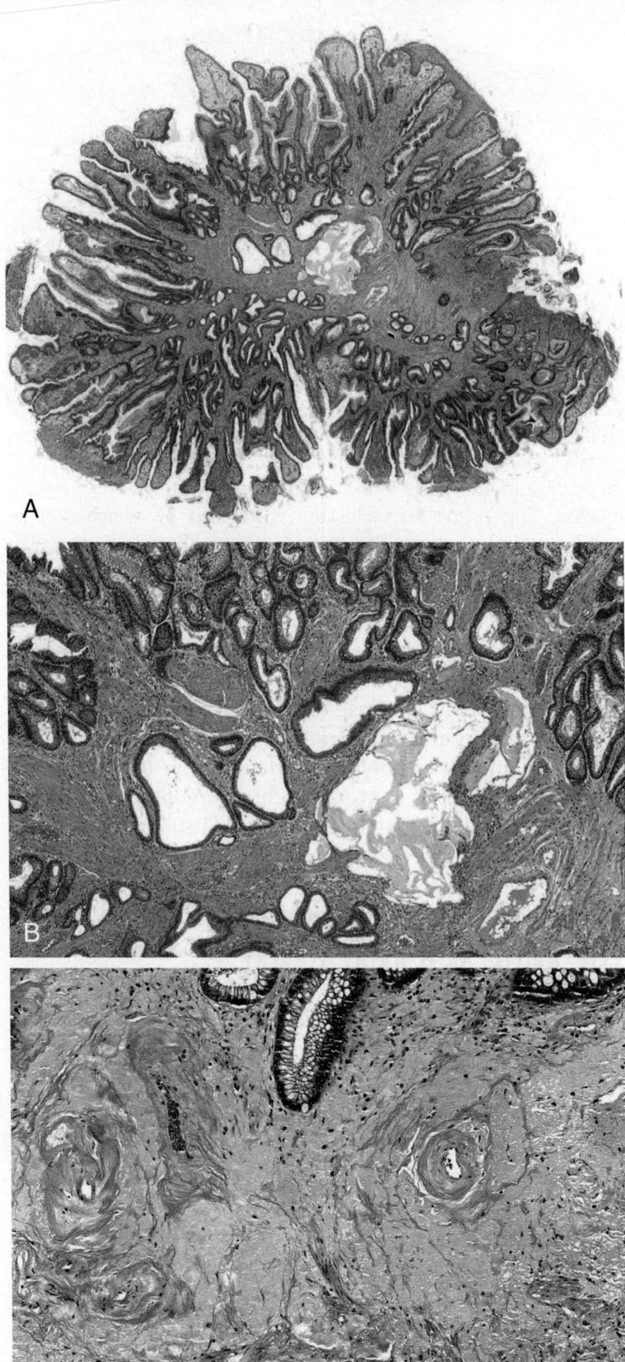

FIGURE 32.5 A, Low-power view of an inflammatory cloacogenic polyp. These lesions have a villiform appearance, incorporate anal squamous epithelium, display prominent crypt distortion, and show reactive epithelial changes. The epithelium often has a serrated architectural appearance that can cause diagnostic confusion with a serrated neoplasm. **B,** High-power view reveals smooth muscle ingrowth between the crypts and misplaced nonneoplastic crypts and acellular mucin. **C,** Stromal deposition of elastin, which is pale staining, among more densely eosinophilic collagen and smooth muscle. The elastin is a helpful clue to chronic trauma-related injury.

inflammatory bowel disease or sporadic).[41] This distinction may be particularly difficult because any type colorectal polyp can undergo secondary prolapse. A low-power view of the polyp often helps one distinguish prolapse

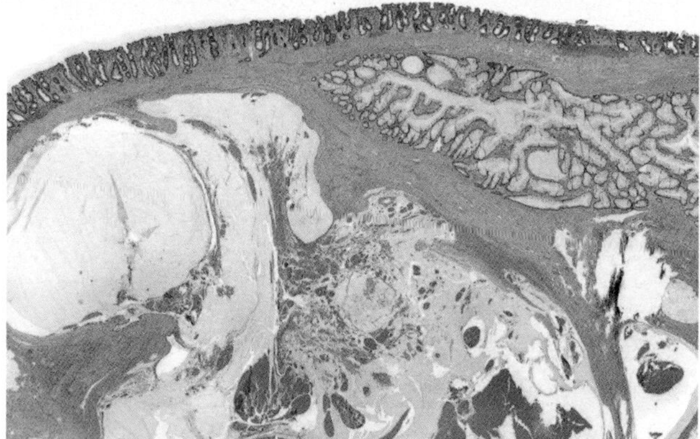

FIGURE 32.6 Low-power view of typical histological findings in proctitis cystica profunda in which well-circumscribed nests of misplaced rectal epithelium and pools of extracellular mucin are seen in the submucosa. This misplaced epithelium is invested by lamina propria, with a surrounding stroma that may show hemorrhage and associated hemosiderin-laden macrophages.

from an injury secondary to a preexisting lesion (often neoplastic). Also, it is important to note that ICPs show muscularization in the base of the polyp, whereas juvenile or inflammatory polyps do not show this feature. Furthermore, inflammatory polyps in inflammatory bowel disease usually occur in the context of chronic colitis in adjacent mucosa. Simple excision of ICPs is usually curative.[39] Recurrences are uncommon.

INFLAMMATORY DISORDERS OF THE ANUS AND ANAL CANAL

Anal Tears, Fissures, and Ulcers

Clinical Features

Acute anal fissures are common, although the exact incidence is unknown because most patients do not present for clinical evaluation.[43] Chronic anal fissures affect men and women equally, and they account for up to 10% of patients who are seen in colorectal clinics. Although there are no uniform criteria, most define *chronicity* of an anal fissure by persistence for at least 6 weeks and with visible transverse internal anal sphincter fibers on anoscopy. Other features of chronicity include an indurated edge and the presence of a hypertrophic anal papilla (Fig. 32.7A). When a fissure becomes large, deep, and chronic, it is often referred to as an *anal ulcer*. Patients typically present with intense pain, particularly after defecation.[44]

Pathogenesis

The term *anal tear* refers to an acute linear tear in the mucosa of the anal canal. Although most anal tears heal spontaneously, the development of an anal fissure is associated with spasm of the internal anal sphincter and a reduction in mucosal blood flow that leads to delayed or failed healing of the initial mucosal injury.[45] Chronic anal fissures are further propagated by an increased resting internal anal sphincter tone. In patients with a normal sphincter tone, other factors have been linked to the development of an anal fissure, such as HIV infection, anal receptive intercourse, sexual abuse, Crohn's disease, and previous obstetric operations or anorectal malformation repair.[43]

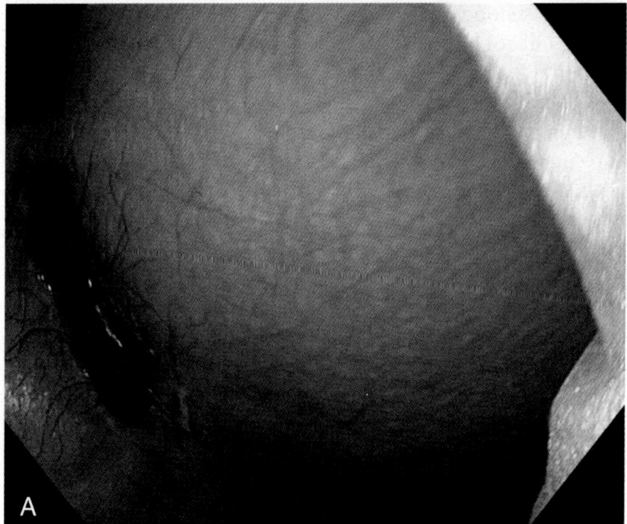

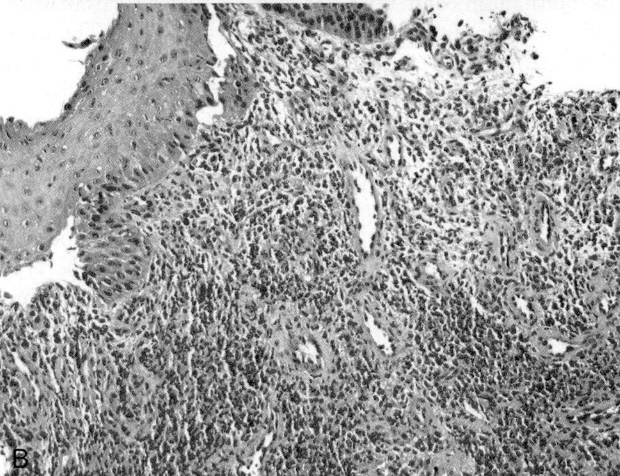

FIGURE 32.7 A, Chronic anal fissure at anoscopy. **B,** Typical histological findings in anal tear/fissure/ulcer. A mucosal break leads to inflammation and reactive changes of the overlying squamous epithelium *(upper left)* and intensely inflamed granulation tissue at the base of the break.

Pathology

Anal fissures typically extend from the dentate line to the anal verge in the posterior midline of the anal canal overlying the lower portion of the internal sphincter. Histologically, anal fissures/ulcers are characterized by nonspecific acute and chronic inflammation, granulation tissue, and reactive changes of the squamous epithelium at the edges of the fissure (Fig 32.7B). Chronic fissures are also frequently associated with hypertrophy of the anal papillae at the proximal end of the lesion,[45] Histologically, hypertrophic anal papillae are similar to other types of benign fibroepithelial polyps.

In cases in which a fissure is located in an unusual location or fails to heal after treatment, inflammatory bowel disease (most often Crohn's disease), neoplasm, or infectious processes should be considered.[46-48]

Prognosis and Treatment

Most acute fissures are superficial and heal quickly. Healing may be facilitated by increased dietary fiber and water, stool softeners, and warm sitz baths. For nonhealing acute anal fissures or chronic anal fissures, medical management is recommended for first-line treatment with the aim of reducing internal anal sphincter resting pressure.[43,49,50] Current medical treatments include use of topical calcium channel blockers (nifedipine or diltiazem) to reduce anal sphincter tone; nitric oxide donors, such as topical glyceryl trinitrate (GTN), to increase anodermal blood flow; and botulinum toxin to reduce resting internal anal sphincter tone. All three of these methods have been associated with similar healing rates, but topical calcium channel blockers are reported to have the benefits of fewer side effects than topical GTN and lower cost than botulinum toxin.[51] If these methods fail or if the fissures recur, surgical management may be indicated using approaches such as anal dilation, internal sphincterotomy, or fissurectomy.[45] Surgical management permits healing of chronic fissures in up to 100% of patients with low rates of recurrence.[43] Patients with recurrent anal fissure after surgical management should be evaluated for alternative causes, such as Crohn's disease, sexually transmitted disease, sexual abuse, or HIV infection.

Anal Abscesses and Fistulas

Most anal fistulas or abscesses are idiopathic, although they may occur in patients with Crohn's disease or carcinoma in this region.[52] Anorectal abscesses may also be found in patients with hidradenitis suppurativa.[53-55] In hidradenitis patients, wound healing is often complicated by coexistent obesity and diabetes.

Anal abscesses and fistulas represent different stages of anorectal suppurative disease. The majority of suppurative processes in this location are believed to arise after infection of an anal duct/gland, which provides a pathway from the anal canal to perineal soft tissues.[56,57] In the acute phase, an abscess may form, whereas a fistula represents the chronic phase of infection, occurring in 20% to 50% of patients with an anal abscess.[44,58,59] There are no reliable ways to predict which patients will progress to a fistula. Fistulas are usually classified according to their relationship to the external anal sphincter (i.e., intersphincteric, transsphincteric, suprasphincteric, or extrasphincteric; Figure 32.8).

Histological specimens obtained from fistulas show nonspecific acute and chronic inflammation, fibrosis, and granulation tissue. Foreign-body giant cell reaction to fecal matter may also be seen in specimens from fistula tracts of the anus and should not be confused with the well-formed, sarcoid-like granulomatous reaction typical of Crohn's disease. In patients with hidradenitis suppurativa, the histological findings in the anal canal are identical to those found in other affected locations.

Any cause of infection or fistula formation should be considered in the differential diagnosis of an anal abscess or fistula. A thorough histological examination, including multiple sections, should be conducted to rule out an underlying neoplasm, and special stains for acid-fast bacilli, fungal forms, or other infectious organisms should be performed, particularly if granulomatous inflammation is found. A careful review of the patient's clinical history, including the presence of inflammatory bowel disease, should be obtained.

Antibiotics are often ineffective because of poor penetration into inflamed areas. Incision and drainage remains the primary method of treatment modality for anal abscesses, but recurrences are relatively common.[59] Wide surgical excision is curative in most cases of idiopathic anal abscess or fistula.

Common Infections of the Anal Canal

Clinical Features and Etiology

Individuals who engage in unprotected anal intercourse are at greatest risk for acquiring anorectal infections. Thus anorectal infections are most common among men who have sex with men (MSM). The symptoms of an anorectal infection may vary depending on the specific infection or pathological process, but they are often indistinguishable from those of inflammatory bowel disease. The most common symptom is a frequent or continuous urge to have a bowel movement. Other symptoms include anorectal pain or discomfort, anal discharge (which may be purulent, mucoid, or blood-stained), tenesmus, urgency of defecation, rectal bleeding, and constipation. Systemic symptoms, such as fever, may also occur. However, many patients are asymptomatic.[60]

Infections of the anal canal are most often caused by sexually transmitted pathogens. The most common agent identified is *Neisseria gonorrhoeae* (gonorrhea), found in 30% of patients, followed by *Chlamydia trachomatis* (19%), herpes simplex virus (HSV) type 2 (16%), and *Treponema pallidum* (syphilis; 2%). HSV type 1 accounts for 13% of anorectal herpes infections and likely represents ano-oral transmission.[60] The incidence of anorectal disease caused by *C. trachomatis*, the causative agent of lymphogranuloma venereum (LGV), is increasing.[61,62] More than one infection may be present in a single individual.

Pathology

Different pathogens typically infect different types of mucosa. HSV and *T. pallidum* infect the stratified squamous epithelium of the perianal area and anal verge, although syphilitic proctitis also occurs.[63,64] As in other sites, HSV infections are associated with small vesicles that

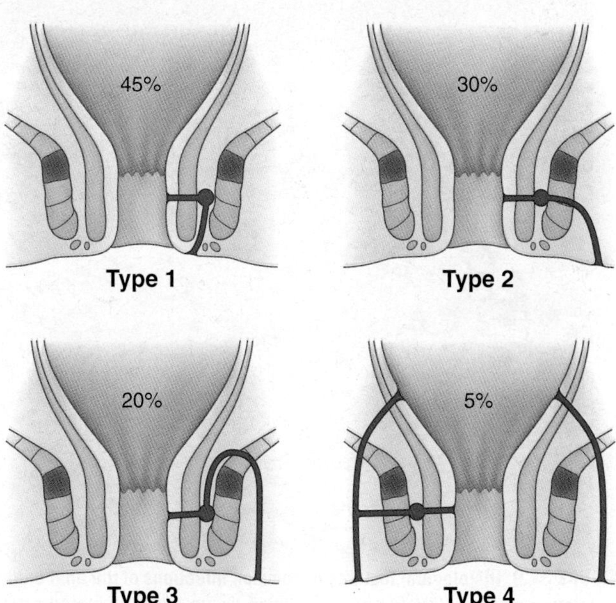

FIGURE 32.8 Anatomical classification of the four main types of fistulas, including intersphincteric (type 1), trans-sphincteric (type 2), suprasphincteric (type 3), and extrasphincteric (type 4). (From Parks AG, Gordon PH, Hardcastle JD. A classification of fistula-in-ano. Br J Surg. 1976;63(1):1-12.)

ulcerate and are seen histologically as mucosal ulcerations with associated acute and chronic inflammation and granulation tissue. Virally infected multinucleated cells with smudged chromatin may be seen in routine hematoxylin and eosin (H&E) sections, although immunohistochemical stains are of great value in confirming the presence of virally infected cells (Fig. 32.9A,B). In contrast, syphilis is commonly associated with a chronic inflammatory infiltrate rich in plasma cells and may also show associated granulomatous inflammation (Fig. 32.9C–E). Dark-field microscopy of

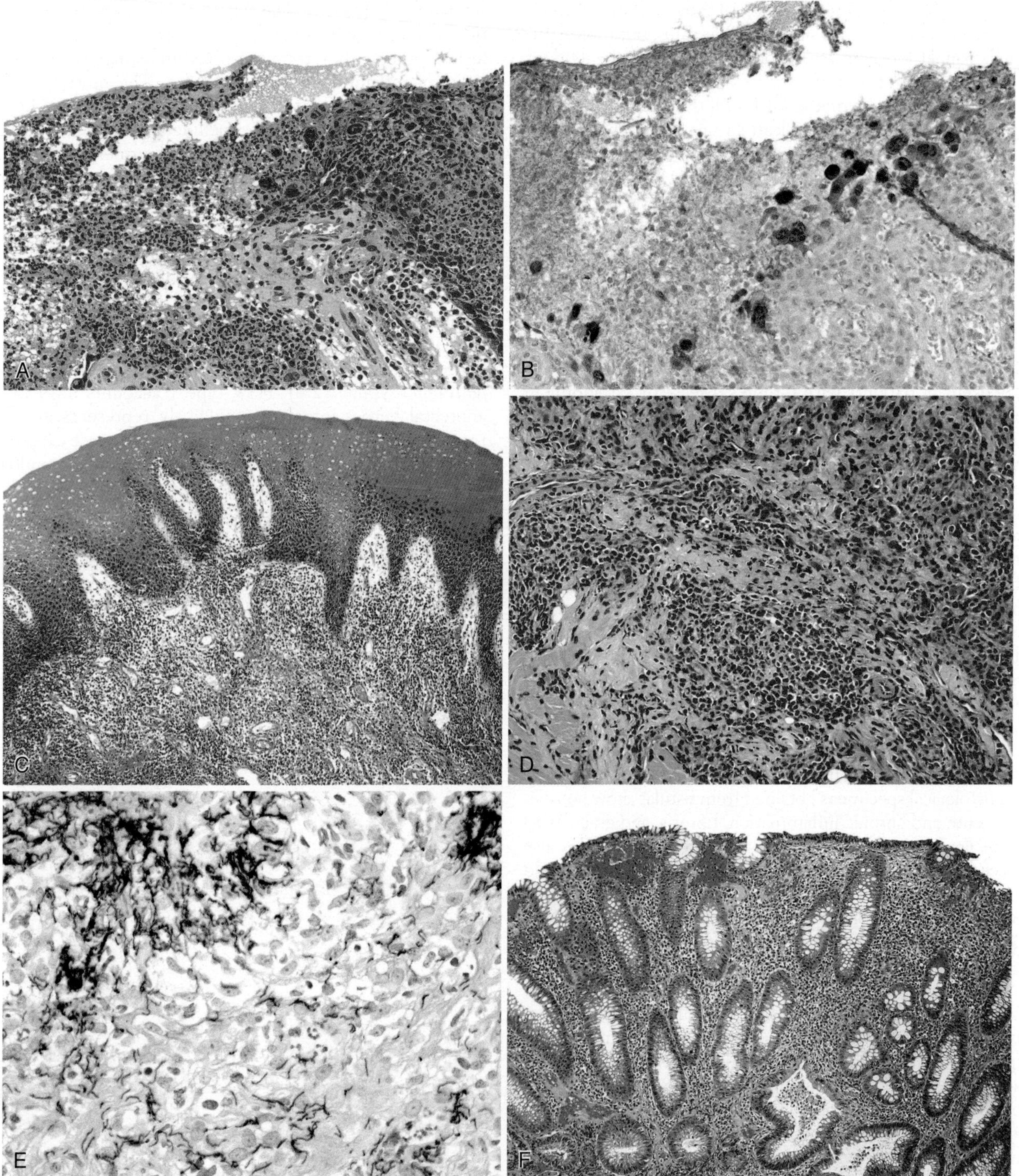

FIGURE 32.9 Histological features of common infections of the anal canal. A, Herpes ulcer of the anal canal mucosa. Mucosal ulcers contain an acute fibroinflammatory infiltrate and granulation tissue. Virally infected cells are best seen at the ulcer edge, characterized by the nuclear "*M*'s": multinucleation, nuclear molding, and chromatin margination. **B,** Herpes viral particles can be demonstrated by use of a herpes immunostain. **C,** Syphilis infection of the anal canal. At low power, an intense, bandlike chronic inflammatory infiltrate is present. **D,** High-power view shows the inflammatory infiltrate in **C** to comprise lymphocytes and plasma cells. **E,** Immunohistochemical stain for *Treponema pallidum* revealing copious spirochete organisms. **F,** Severe active inflammation, crypt abscesses, and chronic inflammation with associated reactive changes of the columnar mucosa of the lower rectum/upper anal canal characteristic of gonorrheal infection.

exudates from anorectal ulcers may be inaccurate as a result of contamination from commensal spirochetes found in the normal flora of the colorectum; however, *T. pallidum* immunohistochemical stains have become a useful tool for surgical pathologists (Fig. 32.9E).[65] Demonstration of antibodies in the serum is the gold standard of syphilis diagnosis. Serological tests consist of two main types of nonspecific cardiolipin antigen test: the Venereal Disease Research Laboratory slide test and the rapid plasma reagin test. These tests can be used to diagnose primary and secondary syphilis and to monitor treatment response. The specific treponemal antigen tests (i.e., enzyme immunoassay, *T. pallidum* hemagglutination assay, *T. pallidum* particle agglutination assay, fluorescent treponemal antibody absorption test) stay positive even after treatment and can detect latent syphilis in untreated adults. Infections occurring between the anal verge and the dentate line tend to be extremely painful because of the abundance of sensory nerve endings in this area. Chlamydial infections and gonorrhea target the columnar epithelium of the rectum. One may see evidence of cryptitis, crypt abscesses, and reactive epithelial changes in affected individuals (Fig. 32.9F), but the degree of activity and chronic injury is characteristically less than untreated inflammatory bowel disease.[63,64] Granulomas are not uncommon. Polymerase chain reaction amplification for C. *trachomatis* DNA is the standard diagnostic test for anorectal chlamydial infection. The rectum itself has few sensory nerve endings, so infections that spare the anus may be painless.[60]

Differential Diagnosis

Solitary anal ulcers, as in HSV infection, may be misdiagnosed clinically as a chronic anal fissure. Granulomatous inflammation can lead to the formation of a rectal mass in both primary and secondary syphilis, and this must be differentiated from other causes of a rectal mass, such as a neoplasm. Condylomata lata occurring in the perianal region in syphilis patients appear as moist, wartlike lesions and may be confused for human papillomavirus (HPV) infection. The pain, tenesmus, bloody discharge, and constipation of untreated LGV may mimic Crohn's disease. In the tertiary stage, anorectal fistulas and strictures may also occur in LGV.

Inflammatory Bowel Disease

The histopathological features of inflammatory bowel disease are covered in detail in Chapters 16 and 17. However, involvement of the anal canal is sufficiently frequent to warrant additional comments here, particularly because neoplastic disorders may present with similar findings in this region.

Clinical Features and Pathogenesis

In ulcerative colitis, involvement of the anus is typically nonspecific and indistinguishable from the appearance in patients without colitis. In contrast with ulcerative colitis, at least 50% of patients with Crohn's disease have perianal or anal disease.[66] The anal canal is involved in approximately 25% of patients with small-intestinal Crohn's disease, more than 40% of patients with large-bowel disease and rectal sparing, and more than 90% of patients with large-bowel disease that includes the rectum.[67] In some patients, anal involvement is the first or only clinical manifestation of Crohn's disease.[68]

The clinical features of Crohn's disease involving the anus have been well characterized.[68,69] Symptoms include recurrent sepsis, local pain, discharge, ulceration, fecal incontinence, sleep disruption, psychological disturbance, and sexual dysfunction.[70] Signs most characteristic of Crohn's disease affecting the anus are chronic inflammatory changes, induration of the anal skin, multiplicity of lesions, and skin discoloration. Anal canal lesions include fissures, ulcers, strictures, perianal fistulas that open into or near the anal canal, abscesses, rectovaginal fistulas in women, and cancer.[66] Anal skin lesions are usually perianal skin tags or hemorrhoids. Anal skin tags are the most frequent finding and tend to be larger than those in patients without Crohn's disease. Fissures and fistulas are the next most common finding.[66] Fissures in Crohn's disease tend to be large, deep, and located more atypically compared with traumatic anal fissures. Most fistulas in anal Crohn's disease are classified as *simple*, although in some patients they may contain multiple openings, some at a considerable distance from the anal canal ("watering-can" perineum).[68] The etiology of Crohn's perianal fistulas is uncertain, but in some patients it is thought to be caused by a fistula-in-ano arising from inflamed or infected anal glands or by penetration of fissures or ulcers in the rectum or anal canal.[68]

Pathology

In ulcerative colitis, chronic active inflammation tends to involve rectal mucosa in the proximal anal canal.[71] If histological findings are encountered more distally in the anal canal, they are limited to nonspecific chronic inflammation of the submucosal tissues with associated mild reactive changes of the squamous or transitional epithelium. Anal fissures, abscesses, or fistulas are also occasionally found, but these more severe changes would prompt clinical consideration of Crohn's disease. The anal findings in Crohn's disease are variable. They include anal fissures, fistulas, ulcers, abscesses, and tags.[68] Unfortunately, the histological features seen in the fissures and fistulas in patients with Crohn's disease are the same as those seen in the fissures and fistulas in patients without Crohn's disease. A feature supporting the diagnosis of anal Crohn's disease is the presence of sarcoid-like (noncaseating) granulomatous inflammation close to the anal mucosa, particularly in a young patient with no other obvious reason for an inflammatory disorder of the anal canal (Fig. 32.10). Thus, as in other gastrointestinal sites, a diagnosis of Crohn's disease requires correlation of the histological changes with all available clinical, endoscopic, and radiological information.

Differential Diagnosis

The differential diagnosis of granulomatous inflammation in the anal canal includes foreign body reaction to nonspecific fistulas, sarcoidosis, tuberculosis, granuloma inguinale caused by *Calymmatobacterium granulomatis*, or LGV caused by sexual transmission of C. *trachomatis*, among others.[60,72-74] Tuberculous granulomas are typically caseating. Stains for acid-fast bacilli and other microbiological studies are helpful. Patients with tuberculosis of the anal canal invariably also have pulmonary disease. The finding of

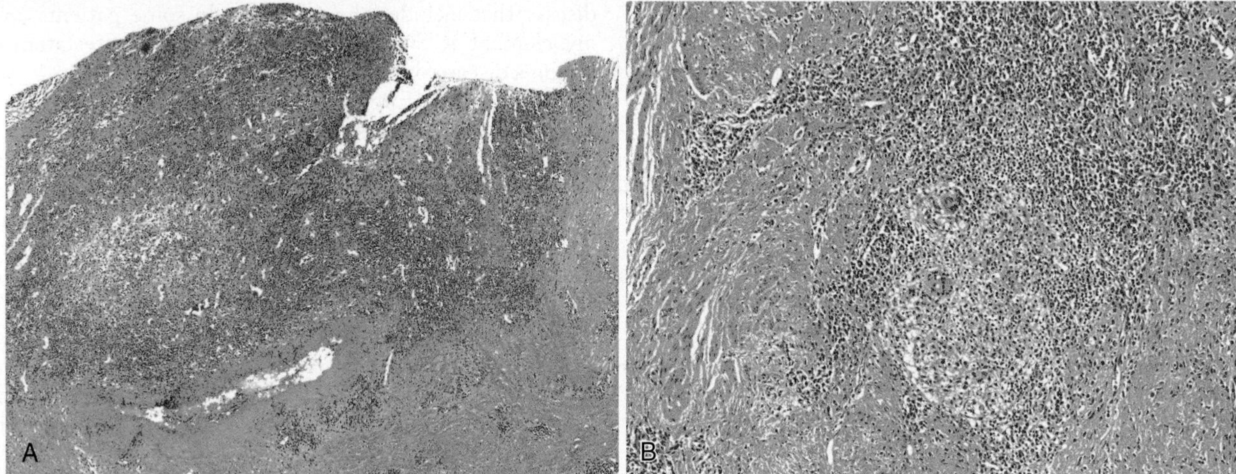

FIGURE 32.10 Histological findings in perianal Crohn's disease. A, Ulcer with granulation tissue, fibrosis, and chronic inflammation. The findings are nonspecific and similar to fistulas in patients without Crohn's disease. **B,** In this patient with perianal Crohn's disease, a helpful clue to the cause of the inflammation is the presence of granulomatous inflammation with giant cells.

Donovan bodies in a Warthin-Starry stain supports a diagnosis of granuloma inguinale, whereas the finding of follicular lymphohistiocytic and plasma cell infiltrates in association with neural hyperplasia may suggest chlamydial infection.[75] Hidradenitis suppurativa (Fig. 32.11), which presents as painful, purulent or suppurative lesions of the skin that bears apocrine glands and hair follicles,[76] may be confused with complex fistulizing perianal Crohn's disease. Healing of hidradenitis may lead to tunneling or scarring that mimics Crohn's-type fistulas. A correct diagnosis of hidradenitis can often be made with examination under anesthesia, by probing the cutaneous tracts and demonstrating that they traverse only to the subdermal space and do not communicate with the rectum or other parts of the digestive tract, as would be expected in Crohn's-related fistulas.[77]

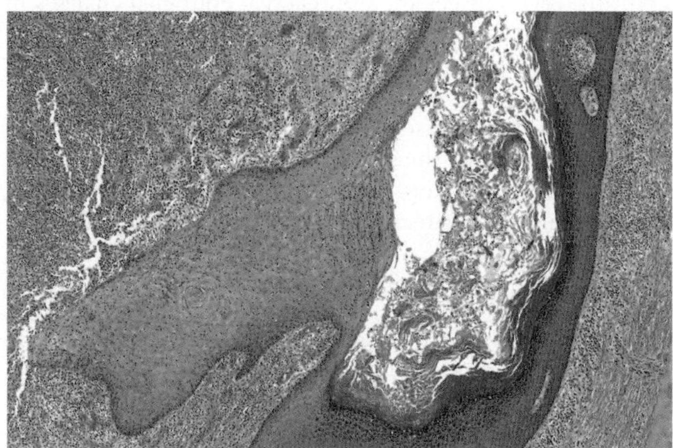

FIGURE 32.11 Histological features common to hidradenitis suppurativa include dilated hair follicles with intraluminal keratinous and inflammatory debris as well as associated perifolliculitis, which may include frank abscess formation.

Prognosis

The prognosis for patients with anal Crohn's disease is related to the extent of involvement, and for most patients it is excellent.[78] A variety of classification schemes for perianal Crohn's disease have been proposed, although most are not widely used because they have not shown a reproducible relationship to meaningful clinical outcomes, such as fistula formation.[68,79] Thus most clinicians use a simpler system to classify perianal disease into "simple" and "complex." Proper classification involves a thorough evaluation of the perianal area for involvement by skin tags, fistulas, fissures, abscesses, and stricturing disease as well as an endoscopic examination of the rectum to assess for inflammation. Fistulas classified as *simple* indicate that the fistula tract arises below the external sphincter, has a single external opening, has no pain or fluctuation to suggest perianal abscess, is not a rectovaginal fistula, and has no evidence of anorectal stricture. In contrast, fistulas classified as *complex* arise above the external anal sphincter and may contain one or more of the aforementioned features. Rectal Crohn's disease may make a simple fistula more complicated to manage, but patients with Crohn's disease and simple fistulas generally have higher rates of healing than non-Crohn's patients with complex fistulas.[80] Combined with small bowel disease, perianal Crohn's disease serves as an absolute contraindication to restorative proctocolectomy (ileal pouch anal anastomosis) in the well-motivated subset of Crohn's patients seeking a continence-preserving procedure.[81]

Treatment

Management of perianal Crohn's disease includes both medical and surgical treatment. Short-term therapy is aimed at abscess drainage and symptom reduction. Long-term treatment goals include healing the fistula, preserving continence, and avoiding proctectomy/stoma.[82] In the absence of pelvic sepsis/abscess, which must be addressed immediately, treatment often begins with conservative medical treatment that includes antibiotics, thiopurines, and anti–tumor necrosis factor-α agents. These agents are used in an attempt to reduce the number of draining fistulas and are most effective in simple perianal disease.[68,80] Surgical management is reserved for patients with complex fistulizing disease, abscesses, or severe/refractory proctitis. Up to 50% of patients require surgical management of their perianal disease, ranging from local procedures such as sepsis drainage and seton placement, to segmental resections such as proctectomy with ostomy creation.[68,80]

BENIGN TUMORS OF THE ANUS AND ANAL CANAL

Adnexal Tumors

Clinical Features

A wide variety of adnexal tumors have been described in the perianal skin, but all are uncommon.[83] Probably the most frequently encountered lesion is hidradenoma papilliferum.[84,85] Hidradenoma papilliferum occurs almost exclusively in women, over a broad age range. In most patients, it presents as a solitary, painless mass of the perianal skin or perineum, although ulceration of the overlying skin has been reported in some cases.[85] More rarely, trichoepitheliomas or apocrine gland adenomas may arise in the perianal skin.[86,87] Trichoepitheliomas occur in both sexes and may reach several centimeters in diameter when they occur in the perianal skin, unlike trichoepitheliomas of other skin regions.[86]

Most adnexal tumors of the perianal skin are of apocrine or sweat gland origin, although trichoepitheliomas are derived from hair follicles. Immunolabeling for estrogen and progesterone receptors has been shown to be a reliable marker for anogenital sweat glands in women, but not conventional sweat glands, in keeping with the fact that benign tumors of apocrine gland origin occur almost exclusively in the female anogenital region.[85] Further, the native glands (as well as associated tumors such as hidradenoma papilliferum, primary extramammary Paget's disease, and invasive mammary-type carcinomas) bear striking morphological, immunohistochemical, and molecular similarities to primary breast such that they have been dubbed anogenital mammary-like glands.[88-93]

Pathology

Grossly, perianal adnexal tumors appear as solitary subcutaneous nodules with a smooth red to tan surface, although cases of ulceration mimicking a more aggressive lesion have also been reported.[94] In the case of hidradenoma papilliferum, pathological examination reveals a complex papillary glandular pattern characterized by the presence of a prominent myoepithelial layer. Some stratification of the epithelial cells and mild pleomorphism may be seen as well (Fig. 32.12A,B). Rare hidradenomas have been reported to have oncocytic differentiation (Fig. 32.12C).[95] Like mammary-type intraductal papillomas, hidradenoma papilliferum has been shown to harbor activating mutations in either *PIK3CA* or *AKT1* in a majority of cases.[96,97] Trichoepitheliomas often appear as a solid mass without ulceration of the overlying skin (Fig. 32.13). Histological examination reveals uniform eosinophilic cells with centrally located, minimally atypical nuclei. The epithelial cells form tracts throughout the supportive stroma that are two or more cells thick and also form pseudopapillae in regions of loose matrix, reminiscent of abortive pilar differentiation.[98] Local excision is usually curative.

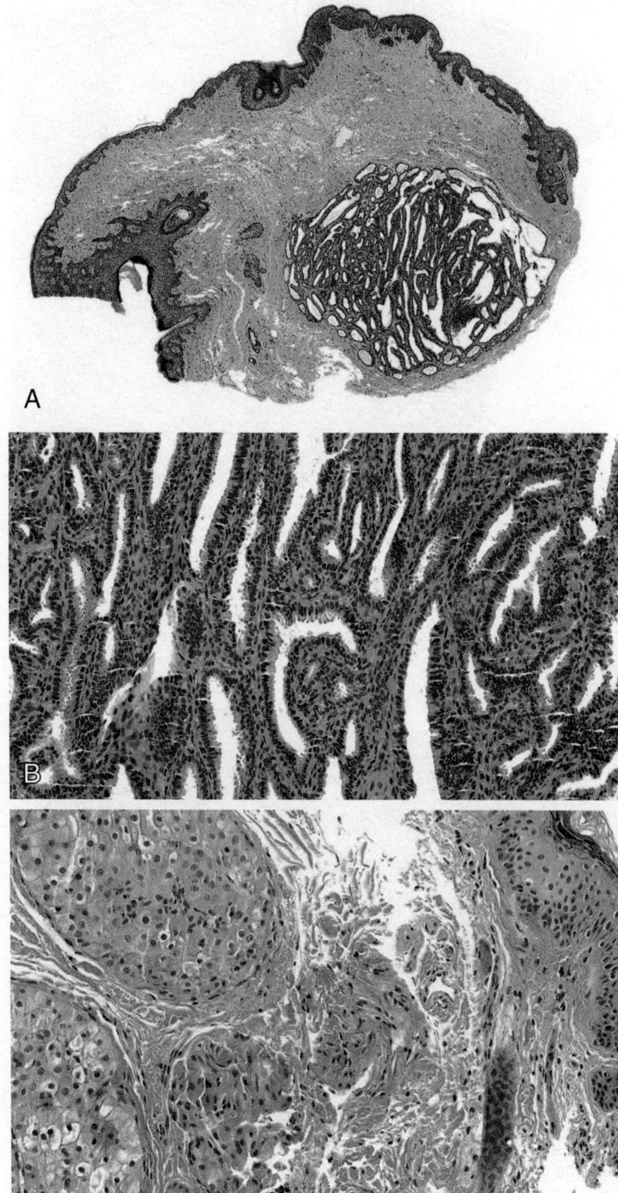

FIGURE 32.12 A, Hidradenoma papilliferum of the perianal skin. This lesion is identical to its vulvar counterpart and is thought to arise from anogenital mammary-like glands. **B,** High-power view demonstrates its glandular appearance and the two cell layers of the epithelial lining. **C,** Oncocytic differentiation demonstrates larger cuboidal cells with granular eosinophilic cytoplasm.

Differential Diagnosis

In the case of hidradenoma papilliferum, the finding of a solitary perianal mass with ulceration may indicate a more aggressive lesion, such as an infiltrating squamous carcinoma. The main differential diagnosis of a trichoepithelioma is basal cell carcinoma because both of these lesions consist of a proliferation of basaloid cells. The formation of pseudopapillae is characteristic of trichoepitheliomas, whereas peripheral nuclear palisading and retraction artifact are important features of basal cell carcinomas (Fig. 32.14).[98,99]

Granular Cell Tumors

Clinical Features and Pathogenesis

Granular cell tumors are common benign lesions that originate from Schwann cells. They occur in a variety of locations, including the gastrointestinal tract. When the gastrointestinal

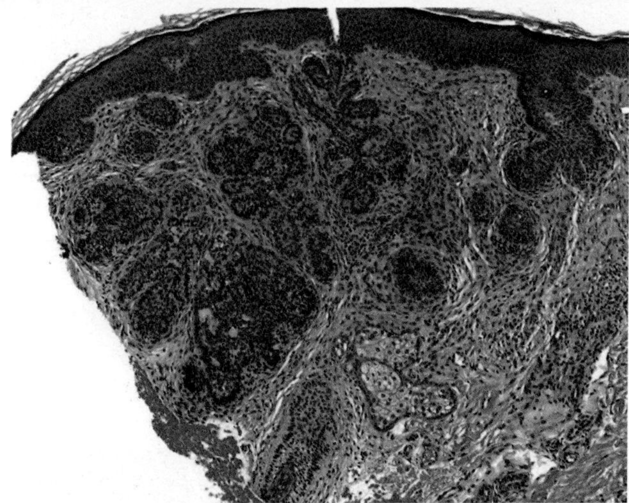

FIGURE 32.13 Low-power view of typical histological findings in trichoepithelioma in which lobules and nests of bland basaloid-appearing cells are set in a fibrotic and cellular stroma. These structures often resemble hair papillae or abortive hair follicles. Notice that, while there is stromal cracking, there is no evidence of cleft spaces between the tumor and stroma (retraction artifact).

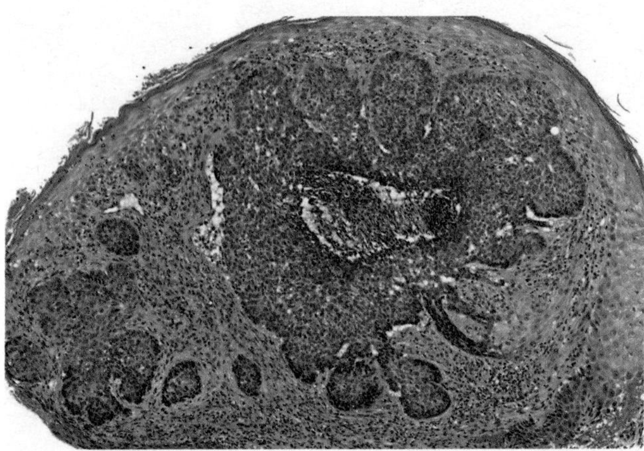

FIGURE 32.14 Basal cell carcinoma is the main differential of trichoepithelioma. Features frequently identified in basal cell carcinoma that are typically lacking in trichoepithelioma include multiple attachments of tumor to overlying epithelium, prominent peripheral nuclear palisading in tumor nests, tumor-stromal clefting (retraction artifact), and mucinous stroma surrounding the tumor.

tract is involved, the perianal region is a common site (21% in a large series).[100,101] They are most commonly diagnosed in adults in the fifth decade of life and are more common in women. The most common presentation is an incidental asymptomatic, solitary mass.[100]

Grossly, granular cell tumors appear as firm, solitary subcutaneous nodules that are white or yellow on cut section. Histologically, these lesions are composed of sheets of cells with small, uniform, hyperchromatic nuclei and with characteristic eosinophilic granular cytoplasm that is diastase resistant by periodic acid–Schiff (PAS) stain. The granularity of the cytoplasm corresponds to vacuoles that contain cellular debris, easily evident by electron microscopy.

The histological features of a granular cell tumor are distinctive enough to distinguish it from other subcutaneous perianal masses. A positive immunostain for S100 protein or SOX10 may be used to support the diagnosis of a granular cell tumor. These tumors are also strongly positive for CD68 (KP-1). Of particular significance is the occurrence of pseudoepitheliomatous hyperplasia of the epithelium overlying granular cell tumors in up to 50% of cases, which may be mistaken for an infiltrating squamous carcinoma (Fig. 32.15).[100] The presence of S100 protein–positive granular cells located immediately beneath the "atypical" epithelium should help indicate its benign nature. Local excision is usually curative.

SQUAMOUS NEOPLASIA OF THE ANUS AND ANAL CANAL

Nomenclature of Preinvasive Anal Squamous Neoplasia

Over the past several decades, various terms have been used to describe the same anal squamous pathology. Consensus groups such as the American Joint Committee on Cancer (AJCC), the Bethesda system, and the World Health Organization (WHO) all have employed somewhat different nomenclature; however, the nomenclature recently has become more and more similar. This chapter utilizes the WHO nomenclature, which adopts the two-tier Lower Anogenital Squamous Terminology (LAST) system in their most recent (fifth) edition. A brief discussion of the most recent attempt at unifying squamous neoplasia nomenclature is warranted (see Table 32.2 for a comparison of common nomenclature). In 2012, the College of American Pathologists and the American Society for Colposcopy and Cervical Pathology (CAP-ASCCP) released the product of a joint LAST Project in which the group reported their recommendations for a unified terminology for all HPV-related squamous lesions in the lower anogenital tract.[102] The authors contended that the clinical, epidemiological, and biological similarities among the various anogenital sites justify the use of a single nomenclature for HPV-associated lesions. When presented with a lesion, it is essentially impossible for a pathologist to reliably predict from which site it was derived (e.g., cervix, vagina, anus) or even whether it came from a male or a female. Furthermore, there are no differences in the molecular or biomarker phenotypes in the various HPV-related lower anogenital sites. The CAP/LAST authors therefore contend that HPV interacts with all of the anogenital squamous epithelium in two basic mechanisms: (1) squamous cells transiently support the virus, which manifests as a low-grade squamous intraepithelial lesion (LSIL), and (2) precancerous lesions resulting from viral oncogene expression cause a clonal proliferation of relatively undifferentiated cells, or a high-grade squamous intraepithelial lesion (HSIL). With time, persistent HPV infection results in a substantial risk of malignancy. In the LAST nomenclature, additional pathological descriptors such as *anal squamous intraepithelial neoplasia* (ASIN), *condyloma acuminatum*, or *Bowenoid papulosis* may be added in parentheses as needed.

Some investigators and clinicians are skeptical of applying the cervix HPV screening and treatment paradigm to anal pathology. They cite reasons such as unclear natural history data for anal HPV infection. In addition, many of the studies in anal squamous neoplasia focus on MSM, which

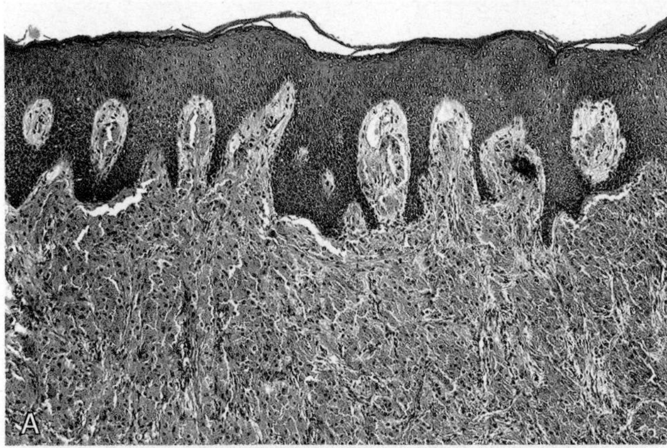

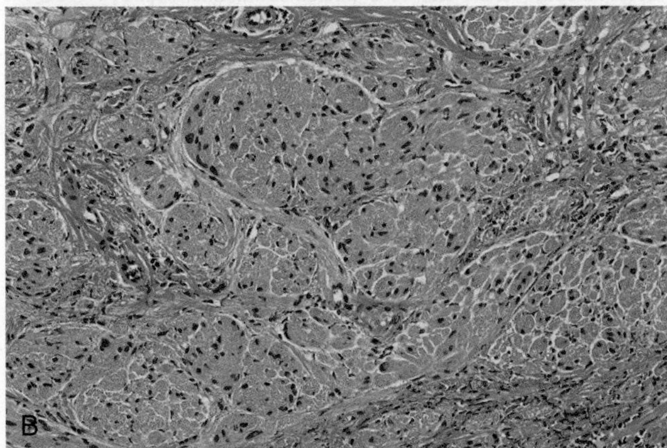

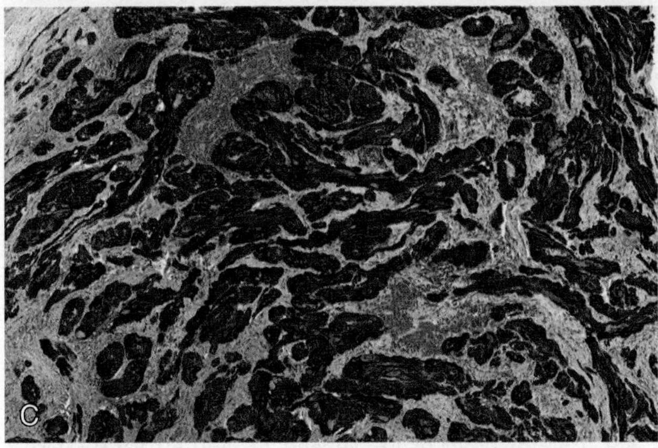

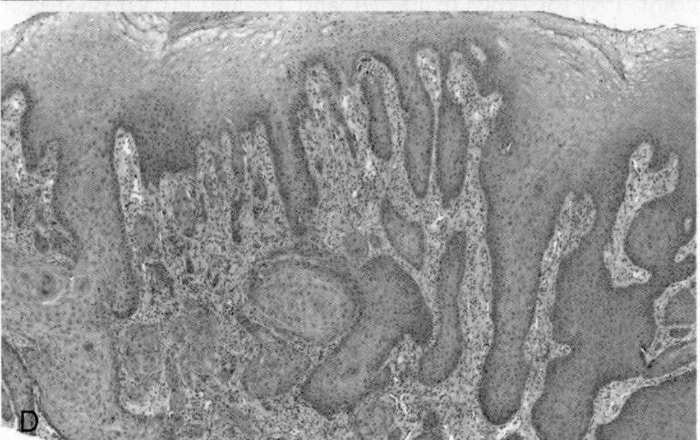

FIGURE 32.15 A, Low-power view of a granular cell tumor arising in the perianal skin. Note the presence of pseudoepitheliomatous change in the overlying epithelium. **B,** High-power view demonstrating the granular appearance of the cytoplasm and small, hyperchromatic nuclei. **C,** Granular cell tumors are characteristically diffusely positive for S100 protein by immunohistochemistry. **D,** Marked pseudoepitheliomatous hyperplasia overlying granular cell tumor is a histological mimic of invasive squamous cell carcinoma, as seen in this low-power image.

may be a significantly different population than women with cervical neoplasia. For example, HPV infection and anal intraepithelial neoplasia tends to persist in MSM as the population ages, whereas cervical HPV infection and intraepithelial neoplasia dramatically decrease with age.[103] Second, some report high-grade anal squamous dysplasia/intraepithelial neoplasia (ASD/IEN) with a relatively high risk of progression to invasive carcinoma (Scholefield et al. estimate 10% at 5 years),[104] whereas one meta-analysis estimates the risk to be much lower, at 0.15% per year for HIV-positive MSM and 0.02% per year for HIV-negative MSM.[103] Finally, there are no randomized trials that have investigated the benefits (and risks) of managing ASIN.

Risk Factors and Pathogenesis

Risk factors for squamous tumors and neoplasms of the anal canal include receptive anal intercourse, heavy smoking, a history of sexually transmitted diseases, HIV-positive status, and immunosuppression.[105-109] In one study, 92% of HIV-positive MSM demonstrated evidence of anal HPV infection, compared with 66% of those MSM who were HIV negative. In women, the presence of lower genital tract squamous neoplasia is also a risk factor, and numerous similarities to the incidence and epidemiology of cervical and vulvar neoplasia have been noted.[110] Women with multifocal genital intraepithelial neoplasia demonstrate a 16-fold increase in the rate of anal canal intraepithelial neoplasia.[109] In solid organ transplant patients, there is a 10- to 100-fold increased risk of anogenital neoplasia.

There are over 200 subtypes of HPV, of which approximately 30 infect the anogenital tract, most often types 6, 11, 16, and 18.[111] The finding of HPV in an anal carcinoma is related to the sensitivity of the technique used,[112] but some evidence suggests geographic or population differences in HPV genotypes associated with anal cancers because the prevalence of HPV16- associated anal squamous cell carcinoma was found to be significantly lower in India and South Africa compared with more developed countries.[113] Although HPV infection is identified in more than 80% of anal squamous cell carcinomas[103] (up to 97% according to the Centers for Disease Control and Prevention[114]), it is not sufficient to cause malignancy by itself. Evidence for this claim is largely related to two phenomena. First, HPV infection is highly prevalent in sexually active individuals, but most patients infected with high-risk genotypes (see the list of high-risk genotypes in the next paragraph) do not develop cancer.[115,116] In most patients, cell-mediated immunity is responsible for clearance of the infection, and neutralizing antibodies prevent subsequent infections.[117] Second, in experimental studies, infection with high-risk ("oncogenic") HPV genotypes is insufficient to induce transformation and tumor progression.[118,119] This may result from the inability of HPV to integrate into the host genome. For example, in benign lesions, the viral genome replicates as an extrachromosomal episome, whereas in malignant tumors, the viral genome becomes integrated into the host cell chromosomes.[120-123] Viral integration does not appear to occur randomly. In a systematic review of known HPV integration sites, integration at 8q24, the location of the *MYC* oncogene, and 3p14, the location of the *FHIT* tumor suppressor gene, were the most common sites reported.[124]

High-risk HPVs, most commonly genotypes HPV16 and HPV18, but also types 31, 33, 35, 39, 45, 50, 51, 53, 56,

TABLE 32.2 Nomenclature for Preinvasive Anal Squamous Lesions

Lesion	AIN*	ASD/IEN (WHO)	HSIL/LSIL (CAP/LAST)
Condyloma acuminatum	Condyloma acuminatum	Anal condyloma	LSIL (condyloma acuminatum)
Mild dysplasia	I	Low-grade ASD/IEN	LSIL
Moderate dysplasia	II	High-grade ASD/IEN	HSIL
Severe dysplasia	III	High-grade ASD/IEN	HSIL
Carcinoma in situ	III	High-grade ASD/IEN	HSIL
Bowen's disease	N/A	High-grade ASD/IEN	HSIL
Bowenoid papulosis	N/A	High-grade ASD/IEN (Bowenoid papulosis)	HSIL (Bowenoid papulosis)

*Fenger C, Nielsen VT. *Precancerous changes in the anal canal epithelium in resection specimens.* Acta Pathol Microbiol Immunol Scand A. *1986;94A(1-6):63-69.*

AIN, *Anal intraepithelial neoplasia;* ASD/IEN, *anal squamous dysplasia/intraepithelial neoplasia;* CAP/LAST, *College of American Pathologists/ Lower Anogenital Squamous Terminology Project;* HSIL, *high-grade squamous intraepithelial neoplasia;* LSIL, *low-grade squamous intraepithelial neoplasia.*

58, 59, 68, and others, encode for at least three oncoproteins that are growth stimulating and have transforming properties, known as *E5*, *E6*, and *E7*. With integration of HPV DNA into the host genome, a subsequent increase in E6 and E7 expression occurs.[125] The E6 protein binds to the p53 tumor suppressor protein, which is encoded by the *TP53* gene and is a critical regulator of cell growth and response to stress.[126,127] E6-p53 binding leads to rapid degradation of p53.[127] Similarly, E7 protein binds to and inactivates the retinoblastoma-associated protein (pRb) tumor suppressor protein, which normally acts to restrict cell proliferation to the basal layer.[128-130] In most human cancers with defects in *TP53* or *RB1*, *TP53* and *RB* are inactivated by genetic mutation; however, *TP53* and *RB1* genes are commonly wild type in anogenital cancers.[131-134] Thus, by inactivating p53 and pRb and deregulating cellular growth, the action of E6 and E7 on these tumor suppressor proteins appears functionally equivalent to genetic mutations and acts to increase the risk of anogenital cancer. Consistent with this notion, HPV-negative cervical and anal cancers have been shown to harbor inactivating mutations in *TP53* and *RB1*.[134,135]

HPV integration also promotes more general changes of the host genome, such as chromosome instability. The degree of chromosome instability is highly correlated with levels of E7 overexpression, although whether the instability precedes or is subsequent to viral integration is unclear.[136-138] Regardless, recurrent chromosomal alterations associated with chromosome instability have been described in anal squamous carcinoma and include deletion of chromosome arms 11q, 3p, 4p, 13q, and 18q and nonrandom copy number increases of chromosomes 17 and 19.[139,140] In contrast, chromosome instability is relatively uncommon among anal carcinomas from HIV-positive patients, suggesting that immunosuppression may promote carcinogenesis through an alternate pathway.[141,142]

There is no known association between any HPV subtype and specific tumor morphology. That said, HPV6 and HPV11 are most likely to be associated with condyloma acuminatum; however, HPV16 and HPV18 are also found in a significant minority of conventional condylomata as well as those with high-grade dysplasia.[112,143-145] Verrucous carcinoma is also most commonly associated with HPV6 and HPV11 infection, although HPV16 and HPV18 are occasionally found in these lesions.[146-148] Similar to the documented progression of HPV-associated premalignant conditions of the uterine cervix, epidemiological studies indicate that the development of anal canal intraepithelial neoplasia is also associated with HPV16 and HPV18 infection, and less commonly HPV6 and HPV11.[149,150]

Evidence in support of the precursor potential of ASD/IEN lies in its close similarity to dysplasia of the uterine cervix, including histological similarities between the preinvasive and invasive lesion, its occurrence at a younger average age compared with its invasive counterpart, and its common occurrence adjacent to invasive cancers, particularly those associated with HPV infection in MSM.[107,109] Perianal intraepithelial neoplasia, including Bowenoid papulosis and Bowen's disease, also show an association with HPV infection; in particular, HPV16 has been demonstrated in Bowenoid papulosis and in Bowen's disease.[151,152] Three HPV vaccines have been developed to protect recipients against HPV types 16 and 18: HPV2 (Cervarix, GlaxoSmithKline Biologicals, Rixensart, Belgium) for types 16 and 18; HPV4 (Gardasil, Silgard; Merck & Company, West Point, PA) for types 6, 11, 16, and 18; and HPV9 (Gardasil 9; Merck & Company) for types 6, 11, 16, 18, 31, 33, 45, 52, and 58.[153] Currently, only the 9-valent vaccine is available in the United States. A vast body of evidence supports HPV vaccination in preventing HPV-associated cancerous and precancerous squamous lesions in the anogenital tract[153]; however, there may be some gender- and site-specific differences.[154] Efficacy is maximized in HPV-naïve patients such that advocacy groups argue for vaccination before sexual activity.[155]

Anal Condyloma

Clinical Features

Anal condyloma (condyloma acuminatum or common anogenital wart) is the most common tumor of the anal and perianal region.[143] These lesions typically grow on warm, moist mucosal regions, characteristic of the anogenital skin. Up to 1% of sexually active people have anal condylomata, and they often occur in association with other sexually transmitted diseases.[112] Anal condylomata may be seen in association with penile warts in men or vulvar warts in women, but they may also occur as the sole area of infection, particularly in the MSM population. Nonsexual transmission may occur, particularly in children.[156] The most recent WHO classification separates giant condylomas of Buschke-Lowenstein (HPV positive) from verrucous carcinoma (HPV negative) based on HPV status.[157,158]

Pathology

The perianal skin is the most commonly affected area, although condylomata located solely within the anal canal may occur. Grossly, condylomata are soft, fleshy, tan, gray, or pink papillomatous growths that often occur in groups or clusters (Fig 32.16). Histologically, the papillomatous appearance is best appreciated at low magnification (Fig. 32.17A). The squamous epithelium shows marked acanthosis and a variable expansion of the stratum corneum layer. Surface parakeratosis is common. The rete pegs may appear elongated with broad bases. On higher magnification, the surface epithelium contains squamous cells with an enlarged, irregular, and hyperchromatic nucleus and an accompanying perinuclear halo. These cells, known as *koilocytes*, are the histological hallmark of HPV infection (Fig. 32.17B). Dyskeratotic cells (Fig. 32.17C) are usually easily found, as well as multinucleated cells, which are also characteristic of HPV infection. Basal cell hyperplasia is typically seen in association with orderly and progressive maturation of the epithelium. The squamous epithelium is well delineated from the underlying stroma, the latter of which often contains chronic inflammation, edema, and vascular dilation. The level of atypia/dysplasia in condyloma is graded similarly to LSILs and HSILs that develop in flat mucosa and are not associated with condyloma (see later). All condylomas contain, at minimum, LSIL-like atypia, but few may develop high-grade changes (see later discussion on HSILs).

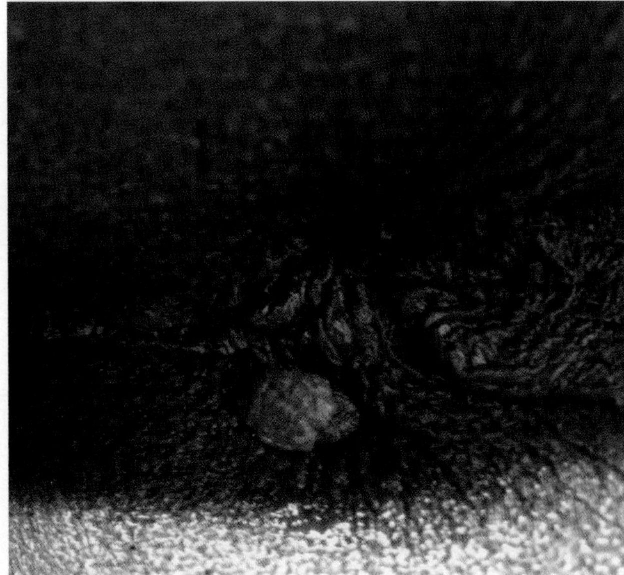

FIGURE 32.16 Anal condyloma with a soft, fleshy, papillomatous appearance.

Differential Diagnosis

The differential diagnosis of condyloma includes verrucous carcinoma on one end of the spectrum and benign anal/perianal lesions, such as seborrheic keratosis, fibroepithelial polyp, and prolapse-type polyp, on the other end. Purely on histological grounds, condyloma acuminatum may be impossible to distinguish from verrucous carcinoma, particularly in biopsy samples or in cases in which the clinical impression is not provided. Verrucous carcinomas are typically larger than condylomata acuminata, and verrucous carcinomas display both an exophytic and endophytic growth pattern, whereas condylomata are generally only exophytic. According to the WHO classification, HPV status is now a critical adjunct to the differential diagnosis of condyloma and verrucous carcinoma, as verrucous carcinoma is HPV negative. Separating condyloma from another type of benign lesion rests on identifying HPV cytopathic effect in the condyloma or the characteristic histological features in the other benign lesions. Immunohistochemistry or in situ hybridization studies for HPV can be quite helpful in equivocal cases.

Prognosis

There is controversy regarding the malignant potential of condylomata. Although they generally harbor low-risk HPV genotypes, up to 35% demonstrate high-risk HPV, most commonly genotypes 16 and 18.[145] Furthermore, high-grade intraepithelial neoplasia, which is diagnosed in an identical manner as its non-warty counterparts (see Anal Squamous Dysplasia/Intraepithelial Neoplasia), has been described in up to 20% of HIV-infected patients with condylomata, and cases of invasive squamous carcinoma arising in an anal condyloma have also been reported.[144]

Treatment

The most common treatments for anal condylomata are either ablative or cytodestructive.[159] Methods of ablative treatment include cryotherapy, local excision, electrocautery, and laser therapy. Cytodestructive therapies include podophyllotoxin and trichloroacetic acid. Both forms of treatment are associated with a high recurrence rate believed to be caused by the presence of latent HPV in clinically unremarkable adjacent epithelium. Immunosuppression is also associated with an increased rate of recurrence after surgical removal.[160] More recently, the immunomodulatory agent imiquimod has been shown to have potent antiviral and antitumoral activity, but without the common side effects associated with the other forms of treatment.[161]

Anal Squamous Dysplasia/Intraepithelial Neoplasia

Clinical Features

ASD/IEN may be found in tissues removed for a variety of disorders.[162] Similar to its cervical counterpart, ASD/IEN has been identified in anal mucosa adjacent to invasive carcinomas of the anal canal as well as an incidental finding in resection specimens from this region.[163] The demographics, symptoms, and signs are similar to those described earlier in the discussion on HPV-related lesions. Its prevalence in the general population is estimated at 2 to 3 per 1000 individuals, but its prevalence is much higher in at-risk populations, such as MSM, HIV-positive individuals, women with cervical or vaginal squamous carcinoma, or immunocompromised individuals.[162,164] ASD/IEN has been documented at much greater frequencies in HIV-positive MSM compared with HIV-negative MSM. For example, one study found ASD/IEN in 36% of HIV-positive men and 7% of HIV-negative men.[165] The difference also seems to hold true for high-grade ASD/IEN, where 49% of HIV-positive MSM had high-grade ASD/IEN and 17% of HIV-negative MSM had high-grade ASD/IEN in one study.[166] Clinically, ASD/IEN may appear as raised, scaly, white, erythematous, pigmented, fissured, or ulcerated areas in the anal canal, although it is often subclinical and presents as an unanticipated incidental finding.[167] ASIN may also be identified as acetowhite epithelium, which contrasts with iodine-positive nonneoplastic mucosa by anal colposcopy.

Pathology

ASD/IEN is characterized by cells with enlarged nuclei, irregular nuclear membranes, and an increased nuclear-to-cytoplasmic ratio, with lack of cytoplasmic maturation toward the luminal surface.[102] Mitotic figures may be encountered beyond the normal regenerative basal zone of the squamous epithelium. Individual cell keratinization and dyskeratosis are common and may represent markers of HPV infection. These changes typically occur in the absence of inflammation. ASD/IEN is divided into two grades, primarily based on the level at which orderly cytoplasmic maturation begins and the level at which mitotic activity stops. In low-grade ASD/IEN (Fig. 32.18A), mitotic figures and cellular pleomorphism are predominantly located in the basal third of the epithelium, with evidence of surface maturation in the upper two-thirds and/or evidence of HPV cytopathic effect (i.e., koilocytic atypia). In contrast, high-grade ASD/IEN is characterized by cellular pleomorphism, mitotic figures, and lack of cytoplasmic maturation extending into the middle and superficial thirds of the epithelium (Fig. 32.18B). These preinvasive changes may colonize the underlying anal ducts and glands as well, which may not be detected or excised during treatment. High-grade ASD/IEN is graded in the ducts similar to the neighboring

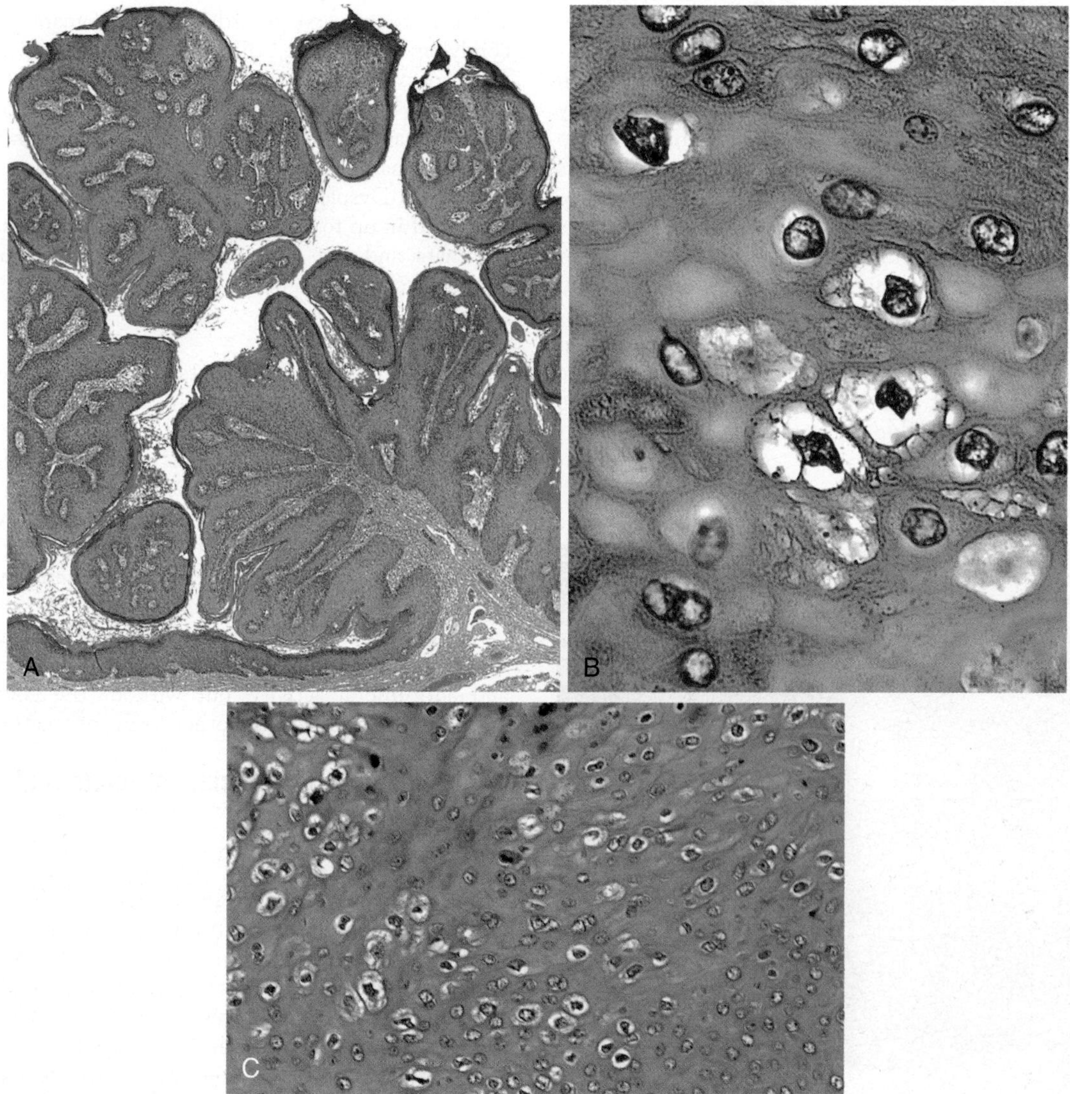

FIGURE 32.17 **A,** Low-power view of condyloma acuminatum. Note the papillary formations and acanthosis of the epithelium compared with normal squamous epithelium, which is present at the *bottom left* of the image. **B,** High-power view demonstrates koilocytotic changes. **C,** High-power view demonstrates dyskeratotic cells among koilocytic changes.

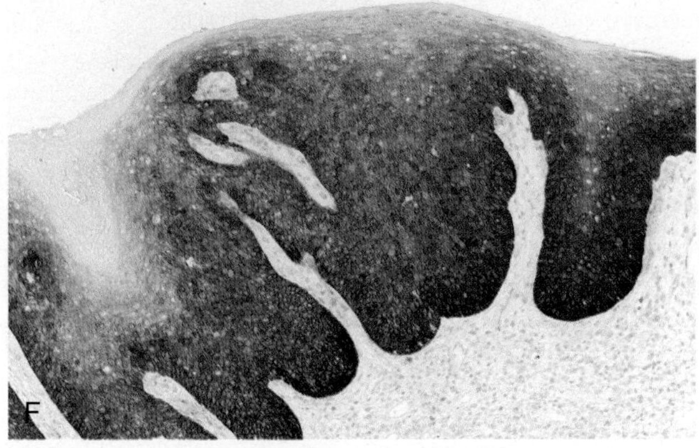

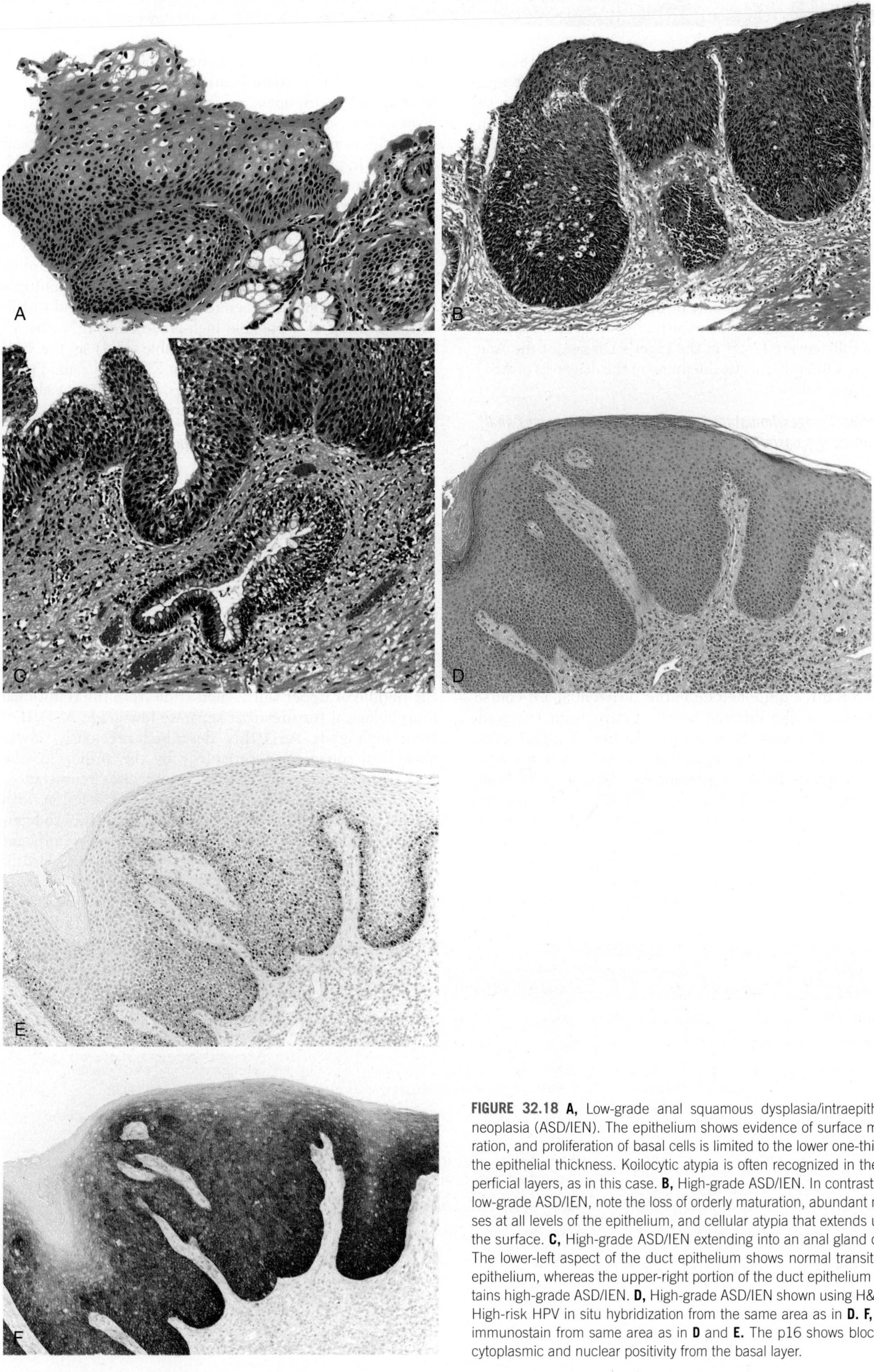

FIGURE 32.18 A, Low-grade anal squamous dysplasia/intraepithelial neoplasia (ASD/IEN). The epithelium shows evidence of surface maturation, and proliferation of basal cells is limited to the lower one-third of the epithelial thickness. Koilocytic atypia is often recognized in the superficial layers, as in this case. **B,** High-grade ASD/IEN. In contrast with low-grade ASD/IEN, note the loss of orderly maturation, abundant mitoses at all levels of the epithelium, and cellular atypia that extends up to the surface. **C,** High-grade ASD/IEN extending into an anal gland duct. The lower-left aspect of the duct epithelium shows normal transitional epithelium, whereas the upper-right portion of the duct epithelium contains high-grade ASD/IEN. **D,** High-grade ASD/IEN shown using H&E. **E,** High-risk HPV in situ hybridization from the same area as in **D. F,** P16 immunostain from same area as in **D** and **E.** The p16 shows blocklike cytoplasmic and nuclear positivity from the basal layer.

squamous epithelium, as described earlier (Fig. 32.18C). Of course, using the degree of dysplasia in the adjacent squamous epithelium as a clue to the degree of dysplasia in the ducts is helpful in difficult cases. Further, p16 staining results can be quite helpful, particularly if one is attempting to separate tangential sectioning from high-grade ASD/IEN.

Differential Diagnosis

The differential diagnoses of ASD/IEN include other neoplasms within the squamous epithelium such as melanoma and primary or secondary Paget's disease. In particular, some high-grade ASD/IEN may demonstrate a pattern of pagetoid spread that can only be differentiated from Paget's disease by immunohistochemistry.[168] This differential is more fully covered later in the Paget's Disease of the Anus section. Other diagnostic dilemmas in the diagnosis of ASD/IEN are as follows:

Reactive Changes/Immature Squamous Metaplasia versus Anal Squamous Dysplasia/Intraepithelial Neoplasia

Distinguishing reactive changes from low-grade ASD/IEL in biopsy material is fraught with high observer variability.[169] Practically speaking, low-grade lesions, with or without warty growth, are characterized by HPV cytopathic effect in the form of koilocytes, whereas reactive atypia is usually associated with acute inflammation; spongiosis of the squamous epithelium with visible intercellular bridges; and round, uniform nuclei with open chromatin and single, prominent nucleoli. In these borderline cases, particularly in patients with a non-warty growth pattern or those without a history HPV infection, HPV chromogenic in situ hybridization is often quite helpful in this differential. Of course, discussion of the differential of reactive from low-grade lesion implies that there are no features of a high-grade lesion. In fact, reliably separating a reactive lesion from a high-grade ASD/IEN, a precancerous lesion, is clinically important and more feasible. Although both reactive changes/immature squamous metaplasia and high-grade ASD/IEN may show immature cells located beyond the basal layer, high-grade ASD/IEN demonstrates a more disorganized, or "jumbled," arrangement to the epithelium, in contrast with reactive processes, which tend to retain an orderly configuration of squamous epithelial cells (Table 32.3; Fig. 32.19). Identification of inflammation and/or regular nuclei with open chromatin and prominent nucleoli favor a reactive process, whereas high-grade ASD/IEN generally shows nuclear hyperchromasia and irregular nuclear contours. In practice, when this differential is encountered, p16 immunohistochemistry often becomes critical to separating reactive processes from high-grade ASD/IEN. Weak and patchy immunoreactivity favors a nonneoplastic process, whereas diffuse, strong, and block positivity argues in favor of high-grade ASD/IEN (see Table 32.3).[102] The most recent recommendations argue against using multiple adjunctive immunohistochemical tests (e.g., p16 and Ki-67) in the workup of a possible high-grade ASD/IEN case.[102] Current evidence supports p16 (Table 32.4) as the best marker for high-grade ASD/IEN, but Ki-67[170-172] and ProEx C (Becton Dickinson, Franklin Lakes, NJ)[173-175] may also be useful when difficulties with p16 arise.

Low-Grade versus High-Grade Anal Squamous Dysplasia/Intraepithelial Neoplasia

The natural history of low-grade squamous lesions in immunocompetent hosts is almost always transient and not precancerous, although this is often not the case in immunocompromised patients. Since the defining feature of low-grade lesions, the koilocyte, may be present in high-grade lesions as well, one must judge the level of dysmaturation, cells with high nuclear-to-cytoplasmic ratios, hyperchromasia, mitotic activity, and irregular nuclear membranes within the epithelium (see Table 32.3; Fig. 32.20). If the atypical squamous proliferation extends into the middle or upper third, then aside from the traditional morphological features that separate low-grade ASD/IEN from high-grade ASD/IEN described previously, lower anogenital squamous terminology by the authors of the LAST project identifies at least two special circumstances in which one may consider "bumping up" a lesion with cytoarchitectural features of low-grade ASD/IEN to high-grade ASD/IEN: (1) atypical mitotic figures or significant nuclear atypia (even if restricted to the basal one-third of the epithelium) beyond that expected in typical low-grade ASD/IEN and (2) thin ASD/IEN, which consists of

TABLE 32.3 Differential Diagnosis of Anal Intraepithelial Neoplasia and Separation from Reactive Lesions

Feature	Reactive	Low-Grade ASD/IEN	High-Grade ASD/IEN
N:C ratio	Low	Low	High
Koilocytes	No	Yes	Often
Nuclear features	Open chromatin; single prominent nucleolus	Only mild pleomorphism (excluding koilocytes/multinucleate cells)	Hyperchromasia and pleomorphism throughout the epithelium
Mitotic activity	Basal layer(s) only	Lower one-third of mucosa	Upper two-thirds of mucosa (may have abnormal mitotic figures)
Maturation	Orderly	Dysmaturation/nuclear overlapping in lower one-third of mucosa only	Dysmaturation/nuclear overlapping in upper layers to full-thickness
Cell polarity	Normal polarity	Relatively well-maintained polarity	Loss of polarity
Proliferation	Basal layers	Lower one-third of epithelium	Throughout epithelium
p16 staining	Negative or patchy positivity	Variable	Blocklike positivity (nuclear and cytoplasmic)

ASD/IEN, *Anal squamous dysplasia/intraepithelial neoplasia.*

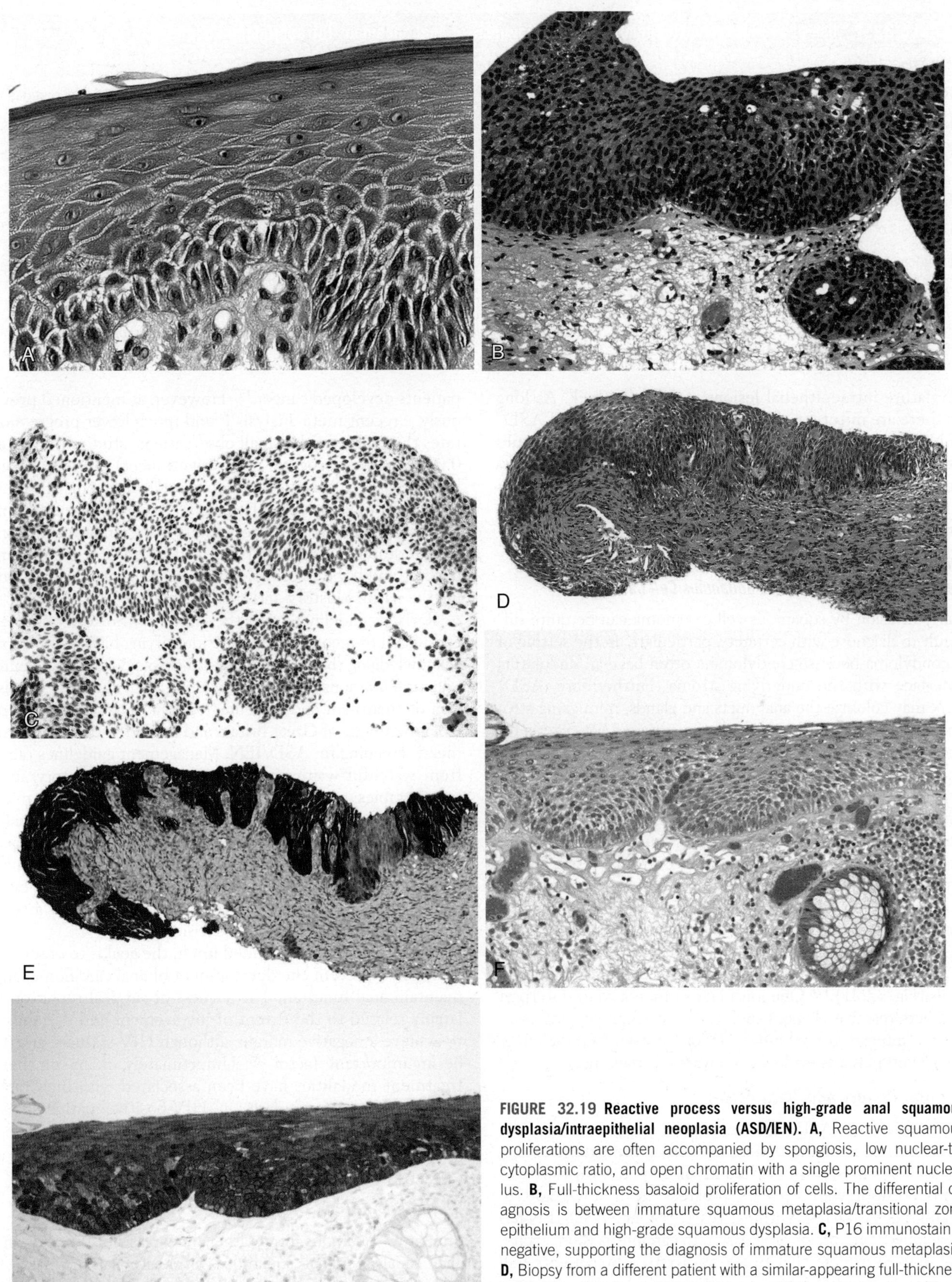

FIGURE 32.19 Reactive process versus high-grade anal squamous dysplasia/intraepithelial neoplasia (ASD/IEN). A, Reactive squamous proliferations are often accompanied by spongiosis, low nuclear-to-cytoplasmic ratio, and open chromatin with a single prominent nucleolus. **B,** Full-thickness basaloid proliferation of cells. The differential diagnosis is between immature squamous metaplasia/transitional zone epithelium and high-grade squamous dysplasia. **C,** P16 immunostain is negative, supporting the diagnosis of immature squamous metaplasia. **D,** Biopsy from a different patient with a similar-appearing full-thickness basaloid proliferation to **A. E,** In this case, p16 immunostain is positive in a diffuse, blocklike pattern, which supports the diagnosis of high-grade squamous intraepithelial neoplasia. **F,** Subtle example of high-grade ASD/IEN, confirmed by p16 immunostain (**G**).

TABLE 32.4 Use of p16 Immunohistochemistry in the Diagnosis of Anal Squamous Intraepithelial Neoplasia

Situation	p16 Recommended?	Interpretation/Reasoning
Reactive vs. high-grade ASD/IEN	Yes	Block-positive staining supports high-grade ASD/IEN diagnosis
Low-grade vs. high-grade ASD/IEN	Yes	Block-positive staining supports high-grade ASD/IEN diagnosis
Professional disagreement of histological diagnosis (provided that high-grade dysplasia is in differential)	Yes	Block-positive staining supports high-grade ASD/IEN diagnosis
Diagnosis of negative/reactive on histology	No	Staining may be confusing
Diagnosis of low-grade ASD/IEN on histology	No	Staining may be confusing
Diagnosis of high-grade ASD/IEN on histology	No	Staining may be confusing

ASD/IEN, *Anal squamous dysplasia/ intraepithelial neoplasia*
From Darragh TM, Colgan TJ, Cox JT, et al. The Lower Anogenital Squamous Terminology Standardization Project for HPV-Associated Lesions: background and consensus recommendations from the College of American Pathologists and the American Society for Colposcopy and Cervical Pathology. Arch Pathol Lab Med. *2012;136(10):1266-1297.*

immature intraepithelial lesions < 10 cells thick. As long as there are mitotic figures or cytological features of ASD/IEN above the basal layer, "thin" ASD/IEN lesions should be considered high-grade ASD/IEN. In both of these circumstances, a diffuse, strong, and blocklike positivity for p16 immunohistochemistry would help confirm high-grade ASD/IEN.[102]

High-Grade Anal Squamous Dysplasia/Intraepithelial Neoplasia versus Superficially Invasive Squamous Cell Carcinoma

Early invasion by squamous cell carcinoma can be quite difficult to diagnose with certainty, particularly in the setting of a condyloma because condylomata often have an undulating interface with the underlying stroma. Furthermore, ASD/IEN may colonize the anal ducts and glands, mimicking stromal invasion. Therefore it is best to maintain strict criteria for stromal invasion by a squamous carcinoma. Invasive carcinomas tend to arise in mucosa extensively involved by high-grade intraepithelial neoplasia. Features supporting the diagnosis of invasion include: (1) irregular and angulated downward extension of the neoplastic squamous cells with an accompanying reactive or desmoplastic stromal response; (2) small nests or individual cells, often acquiring more abundant eosinophilic cytoplasm ("paradoxical maturation") with prominent nucleoli that are clearly separate from the main lesion; and (3) blurring of the epithelial-stromal interface with loss of the regular arrangement of the squamous basal cells (Fig. 32.21).[176] One must be careful not to misinterpret artifacts/reactive changes such as those accompanying prior biopsy, intense stromal inflammation, or pseudoepitheliomatous hyperplasia as evidence of invasive carcinoma.

Natural History and Treatment

Progression of ASD/IEN is largely dependent on the immune status of the patient as well as the extent of disease.[177] Small series have found that up to two-thirds of immunosuppressed patients progress from low-grade to high-grade ASD/IEN within 2 years.[165] Once ASD/IEN has developed, the rate of progression to carcinoma is uncertain, but some estimate that up to 5% to 10% of patients will ultimately progress to invasive disease.[167] In one long-term surveillance study of 35 patients with high-grade ASD/IEN, 3 of 6 immunosuppressed patients (all with multifocal disease) developed invasive carcinoma in the follow-up period, but none of the remainder of the immunocompetent patients developed cancer.[177] However, as mentioned previously, a recent meta-analysis found much lower progression rates than some of the small observational studies (as low as 0.02% per year progress to invasive cancer). Society guidelines regarding specific screening and treatment of ASD/IEN, even in at-risk populations, are based on expert opinion or low-quality science rather than randomized controlled studies. The ANCHOR and SPANC[178] studies are ongoing and hope to provide much more robust data regarding the natural history and treatment of ASD/IEN.

Revised guidelines from the American Society of Colon and Rectal Surgeons[179] advocate identifying high-risk groups, acknowledging the imperfections of cytology-based screening recommendations, and implementing individualized discussion of treatment and screening options. The Association of Coloproctology of Great Britain and Ireland[104] do not recommend screening for ASD/IEN. Management guidelines range from watchful waiting to topical immunomodulatory/ablative therapies, to surgical excision or fulguration. Again, management of ASD/IEN should probably be individually tailored, taking into account the immune status, the size and focality of the disease, and the symptoms of the patient.[104] Of course, highly suspicious lesions or masses should be evaluated thoroughly with some combination of clinical assessment, cytology, and/or biopsy/excision.[180]

When treatment is decided upon, the goal is to eradicate ASD/IEN, prevent the development of anal carcinoma, and maintain anal function. The success of surgical resection is largely related to the extent of involvement and the ability to achieve a negative margin, although HIV status seems to be an important factor.[167] Unfortunately, many of these treatment modalities have been associated with high rates of recurrence, particularly in HIV-positive patients and those with extensive/multifocal disease.[181]

Perianal Squamous Intraepithelial Neoplasia

Clinical Features

Similar to squamous intraepithelial neoplasia of the anus and anal canal, perianal squamous intraepithelial neoplasia is HPV-related and is incorporated under the LAST nomenclature reviewed earlier. Many of the previously discussed clinical and pathological principles for ASIN apply to perianal lesions as well; however, two perianal-specific terms are worthy of additional review, namely *Bowenoid papulosis* and

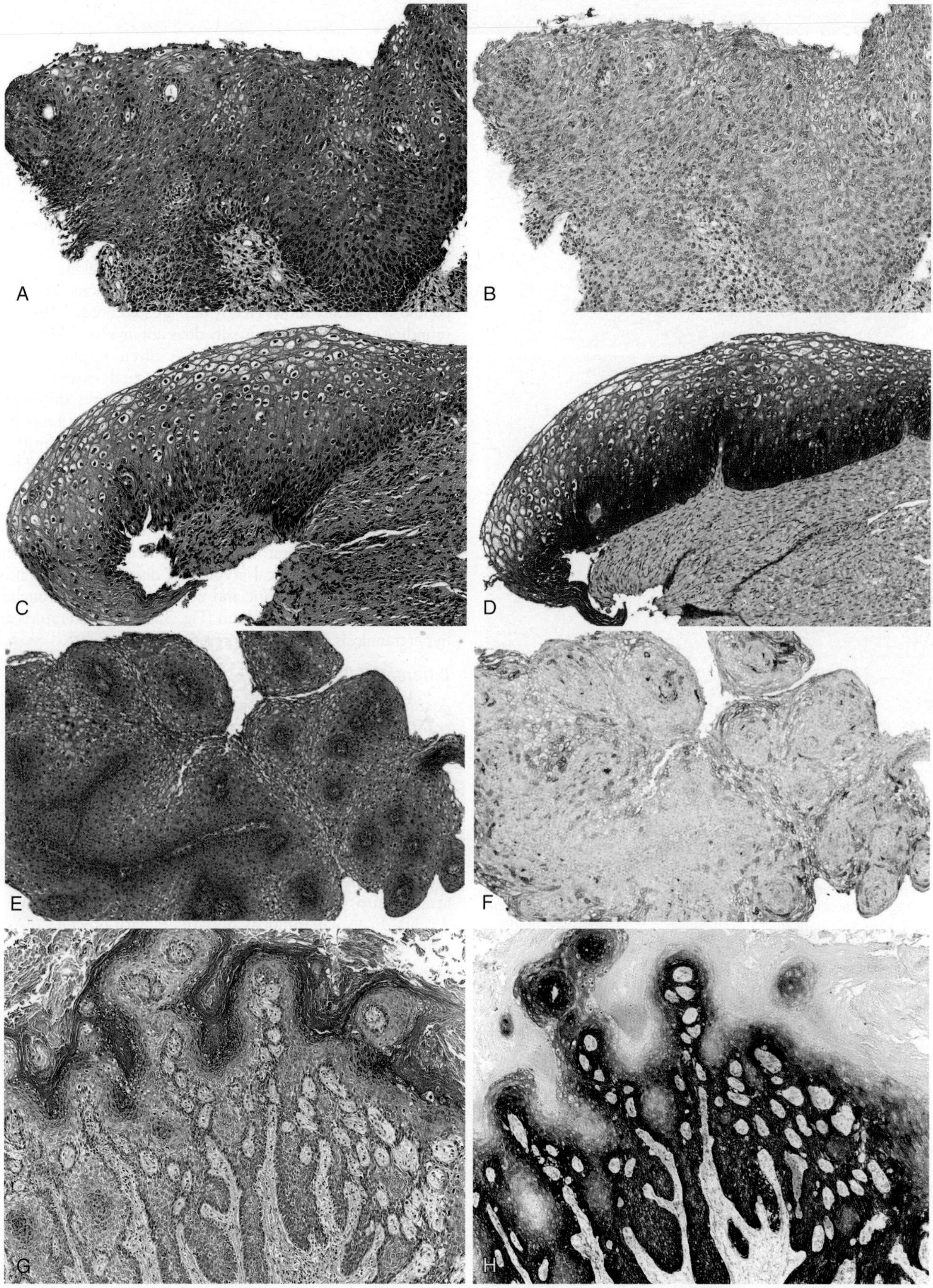

FIGURE 32.20 Low-grade anal squamous dysplasia/intraepithelial neoplasia (ASD/IEN) versus high-grade ASD/IEN. A, Biopsy demonstrating surface maturation and unequivocal koilocytic atypia and a proliferation of basaloid cells beyond the normal basal layer. The differential diagnosis is between tangential sectioning of low-grade ASD/IEN and high-grade ASD/IEN. **B,** P16 immunostain is negative, supporting the diagnosis of low-grade ASD/IEN. **C,** Similar-appearing biopsy reveals a proliferation of basaloid cells extending nearly one-half of the epithelial thickness. **D,** P16 immunostain is positive in a diffuse, blocklike pattern, which argues in favor of high-grade ASD/IEN. **E,** Condyloma acuminatum in which there is koilocytic change indicative of HPV infection and tangential sectioning, raising concern for a high-grade lesion. **F,** P16 immunostain lacks a high-grade pattern, supporting the diagnosis of a low-grade lesion. **G,** Warty growth of a full-thickness atypical keratinizing squamous proliferation, raising concern for a high-grade lesion. **H,** P16 immunostain diffuse block positivity in cytoplasm and some nuclei extending from the basal layer.

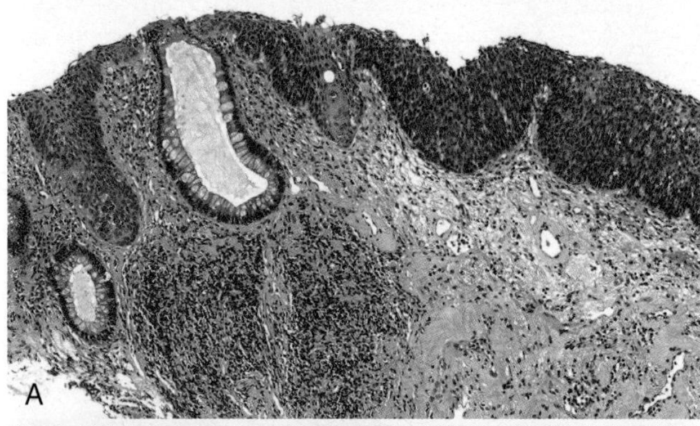

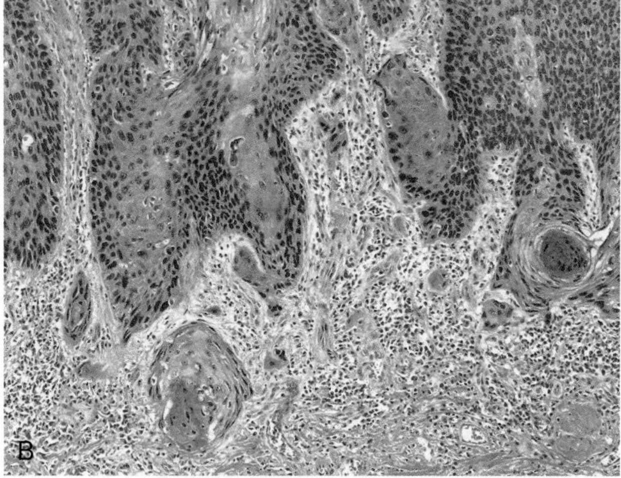

FIGURE 32.21 High-grade anal squamous dysplasia/intraepithelial neoplasia (ASD/IEN) versus superficially invasive squamous cell carcinoma (SCC). A, High-grade ASD/IEN maintains a smooth interface with the underlying stroma. In particular, the basal nuclei show an orderly arrangement, and their long axis should be perpendicularly oriented to the basement membrane. **B,** In superficially invasive SCC, the smooth epithelial-stromal interface is characteristically lost. Instead, there is a jagged, irregular arrangement to the basal epithelial cells, often with small nests and single atypical squamous cells. The basal cells also lose their regular perpendicular arrangement to the basement membrane and acquire abundant dense eosinophilic cytoplasm and/or produce keratin, so-called *paradoxical maturation.*

Bowen's disease. The use of both *Bowenoid papulosis* and *Bowen's disease* has been discouraged in anal pathology by some because they have engendered confusion with regard to their cutaneous counterparts, and the WHO no longer encourages the use of *Bowen's disease* at this anatomical site.

Both Bowenoid papulosis and Bowen's disease are conditions considered HPV-related in the vast majority of cases, and they should be approached as such. Clinically, Bowenoid papulosis appears as slightly raised, firm, red to brown papules that may be scaly in appearance and are usually located on the perianal skin. Most patients are asymptomatic, although occasional patients complain of pruritus in association with areas of involved perianal skin. In contrast with clustered small papules of Bowenoid papulosis, Bowen's disease is typically composed of large and often multifocal plaques. While Bowen's disease terminology is no longer encouraged, the clinicopathologically defined Bowenoid papulosis may continue to have diagnostic relevance because of its more indolent clinical course.

Pathology

Though the WHO has seemingly eliminated low-grade perianal squamous intraepithelial neoplasia, low-grade squamous intraepithelial lesions, especially in the form of condylomata acuminate, do occur. It may be that the "flat" low-grade lesions are exceedingly difficult to reproducibly recognize, akin to the vulva, hence the lack of emphasis on this diagnostic entity.[182] Bowen's disease and Bowenoid papulosis are two forms of high-grade squamous dysplasia/intraepithelial neoplasia and cannot be reliably separated based on histology alone.

In addition to their varied clinical presentations, Bowenoid papulosis typically shows clearly demarcated borders from surrounding normal skin and usually does not involve skin appendages. In contrast, Bowen's disease often requires formal histological mapping to discern the actual extent of disease.[183,184] Bowen's disease is also included in the differential diagnosis of Paget's disease and melanoma. Distinction of high grade squamous intraepithelial neoplasia from these entities is discussed further later and in Table 32.5. The histology of both Bowenoid papulosis and Bowen's disease is similar to conventional high-grade squamous intraepithelial neoplasia. The squamous epithelium is typically acanthotic, and the surface of the epithelium is hyperkeratotic. At higher magnification, the epithelium shows cytological atypia and disordered maturation, with scattered dyskeratotic and mitotic cells seen throughout the thickness of the epithelium (Fig. 32.22). Parakeratosis and hypergranulosis may also be present.

Differential Diagnosis

A summary of squamous lesions that may cause diagnostic confusion with, or progress to, invasive squamous cell carcinoma is summarized in Table 32.6.

Natural History and Treatment

Bowen's disease of the anus is a chronic and slowly progressive condition that tends to spread intradermally. It is prone to local recurrence after wide excision if negative margins are not achieved.[184,185] Even when negative margins are attained, up to 25% of patients show recurrence within 3 to 4 years. In a small minority of patients with Bowen's disease who are not managed adequately by wide local excision, transformation to invasive disease may occur.[185] In the past, the standard form of treatment of Bowen's disease is histological mapping followed by wide local excision to achieve negative margins.[183,184] However, despite preoperative mapping, recurrence may occur in up to 63% of patients within 1 year after wide local excision.[186] Topical 5-fluorouracil or imiquimod has been reported to be effective for patients with extensive disease.[187,188]

Bowenoid papulosis was initially described as a lesion of the genitalia of young adults, most often in the third decade of life. In addition to its common occurrence on the penis and vulva, anal lesions may occur.[33] Clinically, Bowenoid papulosis is characterized by the presence of one or more small reddish-brown papules in the anogenital region (which may be scaly in appearance) that persist for a few weeks to several years.[189] Most cases resolve spontaneously without treatment, although in some patients, it is chronic and slowly progressive. Generally, these lesions are sharply circumscribed from surrounding uninvolved skin and are most easily treated by excision. These papules rarely exceed a few millimeters in diameter.

TABLE 32.5 Immunohistochemistry of Intraepithelial Lesions of the Anus with Possible Pagetoid Cell Spread

Lesion	CK7	CK20	GCDFP15	CDX2	S100 protein/ SOX10	HMB45 and Melan-A	CK5, CK6, and p63
Primary Paget's disease	+	–	+	–	–	–	–
Secondary Paget's disease/rectal carcinoma	–/+	+	–	+	–	–	–
Anal gland carcinoma	+	–	–	–	–	–	–
Melanoma	–	–	–	–	+	+	–
HSIL	–/+	–	–	–	–	–	+

CK, *Cytokeratin;* GCDFP, *gross cystic disease fluid protein;* HSIL, *high grade squamous intraepithelial lesion.*

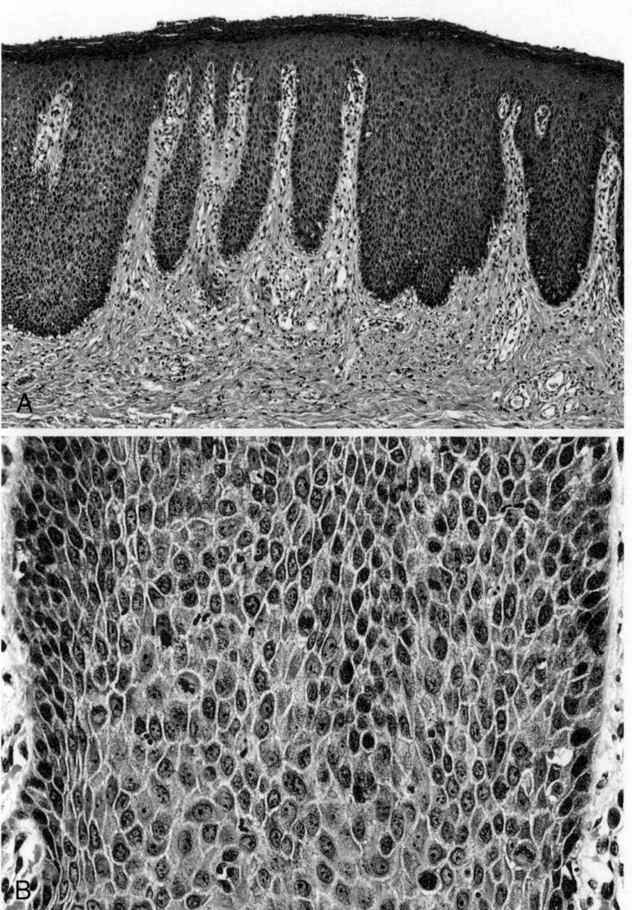

FIGURE 32.22 A, High-grade perianal squamous dysplasia/intraepithelial neoplasia. The epithelium is acanthotic and hypercellular and shows loss of surface maturation. Parakeratosis is also present. **B,** At higher power, numerous mitoses are seen, and significant nuclear crowding and hyperchromasia is evident.

Anus and Anal Canal Squamous Cell Carcinoma

Clinical Features

Carcinomas of the anal canal are rare but increasing in frequency. About 9100 new cases of anal cancer are expected in 2021 in the United States, which corresponds to about 5% of all cancers involving the colon, rectum, and anus.[190] The incidence of anal cancer is greater in women than in men (2:1 male-to-female ratio) and is also slightly higher in African Americans.[191] Anal squamous neoplasia is increasing in incidence, particularly in MSM, either with or without HIV/AIDS, and in women with multifocal anogenital neoplasia. About 80% to 90% of anal squamous cell carcinomas are associated with HPV infection.[164,192]

Carcinomas that develop above (proximal to) the dentate line are two to three times more common in women than in men, with an average age at diagnosis in the sixth decade of life. The clinical presentation of neoplasms in this location includes bleeding, pain, change in bowel habits, and pruritus ani. Carcinomas in this location often arise in the absence of any known preexisting condition. In contrast, carcinomas that develop below (distal to) the dentate line are four times more common in men than in women. Coexisting conditions are more common for carcinomas in this region and include anal condyloma, high-grade squamous dysplasia (intraepithelial neoplasia), chronic fistula (as in patients with Crohn's disease), chronic pruritus, or a history of radiation treatment. The clinical presentation of carcinomas at this location ranges from small, firm nodules for early-stage lesions to large, ulcerated tumors in advanced-stage lesions (Fig. 32.23). A summary of the clinicopathological features of anal cancers in relation to their anatomic location is shown in Table 32.7.

Pathology

The WHO previously recognized several types of malignancies of the anal canal, including squamous cell carcinoma, adenocarcinoma, neuroendocrine carcinoma, and mixed neuroendocrine–nonneuroendocrine neoplasm (MiNEN)[193] (Box 32.2). Each carcinoma is associated with several histological patterns, which is probably a reflection of the histological complexity of the anal canal. The locations of the most common tumors of the anal canal are illustrated in Figure 32.24. The vast majority of malignant neoplasms of the anal canal are squamous cell carcinomas (about 90% to 95%), which are often histologically heterogeneous.[194] In the past, anal squamous cell carcinoma had been subclassified into large cell keratinizing, nonkeratinizing, and basaloid types[195]; however, the current and previous WHO classifications have eliminated this category, primarily because anal canal invasive squamous cell carcinomas are most often treated with combination chemotherapy and radiation after diagnostic biopsy rather than primary resection.[157] Anal canal squamous cell carcinomas are also often heterogenous, so biopsies are insufficient at completely

TABLE 32.6 Clinical and Pathological Features of Noninvasive HPV-Associated Anal Squamous Lesions

Lesion	Clinical Presentation	Gross Features	Microscopic Features	Molecular Features	Treatment	Outcome
Condyloma acuminatum	Sexually active patients Increasing in MSM and HIV+ patients	Exophytic papillomatous lesions 1-20 mm (giant condyloma much larger) Often multiple	Papillary proliferation of acanthotic squamous epithelium with orderly maturation Prominent granular cell layer and koilocytes	HPV subtypes 6 and 11 most common Significant minority with HPV subtypes 16 and 18	Optional: Topical podophyllin or imiquimod (patient applied); cryotherapy, podophyllin resin, TCA, curettage intralesional interferon (provider applied) Surgical excision for large, persistent, or primarily intraanal lesions	Generally benign course Immunosuppressed patients have high risk of recurrence, including high-grade intraepithelial neoplasia or carcinoma
Verrucous carcinoma	Males > females Mean age: fifth decade No association with sexual orientation Very rare in children	Large, bulky cauliflower-like mass Prone to ulceration and bleeding	Very well-differentiated squamoproliferative lesion No koilocytes Broad, pushing invasive front	HPV negative	Wide local excision Radiochemotherapy if complete resection not possible	Generally favorable Morbidity and mortality related to extensive disease with locally destructive growth
ASD/IEN	Young, sexually active MSM and women with anogenital HPV-associated lesions Often incidental	Usually flat High-resolution anoscopy with application of 3% acetic acid and Lugol iodine solution helps identify lesions	Low-grade lesions are usually recognized by koilocytes (HPV effect) High-grade lesions are indistinguishable from PSIN-H (see above)	HPV subtypes 16 and 18 most common	Watchful waiting (especially low-grade) Topical therapy (5-FU, TCA, imiquimod) Anoscopy-directed ablation Surgical excision	Rate of progression to invasive carcinoma is variable (up to 10% at 5 years for high-grade); high-risk patients include immunosuppressed (HIV+), infected with HPV subtypes 16 and 18, and those with extensive disease
High-grade ASD/ IEN (Bowenoid papulosis)	Young, sexually active patients	Small, smooth papules < 5 mm	Disordered organization Basaloid proliferation of atypical cells with mitotic figures beyond the lower half of the epithelium	HPV subtypes 16 and 18 most common	Generally conservative; spontaneous resolution reported in some patients	Generally excellent

ASD/IEN, *Anal squamous dysplasia/ intraepithelial neoplasia;* 5-FU, *5-fluorouracil;* MSM, *men who have sex with men;* TCA, *trichloroacetic acid.*

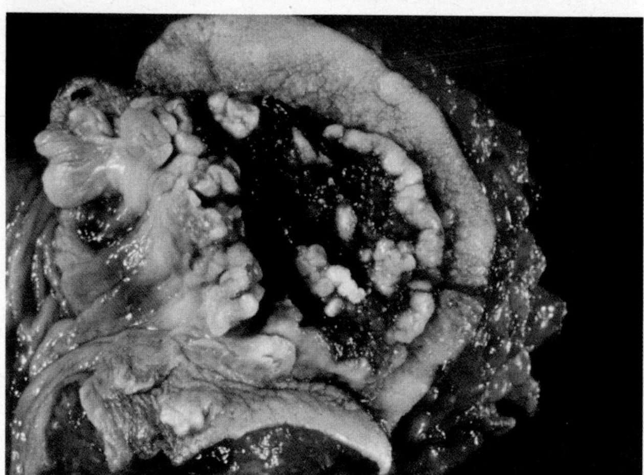

FIGURE 32.23 Infiltrating squamous cell carcinoma arising in the anal canal. Note the transition of colorectal-type mucosa *(left)* to squamous mucosa, which corresponds to the dentate line immediately above the large ulcerated mass. (*Courtesy of Dr. Carolyn Compton, National Institutes of Health, Bethesda, MD.*)

subclassifying them. Furthermore, subclassifying conventional anal squamous cell carcinoma has not yielded consistent prognostic groups.

Squamous cell carcinomas located above the dentate line are believed to arise from the anal transitional epithelium. The majority of these tumors are nonkeratinizing squamous cell carcinomas that are similar in appearance to nonkeratinizing squamous cell cancers in other anatomical locations. Basaloid features may predominate (Fig. 32.25). Microscopically, basaloid zones of anal canal squamous cell carcinoma frequently show an irregular, angulated, nested, or trabecular pattern composed of relatively small cells without intercellular bridges. Central necrosis is a common histological feature, and mitotic figures are also frequently observed. Some basaloid zones also contain small cystic foci lined by mucin-producing cells, formerly considered *mucoepidermoid carcinoma* or *squamous cell carcinoma with mucinous microcysts*. Some pathologists require prominent peripheral palisading within the tumor cell nests, similar to cutaneous basal cell carcinomas, to consider a tumor to have basaloid features. Not uncommonly, a single tumor shows a mixture of histological patterns, including foci of squamous differentiation.

Tumors in this region may extend either proximally or distally, which often obscures their precise site of origin. The adjacent mucosa may show squamous dysplasia/intraepithelial neoplasia. Squamous cell carcinomas, with or without basaloid features, may occasionally arise from anal duct epithelium, which reflects the common embryological origin with anal transitional epithelium. In some instances, dysplasia/intraepithelial neoplasia may involve both the surface mucosa and anal duct epithelium.[196]

Carcinomas that arise below the dentate line are virtually all typical squamous cell carcinomas, and they tend to be better differentiated and show more keratinizing features than those that arise above the dentate line.[197] Of importance, it is often difficult to ascertain the precise site of origin of any neoplasm, either grossly or endoscopically, because carcinomas often destroy the normal anatomic landmarks (see Embryology and Anatomy of the Anus and Anal Canal at the beginning of this chapter). Preoperative radiochemotherapy of anal canal carcinomas may also affect the ability to determine the correct site of origin of the neoplasm.[149]

Special Subtypes

Although the WHO 2019 classification[157] downplays the importance anal carcinoma subtypes, two subtypes bear brief mentioning. First, the rare small cell anaplastic carcinoma (Fig. 32.26) is of particular importance because of its poor prognosis. For instance, Shepherd et al. found that 2 of 2 patients with this histological subtype, which is characterized by basaloid features, diffuse infiltration, nuclear molding, abundant single cell necrosis, and frequent mitoses, died of their disease within 14 months after surgical resection.[198] Although the WHO (and the College of American Pathologists) suggest that these tumors should be differentiated from small cell neuroendocrine carcinomas, no guidelines have been offered on how to do this. Practically speaking, both small cell anaplastic carcinoma and small cell neuroendocrine carcinoma of the anal canal have a dismal prognosis and may, in fact, represent the same neoplasm.

Squamous cell carcinomas may show microcyst formation, including Alcian blue/PAS-positive mucin production in some cases. These tumors are rare. Shepherd et al.[198] found that 10 of 235 cases showed microcyst production in addition to conventional squamous cell carcinoma features. Of these 10 cases, 4 revealed histochemically confirmed mucin production. The prognosis of these tumors appears poor because 6 of 10 patients died of their disease at the time of publication.

Differential Diagnosis

Squamous cell carcinomas of the anal canal should be differentiated from other malignancies, both primary and metastatic, including low rectal adenocarcinoma, anal gland carcinoma, melanoma, and small cell (neuroendocrine) carcinoma, among others. Distinction is greatly aided by judicious use of immunohistochemical stains, particularly for poorly differentiated malignant neoplasms (see Table 32.5).

Prognosis

Staging of anal carcinomas should be performed in accordance with the criteria set forth by the AJCC.[12] The most important prognostic indicators of anal carcinoma are size, depth of invasion, and extent of tumor spread. Carcinomas located above the dentate line commonly spread to the lower rectum and involve perirectal and inguinal lymph nodes. The specific histological type of squamous carcinoma from this region has not been shown to be a significant predictor of survival, although nonsquamous carcinomas tend to have a 5% to 15% poorer 5-year survival, stage-for-stage, compared with anal canal squamous cell carcinoma. Furthermore, the degree of differentiation has been shown to correlate with the presence of lymph node metastases.[198] Poorer survival has been observed among patients with node-positive tumors versus node-negative tumors.[199,200] Carcinomas of the perianal region often grow more slowly than proximally located tumors and are more frequently diagnosed at an early stage; therefore the prognosis tends to be considerably more favorable. Small perianal carcinomas are usually treated with surgical excision and wide margins

TABLE 32.7 Clinical and Histological Features of Squamous Cell Carcinoma and its Variants

Variant	Demographics	Clinical Features	Location	Histology	Ancillary Tests	Treatment	Survival
Conventional SCC	Equal sex distribution or M > F Younger age	Variable size May present as large, ulcerated mass with bleeding Pain	Tend to occur below dentate line	Often keratinizing May be mixed with nonkeratinizing, mucus-producing areas	Often preceded by HPV-associated lesions High-risk HPV subtypes (16, 18)	Chemoradiation for anal SCC; abdominoperineal resection for salvage Wide local excision for small perianal SCC (T1)	70% to 90% cured with radiochemotherapy alone; salvage surgery cures up to an additional 70%
Nonkeratinizing and basaloid SCC	F > M Older age	Bleeding Pain Pruritus Change in bowel habits	Tend to occur above dentate line	No or little keratin Basaloid: prominent peripheral palisading May have mucus-producing areas	Less often associated with HPV Express p63 and CK5/6 by immunohistochemistry	Chemoradiation for anal SCC; abdominoperineal resection for salvage	70% to 90% cured with radiochemotherapy alone; salvage surgery cures up to an additional 70%
Verrucous SCC	M > F Middle age	Bulky, space-occupying May be strikingly exophytic	Tend to occur below dentate line and in anogenital skin	Very well-differentiated Surface maturation and hyperparakeratosis Broad, pushing invasive front; no koilocytes	No HPV	Wide local excision; radiochemotherapy if excision not possible	Rare tumor-related deaths

CK, *Cytokeratin;* HPV, *human papillomavirus;* SCC, *squamous cell carcinoma.*

(at least 1 cm) rather than radiochemotherapy; however, larger tumors may require radiochemotherapy. Outcome of perianal skin squamous cell carcinomas also depends on the tumor size and locoregional spread; metastases to inguinal lymph nodes may occur, but visceral metastases are uncommon.

Features that have been shown to have an impact on local control of anal canal carcinoma include advanced tumor stage, older age at diagnosis, lower radiation dose, and reduced overall treatment time (see Eng[201] for review). In HIV-positive patients, CD4+ T-cell counts of less than 200/mm^3 have also been reported as a negative prognostic indicator of local control, although possible differences in the molecular biology of HIV-positive anal cancers may affect outcome.[141,202,203] Highly active antiretroviral therapy (HAART) has revolutionized HIV therapy, but its benefit in anal HPV infection and intraepithelial neoplasia is still debated. Although some larger studies[204-206] have found a beneficial effect of HAART on the prevalence of HPV infection, ASD/IEN, or both, others have not.[207,208] Furthermore, recent studies suggest that HAART does not affect the high incidence of anal carcinoma in HIV-positive patients.[209,210] With respect to tumor stage, 5-year survival rates are 77% for stage I squamous cell carcinoma (71% for non–squamous cell carcinoma), 67% for stage II squamous cell carcinoma (59% for non–squamous cell carcinoma), 58% for stage IIIA squamous cell carcinoma (50% for non–squamous cell carcinoma only), 51% for stage IIIB squamous cell carcinoma (35% for non–squamous cell carcinoma only), and 15% for stage IV squamous cell carcinoma (7% for non–squamous cell carcinoma only).[12]

BOX 32.2 World Health Organization Classification of Epithelial Tumors of the Anal Canal

PREMALIGNANT LESIONS
- Squamous dysplasia (intraepithelial neoplasia), low-grade
- Squamous dysplasia (intraepithelial neoplasia), high-grade

MALIGNANT EPITHELIAL TUMORS
- Squamous cell carcinoma NOS
  - Verrucous carcinoma
- Adenocarcinoma NOS
- Neuroendocrine tumor NOS
- Neuroendocrine tumor G1
- Neuroendocrine tumor G2
- Neuroendocrine tumor G3

NEUROENDOCRINE CARCINOMA (NEC)
- Large cell NEC
- Small cell NEC
- Mixed Neuroendocrine-Nonneuroendocrine Neoplasms (MiNENs)

Data from World Health Organization & International Agency for Research on Cancer. Digestive System Tumours. 2019.

Treatment

Before the 1970s, patients with anal cancer were managed primarily by radical surgery, resulting in an abdominoperineal resection and a permanent colostomy, with a 5-year survival rate of 40% to 70%. However, current management protocols for patients with anal cancer include combined radiochemotherapy. The National Comprehensive Cancer Network (NCCN) guidelines for anal canal cancer now recommend combination mitomycin C and 5-flurouracil (or capecitabine) chemotherapy and multifield radiotherapy as primary therapy for localized invasive anal canal squamous cell carcinoma.[211] With this approach, 70% to 90% of patients have a complete clinical response, with no tumor found on subsequent biopsies after 6 weeks.[212] Furthermore, one trial found that 29% who did not demonstrate an early complete response (by 11 weeks) demonstrated a complete response by week 26, arguing for conservative management within 6 months of completing radiochemotherapy.[213] This remarkable improvement in local control with primary radiochemotherapy allows for preservation of the anal sphincter and an improved quality of life. Local excision is generally reserved for small (T1/2, N0) well-differentiated perianal squamous cell carcinomas that do

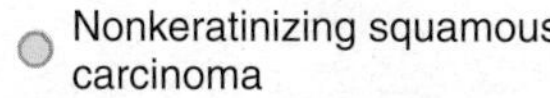
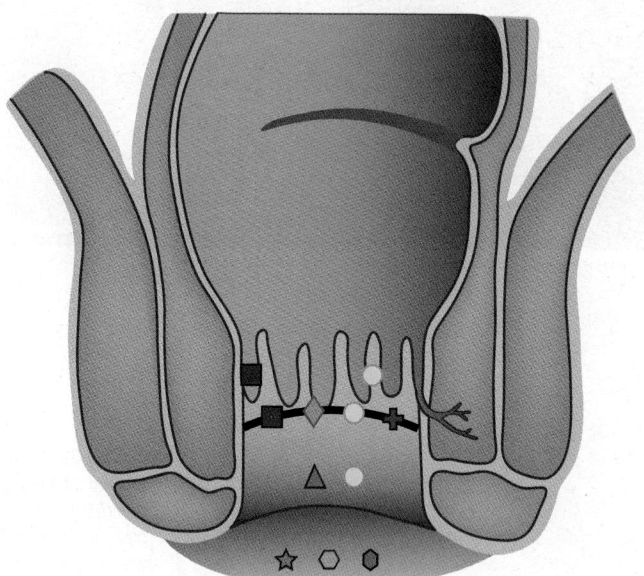

FIGURE 32.24 Most common locations of anal canal neoplasms.

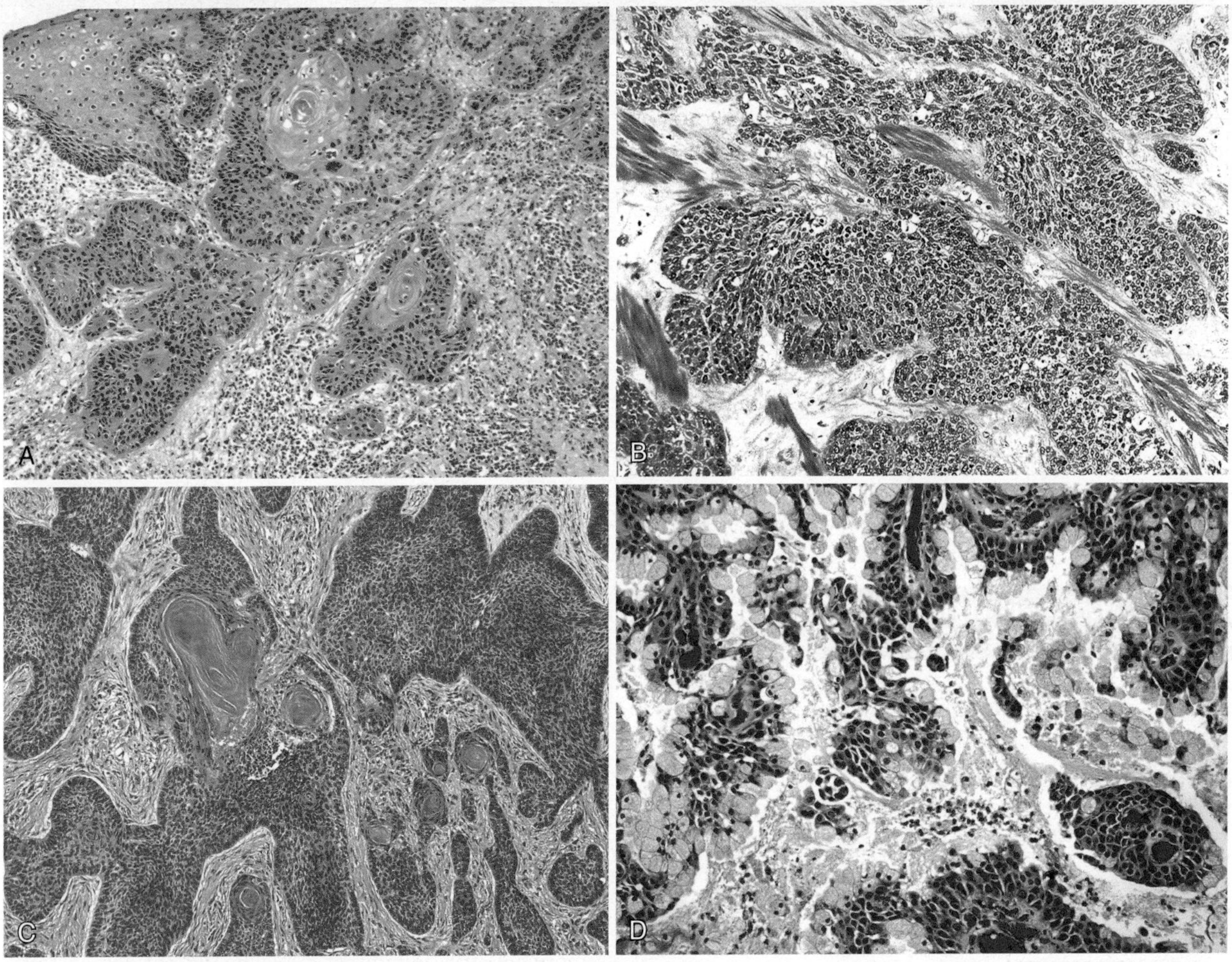

FIGURE 32.25 Morphological appearances of squamous cell carcinoma of the anus. A, Infiltrating keratinizing squamous cell carcinoma of the anus. **B,** Squamous carcinoma with basaloid features comprising small, hyperchromatic cells arranged in a trabecular or nested pattern. **C,** Infiltrating keratinizing squamous cell carcinoma of the anus with basaloid features **D,** Squamous carcinoma with mucinous features.

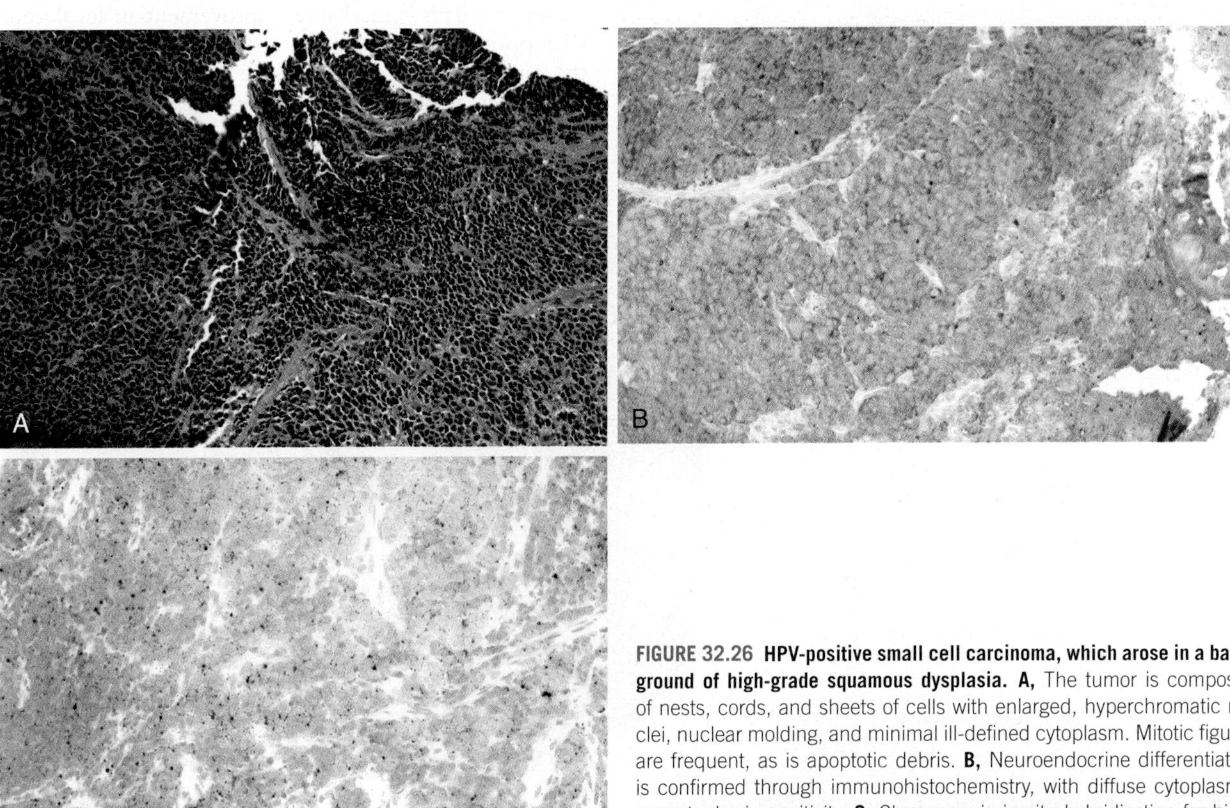

FIGURE 32.26 HPV-positive small cell carcinoma, which arose in a background of high-grade squamous dysplasia. A, The tumor is composed of nests, cords, and sheets of cells with enlarged, hyperchromatic nuclei, nuclear molding, and minimal ill-defined cytoplasm. Mitotic figures are frequent, as is apoptotic debris. **B,** Neuroendocrine differentiation is confirmed through immunohistochemistry, with diffuse cytoplasmic synaptophysin positivity. **C,** Chromogenic in situ hybridization for high-risk HPV subtypes demonstrates punctate staining, confirming the presence of E6/E7 HPV mRNA.

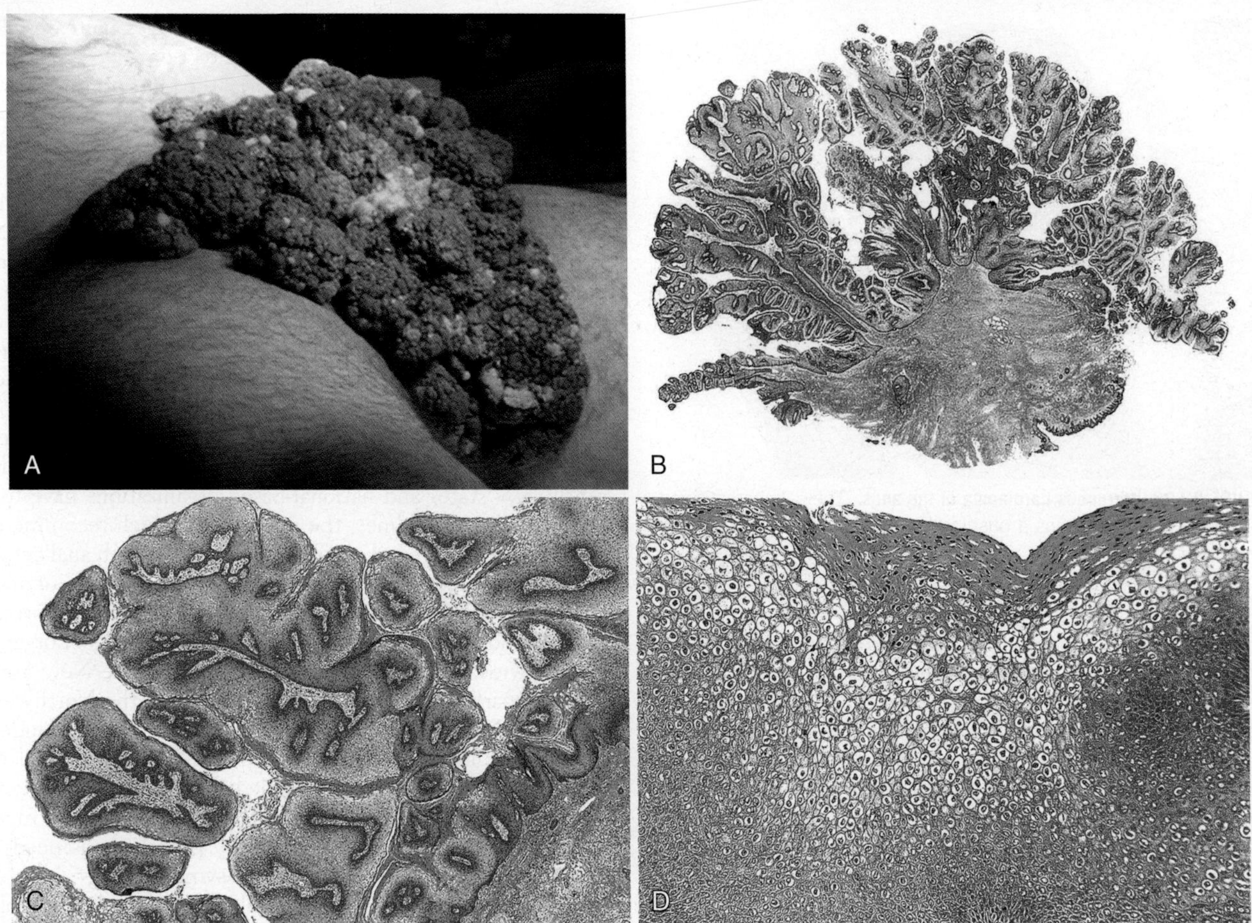

FIGURE 32.27 Giant condyloma acuminatum of Buschke-Löwenstein. A, In this dramatic example, the condyloma extensively involves the external genitalia and the perineum and extends to the perianal skin. **B,** Whole-mount view of a giant condyloma demonstrates its striking papillary architecture. **C,** Papillary fronds lined by acanthotic and hyperkeratotic epithelium are characteristic of this lesion. **D,** High-power view demonstrates koilocytotic changes and surface parakeratosis. (*Courtesy of Dr. Keith Volmar, University of North Carolina, Chapel Hill, NC.*)

not invade the sphincter or superficially invasive anal squamous cell carcinoma (≤3 mm depth of stromal invasion and ≤7 mm horizontal spread).[214,215] In our practice, local excisions of anal/perianal squamous cell carcinoma remain quite uncommon.

The risk of local failure after treatment is greatest within the first 3 years after treatment.[199,216-218] Residual disease is defined as persistent disease within 6 months of completion of radiochemotherapy, and recurrent disease is defined as carcinoma diagnosed 6 or more months after a complete clinical response. Because additional medical therapy is unlikely to provide a cure in this setting, the preferred method of treatment for locally residual or recurrent disease is abdominoperineal resection.[216-218] Up to 70% of patients are cured after salvage surgery. Positive surgical margins are the best predictor of a poor outcome.[218]

Verrucous Carcinoma and Giant Condyloma of Buschke-Löwenstein

Once considered synonymous, verrucous carcinoma and giant condyloma acuminatum (Buschke-Löwenstein tumor) are now considered separate entities, according to the most recent WHO classification.[157] This new separation is based on relatively limited but fairly convincing data, the most important being giant condylomas are HPV-related and verrucous carcinomas are not.[158] As the separation of these two entities is a recent development, there does not yet exist enough peer-reviewed medical literature to meaningfully draw distinctions among clinical presentation, prognosis, and treatment of these two entities. Both of these lesions are characterized by bulky exophytic growth and tumor size that often exceeds 10 cm in greatest diameter (Fig. 32.27). Despite their inability to metastasize (unless containing conventional invasive squamous carcinoma), verrucous carcinomas are locally invasive and, hence, are considered malignant tumors.[219,220] They are more common in men, and the incidence in men is even greater in patients younger than 50 years of age. The clinical presentation includes a perianal mass and pain, abscess, or fistula. Because of their large size, these tumors have a propensity to ulcerate, and bleeding is a common complaint.

Their histological appearance is, paradoxically, benign. Giant condylomas are exophytic tumors that lack destructive invasion. Giant condylomas must show HPV-related changes (e.g., koilocytosis or HPV nucleic acids). Both of these tumors appear as very well-differentiated squamoproliferative lesions on microscopic examination (see Figs. 32.27 and 32.28). Verrucous carcinomas contain minimal cytological atypia and lack HPV cytopathic effect, but they

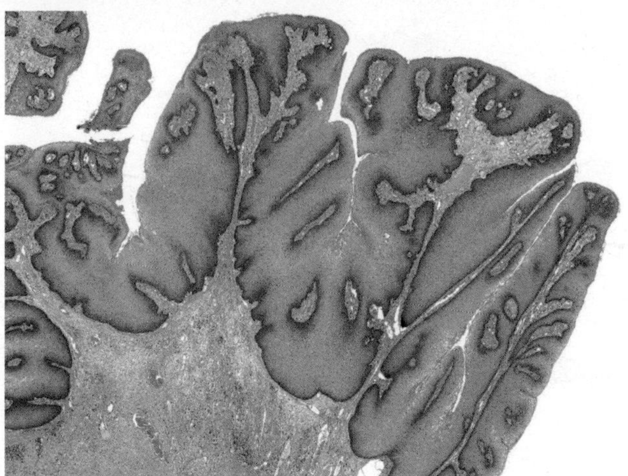

FIGURE 32.28 Verrucous carcinoma of the anus. The carcinoma is very well differentiated and has a pushing border into the submucosal tissues and lacks koilocytes.

must show a broad invasive front and downward growth. They are typically locally invasive into adjacent chronically inflamed stromal tissue and reveal a pushing, rather than an infiltrating, tumor margin. The epithelium often shows evidence of surface maturation and extensive crater-like keratinization. Treatment strategies for giant condyloma/verrucous carcinoma are variable and include topical chemotherapy, wide local excision, abdominoperineal resection, and adjuvant and neoadjuvant systemic chemotherapy and radiation therapy.[221,222] Recurrences are common after surgical resection. Up to 20% of patients die of their disease.[219] Because of their slow growth, local excision is the preferred method of management, although for large and bulky tumors that are locally destructive, radiochemotherapy, cryotherapy, and more extensive surgical management may be required.[223]

Anal Cytology

Anal Cancer Screening

At the time of this writing, national cancer screening guidelines for anal carcinoma have not been established in the United States. To date, no prospective studies have been conducted to demonstrate that the identification and treatment of high-grade anal intraepithelial neoplasia reduces the incidence of anal carcinoma.[224] Importantly, the National Cancer Institute of the National Institutes of Health partnered with the AIDS Malignancy Consortium is currently conducting the first prospective randomized controlled trial to investigate this query, called the Anal Cancer HSIL Outcome Research (ANCHOR) Study (NCT02135419). Forthcoming results will certainly inform national standardized guidelines in years to come. Although standardized screening guidelines do not yet exist, the International Anal Neoplasia Society (IANS), with input from the American Society for Colposcopy and Cervical Pathology (ASCCP), released Guidelines for Practice Standards in the Detection of Anal Cancer Precursors in 2016.[225] These recommendations established quality metrics for anal cancer screening procedures and highlighted the complementary nature of anal cytology and high-resolution anoscopy (HRA) with biopsy, in that the combination of both screening methodologies increases the sensitivity of anal cancer precursor detection.[225]

In contrast with cervical neoplasia, the rates of progression to squamous cell carcinoma for low- and high-grade anal dysplasia are not yet well-established.[224] Despite this, the natural history of anal neoplasia secondary to HPV infection is presumed to closely mirror that in the cervix. Based on this presumption, it is posited that specific patient cohorts may benefit from anal cancer screening, though data are still being collected on the efficacy of such programs.[226,227] As it has been well-established that specific patient populations are at substantially increased risk of developing anal carcinoma compared with the general population, particularly immunocompromised patients and those with a history of lower genital tract epithelial dysplasia, screening programs have been enacted selectively throughout the United States.[227,228] Currently, few state- and national-based organizations have formal screening guidelines, the majority of which recommend annual digital anorectal examination (DARE) with anal cytology in HIV-infected MSM, any patient with a history of anogenital condyloma, and HIV-infected women with abnormal cervical and/or vulvar histology.[224,228,229] Examples of organizations with such recommendations include the New York State Department of Health AIDS Institute, the Northwest Pennsylvania Rural AIDS Alliance, and the now defunded National Guideline Clearinghouse.[229] Informally, annual or biannual screening is recommended for "high-risk" patients by various experts.[229] Outside of these patient cohorts, most anal cancer screening is conducted by physicians as needed based on patient presentation and/or symptomology.

Anal cancer screening methodologies currently available include DARE, anal cytology, and HRA. Histology serves as the diagnostic gold standard. Importantly, anal cytology frequently underestimates the severity of disease identified on subsequent histology.[228,230] Of course, the specificity and positive predictive value of a cytological interpretation of HSIL, particularly in MSM, is very high (93% and 89%, respectively).[224] It is not recommended that anal cytology be offered to patients unless HRA, biopsy, and accompanying ablative therapies are also available.[231]

Sample Collection and Adequacy

Anal cytology sample collection is generally performed with a moistened Dacron swab and without direct visualization of the anal canal.[228] The goal is to sample the entire anal canal, including both keratinized and nonkeratinized squamous mucosa as well as the anal transition zone.[230] When feasible, liquid-based cytology (LBC) is preferred over conventional smears as it minimizes drying artifact, optimizes cellular dispersion, and reduces the rate of cellular obscuration. Of note, some authors have shown similar performance of conventional and liquid-based preparations; thus direct smears are still of utility in resource-limited settings.[232] The cellularity necessary to deem a conventional or LBC anal pap test as adequate, barring no identified abnormality, is 2000 to 3000 well-visualized, nucleated squamous cells.[233] Unsatisfactory anal cytology samples may consist nearly exclusively of anucleate squamous cells, or the present nucleated squamous cells may be visually obscured by bacteria, fecal matter, lubricant, or other foreign material.

Interpretation

Anal cytology was first included in the Bethesda system in 2001, and it is still recommended that Bethesda terminology be used for anal cytology interpretation (Table 32.8). The cells that compose an anal cytology specimen closely mirror those seen in cervical/vaginal cytology specimens: superficial and intermediate squamous cells, metaplastic squamous cells, columnar glandular cells from the anal transition zone, and anucleate squamous cells from the more distal anal canal. As is true for cervical cytology, the presence of a transformation zone is reported as a quality indicator but is not necessary to deem an anal cytology specimen as satisfactory for evaluation.[233] The dysplasia terminology and cytomorphological criteria used in cervical/vaginal cytology are directly applicable to anal cytology specimens as well. Recommended diagnostic interpretations include (Fig. 32.29): negative for intraepithelial lesion or malignancy (NILM), atypical squamous cells of undetermined significance (ASCUS), atypical squamous cells cannot exclude HSIL (ASC-H), LSIL, HSIL, and squamous cell carcinoma. Rarely, other epithelial abnormalities, such as glandular abnormalities, may be identified. Related interpretations include atypical glandular cells (AGCs) and adenocarcinoma.[233]

NILM anal cytology specimens (Fig. 32.29B) are largely similar to negative cervical cytology specimens, with a few caveats. Abundant anucleate squamous cells are more common in the anal canal than in the cervix, and this hyperkeratosis should not raise alarm.[230]Additionally common in the anal canal are keratotic changes as well as reactive changes. Interestingly, streaming reparative-type atypia is actually less common. Parakeratosis spans the spectrum of normal, reactive-type changes to atypical, lesional alterations. Similar to the gynecological cytology, HPV infection is associated with atypical parakeratosis.[233]

TABLE 32.8 Bethesda Classification for Interpretation of Anal Cytology

Category	Features
NILM	Reactive changes, fecal contamination, keratosis, and parakeratosis common, repair uncommon
ASC-US	Enlarged nuclei with smooth contours and smudgy chromatin
ASC-H	Hyperchromatic nuclei with high N:C ratios
LSIL	Nuclear enlargement, hyperchromasia, nuclear membrane irregularities; Perinuclear halos with low N:C ratios
HSIL	Similar nuclei to LSIL with marked increase in N:C ratios
SCC	Difficult to distinguish from HSIL. Look for clinging tumor diathesis

ASC-US, *Atypical squamous cell of undetermined significance;* ASC-H, *atypical squamous cell, cannot exclude high-grade lesion;* LSIL, *low-grade squamous intraepithelial lesion;* HSIL, *high-grade squamous intraepithelial lesion;* NILM, *negative for intraepithelial lesion or malignancy;* SCC, *squamous cell carcinoma.*

From Nayar R, Wilbur DC. Ohio Library and Information Network. The Bethesda System For Reporting Cervical Cytology: Definitions, Criteria, And Explanatory Notes, 3rd ed; 2014.

Data from World Health Organization & International Agency for Research on Cancer. Digestive System Tumours. 2019.

LSIL cells (Fig. 32.29C) are typically the size of intermediate or superficial squamous cells and have nuclei that are enlarged to three times greater or more in size when compared with a typical intermediate cell nucleus. Nuclei are generally hyperchromatic, with irregular nuclear membranes. Binucleation and multinucleation are relatively common, whereas nucleoli are infrequent. Complete cytoplasmic koilocytosis is seen, in which the perinuclear clearing is sharply delineated throughout its entire circumference, with cytoplasmic "condensation," or increased cytoplasmic density, along its peripheral rim.[233]

HSIL cells (Fig. 32.29D) are generally smaller than LSIL cells, though their overall size is variable. The nuclei in HSIL cells are also more variable in size than those of LSIL, though typically they enlarged to a size similar to LSIL nuclei. Of course, the cytoplasmic area in HSIL cells is much reduced, resulting in a significantly increased nuclear-to-cytoplasmic ratio. The nuclei in HSILs are generally hyperchromatic and have irregular nuclear membranes with frequent prominent indentations. Nucleoli are uncommon and raise the possibility of a squamous cell carcinoma when seen. The scant cytoplasm itself is variable in content, ranging from frothy and immature to densely metaplastic to keratinized.[233]

Squamous cell carcinoma of the anus can be keratinizing or nonkeratinizing (Fig. 32.29E–H). Generally, the cytomorphological presentation is that of predominantly isolated single cells that demonstrate marked variation in cellular shape and size. Syncytial aggregates are more common in the nonkeratinizing variant. Caudate and spindled cells may be identified, often with densely keratinized, orangeophilic cytoplasm. The nuclei are generally markedly atypical, with coarse and irregular nuclear chromatin, nuclear membrane irregularity, and variably prominent nucleoli. In the background, tumor diathesis clinging to malignant cells is a useful feature supporting the diagnosis of carcinoma. In general, in the anus, keratinizing squamous lesions are more common than in the gynecological tract.[233]

ASCUS (Fig. 32.29I) and ASC-H (Fig. 32.29H) diagnoses should be rendered in samples in which the cytomorphological alterations fall short of the definitions of LSIL and HSIL, respectively. For ASCUS cells, their nuclei are usually 2.5 to 3 times the size of a normal intermediate cell nucleus or twice the size of a normal metaplastic cell nucleus. There is an associated mild increase in the nuclear-to-cytoplasmic ratio. Other minimal changes that may be identified include nuclear chromatin alterations, nuclear irregularity, and incomplete cytoplasmic koilocytosis. Atypical parakeratosis, without accompanying cells diagnostic of LSIL, also falls within the diagnostic spectrum of ASCUS. For ASC-H, cells are typically the size of metaplastic cells and have nuclei that are 1.5 to 2.5 times larger than a normal metaplastic cell, with an increased nuclear-to-cytoplasmic ratio that closely mirrors that of HSIL.[233]

Finally, one must remember to consider diagnostic abnormalities outside of the realm of epithelial abnormalities. It is not uncommon to encounter microorganisms in anal cytology samples. Similar to cervical cytology, a myriad of microorganisms can be identified, including fungi, viruses, protozoa, and helminths. The fungi and viruses are identical to those seen in gynecological cytology, including *Candida* sp. and herpes virus. Protozoa include trichomonas and amebiasis (*Entamoeba histolytica*). Of the helminths, pinworms (*Enterobius vermicularis*), particularly their eggs, are most commonly identified.[230,233]

ANAL ADENOCARCINOMA

Clinical Features and Pathogenesis

Primary adenocarcinomas of the anal canal are quite uncommon and are thought to compose about 5% of anal malignancies.[234,235] Most adenocarcinomas in this region result from secondary involvement by a distal rectal tumor. The mean age at diagnosis of primary adenocarcinomas is in the seventh decade, and men may be more frequently affected than women.[8,191] The clinical presentation is often due to a painful mass of the buttock accompanied by a mucin-like discharge. Anorectal bleeding or obstruction is not common.

Primary adenocarcinomas of the anal canal (not from the rectum) historically have been placed into one of two categories: those that arise in preexisting anorectal sinuses or fistulae and those that presumably arise from anal glands (essentially in the absence of fistulae). The WHO has classified primary anal adenocarcinoma into two types as mucosal (intestinal-type that is indistinguishable from rectal carcinoma) and extramucosal, which has three subtypes: fistula-associated, anal gland, and neither fistula-associated or anal gland type.[157] Patients with Crohn's disease have been identified as an important risk group for developing a

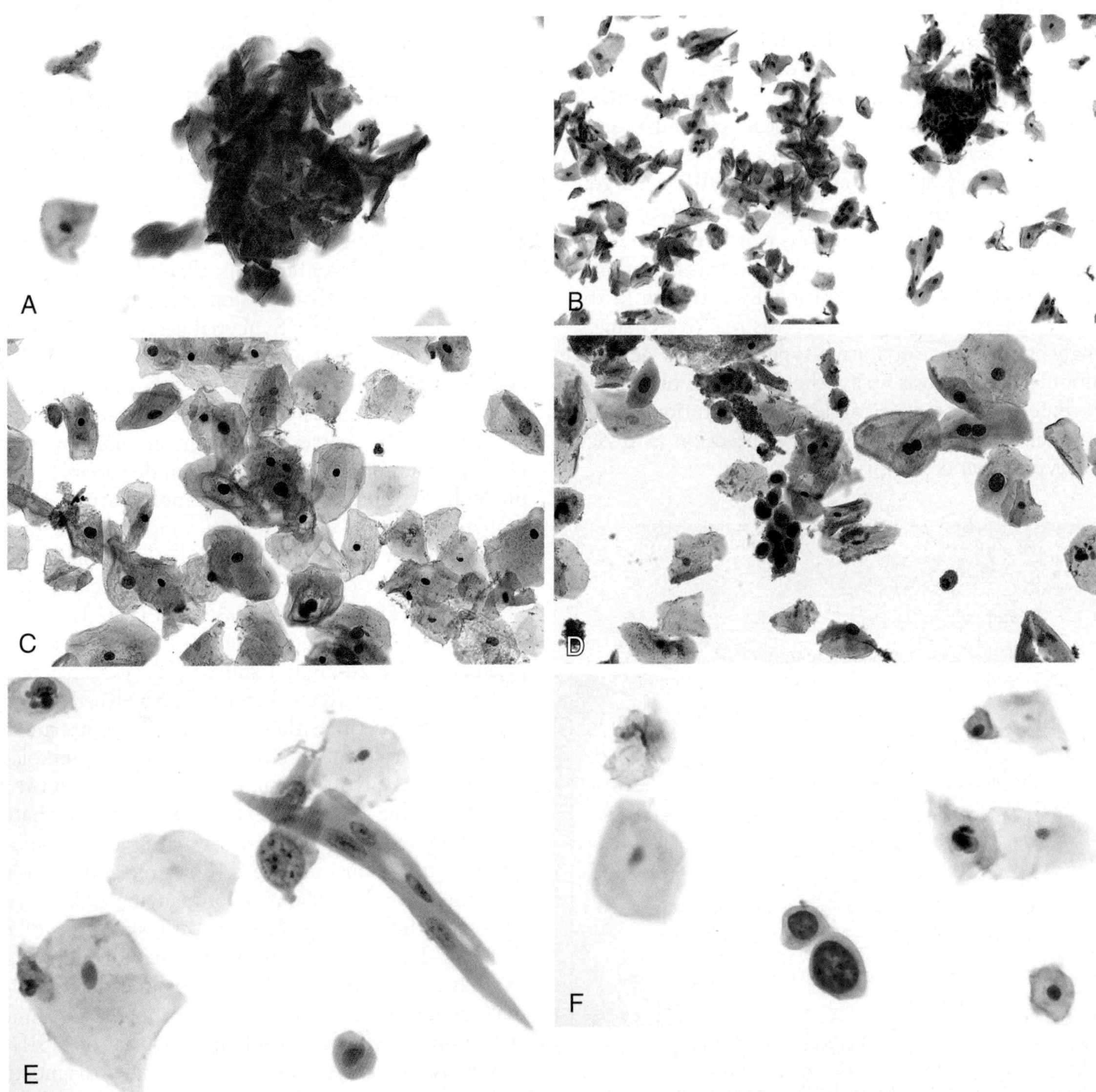

FIGURE 32.29 A, Unsatisfactory anal cytology specimen in which the specimen is composed of anucleated squamous cells only. **B,** Anal cytology interpreted as NILM, demonstrating unremarkable intermediate, superficial, and metaplastic squamous cells as well as glandular epithelium, consistent with the anal transition zone. In the background, scattered anucleated squamous cells can be seen. **C,** Anal cytology demonstrating LSIL, characterized by an HPV cytopathic effect manifesting as perinuclear halos accompanying nuclear abnormalities including enlargement, membrane irregularity, hyperchromasia, and binucleation. **D,** Anal cytology demonstrating HSIL, characterized by variably sized cells with increased nuclear-to-cytoplasmic ratios, nuclear membrane irregularity, and nuclear hyperchromasia. **E–H,** Anal cytology demonstrating squamous cell carcinoma. **E,** Atypical keratinizing spindled cells with coarse nuclear chromatin and irregular nuclear membrane. **F,** Marked variation in cell size.

Continued

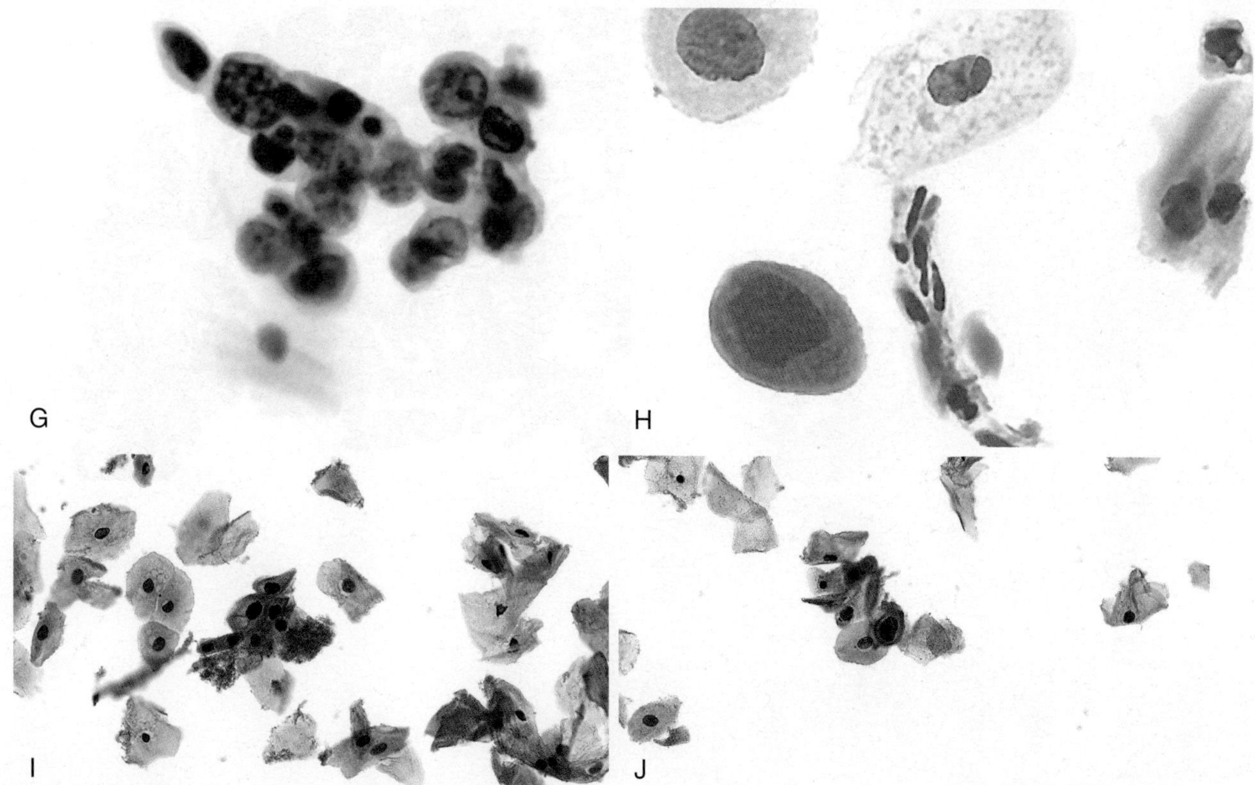

FIGURE 32.29 cont'd G, An aggregate of malignant cells with variable size and shape, coarse nuclear chromatin, and variably prominent nucleoli. **H,** Marked pleomorphism of malignant cells, including cells with cytoplasmic keratinization, as well as minute fragments of clinging tumor diathesis. **I,** Anal cytology demonstrating ASCUS, characterized by atypical squamous cells that have moderately enlarged nuclei with hyperchromatic nuclear chromatin and vague, ill-defined perinuclear clearing, suggestive of incomplete koilocytosis. **J,** Anal cytology demonstrating ASC-H, characterized by a single cell with an increased nuclear-to-cytoplasmic ratio, an enlarged, hyperchromatic nucleus with nuclear membrane irregularity, and keratinized cytoplasm.

fistula-associated tumor.[236] The causal relationship between perianal fistulae and abscesses and the subsequent development of carcinoma is a subject of debate. Some authorities have proposed that the inflammatory process precedes the neoplasm, whereas others believe that these rather slow-growing neoplasms undergo secondary fistulization with time. An association of anal adenocarcinoma (and other lower genital sites) with HPV infection has also been described, similar to that observed for endocervical adenocarcinomas (Fig. 32.30).[196,237]

Pathology

Primary adenocarcinoma of the anal canal characteristically arises in the deep perianal tissues without evidence of surface mucosal involvement (Fig. 32.31). On cut section, these tumors typically appear as an infiltrative mass with an epicenter located deep within the soft tissues and involvement of the adjacent structures of the anal canal. Most primary anal gland adenocarcinomas are well-differentiated, comprising haphazardly dispersed, small glands with scant mucin production (Fig. 32.31D,E), although rare cases may be poorly differentiated or within mucin pools.[238] These carcinomas typically show an anal gland immunophenotype, being CK7+ and CK20–.[8] Presumably, these carcinomas are also CDX2–, like their benign glandular counterparts, although the literature is quite limited in these very rare tumors. Carcinomas arising within fistulae are usually associated with abundant mucin production (Fig 32.31B,C), and some have termed them *perianal mucinous (colloid) adenocarcinomas*.[8,239] Perianal mucinous adenocarcinomas are more commonly associated with fistulas and may be more often associated with a rectal phenotype (CK20+ and CDX2+).[240] Multiple deep biopsies are often required to establish a diagnosis of colloid carcinoma because the abundance of mucin and low-grade–appearing epithelium may make identification of tumor cells difficult.[241,242] The most recent addition to the anal adenocarcinoma subtype family is the non–anal gland type and non–fistula-associated extramucosal anal adenocarcinoma. The few case reports in the literature describe this tumor as harboring an intestinal phenotype (CDX2+) without precursor mucosal neoplasia, and its authors have proposed the name primary *perianal adenocarcinoma of intestinal type*,[243] which seems like a less cumbersome name than the WHO's attempt. Before rendering a diagnosis of this rare variant, exclusion of metastasis from an intestinal tract primary tumor is certainly paramount.

Differential Diagnosis

The main differential diagnosis of a primary anal adenocarcinoma is a distal rectal cancer that extends into the anal

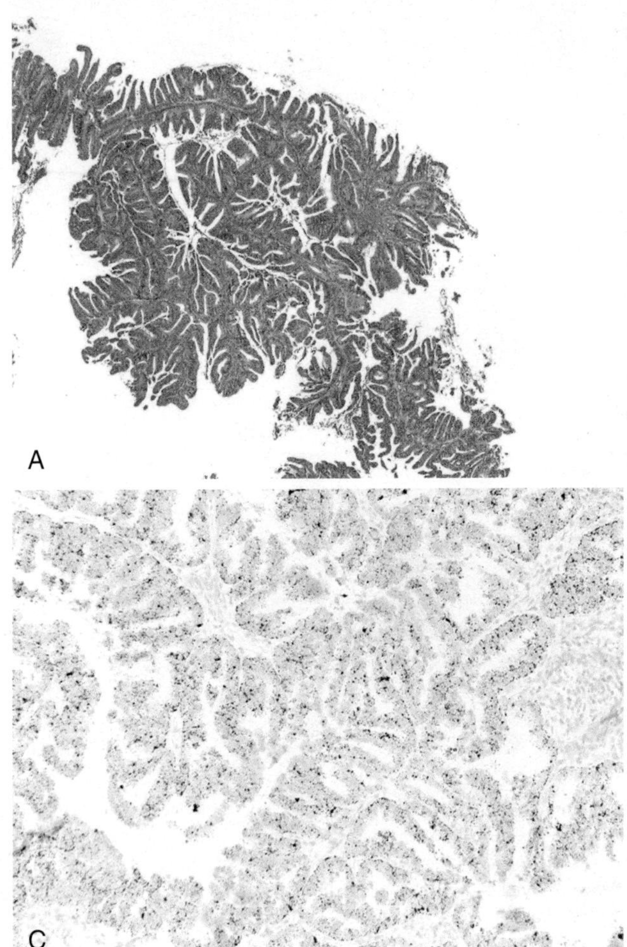

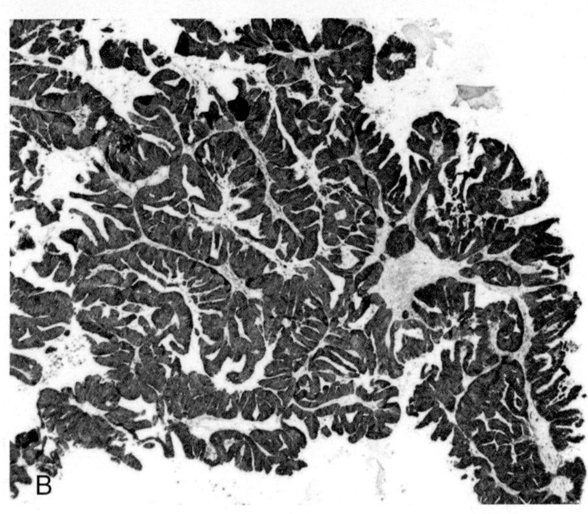

FIGURE 32.30 HPV-related adenocarcinoma of the anorectum. A, These adenocarcinomas are characterized by a papillary or villiform architecture. **B,** Strong and diffuse (block-type) p16 staining supports a diagnosis of HPV-associated neoplasia. **C,** In situ hybridization (ISH) for high-risk HPV demonstrates the presence of high-risk HPV RNA within the adenocarcinoma.

canal (Table 32.9). Demonstration of a precursor adenomatous component in rectal mucosa is helpful to demonstrate its origin in rectal columnar epithelium. Immunohistochemical labeling for CK7 and CK20 may also be useful because primary anal gland adenocarcinomas are probably universally CK7+, whereas most rectal tumors are CK7– and CK20+. A significant minority of rectal carcinomas are CK7+ (10% to 20%),[5,244,245] so CK7 positivity does not exclude the possibility of a rectal primary tumor. CDX2 (and probably SATB2) are extremely useful markers of intestinal, rather than anal gland, phenotype[246]; however, as mentioned previously, fistula-associated adenocarcinoma may more commonly demonstrate a rectal phenotype rather than an anal gland phenotype[240] (see Table 32.9).

Prognosis and Treatment

Primary adenocarcinoma of the anal canal is considered a more aggressive tumor than squamous cell carcinoma in this location.[235] Patients are at higher risk for both local and distant recurrence.[247] Tumor stage, lymph node status, and differentiation status have all been shown to be independently associated with outcome. Treatment of primary adenocarcinomas of the anal canal is similar to that of rectal cancer and usually includes both surgical resection and aggressive radiochemotherapy. Historically, the overall 5-year survival rate was approximately 30%[247,248]; however, a recent study of 1183 anal adenocarcinoma patients using the National Cancer Data Base reported a median overall survival of 72.5 months. That said, the prognosis still greatly lags behind anal squamous carcinoma patients, who, in the same registry, had a median overall survival of 143.8 months.[235]

PAGET'S DISEASE OF THE ANUS

Clinical Features

Primary (extramammary) Paget's disease of the anal canal is rare. Among patients with primary anal Paget's disease, men and women are equally affected, and most patients are diagnosed in the fifth to seventh decades of life.[249] The clinical appearance of extramammary Paget's disease is well described.[250,251] Typical lesions consist of erythematous patches or plaques that may be scaly, eroded, or ulcerated and located anywhere between the dentate line and the perianal skin.[249] Pruritus is also a frequent clinical complaint. Lesions can be quite variable in size. In fact,

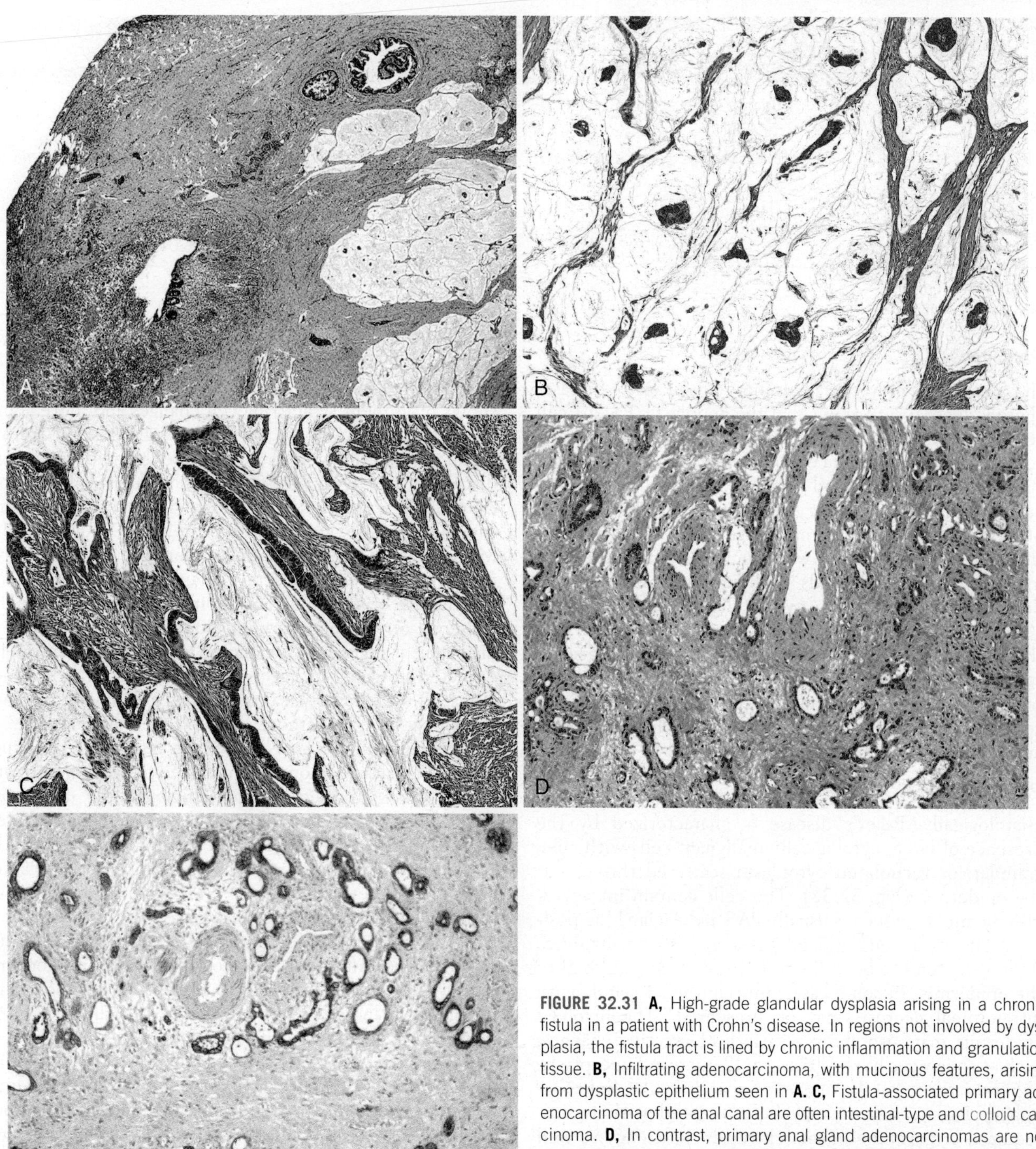

FIGURE 32.31 **A,** High-grade glandular dysplasia arising in a chronic fistula in a patient with Crohn's disease. In regions not involved by dysplasia, the fistula tract is lined by chronic inflammation and granulation tissue. **B,** Infiltrating adenocarcinoma, with mucinous features, arising from dysplastic epithelium seen in **A. C,** Fistula-associated primary adenocarcinoma of the anal canal are often intestinal-type and colloid carcinoma. **D,** In contrast, primary anal gland adenocarcinomas are not associated with a chronic fistula. Microscopically, they are characterized by simple glands and minimal mucin production. **E,** Anal gland carcinomas are typically diffusely positive for CK7 by immunohistochemistry.

regions of involvement by neoplastic cells may extend well beyond the gross impression of involvement. Secondary anal or perianal Paget's disease may occur in association with a distal adenocarcinoma of the rectum, the latter of which may be diagnosed before the anal Paget's disease, at the same time, or later.[250-253] About one-half of cases of Paget's disease of the anus are secondary, associated with a visceral malignancy such as rectal adenocarcinoma. The remaining half are primary (extramammary) Paget's disease. Perianal Paget's disease may also develop as an extension of perineal Paget's disease, particularly in postmenopausal White women.[254] In this instance, the finding of Paget cells likely represents migration of malignant cells into the anal epidermis from an associated rectal adenocarcinoma or extramammary Paget's disease of the perineum.[255] Thus these varied patterns of occurrence of anal Paget's disease suggest that it has multiple potential etiologies (see the next section).[252]

TABLE 32.9 Distinguishing Features of Primary Rectal and Primary Anal Adenocarcinomas

Features	Rectal Adenocarcinoma	Anal Gland Carcinoma	Fistula-Associated Adenocarcinoma
Clinical presentation	Change in bowel habits, rectal bleeding	Painful buttock mass	Mucoid discharge
Typical histology	Intestinal-type adenocarcinoma	Simple glands with minimal mucin production	Mucinous (colloid) adenocarcinoma
Coexisting conditions	Uncommon	Uncommon	Fistula, Crohn's disease
Immunohistochemistry	CK7–/+, CK20+, CDX2+	CK7+, CK20–, CDX2–	CK7–/+, CK20+, CDX2+

CK, *Cytokeratin.*

Pathogenesis

In cases of primary extramammary anal Paget's disease, there is general agreement that the neoplastic Paget's cell represents a secretory (glandular) epithelial cell. Although some authorities favor an eccrine sweat gland origin, most support an apocrine gland origin of Paget cells.[256,257] So-called *anogenital mammary-like glands* may be a source of at least rare extramammary Paget's disease cases, particularly those associated with ductal carcinoma in situ–like changes in these glands.[89] The immunohistochemical demonstration of gross cystic disease fluid protein (GCDFP) expression, which is a marker of apocrine epithelium, in many cases of extramammary Paget's disease supports this viewpoint. Paget cells may also be positive for epithelial membrane antigen, carcinoembryonic antigen, androgen receptors, and low-molecular-weight keratins.

Pathology

Histologically, Paget's disease is characterized by the presence of large, cytologically malignant cells with pale, granular, or vacuolated cytoplasm scattered throughout the epidermis (Fig. 32.32). The cells contain intracytoplasmic mucin, which is usually PAS and Alcian blue positive. The cutaneous appendages may also be involved. Paget cells tend to be more numerous in the basal half of the epidermis. In some cases, intraepithelial glands with intraluminal necrosis may be present.[244] The involved epidermis may also show a variety of reactive changes, such as squamous hyperplasia, papillomatous hyperplasia, hyperkeratosis, parakeratosis, or acanthosis.[258] Extramammary Paget's disease may be associated with tumor-acquired or germline mismatch repair deficiency as well as *HER2* amplification.[259,260]

Differential Diagnosis

The differential diagnosis of anal Paget's disease is pagetoid spread by a primary rectal adenocarcinoma, malignant melanoma, and squamous intraepithelial neoplasia (see Tables 32.5 and 32.10). Fortunately, a limited panel of immunohistochemical studies can help establish a correct diagnosis in most cases. A CK20+, CDX2+, and GCDFP– immunophenotype is typical of Paget's disease associated with a coexistent rectal cancer, whereas a CK7+, CK20–, and GCDFP+ immunophenotype is typical of primary anogenital Paget's disease [244]. Ber-Ep4 *(EPCAM)* is not of utility in distinguishing these two entities as it is typically positive in both. Morphologically, Paget's disease caused by rectal adenocarcinoma usually shows prominent signet ring cell changes and more abundant cytoplasmic mucin. Also, the cells derived from a rectal adenocarcinoma tend to invade the epidermis more discretely and with less predilection for the basal portions of the epithelium. Stains for markers of melanoma can also be of value. S100 protein/SOX10, HMB45, Melan-A, and other melanocyte markers will be positive in most, if not all, anorectal melanomas, but not in Paget's disease or squamous intraepithelial neoplasia.[261] The presence of melanin pigment alone does not establish a diagnosis of malignant melanoma because melanin can be detected not only in Paget cells, but in normal melanocytes, which may be scattered among neoplastic keratinocytes in cases of squamous intraepithelial neoplasia.[262]

Approximately 5% of high-grade intraepithelial squamous neoplasias demonstrate a nested or pagetoid growth pattern, often termed *pagetoid squamous cell carcinoma* (Fig. 32.33). A minority of these cases have been reported to be strongly and diffusely positive for CK7, which traditionally has been considered a sensitive and specific marker of primary Paget's disease.[168,263] Ber-Ep4 is another sensitive marker of primary Paget's disease, which is negative in pagetoid squamous cell carcinoma.[264] Florid Paget's disease replacement of the squamous epithelium also occurs, closely mimicking high-grade squamous intraepithelial neoplasia, including p16 positivity.[258,265] Findings supporting pagetoid squamous cell carcinoma in situ include areas of unequivocal full-thickness squamous cell intraepithelial neoplasia and features of HPV cytopathic effect (multinucleated giant cells and koilocytes). Pagetoid squamous cell carcinoma cells should also coexpress p63, CK5, and CK6. GATA3 is typically positive in secondary Paget's disease from a urothelial primary tumor or a primary Paget tumor, so it is less helpful in that distinction.[266] GATA3 is often helpful in differentiating rectal adenocarcinoma from urothelial carcinoma, however.[267] Findings that support Paget's disease include signet ring cells and the presence of intraepithelial mucin.[168] Finally, immunostaining for p16 is a useful surrogate marker of HPV infection and is highly associated with anogenital squamous intraepithelial neoplasia, but generally not with Paget's disease or melanoma.[268-270] A recent small series does highlight the pitfalls in relying too heavily on p16 alone because the authors documented p16+ Paget's disease cells, which were sometimes diffusely and strongly positive.[265]

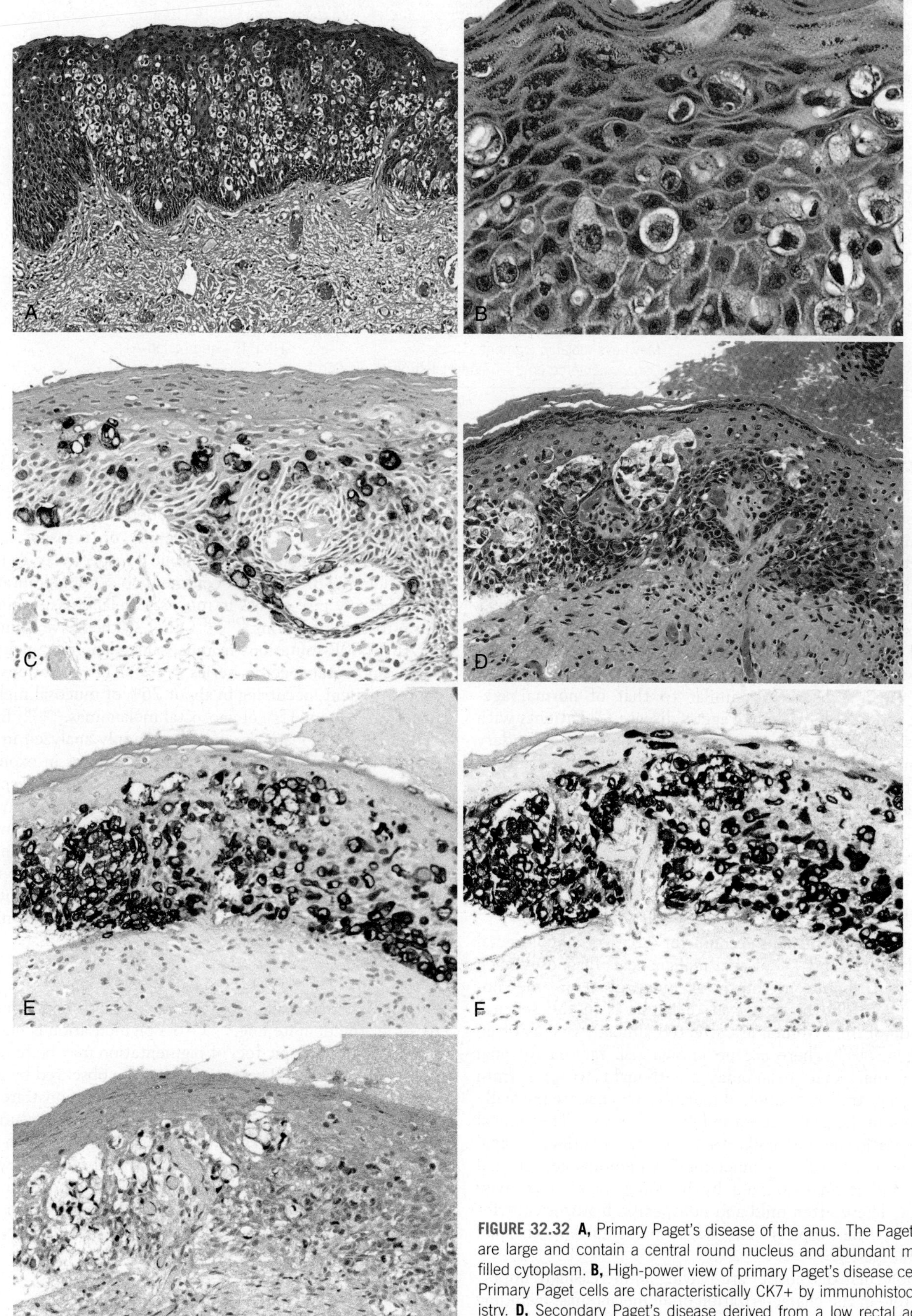

FIGURE 32.32 **A,** Primary Paget's disease of the anus. The Paget cells are large and contain a central round nucleus and abundant mucin-filled cytoplasm. **B,** High-power view of primary Paget's disease cells. **C,** Primary Paget cells are characteristically CK7+ by immunohistochemistry. **D,** Secondary Paget's disease derived from a low rectal adenocarcinoma. These cells often demonstrate signet ring morphology. **E,** Secondary Paget's disease may also be CK7+. The use of CK20 (**F**) and CDX2 (**G**) is helpful in differentiating CK7+ Paget's disease.

TABLE 32.10 Pathological Features of Intraepithelial Lesions of the Anus with Possible Pagetoid Cell Spread

Lesion	Histology	Ancillary Studies
Primary Paget's disease	Large, cytologically malignant cells most prominent in basal half of epithelium Glands with luminal necrosis May involve cutaneous appendages	CK7+, GATA3+, and GCDFP15+ CK20– and CDX2– MUC1+ and MUC5AC+
Pagetoid spread by rectal adenocarcinoma	Less predilection for basal half of epithelium Often signet ring morphology May involve cutaneous appendages	CK7–/+ and GATA3/GCDFP15– CK20+ and CDX2+ MUC2+
High-grade anal squamous intraepithelial neoplasia	Usually diffuse proliferation of disordered atypical squamous cells Pagetoid pattern in about 5%	CK7– (rare +, especially in pagetoid pattern) High-risk HPV+ Diffuse, blocklike p16+
Anal melanoma	Nests and single cytologically malignant cells with prominent nucleoli and dusky cytoplasm May have melanin pigment Usually centered on the epidermal-stromal junction	CK7– and CK20– S100 protein positive and SOX10+ HMB45+ and Melan-A+

CK, *Cytokeratin;* MUC, *mucin.*

Prognosis and Treatment

Not surprisingly, whether or not there is a coexisting invasive carcinoma associated with Paget's disease has a dramatic effect on outcome. Noninvasive primary anal Paget's disease tends to follow an indolent course, although as much as 60% of patients managed by wide local excision develop recurrence of disease within 5 years. Recurrences are also frequently managed by wide local excision. Despite a tendency for recurrence, the long-term survival of patients with primary noninvasive anal Paget's disease is similar to that of normal age-matched people without Paget's disease.[249] Patients with an associated invasive carcinoma (primary vs. secondary often not distinguished in series) tend to suffer similar recurrences but significantly poorer disease-specific and overall survival.[271-273]

ANORECTAL MALIGNANT MELANOMA

Clinical Features and Pathogenesis

Melanomas of the anus account for 0.05% of all colorectal malignancies and 1% of anal malignancies diagnosed each year and about one-fourth of mucocutaneous melanomas.[274,275] The mean age at diagnosis is in the seventh decade of life. Women are affected almost twice as often as men.[274,276] There are no known risk factors for anal melanoma. Anal melanomas are thought to arise from malignant transformation of melanocytes that are normally present in the anal mucosa and transition zone. The clinical presentation is not unlike that seen for a variety of anal lesions, even those as innocuous as hemorrhoids or anal tags, and is characterized by bleeding, pain, or a mass lesion. These often mild and nonspecific features contribute to the typical late-stage presentation of anal melanomas.[277,278]

Molecular diagnostics are playing an increasingly important role in the characterization of all melanomas, including anorectal melanoma. There is a particular focus on treatment-determining somatic mutations. Most, if not all, of the clinically significant tests can be performed on formalin-fixed, paraffin-embedded tissue. The two most treatment-specific mutations tested in melanoma are *BRAF* and *KIT,* the results of which may determine therapy with BRAF inhibitors (e.g., vemurafenib) or tyrosine kinase inhibitors (e.g., imatinib or sunitinib), respectively. Activating codon 600 *BRAF* (most commonly p. V600E) mutations are relatively rare events in mucosal melanomas, occurring in up to 11% of lesions.[279-281] Other studies have found no *BRAF* V600E mutations in mucosal melanomas, including some anorectal-specific series.[282-285] *KIT* mutations are more frequent, occurring in about 26% of mucosal melanomas[286] and about 15% of anorectal melanomas.[285,287] Exons 9, 11, 13, and 17 are the most commonly analyzed in *KIT* mutation testing, and it seems that mutations in exons 11 and 13 may have the best possibility of treatment response to tyrosine kinase inhibitors.[288] Other driver mutations in *NF1* and *RAS* family occur in <10% of cases.[281] Immunotherapy has greatly advanced the treatment of cutaneous melanoma and has shown clinically relevant response rates in mucosal melanoma, albeit less commonly than in cutaneous melanoma, possibly resulting from lower tumor mutational burden.[289-292]

Pathology

Anal melanomas usually arise as a polypoid mass adjacent to, or at, the dentate line.[274] Gross pigmentation is uncommon, but microscopic foci of pigmentation may be found in up to 80% of cases. Pigmentation may be obscured by hemorrhage in the lesion. Anal melanomas demonstrate the same immunohistochemical and ultrastructural features as their cutaneous counterpart.[261,293] However, similar to melanomas that arise in other mucous membranes, they are typically of the acrolentiginous type. Invasive melanomas in this region are commonly epithelioid, although sarcomatous and desmoplastic melanomas have also been described[261] (Fig. 32.34).

Differential Diagnosis

The differentiation of anal melanomas from primary anal Paget's disease is discussed in the Paget's Disease of the Anus section earlier in this chapter. Similar to melanomas

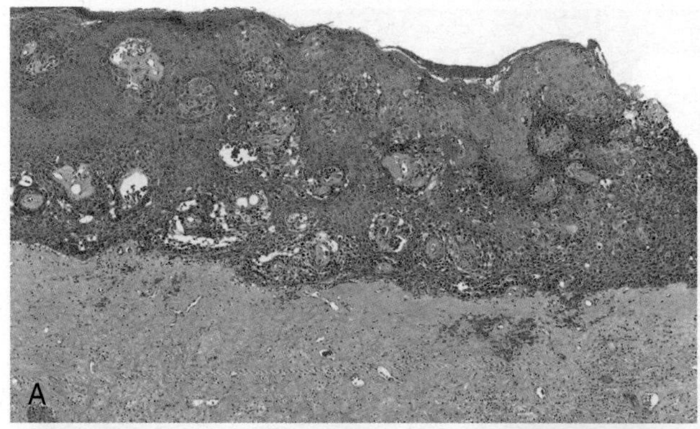

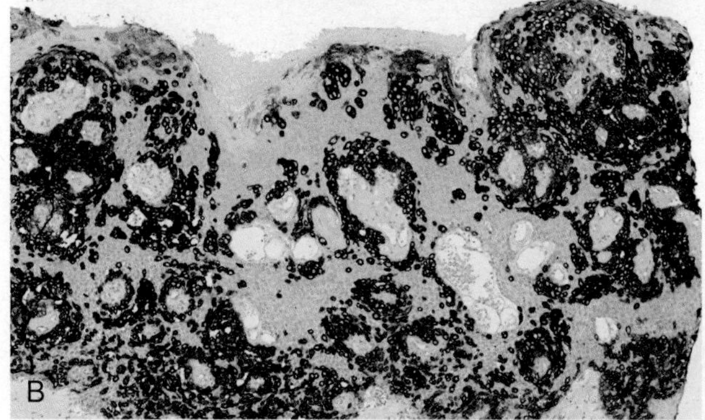

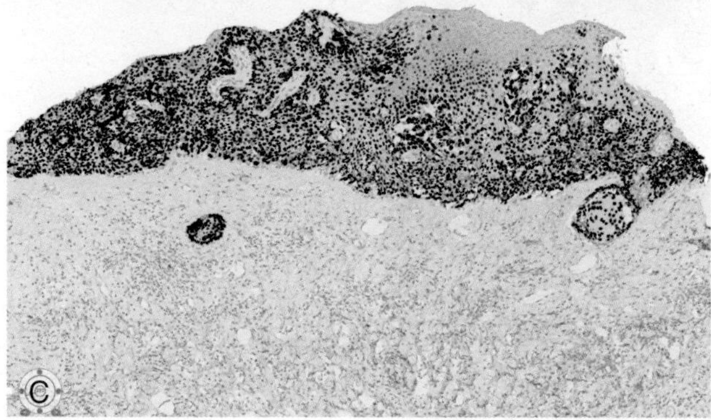

FIGURE 32.33 A, Pagetoid high-grade anal squamous intraepithelial neoplasia reveals enlarged, cytologically malignant epithelioid cells that are scattered singly or dispersed in small nests throughout squamous epithelium. These cells can have abundant pale eosinophilic cytoplasm, similar to primary and secondary Paget's disease of the anus. Often, differentiation can only be discerned through immunohistochemistry. **B,** Pagetoid squamous intraepithelial neoplasia can be CK7+, which is a diagnostic pitfall. **C,** It is also positive for squamous markers such as p63. These tumor cells were negative for mucin, PAS/D, CEA, GCDFP-15, and CK20.

that occur elsewhere, the histological features in support of an anal melanoma are the presence of a nested growth pattern as well as asymmetrical junctional changes in association with the appropriate immunohistochemical labeling pattern (positive for S100 protein/SOX10, HMB45, Melan-A, and other melanocytic markers, and negative for cytokeratins).[261,293] Junctional changes, although useful when present, may be obscured by ulceration. Furthermore, because melanomas may also extend proximally into the rectum, they may infiltrate colorectal mucosa in a manner analogous to lymphoma at that site. Negative immunohistochemical labeling for lymphoid markers (i.e., CD20, CD3, and CD45) should be helpful in ruling out this possibility.

Prognosis and Treatment

The prognosis of anal melanoma is poor. Reported 5-year survival rates range from 15% to 35%.[274,276,278,294,295] Survival rates are better in younger patients (i.e., 25 to 44 years of age).[274] The specific histological type of anal melanoma or lymph node status has not been shown consistently to correlate with survival; however, the thickness of the tumor (as measured from the top of the overlying intact mucosa or ulcerated tumor) and the presence of perineural invasion have been shown to be related to outcome.[293,295,296] Anal melanomas that measure 2 mm or less in thickness have a much more favorable prognosis than those that measure greater than 2 mm in thickness. There is no relationship between the type of surgical management (abdominoperineal resection vs. wide local excision) and either local recurrence or outcome, so current practice is to perform wide local excision if technically feasible.[294,295] Given the lack of benefit of radical surgery in the absence of large/bulky tumors, disease-free survival appears to be a function of distant spread rather than local control.[297]

OTHER RARE NEOPLASMS OF THE ANAL CANAL

Basal cell carcinoma may arise, rarely, from the perianal skin (Fig. 32.35A).[298,299] These are usually in the form of an ulcerated nodule with raised, pearly margins, similar to its cutaneous counterpart. The prognosis of basal cell carcinomas of this region is distinctly more favorable than that for squamous cell carcinomas of the anal canal, so differentiation of this tumor from a well-differentiated basaloid squamous carcinoma of the anal canal is clinically important. Basal cell carcinomas are quite characteristic from low power. They are often seen budding off the basal layer of the squamous epithelium rather than emerging from full-thickness squamous dysplasia in squamous cell carcinoma. Basal cell carcinomas also demonstrate peripheral palisading of the nuclei, often associated with artifactual clefts and/or mucinous-type stroma. Ber-EP4 immunohistochemical stain is typically positive in basal cell carcinoma and negative in squamous cell carcinoma.[300] Histologically, anal canal carcinomas with basaloid features often have more pronounced cytological atypia, greater numbers of mitoses, and, most importantly, lack defining features of basal cell carcinoma (Fig. 32.35B).

Other rare tumors of the anal region include apocrine adenocarcinoma, embryonal rhabdomyosarcoma, and malignant fibrous histocytoma.[301-303] Tumors from other sites may also involve the anus as a result of metastasis or direct extension. The most common source of metastatic tumor is colorectal carcinoma, although rare cases of renal, lung, or breast carcinoma metastatic to the anus have been reported.[29,304,305]

The full reference list may be accessed online *at Elsevier eBooks for Practicing Clinicians*.

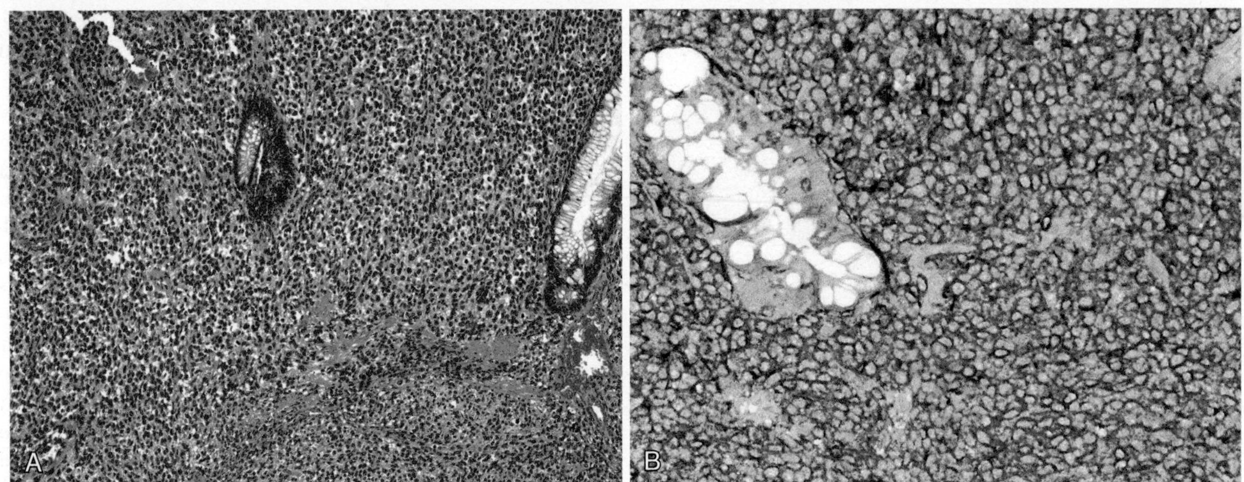

FIGURE 32.34 Anorectal melanoma. A, The mucosa of the upper anal canal/lower rectum is replaced by sheets and nests of atypical epithelioid cells. **B,** HMB45 is diffusely positive in this melanoma.

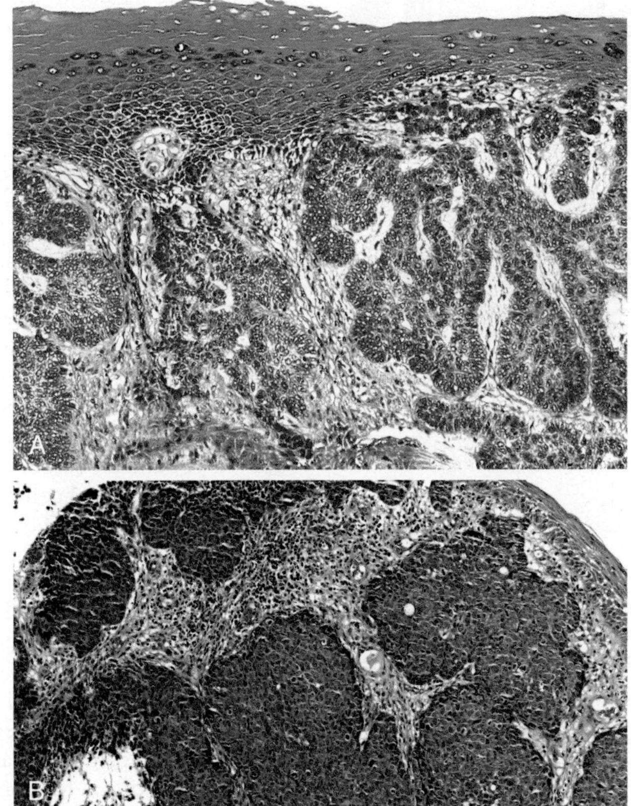

FIGURE 32.35 A, A true basal cell carcinoma of the distal anal canal/perianal skin. These exceedingly rare tumors are identical to basal cell carcinoma in sun-exposed skin, with prominent palisading of peripheral cells. **B,** Basaloid squamous cell carcinomas of the anus typically demonstrate more pronounced cytological atypia, a greater number of mitoses, and a lack of histological features classic of basal cell carcinoma.

PART 2

GALLBLADDER, EXTRAHEPATIC BILIARY TRACT, AND PANCREAS

CHAPTER 33

Algorithmic Approach to Diagnosis of Pancreatic Disorders

Natalie Ciomek, Robert D. Odze

Contents

INTRODUCTION

Normal Histology

Microscopically, the pancreas is composed of epithelium (acini, islets, and ducts), connective tissue, and lymphoid tissue. These components may be variably present within any individual pancreatic biopsy, depending on the location and adequacy of the tissue sample. The parenchyma is divided into lobules separated by loose connective tissue septa. Because the pancreas functions as both an exocrine (secretory) and endocrine organ, its parenchyma includes both exocrine and endocrine elements intimately mixed. The exocrine glands (acini) and their associated duct system comprise the majority of the lobular parenchyma and up to 85% of the total volume of the adult pancreas. The exocrine glands are composed of a single layer of triangular-shaped cells radially arranged to form spherical or tubular acini that each surround a central lumen. These acinar cells have round, basally-located nuclei with evenly distributed chromatin and small nucleoli. The cells appear granular because of their cytoplasmic secretory granules, including the basophilic basally located granules and the eosinophilic granules concentrated toward the lumen.

The duct system transports the luminal acinar secretions to the duodenum. This system begins with the intercalated ducts that drain each acinus. These ducts then fuse to form the intralobular ducts. The intralobular ducts converge to form the interlobular ducts and ultimately the large main pancreatic ducts. All of these ducts demonstrate a smooth and regular contour without angulation and vary in their epithelial lining. The intercalated ducts are lined by a single layer of cuboidal epithelium lacking mucin that transitions to columnar, mucinous epithelium within the larger pancreatic duct. Accessory mucous glands surround larger pancreatic ducts. The duct epithelial nuclei are round, basally located, and have evenly distributed chromatin.

The endocrine component is present primarily within the islets of Langerhans cells, which are randomly distributed throughout the pancreas. The islets are usually found as single, compact clusters of cells associated with a rich capillary network. They can also be seen as diffuse islets with ill-defined borders in the inferior portion of the pancreatic head. The cells within the islets are a mixed population of four major types, including beta, alpha, delta, and pancreatic polypeptide (PP) cells, each of which secrete a different hormone. These endocrine cells typically contain nuclei with coarsely clumped chromatin and abundant cytoplasm.

Variable amounts of connective tissue, including collagen and adipose tissue, are present within and outside the pancreas. In fact, the pancreatic parenchyma is divided into lobules by loose connective tissue septa supporting ducts, vessels, and nerves. The interlobular and main pancreatic ducts are surrounded by a thicker layer of collagen than the smaller ducts. Adipocytes can be scattered within the pancreas and are usually most abundant in the surrounding peripancreatic tissue. The distribution of collagen and fat in the pancreas is important to keep in mind when considering the location of a particular biopsy and whether it represents intraparenchymal or extraparenchymal tissue in the biopsy sample.

Lymphoid tissue may be present within the pancreas as intrapancreatic lymph nodes, lymphoid follicles, or small aggregates of lymphocytes. The lymphoid follicles include mucosa-associated lymphoid tissue (MALT). The follicles can be unstimulated primary follicles or secondary follicles with a germinal center. Small and mature lymphocytes, specifically T-lymphocytes, are the predominant cell population within the lymphoid tissue.

Plasma cells may be present within the lymphoid tissue as well. Normal, mature plasma cells show abundant deep blue cytoplasm and one to two nuclei with a coarse "clock face" chromatin pattern. A perinuclear clearing, or "hof," representing the prominent Golgi apparatus may be visible as well. Occasionally, intracellular or extracellular immunoglobulin in the form of a variably sized and well-circumscribed round pink structure may be present. The coarse nuclear chromatin pattern and abundant cytoplasm of the plasma cell may appear similar to the endocrine cell histology described earlier. Anecdotally, endocrine cells and plasma cells can be difficult to distinguish from each other, particularly during an intraoperative frozen-section consultation. In scenarios in which neoplastic plasma cells are suspected and cannot be confirmed immediately, fresh tissue may be processed or held for immediate or future flow-cytometry studies, respectively.

Inflammation of the Pancreas

Inflammatory cells found outside of normal lymphoid tissue are considered abnormal, especially in the setting of active epithelial injury (such as in acute pancreatitis) and/or the chronic reactive changes of stromal fibrosis (chronic pancreatitis). In acute pancreatitis, destruction of acinar parenchyma is accompanied by varying amounts of necrosis and acute inflammation including neutrophils and/or eosinophils. Chronic pancreatitis is believed to occur secondary to multiple episodes of acinar cell destruction followed by an associated inflammatory response. This response stimulates repeated tissue reactions, leading to increased stromal fibrosis and changes to the residual ductal epithelium. These ducts retain a lobular configuration despite the atrophic or absent parenchyma in chronic pancreatitis. They are arranged in lobules such that a larger branched duct is surrounded by smaller round ductules. The stroma between lobules is denser than within the lobules. These residual ducts demonstrate smooth contours without sharp angles and a complete epithelial lining. The lining is made of relatively uniform cells without significant variations in their nuclear sizes. Histologically, the inflammation present in a biopsy of chronic pancreatitis is typically composed of a lymphocytic or lymphoplasmacytic population of cells. If clinically significant inflammation is present in a benign biopsy, the predominant inflammatory cell type and assessment of the type and degree of connective tissue often helps pathologists subclassify the type of pancreatitis. Accurate subclassification of an inflammatory process is clinically important because some diseases, such as autoimmune pancreatitis (AIP), are steroid responsive.

APPROACH TO THE INTERPRETATION OF PANCREATIC BIOPSIES

General Comments

Pancreatic biopsies are most often performed for evaluation of a tumor, mass, or ill-defined lesion on imaging. Thus the main primary differential diagnosis of a pancreatic lesion typically includes neoplasia versus an inflammatory process that may, both clinically and radiologically, mimic a neoplasm. As discussed previously, chronic pancreatitis–associated lesions are believed to develop as a result of multiple repeated episodes of acinar cell destruction and subsequent inflammatory response within the parenchyma. Inflammation then stimulates repeated tissue reactions that lead to increased levels of stromal fibrosis. This stromal fibrosis can appear as a lesion radiologically, which ultimately leads to tissue sampling.

Biopsies of the pancreas can be obtained via endoscopic retrograde cholangiopancreatography or endoscopic ultrasound. Endoscopic ultrasound evaluates the pancreatic head and uncinate process through the duodenum. The pancreatic body and tail are imaged via the stomach. If clinically indicated, these areas of the pancreas can be sampled along with the proximal lymph nodes. As noted earlier, these biopsies can vary in the amount of pancreatic epithelium, connective tissue, and lymphoid tissue present.

An artifact to consider related to the tissue acquisition procedure and subsequent laboratory processing is poor fixation caused by pancreatic autolytic enzymes. Reasons for additional variations of normal pancreatic histology include patient age and the precise anatomical location of the biopsy. For example, the endocrine component is relatively increased in neonates compared with adults and can compose up to 20% of the organ. Also, diffuse islets of Langerhans can mimic a neoplastic process and are concentrated in the inferior portion of the pancreatic head.

In this chapter, we suggest an approach to pancreatic biopsies based broadly on the type and degree of the cellular and inflammatory components of the sample (Fig. 33.1). With this approach, one can often place a biopsy into one of several major histological patterns of injury from which a more narrow differential diagnosis can be generated, often with the help of additional clinical or serological studies. When evaluating a biopsy, major patterns of disease include the presence of (1) normal or near-normal–appearing tissue, (2) acute pancreatitis–like changes, (3) granulomatous inflammation, and (4) chronic pancreatitis–like changes. These patterns of disease are discussed more thoroughly and individually in the remainder of this chapter.

Because most pancreatic biopsies are performed for evaluation of a targeted lesion, the first step of a pathologist is to determine whether a biopsy is simply benign (inflammatory) or malignant. This can be challenging when a tumor, specifically carcinoma, is desmoplastic and/or the inflammatory process is quite fibrotic, as in some forms of chronic pancreatitis, particularly the autoimmune types. Relative to the normal highly cellular acinar/endocrine parenchyma, the normal pancreas contains only a minimal amount of stromal connective tissue. This connective tissue includes varying amounts of collagen organized around pancreatic ducts, between lobules, and within the peripancreatic tissue. Thus it is histologically "striking" when one sees an increase in paucicellular connective tissue relative to atrophic or absent parenchyma on a biopsy, and this should always raise concern for a malignant tumor.

Increases in connective tissue can be present in both epithelial malignancies and chronic pancreatitis. The most common epithelial malignancy of the pancreas, pancreatic ductal adenocarcinoma, typically displays desmoplastic stroma. Chronic inflammatory, or "chronic pancreatitis-like," diseases can demonstrate a "fibroinflammatory" histological pattern, which includes significant stromal fibrosis

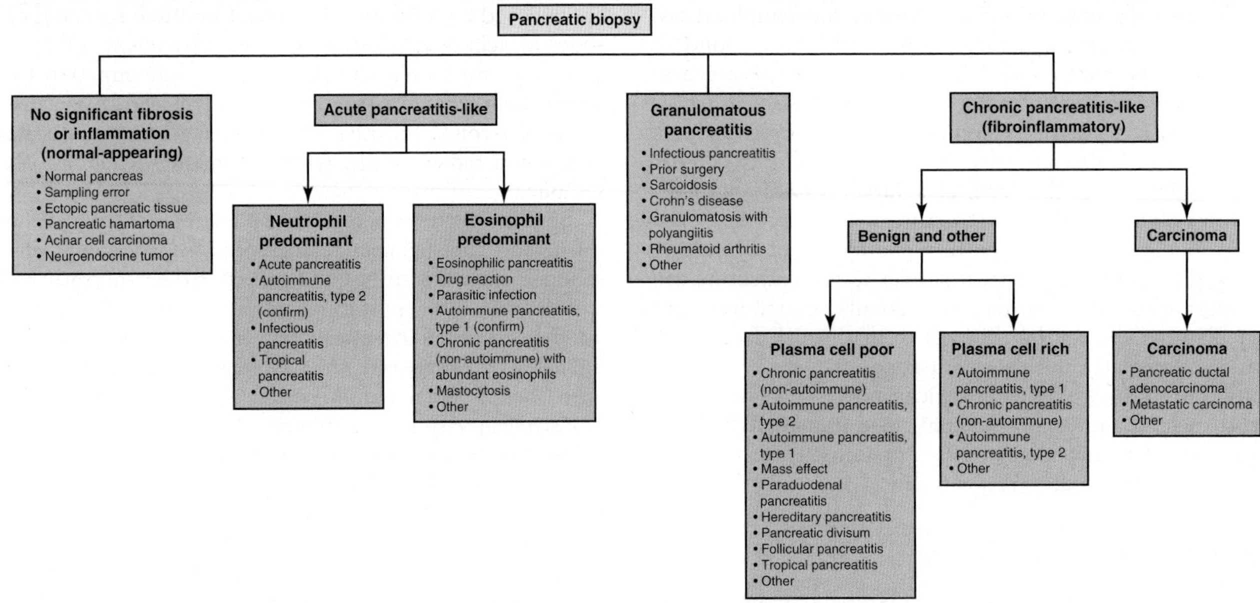

FIGURE 33.1 Algorithmic approach to the diagnosis of inflammatory disorders of the pancreas.

accompanied by variable amounts of inflammation. Thus an initial assessment of connective tissue may be the first step in assessing a biopsy as benign or malignant.

After an epithelial malignancy, such as pancreatic ductal adenocarcinoma or metastatic carcinoma, is excluded, the presence, type, and amount of inflammation relative to fibrosis, if present, will help further subclassify the biopsy. Inflammation in the pancreas may include neutrophils, eosinophils, histiocytes (and granulomas), lymphocytes, and plasma cells. Active inflammation without granulomas or increased stromal fibrosis suggests acute pancreatitis or an "acute pancreatitis–like pattern" of injury. The inflammatory cells in an acute pancreatitis–like pattern are typically neutrophils and/or eosinophils. A fibroinflammatory pattern, as described later in this chapter, consists of increased fibrosis relative to inflammation. The chronic inflammatory cells are typically lymphocytes with variable amounts of plasma cells. Biopsies without significant inflammation, granulomas, or stromal fibrosis are considered *normal* or *near-normal*.

The Normal (or Near-Normal)–Appearing Biopsy

One of the biggest initial challenges for a pathologist when evaluating a pancreatic biopsy is the determination of whether a biopsy represents normal parenchyma and thus may not be representative of the patient's "lesion." Therefore knowledge of the normal anatomy, location of the biopsy, and artifacts or variations of tissue that can lead to confusion is important. For the most part, if the biopsy demonstrates normal parenchymal histology without desmoplastic stroma, stromal fibrosis, and significant inflammation, it can be considered normal or near-normal appearing.

A normal-appearing biopsy can represent a normal pancreas, sampling error, or other disorders such as ectopic pancreatic tissue or rarely, a pancreatic hamartoma. An *ectopic pancreas* refers to benign pancreatic tissue that is present outside of its normal anatomical location. Pancreatic hamartomas are disorganized proliferations and disordered arrangements of normal, benign pancreatic epithelial and connective tissue elements (see Chapter 40 for further details).

However, even when a biopsy lacks overt desmoplastic or fibrotic stroma, malignant entities to consider in the differential include acinar cell carcinoma and neuroendocrine tumor. Acinar cell carcinomas (Fig. 33.2) are highly cellular neoplasms that lack a desmoplastic stromal response typical of ductal adenocarcinomas. The tumor cells appear monotonous and well organized, and they are arranged in acinar structures that may closely resemble normal pancreatic parenchyma. On high-power view, atypical prominent large nucleoli and mitoses may be present. Pancreatic neuroendocrine tumors can also demonstrate a range of morphological patterns, some of which include an organized glandular differentiation of normal, or almost normal-appearing, endocrine cells without desmoplastic stroma. Most benign (normal) islets of Langerhans are compact structures that contain a heterogeneous population of its four major cell types. The four major cell types in decreasing order of frequency within the islet are beta, alpha, delta, and pancreatic polypeptide (PP) cells. Beta cells comprise the majority of the islets and produce insulin. Alpha cells secrete glucagon, delta cells produce somatostatin, and PP cells contain a unique type of pancreatic polypeptide. The presence of larger, more confluent, or diffuse collections of endocrine cells that appear more homogeneous in type suggests a neoplastic process. Immunohistochemistry for the specific endocrine peptides may be used to identify the type, extent, and location of endocrine cells in a suspected lesion to try and differentiate a clonal population of neoplastic cells from normal or hyperplastic islets (see Chapters 29 and 41 for further details). Of note is that diffuse collections of islets of Langerhans can mimic a neoplastic process, and these are typically concentrated in the inferior portion of the pancreatic head.

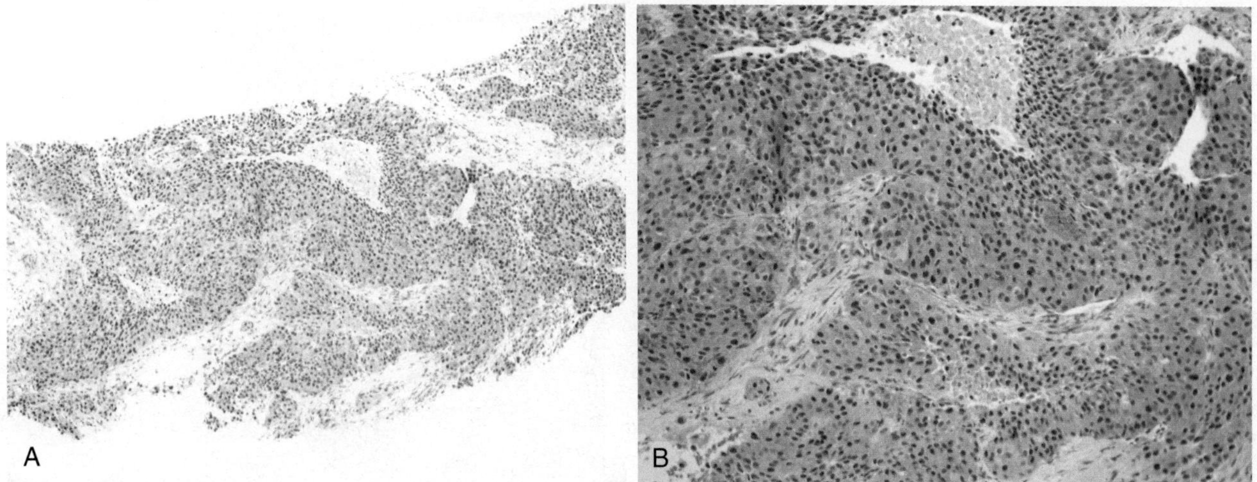

FIGURE 33.2 Acinar cell carcinomas demonstrate a solid growth pattern of monotonous tumor cells **(A)** and typically lack a desmoplastic stroma **(B)**.

Acute Pancreatitis-Like Pattern of Injury

Patients with acute pancreatitis may undergo biopsy, especially if a cyst or masslike lesion (such as an abscess) is identified clinically, and a malignant process cannot be ruled out. An acute pancreatitis-like pattern of injury is characterized by the presence of significant active inflammation (composed of neutrophils, eosinophils, or both), either with or without tissue necrosis, but typically without an increase in stromal fibrosis. Acute pancreatitis is usually diagnosed clinically and only rarely by tissue alone. Nevertheless, biopsies or even small residual pancreatic fragments noted during surgery (e.g., pancreatic necrosectomy) may be submitted for histological examination to rule out metastasis. In addition, rarely, pancreatic neoplasms can present clinically with symptoms and signs of acute pancreatitis. Microscopic foci of resolving acute pancreatitis can be seen adjacent to a pancreatic neoplasm.

In acute pancreatitis, the tissue usually demonstrates variable necrosis accompanied by neutrophil- or eosinophil-predominant acute inflammatory infiltrates. When this pattern of injury is noted in biopsies, it is often helpful to formulate the differential diagnosis based on the predominant inflammatory cell (neutrophilic vs. eosinophilic).

Neutrophil-Predominant Acute Pancreatitis

A neutrophil predominant acute pancreatitis pattern of inflammation and injury is most commonly seen in patients with acute pancreatitis secondary to obstructive or toxic causes. The pancreas can demonstrate a variable degree of tissue necrosis. The amount of necrosis is often proportional to the severity of the inflammation, with milder inflammation present focally in the interlobular septa and severe inflammation demonstrating diffuse necrosis of both acinar and ductal tissue. Damage to the vasculature can also result in diffuse hemorrhage, or "hemorrhagic pancreatitis." The most common etiologies of neutrophil-predominant acute pancreatitis are duct obstruction secondary to gallstones or a neoplasm, or toxic causes such as alcohol and drugs. Prominent neutrophils can also be seen in cases of AIP, particularly AIP type 2. Though classified as chronic pancreatitis, AIP type 2 demonstrates increased neutrophils within its characteristic granulocytic epithelial lesions associated with ductal ulceration and ductular and lobular abscesses. Additionally, it features a dense periductal lymphoplasmacytic infiltrate that distinguishes it from other forms of chronic pancreatitis.

Lastly, infectious pancreatitis and other rare entities, such as tropical pancreatitis, may also manifest as a neutrophil-predominant acute pancreatitis–like pattern of injury. Infectious pancreatitis is rare in immunocompetent hosts but may be seen in immunocompromised patients. Infectious pancreatitis may be caused by a variety of microorganisms, including viruses, fungi, and parasites. The most common viruses include hepatotropic viruses in post–liver transplant patients, Coxsackie virus type B, cytomegalovirus, and HIV. A rare case of aspergillus was reported as a cause for acute pancreatitis at autopsy. Candida has been previously associated with acute pancreatitis, but is postulated to complicate acute necrotizing pancreatitis rather than cause it. Lastly, parasites such as *Ascaris lumbricoides and Clonorchis sinensis* can cause acute pancreatitis.[1] The infiltrate usually contains neutrophils, but it can also present with increased eosinophils typical of a parasitic infection. Tropical pancreatitis usually presents with significant intralobular and interlobular fibrosis, with large intraductal calculi at an advanced stage. If a biopsy is performed at an earlier stage, neutrophils may comprise a more significant proportion of the inflammatory infiltrate.

Eosinophil-Predominant Acute Pancreatitis

An eosinophil-predominant acute pancreatitis can develop as a primary pancreatic process or secondary to a systemic disease. When this pattern is noted on biopsy, it can be further evaluated by noting the presence or absence of accompanying mixed inflammation and/or infiltration present predominantly as eosinophilic microabscesses. For instance, diffuse inflammation composed exclusively, or almost exclusively, of eosinophils raises the possibility of eosinophilic pancreatitis. Histologically, the dense eosinophilic infiltrate is present around ducts, acini, and interlobular septa. Eosinophilic phlebitis and arteritis may also be present. Rarely, a mature eosinophilic infiltrate may secondarily involve the pancreas in hypereosinophilic syndrome and clonal myeloid neoplasms with eosinophilia, such as chronic eosinophilic leukemia.[2]

If eosinophilic microabscesses are the primary pattern of eosinophilic infiltration, parasitic infections, and hematopoietic entities such as Langerhans cell histiocytosis (LCH) and Kimura disease should be considered. Parasitic infections can be accompanied by increased peripheral blood eosinophilia in addition to tissue infiltration. *Ascaris lumbricoides* is an example of a parasite that may enter the pancreas via the pancreatic duct system and cause necrosis, abscess formation, and granulomatous inflammation. Though typically presenting in the neck, Kimura disease, an IgG4-related disease, can affect the pancreas. It is a benign idiopathic chronic inflammatory disorder in which eosinophilic microabscesses are present in a background of mixed inflammation. Collections of eosinophils can accompany the grooved Langerhans cells of LCH.

Inflammatory processes composed of increased eosinophils relative to the presence of other inflammatory cell types include hypersensitivity and allergic illnesses. Both can present with an eosinophil-predominant mixed inflammatory infiltrate, typically without overt microabscesses.

Eosinophils may also represent a significant proportion of the inflammatory reaction in patients with AIP, particularly AIP type 1, and chronic pancreatitis, mainly the nonautoimmune type. Eosinophils are identified in virtually every case of AIP type 1. Some cases demonstrate such a marked eosinophilic infiltrate, which suggests the possibility of eosinophilic pancreatitis. However, the presence of other histological features, such as a dense lymphoplasmacytic infiltrate including increased IgG4-positive plasma cells, storiform-type fibrosis, and obliterative phlebitis, can help separate the former from the latter disorders. Chronic pancreatitis, especially of the nonautoimmune type, may also present with increased eosinophils that accompany the predominant lymphocytic or lymphoplasmacytic inflammation.

Granulomatous Pancreatitis

Although not a common pattern of injury seen in pancreatic biopsies, granulomatous inflammation in the pancreas (Fig. 33.3) raises the possibility of disorders that often have systemic implications. Common causes include infections, the effects of prior surgery, and rarely other disorders such as Crohn disease, sarcoidosis, rheumatoid arthritis, granulomatosis with polyangiitis (formerly known as *Wegener granulomatosis*), and others.

Infectious agents that may cause granulomatous pancreatitis include tuberculosis, fungus, and parasites such as *Ascaris lumbricoides*. Tuberculosis pancreatitis demonstrates necrotizing granulomatous inflammation and presence of the mycobacterium bacteria by acid-fast stain on histochemistry, a positive culture, and/or diagnostic polymerase chain reaction (PCR) testing. Rare fungal infections, such as aspergillus, can manifest in the pancreas.[3] Parasites such as *Ascaris lumbricoides* can enter the organ via the pancreatic duct system and cause necrosis, abscess formation, granulomatous inflammation, and fibrosis.

Noncaseating granulomas including foreign-body giant cell reactions can be present in biopsies in patients who have had prior surgery in the area. Crohn disease can show epithelioid granulomas accompanied by chronic inflammation. These patients invariably have a documented history of disease in the gastrointestinal tract. Systemic inflammatory diseases featuring granulomas include sarcoidosis, granulomatosis with polyangiitis, and rheumatoid arthritis. Sarcoidosis features confluent granulomas and adjacent lymphadenopathy. Granulomatosis with polyangiitis demonstrates "dirty" necrosis, giant cells, and poorly formed granulomas. Vasculitis is seldom seen on pancreatic biopsy. Rheumatoid arthritis can rarely affect the pancreas and shows rheumatoid nodules composed of central areas of necrobiosis, palisading histiocytes, and a dense lymphoplasmacytic infiltrate at the rim of the nodule.

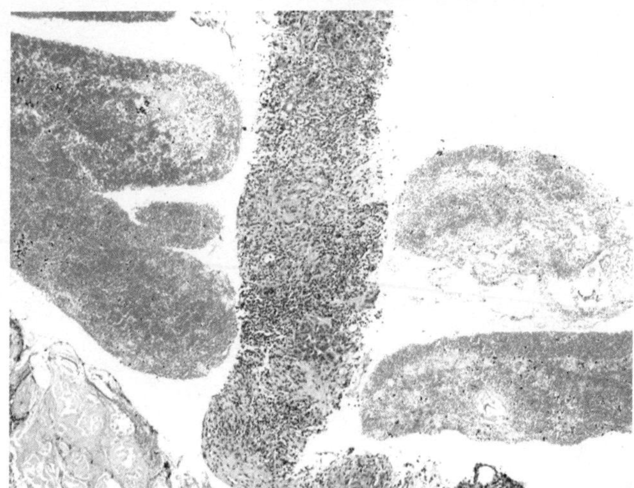

FIGURE 33.3 Idiopathic granulomatous pancreatitis demonstrating a poorly formed granuloma in a background of chronic inflammation.

Chronic Pancreatitis-like ("Fibro-inflammatory") Pattern of Injury

Chronic pancreatitis is a fibroinflammatory disorder in which the pancreatic acinar compartment of the pancreas becomes replaced by interlobular and/or intralobular fibrosis (Fig. 33.4). As previously discussed, increases in stromal fibrosis can appear clinically and radiologically as a pancreatic mass or lesion and thus mimic a malignant tumor, most often ductal adenocarcinoma. Additionally, increases in connective tissue ("desmoplasia") can be prominent in some pancreatic ductal adenocarcinomas, and this may also be accompanied by a variable degree of mostly lymphocytic inflammation.

Thus the first step in the approach of a biopsy that shows a fibroinflammatory infiltrate, particularly in a patient with a mass lesion, is to exclude a malignancy such as pancreatic ductal adenocarcinoma, the most common epithelial primary pancreatic malignancy. This is discussed more thoroughly in the next section and in Chapter 41.

Benign (And Other) Versus Malignant Epithelial Neoplasms

Increases in connective tissue can be present in both epithelial malignancies and chronic pancreatitis (see Chapter 40 and 41 for further details). The most common epithelial malignancy of the pancreas, pancreatic ductal adenocarcinoma, typically displays desmoplastic stroma (Fig. 33.5). Chronic inflammatory, or "chronic pancreatitis-like," diseases can demonstrate a "fibroinflammatory" histological

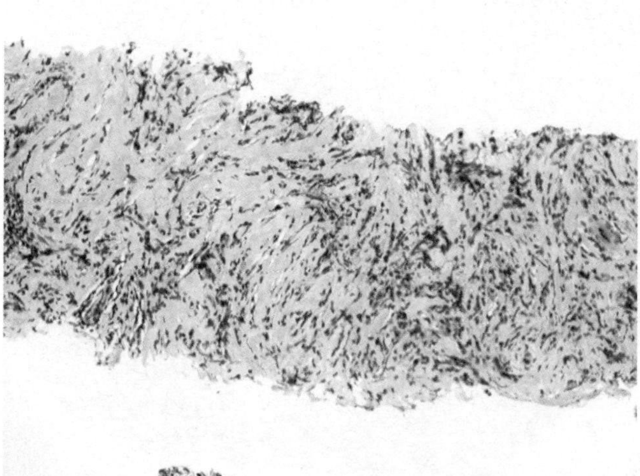

FIGURE 33.4 Chronic pancreatitis, nonautoimmune type, featuring lymphocytic inflammation and increased stromal fibrosis.

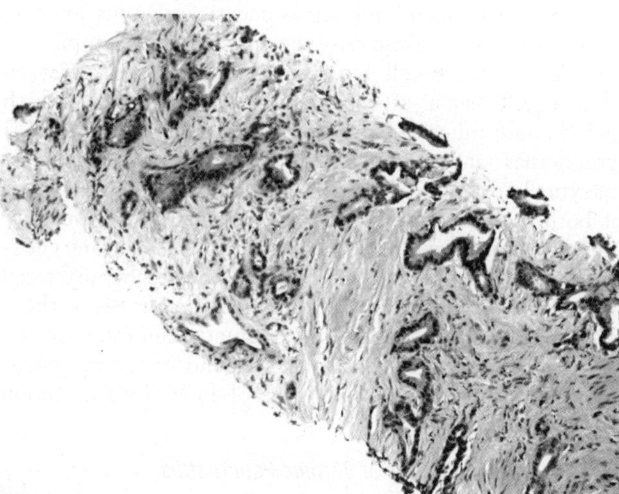

FIGURE 33.5 Pancreatic ductal adenocarcinoma with prominent stromal desmoplasia.

pattern, which includes significant stromal fibrosis accompanied by variable amounts of inflammation. Thus initial assessment of connective tissue may be the first step in assessing a biopsy as benign or malignant. However, differentiating between desmoplasia and stromal fibrosis alone can be difficult. Assessment of the epithelium in these biopsies is helpful in determining whether an epithelial malignancy is present.

The ductal epithelium in ductal adenocarcinoma can appear deceptively bland, whereas the ducts in chronic pancreatitis may appear "invasive." Assessment of the organization of the epithelium within the stroma, location of the glands relative to other tissue structures, and cytological features is helpful.[4-6] The lobular acinar parenchyma can be atrophic or absent in fibroinflammatory chronic pancreatitis. However, ducts remain and will feature some sort of organization, in contrast with the typically haphazard neoplastic growth of ductal adenocarcinoma. Residual benign ductules still retain a lobular configuration, such that a larger, branched, and dilated duct is surrounded by smaller round ductules. The stroma within each lobular cluster is less dense than the stroma between separate lobules. In contrast, invasive glands lack an organized lobular growth pattern and are distributed irregularly. Invasive glands can be located near or within nerves, vascular stroma, and adipose tissue, all of which are atypical findings not normally present in chronic pancreatitis.

The ducts of chronic pancreatitis demonstrate regularity, relatively smooth contours without sharp angles, and a complete lining. In contrast, carcinomatous ductal epithelium can be incomplete, lining only part of the neoplastic lumen, and often with sharp angulations. Cytologically, the ductal cells of chronic pancreatitis demonstrate uniform cells relative to a preserved nuclear-to-cytoplasm ratio and nuclear size, basophilic cytoplasm, and no bizarre nuclear morphology. In contrast, nuclear enlargement, variation of nuclear volume among cells greater than a ratio of 4:1, and acidophilic cytoplasm are suspicious for carcinoma. Additionally, individual and morphologically atypical cells within the stroma of the pancreas are much more likely to be carcinoma, as the fibrous stroma of a chronic pancreatitis contains rare bland fibroblasts.

When the pathologist has confirmed that the biopsy under consideration is "benign" (inflammatory), and thus most likely represents a form of chronic pancreatitis, the next step in the evaluation process is to determine the cause of pancreatitis as best as possible within the limits of an individual biopsy sample. Of course, this often requires clinical and serological correlation and even consultation with the treating physician to narrow down the differential diagnosis. In this differential diagnosis, we find it helpful to evaluate the type and degree of inflammation in the biopsy to help determine the most likely cause of the patient's inflammatory condition.

Most cases of chronic pancreatitis are accompanied by lymphoplasmacytic inflammation composed of variable proportions of small lymphocytes and plasma cells. The degree of plasma cell infiltration assists in further subclassifying the patient's chronic pancreatitis. For instance, a biopsy that shows increased plasma cells relative to lymphocytes (considered *plasma cell–rich* in our algorithm) raises the likelihood of certain types of chronic pancreatitis in contrast with those that are plasma cell–poor compared with lymphocytes. This is discussed more thoroughly in the next section.

Plasma Cell–Rich Forms of Chronic Pancreatitis

Plasma cell–rich chronic pancreatitis patterns can be present in biopsies of a variety of disorders, but it is more common in some compared with others. For instance, AIP (more commonly in type 1 than type 2), chronic pancreatitis (nonautoimmune), and hematopoietic neoplasms are all conditions that should be considered in this differential diagnosis and are ranked generally in order of prevalence. Plasma cell–rich chronic pancreatitis most commonly represents AIP type 1, the pancreatic manifestation of IgG4-related disease (Fig. 33.6). In this type of AIP, the plasma cells appear mature, contain one to two nuclei, are polyclonal, and have a background of storiform fibrotic stroma often accompanied by obliterative phlebitis. The plasma cells are predominantly of the IgG4 type, which can be assessed by immunohistochemistry. Typically, greater than 50 IgG4-positive plasma cells per high-power field are present in

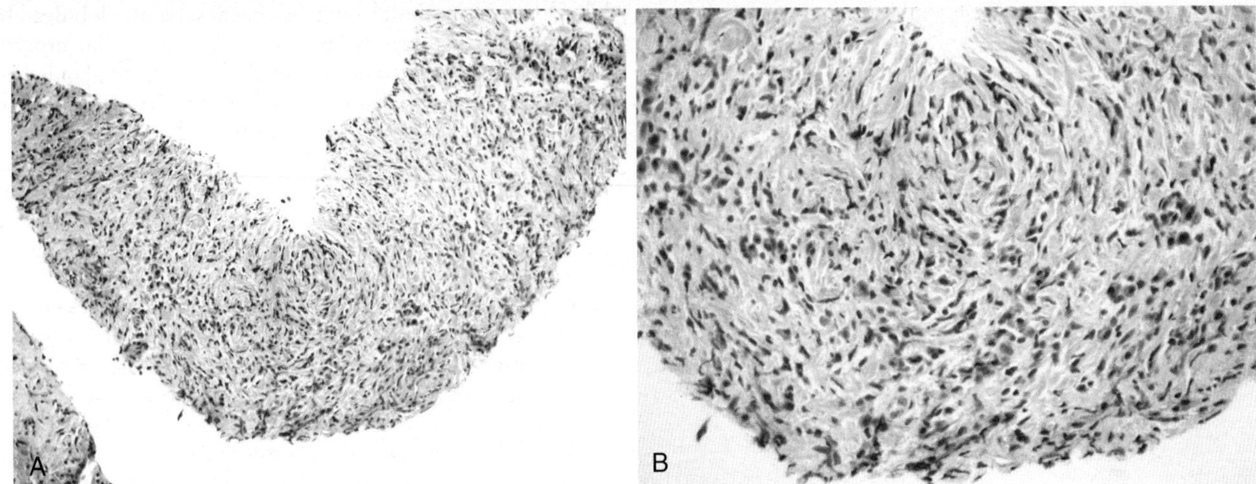

FIGURE 33.6 Autoimmune pancreatitis, type 1, with increased stromal fibrosis **(A)** and a plasma cell–rich chronic pancreatitis-like pattern **(B)**.

AIP type 1. However, this interpretation may be limited by the smaller sampling of a biopsy and a possible patchy distribution of disease. Clinically, serum IgG4 levels are also increased. A concentration of greater than 135 mg/dL has been accepted as the minimum value for a diagnosis for IgG-related disease; however, the specificity of this test is improved when the threshold is set at two times normal, at 280 mg/dL. In AIP type 2, plasma cells may also be present, albeit much less than in AIP type 1. Unlike AIP type 1, IgG4-positive plasma cells are not increased or predominant by immunohistochemistry, and serum IgG4 levels are not increased in AIP type 2. Plasma cells may be rarely increased in other forms of chronic pancreatitis (nonautoimmune). Usually, such plasma cells are present in the late stage of alcoholic chronic pancreatitis. IgG4-positive plasma cells are not increased by immunohistochemistry, and serum IgG4 levels are not increased in chronic nonautoimmune pancreatitis.

Markedly increased plasma cells can be seen in a variety of other disorders more rarely, for instance, hematopoietic neoplasms including plasma cell neoplasms and lymphoma. Plasma cell neoplasms are composed of atypical and clonal plasma cells. Plasma cells can demonstrate atypical morphologies including multinucleation and the presence of three or more nuclei, increased nuclear-to-cytoplasm ratio (most dramatically in plasmablasts that feature a high nuclear-to-cytoplasm ratio), and increased immunoglobulin deposition. Clonality of the plasma cells can be determined in several ways. If fresh tissue is available, flow cytometry for surface or cytoplasmic kappa and lambda light-chain expression can be performed. On formalin-fixed tissue, immunohistochemistry or fluorescence in situ hybridization (FISH) for kappa and lambda light chains can assess for light-chain restriction. Kappa or lambda light-chain restriction is designated when the kappa-to-lambda ratio is significantly greater than 4 (kappa light-chain restriction) or less than 1 (lambda light-chain restriction). Additionally, amyloid deposition can mimic stromal fibrosis and be accompanied by increased plasma cells. Demonstrating Congo red birefringence under polarized light can confirm the presence of amyloid. Mass spectrometry can further subtype the amyloid deposition.

Finally, significant lymphoplasmacytic inflammation may be so extensive as to also raise the possibility of a lymphoma. Several mature B-cell lymphomas can feature increased plasma cells such as marginal zone lymphomas, which include both mucosa-associated lymphoid tissue ("MALT") lymphomas and extranodal subtypes, and lymphoplasmacytic lymphomas (LPLs). The atypical B-lymphocytes of both marginal-zone lymphomas and LPLs demonstrate nonspecific immunohistochemical profiles. Aberrant coexpression of CD43 and BCL2 by immunohistochemistry can be present on nongerminal-center B-lymphocytes in these lymphomas. Additionally, flow cytometry can establish the monoclonality of the B-lymphocytes and/or the accompanying plasma cells. Demonstration of an *MYD88* mutation is diagnostic of LPL.

Plasma Cell–Poor Forms of Chronic Pancreatitis

A biopsy that shows increased stromal fibrosis accompanied by lymphocytic inflammation, but without a significant plasma cell population, is typically seen in nonautoimmune cases of chronic pancreatitis, AIP type 2, paraduodenal ("groove") pancreatitis, and tropical pancreatitis. Additionally, similar histological features can be present related to a mechanical effect on the pancreas, including "mass effect" (or tissue in the proximity of a mass). A marked, diffuse lymphocytic infiltrate raises the possibility of a lymphoma.

Chronic (nonautoimmune) pancreatitis, most often secondary to obstructive and toxic causes, demonstrates relatively acellular fibrosis and variable lymphocytic inflammation. Most of the inflammation is caused by small lymphocytes in the tissue and within lymphoid aggregates. Plasma cells are usually rare in these types of chronic pancreatitis. AIP type 2 demonstrates a dense periductal lymphoplasmacytic infiltrate but with typically fewer plasma cells than type 1, in which IgG4-positive plasma cells are the predominant inflammatory cell type. Paraduodenal pancreatitis *(groove pancreatitis)* features a sparse lymphocytic infiltrate with marked fibrosis extending from the duodenal wall (see Chapter 40 for details). Increased smooth muscle cells or myofibroblasts can be associated with the fibrosis. Usually, multiple cysts with proteinaceous material are present. Tropical pancreatitis

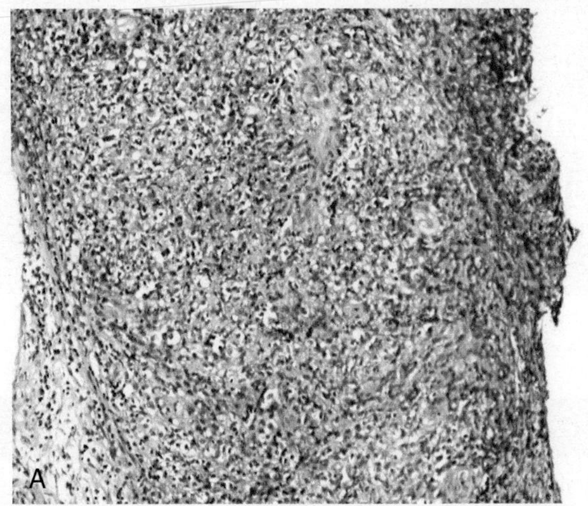

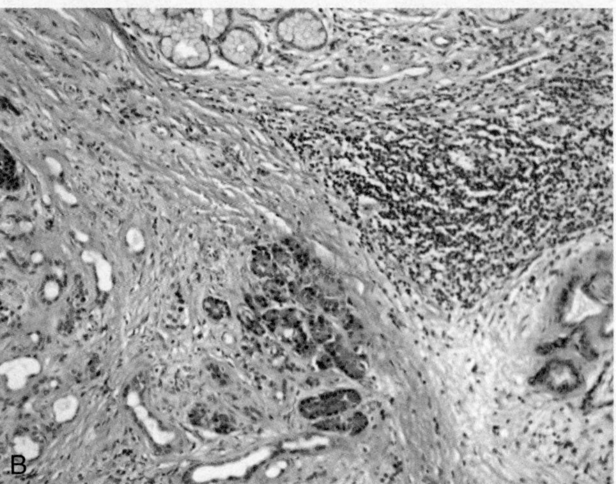

FIGURE 33.7 Diffuse large B-cell lymphoma of the pancreas **(A)** featuring a diffuse infiltrate of atypical lymphocytes in contrast to the well-circumscribed lymphoid aggregates that may be present in benign pancreatic biopsies, such as chronic pancreatitis **(B).**

can resemble chronic pancreatitis (nonautoimmune) with intralobular and interlobular fibrosis and a sparse inflammatory infiltrate. However, large intraductal calculi will be present in the main duct, and the disease will manifest in a younger age group than that of chronic pancreatitis secondary to toxic or obstructive causes. "Mass effect," or tissue in the proximity of a mass, includes marked fibrosis and a mixed inflammatory infiltrate composed of lymphocytes admixed with acute inflammatory cells including neutrophils.

A differential diagnosis of lymphoma is raised when small lymphocytes are markedly increased and are the predominant cell population. B-cell lymphomas are more common than T-cell lymphomas. Secondary involvement of the pancreas by a lymphoma arising in another location is more common than a primary pancreatic lymphoma. The most common primary pancreatic lymphoma is diffuse large B-cell lymphoma (DLBCL),[7] which presents with atypical, enlarged medium- to large-sized lymphocytes with prominent nucleoli (Fig. 33.7). In contrast, when a monotonous population of small lymphomas are present, the differential diagnosis includes small lymphocytic leukemia/lymphoma (CLL/SLL), follicular lymphoma, mantle cell lymphoma, and marginal zone lymphomas including the previously described MALT and extranodal lymphomas. All B-lymphocytic lymphomas will demonstrate clonal B-lymphocytes by flow-cytometry studies. Additionally, some lymphomas will have a typical immunophenotype to that entity that can be further assessed by flow cytometry and/or immunohistochemistry. The B-lymphocytes of CLL/SLL will typically aberrantly coexpress CD5 and CD23 by flow cytometry and immunohistochemistry. Follicular lymphoma is composed of B-lymphocytes that are positive for CD10 and BCL6 and aberrantly coexpress BCL2, the product of the t(14;18) translocation that can be assessed by FISH studies. Mantle cell lymphomas features atypical B-lymphocytes that coexpress CD5 and cyclin D1. Cyclin D1, also known as *BCL1*, is a product of the diagnostic t(11;14) translocation that can be assessed by FISH studies to confirm mantle cell lymphoma.

ACKNOWLEDGMENTS

The authors thank Dr. Kimberly Kado, MD, for providing all figures in this chapter.

The full reference list may be accessed online at *Elsevier eBooks for Practicing Clinicians*.

CHAPTER 34

Gallbladder, Extrahepatic Biliary Tract, and Pancreas Tissue Processing Techniques and Normal Histology

James M. Crawford

Chapter Outline

INTRODUCTION

Disorders of the biliary tract affect a significant portion of the world's population. More than 95% of biliary tract disease is attributable to cholecystitis and cholelithiasis (i.e., gallstones). It is estimated that about 20 million persons in the United States have gallstones.[1] The annual cost of treatment for gallbladder disease was estimated in 2014 to exceed $4 billion, representing approximately 0.1% of the national health care budget.[2] More than 900,000 cholecystectomies are performed annually in the United States, making it one of the most common abdominal operations performed.[3,4] There are 1200 deaths per year in the United States from cholelithiasis and its complications[2]; the presence of gallstones imparts an increased risk of death in individuals with other morbidities such as cardiovascular disease and cancer.[5]

Carcinoma of the pancreas is the fifth most frequent cause of death from cancer in the United States. Its incidence has remained unchanged during the past 50 years. The 5-year survival rate remains a dismal 5%, and there are more than 47,000 deaths per year in the United States from pancreatic cancer.[2,6]

This chapter presents an approach to the processing of surgical specimens of the gallbladder, extrahepatic biliary tract, and pancreas. Guidelines for handling intraoperative frozen section specimens are also discussed.

NORMAL ANATOMY AND HISTOLOGY

Gallbladder and Extrahepatic Biliary Tract

The liver secretes as much as 1 L of bile per day. Between meals, bile is stored in the gallbladder, which in adults has a capacity of approximately 50 mL. Bile is concentrated 5- to 10-fold in the gallbladder through active absorption of electrolytes combined with passive movement of water. After ingestion of food that stimulates cholecystokinin and neural activation, the gallbladder contracts and propels the concentrated bile into the tubal gut through the extrahepatic biliary system. The gallbladder is not considered essential for adequate biliary function because humans do not suffer from maldigestion or malabsorption of fat after cholecystectomy.

The gallbladder is an elongated sac that lies in a fossa on the inferior surface of the right hepatic lobe. In adults, it is 7 to 10 cm long and 3 cm at its widest part. It is covered by peritoneum over its inferior aspect, but it is directly apposed to the surface of the liver along its superior aspect. The domelike fundus projects beyond the inferior border of the liver and slightly downward, and it is covered entirely with peritoneum. The body projects upward, backward, and to the left, approaching the porta hepatis. The neck corresponds to the tapered portion of the gallbladder. It curves backward and abruptly downward to enter the delicate connective tissue investment of the porta hepatis.

At the most proximal end of the cystic duct, there is a discrete area of narrowing that helps regulate the flow of bile into and out of the gallbladder. The cystic duct is approximately 3 to 4 cm long and joins the common hepatic duct to form the common bile duct. This junction lies at the lowest region of the porta hepatis. The common bile duct then courses downward about 7 cm, passes behind the superior part of the duodenum, and enters the pancreas. In 80% to 90% of individuals, the common bile duct and main pancreatic duct unite and emerge as a common channel through

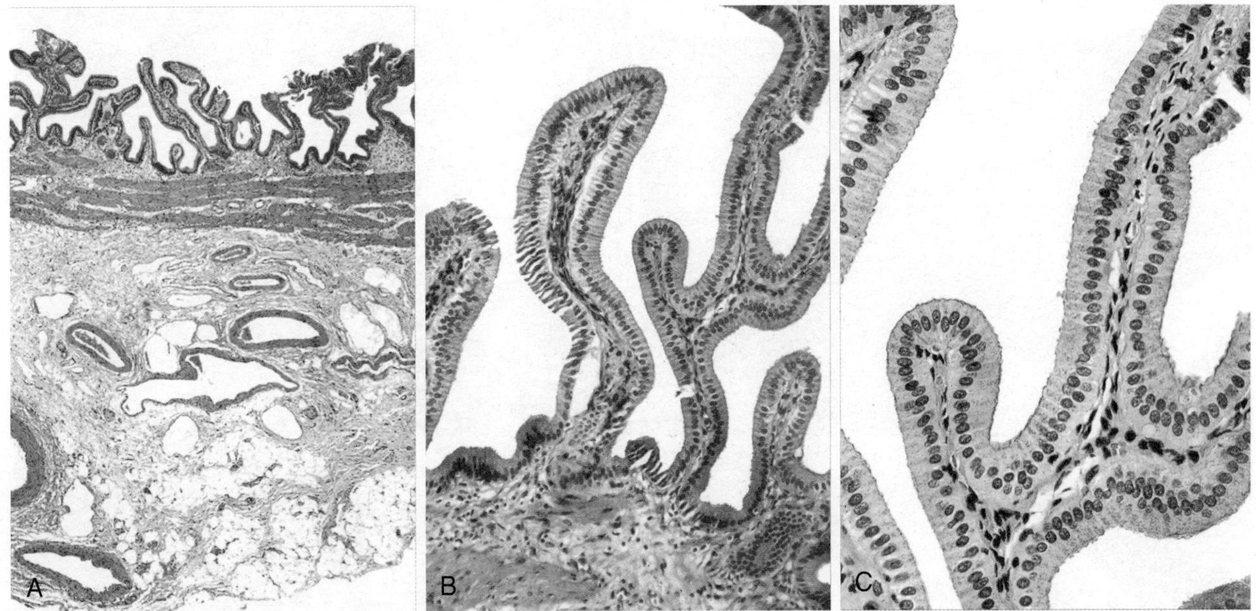

FIGURE 34.1 Histology of the normal gallbladder. A, Low-power image shows the mucosa, the single fibromuscular layer, and perihilar subserosal soft tissue. **B,** Medium-power image shows the folds of the mucosa. **C,** High-power image shows the absorptive columnar epithelium of the mucosa.

the ampulla of Vater. However, in a minority of individuals, the common bile duct and pancreatic duct remain separate when they pass through the pancreas and ampulla.[7]

The common bile duct is the most anterior structure of the three major structures of the porta hepatis: common bile duct, portal vein, and hepatic artery. The common bile duct lies at the edge of the peritoneal reflection, which is the anterior edge of the epiploic foramen, the orifice between the greater and lesser peritoneal cavity located behind the stomach. The portal vein lies posterior to and to the left of the common bile duct. The hepatic artery and peripheral nerves lie most posteriorly. There may be marked variation in the relationship of the biliary tree to the portal vein and hepatic artery where these structures approach the porta hepatis and enter the liver.[8] These variations include the topological layering of bile duct, portal vein and hepatic artery, aberrant hepatic artery location, agenesis or duplication of the gallbladder, and aberrant courses of the hepatic bile ducts.

Unlike the remainder of the gastrointestinal tract, the gallbladder lacks a discrete muscularis mucosae and submucosa. It consists only of a mucosal lining with a single layer of simple columnar cells; a fibromuscular layer; a layer of subserosal fat with arteries, veins, lymphatics, nerves, and paraganglia; and a peritoneal covering, except where the gallbladder lies adjacent to or is embedded in the liver (Fig. 34.1). The epithelium is arranged in numerous interlacing folds, which imparts a honeycombed pattern to the surface. In the neck of the gallbladder, these folds coalesce to form the spiral valves of Heister, which extend into the cystic duct. In combination with cystic duct muscle action, the valves of Heister assist in retaining bile between meals. The rapid tapering of the gallbladder neck just proximal to the cystic duct is the primary site of gallstone impaction.

Small tubular channels are occasionally found buried in the gallbladder wall subjacent to the liver. These "subvesical bile ducts" occur in approximately 4% of gallbladders.[9] Although their anatomy is quite variable, approximately half originate in the biliary tree of the right lobe of the liver and drain directly into the gallbladder; the remainder traverse the mesenchyme but do not directly communicate with the gallbladder lumen.

Small outpouchings of the gallbladder mucosa (i.e., Rokitansky-Aschoff sinuses) may penetrate into and occasionally through the muscle layer. Their prominence in the setting of inflammation and gallstone formation suggests that they are a type of acquired herniation.

Scattered along the length of the intrahepatic and extrahepatic biliary tree are mucin-secreting submucosal glands. They become prominent near the terminus of the common bile duct, appearing as microscopic outpouchings that interdigitate with the spiraling smooth muscle of the ampullary sphincter. To the unwary, buried glands may be mistaken for invasive cancer, especially when there is inflammation and fibrosis.

Pancreas

In adults, the average length of the pancreas is approximately 15 cm, and the average weight is 60 to 140 g. Embryologically, the pancreas arises from the duodenum as a dorsal bud and a smaller ventral bud. Fusion of the two creates the composite head; the dorsal bud is the primary source of the tapering body and tail. Fusion of the ventral duct and distal portion of the dorsal duct creates the main pancreatic duct (i.e., duct of Wirsung). Occasionally, the proximal portion of the dorsal duct persists as the accessory duct of Santorini.

The head represents the residuum of the embryological ventral bud of the pancreas, having fused with the dorsal bud that constitutes the body and tail. From the ampulla of Vater, the main pancreatic duct traverses diagonally upward through the pancreatic head to the angle of the pancreatic duct of the body and tail, representing the duct of the embryological dorsal bud. The bulbous head of the pancreas

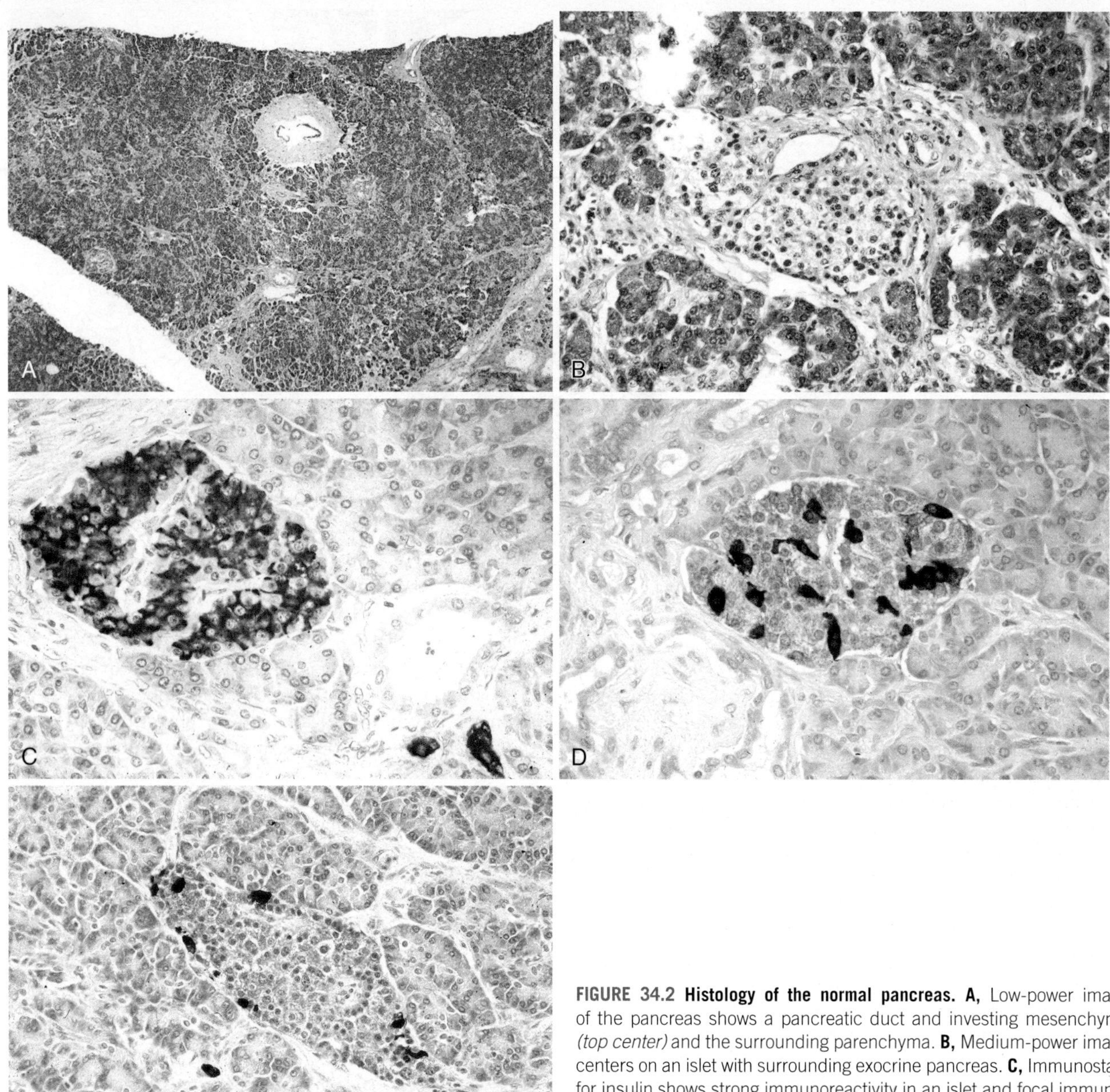

FIGURE 34.2 Histology of the normal pancreas. A, Low-power image of the pancreas shows a pancreatic duct and investing mesenchyme *(top center)* and the surrounding parenchyma. **B,** Medium-power image centers on an islet with surrounding exocrine pancreas. **C,** Immunostain for insulin shows strong immunoreactivity in an islet and focal immunoreactivity adjacent to a duct *(lower right).* **D,** Immunostain for glucagon shows scattered immunoreactive cells in the islet. **E,** Immunostain for somatostatin reveals rare immunoreactive cells in the islet.

is situated in the curve of the duodenum and is the widest portion of the pancreas. The uncinate process is the portion of the pancreatic head that is most caudad and imparts a comma shape to the pancreas.

The body of the pancreas normally has a uniform diameter and a prismoid cross section with three surfaces; the posterior surface is the most vertical. The tail of the pancreas consists of the terminal few centimeters. It tapers gently to a point in the splenorenal ligament that contains the splenic artery and vein.

The pancreas is a pinkish-tan organ with grossly distinct, coarse lobulations, which result from delicate collagen septa that subdivide the parenchyma into macroscopic lobules. Histologically, the pancreas has two separate glandular components, the exocrine and endocrine glands (Fig. 34.2). The exocrine portion, which constitutes 80% to 85% of the organ's volume, is composed of numerous small glands (i.e., acini) that contain columnar to pyramidal epithelial cells oriented in a radial fashion in the individual glands. The fine duct channels that drain each secretory acinus progressively converge to form the main pancreatic ductal system. The epithelium lining the smallest ducts is cuboidal but gradually evolves into a tall, columnar epithelium in the main duct. The main duct's epithelium secretes electrolytes and mucin. Surrounding the larger pancreatic ducts are numerous accessory mucous glands.

The endocrine pancreas consists of approximately 1 million microscopic clusters of cells, the islets of Langerhans. Most islets are 100 to 200 μm in diameter and consist of four major and two minor cell types. The four main types are beta, alpha, delta, and pancreatic polypeptide (PP) cells. They make up approximately 68%, 20%, 10%, and 2%, respectively, of the adult islet cell population. Beta cells produce insulin, alpha cells secrete glucagon, delta cells produce somatostatin, and PP cells contain a unique type of pancreatic polypeptide. There are rare cell types referred to as *D1 cells* and *enterochromaffin cells*. D1 cells elaborate vasoactive intestinal polypeptide. Enterochromaffin cells synthesize serotonin and are the progenitors of pancreatic endocrine tumors that cause the carcinoid syndrome.

The only surfaces of the pancreas that are covered by peritoneum are the most anteroinferior aspect of the head, the anterosuperior surface of the body and tail, and the portion of the anteroinferior surface of the body and tail that is not apposed to the transverse mesocolon. The remainder of the pancreas is devoid of peritoneum and is apposed to some of the most vital structures of the mesenteric root and retroperitoneum.

Depending on the body mass of the host, the pancreas may lie in a bed of adipose tissue. This has relevance in determining where the corpus of the pancreas ends. The mesenchyme of the pancreas corpus consists of delicate connective tissue septa that separate the pancreatic parenchyma into lobules and a delicate sheath of connective tissue, vasculature, and nerves that travels along the pancreatic ductal system. Scattered adipocytes are located within these connective tissue septa, even in the normal pancreas of a lean individual. When the pancreas becomes damaged, inflamed, scarred, or atrophied, the boundaries of residual pancreatic exocrine glandular tissue with the peripancreatic mesenchymal adipose tissue may be difficult to establish with certainty. Pancreatic exocrine atrophy may leave residual islets of Langerhans, giving the impression that they are floating in adipose tissue.

GALLBLADDER

Gallstones afflict 10% to 20% of the adult population in developed countries. More than 80% of gallstones are clinically silent. Most individuals remain free of biliary pain or gallstone complications for decades, but biliary colic develops in approximately 25% over 10 years.[10,11] Each year in the United States, approximately 1,000,000 symptomatic patients are found to have gallstones, ensuring a steady future population for the 900,000 cholecystectomies performed annually. Complication rates for gallstones are higher in older people and in some ethnic groups and are influenced by socioeconomic factors.[12,13]

Gallbladder cancer arises most frequently in the setting of long-standing cholecystitis with gallstones. The symptoms associated with gallbladder cancer usually mimic those of chronic cholecystitis, and the cancer may be advanced at the time of diagnosis. Occasionally, previously undetected gallbladder cancer is found only on examination of a specimen resected for gallstones. Gallbladder lesions identified by endoscopic retrograde cholangiopancreatography (ERCP) may be amenable to endoscopic biopsy,[14] and percutaneous fine-needle aspiration of the gallbladder may be performed.[15-17] However, most often, gallbladder cancer is encountered in cholecystectomy specimens.

Gallbladders removed during laparoscopic cholecystectomy or open laparotomy are common specimens. Standard of care is that resected gallbladder specimens are examined both macroscopically and microscopically by pathology. Argument has been made that selective pathological examination of gallbladder specimens is more efficient, based on the premises that (1) gross examination by the surgeon will be sufficient to identify suspicious lesions, and (2) if an early neoplastic lesion is identified, the patient will have received appropriate care regardless.[18,19] A meta-analysis of 73 studies involving 232,155 patients demonstrated a 0.32% incidence of incidental gallbladder cancer (IGBC) in low-incidence countries and a 0.83% incidence of IGBC in high-incidence countries.[20] If surgeons systematically examined the gallbladder specimens, the pooled incidence of IGBC was less than 0.1%. The incidental cancers were consistently T1a category or less by TNM staging, for which no additional treatment would be indicated. The counterargument is that failure to identify T1b or T2 gallbladder cancer may have a negative impact on patients who are then at risk for residual disease requiring additional surgery.[21-24] This premise of "selective histopathology" is currently being examined by a Dutch multicenter prospective observational study, with the goal of assessing oncological safety and potential cost savings.[20]

A separate consideration is subtotal cholecystectomy, defined as leaving behind any portion of gallbladder other than the cystic duct. This is a consideration during laparoscopic cholecystectomy, when either variant anatomy or complicated cholecystitis or fibrosis obscures the operative field with a high risk of biliovascular injury, and conversion to an open procedure is not preferred. In a recent series of more than 600 patients in India, almost 12% underwent subtotal cholecystectomy[25]; this incidence is 0.4% in a large series from the United States.[26] In the former study, bile leak and surgical site infection did occur in a subset of patients, but long-term follow-up was satisfactory.[25] In the latter study, subtotal cholecystectomy patients are subject to prolonged hospital length of stay, greater total direct cost, higher readmission rates, and higher mortality rates; the contribution of preexisting patient factors to these statistics cannot be excluded.[26] There is about a 10% incidence of patients developing symptoms and seeking medical advice following the subtotal cholecystectomy, including symptoms from recurrent cholelithiasis in the gallbladder stump.

Gallstones

The two main types of gallstones are cholesterol stones and pigment stones. In the West, approximately 80% are cholesterol stones, which contain more than 50% crystalline cholesterol monohydrate. The remainder are pigment stones, which are composed predominantly of bilirubin calcium salts. There is a greater preponderance of pigmented gallstones in Asia because of the high prevalence of fluke infections of the biliary tract.

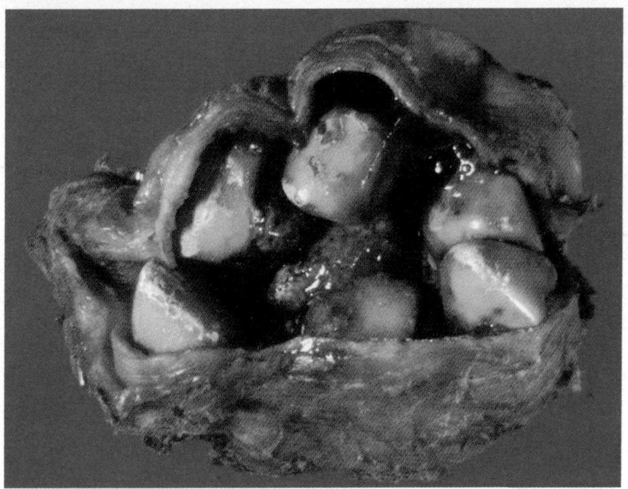

FIGURE 34.3 In a partially opened gallbladder, the cholesterol gallstones are yellow-white, faceted, few in number, and uniform in size.

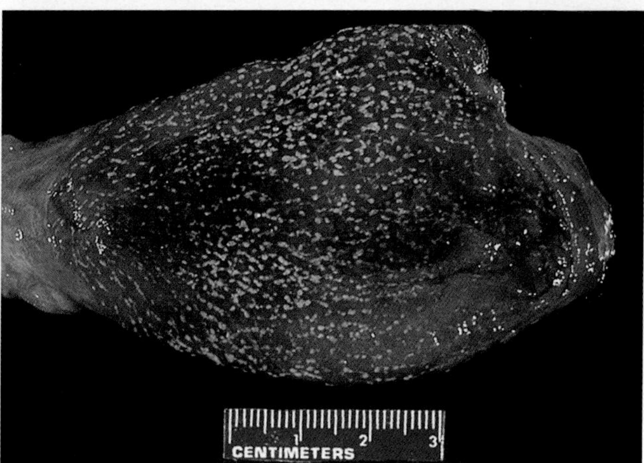

FIGURE 34.4 Gallbladder with cholesterolosis has bright yellow flecks throughout the mucosa.

Cholesterol Stones

Cholesterol stones develop exclusively in the gallbladder and are composed of various amounts of cholesterol, ranging from 100% (which is rare) to approximately 50%. Pure cholesterol stones are pale yellow and round to ovoid, and they have a finely granular, hard external surface (Fig. 34.3), which on transection reveals a glistening, radiating crystalline palisade. With increasing proportions of calcium carbonate, phosphates, and bilirubin, the stones exhibit discoloration and may be lamellated and grayish-white to black on transection.

Most often, multiple stones may range as large as several centimeters in diameter. Rarely, there is a single, large stone that may fill the entire fundus or obstruct the gallbladder neck. The surfaces of stones may be rounded or faceted; the latter results from tight apposition when they occur in multiples.

Cholesterol stones are gross-only specimens. Regardless of their color, they are hard and cannot be crushed easily between the thumb and forefinger, unlike pigmented gallstones. Larger stones may be crushed intraoperatively during laparoscopic cholecystectomy to minimize the size of the abdominal wall incision required to remove the gallbladder. In this situation, the lamellated interior of the stones is usually evident. Chemical analysis of stones is not required for clinical care and is of value for research purposes only.

Cholesterolosis is an incidental finding pertinent to cholesterol biology but not directly related to gallstone formation. Cholesterol normally enters the gallbladder mucosa by free exchange with the lumen and is esterified by acyl-coenzyme A:cholesterol acyltransferase. Cholesterol hypersecretion by the liver promotes excessive accumulation of cholesterol esters in the lamina propria of the gallbladder. The mucosal surface may be studded with minute, yellow flecks, giving a strawberry appearance to the gallbladder mucosa (Fig. 34.4).

Pigment Stones

Pigment gallstones are a complex mixture of insoluble calcium salts of unconjugated bilirubin combined with inorganic calcium salts. Pigment gallstones are classified as black or brown. Black pigment stones usually are found in sterile gallbladder bile, and brown stones are found in infected intrahepatic or extrahepatic ducts. Black pigment stones contain oxidized polymers of calcium salts of unconjugated bilirubin; lesser amounts of calcium carbonate, calcium phosphate, and mucin glycoprotein; and a modicum of cholesterol monohydrate crystals. Brown pigment stones contain pure calcium salts of unconjugated bilirubin, mucin glycoprotein, a substantial cholesterol fraction, and calcium salts of palmitate and stearate.

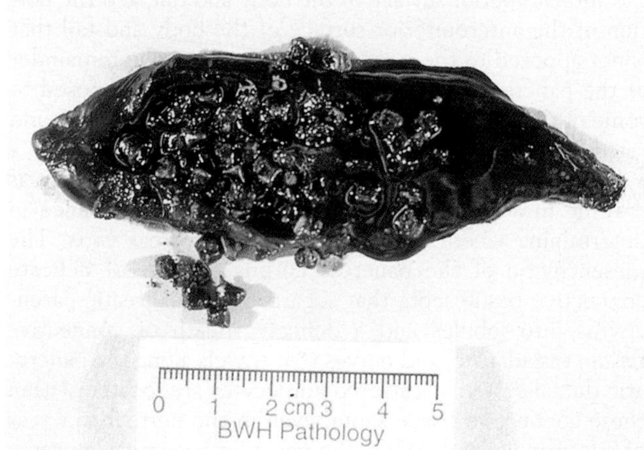

FIGURE 34.5 The pigment gallstones in an opened gallbladder are black, small, and numerous, and they do not have a uniform shape.

Black stones are rarely greater than 1.5 cm in diameter and almost invariably occur in large numbers (with an inverse relationship between size and number) (Fig. 34.5). Their contours are usually spiculated and molded. Brown stones tend to be laminated and soft, and they may have a soaplike or greasy consistency, resembling fecal material.

Pigment stones are gross-only specimens. Black and brown stones crumble or crush easily between the thumb and forefinger, which constitutes the primary confirmatory finding for distinguishing true pigment stones from darkly pigmented cholesterol stones, which do not crush.

Processing Gallbladder Specimens

Cholecystectomy is performed for gallstone disease, cholecystitis, cancer or presumed neoplasia, or incidental findings. Gallbladders removed at open laparotomy usually are intact. Because those removed during laparoscopic cholecystectomy may be torn or incomplete, spillage of bile and gallstones into the abdominal cavity is a complication of this procedure.

Cholecystitis

Acute cholecystitis may be acalculous (without stones) or calculous (with stones). Chronic cholecystitis almost always occurs in the setting of gallstones. In acute cholecystitis, the gallbladder is usually enlarged and tense, and it may assume a bright red or blotchy, violaceous to green-black discoloration because of subserosal hemorrhages. The serosal covering is frequently layered by fibrin and, in severe cases, by a suppurative, coagulated exudate. There are no specific morphological differences between acute acalculous and calculous cholecystitis, except for the absence of macroscopic stones in the former. In the latter, an obstructing stone is usually found in the neck of the gallbladder or the cystic duct.

In addition to gallstones, the gallbladder lumen is usually filled with cloudy or turbid bile that may contain large amounts of fibrin, pus, and blood. When the exudate is composed of pure pus, the condition is referred to as *empyema of the gallbladder*. In mild cases of cholecystitis, the gallbladder wall is thickened, edematous, and hyperemic. In more severe cases, the organ is green-black and necrotic, with or without perforation; this condition is called *gangrenous cholecystitis*. The inflammatory reactions are not histologically distinctive and consist of the usual patterns of acute inflammation (i.e., edema, leukocytic infiltration, vascular congestion, frank abscess formation, or gangrenous necrosis).

The morphological changes in chronic cholecystitis are extremely varied and sometimes minimal. The serosa is usually smooth and glistening, but it may be dulled by subserosal fibrosis. Dense fibrous adhesions may remain as a sequela of preexistent acute inflammation. On tissue sectioning, the wall is thickened to some degree but rarely to more than three times normal. The wall of the gallbladder has an opaque gray-white appearance and may be less flexible than normal. In uncomplicated cases, the lumen contains fairly clear, greenish-yellow, mucoid bile and usually contains stones. The mucosa typically is well preserved.

In rare instances, extensive dystrophic calcification in a chronically inflamed gallbladder wall may produce a porcelain gallbladder, which is associated with a markedly increased incidence of cancer. Xanthogranulomatous cholecystitis is a rare condition in which the gallbladder is shrunken, nodular, and chronically inflamed with foci of necrosis and hemorrhage. Gallstones are usually found. This rare condition can be confused macroscopically with a malignant neoplasm. An atrophic, chronically obstructed gallbladder may contain only clear secretions, a condition known as *hydrops of the gallbladder*.

Carcinoma of the Gallbladder

Carcinomas of the gallbladder exhibit two patterns of growth: infiltrating or exophytic. The infiltrating pattern is more common and usually appears as a poorly defined area of diffuse thickening and induration of the gallbladder wall that may cover several square centimeters or may involve the entire gallbladder. Deep ulceration may cause direct penetration of the gallbladder wall or fistula formation into adjacent viscera. These tumors are scirrhous and have a very firm consistency.

The exophytic pattern grows into the lumen as an irregular, cauliflower-shaped mass, but it may also invade the underlying gallbladder wall. The luminal portion may be necrotic, hemorrhagic, and ulcerated. The most common sites of involvement are the fundus and neck; approximately 20% of cases involve the lateral walls. By the time these neoplasms are discovered, most have invaded the liver centrifugally, and many have extended to the cystic duct, adjacent bile ducts, and portohepatic lymph nodes.

Specimen Appearance

Perforations or tears in the gallbladder specimen, as well as the anatomic completeness, should be documented. The serosa should be evaluated for its color and consistency. Inflammation usually imparts a dull and irregular appearance to the serosa. Adhesions may be evident, particularly in the region adjacent to the liver bed. In many cases, adherent cauterized liver tissue may be included with the gallbladder specimen. The finding of a fibrinous or purulent exudate points to a severe form of acute cholecystitis. Gangrenous gallbladders are blue-black, typically with a green bile discoloration; gross necrosis and perforation also are seen. The wall of a gallbladder with chronic cholecystitis may be markedly thickened. With extensive calcification, the gallbladder may take on a shiny, white, and hard porcelain appearance (Fig. 34.6).

Carcinoma in a gallbladder specimen may be evident on external examination as a dense mass bulging out of or penetrating into the gallbladder wall. Given the frequent advanced nature of gallbladder cancer at the time of diagnosis or resection, the tumor may be grossly transected at the specimen margin. This is particularly of concern on the side of the gallbladder apposing the liver,[24] as re-resection improves patient outcomes if there is residual cancer.[27] Lymph nodes in the vicinity of the cystic duct should be identified and evaluated for metastasis. Serosal tumor implants from elsewhere in the abdominal cavity may also be found by the surgeon.

Definitive surgical resection of advanced gallbladder cancer consists of resection of liver segments 4b and 5, en bloc cholecystectomy, and lymph node dissection including the hepatic pedicle (D1) and the celiac and retropancreatic area (D2).[28] The number of retrieval lymph nodes may range from 1 to more than 30, with a median of 7 lymph nodes, with a strong impact on prognosis based on the number of lymph nodes positive for cancer.[29]

Specimen Dissection

The length of the gallbladder should be measured, and it should be opened longitudinally. The luminal contents are documented, including their volume and color, mucin content, and the presence or absence of sludge or stones. Biliary sludge consists of microcrystalline aggregates suspended in the mucinous fluid. The gallbladder wall thickness and circumference should be measured. The cystic duct is often tortuous and difficult to open, but an attempt should be made to examine the cystic duct margin at minimum. Gallstones in the gallbladder lumen, gallbladder neck, or cystic

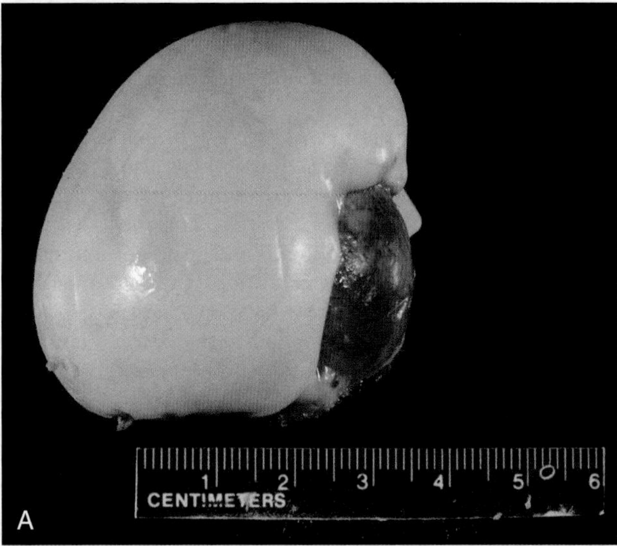

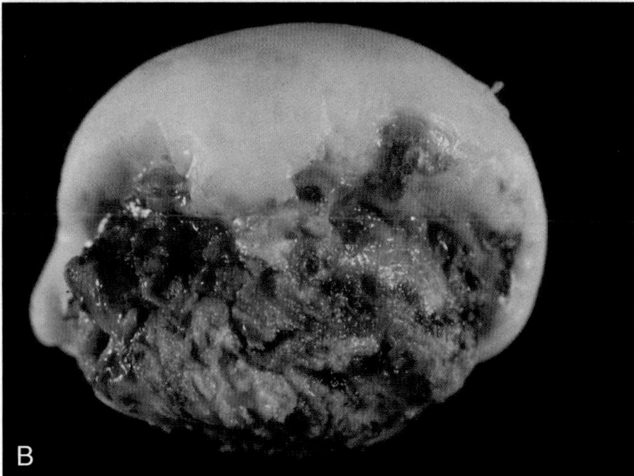

FIGURE 34.6 Porcelain gallbladder. A, Exterior aspect of the fundus of the gallbladder. **B,** Opened specimen shows eccentric, massive thickening of the gallbladder wall.

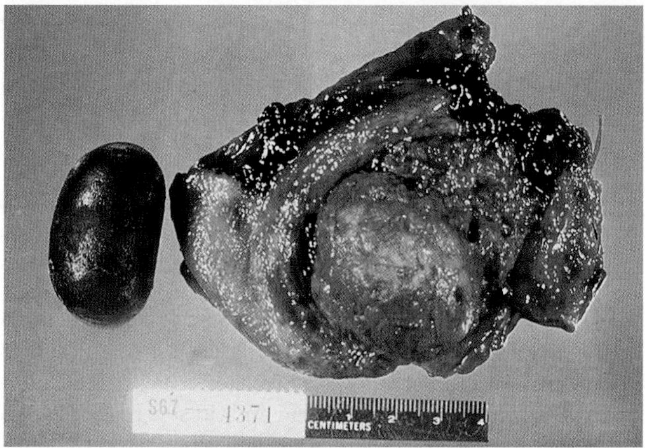

FIGURE 34.7 The opened gallbladder has a single cholesterol stone, which is darkly pigmented because of entrapped bilirubin pigments, and a 5-cm gallbladder adenocarcinoma bulging into the lumen.

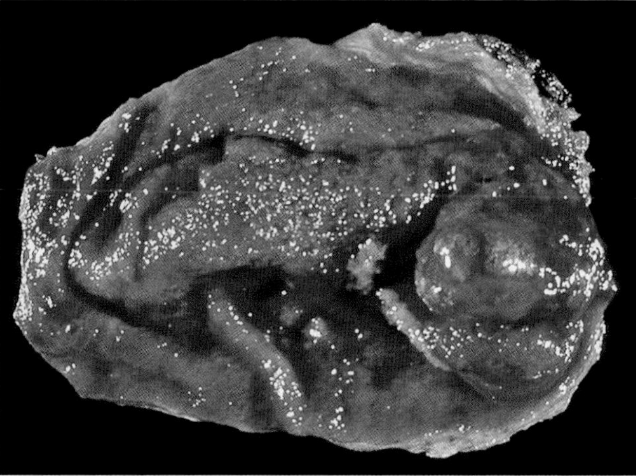

FIGURE 34.8 The opened gallbladder shows a bulging mural mass (adenomyosis) in the fundus *(right)*.

duct should be reported. Their gross features should be specifically described.

Occasionally, gallstones are returned to the patient. This should be done in a sealed container without formalin because formalin is a chemical biohazard. If the gallstones have been immersed in formalin, they should be rinsed in water before release to the patient. If chemical analysis is requested, the gallstones should be placed in a dry, sterile container and forwarded to the appropriate laboratory.

The mucosa of the gallbladder should be inspected and described. Normal mucosa has a honeycomb appearance and is tan and velvety. In cases of acute or chronic cholecystitis, the mucosa becomes effaced and loses its velvety appearance; it may be ulcerated and friable or flattened and atrophic, respectively. Cholesterolosis produces diffuse, small, yellow flecks on the mucosal surface.

Mucosal polyps are usually delicate, protuberant, papillary structures that are easily disrupted. Alternatively, flat areas of mucosal dysplasia or adenocarcinoma may appear as firm, plaquelike elevations of the mucosa or exophytic tumors (Fig. 34.7) with effacement of the layers of the gallbladder wall in cases of invasive carcinoma. Invasive carcinoma should not be confused with adenomyosis, which is displacement of benign glandular epithelium into the gallbladder wall and which is usually associated with marked muscular hypertrophy. Adenomyosis may appear as a dense, focal, tumor-like thickening of the gallbladder wall (Fig. 34.8). Massively dilated Rokitansky-Aschoff sinuses in chronic cholecystitis may impart tumor-like thickening of the gallbladder wall.

Specimen Sectioning

Cross sections of the gallbladder fundus and lateral wall should be submitted along with a section through the neck of the gallbladder and cystic duct, including its margin. Gross lesions, whether nonneoplastic or neoplastic, should be sampled thoroughly, with particular attention paid to the surgical margins of resection. Accompanying lymph nodes should be submitted and evaluated histologically.

If a neoplastic lesion is identified on gross examination, that entire portion of the gallbladder should be submitted for histological evaluation. If neoplasia is identified on histological review of standard sections obtained from a gallbladder specimen, the specimen should be revisited and the entire area of interest submitted for histological evaluation, which often involves submission of the entire gallbladder specimen.

EXTRAHEPATIC BILIARY TRACT

The extrahepatic biliary tract consists of the common bile duct, cystic duct, gallbladder, and common hepatic duct. In approximately 60% to 70% of individuals, the common hepatic duct bifurcates into the right and left hepatic ducts before entry into the liver.[30] The most common anatomic variation is congenital absence of the right hepatic duct. Instead, the posterior and anterior branches of the bile ducts that supply the right portion of the liver arise from a hilar confluence with the left hepatic bile duct. This occurs in the form of a three-way branch point with the left hepatic bile duct or by a two-way confluence of the anterior or posterior branches with the left hepatic duct.[30] Although the common hepatic duct and its branches lie ventral to the portal vein system, the right posterior bile duct may be situated in an inferior-ventral or superior-dorsal fashion around the right portal vein.

In two situations, the extrahepatic biliary tract should be submitted for surgical pathology analysis. The first is for resection of lesions that are primary to the biliary tree, particularly bile duct cancer[31] and choledochal cysts. The second is for resection of the biliary tree as part of a pancreas or liver resection specimen. Pancreaticoduodenectomy (Whipple) specimens are discussed later.

Processing Biliary Tract Specimens

Isolated resection of the extrahepatic biliary tree is performed as part of procedures designed to reconstruct the biliary system. Biliary tract reconstruction in situ is not usually possible except in cases of small perforations or strictures, such as those that occur accidentally during laparoscopic cholecystectomy.[32]

The most common surgical procedure of the extrahepatic biliary tract is resection combined with the performance of a Roux-en-Y choledochojejunostomy. In this procedure, a blind loop of jejunum is anastomosed end to side or end to end with the remaining common bile duct. This type of reconstructive procedure is a routine part of pancreaticoduodenectomy. Because patients with primary sclerosing cholangitis are not treated with surgery, except for those undergoing liver transplantation, the primary indications for biliary tract extirpation and choledochojejunostomy are biliary tract cancer and bypass and resection of a choledochal cyst. If the transection of the extrahepatic biliary tree is more proximal to the porta hepatis, the roux intestinal segment may have to be affixed to the porta directly, rather than to bile duct structures.

Biliary Tract Cancer

For patients with bile duct cancer, the resection specimen usually consists of the extrahepatic biliary tree, gallbladder, and accompanying soft tissue with lymph nodes. The surgeon should provide anatomic orientation by applying suture tags at the proximal and distal duct margins. Consultation with the surgeon is mandatory if there is any uncertainty with regard to anatomic orientation. En face sections should be obtained of the proximal (toward the liver) and distal (toward the pancreas) bile duct margins. The soft tissue margins should be marked with ink. However, disruption of anatomic planes during operative dissection may make identification of the true soft tissue margins difficult. The biliary system should be opened in the fresh state and examined for the intraluminal extent of tumor. The specimen should then be fixed in formalin overnight.

After fixation, optimal tissue sections for histological evaluation include cross sections along the length of the biliary tree and all soft tissue margins: anterior, left lateral, posterior, and right lateral. Depending on the amount of soft tissue, lymph nodes may be included with the cut sections through the biliary tree or may be separately dissected from the soft tissue and submitted for histological evaluation. Lymph node groups should be submitted in separate cassettes as follows: periductal (i.e., along the common bile duct), perihilar, peripancreatic, subpyloric, and celiac and preaortic.

Choledochal Cyst

Congenital cystic dilations of the common bile duct (i.e., choledochal cyst) are nonheritable, extrahepatic lesions (see Chapter 36). Although they may be associated with cystic dilation of the intrahepatic biliary tree, extrahepatic choledochal cysts do not arise from ductal plate malformations. Cystic dilations of the extrahepatic biliary tract are classified as cylindrical dilations of the common bile duct, cystic diverticula, intrapancreatic dilations, or lesions protruding into the gut lumen at the ampulla of Vater.

Choledochal cysts are more common in Asian than in Western countries,[33] and they are more common among females. Approximately 60% of patients are diagnosed before the age of 10 years, but cyst identification in adulthood also occurs. Ascending cholangitis and obstruction are possible underlying causes of symptoms. Complications other than obstruction include stone formation (approximately 8% of patients), pancreatitis (infrequent), carcinoma (approximately 4% of patients), and perforation (rare).[34] Surgical resection of choledochal cysts is the preferred method of treatment because of the risk of carcinoma, which increases progressively with age.[35-37] The risk of malignancy in adult patients with choledochal cysts is more evident in Asian patients than in the Western population.[33] However, the risk of malignancy in Western adults is still appreciable, reported as 11% at the time of surgical resection of the choledochal cyst.[38]

Dissection of the resection specimen requires careful attention to the anatomy and the sites and nature of the cystic dilatation. The cyst walls may be thin and delicate. The specimen's anatomy may be easily disrupted by the surgeon or pathologist. If the cystic dilatation cannot be identified at gross examination, consultation with the surgeon is appropriate. Because of the risk of carcinoma, the mucosal surfaces of the cyst should be examined carefully, and areas exhibiting plaquelike thickening; a thickened, velvety texture; or effacement of the underlying tissue layers should be submitted for histological examination. The proximal and distal bile duct margins (including the region of the ampulla if a Whipple procedure was performed) should be sampled, along with soft tissue margins adjacent to suspect areas. The region of cystic dilatation can be submitted entirely or representatively; histological examination will be important both for delineation of the underlying mural anatomy, as well as to evaluate the mucosa for metaplasia and epithelial neoplasia.[39]

Extrahepatic Biliary Atresia

The salient features of extrahepatic biliary atresia include inflammation and fibrosing strictures of the common hepatic duct and common bile duct, with secondary periductal inflammation of intrahepatic bile ducts and progressive destruction of the intrahepatic biliary tree. There is considerable variation in the anatomy of patients with biliary atresia. When the disease is limited to the common (type I) or hepatic (type II) bile ducts with patent proximal branches, it is considered surgically correctable. Unfortunately, 90% of patients have type III biliary atresia, in which there also is obstruction of bile ducts at or above the porta hepatis. The latter group includes early, severe biliary atresia, in which the intrahepatic biliary tree does not form properly, and there is no patency to the intrahepatic biliary tree.[37] Cases with severe obliteration of the intrahepatic biliary tree are not surgically correctable except by liver transplantation. In most patients with biliary atresia, bile ducts in the liver may be patent initially, but they are progressively destroyed with time.

In infants with type I or type II extrahepatic biliary atresia, biliary tract resection with a portoenterostomy (i.e., Kasai procedure) is the first surgical option. Biliary drainage is reestablished by connecting a portion of the jejunum with the hilum of the liver by a Roux-en-Y procedure.[40] The primary responsibility of the pathologist is to obtain cross sections of the resected biliary tree, with particular attention to the most proximal portion. The diameter of the residual bile duct lumina at the porta hepatis correlates with long-term functionality of the portoenterostomy.[41] If a liver transplantation is performed some time after a Kasai procedure, the resected liver specimen usually reveals a segment of jejunum anastomosed to the porta hepatis.

Hepatectomy Specimens

In this brief section, consideration is given to examination of livers partially or completely resected for diseases affecting the extrahepatic biliary tree. After initially assessing the overall specimen macroscopically, the first goal on dissection is to delineate the anatomy of the porta hepatis, or that portion of a smaller specimen containing the major portal vein, hepatic artery, and bile duct structures. Whether the biliary tract accompanies complete liver explants or partial hepatectomy specimens, a second fundamental goal of dissection is to identify the anatomy of the extrahepatic and intrahepatic biliary tree. Livers explanted for diseases that affect the extrahepatic biliary tree, particularly biliary atresia or primary sclerosing cholangitis, likely have a partially or completely obliterated extrahepatic bile duct system. Cross sections of the biliary tree are the best method to document the extent of disease. In patients with primary sclerosing cholangitis, attention should be given to the possibility of a coexistent bile duct carcinoma. Sections should be submitted of hilar or extrahepatic areas that are diffusely effaced by white, sclerotic tissue. In all instances, a cross section of the most distal margin of the extrahepatic biliary tree should be obtained.

Partial hepatectomy specimens for known biliary tract cancer, especially for those involving the confluence of the right and left hepatic bile ducts (i.e., Klatskin tumor), should be examined carefully.[42] This examination includes obtaining sections of the distal surgical margins (i.e., bile duct, portal vein, and hepatic artery samples), all regional lymph nodes, soft tissue margins, and the liver margin. The main tumor mass should be well sampled, with specific attention to its relationship to the major bile ducts. The major ramifications of the intrahepatic portal tree should be sampled because cancer cells can track for a considerable distance up the vasculature, lymphatics, bile ducts, and mesenchyme of portal tracts. This may be evident grossly as white, thickened portal tracts extending well into the liver corpus. As a result, hepatic resection margins may contain invasive cancer at sites where portal tracts have been transected (Fig. 34.9). Major portal tracts at the hepatic resection margin should be sampled generously. The liver parenchyma well away from the tumor also should be sampled to gain insight into the obstructive changes in the liver tissue.

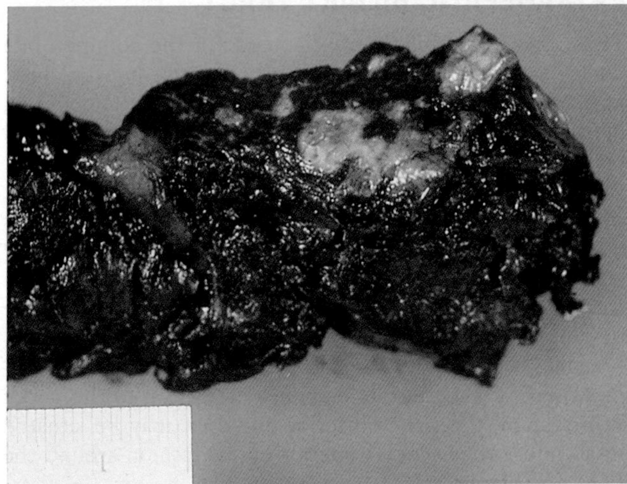

FIGURE 34.9 En face liver surface specimen represents the resection margin of a left hepatic lobectomy and resection of the upper portion of the extrahepatic biliary tree for a Klatskin tumor. The liver parenchyma is darkly pigmented because of obstructive cholestasis. Yellow-white portal tracts are massively expanded by invasive bile duct adenocarcinoma (i.e., cholangiocarcinoma), tracking up the portal tract system from the main tumor mass at the confluence of the right and left hepatic bile ducts. These malignant portal tracts were 5 cm upstream and were not evident on preoperative imaging studies.

Distal carcinomas of the extrahepatic biliary tree down to and including the ampulla of Vater are uncommon and are most often treated with a pancreaticoduodenectomy. A subgroup of biliary tract carcinomas arises in the immediate vicinity of the ampulla of Vater. Tumors of this region also include adenomas of the duodenal mucosa and pancreatic carcinoma. Collectively, these tumors are referred to as *periampullary* carcinomas, and all are treated by surgical resection.

PANCREAS

Surgical resection of the pancreas typically generates two classes of specimens: pancreaticoduodenectomy specimens and distal pancreatectomy specimens. Needle biopsies may be obtained during surgery by ERCP (often as brushings), through the gastric wall during endoscopy, or during radiographic localizing procedures.[43,44] Biopsy of biliary or pancreatic tissue during ERCP uses standard or specially designed small biopsy forceps.[45]

Processing Pancreaticoduodenectomy Specimens

Pancreaticoduodenectomy (i.e., Whipple procedure) usually is performed for resection of neoplasms of the pancreas, distal bile duct, ampulla of Vater, and duodenum.[46] The intent of the operation (palliative vs. curative) is a key prognostic indicator.[47] If it is meant to be curative, the intraoperative goal is to obtain surgical margins that are free of tumor.

Whipple specimens consist of duodenum from the pylorus to the ligament of Treitz, the head of the pancreas, and the distal extrahepatic biliary tract (Fig. 34.10). The most distal portion of the stomach also may be included. The gallbladder is usually submitted as a separate specimen. Proper anatomic orientation must be maintained at all times during processing of a Whipple resection specimen. On initial examination of the fresh specimen, several anatomic structures should be identified: common bile duct margin, pancreatic tissue margin (with main pancreatic duct), proximal tubal gut margin (stomach or duodenum), and the distal duodenal margin. The common bile duct, pancreatic, and selected peripancreatic soft tissue margins should be inked before processing. At least two en face sections of the pancreatic resection margin, including the pancreatic duct, should be performed at the outset to assess the pancreatic margin. If tumor appears close to the pancreatic margin, sampling of the pancreatic margin can be delayed until after overnight fixation. This approach allows perpendicular margins, which help to establish the precise distance of tumor to the pancreatic margin. The common bile duct margin, which is usually located posterior to the duodenum, should be cut in cross section and submitted en face for microscopic examination of the tissue margin.

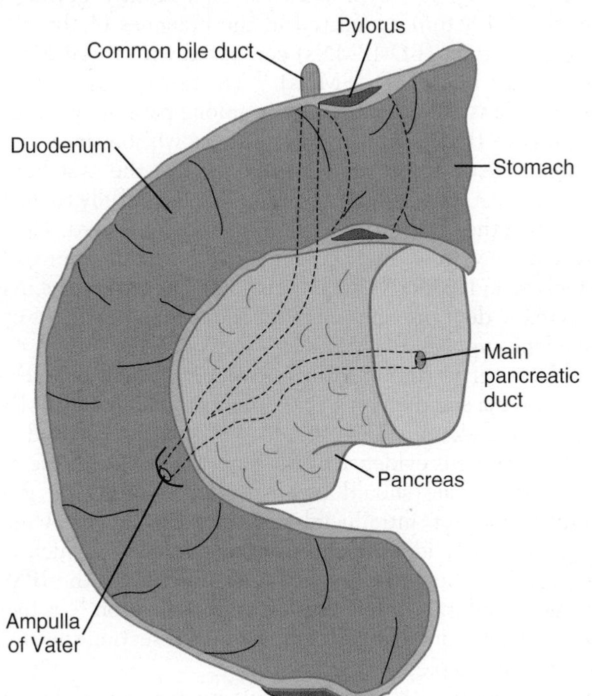

FIGURE 34.10 Drawing of a pancreatoduodenectomy (Whipple) specimen.

For further dissection of the fresh specimen, the following protocol is recommended. The specimen should be opened along the greater curvature of the stomach, the anterior wall of the pylorus, and the greater curvature of the duodenum. The contents of the lumen should be rinsed with saline, and any mucosal lesions, particularly those surrounding the ampulla, should be documented. Photographs of lesions should be obtained after the specimen is opened (Fig. 34.11).

A probe should then be placed in the common bile duct (proximal end) and advanced carefully toward the ampulla. Similarly, a probe should be placed in the main pancreatic duct at the pancreatic margin and advanced gently and carefully toward the ampulla. The ducts may then be opened along the longitudinal paths of the probes with fine blunt scissors. This method of dissection permits evaluation of the relationship of biliary or intrapancreatic tumors to the ductal system and provides an opportunity for specimen photography (Fig. 34.12).

Snap-freezing a portion of tumor should be considered because molecular analysis of pancreatic cancer can provide useful prognostic information.[48-50] Samples of tumors also can be placed in glutaraldehyde-based fixative for subsequent electron microscopy.

Delineation of the anatomy of the common bile duct and pancreatic duct is done to determine the precise anatomic location and origin of the tumor.[51] After initial dissection, it is best to fix the specimen in 10% buffered formalin

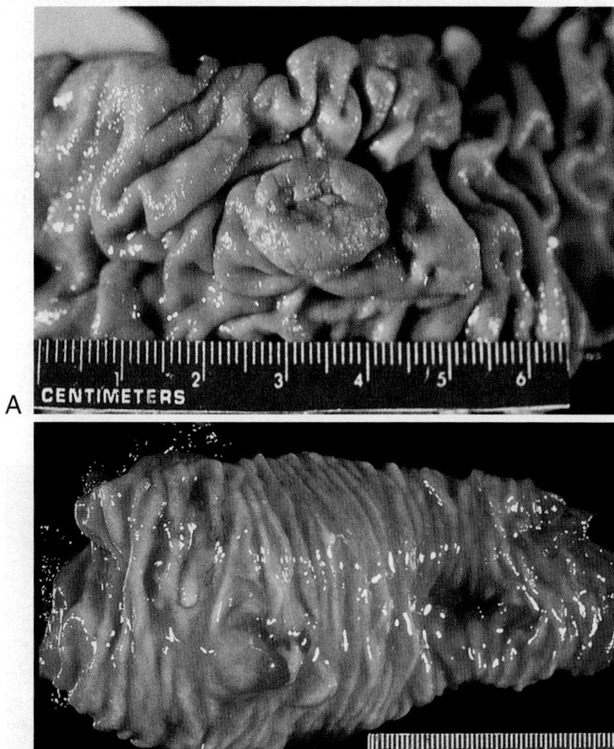

FIGURE 34.11 Pancreatoduodenectomy (Whipple) resections of periampullary tumors. A, Examination of the ampulla of Vater identifies a protuberant villous adenoma of the intestinal mucosa that circumferentially involved the ampullary orifice. **B,** Sweep of the duodenum in a different specimen, showing an ampulla of Vater bulging toward the lower left. A common bile duct cancer subjacent to the ampulla caused this protrusion.

overnight before further dissection of the tumor, intrapancreatic ductal system, extrapancreatic common bile duct, and the ampulla of Vater. Attention also should be given to possible patency of the accessory duct of Santorini.

The cut sections of the fixed pancreas should be evaluated for color, consistency, and texture and for tumors, nodules, cysts, and dilation of the pancreatic duct system. In addition to the initial tissue sections obtained from the fresh specimen (e.g., pancreatic margin, common bile duct margin), recommended sections for histological analysis include the relationship of the tumor to the pancreas and representative sections of the common bile duct and pancreatic ducts, ampulla, duodenum, pancreatic tissue margin, and common bile duct margin. Perpendicular sections also should be obtained through the nearest superior, posterior, inferior, and anterior soft tissue margins. The uninvolved pancreas, ampulla in longitudinal section (if not previously sampled), and proximal gastric and distal duodenal margins (i.e., en face and full thickness) should be sampled.

All regional lymph nodes should be submitted. This includes lymph nodes superior, anterior, inferior, and posterior to the pancreas; retroperitoneal lymph nodes; and lymph nodes from the lateral aortic, hepatic artery, superior mesenteric, subpyloric, and celiac areas.

Pancreatic adenocarcinomas of ductal or acinar origin may be difficult to appreciate on gross examination. In some instances, the predominant indicator of tumor extent is effacement of the lobular architecture of the pancreas by dense, white fibrous tissue. However, chronic pancreatitis may obscure the macroscopic relationship of invasive tumor to the surrounding pancreatic parenchyma. Some infiltrative tumors may secrete mucin. Many desmoplastic lesions therefore appear as gritty, gray-white, hard masses. Early-stage pancreatic tumors are confined to the pancreas. In more advanced stages, tumor extends into the peripancreatic soft tissue and into adjacent peripancreatic structures. The goal in obtaining samples for microscopic sections is to maximize the pathologist's ability to characterize the histological features of the tumor, determine its relationship to the surrounding pancreatic parenchyma and soft tissues, and establish its anatomic origin and extent.

For endocrine tumors, cystic tumors, and other mass lesions of the pancreas, the same dissection principles usually apply. Cystic neoplasms are usually multicystic and contain serous or mucinous fluid. Cystic cavities should be opened and examined closely for areas of thickening, nodularity, ulceration, tumors, or effacement of adjacent tissue. Cyst walls should be generously sampled up to and including the entire epithelial lining in mucinous tumors.

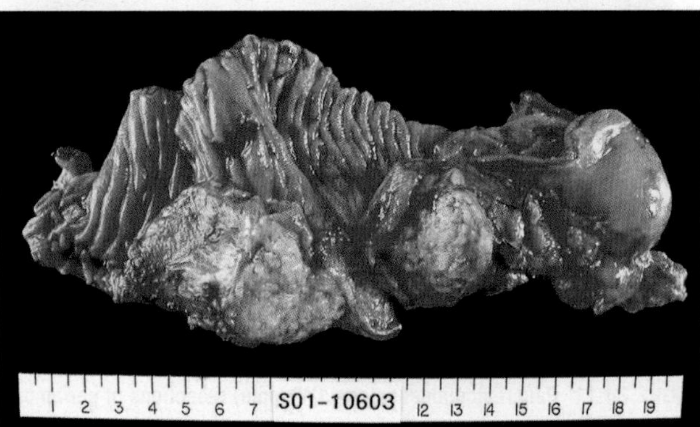

FIGURE 34.12 Pancreatoduodenectomy (Whipple) resection is performed to remove a pancreatic carcinoma located in the head of the pancreas. The ampulla was opened longitudinally, revealing an ill-defined mass expanding the head of the pancreas.

Intraductal Papillary Mucinous Neoplasms

Intraductal papillary mucinous neoplasms (IPMNs) are a unique category of pancreatic neoplasia as defined and classified by the World Health Organization[52] (WHO) (see Chapter 41). They may contain dysplasia ranging from minimal mucinous hyperplasia to invasive carcinoma,[53] and they may involve the main pancreatic duct (MD-IPMNs), its branch ducts (BD-IPMNs), or a mixed pattern.

In the most florid form, the IPMN manifests as a massive dilation of the intrapancreatic ductal system, and this appearance may extend throughout the length of the pancreatic ductal system. This type of neoplasm may be suspected on the basis of cytology or radiographic imaging.[54] The type of surgical procedure often is chosen preoperatively: a pancreaticoduodenectomy for tumors located in the head, neck, or uncinate process of the pancreas or a distal pancreatectomy or partial pancreatectomy for tumors located in the body or tail. Rarely, total pancreatectomy may be considered.

Preoperative findings and gross examination of the resected specimen are critical in evaluating possible IPMNs, although the final diagnosis is ultimately established by histological evaluation.[55] Adequate tissue sampling of the specimen includes the pancreatic resection margin, extensive sampling along the pancreatic duct system (i.e., main duct and its branches), and any cystic lesions or mural nodules identified in the pancreatic parenchyma. When mural nodules are identified outside of the duct system, their relationship to the duct system should be described carefully.[56]

The postoperative prognosis is significantly better for patients with tumors located in the branches of the main pancreatic duct (BD-IPMNs) compared with those tumors in the main duct (MD-IPMNs).[55] The rate of postoperative recurrence is considerably higher among patients who have an invasive IPMN compared with those without invasion.[57] When a cystic tumor is identified grossly, the cyst lumen and pancreatic duct should be cannulated carefully to determine whether these two structures are connected. Continuity between the duct system and the cyst lumen usually indicates an IPMN. A cyst lumen not connected to the main pancreatic duct provides more evidence for a mucinous cystic neoplasm or BD-IPMN.

Multicentric tumor with intervening normal pancreatic parenchyma and ducts is a concern when evaluating IPMNs. The gross examination should be sharply focused on whether there is evidence of invasion.[58] The entire resected pancreatic tissue should be inspected carefully on gross examination for intraductal and invasive cancer. Unless there is grossly identifiable invasive carcinoma, which can be sampled, the entire lesional area affected by the IPMN should be submitted for histological examination.[58] A focus of invasive carcinoma may be missed if a resection specimen is not well sampled.

For patients with negative pancreatic tumor margins who have subsequent recurrence, metachronous multicentric

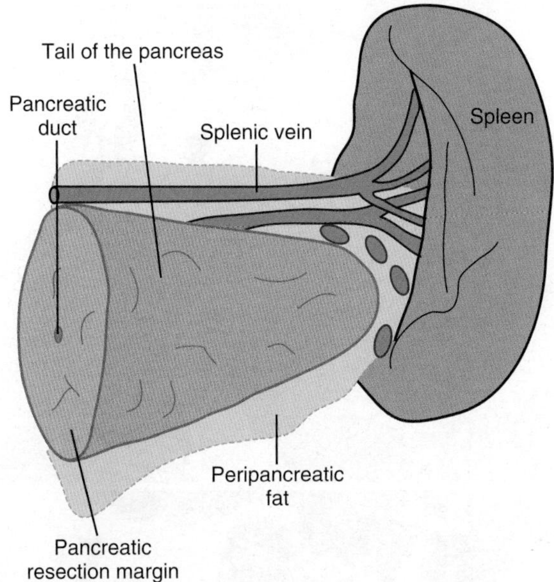

FIGURE 34.13 Drawing of a distal pancreatectomy specimen.

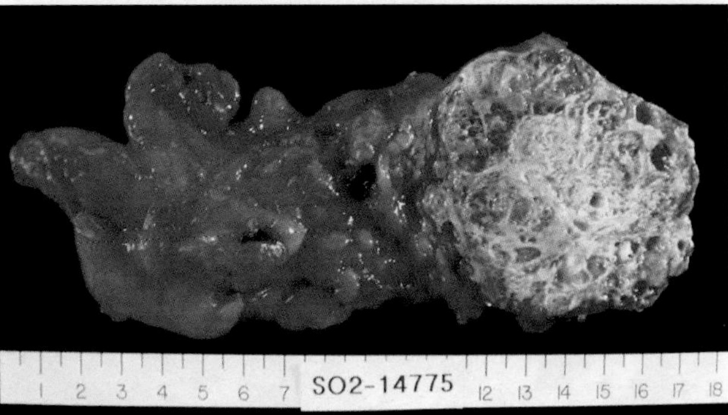

FIGURE 34.14 After a distal pancreatectomy, a cross section showed a cystic tumor.

tumor is often considered a plausible explanation. These tumors are more likely to occur after distal pancreatectomy for an IPMN compared with proximal pancreaticoduodenectomy.[55] Discontinuous IPMNs have been documented in 6% of specimens in two surgical series.[59,60]

Distal Pancreatectomy for Tumor

When neoplasia is located in the body or tail of the pancreas, a distal pancreatectomy usually is performed. It typically includes the tail and some portion of the body of the pancreas, the spleen, and the accompanying splenic vein along the superior aspect of the pancreas and peripancreatic fat (Fig. 34.13). Ductal carcinomas of the body and tail of the pancreas do not impinge on the biliary tract and often remain clinically silent for some time. At the time of discovery, these tumors may be large and widely disseminated, often with extension into the retroperitoneal soft tissue and adjacent nerves. Occasionally, they may invade the spleen, adrenal glands, vertebral column, transverse colon, and stomach. Peripancreatic, gastric, mesenteric, omental, and portohepatic nodes are frequently involved.

Other pancreatic tumors in the body and tail with life-limiting potential include acinar cell carcinoma and cystic or solid epithelial neoplasms of the exocrine pancreas. Islet cell tumors of the endocrine pancreas (i.e., endocrine tumors) in the body or tail also are resected by distal pancreatectomy.

The following guidelines describe appropriate dissection and sampling of a distal pancreatectomy specimen[17]:

- The specimen should be oriented according to its anterior, posterior, superior, inferior, lateral, and medial aspects. The organ anatomy (i.e., spleen and pancreas), pancreatic resection margin, and main pancreatic duct should be identified.
- Photographs of the entire specimen and cross sections should be obtained as needed. The critical surgical margins should be marked with ink before transection of the specimen for photography and further dissection.
- The outer appearance of the specimen should be documented, and the pancreatic parenchyma should be examined.
- The proximal pancreatic resection margin should be sectioned en face for histological processing.
- The pancreas should be serially sectioned perpendicular to its long axis. Lesions should be described in detail, with their relationship to the tissue margins.
- If it is not directly involved by tumor, the spleen should be separated and thinly sectioned to help locate potential lesions. The splenic vein should be examined for thrombosis or invasive tumor.
- After overnight specimen fixation in formalin, sections should be obtained of solid tumor or lesions suspected to be tumor and of the closest approach of the tumor to the superior, posterior, inferior, and anterior soft tissue margins using perpendicular sections.
- Cystic tumors (Fig. 34.14) should be sampled as described for Whipple specimens.
- The peripancreatic soft tissue should be carefully examined for lymph nodes. Peripancreatic lymph nodes should be submitted separately from the splenic nodes. If found in the specimen, perigastric nodes and pericolic nodes should be submitted separately because they are considered distant nodal metastasis if found to be positive for tumor.

Pancreatectomy for Pancreatitis

Partial resection of the pancreas for acute pancreatitis and pancreatic necrosis is considered a final, desperate procedure for patients with severe, hemorrhagic, acute pancreatitis.[61] In these cases, the pancreatic parenchyma is extensively necrotic and hemorrhagic (Fig. 34.15). Dissection and tissue processing are done primarily to document the severity of pancreatic injury and the presence or absence of microorganisms.

Partial resection of the pancreas for chronic pancreatitis is an established procedure for alleviation of intractable pain. The main goals of dissection and tissue processing are to establish an accurate diagnosis of pancreatitis and to exclude the possibility of unsuspected pancreatic carcinoma. Accordingly, attention should be given to the surgical margins of resection as described previously. Total pancreatectomy with islet cell autotransplantation for recurrent acute pancreatitis or for chronic pancreatitis now also is a treatment option.[62,63] Because the resected pancreas is digested with collagenase for isolation of islets, a pancreas specimen is not submitted for pathological examination.

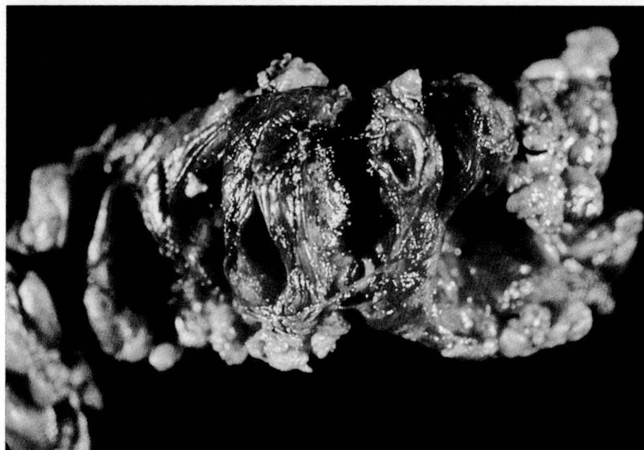

FIGURE 34.15 Acute hemorrhagic pancreatitis is seen in a pancreaticoduodenectomy specimen from a patient who was bleeding heavily from the accessory duct of Santorini. The specimen was processed by breadloafing to reveal the dusky, hemorrhagic pancreatic corpus.

FROZEN SECTIONS AND INTRAOPERATIVE CONSULTATION

For extrahepatic bile duct cancer and pancreatic cancer, positive surgical margins constitute a strong risk factor for postoperative recurrence.[64-67] Frozen section confirmation of lymph node metastasis at the time of surgery may help the surgeon to decide against resection.[68,69] The pathologist commonly plays a key role in intraoperative decision making in the following situations:

- Distal common bile duct margin of a partial hepatectomy procedure for biliary tract cancer (i.e., Klatskin tumor) or for a suspect lesion of the biliary tree
- Proximal and distal bile duct margins of a limited resection of an extrahepatic biliary tract tumor
- Proximal common bile duct margin of a pancreaticoduodenectomy (Whipple) procedure for tumors of the distal common bile duct, pancreas, ampulla, or periampullary region
- Pancreatic margin of a pancreaticoduodenectomy or distal pancreatectomy procedure

The main intraoperative decision is whether to extend the surgical resection. False-negative rates for intraoperative interpretation of surgical margins range as high as 10% in some series.[65] The value of using frozen section of the pancreas parenchymal margin to extend the surgical resection has been questioned, as survival benefit from doing so has not been established.[70]

Occasionally, an intraoperative frozen section is requested to confirm a biliary or pancreatic lesion as malignant.[71-73] Specimens may be obtained by an intraoperative incisional biopsy or, in the case of the pancreas, a needle biopsy. The intraoperative decision in these instances (e.g., biliary tract cancer versus benign lesions, pancreatic carcinoma versus chronic pancreatitis) depends heavily on preoperative staging and intraoperative surgical judgment. This is owing to the fact that while the positive predictive value of such frozen sections is high, the negative predictive value may be as low as 50% and malignant lesions may not be successfully identified on frozen section.[74]

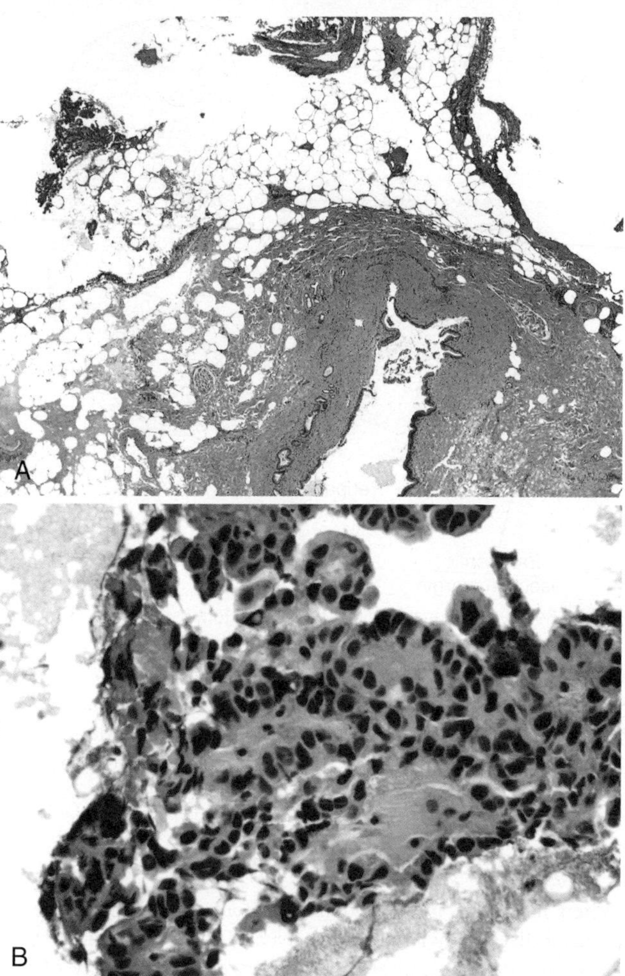

FIGURE 34.16 Bile duct adenocarcinoma is identified at a distal hepatic bile duct margin of a resection specimen (frozen section) for a Klatskin tumor. Low-power **(A)** and high-power **(B)** images show a focus of adenocarcinoma in the periductal soft tissue (**A,** *upper left*).

Bile Duct Margins

Hilar Resections or Partial Hepatectomy

Distal Bile Duct Margin

Intraoperative frozen section evaluation of the distal bile duct stump is frequently performed for resections of a carcinoma of the proximal extrahepatic (i.e., Klatskin tumor) or intrahepatic biliary tract.[75] A distal tumor-free surgical margin of at least 0.5 cm is desirable.[76] Because the distal portion of the biliary tract is normally not obstructed in patients with Klatskin tumor, obstructive changes of the bile duct epithelium and peribiliary glands are normally not found.

One task is to determine the presence or absence of a malignant tumor (Fig. 34.16). Well-differentiated tumors may be difficult to identify because they exhibit well-formed glandular structures with ample mucin and have regularly shaped, inconspicuous nuclei.[75,77-80] The location of glandular structures in the stroma and wall of the bile duct is critical to help determine malignancy. In contrast, moderately differentiated tumor exhibits a predominantly cribriform growth pattern of tumor cells. Poorly differentiated tumors exhibit solid strands of tumor cells or single,

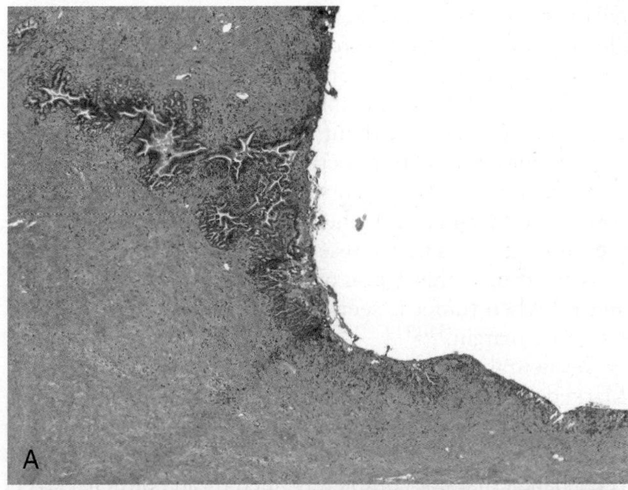

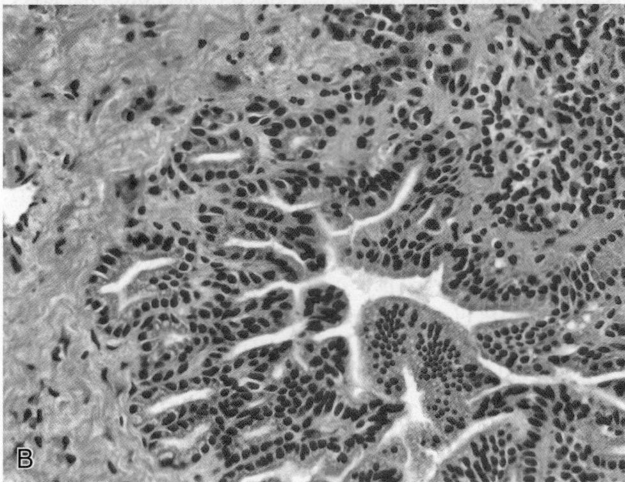

FIGURE 34.17 Reactive bile duct changes are seen at a proximal common bile duct margin of a Whipple specimen (frozen section) of periampullary adenocarcinoma. Low-power **(A)** and high-power **(B)** images of the dilated common bile duct show hyperplastic and reactive ductal epithelium, including the complexity of epithelial folds.

infiltrating malignant cells. In moderately and poorly differentiated tumors, the nucleus-to-cytoplasm ratio is high, and the nucleus is large, irregularly shaped, and hyperchromatic. A signet ring configuration may be prominent. Specific attention should be given to identifying perineural invasion, which always implies malignancy.

Proximal Bile Duct Margin

The surgeon may request frozen section evaluation of the proximal resection margin of hilar cholangiocarcinoma (i.e., Klatskin tumor). The same criteria for malignancy should be applied, and the invasive carcinoma within the wall of a bile duct should be distinguished from dysplasia. The inflammatory and reactive changes of downstream biliary obstruction should not be confused with neoplasia (Fig. 34.17).

The ultimate value of frozen sections for proximal bile duct margins is controversial.[81] The accuracy, sensitivity, and specificity for invasive carcinoma have been reported as only 57%, 75%, and 47%, respectively.[82] In 9% of cases, proximal margins deemed negative for invasive carcinoma at the time of frozen section evaluation are found to have invasive carcinoma in the permanent histological section.[83] A more recent report examining concordance between frozen section diagnosis and permanent section diagnosis showed 68% confidence for neoplasia in the epithelial layer, and 98% for neoplasia in the subepithelial layer.[84] Performance of intraoperative cytological evaluation of the bile duct resection margin (with the cytology sample obtained immediately before obtaining the frozen section sample) has been advocated as an adjunct to frozen section interpretation,[85] but has not found regular use as further evidence has not emerged to evaluate its adjunct utility.

From a surgical standpoint, extension of a proximal margin of resection found to be positive for invasive cancer on frozen section is technically difficult, regardless of whether the resection is of a proximal extrahepatic tumor or is a partial hepatectomy with further sacrifice of a major portion of the liver. Even if the new margin of resection is negative, there is inconsistent evidence about whether survival is improved compared with that of patients for whom a positive proximal margin was not extended.[86,87]

Prognostic Considerations

For extrahepatic bile duct margins (distal or proximal) for resection of cholangiocarcinoma, high-grade dysplasia at the bile duct resection margin, inclusive of what is known as biliary intraepithelial neoplasm (BilIN) and intraductal papillary neoplasm of the bile duct (IPNB),[88,89] does not have a strong adverse effect on patient survival.[90] Whether the morphology is nonpapillary (BilIN) or papillary (IPNB), the epithelium shows nuclear pseudostratification, a high nuclear-to-cytoplasmic ratio, and enlarged atypical nuclei, but it remains confined to the basement membrane and does not invade the underlying stroma. Extension of the proximal or distal surgical resection margins for a frozen section finding of high-grade dysplasia (including carcinoma in situ) decreases the risk of local recurrence[91]; but progression of residual in situ lesions seems to take several years[90] and does not have significant impact on overall patient survival.[91]

In contrast, invasive carcinoma at the duct margin of a surgical specimen resected for distal cholangiocarcinoma occurs in up to 70% of cases,[92] and is a poor prognostic indicator with early local recurrence of invasive carcinoma.[93] False-negative detection of such invasive carcinoma at intraoperative frozen section may be 5% to 16%,[94,95] and reliable detection of invasive carcinoma at the time of frozen section remains difficult. Positive identification by intraoperative frozen section of invasive carcinoma is justification for additional resection, in patients who can tolerate the more extended surgery.[96] If surgery is extended, 54% to 83% of patients can achieve a negative resection margin,[97] with improvement in survival.[98,99] Nevertheless, intraoperative frozen section of bile duct margins remains highly challenging for pathologist and surgeon both, because of the risk of false-negative results and relatively low rate of secondary obtained tumor-free resection margins.[94]

Surgical intervention for highly suspect hilar masses is justified because there are patients for whom a definitive preoperative diagnosis of malignancy cannot be made with certainty.[71,100-103] In this instance, intraoperative frozen sections of the mass may confirm invasive carcinoma, or instead document fibrosing cholangitis, erosive inflammation, a benign granular cell tumor, granulomatous disease, or lymphoplasmacytic sclerosing cholangitis.[104-106]

Pancreaticoduodenectomy (Whipple) Procedure

Intraoperative frozen section evaluation of proximal bile duct margins is common during resection of tumors of the middle or distal biliary tract, pancreas, or ampullary region.[81] For patients undergoing a pancreaticoduodenectomy for carcinoma of the distal common bile duct (cholangiocarcinomas), the initial frozen section of the proximal bile duct margin is negative for invasive carcinoma in 50% to 85% of cases; intraoperative extension of the proximal bile duct margin can bring the final negative rate to 90% and improves patient survival.[107] Invasive carcinoma may be identified in the stroma or muscle layer of the wall of the bile duct, with criteria similar to those used to examine the distal bile duct margin of a proximal tumor resection. Anatomic peribiliary glands nestled within the muscle wall should not be confused for invasive carcinoma.

Unfortunately, obstructing tumors in the middle and distal biliary tract often lead to dilation and inflammation of the proximal common bile duct. The bile duct epithelium may become markedly reactive and inflamed, showing loss of maturation, elongation and stratification of cell nuclei, and increased mitoses (see Fig. 34.17). If the common bile duct has been stented before surgery, ulceration, epithelial metaplasia, increased nuclear atypia, increased wall thickness, nerve entrapment, and smooth muscle hyperplasia may be seen.[108] The peribiliary glands also may show hyperplasia, inflammation, and edema. In contrast, the finding of in situ carcinoma or high-grade dysplasia at the proximal bile duct margin of a pancreaticoduodenectomy specimen performed for distal cholangiocarcinoma may not necessarily impart a significant negative impact on postoperative outcome.[81]

The proximal bile duct margin of a pancreaticoduodenectomy performed for pancreatic cancer is expected to be negative and is best assessed by permanent section without need for intraoperative frozen section consultation.[109]

Pancreatic Margins

Pancreatic Ductal Adenocarcinoma

The most powerful independent predictors of favorable long-term survival after pancreaticoduodenectomy for pancreatic ductal adenocarcinoma are a tumor diameter less than 3 cm, a negative resection margin at the time of initial frozen section evaluation of the pancreatic margin,[110] negative resection margins overall on evaluation of permanent sections, absence of lymph node metastases, well-differentiated histology, and lack of postoperative complications.[46] Some have made a strong argument that the surgical pancreatic margin should be assessed intraoperatively to look for adenocarcinoma,[111-113] although the ultimate impact of intraoperative frozen section evaluation of the pancreatic margin on patient survival remains controversial.[114]

At the time of intraoperative frozen section consultation, when special immunohistochemical or molecular studies are not readily available, several features help to determine whether a proliferation of glands detected at a parenchymal margin is malignant[115,116] (see Chapter 41). Even in the setting of fibrosis and inflammation, nonneoplastic glands retain a lobular architecture, exhibit a maximum nuclear size variation of 3:1, and reveal an absence of mitoses and enlarged, irregular nucleoli. Cancerous glands are usually arranged in a haphazard fashion. Cancerous glands are larger than benign ducts, are more irregularly distributed, may show irregular branching, and may be located adjacent to muscular arteries without intervening pancreatic parenchyma. For either frozen section diagnosis or interpretation of permanent sections, current terminology designates a pancreatic margin as R0 when no malignant tumor cells are identified at the surgical resection margin, R1 when tumor cells are at or within 1 mm of the surgical resection margin, and R2 when tumor is seen macroscopically at the surgical resection margin.[110,114]

Perineural or vascular invasion always implies malignancy. Marked variability in nuclear size, exceeding 4:1 among cells, and the finding of necrotic debris in the lumen of a gland are features of malignancy. Incomplete gland lumens (i.e., glands that not completely lined by an epithelial layer) and glands that are in direct contact with adipose tissue without intervening stroma indicate malignancy.

Three grades of pancreatic intraepithelial neoplasia (PanIN) are recognized on the basis of architectural and nuclear atypia (see Chapter 41). At the time of frozen section evaluation, PanIN may be identified in more than 50% of resections for pancreatic ductal adenocarcinoma.[117] Authorities have substantially agreed that extension of the pancreatic surgical resection is not indicated when low-grade lesions (PanIN-1 or PanIN-2) are identified at a surgical margin.[118] However, it has been demonstrated that even the finding of high-grade PanIN (PanIN-3) at a frozen section parenchymal margin does not negatively affect postoperative survival.[117]

Invasive carcinoma identified at a frozen section margin is a negative prognostic indicator of postoperative survival; initial frozen section histology may be positive for carcinoma in approximately 10% of patients.[110] Although the pancreatic surgical resection margin may be extended with achievement of R0 status in about one-half to two-thirds of patients,[110,119] the postoperative survival rate remains substantially lower[109,120,121] or does not improve at all[70,110,122-124] when compared with patients in whom the initial pancreatic frozen section margin was negative for carcinoma. Separately, neoadjuvant therapy decreases tumor diameter but has not been shown to decrease the rate of positive pancreatic margins at the time of intraoperative frozen sections.[109,114]

Intraductal Papillary Mucinous Neoplasms

IPMNs of the pancreas may be suspected before surgery on the basis of endoscopic, cytological, or radiographic findings. However, preoperative imaging is not reliable for precise evaluation of tumor extension, and preoperative biopsies often underestimate tumor grade.[125-127]

At the time of pancreaticoduodenectomy or distal pancreatectomy, intraoperative frozen section consultation is often performed.[58] On receiving a request to perform a frozen section analysis of a tissue margin in a patient with an IPMN, the pathologist should determine whether the ductal epithelium is normal or exhibits adenomatous, borderline, or carcinoma in situ features[53] (see Chapter 41). The pancreatic parenchyma should also be examined for the presence or absence of invasive carcinoma. Long-term survival of patients without invasive tumor is excellent, but invasive carcinoma carries a

5-year survival rate of approximately 65% and a 10-year survival rate of approximately 35%.[55]

The histological classification of IPMNs is provided in Chapter 40. In brief, four types are recognized: intestinal type, pancreaticobiliary type, gastric foveolar type, intraductal papillary oncocytic neoplasm, and intraductal tubulopapillary neoplasm.[58,128] The most common type, the intestinal type, shows a villous growth pattern similar to that of villous adenoma of the colon. When this type of IPMN becomes invasive, the invasive component resembles mucinous (colloid) carcinoma, with pools of extracellular mucin containing single cells or strands of neoplastic glandular epithelium with or without signet ring cells. The pancreaticobiliary type of IPMN shows complex, arborizing intraductal papillae, and its invasive component resembles conventional pancreatic ductal adenocarcinoma. The oncocytic type of IPMN shows complex intraductal papillae similar to the pancreaticobiliary type, but the lining cells have a granular eosinophilic cytoplasm. Numerous goblet cells may be seen. The gastric type exhibits papillary projections lined by epithelial cells resembling gastric surface epithelial cells and shows pyloric gland–like structures at the base of the papillae. The gastric type has been reported only in BD-IPMNs.[128] The fifth type of intraductal tubulopapillary neoplasm is the most recently recognized, associated with dilated pancreatic ducts and predominant tubulopapillary growth of neoplastic cells.

IPMNs may exhibit low-, intermediate-, or high-grade dysplasia, or they may harbor invasive adenocarcinoma. The criteria for invasive carcinoma are the same as those stated previously for ductal adenocarcinoma. MD-IPMNs have a higher risk of associated invasive adenocarcinoma than BD-IPMNs. However, if untreated, both forms of IPMN may progress to invasive carcinoma and eventually metastasize. Complete surgical resection of the IPMN is considered the best approach to prevent the development of an invasive cancer.[58] Frozen section evaluation of the pancreatic resection margin is performed to secure complete resection of the IPMN lesion.

The pancreatic surgical resection margin should be extended if there is high-grade dysplasia or invasive carcinoma.[129-135] Extension of the margin occurs in approximately 30% of cases examined by frozen section.[136,137] However, there are no management standards for IPMNs with low- or intermediate-grade dysplasia (also referred to as *adenoma* or *borderline* in the literature) found at frozen section evaluation of the pancreatic resection margin,[58] because the frequency of recurrence of invasive cancer in the remnant pancreas is low (0% to 8%).[138,139] The decision to resect more pancreas if the resection margin shows only low- or intermediate-grade dysplasia may rest on clinical factors such as patient comorbidities and age and the preferences of the surgeon and patient.

A second consideration is the discontinuous nature of IPMNs. Intraoperative pancreatoscopy (i.e., wirsungoscopy)—endoscopic examination of the intact pancreatic duct—is performed in some highly specialized medical centers.[140,141] Staged biopsies of duct epithelium are performed, permitting detection of discontinuous intraductal lesions. However, this technique is feasible only when the main pancreatic duct is dilated. A more feasible technique is intraoperative cytology, for which samples are obtained from residual pancreas even if the frozen section margin is histologically negative for IPMN.[142] Cytological positivity for carcinoma in a sample obtained from residual pancreatic tissue is justification for extension of the surgical resection, potentially up to a total pancreatectomy.[142,143]

The pathologist should be aware that small intraductal mucin-producing lesions are almost always present in the older adult patient. An incidental PanIN lesion identified on frozen section should not be confused with continuity of an IPMN extending into small ducts.[58] The gross features of the specimen can be helpful in distinguishing whether an intraepithelial mucinous lesion is an incidental PanIN or part of a more worrisome IPMN lesion.[58] The goal of intraoperative frozen section evaluation of pancreatic margins is not to overreact, but to guide resection of grossly visible lesions that exhibit a high-grade IPMN or invasive carcinoma at the surgical resection margin.

Intraoperative Pancreatic Biopsy

Differentiating pancreatic carcinoma from chronic pancreatitis may be requested for an intraoperative specimen obtained in a cutting-needle biopsy or an incisional biopsy. The sensitivity, specificity, and positive predictive value for intraoperative frozen section determination of malignancy is reported as 97%, 95%, and 97%, respectively.[144] Distinguishing benign from malignant glands in frozen section specimens is discussed in Chapters 40 and 41.[73,145,146]

Gallbladder

Frozen section assessment of the gallbladder is rare and indicated only for the unexpected finding of a polypoid mucosal lesion or a suspicious thickening of the gallbladder wall.[147] Identification of a malignant lesion determines conversion from a laparoscopic cholecystectomy to an open procedure to allow lymph node exploration and resection of the liver bed.[148] Frozen section diagnosis is most reliable for mural lesions, with concurrence with permanent section findings in more than 95% of cases.[149] Frozen section assessment of polypoid or exophytic lesions for carcinoma is less reliable.[149,150] Fortunately, simple cholecystectomy should be curative for superficial lesions. Determining the depth of invasion is best done by permanent sections.

The full reference list may be accessed online at Elsevier eBooks for Practicing Clinicians.

CHAPTER 35

Molecular Genetics of Pancreatobiliary Neoplasms

Laura D. Wood, Ralph H. Hruban*

Chapter Outline

INTRODUCTION

Cancer is fundamentally a genetic disease caused by inherited germline variants coupled with the accumulation of somatic mutations in oncogenes and tumor suppressor genes. Some patients inherit gene mutations that predispose them to cancer, while others acquire all alterations somatically. In both inherited and sporadic cancers, neoplasms acquire numerous somatic alterations throughout their development; some are driver alterations that play crucial roles in tumorigenesis while others are passenger alterations with no known functional consequences. Knowledge of the genetic drivers of neoplasia has greatly advanced our understanding of basic tumor biology and has revolutionized the practice of oncological pathology, with mutation-specific diagnostic and treatment strategies in multiple tumor types.

Pancreatobiliary neoplasms are among the best genetically characterized tumors, and studies of their molecular features have shown that molecular changes match morphologically defined entities: genetics mirrors morphology. With this newly reached understanding of the molecular biology of pancreatobiliary neoplasms, the field has moved into an era of genomic medicine. In the coming decades, knowledge of the molecular underpinnings of a neoplasm will be crucial for a given patient's clinical care, and pathologists will play an even greater role in patient care. Therefore a sound understanding of the molecular genetics of pancreatobiliary neoplasms is required to care effectively for patients.

*Dr. Ralph Hruban has the potential to receive royalty payments from Thrive Earlier Diagnosis for the GNAS invention in a relationship overseen by Johns Hopkins University.

PANCREATIC NEOPLASMS

Ductal Adenocarcinoma

Ductal (tubular) adenocarcinomas are malignant invasive gland-forming epithelial neoplasms.

Germline Alterations

Approximately 10% of pancreatic ductal adenocarcinomas have a familial basis, and several germline variants have been identified that lead to an increased risk of pancreatic cancer (Table 35.1).[1,2] These germline variants are important to recognize for two reasons. First, they can be used to quantify cancer risk.[2] Second, some cancers that arise in patients with a germline variant are remarkably sensitive to specific therapies.[3,4] Although a strong family history of cancer suggests an increased likelihood of a deleterious germline variant, many individuals with a germline variant do not have a family history of cancer.[5,6] The National Comprehensive Cancer Network (NCCN) has therefore updated its guidelines to recommend that all patients with pancreatic cancer should be offered germline testing.[7] Although germline testing is powerful, it should also be noted that the genetic basis for the majority of familial pancreatic cancer remains unknown.[1]

Germline mutations in genes in the Fanconi anemia pathway, which encode proteins involved in repair of DNA cross-linking damage, have been strongly associated with familial pancreatic cancer.[1,8-10] Germline mutations in *BRCA2*, a crucial component of the Fanconi anemia pathway, result in increased risk of breast, ovarian, pancreatic, and other cancers.[2,11] In addition to germline *BRCA2* mutations, germline alterations in other genes in the Fanconi pathway also play important roles in familial pancreatic cancer. The gene *PALB2* (also known as *FANCN*) encodes a protein that

TABLE 35.1 Genes with Germline Alterations Causing Increased Risk of Pancreatobiliary Neoplasia

Gene	Chromosome	Syndrome	Neoplasm
APC	5	Familial adenomatous polyposis (FAP)	SPN, PB
ATM	11	Ataxia-telangiectasia	PDA
BRCA1	17	Familial breast cancer	PDA
BRCA2	13	Familial breast cancer	PDA, acinar, cholangio
FANCC, FANCG	Multiple	Fanconi's anemia pathway	PDA (?)
Highly imprinted area: effects IGF2 and CDKN1C expression	11	Beckwith-Wiedemann syndrome (BWS)	PB
hMSH2, hMLH1, hPMS1, hPMS2, hMSH6/GTB	Multiple	Lynch syndrome/hereditary nonpolyposis colorectal cancer (HNPCC)	PDA (medullary variant), PanNETs, cholangio
MEN1	11	Multiple endocrine neoplasia type 1 (MEN1)	PanNET
NF1	17	Neurofibromatosis type 1 (NF1)	PanNET
P16/CDKN2A	9	Familial atypical multiple mole melanoma syndrome (FAMMM)	PDA
PALB2 (FANCN)	16	Familial breast cancer	PDA
PRKAR1A	17	Carney complex	Acinar
PRSS1, SPINK1	7, 5	Hereditary pancreatitis	PDA
STK11/LKB1	19	Peutz-Jeghers syndrome (PJS)	PDA, IPMN
TSC1, TSC2	9, 16	Tuberous sclerosis complex (TSC)	PanNET
VHL	3	von Hippel-Lindau syndrome (VHL)	SCA, PanNET

Cholangio, *Cholangiocarcinoma;* IPMN, *intraductal papillary mucinous neoplasm;* PanNET, *well-differentiated pancreatic neuroendocrine tumor;* PB, *pancreatoblastoma;* PDA, *pancreatic ductal adenocarcinoma;* SCA, *serous cystadenoma;* SPN, *solid-pseudopapillary neoplasm;* (?), *weak or questionable association.*

interacts with the BRCA2 protein, and germline mutations in *PALB2* account for a subset (approximately 3%) of patients with familial pancreatic cancer.[1,2,10] Germline mutations in other Fanconi pathway genes, including *BRCA1*, also predispose to familial pancreatic cancer.[2,8]

In addition to syndromes associated with germline mutations in Fanconi pathway genes, increased risk of pancreatic cancer is also a key feature in several other inherited syndromes (see Table 35.1). Germline mutation in *p16/CDKN2A* cause familial atypical mole melanoma syndrome (FAMMM); patients with this syndrome have an increased risk of melanoma (with multiple nevi and atypical nevi) and pancreatic cancer.[2] Individuals with germline mutations in *p16/CDKN2A* without a history of melanoma also have an increased risk of developing pancreatic cancer, and smoking appears to significantly increase risk in gene carriers.[12] Germline mutations in *STK11/LKB1* are associated with Peutz-Jeghers syndrome (PJS), a syndrome associated with gastrointestinal hamartomas and pigmented macules on the lips and buccal mucosa, as well as cancer predisposition, including an increased risk of pancreatic cancer.[13,14] Pancreatic ductal adenocarcinomas in these patients show somatic loss of the wild-type *STK11/LKB1* allele, indicating the importance of biallelic inactivation of the gene for carcinoma development in these patients.[15] Patients with hereditary pancreatitis are also at a markedly increased risk of pancreatic cancer.[16,17] In contrast to germline mutations in tumor suppressor genes, the increased risk of cancer in these patients appears to be the result of repeated bouts of inflammation and repair, and importantly, the increased cancer risk is limited to the pancreas.

Hereditary nonpolyposis colorectal cancer (HNPCC, or Lynch syndrome) is caused by germline mutations in *hMSH2, hMLH1, hPMS1, hPMS2*, or *hMSH6/GTB*, leading to defects in DNA mismatch repair (and thus microsatellite instability), as well as markedly increased risk of carcinomas of the colon and other sites. There is a slight, but real, increased risk of pancreatic cancer in patients with HNPCC.[11,18-20] Some, but not all, pancreatic cancers with microsatellite instability have a characteristic "medullary" morphology.[19] Germline mutations in the *ATM* gene, which encodes a protein with roles in DNA damage response as well as cell cycle regulation, also rarely occur in familial pancreatic cancer kindreds.[2,11,21] Although bi-allelic germline mutations in *ATM* cause ataxia-telangiectasia, a syndrome characterized by cerebellar ataxia, sensitivity to ionizing radiation, and increased frequency of multiple malignancies, germline heterozygous *ATM* mutations have been reported in approximately 2% of patients with familial pancreatic cancer.[2,11,21]

As noted earlier, these germline variants are important to recognize for two reasons. First, they have implications for other family members who may have a significantly increased risk of developing cancer.[2] Decisions can be made on whether or not to screen for pancreatic and extrapancreatic neoplasms, and some patients with an extremely high risk of cancer and minimal pancreas function, such as cigarette smokers with familial pancreatitis, even chose prophylactic surgery. Second, cancers that arise in patients with some of these germline variants, particularly those that code for proteins in the Fanconi anemia and DNA mismatch repair pathways, are exquisitely sensitive to specific forms of treatment.[3,22,23] Cancers with microsatellite instability respond particularly well to immunotherapy, whereas cancers with mutations in a gene coding for a protein in the

Fanconi anemia are often responsive to poly (ADP-ribose) polymerase (PARP) inhibitors.[4,24]

Somatic Alterations

The exomes and even genomes of several large well-characterized series of ductal adenocarcinomas have been sequenced and somatic alterations clearly play a crucial role in tumorigenesis (Table 35.2).[25-29] The somatic alterations driving pancreatic tumorigenesis are remarkably uniform, with four main driver genes (*KRAS*, *TP53*, *SMAD4*, and *p16/CDKN2A*). Superimposed on these common genetic drivers are less prevalent alterations in a longer list of oncogenes and tumor suppressor genes (see Table 35.2).

KRAS is the most commonly altered oncogene in ductal adenocarcinoma, with somatic *KRAS* mutations in more than 90% of cancers, clearly indicating that this gene is a driver of tumorigenesis in the pancreas.[25-30] *KRAS* codes for a small GTPase that mediates downstream signaling from growth factor receptors, and somatic mutations in *KRAS* cluster in a few specific hotspots (most commonly in codon 12), confirming the role of *KRAS* as an oncogene. Mutations have been reported in other oncogenes in the same cell-signaling pathway (including *BRAF*) in rare *KRAS* wild-type carcinomas.[25,28,29,31] Recently, germline mutations in the *RABL3* gene, which encodes for a protein that regulates RAS prenylation, have been associated with hereditary pancreatic cancer.[32]

Several frequently inactivated tumor suppressor genes have also been identified in ductal adenocarcinoma of the pancreas, including *p16/CDKN2A*, *TP53*, and *SMAD4*; these genes also represent drivers in pancreatic tumorigenesis.[25-29,33] *P16/CDKN2A* is the most frequently altered tumor suppressor gene in ductal adenocarcinoma, with loss of p16 protein function in more than 90% of carcinomas.[25-29,34] Multiple genetic and epigenetic mechanisms underlie this loss of p16 protein expression, including intragenic mutation coupled with loss of the second allele, homozygous deletion of both copies of the gene, and promoter methylation.[35] Loss of p16 results in cell cycle dysregulation, as this protein normally blocks cell cycle progression by preventing inactivation of Rb, another important cell cycle regulator. Immunolabeling for the p16 protein has been reported, but the labeling is often hard to interpret and therefore not useful in clinical practice.

TP53, which encodes a protein with a pivotal role in the cellular stress response, is another key tumor suppressor gene in ductal adenocarcinoma of the pancreas, with somatic mutations reported in approximately 75% of cases.[25-29,33] These somatic mutations almost always occur through intragenic mutation followed by loss of the wild-type allele. Immunolabeling for the p53 protein can be useful, as overexpression or complete loss of labeling correlates with the presence of *TP53* gene mutations.[36]

Somatic inactivation of *SMAD4* also occurs frequently in invasive ductal adenocarcinomas, with homozygous deletion or intragenic mutation followed by loss of the wild-type allele occurring in approximately 55% of carcinomas.[25-29,33,37] The Smad4 protein mediates cellular signaling downstream of the transforming growth factor beta (TGF-β) receptor, and less frequent somatic mutations occur in other components of the same signaling pathway, including *TGFBR2* and *ALK5*.[25,28,29,38] Immunolabeling for the Smad4 protein can be useful, as complete loss of labeling correlates with the presence of *SMAD4* gene mutations.[39] Of all of the genes targeted in pancreatic cancer, loss of *SMAD4* has been the most closely tied to poor prognosis.[40]

In addition to these known driver genes, somatic mutations are present at low prevalence in numerous other genes in pancreatic ductal adenocarcinoma.[25-29] The role of these genes as drivers or passengers is more difficult to establish when only a few mutations are identified; however, some are likely to play a functional role and can be important in the individual patients in whose cancers they are targeted. For example, *ARID1A* and other chromatin-regulating genes, such as *MLL2* and *MLL3*, are mutated in a minority of pancreatic cancers, but these mutations may have prognostic significance and some may be therapeutically targetable.[25-29,41,42]

In addition to small somatic mutations, large chromosomal gains and losses as well as complex chromosome rearrangements also occur frequently in ductal adenocarcinoma. Some alterations target known driver genes, while many others may be a manifestation of widespread chromosomal instability. Chromothripsis, the cataclysmic shattering and abnormal reassembling of selected chromosomes, has also been described in pancreatic cancer.[43] Notta et al. have suggested that chromothripsis may lead to abrupt progression of disease; however, most chromothriptic events do not target known driver genes.[43]

The expression of mRNAs and of proteins also changes as neoplastic cells progress to invasive carcinoma, and the patterns of gene expression have been used to define subtypes of ductal adenocarcinoma.[25,44-46] Although several studies establishing these subtypes were confounded by the inclusion of mRNAs expressed in contaminating nonneoplastic stroma, at least two subtypes appear to be reproducible. The "squamous" and "basal-like" subtypes correlate well with squamous differentiation by light microscopy and with decreased *GATA6* expression.[44,47] The second subtype, the "classical" subtype, is associated with a better prognosis.[25,44,45,47] Rather than relying on a single marker, a panel of immunomarkers that includes GATA6, p40 (deltaN-p63), cytokeratin 5 (CK5), and claudin 18 may be most useful in separating these subtypes.

Ductal adenocarcinomas also express microRNAs, small noncoding RNAs that regulate gene expression. Differential expression of multiple microRNAs has been reported in ductal adenocarcinoma compared with nonneoplastic pancreatic tissue.[48]

Although pancreatic intraepithelial neoplasia (PanIN) was recognized histologically for years, data on the genetic alterations in PanIN lesions firmly established them as noninvasive precursors to ductal adenocarcinoma.[49,50] Just as PanINs acquire increasing cytological and architectural abnormalities with increasing grade, they also acquire the same genetic alterations that occur in invasive carcinoma. Although some molecular changes occur early and are present in low-grade PanINs, other alterations are limited to severely dysplastic and invasive lesions. *KRAS* mutation and loss of p16 expression are early events that are present in even low-grade PanINs. When extremely sensitive techniques are employed, *KRAS* mutations are present in more than 90% of even low-grade PanINs, suggesting that *KRAS* mutations may represent a key initiating step in pancreatic

TABLE 35.2 Somatic Mutation Prevalence of Commonly Altered Genes in Pancreatobiliary Neoplasms

Neoplasm	Gene	Chromosome	Alteration Prevalence	Mechanisms of Alteration
PDA	*KRAS*	12	95%	Missense mutation
	P16/CDKN2A	9	95%	Missense mutation with LOH, homozygous deletion, promoter methylation
	TP53	17	75%	Missense mutation with LOH
	SMAD4/DPC4	18	55%	Missense mutation with LOH, homozygous deletion
IOPN	*PRKACA*	19	45%	Gene fusions
	PRKACB	1	55%	Gene fusions
IPMN	*KRAS*	12	80%	Missense mutation
	RNF43	17	75%	Missense mutation or nonsense mutation with LOH
	GNAS	20	60%	Missense mutation
	P16/CDKN2A	9	Increase with dysplasia	Missense mutation with LOH, homozygous deletion, promoter methylation
	TP53	17	only in HGD/carcinoma	Missense mutation with LOH
	SMAD4/DPC4	18	only in HGD/carcinoma	Missense mutation with LOH, homozygous deletion
	PIK3CA	3	10%	Missense mutation
MCN	*KRAS*	12	80%	Missense mutation
	RNF43	17	40%	Missense mutation or nonsense mutation with LOH
	P16/CDKN2A	9	Increase with dysplasia	Missense mutation with LOH, homozygous deletion, promoter methylation
	TP53	17	only in HGD/carcinoma	Missense mutation with LOH
	SMAD4/DPC4	18	only in HGD/carcinoma	Missense mutation with LOH, homozygous deletion
SCA	*VHL*	3	50%	Missense mutation with LOH
PanNET	*MEN1*	11	45%	Missense mutation with LOH
	DAXX/ATRX	6/X	45%	Missense or nonsense mutation with LOH
	mTOR pathway	Multiple	15%	Multiple
	VHL	3	25%	Promoter methylation
SPN	*CTNNB1*	3	95%	Missense mutation
ACC	*cMYC*	8	50%	Amplified
	BRAF	7	25%	Rearrangements
	APC	5	15%	Inactivating/truncating mutation with LOH
	CTNNB1	3	5%	Missense mutation
PB	Imprinted locus	11	85%	Loss of heterozygosity
	CTNNB1	3	55%	Missense mutation
	APC	5	10%	Inactivating/truncating mutation with LOH
Cholangio	*P16/CDKN2A*	9	85%	Missense mutation with LOH, homozygous deletion, promoter methylation
	TP53	17	50%	Missense mutation with LOH
	SMAD4/DPC4	18	50%	Missense mutation with LOH, homozygous deletion
	FGFR2	10	45%	Fusions, often with *PPHLN1*
	IDH1/IDH2	2/15	20%	Missense mutation
	PIK3CA	3	Variable	Missense mutation
	Chromatin remodeling genes *(ARID1A, BAP1, PBRM1,* etc.)	Multiple	Variable	Missense mutation with LOH
	KRAS	12	Variable	Missense mutation

TABLE 35.2 Somatic Mutation Prevalence of Commonly Altered Genes in Pancreatobiliary Neoplasms—cont'd

Neoplasm	Gene	Chromosome	Alteration Prevalence	Mechanisms of Alteration
GBC				
	P16/CDKN2A	9	75%	Missense mutation with LOH, homozygous deletion, promoter methylation
	TP53	17	60%	Missense mutation with LOH
	BRAF	7	30%	Missense mutation
	KEAP1	19	30%	Inactivating/truncating mutation with LOH
	SMAD4/DPC4	18	20%	Missense mutation with LOH, homozygous deletion
	PIK3CA	3	10%	Missense mutation
	CTNNB1	3	10%	Missense mutation
	KRAS	12	Variable	Missense mutation

ACC, *Acinar cell carcinoma;* carcinoma, *invasive carcinoma;* CCA, *cholangiocarcinoma;* GBC: *gallbladder carcinoma;* HGD, *high-grade dysplasia;* IOPN, *intraductal oncocytic papillary neoplasm;* IPMN, *intraductal papillary mucinous neoplasm;* LOH, *loss of heterozygosity;* MCN, *mucinous cystic neoplasm;* PanNET, *well-differentiated pancreatic neuroendocrine tumor;* PB, *pancreatoblastoma;* PDA, *pancreatic ductal adenocarcinoma;* SCA, *serous cystadenoma;* SPN, *solid-pseudopapillary neoplasm.*

neoplasia.[51] In contrast, loss of Smad4 and *TP53* mutation are late events, occurring only in high-grade PanIN and invasive carcinoma.[50] Alterations other than those in known driver genes also occur in PanINs; telomere shortening is one of the most common early events in pancreatic tumorigenesis, with shortening in approximately 90% of low-grade PanINs.[52] Early telomere shortening may make the cells susceptible to chromosomal fusion and anaphase bridges, which may produce some of the chromosomal abnormalities observed in invasive pancreatic cancer.

In addition to expanding our knowledge of precursors to ductal adenocarcinoma, detailed study of somatic mutations in primary tumors and metastases has deepened our understanding of the process of clonal evolution within tumors, enabling the estimation of evolutionary time in tumors.[53,54] These studies suggest a time window of approximately 15 years between tumor initiation and the acquisition of metastatic ability, providing a broad time window for early detection and subsequent clinical intervention.[53,54]

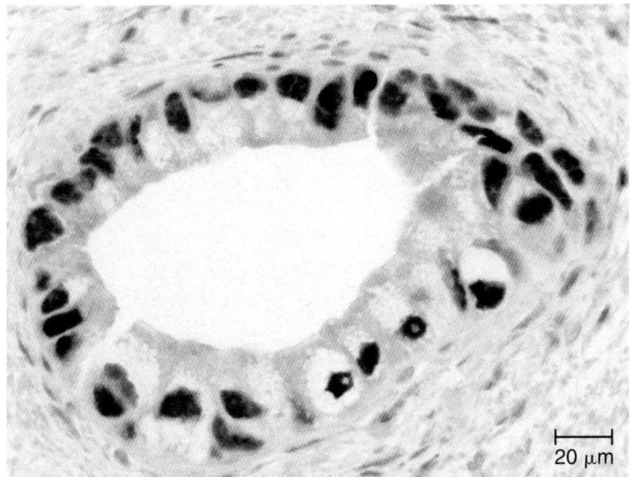

FIGURE 35.1 p53 immunohistochemistry in pancreatic ductal adenocarcinoma. Immunohistochemical labeling for p53 protein shows aberrant strong nuclear labeling in this neoplastic gland of pancreatic ductal adenocarcinoma, while the associated nonneoplastic stroma is negative.

Implications for Pathology

Knowledge of the genetic underpinnings of familial pancreatic cancer has direct clinical implications for pathologists in several ways. First, the pathologist will be the first to recognize subtypes of pancreatic cancer (such as "medullary" carcinoma) that are associated with specific familial syndromes.[19] When a pathologist diagnoses a medullary carcinoma, he or she should suggest clinical germline testing. The reality, however, is that there is not a specific histological phenotype for cancers caused by germline variants, and universal consideration of germline testing is therefore now recommended for all patients with pancreatic cancer.[55] Second, as noted earlier, some familial syndromes have specific treatment implications, highlighting the importance that they be clinically recognized at the time of diagnosis. For example, carcinomas in patients with germline alterations in the Fanconi anemia pathway *(BRCA2, BRCA1, PALB2)* are exquisitely sensitive to drugs that target their specific DNA repair defect, such as PARP inhibitors.[4,24] Carcinomas in patients with HNPCC also possess specific recommendations for treatment: tumors with microsatellite instability are resistant to fluorouracil-based chemotherapy but extremely sensitive to immune checkpoint blockade.[3,24,56] Finally, clinical recognition of familial pancreatic cancer syndromes will lead to increased screening of at-risk patients.[57] The screening for select extrapancreatic neoplasms can be guided by the specific germline variant identified.

Somatic alterations in sporadic pancreatic cancer also impact pathology practice. Immunohistochemistry can be used to demonstrate protein expression alterations indicative of characteristic gene mutations. For example, *TP53* mutations result in strong diffuse or complete loss of p53 nuclear labeling by immunohistochemistry, providing a histological surrogate for the genetic alteration and a potential technique for the identification of neoplastic pancreatic cells (Fig. 35.1).[36] In addition, loss of Smad4 protein expression by immunohistochemistry is correlated with genetic alterations in the *SMAD4* gene (Fig. 35.2).[58] This technique can

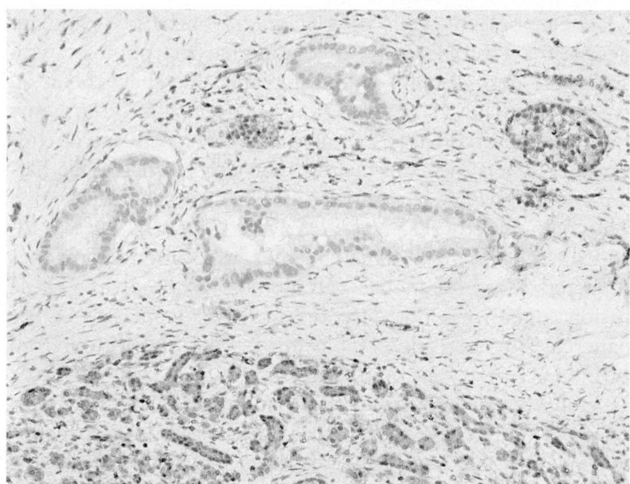

FIGURE 35.2 Smad4 immunohistochemistry in pancreatic ductal adenocarcinoma. Immunohistochemical labeling for Smad4 protein shows loss of expression in the neoplastic glands of pancreatic ductal adenocarcinoma, while the associated nonneoplastic stroma retains normal nuclear labeling.

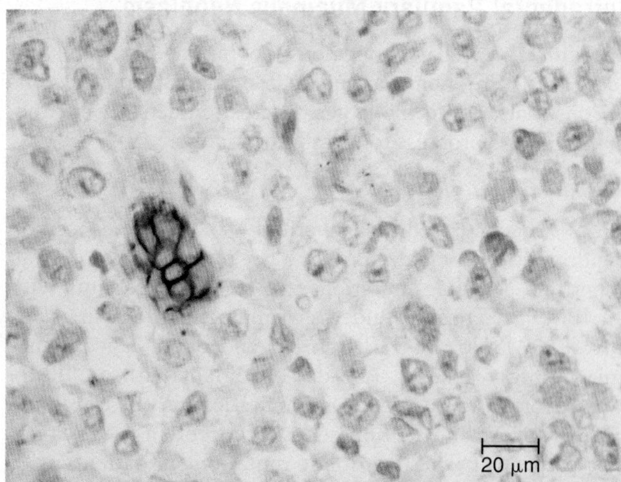

FIGURE 35.3 E-cadherin immunohistochemistry in undifferentiated pancreatic carcinoma. Immunohistochemical labeling for E-cadherin protein shows loss of expression in this undifferentiated pancreatic carcinoma, while the entrapped better-differentiated component retains membranous E-cadherin labeling.

be used to distinguish ductal adenocarcinoma (with loss of Smad4) from atypical, but reactive, nonneoplastic pancreatic diseases (with retention of Smad4), and to suggest that a metastatic adenocarcinoma is of pancreatobiliary origin.[39,58] Although extremely promising, somatic mutations have, to date, not had a great impact on guiding therapy. The two largest trials of personalized therapy based on somatic mutations, IMPACT and COMPASS, both proved disappointing.[47,59]

In addition, molecular studies interrogating genetic alterations also demonstrate clinical utility. For example, molecular analyses of *KRAS*, *TP53*, and *SMAD4* can be used to supplement morphological diagnosis in cytology specimens to increase sensitivity of fine-needle aspiration.[60] In addition, with the continuous development of targeted therapies, molecular studies will likely serve a critical role in determining eligibility for therapy.

Variants of Ductal Adenocarcinoma

There are multiple uncommon morphological variants of ductal adenocarcinoma. While some share the molecular features of ductal adenocarcinoma, others harbor unique genetic alterations, and these entities have clinical implications.

Adenosquamous carcinoma has molecular features similar to those of ductal adenocarcinoma, with prevalent alterations in *KRAS*, *p16/CDKN2A*, *SMAD4*, and *TP53*, but it is an aggressive neoplasm with a poor prognosis.[61] As noted earlier, *GATA6* expression is decreased in these carcinomas compared with carcinomas of the "classical" subtype.[44,47,61] It has been suggested that adenosquamous carcinomas respond best to platinum-based chemotherapies.[62]

Colloid carcinoma (mucinous noncystic carcinoma) has a better prognosis than pure ductal (tubular) adenocarcinoma of the pancreas.[63] These carcinomas almost always arise in association with an intestinal-type intraductal papillary mucinous neoplasm (IPMN), and, not surprisingly, the pattern of genetic alterations in colloid carcinomas parallels that of IPMNs.[64-66] Colloid carcinomas, in addition to frequently harboring mutations in the genes targeted in ductal adenocarcinomas (*KRAS*, *TP53* etc.), also often harbor mutations in *GNAS*, an oncogene frequently altered in intraductal papillary mucinous neoplasms.[64-66]

Medullary carcinoma, another variant with a better prognosis than ductal adenocarcinoma, has a high prevalence of microsatellite instability and lacks somatic mutations in *KRAS*, though oncogenic *BRAF* mutations have been reported.[19,67] As noted earlier, these cancers with microsatellite instability may be exquisitely sensitive to immunotherapy.[3,24]

Undifferentiated carcinoma is an aggressive neoplasm with a poor prognosis; in addition to prevalent *KRAS* mutations, these carcinomas also exhibit frequent loss of E-cadherin protein expression, providing a possible explanation for the carcinoma's poorly cohesive morphology (Fig. 35.3).[68,69] *Undifferentiated rhabdoid carcinomas* have been described, and the monomorphic variants of this carcinoma have *SMARCB1* loss.[70,71]

Undifferentiated carcinoma with osteoclast-like giant cells, another aggressive carcinoma with poor prognosis, contains two distinct cell populations: while the neoplastic mononuclear cells contain frequent *KRAS* mutations and p53 overexpression, the osteoclast-like giant cells are nonneoplastic and contain only mutant *KRAS* from phagocytized neoplastic mononuclear cell DNA.[72,73] Indeed, recent whole exome sequencing has highlighted that undifferentiated carcinomas with osteoclast-like giant cells are genetically very similar to invasive ductal adenocarcinomas.[72]

Thus careful integration of molecular findings with histopathology has helped explain some of the morphological variants of ductal adenocarcinoma and is forming the basis for a new classification of pancreatic neoplasia, one that integrates molecular genetics together with tumor histopathology. In contrast to those in other organs, molecular findings have tended to support, and not supplant, existing morphological classifications.

Intraductal Papillary Mucinous Neoplasm

Intraductal papillary mucinous neoplasms (IPMNs) are large (≥1.0 cm), noninvasive mucin-producing precancerous lesions that arise in the larger pancreatic ducts. Over time, some IPMNs progress to invasive carcinoma.

Germline Alterations

IPMNs occur rarely in inherited cancer predisposition syndromes (see Table 35.1).[74,75] For example, Skaro et al. identified germline mutations in 7% of 315 patients with an IPMN.[74] These included germline mutations in *ATM*, *BRCA2*, *MSH6*, *BUB1B*, *PALB2*, and other Fanconi anemia pathway genes.[74] A 3-day-old infant with an IPMN was reported to have germline mutations in the *SKIL* and *TUBB5* genes, and *TUBB5* codes for a protein in the Robo-Slit pathway.[76] These germline mutations in patients with IPMNs are important for the same reasons given earlier for germline mutations in patients with invasive carcinoma. In addition, patients with a surgically resected IPMN with a germline mutation are more likely to have concurrent invasive pancreatic carcinoma than are IPMN patients without a germline mutation.[74]

Somatic Alterations

Many of the genes mutated in IPMNs are the same genes commonly mutated in pancreatic ductal adenocarcinoma (see Table 35.2).[64,65] These include somatic mutations in *KRAS*, *p16/CDKN2A*, *TP53*, and *SMAD4*.[64,65,77,78] *KRAS* mutations occur early, in lesions with low-grade dysplasia, *p16/CDKN2A* an intermediate event, and *TP53* and *SMAD4* inactivation are late events.[64,65,77] In addition to alterations in genes frequently altered in ductal adenocarcinoma, IPMNs also contain mutations in genes unique among pancreatic neoplasms (see Table 35.2). Somatic mutations in *GNAS* have been reported in approximately 60% of IPMNs.[64,65,77,79] Intriguingly, the *GNAS* mutations in IPMNs all occur in a previously described oncogenic hotspot (codon 201), providing strong evidence for their functional importance in IPMNs. Mutations in *GNAS* are most prevalent in intestinal-type IPMNs but occur in most other histological subtypes, with the possible exception of oncocytic IPMNs.[64,65,77] In IPMNs with associated invasive carcinoma, *GNAS* mutations can be identified in both the noninvasive and invasive components, providing further genetic evidence that IPMNs give rise to invasive carcinoma.[64,65,77]

The gene *RNF43* is also frequently altered in IPMNs: up to 75% of IPMNs contain somatic mutations in *RNF43*, which encodes an E3 ubiquitin ligase.[64,65,77] The majority of these alterations are nonsense substitution mutations, leading to the insertion of stop codons and thus loss of function of the encoded protein. This mutation pattern, along with frequent loss of heterozygosity at the *RNF43* locus on chromosome 17q, provides strong evidence that *RNF43* is a tumor suppressor gene in IPMNs.

In addition, approximately 10% of intestinal-type IPMNs contain somatic mutations in *PIK3CA*, the catalytic component of a crucial cell signaling pathway known to be an oncogene in several other tumor types, and some somatic mutations in IPMNs occur at previously described oncogenic hotspots in *PIK3CA*.[64,65,77] Other less commonly targeted genes include *STK11/LKB1* (the locus of PJS), *EGFR*, and *ERBB2*.

The neoplastic cells of intraductal oncocytic papillary neoplasms (IOPNs) have a distinctive morphology with abundant eosinophilic cytoplasm, and they have been an enigma, as they lack the genetic alterations commonly found in other IPMNs.[80] Singhi et al. recently solved this mystery when they discovered that almost all IOPNs harbor recurrent *PRKACA* or *PRKACB* gene rearrangements.[81] These included *ATP1B1-PRKACB*, *DNAJB1-PRKACA*, and *ATP1B1-PRKACA* fusion genes, the same fusion genes reported in fibrolamellar carcinomas of the liver. These fusion genes were not detected in other neoplasms of the pancreas but were detectable in cyst fluid aspirated from IOPNs.

Genetic mechanisms other than somatic mutation also play a role in the development of IPMNs. Promoter hypermethylation occurs in several genes in IPMNs, including p16/CDKN2A hypermethylation, and the expression of a number of microRNAs is altered in IPMNs.[82,83]

Implications for Pathology

These genetic data provide strong evidence for the role of IPMNs as a precursor to invasive adenocarcinoma, a role strongly supported by clinical data as well. Knowledge of the genetic drivers of IPMNs can be utilized in the development of diagnostic assays. For example, mutations shed from neoplastic cells can be detected in aspirated cyst fluid, indicating that molecular analyses of cyst fluid may be useful as a preoperative diagnostic tool in pancreatic cysts.[64,84-88] In specific, more than 95% of IPMNs contain a somatic mutation in either *KRAS* or *GNAS*, suggesting that a molecular assay involving these two genes would be a highly sensitive assay for the identification of IPMNs.[84,85,87] Similarly, as described later, *VHL* gene mutations in cyst fluid are highly suggestive of a serous cystadenoma. It is likely that a combination of markers, one that includes clinical information as well as genetic analyses, will be the most useful in preoperative cyst classification.[84]

Genetic analyses have also provided novel insights into the heterogeneity of IPMNs. Co-occurring IPMNs and invasive cancers sometimes have distinct somatic mutations, establishing that while IPMNs can progress to invasive cancer, not all invasive cancers arise from the IPMN that they happen to be adjacent to.[89] Complicating things even more, IPMNs appear to be genetically very heterogeneous and some even have a polyclonal origin.[90] This heterogeneity needs to be considered when interpreting tests of cyst fluid.

Mucinous Cystic Neoplasm

Mucinous cystic neoplasms (MCNs) are mucin-producing epithelial neoplasms that do not communicate with the duct system. They are characterized by a distinctive ovarian-type stroma.

Germline Alterations

There is no known genetic predisposition or association with particular genetic syndromes for mucinous cystic neoplasms.

Somatic Alterations

The exomes of MCNs have been sequenced, and, like IPMNs, many of the same genes targeted in ductal adenocarcinomas *(KRAS*, *p16/CDKN2A*, *TP53)* are also

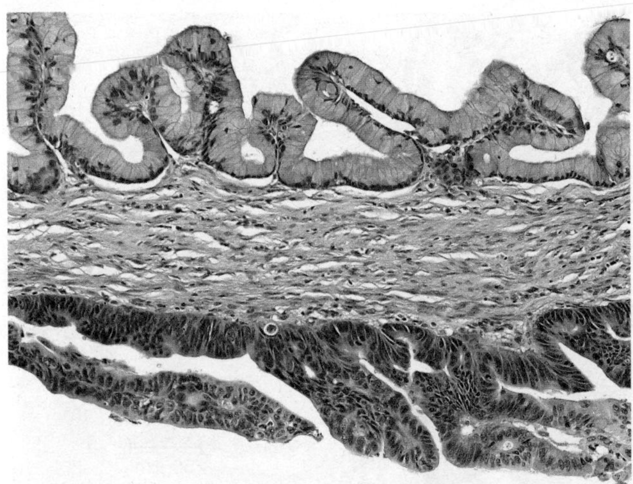

FIGURE 35.4 Mucinous cystic neoplasm. Note how two adjacent locules can have very different degrees of dysplasia.

targeted in MCNs (see Table 35.2).[64,84] Somatic mutations in *KRAS* oncogenic hotspots are common in MCNs, with mutation prevalence that correlates with degree of dysplasia (approximately 30% *KRAS* mutation prevalence in MCNs with low-grade dysplasia vs ~80% *KRAS* mutation prevalence in MCNs with high-grade dysplasia or with an associated invasive carcinoma).[64,90,91] *KRAS* mutations are also identified in areas of MCNs that are lined by flat, non-mucinous epithelium.[92] Somatic mutation of *TP53* as well as p53 protein overexpression are limited to MCNs with high-grade dysplasia.[64,84] Loss of Smad4 protein expression, indicating somatic mutation in the *SMAD4* gene, has been reported primarily in invasive carcinomas associated with MCNs; this loss of Smad4 expression occurs in only 14% of MCN-associated invasive carcinomas, a far lower prevalence than in invasive carcinomas not associated with MCNs.[64,93] The *p16/CKDN2A* gene is also infrequently altered in MCNs: somatic mutation has been reported in a neoplasm with high-grade dysplasia, and hypermethylation of the *p16/CKDN2A* promoter occurs in approximately 15% of MCNs.[64,84,94]

These findings suggest a stepwise genetic progression in MCNs from low-grade dysplasia to invasive carcinoma, in which *KRAS* mutation is an early event and loss of Smad4 is a late event. The dysplasia can progress at different rates in different cyst locules, and so the sampling of one locule cannot be used to define the degree of dysplasia in all locules (Fig. 35.4).

In addition to mutations in genes frequently altered in ductal adenocarcinoma, MCNs also share alterations in genes unique to mucin-producing cyst-forming neoplasms of the pancreas (see Table 35.2). Like IPMNs, MCNs often contain alterations in *RNF43*: approximately 40% of MCNs harbor somatic mutations in *RNF43*, and these mutations are enriched for nonsense substitutions.[64] *PIK3CA* can also be somatically altered in MCNs.[95]

Molecular studies have also provided insight into the biphasic nature of MCNs. Gene expression studies suggest different expression profiles in the epithelial and stromal components, with activation of the Notch pathway (*JAG1* and *HES1*) in the epithelial component and activation of estrogen metabolism (*STAR* and *ESR*) and markers of primordial germ cells in the stromal component.[96,97] The genetic or epigenetic basis for these differences remains unclear. In exceedingly rare mixed malignant neoplasms with both epithelial and high-grade "sarcomatous" components, studies of loss of heterozygosity suggest a monoclonal origin for the two components with subsequent genetic and morphological divergence.[98]

Implications for Pathology

As in other pancreatic neoplasms, immunohistochemical labeling for p53 and Smad4 can facilitate identification of neoplastic cells in MCNs, though the prevalence of alterations in these genes is far lower in MCNs than in ductal adenocarcinoma. Like IPMNs, identification of mutations in DNA from cyst fluid (including mutations *KRAS* and *RNF43*) represents a promising preoperative diagnostic test to determine the likelihood of a preinvasive mucin-producing cyst.[84,87]

Serous Cystadenoma

Serous cystadenomas (SCAs) are benign neoplasms composed of cysts lined by uniform glycogen-rich cuboidal cells.

Germline Alterations

Almost all patients with von Hippel-Lindau (VHL) syndrome have cysts in their pancreas, including serous cystadenomas, simple cysts, and cystic neuroendocrine tumors (see Table 35.1).[99-101] VHL is caused by germline mutations in the *VHL* gene on chromosome 3p, which encodes a regulator of the hypoxia-inducible factor 1 (HIF1α) pathway.[102] The SCAs that occur in this syndrome are often combined serous-neuroendocrine neoplasms.[101]

Somatic Alterations

Whole exome sequencing of sporadic SCAs identified only a handful (average of 10) of nonsynonymous somatic alterations per tumor, approximately half the number of alterations in IPMN and far fewer than in invasive ductal adenocarcinoma.[64] Importantly, SCAs lack somatic alterations in genes frequently mutated in invasive ductal adenocarcinoma, such as *KRAS*, *SMAD4*, and *TP53* (see Table 35.2). The main genetic driver of SCAs instead is somatic mutation of the *VHL* gene, which has been reported in as many as 50% of SCAs.[64] Loss of heterozygosity at the *VHL* locus on chromosome 3p also occurs in a large proportion of sporadic SCAs[64,103]

Implications for Pathology

The prevalence of SCAs in patients with VHL syndrome requires a high index of suspicion when examining pancreata from patients with VHL. Conversely, the finding of multiple SCAs or a combined serous-neuroendocrine neoplasm should raise the suspicion that the patient has VHL. In addition, *VHL* mutations have been identified in DNA from cyst fluid aspirated from SCAs.[84,87,104] The specificity of these mutations for SCAs suggest that molecular assays to identify *VHL* mutations in cyst fluid may provide a useful preoperative diagnostic test, separating cysts with a risk of malignant progressions (IPMNs and MCNs) from entirely benign cysts (SCAs).[84]

Solid-Pseudopapillary Neoplasm

Solid-pseudopapillary neoplasms (SPNs) are malignant neoplasms composed of poorly cohesive cells surrounding thin blood vessels. They characteristically form solid masses with prominent cystic degeneration.

Germline Alterations

A solid-pseudopapillary neoplasm occurring in a patient with familial adenomatous polyposis has been reported, but the vast majority of SPNs are sporadic.[105]

Somatic Alterations

The β-catenin gene *(CTNNB1)* is somatically mutated in 95% of SPNs, and in the vast majority of these neoplasms *CTNNB1* is the only gene mutated (see Table 35.2).[64,106-108] SPNs lack alterations in genes commonly altered in pancreatic ductal adenocarcinoma, such as *KRAS*, *TP53*, and *SMAD4*, as well as those mutated in other pancreatic cysts such as *GNAS*, *VHL*, and *RNF43*.[64] The *CTNNB1* mutations in SPNs are activating mutations that lead to the abnormal nuclear accumulation of β-catenin protein in almost 100% of SPNs.[106,107] This protein has diverse functions in normal cells, regulating cell adhesion through its interaction with E-cadherin as well as serving as an important target of Wnt signaling: β-catenin is normally targeted for degradation by APC and GSK-3β, but when degradation of β-catenin is inhibited by Wnt signaling, the protein translocates to the nucleus, leading to transcription of target genes.[109] The somatic mutations in *CTNNB1* frequently affect key phosphorylation sites, preventing degradation of the β-catenin protein and leading to nuclear translocation of β-catenin and transcriptional activation.[106,107] Somatic mutations in *CTNNB1* in SPNs lead to overexpression of cyclin D1, a key cell cycle regulator and important downstream target of β-catenin.[106,107] In addition, the expression of the E-cadherin protein is also dramatically altered in SPNs: expression of the extracellular domain of E-cadherin is lost in these neoplasms, while the intracellular component of the E-cadherin protein is abnormally expressed in the nucleus of neoplastic cells.[110-112] Importantly, the other common pancreatic neoplasms (including invasive ductal adenocarcinoma and PanNET) typically lack somatic mutations in *CTNNB1*.

Amato et al. have reported additional somatic mutations beyond *CTNNB1* mutations in SPNs that had metastasized, but it is unclear if these were drivers of metastasis, or if they were treatment induced, as many of the metastases were sampled after the patient received chemotherapy.[113]

Implications for Pathology

Importantly, discovery of an almost universal genetic alteration in SPNs (*CTNNB1* mutation) has led to the development of a diagnostic test (β-catenin immunohistochemistry) that, when combined with routine histopathology and other immunohistochemical markers, helps distinguish this neoplasm from other solid cellular neoplasms of the pancreas (Fig. 35.5). In the appropriate setting, immunohistochemical labeling for β-catenin to identify aberrant nuclear labeling represents a key step in the diagnostic algorithm for solid-pseudopapillary neoplasm. In addition, the abnormalities in E-cadherin expression may explain this lesion's discohesive morphology.

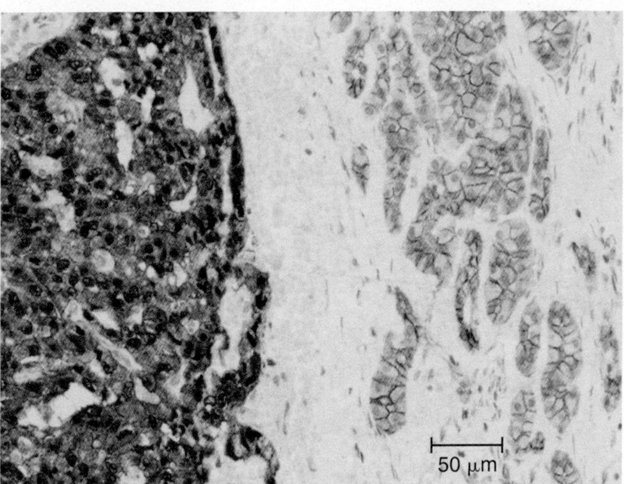

FIGURE 35.5 β-catenin immunohistochemistry in solid pseudopapillary neoplasms. Immunohistochemical labeling for β-catenin protein shows aberrant nuclear and cytoplasmic staining in the neoplastic cells of a solid pseudopapillary neoplasm *(left)*, while the adjacent nonneoplastic pancreas shows normal membranous labeling *(right)*.

Pancreatic Neuroendocrine Tumor

Well-differentiated pancreatic neuroendocrine tumors (PanNETs) are epithelial neoplasms characterized by organoid or trabecular growth, nuclear and cytoplasmic features that resemble nonneoplastic islet cells, and the expression of markers of neuroendocrine differentiation. All neuroendocrine tumors ≥0.5 cm are considered malignant.

Germline Alterations

Pancreatic neuroendocrine tumors occur as key features of multiple inherited syndromes (see Table 35.1). PanNETs occur in 60% to 70% of patients with multiple endocrine neoplasia syndrome, type 1 (MEN1), an autosomal dominant syndrome characterized by neuroendocrine lesions of the parathyroid, pituitary, pancreas, duodenum, and adrenal.[114,115] MEN1 is caused by germline mutations in the *MEN1* gene on chromosome 11q.[116] PanNETs also occur in 5% to 10% of patients with VHL syndrome, which is caused by germline mutations in the *VHL* gene on chromosome 3p. Patients with VHL syndrome are predisposed to neoplasms in various organs, including the adrenal, kidney, and pancreas, many of which are composed of optically clear neoplastic cells.[117]

In addition, PanNETs occur rarely in other genetic syndromes. Tuberous sclerosis complex is caused by germline mutations in *TSC1* on chromosome 9q or *TSC2* on chromosome 16p.[118] This autosomal dominant clinical syndrome is characterized by hamartomas and a variety of neoplasms, including, rarely PanNETs. Neurofibromatosis type 1 (NF1) is an autosomal dominant clinical syndrome characterized most prominently by nervous system abnormalities. PanNETs expressing somatostatin (somatostatinomas) are a rare finding in this syndrome, which is caused by germline mutations in the tumor suppressor gene *NF1* on chromosome 17q.[119] The second, wild-type, allele of *NF1* is somatically inactivated in these tumors.[119] Although pancreatic neoplasms have been reported, somatostatinomas occur more frequently in the duodenums of patients with NF1.[119]

Whole-genome sequencing of PanNETs has also revealed rare germline mutations in DNA repair genes (*MUTYH*, *CHEK2*, and *BRCA2*) as well as the expected germline mutations in *MEN1*, *VHL*, and *CDKN1B*.[120]

Somatic Alterations

The somatic genetic alterations in sporadic well-differentiated PanNETs have been well characterized (see Table 35.2).[120-122] Somatic mutations in the *MEN1* gene occur in 45% of sporadic PanNETs.[120-122] Loss of heterozygosity at the *MEN1* locus also frequently occurs in PanNETs, establishing *MEN1* as a bona fide tumor suppressor gene in this tumor type.[120-122] Somatic mutations in *MEN1* cause defects in menin protein function, with loss of expression or aberrant localization.[123] Loss of menin expression appears to be an early event in these tumors.[124]

Somatic mutations in the *ATRX* and *DAXX* genes are also common in sporadic PanNETs.[120-122] These somatic mutations, which occur in approximately 45% of sporadic PanNETs, inactivate the encoded proteins that function in chromatin remodeling.[120-122] The proteins encoded by *ATRX* and *DAXX* are components of a complex involved in telomere maintenance; these inactivating mutations in PanNETs are associated with the telomerase-independent telomere maintenance mechanism termed "alternative lengthening of telomeres (ALT)."[120-122] Therefore inactivating mutations in *ATRX* and *DAXX* are associated with the acquisition of the ALT phenotype, indicating that the telomeres of many PanNETs are fundamentally different from the telomeres of ductal adenocarcinoma, which exhibit telomere shortening and reactivation of telomerase.[52] Moreover, mutations in *ATRX* and *DAXX* (as well as the ALT phenotype) occur late in the development of PanNETs, as they occur only in large tumors (>3 cm) and are absent from microadenomas.[124,125]

Genes coding for members of the mammalian target of rapamycin (mTOR) cell signaling pathway are also altered in some PanNETs; mutations in components of this pathway (including *PIK3CA*, *PTEN*, *DEPDC5*, *TSC1*, and *TSC2*) occur in approximately 15% of sporadic PanNETs.[120-122] Chromosomal rearrangements occur in PanNETs, and some of these inactivate tumor suppressor genes, including *MTAP*, *ARID2*, *SMARCA4*, *MLL3*, *p16/CDKN2A*, and *STED2*.[120]

Well-differentiated PanNETs almost always lack alterations in genes commonly mutated in pancreatic ductal adenocarcinoma, including *KRAS*, *TP53*, and *SMAD4*.[120-122,126] Mutations in *TP53* are very rare in well-differentiated PanNETs, occurring in only approximately 3% of neoplasms, a far lower prevalence than in ductal adenocarcinoma.[120-122]

The genetic alterations in small and large cell neuroendocrine carcinomas of the pancreas are distinct from those in well-differentiated PanNETs. In contrast to well-differentiated PanNETs, *TP53* (95%) and *RB* (75%) alterations are common in small and large cell neuroendocrine carcinomas.[127] Conversely, the genes frequently targeted in well-differentiated neuroendocrine tumors (*DAXX*, *ATRX*, etc.) are not targeted in small and large cell neuroendocrine carcinomas.[127] As described later, these genetic differences helped in the establishment of a revised grading system for PanNETs, one that clearly separates well-differentiated tumors from the higher grade neuroendocrine carcinomas.[128]

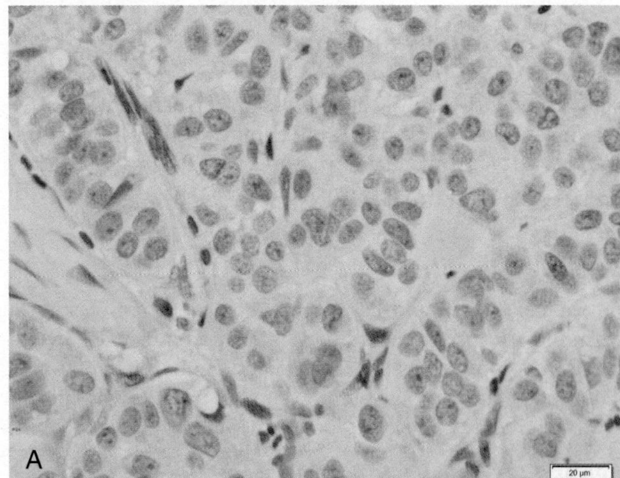

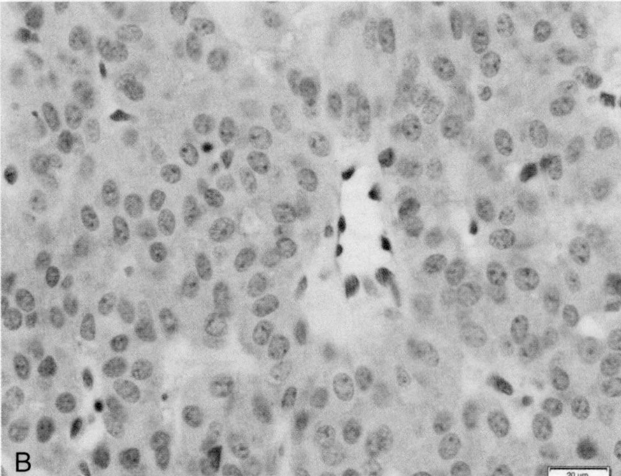

FIGURE 35.6 ATRX and DAXX immunohistochemistry in well-differentiated pancreatic neuroendocrine tumors (PanNET). Immunohistochemical labeling for ATRX **(A)** and DAXX **(B)** proteins show loss of expression in the neoplastic cells of PanNETs, while normal nuclear labeling is retained in associated nonneoplastic endothelial cells.

Implications for Pathology

Knowledge of the genetic syndromes predisposing to PanNETs (including MEN1 and VHL) allows recognition of these neoplasms in syndromic patients. In particular, pathologists need to carefully examine the duodenum in patients with MEN1, as small duodenal neuroendocrine tumors (gastrinomas) in these patients can metastasize to a peripancreatic lymph node and mimic a primary pancreatic neoplasm.[129] In addition, some somatic alterations, including mutations in *MEN1*, *ATRX*, and *DAXX*, have prognostic implications.[130-132] Immunohistochemistry can be utilized to show loss of ATRX or DAXX protein expression in mutant cases (Fig. 35.6). Prognostic groups have been identified based on the somatic genetic alterations inPanNETs.[120,133] Finally, the genetic alterations may influence therapy; the alterations in the mTOR pathway may have profound clinical significance, as drugs targeting the mTOR pathway have already been developed for clinical use and these drugs may be specifically efficacious in patients with somatic alterations in this cellular pathway.[134] Patients with high-grade neuroendocrine carcinomas (small and large cell carcinomas) are often treated with platinum-based chemotherapy.[135]

Acinar Cell Carcinoma

Acinar cell carcinomas (ACCs) are malignant epithelial neoplasms with significant expression of secreted digestive enzymes including trypsin and chymotrypsin. The neoplastic cells often form acinar structures or grow in sheets, they can have granular cytoplasm, and often have nuclei with single prominent nucleoli.

Germline Alterations

Acinar cell carcinoma has been reported in patients with germline *BRCA2* gene mutations, in patients with Lynch syndrome, in patients with familial adenomatous polyposis, in patients with Carney complex, and in patients with germline variants in the *PRKAR1A* gene.[136-144]

Somatic Alterations

Recurrent somatic alterations of few genes have been identified in ACCs (see Table 35.2).[138,145,146] Somatic mutations in the APC/β-catenin pathway occur in 20% to 25% of ACCs; both activating mutations in *CTNNB1* and inactivating mutations in *APC* have been reported.[145,146] Importantly, ACCs lack frequent alterations in genes commonly mutated in ductal adenocarcinoma. *KRAS* mutations are extremely rare in ACC, and mutations of *TP53*, *SMAD4*, and *p16/CDKN2A* are less prevalent than they are in ductal adenocarcinomas.[138,145,146] Interestingly, a subset of ACCs exhibits microsatellite instability.[138,141,145,146] *CMYC* is amplified in close to half of the cases, and PRKAR1A, the gene associated with Carney complex, is targeted in approximately 10% of the cancers.[139,147,148]

Rearrangements involving the *BRAF* gene that create novel *BRAF* fusion genes *(SND1-BRAF)* that activate the gene product are common in ACC, and fluorescence in situ hybridization (FISH) probes have been developed that can detect these fusions in clinical samples.[138,149]

Implications for Pathology

Immunohistochemical labeling for β-catenin shows the characteristic abnormal nuclear accumulation in a subset of acinar cell carcinomas.[146] However, immunohistochemistry for β-catenin must be interpreted in the context of other immunohistochemical, morphological, and clinical data to avoid confusion with other neoplasms with aberrant β-catenin staining, particularly solid-pseudopapillary neoplasms. The FISH assay to detect *BRAF* gene rearrangements has been used to identify acinar-type neoplasms.[150]

One thing that stands out about the mutations identified in ACC is that many are potentially therapeutically targetable. For example, ACCs with microsatellite instability may be susceptible to immunotherapy, ACCs with *BRCA2* gene inactivation to PARP inhibitors, and ACCs with *BRAF* fusions to selective kinase inhibitors.[22,145,151]

Pancreatoblastoma

Pancreatoblastomas are malignant epithelial neoplasms with acinar differentiation and distinctive squamoid nests.

Germline Alterations

Several cases of pancreatoblastoma have been reported in patients with Beckwith-Wiedemann syndrome, a disorder of organ overgrowth and predisposition to embryonal tumors associated with dysregulation of a highly imprinted region on chromosome 11p (see Table 35.1).[152,153] In addition, pancreatoblastomas have been reported in patients with familial adenomatous polyposis.[143,154,155]

Somatic Alterations

Sporadic pancreatoblastomas show frequent allelic loss at chromosome 11p, occurring in 86% of cases in one study (see Table 35.2).[154-157] Intriguingly, loss of 11p has also been reported in other embryonal neoplasms, such as hepatoblastoma and Wilms tumor, suggesting the possibility of a common genetic pathway in embryonal tumors.[158-160] In addition, the majority of pancreatoblastomas have somatic alterations in the APC/β-catenin pathway, including activating mutations in *CTNNB1* as well as inactivating mutations in *APC*.[154] These alterations lead to abnormal nuclear accumulation of β-catenin as well as overexpression of cyclin D1, both of which often occur in a patchy fashion, sometimes involving the squamoid nests of pancreatoblastoma.[156,161] Pancreatoblastomas lack frequent alterations in genes commonly mutated in ductal adenocarcinoma; although rare loss of Smad4 expression has been reported, no *KRAS* mutations or alteration of p53 expression have been identified in pancreatoblastoma.[154,156,157] Methylation of the promoter of the *RASSF1A* gene has also been reported.[162,163]

Implications for Pathology

Due to germline predisposition to pancreatoblastoma, this tumor should be suspected in patients with Beckwith-Wiedemann syndrome. In addition, due to genetic alterations in the APC/β-catenin pathway, many pancreatoblastomas show abnormal nuclear accumulation of β-catenin that can be detected by immunohistochemistry.[154,156,157] Although this nuclear β-catenin labeling may be useful diagnostically, if other histopathological features are not considered, it can also create confusion in the differential diagnosis with solid-pseudopapillary neoplasm and other neoplasms with aberrant β-catenin labeling: a perfect example of how molecular genetics has added to, not replaced, histology in the pancreas!

BILIARY NEOPLASMS

Cholangiocarcinoma

Germline Alterations

Germline variants in Fanconi anemia pathway genes, including *BRCA2* and *BRCA1*, have been reported in patients with cholangiocarcinoma, and, as is true for other neoplasms, these cancers appear to be sensitive to PARP inhibitors.[164-166] Germline mutations in the DNA mismatch repair genes, including *MLH1* and *MSH2* have also been reported.[166,167] The therapeutic implications of the resultant microsatellite instability were discussed previously.

Somatic Alterations

The term *cholangiocarcinoma* refers to carcinoma of the biliary tract, including the intrahepatic, hilar, and extrahepatic bile ducts. Although some studies do not separately assess these neoplasms based on site, more recent studies have made it clear that somatic alterations in cholangiocarcinoma vary by anatomic location within the body, and underlying carcinogenic etiology including geographic location of the patient.[168] Still, further studies that directly compare different subgroups of cholangiocarcinoma will be necessary to understand better their unique genetic features.

Recent comprehensive genomic analyses of cholangiocarcinomas highlighted some genetic features that are distinct from those found in pancreatic neoplasms. A significant number of mutations in isocitrate dehydrogenase 1 and 2 (*IDH1* and *IDH2*) have been reported in intrahepatic cholangiocarcinoma.[166,168-171] These genes encode metabolic enzymes and are frequently altered in tumors of the central nervous system, but intrahepatic cholangiocarcinoma is unique among pancreatobiliary cancers in somatic mutations in *IDH1* and *IDH2*.[170,172] In addition, mutations in genes that encode chromatin remodelers, including *ARID1A*, *BAP1*, and *PBRM1*, occur frequently in intrahepatic cholangiocarcinomas.[169] Recurrent chromosomal rearrangements resulting in gene fusions of the *FGFR2* gene have also been documented in intrahepatic cholangiocarcinoma, occurring in more than 10% of these cancers.[173]

In addition to these unique genes, sporadic cholangiocarcinomas also contain somatic alterations in many of the driver genes altered in pancreatic ductal adenocarcinoma (see Table 35.2).[166,168,169,171] Oncogenic hotspot mutations in *KRAS* are frequent in cholangiocarcinomas.[166,168,169,174,175] Interestingly, the prevalence of *KRAS* mutations reported in different studies varies significantly, including variation related to the country of origin of the patient, suggesting either methodological differences, or a significant environmental impact driving these gene mutations.[174,175] For example, a high prevalence of *KRAS* mutations has been reported in cholangiocarcinomas in patients with pancreatobiliary maljunction: the prevalence of *KRAS* mutation is approximately 60% in these patients.[176] Alterations in *p16/CDK2NA* have been reported in 55% to 85% of cholangiocarcinomas by mechanisms including intragenic mutation, homozygous deletion, and promoter methylation.[166,168,169] Many cholangiocarcinomas harbor alterations in the *TP53* tumor suppressor gene, with aberrant expression reported in 25% to 50% of carcinomas.[166,168,169] Complementing *TP53* inactivation, *MDM2* amplification is seen in approximately 10% of cholangiocarcinomas.[177] Loss of Smad4 also frequently occurs in cholangiocarcinoma.[178] The prevalence of *SMAD4* mutations in these genes varies depending on the location of the tumor within the biliary tree, with increased prevalence in carcinomas of the more distal biliary tree.[178]

Cholangiocarcinomas also contain less prevalent mutations in a large number of genes (see Table 35.2).[166,168,169] The PI3K pathway has been reported to be altered in cholangiocarcinoma, but the overall significance of this pathway remains controversial. Prevalence of oncogenic mutations in *PIK3CA* in cholangiocarcinoma varies widely among studies: whereas some fail to identify any mutations, others identify a prevalence of greater than 30%.[166,168-170] In addition, rare mutations in *PTEN* and *AKT1*, the protein products of which act in the same pathway as *PIK3CA*,have also been reported in cholangiocarcinomas.[170] Rare mutations in *EGFR* kinase as well as in *CDH1* (E-cadherin gene) have also been reported, as has a homozygous deletion of *STK11/LKB1*.[166,168-170,179,180] In addition, infrequent amplification of *ERBB2*, *CCND1*, and *EGFR* has been documented.[181-183]

Environmental factors shape the mutational patterns observed in cholangiocarcinoma.[184,185] For example, liver fluke infection (*Opisthorchis viverrini* and *Clonorchis sinensis*) is a known risk factor for cholangiocarcinoma in parts of Asia. Analysis of a large cohort of cholangiocarcinoma patients revealed unique molecular subtypes that correlated with underlying etiology (sporadic vs liver fluke), and smaller studies of cholangiocarcinomas related to liver fluke infection revealed unique genetic features.[186-188] In particular, fluke-associated cholangiocarcinomas were enriched for *TP53* mutations and *ERBB2* amplifications, while fluke-negative cholangiocarcinomas contained alterations in chromatin remodeling genes, *IDH1/2*, and in *FGFR*. Thus this cholangiocarcinoma subtype initially defined by its unique underlying infection also constitutes a distinct genetic subset of this cancer.

Implications for Pathology

Like pancreatic ductal adenocarcinoma, immunohistochemical labeling for p53 and Smad4 have clinical utility in their ability to identify tumors with mutations in these genes. The development of diagnostic assays and therapeutic approaches based on *IDH1* mutations will be applicable to cholangiocarcinomas as well as neoplasms of the central nervous system (which also contain prevalent *IDH1* mutations).[189] In addition, cholangiocarcinomas also infrequently contain alterations in *ERBB2*, *FGFR1*, *FGFR2*, *FGFR3*, and *EGFR*, each of which are targets for mutation-specific therapies.[185,190,191] Assays identifying tumors with these alterations will help to identify patients most likely to benefit from targeted therapies. Even small biopsies from the duct system can be sequenced, opening the door to a broad array of biosamples for clinical use.[192]

Gallbladder Carcinoma

Gallbladder carcinoma is a malignant epithelial neoplasm that arises in the gallbladder.

Germline Alterations

Although gallbladder carcinoma is not associated with a known genetic syndrome, a small fraction of patients with gallbladder cancer have, on sequencing, been found to harbor a deleterious germline mutation in cancer-associated genes.[193-195] These include germline variants in Fanconi anemia pathway genes.

Somatic Alterations

Sporadic gallbladder carcinomas contain somatic alterations in many of the driver genes altered in pancreatic ductal adenocarcinoma (see Table 35.2).[169,193,196,197] The prevalence of somatic mutations in *KRAS* is lower in gallbladder carcinoma than in other pancreatobiliary carcinomas, in the range of only 10% to 20%.[169,193,196,197] Oncogenic mutations in *KRAS* also occur and can also be found in the precursors to gallbladder carcinoma, including 25% of gallbladder adenomas.[198,199] However, some experts argue that the difference in *KRAS* mutation prevalence between adenomas and carcinomas provides evidence for the model of multiple tumorigenic pathways in the gallbladder, a more common pathway in which carcinoma arises from flat dysplasia and a less common pathway in which carcinoma arises from an adenoma (which on its own has low malignant potential). Interestingly, in addition to *KRAS* mutations, somatic mutations at a previously described oncogenic hotspot in *BRAF* also occur frequently in gallbladder carcinoma, occurring in more than 30% of carcinomas in one study.[200]

Somatic mutations in tumor suppressor genes also occur in gallbladder carcinoma. *P16/CDKN2A* alterations are common in gallbladder carcinoma, occurring in 60% to 75% of carcinomas by mechanisms including point mutation, chromosomal loss, and promoter methylation.[169,193,196,197,201] Loss of expression of pRB, a protein that functions in the same cell cycle control pathway as p16, occurs infrequently in gallbladder carcinomas, with loss in only 4% of carcinomas.[201] Alterations in *TP53* are common, with abnormal p53 protein expression in approximately 60% of carcinomas.[169,193,196,201] Intriguingly, both *TP53* loss and mutation have been identified in dysplastic gallbladder mucosa as well as histologically normal mucosa adjacent to an invasive carcinoma, and different mutations have been reported in carcinomas and adjacent nonneoplastic mucosa, suggesting the possibility of a "field effect" in this tumor type.[202] Loss of Smad4 expression also occurs in gallbladder carcinomas, though less frequently than in other tumor types: fewer than 20% of gallbladder carcinomas show loss of this protein.[201,203]

The ErbB signaling pathway (including *EGFR*, *ERBB2*, *ERBB3*, and *ERBB4*) is targeted in close to 40% of gallbladder cancers.[197] Somatic mutations in *CTNNB1* occur in fewer than 10% of gallbladder carcinomas.[204] Gallbladder adenomas exhibit a much higher *CTNNB1* mutation prevalence (approximately 60%) than carcinomas, providing further evidence for the model of separate genetic pathways underlying adenomas and invasive carcinomas of the gallbladder.[204] Activating somatic mutations in the oncogene *PIK3CA* occur in approximately 10% of gallbladder carcinomas.[170] Somatic mutations in *KEAP1*, a regulator of the cellular response to oxidative stress, have been reported in several gallbladder carcinomas, with a mutation prevalence of approximately 30%.[205] A few amplifications with known target genes have been identified: a small number of gallbladder carcinomas (less than 5%) exhibit amplification of the *MYC* oncogene.[206-208]

Implications for Pathology

Like other pancreatobiliary neoplasms, immunohistochemical assays for p53, Smad4, and β-catenin have clinical utility in gallbladder carcinoma; these assays reliably identify tumors with gene mutations. In the case of β-catenin, immunolabeling for this protein may separate carcinomas that occur through a separate tumorigenic pathway, as mutations in *CTNNB1* are much more common in gallbladder adenomas; however, the precise clinical relevance of this distinction remains to be determined.[204] As in cholangiocarcinoma, identification of patients with gallbladder cancer with alterations in *ERBB2* or *EGFR* may help to identify patients likely to benefit from specific targeted therapies.

High-Grade Neuroendocrine Carcinoma

High-grade neuroendocrine carcinoma (small cell carcinoma) of the gallbladder is a distinct clinical, histological, and molecular entity. These neoplasms, which have similar histological features to small cell carcinomas in other organs, have a dismal prognosis and frequently occur as one component of a mixed neoplasm combined with more conventional adenocarcinoma.[209] In contrast to conventional gallbladder adenocarcinoma, high-grade neuroendocrine carcinomas of the gallbladder have inactivation of the p16/pRB pathway, with two-thirds of tumors showing loss of RB and the remaining third showing loss of p16.[201,210] These neoplasms also have a very high prevalence of *TP53* alterations, with abnormal p53 protein expression in 80%.[201] By contrast, *KRAS* mutation and loss of Smad4 have not been identified in small cell carcinoma of the gallbladder, demonstrating significant differences in the molecular features of this tumor type compared with conventional gallbladder adenocarcinoma. The recognition of small cell carcinoma of the gallbladder as a morphologically and genetically distinct entity will facilitate the identification of a subset of patients with gallbladder carcinoma with a far worse prognosis.

CONCLUSION

Pancreatobiliary neoplasms encompass a broad range of clinical and morphological entities. As some of the best characterized neoplasms on a genetic level, these neoplasms provide a unique opportunity for the integration of clinical, morphological, and genetic data. Pathologists will be at the forefront of this integration. As the fields of pathology and oncology move into the era of genomic medicine, pathologists must combine morphological and molecular data in their assessment of pancreatobiliary specimens. These combined data will allow clinicians to provide the best possible care for patients with pancreatobiliary neoplasms, including diagnosis and treatment based on the specific genetic alterations in an individual patient's tumor.

The full reference list may be viewed online at Elsevier eBooks for Practicing Clinicians.

CHAPTER 36

Diagnostic Cytology of the Biliary Tract and Pancreas

Barbara A. Centeno, Michelle D. Reid

Contents

INTRODUCTION

Brushing cytology and fine-needle aspiration (FNA) are used to sample lesions in the biliary tract and pancreas. Endobiliary brushing is currently the preferred method of sampling the pancreatobiliary system in patients with a stricture or obstruction without an associated mass. It is also used to screen patients with primary sclerosing cholangitis (PSC). FNA is the most effective procedure for sampling solid and cystic masses of the pancreatobiliary tract.

The primary challenge for the pathologist in pancreatobiliary cytology specimens is the distinction of benign and reactive processes from adenocarcinoma. Other challenges include the diagnosis of nonductal neoplasms of the pancreas, the identification of subtypes of ductal adenocarcinoma, and the diagnosis of metastases. This chapter reviews the cytomorphology of the biliary tract and pancreas and discusses cytological differential diagnoses and the application of ancillary studies.

Guidance Methods

Guidance methods for endobiliary brushing include endoscopy, endoscopic retrograde cholangiopancreatography (ERCP), and percutaneous transhepatic cholangiopancreatography (PTC). Guidance techniques for FNA include intraoperative palpation and direct visualization, transabdominal ultrasound (TUS), intraoperative ultrasound, computed tomography (CT), and endoscopic ultrasound (EUS). EUS has become the preferred imaging technique at many academic centers and large community hospitals. Briefly, a biopsy needle is passed through the biopsy chamber of an echoendoscope, which consists of a linear array transducer mounted distal to the end of the viewing optical component of the endoscope. The needle is passed through either the duodenum, or stomach, into the pancreatobiliary mass, under real-time imaging.

Indications for Cytological Sampling of the Pancreatobiliary Tract

Indications for sampling of the biliary and pancreatic ducts using brushing cytology include the presence of a stricture or obstruction. The biliary tree is also sampled using brushing cytology to monitor patients with primary sclerosing cholangitis (PSC)[1, 2] who are at risk of developing cholangiocarcinoma. FNA is indicated for the sampling of solid or cystic masses of the pancreatobiliary tract.

Contraindications to Cytological Sampling of the Pancreatobiliary Tract

Contraindications to brushing of the biliary tract or pancreatic ducts include the contraindications to the techniques used to guide ERCP and PTC. Absolute contraindications to ERCP include patient refusal to undergo the procedure; unstable cardiopulmonary, neurological, or cardiovascular status; and existing bowel perforation. Relative contraindications include structural abnormalities of the esophagus, stomach, or small intestine. PTC is contraindicated in patients with bleeding diatheses and significant ascites.

Contraindications to EUS-FNA include an uncorrectable bleeding disorder or lack of a safe needle access route.[3] Gastrointestinal (GI) obstruction is an absolute contraindication for EUS-FNA because of the risk of intestinal perforation.[4]

Rapid On-Site Evaluation

The role of rapid on-site evaluation (ROSE) is not clearly established for brushing cytology. However, if smears are going to be prepared on-site, then it is preferable that they be prepared by an experienced cytotechnologist or pathologist.

ROSE, performed by either a cytotechnologist or pathologist, is probably the single greatest factor responsible for improving the diagnostic accuracy of FNA for solid masses of the pancreatobiliary tract. ROSE of selected smears ensures specimen adequacy and reduces the number of inadequate specimens due to poor localization of the lesion, scant cellularity, obscuring blood, as well as poor sample preparation or preservation. Thus ROSE produces significant cost savings and may spare the patient additional procedures.[5-10] ROSE also allows the interpreter to determine the need for adjunctive studies, such as flow cytometry, immunohistochemistry, or microbiology. ROSE is not indicated for purely cystic masses but can be performed on the solid component of a cystic mass.

Sensitivity and Specificity

Biliary Brushing Cytology

Prospective and retrospective studies documented a higher level of sensitivity of biliary brushings over exfoliative cytology for the detection of biliary carcinomas.[11] Duct brushing cytology has an overall sensitivity of 26% to 88.9%, a specificity of 80% to 100%, and an overall accuracy of 48.1% to 96%. In PSC, the sensitivity has been 60%, with a specificity of 89%. The sensitivity of bile duct brushings has been shown to increase after repeated attempts.[12,13] In fact, the probability of a patient having a carcinoma is less than 6% after three negative brushings.[14] Predictors of positive yield include the presence of a true stricture, older age, mass size >1 cm, and stricture length of >1 cm.[15,16] The presence of stones correlates with benign cytology.[17]

Most false negatives occur because of sampling error,[12,13] which may occur when the tumor does not invade biliary mucosa. In addition, tumors with sclerotic desmoplastic stroma do not exfoliate cells as readily as tumors without desmoplasia, and thus may not be detected with brushings. Poor visualization of the area by the endoscopist may negatively impact the sampling. Interpretation errors (17%) and technical errors (17%) are the second most frequent causes of false-negative results. Most interpretative errors result from underinterpretation of adenocarcinoma due to the difficulty of distinguishing adenocarcinoma from reactive changes.[18] The converse is also true: reactive changes can mimic adenocarcinoma, and lead to false-positive results. Degeneration of malignant cells is also a source of false negatives. False positives commonly result from overinterpretation of reactive and degenerative changes[19] or adenomatous epithelium from villous tumors of the ampulla[20] or bile duct. Intraductal neoplasms and dysplasia within the biliary ductal system may also lead to false positives.

FNA Cytology

The reported sensitivity for percutaneous pancreatic FNA, with the use of a variety of guidance techniques, ranges from 45% to 97%. The specificity is nearly 100%. Diagnostic accuracy ranges from 75% to 100%.[21] The low sensitivity and low negative predictor values are cited as major limitations of pancreatic fine-needle aspiration biopsy (FNA).[21] However, in our experience, the sensitivity for a diagnosis of adenocarcinoma is greater than 90% when ROSE is performed to ensure specimen adequacy.[9] The sensitivity for EUS-FNA ranges from 60% to 96%, with a specificity of nearly 100%.[22-26]

Factors that affect the accuracy of the procedure include (1) accurate localization of the mass by the operator, (2) adequate sampling of the mass, (3) correct sample preparation, and (4) correct interpretation by the pathologist. Accurate localization and adequate sampling are highly dependent on the skill of the operator. The sample should be representative of the intended target and should contain a sufficient number of cells for proper interpretation. Certain lesions may not yield diagnostic material regardless of the skill of the operator. These include most cystic lesions and sclerotic, vascular, or necrotic tumors. Aspiration of the periphery of necrotic tumors may help obtain better-preserved material. Poor sample preparation also hinders accurate interpretation by the pathologist. Factors that affect interpretation include blood, air-drying artifact on smears intended for alcohol fixation, crush artifact, and smears that are spread too thick.

Specimen Preparation

Preparation of Pancreatobiliary Tract Brushing Specimens

The traditional method is to prepare smears from the brushing and make both air-dried smears for on-site evaluation and alcohol fixed smears for Papanicolaou stains. The brush may also be collected in Cytolyt (Hologic, Marlborough, MA) and the sample prepared as a ThinPrep (Hologic, Marlborough, MA). Although the latter shows great sensitivity,[17] another potential method involves vortex-mixing the brush and then cutting the sheath and guidewire into 5 cm pieces, vortex-mixing these separately, and preparing a cytospin. This procedure may significantly increase cellularity.[27]

Preparation of FNA Specimens

Preparation methods used for FNA samples include direct smears, cytospins (Thermo-Shandon Instruments), liquid-based preparations, such as ThinPrep (Cytyc Corporation, Marlborough, MA) or SurePath Prep (TriPath, Inc., Burlington, NC), and cellblocks. Guidelines for preparation of different sample types are as follows.

Samples from Cystic Lesions

Current cyst fluid protocols include analysis of carcinoembryonic antigen (CEA) and amylase and molecular studies, in addition to cytology. Proper triage of the specimen is necessary to ensure that all necessary studies may be performed. The sample for the molecular studies should be submitted from the neat fluid (fluid before it is centrifuged); usually only 0.3 mL is required. CEA and amylase may be measured from the supernatant after the fluid is centrifuged. If the sample is insufficient, it may be diluted and then the final CEA and amylase values corrected by the dilution ratio.[28] The cell pellet is used to prepare the cytology sample using either cytospins or other concentration technique and cell block.

Triage of pancreatic cyst fluid is volume dependent. Usually, with volumes greater than 1 mL, all of the studies can be performed. If the volume is 0.5 mL or less, triage will depend on the clinical question. If the question is whether the cyst is mucinous or nonmucinous, then priority should be given to CEA. If the question is whether it is a low- or high-grade lesion with a greater risk of malignancy, then DNA analysis should be given priority.[29]

Some laboratories use ThinPrep to prepare their cyst fluids. A concern is that mucin may be attenuated using ThinPrep. At the Moffitt Cancer Center practice, we receive pancreatic cyst fluids prepared using ThinPrep and have noticed the mucin is retained.

Samples from Solid Masses

FNA of solid masses may be assessed by ROSE. Typically, air-dried and alcohol-fixed smears are prepared from an aliquot of each pass sample and the remainder of the material in the needle and syringe is rinsed in a preservative for cell block. The air-dried smear is stained with Diff-Quik or other Romanowsky stain and the alcohol-fixed smear is stained with Papanicolaou. There are a number of alternative staining methods for ROSE, which are beyond the scope of this chapter.

Papanicolaou Society of Cytopathology Terminology and Reporting for Pancreatobiliary Cytopathology

The Papanicolaou Society of Cytopathology terminology system for reporting pancreatobiliary cytology specimens (PSCSRPBC) is a standardized terminology scheme for reporting pancreatobiliary specimens that includes diagnostic criteria. The PSCSRPBC created six reporting categories: Nondiagnostic, Negative (for malignancy), Atypical, Neoplastic, Suspicious (for malignancy), and Positive/Malignant.[30] These categories are for use in laboratories where the information system requires a diagnostic category for reporting cytology specimens; otherwise samples may be reported with only a diagnosis line.

Correlation of cytology findings with clinical, imaging, and ancillary findings is required to determine sample adequacy. If a sample does not meet adequacy criteria, it is categorized as nondiagnostic. Adequacy criteria are summarized in Box 36.1. The term *nondiagnostic* is preferred to *unsatisfactory* because *unsatisfactory* implies that the sample could not be evaluated microscopically.

The negative category is used when the sample is representative of a nonneoplastic process, such as acute or chronic pancreatitis (Table 36.1). The atypical and suspicious categories are both indeterminate categories, and criteria for these are summarized in Boxes 36.2 and 36.3, respectively. In general terms, these categories are used when the sample shows abnormal cells, which cannot be classified as definitely benign or definitely malignant, because of either a scant number of representative cells or artifact precluding evaluation. These categories should be used sparingly. The positive/malignant category is used for samples with high-grade and aggressive neoplasms, such as ductal adenocarcinoma (see Table 36.1).

The neoplastic category is further subdivided into *Neoplastic: Benign* and *Neoplastic: Other*. Neoplastic: Benign includes benign neoplasms such as serous cystadenoma or lymphangioma. The Neoplastic: Other category includes neoplastic processes that are preinvasive precursor lesions for

BOX 36.1 Cytological Criteria for Nondiagnostic Pancreatobiliary Specimens

- Preparation artifact or obscuring artifact precludes evaluation of the cellular component
- Gastrointestinal epithelium only
- Normal pancreatic tissue in the setting of a clearly defined solid or cystic mass by imaging
- Acellular aspirates of a solid mass or pancreatobiliary brushing
- Acellular aspirate of a cyst without evidence of a mucinous etiology

TABLE 36.1 Diagnostic Entities in the Negative, Neoplastic, and Positive/Malignant Categories of the Papanicolaou Society of Cytopathology Reporting System for Pancreatobiliary Cytology

Category	Diagnostic Entity
Negative	Acute pancreatitis Chronic pancreatitis Autoimmune pancreatitis Para duodenal pancreatitis Ectopic spleen Lymphoepithelial cyst Pseudocyst
Neoplastic: Benign	Serous cystadenoma Lymphangioma
Neoplastic: Other	Intraductal papillary mucinous neoplasm Mucinous cystic neoplasm Pancreatic neuroendocrine tumor Solid pseudopapillary neoplasm
Positive/Malignant	Adenocarcinoma Lymphoma Sarcoma Metastatic malignancies Neuroendocrine carcinoma Acinar cell carcinoma

adenocarcinoma, such as mucinous cystic neoplasm (MCN) and intraductal papillary mucinous neoplasm (IPMN), with low- and high-grade dysplasia. Pancreatic neuroendocrine tumor (PanNET) is included under the Neoplastic: Other category but this decision remains controversial. It is recognized that PanNET > 0.5 cm have malignant potential. The decision to categorize them as Neoplastic: Other was the fact that some PanNET in elderly patients with comorbid conditions may be managed expectantly and to maintain the classification consistent with the term "tumor." Solid pseudopapillary neoplasm is also categorized as Neoplastic: Other. The categories and corresponding diagnostic entities are listed in Table 36.1.

Any cyst classified as mucinous, based on the presence of background mucin, CEA levels, or *KRAS* or *GNAS* mutations is categorized as Neoplastic: Other.[30] A key caveat is that it is never acceptable to interpret the cytology of a pancreatic cyst as consistent with cyst contents.

Contaminants

Contaminants from the duodenum may occasionally be seen with ERCP-guided brushing cytology of the pancreatobiliary tree and contaminants from other sites may be obtained with FNA of either the biliary tract or pancreas (Box 36.4).

BOX 36.2 Cytological Criteria for Atypical Pancreatobiliary Specimens

- Atypia is not clearly recognized as benign/reactive, less than that considered sufficient for suspicious.
- Mild alteration of the honeycomb pattern in the epithelial sheets and nuclear crowding with minor degrees of nuclear overlapping are observed.
- Cell balls with marked nuclear overlap obscuring underlying nuclei are not seen and true nuclear molding is absent.
- Nucleoli are often enlarged, but true macronucleoli are absent.
- A near-normal nuclear cytoplasmic ratio is maintained.
- Slight membrane irregularities are present.
- Parachromatin clearing is observed without other features of adenocarcinoma such as nuclear membrane abnormalities, 4:1 anisonucleosis, and true "drunken honeycomb."
- The smear background is either clean or contains red blood cells.

BOX 36.3 Cytological Criteria for Suspicious Pancreatobiliary Specimens

- Significant alterations in architectural and individual cell morphology are present that may be qualitatively or quantitatively insufficient for a definitive diagnosis of any type of malignancy.
- Some, but not all features of adenocarcinoma are present, such as crowed groups and nuclear overlapping.
- Hyper- or hypochromasia, irregular nuclear membranes, macronucleoli, increased nuclear-to-cytoplasmic ratio, and significant anisonucleosis (4:1) are present.
- Tumor diathesis is highly suggestive of malignancy.

Mesothelial Cells

Mesothelial cells are polygonal cells arranged in flat sheets and show round to oval nuclei and intercytoplasmic "windows" (Fig. 36.1). They may be mistaken for benign ductal cells or squamous cells.

Hepatocytes

Normal hepatocytes are large polygonal cells with dense, sharply defined cytoplasmic borders and round, central, or eccentric nuclei with prominent nucleoli (Fig. 36.2).

Gastrointestinal Epithelium

GI epithelium is a frequent contaminant in EUS-FNA samples.

BOX 36.4 Cytological Characteristics of Contaminants

MESOTHELIAL CELLS
Round nuclei, even chromatin
Flat, evenly spaced sheets, sometimes folded over
Intracytoplasmic windows

HEPATOCYTES
Polygonal cells with well-defined, granular cytoplasm
Cells may occur singly; as small clusters; or as jagged, irregular groups
Round nuclei with small nucleoli
Cytoplasmic inclusions including fat, lipofuscin, bile

GASTRIC EPITHELIUM
Flat, monolayered, honeycomb sheets or columnar cells on edge with basally located nuclei
Foveolar mucinous cells with mucin in upper two-thirds of cytoplasm or involving the entire cytoplasm
Stripped nuclei in a background of mucin
Parietal cells and chief cells

SMALL INTESTINAL EPITHELIUM
Flat sheets in a honeycomb pattern with distinct cytoplasmic borders or picket fence arrangement with basally located nuclei
Columnar enterocytes with microvillus brush border
Goblet cells
Paneth cells
Background mucin

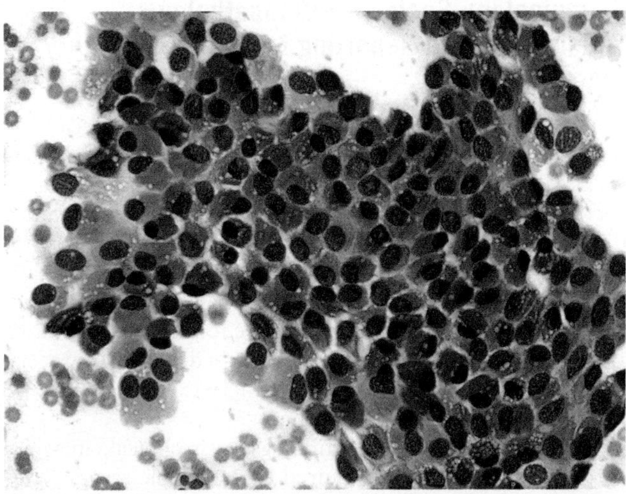

FIGURE 36.1 Mesothelial cells. The mesothelial cells are arranged in a flat, loosely cohesive sheet with intercellular windows. Diff-Quik, 40×.

Gastric Epithelium

The surface mucus cells of the gastric epithelium are columnar cells that are typically arranged in large folded sheets, with palisaded rows or single cells, usually associated with background mucin. Typically, a luminal border may be seen along one edge of the cellular aggregates. The sheets are typically monolayered, but occasionally may be folded or thick (Fig. 36.3A,B). The gastric pits may appear as rosettes in the center of a cellular sheet. The mucus glands of the cardia or pylorus are indistinguishable from the foveolar surface mucous cells. The cells derived from the foveolae and mucous glands display mucinous cytoplasm, often contained in the upper third of the cytoplasmic compartment (Fig. 36.4), although the mucin may extend to the nucleus. Gastric epithelium may also appear as stripped, bland, slightly elongated nuclei within a background of mucin (Fig. 36.5).[31,32] Chief and parietal cells may be noted if the needle traverses the gastric fundus or body (Fig. 36.6). Intact fragments may show attachment of the surface epithelium to the lamina propria. Gastric epithelium is associated with abundant watery mucin that may contain degenerated cells if there is an inflammatory process.

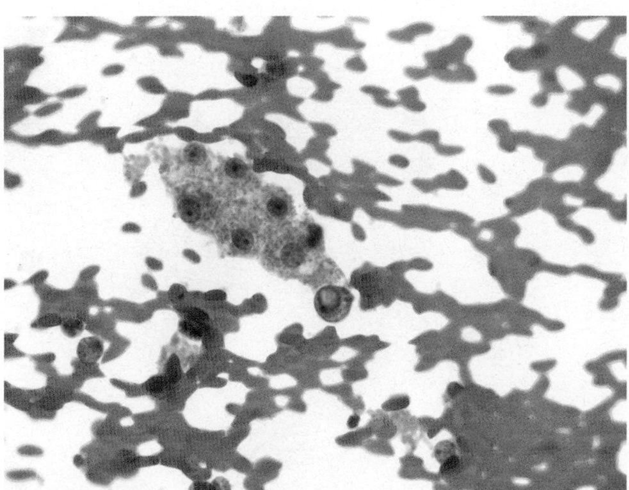

FIGURE 36.2 Benign hepatocytes with granular well-defined cytoplasm. One nucleus shows degenerative, intranuclear inclusion. Papanicolaou, 60×.

Small Intestinal Epithelium

Small intestinal epithelium has a similar architectural appearance to the surface mucous epithelium of the stomach, but the epithelial component is composed of a dual population of absorptive enterocytes with interspersed pale goblet cells and is also associated with background mucin (Fig. 36.7A). The brush border is visible when the cells are seen on edge (Fig. 36.7B). The epithelium may contain lymphocytes, which appear as darker, small cells within the epithelium.[31,32] Paneth cells are occasionally seen and are identified by the presence of coarse eosinophilic granules in the cytoplasm.

Both the small intestinal epithelium and gastric epithelium may produce abundant degenerated material that should not be confused with neoplastic cells. Both may also be associated with lamina propria that may resemble a stromal neoplasm.

CYTOLOGY OF THE BILIARY TRACT

Because brushing cytology is the most frequent technique used to sample the biliary tract, the cytological descriptions in this section pertain to brushing cytology. The cytological criteria for the FNA diagnosis of benign and malignant entities in the biliary tract are similar to those in the pancreas.

Normal Biliary Tract

Normal bile duct epithelial cells are tall columnar or cuboidal in appearance and are typically arranged in flat monolayer sheets (Fig. 36.8A), or in a picket fence arrangement with basally located nuclei (Fig. 36.8B).

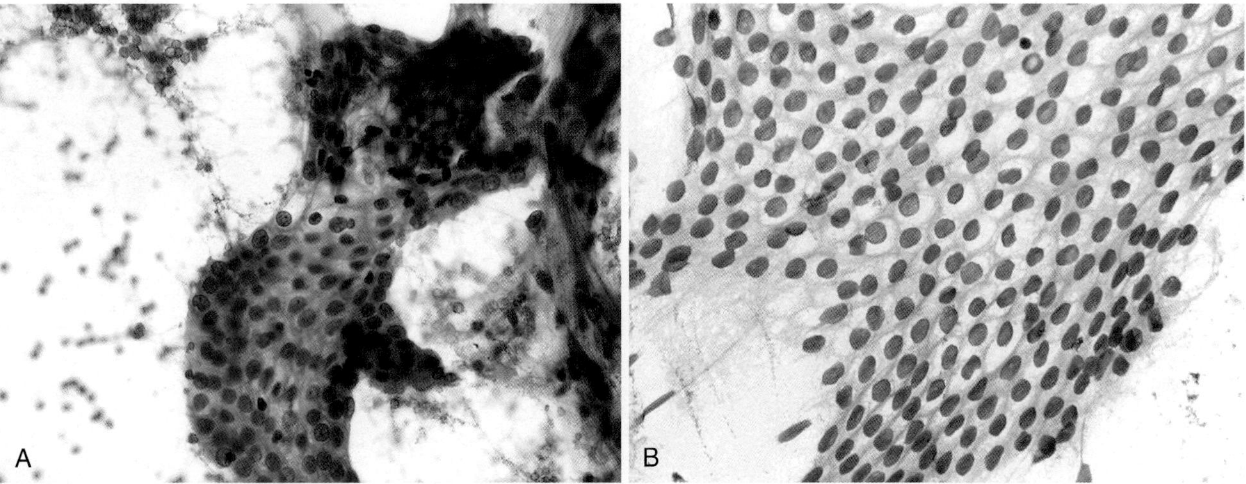

FIGURE 36.3 **A,** Gastric epithelium., Monolayered sheet with cells having well-defined cytoplasmic borders with mucin. The nuclei are round and fairly uniform in size. The group is associated with background mucin and single cells. Papanicolaou, 40×. **B,** Gastric epithelium. Large, flat monolayered group with well-defined cytoplasmic borders. The nuclei are relatively monomorphic, but do show subtle grooves. Diff-Quik, 40×.

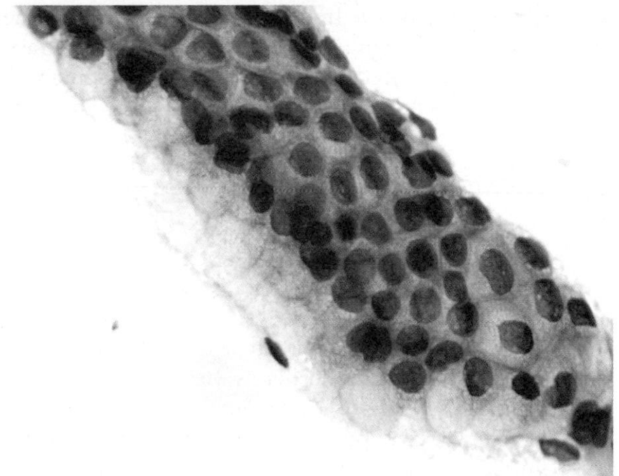

FIGURE 36.4 Gastric epithelium. Group showing cup shaped cytoplasmic mucin in the upper two-thirds of the cytoplasm. Diff-Quik, 60×.

Nuclei are round to oval, and cytoplasmic borders are distinct (Box 36.5).

Reactive Changes

Inflammation of the biliary system results from choledocholithiasis, primary sclerosing cholangitis, acute cholangitis, infections, calculi, stents, or instrumentation. The changes induced by inflammation include loss of surface structures, cytoplasmic vacuolization, nuclear enlargement, coarse hyperchromasia, and multinucleation[33] (Fig. 36.9). The epithelium remains monolayered and lacks pseudoacinar structures. Increased numbers of mitoses may be seen but these are normal in appearance. Reactive ductal cells may undergo degeneration including single-cell necrosis with resultant apoptotic and necrotic debris in the smear background. Necrosis alone is therefore insufficient for a diagnosis of malignancy.[34] In inflammation or injury, the epithelial lining may undergo mucinous metaplasia or squamous metaplasia (Box 36.6).

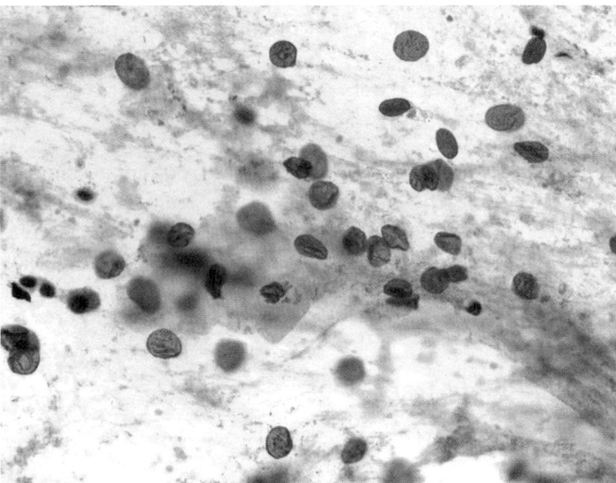

FIGURE 36.5 Gastric epithelium. Stripped nuclei with subtle nuclear membrane irregularities and grooves with background mucin. Papanicolaou, 60×.

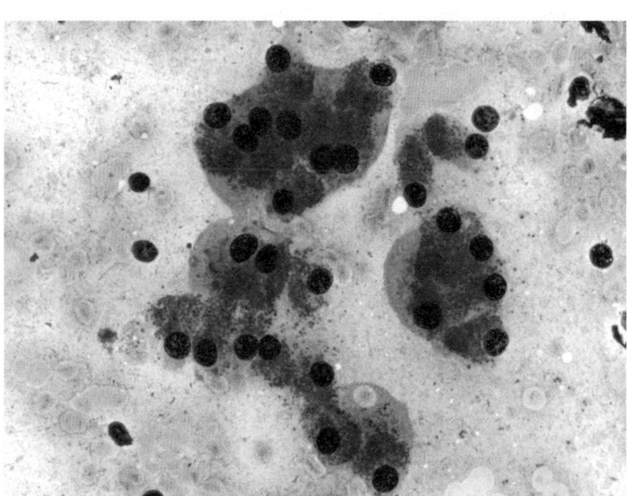

FIGURE 36.6 Gastric epithelium. Chief cells with well-defined cytoplasm showing cytoplasmic granules and adjacent parietal cells with well-defined, pink cytoplasm. Diff-Quik, 60×.

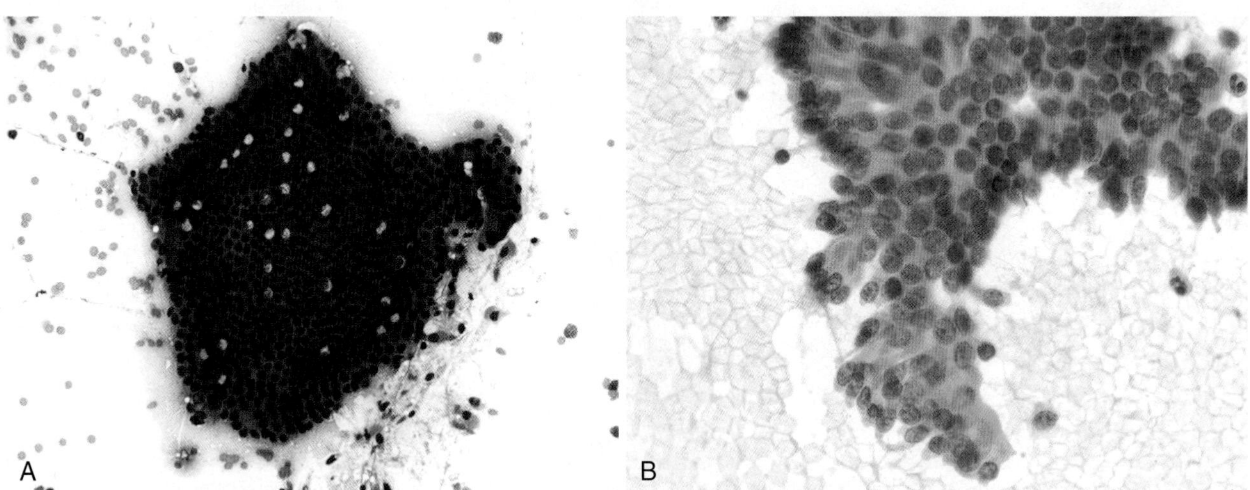

FIGURE 36.7 **Duodenal epithelium. A,** Flat sheet of duodenal epithelium showing goblet cells interspersed with enterocytes. Diff-Quik, 20×. **B,** Duodenal cells seen on edge, with basally located nuclei. A terminal bar and brush border are visualized along the edge. Papanicolaou, 60×.

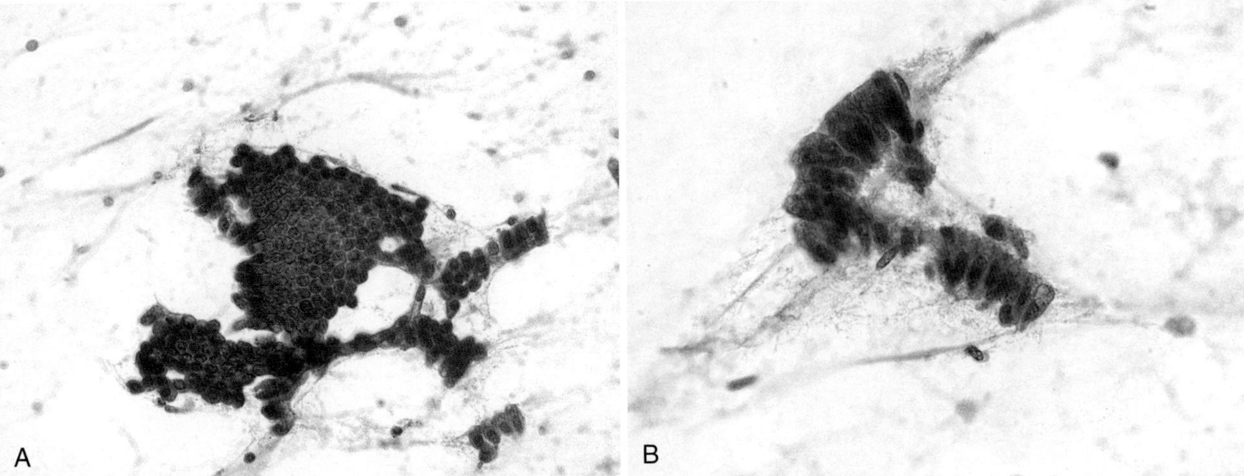

FIGURE 36.8 Normal biliary tract epithelium. A, Flat, monolayered, honeycomb group. Papanicolaou, 60×. **B,** Normal biliary tract epithelium. Benign cells seen in a picket fence arrangement, with basally located nuclei, and columnar, nonmucinous cytoplasms. Papanicolaou, 40×.

BOX 36.5 Cytological Characteristics of Benign Biliary Tract Epithelium

Flat, monolayered, honeycomb sheets or picket fence arrangement with basally located nuclei
Round to oval, uniformly sized and spaced nuclei

BOX 36.6 Cytological Characteristics of Normal and Reactive Biliary Tract Epithelium

Less orderly groups
Loss of surface structures
Vacuolization of the cytoplasm
Minimal nuclear enlargement and anisonucleosis
Coarse hyperchromasia
Multinucleation
Squamous or mucinous metaplasia

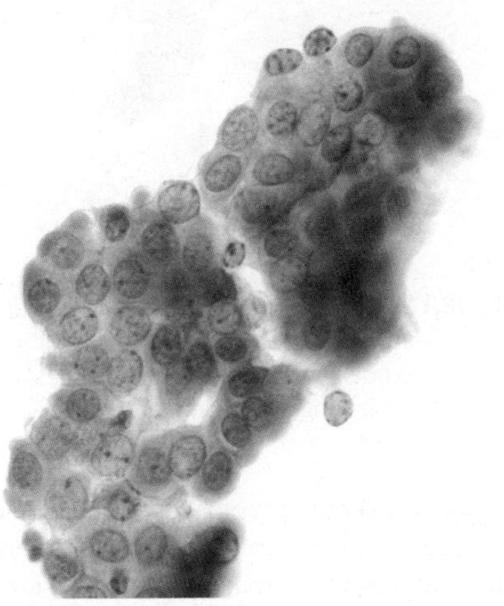

FIGURE 36.9 Group showing subtle nuclear enlargement and anisonucleosis. This reactive group retains a relatively monolayered appearance. Papanicolaou, 60×.

BOX 36.7 Cytological Characteristics of Adenoma

Loosely cohesive sheets, clusters, or single cells
Columnar cells, with elongated, basally located nuclei
Nuclei occupy approximately one-third of the cell
Fine, granular chromatin
Prominent nucleoli

Dysplasia or Adenoma of the Biliary Tract and Ampulla

Adenomatous epithelium with low-grade dysplasia appears as slender, elongated columnar cells arranged singly or in small sheets and clusters. The long, thin, basally oriented nuclei occupy about one third of the cell. The chromatin is typically fine and granular with one or more small nucleoli.[35] Brushings from these may be difficult to separate from adenocarcinoma or dysplasia (see Box 36.7). Premalignant lesions of the bile ducts have historically been called biliary dysplasia or atypical biliary epithelium. The original 3-tier classification of Biliary Intraepithelial Neoplasia (BilIN) that was published in 2007[36] has been replaced by a more reproducible 2-tier system of low- and high-grade dysplasia. Low-grade BilIN encompasses BilIN grade 1 and 2, while high-grade BilIN represents severe or grade 3 dysplasia.[37] The diagnostic histopathological criteria are similar to those used for other intraepithelial lesions, but the diagnostic cytopathological criteria for these lesions have not been defined. However, it can be assumed that their cytological features will be similar to what has been described as dysplasia in the biliary tract,[33] with low-grade (grade 1 and 2) lesions causing atypia on bile duct brushings, previously referred to as low-grade dysplasia,[2] and grade 3 lesions causing atypia previously referred to as high-grade dysplasia (grade 3).

Low-grade dysplasia or BilIN is characterized by sheets and clusters of cells that show nuclear crowding and overlapping, smooth nuclear membranes, and a moderate increase in nuclear-to-cytoplasmic (N/C) ratio (Fig. 36.10A).[33] Chromatin is characteristically clear and granular, with mild clumping. Low-grade dysplastic cells may have one or two distinct nucleoli. More pronounced nuclear crowding and overlapping occurs in high-grade dysplasia/BilIN (grade 3). In these cases,

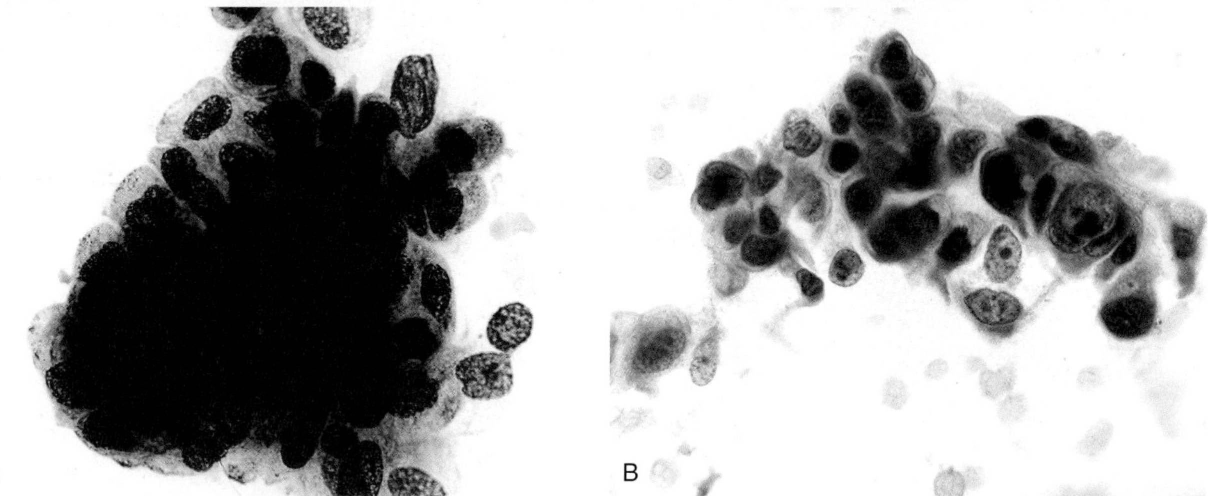

FIGURE 36.10 **A,** Low-grade biliary dysplasia. Cells with nuclear crowding, smooth nuclear membranes and overlapping. **B,** High-grade biliary dysplasia. The groups are 3-dimensional, with enlarged, crowded nuclei, and coarse chromatin.

BOX 36.8 Cytological Characteristics of Biliary Tract Dysplasia (Intraepithelial Neoplasia)

LOW-GRADE DYSPLASIA (BILIN 1 AND 2)
Sheets and clusters with nuclear crowding and overlapping
Smooth nuclear membrane
Moderately increased nuclear-to-cytoplasmic ratio
Minimal nuclear enlargement

HIGH-GRADE DYSPLASIA (BILIN 3)
Three-dimensional, crowded groups with nuclear overlapping
Nuclear enlargement
Nuclear membrane irregularities
Coarse chromatin

nuclear membranes are irregular and the N/C ratio is significantly increased, with coarse or pale chromatin and distinct and/or prominent nucleoli (Fig. 36.10B [33]; Box 36.8).

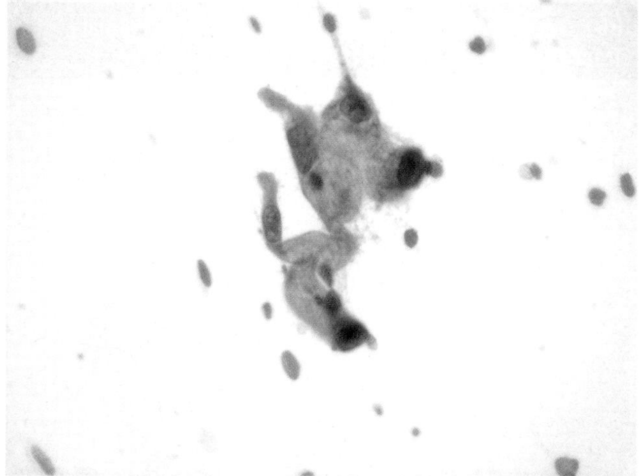

FIGURE 36.11 Atypical mucinous cells in a biliary tract brushing. The cells are columnar, with abundant cytoplasmic mucin. Nuclear atypia, such as subtle nuclear membrane irregularities, nucleoli, and abnormal parachromatin clearing are evident. Papanicolaou, 60×.

Intraductal Neoplasms of the Biliary Tract

Intraductal papillary neoplasms of the bile ducts (IPN-Bs) correspond to lesions previously referred to as biliary papillomatosis, or cystic or mucinous lesions of the biliary tract,[38] similar to intraductal papillary mucinous neoplasms of the pancreas (IPMN-P).[39] The role of cytology in diagnosing these lesions is not established. What has been previously described as atypical papillary or mucinous cells indicative of well-differentiated adenocarcinoma are probably derived from these lesions.[15] Cytological features of papillary differentiation include cell groups with crowding and overlapping, papillae formation, and elongated nuclei. IPN-B may or may not contain intracytoplasmic mucin depending on their lining epithelium (Fig. 36.11).

Adenocarcinoma

Cytology preparations of adenocarcinoma tend to be cellular and contain both cohesive groups and singly dispersed cells. In well-differentiated examples, groups of cells may be arranged in crowded overlapping "drunken honeycomb" sheets with minimal loss of polarity. However, 3-dimensional clusters of markedly atypical cell are more common in poorly differentiated carcinoma. Other characteristics that are frequent in adenocarcinoma include (from greatest to least common) changes in chromatin pattern (both hypochromasia and hyperchromasia), nuclear membrane irregularity, pleomorphism, two-cell populations, high N/C ratio, and cytoplasmic mucin vacuoles[34] (Figs. 36.12 and 36.13). Other nonspecific and less common changes that can be seen in malignancy include dyscohesion of cells with high N/C ratio, specimen hypercellularity, prominent nucleoli, and necrosis. In poorly differentiated or high-grade carcinomas nuclei are less rounded and become rectangular, pointed, or angulated with convolutions and notches and have more prominent nucleoli. Pseudoacinar formations are another feature of adenocarcinoma (Fig. 36.14; Box 36.9). Some adenocarcinomas are rich in acute inflammatory cells, which may lead to misinterpretation as representing reactive atypia. Usually in reactive atypia there is no nuclear membrane folding.[34]

Mucinous and papillary differentiation have been described as subtle findings in well-differentiated

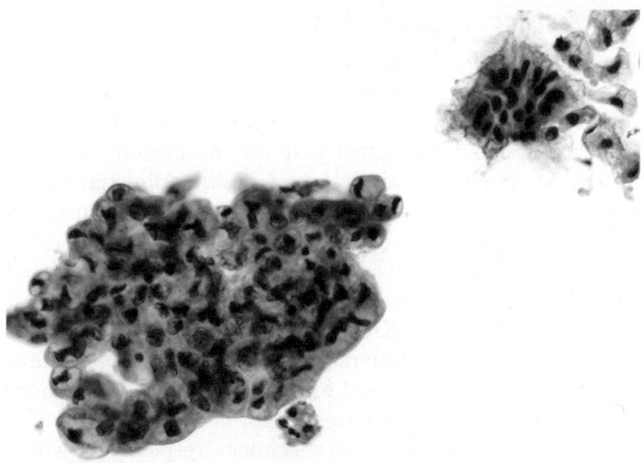

FIGURE 36.12 Adenocarcinoma. Liquid-based preparation showing larger, malignant group *(bottom left)* and benign group *(top right)*. The malignant group shows nuclear enlargement compared with the benign group. Anisonucleosis and nuclear membrane irregularity are significant. In addition, the malignant group shows loss of polarity and crowding. Papanicolaou, 40×.

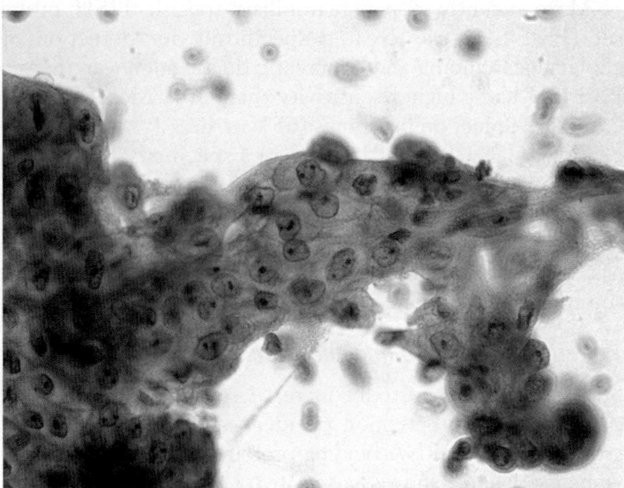

FIGURE 36.13 Adenocarcinoma. The group shows loss of polarity, irregularly spaced nuclei, and the beginning of a pseudoacinar formation. The nuclei are angulated and pointed, with subtle grooves and foldings. Anisonucleosis is significant. Small nucleoli are present in the cells. Papanicolaou, 60×.

adenocarcinoma,[15] and it was once recommended that pathologists report any mucinous change as possibly representative of a mucinous neoplasm, and any papillary change as suggestive of a papillary neoplasm. It now seems that these morphological patterns are derived from IPN-B if identified on a brushing as previously described in this chapter. If these findings are identified on an FNA of a solid mass they are more likely to correlate with an invasive process.

One major pitfall in the interpretation of biliary tract cytology samples is the presence of papillary pattern because normal bile epithelium may form pseudopapillary clusters. Papillary clusters in normal duct cells are 2-dimensional while the cell clusters in true papillary lesions are crowded, and nuclei are haphazardly arranged. The nuclei of true papillary lesions are also more angulated and elongated, in contrast to normal cells, which remain round to oval in

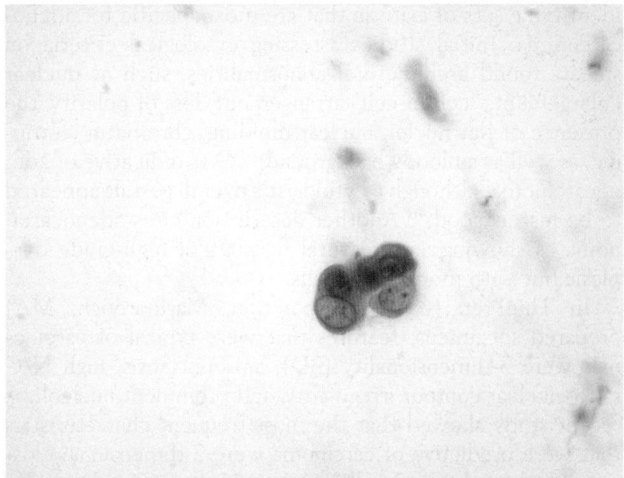

FIGURE 36.14 Adenocarcinoma. Small cluster of cells with nuclear enlargement, high nuclear-to-cytoplasmic ratio, and anisonucleosis. Papanicolaou, 60×.

BOX 36.9 Brushing Cytology of Biliary Tract Adenocarcinoma

- Cellular smears
- Two-cell populations
- Crowded groups of cells with nuclear overlapping and loss of polarity
- Dyshesion
- Excessive mucinous cytoplasm
- Anisonucleosis
- Nuclear membrane irregularities
- Increased nuclear size
- Increased nuclear-to-cytoplasmic ratio

shape. Occasionally, the nuclei of benign epithelium may also appear elongated, but again, the architectural arrangement is key. Carcinomas show a greater degree of architectural abnormalities and the presence of hyperchromatic or hypochromatic, transparent nuclei.

Secondary Tumors

Secondary tumors may also involve the biliary tree and lead to positive brushings. These may represent biliary tract extension of nearby nonductal cancers such as hepatocellular carcinoma or gallbladder carcinoma.[40] They also include metastatic neoplasms such as neuroendocrine neoplasms, lymphoma, and metastases from lung, esophageal, and colonic adenocarcinoma.[17,41-43] In patients without a known history of prior malignancy these malignant cells may be misinterpreted as primary pancreatobiliary carcinomas. A high index of suspicion is therefore warranted, along with ancillary studies (immunohistochemistry and flow cytometry) whenever this is suspected.

Differential Diagnosis: Reactive Processes vs. Adenocarcinoma in the Biliary Tract

The key problem when assessing pancreatobiliary brushing cytology specimens is differentiating a reactive process from adenocarcinoma. A number of studies have focused on identifying sets of criteria that are most specific for adenocarcinoma. Initial studies assessing cytological criteria on smears found architectural abnormalities, such as nuclear enlargement, "cell-in-cell" arrangement, loss of polarity, the presence of flat nuclei, nuclear molding, chromatin clumping, as well as a bloody background,[44-46] as indicative of adenocarcinoma, although a cytologist's overall gestalt appeared to be just as good.[46] Another description cites adenocarcinoma as showing architectural features of high-grade dysplasia but with more single cells.[33]

In ThinPrep (Cytyc Corporation, Marlborough, MA) prepared specimens; features that were typical of carcinomas were 3-dimensionality (3D), anisonucleosis, high N/C ratio, nuclear contour irregularity, and prominent nucleoli. A recent study showed that the most frequent characteristics that were predictive of carcinoma were 3-dimensional clusters, pleomorphism, 2-cell population, change in chromatin pattern (hypo/hyperchromasia), high N/C ratio, cytoplasmic mucin vacuoles, nuclear irregularity, cellular dyscohesion, hypercellularity, nuclear molding, and prominent nucleoli.[34] Most malignant brushings had ≥3 malignant characteristics, while 77% of benign brushings had none. Cytomorphological features that are not helpful in distinguishing malignant and benign cases are single naked nuclei, inflammation, and necrosis.[34,47,48] Table 36.2 summarizes these criteria.

Ancillary Studies

A number of technologies have been applied to indeterminate bile duct cytology specimens to improve sensitivity and specificity. The ancillary techniques employed include next-generation sequencing (NGS), fluorescent in situ hybridization (FISH), protein analysis, and immunocytochemistry.

Molecular

NGS was recently used to identify driver gene mutations in 30% of bile duct brushings, including mutations in *KRAS* (88%), *TP53* (58%), *SMAD4* (25%), and *CDKN2A* (17%).[49]

TABLE 36.2 Biliary Tract: Reactive Processes vs. Adenocarcinoma

Criterion	Reactive	Adenocarcinoma
Architecture	Retain honeycomb pattern, 2-dimensionality	Lose honeycomb pattern, 3-dimensionality
Loss of polarity	Absent	Present
Nuclear molding	Absent	Present
Nuclear-to-cytoplasmic ratio	Low	Increased
Nuclear membrane irregularities	Minimal	Loss of roundness, nuclei become angulated
Anisonucleosis	Minimal	>4:1
Nuclear enlargement	Absent to minimal	Present
Chromatin	Finely dispersed	Coarse or hypochromatic
Cell population	Range of atypia	Two-cell population
Single, malignant cells	Absent	Present

Fluorescence In Situ Hybridization

Initial studies showed that both digital image analysis (DIA) and FISH improved the sensitivity of brushing cytology in the diagnosis of adenocarcinoma in pancreatobiliary strictures.[50] The UroVysion FISH panel that was developed to detect urothelial carcinoma and consists of 4 probes directed against chromosomes 3, 7, 9p21, and 17 increases the sensitivity of routine cytology in detecting carcinoma,[51,52] In another study, UroVysion FISH had a sensitivity of 94% compared with a sensitivity of 81% using routine cytomorphology.[53] Combining NGS for *KRAS* mutation with FISH analysis increases cancer detection rates in pancreatobiliary strictures beyond that of cytology and FISH alone.[54] *KRAS* mutations and positive FISH results were identified in 69% and 63% of pancreatic adenocarcinoma specimens, respectively, with a combined sensitivity of 86%. *KRAS* mutations and polysomic FISH results were identified in fewer cholangiocarcinoma cases (29% and 41%, respectively) and had a combined sensitivity of 54%. In an analysis of 81 brushings, where cytology had a sensitivity of 67% (95% CI, 48% to 82%) and a specificity of 98% (95% CI, 89% to 100%), NGS and UroVysion FISH both increased test sensitivity (85% [95% CI, 68% to 95%] and 76% [95% CI, 58% to 89%], respectively).[49]

More recently, a pancreatobiliary-specific FISH probe set (PB-FISH) was created specifically for detection of cholangiocarcinoma and pancreatic ductal adenocarcinoma. PB-FISH had a higher sensitivity than UroVysion FISH for detecting cancer on brushings (65% vs 46%; $P < 0.001$) and cytology (19%; $P < 0.01$) but had a specificity (93%) that was similar to both (UroVysion, 91%; cytology, 100%). The PB-FISH probes identify polysomy of multiple oncogenes (*MCL1* on chromosome 1q, *EGFR* on chromosome 7p, and *MYC* on chromosome 8q) and deletion of p16/*CDKN2A* tumor suppressor gene on the 9p21 locus.[55]

Protein Analysis and Immunocytochemistry

Some proteins reportedly increase sensitivity of brushing cytology for the detection of adenocarcinoma. Insulin-like growth factor mRNA-binding-protein-3 (IMP3 cytology), when used alone, showed a sensitivity of 64.1% for the diagnosis of adenocarcinoma and 74.1% when combined with cytology, while cytology alone showed a sensitivity of 33.3%.[56] S100P is upregulated in cholangiocarcinoma.[57] Analysis of S100P expression using reverse transcription-polymerase chain reaction (RT-PCR) showed that this protein was frequently expressed in adenocarcinomas of the biliary tract but not in normal tissues. Tumor cells of cholangiocarcinoma show loss of von Hippel-Lindau protein (pVHL) and are positive for S100P, IMP3, and monoclonal CEA immunostains, whereas reactive biliary epithelium shows opposite results.[58]

CYTOLOGY OF THE PANCREAS

Assessment of the pancreatic FNAB sample begins before the review of slides and requires an integrative approach that incorporates the clinical history, radiological findings, cytological findings, and ancillary studies yields. This combined approach ensures the most clinically relevant interpretation of the aspirate material (Box 36.10).

Age and gender are important, as some neoplasms show specific gender and age predilections. Because metastases from known primaries may occur to the pancreas, it is important to obtain a history of any previous malignancies. A prolonged history of pancreatitis without an underlying cause may suggest intraductal papillary mucinous neoplasm. A cyst associated with a history of alcohol-induced pancreatitis may suggest pseudocyst.

Most crucial are the imaging findings indicating whether the mass is solid or cystic, as this information will determine the cytopathological algorithm. Different entities are considered depending on whether the imaging studies show a mass that is solid, solid and cystic, purely cystic, or cystic with a connection to the ductal system (an intraductal lesion). Chronic pancreatitis, lobular atrophy, ductal adenocarcinoma, pancreatic neuroendocrine tumor, acinar cell carcinoma, and metastases are among the entities that would be considered if the lesion is solid. Solid and cystic lesions include any solid tumor that has undergone cystic degeneration, such as pancreatic neuroendocrine tumor, and also solid pseudopapillary neoplasm. Purely cystic appearing lesions include mucinous cystic neoplasms (MCN), serous cystadenoma, side branch intraductal papillary mucinous neoplasms (IPMNs, and pseudocysts.

A stepwise analysis of the aspirate sample begins with an evaluation of the gross sample. This is particularly informative for cystic lesions. At low power, assessment of cellularity, architectural features, and background yields a great deal of information, which may in itself be diagnostic. At intermediate power, architectural features can be assessed in greater detail. At high power, the nuclear, cytoplasmic, and mitotic features are appreciated.

Ancillary studies include immunohistochemistry, flow cytometry for suspected lymphoma, and cyst fluid analysis for CEA and amylase levels, and mutational analyses. Ancillary studies are most routinely used for the differential diagnosis of nonductal neoplasms and metastases, and in the workup of pancreatic cyst fluid.

Normal Pancreas and Contaminants

Table 36.3 summarizes the cytological features of normal pancreatic epithelia.

BOX 36.10 Approach to Evaluation of Pancreatic Aspirates

Evaluate clinical information
Evaluate radiological information
Evaluate cytological features
Evaluate ancillary studies
Correlate all of above

Ductal Cells

The epithelium lining the large pancreatic ducts is composed of columnar epithelium arranged in flat, honeycombed, 2-dimensional sheets of cells with centrally located nuclei (Fig. 36.15A,B). The ductal cells may also be present in a palisaded "picket fence" arrangement, in which the nuclei are basally located. In contrast to the epithelium of the large ducts, intralobular duct epithelium is composed of cuboidal-shaped cells with scant basophilic cytoplasm and are usually present as flat sheets, small clusters, or tubular structures.

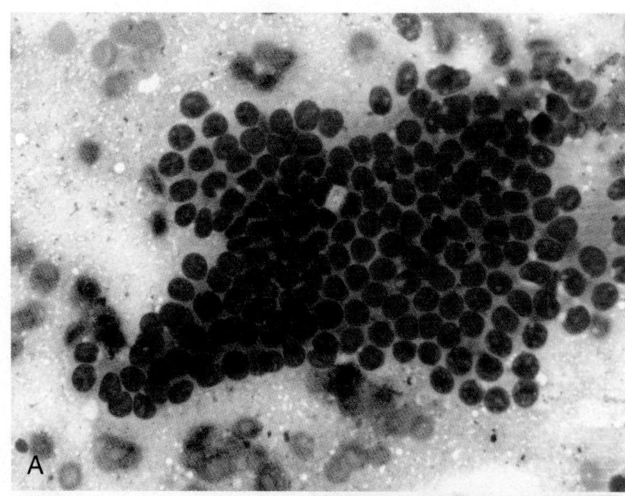

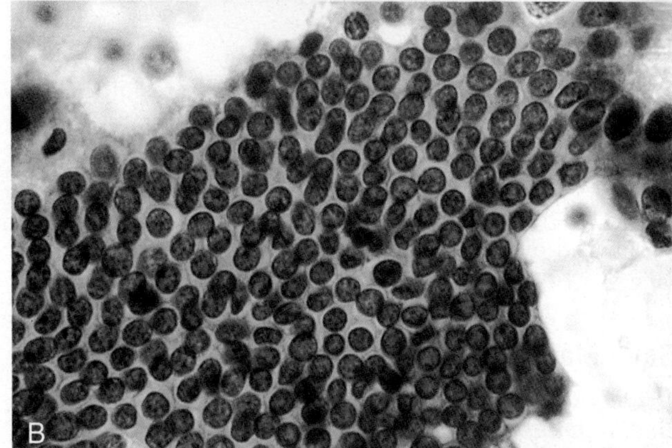

FIGURE 36.15 Normal duct. A, The cells are arranged in a monolayered sheet. The nuclei are uniform in size and shape. Diff-Quik, 60×. **B,** The cells are uniform in size and shape and have scant cytoplasm without mucin. Papanicolaou, 60×.

TABLE 36.3 Cytological Characteristics of Pancreatic Epithelia

Epithelium	Cytoplasm	Nuclei	Architectural features
Ductal epithelium	Tall columnar or cuboidal, with mucin	Round to oval	Flat, honeycomb sheets or palisade columns of cells
Acinar epithelium	Pyramidal, abundant, well-defined, contains zymogen granules	Round, with prominent nucleoli	Acinar groups of cells or singly dispersed
Islet cells	Scant and variable, amphophilic, contains neurosecretory granules	Round to oval with salt and pepper chromatin	Loosely cohesive groups of cells

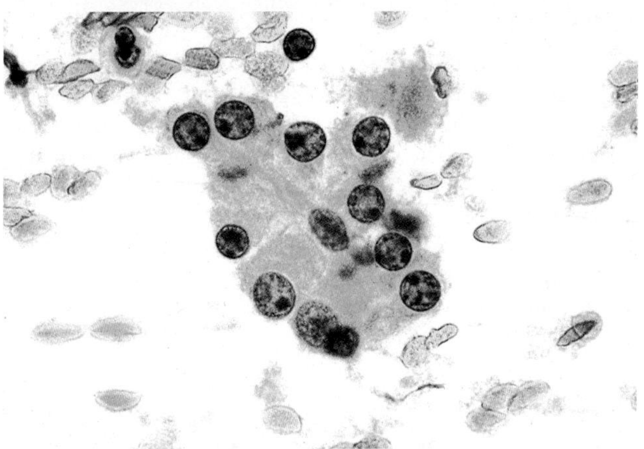

FIGURE 36.16 Acinar cells. Group of acinar cells forming an acinar group. The nuclei are peripherally located. The cytoplasm is pyramidal with cytoplasmic granules. The nuclei are round with prominent nucleoli. Papanicolaou, 100×.

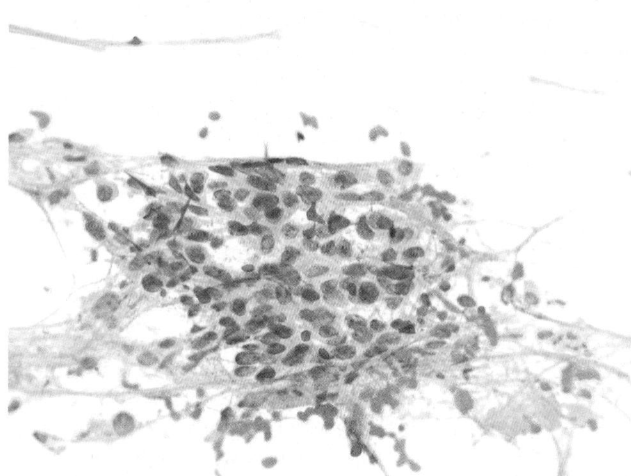

FIGURE 36.17 Islet cells. Loosely cohesive group of islet cells with scant, wispy cytoplasm and oval nuclei with finely stippled chromatin. Papanicolaou, 60×.

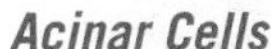

Acinar Cells

Aspirates of the normal pancreas consist predominantly of acinar type epithelium, which is typically arranged either singly or in small acinar-shaped structures without lumina (Fig. 36.16). The cells are pyramidal or triangular in shape and contain abundant, granular cytoplasm with numerous cytoplasmic zymogen granules. The nuclei are round and centrally or eccentrically located and have a granular chromatin pattern with nucleoli that may or may not be prominent.

Islet Cells

Islet cells are only rarely detected in aspirates of the normal pancreas. More often, they are seen in aspirates from patients with chronic pancreatitis with islet cell hyperplasia. When present, they occur as loose aggregates of cells that contain wispy, ill-defined amphophilic cytoplasm and oval nuclei with a stippled chromatin pattern (Fig. 36.17).

Solid Masses

Cytological Approach to Aspirates of Solid Masses: Ductal pattern vs. Solid Cellular Pattern

Primary neoplasms of the pancreas presenting as solid masses have predominantly two distinct morphological patterns. The first is the typical histopathological pattern of ductal neoplasms, which shows ductal type groups with significant pleomorphism, associated with abundant desmoplastic stroma. Aspiration may be difficult because of the fibrous stroma, and sometimes the stroma causes scantly cellular samples. The differential is usually with pancreatitis. The other pattern is that of the solid, cellular neoplasm with a frequent back-to-back arrangement of sheets of tumor cells and scant intervening stroma. Pancreatic neuroendocrine neoplasms, acinar cell carcinoma, solid pseudopapillary neoplasm, and pancreatoblastoma fall within this category. The cytology smears are diffusely cellular, with numerous single cells and loose groups. These neoplasms may also be vascular.

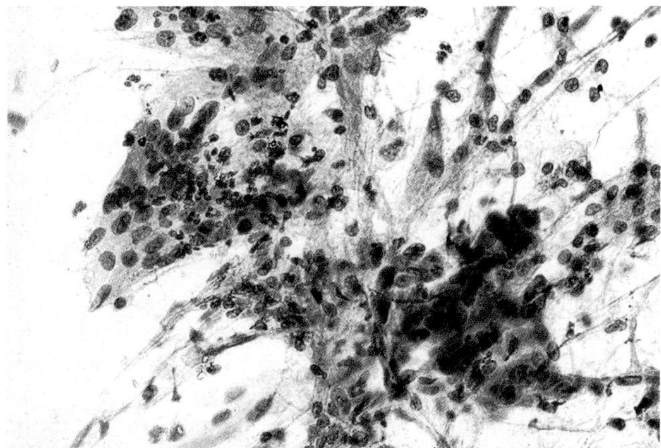

FIGURE 36.18 Acute pancreatitis. Degenerated residual ductal cells infiltrated by acute inflammation with foamy macrophages. Hematoxylin and eosin, 40×.

Reactive Processes

Reactive processes of the pancreas that may be sampled by FNA include acute and chronic pancreatitis and autoimmune pancreatitis. The role of FNA is to rule out adenocarcinoma or other neoplasms. Occasionally, the FNA may sample a reactive process adjacent to a neoplasm; therefore clinical follow-up and further evaluation are always indicated in patients with clinical and imaging findings suspicious for adenocarcinoma or neoplasia (Box 36.10).

Acute Pancreatitis

Typical smears of patients with acute pancreatitis show dirty, necrotic, background cells; cellular debris; and fat necrosis with saponification. Acute inflammation may be prominent. The normal pancreatic elements, when present, may show evidence of necrosis and degeneration (Fig. 36.18). Pancreatic ductal epithelium may show various degrees of reactive atypia as well (Box 36.11).

Chronic Pancreatitis

Aspirates of chronic pancreatitis are not typically very cellular and consist of varying amounts of inflammatory cells, ductal

BOX 36.11 Cytology of Reactive Processes in the Pancreas

ACUTE PANCREATITIS
Acute inflammation
Necrotic debris with degenerating cells
Foamy histiocytes
Fat necrosis

CHRONIC PANCREATITIS
Background mixed inflammation and histiocytes
Fat necrosis
Calcific debris
Epithelial groups with only slightly crowded nuclei
Absent or only rare isolated atypical cells
Enlarged cells <4:1 in a single sheet with low nuclear-to-cytoplasmic ratio
Round to oval nucleus and smooth nuclear membranes
Prominent nucleoli common

AUTOIMMUNE PANCREATITIS
Cellular stromal fragments
Lymphoplasmacytic infiltrate with eosinophils

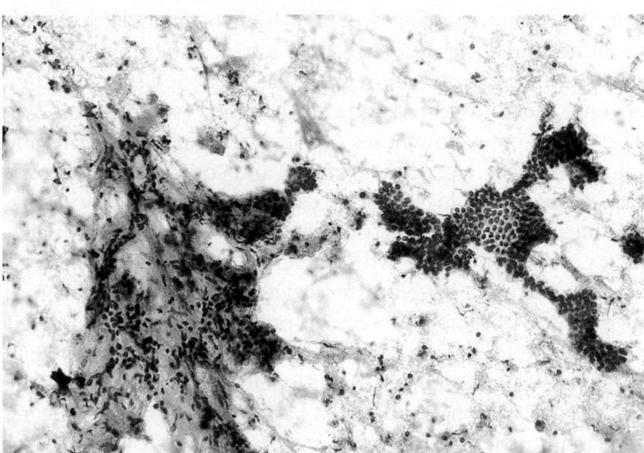

FIGURE 36.19 Chronic pancreatitis. Low-power view demonstrating an aspirate composed mostly of fibrous tissue fragments infiltrated by lymphocytes and few residual ductal epithelial cells. Papanicolaou, 20×.

cells, acinar cells, calcifications, fibrous tissue fragments (Fig. 36.19), and debris.[59] Islet cells are sparse if present. The inflammatory component usually consists of mononuclear cells and histiocytes. Acinar cells may be associated with inflammation and fibrosis. The ductal cells show mild atypia but remain monolayered and organized (see Box 36.11).

Autoimmune Pancreatitis

FNA smears show a paucity of ductal epithelium and are composed of inflammatory cells and stromal fragments. The key feature that helps distinguish this process from others is the presence of cellular stromal fragments with embedded lymphocytes.[60] A dense plasmacytic infiltrate, and eosinophils, are also common components of this process, but a lymphocytic background is rare.

Reactive Atypia

Reactive atypia induced by pancreatitis or other processes shows a spectrum of changes (Fig. 36.20). When severe, the atypia may mimic adenocarcinoma. A key feature is that the atypical groups are fewer in number than the number of groups associated with ductal adenocarcinoma. Another feature is that there is usually a range of atypia in the ductal groups. The differential diagnosis of benign and reactive processes from adenocarcinoma will be discussed at the end of the discussion on adenocarcinoma.

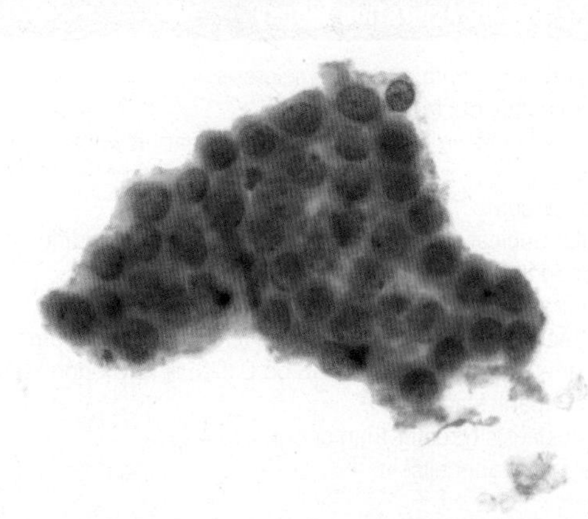

FIGURE 36.20 Reactive atypia. An example of reactive ductal cells with mild nuclear enlargement and minimal anisonucleosis. The sheet is relatively monolayered. Papanicolaou, 40×.

Ductal Adenocarcinoma, NOS

Diagnosis of pancreatic ductal adenocarcinoma (PDAC) based on FNA samples is usually straightforward. Occasionally, the distinction between benign lesions and adenocarcinoma or between reactive lesions and adenocarcinoma may be difficult. Several studies have evaluated a number of cytomorphological criteria in pancreatic FNA specimens in an effort to identify a set of minimal cytological criteria that could reliably separate benign processes from adenocarcinoma.[61-63] Although the criteria identified as being most accurate vary among these studies, and the accuracy of these sets of criteria has not been proven in a prospective study, it is clear that a systematic approach incorporating these criteria leads to improved diagnostic accuracy. The criteria can be categorized into cellular composition and cellularity, background, architectural features, cytoplasmic features, nuclear features, and mitotic activity (Box 36.12).

Cellular Composition

Benign pancreas is composed of a mixture of ductal cells and acinar cells, whereas PDAC is often predominantly composed of ductal type cells (Fig. 36.21). However, benign acinar and ductal cells may be seen in the smear background in PDAC. Care must be taken in EUS-FNA–guided biopsies not to misinterpret GI contaminants that may also be present as lesional.

Cellularity

Although adenocarcinoma tends to produce cellular smears (see Fig. 36.21), tumors with a sclerotic stroma or necrosis may yield paucicellular samples. In this case, close attention

BOX 36.12 Criteria of Pancreatic Ductal Adenocarcinoma on Fine-Needle Aspiration Biopsy

Cellularity varies with degree of sclerosis
Predominantly ductal population
Loss of honeycomb architecture with nuclear crowding, overlapping, loss of polarity and uneven spacing ("drunken honey-comb")
Irregular nuclear membranes; may be subtle in well-differentiated carcinoma
Hyperchromasia generally, but often hypochromasia with parachromatin clearing in well-differentiated carcinoma
Nuclear enlargement (1.5× RBC on Diff-Quik, 2.5× normal nucleus on Papanicolaou stain)
Anisonucleosis (greater than or equal to 4:1)
Single malignant cells[110-112]
Mitoses
Necrosis

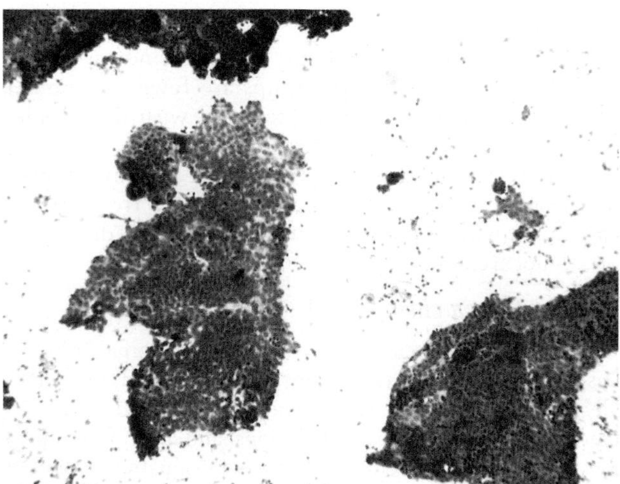

FIGURE 36.21 Adenocarcinoma. Cellular field of a well-differentiated adenocarcinoma. The malignant groups are forming acinar structures. The nuclei are subtly enlarged, and angulated. Diff-Quik, 20×.

to the atypia of particular groups is needed. Preparation of a cellblock from the collected material is helpful as it may contain diagnostic tissue, and even tissue fragments or cores with infiltrative glands or single cells, when the smears are scant and indeterminate.

Architectural Features

Architectural features are the most helpful. Malignant groups lose the normal, honeycomb, 2-dimensional patterns of normal ductal epithelium. Architectural atypia is manifested as 3-dimensionality, crowding, and overlapping of the nuclei (Fig. 36.22A,B), or an exaggerated (drunken) honeycomb sheet arrangement (Fig, 36.22C). Cribriforming is also a feature of malignancy. Cells may be arranged either in sheets, or small clusters or groups. Other helpful features include loss of polarity and nuclear molding (Fig. 36.22A,B). Loss of cohesion and single intact cells (Fig. 36.22D) are also features of malignancy, but well-differentiated carcinomas may retain their cohesion with a predominance of sheets (Fig. 36.22A-C) and may not have any malignant single cells.

Background

Coagulative necrosis is typical of malignancy but is more frequent in higher-grade carcinomas (Fig. 36.23A). Well-differentiated carcinomas may have a clean background (see Fig. 36.22A-C). Other features that can be assessed as part of the background are inflammation (Fig. 36.23B), secretory products, and cellular dyscohesion.

Cytoplasmic Features

Because normal pancreatic ductal cells do not display visible cytoplasmic mucin, the presence of abundant cytoplasmic mucin (as in Fig. 36.22C) is a feature of a neoplastic process. In the setting of a radiologically detected mass lesion, it is a feature that supports a malignant interpretation. The cells may appear as columnar cells seen on edge with a column of mucin containing cytoplasm (Fig. 36.24A) or the cells may show abnormal more rounded cytoplasmic mucin vacuoles (Fig. 36.24B) with or without central targetoid droplets.

Nuclear Features

Nuclear features include changes in nuclear size, membrane profile, and distribution of chromatin. Normal nuclei are round and uniform with an even chromatin distribution in all four quadrants (see Fig. 36.15A). Malignant nuclei lose that roundness and develop irregular nuclear membranes with angulated, sharp edges or rectangular, flattened sides, or they become more elongated and carrot shaped (see Fig. 36.22B). The nuclei may show noses or blebs and nuclear membrane folding (see Fig. 36.22C). Notches and convolutions become more apparent in higher-grade carcinomas (see Fig. 36.23A). An uneven chromatin distribution is more common in malignancy. Hypochromasia with parachromatin clearing is more often a feature of well-differentiated adenocarcinoma (see Fig. 36.23B) but can be seen in poorly differentiated carcinoma as well. Hyperchromasia is a more apparent feature in higher-grade carcinomas. Additionally, while tumor nuclei may be more hypochromatic on Papanicolaou stained smears, the same nuclei can be more hyperchromatic on the corresponding hematoxylin and eosin-stained cellblock.

Nuclear Enlargement

Carcinoma nuclei are about 1.5 times (or greater) the size of a red blood cell on Romanowsky stain or are twice the size of normal ductal cells (see Fig. 36.24A).

Anisonucleosis

Variation in nuclear size of greater than 4:1 is a feature of malignancy but is more frequent in poorly differentiated than well-differentiated PDAC (see Fig. 36.23B).

Mitoses

Abnormal mitotic figures are diagnostic when identified (see Fig 36.22C,D).

Comparison of the cytological criteria distinguishing benign/reactive changes from adenocarcinoma are summarized in Table 36.4. A comparison of the cytological criteria distinguishing well-differentiated and high-grade PDAC is outlined in Table 36.5.

Undifferentiated (Anaplastic) Carcinoma

Undifferentiated carcinomas of pancreas are morphologically heterogeneous. The cytological features (Box 36.13)

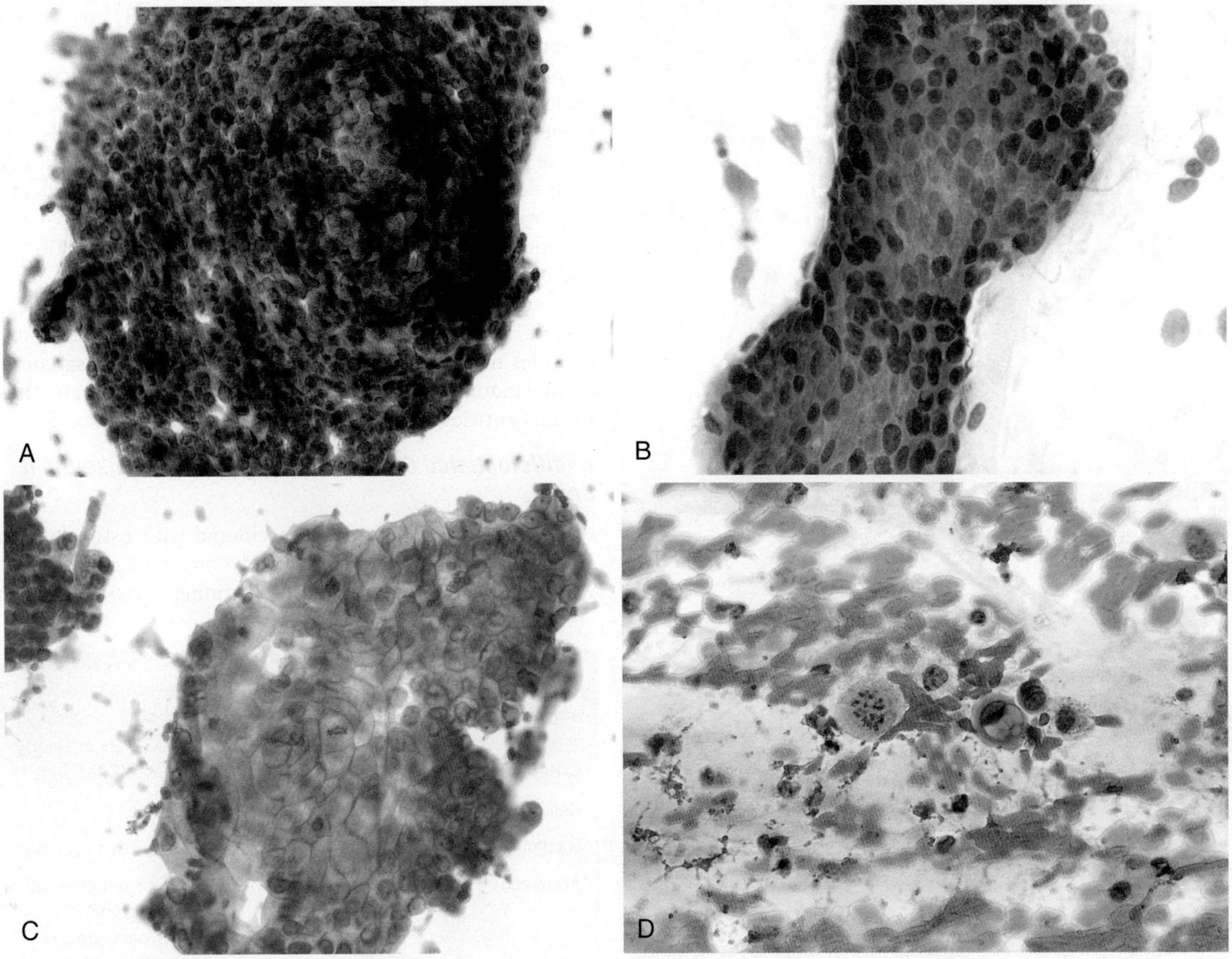

FIGURE 36.22 Adenocarcinoma. A, Hypercellular, crowded group. The cytoplasmic borders are no longer definable. Diff-Quik, 40×. **B,** Hypercellular, crowded group, with loss of polarity. Papanicolaou, 40×. **C,** Adenocarcinoma. Malignant group showing an exaggerated honeycomb pattern due to excessive cytoplasmic mucin. The cells appear to have a very low nuclear-to-cytoplasmic ratio. There is also a pseudoacinar formation in the group. Papanicolaou, 40×. **D,** Single malignant cell with abnormal cytoplasmic mucin vacuoles. Papanicolaou, 40×.

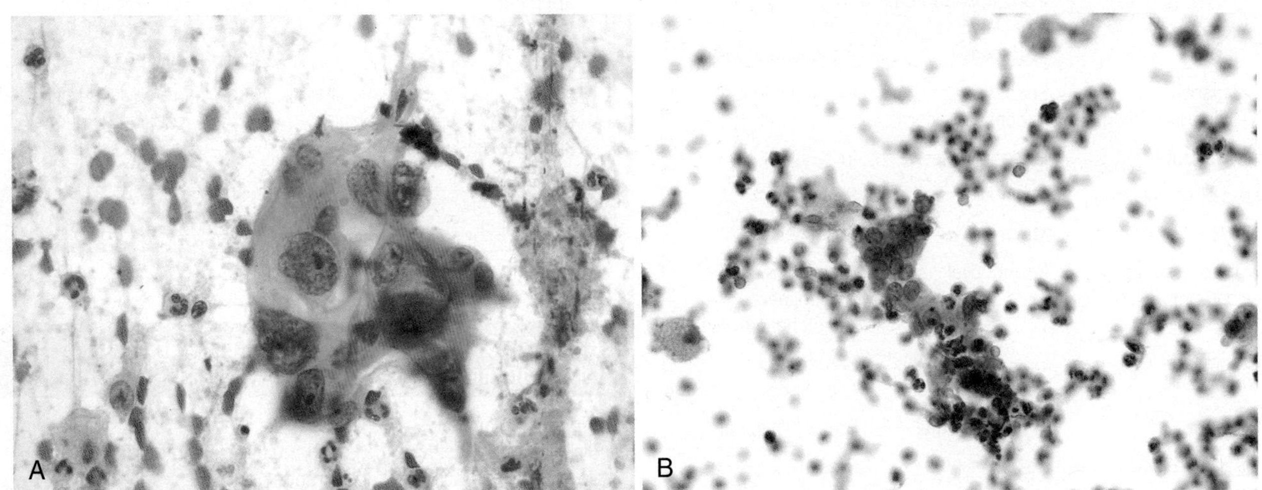

FIGURE 36.23 Adenocarcinoma. A, Poorly differentiated adenocarcinoma with marked anisonucleosis; nuclear angulations, notches, and blebs; abnormal parachromatin clearing; and prominent nucleoli. Papanicolaou, 60×. **B,** Adenocarcinoma partially obscured by inflammation. The nuclear membrane abnormalities are not as pronounced in these cells compared with the cells in **A**. Features of malignancy in these cells include a high nuclear-to-cytoplasmic ratio, anisonucleosis, pale chromatin, and subtle grooves. Papanicolaou, 60×.

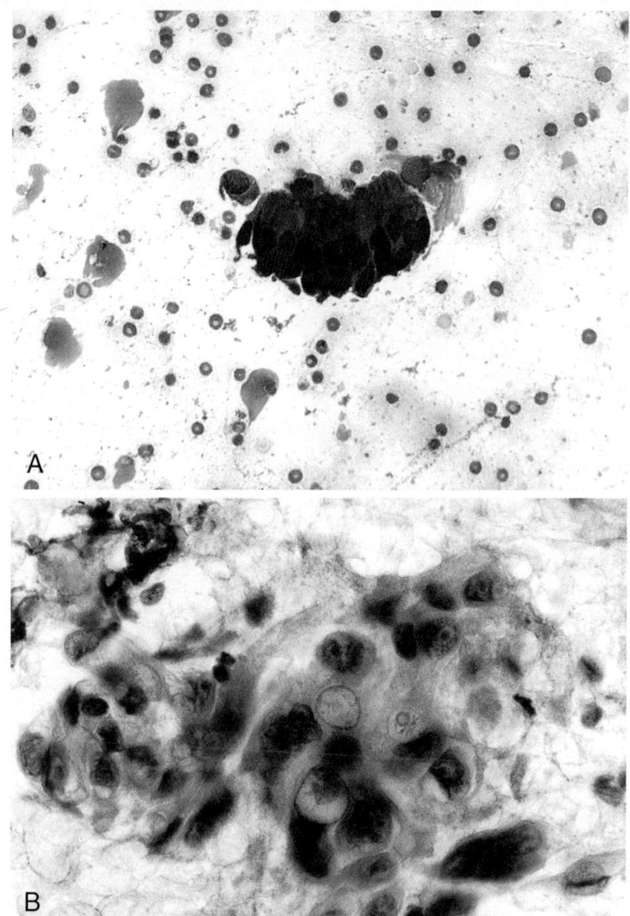

FIGURE 36.24 Adenocarcinoma. A, The cells have abundant cytoplasmic mucin. The nuclei are enlarged as compared with the background red blood cells and show nuclear size variation in a range of 1:3. The nuclear membranes show focal elongated or flattened edges. The nuclei are pseudostratified and crowded. Diff-Quik, 60×. **B,** Group of malignant cells with mucin vacuoles in the cytoplasm. Papanicolaou, 40×.

TABLE 36.4 Benign Processes vs Adenocarcinoma Using FNA

Feature	Benign Epithelium and Reactive Processes	Adenocarcinoma
Cellularity	Scant (except GI contamination)	Moderate to high
Architecture	Flat and cohesive	Irregular
Loss of polarity	Minimal	Prominent
Nuclear crowding	Minimal	Prominent
Nuclear membrane contour	Round, oval	Angulation, elongation, notches, grooves
Chromatin	Fine, granular	Parachromatin clearing
Mitoses	Minimal/normal	Present/atypical
Single atypical cells	Absent	Present
Nuclear enlargement	Minimal	1.5× RBC, or 2-3× neutrophil
Nuclear size variation	Minimal	4:1

of undifferentiated adenocarcinoma, NOS, are poorly described. Smears are usually cellular. The carcinoma is composed of mononuclear and multinucleated cells. The mononuclear cells appear singly or in small clusters and can range from medium-sized polygonal epithelioid cells with dense or clear cytoplasm to large bizarre sarcomatoid cells with dense and/or spindled cytoplasm. The multinucleated tumor cells form bizarre, giant cells (Fig. 36.25).[64,65] Cytophagocytosis, tumor necrosis, and marked inflammation are additional common findings.

Undifferentiated carcinomas are usually easily recognizable as malignant. However, the differential diagnosis includes metastatic undifferentiated carcinomas, sarcomas, or melanomas. Immunohistochemistry will separate these various entities.

Undifferentiated Carcinoma with Osteoclast-Like Giant Cells

Undifferentiated pancreatic carcinoma with osteoclast-like giant cells (UOC) is an extremely rare pancreatic cancer with a preponderance of entity-defining osteoclastic giant

TABLE 36.5 Comparison of Well-Differentiated to Moderately and Poorly Differentiated Adenocarcinomas

Criteria	Well-Differentiated	Moderately or Poorly Differentiated
Cellularity	Variable	Variable
Background	Clean or bloody	Coagulative necrosis
Architecture	Large, folded groups, crowding and nuclear overlapping	More 3-dimensional groups, smaller atypical groups
Dyshesion	Infrequent, cohesion more typical	Present
Anisonucleosis	Present as defined but subtle	More variable
Nuclear enlargement	Minimal as defined	Larger and more variable
Chromatin appearance	More often hypochromatic	Hyperchromasia and abnormal parachromatin clearing
Nuclear membrane abnormalities	Elongations and angulation	More obvious notches and convolutions
Mitoses	Infrequent	More apparent
Macronucleoli	Absent	More apparent

BOX 36.13 Cytological Features of Undifferentiated Adenocarcinoma

Highly cellular
Bizarre, mononucleated cells and multinucleated cells
Cells have a sarcomatoid appearance
Cytophagocytosis
Tumor necrosis
Prominent inflammatory infiltrate

cells showing all the characteristics of osteoclasts of bone. It is characterized by three cell types that include (1) malignant, mononuclear, epithelial cells; (2) smaller spindled or histiocytoid cells; and (3) benign appearing osteoclast-type giant cells containing variable numbers (typically > 10) of round to oval nuclei, some with prominent nucleoli (Box 36.14; Fig. 36.26).[66-71] All three cell types may be seen, in variable quantity, on aspiration.[71] The osteoclast-like giant cells express histiocytic markers CD68 and CD163, and are negative for keratin and p53. The truly malignant cells in this tumor (i.e., the pleomorphic tumor giant cells, and the spindled or histiocytoid cells that are often overlooked in the background), strongly express vimentin, and variably, but typically, express keratin, have a mutant p53 staining pattern (with strong diffuse positivity) and elevated Ki-67 proliferation index. A recent cytological analysis of 15 tumor samples revealed that, in addition to the 3 cell types described earlier, a conventional adenocarcinoma component is seen in 73%.[71] Because UOC may arise in mucinous cysts (intraductal papillary mucinous neoplasm and mucinous cystic neoplasm) one should carefully examine the smear background for features suggestive of a mucinous cystic component (discussed in more detail later).

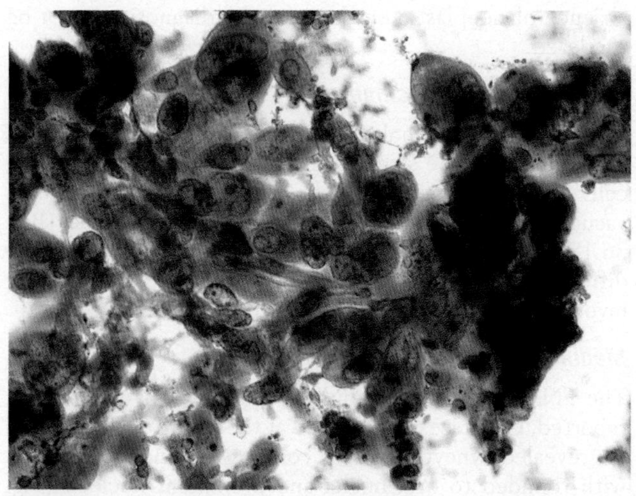

FIGURE 36.25 Undifferentiated carcinoma. The carcinoma is composed of bizarre mononucleated cells and pleomorphic bi- or multinucleated cells. Papanicolaou, 60×.

Undifferentiated/Rhabdoid Carcinoma with SMARCB1 (INI-1) Loss

This is an extremely rare (1%) aggressive undifferentiated pancreatic malignancy that is predominantly (>50%) composed of rhabdoid cells. Tumors are of two subtypes: (1) the pleomorphic giant cell type with *KRAS* mutations and/or amplification (on PCR/sequencing and FISH), and intact immunohistochemical expression of *SMARCB1*, which is a highly sensitive and specific marker, and (2) the monomorphic anaplastic type that lacks *KRAS* alterations and shows loss of nuclear *SMARCB1* (INI-1), which is a highly sensitive and specific marker for intact *SMARCB1* locus[72] (Box 36.15). Pleomorphic giant cell undifferentiated carcinoma with rhabdoid morphology is composed of loosely cohesive large pleomorphic tumor cells with abundant eosinophilic cytoplasm and eccentric nuclei. Some examples show more clusters or sheets of cells. In monomorphic anaplastic type undifferentiated carcinoma, tumor cells are loosely cohesive or singly dispersed and monomorphic with high N/C ratio and strikingly dense cytoplasmic protein inclusions (magenta-colored on Diff-Quik or eosinophilic on hematoxylin and eosin), or gray-green on Papanicolaou stain representing paranuclear cytoplasmic filamentous inclusions of intermediate filaments that displace the nuclei peripherally (Fig. 36.27A). These tumors may also harbor a conventional adenocarcinoma component.

BOX 36.14 Cytological Features of Undifferentiated Carcinoma with Osteoclast-Like Giant Cells

- Bizarre, mononucleated cells as for undifferentiated adenocarcinoma
- Osteoclast type giant cells

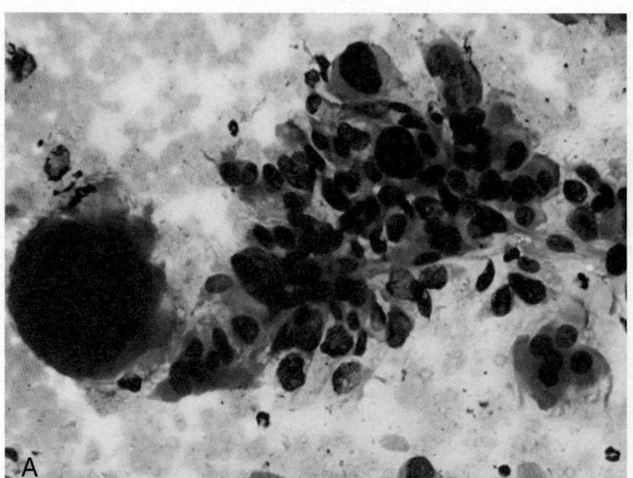

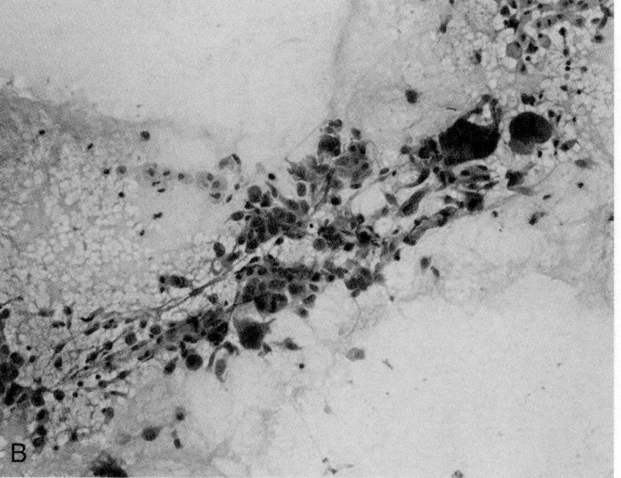

FIGURE 36.26 Undifferentiated osteoclastic giant cell carcinoma. A, Clusters and singly dispersed malignant cells with high nuclear-to-cytoplasmic ratio and irregular nuclear borders amid scattered multinucleated osteoclast-like giant cells. Diff-Quik, 40×. **B,** Singly dispersed tumor giant cells are surrounded by multinucleated benign-appearing giant cells resembling osteoclasts. Papanicolaou, 40×.

Undifferentiated rhabdoid carcinoma coexpresses cytokeratin and vimentin, and in the monomorphic subtype shows loss of nuclear SMARCB1/INI-1. *SMARCB1* is a member of the SWI/SNF chromatin remodeling complex on chromosome 22q11.2, and deletions/mutations result in loss of nuclear staining with the gene product INI-1 (Fig. 36.27B). Tumor cells also show loss of membranous e-cadherin and β-catenin staining, have a high Ki-67 index and overexpress nuclear p53.

Ductal Carcinoma Variants

Adenosquamous Carcinoma

Adenosquamous carcinoma is the most common variant of ductal adenocarcinoma. These tumors are typically high grade. Aspirate smears show moderate to high cellularity, and necrosis. The squamous component may predominate, with focal intracellular mucin or glandular groups of cells as evidence of glandular differentiation. Atypical, keratinized squamous cells may represent the only evidence of squamous differentiation in a predominantly glandular tumor (Fig. 36.28).[73] Without keratin, the squamous cells show dense cytoplasm. The cell block may show classic components as well (Box 36.16). The differential diagnosis includes metastatic squamous cell carcinoma.

BOX 36.15 Undifferentiated/Rhabdoid Carcinoma with *SMARCB1* (INI-1) Loss

1. Pleomorphic giant cell type with *KRAS* mutations and/or amplification (on PCR/sequencing and FISH), and intact immunohistochemical expression of *SMARCB1*
   - Loosely cohesive large pleomorphic tumor cells; some show more clusters or sheets of cells
   - Abundant eosinophilic cytoplasm
   - Eccentric nuclei
2. Monomorphic anaplastic type that lacks *KRAS* alterations and shows loss of nuclear *SMARCB1* or INI-1
   - Loosely cohesive or singly dispersed
   - Monomorphic with high nuclear-to-cytoplasmic ratio
   - Strikingly dense cytoplasmic protein inclusions that displace the nuclei peripherally
   - Tumors may also contain a conventional adenocarcinoma component

Colloid (Mucinous Noncystic) Carcinoma

The classic cytomorphological appearance is that of malignant glandular cells floating in thick, background mucin (Fig. 36.29; Box 36.17). Difficulty in diagnosis may occur in distinguishing this carcinoma from metastases of similar tumors from the lung, colon, or breast, particularly in patients with a history of carcinoma at these sites, or from intracystic/intraductal mucinous neoplasms. When the FNA is obtained from a solid mass, the diagnosis of this invasive process can be made. Uncertainty may occur if a similar pattern is found in material aspirated from what is described as a cyst or dilated duct, in which case, the differential includes MCN or IPMN. The background mucin and malignant features of the glandular epithelium will distinguish this process from GI contamination. In the absence of neoplastic epithelium, the diagnosis cannot be rendered.

Signet-Ring Cell Carcinoma

The FNA cytomorphology of signet ring cell carcinoma in the pancreas is the same as that in other sites. Signet ring cells are single malignant cells with a cytoplasmic mucin vacuole that distends and compresses the nucleus (Box 36.18). These should be recognized as malignant, but the differential diagnosis will include metastatic or secondary involvement by gastric signet ring cell carcinoma.

Medullary Carcinoma

The FNA features of medullary carcinoma have not been reported. One case encountered at the Moffitt Cancer Center revealed syncytial groups composed of neoplastic cells with rounded to oval nuclei and prominent nucleoli (Fig. 36.30). Lymphocytes and plasma cells were associated with the neoplastic cells (Box 36.19).

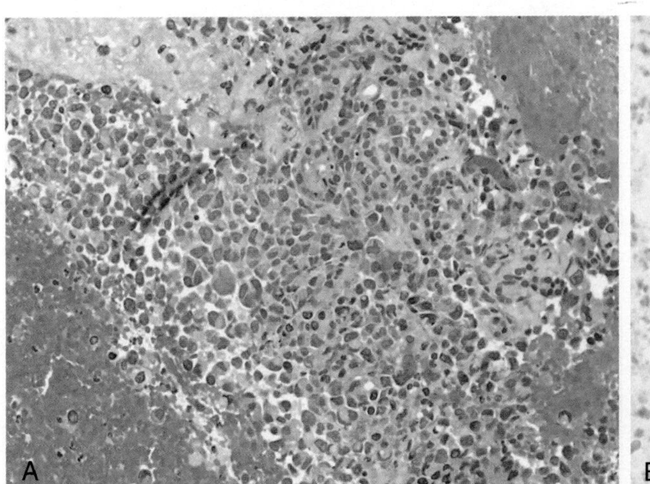

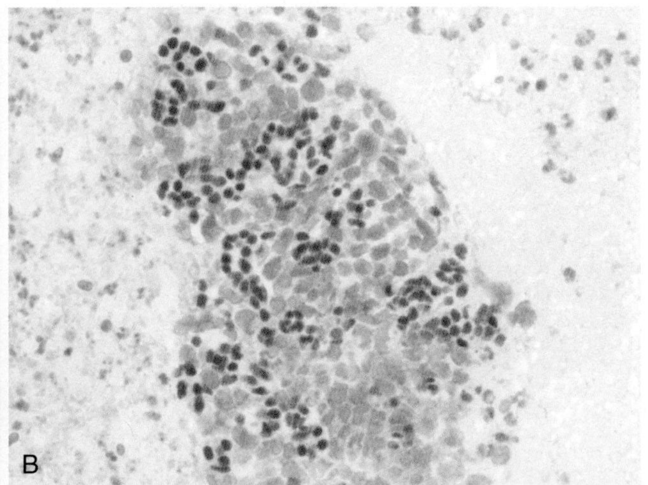

FIGURE 36.27 Undifferentiated carcinoma with rhabdoid morphology. A, Cell block is composed of loosely cohesive sheets of monotonous rhabdoid cells with high nuclear-to-cytoplasmic ratio and brightly eosinophilic intracytoplasmic globoid proteinaceous material displacing the nuclei peripherally. Hematoxylin and eosin, 40×. **B,** Tumor cells show loss of INI-1, but nuclear staining is preserved in residual benign ductal cells, 40×.

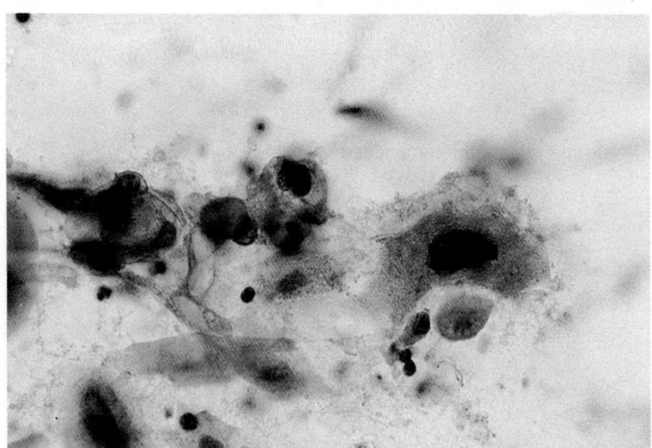

FIGURE 36.28 Adenosquamous carcinoma. Keratinized malignant squamous cells with vacuolated malignant glandular cells. Papanicolaou, 60×.

BOX 36.16 Cytological features of Adenosquamous Cell Carcinoma

Combined glandular and squamous differentiation
Squamous component may consist of atypical, keratinized cells or cells with dense cytoplasm
Glandular component may be typical adenocarcinoma, or few cells with vacuolated cytoplasm
Necrosis is common

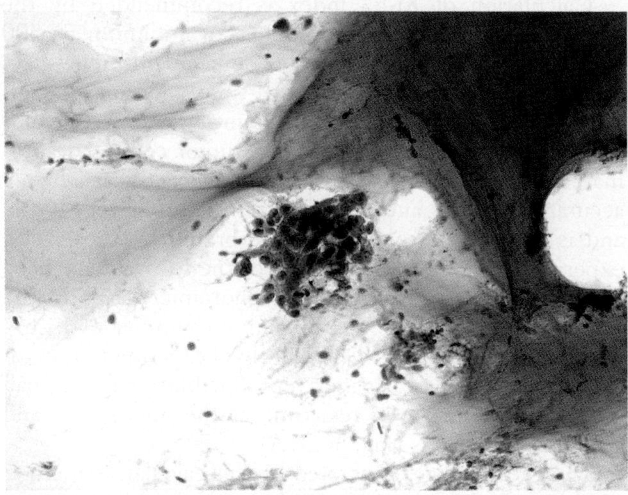

FIGURE 36.29 Mucinous carcinoma. Adenocarcinoma cells floating in abundant, thick, background mucin. Papanicolaou, 60×.

Differential Diagnosis and Pitfalls

Key diagnostic problems include differentiating adenocarcinoma from benign or reactive epithelium (see Table 36.4) and differentiating primary from metastatic disease. Identification of well-differentiated adenocarcinoma may be particularly problematic, as the cytomorphological features of these tumors are subtle. Crowded, hypercellular groups are the most frequent finding. The cells will show nuclear enlargement and significant loss of polarity. Moderately and poorly differentiated adenocarcinomas are easier to diagnose

BOX 36.17 Cytological Features of Mucinous Noncystic Carcinoma

Abundant background mucin
Malignant glandular cells

BOX 36.18 Cytological Features of Signet Ring Cell Carcinoma

Mostly dyshesive cell population
Cells with cytoplasmic mucin vacuoles compressing the nucleus

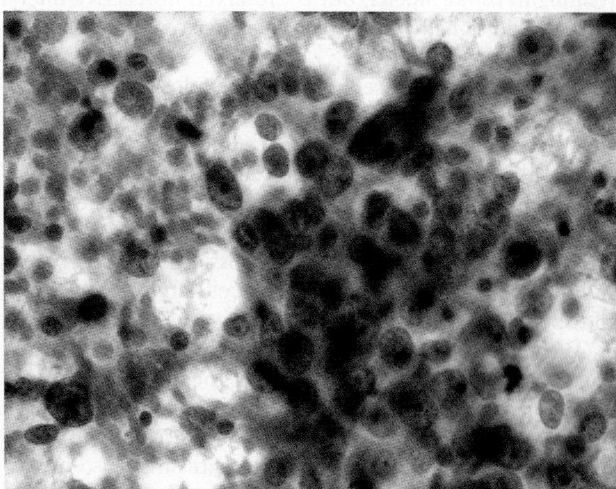

FIGURE 36.30 Medullary carcinoma. Syncytial group of malignant cells with round nuclei with prominent nucleoli, and a lymphocytic infiltrate. Hematoxylin and eosin, 60×.

BOX 36.19 Cytological Features of Medullary Carcinoma

Syncytial group
Scant, ill-defined cytoplasm
Round to oval nuclei with prominent nucleoli
Lymphocytic infiltrate

(see Table 36.5), although in an inflamed smear, the differential may include reactive ductal groups. Variants of ductal adenocarcinoma are usually recognized as malignant; the differential diagnosis is with metastatic disease from other sites that produce carcinomas with similar features. In this case, immunohistochemistry is indicated.

Ancillary Studies

Indications for the use of ancillary studies when dealing with ductal type neoplasms are to differentiate benign from malignant disease, or to differentiate primary from metastatic disease.

Ancillary Studies to Differentiate Benign from Malignant Ductal Cells

Four key driver gene mutations (*KRAS*, *TP53*, *p16/CDKN2A*, and *SMAD4/DPC4*) orchestrate PDAC development, and their identification in tissues, fluid, and cytological samples can be very helpful diagnostically. *KRAS* was the first mutation analyzed in PDAC and is the most frequently assessed in small biopsy samples. The addition of *KRAS* mutation analysis to standard FNA cytomorphology increases the detection of adenocarcinoma.[74,75] *KRAS* lacks specificity since it is expressed in early lesions before significant morphological alterations occur, leading to false positives. The p53 and Dpc4 immunostains are surrogate markers for their respective gene mutations.[76] Somatic *TP53* mutations lead to diffuse nuclear positivity for p53 protein in PDAC. Wild-type p53 may cause weak to moderate nuclear labeling in reactive ductal cells and GI epithelium, a potential diagnostic pitfall. *SMAD4/DPC4* inactivation (seen in 55% of PDACs) results in loss of Dpc4 staining in tumor nuclei, but is preserved in reactive ductal cells.[77] Additionally, Dpc4 loss is associated with disseminated metastasis of PDAC.[78]

In recent years, there has been an explosion in the identification of genes and their related proteins involved in pancreatic carcinogenesis.[79,80] Placental S100 (S100P) and insulin-like growth factor II messenger RNA–binding protein-3 (IMP-3) are positive in malignant cells while pVHL protein is lost.[81-85] The use a panel of markers, such as analysis of *KRAS* mutations, along with loss of Dpc4 and pVHL and overexpression of p53 in tumor cells are more sensitive and specific.[76]

The pancreas is a site of metastasis, and therefore the immunohistochemical workup may need to be geared toward differentiating primary from metastatic disease. This may be more of an issue with the variants of PDAC, although adenocarcinoma from other sites may also metastasize to the pancreas and create a diagnostic dilemma.

Cytological Diagnosis of Nonductal Pancreatic Neoplasms

Included in this category are pancreatic neuroendocrine neoplasms (including well and poorly differentiated examples), acinar cell carcinoma (ACC), solid pseudopapillary neoplasm (SPN), and pancreatoblastoma (PB). These tumors are typically solid and circumscribed fleshy masses (unlike PDAC, which is typically solid, ill defined, and scirrhous) and on histological evaluation are characterized by cellular tumors with a back-to-back arrangement of tumor cells with a stroma-deficient background. The low-power cytopathological picture in these tumors is typically that of a very cellular, monomorphic appearing aspirate, with numerous intact single cells, stripped nuclei, and loosely or tightly cohesive clusters. These neoplasms are vascular and may demonstrate this hypervascularity on the cytology samples. Branching vascularity is a key cytological feature of solid pseudopapillary neoplasm.

Neuroendocrine Neoplasms

Neuroendocrine neoplasms are thought to arise from islet cells and are classified as well or poorly differentiated grade 1–3 neoplasms, per current (2019) WHO guidelines.[86,87] This subclassification was based in part on morphology as well as proliferative activity, which is typically measured by mitotic activity and Ki-67 index calculation (Table 36.6).[86,87]

TABLE 36.6 Grading of Pancreatic Neuroendocrine Neoplasms per WHO 2019 Guidelines

	Mitoses	Ki-67 Index
Well-differentiated Neuroendocrine Tumor		
Grade 1	<2/10 HPF	<3%
Grade 2	2-20/10 HPF	3%-20%
Grade 3	>20/10 HPF	>20%
Poorly Differentiated Neuroendocrine Carcinoma		
Grade 3	>20/10 HPF	>20%
Small cell type		
Large cell type		
Mixed neuroendocrine-nonneuroendocrine neoplasm	Variable	Variable

HPF, *High-power field.*

Grade 1 (well-differentiated, low-grade) pancreatic neuroendocrine tumors (WDPanNETs) are defined as tumors whose Ki-67 index is <3%, whereas in grade 2 (intermediate grade) WDPanNETs it is 3% to 20%. Grade 3 NENs are subdivided into two groups: (1) those that are morphologically well-differentiated tumors (WDPanNET) but have high proliferative activity (with a Ki-67 index that is >20% but often <55%) and (2) those that are morphologically poorly differentiated, high-grade carcinomas (of small or large cell type), and have a Ki-67 index that is >20% (and often >55%).[86,87]

Calculation of Ki-67 index is recommended by the WHO and requires the counting of a minimum of 500 tumor cells. Calculation can be done in different ways including eyeball estimation, real-time counting of cells at the light microscope, manual counting on a static color photomicrograph of Ki-67–stained tumor cells, and automated counting systems.[88] Although advocated as a highly accurate test, the automated system is often very costly and is prone to errors if not interpreted by those with experience.[88] Manual calculation of the Ki-67 index using a printed image of a static color photomicrograph of the tumor hot spots (area with maximum number of Ki-67-positive tumor cells) is significantly cheaper and on cytological material has a higher reproducibility than eyeball estimation, counting in real time at the microscope and automated methods (Fig. 36.31A).

The Ki-67 indices generated by this calculation method can be performed on cytological samples and gives results that are comparable to those on corresponding resections.[89] False low/high indices may occur in specimens with low cellularity, abundant hemosiderin-laden macrophages, and increased background lymphocytes, which may also stain with Ki-67, thus leading to overestimation of the Ki-67 index. The inclusion of a comment in cytology reports stating that "the grade and index may change on the resection specimen" is therefore advocated.

Well-Differentiated Pancreatic Neuroendocrine Tumors (WDPanNET)

Aspirates of WDPanNET are very cellular and composed of a monomorphic, dyshesive population of cells occurring most often as single cells, but also in loosely

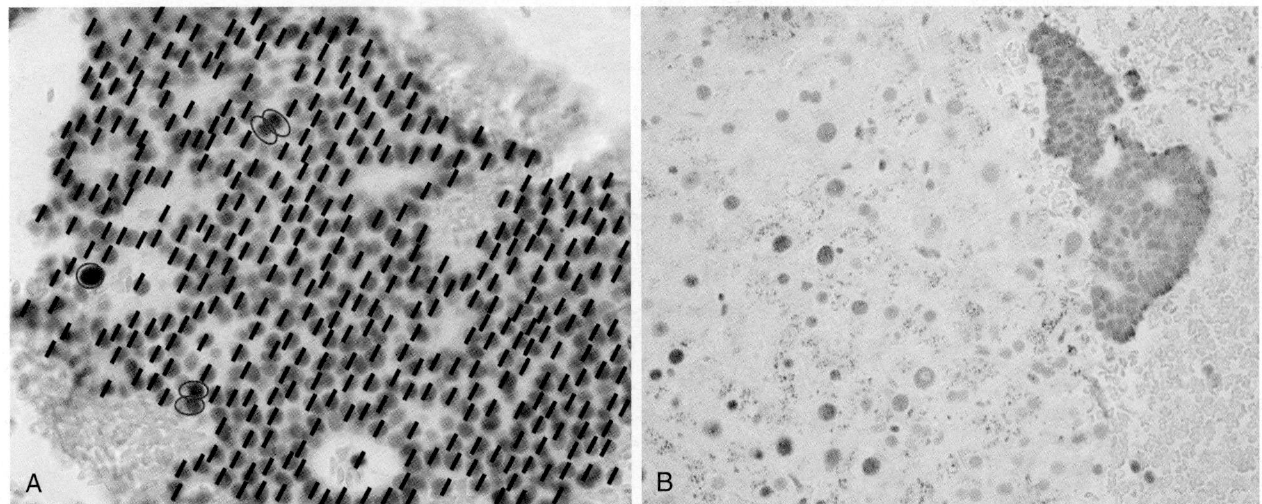

FIGURE 36.31 Well-differentiated neuroendocrine tumor. A, Camera-captured photomicrographic image of cell block showing scattered Ki-67 stain positive brown cells and Ki-67-negative cells highlighted in black lines, 40×. **B,** Fine-needle aspiration of liver showing loss of nuclear DAXX in a metastatic well-differentiated neuroendocrine tumor with retained nuclear staining in benign hepatocytes, 20×.

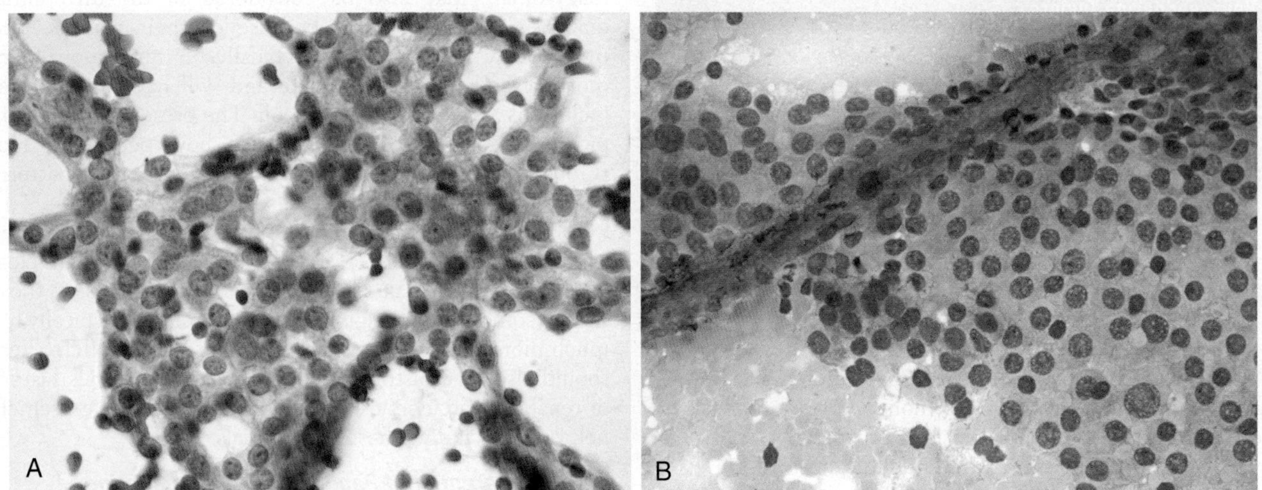

FIGURE 36.32 Pancreatic neuroendocrine tumor. A, Loosely cohesive group of neoplastic cells with scant, amphophilic cytoplasm and monotonous nuclei with round, smooth nuclear membranes and finely granular, evenly distributed chromatin. Small nucleoli are evident. Papanicolaou, 60×. **B,** Neoplastic cells adherent to a fibrovascular core. Diff-Quik, 40×.

cohesive clusters (Fig. 36.32A), that may occasionally form pseudorosettes. These patterns are often accompanied by stripped nuclei. The nuclei are round to oval and eccentrically located, and the chromatin pattern has a characteristic salt-and-pepper appearance on Papanicolaou stain. Nucleoli are of variable size but are usually small, although they may be prominent which may lead to misdiagnosis as carcinoma or lymphoma. The cytoplasm varies in quantity but is usually scant. In some examples, tumor cells may be more pleomorphic, rhabdoid, or can have abundant cytoplasmic microvesicles (lipid-rich variant) (Fig. 36.33A), or granular, oncocytic cytoplasm (Fig. 36.33B).[83,90] Oncocytic WDPanNET has been shown to be more aggressive and associated with larger, more mitotically active, higher-stage tumors, with more frequent lymph node and distant metastases. As mentioned, WDPanNET are vascular neoplasms, and this vascularity may be seen on the corresponding cytology smears and is characterized by vascular cores with loosely attached neoplastic cells (see Fig. 36.32B; Box 36.20).

The immunoprofile of WDPanNET is characterized by expression of cytokeratins, and markers of neuroendocrine differentiation, including synaptophysin, chromogranin, neural cell adhesion molecule (CD56), and insulinoma-associated protein 1 (INSM1). INSM1 is a transcription factor expressed in developing and mature neuroendocrine tissue. It has recently been shown to be a sensitive and specific marker for neuroendocrine neoplasms of all sites (GI, pancreatobiliary, lung, and skin), and in histological and cytological samples.[91,92] Chromogranin A is also a specific (but less sensitive) neuroendocrine marker. PAX8, Cytokeratin 19 (a pancreatic ductal lineage marker), and CD117 may be positive in WDPanNETs, and have been proposed as adverse prognostic markers, but are not used routinely.[93] Ki-67 index is a critical parameter used in the grading of all pancreatic NENs (see discussion earlier) (see Fig. 36.31A).

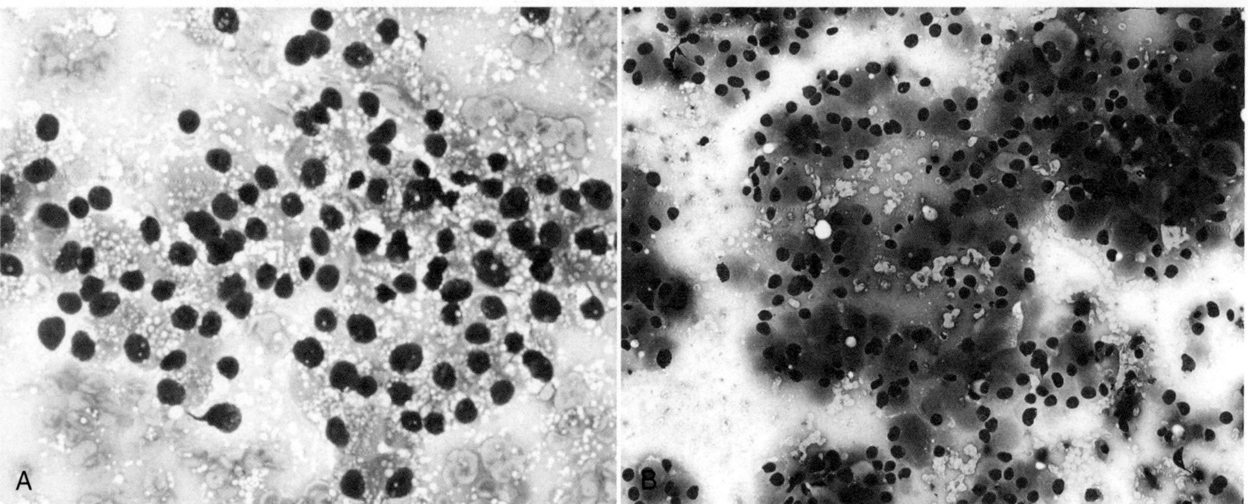

FIGURE 36.33 Variants of well-differentiated neuroendocrine tumor. A, Lipid-rich variant has abundant cytoplasmic and background clear vesicles, Diff-Quik. **B,** Oncocytic variant with pleomorphic cells containing abundant dense granular cytoplasm and low nuclear-to-cytoplasmic ratio, Diff-Quik.

BOX 36.20 Cytological Features of Well-Differentiated Neuroendocrine Tumors

Cellular smears; monomorphic, dyshesive cells
Cells arranged singly or in loose clusters and pseudorosettes
Naked nuclei are common
Basophilic, wispy, and ill-defined, but may be dense and well-defined cytoplasm
Finely stippled chromatin (a salt-and-pepper appearance), small nucleoli
Binucleation or multinucleation common
Plasmacytoid cells with eccentric nucleus and dense cytoplasm

WDPanNETs may express a variety of hormones, but immunohistochemical analysis for hormone expression does not add further value to the diagnosis or prognosis.

The key entities in the differential diagnosis of WDPanNET include islet cell hyperplasia and a number of neoplasms, specifically acinar cell carcinoma (ACC), solid pseudopapillary neoplasm (SPN), adenocarcinoma (PDAC), lymphomas, and metastases to the pancreas, such as melanoma and renal cell carcinoma. Because WDPanNET, ACC, SPN, and PB have many characteristics in common, their differential diagnosis will be summarized at the end of this section and in Table 36.7.

WDPanNET may occasionally be mistaken for adenocarcinoma, if the nuclei have prominent nucleoli, and show significant size variation or pleomorphism, and the groups are cohesive with crowding or some pseudorosettes. Features that will distinguish WDPanNET from PDAC include rounded or oval nuclei and absence of nuclear angulations, sharpness, and convolutions in WDPanNET, features that are seen in PDAC. PDAC tumor cells also tend to be more cohesive, particularly when well differentiated, and show evidence of glandular differentiation.

The stripped nuclei and dyshesive pattern of WDpanNET raises the differential diagnosis of non-Hodgkin's lymphomas (NHL). Lymphomas are characterized by lymphoglandular bodies in the smear background on modified Giemsa or Diff-Quik stain. Flow cytometry may identify a monoclonal lymphoid population. Melanoma[94] and plasmacytoma[95] may also be considered in the differential diagnosis of WDPanNET because of their plasmacytoid morphology. Melanoma will typically be much more pleomorphic and mitotically active and will have intranuclear inclusions and prominent nucleoli. The presence of melanin pigment is diagnostic. Plasmacytoma shows perinuclear Hof (Golgi zone) and a clock face nuclear chromatin pattern, which will distinguish these cells from WDPanNET.

The pancreas is a common site for metastases by renal cell carcinoma, which is also a vascular tumor that may have clear lipid-rich cytoplasm and branching capillaries similar to those seen in some WDPanNETs. Renal cell carcinoma typically has much more nuclear pleomorphism than WDPanNET. There should also be a history of a renal mass or previous history of renal cell carcinoma. Immunohistochemistry is extremely helpful in excluding these differentials.

Poorly Differentiated Pancreatic Neuroendocrine Carcinoma

These neoplasms resemble poorly differentiated small cell and large cell neuroendocrine carcinomas from other sites (Box 36.21). The cytomorphological features are those of fusiform, small cells with molding, high-grade morphology, high N/C ratio, brisk mitoses, and necrosis (Fig. 36.34). These neoplasms are as aggressive as pulmonary small cell carcinomas. Large cell neuroendocrine carcinomas show vesicular nuclei, prominent nucleoli, more abundant cytoplasm, and prominent mitotic activity.

Mixed Neuroendocrine-Nonneuroendocrine Neoplasm

MiNENs may be admixed with a nonneuroendocrine component, including adenocarcinoma and acinar cell carcinoma. Diagnosis of MiNEN requires an adequate cytological sample and a high index of suspicion of a mixed neoplasm. Tumors show multiple lines of differentiation on immunohistochemistry and can have variable cytology. The diagnosis of MiNEN should be made with caution on cytological samples because of the limited cellularity of cytology samples and the strict quantitative criteria required for making this diagnosis.

TABLE 36.7 Differential Diagnosis of WDPanNET, ACC, SPN, and PB

Criteria	WDPanNET	ACC	SPN	PB
Nuclei	Salt-and-pepper chromatin Round and oval –/+ nucleoli	Round to oval Prominent nucleoli	Grooves Uniform Small nucleoli	Variable amounts of acinar, squamous, endocrine, ductal and primitive component
Cytoplasm	Scant and wispy Plasmacytoid Oncocytic Clear	Dense, well-defined Zymogen granules Negative image	Scant Tail-like Inclusions	
Stroma	Vascular	Vascular	Mucoid fibrovascular stroma	Variable, may be cartilage or bone
Architecture	Single cells Pseudorosettes Loose clusters	Single cells Stripped nuclei Grapelike clusters	Papillary fronds Single cells	
Immunoprofile	Cytokeratin + INSM1+ Synaptophysin+ Chromogranin+	Cytokeratin+ Bcl10+ Trypsin+ Chymotrypsin+	NSE+ Vimentin+ Cytokeratin+/– CD 10+ PR+ AR+ e-Cadherin– β-Catenin+ N/C CD99+ perinuclear dotlike pattern Cyclin D1+	As for components Squamoid corpuscles: β-catenin N/C Cyclin D1 CK8, 18,19, EMA+

ACC, *Acinar cell carcinoma;* AR, *androgen receptor;* EMA, *epithelial membrane antigen;* INSM1, *insulinoma-associated protein 1;* N/C, *nuclear/cytoplasmic;* PB, *pancreatoblastoma;* PR, *progesterone receptor;* SPN, *solid pseudopapillary neoplasm;* WDPanNET, *well-differentiated pancreatic neuroendocrine tumor.*

BOX 36.21 Cytological Features of Poorly Differentiated Neuroendocrine Carcinoma

Small cell type: small, fusiform cells, apoptosis, mitotic activity
Large cell neuroendocrine carcinoma: large, vesicular nuclei, more cytoplasm

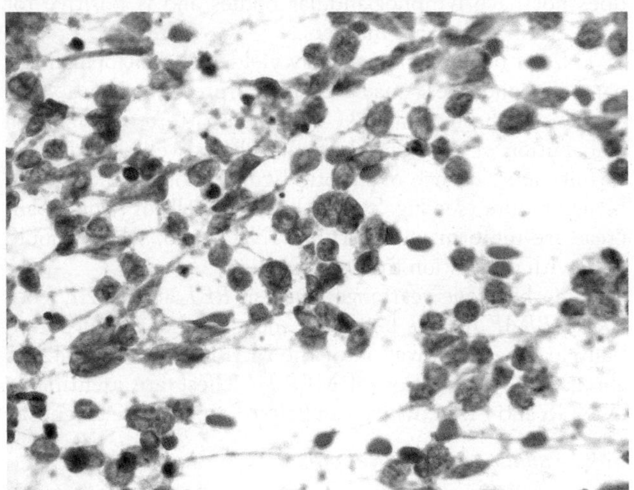

FIGURE 36.34 Small cell carcinoma. Small, fusiform cells with nuclear molding and apoptosis. Papanicolaou, 60×.

Ancillary Studies in Neuroendocrine Neoplasms

The most common (45%) recurring mutations in WDPanNETs involve the death domain–associated protein *(DAXX)* and the α-thalassemia/mental retardation X-linked *(ATRX)* genes.[96,97] These nuclear proteins are involved in telomere maintenance, and mutation results in loss of/negative tumor cell staining with retention in nonneoplastic tissue (see Fig. 36.31B). DAXX or ATRX loss is associated with increased risk of metastasis and shorter survival in WDPanNETs.[96,97] WDPanNETs may rarely show *TP53* mutation resulting in overexpression of p53. The mammalian target of rapamycin (mTOR) cell signaling pathway is rarely mutated (15%) and involves somatic mutations in *PIK3CA*, *PTEN*, and *TSC2*.[96] Sporadic or syndrome-associated WDPanNETs may also show mutation in *MEN* and *VHL* genes.

PDPanNECs (high-grade neuroendocrine carcinomas of small cell or large cell type), on the other hand, are infrequently associated with MEN1 and do not show *DAXX/ATRX* mutations, hence retained DAXX and ATRX immunoreactivity.[98,99] More than 50% of PDPanNECs are diffusely positive for p53, consistent with mutated *TP53*. The retinoblastoma *(RB-1)* gene is also frequently mutated (50%) in PDPanNEC and is associated with nuclear loss of Rb protein in 60-90%. Rb-positive PDPanNECs often show concurrent p16 protein loss, suggesting mutually exclusive roles in pathogenesis.[99] Conversely, WDPanNETs retain p53, Rb, and p16. BCL2 protein, which is overexpressed in pulmonary small cell carcinoma, is also overexpressed in PDPanNECs (100% in small cell and 50% in large cell tumors), but it is typically negative in WDPanNETs.[99]

Acinar Cell Carcinoma

Acinar cell carcinoma (ACC) is a pancreatic tumor of acinar lineage that occurs primarily in older adults.[100] Tumors have characteristic cytomorphology (acinar or rosette-like

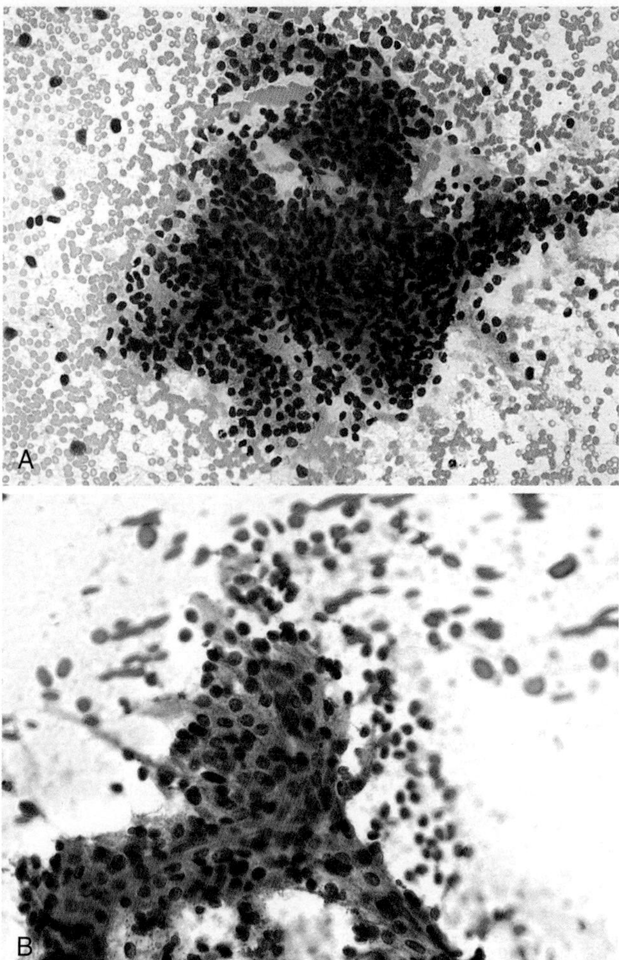

FIGURE 36.35 Acinar cell carcinoma. A, Grapelike cluster showing nuclear overlapping. The cytoplasm is vacuolated. Diff-Quik, 40×. **B,** Group with central, fibrovascular core. The cytoplasm is granular. Some of the cells have prominent nucleoli. The background has stripped nuclei. Papanicolaou, 40×.

pattern, or diffuse monotonous round cells with single prominent nucleoli and basophilic cytoplasm) and immunohistochemical features (expression of enzyme markers, especially trypsin); however, cytohistological misdiagnosis (particularly as NEN) is not uncommon.

On Diff-Quik stained smear, ACC typically produces moderately cellular smears with cohesive, syncytial clusters and singly dispersed basophilic cells as well as stripped nuclei.[101] The smear background may contain blue (Diff-Quik stain) or red (Papanicolaou stain) cytoplasmic granules from the stripped cytoplasm of tumor cells. Tumors typically have 3-dimensional, acinar, and organoid clusters of tumor cells (Fig. 36.35A) and are also quite vascular, with thin-walled capillaries traversing epithelial groups (Fig. 36.35B). Tumor cells are polygonal, of uniform size and shape and have low N/C ratio with abundant zymogen-rich, granular cytoplasm. On Diff-Quik smear these zymogen granules are dark blue in color or may appear as vacuoles or negative images. Nuclear chromatin is generally coarse but may be pale and vesicular, and usually one or two prominent nucleoli are seen. In more poorly differentiated examples there is more nuclear pleomorphism; single-cell necrosis; nuclear membrane irregularity; large, sometimes cherry red nucleoli; and brisk mitotic activity (Box 36.22).

BOX 36.22 Cytological Features of Acinar Cell Carcinoma

- Richly cellular
- Mixture of large and small clusters of cells, single cells, stripped nuclei
- Uniform cells that resemble normal acinar cells
- Round to oval, central or eccentric euchromatic nuclei with smooth nuclear contour and prominent nucleoli (1-2)
- Scant to moderate granular cytoplasm (Romanowsky stain, periodic acid–Schiff with diastase)

The immunoprofile of ACC is characterized by expression for cytokeratins, trypsin, chymotrypsin, and bcl10, a monoclonal antibody directed against the COOH-terminal portion of pancreatic carboxyl ester lipase, a highly specific marker of acinar differentiation that is positive even in trypsin-negative cases.[102] Use of two or more acinar markers increases the likelihood of accurate diagnosis. Tumor cells may also express CK7 and CK19, show focal nuclear β-catenin positivity, and occasionally stain with markers of hepatocellular carcinoma (including Hep Par-1, glypican-3, and albumin mRNA [by in situ hybridization]).

The cytological differential diagnosis includes WDPanNET, PB, SPN, and nonneoplastic acinar parenchyma. The differential diagnosis with WDPanNET, SPN, and PB will be discussed at the end of this section. ACC may resemble the tumor cells of WDPanNET and PDPanNEC. Cytoplasmic neurosecretory granules of NENs that are red on Papanicolaou stain may resemble red cytoplasmic zymogen granules of ACC. These tumors can be distinguished by trypsin and bcl10 stains, which are negative in neuroendocrine neoplasms. Bcl10 is negative in SPN. The stripped nuclei of ACC may resemble those of non-Hodgkin's lymphoma (NHL). However, unlike NHL, ACC smear background does not have lymphoglandular bodies and is positive for cytokeratin and acinar markers.

FNA of benign pancreas may yield abundant benign acinar cells, and these may be misinterpreted as ACC. The organoid, cohesive grapelike clustered pattern or single cell distribution of the normal acinar cells as well as their uniformity and absence of mitotic figures should hint at their benign nature (see Fig. 36.34A). Acinar cells of benign pancreas are uniform with very low N/C ratio, which should help with distinction from ACC.

ACC has gene rearrangements in *RET* and *BRAF*, with *SND1-BRAF* fusions being the most frequent, and potentially leading to activation of the MAPK pathway, which is abrogated by inhibition of MEK.[103] These are identifiable by NGS and FISH, which can help to support the diagnosis.

Solid Pseudopapillary Neoplasm

SPN of the pancreas has a characteristic cytological picture. Smears are typically quite cellular and contain numerous branching papillary-like groups of epithelial cells with a central fibrovascular core. The papillary fronds have three layers: a central vessel, an outer myxoid stromal layer, and an outer neoplastic layer (Fig. 36.36A). The outermost layer is composed of monomorphic neoplastic cells with round

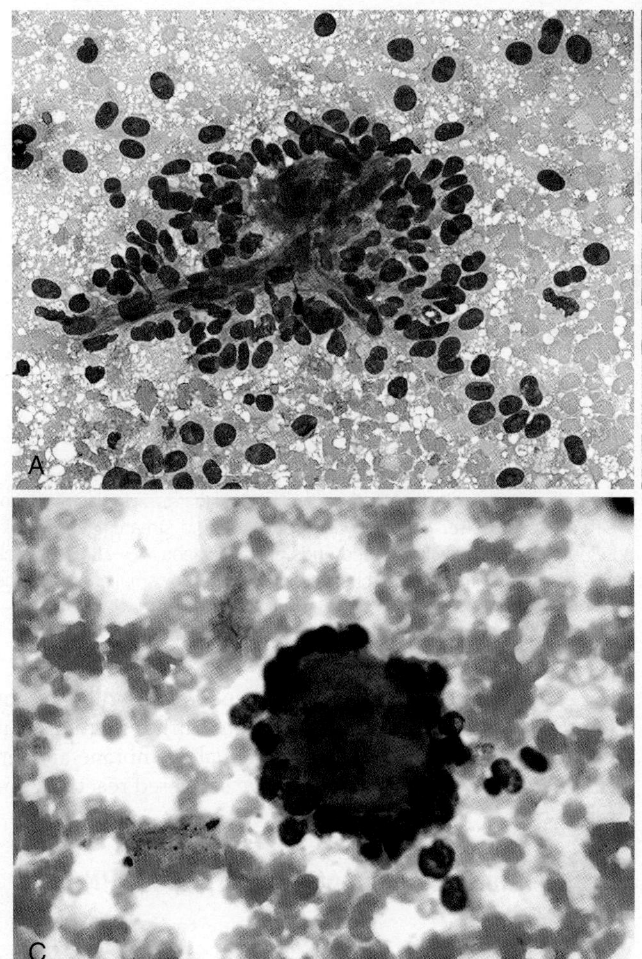

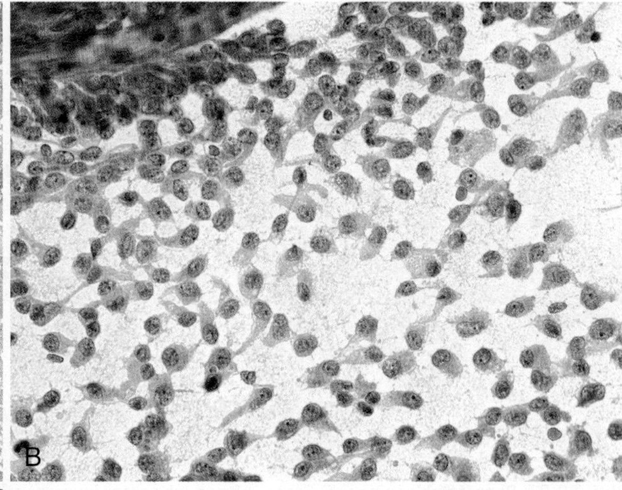

FIGURE 36.36 Solid pseudopapillary neoplasm. A, Group with fibrovascular core showing middle capillary, second layer of mucinous stroma, and outer layer of neoplastic cells. Diff-Quik, 40×. **B,** Neoplastic cells with cytoplasmic tails. The cytoplasm is vacuolated in some cells. The nuclei are relatively monomorphic, and some show small nucleoli and grooves. Papanicolaou, 40×. **C,** Balls of mucoid stroma are pathognomic. Diff-Quik, 40×.

BOX 36.23 Cytology of Solid Pseudopapillary Neoplasm

Cellular, branching groups of cells
Papillary fronds composed of a central fibrovascular core, surrounded by a myxoid layer of stroma, and an outer layer of neoplastic cells
Neoplastic cells with bland nuclei and scant amphophilic cytoplasm that occasionally contains periodic acid–Schiff-positive granules
"Balls" of mucoid stroma, +/– rim of neoplastic cells

to oval nuclei, finely dispersed chromatin, nuclear indentations or grooves, and small nucleoli. The cytoplasm of these cells is basophilic, varies in shape and quantity, may be vacuolated, or may contain periodic acid-Schiff (PAS)-positive granules, and may demonstrate cytoplasmic tails (Fig. 36.36B). The pathognomonic feature is "balls" of myxoid stroma that may or may not contain a rim of neoplastic cells (Fig. 36.36C; Box 36.23).[104]

The characteristic immunohistochemical profile is strong and diffuse nuclear and cytoplasmic expression for β-catenin, and strong and diffuse expression for vimentin, progesterone receptor (PR), androgen receptor (AR), cyclin D1, and CD10. Tumor cells are typically negative for cytokeratins but may show focal weak positivity. Tumor cells also show either complete loss of expression for e-cadherin or partial nuclear expression for e-cadherin.[105] Lymphoid enhancing binding factor 1 (LEF1) and transcription factor for immunoglobulin heavy-chain enhancer 3 (TFE3), both of which are proteins in the β-catenin pathway, are also expressed in SPN and have been tested in cytology specimens.[106] CD99 positivity in a dotlike pattern is reproducible, and apparently unique to this neoplasm, compared with the other nonductal neoplasms.[107,108] Synaptophysin may be focally positive.

PanNET, ACC, and PB are the key entities in the differential diagnosis, which will be discussed at the end of this section.

Pancreatoblastoma

Pancreatoblastoma (PB) is a rare malignancy that is most frequently seen in childhood but may occur in adults. Tumors show multilinear differentiation and entity-defining squamoid morules. On aspiration, PB produces cellular smears composed of clusters and singly dispersed cells whose appearance varies depending on the direction of differentiation.[109-112] The most characteristic cells are small and blastlike with

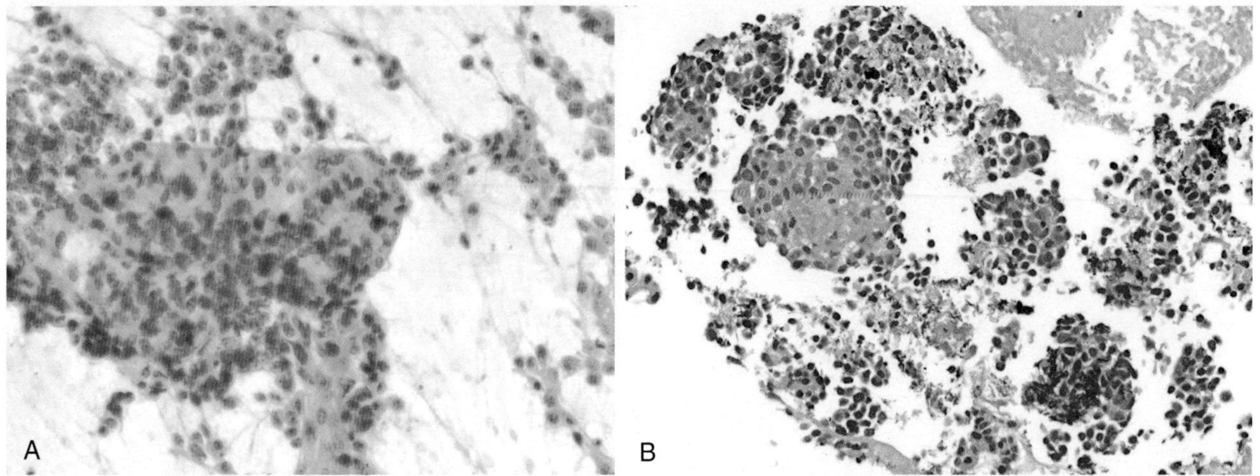

FIGURE 36.37 Pancreatoblastoma. A, Smear shows a two-cell population of small primitive blastlike cells with high nuclear-to-cytoplasmic ratio, smooth nuclear contours, distinct central nuclei, and immature chromatin with adjacent *(lower left)* syncytial group of bland streaming squamoid cells with abundant granular cytoplasm, low nuclear-to-cytoplasmic ratio and elongated, nuclei with blunted ends. Papanicolaou, 40×. **B,** Cell block shows intermediate poor image of central cluster of eosinophilic epithelioid cells consistent with squamoid morule, surrounded by smaller round blue blastlike cells. Hematoxylin and eosin, 40×.

BOX 36.24 Cytological Features of Pancreatoblastoma

Highly cellular smears
Single cells > clusters
Primitive "blastema"-type epithelial cells
Eccentric nuclei
Evenly distributed chromatin
Second population of squamoid cells with elongated blunted nuclei and dense cytoplasm

high N/C ratios, fine immature chromatin, and small but distinctive nucleoli. A second population of larger streaming or whorled cells with more abundant, dense, squamoid cytoplasm, low N/C ratio, and elongated, oval nuclei with evenly distributed chromatin and without nucleoli may also be seen. These cells represent squamoid morules, and although best seen on cell block, they are also visible on smear (Fig. 36.37A). The cells of the squamoid morules may also have optically clear nuclei. Additionally, cells with acinar differentiation showing oval to cuboidal shape, moderate granular cytoplasm resembling ACC, round central to eccentric nuclei, and one or more small nucleoli may also be seen (Fig. 36.37B). These cells are cytologically indistinguishable from ACC. In cases with neuroendocrine differentiation tumor cells are more plasmacytoid with coarse chromatin, higher N/C ratio, denser, less granular cytoplasm, and less conspicuous nucleoli. Stromal fragments may be scant or prominent with traversing capillaries (Box 36.24).

PBs show aberrant Wnt pathway activation manifested as somatic *CTNNB1* mutations (in 90% of cases), and loss of heterozygosity (LOH) of *APC* (in 10%). APC/β-catenin pathway alterations are seen in patients with and without FAP. *CTNNB1* mutation leads to nuclear overexpression of β-catenin immunostain in squamoid morules. β-Catenin highlights even subtle or microscopically invisible morules, and can be diffuse in some cases.[109] Tumor cells are also positive for cytokeratin and show variable expression of acinar, neuroendocrine, and ductal immunohistochemical markers, depending on differentiation. The squamoid morules do not express typical markers of squamous differentiation, but instead express CK8, 18, 19; epithelial membrane antigen (EMA); and cyclin D1 and may have scattered reactivity for CK 5/6.

Differential Diagnosis of PanNET, ACC, SPN, and PB

These neoplasms can be differentiated based on assessment of their cytomorphological features and immunohistochemical studies (see Table 36.7). The cytomorphological features to consider are nuclear, cytoplasmic, and stromal. The nuclei of WDPanNET show a salt-and-pepper chromatin pattern; the nuclei of SPN are subtly more irregular and pale, with longitudinal grooves, fine chromatin, and micronucleoli; and the nuclei of ACC and PB with acinar differentiation are round and uniform and may both show prominent nucleoli. The cytoplasm of WDPanNET is variable in amount and quantity, but when plasmacytoid, this neoplasm may be more readily recognized. The cytoplasm of ACC shows granularity due to zymogen granules. The cytoplasm of PB may be similar to that of ACC if acinar differentiation predominates. The cytoplasm of SPN may show tails or vacuoles, which are unique to this neoplasm. Cytoplasmic inclusions have been described as a feature of SPN, but these are not unique to SPN, and may be seen in PanNET.

All of these neoplasms are vascular, and a vascular stromal component is present on the smears to a variable extent. However, only SPN shows a layer of myxoid stroma surrounding the capillaries in the fibrovascular cores. This myxoid stroma, when identified, is virtually pathognomonic of SPN.

When the cytomorphological features do not provide a clear diagnosis, immunohistochemical studies are indicated. A panel consisting of cytokeratins, neuroendocrine markers, pancreatic enzymes, progesterone or androgen receptor, e-cadherin, and β-catenin can differentiate these tumors (see Table 36.7).

Pancreatic Cysts

Many pancreatic cysts are discovered incidentally, as part of the workup for abdominal pain or other reasons. In contrast to other organs, in which an incidentally discovered mass is more likely to be benign, in the pancreas, they are more likely to represent either a preinvasive or invasive neoplasm. In fact, 78% of all incidentally discovered masses in the pancreas are either premalignant or malignant.[113] Among incidentally discovered cysts, preinvasive neoplasms account for more than 50% of cases.[114]

FNAB is performed to answer two questions:

1. Is the cyst neoplastic or nonneoplastic?
2. If it is neoplastic, does it contain a neoplasm that is indolent or unlikely to progress, or a neoplasm with a high potential to progress to invasion?

Cytology has excellent specificity, but poor sensitivity, for diagnosis of cystic neoplasms of the pancreas. Therefore an integrative approach, as described at the beginning of this chapter, which includes correlation of the clinical, radiological, cytological, and ancillary studies, is even more necessary for assessing pancreatic cysts.

Analysis of the cytological specimen needs to begin with assessment of the gross appearance of the pancreatic cyst fluid (PCF) aspirated, as this can provide critical information about the nature of the cyst.[115] The approach should then assess background, cellular components, architectural appearance of groups, cytoplasm, and nuclear features. Ancillary studies are essential for the workup of pancreatic cysts.

Ancillary Studies

Mucin Stains

Mucicarmine and Alcian blue stains aid in identifying background material as mucinous when its nature is questionable. However, mucin from GI contaminants may lead to false-positive interpretation.[116] The presence of abundant, thick background mucin or cells containing mucin will lead in the direction of a MCN or IPMN and excludes serous cystadenoma and pseudocyst. If the sample is obviously mucinous, mucin stains are not indicated.

Glycogen Stains

PAS with and without diastase detects glycogen. The glycogen granules are positive with PAS but are digested by diastase. This is useful for the diagnosis of serous cystadenoma.

Cyst Fluid Viscosity

The original studies published on this topic utilized viscosity measurements as a means of distinguishing between nonmucinous and mucinous lesions. The string sign is measured at the time of FNA by the endoscopist. It is performed by placing a drop of fluid between the thumb and index finger and measuring the maximum length of stretch before disruption of the mucus string.[117] This serves as a surrogate for viscosity. While this is a useful and quick test to determine whether a cyst is mucinous or not, preference should be given to processing the PCF for CEA, amylase, cytology, and molecular studies if the amount of aspirated fluid is scant.

Tumor Markers

Current PCF protocols, recommend analysis of CEA, as an elevated CEA level correlates with the presence of a cystic mucinous neoplasm. Serous cystadenomas and pseudocysts typically have low levels of CEA. A cutoff level of 192 ng/mL was established in a prospective, multiinstitutional series as being indicative of the presence of a mucinous type neoplasm, either MCN or IPMN. Since then, there have been a number of studies evaluating the optimum CEA level in cystic mucinous neoplasms, with results ranging from 50 ng/mL to 800 ng/mL. PCF CEA level <5 ng/mL is suggestive of a serous cystadenoma or pseudocyst. However, it is recommended that each laboratory establish its own threshold. CEA levels do not correlate with the grade of dysplasia in a mucinous cyst.[118]

Benign entities, such as enteric duplication cysts,[119] mesothelial inclusion cysts,[120] and lymphoepithelial cyst of the pancreas (LECP) may also produce elevated CEA levels.[121,122] Therefore CEA levels should not be used as the sole criterion for the diagnosis of a cystic mucinous neoplasm.

Enzymes

Elevated amylase levels are associated with a pseudocyst, but elevated amylase levels may also be encountered in neoplasms, such as IPMN, and even LECP.[122] An amylase level <250 units/L excludes pseudocyst.

Mutations

The molecular landscape of pancreatic cystic neoplasms has been defined in recent years. *KRAS* mutations are identified in both MCN and IPMN.[123] *GNAS* mutations are identified in IPMN. Neither of these mutations identifies high-grade dysplasia.[124] Mutational allelic frequency of *GNAS* >55%, or detection of alteration in *TP53//PIK3CA/PTEN*, or mutations in *p16* or *SMAD4*, are associated with advanced neoplasia. Molecular analysis adds value to PCF analysis by identifying a cyst as mucinous, further subclassifying a cyst as IPMN and defining if it is high risk. Serous cystadenomas are characterized by mutations in *VHL*, and solid pseudopapillary neoplasm has mutations in *CTNBB1*. The type of molecular analysis performed is laboratory dependent and may be an in-house test or a send-out commercial test.

Nonneoplastic Cysts

Pseudocysts

Pseudocysts are the most common nonneoplastic cyst of the pancreas. Aspiration of a pseudocyst typically obtains an abundant amount of turbid, brown fluid. The cytology sample demonstrates hemosiderin laden macrophages, few acute inflammatory cells or lymphocytes, fibrin, debris, and bile pigment (Fig. 36.38) and lacks neoplastic lining epithelium (Box 36.25).[125,126] These cysts should not have background mucin, although thin watery mucin may be obtained as a contaminant from the GI epithelium.[116] Benign cells from adjacent pancreatic parenchyma[126] may be aspirated and represent a potential pitfall.

The cyst fluid aspirated from pseudocysts will be thin and not viscid.[117] Pseudocyst fluid will show elevated levels of amylase and low levels of CEA.[28,123,127,128] *KRAS* mutations should not be detectable[123]; however, if adjacent pancreatic parenchyma containing pancreatic intraepithelial neoplasia or IPMN is sampled, *KRAS* mutations may be detected in the fluid (personal unpublished data).

The differential diagnosis of pseudocysts includes other types of inflammatory or infectious cysts, as well as true cysts and cystic neoplasms. Secondary bacterial infection may produce cyst fluid that contains abundant neutrophils and proteinaceous background debris.[125] Cultures of the fluid are usually positive. Hydatid cyst is a rare cause of cysts in the pancreas and should be considered a possibility in endemic regions.[129-131] Diagnosis is usually suspected preoperatively based on imaging findings and serologies, and aspiration is contraindicated,[132] but some patients do not present with positive serology.[131] Cytology aspirates will show scoliosis, hooklets, and laminated fragments.[130] The presence of a neoplastic lining epithelium, or background mucin, excludes a diagnosis of pseudocyst, although false-positive mucin stains occur due to GI contamination.[116]

Ciliated Foregut Cyst

Aspirates are characterized by ciliated columnar cells and detached ciliary tufts. The background fluid contains amorphous debris and rare macrophages.[133] The differential diagnosis includes cystic neoplasms. The presence of ciliated cells is diagnostic of this entity.

Lymphoepithelial Cyst of the Pancreas

Lymphoepithelial cyst of the pancreas (LECP) is typically discovered incidentally. These lesions have a very typical CT scan appearance. The clinical and imaging features are described in Chapter 40. Endoscopic ultrasound imaging shows a hypoechoic, unilocular or multilocular mass, possibly with hyperechoic, sludgelike material in the cyst.[134] Aspirates of LECP usually yield a variable amount of pasty, yellow-gray or yellow-white material.[135] The characteristic smear pattern shows abundant anucleated squames, keratinous debris, and few nucleated squamous cells with background cholesterol crystals and clefts. Lymphocytes, histiocytes, and background debris are variable (Fig. 36.39A).[136,137] The cell block may show squamous cells with a preserved granular layer (Fig. 36.39B). These cytological findings are diagnostic (Box 36.26).

Measurement of cyst fluid levels may lead to misinterpretation as an MCN or IPMN, as LECP may produce high levels of cyst fluid CEA and CA 19-9. The reported range of CEA levels is 2700 to 35,028 ng/ mL.[122,137-139] The cyst fluid amylase levels range from normal to 480 units/L.[122,137,140,141] The cyst fluid CA 19-9 may be elevated[139,140] and has been reported as high as greater than 5 × 10.[6,122] The wide range of these test results helps

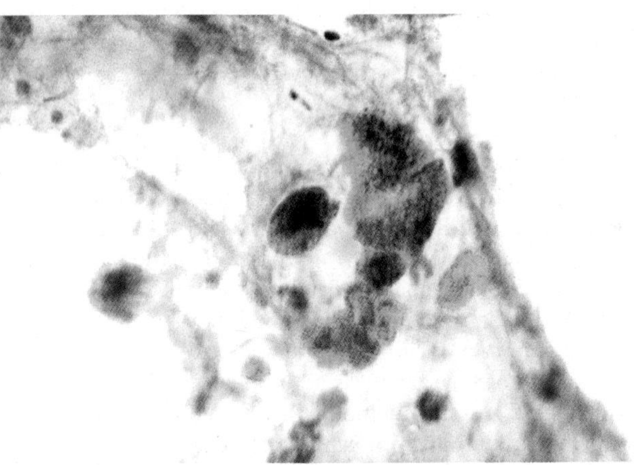

FIGURE 36.38 Pseudocyst. Dirty background with bile pigment and histiocytes. Papanicolaou, 60×.

BOX 36.25 Cytological Features of Pseudocysts

- Abundant, turbid, brown fluid
- Variable number of inflammatory cells, including neutrophils and histiocytes
- Hemosiderin-laden macrophages
- Granular debris, fibrin, bile, or hematoidin pigment
- Absence of cyst lining epithelial cells
- Normal pancreatic cells, fibroblasts, mesothelial cells, and metaplastic cells as contaminants

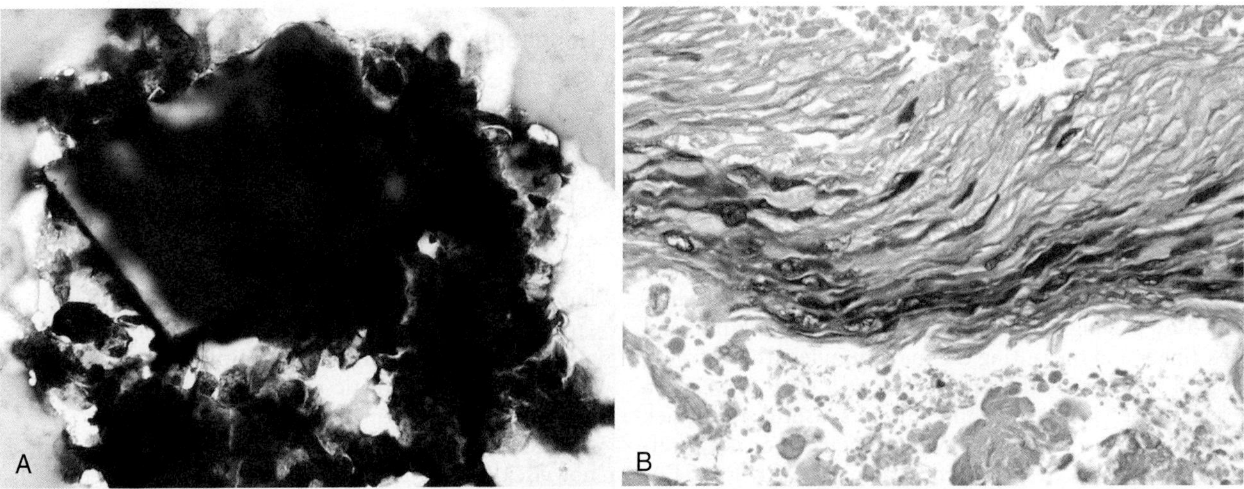

FIGURE 36.39 Lymphoepithelial cyst of the pancreas. A, Anucleated squamous cells with cholesterol crystals, Diff-Quik 60×. **B,** Cell block showing cohesive sheet of squamous cells with a granular cell layer and keratinous debris. Hematoxylin and eosin, 40×.

emphasize why cytology is considered the gold standard diagnostic method.

The differential diagnosis includes pseudocysts and cystic neoplasms. The presence of abundant squamous material within the cytology sample helps exclude these other entities. The morphological differential diagnosis includes any other entity with a squamous component including squamous metaplasia, squamous cyst of the pancreas, dermoid cyst, epidermoid cyst involving intrapancreatic accessory spleen, adenosquamous carcinoma, and metastatic squamous cell carcinoma. Squamous metaplasia occurs mainly in association with chronic pancreatitis and is unlikely to produce a cystic mass lesion. It may be difficult on cytological features alone to differentiate dermoid cyst of the pancreas and splenic epidermoid cyst from LECP. Epidermoid cyst arising in intrapancreatic accessory spleen shows mostly macrophages and debris.[142] The lack of malignant epithelium helps exclude adenosquamous and squamous cell carcinoma.

Lymphangioma

Lymphangioma may present as a cystic mass in or extrinsic to the pancreas. The fluid will be thin and not viscous. The cytology shows a population of small T lymphocytes without atypia. The CEA is typically in the low range and CA 19.9 and CA 72.4 will be within normal range[143] (see Box 36.27).

Cystic Neoplasms

Cystic neoplasms can be either inherently cystic neoplasms, such as serous cystadenomas and mucinous cystic neoplasms; intraductal neoplasms presenting as cysts, such as intraductal papillary mucinous neoplasms; or solid neoplasms with cystic degeneration, such as neuroendocrine neoplasms or SPN.

Serous Cystic Neoplasm (Serous Cystadenoma/Serous Cystadenocarcinoma)

Aspiration of a serous cystadenoma is generally nondiagnostic due to scant cellularity.[123] Typically, a scant amount of clear, thin fluid is aspirated. The background is usually watery and may contain fibrovascular stromal fragments that are stripped of epithelial cells. The cells are usually arranged in flat, monolayered sheets, or as dispersed single cells or stripped nuclei (Fig. 36.40A,B). The nuclei are round and uniform in shape but may vary in size and lack nucleoli and mitoses.[144] Aspirates may contain only a few cuboidal cells or histiocytes.[145] Since the stroma is typically quite vascular, these cysts may hemorrhage, in which case the aspirate may reveal blood and hemosiderin laden macrophages. The cytological features of serous cystic neoplasms are summarized in Box 36.28.

Cytology lacks sensitivity for serous cystic neoplasms due to difficulty in obtaining cells from these neoplasms.[144] Thus knowledge of the radiological findings is essential. If imaging studies are interpreted as characteristic of serous cystadenoma, then the pathologist should evaluate the sample carefully for diagnostic cells. A few cells are sufficient if there are appropriate clinical and imaging findings.

Oligocystic and solid variants of serous cystic neoplasms occur as well. The solid variant may be interpreted as a neuroendocrine tumor on imaging. The pathologist should be aware of any neoplasm presenting as a NET that is negative for neuroendocrine markers and work it up for serous cystadenoma (see Fig. 36.40A).

A diagnosis of cystadenocarcinoma depends primarily on histological identification of tissue invasion. There are no reliable differences in the cytological appearance between

BOX 36.26 Cytological Features of Lymphoepithelial Cyst of the Pancreas

Pasty, yellow-gray or yellow white material
Abundant nucleated anucleated squamous cells
Mature squamous cells, occasionally with a granular layer
Keratinous debris
Lymphocytes and histiocytes
Cholesterol clefts and crystals

BOX 36.27 Cytological Features of Lymphangioma

Small, mature appearing lymphocytes
Nonmucinous background
Lacks epithelial cyst lining cells

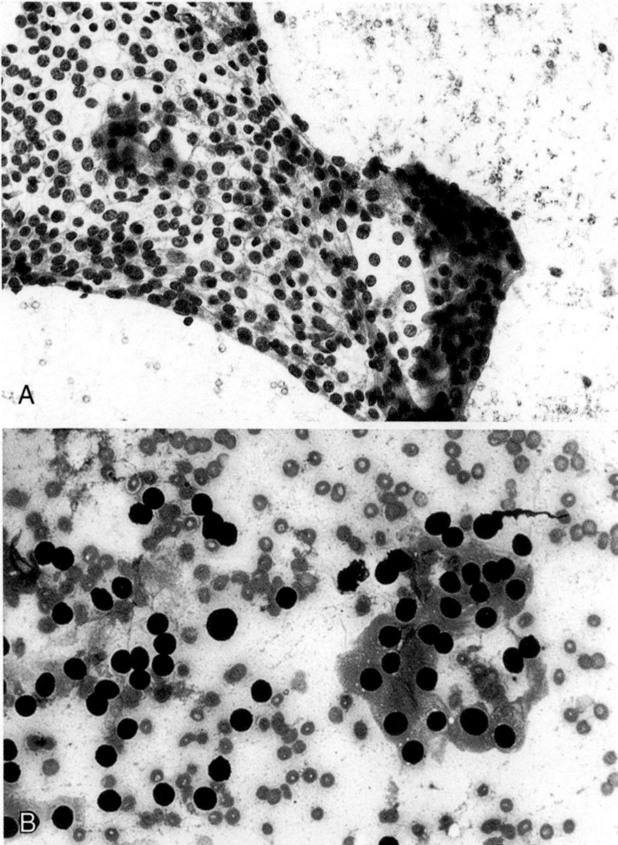

FIGURE 36.40 Serous cystadenoma. A, Sheet of cells with well-defined, clear, cuboidal cytoplasm and uniform, rounded nuclei. Papanicolaou, 60×. **B,** Cohesive sheet of cells with well-defined, clear, cuboidal cytoplasm. The nuclei show some size variation and binucleation. Stripped nuclei are seen. Diff-Quik, 40×.

benign and malignant serous neoplasms as there are no reliable differences in histopathological specimens.[146]

The PAS stain, with and without diastase, may be performed on cytology samples to demonstrate the presence of cytoplasmic glycogen, a characteristic feature of serous cystadenomas. CEA and amylase levels in the cyst fluid will be low.[28,123,128] Immunohistochemistry for MUC6 and inhibin will be positive in the neoplastic cells (Fig 36.40B).[147] These neoplasms will be negative for *KRAS* and *GNAS* mutations.[124] Somatic mutation of *VHL* is common in these tumors.

The differential diagnosis includes pseudocyst, mucinous cystic neoplasm, and solid neoplasms presenting as a cyst (Table 36.8).

BOX 36.28 Cytological Features of Serous Cystadenoma

Scant amount of serous fluid
Smears with low cellularity, rich in protein
Epithelial cells arranged in flat sheets or singly
Stripped nuclei
Clear cytoplasm
Cytoplasmic borders well defined.
Round nuclei, evenly distributed chromatin

Neoplastic Mucinous Cysts

Neoplastic mucinous cysts include MCN and IPMN, which have overlapping cytological features.

Mucinous cystic neoplasm (MCN) presents as a solitary unilocular or multilocular cyst in the distal pancreas in middle-aged women.[148] Histology is characterized by columnar, mucinous cyst lining cells surrounded by ovarian type stroma. [117,123] The diagnosis of intraductal papillary mucinous neoplasm (IPMN) may be suggested on the imaging studies if the cyst is associated with a dilated main pancreatic duct, connecting to the main pancreatic duct, or multiple cysts. A connection to the ductal system is not always identified.

TABLE 36.8 Cytological, Immunohistochemical, Biochemical, and Molecular Features of Most Common Pancreatic Cysts

Cyst	Cytology	Immunohistochemical	Biochemical	Molecular
PC	Hematoidin yellow pigment Background debris Histiocytes Lacks neoplastic epithelium	N/A	Amylase >250 units/L, usually >1000 units/L CEA low	None
LECP	Anucleated squames Benign squames Granular layer Cholesterol crystals	N/A	CEA elevated Amylase elevated	None
Lymphangioma	Benign lymphocytes Lacks neoplastic epithelium and mucin	N/A	CEA low Amylase low	None
SCA	Scantly cellular Lacks background mucin Uniform cuboidal cells with round nuclei, smooth nuclear membranes Finely vacuolated cytoplasm that contains glycogen Stripped nuclei Hemosiderin laden macrophages (surrogate markers) Fibrous septae	MUC6 + Inhibin +	CEA low (<5 ng/mL) Amylase low (<250 units /L)	*VHL* deletions and/or mutations
MCN	Thick, colloid-like mucin or thin mucin with oncotic debris Variable cellularity Neoplastic mucinous glandular epithelium	N/A	CEA elevated Amylase variable	*KRAS*, *RNF 43* mutations
IPMN	Thick, colloid-like mucin or thin mucin with oncotic debris Variable cellularity Neoplastic mucinous glandular epithelium	MUC5 + MUC2, CDX2 + (intestinal type) MUC1+ (pancreatobiliary type)	CEA elevated Amylase variable DAS1 elevated (high-risk cysts)	*KRAS, RNF43,* and *GNAS* mutations
IOPN	Background mucin Papillary fronds Oncocytic neoplastic cells	MUC6+ HepPar+	CEA elevated	*PRKACA* and *PRKACB*-related oncogenic fusions *(DNAJB1-* and *ATP1B1-PRKACA)*

CEA, *Carcinoembryonic antigen;* IOPN, *intraductal oncocytic papillary mucinous neoplasm;* IPMN, *intraductal papillary mucinous neoplasm;* LECP, *lymphoepithelial cyst of pancreas;* MCN, *mucinous cystic neoplasm;* N/A, *not applicable;* PC, *pseudocyst;* SCA, *serous cystadenoma.*

Cytology

Aspiration of fluid from an MCN/IPMN may be difficult because the fluid is often extremely viscous. Gross examination of the fluid often reveals highly viscous fluid or clear fluid with strands of mucus plugs. In fact, the material may be expressed from the needle as a "plug" of mucin. This feature is considered diagnostic of a mucinous cyst, regardless of the cellularity of the aspirate.

The classic cytomorphological appearance is the presence of thick background mucin combined with neoplastic mucinous epithelium. Assessment, therefore, includes a stepwise approach of the background and the cellular component.

The key feature is the presence of background mucin, which can be variable in quantity. The most diagnostic appearance is when the mucin covers the entire slide, and forms a thick film, similar to colloid from thyroid aspirates. On Papanicolaou stain, the mucin has a characteristic pink hue (Fig. 36.41). When not diffuse, it may be aggregated or clumped (Fig. 36.41B). The mucin is usually accompanied by degenerated cells, called oncotic cells,[149] and macrophages (Fig. 36.41A). The mucin may present as thick, inspissated, fibrillary or fanlike material (Fig 36.41C). Psammomatous calcification may occur with IPMN. The presence of thick background mucin with these characteristics indicates the presence of MCN/IPMN. A cytology specimen from a cyst of the pancreas showing characteristic mucin is diagnostic of a mucinous cyst and should be included in the Neoplastic: Other category.

The cellularity is variable and consists of neoplastic mucinous epithelium with varying degrees of cytological atypia, dependent on the degree of dysplasia of the cyst lining epithelium.[150] The evaluated neoplastic cells are either cells that have sloughed into the cyst fluid, or are cells picked up when the needle traversed the cyst wall. A caveat is the cells in the fluid may not be representative of the entire cyst lining and will not be representative of an adjacent mural nodule, or a separate cyst.

The cells may be arranged singly, on edge, in sheets, of papillary clusters, or small papillary tufts. The sheets or groups do not form a honeycomb pattern, but rather are subtly hypercellular and crowded (Fig. 36.42A,B).

Architectural features of neoplastic mucinous epithelium are crowding of the sheets of cells, with nuclear overlap. The nuclei may be hypochromatic with small, peripherally located nucleoli, similar to those seen in papillary thyroid carcinoma. Nuclear grooves and pseudo inclusions become more evident and are evidence of IPMN.

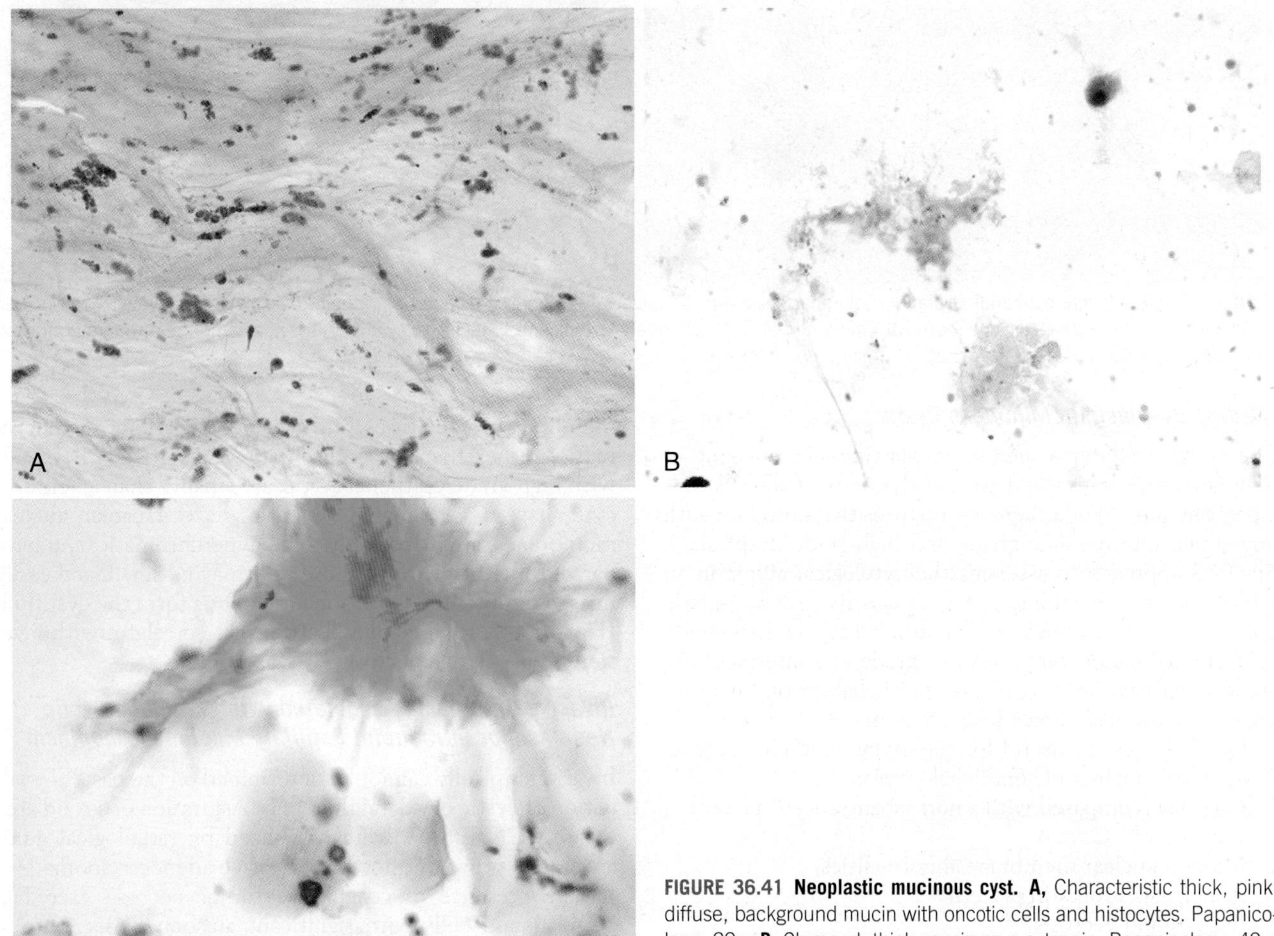

FIGURE 36.41 Neoplastic mucinous cyst. A, Characteristic thick, pink, diffuse, background mucin with oncotic cells and histocytes. Papanicolaou, 20×. **B,** Clumped, thick mucin on a cytospin. Papanicolaou, 40×. **C,** Thick, fibrillary material and single calcification. Papanicolaou, 20×.

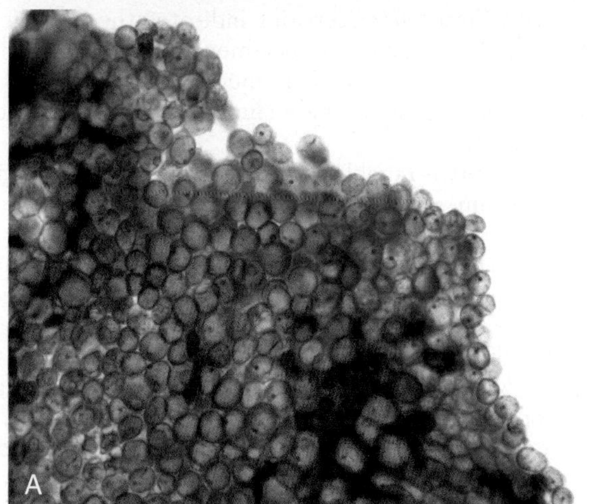

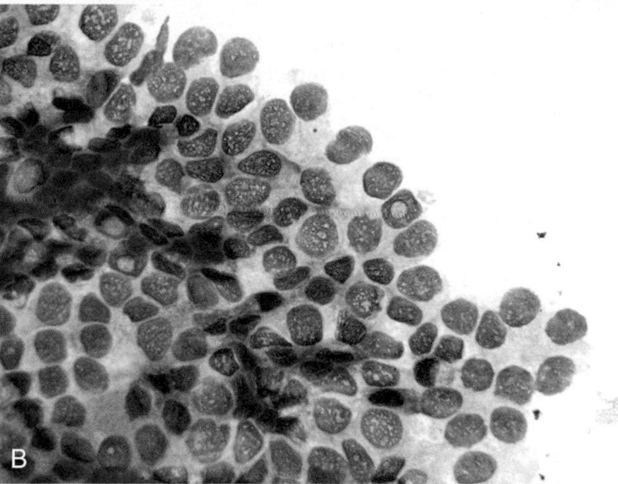

FIGURE 36.42 Intraductal papillary mucinous neoplasm. A, Crowded, 3-dimensional sheet of cells. The chromatin is pale. Many of the nuclei contain intranuclear pseudoinclusions; small, peripherally located nucleoli and grooves. Anisonucleosis is evident. Papanicolaou, 60×. **B,** Crowded sheet with nuclear atypia and intranuclear inclusions. Diff-Quik, 60×.

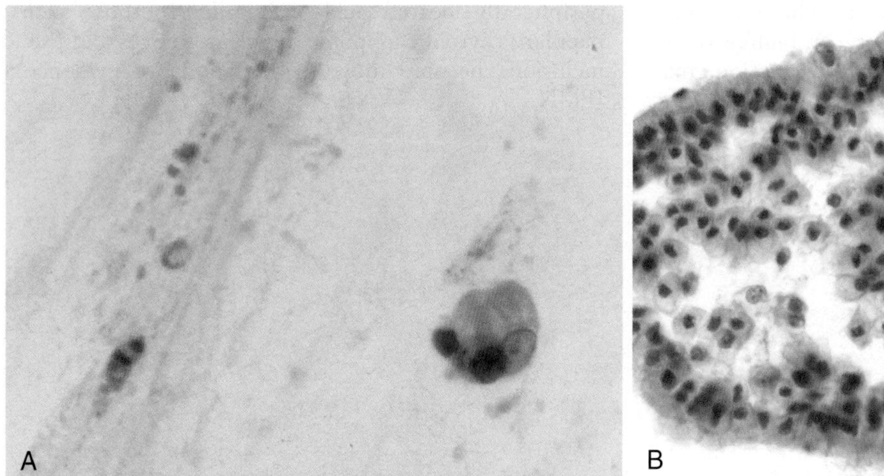

FIGURE 36.43 Low-grade epithelial atypia. A, Columnar cells seen on edge with abundant cytoplasmic mucin, basally located nuclei, low nuclear-to-cytoplasmic ratio, size of an enterocyte. **B,** Sheet of cells with abundant cytoplasmic mucin, low nuclear-to-cytoplasmic ratio, minimal nuclear membrane irregularity, evenly distributed chromatin. Papanicolaou, 40×.

Grading Dysplasia in Mucinous Cysts

The cytological atypia seen in neoplastic mucinous epithelium correlates with the degree of dysplasia of the cyst lining epithelium. While there are features that correlate with low-grade, intermediate-grade, and high-grade dysplasia, a practical approach to assessing the cytological atypia in an aspirate from a mucinous cyst is to classify it as low-grade epithelial atypia and high-grade epithelial atypia. Low-grade epithelial atypia encompasses low-grade and intermediate-grade dysplasia, and high-grade epithelial atypia includes high-grade dysplasia and adenocarcinoma.[151]

Five features are useful for classifying epithelial cells as low-grade or high-grade epithelial atypia:

1. Cell size (compared with a normal enterocyte 12 μm)
2. Increased N/C ratio
3. Marked nuclear membrane abnormalities
4. Abnormal chromatin pattern
5. Background necrosis

Cells of low-grade epithelial atypia are larger than an enterocyte; retain a low N/C ratio, show minimal nuclear membrane irregularities, and are euchromatic or hypochromatic, rather than hyperchromatic (Fig. 36.43A,B). Cells with high-grade epithelial atypia are smaller than an enterocyte, have a very high N/C ratio, have irregular nuclear membranes, are more likely to be hyperchromatic, and have parachromatin clearing. These cells may be small, and easily missed or obscured by the oncotic debris form the cyst fluid (Fig. 36.44A,B). The only feature that correlates with invasion is coagulative necrosis[151] (Box 36.30).

Invasive Carcinoma Associated with Mucinous Cystic Neoplasm or Intraductal Papillary Mucinous Neoplasm

Invasion typically cannot be determined on the basis of evaluation of cystic or ductal fluid only. Aspiration of a solid area of an MCN/IPMN, when visualized by radiological guidance, may prove diagnostic of invasive adenocarcinoma.[152]

The presence of coagulative tumor necrosis (see Fig. 36.44B) and cells with significant anisonucleosis, mitotic features, and other criteria of adenocarcinoma may indicate the presence of an invasive ductal carcinoma component.

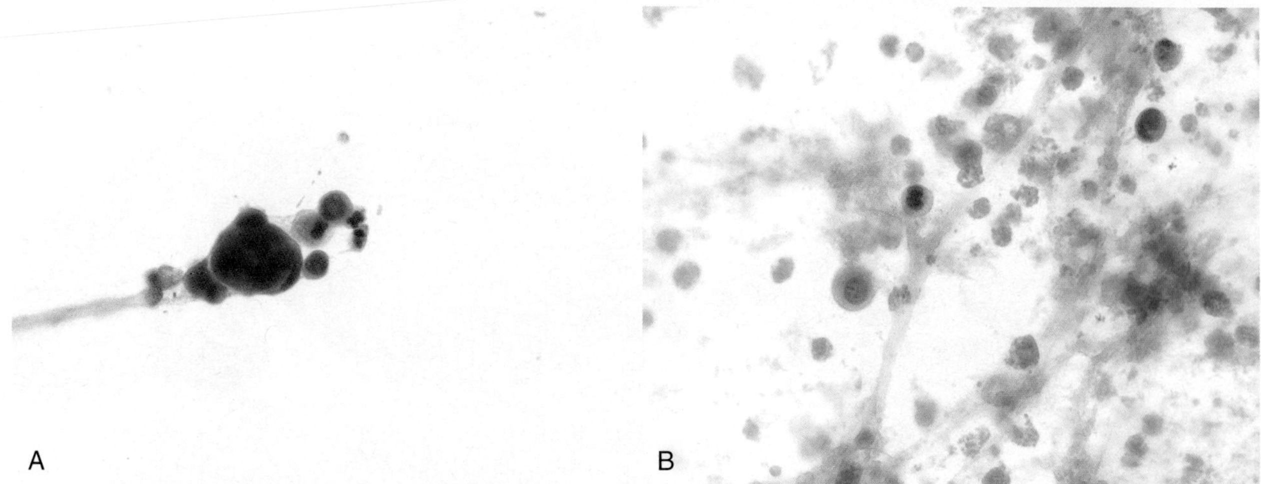

FIGURE 36.44 High-grade epithelial atypia. A, Papillary, 3-dimensional tuft and single cells. The cells have a high nuclear-to-cytoplasmic ratio and angulated, irregular nuclei. Papanicolaou, 60×. **B,** Single cells, and background necrosis, suggestive of invasion. Papanicolaou, 60×.

BOX 36.29 Cytological Features of Neoplastic Mucinous Cysts

Highly viscous fluid
Tenacious mucin in background, which is pink on Papanicolaou, and resembles colloid
Degenerated cellular debris and histiocytes in mucin
Neoplastic glandular epithelium with variable cytoplasmic mucin
Hypochromatic pale nuclei, with small peripheral nucleoli, mild nuclear folding and irregularity or more pronounced nuclear abnormalities, such as hyperchromasia and abnormal parachromatin clearing, intranuclear grooves and inclusions
Papillary clusters with fibrovascular cores (in intraductal papillary mucinous neoplasm)

BOX 36.30 Cytological Features of Low-Grade and High-Grade Epithelial Atypia

LOW-GRADE EPITHELIAL ATYPIA
Size ≥ 0.12 μm
Low nuclear-to-cytoplasmic ratio
Minimal nuclear membrane irregularities
Euchromatin or hypochromasia

HIGH-GRADE EPITHELIAL ATYPIA
Small size < 0.12 μm
Increased nuclear-to-cytoplasmic ratio
Irregular nuclear membranes
Hyperchromasia and abnormal chromatin distribution

The intestinal type of IPMN is associated with colloid carcinoma.

Intraductal Oncocytic Papillary Neoplasms and Invasive Oncocytic Carcinomas

Intraductal oncocytic papillary neoplasm is an intraductal neoplasm that has morphological and clinical features that overlap with those of IPMN.[153,154] Although typically cystic, these tumors may have a solid appearance on imaging. Aspirates from these may yield viscous fluid although this is less common. Cytology smears show cells that are usually arranged in papillary clusters with or without thick background mucin, rich in macrophages and cell debris (Box 36.31). However, the most distinctive feature of the smears of IOPN is the predominance of oncocytic cells (Fig. 36.45A). These are large and polygonal with abundant granular cytoplasm, low N/C and large central oval to irregular nuclei with prominent eccentric nucleoli (Fig. 36.45B). Despite their large size and presence of thick mucin in the smear background of some examples, intracytoplasmic mucin vacuoles are infrequently seen in IOPN. Instead, tumor cells are crowded, and pseudostratified with interspersed punched out empty intercellular spaces. Tumor cells may show increased and abnormal mitoses and well as degenerative atypia and necrosis, which may be extensive (Box 36.31). Invasive carcinoma may develop in IOPN and may be of conventional tubular pancreatobiliary type or be more oncocytic in appearance. Aspirate smears from invasive carcinoma show features of malignancy including 3-D clusters, pleomorphism, high N/C ratio cells, and nuclear membrane irregularity.

Oncocytic neoplasms lack *KRAS* mutations,[155] but instead show *PRKACA* and *PRKACB*-related oncogenic fusions (DNAJB1- and ATP1B1-PRKACA), previously reported only in fibrolamellar hepatocellular carcinoma.[156,157] The differential diagnosis of IOPN includes ACC, oncocytic WDPanNET, and hepatoid pancreatic ductal adenocarcinoma. Immunohistochemistry will assist with these differential diagnoses as ACC expresses trypsin, chymotrypsin, and bcl10 and WDPanNET expresses neuroendocrine markers, which are not present in IOPNs or their invasive counterparts. The distinction between invasive adenocarcinoma with oncocytic features and hepatoid carcinoma is more challenging on cytology, with the former typically showing MUC6[158] expression and the latter showing Hep Par1, glypican 3, and AFP positivity, along with glandular differentiation, which are negative in conventional PDAC. Furthermore, the invasive carcinoma that develops in IOPN shows background features of IOPN that may be helpful in this distinction.

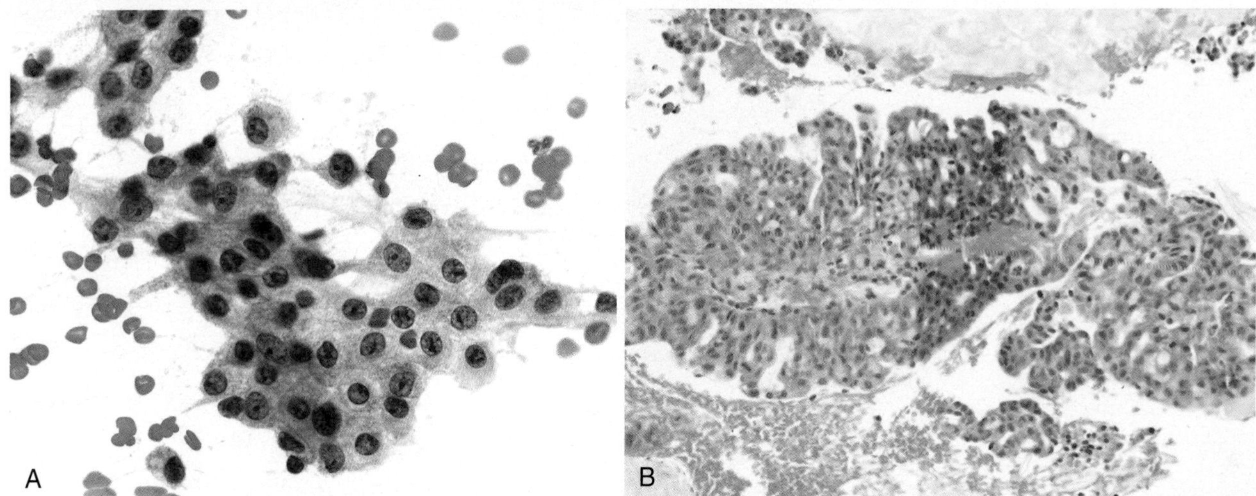

FIGURE 36.45 Intraductal oncocytic papillary neoplasm. A, Cells are large with abundant granular cytoplasm and large oval shaped nuclei with vesicular chromatin and prominent mostly eccentric nucleoli. Note absence of cytoplasmic mucin. Papanicolaou 40x. **B,** Cell block highlights large papilla with central fibrovascular core lined by pseudostratified eosinophilic, oncocytoid cells with punched out intercellular spaces, and scant cytoplasmic mucin. Hematoxylin and eosin.

BOX 36.31 Cytology of Intraductal Papillary Oncocytic Neoplasm

Papillary fronds
Oncocytic cells and mucinous cells
Background mucin

Role of Cytology in the Management of Mucinous Cysts

Preoperative assessment of patients with suspected IPMN now focuses on identifying patients who are at high risk of harboring high-grade dysplasia or invasive carcinoma using a combination of clinical history, gender, imaging characteristics, cytology, and cyst fluid biochemical and mutational analysis. The 2017 revisions of international consensus Fukuoka guidelines for the management of IPMN of the pancreas define high-risk stigmata for the presence of malignancy and features as worrisome for malignancy (Box 36.32).[159] If worrisome features are present, the patient is referred for EUS assessment with FNA. It is at this juncture that cytology becomes critical because the patient will be referred for surgery if the aspirate is suspicious or positive for malignancy. In this context, cytology is considered a screening test for pancreatic cysts,[160] and it should be assessed with an eye toward identifying cells that indicate the presence of at least high-grade dysplasia, if not invasive carcinoma. The cytological features that are predictive of high-grade dysplasia or adenocarcinoma have been grouped together as "high-grade epithelial atypia" because outright features of malignancy are infrequently present, and there is significant overlap between the features of high-grade dysplasia and invasive carcinoma. The specific cytological features that warrant classifying a cyst as showing high-grade atypia are discussed under the description of cytology for mucinous cysts (see Box 36.30).

BOX 36.32 Summary of 2017 International Consensus Guidelines

HIGH-RISK STIGMATA FOR MALIGNANCY[167]
Obstructive jaundice in a patient with a cyst in the head of the pancreas
Enhancing solid component within the cyst
Main pancreatic duct ≥10 mm

WORRISOME FEATURES FOR MALIGNANCY
Cyst ≥ 3 cm
Thickened, enhancing cyst walls
Main duct size 5-9 mm
Mural nodule
Abrupt change in caliber of pancreatic duct with distal pancreatic atrophy

ENDOSCOPIC ULTRASOUND FEATURES THAT ARE WORRISOME
Definite mural nodule
Main duct features suspicious for involvement
Cytology suspicious or positive for malignancy

Acinar Cell Cystadenoma and Cystadenocarcinoma

Acinar cell cystadenoma is misdiagnosed on cytology, according to case reports. Recently, a case of acinar cell cystadenoma was described that was correctly diagnosed using Moray forceps.[161] The small biopsy showed a cyst lined by benign acinar cells. The cytological features of acinar cell cystadenocarcinoma have not been described.

Cystic Pancreatic Neuroendocrine Tumors

WDPanNET may present as cystic or partially cystic masses on imaging. The cytological features are similar to those of their solid counterpart. Cyst fluid CEA and amylase are low, and they lack *KRAS* and *GNAS* mutations.[162] A pitfall is that the aspirates may be scantly cellular. Therefore a lower threshold is needed to diagnose these.

Differential Diagnosis and Pitfalls

Neoplastic Mucinous Epithelium vs. GI Contaminant

The main pitfall in the evaluation of pancreatic cysts is distinguishing benign gastric or duodenal epithelium from cystic mucinous neoplasms, MCN or IPMN. GI epithelium mimics the epithelium derived from these neoplasms because it consists of glandular, mucin containing epithelium and background mucin.

An approach to differentiating GI epithelium from neoplastic mucinous epithelium will incorporate assessment of the following:

1. Gross appearance of the fluid
2. Appearance of mucin on smears
3. Cytomorphological features of the cells

It is also critical to know where the mass is located, since aspirates of the pancreatic head and uncinate process will traverse the duodenum and aspirates of the neck, body and tail will traverse the stomach. This will determine what type of contaminant one is trying to identify. In general, duodenal epithelium is easier to recognize because of the goblet cells and enterocytes.

Gastric and duodenal contents are usually watery and thin in contrast to the mucin from MCN/IPMN, which is viscous. The mucin of GI epithelium appears thinner and wispier on smears and is associated with the GI epithelium. The mucin of neoplasms contains histiocytes and oncotic cells.[149] Mucin from GI epithelium may contain degenerated cells.[31]

Key to the diagnosis of a neoplasm is evaluation of the cytological features. Gastric and duodenal epithelium will retain a 2-dimensional architecture in which the nuclei are evenly spaced within the sheets. Epithelium from MCN/IPMN will show crowding and nuclear overlap, which may be subtle. The nuclei will be irregularly distributed.

Both gastric and duodenal epithelium may yield single cells. The mucin in foveolar cells typically does not fill the entire cytoplasm, but instead appears as a cup-shaped mucin vacuole sitting above the nucleus. In neoplastic cells, the mucin reaches the nucleus. Single cells with a brush border are enterocytes and are derived from the duodenum. Goblet cells are seen in IPMN and MCN, but these will be less uniform, and unevenly distributed, in contrast to the goblet cells in the duodenum.

The nuclei from GI epithelium will be round and uniform. Neoplastic nuclei are subtly atypical, with nuclear membrane irregularities. Pseudoinclusions and grooves are typical of neoplastic epithelium, although gastric epithelium may also exhibit grooves and inclusions as a result of degeneration. Gastric epithelium frequently produces stripped nuclei with atypia and grooves in a background of mucin; this pattern should be recognized as part of the spectrum of gastric epithelium.

Even using these criteria, it can be difficult to differentiate GI epithelium, particularly gastric epithelium, from neoplastic epithelium. Fortunately, as discussed previously, it is not as crucial to differentiate gastric epithelium from low-grade, foveolar-type neoplastic epithelium. What is crucial is identifying the features that indicate the presence of high-grade dysplasia or invasive carcinoma

Pancreatic Metastases

FNA biopsy is also useful in the evaluation of secondary pancreatic tumors.[163]

The most commonly encountered metastases on FNA are kidney, lung, skin, and breast carcinoma. Immunohistochemical studies often provide helpful information in the differential diagnosis of these tumors, and an approach to using immunohistochemistry on cytology samples to analyze neoplasms of unknown origin is summarized by Cowan and VandenBussche.[164] Breast, colon, and gastric adenocarcinomas have cytomorphological features that suggest their site of origin. Metastatic lung adenocarcinoma is difficult to distinguish from pancreatic carcinoma due to similar morphology. Both tumors may demonstrate squamous differentiation. Immunostains for napsin and TTF1 assist with the differential diagnosis, as pancreatic carcinoma is negative for these markers.[165]

Malignant melanoma is one of the most common metastases to the pancreas. The presence of melanin pigment is diagnostic but is not always present. In the absence of melanin pigment, diagnostic ancillary workup should include SOX10, S-100, HMB 45, MART-1, and MITF1.[164]

Renal cell carcinoma is the most common metastasis to the pancreas.[163] The characteristic appearance is a uniform population of clear cells with central round nuclei and prominent nucleoli. Stripped nuclei, which occur in renal cell carcinoma, are not characteristic of ductal adenocarcinoma of the pancreas. The differential diagnosis includes PanNET with clear cell features or lipid rich cytoplasm.[166] Both tumors may occur in association with von Hippel-Lindau's disease. PAX8 is expressed by both WDPanNET and RCC; therefore if WDPanNET is included in the differential diagnosis of a clear cell neoplasm in the pancreas, the panel needs to include neuroendocrine markers and other markers for renal cell carcinoma.

The full reference list may be viewed online at Elsevier eBooks for Practicing Clinicians.

CHAPTER 37

Developmental Disorders of the Gallbladder, Extrahepatic Biliary Tract, and Pancreas

Alyssa M. Krasinskas

Chapter Outline

INTRODUCTION

Developmental, congenital, hereditary, and structural disorders that can affect the gallbladder, extrahepatic biliary tract, and pancreas are listed in Box 37.1. This chapter focuses primarily on the few disorders that are encountered peripherally or directly in surgical pathology. Hereditary pancreatitis is discussed in Chapter 40.

STRUCTURAL DEVELOPMENT OF THE GALLBLADDER, EXTRAHEPATIC BILIARY TRACT, AND PANCREAS

Some disorders of the gallbladder, extrahepatic biliary tract, and pancreas are easier to conceptualize if the embryological development of these structures is understood. The liver, gallbladder, biliary tract, and pancreas bud from the endodermal epithelium of the foregut (i.e., duodenum) at approximately the third week of gestation. A small caudal portion of the liver bud (i.e., caudal foregut diverticulum) expands to form the gallbladder. While the diverticulum enlarges, its connection with the intestine narrows to form the biliary tree. Early in this process, these structures form hollow cylinders that become solid cords because of epithelial cell proliferation. They subsequently develop a lumen by a process known as *cellular vacuolization* at approximately the seventh week of gestation.

The pancreas arises from the dorsal and ventral diverticula, which first appear at approximately the fourth week of gestation. The dorsal bud elongates to form part of the head, body, and tail of the pancreas. The ventral bud develops at the base of the hepatic diverticulum. The left segment of this structure atrophies, and the right rotates posteriorly with the rotation of the duodenum to fuse with the dorsal bud. Portions of the pancreas derived from either diverticulum are histologically indistinguishable. Because of the direct association of the development of the common bile duct with the ventral portion of the pancreas, they share a common outflow tract, the ampulla of Vater. Although the length of this common channel varies from person to person, it is less than 3 mm in most people, and in some, the two ducts do not converge but drain into the duodenum through two adjacent but separate orifices.[1]

When the two pancreatic buds merge at the sixth to seventh week, their duct systems also coalesce to form the main pancreatic duct of Wirsung. A remnant of the dorsal bud duct persists as the accessory duct of Santorini in

BOX 37.1 Developmental Disorders and Structural Abnormalities of the Gallbladder, Extrahepatic Biliary Tract, and Pancreas

- Gallbladder
  - Agenesis
  - Hypoplasia
  - Duplication or multiple gallbladders
  - Septation
  - Phrygian cap
  - Diverticulum
  - Anomalous location
  - Heterotopias
- Extrahepatic biliary tract
  - Choledochal cysts
  - Biliary atresia
- Pancreas
  - Agenesis
  - Duct abnormalities
  - Pancreas divisum
  - Annular pancreas
  - Heterotopic pancreas
  - Congenital cysts
  - Cystic fibrosis
  - Pancreatic exocrine deficiencies
    - Shwachman-Diamond's syndrome
    - Johanson-Blizzard's syndrome
    - Sideroblastic anemia and exocrine pancreatic insufficiency
    - Enzymatic deficiencies
- Diabetes mellitus
- Hereditary pancreatitis*
- Neonatal islet cell hypertrophy and hyperplasia
  - Maternal diabetes
  - Beckwith-Wiedemann's syndrome
- Persistent hyperinsulinemic hypoglycemia of infancy (i.e., nesidioblastosis)

*See Chapter 34.

approximately 40% of people, with its opening in the minor papilla of the duodenum (Fig. 37.1).[1-3]

STRUCTURAL AND DEVELOPMENTAL ANOMALIES OF THE GALLBLADDER

Congenital abnormalities of the gallbladder are rare. They are traditionally classified according to their number, form, and location.

Agenesis

Gallbladder agenesis was originally described in 1701. It occurs in less than 0.1% of the population. Autopsy series report an equal sex distribution.[4] Some patients have a variety of disparate congenital anomalies and syndromes.[4-9] Rare familial associations have also been described.[10,11] As with many structural anomalies of embryogenesis, the cause of gallbladder agenesis is unknown.[12,13] It may result from a complete lack of bud formation or lack of recanalization of the bud during its growth. A compensatory secondary dilation of the right hepatic bile duct that takes on a bile storage function develops in some patients. Patients with gallbladder agenesis who are symptomatic are likely to be women in their fourth or fifth decade who have right upper quadrant symptoms.[14] Possible mechanisms responsible for symptoms include abnormalities of the biliary tree, primary duct stones, biliary dyskinesia, and nonbiliary disorders.[12]

Hypoplasia

Hypoplasia of the gallbladder is classically associated with biliary atresia and cystic fibrosis. Some cases of gallbladder hypoplasia presumably have a cause similar to that of gallbladder agenesis. Gallbladder hypoplasia is associated with rare genetic syndromes and structural anomalies.[15,16] This entity likely is underdiagnosed because the main differential diagnosis of gallbladder hypoplasia is fibrotic retraction caused by chronic cholecystitis.

Gallbladder Duplication

Double or triple gallbladders are seldom encountered in clinical practice, although more than 200 cases have been reported. A female predominance is documented among symptomatic patients, whereas an equal sex distribution is seen for asymptomatic individuals.

Multiple gallbladders have been classified according to whether each of the gallbladders has a separate cystic duct insertion into the biliary tree ("H" configuration) (Fig. 37.2) or a common cystic duct insertion ("Y" configuration). This distinction is of vital importance for intraoperative surgical management.[17]

The spectrum of disease identified in patients with multiple gallbladders is similar to that found in patients with a single gallbladder.[17] In the absence of symptoms, prophylactic cholecystectomy is not routinely advocated, although removal of all gallbladders is indicated if only one is found to be pathological.[18]

Septation

Septation of the gallbladder (Fig. 37.3) is often diagnosed on preoperative ultrasonography. It most commonly results from cholelithiasis and inflammation, an association that is supported by prominent inflammation and fibrosis in most of the specimens. Congenital gallbladder septation also has been attributed to incomplete cavitation of the developing gallbladder bud.[19]

Septations may be single or multiple. Rare multiseptate gallbladders occurring as part of a constellation of congenital abnormalities of the hepatobiliary-pancreatic tree offer the best evidence for septation as a congenital event, at least in some patients.[20-22] They may occur in the pediatric population and commonly without gallstones. Each septation may contain a mucosal surface with interdigitating muscle fibers. Various amounts of chronic inflammation and secondary cholelithiasis have been described in these specimens.

The term *hourglass gallbladder* describes a transverse septum that divides the gallbladder into two compartments. This lesion may be congenital or acquired.

Phrygian Cap

The most exotically named congenital lesion of the gallbladder is the Phrygian cap. It occurs when the fundus of the

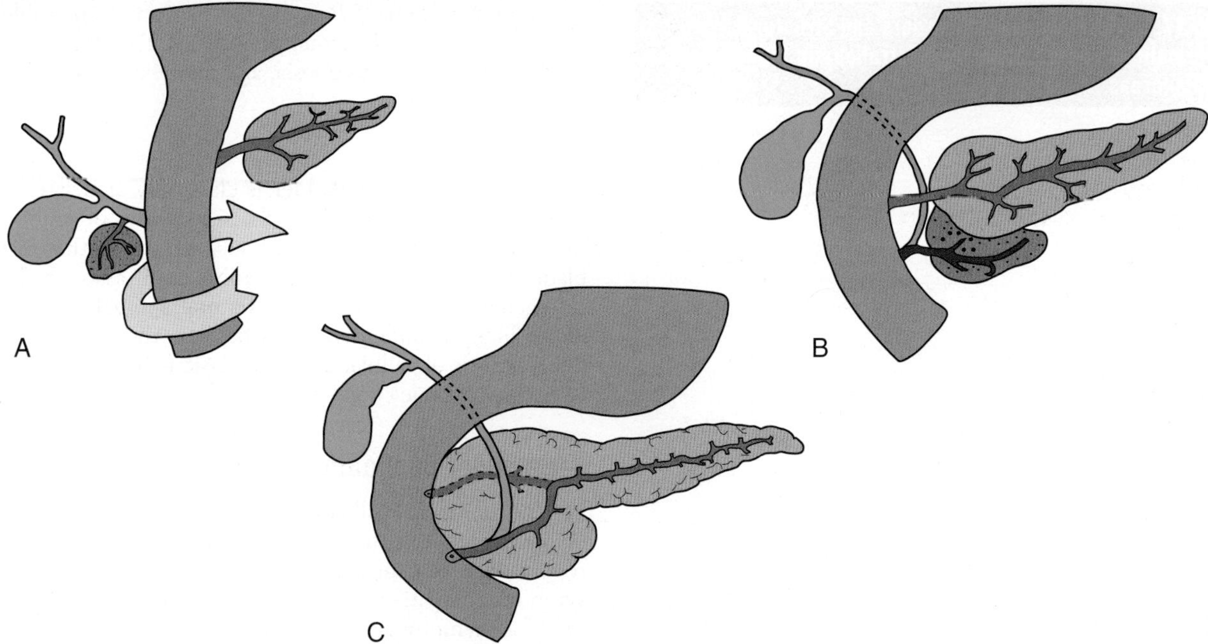

FIGURE 37.1 Embryology of the pancreas. A, Separate dorsal and ventral pancreatic anlagen developing from the gut tube at approximately 5 weeks' gestation. With subsequent midgut rotation, the ventral bud and its closely related biliary ducts migrate posteriorly *(arrow)*. **B,** After midgut rotation, the dorsal and ventral anlagen are closely opposed and eventually fuse. Note the separate dorsal and ventral pancreatic ducts at this time. **C,** Eventually, the pancreatic ducts fuse. The main pancreatic duct is formed from the distal portion of the dorsal duct of the ventral pancreas; it enters the duodenum with the common bile duct at the ampulla of Vater. The proximal portion of the duct of the dorsal pancreas may become obliterated *(dashed line)*, but it may persist and enter the duodenum separately through the minor papilla that is located approximately 2 cm proximal to the major papilla. (*From Dahms BB. Gastrointestinal tract and pancreas. In: Gilbert-Barness E, ed. Potter's Pathology of the Fetus and Infant. Vol 1. St. Louis: Mosby; 1997:774-822.*)

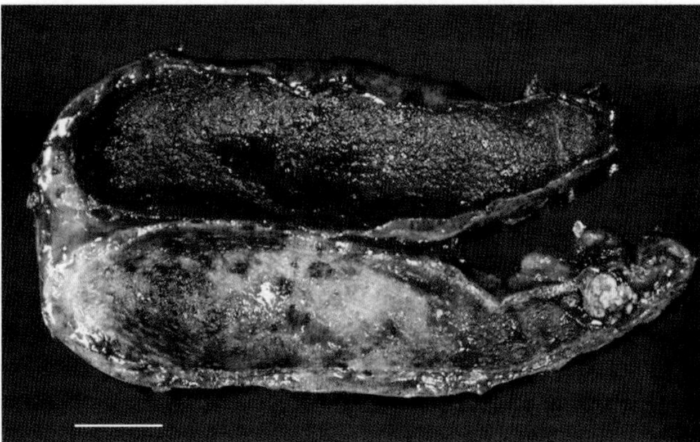

FIGURE 37.2 Duplicated gallbladders. These fused gallbladders were removed from a 69-year-old woman who had symptomatic cholelithiasis. Each gallbladder has its own cystic duct insertion into the biliary tree. The cystic duct of the gallbladder on the bottom is obstructed by a stone. *Line* = 1 cm.

gallbladder folds over its body. It is a common radiological finding, occurring in approximately 4% of the general population (Fig. 37.4). The term *Phrygian cap* refers to the shape of a soft, conical cap worn with the top curled forward by the inhabitants of the Bronze Age country of Phrygia, a region that is now known as Turkey. The lesion is important mainly from a radiological perspective because it may lead to an erroneous diagnosis of cholelithiasis or pathological septum.[23]

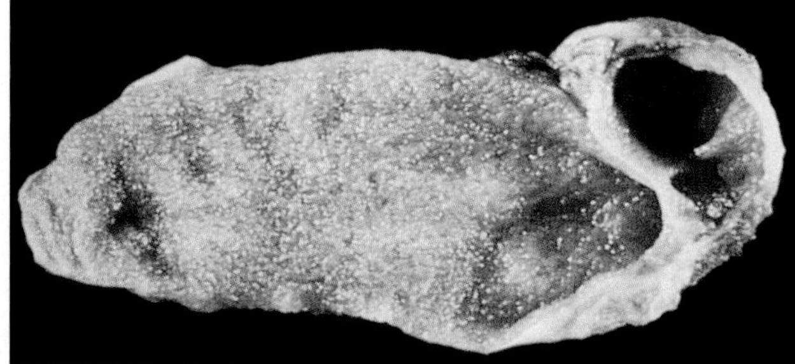

FIGURE 37.3 Septate gallbladder. Because the septation is close to the fundus, it may represent a Phrygian cap. (*From Jessurun J, Albores-Saavedra J. Gallbladder and extrahepatic biliary ducts. In: Damjanov I, Linder J, eds. Anderson's Pathology. Vol. 2, 10th ed. St. Louis: Mosby; 1996.*)

Diverticulum

A congenital gallbladder diverticulum is identified in as many as 1% of cholecystectomies. They are distinguished from acquired lesions by mucosa and smooth muscle in the wall of the outpouching. This finding differentiates them from acquired Rokitansky-Aschoff sinuses. They may be single or multiple, and they rarely may cause symptoms.[24]

Anomalous Location

Anatomic variations of position of the gallbladder may occur. Gallbladders occurring outside of the line of the middle hepatic vein on the visceral surface are referred to as

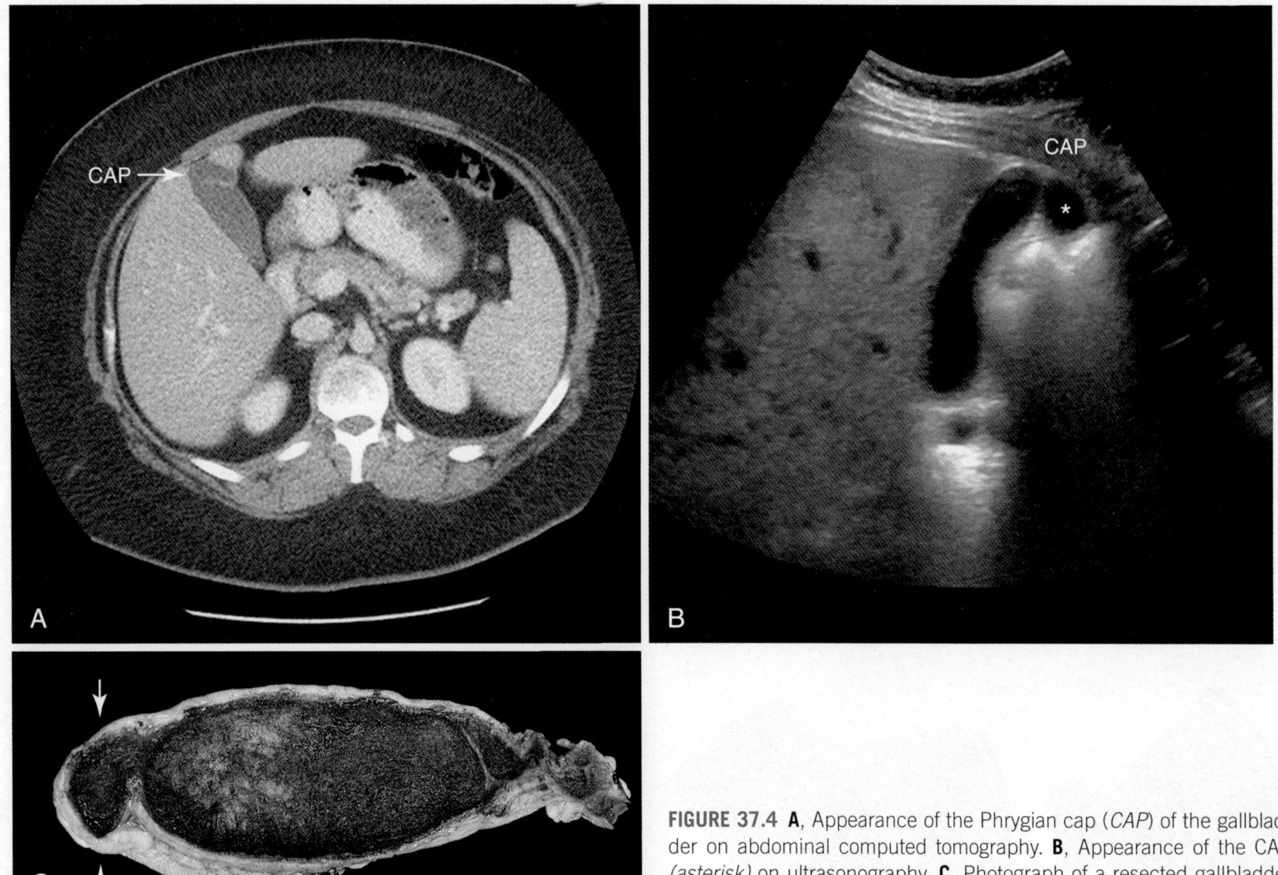

FIGURE 37.4 **A**, Appearance of the Phrygian cap (*CAP*) of the gallbladder on abdominal computed tomography. **B**, Appearance of the CAP (*asterisk*) on ultrasonography. **C,** Photograph of a resected gallbladder with a CAP (*arrows*).

aberrant gallbladders. These sites are classified as intrahepatic, left sided (i.e., an isolated finding or associated with situs inversus), transverse, and retrodisplaced.[25,26] Rarely, they may be associated with anomalies of the liver.[27] A gallbladder with little or no connection to the liver may wander or float in the peritoneal cavity. It may be completely surrounded by peritoneum or have abundant mesentery. Its mobility may allow twisting of the vascular supply and subsequent infarction of the gallbladder.

Heterotopias of the Gallbladder and Biliary Tree

Rarely, heterotopias consisting of pancreas, gastric or intestinal mucosa, liver, adrenal gland, and thyroid tissue have been described in the biliary tree and gallbladder.[28] Of these, pancreatic heterotopia in the gallbladder is the most common.[29] Most heterotopic lesions are found incidentally at the time of surgery. However, in some patients, classic biliary-type symptoms have been attributed to heterotopia.[30]

STRUCTURAL AND DEVELOPMENTAL ANOMALIES OF THE EXTRAHEPATIC BILIARY TRACT

With rare exceptions, anomalies of the extrahepatic biliary tract, apart from choledochal cysts, are usually diagnosed as incidental findings.[31] These anomalies are relevant for clinical and radiological diagnoses and for the prevention of surgical misadventures, such as injury to the extrahepatic biliary system.[32]

Choledochal Cyst

Cystic dilation of the biliary tree was described as early as 1723. Not until the modern era was there significant improvement in understanding the pathophysiology of choledochal cysts. These cysts are uncommon, occurring in approximately 1 of 100,000 to 150,000 live births. Most patients are diagnosed in infancy and childhood; only 20% to 30% of patients are identified as adults.[33,34] Table 37.1 summarizes the common presenting features.

Etiology

Choledochal cysts can be caused by a diverse set of abnormalities that predispose to reflux of pancreatic secretions into the common bile duct or obstruction of the distal common bile duct. Its predominance in pediatric populations, gender distribution, greater incidence among Asian populations, and rare association with other anomalies are consistent with a congenital origin.[35-37] Most patients have an identifiable anomalous pancreaticobiliary junction between the common bile duct and the duct of Wirsung.[38,39]

Although the mean length of the common channel increases with age, a common channel more than 6 mm long in adults is considered abnormal (Figs. 37.5 and 37.6).[40,41]

TABLE 37.1 Choledochal Cysts in Adults and Children

Feature	Pediatric Patients[39,48]	Adult Patients[49,50,56]
Overall occurrence	75%	25%
Male-to-female ratio	1:4	1:4
Median age at diagnosis	2.2 yr[48]	37 yr[49]
Symptoms	Obstructive jaundice Pain Abdominal mass	Abdominal pain Cholangitis Jaundice Fever Pancreatitis
Differential diagnosis	Infants Biliary atresia Prolonged neonatal jaundice Children Congenital hepatic fibrosis Congenital biliary stricture	Biliary stones Hepatitis Chronic pancreatitis
Most common type	I*	IV*

These types may represent a spectrum of the same disease, with intrahepatic disease resulting from biliary obstruction in older patients.[50]

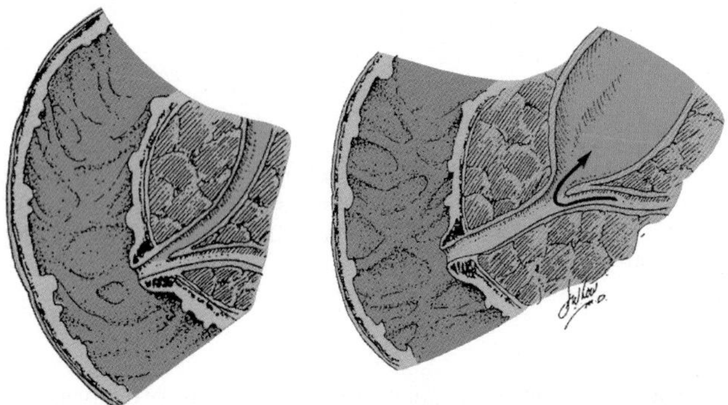

FIGURE 37.5 Schematic diagram of normal anatomy *(left)* is contrasted with the anomalous common channel anatomy *(right, arrow)* thought to be responsible for reflux of pancreatic enzymes during cyst formation in utero. (*From O'Neill JA Jr. Choledochal cyst. Curr Probl Surg. 1992;29:361-410.*)

The formation of this elongated common channel is thought to predispose to pancreaticobiliary reflux, with subsequent in utero dilation of portions of the extrahepatic biliary tract.

Possible mechanisms of distal common bile duct obstruction attributed to choledochal cyst formation include sphincter of Oddi dysfunction,[42,43] autonomic innervation abnormalities,[44] and other problems of embryogenesis.[45] Different pathogenic mechanisms are probably responsible for different types of choledochal cysts. Even in adults, choledochal cysts are thought to be mostly congenital in origin. Uncommonly, adults have a dilated common bile duct after extrahepatic biliary tract surgery with normal results on initial intraoperative cholangiograms. These cases are probably derived in part from secondary stricture formation, although even in these patients, an anomalous pancreaticobiliary junction is common.[46]

Classification

Todani and colleagues[47] classified choledochal cysts into five major types according to their anatomic location (Table 37.2 and Fig. 37.7). Ninety-two percent of choledochal cysts in children are classified as type I.[48] This cyst has a fusiform or saccular dilation of the common bile duct (see Fig. 37.6). Infants commonly have a complete obstruction of the distal common bile duct. Type IV choledochal cysts are the most common type encountered in adults (Fig. 37.8).[49] In adults, the distal common bile duct is most commonly patent. Rarely, choledochal cysts may be entirely intraduodenal (i.e., choledochocele) or consist of multiple intrahepatic cysts (i.e., Caroli's disease).

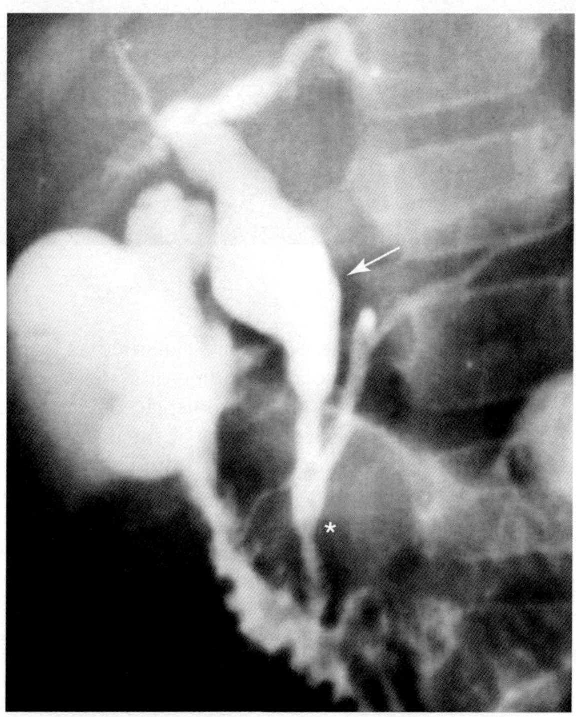

FIGURE 37.6 Endoscopic retrograde cholangiopancreatography shows anomalous pancreaticobiliary union *(asterisk)* in a 4-year-old girl with a choledochal cyst *(arrow)*. (*From Guelrud M, Morera C, Rodriguez M, et al. Normal and anomalous pancreaticobiliary union in children and adolescents. Gastrointest Endosc. 1999;50:189-193.*)

Cystic malformations of the gallbladder probably share a common etiological basis with choledochal cysts. Most patients are diagnosed with a variety of standard and invasive radiological procedures.[49]

The Todani classification has been criticized. Visser and colleagues[50] made a strong case that the current nomenclature incorrectly groups four distinct diseases together as one entity and that types I and IV are artificially separated. They observed marked dissimilarities between Caroli's disease and choledochocele and the remaining lesions classified by Todani as choledochal cysts.[50]

TABLE 37.2 Todani Classification of Choledochal Cysts

Type	Description
I	Fusiform dilation of the extrahepatic duct
II	Focal saccular dilation or diverticulum of the extrahepatic duct
III	Cystic dilation of the bile duct confined to the duodenal wall (choledochocele)
IVa	Combined intrahepatic and extrahepatic dilation of the bile duct
IVb	Multiple dilations of the extrahepatic bile duct
V	Multiple intrahepatic biliary cysts (Caroli's disease)

Pathology

Grossly, a choledochal cyst may contain as much as 2 L of bile. The surface is typically coarsely granular. The wall is normally fibrotic, and distal narrowing is a common feature. Microscopic findings tend to vary with patient age. Intact surface columnar epithelium is characteristic of younger patients, and an increasing degree of chronic inflammation and adhesions to adjacent structures is characteristic of older patients (Fig. 37.9). The cyst wall usually is composed of dense fibrous tissue with various amounts of smooth muscle.[37]

Complications and Treatment

Delayed diagnosis may be associated with untoward complications such as pancreatitis, spontaneous perforation, cholelithiasis, cholangitis, secondary biliary cirrhosis, and portal hypertension. A significant risk of carcinoma is associated with choledochal cysts; this risk increases with age. The risk for children younger than 10 years of age is less than 1%, but the reported risk is as high as 30% to 43% for

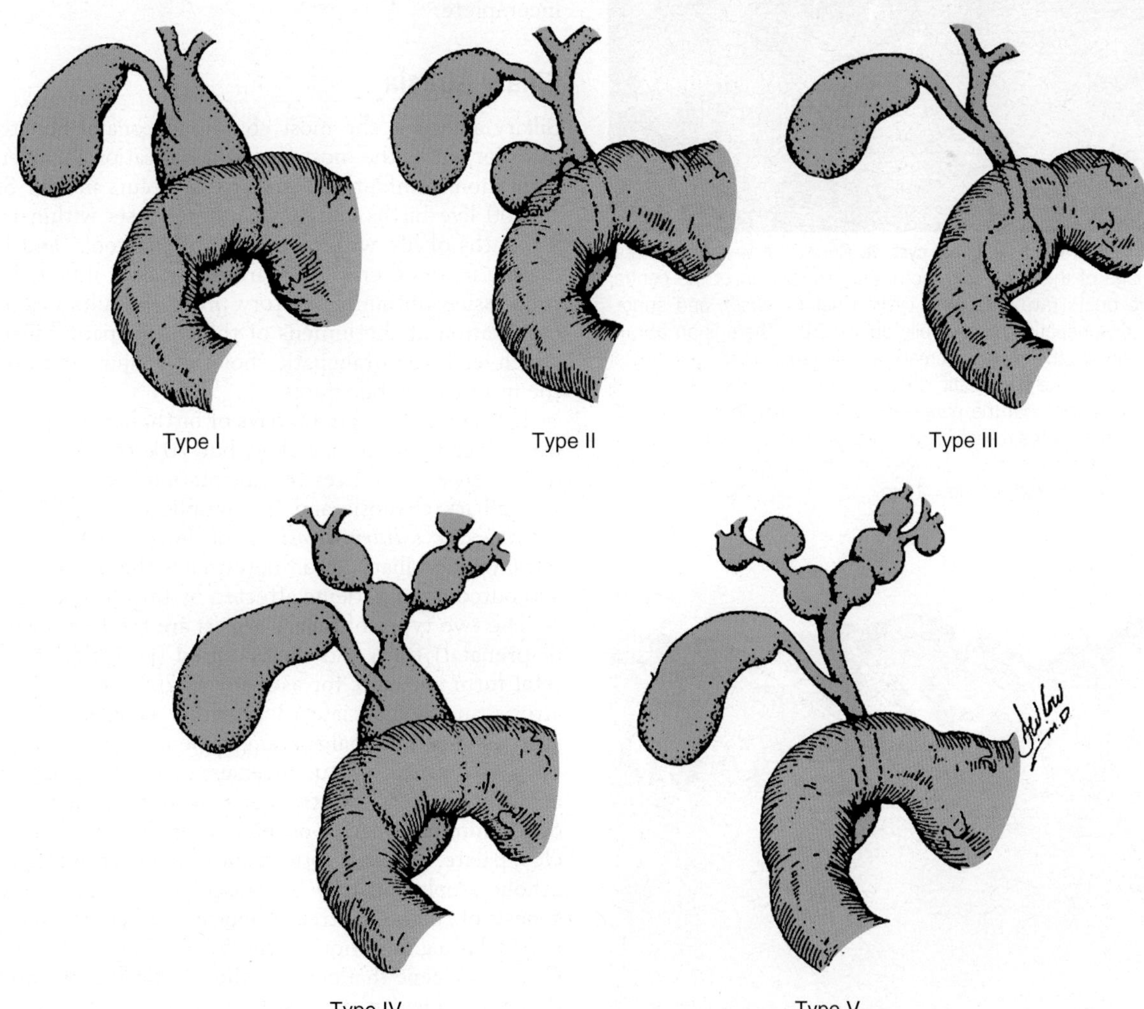

FIGURE 37.7 The five types of choledochal cyst that can be found by cholangiography were originally described by Todani. (*From O'Neill JA Jr. Choledochal cyst. Curr Probl Surg. 1992;29:361-410.*)

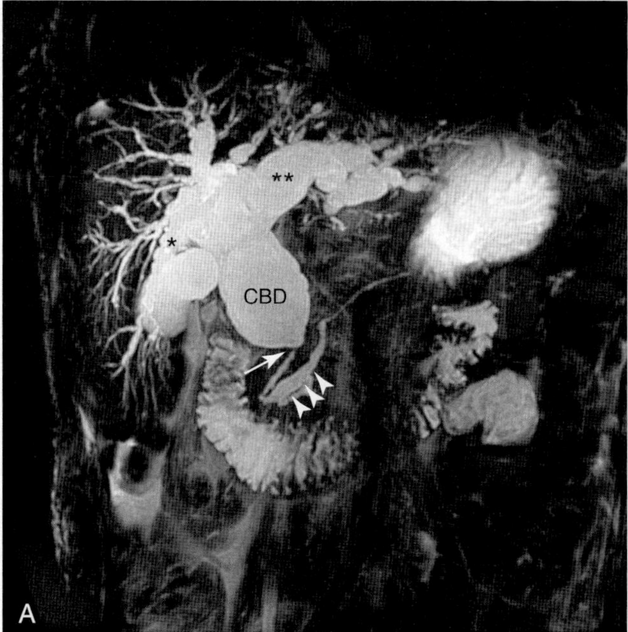

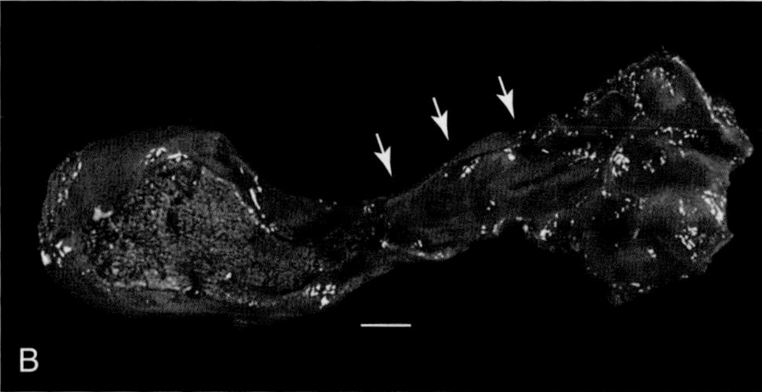

FIGURE 37.8 Type IV choledochal cyst. A, Coronal view magnetic resonance image of the abdomen shows marked dilation of the central intrahepatic ducts *(two asterisks)*, cystic duct *(asterisk)*, and suprapancreatic extrahepatic common bile duct (CBD). There is an abrupt transition between the suprapancreatic and intrapancreatic portions of the CBD *(arrow)*. The pancreatic duct in the head of the pancreas is dilated *(arrowheads)*, but the pancreaticobiliary junction is normal. **B,** Gross appearance of the resected cyst. The gallbladder *(left)* drains into a markedly dilated cystic duct *(arrows)*, which communicates with the choledochal cyst *(far right)*. *Line* = 1 cm.

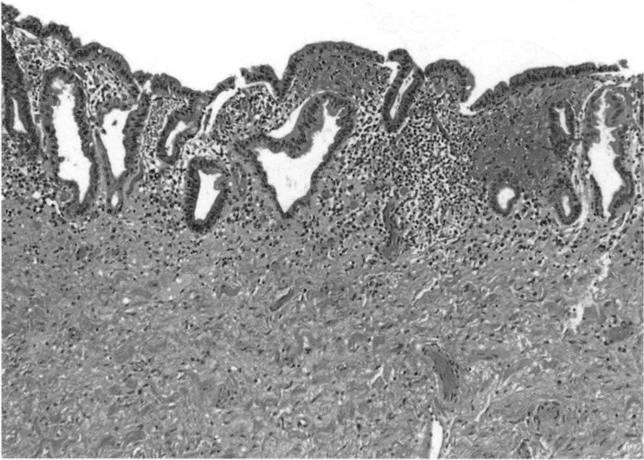

FIGURE 37.9 The choledochal cyst lining has biliary-type mucosa with a chronic inflammatory infiltrate, hemorrhage, and reactive epithelial atypia.

adults.[51,52] Reflux of pancreatic enzymes into the common bile duct and abnormal bile composition may predispose to neoplastic change. For unknown reasons, the neoplasms have a predilection for the posterior wall of the cyst. Most commonly, the tumors are adenocarcinomas (Fig. 37.10),[50] although squamous cell carcinomas and anaplastic carcinomas also occur.[53,54] Other types of neoplasms are rare.[55] These patients also have an increased incidence of gallbladder carcinoma.

Surgical treatment of choledochal cysts involves complete resection when possible, although specific surgical approaches are usually tailored to the findings in a patient.[50,56] Resection has been reported to be safe, even in small infants.[48] Until recently, Roux-en-Y cystojejunostomy was the surgical treatment of choice. However, long-term follow-up of patients treated in this manner identified a significant lifetime risk of anastomotic stricture formation and development of cholangiocarcinoma. Some published series identified patients previously treated by Roux-en-Y cystojejunostomy who underwent radical excision of their choledochal cysts in an attempt to decrease their risk of cancer. This approach was associated with low long-term morbidity and mortality rates.[50,51] Rarely, adenocarcinoma may develop at the site of choledochal site excision. In most cases, the previous surgical excision was found to be incomplete.[52]

Biliary Atresia

Biliary atresia is the most common neonatal hepatobiliary disorder and is the most frequent indication for liver transplantation in infants. Biliary atresia occurs in 1 of 8000 to 18,000 live births and typically manifests within the first 3 months of life with jaundice, acholic stools, and hepatomegaly in an otherwise apparently healthy infant.[57-59] This progressive fibroinflammatory process results in complete obliteration of the lumens of the extrahepatic biliary tree, which leads to intrahepatic cholestatic injury and fibrosis of the intrahepatic bile ducts.

If diagnosed within 60 days of birth, hepatic portoenterostomy can restore bile flow, but 70% to 80% of patients ultimately require liver transplantation because of progressive biliary cirrhosis and its complications.[58,59] The term *extrahepatic biliary atresia* is no longer used because the intrahepatic biliary lesion determines the overall prognosis and outcome of patients affected by this disease.

The two types of biliary atresia are the fetal (syndromic or prenatal) form and the acquired (perinatal) form. The fetal form accounts for as many as 20% of cases of biliary atresia and is associated with other congenital anomalies such as intestinal malrotation; asplenia or polysplenia; portal vein anomalies; situs inversus; congenital heart disease; annular pancreas; Kartagener's syndrome; atresia of the duodenum, esophagus, or jejunum; polycystic kidneys; and cleft palate.[57,59] This form manifests earlier in infancy with acholic stools and may be caused by a defect in morphogenesis of the biliary tree. Abnormal Notch pathway signaling, including mutations in the *Jagged 1* (*JAG1*) gene and in *CFC1*, the gene that encodes the cryptic family 1 protein, is thought to play an etiological role in biliary atresia.[60]

The more common acquired form of biliary atresia usually manifests with cholestatic jaundice between 1 and 2 months

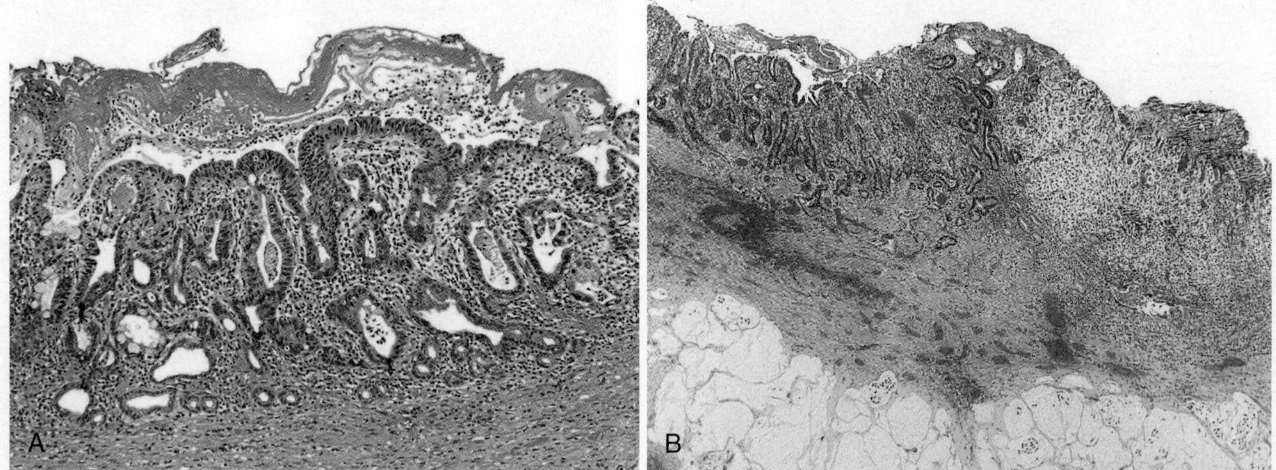

FIGURE 37.10 Malignant transformation in a choledochal cyst. A, High-grade dysplasia. **B,** Invasive adenocarcinoma with a prominent mucinous component.

of age and does not have coincident congenital anomalies. Several etiological factors have been proposed, including infectious, vascular, toxic, and immune factors.[57,58]

STRUCTURAL AND DEVELOPMENTAL ANOMALIES OF THE PANCREAS

Complete and Partial Pancreatic Agenesis

Complete and partial forms of pancreatic agenesis constitute a rare group of structural anomalies, many of which go undetected because they may not be associated with pancreatic insufficiency. Agenesis of the pancreas is a rare lethal anomaly that sometimes is associated with gallbladder agenesis.[61] Partial agenesis, which may be familial in origin, is associated with complete absence of dorsal pancreatic parenchyma and has only rarely been reported.[62] Patients may have pancreatitis of the remaining ventral pancreas. A linkage between two families demonstrating pancreatic and cerebellar agenesis and mutations in the *PTF1A* gene encoding pancreas transcription factor 1A has been described.[63]

Duct Abnormalities

Because pancreatic development is complex, variations in duct anatomy are relatively common. A detailed autopsy study by Berman and associates,[64] in which vinyl acetate casts of postmortem pancreas specimens were used, revealed the previously described pattern of duct arrangement in approximately 90% of specimens. Although several ductal anatomic patterns of development were seen, the most common aberrant finding was insertion of the main pancreatic duct into the common bile duct 5 to 15 mm proximal to the ampulla of Vater. This formation is known as the *common channel* or the *anomalous pancreaticobiliary junction*. In endoscopic retrograde cholangiopancreatography (ERCP) series, this variation in duct anatomy has been identified in 0.9% to 28% of patients (depending on patient selection) and is associated with an increase in pancreaticobiliary disease.[42,65]

Pancreas Divisum

Pancreas divisum is the most common congenital anomaly of the pancreas, occurring in 5% to 10% of the population.[66] Variations in the prevalence rate based on ethnicity have been reported.[67] Since its identification in the 1970s with the introduction of ERCP, the significance of pancreas divisum has been intensively studied. Pancreas divisum has been identified in 12% to 26% of patients with idiopathic pancreatitis, and the pancreatitis was confined to the dorsal portions of the pancreas in some of these patients.[2,68] Conversely, some studies have not shown a significant association between pancreas divisum and increased pancreatic disease.[67,69-71]

The classic or complete type of pancreas divisum arises from a lack of fusion of the two embryological portions of pancreas. As a result, the main portion of the pancreas is drained by a patent duct of Santorini into the minor duodenal papilla (Fig. 37.11), and the inferior portion of the pancreatic head drains through the major papilla. An associated stenosis of the minor orifice in a subset of patients with pancreas divisum probably influences the predisposition to pancreatitis. A partial or incomplete type of divisum occurs when a small communication exists between the ventral and dorsal ducts. Several variants of this type have been elucidated.[72]

Three main clinical manifestations are associated with pancreas divisum: acute relapsing pancreatitis, chronic pancreatitis, and abdominal pain without evidence of pancreatitis. Inflammation has been attributed mainly to mechanical or obstructive problems in pancreas divisum. Evidence supporting aberrant functioning of the cystic fibrosis transmembrane conductance regulator as a cause of pancreatitis in these patients has been reported.[73,74]

The role of endoscopic and surgical interventions is controversial. Several excellent synopses of the issues involved have been published.[67,71,75]

Rare cases of pancreatic neoplasia developing in patients with pancreas divisum have been reported.[76-80] At least one single-institution series reported that patients with pancreas divisum have an increased relative risk of pancreatic neoplasia.[81]

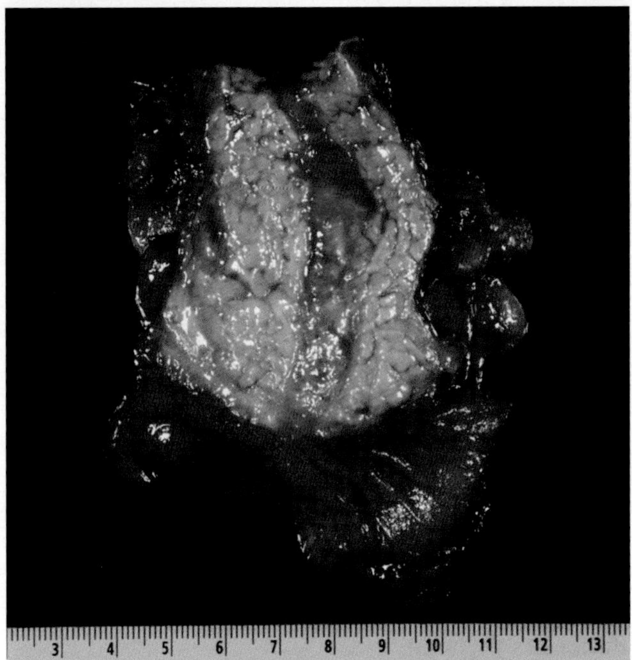

FIGURE 37.11 Pancreas divisum. This gross specimen has a widely patent and dilated accessory duct of Santorini coursing from the pancreatic neck resection margin *(top, yellow)* to the minor duodenal papilla. The bile duct opens into the major papilla (not visible in this section), and the main pancreatic duct of Wirsung is not identified.

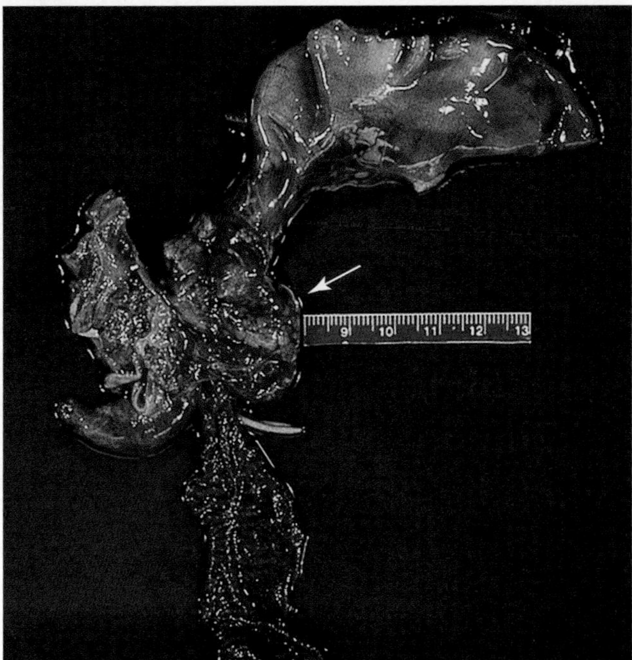

FIGURE 37.12 Annular pancreas *(arrow)* involves the second portion of the duodenum with distended duodenal bulb.

Annular Pancreas

Annular pancreas, which was originally identified at an autopsy in 1818, is a congenital malformation characterized by a ring of pancreatic tissue that encircles the descending portion of the duodenum to various degrees. It is a rare anomaly. A prevalence of approximately 1 in 2000 pancreatic or periduodenal endoscopic ultrasonographic scans was found in one series of adults.[82] In their extensive review, Kiernan and colleagues stated that approximately one-half of all patients diagnosed with annular pancreas are in the pediatric age group, with most identified in the neonatal period. Upper gastrointestinal (GI) tract obstruction is the most common initial finding.[83] Peptic ulceration, pancreatitis, and more nonspecific symptoms tend to occur in adults.[84]

The embryological sequence that leads to annular pancreas is unclear, and several theories have been proposed. One early theory posited that ventral and dorsal segment hypertrophy encircled the duodenum. Hypertrophy of the dorsal segment repositions the main duct anteriorly. Fixation of the tip of the ventral bud before rotation of the duodenum with subsequent persistence of the ventral lobe after rotation is plausible for most cases. However, it is likely that annular pancreas has a diverse set of causes related to anomalies of the ventral and dorsal pancreatic buds and the duodenum.[85]

Most commonly, the lesion is composed of a flat band of pancreatic tissue circumferentially surrounding the second part of the duodenum (Fig. 37.12). Histologically, pancreatic parenchyma is characteristically found intertwined with the muscularis mucosae. Only rarely is the anterior wall of the duodenum spared. The ductal system most commonly drains around the right side of the duodenum in an anterior to posterior direction, and it merges with the left duct. However, the right duct may pass anteriorly, or there may be multiple small ducts that penetrate the wall of the duodenum and empty directly into the duodenum. Concomitant duodenal atresia or stenosis is often found.[2]

Annular pancreas is often associated with other anomalies, such as duodenal bands, intestinal malrotation, Meckel's diverticulum, imperforate anus, cryptorchidism, and heart and spinal cord defects. Down's syndrome has been identified in as many as 20% of these patients. A familial predisposition has also been documented.[86,87]

Heterotopic Pancreas

Pancreatic tissue that lacks anatomic or vascular continuity with the main body of the pancreas has been identified in 1% to 15% of autopsies.[2] Most cases of heterotopic pancreas occur in the upper portions of the GI tract, especially in the prepyloric region of the stomach along the greater curvature, although other intraabdominal sites, including Meckel's diverticulum, liver, gallbladder, small intestine, appendix, colon, omentum, and spleen, have been identified. Rarely, pancreatic tissue may arise in extraabdominal sites such as the lung and umbilicus.

Congenital Cyst of the Pancreas

Most cysts of the pancreas, even in the pediatric age group, are pancreatic pseudocysts that form due to pancreatitis. Fewer than 30 cases of true congenital cysts have been reported in the literature.[88]

Congenital cysts may be solitary or multiple. Solitary cysts have been identified in all age groups, from fetuses to adults, and there is predominance among female patients. These cysts are thought to arise by developmental errors of pancreatic ducts presumably related to localized obstruction of the duct in utero. Various sizes of cysts in the region of dominant cysts have been cited as further evidence to support this theory of pathogenesis.[89] Pancreatic cysts rarely have been associated with polyhydramnios.

Symptoms of congenital pancreatic cysts occur usually in patients younger than 2 years of age. Newborns may have an abdominal mass or an upper GI or biliary obstruction. These true cysts are localized in the tail or neck of the pancreas in 62% of cases. Associations with other anomalies, including renal tubular ectasia, polydactyly, anorectal malformations, and thoracic dystrophy, have been described. Multicystic lesions of the pancreas are usually associated with von Hippel-Lindau's disease[90] or, rarely, with autosomal dominant polycystic kidney disease.

Solitary pancreatic cysts are usually small (1 to 2 cm). Multiple cysts such as those seen in von Hippel-Lindau's disease may diffusely efface the pancreas, although the spectrum of changes in these patients is broad. The cysts are lined by non–mucin-producing cuboidal, columnar, or flattened (atrophic) cells with an adjacent fibrous wall (Figs. 37.13 and 37.14).[91,92] These lesions should not be confused with intrapancreatic enteric cysts, which most commonly contain gastric mucosa in the cyst wall, although they may rarely contain small intestinal, ciliated, or respiratory-type epithelium.[93]

Cystic Fibrosis

Cystic fibrosis (CF) is a multisystem disease with many GI tract manifestations. The pancreas was the first organ to be identified as significantly affected in this disease,[94] and its name is derived from the characteristic pathological findings of cysts and fibrosis in the pancreas.

CF, an autosomal recessive disease, is the most common hereditary disorder among whites, affecting 1 of 2000 in this population. CF also occurs in Hispanics, African Americans, and some Native Americans, but it is rare in people of Asian and Middle Eastern origin.

The genetic abnormality associated with CF is located on chromosome 7q31.[95] This region is responsible for expression of cystic fibrosis transmembrane conductance regulator (CFTR) protein, which functions as a chloride ion channel in epithelial cells. Defective chloride transport, which is associated with decreased bicarbonate secretion, causes mucus, sweat, and digestive juice secretions to become thick and tenacious. In the pancreas, precipitation of acinar secretions into pancreatic ducts leads to obstruction and chronic pancreatitis.[96]

Many of the clinical and histopathological findings in patients with CF result from obstruction of exocrine ducts. The hallmark clinical features of CF include pancreatic insufficiency (manifested as steatorrhea), pulmonary disease, elevated levels of sweat electrolytes (i.e., sodium and chloride), meconium ileus, and failure to thrive. Pathological abnormalities of the pancreas can be recognized as early as 32 to 38 weeks' gestation, and they progressively worsen with age. Malabsorption resulting from pancreatic insufficiency occurs in early infancy in 85% of patients with CF. Pancreatic insufficiency develops in most of the remaining patients at some stage during the course of their illness. Newborns with CF have a higher connective tissue–to–acinar gland ratio, with more prominent acinar and ductal lumens.

Grossly, the pancreas is often small, hard, and nodular. The parenchyma has a granular appearance due to extensive fibrosis, and cystic spaces are often apparent (Fig. 37.15). The earliest histological finding is that of abundant eosinophilic concretions, which may be laminated or calcified, within ectatic pancreatic ducts (Fig. 37.16A). The secretions represent mucoprotein and react with stains for acid mucopolysaccharides. Desquamated epithelial cells and inflammatory cells are usually admixed with the intraluminal secretions. Secondary changes of obstruction include flattening, atrophy, and dilation of acinar and ductal epithelia. Duct dilation with eventual cyst formation and parenchymal fibrosis occurs at an early age in most patients (Fig. 37.16B). An inflammatory cell infiltrate, including polymorphonuclear leukocytes and abundant lymphocytes, may be seen in the intralobular fibrous tissue within and surrounding the ducts and acini. Intraductal papillary hyperplasia and goblet cell metaplasia may also be evident.

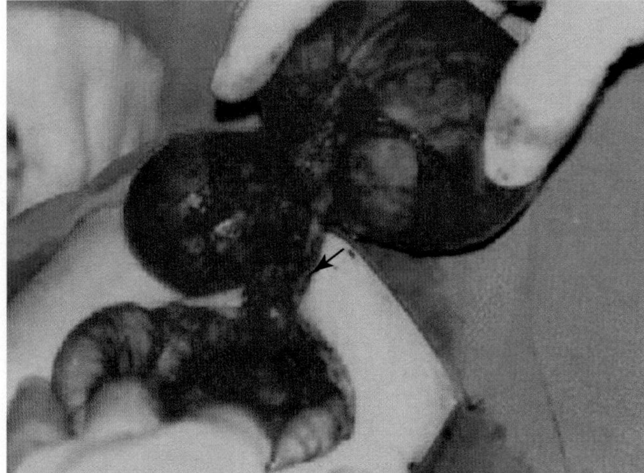

FIGURE 37.13 Congenital pancreatic cyst. A bilocular cystic mass shows continuity toward the tail of the pancreas *(arrow)*. (*From Kazez A, Akpolat N, Kocakoc E, et al. Congenital true pancreatic cyst: a rare case. Diagn Interv Radiol. 2006;12:31-33.*)

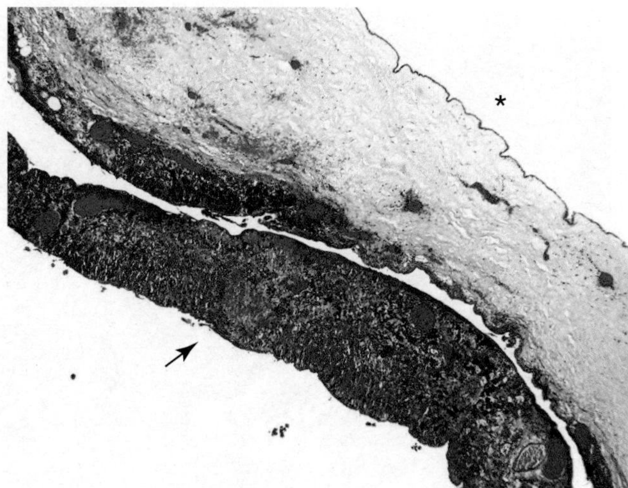

FIGURE 37.14 Congenital cyst of pancreas with attenuated cuboidal epithelium *(asterisk)* and adjacent pancreatic parenchyma *(arrow)*.

Continued involution of acinar tissue occurs during childhood, initially with a proliferation of fibroblasts, but subsequently by fatty replacement of the entire pancreas (Fig. 37.17). By the end of the first decade of life, the pancreas is replaced by fat, even though the normal gross architecture of the organ is usually well maintained.[97] Islets of Langerhans are usually well preserved initially, but as parenchymal damage progresses, insulin-dependent diabetes mellitus develops in approximately 25% of patients with CF (mostly adults), caused by an overall decrease in the number of insulin-producing islet cells.[98] Sporadic cases of adenocarcinoma of the pancreas arising in patients with CF have been reported, raising concern about a possible association between these two entities.[99]

In some patients with CF, common bile duct stenosis occurs as a direct result of pancreatic fibrosis affecting the intrapancreatic bile duct. This can occur even in patients with CF without pancreatic insufficiency.[100] Sclerosing cholangitis, common bile duct strictures, and extrahepatic cholangiocarcinoma (rare) have been reported.[101] Increased

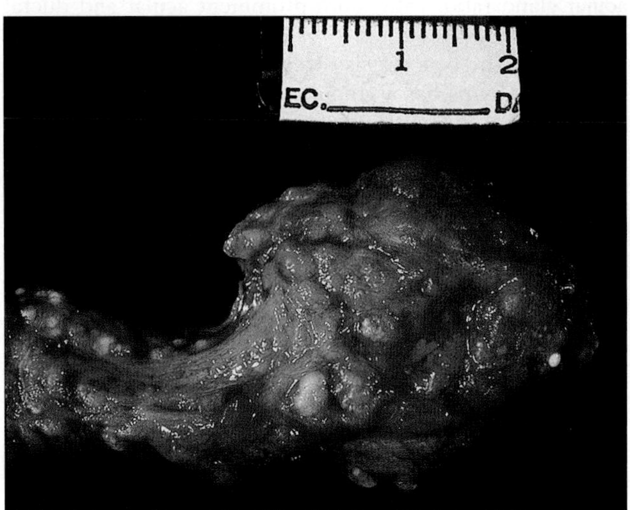

FIGURE 37.15 Pancreas from a 6-year-old patient with cystic fibrosis. Note the accentuated lobular parenchyma with prominent fibrosis.

fecal bile acid loss caused by malabsorption renders the bile lithogenic. At least one-third of older patients with CF have cholelithiasis. Microgallbladders (i.e., gallbladder hypoplasia), mucinous metaplasia, and cystic duct stenosis have been described.[100]

Congenital Pancreatic Exocrine Deficiencies

Shwachman-Diamond's syndrome (i.e., Shwachman-Bodian-Diamond's syndrome), originally described in 1964, is a rare, autosomal recessive, multisystem disorder linked to the *SBDS* gene on chromosome 7.[102] Infants usually have low birth weight and commonly fail to thrive. They often have feeding problems, diarrhea, and hypotonia. Virtually all patients are symptomatic by 4 months of age, and most have pancreatic insufficiency. After CF, this syndrome accounts for the most cases of primary pancreatic insufficiency in childhood.

The characteristic finding in the pancreas is diffuse fatty replacement of pancreatic parenchyma early in the disease course. The high mortality rate results from a constellation of problems involving bone marrow abnormalities (including aplasia with a high risk of leukemia), recurrent bacterial infections, myocardial inflammation, and multisystem anomalies.[103-106] Other rare causes of pancreatic exocrine deficiency include Johanson-Blizzard's syndrome,[107] exocrine pancreatic dysfunction with refractory sideroblastic anemia, and isolated enzyme deficiencies.[108]

Diabetes Mellitus

Diabetes mellitus is characterized by high blood glucose levels that result from defects in the body's ability to produce and use insulin. Symptoms include frequent urination, lethargy, excessive thirst, dehydration, and hunger.

Diabetes mellitus is separated into two types. Type 1, previously known as *juvenile diabetes*, is usually diagnosed in children and young adults and develops because the body does not produce insulin. Patients with type 1 diabetes are dependent on insulin therapy. Only 5% of diabetics have type 1 disease. Type 1 diabetes is associated with a genetic

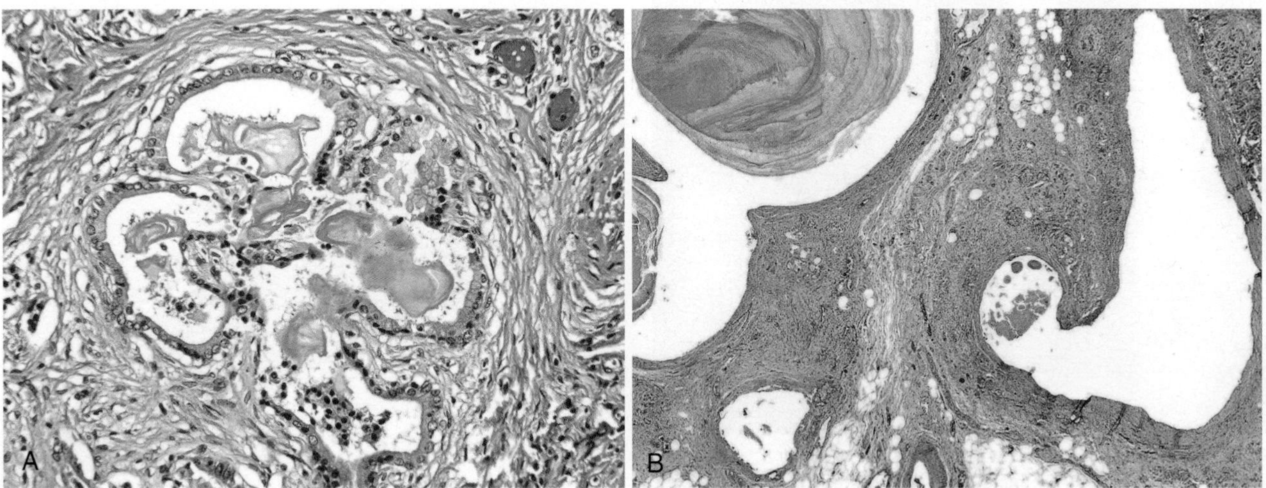

FIGURE 37.16 Histological features of cystic fibrosis. A, Eosinophilic concentric concretions are seen within a dilated ductal structure with surrounding fibrosis. **B,** Large cysts containing eosinophilic secretions are associated with parenchymal atrophy and intraparenchymal fat.

predisposition and autoimmunity, which leads to a severe loss of islet beta cells. Other possible causes include viral infection and the toxic effects of drugs or chemicals.

In type 2 diabetes, the most common form, the body does not produce enough insulin or the body's cells ignore the insulin that is produced. Type 2 diabetes occurs mainly in adults, is usually treated by diet and hypoglycemic medication, and is associated with obesity and a family history of diabetes. Type 2 diabetes is more common among African Americans, Latinos, Native Americans, Asian Americans, and Pacific Islanders.

Diabetes is associated with few gross alterations in the pancreas. Microscopically, in type 1 diabetes, the islets often show distinctive changes, even in cases of recent onset. The islets may be small and inconspicuous by hematoxylin and eosin staining (Fig. 37.18). Although some islets in some lobules may appear normal, islets in other lobules may be composed of small, irregular nests of cells with or without fibrosis (i.e., islet fibrosis) and may show continuity between the endocrine and acinar cells (i.e., neotransformation).[109]

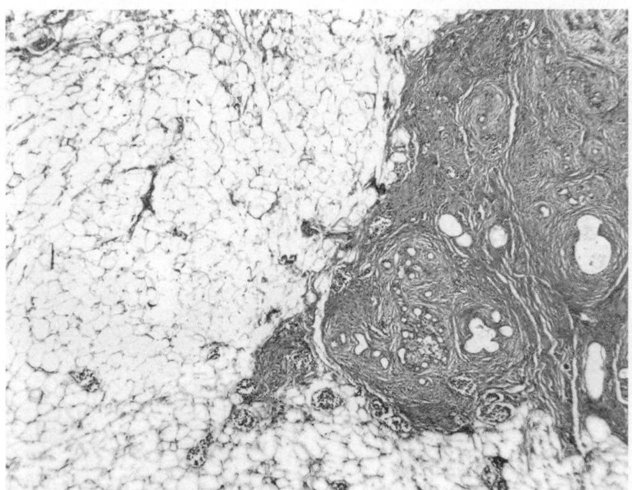

FIGURE 37.17 Diffuse fatty replacement and end-stage lobular fibrosis of a pancreas from a 23-year-old patient with cystic fibrosis.

An inflammatory cell infiltrate is often seen in some islets, a finding called *insulitis*.[110] The infiltrate consists predominantly of CD8+ T cells but may also contain CD4+ T cells, B lymphocytes, and macrophages.[111] Insulitis tends to occur in young (≤14 years) type 1 diabetic patients with a short (≤1 month) duration of the disease; it is infrequently encountered in older patients and patients with a disease duration longer than 1 year.[110] Insulitis preferentially affects islets, which contain beta cells, and after the beta cells have been destroyed, the inflammation subsides.[112] Immunohistochemical evaluation can reveal the loss of beta cells, but this may not be a uniform finding.

Islet amyloidosis is a rare feature of type 1 diabetes. Alterations in the exocrine pancreas include acinar cell atrophy and interacinar and interlobular fibrosis. Vascular changes include atherosclerosis of the large arteries and diabetic microangiopathy of smaller arterioles.

In type 2 diabetes, the islets are essentially normal in appearance, and in some patients there are few or no morphological differences compared with the islets in nondiabetic patients. However, some patients show as much as a 50% reduction in islet cell mass because of a decrease in the total number of insulin-producing beta cells. Islet amyloidosis (Fig. 37.19) is a characteristic histopathological feature of type 2 diabetes and affects islets containing insulin-producing beta cells, although it is not specific for type 2 diabetes. Both in vitro and in vivo studies have reported that amyloid formation causes the death of islet beta cells.[113]

Additional alterations in type 2 diabetes include islet fibrosis and fatty infiltration of the pancreas. Insulitis is a rare feature in type 2 diabetes.

Neonatal Islet Cell Hypertrophy and Hyperplasia

Marked variation in the size and number of islets of Langerhans in neonates and young adults has been well documented. The causes are listed in Box 37.2. An assessment of the significance of islet size and number can be made only in conjunction with knowledge of the gestational age at birth.[114] The most common cause of islet hypertrophy is maternal diabetes. In addition to hypertrophy and

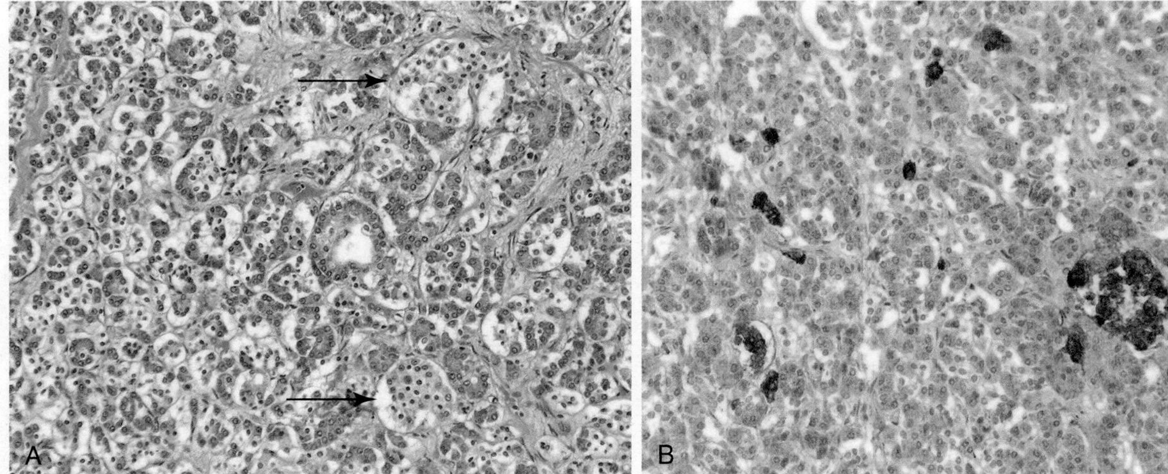

FIGURE 37.18 Specimens from an autopsy of a 47-year-old man with chronic type 1 diabetes. A, Some islets may appear normal or small *(arrows)*. **B,** Islets that are inconspicuous on hematoxylin and eosin staining can be highlighted with a neuroendocrine marker. One obvious islet and several smaller ones are highlighted by the synaptophysin stain.

hyperplasia, the islets in infants of diabetic mothers may show increased islet cell volume, pleomorphic nuclei of beta cells, fibrosis, and eosinophilic infiltrates with or without Charcot-Leyden crystals (Fig. 37.20). Alpha cell and pancreatic polypeptide (PP) cell hyperplasia may occur concomitantly with the marked hyperplasia of beta cells.[115-117]

Beckwith-Wiedemann's syndrome is a congenital, generalized, somatic overgrowth syndrome with various phenotypes, including prenatal and postnatal overgrowth, macroglossia, and anterior abdominal wall defects, most commonly exomphalos. It is usually a sporadic disorder, with only 10% to 15% of cases having a familial origin. It results from dysregulation of imprinted genes on chromosome 11p15.5.[118]

Beckwith-Wiedemann's syndrome is associated with hypoglycemia caused by islet cell hyperplasia and hyperinsulinism in 50% of cases. Islets are enlarged, and smaller clusters of endocrine cells occur in the form of nodular aggregates (Fig. 37.21). Immunohistochemical staining reveals a marked increase in beta cells and a slight increase in alpha cells. The number of PP cells is decreased. Rarely, pancreatoblastoma and cystic dysplasia of the pancreas may be identified in these patients.[119,120] They have an increased incidence of nonpancreatic cancers, especially Wilms tumor.

Persistent Hyperinsulinemic Hypoglycemia of Infancy

Persistent hyperinsulinemic hypoglycemia of infancy (PHHI) is the most common cause of severe, prolonged neonatal hypoglycemia, occurring in 1 of 27,000 to 50,000 births.[121] Although an excellent argument for the designation *PHHI* has been made, the term *nesidioblastosis* is more commonly used.

PHHI is caused by mutations in genes that regulate insulin secretion, most commonly autosomal recessive mutations in the sulfonylurea receptor gene, *SUR1* (official symbol, *ABCC8*). Other causes include mutations of the *ABCC8*-associated inward rectifier gene, *Kir6.2* (now called *KCNJ11*). The ABCC8 and KCNJ11 proteins are the main constituents of an adenosine triphosphate–sensitive potassium channel. Autosomal dominant

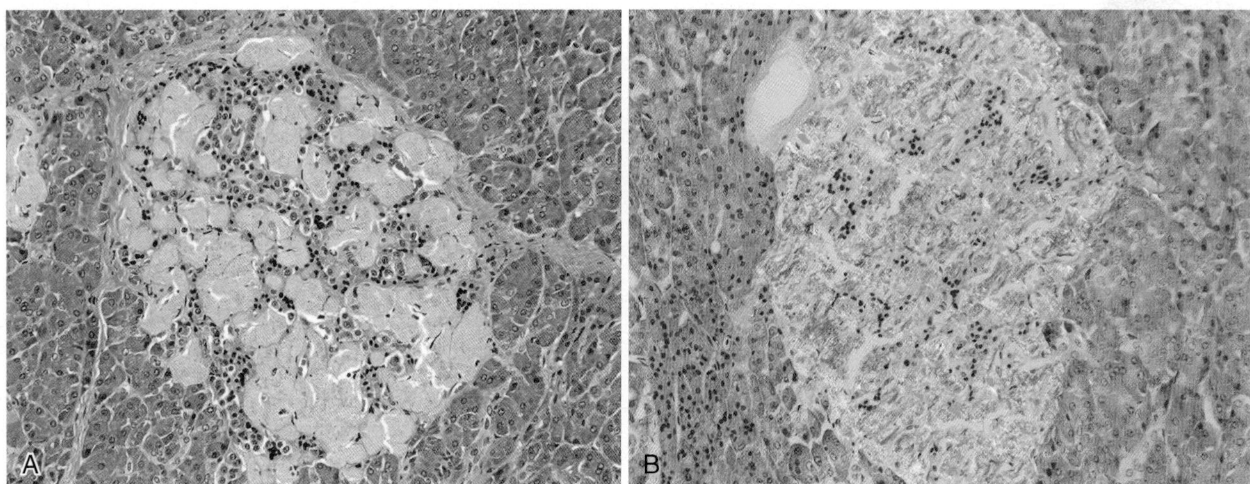

FIGURE 37.19 Type 2 diabetes. A, Hematoxylin and eosin staining shows a few residual islet cells compressed by amorphous pink amyloid. **B,** Congo red staining shows apple-green birefringence.

BOX 37.2 Conditions Associated with Hypertrophy and Hyperplasia of the Islets of Langerhans

- Infant of a diabetic mother
- Beckwith-Wiedemann's syndrome
- Erythroblastosis fetalis
- Nesidioblastosis and focal adenomatosis
- Zellweger's syndrome
- Donohue's syndrome
- Tyrosinemia
- Cyanotic congenital heart disease
- Long-term total parenteral nutrition
- Multiple endocrine neoplasia type II

Data from Dahms BB. Gastrointestinal tract and pancreas. In: Gilbert-Barness E, ed. Potter's Pathology of the Fetus and Infant. *Vol. 1. St. Louis: Mosby; 1997:774-822.*

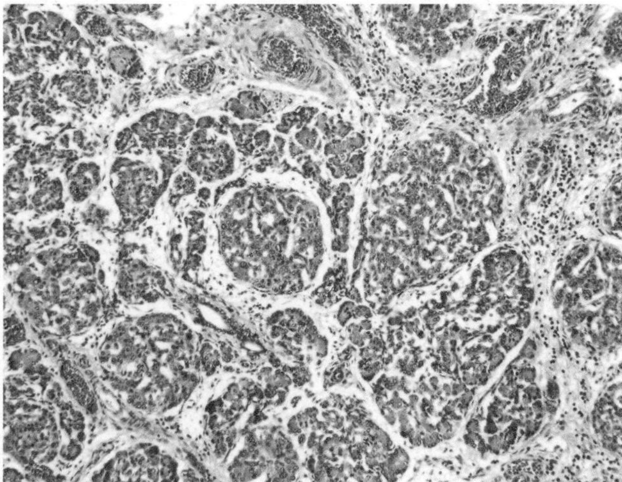

FIGURE 37.20 Diffuse islet cell proliferation in a fetus resulting from maternal diabetes mellitus.

mutations of glucokinase and glutamate dehydrogenase are uncommonly associated with PHHI (Fig. 37.22).[121] Rarely, other causes of congenital hyperinsulinism have been described.[122]

The disease is characterized by diffuse or focal abnormalities of the islets of Langerhans. Histological features associated with PHHI include islets that are irregular in size and shape (Fig. 37.23), enlargement of beta cell nuclei (i.e., three to four times the size of normal endocrine nuclei) (Fig. 37.24), ductulo-insular complexes (i.e., budding of endocrine cells from duct epithelium) (Fig. 37.25), centroacinar cell proliferation (i.e., ductal cells with pale cytoplasm in centroacinar regions), septal islets (i.e., islets within fibrous septa), and nesidiodysplasia, a subtle increase in endocrine cell aggregates randomly distributed in pancreatic lobules. Adenomatosis, which is excess islet cell proliferation defined as more than 40% of a low-power microscopic field, is found less commonly than diffuse islet cell changes.[114,116,123,124] Diffuse hyperinsulinism, which is characterized by enlarged islet cell nuclei throughout the pancreas, most commonly results from recessive mutations in *ABCC8* and *KCNJ11*. Focal-type congenital hyperinsulinism develops in patients with a germline mutation in the paternal allele of *ABCC8* or *KCNJ11*.[121,125]

Extensive pancreatic resection is often required to control hypoglycemia. Conflicting data have emerged concerning the likelihood of diffuse pancreatic islet cell abnormalities in the

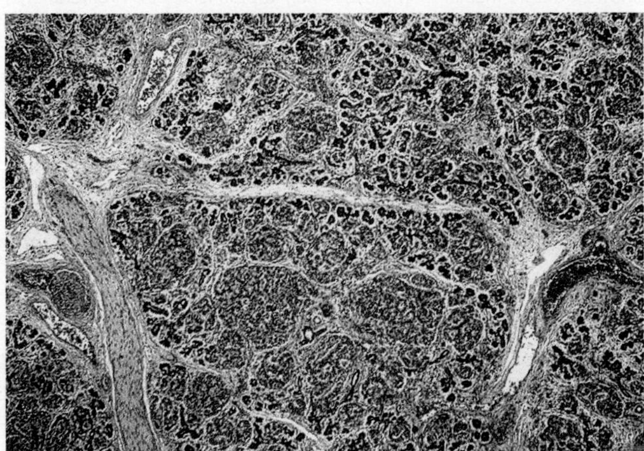

FIGURE 37.21 Beckwith-Wiedemann's syndrome is characterized by enlarged and closely packed islets of Langerhans.

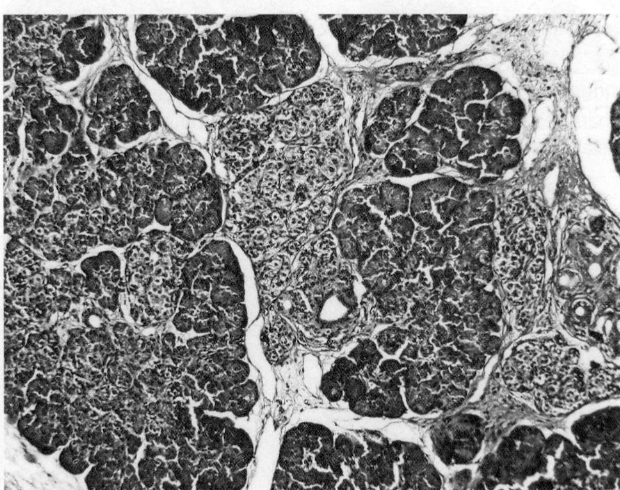

FIGURE 37.23 Persistent hyperinsulinemic hypoglycemia of infancy is characterized by islets of irregular size and shape.

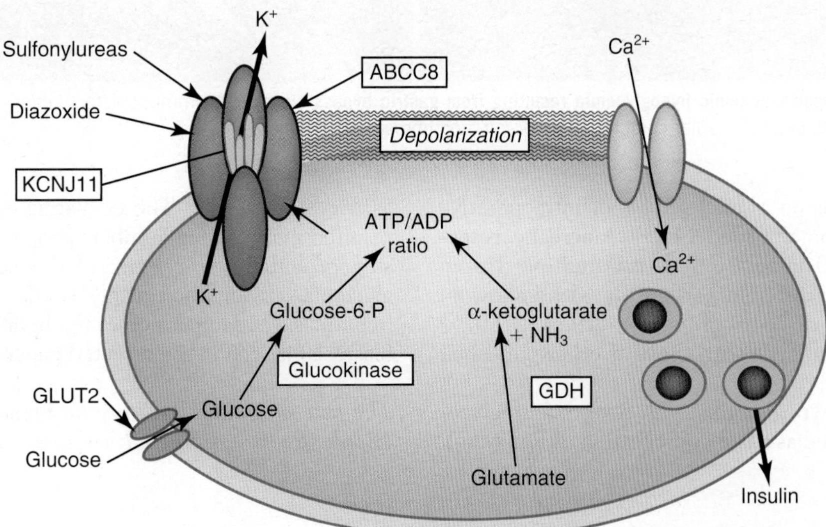

FIGURE 37.22 The major pathways responsible for glucose regulation of insulin secretion. Hyperinsulinism can be caused by mutations in the genes encoding four proteins *(boxes)*. The adenosine triphosphate (ATP)–sensitive potassium channel (K_{ATP}) is composed of four molecules of ABCC8 and four of KCNJ11. Glucokinase, an enzyme that facilitates phosphorylation of glucose to glucose-6-phosphate (Glucose-6-P), is the rate-limiting step in the metabolism of glucose, and it regulates changes in the intracellular ATP/adenosine diphosphate (ADP) ratio in response to extracellular glucose concentrations. The mechanism by which activating mutations in the gene for glutamate dehydrogenase (GDH) cause unregulated insulin secretion has not been confirmed experimentally. (*From Glaser B, Thornton P, Otonkoski T, Junien C. Genetics of neonatal hyperinsulinism. Arch Dis Child Fetal Neonatal Ed. 2000;82:F79-F86.*)

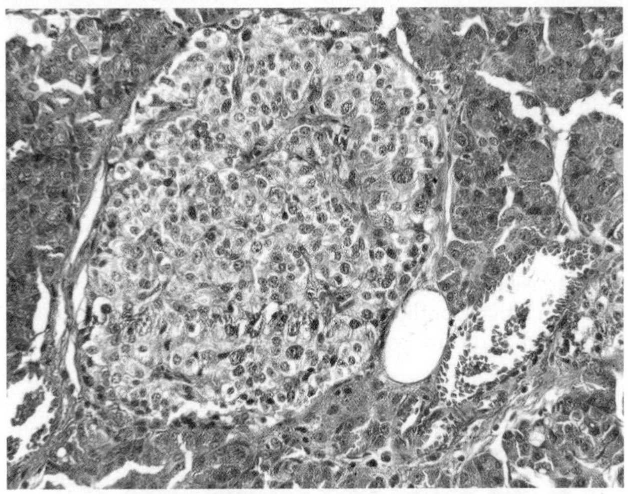

FIGURE 37.24 Persistent hyperinsulinemic hypoglycemia of infancy is characterized by enlarged, irregular islets of Langerhans containing beta cells with nuclear pleomorphism.

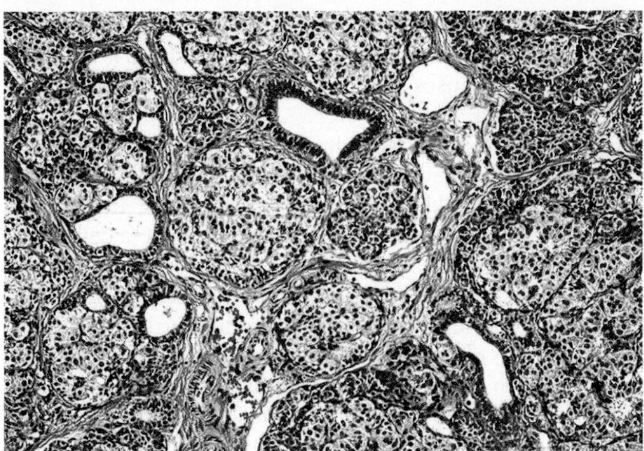

FIGURE 37.25 Persistent hyperinsulinemic hypoglycemia of infancy shows ductulo-insular complexes (i.e., tubulo-islet cell proliferations) characterized by large aggregates of neuroendocrine cells with intermixed ductal proliferation.

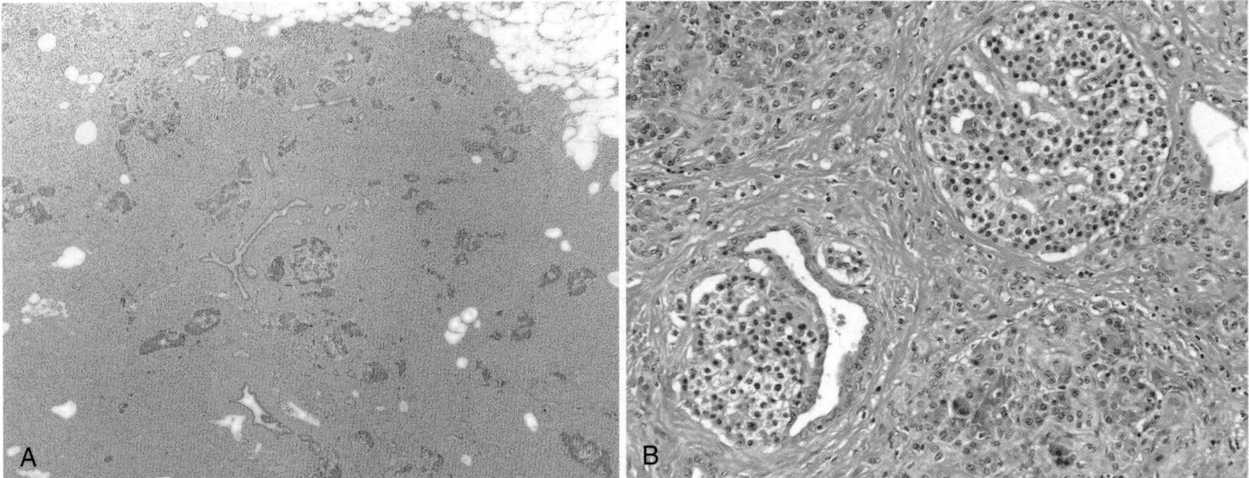

FIGURE 37.26 Acquired hyperinsulinemic hypoglycemia resulting from gastric bypass surgery. A, Immunohistochemical stain for insulin shows an expanded beta cell mass. **B**, Ductulo-insular complexes *(lower left)* and fibrosis can be seen.

setting of adenomatosis on a small sample of intraoperative frozen pancreas section obtained before pancreatic resection. One study of 20 infants found that multiple frozen sections obtained from different parts of the gland allow an accurate intraoperative diagnosis of focal or diffuse PHHI.[126] These findings are at variance with those of other published series.[114,124]

Hyperinsulinemic hypoglycemia with severe neuroglycopenia has been identified as a late complication of Roux-en-Y gastric bypass.[127,128] The escalating epidemic of obesity has resulted in increasing numbers people who have had bariatric surgery and the emergence of this acquired form of hypoglycemia. Histopathologically, similar to PHHI, diffuse islet hyperplasia and expansion of the beta cell mass (i.e., nesidioblastosis) is seen in the resected pancreata (Fig. 37.26).[127,128]

The full reference list may be viewed online at Elsevier eBooks for Practicing Clinicians.

CHAPTER 38

Infectious and Inflammatory Disorders of the Gallbladder and Extrahepatic Biliary Tract

Jose Jessurun, Lihui Qin

Chapter Outline

INTRODUCTION

The gallbladder is a surgical pathology specimen normally obtained by laparoscopic cholecystectomy or laparotomy. Historically, surgical pathologists have dedicated little time to the gross and microscopic examination of the gallbladder because they have believed that the information derived from them is not relevant to patient care. This persistent lack of interest has hampered our understanding of the broad range of inflammatory conditions of this organ. This chapter describes the pathological features of nonneoplastic disorders of the gallbladder and extrahepatic bile ducts, including the epidemiology and physiopathology of gallstones.

GALLSTONES

Gallstones are a common cause of morbidity worldwide. The incidence of gallstones is very high in Native American populations in North America. Compared with the incidence of gallstones of 16.6% and 8.6% among non-Hispanic white women and men in the United States, respectively, the estimated incidence for Canadian Indians is 62%; for young Pima Indian women it is roughly 70% to approximately 80% in South American Indians.[1] Approximately 700,000 cholecystectomies are performed each year in the United States.[2] In 2015, biliary disorders were among the most expensive of all digestive diseases, accounting for 10.3 billion of the 135.9 billion dollars of annual health care expenditures for gastrointestinal (GI) diseases.[3] If inpatient physician services and hospital costs are considered in the equation, cholelithiasis is one of the most costly digestive disorders.[4,5] Further improvements in therapy and prevention can be derived from a better understanding of the epidemiology and pathophysiology of gallstone formation.

Historical Perspective

Since antiquity, gallstones have been of keen interest to physicians. Historical accounts of Alexander the Great's illness that preceded his death in 323 BC strongly suggest that he suffered from gallstones and cholecystitis. Galen, in his description of obstructive jaundice, mentioned small foreign bodies similar to grain, fig, and pomegranate seeds within the common bile duct.

The first description of gallstones as "dried up humors concreted like stones" and their relationship to hepatic obstruction is ascribed to the Greek physician Alexander of Tralles (5th century AD). The 14th century physician Gentile da Foligno first postulated a relationship between cholecystitis and gallstones based on autopsy findings. Antonio Benivieni successfully diagnosed gallstone disease in a patient with abdominal pain. His clinical impression was confirmed at autopsy. However, it was Jean Fernel (1497-1558), physician to the king of France, who provided the most accurate clinical description of symptoms associated with cholelithiasis. In his masterpiece, *De Sedibus et Causis Morborum per Anatomen Indagatis* (1761), Giovanni Battista Morgagni described gallstones in great detail. He noticed an increased frequency of this condition with age, occurrence in a preponderance of women, and an association with a sedentary lifestyle.

Gallstones were removed from a living patient for the first time in 1618 by the German surgeon Wilhelm Fabry. Two and a half centuries later, another German physician, Carl Langenbuch, performed the first cholecystectomy.

The composition of gallstones was essentially unknown until the end of the 18th century. It was through the excellent work of researchers such as Antonio Vallisneri, Francois Poulletier de la Salle, and Félix Vicq d'Azyr that the chemical composition and variability in the components of gallstones were determined.[6]

Gallstone Classification

Gallstones are composed predominantly of cholesterol, bilirubin, and calcium salts, with lesser quantities of other constituents. The most widely used classification system is based on the relative amount of cholesterol in the stones. There are two main categories: cholesterol and noncholesterol (pigment) stones (Fig. 38.1). The latter are further classified as black or brown pigment stones.[7–9] Cholesterol gallstones constitute more than 80% of stones in industrialized nations. They are composed predominantly of cholesterol crystals. Noncholesterol gallstones are far more common in other parts of the world, such as Asia.

Black pigment stones are formed from calcium salts of unconjugated bilirubin in a polymerized matrix. Brown pigment stones may form within bile ducts (i.e., primary bile duct stones) and contain the bacterial degradation products of biliary lipids, calcium salts of fatty acids, unconjugated bilirubin, and precipitated cholesterol. Because the pathogenesis and epidemiology of gallstones are considerably different, they are discussed separately (Table 38.1).

Cholesterol Gallstones

Pathogenesis

The major lipid components of bile are bile salts (67% of solutes by weight), phospholipids (22%), and cholesterol (4%). Hepatocytes express specific adenosine triphosphate (ATP)–binding cassette transport proteins (i.e., ABC transporters) for each of the three types of lipids at the canalicular membrane domain. The bile salt export pump is the ABCB2 transporter. The one for the major biliary phospholipid, phosphatidylcholine (i.e., lecithin), is the ABCB4 transporter. The one for cholesterol secretion is the obligate heterodimer ABCG5/ABCG8.[1]

Because cholesterol is insoluble in water, it requires a solubilizing system, which is provided by the detergent action of phospholipids and bile salts. After being cosecreted by hepatocytes, cholesterol and phospholipids form spherical structures composed of a double layer of phospholipids (mainly lecithin). These vesicles are soluble by virtue of the outward orientation of the hydrophilic (water-loving)

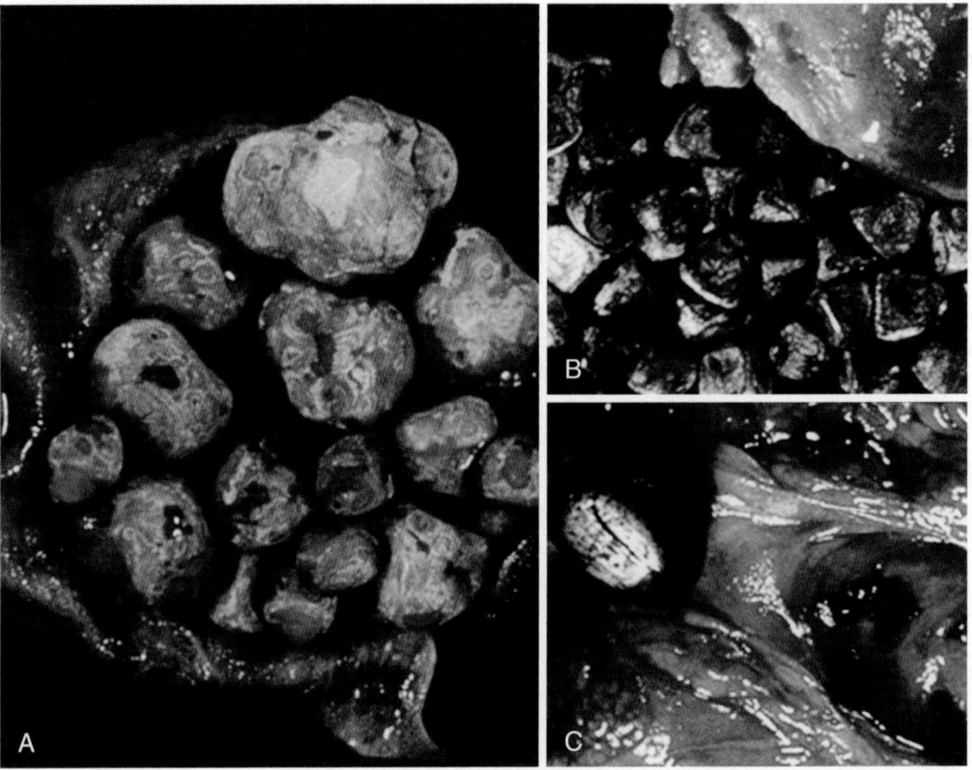

FIGURE 38.1 Cholesterol gallstones **(A),** black stones **(B),** and brown stones **(C)** within bile ducts.

TABLE 38.1 Types of Gallstones

Characteristics	Cholesterol Gallstones	Noncholesterol (Pigmented) Gallstones	
		Black	*Brown*
Epidemiology	Western countries > Africa and Asia	Africa and Asia > Western countries	Asia > Africa > Western countries
Appearance	Small or large, yellow; single or multiple	Small, black, firm, multiple	Large, brown, soft, single or few > multiple
Composition	Cholesterol Phospholipids Bile salts	Calcium bilirubinate Calcium phosphate Calcium carbonate Low cholesterol level	Calcium bilirubinate Palmitate Cholesterol
Associated conditions	Usually none	Hemolysis Alcoholism Crohn's disease Cirrhosis	Biliary infections

choline groups, which allows cholesterol to be inserted into the hydrophobic (water-fearing) milieu provided by the fatty acid chains.[9-11]

Liver cells secrete bile acids through a different transport mechanism. Although soluble in water, bile salt monomers self-aggregate into simple micelles after they surpass the critical micellar concentration (≈0.5 to 5 mM). The amphophilic properties of bile acids produce an extremely water-soluble structure because of orientation of the hydrophobic portions of the molecules away from water and exposure of the hydrophilic surfaces to the aqueous environment. As detergents, bile acids can dissolve portions of vesicles and incorporate them into mixed micelles. The resulting structures are disks composed of cholesterol and phospholipids surrounded by bile acids.[11-13]

As the concentration of cholesterol increases, more of it is carried in vesicles. A higher cholesterol concentration increases cholesterol transfer from vesicles to micelles during the micellation process. The resulting cholesterol-enriched unilamellar vesicles are unstable and fuse into large, multilamellar vesicles. When the cholesterol-to-phospholipid ratio exceeds 1, cholesterol crystallizes at the surface. Crystallization is enhanced by the concentration of solutes in bile, because aggregation occurs more efficiently when cholesterol carriers are close to each other.[10,12,14]

Cholesterol is most soluble in a mixture of lipids that contains at least 50% bile acids and lesser amounts of phospholipids. Supersaturation occurs when a solution contains more cholesterol molecules than can be solubilized. Theoretically, bile supersaturation may be caused by hypersecretion of cholesterol, hyposecretion of bile acids, hyposecretion of phospholipids, or a combination of these mechanisms. An increase in biliary cholesterol output resulting from increased synthesis or increased uptake is the most common cause of supersaturation and subsequent stone formation. Increased uptake by hepatocytes may involve endogenous cholesterol (transported by low-density lipoprotein) or exogenous cholesterol (transported by chylomicrons).

Cholesterol supersaturation may result from bile acid hyposecretion. However, most patients with gallstones have normal biliary acid secretion. Adequate bile acid secretion depends on the integrity of the enterohepatic circulation. Approximately 90% of bile acids are resorbed from the terminal ileum and returned to the liver by the portal system 3 to 12 times per day. Bile acids are reused by hepatocytes after passive and active reuptake. Theoretically, interference with this recycling mechanism contributes to bile acid hyposecretion and subsequent cholesterol supersaturation.[11-13]

A study of first-degree relatives of gallstone carriers has provided clues that bile lipid secretion may be under genetic control.[14] Most information is based on animal models. Knockout mice deficient in the multiple drug–resistant gene 2 maintain normal bile acid secretion but are incapable of secreting phospholipids and cholesterol into bile as a result of the absence of a protein that flips phospholipids from the inner to the outer half of canalicular membranes.[15] In other models, mice fed a lithogenic diet developed gallstones at a frequency that varied according to the presence of the *Lith1*, *Lith2*, or *Lith3* genes and other genes.[3] The importance of a genetic background in the pathogenesis of gallstones is suggested by the finding of gallstones in certain families and ethnic groups and the presence of specific gene polymorphisms.[16]

Supersaturation of cholesterol is necessary, but not sufficient, for the formation of cholesterol gallstones. For any degree of cholesterol saturation, patients with gallstones form cholesterol crystals more rapidly than individuals without gallstones. This observation led to the theory that stone formation probably involves a nucleation process. The tendency of bile to nucleate cholesterol depends on a balance between substances that promote and prevent nucleation. Pronucleating agents are mostly heterogeneous mucin gels. Other biliary proteins have been postulated as promoters (e.g., nonmucin glycoproteins, mainly immunoglobulins) or inhibitors (e.g., apolipoproteins A-I and A-II, other glycoproteins) of cholesterol precipitation in bile.[17-21] However, their participation is most likely nonspecific, and their relevance remains controversial.

Abnormal gallbladder motility contributes to gallstone formation. By causing incomplete emptying of supersaturated and crystal-containing bile, gallbladder hypomotility promotes the formation of gallstones.[22]

Biliary sludge is a viscous gel composed of mucin and microscopic precipitates of multilamellar vesicles, cholesterol monohydrate, and calcium bilirubinate. Because mucin is at the center of almost all gallstones, it was suggested that the formation of biliary sludge precedes the formation of macroscopic cholesterol gallstones.

Bacteria may contribute to the formation of gallstones as well. Using polymerase chain reaction (PCR) amplification, Swidsinski and colleagues identified bacteria in cholesterol gallstones.[23] *Pseudomonas* and *Escherichia coli* were initially thought to be the main responsible organisms, but bile-resistant *Helicobacter* species and *Helicobacter pylori* are also thought to participate in the formation of mixed cholesterol gallstones.[24,25] Whether these organisms are innocent bystanders or play a role in the formation of gallstones awaits further studies.

Epidemiology and Risk Factors

The prevalence of cholesterol gallstones depends on the age, gender, country of residence, and ethnicity of the population. Geographic differences are most likely related to interaction of genetic and environmental factors. In the United States, it is estimated that 20 to 30 million people have gallstones.

The prevalence rate increases with age. Cholelithiasis in children is rare; however, recent studies have shown a substantial increase in the incidence during childhood, which is attributed to obesity, physical inactivity, diabetes, and early pregnancy.[16] After 20 years of age, the prevalence of gallstones increases with each decade of life: 7% to 11% for those younger than 50 years, 11% to 30% for individuals between 60 and 70 years, and 33% to 50% for people older than 90 years of age.[26] Gallstones develop more frequently in women than in men. For reproductive-age women, the risk of cholelithiasis is two to three times higher than for men. Increased risk of gallstones is associated with pregnancy, multiparity, estrogen replacement therapy, oral contraceptive use, obesity, and rapid weight loss.[27] In addition to estrogens, other drugs that increase the risk of cholelithiasis are prednisolone, cyclosporine, azathioprine, octreotide (Sandostatin), clofibrate, and nicotinic acid.[28] Whether diabetes predisposes to gallstone formation remains controversial. Substantial evidence suggests that alcohol intake protects against gallstone formation.[29,30]

As mentioned previously, the prevalence of cholelithiasis is influenced by the genetic composition of the population. Patients who have a relative who had gallstones have a two to four times higher rate of gallstones.[28] In the United States, the highest prevalence of gallstones is observed among Native Americans, with a progressively lower risk among whites, blacks, and some Asian groups.[31] The prevalence of gallstones among Mexican American women is higher compared with that among other Hispanic women.[32,33] Gallstones are extremely common in Chile and in Scandinavian countries, but the incidence is much lower in Asia and Africa.[34,35]

Epidemiological data from North America suggest that populations with a high rate of gallstones carry dominant Amerindian lithogenic genes transmitted by common ancestral Asians who colonized America more than 20,000 years ago. In support of this hypothesis, an epidemiological study from Chile found a positive correlation between Native American genes (measured by ABO blood group distribution and determination of mitochondrial DNA polymorphisms) and the prevalence of gallstones in young women.[36] In this study, the highest prevalence of gallstone disease was detected among the indigenous Mapuche (35.2%), followed by residents of urban Santiago (27.5%) and the Maoris of Easter Island (20.9%).[36] The high prevalence among Native American and Mexican American women also supports this hypothesis.

The specific genes associated with gallstone susceptibility have been partially characterized in animal models. Undoubtedly, the corresponding human genes and their products will be elucidated soon. Knowledge of the function of gene products involved in lithogenesis and the potential relevance of genetic polymorphism in their synthesis or functionality will elucidate their complex interactions with environmental (dietary) factors. Based on this information, specific prevention strategies can be tailored to populations with a high prevalence of cholesterol gallstones.

Pigment Gallstones

Pathogenesis

There are two types of pigment stones: black and brown. This distinction is important because they differ in their pathophysiology, associated clinical conditions, morphology, and chemical composition. Black stones are composed of calcium bilirubinate, phosphate, and carbonate embedded in a glycoprotein and have a very low cholesterol concentration. Brown stones contain calcium salts of bilirubin and fatty acids (palmitate) in a glycoprotein matrix and have a higher concentration of cholesterol. Calcium carbonate and phosphate are usually absent.[37] Black stones are small, black, and multiple. Brown stones are soft, brownish-green, and large.

Because it is a precursor of calcium bilirubinate, unconjugated bilirubin plays a central role in the formation of brown and black pigment stones. Unconjugated bilirubin is solubilized by bile salts in mixed micelles and then combines with calcium to form calcium bilirubinate. Any condition that results in elevated levels of unconjugated bilirubin may predispose to stone formation. Biliary infections that contribute to bile stasis are common causes of brown stones, because bacterial overgrowth generates hydrolases that form free bile acids from conjugated bile salts. Bacteria elaborate phospholipase A, which cleaves phospholipids to form lysolecithin and free fatty acids. Free fatty acids (mainly palmitic and stearic) combine with free bile salts generated by bacterial hydrolases and precipitate as calcium salts. It is therefore not surprising that bacteria are found within the matrix of most brown stones.[37]

Black pigment stones are not associated with bacterial infection. An increased concentration of unconjugated bilirubin originates from an increase in the secretion of bilirubin conjugates, as in patients with hemolysis and chronic alcoholism, followed by nonbacterial enzymatic or nonenzymatic hydrolysis. An analogous effect occurs if the secretion of bile salts is decreased, as in patients with cirrhosis, because these compounds are required to solubilize unconjugated bilirubin and buffer ionized calcium.[16] Phospholipids also play an important role in pigment sludge formation. Calcium bilirubinate sludge contains an increased amount of phospholipids, and these compounds occur in the core of pigment gallstones. Carbohydrate-rich diets stimulate enzymes that are important in the synthesis of phospholipids, such as fatty acid synthetase. Increased activity of these enzymes helps explain the higher hepatic bile phospholipid concentrations found in some clinical situations, such as total parenteral nutrition.

The gallbladder mucosa plays a role in lithogenesis. Biliary epithelium acidifies bile, increasing the solubility of calcium carbonate. Mucosal inflammation interferes with the ability of the epithelium to perform its acidifying role, which results in increased biliary pH and subsequent calcium carbonate precipitation. Reparative metaplastic changes in the mucosa (discussed later) increases the concentration of biliary glycoproteins, which promotes gallstone formation.[38]

In adult and fetal gallbladders, *MUC1*, *MUC2*, *MUC3*, *MUC5AC*, *MUC5B*, and *MUC6* gene expression has been found; the most prominently expressed is *MUC5B*.[39,40] With the exception of *MUC2*, all of these mucin genes appear to be expressed in the gallbladder epithelium of gallstone patients. *MUC5AC* gene expression is elevated in patients with cholecystitis, particularly those with brown stones. Inflammation does not affect the expression of other mucins.[41]

Brown stones are strongly associated with infection, and they may be found within the bile ducts and gallbladder. The β-glucuronidase produced by bacteria deconjugates bilirubin to its water-insoluble form. Calcium salts of unconjugated bilirubin (i.e., deconjugated bile acids and saturated long-chain fatty acids) are generated, which leads to the formation of brown stones. Organisms implicated in the formation of these stones include *E. coli*, *Clonorchis sinensis*, *Opisthorchis viverrini*, and *Ascaris lumbricoides*.[42]

Epidemiology

Pigment gallstones occur in patients worldwide. Although they account for only 20% to 25% of gallstones in the United States, they are much more common in other parts of the world, such as Asia. Similar to cholesterol gallstones, pigment stones develop more frequently in women. The incidence increases with age. Race is not a factor.

Clinical conditions associated with black gallstones include hemolytic anemia, cirrhosis, alcoholism, malaria, pancreatitis, total parenteral nutrition, and older age. Black pigment stones develop more frequently in patients with Crohn's disease, particularly those with extensive ileitis, and those who have had an ileal resection. The predilection for stone formation in patients with ileitis or in those who have had an ileal resection stems from decreased or absent functionality of the terminal ileum, which is the site of 90% of bile salt resorption. In normal individuals, unconjugated bilirubin precipitates in the colon as calcium bilirubinate or other bilirubinates. In contrast, impaired or absent resorptive function in the ileum in patients with Crohn's disease leads to increased levels of bile salts in the colon, where salts solubilize unconjugated bilirubin.[43] Subsequent increased resorption of unconjugated bilirubin in the colon leads to supersaturation of bile (as much as three times normal levels), and stone formation.

Histology of the Gallbladder

The normal histology of the gallbladder is described in detail in Chapter 34. However, a brief description of the most salient features that are important to know when evaluating cholecystectomy specimens for chronic diseases is warranted here. A single layer of columnar epithelial cells containing eosinophilic cytoplasm and basally located nuclei line the luminal folds. Except for the presence of occasional small apical vacuoles, these cells do not contain mucin. When mucin is present, it should be regarded as a metaplastic change and thus a reflection of inflammation. Mucin-producing tubule-alveolar glands are, in fact, found exclusively in the neck of the gallbladder. When found in other locations of the gallbladder, these glands should be interpreted as antral/pyloric metaplasia. Inflammatory cells are not a constituent of the normal lamina propria. The muscularis (without further qualification) bears closer similarity to intestinal muscularis mucosae than to muscularis propria. This structure is formed of three or four layers of smooth muscle bundles, with evenly spaced "gaps" (similar to the intestinal muscularis mucosae). When there is increased intraluminal pressure, the epithelium may herniate through gaps, and give rise to Rokitansky-Aschoff sinuses. Penetration into the deep layers of the wall through the muscularis is, almost invariably, accompanied by hyperplasia/hypertrophy of the muscle fibers, as expected in conditions that are associated with outflow obstruction (e.g., gallstones, chronic bile duct disease, or biliary dyskinesia).

CHOLECYSTITIS

Inflammatory diseases of the gallbladder are a frequent cause of morbidity in Western countries. The term *cholecystitis* encompasses a group of disorders that have different pathological, pathogenetic, and clinical characteristics. As in other organs of the GI tract, most inflammatory diseases of the gallbladder produce nonspecific histological features because they elicit a nondistinctive type of cellular inflammatory infiltrate. However, characterization of specific inflammatory patterns helps establish pathological diagnoses and provides insight into the pathogenesis of disease. Recognition of different patterns of inflammation can render clinically useful histological diagnoses (Box 38.1).

Acute Cholecystitis

Clinically, acute cholecystitis is defined as an episode of acute biliary pain accompanied by fever, right upper quadrant tenderness, guarding, persistence of symptoms beyond 24 hours, and leukocytosis.[44] Approximately 90% of cases

BOX 38.1 Classification of Cholecystitis

ACUTE CHOLECYSTITIS

- Calculous
- Acalculous
- Gangrenous
- Emphysematous

CHRONIC CHOLECYSTITIS

- Calculous
  - Not otherwise specified
  - Follicular
  - Hyalinizing
  - Xanthogranulomatous
- Acalculous
  - Lymphoeosinophilic
  - Eosinophilic
  - Granulomatous
  - Diffuse lymphoplasmacytic
  - Lymphocytic

are associated with gallstones. Ultrasonography often demonstrates thickening of the gallbladder wall or pericholecystic fluid. The diagnosis is also supported by failure to visualize the gallbladder during a hepatobiliary scintigram.[45] Because of unique clinical and pathological characteristics, the three types of acute cholecystitis—acute calculous cholecystitis, acute acalculous cholecystitis, and emphysematous cholecystitis—are discussed separately.

Acute Calculous Cholecystitis

Clinical Features

Most patients in whom acute calculous cholecystitis develops are women between 50 and 70 years of age. Typical symptoms are right upper quadrant pain of recent onset, accompanied by abdominal guarding and local tenderness. Anorexia, nausea, and vomiting are common. A history of similar episodes in the past that resolved spontaneously is frequently obtained. In the elderly, symptoms may be deceptively mild or even absent. Occasionally, an enlarged gallbladder may be palpated. Pain may be elicited upon palpation of the right upper quadrant when the patient inhales deeply (i.e., Murphy's sign). Some patients may be febrile. Rarely, jaundice develops. Most patients have leukocytosis.

Because the clinical features are nonspecific, imaging techniques, such as ultrasonography, are used to confirm the clinical diagnosis. Preoperative clinical findings of acute cholecystitis are highly reliable for predicting intraoperative gross findings. However, intraoperative findings of acute cholecystitis are commonly found in the absence of preoperative clinical signs. For unknown reasons, correlation between pathological and intraoperative findings is poor.[45]

A rare complication that results from compression of the common bile duct by gallstones lodged in the cystic bile duct is termed Mirizzi's syndrome. Imaging techniques may help to confirm the extrinsic nature of the bile duct obstruction and help plan the appropriate surgical procedure.

Pathogenesis

The main precipitating event in the development of acute calculous cholecystitis is occlusion of the neck of the gallbladder (i.e., cystic duct) by gallstones. The resulting increase in intraluminal pressure dilates the gallbladder and causes mural edema. However, outflow obstruction does not always cause acute cholecystitis. Animal models in which the cystic duct has been ligated or obliterated experience shrinkage of the gallbladder but not acute cholecystitis.[46] Factors contributing to the development of acute cholecystitis include mucosal ischemia resulting from visceral distention and external compression of the cystic artery by an impacted stone.

Formation of inflammatory mediators, such as lysolecithin and prostaglandins, and mucosal damage by concentrated bile, cholesterol, or gallstones may also contribute to mucosal injury.[47] Trauma to the mucosa caused by stones may release phospholipase from lysosomes that normally reside in mucosal epithelial cells. This enzyme converts lecithin to lysolecithin, an active detergent that is toxic to the mucosa.[48] Phospholipids can damage biliary cells. Bile from patients with gallstones contains lysophosphatidylcholine, which induces mucosal necrosis and inflammation of the gallbladder.[38]

When bile cultures are obtained within 48 hours of onset, bacteria are identified in 42% to 72% of cases. The predominant organisms are *E. coli*, other gram-negative aerobic rods, enterococci, and anaerobes (20% of cases).[49,50] Most authorities agree that infection is a secondary, and not the principal, etiological factor of acute cholecystitis.

Pathological Features

Acute cholecystitis may be identified at the time of laparoscopy or laparotomy by gross visualization of signs of acute inflammation, such as omental adhesions to the gallbladder wall, edema, friability, pericholecystic fluid, and frank gangrene. The gallbladder is usually enlarged and the wall thickened by edema, vascular congestion, and hemorrhage, or it may appear necrotic (Fig. 38.2). The serosa is usually dull and often covered by patches of fibrinopurulent exudate. A gallstone is frequently found obstructing the lumen of the cystic duct. Pus may fill the lumen, and it may be mixed with thick, cloudy bile. Depending on the severity of the inflammatory response, mucosal changes range from edema and congestion to widespread ulcers and necrosis.

Histological evaluation invariably identifies ischemic changes, which may be the predominant findings. An acute inflammatory reaction, characterized by edema, vascular congestion, hemorrhage, neutrophilic infiltration, and mucosal necrosis, predominates in specimens obtained early in the course of disease (Fig. 38.3). In the early phases, the inflammatory and necrotic changes are confined to the mucosa. As the pathological process evolves, transmural inflammation, secondary acute vasculitis, and transmural necrosis follow. Fibrinous pseudomembranes (i.e., pseudomembranous cholecystitis) may develop over necrotic-appearing mucosa (Fig. 38.4). After the first week, lymphocytes, plasma cells, macrophages, and eosinophils appear. Granulation tissue and collagen then replace previously ulcerated or necrotic tissue.

Gangrenous cholecystitis is a severe form of acute cholecystitis that occurs most frequently in patients with other comorbidities such as cardiovascular disease, diabetes, and trauma. The gallbladder is characteristically distended and

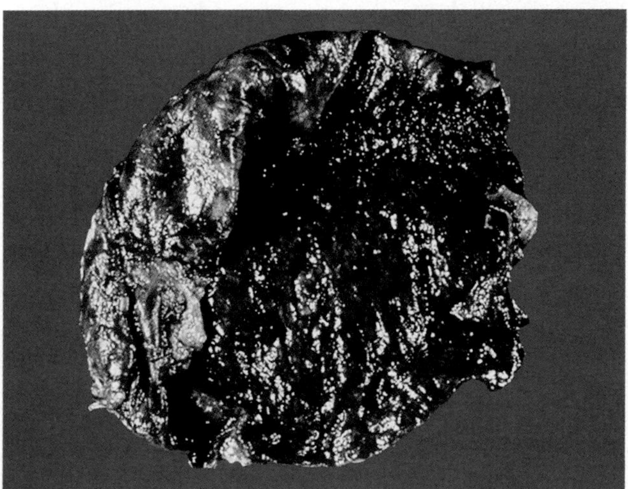

FIGURE 38.2 Acute gangrenous cholecystitis. The gallbladder is distended and contains numerous stones. The mucosa has a necrotic and hemorrhagic appearance.

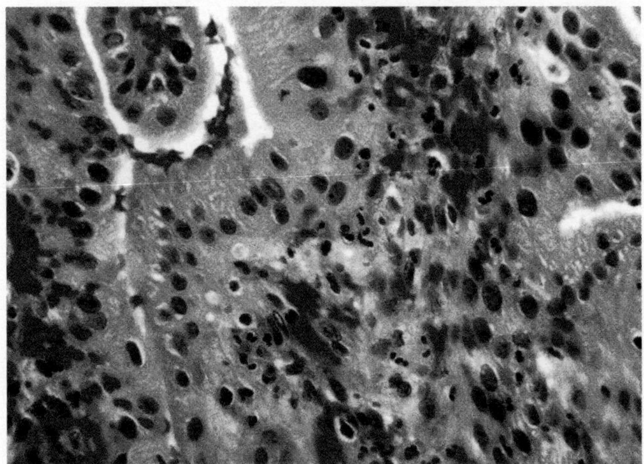

FIGURE 38.3 In the early phases of acute cholecystitis, neutrophils predominate, and the lamina propria is frequently hemorrhagic.

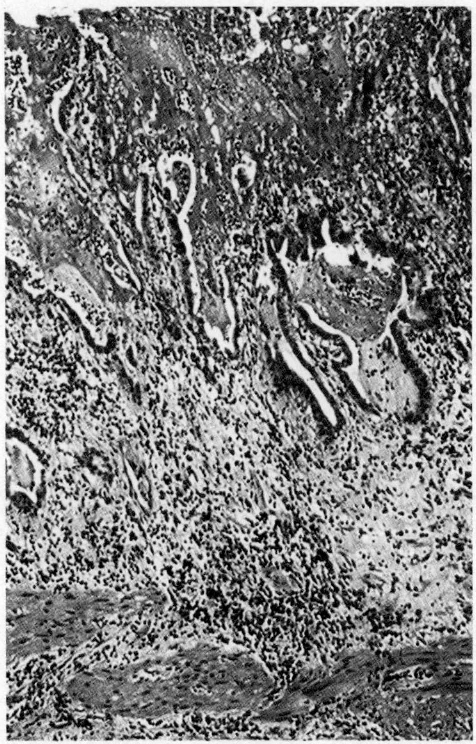

FIGURE 38.4 In acute pseudomembranous cholecystitis, thick, fibrinous pseudomembranes are firmly attached to necrotic biliary epithelium and appear to merge with the underlying edematous and inflamed lamina propria.

has a hemorrhagic to black-colored wall indicative of ischemia. Histologically, the mucosa and muscularis often are absent and replaced by necrotic debris, neutrophils, and granulation tissue.

Areas of perforation are commonly sealed off by the omentum, inducing formation of pericholecystic adhesions or abscesses. Severe complications include life-threatening bacteremia and sepsis.[44] Correlation between the pathophysiological events leading to acute cholecystitis and the pathological patterns of injury are summarized in Table 38.2.

TABLE 38.2 Pathophysiological and Pathological Manifestations of Acute Cholecystitis

Cause	Mechanism of Injury	Type of Injury
Obstruction of the outflow tract and/or compression of the cystic artery by a gallstone	Distention of the gallbladder	Ischemic necrosis
Mechanical and inflammatory injury to biliary cells	Formation of inflammatory mediators and chemical injury by detergents	Mucosal injury or necrosis and inflammation
Secondary bacterial infection	Inflammatory response	Mucosal injury or necrosis and inflammation

Natural History and Treatment

Most patients treated medically have symptomatic remission within a few days. Cholecystectomy is the treatment of choice for patients with complications. Because most patients with acute cholecystitis experience at least one recurrence, surgical treatment is recommended for all patients whenever possible. Cholecystectomy should be performed preferably within 2 to 3 days of the onset of symptoms, a time frame that is referred to as the "golden period."[51,52] After inflammation has persisted for more than 72 hours, the development of fibrous adhesions and transmural inflammation makes surgery more laborious and prone to complications.

Acute Acalculous Cholecystitis

Clinical Features and Pathogenesis

Acute acalculous cholecystitis occurs in approximately 2% to 15% of all patients who have undergone a cholecystectomy.[53,54] Affected individuals often have associated conditions, such as a history of trauma or a nonbiliary surgical procedure, sepsis, burns, parenteral nutrition, mechanical ventilation, multiple blood transfusions, or prior use of narcotics or antibiotics. However, this disorder may occur, de novo, in patients without any predisposing factors.[55] In these cases, the pathogenesis is probably multifactorial. Visceral hypoperfusion, ischemia, reperfusion injury, and bile stasis have all been postulated as possible mechanisms.[27]

Increased bile viscosity from stasis, with subsequent obstruction of the cystic duct, has been suggested as a contributing factor as well. It may help to explain the association of acalculous cholecystitis with a clinical history of fasting, narcotic use, dehydration, or recent anesthesia, all of which may result in bile stasis.

Mucosal ischemia plays a major role in patients with underlying cardiovascular disease and those who develop acute acalculous cholecystitis after trauma, sepsis, or a surgical procedure. There is a high mortality rate, as high as 45%, for this group of patients.

Prostanoid and bile salts may contribute to the development of acalculous cholecystitis. Prostaglandins are involved in gallbladder contraction, water absorption, inflammation, and pain associated with gallbladder disease. Prostaglandins have various roles in acute inflammatory conditions of the gallbladder. Prostaglandin E (PGE) levels correlate positively with the degree of inflammation. The levels of this prostaglandin are increased sevenfold in patients with acute acalculous cholecystitis. Tissue anoxia may result from shock, bacterial contamination and invasion, stasis, and changes in bile salt concentration, all of which can injure gallbladder mucosa. As a consequence, inflammation, distention, atonicity, and pain develop.[55,56]

In animal models, platelet-activating factor (PAF) plays a role in the induction of acute acalculous cholecystitis. PAF is released by basophils, eosinophils, neutrophils, macrophages, monocytes, mast cells, vascular endothelial cells, and smooth muscle cells. It increases vascular permeability and induces neutrophil aggregation and degranulation. Indirectly, PAF may cause acalculous cholecystitis by stimulating and releasing interleukin-1, tumor necrosis factor, and interleukin-6. PAF may also be associated with the development of arteriolar thrombosis and ischemia.[56]

Secondary infection of the gallbladder during sepsis may cause acute acalculous cholecystitis. This situation has been reported for patients with disseminated candidiasis, leptospirosis, chronic biliary tract carriage of typhoidal and nontyphoidal *Salmonella,* cholera, *Campylobacter* enteritis, tuberculosis, malaria, brucellosis, Q fever, and dengue fever. Hepatitis A and B and Epstein-Barr virus infections have been associated with this condition. Obstruction of extrahepatic bile ducts by ascariasis and echinococcal cysts also may cause acute acalculous cholecystitis.[57] This condition has also been described in patients with autoimmune disorders, such as lupus erythematosus.[58]

Acalculous cholecystitis is the most common form of cholecystitis in children. It accounts for 50% to 70% of all cases of cholecystitis in this age group. Dehydration, bacterial, viral, and parasitic infections, and immune-mediated disorders are the most frequent associated conditions.[59] Recently, acalculous cholecystitis has been reported in patients who have received immune checkpoint inhibitor therapy and in patients with COVID-19.[60,61] The gallbladder epithelial cells, and bile duct cells, express angiotensin-converting enzyme 2 receptor, which is also the receptor for the novel SARS-CoV-2 virus.[62]

Pathological Features

The gallbladder is frequently distended, and the serosa appears congested. The appearance of the mucosa varies from normal to hyperemic and necrotic. By definition, gallstones are absent.

Common histological features of acute acalculous cholecystitis include bile infiltration, leukocyte margination within blood vessels, neutrophilic and mononuclear cell infiltration of the lamina propria and biliary epithelium, edema, and lymphatic dilatation (Fig. 38.5). Compared with calculous cholecystitis, bile infiltration of the gallbladder is typically wider and deeper, as is the extent of necrosis of the muscularis.[27] Similarly to calculous cholecystitis, mucosal ischemic changes are frequently observed (Fig. 38.6). Ischemic changes are particularly prominent in postsurgical patients, and in those hospitalized for trauma or another type of critical illness.

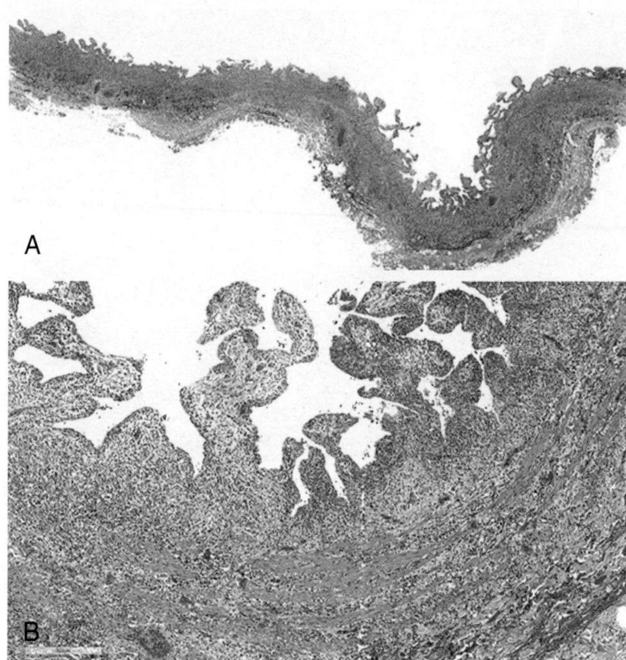

FIGURE 38.5 Five-year-old boy who developed acute acalculous cholecystitis following a viral-like illness. A, The gallbladder is slightly edematous and diffusely infiltrated by inflammatory cells. **B,** Dense mixed inflammatory cell infiltrate composed of lymphocytes, neutrophils, and plasma cells with injury to biliary cells.

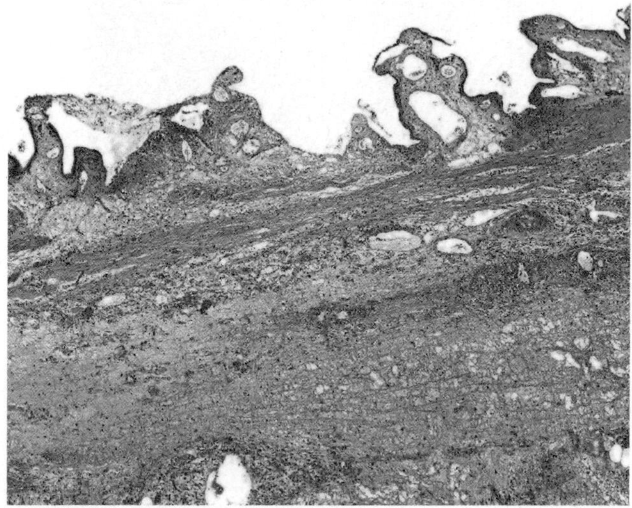

FIGURE 38.6 Acute acalculous cholecystitis is characterized by edema of the lamina propria, focal necrosis of the biliary epithelium, and lymphatic dilation. The muscularis is not thickened. The inflammatory process involves the pericystic tissues.

Specific histological differences between acute calculous cholecystitis and acalculous cholecystitis are lacking. A possible drug-induced injury should be suspected when there is a predominance of eosinophils within the lamina propria in the setting of acute cholecystitis.

Acute Emphysematous Cholecystitis

Clinical Features and Pathogenesis

Acute emphysematous cholecystitis is an uncommon variant of acute cholecystitis caused by bacterial infection with

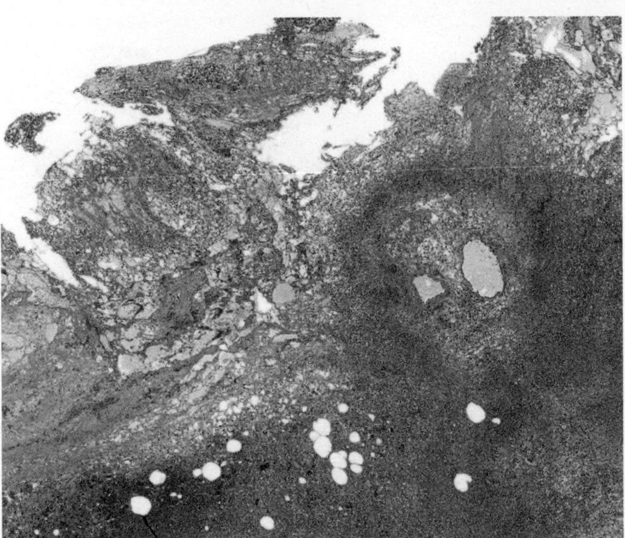

FIGURE 38.7 In acute emphysematous cholecystitis, transmural necrosis and inflammation are apparent. The empty spaces represent gas bubbles.

gas-producing organisms. Diabetic patients and those with peripheral atherosclerotic disease are at particular risk. The diagnosis is usually established with the use of radiographic studies. A computed tomography (CT) scan is the most sensitive method to demonstrate gas within the gallbladder lumen or wall. Diagnostic delay results in a high incidence of complications, such as gangrene and perforation, which explains the high overall mortality rate for patients with this condition (15% vs. 4.1% for acute calculous cholecystitis).

Approximately 50% of patients have a positive blood culture for clostridial organisms. Tests reveal *E. coli*, *Bacteroides fragilis*, *Klebsiella* species, and anaerobic streptococci infection in a lower percentage of patients.[63] Occlusion of the cystic artery or its branches, by atherosclerosis and small vessel disease (both frequent complications of diabetes mellitus), is a major contributing factor. Other ischemic events, such as arterial embolism, vasculitis, and systemic hypoperfusion, also predispose to this condition.[64-66]

Pathological Features

At the time of cholecystectomy, the gallbladder may appear distended, tense, or encased by omentum and may have fibrous adhesions or a pericholecystic abscess, or both. A necrotic, friable wall frequently is the cause of fragmentation of the gallbladder during an attempt at removal. On opening the gallbladder, gas and a foul-smelling purulent exudate may escape from the lumen. Gallstones, typically of the pigment type, are detected in 70% of cases. The mucosa usually appears necrotic, congested, and hemorrhagic.

Microscopically, necrotic and acutely inflamed mucosa often contains colonies of gram-positive bacilli. The inflammatory infiltrate is composed predominantly of neutrophils admixed with necrotic debris. Inflammation of the mural and blood vessels, which can include fibrinous necrosis of the wall, is common and should not be interpreted as a primary vasculitis. Gas bubbles occasionally occur within the wall of the gallbladder or subserosal connective tissue. Perforation and bile peritonitis occur in approximately 10% of cases (Fig. 38.7).

Chronic Cholecystitis

Chronic Calculous Cholecystitis

Clinical Features and Pathogenesis

Chronic cholecystitis is better defined by its gross and histological features than by its clinical characteristics. There is uncertainty regarding symptoms associated with gallstone disease and chronic cholecystitis. Most patients with gallstones never experience attacks of pain. In some cases, the only symptom related to gallstones may be episodic, mild upper abdominal pain.[67] Dyspeptic symptoms, belching, bloating, abdominal discomfort, heartburn, and food intolerances are frequently attributed, by patients and physicians, to cholelithiasis and chronic cholecystitis. However, most of these symptoms are probably unrelated to gallstone disease, and some persist after cholecystectomy. Because chronic cholecystitis typically is associated with cholelithiasis, the demographic characteristics of these patients, and risk factors, are the same as for patients with cholesterol gallstones.

The most common symptom is episodic, nonintermittent abdominal pain (erroneously referred to as biliary colic) that is typically located in the epigastrium or right upper quadrant. Pain may be precipitated by ingestion of food, but in most instances, it occurs spontaneously without an inciting event. On physical examination, mild to moderate tenderness may be elicited when palpating the gallbladder, particularly during a pain attack. Ultrasound examination of the gallbladder is the method of choice to demonstrate stones and abnormalities in the gallbladder wall resulting from inflammation or fibrosis, or both.

Chronic cholecystitis typically is associated with gallstones. The pathogenesis of this common disorder is poorly understood. It has been suggested that chronic cholecystitis results from recurrent attacks of mild acute cholecystitis, but few patients provide a clinical history that supports this hypothesis. The inflammatory and reparative changes may be explained in part by repetitive mucosal trauma and inflammation produced by gallstones, although other factors likely play a role as well.

Because of poor correlation between the severity of the inflammatory response and the number and volume of stones, it is possible that the intensity of the inflammatory response induced by gallstones in different populations is genetically determined.[68] One hypothesis is that a copious inflammatory response provides a protective effect in some patient populations whose ancestors resided in geographic areas with a high incidence of parasitic biliary infections.

Some scientists have postulated that cholelithiasis and chronic cholecystitis are caused by an abnormal composition of bile, which leads to stone formation and chemical injury to the mucosa. At variance with a high percentage of positive bile cultures for patients with acute cholecystitis is that bacteria, mostly *E. coli* and enterococci, are cultured in less than one-third of cases of chronic cholecystitis.[69] DNA from *Helicobacter* species has been identified in biliary tract specimens from patients with cholecystitis.[70,71] However, this association has not been confirmed in all studies.[72]

Pathological Features

In chronic cholecystitis, the varied appearance of the gallbladder reflects the degree of inflammation and fibrosis.

The gallbladder may be distended or shrunken and atrophic. Fibrous serosal adhesions suggest previous episodes of acute cholecystitis. On gross examination, the wall is usually thickened, but it may be thin in some cases. The mucosa may be intact with preservation or accentuation of its folds, or it may be flattened with outflow obstruction. Mucosal erosions or ulcers are frequently associated with impacted stones (Fig. 38.8).

The presence of gallstones is neither necessary nor sufficient for a diagnosis of chronic cholecystitis. The diagnosis is based on three major histological characteristics: a predominantly mononuclear inflammatory infiltrate in the lamina propria, either with or without extension into the muscularis and pericholecystic tissues, fibrosis, and metaplastic changes. The degree of inflammation varies. The infiltrate may be located exclusively in the mucosa, or it may extend into the muscularis and serosa. The inflammatory infiltrate may be distributed focally or diffusely. More commonly, lymphocytes predominate over plasma cells and histiocytes. Sparse, focally distributed lymphoid cells may be found in normal gallbladders obtained from healthy individuals who have died of trauma and whose livers were used for transplantation[73] (Fig. 38.9). Occasionally, lymphoid follicles arise in a background of chronic inflammation. Most lymphoid follicles are located in the lamina propria, but they may be identified within the gallbladder wall as well. When abundant, the term *follicular cholecystitis* has been used to describe this condition[74] (Fig. 38.10). In fact, a recent study has shown that this histological pattern is strongly associated with extrahepatic biliary obstruction distal to the gallbladder.[75] A minor component of eosinophils and neutrophils may also be present. When neutrophils are found predominantly within the epithelium in the setting of chronic cholecystitis, the disorder should be termed *chronic active cholecystitis* rather than *mixed acute and chronic cholecystitis* or *subacute cholecystitis* (Fig. 38.11).

When bile penetrates into the subepithelial mesenchyme through mucosal ulcers or fissures, it frequently elicits an inflammatory reaction composed of closely packed histiocytes with pale cytoplasm containing abundant brown-pigmented granules (Fig. 38.12). In addition to its color, the ceroid pigment is characterized histochemically by

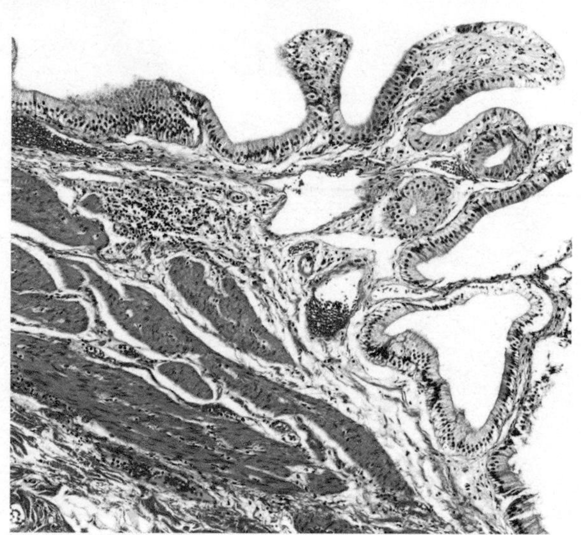

FIGURE 38.9 Focal lymphoid aggregates in the lamina propria *(left)* are frequently seen in normal gallbladders excised from the livers of donors who died of traumatic injuries.

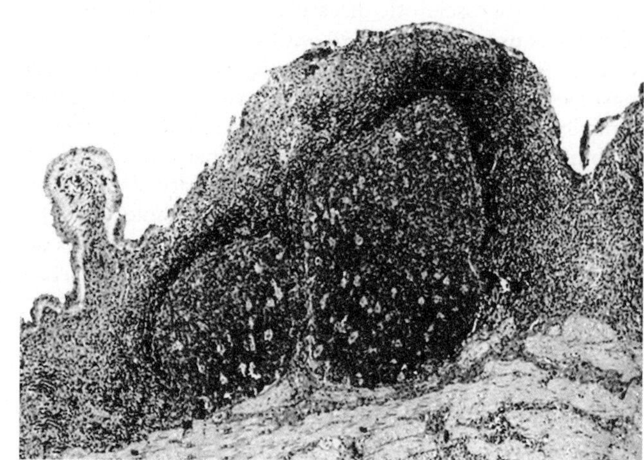

FIGURE 38.10 Reactive lymphoid follicles with prominent germinal centers characterize chronic follicular cholecystitis.

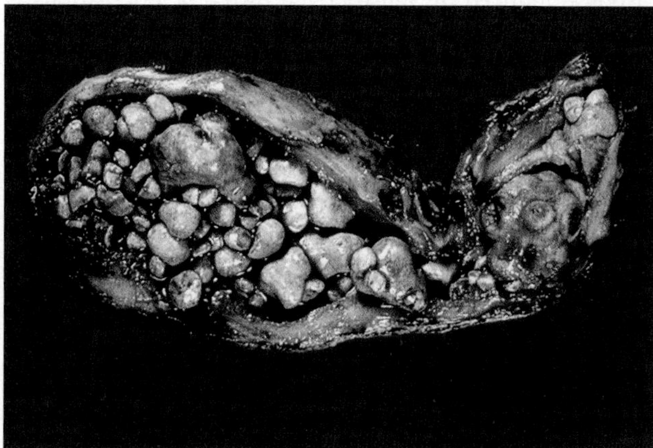

FIGURE 38.8 In a case of chronic calculous cholecystitis, the wall of the gallbladder is thickened, and the lumen contains innumerable cholesterol stones.

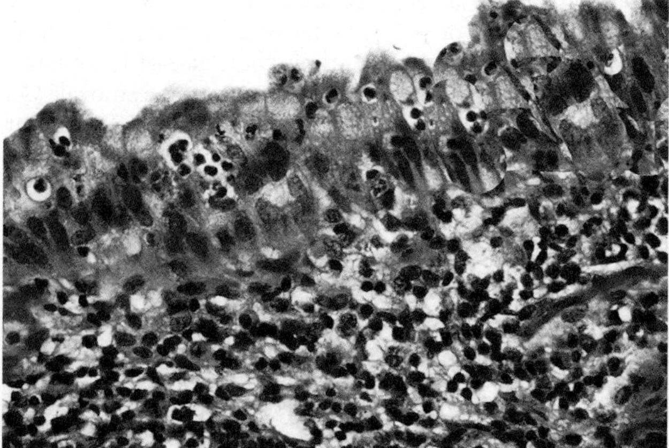

FIGURE 38.11 The dense lymphoplasmacytic infiltrate in the lamina propria defines this as chronic active cholecystitis. Intraepithelial neutrophils are the hallmark of activity.

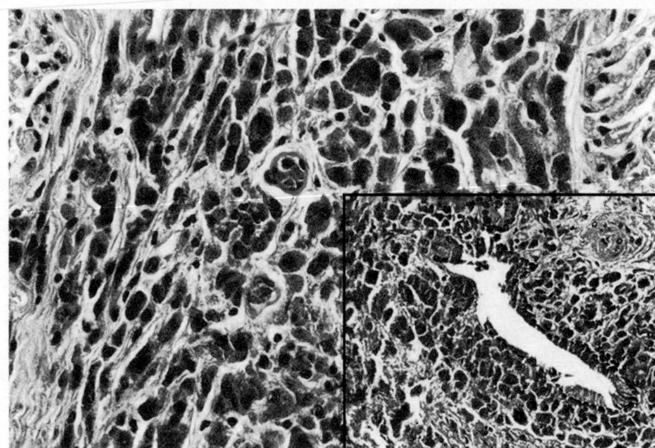

FIGURE 38.12 Ceroid granulomas, which are aggregates of histiocytes with pale cytoplasm containing dusky-brown–pigmented granules, are frequently encountered. They result from penetration of bile into the lamina propria. Ceroid granuloma surrounding Rokitansky-Aschoff sinus *(inset)*.

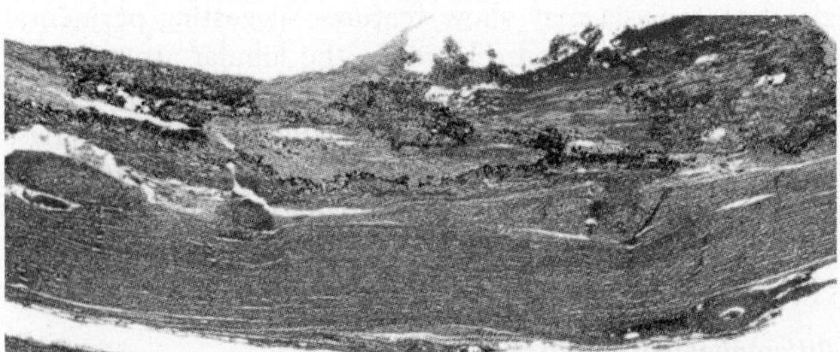

FIGURE 38.13 In hyalinizing chronic cholecystitis, dense, fibrous tissue with sparse inflammation and dystrophic calcifications replace the gallbladder wall.

acid fastness and diastase-resistant periodic acid–Schiff (PAS) positivity. A sparse lymphocytic reaction usually accompanies the histiocytes.[76] Ceroid granulomas trigger a reparative response that often leads to deposition of dense collagen. Fibrosis eventually replaces areas previously involved by the inflammatory process and may replace the entire gallbladder. Dystrophic calcifications are often associated with this fibrous reaction, and when diffuse, they may produce a *porcelain gallbladder*. Although previously thought to be associated with a higher incidence of carcinoma than other forms of cholecystitis,[77] not all studies support this contention.[78]

The term *hyalinizing cholecystitis* has been proposed for a type of chronic cholecystitis characterized by the presence of dense hyaline fibrosis, with relatively sparse inflammation, that transforms the gallbladder wall into a thin, uniform shell. Various degrees of dystrophic calcification are often identified. This type of cholecystitis is thought to be associated with a higher incidence of carcinoma, particularly in cases with scant or no calcifications[79] (Fig. 38.13).

In addition to ceroid granulomas, foreign body–type granulomas, characterized by aggregates of multinucleated giant cells and foamy histiocytes, may be present around clefts that contain cholesterol crystals or concretions of bile. Foamy histiocytes are predominant in xanthogranulomas, which are associated with plasma cells, giant cells,

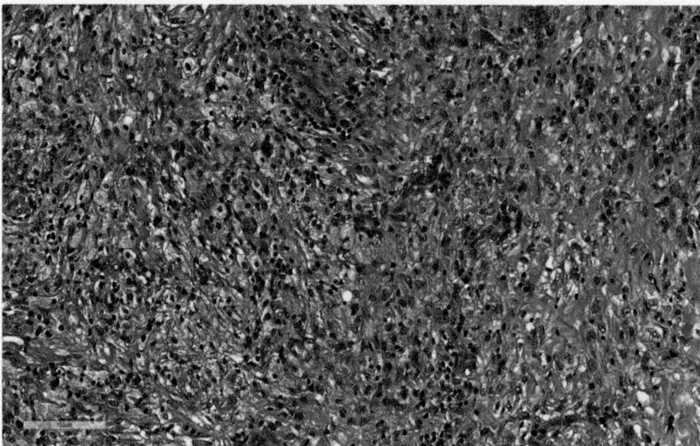

FIGURE 38.14 In addition to the characteristic aggregates of foamy macrophages that are typical of xanthogranulomas, plasma cells and various degrees of fibrosis are common.

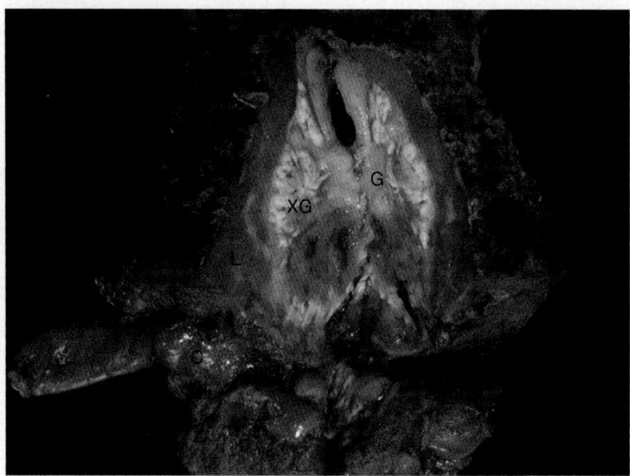

FIGURE 38.15 Xanthogranulomatous cholecystitis. The gallbladder (G) wall is replaced by a firm, yellow tissue (XG) that extends into the hepatic bed (L) and adjacent colon (C).

or ceroid-containing histiocytes (Fig. 38.14). The cells can form a tumor-like aggregate that may be confused with a neoplasm (i.e., xanthogranulomatous cholecystitis)[80-83] (Fig. 38.15). A granulomatous reaction caused by infection rarely occurs in the gallbladder (Fig. 38.16).

Rokitansky-Aschoff sinuses are pathological herniations of the mucosa either into, or through, the muscularis, analogous to intestinal diverticula (i.e., pseudodiverticula) (Fig. 38.17). They form in response to increased intraluminal pressure and are commonly associated with hypertrophic muscularis. In the absence of other features of chronic cholecystitis (i.e., inflammation or metaplastic changes), their occurrence is not considered sufficient to diagnose chronic cholecystitis. They are, in fact, a type of *mucosal herniation*, which is a consequence of outflow obstruction that is most frequently caused by gallstones. Rokitansky-Aschoff sinuses may be the only pathological change detected in patients with biliary dyskinesia, a condition that is not normally associated with gallstones.[73]

As in other organ systems, chronic injury to the gallbladder mucosa may cause a variety of metaplastic changes.[84-87] The most common type of metaplasia—antral or pyloric metaplasia—is characterized by the presence of tubular-shaped

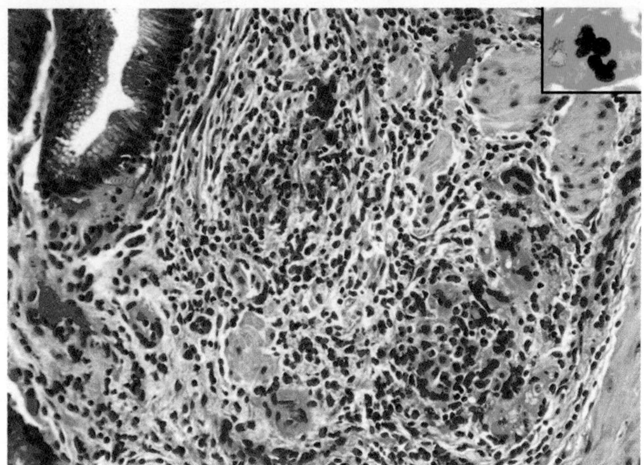

FIGURE 38.16 In granulomatous cholecystitis, the granulomas are composed of epithelioid histiocytes, giant cells, lymphocytes, and numerous eosinophils. *Inset*, Silver stains demonstrated fungal elements. Cultures were positive for *Trichophyton* species.

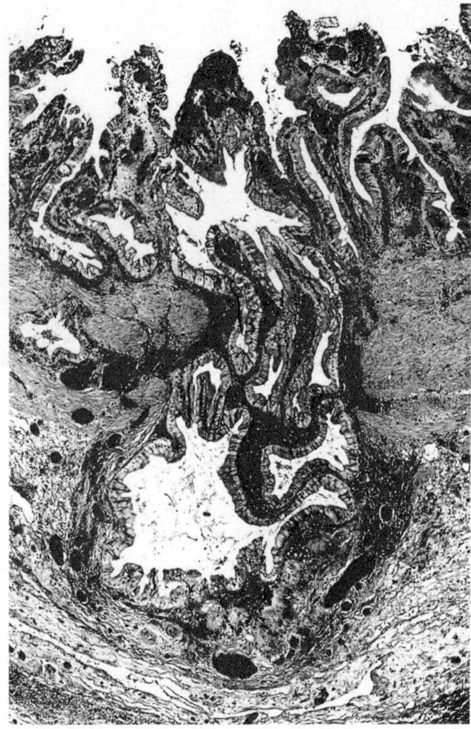

FIGURE 38.17 Rokitansky-Aschoff sinuses are herniations of the mucosa through the discontinuous muscle bundles of the muscularis of the gallbladder. A consequence of increased intraluminal pressure, the herniations are commonly seen when there is obstruction of the outflow tract, which in most instances is caused by gallstones.

glands in the lamina propria composed of clear cells with abundant mucin vacuoles. The glands are similar to those in the gastric antrum (Fig. 38.18). The surface epithelium frequently undergoes mucinous columnar metaplasia of the gastric type. This change is characterized by focal or diffuse replacement of the columnar epithelium of the gallbladder by tall, mucin-rich, PAS-positive columnar cells. When metaplastic pyloric glands proliferate and permeate smooth muscle fibers, their histological appearance may

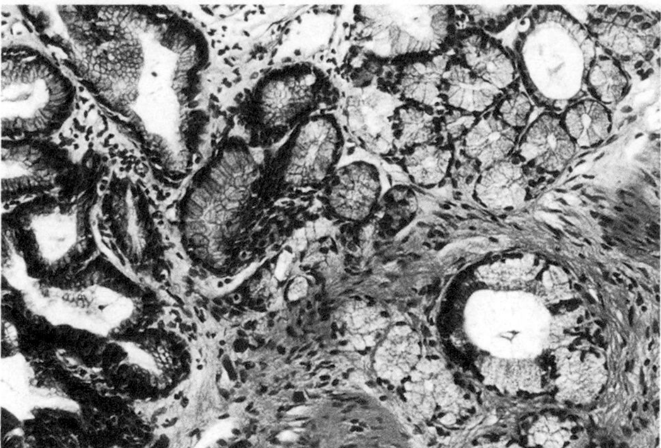

FIGURE 38.18 Antral metaplasia is composed of mucin-secreting antral-type glands, and it is the most common type of metaplasia encountered in cholecystectomy specimens from patients with chronic calculous cholecystitis.

be confused with an adenocarcinoma. Rarely, florid pyloric gland metaplasia may show features suggesting perineural or intraneural invasion. However, the lobular arrangement of the glands combined with the bland cytological features helps distinguish this reaction from adenocarcinoma.[87] Less frequently, intestinal metaplasia may occur. It is identified as epithelium with an intestinal phenotype containing goblet cells, absorptive columnar cells, Paneth cells, and endocrine cells. Infrequently, squamous metaplasia may develop.

Differential Diagnosis

The differential diagnosis of invasive well-differentiated adenocarcinoma of the gallbladder and reactive atypia is summarized in Table 38.3. Dysplasia involving Rokitansky-Aschoff sinuses may also mimic invasive adenocarcinoma. Rokitansky-Aschoff sinuses usually have a perpendicular orientation to the surface, whereas adenocarcinoma glands proliferate haphazardly, are more abundant, and are frequently oriented parallel to the mucosa (Fig. 38.19). Although the finding of desmoplasia supports a malignant process, dense fibrosis is common in the stroma surrounding inflamed Rokitansky-Aschoff sinuses (Fig. 38.20). Cytological atypia and mitoses favor a malignant tumor. Immunostains for p53 and Ki-67 are of little value in making this distinction.

Treatment

In the United States, laparoscopic cholecystectomy has become the preferred method of treatment for patients with cholelithiasis.[88-90] The minimally invasive surgical procedure offers the advantage of shorter hospitalization, limited postoperative pain, diminished disability, and improved cosmesis. In most instances, the gallbladder is easily removed through the umbilical puncture wound, although difficulties may arise when either bile or gallstones distend the gallbladder or when inflammation and fibrosis give rise to a thick, noncollapsible wall. This problem is usually solved by extending the umbilical incision or by removing bile and stones after the neck of the gallbladder has been pulled through the skin and amputated. Mechanical devices, ultrasound, or laser energy may be used to pulverize large stones.[90]

TABLE 38.3 Differential Diagnosis between Rokitansky-Aschoff Sinuses with Atypia and Well-Differentiated Adenocarcinoma

Feature	RAS with Reactive Atypia	Well-Differentiated Adenocarcinoma
Orientation of the glands	Perpendicular to surface	Frequently parallel to surface
Glandular crowding	Usually absent	Often present
Glands adjacent to muscular vessels	Usually absent	May be present
Glandular necrotic debris	Absent	May be present
Dysplastic epithelium in the mucosa	Usually absent*	Frequently present
Presence of luminal bile	May be present	Absent
Inflammatory cells	Frequently present	Usually absent
Intravascular invasion	Absent	May be present
Perineural invasion	Absent†	May be present
Nuclear pleomorphism	Absent	Present, may be mild
Immunolabeling for CEA	Usually absent	May be present
Loss of DPC4 nuclear staining	Absent	Present in one half of cases

CEA, *Carcinoembryonic antigen;* DPC4, *mediator of intracellular signaling, with loss associated with a poor prognosis;* RAS, *Rokitansky-Aschoff sinuses.*

**Dysplastic epithelium may extend into the RAS and should not be interpreted as representing invasive carcinoma.*

†Although perineural invasion is not seen in relation to RAS, it may occur in chronic cholecystitis with extensive pyloric metaplasia and should not be interpreted as unequivocal evidence of malignancy.

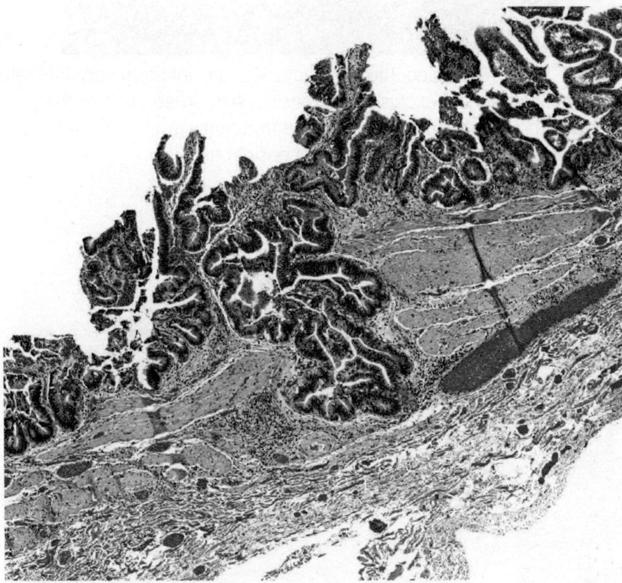

FIGURE 38.19 Rokitansky-Aschoff sinuses with dysplastic epithelium. The perpendicular orientation of the sinuses to the lumen help to differentiate this condition from invasive adenocarcinoma, even in sections in which the connection to the lumen is not apparent.

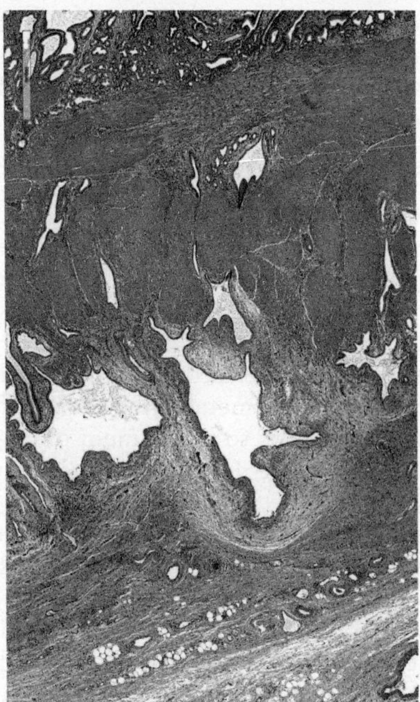

FIGURE 38.20 Fibrosis surrounding Rokitansky-Aschoff sinuses is a common finding and should not be confused with tumor desmoplasia.

Chronic Acalculous Cholecystitis

Approximately 12% to 13% of patients with chronic cholecystitis do not have gallstones.[91] In some instances, the inflammation is a consequence of postinflammatory stenosis or anatomic abnormalities of the cystic duct that may impede normal emptying of the gallbladder. Other patients with biliary symptoms do not show gallstones in imaging studies. The type of disorders associated with this condition varies. In some patients, the disease may be confined to the gallbladder, but in others, it may be a manifestation of a generalized extrahepatic bile duct disorder. Although the inflammatory pattern in some patients with chronic acalculous cholecystitis is nonspecific, judicious analysis of the type of inflammatory cells, and their distribution in cholecystectomy specimens, may provide clues regarding the nature of the disease in others. Three histological patterns of chronic acalculous cholecystitis have recently been described (see later). These include lymphoeosinophilic and eosinophilic cholecystitis, diffuse lymphoplasmacytic acalculous cholecystitis, and lymphocytic cholecystitis.

Some patients have a dysmotility disorder of the gallbladder known as *biliary dyskinesia*. Patients who may benefit from cholecystectomy are identified by a cholecystokinin provocation test. A positive test result consists of reproduction of pain within 5 to 10 minutes after an intravenous injection of cholecystokinin.[92,93] Incomplete emptying of the gallbladder can be documented when this test is performed at the same time as oral cholecystography.

At the time of surgery, a normal, distended, or thickened gallbladder may be found. Microscopic examination may be unremarkable or demonstrate changes consistent with outflow obstruction or inflammation, or both. Rokitansky-Aschoff sinuses and thickening of the muscularis propria are characteristic features of outflow obstruction. Gallbladders excised from patients with biliary dyskinesia may show abundant Rokitansky-Aschoff sinuses in the absence of inflammation[73] (Fig. 38.21). Other patients may have a normal-appearing gallbladder or nonspecific chronic cholecystitis.

Lymphoeosinophilic and Eosinophilic Cholecystitis

Inflammatory infiltrates in patients with acalculous cholecystitis typically contain a higher percentage of eosinophils than in patients with gallstones. Lymphoeosinophilic cholecystitis is diagnosed when eosinophils comprise more than 50% of the total number of inflammatory cells. It has been hypothesized that abnormal biliary contents or certain hepatic metabolites evoke a hypersensitivity reaction that leads to recruitment of large numbers of eosinophils that cause mucosal damage and gallbladder dysmotility.[94]

True eosinophilic cholecystitis is rare, and it is characterized histologically by an inflammatory infiltrate composed almost exclusively of eosinophils (Fig. 38.22). In this condition, eosinophilic infiltrates commonly involve the extrahepatic bile ducts in addition to the gallbladder. At presentation, these patients often have obstructive jaundice that mimics a neoplasm.[95] This disorder is discussed further under the heading of Eosinophilic Cholangitis.

Diffuse Lymphoplasmacytic Acalculous Cholecystitis

Some cases of chronic cholecystitis, which are characterized by diffuse lymphoplasmacytic infiltrates confined to the lamina propria either with or without active lesions (i.e., intramucosal neutrophilic infiltrates) (Fig. 38.23), occur in patients with extrahepatic bile duct obstruction.[96] In the absence of gallstones, this form of chronic cholecystitis was initially thought to be relatively specific for primary sclerosing cholangitis (PSC).[96] However, comparative studies that included controls with various types of extrahepatic bile duct obstruction, showed that diffuse lymphoplasmacytic acalculous chronic cholecystitis was specific for extrahepatic biliary tract disorders, but did not differentiate primary from secondary cholangiopathies.[97,98]

Acalculous cholecystitis with superficial or deep lymphoplasmacytic infiltrates has been described in patients with autoimmune pancreatitis.[99] As in the pancreas, there typically are numerous plasma cells that express immunoglobulin G4 (IgG4). This condition is discussed in further detail in the section Inflammatory Disorders of the Extrahepatic Bile Ducts.

Lymphocytic Cholecystitis

During the years, we have encountered four cases with a unique inflammatory pattern of cholecystitis characterized by an increased number of intraepithelial CD3-positive lymphocytes within biliary epithelium. All cases were accompanied by an inflammatory process within the lamina propria, similar to diffuse lymphoplasmacytic acalculous cholecystitis. The inflammatory changes primarily

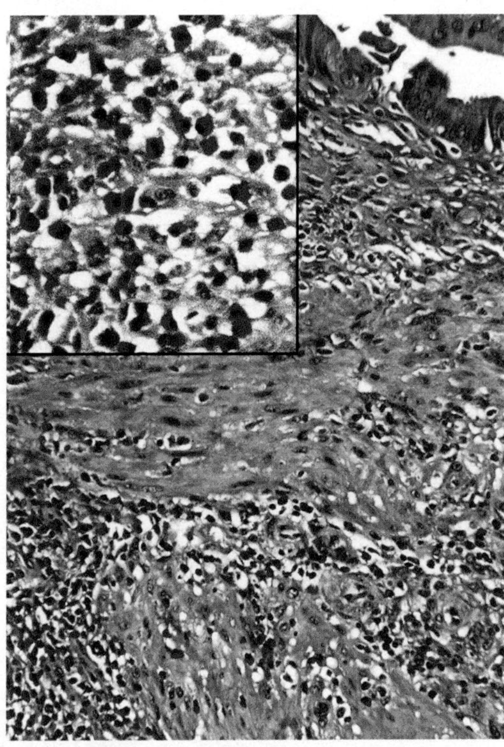

FIGURE 38.22 In eosinophilic cholecystitis, the inflammatory infiltrate is composed almost exclusively of eosinophils. In addition to the gallbladder, the extrahepatic bile ducts are frequently involved. *Inset*, High-power view shows a predominance of eosinophils.

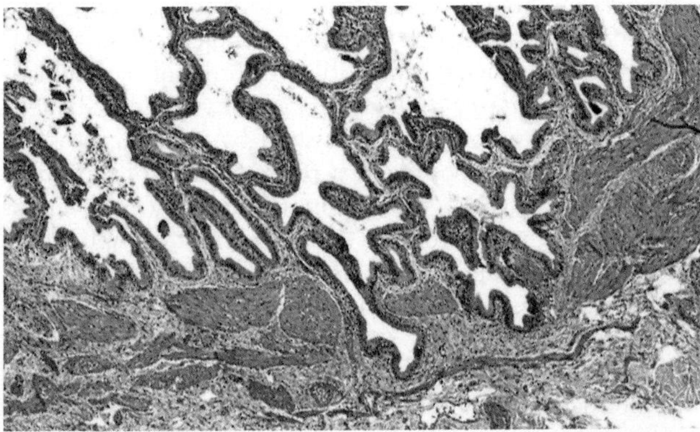

FIGURE 38.21 The formation of superficial and contiguous Rokitansky-Aschoff sinuses and the absence of inflammation are common features in gallbladder specimens from patients with biliary dyskinesia. Thickening of the muscularis develops in chronic cases as a consequence of functional outflow obstruction.

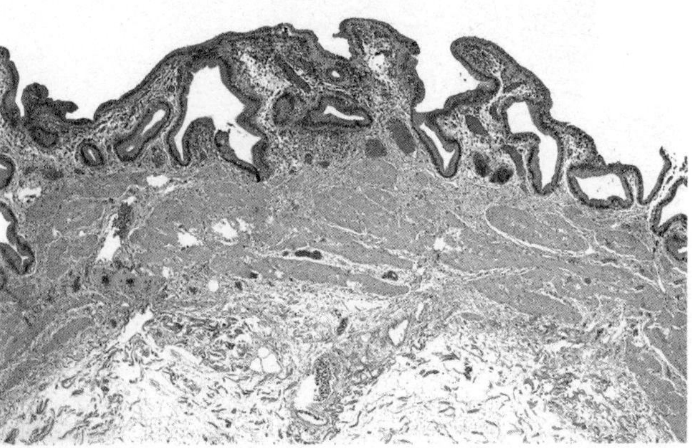

FIGURE 38.23 Cholecystitis in a patient with primary sclerosing cholangitis. The inflammatory infiltrate is confined to the mucosa, has a diffuse distribution, and is composed of plasma cells and lymphocytes.

affected the infundibulum and were associated with epithelial hyperplasia. Because of its resemblance to lymphocytic colitis or gastritis, we proposed the term *lymphocytic cholecystitis* for this condition. All patients were adults and none had cholelithiasis. In three patients, cholecystitis was the predominant disease. The other patient had other medical problems[100] (Fig. 38.24).

Xanthogranulomatous Cholecystitis

Xanthogranulomatous cholecystitis, an uncommon form of chronic cholecystitis, typically is associated with gallstones, and is frequently accompanied by at least some degree of fibrosis. The incidence ranges from 0.7% to 1.8% of excised gallbladders, although one study reported an incidence of 9.0% in Japan and India.[101-103]

The pathogenesis of this condition is uncertain. It has been proposed that xanthogranulomas form as a reaction to penetration of bile into the gallbladder wall from mucosal ulcers or ruptured Rokitansky-Aschoff sinuses in conjunction with outflow obstruction by calculi and infection.[103,104] Bile cultures are positive, mostly for enterobacteria, in about 50% of patients.

Xanthogranulomatous cholecystitis may be difficult to distinguish from other forms of cholecystitis clinically. However, in contrast to chronic cholecystitis, a history of at least one previous episode of acute cholecystitis is obtained from most patients. Some patients have a clinical picture that suggests acute cholecystitis. Imaging studies demonstrate a thickened wall. Gallstones are found in most patients.

This condition is confused clinically with carcinoma because the inflammatory process frequently extends to adjacent organs, and the serum CA 19-9 level may be elevated. Pathologically, the areas involved by the xanthogranulomatous process may appear as firm, yellow masses that resemble carcinoma clinically and macroscopically.

Histological examination shows round to spindle-shaped, lipid-laden macrophages, plasma cells, and fibrosis. Cholesterol clefts, foreign body– and Touton-type giant cells, and other types of inflammatory cells (i.e., lymphocytes, eosinophils, and neutrophils) are commonly found as well. Frequently, the xanthogranulomatous reaction occupies only a limited portion of the gallbladder, whereas the remainder shows conventional chronic cholecystitis, often with lymphoid follicles. Although abundant IgG4 plasma cells may be present in this condition, it should not be considered diagnostic of an IgG4-related disorder in the absence of other features such as storiform fibrosis or obliterative phlebitis. [105]

Xanthogranulomatous inflammation should be differentiated from malakoplakia. The characteristic microscopic findings of malakoplakia consist of a diffuse proliferation of histiocytes with abundant eosinophilic granular cytoplasm, some of which contain spherules (i.e., Michaelis-Gutmann bodies) that are positive for PAS and von Kossa (calcium) stains (Fig. 38.25).

FIGURE 38.24 In a specimen from a patient with lymphocytic cholecystitis, there are numerous intraepithelial lymphocytes, and the lamina propria shows lymphoplasmacytic inflammation. *Inset,* CD3 immunoperoxidase stain shows numerous positive cells.

Cholecystitis in Patients with Acquired Immunodeficiency Syndrome

Chronic acalculous cholecystitis may occur as a complication of human immunodeficiency virus (HIV) infection.[106-109] *Cryptosporidium* is the most common cause of acquired immunodeficiency syndrome (AIDS)–related infection of the extrahepatic bile ducts and gallbladder. This organism has been found in the bile ducts or stools in as many as 62% of patients with symptoms of AIDS-related cholangitis. *Cryptosporidium* colonizes, but does not invade, biliary epithelial cells and elicits an inflammatory response of variable intensity, but it is mostly mild in cases not associated with other organisms.

Cytomegalovirus (CMV) infection is the second most common type of infection in AIDS-related cholecystitis.

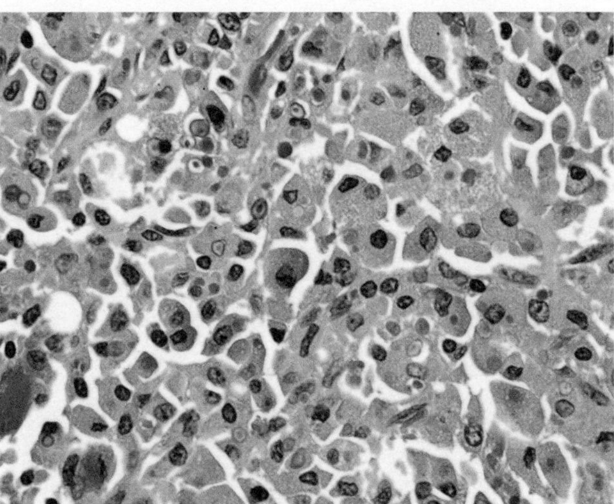

FIGURE 38.25 Characteristic findings of malakoplakia include a diffuse inflammatory cell infiltrate composed of epithelioid histiocytes, several of which contain intracytoplasmic calcified spherules (i.e., Michaelis-Gutmann bodies).

Biliary involvement develops in as many as 10% of AIDS patients with CMV.[106,107] CMV infection is associated with mucosal ulcers and mixed inflammatory infiltrates. Intranuclear and intracytoplasmic inclusions are found in endothelial and epithelial cells. Occasionally, CMV coexists with other infectious organisms in the same gallbladder (Fig. 38.26).

Rare instances of infection with *Mycobacterium avium-intracellulare* complex have been reported. The diffuse histiocytic proliferation in this condition may mimic xanthogranulomatous cholecystitis and malakoplakia. Other organisms in HIV patients that may involve the gallbladder include intracellular parasites of the Microsporida order, particularly *Enterocytozoon bieneusi*.[108]

Cystoisospora belli, formerly known as *Isospora belli*, has been reported in immunocompetent and immunosuppressed individuals in both the gallbladder and bile ducts.[110] However, recent studies based on ultrastructural observations have questioned the interpretation of intracytoplasmic structures in the gallbladder epithelium as *Cystoisospora*[111,112] (Fig. 38.27).

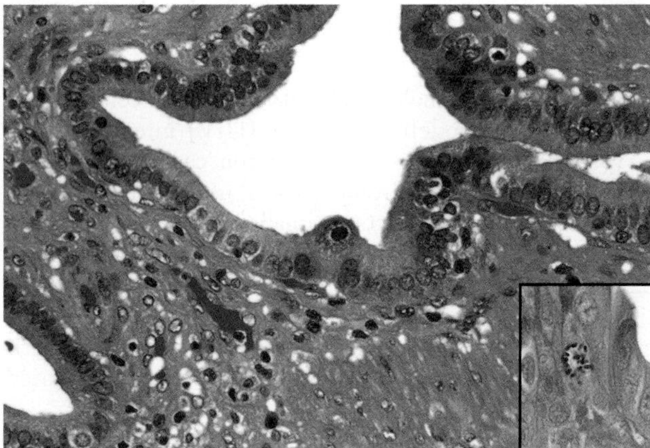

FIGURE 38.26 Cholecystitis in a patient with AIDS. Cytomegalovirus inclusion and microsporidiosis were identified in this gallbladder from a human immunodeficiency virus-infected patient. *Inset,* The sample with Brown-Brenn stain illustrates the importance of performing special stains to look for multiple causative agents, even when one of them is obvious on initial histological inspection.

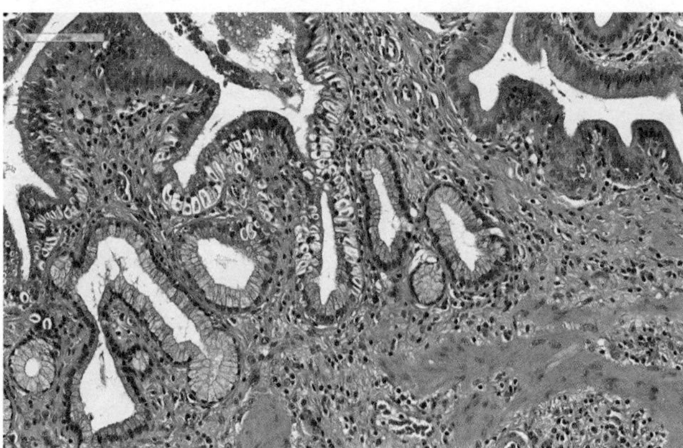

FIGURE 38.27 Epithelial inclusions representing aggregates of degenerating cytoplasmic structures simulating *Cystoisospora*.

PARASITIC INFESTATION

Infestation of the gallbladder with *Fasciola hepatica* and the liver flukes C. *sinensis* and O. *viverrini* causes chronic infection of the bile ducts and may cause acute acalculous cholecystitis. These organisms may induce an inflammatory response rich in lymphocytes and eosinophils, usually accompanied by hyperplasia of metaplastic pyloric-type glands. Granulomatous cholecystitis has been described in association with the ova of *Schistosoma mansoni*, *Paragonimus westermani*, and *A. lumbricoides*.[113]

POLYARTERITIS NODOSA AND OTHER TYPES OF VASCULITIS

Histological changes of classic polyarteritis nodosa may be detected in the gallbladder in two main clinical settings: in patients with isolated gallbladder involvement and in patients with systemic disease, such as scleroderma, systemic lupus erythematosus, or antiphospholipid syndrome.[114-116] The localized form of polyarteritis nodosa may, rarely, progress to systemic disease, especially in patients with serum autoantibodies (e.g., rheumatoid factor, antinuclear antibodies). Other forms of vasculitis include granulomatous vasculitis of the gallbladder in patients with Churg-Strauss syndrome or temporal giant cell arteritis. Rarely, idiopathic lymphocytic phlebitis may be confined to the gallbladder, which shows histological features similar to those reported in cases of idiopathic enterocolic lymphocytic phlebitis.[117,118] Lymphocytic vasculitis may be identified in patients with Behçet's disease as well (Fig. 38.28).

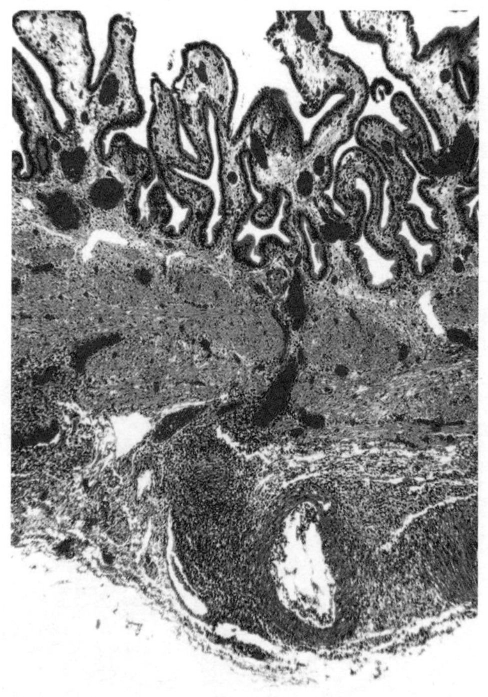

FIGURE 38.28 Lymphocytic phlebitis may be confined to the gallbladder, but venular lesions identical to the ones in the gallbladder were found in sections of the small bowel from a patient with Behçet's disease.

CHOLESTEROLOSIS

Cholesterolosis is characterized by aggregates of lipid-containing macrophages in the lamina propria of the gallbladder. Autopsy and surgical studies have demonstrated a prevalence rate of 12% and 9% to 26%, respectively.[119,120]

The cause and pathogenesis of cholesterolosis are poorly understood. Accumulation of cholesterol esters and triglycerides may reflect increased hepatic synthesis of lipids or an increased absorption and esterification by the gallbladder mucosa. The normal gallbladder absorbs free and nonesterified cholesterols from the bile. Cholesterol is esterified in the endoplasmic reticulum and forms lipid droplets that are released into the intercellular space, where they are phagocytized by macrophages.[121] Patients with cholesterolosis and patients with cholesterol stones have supersaturated bile; as expected, these conditions frequently coexist. Cholesterolosis likely results from increased cholesterol uptake from supersaturated bile.

Almost a century after the first description of this entity, the clinical relevance of cholesterolosis remains a subject of debate. Some studies have suggested that cholesterolosis is associated with symptoms in patients who have acalculous biliary disease, with colicky abdominal pain and selective food intolerance as the most common complaints. Some patients with biliary dyskinesia have cholesterolosis, in which case resolution of symptoms after is more likely caused by eradication of dyskinesia than removal of cholesterolosis. Evidence suggests a possible relationship between cholesterolosis and acute pancreatitis. Temporary impaction of cholesterolosis polyps at the sphincter of Oddi may produce recurrent attacks of acute pancreatitis.[122]

If the prevalence of cholesterolosis derived from autopsy studies reflects the frequency in the general population, symptoms do not develop in most individuals with cholesterolosis. One recent study did not find any association between cholesterolosis and elevated serum cholesterol, depressed ejection fraction, or an increased risk of pancreatitis.[123] A negative association between cholesterolosis and gallbladder carcinoma has been reported.[124]

On gross examination, lipid deposits appear as yellow flecks against a dark green background, earning the sobriquet *strawberry gallbladder.* When extensive, lipid deposits may form polypoid excrescences that project into the lumen. Commonly referred to as *cholesterol polyps*, but more properly called *polypoid cholesterolosis*, these lesions are usually small in size but may be large enough to be detected by radiological imaging. Cholesterol gallstones are associated with cholesterolosis in approximately 50% of surgical cases and 10% of autopsies (Fig. 38.29).

Microscopically, the diagnostic feature of cholesterolosis is accumulation of foamy macrophages within an expanded lamina propria, resulting in the development of thickened folds or polyps, or both (Fig. 38.30). The adjacent mucosa may be normal or inflamed. However, inflammation occurs almost exclusively in patients with coexistent stones.

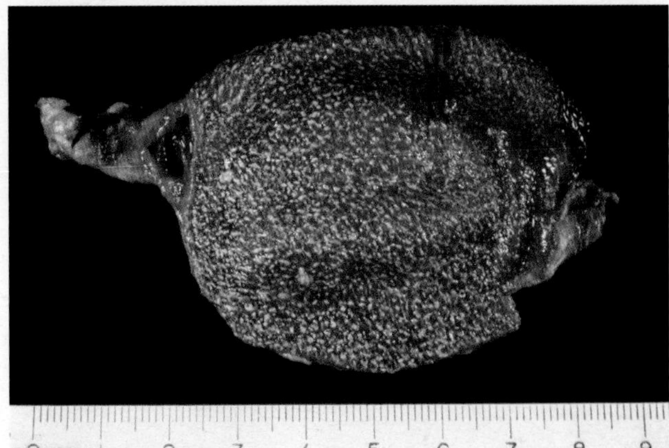

FIGURE 38.29 Strawberry gallbladder. The diffusely distributed yellow streaks characteristic of cholesterolosis have been compared by imaginative observers to strawberries.

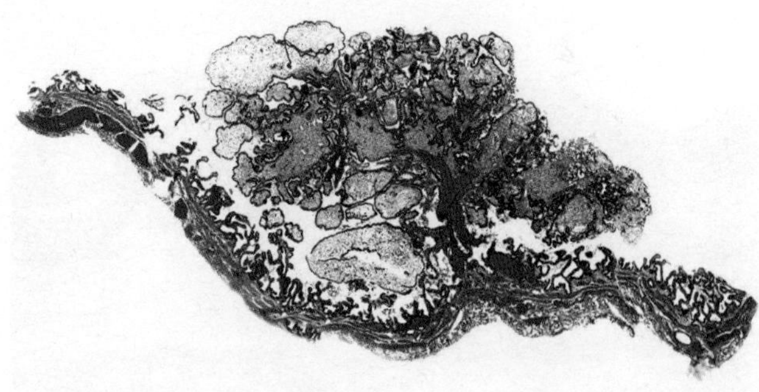

FIGURE 38.30 Polypoid cholesterolosis is characterized by abundant foamy macrophages within the lamina propria that form an intraluminal polyp.

HYDROPS AND MUCOCELE

Gallbladders distended by clear, watery fluid (i.e., hydrops) or mucus (i.e., mucocele) account for 3% of cholecystectomy specimens in adults.[125] In this age group, the most common cause is an impacted stone in the neck of the gallbladder or cystic duct. Less common causes include cystic fibrosis, tumors, fibrosis, kinking of the cystic duct, and external compression by an inflammatory or neoplastic mass. In children, these conditions are usually acute and associated with infectious or inflammatory disorders of unknown origin, such as streptococcal infection, mesenteric adenitis, typhoid, leptospirosis, viral hepatitis, familial Mediterranean fever, or Kawasaki's syndrome. Symptoms may resolve with conservative treatment.[124,125]

Hydropic gallbladders show considerable distention and may contain more than 1500 mL of fluid or inspissated mucin. When associated with numerous stones, the wall is usually thickened. The wall is usually thin when there is a single stone that obstructs the cystic duct or in acute childhood cases (Fig. 38.31). Microscopic examination usually reveals flattened mucosa lined by low columnar or cuboidal cells or metaplastic mucin-producing cells (Fig. 38.32). As a result of increased intraluminal pressure, Rokitansky-Aschoff sinuses may be plentiful. In some cases, mucin spills into the peritoneal cavity, simulating a mucinous adenocarcinoma. Inflammatory cells may be sparse or abundant. Acute cholecystitis, with edema of the lamina propria and abundant neutrophils, occurs in some patients with Kawasaki's syndrome.[126]

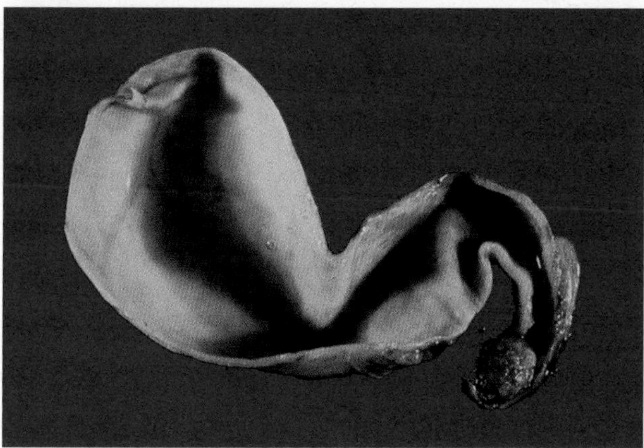

FIGURE 38.31 The gallbladder is distended and displays a smooth mucosa. The cystic duct is obstructed by a gallstone.

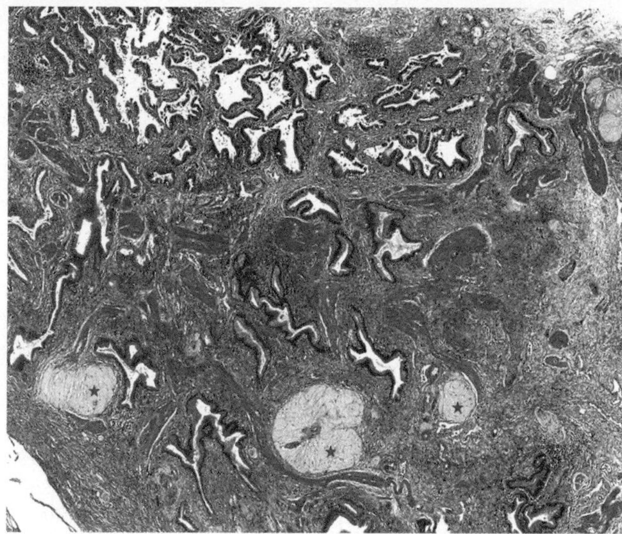

FIGURE 38.33 Adenomyomatous hyperplasia. Mucosal herniations representing Rokitansky-Aschoff sinuses are intermixed with hyperplastic muscle derived from the muscularis. Mucosal entrapment may give rise to "mucin pools" *(stars).*

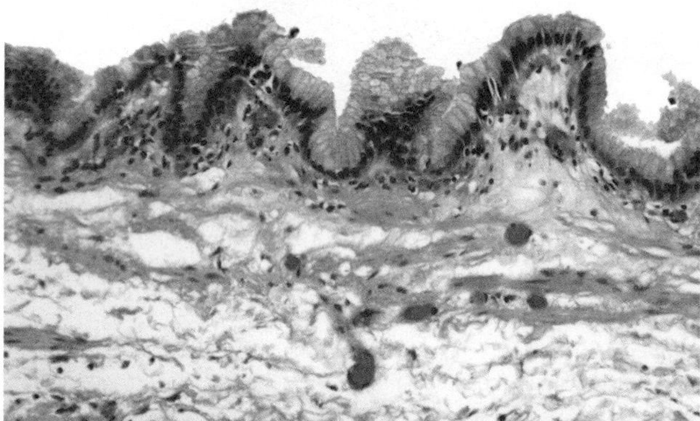

FIGURE 38.32 Mucocele: the biliary cells are replaced by metaplastic mucin-producing cells.

DIVERTICULAR DISEASE

Congenital and traction diverticula are the two types of "true" diverticula that occur in the gallbladder. Congenital lesions are discussed in Chapter 37. Constituents of the wall of diverticula differentiate them from the more common acquired pseudodiverticula. True diverticula contain all elements of the normal gallbladder wall, whereas pseudodiverticula contain little or no smooth muscle.

Traction diverticula are caused by the pulling action of postinflammatory fibrous adhesions, which anchors the serosa of the gallbladder to adjacent structures. Erosion by stones, healing fistulas, widespread peritonitis of any cause, or previous intraabdominal surgery precede their formation. Traction diverticula are distinguished from congenital outpouchings principally by their relationship with other intraabdominal lesions in the vicinity of the gallbladder and by the predominance of serosal (rather than mucosal) inflammation and fibrosis. In some cases, however, distinction between the two types of true diverticula may be impossible.

Acquired pseudodiverticula are mucosal herniations within the smooth muscle of the gallbladder wall that should be regarded as prominent Rokitansky-Aschoff sinuses. Acquired pulsion diverticula typically are associated with stones and chronic cholecystitis or with outflow obstruction. Analogous to diverticular disease of the colon, the intervening smooth muscle is usually hypertrophic. The mucosal outpouchings combined with prominent smooth muscle hypertrophy/hyperplasia may form a localized tumor-like lesion commonly referred to as *adenomyoma* (i.e., localized adenomyomatous hyperplasia), or it may diffusely thicken the gallbladder wall (i.e., diffuse adenomyomatous hyperplasia)[127,128] (Fig. 38.33). The epithelial lining of mucosal herniations is usually normal, but it may rarely have gastric foveolar metaplasia or dysplastic or neoplastic changes. Perineural involvement has rarely been observed in cases of adenomyomatous hyperplasia and should not be confused with adenocarcinoma.[86]

ISCHEMIC DISEASES

Deprivation of arterial blood flow or obstruction to venous drainage may result in infarction of the gallbladder. Atherosclerosis and thrombosis are the usual causes of deficiency of arterial blood flow. Emboli may occur as a complication of valvular heart disease or bacterial endocarditis. Rarely, dissecting aneurysms may extend into the celiac artery, occluding the origin of the hepatic artery. External compression of the arteries or interference of the venous drainage may result from impingement on blood vessels by gallstones or tumors, or iatrogenic injury may be caused by surgical ligation.[129]

Gallbladders with a high degree of mobility (i.e., floating gallbladders) may twist on their pedicle and cause torsion or volvulus. Floating gallbladders lack a firm attachment to the liver and are completely surrounded by peritoneum (see Congenital Abnormalities in Chapter 9). Torsion in developmentally normal gallbladders may also result from loosening of the suspensory connective tissue, as in normal aging, or from shrinkage of the liver (i.e., cirrhosis), leading to detachment of the gallbladder from its bed and visceroptosis.[124] Ischemic disease may also result from vasculitis. Most cases of ischemic cholecystitis occur in patients older than

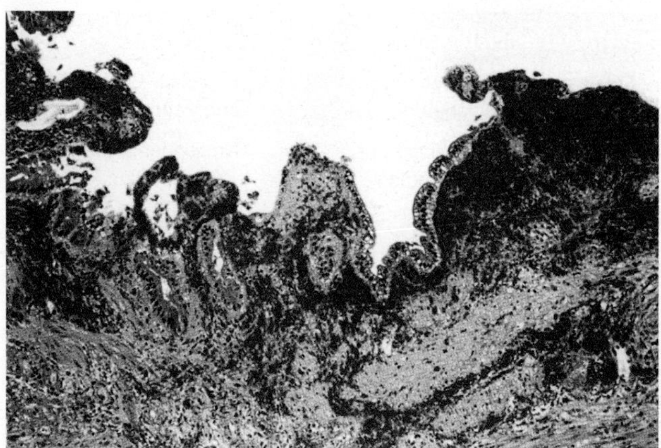

FIGURE 38.34 Hemorrhage within the lamina propria, epithelial cell necrosis, and paucity of inflammatory cells characterize ischemic cholangiopathy.

60 years. The correct clinical diagnosis is rarely established before surgery, because the symptoms mimic those of acute cholecystitis.

The gallbladder wall in ischemic disease is usually thickened, congested, and hemorrhagic. Microscopic examination may reveal partial or complete loss (e.g., necrosis) of the epithelium, edema, or hemorrhage in the lamina propria (Fig. 38.34). When occlusion to venous outflow predominates, there is usually extensive and often transmural hemorrhagic infarction. Ischemic lesions associated with primary vasculitis are often focal and typically confined to the mucosa. In patients with calculous cholecystitis, superimposed ischemic damage, caused by secondary vasculitis or small vessel thrombosis, is often found. Healed ischemic lesions may cause fibrous replacement and dystrophic calcifications of the gallbladder wall.

TRAUMATIC CONDITIONS AND CHEMICAL CHOLECYSTITIS

The gallbladder is seldom damaged by abdominal trauma because it is partially protected by the ribs and liver. Occasionally, blunt abdominal trauma may disrupt a distended gallbladder, causing contusion, laceration, torsion, avulsion, or intraluminal hemorrhage.[130] Penetrating wounds may damage the gallbladder, usually in association with injury to adjacent organs.

Iatrogenic injury can result from liver biopsy or percutaneous transhepatic cholangiography. Acute cholecystitis with mucosal necrosis and fibrosis may result from repeated infusion of chemotherapeutic agents through a catheter placed in the hepatic artery.[131]

BILIARY FISTULAS

In most cases, fistulas between the biliary tract and adjacent organs are a consequence of gallstone-associated necrosis with inflammation of the gallbladder or bile ducts, or both. Inflammatory adhesions precede fistula formation. These lesions may form a mass lesion that can resemble a neoplasm. Cholecystectomy in the setting of a fistula carries a high risk of injury to the bile ducts. The most common fistulas are cholecystoduodenal, followed by cholecystocolic and

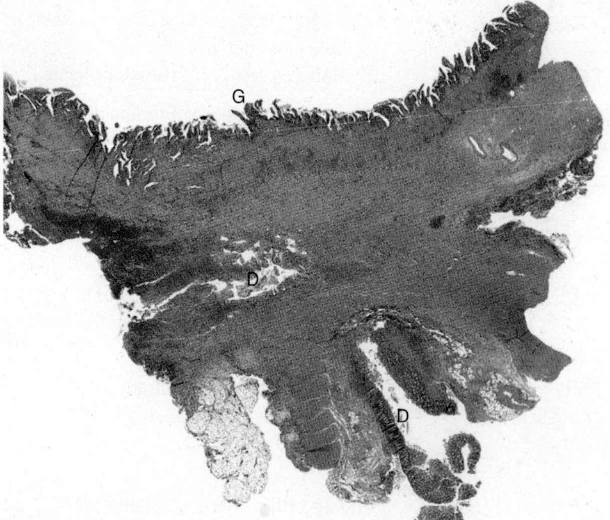

FIGURE 38.35 Chronic calculous cholecystitis with a fistulous tract between the gallbladder *(G)* and duodenum *(D)*.

choledochoduodenal (Fig. 38.35). Biliobiliary fistulas form between the gallbladder and the common bile duct. This complication should be suspected in patients with cholelithiasis and jaundice.[132]

METACHROMATIC LEUKODYSTROPHY

Metachromatic leukodystrophy is an inborn error of metabolism associated with a deficiency of aryl sulfatase. The disease is characterized by diffuse breakdown of myelin in the central and peripheral nervous systems. Microscopic changes in the gallbladder consist of papillary hyperplasia (i.e., papillomatosis) and expansion of the lamina propria by macrophages containing abnormal metachromatic material (i.e., sulfatides). The metachromatic material also is found within epithelial cells, and it may be responsible for the hyperplastic epithelial changes.[133]

INFLAMMATORY DISORDERS OF THE EXTRAHEPATIC BILE DUCTS

With the exception of PSC, the pathological features of most types of inflammatory conditions of the bile ducts have been poorly studied. Clinically, these conditions mimic an obstructive tumor, because silent cholestasis is a common complication.

One useful clinical and pathological classification of cholangitis used by the authors of this chapter includes seven categories: (1) simple obstructive cholangitis, (2) primary hepatolithiasis, (3) PSC, (4) IgG4-associated cholangitis, (5) follicular cholangitis and pancreatitis, (6) eosinophilic cholangitis, and (7) other conditions. The features of these disorders are summarized in Table 38.4.

Simple Obstructive Cholangitis

Clinical Features

The classic symptoms associated with acute obstructive cholangitis are known as the Charcot triad: intermittent abdominal pain, fever, and jaundice. This triad of symptoms

TABLE 38.4 Comparison of Types of Cholangitis with Lymphoplasmacytic Inflammation

Features	Simple Obstructive Cholangitis	Primary Hepatolithiasis	Primary Sclerosing Cholangitis	IgG4-Related Cholangitis	Follicular Cholangitis and Pancreatitis
Epidemiology	All ethnic groups Women > men	Predominantly Asians No gender predilection	Predominantly whites Men > women	All ethnic groups Men > women	No gender or ethnic predilection
Presence and type of gallstone	Cholesterol	Pigmented	Usually none	None	None
Associated conditions	Cholelithiasis; obstructive conditions	Infections? Malnutrition?	Ulcerative colitis	Pancreatitis; other IgG4-related conditions	Pancreatitis
Predominant site of obstruction	Common bile duct	Intrahepatic ducts	Intrahepatic and extrahepatic ducts	Intrapancreatic segment of common bile duct and hilar or large intrahepatic bile ducts	Hilar and intrapancreatic bile ducts
Pathological aspects	NSI and PIF	NSI and PIF Adenomatous hyperplasia	Mucosa-based NSI and PIF	Deep > mucosal inflammation IgG4-positive plasma cells OP, SF	Inflammation with abundant lymphoid follicles and PIF Few IgG4 plasma cells No OP or SF
Predisposition to dysplasia and cholangiocarcinoma	Rarely	Yes	Yes	No	Unknown

IgG4, *Immunoglobulin G4;* NSI, *nonspecific inflammation;* OP, *obliterative phlebitis;* PIF, *postinflammatory fibrosis;* SF, *storiform fibrosis.*

is identified in 20% to 70% of affected patients. Most patients have leukocytosis and abnormal liver function test results, mainly hyperbilirubinemia, with an elevated alkaline phosphatase level and a mild to moderate elevation of aminotransferases. Serum concentration of amylase is increased in 40% of patients, but this does not necessarily indicate concomitant pancreatitis. Blood cultures positive for enteric organisms suggest biliary sepsis.

A particularly severe form of this illness associated with a high mortality rate has been termed *acute suppurative* or *toxic cholangitis*. The typical symptoms associated with this condition constitute the Reynolds pentad: abdominal pain, fever, jaundice, shock, and delirium. The risk of progression to toxic cholangitis is increased in patients who do not respond to antibiotic management and in those who have a congenital or malignant obstruction. Acute renal failure and intrahepatic abscesses are the two most common complications of acute cholangitis. Renal failure may develop as a result of hypoperfusion from sepsis, endotoxemia, and tubular injury from bile pigments.[134-136]

Risk Factors and Pathogenesis

Biliary obstruction is caused by disorders that primarily affect the bile ducts and diseases of other organs that produce secondary obstruction. Among the former are choledocholithiasis, bile duct cysts, diverticula, tumors, fistulas, and complications from previous surgical procedures (e.g., nonabsorbable sutures, metal clips, plugged T-tubes, stents). Extrinsic obstruction of the bile ducts may be a complication of pancreatic tumors, chronic pancreatitis, ampullary lesions, and gallstones within the cystic duct with secondary compression of the common bile duct (i.e., Mirizzi's syndrome).

In Western countries, migration of cholesterol gallstones from the gallbladder into the bile ducts is the most frequent cause of obstruction.[137] Most cholesterol gallstones do not harbor bacteria and are not associated with infected bile. In a few cases, the organisms most commonly found are enteric bacteria, such as *E. coli*, *Streptococcus faecalis*, *Clostridium*, *Klebsiella*, *Enterobacter*, *Pseudomonas*, and *Proteus*.[137] The route by which bacteria colonize the biliary system remains unknown. Contamination from an infected gallbladder, duodenal reflux, and lymphatic, hepatic arterial, or portal venous bacteremia has been proposed.

Approximately 15% of patients with cholelithiasis have stones within the bile ducts; 15% to 20% are asymptomatic. Because severe symptomatic diseases such as acute cholangitis, chronic obstruction with hepatic fibrosis, and gallstone pancreatitis may develop in patients with ductal stones, stone removal is recommended at the time of cholecystectomy by endoscopic stone extraction.

Gallstones that form within the bile duct (i.e., primary bile duct stones) are usually brown pigment stones. At variance with the sterile nature of most cholesterol gallstones, brown stones are frequently associated with infection of the biliary tract. In Asia, primary bile duct stones often are associated with a high incidence of intrahepatic bile duct infections. Conditions that predispose to primary stone formation include obstructive diseases such as fibrosis resulting from prior biliary surgery, iatrogenic strictures, biliary-enteric anastomosis, sclerosing cholangitis, stenosing papillitis, periampullary duodenal diverticula, parasitic infections, Caroli disease, indwelling biliary endoprostheses, and use of nonabsorbable suture material or metal clips.[138] The bacteria most commonly found are β-glucuronidase–producing, gram-negative organisms, such as *E. coli* and *B.*

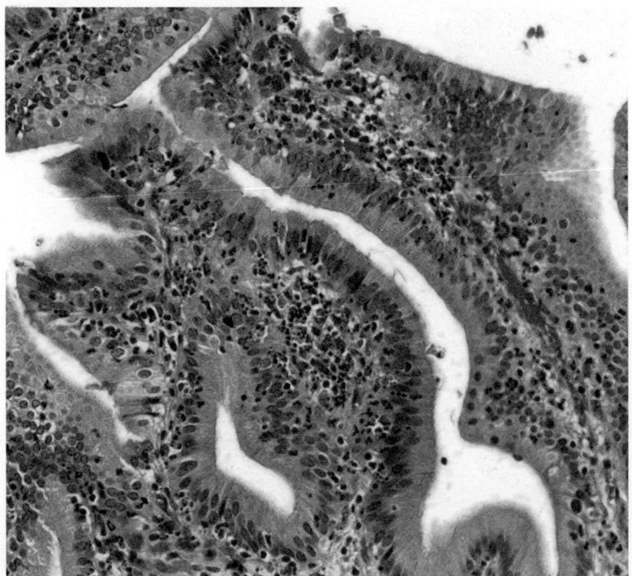

FIGURE 38.36 In simple obstructive cholangitis, neutrophils within lamina propria focally infiltrate bile duct epithelium. Notice the similarity of these lesions with the inflammatory pattern observed in liver biopsy specimens of patients with ascending cholangitis.

fragilis. Biliary sludge within the bile ducts has the same clinical significance as bile duct stones and predisposes to recurrent choledocholithiasis.[139] A xanthogranulomatous reaction similar to xanthogranulomatous cholecystitis may be encountered in bile ducts in the absence of other lesions. This type of cholangitis may be confused with a malignant tumor on imaging studies or cytology.[140,141]

Pathological Features

In acute cholangitis, examination of the extrahepatic bile ducts reveals edema, a predominantly neutrophilic infiltrate in the lamina propria, and focal infiltration of the epithelium (Fig. 38.36). Ulcers and erosions containing fragments of gallstones may be seen. The biliary epithelium usually shows degenerative and regenerative changes. Extravasation of bile into the lamina propria elicits an intense histiocyte-rich inflammatory reaction that may be followed by fibrosis. As the disorder evolves, lymphocytes and plasma cells become more abundant.

Treatment

Most symptomatic stones may be removed endoscopically either with or without mechanical lithotripsy. Shock wave and laser lithotripsy may be used before endoscopic removal of large stones. The role of ursodeoxycholic acid remains controversial.[142]

Primary Hepatolithiasis

Clinical Features and Epidemiology

Recurrent attacks of ascending cholangitis caused by intrahepatic stone formation characterize the syndrome of recurrent pyogenic cholangitis, also known as Oriental cholangiohepatitis, intrahepatic pigment stone disease, biliary obstruction syndrome of the Chinese, and primary hepatolithiasis. *Primary hepatolithiasis* is the preferred term because it distinguishes this form of hepatolithiasis from the Western type of cholangitis that complicates cholecystitis and cholelithiasis.

First described in Chinese patients in Hong Kong, the disorder is recognized as a serious health problem in China, Taiwan, Japan, Korea, Singapore, Vietnam, Malaysia, and the Philippines.[143] It is the main cause of acute abdominal pain in Hong Kong emergency rooms.[144] Sporadic cases have been reported in Europe, South Africa, and Australia. In the United States and Canada, the disease is largely limited to Asian immigrants.[145,146] The estimated incidence in the Far East is 4% to 52%, whereas in the West, it is 0.6% to 1.3%. With the exception of Korea, the incidence of this disorder appears to be decreasing in recent decades.[146]

Most cases of primary hepatolithiasis (i.e., recurrent pyogenic cholangitis or Oriental cholangiohepatitis) are diagnosed in patients 20 to 40 years of age. There is no sex predilection. There is a strong association with lower socioeconomic class. A history of recurrent attacks is common, and cases are characterized by abdominal pain, nausea, vomiting, fever, shaking chills, and jaundice. The findings on physical examination include epigastric tenderness and rigidity, enlargement of the liver, and a palpable gallbladder.

Laboratory findings include leukocytosis and an elevated serum alkaline phosphatase level. Most patients have bile cultures positive for enteric bacteria. Imaging studies demonstrate a characteristic pattern of ductal dilation with tight proximal stenosis and subsequent dilation and parenchymal atrophy, producing an arrowhead sign on CT.[143]

Pathogenesis

The cause of this disease is unknown. The two most accepted theories include infection and malnutrition. The former postulates that inflammatory and fibrosing changes result from chronic infestation of the biliary tract with endemic parasites, such as C. *sinensis* and *A. lumbricoides*. Interference with bile flow caused by adult flukes or eggs, produces stagnation that leads to secondary bacterial infection, pigment stone formation, and pyogenic cholangitis.[147] Demonstration of ova or fragments of parasites within stones provides support for this theory. However, patients with recurrent cholangitis have only a slightly higher rate of infestation by C. *sinensis* than the general population in endemic areas, where numerous individuals are infected with liver flukes without ever experiencing cholangitis. In other areas where parasitic infection is much less common, such as Taiwan, the incidence of recurrent cholangitis and hepatolithiasis is high. In Japan, primary hepatolithiasis persists despite eradication of intestinal parasites.[148]

The second theory postulates that recurrent infectious gastroenteritis in malnourished people causes frequent episodes of portal bacteremia. Calcium bilirubinate precipitates formed by deconjugation of bilirubin glucuronide by β-glucuronidase produced by *E. coli* infection initiates the formation of brown stones. A protein-poor diet is believed to be associated with a deficiency of glucaro-1:4-lactone, a natural inhibitor of the enzyme in bile. The formation of biliary sludge converts an otherwise innocuous portal bacteremia into an infection. This theory explains the much higher incidence of disease in patients from low socioeconomic classes and in rural areas. However, it does not explain why this disorder is uncommon in other geographic areas, where the population also suffers from chronic malnourishment.

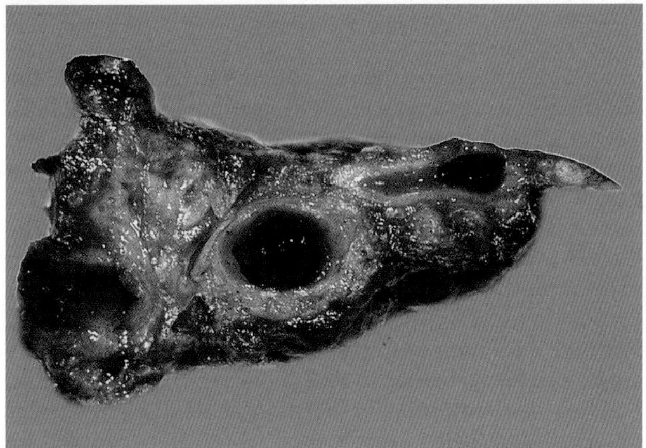

FIGURE 38.37 A cross section of the left and right intrahepatic ducts of a patient with recurrent pyogenic cholangitis reveals firm and thickened walls.

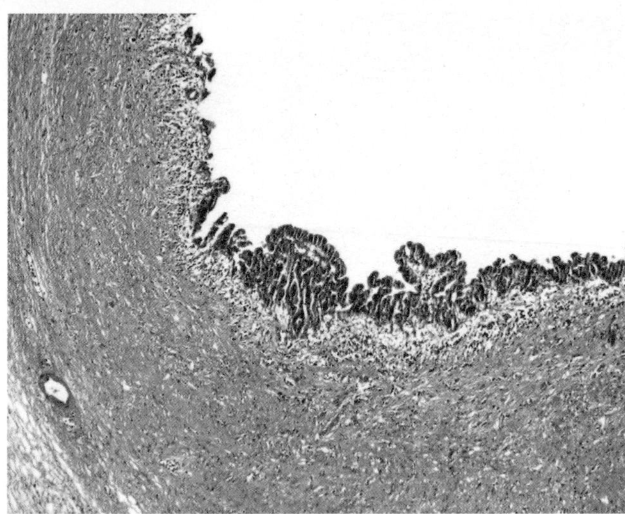

FIGURE 38.38 Recurrent pyogenic cholangitis is characterized by fibrosis and mucosal inflammation. The biliary epithelium shows dysplastic features.

Pathological Features

The intrahepatic ducts, which are proximal to the confluence of the right and left hepatic ducts, and the extrahepatic bile ducts may be affected. The left lateral segmental duct is more frequently affected, followed by the posterior segmental duct of the right lobe. This distribution is thought to be related to the angulation of these ducts, which is more marked than in other segments.[146] The liver may be enlarged, display irregular scarring, and have capsular adhesions. After multiple attacks, it may become shrunken, especially the lateral segment of the left lobe. The intrahepatic bile ducts show alternating areas of stricture and dilation (Fig. 38.37). An unusual feature is abrupt tapering toward the periphery of the dilated segments. This contrasts sharply with diffuse dilation seen in patients with other causes of obstruction. Pigment stones and secretions are usually found within the lumen.

In most cases, the extrahepatic ducts are not stenotic, except for the most distal segment, where repeated passage of stones through the sphincter of Oddi may cause inflammation and postinflammatory strictures of the papilla, a condition known as *stenosing papillitis*. The dilated segments are not strictly related to the location of the stones.[149] Bile duct stones occur in 75% to 80% of cases. Histological changes in the extrahepatic ducts include a mixed inflammatory infiltrate, sometimes with the formation of lymphoid follicles, some degree of fibrosis, and epithelial changes that range from loss of cells to adenomatous hyperplasia and dysplasia. The term *chronic proliferative cholangitis* is sometimes used for the latter type of lesions. The neutral and acid mucins produced by metaplastic glands participate in the formation of the stones.

Portal tracts in the liver show a characteristic cluster of changes of bile duct obstruction: proliferation of bile ducts, inflammatory cells (mainly neutrophils), and some degree of edema. Periductal fibrosis is frequently identified. The hepatic parenchyma adjacent to intrahepatic stones is commonly atrophic. However, postobstructive cirrhosis is rare.

Cholangiocarcinoma develops in 2.4% to 4.9% of patients with recurrent pyogenic cholangitis.[150] It has been suggested that continuous inflammation caused by the concerted action of persistent infection and mechanical irritation by stones leads to adenomatous hyperplasia, dysplasia, and cholangiocarcinoma[151] (Fig. 38.38).

Treatment

Several treatment options are available. Ideally, complete removal of stones and elimination of bile stasis and infection should be attempted to eliminate the inflammatory process and prevent the development of cholangiocarcinoma. Nonsurgical procedures such as percutaneous transhepatic cholangioscopic lithotripsy, and extracorporal shock wave lithotripsy have been tried with suboptimal results due to a high prevalence rate of residual and recurrent stones. Poor results have also been reported with conservative surgical treatments, such as biliary-enteric anastomosis or T-tube insertion. Hepatic resection provides a definitive solution for patients who do not have bilateral disease.[152]

Primary Sclerosing Cholangitis

Clinical Features

Primary sclerosing cholangitis is a chronic progressive disorder that if left untreated may progress to bile duct fibrosis, cholestasis, and biliary cirrhosis. Most patients with PSC are male and younger than 45 years of age. Fifty percent of patients also have a history of inflammatory bowel disease, usually ulcerative pancolitis. Other diseases associated with PSC include thyroiditis, pancreatitis, insulin-dependent diabetes mellitus, celiac disease, thymoma, sicca syndrome, retroperitoneal and mediastinal fibrosis, Peyronie's disease, pseudotumor of the orbit, sarcoidosis, histiocytosis X, angioimmunoblastic lymphadenopathy, Weber-Christian's disease, rheumatoid arthritis, autoimmune hemolytic anemia, systemic lupus erythematosus, and a variety of immunodeficiency syndromes. [153-155]

Approximately 25% of patients with PSC are asymptomatic at presentation. They are diagnosed by abnormal liver test results and retrograde cholangiopancreatography. Typically, symptoms appear insidiously, and the most common are fatigue, pruritus, and jaundice. Cholangitis may occur with the development of advanced liver disease and ductal stenosis. Liver function tests typically reveal a cholestatic profile. The alkaline phosphatase level is always elevated, usually at least three to five times over its normal value. Serum aminotransferase and bilirubin levels are usually only mildly elevated at presentation but increase with disease progression.

There are no reliable serological markers that are useful for the diagnosis of this disorder. Less than 50% of patients have positive test results for antinuclear and smooth muscle antibodies. Antineutrophilic cytoplasmic antibodies are detected in 87% of patients. However, they are not disease specific.[156]

Cholangiographic studies demonstrate multifocal strictures involving, in most instances, intrahepatic and extrahepatic ducts. Strictures are typically short, annular, and alternate with normal or dilated segments.

Risk Factors and Pathogenesis

PSC occurs primarily in young men and has an estimated prevalence rate of 20 to 60 cases per 1 million people.[153] The disorder is characterized by persistent chronic inflammation and fibrosis of the intrahepatic and extrahepatic bile ducts, with a gradual onset of progressive fatigue and pruritus, followed by jaundice and slow progression to cirrhosis.

PSC usually has a cholestatic biochemical profile. Approximately 70% of patients with PSC either have or eventually develop ulcerative colitis.[153] It is less commonly associated with Crohn's disease. Inflammatory bowel disease may precede PSC by many years (median, 9 years). When PSC is the presenting disorder, inflammatory bowel disease can develop many years later. Most patients with PSC develop ulcerative colitis with diffuse involvement of the colon or Crohn's disease with colonic involvement.[154]

Designation of PSC as an "autoimmune" disease is based on its common association with an autoimmune haplotype (HLA-A1-B8-DR3) and the presence of autoantibodies against peptides shared by the colonic and biliary epithelial cells.[155] Additional evidence is provided by the finding of antineutrophilic cytoplasmic antibodies at high titer in most patients with PSC and its strong association with ulcerative colitis and other autoimmune disorders (e.g., insulin-dependent diabetes mellitus, systemic lupus erythematosus, Sjögren's syndrome, celiac disease).[156]

Chronic portal bacteremia may play a role in the pathogenesis of this disease. Chronic absorption of toxins and bacterial products in patients with ulcerative colitis may cause release of inflammatory cytokines into the biliary mucosa. Observations in animal models support this hypothesis.[157]

Pathological Features

Both the intrahepatic and extrahepatic bile ducts are affected in most patients with PSC. The disorder remains confined to the intrahepatic biliary tract in only approximately 20% of patients. The intrahepatic and extrahepatic bile ducts usually reveal alternating areas of stricture formation with normal lumen or slightly dilated segments, producing a characteristic beaded pattern on cholangiographic studies. Diverticulum-like outpouchings are found in approximately 25% of cases.

Microscopically, bile ducts show expansion of the lamina propria by a plasma cell–rich infiltrate that is diffuse and even present in segments that are grossly normal (Fig. 38.39). This diffuse pattern of mucositis mimics the features of colonic mucosa in ulcerative colitis. The resemblance to ulcerative colitis is further reinforced by the presence of active lesions, characterized by neutrophilic infiltration of the biliary epithelium and glands, with formation of microabscesses, erosions, and ulcers. Changes in the biliary epithelium ranges from atrophy to regenerative hyperplasia and true dysplasia (Fig. 38.40).[158] Cholangiocarcinoma develops in 4% to 20% of patients with PSC.[158]

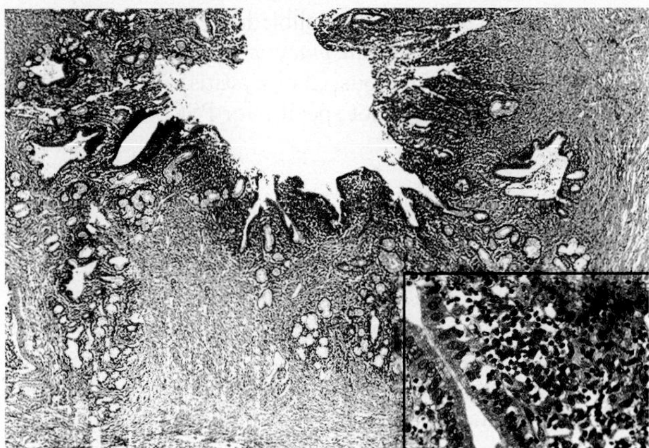

FIGURE 38.39 A diffuse mucositis characterizes primary sclerosing cholangitis. Intraepithelial neutrophils (active lesions) are common. Partial obliteration of the lumen by fibrous tissue is common in late stages. *Inset,* The lamina propria is distended by an inflammatory infiltrate composed of lymphocytes and plasma cells.

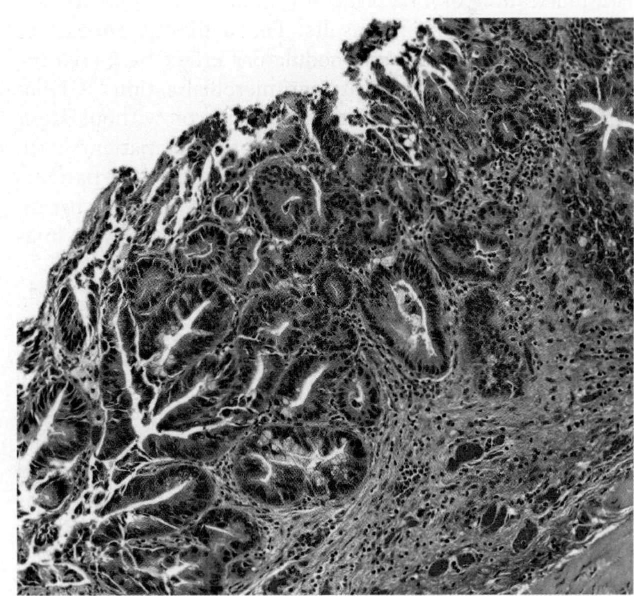

FIGURE 38.40 A focus of high-grade dysplasia was found in sections of the right hepatic duct in a hepatectomy specimen of a patient who underwent liver transplantation for cirrhosis due to primary sclerosing cholangitis.

Fibrosis is typically found in strictured segments. Biliary stones develop in areas proximal to the stenosis, and if the clinical and pathological features support a diagnosis of PSC, the presence of stones should not be used to exclude the diagnosis. Cholelithiasis is usually absent, except in patients with cirrhosis. The inflammatory pattern in the bile ducts often occurs in the gallbladder, as well, a disorder known as *diffuse lymphoplasmacytic acalculous cholecystitis* (see Chronic Acalculous Cholecystitis). However, this inflammatory pattern is not specific for PSC.

Natural History

The natural history of PSC has not been clearly defined. The clinical course of patients with PSC is quite variable. Some patients remain stable for many years, whereas in others, it evolves rapidly to liver failure. In most instances, the disease progresses to biliary cirrhosis within 10 to 15 years. The average survival time is 10 to 12 years. The most common cause of death is liver failure, followed by cholangiocarcinoma.[153,154]

Treatment

There is no effective medical treatment available for PSC. Novel ursodeoxycholic acid derivatives and monoclonal antibodies against integrins that prevent mucosal homing of T lymphocytes are in the presence of clinical trials. Administration of oral vancomycin is a new therapeutic strategy with promising results. This antibiotic appears to be effective in its immunomodulatory effect by increasing regulatory T cells, and in its antimicrobial action.[159] Dilation of dominant strictures, either with or without stent placement, is recommended for symptomatic patients with complications. Liver transplantation is offered to patients with end-stage liver failure, refractory pruritus, or recurrent bacterial cholangitis. PSC recurs in transplanted livers in as many as 20% of patients after a median of 4.6 years.[154]

Immunoglobulin G4–Associated Cholangitis and Cholecystitis

IgG4-associated cholangitis and cholecystitis have clinical and pathological features that separate them from the disorders discussed earlier in this chapter. They are included among the expanding group of fibroinflammatory conditions referred to as *IgG4-related diseases*. The prototype of these disorders is autoimmune pancreatitis, but IgG4-related conditions have been described in other organs, such as the biliary tract, gallbladder, salivary glands, periorbital tissues, kidneys, lungs, lymph nodes, meninges, aorta, breast, prostate, thyroid, pericardium, and skin.[160]

Clinical Features

IgG4-associated cholangitis predominantly affects patients older than 50 years of age. It has a male-to-female predominance of approximately 2.8 to 1.

Biliary tract involvement is referred to as IgG4 sclerosing cholangitis. Bile duct involvement is present in about 60% to 80% of patients with type 1 autoimmune pancreatitis as well. However, in approximately 8% of cases, the pancreas is not involved.[161] The predominant clinical manifestation of IgG4-associated cholangitis is obstructive jaundice resulting from hilar bile duct strictures, or a pancreatic head mass mimicking carcinoma. At presentation, most patients have a chemical cholestatic pattern, including hyperbilirubinemia; mild transaminasemia; elevated levels of alkaline phosphatase, γ-glutamyltransferase, and CA 19-9; and bile duct or pancreatic duct strictures seen on imaging studies.[162] Elevated IgG and IgG4 serum levels and autoantibodies (e.g., rheumatoid factor, antinuclear antibodies) are common but not always present.

PSC tends to occur in younger patients (30 to 40 years old), and the clinical presentation usually is less symptomatic, with disease progression occurring over the course of several years. Patients with IgG4-associated cholangitis are a decade or two older and have an acute presentation with a shorter duration of symptoms. Extrabiliary disease, especially pancreatic and kidney disorders, supports a diagnosis of an IgG4-related condition.[163]

Pathological Features

The most frequently affected segments of the biliary tract are the intrapancreatic portion of the common bile duct, and the hilar or intrahepatic large caliber bile ducts. The common hepatic duct and the extrapancreatic portion of the common bile duct usually are spared. This anatomic distribution of disease probably reflects the abundance of peribiliary glands in these locations.[164] Examination of the involved bile ducts reveals thickening of the wall, which is partially replaced by a white, fleshy tissue that merges with periductal tissues, and luminal stenosis with dilation of the proximal segments.

Histologically, the classic triad of IgG4-related diseases—dense lymphoplasmacytic inflammation, fibrosis with a storiform pattern, and obliterative phlebitis—is characteristic, although the phlebitis is sometimes absent. Lymphoid follicles and tissue eosinophils may be present as well. The inflammatory infiltrate tends to be more abundant in the peribiliary glands than in the lamina propria, the latter of which tends to be relatively spared (Fig. 38.41). The distribution of inflammation contrasts sharply with PSC, in which the infiltrate predominates in the luminal portion of the mucosa. In PSC, the biliary epithelium is inflamed, shows degenerative changes, and is frequently ulcerated. Extension of the inflammatory process into the soft tissues surrounding the bile ducts is common in IgG4-associated

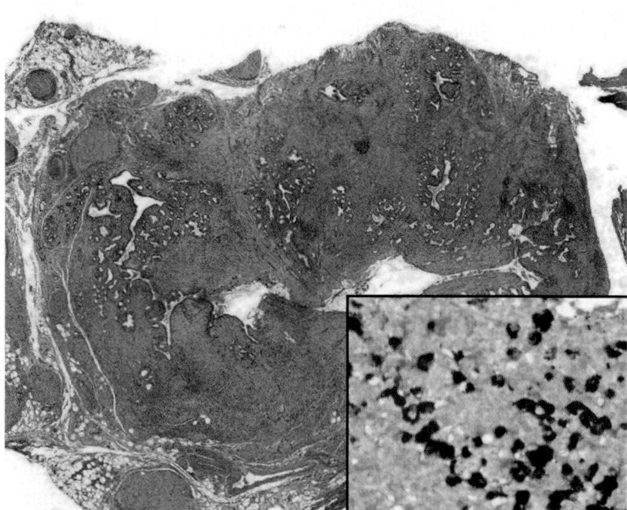

FIGURE 38.41 Immunoglobulin G4 (IgG4)–associated cholangitis. Most of the inflammatory cell infiltrates are located around the biliary glands, with relative sparing of the lamina propria. An IgG4 immunohistochemical stain shows numerous positive cells *(inset)*.

cholangitis. Immunohistochemically, most plasma cells express IgG, and most are positive for IgG4. The specificity of this type of infiltrate is high when the IgG4-to-IgG ratio is 0.47 or higher, and the number of IgG4-positive plasma cells exceeds 10 per high-power field.[165]

The gallbladder is universally involved in patients with IgG4-associated cholangitis. The distribution and characteristics of the inflammatory infiltrate is similar to those of PSC. Diffuse lymphoplasmacytic inflammatory infiltrates expand the lamina propria. Active lesions (i.e., neutrophils within the epithelium) are common in patients with bile duct obstruction. However, one noticeable difference is an increase in transmural infiltration in IgG4-associated cholangitis, which contrasts with most cases of PSC in which the inflammation is mainly mucosal. In addition to the identification of IgG4-positive plasma cells, important findings are phlebitis and inflammatory nodules, particularly when located in perivesical tissues.[165,166]

IgG4-positive plasma cells may be observed in other conditions, such as suppurative granulation tissue, pancreatic carcinoma, and cholangiocarcinoma, PSC, and autoimmune hepatitis.[167] A diagnosis of carcinoma in patients with a biliary or pancreatic mass should not be excluded solely because cholecystectomy or biliary biopsy specimens show a histological pattern of injury that mimics IgG4-associated cholangitis, including abundant IgG4-positive plasma cells.

Treatment

Differentiating this type of cholangitis from PSC is important because IgG4-associated cholangitis is steroid responsive, whereas PSC usually is not.[160] Spontaneous resolution has been described. The disease may recur during the tapering phase or after discontinuation of steroid therapy. Most relapses occur within the first 3 years. Increased alkaline phosphatase and IgG4 levels, and proximal bile duct involvement, have been associated with disease relapse. Other immunosuppressive drugs have been used when the disorder recurs or is refractory to steroid therapy.[168] Patients with IgG4-associated cholangitis do not appear to have an increased risk of cholangiocarcinoma, as in patients with PSC.

Eosinophilic Cholangitis

Clinical Features

Inflammatory diseases of the bile ducts account for approximately 10% of patients who undergo surgery for hepatic hilar strictures. One condition that closely mimics the presentation of a biliary tumor is eosinophilic cholangitis. This uncommon condition has a slight male predominance (1.6 to 1), and the mean age at presentation is 35.4 years.

Most patients have abdominal pain followed by jaundice, and 70% have peripheral eosinophilia. Ultrasound and contrast-enhanced CT studies commonly show thickening of the bile duct wall either with or without biliary dilation. Brush cytology and biopsies may help to diagnose this condition and exclude cholangiocarcinoma.[169] The gallbladder is frequently involved. This condition may be confined to the biliary tract, or it may be a component of a systemic disorder with eosinophilia, such as the idiopathic hypereosinophilic syndrome or eosinophilic gastroenteritis.

Pathological Features

In patients with eosinophilic cholangitis, segmental thickening of the bile duct wall results in the development of grossly apparent white, fleshy tissue usually with various degrees of obliteration of the lumen. Microscopic examination of cases reveals a dense inflammatory cell infiltrate composed almost exclusively of eosinophils within the mucosa and muscular layer, and some degree of fibrosis and luminal obliteration. Liver biopsy specimens show an obstructive pattern with abundant eosinophils (Fig. 38.42).

Treatment

The disease may resolve after surgery or with corticosteroid therapy. A diagnostic trial of oral corticosteroids may provide support for the diagnosis of eosinophilic cholangitis before surgical intervention.[170]

Follicular Cholangitis and Pancreatitis

Clinical Features

Follicular cholangitis and pancreatitis constitute a specific pathological condition. It affects adult elderly patients without a gender predilection. The predominant clinical manifestations are related to hilar bile duct strictures or a bulky pancreatic head mass that mimics carcinoma. Most patients have hyperbilirubinemia; mild transaminasemia; elevated levels of alkaline phosphatase, γ-glutamyltransferase, and CA 19-9; and bile duct or pancreatic duct strictures seen on imaging studies.[171]

Pathological Features

Gross examination shows bile duct wall thickening or an ill-circumscribed mass in the head of the pancreas. Histologically, there is a duct-centered lymphoplasmacytic infiltrate, with lymphoid follicles, containing mitotic figures and tangible body macrophages within the germinal centers.

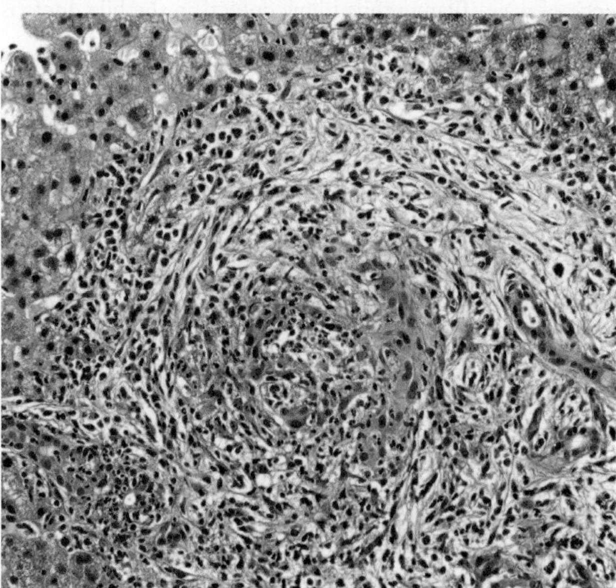

FIGURE 38.42 Liver biopsy from a patient with eosinophilic cholangitis. The obstructive pattern consists of bile ductular proliferation, edema, and inflammation. In addition to neutrophils, there are abundant eosinophils. Extrahepatic bile duct obstruction was confirmed by imaging studies. The patient had a dramatic response to steroid therapy.

Nonstoriform collagen is deposited in the bile ducts or pancreatic ducts, or both. Within the interfollicular areas, there is a dense plasmacytic infiltrate with occasional eosinophils. Lymphoid follicles are usually found in the gallbladder, mimicking follicular cholecystitis. Nonobliterative phlebitis may be identified. IgG4-positive plasma cells are usually present, but they represent only 2% to 15% of the plasma cell population.

Based on the absence of numerous IgG4-positive plasma cells, obliterative phlebitis, storiform-type periductal fibrosis, and granulocytic epithelial lesions (seen in type 2 autoimmune pancreatitis), it has been proposed that this entity is probably different from or represents a variant of autoimmune pancreatitis or cholangitis.[171]

Parasitic Infections of the Biliary Tract

Clonorchis sinensis

Worldwide, an estimated 19,000,000 persons are infected with C. *sinensis*; most live in the Far East.[172] Infected persons can harbor the organism inside the biliary system for as long as 30 years. Routine stool screening of Chinese immigrants to the United States has demonstrated active infection in 25%.[173]

Two intermediate hosts are needed for transmission to humans: various species of snails (not found in the United States) and freshwater fish. The infection is acquired by eating raw freshwater fish infected with the metacercariae of this parasite. In humans, the metacercariae excyst in the duodenum, and the worms migrate into the bile ducts and lodge in the peripheral bile ducts, where they mature.

Symptoms are related to the burden of flukes. Persons with fewer than 100 flukes are usually asymptomatic, whereas those with 100 to 1000 flukes usually have anorexia, nausea, epigastric pain, and diarrhea. A higher fluke load is accompanied by biliary colic and right upper quadrant tenderness. On cholangiographic studies, the presence of wavy, filamentous filling defects in the bile ducts is pathognomonic for clonorchiasis.

The pathological findings in patients with C. *sinensis* infection are variable. Since the parasite does not invade bile ducts, there is little inflammatory response. Initially, the biliary mucosa is edematous and has an intact or desquamated epithelium. With persistent infection, the epithelium undergoes mucinous metaplasia and becomes hyperplastic (Fig. 38.43). Periductal fibrosis is the hallmark of long-standing infection. At this stage, it is common for organisms to be absent and for mucinous metaplasia to disappear. Uncomplicated lesions contain either few or no inflammatory cells. When complicated by pyogenic cholangitis, a heavy neutrophilic response suggests bacterial superinfection, usually by *E. coli*. As a result of disruption of the eggs by inflammatory cells, granulomas rich in eosinophils may develop. Secondary biliary cirrhosis is a long-term consequence of chronic cholangitis and fibrosis. Adenomatous hyperplasia may evolve into biliary dysplasia and adenocarcinoma.

Ascaris lumbricoides

The nematode *A. lumbricoides* is the most prevalent type of helminthic infestation in the world. Up to 60% of the general population may be infected in endemic areas of South Africa, Asia, India, and South America. In the United States, *A. lumbricoides* accounts for less than 1% of all helminthic infections. After ingestion of *Ascaris* eggs, the larva hatches in the jejunum, penetrates the lymphatic vessels and portal circulation, and then migrates through the liver to the lungs. The larvae are then swallowed, and then mature to adult worms in the gut. The worms may migrate from the intestine into the bile ducts, producing obstruction. Bacterial superinfection may cause recurrent cholangitis. The worms are usually easily visualized by imaging techniques, such as cholangiogram and ultrasound.[174,175]

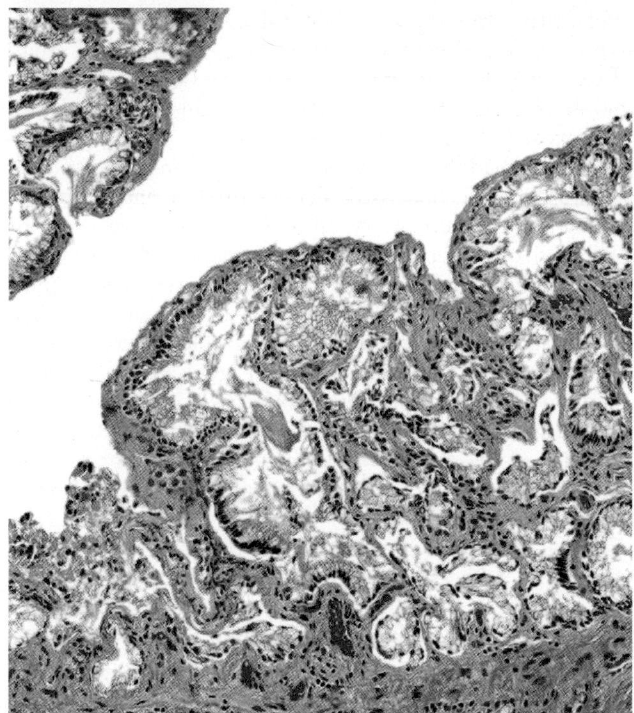

FIGURE 38.43 Hyperplastic biliary glands with mucinous metaplasia of the bile ducts were obtained from a Chinese patient with suspected *Clonorchis sinensis* infection.

Fasciola hepatica

Fasciola hepatica is another parasite that can produce biliary obstruction and cholangitis and, rarely, cholecystitis. Infection occurs more frequently in Europe, Asia, Africa, and South America. It is acquired by ingestion of water plants that contain encysted metacercariae. In the duodenum, metacercariae hatch and migrate through the wall of the intestine, penetrate the Glisson capsule, burrow through the parenchyma of the liver, and invade bile ducts and occasionally the gallbladder (Fig. 38.44). In the acute phase, an inflammatory infiltrate rich in eosinophils may be seen, followed by regenerative hyperplasia of the biliary epithelium and fibrosis.[174,175]

AIDS-RELATED LESIONS

The therapeutic efficacy of current antiretroviral therapy has dramatically improved outcomes for HIV-infected patients. The biliary problems that afflict these individuals on therapy are identical to those that occur in immunocompetent patients. The most prevalent condition in this population is cholelithiasis, and when it is associated with biliary

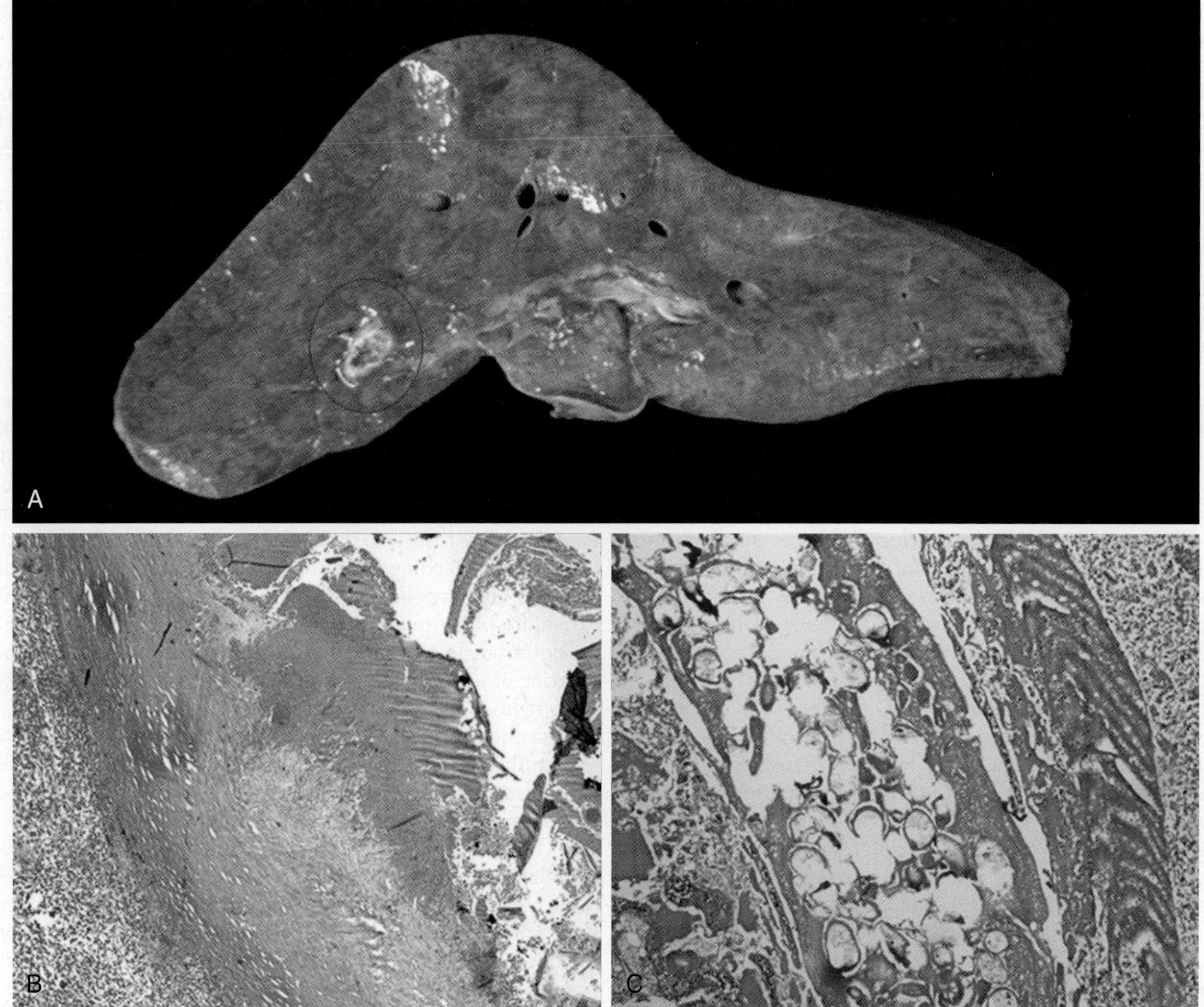

FIGURE 38.44 ***Fasciola hepatica.*** **A,** Liver autopsy specimen from an adult Dominican woman who died of COVID-19 showing a dilated bile duct *(circle)*. **B,** Microscopic section of the bile duct showing an inflamed fibrotic wall devoid of epithelium. **C,** Poorly preserved parasite structures most likely representing ovarian tubules.

colic, cholecystectomy may result in pain relief if HIV cholangiopathy is absent. The term *HIV cholangiopathy* refers to several types of bile duct disorders unrelated to gallstones, malignant disease, or previous surgery. These conditions are seen mostly in severely immunosuppressed patients and include papillary stenosis, a sclerosing cholangitis–like disorder, a combination of papillary stenosis and sclerosing cholangitis, and long extrahepatic bile duct strictures.[176]

Patients with HIV-associated cholangiopathy experience right upper quadrant or epigastric pain and fever. Most have an elevated serum alkaline phosphatase level, but only 15% have elevated bilirubin levels. Endoscopic retrograde cholangiopancreatography frequently demonstrates duct irregularities and a beaded appearance. In patients with papillary stenosis, relief of pain typically follows endoscopic sphincterotomy. However, because of ongoing intrahepatic duct disease, serum alkaline phosphatase levels usually continue to increase.

The pathogenesis of AIDS-related cholangitis, although unknown, may be similar to that for PSC. The altered immune status of HIV-infected patients may contribute to the pathogenesis of bile duct damage, as in some patients with congenital immunodeficiencies. Particularly attractive is the hypothesis that enteric infections in AIDS patients may lead to portal bacteremia, bile duct injury, and destruction. Some cases may be related to CMV or *Cryptosporidium* infection. However, by itself, *Cryptosporidium* is an unlikely candidate, because it usually elicits only a very mild inflammatory response. Histological changes associated with CMV infection vary from mild to severe. In the neonate, this organism may infect bile duct epithelium and cause obliterative cholangitis and paucity of bile ducts.[177] Its propensity to infect endothelial cells may induce vasculitis and ischemic damage. Infection of the biliary tract with *E. bieneusi* is associated with and may be a cause of AIDS-related cholangitis.[178-180]

Pathological lesions that characterize these conditions have not been adequately studied. In most cases, the extrahepatic bile ducts show nonspecific mixed inflammatory infiltrates and fibrosis. In most instances, organisms are not identified. The organisms that have been reported in the extrahepatic bile ducts are CMV, *Cryptosporidium*,

Cystoisospora, *M. avium* complex, *Pneumocystis carinii*, and *E. bieneusi*. *E. bieneusi* organisms may be seen on sections stained with hematoxylin and eosin within the cytoplasm of biliary cells, but they are easily missed, even by experienced pathologists. A Giemsa stain may help in their identification, and in some cases, electron microscopy is required.

In the liver, the portal tracts show increased fibrous tissue and sparse lymphocytic inflammation. Interlobular bile ducts are absent or show degenerative epithelial changes. Inflammatory cells are characteristically sparse. Lymphoma and Kaposi's sarcoma are rare complications that may cause cholangitis.[176]

CHOLANGIOPATHY

Ischemic Cholangitis

Damage to the blood vessels that nourish the bile ducts may result in necrosis and fibrous occlusion. Unlike the dual (portal and arterial) blood supply of the hepatic parenchyma, the biliary system is nourished exclusively by arterial blood flow. As in other segments of the GI tract, ischemia may be related to luminal occlusion of the blood vessels (e.g., thrombosis, vasculitis), external compression, or hypoperfusion. Ischemic cholangitis accounts for about 2% to 19% of nonanastomotic strictures in liver transplant recipients.[181] Posttraumatic ischemia of the bile ducts causes jaundice in patients hospitalized for life-threatening trauma, or blunt abdominal injury, and in patients who suffer inadvertent damage to blood vessels during abdominal surgery. Another important cause is hepatic artery infusion of chemotherapeutic agents such as floxuridine, 5-fluorouracil, mitomycin C, and *cis*-platinum.[182]

Ischemic changes may be confined to one segment of the bile duct or affect multiple segments in a discontinuous fashion. Injury to the biliary epithelium varies according to the cause of hypoperfusion. When the ischemic event occurs abruptly, edema and hemorrhage of the lamina propria and sloughing of necrotic biliary epithelial cells obliterate the lumen of the duct. Necrotic biliary cells admixed with fibrinous exudate and bile components may form a biliary cast. Full-thickness necrosis of the bile duct wall may occur with spillage of bile into the liver parenchyma, peritoneum, or retroperitoneum. In patients with less severe hypoperfusion or progressive arterial occlusion, fibrosis of the bile ducts may obliterate the lumen. Inflammatory cell infiltrates are usually sparse except in cases of superimposed infection.

The development of secondary sclerosing cholangitis in critically ill patients (SSC-CIP) following prolonged hospitalizations involving intensive care unit care is covered in Chapter 52.

Other Nonneoplastic Biliary Strictures

More than 80% of bile duct strictures occur after cholecystectomy. Two cases of this complication occur per 1000 operations. Inadvertent damage of the bile ducts may result from failure to recognize unexpected anatomic variations or poor visualization because of encasement of the ducts by an abscess or fibrous tissue. Attempts to gain hemostasis because of bleeding from the cystic or hepatic arteries may lead to bile duct injury. Even in expert hands, the extreme friability of acutely inflamed tissue makes dissection of the Calot triangle a formidable task. Cholecystectomy in the setting of a biliobiliary fistula carries a high risk of injury to the right or common hepatic duct. Other conditions that affect the biliopancreatoduodenal area that may give rise to postinflammatory bile duct strictures include subhepatic abscesses, chronic duodenal ulcers, chronic pancreatitis, and granulomatous lymphadenitis.

The location of the stricture influences the choice of surgical technique and likely outcome of the repair.[183-185] Uncommon causes of biliary strictures include Langerhans cell granulomatosis (i.e., histiocytosis X), sarcoidosis, amyloidosis, congenital biliary anomalies, and cystic fibrosis.[182] Extrinsic compression of the bile ducts from cirrhotic nodules, cysts, tumors, and adhesions may mimic a primary biliary disorder.

The full reference list may be viewed online at *Elsevier eBooks for Practicing Clinicians.*

CHAPTER 39

Benign and Malignant Tumors of the Gallbladder and Extrahepatic Biliary Tract

Olca Basturk, N. Volkan Adsay

Contents

INTRODUCTION

As discussed in other chapters, gallstones and inflammatory disorders constitute the vast majority of biliary tract pathology. Neoplasms and tumor-like lesions (pseudotumors) are relatively rare but form an important category with challenging diagnostic issues. As a result of advances in radiographic modalities and widespread use of laparoscopic cholecystectomy, the frequency of gallbladder and biliary tumors that have come to clinical attention has increased in recent years. These techniques have also led to an increase in the diagnosis of mass-forming lesions that would have otherwise gone undetected, including incidentalomas such as cholesterol polyps. Nevertheless, a significant proportion of gallbladder neoplasms, including adenocarcinomas, are detected as "clinically unapparent" in cholecystectomies performed for cholecystitis.

Recent work has focused on reevaluation of the terminology used for gallbladder and bile duct tumors and, in particular, for preinvasive neoplasms. This was done to standardize the approach to tumors across the entire pancreatobiliary system.

SAMPLING OF GALLBLADDER SPECIMENS

A significant proportion of gallbladder carcinomas are unapparent both clinically and grossly,[1] discovered only after microscopic examination of cholecystectomy specimens performed for cholecystitis.[2-10] Therefore a sampling protocol addressing this possibility should be utilized routinely.[2,8] Our approach is the following[8,11]: The cystic duct margin is sampled en-face and unopened. The serosal and hepatic surfaces of the gallbladder are inked in different colors, and the gallbladder is opened from the serosal aspect. If no overt lesions are noted, a through-and-through section, proceeding from the fundus to the cystic duct, is taken, rolled up, and submitted in the same cassette along with the cystic duct margin. If a lymph node is present, this is also included in the same cassette, if possible.

If epithelial atypia or low-grade dysplasia is identified in this random sample, four additional tissue blocks with multiple strips are obtained. If high-grade dysplasia is identified, then the entire gallbladder is examined because of its association with invasive carcinoma. The prognosis changes dramatically if a patient has invasive carcinoma rather than high-grade dysplasia. Similarly, if a pTis, pT1a, or pT1b carcinoma is identified, then the entire gallbladder should be examined to rule out a pT2 carcinoma (invasion through the tunica muscularis) because the clinical outcome of the latter-stage tumor is far worse.[12] In fact, a diagnosis of early gallbladder cancer (pTis or pT1) must not be rendered unless the entire gallbladder is examined.[10,13] It has been recently shown in an analysis from a high cancer-risk population that although high-grade dysplasia and invasive carcinoma are likely to be identified in initial sections, accurate staging requires total sampling.[14]

If a polyp or papillary lesion is present, it is submitted entirely for microscopic examination. If it is neoplastic, a minimum of four tissue blocks with multiple strips are obtained from the uninvolved gallbladder to evaluate any other dysplastic lesions.[15] If the polyp shows high-grade dysplasia, then the entire gallbladder should be examined because of its association with invasive carcinoma as mentioned earlier.[14]

TABLE 39.1A Intracholecystic Neoplasms

Mass-Forming Lesion	Authors' Approach	Old Literature	2019 WHO Classification
Polypoid pyloric gland collections in the mucosa	<1 cm, not well demarcated, and without atypia: polypoid pyloric gland metaplasia ≥1 cm and distinct from the neighboring mucosa: Intracholecystic papillary-tubular neoplasm (ICPN), exclusively pyloric phenotype[15]	Pyloric gland adenoma	<0.5 cm and not well demarcated: polypoid pyloric gland metaplasia Distinct from the neighboring mucosa: pyloric gland adenoma
Papillary, tubulopapillary, or tubular and mucinous preinvasive neoplasm in the mucosa (including gastric pyloric, gastric foveolar, biliary, intestinal, and oncocytic cell types, which often occur in a mixture)	Intracholecystic papillary-tubular neoplasm (ICPN)[15] Document: • Predominant cell type (if possible) • Extent of high-grade dysplasia (in percentage)	Biliary adenoma Intestinal type adenoma Tubular adenoma Tubulopapillary adenoma Papillary adenoma Papillary neoplasm Papillary carcinoma	Pyloric gland adenoma *or* Intracholecystic papillary neoplasm
Complex tubular and nonmucinous preinvasive neoplasm	Intracholecystic tubular nonmucinous neoplasm (ICTN)[17]	Pyloric gland adenoma Tubulopapillary adenocarcinoma	No specific information
Cystic papillary/tubular and mucinous lesion on the wall (arising in adenomyoma)	Mural intracholecystic neoplasm arising in adenomyomatous nodule[18]	Mural IPMN-like tumor[192]	No specific information

Modified from Roa JC, Basturk O, Adsay V. Dysplasia and carcinoma of the gallbladder: pathological evaluation, sampling, differential diagnosis and clinical implications. Histopathology. *2021;79(1):2-19.*

For a pT2 or greater carcinoma, documentation should include, in addition to the cystic duct margin, the presence or absence of spread to the serosal versus hepatic surfaces, respectively. Typically, proper documentation of the deepest region requires at least 12 tissue blocks with multiple strips because foci of carcinoma are often grossly unapparent.

For high-risk lesions, such as hyalinizing cholecystitis or xanthogranulomatous cholecystitis, which are notorious for being associated with grossly unapparent carcinomas, extensive sampling (minimum 20 sections) should be performed. If there is pancreatobiliary maljunction (anomalous union of pancreatobiliary ducts where the common bile duct and main pancreatic duct adjoin above the sphincter of Oddi and thus lead to reflux and cancers), the entire gallbladder should be examined, irrespective of gross findings.[16]

Patients with a clinical history of high-risk disease for carcinoma, such as primary sclerosing cholangitis, should also be sampled more extensively, preferably with at least four tissue blocks with multiple strips during the initial random sampling procedure.[8,11]

GALLBLADDER

Tumoral Intraepithelial Neoplasms

Similar to the remainder of the pancreatobiliary tract, mass-forming (>1 cm), preinvasive neoplastic lesions also occur in the gallbladder.[11,15,17-20] As such, these lesions represent gallbladder counterparts of *intraductal neoplasms* of the pancreas[21-29] and bile ducts,[30-32] or *intra-ampullary papillary tubular neoplasms*[33,34] and *duodenal surface adenomas*[35] of the ampulla, and much of the information elucidated about these tumors is also applicable to the gallbladder. Of course, there are also organ-specific characteristics.[11,15,17,18] In essence, these are gallbladder examples of what is known in other organs as *adenoma-carcinoma sequence*. Because they are relatively rare and the experience with them is relatively limited, the views about these tumors have been in flux. However, at the same time, there are numerous characteristics that have been delineated and agreed on in the past decade. They are all considered premalignant, although the risk of invasive carcinoma may vary greatly by subtype (discussed later).

In the past, various terms have been employed for these lesions (Table 39.1A). In the 2019 World Health Organization (WHO) classification of tumors of the digestive system, these lesions are regarded in two broad categories of *intracholecystic papillary neoplasm*[19] and *pyloric gland adenoma*[20] (Box 39.1). However, *intracholecystic papillary neoplasm*–type lesions often show areas of pyloric gland differentiation, and *pyloric gland adenoma*–type lesions often have papillary architecture or even mixed components. In addition, in the pancreatobiliary tract, *pyloric gland adenoma*–type lesions are now classified as *intraductal papillary mucinous neoplasms* (IPMNs) and intraductal papillary neoplasms of the bile ducts [IPNBs]).[29,32] Therefore we have proposed a unifying term of intracholecystic papillary-tubular neoplasms (ICPNs) for these lesions.[15] Recently, new entities, namely *intracholecystic tubular nonmucinous neoplasm (ICTN)*[17] and *mural intracholecystic neoplasm arising in adenomyomatous nodules*,[18] have been described. In this text, all of these entities are collectively referred to as *intracholecystic neoplasms,* and distinct subtypes are discussed in the following sections.

BOX 39.1 WHO Classification of Tumors of the Gallbladder/ Extrahepatic Bile Ducts

BENIGN EPITHELIAL TUMORS AND PRECURSORS
Adenoma
Biliary intraepithelial neoplasia (dysplasia) (BilIN)
Intracholecystic papillary neoplasm (gallbladder)
Intraductal papillary neoplasm (bile ducts)
Mucinous cystic neoplasm

MALIGNANT EPITHELIAL TUMORS
Carcinomas
- Adenocarcinoma, pancreatobiliary type
- Adenocarcinoma, intestinal type
- Adenocarcinoma, clear cell type
- Poorly cohesive carcinoma
- Mucinous carcinoma
- Adenosquamous carcinoma
- Squamous cell carcinoma
- Intracholecystic papillary neoplasm with associated invasive carcinoma
- Intraductal papillary neoplasm with associated invasive carcinoma
- Mucinous cystic neoplasm with associated invasive carcinoma

NEUROENDOCRINE NEOPLASMS
Well differentiated neuroendocrine tumor (NET G1, G2, and G3)
Poorly differentiated neuroendocrine carcinoma
- Large cell neuroendocrine carcinoma
- Small cell neuroendocrine carcinoma

Mixed neuroendocrine–nonneuroendocrine neoplasm (MINEN)

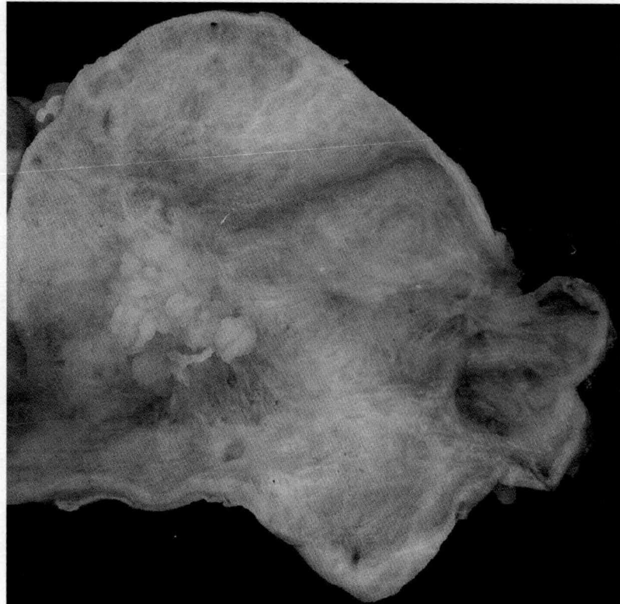

FIGURE 39.1 Intracholecystic papillary-tubular neoplasms are exophytic (papillary or polypoid) gallbladder lesions distinct from neighboring mucosa.

Intracholecystic Papillary-Tubular Neoplasms

Clinical Features

Clinically significant (>1 cm) ICPNs have certain recognized characteristics.[15] They occur in older adults who are typically in their early 60s at the time of diagnosis. Patients may present with abdominal pain, or the tumor may be detected incidentally. Gallstones in these patients are less common compared with patients with other types of gallbladder tumors. Rarely, patients have Peutz-Jeghers syndrome,[36,37] Gardner syndrome,[38,39] or an anomalous union of pancreatobiliary ducts.[16] Some cases are associated with a Brunner gland hamartoma of the duodenum.

Radiologically, nearly 50% of cases are classified as *cancer* because of the mucosal mass that defines these tumors, whereas others are classified as *polypoid tumors*. About 10% are not detected clinically, presumably because they are mistaken for stones or sludge.

There are geographic differences in the incidence and association with invasive carcinoma. For instance, both the overall incidence of ICPNs and its relative proportion in intraepithelial neoplasia is higher in the East than in the West (ICPNs constitute 52.5% of gallbladder intraepithelial neoplasia in the East and only 26% in the West). Moreover, ICPNs, although lower in relative frequency, may be more prone to advance to invasive carcinoma in the West (ICPN-associated invasive carcinomas constitute 42% of the gallbladder carcinomas in the West and 29% in the East).[40]

Pathological Features

ICPNs are characterized by the presence of large, papillary (or villous) growths with a feathery pattern or by smooth-surfaced polypoid projections that may be pedunculated or sessile (Fig. 39.1).[15,19] They occur more commonly in the body or fundus of the gallbladder. They may grow up to 8 cm in the maximum dimension and even fill the entire gallbladder in some cases. A substantial proportion, especially predominantly papillary examples, present as multifocal sessile lesions and have a field effect risk to the remainder of the biliary tract, with some noninvasive cases developing biliary tract cancers several years after the cholecystectomy.[15] Of note, ICTNs (discussed later) invariably form unifocal pedunculated lobulated polyps that easily detach from the surface and present as debris in the lumen.[17] Similarly, *intracholecystic neoplasms arising in adenomyomatous nodules* (discussed later) are localized mural nodular tumors that typically do not even show significant involvement of the gallbladder mucosa and remain mostly confined to the adenomyomatous nodule on the wall.[18]

The lesions are overtly exophytic and distinct from neighboring tissues. They may be predominantly papillary (or villous) or predominantly tubular, but a significant proportion show a mixed pattern of growth (Fig. 39.2).[15]

On the basis of the highest degree of cytoarchitectural atypia in the epithelium, dysplasia in ICPNs is classified as *low-grade* or *high-grade*. ICPNs with low-grade dysplasia reveal only mild architectural and cytological atypia. Relatively uniform but enlarged and hyperchromatic atypical nuclei are still mostly confined to the lower aspect of the epithelium (Fig. 39.3). High-grade dysplasia, which is present in a significant proportion of ICPNs that are >1 cm in size, are characterized by severe architectural and cytological atypia, and they may present in different patterns. In most cases, the main histological finding is pseudostratification of cells with loss of polarity and nuclear pleomorphism. Others exhibit a cribriform arrangement

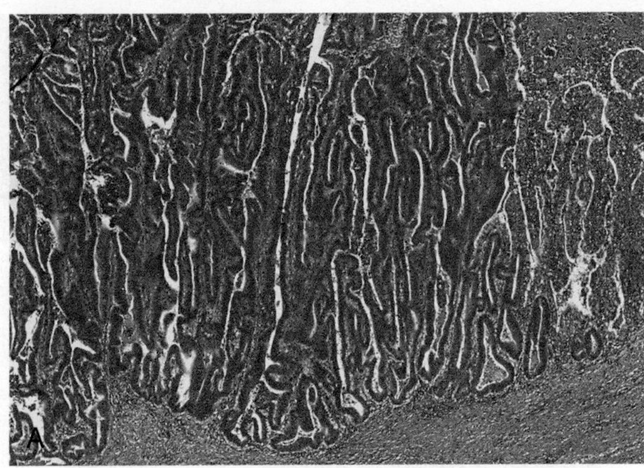

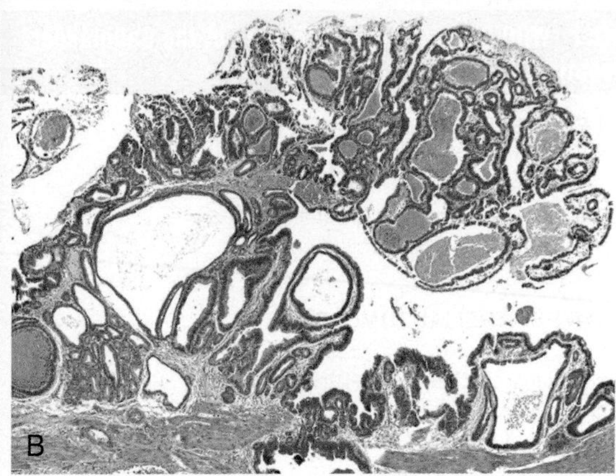

FIGURE 39.2 Intracholecystic papillary-tubular neoplasms are characterized by intraluminal growth of back-to-back epithelial units, either in a papillary **(A)** or tubular **(B)** configuration or both, with minimal or no intervening stroma.

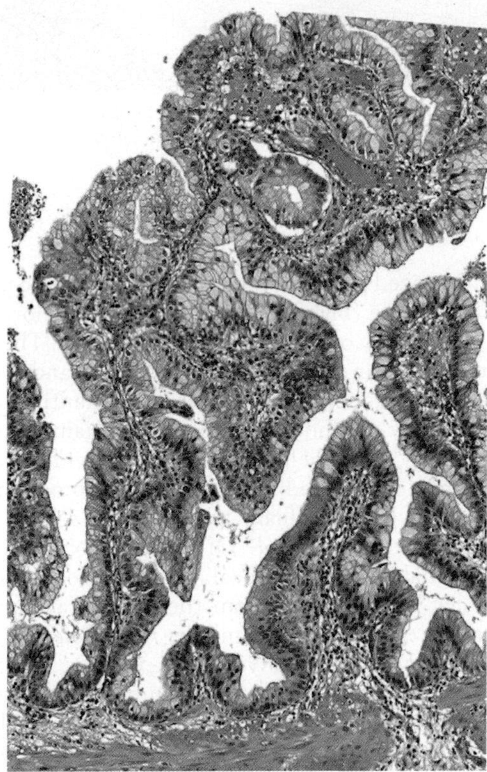

FIGURE 39.3 Intracholecystic papillary-tubular neoplasms with low-grade dysplasia reveal subtle cytoarchitectural changes. The nuclei are still small, relatively uniform, and mostly confined to the lower aspect of the epithelium.

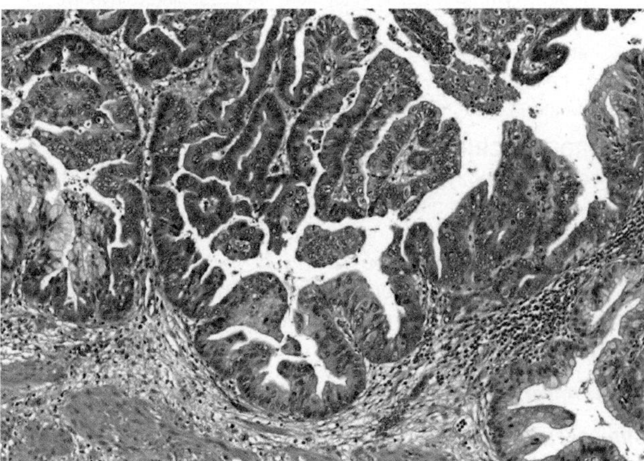

FIGURE 39.4 High-grade dysplasia in intracholecystic papillary-tubular neoplasms is characterized by stratification, loss of polarity, mucin depletion, disorganization, and nuclear enlargement.

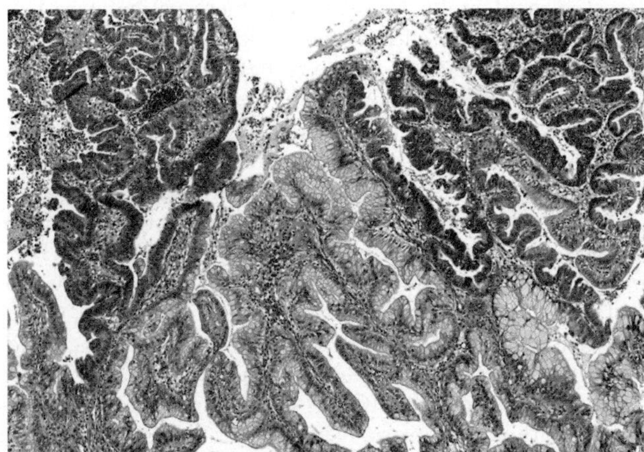

FIGURE 39.5 Transition from low-grade dysplasia *(center)* to high-grade dysplasia *(left and right upper corners)* is common in intracholecystic papillary-tubular neoplasms.

of cells, either with or without clear cell features, or a single layer of epithelium with centrally located and markedly abnormal nuclei (Fig. 39.4). A transition from low-grade dysplasia to high-grade dysplasia is common in these tumors (Fig. 39.5).[19,41]

Intracholecystic Papillary-Tubular Neoplasms with a Predominantly Papillary Growth Pattern. Once intracholecystic neoplasms[15,17,18] as well as polypoid pyloric metaplasias and fibromyoglandular polyps[15,42,43] were better characterized, ICPNs with a predominantly papillary growth pattern became the most common among mass-forming (>1 cm) preinvasive neoplasias in the gallbladder. As mentioned earlier, these are recognized in the 2019 WHO classification as *intracholecystic papillary neoplasms*[19] and are distinguished from *pyloric gland adenomas*[20]; however, they often exhibit gastric pyloric–type (or Brunner gland–like) mucinous glands as well.

TABLE 39.1B Clinicopathological Features of Intracholecystic Neoplasms

Authors' Classification	Key Features
Intracholecystic papillary-tubular neoplasm (ICPN), exclusively pyloric phenotype	• Distinct from the neighboring mucosa • Uniform mucinous glands with abundant apical mucinous cytoplasm and well-polarized nuclei • Express MUC6 • Reveal predominantly low-grade dysplasia • Associated invasive carcinoma uncommon
Intracholecystic papillary-tubular neoplasm (ICPN), predominantly foveolar phenotype	• Tall columnar cells with abundant, pale, mucinous cytoplasm • Express MUC5AC • Associated invasive carcinoma common
Intracholecystic papillary-tubular neoplasm (ICPN), predominantly biliary phenotype	• Cuboidal cells with prominent nucleoli • Express MUC1 • Reveal high-grade dysplasia • Associated invasive carcinoma common
Intracholecystic papillary-tubular neoplasm (ICPN), predominantly intestinal phenotype	• Tubular and/or villous architecture pseudostratified columnar cells with cigar-shaped nuclei • Express CDX2 and MUC2 • May reveal low- or high-grade dysplasia • Associated invasive carcinoma common
Intracholecystic papillary-tubular neoplasm (ICPN), predominantly oncocytic phenotype	• Arborizing papillae • Lined by two to five cell layers of oncocytic cells with abundant acidophilic granular cytoplasm and single prominent nucleoli • Express MUC1 • Associated invasive carcinoma common
Intracholecystic tubular nonmucinous neoplasm (ICTN)	• Lobulated, complex tubular pattern of small, back-to-back glandular units • Lined by cuboidal cells without overt intracytoplasmic mucin • Express MUC6 • Reveal predominantly high-grade dysplasia • Not associated with invasive carcinoma
Mural intracholecystic neoplasm arising in adenomyomatous nodules	• Confined to the adenomyomatous nodule region • Lined by gastric/endocervical-like mucinous epithelium • Express MUC5AC • Reveal predominantly low-grade dysplasia • Associated invasive carcinoma uncommon

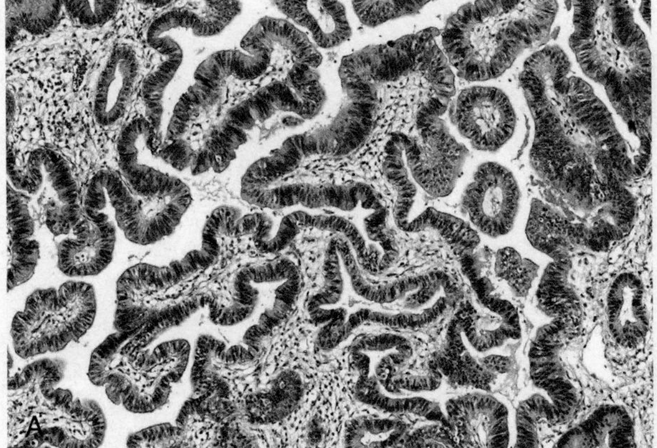

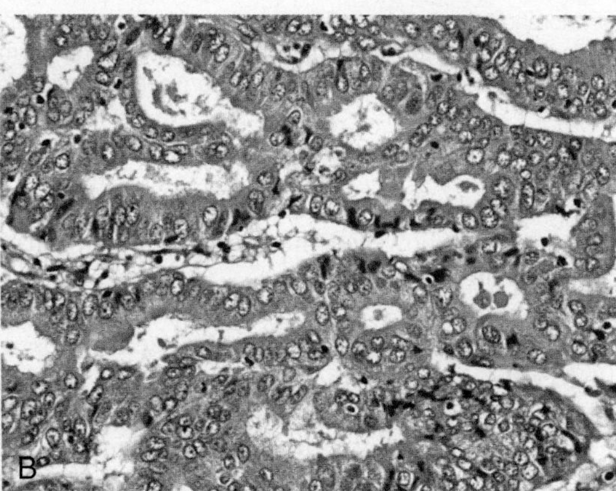

FIGURE 39.6 Biliary phenotype in intracholecystic papillary-tubular neoplasms. Morphologically it is similar to gallbladder epithelium, characterized by nondescript cuboidal cells **(A)** and is associated with high-grade dysplasia **(B).**

There are also different cell lineages observed in this group of ICPNs (Table 39.1B).[15] The majority exhibit *biliary* phenotype (Fig. 39.6), characterized by round cuboidal cells with prominent nucleoli and thus by nature, dysplasia is classified as high-grade. These lesions commonly express MUC1 and are often associated with invasive carcinoma. That is why they were classified as *papillary adenocarcinomas* in the past. Prominent lymphoplasmacytic and neutrophilic inflammation may involve the papillary cores and the epithelium. Follicular cholecystitis may also occur in patients with this type of tumor.[15,44]

Some ICPNs have a *gastric foveolar* phenotype (Fig. 39.7), which is characterized by the presence of tall columnar cells that have abundant, pale, mucinous cytoplasm and MUC5AC expression. These lesions may be analogous to the foveolar dysplasia that is being increasingly recognized.[45-47]

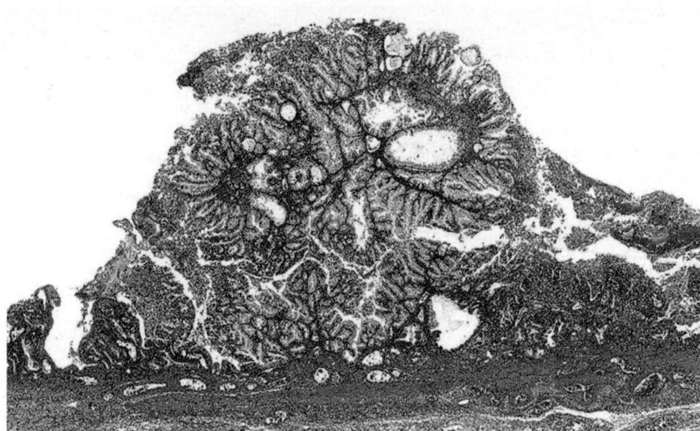

FIGURE 39.7 The gastric foveolar phenotype in intracholecystic papillary-tubular neoplasm is characterized by ill-formed papillae or elongated, interconnecting tubules lined by tall columnar cells with abundant pale mucin.

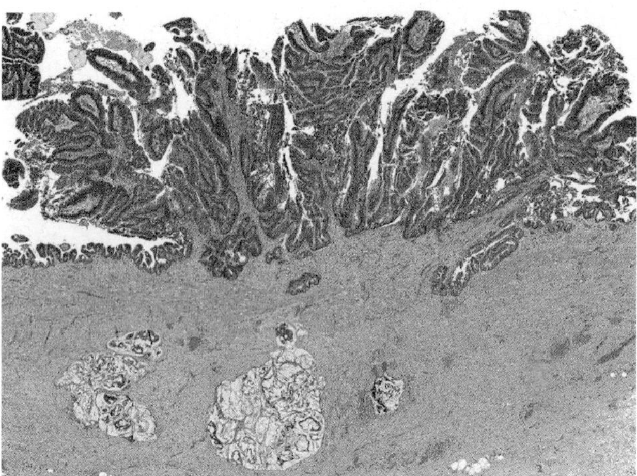

FIGURE 39.8 Intestinal phenotype in intracholecystic papillary-tubular neoplasms. Morphologically it is similar to colonic adenomas, showing pseudostratified cigar-shaped nuclei and overall basophilia. This example even reveals an associated invasive colloid carcinoma component *(bottom)*.

In the gallbladder, they appear very innocuous and do not seem overtly atypical; however, their association with invasive carcinoma is high.[15]

A small percentage of ICPNs resemble *intestinal*-type adenomas (Fig. 39.8). They are characterized by pseudostratified columnar epithelium with cells that contain cigar-shaped nuclei with conspicuous nucleoli, arranged in a tubular and/or villous architecture. In low-grade foci, the neoplastic cells are well oriented, have small and uniform nuclei, lack nucleoli, and have atypical mitoses (Fig. 39.9). High-grade foci are characterized by severe atypia with irregular branching papillae and budding of cell clusters into the lumen, cuboidal-shaped cells with stratification, loss of polarity, pleomorphism, and prominent nucleoli; mitoses are frequent (Fig. 39.10). As expected, these tumors are commonly positive for CK20, CDX2, and MUC2. Of note, goblet cells may be found in any type of ICPN.[15,20]

Rare cases may be *oncocytic* (Fig. 39.11), revealing features similar to those of intraductal oncocytic papillary neoplasms of the pancreas and bile ducts,[15,20] although

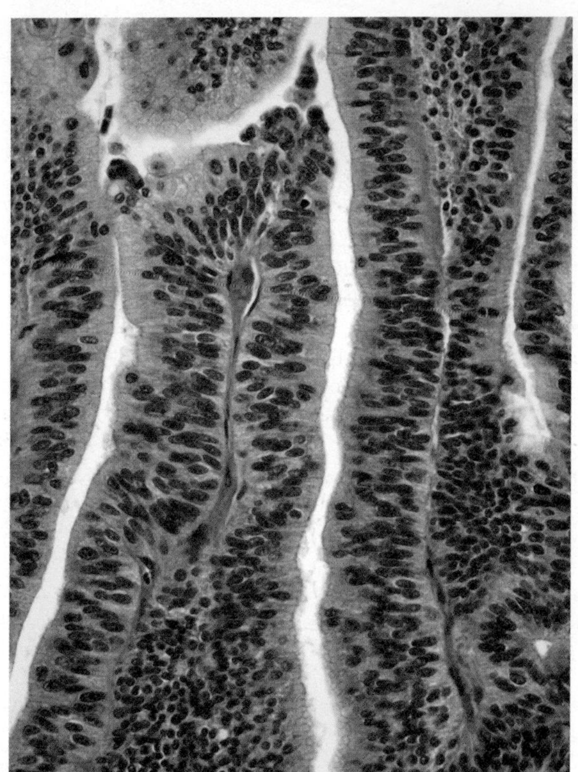

FIGURE 39.9 In low-grade foci of intracholecystic papillary-tubular neoplasms with the intestinal phenotype, the neoplastic cells are well oriented and have relatively small and uniform nuclei.

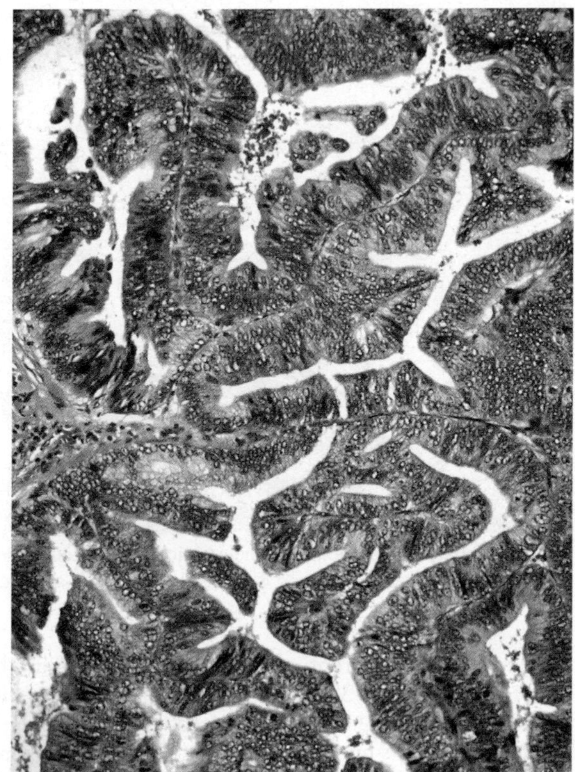

FIGURE 39.10 High-grade foci are characterized by irregular branching papillae and budding of cell clusters into the lumen, cuboidal-shaped cells with stratification, loss of polarity, pleomorphism, and prominent nucleoli.

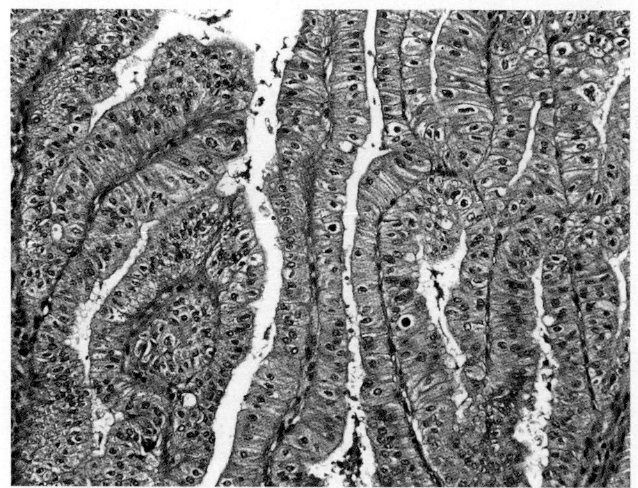

FIGURE 39.11 The oncocytic phenotype in intracholecystic papillary-tubular neoplasms is characterized by arborizing papillae lined by several layers of cells with abundant acidophilic granular cytoplasm and single prominent nucleoli. Intraepithelial lumen formation can also be encountered.

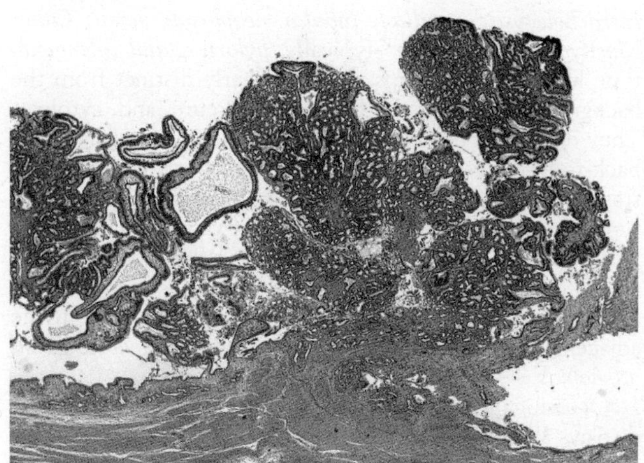

FIGURE 39.12 An intracholecystic papillary-tubular neoplasm with an exclusively gastric pyloric phenotype (also called *pyloric gland adenoma of the gallbladder*). Tightly packed, predominantly tubular and bland-appearing pyloric-type or Brunner-like glands are characteristic.

these are more prone to have intracytoplasmic hyaline globules.[48] Interestingly, oncocytic morphology in ICPNs does not correlate with the characteristic immunoprofile of intraductal oncocytic papillary neoplasms in the pancreas.[21,24,25,49] Instead, there is diffuse MUC1 expression and an absence of MUC6.[15]

Intracholecystic Papillary-Tubular Neoplasms with an Exclusively Pyloric Gland Phenotype (Pyloric Gland Adenomas). As mentioned earlier, ICPNs that are composed almost entirely of gastric pyloric–type (or Brunner gland–like) mucinous glands are classified as a separate category of *pyloric gland adenomas* (Fig. 39.12). However, these often have papillary architecture or even mixed components.

In the older literature, *pyloric gland adenoma*-type lesions were regarded as the most common type of "adenomatous" process in the gallbladder, but this was because noninvasive papillary neoplasms were regarded as part of

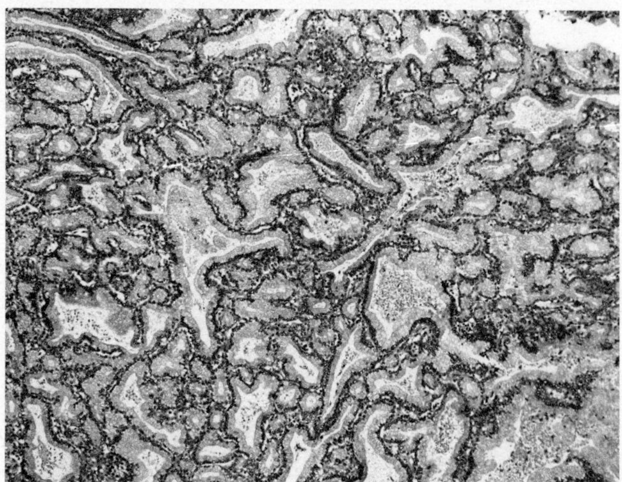

FIGURE 39.13 An intracholecystic papillary-tubular neoplasm with an exclusively gastric pyloric phenotype (also called *pyloric gland adenoma of the gallbladder*). Most cases reveal uniform glands with abundant mucinous cytoplasm and well-polarized nuclei located at the periphery of the cell cytoplasm and are classified as *low-grade.*

adenocarcinomas.[15,20,50] Moreover, the older literature is mostly based on series that included cases as small as 2 mm in largest dimension (mean size ranged from 0.6 to 0.9 cm).[51-53] It is now well known that pyloric gland metaplasia is seen in 60% of cholecystitis patients, and these lesions often form polypoid collections. It appears that a significant proportion of the lesions reported as *pyloric gland adenomas* actually represent exuberant polypoid examples of pyloric gland metaplasia, rather than true adenomas.[15,43] Perhaps as importantly, fibromyoglandular polyps of the gallbladder often have prominent collections of pyloric glands, and we have seen these polyps also designated erroneously as *pyloric gland adenomas*. To address these issues, the 2019 WHO classification recommends that small (<0.5 cm) pyloric gland nodules arising in a background of pyloric gland metaplasia in the adjacent mucosa should not be designated as *pyloric gland adenomas*.[20]

A true *adenoma* typically forms a true polyp and is sharply distinct from the neighboring mucosa. By definition, the majority of the lesions reveal uniform mucinous glands with abundant apical mucinous cytoplasm and well-polarized nuclei located at the periphery of the cell cytoplasm, and they are thus classified as *low grade* (Fig. 39.13). However, in large (>1 cm) *pyloric gland adenomas*, foci of high-grade dysplasia, characterized by cytoarchitectural complexity (disorganized appearance and highly atypical nuclei), may be present (Fig. 39.14). These cases are occasionally associated with invasive carcinoma.[15,20]

Intracholecystic Papillary-Tubular Neoplasms with an Associated Invasive Carcinoma. Regardless of the subtype, the most important task in a patient with ICPN is to rule out invasive carcinoma. In fact, in the presence of invasive carcinoma, typing of the preinvasive lesion becomes much less significant. Invasive carcinoma is difficult to detect in the gallbladder in general. This becomes even a bigger issue in patients with ICPNs, where invasive elements can be masked, in addition to inflammatory reactive changes, by the preinvasive dysplastic process. Moreover, especially

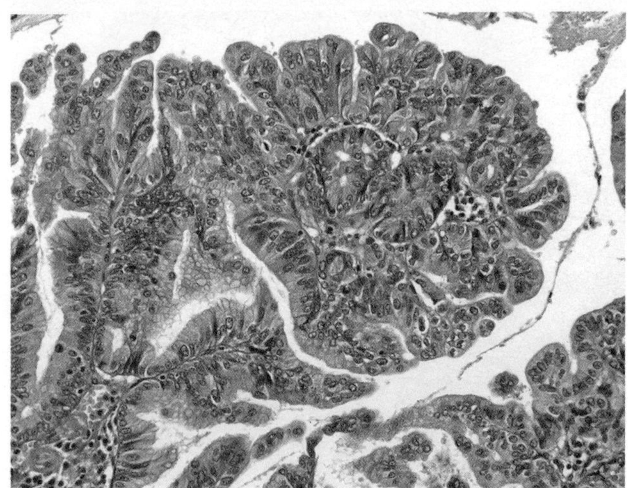

FIGURE 39.14 Foci of high-grade dysplasia may be seen in rare intracholecystic papillary-tubular neoplasms with a gastric pyloric phenotype (also called *pyloric gland adenoma of the gallbladder*).

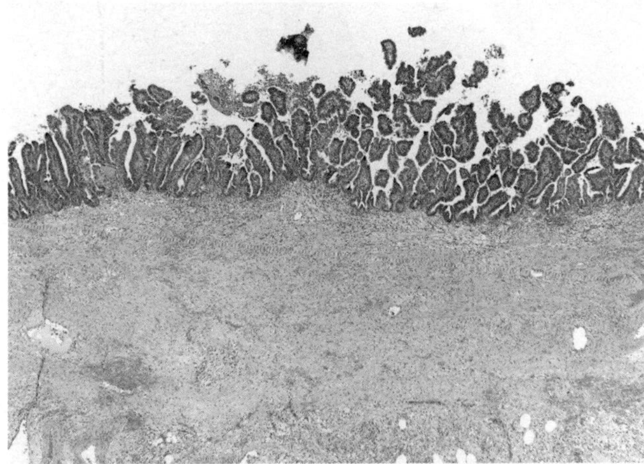

FIGURE 39.15 Ordinary nontumoral (flat) dysplasia of the gallbladder may reveal numerous papillary structures, mimicking an intracholecystic papillary-tubular neoplasm. However, these are microscopic lesions and do not form a grossly visible, distinct mass.

in patients with predominantly papillary ICPNs, invasive carcinoma can be hidden away from the main lesion. For this reason, it is imperative that extensive, if not entire, sampling is employed before a case can be classified as noninvasive. If an invasive carcinoma is identified, its size, extent, and type should be documented separately. Most invasive carcinomas that arise in patients with these tumors are ordinary tubule-forming adenocarcinomas (pancreatobiliary type), although unusual types such as mucinous (colloid), squamous, and neuroendocrine carcinomas may also occur and may in fact be proportionally more common.[15] If invasive carcinoma is not found, it is helpful to document the extent of high-grade dysplasia, the amount of papillary growth, and the cell lineages (especially biliary and gastric foveolar phenotypes) because these parameters have been found to be associated with a higher incidence of invasive carcinoma elsewhere in the biliary tract and with disease progression.[15,54]

Immunohistochemical and Molecular Features of Intracholecystic Papillary-Tubular Neoplasms. The immunophenotype of ordinary ICPNs corresponds to their line of differentiation. Most are cytokeratin 7 (CK7) positive, and many express mucin-related glycoproteins and oncoproteins, including carcinoembryonic antigen (CEA). The MUC1 response is typically confined to the apical membrane of cells in areas of biliary differentiation or high-grade dysplasia. MUC2 is expressed in intestinal areas, MUC5AC in gastric foveolar areas, and MUC6 in gastric pyloric or Brunner gland–like areas.[15,19]

Current evidence indicates that molecular alterations of ICPNs are different from those observed in the conventional dysplasia-carcinoma sequence in the gallbladder. They are more similar to those described in intraductal neoplasms of the intrahepatic and extrahepatic bile ducts.[55] Although *KRAS* mutations are common,[56,57] the *GNAS* codon 201 mutation, which is seen in about two-thirds of pancreatic IPMNs,[58] is rarely seen in ICPNs.[59-61] This disparity is presumably related to the rarity of the intestinal variant, which appears to be linked with this mutation.

Differential Diagnosis

Intracholecystic papillary-tubular neoplasms versus Other *Mostly Benign Lesions.* Typically, *pyloric gland adenoma*–type lesions form polyps that are clearly distinct from the background mucosa, both in architecture and cytology. They display large (usually >1 cm) collections of uniform, back-to-back glands without intervening stroma. In contrast, polypoid metaplasia and fibromyoglandular polyps are typically composed of smaller focus of variably sized glands with intervening stroma. The 2019 WHO classification recommends that small (<0.5 cm) pyloric gland nodules arising in a background of pyloric gland metaplasia in the adjacent mucosa should not be designated as *pyloric gland adenomas*.[20]

Occasionally, an ICPN that is smaller than 1 cm but that displays all characteristics of the larger examples (including clear-cut evidence of dysplastic changes) are encountered in a gallbladder. These should prompt total sampling of the gallbladder if this has not been performed. If no other lesions are discovered, then the case can be classified as an *incipient ICPN* with proper descriptions, as has been employed in the pancreatobiliary tract.[62] These do not appear to imply the field effect risk that larger and more extensive ICPNs signify.

ICPNs also should be distinguished from ordinary nontumoral (flat) dysplasia, which often reveals papillary structures or tubular units forming small collections. In some cases, these papillae may be tall and exuberant, but these cases should not be regarded as ICPNs unless they form a distinct clinically evident mass (Fig. 39.15).

Intracholecystic Papillary-Tubular Neoplasms versus Invasive Carcinoma. Recognition of the presence or absence of invasive carcinoma within or under polypoid tumors may be problematic because of architectural complexity and tangential sectioning. Features that favor carcinoma include wide separation of glandular units, their irregular contours (Figs. 39.16 and 39.17), cytological differences from the surface lesion (including paradoxical differentiation with more abundant cytoplasm and tubule formation), and foamy gland features and cell clusters that reside in clefts.[15,63] Extension of dysplastic epithelium into Rokitansky-Aschoff sinuses creates a pseudo-invasive appearance (Fig. 39.18, Table 39.2).[64] The distribution of the units, their spatial connection to the overlying mucosa, and the finding of remnant normal epithelium are helpful clues in determining that the lesion is not invasive. Unlike invasive adenocarcinomas, Rokitansky-Aschoff sinuses are often flask-shaped or elongated, with the longitudinal axis oriented perpendicular to the surface (Fig. 39.19). Paradoxically, these sinuses often have concentric bands of loose stroma that resembles desmoplasia (Fig. 39.20). Most gallbladder adenocarcinomas do not exhibit significantly desmoplastic stroma.

Natural History and Prognosis

Small (<1 cm) noninvasive ICPNs are typically clinically inconsequential.[51-53] However, when larger (≥ 1 cm) ICPNs are analyzed separately, even the *pyloric gland adenoma*–type lesions (previously thought to be innocuous) may be associated with or progress to invasive carcinoma.[15] In our experience, invasive carcinomas occur in about 65% of ≥1-cm ICPNs with prominent papillary architecture.[15] Biliary and foveolar cell phenotypes seem to be more frequently (60% to 70%) associated with invasive carcinoma, but the incidence of invasion is low (approximately 15%) in *pyloric gland adenoma*–type lesions.[15] From the opposite perspective, 6% of invasive gallbladder carcinomas arise in association with tumoral intraepithelial neoplasms.[65,66] This association seems to be even stronger in patients with chemical carcinogenesis, as exemplified in pancreatobiliary maljunction cases. In pancreatobiliary maljunction cases, the reflux of the pancreatic acinar enzymes leads to reflux cholecystopathy and ultimately to invasive carcinoma. One fourth of the pancreatobiliary maljunction–associated gallbladder carcinomas proved to be through the ICPN pathway.[67]

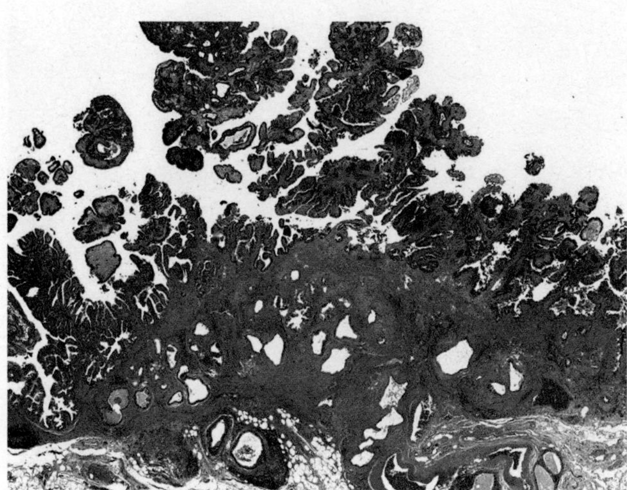

FIGURE 39.16 About 6% of gallbladder carcinomas arise from intracholecystic papillary-tubular neoplasms.

The 3-year survival rate for noninvasive ICPNs is 90%, compared with 60% for invasive tumors. Some noninvasive cases are found to have recurrences and metastases on long-term follow-up that cannot be explained by undersampling or missed invasion. This suggests that there may be a field-effect phenomenon responsible for the development of new biliary tract carcinomas years after the original gallbladder tumor was diagnosed. Thus these cases, especially the papillary and extensive/multifocal examples, should not only be carefully evaluated for the presence of invasion, but they also should be placed on a surveillance protocol, although currently there are no specific guidelines for this. Of note, ICTNs (discussed later)[17] and *intracholecystic neoplasms arising in adenomyomatous nodules* (discussed later)[18] seem to lack the field-effect phenomenon.

There is some evidence that, similar to the intraductal neoplasms of the pancreas/biliary tract, invasive carcinomas that arise from ICPNs have a more favorable survival rate than those that arise from flat dysplasia (3-year survival, 60% vs. 30%). This survival advantage is maintained even in stage-matched cases.[15]

Intracholecystic Tubular Nonmucinous Neoplasms

These cases are viewed differently by different experts. Some authors (especially in Asia and South America) typically classify these as *tubular adenocarcinomas.* Although they are not mucinous, because of some morphological

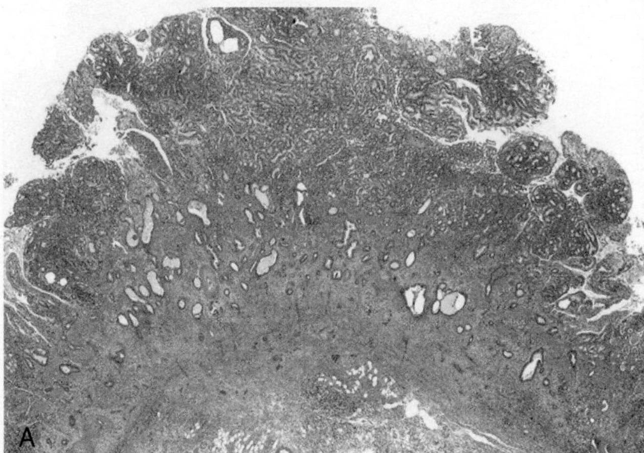

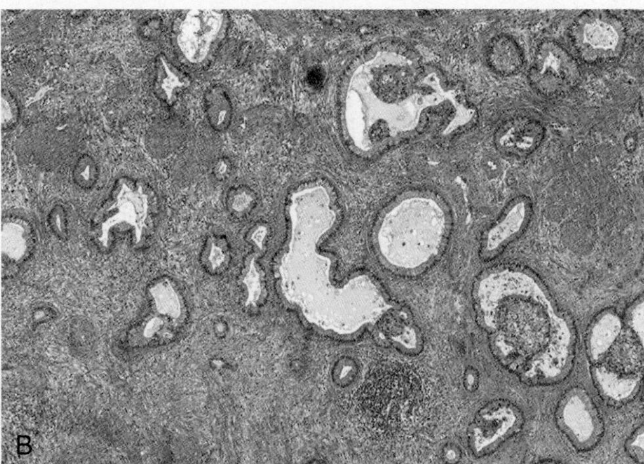

FIGURE 39.17 An invasive carcinoma component is characterized by wide separated glandular units with irregular contours (**A**) and usually reveals paradoxical differentiation with tubule formation and abundant intracytoplasmic mucin (**B**).

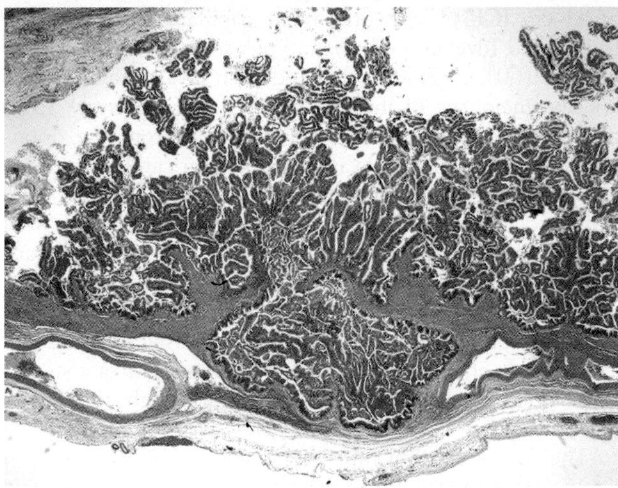

FIGURE 39.18 In intracholecystic papillary-tubular neoplasms, extension of dysplastic epithelium into Rokitansky-Aschoff sinuses may create a pseudo-invasive appearance.

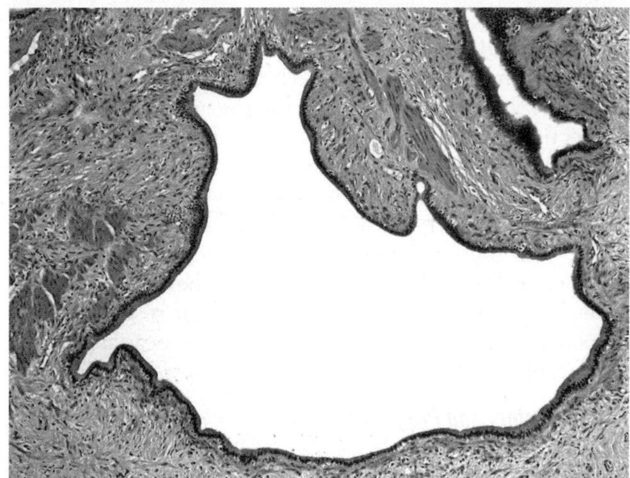

FIGURE 39.19 Rokitansky-Aschoff sinuses often appear as flask-shaped invaginations with their axis perpendicular to the surface. They are lined by columnar epithelium with basally oriented nuclei and acidophilic cytoplasm.

TABLE 39.2 Invasive Carcinoma versus Involvement of Rokitansky-Aschoff Sinuses by Neoplastic Epithelium

Invasive Carcinoma	Involvement of Rokitansky-Aschoff Sinuses by Neoplasia
Small to medium-sized round, dispersed glands	Long tubular units; flask shaped
Perineural invasion	Absence of perineural invasion
Longitudinal axis parallel to surface	Longitudinal axis perpendicular to surface
Cuboidal epithelium with either attenuated or foamy cells	Columnar epithelium with basally located nuclei and acidophilic cytoplasm
Glands without a connection to surface	Invaginations revealing connection to surface
Absence of a mixture of normal and neoplastic cells within glands	Mixture of normal and neoplastic cells within invaginations
Absence of inspissated bile within long dilated spaces	Inspissated bile within long dilated spaces

FIGURE 39.20 Unlike invasive adenocarcinomas, Rokitansky-Aschoff sinuses often have concentric bands of loose stroma that resembles desmoplasia.

similarities to *pyloric gland adenomas* and MUC6 positivity, we and some others have regarded these as a peculiar form of pyloric gland lesion in the past.[15,65] However, more analyses disclosed that they have several features clearly distinguishing them from other intracholecystic neoplasms and warranting their separate classification as ICTNs,[17] akin to intraductal tubulopapillary neoplasms (ITPNs) of the pancreas[26-28] and bile ducts.[30]

Unlike ICPNs, these form pedunculated polyps with very thin stalks, and they often become detached from the mucosa and can be easily dismissed as "debris" during gross examination. We have seen several examples in which a revisit to the specimen container brought in the main diagnostic material.[17]

Microscopically they are characterized by the presence of a distinctive lobulated, complex tubular pattern of small, back-to-back, round, or compressed glandular units with minimal lumen formation (Fig. 39.21). The lobules are

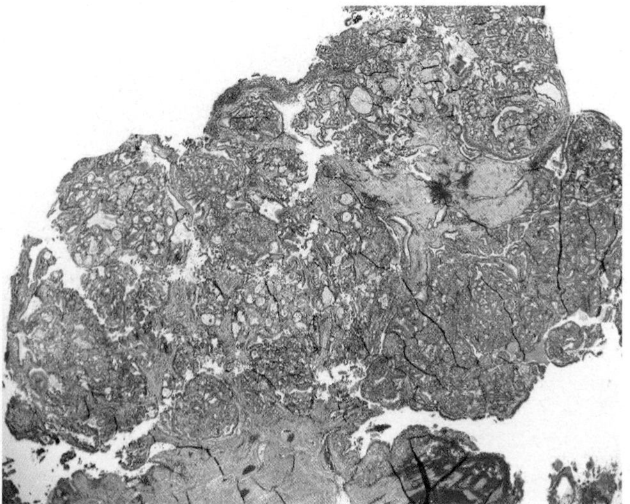

FIGURE 39.21 Intracholecystic tubular nonmucinous neoplasms are characterized by large pedunculated polyps with a thin stalk and multilobulated growth, typically in the background of a relatively unremarkable gallbladder.

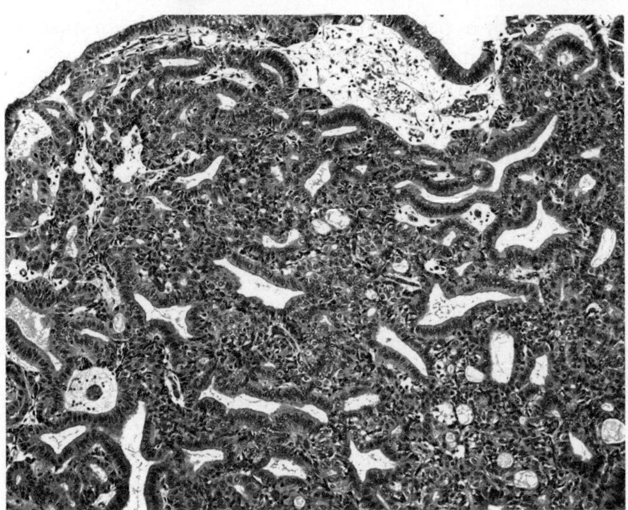

FIGURE 39.22 Intracholecystic tubular nonmucinous neoplasms are composed of tightly packed small- to medium-sized tubules, some showing cystic dilation. These show diffuse labeling with the pyloric marker MUC6.

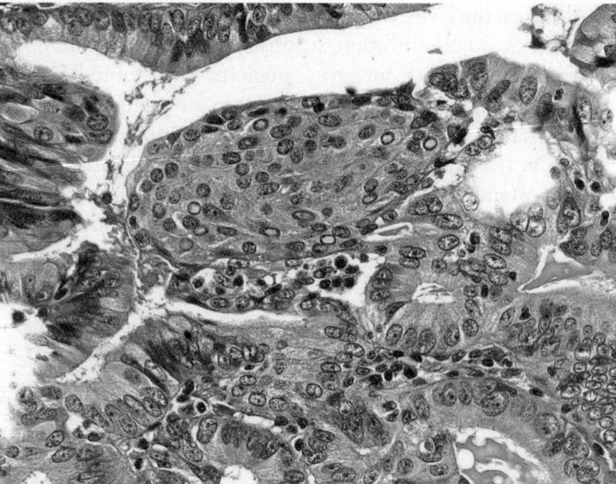

FIGURE 39.24 Morules composed of whorled, plump spindle cells are commonly seen in intracholecystic tubular nonmucinous neoplasms. The nuclei in these morules are large and often clear as a result of intranuclear biotin; nucleoli are usually absent.

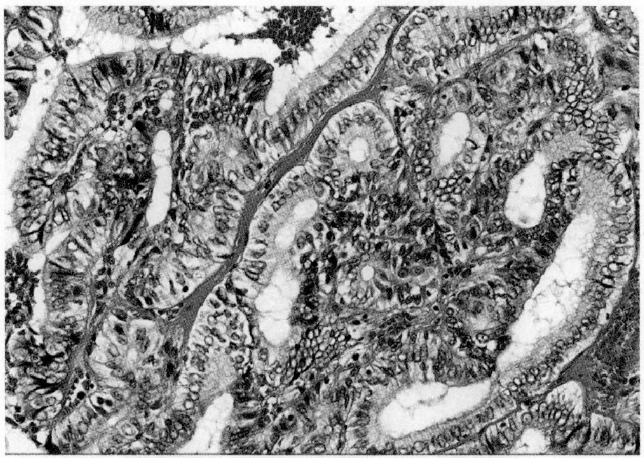

FIGURE 39.23 In many intracholecystic tubular nonmucinous neoplasms, clearing of the nuclear chromatin combined with the nuclear overlapping and elongated nature of the cells creates a picture highly reminiscent of papillary thyroid carcinomas.

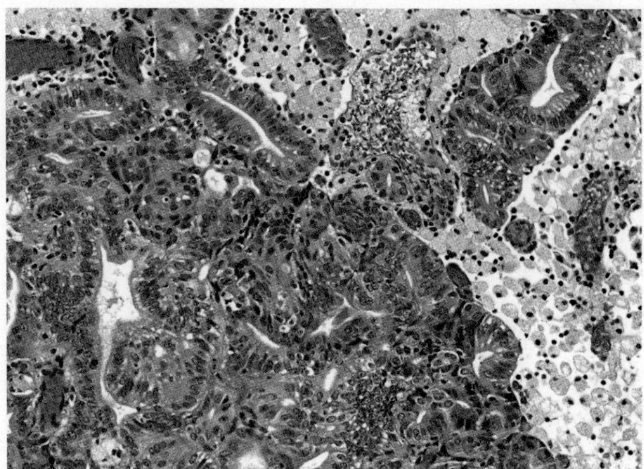

FIGURE 39.25 Cholesterolosis within the polyp as well as in the uninvolved gallbladder is a common finding in intracholecystic tubular nonmucinous neoplasms.

often covered by unremarkable gallbladder epithelium, and scattered cystically dilated glands with acidophilic granular secretions are often evident within the lobules. The glands are lined by cuboidal cells without overt intracytoplasmic mucin formation (Fig. 39.22). Paneth cells and neuroendocrine cells may also be identified.[17]

In some examples, the nuclei are more elongated and reveal overlapping features and chromatin clearing, which creates a pattern reminiscent of papillary thyroid carcinomas, which is not seen in other intracholecystic neoplasms (Fig. 39.23). In addition, morules composed of squamoid to spindle cells in a vague whorled pattern, similar to the squamoid morules found in pancreatoblastoma, pulmonary blastoma, cribriform-morular thyroid carcinoma, or endometrioid adenocarcinoma, are seen in more than 66% of ICTNs. The nuclei in these morules often have biotin-rich, optically clear pseudoinclusions (Fig. 39.24).[17] These morules are not seen in other intracholecystic neoplasms other than rare pyloric gland adenoma–type lesions, which often show transition to ICTNs. This kinship to other morule-forming tumors, also known as *biotin-rich, optically clear nuclei [BROCN]-forming tumors,*[68,69] also involves expression of estrogen receptors and mutations in β-catenin.[61,70] Recently it has been reported that ICTNs appear to be driven by the Notch and Wnt/CTNNB1 signaling pathways, bearing mutations in *APC2* and *MLL2* (two known regulators of β-catenin signaling) and demonstrate aberrant nuclear CTNNB1 protein expression.[71,72]

Another important distinguishing feature of ICTNs is the association with cholesterol polyps. The overall cauliflower-like architecture, which is consistent in every case, is something that is highly characteristic of a cholesterol polyp (Fig. 39.25).[15,17,61,66] The fact that the lobules are typically outlined by normal epithelium, combined with the common presence of cholesterolosis in the stroma and the lack of significant injury in the remainder of the gallbladder[17,61,66] (a common feature in patients with cholesterol polyps),[43] makes this association even more impressive.

Although the level of cytoarchitectural atypia warrants a *high-grade dysplasia* classification, surprisingly ICTNs do not appear to be associated with invasive carcinoma (undoubtedly, there must be cases, but we have not yet seen an example).[17] From the opposite perspective, we also have not identified this growth pattern in the background of invasive adenocarcinomas.[17] It is also important to note that the dysplastic process is largely confined to the polypoid lesion and does not show multifocality. More importantly, unlike ICPNs, ICTNs do not seem to pose any field-effect risk for the remainder of the biliary tract.[17]

Mural Intracholecystic Neoplasms Arising in Adenomyomatous Nodules

Intracholecystic neoplasms arising in adenomyomatous nodules also appear to form a distinct category (see Table 39.1B).[18] They are typically discovered in elderly patients. Unlike other intracholecystic neoplasms, they form distinct mural nodules on the gallbladder wall in the fundic region, mostly preserving the surface mucosa. Microscopically, they are characterized by papillary proliferations lined by gastric/endocervical-like mucinous epithelium (Figs. 39.26 and 39.27). Focal intestinal-type epithelium may also be seen (16%; Fig. 39.28). They predominantly reveal low-grade dysplasia (see Fig. 39.27), have a low incidence of associated invasive carcinoma (16%), and do not appear to bear risk for the remainder of the biliary tract.[18] As such, they have some analogy to pancreatic branch duct–type IPMNs, which are more innocuous, typically of gastric phenotype, and progress to invasive carcinoma in only 15% of cases. In contrast, surface intracholecystic neoplasms (ICPNs and ITPNs) are like pancreatic main duct–type IPMNs, which tend to be much more complex, extensive, and multifocal, and show high (>50%) propensity for invasion and dissemination.[73,74]

Mucinous Cystic Neoplasms

Hepatobiliary mucinous cystic neoplasms (with ovarian-type stroma) is another type of tumoral intraepithelial neoplasm that is worth mentioning. On careful scrutiny, the majority of mucinous cystic neoplasms identified in the gallbladder originate in the bile ducts and liver (discussed later). They secondarily involve the gallbladder. Convincing cases that originate in the gallbladder mucosa/wall independent of the large bile ducts of the liver are extremely rare.[75-78] In a few cases, adenomyomatous nodules with hypercellular stroma have also been misconstrued as mucinous cystic neoplasms.

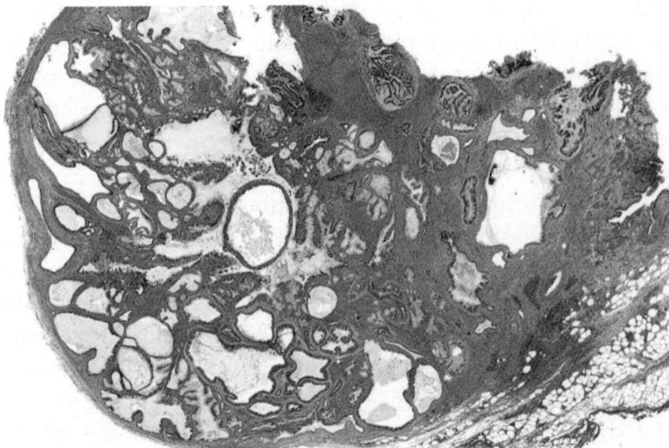

FIGURE 39.26 Mural intracholecystic neoplasms arising in adenomyomatous nodules of the gallbladder are characterized by a compact multilocular, demarcated, cystic lesion with a mucinous epithelial lining and at least some degree of papillary proliferation.

Nontumoral ("Flat") Intraepithelial Neoplasms (Dysplasia)

Definition and Terminology

As in the pancreas and the bile ducts, there are microscopic forms of dysplasia that occur in the gallbladder, discovered either incidentally or adjacent to invasive carcinomas. Essentially these are the gallbladder counterparts of *pancreatic intraepithelial neoplasia* (PanIN)[79] and *biliary intraepithelial neoplasia* (BilIN).[80] In fact, *BilIN*, a term originally proposed for the bile ducts,[81] is now used synonymously for the gallbladder as well, as depicted in the 2019 WHO classification.[80] However, many authorities prefer the term *dysplasia* for the gallbladder, and this is considered acceptable as well.

These nontumoral ("flat") forms of intraepithelial neoplasms (dysplasia) have many characteristics that distinguish them from the tumoral (mass-forming) intraepithelial neoplasms discussed previously. These will be presented in detail in the following sections. However, it should be noted that dysplasia often has a microscopic papillary

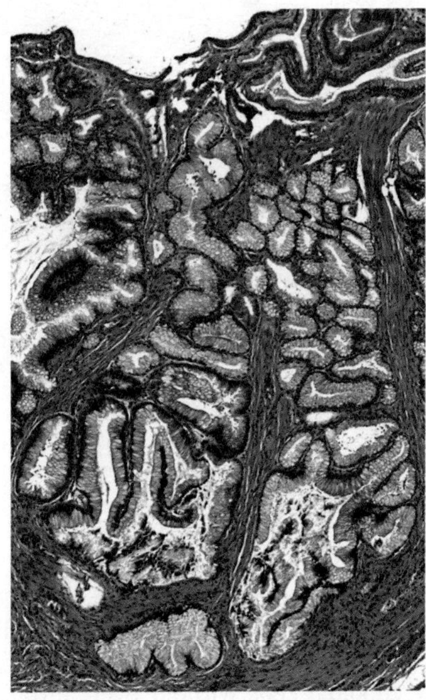

FIGURE 39.27 The lining of mural intracholecystic neoplasms arising in adenomyomatous nodules is often composed of gastric/endocervical-like mucinous epithelium.

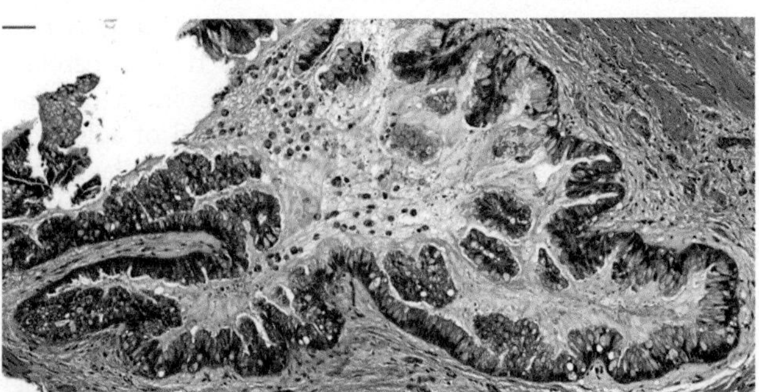

FIGURE 39.28 Focal intestinal-type epithelium may also be seen in mural intracholecystic neoplasms arising in adenomyomatous nodules.

configuration as well as zones of tubule formation, and it may not be distinguishable from the tumoral intraepithelial neoplasm if taken in isolation (on high-power examination). However, by definition, dysplasia does not form a grossly or radiographically recognizable mass lesion.[80,81]

Clinical Features

Patients with dysplasia are identified mainly in their 50s to 60s. Dysplasia cases without invasive carcinoma are diagnosed at a mean age of 57 years compared with 66 years for dysplasia cases with invasive carcinoma.[82]

All risk factors that have been established for gallbladder adenocarcinoma (see later), including geography, gallstones, sclerosing cholangitis, and anomalous union of pancreatobiliary ducts, are considered risk factors for dysplasia as well.

Dysplastic lesions are normally detected incidentally in gallbladder specimens removed for other disorders because dysplasia is clinically unapparent.[83-86] Low-grade dysplasia, which is subjective and difficult to define, is more likely to be detected when multiple sections of the gallbladder are examined, whereas high-grade dysplasia is often extensive at the time of diagnosis.[14] The overall incidence of dysplasia varies greatly among different populations, but it parallels the incidence of adenocarcinoma. In one North American population, routine cholecystectomies for gallstones and morbid obesity contained low-grade dysplasia in less than 5% of cases, high-grade dysplasia in less than 1%, and frank carcinoma in less than 0.2%.[87] The rate approaches 15% in high-risk regions such as Mexico and Chile.[14] Dysplasia is associated with 40% to 60% of invasive gallbladder carcinomas. However, it is sometimes difficult to distinguish true dysplasia from colonization of the surface epithelium by invasive carcinoma cells. This makes analysis of dysplasia in invasive carcinoma cases more difficult.[88]

Pathological Features

By definition, gallbladder dysplasia is difficult to appreciate grossly.[89] Some cases, especially those with a prominent papillary configuration, may reveal granularity or a feathery change to the mucosa, but most appear hyperemic or are entirely normal by macroscopic examination.

Grading. Microscopically, gallbladder dysplasia is graded based on the highest degree of cytoarchitectural atypia in the epithelium as either *low-grade* or *high-grade*. The terms *high-grade dysplasia* and *carcinoma in situ* (CIS) are interchangeable, but the former is recommended.[41] The 2019 WHO classification also advocates use of the term *high-grade dysplasia*.[80] Of note, cases are categorized as *indefinite* if the cytological features approach but do not quite reach those of definite dysplasia or if the epithelium shows atypical features suggesting dysplasia, but a definitive diagnosis cannot be established because of ulceration, inflammation, or technical reasons.

Low-grade dysplasia is characterized by columnar cells that show mild pseudostratification, nuclear enlargement, an increased nucleus-to-cytoplasm (N:C) ratio, and nuclear irregularity. In low-grade dysplasia, the nuclei are usually limited to the basal portion of the cell cytoplasm, and there is only a minimal amount of architectural distortion and loss of nuclear polarity. Mitoses are increased in number, but atypical mitoses are rare (Fig. 39.29). Similar to the esophagus, if the surface epithelium lining the tips of the mucosal folds are not involved, then the diagnosis of dysplasia should be regarded dubious. *High-grade dysplasia* is characterized by cells with loss of polarity, marked nuclear enlargement, a markedly increased N:C ratio, significant nuclear irregularity, and hyperchromasia (Fig. 39.30). Mitotic activity is brisk, but it should be kept in mind that mitotic activity also can be brisk in some cases of regeneration. High-grade dysplasia is most commonly characterized by nuclei that appear round, but some cases have a more elongated and pencillate appearance.

Because of a lack of prospective (outcome) studies, it is difficult to determine the biological and clinical significance of low-grade dysplasia in the gallbladder. However, it is clear that high-grade dysplasia is often associated with invasive carcinoma. Therefore thorough sampling is crucial in any case of high-grade dysplasia. Recurrences and metastasis seen in some patients with high-grade dysplasia are attributable to missed areas of invasion and/or a field-effect phenomenon. In fact, a case should not be classified as mere *high-grade dysplasia* only (noninvasive) unless total sampling is performed.[11]

Growth Patterns. Gallbladder dysplasia has various growth patterns,[90] and any one case may have multiple growth patterns (Fig. 39.31). However, the diagnosis is established

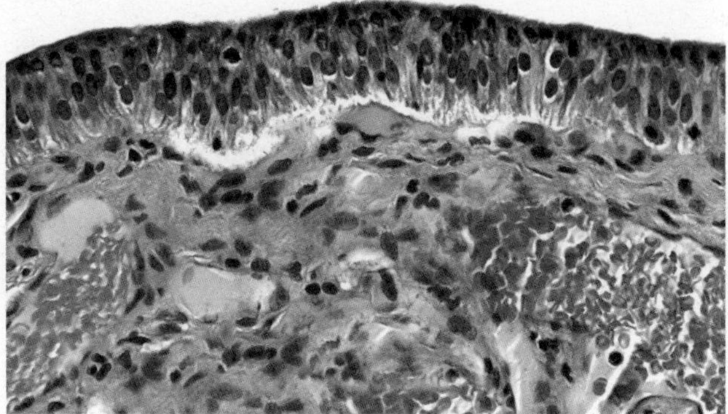

FIGURE 39.29 Low-grade dysplasia. There is mild nuclear enlargement and slight hyperchromasia with clumping of chromatin.

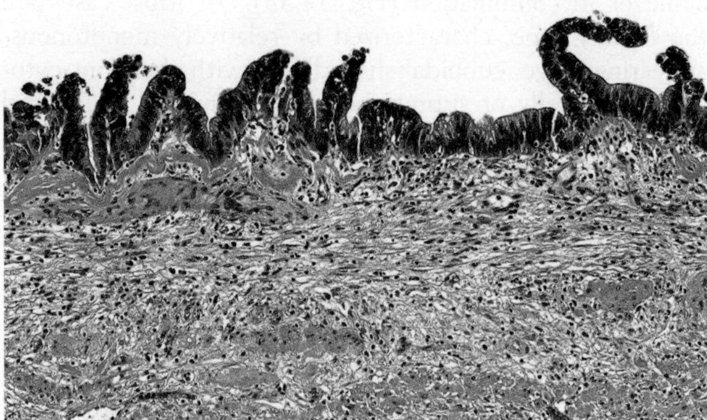

FIGURE 39.30 High-grade dysplasia. In this case, the cells show marked cytological atypia including a high nucleus-to-cytoplasm ratio compared with reactive epithelium. The cells show stratification with tuft formations.

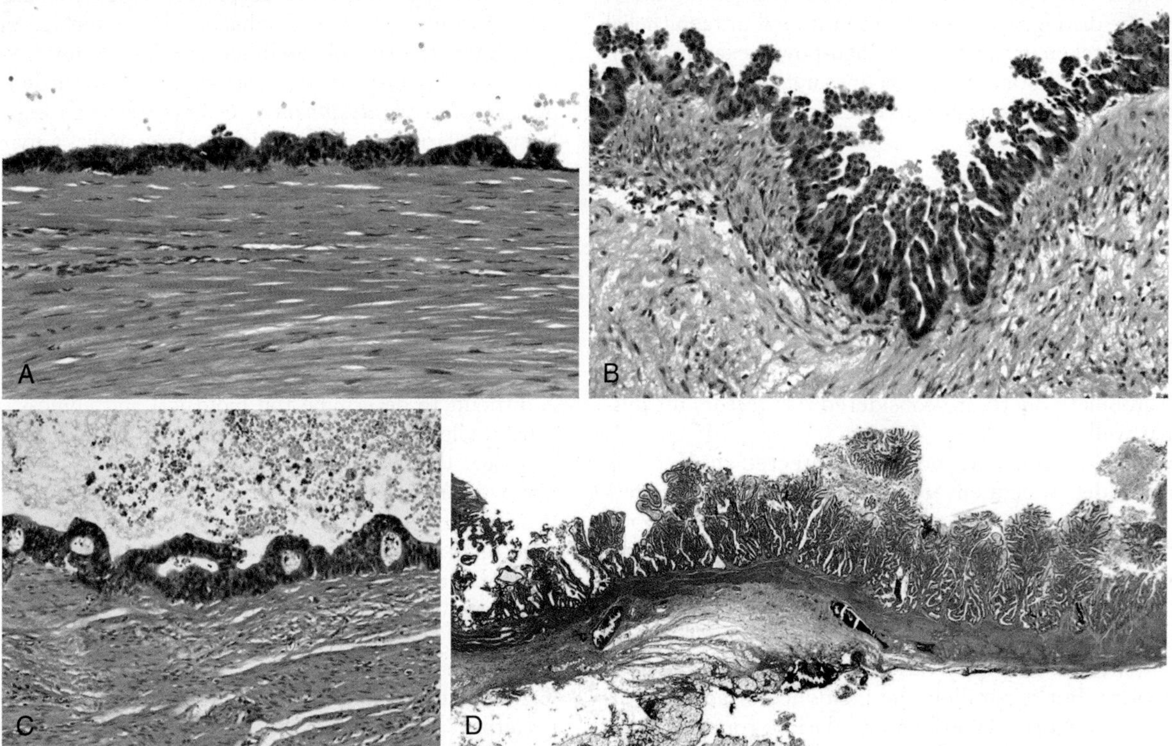

FIGURE 39.31 Nontumoral (flat) dysplasia has various growth patterns that can be seen in combination in any given case, ranging from flat/undulating **(A)** to micropapillary/tufting **(B)** to tubular **(C)** to tall papillary **(D)**.

solely on the basis of cytological findings rather than architecture. The *tubular* pattern can be difficult to distinguish from invasive well-differentiated adenocarcinomas (see Fig. 39.31). The *tall papillary* pattern is seen in about 25% of cases (see Fig. 39.31). If the papillae form is a grossly visible, compact polypoid mass, the lesion is best classified as an *intracholecystic neoplasm* (discussed earlier).[9]

In some cases, the glands reveal partially preserved nonneoplastic epithelium, indicating that the dysplasia represents pagetoid involvement of nonneoplastic glands by dysplastic cells (Fig. 39.32). Unusual types of carcinoma, such as adenosquamous, squamous cell, and neuroendocrine, also can have intramucosal components.

Types of Dysplasia. Adsay and his colleagues reported that gallbladder dysplasia reveals different cell lineages, either alone or in combination (Fig. 39.33).[82,91] Most cases are the *biliary* type, characterized by relatively monotonous-appearing, large, cuboidal-shaped cells with abundant cytoplasm; centrally or suprabasally located nuclei; cherry-red macronucleoli; and relatively fine chromatin. The cytoplasm may reveal clear cell (centrally located nuclei and nuclear contour irregularities), chromophobe-like (perinuclear cytoplasmic clearing), or oncocytoid (abundant acidophilic granular cytoplasm) features (Fig. 39.33A). The latter two often contain smoother nuclear contours. Some cases are the *intestinal* type, showing features similar to those of colonic adenomas, such as basophilia and pseudostratified, cigar-shaped nuclei (Fig. 39.33B). *Gastric foveolar*–type dysplasia reveals abundant, apical, pale cytoplasm and basally located, mildly enlarged nuclei with marked nuclear irregularity and hyperchromasia or prominent nucleoli (Fig. 39.33C). This is not to be confused with pyloric gland metaplasia that forms small antral-type (or Brunner-like) glandular units in the subsurface. Gastric foveolar–type dysplasia is characterized by an alteration in the surface epithelium.[91,92] The clinical significance of these cell types has not yet been determined, therefore it is not imperative to determine the type for diagnostic or clinical purposes.[82,91]

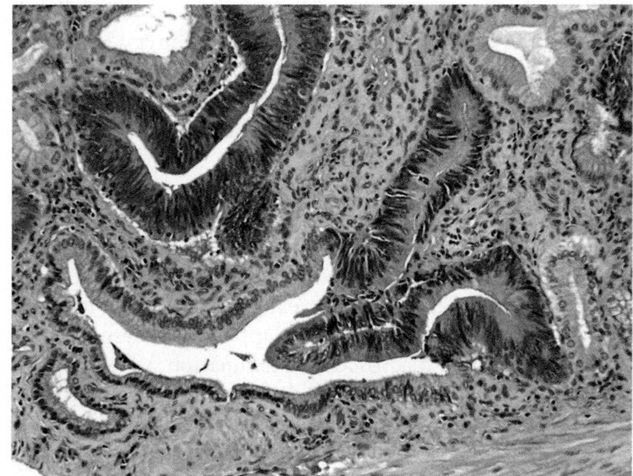

FIGURE 39.32 Pagetoid involvement by dysplastic cells. The glands are still partially lined by nonneoplastic epithelium.

Differential Diagnosis

Dysplasia versus Reactive Changes. The differential diagnosis of dysplasia and reactive changes is a well-known

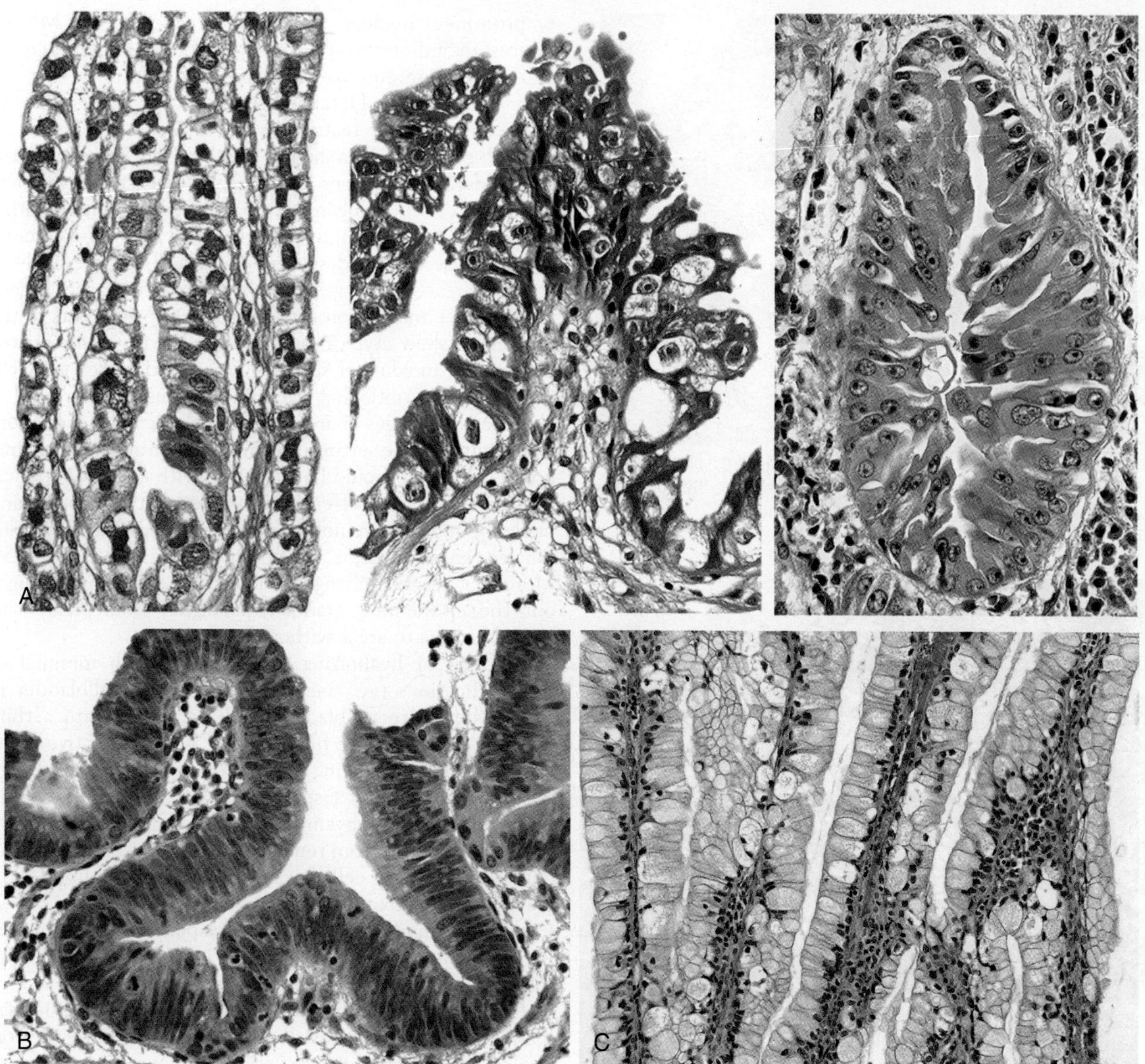

FIGURE 39.33 A, Cellular phenotypes in gallbladder dysplasia. The biliary-cuboidal phenotype is characterized by monotonous round cells with centrally/suprabasally located large nuclei (2 to 3× normal), relatively even and fine chromatin, and often prominent cherry-red nucleoli. Abundant cytoplasm may reveal variable (clear, *left;* chromophobe-like, *center;* or eosinophilic/oncocytoid, *right*) textures. **B,** Intestinal-type dysplasia has features similar to those of colonic adenomas, such as basophilia and pseudostratified cigar-shaped nuclei. **C,** Deceptively bland-appearing gastric foveolar–type has abundant apical pale cytoplasm, basally located mildly enlarged nuclei, and open chromatin. Nuclear irregularities (raisinoid) or nucleolar prominence is also present.

problem in gallbladder pathology (Figs. 39.34 and 39.35; Table 39.3).[93] Molecular studies to document abnormalities in cancer-associated genes (findings that could help establish the neoplastic nature of morphologically defined lesions) have been limited. Therefore dysplasia is defined and distinguished from other epithelial lesions based primarily on morphological principles, drawing in part from experience with early neoplastic changes in the pancreatobiliary tract.

The architectural growth pattern, such as a tall papillary configuration with cytological atypia, micropapillary or tufting pattern, cribriform arrangements, fused units, piled cells, and severe dispolarity of cells, is very helpful in diagnosing dysplasia (see Fig. 39.31). These patterns of growth are unusual in reactive lesions, although there are always exceptions. In the biliary type, cells typically lose their columnar shape and often acquire a monotonous appearance. Nuclear enlargement (two or three times normal) and prominent, cherry-red nucleoli are characteristic features of dysplasia, not seen in reactive lesions (see Fig. 39.33A).[91] Some cases are associated with abundant neutrophils, so inflammatory cells should not always be regarded as definite evidence of reactive changes (Fig. 39.36). The gastric foveolar type of dysplasia is typically composed of a single layer of innocuous-appearing cells on the tips of the folds, with pale cytoplasm and eccentric nuclei. Some cases have foamy or microvesicular cytoplasm. Nuclei are hyperchromatic when compressed at the periphery, but they typically have a raisinoid appearance

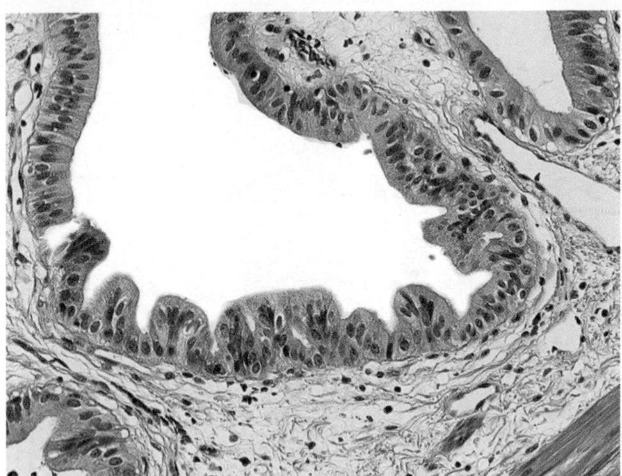

FIGURE 39.34 Reactive epithelial changes mimicking dysplasia. There is mild atypia and disorganization of the cells. However, the nuclei are relatively hypochromatic and show single, small nucleoli.

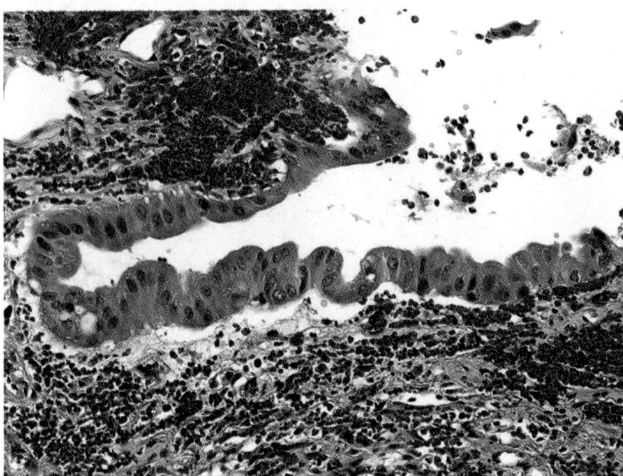

FIGURE 39.35 Reactive epithelial changes mimicking dysplasia. The nuclei show mild atypia and pseudostratification. However, the nuclei exhibit fine chromatin and a smooth contour. There is marked congestion in the stroma, indicating that this is a focus of injury.

or prominent nucleoli when they are suprabasal. Mitotic figures, including atypical forms, can be prominent in areas of regeneration and are therefore not helpful in this differential diagnosis. Detached reactive cells can also exhibit signet ring cell–like features (Fig. 39.37).[94]

High-grade dysplasia shows a "wildfire" phenomenon in the gallbladder, which means it is typically extensive at the time it is detected and involving a significant proportion of epithelium.[14,82,90,91] However, focal epithelial atypia in a background of well-preserved nondysplastic epithelium is more likely to represent reactive changes. Moreover, reactive changes usually show surface maturation (Fig. 39.38). Deeper aspects of the epithelium show atypical basophilic cells with an attenuated appearance, molding of slightly disorganized nuclei, and cells with a high N:C ratio, but the surface is usually mature.

Reactive changes in areas of ulceration can be even more challenging. In the setting of hemorrhage in adjacent stroma, epithelial atypia should be evaluated with caution. Atypical cells in these areas often have washed-out chromatin and nucleoli, but they are not as large as in high-grade dysplasia. Nuclear enlargement is also not as striking (see Fig. 39.35). Moreover, reactive changes tend to wax and wane throughout the epithelium, gradually changing from areas with marked atypia to areas without atypia.

In cases of hyalinizing cholecystitis[9] with minimal or no calcifications (i.e., incomplete porcelain gallbladder in which the entire gallbladder wall transforms into a thin, uniform, paucicellular, fibrotic band with distinctive clefting), any type of "clinging" epithelium on the surface should be regarded as highly suspicious for dysplasia. However, in well-preserved (nonhyalinized) gallbladders, the pathologist should refrain from rendering a diagnosis of dysplasia in detached epithelial cells because they often acquire degenerative changes that resemble dysplasia.[81]

Cancerization of Mucosa versus Dysplasia. In gallbladders with invasive carcinoma, secondary involvement of the epithelium, referred to as *cancerization* or *colonization*, may be difficult or even impossible to distinguish from true dysplasia. If the process has direct continuity with and morphological similarity to an underlying invasive carcinoma, it is best regarded as cancerization rather than dysplasia.

TABLE 39.3 Features Helpful in Distinguishing Reactive Changes from Dysplasia

Feature	Reactive Changes	Low-Grade Dysplasia	High-Grade Dysplasia
Architectural growth pattern, such as tall papillary, micropapillary/tufting, cribriform arrangements	–	–	+
Nuclear chromasia	Hyperchromatic/hypochromatic	Hyperchromatic	Hyperchromatic
Nuclear enlargement	–	+	++
Very large, prominent "cherry-red" nucleoli	–	–	+/–
Surface maturation	+	–	–
Dislodged stone– related changes	+	+/–	+/–
Inflammatory cells	++	+/–	+/–
Stromal hemorrhage and edema	++	–/+	–/+
Goblet cells	–/+	++	++
Mitotic figures	++	+/–	++
Loss of polarity	–	+/–	++

+, Present; –, not present; +/–, may be present.

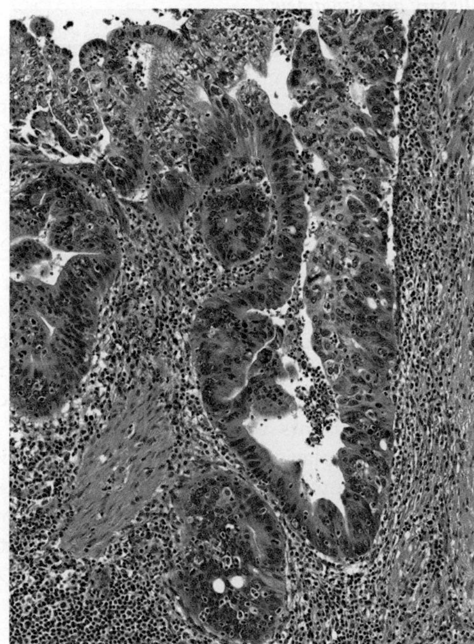

FIGURE 39.36 Examples of dysplasia that attract neutrophils, as shown here, may be difficult to distinguish from reactive atypia associated with inflammation. Nuclear enlargement (size, 2 to 3x normal) along with the presence of prominent, cherry-red nucleoli seen in dysplasia is unusual in reactive atypia.

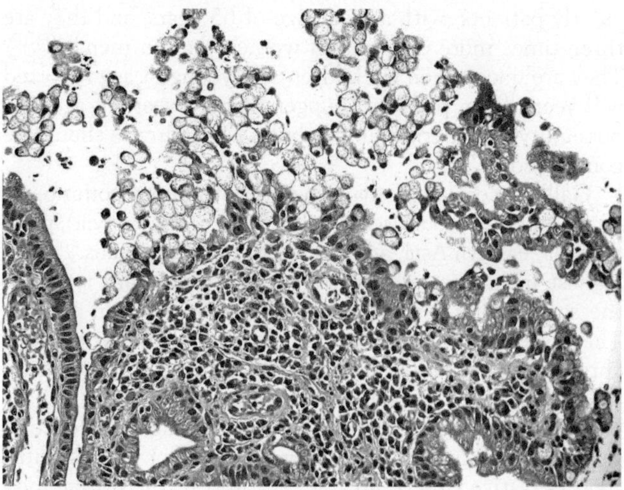

FIGURE 39.37 Signet ring cell–like degeneration of detached gallbladder epithelial cells. This is a rare and peculiar phenomenon that easily can be mistaken for a signet ring cell carcinoma. The fact that only the detached cells show signet ring cell morphology is helpful to indicate that this is a degenerative process.

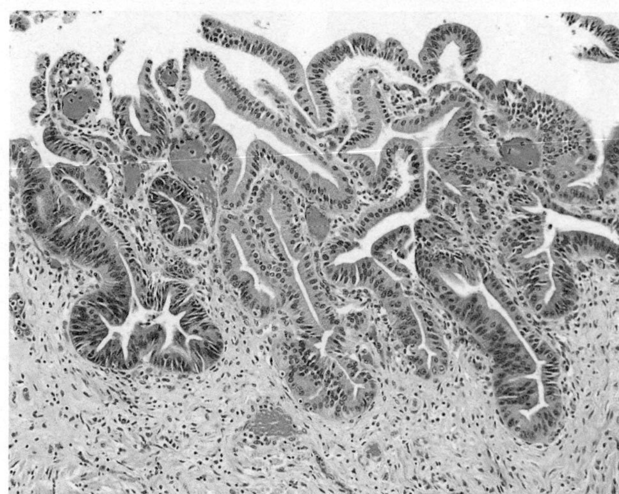

FIGURE 39.38 Although the deeper aspect of the epithelium is "darker" as a result of atypical basophilic cells, toward the surface, reactive atypia often displays maturation. Evenness of nuclear chromatin, the presence of sharp and smooth chromatin, and lack of marked nuclear enlargement are also helpful.

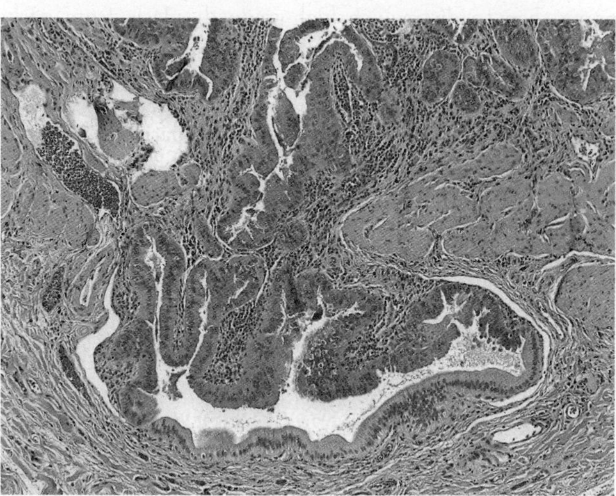

FIGURE 39.39 Cancerization of the gallbladder epithelium. The cytological features of the malignant cells within the epithelium are identical to those in the invasive component of the tumor. Note the abrupt transition between the malignant cells and normal cuboidal epithelium.

Abrupt transition from normal epithelium to atypical cells also favors cancerization (Fig. 39.39).

High-Grade Dysplasia versus Early Invasive Carcinoma. For early gallbladder carcinomas (i.e., pTis, pT1a with lamina propria invasion, and pT1b with tunica muscularis invasion), it may be difficult to distinguish "in situ" changes from true early invasive carcinomas, if the dysplastic changes occur in areas of the gallbladder with peribiliary mucous glands (i.e., neck and cystic duct region), in areas with pyloric gland metaplasia (i.e., common in injured gallbladders and seen in up to 60% of cholecystectomy specimens), or in areas with Rokitansky-Aschoff sinuses.[10] The gallbladder epithelium normally shows undulations, and there is no muscularis mucosa to separate the mucosa from the submucosa. More importantly, the tunica muscularis (there is no muscularis propria in the gallbladder) is highly irregular and porous in normal gallbladders.[95] Dysplastic glands can often be seen lying within or deep to the tunica muscularis (Fig. 39.40). There are no basal or myoepithelial cells that can help distinguish native epithelium from invasive carcinoma. Nevertheless, features that favor true invasive carcinoma include invasion of nerves or blood vessels, a monotonous population of atypical glands (rather than a mixture of neoplastic and benign or metaplastic glands), a haphazard infiltrative pattern, variable size and shape of the glands, angulated contours, lack of luminal bile, and lack of a connection to benign epithelium at the surface or adjacent submucosal glands (see Figs. 39.42 to 39.48). Fortunately, this distinction may not be clinically significant because data from high-risk regions have concluded that cases classified as *early gallbladder cancer* (i.e., pTis, pT1a, and pT1b) have a very good long-term survival rate, much more favorable than those with advanced carcinomas.[10]

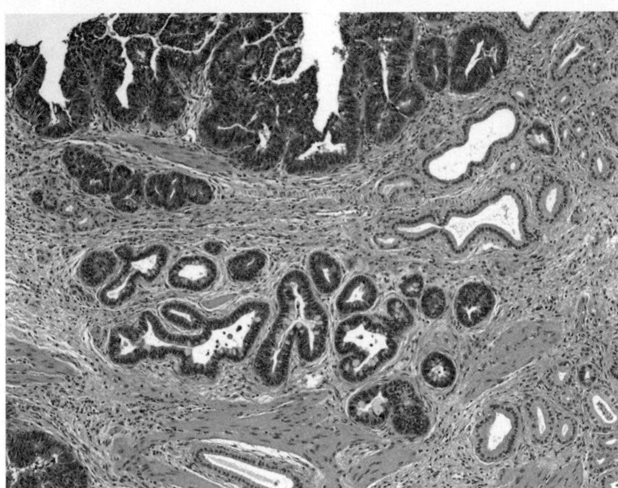

FIGURE 39.40 High-grade dysplasia (carcinoma in situ) involving complex glandular units and abutting tunica muscularis in a pseudoinfiltrative pattern.

It is far more important to exclude an advanced carcinoma than to distinguish high-grade dysplasia from early gallbladder carcinoma. In fact, a case should not be classified as pTis, pT1a, or pT1b unless complete sampling of the gallbladder is performed. The reported differences in survival rates of pT1 cases in Western populations compared with high-risk regions, such as Chile and Southeast Asia, may be caused by undersampling in the West, resulting in downstaging of pT2 carcinomas. For cases of early gallbladder carcinoma identified by a thorough sampling of the gallbladder with the protocol established by Roa and colleagues, in which advanced carcinomas are definitely ruled out, the 10-year survival rate approaches 90%.[8,10]

Immunohistochemical and Molecular Features

Immunohistochemically, mCEA and MUC1 typically show a linear pattern on staining at the apical border of dysplastic cells. In high-grade dysplasia, intercellular membranes may also be accentuated by CEA; however, intracytoplasmic labeling with mCEA and MUC1 is uncommon. Therefore dense intracytoplasmic staining favors cancerization over dysplasia. TP53 nuclear staining occurs in more than 30% of cases of dysplasia and tends to be more common (and stronger) in high-grade lesions.[56] However, it should be kept in mind that it can also be seen in areas of regenerative changes.[96] Similarly, although the Ki67 labeling index is high in cases of dysplasia and increases by grade, it can also be high in areas of regenerative changes.

Analysis of normal and dysplastic gallbladder epithelium has shown that allelic losses of chromosome 8p occur in normal mucosa.[56] In low-grade dysplasia, allelic loss of chromosome 3p is common and regarded as an intermediate change, which also corresponds to progressive loss of fragile histidine triad (FHIT) protein in dysplastic lesions of increasing grade. Loss of heterozygosity of 5q has been found in various grades of dysplasia.[97] Oncogenic mutations of the *KRAS* gene is uncommon in upper biliary (gallbladder and proximal bile duct) dysplasia.[98,99] Telomere shortening is very common in dysplasia, similar to invasive carcinomas, and it is typically absent in normal epithelium.[100] However, metaplastic changes also commonly show telomere shortening.

Natural History and Prognosis

Prognostic data are limited for dysplasia cases not accompanied by invasive carcinoma. The only information available has been from the Surveillance, Epidemiology and End Results (SEER) database sponsored by the National Cancer Institute (NCI), which is itself limited by the lack of pathological review or standardized sectioning of specimens. Nevertheless, a 2014 analysis of cases recorded as *carcinoma in situ* in the SEER database revealed age-adjusted 5- and 10-year survival estimates as 87% and 79%, respectively.[101] It is presumed that the early mortalities represent missed invasive carcinomas, and the late ones represent a field-effect phenomenon resulting in the development of new cancers in the biliary tract.[101,102] Appropriate clinical management for patients with a cholecystectomy specimen that reveals dysplasia without invasive carcinoma has not been defined. However, involvement of the cystic duct margin by high-grade dysplasia raises concern about the status of the distal cystic duct and other extrahepatic bile ducts.

Invasive Epithelial Neoplasms

Adenocarcinoma

Clinical Features

Most adenocarcinomas of the biliary tract occur in the gallbladder.[12] Gallbladder carcinomas occur predominantly in elderly patients, with a mean age of 65 years, and they are three times more common in women than in men.[9,103-106] They are uncommon in children; the youngest age reported is 9 years.[107] In patients younger than 20 years of age, the possibility of hyperimmunoglobulin M syndrome should be considered.

Gallbladder carcinoma is significantly more common in Latin American countries (Chile, Mexico, and Bolivia), parts of India, eastern Asia, and among Native Americans.[108] The highest incidence rates in the United States are found in the southwestern, north central, and Appalachian regions. The association of gallbladder adenocarcinoma with prior chronic inflammation has been well established, mostly by epidemiological data showing a high incidence of gallbladder cancer in populations with a very high incidence of gallstones (particularly cholesterol stones) or cholecystitis, such as Native Americans.[103,109] However, the overall incidence of gallbladder cancer among patients with gallstones is <0.2%. Aflatoxin B1, found in food not properly stored, and *Salmonella typhi* have also been implicated as triggers of the inflammatory cascade. Another established and underappreciated risk factor is pancreatobiliary maljunction (also called *anomalous union of pancreatobiliary ducts* or *long common channel*), which is the supra-Oddi union of the common bile duct with the main pancreatic duct.[12,110,111] This anomaly leads to reflux of pancreatic enzymes to the biliary system and presents a very high risk of mucosal abnormalities and cancerous transformation.[67] Previously thought to be mostly a disorder in Asian populations, we recently found that close to 10% of gallbladder carcinomas in the West are also attributable to this condition.

The most common symptoms of gallbladder cancer are upper quadrant pain and fever. Laboratory abnormalities include increased serum alkaline phosphatase levels. At clinical

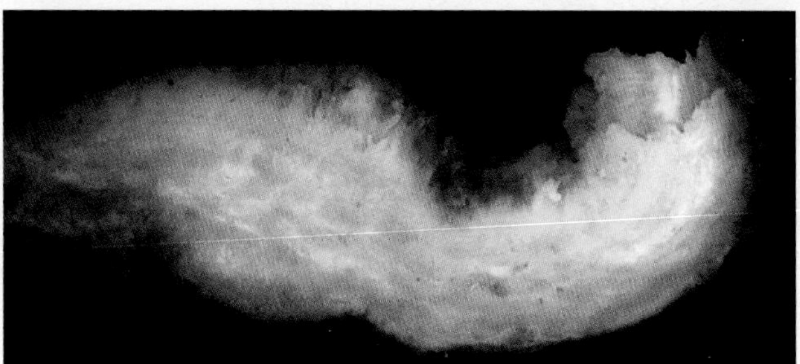

FIGURE 39.41 Gallbladder carcinomas are typically scirrhous tumors. However, they can be almost impossible to distinguish from chronic cholecystitis both clinically and pathologically, and therefore a significant proportion of patients present with "inapparent" cancers.

presentation, many patients with gallbladder adenocarcinoma have cholecystitis. Because their gallbladders usually contain gallstones, the organ is typically removed by a routine cholecystectomy (including laparoscopic cholecystectomy) with the clinical intent of treating cholecystitis and cholelithiasis. In fact, more than one third of gallbladder carcinomas are *clinically unapparent* (i.e., detected incidentally).[1]

Pathological Features

Most (70%) gallbladder adenocarcinomas arise in the fundus. They are firm, white, gritty, and ill-defined tumors that typically grow diffusely and have a propensity to infiltrate surrounding tissues in an insidious fashion (Fig. 39.41). Therefore it is often difficult to distinguish carcinoma from chronic cholecystitis.[2-4,112] In fact, even on careful macroscopic evaluation of the gallbladder, more than one third of advanced gallbladder carcinomas (pT2 stage or higher) are missed at the time of gross examination. This figure increases to 70% for superficial cancers.[2-4] As such, if any evidence of high-grade dysplasia or carcinoma is detected in random sampling of the gallbladder, extensive sampling should follow for proper identification and staging of the carcinoma. It is also important to orient the hepatic and nonhepatic serosal surfaces to comply with the current staging requirements (see later).

Some cases are associated with a grossly detectable intraepithelial component (i.e., intracholecystic neoplasm) (see Fig. 39.16). These often appear tan, granular, and soft, and they often become detached from the surface because they are friable. Because they are usually admixed with necrotic material, they also may be disregarded as debris by the prosector.

Carcinomas that arise from hyalinizing cholecystitis (i.e., incomplete porcelain gallbladder) warrant special attention. Most invasive carcinomas in this setting are difficult to recognize grossly because they often are hidden within the thin, uniform band of the fibrotic wall of the gallbladder. However, some form subserosal or subhepatic nodular infiltrates.[9]

Rare carcinoma types may exhibit subtle differences in gross appearance. For instance, in some cases, mucinous carcinoma is associated with acute cholecystitis and has a gelatinous appearance.[104] Undifferentiated carcinomas often have a fleshy appearance and may have a polypoid contour.[113] Some poorly cohesive carcinomas have a linitis plastica pattern in which the wall of the gallbladder and its layers are thickened but relatively well preserved.[114]

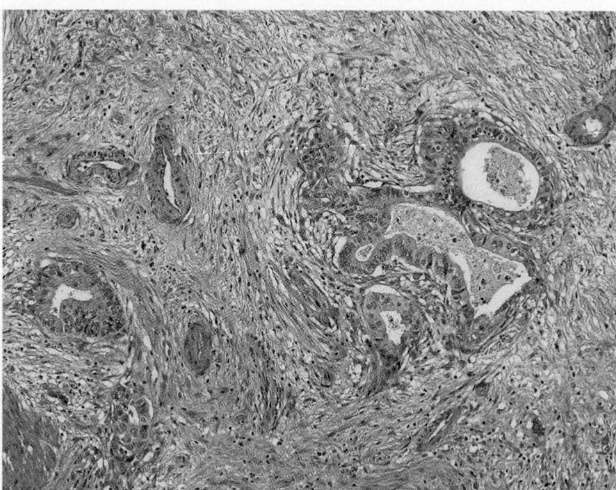

FIGURE 39.42 Adenocarcinoma of the cystic duct, usual (pancreatobiliary) type. There are scattered, well-formed, but irregular glandular units associated with desmoplastic stroma.

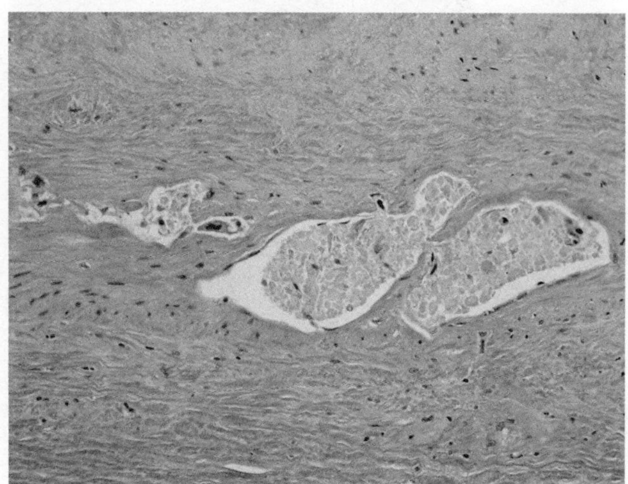

FIGURE 39.43 Adenocarcinoma within an incomplete porcelain gallbladder. Many glands have partially attenuated epithelium. The luminal contents are often seen to merge with the stroma, sometimes leaving distinctive granular debris, which can be the only evidence of carcinoma in some sections.

Microscopically, most gallbladder adenocarcinomas display features typical of pancreatobiliary adenocarcinomas, such as the presence of widely separated, well-formed glands and small clusters of cells embedded within a densely fibrotic stroma.[50,103,115] In most cases, the glands are simple, lined by cuboidal cells, and have dilated, round lumina (Fig. 39.42). Hyalinizing cholecystitis (i.e., incomplete porcelain gallbladder) often shows plaquelike lesions with glands embedded within thin bands of paucicellular sclerotic stroma (Fig. 39.43).[9] These glands are often arranged horizontally on cross-section of the gallbladder. Architecturally, malignant glands are normally arranged in a random or haphazard pattern, which contrasts sharply with the organoid clusters of benign ductules normally located in the wall of the bile ducts. Often, the nuclear grade is high compared with the degree of glandular differentiation. The cytoplasm may be acidophilic and granular in some cases or pale to clear in others (Fig. 39.44). Various amounts of

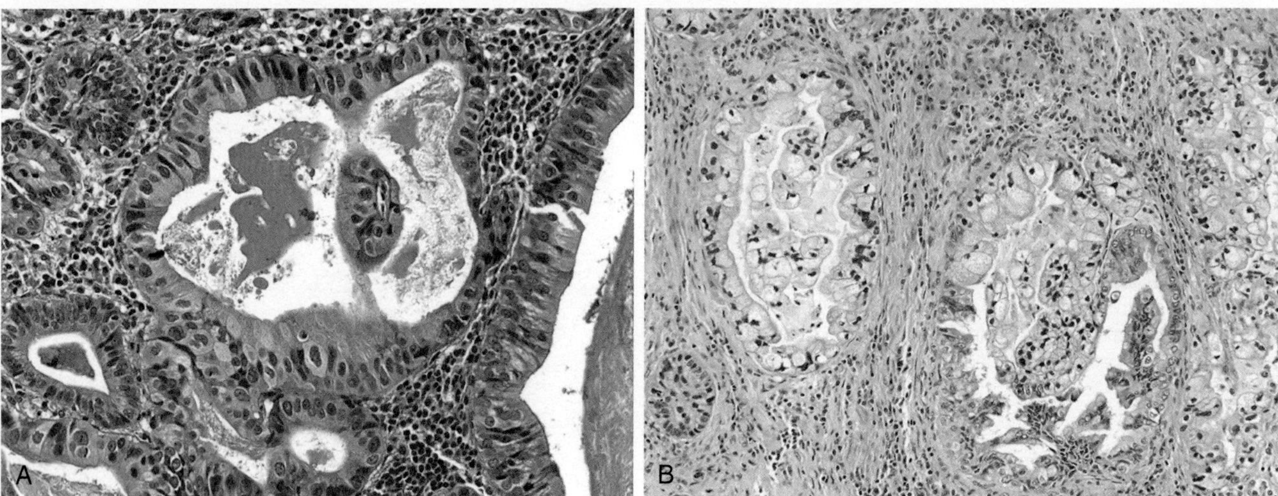

FIGURE 39.44 Gallbladder adenocarcinomas may reveal different histopathological features. The cytoplasm may be acidophilic and granular (**A**) or pale to clear in others (**B**).

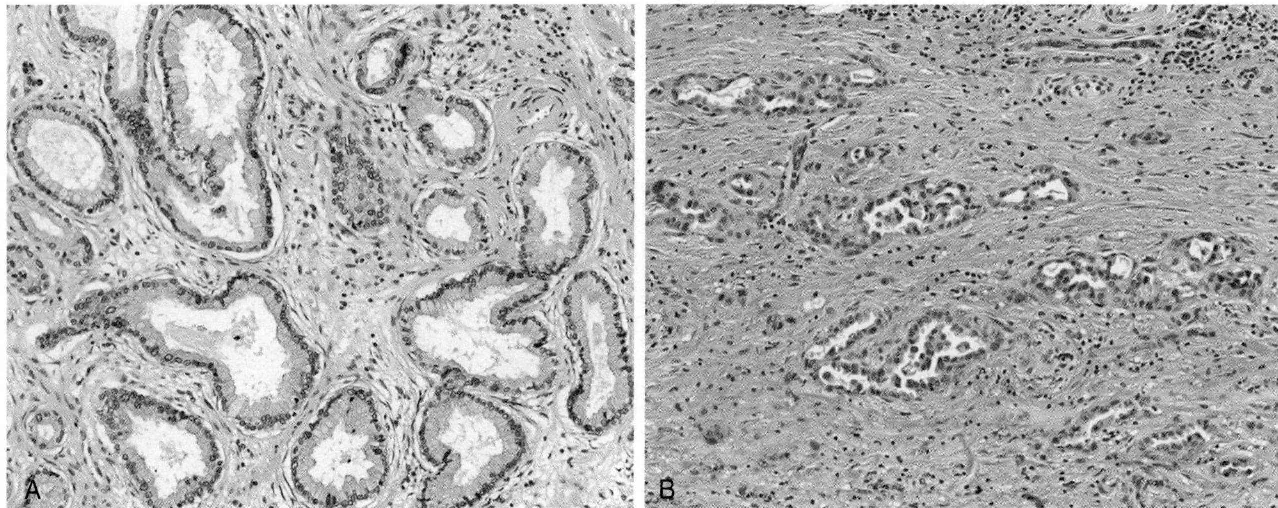

FIGURE 39.45 The glands may reveal abundant (**A**) or minimal (**B**) intracytoplasmic and intraluminal mucin.

intracytoplasmic and intraluminal mucin may be seen (Fig. 39.45). In some cases this is evident by routine histological examination, and in others it is demonstrable only by special stains. Goblet, Paneth, and neuroendocrine cells may occur randomly in some tumors and are more common in carcinomas with an intestinal appearance.[103,116] Perineural and vascular invasion are common and can be prominent in some cases. Extensive intravascular spread through the subserosal or subhepatic vasculature may cause a plaquelike growth within perimuscular tissue. Tumor-infiltrating inflammatory cells may consist of various amounts of lymphocytes, plasma cells, neutrophils, and eosinophils. Follicular cholecystitis is associated with some tumors.[18,44]

In addition to the characteristics previously described, adenocarcinomas of the gallbladder may exhibit unusual patterns of growth that typically are mixed with the conventional pattern. Some tumors reveal a fair amount of cytoplasm that may appear clear, foamy, or microvesicular (Fig. 39.46).[117] This pattern is typically associated with distinct cytoplasmic borders, an apical cuticle-like cytoplasmic condensation, and raisinoid or round nuclei with prominent nucleoli. Conversely,

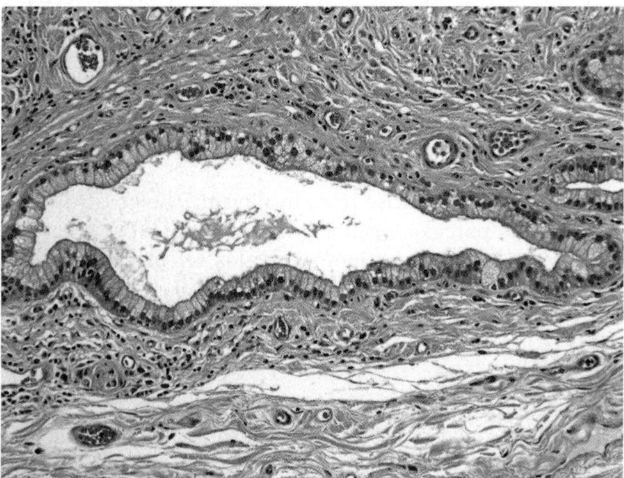

FIGURE 39.46 Pancreatobiliary-type adenocarcinoma with a foamy gland pattern. The glands are well-formed and show nuclei polarized toward the periphery of the cell cytoplasm. The cells have abundant pale, microvesicular mucin resembling pyloric or endocervical glands. The nuclei are hyperchromatic and raisinoid.

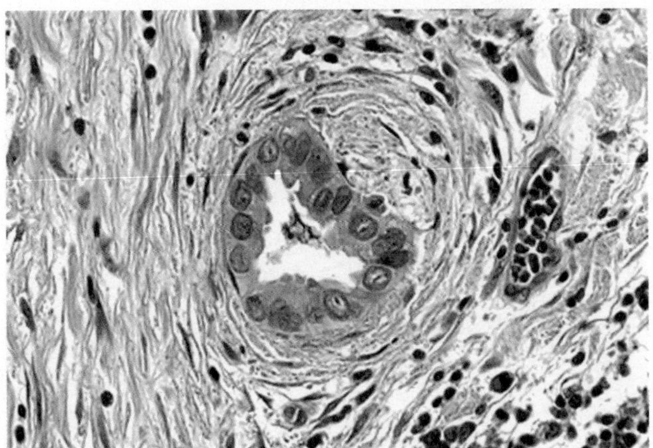

FIGURE 39.47 Pancreatobiliary-type adenocarcinoma. This case reveals a deceptively benign-appearing variant of adenocarcinoma in which the glands look atrophic. The presence of nuclear grooves is a clue to the diagnosis.

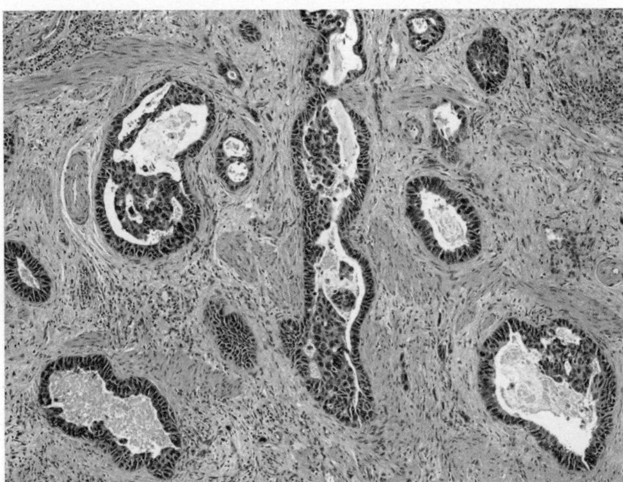

FIGURE 39.48 This gallbladder adenocarcinoma reveals a complex glandular arrangement with cribriforming that resembles intestinal-type carcinoma. This is not a common finding in tumors of this anatomic region.

some well-differentiated tumors exhibit atrophic-appearing glands consisting of attenuated cells with a minimal amount of cytoplasm and small, bland-appearing nuclei, resembling a tubular carcinoma of the breast (Fig. 39.47). However, these benign-appearing cells often have nuclear grooves. Some tumors reveal substantial intraglandular architectural complexity, including papillary units and cribriform arrangements (Fig. 39.48).

The well-differentiated appearance of gallbladder carcinomas is commonly retained in metastatic sites. The degree of differentiation may become even more pronounced in some sites, such as the ovaries, where metastatic biliary carcinomas may form cystic tumors that are often mistaken as a primary ovarian mucinous tumor that is either benign or borderline. Some metastatic biliary carcinomas in the lung resemble primary mucinous bronchioloalveolar carcinoma.

Poorly differentiated adenocarcinomas may also exhibit various patterns of growth. In some carcinomas, the cells form cords or nests or infiltrate as single cells. A diffuse sheetlike arrangement may be seen in others. Occasionally, carcinoma cells form compressed units with central clefts

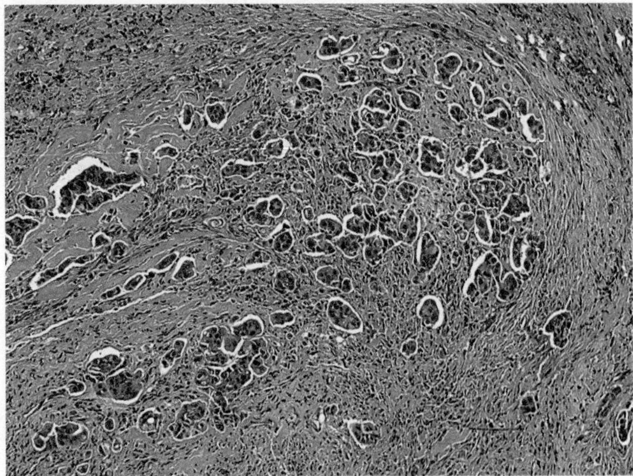

FIGURE 39.49 Invasive micropapillary carcinoma, characterized by the presence of clusters of cells within artifactual clefts. Invasive micropapillary carcinomas of this anatomic region are often accompanied by prominent neutrophilic infiltrates, as in this case.

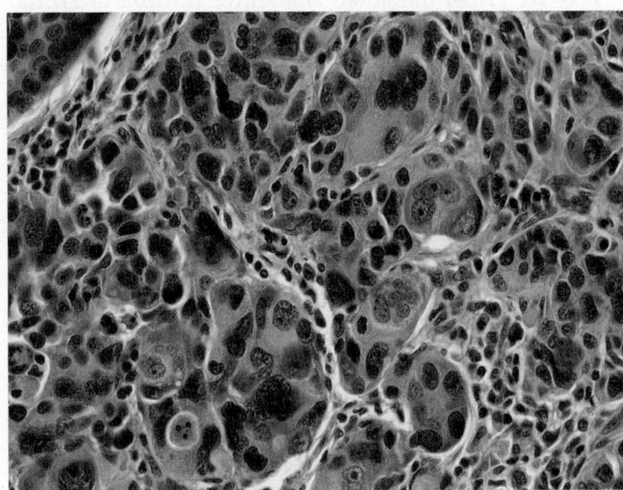

FIGURE 39.50 Adenocarcinoma (poorly differentiated) with pleomorphic giant cells. These cells should not be confused with osteoclast-like giant cells (see Fig. 39.58).

and acantholysis in a pseudoangiomatous pattern. Some cases have a characteristic micropapillary pattern (Fig. 39.49). Poorly differentiated adenocarcinomas may show significant pleomorphism, bizarre nuclei, and even multinucleated giant cells, which are true tumor giant cells (Fig. 39.50). Focal choriocarcinoma-like areas may be seen as well.

The histological grading system used for gallbladder adenocarcinomas is based on the degree of glandular differentiation, similar to other GI tumors. More than 95% differentiation is graded as *well differentiated,* 50% to 95% is *moderately differentiated,* and less than 50% is *poorly differentiated.*[103]

Histochemical, Immunohistochemical, and Molecular Features

Adenocarcinomas of the gallbladder have various amounts of mucin that range from pale shades detectable only by mucin stains or molecular analysis of glycoproteins to scattered intraluminal globules that are easily identified by light microscopy. Stromal mucin deposition occurs in some cases.

The mucin type more commonly associated with neoplasia is sialomucin, whereas benign reactive conditions tend to produce sulfomucin. In some studies, MUC1 expression has been associated with a higher rate of metastasis and a poorer prognosis.[118]

The immunoprofile of gallbladder carcinomas is of the classic foregut type. Tumors are typically positive for CK7.[119] CK20 may also be positive, but staining is usually focal. The latter pattern contrasts with intrahepatic (peripheral) cholangiocarcinomas, which tend to be negative for CK20. Several mucin-related glycoproteins and oncoproteins, such as mCEA, MUC1, MUC5AC, TAG72 (B72.3), and CA 19-9, are usually expressed, although focally in some specimens.[50,103,115,120] For some markers, such as mCEA and MUC1, there is a progressive increase in the level of expression from preinvasive to well-differentiated to poorly differentiated carcinomas, with dense intracytoplasmic expression detected mostly in advanced tumors.

More than half of gallbladder cancers harbor *TP53* alterations.[121] Other common alterations involve *CDKN2A* or *CDKN2B* (19%), *ARID1A* (13%), *PIK3CA* (10%), and *CTNNB1* (10%) mutations and *HER2* (*ERBB2* or *HER2/NEU*, 16%) amplifications.[122,123] The incidences of *KRAS* oncogenic mutation and loss of SMAD4 (DPC4) protein expression are far less common than in pancreatic tumors.[124] Microsatellite instability has been reported in up to 10% of cases.[125]

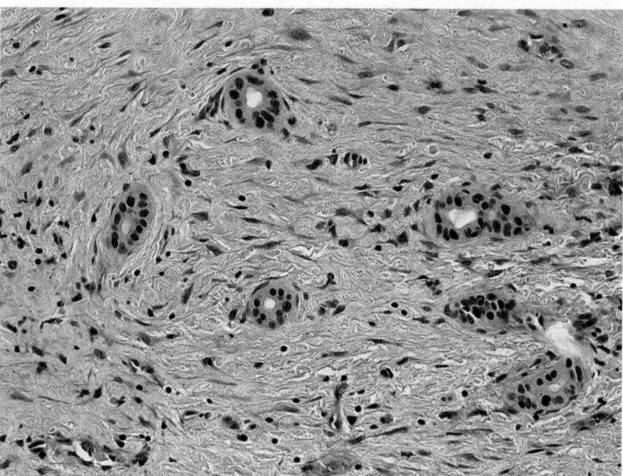

FIGURE 39.51 Benign biliary-type ducts, referred to as *Luschka's ducts*, are present commonly in the perimuscular tissue at the hepatic surface of the gallbladder.

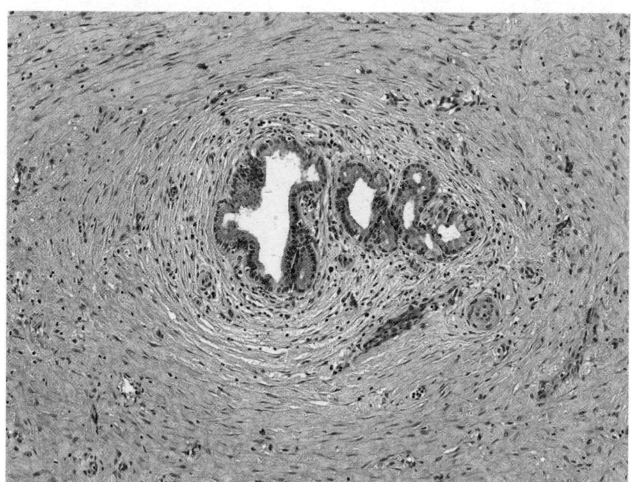

FIGURE 39.52 Lobular arrangement of peribiliary mucous glands is the most helpful feature in establishing that these glands are not malignant.

Differential Diagnosis

Most of the difficulties in distinguishing dysplasia from reactive changes at the cytological level also apply to differentiating invasive carcinoma from benign processes because carcinoma cells can appear deceptively benign. Moreover, architecturally, well-differentiated adenocarcinomas often show exceedingly well-organized glandular formations, which can be difficult to distinguish from peribiliary mucous glands in the neck and cystic duct region, Luschka ducts in the subhepatic or subserosal tissues (Fig. 39.51), Rokitansky-Aschoff sinuses (see Fig. 39.19), or metaplastic glands.[126-128]

Peribiliary mucous glands normally have a lobular architecture and are composed of uniform and evenly sized tubules (Fig. 39.52), whereas invasive carcinomas are typically composed of dispersed, haphazardly arranged tubular units (Table 39.4).

Luschka ducts, which are remnants of hepatic biliary ductules located on the outside of the gallbladder wall (see Fig. 39.51), may have a highly proliferative atypical and pseudoinfiltrative appearance, especially in the setting of acute cholecystitis.[127] However, this process often forms a discernible band confined to the subhepatic or subserosal surface of the gallbladder.

Rokitansky-Aschoff sinuses can be more difficult to distinguish from carcinoma because they do not have a lobular arrangement and can be found in any portion of the gallbladder wall and surrounding adipose tissue.[128] The epithelium of Rokitansky-Aschoff sinuses may be continuous with the surface epithelium. The sinuses are usually oriented perpendicular to the surface, have an undulating contour, and may appear flask shaped in the muscularis layer. Luminal bile may be present. In contrast, malignant glands are usually smaller in size and often have open, round lumina or angulated contours, and they may be oriented parallel to the mucosal surface. Also, carcinomas are usually more densely packed than Rokitansky-Aschoff sinuses or adenomyomatous hyperplasia. Stromal changes may not be helpful because Rokitansky-Aschoff sinuses and adenomyomatous hyperplasia are often associated with fibrotic, desmoplastic-like stroma. However, if these glands rupture as a result of increased pressure, the mucin in the stroma may induce reactive changes and an infiltrative appearance to the glands.

In some cases, proliferating metaplastic glands can exhibit dispersion and may be accompanied by intervening stroma, creating a pseudoinfiltrative appearance. They may also impinge on nerves, mimicking perineural invasion. However, metaplastic glands typically form a band confined to the mucosa and superficial muscularis, rather than showing vertical spread.

In general, perineural or vascular invasion, open lumina, intraglandular necrosis with neutrophils, microvesicular cytoplasm with a distinct, thin apical chromophilic band, nuclear enlargement, nuclear irregularities, hyperchromatism, loss

TABLE 39.4 Features Helpful in Distinguishing Malignant Glands from Benign Peribiliary (Normal) Glands in Gallbladder and Bile Duct Specimens

Feature	Benign Glands	Malignant Glands
Lobular arrangement of glands	++	–
Haphazard infiltrative pattern	–	+
Irregular glands, variable size and shape, angulated contours	–	+
Uniformity of glands	++	–/+
Mitoses	+/–	+
Necrosis (intraluminal)	–	+
Cytological atypia (pleomorphism, hyperchromicity, loss of polarity)	– to +	+ to ++
Infiltrative single cells or clusters of cells	–	+/–
Perineural invasion	–	+
Concentric periglandular fibrosis	+/–	+
MCEA positivity	+/– (apical)	+ (cytoplasmic)
p53 positivity	+/– (weak)	+/– (strong)

+, Present; –, not present; +/–, may be present.

of polarity, mitotic figures, and apoptotic cells are findings that favor carcinoma. Subtle nuclear grooves can be helpful in recognizing extremely well-differentiated adenocarcinomas (see Fig. 39.47).

TP53 protein overexpression, a high Ki67 labeling index, and dense cytoplasmic positivity for glycoproteins such as mCEA and MUC1 are significantly more common in carcinomas than in benign conditions.[50,103,115] However, the high degree of overlap prevents effective use of these markers in daily clinical practice.

Natural History and Prognosis

Gallbladder adenocarcinomas are highly aggressive neoplasms, and unfortunately in many cases the tumor shows invasion into neighboring organs and/or has metastasized to the regional lymph nodes at the time of presentation.[129] However, data from high-risk geographic regions such as Chile and Southeast Asia have revealed that cases classified as *early gallbladder cancer* (i.e., pTis, pT1a with lamina propria invasion, and pT1b with tunica muscularis invasion) by entire sampling of the gallbladder have a very favorable prognosis, with 10-year survival rates close to 90%.[10] Nevertheless, it should be kept in mind that a small percentage of such cases develop recurrence many years after cholecystectomy. Data suggest that if there is Rokitansky-Aschoff involvement, the risk of recurrence is higher.[10] Therefore some groups advocate a more radical operation for cases with early gallbladder cancer involving Rokitansky-Aschoff sinuses.[10]

The 5-year survival rate of patients with pT2 carcinoma is approximately 45%, and it is lower (40%) in the West and higher (>70%) in Japan and Korea.[13] The survival advantage in the East has been shown not to be related to definitional or histopathological examination differences.[13] Therefore it is presumably populational or health care related. For pT2 carcinomas, the location of the carcinoma (serosa vs. hepatic surface) was also found to be associated with survival differences.[130] As a result, this parameter is now part of the TNM staging system as *T2a* and *T2b*.[131] However, this is based on only one study, and more recent studies have failed to confirm this.[132]

Radical surgery with lymphadenectomy and right hepatic lobectomy is typically performed for resectable cases.[133-136] However, most gallbladder carcinomas are incidental (clinically inapparent), being diagnosed in cholecystectomy specimens performed for a presurgical diagnosis of cholecystitis or cholelithiasis.[1] A further hepatic resection and lymphadenectomy may still benefit these patients if the tumor is relatively localized (pT2).[137] This method of treatment is controversial for more advanced (pT3) cancers.[138] Similarly, the management of pT1b cases remains controversial. In the West, radical surgery is performed in most cases. However, emerging evidence suggests that this may not be necessary because if pT2 carcinoma is ruled out by total sampling, pT1 carcinomas are cured in most cases.[10,139]

Although there is growing consensus regarding the role of adjuvant chemotherapy in the management of biliary tract cancer,[137,140] the type of chemotherapy protocol that is most beneficial remains a subject of debate.[141,142] Major academic centers typically administer a chemotherapy protocol that is similar to pancreatic adenocarcinoma.[141] The role of radiotherapy is also a subject of debate.

Other Types of Carcinoma

So-Called Papillary Carcinoma

Cases previously classified as *papillary* (adeno)carcinoma encompass a spectrum of tumors that ranges from predominantly papillary ICPNs to invasive adenocarcinoma with a papillary configuration (see Figs. 39.2, 39.16, and 39.31D).[15,143] ICPNs were discussed earlier. Invasive adenocarcinoma with prominent papilla formation should ideally be classified as a *well-differentiated invasive adenocarcinoma*. This tumor should not be confused with carcinomas with a *micropapillary* pattern (see Fig. 39.49), which is composed of clusters of cells with surrounding cleft formation.

Intestinal-Type Adenocarcinoma

Some conventional pancreatobiliary-type gallbladder adenocarcinomas may consist of columnar cells with pseudostratification and, as such, resemble an intestinal-type adenocarcinoma. Frank intestinal-type adenocarcinoma, a tumor that contains all characteristics of colonic adenocarcinomas, such as cellular basophilia, pseudostratification, central necrosis, and goblet cell–like intestinal mucin, is uncommon in the gallbladder. As such, this finding should raise suspicion of metastatic involvement by a colonic adenocarcinoma when it is diagnosed.[103,144,145]

Mucinous Carcinoma

Gallbladder carcinomas often contain intracytoplasmic and/or intraluminal mucin within the invasive glands. However, stromal mucin deposition is present in only

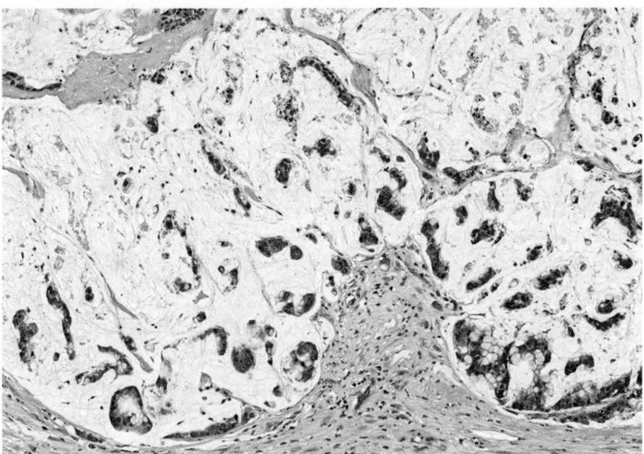

FIGURE 39.53 Colloid carcinoma (pure mucinous carcinoma) characterized by the presence of well-defined pools of mucin containing detached clusters of carcinoma cells. This type of tumor is highly uncommon in the gallbladder and extrahepatic bile ducts.

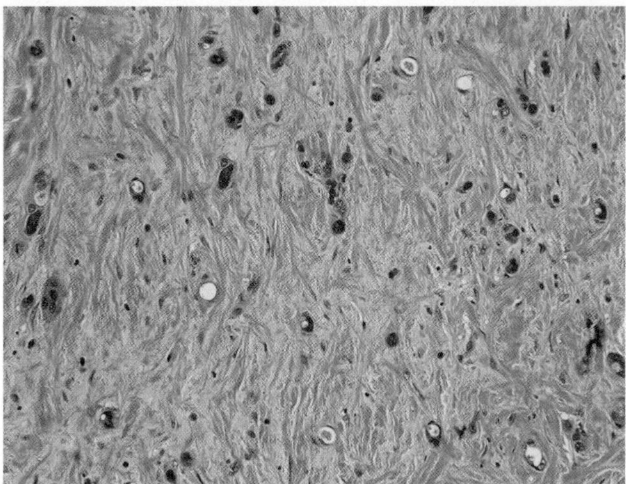

FIGURE 39.54 A diffuse infiltrative type of carcinoma with signet ring cells *(poorly cohesive cell carcinoma)*. The tumor is composed of cords of cells and individual cells, some with signet ring cell morphology, infiltrating the muscle.

about 7% of cases.[104] About one third of these tumors qualify as a *mucinous carcinoma* as defined by the 2019 WHO classification (>50% of the tumor composed of stromal mucin).[12] These tumors are often large and typically manifest with symptoms reminiscent of acute cholecystitis. Most tumors are mixed with other nonmucinous adenocarcinoma components. Pure colloid-type mucinous carcinoma, characterized by infiltrating epithelial elements suspended in abundant stromal mucin, is exceedingly uncommon in the gallbladder (Fig. 39.53).[104] Calcifications may be prominent in this type of tumor.[146] Immunophenotypically, mucinous gallbladder carcinomas reveal prominent MUC2 expression, which differentiates them from conventional gallbladder adenocarcinomas.[104] They differ from tubular GI tract mucinous carcinomas by having an inverse CK7/20 profile and from pancreatic mucinous carcinomas by not revealing CDX2 labeling. These tumors are microsatellite stable.[104]

Mucinous carcinomas are typically diagnosed at an advanced stage at the time of diagnosis. They also usually exhibit more aggressive behavior than conventional gallbladder adenocarcinomas.[104]

Poorly Cohesive Carcinoma (with or without Signet Ring Cells)

Diffusely infiltrative carcinomas occur very rarely in the gallbladder (about 4% of gallbladder carcinomas) and show a striking predilection for females, even more than conventional gallbladder adenocarcinomas.[114]

Grossly, these tumors often have a linitis plastica configuration, which is characterized by infiltration of cells between the tissue planes, similar to diffuse-type gastric carcinoma, mammary lobular carcinoma, or urothelial plasmacytoid cell carcinoma.[147] They are composed of cords or individual cells (i.e., they have a poorly cohesive cell pattern) (Fig. 39.54). Some cases have prominent signet ring morphology, but in most, signet ring cells with abundant intracytoplasmic mucin occur only focally or may be entirely absent.[86,103] Some cases are associated with stromal mucin production (see Mucinous Carcinoma).

The clinical course of poorly cohesive carcinoma appears to be more aggressive than conventional adenocarcinomas.[114]

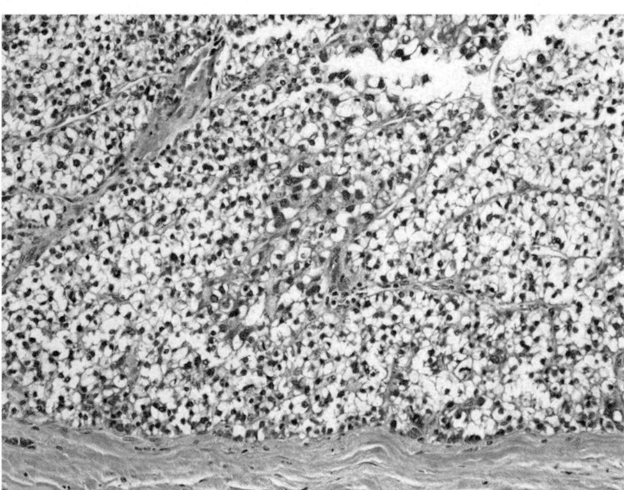

FIGURE 39.55 Clear cell component of an adenocarcinoma of the pancreatobiliary type. The cells contain abundant clear cytoplasm, centrally located nuclei, and distinct cytoplasmic borders. Some cases show a more solid and alveolar growth pattern, mimicking clear cell carcinoma of the kidney.

Clear Cell Carcinoma

A clear cell *(hypernephroid)* pattern characterized by sheets of clear cells in an alveolar arrangement and separated by sinusoid vessels has been described in gallbladder carcinomas, but it is exceedingly uncommon.[94,117,148] If such a tumor is encountered in this region, the pathologist should consider a metastatic renal cell carcinoma, which may also be polypoid. The latter tumor is significantly more common than the true primary clear cell carcinoma of the gallbladder. However, in rare cases, a carcinoma with prominent hypernephroid features (Fig. 39.55) is associated with a conventional pancreatobiliary-type adenocarcinoma or preinvasive neoplasia. It should be kept in mind that conventional adenocarcinomas of the gallbladder, characterized by a foamy gland pattern and endocervical-like glands, may also appear to have clear cytoplasm as a result of the presence of ample mucin, but these tumors should not be classified as

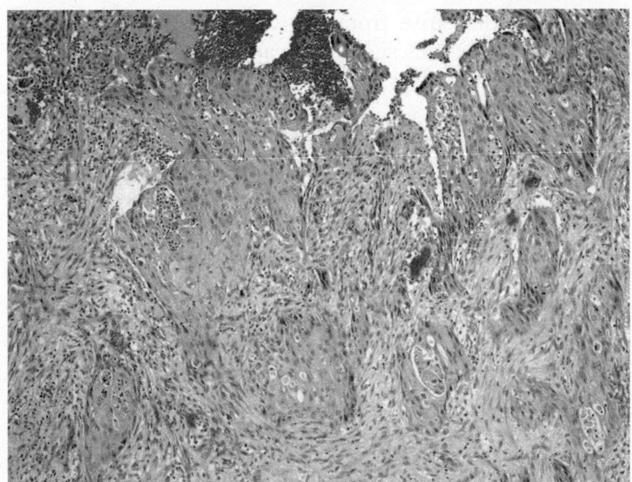

FIGURE 39.56 Pure squamous cell carcinoma with keratinization.

clear cell carcinomas. The prognosis of clear cell carcinoma is poor and mainly related to the pathological stage.[117]

Adenosquamous and Squamous Cell Carcinomas

Focal squamous differentiation is detected in approximately 5% of all gallbladder carcinomas.[105] If squamous elements constitute a substantial part of the tumor (>25%), the neoplasm is best classified as an *adenosquamous carcinoma*.[12,105,149] Glandular and squamous components of the tumors have immunophenotypes that correspond to their respective lines of differentiation. For example, squamous areas often show nuclear tumor protein p63 (TP63) expression and positivity with high-molecular-weight keratins, whereas glandular areas express mCEA and tumor-associated glycoprotein 72 (TAG72 [clone B72.3]).

Pure squamous cell carcinomas constitute less than 1% of all gallbladder carcinomas.[105] They often show overt and abundant keratinization (Fig. 39.56). They are usually associated with gallstones. Intramucosal components of the carcinoma may also be entirely squamous, or there may be squamous metaplasia. Mucin stains to identify foci of glandular differentiation may be performed to exclude an adenosquamous carcinoma with predominant squamous differentiation. Any amount of glandular differentiation is considered sufficient for a diagnosis of adenosquamous carcinoma.

Similar to their counterpart in the breast, some squamous cell carcinomas have a spindle cell pattern and may be difficult to distinguish from a high-grade sarcoma. In these cases, the finding of a more conventional squamous pattern may be helpful. Immunohistochemical stains may not be helpful because many spindle cell carcinomas are keratin negative, and, conversely, some sarcomas may show weak keratin expression.

Squamous cell carcinomas tend to present initially at a higher stage. They have more adverse outcomes than conventional adenocarcinomas when compared stage by stage.[105]

Undifferentiated Carcinoma

Undifferentiated carcinomas of the gallbladder can be divided into two broad categories (*sarcomatoid/spindle cell type* and *epithelioid type*). In both, a conventional adenocarcinoma component often coexists.

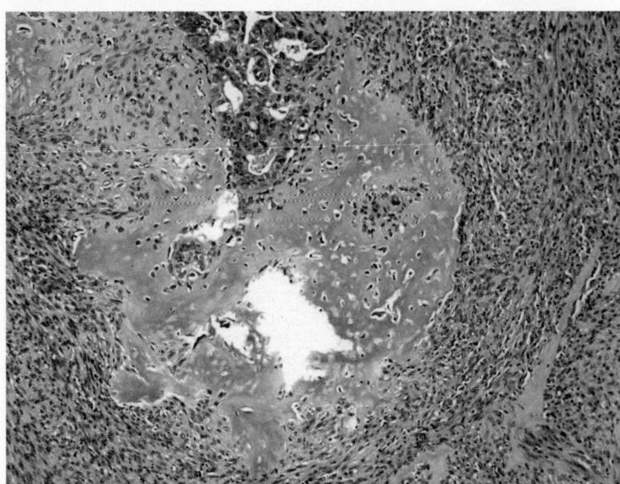

FIGURE 39.57 Sarcomatoid carcinomas may reveal evidence of heterologous differentiation (bone formation is depicted here).

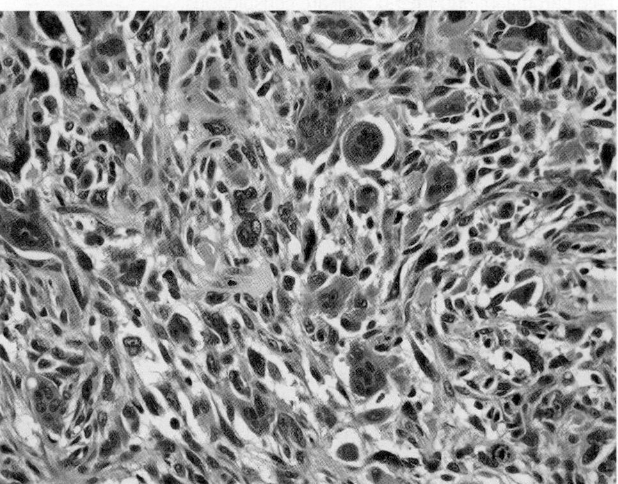

FIGURE 39.58 Undifferentiated carcinoma with osteoclast-like giant cells. Osteoclastic-like giant cells are of histiocytic origin and are, presumably, reactive in nature.

Sarcomatoid/Spindle Cell Type. Although these are characterized by spindle-shaped cells, some cases may also reveal epithelioid cells. The two components may appear distinct in some cases, however, there is overwhelming evidence that both components are of epithelial origin. The spindle-shaped component may be very subtle and fibroblast-like, but it is more commonly pleomorphic or shows evidence of heterologous differentiation (i.e., skeletal muscle, bone, and cartilage; Fig. 39.57).[113] An angiosarcoma-like pattern also occurs. Tumors with abundant osteoclast-like giant cells (i.e., *undifferentiated carcinoma with osteoclast-like giant cells*[150,151]) in which nonneoplastic, histiocytic, multinucleated cells are suspended among dyshesive, pleomorphic, spindle- to epithelioid-shaped neoplastic cells (Fig. 39.58) are uncommon in the gallbladder compared with the bile ducts or the pancreas.[94,103,113,152,153] Patients present with large/advanced-stage tumors. Limited data suggest that these sarcomatoid/spindle cell–type undifferentiated carcinomas are aggressive tumors with rapid mortality.[113]

Epithelioid Type. Some undifferentiated carcinomas resemble *medullary carcinomas* of the GI tract or

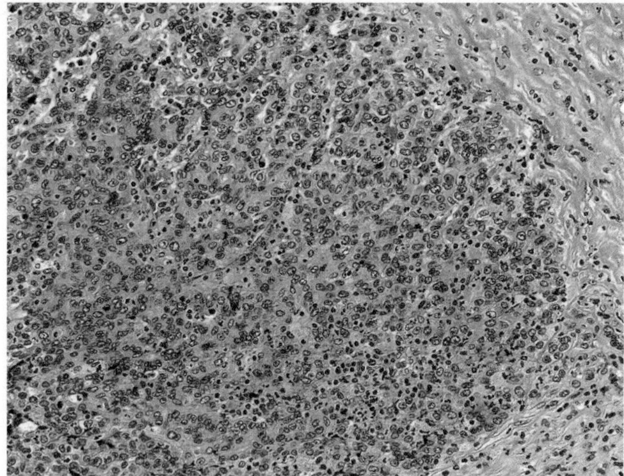

FIGURE 39.59 Poorly differentiated carcinoma, medullary type. This tumor is characterized by a syncytial growth pattern of cells and a pushing border. There is no glandular differentiation. The nuclei have vesicular, pale chromatin, and the nucleoli are conspicuous.

lymphoepithelioma-like carcinomas of the upper aerodigestive tract (Fig. 39.59).[154-156] They are characterized by a nodular growth pattern with pushing borders. The tumor cells are large, round to ovoid with vesicular chromatin and single prominent nucleoli. Lymphoplasmacytic infiltrates are prominent in some (i.e., lymphoepithelioma-like lesions). Loss of mismatch repair protein expression may be detected. Evidence of Epstein-Barr virus was found in these tumors in some studies, but it was lacking in others.[156]

Hepatoid Carcinoma

Gallbladder carcinomas with *hepatoid* features should always raise concern for a primary hepatocellular carcinoma, especially considering hepatocellular carcinomas can invade the gallbladder or the extrahepatic bile ducts and extend, in a finger-like fashion, into the lumen. However, rarely, *hepatoid* carcinomas may originate within the gallbladder or the extrahepatic bile ducts,[154,155,157] and an accompanying preinvasive lesion may be identified within the mucosa. These tumors have a trabecular or sheetlike arrangement of polygonal-shaped cells that have abundant cytoplasm, fine granularity, and round nuclei with prominent nucleoli. They may even express hepatocytic markers and a canalicular pattern of staining for polyclonal CEA or CD10. However, unlike primary hepatocellular carcinomas, they also often express CK19 and CK20. More studies are needed to determine the true nature of these tumors. About 10% of hepatoid carcinomas have microsatellite instability.[158]

Adenocarcinomas Arising in Specific Risk Groups

Adenocarcinomas that arise in certain clinical settings *(intracholecystic neoplasms, hyalinizing cholecystitis,* or *anomalous union of pancreatobiliary ducts)* may have some distinctive features and thus warrant special attention.

Carcinoma Associated with Intracholecystic Neoplasms

Carcinomas associated with intracholecystic neoplasms (discussed earlier) constitute about 6% of all invasive gallbladder carcinomas.[15,29] They should be recognized because their biological behavior appears to be better than that of carcinomas that arise from flat dysplasia (3-year survival, 60% vs. 30%).[15] This survival advantage is maintained even in stage-matched cases.[15]

Carcinoma Associated with Hyalinizing Cholecystitis

The association of porcelain gallbladder with cancer has long been the subject of debate. Some studies have shown that diffusely calcific gallbladders *(complete porcelain gallbladder)* are not associated with carcinoma. However, a distinctive variant of chronic cholecystitis characterized by diffuse effacement of the gallbladder wall by a thin band of paucicellular, hyaline, fibrous tissue with a peculiar clefting pattern and minimal or no calcifications (*incomplete porcelain gallbladder*, also known as *hyalinizing cholecystitis;* see Fig. 39.43) has a strong association with carcinoma.[9,159,160]

Carcinomas that arise in this setting often have a subtle appearance. Extensive sampling is crucial to reveal the presence and extent of carcinoma. If there is a substantial amount of preserved mucosa and tunica muscularis or the calcifications are extensive, the likelihood of carcinoma is much lower.[159,160] In established cases, in which the entire wall is replaced by hyaline fibrosis, glands within the areas of fibrosis or overlying it should alert the pathologist to the possibility of invasive or in situ carcinoma. We recommend a thorough examination of the gallbladder in these cases. Invasive glands often form elongated tubules aligned with their longitudinal axes that are oriented perpendicular to the surface. They typically have clear cytoplasm, distinct cytoplasmic borders, and nuclei that are small, pushed to the periphery, and raisinoid or, if enlarged, contain prominent nucleoli. Some cases exhibit large, cystically dilated glands. Many glands reveal partially attenuated epithelium, and the luminal contents often merge with the stroma, sometimes leaving distinctive granular debris (see Fig. 39.43) as the only sign of carcinoma in some sections.

These cases are also challenging for staging purposes because in well-established cases, the layers of the gallbladder, including the epithelium and the tunica muscularis, have been replaced by fibrous tissue. However, they should best be regarded as at least pT2 by default because they are no longer delimited by the muscularis.

Their median survival and 5-year overall survival is reported as 7 months and 18%, respectively (compared with 12 months and 36%, respectively, for ordinary carcinomas). The aggressive behavior of hyalinizing cholecystitis–associated carcinomas may be partially attributable to the advanced stage of the carcinoma at diagnosis.[9]

Carcinoma Associated with Anomalous Union of Pancreatobiliary Ducts

Pancreatobiliary maljunction is an anomalous union of the main pancreatic duct and common bile duct outside the sphincter of Oddi with a 200 times risk of gallbladder cancer, attributed to reflux of pancreatic enzymes to the gallbladder. Carcinomas that arise in the setting of pancreatobiliary maljunction have been mostly regarded as a disorder that occurred in only Asian populations. However, they recently were shown to be as common in the West (pancreatobiliary maljunction accounts for 8% of gallbladder cancer both in the East and West).[16] These carcinomas appear to have distinct clinicopathological characteristics as

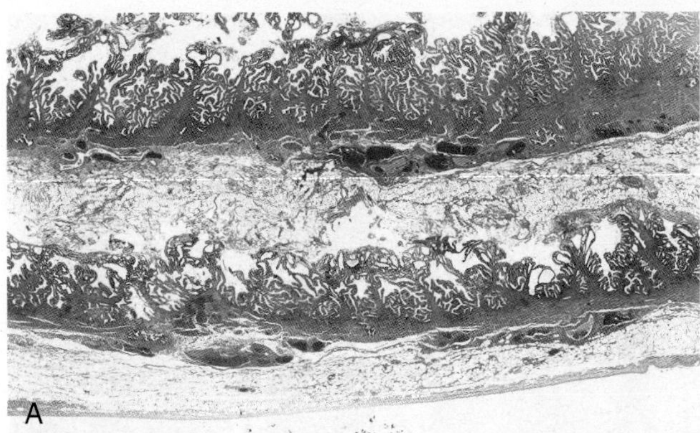

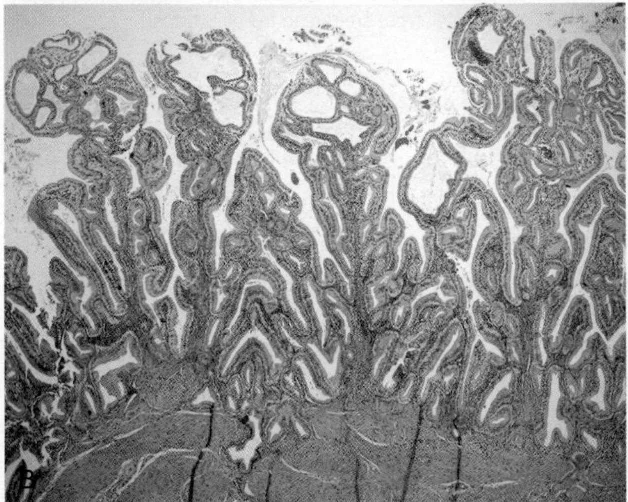

FIGURE 39.60 Mucosal hyperplasia of pancreatobiliary maljunction has distinctive features. A, The thick hyperplastic mucosa continuously abuts and pushes into the tunica muscularis and is associated with multiple Rokitansky-Aschoff sinuses. **B,** Bulbous dilation of the tips of the mucosal folds is characteristic.

they are uncommonly associated with gallstones and tend to manifest in relatively young female patients (<50 years of age), often through adenoma-carcinoma sequence, leading to unusual carcinoma types.[16,161]

It should also be kept in mind that gallbladders in patients with pancreatobiliary maljunction display a distinctive pattern of mucosal hyperplasia with distinguishing features termed *reflux cholecystopathy*.[67] It is characterized by significantly thickened, stroma poor mucosa composed of tall projections with bulbous dilation of the tips of the mucosal folds (Fig. 39.60). Recognition of the pathological characteristics of this entity is important so that investigation, treatment, and prevention of pancreatobiliary maljunction–associated complications (biliary tract cancers and pancreatitis) can be instituted.[67]

Neuroendocrine Neoplasms

By definition, neuroendocrine neoplasms of the gallbladder and the bile ducts show neuroendocrine differentiation, but they represent a broad and heterogeneous group of neoplasms with diverse clinical and pathological characteristics. According to the 2019 WHO classification, they can be categorized as *well-differentiated neuroendocrine tumors*, *poorly differentiated neuroendocrine carcinomas*, and *mixed neuroendocrine–nonneuroendocrine neoplasms*.

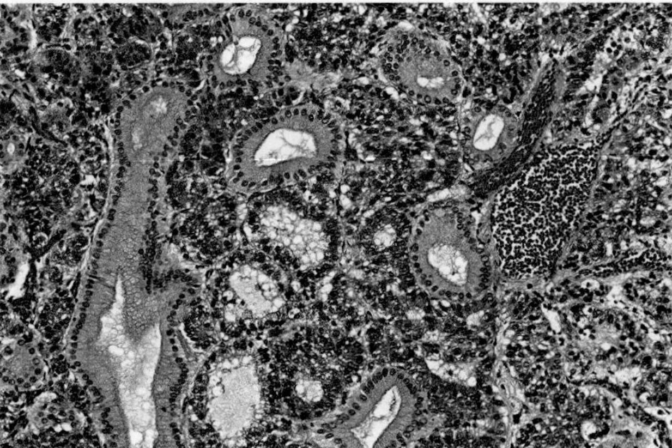

FIGURE 39.61 WDNETs reveal an insular or tubular pattern of growth. The cells have a moderate amount of cytoplasm and round, uniform nuclei with finely stippled chromatin.

Well-Differentiated Neuroendocrine Tumors

Well-differentiated neuroendocrine tumors (WDNETs) of the gallbladder and the bile ducts are extremely rare.[103,162-166] They typically manifest with nonspecific symptoms or are discovered incidentally. Some may be associated with genetic syndromes, such as von Hippel-Lindau syndrome[167] or multiple endocrine neoplasia type I (MEN I) syndrome.[103] Zollinger-Ellison syndrome has also been reported.[103] The mean age at presentation is 60 years. These tumors are slightly more common among females than males.[162]

WDNETs typically form nodular or polypoid lesions. They are usually white-yellow in color and homogenous. Microscopic examination usually reveals an insular or tubular pattern of growth.[168-170] Cytologically, the tumors exhibit typical features of low-grade neuroendocrine neoplasms, including the presence of round, uniform nuclei with finely stippled chromatin and a moderate amount of cytoplasm (Fig. 39.61). Tumors associated with von Hippel-Lindau syndrome may have clear cell features and commonly express inhibin.[167,171] By definition, these tumors have minimal or no necrosis. Rarely, gland formation in a WDNET can cause confusion with an adenocarcinoma.

Immunohistochemically, WDNETs are normally positive for chromogranin, synaptophysin, and CD56. The hormones most commonly detected are serotonin and somatostatin.

Current data indicate that WDNETs of the biliary tract have a biological behavior similar to those in other portions of the GI tract. They are relatively indolent tumors. Small tumors may remain clinically silent for a long period. Tumors larger than 2 cm in size are prone to metastasize. In the SEER database, the 10-year overall survival rate was 36% for gallbladder tumors and 80% for extrahepatic bile duct tumors[162]; however, it is not clear what percentage of these cases would be called *WDNETs* with the current criteria.

Poorly Differentiated Neuroendocrine Carcinoma

Focal neuroendocrine differentiation in the form of scattered chromogranin-positive cells can be seen in many conventional adenocarcinomas and has no clinical significance. However, diffuse neuroendocrine differentiation or poorly differentiated neuroendocrine carcinomas (PDNECs) with small (Fig. 39.62) or large cell

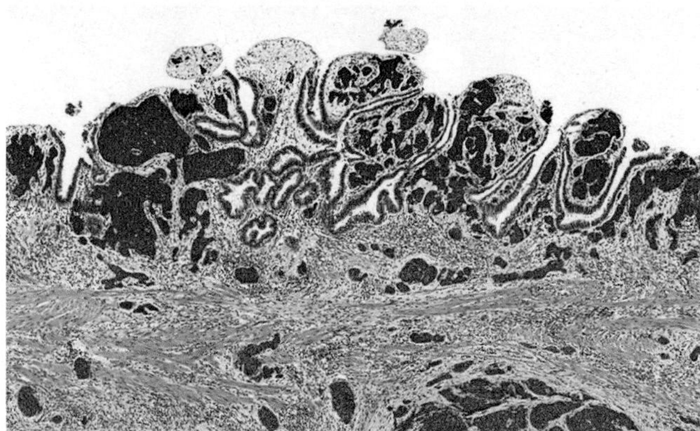

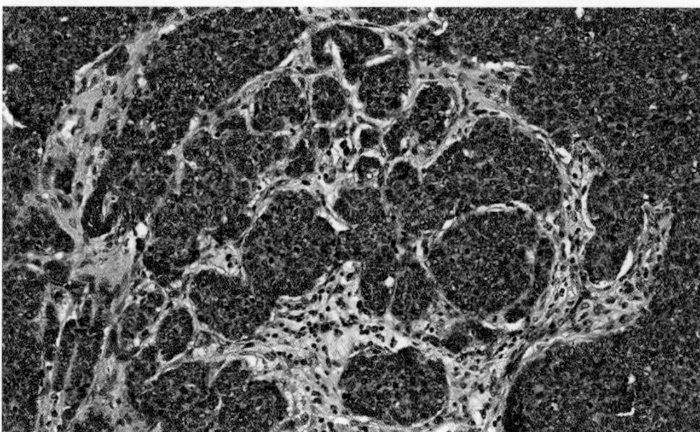

FIGURE 39.62 Small cell carcinomas (poorly differentiated neuroendocrine carcinomas of small cell type) are rare in the gallbladder.

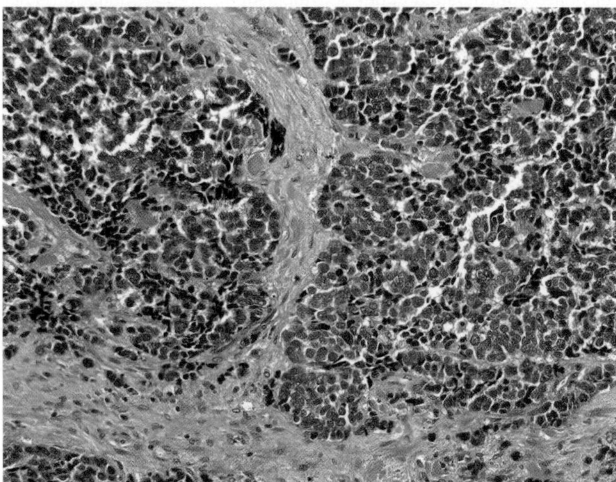

FIGURE 39.63 Small cell carcinoma (poorly differentiated neuroendocrine carcinoma of small cell type). Diffuse and nested growth of small *blue* cells with high nucleus-to-cytoplasm ratio and nuclear molding.

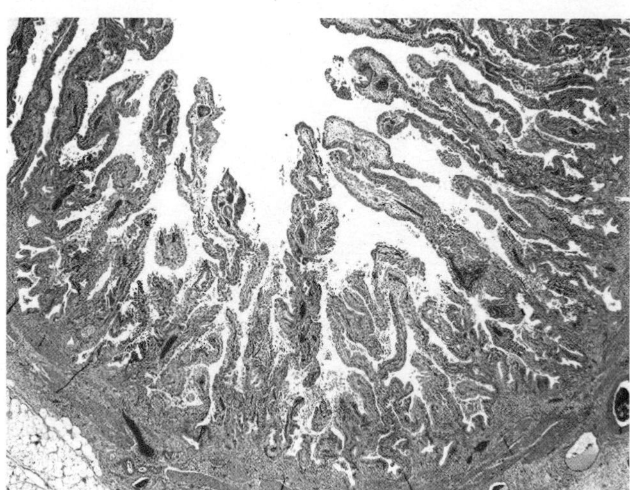

FIGURE 39.64 Primary papillary hyperplasia is a rare phenomenon in which there is prominent thickening of the mucosa characterized by villous-like folds that are taller than normal and closer together without any distinct nodule formation. The epithelium is composed of unremarkable biliary-type cells.

morphology, similar to those seen in the lung, are rare in the biliary tract. They constitute less than 4% of all gallbladder cancers[172] and may be associated with a paraneoplastic syndrome.[173,174] The mean age of patients with PDNECs is slightly younger than that of those with conventional adenocarcinomas.[172,175]

A diffuse or nested growth pattern, high N:C ratio, finely stippled chromatin, high mitotic activity (>20 mitoses per 10 high-power fields [HPF]), and necrosis are characteristic features. Focal rosette formation may be present.[176] Most cases have typical small cell carcinoma features, such as molding of nuclei and inconspicuous nucleoli (Fig. 39.63).[177] Some cases have a large cell phenotype (i.e., large cell neuroendocrine carcinomas).[178] One half of small cell carcinomas are pure, but large cell neuroendocrine carcinomas are typically admixed with another carcinoma component, such as adenocarcinoma or squamous cell carcinoma. If both components are substantial (≥30% of the neoplasm), the tumors are classified as *mixed neuroendocrine–nonneuroendocrine neoplasms* (MiNENs).[172,179]

Immunohistochemical expression of neuroendocrine markers, particularly chromogranin, may be focal or weak and may appear only as fine granules in the cytoplasm. Small cell carcinomas are defined mainly by their morphological features, without the necessity of proving neuroendocrine differentiation by immunohistochemistry. However, staining for neuroendocrine markers is required to separate a large cell neuroendocrine carcinoma from a poorly differentiated adenocarcinoma or squamous cell carcinoma. Inactivation of the CDKN2A/RB1 pathway is typical of small cell carcinomas.[180]

These are highly aggressive neoplasms; more than one half of all patients have disseminated disease at the time of diagnosis.[172,176,181-183] The median survival is less than 1 year, and the 5-year survival rate is 20%.[162,182-184] Patients with small cell carcinoma appear to be responsive to cisplatin-based chemotherapy as well as radiotherapy.

Pseudoneoplastic Lesions

Epithelial Alterations Mimicking Intraepithelial Neoplasia

Primary papillary hyperplasia is an uncommon phenomenon (Fig. 39.64). It consists of thickening of the mucosa with villous-like folds that are taller and more closely spaced than normal. In contrast with ICPNs, these lesions do not reveal distinct nodular formation or cytological atypia. The few patients reported were all young females (between 10 and 40 years of age). Its clinical significance and associations

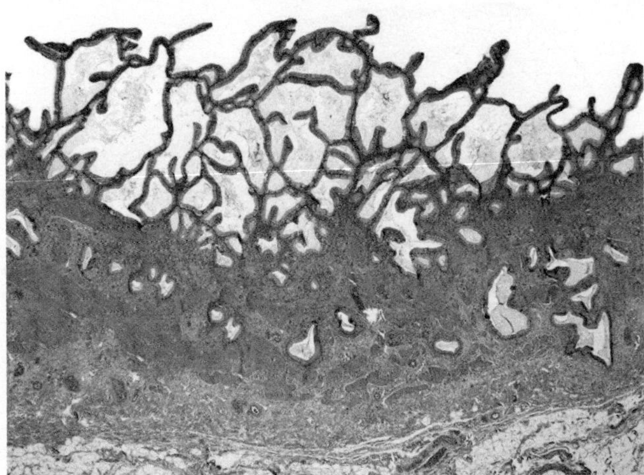

FIGURE 39.65 Combination of hyperplasia with delicate fusion of mucosal projections and tangential sectioning creates a complex architecture referred as *spongioid hyperplasia*. Although mostly localized, it may be more diffuse in some cases.

have not been determined. Villous-papillary proliferations described in patients with metachromatic leukodystrophy can be regarded as a form of primary papillary hyperplasia, although some are probably ICPNs. In some cases with gallbladder injury, regenerating mucosa may form folds, creating a more complex architecture referred as *spongioid hyperplasia* (Fig. 39.65).

More importantly, gallbladders in patients with pancreatobiliary maljunction display a distinctive pattern of mucosal hyperplasia with distinguishing features.[67] It is characterized by significantly thickened, stroma-poor mucosa composed of tall projections with bulbous dilation of the tips of the mucosal folds (see Fig. 39.60). As mentioned earlier, recognition of the pathological characteristics of this entity is important so investigation, treatment, and prevention of pancreatobiliary maljunction–associated complications (biliary tract cancers and pancreatitis) can be instituted.[67]

Metaplasia is a common manifestation of chronic injury in the gallbladder.[103] Gallbladders with gallstones or cholecystitis commonly exhibit metaplasia (60% to 75% of cases), especially pyloric gland type.[185] *Pyloric gland metaplasia* can be extensive and diffusely involve the mucosa. Occasionally, metaplastic glands form microscopic polyps or nodules. Unless these form ≥1 cm distinct lesions and/or have convincingly dysplastic epithelium, they should not be considered *neoplastic* (see Intracholecystic Neoplasms). *Intestinal metaplasia* is far less common than pyloric gland metaplasia.[88] It is characterized by goblet cells and very rarely, by intestinal-type absorptive cells (Fig. 39.66). The latter are difficult to distinguish from biliary surface epithelial cells because brush-border formation is often not very evident.[103] Basal nuclear pseudostratification may occur in intestinal metaplasia. However, full-thickness pseudostratification favors a diagnosis of dysplasia. As in the stomach, intestinal metaplasia is believed to be a precursor to carcinoma.[186,187] Epidemiological studies support this notion. In fact, intestinal metaplasia often accompanies high-grade dysplasia or invasive carcinoma.[21] Goblet cells are less common in gallbladders that lack dysplasia.[91,185]

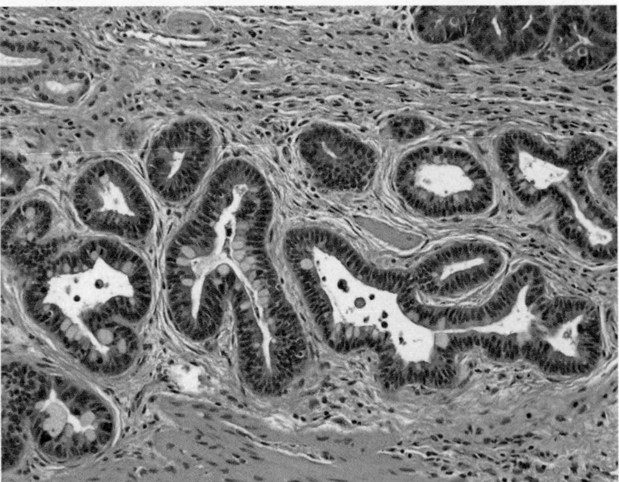

FIGURE 39.66 Intestinal metaplasia associated with dysplasia. There are scattered goblet cells among atypical-appearing epithelial cells.

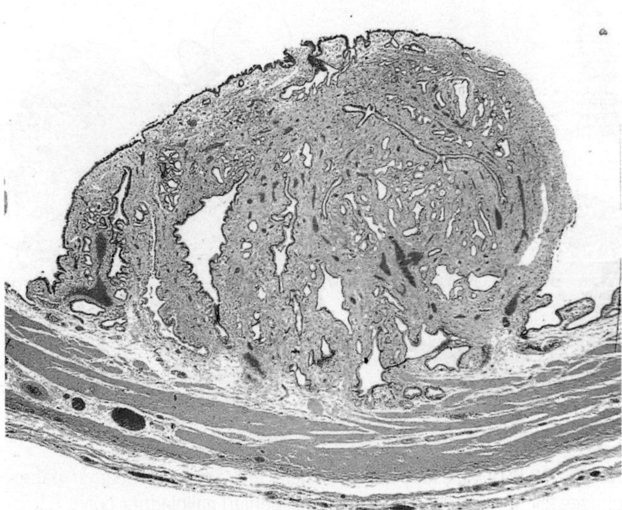

FIGURE 39.67 Benign fibroepithelial polyp with myoglandular features. There are multiple glandular elements some showing cystic dilation dispersed within a myoid stroma in a hamartoma-like pattern. These are presumed to represent a regenerative lesion.

Pseudotumors Clinically Mimicking Neoplasia

A variety of nonneoplastic lesions in the gallbladder may occasionally form a polyp or mass lesion that clinically mimics a neoplasm. Although most neoplastic polyps are larger than 1 cm in diameter, only approximately 5% of nonneoplastic polyps are larger than 1 cm.[42,43] Nonneoplastic polyps typically do not cause diagnostic problems at the pathological level if they are resected.

Fibromyoglandular Polyps

A significant proportion of nonneoplastic polyps develop as a result of reparation of mucosal injury or as a sequela of cholecystitis. One example of this phenomenon is the *fibromyoglandular polyp* (Fig. 39.67). It occurs in a background of chronic cholecystitis and is almost always (98%) gallstone associated.[43] Most fibromyoglandular polyps are small lesions that are characterized by broad-based (myo) fibroblastic tissue containing scattered glandular units.[43]

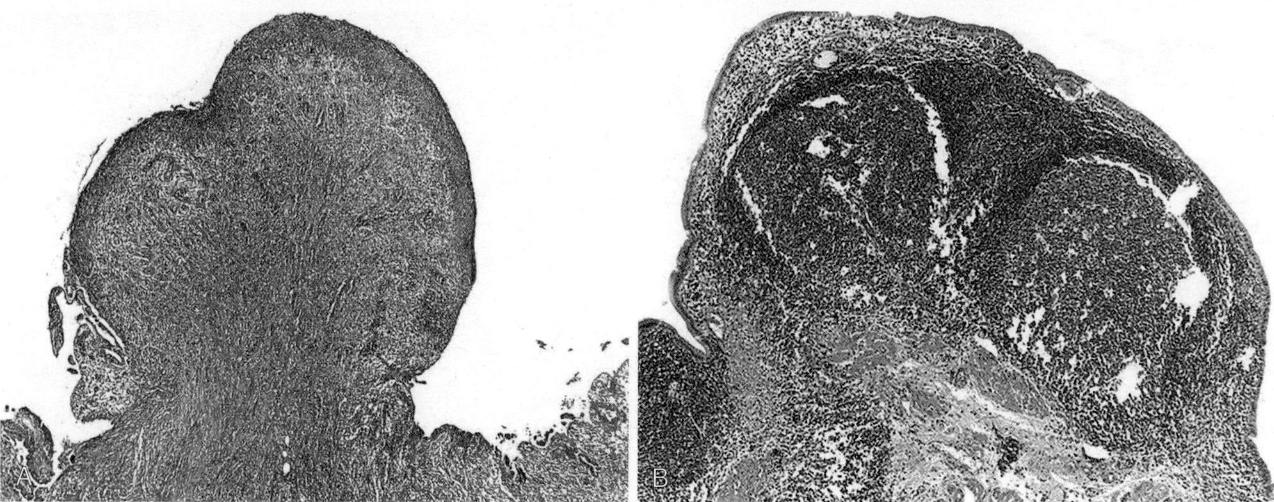

FIGURE 39.68 Inflammatory polyps of the gallbladder are composed of various types of inflammatory processes, including granulation tissue **(A)** and lymphoid aggregates **(B).**

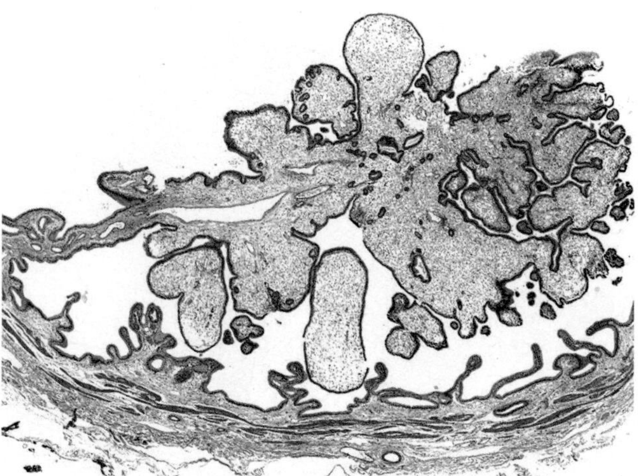

FIGURE 39.69 Cholesterol polyp. There are abundant foamy macrophages filling the lamina propria of this benign gallbladder polyp.

Inflammation-Associated Polyps

Other injury-related polyps include *granulation tissue polyps, xanthogranulomatous polyps*, and *lymphoid polyps* (Fig. 39.68). Lymphoid polyps are composed of prominent lymphoid tissue. They may be single or multiple.[43] Miniature versions of these are common in follicular cholecystitis.[44]

Cholesterol Polyps

Cholesterol polyps are unrelated to gallbladder injury; therefore they are characterized by absence of significant inflammation in the adjacent gallbladder. They often present as small mucosal bumps in the setting of widespread cholesterolosis. However, well-developed cholesterol polyps have a distinctive pedunculated cauliflower architecture (Fig. 39.69). It should be kept in mind that *cholesterol polyps* can be devoid of cholesterol-laden macrophages in 15% of cases, with the cores showing only edema (Fig. 39.70).[43] A subtle form of low-grade and clinically inconsequential dysplasia can be seen in 3% of cholesterol polyps.[43]

Hamartomatous Polyps

Hamartomatous polyps composed of disorganized and focally cystic epithelial elements have been described in Peutz-Jeghers syndrome and Cowden disease.[103]

Heterotopia

Heterotopic tissue, particularly gastric, pancreatic, or adrenocortical types, may form a mass up to 2 cm in diameter. Gastric heterotopia (Fig. 39.71) may be associated with secretory activity and lead to cholecystitis or ulcers.[188]

Adenomyomas

Adenomyomatous nodule or hyperplasia is characterized by a mural collection of cystically dilated glands forming a small solitary mass or a band of trabeculated thickening of the gallbladder wall with sievelike configuration (Fig. 39.72).[189] The majority of lesions are located in the fundus.[190] *Adenomyomatosis* refers to the more diffuse form of this condition, which is very uncommon (Fig. 39.73).

This process is not neoplastic, but rather appears to be developmental in origin. Some regard it as an exaggerated form of Rokitansky-Aschoff sinuses. However, in many cases, there is no evidence of tissue injury, no other sinuses elsewhere, no overt communication with the surface mucosa, and the configuration of the glands is not typical of Rokitansky-Aschoff sinuses. Additionally, although the terminology indicates a "myoid" process, many cases lack a significant myoid component and contain a more fibrotic stroma (see Fig. 39.72).

Low- and/or high-grade dysplasia may be seen in adenomyomatous nodules, but this usually represents pagetoid involvement by dysplasia elsewhere in the gallbladder. However, in some cases, the neoplastic process is largely confined to the adenomyomatous nodule and is characterized by papillary proliferations predominantly lined by gastric/endocervical-like mucinous epithelium. These lesions are regarded as *intracholecystic neoplasms arising in adenomyomatous nodules*, as discussed earlier (see Figs. 39.27 and 39.28).[18,191,192]

EXTRAHEPATIC BILE DUCTS

Tumoral Intraepithelial Neoplasms

Mass-forming, preinvasive neoplastic lesions of the extrahepatic biliary tract may be classified into two categories: (1) intraductal papillary, tubular, and tubulopapillary neoplasms, such as *intraductal papillary neoplasms of the bile ducts*,[32,60,193]

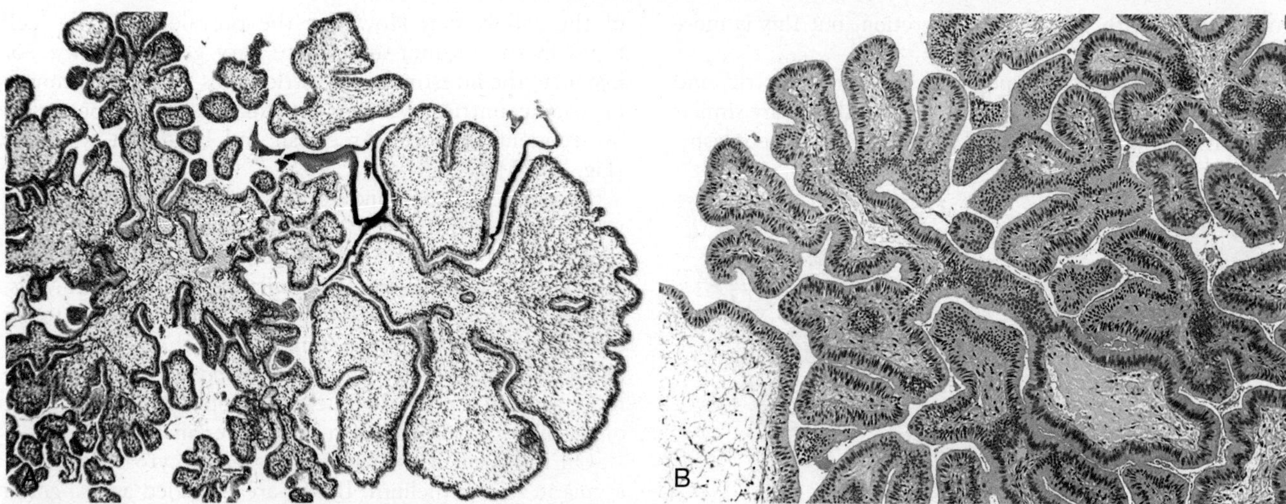

FIGURE 39.70 Cholesterol polyps are characterized by the cauliflower architecture **(A)**, even when the polyp is devoid of lipid-laden macrophages **(B)**.

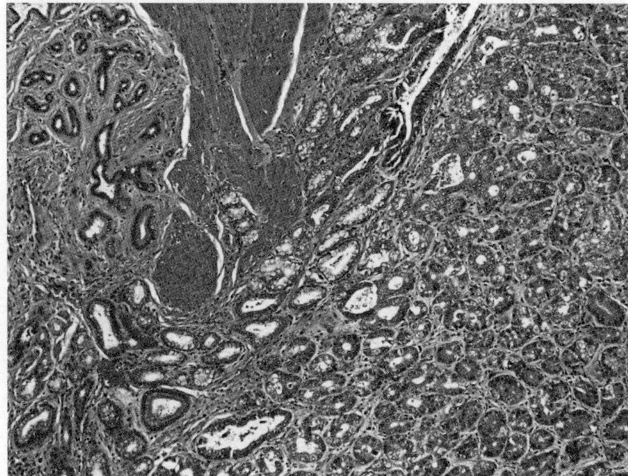

FIGURE 39.71 Heterotopic tissue is not that uncommon and may form a mass. Gastric heterotopia is depicted here.

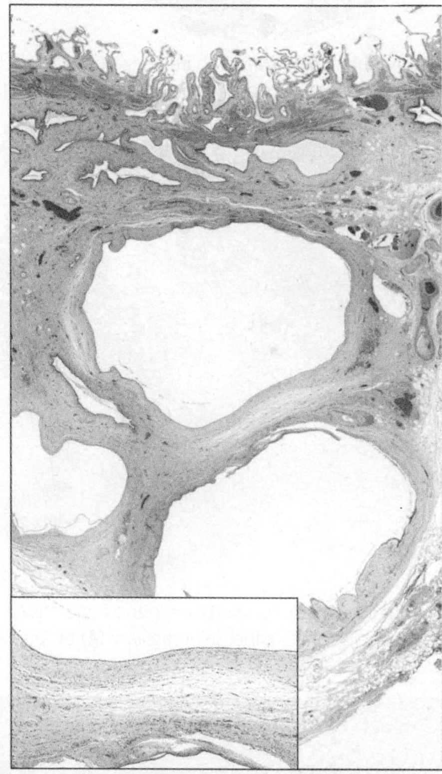

FIGURE 39.72 Adenomyomatous nodule of the gallbladder. In some cases, this process results in the formation of a distinct nodule composed of glandular elements with cystic dilation admixed with hyperplastic bundles of smooth muscle.

intraductal oncocytic papillary neoplasms of the bile ducts, and *intraductal tubular*[194] *or tubulopapillary neoplasms of the bile ducts,*[30] and (2) mucinous cystic neoplasm with ovarian-type stroma.[78] All of these lesions may show a spectrum of neoplastic changes, from low- to high-grade dysplasia and to invasive carcinoma.

Intraductal Papillary Neoplasms of the Bile Ducts

The 2019 WHO classification endorses the category of *intraductal papillary neoplasms of the bile ducts* (IPNBs), which encompasses all tumors that were previously termed *papillary adenomas, papillomas, papillomatosis, biliary intraductal "papillary" mucinous neoplasms,* or *papillary adenocarcinomas* (Fig. 39.74A).[32] For all practical purposes, these are the biliary counterparts of pancreatic IPMNs. Of note, tubular and tubulopapillary versions of these neoplasms are also increasingly being recognized and classified separately under the term *intraductal tubulopapillary neoplasm* (ITPN; see Fig. 39.74B).[60,194]

Clinical Features

IPNBs account for 10% to 38% of all bile duct tumors in Eastern Asia, but only 7% to 12% of all bile duct tumors in North American and European countries.[32] Patients are usually in their early 60s at the time of diagnosis. Intermittent abdominal pain and cholangitis are the main symptoms and signs, but some cases are detected incidentally. IPNBs may be associated with primary sclerosing cholangitis, hepatolithiasis,[195] and liver fluke infections, especially *Opisthorchis viverrini.*[196,197]

Pathological Features

Some IPNBs are isolated papillary lesions, whereas others appear as multiple contiguous lesions; cases previously called *papillomatosis* are now included in this category. They may present with mucus hypersecretion, but this is more common in Asian patents.[198]

In terms of the cell types (i.e., intestinal, gastric, and biliary) that compose most of the lesions, IPNBs are similar to IPMNs of the pancreas and intracholecystic neoplasms of the gallbladder. However, the prevalence of the cell types in each tumor appears to vary geographically. For instance, the intestinal and gastric types are more common in Asian countries, whereas the biliary type is reported to be frequent in North American and European countries (Fig. 39.75)[32,193,199]

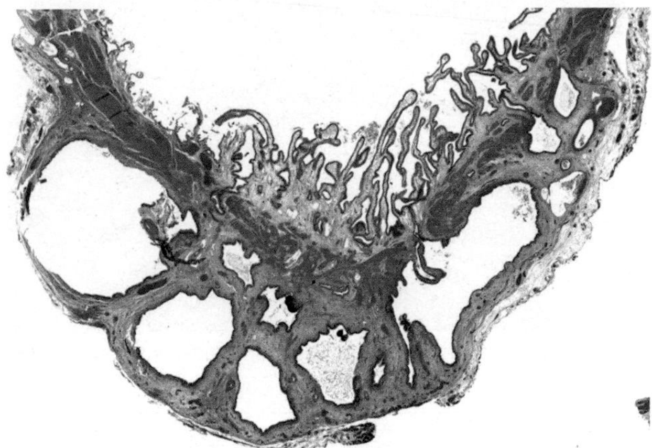

FIGURE 39.73 Adenomyomatosis is characterized by diffuse wall thickening with numerous cystic spaces within the gallbladder wall.

Recently, in Japan and Korea, a different classification was proposed, dividing IPNBs into type 1 and type 2 categories based on their similarity to pancreatic IPMNs: type 1 IPNBs are morphologically similar to pancreatic IPMNs, whereas type 2 IPNBs differ from them. The latter is described as "having more complex branching architecture or foci of solid-tubular components" and are reported to be more aggressive.[200] Reproducibility, applicability, and value of this new classification require further analysis.

On the basis of the highest degree of cytoarchitectural atypia in the epithelium, IPNBs are classified as *low grade* or *high grade*. Foci with low-grade dysplasia reveal only mild architectural and cytological atypia. Relatively uniform nuclei are still mostly confined to the lower aspect of the epithelium. High-grade dysplasia is characterized by pseudostratification of cells with loss of polarity and nuclear pleomorphism. A majority of IPBNs typically reveals

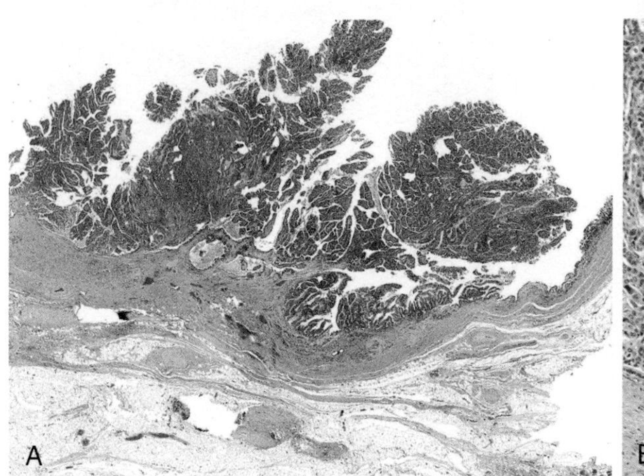

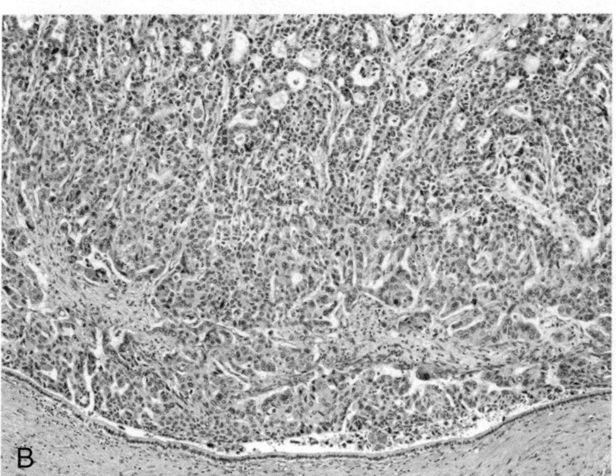

FIGURE 39.74 Just like their counterparts in the pancreas, intraductal neoplasms of the bile ducts are also characterized by intraluminal growth of back-to-back epithelial units, either in a papillary **(A)** or tubular/tubulopapillary **(B)** configuration.

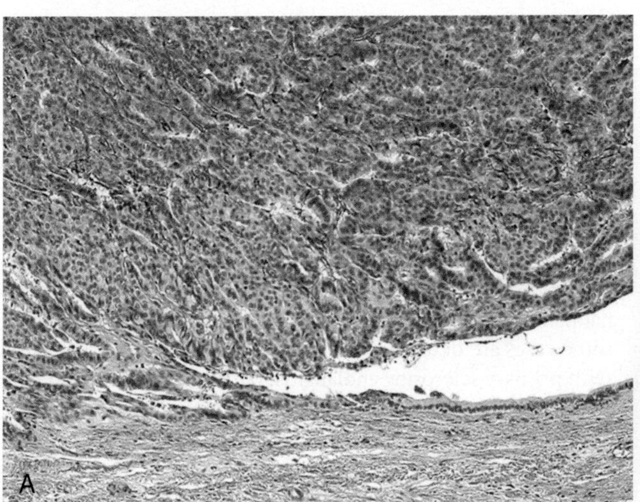

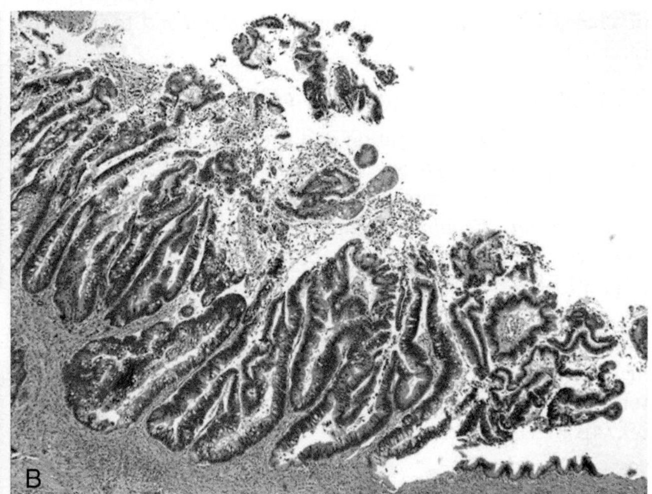

FIGURE 39.75 Intraductal neoplasms of the bile ducts, similar to pancreatic intraductal papillary mucinous neoplasms and intracholecystic papillary-tubular neoplasms of the gallbladder, may reveal different cellular phenotypes. Biliary **(A)** and intestinal **(B)** ones are depicted here.

extensive high-grade dysplasia, and invasive carcinomas are commonly associated with these lesions.[31] Most carcinomas that arise from these tumors are tubular (pancreatobiliary type) adenocarcinomas composed of well to poorly formed glandular/ductal structures surrounded by remarkably desmoplastic stroma. Colloid carcinoma, characterized by large mucin pools of mucin that are partially lined by neoplastic cells or contain suspended neoplastic cells, and other rare carcinoma variants, such as poorly differentiated neuroendocrine carcinomas, may also occur.[31,55,201]

Immunohistochemical and Molecular Features

The immunoprofile of IPNBs parallels their specific type of cell differentiation. The intestinal type expresses MUC2, CK20, and CDX2; the gastric type expresses MUC5AC, MUC6, and CK7; and the biliary type expresses MUC1.[31,195] Similar to pancreatic IPMNs, SMAD4 (DPC4) expression is normally retained.[55,202] In one study, nuclear β-catenin expression was reported in 25% of the cases.[203] Microsatellite instability can be identified in 10%.[203,204] Allelic loss of chromosome 18q is detected in one third of the cases[203]; there have been no reported 17p allelic losses or *TP53* alterations.[203,204] Except for the gastric type, *KRAS* mutations are uncommon in IPNBs.[31,55] Similarly, *GNAS* mutations are seen in the intestinal type.[60]

Differential Diagnosis

The main differential diagnosis of IPNBs is determining the location of the tumor (i.e., whether a lesion is primary to the bile duct, gallbladder, or pancreas). Rarely, a pancreatic IPMN may develop a fistula to the common bile duct and show intramucosal spread mimicking an IPNB.

Regarding cystic components of the tumor, it may occasionally be difficult to distinguish a primary tumor from other cystic lesions, such as choledochal cysts and Caroli disease. In addition, congenital cysts or duplication cysts in this region occasionally develop carcinoma in situ that is indistinguishable from an IPNB.[205] This situation may require careful sampling to determine the underlying congenital epithelium associated with normal structures or cilia formation or a muscular coat in some cases.[193]

Natural History and Treatment

Not surprisingly, IPNBs have a significantly more favorable prognosis than conventional cholangiocarcinomas.[206] Minimally invasive examples also have a better clinical course.[207] In contrast, widely invasive (advanced-stage) cases often have an aggressive clinical course. Even in the absence of significant high-grade dysplasia or invasive carcinoma, these tumors may recur and metastasize, possibly because of an undetected focus of invasive carcinoma or a field-effect phenomenon that predisposes the remaining segments of the biliary tract to development of carcinoma.[32]

Intraductal Oncocytic Papillary Neoplasms of the Bile Ducts

Intraductal oncocytic papillary neoplasms of bile ducts[208] are virtually identical to their more common pancreatic counterparts.[21,23,25] Clinically, they present as complex cystic neoplasms that often get the preoperative diagnosis of a *cystadenocarcinoma* because their intraductal nature is often obscured. The associated inflammation and fibrosis also contribute to the radiological impression of *infiltrative malignant mass.* On histological examination, they are characterized by arborizing papillary architecture. The papillae are lined by two to five cell layers of oncocytic cells showing abundant acidophilic granular cytoplasm and round nuclei with single prominent eccentric nucleoli. The lesions are indeed very complex, especially the intrahepatic lesions, which also extend to the smaller ductules and create an invasive appearance. However, overt invasion is fairly uncommon in these tumors. More importantly, even when these tumors are invasive, they are highly indolent despite their highly complex nature, with very few leading to mortality. Immunohistochemically they are often MUC6 positive.[208] In limited studies, their molecular phenotype was also found to be different from that of ordinary IPNBs.[209]

Intraductal Tubular or Tubulopapillary Neoplasms of the Bile Ducts

Intraductal neoplasms with a tubular or tubulopapillary growth pattern composed of nonmucinous or minimally mucinous cells are increasingly recognized as a separate entity.[30,194] They occur predominantly in women and are more commonly intrahepatic in location.[30,194]

Microscopically, in addition to a tubular pattern, solid sheets of cells and comedo-like necrotic areas are common. The tumor cells are cuboidal, lacking apparent intracellular mucin. They contain round and atypical nuclei and prominent nucleoli.[30,194] Using the dysplasia grading criteria in the pancreatobiliary tract, all cases ultimately qualify as high-grade dysplasia. This is because although there is cytological uniformity in most cases, there is also at least some foci with striking architectural complexity (see Fig. 39.74B).

Immunohistochemically, the tumor cells are positive for CK19, CA 19-9, MUC1, and MUC6 in most cases, whereas they are negative for CA 125, MUC2, MUC5AC, HepPar1, synaptophysin, and chromogranin. SMAD4 is normally retained.[30,194] Of these, MUC5AC has been used as a criterion of exclusion to distinguish these tumors from their kindreds, IPNBs. The molecular alterations observed include *CDKN2A/p16* and *TP53* mutations seen in 44% and 17% of cases, respectively. *KRAS, PIK3CA* mutations and loss of SMAD4/DPC4 are rare.[30,55]

Associated invasive carcinomas are common (identified in 80% of cases) and mostly tubular (pancreatobiliary type) adenocarcinomas. They are virtually indistinguishable from ordinary cholangiocarcinomas and are composed of relatively small tubular units infiltrating into desmoplastic stroma. However, similar to IPNBs, their clinical course is typically relatively indolent. In fact, even some invasive cases have a long protracted clinical course. Metastases and recurrences may occur several years after the original diagnosis.[30,194]

Biliary Mucinous Cystic Neoplasms

Mucinous cystic neoplasms (i.e., cystadenoma and cystadenocarcinoma) with ovarian-type stroma,[210] similar to those that occur in the pancreas, occur in the biliary tract as well, but most are intrahepatic in location.[75,78,210-213]

Clinical Features

Once defined by the presence of ovarian-type stroma, essentially all patients are women, typically of perimenopausal age group.[210] Very few men have mucinous cystic neoplasms defined by the presence of ovarian-type stroma.[115] At clinical presentation, most tumors have a multilocular cystic appearance that may grow up to 20 cm in diameter. Although most tumors arise within liver parenchyma or in perihepatic soft tissue and do not directly involve the major bile ducts, some may extend to the bile ducts and exhibit an intraductal growth pattern in that location as well.[78,103,210,214]

Pathological Features

Mucinous cystic neoplasms typically are multilocular, thick-walled cysts that contain seromucinous fluid. The cyst wall may be 0.1 to 3.0 cm thick. Polypoid projections may be identified in the cyst lumina, and these areas should be examined carefully for malignant change.[103,215] The cysts are lined by tall columnar mucinous epithelium resembling endocervical epithelium, or it may appear to be low cuboidal in areas. Although they are termed *mucinous*, a substantial proportion have a predominantly nonmucinous biliary lining, and some may totally lack mucinous epithelium.[216] In some cases, the epithelium may become attenuated. Scattered goblet cells, endocrine cells, and Paneth cells may be identified in these tumors.[75,210-212,217,218]

Hypercellular mesenchyme characteristically has the morphological and immunophenotypic features of ovarian stroma and typically forms discrete layers surrounding the cysts.[75,211,212,217,218] This stroma probably represents a recapitulation of periductal fetal mesenchyme that is hormone sensitive, as has been proposed for other biphasic tumors with ovarian-type stroma.[219] The density and distribution of stroma may vary in different areas of the same tumor. A band of paucicellular dense fibrous tissue may separate the stroma from the epithelium. In some tumors, the stroma may be located immediately adjacent to the epithelium. Per the WHO classification, ovarian-type stroma is a requisite feature for the diagnosis of *mucinous cystic neoplasm* as in the pancreas.[78,115,210]

Most cases lack significant cytoarchitectural atypia and are classified as *mucinous cystic neoplasm with low-grade dysplasia*.[210] However, in <10%, malignant transformation is evident in the form of highly atypical cells with enlarged, pleomorphic, and irregular nuclei and hyperchromatism that typically form papillary structures and are classified as *mucinous cystic neoplasm with high-grade dysplasia*.[210] If invasive carcinoma is identified, it should be reported as an *invasive carcinoma arising in a mucinous cystic neoplasm*.[75,211,212,217,218,220] The associated invasive carcinoma is often conventional tubular adenocarcinoma (50%), virtually indistinguishable from ordinary cholangiocarcinomas, composed of relatively small tubular units infiltrating into desmoplastic stroma. The invasive component may be focal, therefore these neoplasms must be sampled extensively, if not entirely.

Immunohistochemical and Molecular Features

Ovarian stroma that characterizes these tumors indeed show all features of true ovarian stroma including molecular pathways involved in hormone production.[221] Immunohistochemically, actin and desmin labeling and nuclear expression of progesterone receptors are typical. Calretinin, inhibin, and CD99 may be positive as well.

The epithelium shows CK7 expression, whereas CK20 is usually only focal. The epithelium is mostly negative for the progesterone receptor.[182,187] Neuroendocrine markers may reveal scattered neuroendocrine cells in some cases.

KRAS mutations are identified in 20% of mucinous cystic neoplasms, especially in cases with high-grade dysplasia. However, *GNAS*, *RNF43*, and *PIK3CA* are wild type in 100% of cases.[210,222]

Differential Diagnosis

Congenital and acquired cystic lesions, such as cystic biliary hamartomas, can mimic mucinous cystic neoplasms, especially when they are inflamed and accompanied by granulation tissue.[220] Immunohistochemical stains for progesterone receptors can help clarify the nature of the stroma in these cases.

Moreover, different types of intraductal neoplasms may manifest as complex cystic masses and may clinically be designated as *cystic neoplasms*. Ovarian-type stroma may be the only distinguishing feature.[210] Also, oncocytic (characterized by MUC6 expression) and intestinal differentiation (characterized by MUC2 and CDX2 expression) are not features of mucinous cystic neoplasms.

Natural History and Treatment

Data suggest that if the tumor is sampled thoroughly and high-grade dysplasia and invasive carcinoma have been excluded, it invariably behaves in a benign fashion.[210] Cases treated with incomplete resections may recur.[210] Cases with high-grade dysplasia and invasive carcinoma, which are very uncommon once the entity is defined by the ovarian-type stroma, are prone to recurrence and metastasis. The prognosis of invasive carcinoma depends on the extent of invasion.[78,210]

Nontumoral ("Flat") Intraepithelial Neoplasms (Biliary Intraepithelial Neoplasia)

Microscopic, incidental, preinvasive neoplasms of the bile ducts are considered *flat* lesions,[81] which distinguishes them from mass-forming preinvasive neoplasms.[15] Flat lesions may have some early papilla formation, but by definition, they do not form a grossly or radiographically recognizable mass.[81]

The 2019 WHO classification endorses the term *biliary intraepithelial neoplasia* (BilIN) for flat lesions, based on the approach used for other organs such as the pancreas (i.e., PanINs).

Clinical Features

BilIN can occur anywhere within the biliary tree or the gallbladder but mostly involves larger bile ducts. Given their microscopic nature, BilINs are typically found incidentally in bile duct specimens resected for other reasons or adjacent to invasive carcinomas. *High-grade* BilIN is detected in 40% to 60% of patients with invasive carcinoma. It is also well established that BilIN is more common in clinical conditions normally associated with a greater risk of carcinoma, such as primary sclerosing cholangitis, choledochal cysts, and anomalous union of the pancreatic and biliary ducts.[110,205,223-225]

Pathological Features

Because of the inaccessibility of the region and frequent association with invasive carcinoma, follow-up and correlative clinical studies of BilIN are difficult to perform. However, an association between intestinal metaplasia and BilIN has been documented.[189]

BilIN is difficult to appreciate grossly. Some cases manifest as mucosal granularity, but most appear hyperemic or even entirely normal to the naked eye. Microscopically, BilIN is characterized by disorderly, atypical columnar or cuboidal biliary-type cells. It is graded based on the highest degree of cytoarchitectural atypia as either *low grade* or *high grade.* This two-tier classification has replaced the former three-tier classification (the former BilIN-1 and BilIN-2 categories are now classified as *low grade*, and the former BilIN-3 category is now classified as *high grade*).[80] In *low-grade* lesions, the cells show mild pseudostratification, inconspicuous nuclear enlargement, and minimal nuclear irregularities (Fig. 39.76A). *High-grade* lesions show marked nuclear enlargement, irregularity, hyperchromasia, and loss of polarity (Fig. 39.76B). Architectural changes, such as fusion of the epithelium or cribriform architecture, may occur in *high-grade* cases as well.

It is important to recognize BilIN of especially high-grade lesions in resections performed for reasons other than invasive cancer.[205] High-risk conditions like primary sclerosing cholangitis, choledochal cyst[205] and pancreatobiliary maljunction[16] should be sampled entirely to rule out BilIN and invasive carcinoma. If high-grade BilIN is discovered, the patient should be placed under close surveillance.

Differential Diagnosis

Differentiating BilIN from reactive changes can be challenging for pathologists. *Low-grade* BilIN may be difficult to distinguish from regenerating and hyperplastic epithelium, especially when thick sections impart a multilayered appearance to the cells. In addition, the biliary tract may form stratified epithelium normally, but these areas do not show the nuclear enlargement and coarse chromatin that are typical features of BilIN. There is also a type of biliary epithelium, probably a form of hyperplasia, that can closely mimic low-grade BilIN.[205] It is typically encountered in transition regions like the cystic duct or the distal common bile duct and is characterized by subtle stratification of thin, slender pencillate-shaped nuclei with homogenous but dense chromatin. However, unlike dysplasia, this is typically confined to the lower part of the epithelium (i.e., does not reach to the surface).

For differentiating *high-grade* BilIN from reactive changes, several features are helpful: loss of polarity, nuclear stratification, enlargement, irregularity, and hyperchromasia (see Table 39.3).[226,227] It is highly unusual for reactive epithelium to show all of these features, but one or two may be seen in individual cases. Degenerating cells may appear nonpolarized and atypical. However, the nuclear chromatin is usually fine and pale. Maturation toward the surface, evenness of nuclear chromatin, and lack of marked nuclear enlargement favor reactive changes. In contrast, prominent tufting of irregularly shaped nuclei with apoptosis favors BilIN. Nuclear TP53 staining occurs in more than 30% of BilIN cases and tends to be stronger in high-grade lesions.[202,228] Although TP53 expression is significantly less common in nonneoplastic epithelium, it can be seen in areas of regenerative changes as well, which limits the value of this marker in the differential diagnosis of reactive versus neoplastic lesions. Similarly, although the Ki67 labeling index is substantially higher for dysplastic lesions, it can also be high in areas of regenerative change. It has been

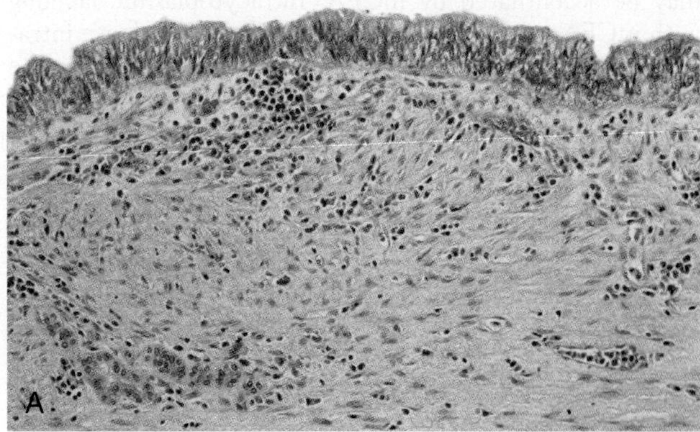

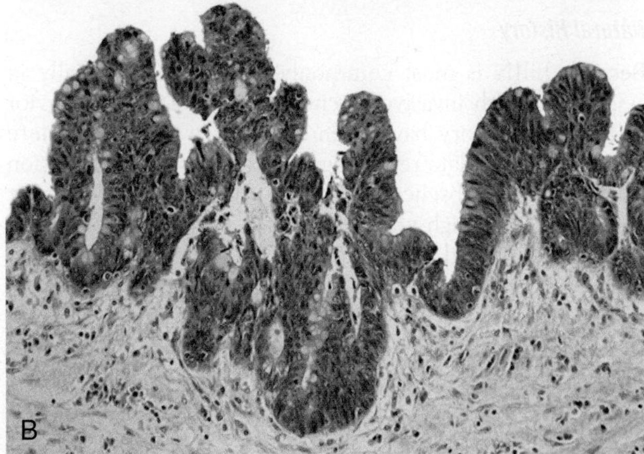

FIGURE 39.76 A, Low-grade BilINs (formerly BilIN-1 or 2) are characterized by mild pseudostratification of nuclei that have mild to moderate cytological abnormalities. Nuclear enlargement is usually inconspicuous. **B,** In contrast, high-grade BilINs (formerly BilIN-3) are characterized by complete loss of polarity and significant nuclear atypia, such as marked nuclear enlargement, irregularity, and hyperchromasia. True cribriforming or budding of cell clusters into the duct lumen may be present.

suggested that S100P expression increases during the multistep carcinogenesis process and may be used as an adjunct to distinguish high-grade dysplasia from reactive changes; however, the results are not conclusive.[229-231]

In areas of active inflammation or ulceration, pathologists should refrain from establishing a diagnosis of BilIN because regenerative changes may show substantial cellular alterations, including nuclear crowding, enlargement, and hyperchromasia. A history of instrumentation or stent placement should also raise the bar significantly for a diagnosis of BilIN.[232] On the other hand, it should be kept in mind that some forms of high-grade dysplasia are associated with neutrophilic infiltrate in the dysplastic epithelium.

BilIN that extends into accessory (peribiliary) mucous glands can result in a pseudoinfiltrative appearance. However, preservation of lobular architecture favors a noninvasive lesion. Peribiliary glands tend to have a small, round appearance with narrow lumina (see Fig. 39.52), whereas invasive glands normally vary considerably in size and shape, show contour irregularity, and have open and round lumina or elongated and cordlike forms.

Immunohistochemically, MUC1 and mCEA typically stain the apical border of BilIN cells and highlight the luminal membrane. In high-grade BilIN, intercellular membranes may be accentuated by mCEA. Intracytoplasmic labeling with mCEA is uncommon in high-grade BilIN; dense intracytoplasmic staining favors cancerization over high-grade BilIN.

Molecular Features

KRAS mutations are identified in about 40% of cases. *KRAS* mutation represents an early molecular event during the progression of BilIN, whereas *TP53* mutation represents a late molecular event.[59,202] Alterations in cell cycle proteins, including cyclin-dependent kinase inhibitor 1A (CDKN1A), cyclin D1 (CCND1), and SMAD4 (DPC4), are detected in some cases.[202] Claudin 18 (CLDN18) abnormalities are also common.[233]

Natural History

Because BilIN is most commonly detected incidentally in association with invasive carcinoma, its biological behavior and natural history have been difficult to evaluate. There are no concrete data regarding the exact risk of progression of BilIN in the absence of invasive carcinoma; however, it is believed that high-grade BilIN is a disease that warrants close attention and follow-up.

Malignant Epithelial Tumors

Adenocarcinoma

Clinical Features

The most common symptom is upper quadrant pain.[50] Unlike gallbladder carcinomas, extrahepatic bile duct carcinomas usually present with obstructive jaundice. Weight loss and pruritis may also be present. Serum alkaline phosphatase levels are usually elevated.

Clinically, extrahepatic bile duct carcinomas are separated into thirds for therapeutic and prognostic purposes: upper third (i.e., above the cystic duct junction, including the right and left hepatic ducts, the common hepatic duct, and the cystic duct), middle third (i.e., upper half of the common bile duct), and lower third (i.e., distal half of common bile duct).[234-238] Most extrahepatic bile duct carcinomas occur in the upper third and arise within 5 mm of the cystic duct. Those that occur at the confluence of the right and left hepatic ducts are termed *Klatskin tumors*.[239] Tumors that arise in the perihilar region have been further classified according to their pattern of involvement of the hepatic ducts (i.e., Bismuth-Corlette classification). Those that occur below the confluence of the left and right hepatic ducts are classified as type I, those that reach the confluence are type II, and those that occlude the common hepatic duct and the right or left hepatic duct are considered types IIIA and IIIB, respectively. Those that are multicentric or involve the confluence of the right and left hepatic duct are classified as type IV.[240] Of note, these carcinomas, regardless of the location, are similar microscopically.

Extrahepatic bile duct carcinomas do not have a female predominance characteristic of gallbladder carcinomas, presumably because of a lack of association with gallstones. However, the risk of extrahepatic bile duct carcinoma is high among patients with primary sclerosing cholangitis.[110,232,241-243] A lifetime risk of 10% has been documented for patients with primary sclerosing cholangitis.[240] The association of intrahepatic cholangiocarcinomas with parasites (e.g., *Clonorchis sinensis* and *Opisthorchis viverrini*)[244-246] and hepatolithiasis[247-249] and of extrahepatic adenocarcinoma with choledochal cysts[224,225] is also a reflection of long-standing chronic inflammation. Congenital anomalies of the hepatobiliary region,[251] such as polycystic disease, Caroli disease, and congenital hepatic fibrosis are other known risk factors for extrahepatic bile duct carcinoma. Metabolic conditions such as type 1 diabetes, chronic pancreatitis, gout, smoking,[252] and occupational exposure to 1,2-dichloropropane and dichloromethane in the printing industry[253] have also been reported as risk factors.

As discussed earlier, pancreatobiliary maljunction (an anomalous union of the main pancreatic duct and common bile duct outside the sphincter of Oddi) is also associated with a high incidence of dysplasia and carcinoma in the biliary tract[16,250] (see Carcinoma Associated with Anomalous Union of Pancreatobiliary Ducts section).

More importantly, recent studies have disclosed that low-level union of the cystic duct with the common hepatic duct, in which the cystic duct joins the hepatic duct within or immediately adjacent to the pancreas, is frequently associated with pancreatobiliary neoplasia, especially with distal bile duct carcinomas (seen in more than 70% of the cases).[254]

Pathological Features

Macroscopically, extrahepatic bile duct carcinomas can present as either nodular, papillary, or sclerotic tumors. As a matter of fact, most nodular or papillary tumors are intraductal papillary or tubulopapillary neoplasms.[193] On cut section, if present, the invasive component reveals a firm, white, gritty appearance because of an abundance of desmoplastic stroma.

Carcinomas often invade deeply into or through the wall of the bile ducts into adjacent soft tissue, liver, or pancreas.[255,256] Often, the gross boundaries of the carcinoma are difficult to determine with certainty. The tumor may merge with adjacent areas of inflammation and fibrosis. The margins of surgical resection specimens may be difficult to evaluate grossly, which necessitates frozen-section analysis.

Microscopically, most carcinomas are pancreatobiliary-type adenocarcinomas, characterized by widely spaced, well-formed, irregular glands and small clusters of cells associated with a desmoplastic stroma.[50,115] The spectrum and variants described for pancreatobiliary-type adenocarcinomas discussed earlier in the Gallbladder section are valid for extrahepatic bile duct carcinomas.

Immunohistochemical and Molecular Features

TP53 protein overexpression is seen in nearly 50% of cases. The highest frequency is reported for tumors of the distal common bile duct.[257] Some immunohistochemical studies have found that TP53 expression is specific for carcinoma rather than nonneoplastic changes associated with primary sclerosing cholangitis.[257,258] Similar to TP53 expression, frequency of loss of SMAD4 (DPC4) expression and *KRAS* mutations increase from the proximal to the distal portions of the biliary tract. However, even in the distal common bile duct, these are less common compared with the pancreas, where they occur in 50% and more than 90% of cases, respectively.[124,259] The rate of *KRAS* mutations is high among patients with anomalous union of pancreatobiliary ducts.[260,261] This supports the hypothesis that *KRAS* mutations may be related to exposure to pancreatic juice. In patients with primary sclerosing cholangitis, *KRAS* mutations in bile samples were found to be an indicator of subsequent progression to dysplasia and invasive cancer.[262] Recently, *ELF3* and *ARID1B* mutations and *PRKACA/PRKACB* fusion have been reported as extrahepatic bile duct carcinoma–specific alterations.[263,264]

Staging

For staging purposes, the AJCC/TNM system divides bile duct cancers into several categories based on location[131]:

1. *Intrahepatic,* which is usually resected with a segment of liver
2. *Perihilar,* which can be resected segmentally or with a portion of liver or gallbladder
3. *Distal* (includes the region between the cystic duct and the ampulla), which is typically removed by pancreatoduodenectomy

Of note, the cystic duct is often resected with the gallbladder and staged according to the gallbladder protocol. Some of the AJCC/TNM staging parameters rely heavily on radiological and intraoperative findings, such as involvement of the hepatic artery and its branches.[10] They require close clinicopathological correlation.[265]

Natural History and Prognosis

The primary form of management of extrahepatic bile duct carcinomas is radical surgery.[266,267] Adjuvant chemotherapy is also commonly provided, but the most efficacious chemotherapy protocol remains a subject of debate.[141]

The stage of disease at presentation and its resectability are the most important factors associated with patient outcome. The 5-year overall survival rate is estimated to be 20% to 30% for resectable cancers, but it is almost 0% for unresectable cases.[130,268] High tumor grade and lymphovascular and perineural invasions are also associated with poor prognosis.[269]

Other Types of Carcinoma

Other types of carcinoma that occur in the gallbladder, including *mucinous, poorly cohesive* (with or without signet ring cells),[270] *adenosquamous,*[271,272] *squamous cell, undifferentiated,* and *neuroendocrine*[273,274] carcinoma, also occur in the extrahepatic bile ducts (see definitions and descriptions in the Gallbladder section). These carcinomas are often mixed with some degree of pancreatobiliary-type adenocarcinoma. Among these carcinomas, undifferentiated carcinomas with osteoclast-like giant cells, tumors that are typically of pancreatic origin,[150,151] are significantly more common in the bile ducts than in the gallbladder.[150] Another rare tumor that is more common in the bile ducts is *tubulocystic carcinomas* (Fig. 39.77).[228] This entity may be related to intraductal tubular/tubulopapillary neoplasms.

Neuroendocrine Neoplasms

Well-differentiated neuroendocrine tumors are uncommon in the biliary tract.[162] However, the distal common bile duct is the most common site,[275,276] followed by the cystic duct. They often manifest with symptoms of biliary obstruction, but may also be discovered incidentally.[277,278] Some tumors may be associated with genetic syndromes, such as von Hippel-Lindau or MEN I syndromes. Zollinger-Ellison syndrome has also been reported.[103] Most patients are middle age at time of clinical presentation.

These neuroendocrine tumors usually form nodular or polypoid lesions. The white-yellow cut surface of the tumor is typically homogenous. Microscopic examination of these tumors reveals an insular or nested growth pattern.[168-170] Cytologically, they exhibit typical features of low-grade neuroendocrine neoplasms, including the presence of round, uniform nuclei with finely stippled chromatin and a moderate amount of cytoplasm (Fig. 39.78). Immunohistochemically, these tumors are commonly positive for chromogranin, synaptophysin, CD56, and hormones to a variable degree. However, hormone expression has not been correlated with serological activity. The data on their

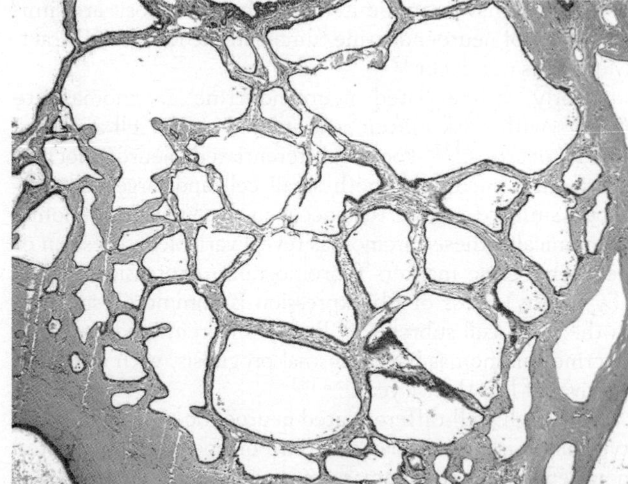

FIGURE 39.77 Tubulocystic carcinomas are composed of a conglomerate of back-to-back, variably sized cysts that form a microcystic pattern.

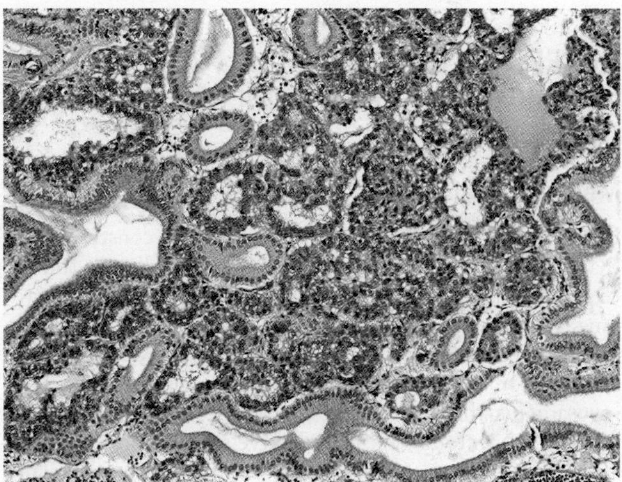

FIGURE 39.78 A well-differentiated neuroendocrine tumor (carcinoid) of the common bile duct composed of nests of relatively uniform cells.

biological behavior are limited, but their prognosis are similar to that of neuroendocrine tumors in the tubular GI tract. Metastasis can occur.[177]

Poorly differentiated neuroendocrine carcinomas are tumors with brisk mitotic activity and single-cell and confluent necrosis.[177] Poorly differentiated neuroendocrine carcinomas encompass both small cell and large cell subtypes, similar to those that occur in the lung. Immunohistochemically, these carcinomas reveal variable expression of neuroendocrine markers (chromogranin expression is usually patchy). Loss of Rb expression is common, especially in the small cell subtype.[180] Poorly differentiated neuroendocrine carcinomas have a dismal prognosis, with a median survival of less than 1 year.[182,183]

Although well-differentiated neuroendocrine tumors are typically pure, more than one third of poorly differentiated neuroendocrine carcinomas are accompanied by an adenocarcinoma component. They often arise from an intraductal neoplasm. The presence and extent of poorly differentiated neuroendocrine component should be reported because this feature correlates with outcome.[182,279]

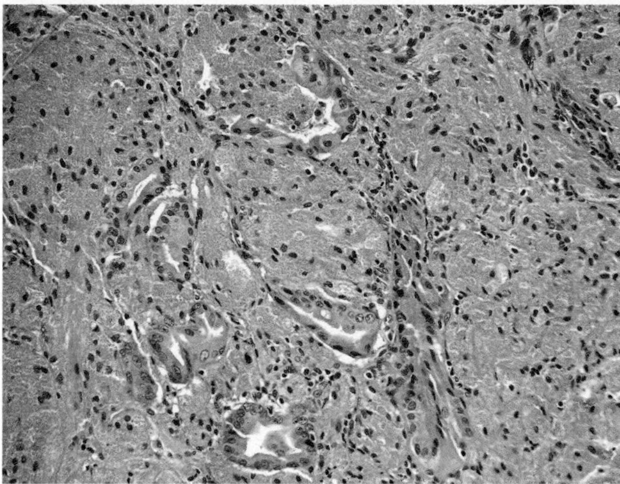

FIGURE 39.79 Granular cell tumor of the common bile duct. Sheets of cells with abundant eosinophilic granular cytoplasm are characteristic features of a granular cell tumor. Pseudoinfiltrative clusters of glandular epithelial elements are admixed with the granular tumor cells.

NONEPITHELIAL TUMORS OF THE GALLBLADDER AND EXTRAHEPATIC BILE DUCTS

Mesenchymal Tumors

Benign and malignant mesenchymal tumors constitute less than 1% of all biliary tract tumors. A variety of benign tumors (e.g., hemangioma, lymphangioma, leiomyoma, lipoma, osteoma, ganglioneuroma, neurofibroma, schwannoma, infantile myofibromatosis, solitary fibrous tumor, perivascular epithelioid cell tumor) and many sarcomas (e.g., angiosarcoma, leiomyosarcoma, rhabdomyosarcoma, chondrosarcoma, malignant fibrous histiocytoma, peripheral nerve sheath tumors, Kaposi sarcoma, AIDS-related and Epstein-Barr virus–associated smooth muscle tumors, CD117-positive GI stromal tumors) have been reported in the biliary system.[50,115,280,281] Lipomas may be associated with MEN I syndrome. All of these entities have histological features similar to those that occur in soft tissues elsewhere in the body. However, it is important to note that *sarcomatoid carcinoma* should be excluded in any case of a stromal sarcoma. A preinvasive component is typically diagnostic of the former.

The biliary tract, especially the distal common bile duct, is a preferred site for *granular cell tumors* (Fig. 39.79).[282,283] They are the most common nonepithelial tumor of the extrahepatic bile duct.[284] Granular cell tumors may be multicentric.[285] They manifest with obstructive symptoms and are associated with proliferation of surface epithelium or accessory ducts. Otherwise, the morphological features of granular cell tumors are similar to those that occur elsewhere in the body. They are composed of sheets of cells with abundant acidophilic granular cytoplasm and occasional globules. Cells show strong labeling for S100, CD68, nestin, calretinin, and CD68.[285]

Embryonal rhabdomyosarcoma in the extrahepatic bile duct is the most common malignant tumor of this region in children. However, less than 1% of rhabdomyosarcomas develop in the biliary tree.[280,286] The common bile duct is the most common location. Patients typically are diagnosed at 3 to 4 years of age.[287-289] Rhabdomyosarcomas form polypoid tumors and may exhibit the classic botryoid growth pattern. Tumors may be up to 14 cm in the greatest dimension. They often have a cambium layer, which represents a condensation of sarcoma cells beneath the epithelium. Muscle differentiation is demonstrable by immunohistochemical markers, including actin, desmin, myogenin, and myogenic differentiation 1 (MYOD1). Ultrastructural examination reveals the presence of thick and thin filaments. Multimodality treatment, including chemotherapy and radiotherapy, has produced long-term survival in some cases.[290] However, the prognosis usually is poor. Metastases occur in 40% of cases. Death usually results from local complications of the tumor.[288]

Paragangliomas

Paragangliomas may occur in the gallbladder. They are usually asymptomatic and detected incidentally, although patients occasionally are diagnosed because of complications.[291] They are typically less than 1 cm in diameter and located in the perimuscular connective tissue, where normal paraganglia reside. Paragangliomas of this region show small, tight clusters of polygonal cells (i.e., zellballen pattern) with endocrine properties (i.e., chromogranin and synaptophysin positive), surrounded by S100-positive sustentacular cells.[292-294] Paragangliomas are rare in the bile ducts.

SECONDARY TUMORS OF THE GALLBLADDER AND EXTRAHEPATIC BILE DUCTS

The gallbladder may be involved by lymphoma, leukemia, myeloma, or mast cell tumors as part of a systemic disease. Rarely, the malignancy initially manifests in the gallbladder.[295-301] The extrahepatic bile ducts are seldom involved by these tumors.[302]

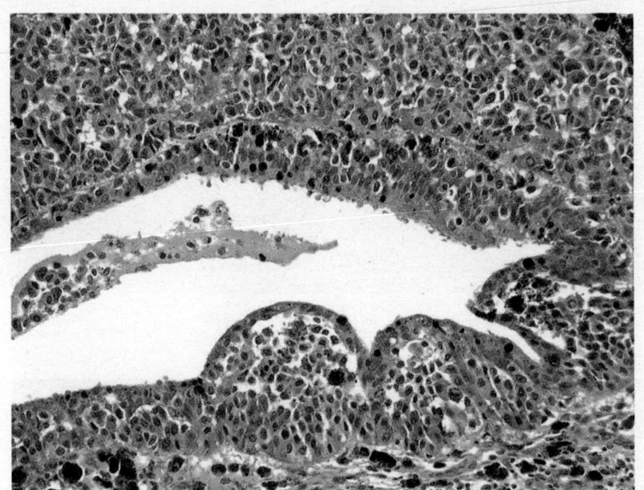

FIGURE 39.80 Metastatic malignant melanoma of the gallbladder. Pigmentation is prominent. Melanoma cells also involve the biliary epithelium. Secondary melanomas can display a pagetoid pattern of involvement of the biliary epithelium. This patient was known to have a primary melanoma in the abdominal skin.

Metastatic melanomas may occur in the biliary tract, particularly in the gallbladder. These tumors often form a polyp or nodule. A melanoma in this region is considered metastatic unless proven otherwise (Fig. 39.80). However, it rarely may be a primary and associated with an intraepithelial component.[303-307]

ACKNOWLEDGMENT

We thank Drs. Kerem Ozcan and Aslihan Yavas for their contributions in the preparation of this chapter.

The full reference list may be accessed online at Elsevier eBooks for Practicing Clinicians.

CHAPTER 40

Inflammatory and Other Nonneoplastic Disorders of the Pancreas

Vikram Deshpande

Contents

INTRODUCTION

This chapter discusses a range of inflammatory and other nonneoplastic diseases of the pancreas, with a focus on variants of chronic pancreatitis that mimic pancreatic neoplasia including autoimmune pancreatitis (AIP) and paraduodenal pancreatitis. In the past, a generic diagnosis of chronic pancreatitis was often sufficient, but with the recent recognition of unique variants, some steroid responsive, the pathologist is required to further subclassify this disorder.

A brief review of the pancreatic duct system is in order before a discussion of pancreatitis. The anatomy of the pancreatic ductal system is unpredictable because of developmental variability. The main pancreatic duct, the duct of Wirsung, carries the bulk of pancreatic secretions and drains into the duodenum at the papilla of Vater. The accessory pancreatic duct, also known as the *duct of Santorini*, drains into the duodenum through a separate minor papilla that is typically 2 cm cephalad to the papilla of Vater. In most individuals, the accessory pancreatic duct is nonfunctional. The minor papilla may appear as a nodule in the second part of the duodenum, and the endoscopist could mistake this for a polyp. Histologically, the relatively narrow accessory pancreatic duct is accompanied by pancreatic acinar and occasionally endocrine elements, which are often found within the submucosa of the duodenal wall.

ACUTE PANCREATITIS

Acute pancreatitis is an inflammatory disease of the pancreas that is characterized clinically by acute abdominal pain and elevated serum amylase and lipase.[1,2] The incidence of this disease has increased in the past two decades, and acute pancreatitis accounts for more than 200,000 hospital admissions every year in the United States. Eighty percent of these episodes are mild and resolve without serious morbidity, but in 20% of cases, the episodes are more severe and are associated with substantially increased morbidity and mortality.[1,2] Although frequently encountered at autopsy, acute pancreatitis is seldom seen by the surgical pathologist. In rare instances, pancreatic neoplasms could present as acute pancreatitis, and microscopic foci of resolving acute pancreatitis may be seen adjacent to neoplasms of the pancreas.

Clinical Features

There is a wide spectrum of severity, with some episodes of acute pancreatitis being mild and self-limited, requiring only brief hospitalization, and those most severely affected developing persistent hypovolemia and multiorgan dysfunction. The diagnosis of acute pancreatitis requires at least two of the following three features: (1) abdominal pain, (2) serum lipase and/or amylase levels at least three times that of normal, and (3) evidence of acute pancreatitis on imaging.[1,2]

Etiology and Pathogenesis

The two most common triggers of acute pancreatitis, obstruction of the common bile duct by stones and alcohol abuse, together account for approximately 80% of cases of acute pancreatitis in Western countries (Box 40.1).[1,2] Bile stone–induced pancreatitis typically affects elderly women and is caused by gallstone migration and subsequent pancreatic duct obstruction. Although gallstones are the most common cause of biliary obstruction, other forms of obstruction, such as periampullary tumors and neoplasms involving the head of the pancreas, may also provoke acute pancreatitis. Alcohol-related acute pancreatitis is more frequently seen in middle-aged men. Experimental studies have implicated alcohol in transient increases in pancreatic exocrine secretions, direct toxic injury to acinar cells, and contraction of the sphincter of Oddi. However, the relationship between alcohol and acute pancreatitis is not completely understood because acute pancreatitis develops in only a small fraction of patients who abuse alcohol.[3] Clearly, other genetic and environmental factors play a major role in the development of alcohol-related acute pancreatitis.

Drugs appear to account for about 5% of all cases of acute pancreatitis. The drugs most often associated with this disorder include azathioprine, 6-mercaptopurine, valproic acid, angiotensin-converting enzyme inhibitors, and mesalamine.

In a substantial minority of cases, the cause of acute pancreatitis is unexplained. Genetic testing for mutations, including the cationic trypsinogen *(PRSS1)*, serine protease inhibitor Kazal type I *(SPINK1)*, or cystic fibrosis transmembrane conductance regulator *(CFTR)* gene, may provide an explanation for recurrent acute pancreatitis because these may provide cofactors that precipitate acute pancreatitis (see later discussion).

Although the precise pathogenesis is controversial, it is nonetheless believed by most investigators that acute pancreatitis is caused by unregulated activation of pancreatic trypsin, and this enzyme leads to both autodigestion and local inflammation. After activation of trypsinogen to active trypsin, other pathways and enzymes in the pancreas such as elastase, complement, and kinin systems are activated. The inflammation is further propagated by the production of mediators such as interleukin 1 (IL-1), IL-6, and IL-8, which are produced by neutrophils, macrophages, and lymphocytes that are attracted to the diseased pancreas.

BOX 40.1 Causative Factors for Acute Pancreatitis

TOXIC AGENTS
Alcohol*
Cigarette smoke
Drugs: valproate, phenacetin, thiazide, estrogen, and azathioprine

OBSTRUCTION OF MAIN PANCREATIC DUCT
Gallstones*
Pancreatic neoplasms

ENDOGENOUS CAUSES
Hypercalcemia, hyperparathyroidism
Hyperlipidemia, lipoprotein lipase deficiency
Chronic renal failure

INFECTION OR INFESTATION
HIV, mumps virus, coxsackie-virus

GENETIC INCLUDING HEREDITARY PANCREATITIS
CFTR mutation
PRSS1 mutation
SPINK1 mutation
CTRC mutation

AUTOIMMUNE
Autoimmune pancreatitis (rare)

MISCELLANEOUS
After transplantation
After irradiation
Vascular disease: atheroembolism
Tropical pancreatitis

* *Alcohol and bile stones are the two most common causes of acute pancreatitis.*

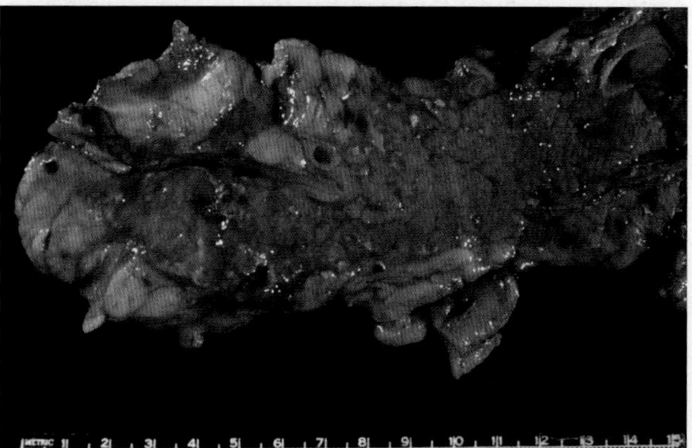

FIGURE 40.1 Acute pancreatitis. This cross section of the pancreas shows yellow specks in the fat, consistent with fat necrosis.

Pathological Features

The pancreas typically appears swollen and pale. With mild acute pancreatitis, multiple tiny spots of opaque white fat necrosis are seen on the surface of the pancreas (Fig. 40.1).[4] The amount of intrapancreatic fat varies considerably among individuals, and the presence of intraparenchymal fat necrosis is appreciable only in those with a moderate amount of intrapancreatic fat. In cases of severe acute pancreatitis, confluent areas of necrosis and hemorrhage are identified.

Histologically, the changes of acute pancreatitis are best characterized in autopsy material. In mild forms of acute pancreatitis, the disease is concentrated in the interlobular

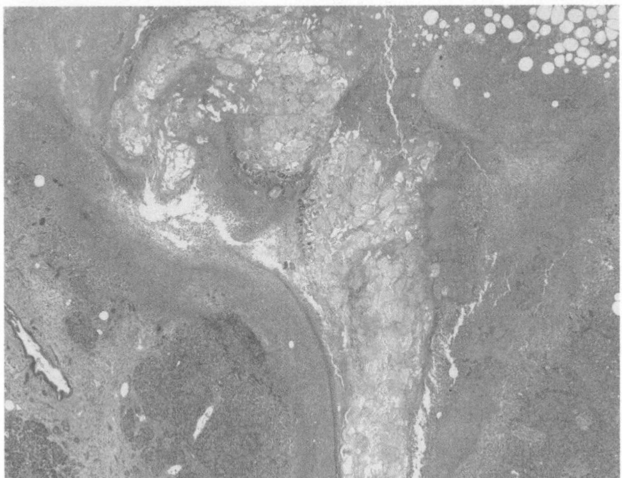

FIGURE 40.2 Acute pancreatitis. The central portion of the image shows areas of fat necrosis.

septa.[4] With time, these foci of fat necrosis are replaced by foamy macrophages and, ultimately, by fibrosis (Fig. 40.2). In the more severe examples of acute pancreatitis, there is diffuse necrosis involving the acinar and ductal tissue accompanied by acute inflammatory cells. Infected acute pancreatitis is associated with high mortality. Damage to the vasculature results in diffuse hemorrhage (hemorrhagic pancreatitis). Well-characterized examples of acute pancreatitis triggered by atheroembolism have also been reported.[5]

Therapy

The treatment for mild forms of the disease is largely supportive and includes fluid resuscitation.[1,2] More severe cases require aggressive fluid resuscitation and antibiotics.

CHRONIC PANCREATITIS

Chronic pancreatitis is a fibroinflammatory disorder in which the pancreatic acinar compartment is replaced by fibrosis, eventually leading to exocrine insufficiency.[6-8]

The annual incidence rate ranges from 5 to 14 per 100,000 individuals, and the prevalence ranges from approximately 30 to 50 per 100,000 individuals. Recent studies seem to indicate an increasing incidence of chronic pancreatitis. The median age of patients ranges from 51 to 58 years. Chronic pancreatitis is up to five times more common among men than women.

Patients with chronic pancreatitis typically show steatorrhea, diabetes mellitus, and pancreatic calcification on abdominal imaging. However, these diagnostic criteria are insensitive in the early phase of the disease and are fulfilled only when the pancreas is essentially destroyed. Pain is often the leading symptom in patients with chronic pancreatitis.

The diagnosis of chronic pancreatitis typically involves: (1) recurrent bouts of abdominal pain with or without greater than threefold elevation of amylase and lipase levels, (2) radiological evidence of strictures and dilation of the pancreatic duct and branches with or without calcification, and (3) histological proof of chronic pancreatitis, typically in the form of endoscopic ultrasound (EUS)-guided biopsy.

A number of classification schemes for chronic pancreatitis have been proposed, including the Marseille classification of 1963, the revised Marseille classification of 1984, the Marseille-Rome classification of 1988, the Cambridge classification of 1984, the Zurich classification of 1997, and the Japan Pancreas Society classification of 1997.[7] However, there is no single widely accepted system, and most of these schemes are not helpful in clinical practice. Furthermore, many of them focus on the distinction between acute and chronic pancreatitis and pay little attention to histopathological changes; hence they are of limited interest to the anatomical pathologist. Of note, the composition of the inflammatory infiltrate and the pattern of fibrosis provide clues to the etiology of the disease.

BOX 40.2 Common Causes of Chronic Pancreatitis

Alcohol and tobacco
Paraduodenal pancreatitis
Autoimmune pancreatitis
Tropical pancreatitis
Hereditary pancreatitis
Cystic fibrosis–related pancreatitis

Pathogenesis

Etiological factors include toxic metabolic injuries such as those caused by alcohol abuse, tobacco smoking, hypercalcemia, hyperlipidemia, medications, and other toxins. The most common cause of chronic pancreatitis in developed nations is alcohol ingestion, which accounts for approximately 70% to 95% of cases (Box 40.2).

The pathogenesis of chronic pancreatitis is not well defined, although five mechanisms have been implicated in the development the disease[9]: (1) the necrosis-fibrosis sequence argues that chronic pancreatitis develops through multiple episodes of acute pancreatitis, (2) the sentinel acute pancreatitis event that advocates the chronic pancreatitis is triggered by a single attack of acute pancreatitis, (3) the direct toxic metabolic effect is caused by environmental factors, most typically alcohol and tobacco, (4) free radicals contribute to oxidative stress and the expression of transcription factors and release of cytokines, and (5) ductal dysfunction occurs, leading to protein plugs and ductal obstruction. Pancreatic stellate cells are activated and play a critical role in the development of fibrosis.

Pathological Features

The hallmark of chronic pancreatitis is fibrosis, although in the early stages it may be unevenly distributed. Most surgical specimens show diffuse fibrosis and significant induration.[10-12] The gland may appear enlarged, but in the late phase of the disease the pancreas is shrunken. Cysts of varying sizes are identified both within and outside the pancreas. The extrapancreatic cysts invariably represent pseudocysts; the intrapancreatic cysts are either pseudocysts or retention cysts.[10] Another hallmark of alcoholic chronic pancreatitis is calcification, both within the main pancreatic duct and in the parenchyma. The main pancreatic duct may be obstructed and dilated, although strictures may also be identified. Tapering stenosis of the common bile duct is present in a minority of cases.

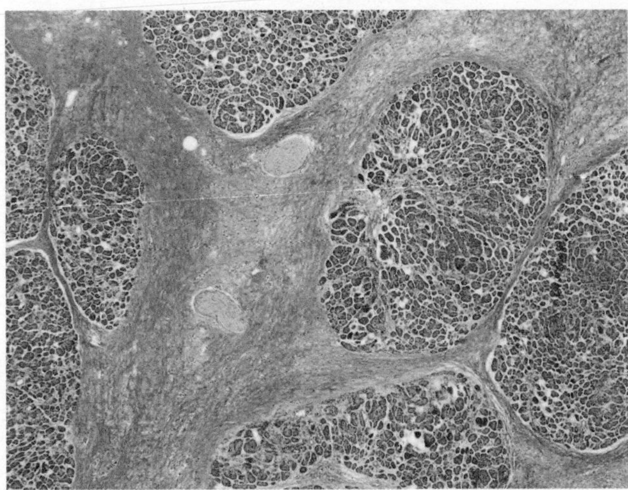

FIGURE 40.3 Alcoholic chronic pancreatitis. Dense interlobular fibrosis with preserved zones of acinar cells between the septa are seen. In comparison with autoimmune pancreatitis, the stroma is relatively acellular and lacks an inflammatory infiltrate.

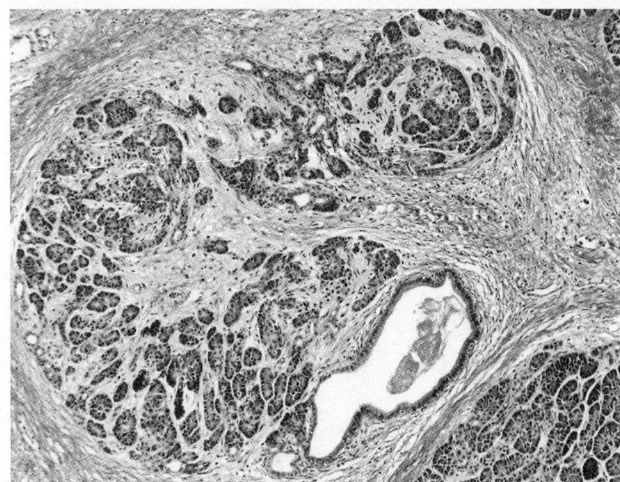

FIGURE 40.4 Alcoholic chronic pancreatitis. The dilated duct is filled with inspissated proteinaceous material. Also notice the presence of interlobular and intralobular fibrosis.

Histologically, alcohol-related pancreatitis exhibits varying degrees of atrophy of the exocrine and endocrine components along with calcification and fibrosis (Fig. 40.3).[10-12] In the late phase of the disease, overt interlobular fibrosis is seen, and intralobular fibrosis is also invariably present. The fibrosis is relatively acellular, but occasional fibroblasts and myofibroblasts are seen. Although much of the acinar component may be depleted, foci of well-preserved acinar tissue are seen interspersed. Some of the pancreatic ducts are dilated; they are filled with proteinaceous material and sometimes calculi (Figs. 40.4 and 40.5).

An inflammatory component is invariably identified, but the degree of inflammation is significantly less than that seen in AIP. Most of the inflammatory cells are small lymphocytes, and lymphoid aggregates are also occasionally present. The inflammatory infiltrate often surrounds peripheral nerve twigs. Plasma cells are usually inconspicuous. In contrast with AIP, periductal lymphocytic accentuation is rarely identified. Intraneural and perineural lymphocytic aggregates are usually prominent. The small lymphocytes are predominantly T cells, although scattered B cells are also present. When neutrophils are identified, they are usually seen adjacent to pseudocysts and residual foci of acute pancreatitis; intraductal aggregates of neutrophils are uncommon.

In the early stages of chronic pancreatitis, the islets of Langerhans are usually normal in appearance. In the late phase, the pancreatic islets may appear remarkably prominent. This apparent prominence of the endocrine component is primarily related to the preferential loss of acinar tissue. It may occasionally be difficult to distinguish this "pseudohypertrophy" of the endocrine component from a pancreatic endocrine microadenoma. Immunohistochemical stains for insulin and glucagon can assist in making this distinction: pseudohypertrophic islets show an intimate admixture of insulin- and glucagon-producing cells, whereas a microadenoma is entirely negative for both markers or may show diffuse reactivity for glucagon. Ductular-insular complexes may be seen, but this is a relatively nonspecific finding. In the very late phase of the disease, there is an appreciable decrease in the endocrine component.

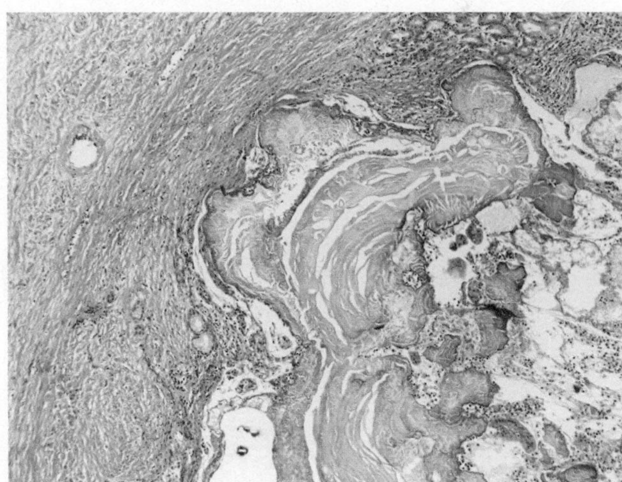

FIGURE 40.5 Alcoholic chronic pancreatitis. An impacted stone is present in a markedly dilated duct.

Lesions of pancreatic intraepithelial neoplasia (PanIN) are frequently identified in resections from patients with chronic pancreatitis. Most of these are low grade (grade 1 and grade 2); PanIN3 lesions are distinctly uncommon. The risk of carcinoma in the setting of chronic pancreatitis is discussed later.

Differential Diagnosis

Chronic Pancreatitis versus Pancreatic Adenocarcinoma

Distinguishing a well-differentiated pancreatic adenocarcinoma from chronic pancreatitis can be one of the most difficult decisions a pathologist encounters.[13] Making this distinction on the basis of a frozen-section or needle biopsy specimen exponentially increases the level of difficulty. Attention to the following four features is key to making the distinction of benign ducts from ductal neoplasia (Table 40.1).

Location of Ducts and Glands. As a general rule, ducts organized in well-circumscribed lobules are benign, whereas atypical ducts scattered in the interlobular septa or suspended within peripancreatic fat are concerning for

TABLE 40.1 Features to Distinguish Chronic Pancreatitis from Well-Differentiated Adenocarcinoma

	Chronic Pancreatitis	Invasive Ductal Adenocarcinoma
Lobular architecture maintained	Yes	No
Nonlobular distribution of glands	No	Yes
Nuclear variation >4:1 within a gland	No	Yes
Nuclear membrane irregularities	No	Yes
Cytoplasm	Frequently dense, eosinophilic	Frequently pale, vacuolated
Perineural invasion	No	Yes
Association of ducts with arteries	No	Yes

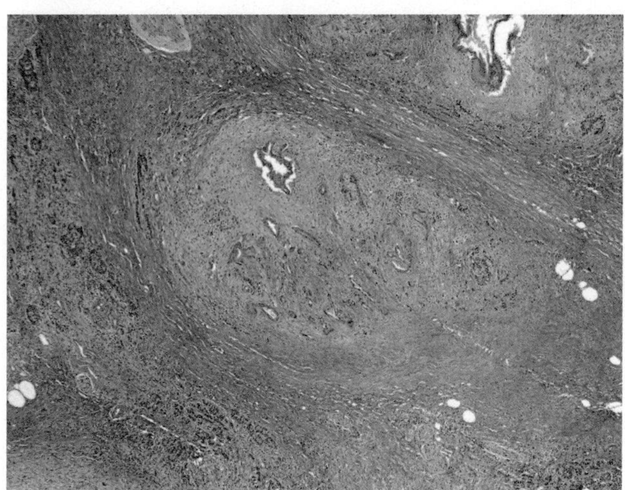

FIGURE 40.6 Chronic pancreatitis. The presence of ductal structures in a lobular configuration virtually rules out the diagnosis of pancreatic adenocarcinoma.

a malignant process (Fig. 40.6). Glands located within lobules, regardless of the degree of atypia, should suggest a "benign" interpretation (Fig. 40.7). Other than an occasional large-caliber duct, ducts within the interlobular septa should be viewed with suspicion. Furthermore, unlike ducts in the liver, those in the pancreas do not accompany arteries, so the presence of a duct adjacent to an artery is highly suspicious for a pancreatic adenocarcinoma.[14] The presence of perineural invasion is diagnostic for carcinoma, although it is important to ensure that the gland is actually infiltrating the perineural space. An additional caveat of significance is that pancreatic islets may be identified adjacent to islets. Vascular invasion is also diagnostic for carcinoma. Of note, veins may be inconspicuous on hematoxylin and eosin stain. An elastic stain greatly increases the sensitivity and specificity for detecting venous invasion.

Desmoplastic Stroma. The desmoplastic reaction, a peculiar mesenchymal proliferation composed of fibroblasts suspended within a basophilic stroma, is an important feature of ductal adenocarcinoma. However, distinguishing desmoplastic stroma from the stroma of chronic pancreatitis can be quite subjective.

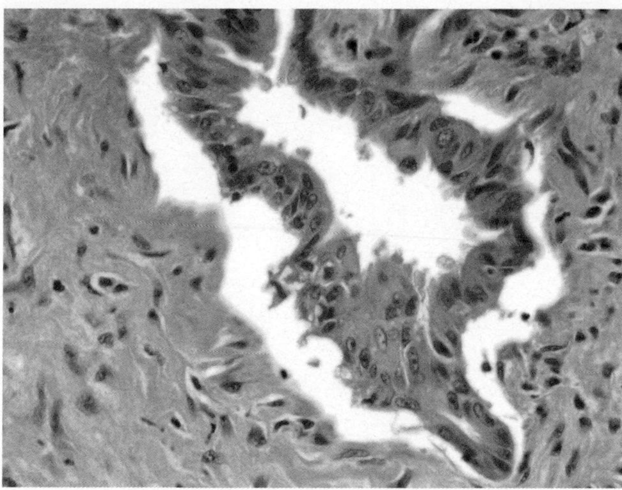

FIGURE 40.7 Chronic pancreatitis with cytological atypia. In isolation, the anisonucleosis and nuclear atypia raise the possibility of a pancreatic adenocarcinoma. However, this duct is located within a lobule (shown in Fig. 40.6), supporting a benign interpretation.

Cytoplasmic Features. The identification of cytoplasmic features is underemphasized in the diagnosis of malignancy. Benign ducts show a dense eosinophilic cytoplasm, whereas many (but not all) adenocarcinomas, especially the well-differentiated carcinomas, show abundant pale cytoplasm, giving the cells a low nucleus-to-cytoplasm (N:C) ratio. A low N:C ratio is a common finding in pancreatic ductal adenocarcinoma.

Nuclear Features. The two most reliable nuclear features of pancreatic ductal adenocarcinoma are markedly irregular nuclear outlines and anisonucleosis (>4:1 variation in nuclear size), the latter within a glandular unit. The variation in nuclear size is appreciable on paraffin and frozen sections, but the nuclear irregularities are less obvious on these preparations. Both features, however, are reliably identified on cytology preparations.

A number of immunohistochemical and molecular markers can help with this distinction, and these are covered in great detail in Chapter 41.

Chronic Alcoholic Pancreatitis versus Autoimmune Pancreatitis

The type 2 variant of AIP is most likely to be confused with alcoholic chronic pancreatitis. The two hallmarks of type 2 AIP (a dense periductal lymphoplasmacytic infiltrate and granulocytic epithelial lesions) are seldom seen in alcoholic chronic pancreatitis. It is important to emphasize that type 2 AIP is not an immunoglobulin G4 (IgG4)-related disease and is not associated with elevated serum or tissue levels of IgG4, although mild elevations may be seen. An immunohistochemical stain for programmed death-ligand 1 (PD-L1), expressed by involved ducts in type 2 AIP, may assist in this distinction (see later in this chapter).[15]

In contrast, distinguishing the type 1 variant of AIP from alcoholic pancreatitis is relatively straightforward. Histologically, virtually all cases of type 1 AIP demonstrate a triumvirate of histological features: (1) a dense and diffuse lymphoplasmacytic infiltrate, unlike the patchy lymphocytic infiltrate of alcoholic pancreatitis; (2) storiform-type

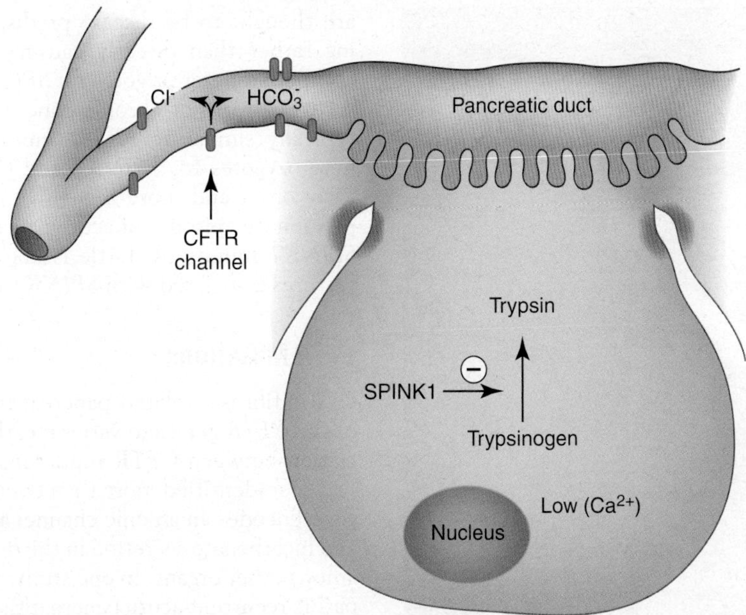

FIGURE 40.8 Mutations in *PRSS1* (trypsinogen gene), *SPINK1*, and *CFTR* (a gene involved in cystic fibrosis) have been implicated in pancreatitis. Activation of trypsinogen to trypsin is a key event in the initiation of pancreatitis and is inhibited by *SPINK1*. Mutations in *CFTR* result in decreased luminal secretion of chloride ion (Cl^-), which ultimately results in reduced surface fluid in the ducts. Ca^{2+}, calcium ion; HCO_3^-, bicarbonate ion. (*Modified from Braganza JM, Lee SH, McCloy RF, et al. Chronic pancreatitis. Lancet. 2011;377:1184-1197.*)

fibrosis, unlike the acellular fibrosis of chronic alcoholic pancreatitis; and (3) obliterative phlebitis. Furthermore, almost all cases of type 1 AIP show greater than 50 IgG4-positive plasma cells per high-power field (HPF). However, difficulties arise when interpreting needle biopsy specimens. Patchy involvement of the pancreas is common, and some biopsies may not demonstrate the full spectrum of histological findings. In such cases, correlation with clinical and radiological features as well as serum IgG4 levels is required.

Risk of Cancer

Chronic pancreatitis has consistently been shown to be a risk factor for pancreatic cancer. One of the concerns with many studies evaluating the association between chronic pancreatitis and pancreatic carcinoma is the potential for misdiagnosis of pancreatic cancer as chronic pancreatitis, which inflates the risk of malignancy. However, even after excluding cancer within in the first 2 years following the diagnosis of chronic pancreatitis, the risk of pancreatic cancer is elevated 16-fold. Notably, the risk declines over time, but is still eightfold increased when the analysis is limited to cases that are greater than 5 years from the diagnosis of chronic pancreatitis.[16] In comparison with chronic alcoholic pancreatitis, hereditary pancreatitis carries a far higher risk of pancreatic cancer (approximately 35% during a lifetime).

Therapy

The goals of treatment are to relieve pain, prevent recurrent attacks of acute pancreatitis, and manage the metabolic consequences such as maldigestion and diabetes. Surgery or endoscopic intervention is required to relieve intractable pain or to address specific complications such as pseudocysts. The objective of surgery (pancreatojejunostomy) is to decompress the pancreatic duct (which relieves pain) and to preserve as much of the pancreas as possible (to preserve pancreatic islets).

GENETICS OF RECURRENT ACUTE AND CHRONIC PANCREATITIS

There is growing evidence that a significant proportion of patients with apparently idiopathic recurrent acute or chronic pancreatitis have underlying genetic abnormalities. Among the genes that predispose an individual to chronic pancreatitis, three are associated with defects in the activation of trypsinogen: *PRSS1*, *SPINK1*, and chymotrypsin C *(CTRC)*.[17-21] This is not surprising because one of the fundamental events in the development of pancreatitis is the activation of trypsinogen to trypsin (Fig. 40.8). Trypsin is associated with some unique enzymatic features because it can both self-activate and deactivate itself. The mutations in *PRSS1* that are associated with the development of chronic pancreatitis either cause premature activation of this enzyme or abrogate the inactivation.[21] The most common mutation in *PRSS1*, R122H, abrogates the ability of trypsin to inactivate itself and also enhances trypsinogen autoactivation. The *SPINK1* gene encodes for a trypsin inhibitor, and loss-of-function mutations of this gene abrogate the ability of the protein to inhibit activation of trypsin.[19] Other genes implicated in chronic pancreatitis are calcium-sensing receptor, such as calcium-sensing receptor *(CASR)*, Claudin-2 *(CLDN2)*, *CTRC*,[20] and *CFTR*.[22] The *PRSS1* gene carries an 80% penetrance, while that for most other genes is less than 1%. It should be noted that in many cases, hereditary pancreatitis is a complex multigene and a multifactorial disease, one that includes gene-environment interactions and interactions among various pathogenic gene variants.

With rapid advances in technology, it is relatively easy to identify mutations in genes that contribute to the development of pancreatitis. Although mutations in each of these genes have unequivocally been linked to pancreatitis, many

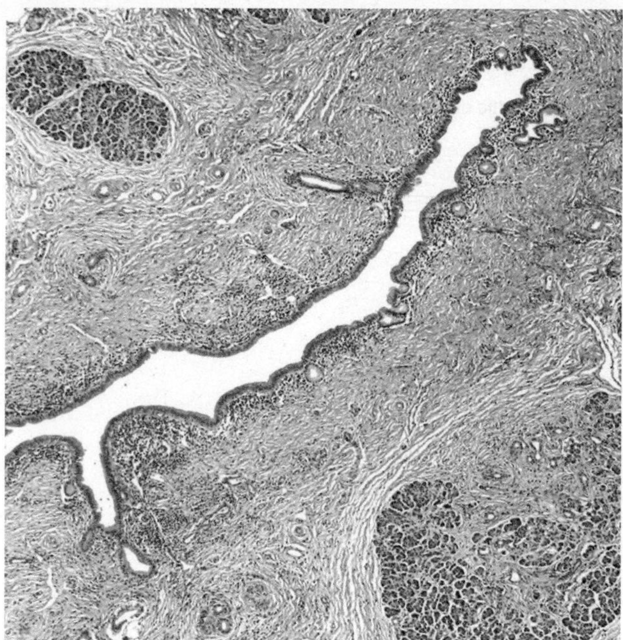

FIGURE 40.9 Chronic pancreatitis. This pancreas was resected from a 25-year-old male patient with a cationic trypsinogen mutation. Note the periductal inflammation.

of the mutations are disease-neutral, and some could even be protective. Furthermore, the penetrance is extremely low—in some cases, less than 1%. Therefore the interpretation of these genetic tests is complex. With some exceptions (discussed later), testing for mutations in unselected patients with suspected pancreatitis is not recommended.[18]

Current guidelines, based largely on expert consensus reviews, recommend the use of genetic testing in the following individuals: (1) recurrent acute pancreatitis or chronic pancreatitis of uncertain cause, (2) idiopathic chronic pancreatitis in individuals younger than 25 years of age, (3) family history of idiopathic chronic pancreatitis, or recurrent acute pancreatitis, and (4) at-risk family members of individuals with a positive pathogenic mutation.

Trypsinogen Mutations

Since the discovery of the *PRSS1* gene, more than 20 mutations have been identified (Fig. 40.9). The clinical relevance of the R122H mutation is supported by data from a transgenic model.[23] Gain-of-function mutations, especially R122H and N29I, show a high penetrance (80%). This, coupled with the increased risk of pancreatic cancer (35-fold), supports the use of diagnostic testing for these mutations in young patients with acute or chronic pancreatitis.[18]

SPINK1 Mutations

The enzyme protects the pancreas against premature trypsinogen activation. The most common *SPINK1* mutation, N34S, has a high frequency (approximately 2%) in the general population and is associated with a very low disease penetrance.[19] Less than 1% of heterozygous *SPINK1* carriers develop chronic pancreatitis in the absence of other contributory factors. Consequently, *SPINK1* mutations are thought to be disease predisposing or disease modifying rather than directly causing disease. Homozygous or compound heterozygotes for *SPINK1* leads to an autosomal recessive form of chronic pancreatitis that may be phenotypically similar to *PRSS1* mutation carriers. Compound heterozygotes for *SPINK1* and *CFTR* are associated with early onset and more aggressive pancreatitis. Alcohol may precipitate episodes of acute pancreatitis in individuals with *SPINK1* mutations. Little is known about the histological features associated with *SPINK1* mutations.

CFTR Mutations

Cystic fibrosis–related pancreatitis is caused by alterations of the *CFTR* gene and varies greatly in its severity. The association between *CFTR* mutations and chronic pancreatitis was first identified more than two decades ago.[22] The *CFTR* gene encodes an anionic channel and is involved in chloride and bicarbonate secretion in the ductal cells of the pancreas, among other organs. In one study, 43% of patients with idiopathic recurrent acute pancreatitis and 11% of patients with chronic pancreatitis carried *CFTR* mutations in one or both genes.[17] F508 mutations account for approximately 40% of *CFTR* variants in patients with hereditary pancreatitis.

Although chronic pancreatitis develops in a substantial majority of patients with cystic fibrosis, a small but distinct group of mutations is associated with isolated involvement of the pancreas (i.e., without pulmonary and other typical manifestations). The mutations seen in this setting are distinct from those associated with cystic fibrosis, and the patients typically do not show other clinical features of cystic fibrosis. Furthermore, their sweat chloride levels are normal.[8,17,22] Unlike patients with cystic fibrosis, these patients are diagnosed in adulthood.

Morphologically, in addition to fibrosis, patients with *CFTR* genetic alterations show ductal protein plugs.

Hereditary Pancreatitis

Clinical Features

This is an uncommon cause of chronic pancreatitis, accounting for fewer than 2% of all cases. Hereditary pancreatitis is an autosomal dominant disease that typically manifests with recurrent attacks of acute pancreatitis in childhood, typically in the first and second decades of life.[21] A diagnosis of hereditary pancreatitis should be suspected in any individual in whom chronic pancreatitis develops at an early age (<25 years). The disease affects men and women equally.

In 80% of cases, hereditary pancreatitis is caused by a gain-of-function mutation in the *PRSS1* gene (see earlier discussion). Although 20 mutations have been identified, the 2 most common mutations are *R122H* and *N29I*. The penetrance of these mutations is high, and approximately one-half of these patients progress to chronic pancreatitis. The estimated cumulative risk of pancreatic cancer to 70 years of age in patients with hereditary pancreatitis approaches 40%.[24-26] The type of genetic mutation does not correlate with the risk of cancer.[24]

Pathological Features

The disease is characterized by fatty replacement of the pancreas.[27] Fibrosis, typically mild, is significantly less than that seen in alcohol-related chronic pancreatitis. Periductal inflammation may be observed. In older patients, PanIN is often seen.

PANCREATIC DIVISUM

During development, the dorsal and ventral pancreatic ducts fuse, with the major pancreatic drainage occurring through the duct of Wirsung (the ventral duct), with little or no drainage through the duct of Santorini (the dorsal duct). In about 10% of the population, the duct of Santorini and duct of Wirsung fail to fuse, a condition referred to as *pancreatic divisum.*[28]

Three forms of pancreatic divisum are recognized: (1) type 1 or classic pancreatic divisum, characterized by complete absence of communication between the ducts of Wirsung and Santorini (70% of cases); (2) type 2 (25% of cases), defined by the complete absence of the duct of Wirsung, with the entire drainage occurring through the duct of Santorini and the minor papilla; and (3) type 3 (5% of cases), characterized by a narrow and inadequate communication between the ventral and dorsal pancreatic ducts.[29]

Most individuals with pancreatic divisum are asymptomatic, and pancreatitis develops in only a minority of patients. The disease manifests primarily in adults, and both sexes are affected. Pancreatic disease in the form of acute or chronic pancreatitis is in part caused by inadequate pancreatic drainage through a narrow dorsal pancreatic duct. Endoscopic retrograde cholangiopancreatography (ERCP) often reveals a short ventral duct and a main pancreatic duct that communicates with the dorsal duct and drains into the duodenum near the minor papilla.

One of the most controversial aspects of this disease is the difficulty in demonstrating a causal relationship between pancreatitis and this anatomical variation of the ductal system. There is increasing evidence to suggest that pancreatic divisum alone is insufficient to precipitate pancreatitis.[30] Some studies have shown no difference in the prevalence of pancreatic divisum between patients with idiopathic pancreatitis and a control population, 5% and 7%, respectively.[31] However, this group of authors also found that the prevalence of pancreatic divisum in patients with pancreatitis and mutations in *CFTR*, *SPINK1*, or *PRSS1* was 47%, 16%, and 16%, respectively.[31] Therefore only a small proportion of patients with pancreatic divisum would benefit from decompression of the dorsal pancreatic duct, a procedure that can be performed endoscopically. Histologically, the pancreas may show features similar to obstructive chronic pancreatitis.

AUTOIMMUNE PANCREATITIS

Definition and Historical Aspects

AIP is a mass-forming inflammatory lesion of the pancreas that may mimic pancreatic carcinoma.[32-34] It is only in the past two decades that this disease has received the attention it richly deserves. Previously, these cases were diagnosed nonspecifically as chronic pancreatitis. In retrospect, approximately 25% of pancreatic resections that lack histological evidence of malignancy may represent AIP.[35]

AIP was first described by Sarles and colleagues in the 1960s.[36] They described four cases of chronic pancreatitis in patients presenting with steatorrhea and obstructive jaundice. Histologically, the pancreas showed a dense lymphoplasmacytic infiltrate. Although the histological description was brief, it is likely that these cases represented AIP. Little progress was made in the subsequent 3 decades, although there were similar sporadic case reports in the literature. Kawaguchi and coworkers are credited with the first modern histopathological description of type 1 AIP.[37] They described two men with obstructive jaundice and histological features that are now considered typical for AIP.[37] The term *autoimmune pancreatitis* was coined by Yoshida and colleagues in a case report in 1995, and this term is now the preferred designation for this disease.[38,39]

A major milestone in understanding of this disease came with the apparently serendipitous discovery of its association with elevated levels of serum IgG4.[40] Shortly thereafter, it was established that the inflamed pancreas shows a substantial increase in IgG4-positive plasma cells.[41-44] It was subsequently realized that a sizeable number of patients with AIP also exhibit either synchronous or metachronous fibroinflammatory mass lesions in other organs, including the liver and biliary tract.[43,45] This multifocal systemic fibroinflammatory disease is now termed IgG4-related disease.[33] Notably, AIP is only one manifestation of IgG4-related disease, and in an attempt to highlight this relationship, some authorities advocate use of the term *IgG4-related pancreatitis.*[38]

Subtypes

AIP is not a homogenous entity because the disease can be clearly segregated into two distinct clinicopathological subtypes: AIP type 1 and AIP type 2.[33,46-51] Type 1 AIP is the pancreatic manifestation of IgG4-related disease, whereas the type 2 variant is a distinct and non–IgG4-related disease. Although there is some overlap in the clinical and radiological aspects of these two variants (see later discussion), the two entities are biologically distinct, and some authors prefer to use the term *idiopathic duct-centric pancreatitis* when referring to type 2 AIP in an attempt to draw a clear distinction between the diseases.[33,46-50,52]

Clinical Features

AIP is an uncommon disorder. A recent nationwide survey in Japan identified an overall prevalence rate of 45.1 cases per 100,000 patients, with a threefold increase in the number of cases during a decade.[53] Although no data are available from North America, it is important to emphasize the fact that this disease is significantly less common than pancreatic carcinoma.

Both the gender ratio and the mean age at presentation vary according to the histological subtype. Patients with type 1 AIP tend to be older (in their seventies) than patients with the type 2 variant (in their fifties).[32,34,41,46,47,50,52-54] Most patients with type 1 AIP are male, whereas the gender ratio for type 2 AIP is approximately 1:1. There is considerable overlap between the demographic and clinical features of alcoholic chronic pancreatitis and those of the type 2 variant of AIP, although the former entity tends to be more common in men.

BOX 40.3 Solid Nonneoplastic Lesions That Mimic Primary Pancreatic and Ampullary Malignancies

Autoimmune pancreatitis, type 1 and type 2
Paraduodenal pancreatitis
Alcoholic pancreatitis (extremely uncommon mimic of carcinoma)
Lipomatous pseudohypertrophy
Adenomyomatous hyperplasia of the Vaterian system
Intrapancreatic spleen
Pancreatic hamartoma
Infectious pancreatitis-tuberculosis
Sarcoidosis

There appear to be geographic variations in the incidence of the two subtypes: the type 2 variant is relatively uncommon in Asia but constitutes almost one-half of all patients of AIP in series from Europe and North America.[46,52,55]

Obstructive jaundice and weight loss are characteristic features of type 1 AIP.[46-48,50,52,54,56,57] These symptoms, along with a mass on imaging, make the clinical distinction of this disease from pancreatic ductal adenocarcinoma extremely problematic. Other nonneoplastic pancreatic lesions that mimic pancreatic cancer are listed in Box 40.3. Other presenting symptoms of patients with type 1 AIP include fatigue and recent onset of diabetes mellitus. Some patients may complain of vague abdominal pain. Patients with type 1 AIP may have other manifestations of IgG4-related disease, either synchronously or metachronously, and the involvement of these organs represents one of the most valuable clues to the diagnosis of this inflammatory pancreatic disease.[46-48,50,52,54,56,57] One of the more common extra-pancreatic manifestations of type 1 AIP is a painless unilateral and, more often, bilateral swelling of the submandibular salivary gland. In fact, in an individual with painless obstructive jaundice, bilateral enlargement of the submandibular salivary glands is strongly suggestive of IgG4-related disease (AIP).[58] Other sites commonly involved by IgG4-related disease include the biliary system, lung, kidney, and retroperitoneum.

Patients with type 2 AIP often present with abdominal pain, although the pain is rarely severe enough to suggest acute pancreatitis.[46-48,51,53,54,56,57] In comparison with type 1 disease, a smaller proportion of patients with type 2 AIP have obstructive jaundice at presentation. The disease is confined to the pancreas, and extrapancreatic involvement is type 2 AIP.

Although AIP is an uncommon cause for either acute or chronic pancreatitis, more than 33% of patients with this disease have symptoms that mimic other forms of acute or chronic pancreatitis.[56]

Serum Markers

Type 1 Autoimmune Pancreatitis

Elevated serum IgG4 is the most robust biomarker for this disease.[40,59] Elevated serum IgG4 is fairly sensitive (80%) for type 1 AIP, but its specificity, particularly in an unselected population, is low.[34,48,59] In one survey, only 10% of patients with elevated levels of serum IgG4 had evidence of IgG4-related disease.[60] An even more worrisome observation is that approximately 10% of patients with pancreatic cancer show elevated levels of serum IgG4. Further compounding this challenge is that the pretest probability of AIP is relatively low. Nevertheless, in general, the higher the serum IgG4, the more likely the patient has type 1 AIP. Thus specificity of this test is improved when the threshold is set at 280 mg/dL (two times normal).

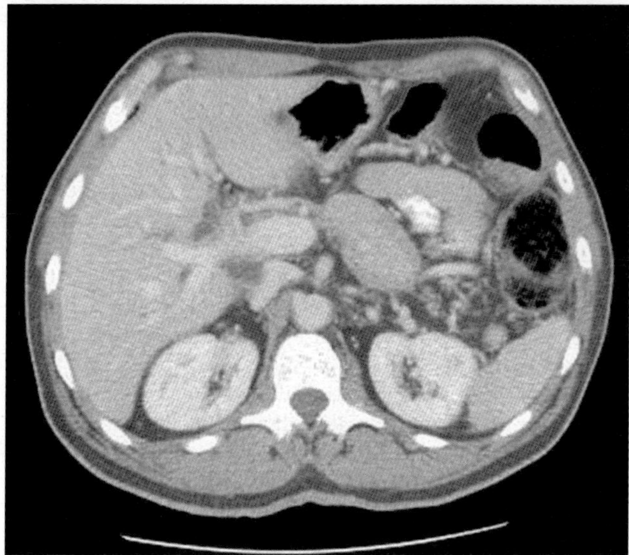

FIGURE 40.10 CT image from a patient with autoimmune pancreatitis. Note the enlarged, "sausage-shaped" pancreas and the presence of a "halo," also known as *Saran wrap sign,* around the pancreas.

Many other serological immunological abnormalities are identified in patients with AIP. These include positive antinuclear antibody, rheumatoid factor, and elevated gamma globulin levels. A variety of other antibodies have been identified, including antilactoferrin and anti–carbonic anhydrase antibodies, although these are not specific and are not used in clinical practice.[32,61]

An autoantibody against a plasminogen-binding protein peptide, originally reported to be a highly specific and sensitive test for AIP, has been refuted by recent studies.[61,62]

Type 2 Autoimmune Pancreatitis

Patients with type 2 AIP only rarely show elevated levels of serum IgG4, and there is currently no reliable biomarker for the recognition of this variant.[49]

Radiology

During the past decade, radiologists have greatly improved their ability to identify AIP and distinguish it from pancreatic carcinoma.

On imaging, three patterns of AIP are recognized: diffuse, focal, and multifocal.[63-65] The diffuse form of the disease (Fig. 40.10) is the most common type; the pancreas appears enlarged and "sausage shaped." Among these patterns, the focal form of disease is most likely to be confused with pancreatic carcinoma.

The affected regions of the pancreas are hypoechoic on ultrasonography and hypointense on CT. On contrast-enhanced CT, there is decreased enhancement of the mass in the arterial phase and delayed enhancement in the late phase.[63,65] A small, hypodense rim is often identified around

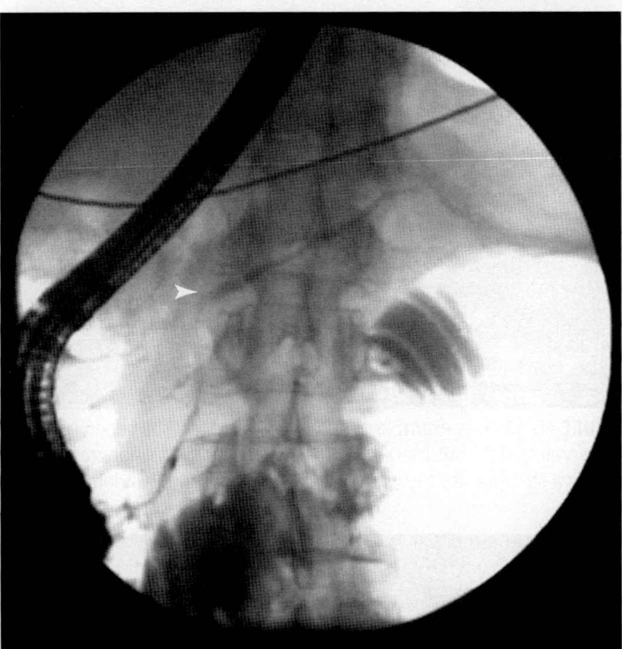

FIGURE 40.11 A pancreatogram from a patient with autoimmune pancreatitis. The pancreatic duct *(arrow)* is narrow and irregular.

the lesion—the so-called *halo sign*. On MRI, the pancreas is diffusely hypointense on T1-weighted images and slightly hyperintense on T2-weighted images. The main pancreatic duct is usually narrow, and upstream dilation of the pancreatic duct should raise concern for pancreatic carcinoma. Both the bile duct and the pancreatic duct may be narrowed (double duct sign), a feature that is otherwise suggestive of pancreatic carcinoma.

An irregularly narrowed main pancreatic duct is very characteristic of AIP (Fig. 40.11). On ERCP, the following four features help distinguish AIP from pancreatic adenocarcinoma: (1) a long stricture involving more than one-third of the main pancreatic duct, (2) lack of upstream dilation, (3) side branches arising from a strictured segment, and (4) the presence of multiple strictures involving the main pancreatic duct.[66] The presence of all four features is highly specific but only moderately sensitive for AIP.[66] Although the Japanese and Korean diagnostic criteria are highly dependent on pancreatography, those published from the United States do not require imaging of the pancreatic duct.[67-69]

Within 1 to 2 weeks of initiation of steroid therapy, there is a dramatic shrinkage of the mass with partial to complete normalization of the main pancreatic duct, a finding that helps reaffirm the diagnosis of AIP. In the late phase of this disease, the pancreas appears shrunken and atrophic.

Type 1 Autoimmune Pancreatitis

Etiology

The exposure of genetically susceptible individuals to environmental or intrinsic risk factors triggering a stereotypical orchestral immune reaction represents a likely pathogenetic mechanism for type 1 AIP. It is notable that unlike classic autoimmune diseases, type 1 AIP affects elderly men.

Genetic Risk Factors

The strongest genetic risk relates to human leukocyte antigen (HLA),[70] with minor associations involving polymorphisms of immune-related genes (e.g., *CTLA4, FCRL3*).[71,72] The genetic susceptibility factors that have been identified in the Japanese population include the HLA serotypes *DRB1*0405* and *DQB1*0401*.[70]

Role of T Cells

T cells play a prominent role in IgG4-related disease. [73] Although B cells and IgG4-positive plasma cells are often emphasized, the T cell is the dominant cell type in IgG4-related disease. Early observations suggested that T cells in type 1 AIP show a Th2 bias.[74] In theory, Th2 cytokines such as IL-4, IL-5, and IL-13 could account for tissue and/or serum eosinophilia and elevated serum IgE levels, characteristic findings in patients with type 1 AIP.[48] However, recent evidence suggests that the Th1 reaction is not fully suppressed and occasional T cells express IFN-γ, the latter a defining feature of Th1 bias.[74,75] Unlike classic autoimmune diseases in which regulatory immune pathways are suppressed, AIP shows an increased proportion of regulatory T cells (Tregs), both within tissue and peripheral blood.[74,76] IL-10 produced by Tregs may guide IgG4 class-switching.[77] Recent studies have also implicated oligoclonal CD4+ cytotoxic T cells that secrete of IFN-γ, IL-1β, and TGF-β.[78]

Recent studies on IgG4-related sialodacryoadenitis support a role for Tfh cells in IgG4-related disease.[79] Tfh cells, a distinct subset of CD4+ T-helper cells, are involved in germinal center formation, B-cell differentiation, and antibody maturation;[78] these processes are partly mediated by IL-4 and IL-21 produced by Tfh cells. Circulating Tfh2 cells are preferentially expanded in IgG4-related disease with their quantities positively correlating with the number of affected organs, disease activity scores, and serum IgG4 levels.[79]

B Cell in IgG4-Related Disease

The role of B cells in the pathogenesis of type 1 AIP is highlighted by the observation that rituximab, a B-cell–depletion therapy, is effective for type 1 AIP.[80] The expanded plasmablast population in patients with IgG4-related disease decreased on treatment.[78,81,82] Plasmablast represents precursors of plasma cells. An analysis of the plasmablast B-cell receptor repertoire also noted the oligoclonal nature of this expansion.[78,81-83] Interestingly, the dominant clones vary between patients, and novel clones emerge on relapse.[78,81,82]

Serum IgG4 and IgG4 Plasma Cells

IgG4 is generally regarded as a noninflammatory antibody because of its relative inability to fix complement and its limited capacity to bind Fc receptors.[84-86] A conformational change accounts for its antiinflammatory nature, the so-called *Fab-arm exchange*, wherein a pair of heavy and light chains are exchanged between two IgG4 antibody molecules.[87] As a result of the unusual structural alteration, the antibody loses its ability to cross-link antigens and form large immune complexes. Collectively, IgG4 may be secondarily induced in type 1 AIP, and may represent an attempt to dampen excess inflammatory reaction. A recent murine model lends credence to this hypothesis.[88]

Autoantibodies in IgG4-Related Disease

Autoantibodies are detected in ~40% of patients.[73,89] These antibodies recognize pancreatic enzymes or secretory proteins (antilactoferrin and anti–carbonic anhydrase II) and are considered nonspecific and nondrivers of the disease.[73,89] A recent study identified an autoantibody against laminin 511-E8; laminin is an extracellular matrix protein, and the antibody is against a truncated form of laminin 511. Anti–laminin 511-E8 IgG was identified in 26 of 51 AIP patients (51.0%), but in only 2 of 122 controls (1.6%).[90] Annexin A11 is another potential novel autoantigen in IgG4-related disease. Annexin A11 is targeted by both IgG4 and IgG1 antibodies in patients with IgG4-related disease.[91]

Extrinsic Factors

Homology has been demonstrated between the plasminogen-binding protein of *Helicobacter pylori* and the ubiquitin-protein ligase E3 component n-recognin, a protein expressed in pancreatic acinar cells,[62] raising the possibility that a protein mimicry may incite the production of autoantibodies. The same study identified an anti–plasminogen binding protein antibody in the serum of patients with AIP.[62] Other hypotheses include chronic exposure to chemicals or microbes, allergic reactions, and paraneoplastic syndrome.[62,92]

Pathology

Gross Evaluation

The disease can involve any part of the pancreas. In the active phase, the pancreas is enlarged, but in the late phases of the disease, the pancreas may appear shrunken and fibrotic. On gross evaluation, the pancreas is generally bulky and feels firm to hard, although serial sections usually fail to identify a distinct tumor (Fig. 40.12). Occasionally, a distinct mass is identified, in which case the gross appearance is indistinguishable from a pancreatic neoplasm (Fig. 40.13). The main pancreatic duct is typically narrow, and dilation of the main pancreatic duct is uncommon. Stigmata of alcoholic pancreatitis, such as pseudocysts and calcification, are uncommon as well, although their presence does not exclude the diagnosis of AIP.

Although the principal changes in type 1 and type 2 AIP are fibrosis and inflammation, the pattern of fibrosis and the type and degree of inflammation are so markedly different that they are discussed separately here.

Microscopic Evaluation

Type 1 AIP. Histologically, the type 1 variant of AIP is a prototypical IgG4-related disease that is characterized by a triumvirate of histological features: dense lymphoplasmacytic infiltrate, storiform-type fibrosis (Figs. 40.14 and 40.15), and obliterative phlebitis (Figs. 40.15 and 40.16).[11,37,41,42,44,46,51,55,93-97]

Although in some areas the fibrosis is organized in a patternless pattern, careful evaluation invariably reveals storiform-type fibrosis (see Figs. 40.14 and 40.15). The fibroinflammatory infiltrate also extends into the peripancreatic adipose tissue. The collagen in the zones of fibrosis is accompanied by benign-appearing spindle-shaped cells, representing either fibroblasts or myofibroblasts.

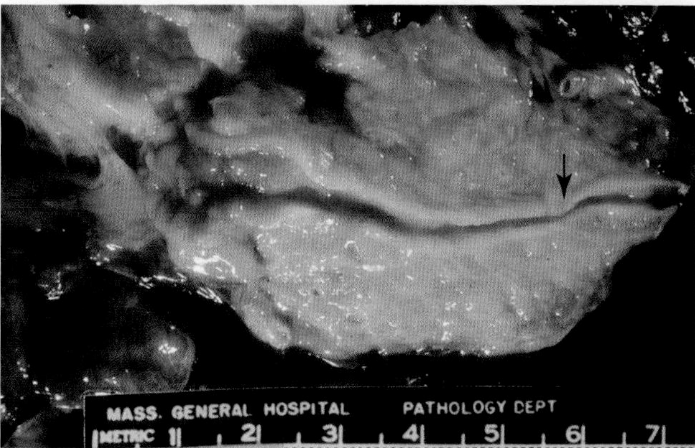

FIGURE 40.12 This example of autoimmune pancreatitis does not show a discrete mass, but marked fibrosis is present. The pancreatic duct shows a stricture *(arrow)* with mild dilation distal to the stricture.

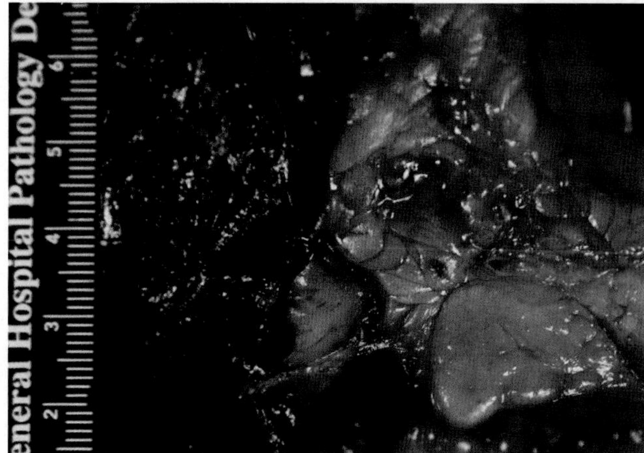

FIGURE 40.13 Autoimmune pancreatitis. Gross image of a distal pancreatectomy specimen shows a discrete mass in the distal end of the pancreas. The preoperative diagnosis was a neuroendocrine tumor.

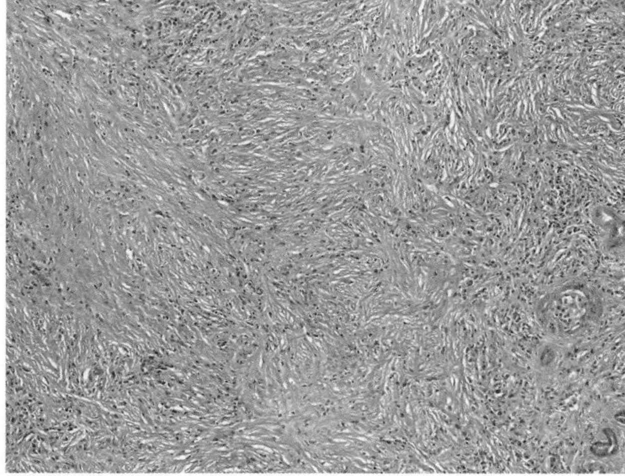

FIGURE 40.14 Type 1 autoimmune pancreatitis shows storiform-type fibrosis.

The disease is characterized by a dense and diffuse lymphoplasmacytic infiltrate, one rich in IgG4-positive cells. Absence of IgG4-positive cells is generally considered incompatible with a diagnosis of type 1 AIP, although bonefide examples of type 1 AIP have been reported.[98] Although

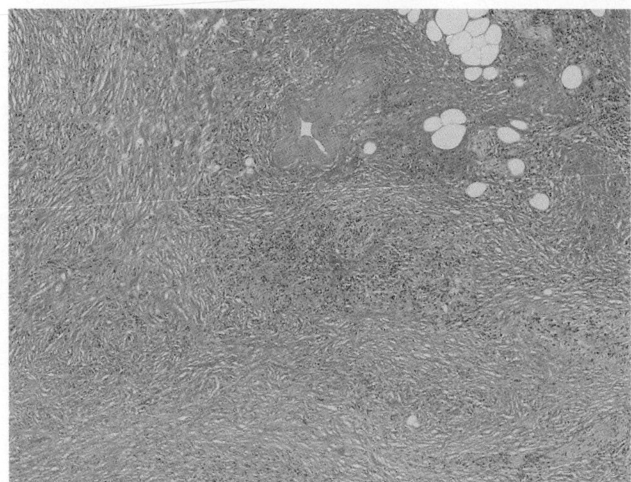

FIGURE 40.15 Type 1 autoimmune pancreatitis shows storiform-type fibrosis. Also note the focus of obliterative phlebitis. The obliterative phlebitis could easily be overlooked; however, the adjacent arterial channel provides a clue to its presence.

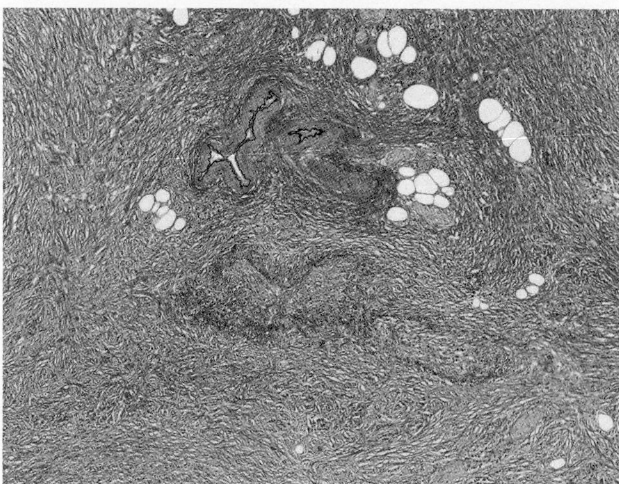

FIGURE 40.16 The obliterative phlebitis depicted in Fig. 40.15 is highlighted on an elastic stain.

counterintuitive, it should be recalled that IgG4 does not appear to be the primary driver behind the disease. Eosinophils are identified in virtually every case, with occasional cases showing a marked infiltrate, sufficient to raise the possibility of "eosinophilic pancreatitis."

Obliterative phlebitis is readily identified, but the vein may be camouflaged by the dense and diffuse inflammatory infiltrate. It is often difficult to identify totally obliterated veins, and an elastic stain may help uncover these venous channels (see Figs. 40.15 and 40.16). However, an elastic stain is not mandatory: medium-sized venous channels are usually accompanied by arteries, which are less likely to be affected by the inflammatory process, and can therefore serve as guideposts for identification of the veins. A less widely acknowledged feature of type 1 AIP is obliterative arteritis. As in obliterative phlebitis, the lumen and the wall of the vascular channel are infiltrated by lymphocytes and plasma cells. The presence of necrotizing inflammation involving either the vein or the arteries virtually excludes the diagnosis of AIP.

The ductal epithelium is typically preserved and often adopts a star-shaped profile (Fig. 40.17). Notably, the ducts are not associated with neutrophils, and erosion and ulceration of the duct-lining epithelium are distinctly uncommon. Although the inflammatory cells tend to aggregate around ducts, this periductal infiltrate is seldom as prominent as in the type 2 variant of the disease. The intrapancreatic portion of the bile duct is typically involved, and the IgG4-rich plasma cell infiltrate involves the full thickness of the bile duct (Fig. 40.18).

Long-standing examples of AIP exhibit extensive atrophy of the exocrine component, although the endocrine component is usually preserved, at least in the initial phases of the disease.

After steroid therapy, there is a rapid depletion of the inflammatory component, leaving behind only a sparse lymphoplasmacytic infiltrate, and IgG4-bearing plasma cells typically are not identified. Such cases do not fulfill the minimum diagnostic criteria for AIP. Nonetheless, a storiform pattern of fibrosis may be recognizable and may provide the only clue to the existence of AIP in the specimen.

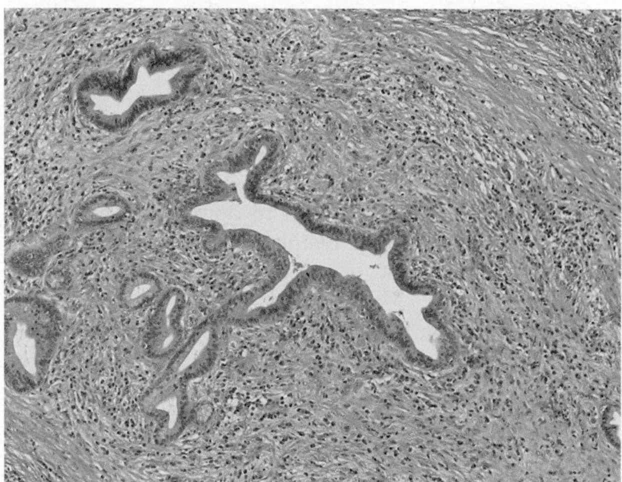

FIGURE 40.17 Type 1 autoimmune pancreatitis. The ductal epithelium is preserved, and the duct shows a star-shaped profile.

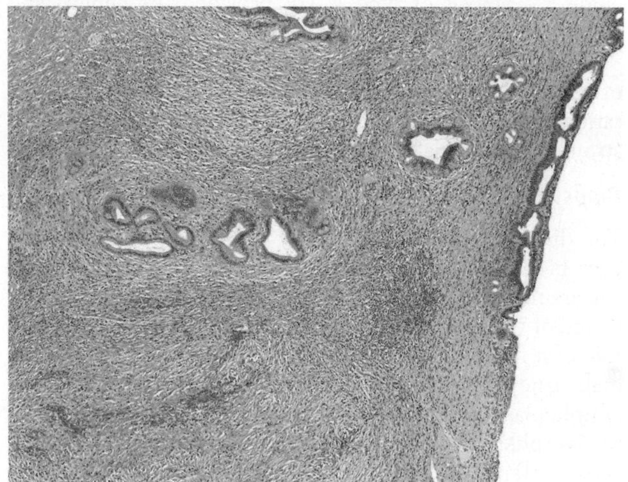

FIGURE 40.18 Type 1 autoimmune pancreatitis involving the intrapancreatic portion of the bile duct. Note the fibroinflammatory infiltrate involves the full thickness of the bile duct.

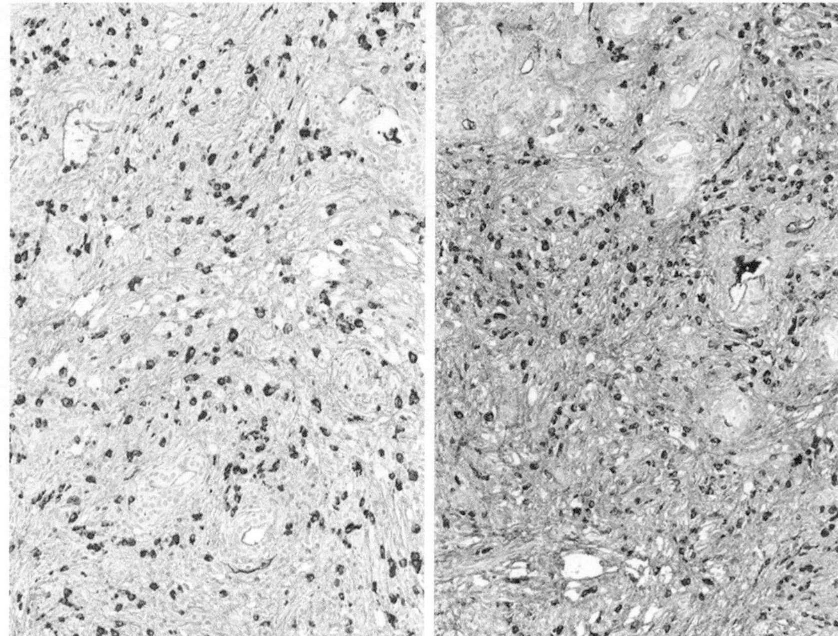

FIGURE 40.19 Type 1 autoimmune pancreatitis invariably shows a diffuse infiltrate of immunoglobulin 4 (IgG4)-positive plasma cells, as seen here with IgG4 immunostain (*left*). The IgG4-to-IgG ratio is >40%.

Immunohistochemistry

Both variants of AIP show an admixture of B cells and T cells, although the T cells tend to dominate. The B cells are typically organized as lymphoid aggregates. By definition, both the lymphocyte and the plasma cell populations are polyclonal.

Virtually every case of type 1 AIP shows a markedly elevated number of IgG4-positive plasma cells (Fig. 40.19),[41,44,46,96,99] with a minimum requirement of 50 IgG4-positive plasma cells per HPF on a resection specimen and 10 cells per HPF on a biopsy sample.[49,100] Typically, the IgG4-positive plasma cells are diffusely distributed, although focal accentuations around venous channels and ducts may be appreciable. Although documentation of IgG4-bearing cells is an important component of the diagnostic algorithm, the paucity of such cells should not preclude a diagnosis of type 1 AIP, provided the clinical and histological features support the diagnosis.

The consensus document on the histological diagnosis of IgG4-related disease emphasizes the importance of the ratio of IgG4 to total IgG, with a ratio of greater than 40% strongly supporting the diagnosis of type 1 AIP.[100]

Biopsy Diagnosis

The diagnosis of AIP is generally based on an EUS-guided core biopsy. Although the cellular material on cytological smears may suggest a diagnosis of type 1 AIP, the findings, in and of themselves, are seldom diagnostic.[101] The primary role of a fine-needle aspiration (FNA) biopsy is to rule out malignancy. The diagnosis requires the presence of a dense lymphoplasmacytic infiltrate, storiform type fibrosis, obliterative phlebitis, and increased numbers of IgG4-positive cells (>10 per HPF on a biopsy). However, classic storiform type fibrosis may not be observed on a biopsy, and obliterative phlebitis is typically absent (Figs. 40.20 to 40.22). An elastic stain may assist in uncovering obliterated veins.

Given the inherently patchy nature of the disease, a biopsy may prove nondiagnostic. It should be noted that the current diagnostic algorithms do not mandate a biopsy, and the presence of the following features may obviate the need of tissue: (1) imaging findings supportive of AIP, (2) elevated serum IgG4, and (3) involvement of organs typically affected by IgG4-related disease. In selected circumstances, a trial of steroid is utilized as a diagnostic measure: a rapid clinical and radiological response is indicative of AIP.

Type 2 Autoimmune Pancreatitis

Pathogenesis

The immunological aspects of type 2 AIP are largely unknown. In this context, it is notable that up to one-third of patients report inflammatory bowel disease, particularly ulcerative colitis.[34] Unlike type 1 AIP, cytokine expression in pancreatic tissue samples from patients with type 2 AIP revealed almost undetectable levels of IL-4, IL-10, and TNFA mRNA; however, higher expression of IL-8 mRNA is observed in type 2 AIP, 13-fold higher than type 1 disease.[102] Notably, IL-8 is a known chemotactic factor for neutrophils. The ductal epithelium from patients with type 2 AIP express PD-L1 and IDO1, checkpoint proteins, a finding generally not observed in mimics of the disease, including type 1 AIP. Expression of these checkpoint proteins may represent a defense mechanism that limits tissue destruction in type 2 AIP.[15]

Pathology

Histologically, type 2 AIP has little in common with the type 1 variant; instead, the morphological features overlap with other forms of chronic pancreatitis (Table 40.2). The most distinctive feature of this variant is a dense periductal collar of lymphocytes and plasma cells, accompanied by neutrophilic microabscesses within the lumen of the duct, the so-called *granulocytic epithelial lesion* (Fig. 40.23).[11,37,41,42,44,46,51,55] Erosion and ulceration of the duct lining are frequently seen, occasionally accompanied by complete destruction of the duct. Another characteristic feature of this variant is the presence of neutrophils within acinar units. Storiform-type fibrosis is typically not prominent. Although some veins may be focally involved by the lymphoplasmacytic infiltrate (i.e., phlebitis), overt obliterative phlebitis is uncommon.

Immunohistochemistry

The number of IgG4-positive cells is typically fewer than 10 per HPF on needle biopsy and fewer than 50 per HPF on a resection specimen, although occasional pockets of IgG4-positive plasma cells may be observed. However, type 2 AIP typically lacks the diffuse increase in IgG4-positive cells seen in type 1 AIP. The pancreatic ductal epithelium in patients with type 2 AIP show a membranous pattern of PD-L1 reactivity. The sensitivity of PD-L1 as a marker of type 2 AIP is 70%, and although relatively specific, a small proportion of pancreatic ductal adenocarcinomas may also show similar reactivity.[15]

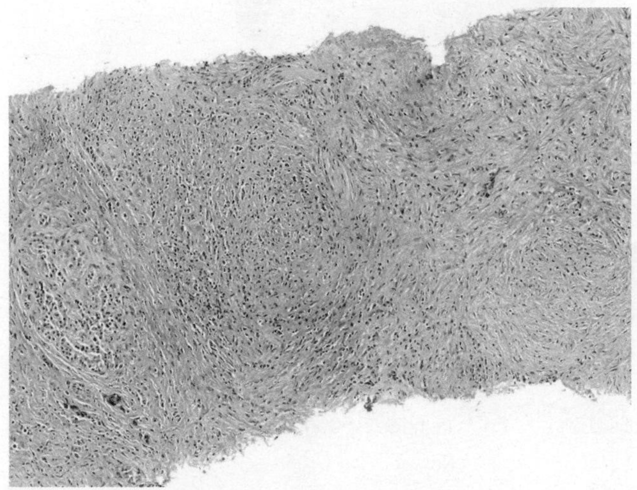

FIGURE 40.20 Needle biopsy from a patient with type 1 autoimmune pancreatitis. Note the dense fibroinflammatory and storiform type fibrosis.

Biopsy Diagnosis

Like the interpretation of type 1 AIP, the type 2 variant may also be challenging. On biopsy material, the sine qua non lesion, granulocytic epithelial lesions, may not be represented on biopsy. Notably, because ducts may not be sampled, the diagnosis often relies on the presence of neutrophils within acinar units (Figs. 40.24 and 40.25). Duct or acinar-based neutrophils may be seen in the peritumoral region of patients with pancreatic ductal adenocarcinoma and constitutes a potential pitfall on needle biopsy.

Risk of Malignancy

The development of synchronous and metachronous pancreatic adenocarcinomas in patients with AIP has been described.[111-114] Almost all of these malignancies have arisen on a background of type 1 AIP. Recent data have shown that pancreata from patients with AIP, compared with chronic alcoholic pancreatitis, have at least an equivalent number of PanIN lesions and a comparable number of high-grade PanIN lesions (grades 2 and 3).[114] These findings, although far from conclusive, do raise the possibility that patients with AIP may have an elevated risk of malignancy, and the level of this risk may be equal to that in patients with chronic alcoholic pancreatitis.

Unclassified Autoimmune Pancreatitis

Not all cases of AIP fit into the aforementioned subtypes. Some cases demonstrate the histological triumvirate of type

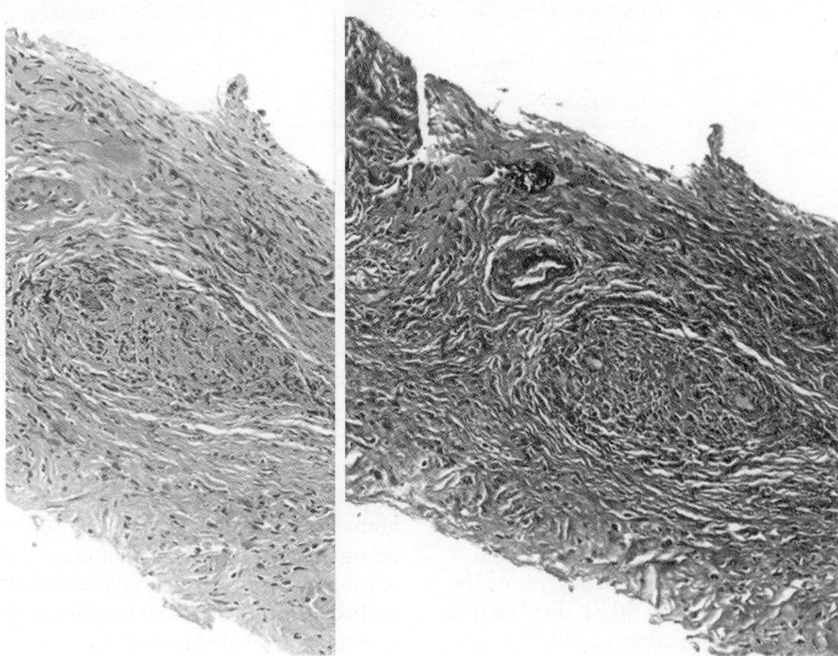

FIGURE 40.21 Obliterative phlebitis in present in this needle biopsy from a patient with type 1 autoimmune pancreatitis, a finding supported on an elastic stain *(right)*.

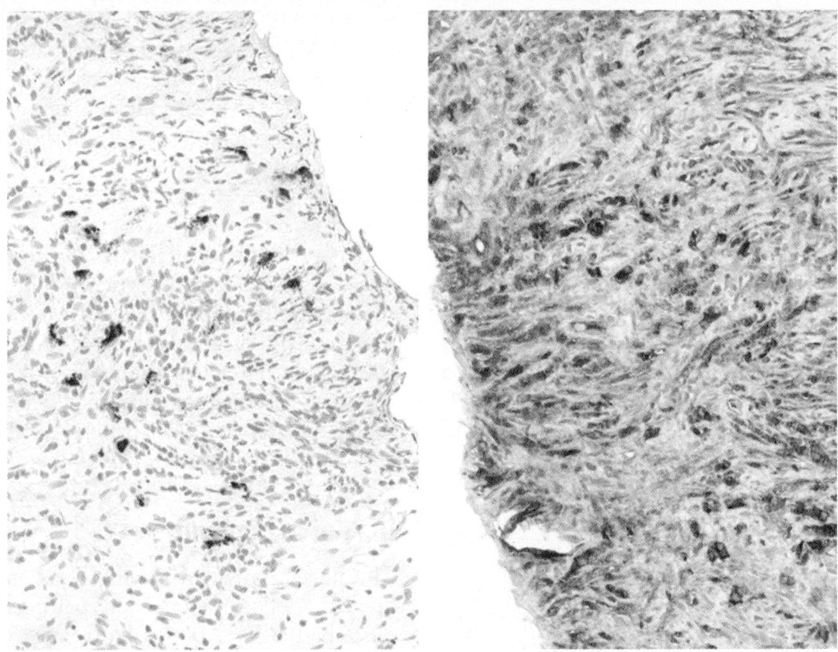

FIGURE 40.22 Biopsies from a patient with type 1 autoimmune pancreatitis depicted in Figs. 40.20 and 40.21 show a mild elevation in IgG4-positive cells and an IgG4-to-IgG ratio of >40%.

TABLE 40.2 Differences Between Type 1 and Type 2 Autoimmune Pancreatitis

	Type 1 AIP	Type 2 AIP
Age	Elderly, seventh decade of life	Middle age, fifth decade of life
Sex	Predominantly male	Males and females equally affected
Presentation	Jaundice (75%), acute pancreatitis (15%)	Jaundice (~50%), acute pancreatitis (~33%)
Systemic disease	Yes	No
Elevated serum immunoglobulin G4	80%	Uncommon
Inflammatory bowel disease	No association	Present in 16%-30% of cases
Histopathology	Periductal inflammation with one or more of the following features: 1. Storiform fibrosis 2. Obliterative phlebitis	Periductal inflammation with one or more of the following features: 1. Ductal/lobular abscesses 2. Ductal ulceration with neutrophils
Long-term outcome	Frequent relapses	Rare relapses (<10%)

AIP, *Autoimmune pancreatitis.*

1 disease (i.e., dense lymphoplasmacytic inflammation, storiform-type fibrosis, and obliterative phlebitis), but in addition show more than an occasional intraductal aggregate of neutrophils. Others show typical type 2 disease but with diffuse infiltrates of IgG4-positive plasma cells, more than 50 per HPF. For now, it is prudent not to subcategorize such cases but instead to label them as *unclassified* variants of AIP.

Differential Diagnosis

Autoimmune Pancreatitis versus Pancreatic Carcinoma

In its most common manifestation, AIP mimics pancreatic cancer; therefore a correct diagnosis of AIP can prevent the patient undergoing major surgery (Table 40.3). Two factors make this an extremely challenging diagnosis: (1) The incidence of AIP is far lower than that of pancreatic cancer, and (2) there is no single diagnostic clinical feature or test that can identify the full spectrum of AIP. The most feared scenario is misdiagnosis of AIP in a patient with pancreatic adenocarcinoma because a delay in diagnosis may close the already narrow surgical window.

Usually, the diagnosis of AIP (particularly type 1) is established on clinical and radiological grounds alone, and a biopsy is performed only in a minority of cases. For the surgical pathologist, the distinction is generally not a challenge. Although the ducts involved by AIP may show mild reactive atypia, they are unlikely to be mistaken for an adenocarcinoma. On FNA biopsy, however, these "atypical" ducts may be mistaken for adenocarcinoma.[101] A substantial minority of biopsy specimens from patients with AIP are nondiagnostic because they lack the key histological features, probably because the involvement of the pancreas is patchy. A minority of pancreatic adenocarcinomas show a dense intratumoral and peritumoral lymphoplasmacytic infiltrate that is

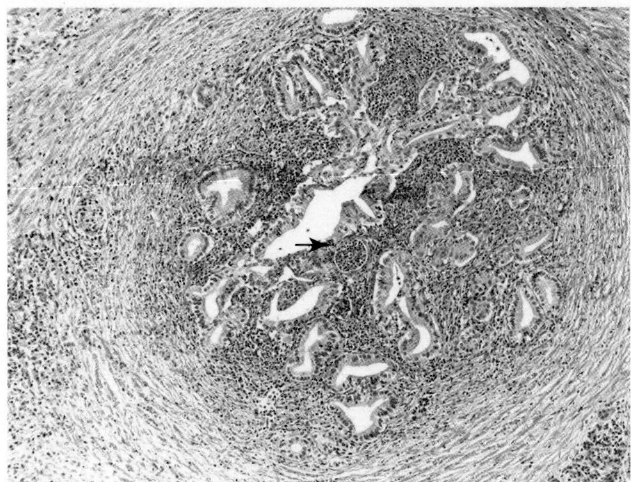

FIGURE 40.23 Type 2 autoimmune pancreatitis. The pancreatic duct is surrounded by a robust lymphoplasmacytic infiltrate. Note the presence of neutrophils infiltrating the duct *(arrow)*—the so-called *granulocytic epithelial lesion.*

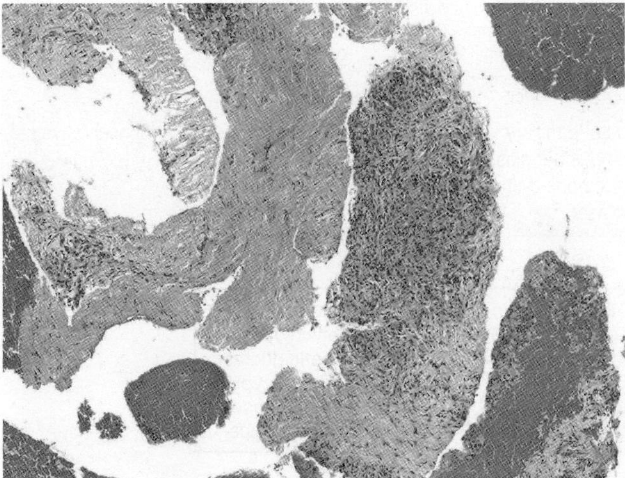

FIGURE 40.24 Needle biopsy from a patient with type 2 autoimmune pancreatitis shows prominent fibrosis and inflamed acinar tissue.

also rich in IgG4-bearing plasma cells[41]; because the number of IgG4-positive plasma cells may be elevated, these lesions may be mistaken for AIP. To avoid this diagnostic trap, an elevated number of IgG4-positive plasma cells should not be used as the sole criterion to diagnose AIP, instead the diagnosis requires careful correlation with clinical, radiological, and serological features (Fig. 40.26). An immunohistochemical stain for PD-L1 can aid in the distinction of type 2 AIP from pancreatic adenocarcinoma. A membranous pattern of PD-L1 reactivity is seen in 70% of patients with type 2 AIP, including core biopsy material.[15] However, although the specificity is >95%, rare examples of pancreatic adenocarcinoma also stain positive for PD-L1.

Autoimmune Pancreatitis versus Other Forms of Chronic Pancreatitis

Histologically, type 1 AIP is unlikely to be mistaken for any other form of pancreatitis. However, the histological features of type 2 AIP may overlap with those of chronic alcoholic pancreatitis. Alcohol-related pancreatitis is typified by the presence of dense acellular fibrosis, calcification, and dilated ducts filled with inspissated proteinaceous material, uncommon histological features in the type 2 variant. Furthermore, alcoholic chronic pancreatitis shows only a mild inflammatory infiltrate, composed predominantly of lymphocytes. Nonetheless, some pancreata from patients with alcohol abuse show a periductal lymphoplasmacytic infiltrate associated with intraepithelial neutrophils.

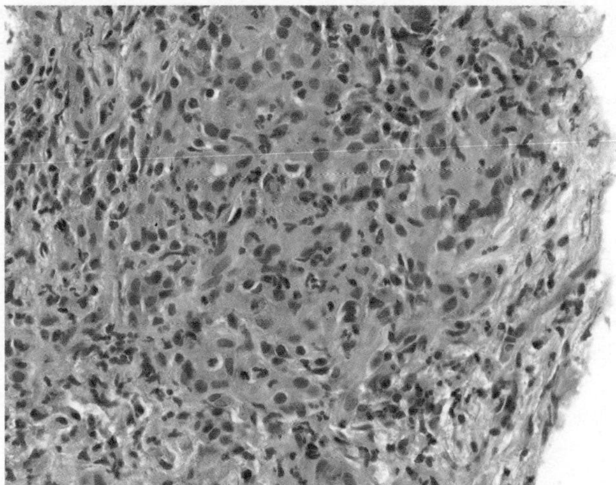

FIGURE 40.25 Needle biopsy from a patient with type 2 autoimmune pancreatitis. Neutrophils are present within acinar tissue.

Other Diseases That May Mimic Autoimmune Pancreatitis

Additional diseases that should be ruled out include lymphoma, inflammatory myofibroblastic tumor, infectious diseases, and other inflammatory diseases such as granulomatosis and polyangiitis (Wegener granulomatosis).[100] The morphological features of AIP do not overlap with these diseases. However, several of these diseases, including infections, may be associated with elevated numbers of IgG4-bearing plasma cells.[103-105]

Diagnostic Criteria

Histology is the gold standard for the diagnosis of AIP, but this statement applies primarily to a resection specimen. On biopsy material, a diagnosis of AIP should not be rendered in a clinical vacuum: Close collaboration among clinician, radiologist, and pathologist is vital. An international consensus document on the diagnostic criteria of AIP has codified this collaborative effort.[95] A modified version of this algorithm is shown in Fig. 40.26.

Diagnostic Value of an Ampullary or Bile Duct Biopsy

A random biopsy specimen from either the ampulla of Vater or the bile duct may provide diagnostically valuable information. In one study, a cutoff value of 10 IgG4-positive plasma cells per HPF was used; the sensitivity and specificity were 52% and 89%, respectively, for ampullary biopsy and 52% and 96%, respectively, for bile duct biopsy.[106] The results of other studies have been similar, although they have reported higher specificity and sensitivity values.[107,108]

TABLE 40.3 Noninflammatory and Nonneoplastic Lesions of the Pancreas That Mimic Pancreatic Neoplasms

	Mean Age/Gender Prediction	Imaging	Differential Diagnosis on Clinical Features and Imaging	Pathology	Treatment
Intrapancreatic accessory spleen	52/M	Solid round to oval	Pancreatic neuroendocrine tumor	Similar to normal spleen	Conservative
Epidermoid cyst in intrapancreatic accessory spleen	50s/none	Cystic lesion with solid component	Mucinous cystic neoplasm	Keratinized epithelium surrounded by splenic tissue	Conservative
Lipomatous pseudohypertrophy	41/none	Adipose tissue	Well-differentiated liposarcoma	Mature adipose tissue	Conservative
Pancreatic hamartoma	Neonates and adults	Solid to cystic lesion	A range of pancreatic solid and cystic neoplasms	Disorganized pancreatic tissue, may show prominent stromal component	Conservative
Adenomyomatous hyperplasia of the Vaterian system	63/M	Distal bile duct mass lesion	Ampullary carcinoma	Benign glandular units with smooth muscle proliferation	Conservative
Lymphoepithelial cyst of the pancreas	55/M	Cystic lesion	Intraductal papillary mucinous neoplasm or mucinous cystic neoplasm	Cyst lined by squamous epithelium and lymphoid tissue	Conservative
Squamoid cyst of the pancreas	63/none	Cystic lesion	Intraductal papillary mucinous neoplasm	Cyst lined with squamous epithelium	Conservative
Enteric duplication cyst	Adult/none	Cystic lesion	Intraductal papillary mucinous neoplasm or mucinous cystic neoplasm	Bilayered muscle wall, columnar lining epithelium	Conservative

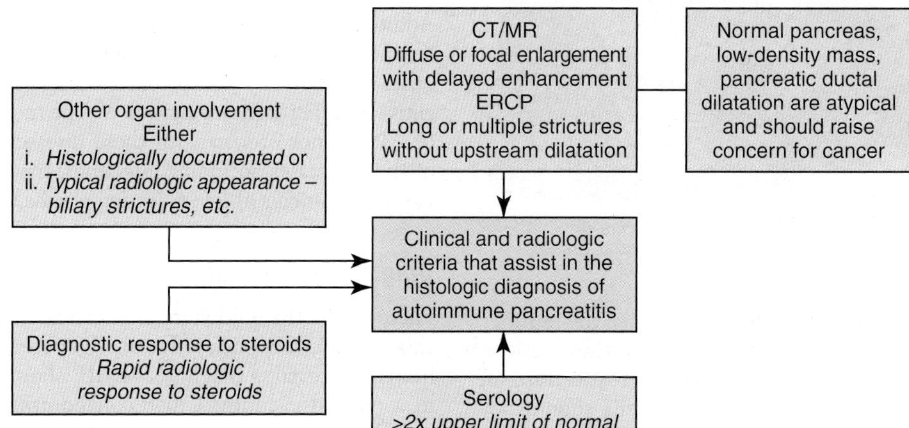

FIGURE 40.26 A diagnosis of autoimmune pancreatitis should not be made in a clinical vacuum. Integration of clinical, radiological, and serological information is crucial. *CT/MR*, Computed tomography/magnetic resonance imaging; *ERCP*, endoscopic retrograde cholangiopancreatography. (*Data from Shinagare S, Shinagare AB, Deshpande V. Autoimmune pancreatitis: a guide for the histopathologist. Semin Diagn Pathol. 2012;29:197-204.*)

Although the presence of more than 10 IgG4-bearing plasma cells per HPF provides another tool for distinguishing AIP from pancreatic carcinoma, several caveats should be considered when interpreting these results:

1. Ampullary biopsy specimens typically lack the characteristic morphological features of IgG4-related disease, and excessive reliance on IgG4-positive plasma cell counts is generally unwise. Of note, an ampullary biopsy specimen from a patient with pancreatic adenocarcinoma may show elevated numbers of IgG4-positive plasma cells. Storiform-type fibrosis, however, is seen in a minority of bile duct biopsies, and identification of this feature greatly strengthens the diagnosis of AIP.
2. It is not unusual for the endoscopist to biopsy the adjacent duodenum instead of the ampulla, and the diagnostic value of a random duodenal biopsy is unknown.
3. Virtually all studies evaluating the diagnostic value of ampullary biopsies in AIP are from Japan. It is very likely that the diagnostic yield in Western countries is significantly lower, primarily because of the high prevalence of type 2 AIP, a disease associated with low to absent IgG4-positive plasma cells. Notably, an ampullary biopsy does not aid in the diagnosis of type 2 AIP.

Therapy

Type 1 AIP responds dramatically and swiftly to immunosuppressive therapy.[96,109] The response to steroids provides additional reassurance of a benign disease. For induction of remission, steroid is the first-line agent in all patients with active untreated AIP. Prednisone is used at an initial dose of 0.6 to 1.0 mg/kg/day. Steroids are usually tapered by 5 to 10 mg/day every 1 to 2 weeks until a daily dosage of 20 mg, followed by tapering with 5 mg every 2 weeks. The use of maintenance therapy following successful induction therapy remains controversial. Patients with type 1 AIP with low disease activity before treatment do not need maintenance treatment.[110] Although risk factors for relapse remain poorly understood, patients with the following features are considered at a high risk for relapse: (1) high serum IgG4 levels (>4× upper limit of normal), (2) persistently high serum IgG4 levels after steroid treatment, (3) diffuse enlargement of the pancreas, (4) proximal type IgG4-related sclerosing cholangitis, and (5) extensive multiorgan involvement. The lesions in some patients with AIP (about 10% to 25%) improve spontaneously without intervention or steroid treatment, thus "watchful waiting" may be appropriate in some asymptomatic patients. Relapse of disease is also treated with steroid therapy, although data support the use of rituximab in treating relapses.[38]

Type 2 AIP also responds to steroids, although, long-term immunosuppression is not recommended, given that the risk of relapse is <10%.[34]

FOLLICULAR PANCREATITIS

This is an uncommon form of pancreatitis and far less common than AIP. Although the term *follicular pancreatitis* was first used in 2012, histologically similar cases had been reported before that date.[75,115-121]

The disease typically affects adults who are older than 50 years of age, with a slight male predominance (60%). Although some patients present with abdominal pain, many patients are asymptomatic, and like most serendipitously detected lesions, follicular pancreatitis is initially detected on cross-sectional imaging performed for an unrelated illness.[75,116-118]

On imaging, most patients show a mass lesion, mimicking a solid pancreatic neoplasm. A less common form of disease is characterized by a dilated main pancreatic duct, an appearance that resembles an intraductal papillary mucinous neoplasm. There are no clinical or serological clues to a diagnosis of follicular pancreatitis.

Pathogenesis

Little is known regarding the etiopathogenesis of this disorder. It has been argued that the disease is T-cell mediated with the T-cell population skewed toward the Th17 pathway.[121] Interestingly, a histologically similar disease has been reported to involve the bile duct and gallbladder, the so-called *follicular cholangitis* and *follicular cholecystitis*.

Pathological Findings

Follicular pancreatitis is characterized by lymphoid follicle formation, often with periductal accentuation.[75,116,118]

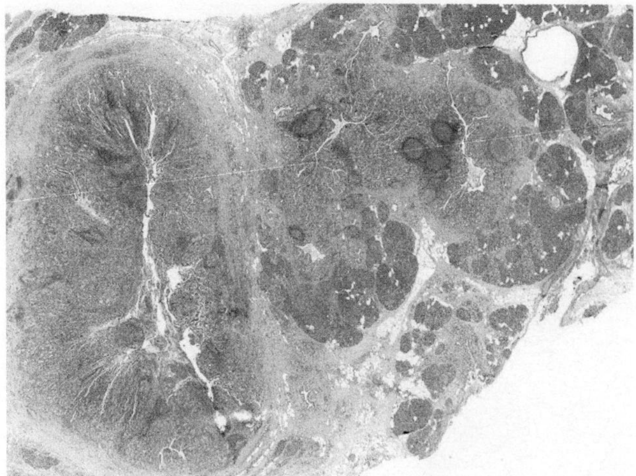

FIGURE 40.27 Follicular pancreatitis. The main pancreatic duct is surrounded by reactive germinal centers.

Many lymphoid follicles are accompanied by germinal centers that display a prominent reactive appearance (Figs. 40.27 and 40.28). Extension of these lymphoid aggregates into the pancreatic parenchyma is also observed. The pancreatic ducts are intact and lack evidence of injury. Fibrosis, although present, is generally not as conspicuous as that seen in AIP.

Differential Diagnosis

When confronted by a pancreas with a prominent infiltrate of lymphoid follicles, a broad range of inflammatory and neoplastic diseases must be considered. Follicular pancreatitis is readily distinguished from a follicular lymphoma because the germinal centers appear overtly reactive. Although lymphoid aggregates and reactive geminal centers are present in type 1 AIP, follicular pancreatitis lacks storiform fibrosis and obliterative phlebitis. Furthermore, IgG4-positive plasma cells in follicular pancreatitis are sparse, and the IgG4/IgG-positive plasma cell ratio is less than 40%.

Therapy

Most reported cases were diagnosed by histological examination of the resected pancreas, hence the efficacy of immunosuppressive agents has not been investigated; however, the one case of follicular pancreatitis treated with steroids showed a 50% reduction in the size of the pancreatic mass.[116]

PARADUODENAL PANCREATITIS ("GROOVE" PANCREATITIS)

Definitions and Terminology

Paraduodenal pancreatitis is a distinct form of chronic pancreatitis that involves paraduodenal pancreatic tissue and the duodenum itself, and it is typically centered on the minor papilla.[122] A multitude of other terms have been used to describe this entity, including cystic dystrophy of heterotopic pancreas,[123] pancreatic hamartoma of duodenal wall,[124] periampullary or periduodenal wall cyst,[125] adenomyoma/myoadenomatosis,[126] and groove pancreatitis.[127] Each of these terms describes one facet of this multifaceted

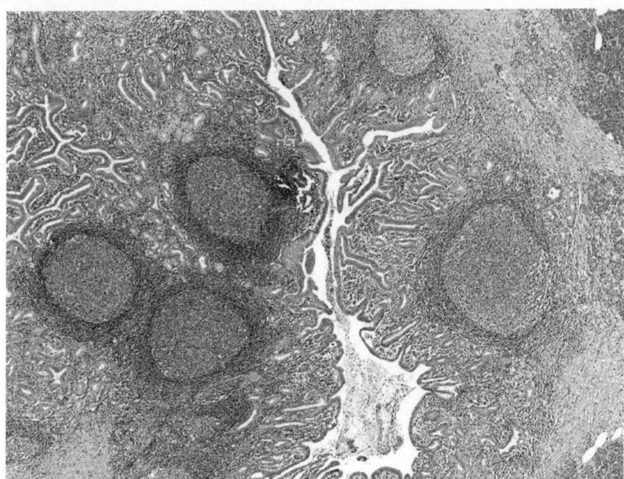

FIGURE 40.28 Follicular pancreatitis. High-power view of the reactive germinal centers.

disease. The designation *groove pancreatitis* is based on the fact that the pancreatitis is located in the groove between the common bile duct and duodenum. *Paraduodenal pancreatitis* has been proposed as a unifying term for this entity.[122]

Clinical Features

In one North American study, patients with groove pancreatitis constituted 5% of all pancreatoduodenectomies.[128] This disease manifests most commonly in the fourth decade of life and predominantly affects males.[11,122,129,130] Most patients report a history of alcohol abuse and often a history of smoking. The most common clinical symptoms are abdominal pain, vomiting, and weight loss.[130,131] Similar to AIP, paraduodenal pancreatitis often forms a tumefactive lesion in the head of the pancreas and thus mimics pancreatic carcinoma. Other symptoms relate to upper gastrointestinal obstruction, a consequence of duodenal stenosis. The disease can also narrow the common bile duct, resulting in obstructive jaundice.

Radiological Features

Radiologically, the disease may be limited to the duodenal wall or involve the adjacent pancreas.[132] On CT, a poorly enhancing, hypodense lesion is often identified in the groove between the common bile duct and the duodenum.[129] The duodenal wall is invariably thickened, and cysts are commonly found.[130,133] Luminal narrowing of the distal common bile duct and the main pancreatic duct may be seen. However, an abrupt pancreatic and bile duct cutoff, as seen in pancreatic carcinoma, is not a feature of paraduodenal pancreatitis. Radiologically, the disease may be mistaken for a host of neoplastic entities, including solid pancreatic neoplasms such as pancreatic and duodenal adenocarcinomas, neuroendocrine tumors, and cystic pancreatic neoplasms including intraductal papillary mucinous neoplasm.[134]

Pathogenesis

Any hypothesis that attempts to explain the disease must take into account two factors: (1) The disease is centered on the accessory pancreatic duct, and (2) a strong association with alcohol abuse.[11,122] Therefore one could speculate that a partially obstructed accessory pancreatic duct precipitates paraduodenal pancreatitis in an individual susceptible to alcoholic pancreatitis.

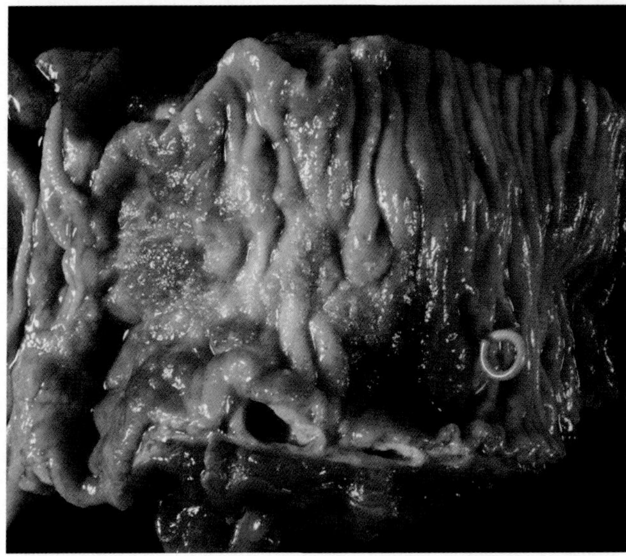

FIGURE 40.29 Groove pancreatitis. The duodenal mucosa immediately distal to the gastroduodenal junction is abnormal. The duodenal mucosal folds are thickened and granular.

Pathological Findings

Gross Features

The gross evaluation of the pancreaticoduodenectomy specimen plays a critical role in establishing a diagnosis of paraduodenal pancreatitis.[11,122,128] The disease is centered either in the duodenal wall or at the interface between the duodenum and the pancreas. It is also relevant to document the involvement of the minor papilla: the minor papilla is identified approximately 2 cm proximal to the major papilla. The duodenal wall is thickened, and the mucosal surface appears granular (Fig. 40.29).[123] The lobular architecture of the paraduodenal pancreas is replaced by a gray-white fibrotic lesion (Fig. 40.30). The diseased tissue is invariably associated with cysts that contain clear fluid[123]; cysts as large as 10 cm in diameter have been described. Although the lesion is often centered on the accessory pancreatic duct, it is frequently difficult to identify this duct grossly. The scarring process can narrow both the duodenum and the distal common bile duct.

Microscopic Features

Histologically, no single feature is diagnostic of this disease. However, a constellation of features, when viewed collectively, allude to a diagnosis of paraduodenal pancreatitis.[11,122,123,129]

1. Marked fibrosis of the duodenal wall extends into the adjacent pancreas (Fig. 40.31). Much of the muscularis propria is replaced by fibrosis. Multiple sections are required to demonstrate an accessory pancreatic duct surrounded by fibrosis.
2. Multiple cysts are identified within the zones of fibrosis. Some of these cysts may be lined by ductal epithelium. The larger cysts are lined by granulation tissue and may contain proteinaceous material.
3. The diseased tissue may also show a proliferation of myoid cells, either smooth muscle cells or myofibroblasts,

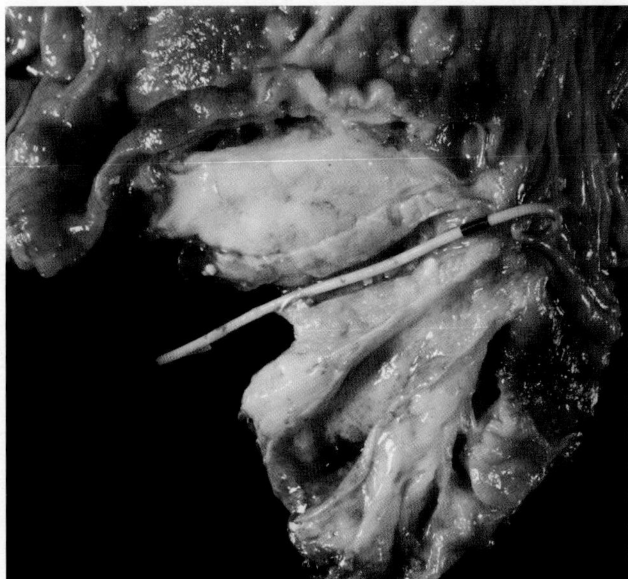

FIGURE 40.30 Groove pancreatitis. The pancreas depicted in Fig. 40.29 has been dissected. Both the bile duct and pancreatic duct (with stent) are dilated. The paraduodenal pancreas shows extensive fibrosis.

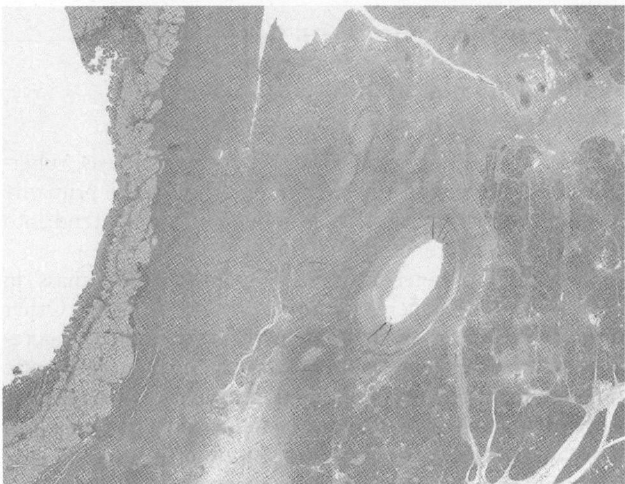

FIGURE 40.31 Paraduodenal pancreatitis shows marked Brunner gland hyperplasia and fibrosis in the zone between the duodenum and pancreas.

particularly in the immediate vicinity of the duodenum. In fact, some examples of this entity may have been diagnosed as *leiomyoma.*
4. Most cases demonstrate prominent Brunner gland hyperplasia.
5. The inflammatory infiltrate is generally sparse and is composed mostly of lymphocytes. Stigmata of alcoholic chronic pancreatitis may also be identified in the pancreas.

Differential Diagnosis

Although the radiological features of paraduodenal pancreatitis may mimic carcinoma, histological evaluation readily excludes ampullary or duodenal adenocarcinoma. However, a relatively small periampullary carcinoma may be associated with a paraduodenal pancreatitis–like lesion. Therefore a thorough evaluation to exclude the possibility of a carcinoma is necessary.

Therapy

Conservative therapeutic options include alcohol abstinence and smoking cessation. However, it has been argued that surgery is the treatment of choice in symptomatic patients.[131]

EOSINOPHILIC PANCREATITIS

Eosinophilic pancreatitis, in which the inflammatory infiltrate is predominantly or exclusively composed of eosinophils, is an extraordinarily rare condition.[35] A more common cause of pancreatic tissue eosinophilia is AIP.[39,40,46,100] Most cases of eosinophilic pancreatitis were reported before the recognition of AIP, and in retrospect, it is likely that some of these cases in the literature represent examples of AIP with prominent eosinophilia.

Clinical Features

The presenting symptoms vary from abdominal pain to obstructive jaundice.[35,135,136] Some patients show peripheral eosinophilia. A prior history of allergic symptoms is not uncommon. Imaging reveals a pancreatic mass in most cases and may demonstrate stricture of the bile duct.[137] Pseudocyst formation is occasionally seen.[1] Hypereosinophilic syndrome develops in some of these patients.[35,138]

Pathological Findings

Grossly, the pancreas may be enlarged and fibrotic. Histologically, a diffuse eosinophilic infiltrate is seen around ducts, acini, and interlobular septa.[139] In addition, eosinophilic phlebitis and arteritis may be seen.[35] Although lymphocytes and plasma cells are also present, they do not dominate the picture. In addition to this diffuse form of involvement, focal involvement of the pancreas, particularly adjacent to a pseudocyst, has been reported.[35] The eosinophilia can also involve the gastrointestinal tract, particularly the duodenum. Involvement of the biliary tract in the form of multiple biliary strictures has also been reported.[35]

Differential Diagnosis

A diverse group of diseases is associated with increased numbers of eosinophils in the pancreas, including AIP, malignancy, parasitic infections, hypersensitivity reaction to drugs, inflammatory myofibroblastic tumors, and systemic mastocytosis.[35] As mentioned previously, the most common concern in the differential diagnosis of eosinophilic pancreatitis is AIP. Findings of elevated levels of serum IgG4, multiorgan tumefactive lesions, the presence of storiform fibrosis, and elevated numbers of IgG4-positive plasma cells favor of a diagnosis of AIP. The mainline therapy for both diseases is steroid therapy.

TROPICAL PANCREATITIS

Tropical pancreatitis is a variant of chronic pancreatitis that is seen in tropical regions such as the Indian subcontinent and certain parts of Africa.[140,141] It is also been referred to as *Afro-Asian pancreatitis, juvenile pancreatitis syndrome, chronic calcific pancreatitis of the tropics, nonalcoholic tropical pancreatitis,* and *nutritional pancreatitis.* In southern India, where the disease is endemic, the prevalence is 126 cases per 100,000 individuals.[141] Tropical pancreatitis occurs predominantly in children and young adults and is characterized by pain, pancreatic calcification, and diabetes. Older patients with tropical pancreatitis have also been reported. The disease affects both men and women.

Etiology and Pathogenesis

Historically, suspected causative factors for tropical pancreatitis have included malnutrition and cyanogenic glycosides from consumption of cassava.[141] Mutations and polymorphisms in *SPINK1*, *CFTR*, and *cathepsin B (CTSB)* appear to increase the susceptibility to this disease.[19,142,143] It is likely that the disease involves an interplay between genetic and environmental factors, and the genes implicated are likely to be disease modifiers rather than the direct cause of tropical pancreatitis.[19,142,143] Similar to other forms of pancreatitis, tropical pancreatitis is associated with an increased risk of malignancy—a fivefold increase.[144]

Pathological Features

The pathological features depend on the duration and severity of disease. At an advanced stage, the pancreas appears shrunken. The most characteristic feature of tropical pancreatitis is the presence of large intraductal calculi in the main duct. Histologically, there appears to be little difference between tropical pancreatitis and alcoholic pancreatitis. The disease shows both intralobular and interlobular fibrosis and a sparse inflammatory infiltrate. It is distinguishable from alcoholic chronic pancreatitis by younger patient age at presentation and by the presence of large intraductal calculi.

PANCREATIC INVOLVEMENT IN SYSTEMIC CONDITIONS

Symptomatic involvement of the pancreas is uncommon in systemic inflammatory conditions. Granulomatosis with polyangiitis, formally known as *Wegener's granulomatosis*, is one of the more common diseases with pancreas involvement and may exhibit mass-forming pancreatitis or present as acute pancreatitis.[145-147] In patients with extensive systemic disease, the diagnosis is straightforward; however, those with isolated pancreatic involvement may pose a diagnostic challenge. On needle biopsy, the diagnosis of granulomatosis with polyangiitis may be difficult, particularly in patients with a low index of suspicion. The histological features of granulomatosis with polyangiitis include "dirty" necrosis, giant cells, and poorly formed granulomas. Vasculitis is seldom seen on needle biopsy.[148,149] Granulomatosis with polyangiitis may be associated with increased numbers of IgG4-positive cells, a finding that may raise concern for type 1 AIP.

Rheumatoid arthritis may rarely affect the pancreas, and these patients may present with a pancreatic mass lesion. Like granulomatosis with polyangiitis, the diagnosis is rarely considered clinically and thus presents a diagnostic challenge for the pathologist. Histologically, the pancreas shows rheumatoid nodules that are characterized by central areas of necrobiosis, palisading granulomas, and a dense lymphoplasmacytic infiltration at the rim of the nodule.

OBSTRUCTIVE PANCREATITIS

A variety of neoplastic and nonneoplastic diseases are associated with obstruction of large-caliber pancreatic ducts. There is extensive loss of acinar tissue distal to the obstruction, although the islets are preserved. Eventually, extensive interlobular and intralobular fibrosis are observed (Fig. 40.32).

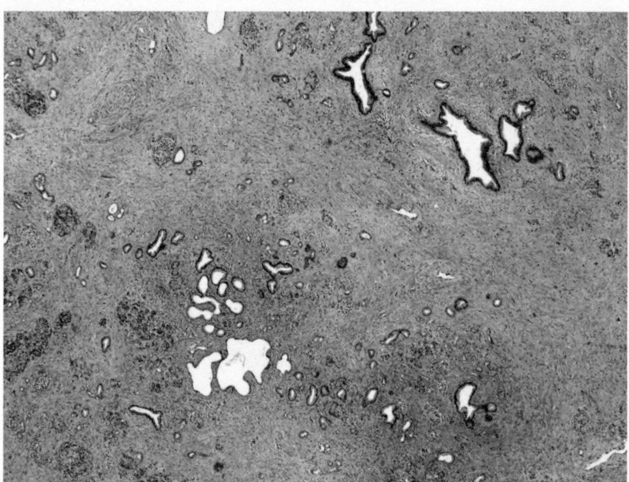

FIGURE 40.32 Obstructive pancreatitis. The image shows marked interlobular and intralobular fibrosis.

INFECTIOUS CAUSES OF PANCREATITIS

Tuberculous Pancreatitis

Clinical Features

Similar to other infectious diseases of the pancreas, tuberculosis of the pancreas is uncommon. The disease primarily involves peripancreatic lymph nodes but may extend into the pancreatic parenchyma.[150]

Tuberculous pancreatitis may manifest as a mass in the head of the pancreas, mimicking carcinoma.[150] Other forms of presentation include obstructive jaundice, pancreatic abscess, and acute and chronic pancreatitis. Pancreatic tuberculosis should be considered in patients who have lived in or traveled to areas that are endemic for tuberculosis. In most cases, the disease is present in other organs; primary pancreatic tuberculosis is exceptionally rare.

Pathological Findings

Intrapancreatic tuberculosis manifests as a tumefactive mass that may be focally cystic (Fig. 40.33). A surgical biopsy or FNA of peripancreatic lymph nodes or the pancreas itself reveals necrotizing granulomatous inflammation (Fig. 40.34). Documentation of the presence of acid-fast bacilli, positive culture, or polymerase chain reaction (PCR) testing is necessary to confirm a diagnosis of mycobacterial infection. Other causes of granulomatous inflammation in the pancreas include sarcoidosis (a disease that may also present as a tumefactive lesion),[151] Crohn's disease, and type 2 AIP.[41]

Other Infections

Infection as a cause of pancreatic disease is extremely uncommon in immunocompetent hosts but may be seen in immunocompromised individuals.

A wide variety of infectious pathogens can affect the pancreas, including viruses, parasites, bacteria, and fungi. Other

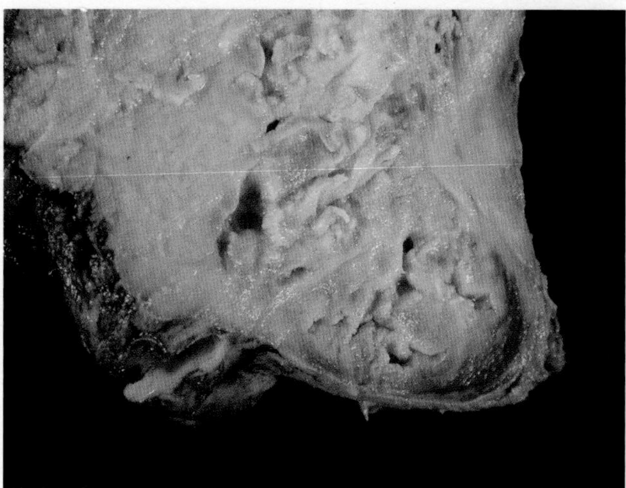

FIGURE 40.33 Tuberculous pancreatitis. A mixed solid and cystic pancreatic mass was seen on imaging. This image shows a large area of intrapancreatic necrosis with cystic changes and necrosis.

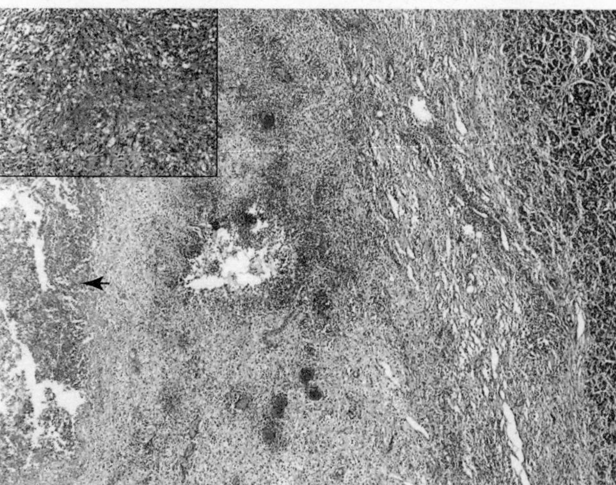

FIGURE 40.34 Tuberculous pancreatitis with intrapancreatic abscesses *(arrow)*. Necrotizing granulomas were identified in the adjacent lymph nodes *(inset)*.

forms of infectious pancreatitis include *Ascaris lumbricoides*,[152] cytomegalovirus,[153] and *Strongyloides stercoralis*.[154] *A. lumbricoides* may enter the pancreas via the pancreatic duct system and cause necrosis, abscess formation, granulomatous inflammation, and fibrosis.

SOLID NONNEOPLASTIC LESIONS THAT MIMIC PANCREATIC NEOPLASMS

Intrapancreatic Accessory Spleen

Accessory spleen (AS), a congenital abnormality, develops through fusion failure of multiple splenic anlages. An accessory spleen is identified in approximately 10% of the population. The majority of these are located close to the splenic hilum. The pancreas is the second most frequent site, with 20% located in the tail of the pancreas.[155] This developmental abnormality is asymptomatic but has recently received attention because of the widespread use of cross-sectional imaging. An intrapancreatic accessory spleen may be associated with an intrasplenic epidermoid cyst (see later).

Clinical Features

The mean patient age at detection is 52 years, and there is a slight male predilection.[156,157] The contrast enhancement pattern on CT and the signal intensities on MRI are similar to those of the normal spleen.[156,157] On EUS, CT, and MRI, an intrapancreatic spleen could be mistaken for a solid pancreatic neoplasm, typically a pancreatic endocrine neoplasm.[156,158]

Pathological Features

Grossly, these are well circumscribed, solid lesions with color and texture identical to spleen—a firm, beefy-red nodule (Fig. 40.35). A preoperative diagnosis of an intrapancreatic spleen is often based on imaging and FNA biopsy.[159,160] Histologically, these lesions are identical to the native spleen, composed of white pulp and red pulp (Fig. 40.36).

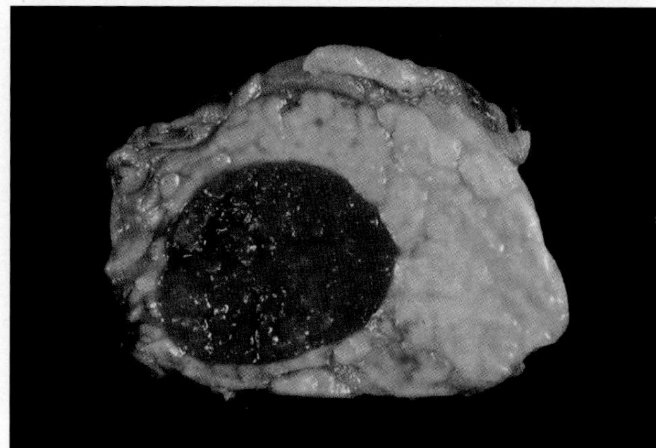

FIGURE 40.35 Intrapancreatic spleen. The nodule is remarkably similar to splenic tissue.

Therapy

An incidentally detected accessory spleen does not require surgical intervention.

Epidermoid Cyst in Intrapancreatic Accessory Spleen

This cystic lesion is encased within an intraductal accessory spleen. Although an extremely uncommon entity, its importance lies in the difficulty in distinguishing this lesion from a mucinous cystic neoplasm.[161]

Clinical Features

Most patients are diagnosed between 40 and 65 years of age, and there is no gender predilection. Most lesions are detected incidentally, although some patients may report nonspecific abdominal symptoms, often unrelated to the pancreatic lesion. On imaging, an epidermoid cyst in the intrapancreatic accessory spleen appears as a solitary monolobular/multilobular cystic lesion in the pancreatic tail, with a thickened cystic wall or with a varying amount of solid component. Serum carbohydrate antigen 19-9 (CA19-9) and carcinoembryonic antigen (CEA) may be elevated.[161]

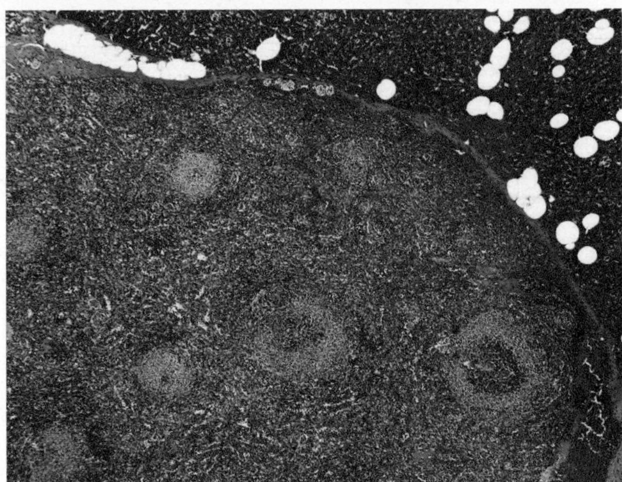

FIGURE 40.36 Intrapancreatic spleen. Note the red and while pulp.

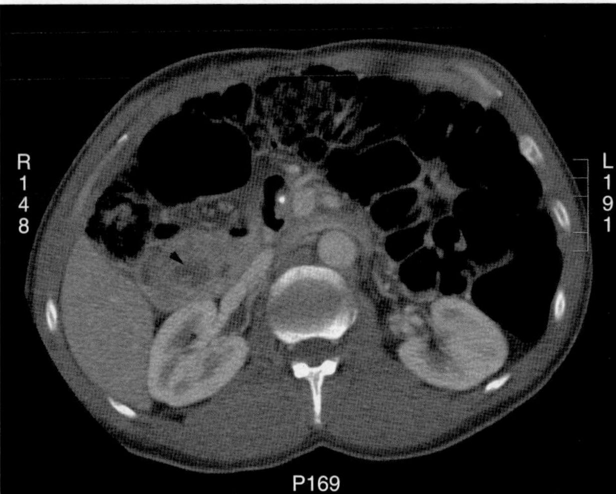

FIGURE 40.37 Lipomatous pseudohypertrophy. On this CT scan the distal pancreas is enlarged and contains significant amounts of intrapancreatic fat.

Surgical intervention is driven by concern for malignant transformation of a mucinous cystic neoplasm or intraductal papillary mucinous neoplasm. Other preoperative clinical and radiological considerations include solid pseudopapillary tumor or cystic pancreatic neuroendocrine tumor. On imaging, recognition of the surrounding ectopic splenic tissue is a key factor in diagnosing epidermoid cyst in an intrapancreatic accessory spleen.

Pathology

Macroscopic evaluation reveals a cyst with either serous or nonserous fluid. Histologically, the cyst is lined with keratinized and nonkeratinized stratified squamous epithelium surrounded by normal splenic tissues.[162,163]

Differential Diagnosis

The absence of skin appendages and mature lymphoid tissues help distinguish an epidermoid cyst in an intrapancreatic accessory spleen from a dermoid or lymphoepithelial cyst.

Therapy

Epidermoid cysts with accessory spleens do not require surgical intervention.

Lipomatous Pseudohypertrophy

Lipomatous pseudohypertrophy is associated with a marked increase in intrapancreatic mature adipose tissue.[164-167] By definition, this diagnosis excludes other pathologies associated with a significant increase in intrapancreatic fat, such as morbid obesity, diabetes mellitus, and chronic pancreatitis. It should be noted that the quantity of intrapancreatic fat increases with age and basal mass index.[168] This entity is extremely uncommon, yet noteworthy, because it may mimic a malignant fatty neoplasm.

Clinical and Radiological Features

The mean patient age at presentation is 41 years, and the disease affects both women and men without a distinct difference in sex distribution.[164] The presenting symptoms are variable, and a significant percentage of patients are identified on cross-sectional imaging performed for symptoms unrelated to the pancreas (Fig. 40.37). However, patients may also have symptoms related to a mass lesion, such as abdominal pain and biliary obstruction. Cross-sectional imaging reveals an intrapancreatic fatty neoplasm. Approximately two-thirds of cases show diffuse involvement of the pancreas, and the remaining one-third demonstrates a focal intrapancreatic fatty mass. These tumefactive lesions are typically large, and tumors as large as 24 cm have been recorded.[164]

Pathogenesis

Little is known about the pathogenesis of this lesion. One plausible hypothesis is that it represents an extremely infiltrative lipoma, although some authors have argued persuasively against this possibility.[164]

Pathological Features

In cases with diffuse involvement, a massive increase in adipose tissue is identified throughout the pancreas. In individuals with focal involvement, a sharp demarcation between the fatty deposition and adjacent pancreas is noted. The lesion may compress the common bile duct.

The tumefactive lesion is composed almost entirely of mature adipose tissue, within which scattered pancreatic elements are identified (Fig. 40.38). Apart from the "dilution" of the pancreatic parenchyma by adipose tissue, the pancreas itself is histologically unremarkable and does not show evidence of either acute or chronic pancreatitis.

Differential Diagnosis

Before a diagnosis of lipomatous pseudohypertrophy is considered, a well-differentiated liposarcoma should be excluded. Well-differentiated liposarcomas are located mainly in the retroperitoneal region and typically do not manifest as a primary pancreatic mass. Microscopically, large single atypical stromal cells are seen within fibrous septa. Nonetheless, on core biopsy, it may not be possible to unequivocally distinguish lipomatous pseudohypertrophy from a lipoma-like well-differentiated liposarcoma without resorting to special studies. Careful attention to the presence of atypical stroma cells may distinguish the two entities. Immunohistochemistry for MDM2 is notoriously

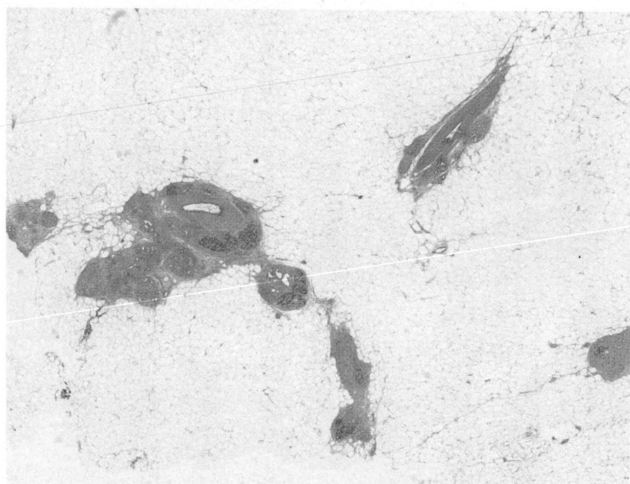

FIGURE 40.38 Lipomatous pseudohypertrophy. Histologically, the pancreas is almost completely replaced by mature adipose tissue.

insensitive for well-differentiated lipoma, and MDM2 amplification on FISH is widely considered to be the gold standard for diagnosis of this entity.[169]

Lipomatous pseudohypertrophy has been associated with Shwartzman-Diamond syndrome, Bannayan syndrome, Johnson-Blizzard syndrome, and the juvenile variant of Parkinson disease. Some hamartomatous lesions may also show abundant intralesional adipose tissue.[170]

Therapy

Asymptomatic cases may be managed conservatively, without resection, provided a secure diagnosis can be established. Resection is required in symptomatic patients.

Pancreatic Hamartoma

A variety of terms have been used to designate this entity, including multicystic pancreatic hamartoma, solid pancreatic hamartoma, and pancreatic solid and cystic hamar toma.[129,143,171-174] Pancreatic hamartoma is histologically characterized by a disorganized proliferation of acinar, endocrine, and ductal cells.[171,174,175] These lesions have been identified predominantly in neonates, although bona fide examples are reported in adults.

Pathological Features

Pancreatic hamartomas have ranged in size from 1 to 11.5 cm. Grossly, these lesions vary from homogenous white, solid nodules to solid and cystic lesions (Fig. 40.39).[171,174-180] The lesion is composed of mature pancreatic tissue (predominantly mature ducts and acini), albeit disorganized, thus fulfilling the definition of a hamartoma. It is notable that the reported cases of pancreatic hamartoma vary widely in their histological appearance (Fig. 40.40). Pancreatic hamartomas in the neonatal period are often dominated by large dilated cysts lined by low cuboidal epithelium.[171,177,179] Neither the acinar nor the ductal elements show atypia. The stromal component, composed of collagenous stroma and spindled cells, is generally prominent. Although scattered endocrine cells are detected, well-formed islets are absent. A paucity of nerve twigs has been observed. Examples dominated by mature adipose tissue have also been reported.[170]

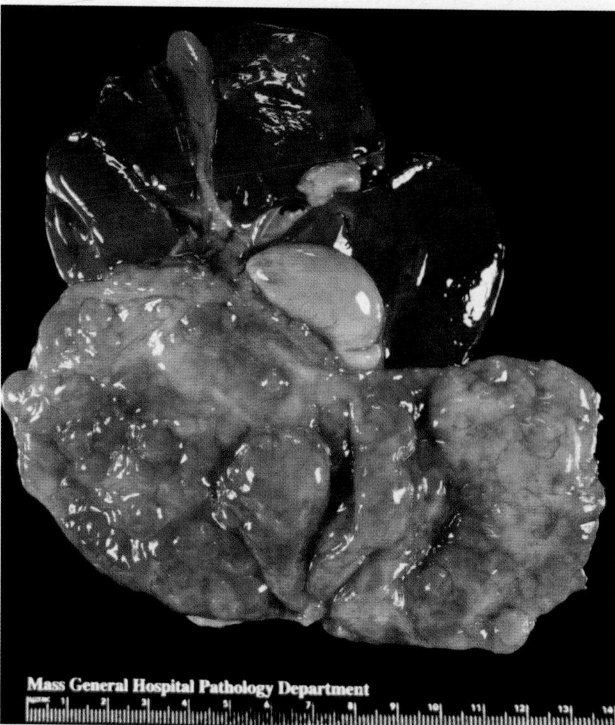

FIGURE 40.39 Pancreatic hamartoma. Large solid and cystic pancreatic lesion in a 24-week-old fetus.

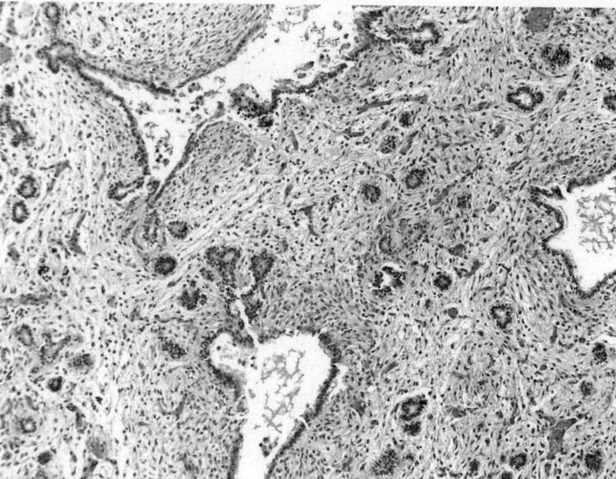

FIGURE 40.40 Pancreatic hamartoma. Notice the disorganized and dilated pancreatic ducts. This lesion was identified in a 24-week-old fetus.

Given the prominent stromal component, other forms of pancreatitis, including AIP, should be excluded. Similar to chronic pancreatitis, pancreatic hamartomas are associated with an increased amount of pancreatic stroma. The mesenchymal cells within this stroma may be positive for CD34 and CD117; the latter reactivity is generally weak.[173,176]

Adenomyomatous Hyperplasia of the Vaterian System

Adenomyomatous hyperplasia of the Vaterian system is a benign, nonneoplastic proliferation of glands and mesenchymal elements involving the distal portion of the bile duct and the ampullary region.[181] Synonyms used to describe

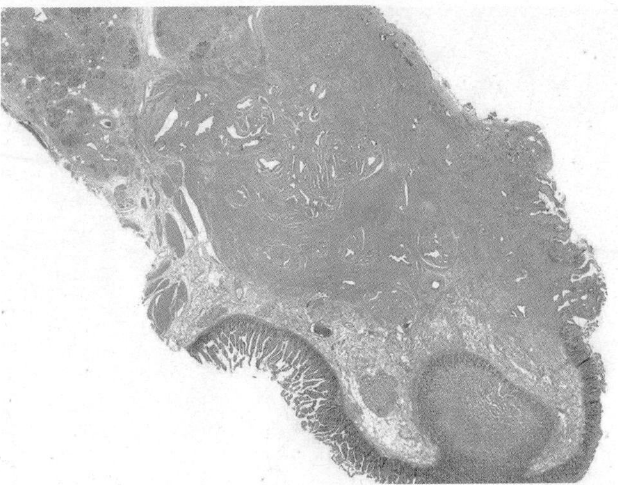

FIGURE 40.41 Adenomyomatous hyperplasia. This section is from the distal end of the bile duct. The ducts are organized in lobular units.

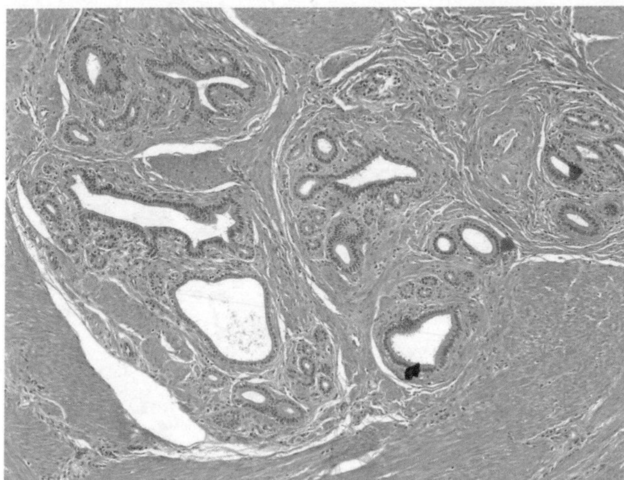

FIGURE 40.42 Adenomyomatous hyperplasia. High-power view of the image shown in Fig. 40.41. The ducts are organized in lobular units and surrounded by smooth muscle.

this entity include *adenomyoma, adenomyomatosis, myoepithelial hamartoma,* and *adenomyomatous hyperplasia.* The term *adenomyomatous hyperplasia* is preferable, because the term *adenomyoma* has a neoplastic connotation. This lesion is benign without malignant potential, and its importance lies in its ability to mimic an ampullary malignancy.

Clinical Features

The mean patient age in one series was 63 years, with males and females affected equally.[181] Patients typically have symptoms related to obstruction of the pancreaticobiliary tract, such as jaundice and abdominal pain. On endoscopy, an enlarged ampulla is identified; endosonographically, an ampullary lesion is typically noted.

Pathological Features

On macroscopic evaluation, a firm, nodular lesion is identified in the terminal portion of the bile duct and ampulla. The mucosa overlying the lesion is normal and typically lacks ulceration. Histologically, this lesion is characterized by lobules of small glands that often surround a larger duct (Figs. 40.41 and 40.42).[181] The lobular pattern of organization helps distinguish this lesion from an invasive pancreaticobiliary carcinoma. The lobules are, in turn, surrounded by a robust mesenchymal proliferation composed of fibroblasts, myofibroblasts, and scattered smooth muscle cells. Heterotopic pancreatic tissue may be identified adjacent to the lesion.

NONNEOPLASTIC CYSTIC LESIONS OF THE PANCREAS

A variety of nonneoplastic pancreatic cysts mimic neoplastic cysts of the pancreas. Although the goal is to avoid resecting these cysts, in many instances such lesions cannot be distinguished clinically and radiologically from their neoplastic counterparts. Therefore surgical pathologists occasionally encounter such cysts (Box 40.4).

BOX 40.4 Benign and Nonneoplastic Intrapancreatic Cysts That May Mimic Malignant and Potentially Malignant Pancreatic Cysts

Lymphoepithelial cysts
Epidermoid cysts in an intrapancreatic accessory spleen
Cysts associated with paraduodenal pancreatitis
Squamoid cysts
Cystic acinar transformation (acinar cell cystadenoma)
Infectious cysts; *Echinococcus* cysts
Pseudocysts
Cystic examples of pancreatic hamartoma
Enteric duplication cysts

Pseudocyst

A pseudocyst lacks a lining epithelium and contains amylase-rich fluid. Historically, pseudocysts were the most common cysts of the pancreas. More recently, with the increased detection of asymptomatic nonneoplastic and neoplastic pancreatic cysts, the relative percentage of pseudocysts by the surgical pathologist has declined. Nonetheless, they continue to constitute a great majority of cysts seen in clinical practice, although because they are seldom resected, the surgical pathologist is more likely to encounter a neoplastic pancreatic cyst than a pseudocyst. A pseudocyst can arise both within the pancreas and in peripancreatic tissue.

Clinical and Imaging Features

Pseudocysts are a consequence of pancreatitis or trauma.[10,12,182] The most common underlying trigger for pseudocyst is alcoholic pancreatitis, and pseudocysts are more common in young to middle-aged men than in women. Nonetheless, almost any form of acute or chronic pancreatitis can trigger the development of a pseudocyst.

EUS plays a major role in both the diagnosis and treatment of pseudocysts. Imaging demonstrates a unilocular cyst filled with debris but without a mural nodule. Analysis of the cyst fluid demonstrates an elevated amylase level (>250 IU/mL) and a low level of carcinoembryonic antigen (typically <200 IU/mL). The cytology specimen is typically hypocellular and usually shows a few inflammatory cells only.[183] In addition, a large amount of acellular debris associated with blood pigment and hemosiderin is frequently seen.[183]

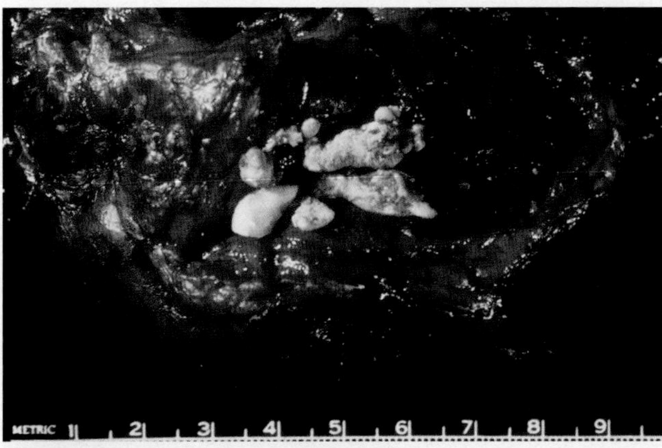

FIGURE 40.43 Pancreatic pseudocyst. Large calculi were found in the adjacent ducts.

Pathological Features

Pseudocysts are for the most part unilocular and contain turbid, sometimes blood-tinged fluid. These cysts can measure greater than 20 cm in size. The wall of the pseudocyst is typically thick and fibrotic (Fig. 40.43). By definition, the cyst lacks a lining epithelium.[10-12,182] However, intrapancreatic pseudocysts may show large-caliber pancreatic ducts at the interface between the cyst and adjacent pancreas, and they should not be mistaken for lining epithelium (Fig. 40.44). Pseudocysts instead show a wall composed of granulation tissue and fibrosis. If adjacent pancreatic tissue is present, stigmata of resolving acute pancreatitis or evidence of chronic pancreatitis may be seen.

Differential Diagnosis

When considering the diagnosis of a pseudocyst, it is prudent to histologically examine the entire cyst wall to rule out a cystic neoplasm. Cystic pancreatic neoplasms in which significant denudation of the lining epithelium may be seen include serous cystadenoma, mucinous cystic neoplasm, and, very occasionally, intraductal papillary mucinous neoplasm. Mucinous cystadenomas with total denudation of the lining epithelium will nonetheless show ovarian-type stroma, a feature not seen in a pseudocyst. Serous cystadenomas, particularly the unilocular variant, may exhibit complete loss of lining epithelium. However, this cystic neoplasm shows a unique subepithelial network of delicate capillary channels.[184] Virtually all patients with pseudocysts report a prior episode of acute pancreatitis, and in the absence of such a history, a diagnosis of a pseudocyst should be made with caution.

Therapy

A significant percentage of pseudocysts resolve spontaneously; others progressively increase in size. The available treatment options include medical management, surgical treatment, and percutaneous or endoscopic drainage. The vast majority of pseudocysts are now treated endoscopically.

Lymphoepithelial Cyst of the Pancreas

A lymphoepithelial cyst of the pancreas is a benign pancreatic cyst that is lined by squamous epithelium and surrounded by reactive lymphoid tissue.[185]

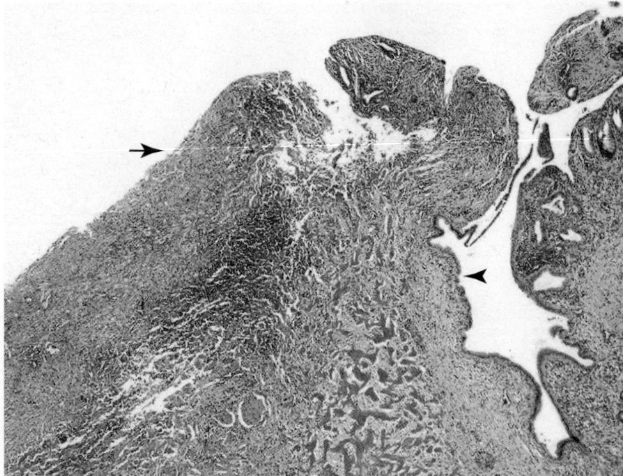

FIGURE 40.44 Pancreatic pseudocyst. The cyst is lined by fibrosis and granulation tissue. Notice the dilated pancreatic duct *(ar)* that communicates with the lumen of the cyst *(arrow)*.

Clinical Features

The mean patient age at diagnosis is 55 years, and this pancreatic cyst is more common in men than in women (male-to-female ratio, 4:1). In one series, these lesions constituted 0.5% of all resected pancreatic cysts.[185] In most contemporary series, patients had been asymptomatic, and the lesions were detected on cross-sectional imaging. Larger cysts may present with abdominal pain.

Pathogenesis

A number of hypotheses have been proposed to rationalize the presence of both lymphoid and epithelial tissue, including (1) origin from epithelial remnants in a lymph node, (2) cystic transformation and squamous metaplasia of pancreatic ducts, and (3) derivation from a branchial cleft cyst that is misplaced and fused with the pancreas during embryogenesis.[185]

Pathological Features

The diagnosis could be made on FNA biopsy; aspirates typically show anucleate squames.[130] However, it should be noted that the cyst fluid CEA may be elevated, thus mimicking a mucinous cystic neoplasm or intraductal papillary mucinous neoplasm.[186,187] The cysts vary from unilocular to multilocular and arise anywhere within the pancreas. The largest cyst in one study was 17 cm.[185] The cysts are typically filled with cheesy-brown contents (Fig. 40.45), although serous-like fluid may also be identified. A dominant mural nodule is not present. Microscopically, the cyst is lined by squamous epithelium and shows a dense subepithelial rind of reactive lymphoid tissue (Fig. 40.46).[163] The squamous epithelium typically shows prominent keratinization, and keratinaceous debris is present within the cyst contents. Columnar mucinous cells may be detected, albeit uncommonly. Occasionally, sebaceous differentiation is present.[188] The lymphoid tissue typically shows numerous reactive germinal centers.

Differential Diagnosis

Entities that should be considered in the differential diagnosis of a lymphoepithelial cyst include dermoid cyst,

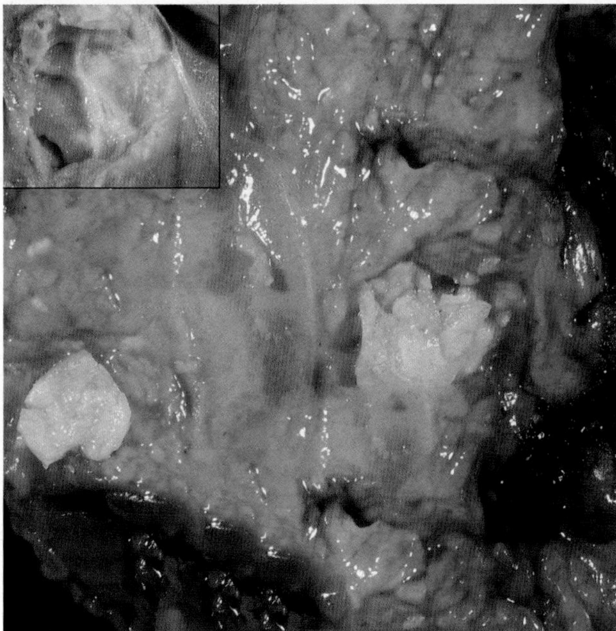

FIGURE 40.45 Lymphoepithelial cyst. This cyst in the head of the pancreas is adjacent to the bile duct and is filled with cheesy white material. *Inset,* After removal of the contents, the cyst is shown to be unilocular, although trabeculations are seen in the wall.

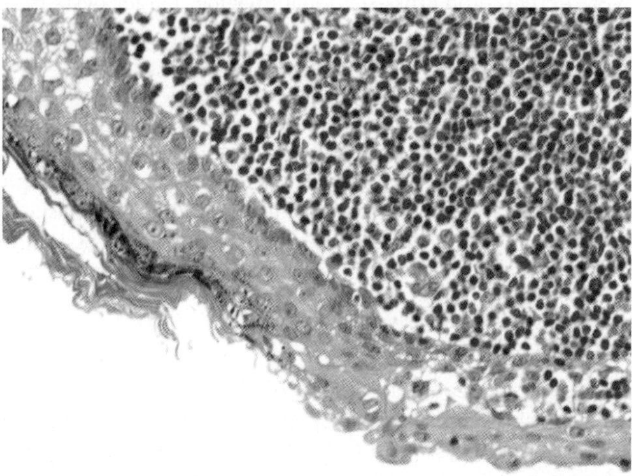

FIGURE 40.46 Lymphoepithelial cyst. The squamous lining shows keratinization and a granular layer. Subepithelial lymphoid tissue is also seen.

epidermoid cyst within intrapancreatic accessory spleen, and squamoid cyst of the pancreas. A diagnosis of dermoid cyst should not be solely based on the presence of sebaceous tissue; instead, this diagnosis requires the presence of elements such as cartilage, hair follicles, and neural tissue. Squamoid cysts of the pancreas lack keratinization and, more crucially, lack lymphoid tissue. Lymphangioma, another lesion associated with prominent lymphoid tissues, demonstrates ectatic vascular structures lined by endothelial-type cells.

Therapy

The FNA biopsy typically allows a conservative approach,[159] although symptomatic lymphoepithelial cysts require resection.

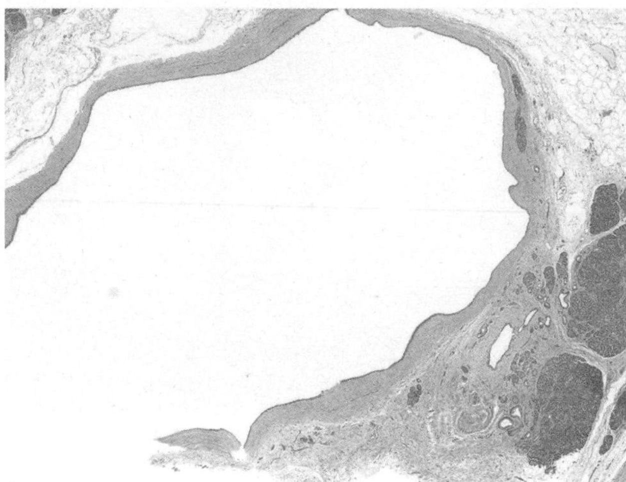

FIGURE 40.47 Squamoid cyst of the pancreas. This unilocular cyst is lined by squamous epithelium and lacks keratinization.

Squamoid Cyst of the Pancreas

A squamoid cyst of the pancreas is an uncommon nonneoplastic cyst that is lined exclusively by squamous epithelium.[189] These cysts have come to attention primarily because of the widespread use of cross-sectional imaging. The mean age of patients in one series was 63 years, and the male-to-female ratio was 1:1. The cysts range from 0.8 cm to 9 cm in diameter, with a median size of 1.5 cm.[189]

Pathology

Grossly, these unilocular cysts are well demarcated and surrounded by a thin fibrotic wall. Like most other benign cysts of the pancreas, they are devoid of solid areas. The cysts are reported to contain clear fluid, although white flaky material may also be identified.[189]

Histologically, the lesion is characterized by the presence of squamous epithelium that can vary from an attenuated layer to a well-developed layer of stratified squamous epithelium (Fig. 40.47 and 40.48). Multilayered epithelium with a transitional appearance is frequently seen, but keratinization is uncommon. The lining epithelium lacks cytological atypia. By definition, the lesion lacks mucinous or acinar epithelium. On immunohistochemistry, the squamous epithelium is positive for P63 and cytokeratin 5/6.

Differential Diagnosis

Squamoid cysts are easily distinguished from lymphoepithelial cysts by the absence of lymphoid tissue. Additionally, lymphoepithelial cysts invariably show keratinization and a prominent granular layer, features not seen in squamoid cysts of the pancreas. Squamous metaplasia, such as in acinar cell cystadenoma, may occasionally be identified in other cysts of the pancreas.[190] However, acinar cell differentiation, a characteristic feature of cystic acinar transformation, is absent in squamoid cysts of the pancreas.

Microscopic incidental cysts lined by squamous epithelium are not uncommon in the pancreas; one study identified such cysts in 10 of 110 pancreatectomy specimens.[189] Such incidental cysts should not be designated as squamoid cysts. In contrast with squamoid cysts of the pancreas, cystic squamous cell carcinomas always show high-grade cytological atypia.

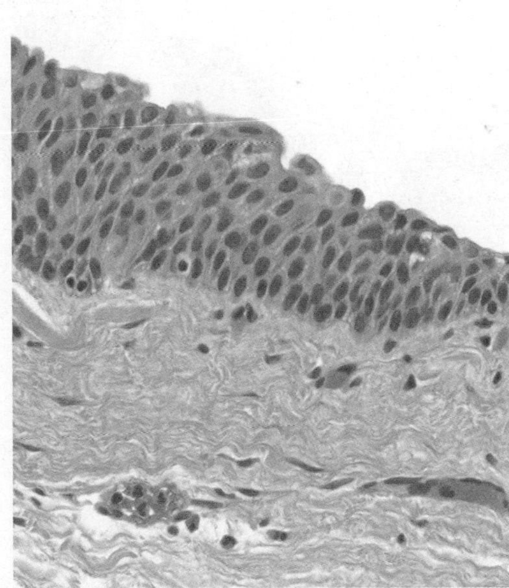

FIGURE 40.48 Squamoid cyst of the pancreas. High-power view of the image shown in Fig. 40.47.

Cystic Acinar Transformation (Acinar Cell Cystadenoma)

This cystic lesion of the pancreas, described in 2002, is lined by benign-appearing acinar cells.[191]

Clinical Features

This lesion is seen in young individuals (mean age, 41 years) and shows a distinct female predominance (male-to-female ratio, 1:3).[190-193] They are distributed throughout the pancreas. A substantial proportion of patients are asymptomatic, but some report abdominal pain. This is a benign neoplasm, and transformation to a malignant neoplasm has not been reported.

Etiopathogenesis

There is continuing debate as to whether this lesion represents a neoplastic entity.[190,193] The term *acinar cystic transformation of the pancreas* advocates a nonneoplastic alteration of the pancreas,[192] a contention supported by the detection of incidentally detected microscopic cysts lined by acinar cells. However, the presence of solid nodules composed of acinar cells and the presence of chromosomal aberrations on microarray-based comparative genomic hybridization suggest that at least a subset of these cysts are neoplastic.[190] Common genetic alterations associated with pancreatic ductal adenocarcinoma and its cystic precursor neoplasms have not been reported in these lesions.[194]

Pathological Findings

Either a single unilocular cyst is identified, or multiple cysts are seen (Fig. 40.49), sometimes involving most of the pancreas. The cyst wall is typically thin and translucent, filled with clear fluid, and lined with a single layer of cuboidal epithelium.[190-193] In part, the lining epithelium is nondescript, with basally placed nuclei and pale apical cytoplasm, often resembling normal ductal cells. The diagnosis relies on identification of acinar cell differentiation,[185,189-193] which can be revealed on hematoxylin and eosin stain by the presence of apical acinar granules and architectural evidence of acinar differentiation, either abortive or overt (Fig. 40.50). In a minority of cases, the proliferating acinar cells form intramural nodules. When overt acinar differentiation is identified, the lesional epithelium is readily distinguished from normal acinar cells by the presence of an irregular anastomosing pattern and the lack of intervening ductal structures or islets. Some cases also show intracystic, club-like, pseudopapillary structures with a fibrous stalk. The lining epithelium may be mucinous or squamous, albeit only focally. Within the lumen, eosinophilic lamellar concretions are frequently present.

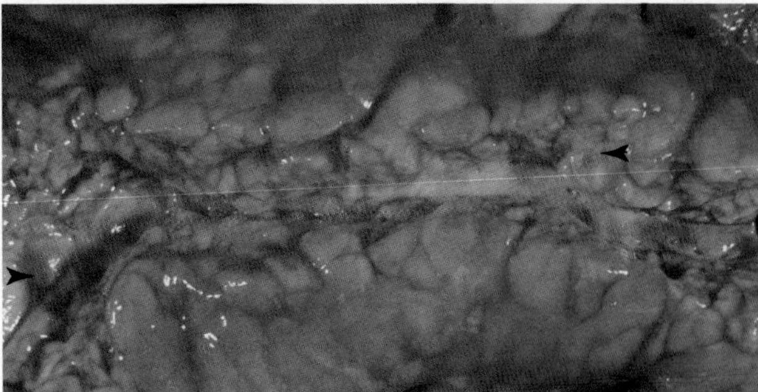

FIGURE 40.49 Acinar cystic transformation of the pancreas. Multiple thin-walled cysts *(arrowheads)* are seen adjacent to the main pancreatic duct. The cysts did not communicate with the main pancreatic duct.

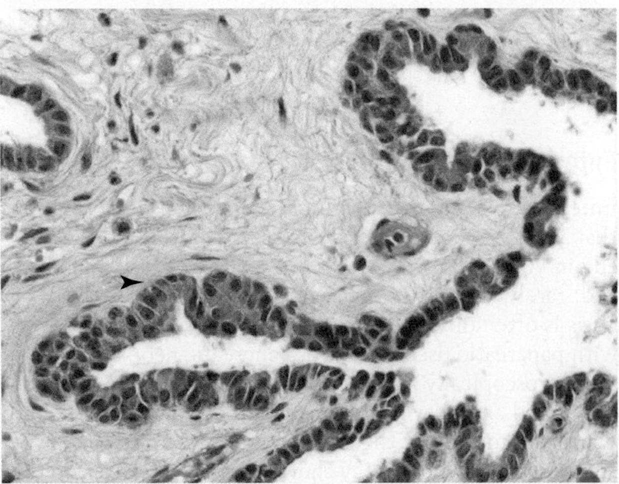

FIGURE 40.50 Acinar cystic transformation of the pancreas. A single layer of lining epithelial cells is seen. Occasional cells show apical red granules. Notice also the abortive acinar structures *(arrow)*.

Differential Diagnosis

Acinar cystic transformation is often confused with serous cystadenoma. The lining epithelial cells of a serous cystadenoma show clear cytoplasm and distinct cytoplasmic membranes. Additionally, the cells lining cystic transformation of the pancreas will stain for markers of acinar cell differentiation; staining for trypsin, chymotrypsin, and BCL10 ranges from focal to diffuse and is identified in the apical compartment of the cell.

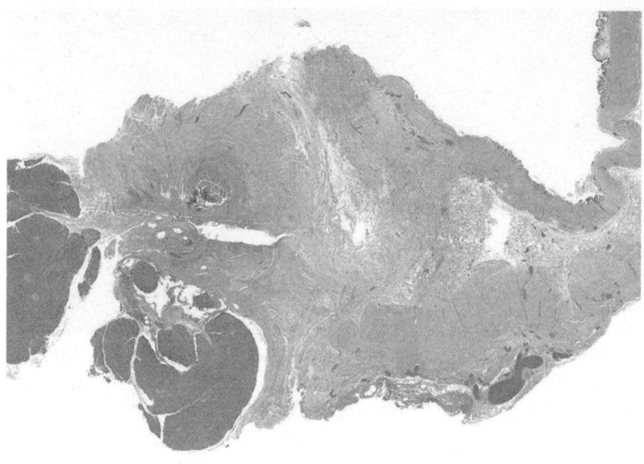

FIGURE 40.51 Enteric duplication cyst of pancreas. Note the two layers of smooth muscle surrounding the cyst.

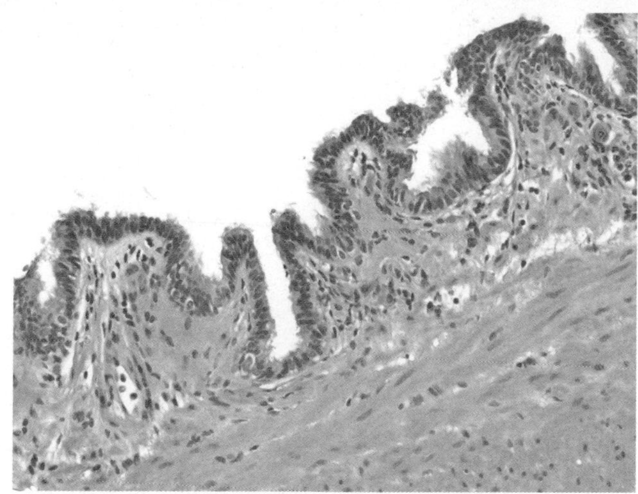

FIGURE 40.52 Enteric duplication cyst of pancreas. The cyst is lined by a single layer of columnar epithelium.

Enteric Duplication Cyst

Enteric duplication cysts are rare congenital malformations that are most commonly diagnosed in children and occasionally in young adults. Patients are seen with abdominal pain and, rarely, with acute pancreatitis. The preoperative diagnosis is often difficult because these cysts may be confused with pancreatic pseudocysts or pancreatic neoplasms.[195]

Microscopically, enteric duplication cysts show a well-developed and bilayer muscular wall. The lining epithelium varies and may be of the gastric type or the intestinal type. Alternatively, the cyst may show a simple columnar epithelium (Figs. 40.51 and 40.52).[196]

CONGENITAL AND HEREDITARY ABNORMALITIES OF THE EXOCRINE PANCREAS

There are a variety of congenital abnormalities of the exocrine pancreas—including cystic fibrosis; annular pancreas; aplasia, hypoplasia, and dysplasia of the pancreas; and congenital cysts—all of which are covered in Chapter 37.

The full reference list may be accessed online at *Elsevier eBooks for Practicing Clinicians.*

CHAPTER 41

Tumors of the Pancreas

David S. Klimstra, Olca Basturk, N. Volkan Adsay

Contents

INTRODUCTION AND CLASSIFICATION

Probably the most common problems in the diagnosis of pancreatic neoplasms are the distinction of invasive ductal adenocarcinoma from its mimics and the preoperative evaluation of cystic lesions, which are increasingly recognized. Solid, cellular pancreatic neoplasms present a different type of diagnostic challenge. The relative inaccessibility of the pancreas and the potential for complications from biopsies mean that small tissue samples (core biopsy or fine-needle aspiration [FNA] biopsy) are commonly the only specimens available for diagnosis, and for many patients, it is a biopsy of metastatic disease that is the basis for the diagnosis. This has become even more crucial with neoadjuvant therapy being more widely employed. Recent work has helped clarify the diagnostic features of cystic and intraductal neoplasms, neuroendocrine neoplasms, acinar cell neoplasms and related entities, as well as rare variants of ductal adenocarcinoma. A range of ancillary diagnostic tools are available to aid in accurate diagnosis, and correlation with clinical and radiographic findings is also helpful.

Through increased use of sensitive imaging techniques, such as spiral CT scanning, endoscopic ultrasound, magnetic resonance cholangiopancreatography (MRCP), and functional imaging, there has been an increase in detection of less common types of pancreatic tumors. In addition, advances in surgical techniques and improvements in postoperative care have rendered pancreatectomy a relatively commonplace operation, with markedly decreased mortality and morbidity. The past few decades have witnessed the characterization of several previously unrecognized types of pancreatic neoplasms and tumor-like lesions (such as autoimmune pancreatitis). The classification of pancreatic neoplasms and the delineation of the mechanisms of pancreatic neoplasia also have changed somewhat with the publication of the new World Health Organization classification in 2019.[1] In the following sections, the pathology of pancreatic neoplasms and tumor-like lesions is presented.

The current classification of pancreatic neoplasms is outlined in Box 41.1.[1,2] The classification system is based on three general features: (1) the line(s) of cellular differentiation reflected in the neoplasm,[3] (2) the gross configuration of the tumor (solid vs. cystic vs. intraductal), and, for the subgroup of potentially noninvasive neoplasms, (3) the degree of dysplasia (low- or high-grade).

The line of differentiation refers to the cellular phenotype of the neoplasm.[4] Most pancreatic tumors recapitulate one or more of the normal epithelial cell lines of the pancreas: ductal, acinar, or neuroendocrine (Fig. 41.1). The

BOX 41.1 Classification of Pancreatic Neoplasms

INVASIVE DUCTAL ADENOCARCINOMA
Tubular (conventional) adenocarcinoma
Colloid (mucinous noncystic) carcinoma
Medullary carcinoma
Adenosquamous carcinoma
Signet ring cell carcinoma
Hepatoid carcinoma
Undifferentiated carcinoma
- Anaplastic (giant cell) carcinoma
- Sarcomatoid carcinoma
- Carcinosarcoma

Undifferentiated carcinoma with osteoclast-like giant cells
Mixed ductal-neuroendocrine carcinoma

PANCREATIC INTRAEPITHELIAL NEOPLASIA (PanIN)
Low-grade PanIN
High-grade PanIN

INTRADUCTAL NEOPLASMS
Intraductal papillary-mucinous neoplasms
- Intraductal papillary-mucinous neoplasm with low-grade dysplasia
- Intraductal papillary-mucinous neoplasm with high-grade dysplasia (carcinoma in situ)
- Intraductal papillary mucinous neoplasm with an associated invasive carcinoma

Intraductal oncocytic papillary neoplasms
- Intraductal oncocytic papillary neoplasm
- Intraductal oncocytic papillary neoplasm with an associated invasive carcinoma

Intraductal tubulopapillary neoplasms
- Intraductal tubulopapillary neoplasm
- Intraductal tubulopapillary neoplasm with an associated invasive carcinoma

SEROUS NEOPLASMS
Microcystic serous cystadenoma
Macrocystic serous cystadenoma
Solid serous adenoma
Serous cystadenocarcinoma

MUCINOUS CYSTIC NEOPLASMS
Mucinous cystic neoplasm with low-grade dysplasia (mucinous cystadenoma)
Mucinous cystic neoplasm with high-grade dysplasia (carcinoma in situ)
Mucinous cystic neoplasm with an associated invasive carcinoma

ACINAR CELL NEOPLASMS
Acinar cell carcinoma
Cystic and intraductal acinar cell carcinomas
Cystic acinar transformation
Mixed acinar-neuroendocrine carcinoma
Mixed acinar-ductal carcinoma
Mixed acinar-neuroendocrine-ductal carcinoma

PANCREATOBLASTOMA

PANCREATIC NEUROENDOCRINE NEOPLASMS
Neuroendocrine microtumor
Well-differentiated pancreatic neuroendocrine tumor
- Functional
  - Insulinoma
  - Glucagonoma
  - Somatostatinoma
  - VIPoma
- Nonfunctional
  - PPoma
  - Not otherwise specified

Poorly differentiated neuroendocrine carcinoma
- Small cell carcinoma
- Large cell neuroendocrine carcinoma

SOLID PSEUDOPAPILLARY NEOPLASM

MESENCHYMAL NEOPLASMS
Lymphoma
Secondary neoplasms

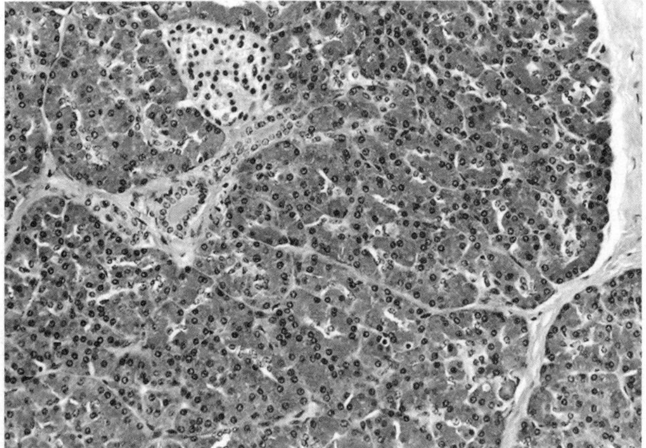

FIGURE 41.1 The normal pancreas. Most of the epithelial elements in the pancreas are acinar cells, which drain their secretions into the terminal portion of the ductal system (lined by centroacinar cells) and then into increasingly larger ducts. In the normal pancreas, the ducts are relatively inconspicuous and are lined by a single layer of cuboidal epithelial cells without obvious mucin. The third epithelial component, (neuroendocrine cells) are largely contained within the islets of Langerhans.

defining pathological features of each of these cell types are reflected, to various degrees, in their corresponding neoplasms (Table 41.1).

Ductal differentiation in pancreatic neoplasms is defined as recapitulation of the characteristics of normal ducts, that is, gland or tubule formation and mucin production. Mucin can be demonstrated histochemically with stains such as periodic acid–Schiff (PAS), mucicarmine, or high iron diamine and Alcian blue, and it is regarded as a hallmark of ductal differentiation in the pancreas, although it is not invariably present in neoplasms of ductal type. Immunohistochemical markers of ductal differentiation such as CA19-9, carcinoembryonic antigen (CEA), B72.3, DUPAN-2, and MUC1,[5] many of which detect mucin-related antigens or oncoproteins, are often helpful.[6] In addition, mutations at codon 12 of the *KRAS* oncogene are common (>90%) in ductal adenocarcinomas and are also present in many related carcinomas and preinvasive neoplasms of ductal type. Because *KRAS* mutations are not usually present in nonductal neoplasms, they may also be considered as evidence of ductal differentiation in certain situations. Expression of specific keratin subtypes, including cytokeratins 7 and 19 (CK7 and CK19), is characteristic of ductal neoplasms, but not lineage specific.

TABLE 41.1 Characteristics of Pancreatic Epithelial Cells and Corresponding Neoplasms

Cell Line	Light Microscopy	Histochemistry	Immunohistochemistry	Ultrastructure	Genetic Changes
Ductal	Glands, papillae, lumina, mucin	Mucin stains positive	Glycoprotein markers (B72.3, CEA, DUPAN2, MUC1, CA19-9)	Mucigen granules	*KRAS, TP53, DPC4, p16*
Acinar	Solid sheets, nests, acini; granular eosinophilic cytoplasm; prominent nucleoli	d-PAS positive granules	Enzyme markers (trypsin, chymotrypsin, lipase)	Zymogen granules, irregular fibrillary granules	APC/β-catenin pathway
Neuroendocrine	Nested, trabecular, gyriform patterns; cytological uniformity; salt-and-pepper chromatin	Argyrophil (Grimelius)-positive granules	Neuroendocrine markers (chromogranin, synaptophysin)	Neurosecretory granules	*MEN1* gene, *DAXX/ATRX* genes, mTOR pathway genes

Neuroendocrine differentiation is defined as the production of peptide hormones or bioamines by tumor cells.[3] In addition, well-differentiated pancreatic neuroendocrine tumors (PanNETs) often have an organoid growth pattern and a characteristic appearance of the nuclear chromatin. Neuroendocrine differentiation is documented mainly by immunohistochemistry. The general neuroendocrine markers, chromogranin A and synaptophysin, are considered most specific. Other neuroendocrine markers include neuron-specific enolase (NSE), Leu7 (CD57), and neural cell adhesion molecule (CD56), but the specificity of these has been questioned, and they are no longer recommended for the diagnostic confirmation of neuroendocrine differentiation.[7] A novel marker, insulinoma-associated protein 1 (INSM1), is still being assessed but appears to be quite specific.[8] The production of specific peptides or bioamines may also be demonstrable in certain PanNETs, but it is not necessary diagnostically. Electron microscopy may be used to identify dense core secretory granules, but this technique has been largely supplanted by immunohistochemistry.

Despite the preponderance of acinar cells among the epithelial elements of the pancreas, pancreatic neoplasms with acinar differentiation are uncommon.[3] In addition to having characteristic light microscopic features, acinar cell neoplasms produce zymogen granules containing pancreatic enzymes that can be detected by immunohistochemistry. Antibodies directed against trypsin and chymotrypsin are the most widely used,[9] and lipase, elastase, and a few others can also be detected.[9] The antibody BCL10 cross-reacts with carboxyl ester hydrolase and therefore also detects lipase and can verify acinar differentiation.[10] Zymogen granules can be demonstrated with PAS stain, which shows resistance to diastase (d-PAS) and typically reveals small, positive cytoplasmic granules. Zymogen granules can be visualized ultrastructurally as well. A second granule type, termed *irregular fibrillary granule,* is considered a highly specific ultrastructural feature of acinar cell neoplasms.[9]

Many primary tumors of the pancreas have a characteristic radiographic and gross appearance. Thus most can be divided into primarily solid or primarily cystic categories (Table 41.2). Several types of tumors are inherently cystic, with each locule lined by neoplastic epithelial cells. Others develop cystic change through a process of degeneration, necrosis, or both; this feature is characteristic of some entities, but it may occur in typically solid tumor types as well. Finally, intraductal tumors often appear cystic because of the presence of dilation of the native pancreatic ducts.

DUCTAL ADENOCARCINOMA AND VARIANTS

The ductal system of the pancreas, which is responsible for carrying acinar secretions to the duodenum, is not the most abundant epithelial component of the organ. However, most pancreatic neoplasms (>90%) are of ductal origin, and most of these (80% to 90%) are invasive ductal adenocarcinomas.[11] In general, the term *pancreas cancer* is used synonymously with ductal adenocarcinoma, despite the fact that there are many other carcinoma types that arise within this organ. It is this type of neoplasm that imbues pancreatic cancer with such a dismal outlook. The diagnosis of ductal adenocarcinoma remains problematic for pathologists.

Pancreatic carcinomas of ductal type are separated into the following three general categories:

1. Conventional ductal adenocarcinoma, which consists of small, tubular glands with luminal and intracellular mucin, associated with marked stromal desmoplasia.
2. Unusual histological variants of conventional ductal adenocarcinoma, such as foamy gland pattern, large duct pattern, vacuolated pattern, and lobular carcinoma-like pattern.
3. Other carcinomas of ductal origin, such as colloid carcinoma, adenosquamous carcinoma, squamous cell carcinoma, medullary carcinoma, hepatoid carcinoma, and undifferentiated carcinomas. Carcinomas in this last category often have an associated conventional ductal adenocarcinoma component, which provides evidence of their ductal origin.

Invasive Ductal Adenocarcinoma (Conventional Ductal Adenocarcinoma, Tubular Adenocarcinoma)

Clinical Features

This is the most common type of pancreatic neoplasm and is one of the most lethal of all human cancers. According to the American Cancer Society, it is estimated that there will

TABLE 41.2 Solid and Cystic Pancreatic Neoplasms

Typically Solid Neoplasms	Typically Cystic Neoplasms
Ductal adenocarcinomas (and variants)	Serous cystic neoplasms
Pancreatic endocrine neoplasms	Mucinous cystic neoplasms
Acinar cell carcinomas	Intraductal papillary mucinous neoplasms
Pancreatoblastomas	Solid pseudopapillary neoplasms
	Lymphoepithelial cysts

be 60,430 new cases and 48,220 deaths in the United States in 2021, and the number of new cases appears to have risen significantly over the past few decades. The age-adjusted incidence rate is 11 per 100,000 individuals.[12] Pancreatic cancer is the third leading cause of death from cancer in the United States and accounts for 7% of cancer deaths. Affected patients are usually between 60 and 80 years of age; occurrence in patients younger than 40 years of age is unusual.[13] Patients usually present with jaundice (caused by invasion and obstruction of the common bile duct) when the carcinoma is in the head of the pancreas, or they present with nonspecific symptoms such as back pain and weight loss.[14] The cause of ductal adenocarcinoma is complex and probably multifactorial. Smoking and high intake of dietary fat are considered risk factors.[15-18] Whether acquired chronic pancreatitis and diabetes mellitus constitute risk factors is a subject of ongoing debate, although patients with hereditary chronic pancreatitis and tropical calcifying pancreatitis are considered at increased risk.[19-22] Although most ductal adenocarcinomas are sporadic, pancreatic cancer is familial in about 10% of cases. The genetic basis for most (80%) familial cases is unknown, but heritable genetic syndromes that increase the risk of pancreas cancer are known, such as hereditary breast cancer syndrome (resulting from *BRCA2* or, less commonly, *BRCA1* mutations), FAMMM (familial atypical multiple-mole melanoma) syndrome (resulting from *CDKN2A* mutations), Peutz-Jeghers syndrome (resulting from *STK11/LKB1* mutations), familial pancreatitis (resulting from *PRSS1* mutations), hereditary nonpolyposis colorectal cancer (HNPCC) syndrome (resulting from mutations in DNA mismatch repair genes), and Fanconi's anemia (resulting from *FANC-C* and *FANC-G* mutations).[23-30] Some families also carry germline mutations in *PALB2* and *ATM*.[31-33] Patients with familial pancreatic carcinoma also appear to develop intraductal papillary mucinous neoplasms (IPMNs) at an increased frequency.[34,35] Recently, an anatomic variation normally seen in 10% of the population, low union, in which the cystic duct adjoins the common bile duct in the intrapancreatic location or immediately above the pancreas border, has been detected in 42% of ordinary ductal adenocarcinomas of the head and 73% of distal common bile duct (CBD) cancers.[36] This, combined with the fact that most pancreatic adenocarcinomas occur in the head, has led to the speculation that change in flow pattern and chemical composition of bile may be a factor in the ductal carcinogenesis. It is believed this may also be linked to the other peculiar risk factors identified in epidemiological studies such as history of cholecystectomy, peptic ulcer disease, and periodontal conditions.

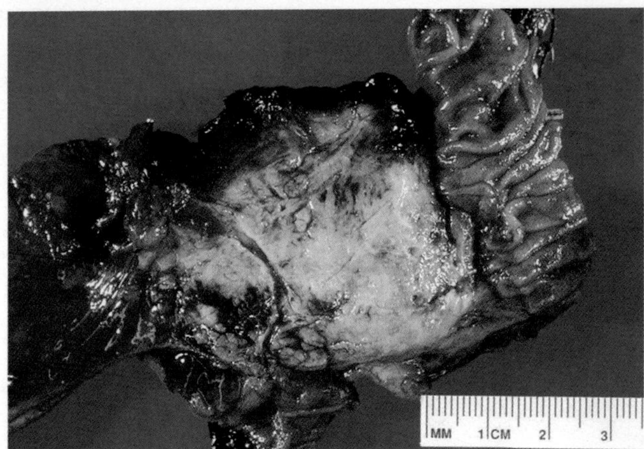

FIGURE 41.2 Gross appearance of ductal adenocarcinoma. The tumor is solid, white to yellow, and ill-defined, occupying much of the head of the gland.

Most ductal adenocarcinomas (>75%) are solid tumors, and 60% to 70% develop in the head of the pancreas.[37] Possibly because of the lack of a capsule surrounding the pancreas, ductal adenocarcinomas typically involve surrounding structures, especially the common bile duct, duodenum, and peripancreatic soft tissues, early in the course of the disease, when the tumors are relatively small. Ductal adenocarcinomas that develop in the tail of the pancreas may spread to surrounding organs (spleen, kidney, stomach, and colon).[37] In fact, if a solid pancreatic tumor measures larger than 5 cm and is still resectable, it is unlikely to represent a ductal adenocarcinoma. Most cases (close to 80%) are unresectable at the time of diagnosis,[38] largely because of encasement of major mesenteric vessels[39] or metastases to the liver, peritoneum, or other sites. Many ductal adenocarcinomas disseminate very early in the course of disease, although some data suggest that the subset of cases lacking mutations in *SMAD4* (*DPC4*) remains more localized to the pancreas and adjacent structures.[40]

Pathological Features

Grossly, most ductal adenocarcinomas are solid, firm, infiltrative tumors (Fig. 41.2) with ill-defined borders. The cut surface is often gritty or slightly gelatinous.[41,42] Less commonly, gross areas of necrosis may be present. It is often difficult to distinguish a carcinoma from adjacent areas of fibrosing chronic pancreatitis, which commonly coexists. For tumors in the head of the gland, direct invasion of the common bile duct and duodenum is common. The major pancreatic ducts coursing through the carcinoma are usually narrowed or even completely obliterated. Recognition that the center of the tumor is grossly located within the head of the pancreas is helpful in distinguishing pancreatic ductal adenocarcinomas (PDACs) from primary carcinomas of the common bile duct, duodenum, or ampulla of Vater. Some ductal adenocarcinomas exhibit cystic change, either from necrosis with cystic degeneration, as a result of cystic dilation of obstructed ducts (retention cyst formation), or because of cystic dilation of the neoplastic glands themselves (large duct pattern; see later discussion).[43] In

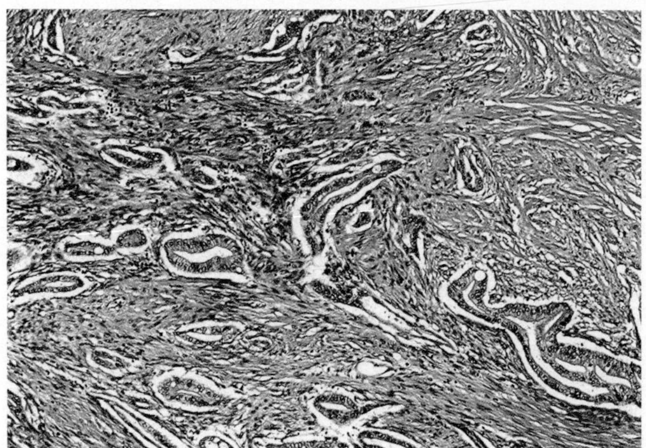

FIGURE 41.3 Ductal adenocarcinoma. The tumor consists of variably sized, well-formed glands surrounded by abundant desmoplastic stroma.

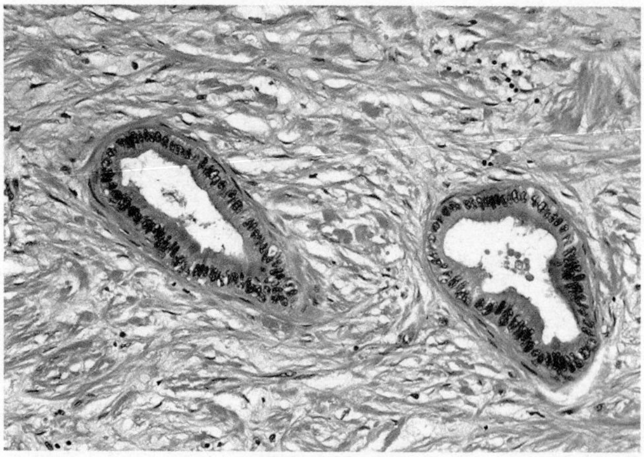

FIGURE 41.4 Well-differentiated ductal adenocarcinoma. Some infiltrating carcinomas consist of remarkably well-formed glands and exhibit relatively minimal cytological atypia, mimicking benign ductules.

some cases, invasive ductal adenocarcinomas may be associated with a preexisting noninvasive cystic or intraductal neoplasm, such as a mucinous cystic neoplasm (MCN) or an intraductal papillary mucinous neoplasm. Some ductal adenocarcinomas have central necrosis and form a more demarcated tumor similar to centrally necrotizing/hyalinizing carcinomas described in the breast, and this seems to be more commonly associated with high-grade carcinomas showing metaplastic changes including sarcomatoid and squamoid.

Microscopically, in its conventional form, ductal adenocarcinoma is characterized by small tubular structures lined by cuboidal mucinous cells associated with abundant desmoplastic stroma[44] (Fig. 41.3). In well-differentiated ductal adenocarcinomas, the growth pattern and cytological appearance of the cells may be deceptively benign, closely mimicking nonneoplastic ductules characteristic of chronic pancreatitis (Fig. 41.4). Malignant glands usually replace the normal lobular arrangement of benign ducts with haphazardly arranged tubules. The cells that line malignant glands typically form a single regular layer, but stratification and irregular papillae may be prominent in some cases as well. The cytoplasm of the tumor cells may be abundant and generally contains mucin; clear cell change is also common. Some nuclei retain basal orientation within the cells, but loss of polarity in some of the glands is typical. The nuclei typically vary in size, shape, and intracellular location between cells within each gland (Fig. 41.5). A variation in size of more than fourfold between adjacent nuclei is a feature considered highly suggestive of carcinoma. Perineural invasion and vascular invasion are common and diagnostically useful, although these features often are not detected in core needle biopsies. In some cases, tumor cells infiltrate adjacent normal islets. Invasion into peripancreatic adipose tissue is also common. In fact, the finding of immediate juxtaposition of a gland with an adipocyte (without intervening stroma, so-called *naked glands* in fat) is a strong sign of malignancy.[45] Another helpful feature in the differential diagnosis of benign from malignant glands is the finding of glands situated adjacent to muscular blood vessels because normal pancreatic ducts are usually separated from large blood vessels by a considerable amount of acinar

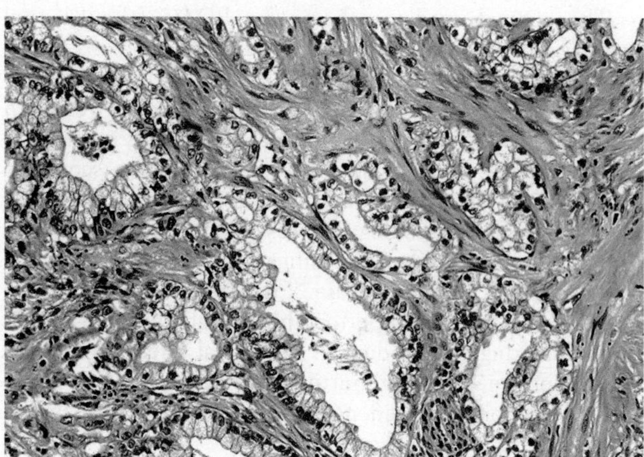

FIGURE 41.5 Moderately differentiated ductal adenocarcinoma. The nuclei show variability in size, shape, and location within the cells.

parenchyma.[46,47] This feature is less helpful when the pancreas is profoundly atrophic, however. In poorly differentiated ductal adenocarcinomas, the neoplastic glands are usually admixed with small clusters of cells with ill-formed lumina, pleomorphic nuclei, and abundant mitotic figures (Fig. 41.6). In fact, it is common for ductal adenocarcinomas to exhibit a mixture of very-well-formed glands along with individual cells or solid clusters.

The periphery of ductal adenocarcinomas is often quite indistinct, such that neoplastic glands may be present well beyond the apparent gross extent of the tumor. The finding of isolated glands within otherwise normal peripancreatic adipose tissue, several millimeters from the nearest edge of the carcinoma, confounds the measurement of the tumor and the evaluation of the soft tissue margins.[45] Invasion of preexisting epithelial structures, such as the common bile duct, duodenal mucosa, blood vessels, or native pancreatic ducts, can result in colonization of the basement membrane of the invaded structure,[48] which may simulate a preinvasive neoplasm, such as a duodenal adenoma or pancreatic intraepithelial neoplasia (PanIN). Continuity of intraductal neoplastic cells with frankly invasive elements supports an interpretation of colonization.

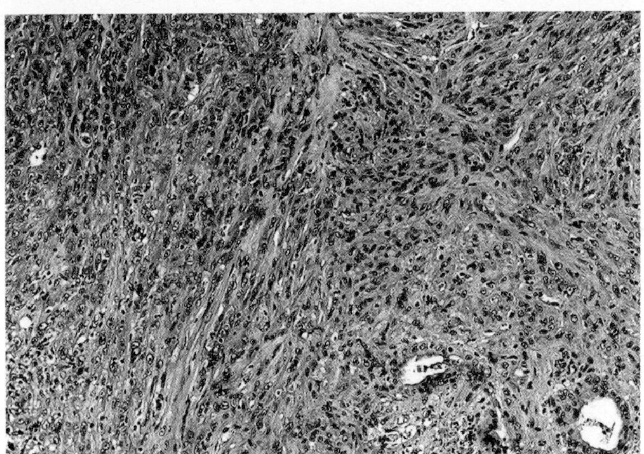

FIGURE 41.6 Poorly differentiated ductal adenocarcinoma. The tumor exhibits minimal gland formation, instead growing as clusters and individual cells with marked cytological atypia.

The current grading scheme for PDAC (the Kloppel grading scheme, also endorsed by the WHO) entails evaluation of glandular differentiation, mucin production, mitoses, and nuclear atypia.[49] This scheme correlates well with prognosis but is rather cumbersome; hence, it is not widely used. Another proposal advocates assigning two scores to the most prevalent and second most prevalent patterns, mirroring Gleason grading for prostate carcinoma; this system is more independently significant in predicting outcome but is also not in common use.[50] In fact, most pathologists grade PDAC based simply on the extent of gland formation, mirroring the grading of colorectal adenocarcinoma. The American Joint Committee on Cancer (AJCC) staging parameters for ductal adenocarcinoma are available in the AJCC staging manual.[51]

Chronic pancreatitis (interstitial fibrosis, atrophy, and modestly dense inflammation) is often present in the pancreatic tissue adjacent to ductal adenocarcinomas. Distinction of chronic pancreatitis from carcinoma is discussed later (see Differential Diagnosis). In addition, the lining of native pancreatic ducts may show proliferative changes (PanIN, see later). Squamous, transitional, intestinal, and rarely, oncocytic[52] metaplasia may be seen within the nonneoplastic ducts.[53]

Ancillary Diagnostic Tests and Molecular Properties

Mucin histochemical stains and immunohistochemical markers of ductal differentiation (glycoproteins) invariably show at least focal positivity within conventional ductal adenocarcinomas. In addition, stains for cytokeratins (CKs) 7, 8, 18, and 19 and epithelial membrane antigen (EMA) are usually positive. CK20 is detected in about 25% of cases, and its expression is usually less widespread and intense than that of CK7. The exception to this cytokeratin expression pattern is colloid carcinoma, in which CK20 expression is strong and diffuse (see later discussion).[54,55] Immunohistochemical markers of glycoproteins often detectable in ductal adenocarcinoma include CA19-9, CEA, B72.3, CA125, and DUPAN-2. Of these, CEA, B72.3, and CA125 are regarded as tumor-associated glycoproteins that are not significantly expressed in normal ductal cells, and they are expressed only to a limited degree in low-grade PanIN.[56] The MUC proteins are also expressed in different types of ductal neoplasms to varying degrees. Most conventional ductal adenocarcinomas express MUC1, MUC3, MUC4, and MUC5AC.[55,57-60] In contrast, MUC2 is not expressed in ductal adenocarcinomas other than those with intestinal differentiation, such as colloid carcinoma (see later discussion). MUC6, a marker of pyloric gland differentiation, is expressed in 35% of ductal adenocarcinomas.[61] Stains for chromogranin or synaptophysin may demonstrate a minor neuroendocrine cell component associated with the neoplastic glands. Some neuroendocrine cells are nonneoplastic islet cells entrapped within the tumor because ductal adenocarcinomas have a propensity to invade islets. However, neoplastic neuroendocrine cells also occur within ductal adenocarcinomas.[62,63]

The molecular alterations in ductal carcinomas have been studied extensively in past decades. A comprehensive genomic analysis of over 20,000 genes disclosed that most cases have primarily point mutations, which average 63 per tumor.[64] Twelve core signaling pathways were altered in 67% to 100% of the tumors. The most commonly mutated genes include *KRAS*, *p16/CDKN2A*, *TP53*, and *SMAD4*.[65,66] Mutations in codon 12 of the *KRAS* oncogene are detected in more than 90% of ductal adenocarcinomas, and *TP53* mutation occurs in 50%. Most ductal adenocarcinomas also harbor abnormalities in *CDKN2A*, through either mutation or hypermethylation of the promotor region of DNA.[67] Loss of SMAD4 (DPC4) is also found in 55% of invasive ductal adenocarcinomas.[68,69] There are many other molecular abnormalities in ductal adenocarcinoma,[67] but this previously mentioned constellation of genetic changes is characteristic and distinguishes ductal adenocarcinomas from pancreatic neoplasms of other cell lineages. Other pathways commonly altered include apoptosis, regulation of the G1/S phase transition, hedgehog signaling, DNA damage control, cell adhesion, integrin signaling, JNK signaling, control of invasion, GTPase signaling, transforming growth factor (TGF)-β signaling, and notch signaling.[64] Mutations in mismatch repair genes, *BRCA2*, *STK11/LKB1*, *BRAF*, *TGFBR2*, and *MAP2K4* are less common, but some of these underly the hereditary cases of pancreatic ductal carcinoma.[66] Analysis of gene expression has revealed a number of other overexpressed molecules within ductal adenocarcinomas (e.g., fascin, mesothelin, claudin-4, S100AP, S100A6, and S100P), some of which have been used as potential immunohistochemical markers to help distinguish reactive (nonneoplastic) glands from carcinoma.[70-76] Strong immunoexpression of p53, or complete loss of immunoexpression of DPC4, can be used to support a diagnosis of carcinoma, although both of these markers lack a high degree of sensitivity.

Differential Diagnosis Including Chronic Pancreatitis versus Carcinoma

The main diagnostic consideration for conventional ductal adenocarcinoma is the distinction of a well-differentiated carcinoma from benign ductules in areas of atrophic chronic pancreatitis.[77] Ductal adenocarcinoma may appear deceptively bland, and ductules in chronic pancreatitis may appear infiltrative. On low-power examination, ductules in areas of chronic pancreatitis retain the original lobular configuration of the normal pancreas because they represent the residual intralobular ductules remaining after the loss of acinar

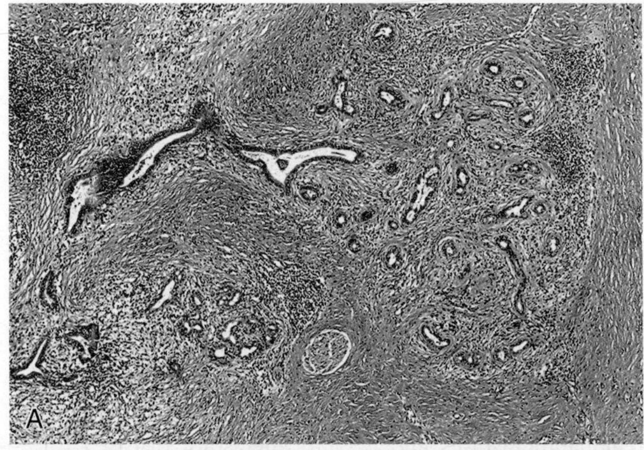

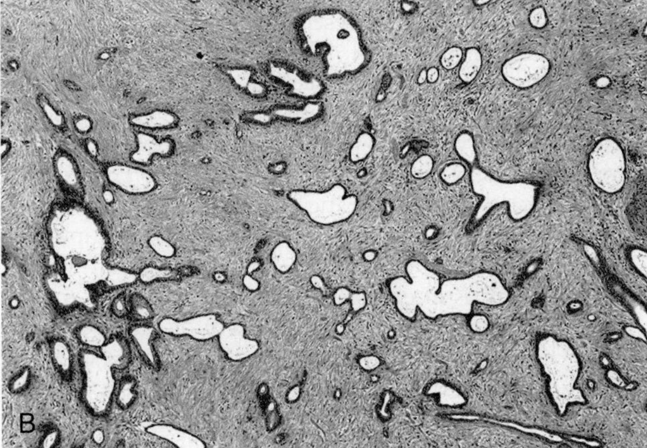

FIGURE 41.7 Comparison between atrophic chronic pancreatitis and well-differentiated ductal adenocarcinoma. In these low-power images, the example of chronic pancreatitis **(A)** shows retention of the lobular architecture of the gland, with larger, dilated central ducts surrounded by smaller round ductules. The stroma separating each lobule is somewhat denser than the intralobular stroma. In contrast, adenocarcinoma **(B)** shows a haphazard arrangement of neoplastic glands, and lacks a lobular configuration.

elements during atrophy. Each lobular cluster of ductules contains a central larger, branched, slightly dilated duct surrounded by small round ductules (Fig. 41.7). The stroma within each lobule often is less dense than that between lobules. In contrast, invasive glands lack a lobular growth pattern and are usually distributed more haphazardly (see Fig. 41.7). The contours of individual glands are also usually irregular and angulated. Some glands may be incomplete, with epithelium lining only part of the neoplastic lumen and stroma lining the rest. Cytologically, nuclear enlargement, nuclear contour irregularities, and loss of nuclear polarity are important clues to a diagnosis of carcinoma. Variation in size, shape, and intracellular location between adjacent nuclei within individual glands indicates malignancy. The finding of a nuclear volume variation of 4:1 is considered highly suspicious for carcinoma. Dense acidophilic cytoplasm is more common in carcinoma compared with benign conditions. Unlike other sites where reactive stromal cells may display significant atypia, pleomorphism and bizarre nuclei are uncommon in the stroma of inflammatory conditions of the pancreas. Thus individual atypical cells within the stroma of the pancreas are much more likely to be cancer cells, especially if they contain dense acidophilic cytoplasm.

The finding of atypical glands in abnormal locations is also helpful. For instance, perineural or vascular invasion, invasion of the duodenal muscularis propria, invasion of stroma closely adjacent to a muscular vessel,[46,47] and immediate juxtaposition of duct to adipocytes[45] are all features considered nearly 100% diagnostic of carcinoma (Fig. 41.8). Familiarity with the morphological spectrum of ductal adenocarcinomas including those of the variants such as foamy gland,[78] large duct,[79] and vacuolated[80] (see the Morphological Patterns of Ductal Adenocarcinoma section) may also aid in this differential.

Invasive ductal adenocarcinoma should also be differentiated from noninvasive PanIN (see later), which can be challenging because high-grade PanIN displays most of the cytological abnormalities of invasive carcinoma. Evaluation of the number, distribution, and location of the individual glandular units (in relation to the lobular architecture) is helpful in this pathological distinction. Furthermore, the presence of desmoplastic stroma and irregularity of ductal contours are features of invasive carcinoma. Pancreatic ducts do not contain a basal or myoepithelial cell layer, and many of the abnormalities of invasive carcinoma are also present in high-grade PanIN; therefore no immunohistochemical stains can reliably determine whether a specific atypical gland is invasive. When the differential diagnosis on a core needle biopsy includes high-grade PanIN and invasive carcinoma, it is worth considering that high-grade PanIN is rarely encountered in the absence of invasive carcinoma somewhere in the gland, especially when there is a pancreatic mass.

Another potential pitfall in the differential diagnosis of ductal adenocarcinoma is aggregation of islets in atrophic chronic pancreatitis[81] (Fig. 41.9). Clustered islets may form small irregular nests or cords of cells that have an infiltrative appearance. Occasionally these islet cells are situated around small nerve fibers, simulating perineural invasion by carcinoma. However, the uniformity of cells, the presence of round nuclei with neuroendocrine-type chromatin, and lack of glandular lumina all help point toward a benign reactive process. Immunolabeling for neuroendocrine markers (chromogranin and synaptophysin) can be helpful in problematic cases.

Adenocarcinomas of other organs can resemble PDAC, especially carcinomas arising in the biliary tree or upper gastrointestinal tract. Metastases to the pancreas from sites such as the lung, breast, or gynecological organs can be confused for pancreatic primary tumors, but more commonly, it is the liver or peritoneal metastasis for which a pancreatic primary tumor is considered, along with multiple other organs.[82] Although the immunophenotype and molecular profile of PDAC mentioned earlier is characteristic, it is not sufficiently specific to be useful in the distinction from adenocarcinomas of other sites. Coexpression of CK7, CK19, CEA, CA19-9, B72.3, and CA125 can occur among multiple primary adenocarcinomas, and the lack of expression of lung markers (TTF1, Napsin-A) or hormone receptors does not exclude origin in the lung, breast, or gynecological tract. It should be noted here that the differential diagnosis of adenosquamous carcinoma as a primary versus secondary tumor could be the most problematic, and adenosquamous carcinoma originating from the lung may lack TTF1. Clinical and radiographic correlation is often needed to define

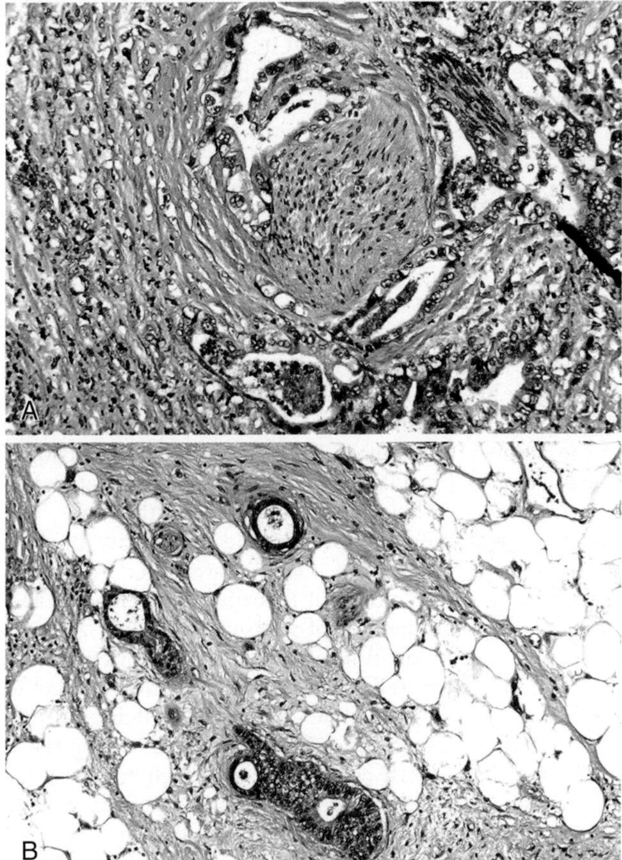

FIGURE 41.8 Findings diagnostic of ductal adenocarcinoma. Perineural invasion **(A)** is virtually diagnostic of invasive carcinoma, provided the epithelial structures are gland forming. Immediate juxtaposition of ducts to adipocytes **(B)** is also a very helpful finding.

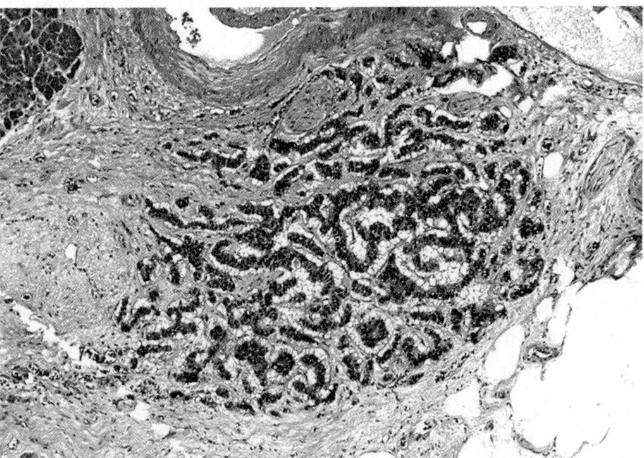

FIGURE 41.9 Pancreatic atrophy with aggregation of islets. The neuroendocrine cells in this focus exhibit a trabecular configuration, suggesting they originated from the diffuse islets located in the posterior head of the pancreas. The pseudoinfiltrative nature of these neuroendocrine cells may simulate an invasive carcinoma.

the primary site in these cases. In the distinction between metastatic pancreatic carcinoma and primary cholangiocarcinoma, in situ hybridization for albumin may be helpful because the small duct (peripheral) type of cholangiocarcinoma is positive, and pancreatic carcinomas are negative.[83]

Natural History

As mentioned earlier, the prognosis of patients with PDAC is dismal.[84] The overall 5-year survival rate is about 10%.[85] Its biological properties including its ability for insidious spread, common neural involvement, and vascular involvement early on are all believed to play a role in its highly aggressive behavior. A major contributor to the poor prognosis is the advanced stage at presentation for most patients: 49.6% of cases of newly diagnosed pancreatic carcinomas present with distant metastases, 29.1% present with regional lymph node involvement, and only 10.8% have tumors that are localized solely within the pancreas (Surveillance Epidemiology and End Results (SEER)-21, 2008–2017). Survival rates are stage-dependent: 39.4% for localized disease, 13.3% for regional metastases, and 2.9% for metastatic disease (SEER-18, 2010–2016). Surgical resection is considered the best hope for long-term survival.[86] However, only about 30% of ductal adenocarcinomas are resectable at the time of diagnosis. In addition to high-resolution CT scanning, laparoscopy is used to identify radiographically occult metastatic disease before laparotomy.[38] Over time, the proportion of patients with very-early-stage pancreatic carcinoma (stage IA and IB) has increased, and the survival of these patients has improved. The 5-year survival for stage IA (node-negative, measuring less than 2 cm) is in excess of 80%.[87] Note, however, that the survival for other resectable stages of disease (stage IIA and IIB) has improved only marginally, emphasizing the need to diagnose pancreatic carcinoma very early; only 1.8% of the patients in this SEER analysis were diagnosed at stage I. Survival beyond 7 to 8 years is exceedingly uncommon, and patients may still die of their pancreatic carcinoma after 5 years.[88] Some authors advocate adjuvant therapy (chemotherapy and radiation) after surgery, and neoadjuvant treatment is increasingly used before surgery. Cases that are unresectable are usually treated with chemotherapy. Current chemotherapy protocols include mainly gemcitabine or 5-FU, often in combination with other agents.[89]

Morphological Patterns of Ductal Adenocarcinoma

Ductal adenocarcinoma of the pancreas includes, in addition to its conventional tubular pattern, several morphological variations. The clinical and biological characteristics of these patterns do not differ significantly from those of conventional ductal adenocarcinoma, but the morphological features are distinctive and may raise differential diagnostic issues. These patterns are often found focally within otherwise typical ductal adenocarcinomas.

Foamy Gland Pattern

This pattern represents a subtle, well-differentiated carcinoma that mimics benign glands with low-grade PanIN.[78] This variant is characterized by infiltrating, well-formed glands lined by fairly well polarized columnar cells that contain abundant, pale microvesicular cytoplasm. The nuclei are typically confined to the base but wrinkled in appearance, with indentations caused by the cytoplasmic contents (Fig. 41.10). The most characteristic features that help distinguish this variant from low-grade PanIN are the presence of foamy, microvesicular, pale cytoplasm with vesicles that are small, fine, and evenly sized, and apical chromophilic condensation of the cytoplasm that forms a thin, well-delineated

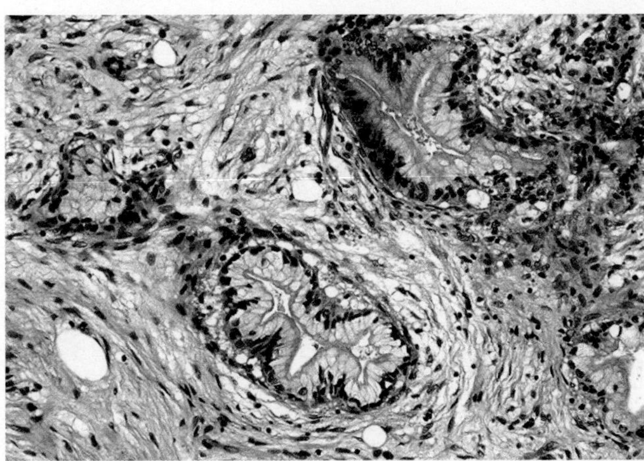

FIGURE 41.10 Ductal adenocarcinoma with a foamy gland pattern. The tumor exhibits well-formed ductal structures, simulating a low-grade intraductal proliferation. There is abundant, foamy cytoplasm with thick apical cytoplasmic condensation. Only subtle nuclear abnormalities are present.

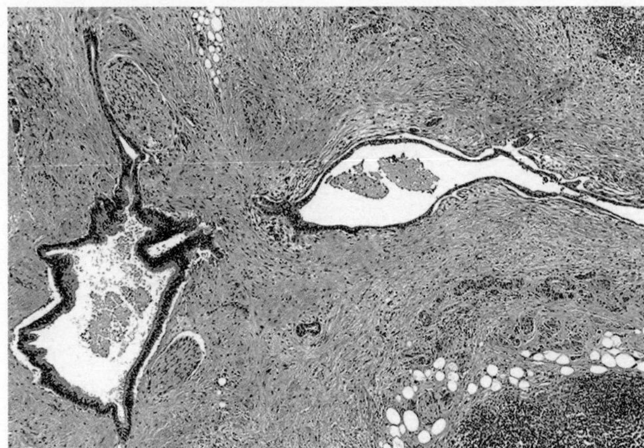

FIGURE 41.11 Ductal adenocarcinoma with a large duct pattern. The invasive neoplastic glands are ectatic, resembling dilated native ducts, but the configuration is irregular, and smaller, more typical infiltrating glands also are present.

band reminiscent of a brush border. Although the apical condensation is strongly positive with mucin markers, the microvesicular component of the cytoplasm is typically negative (in contrast with ducts involved by PanIN that are often PAS positive). p53 is also often abnormally expressed in the nuclei of these malignant glands.

Large Duct Pattern

Occasionally, invasive tubular adenocarcinomas show a microcystic appearance because of ectasia of infiltrating neoplastic glands (Fig. 41.11).[79] For unclear reasons, this phenomenon may be particularly pronounced in regions of the tumor infiltrating the muscularis propria of the duodenum. Although microcystic glands may be detected grossly, cystic change is generally not pronounced enough to be detected radiographically as a "cystic mass." The cytological appearance of the epithelium may be deceptively bland. They also often have a cribriform pattern and papilla or micropapilla formation that creates a picture indistinguishable from IPMN or PanIN, especially if a given duct is examined out of context. Patients with tumors that contain a large duct pattern have only a slightly longer survival rate compared with patients who have conventional ductal adenocarcinoma. Thus it is important to distinguish cystic dilation of an invasive gland from a noninvasive component of an MCN or intraductal neoplasm, both of which have a much more favorable prognosis. Features that favor large duct–type adenocarcinoma are the presence of clustering of glands, haphazard distribution, angulations and irregularity of the contour of the ducts, and the presence of a desmoplastic stroma. Tumor cells also often contain intraluminal necrotic debris with neutrophils.

Vacuolated Pattern

This pattern reveals a gland-in-gland architecture in which tumor cells form cribriformed nests punctuated by multiple large vacuoles (or microcysts) that contain cellular debris and mucin (Fig. 41.12). These vacuoles apparently form by the merging of multiple intracytoplasmic lumina that punctate a nest or cluster of cells. This is different than the cribriform pattern displayed by colonic adenocarcinomas, which typically have polarization of cells that create glands and rosettes. Focally, vacuolated cells have the morphological features of adipocytes or signet ring cells.[80] This pattern may be helpful in the differential diagnosis of metastatic tumors of unknown origin because it is seen only rarely in other types of adenocarcinoma.

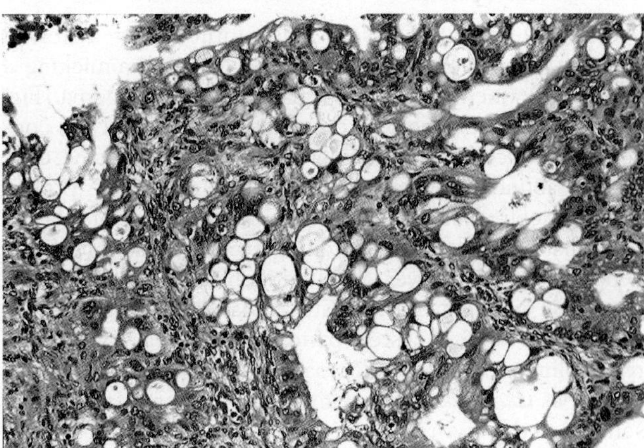

FIGURE 41.12 Ductal carcinoma with a vacuolated pattern. Solid nests of cells are punctuated by multiple large empty vacuoles.

Poorly Cohesive Cell Pattern

Occasionally, ductal adenocarcinoma may display a focal pattern of growth similar to that of mammary lobular carcinoma.[90,91] Instead of forming tubules, the tumor cells form cords and may have an "Indian-file" appearance (Fig. 41.13). Targetoid patterns, as well as individual cell infiltration, may also be present, often with signet ring cell formation.[92] This growth pattern may remotely mimic diffuse-type gastric adenocarcinoma and is often associated with conventional tubular-type ductal adenocarcinoma elsewhere in the tumor. However, it is almost never of the type that is seen in true poorly cohesive cell carcinomas. In fact, a true signet ring carcinoma or poorly cohesive cell carcinoma occurring in this region should be considered secondary from either ampulla or stomach before it can be classified as a pancreatic primary tumor.[93]

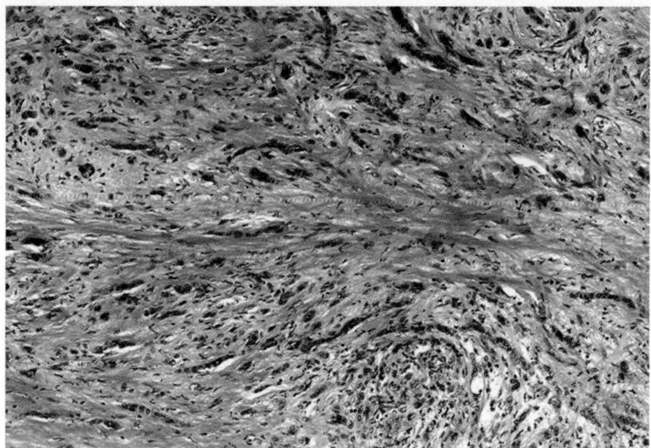

FIGURE 41.13 Ductal carcinoma with a poorly cohesive cell pattern. Small neoplastic cells are arranged in thin cords without lumen formation, resembling mammary lobular carcinoma.

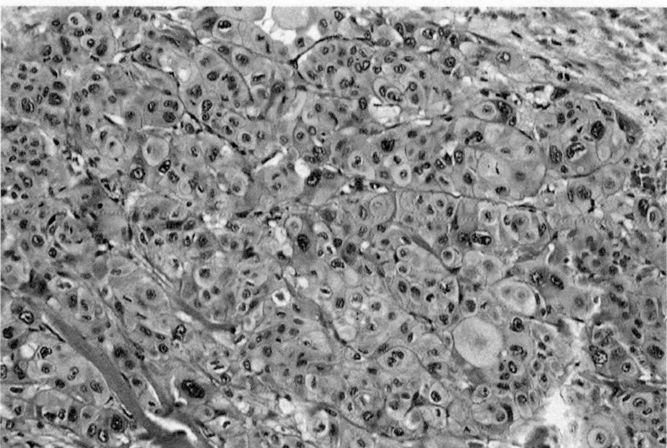

FIGURE 41.14 Ductal carcinoma with a solid nested pattern. There are large cells with pleomorphic nuclei and abundant eosinophilic cytoplasm.

Solid Nested Pattern

Poorly differentiated PDACs may infiltrate in a nested pattern without prominent gland formation, mimicking a neuroendocrine neoplasm or squamous cell carcinoma (Fig. 41.14). However, most of these cases contain foci of conventional ductal adenocarcinoma. In some cases, the cells display abundant acidophilic cytoplasm and single prominent nucleoli. This creates a picture reminiscent of a hepatocellular carcinoma (hepatoid pattern) or an oncocytic neoplasm.[94,95] However, the immunohistochemical staining pattern is different from hepatocellular carcinoma. In some cases, cells with a nested pattern show clear cytoplasm, resembling renal cell carcinoma. Some authors refer to this variant as *clear cell carcinoma.*[96,97] In a recent study, these solid-nested growth patterns were found to be a part of the centrally necrotic/hyalinizing carcinomas, akin to those in the breast.[98,99]

Micropapillary Pattern

Some poorly differentiated ductal adenocarcinomas exhibit a micropapillary pattern, with solid clusters of cells suspended in lacunar spaces (Fig. 41.15). The micropapillary pattern is generally a focal finding within an otherwise conventional ductal adenocarcinoma, but it can be extensive. Infiltration of neutrophils in regions with the micropapillary pattern has been noted.[100] As in other anatomic locations, pancreatic carcinomas with a micropapillary pattern are particularly aggressive.

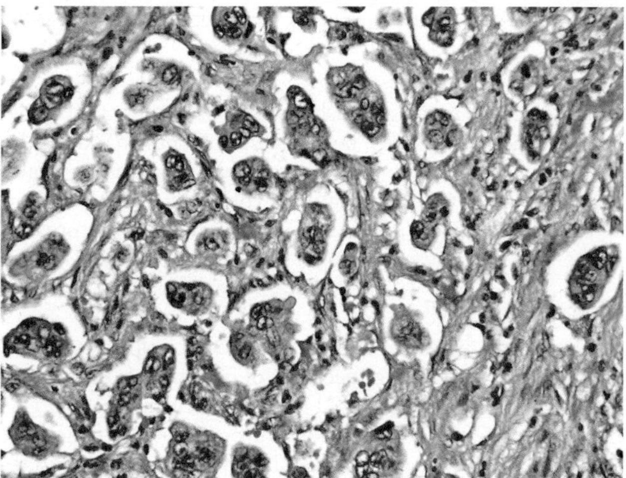

FIGURE 41.15 Ductal carcinoma with a micropapillary pattern. Clusters of tumor cells are suspended in lacunar spaces.

Other Pancreatic Carcinomas of Ductal Origin

Colloid Carcinoma

Colloid carcinoma is a clinically and biologically distinct type of pancreatic adenocarcinoma of ductal lineage, but it has to be viewed differently than ordinary ductal adenocarcinomas.[101] Whereas the tumor types discussed earlier are clinically aggressive, colloid carcinomas have a more indolent clinical course. Colloid carcinoma, previously referred to as *mucinous noncystic carcinoma,* is characterized by stromal pools of mucin containing scant malignant epithelial cells arranged as strips, stellate or cribriform clusters, small tubules, or individual signet ring cells (Fig. 41.16).

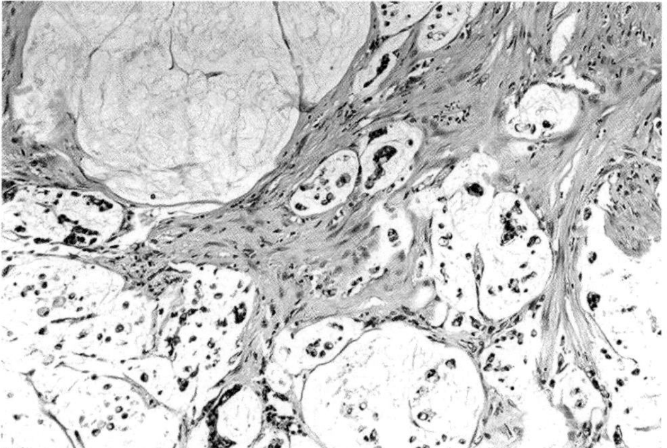

FIGURE 41.16 Colloid carcinoma (mucinous noncystic carcinoma). The tumor is composed of large stromal mucin lakes in which are suspended relatively scanty strips and clusters of cells, with individual cells having a signet ring configuration.

Colloid carcinomas are usually associated with an intraductal papillary mucinous neoplasm of intestinal type.[102] Colloid carcinomas have a more favorable clinical course than invasive carcinomas of conventional ductal type. The 5-year survival rate is 55%, compared with 12% to 15% for conventional ductal adenocarcinomas.[101,103] Some patients died of thromboembolic complications. In one study, all patients who died had a history of an incisional biopsy, which raises the possibility that disruption of the integrity of the tumor may cause dissemination of these highly mucinous lesions.[101] Colloid carcinomas share intestinal differentiation (expression of CK20, MUC2, and CDX2) with IPMNs of intestinal types.[104] Although these tumors harbor similar molecular abnormalities as conventional ductal adenocarcinoma (mutations in *KRAS* and *TP53*), they are less frequent in colloid carcinomas. Furthermore, loss of DPC4 essentially never occurs in colloid carcinomas.[101,105]

Medullary Carcinoma

Similar to medullary carcinomas in the breast and large intestine, medullary carcinoma of the pancreas is defined as having broad sheets of poorly differentiated cells with a syncytial pattern of growth. They are much more common in the ampulla. In fact, before a case of medullary carcinoma can be classified as primary, the possibility of an ampullary origin must be ruled out with thorough evaluation. Of note, the differences in the frequency of microsatellite instability (and PDL1) reported for "pancreatic" cancers may partly be attributed to the inclusion of ampullary cancers as pancreatic.[106-108] As described in other organs, the periphery has pushing borders, and the tumor is mostly devoid of a desmoplastic reaction but can exhibit tumor-infiltrating lymphocytes (Fig. 41.17).[109,110] Experience with these tumors is limited. Their natural history and prognosis are poorly understood, but they do not appear to be significantly different from conventional ductal adenocarcinomas. In contrast with conventional ductal adenocarcinoma, some medullary carcinomas are associated with genetic alterations commonly seen in medullary carcinomas of the colon (microsatellite instability), and the rate of *KRAS* mutations is low.[109] Some patients have a personal or family history of colon cancer, which raises the possibility of an associated inherited cancer syndrome.

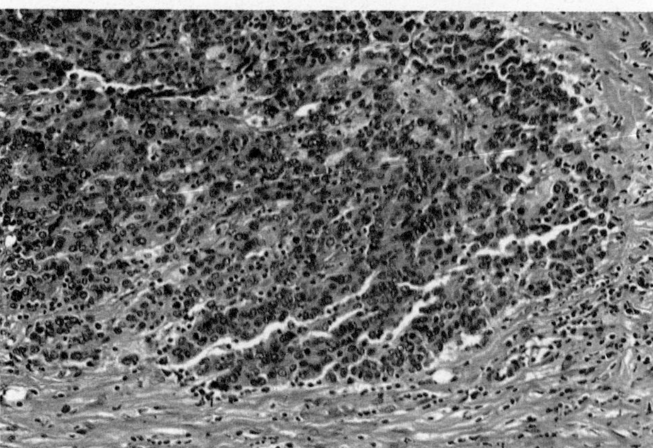

FIGURE 41.17 Medullary carcinoma. The tumor is poorly differentiated, lacks gland formation, and has a pushing growth pattern at the periphery. The tumor cells are large and appear syncytial. There is a lymphocytic infiltrate between tumor cells.

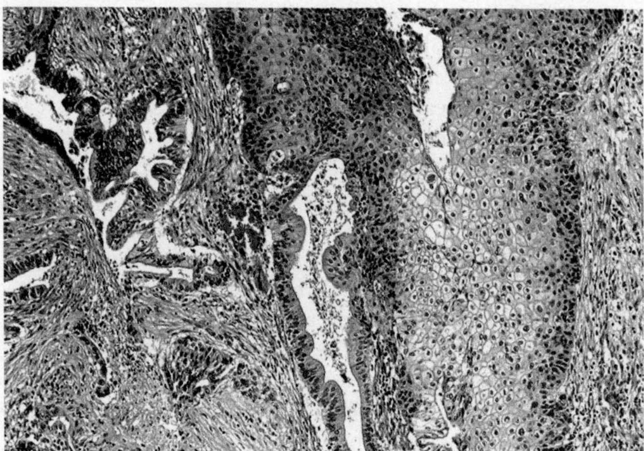

FIGURE 41.18 Adenosquamous carcinoma. The tumor contains neoplastic glands resembling conventional ductal adenocarcinoma as well as large nests of cells with squamous differentiation.

Squamous Cell Carcinoma and Adenosquamous Carcinoma

These tumors constitute approximately 2% of all pancreatic cancers.[111-113] They are more prevalent in the tail of the pancreas.[37] Some cases reveal an adenoacanthoma appearance (adenocarcinoma with benign-appearing squamous elements), whereas others may show a combination of adenocarcinoma with either a well-differentiated keratinizing squamous cell carcinoma, poorly differentiated squamous carcinoma without keratinization, or basaloid squamous cell carcinoma. Because small foci of squamous differentiation are not uncommon in ductal adenocarcinomas, an arbitrary squamous component of 30% has been proposed for a carcinoma to be regarded as adenosquamous.[2] Pure squamous cell carcinoma (without a glandular component) is exceedingly rare. Most cases contain a glandular component (e.g., adenosquamous carcinoma) on careful histological examination (Fig. 41.18), and any amount of glandular differentiation is sufficient for a predominantly squamous carcinoma to be regarded as adenosquamous. The clinical outcome of these tumors is proving to be even poorer than that of conventional ductal adenocarcinoma. There is an evolving impression that they are more resistant to the mainline PDAC treatments as well. Adenosquamous carcinomas share many genomic alterations with conventional ductal adenocarcinoma but also may have *UPF1* mutations.[114] In a recent study, a group of cases characterized by central necrosis/hyalinization (also often showing more demarcated growth) commonly exhibit squamoid morphology even in the absence of squamous markers. This entity typically also shows other metaplastic and anaplastic differentiation and sarcomatoid change.

Hepatoid Carcinoma

Extremely rarely, pancreatic carcinomas may show bona fide hepatocellular differentiation. Hepatoid carcinomas have a solid, nested, or trabecular architecture and are composed of polygonal-shaped cells with granular eosinophilic cytoplasm, centrally located nuclei, and prominent nucleoli.[115-118] Bile pigment may be present. Stains for hepatocellular differentiation are typically positive, including hepatocyte paraffin-1, polyclonal CEA (canalicular), and CD10 (canalicular). Alpha-fetoprotein (AFP) also may be expressed in these tumors. The differential diagnosis of hepatoid carcinoma includes acinar cell carcinoma and pancreatoblastoma, both of which can also express AFP,[119] and intraductal oncocytic papillary neoplasm, which consistently stains for hepatocyte paraffin-1 but is not believed to possess true hepatocellular differentiation.[120] This is exceedingly uncommon, and for a case with pure hepatoid morphology without ordinary ductal adenocarcinoma component the possibility of a metastasis from a primary hepatic carcinoma or a hepatoid PanNET[121] must be excluded first.

Undifferentiated Carcinoma

Like other organs, the pancreas may give rise to a family of neoplasms that show little or no morphological evidence of epithelial differentiation. In theory, undifferentiated carcinomas may arise from any of the epithelial cell lines within the pancreas. However, most undifferentiated carcinomas are believed to represent ductal neoplasms. Often, evidence for ductal origin stems from the finding of a ductal adenocarcinoma component within an otherwise undifferentiated carcinoma. In some cases, mutations in oncogenes typical of ductal carcinomas (such as *KRAS*) have been identified in undifferentiated carcinomas.[122,123] There are several histological types of undifferentiated carcinomas, such as spindle cell (sarcomatoid) carcinoma, carcinosarcoma, anaplastic giant cell carcinoma,[124] and undifferentiated carcinoma with osteoclast-like giant cells (discussed later). The histological features of the first three of these tumors overlap, with the sarcomatoid components consisting of either anaplastic giant cells or spindle cells (Fig. 41.19), sometimes containing heterologous stromal differentiation (e.g., bone, cartilage, skeletal muscle).[125] The designation *carcinosarcoma* is used when a separate glandular component is also present, which results in a biphasic appearance (Fig. 41.19B). In some cases, the undifferentiated elements retain immunohistochemical positivity for epithelial markers, such as keratin or EMA. In others, evidence of epithelial differentiation is absent, even at the immunohistochemical level. If these tumors lack an associated glandular component, they are essentially indistinguishable from undifferentiated sarcoma. Cases that reveal differentiation along a definable mesenchymal line may, in fact, be classified as primary sarcomas of the pancreas, even though they may have originated from an epithelial precursor. A recently recognized variant of undifferentiated carcinoma of the pancreas has prominent rhabdoid features and is associated with frequent abnormalities in genes in the SWI/SNF complex, such as *SMARCA4* or *SMARCB1*.[126] With the possible exception of undifferentiated carcinoma with osteoclast-like giant cells, the prognosis of undifferentiated carcinomas is extremely poor, possibly even poorer than that of conventional ductal adenocarcinoma.

Undifferentiated Carcinoma with Osteoclast-like Giant Cells

This type of undifferentiated carcinoma shares histological features with certain poorly differentiated neoplasms of other epithelial organs, sarcomas, and even melanoma. However, most striking examples of this tumor type are seen in the pancreas.[127] In all of these situations, undifferentiated neoplasms occur that contain a combination of neoplastic plump spindle cells and nonneoplastic osteoclast-like giant cells.[128-132] Within the pancreas, many undifferentiated carcinomas with osteoclast-like giant cells

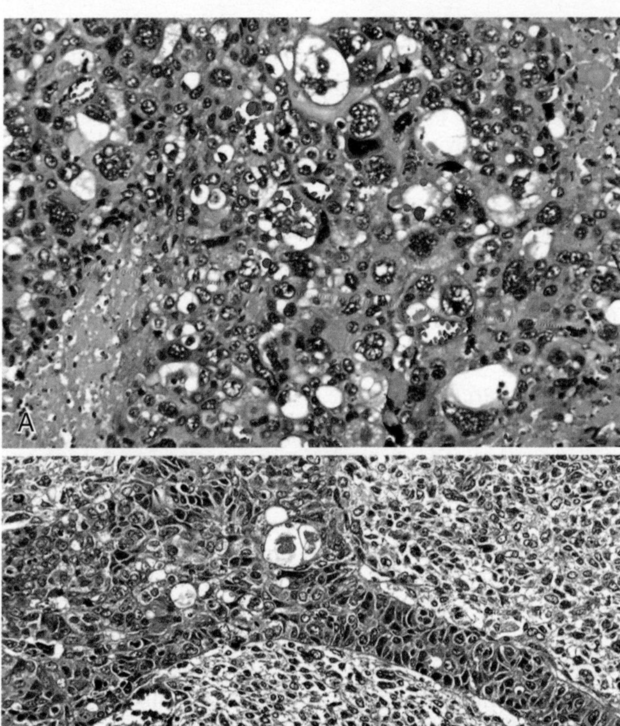

FIGURE 41.19 Undifferentiated carcinoma. Patterns of undifferentiated carcinoma include anaplastic giant cell carcinoma **(A),** with enormous tumor cells growing in solid sheets and having markedly atypical nuclei, and carcinosarcoma **(B),** in which the tumor exhibits a biphasic pattern of glandular epithelium and sarcomatoid elements.

contain a separate glandular component or are associated with a preinvasive neoplasm, such as an MCN[133,134] or PanIN. The neoplastic elements are usually moderately to markedly atypical, noncohesive, and somewhat epithelioid in shape. A variable number of osteoclast-like giant cells, with multiple nuclei showing only mild atypia (Fig. 41.20), are typically scattered randomly among the neoplastic elements. A component of mononuclear histiocytic cells is also present within these tumors.[135] Some cases also contain anaplastic giant tumor cells in addition to osteoclast-like giant cells. The osteoclast-like cells have phagocytic capability and may contain engulfed neoplastic cells within the cytoplasm. The giant cells are of histiocytic origin, as demonstrated by positive immunohistochemical staining for CD68 (see Fig. 41.20B).[136,137] Anaplastic giant cells and mononuclear neoplastic cells are generally undifferentiated at the immunohistochemical level, with keratin expression often restricted to only the associated glandular component, if present. Interestingly, mutations in the *KRAS* oncogene have been detected within the neoplastic elements of undifferentiated carcinomas with osteoclast-like giant cells.[136,137] The molecular profile of these tumors appears to be different from the other undifferentiated carcinomas of the pancreas.[138]

Some cases have a less aggressive clinical course than conventional ductal adenocarcinoma, with a 5-year survival

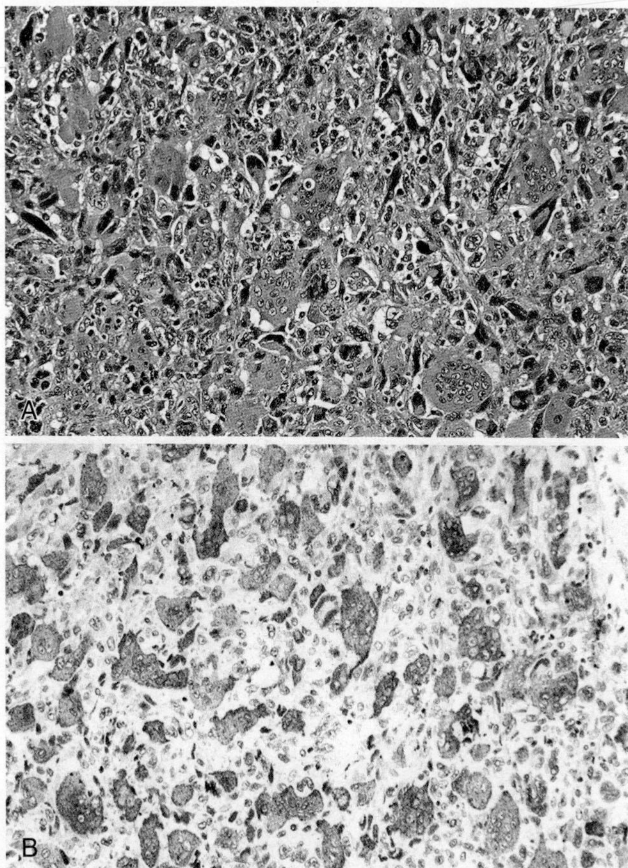

FIGURE 41.20 Undifferentiated carcinoma with osteoclastic giant cells (osteoclastic giant cell carcinoma). This tumor contains neoplastic undifferentiated cells that vary from epithelioid to spindle in shape, mixed with varying numbers of nonneoplastic multinucleated osteoclasts **(A).** Immunohistochemical staining for CD68 **(B)** demonstrates the histiocytic nature of the osteoclast-like giant cells.

rate as high as 59%.[127] This protracted course appears to be more common in examples with abundance of osteoclasts and paucity of ductal component.

PANCREATIC INTRAEPITHELIAL NEOPLASIA

Precursors of ductal adenocarcinoma have been identified as a series of increasingly atypical proliferative changes within the epithelium of the pancreatic ducts. Many of these lesions have long been recognized, but only reported with descriptive terminology.[139-142] Early lesions, those with minimal cytological atypia, were not originally regarded as neoplastic, and instead were designated as *hyperplasia* or *metaplasia*. However, more recent molecular data have established most ductal proliferative lesions as neoplastic.[140] Thus the entire spectrum of ductal proliferative lesions is now commonly referred to as *PanIN*,[140] which originally was graded on a three-tier scale (PanIN1A, 1B, 2, and 3), but is now more simply designated as *low-grade* or *high-grade* PanIN (the prior PanIN2 category regarded to be low-grade).[143]

All PanIN lesions contain cytoplasmic mucin, which is not normally observed in pancreatic ductal cells, except occasionally in the largest interlobular ducts. Low-grade PanIN encompasses a range of histological changes previously designated *mucinous metaplasia* or *mucous cell hypertrophy, papillary hyperplasia,* and *atypical hyperplasia* (Fig. 41.21A–C). Because low-grade PanIN lesions harbor clonal mutations in the *KRAS* oncogene,[144,145] they are regarded as neoplastic. Low-grade PanIN reveals replacement of the normal nonmucinous cuboidal epithelium with mucinous columnar cells, either with a flat, undulating, or papillary architecture. The earliest lesions have well-polarized nuclei lacking atypia or loss of polarity. PanIN lesions with full-thickness nuclear stratification and mild nuclear atypia are also low-grade PanIN, but were previously considered PanIN2 (see Fig. 41.21C). High-grade PanIN (previously termed *carcinoma in situ* or *severe dysplasia*) shows significant loss of polarity, tufting of cells into the lumen, marked irregularity of nuclei, increased mitotic figures, and sometimes necrosis (see Fig. 41.21D). Most of the molecular abnormalities identified in invasive ductal adenocarcinomas have also been detected in PanIN, particularly in high-grade lesions. Some molecular changes occur early in the sequence (*KRAS* mutations), some in the middle stages (*CDKN2A* loss), and others only in the late stage (*DPC4* and *TP53* mutations).[144,146,147]

PanIN is a relatively frequent incidental finding. Nearly 50% of older adults have foci of low-grade PanIN in their pancreas.[148] High-grade PanIN is significantly more common in pancreata that contain invasive ductal carcinoma and is rare as an isolated finding. Foci of PanIN found in association with other tumor types or in pancreata without neoplasms are most often low grade.[149] In fact, high-grade PanINs are so uncommon to encounter in the absence of invasive adenocarcinoma that it becomes difficult to ascertain colonization (ductal spread of invasive carcinoma) from a true precursor lesion.[143] The natural history of these lesions is essentially unknown, especially because of the difficulty of detecting PanIN in other than pancreas resection specimens. Only rare cases have been documented in which a PanIN lesion was identified before the development of invasive carcinoma.[150] Thus treatment recommendations have been challenging to develop.[151] Although it is difficult to determine its biological significance, foci of high-grade PanIN identified in a pancreas resection specimen should be reported, particularly in cases that lack invasive carcinoma. Low-grade PanIN is extremely common and is generally considered an incidental finding with a very low risk for progression to carcinoma and therefore of negligible clinical significance.[152] Ideally, detection of pancreatic neoplasia at the high-grade PanIN stage would provide an opportunity for cure that is, essentially, lost once the affected patient develops overt clinical symptoms. Efforts to screen patients for high-grade PanIN have been thwarted by the lack of serum biomarkers and reproducible radiographic findings, although in patients with a strong family history of pancreatic carcinoma, there may be subtle radiographic findings of localized lobular atrophy that can herald the presence of PanIN.[34]

PanIN should be distinguished from well-differentiated invasive ductal adenocarcinoma, which may be difficult on the basis of a biopsy specimen in which the underlying ductal architecture is challenging to recognize. In addition, PanIN shares many cytological features with IPMNs (see Intraductal Papillary Mucinous Neoplasms). Although most IPMNs are larger than PanINs and involve cystically

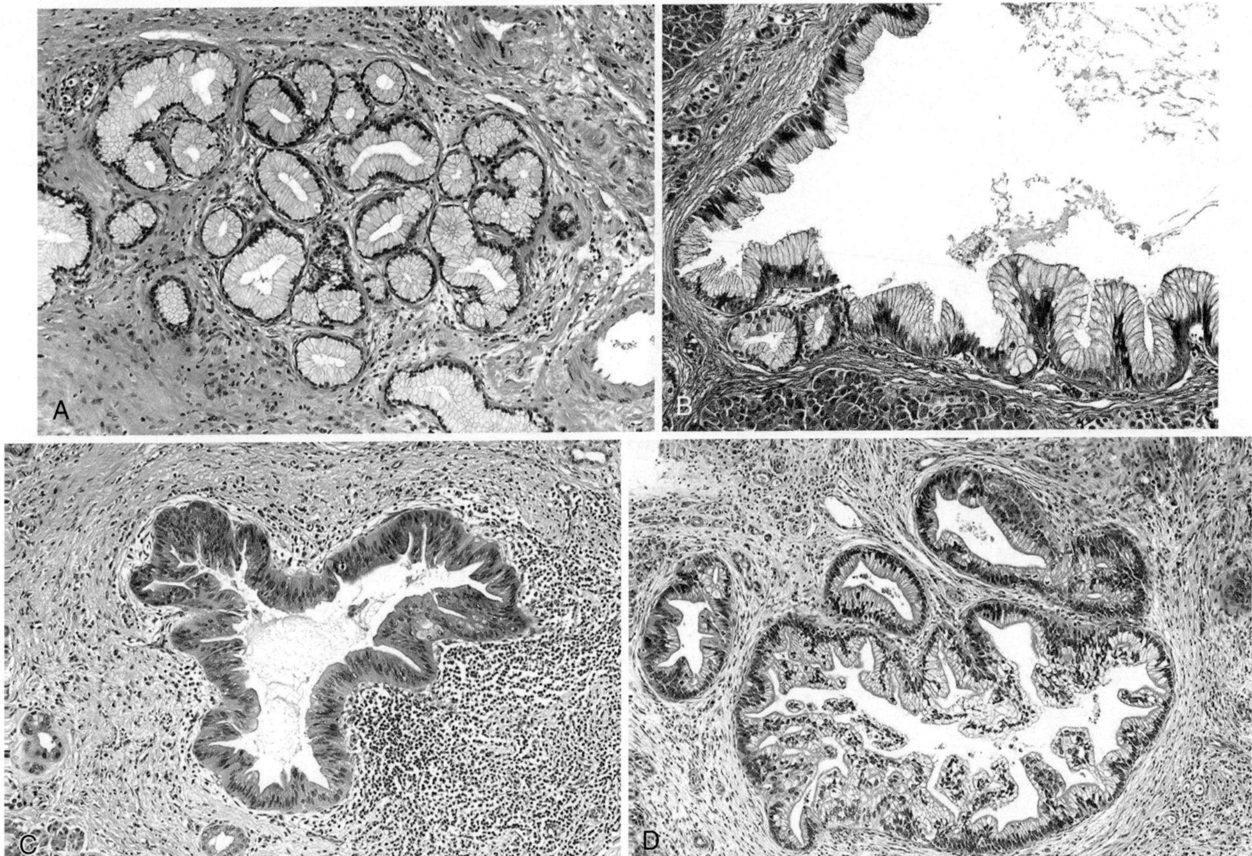

FIGURE 41.21 Pancreatic intraepithelial neoplasia (PanIN). In low-grade PanIN **(A)**, small ductules are usually lined by tall, columnar mucinous epithelial cells without loss of polarization or nuclear atypia, but some lesions **(B)** may have papillae and micropapillae or **(C)** exhibit full-thickness nuclear pseudostratification and mild to moderate nuclear atypia. High-grade PanIN **(D)** exhibits more substantial cytoarchitectural abnormalities, including complete loss of polarity with budding of unsupported epithelial tufts into the gland lumen. Marked nuclear atypia is also present.

dilated ducts that measure at least 1 cm in diameter, distinction of these two types of intraductal neoplasms may be nearly impossible in some cases. Furthermore, both PanIN and IPMN may be present within the same pancreas.[151,153,154]

INTRADUCTAL NEOPLASMS

Intraductal neoplasms have rapidly become one of the most widely studied groups of pancreatic tumors, and they are being detected much more frequently in recent years because of the increased use of cross-sectional imaging.[155-171] The vast majority of "incidentaloma" cysts discovered in the pancreas prove to belong to this category if resected. These tumors have very distinctive clinical and radiographic findings. In addition, they often lack a component of invasive carcinoma and are therefore amenable to surgical resection. Many cases appear radiographically cystic, and the preoperative distinction of an intraductal neoplasm from true cystic neoplasms, such as serous or MCNs, can be difficult.[78] Most important, intraductal neoplasms exhibit a spectrum of neoplastic progression,[155] from the earliest neoplastic changes to invasive carcinoma, but unlike PanIN lesions associated with conventional ductal adenocarcinomas, intraductal neoplasms are clinically detectable, providing an excellent model of preinvasive neoplasia in the pancreas.[104,171]

Intraductal Papillary Mucinous Neoplasms

Clinical Features

IPMNs are grossly and radiographically visible tumors characterized by an intraductal proliferation of mucin-producing cells, usually (but not always) arranged in a papillary pattern.[156-160] These tumors are usually associated with intraluminal mucin accumulation and cystic dilation of the ducts, and they can either be localized or involve the entire ductal system. Mucin spillage into the duodenum through the ampulla of Vater is an endoscopic finding virtually diagnostic of IPMN but is seen in only a small percentage of cases.[161,172] Depending on the location of the primary process and subsequent mechanical changes within the pancreatic ducts, IPMNs may present as a multilocular cystic mass or as abundant papillary nodules. Papilla formation may be microscopic or macroscopic, the latter appearing as large nodular masses within the dilated ducts. The various patterns that can occur in IPMNs led to a wide variety of designations for this group of tumors before their unification under the term *IPMN*. Previous terms include *mucinous duct ectasia (ductectatic mucinous cystadenoma)*[163,164] *mucin-producing tumor, villous adenoma of the pancreatic duct*,[167] and *intraductal papillary tumor*, each describing a different facet of this tumor type.[168,171] IPMNs are the most common cystic neoplasm of the pancreas. The larger and more complex examples that manifest clinically are typically seen in the seventh to eighth decades of life. A history of pancreatitis is noted in some patients. IPMNs in asymptomatic patients are often detected incidentally during abdominal imaging performed for other indications. Endoscopic findings (mucin extrusion through the ampulla of Vater) and radiographic findings (ectasia of the ducts) are diagnostic features. IPMNs occur mainly (80%) in the head of the pancreas. IPMNs are separated based on the extent of involvement of the ductal system into main duct and branch duct types, which is valuable in the preoperative management algorithm (discussed further later).[171]

Pathological Features

Careful macroscopic examination is imperative to document the intraductal nature of the tumor. The extent of ductal dilation and the amount of gross papilla formation vary from case to case and even regionally within an individual case (Fig. 41.22).[171] The tumor can primarily involve the major pancreatic ducts (main duct type). However, other cases are limited to involvement of the secondary ducts (branch duct type), particularly in the uncinate process and in the body and tail of the pancreas.[169,170,173] Branch duct IPMNs may appear as multiple separate small cysts both grossly and radiographically because of the tortuous nature of the dilated ducts. In fact, in these cases, connection to the ductal system may be difficult to demonstrate grossly. Preoperative separation of IPMNs into main duct and branch duct types is of clinical importance because the main duct type has a greater likelihood of harboring high-grade dysplasia or invasive carcinoma, and small (<3 cm) branch duct IPMNs may not require surgical resection if they lack other worrisome findings such as mural nodules and interval growth during follow-up.[171,173-175]

IPMNs may be localized, multicentric, or rarely the entire ductal system of the organ may be involved. High-grade dysplasia and invasive carcinoma may be focal, so it is vital to thoroughly sample the specimen to search for carcinoma, which is present in about 35% of resected cases.[176]

Microscopically, mucinous cells with various degrees of atypia line the cystically dilated ducts (Fig. 41.23). Three different papillary patterns have been described.[104,156,177,178] The intestinal type (35% of resected cases) is morphologically similar to villous adenomas of the GI tract,[104,171] the gastric type (50%) is characterized by cells that resemble the foveolar epithelium of the stomach,[104,171] and the pancreatobiliary type (15%) has more complex papillae composed of cuboidal-shaped cells (Fig. 41.24).[104,171,179] A fourth pattern, oncocytic, was briefly included as an IPMN type in the WHO classification,[180] but recently this variant was separately classified as intraductal oncocytic papillary neoplasm (see later).[1] The papillae in intestinal-type IPMNs show diffuse MUC2 and CDX2 expression and are typically long and villiform, although some branching may be present. The nuclei are elongated and show a variable degree of pseudostratification and intracellular mucin, depending on the degree of dysplasia (see later). Gastric papillae reveal predominantly a single layer of cells with basally oriented nuclei and abundant mucinous cytoplasm that closely resemble gastric foveolar cells. These often show less exuberant papilla formation. This is the type of epithelium that may also be seen in the background cystic areas of other IPMNs as well and thus regarded as the

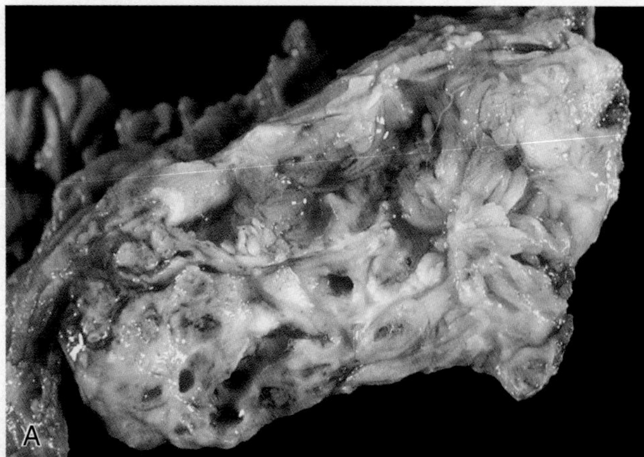

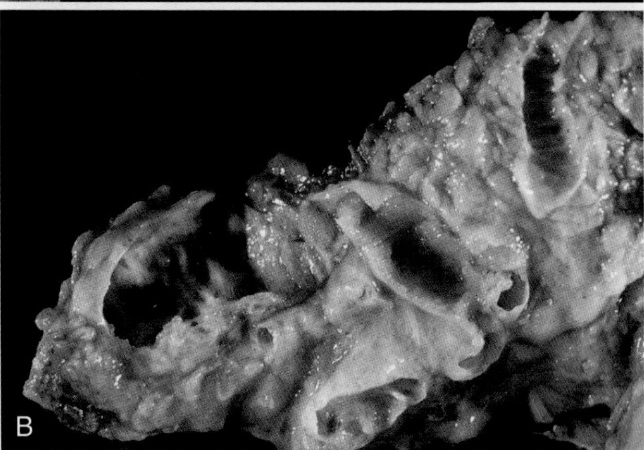

FIGURE 41.22 Gross appearance of intraductal papillary-mucinous neoplasm. The pancreatic ducts are significantly dilated. In some examples, obvious gross papilla formation is noted **(A)**, with extensive involvement of the main pancreatic ducts and cystic dilation of branch ducts. In other examples **(B)**, intraductal papillae are inconspicuous, the lesion appearing largely as cystic dilation of branch ducts.

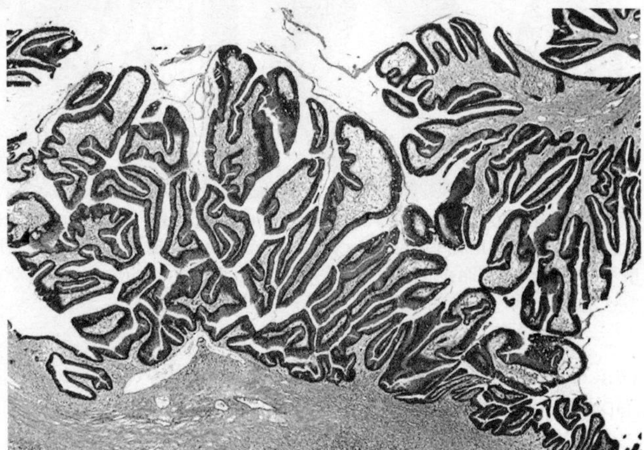

FIGURE 41.23 Intraductal papillary mucinous neoplasm. At low power, the ducts are filled with variably complex papillary projections lined by tall, columnar mucinous epithelial cells.

"null" type. Some cystic ducts may not contain any papillae and instead are lined by a flat layer of mucinous epithelium. A tubular pattern, with back-to-back simple glands, has been reported as pyloric gland adenoma of the pancreas (or intraductal tubular adenoma, pyloric gland type) but is now considered a variant of gastric-type IPMN, with

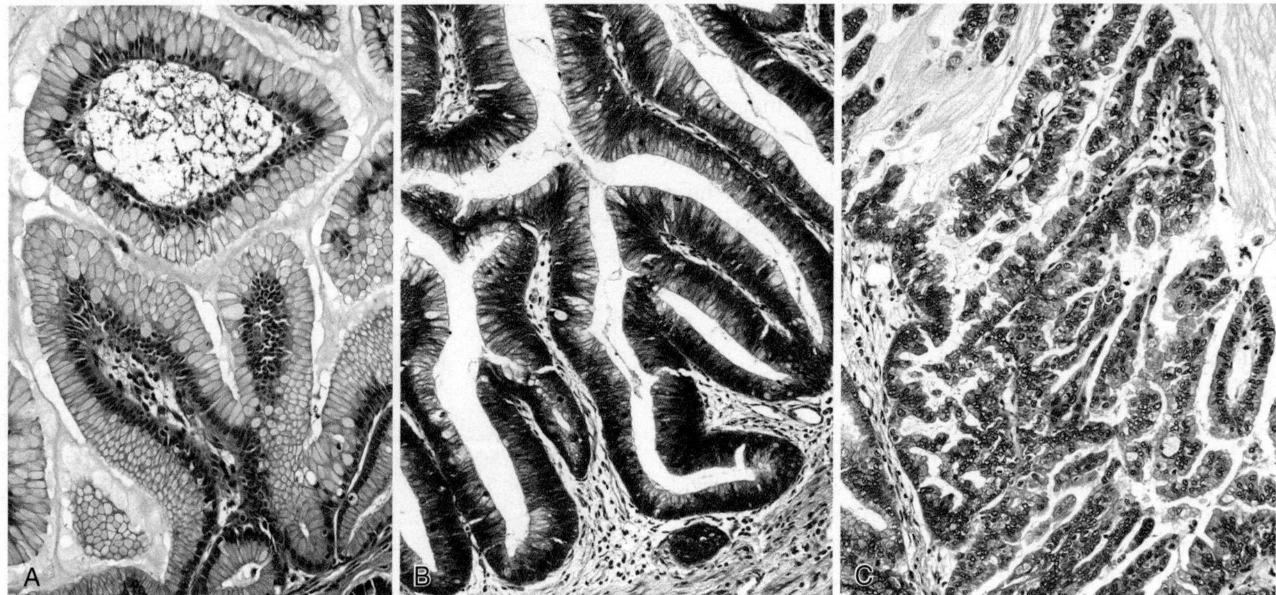

FIGURE 41.24 Intraductal papillary-mucinous neoplasm. Different types of papillae may be found. Gastric-type papillae have uniform columnar cells with abundant apical mucin **(A).** Some cases exhibit intestinal-type papillae **(B),** which resemble the papillae of villous adenomas of the large bowel. Less commonly, intraductal papillary-mucinous neoplasms exhibit pancreatobiliary papillae **(C)** in which the lining epithelium shows marked architectural complexity, with cribriforming and micropapilla formation, and the nuclei are round and lack significant pseudostratification.

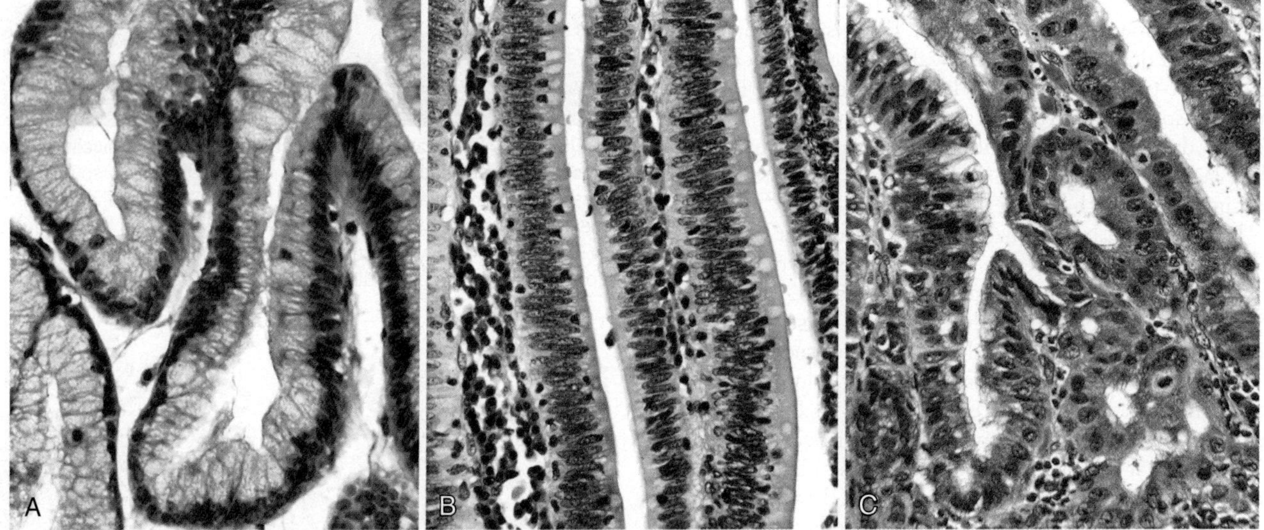

FIGURE 41.25 Various grades of dysplasia in intraductal papillary-mucinous neoplasms. Low-grade dysplasia either **(A)** displays uniform, basally oriented nuclei and minimal architectural complexity or **(B)** is characterized by loss of polarity and moderate nuclear atypia and architectural complexity. In high-grade dysplasia **(C),** there is marked cytoarchitectural complexity.

which it may be associated.[1,181-184] The cells that line the papillae of pancreatobiliary-type IPMNs show the most pronounced degree of cytological atypia and architectural complexity, with numerous branched papillae, micropapillae, and cribriformed areas.[171] The nuclei are typically not pseudostratified but show marked variation in size and shape and have irregular contours and prominent nucleoli. Loss of nuclear polarity is common in these lesions. Both the intestinal and pancreatobiliary type of IPMNs also may show areas of gastric foveolar morphology. However, it is generally uncommon for an individual IPMN to reveal both intestinal and pancreatobiliary morphology in the same tumor.

Like MCNs, the dysplasia in IPMNs is graded as low grade or high grade, a change from the prior three-tier grading system first proposed in 2015, when the prior low- and intermediate-grade dysplasia categories were collapsed into low-grade dysplasia.[143] Grading is based on the most severely dysplastic region (Fig. 41.25), emphasizing the need for extensive, if not complete, histological sampling for proper diagnostic evaluation. In fact, some IPMNs may exhibit a lesser degree of dysplasia within the grossly cystic regions than in the nondilated ducts in the surrounding pancreas, and discontinuous foci of invasive carcinoma may also occur. These observations argue for careful gross and histological examination of the noncystic regions of the pancreas as well. The morphological changes within this dysplasia spectrum parallel those seen in PanIN or MCN.

The different types of papillae (intestinal, gastric, pancreatobiliary) characteristically reveal different degrees of dysplasia.[171] For example, gastric foveolar IPMNs usually have low-grade dysplasia; intestinal ones are more moderate to high-grade; and pancreatobiliary-type IPMNs are almost by default high grade. Invasive carcinoma, which is present in up to one-third of resected cases, is usually either of the colloid[101] or tubular (conventional ductal) type (Fig. 41.26), each representing about 50% of the invasive carcinomas arising in IPMNs. When colloid carcinomas are found, the IPMN is usually of the intestinal type[101,102,171]; tubular type invasive carcinoma may arise in association with any of the papilla types.[103] It is important to make the distinction because colloid carcinoma has a very favorable prognosis,[101] whereas IPMN-associated tubular/ductal carcinomas are aggressive. The latter may have a morphology slightly different than ordinary ductal adenocarcinomas, but some are indistinguishable. It may be important to note here that about 5% of ordinary ductal adenocarcinomas appear to arise from IPMNs.[185] Invasive carcinoma in IPMNs is usually associated with high-grade dysplasia.[59,156] When present, invasive carcinoma may be focal or multifocal, or it may represent the majority of the tumor mass. The presence of invasive carcinoma should always be mentioned in the diagnosis *(IPMN with an associated invasive carcinoma)*, and the type and extent of invasive carcinoma should also be specified.[171]

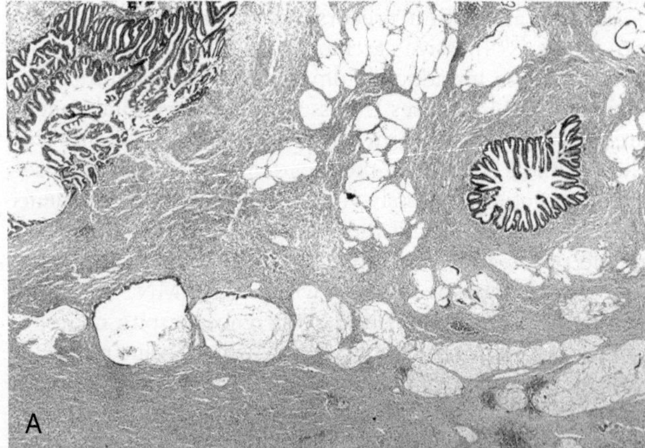

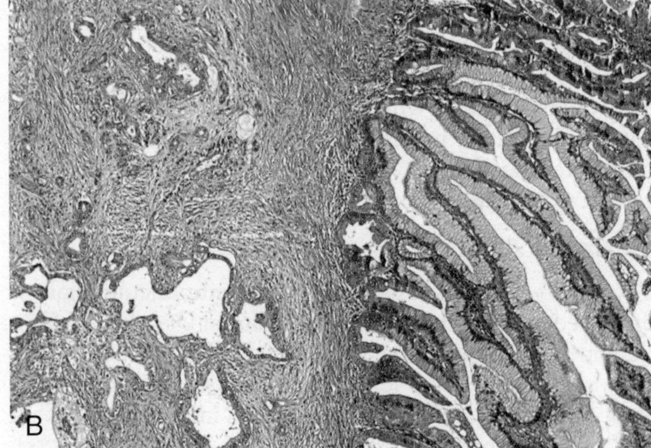

FIGURE 41.26 IPMN with an associated invasive carcinoma. Two distinct types of invasive carcinoma may arise from intraductal papillary mucinous neoplasms. Colloid carcinomas **(A)** consist of paucicellular stromal mucin pools with strips and clusters of floating epithelial cells. In other cases, the invasive component is of tubular type **(B)**, resembling conventional ductal adenocarcinomas.

Special Studies and Molecular Features

By immunohistochemistry, IPMNs express keratins, including CK7, CK8, CK18, and CK19, with variable staining for CK20, depending on the type of papillae.[160,186] Most IPMNs express CEA, CA19-9, and MUC5AC.[164,186] Expression of MUC1 and MUC2, however, varies with the type of papillae.[59,104,178,187] MUC5AC is commonly expressed in all types of IPMNs. Expression of MUC1 (mammary-type mucin) is more common in the pancreatobiliary type. In contrast, diffuse MUC2 and CDX2 expression is virtually exclusive to the intestinal type. Gastric-type IPMNs do not normally express MUC1 or MUC2. MUC6 is preferentially expressed in pancreatobiliary-type IPMNs, suggesting the presence of pyloric differentiation.[61] These findings demonstrate that there is a separate intestinal pathway of carcinogenesis in the pancreas, which is exemplified by an intestinal-type IPMN and the development of colloid carcinoma,[104] which also reveals intestinal differentiation and a more favorable prognosis than other ductal adenocarcinoma variants (see earlier). Carcinomas that develop within pancreatobiliary-type IPMNs are usually conventional ductal adenocarcinoma.

Many of the molecular alterations in IPMNs are similar to those of ductal adenocarcinomas. More molecular abnormalities are present in IPMNs with high-grade dysplasia. However, mutations in *KRAS* and *TP53* are less frequent than in ductal adenocarcinoma. Inactivation of *p16* occurs in some tumors.[188] In contrast with ductal adenocarcinoma, DPC4 is typically retained in IPMNs.[105] Inactivation of the Peutz-Jeghers gene *(STK11/LKB1)* is found in about 25% of IPMNs,[189] but not in ductal adenocarcinomas. Two novel genes altered in IPMNs have been described. *GNAS* is mutated in 60% of IPMNs, and *RNF43*, a gene coding for a protein with intrinsic E3 ubiquitin ligase activity, is mutated in 75%.[190,191] *APC* is mutated in about 25% of IPMNs. None of these three genes is commonly altered in conventional ductal adenocarcinomas, although *RNF43* mutations do occur in MCNs.[190] The frequency of mutations varies according to the papilla type, with *GNAS* mutations being more frequent in IPMNs with intestinal-type papillae.[192] The detection of mutations in IPMNs can be used for preoperative diagnosis to help distinguish these neoplasms from other cystic lesions of the pancreas.[147,193]

Natural History and Treatment

The overall 5-year survival rate of patients with IPMN is relatively good.[103,175] More than 75% of patients are free from disease 5 years after resection, although longer follow-up has shown recurrences in greater numbers of patients.[194] Even patients with an associated invasive carcinoma have a favorable prognosis, particularly if the carcinoma is of the colloid type, or the amount of invasive carcinoma is small. Invasive carcinomas measuring less than 0.5 cm (AJCC stage pT1a) have been designated *minimally invasive* and have an excellent prognosis.[195] Cases with a significant component of invasive tubular type adenocarcinoma pursue an aggressive course, similar to that of conventional ductal carcinoma that arises without a preexisting IPMN.[196]

IPMNs are both a precursor and a marker of invasive carcinoma.[156] Invasive carcinoma may occur within or distant from the intraductal component.[197] The multicentric nature of IPMNs raises the issue of whether total pancreatectomy is the best form of management for patients with these tumors. However, most patients managed by conservative resection of grossly visible disease do not experience local recurrence, even if the intraductal component extends to the pancreatic ductal margin, with recurrence rate tied more to the grade of dysplasia within the IPMN.[103,175] Conversely, some patients suffer recurrence despite complete resection (with negative margins), which again raises the possibility of tumor multicentricity, as does the observation that patients with IPMNs under surveillance may develop invasive carcinoma distant from the cystic lesion.[198] Additional long-term follow-up is needed to determine the optimal form of management for patients with a positive ductal margin. Different approaches are being applied in different institutions, most of which are largely individualized to the patient. However, patients with invasive carcinoma should be treated similarly to patients with conventional ductal adenocarcinoma.

Differential Diagnosis

The differential diagnosis of cystic and intraductal lesions is discussed in detail later in the Differential Diagnosis of Cystic and Intraductal Lesions section. IPMNs should be distinguished from lesser lesions like PanIN, small incidental ectatic ducts,[199] and pseudo-IPMNs,[185] in particular, retention cysts (secondary cystic dilation of obstructed ducts), all of which are intraductal processes that may contain cells with mucinous lining. Small IPMNs are essentially indistinguishable from large foci of PanIN. Criteria offered to separate these two related types of preinvasive neoplasms are admittedly arbitrary and allow for some degree of overlap.[151] If there is villous-intestinal epithelium or florid complex pancreatobiliary-type papilla filling a duct, then it is IPMN. Typically, such cases will reveal much larger tumors in other sections. However, if the process has gastric (or endocervical-like) epithelium, then the distinction becomes a challenge. PanINs are usually incidental, microscopic (not radiographically detectable) lesions that measure less than 0.5 cm in maximal diameter, whereas IPMNs are defined by radiographically or macroscopically detectable masses or cysts and measure more than 1.0 cm.[171] In essence, IPMNs represent mass-forming preinvasive neoplasms (adenoma-carcinoma sequence; tumoral intraepithelial neoplasms).[143,200] It is relatively common for mucinous lesions to be found in small ducts near or distant from ducts involved by IPMNs. In some cases, the morphology of the epithelium in the small ducts is distinct from that of IPMN, arguing that additional foci or PanIN are present in the surrounding pancreas. However, it is often difficult to determine whether the small duct lesion represents extension of the IPMN. Comparative mutational studies suggest that two adjacent ducts are more likely to have the same *KRAS* and *GNAS* mutations (and therefore reflect involvement by a single neoplasm) compared with topographically separate locules, which often contain genetically distinct lesions.[191]

Another diagnostic challenge with regard to IPMNs relates to the recognition of focal invasive colloid carcinoma and its distinction from benign leakage of mucin into the surrounding stroma, which is presumably related to rupture of the involved pancreatic ducts. When mucin leakage occurs, it is usually very limited in amount. The mucin in these cases is typically located adjacent to an involved duct, and it is devoid of free-floating neoplastic epithelial cells. If epithelium is present, it is usually present in continuity with the epithelium of the intraductal component. Mucin leakage also is more likely to produce an inflammatory reaction compared with mucin associated with an invasive colloid carcinoma, although this is not entirely specific. When acellular mucin pools lacking an inflammatory response are found in the stroma in cases of IPMN, a careful search with multiple histological levels should be undertaken to search for diagnostic evidence of invasive colloid carcinoma. The presence of perineurial invasion and, of course, lymph node metastasis is helpful in this regard.

Intraductal Oncocytic Papillary Neoplasm

Intraductal oncocytic papillary neoplasm (IOPN) is a distinctive intraductal tumor type.[201] These tumors often present as large complex lesions that are designated as *cystadenocarcinoma* radiologically or diagnosed as *cystic ductal adenocarcinoma*. Because of the accompanying inflammation, they also often give the impression of tumors infiltrating neighboring sites including the large vessels, and they may be deemed unresectable, although a resection proves curative in the vast majority of cases. In some cases, IOPNs present with many clinicopathological similarities to IPMN.[120,202-204] In the 2010 WHO classification of pancreatic neoplasms, IOPN was regarded as the oncocytic variant of IPMN,[178,180] although in the 2019 classification, it was again separated as a distinct entity.[1] Grossly, IOPNs exhibit cysts that contain large, tan, and friable mural tumor nodules. The neoplasms are usually relatively large (mean, 5.2 cm) at the time of diagnosis, and their intraductal nature may be difficult to demonstrate because of the marked extent of cystic change.[171] Histologically, IOPNs are characterized by a florid intraductal papillary growth pattern frequently associated with mucin production, as well as multilocular cystic transformation of the ductal system similar to IPMN. However, in IOPN, the cells are oncocytic in appearance. They display an architecturally distinctive papillary growth pattern consisting of exuberant, arborizing papillae lined by one to five layers of cuboidal-shaped cells (Fig. 41.27). Large nuclei contain single, prominent, and eccentric nucleoli.[205] A distinctive feature that is relatively specific for IOPN is the presence of mucin-containing intraepithelial lumina that appear as round, punched-out spaces within the epithelium, imparting a cribriformed architecture to the tumor.[171] In some cases, the papillae may fuse, producing a solid pattern of intraductal tumor that may be difficult to distinguish from a solid invasive carcinoma. IOPNs share with pancreatobiliary-type IPMNs the immunoexpression of MUC6 and also stain focally for MUC1.[61] Interestingly, there is also consistent expression of Hepatocyte Paraffin 1 (HepPar1) in most cases.[206] Most IOPNs exhibit high-grade dysplasia. Invasive carcinomas may develop in association with IOPN in 30% of cases, some of which produce abundant extracellular mucin.[207] However, most invasive carcinomas retain oncocytic features, which is a highly unusual pattern for invasive carcinomas in the pancreas. The

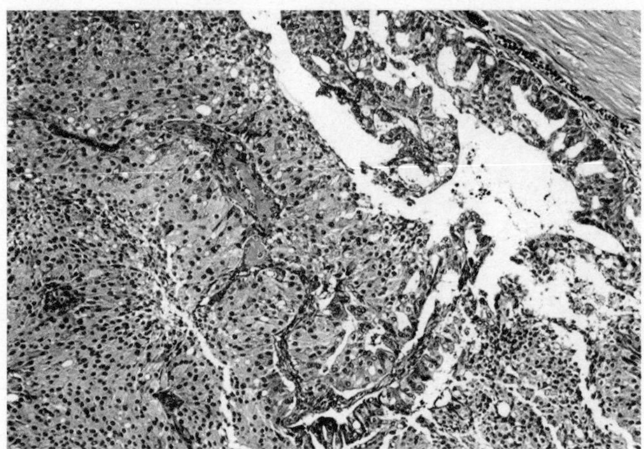

FIGURE 41.27 Intraductal oncocytic papillary neoplasm. These intraductal tumors exhibit markedly complex papillae, with cribriformed areas and fusion of papillae to form solid sheets. The tumor cells also exhibit intracellular lumina and contain abundant eosinophilic cytoplasm.

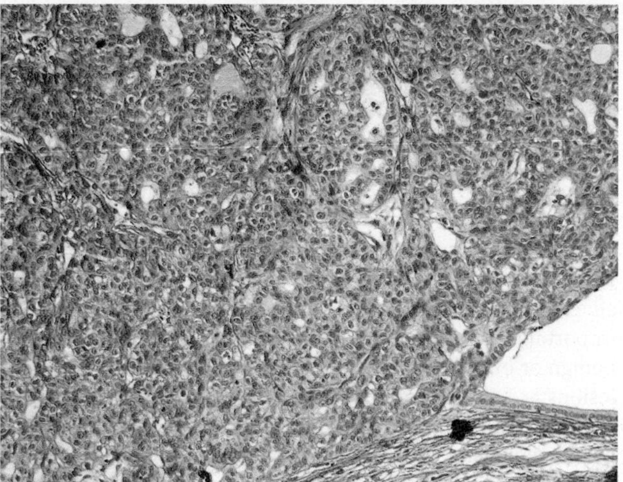

FIGURE 41.28 Intraductal tubulopapillary neoplasm. The intraductal neoplasm is composed of irregular tubules forming a large cribriformed mass. The nuclei are moderately atypical.

prognosis of IOPNs lacking invasive carcinoma is excellent, although local recurrence within residual ducts has been observed, sometimes many years after the initial resection. Even the invasive carcinomas have a nearly 100% 5-year survival.[207]

IOPNs have distinctive molecular alterations that differ from those in IPMNs and ductal adenocarcinomas. For instance, IOPNs generally lack mutations in *KRAS, GNAS, TP53, SMAD4,* and *CDKN2A,* and *RNF43* mutations are rare.[204,206,208,209] Instead, recurrent mutations have been described in *ARHGAP26, ASXL1, EPHA8,* and *ERBB4*.[208] In addition, there are *DNAJB1-PRKACA* fusions, which had been thought to be specific for a diagnosis of fibrolamellar hepatocellular carcinoma.[210]

Although IOPNs are distinct from IPMNs with intestinal-type papillae, IOPNs with pancreatobiliary-type papillae represent a "transition" between these two entities. IOPNs can be distinguished from IPMNs by the presence of marked architectural complexity, distinctive intraepithelial lumina, and the predominance of oncocytic cells.

Intraductal Tubulopapillary Neoplasm

An additional family of intraductal neoplasms exhibits a predominantly tubular, rather than papillary, architecture.[211-214] They often present as nodular masses in the pancreas that may be interpreted as ordinary ductal adenocarcinoma or some of the nonductal tumors, although some have features similar to IPMNs.[171] Intraductal tubulopapillary neoplasms (ITPNs) usually have high-grade dysplasia, manifested as significant architectural complexity within the intraductal tumor, and they may be associated with invasive carcinoma. In these cases, the intraductal component typically fills the entire duct, resulting in the formation of large nodules of circumscribed tumor that may be difficult to recognize as intraductal unless continuity with the normal ductal epithelium can be identified (Fig. 41.28). These intraductal tumors are composed of sheets of tubular structures, irregular papillae (but less prominent than IPMNs), and solid sheets of cells. The nuclei are moderately to markedly atypical, and mitotic activity is usually brisk. The tumor cells contain minimal cytoplasm without obvious intracellular mucin, another key difference from IPMNs. Although the name bears the term *papillary,* most cases are almost exclusively tubular, and papilla formation is either focal or abortive. In fact, the overall histomorphology is highly similar to acinar cell carcinomas rather than any type of IPMN, and the possibility of an acinar cell carcinoma must be excluded with careful evaluation before a case is classified as ITPN. Invasive carcinomas are usually of the tubular type and are characterized by irregular, angulated infiltrating glands associated with a desmoplastic stromal response.

Intraductal tubulopapillary neoplasm typically stains with CK7 and CK19. Glycoprotein markers are also expressed in these tumors, including CA19-9 and MUC1; MUC6, which is a marker of pyloric glands, is also positive in about 50% of cases.[171,212] An important difference from pancreatobiliary-type IPMNs is that ITPNs lack MUC5AC expression in essentially every case.[215] Molecular analysis of ITPNs reveals distinctive genetic characteristics compared with those of other intraductal tumors of the pancreas and PDACs. Mutations in *KRAS, GNAS,* and *RNF43* are not seen. In contrast with most ductal neoplasms of the pancreas, MAP-kinase pathway alterations are not present. Certain chromatin remodeling genes such as *MLL1, MLL2, MLL3, BAP1, PBRM1, EED,* and *ATRX* are mutated in 32% of ITPNs, and 27% of cases harbor mutations in phosphatidylinositol 3-kinase (PI3K) pathway–related genes (*PIK3CA, PIK3CB, INPP4A,* and *PTEN*).[171,216] *FGFR2* fusions with various fusion partners are observed in 18%. Ten percent of the cases do not have any detectable molecular alterations.[171,211,217]

As mentioned previously, the main differential is with acinar cell carcinomas.[218] Intraductal tubulopapillary neoplasms fail to express acinar cell markers (trypsin and chymotrypsin) and are negative for chromogranin and synaptophysin, which helps rule out the other main differential diagnostic possibility, PanNET. Intraductal tubulopapillary neoplasms appear to be less aggressive than conventional ductal adenocarcinomas, even when there is a component of invasive carcinoma.[212]

CYSTIC NEOPLASMS

Advents in the radiology field have placed pancreatic cysts as a common incidental finding. More than 10% of the detailed radiological analysis of the region performed in older adult patients reveal incidental cysts in the pancreas. Most of these are presumed to be innocuous form of IPMNs, which are discussed later. However, cystic neoplasms of the pancreas are less commonly geared to surgery than ductal adenocarcinomas, representing 5% to 10% of all pancreatic neoplasms resected, but they constitute an important subset because many cystic tumors are either benign or only low-grade malignant neoplasms.[219,220] Cystic lesions are also being detected more commonly because of the increased use of sensitive imaging techniques. Most true cystic neoplasms of the pancreas represent cystic dilation of IPMNs (and their kindreds, intraductal oncocytic papillary neoplasms and intraductal tubulopapillary neoplasms) followed by either serous cystadenomas or MCNs. However, a variety of other less common cystic tumors may occur in the pancreas as well. Typically solid tumors also may develop cystic changes.[221]

Serous Cystic Neoplasms

Clinical Features

Serous cystic neoplasms are a highly distinctive and virtually pancreas-specific tumor that are believed to arise from centroacinar cells.[222-227] Serous cystic neoplasms are further classified based on the size of the individual cyst locules as *microcystic serous cystadenoma* (formerly known as *microcystic adenoma* or *glycogen-rich adenoma*) and *macrocystic serous cystadenoma* (formerly known as *oligocystic serous cystadenoma*).[223,228,229] A rare solid variant (solid serous adenoma) has no cystic changes but features histologically similar epithelium.[230,231] Microcystic serous cystadenomas are the most common (75%)[223] and are composed of numerous small cysts, each ranging from less than 1 mm to about 1 cm, ultimately forming a well-demarcated tumor mass. Microcystic serous cystadenomas are usually relatively large, measuring up to 25 cm, and they arise mostly in the body or tail of the pancreas, predominantly in women (female-to-male ratio, 3:1). The mean age of patients is 66 years. Patients with von Hippel-Lindau syndrome may develop histologically similar appearing cysts (often multiple),[232-234] although most patients with microcystic serous cystadenomas have no other associated diseases. However, this association provides some insight into the molecular biology of these neoplasms. Other concurrent pancreatic tumors found in about 13% of patients[223] with microcystic serous cystadenomas include ductal adenocarcinoma[223,235] and PanNETs.[236] By imaging, macrocystic serous cystadenomas are more likely to be mistaken for other macrocystic lesions such as IPMNs of branch duct type. The macrocystic variant was initially reported to be more common in men, but recent studies have shown that they are also more prevalent in women. Solid examples are often mistaken as neuroendocrine tumors both radiologically and grossly.

Pathological Features

Grossly, microcystic serous cystadenomas are usually well circumscribed and often contain a central, stellate fibrous scar. The innumerable cysts produce a gross appearance resembling that of a sponge (Fig. 41.29), and this is pathognomonic for this entity. In some regions, the cysts may be so small that the tumor appears solid. Degenerative changes, including hemorrhage and macrocystic degeneration, may be prominent in some cases,[237] mimicking the gross appearance of a pseudocyst. Hemorrhagic ones may be more prone to show adhesions to neighboring organs.

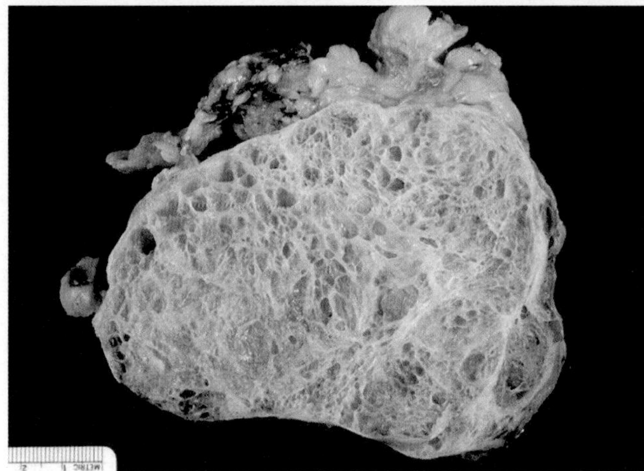

FIGURE 41.29 Gross appearance of microcystic serous cystadenoma. The lesion is well circumscribed and composed of small cysts, each measuring less than 1 cm, separated by thin, translucent septa.

Microscopically, the cysts of microcystic serous cystadenomas have a very characteristic and specific cytology composed of a single layer of flat to cuboidal cells with clear cytoplasm, well-defined cytoplasmic borders, and small, round nuclei with dense, hyperchromatic chromatin (Fig. 41.30). The cytoplasmic clearing is caused by accumulation of glycogen; mucin is not present. Also characteristic is the presence of a rich capillary network hugging the epithelium, a feature that they share with other vHL-associated neoplasms such as renal cell carcinomas and hemangioblastomas.[238] In rare cases, the cells are more columnar in shape or contain acidophilic, granular cytoplasm. Blunt papillary projections may be found focally as well; however, well-formed or complex papillae are unusual. The stroma between cysts is hyalinized and may contain entrapped islets and may also harbor calcifications.

These characteristic cytological features of serous neoplasms of the pancreas are present not only in microcystic serous cystadenomas, but also in the less common types of serous tumors, such as macrocystic serous cystadenoma and solid serous adenoma.[223,231] The boundaries of macrocystic serous cystadenomas are often less defined, the individual locules range from one to several centimeters in size, and a central scar is usually absent (Fig. 41.31). Microscopically, the lining of the cysts is identical to that of the microcystic type, with glycogen-rich clear cells arranged in a single flat layer without atypia or mucin production (Fig. 41.32). Solid serous adenomas are composed of back-to-back small glands with cytological features otherwise typical of a serous neoplasm (Fig. 41.33). The subepithelial capillary network is present in both variants.

Both histologically and immunophenotypically, all these types of serous neoplasms appear to recapitulate centroacinar cells.[226] For instance, they express low-molecular-weight

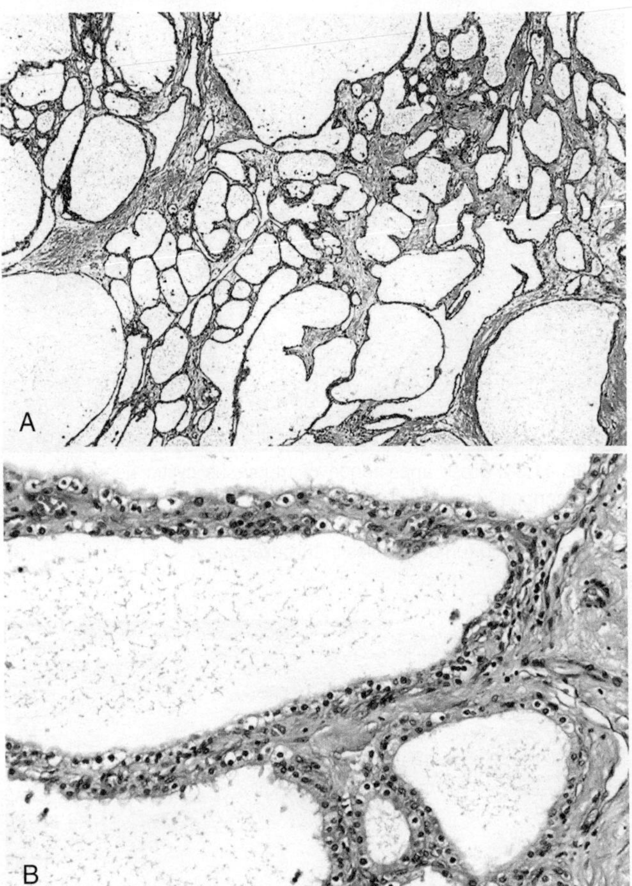

FIGURE 41.30 **Microcystic serous cystadenoma.** At low power **(A),** each small cyst is lined by a flattened layer of epithelium. Cytologically **(B),** the lining cells show clear cytoplasm and small, uniform, hyperchromatic nuclei.

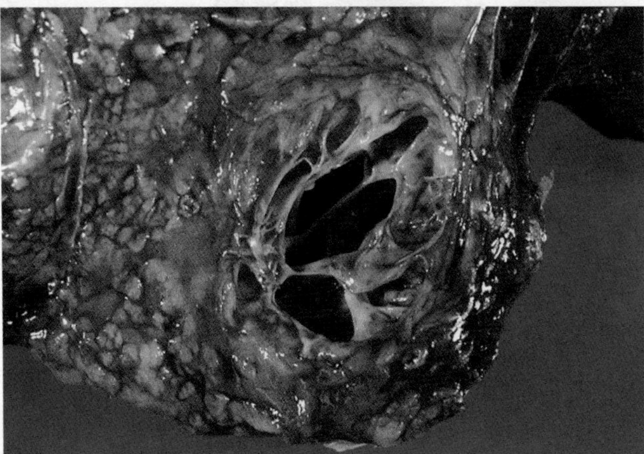

FIGURE 41.31 Gross appearance of macrocystic serous cystadenoma. The cysts are much larger than those of the microcystic counterpart.

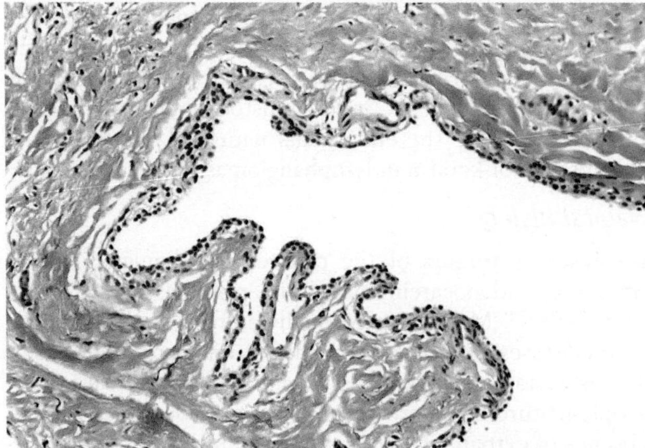

FIGURE 41.32 Macrocystic serous cystadenoma. Despite the large size of the cysts, the lining epithelium is identical to that of microcystic serous cystadenomas, with clear cells having round, hyperchromatic nuclei.

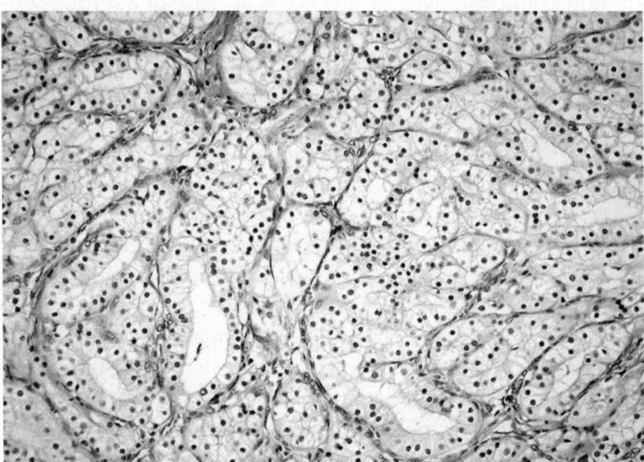

FIGURE 41.33 Solid serous adenoma. There is no cyst formation, with back-to-back glands exhibiting the same cytological features as the cystic members of the serous tumor family.

keratins (in addition to broad-spectrum keratins), EMA, inhibin, and MART-1.[239,240] HMB-45 is typically negative in these tumors. Ductal mucin markers (B72.3, MUC1, CA19-9, and CEA) are either negative or only focally positive, although MUC6 is usually positive.[239] Molecular genetic alterations include those associated with the *VHL* gene (chromosome 3p25 and 10q).[190,241] As is true of other neoplasms arising in patients with VHL, serous neoplasms express CA-IX, HIF-1α, vascular endothelial growth factor (VEGF), and Glut-1.[238] Overexpression of the glucose transporter Glut-1 may help explain the accumulation of cytoplasmic glycogen in serous tumors.[242] Genetic abnormalities typical of ductal adenocarcinoma (such as *KRAS* and *TP53* mutations) have not been identified in serous tumors, nor have mutations in *GNAS* or *RNF43*, which are found in other cystic or intraductal pancreatic neoplasms.[190,191]

Differential Diagnosis

The differential diagnosis of serous neoplasms includes other cystic tumors of the pancreas (see Differential Diagnosis of Cystic and Intraductal Lesions later). In addition, the clear cell nature of the cytoplasm raises the possibility of metastatic renal cell carcinoma, a tumor that may involve the pancreas as the sole site of metastasis and also may reveal cystic change, and which is also common in patients with VHL syndrome. The presence of solid and acinar regions and prominent nuclear atypia, combined with a more pronounced sinusoidal vascular pattern, favors a diagnosis of renal cell carcinoma. Lymphangiomas also resemble serous cystic neoplasms,[243] particularly when the latter have a more attenuated epithelial lining. Lymphangiomas typically occur in peripancreatic tissue rather than within the pancreas and contain lymphoid aggregates between the cystic spaces. In difficult cases, immunohistochemical staining can help demonstrate the endothelial nature of the lining and the absence of keratin in lymphangiomas.

Natural History

Most serous tumors of the pancreas are benign.[223,244,245] Serous cystadenocarcinoma of the pancreas is extremely rare.[223,246-248] Malignancy is usually defined by the presence of metastases. In both the primary tumor and metastases, serous cystadenocarcinomas usually exhibit typical microscopic features of microcystic serous cystadenomas with an absence of cytoarchitectural atypia or any other morphological findings suggestive of malignancy. Thus some authorities have questioned the malignant potential of these rare cases and have suggested instead that they developed as a form of parasitic growth of a benign neoplasm or as a manifestation of multicentricity. Suffice it to say that in the absence of demonstrable metastases, any "typical" case of a serous neoplasm should be considered benign. In fact, if a definitive diagnosis can be achieved preoperatively and the tumor is asymptomatic, treatment by clinical observation and follow-up is considered a viable option.[249]

Recently, another type of malignancy has been reported in serous neoplasms. In rare cases, a cytologically obvious carcinoma may arise within a microcystic serous cystadenoma *(carcinoma* ex *microcystic adenoma)*.[250] The carcinomas in these cases are composed of nests or clusters of clear cells, some with large cytoplasmic vacuoles producing a sievelike pattern. The nuclei are enlarged and atypical, relative to the residual benign serous elements, and there can be increased mitotic activity and necrosis. The biological behavior of these rare cases is yet to be defined.[250]

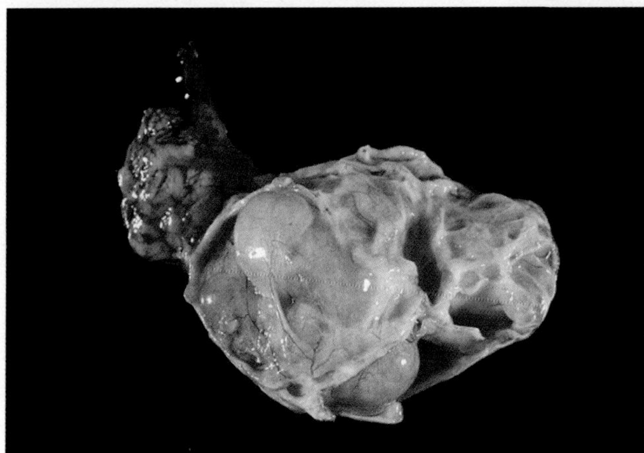

FIGURE 41.34 Gross appearance of mucinous cystic neoplasm. The circumscribed tumor involves the tail of the pancreas and contains numerous large (1 to 5 cm) cysts. The septa are fibrotic and show no gross evidence of solid tumor nodules in this example.

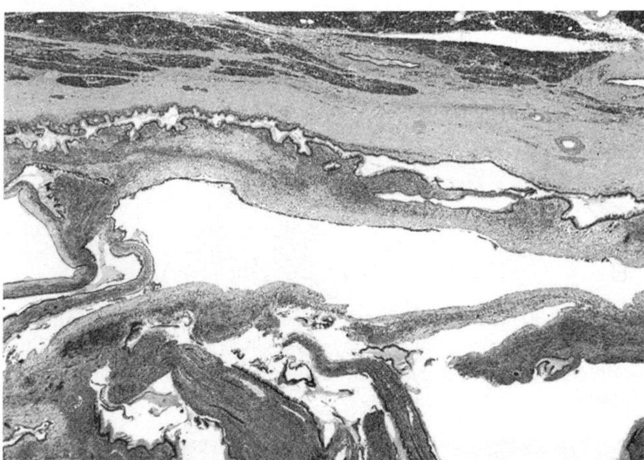

FIGURE 41.35 Mucinous cystic neoplasm. At low power, the lesion is surrounded by a thick, fibrous capsule. The large cysts are lined by mucinous epithelium, and the stroma of the septa is hypercellular.

Mucinous Cystic Neoplasms

Clinical Features

MCNs represent the other major type of "true" cystic neoplasm of the pancreas.[251-254] In contrast with most serous cystadenomas, MCNs are consistently macrocystic, and when defined strictly by the presence of ovarian-type stroma (see later), they have very distinctive clinicopathological characteristics.[171,255] They are seen almost exclusively (97%) in females (only rare examples have been documented in males) in the fifth to sixth decades of life (mean age, 50 years), and the tumor is nearly always located in the tail of the pancreas.[255] Presenting symptoms are nonspecific and reflect the effects of an enlarging mass.

Pathological Features

Macroscopically, MCNs are typically single multilocular cysts surrounded by a thick fibrotic pseudocapsule (Fig. 41.34). They are often relatively large by the time of diagnosis, often greater than 10 cm.[255] Unless there is fistula formation, these tumors do not communicate with the pancreatic ductal system. The septa between individual cysts are usually thin and may show velvety papillations; some appear trabeculated and thickened. The cyst contents are often mucoid, but a more watery consistency also may be noted in some cases. Solid areas within the cysts or within the peripheral capsule may harbor an invasive carcinoma component. Papillary nodules represented as soft, tan, friable polypoid projections can be seen.[255] Degenerative changes with hemorrhage may occur, simulating the gross appearance of a pseudocyst.

Histologically, MCNs are lined by columnar cells with abundant apical cytoplasmic mucin, although cuboidal cells that lack obvious mucin may also be present in some cases, or they may predominate (Figs. 41.35 and 41.36).[256] Those with predominantly nonmucinous cells tend to be smaller and devoid of cancerous transformation.[256] Some cases reveal intestinal-like epithelium with goblet cells, but villiform papillae typical of intestinal-type IPMNs are very unusual.[220] Neuroendocrine cells and Paneth cells may be detected. The epithelium may display a wide range of cytological atypia. Some MCNs have only low-grade dysplasia and are largely bland in appearance, containing mostly uniform, basally oriented nuclei and displaying minimal architectural complexity. Others have high-grade dysplasia, with abundant papillary formations, pseudostratified hyperchromatic nuclei, and a cribriform architecture. High-grade

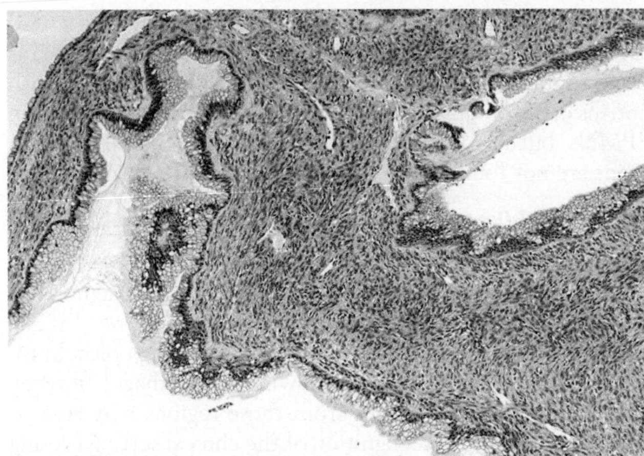

FIGURE 41.36 Mucinous cystic neoplasm. At higher magnification, the epithelial lining is composed of tall, columnar, mucin-containing cells. In this region, there is no significant nuclear atypia, loss of polarity, or architectural complexity (mucinous cystic neoplasm with low-grade dysplasia). The subepithelial stroma is hypercellular, resembling the stroma of the ovary.

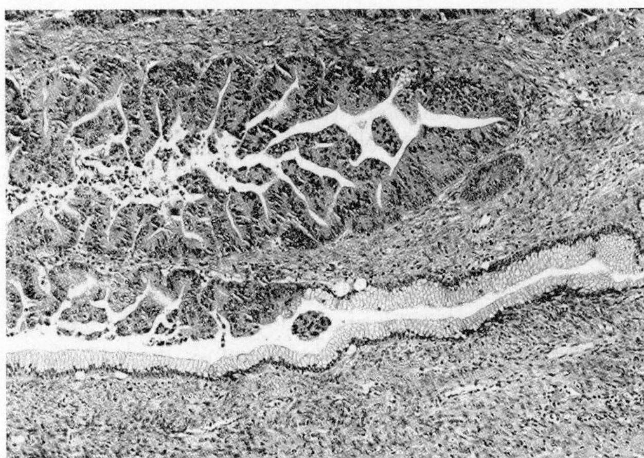

FIGURE 41.37 Mucinous cystic neoplasm. High-grade dysplasia may be focal, with an abrupt transition from bland mucinous epithelium. In this case, there is marked nuclear atypia and complete loss of polarity but no invasive carcinoma (mucinous cystic neoplasm with high-grade dysplasia).

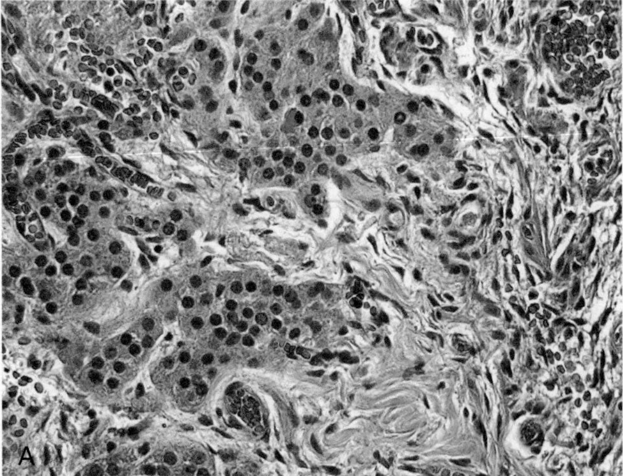

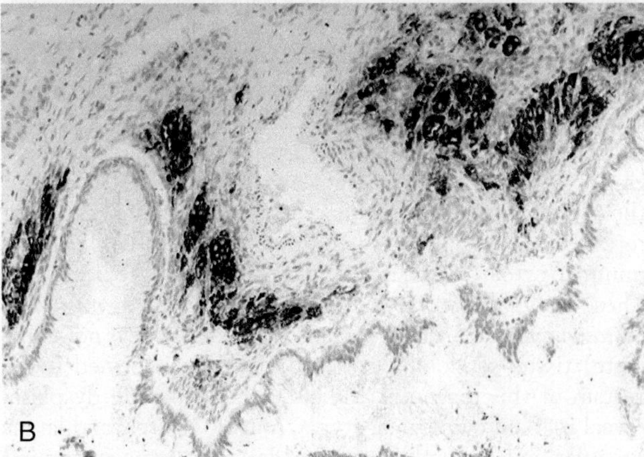

FIGURE 41.38 Stroma of mucinous cystic neoplasm. In addition to the hypercellular spindle cell component, there may be clusters of epithelioid cells resembling the luteinized stroma of the ovary **(A).** Immunohistochemical staining for inhibin **(B)** is positive in the epithelioid cell nests.

dysplasia may be focal, and numerous sections are required to properly evaluate these neoplasms (Fig. 41.37).

A prerequisite for the diagnosis of MCN is the presence of distinctive subepithelial hypercellular spindle cell stroma (referred to as *ovarian-type stroma*), which is found, at least focally, in all *bona fide* examples of this neoplasm. In addition to spindle cell elements, the stroma often contains nests of epithelioid cells with changes suggestive of luteinization (Fig. 41.38). Occasionally, there may be large circumscribed regions of stromal hyalinization resembling corpora albicantia. The stromal cells frequently express estrogen and progesterone receptors as well as inhibin and A103,[254,257,258] the last two being intensely expressed in the epithelioid, lutea-like cells (see Fig. 41.38B). A plausible explanation for the presence of ovarian-type stroma in MCNs has not yet been proven, although the fetal pancreas contains similar hypercellular stroma surrounding developing pancreatic ducts, so some authorities have suggested that the stroma of MCNs represents recapitulation of the fetal periductal mesenchyme.[259] The epithelium of MCNs expresses keratin as well as glycoprotein markers, such as CEA and CA19-9.[252,254,260] MUC5AC is expressed diffusely, whereas MUC2 typically only stains scattered goblet cells.[261] MUC1 is generally present only in the papillary high-grade dysplasias as a luminal membranous labeling, or in invasive carcinomas. Intestinal differentiation, other than goblet cells, is not commonly found. For instance, stains for CK20 and CDX2 are usually negative in these tumors.

Invasive carcinoma develops within 15% of MCNs.[255,262] In cases with high-grade dysplasia, this is of particular concern because the invasive component may be focal and grossly inapparent. Thus it is highly recommended that any solid areas of the tumor and the interface with adjacent tissues should be sampled generously and carefully. Invasive carcinoma arising in MCNs is mostly (90%) tubular type and resembles conventional PDAC.[255] However, other types may also occur, such as sarcomatoid carcinoma or undifferentiated carcinoma with osteoclast-like giant cells,[127,255] although colloid carcinoma (a common subtype arising in association with IPMNs) is rare[255] (Fig. 41.39). Reports of apparent sarcomatous transformation of the cellular subepithelial stroma exist, although genetic analysis of these cases suggests that the sarcomatoid elements were of epithelial derivation and, thus, represent sarcomatoid

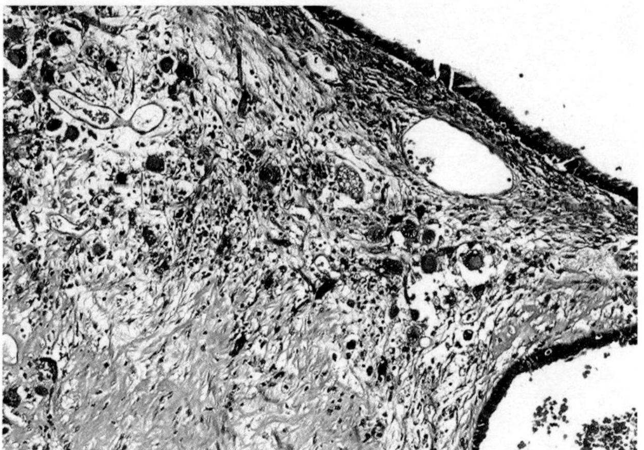

FIGURE 41.39 Mucinous cystic neoplasm with invasive carcinoma. Within a septum of this tumor, there is a component of undifferentiated anaplastic giant cell carcinoma, one of several types of invasive carcinoma that may arise in mucinous cystic neoplasms.

carcinoma rather than true sarcoma.[263-265] The degree of dysplasia in MCNs should be graded (low grade or high grade) based on the most severely dysplastic region, and the presence or absence of an invasive carcinoma should be reported as well. In cases with low-grade dysplasia, there is minimal cytoarchitectural atypia of the lining epithelium. These tumors have previously been designated as *mucinous cystadenoma,* but it is important that extensive (if not complete) tissue sectioning of the tumor be performed to be certain of this diagnosis. MCNs with high-grade dysplasia reveal marked cytological atypia, mitotic figures, and larger irregular and hyperchromatic nuclei, usually accompanied by significant architectural complexity. In cases of MCN with an associated invasive carcinoma, the histological type of invasive carcinoma should be reported, and the size and extent of invasion (intratumoral or extratumoral) should be determined. Unfortunately, the clinical relevance of this classification system is a matter of debate. Early reports of metastasis from tumors that lacked an obvious invasive carcinoma (or even significant cellular atypia) have been explained based on inadequate sampling for histology,[251,252] and studies in which MCNs have been thoroughly sectioned revealed no recurrences in cases that lacked a significant component of invasive carcinoma at the time of resection (i.e., invasion extending into or through the peripheral pseudocapsule of the tumor).[254,266,267] However, larger more recent studies have documented cases in which metastases arose from very small invasive carcinomas that were limited to the septa of the cyst,[255] again emphasizing the need for thorough histological sampling of MCNs.

Overall, the rate of invasive carcinoma in MCNs is approximately 15%.[255,262,268] It has been suggested that invasive carcinomas arising in MCNs are less aggressive than conventional PDACs, although the differences may be stage-related. In some studies, even small invasive carcinomas have been found to behave aggressively;[255] however, other studies found microinvasive carcinomas to be more benevolent.[267] Invasion is seldom seen in small (<3 cm) and noncomplex examples. Nevertheless, surgical resection is recommended for all patients with an MCN.

Molecular analysis of MCNs has disclosed mutations (or promoter methylation) in many of the genes known to be abnormal in ductal adenocarcinomas, including *KRAS, TP53, DPC4,* and *CDKN2A*. Additionally, about one-half of MCNs have mutations in *RNF43,* which codes for a protein with intrinsic E3 ubiquitin ligase activity that is also mutated in IPMNs, but not in ductal adenocarcinoma.[190] *GNAS* mutations are not found in MCNs, in contrast with IPMNs.[190]

Differential Diagnosis

The differential diagnosis of MCNs of the pancreas is discussed later in this chapter in the "Differential Diagnosis of Cystic and Intraductal Lesions" section. Sometimes MCNs may develop extensive denudation of the lining epithelium, with the underlying stroma showing hemorrhage, fibrosis, and inflammation. Biopsies from these regions may resemble pseudocysts.[269] Recognition of the clinical setting (young female, usually without a history of pancreatitis or any other cause for a pseudocyst, and an otherwise normal-appearing pancreas) can help direct the pathologist to examine other regions of the cyst to find the characteristic mucinous lining. Also, elements of ovarian-type stroma may persist in denuded areas and can be demonstrated immunohistochemically. One other important consideration is to avoid use of the term *mucinous cystadenocarcinoma* for a ductal adenocarcinoma that shows ectatic glands (large duct pattern), unless there is evidence that the tumor arose from a preexisting MCN. Some cystic lesions of the pancreas have a mucinous lining resembling MCN but lack any evidence of cellular, ovarian-type stroma. Most such lesions represent either branch duct-type intraductal papillary-mucinous neoplasm or retention cyst with superimposed PanIN (simple mucinous cyst[270]). Because the stromal component is regarded as critical for the diagnosis of MCN, the diagnosis should be made with great caution in its absence. The examples of the entity recently named as *simple mucinous cyst*[271] that occur in older adult females raise the question of whether they may be burned-out versions of MCN; however, currently they are classified separately if no convincing ovarian stroma is identified.

Cystic Change in Typically Solid Tumors

Cystic Change in Ductal Adenocarcinoma

This uncommon phenomenon may occur via three mechanisms.[43] A large, radiographically detectable cyst may develop as a result of central necrosis of the carcinoma.[272] Such cases with central necrosis often have a more demarcated growth and histologically prove to show various metaplastic features including squamoid, sarcomatoid, and undifferentiated epithelioid patterns.[98] This can be clinically challenging, but the presence of residual carcinoma at the periphery of the cystic cavity is usually obvious histologically. In other cases, the presence of a ductal adenocarcinoma can lead to cystic dilation of distally located obstructed ducts, which results in the development of one or more ductal retention cysts that can be misinterpreted as the main disease process on imaging or gross pathological evaluation. Finally, in the large duct pattern of ductal adenocarcinoma, infiltrating tubular units are cystically dilated and may achieve a size sufficient to be visible grossly.[79] Cystic glands may appear noninvasive, mimicking foci of PanIN or even IPMN, especially when the cystic change occurs within pancreatic parenchyma.

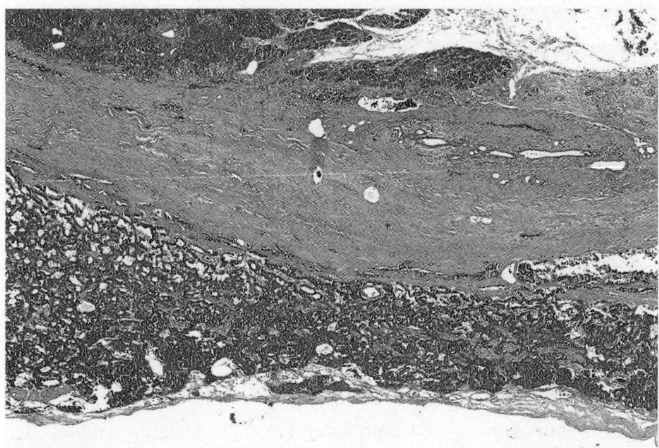

FIGURE 41.40 Pancreatic neuroendocrine tumor with central cystic degeneration. A rim of viable tumor covered by fibrin is present between the fibrotic capsule of the tumor and the central region of cystic change.

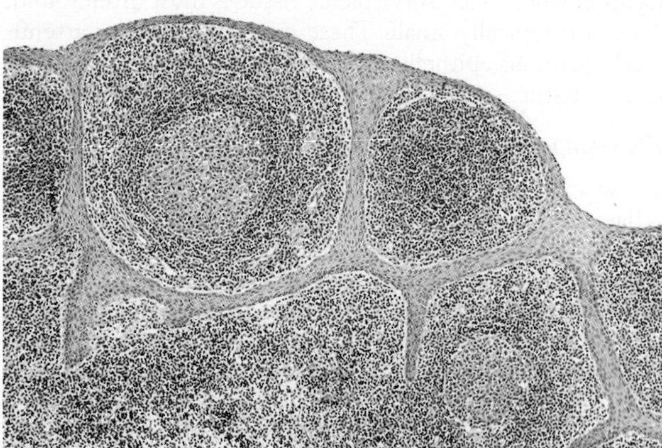

FIGURE 41.41 Lymphoepithelial cyst. The wall of the cyst is lined by squamous epithelium without keratinization in this region. Underlying the epithelium is a dense band of lymphocytes containing germinal centers.

Cystic Pancreatic Neuroendocrine Tumor

This is a rare occurrence and usually consists of a single unilocular cyst that occupies the majority of the tumor.[273-275] Cysts that develop within well-differentiated PanNETs are usually centrally located and solitary and are typically lined by a cuff of well-preserved tumor with overlying fibrin (Fig. 41.40). The cyst cavity is typically filled with clear fluid instead of necrotic debris. Presumably, the most cystic changes in PanNETs are degenerative in nature, although in some cases, the cyst is partially lined by nonneoplastic ductal epithelium, suggesting the cyst may occur as a result of dilation of a duct surrounded by the neoplasm. Some cysts may reach a significantly large size (up to 25 cm). A pathological diagnosis of cystic neuroendocrine tumor is relatively simple if careful attention is paid to the cytological features of the tumor cells.

Cystic Acinar Neoplasms

Acinar cystic transformation (acinar cell cystadenoma) and acinar cell cystadenocarcinoma are discussed later in this chapter.

Lymphoepithelial Cysts

Lymphoepithelial cyst occurs predominantly, but not exclusively, in men in the fifth to sixth decades of life.[276] Lymphoepithelial cysts do not appear to be associated with autoimmune conditions, HIV infection, lymphoma, or carcinoma, all of which have been documented in association with salivary lymphoepithelial cysts. Most lymphoepithelial cysts arise in the periphery of the pancreas, generally in the body or tail; some appear to be peripancreatic, and the connection to the organ may be difficult to recognize. The cyst contents vary from serous to caseous, depending on the degree of keratin formation. The cyst wall and trabecula are usually thin. The inner lining of the cyst is smooth, sometimes with focal nodularity. The lymphoid tissue is not prominent grossly because it is usually limited to a thin band underlying the epithelium. Microscopically, the cysts are lined by stratified squamous epithelium that may or may not reveal prominent keratinization (Fig. 41.41). In some cases, the lining epithelium may be transitional in appearance focally; in others, it may be cuboidal or focally denuded. Sebaceous elements and mucinous cells are uncommon but can be found, usually very limited in amount; their presence should raise consideration of a teratoma, and pilar structures clearly suggest this diagnosis. The squamous lining is surrounded by dense lymphoid tissue composed of mature T lymphocytes. Germinal centers formed by B cells are abundant in some cases. Lymphocytes within the epithelium are uncommon. Solid lymphoepithelial islands (microscopic clusters of epithelial cells admixed with lymphocytes, akin to the so-called *epimyoepithelial islands* in salivary gland counterparts) may be present in some cases. The uninvolved pancreas is usually unremarkable. Lymphoepithelial cysts are benign.

Miscellaneous Epithelial Cysts

Squamoid Cyst of Pancreatic Ducts

These cysts average 2.5 cm and arise in adults.[277] They are lined by flat epithelium composed of immature squamous or transitional cells that can be simple or stratified. Preoperative cyst evaluation may yield high CEA and CA19-9 levels, leading to the suspicion of mucinous cyst. Keratinization is not found. The cells in the basal layers express p63, and the cells bordering the cyst lumen are positive for MUC1 and MUC6. These cysts appear to represent dilated pancreatic ducts involved by squamous (multilayered) metaplasia. In some cases, there is a transition to cystic acinar transformation making it difficult to determine which category to place the lesion.

Dermoid Cyst (Mature Cystic Teratoma)

These are exceedingly rare in the pancreatic region.[278] They have been reported in young patients (second to third decade of life) and are morphologically similar to teratomas that develop in other sites of the body.

Epidermoid Cyst in Intrapancreatic Accessory Spleen

These are also very rare lesions[278] that are seen mainly in younger patients (second to third decade of life). They occur almost exclusively in the tail of the pancreas, a location where accessory splenic tissue is most often found. They are typically small. These cysts are lined by attenuated squamous epithelium surrounded by normal-appearing splenic tissue.

Para-Ampullary Duodenal Wall Cysts

These cysts occur as a consequence of chronic fibrosing inflammation within the periampullary region, between the duodenum and the distal common bile duct.[279] Accessory pancreatic ducts may form the cysts in the duodenal wall and underlying pancreas, mimicking duodenal duplication cysts. The cyst wall is lined partially by ductal epithelium and partly by inflammation and granulation tissue and is surrounded by hypercellular spindle cells with smooth muscle features, possibly derived from the muscularis propria of the duodenum. The process is closely related to so-called *groove pancreatitis*, also known as *paraduodenal pancreatitis*.[280-283]

Simple Mucinous Cysts

Simple mucinous cysts closely resemble gastric-type branch duct IPMNs, which can have minimal papilla formation in the most cystic regions of the neoplasm.[143,271] In fact, the distinction between these two entities is largely semantic. Features favoring a diagnosis of IPMN include papilla formation, multiple cysts, specialized (intestinal or oncocytic) epithelium, and lack of nonneoplastic ductal epithelium lining part of the cystic duct. Simple mucinous cysts can have an array of molecular alterations, supporting their neoplastic nature, but they rarely share mutations typical of IPMNs, more commonly showing mutations in *MLL3* (62%).[270] Examples that occur in elderly women also often show a subtle stromal band that raises the question of atrophic ovarian stroma, but by definition does not qualify as ovarian stroma or express progesterone receptor.

Retention Cysts and Secondary Cystic Dilation

Retention cysts come in two flavors. Some are unilocular cysts that presumably develop as a result of obstruction of a pancreatic duct,[151,279,284] and these overlap with the *simple mucinous cysts* discussed earlier. A cause for ductal obstruction should be investigated, especially to ensure that there is no pancreatic carcinoma or other neoplasm upstream of the cystic region. Sometimes, a simple cyst is partially or completely lined by flat nonpapillary mucinous epithelium lacking significant atypia. This finding has been interpreted as a retention cyst with superimposed PanIN.[285] However, a recent consensus recommends terming these *simple mucinous cysts*.[143,271] Retention cysts may be multiple. As such, these constitute the most common source of pseudo-IPMN[185] (see later). These often form a chain of round cysts at the periphery of the pancreatic parenchyma that creates a pattern similar to that of polycystic ovary. These are usually lined by normal-appearing ductal epithelium but may show mucinous changes, and, more importantly, they are often colonized by the carcinoma in patients with ductal adenocarcinoma and thus misinterpreted as IPMN.[185]

Other Cysts

Other rare cysts that can occur in the pancreas include parasitic cysts, endometriotic cysts, and congenital foregut (intestinal-type) cysts.

TABLE 41.3 Features of Mucinous Cystic Neoplasms and Intraductal Papillary Mucinous Neoplasms

	Intraductal Papillary Mucinous Cystic Neoplasm	Mucinous Neoplasm
Age	50-75 years	40-50 years
Gender	Male > female	Female preponderance
Location	Head > tail	Tail >>> head
Intraductal	Yes	No
Cyst configuration	Multiple	Single, multilocular
Papilla formation	Usually extensive	Usually minimal
Ovarian-type stroma	Absent	Present
ER/PR in stroma	No	Yes
Intestinal differentiation	May be prominent	Usually limited

ER, *Estrogen receptor;* PR, *progesterone receptor.*

DIFFERENTIAL DIAGNOSIS OF CYSTIC AND INTRADUCTAL LESIONS

Because of radiographic similarities between many types of cystic and intraductal neoplasms of the pancreas, it is best to consider their differential diagnosis together (Table 41.3).[286] From the outset, the clinical, radiological, and macroscopic findings are helpful to distinguish the various types of pancreatic lesions presenting as cysts. In addition, biochemical or molecular analysis of cyst fluid for tumor markers has been successfully used as a diagnostic aid in the preoperative evaluation of some types of cystic pancreatic lesions, although all such techniques have limitations in predicting the specific diagnosis or even in stratifying patients between operative and nonoperative management.[193,287-291]

Nearly all microcystic tumors of the pancreas (i.e., those with spongelike configuration) are microcystic serous cystadenomas and are therefore benign. Thus evaluation of the size of the tumor cysts is critical in the differential diagnosis process. Radiographically, the presence of a central stellate scar is typical of serous cystadenomas, although the individual small cysts may not be well visualized. These tumors lack mucinous epithelium; thus the finding of columnar, mucin-containing cells in a cystic lesion rules out a serous neoplasm. Macrocystic serous cystadenomas may simulate an MCN or IPMN (particularly the branch duct type) grossly, but the presence of a clear-cell nonmucinous epithelial lining and the peculiar, extensive, but subtle capillarization in serous cystadenomas helps in this distinction. A common problem involves distinction of an MCN from an IPMN, because both neoplasms may appear macrocystic and contain mucinous epithelium. Ovarian stroma that is pathognomonic (and sine qua non) for MCN is unfortunately not recognizable radiologically and is almost never detectable in FNA specimens. Helpful criteria are summarized in Table 41.3. In general, MCNs develop predominantly in middle-aged women and are located mainly in the tail of the pancreas, whereas IPMNs affect both sexes equally, occur in older patients, and are located predominantly in the head of the pancreas. Involvement of the pancreatic ducts is the hallmark of IPMN, whereas MCNs do not communicate with the ductal system unless there is fistula formation. In the Japanese literature, the cysts of IPMN are described as *cyst-by-cyst*, whereas MCNs are described as *cyst-in-cyst*. Microscopically, the extension of mucinous epithelium into tributary ducts and the absence of ovarian-type stroma are features that help distinguish a cystically dilated duct of an IPMN from de novo true cysts of an MCN. The cytoarchitectural features of these two entities overlap. However, extensive papilla formation is less common in MCNs. Villous intestinal pattern, in the form of elongated papillae resembling those of colorectal villous adenomas, and diffuse immunoreactivity for MUC2 favor a diagnosis of intestinal-type IPMN. MCNs often have goblet cells, but the papillae do not have this villous architecture and are instead more complex and pancreatobiliary. Finally, the presence of subepithelial ovarian-type stroma is considered entirely specific for an MCN.

A problematic differential diagnosis occurs when relatively simple cysts are found that contain mucinous epithelium without significant papilla formation, now designated *simple mucinous cyst*.[143,271] The size range of many of these lesions exceeds that proposed as the upper limit for PanINs (<1.0 cm), and some authorities recommend diagnosing larger cystic ducts with mucinous epithelium as IPMNs, even when papillae are scant. Other alternative diagnoses include *retention cyst with superimposed PanIN* or *simple mucinous cyst*, a term endorsed by a recent consensus group.[292] Simple mucinous cysts are defined to have only low-grade dysplasia, with a flat, simple mucinous lining lacking papillae. If either papillae or high-grade dysplasia are found, the preferred diagnosis is IPMN.[292]

In cases with resected PDAC, cysts >1 cm are encountered in 10% of the cases.[185] Careful inspection with the current criteria, more than one-third of these prove to be pseudo-IPMNs, that is, lesions that have ductal structures with mucinous or carcinoma lining. Most of these are secondary ectasias that can be recognized by their round appearance and location at the periphery.[185] In the large duct variant of ductal adenocarcinoma (discussed earlier), the infiltrating units are not only large but also often have papillary elements and thus closely mimic PDAC. Haphazard distribution, contour irregularities, and transition to more convincing small tubular pattern help distinguish these from IPMNs. Paraduodenal wall cysts of paraduodenal pancreatitis often have ducts lined by mucinous epithelium, but the context of myo-fibroinflammatory infiltrates, location, and other characteristic features of paraduodenal pancreatitis[280,293] allow it to be recognized. Congenital and duplication cysts may also accompany PDACs and mimic IPMN, but careful inspection reveals the muscular coat of the cyst or a distinguishing epithelium (i.e., respiratory).[185]

Acinar cell carcinomas may exhibit prominent intraductal growth,[218] and such cases can also show papillary elements, creating a picture highly reminiscent of IPMNs. Acinar cytology (round, uniform nuclei with single prominent nucleoli), presence of intraluminal crystals, and trypsin, chymotrypsin, and BCL10 expression can be diagnostic.

ACINAR CELL CARCINOMA, PANCREATOBLASTOMA, AND RELATED ENTITIES

Defined by the presence of enzyme production by the neoplastic cells, acinar differentiation is the predominant feature of a variety of uncommon pancreatic neoplasms, such as acinar cell carcinoma, pancreatoblastoma, and some carcinomas with mixed differentiation. These tumors all differ substantially from ductal adenocarcinoma at the histological, immunohistochemical, and genetic levels.

Acinar Cell Carcinomas

Clinical Features

Acinar cell carcinoma of the pancreas is an uncommon neoplasm, accounting for less than 2% of all pancreatic carcinomas.[9,294] Most patients are adults in the seventh decade of life, and there is a male predominance. Rare pediatric cases also have been described.[295-297] The presenting symptoms are generally nonspecific, and in contrast with ductal adenocarcinoma, jaundice is rare. A minority of patients develop a syndrome of lipase hypersecretion[298] characterized by markedly elevated serum lipase levels with consequent subcutaneous (and intraosseous) fat necrosis, polyarthralgia, and occasionally eosinophilia, which usually occurs only in the presence of metastatic disease. [299] Thrombotic endocarditis may be present as well.[300,301] Most patients with acinar cell carcinoma have metastases early in the course of their disease. Regional spread to the lymph nodes and liver is most common, but some patients also develop distant metastases to sites such as the ovary.[302] The long-term survival for patients with acinar cell carcinoma is poor[303]; however, several studies have shown that the clinical course is less rapidly fatal than that of ductal adenocarcinoma.[304,305] Data from the SEER program of the National Cancer Institute also shows a median survival for all patients of 47 months and a postresection survival rate of 72% at 5 years, with a median survival of 123 months.[306] Favorable responses to chemotherapy have been noted.[307,308]

Pathological Features

Grossly, acinar cell carcinomas are usually large, solid, well-circumscribed tumors. Occasionally, they show extensive necrosis, cystic degeneration, or both. The absence of a prominent stromal component imparts a soft consistency to these tumors.

Microscopically, acinar cell carcinomas are highly cellular neoplasms that form large nodules of tumor cells and lack the desmoplastic stromal response so characteristic of ductal adenocarcinomas. In fact, many cases contain little or no stroma within the tumor nodules, other than thin, wispy, fibrovascular bands surrounding the nodules of tumor. The tumor cells are typically monotonous in appearance and usually arranged in solid sheets and nests punctuated by acinar and small glandular spaces (Fig. 41.42). Occasionally, a trabecular pattern may be present, which mimics the architectural pattern of neuroendocrine tumors. The cells often exhibit basal nuclear polarization, even in solid areas (Fig. 41.43). The cytoplasm is moderate to focally abundant and characteristically shows eosinophilic granularity in the apical

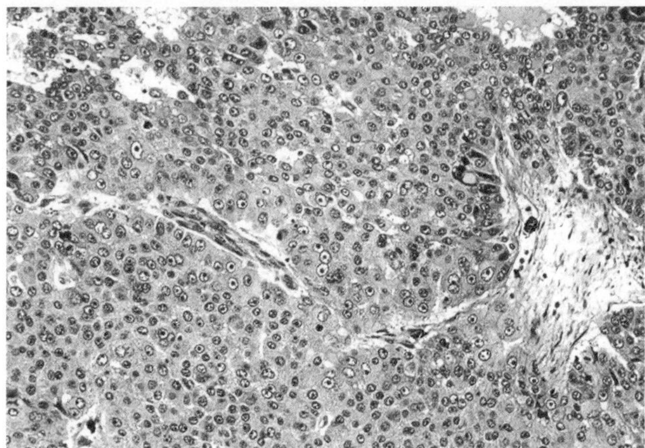

FIGURE 41.42 Acinar cell carcinoma. These tumors commonly exhibit a solid growth pattern, with sheets and nests of cells having moderate amounts of amphophilic cytoplasm and minimal lumen formation.

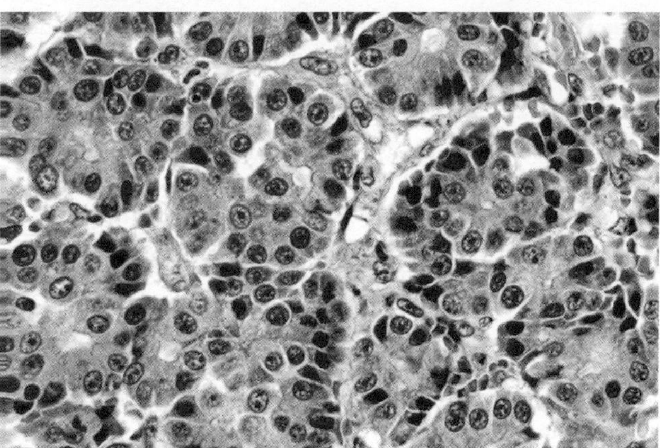

FIGURE 41.44 Acinar cell carcinoma. At high power, the acinar structures of this tumor are evident, with pinpoint lumina and basally located nuclei. Prominent nucleoli are also a characteristic feature.

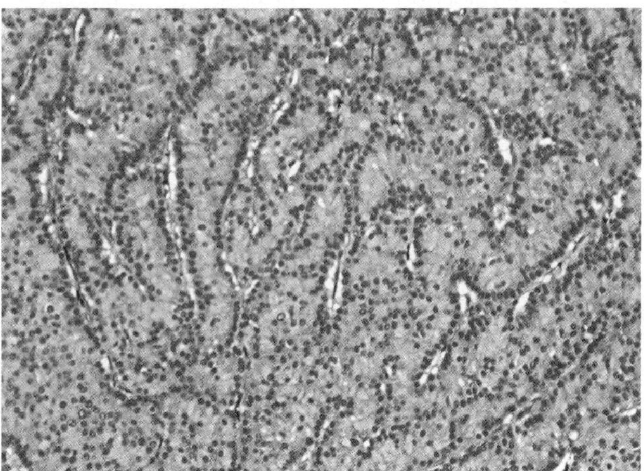

FIGURE 41.43 Acinar cell carcinoma. In some examples, there is pronounced basal polarization of the nuclei where the tumor cell nests interface with the minimal vascular stroma.

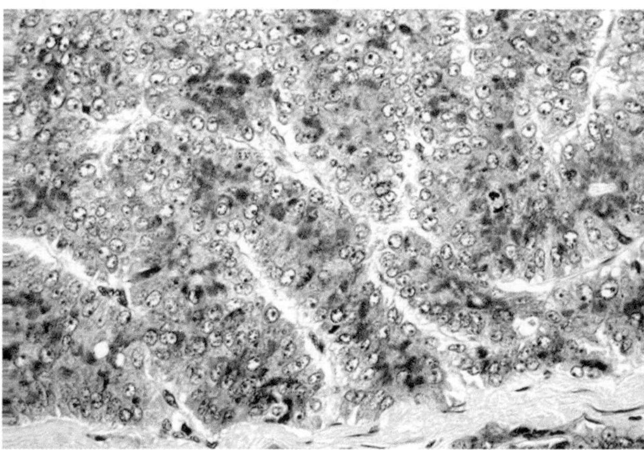

FIGURE 41.45 Acinar cell carcinoma: immunohistochemical staining for trypsin. Apical cytoplasmic positivity for this pancreatic enzyme is found in most examples of this tumor.

region caused by aggregates of zymogen granules, although in some cases, granules are difficult to appreciate histologically. The nuclei are usually only moderately atypical, although occasional cases may show marked nuclear atypia.[309] The presence of prominent single nucleoli is a characteristic feature of acinar cell carcinoma and is a helpful clue to the correct diagnosis when present (Fig. 41.44).[310] The mitotic rate of these tumors is variable but is often quite high.

Documentation of enzyme production is important to confirm a diagnosis of acinar cell carcinoma. Zymogen granules stain positively with PAS and are resistant to diastase. In well-granulated cases, a positive PAS stain can suggest a diagnosis of acinar cell carcinoma, provided that the presence of cytoplasmic mucin is excluded. However, immunohistochemical staining for specific enzymes (trypsin, lipase, and chymotrypsin) is a much more sensitive and specific method of confirming the diagnosis; 95% of acinar cell carcinomas express one or more of these enzymes by this technique (Fig. 41.45). BCL10 is a more recently described immunohistochemical marker as well.[295] Finally, ultrastructural demonstration of zymogen granules can be used to establish the diagnosis, although this technique is now rarely performed.[9] The ultrastructural morphology of zymogen granules in neoplastic cells differs from that of zymogen granules in nonneoplastic acinar cells, and their large size distinguishes them from neurosecretory granules. Irregular fibrillary granules also are detected in pancreatic acinar neoplasms and are more specific than round dense granules for confirmation of acinar cell lineage.[9]

The molecular changes of acinar cell carcinoma are becoming better understood.[311] In contrast with ductal adenocarcinoma, acinar cell carcinomas typically lack mutations in *KRAS*.[220] Alterations in the MAP kinase pathway do occur, usually as fusions involving *BRAF* or *RAF1*, which are found in 25% of cases and are mutually exclusive with alterations in DNA repair genes.[312,313] However, alterations in the wnt pathway, such as *APC* or β-catenin mutations, losses, or promoter methylation, are present in 60% to 70% of acinar cell carcinomas.[314-316] Other genes altered in acinar cell carcinoma include *CDKN2A/B* (15% to 50%), *TP53* (25% to 50%), and *SMAD4* (15% to 25%). Mutations in *ATM* and DNA repair genes are found in 45% of cases.[312] Mismatch repair gene abnormalities are more common than in ductal adenocarcinomas.[308]

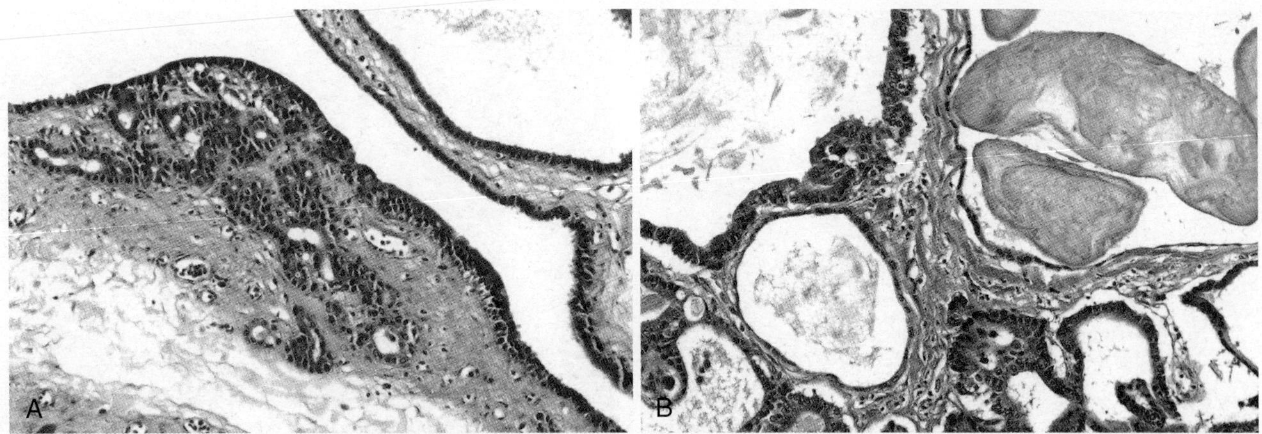

FIGURE 41.46 Acinar cell cystic neoplasms. In acinar cystic transformation (previously termed *acinar cell cystadenoma*) **(A)**, variably sized cysts are lined by a single layer of acinar or ductlike cells, with clusters of acinar cells projecting into the adjacent fibrotic stroma. Acinar cell cystadenocarcinoma **(B)** is an infiltrative neoplasm composed of cystic spaces lined by cytologically atypical acinar cells.

The main differential diagnosis of acinar cell carcinoma is PanNET. In fact, in some cases, these two tumor types may be nearly indistinguishable histologically. Pancreatoblastoma and solid pseudopapillary tumor should also be excluded. The distinguishing features of all the solid, cellular pancreatic tumors are discussed later in this chapter.

Cystic Acinar Cell Neoplasms and Lesions

Cystic and Intraductal Acinar Cell Carcinomas

Most pancreatic acinar cell neoplasms are solid acinar cell carcinomas. However, they may have cystic degeneration or necrosis. Additionally, a small proportion of acinar cell carcinomas may form true cysts (Fig. 41.46B). These very rare acinar cell cystadenocarcinomas show microcysts and macrocysts lined by atypical acinar cells, commonly with invasion into adjacent structures, and they have a prognosis similar to solid acinar cell carcinomas.[231,232] Pancreatic exocrine enzymes can be detected by immunohistochemistry.[2]

Moreover, there are also rare examples in which the acinar elements become extensively dilated and create microcystic pattern. Additionally, some acinar cell carcinomas have prominent intraductal growth that leads to cystic dilation of the ductal system and closely resemble IPMNs.[218] Some studies have found these cases to be slightly less aggressive than their solid counterparts.[218] Apart from the cystic and intraductal growth patterns, these carcinomas are identical morphologically to solid acinar cell carcinomas cytologically and immunophenotypically.

Cystic Acinar Transformation

Reported initially under the term *acinar cell cystadenoma*,[317-319] this entity is now largely regarded as a nonclonal, nonneoplastic cystic transformation in the pancreas lined at least partially by innocuous acinar cells and thus termed *cystic acinar transformation* (Fig. 41.46A).[320] Some have atypical foci formed by mural nodules that raise the concern of a neoplastic transformation, but the nature of such cases has yet to be clarified.[319] These are often incidental microscopic findings, although extensive involvement of the gland may also occur, mostly patchy but occasionally diffuse. The lining of the cysts may have more ductal elements as well as some squamoid areas, creating a challenge diagnostically. Fundamentally, this lesion displays gradual cystic changes involving the terminal ductal elements and acinar cells, and some of the cystic spaces are lined by flattened ductal-type cells. The acinar elements appear as multilayered strips and nests along the edge of the cysts, budding into the adjacent fibrotic stroma. In some incidental microscopic cases, there is obvious transition from ductal to acinar epithelium within a native ductal structure, suggesting a metaplastic process.[46] In fact, some cases give the impression of a reactive secondary cystic process.[321] There is often interposition of neoplastic cysts among nonneoplastic parenchymal elements, which is an additional feature that helps distinguish these lesions from acinar cell cystadenocarcinoma.[322]

Mixed Acinar Carcinomas

Scattered neuroendocrine cells are present in up to 40% of acinar cell carcinomas.[9] A minor element of ductal differentiation can also be detected by staining for mucin or for glycoproteins, such as mCEA. These findings do not change the diagnostic classification. However, rare pancreatic neoplasms with acinar differentiation also contain substantial amounts of neuroendocrine and/or ductal cell types.[323-327] These *mixed* carcinomas have been arbitrarily defined to have 30% of each line of differentiation.[322,324] All different combinations of mixed tumors have been reported, including *mixed acinar-neuroendocrine*, *mixed acinar-ductal*, *mixed ductal-neuroendocrine*, and *mixed acinar-neuroendocrine-ductal* carcinomas.[327] Mixed ductal-neuroendocrine tumors are discussed elsewhere in this text. Most other mixed tumors exhibit predominantly acinar differentiation, and mixed acinar-neuroendocrine carcinoma is the most common combination.[324,328] In rare cases, histologically distinct elements of each line of cellular differentiation may be found in a single tumor (Fig. 41.47), which qualifies it for the conceptual category of *mixed neuroendocrine non-neuroendocrine neoplasm* (MiNEN) and is included in the 2019 WHO classification.[1] Usually, however, there are more subtle areas of histological transition among various cell types within the tumor. In such cases, immunohistochemistry is needed to fully recognize the type and

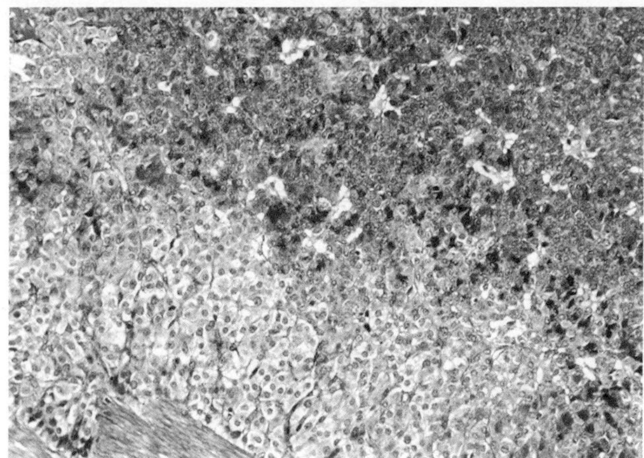

FIGURE 41.47 Mixed acinar-neuroendocrine carcinoma: Periodic acid-Schiff (PAS) stain after diastase pretreatment. In this example, two morphologically separate cell populations are identifiable: the diastase PAS (d-PAS)-positive elements representing the acinar component and the pale-staining peripheral elements representing the endocrine component.

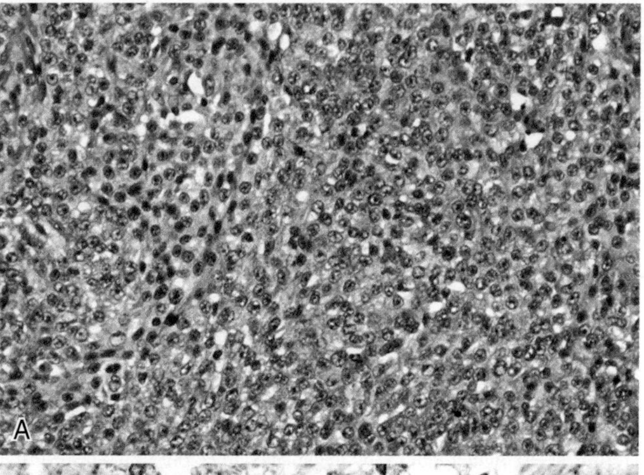

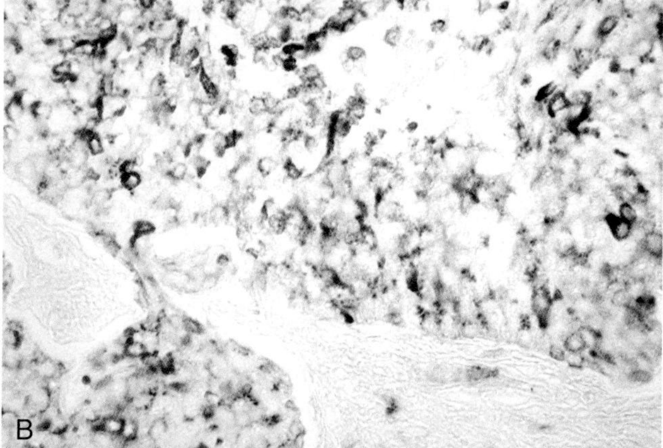

FIGURE 41.48 Mixed acinar-neuroendocrine carcinoma. In most examples of mixed tumors, the dual cell population is difficult to recognize by routine microscopy **(A)**. Immunohistochemical staining **(B)** demonstrates that each component represents more than 30% of the tumor cell population (double immunohistochemical staining for trypsin [blue reaction product] and chromogranin [brown reaction product]).

extent of each line of cellular differentiation (Fig. 41.48). Mixed acinar-neuroendocrine carcinomas are usually solid, with some areas showing acinar structures or eosinophilic granular cytoplasm. If only neuroendocrine staining is performed, these cases can be misinterpreted as pure neuroendocrine tumors. Mixed acinar-ductal carcinomas can have intracellular and extracellular mucin, providing strong evidence of ductal differentiation (Fig. 41.49).[323] Other cases have a combination of histologically typical acinar cell carcinoma with an infiltrating gland-forming component associated with stromal desmoplasia and individual glands, more typical of ductal-type carcinomas, which also show immunohistochemical evidence of ductal differentiation in the form of glycoprotein and ductal-type keratin (CK7, CK19) expression.

Because most cases of mixed acinar carcinomas are predominantly acinar, it follows that the molecular phenotype of mixed acinar carcinomas resembles that of pure acinar cell carcinomas, including *BRAF* fusions.[312] A few cases of mixed acinar-ductal carcinoma additionally have mutations characteristic of ductal carcinoma *(TP53, KRAS)*.

Most mixed acinar carcinomas behave clinically similar to pure acinar cell carcinomas. Importantly, mixed acinar-neuroendocrine carcinomas are more aggressive than PanNETs. Thus, for treatment purposes, mixed acinar carcinomas are best classified as variants of acinar cell carcinoma.[328]

Pancreatoblastomas

Pancreatoblastomas are uncommon but represent the most frequent type of pancreatic neoplasm in early childhood.[329,330] Most occur in the first decade of life, with a mean age of 4 years. However, there is a second peak in the early thirties, and such cases often create a diagnostic challenge because of a lack of awareness.[331] Some pancreatoblastomas are congenital in origin, and an association with the Beckwith-Wiedemann syndrome has been described.[332]

Pancreatoblastoma is defined as an epithelial tumor that exhibits acinar differentiation and often a lesser degree of neuroendocrine and ductal differentiation. These tumors contain "squamoid nests," which are pathognomonic for this entity, not seen in other tumor types (see later). Pancreatoblastomas share the solid, highly cellular appearance typical of acinar cell carcinomas. They are usually lobulated, with a geographic low-power appearance, and the lobules are separated by hypercellular stromal bands (Fig. 41.50). In some cases, the stroma may appear neoplastic, and heterologous bone or cartilage formation uncommonly occurs. The neoplastic epithelial cells are typically arranged in solid sheets and small acini. The tumor cells contain a modest amount of cytoplasm and prominent nucleoli.

Squamoid nests are the histological hallmark of pancreatoblastomas and should be present to establish the distinction from acinar cell carcinoma, which can also occur in children. These are distinctive structures[333] composed of a loose aggregate of large spindle-shaped cells resembling meningothelial whorls, and occasionally frankly squamous in appearance, either with or without keratinization. They form small distinct clusters that may be prominent but, in some cases, it is very subtle and can be recognized as small zones of pallor in the sea of blue. They also closely resemble the morules seen in endometrial carcinomas, cribriform morular thyroid carcinomas, and intracholecystic tubular neoplasms of the gallbladder.[334] Because they also often

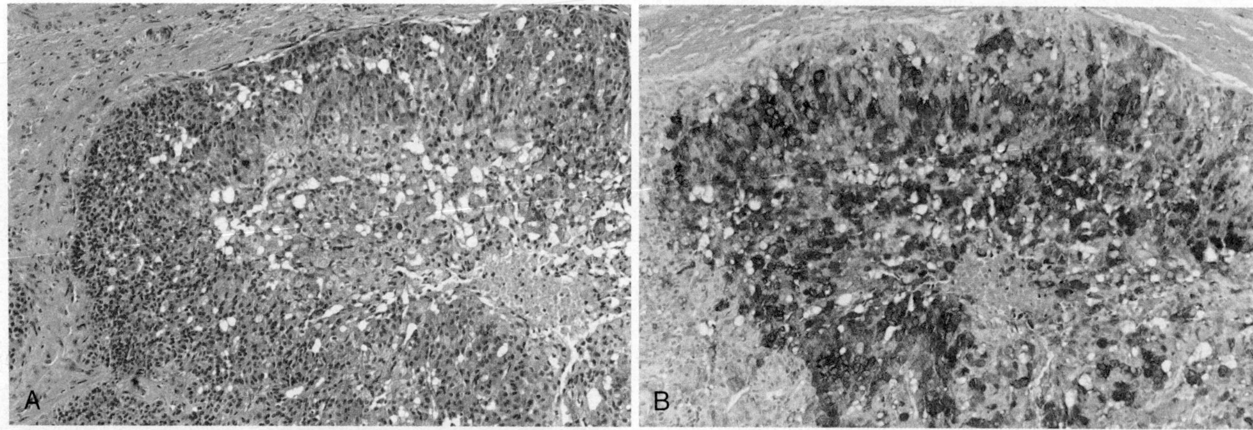

FIGURE 41.49 Mixed acinar ductal carcinoma. The tumor has a solid, nested growth pattern. The central areas have granular eosinophilic cytoplasm containing zymogen granules, while the peripheral cells have cytoplasmic mucin **(A).** Double staining with immunohistochemistry for trypsin (brown reaction product) and histochemical staining with Alcian blue for mucin (blue reaction product) highlight the dual differentiation **(B).**

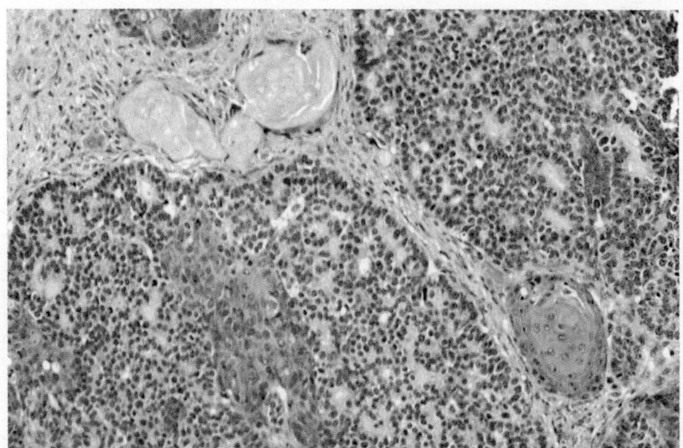

FIGURE 41.50 Pancreatoblastoma. Solid nests with acinar lumina are formed from small cells with hyperchromatic nuclei. Several squamoid nests are present, composed of larger cells with less dense nuclei; focal keratinization is present in this example.

contain intranuclear inclusion of biotin and show nuclear β-catenin pathway expression, they are now classified in the BROCN (biotin-rich optically clear nuclei) family of tumors, which share APC/β-catenin pathway alterations.

Acinar differentiation is detected in nearly all cases of pancreatoblastoma, as documented by histochemical and immunohistochemical positivity for pancreatic enzymes (e.g., trypsin and chymotrypsin) or by the presence of zymogen granules and irregular fibrillary granules by electron microscopy. In addition, a variable but usually minor amount of neuroendocrine and ductal differentiation is common in pancreatoblastomas and can be confirmed by immunohistochemistry.[330] Alpha-fetoprotein production also has been reported in pancreatoblastoma, similar to acinar cell carcinomas in childhood, and it can be detected in serum and in tissue by immunohistochemistry.[119]

The molecular alterations of pancreatoblastomas share with acinar cell carcinomas alterations in the wnt pathway,[335] although almost all cases have *CTNNB1* mutations, and there is also imprinting dysregulation of *IGF2* through a variety of genomic mechanisms, which may be the only detectable genomic alterations.[336] Typical genetic changes of ductal adenocarcinoma are absent, as are the *BRAF* fusions and DNA repair gene mutations of acinar cell carcinomas. Immunolabeling for β-catenin often shows abnormal nuclear staining, particularly localized within the squamoid nests.

The behavior of pancreatoblastomas differs in infants versus adults. In childhood, most cases that are detected before the occurrence of metastases are curable by surgery. Responses to preoperative chemotherapy have been reported.[337-339] The prognosis has been poor in patients with metastases. In adults, almost all cases of pancreatoblastoma are fatal, similar to the prognosis of acinar cell carcinomas in this age group.

The differential diagnosis of pancreatoblastoma includes other solid, cellular tumors of the pancreas (see later). In particular, pancreatoblastomas share many histological features with acinar cell carcinomas.[340] Some authorities consider pancreatoblastoma a pediatric form of acinar cell carcinoma. Because both tumors show similar lines of cellular differentiation, the presence of squamoid nests is important to distinguish them. In fact, it is advisable to carefully check for these squamoid nests in every acinar and neuroendocrine neoplasm because the behavior and genetic/familial association of pancreatoblastomas are vastly different.

PANCREATIC NEUROENDOCRINE NEOPLASMS

Pancreatic neuroendocrine neoplasms are covered in detail in Chapter 29. The classification of pancreatic neuroendocrine neoplasms recognizes the fundamental distinction between well-differentiated PanNETs and poorly differentiated pancreatic neuroendocrine carcinomas (PanNECs). PanNETs usually bear a strong resemblance to nonneoplastic islet cells and to other well-differentiated neuroendocrine neoplasms, and they strongly express immunohistochemical markers of neuroendocrine differentiation such as chromogranin A and synaptophysin. When they measure less than 0.5 mm, they are designated *pancreatic neuroendocrine microtumors*. PanNETs are separated into three grades (G1, G2, and G3) based on their proliferative rate, assessed by counting mitoses and the Ki67 labeling index. PanNECs, on the other hand, are high grade by definition and are separated into small cell carcinoma and large cell neuroendocrine carcinoma based on their specific cytological features. They express neuroendocrine differentiation immunohistochemically, but often less intensely than PanNETs. PanNECs are genetically related to ductal adenocarcinomas and also to small cell carcinomas of the lung and other organs, and they are distinct from PanNETs. A category of MiNENs also occurs in the pancreas. Almost all are a combination of ductal adenocarcinoma with poorly differentiated neuroendocrine carcinoma, but rarely the neuroendocrine component may be well differentiated.

SOLID PSEUDOPAPILLARY NEOPLASMS

Clinical Features

Solid pseudopapillary neoplasms (SPNs)[341] are tumors of uncertain cellular differentiation.[342] This is reflected in the various descriptive names previously used for this tumor, such as *solid tumor, cystic tumor, solid epithelial neoplasm, papillary epithelial neoplasm,* and *papillary-cystic tumor.*[342-345] Clinically, SPNs are significantly more common in women (male-to-female ratio, 1:9) with a mean age of 30 years. In men, they seem to occur more in children or late adulthood, but they have been described in all age groups. It is virtually nonexistent in other organs with the exception of the ovary,[346] and an analogous tumor has been described in the testis.[347] Symptoms are nonspecific, and some cases are detected only incidentally after trauma or during gynecological or obstetrical examinations. SPNs often reach large sizes before clinical detection, and the average case measures more than 10 cm in size.

Pathological Features

SPNs are solid tumors that commonly undergo cystic degeneration upon growth. Grossly, these tumors usually appear well circumscribed. They are typically yellow-brown and hemorrhagic. Most cases are soft and friable, but some may be densely fibrotic. When present, the cysts are typically quite irregular and lined by shaggy debris (Fig. 41.51). Marked cystic change may simulate the appearance of a pseudocyst.

A diagnosis of SPN is essentially based on routine histology or cytopathology.[348] The basic architecture is that of solid nests of cells surrounded by abundant small blood vessels. The tumor cells are noncohesive, as they have defects in intercellular adhesion molecules. Cells located distant from the blood vessels tend to degenerate; thus a cuff of viable cells surrounding each blood vessel imparts the characteristic pseudopapillary architecture to these tumors (Fig. 41.52). True intercellular luminal spaces are not present, although cytoplasmic vacuolization may be prominent. Variable degrees of stromal hyalinization may be present, and some cases exhibit balls of stroma within tumor cell nests, which results in a cylindromatous pattern. The cytoplasm of the tumor cells is usually moderate in amount and eosinophilic; it may appear oncocytic in some cases.[349] Clear cell change may occur.[350] Large eosinophilic hyaline globules are usually found in the cell cytoplasm, typically within clusters of adjacent cells (Fig. 41.53). The tumor nuclei are relatively uniform and characteristically contain longitudinal grooves. This creates a pattern that mimics granulosa cell tumors of the ovary. In typical cases, mitotic figures are essentially undetectable, and Ki67 is typically very low (<1%). Despite the grossly well-circumscribed nature of these tumors, a microscopic infiltrative growth pattern into adjacent nonneoplastic pancreatic tissue is common. At the interface with the nonneoplastic tissue, an intimate juxtaposition between normal acinar elements and tumor cell nests is apparent. A subset of SPNs show substantial symplastic degenerative atypia composed of markedly atypical-appearing pleomorphic cells,[351] similar to those seen in symplastic leiomyomas, ancient schwannomas, and some PanNETs, and they are believed to be biologically inconsequential.[121]

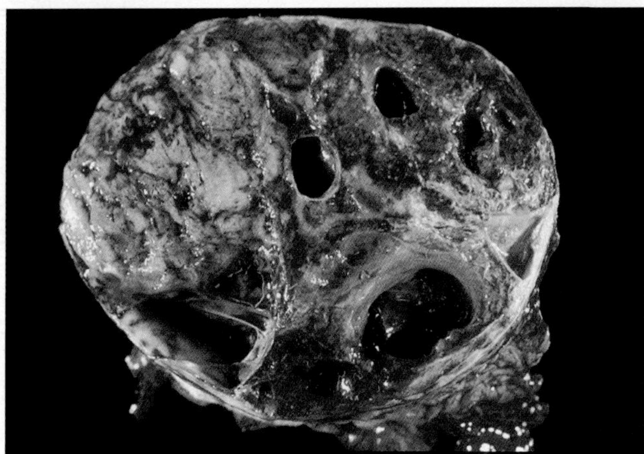

FIGURE 41.51 Gross appearance of solid pseudopapillary neoplasm. The tumor appears circumscribed and consists of soft, friable, hemorrhagic tissue with multiple large areas of cystic degeneration.

Despite intensive study, the line of cellular differentiation of SPNs remains unknown. Some cases appear to exhibit neuroendocrine differentiation, based on consistent staining for CD56 (neural cell adhesion molecule) and occasional staining for synaptophysin. However, chromogranin A is typically negative in these tumors. Both acinar and ductal markers are also consistently negative. In fact, the absence of keratin expression in more than 50% of cases is unusual for any type of epithelial neoplasm or normal epithelial cell type of the pancreas. Because SPNs almost always harbor *CTNNB1* mutations,[352] they show diffuse abnormal nuclear immunoexpression of β-catenin protein, a finding that can be useful diagnostically (Fig. 41.54). Membranous E-cadherin expression is also lost in this tumor, presumably reflecting downstream effects of the *CTNNB1* mutations.[353] Consistently positive immunohistochemical stains in these tumors include vimentin; α_1-antitrypsin, not to be confused with trypsin and α_1-antichymotrypsin; CD10; Cyclin D1; TFE3; LEF1; CD117; and progesterone receptors (but not estrogen receptors),[341,354,355] none of which are specific for any particular line of cellular differentiation. By electron microscopy, the most striking finding is the presence of large electron-dense granules, generally containing complex internal membranous and granular inclusions.[341,356] Initially interpreted to represent either zymogen granules or neurosecretory granules, these structures are now believed to resemble complex secondary lysosomes. They contain α_1-antitrypsin immunohistochemically.

Natural History

SPNs are regarded as very-low-grade malignancies, with the vast majority of the cases following a benevolent course with resection. Earlier literature cited malignancy in about

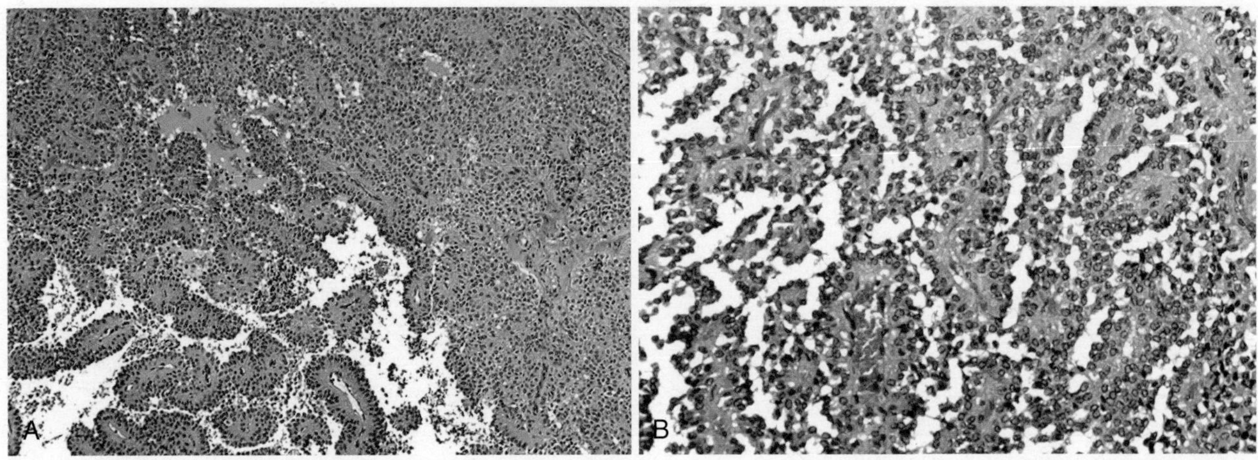

FIGURE 41.52 Solid pseudopapillary neoplasm. The solid, cellular regions of this tumor are punctuated by numerous small vessels. In some areas, the tumor cells between the vessels are discohesive and have degenerated, resulting in the formation of pseudopapillae **(A).** At higher magnification **(B),** the central vessel of each pseudopapilla can be seen with a rim of cytoplasm separating it from the surrounding nuclei. The nuclei are oval, bland, and contain longitudinal grooves.

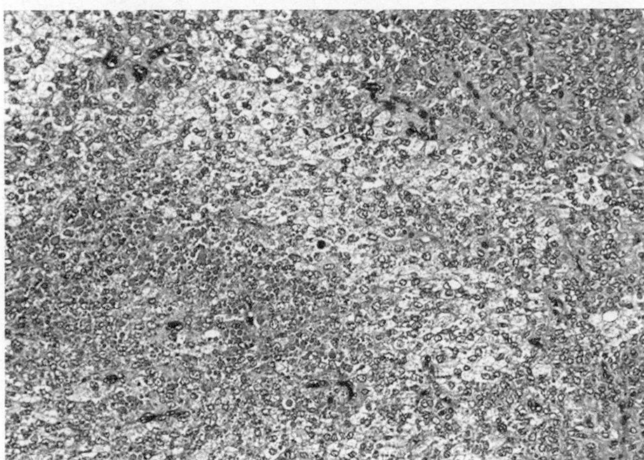

FIGURE 41.53 Solid pseudopapillary neoplasm. Some cells show foamy cytoplasm, and others contain numerous large hyaline globules.

10% of cases[341,352,357,358]; however, more recent studies scrutinizing its behavior and utilizing the more reliable diagnostic criteria reveal that metastasis and malignant behavior are in fact very uncommon in these neoplasms.[359] Metastases, if present, are almost exclusively reported either in the liver or peritoneum; nodal metastases are extremely rare. Metastases are more common in cases with even slightly notable mitotic activity. Most patients who do not exhibit metastases at the time of initial presentation do not develop them after surgical resection.[360] Interestingly, even patients with metastatic disease often survive for many years (even decades) with few symptoms. In fact, only rare deaths have been attributed to the direct effect of this neoplasm.

Two isolated cases have been reported in which an SPN underwent high-grade malignant transformation, showing elements of undifferentiated carcinoma (in one case with focal sarcomatoid differentiation).[361] The undifferentiated elements showed a sheetlike arrangement of more atypical cells, with an increased mitotic rate. Both patients died of disease within a short period.

The differential diagnosis of SPNs is discussed later. In addition to other primary pancreatic tumors, SPNs should be distinguished from adrenal cortical neoplasms, which may also exhibit a pseudopapillary pattern as a result of cellular degeneration. Both of these tumors share vimentin positivity, frequent keratin negativity, and staining for synaptophysin. Staining for inhibin (positive in adrenal cortical neoplasms) and α_1-antitrypsin (positive in SPNs) is helpful in this differential diagnosis.

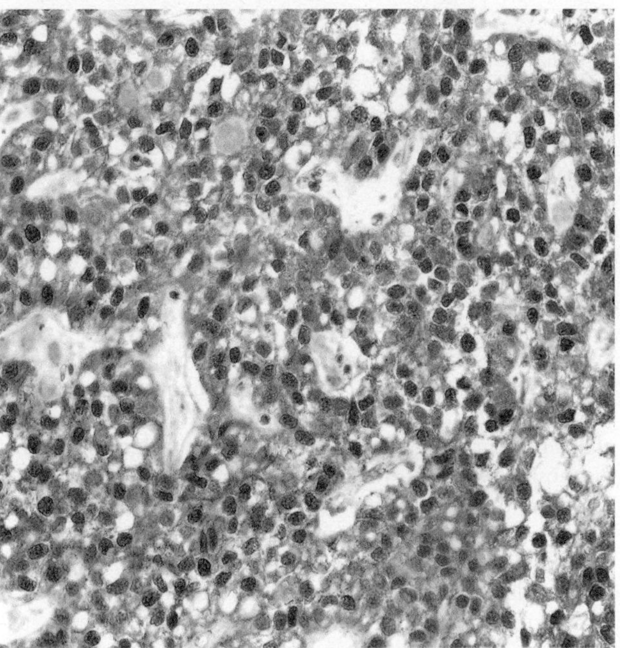

FIGURE 41.54 Solid pseudopapillary neoplasm: immunohistochemical staining for β-catenin. There is labeling of the cytoplasm and nuclei, in contrast with the normal cell membrane pattern found in the nonneoplastic pancreatic epithelium.

DIFFERENTIAL DIAGNOSIS OF SOLID CELLULAR NEOPLASMS

The group of neoplasms that includes acinar cell carcinoma, mixed acinar carcinomas, pancreatoblastoma, PanNET, and SPN all share a relatively solid, cellular appearance, which is distinct from that of conventional ductal adenocarcinoma

TABLE 41.4 Clinical and Pathological Features of Solid, Cellular Pancreatic Tumors

	Acinar Cell Carcinoma	Mixed Acinar-Neuroendocrine Carcinoma	Pancreatoblastoma	Pancreatic Neuroendocrine Tumor	Solid Pseudopapillary Neoplasm
Age (years)	50-80	18-75	0-9	30-80	15-45
Gender	M > F	M > F	M > F	M = F	F >>> M
Symptoms	Pain, lipase hypersecretion	Pain	Pain	Pain, neuroendocrine paraneoplastic syndrome	Pain
Histology	Solid nests, acini, scant stroma	Solid nests, acini, variable stroma	Solid nests, acini, squamoid corpuscles, cellular stroma	Solid nests, trabeculae, hyalinized stroma	Pseudopapillae, no lumina, variable stroma

TABLE 41.5 Immunohistochemical Findings of Solid, Cellular Pancreatic Tumors

	Acinar Cell Carcinoma	Mixed Acinar-Neuroendocrine Carcinoma	Pancreatoblastoma	Pancreatic Neuroendocrine Tumor	Solid Pseudopapillary Neoplasm
Keratin	++	++	++	++	–/+
Trypsin/chymotrypsin	++	++	++	–	–
Chromogranin	–	++	+	++	–
Synaptophysin	–	++	+	++	–/+
β-Catenin (nuclear)	–	–	+ *	–	++

*–, Usually negative; –/+, usually negative, may be positive; +, often positive; ++, consistently positive; * within squamoid nests.*

and most cystic neoplasms.[4,362] Macroscopically they form relatively demarcated and round and solid neoplasms that can protrude into the surrounding soft tissues. Certain clinical features (age, gender) are helpful in this differential diagnosis (Table 41.4). In childhood, pancreatoblastoma is most common in patients younger than 10 years of age, but SPNs are more prevalent in teenagers. The latter type of tumor is far more frequent in females, whereas all other solid, cellular tumors affect both sexes equally.

Specific histological features are helpful, such as squamoid nests in pancreatoblastoma (see Table 41.4). However, immunohistochemistry is widely considered the most helpful diagnostic technique and may be essential to recognize certain entities (e.g., mixed carcinomas).[9,324,330,341,361,363] By combining intermediate filament markers, neuroendocrine markers, enzyme markers, and selected other stains (Table 41.5), a specific diagnosis can usually be rendered. A smartly employed panel that includes trypsin, keratin, chromogranin, synaptophysin, Ki67, and β-catenin combined with a careful morphological assessment typically leads to an accurate diagnosis.

MESENCHYMAL AND LYMPHOID NEOPLASMS

Primary mesenchymal neoplasms of the pancreas are rare.[364] A review of the literature reveals only occasional examples of pancreatic soft tissue tumors, and although they present radiographically as pancreatic masses, many of these involve adjacent tissue structures, such as the retroperitoneum or duodenum, from which they may have primarily arisen.

Examples of benign pancreatic soft tissue tumors include schwannoma and lymphangioma.[365] The former may mimic MCN because of the presence of spindle cell stroma, and the latter may simulate a serous cystadenoma, but contains aggregates of lymphocytes in the cyst walls and lacks keratin immunoexpression. Solitary fibrous tumors may arise in the pancreas. They are histologically typical, containing alternating areas of hypocellular and hypercellular spindle cell elements, a variable degree of collagenization, and hemangiopericytoma-like vascular spaces. Entrapped areas of nonneoplastic pancreatic parenchyma may be extensive (Fig. 41.55). Another recently described pancreatic tumor is the benign sugar tumor (angiomyolipoma), a neoplasm of perivascular epithelioid cell origin related to renal angiomyolipoma and pulmonary sugar tumor (Fig. 41.56).[366] Similar to these other entities, pancreatic sugar tumors typically express HMB-45 immunohistochemically.

Soft tissue sarcomas also have been reported in the pancreas, such as liposarcoma, leiomyosarcoma, synovial sarcoma, and sclerosing epithelioid fibrosarcoma. Of these, leiomyosarcoma is the most frequent. GI stromal tumors also may involve the pancreas, but these presumably originate from the duodenum. Critical to the diagnosis of a primary pancreatic sarcoma is exclusion of a sarcomatoid carcinoma[125] or carcinosarcoma. Because some of these fundamentally epithelial tumors may exhibit heterologous mesenchymal differentiation, it is important to evaluate for the presence of epithelial differentiation by immunohistochemistry within the more generic spindle cell elements. Primitive neuroectodermal tumors also affect the pancreas

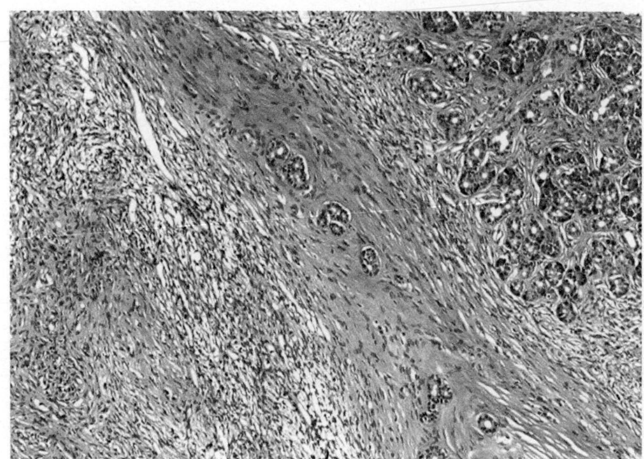

FIGURE 41.55 Solitary fibrous tumor. This spindle cell tumor exhibits variable cellularity and ectatic, hemangiopericytoma-like vasculature. The tumor surrounds clusters of nonneoplastic acini.

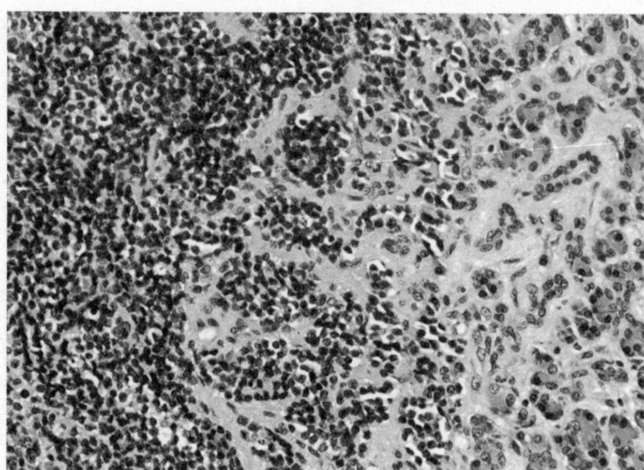

FIGURE 41.57 Primitive neuroectodermal tumor. Dense cellularity and uniform, small, round cells characterize pancreatic primitive neuroectodermal tumors.

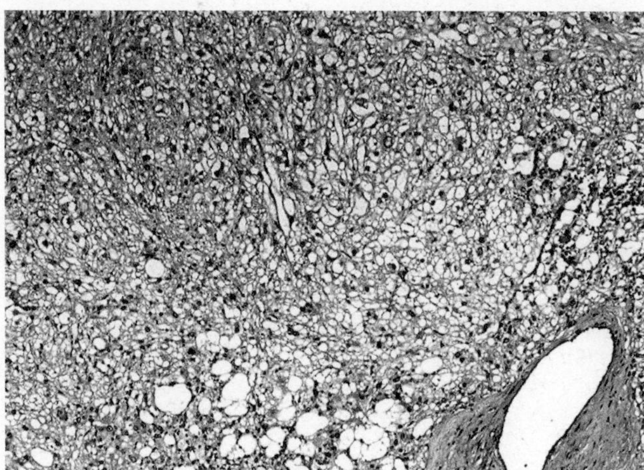

FIGURE 41.56 Sugar tumor (perivascular epithelioid cell tumor; angiomyolipoma). The tumor is composed of epithelioid spindle cells with cytoplasmic vacuolization and focally prominent vessels, resembling cellular angiomyolipoma of the kidney.

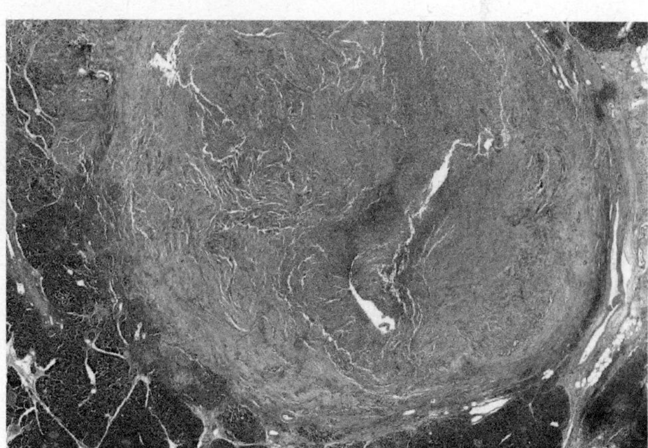

FIGURE 41.58 Sclerosing epithelioid mesenchymal neoplasm of the pancreas. The tumor is well-circumscribed and characterized with the geographic appearance of hypocellular and hypercellular areas and dense lymphoid aggregates at the periphery.

rarely.[367] Most patients are relatively young. The histological appearance resembles that of PanNETs, although primitive neuroectodermal tumors are more infiltrative and have smaller-sized cells than well-differentiated PanNETs (Fig. 41.57). One potential confounding feature in this differential diagnosis is the fact that pancreatic primitive neuroectodermal tumors commonly express keratin in a strong and diffuse manner.[367] Furthermore, well-differentiated PanNETs often express CD99 (similar to normal pancreatic islet cells).[368,369] Thus it is helpful to confirm the diagnosis of a pancreatic primitive neuroectodermal tumor by demonstrating involvement of *EWSR1*, which is found in almost all of these tumors.

Recently, a pancreatic neoplasm with unique morphological and immunophenotypic features, named *sclerosing epithelioid mesenchymal neoplasm of the pancreas*, has been reported.[370] The neoplasm presents as a solid, relatively well-circumscribed tumor (Fig. 41.58) composed of epithelioid to spindled cells with moderately atypical nuclei and occasional mitotic figures (Fig. 41.59A,B). There is a variable degree of collagenization, including cellular fibrous bands (see Fig. 41.59C). Dense lymphoid aggregates are also present at the tumor periphery. It only expresses vimentin, CD99, and cytokeratin and appears to lack abnormalities in any of the key genetic drivers except activation/enrichment of certain pathways including extracellular matrix, tight junctions, adherens junctions, and TGFβ-signaling by Gene Set Enrichment Analysis pathways that typify cells of mesenchymal origin. Methylation profiling also demonstrates a distinct methylation signature.[370]

Involvement of the pancreas by lymphoma is not uncommon in patients with widespread disease. Primary involvement of the organ or direct extension from adjacent involved lymph nodes are other forms of pancreatic involvement by lymphoma. However, primary origin of lymphoid neoplasms in the pancreas is rare. A number of the previously reported cases in fact represent plasmacytomas. Other types of non-Hodgkin lymphoma also may arise in the pancreas, but rarely.

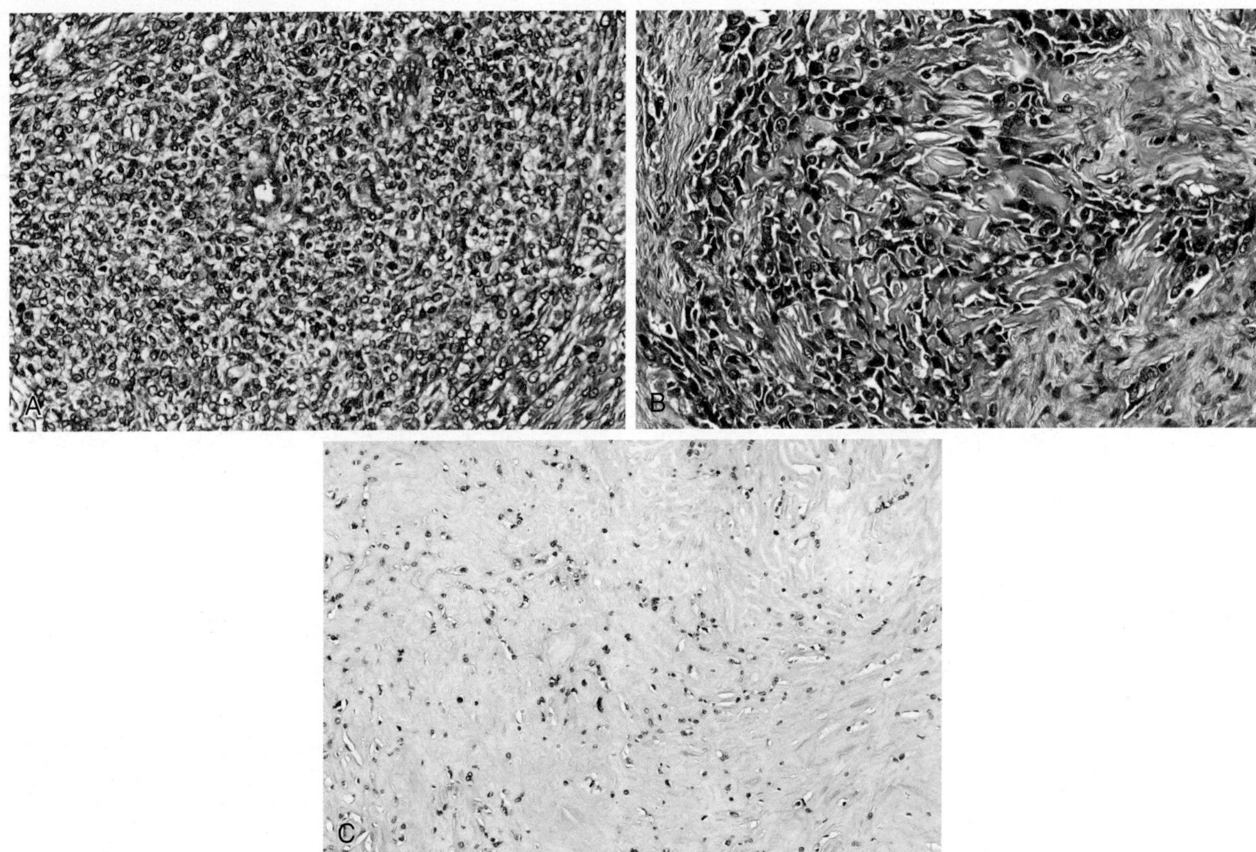

FIGURE 41.59 Sclerosing epithelioid mesenchymal neoplasm of the pancreas. The tumor cells reveal variable morphology. Most tumor cells are epithelioid to spindled and contain scant cytoplasm and round to oval nuclei with open chromatin **(A).** Others display more irregular, hyperchromatic nuclei **(B).** In some areas, scattered tumor cells are surrounded by dense hyaline fibrosis **(C).**

TUMOR-LIKE LESIONS

Various types of inflammatory processes may result in the development of a pancreatic mass and simulate a neoplastic process.[371] In some studies, 5% of pancreatectomies performed for a preoperative diagnosis of carcinoma eventually proved to be nonneoplastic on pathological examination.[371] These cases have been termed *pseudotumoral pancreatitis,* and they constitute a variety of entities with different etiologies. Among these, two are notorious for mimicking carcinoma, autoimmune pancreatitis, and paraduodenal (groove) pancreatitis (see later). In some cases, conventional chronic pancreatitis[372] (alcohol- or gallstone-related) may also develop an exaggerated focus of fibrosis that mimics carcinoma clinically. In other cases, pancreatitis and pseudotumor formation may represent autoimmune disease or a manifestation of multifocal fibrosclerosis. Cases of pancreatitis limited to the groove region (in the head of the pancreas between the bile duct and the duodenum) may resemble both solid and cystic neoplasms. These cases have been termed *groove pancreatitis, para-ampullary duodenal wall cyst,* or *paraduodenal pancreatitis.* Most occur in patients with alcohol abuse and are etiologically related to obstruction of the duct of Santorini at the minor papillae. In addition to inflammation and fibrosis, there is often formation of cysts with a partial ductal epithelial lining surrounded by hypercellular stroma derived from the duodenal muscularis.

Type 1 autoimmune pancreatitis[373,374] is another distinctive type of pseudotumoral pancreatitis that is sometimes associated with other autoimmune diseases or multifocal fibrosclerosis (e.g., retroperitoneal fibrosis, mediastinal fibrosis, Riedel thyroiditis, inflammatory pseudotumor of the orbit). These cases are characterized by a dense lymphoplasmacytic inflammatory infiltrate centered on medium- to large-sized pancreatic ducts, duct epithelial destruction, inflammatory aggregates within and surrounding small veins (obliterative venulitis), fibrosis with a storiform pattern, and atrophy (Fig. 41.60). Many patients with autoimmune pancreatitis do not exhibit an associated autoimmune disease.[373] Radiographic findings may closely mimic pancreatic carcinoma,[375] including the presence of bile duct involvement, with biliary obstruction. If the diagnosis of type 1 autoimmune pancreatitis is suspected, serum levels of IgG4 may be elevated, which is helpful for the diagnosis. Immunohistochemical staining for IgG4 also reveals increased numbers of positive plasma cells in the periductal infiltrates in many cases, and this finding may be diagnostically helpful in the evaluation of core needle biopsies.[376] The number of positive cells required to support a diagnosis of autoimmune pancreatitis varies in different studies, but a threshold of greater than 50 per high-power field is considered most specific.[376] A favorable response to steroid therapy occurs in some patients.

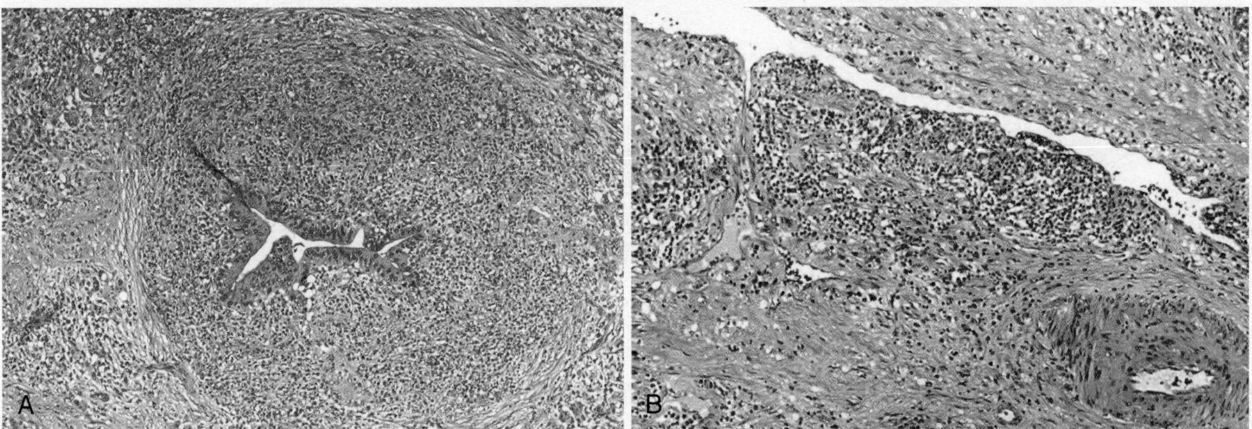

FIGURE 41.60 Autoimmune (lymphoplasmacytic sclerosing) pancreatitis, type 1. There is dense inflammation centered around pancreatic ducts **(A)**, composed predominantly of lymphocytes, plasma cells, and scattered eosinophils. Involvement of the walls of small veins (obliterative venulitis) is a typical feature of this type of pancreatitis **(B)**.

Type 2 autoimmune pancreatitis shares the periductal inflammation of type 1 but also has distinctive features, including younger age of onset, lack of serum IgG4 elevation, and different histological findings, including neutrophilic infiltrates in the ducts (so-called *granulocytic epithelial lesions*) less fibrosis, and lobular edema.[377] The diagnosis may be more difficult to establish based on biopsy specimens because immunolabeling for IgG4 is negative.[376]

SECONDARY TUMORS

Secondary tumors of the pancreas are uncommon.[82,310-313,378,379] In one analysis of 4955 autopsies, 82 of 190 presumably primary tumors of the pancreas were secondary.[82] Lung cancer was the most common source of metastasis to the pancreas, followed by lymphoma and carcinomas of the gastrointestinal tract, kidney, and breast. However, biopsy is rarely performed for these cases because they occur mainly in patients with established widespread disease.

In contrast, among resected pancreatic specimens, lymphomas are the most common secondary tumor of the pancreas, followed by gastric adenocarcinoma and renal cell carcinoma. The majority of gastric carcinomas involve the pancreas by direct extension. Lymphomas and renal cell carcinomas are prone to preoperative misdiagnosis as a primary pancreatic carcinoma. Pancreatic metastases from renal cell carcinoma may be solitary and may form polypoid masses within the pancreatic ducts in the ampulla. They may manifest years (even decades)[380] after the original diagnosis was established; furthermore, the pancreas may be the only site of recurrence. Resection of some of these secondary tumors, particularly renal cell carcinoma, is associated with relatively favorable survival rates.[381,382] Secondary tumors of the pancreas may mimic primary neoplasms not only clinically, but also microscopically; some may even grow within the ducts, simulating a primary intraductal neoplasm.

ACKNOWLEDGMENT

The authors are indebted to Drs. Kerem Ozcan and Hulya Sahin Ozkan for their contributions in the preparation of this chapter.

The full reference list may be accessed online at Elsevier eBooks for Practicing Clinicians.

CHAPTER 42

Tumors of Major and Minor Ampullae

Olca Basturk, N. Volkan Adsay

Contents

INTRODUCTION

Since both the distal common bile duct and the main pancreatic duct converge at the level of the ampulla, ampullary tumors (Box 42.1) may obstruct two organs, which may lead to early onset of symptoms. However, the potential for early detection has improved the prognosis for neoplasms of the ampulla, especially in comparison with other pancreatobiliary tumors. New techniques that are being used for local treatment, such as endoscopic polypectomy and transduodenal ampullectomy,[1-3] have created challenges with regard to pathological analysis of ampullary tumors. These are discussed more thoroughly in the following sections.

ANATOMICAL AND HISTOLOGICAL CONSIDERATIONS

In this chapter, the term *ampulla* refers to the entire ampullary structure, which includes all four compartments (Table 42.1). The word *papilla* is discouraged so it is not confused with papilla-forming neoplasms, but when it is used, it typically refers to the pinnacle (edge) of the ampullary prominence (Figs. 42.1 to 42.3). For lesions that arise from or are localized preferentially at the duodenal surface of the ampulla, the term *ampullary duodenum* should be used. Although the term *periampullary duodenum* has also been used in publications to describe this particular anatomical region,[4] it is not used in this chapter to avoid confusion.

The anatomy of the ampulla of Vater (major ampulla) can vary considerably among individuals. In most people, the common bile duct and the main pancreatic duct join into a common channel within the wall of the duodenum. Flow of luminal material through the ampulla is regulated by dense fascicles of smooth muscle, called the *sphincter of Oddi* (see Fig. 42.1A). The mucosa forms folds called *plicae*. Although the length of the common channel varies,[5] it is less than 3 mm long in most individuals. In some individuals, the common bile duct and the main pancreatic duct are separated by a septum. These anatomical variations are difficult to demonstrate in routine examination of surgical specimens[6] unless dye injection or specimen radiographs are performed.

The minor ampulla (accessory ampulla) is also subject to anatomical variations. It is typically located 2 cm proximal and anterior to the ampulla of Vater (major ampulla) within the duodenum (see Fig. 42.2A). It can be mistaken for a polyp endoscopically. The dorsal pancreatic duct (Santorini) drains through the minor ampulla. Although this duct usually regresses with fetal maturation, residual duct elements often remain in the submucosa of the duodenum. The minor ampulla is patent in approximately 40% of the population.[7,8] The composition of the minor ampulla varies among individuals.

The epithelium of both ampullae is small intestinal–type on the duodenal surface. At the edge of the ampullae, where the ducts open to the duodenum (i.e., the papilla), a specialized epithelium with features that resemble gastric-foveolar epithelium with scattered goblet cells is often present (see Figs. 42.1B and 42.3B). Because of the presence of mucinous epithelium, biopsy specimens from this area can be mistaken for peptic injury. Pancreatobiliary-type ductules lie within the wall of the ampullae (see Fig. 42.1B). These structures are usually embedded in dense myoid tissue of the sphincter of Oddi or duodenal musculature (see Fig. 42.1B).[9] Pancreatic acinar lobules often reside in the wall of the ampullae as well (see Fig. 42.3C). They may contain islets of Langerhans. Clusters of neuroendocrine cells may also occur in the minor ampulla, but only rarely in the ampulla of Vater.[10]

BOX 42.1 Classification of Ampullary Tumors

PRECURSORS
Adenomas of ampullary duodenum
Intraampullary papillary-tubular neoplasm
Flat dysplasia

CARCINOMAS
Pancreatobiliary-type adenocarcinoma
Intestinal-type adenocarcinoma
Mucinous (colloid) carcinoma
Poorly cohesive carcinoma (with/without signet-ring cells)
Adenosquamous carcinoma
Medullary carcinoma
Micropapillary carcinoma
Undifferentiated carcinoma

NEUROENDOCRINE NEOPLASMS
Well-differentiated neuroendocrine tumor
  Not otherwise specified
  Gastrinoma
  Somatostatinoma (glandular psammomatous carcinoid)
Poorly differentiated neuroendocrine carcinoma
  Small cell neuroendocrine carcinoma
  Large cell neuroendocrine carcinoma
Mixed neuroendocrine–nonneuroendocrine neoplasm (MiNEN)
  Gangliocytic paraganglioma

MESENCHYMAL NEOPLASMS
TUMOR-LIKE LESIONS
Paraduodenal pancreatitis
Adenomyomatous hyperplasia ("adenomyoma")
Others

CLASSIFICATION OF AMPULLARY TUMORS

Various criteria to determine whether a particular tumor originates in the ampulla or in the nonampullary duodenum have been described in the literature. Inconsistent use of the term *periampullary* has further complicated the issue. In some publications, it refers to the ampullary region proper, whereas in others it is used to describe the nonampullary segment of the duodenum.[11,12]

A more specific definition of the ampulla is as follows[4,13,14]: Tumors are defined as *ampullary* if more than 75% of the tumor is either localized to, or engulfed by, the ampulla and the preinvasive component (if present) is located within one of the four compartments of the ampulla. The four subtypes of ampullary carcinomas are classified according to their primary site of growth: ampullary, not otherwise specified (AMP-NOS); intraampullary papillary-tubular neoplasm (IAPN)-associated; ampullary duct; and ampullary duodenum[4,13,14] (Table 42.2; see Figs. 42.2 and 42.4 to 42.6):

1. AMP-NOS carcinomas involve the edge of the ampullary orifice (i.e., the papilla of Vater) (Fig. 42.7; see Figs. 42.1B and 42.3B), which is lined by mixed epithelia including intestinal-type, pancreatobiliary-type, and specialized epithelium with mucinous features resembling gastric-foveolar epithelium as well as scattered goblet cells.
2. IAPN-associated carcinomas arise from the distalmost ends of the common bile duct and pancreatic duct, which are lined by simple cuboidal to columnar epithelium (see Figs. 42.1A and 42.5).
3. Carcinomas of the ampullary duct involve the wall of the papilla of Vater. The wall is composed of pancreatobiliary-type ductules, peribiliary mucous glands, and myoid tissue of the sphincter of Oddi complex, which merges with the duodenal musculature (see Fig. 42.1).
4. Carcinomas of the ampullary duodenum arise from the duodenal surface of the prominence (see Figs. 42.1A and 42.5).

TABLE 42.1 Terminology

Term	Synonyms Used in This Chapter	Description
Ampulla of Vater (see Fig. 42.1)	Major ampulla	Protuberance in the second portion of the duodenum composed of (1) duodenal mucosa, (2) papilla of Vater lined by mixed epithelia, (3) pancreatobiliary-type ductules embedded in myoid tissue of the sphincter of Oddi or duodenal musculature, and (4) distal ends of the common bile and pancreatic ducts
Ampullary duodenum (see Fig. 42.5)	Duodenal surface of ampulla	Duodenum-facing surface of the ampulla, which is mostly lined by intestinal-type epithelium
Papilla of Vater (see Figs. 42.1 and 42.3)	None	Refers specifically to the protuberance (edge of the pinnacle) of the ampulla, lined by mixed epithelia including specialized epithelium with mucinous features and scattered Goblet cells. Its wall is composed of pancreatobiliary-type ductules embedded in myoid tissue of the sphincter of Oddi or duodenal musculature
Ampullary duct (see Figs. 42.2 and 42.6)	None	Refers to pancreatobiliary-type ductules and peribiliary mucous glands as well as the duct epithelium of the very distal segments of the common bile duct and the main pancreatic duct
Minor ampulla (see Fig. 42.3)	Accessory ampulla	Located 2 cm proximal and anterior to the ampulla of Vater (major ampulla), within the duodenum

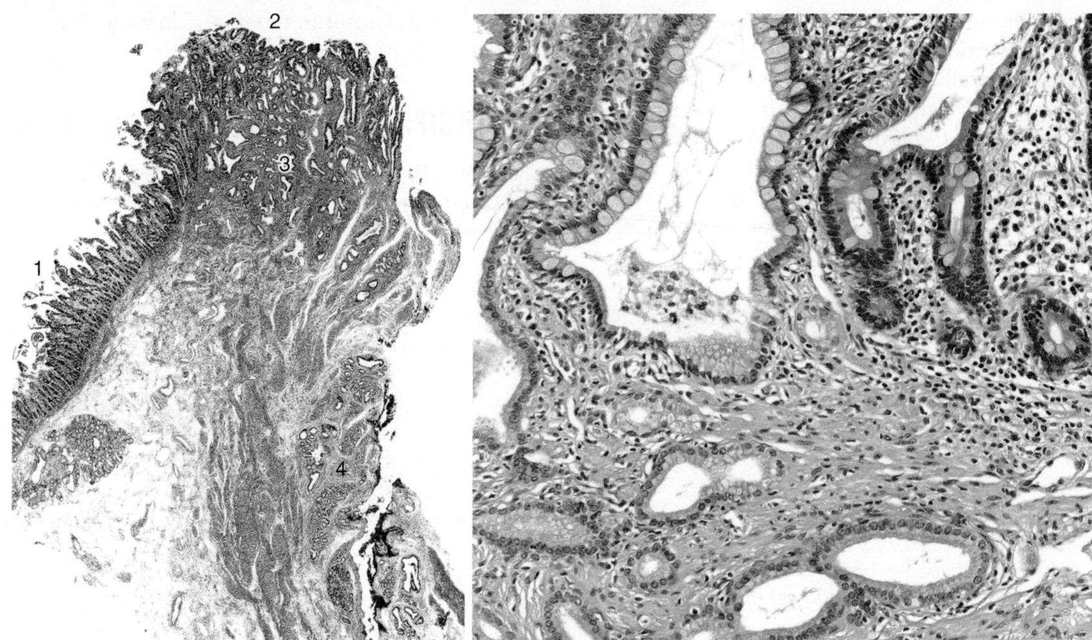

FIGURE 42.1 Histological constituents of the ampulla pertinent to tumor classification. The duodenal surface of the ampulla *(1)* is lined by intestinal epithelium. The papilla of Vater *(2),* which is the prominence where the tips of the two ducts transition into duodenal mucosa, exhibits mixed epithelia, including specialized epithelium with mucinous features and scattered goblet cells (see Fig. 42.3). In the wall of the ampulla, pancreatobiliary-type ductules *(3)* are embedded in the dense musculature of the sphincter of Oddi. The very distal segments of the common bile duct and the main pancreatic duct contain various amounts of tributary ductules or peribiliary mucous glands *(4).*

PREINVASIVE NEOPLASMS

Adenomas of the Ampullary Duodenum

Clinical Features and Definition

Adenomas of the intestinal type, similar in appearance to colorectal adenomas, may arise and grow in the ampullary duodenum (i.e., duodenal surface of the ampulla).[15] In the small intestine, the ampulla is a particularly common site of adenoma development,[16] presumably because this is an anatomical site that is prone to chemical or physical injury. Most ampullary adenomas are sporadic, but the ampullary and other parts of the duodenum are the most common sites of extracolonic adenomas in patients with familial adenomatous polyposis (FAP).[17-21] Between 80% and 90% of patients with FAP develop multiple adenomas in the duodenum, and 25% occur in the ampullary duodenum. Symptomatic adenomas are usually detected within 10 to 15 years of colectomy in FAP patients.[20] Fortunately, because FAP screening protocols include periodic endoscopic surveillance of the duodenum, adenomas are increasingly detected at an earlier stage of development, while they are still asymptomatic.[22]

Adenomas of ampullary duodenum often extend inside the ampulla and involve its distal common bile duct/main pancreatic duct segments. By definition, more than 75% of the lesion should be located on the duodenal surface of the ampulla for it to be classified as an adenoma of the ampullary duodenum. Tumors with complete or near-complete intrapapillary growth are classified as IAPNs.

Patients with sporadic adenomas of the ampullary duodenum are an average of 60 years of age. In contrast, FAP patients are typically 20 years younger at the time of diagnosis.[16,23-26] Sporadic cases have a female predilection, whereas both sexes are affected equally by FAP.[17,18,20,22] Clinical symptoms vary. Larger adenomas may cause bile duct obstruction with jaundice, abdominal pain, and pancreatitis.[26] Smaller adenomas are often asymptomatic. Gastrointestinal (GI) hemorrhage is rare and raises concerns regarding the existence of an invasive carcinoma. However, invasive carcinomas that arise in adenomas are often hidden at the base of the polyp and are difficult to detect in surface biopsies.[27] Of note, adenomas of the ampullary duodenum are more likely to harbor an invasive carcinoma than similarly sized colorectal adenomas. The prevalence of carcinoma increases proportionately with the size of the polyp.[17,18,20,22]

Pathological Features

Adenomas are classified as tubular, tubulovillous, or villous, depending on the amount of glandular and papillary architecture. Tubulovillous adenomas contain more than 25% villi,[15] and villous adenomas contain more than 75% villi. Tubular, villous, and tubulovillous adenomas occur with equal frequency in sporadic cases. However, tubular adenomas are more common in patients with FAP.[17-22] Villous adenomas tend to be larger than tubular or tubulovillous adenomas, and they are more likely to harbor a carcinoma.

Grossly, most tubular adenomas of the ampullary duodenum are bosselated in appearance, whereas most villous adenomas have a feathery or papillary appearance (Fig. 42.8).[28,29] A firm texture or the presence of surface ulceration should always raise concern of an invasive component.[17-22]

Microscopically, adenomas of the ampullary duodenum are similar to those that occur in the large intestine. They are composed of tubules and/or villi (papillae) lined by columnar cells with elongated, hyperchromatic, pencil-shaped nuclei and nuclear pseudostratification. The amount of cytoplasmic

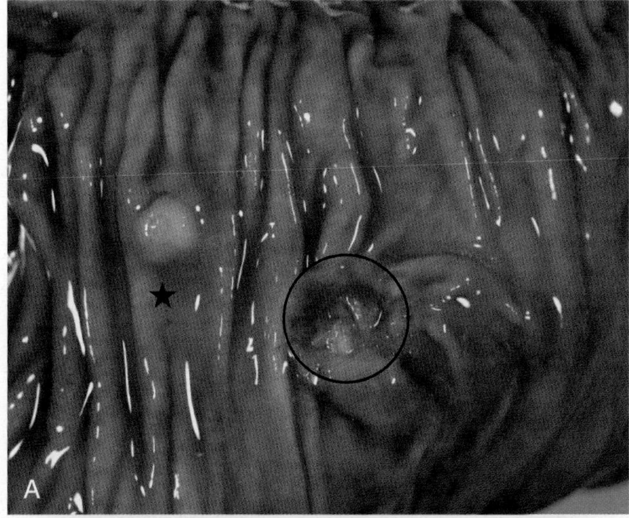

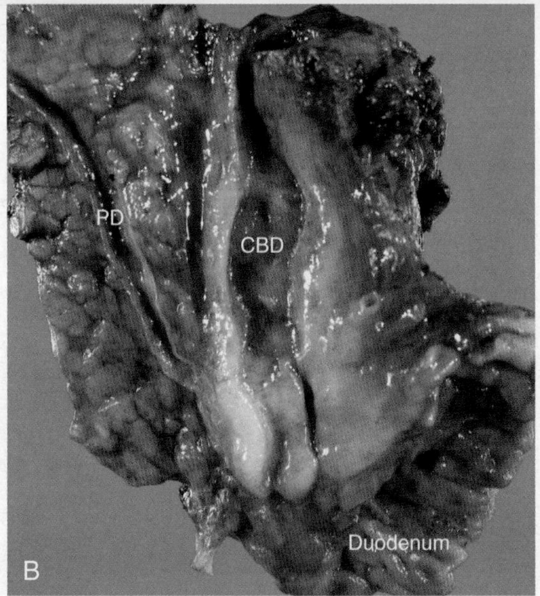

FIGURE 42.2 **A,** Ampullary duct carcinomas *(circle)* are characterized by relatively subtle changes from the duodenal perspective. The mucosal-covered elevation may be irregular or ulcerated. Note the minor ampulla *(star)*. **B,** On sectioning, ampullary duct carcinomas typically reveal plaquelike firmness in the wall of the ampulla. *CBD*, Distal end of the common bile duct; *PD*, the main pancreatic duct.

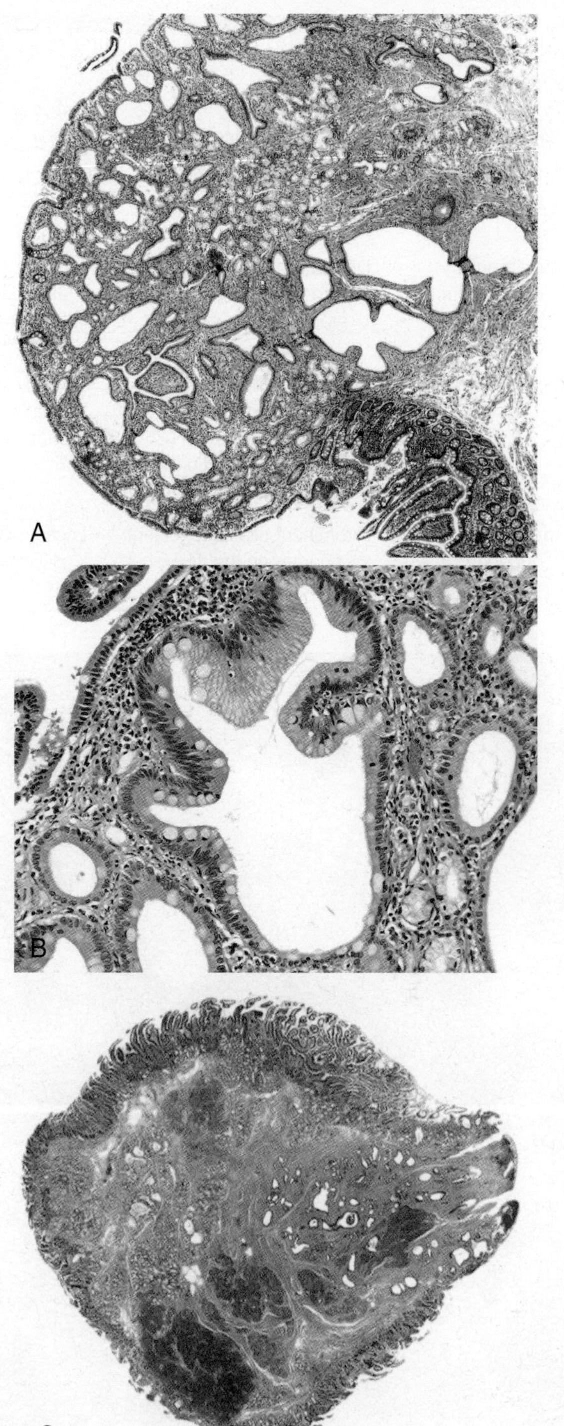

FIGURE 42.3 The minor papilla is similar to the major papilla morphologically. It shows intestinal-type mucosa that transitions into a papilla, which is composed of pancreatobiliary-type ductules **(A)** and specialized epithelium with mucinous features and scattered goblet cells **(B).** Pancreatic lobules **(C)** and clusters of neuroendocrine cells may be seen on the wall of the minor papilla.

mucin varies. Goblet cells may be present, but they are not usually numerous. Some FAP-associated cases may be quite subtle, in some cases showing surface maturation.[17-22]

By definition, all adenomas are dysplastic. Dysplasia is categorized as low grade or high grade, depending on the degree of cytological and architectural atypia. Low-grade dysplasia consists of pseudostratified, relatively monotonous columnar cells with cigar-shaped, elongated nuclei. The nuclei are mostly lined up in the basal aspect of the cell cytoplasm, and there is no, or only mild, pleomorphism and loss of nuclear polarity. High-grade dysplasia is characterized by marked nuclear pleomorphism, loss of polarity, increased nucleus-to-cytoplasm ratio, and increased mitoses combined with architectural complexity, such as cribriforming, back-to-back glands, and micropapillae formation.

Paneth cells and neuroendocrine cells are particularly common in all ampullary adenomas, and in some cases they can form more than 50% of the neoplastic cell population, particularly in FAP.[30] Rare cases contain independent clusters of neuroendocrine cells at the base of the adenoma. Immunohistochemical staining reveals intestinal differentiation, such as positivity for cytokeratin (CK)20, CDX2, and MUC2.[27,31] CK7 is also commonly positive in these

TABLE 42.2 Macroscopic Properties of Ampullary Tumors[13,14]

Subtype of Ampullary Carcinoma	Luminal Findings	Status of Ampullary Orifice	Cut Section Appearance	Findings in the Distal Segments of the Common Bile and Pancreatic Duct
Ampullary-NOS (papilla of Vater)	Ulceration and/or polypoid lesion localized in the ampulla	Centrally located	White, firm lesion involving the papilla of Vater	Nondescript tumor involvement of the distal tips
Intraampullary papillary-tubular neoplasm associated	Dilated ampullary orifice with protruding polypoid granular material	Centrally located; dilated orifice, easily probable	Preinvasive (polypoid/granular) exophytic lesion *within* ampullary channel and distal segments of the ducts	Filled with papillary nodular or granular material; often significantly dilated
Ampullary duct	Minimal changes; button-like mucosal-covered elevation or subtle ulceration or minimal granulation	Centrally located; often relatively difficult to probe	Scirrhous, plaquelike, constrictive, and often subtle lesion on the wall of the papilla of Vater and distal segments of the ducts	Scarlike firmness on the walls, often concentric
Ampullary duodenum	Prominent ulcero-vegetating nodules on the duodenal surface of the ampulla	Eccentrically located; difficult to probe in some cases	Granular, nodular tumor on the duodenal surface, pushing into the inner structures	Variable secondary destruction by invasion of the duodenal surface lesion

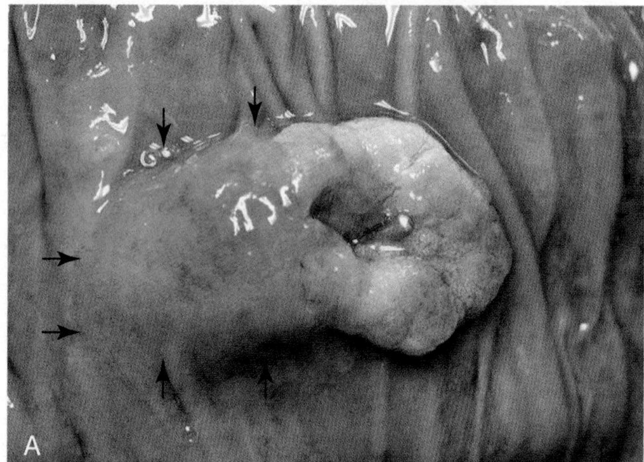

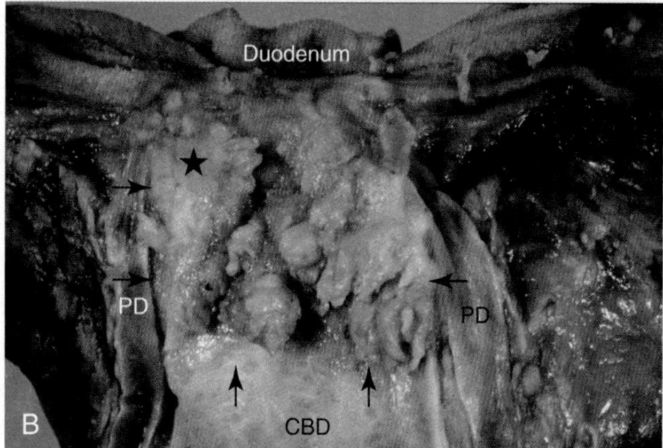

FIGURE 42.4 Intraampullary papillary-tubular neoplasm–associated invasive carcinoma.[6,13,14] **A,** The ampullary orifice is markedly dilated. White, granular mucosa involves the papilla of Vater and protrudes into the duodenum. The probe in the common bile duct indicates the ampullary orifice. The bulge on the left, which is covered by duodenal mucosa *(arrows),* is caused by the underlying tumor that fills the ampullary channel. **B,** On sectioning, the bulk of the lesion was found to be localized within the distal segment of the common bile duct *(CBD)* and the main pancreatic duct *(PD),* forming a granular, polypoid, exophytic lesion *(arrows).* The duodenal mucosa was mostly uninvolved. Beige-tan areas of this polypoid or nodular lesion represented preinvasive neoplasm, whereas the white-gray area *(star)* was found to be invasive carcinoma on microscopic examination.

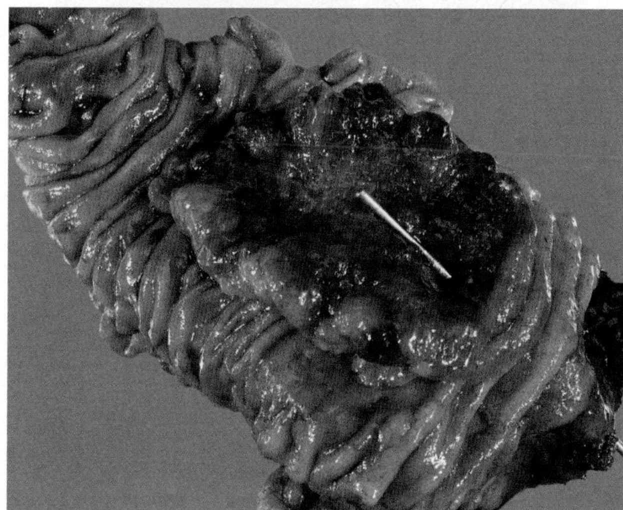

FIGURE 42.5 Carcinomas of the ampullary duodenum manifest as ulcerovegetative tumors. The ampullary orifice is located eccentrically *(probe).*

tumors.[31,32] Paneth cells label for lysozyme, and the neuroendocrine cell component can be detected with chromogranin and/or synaptophysin.[20,31,33,34]

Differential Diagnosis

Extension of adenomatous epithelium into ductules located in the wall of the papilla can simulate invasive carcinoma, particularly where continuity with the normal surface epithelium is lost and high-grade dysplasia is present. Because of the complexity of ductular structures, it may be difficult or even impossible to distinguish a preinvasive lesion from true invasion in some cases (Fig. 42.9). Findings such as paradoxical differentiation (i.e., different cytomorphology in preinvasive vs. invasive components), cuboidal epithelium, dispersion in a nonlobular and nonorganoid fashion, formation of complex micropapillary tufts or markedly elongated gland units, marked contour irregularities, and severe cytological atypia all favor invasive carcinoma (Table 42.3). Budding and vascular or perineural invasion are also helpful findings for a diagnosis of invasion. Unfortunately, in some cases invasion can be

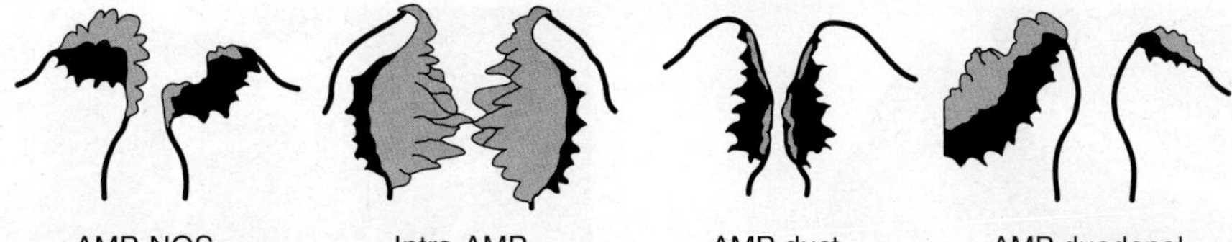

FIGURE 42.6 Subtypes of ampullary carcinoma can be determined by careful gross examination.[6,13,14] The diagrams indicate preinvasive tumor *(gray)* and invasive tumor *(black)* areas. Arising in the papilla of Vater, ampullary carcinoma may be classified as not otherwise specified *(AMP-NOS)*. Intraampullary papillary-tubular neoplasm associated carcinomas *(Intra-AMP)* are characterized by a prominent preinvasive neoplasm that grows predominantly as an exophytic mass within the ampullary channel (i.e., distal ends of the common bile duct and the main pancreatic duct). In contrast, ampullary duct (AMP duct) carcinomas show minimal or no preinvasive lesion, and instead form a plaquelike stricture at the distal ends of the ducts. Ampullary duodenum carcinomas *(AMP duodenum)* form ulcerovegetative tumors that grow predominantly (>75%) on the duodenal surface of the ampulla.

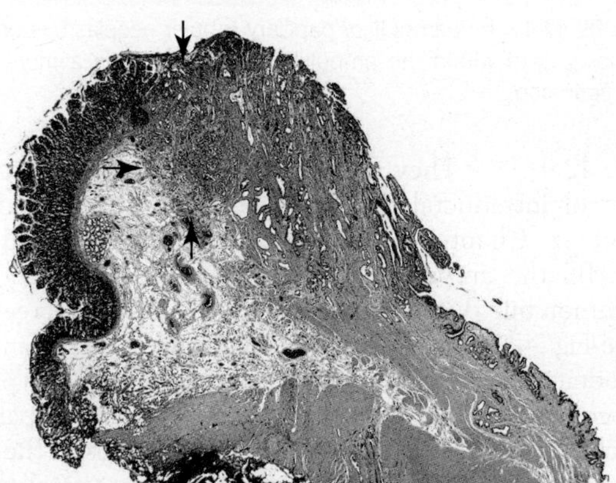

FIGURE 42.7 Early-stage ampullary adenocarcinoma arising in the papilla of Vater (i.e., ampullary carcinoma, not otherwise specified). This relatively small carcinoma *(arrows)* invades through the sphincter of Oddi into duodenal submucosa. The American Joint Committee on Cancer tumor-node-metastasis classification (2017) regards this as a T1b tumor.

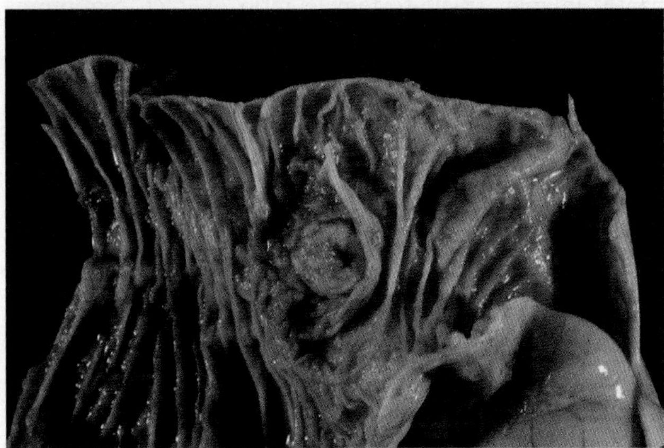

FIGURE 42.8 Gross appearance of an ampullary adenoma. In a patient with familial adenomatous polyposis, the ampulla is prominent and granular, and there are multiple, small polyps in the surrounding duodenal mucosa.

expansile (i.e., nodular or pushing border), without evidence of a conventional infiltration pattern.

Another diagnostic dilemma arises when an underlying invasive carcinoma of the pancreas or bile duct involves the ampullary epithelium by colonization ("cancerization") of the mucosal basement membrane, which simulates a preinvasive component (Fig. 42.10). This process is termed *pseudoadenomatous transformation*. This process can be very innocuous.

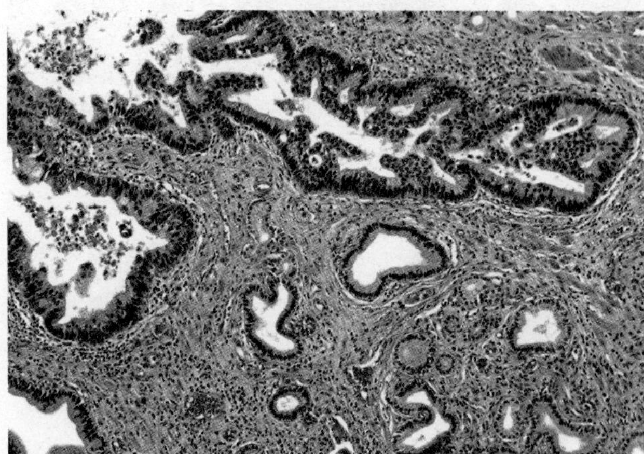

FIGURE 42.9 Adenomatous epithelium extends into biliary-type ductules in the duodenal wall.

TABLE 42.3 Morphological Characteristics of Invasive Carcinomas and Preinvasive Lesions

Findings	Invasive	Preinvasive
Dispersion of glands	+++	–
Lobularity	–	+++
Clustering of evenly shaped glands	–	+++
Cytological discrepancy with the surface component	++	–
Loss of cell polarity	++	±
Contour irregularities	++	–

It often forms scattered units that appear to be out of context. In these cases, immunohistochemical stains may help demonstrate that both components have the same type of pancreatobiliary (rather than intestinal) differentiation and are positive for only CK7 (rather than both CK7 and CK20) and for MUC1 (rather than MUC2 and CDX2).[31]

Reactive changes associated with inflammatory processes of the ampulla can also mimic an adenoma (Fig. 42.11). However, in addition to having associated inflammation, reactive changes usually lack the degree of nuclear elongation and pseudostratification characteristic of dysplasia. Paradoxically, reactive nuclei occasionally show more severe atypia than low-grade dysplasia, in the form of nuclear enlargement and macronucleoli. Reactive epithelium may also reveal a higher degree of cytoplasmic eosinophilia than dysplasia, presumably because it does not contain abnormal mucins. Nevertheless,

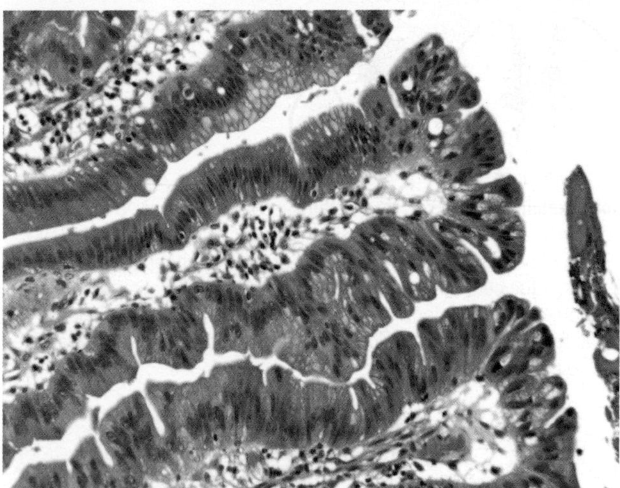

FIGURE 42.10 Mucosal colonization by an underlying invasive ductal adenocarcinoma of the pancreas. The malignant cells grow along the basement membrane, resembling the pattern of a primary ampullary adenoma (i.e., pseudoadenomatous transformation).

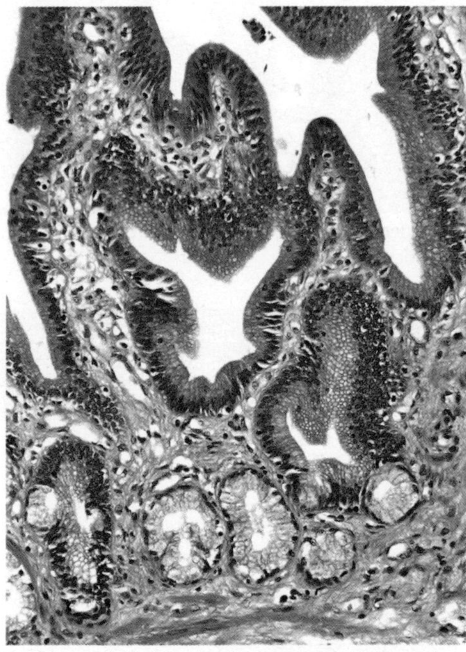

FIGURE 42.11 Reactive hyperplastic changes in the ampullary mucosa can manifest as columnar cells with pseudostratification that can resemble adenomatous (dysplastic) epithelium. Unlike dysplasia, these reactive foci usually retain their cellular maturity, basal location of the nuclei, and the cytoplasmic texture and color of normal mucosal epithelium.

architectural complexity, a characteristic feature of high-grade dysplasia, is not seen in reactive epithelium.

Adenomatous lesions that occur within the papilla and distal common bile duct (i.e., IAPNs) have several distinctive characteristics that distinguish them from adenomas of the ampullary duodenum as discussed in the following sections.

Intraampullary Papillary-Tubular Neoplasms

Clinical Features and Definition

IAPNs are adenomatous (tumoral, intraepithelial, neoplastic) lesions that occur almost exclusively in the ampulla (see Fig. 42.4).[14,35] They represent the intraampullary counterpart of intraductal neoplasms of the pancreas and biliary tract (see Chapters 38 and 40). Papillary or polypoid tumors can fill the ampullary channel and distal segment of the common bile duct, or they can fill the main pancreatic duct (see Fig. 42.4). By definition, involvement of the ampullary duodenum and intramucosal extension into the proximal aspect of the common bile duct and the main pancreatic duct is minimal (<25%). Although adenomas of the ampullary duodenum are almost invariably of intestinal type and are morphologically identical to colonic adenomas, IAPNs commonly exhibit nonintestinal phenotypes.[36]

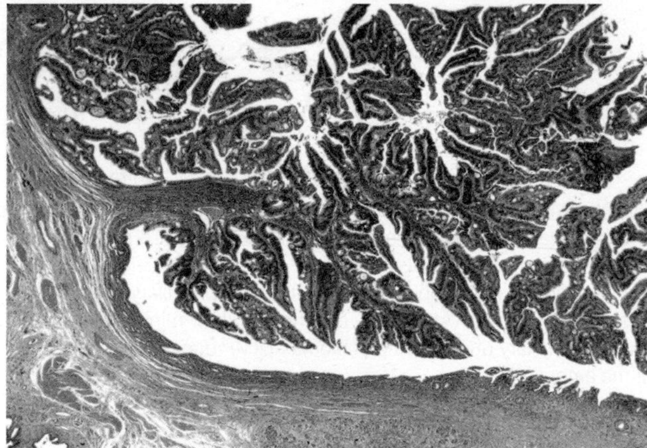

FIGURE 42.12 Intraampullary papillary-tubular neoplasm is preinvasive tumor growth within the ampulla. This case shows a more papillary configuration.

These tumors account for one-third of all pancreatoduodenectomies performed for a clinical diagnosis of an ampullary tumor. The mean age of affected patients is 64 years (range, 27 to 85 years), and these tumors occur predominantly in men (male-to-female ratio of 2.2). Symptoms (e.g., jaundice, pruritus, light stool, dark urine) are usually related to obstruction of the common bile duct, but patients also may have nonspecific symptoms such as abdominal pain and weight loss.

Pathological Features

Gross examination of the ampullary duodenum[6] typically reveals a hemispheric elevation of intact mucosa, often with a patulous papilla orifice from which nodules of friable granular material protrude into the duodenal lumen (see Fig. 42.4A). A probe inserted into the common bile duct or the main pancreatic duct typically extends into the center of the lesion. Ulceration may be evident, but overt mucinous discharge, characteristic of pancreatic intraductal neoplasms, is seldom encountered. On sectioning the ampullary channel, the tumors are characterized by a prominent exophytic growth pattern in the dilated distal bile and pancreatic ducts (see Fig. 42.4B). Obstructive polypoid and light tan, granular nodules, which are often associated with dilation of upstream biliary or pancreatic ducts, may be present (see Fig. 42.4B). Although not very impressive from the duodenal perspective, they are often quite large within the ampulla, with a mean tumor diameter of 2.9 cm.

Microscopically, IAPNs show various degrees of papillary or tubular growth (Figs. 42.12 to 42.14). Most show a mixture of these patterns. They exhibit a spectrum of dysplasia; most cases show a mixture of low- and high-grade dysplasia.

The criteria used for low- and high-grade dysplasia is the same as that used for adenomas of the ampullary duodenum (discussed earlier). However, a significant proportion of cases reveal hybrid morphology, and some even exhibit gastric differentiation (see Fig. 42.14) similar to that of intraductal and intracholecystic tumors of the pancreatobiliary tract as well as foveolar and pyloric adenomas of the stomach. These cases may lack overt cytological atypia characteristic of intestinal-type adenomas. In most cases, foci of high-grade dysplasia are present. High-grade dysplasia correlates positively with a papillary configuration. Unlike adenomas of the ampullary duodenum, approximately 50% of IAPNs show mixed (intestinal, gastric, pancreatobiliary) differentiation.

Unlike adenomas of the ampullary duodenum, IAPNs are often invasive. Approximately 75% are associated with invasive carcinoma at the time of diagnosis, but the invasive component is usually less than 1 cm in diameter. Invasion is mostly tubular and often shows a mixture of intestinal (Fig. 42.15) and pancreatobiliary features (Fig. 42.16). The histological type of invasive carcinoma parallels that of the preinvasive component in many, but not all, cases.

The hybrid nature of these lesions is reflected in their immunophenotype. More than 50% of cases coexpress CK7 and CK20. Immunostaining for MUC2 and CDX2 is positive in cases with intestinal differentiation. MUC1, MUC5AC, and MUC6 are positive in cases with gastropancreatobiliary differentiation. However, a significant proportion of the cases reveal a mixed immunophenotype.[14]

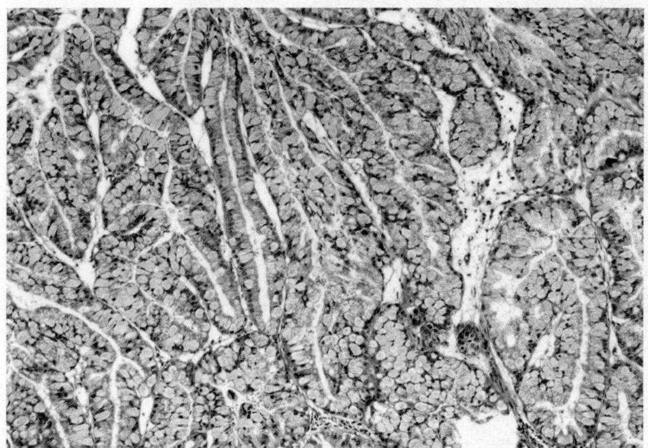

FIGURE 42.13 Intraampullary papillary-tubular neoplasm. This case has a markedly complex growth pattern.

Differential Diagnosis

The most challenging aspect of these lesions is to differentiate invasion from pseudoinvasion. The preinvasive component of these lesions often involves ductules in the wall of the ampulla. The criteria for identifying invasion in adenomas of the ampullary duodenum are also applicable in these cases (see Table 42.3).

Differentiating IAPNs from their pancreatic and biliary counterparts, or adenomas of the ampullary duodenum, requires knowledge of the location and distribution of the neoplastic lesion. A nonintestinal phenotype is helpful in distinguishing these lesions from adenomas of the ampullary duodenum because the latter invariably reveal intestinal differentiation.

Natural History and Prognosis

Noninvasive cases have an excellent prognosis. However, cases with extensive high-grade dysplasia but without invasion may recur. Lymph node metastasis occurs, not uncommonly, even in cases that are minimally invasive. Long-term follow-up is warranted, even in noninvasive cases.[14]

Cases with invasive carcinoma are associated with better survival than conventional (invasive) ampullary carcinomas unaccompanied by an IAPN (3-year survival of 69% vs. 44%).[14] This survival advantage is likely attributable to early detection of invasion, but likely also reflects differences in tumor biology.[4,14,37]

Flat Dysplasia

Some ampullary carcinomas arise from flat dysplasia instead of developing from an adenomatous polyp.[15] In rare cases, dysplastic epithelial cells grow along the ducts at the periphery of an invasive carcinoma. Flat dysplasia of the ampulla in the absence of invasive carcinoma is rarely seen, presumably because these lesions do not obstruct the ampulla and are usually asymptomatic.

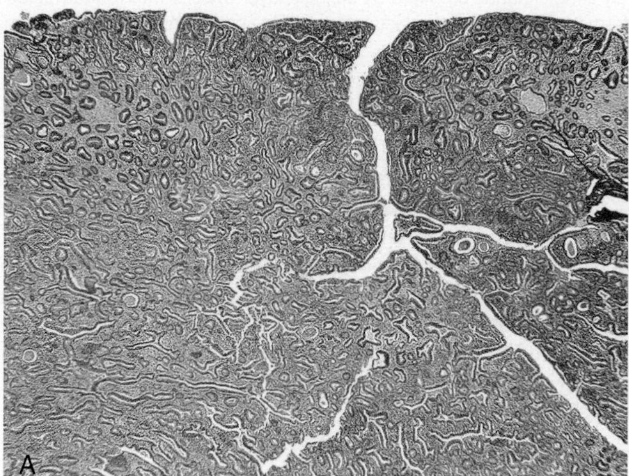

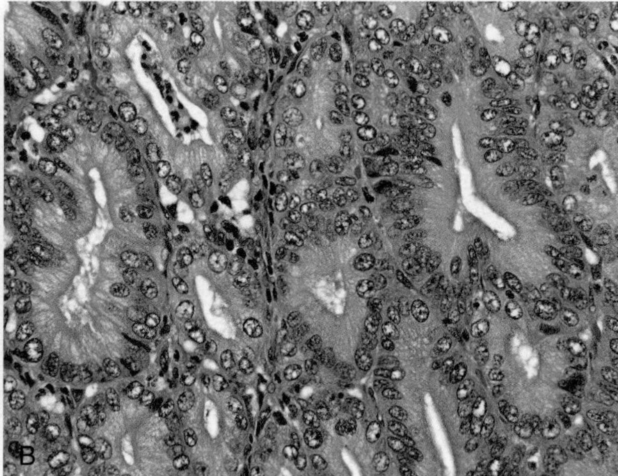

FIGURE 42.14 **A** and **B,** This case of an intraampullary papillary-tubular neoplasm shows a prominent tubular configuration of gastric-like glands.

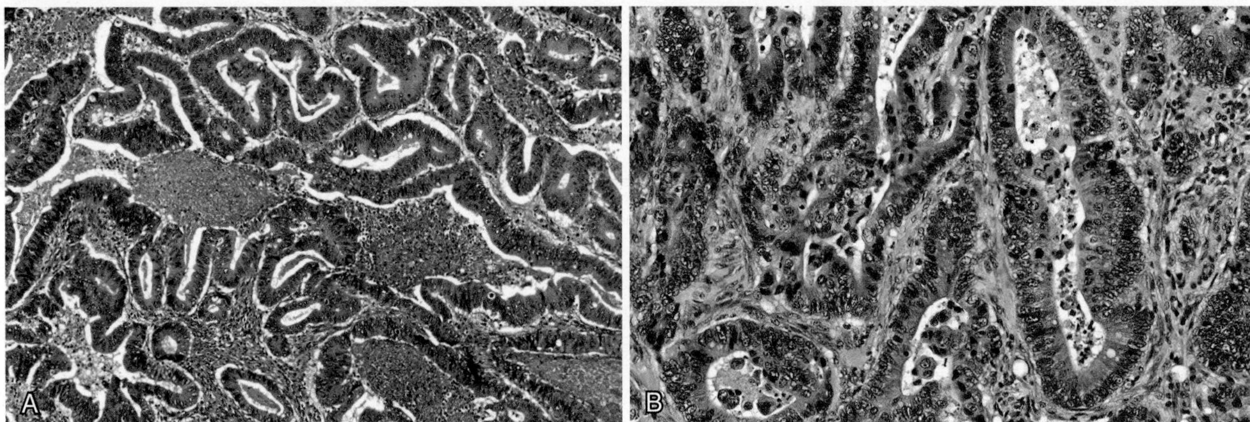

FIGURE 42.15 Intestinal-type ampullary adenocarcinoma. A, The tumor has a glandular pattern with abundant necrosis that resembles colorectal adenocarcinoma. **B,** On high power, the nuclei are pseudostratified, the glands are complex, and there is a modest amount of desmoplastic stroma.

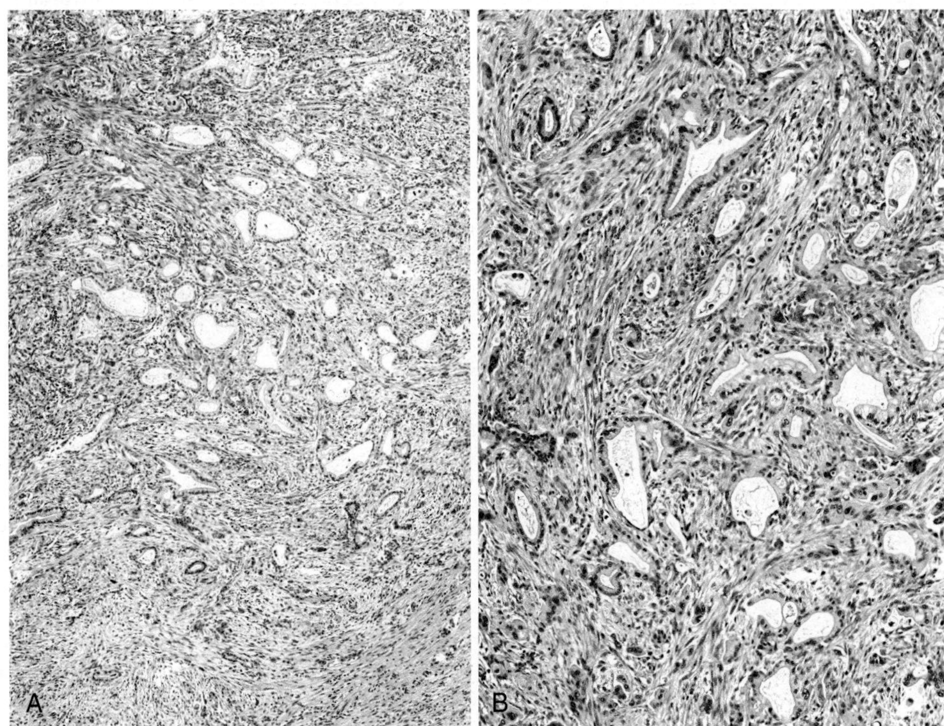

FIGURE 42.16 Pancreatobiliary-type ampullary adenocarcinoma. A, Relatively simple glands are lined by a single layer of cells with round nuclei. **B,** Some glands have abundant mucinous cytoplasm and are remarkably well formed. There is desmoplastic stroma. This pattern resembles carcinomas of the pancreas and bile ducts.

INVASIVE ADENOCARCINOMAS

Because of the proximity of anatomical structures in the ampulla, it is often difficult to grossly and microscopically distinguish tumors that arise in the distal common bile duct from those that arise in the duodenum, pancreatic head, or true ampulla. Published data regarding ampullary neoplasms often contain references to periampullary tumors. In some studies, the term *periampullary* is used to define all tumors located in pancreatoduodenectomy specimens, whereas in others, the term is used specifically for pure ampullary tumors. In other publications, the term *periampullary* refers only to the nonampullary segments of the duodenum.[12,38-41]

Classification

The synoptic reporting document of the College of American Pathologists recognizes three categories of ampullary tumors: intraampullary, periampullary/ampullary duodenal (arising from duodenal surface of the papilla), and mixed intraampullary and periampullary (mixed type).[38] The intraampullary category is further divided into two groups (those that arise from an IAPN or from an ampullary duct). The defining characteristics of these categories are as follows:

I. Primary ampullary carcinomas (Table 42.4; see Table 42.1)
   A. IAPN-associated carcinomas are, essentially, the intraampullary counterpart of intraductal neoplasms, such as intraductal papillary mucinous neoplasms.

TABLE 42.4 Clinicopathological Features of Ampullary Carcinomas[1-3]

Feature	AMP-NOS	Intra-AMP	AMP Duct	AMP Duodenum
Percentage	55	25	15	5
Baseline Demographics				
Mean age (years)	65	64	69	59
Male/female ratio	1.5	2.2	0.9	1
Clinical Characteristics				
Overall tumor size (cm)	2.5	2.9	1.9	4.7
Invasive tumor size (cm)	1.8	1.5	1.7	3.4
Invasive tumor histology (intestinal/ nonintestinal)	0.4	1.2	0.06	3
Lymph node metastasis (%)	42	28	41	50
T stage (T1+T2/T3+T4)	1.6	5.8	0.6	2
Survival Rates				
1 yr	80	88	80	80
3 yr	54	73	41	69
5 yr	39	53	29	55

AMP duct, Ampullary duct carcinoma; *AMP duodenum,* ampullary duodenum carcinoma; *AMP-NOS,* ampullary carcinoma, not otherwise specified; *intra-AMP,* intraampullary papillary-tubular neoplasm associated; *T,* tumor stage.

They are characterized by preinvasive nodules located in the ampullary channel (i.e., distal tip of the common bile duct and main pancreatic duct). From the duodenal perspective, these tumors are often underwhelming. They show a dilated orifice, from which granular material often protrudes into the lumen of the bowel. Probes placed into the common bile duct and pancreatic duct typically exit into the center of the lesion. Microscopic examination often reveals only a small invasive carcinoma. The prognosis is relatively favorable, especially if there is no invasive carcinoma or if invasion is limited to a small amount.

B. Carcinomas of ampullary ducts are also "intraampullary," forming only minimal changes visible from the duodenal perspective. These "scirrhous" lesions circumferentially constrict the distal end of the common bile duct and pancreatic duct, and they show preservation of the papilla of Vater and ampullary duodenal mucosa. In essence, they represent the ampullary counterpart of cholangiocarcinomas. From the duodenal perspective, these tumors typically show a button-like elevation of mucosa or the presence of a subtle, ulcerating lesion (see Fig. 42.2). Microscopically, they often prove to be pancreatobiliary-type carcinomas. Although these tumors are usually less than 2 cm in diameter, they have an aggressive behavior, the worst among the ampullary carcinoma subtypes, but significantly better than pancreatic ductal adenocarcinomas.

C. Carcinomas of the ampullary duodenum (i.e., periampullary-duodenal tumors) arise from the ampullary duodenum, usually from an adenoma of the ampullary duodenum. They form bulky lesions in which the ampullary orifice is often eccentrically located (see Fig. 42.5). They typically have an intestinal (see Fig. 42.15) or mucinous-intestinal phenotype. Although they are usually very large and produce lymph node metastases, their behavior is often better than expected.

D. AMP-NOS carcinomas are, essentially, those tumors that cannot be placed into one of the categories A, B, or C. It also includes tumors that are presumed to arise from the papilla of Vater (i.e., the edge of mucosa where the common bile duct and the main pancreatic duct merge into the duodenal mucosa) (see Fig. 42.7). With improved gross examination skills and careful evaluation, the percentage of cases that ultimately fall within this category decreases significantly.

II. Secondary ampullary carcinomas
   A. Duodenal
   B. Common bile duct
   C. Pancreatic duct

III. Mixed or undetermined origin

It should also be noted that a whole host of neoplasms arise from the minor papilla (accessory ampulla). These are documented separately from the main ampulla.[42]

Clinical Features

Most malignant neoplasms of the ampulla of Vater are adenocarcinomas. The ampulla is the most common site of all small-intestinal adenocarcinomas.[23] Overall, approximately 5% of GI carcinomas arise from the ampulla.[43]

Adenocarcinomas develop mainly in adults (mean age, 62 years) and are more common in men than in women.[43] The estimated lifetime incidence of an ampullary carcinoma is 0.01% to 0.04%.[44] Ampullary adenocarcinomas in patients with FAP are diagnosed in younger patients (mean age, 47.5 years). In FAP cases, ampullary adenocarcinomas usually are associated with other neoplasms. Almost 20% of these patients have multiple primary neoplasms.[15]

Most patients with an ampullary adenocarcinoma have symptoms of biliary obstruction. Jaundice accompanied by

TABLE 42.5 Microscopic Features of Ampullary Carcinomas

		Intestinal Type	Pancreatobiliary Type
Applicable to both preinvasive and invasive components	Stratification	Common, pseudostratified	Often single to two cell layers
	Chromophilia	Overall basophilia	Acidophilic
	Nuclei	Columnar, cigar shaped nuclei	Cuboidal, round nuclei
	Immunoprofile	CDX2 and MUC2	MUC1 and MUC5AC
	Preferential location	Any site of ampulla; Most ampullary-duodenal (surface) lesions are of intestinal type	Any site of ampulla; Most ampullary-ductal carcinomas are of pancreatobiliary type
Applicable to invasive component only	Dispersion of glands	May have compact growth	Often widely separated
	Tubules	Large interconnecting, some anastomotic	Small, dispersed
	Intraluminal debris/ necrosis	Common, proteinaceous fibrinoid	Less common, often with prominent nuclear debris

a palpable, distended gallbladder (i.e., Courvoisier sign) is a classic presentation of ampullary adenocarcinomas, although this constellation of symptoms affects only 15% of patients with these tumors.[44-46] Other common symptoms include abdominal pain, weight loss, nausea, and acute or chronic pancreatitis.[15] Because even small tumors may obstruct the bile duct, ampullary carcinomas often are less than 2 cm in diameter at the time of diagnosis.[47,48]

Pathological Features

The gross findings of ampullary carcinomas vary according to each subtype [4,6,14] (see Fig. 42.2 and Figs. 42.4 to 42.6). IAPN-associated carcinomas are characterized by granular, polypoid material that fills the ampullary channel (i.e., distal segments of the common bile duct and the main pancreatic duct). These tumors may protrude into the duodenal lumen through a dilated orifice (see Fig. 42.4).

Carcinoma of the ampullary duodenum usually manifests as a large, polypoid, and ulcerovegetative mass on the duodenal surface of the ampulla. The orifice of the ampulla is usually located eccentrically in the proximal aspect of the tumor (see Fig. 42.5). In contrast, ampullary duct carcinomas show minimal changes (from the duodenal perspective) such as a button-like mucosal-covered elevation or a small, flat ulcer, and some show subtle and relatively small, plaquelike areas that circumferentially constrict the distal segments of the common bile duct and the main pancreatic duct (see Fig. 42.2).

Ampullary carcinomas are often associated with dilation of the common bile duct and sometimes also the main pancreatic duct. Ductal dilation is usually most striking in cases with a prominent preinvasive component, particularly in IAPNs or tumors of the ampullary duodenum. It is least prominent in ampullary duct tumors. Most ampullary carcinomas are resected by pancreatoduodenectomy. The margins are not usually involved. Extensive ampullary carcinomas are typically unresectable because of distant metastases.

Microscopically, ampullary adenocarcinomas are highly variable in their morphological appearance. The microscopic appearance of ampullary adenocarcinomas reflects their origin in intestinal and biliary epithelium; thus hybrid phenotypes are not uncommon (see Figs. 42.1B and 42.3B). Most invasive adenocarcinomas are tubular.[49] Some are

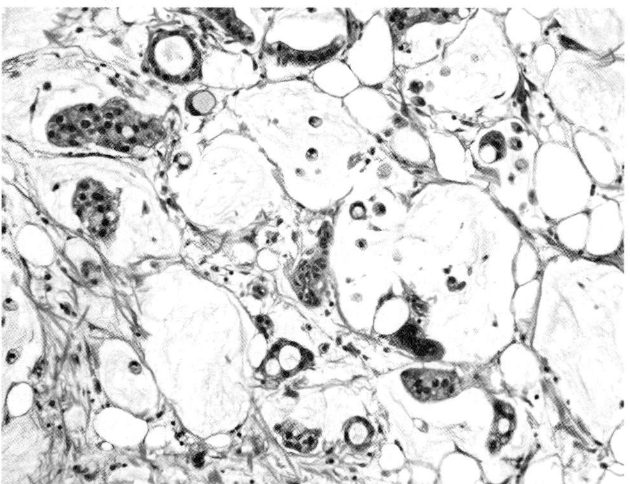

FIGURE 42.17 Mucinous-type ampullary adenocarcinoma. Abundant extracellular mucin contains sparse neoplastic glandular cells.

intestinal-type tumors[43,50-52] that are similar to conventional colonic adenocarcinomas (see Fig. 42.15). Those that resemble pancreatic or bile duct adenocarcinomas are termed *pancreatobiliary-type* adenocarcinomas (Table 42.5, see Fig. 42.16). However, a substantial proportion of the cases have mixed features between these two.[53,54] Other histological types of carcinoma (discussed later) include mucinous (colloid) carcinoma (Fig. 42.17), poorly cohesive carcinoma (with or without signet-ring cells) (Fig. 42.18),[55] micropapillary adenocarcinoma (Fig. 42.19),[56] clear cell carcinoma, adenosquamous carcinoma, and poorly differentiated and undifferentiated carcinomas (Fig. 42.20).[15]

Intestinal-type adenocarcinomas are commonly associated with intestinal-type adenomas. Although they may have any type of gross pattern, most carcinomas of the ampullary duodenum are the intestinal type. Histologically, they are composed of individual glands and cribriform nests of tumor cells with an associated desmoplastic stromal response (see Fig. 42.15). Luminal necrosis is a common feature. The neoplastic glands are often elongated and branched. Many cases exhibit an expansile growth pattern. The cells are columnar and have various amounts of cytoplasmic mucin. Well-differentiated cases may also contain goblet cells. The nuclei are typically elongated, pseudostratified, and have moderate

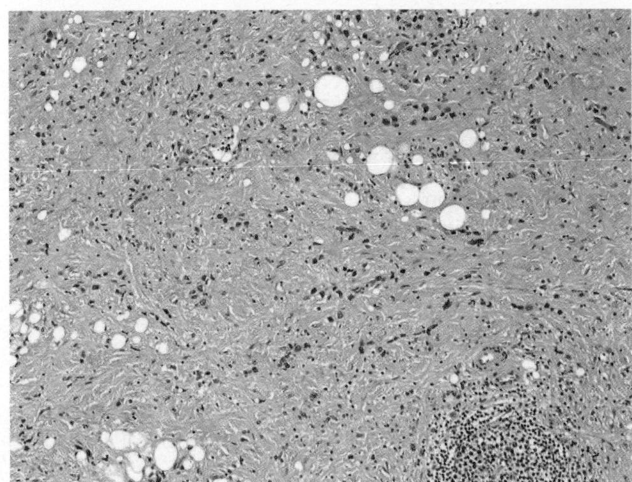

FIGURE 42.18 Poorly cohesive carcinoma is characterized by a subtle infiltration composed of individual malignant cells invading in an insidious fashion.

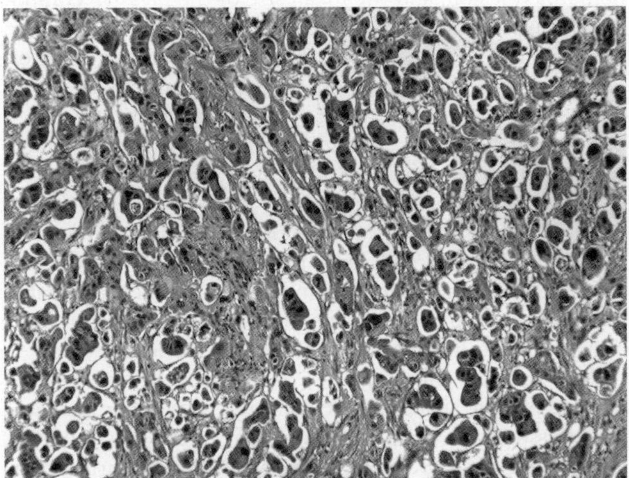

FIGURE 42.19 Micropapillary carcinomas are characterized by small clusters of cells lying in clefts. This pattern commonly is associated with neutrophils in the vicinity of the cells.

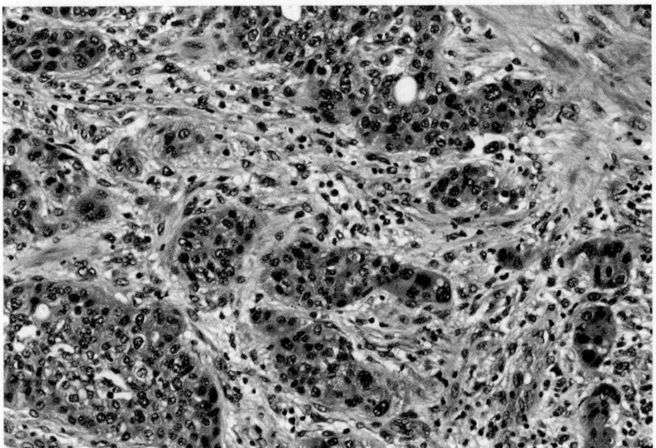

FIGURE 42.20 Poorly differentiated carcinoma, not otherwise specified, of the ampulla. Some adenocarcinomas have a predominantly solid growth pattern and cannot be further subclassified as intestinal or pancreatobiliary types based on histology.

to marked pleomorphism.[49] Rarely, Paneth cell differentiation may be seen,[57] and extracellular mucin pools may be identified. An extensive mucinous component (>50% of the tumor volume) justifies a diagnosis of mucinous adenocarcinoma (see Fig. 42.17). Solid nests of cells and single cells are characteristic of poorly differentiated cases (see Fig. 42.20).

Pancreatobiliary-type adenocarcinomas are more commonly associated with an ampullary duct preneoplastic component, usually the flat type,[4] consistent with the hypothesis that they arise from the terminal pancreatic or biliary ducts. Some arise from IAPNs, adenomas of the papilla of Vater, or duodenal adenomas.

Examination of pancreatobiliary-type adenocarcinomas usually reveals a proliferation of individual glands that are relatively small, remarkably well formed, and widely separated and that infiltrate within an extensively desmoplastic stroma (see Fig. 42.16). Some glands are more complex, showing papillary or micropapillary projections. Cribriform glands also may be present. The cytoplasm of tumor cells contains mucin that, in some cases, may impart a foamy, clear cell appearance to the tumor. The nuclei are round and moderately atypical. They usually lack the characteristic pseudostratification pattern of intestinal-type adenocarcinomas.[49]

Because the ampulla is a transitional region, it is not surprising that many ampullary carcinomas have a mixed phenotypical appearance.[53] In fact, a significant proportion of cases are difficult to place into one of the categories as intestinal or pancreatobiliary, and there is also significant interobserver variability.[14,53] Different regions of a single tumor may show different patterns of growth. Budding is common in all ampullary carcinomas, and areas of budding often exhibit pancreatobiliary-like morphology.[58]

Ancillary Diagnostic Tests and Molecular Properties

With immunohistochemical staining, ampullary adenocarcinomas express keratins and glycoproteins, some of which vary according to the particular histological type of tumor. Intestinal-type adenocarcinomas express markers of intestinal differentiation, such as CDX2 and MUC2; CK7 expression varies, and MUC1 staining is usually negative.[59] The immunophenotype of pancreatobiliary-type adenocarcinomas resembles that of pancreatic and biliary carcinomas, showing consistent expression of CK7, CK19, and MUC1, whereas staining for MUC2 and CDX2 is usually negative or weak.[59] Hybrid (transitional) tumors show a mixed immunophenotype.

Some studies have advocated a combination of the aforementioned markers in a panel format to assist in this classification[60,61]; however, others have failed to confirm the applicability and prognostic value of these panels.[53,54] In one study, MUC5AC was found to be an independent predictor of poor survival in both pancreatobiliary- and intestinal-type ampullary carcinomas by multivariate analysis.[54] Stains for chromogranin or synaptophysin may reveal scattered neuroendocrine cells in all subtypes.[49]

Other histological types of carcinoma have an immunophenotype that corresponds to the predominant line of differentiation. For instance, squamous areas within adenosquamous carcinomas express squamous lineage markers such as P63 and K903. Mucinous carcinomas may acquire

MUC2 and MUC6 expression. Poorly cohesive carcinomas (with or without signet-ring cells) show strong MUC5AC positivity, as some do for MUC6, but they typically lack intestinal differentiation, as indicated by MUC2 and CDX2 positivity.[55] Micropapillary adenocarcinomas show CK7 positivity and reversal of cell polarity with MUC1 (i.e., stroma-facing surface of the cells are positive).[56] Undifferentiated and sarcomatoid carcinomas lose cytokeratin expression but acquire vimentin positivity.

Molecular Features

Ampullary carcinomas reveal molecular alterations similar to those of ductal adenocarcinomas of the pancreas and colorectum.[62] *KRAS* mutations are found in approximately 40% of cases. Increased expression of TP53 is detected in 70% of cases.[63-67] Sixty-four percent of ampullary carcinomas that arise in FAP contain *APC* gene mutations, but only 17% of sporadic ampullary carcinomas have mutations in this gene.[68] Mutations of the β-catenin gene *(CTNNB1)* are also uncommon.[69] Alterations of the *SMAD4 (DPC4)* gene are rare in ampullary carcinomas.[70]

Recently, a 92-gene signature has been proposed as an unbiased standardized molecular-based approach to stratify ampullary carcinomas, which may potentially be used to classify unresectable tumors in which the anatomical source of the cancer (pancreatic vs. biliary vs. duodenal vs. ampullary) cannot be determined.[71] Moreover, it has been reported that gene amplification and immunohistochemical overexpression of ERBB2 occur in 13% of all ampullary carcinomas, therefore providing a potential target for anti-HER2 therapy in these tumors.[72]

A small proportion of poorly differentiated ampullary carcinomas with morphological features that resemble medullary carcinomas of the large bowel demonstrate microsatellite instability.[73] In fact, a recent study[73] has shown that loss of DNA mismatch repair proteins may be as common as in colorectal cancers, although the earlier literature showed conflicting results.[59,74] In most of these studies, carcinomas arising in different compartments of the ampulla and those with various histological types, including intestinal and pancreatobiliary, have been analyzed indiscriminately.

Differential Diagnosis

The differential diagnosis of ampullary tumors includes primary tumors of adjacent structures. Gross evaluation is critical to determine the primary site of origin of any tumor of this region, and some guidelines for this have been proposed recently.[6] With the principle that most tumors expand uniformly from their site of origin, it is presumed that the center of a neoplasm represents the true primary site. Careful examination of the luminal aspect of the duodenum and well-oriented tissue sections of the ampulla helps determine the relationship of the tumor to normal anatomical structures.

When distinguishable from mucosal colonization by an underlying invasive carcinoma (see Fig. 42.10), the location of a residual preinvasive neoplasm suggests its site of origin. Well-developed intestinal differentiation in tumors suggests an ampullary origin because this feature is virtually nonexistent in primary pancreatic and common bile duct carcinomas. However, there is extensive overlap in the histological, immunophenotypical, and molecular alterations among carcinomas of the ampulla, pancreas, and bile duct. Therefore careful dissection and sampling of the pancreatoduodenectomy specimen is crucial for determining the precise origin of the tumor.[6]

Natural History and Treatment

Ampullary carcinomas have an overall survival rate far better than pancreatic and distal common bile duct cancers. The 5-year survival rate is approximately 40%.[4,13,53,75] Rates of survival appear to be even better than for nonampullary duodenum cancers.[76] This rate may be the result of early detection. Some studies have shown a more favorable outcome for stage-matched pure ampullary carcinomas compared with pancreatic tumors.[77] However, this may not be an accurate comparison because the staging parameters used for the two tumors are quite different. Nevertheless, ampullary carcinomas are commonly diagnosed early. Their strategic location at the junction of the common bile duct and the main pancreatic duct causes symptoms early in the course of disease.

Ampullary carcinomas often arise from a precursor (adenomatous) lesion, and the mean size of the invasive component is usually significantly smaller than primary pancreatic carcinomas.[78] Surgical resectability is an important factor. Positive margins occur in less than 5% of ampullary carcinomas, compared with at least 35% of pancreatic tumors.[53] Tumor cell biology may also be a factor in survival rates for ampullary and pancreatic tumors. Some studies have shown that pancreatobiliary-type adenocarcinomas of the ampulla have a poorer prognosis than tumors with intestinal differentiation.[32,38,61,79] Even pancreatobiliary-type adenocarcinomas that arise in the ampulla have a more favorable prognosis than those that arise from the pancreas or common bile duct, likely because of early detection.[4,13,53]

Site-specific subcategories of ampullary tumors have distinct biological and prognostic properties.[13] For instance, IAPN-associated invasive carcinomas often have only a small invasive component (mean, 1.5 cm). Not surprisingly, they have a more favorable prognosis.[6,13,14] Tumors of the ampullary duodenum are typically associated with a prominent preinvasive component, and although they usually are high stage (i.e., very large size with lymph node metastasis), their prognosis is fairly good. In contrast, ampullary duct tumors often reveal a small (most are <2 cm), invasive carcinoma but still exhibit aggressive behavior. Although ampullary duct tumors are invariably of the pancreatobiliary type, they still have a significantly more favorable prognosis than primary pancreatic or distal bile duct carcinomas.[4,13]

Independent prognostic factors include patient age, vascular and perineural invasion, margin status, tumor budding,[58] lymph node metastasis, and MUC5AC expression.[49,54] Increased tumor proliferation rate and abnormal DNA ploidy also have been associated with a poor prognosis.[59,80-84]

OTHER UNCOMMON INVASIVE CARCINOMAS

Unlike the pancreas, where the vast majority of carcinomas are of the tubular-type, presumably because of its transitional nature, the ampulla can give rise to a spectrum of nontubular carcinomas. In fact, if a specific nontubular adenocarcinoma is encountered in this region, such as mucinous, poorly cohesive, or medullary, it is much more likely to be of ampullary origin than pancreatic. Most uncommon tumors are similar to intestinal- and pancreatobiliary-type carcinomas in terms of their clinical presentation, natural history, and prognosis. The following histological subtypes are important mainly because of their distinct morphological patterns of growth.

Mucin production is noted in about 15% of ampullary carcinomas,[48,85] and 10% qualify as mucinous carcinoma, with >50% stromal mucin deposition (see Fig. 42.17). These are mostly mixed-mucinous carcinomas. True colloid carcinomas, in which the carcinoma cells are almost all floating within mucin, are very uncommon. Mucinous carcinomas of the ampulla are seen more commonly in men and tend to arise from the ampullary duodenum.[15] The carcinoma cells often reveal an intestinal (rather than pancreatobiliary) phenotype, which is also illustrated by frequent positivity of MUC2 and CDX2. A significant proportion of the cases have a mixed ordinary (tubular) adenocarcinoma component. Signet-ring cells may be prominent, either confined within the mucin lakes (mucinous signet-ring cell carcinoma), or sometimes infiltrating as cellular/nonmucinous infiltrates into the stroma. Mucinous carcinomas are often fairly large, and two-thirds have lymph node metastasis at presentation, but their behavior appears to be less aggressive than what would be expected from advanced tumors. Of note, a recent study found that mismatch repair protein alteration was not uncommon in tumors with focal mucin production, but was very uncommon in tumors with more profuse mucin formation.[73,85]

Poorly cohesive cell carcinomas (with or without signet-ring cells) are rare.[55,86,87] Unlike mucinous adenocarcinomas, the signet-ring cells are individually arranged and infiltrate the stroma in a single-file pattern resembling diffuse-type gastric adenocarcinomas (see Fig. 42.18).[55] Significant extracellular mucin pools are absent. A poorly cohesive cell pattern may be found in other types of ampullary adenocarcinomas. However, this diagnosis is applied when more than 50% of the tumor volume consists of these elements. The differential diagnosis includes metastases from the stomach or breast (i.e., lobular carcinoma). The latter can be distinguished by immunohistochemical staining for hormone receptors. These tumors have gastric differentiation; most are positive for MUC5AC, and more than 50% are positive for MUC6. They usually lack intestinal differentiation; most are negative for CDX2, and staining for MUC2 is positive in only a few cases.[55]

Micropapillary carcinomas, as described in the breast, urinary bladder, and other organs (characterized by small clusters of cells lying within clefts) can also occur in the ampulla (see Fig. 42.19).[56,88,89] This can be a focal finding, but it may occasionally be the predominant pattern. In one study, these tumors were found to be more aggressive.[56]

Adenosquamous carcinomas contain glandular and squamous elements. Adenosquamous carcinomas account for 1% to 3% of all ampullary primary tumors.[41,90,91] Although any degree of glandular differentiation (in a predominantly squamous neoplasm) is considered sufficient for a diagnosis of adenosquamous carcinoma, by convention, at least 25% of an adenocarcinoma should exhibit squamous differentiation to qualify.[15] The glandular areas usually resemble a pancreatobiliary-type adenocarcinoma. The squamous elements grow in sheets and nests. They are composed of polygonal-shaped cells with a generous amount of eosinophilic cytoplasm. Keratinization is usually evident. In cases with a predominantly squamous pattern, stains for mucin may help identify areas of glandular differentiation. Squamous areas are often positive for P63 or K903. Adenosquamous carcinomas are much more common in the pancreas.

Medullary carcinomas, akin to their colonic counterparts, may also occur in the ampulla.[76] They are characterized by large, nodular masses with pushing borders and syncytial growth and an associated inflammatory infiltrate, and they appear to have strong association with MSI and PDL1 expression.[73] Similar to the ones in the colon, and despite their large size, they seem to be less aggressive.[49]

Carcinomas with neuroendocrine differentiation can arise in adenocarcinomas of the ampulla.[92] When the neuroendocrine component is substantial (>50%), the lesion is classified as a *poorly differentiated neuroendocrine carcinoma* (discussed later). There is emerging evidence that it may be important to recognize even a small neuroendocrine component in tumors of the GI tract. Cis-platinum based therapy may be considered for such cases.[92]

Rarely, sarcomatoid differentiation may occur in the form of a spindle cell carcinoma (i.e., sarcomatoid carcinoma) or as a biphasic neoplasm showing well-defined glandular elements mixed with distinct sarcomatoid elements (i.e., carcinosarcoma). In both cases, the sarcomatoid region often retains epithelial differentiation (i.e., immunoexpression of keratins). Undifferentiated carcinomas with osteoclast-like giant cells, identical to those that occur in the pancreas, rarely develop in the ampulla.[93]

DUCTAL ABNORMALITIES AND NEOPLASIA

It is becoming increasingly recognized that the ampulla may be both the culprit and a participant in neoplasia associated with pancreatobiliary ductal variations and anomalies.

Pancreatobiliary maljunction is the "anomalous" union of the common bile duct with the main pancreatic duct (Wirsung's) in a supra-Oddi position instead of an intrasphincteric merger.[94,95] This rare anomaly, allowing reflux of pancreatic enzymes to the biliary system, accounts for 5% to 10% of gallbladder carcinomas. Because of this reflux, it also bears a risk for carcinomas in the remainder of the biliary system, including the ampulla.[94,95]

Choledochal cysts also can involve the ampulla. Overall, malignant transformation is detected in about 15% of choledochal cysts.[96]

STAGING OF AMPULLARY CARCINOMAS

The AJCC TNM staging manual of ampullary carcinomas defines parameters for the T stage. In the eighth edition, these parameters have been significantly revised and/or subdivided to account for the three-dimensional spreading pattern of these tumors and to clarify the degree and depth of extension into adjacent structures.[97] A T1a tumor is limited to the ampulla of Vater or sphincter of Oddi. A T1b tumor invades beyond the sphincter of Oddi and/or into the duodenal submucosa. A tumor that invades into the muscularis propria of the duodenum is regarded as T2. A T3a category is now created for tumors that invade the pancreas up to

0.5 cm, and T3b encompasses tumors that are more than 0.5 cm into the pancreas or extend into peripancreatic tissue or duodenal serosa. T4 is reserved for tumors involving the celiac axis, superior mesenteric artery, and/or common hepatic artery, irrespective of size.[97] Unfortunately, invasion into the serosa of the duodenum is not addressed separately from subserosal involvement without extension to serosa, unlike in the reminder of the GI tract. We report these tumors as advanced T3 with a comment.[98,99]

The number of lymph nodes with metastasis has also been incorporated into the N stage because it has been shown to have a significant prognostic value.[100] N1 is defined as metastasis to one to three regional lymph nodes, and N2 is defined as metastasis to four or more regional lymph nodes.[97]

NEUROENDOCRINE NEOPLASMS AND RELATED TUMORS

Neuroendocrine cells are uncommon within the pancreatobiliary portion of the ampulla.[101] The overlying duodenal epithelium contains the same amount of neuroendocrine cells as the surrounding nonampullary duodenal mucosa. Nevertheless, a variety of neuroendocrine neoplasms occur in the ampulla.

Ampullary neuroendocrine neoplasms are divided into well-differentiated and poorly differentiated categories, as is the norm for the remainder of GI and pancreatobiliary tracts. In addition to well-differentiated neuroendocrine neoplasms, NOS, clinically functional gastrinomas may arise within the periampullary region as well as histologically distinctive so-called *glandular psammomatous carcinoids* (also called *ampullary somatostatinomas* because of their common expression of somatostatin at the immunohistochemical level).

A distinct tumor type that has neuroendocrine differentiation as one of its defining characteristics and that is essentially specific to the ampulla (seldom occurring elsewhere) is *duodenal gangliocytic paraganglioma*, a neoplasm that combines features of a "carcinoid tumor" with those of a nerve sheath tumor.

Poorly differentiated neuroendocrine carcinomas include small cell and large cell variants.[102] These are discussed separately in the following sections.

Well-Differentiated Neuroendocrine Tumors

Clinical Features

Well-differentiated neuroendocrine tumors (WDNETs), previously referred to as *carcinoids*, compose approximately 3% of all tumors in the ampulla. They arise in adults in their 40s and 50s and have a male predominance.[103-106] Most are solitary and sporadic, but this region is a common site of WDNETs in multiple endocrine neoplasia (MEN) I, including gastrinomas associated with Zollinger-Ellison syndrome.[107-109] Ampullary somatostatinomas may develop in patients with neurofibromatosis.[110-115]

Most ampullary and duodenal WDNETs are clinically nonfunctional, with the exception of gastrinomas. Somatostatin-producing pseudoglandular tumors are not clinically functional, in contrast with some that occur within the pancreas.[105,114,116,117] Carcinoid syndrome is rare.[105]

The clinical presentation is similar to that of other types of ampullary tumors.[105,106,118] Duodenal gastrinomas may be difficult to identify clinically because of their small size, even when they present with a large peripancreatic lymph node metastasis. In patients with MEN I, it can be difficult to determine which of the multiple, small neuroendocrine neoplasms in the pancreas and duodenum are functional.[119] Because most sporadic gastrinomas arise in the head of the pancreas or duodenum (or, rarely, within the peripancreatic lymph nodes), pancreatoduodenectomy has been advocated for patients with Zollinger-Ellison syndrome to remove the gastrinoma triangle.[107] Because most pancreatic gastrinomas are sizable, the ampulla and duodenum in the gastrinoma triangle are the primary locations for most grossly inapparent tumors.[119]

Pathological Features

WDNETs are usually small (3 cm in diameter or less), well-demarcated, submucosal nodules composed of uniform, tan tissue.[104] Because they readily obstruct the distal pancreatic and bile ducts, they may lead to dilation of both ducts. In fact, for a tumor with minimal symptomatology and massive dilation of both ducts, ampullary NET should always be considered. Histologically, most nonfunctional cases (e.g., gastrinomas) are indistinguishable. They resemble their counterpart from other parts of the GI tract, such as the stomach or pancreas (Fig. 42.21).[104] Typically, nests and ribbons of uniform cells are surrounded by some degree of hyalinized stroma. Despite being well circumscribed, these tumors usually infiltrate the surrounding tissues, entrap periampullary ductules within the tumor, and produce lymph node metastases. Individual cells have a modest amount of pale to eosinophilic cytoplasm. The nuclei are uniform in size and shape and contain stippled chromatin. The proliferative rate is usually low. Most cases have fewer than 10 mitoses per 10 high-power fields (HPF), and many cases have no more than 1 to 2 mitoses per 10 HPF. Necrosis may be focal and punctate, but it is usually absent.[102]

Ampullary somatostatinomas (i.e., glandular psammomatous neuroendocrine tumor of the duodenum) have

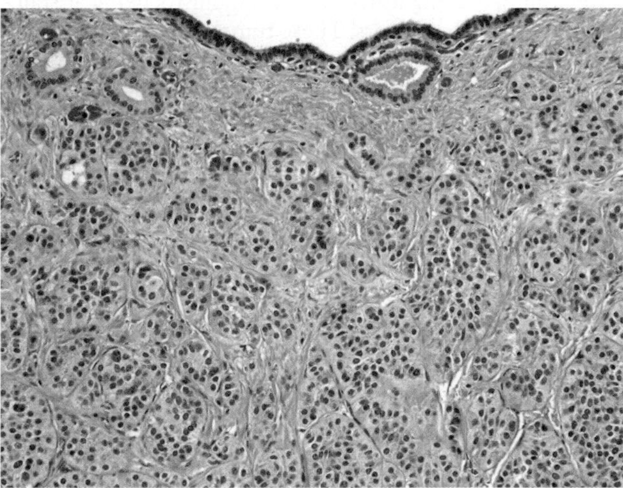

FIGURE 42.21 Well-differentiated neuroendocrine tumor (i.e., carcinoid) of the ampulla. The tumor composed of cells and arranged in nested pattern with uniform nuclei and a low mitotic rate is seen within the duodenal submucosa surrounding the distal bile duct.

distinctive features (Fig. 42.22).[104,111-115,120,121] Although examination of any type of WDNET can reveal focal lumen formation, ampullary somatostatinomas are extensively gland forming. They usually show individual tubular glands that infiltrate the stroma (see Fig. 42.22). Some cribriform glands may also occur. The tumor cells have relatively abundant cytoplasm, which is eosinophilic and finely granular. Psammoma bodies are often found within glandular lumina, and luminal mucin may be seen. However, intracytoplasmic mucin is typically not observed. In some cases, the nuclei are basally oriented and uniform in appearance. The mitotic rate is low. Ampullary somatostatinomas reveal more frequent metastases than other types of duodenal WDNETs in this region.[104] In approximately one-fourth of patients, ampullary somatostatinomas are associated with neurofibromatosis type 1. However, the association may be underreported. In some cases, neurofibromatosis is evident in the resection specimen because of abnormal nerves that have a spectrum of neurofibroma-like changes or because an incidental GI stromal tumor is found.[110,111,113,115,116,120] A distinctive type of sclerotic change within uninvolved blood vessels has been identified in ampullary somatostatinomas.

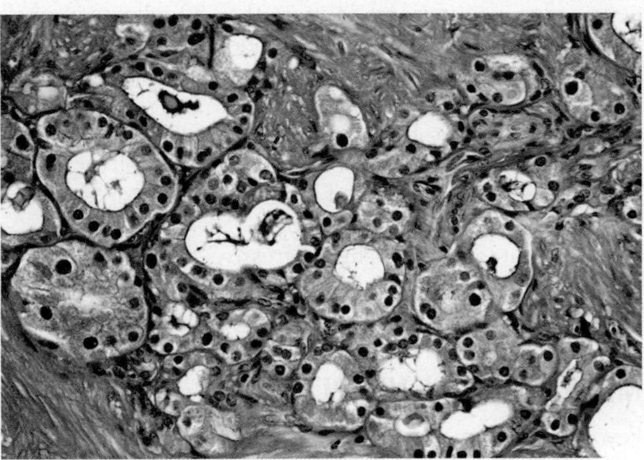

FIGURE 42.22 Ampullary somatostatinoma (i.e., glandular psammomatous neuroendocrine tumor). The tumor grows as individual glands, some with psammoma bodies in the lumina. Abundant, finely granular, pale, acidophilic cytoplasm is characteristic. The nuclei are uniform and have a granular chromatin pattern.

On immunohistochemical staining, all of these tumors express neuroendocrine markers, such as chromogranin and synaptophysin. Staining for keratin is also positive. A variety of peptides and bioamines can be detected, even in cases that are clinically nonfunctional.[104,111,114,122-125] Gastrinomas usually label for gastrin, and somatostatinomas typically express somatostatin.

Differential Diagnosis

The differential diagnosis depends on the specific histology of the tumor. Cases that show a nested or trabecular architecture may be confused with a poorly differentiated neuroendocrine carcinoma, especially in small, poorly preserved biopsies; however, the latter neoplasms have a high mitotic rate (more than 20 mitoses per 10 HPF), extensive necrosis, and nuclear pleomorphism. The Ki67 labeling index is typically greater than 50%.[126] Gland-forming examples, especially somatostatinomas, may resemble adenocarcinomas, but the lack of a high degree of nuclear atypia, mitotic activity, and intracellular mucin helps separate adenocarcinomas from carcinoid tumors. They can also be mistaken for normal Brunner's glands in endoscopic biopsies.

Gangliocytic Paragangliomas

Gangliocytic paragangliomas are rare tumors that occur almost exclusively in the ampullary duodenal region. Patient age at diagnosis varies widely (mean age, 53 years), and men are affected more often than women.[104,127-129] Most gangliocytic paragangliomas are benign, and cases with metastases are rare.

Gangliocytic paragangliomas are usually 1 to 3 cm in diameter, nodular, and occur in the submucosa within a few centimeters of the ampulla. Some are pedunculated.[15] Microscopically, gangliocytic paragangliomas contain three distinct cellular components, although in proportions that vary widely among cases and even within an individual tumor (Fig. 42.23). Carcinoid-like elements form nests and ribbons of cells. They resemble cells of a typical carcinoid tumor or paraganglioma. Scattered, large, ganglion-like cells contain large nuclei with prominent nucleoli and granular cytoplasm. Spindle cells resemble peripheral nerve elements, and they may contain Schwann cells. The neuroendocrine component may also have spindle cell morphology.

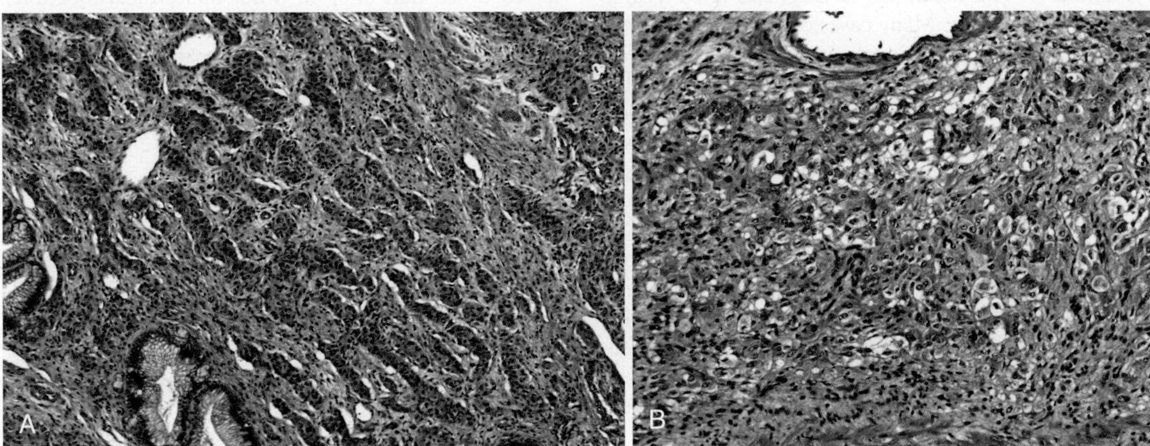

FIGURE 42.23 Gangliocytic paraganglioma. A, The growth pattern is heterogeneous. Some areas have nests of epithelioid cells resembling a carcinoid tumor. **B,** Elsewhere, there are spindle-shaped cells and large, individual ganglion-like cells.

The various cellular components are usually intimately intermixed, although some cases may show a rather sharp segregation between the different cellular elements.

Each component has a different immunohistochemical staining pattern.[130-135] Epithelioid cells are usually keratin positive, although often not as diffusely as typical carcinoid tumors. Staining for chromogranin, synaptophysin, pancreatic polypeptide, and somatostatin is usually positive. Other peptides, such as vasoactive intestinal polypeptide and glucagon, are less frequently positive. Ganglion-like cells express only synaptophysin; staining for keratin and chromogranin is negative. The spindle cell component stains positively for S100 protein and neurofilaments. These findings suggest that gangliocytic paragangliomas contain elements of endodermal (i.e., carcinoid-like cells) and neuroectodermal (i.e., Schwann and ganglion-like cells) origin, which is an unusual combination of findings that has evoked some intriguing hypotheses regarding its possible origin.[128-130,135,136]

Consistent expression of pancreatic polypeptide, which is normally produced by islet cells derived from the embryonic ventral lobe of the gland, and the location of gangliocytic paragangliomas along the course of developmental migration of the ventral pancreas suggest a relationship to pancreatic development. However, it is unknown why these tumors occur only in the duodenum and not in the pancreas. Other investigators have suggested a relationship to an embryonic structure, the sympathetico-insular complex, which contains islet cells and branches of sympathetic nerves, including ganglion cells.[135,137]

Some have proposed that only the epithelial component of gangliocytic paragangliomas is truly neoplastic. The neuroectodermal components may be reactive and derived from the myenteric plexus. However, the observation of Schwann cell elements within metastases argues against this theory. Even when metastatic, these tumors seem to be benevolent.[130,133,138]

Poorly Differentiated Neuroendocrine Carcinomas

Poorly differentiated (high-grade) neuroendocrine carcinomas are categorized as small cell or large cell types. They are uncommon carcinomas of the ampulla but, based on the numbers of reported cases, they are more common in this anatomical location than in the pancreas.[80,92,139-146]

The clinical features are similar to other types of ampullary carcinomas.[146] The mean age at diagnosis is 69 years, and most patients are men. Many cases of poorly differentiated neuroendocrine carcinomas are associated with ampullary adenomas, and an adenocarcinoma component may be found. Therefore conceptually they can be viewed under the category of "MINEN" (*mixed neuroendocrine nonneuroendocrine neoplasm*, previously termed *mixed adenocarcinoma neuroendocrine carcinoma*).

The histological features resemble those that arise in the lung. Small cell carcinomas contain sheets and nests of small cells with minimal cytoplasm, fusiform nuclei, finely granular chromatin, and inconspicuous nucleoli (Fig. 42.24). Focal squamous differentiation may occur.[147] Large cell neuroendocrine carcinomas possess larger cells with moderate amounts of cytoplasm and round to oval nuclei, often with prominent nucleoli (Fig. 42.25).

The high-grade nature of poorly differentiated neuroendocrine carcinomas is reflected in their high proliferation rate,

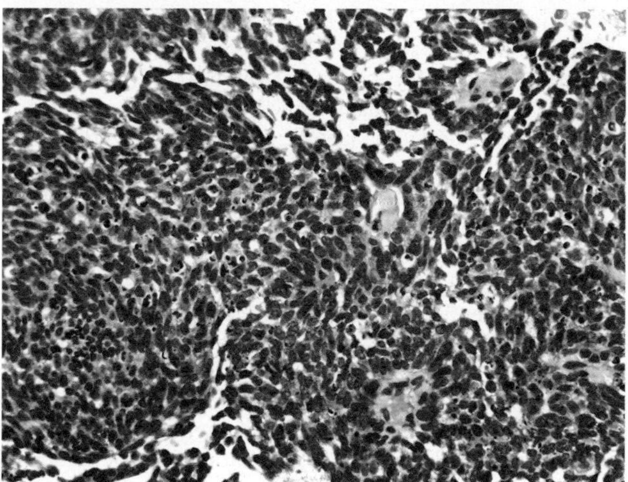

FIGURE 42.24 Small cell type of a poorly differentiated neuroendocrine carcinoma. The tumor is formed of sheets of small cells with minimal cytoplasm, no nucleoli, and a high mitotic rate.

which is usually more than 20 mitoses per 10 HPF (by definition) and often in the range of 40 to 60 mitoses in large cell neuroendocrine carcinoma to more than 80 mitoses in small cell carcinoma. The Ki67 labeling index for these tumors is typically more than 50%.[126] Necrosis is usually extensive. Both types of tumors stain for chromogranin and synaptophysin, although this is typically more focal than in well-differentiated neuroendocrine neoplasms. A diagnosis of small cell carcinoma does not require expression of neuroendocrine markers when classic cytological features are evident.[102]

These tumors are highly aggressive. Rapid dissemination and death from disease usually occur within 2 years of diagnosis.[92,144]

MESENCHYMAL NEOPLASMS

Few types of mesenchymal neoplasms arise specifically in the ampulla. Tumors of the duodenal wall, such as GI stromal tumors or submucosal lipomas, may involve the ampulla secondarily and manifest clinically with obstructive jaundice.[15] Neurofibroma, ganglioneuroma, rhabdomyosarcoma, and Kaposi's sarcoma have been reported in the ampullary region, and their pathological features are similar to those that arise in other anatomical locations.[148-154] Sarcomas should be distinguished from sarcomatoid carcinomas, which are more common and show immunohistochemical evidence of epithelial differentiation (i.e., keratin expression) and a separate, morphologically recognizable carcinoma component.

TUMOR-LIKE LESIONS

A variety of tumor-like lesions can involve the ampulla and simulate a neoplasm clinically, radiographically, and sometimes pathologically.

Paraduodenal (Groove) Pancreatitis

Clinical Features

Paraduodenal pancreatitis is a distinctive form of pancreatitis that is centered in the duodenal wall, especially in the

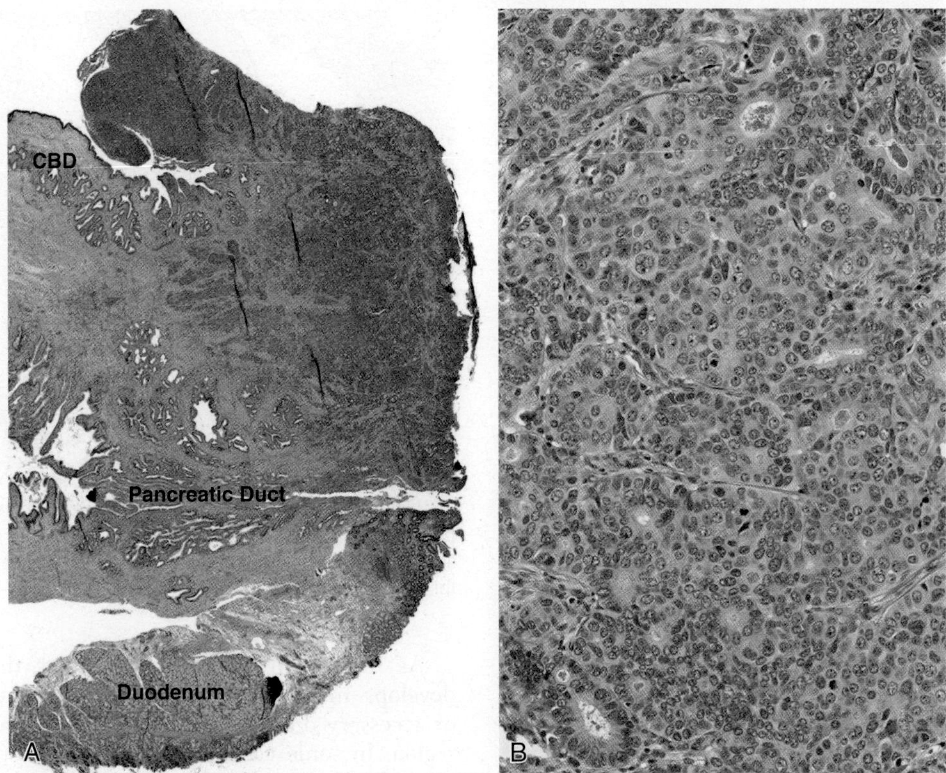

FIGURE 42.25 **A** and **B,** Large cell type of a poorly differentiated neuroendocrine carcinoma. The tumor is characterized by epithelial cells that have moderate amounts of cytoplasm and round to oval nuclei, often with prominent nucleoli. *CBD*, Common bile duct.

accessory ampullary region, and spills into the adjacent pancreatic tissue.[155] The cases included in this category have also been reported as *cystic dystrophy of the heterotopic pancreas* and *myoadenomatosis of the duodenal wall,* and the predominantly cystic examples have also been designated as *paraduodenal wall cyst.*[156-159] All of these names reflect different facets of this distinctive entity. Paraduodenal pancreatitis, along with autoimmune pancreatitis, is the most common cause of a benign condition that is mistaken for cancer.[155] Close to two-thirds of paraduodenal pancreatitis cases are initially diagnosed as periampullary cancer or pancreatic cancer.[155]

Many patients have history of alcohol abuse, but a history of hypertension, diabetes, smoking, and gallstones are also significantly more common than in the general population, suggesting that a combination of vascular compromise and obstructive processes may be involved in its pathogenesis. The fact that the process is often centered in, or at least involving, the accessory ampulla and Santorini's duct (sometimes also forming a "santorinicele") suggests that individuals relying on their ventral pancreas drainage may be more vulnerable to this process.[155]

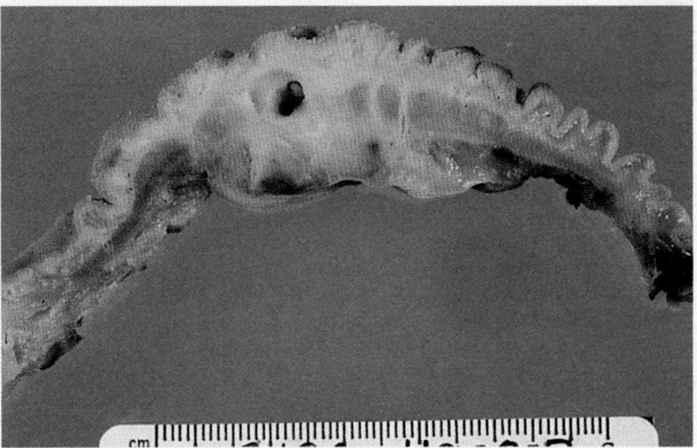

FIGURE 42.26 Paraduodenal (groove) pancreatitis is characterized by a pseudotumor in the vicinity of the minor ampulla and accessory duct. The pseudotumor often involves the duodenal wall and spills over into adjacent pancreas. Thickening of the mucosa (often caused by Brunner's gland hyperplasia) also contributes to nodular changes in the duodenal wall, but the main process is composed of dense, fibrous tissue in the wall of the duodenum that is accompanied by thickening of the musculature. The accessory duct is often dilated.

Pathological Features

Paraduodenal pancreatitis is characterized by a constellation of pathological findings in the duodenal wall in the accessory ampullary region and adjacent pancreas.[155,159] There is often an exuberant myofibroblastic proliferation arranged in fascicles. The process narrows the duodenal lumen and scars the duodenal wall. The duodenal mucosa is thickened, and it often acquires a nodular or cobblestone appearance as a result of Brunner's gland hyperplasia in addition to myoid hyperplasia. On sectioning, the duodenal wall musculature, especially in the vicinity of the minor ampulla, has a trabeculated appearance that is often accompanied by a cystic changes (Figs. 42.26 and 42.27). In some cases, cyst formation may be prominent, forming lesions as large as several centimeters in diameter in some cases (i.e., paraduodenal wall cysts).[155,159]

Microscopic examination often reveals round (well-circumscribed), small lobules of pancreatic tissue (i.e.,

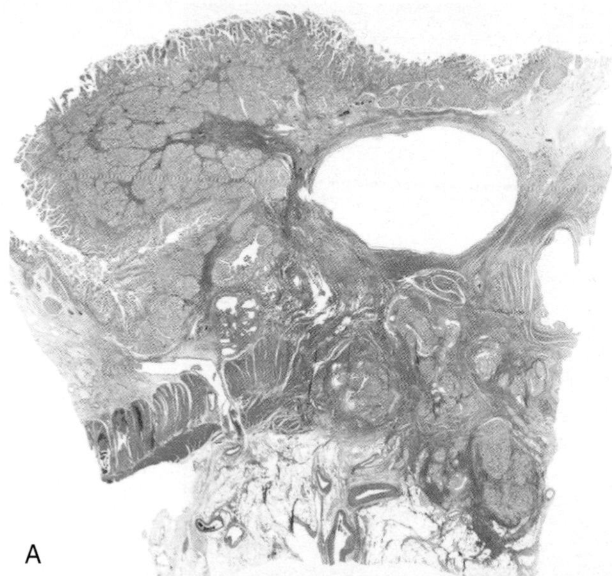

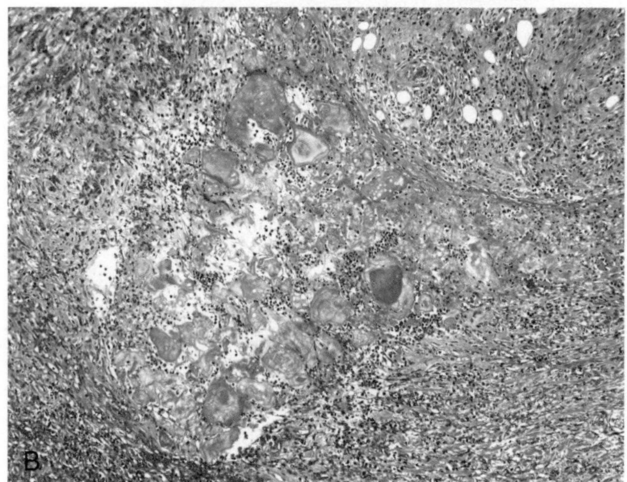

FIGURE 42.27 A, Cystic changes are common in and around the minor ampulla and accessory duct and are typically associated with hyperplasia of the duodenal muscles. It has also been called *cystic dystrophy in heterotopic pancreas.* Brunner's gland hyperplasia is also evident. **B,** Paraduodenal pancreatitis is an inflammatory process.

myoadenomatosis pattern) or various sizes of ducts (i.e., cystic dystrophy in heterotopic pancreas) scattered among myoid stromal cells.[155,159] These ducts may contain inspissated acinar enzymes. Some cysts are devoid of epithelium. Instead, they are lined by a more cellular fibroblastic tissue. Occasionally, the lining fibroblasts may appear epithelioid and raise concern about the possibility of a sarcomatoid carcinoma. The cystic contents may extravasate and cause a foreign-body giant cell reaction and stromal eosinophilia (see Fig. 42.27).[159]

Overall, clinically, the lesion displays several stigmata associated with cancer, including a highly infiltrative appearance, dilation of the common bile duct, and narrowing of portal and mesenteric blood vessels. As mentioned previously, about two-thirds are diagnosed as "periampullary cancers" preoperatively.[155] A tubulocystic change in the vicinity of the accessory duct and duodenal wall (in the minor ampullary region) are highly specific features seen on magnetic resonance imaging.

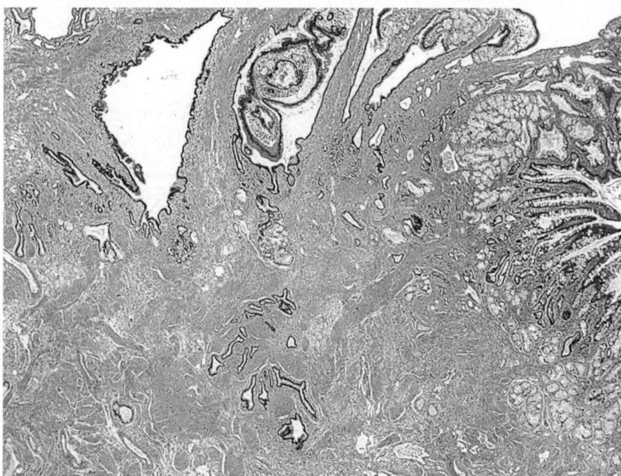

FIGURE 42.28 Adenomyomatous hyperplasia of the ampulla. In this patient with increased intraampullary pressure and clinical signs of obstruction, the only abnormality present is an exaggerated ampulla, with thickened muscle and prominent glands.

As mentioned previously, the fact that this process develops mainly around the minor (accessory) ampulla or accessory duct suggests a selective vulnerability of this region. In some cases, pancreas divisum (i.e., persistence of embryologic-type, dorsal-ventral separation of drainage systems) is suspected. One possibility is occlusion of a functionally overactive accessory duct (by unknown mechanisms), perhaps triggered by alcohol abuse or gallstones and also precipitated by the hypertension and diabetes. Regardless of the mechanisms, the macroscopic and microscopic morphological findings are quite distinctive.

Adenomyomatous Hyperplasia (Adenomyoma)

In some patients, functional obstruction of the ampulla may lead to the development of a masslike effect, including the double duct sign. In these cases, pathological examination reveals only a subtly thickened ampulla that mimics carcinoma, a condition referred as *adenomyomatous hyperplasia of the ampulla* (i.e., adenomyoma). Considering that some studies have claimed that 60% of autopsy cases illustrate this phenomenon,[160] it has become clear that this is a functional problem. Some pathologists define this entity as having at least a 5-mm thickness of the ampullary musculature; however, this is also not helpful. Because the normal ampulla contains tubules within dense muscular tissue (see Fig. 42.1B), it is difficult to determine specific criteria for adenomyomatous hyperplasia. The diagnosis relies heavily on clinical findings, particularly increased intraampullary pressure combined with exclusion of other pathological conditions (Fig. 42.28).

Papillary hyperplasia (Fig. 42.29) is also a similarly poorly characterized type of intraampullary lesion that consists of an exaggeration of the normal papillae.[15] The papillae are lined by biliary-type epithelium and sometimes contain an expanded fibrovascular core. Cases with inflammation may also reveal reactive epithelial changes. However, the degree of nuclear pseudostratification characteristic of intestinal-type adenomas and the marked degree of atypia of true papillary neoplasms are absent in this condition. The diagnosis

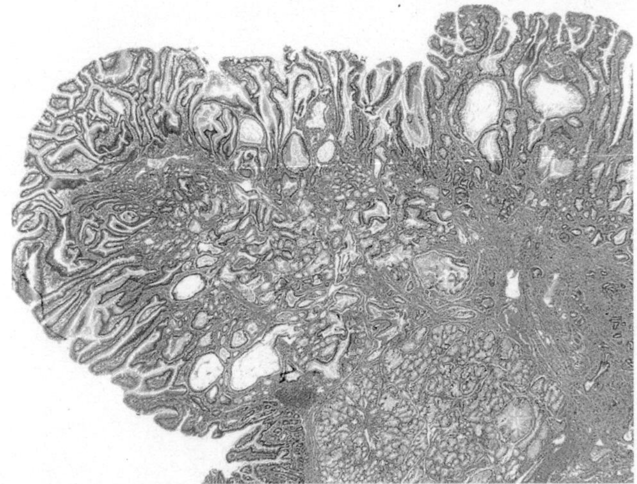

FIGURE 42.29 Papillary hyperplasia is a poorly characterized ampullary lesion that consists of an exaggeration of normal papillae of the ampulla.

rests on recognition that the extent of papilla formation exceeds that normally found in the ampulla, which itself is difficult to define.

Pancreatic heterotopia can occur throughout the upper GI tract, including the ampulla of Vater,[161,162] although symptomatic cases at this anatomical site are rare. Pancreatic acini, ducts, and islets are found adjacent to ducts within the muscularis of the sphincter of Oddi. Pancreatic tissue is commonly associated with the minor ampulla and represents residua from involution of the terminal ventral embryonic pancreatic duct. In some cases, there is no acinar or neuroendocrine tissue, only scattered ducts, which are usually embedded within hyperplastic smooth muscle bundles. Brunner's gland hyperplasia, which consists of nodules of histologically normal Brunner's glands mixed with smooth muscle fibers, also can affect the ampulla.[163-165]

GROSS EVALUATION AND THE SURGICAL PATHOLOGY REPORT

Classification of ampullary tumors and their differentiation from neoplasms of nearby anatomical sites rely heavily on gross examination.[6] Opening the duodenum along the antiampullary side and placing a probe into and through the common bile duct to locate the ampullary orifice in the lesion provides the key findings. For example, ampullary duodenal tumors most often form large, variegated, ulcerovegetative lesions on the duodenal surface of the ampulla with an eccentric location of the orifice. In contrast, IAPNs typically have a centrally located orifice with an evenly distributed and limited amount of granular or polypoid protrusions into the duodenal lumen because the lesion grows predominantly within the ampulla and is not as evident from the duodenal perspective. On the other hand, the ampullary duct cases show minimal changes on the duodenal surface of the ampulla and are often covered by mucosa, and the common bile duct is usually difficult to probe.

Different methods may be used to section the ampulla. Evaluation of the groove region (i.e., posterior aspect of the ampulla that is not covered by pancreatic tissue) usually requires specific attention. Ampullary neoplasms readily infiltrate the periduodenal soft tissues in this groove area, therefore a vertical sampling of this region from the ampulla to this edge is crucial for proper documentation of the stage and extent of the disease.

Standard information should be included in the surgical pathology report for ampullary carcinomas. Site-specific classification should be provided as *ampullary duodenal*, origin, *ampullary ductal*, or *IAPN-associated* tumors (see Fig. 42.6), and those that cannot be placed into one of these categories can be designated as NOS. Histological typing of carcinoma as intestinal (see Fig. 42.15), pancreatobiliary (see Fig. 42.16), or others should be provided separately, if feasible. Cases with unclassifiable patterns should be documented as such. For mixed-pattern cases, the types identified in the diagnostic section and their proportions should be provided in a comment. For cases with a preinvasive (adenomatous) component, the available characteristics should be provided separately, including the location (i.e., ampullary duodenal adenoma or IAPN), size, and cell lineage. If identified, the presence of any ductal abnormality should be documented, including pancreatobiliary maljunction, the supra-Oddi union of the common bile duct and the main pancreatic duct (Wirsung's).[94,95] Similarly, low union (cystic duct adjoining the common bile duct in or immediately adjacent to the pancreas) should also be recorded because it has been found to have an association with ampullary carcinomas.[94]

Reporting of ampullary carcinomas should include all of the conventional parameters for cancer reporting, such as vascular and perineural invasion, margin status, and lymph node status. A pancreatoduodenectomy specimen typically contains more than 12 lymph nodes.[6,166] Orange peeling of the peripancreatic soft tissues before sectioning the pancreatic head can help ensure maximal node recovery because the lymph nodes are typically embedded in the surface indentations of the pancreas and can be difficult to harvest after the specimen has been dissected.[166]

ACKNOWLEDGMENT

We thank Drs. Gokce Askan and Kerem Ozcan for their contributions in the preparation of this chapter.

The full reference list may be accessed online at Elsevier eBooks for Practicing Clinicians.

PART 3

LIVER

CHAPTER 43

Algorithmic Approach to Diagnosis of Medical Liver Disorders

Bita V. Naini

Contents

INTRODUCTION

The goal of this chapter is to provide a structured and efficacious approach to evaluation of nontargeted liver biopsy specimens (i.e., "medical" liver biopsies). The process begins with recognizing the predominant pattern of injury and then, by careful correlation with clinical and laboratory findings, identifying a disease process and/or providing a reliable prioritized differential diagnosis. There is considerable overlap in morphological patterns of injury among the various types of liver diseases, such as those seen in acute hepatitis secondary to viral, drug-induced, or autoimmune hepatitis (AIH). Likewise, more than one pattern of injury may be present in a liver biopsy specimen. For example, drugs and supplements are the most frequent cause of a mixed pattern of liver injury. In addition, some diseases exhibit several different patterns of injury that can mimic other disease processes. Examples include Wilson's disease, α_1-antitrypsin (A1AT) disorder, and drug-induced liver injury (DILI).

Pathognomonic features of certain diseases may be focal and therefore may not be present in one particular liver biopsy specimen. Examples include granulomatous duct destruction characteristic of primary biliary cholangitis (PBC). In such cases, other findings can be helpful in establishing the diagnosis in the correct clinical context.

In this chapter, a systematic approach to interpretation of the different patterns of liver injury is presented that can help pathologists categorize the patterns of injury and then, by correlating with clinical information, propose the most likely etiology.

ASSESSMENT OF HEPATIC ARCHITECTURE

The pathological "thought process" normally begins by assessing the architecture of the liver at low magnification. The liver consists of regularly arranged anastomosing plates of hepatocytes interspersed, at regular intervals, by alternating portal tracts and central veins of various sizes. Fibrous tissue is scarce in normal livers. It is limited to a small amount of collagen that supports the portal tracts and central veins. This amount varies according to the size of these respective structures.

Preservation of normal architecture is typically confirmed by the presence of portal tracts and central veins that occur at regularly spaced intervals. The architecture is considered altered when, for example, portal tracts and central veins are not present in either all or part of a biopsy specimen (indicating a hepatocellular tumor) or are distorted by fibrous tissue (indicating a chronic disorder with fibrosis) or as a result of nodular regeneration. Assessment of architecture is best performed by scanning the tissue at low to medium power magnification. There are several ancillary techniques that may also help in evaluating tissue architecture, and these are summarized in Table 43.1.

IDENTIFICATION OF THE PREDOMINANT PATTERN OF HEPATIC INJURY

After assessing the liver architecture, identifying the predominant pattern of injury is the next most helpful action that can also be performed at low to medium power magnification (Fig. 43.1). The most common general patterns of liver injury include hepatitis, hepatocellular necrosis, biliary disorders, steatosis, and vascular disorders. Examination of the different anatomic compartments in an organized fashion helps establish the predominant pattern of injury, but it may also identify any subtle findings that are missed on low magnification assessment. One sensible approach is to begin in the portal tracts and then view the liver progressively toward the central veins. Table 43.2 summarizes features to evaluate in each of the three main liver compartments: portal tracts, lobules, and central veins.

Portal and Lobular Inflammation

If a biopsy shows inflammation, one helpful method is to first determine the predominant location of the inflammation, which can provide a clue to the underlying etiology (Fig. 43.2). Two major patterns include predominantly portal and predominantly lobular (or mixed portal and lobular). When the inflammation is predominantly portal, it is helpful to determine whether there is accompanying bile duct injury. If there is no significant duct injury, the main diagnostic consideration is chronic hepatitis, whereas if there is bile duct injury, PBC is the main etiological consideration.

Predominantly Portal Inflammation without Significant Bile Duct Injury

Chronic Hepatitis

Hepatitis is defined as an inflammatory process that leads to hepatocyte damage. Clinically, it manifests with elevated transaminases. Hepatitis is categorized as either acute or chronic, based on a variety of clinical and histological features outlined in the following sections. Chronic hepatitis indicates an inflammatory liver dysfunction that has been present for 6 months or more. It is characterized by portal mononuclear inflammation, usually in combination with a variable degree of interface and lobular hepatocyte damage. The most common causes of chronic hepatitis are hepatotropic viruses (such as hepatitis B, C, and E) in which the inflammation often extends beyond the portal tracts into adjacent periportal parenchyma and is associated with hepatocyte injury at the portal tracts/lobular interface, which is termed *interface hepatitis.*[1] There may also be some degree of lobular inflammation associated with hepatocyte necrosis (Fig. 43.3).

In chronic hepatitis, the bile ducts may show mild epithelial damage, but they are not the primary target of injury. Lymphoid aggregates and lymphoid follicles are characteristic features of hepatitis C; however, they are not specific for hepatitis C (Fig. 43.4).[2] In chronic viral hepatitis, necroinflammatory activity is typically present at low levels throughout the natural history of the disease. It may diminish in late stages, and there may occasionally be acute flares (particularly in hepatitis C). Fibrosis may develop with time, regardless of the amount of inflammation (Fig. 43.5).

In chronic hepatitis B, ground-glass hepatocytes help confirm the diagnosis, as it indicates hepatitis B surface antigen (HBsAg) accumulation within the endoplasmic reticulum as a result of viral DNA integration into the host genome. However, ground-glass hepatocytes are not always easy to identify; their appearance is highly variable and dependent on both the quality and type of fixation, as well as staining. In addition, ground-glass hepatocytes are not specific to hepatitis B. They may also be seen in immunosuppressed individuals, especially those receiving multiple medications (see later).[3-4] In hepatitis B infection, an immunostain for HBsAg helps confirm the diagnosis. It may be positive, even in cases without readily apparent ground-glass inclusions (Fig. 43.6).[5] Immunostain with AHBsAg or DNA quantification of HBV can help reveal hepatitis B infections, even if the serological results are negative for hepatitis B infection. For instance, latent infections can occur when viral serology is negative.

If the clinical and serological data confirm chronic viral hepatitis, then the biopsy should be graded and staged accordingly. There are several grading and staging schemes available, and each has advantages and disadvantages. When a particular grading or staging system is used, the name of the system (e.g., METAVIR, Ishak, Batts-Ludwig, modified Ishak) should be stated in the diagnostic report so the clinician is aware and it can be used appropriately for clinical

TABLE 43.1 Stains Used to Evaluate Liver Architecture

Stain	How It Helps
Trichrome	Evaluates for fibrosis and helps distinguish fibrosis from necrosis
Reticulin	Evaluates for regeneration and helps detect collapse of reticulin framework in areas of necrosis
Keratin-7	Highlights bile ducts and thus portal tracts
Glutamine synthetase	Highlights perivenular areas in normal liver
CD34	Highlights portal vessels +/– sinusoids in zone 1 (diffuse staining of sinusoids indicates aberrant expression as a result of abnormal endothelialization of sinusoids, as seen in any etiology that would lead to increased arterial blood flow)

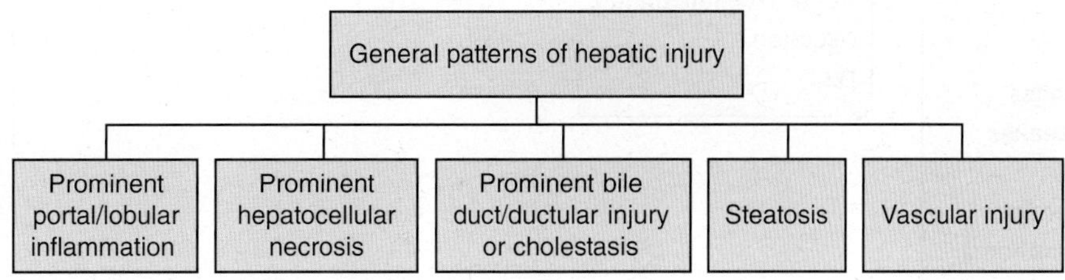

FIGURE 43.1 Algorithm for identification of the predominant pattern of injury.

TABLE 43.2 Systematic Approach for Evaluation of Medical Liver Biopsies

Compartment	Feature to Evaluate	Findings to Look For
Portal tracts	Size	Are they the expected size or expanded? If expanded, is it caused by inflammation, ductular reaction, portal edema, fibrosis, or a combination of these?
	Inflammation	If there is inflammation, which type of inflammatory cells are seen (lymphocytic, lymphoplasmacytic, or mixed)? Are plasma cells or eosinophils prominent? Is the inflammation contained within portal tracts, or does it extend into adjacent parenchyma (i.e., interface hepatitis)? Are there granulomas? If yes, where are they (portal, lobular, or both)?. If portal, are they centered around bile ducts?
	Portal vein	Are they patent or narrowed/sclerosed? Is there perivenular inflammation or endotheliitis?
	Bile duct	Is it present or absent? If present, does it show lymphocytic infiltration and/or epithelial injury (e.g., nuclear overlapping, cytoplasmic vacuolization)? Is there a ductular reaction?
Lobules	Hepatocytes	Are they swollen and injured? Does the cytoplasm appear pale, or is the cellular morphology plantlike?
	Sinusoids	Are they dilated? If yes, is the dilation associated with hepatocyte atrophy? Are they congested? If yes, is there zonal distribution? Do they contain increased inflammatory cells? If yes, which type (lymphocytes, Kupffer cells)? Do they contain abnormal deposits (e.g., amyloid)?
	Steatosis	Do hepatocytes contain fat (steatosis)? If yes, is it microvesicular, macrovesicular, or both? Is there a zonal distribution to steatosis, or is it randomly distributed? If there is steatosis, is it associated with ballooned hepatocytes and/or Mallory-Denk bodies?
	Cholestasis	Is it present or absent? If present, is it canalicular, ductular, hepatocellular or mixed? Is it bland or associated with inflammation?
	Inclusions/Pigments	Do hepatocytes contain abnormal inclusions? Do they show increased pigmentation such as iron, bile, or lipofuscin?
	Inflammation	Is there lobular inflammation? If yes, which type? Is it associated with hepatocyte damage such as apoptosis or necrosis? If necrosis, is it zonal?
Central veins		Are they patent or obliterated? Is there perivenular inflammation or necrosis?

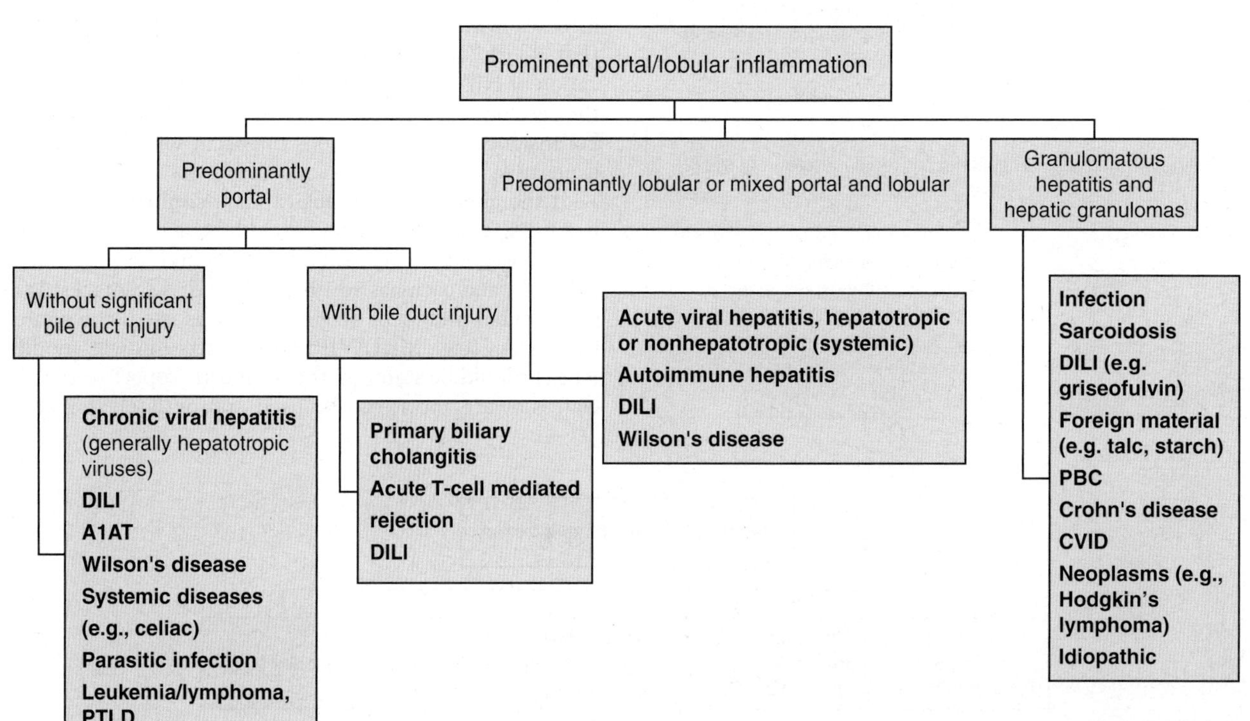

FIGURE 43.2 Algorithm for determining the predominant location of inflammation.

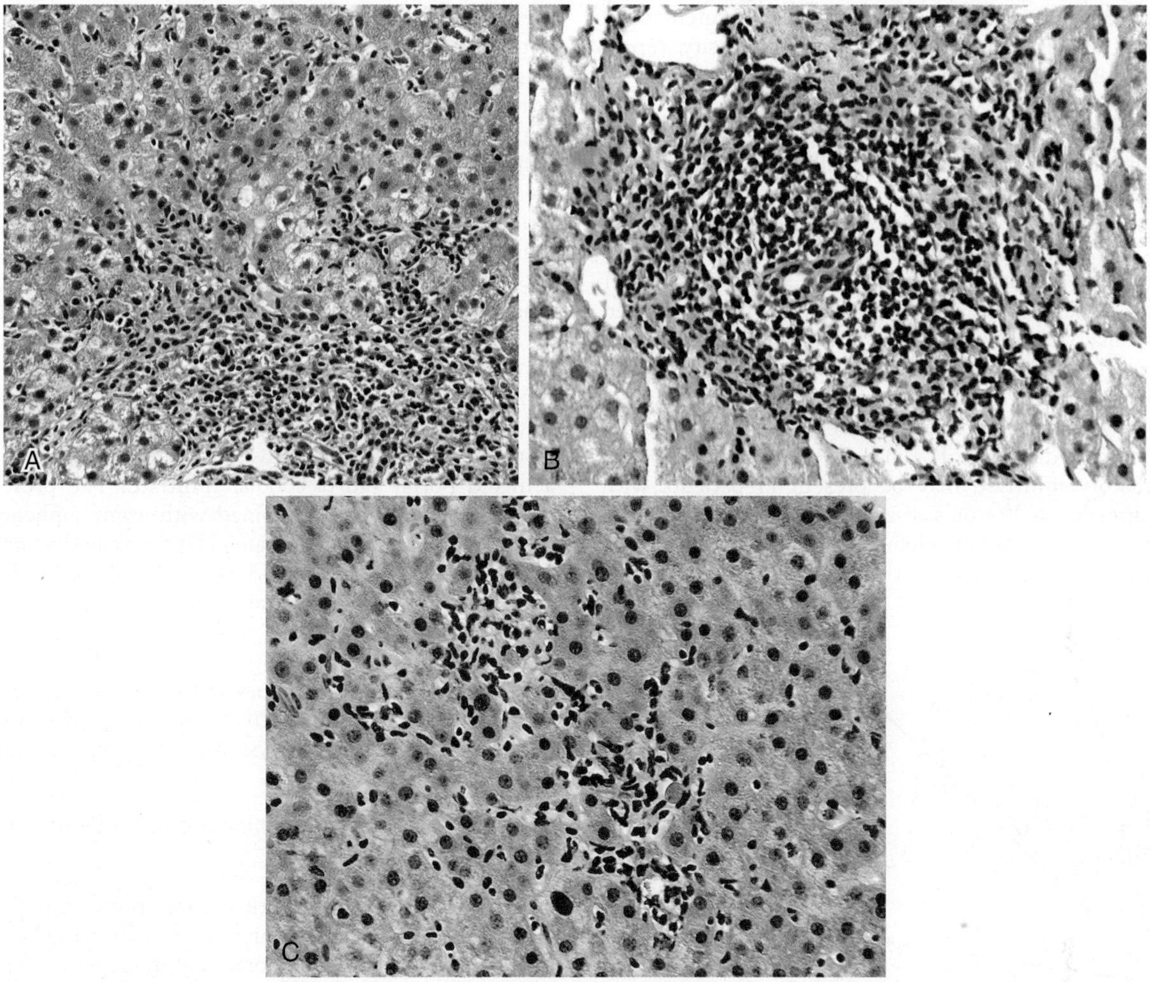

FIGURE 43.3 **A,** Chronic hepatitis B showing interphase activity. The inflammation extends from the portal tract beyond the limiting plate and into the adjacent parenchyma. **B,** Portal inflammation in chronic hepatitis B consists predominantly of lymphocytes surrounding an entrapped bile duct, which is mostly intact. **C,** A variable amount of lobular inflammation associated with hepatocyte damage is also usually present in chronic hepatitis.

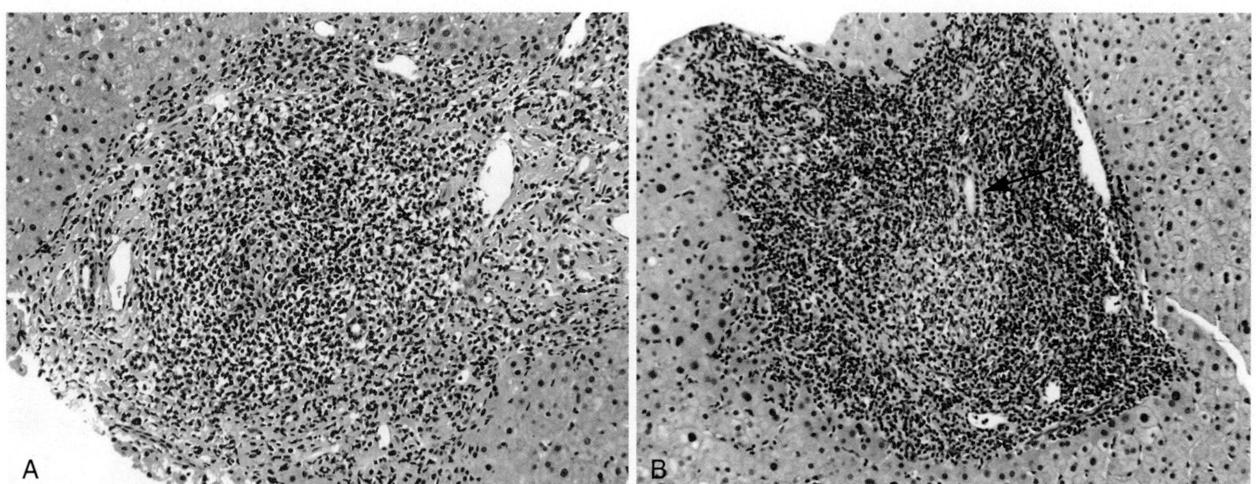

FIGURE 43.4 Lymphoid follicles are often associated with chronic hepatitis C **(A)** but may also be seen in other forms of chronic viral hepatitis, autoimmune hepatitis, and primary biliary cirrhosis (**B**; *arrow* marks bile duct under immune attack).

patient management. This author's personal preference is the Batts-Ludwig system because of its simplicity, reproducibility, and clinical relevance.[6,7]

Portal Inflammation Associated with Other Disease Processes

Although portal inflammation is usually present in chronic hepatitis, it may also occur in a wide variety of other liver diseases, such as acute hepatitis, chronic biliary diseases such as PBC (especially in its early stage), DILI, and certain metabolic diseases, among others. It can also occur in other systemic diseases that do not primarily affect the liver, such as celiac disease.[8] The type of infiltrate, the pattern of involvement (portal predominant or mixed portal and lobular), and the presence or absence of associated findings (e.g., duct injury in chronic biliary diseases) help provide clues to the correct diagnosis. For instance, a prominent portal inflammatory infiltrate may be present in patients with A1AT disorder or Wilson's disease. In the former, characteristic round eosinophilic globules within periportal hepatocytes help provide a clue to the diagnosis. These globules are periodic acid–Schiff (PAS) positive and resist digestion with diastase (Fig. 43.7). However, globules may also represent an acute-phase reaction during concomitant chronic viral hepatitis.[9] Wilson's disease may also resemble chronic hepatitis and show prominent portal lymphocytes. Accompanying findings are relatively nonspecific and include mild steatosis, Mallory-Denk bodies in periportal hepatocytes, binucleated hepatocytes, and clear (glycogenated) nuclei.[10] Demonstration of increased copper deposition in hepatocytes by copper quantification studies helps confirm the diagnosis of Wilson's disease.

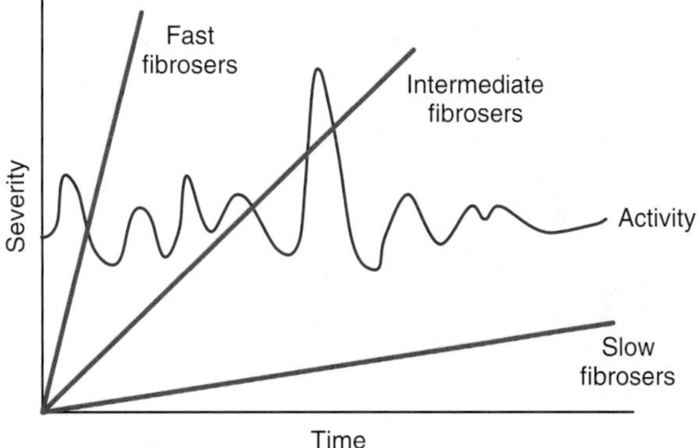

FIGURE 43.5 Patterns of necroinflammatory activity and fibrosis in viral hepatitis. In chronic viral hepatitis, inflammatory activity is variable over time, whereas fibrosis tends to progress linearly. In terms of fibrotic progression, patients fall into three groups: rapid, intermediate, and slow. The degree of activity does not correlate well with the degree of scarring or the likelihood of subsequent scarring.

If the lymphoid infiltrate in portal tracts appears atypical, then the differential diagnosis includes hematopoietic malignancies such as leukemia, lymphoma, and post-transplantation lymphoproliferative disorder.[11] For instance, in Hodgkin's disease involving liver, there may be a mixed portal and/or lobular infiltrate. The presence of Reed-Sternberg cells, combined with immunophenotyping of the inflammatory infiltrate, helps reveal the malignant nature of the lesion (Fig. 43.8). The infiltrate in Epstein-Barr virus (EBV) hepatitis also tends to appear somewhat atypical.

A predominantly eosinophilic portal infiltrate is not a common pattern of liver injury, but when it occurs, parasitic infection should be suspected. Of these, schistosomiasis targets the portal venous system. Larva migrans can cause eosinophilic abscesses.[12]

Predominantly Portal Inflammation with Bile Duct Injury

Primary Biliary Cholangitis

PBC is associated with both chronic portal inflammation and active duct injury/destruction of small to medium-sized bile ducts. The pathognomonic feature of early-stage PBC is termed a *florid duct lesion,* which is defined as a dense portal lymphoplasmacytic inflammation that surrounds a damaged bile duct and characteristically contains a non-necrotizing granuloma. However, the histological changes of PBC are often patchy. Therefore diagnostic bile duct destructive lesions may not always be present in biopsy specimens from patients with PBC.[13] In later stages, PBC

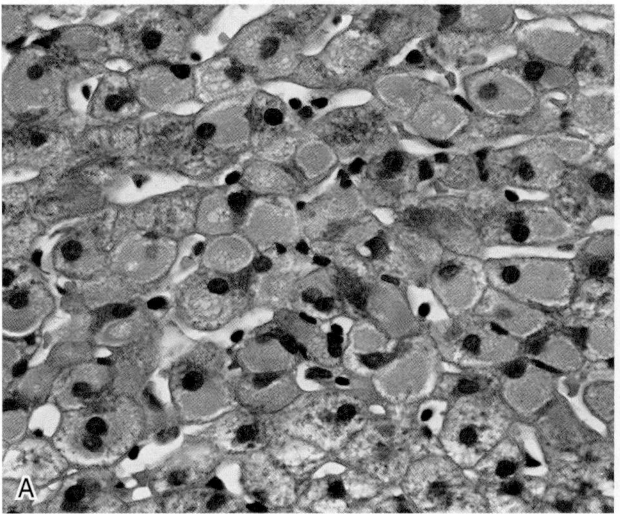

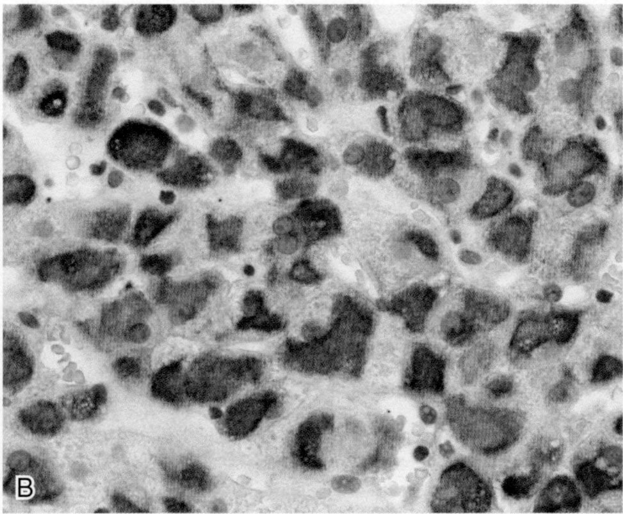

FIGURE 43.6 A, Ground-glass inclusions in chronic hepatitis. These are highlighted by an immunohistochemical stain for hepatitis B surface antigen **(B).**

is associated with a bile ductular reaction that appears to represent a compensatory mechanism to allow for maintenance of bile flow through the hepatic biliary system.[14] As the disease progresses, ductopenia and fibrosis eventually ensue (Fig. 43.9).

Portal Inflammation and Duct Injury Associated with Other Disease Processes

Acute T-cell–mediated rejection represents a prototypical mixed portal inflammatory infiltrate that includes lymphocytes and eosinophils as well as scattered other types of inflammatory cells (Fig. 43.10).[15] This mixed infiltrate is associated with lymphocytic infiltration of bile ducts as well as duct epithelial injury, seen as cytoplasmic vacuolization with nuclear enlargement and overlapping. The findings may closely resemble PBC in native liver. In fact, a challenging differential diagnosis in posttransplant allograft liver biopsies is acute T-cell–mediated rejection versus recurrent PBC. In such cases, other associated findings of rejection such as portal or central vein endotheliitis helps distinguish the two.

DILI may also show portal inflammation with or without duct injury. As DILI is always a diagnosis of exclusion, it is important to histologically and clinically rule out other potential causes. Establishing a temporal relationship between the initiation of the drug or supplement in question and the elevation of liver enzymes (including disappearance of symptoms on withdrawal of the drug and reappearance on rechallenge) is essential in confirming a diagnosis of DILI.

Predominantly Lobular or Mixed Portal and Lobular Inflammation

Acute Hepatitis

Hepatitis is considered acute if the clinical, laboratory, or histological evidence of liver inflammation persists for less than 6 months. It is associated with disease ranging from subclinical to self-limited symptomatic to overt hepatic failure. The characteristic features of acute hepatitis are prominent lobular inflammation with associated disruption of the normal lobular sinusoidal architecture (i.e., lobular "disarray"), hepatocyte injury in the form of cytoplasmic swelling and clearing, as well as apoptosis or necrosis. Necrosis may be patchy, may involve some or all liver zones, or may be confluent (Fig. 43.11). Most types of acute hepatitis are associated with lobular inflammation that is disproportionately high in comparison with portal tracts, but acute

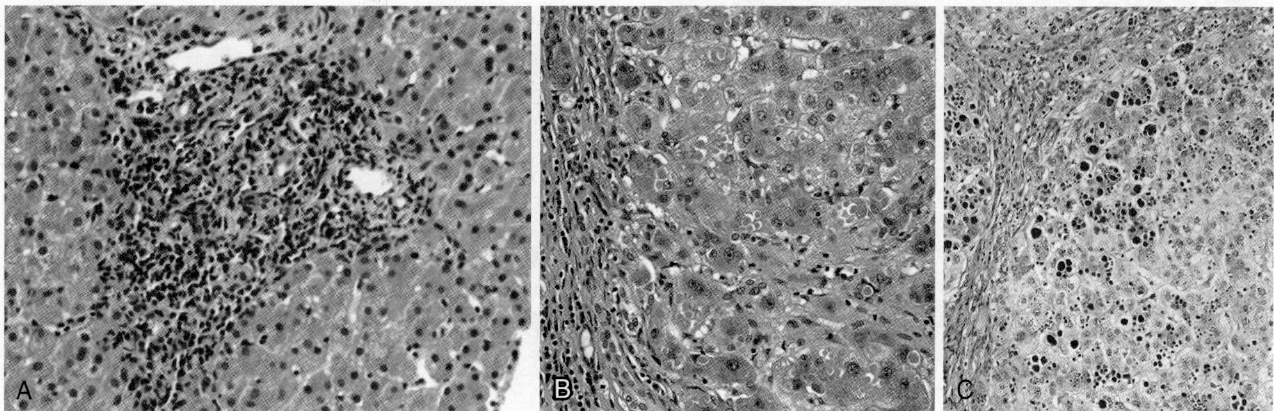

FIGURE 43.7 A, Portal inflammation in a patient with α_1-antitrypsin (A1AT) disorder. **B,** Many intracytoplasmic eosinophilic globules are seen in periportal hepatocytes in this case. **C,** Periodic acid–Schiff (PAS) stain after diastase digestion highlights these globules.

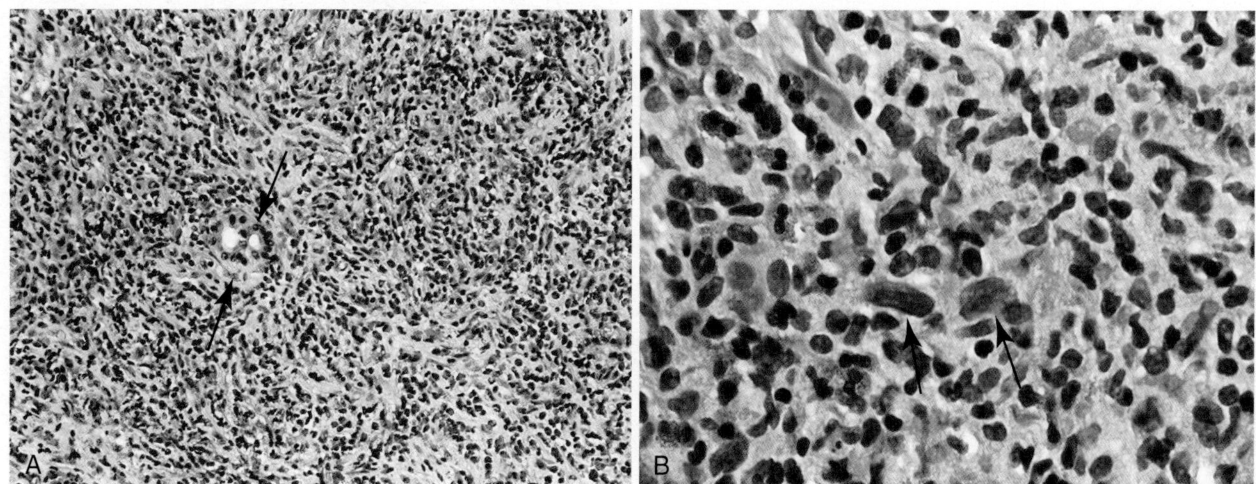

FIGURE 43.8 A, A mixed portal inflammatory infiltrate with prominent eosinophils is seen in a patient with Hodgkin's disease. *Arrows* point to an entrapped bile duct. **B,** Large atypical cells *(arrows)* consistent with Reed-Sternberg cells are present among the inflammatory infiltrate.

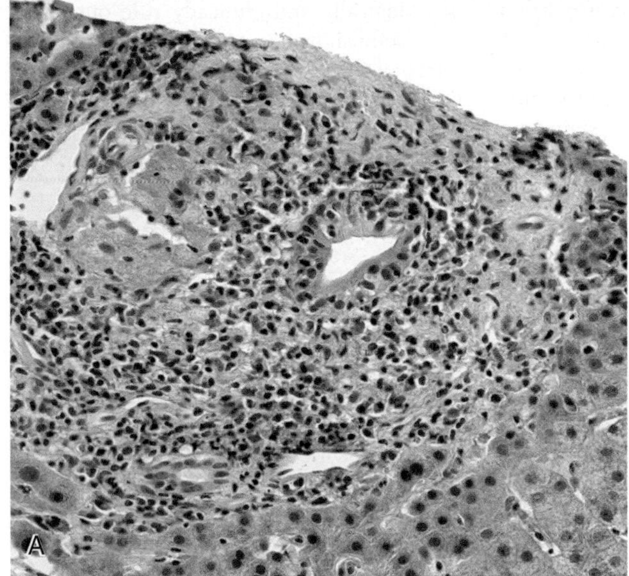

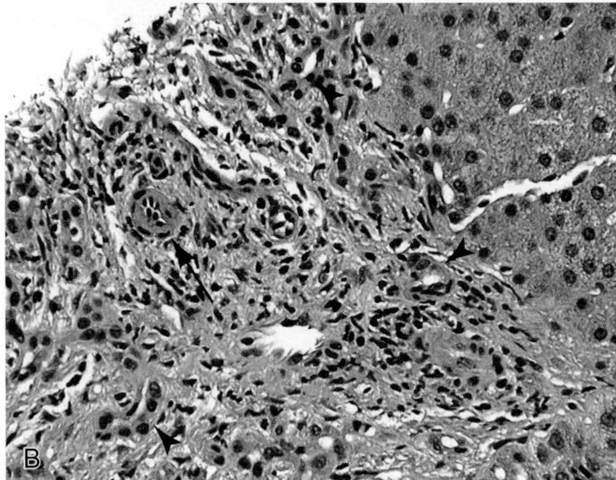

FIGURE 43.9 A, Biopsy of a patient with primary biliary cholangitis *(PBC)* shows prominent portal lymphoplasmacytic infiltrate with a nonnecrotizing granuloma surrounding a markedly damaged bile duct (florid duct lesion). **B,** Other findings in PBC include ductular reaction *(arrowheads)* and unpaired arterioles *(arrow)* in portal tracts that have already lost their interlobular bile duct.

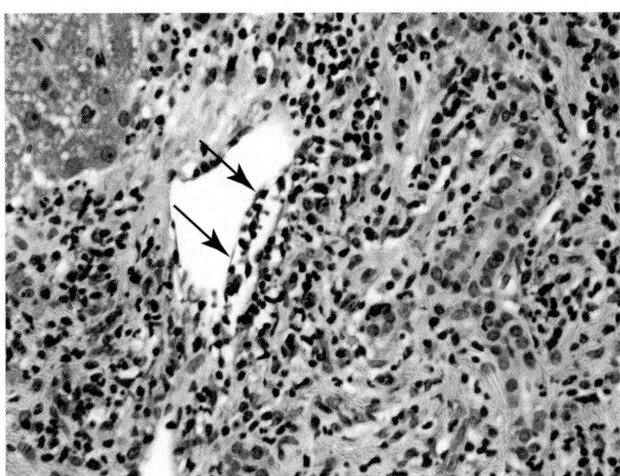

FIGURE 43.10 Acute T-cell–mediated rejection with a mixed inflammatory infiltrate consisting of lymphocytes, neutrophils, and eosinophils. Note the prominent endotheliitis *(arrows)*.

hepatitis is also usually accompanied by a variable degree of portal inflammation, which in some cases can be quite prominent. Similar to chronic hepatitis, acute hepatitis generally causes little to no injury to bile ducts.

The severity of acute hepatitis ranges from scattered apoptotic hepatocytes associated with patchy lobular inflammation to severe lobular inflammation associated with portal-to-portal or portal-to-central "bridging necrosis" and liver parenchymal collapse. The presence of bridging "necroinflammatory" activity is typical of both acute and AIH. If it is present in cases of chronic viral hepatitis, it should trigger an evaluation for other potentially important concomitant diseases (e.g., superinfection with another type of hepatotropic virus) or the presence of an immunodeficiency state (Table 43.3).

The most common etiological agents of acute hepatitis include hepatotropic viruses (hepatitis A, B, C, D, and E viruses),[16] nonhepatotropic viruses, drugs/supplements or toxins, as well as AIH [see later]. There is a considerable overlap in histological findings between viral and nonviral etiologies as well as between drug-induced hepatitis and AIH, and it is only by correlation with serological studies

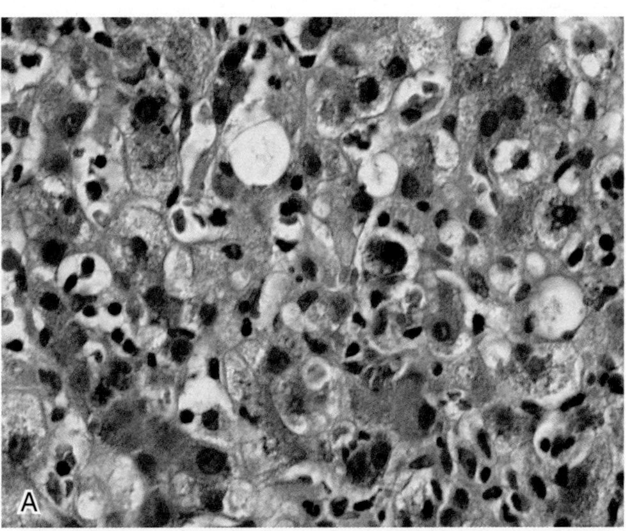

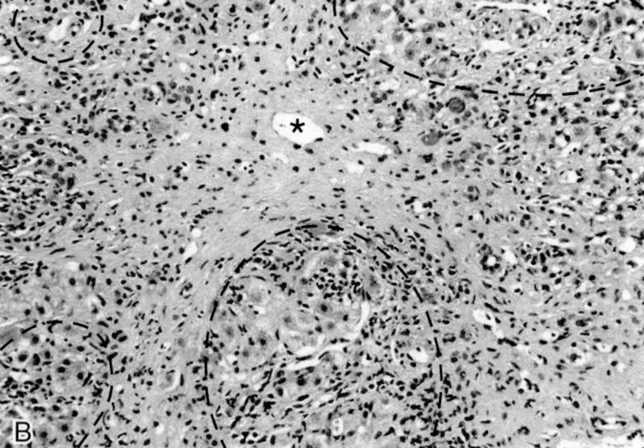

FIGURE 43.11 A, Lobular disarray is characteristic of acute hepatitis. The sinusoids are indiscernible as a result of swollen and injured hepatocytes. **B,** Confluent necrosis in this case of acute hepatitis extends from the central vein *(asterisk)* with areas of surviving parenchyma and/or portal tracts *(dashed circles)*.

that a definite etiology may be confirmed. If viral and serological studies are negative, then DILI or other disorders such as Wilson's disease are entities that should be considered. Ultimately, about 15% of acute hepatitis cases that lead to liver failure remain idiopathic.

Autoimmune Hepatitis

AIH is characterized by the presence of portal inflammation, interface hepatitis, and prominent lobular inflammation. Although plasma cells are characteristic of AIH, they are not always prominent, and this may be dependent on the phase of disease and the treatment status (Fig. 43.12). Some cases show predominant lymphocytic inflammation but without prominent plasma cells.[17] In addition, plasma cells may also be prominent in other conditions, such as hepatitis A or DILI, the latter either as an idiosyncratic drug reaction or as a primary form of drug-induced AIH that is seen with minocycline, nitrofurantoin, and several other drugs.

Most patients with AIH before treatment show a robust hepatitis with severe inflammatory activity. This is characterized by the presence of marked-interface and lobular hepatitis, hepatocyte loss, and confluent necrosis. The latter may be localized around the central veins or may show a central-portal or a portal-portal (bridging necrosis) pattern, or it may involve entire lobules ("total parenchymal collapse") (Fig. 43.13).[6] When the areas of confluent necrosis extend to the portal tracts, a ductular reaction often becomes prominent as well.

Patients with AIH may have bouts of severe activity followed by long periods of inactivity. Fibrosis develops as a result of hepatocyte necrosis/apoptosis, thus progression to cirrhosis is usually swift compared with typical cases of chronic viral hepatitis. As a result, AIH may demonstrate any of the following features[6,17]: (1) cirrhosis with either little or no necroinflammatory activity (*burned out AIH*); (2) intermediate-stage disease associated with moderate to severe activity, often combined with some degree of scarring and nodularity; or (3) early-stage disease associated with marked activity (at least focal confluent necrosis) as well as parenchymal collapse (Fig. 43.14). However, patients with AIH are unlikely to show periods of mild activity combined with either mild or absent fibrosis. Thus biopsies that reveal both mild activity and mild fibrosis are unlikely to represent AIH. In such cases, viral hepatitis or DILI should be considered.

In AIH, the bile ducts may be obscured by the marked degree of portal inflammation, but they do not normally reveal significant lymphocytic inflammation or epithelial damage. If the portal inflammation also shows duct centricity and is associated with moderate or marked epithelial damage, then the possibility of an overlap syndrome with PBC should be considered (see later).[18] In posttransplant allograft biopsies, the presence of a plasma-cell–rich hepatitis is either indicative of recurrent AIH or allograft rejection (i.e., plasma-cell–rich rejection).[19,20]

TABLE 43.3 Possible Implications of Confluent Necrosis in Biopsy Specimens from Patients with Viral Hepatitis

Hepatitis B	Hepatitis C
Acute flare from HBeAg to HBeAb seroconversion Superinfection with HDV Immunocompromised status (HIV-associated or other) Concomitant autoimmune hepatitis Concomitant drug/toxin-induced liver injury	Acute flare Immunocompromise (HIV-associated or other) Concomitant autoimmune hepatitis Concomitant drug/toxin-induced liver injury

HBeAb, *Antibody to the hepatitis B e antigen;* HBeAg, *hepatitis B e antigen;* HDV, *hepatitis D virus;* HIV, *human immunodeficiency virus.*

Primary Biliary Cholangitis–Autoimmune Hepatitis Overlap Syndrome

One frequently encountered problem is identification of a PBC-AIH overlap syndrome versus PBC or AIH alone. Similar to AIH, PBC cases may also show abundant plasma cells[18] as well as mild interface and lobular

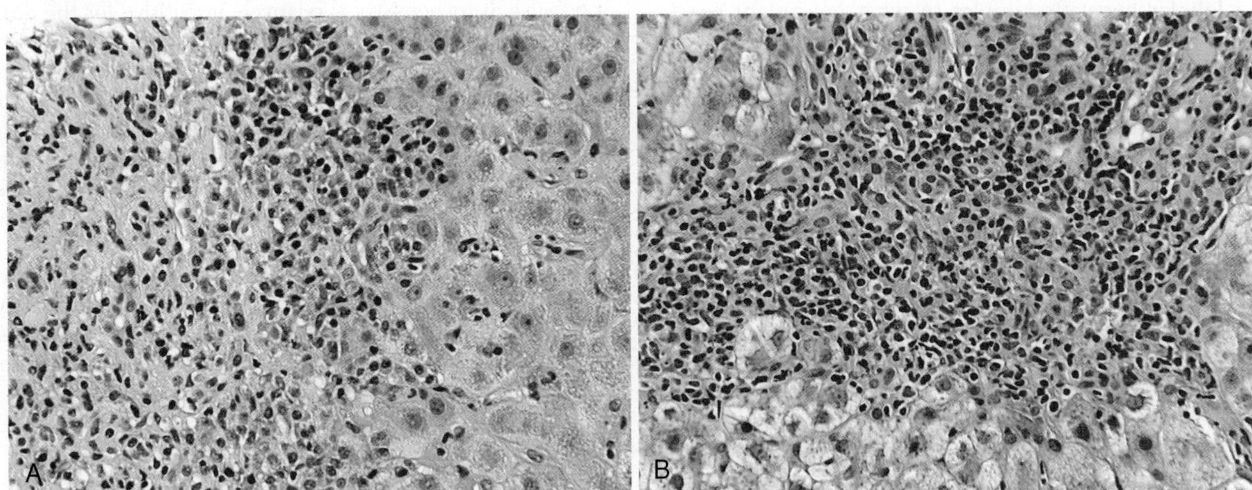

FIGURE 43.12 A, Autoimmune hepatitis showing a portal inflammatory infiltrate rich in plasma cells and prominent interface activity. **B,** Not all cases of autoimmune hepatitis are rich in plasma cells; this case demonstrates a predominantly lymphocytic portal inflammatory infiltrate.

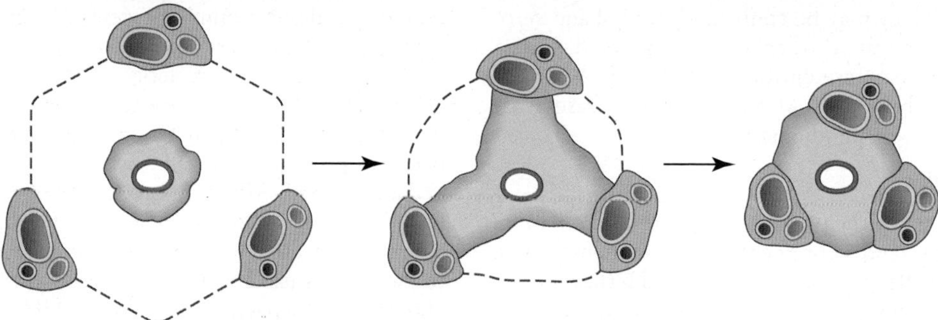

FIGURE 43.13 Confluent necrosis may result in varying degrees of injury: perivenular dropout of hepatocytes *(left)*, bridging necrosis *(middle)*, and parenchymal collapse *(right)*. All of these are considered severe degrees of necroinflammatory activity and typical of acute or autoimmune hepatitis.

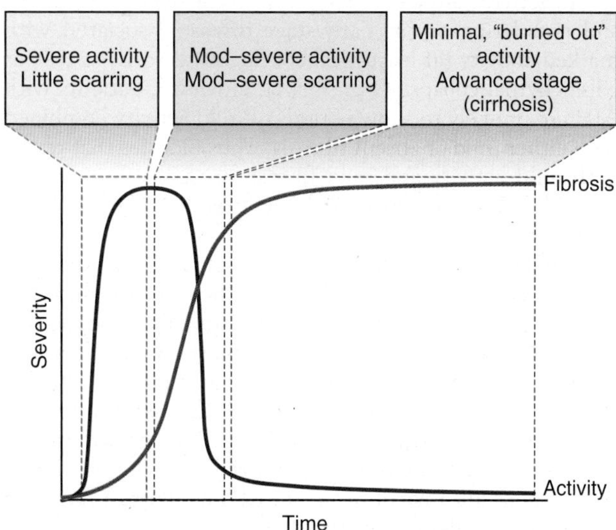

FIGURE 43.14 Pattern of necro-inflammatory activity and fibrosis in autoimmune hepatitis. There is usually an initial wave of severe activity that subsides into a late, "burned out" stage of disease. Scarring takes place directly in response to the activity, often replacing areas of confluent necrosis and parenchymal collapse. In autoimmune hepatitis, only certain combinations of severity of inflammation and fibrotic progression are seen, and no biopsy is likely to show a small degree of both inflammation and fibrosis.

hepatitis. If there are only scattered foci of interface and lobular hepatitis (similar to what one might see in hepatitis C), then the case likely represents only PBC. However, if there is confluent necrosis or widespread interface and lobular hepatitis that is easily recognizable at low magnification, then an overlap syndrome may be considered. This may be suggested on biopsy findings; however, it is ultimately confirmed clinically by showing proof of both serological and biochemical features of PBC and AIH, that is, positive antinuclear antibodies (ANAs) or anti–smooth muscle antibodies (SMAs), markedly elevated transaminases, and elevated alkaline phosphatase. Similarly, AIH alone may show mild bile duct injury or that the duct may be obscured by the brisk inflammation that is present in the portal tract. However, the duct injury would be proportionally mild compared with the amount of interface and lobular hepatitis, and the characteristic conspicuous inflammatory and destructive duct lesion (i.e., florid duct lesion) of PBC will not be present in AIH alone.

Wilson's Disease

As mentioned earlier, Wilson's disease can have different presentations with different histological patterns of injury. The chronic form resembles chronic hepatitis with variable interface and lobular hepatitis and variable fibrosis, as described earlier. However, Wilson's disease may also present acutely with a histological pattern of acute hepatitis including severe hepatitis with bridging necrosis. This form may be the first clinical presentation of the disease. In such cases, accompanying laboratory/clinical features and quantitative copper assay on biopsy are helpful in distinguishing the Wilson's form from other forms of acute hepatitis.

Granulomatous Hepatitis and Hepatic Granulomas

Liver biopsies may contain scattered granulomas, or they may display features of a "granulomatous hepatitis," the latter of which is associated with portal and lobular inflammation accompanied by hepatocyte necrosis. Eosinophils may or may not be prominent. The most common causes include infection (mycobacterial or fungal), drug- and toxin-induced liver injury, sarcoidosis (Fig. 43.15), or other granuloma-associated diseases such as PBC or Crohn's disease.

Caseating granulomas are particularly suspicious for infection. Special stains such as acid-fast bacilli (AFB), Grocott-Gomori's methenamine silver (GMS,) and PAS may be used to detect organisms. However, infectious etiologies remain in the differential, even when the special stains are negative. This is because histochemistry is relatively insensitive for the diagnosis, whereas cultures or serological studies are more sensitive.

Fibrin ring granulomas have a distinctive morphological appearance characterized by the presence of a central fat vacuole surrounded by an eosinophilic ring and an outer layer of macrophages. They are most commonly associated with infection, such as *Coxiella burnetii* (Q fever), EBV, or leishmaniasis. They have also been reported in drug-related injury (such as with griseofulvin or immune checkpoint inhibitors).[21]

In sarcoidosis, granulomas are often confluent showing differing ages of development and degree of cellularity. They may also be sclerotic and/or contain asteroid bodies. In approximately 10% to 15% of cases, a specific cause for hepatic granulomas cannot be ultimately identified.[22]

Other Conditions

Nonhepatotropic Viral Hepatitis

Although most nonhepatotropic viruses (e.g., cytomegalovirus [CMV], herpes simplex virus [HSV], and adenovirus) can

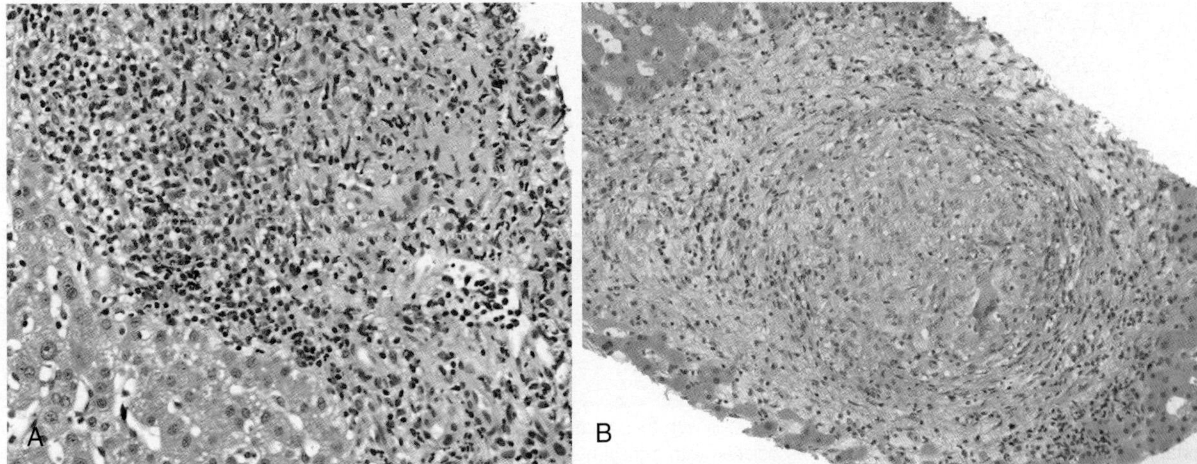

FIGURE 43.15 **A,** Drug (in this case allopurinol)-induced granulomatous hepatitis. Allopurinol may also cause fibrin ring granulomas. **B,** Sarcoidosis with a large, well-formed, nonnecrotizing portal granuloma.

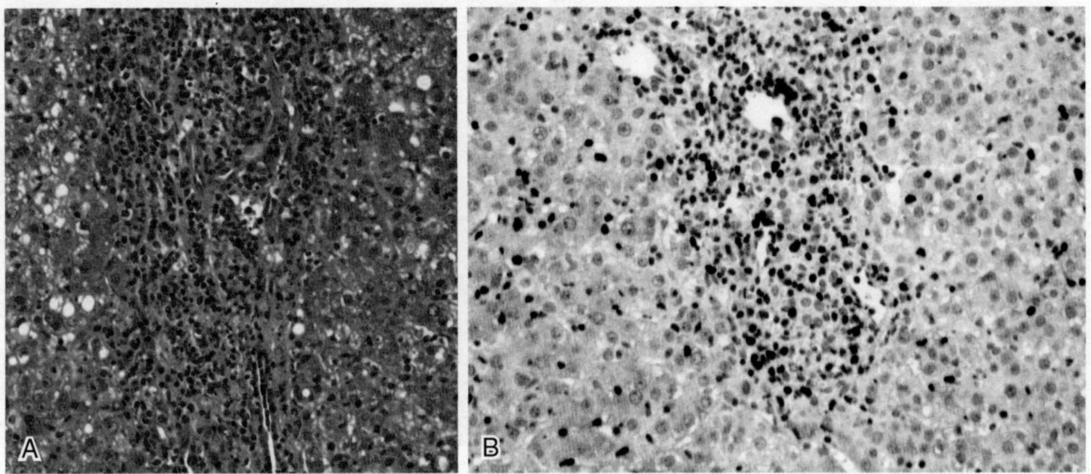

FIGURE 43.16 **A,** Epstein-Barr viral hepatitis can cause portal inflammatory infiltrate, as shown here, or sinusoidal lymphocytic infiltrate. The infiltrating lymphocytes appear slightly atypical and may be highlighted by Epstein-Barr virus–encoded RNA (EBER) **(B).**

cause hepatitis, these organisms are not generally associated with prominent portal or lobular inflammation. HSV and adenovirus hepatitis characteristically show significant hepatocellular necrosis (see later). EBV infection, on the other hand, may be associated with significant inflammatory infiltrate. Hepatic involvement with EBV infection is common but is often subclinical and self-limited. EBV-related hepatitis occurs predominantly in immunocompromised patients and rarely in immunocompetent patients.[23] The characteristic histological findings include a diffuse lymphocytic sinusoidal infiltrate in a "string of beads" pattern, with or without associated apoptotic bodies, as well as expansion of portal tracts by a predominantly lymphocytic infiltrate. The lobular architecture is generally intact. The portal mononuclear infiltration may be to such a degree that it mimics chronic hepatitis B or C in some instances. The infiltrating lymphocytes may appear larger and slightly more atypical than mature lymphocytes. The diagnosis can be confirmed with in situ hybridization for EBV-encoded RNA (EBER) (Fig. 43.16).[24,25]

CMV hepatitis occurs almost exclusively in immunocompromised patients, such as those who have had a bone marrow transplant. Characteristic features include the presence of CMV inclusions, which are eosinophilic inclusions located in both the cytoplasm and nuclei of affected cells. CMV may infect hepatocytes, cholangiocytes, or endothelial cells. CMV-infected cells may be present randomly throughout the lobule, without any particular preferential zone of involvement. Some cases are associated with neutrophilic microabscesses within the liver parenchyma (Fig. 43.17).[26] However, neutrophilic microabscesses are neither a sensitive nor specific finding in CMV hepatitis. CMV hepatitis may also be associated with portal and lobular inflammation, and it may show overlapping features with acute T-cell–mediated rejection in posttransplant cases. Immunostains for CMV help confirm the diagnosis.

Resolving Acute Hepatitis

As mentioned earlier, many types of acute hepatitis resolve. During the resolving period, the inflammation and necrosis subside, and phagocytic activity predominates. If a liver biopsy is taken during this period, it often shows clusters of pigment-laden Kupffer cells, which are silvery-gray on hematoxylin and eosin (H&E) stain but bright magenta with PAS stain after diastase digestion (PASD) (Fig. 43.18). Kupffer cells represent the tissue repair associated with prior hepatocyte injury, such as from acute viral hepatitis, toxins,

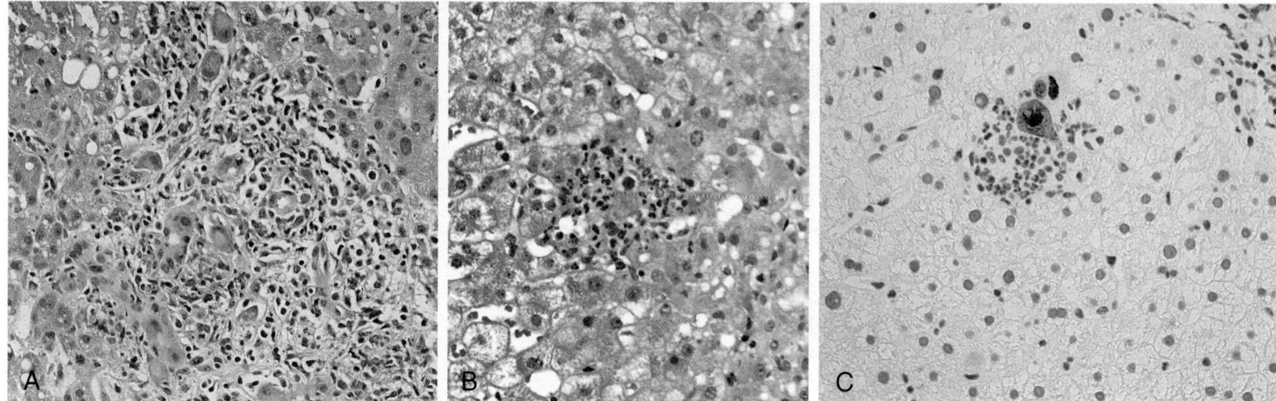

FIGURE 43.17 **A,** Several cytomegalovirus (CMV)-infected cells with their characteristic intranuclear and intracytoplasmic inclusions are seen within this portal tract. **B,** CMV-infected cells are seen in association with a focal neutrophilic inflammation (neutrophilic microabscess); however, neutrophilic microabscesses are not a sensitive or specific finding in CMV hepatitis. **C,** Immunostain highlights CMV-infected cells.

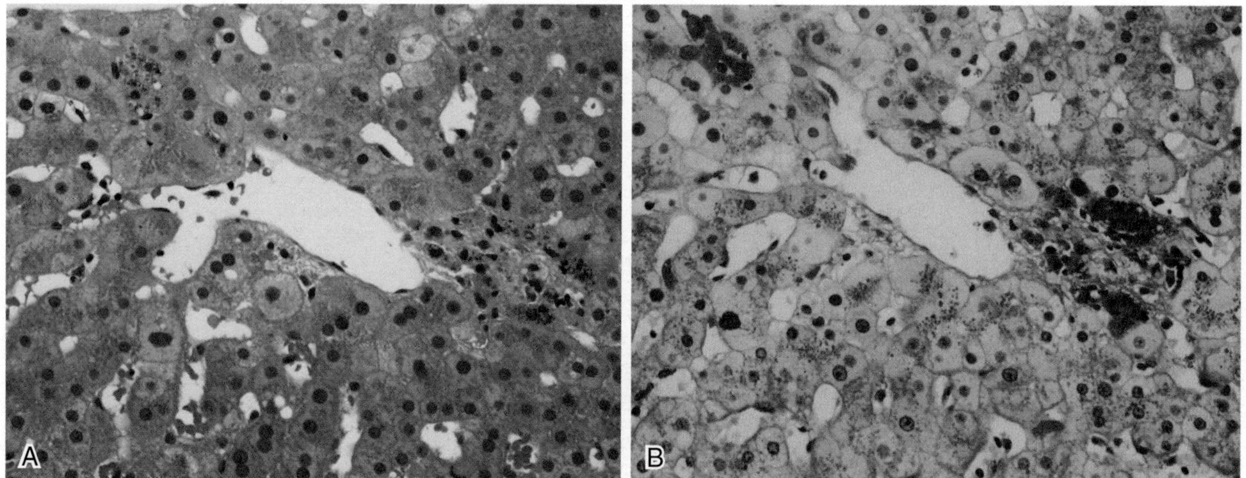

FIGURE 43.18 **Features suggestive of resolving acute or subacute hepatitis.** **A,** Pigment-laden (ceroid) Kupffer cells are present singly and in small clusters in parenchyma that is otherwise normal or shows focal, mild regenerative changes. **B,** Periodic acid–Schiff after diastase digestion (PASD) stain highlights macrophages because the zymogen granules in Kupffer cells contain glycoproteins.

medications, or dietary supplements, and they may be located in the portal tracts or in the lobules. Mild portal and lobular inflammation may also still be present. Other representative tissue responses that help provide evidence of a prior and currently resolving liver injury include hepatocellular regeneration (e.g., increased binucleation, slightly thickened plates) and anisonucleosis. These patients do not typically progress to chronic liver disease or even suffer from recurrences. One appropriate diagnostic statement for such cases is "features of resolving hepatitis/prior parenchymal injury."

Hepatocellular Necrosis

If a liver biopsy reveals necrosis, then attention should be given to the extent and predominant location of necrosis and whether or not there is associated inflammatory activity (Fig. 43.19). This is helpful to narrow the differential diagnosis.

Lobular Necrosis with Significant Inflammatory Activity (and Associated Parenchymal Collapse/Ductular Reaction)

The liver may show confluent hepatocellular necrosis, with associated parenchymal collapse, and a prominent ductular reaction (see Fig. 43.11B). This is often accompanied by prominent portal and pan-lobular inflammation. As mentioned earlier, the differential diagnosis for this pattern of injury includes acute viral hepatitis, AIH, DILI, and Wilson's disease. The distinction among these entities is often not possible based solely on histology, and correlation with clinical and laboratory tests is necessary. It is sometimes difficult to distinguish reticulin collapse associated with parenchymal necrosis from fibrosis secondary to chronic liver disease such as chronic hepatitis (see more on this later).

Lobular Necrosis Without Significant Inflammatory Activity

Predominantly Centrilobular (Zone 3) Necrosis

The leading causes of this pattern of injury are ischemic injury, such as in patients with hypotension or shock (Fig. 43.20) or those with dose-dependent drug injury. The prototypical drug in this category is acetaminophen, which is an intrinsic hepatotoxin that causes dose-dependent toxicity. Although biopsies are not commonly performed during an acute episode of acetaminophen toxicity, the histological changes are characteristic and may be seen in explanted livers. There is confluent and coagulative necrosis that is centered in zone 3,

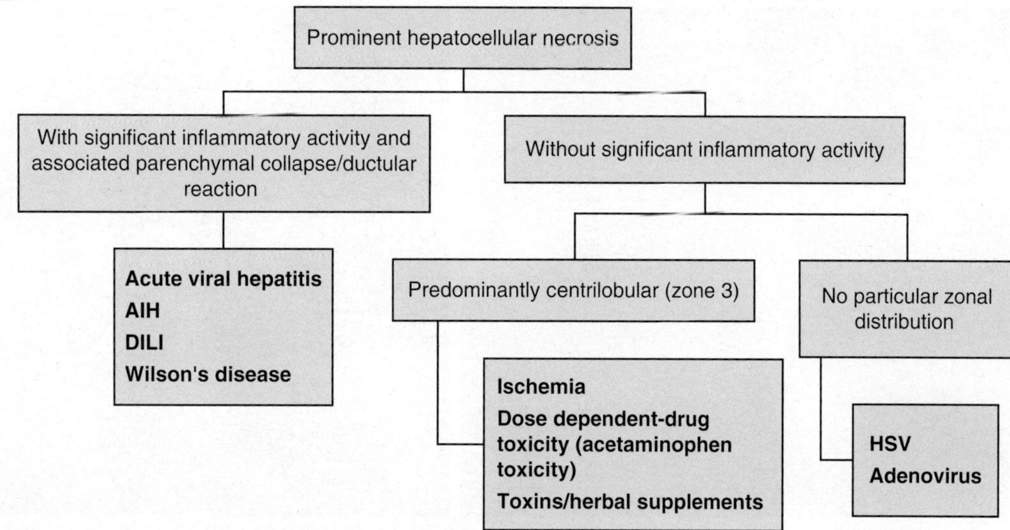

FIGURE 43.19 Algorithm for determining the extent and location of hepatocellular necrosis.

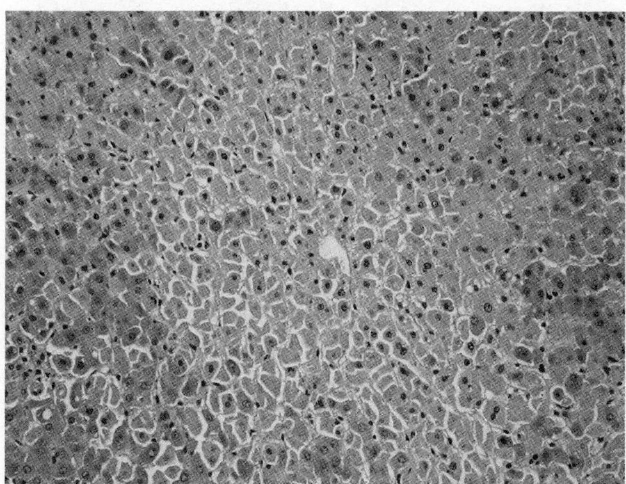

FIGURE 43.20 Pericentral necrosis secondary to severe ischemic injury is seen here in a posttransplant liver biopsy.

but it may also involve other zones of the liver in severe cases. The remaining viable hepatocytes often show steatosis (Fig. 43.21). Some recreational drugs, such as cocaine, may also cause this pattern of injury via secondary vasoconstriction and ischemic injury. Other examples include exposure to organics and toxins such as carbon tetrachloride. The clinical scenario often helps elucidate the etiology.

Necrosis with No Particular Zonal Distribution

HSV and adenovirus infection are the most common causes of this pattern of injury.

Herpes Simplex Virus

HSV infection of the liver is rare. It results in randomly distributed and sharply delineated foci of coagulative necrosis. Necrotic areas may be filled with cellular debris, including macrophages, and may be lined by viable hepatocytes containing characteristic herpes-type nuclear inclusions (nuclear molding, margination, and multinucleation). Immunostain for HSV helps highlight infected cells (Fig. 43.22).

Adenovirus

Most common in children, adenoviral hepatitis may appear similar to HSV infection.[27] Characteristic findings are well-delineated, punched-out areas of nonzonal coagulative necrosis with surrounding viable hepatocytes containing characteristic intranuclear inclusions. Hepatocyte necrosis may range from spotty to massive, and the majority of cases have either no inflammation or only minimal associated inflammation. The inclusions are large and basophilic and impart a smudgy appearance to the cell nuclei. Their presence can be confirmed by immunostaining (Fig. 43.23).[28]

Bile Duct/Ductular Injury or Cholestasis

This pattern of injury involves disorders that primarily affect the biliary system and may be divided into inflammatory destruction of small bile ducts (such as in PBC, see earlier), biliary obstructive pattern (e.g., secondary to primary sclerosing cholangitis [PSC] or mechanical obstruction from stones or strictures), ductopenia, and cholestasis (Fig. 43.24).

Primary Biliary Cholangitis

See earlier discussion.

Biliary Obstructive Pattern

The hallmark of a biliary obstructive pattern of injury is the presence of a ductular reaction. A ductular reaction is defined as the presence of proliferating bile ductules located at the interface of the portal tracts and liver parenchyma. The term *ductular reaction* is preferred to the term *ductular proliferation* because this phenomenon is actually associated with stromal, vascular, and inflammatory changes in addition to ductular proliferation.[29] A ductular reaction develops as a result of either bile duct or hepatocyte injury and is derived from activation of stem cells or progenitor cells.[30] Mild ductular proliferation is also present in other types of nonbiliary disease processes, such as in venous outflow impairment,[31] acute hepatitis in areas of parenchymal collapse, and in late stages of viral hepatitis (e.g., chronic

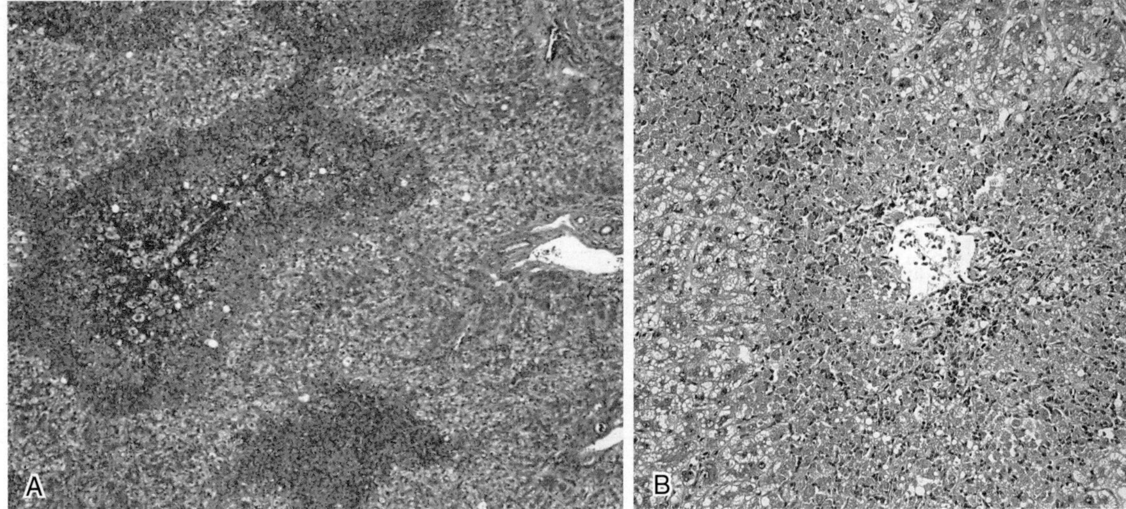

FIGURE 43.21 A, Zonal coagulative necrosis is seen in an explanted liver from a patient who developed acute liver failure secondary to acetaminophen toxicity. **B,** The remaining hepatocytes show fatty changes.

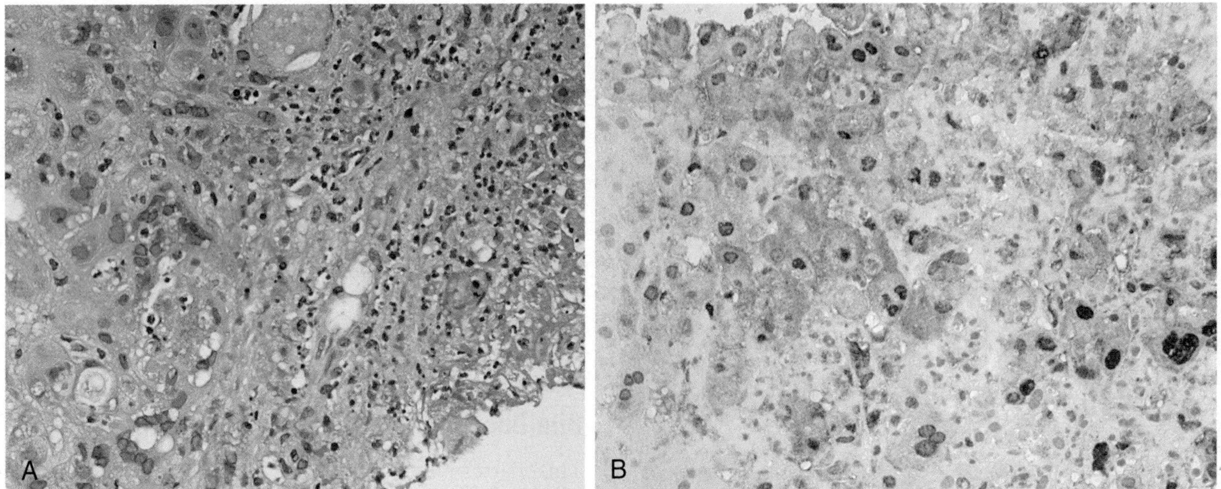

FIGURE 43.22 A, Herpes simplex virus (HSV) hepatitis causing large areas of coagulative necrosis. The adjacent viable hepatocytes show characteristic HSV inclusions with nuclear molding, margination, and multinucleation. **B,** An immunostain highlights numerous HSV-infected cells.

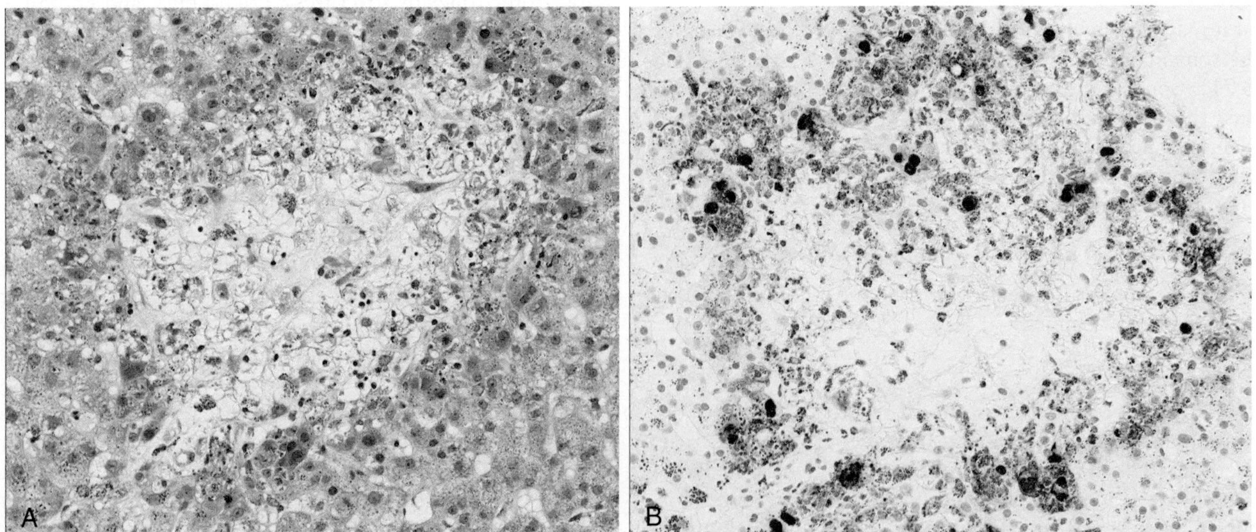

FIGURE 43.23 A, Adenovirus hepatitis typically causes well-delineated, "punched out" areas of coagulative necrosis. Viral inclusions are seen in the surrounding hepatocytes as glassy intranuclear inclusions and are highlighted by immunostain **(B).**

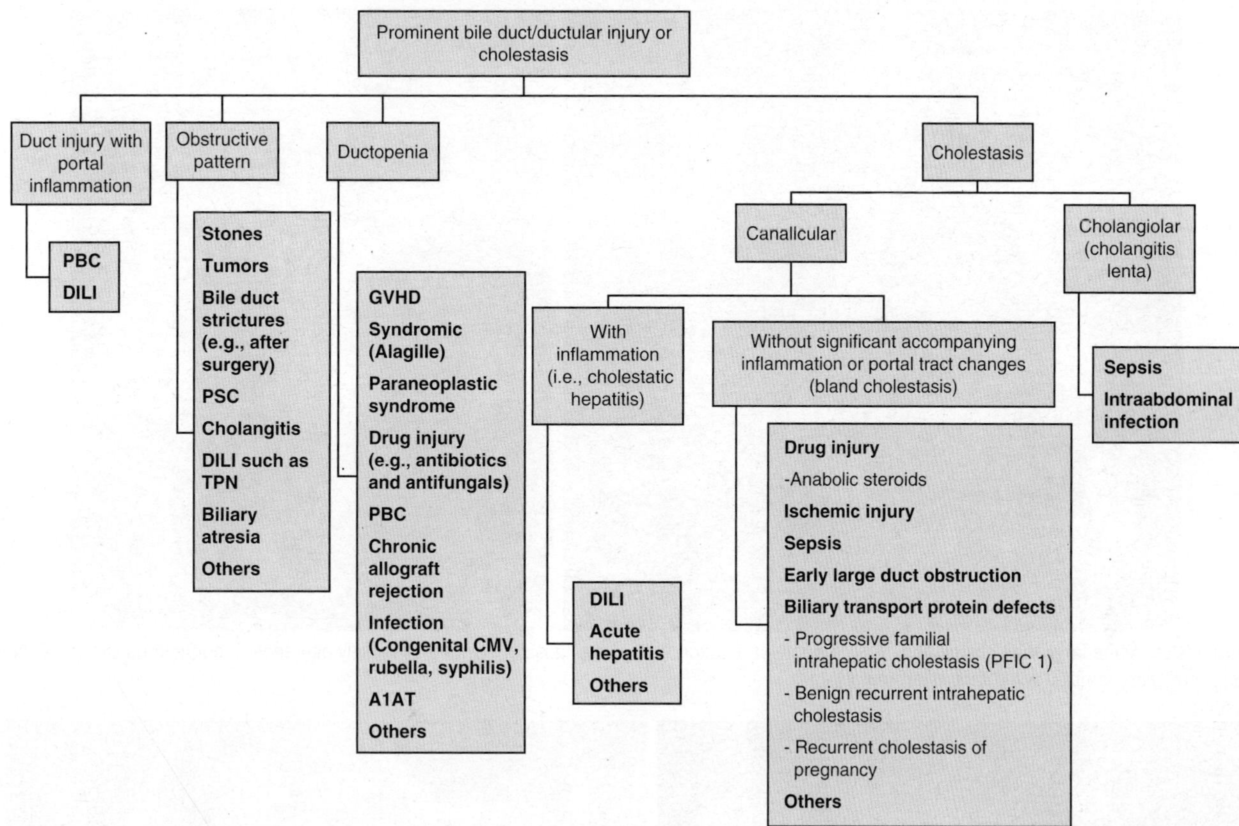

FIGURE 43.24 Diagnostic algorithm for bile duct/ductular injury or cholestasis.

hepatitis C), particularly as fibrous septa become more prominent and cirrhosis begins to develop.

Acute Bile Duct Obstruction

The characteristic features include portal expansion by ductular reaction associated with edematous stroma and neutrophils (Fig. 43.25). This often indicates downstream biliary tract obstructive disease from stones, strictures, tumors, and so on. However, it is not limited to mechanical biliary obstruction. It may be seen in other disease processes such as in chronic biliary disease, vascular outflow disease, or when there is ischemic injury to the biliary tree (e.g., cardiac decompensation with poor hepatic perfusion, sepsis, or severe dehydration, particularly in postsurgical patients). Except in patients who have undergone liver transplantation, the features of acute bile duct obstruction in liver biopsies is rare. In most instances, bile duct obstruction is clinically diagnosed with radiological testing. Patients with extrahepatic bile duct obstruction who have a secondary bacterial infection can develop ascending cholangitis. Acute bile duct obstruction, particularly in patients with acute cholangitis, may also be associated with bile infarcts, which are caused by the degenerating and detergent action of bile on hepatocytes.

Chronic Bile Duct Obstruction

Patients with chronic bile duct obstruction may develop a ductular reaction as well. Ductular reactions associated with chronic bile duct obstruction show scattered mononuclear cells and dense fibrosis, instead of edema and neutrophils. The ductular reaction may link portal tracts in patients with cirrhosis as a result of chronic obstruction. The fibrous septa may show a "halo effect" consisting of a band of edematous stromal tissue located directly beneath the ductular reaction; this may be associated with cholate stasis, defined by the presence of swollen hepatocytes sometimes containing Mallory-Denk bodies (Fig. 43.26). The presence of a halo effect may be observed in many forms of chronic biliary tract injury, including PBC and PSC. Copper accumulation in periportal hepatocytes, highlighted by a copper stain, may help confirm the presence of a chronic biliary disease (Fig. 43.27). However, absence of periportal copper does not exclude biliary disease from the differential diagnosis.

Primary Sclerosing Cholangitis

PSC is characterized by destruction of small, medium, and large-sized bile ducts, both within and outside the liver parenchyma. Extrahepatic bile duct injury leads to the development of acute and chronic bile duct obstruction within the liver parenchyma. Therefore the finding of biliary obstructive features in small portal tracts should raise the possibility of PSC. This can be confirmed by imaging the biliary tree by endoscopic retrograde cholangiopancreatography (ERCP) or magnetic resonance cholangiopancreatography (MRCP). Patients with the small duct variant of PSC may show normal imaging results and therefore are more likely to have a liver biopsy for diagnostic purposes.

The characteristic findings of PSC, such as concentric periductal inflammation, "onion skinning" (i.e., the presence of degenerative bile ducts surrounded by concentric bands of fibrosis) or "tombstone scars" (in which bile ducts are replaced by fibrous scars) may not be present in biopsy

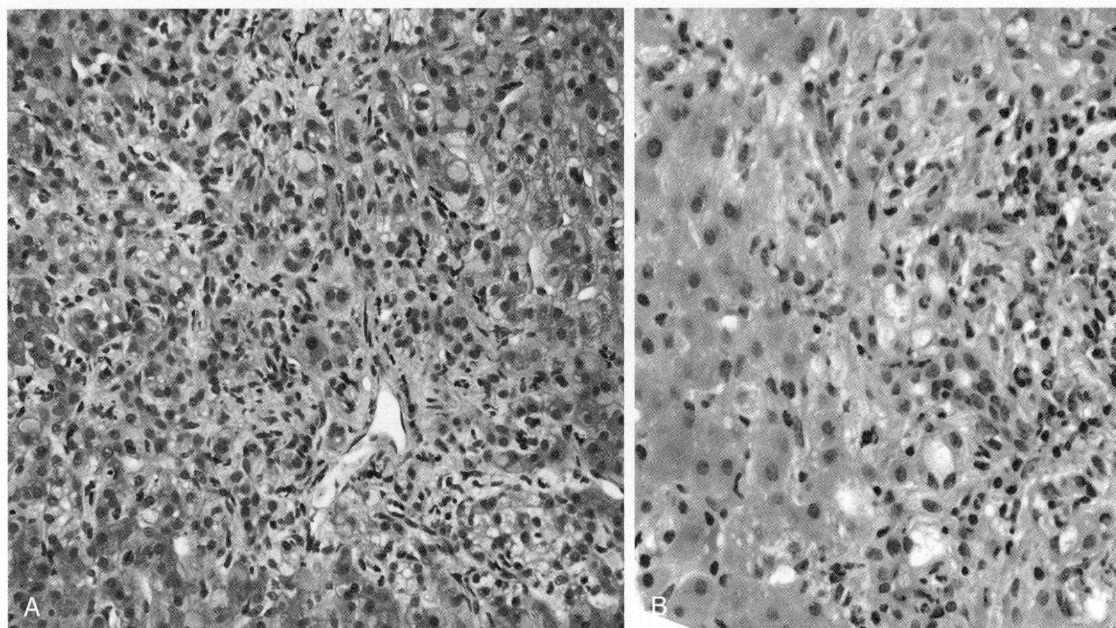

FIGURE 43.25 Acute large duct obstruction. A, The ductular reaction in this setting is surrounded by loosely aggregated, edematous stroma. **B,** Neutrophils are seen admixed with other inflammatory cells.

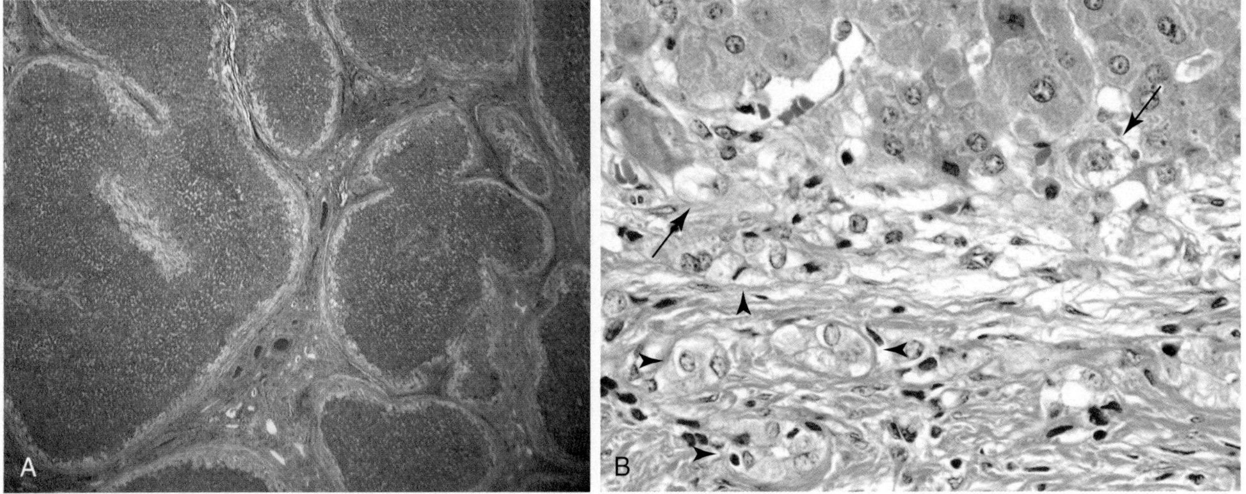

FIGURE 43.26 Biliary cirrhosis. A, The ductular reaction in cirrhosis from chronic biliary disease shows a halo effect surrounding the nodules. **B,** At higher magnification, the halo is composed of stromal edema, ductular reaction *(arrowheads),* and cholate stasis ("feathery degeneration") of cholestatic hepatocytes *(arrows).*

specimens (Fig. 43.28). Often the presence of a ductular reaction is the only histological manifestation of PSC in liver biopsies.

Ductopenia

Ductopenia refers to the absence of bile ducts in more than one-half of the portal tracts. A variety of conditions may lead to ductopenia. See Table 43.4 for the differential diagnosis.

Cholestasis

Cholestasis may be seen accompanying many of the biliary disorders mentioned earlier or in the setting of hepatitis when the hepatocyte injury is severe enough to interfere with bile secretion. It should also be noted that biliary disorders may not always be associated with visible bile in tissue sections. Examples include liver involvement in PSC or early-stage PBC. If the predominant biopsy finding is cholestasis, one helpful clue is to note the predominant location of the bile accumulation (i.e., whether it is mostly within canalicular spaces or ductular/cholangiolar lumen) and whether or not there is accompanying hepatitis and hepatocyte injury (i.e., cholestatic hepatitis).

Canalicular Cholestasis

Cholestatic Hepatitis. Although any form of acute hepatitis may show a mild degree of cholestasis, the term *cholestatic hepatitis* is reserved for a mixed pattern of injury that includes features of both acute hepatitis and conspicuous hepatocellular and/or canalicular cholestasis. Cholestatic hepatitis is clinically and histologically different from other forms of acute hepatitis. Clinically, there is a mixed

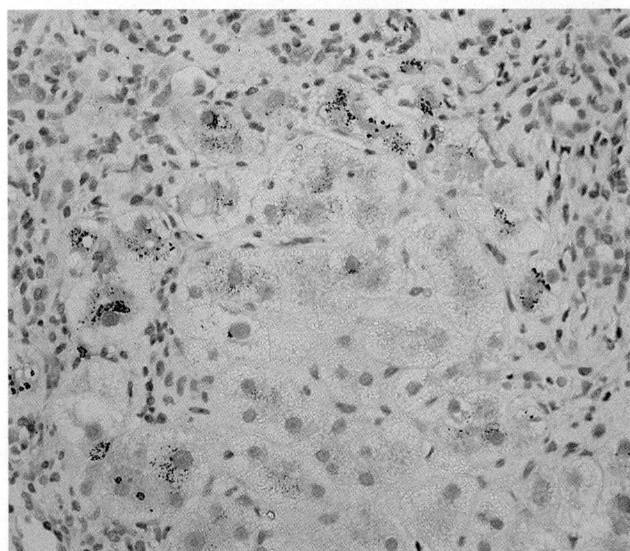

FIGURE 43.27 Copper accumulation in periportal hepatocytes is seen in this case of chronic biliary disease. Copper appears as a course, orange-brown pigment on rhodamine staining.

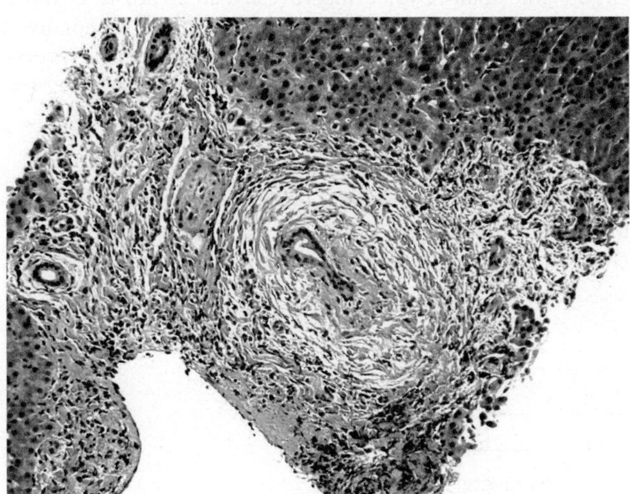

FIGURE 43.28 Primary sclerosing cholangitis shows concentric periductal fibrosis surrounding a damaged and atrophic-appearing bile duct. This lesion is only rarely present in a liver biopsy specimen.

hepatitis/cholestatic pattern of liver enzyme abnormalities. Histologically, the picture is not overwhelmingly dominated by hepatitis; instead the features of acute hepatitis and cholestasis are equally present, or it may even be dominated by cholestasis with only mild hepatocellular injury. The hepatitic component may resemble acute hepatitis, with a predominance of lobular inflammation with or without necrosis, or it may resemble chronic hepatitis in which the portal inflammation stands out over the lobular inflammation. Cholestatic hepatitis is a commonly reported pattern of DILI. Some drug classes have been particularly associated with this pattern, including the antibacterials, antifungals, statins, among several others.

Bland Cholestasis. Canalicular cholestasis may be seen without accompanying inflammation or significant portal tracts or parenchymal changes. This pattern may be seen in ischemic injury, such as in ischemia/reperfusion injury after transplantation, DILI (e.g., anabolic steroid use) (Fig. 43.29), and primary biliary transport protein defects, such as in progressive familiar intrahepatic cholestasis type I (PFIC I), benign recurrent intrahepatic cholestasis, or recurrent cholestasis of pregnancy. Perivenular regions (acinar zone 3) are primarily affected as a result of susceptibility of the zone 3 canalicular bile transport system to ischemia as well as localization of drug-metabolizing enzymes in perivenular hepatocytes.

TABLE 43.4 Differential Diagnosis of Ductopenia

Clinical Setting	Examples
Transplant-related	Chronic allograft rejection, GVHD
Chronic biliary diseases	PBC, PSC
Pediatrics	Syndromic (Alagille syndrome) Nonsyndromic paucity of bile ducts resulting from metabolic diseases (A1AT deficiency, PFIC I and/or 2) or infections (congenital rubella, syphilis, or CMV)
Neoplastic as paraneoplastic syndrome	Hodgkin's disease,[54] peripheral T-cell lymphoma[55]
Drugs/medications	Various drugs, TPN

A1AT, *α_1-antitrypsin disorder;* CMV, *cytomegalovirus;* GVHD, *graft-versus-host disease;* PBC, *primary biliary cholangitis;* PFIC, *progressive familial intrahepatic cholestasis;* PSC, *primary sclerosing cholangitis.*

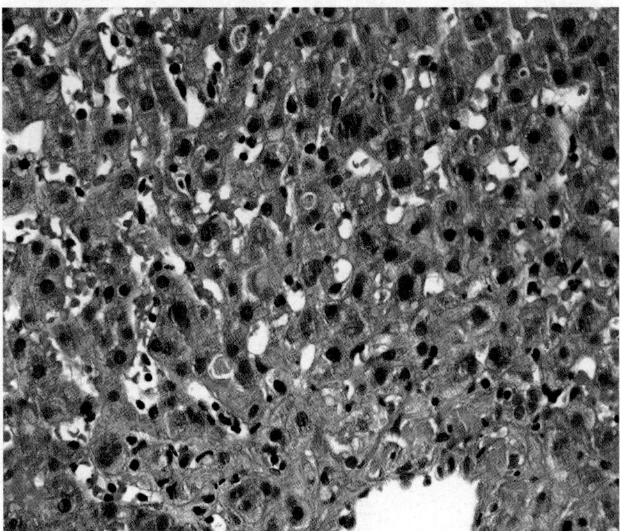

FIGURE 43.29 Bland cholestasis. Prominent canalicular cholestasis is seen in a case of drug-induced liver injury secondary to anabolic steroid use. There is no significant associated portal or lobular inflammation or hepatocyte injury.

Cholangiolar/Ductular Cholestasis (Cholangitis Lenta)

Cholangitis lenta is characterized by the presence of dilated ductules that are located at the portal-lobular interface and contain inspissated biliary concretions (ductular or cholangiolar cholestasis) (Fig. 43.30). It is most often associated with sepsis or intraabdominal infection, and it is believed that this type of ductular cholestasis is caused by circulating endotoxins. The finding of cholangitis lenta in biopsy specimens should prompt the pathologist to notify the clinician of a potentially serious medical disorder that can result in sepsis. In some cases, cholangitis lenta may occur before clinical sepsis, the latter of which may not be evident clinically at the time of the liver biopsy.[32]

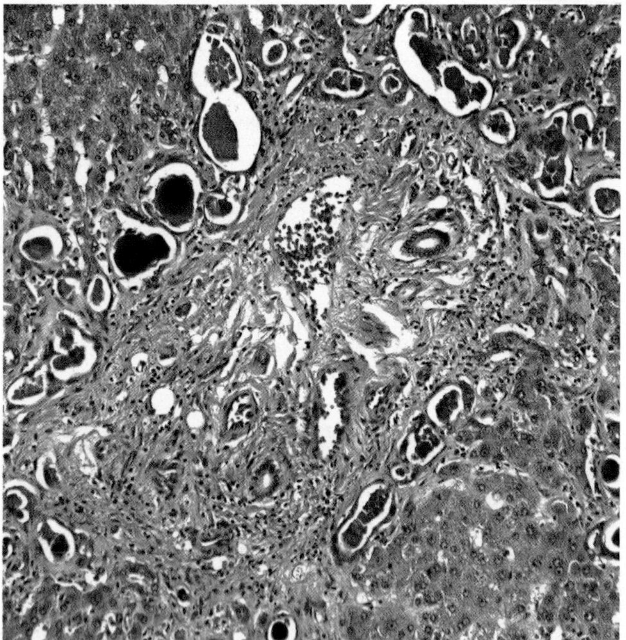

FIGURE 43.30 Cholangitis lenta. The ductules at the margins of the portal tract are markedly dilated and contain concretions of inspissated bile. This lesion may be seen in association with sepsis and should be considered a critical finding.

Steatosis

Steatosis in the liver is categorized into two broad types: macrovesicular and microvesicular. Recognition of the different types of fat is important because microvesicular steatosis has a different differential than purely macrovesicular or a combined macro and microvesicular steatosis (Fig. 43.31). The type and pattern of fat accumulation along with the accompanying histological findings help provide clues to the specific type of disorder. Table 43.5 summarizes the common causes of different types of steatosis.

Macrovesicular Steatosis

Macrovesicular steatosis is further divided into large-droplet and small-droplet types. The large-droplet type is characterized by the presence of one intracytoplasmic lipid vacuole that occupies more than one-half of the cytoplasm of the hepatocyte and results in displacement of the nucleus to the edge of the cell membrane. Small-droplet macrovesicular steatosis refers to the presence of multiple distinct, small fat droplets within the cytoplasm of a hepatocyte that occupies less than one-half of the cytoplasm and does not result in displacement of the nucleus. Differentiation between large- and small-droplet macrovesicular steatosis is most relevant in the context of transplantation and donor liver evaluation.[33,34] Steatosis is believed to represent a reversible type of disorder, whereas steatohepatitis can progress to fibrosis and cirrhosis.

Steatohepatitis

Steatohepatitis is diagnosed when there is evidence of liver injury secondary to fat accumulation. Hepatocyte injury is characteristically seen in the form of ballooning degeneration

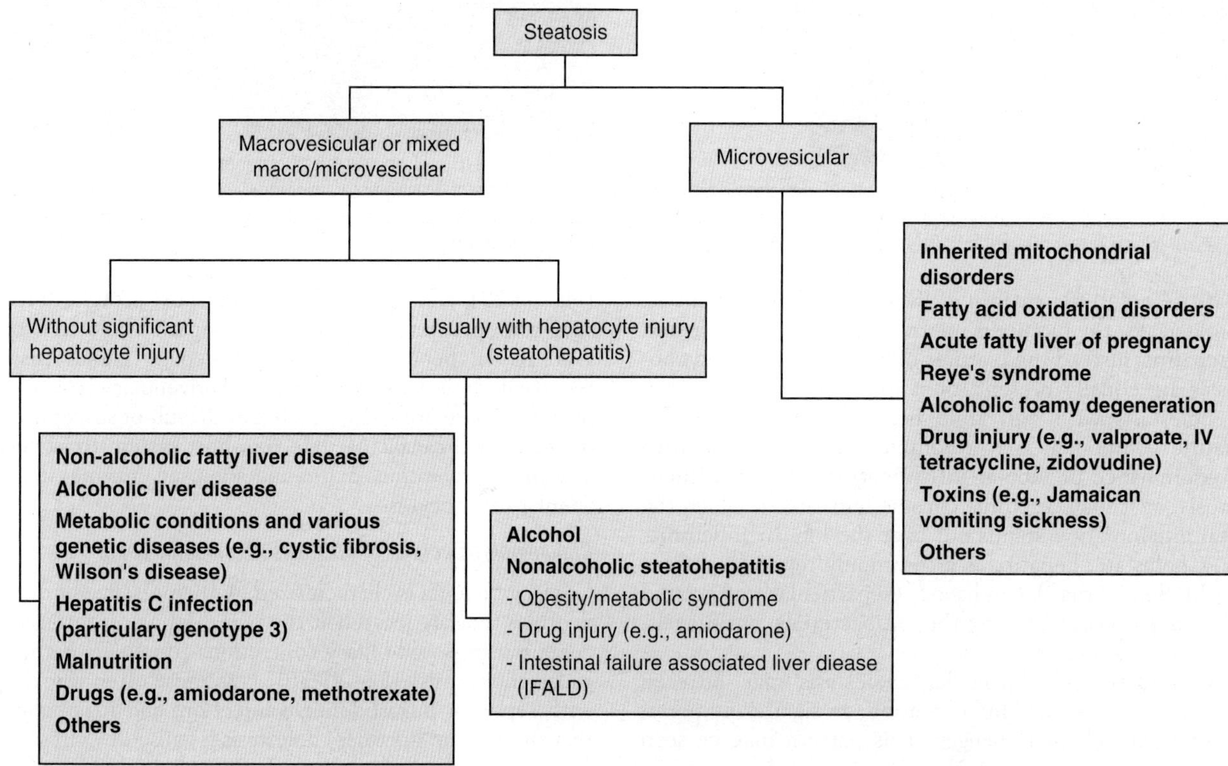

FIGURE 43.31 Diagnostic algorithm for steatosis.

of hepatocytes (often associated with Mallory-Denk bodies) and a variable amount of pericellular/sinusoidal fibrosis (Fig. 43.32). In terms of etiology, steatohepatitis is categorized into two broad groups: alcoholic steatohepatitis (ASH) and nonalcoholic steatohepatitis (NASH). The metabolic syndrome (diabetes, hypertension, hyperlipidemia, insulin resistance, and hyperinsulinemia) usually underlies the development of NASH. NASH is currently a leading cause of liver disease in Western populations, which is related to the increasing incidence of obesity and metabolic syndrome.[35,36]

TABLE 43.5 Differential Diagnosis of Macrovesicular and Microvesicular Steatosis

Macrovesicular	Microvesicular
Alcoholic liver disease	Reye's syndrome
Nonalcoholic liver disease	Drug effect (e.g., tetracycline, valproic acid, nucleoside analogues)
Genetic diseases such as cystic fibrosis, galactosemia, hereditary fructose intolerance, glycogen storage disease I and III, urea cycle defects	Alcoholic foamy degeneration
Rapid weight loss[56] and malnutrition, more commonly protein/calorie deprivation	Mitochondrial diseases
Metabolic diseases such as Wilson's disease	Fatty acid oxidation disorders
Intestinal failure–associated liver disease	Toxins such as Jamaican vomiting sickness
Drug effect (e.g., amiodarone, methotrexate, chemotherapeutic agents such as irinotecan, anti-HIV medications	Acute fatty liver of pregnancy
Infection (e.g., hepatitis C or HIV)	

NASH typically consists of a mixture of macrovesicular and microvesicular steatosis. Portal and lobular inflammation are generally only minimal to mild in severity and predominantly lymphocytic. Apoptotic bodies and giant mitochondria may also be present. In most patients, steatosis and ballooning are present, most notably in the centrilobular region surrounding central veins (zone 3) (Fig. 43.33). However, in drug-induced NASH (e.g. amiodarone), the ballooned hepatocytes and Mallory-Denk bodies are most prominent in periportal hepatocytes (Fig. 43.34). NASH-associated fibrosis typically begins in the centrilobular (perivenular) location and progresses through the sinusoids to create a sinusoidal pattern of fibrosis (see Fig. 43.33B). NASH-associated cirrhosis may be devoid of fat ("burnt out NASH"), and it is thought to account for a large proportion of patients with so-called "cryptogenic" cirrhosis.

NASH in children may reveal a different morphological pattern of injury and is sometimes referred to as *NASH type 2*.[35]

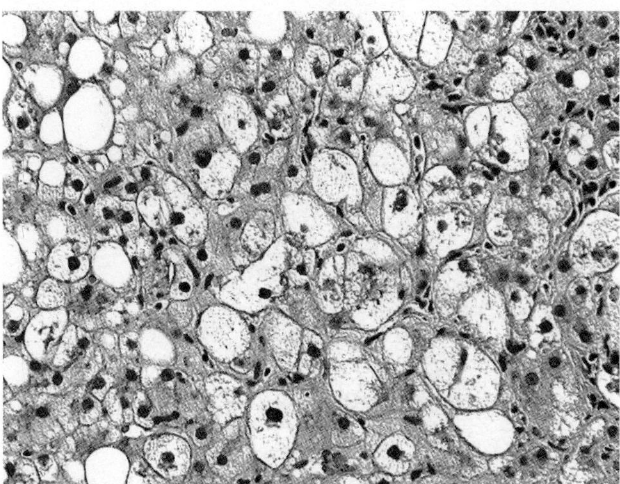

FIGURE 43.32 Steatohepatitis is differentiated from simple steatosis by the presence of damaged hepatocytes. In this image, numerous ballooned hepatocytes appear enlarged and contain pale cytoplasm with some Mallory-Denk bodies. Perisinusoidal fibrosis is also present.

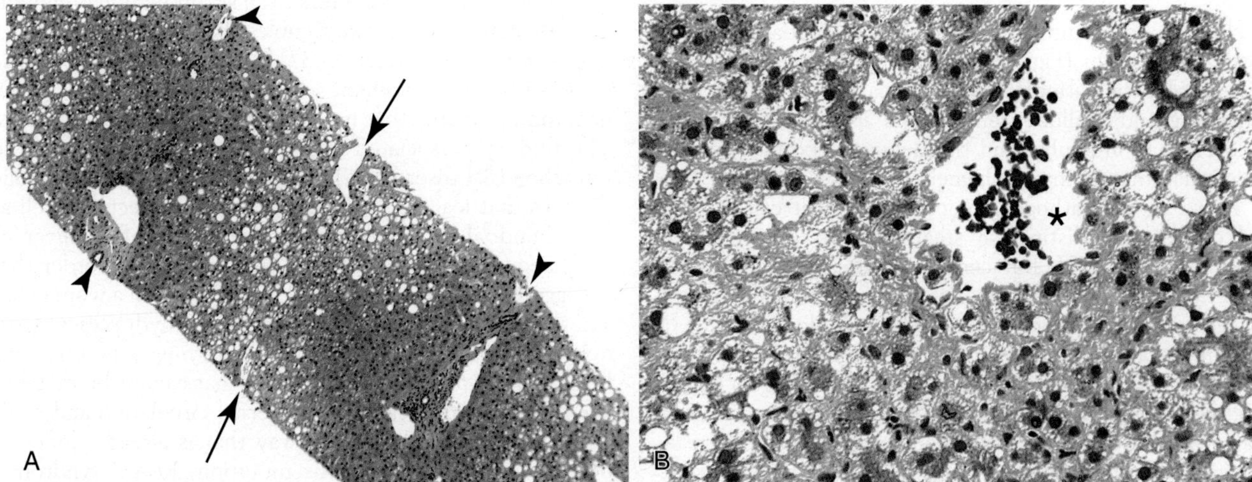

FIGURE 43.33 The pathological features of steatohepatitis, both alcoholic steatohepatitis (ASH) and nonalcoholic steatohepatitis (NASH), begin in the centrilobular region around the central veins *(arrows)*. **A,** Hepatocytes around portal tracts *(arrowheads)* do not contain fat. **B,** Fibrosis in both ASH and NASH also typically begins around the central veins *(asterisk)* and involves the sinusoids in a perisinusoidal fashion (Trichrome stain).

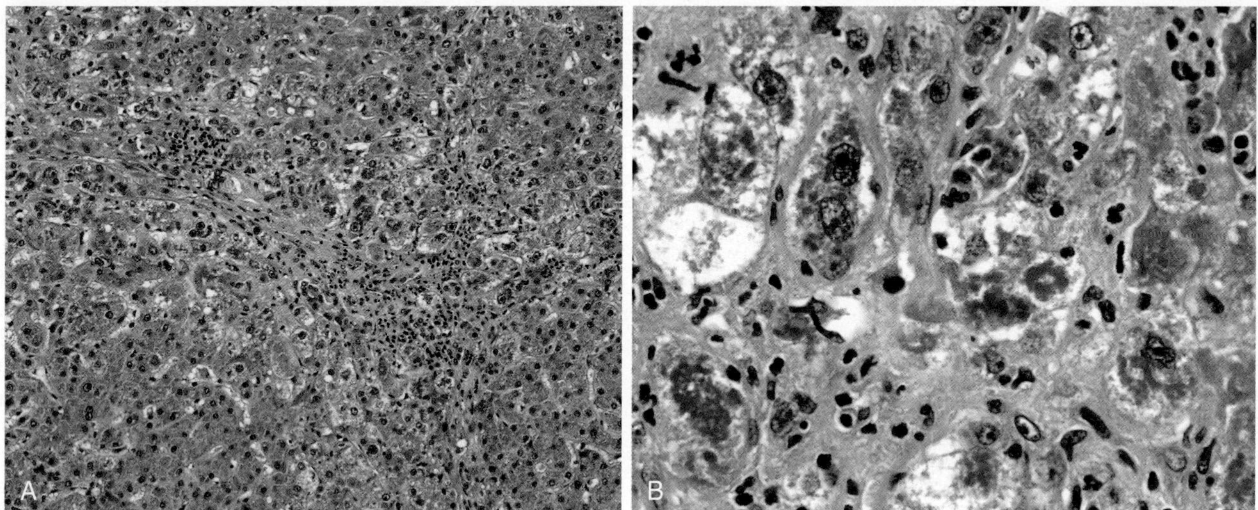

FIGURE 43.34 A, Ballooned hepatocytes with Mallory-Denk bodies are seen in periportal hepatocytes in this case of amiodarone-induced liver injury. **B,** The Mallory-Denk bodies are typically numerous and well-formed in such cases.

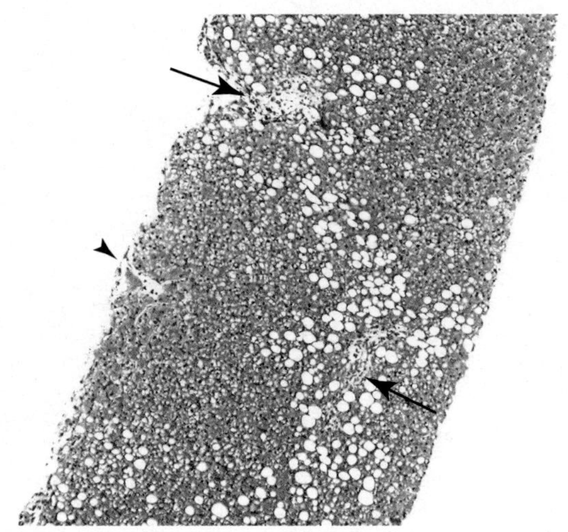

FIGURE 43.35 In children, the features of nonalcoholic steatohepatitis, such as accumulation of fat, may begin around portal tracts *(arrows)* rather than around the central veins *(arrowhead)*.

In children, fat accumulation occurs preferentially in periportal hepatocytes (Fig. 43.35), and fibrosis may preferentially involve the periportal parenchyma as well. Hepatocyte ballooning and Mallory-Denk bodies are less common in children than in adults, and the degree of portal lymphocytic inflammation may be higher.

There are no pathognomonic features that can reliably and consistently distinguish steatohepatitis secondary to alcohol from NASH, but certain features can help favor one etiology over the other. For instance, the severity of changes correlates more consistently with alcohol use.[37,38] The presence of well-formed (thick) or numerous Mallory-Denk bodies, neutrophilic infiltration of the parenchyma, and prominent mitochondria are more suggestive of ASH than NASH. Similarly, perivenular fibrosis tends to be particularly prominent in patients with ASH, in which case it may result in occlusion of the central veins (Fig. 43.36).

A comment about alcohol use in a biopsy report has medicolegal and ethical implications. If the clinician provides a written statement documenting the cause of the fatty liver disease (e.g., long-term alcohol use, morbid obesity, uncontrolled diabetes mellitus, dyslipidemia), then the diagnosis may indicate "compatible with ASH" or "compatible with NASH." However, in the absence of such information, it is best to indicate that the liver disease is "steatohepatitis" that could be compatible with either ASH or NASH.

One common clinical question accompanying liver biopsies is the evaluation for AIH in a patient who has both elevated serum transaminases and positive autoantibodies, such as ANAs and/or SMAs, and is thus suspected of having AIH. However, the biopsy specimens often show negligible interface and lobular hepatitis but instead reveal steatohepatitis. In such cases, the elevated autoantibody levels represent a reflection of the underlying metabolic syndrome. Mild elevations of autoantibodies, such as ANA, SMA, or even AMA, are frequently present in patients with metabolic syndrome and NASH.[39]

Microvesicular Steatosis

Microvesicular steatosis refers to an accumulation of numerous intracytoplasmic lipid vacuoles that gives hepatocytes a foamy appearance. (Fig. 43.37).[33] The presence of diffuse or mixed, but prominent, microvesicular steatosis is an uncommon finding that has a distinct differential diagnosis. This finding is associated with disease processes that lead to mitochondrial disorders. This includes inherited metabolic diseases that lead to fatty acid oxidation defects as well as mitochondrial disorders of the liver. Acute fatty liver of pregnancy is one example of a mitochondrial disorder that is triggered during pregnancy.[40] It occurs when a woman has a heterozygous mutation for long-chain 3-hydroxyacyl-CoA dehydrogenase (LCHAD) and is carrying a homozygous fetus for this mutation. Fatty acids that cannot be metabolized by the fetus reach the maternal circulation and overwhelm the metabolizing pathway that is already deficient because of the heterozygous mutation. Reyes' syndrome, although rare, can lead to diffuse microvesicular steatosis in the liver.[41] Other rare causes are alcoholic foamy degeneration and the effects of drugs such as valproate

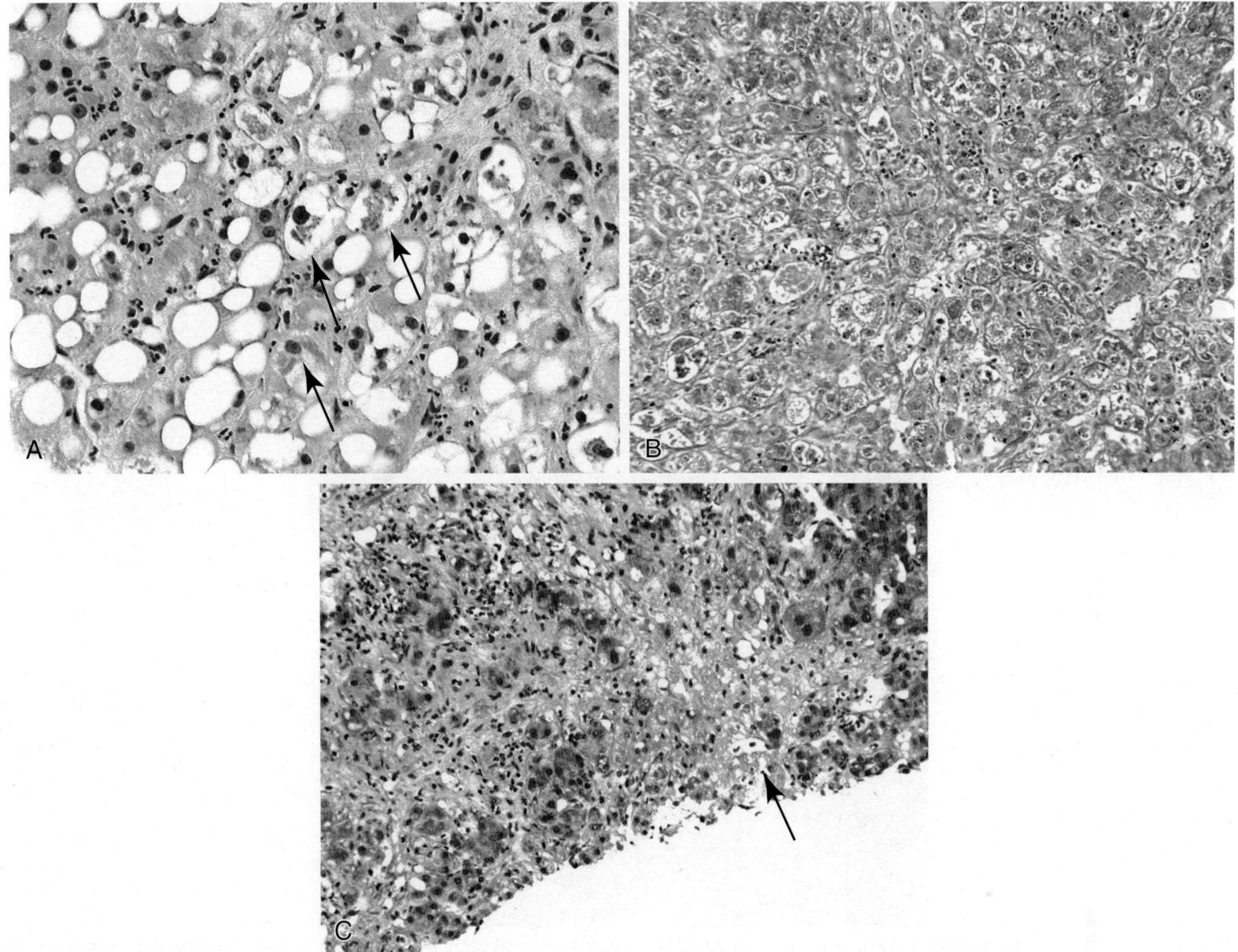

FIGURE 43.36 A, Alcoholic steatohepatitis is characterized by numerous ballooned hepatocytes, well-formed Mallory-Denk bodies *(arrows)*, and prominent neutrophilic infiltrate. **B,** Dense perisinusoidal fibrosis is often seen in alcoholic liver disease, which may lead to central vein sclerosis **(C)**.

and intravenously administered tetracycline. Consumption of unripened ackee fruit, which contains the hepatotoxin hypoglycin A, may also result in diffuse microvesicular steatosis. This is known as *vomiting sickness of Jamaica.*

Vascular Injury

This category of injury involves diseases that affect the vasculature of the liver or disease processes that are not intrinsic to the liver but affect it secondarily (Fig. 43.38). The first helpful evaluation process involves determination of the predominant zone or type of vascular injury such as zonal necrosis, sinusoidal dilation/congestion, or portal vein abnormalities.

Zonal Necrosis

As mentioned earlier, pericentral hepatocellular coagulative necrosis may be a result of ischemic damage. The necrosis may ultimately extend to other zones, depending on the severity of the ischemic injury. Ischemia results from reduced blood flow and may be a result of hepatic artery thrombosis or systemic ischemia (i.e., shock liver).

Sinusoidal Dilation with or without Congestion

Sinusoidal dilation is a hallmark of insufficient venous drainage leading to chronic venous outflow obstruction. This will lead to congestive hepatopathy, which is characterized by sinusoidal dilation with or without congestion, often accompanied by hepatic plate atrophy. There may also be centrizonal fibrosis in chronic cases (Fig. 43.39).

Insufficient venous drainage may result from obstruction or right-sided heart failure. Obstruction can occur at the level of extrahepatic veins, such as in hepatic vein thrombosis (i.e., Budd-Chiari's syndrome) or at the level of interhepatic terminal hepatic venules and sinusoids, such as in sinusoidal obstruction syndrome (SOS)/veno-occlusive disease. The latter can be seen in the setting of stem cell or bone marrow transplant or be secondary to certain chemotherapeutic agents or toxins. In SOS, central veins show subendothelial edema, and there is often centrizonal necrosis too. Fibrin thrombi can also be seen but are uncommon. Sinusoidal dilation is not specific to chronic venous outflow obstruction, however, and it may also be seen in a wide variety of settings (Table 43.6).[42,43]

Portal Vein Stenosis/Obliterative Portal Venopathy

Insufficient venous inflow results from conditions that compromise the portal vein blood flow and may be secondary to obstruction of extrahepatic portal vein (e.g., portal vein thrombosis) or smaller intrahepatic branches of portal vein. Examples of the latter include local portal vein inflammation secondary to parasitic infection, toxic injury (e.g., chronic exposure to

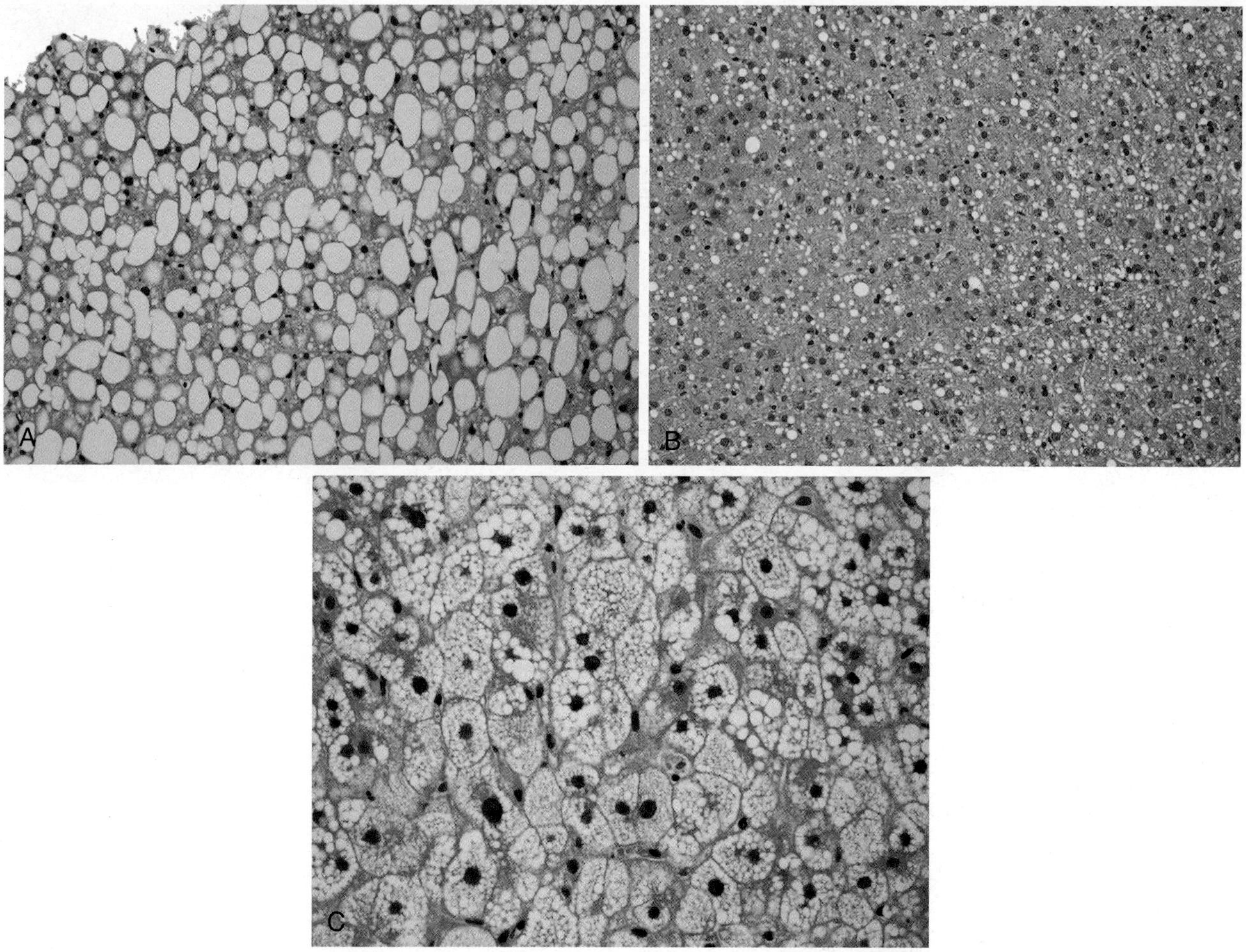

FIGURE 43.37 Macrovesicular steatosis may be either large droplet **(A)** in which a large fat vacuole occupies more than one-half of the cytoplasm of a hepatocyte and pushes the nucleus to one side, or small droplet **(B)** in which small fat droplets occupy the cytoplasm without displacing the nucleus. **C,** Microvesicular steatosis is seen as numerous fat vesicles accumulating in the hepatocyte cytoplasm giving it a foamy appearance.

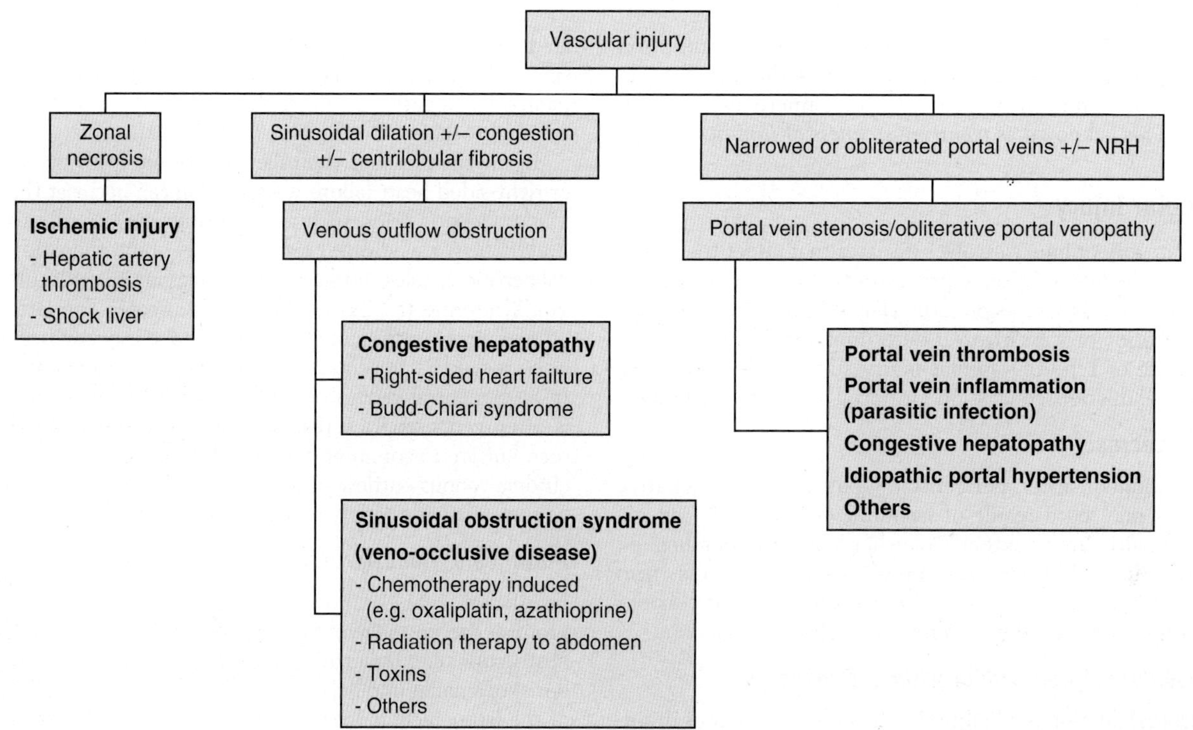

FIGURE 43.38 Diagnostic algorithm for vascular injury.

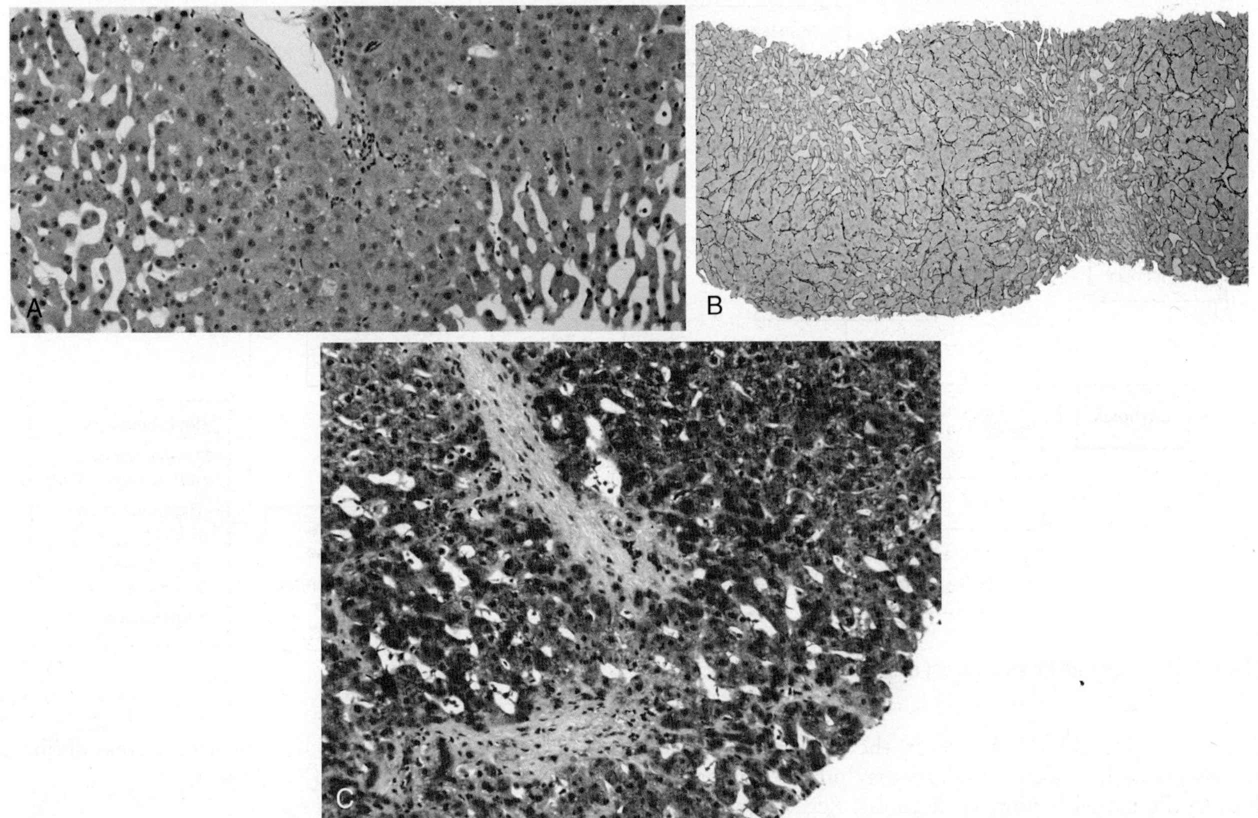

FIGURE 43.39 **A,** Prominent sinusoidal dilation is seen in a patient with venous outflow obstruction secondary to right-sided heart failure. **B,** Reticulin stain highlights marked hepatic plate atrophy in association with dilated sinusoid. **C,** Long-standing compromise of venous outflow may also cause centrilobular fibrosis, as seen here with trichrome stain.

TABLE 43.6 Disorders That May Result in Hepatic Sinusoidal Dilation

Disorder	Examples
Vascular outflow obstruction	Heart disease Budd-Chiari's syndrome
Sinusoidal obstruction syndrome	Chemotherapeutic drugs such as oxaliplatin, leukemia/lymphoma, sickle cell anemia
Systemic diseases	Granulomatous disorders (sarcoidosis, tuberculosis) Crohn's disease Rheumatoid arthritis/Still disease Antiphospholipid syndrome Castleman disease
Drug effect	Estrogen, azathioprine, chemotherapeutic drugs such as oxaliplatin
Systemic infection	HIV, brucellosis
Adjacent mass effect	Hepatic vein stenosis
Paraneoplastic effects	Renal cell carcinoma, Hodgkin's lymphoma

From Kakar S, Kamath PS, Burgart LJ. Sinusoidal dilatation and congestion in liver biopsy: is it always due to venous outflow impairment? Arch Pathol Lab Med. *2004;128(8):901–904.*

arsenic), and congestive hepatopathy. This can be seen as luminal narrowing or even complete obliteration of small intrahepatic portal veins seen in needle biopsies, leading to portal vein stenosis/obliterative portal venopathy (Fig. 43.40). It may or may not be associated with thickening of the vein wall and is often accompanied with nodular regenerative hyperplasia.[44]

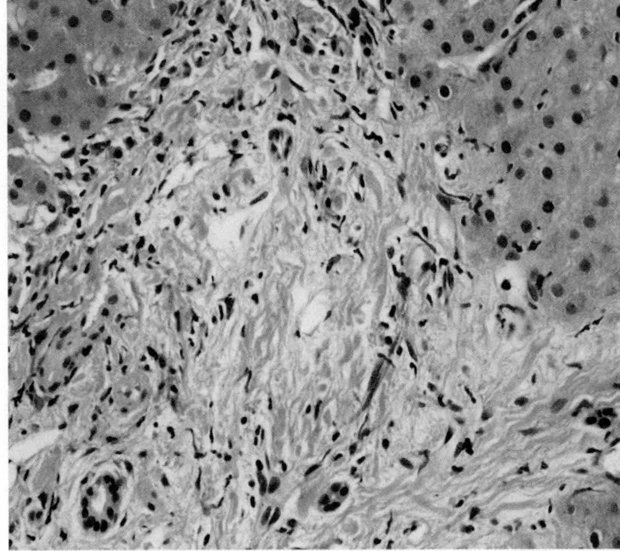

FIGURE 43.40 Complete stenosis of portal vein (also known as *obliterative portal venopathy*) is seen here secondary to portal vein thrombosis.

FIBROSIS AND NODULARITY

Fibrosis, which is the result of most forms of chronic liver disease, is not considered to be a primary pattern of injury

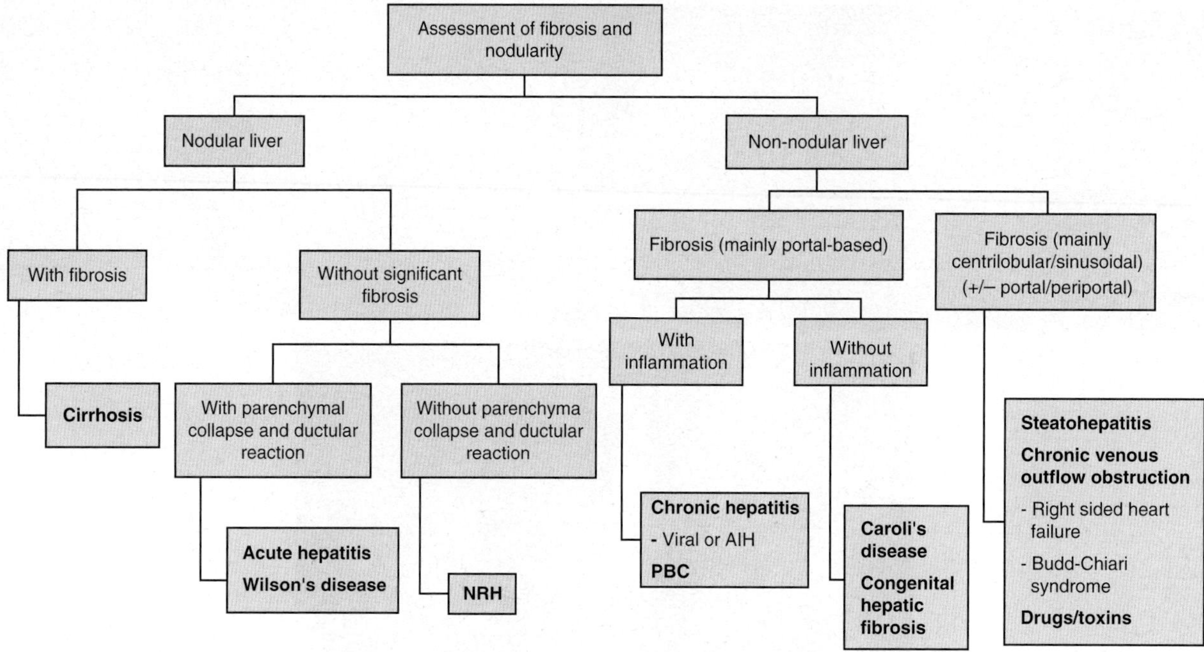

FIGURE 43.41 Algorithm for assessment of fibrosis and nodularity.

of the liver (Fig. 43.41). However, the pattern of fibrosis and associated histological findings may provide important clues to the patient's primary diagnosis. Regeneration may also occur with or without accompanying fibrosis. When evaluating a liver specimen for fibrosis and regeneration, it is helpful to first categorize whether there is nodular regeneration (confirmed by reticulin stain). In cases with nodular regeneration, it is important to determine whether there is also significant accompanying fibrosis. Nodular regeneration with fibrosis is characteristic of a cirrhotic liver. Regeneration without significant accompanying fibrosis may occur with acute liver injury and bridging necrosis or in nodular regenerative hyperplasia.

Differentiating Bridging Necrosis and Parenchymal Collapse from Fibrosis

As mentioned earlier, in liver injury from acute hepatitis, AIH, or Wilson's disease, massive or submassive loss of hepatic parenchyma may occur with resulting bridging necrosis. This is often accompanied by collapse of the normal connective tissue framework of the liver and a ductular reaction, surrounding nodules of remaining hepatocytes that appear regenerative. This appearance of bridging necrosis surrounding regenerating liver nodules may closely mimic true fibrous septa and cirrhosis.[30] A reticulin stain may illustrate collapsed reticulin fibers in areas of necrosis; however, the remaining liver parenchyma often appears regenerative and nodular, making it difficult to distinguish from cirrhosis (Fig. 43.42). A trichrome stain may also be difficult to interpret because both necrosis and fibrous septa stain blue, although fibrosis appear darker blue compared with the pale blue hue of necrosis. A helpful clue is that in bridging necrosis, the ductular reaction is typically located within the necrotic septa rather than at the border with the parenchyma, which is generally seen in bridging fibrosis. In difficult cases, a Victoria blue stain may be helpful as it highlights elastic fibers, which are present in areas of fibrosis but not in areas of necrosis (Fig. 43.43).[45,46]

Differentiating Nodular Regenerative Hyperplasia from Cirrhosis

A common clinical scenario is receiving a liver biopsy of patients who have signs of portal hypertension and the liver appears nodular on imaging. The main differential consideration includes cirrhosis and NRH (i.e., noncirrhotic portal hypertension). Trichrome and reticulin stains are helpful in making this distinction. In contrast with cirrhosis (in which the regenerative nodules are surrounded by fibrosis), trichrome stain with NRH does not reveal significant fibrosis, whereas reticulin stain highlights nodular architecture with alternating atrophic and widened hepatic plates and compression of hepatic plates at the periphery of the nodules (Fig. 43.44).

Fibrosis with No Well-Established Nodularity

In cases of fibrosis, it is helpful to first determine the primary location of fibrosis, that is, whether it is mainly portal based or mainly lobular/sinusoidal. Predominantly portal-based fibrosis is more common in chronic viral hepatitis, AIH, and chronic biliary diseases.[7] All of these disorders are characterized by pathology that is located primarily within the portal tracts and associated with portal and periportal fibrosis in the early stage of disease, before the development of cirrhosis. Chronic biliary disorders may be associated with strands of fibrous tissue that parallel bile ductules.[13] These diseases are associated with cholestasis and are marked by an accumulation of intracellular bile and copper within periportal hepatocytes. As mentioned earlier, cirrhosis associated with chronic biliary diseases may show a halo surrounding cirrhotic nodules. This represents a zone of edematous, lighter-appearing tissue containing proliferating bile ductules and ballooned periportal hepatocytes.

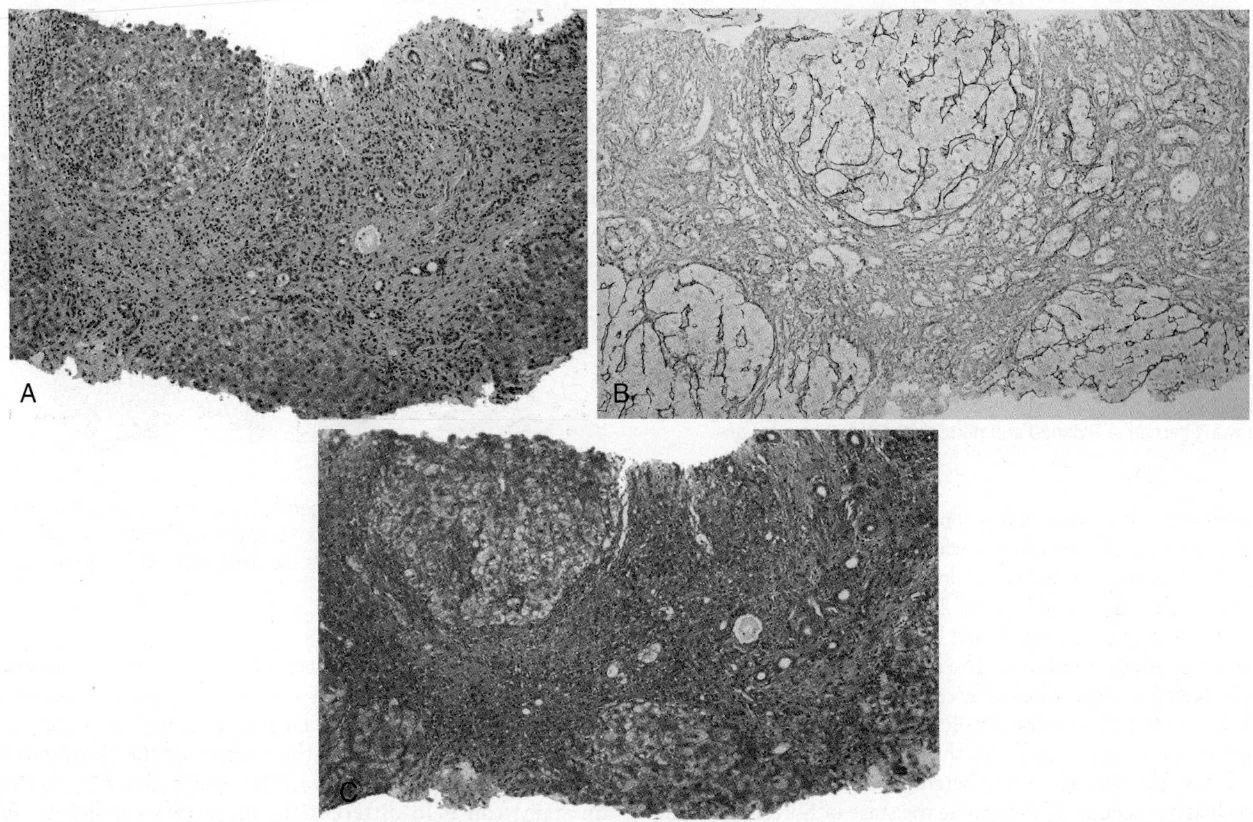

FIGURE 43.42 **A,** Bridging necrosis in a case of acute hepatitis. It is difficult to distinguish this necrosis from bridging fibrosis, particularly because the residual hepatocytes may appear nodular with reticulin stain **(B)**. **C,** Necrotic areas appear more grayish or light blue with trichrome stain as opposed to the densely colored blue of true fibrosis.

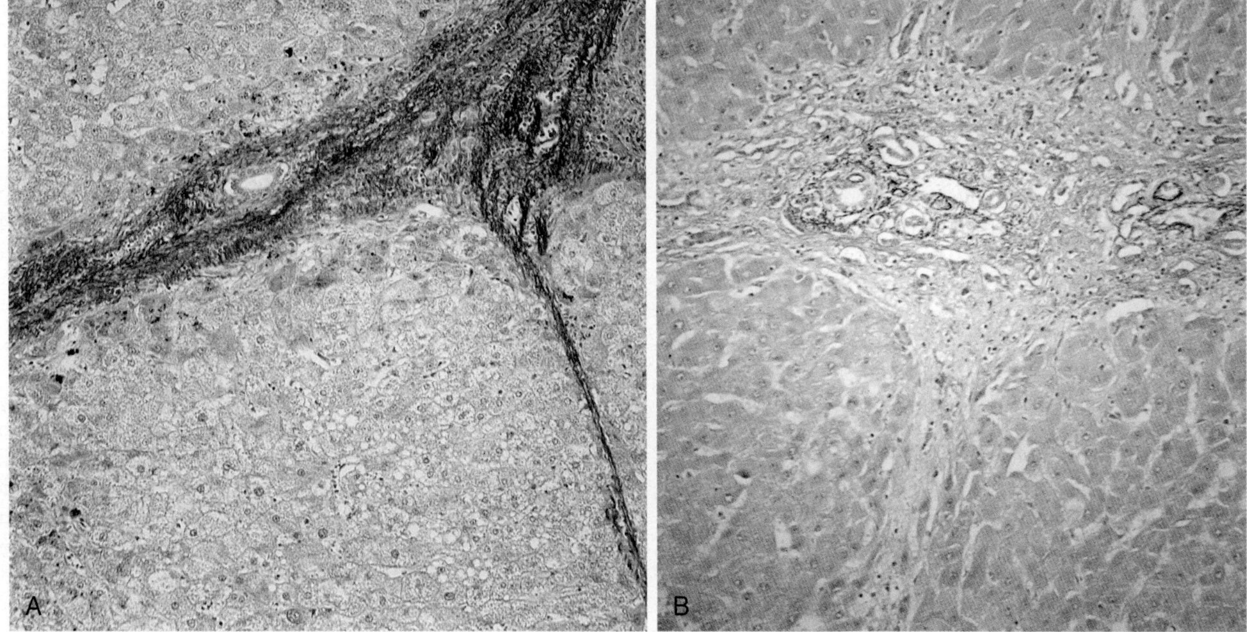

FIGURE 43.43 Victoria blue stain highlights elastic fibers that are formed in true pathological fibrosis **(A)**, but not in areas of bridging necrosis **(B)**.

Disorders of duct plate malformation such as congenital hepatic fibrosis and Caroli's disease can also cause fibrous expansion of the portal tracts, which may result in development of fibrous septa between adjacent portal tracts.[47] Fibrous tissue may contain ductal structures, with open lumina, containing inspissated bile. These are often arranged in a configuration reminiscent of fetal ductal plates.

In contrast, prominent perivenular and sinusoidal/pericellular fibrosis is most commonly associated with steatohepatitis, chronic venous outflow tract obstruction, and a variety of drugs and toxins such as total parenteral nutrition.[48] In cases of chronic

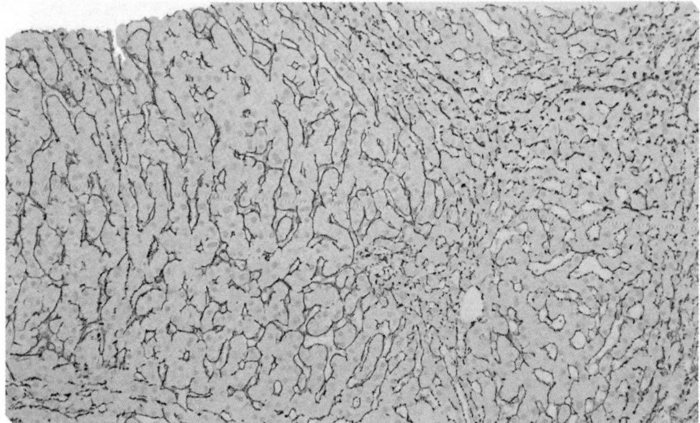

FIGURE 43.44 Reticulin stain highlights nodular regenerative hyperplasia with alternating widened and narrowed plates of hepatocytes.

venous outflow obstruction secondary to right-sided heart failure, liver biopsies are often performed to confirm congestive hepatopathy and to assess the extent of fibrosis. This would affect a patient's candidacy for heart transplantation because patients may require a combined heart and liver transplantation in cases of advanced fibrosis. The majority of these biopsies will show NRH in association with congestive hepatopathy, which would account for the commonly noted nodular appearance of the liver on imaging studies in this setting. Of note, the fibrosis seen in this setting is often heterogeneous in nature, limiting the ability to accurately determine the stage of fibrosis in biopsy specimens. Correlation with complete clinical information and communication with the clinical team is often essential for management decisions in such cases.[49]

Diagnostic Pitfalls

When evaluating liver specimens for fibrosis, pathologists should be aware of several following pitfalls.

Large Portal Tracts

The amount of fibrous tissue in normal portal tracts depends on the size of the tracts. Large portal tracts contain a more significant amount of fibrous tissue that should not be mistaken for true fibrosis. The large size of the duct and artery as well as the presence of nerves within fibrous areas indicate a large portal tract, whereas the presence of neovascularization as well as ductular reaction at the edge of a large fibrous zone indicate true fibrosis.

Subcapsular Biopsy Specimens

The subcapsular region of the liver normally contains fibrous tissue along the subcapsular septa. The portal tracts and central veins may show more prominent fibrous tissue within 5 mm of the liver capsule. In this area, one may see bridges of fibrous tissue between portal tracts or between portal tracts and central veins (Fig. 43.45). Therefore caution should be taken to not overinterpret these as pathological fibrosis in subcapsular biopsies.

Fragmented Biopsy Specimens

Liver tissue that contains bridging fibrosis and regenerating nodules may result in liver biopsy specimens that are fragmented.[50] Therefore biopsies that are received fragmented should always be considered suspicious for cirrhosis.

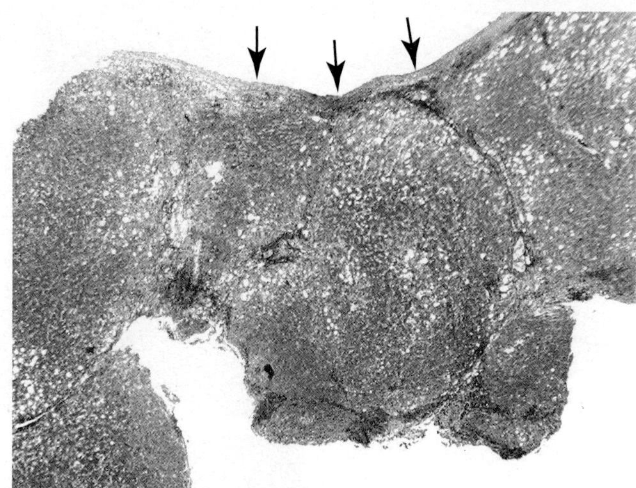

FIGURE 43.45 Subcapsular liver parenchyma may show nodules and fibrous septa bridging portal tracts to other portal tracts and central veins, even in the absence of fibrosis in the deep liver parenchyma. *Arrows* point to liver capsule.

However, fragmentation may also occur in the absence of cirrhosis; for example, it can result from the technical aspects of obtaining a liver biopsy specimen or an artifact of processing. Evaluation of the borders of the fragments of tissue and the architecture of the hepatic plates (by reticulin stain) can help differentiate these two conditions. For instance, the findings of multiple round fragments of liver tissue with wisps of fibrous tissue and portions of portal tracts at the edges of the fragment are more commonly observed in cirrhosis than in artifactual fragmentation.

OTHER FINDINGS

Pigments in the Liver

Lipofuscin

Lipofuscin is a fine, light brown, granular pigment that is often most evident in perivenular hepatocytes (Figs. 43.46 and 43.47). Lipofuscin normally accumulates in the liver with advancing age. Increased lipofuscin deposition may also be seen in any disorder that results in chronic liver injury.[50]

Iron

In contrast with lipofuscin, iron is a refractile pigment that stains positive with Prussian blue or Perls stain. Iron deposition may be primary (hereditary hemochromatosis) or, more often, secondary.[6,51] Although mild hemosiderin may be associated with chronic liver injury of any cause, and particularly in alcoholic steatohepatitis (Fig. 43.48), marked hemosiderin deposition may indicate concomitant hereditary hemochromatosis, and correlation with molecular studies may be recommended to evaluate for this possibility.

Copper

Increased copper deposition within the liver is difficult to identify on routinely stained tissue sections. It is usually present within periportal hepatocytes and can be highlighted with a rhodamine (see Fig. 43.27), Victoria blue, or Orcein stain. These stains highlight copper-associated proteins. Copper accumulation in the liver may occur in a

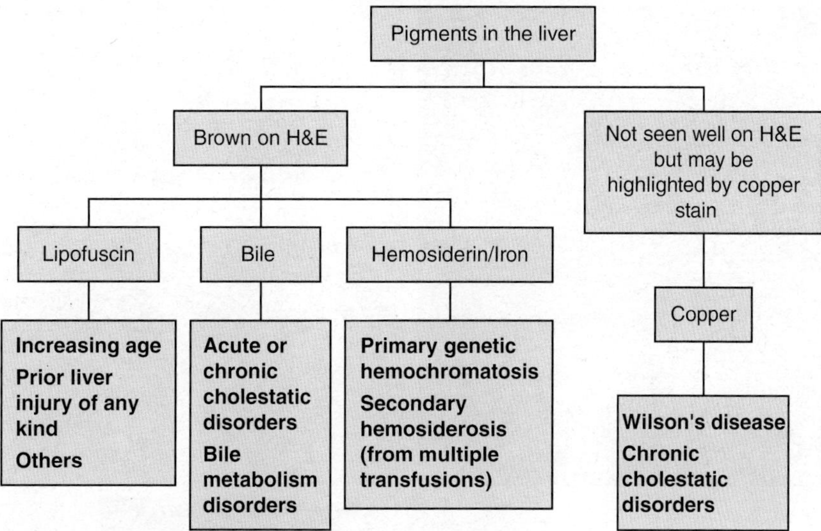

FIGURE 43.46 Diagnostic algorithm for pigments in the liver.

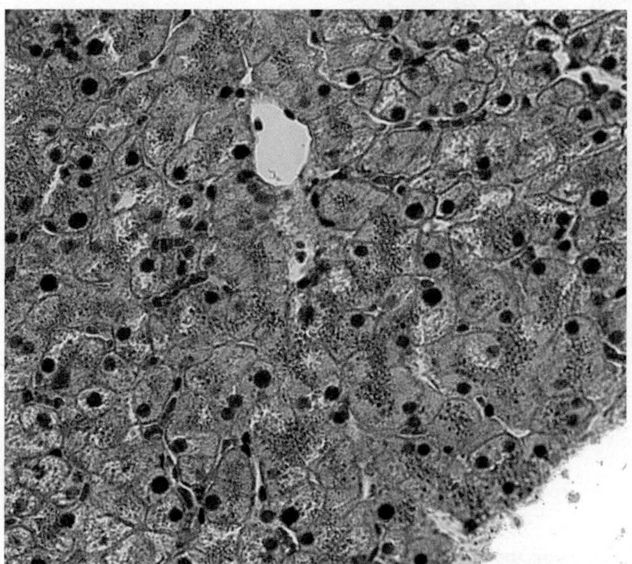

FIGURE 43.47 Lipofuscin pigment appears as fine, light brown, granular intracytoplasmic pigments in perivenular hepatocytes. They often have a pericanalicular distribution, as seen here.

variety of chronic cholestatic disorders or in Wilson's disease. In chronic cholestatic disorders, interference with copper secretion into bile leads to accumulation of the pigment within the liver.

Wilson's disease is protean in its manifestations. Patients with Wilson's disease may show a variety of morphological patterns of liver injury, including steatosis, chronic hepatitis, and even acute liver failure.[52] Other nonspecific features of Wilson's disease include glycogenated hepatocyte nuclei and binucleated hepatocytes. Steatosis associated with Wilson's disease is often mild and of the large-droplet macrovesicular type; it may also be associated with ballooned hepatocytes with Mallory-Denk bodies. Therefore caution should be taken not to misdiagnose Wilson's disease as NASH. A high index of suspicion and confirmation of copper accumulation by quantitative copper analysis from the block can help confirm a diagnosis of Wilson's disease. It should be noted that a copper stain is not reliable for a diagnosis of Wilson's disease because it is neither sensitive nor specific for this disorder. A copper stain can be patchy or even completely negative in Wilson's disease.

Inclusions or Deposits in the Liver

α_1-Antitrypsin (A1AT)

These cytoplasmic globules represent abnormal accumulation of mutant A1AT. They appear as round to oval, eosinophilic globules with a homogeneous appearance and smooth contours. They are strongly PAS positive and diastase resistant and tend to have a periportal or periseptal distribution (see Fig. 43.7). Immunohistochemical stain for A1AT may be used for confirmation. It should be noted that the presence of such globules does not establish a diagnosis of A1AT disease because these globules can be seen in other conditions such as in acute hepatitis resulting from transient defects in secretion. If such globules are noted in liver biopsies, then correlation with protease inhibitor phenotype testing by isoelectric focusing is recommended to help firmly establish the diagnosis of an A1AT disorder.

Ground-Glass/Pseudo–Ground-Glass Hepatocytes

Ground-glass hepatocytes are large, light gray to pink, cytoplasmic inclusions associated with a rim of cytoplasm at the edges of the cells. As mentioned earlier, hepatitis B infection is a common cause in which the inclusions result from surface antigen accumulation within the endoscopic reticulum, and this may be highlighted by immunohistochemistry (see Fig. 43.6). Similar morphology may also be seen in immunosuppressed individuals who are consuming multiple medications, and in those cases, the inclusions are the result of distended endoplasmic reticulum with accumulation of abnormally folded glycogen. These deposits are PAS positive and variably diastase sensitive. Their presence may be associated with mild liver enzyme elevations and rarely with hepatomegaly (Fig. 43.49).[4] Given that these deposits can closely mimic the ground-glass inclusions associated with

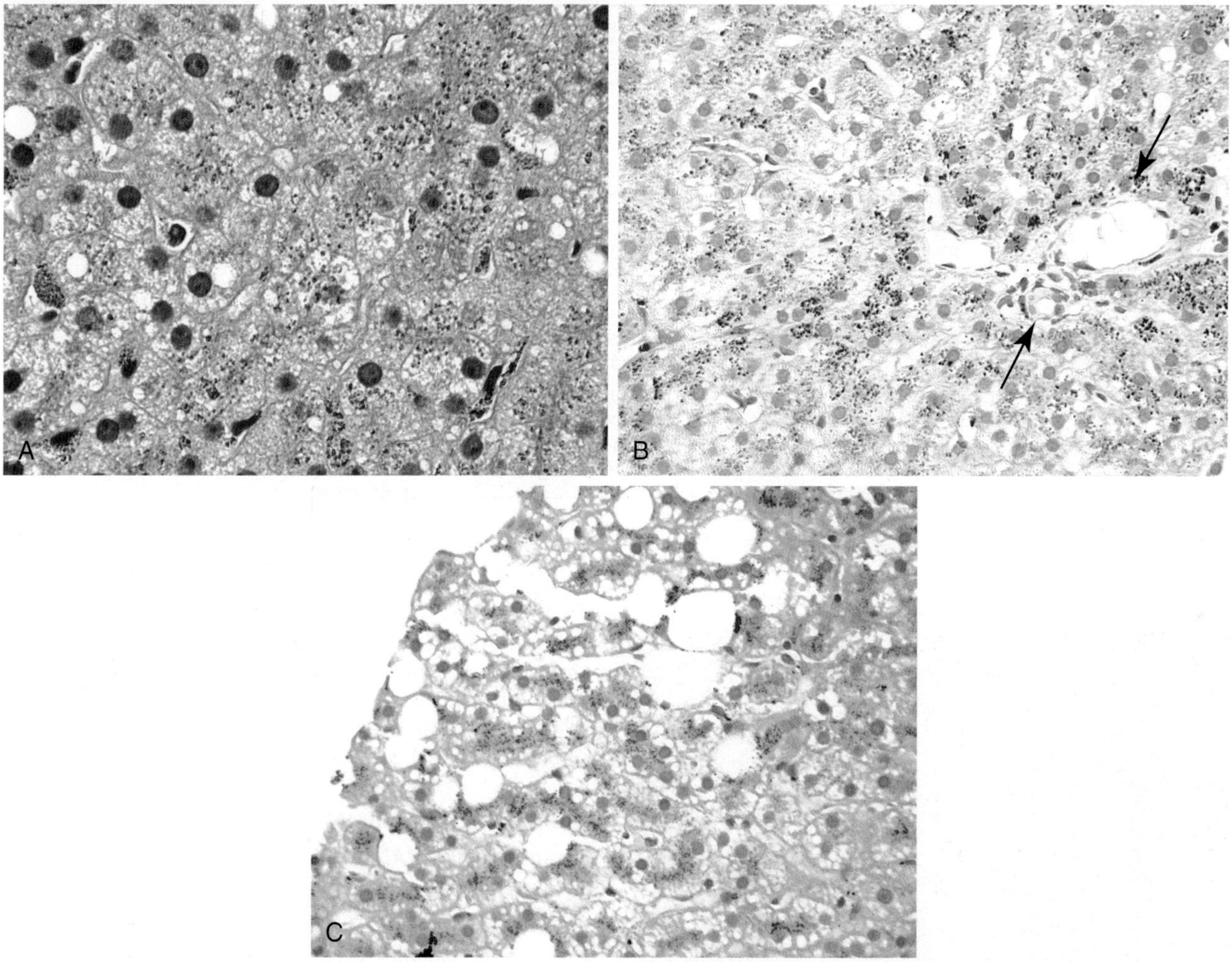

FIGURE 43.48 **A,** Hemosiderin appears as coarse, golden-brown, refractile pigment on hematoxylin and eosin (H&E) stain. **B,** Hemosiderin stains blue with Prussian blue. Accumulation of hemosiderin in hepatocytes begins within periportal hepatocytes *(arrows)*. Accumulation of hemosiderin is prominent in a variety of chronic liver diseases such as chronic hepatitis C or steatohepatitis **(C).**

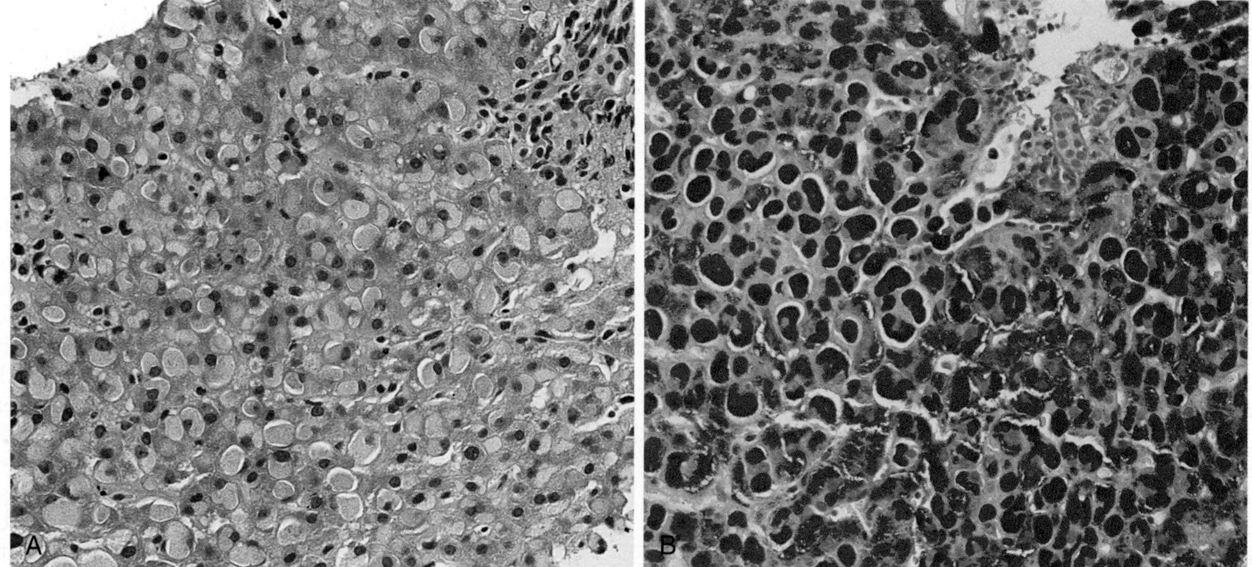

FIGURE 43.49 **A,** Pseudo–ground-glass hepatocytes are seen in this posttransplant liver biopsy. **B,** These cytoplasmic inclusions are associated with accumulation of abnormal forms of glycogen, as highlighted here by periodic acid–Schiff (PAS) stain.

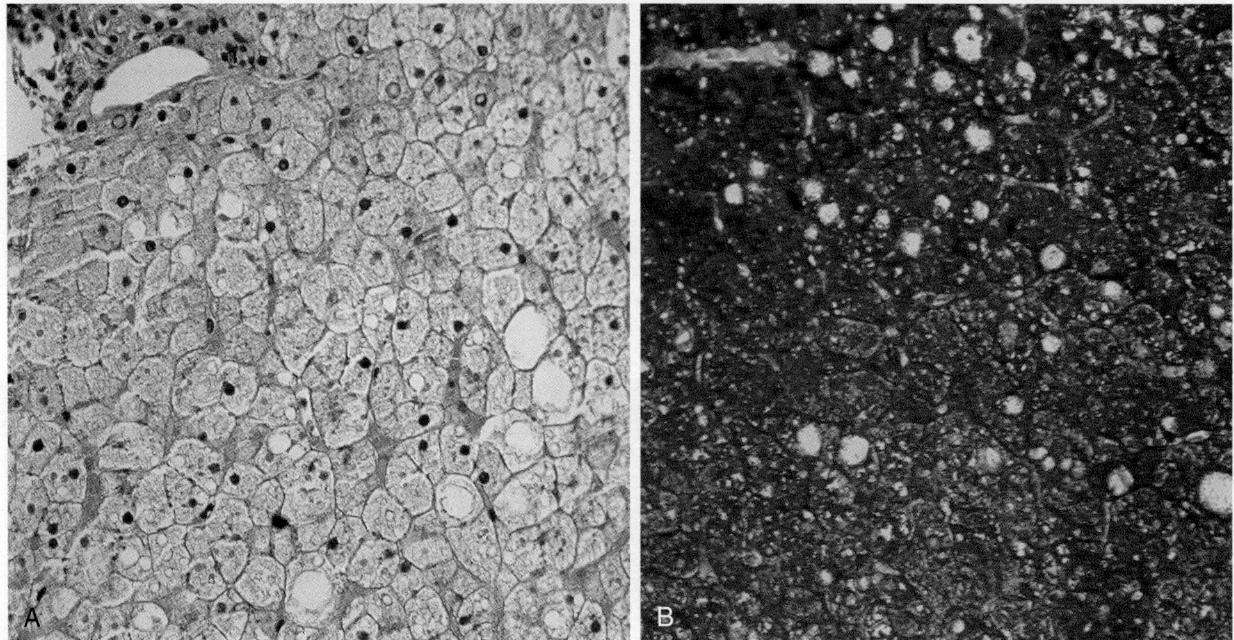

FIGURE 43.50 **A,** The hepatocytes in this liver biopsy of a patient with uncontrolled diabetes show clear cytoplasm with distinct cytoplasmic borders (glycogenic hepatopathy). **B,** Periodic acid–Schiff (PAS) stain highlights the glycogen content within the cytoplasm.

chronic hepatitis B infection, immunostain for HBsAg may be helpful.

Glycogenic Hepatopathy

The term *glycogenic hepatopathy* is used when hepatocytes demonstrate swollen and clear cytoplasm with distinct cytoplasmic borders (plant cell–like appearance). This occurs as a result of increased glycogen accumulation within hepatocytes, and the histological changes are nearly identical to that of inherited glycogen storage diseases. Glycogenic hepatopathy typically occurs in the setting of high and poorly controlled serum glucose levels in diabetic patients, and it is generally responsive to glycemic control. It may be associated with hepatomegaly and often presents with fluctuating transaminases, which can become quite high, raising the possibility of acute hepatitis. There is typically no significant associated inflammation or hepatocyte necrosis. PAS stain helps highlight glycogen within the cytoplasm (Fig. 43.50). Given that normal livers contain PAS-positive glycogen within the cytoplasm, it is the typical H&E appearance that is required to establish a definitive diagnosis of glycogenic hepatopathy.[53]

The full reference list may be accessed online at Elsevier eBooks for Practicing Clinicians.

CHAPTER 44

Liver Tissue Processing and Normal Histology

James M. Crawford

Contents

LIVER BIOPSY SPECIMENS

Histopathological examination of liver tissue by needle biopsy remains an integral part of the management of liver diseases, as morphology is of critical importance for synthesizing clinical and laboratory testing findings into cogent understanding of a patient's liver disease. Liver biopsies were documented in the late 19th century, when Ehrlich and then Lucatello performed liver puncture through a laparoscope, primarily for chemical studies.[1] Schupfer in 1907 is credited with the first application of liver biopsy for the diagnosis of cirrhotic liver disease in humans.

In 1938, the Vim-Silverman needle was introduced. This needle required the patient to hyperventilate for 30 seconds, and then hold his or her breath for the 2 to 6 seconds of needle manipulation within the liver.[2] This procedure carried considerable risk of post-biopsy bleeding.[3] Introduction of the rapid Menghini needle biopsy technique in 1958 dramatically expanded the use of liver biopsy, because it took less than 1 second and was safer and easier to use, while providing adequate tissue for histopathology and other studies.[4] Although fibrotic and cirrhotic liver tissue is more likely to fragment during Menghini biopsy sampling, when compared with use of larger "cutting" needles,[5] the safety profile for Menghini and other rapid needle sampling techniques ensured the latter's popularity for percutaneous access.[6,7] Introduction of transjugular biopsies enabled liver tissue samples to be obtained in patients with suboptimal coagulation indices or with ascites.[8] Open or laparoscopic biopsy such as during bariatric surgery adds to operative time but does not carry increased risk as measured by bleeding complications, length of postoperative stay, morbidity, or death.[9] Intraoperative needle biopsy samples tissue from deeper within the liver, avoiding the risk of misinterpreting anatomically normal subcapsular fibrosis as might be the case with intraoperative wedge biopsy.[10] Endoscopic ultrasound-guided liver biopsy can generate an adequate tissue biopsy for assessment of tumors that are less accessible by a percutaneous route,[11] but the argument is made that percutaneous ultrasound-guided needle biopsy is still the more reliable technique for obtaining adequate biopsies of localized lesions.[12] The various liver biopsy techniques are summarized in Table 44.1.

The indications for liver biopsy are given in Box 44.1. Many liver biopsies are performed for chronic viral hepatitis, steatohepatitis, and allograft dysfunction to assess the degree of liver damage or the response to therapy.[13] Acute hepatitis is usually not an indication for liver biopsy, but if there is doubt about the clinical diagnosis, multifactorial causes of elevated liver enzyme values, or even a mistaken working diagnosis, a biopsy may be indicated. Although surrogate laboratory testing for liver disease and noninvasive imaging techniques (particularly elastometry)[14] and sustained virological response to antiviral therapies[15] argue for decreased frequency of liver biopsy, histological features other than fibrosis stage continue to have an effect on both understanding disease process and provide insight into prognosis and response to therapy.[16] Moreover, many patients with chronic liver disease present with already advanced disease, and histological evaluation is critical to determine the severity of liver damage.[17] Lastly, as the liver is susceptible to insult from multiple agents simultaneously, liver biopsy is valuable for assessing the potential coexistence of different forms of liver

TABLE 44.1 Liver Biopsy Methods

Methods	Technique	Considerations and Risk
Percutaneous (blind)	Suction needle (Menghini, Klatskin, Jamshidi) or cutting needle (Vim-Silverman, Tru-cut)	Most common, least costly, and least invasive liver biopsy. Provides an adequate specimen for histological evaluation and for other ancillary studies. Complications and specimen outcome related to the operator's experience. May rarely result in an inadvertent biopsy of other organs, including kidney, pancreas, lung, gallbladder, and intestine.
Transjugular (transvenous)	Catheter through the internal jugular vein, right atrium, and inferior vena cava	Performed in patients with coagulation disorders, fulminant hepatic failure, gross ascites, or severe obesity. Greater effort and time required compared with percutaneous biopsy. Multiple specimens of good quality can be obtained, especially with experienced operators. Also possible to measure hemodynamics if combined with wedged hepatic pressure and venography. Complications include arrhythmia, contrast-related reaction, and inadvertent biopsy of kidney.
Laparoscopic or open	Providing direct visualization of the liver and peritoneal cavity; needle or wedge biopsy	Wedge biopsy provides a larger specimen, but if too superficial may lead to misinterpretation of liver "fibrosis," owing to penetration of anatomically normal fibrous septa of Glisson's capsule into the immediately subjacent liver parenchyma (to a depth of about 0.5 cm). Needle biopsy is a smaller sample but penetrates deeper into the liver so it can provide better information about the stage of liver fibrosis. Risk of anesthesia and hemorrhage; hemostasis may be monitored visually at the time of biopsy, and Gelfoam plug used if needed. Popularity of laparoscopic bariatric surgery for obesity has increased the number of intraoperative biopsies for evaluation of steatohepatitis and fibrosis.
CT or ultrasound-guided	<1-mm gauge needle typically used (fine-needle aspiration); ultrasound or CT used for visualization of hepatic lesion and to avoid intersecting vessels	For cytological or histological diagnosis of space-occupying lesion or sampling of cystic lesions. Multiple aspirations can be safely performed to ensure an adequate specimen. Immediate assessment of adequacy is possible. Cell block may increase sensitivity and allow additional staining; needle core tissue fragments are fixed and processed for routine histology. Risk of bleeding complications much lower compared with routine percutaneous needle biopsy. Seeding of needle tract by malignant cells is rare; does not appear to worsen prognosis.

CT, *Computed tomography.*

BOX 44.1 Utility of Liver Biopsy

Evaluation of abnormal liver test results
Evaluation of fever of unknown origin
Evaluation of jaundice of unclear origin
Evaluation of portal hypertension and ascites
Evaluation of hereditary or metabolic disease
Evaluation of abnormal serum iron study result
Diagnosis, grading, and staging of chronic hepatitis
Monitoring the effects of new or established therapy
Diagnosis, grading, and staging of chronic biliary disease
Confirmation of fatty liver and grading and staging of steatohepatitis
Diagnosis of space-occupying lesions
Evaluation of donor and posttransplant livers

injury. A key example is the allograft liver, when recurrent disease such as hepatitis C infection may be simultaneously present with organ rejection and/or drug-induced liver injury (see Chapters 49 and 53). Interpretation of the hepatic morphology plays a critical role in guiding clinical management.

Although relatively safe, liver biopsy is an invasive procedure, and the indications, goals, and techniques and their limitations should be carefully considered to avoid performing unnecessary procedures or preparation of a sample that cannot provide the necessary answer. As many as one-third of patients experience right upper quadrant pain or shoulder pain, which may be severe in 1% to 3%.[18] Postprocedure bleeding is the key concern; major hemorrhage occurs in 0.3% of procedures, almost all presenting within 24 hours of biopsy.[19] Less common complications include transient bacteremia, biliary leak with bile peritonitis, or injury to adjacent organs such as the gallbladder, colon, or right lung.[20] The mortality rate associated with different techniques is approximately 0.01%.[21] Rare complications of liver biopsy include hemobilia, pneumoperitoneum, pneumoscrotum, pneumothorax, septic shock, subphrenic abscess, and intrahepatic arteriovenous fistula. Although rare, seeding in the needle track has been reported in cases of hepatocellular carcinoma and metastatic colorectal carcinoma.[22,23] This minimal risk is balanced against the risk of selecting aggressive surgical treatment in a patient who does not have malignancy.[24] The major contraindication to percutaneous liver biopsy is significant coagulopathy. Relative contraindications to percutaneous liver biopsy are morbid obesity and severe ascites. In these conditions, transjugular biopsy is a good alternative.

Fine-needle aspiration (FNA) biopsy guided by ultrasound or computed tomography (CT) has become the preferred method for diagnosis of a space-occupying lesion and confirmation of a suspected malignancy.[25,26] FNA biopsy provides immediate interpretation and assessment of the adequacy of a liver biopsy by using smears or touch preparations. Routine supplementation with a cell block of tissue fragments increases the diagnostic accuracy of FNA, and it provides material for immunohistochemical stains and ancillary studies for primary or metastatic malignant tumors. FNA biopsy can also be used to drain a cyst or abscess for culture and fluid analysis, or it can be followed by therapeutic ablation of malignant tumors. If echinococcal cyst is suspected and ultrasound imaging and serology are inconclusive, FNA sampling of the cyst fluid for evidence of protoscoleces or of antigens specific to *Echinococcus granulosus* may be considered but is best done with an anesthesiologist assisting, owing to the very low but present risk of anaphylaxis.[27]

Specimen Handling

At the time of the biopsy procedure, a needle liver biopsy specimen should be examined immediately for adequacy. It should be at least 1.5 cm long, and if it is not, another pass is recommended because adequate specimen size minimizes sampling error.[28] If a tumor is suspected, a touch preparation from the tissue can immediately determine specimen adequacy or a diagnosis. The specimen is then discharged into a Petri dish lined with lens paper, which has ideally been soaked in normal saline solution to prevent fresh tissue from adhering to it. Artifacts from squeezing or drying of the specimen should be avoided. Biopsy specimens should not be placed on dry gauze, which tends to dehydrate cells, resulting in a prominent nuclear artifact. Tissue squeezing distorts cells and elongates nuclei, which makes cytological evaluation of the specimen difficult.

Gross characteristics of the tissue, such as color, consistency, and tendency to fragment or float in the fixative solution, are documented by the physician. Tumors or granulomas, for example, can be recognized as white areas in otherwise reddish-brown tissue. Gray-black discoloration is seen in Dubin-Johnson syndrome, rusty brown in hemochromatosis, green in cholestasis, yellow in fatty liver, dark red in congested liver, and variegated or dark brown in metastatic melanoma. Fragmentation of specimens, especially in a transjugular biopsy specimen or when a Menghini (suction) needle is used, often indicates advanced fibrosis or cirrhosis.

Unless there are indications for special handling (see later), the liver biopsy cores should then be placed immediately in 10% neutral buffered formalin, which is the routine fixative for liver biopsies. Immersion of biopsies in saline causes discohesion of cells and distortion of the hepatocyte cords. The advantages of routine formalin fixation are that the formalin solution is stable; penetrates and fixes tissues well; is inexpensive; and allows subsequent application of most histochemical, immunohistochemical, and molecular pathology procedures. The characteristics of tissues fixed in formalin are well known. The disadvantage of formalin is the relative lack of cytological detail compared with some other types of fixatives such as Bouin's or Zenker fixatives. However, the latter are contraindicated in this day and age owing to their inclusion of toxic heavy metals and their interference with molecular pathology analytics.

On the basis of the clinical diagnosis or possible differential diagnoses, the clinician determines which additional procedures may be required (Table 44.2): fixation in 3% buffered glutaraldehyde for electron microscopy; fresh, unfixed tissue for viral and mycobacterial cultures; rapid freezing in liquid nitrogen or a mixture of dry ice and isopentane for fat stains, certain immunohistochemical and enzyme activity studies,[29] quantitative studies of hormone receptors, and isolation of genomic and viral DNA and RNA for molecular analyses[30]; and fixation in 1% periodic acid in 10% neutral buffered formalin at 4° C for 48 hours for evaluation of glycogen storage diseases.[31] When RNA recovery is needed, an alcohol-based fixative is better than a formalin fixative. When the patient is a child or a young adult, it may be beneficial to fix tissue in glutaraldehyde fixative in anticipation of possible ultrastructural studies.

TABLE 44.2 Ancillary Studies and Fixatives

Ancillary Studies	Fixative or Procedure
Transmission electron microscopy	3% buffered glutaraldehyde
Viral, bacterial, fungal cultures	Fresh, unfixed tissue or cystic aspirate
Fat stains, enzyme activity, protein analysis, viral DNA and RNA, in situ hybridization	Rapid freezing in liquid nitrogen or mixture of dry ice and isopentane
Glycogen storage diseases	1% periodic acid in 10% neutral buffered formalin at 4° C for 48 hours
Flow cytometry of lymphocytes	Fresh, unfixed tissue in transport media
DNA analysis	10% neutral buffered formalin
RNA analysis	Fresh tissue or fixed alcohol-based fixative (80% ethanol)
mRNA and miRNA analysis	Fresh tissue or fixed 10% neutral buffered formalin
Protein analysis	Fresh or fresh-frozen, unfixed tissue
Laser capture microdissection	Conventional tissue section from paraffin-embedded tissue block

miRNA, *MicroRNA;* mRNA, *messenger RNA.*

As noted, needle liver biopsy specimens should be placed immediately in the desired fixative, because the foundation of a good histological preparation is rapid and complete fixation. Good preservation of tissue can be achieved by following standard guidelines. First, the volume of the fixative should be at least 15 to 20 times the volume of the tissue.[32] When transit to the laboratory is likely to involve much movement, the container should be filled to the brim with fixative to avoid the tissue specimen becoming adherent to a portion of the container that is not bathed in fixative. Second, sufficient time must be allowed for fixation to occur before processing is started. Because formalin penetrates most tissues at approximately 0.5 mm per hour at room temperature, sufficient time must be given for fixative to penetrate the tissue core (16-gauge needles have a nominal internal diameter of 1.19 mm; 18-gauge is 0.84 mm internal diameter). Fixation time may be shortened by application of heat, pressure, vacuum, agitation, or microwave techniques. When a histology slide is examined with the microscope, fragmentation of the central portion of the liver biopsy along the long axis is a sign of insufficient fixation time. Although prolonged formalin exposure (>24 hours) does not result in overfixation (i.e., hardening of tissue), it may reduce the availability of antigen sites for immunohistochemical studies. If there is residual tissue, it may be stored in 10% (or lower) neutral buffered formalin or in 70% alcohol.[33]

Rush liver biopsy specimens should be manually processed to shorten the delay and meet the needs of critically ill or transplant patients; regular specimens are processed in an automated tissue processor. The application of microwave processing has significantly reduced processing time to as little as 15 minutes for a tiny biopsy specimen or to a 60- to 90-minute cycle for a larger biopsy specimen.[34]

Normal Microanatomy of the Liver

The functional unit of the liver is represented by the hepatic lobule of Kiernan or the hepatic acinus of Rappaport.[35,36] A hepatic lobule is viewed as a hexagonal region of the parenchyma, with portal tracts containing a portal vein, hepatic artery, and bile duct occupying three of the six apices of the hexagon, and the effluent "central" hepatic vein at the center of the hexagon. Hepatocyte cords are viewed as being arranged radially around the central vein. The microanatomic regions are referred to as "periportal," "mid-zonal," or "pericentral," terms commonly used in hepatic pathology (Fig. 44.1).

The Rappaport acinus is a more regular, three-dimensional structure in which the portal tract is at one point of the base of an isosceles triangle, and an effluent portal venule penetrates the parenchyma along the base of the triangle. The effluent vein is at the sharp apex of the triangle and is termed the "terminal hepatic vein." Portal vein blood flows from the penetrating portal venule into the sinusoidal channels along a broad front, thence draining into the terminal hepatic vein.

Hepatic arterial blood supplies the plexuses that nourish interlobar, segmental, and sublobular portal veins and bile ducts; these plexuses drain into hepatic sinusoids. Terminal portal veins and interlobular bile ducts do not have an arterial plexus. Arterial blood that reaches the terminal hepatic arteries enters into periportal sinusoids via arteriosinus twigs. Isolated parenchymal arterioles may occasionally be seen within the periportal parenchyma.

The acinus is subdivided into zones 1, 2, and 3, indicative of progressively decreasing tissue oxygenation (see Fig. 44.1). The oxygen gradient, metabolic heterogeneity, and differential distribution of enzymes across the three zones of the acini help explain the zonal distribution of liver damage caused by hypoperfusion or ischemia and by certain toxic substances.

The hepatocyte is a polygonal epithelial cell with one or more centrally located, round nuclei. The number of binucleate forms increases with age (Fig. 44.2). Some nuclei are larger than others, particularly in persons older than 60 years, indicating polyploidy.[37] The significance of polyploidy is unknown. It is usually more prominent in the midzonal areas. Hepatocytes are arranged in one-cell-thick cords in adults, and they are separated by sinusoids, in which blood flows from the portal tracts to the terminal hepatic venules. In keeping with the continued growth of the liver in the early years of life, in children as old as 5 or 6 years, the liver cells are arranged in two-cell-thick plates (Fig. 44.3). In adults, the presence of two-cell-thick hepatocyte plates and rosette formation, along with more uniformly sized nuclei and increased nuclear density, indicates hepatocyte regeneration (Fig. 44.4). Rare eosinophilic bodies or apoptotic bodies indicate normal turnover of hepatocytes in otherwise apparently normal adult livers. Hepatocyte mitotic figures are not usually seen except during hepatic response to parenchymal injury.

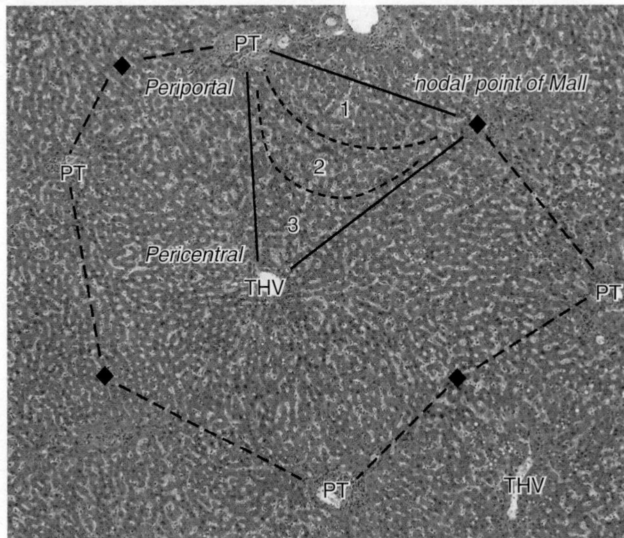

FIGURE 44.1 The normal liver parenchyma, showing portal tracts (PT) and terminal hepatic vein (THV). The concept of the lobule places the THV ("central vein") at the center of an approximately hexagonal lobule; in this image PT are at four of the eight apices of an octagonal lobule, with the watershed areas between portal tracts (the "nodal point of Mall," *black diamond*) occupying four of those apices. The concept of the acinus places a PT and the watershed area (*black diamond*) at the base of an isosceles triangle, with the THV at the apex of the triangle. Blood exiting the penetrating portal venules travels along a broad curvilinear front through zones 1, 2, and 3 of the acinus; note that zone 3 extends partially toward portal tracts. This image of a normal liver makes clear that the geometry of the lobule and acinus is variable.

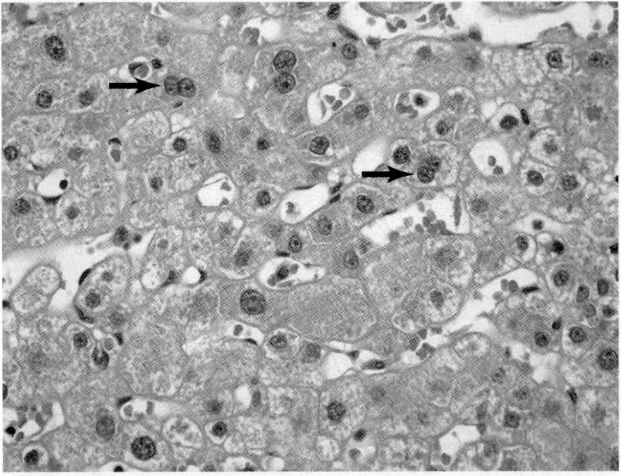

FIGURE 44.2 Liver biopsy from an older individual shows significant polyploidy of hepatocyte nuclei and binucleate forms *(arrows)*.

Glycogen accumulation in hepatocyte nuclei surrounding portal tracts produces a vacuolated appearance and is common in adolescents (Fig. 44.5). In adults, this appearance may be conspicuous in conditions such as Wilson's disease, metabolic syndrome, or diabetes mellitus. Cytoplasmic glycogen is normally present and imparts a fine, reticulated

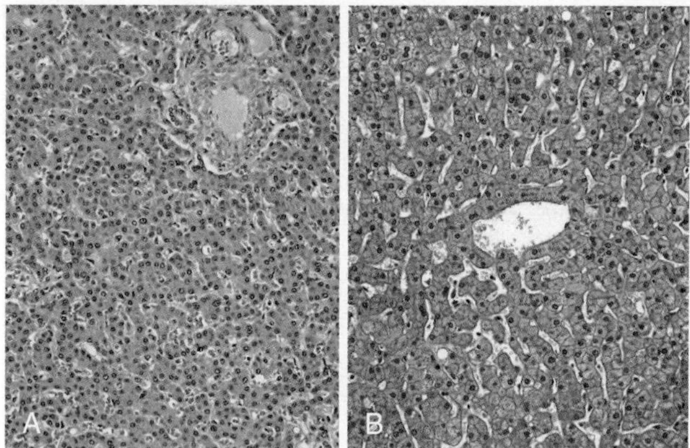

FIGURE 44.3 Comparison of liver parenchyma of a child **(A)** and an adult **(B).** In children, the hepatocytes are arranged less regularly, without a distinct radial arrangement, and in two-cell-thick plates. In adults, the hepatocytes are normally one cell thick and show a more regular radial arrangement around the terminal hepatic venule.

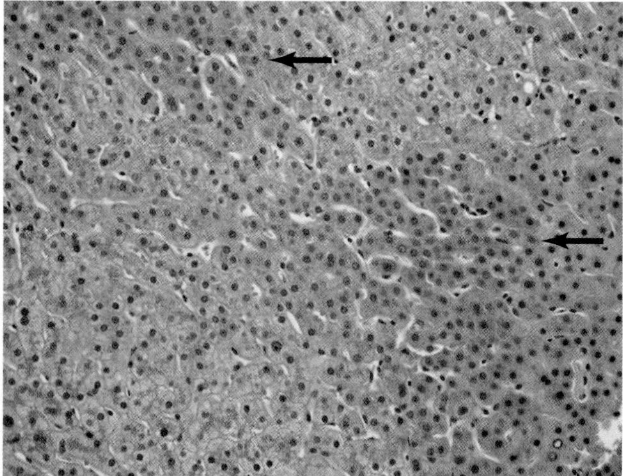

FIGURE 44.4 Dark staining and thickening of hepatocyte cords *(arrows)* indicate hepatocyte regeneration in adults.

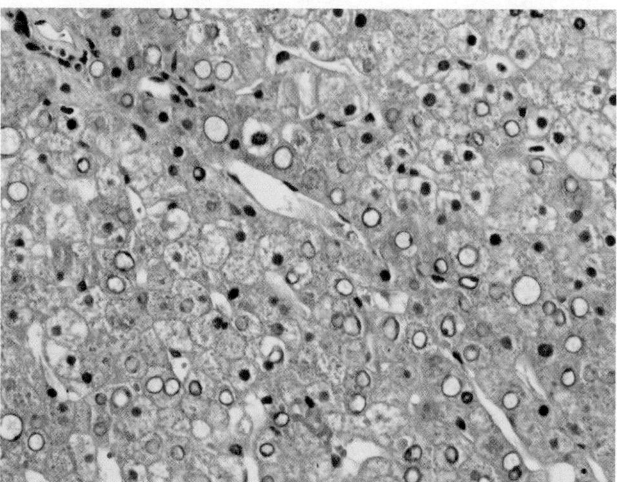

FIGURE 44.5 Glycogen accumulation in hepatocyte nuclei results in a clear, empty appearance.

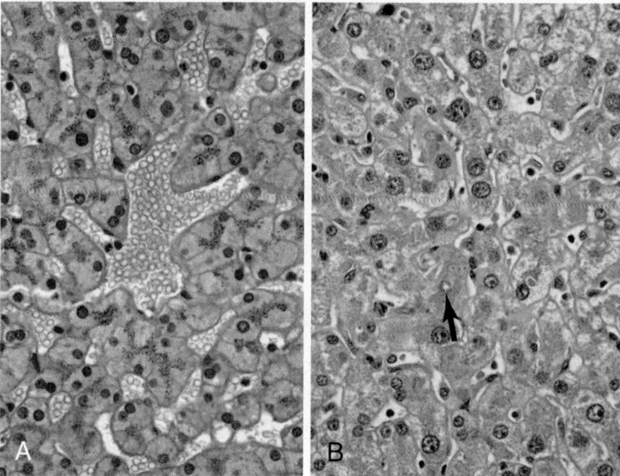

FIGURE 44.6 Lipofuscin pigment **(A)** and cholestasis **(B)** are found predominantly in zone 3 of the acinus. Lipofuscin pigment is fine, well delineated, light brown, and refractile, and is located predominantly at the canalicular pole of hepatocytes. Intracellular bile in cholestasis imparts a brownish hue to the cytoplasm; bile retained in dilated canalicular *(arrow)* may also be visible.

appearance to the cytoplasm. The distribution of glycogen also shows diurnal and diet-related variations. An irregular distribution pattern may be found in biopsies and is not of diagnostic significance. Owing to consumption of hepatocellular glycogen at the time of death, the hepatocytes in autopsy livers are more compact and do not show the reticulated cytoplasm of hepatocytes in liver biopsy specimens.

Lipofuscin pigment is normally seen in variable quantities in the centrilobular areas as fine, light brown granules centered around the canalicular region of the hepatocytes; the periodic acid–Schiff–diastase (PAS-D) stain highlights these granules. There is a progressive increase of lipofuscin in individual hepatocytes with age (Fig. 44.6). The granules represent lysosomes that contain materials that cannot be further degraded; they are not present in recently regenerated hepatocytes. Bile is not visible under normal circumstances. Hepatocellular retention of bile in either obstructive or nonobstructive cholestasis is evident by brown fluid present in dilated bile canaliculi of hepatocytes in zone 3 (see Fig. 44.6); the hepatocyte cytoplasm may also exhibit brown discoloration on hematoxylin and eosin (H&E) stain. Retained bile can be distinguished from lipofuscin by its lack of a granular appearance and lack of refraction when the microscope condenser is lowered.

Large amounts of lipofuscin are difficult to distinguish from Dubin-Johnson pigment microscopically, although Dubin-Johnson pigment is not as refractile as lipofuscin. Compared with lipofuscin, iron and copper are coarser, birefringent, and usually deposited in periportal hepatocytes. Hemosiderin and copper are abundant in the cytoplasm of hepatocytes during the first week of life, then gradually disappear, and should be absent by the age of 9 months. Small quantities of stainable iron are common in normal hepatocytes, particularly in older individuals.

Sinusoidal lining cells consist of specialized fenestrated endothelial cells and specialized macrophages or Kupffer cells, which are usually inconspicuous in normal biopsy specimens. Occasional lymphocytes or neutrophils may be present in the sinusoids. Between the sinusoidal lining cells and the hepatocytes lies the space of Disse, which contains plasma, scanty connective tissue, and perisinusoidal cells such as hepatic stellate cells and pit cells (i.e., natural killer lymphocytes). Hepatic stellate cells are modified resting myofibroblasts that can store fat and vitamin A and produce hepatocyte growth factor and collagen.[38,39] They play a significant role in hepatic fibrogenesis. When activated, hepatic stellate cells contain stainable desmin and actin in their cytoplasm that can be highlighted with an immunohistochemical stain for smooth muscle actin.[40] Elastic fibers and basement membrane material are absent from normal sinusoids.[41,42]

Smaller branches of the sublobular hepatic veins and the terminal hepatic veins are in direct contact with the hepatocyte parenchyma. The terminal hepatic veins have very thin walls lined by endothelial cells. Thickening of the wall of terminal hepatic veins is often part of a pericellular fibrosis reaction and of central hyalin sclerosis in alcoholic liver disease.[43,44] It also may be seen focally in apparently normal individuals.

Portal tracts of different sizes may be seen in biopsy specimens. Defining a portal tract as a focus within the parenchyma containing at least two luminal structures embedded in a connective tissue mesenchyme with a continuous connective tissue circumference,[45] a percutaneous liver biopsy may contain from 3 to more than 20 portal tracts, with the number directly proportional to the length of the biopsy (approximately 6 portal tracts per linear centimeter of tissue core biopsy). On a per specimen basis, in a normal liver, 38% of portal tracts may not contain a portal vein; 9% may not contain a hepatic artery; and 7% may not contain a bile duct. Hepatic arteries and bile ducts almost always travel together as a pair, and the external diameter of the paired structures are comparable. Given the more variable presence of portal veins, portal dyads (hepatic artery:bile duct) are almost as common as portal triads in normal peripheral liver tissue. These numbers reflect the variable anatomy of the terminal ramifications of the portal tree.

The amount of connective tissue and the size of intraportal structures depend on the size of the portal tracts. Pathological processes do not necessarily affect large and small portal tracts to the same extent. Portal tracts normally contain a few lymphocytes, macrophages, and mast cells but do not contain neutrophils or plasma cells. The number of inflammatory cells increases with age and typically varies from one portal tract to another.

The larger intrahepatic or septal bile ducts are lined by tall columnar epithelial cells, and the smaller or interlobular bile ducts are lined by cuboidal or low columnar epithelium. Larger bile ducts have more periductal fibrous tissue than smaller ones. Sizeable bile ducts are often seen in subcapsular liver parenchyma in liver biopsies. Bile ductules are variably located at the peripheral zone of the portal tracts, and they are smaller than interlobular bile ducts. They have a basement membrane and are lined by cuboidal cholangiocytes. These ductules are the connecting conduit between the interlobular bile ducts and canals of Hering, which reside at the portal tract:parenchyma interface and penetrate a short distance into the parenchyma. The bile canalicular channels that course between hepatocytes drain into canals of Hering and thence into the formal biliary tree. Bile canaliculi are not readily recognized microscopically unless

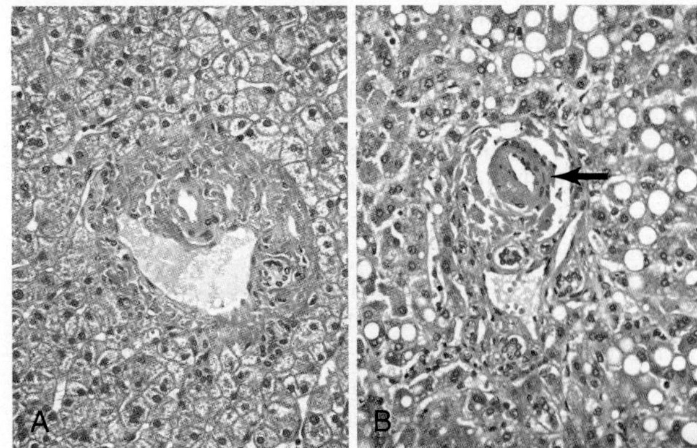

FIGURE 44.7 In older individuals, the portal tracts may contain dense collagen **(A)**, and the hepatic artery may have a thickened wall (**B**, *arrow*).

distended, as in parenchymal cholestasis. Bile ductules and canals of Hering are thought to represent the progenitor cell compartment of the liver.[46] With hepatocellular injury, particularly at the portal tract interface, this progenitor compartment becomes highly replicative, termed "ductular reaction."[47]

Lymphatic channels are not evident in the normal portal tract but may become visible in fibrotic and cirrhotic livers owing to increased lymphatic flow. The meticulous work of Franklin Mall more than a century ago identified interstitial spaces in portal tract stroma of the liver, which were continuous between periarterial, perivenular, and periductal compartments (the "space of Mall").[48] Cenaj et al. have recently demonstrated that this fluid-filled interstitium is indeed a unified network that is in continuity with the vascular (ingress) and lymphatic (egress) fluid systems in the liver.[49]

There are several changes in the liver related to aging, particularly in individuals older than 60 years (Fig. 44.7). There is more variation in the size of hepatocytes and the number of their nuclei (i.e., polyploidy) and an increase in lipofuscin pigment deposition. There may be apparent dilation of sinusoids because of hepatocyte cord atrophy. The portal tracts may contain denser collagen and may contain an increased quantity of mononuclear inflammatory cells. The hepatic arteries may have thickened walls, even in normotensive individuals. These changes are accompanied by alterations in the metabolic function of the liver, including the metabolism of various toxins and drugs.[50]

Interpretation of Liver Biopsies

Histological examination of liver biopsies should conform to a specific routine and include inspection of all tissue fragments and structures of the liver (i.e., architecture, portal tracts, parenchyma, and terminal hepatic veins). A systematic approach ensures that important diagnostic findings are not overlooked, including specific attention to the vasculature, biliary tree, hepatocytes and sinusoids, stroma, and inflammation. A sensible approach is to begin the examination with a low scan magnification to appreciate the lobular architecture, the presence and quantity of the various anatomic structures of the liver, and the presence or absence of normal structures or focal changes. At low magnification, the type and location of inflammation and steatosis can be well appreciated. This should be followed by a careful examination of portal tracts and its anatomic structures, zones 1, 2, and 3 of the acinus and specifically evaluating the presence or absence of hepatocellular steatosis, necrosis, apoptosis, cholestasis, ballooning degeneration, Mallory-Denk bodies, and pigments. The pattern of inflammation must be explicitly observed, including the presence or absence of granulomas. Specific histopathological changes may be easily recognizable, but it is often the cumulative topographical and morphologic relationships of the structures of the liver determined by systematic examination that contribute to a clinically meaningful interpretation.

Two schools of thought pertain to whether the initial histological examination of a liver biopsy specimen is better conducted without knowledge of the clinical and laboratory information, so that observations are unbiased; or with such knowledge, so that the initial histological examination is informed by searching for pertinent positive and negative findings. Regardless, once the morphological changes are appreciated and a generalized pattern of injury has been ascertained, a differential diagnosis can be rendered in combination with the clinical and laboratory information. Clinical information and laboratory data should always be reviewed before submitting a final interpretation, because more often than not, this information is essential in narrowing the differential diagnosis to a specific cause. Moreover, multiple injurious processes may be simultaneously operative, or acute injury from one cause may be superimposed on chronic injury from the same or another cause. The pathologist must consider multiple potential causes of injury, in the context of clinical and laboratory data, so as to avoid being erroneously simplistic in interpretation of the morphological findings.

The liver tends to react similarly to a broad range of injuries. In most instances, the needle biopsy is fairly representative unless portal tracts are underrepresented in a shorter needle core biopsy sample. However, a sampling error, particularly in focal or irregularly distributed disease processes, must always be taken into consideration. For example, in primary sclerosing cholangitis, the characteristic bile duct injury and periductal concentric fibrosis may not be uniformly seen throughout the liver or may not be present at all. All levels must be examined for morphological features, regardless of which histochemical stain and tinctural features any given level may have. Following portal tracts and terminal hepatic veins through these multiple levels may be highly informative. When searching for focal findings such as cytomegalovirus changes, it may be necessary to cut additional serial sections before the typical microabscesses are identified. Biopsy of space-occupying lesions may not show neoplastic cells in every section. In cirrhosis, a small-caliber needle biopsy may not obtain septal fibrosis and may yield only fragments of parenchyma without fibrosis or evident portal tract structures. This is to be distinguished from artefactual fragmentation of sampled tissue into smaller tissue fragments that may occur at the time of histological sectioning, and partial tears in the region of the terminal hepatic vein that may be observed.[45]

Innocent variations that should be considered to avoid erroneous interpretation are subcapsular liver parenchyma and surgery-associated changes. Needle biopsy of the immediate 2-mm subcapsular space often shows parenchyma that mimics cirrhosis (Fig. 44.8) and that may give a false impression of the status of the liver as a whole.[51] The liver capsule may be present in percutaneous liver biopsies at one end of the specimen or in the form of separate pieces of connective tissue. The capsule can be distinguished from most pathological fibrous tissue by its density and maturity, and it often contains blood vessels and bile ducts. Similar artifacts can be found in biopsy samples when the needle enters the liver at an angle close to the capsule or in a wedge biopsy that contains capsular fibrosis tissue on two surfaces.

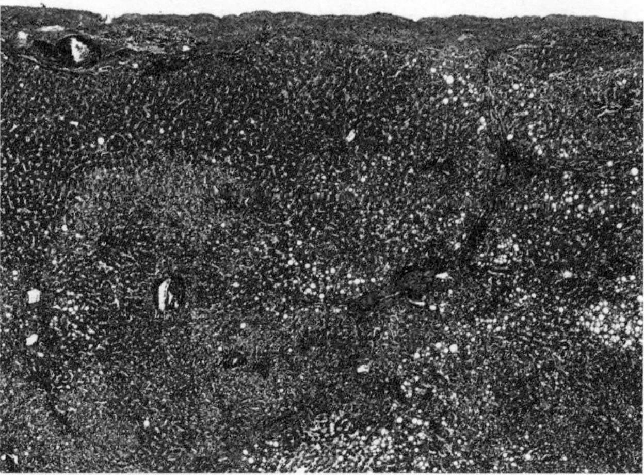

FIGURE 44.8 In the subcapsular liver parenchyma, the mature fibrous framework extends from the capsule (Masson trichrome stain).

In liver biopsy specimens obtained at the end of a long surgical procedure, surgery-associated changes are usually seen as small, tight clusters of neutrophils within or under the hepatic capsule, sinusoids around central venules, portal tracts, and hepatic plates, and they resemble microabscesses (Fig. 44.9).[52]

Other normal variations or innocent hepatic lesions include focal steatosis involving small groups of hepatocytes, fat granulomas from mineral oil deposition in perivenular areas and portal tracts, rare acidophilic bodies in an otherwise normal liver, and unexplained mitoses of hepatocytes that normally have a life span of many years. In biopsies of space-occupying lesions, nonspecific reactive changes also may be seen. These changes are important to observe in biopsies that do not include neoplastic tissue, a cyst, or an abscess. The histological changes, described by Gerber and coworkers as a *histological triad*, consist of a ductular reaction, portal tract edema, and sinusoidal dilation.[53] They may be subtle, are usually focal, and typically involve small portal tracts. These changes most likely occur as a result of local obstruction of blood and bile flow in the setting of an expanding lesion.

LIVER RESECTION SPECIMENS

Partial Hepatectomies

Partial liver resections are usually performed to remove focal lesions. The extent of resection varies from removal of small wedges of tissue to the removal of the entire lobe. In resection specimens, several surfaces may be covered

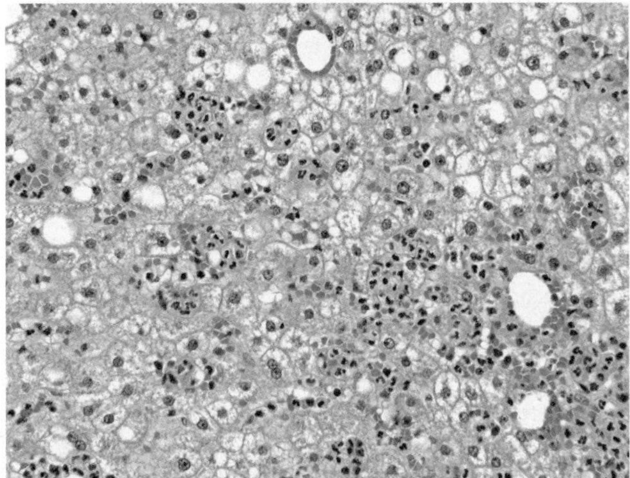

FIGURE 44.9 In intraoperative liver biopsy specimens obtained after a long procedure, clusters of neutrophils may be present (known as *surgical hepatitis*).

by the hepatic capsule. The surface that is not invested by Glisson capsule is the surgical margin and may be designated by the surgeon with different colors of ink or stitches, especially when the lesion is close to a particular margin of concern. After the margin is identified and the specimen is oriented, the specimen should be weighed and measured in each dimension. Often, a bulge in the surface of the liver or retraction of the capsule can help to localize an intraparenchymal mass.

The characteristics of the lesions and of the surrounding liver parenchyma should be described. The presence or absence of involved resection margins, significant fibrosis of the liver parenchyma, or cirrhosis is observed. The specimen should be serially sectioned at 0.5- to 1-cm intervals, with the initial section passing through the center of the tumor to demonstrate the closest approach of the mass to the resection margin. Specimen photographs and representative sections may be taken. Fresh tissue or tissue in fixatives other than formalin should be submitted for additional tests when applicable.

Liver Explants

Explanted livers should be examined carefully and photographed. Careful attention must be given to identifying and examining portal hilar structures for patency of the hepatic artery, portal vein, and bile duct. After the gross examination, several sections from the hilum should be obtained in a plane perpendicular to the long axis of the major hilar structures at 4- to 6-mm intervals, including sections near the margin and the point where these structures branch into the right and left lobes of the liver. Lymph nodes in the hilar soft tissue also should be sampled for histological evaluation.

After the porta hepatis has been carefully examined and sampled, the entire liver parenchyma should be sectioned by using a long and sharp knife in a parallel plane at 0.5- to 1-cm intervals. Because formalin penetrates only superficially into the liver tissue, dissection and serial sectioning of the organ should be performed while the organ is fresh, preferably soon after receipt of the specimen in the dissection suite. Horizontal cross sections of the liver across each of the hepatic lobes reveal the openings of the hepatic veins, which should be carefully examined for patency. This systematic thin sectioning is necessary to avoid missing small hepatocellular carcinomas or dysplastic nodules. All distinct nodules and lesions should be sampled, being particularly attentive to nodules that bulge from the liver surface on sectioning. Routine sampling for histopathology consists of three to five sections each from the right and the left lobes and one section from the caudate lobe. Key samples necessary for histological and special studies should be obtained immediately and immersed in formalin. The tissue slabs can then be fixed overnight in formalin before obtaining the more routine sections.

Photographing tissue slabs individually or serially, along with nodules or lesions, is recommended for all specimens. Proper documentation of the gross specimens is valuable for histological reconstruction and review during the pathology sign-out session. Gross characteristics of the nodules or lesions often correlate well with their key histological features.

ROUTINE AND SPECIAL STAINS

Routine use of H&E stain is the starting point for accurate histological diagnosis in almost all liver biopsy specimens. For assessment of "medical" conditions other than space-filling lesions, other histochemical stains are routinely requested. Table 44.3 lists frequently performed special stains that are helpful in the diagnosis of liver pathology. At a minimum, special stains for connective tissue are needed, such as Masson trichrome[54-56] (Fig. 44.10) or Sirius red[57] (Fig. 44.11) for assessing the overall pattern of fibrosis or the presence of cirrhosis. Additional connective tissue stains include the reticulin stain[58] (Fig. 44.12) for evaluation of the reticular extracellular matrix in the parenchyma and elastin stain (Fig. 44.13) for identification of elastin fibers. Other useful stains are Prussian Blue or Perls iron stain[59,60] (Fig. 44.14), PAS stain for glycogen[61] (Fig. 44.15), PAS-D stain for α_1-antitrypsin[62] (Fig. 44.16) and to identify parenchymal Kupffer cells and portal tract macrophages that are laden with cellular debris (Fig. 44.17), Victoria blue stain for hepatitis B surface antigen[63] (Fig. 44.18), Shikata orcein stain[64] for elastin fibers and copper-binding protein (Fig. 44.19), rhodanine stain[65] for copper (Fig. 44.20), bile stain (Fig. 44.21), and phosphotungstic acid–hematoxylin (PTAH) stain (Fig. 44.22).

IMMUNOHISTOCHEMISTRY

Immunohistochemical staining methods are used in hepatic pathology for several purposes: (1) localization of viral antigens, (2) identification and classification of tumors, (3) determination of prognostic factors in malignant tumors, (4) lymphoma and leukemia immunophenotyping, (5) identification of bile duct epithelium, and (6) assessment of architectural changes. Table 44.4 summarizes the common immunohistochemical stains used for liver pathology diagnosis.[66-99]

Fixation in formalin may reduce the availability of antigen binding sites. When fixed specimens are not embedded in paraffin immediately, they may be stored in 70% alcohol.

TABLE 44.3 Frequently Performed Special Stains in Liver Pathology

Special Stains	Fixatives	Interpretation
Connective and Muscle Tissues		
Masson trichrome	10% NBF	Type I collagen = dark blue; type III, IV (reticular) collagen = light blue. Muscle, keratin, cytoplasm, megamitochondria = red; Mallory-Denk hyalin = red
Sirius red	10% NBF	Type I collagen = red; Mallory-Denk hyalin = greenish orange
Gordon and Sweet reticulin	10% NBF	Type I collagen = pink-brown; type III/IV (reticular) collagen = black
PTAH	10% NBF	Fibrin, nuclei, cytoplasm, mitotic figures, mitochondria = blue; collagen = red
Microorganisms		
Ziehl-Neelsen	10% NBF or Helly fluid	Mycobacterium, lipofuscin, ceroid = red; background = light blue
Shikata orcein	10% NBF	Elastic fibers, hepatitis B surface antigen, copper-binding protein = dark brown
Victoria blue	10% NBF	Elastic fibers, hepatitis B surface antigen, copper-binding protein, lipofuscin, mast cell = blue; cytoplasm, nuclei = red
Ammoniacal silver	10% NBF	Fungi, bacteria, mucin, glycogen, melanin = black; background = green
Pigments and Minerals		
Perls iron	10% NBF	Iron (ferric state) = blue
Hall bile	10% NBF	Bilirubin = green; muscle and cytoplasm = yellow; collagen = red
Rhodanine	10% NBF	Copper = reddish orange
Glycogen		
PAS	10% NBF, absolute alcohol, 10% formalin	Glycogen, fungi = magenta
PAS-D	10% NBF, absolute alcohol, 10% formalin	Glycoprotein, basement membrane, α_1-antitrypsin, atypical mycobacteria, ceroid laden macrophages = magenta; glycogen = digested, no magenta color
Amyloid		
Congo red	10% NBF, absolute alcohol	Amyloid = pink to red (and polarizable); nuclei = blue; elastic fiber = pink
Lipids		
Oil Red O	Frozen section fixed in 10% NBF; xylene processing must be avoided	Fat = red; nuclei = blue

NBF, *Neutral buffered formalin;* PAS, *periodic acid–Schiff;* PAS-D, *Periodic acid–Schiff with diastase digestion;* PTAH, *phosphotungstic acid hematoxylin.*

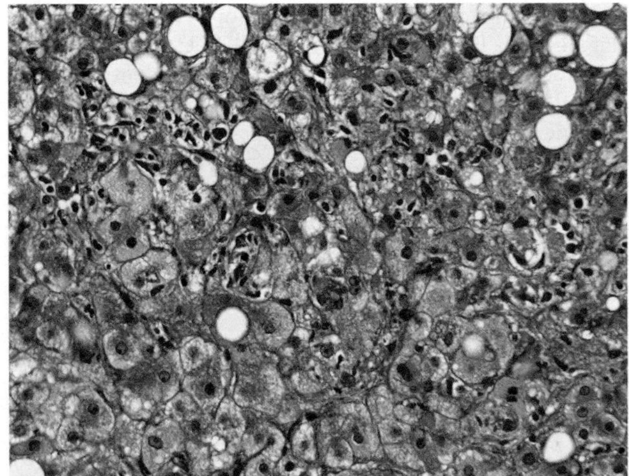

FIGURE 44.10 Masson trichrome stain demonstrates the pericellular "chicken wire" fibrosis in a patient with alcoholic liver disease.

FIGURE 44.11 Sirius red stain demonstrates fibrosis and collagen in red, showing evidence of delicate bridging fibrous septa formation in this liver.

Several modifications in staining procedures are available, but the most common are the peroxidase–antiperoxidase and avidin–biotin–peroxidase complex methods.[100] Liver tissue has significant amounts of endogenous biotin. When an avidin–biotin–peroxidase complex method is used, an augmented background reaction may yield a false-positive result. This can be avoided by applying avidin–biotin blocking reagents before incubating with the biotinylated antibody. Figures 44.23 through 44.32 provide examples of immunohistochemical staining.

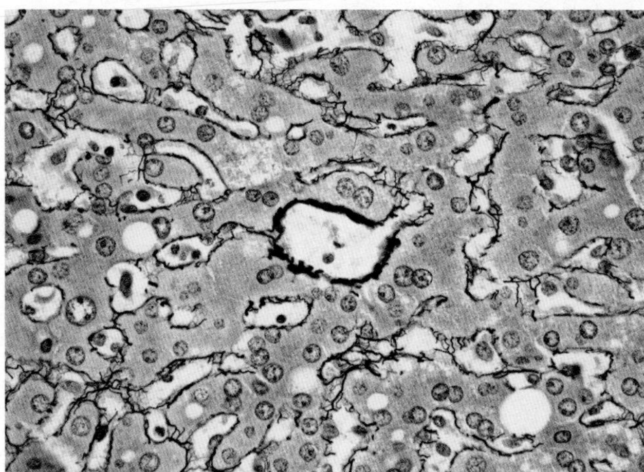

FIGURE 44.12 Reticulin stain of normal liver, showing a terminal hepatic vein with a single sinusoidal channel draining into the vein. The dark rim of extracellular matrix surrounding the vein contains type 1 collagen. The delicate reticulin fibers lining the sinusoids contain types 3 and 4 collagen.

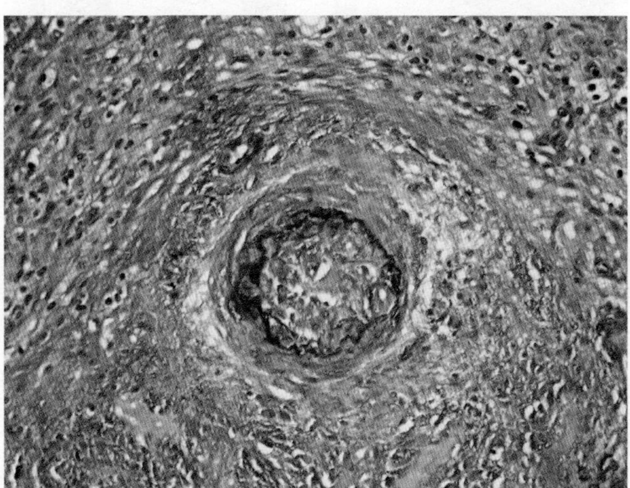

FIGURE 44.13 Elastin stain shows the elastin fibers of a hepatic artery, the lumen of which is obliterated by a thrombotic microangiopathy.

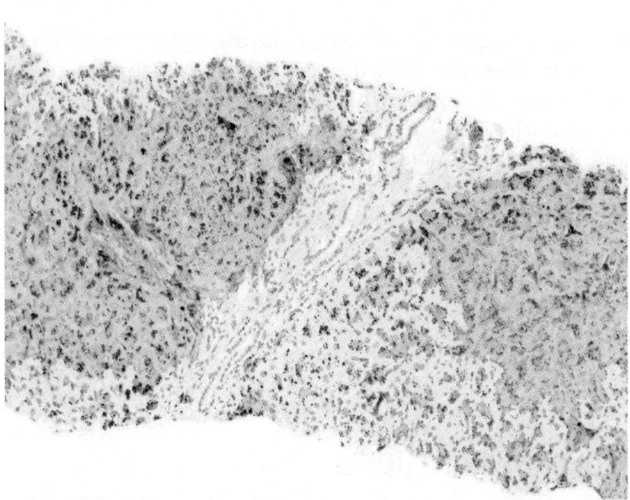

FIGURE 44.14 Perls (Prussian blue) iron stain shows coarse and fine iron granules in the hepatocytes of a cirrhotic liver in a patient with hereditary hemochromatosis. In the center of the image is a larger portal tract with fibrosis, cut in longitudinal section.

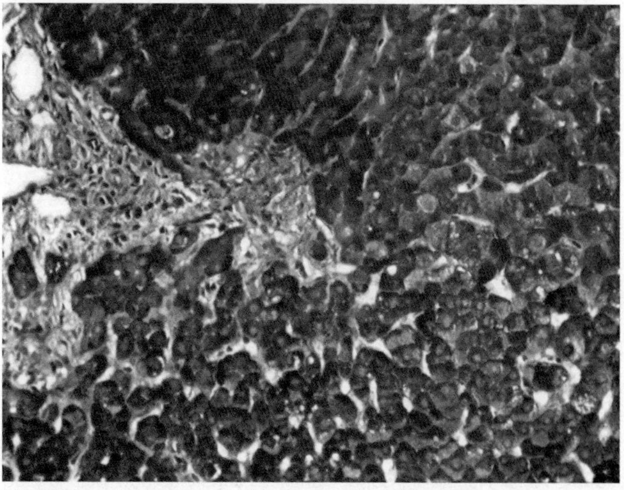

FIGURE 44.15 Glycogen in the cytoplasm of hepatocytes stains a magenta color after a periodic acid–Schiff (PAS) reaction.

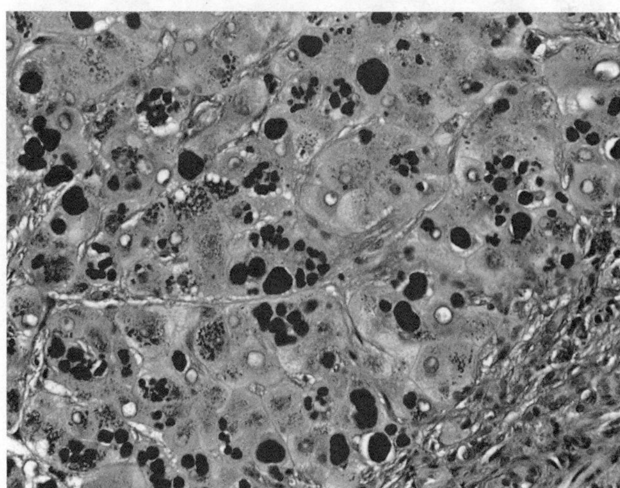

FIGURE 44.16 Diastase digestion abolishes hepatocellular glycogen; in this liver the periodic acid–Schiff–diastase (PAS-D) reaction reveals indigestible intracytoplasmic α_1-antitrypsin globules.

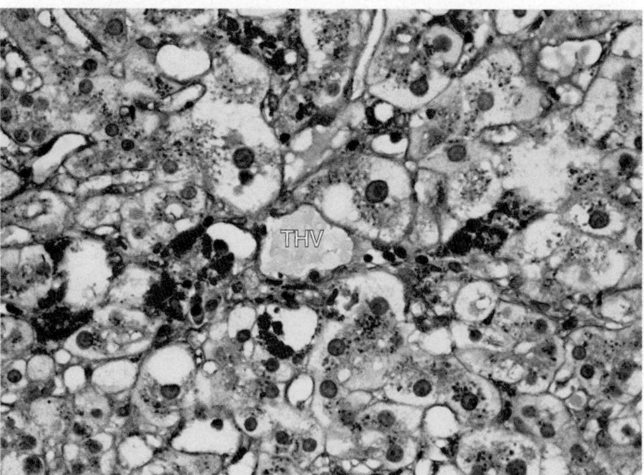

FIGURE 44.17 The periodic acid–Schiff–diastase (PAS-D) reaction also highlights Kupffer cells laden with indigestible cellular debris; in this image in the pericentral region of the lobule near a terminal hepatic vein (THV).

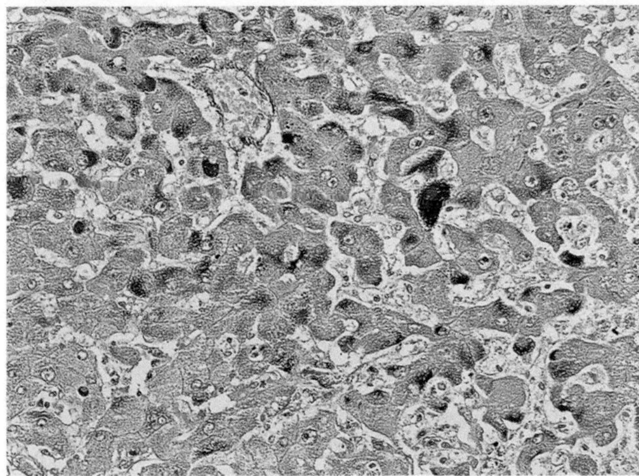

FIGURE 44.18 Hepatitis B surface antigen stains blue with Victoria blue stain.

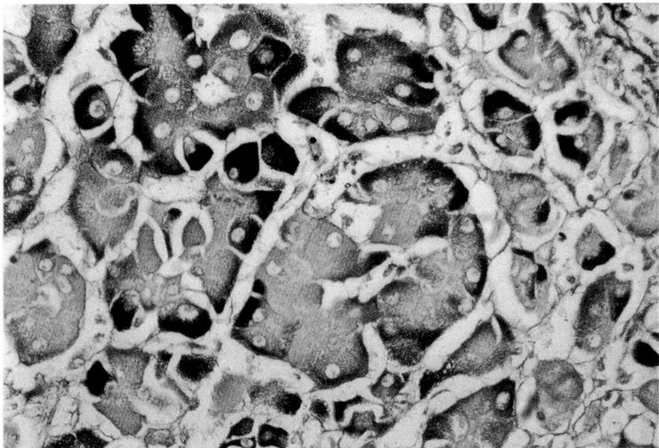

FIGURE 44.19 Hepatitis B surface antigen within ground-glass hepatocytes stains brown with Shikata orcein stain.

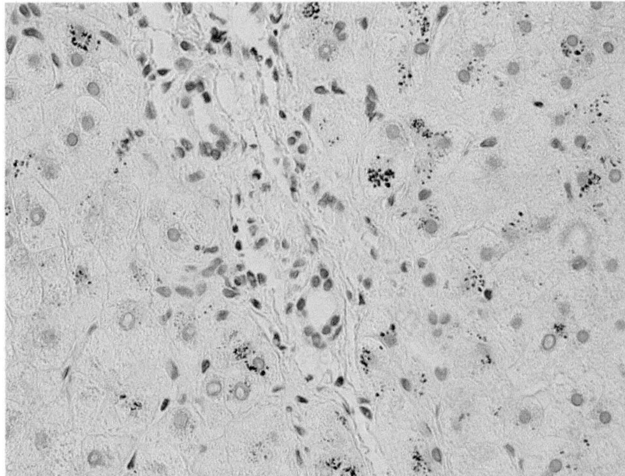

FIGURE 44.20 Orange copper granules in periportal hepatocytes are demonstrated by a rhodanine stain.

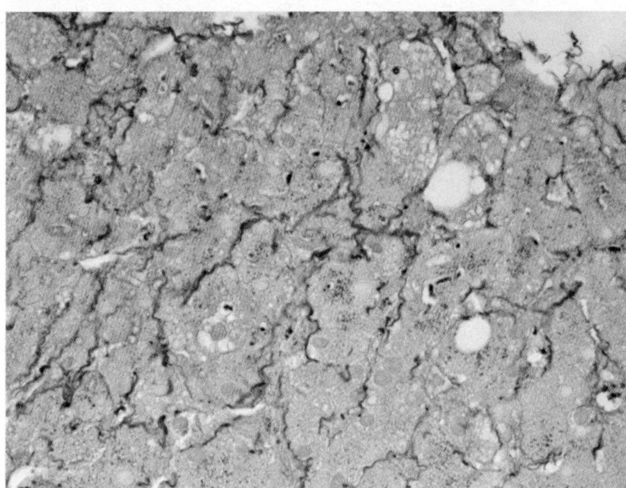

FIGURE 44.21 Green bile in the bile canaliculi of a cholestatic liver is demonstrated by bile stain.

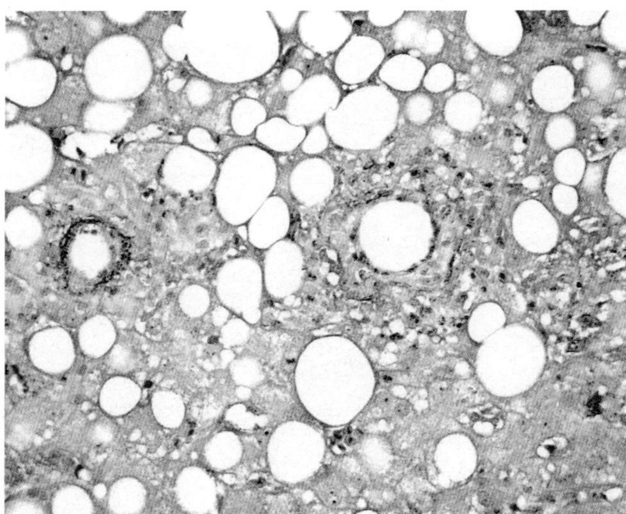

FIGURE 44.22 Fibrin ring granulomas in Q fever are demonstrated by phosphotungstic acid–hematoxylin (PTAH) stain.

ELECTRON MICROSCOPY

Electron microscopy is not routinely performed on liver specimens. However, it has a limited and well-defined role in liver pathology. Submitting tissue in 3% glutaraldehyde for electron microscopy should be considered when investigating genetic and metabolic diseases,[101] viral infection not otherwise identified by light microscopy or serology, tumors of unknown histogenesis, certain drug-induced liver injuries (e.g., amiodarone causing phospholipidosis), and diseases of unclear origin (Table 44.5).[102,103] For this purpose, small pieces as large as 5 mm in length from the liver core should be immersed immediately in ice-cold 3% glutaraldehyde. Reprocessing of formalin-fixed, paraffin-embedded tissue for ultrastructural examination, although not optimal, is often satisfactory, particularly for virus identification, as has been demonstrated recently for identification of SARS-CoV-2 viral particles in human liver.[104]

MOLECULAR STUDIES

Box 44.2 lists applications for molecular studies that are helpful in diagnosing liver diseases in the tissue-processing laboratory. Many of the routine molecular diagnostic applications associated with liver disease are geared toward

TABLE 44.4 Common Immunohistochemical Stains in Liver Pathology

Immunohistochemical Stains	Interpretation
Detection of Viral Antigens	
Hepatitis B surface antigen (HBsAg) and hepatitis B core antigen (HBcAg)	Confirmation of hepatitis B infection and evaluation of status of hepatitis B virus (HBV) replication (HBcAg), especially in combined hepatitis viral infections. Visual aid for identification of ground-glass hepatocytes (HBsAg). Cytoplasmic and membranous HBcAg positivity indicates high levels of viral replication and corresponds to a high level of disease activity.[66,67]
Hepatitis delta (D) virus (HDV)	Confirmation of HDV coinfection or superinfection in HBV-infected patients[68]
Nonhepatotropic viruses (cytomegalovirus [CMV], herpes simplex, Epstein-Barr virus [EBV], adenovirus)	Identification of liver involvement by nonhepatotropic viruses, particularly in immunosuppressed patients and infants[69-71]
Hepatitis C virus	No reliable immunohistochemical stain available
Identification and Classification of Tumors	
Hepatocyte paraffin 1 (Hep Par 1) antigen (carbamoyl phosphate synthase 1); Arginase-1	Hepatocellular differentiation[72-74]
α-Fetoprotein (AFP)	Positive in approximately 40% of hepatocellular carcinomas (HCCs) and in all hepatoblastomas and fetal livers. Hepatocytes in cirrhotic nodules occasionally may show focal positive staining.[75]
Polyclonal carcinoembryonic antigen (pCEA)	Bile canaliculi staining or canalicular differentiation in HCC. Cytoplasmic and membranous staining in adenocarcinoma[76]
CD10, villin	Bile canaliculi staining or canalicular differentiation in HCC[77,78]
Glypican 3	Positive in HCC and negative in nonneoplastic hepatocytes or benign hepatocellular lesions.[79] May be positive in melanoma. Positivity for glypican 3, glutamine synthetase, and heat shock protein 70 distinguishes early HCC from dysplastic nodule.[80]
Glutamine synthetase	Diffusely positive in hepatocellular adenoma and carcinoma, maplike pattern of staining in focal nodular hyperplasia, and positive in centrilobular hepatocytes of normal hepatic parenchyma[81]
Monoclonal carcinoembryonic antigen (mCEA)	Negative in HCC.[78] Positive in 60% of adenocarcinomas
MOC-31 monoclonal antibody	Negative in HCC.[78] Positive in 80% of adenocarcinomas
Cytokeratins (CKs)	Coordinate CK7/CK20 staining is commonly used; both usually are negative in HCC. Hepatocytes are positive for CK8 and CK18.[82] CK7 and CK19 are positive in the presence of cholangiocellular differentiation, either in cholangiocarcinoma or combined HCC-cholangiocarcinoma.
Thyroid transcription factor 1 (TTF-1)	Cytoplasmic staining may indicate hepatocellular differentiation.[83]
Epithelial membrane antigen (EMA)	Negative in HCC. Positive in adenocarcinoma[84]
Factor VIII–related antigen; CD31 and CD34	Vascular tumors.[85] Sinusoidal endothelial cells are positive in immediate periportal sinusoids and negative in the rest of sinusoids in normal liver. Sinusoidal endothelial cells are positive in chronic liver diseases with fibrosis, cirrhosis, and HCC.
Organ-specific antigens	TTF-1 (nuclear staining), gross cystic disease fluid protein 15 (GCDFP-15 or BRST-2), prostate-specific antigen (PSA), estrogen, and progesterone receptors for metastatic lung, breast, prostatic, renal cell carcinoma, and others
Epithelial cell adhesion molecule (EPCAM), CD56	Identification of biliary differentiation in combined or mixed hepatocellular-cholangiocarcinoma[84,86]
Serum amyloid A2 (SAA2)	Positive in inflammatory hepatocellular adenoma and negative in focal nodular hyperplasia[87]
CD68	Positive in fibrolamellar carcinoma but not in the usual HCC[88]
Identification of Bile Duct Epithelium	
Cytokeratin 7 or 19	Identification of bile ducts and ductules. Useful to visualize bile ducts to rule out vanishing bile duct syndrome or chronic ductopenic rejection. Confirmation of the degree of bile ductular reaction in biliary diseases,[89] or loss of biliary elements in bile duct destructive diseases[90]
Prognostic Factors	
Cytokeratin 19	Identification of hepatocellular carcinoma with aggressive behavior or high degree of recurrence[91]
AFP, Ki-67, or proliferating cell nuclear antigen (PCNA)	Differentiation of HCC from high-grade dysplastic nodule or hepatocellular adenoma[92,93]
Smooth muscle actin	Identification of neovascularization in HCC[94]
β-Catenin	Nuclear positivity in HCC and a subset of hepatocellular adenoma with high risk of transformation to HCC[95]

TABLE 44.4 Common Immunohistochemical Stains in Liver Pathology—cont'd

Immunohistochemical Stains	Interpretation
Storage and Hereditary Diseases	
α_1-Antitrypsin	Predominantly periportal intracytoplasmic globules in α_1-antitrypsin deficiency
Fibrinogen	Intracytoplasmic fibrinogen deposition in fibrinogen storage disease
Miscellaneous	
Leukemia or leukemia phenotyping	Differentiating or confirming posttransplantation lymphoproliferative disease (PTLD) from EBV hepatitis or acute rejection[96]
Cytokeratins 8, 18, and 19	Embryonal hepatocytes; expression of CK19 disappears by 10th week of gestation.
Synaptophysin, glial fibrillary acidic protein, and neural cell adhesion molecule	Neural or neuroectodermal differentiation markers can be used to identify resting hepatic stellate cells.[97]
Ubiquitin, cytokeratin 8 and 18, nucleoporin p62	Identification of Mallory-Denk hyalin[98,99]
Vimentin, desmin, and smooth muscle actin	Myofibroblastic differentiation in activated hepatic stellate cells (including vitamin A toxicity)[39,40]

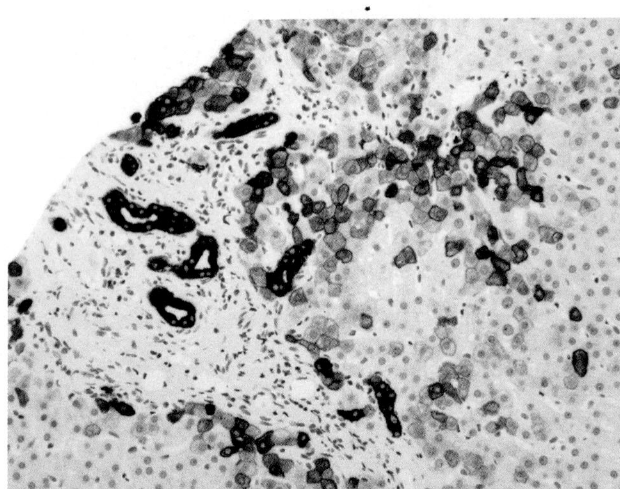

FIGURE 44.23 Bile ducts stained intensely for cytokeratin 7 (CK7). Periportal hepatocytes may also show metaplastic immunoreactivity for CK7, particularly in cholestatic liver disease.

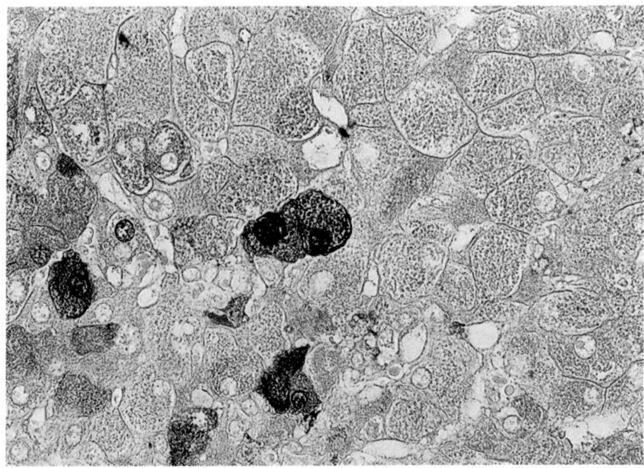

FIGURE 44.25 Immunoperoxidase stain shows nuclear and cytoplasmic hepatitis B core antigen (methylene blue counterstain).

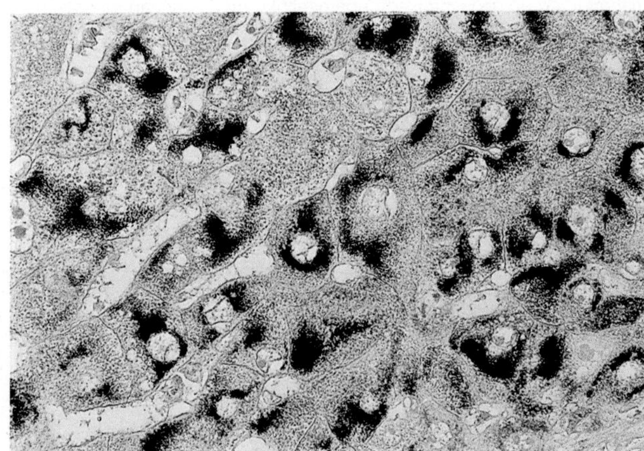

FIGURE 44.24 Immunoperoxidase stain shows hepatocytes positive for hepatitis B surface antigen (methylene blue counterstain).

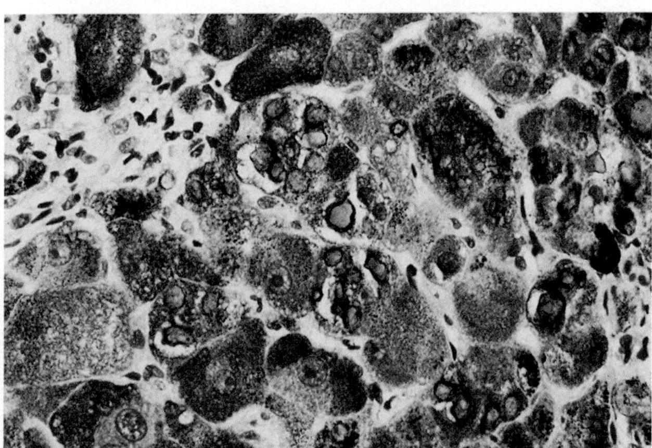

FIGURE 44.26 Hepatocytes filled with α_1-antitrypsin granules and globules in the liver of a patient with α_1-antitrypsin deficiency are shown (immunostain; counterstain with hematoxylin).

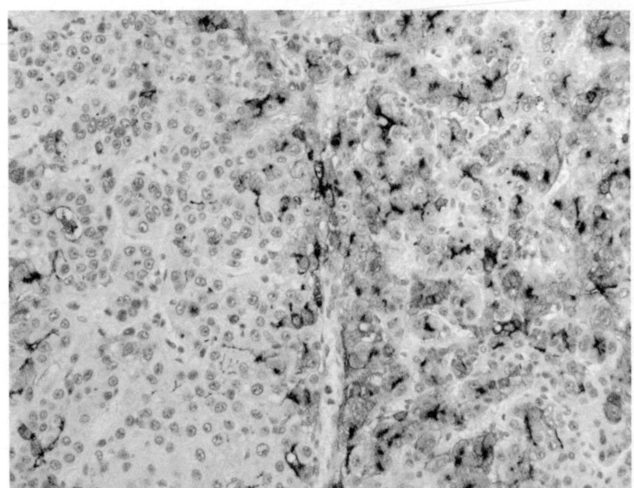

FIGURE 44.27 Canalicular pattern of carcinoembryonic antigen (CEA) staining is characteristic of hepatocellular carcinoma; more poorly differentiated regions may lose their CEA immunoreactivity *(left)*.

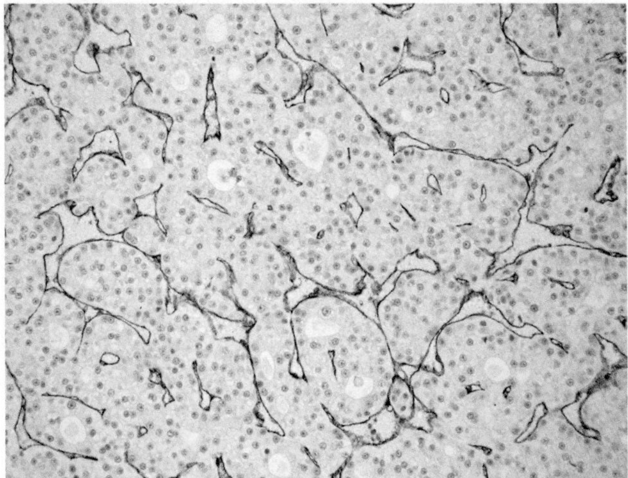

FIGURE 44.28 Thickened trabecular pattern of hepatocellular carcinoma is highlighted by CD31-positive endothelial cells.

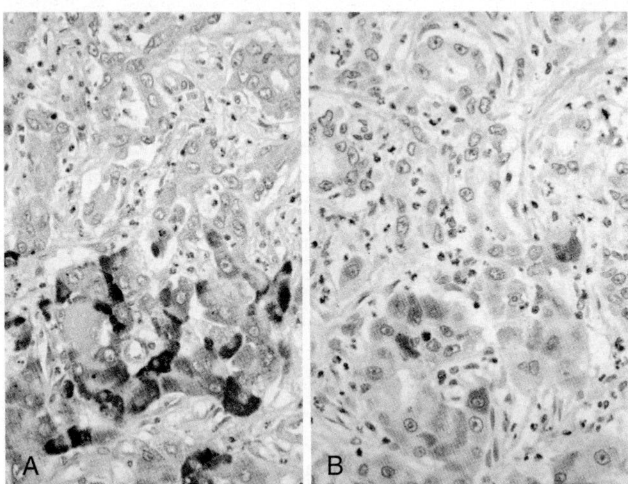

FIGURE 44.29 Hepatocyte paraffin 1 (Hep Par 1) antigen **(A)** and thyroid transcription factor 1 (TTF-1) **(B)** can be used to confirm hepatocellular differentiation. Both show similar patterns of cytoplasmic staining in mixed hepatocellular carcinoma and cholangiocarcinoma (immunostain; counterstain with hematoxylin).

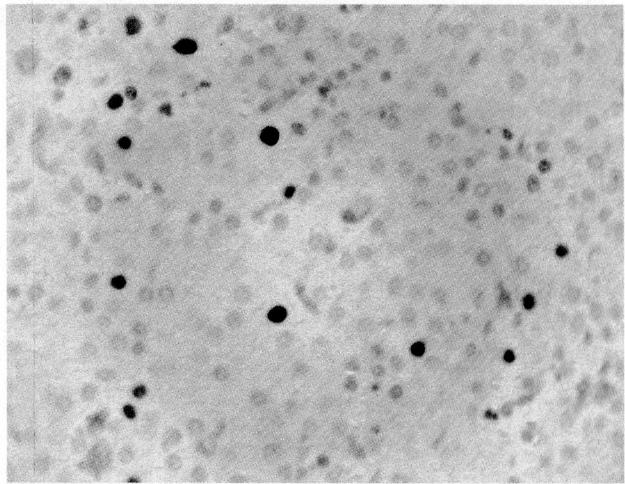

FIGURE 44.30 Ki-67 staining in nuclei of a well-differentiated hepatocellular carcinoma is used to assess the degree of tumor proliferation (immunostain; counterstain with hematoxylin).

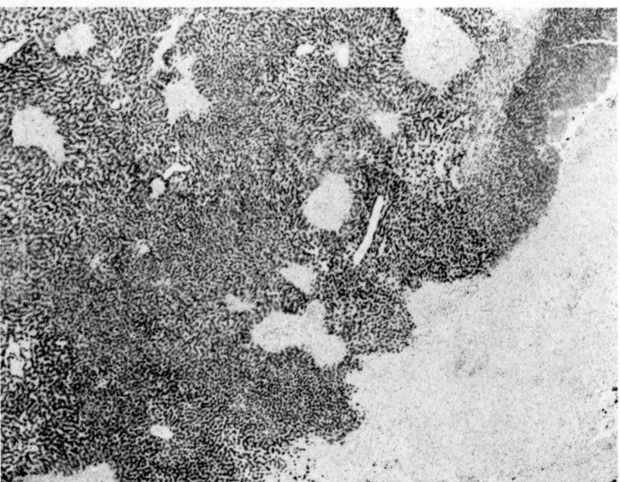

FIGURE 44.31 Inflammatory hepatocellular adenoma is positive for serum amyloid A but not in normal liver parenchyma *(right lower field)* (counterstain with hematoxylin).

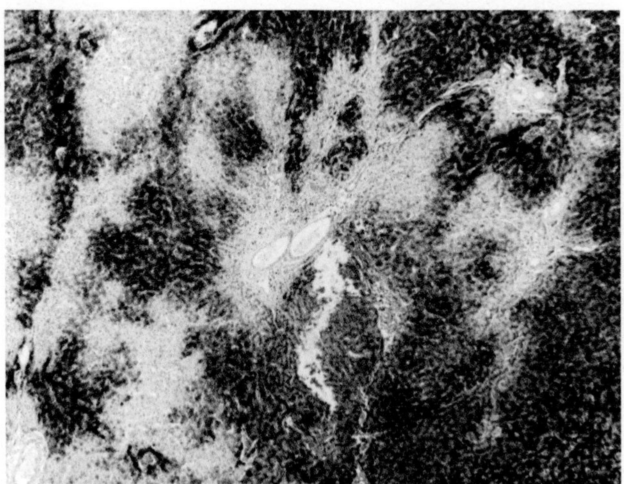

FIGURE 44.32 Glutamine synthetase immunostain shows a maplike pattern of staining of focal nodular hyperplasia.

TABLE 44.5 Electron Microscopy Findings in Liver Diseases

Indication	Interpretation
Establishment of Viral Infection	
Hepatitis B virus	Intranuclear core virus particles, dilated endoplasmic reticulum containing surface antigen
Suspected virus with no serological test or culture	Intranuclear or intracytoplasmic virions
Evaluation of Genetic and Metabolic Disease	
Glycogen storage disease, type II	Lysosome contains glycogen, cytoplasmic glycogen rosettes
Glycogen storage disease, type IV	Undulating, random, delicate fibril inclusions
Myoclonus epilepsy (Lafora disease)	Lafora bodies (fibrillar and granular material)
Hereditary fructose intolerance	Concentric and irregularly disposed membranous arrays and rarefaction of hyaloplasm
Mucopolysaccharidoses	Vacuolated lysosomes containing mucopolysaccharide in hepatocytes and Kupffer cells
Cystinosis	Spaces created by cystine crystals in Kupffer cells
Fibrinogen storage disease	Densely packed tubular structures in fingerprint-like pattern in rough endoplasmic reticulum
Wolman disease	Cholesterol crystals in cytoplasm of hepatocytes
Cholesterol ester storage disease	Triglyceride droplets in cytoplasm of hepatocytes
Gangliosidosis	Membrane bound vacuoles or inclusions
Fabry's disease	Dense and laminated inclusions in hepatocytes and Kupffer cells
Gaucher disease	Cytoplasmic tubular bodies (dense ring in cross section)
Niemann-Pick disease	Whorled lamellar lipid inclusions in lysosomes of hepatocytes and Kupffer cells
Mitochondrial disorders	Densely packed mitochondria separated by small lipid droplets
Dubin-Johnson syndrome	Complex dense bodies
α_1-Antitrypsin deficiency	Finely granular material in the cisternae of dilated endoplasmic reticulum
Wilson's disease	Variation of mitochondria, vacuolation, deposition of crystalline material
Examination of Tumor of Uncertain Histogenesis	
Sarcoma	Intermediate filaments: vimentin, actin
Neuroendocrine tumor	Neurosecretory granules
Melanoma	Melanosomes
Evaluation of Drug-Related Changes	
Phospholipidosis (e.g., amiodarone toxicity)	Enlarged lysosomes containing whorled lamellar and reticular inclusions resembling myelin, in hepatocytes, Kupffer cells, and biliary epithelial cells
Reye syndrome	Abnormal, swollen mitochondria
Hypervitaminosis A	Multivesicular stellate cells with fat droplets

assessment of viral targets such as hepatitis B and C viruses, including the qualitative and quantitative detection and genotyping of the virus. For neoplastic diseases, novel testing applications have been developed for establishing or confirming a diagnosis, molecular profiling and classification of tumors, and demonstrating the potential for response to targeted therapeutic options. In the last instance, analysis of formalin-fixed, paraffin-embedded tissue sections of both primary and metastatic hepatic tumors may provide valuable information regarding treatment response.[105,106]

In Situ Hybridization

For in situ hybridization, radioactively labeled probes for specific RNA or DNA sequences are applied and hybridized to a tissue frozen section. Treated slides are then exposed to photographic emulsion, resulting in distribution of silver grains over cells that contain the target RNA or DNA sequences. The sensitivity of in situ hybridization may be improved if combined with the polymerase chain reaction.

This method has been applied to liver tissue for identification of hepatitis A, B, C, and D viruses; cytomegalovirus; and Epstein-Barr virus (EBV). Most of these viruses, however, can be easily identified by immunohistochemistry, which has become a routine procedure in most laboratories and provides a degree of sensitivity that is similar to that of in situ hybridization.[96] In situ hybridization is particularly useful to detect EBV RNA in paraffin sections of liver with possible EBV hepatitis and to diagnose posttransplantation lymphoproliferative disease with the use of a fluorescein-conjugated peptide nucleic acid (PNA) probe. PNA is detected with an in situ hybridization kit (Dako, Carpinteria, CA).

In situ hybridization for albumin mRNA is highly specific for normal hepatocytes and hepatocellular tumors.[84,107] However, the use of immunohistochemistry to detect albumin

BOX 44.2 Molecular Studies

IN SITU HYBRIDIZATION

Detection of hepatotropic and nonhepatotropic viruses (e.g., HAV, HBV, HCV, HDV, CMV, EBV in PTLD)

Detection of albumin mRNA in hepatocellular tumors

POLYMERASE CHAIN REACTION

Detection and quantification of HBV DNA and HCV RNA level (including genotyping)

Detection of infectious microorganisms (e.g., viruses, bacteria, parasites)

Detection of genetic mutations (e.g., *HFE* in hereditary hemochromatosis, *MDR3* in cholestatic syndromes)

Detection of specific mutations in neoplastic diseases (e.g., microRNAs in hepatocellular carcinoma, *KRAS* or *BRAF* mutation)

LASER CAPTURE MICRODISSECTION

Provides well-defined target cells in inflammatory, infectious, or neoplastic diseases from formalin-fixed paraffin-embedded tissue for other molecular studies

GENE ARRAY ANALYSIS

Provides gene expression profiles for comparative studies of neoplastic and non-neoplastic liver disease (e.g., molecular profiling in carcinoma with an unknown primary)

CMV, *Cytomegalovirus;* EBV, *Epstein-Barr virus;* HAV, *hepatitis A virus;* HBV, *hepatitis B virus;* HCV, *hepatitis C virus;* HDV, *hepatitis D virus;* PTLD, *posttransplantation lymphoproliferative disorder.*

is not considered reliable, because its small molecular size and presence in extracellular fluid may result in its diffusion into the tissue when the tissue is not fixed immediately.

Polymerase Chain Reaction

The polymerase chain reaction can be applied to fresh, unfixed liver tissue, frozen tissue, or formalin-fixed tissue in paraffin.[108] It provides a sensitive diagnostic and research tool for viral, bacterial, parasitic, and genetic diseases. Polymerase chain reaction is the most sensitive and specific method to demonstrate hepatitis B virus DNA, hepatitis C virus RNA, and hepatitis C virus genotypes in liver tissue.

Laser Capture Microdissection

Laser capture microdissection provides well-defined targeted cell populations from formalin-fixed, paraffin-embedded tissue sections for other types of molecular studies, such as the polymerase chain reaction.[108,109]

Gene Array Analysis

Gene array analysis provides gene expression profiles that can be used for comparative studies. Preliminary data from gene array analyses have become available for a wide range of neoplastic and nonneoplastic liver diseases. These data can be used to correlate gene expression with cellular function, with phenotypic alterations in liver diseases, with predisposition or susceptibility to disease, and with therapy and prognosis. For example, deciphering the key host factors implicated in hepatitis C virus pathogenesis helped to improve antiviral therapy.[110] Gene array analysis has increased our understanding of the genetic predisposition for developing hepatocellular carcinoma in nonalcoholic steatohepatitis[111] and has increased our understanding of the mechanisms of hepatocarcinogenesis.[112]

PROGNOSTIC AND THERAPEUTIC INFORMATION FROM LIVER BIOPSIES

Although advances in immunological and serological markers, imaging studies, endoscopy, and molecular and genetic testing have diminished the need for liver biopsy in a variety of circumstances,[113] an accurate diagnosis of liver disease cannot always be made solely on the basis of clinical history, physical examination, laboratory findings, and imaging studies. The histological findings at biopsy support rigorous application of staging and grading systems, adding objectivity to pathology reporting and informing clinical decision-making. This is especially true for viral hepatitis[114-116] and nonalcoholic steatohepatitis.[117,118]

In patients with hereditary hemochromatosis, liver biopsy offers important prognostic information when the stage of the disease is unclear. It also aids in detecting comorbid conditions, such as nonalcoholic steatohepatitis, alcohol abuse, and chronic viral hepatitis. Significant fibrosis or cirrhosis in a patient with hemochromatosis substantially increases the risk of hepatocellular carcinoma,[119] and these patients should be screened periodically. Biopsy may confirm the diagnosis in atypical presentations, including those not associated with any of the classic hereditary hemochromatoses related to mutations of the *HFE* gene.[120]

Although biopsy is not absolutely necessary for the diagnosis of autoimmune hepatitis, it may help to confirm the diagnosis and stage,[121] and it can be used to evaluate the response to therapy. Improvement in the transaminase levels may not correlate with histopathological changes. A firm diagnosis is important because of the implications of long-term immunosuppression. Flare-ups during adequate immunosuppression should arouse suspicion of other disorders, which may be evident in the liver biopsy.

Refinements in imaging studies (specifically endoscopic retrograde cholangiopancreatography and magnetic resonance cholangiopancreatography) have decreased the value of liver biopsy for differentiating intrahepatic from extrahepatic cholestasis.[113] Nevertheless, biopsies in cases of chronic cholestatic diseases, such as primary biliary cholangitis and primary sclerosing cholangitis, are often necessary to assess the stage of disease. An adequate sample is necessary to avoid sampling error, because the pathological changes in the portal tracts are often unevenly distributed throughout the liver. Biopsies may also be helpful in assessing the response to therapy and in confirming the clinical evolution of disease.

Drug-induced liver injury may be clinically obvious when the suspected agent has a known toxicity. However, if the patient takes multiple medications, new medications, or medications without known hepatotoxicity, the liver function test results may be confusing. In these cases, liver biopsy can be helpful, especially if the drug-induced liver injury is superimposed on underlying liver disease of different origin. If a biopsy is considered for assessing drug or herbal hepatotoxicity, an early biopsy is preferred, because after the injury progresses, the risk of liver failure increases, and the histological features become less specific.

The value of serial biopsies to assess hepatotoxicity in patients receiving methotrexate remains controversial.[122] In retrospect, it has become clear that some of the pathological changes described in early studies were the result of chronic viral hepatitis, alcoholic liver disease, or nonalcoholic steatohepatitis.[123] Severe methotrexate-related liver disease is much less common than previously believed.[124]

For patients with acute liver failure, liver biopsy may be of value in identifying an etiology[125] and in assessing potential imminent need for transplantation. However, the potential for sampling error in such patients may limit the prognostic value of liver biopsy.[126] For patients with end-stage decompensated cirrhosis, a liver biopsy is not normally necessary, because knowing the cause rarely affects the need for transplantation. Liver biopsy is less often performed after liver transplantation because of improvements in immunosuppressive medications. However, biopsies are important to evaluate abnormal liver test results for transplant recipients, which can have many causes (see Chapter 53).[127]

For space-occupying lesions, biopsies are performed to distinguish primary from metastatic liver tumors and to demonstrate the potential for a therapeutic response. When patients with cirrhosis are found to have an elevated α-fetoprotein level and a hypervascular tumor on imaging, a liver biopsy is not needed to confirm the presence of hepatocellular carcinoma.[128] Nevertheless, FNA biopsy of hepatocellular carcinoma is often performed for confirmation and to help refine the treatment protocol. As noted earlier, in metastatic diseases (e.g., metastatic colon carcinoma), genomic testing may be of critical value in identifying target genes for drug therapy.

The full reference list may be accessed online at Elsevier eBooks for Practicing Clinicians.

CHAPTER 45

Molecular Pathogenesis and Diagnostics of Hepatocellular Tumors

Prodromos Hytiroglou, Paulette Bioulac-Sage

Contents

INTRODUCTION

Identification of the molecular pathways altered in benign and malignant hepatocellular tumors has significantly increased our understanding of hepatocellular tumorigenesis. The immunohistochemical markers derived from these molecular alterations have been useful in clinical pathology practice, contributing to accurate diagnosis and classification of these tumors in resection and biopsy specimens.[1-3]

BENIGN HEPATOCELLULAR TUMORS

Hepatocellular adenoma (HCA) and focal nodular hyperplasia (FNH) are benign hepatocellular tumors. HCA is a hepatocytic neoplasm, whereas FNH, which is much more frequent, is a hyperplastic hepatocytic response caused by localized hepatic vascular abnormalities.

FNH and HCA occur most frequently in women of childbearing age; these tumors are much less common in men, children, and postmenopausal women.[4] Oral contraceptives are recognized as the main risk factor for HCA, whereas these agents are probably not etiologically implicated in FNH.[5] The epidemiology of HCA has changed in recent years because low-dose contraceptive pills cause fewer cases of HCA than the pills used in the past. However, obesity and the metabolic syndrome are more frequently encountered in women and men with HCA, particularly the inflammatory subtype.[6,7] HCAs also occur in the setting of metabolic disorders such as glycogenosis type 1 and 3,[8] galactosemia, tyrosinemia, and familial diabetes mellitus. Most cases of HCA occurring in men are associated with the administration of anabolic steroids to treat diseases or for bodybuilding.[9]

FNH lesions, especially when multiple, may be associated with hepatic vascular disorders, hemangiomas, and other tumors of the liver or other organs. FNH and HCA usually develop in livers that are otherwise histologically normal, sometimes steatotic,[10] or with features of vascular liver diseases.[11,12]

Focal Nodular Hyperplasia

Molecular Changes

The data regarding molecular aberrations in FNH are limited.[13] Analysis of clonality using the human androgen receptor assay demonstrated the polyclonal nature of the hepatocytes in 60% to 100% of cases.[13-18] Studies of chromosomal gains and losses using comparative genomic hybridization or allelotyping detected alterations in 14% to 50% of cases.[18-20] However, genetic analysis failed to identify somatic gene mutations in *CTNNB1* (which encodes β-catenin), *TP53* (tumor protein 53), *APC* (adenomatous polyposis coli protein), and *HNF1A* (hepatocyte nuclear factor 1α).[18,21,22]

The mRNA expression levels of two angiopoietin genes, *ANGPT1* and *ANGPT2*, involved in vascular maturation are altered in FNH, and the consistently increased ANGPT1/ANGPT2 ratio supports the role of a vascular trigger for this lesion.[18,23] Studies have identified overexpression of genes encoding proteins of the extracellular matrix and cell–matrix adhesion,[24] consistent with the finding of fibrosis in most cases of classic FNH. A twofold overexpression of the *TGFB1* gene was detected, and other key genes involved in the fibrogenesis pathway, such as *PDGFA* and *PDGFRB*, were found overexpressed in FNH. The finding of myofibroblasts expressing smooth muscle actin at the periphery and in the fibrotic areas of FNH is consistent with activation of the transforming growth factor-β (TGF-β) pathway in these cells. The *NTS* gene, which encodes neurotensin, is overexpressed in FNH, resulting in an increased ratio of *NTS* to *HAL*, a periportal area gene that encodes histidine ammonia lyase. This finding can discriminate FNH from other benign tumors.[24]

Alterations in the expression of physiologically zonated genes of the hepatic lobule have been detected in FNH.[24] Thirteen genes of the periportal areas were found to be downregulated, whereas six genes of the perivenous areas were upregulated, indicating altered zonation in FNH. One of the perivenous area genes, *GLUL*, which encodes glutamate-ammonia ligase, also known as glutamine synthetase (GS), is upregulated by β-catenin.[25] GLUL mRNA overexpression correlates with a slight but significant CTNNB1 mRNA overexpression in FNH compared with normal liver parenchyma; this upregulation of the β-catenin signaling pathway is restricted to areas surrounding the veins of FNH nodules and occurs in the absence of *CTNNB1*-activating mutations.

It has been suggested that increased arterial inflow in FNH may contribute to activation of the β-catenin pathway. However, the mechanism of β-catenin activation in FNH remains unresolved, because no alteration of the main known regulators of the WNT signaling pathway have been identified, including a lack of *AXIN1* and *APC* inactivating mutations.[21]

FNH-like nodules are lesions resembling FNH macroscopically and on imaging, but they occur in cirrhotic livers[26,27] or in the setting of vascular hepatic disorders such as Budd-Chiari's syndrome.[12,28,29] The gene expression profile of FNH-like nodules in cirrhosis is significantly different from that of classic FNH.[24] The nodules do not show β-catenin activation, and the β-catenin–induced perivenous genes are significantly downregulated compared with those of nontumorous liver and classic FNH. The periportally zonated genes are not differentially expressed compared with nontumorous liver as determined by quantitative reverse transcription–polymerase chain reaction (RT-PCR), and the NTS/HAL expression ratio is not increased, as observed in classic FNH.[24]

Molecular Diagnostics

As a consequence of the deregulation of the β-catenin pathway, overexpression of GS is heterogeneously distributed in the hepatocytes of the FNH nodules. This can be demonstrated with immunohistochemical techniques, as characteristic staining with relatively large areas anastomosed in "maplike" patterns (Fig. 45.1A,B). The GS-positive areas often predominate at the periphery of FNH, are often centered on veins, and are usually located at a distance from the fibrous bands.[30] This specific pattern of GS staining in FNH contrasts with that of normal liver, in which staining is restricted to a few rows of hepatocytes surrounding the terminal hepatic venules (Fig. 45.1A,C,D). Owing to the absence of β-catenin *(CTNNB1)* mutations, immunohistochemistry using a β-catenin antibody does not show abnormal cytoplasmic or nuclear β-catenin staining, even in hepatocytes overexpressing GS (see Fig. 45.1B, inset *a*). The characteristic GS immunostaining and the lack of aberrant β-catenin expression provide a useful tool for the diagnosis of some FNH lesions that lack typical histological features in surgical specimens or biopsies.[30-32]

As expected from their molecular changes, FNH-like nodules show little or no parenchymal GS immunostaining.[24] When present, GS staining is usually restricted to some persistent venous structures inside the nodules (see Fig. 45.1B, inset *b*). This staining pattern is similar to that of cirrhotic nodules and quite different from that of the large, anastomosing, GS-positive areas of classic FNH.

Hepatocellular Adenoma

HCAs are a heterogenous group of monoclonal tumors in which several recurrent mutations have been identified, leading to a classification based on good genotypic-phenotypic correlations with important consequences for patient management.[33-41] Hemorrhage (20% to 25%) and malignant transformation (4% to 8%) are observed mainly in HCA >5 cm. The risk of malignancy exists particularly for HCA with high activation of the β-catenin pathway, but this occurs rarely in other HCA subtypes (see later). Molecular changes and diagnostics are described for each HCA subtype.

Hepatocellular Adenoma with Inactivating Mutations of the HNF1A Gene

Molecular Changes

The *HNF1A* gene (formerly hepatic transcription factor 1 [*TCF1*]) is located on chromosome 12q24.2 and encodes the hepatocyte nuclear factor 1α protein (HNF1A), a 681-amino acid homeodomain transcription factor that is involved in hepatocyte differentiation.[42] *HNF1A* controls the expression of liver-specific genes, such as those for β-fibrinogen *(FGB)*, α_1-antitrypsin, and albumin *(ALB)*.[43] *HNF1A* is a human tumor suppressor gene involved in liver tumorigenesis.[44]

Biallelic inactivating *HNF1A* mutations have been detected in 30% to 35% of HCAs. In most cases, both mutations are of somatic origin, but in less than 10% of cases, one mutation is germline and the other somatic. Sporadic HNF1A-inactivated HCAs (H-HCAs) with somatic mutations occur almost exclusively in women and usually are associated with oral contraception. Patients with heterozygous germline *HNF1A* mutations are younger than those with somatic mutations, are either male or female, and frequently have a family history of liver adenomatosis or diabetes (usually maturity-onset diabetes of the young type 3 [MODY3]), which is a consequence of heterozygous germline *HNF1A* mutations.[45] The spectrum of *HNF1A* somatic mutations in H-HCA differs significantly from the germline changes in MODY3.[46]

Transcriptomic analysis showed that several metabolic pathways are altered in sporadic H-HCA, including neoglycogenesis repression, glycolysis, and fatty acid synthesis activation.[43] The induction of glycolysis and lipogenesis in H-HCA is linked to HNF1A inactivation and is independent of the activation of sterol regulatory element–binding protein 1 (SREBP1) and MLX interacting protein-like (formerly called carbohydrate response element–binding protein [ChREBP]), leading to the characteristic steatotic phenotype of these tumors. Genes for fatty acid binding protein 1 *(FABP1)* and UDP glucuronosyltransferase 2-B7 *(UGT2B7)* are positively regulated by *HNF1A* and are downregulated in H-HCA.[33,34]

Heterozygous, germline, inactivating mutations of *CYP1B1* have been detected in 15% of women with H-HCA, suggesting that deregulation of the enzyme, which is responsible for the formation of genotoxic metabolites of estrogens, may confer a predisposition to sporadic H-HCA in women. *CYP1B1* mutation modifies the penetrance of the liver adenomatosis phenotype in patients with *HNF1A* germline mutations.[47]

Molecular Diagnostics

Downregulation of the *FABP1* gene leads to a lack of liver-type fatty acid binding protein 1 (LFABP) expression in

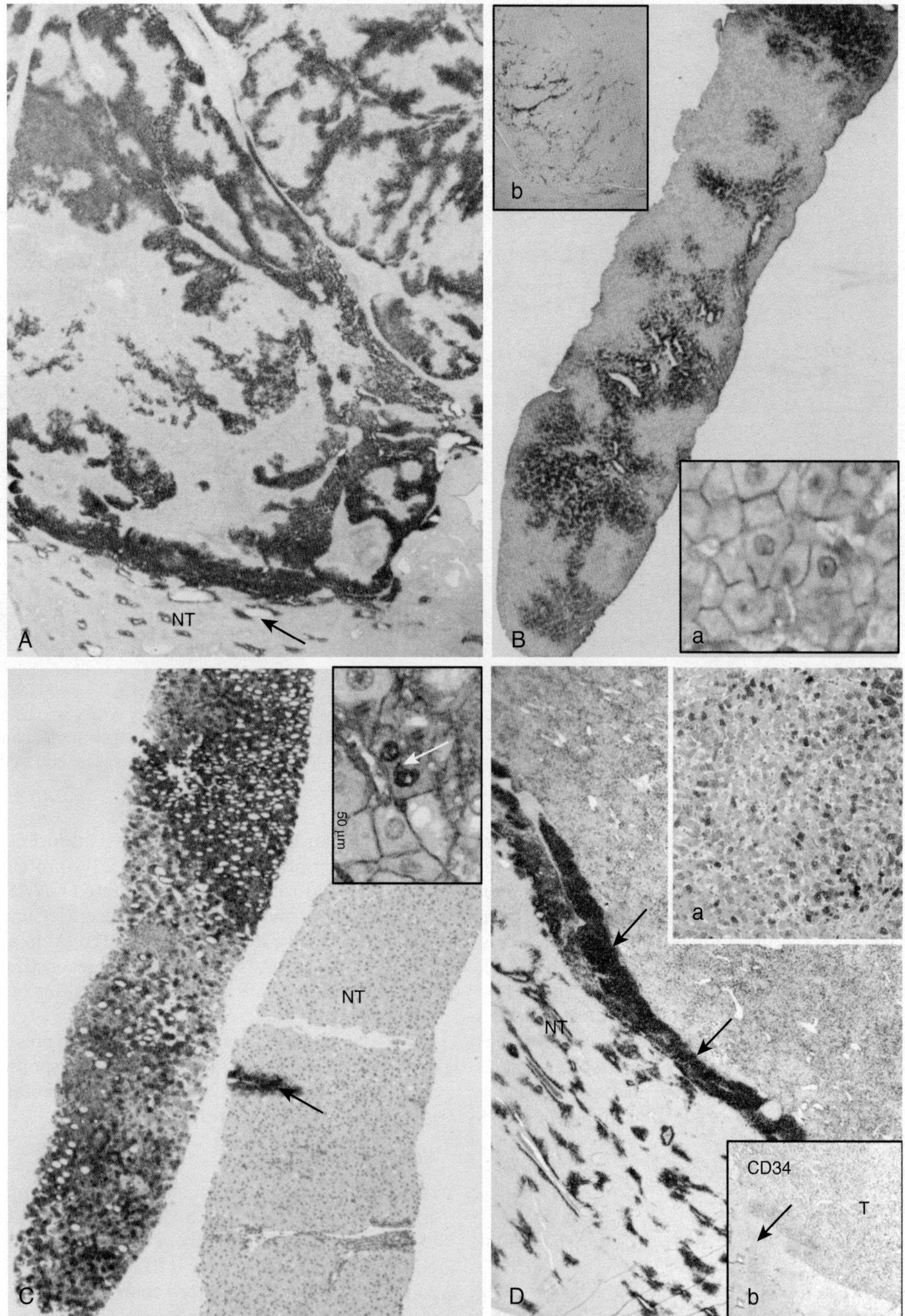

FIGURE 45.1 Characteristic patterns of glutamine synthetase (GS) immunostaining in focal nodular hyperplasia (FNH) **(A, B),** β-catenin–activated hepatocellular adenoma (HCA) **(C, D),** and nontumorous liver **(A, C, D)**. **A,B,** FNH. Large anastomosing GS-positive areas in a "map-like" pattern in resection specimen **(A)** and biopsy sample **(B),** contrasting with nontumorous liver *(NT),* where GS expression is restricted to a few rows of perivenular hepatocytes *(arrow). Inset a,* Normal membranous expression of β-catenin. *Inset b,* Little, nonspecific GS immunostaining in an FNH-like nodule occurring in vascular liver disease. **C,** b-HCA. Strong, diffuse expression of GS in a biopsy sample **(C)** and aberrant nuclear and cytoplasmic β-catenin staining *(inset, arrow),* characteristic of a high level of β-catenin pathway activation (deletions or mutations in exon 3 non S45). **D,** Heterogenous expression of GS in a resection specimen, "starry-sky" pattern *(inset a),* associated with a strong positive rim *(arrows)* adjacent to the nontumorous liver *(NT). Inset b,* CD34 is diffusely expressed in endothelial cells of the tumor *(T)* except at the rim, where GS is strongly expressed *(arrow).* These patterns are characteristic of b-HCA with exon 3 S45 mutation.

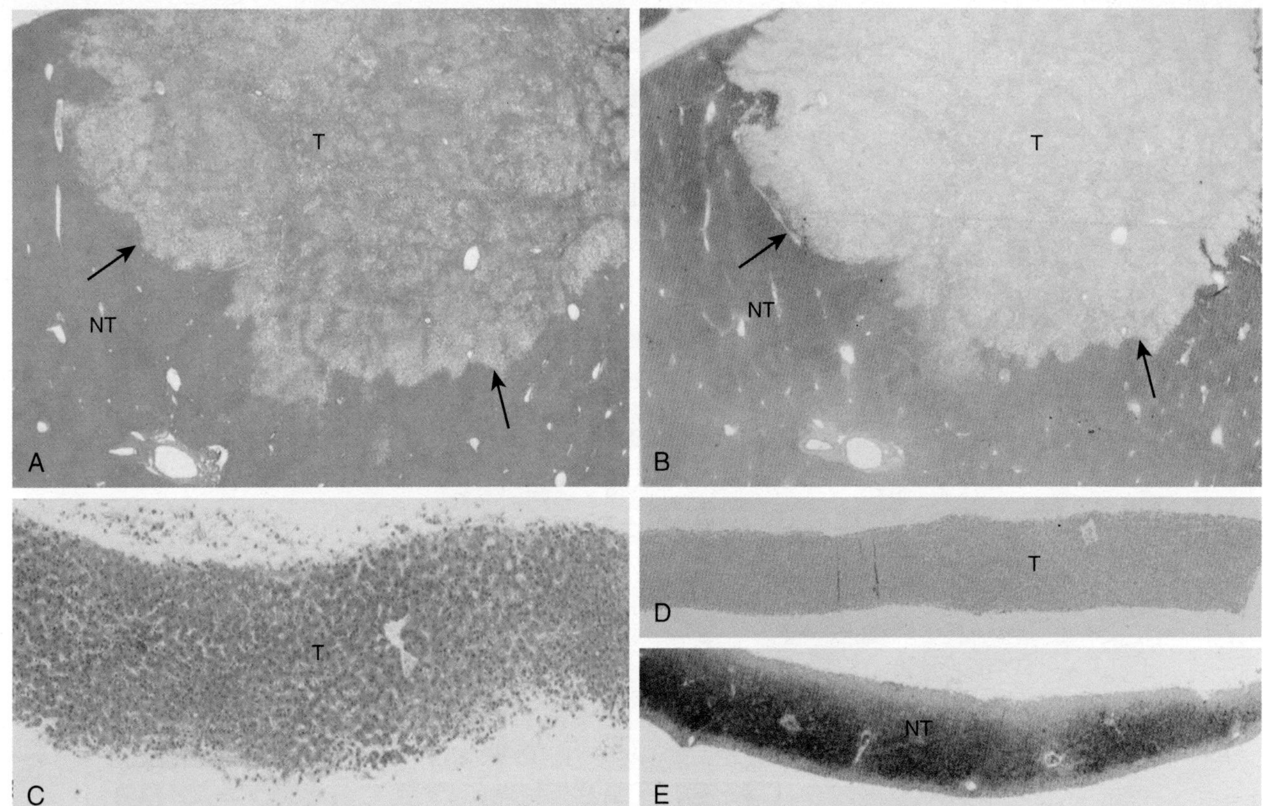

FIGURE 45.2 HNF1A-inactivated hepatocellular adenoma (H-HCA). A, C, Hematoxylin and eosin. **B, D, E,** Lack of liver-type fatty acid binding protein 1 (LFABP) immunostaining. **A, B,** Resection specimen. The steatotic tumor *(T)* has lobulated contours *(arrows)*. **C-E,** Biopsy sample of another nonsteatotic H-HCA. Lack of LFABP staining in *T* contrasted with normal expression in adjacent nontumorous liver *(NT)* in resected **(B)** as well as biopsy **(D, E)** samples.

H-HCA, contrasting with normal expression in the surrounding nontumorous liver as demonstrated by immunohistochemistry.[34] In addition to steatosis, which is common in H-HCA cases, the absence of LFABP expression is an excellent marker for the diagnosis of this subtype of adenoma in resection specimens and biopsy samples (Fig. 45.2), irrespective of the degree of steatosis or size of the lesion. This feature also allows the diagnosis of HNF1A-inactivated adenomatosis to be made when multiple HCAs of various sizes are found throughout the liver. They are often associated with myriad steatotic microadenomas, which can be correctly identified by the lack of LFABP staining.[34,45]

Inflammatory Hepatocellular Adenoma

Molecular Changes

Inflammatory hepatocellular adenomas (IHCAs) account for 35% to 40% of HCAs.

They are characterized by recurrent somatic activating mutations in various genes involved in the IL6/JAK/STAT3 pathway.[48] Approximately 60% of IHCAs have gain-of-function mutations (small, in-frame, somatic deletions) in the interleukin-6 signal transducer gene *(IL6ST)*, causing permanent activation of the IL6/JAK/STAT pathway independent of the ligand. The *IL6ST* gene encodes the signaling coreceptor glycoprotein 130 (GP130), and mutant GP130 constitutively activates STAT3 signaling in the absence of IL6 binding.

In IHCA subsets lacking GP130 mutations, other activating mutations have been identified: *FRK* (10%) coding for an src kinase, *STAT3* (signal transducer and activator of transcription 3, 5%), *GNAS* (G-protein α-subunit gene, 5%), and *JAK1* (2%).[49-51] Mutated *GNAS* is found in various tumors and is known to cause McCune-Albright's syndrome. Finally, less than 20% of IHCA do not have yet identified mutations for explaining the constitutive activation of the IL6/JAK/STAT pathway resulting in the inflammatory phenotype.

All IHCAs are characterized by overexpression of molecules of the acute-phase inflammatory response, including serum amyloid A2 (SAA2) and C-reactive protein (CRP), at the mRNA and protein levels.[34]

Molecular Diagnostics

Positive immunohistochemical staining for inflammation-associated proteins (i.e., SAA and CRP) in tumor cells with a sharp demarcation from the surrounding nontumorous liver is characteristic of IHCAs (Fig. 45.3).[34,38-41] SAA and CRP staining is restricted to hepatocytes, without any staining of the sinusoidal lining and inflammatory cells (see Fig. 45.3E)

Hepatocellular Adenoma with Activating Mutations of the CTNNB1 Gene

Molecular Changes

Approximately 10% of HCAs demonstrate activating mutations of the *CTNNB1* gene encoding β-catenin (b-HCA); in addition, a percentage of IHCAs (corresponding to

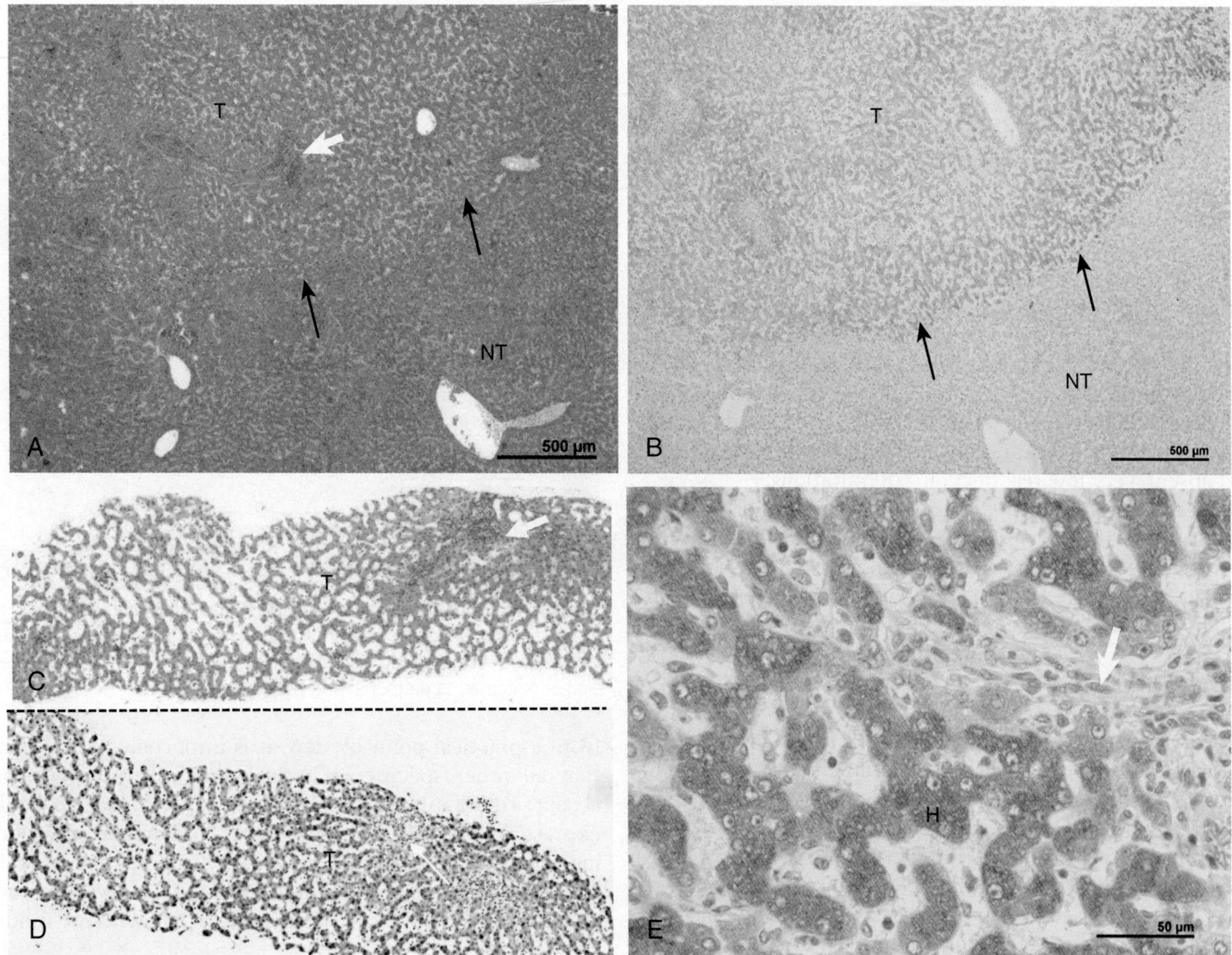

FIGURE 45.3 Inflammatory hepatocellular adenoma (IHCA). Resection specimen **(A, B)** and biopsy sample **(C-E)** of the same IHCA (performed several months before resection). The tumor *(T)* exhibits sinusoidal dilatation and inflammatory infiltrates *(white arrows)*. The contour *(arrows)* of the resected tumor is ill defined on hematoxylin and eosin **(A)** but well limited on C-reactive protein (CRP) immunostaining **(B)**. Overexpression of CRP **(B, D, E)** is restricted to tumor hepatocytes *(H)*, which contrasts with adjacent nontumorous liver *(NT)*.

10% to 15% of HCAs) harbor also mutations of *CTNNB1* leading to activation of the Wnt signaling pathway associated to the inflammatory pathway (b-IHCA). Many malignant tumors, including hepatocellular carcinoma (HCC), can be also β-catenin mutated (see later).

At baseline, β-catenin is associated with a negative regulator complex in the cytoplasm that includes APC, AXIN1, and GSK3B (glycogen synthase kinase 3β) proteins. This complex phosphorylates β-catenin, leading to its cytoplasmic degradation by the proteasome machinery. *CTNNB1* alterations occur mainly in exon 3 and consist of point mutations or deletions that exclude the amino acids normally phosphorylated by GSK3B, leading to an absence of β-catenin phosphorylation and its permanent activation.[33] Unphosphorylated β-catenin is stabilized in the cytoplasm and translocates into the nucleus, promoting the transcription of a large number of genes involved in proliferation, metabolism, and hepatocyte functions.[52] Large deletions and most hot spot mutations occurring in exon 3 of the *CTNNB1* gene lead to high levels of β-catenin activation, whereas mutations in S45 hot spot of exon 3 and mutations in exon 7/8 lead to moderate or weak activation of the pathway, respectively.[53] Activating β-catenin mutations lead to upregulation of two main β-catenin target genes: *GPR49* and *GLUL*, the latter encoding GS, which can be demonstrated by immunohistochemistry.

Molecular Diagnostics

As expected from the molecular changes, GS is overexpressed in β-catenin–activated hepatocellular adenomas (see Fig. 45.1C,D). The GS staining pattern varies according to the levels of β-catenin activation, predicting the types of *CTNNB1* alterations in b-HCA and b-IHCA. The strong and diffuse GS pattern is well correlated with point mutations and deletions in exon 3 non S45 (see Fig. 45.1C); an aberrant nuclear and cytoplasmic expression of β-catenin can be associated, but this staining is usually focal (see Fig. 45.1C, inset), or even absent. Overexpression of GS is easier to interpret than nuclear expression of β-catenin by immunohistochemistry, particularly in small biopsy samples.[32] When mutations occur in exon 3 S45, the GS staining pattern is heterogeneous ("starry-sky" pattern), of variable intensity (see Fig. 45.1D, inset), and occasionally associated with rare aberrant nuclear β-catenin expression. Most HCAs with mutations in exon 7/8 show a weak, patchy GS staining pattern, without any β-catenin nuclear staining. In addition, b-HCAs with mutations in exon 3 S45 or exon 7/8 usually show a strong rim of GS staining (see

Fig. 45.1D), of variable thickness; in these cases, CD34 is usually diffusely expressed in the tumor endothelial cells except at the rim, which separates the tumor from the surrounding nontumorous liver (see Fig. 45.1D, inset). Despite the variations of GS staining in b-HCA, the pattern is usually distinct from the characteristic map-like pattern of FNH (see Fig. 45.1A,B).

Identification of β-catenin–activated HCA is important, because this group of HCAs is more frequently associated with the development of HCC[33,53-56] than other HCA subtypes.[57] In routine practice, GS is a good surrogate marker to identify different types of *CTNNB1* mutations in HCA, in comparison with the molecular gold standard. This is particularly important for evaluation of the HCA malignancy risk, depending on the level of β-catenin activation: high risk in cases with exon 3 mutations (particularly if GS is strong) and absent/very low risk in exon 7/8 mutations.[53]

Because b-HCA can display cytoarchitectural atypias, it can be difficult to distinguish this tumor from well-differentiated HCC (see Chapter 56); the diagnostic difficulties have led to the use of different terms such as "borderline lesion" or "atypical hepatocellular neoplasm."[58,59] Cytogenetic and molecular changes, such as *TERT promoter* mutations, can be found in cases with malignant transformation.[58,59]

Immunopathological features of both IHCA and b-HCA characterize b-IHCAs that have the same risk of malignant transformation as b-HCA.

On the other hand, some HCCs demonstrate GP130-activating mutations of the *IL6ST* gene. These tumors arise in normal liver and accumulate β-catenin–activating mutations.[48] It is reasonable to hypothesize that these HCCs result from malignant transformation of HCAs. These data underline the role of inflammation in hepatic tumorigenesis and suggest that activation of the IL6/JAK/STAT pathway alone promotes benign tumorigenesis, whereas participation of β-catenin activation may lead to malignant transformation.

Hepatocellular Adenoma with Activation of the Sonic Hedgehog Pathway

Molecular Changes

This newly identified HCA subtype (previously included in the group of unclassified HCA [UHCA]) is characterized by activation of the sonic hedgehog pathway due to small somatic deletions of the inhibin beta E chain gene *(INHBE)* that fuse the promoter of *INHBE* with *GLI1*.[40] This subtype, named shHCA, has been characterized in parallel by proteomic analysis showing specific upregulation of the arginine synthesis pathway associated with overexpression of argininosuccinate synthase 1 (ASS1).[60] shHCAs represent 4% to 10% of HCA cases depending on the genetic or proteomic analyses utilized for their characterization respectively[40,60]; this HCA subtype is associated with a high risk of hemorrhage, even when nodules are small, and occurs mainly in obese women.

Molecular Diagnostics

Overexpression of ASS1 in the tumor is a good immunomarker for the diagnosis of this shHCA subtype, provided it is compared with the staining in the nontumorous liver, where ASS1 is expressed at a lower level, usually in periportal and periseptal areas, leading in typical cases to a characteristic "honeycomb" pattern[60] (Fig. 45.4). Furthermore,

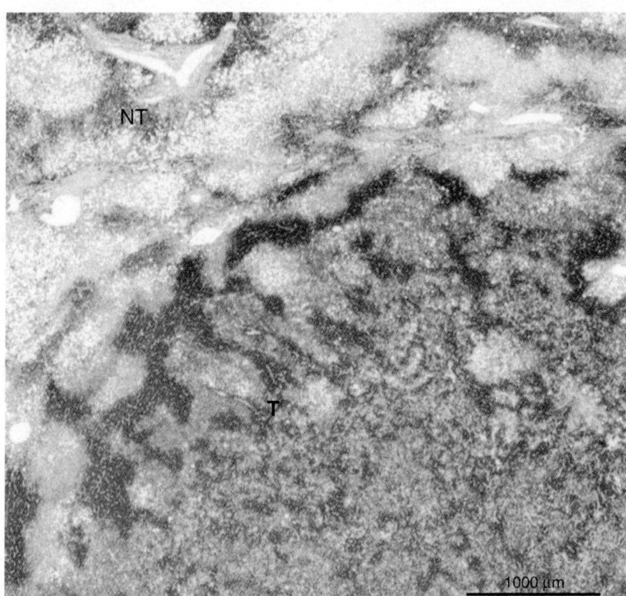

FIGURE 45.4 Sonic hedgehog hepatocellular adenoma (shHCA). The tumor *(T)* overexpresses argininosuccinate synthase 1 (ASS1), in comparison with the steatotic nontumorous liver *(NT)* where ASS1 expression is restricted to periportal and periseptal areas.

from a practical point of view, it is important to underline that all other specific HCA immunomarkers have to be absent, ruling out the other HCA subtypes, which could express ASS1 (but at a lower level than in the surrounding nontumorous liver (as shown by proteomic analysis).[60] The prostaglandin D2 synthase (PTGDS) has also been proposed to identify this new subgroup[40] but without validation for clinical practice.[61,62]

Unclassified Hepatocellular Adenomas

UHCAs account for fewer than 2% of HCA cases. By definition, they do not have *HNF1A* or *CTNNB1* gene mutations, they do not express inflammatory proteins encoded by different genes of the IL6/JAK/STAT pathway, and they do not overexpress ASS1 in the tumor in comparison with nontumorous liver. Therefore this very small number of tumors lacks the immunophenotypic features described for all the other HCA subtypes.

Use of Molecular Diagnostics

Molecular studies of FNH and HCA have significantly clarified the pathogenesis of these tumors and have provided immunohistochemical markers (i.e., LFABP, GS, β-catenin, SAA/CRP, ASS1) for routine diagnostic use. These biomarkers distinguish FNH from HCA and are used to classify HCAs (Table 45.1). An important contribution of these scientific advances was the reclassification of telangiectatic FNH as IHCA.[18,63]

Standard microscopic features (see Chapter 56) often allow accurate differentiation, but because of the significant clinical and prognostic differences among the HCA subtypes, immunophenotyping is considered mandatory to ascertain the subtype in each case and may become an important tool for HCA management in the near future.[64]

In difficult cases, molecular characterization (performed on frozen or formalin-fixed, paraffin embedded tissue)

TABLE 45.1 Genotypic and Immunophenotypic Characteristics of Benign Hepatocellular Tumors, in Comparison with Normal Liver

		Usual Characteristics of Immunohistochemical Markers				
Diagnosis	**Altered Genes**	**GS**	**β-Catenin**	**SAA/CRP**	**LFABP**	**ASS1‡**
Normal liver		+ In only a few rows of hepatocytes around central veins	–	–	+ Diffuse hepatocytic cytoplasmic staining	+ Periportal and periseptal staining
FNH	*CTNNB1* activation without mutations	+, "Maplike" pattern	–	–	+	–
H-HCA 30%-35%†	*HNF1A* biallelic inactivating mutations (90% somatic, 10% germline)	– ¶	–	–	–	–
IHCA 35%-40%†	*IL6ST/JAK/STAT* activation due to activating mutations: *IL6ST* (coding gp130 (60%), FRK (10%), *STAT3* (5%), GNAS (5%), JAK1 (3%), still unknown (20%)	– (Or a few positive hepatocytes around veins, mainly at the periphery)	–	+ Usually diffuse, sharp demarcation from NT	+	–
b-HCA 10%†	*CTNNB1* activating mutations/ deletions (different levels of β-catenin pathway activation according to the type of genetic abnormalities:	+		–	+	–
	-Exon 3 (non S45): high level	Strong/ diffuse	+, Nuclei			
	-Exon 3 S45: moderate to weak level	Heterogenous starry-sky pattern	Rare/absent			
	-Exon 7/8: weak level	Faint* +/– Perivascular staining	Absent			
b-IHCA 10%-15%†	Same as b-HCA and IHCA	Same as b-HCA	Same as b-HCA	Same as IHCA	+	–
shHCA 4%-10%† §	Activation of sonic hedgehog pathway due to small somatic deletions of *INHBE* leading to fusion of *INHBE* and *GLI1*	–¶	–	–	+	+ ‡
UHCA <2%†		–¶	–	–	+	–

FNH, *Focal nodular hyperplasia;* HCA, *hepatocellular adenoma;* H-HCA, *hepatocyte nuclear factor 1A–inactivated HCA;* IHCA, *inflammatory HCA;* b-HCA, *β-catenin–activated HCA;* b-IHCA, *β-catenin–activated inflammatory HCA;* shHCA: *sonic hedgehog HCA;* UHCA: *unclassified HCA;* CRP: *C-reactive protein;* GS: *glutamine synthetase;* LFABP: *liver fatty acid binding protein;* SAA: *serum amyloid A.*

+or –, presence or absence of characteristic features that help to ascertain the diagnosis.

**In S45 and 7/8 b-catenin -mutated HCA, there is usually a GS+ rim; in addition, CD34 is usually diffusely expressed in the tumor endothelial cells except in the rim.*

†Percentage of all HCA.

‡It is important to consider that it is an overexpression of ASS1 in the tumor in comparison with nontumorous liver; warning: ASS1 is not a specific marker; therefore in addition to ASS1 overexpression, all other HCA immunomarkers should be absent to make the diagnosis of shHCA.

§Depending on the genetic or proteomic analyses, respectively.

¶Except for some hepatocytes surrounding a few veins.

remains the gold standard, particularly to detect the different types of b-HCA/b-IHCA that have a higher risk of HCC transformation.

HEPATOCELLULAR CARCINOMA AND ITS PRECURSORS

HCC usually arises in a background of chronic liver disease. In autopsy series, 80% of HCCs are found in livers with cirrhosis[65]; most of the remaining cases arise in chronically diseased rather than normal livers. On a worldwide scale, infection with the hepatitis B virus (HBV) or the hepatitis C virus (HCV) and alcohol use are the most common risk factors.[66,67] In 2015, there were 854,000 incident cases of liver cancer and 810,000 deaths globally. Chronic HBV infection accounted for 265,000 liver cancer deaths (33%), alcohol abuse for 245,000 (30%), chronic HCV infection for 167,000 (21%), and other causes for 133,000 (16%).[67] Nonalcoholic fatty liver disease is now being recognized as a risk factor for HCC of increasing importance.[68] Other risk factors are listed in Box 45.1.

BOX 45.1 Risk Factors for Hepatocellular Carcinoma

Cirrhosis
Chronic hepatitis B
Chronic hepatitis C
Alcohol-induced liver disease
Nonalcoholic steatohepatitis
Diabetes, obesity, metabolic syndrome
Hereditary hemochromatosis
α_1-Antitrypsin deficiency
Hereditary tyrosinemia
Other (rare) metabolic disorders
Aflatoxin B1 exposure (associated with hepatitis B virus infection)
Tobacco smoking
Hepatocellular adenoma, mostly β-catenin–activated hepatocellular adenoma

The direct carcinogenic effects of HBV are illustrated by the fact that HCCs often develop in HBV-infected patients without cirrhosis, whereas HCCs in HCV-infected or alcoholic patients typically occur after cirrhosis is established. Among cirrhotic patients, the highest incidence of HCC is found for those with HCV infection (5-year cumulative incidence of 30% in Japan and 17% in the West), followed by those with hereditary hemochromatosis (5-year cumulative incidence of 21%), and those with HBV infection (5-year cumulative incidence of 15% in regions of high endemicity and 10% in the West).[69] Alcohol abuse appears to be the most common cause of HCC in Western countries, accounting for 32% to 45% of cases in the United States and Italy; the annual incidence of HCC in patients with decompensated alcohol-induced cirrhosis is approximately 1%.[70] HCC may occasionally arise in normal liver. Although some of these cases may be derived from HCA, mostly b-HCA and b-IHCA, recent molecular studies also suggest that some HCCs may be caused by adeno-associated virus type 2 through insertional mutagenesis.[71]

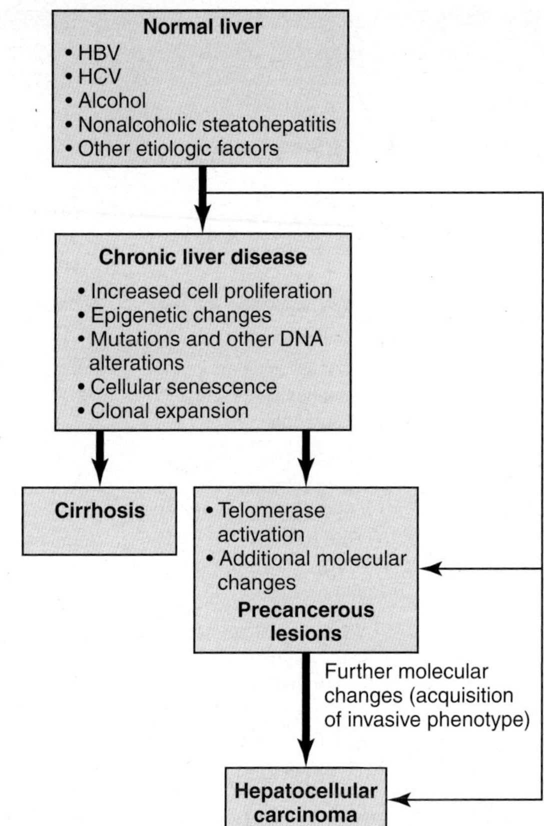

FIGURE 45.5 Hepatocarcinogenesis usually occurs in livers with chronic disease *(thick arrows)*, and most hepatocellular carcinomas emerge after cirrhosis becomes established. Dysplastic foci and dysplastic nodules are precancerous lesions detected in chronically diseased, usually cirrhotic livers. However, hepatocellular carcinoma occasionally arises in the absence of chronic liver disease *(thin arrows)*. Hepatocellular adenoma, especially β-catenin–activated hepatocellular adenoma, is a potential precursor lesion in this setting. *HBV*, Hepatitis B virus; *HCV*, hepatitis C virus.

Molecular Changes in Hepatocarcinogenesis

Many factors favor initiation of hepatocarcinogenesis in chronic liver diseases[72-77]:

- Increased hepatic cell proliferation due to hepatocyte loss
- Oxidative stress resulting from chronic inflammation (e.g., chronic viral hepatitis, steatohepatitis) or accumulation of noxious substances (e.g., hemochromatosis)
- Cellular senescence
- Deregulation of genes due to HBV DNA insertion into the host genome
- Overexpression of growth factors (e.g., TGF-α and insulin-like growth factor 2 [IGF2]) due to inflammatory cytokines and viral transactivation
- Derangements of DNA methyltransferases, causing global DNA hypomethylation and promoter hypermethylation, resulting in silencing of tumor suppressor genes

HBV DNA insertion causes genomic instability and deregulates genes involved in cell signaling and replication, such as human telomerase reverse transcriptase *(TERT)*, platelet-derived growth factor receptor *(PDGFR)*, mixed-lineage leukemia 4 (*MLL4*), cyclin E1 *(CCNE1)*, and calcium signaling–related genes.[78-80] In addition, the HBV X protein acts as an oncoprotein, transactivating various genes involved in signal transduction pathways and inhibiting expression of the tumor suppressor gene *TP53*. On the other hand, a specific *TP53* mutation in codon 249 is characteristic of aflatoxin B1 exposure.[81]

Due to vascular changes causing parenchymal loss in cirrhotic livers, the rate of hepatocyte loss and replication is often significantly enhanced compared with the precirrhotic stages of chronic liver diseases. Simultaneously, hepatocytes become senescent, and hepatic progenitor cells are activated to repopulate the dwindling parenchymal regions.[77,82] In the course of chronic liver diseases, clonal cell populations of increasing size are established,[83] some of which may accumulate genetic and epigenetic changes favoring neoplastic transformation (Fig. 45.5). Clonal cell populations with significant molecular alterations may be identified on microscopic examination as precancerous lesions. The cell of origin of these lesions may be the hepatocyte or the hepatic progenitor cell.[84] Molecular analysis of precancerous lesions and HCCs reveals a sharp increase in structural DNA changes compared with the surrounding hepatic parenchyma.[73]

The molecular changes occurring in HCCs are diverse and include point mutations, chromosomal amplifications and deletions, and epigenetic alterations. The most common cytogenetic abnormalities include gains of 8q and 1q and losses of 8p, 16q, and 17p.[85-87] The cancer-related genes have been identified and validated for several loci; examples include *MYC* (8q), hepatoma-derived growth factor (*HDGF*, 1q), *CCND1* and *FGF19* (11q), *MET* (7q), *RB1* (13q), *CDKN2A* (9p), and *TP53* (17q).[74,76,87] Whole exome and whole genome sequencing studies in HCC have demonstrated 40 to 60 somatic coding mutations per tumor, including 4 to 6 driver mutations.[88] Telomerase reverse transcriptase *(TERT)* promoter mutations have been identified as the most frequent recurrent somatic mutations in this neoplasm, occurring in 60% of cases.[89,90] TERT promoter mutations or other, less frequently occurring mechanisms, including *TERT* amplification, chromosomal rearrangements, and viral insertion into the *TERT* promoter, account for telomerase reactivation and neoplastic cell "immortalization" in up to 90% of HCCs.[91] TERT promoter mutations are considered early events in hepatocarcinogenesis because they have been detected in precancerous nodules and early HCC.[90] They have also been detected in HCCs arising within b-HCAs.[89] Other commonly mutated genes in HCC include *TP53* (12% to 48% of cases), *CTNNB1* (11% to 37%), *AXIN1*, *RB1*, *ARID1A*, *ARID2*, and *NFE2L2*.[87,92]

The molecular changes of hepatocarcinogenesis deregulate important signal transduction pathways. Commonly disrupted pathways include the cell cycle gene and p53 pathway, the WNT/β-catenin pathway, the epidermal growth factor (EGFR)/RAS/mitogen–activated protein kinase (MAPK) pathway, the hepatocyte growth factor (HGF) and IGF signaling cascades, the phosphatidylinositol-3 kinase (PI3K)/AKT/mammalian target of rapamycin (mTOR) pathway, as well as the vascular endothelial growth factor (VEGF) and PDGF signaling cascades.[76,88,93-97] Identification of genomic changes that can be targeted for treatment is a major task of current research. However, to date targeted therapies for HCC are limited to antiangiogenic agents, which have a small contribution to the improvement of prognosis.

Global genomic analysis has provided evidence that certain molecular changes are associated with clinicopathological features and prognosis, providing a basis for molecular classification of HCC. Lee and colleagues[98] identified a subtype of HCC with a poor prognosis that expressed a fetal hepatoblast gene signature, suggesting a progenitor cell origin. Boyault and associates suggested that HCC could be classified in 6 groups (G1 to G6).[99] The primary clinical determinant of group membership was HBV infection, and other major determinants included chromosomal instability (in G1, G2, and G3 tumors but not in G4, G5, and G6 tumors), *CTNNB1* or *TP53* mutations, and parental imprinting. Hoshida and coworkers[100] performed a meta-analysis of gene expression data from studies around the world and suggested that HCC could be grouped in three subclasses (S1, S2, and S3). S1 tumors were characterized by aberrant activation of the WNT/β-catenin pathway due to TGF-β stimulation, S2 tumors were characterized by *MYC* and *AKT* activation, and S3 tumors had gene expression patterns that suggested differentiated hepatocyte function. Nault and associates[101] identified a 5-gene score, based on the combined expression level of *HN1*, *RAN*, *RAMP3*, *KRT19*, and *TAF9*, which was associated with outcomes of patients with HCC treated by surgical resection.

A recent study of HCC from France[102] found that *CTNNB1* and *TP53* mutations are mutually exclusive and define two major groups of tumors characterized by distinct phenotypes: *CTNNB1* mutated tumors, which are large, well-differentiated, cholestatic, with microtrabecular and pseudoglandular patterns of growth, without inflammatory infiltrates, and *TP53* mutated tumors, which are poorly differentiated, with compact pattern of growth, multinucleated and pleomorphic cells, and vascular invasion (Fig. 45.6). *CTNNB1* and *TP53* were detected in 40% and 21% of the tumors examined, respectively. In the same study, characteristic molecular defects were found in two subtypes of HCC, including *TSC1/TSC2* mutations in the scirrhous subtype, and IL6/JAK/STAT pathway activation in the steatohepatitic subtype, while a novel HCC subtype with poor survival was identified. The latter was termed macrotrabecular-massive HCC, and was found to be characterized by *TP53* mutations and *FGF19* amplifications.[102]

Fibrolamellar carcinoma (FLC) is a rare HCC variant with characteristic morphological and immunohistochemical features, which usually occurs in children and young adults without underlying liver disease. FLC has recently been shown to also have a characteristic somatic gene fusion, *DNAJB1-PRKACA*, resulting from deletions on chromosome 19.[103] Increased production of the chimeric transcript is responsible for increased protein kinase A activity in this tumor. Fluorescent in situ hybridization (FISH) for the *PRKACA* rearrangement has been found to be a clinically useful tool to confirm the diagnosis of FLC with high sensitivity and specificity.[104]

Occasionally, hepatic carcinomas exhibit unequivocal morphological features of both hepatocytic and cholangiocytic differentiation. These neoplasms account for 2% to 5% of primary hepatic carcinomas and have been termed combined (or mixed) hepatocellular-cholangiocarcinomas (cHCC-CCAs).[3] The rarity of these tumors, the lack of a universally accepted terminology and classification systems, as well as sampling issues, have all impeded acquisition of adequate and clear molecular data. However, recent studies have provided evidence of a monoclonal origin of the two histological components of these tumors.[105-107] Furthermore, the relatively common development of cHCC-CCA features in HCCs of patients who have undergone transarterial chemoembolization is suggestive of neoplastic cell "plasticity" or "transdifferentiation" in the development of cHCC-CCA.[3,108] Joseph et al.[107] recently demonstrated that cHCC-CCA has a molecular profile similar to that of HCC, even in the CCA component, including recurrent alterations in TERT, *TP53*, cell cycle genes, receptor tyrosine kinase/Ras/PI3-kinase pathway genes, chromatin regulators, and Wnt pathway genes. Alterations of genes that are typically mutated in CCA were not detected in cHCC-CCAs, while TERT promoter mutations were consistently identified in both neoplastic components, incriminating TERT alteration as an early event in cHCC-CCA evolution.[107] Earlier, Moeini et al.[105] showed that cHCC-CCAs with stem cell features were characterized by spaltlike transcription factor 4 positivity, enrichment

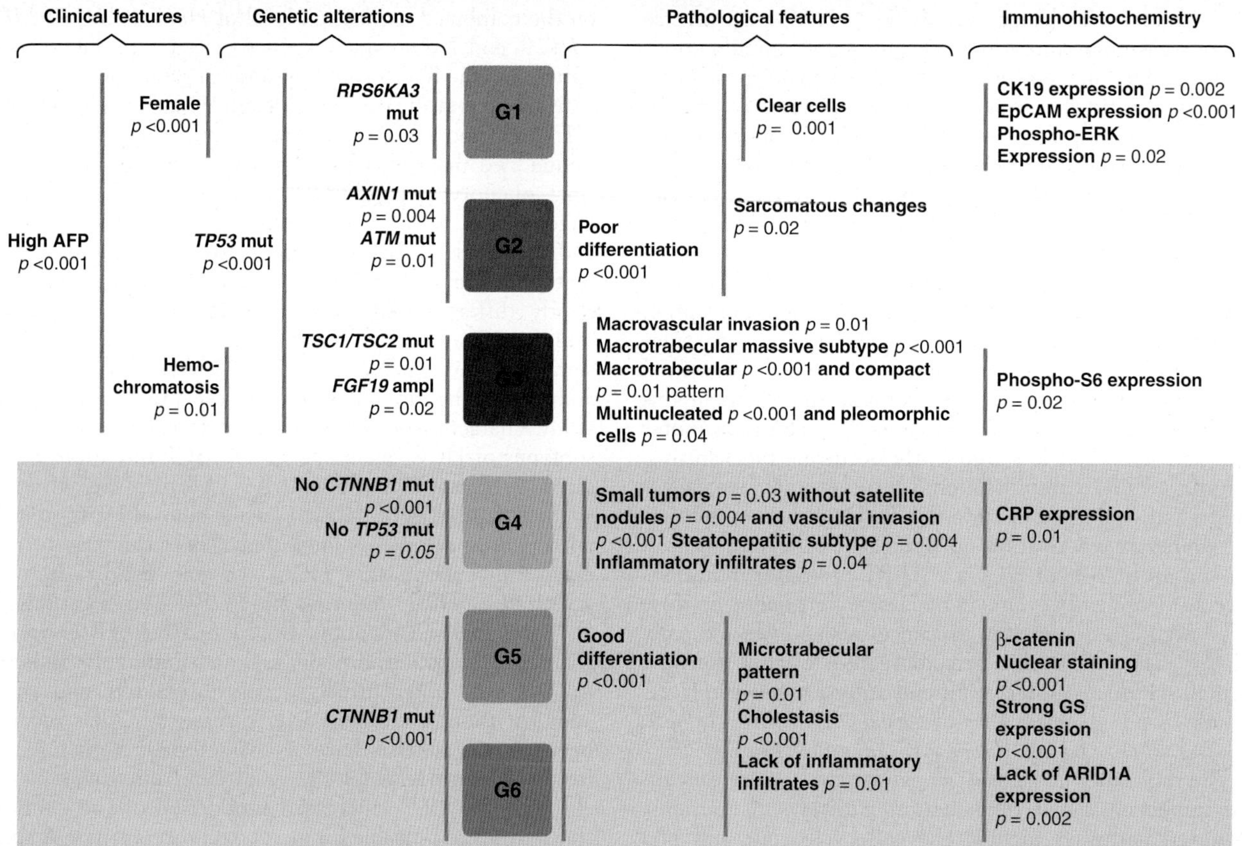

FIGURE 45.6 Integration of clinical, pathological, and molecular features in HCC molecular classification allows differentiation into six groups (G1 to G6). Three of these groups are characterized by *TP53* mutations, and two by *CTNNB1* mutations. *Mut,* Mutation; *ampl,* amplification. (*From Calderaro J, Couchy G, Imbeaud S, et al. Histological subtypes of hepatocellular carcinoma are related to gene mutations and molecular tumour classification. J Hepatol. 2017;67:727-738.*)

of progenitor-like signatures, activation of specific oncogenic pathways, and signatures related to poor clinical outcome. The recently proposed consensus terminology for cHCC-CCA[109] will hopefully facilitate the performance of additional studies that may help elucidate the molecular changes of these unique tumors.

Precancerous Lesions in Hepatocarcinogenesis

In the past 30 years, many studies have investigated the morphological features of candidate HCC precursors in series of resected and explanted livers. The biological nature of these lesions was then investigated by epidemiological, molecular, radiological, and clinical follow-up studies. The terminology for hepatocellular precancerous lesions has been established through international consensus meetings.[110-112]

Two types of lesions are detected in chronically diseased, usually cirrhotic livers, and they are often multiple (Fig. 45.7).[113] *Dysplastic foci* consist of groups of hepatocytes with dysplasia. They are less than 1 mm in diameter and are incidental findings on microscopic examination of hepatic specimens. *Dysplastic nodules* are a few millimeters to a few centimeters in diameter and can be detected on gross examination and sometimes on hepatic imaging. They must be differentiated from HCC, and in all cases, the diagnosis relies on microscopic examination. In patients without chronic liver disease, HCA (mainly b-HCA and b-IHCA) is recognized as a potential HCC precursor (see the section Hepatocellular Adenoma).

Dysplastic Foci

Small cell change (SCC) of hepatocytes, originally described as small cell dysplasia, is the most common cytological change found in dysplastic foci.[114] SCC is characterized by a decreased cell volume, an increased nucleus-to-cytoplasm ratio, mild nuclear pleomorphism and hyperchromasia, and cytoplasmic basophilia (Fig. 45.8A). Hepatocytes with SCC have increased expression of proliferation markers compared with adjacent hepatocytes. They have molecular alterations that indicate a precancerous nature, including chromosomal gains and losses similar to those of adjacent HCCs, telomere shortening, and CDKN1A-regulated cell cycle checkpoint inactivation.[115-117] SCC has great cytological similarity to early HCC.[118]

Iron-free foci have been associated with the development of HCC on follow-up of patients with hereditary hemochromatosis (see Fig. 45.8B).[119] These lesions have increased proliferative activity, as compared with the iron-overloaded parenchyma.[119] In addition to resistance to iron accumulation, iron-free foci may demonstrate SCC or large cell change (LCC) of hepatocytes.

Large Cell Change of Hepatocytes

LCC, originally described as liver cell dysplasia,[120] is characterized by nuclear and cytoplasmic enlargement (with a preserved nucleus-to-cytoplasm ratio), nuclear pleomorphism and hyperchromasia, and multinucleation (Fig. 45.9). LCC is commonly seen in livers with chronic HBV infection or

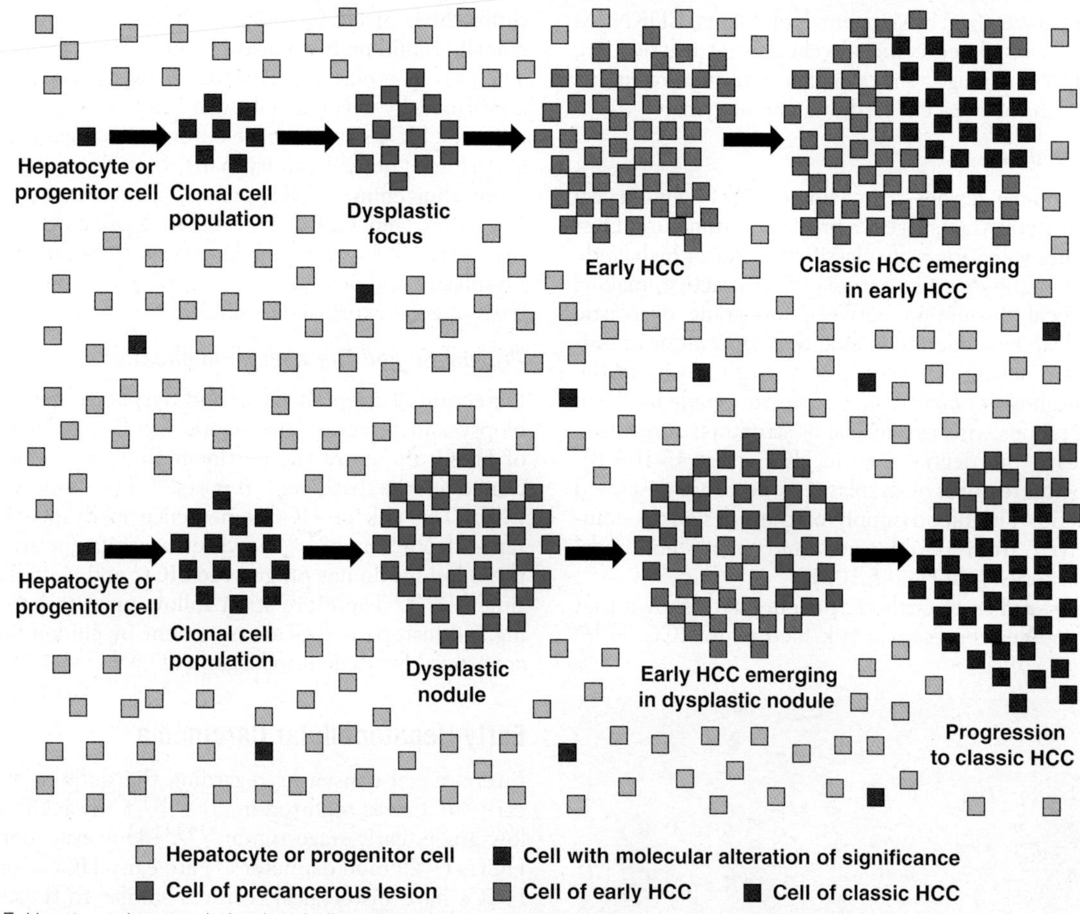

FIGURE 45.7 Hepatocarcinogenesis in chronic liver diseases: accumulating genomic and epigenetic changes, in concert with clonal expansion, lead over time to precancerous lesions, early hepatocellular carcinoma, and ultimately classic hepatocellular carcinoma. *Tan squares,* hepatocyte or progenitor cell; *dark red squares,* cell with molecular alteration of significance; *green squares,* cell of precancerous lesion; *blue squares,* cell of early HCC; *red squares,* cell of classic HCC. (*From Hytiroglou P. Well-differentiated hepatocellular nodule: making a diagnosis on biopsy and resection specimens of patients with advanced stage chronic liver disease. Semin Diagn Pathol. 2017;34:138-145.*)

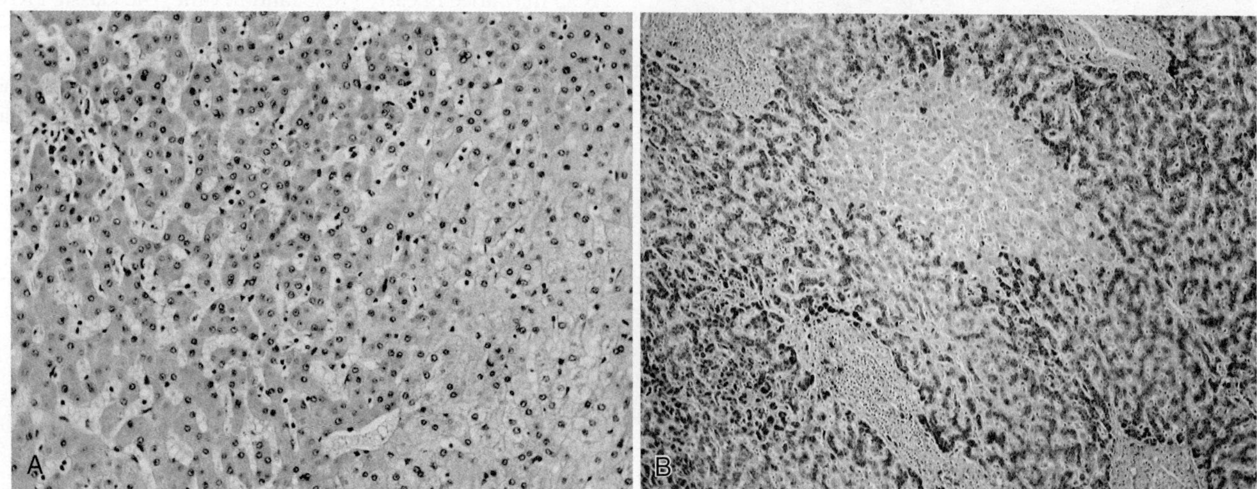

FIGURE 45.8 Dysplastic foci. A, Peripheral portion of a dysplastic focus with small cell change. Adjacent hepatocytes *(right)* have larger size and lower nucleus-to-cytoplasm ratio than dysplastic cells *(left).* **B,** Iron-free focus in a liver with hereditary hemochromatosis (Perl's iron stain). Parts of four portal tracts are also seen. The section is from a hepatic resection specimen with hepatocellular carcinoma (not shown).

cirrhosis of various causes. In cirrhosis due to chronic HBV or HCV infection, LCC is an independent risk factor for HCC.[121,122]

The nature of this cytological change has been disputed, possibly because LCC is biologically heterogeneous. In most cases of cirrhosis, LCC appears to be a degenerative change due to senescence or cholestasis.[123,124] LCC usually occurs diffusely rather than focally, which does not favor a precancerous characterization.[125] However, a subset of LCC in cases of chronic hepatitis B may be precancerous. These lesions are characterized by shortened telomeres, CDKN2A- and CDKN1A-regulated cell cycle checkpoint inactivation, increased DNA damage, and a higher proliferation index compared with the adjacent cirrhotic parenchyma.[126]

Dysplastic Nodules

Dysplastic nodular lesions are characterized by cytological or structural atypia that suggest a precancerous nature. Dysplastic nodules were originally classified as low or high grade on the basis of the degree of atypia.[110] In practice, making the histological distinction between low-grade dysplastic nodules and large regenerative nodules is difficult or impossible,[111] but molecular markers may provide a way in the future. A diagnosis of *high-grade dysplastic nodule* has been assigned to lesions with cytological or structural atypia that does not reach the degree seen in HCC (Fig. 45.10A,B). The histological features of dysplastic nodules are described in Chapter 56. The blood supply of these lesions is commonly derived from portal tracts and small, nontriadal (unpaired) arteries (see Fig. 45.10B).

Follow-up studies of cirrhotic patients have shown that dysplastic nodules represent a risk factor for HCC.[127-129]

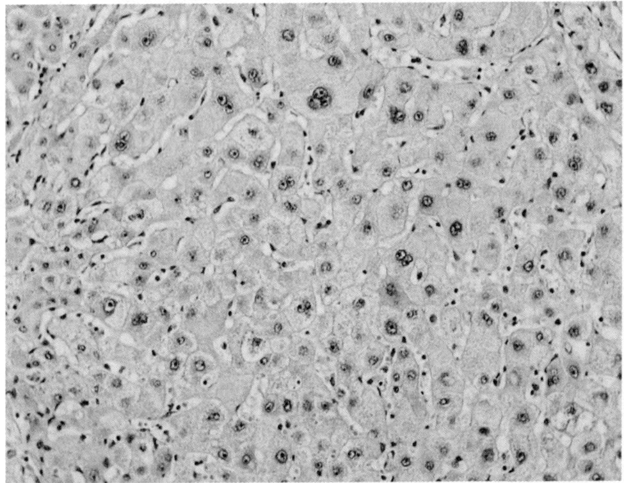

FIGURE 45.9 Large cell change in hepatocytes.

Subnodules of HCC arising in dysplastic nodules are occasionally found on histological examination (Fig. 45.11A).[130] The precancerous nature of the dysplastic nodules has been confirmed by several molecular studies. These lesions and adjacent HCCs had similar chromosomal gains and losses, and a loss of heterozygosity in microsatellite foci.[131-133] Telomere shortening, TERT promoter mutations, telomerase activation, and CDKN1A-regulated cell cycle checkpoint inactivation have been found in dysplastic nodules.[89,90,134-137] Dysplastic nodules can be distinguished from HCC on the basis of gene expression profiles.[138]

Prognostic and Therapeutic Implications

Detection of dysplastic foci and dysplastic nodules in liver biopsy and resection specimens signifies an increased risk of HCC; therefore the pertinent findings should be mentioned in the pathology reports.[84] The same applies for LCC. The risk of HCC emergence in dysplastic nodules ranges from 9% to 31%; however, a significant proportion of these lesions do not progress to HCC and may disappear in time.[3,139,140] Therefore strict follow-up with hepatic imaging and histopathological assessment by guided liver biopsy are crucial for patient management.[3,141]

Early Hepatocellular Carcinoma

International consensus regarding the defining features of early HCC was reported in 2009.[111] Early HCC is a small, low-grade, early-stage tumor.[129,142] However, not all small HCCs (<2 cm in diameter[110]) are early HCCs; some small HCCs have histological features similar to those of larger classic HCCs and are commonly referred to as "small progressed HCCs."[3] The latter may be associated with vascular invasion (27% of cases) and intrahepatic metastases (10% of cases), whereas early HCCs lack the ability to invade vascular structures or metastasize.[142] However, foci of classic HCC may arise in early HCC, and in time, the classic HCC component can replace early HCC.

Most early HCCs consist of small hepatocyte-like neoplastic cells, arranged in irregular, thin trabeculae and pseudoglandular structures (Fig. 45.12A,B).[142-144] Cellular

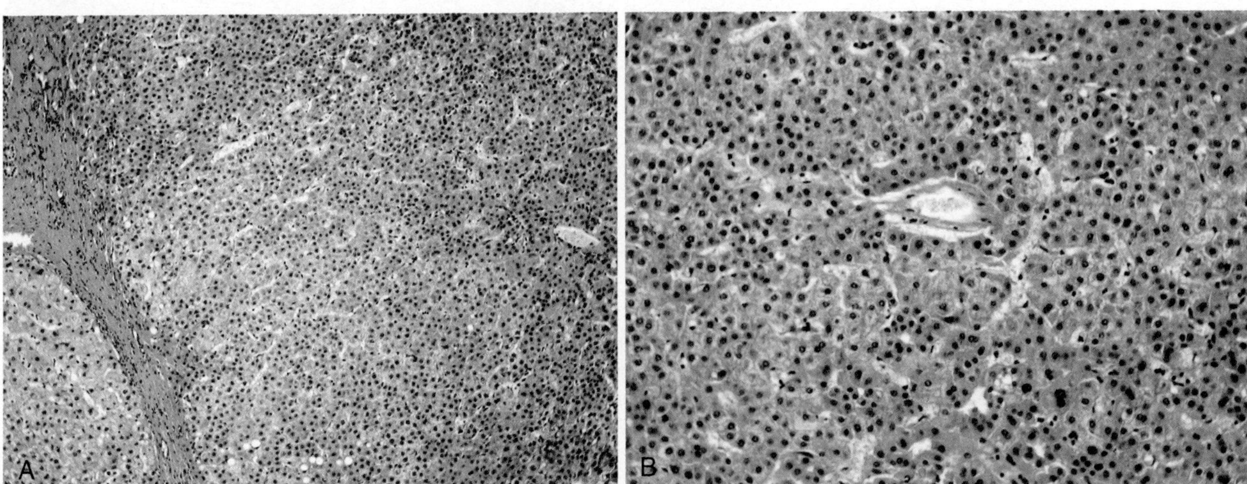

FIGURE 45.10 High-grade dysplastic nodule. A, There is increased cellularity and a higher nucleus-to-cytoplasm ratio compared with the adjacent cirrhotic nodule *(lower left)*. Cell plates are two to three cells thick. **B,** Cytological atypia and an unpaired artery are seen on higher-power magnification.

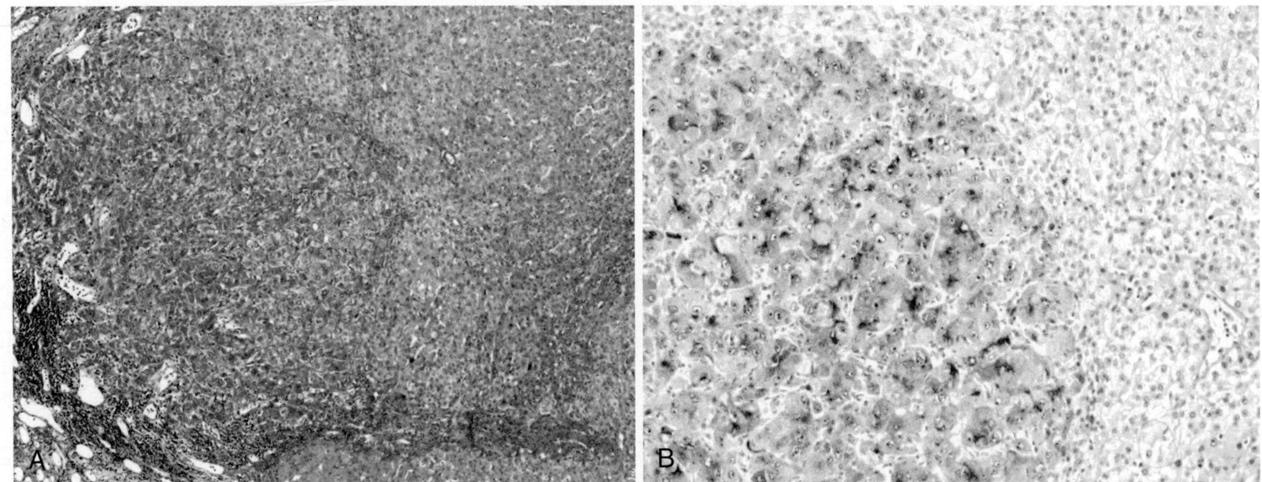

FIGURE 45.11 A, Subnodule of hepatocellular carcinoma *(left)* arises in a dysplastic nodule. **B,** The hepatocellular carcinoma cells exhibit immunopositivity for glypican 3, but the remaining cells of the dysplastic nodule do not.

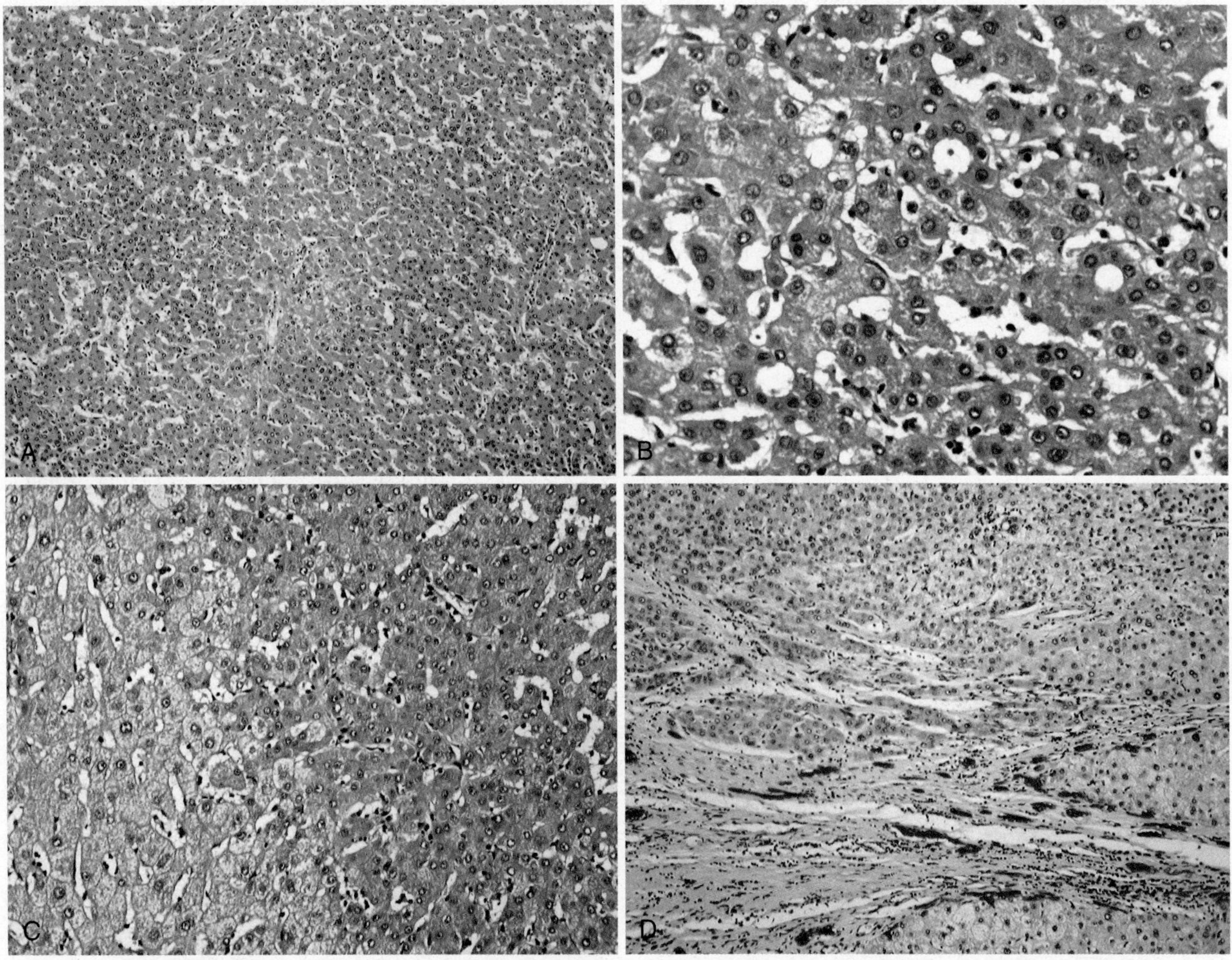

FIGURE 45.12 Early hepatocellular carcinoma. A, High cellularity and a thin trabecular pattern are characteristic features seen on scanning magnification. **B,** Cytological atypia is evident on higher magnification. Small pseudoglandular structures are also evident in this field. **C,** Indistinct margin of the lesion. **D,** Area of stromal invasion *(top)* lacks a ductular reaction. A ductular reaction is seen around adjacent cirrhotic nodules (immunohistochemical stain for cytokeratin 7).

crowding is a characteristic finding on low-power examination of these lesions. Poor circumscription is another characteristic feature. The neoplastic cells at the tumor margin merge imperceptibly with the adjacent hepatocytes (see Fig. 45.12C); this "replacing" growth pattern accounts for the common appearance of these lesions as nodules with indistinct margins on gross examination. Diffuse fatty change is common in early HCC (up to 40% of cases) and has been attributed to insufficient vascular supply.[145]

Similar to a high-grade dysplastic nodule, early HCC may receive its blood supply from the portal tracts and small nontriadal (unpaired) arteries. On the arterial phase of contrast-enhanced imaging studies, early HCCs usually appear isovascular or hypovascular compared with the adjacent hepatic parenchyma. Because of the similarity in imaging findings between dysplastic nodule and early HCC, guided liver biopsy may be required to reach a diagnosis. On the other hand, classic HCCs typically appear hypervascular because of well-developed nontriadal arteries.[111] Therefore lesions consisting of classic HCC arising in early HCC (Fig. 45.13) may provide a characteristic nodule-in-nodule sign on contrast-enhanced imaging studies.

Stromal invasion into the portal tract or septal stroma has emerged as the most important feature distinguishing early HCC from high-grade dysplastic nodules.[111] A ductular reaction is found around noninvasive hepatocellular nodules but is characteristically lacking in areas of stromal invasion by HCC. Immunohistochemical stains for CK7 or CK19 can be used to identify a ductular reaction (see Fig. 45.12D).[146] Other immunohistochemical stains that may be useful in this differential diagnosis are discussed in the following section. TERT promoter mutations have been detected in a majority of early HCCs and in a minority of dysplastic nodules.[90]

Use of Molecular Diagnostics

The diagnosis of HCC is currently based on imaging and histopathological examination; molecular diagnostics are not routinely used. However, molecular analyses can aid in the diagnosis of difficult cases and in the identification of specific HCC subtypes.[3] For example, detection of the PRKACA rearrangement by FISH can confirm the diagnosis of FLC,[104] while certain chromosomal abnormalities, such as gains of 1q and 8q, which can be demonstrated by either FISH or comparative genomic hybridization, may be useful in distinguishing well-differentiated (adenoma-like) HCC from HCA.[147-149] The molecular classifications of HCC have not found their way to clinical care, because they do not provide additional value beyond that obtained by imaging and histology.[3] However, the large-scale studies of gene expression performed in the past 15 years have provided new immunohistochemical markers for the pathologist's armamentarium, presented in the following paragraphs. In addition, CK19 expression (suggesting progenitor cell origin and detected by immunohistochemistry in a minority of HCCs) has been found to confer an adverse prognosis: CK19-positive HCCs have a higher incidence of recurrence, lymph node metastases, and resistance to locoregional therapy than CK19-negative ones.[150-152]

Heat shock protein 70 (HSP70) is significantly upregulated in early and classic HCCs compared with cirrhotic liver and precancerous lesions.[153] Using immunohistochemical methods, approximately 80% of early HCCs are positive for HSP70, compared with only 5% of high-grade dysplastic nodules, making this protein a useful marker in the differential diagnosis. Staining is nuclear and cytoplasmic (Fig. 45.14). Lesions are considered positive when 10% or more of the cells express HSP70.[112] Normal hepatocytes are negative for HSP70, and biliary epithelial cells provide a useful internal positive control.

The oncofetal antigen glypican 3 (GPC3) is an established serum and tissue marker of HCC. Immunohistochemical staining for GPC3 is positive in 70% to 90% of HCCs overall and more often positive in poorly differentiated than well-differentiated tumors.[154-156] Dysplastic nodules occasionally may be positive for GPC3. Nonseminomatous germ cell tumors and malignant melanoma also express GPC3.[149] Staining is usually cytoplasmic, but it may be membranous or canalicular (see Fig. 45.11B).[111] GPC3 is not expressed in HCAs and is therefore a useful marker for distinguishing between well-differentiated HCCs and HCAs.[156] However, negative immunohistochemical results do not rule out HCC.

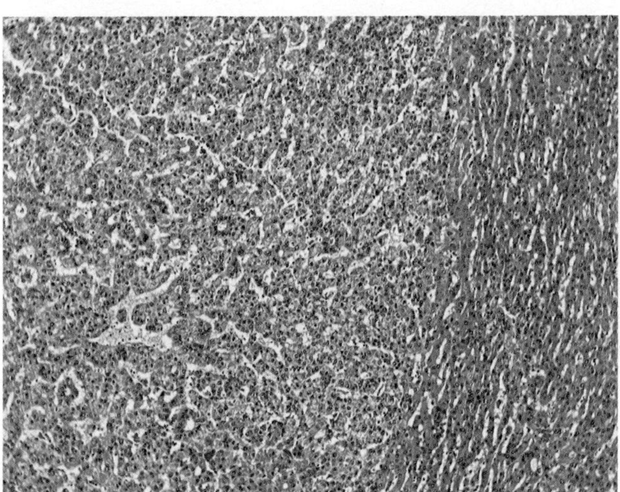

FIGURE 45.13 Subnodule of classic hepatocellular carcinoma arising in an early hepatocellular carcinoma.

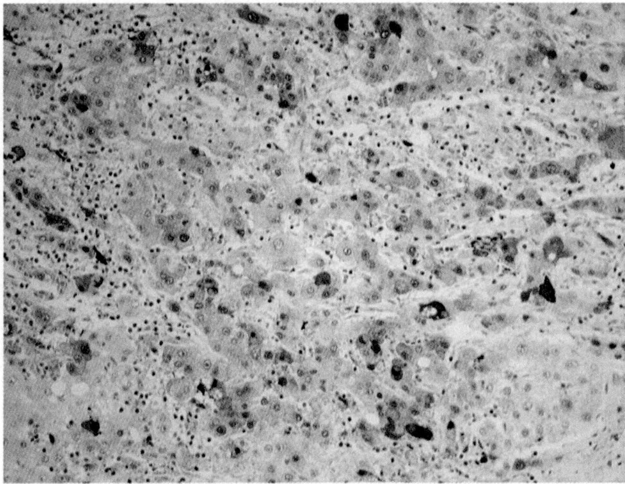

FIGURE 45.14 Positive heat shock protein 70 immunostaining in early hepatocellular carcinoma with stromal invasion.

The GS protein is often detected in HCCs. The characteristic GS immunostaining patterns of normal liver, FNH, and HCA were described earlier (see Benign Hepatocellular Tumors). GS immunopositivity in β-catenin–activated HCCs is usually strong and diffuse and is associated with a variable number of tumor cell nuclei expressing aberrant β-catenin (Fig. 45.15). A small percentage of high-grade dysplastic nodules may also be focally positive.

Assessment of the combination of HSP70, GPC3, and GS in distinguishing between high-grade dysplastic nodules and early or well-differentiated HCCs showed that positivity for any two of the three immunohistochemical markers was a feature of HCC (100% specificity), with modest sensitivity (Table 45.2).[157,158] Although the sensitivity was lower in biopsy (57%) than in resection specimens (72%), the three-stain panel can be useful in this difficult differential diagnosis when stromal invasion is not detected on routine histological examination.[112] Additional diagnostic markers (e.g., clathrin heavy chain[159]) are being developed and tested as molecular data find their way to diagnostic pathology.

Ongoing research relevant to targeted therapies for HCC is likely to provide prognostic and predictive markers in the future. At the present time, early detection still provides the best opportunity for successful HCC treatment. Advances in hepatic imaging methods play a major role in efficient screening of populations at risk.

The full reference list may be accessed online at Elsevier eBooks for Practicing Clinicians.

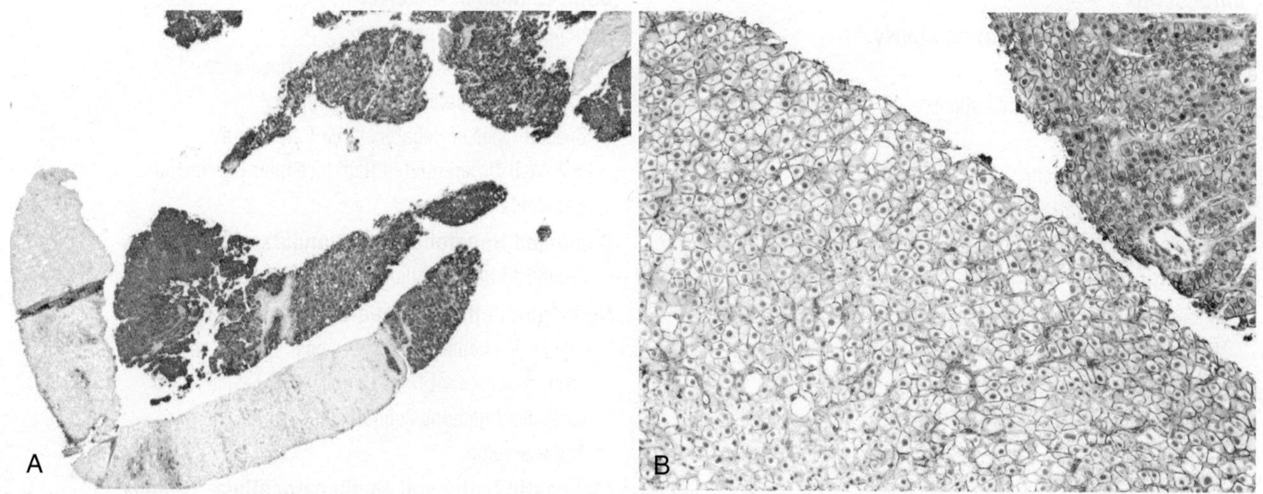

FIGURE 45.15 **A,** Strong and diffuse immunopositivity for glutamine synthetase in a β-catenin–activated hepatocellular carcinoma contrasts with an absence of staining in the nontumorous liver. **B,** Some tumor cells exhibit aberrant nuclear and cytoplasmic expression of β-catenin *(top right).*

TABLE 45.2 Immunohistochemical Stains in the Differential Diagnosis of Hepatocellular Nodules

Protein	HCA	HCC	HGDN
α-Fetoprotein	–	+ or –	– (rarely + in few cells)
Glypican-3*	–	+ or –	Usually –, occasionally +
HSP70*	–	+ or –	Usually –, occasionally +
GS*	– or +[†]	+ or –	Usually –, occasionally +

GS, *Glutamine synthetase;* HCA, *hepatocellular adenoma; HCC, hepatocellular carcinoma;* HGDN, *high-grade dysplastic nodule;* HSP70, *heat shock protein 70.*

**In the differential diagnosis of HCC vs HGDN, positive immunostaining for more than one of these three stains (glypican-3, HSP70 and/or GS) has shown high specificity for HCC diagnosis. The key aspect of this differential diagnosis is detection of stromal invasion, which occurs in HCC but not in HGDN; distinguishing invasive neoplastic cells from entrapped hepatocytes in this setting can be aided by the use of cytokeratin 7 or 19 stains, which highlights ductular reactions.*

[†]Among HCAs, positive GS immunostaining is characteristic of b-HCA and b-IHCA, with different GS patterns according to different CTNNB1 *mutations (see above).*

In the context of overlapping immunohistochemical findings, the differential diagnosis should take into account all clinical, radiological, morphological, and immunohistochemical features.

CHAPTER 46

Diagnostic Cytology of the Liver

Aileen Wee, Martha Bishop Pitman

Contents

INTRODUCTION

As the role of fine-needle aspiration biopsy (FNAB) in the evaluation of focal liver lesions has evolved, it has presented new challenges.[1,2] Advances in dynamic imaging modalities have obviated the need for tissue confirmation in clinically classic cases of hepatocellular carcinoma (HCC).[3-12] Ultrasound surveillance and serum α-fetoprotein (AFP) assessment of high-risk patients have improved the detection of small nodules (≤2 cm in diameter).[13-16] Accurate cytohistological characterization of small, well-differentiated hepatocellular nodules on limited tissue samples is extremely challenging, but it has important therapeutic implications.

Much progress has been made in the molecular characterization of tumors by genomic, microRNA, and proteomic methods. Promising new tools for tumor diagnosis are available for predicting the prognosis and progression of disease and for personalized, molecularly targeted anticancer therapies and chemopreventive strategies.[17-26] Because FNAB is the least invasive tool for tissue procurement, it is predicted that it will become a point of care in the management algorithm of HCC for diagnostic, therapeutic, and prognostication purposes.[27]

USE OF FINE-NEEDLE ASPIRATION BIOPSY

Guidance Systems

Percutaneous (transabdominal) FNAB performed with ultrasound or CT guidance is a safe, efficacious, and cost-effective outpatient procedure for the diagnosis of focal liver lesions.[28-30] Aspiration can also be performed during laparotomy or laparoscopy under palpation or direct vision. Endoscopic ultrasound-guided fine-needle aspiration (EUS-FNA) is the latest diagnostic and staging tool and is used primarily for left hepatic lobe lesions and hilar or perihilar masses in which the needle traverses the wall of the gastrointestinal tract.[31] Factors influencing the choice of guidance system include the size and location of the lesion, operator expertise and preference, and availability of imaging technologies.[27-29]

Ultrasonography provides rapid localization, flexible patient positioning, and imaging of the lesion without radiation. It is typically used for initial guidance, particularly when there are multiple lesions or large, relatively superficial lesions. CT allows optimal resolution of small lesions or lesions that are not visible with ultrasound, accurate localization of the needle tip immediately before sampling,

BOX 46.1 Fine-Needle Aspiration Biopsy of the Liver: Indications, Contraindications, and Complications

INDICATIONS
- Evaluating a mass or cystic lesion
- Draining a cyst or abscess

CONTRAINDICATIONS
- Uncorrectable bleeding diathesis
- Lack of safe access route
- Uncooperative patient
- Intestinal obstruction (for endoscopic ultrasound-guided fine-needle aspiration biopsy)

COMPLICATIONS
- Bleeding
- Needle tract seeding
- Tumor recurrence and post-transplantation tumor recurrence

improved definition of tissue components and vascularity, and more precise demonstration of the anatomic relationships of a given lesion.

EUS-FNA is a safe, accurate, and versatile technique, but it is highly operator dependent.[32-36] It allows concurrent sampling of pancreas and liver lesions, which can confirm primary and metastatic lesions in one diagnostic encounter. The technique is useful for small and deep-seated left lobe lesions that are below CT or magnetic resonance imaging (MRI) resolution or lesions that are not easily accessible by percutaneous FNAB. It improves staging of liver metastases, is good for early detection of multifocal HCC in cirrhosis, and can assess the accurate number of lesions (e.g., intrahepatic staging of HCC) for transplantation eligibility.[37,38]

Percutaneous FNAB techniques include individual puncture, coaxial biopsy, and tandem needle biopsy techniques.[39] Multiple aspirations (as many as four passes) usually can be performed with minimal morbidity. The needle size is between 20 and 22 gauge. Aspiration needles with a guillotine mechanism enable microbiopsy cores to be procured at the same sitting. Concomitant core-needle (18-gauge) biopsies may also be performed.

Indications and Contraindications

FNAB is the diagnostic procedure of choice for focal liver lesions, especially to confirm a suspected malignancy (Box 46.1). It is particularly advantageous for advanced malignancies and patients who are poor surgical candidates. Another indication is drainage of a cyst or abscess for culture and therapeutic ablation.[40] Early affirmative diagnosis leads to cost savings in terms of further investigational tests and hospitalization.

Contraindications for percutaneous FNAB include an uncorrectable bleeding diathesis, lack of a safe access route (i.e., biopsy through a vascular structure), and an uncooperative patient for whom awkward positioning or maintenance of strict breath control is necessary to ensure proper needle placement.[28] For EUS-FNA, gastrointestinal obstruction is an absolute contraindication because of the risk of perforation.[34]

Complications

Complications from FNAB are uncommon.[39] There may be bleeding, which is mostly associated with cirrhosis and coagulopathy but may relate to the size of needle used, particularly in vascular lesions and in large superficial tumors not covered by normal parenchyma (see Box 46.1).[12] Needle tract seeding is rare, with an incidence of 0.003% to 0.009% for malignancy in general and 0.003% to 5% for HCC; if a small (22-gauge), noncutting needle is used, the rate for HCC is approximately 0.11%.[11,41-44] A higher incidence of HCC recurrence in the transplanted liver has been reported in transplantation cases with preoperative FNAB.[45] Death, usually resulting from bleeding, is rare, with a reported mortality rate of 0.018%.[42]

Clinical Considerations

There is much debate regarding the use of preoperative FNAB for the diagnosis of HCC.[27] Several reasons are cited for opposing FNAB[46-48]:

- Sufficiently sensitive advances in dynamic imaging modalities for establishing an HCC diagnosis[3,8,10,11,49]
- Risk of needle tract seeding[11,41-44,50]
- Risk of intraperitoneal bleeding[12]
- Risk of intraprocedural hematogenous dissemination, which results in a higher incidence of tumor and post-transplantation recurrence[41,45]
- Adoption of a wait-and-watch policy for hepatocellular nodules that are less than 1 cm in diameter[4,5]
- Indeterminate cytohistological reports rendered for well-differentiated hepatocellular nodules[51,52]

Several reasons are cited for favoring FNAB[53,54]:

- Serum AFP has a low sensitivity (<50%).[55,56]
- Use of the coaxial biopsy technique to reduce the risk of seeding[57]
- Decreased costs of long-term imaging surveillance
- Avoids futile transplantation in false-positive imaging cases[7]
- Allays patient anxiety after a liver nodule has been detected on imaging
- Confirms HCC, which increases eligibility for liver transplantation
- Immediate institution of anti-HCC therapy when the lesion is less than 2 cm in diameter
- Excludes other types of primary liver carcinomas

According to the European Association for the Study of the Liver (EASL) 2000 Conference and the American Association for the Study of Liver Disease (AASLD) guidelines, nodules more than 2 cm in diameter in cirrhotic livers are diagnosed as HCC if they show an intense arterial profile with contrast washout in delayed venous phase on one dynamic imaging modality.[4,5] Nodules between 1 and 2 cm in cirrhotic livers require concurrence of two coincidental imaging modalities; otherwise, biopsy is recommended.[49] For nodules less than 1 cm in diameter, the EASL guidelines recommend a wait-and-watch policy with surveillance every 3 months. Approximately 68% of nodules less than 1 cm in diameter in cirrhotic livers are HCCs.[58] In skilled hands and with an expert reader, ultrasound-guided FNAB of hepatic nodules less than 1 cm in diameter can yield correct

BOX 46.2 Prerequisites for Optimal Fine-Needle Aspiration Biopsy Results

- Dedicated and experienced aspirator and reader team
- Image-guided representative sampling for heterogeneous focal liver lesions
- On-site cytology service to assess specimen adequacy, retrieve material for cell blocks, and triage specimen for microbiological studies, flow cytometry, electron microscopy, molecular analysis, and other ancillary tests
- Combined cytohistological approach
- Judicious use of immunohistochemistry
- Clinicopathological correlation

a diagnosis in 90% of cases.[41] The conundrum is to balance the risk of unnecessary surgery (2.5%) against the risk of seeding.[9,11,53,54]

Specimen Preparation

The types of small tissue samples from liver FNAB include direct smears, needle rinses, core imprints, cell blocks, microbiopsies, and core-needle biopsies. Smears may be air-dried and stained with Diff-Quik or May-Grünwald-Giemsa stain or fixed in 95% alcohol and stained using the Papanicolaou method. Rapid touch preparations (imprints) can be performed to assess the adequacy of tissue cores.[59] If well-fixed, adequately smeared slides are difficult to obtain, the aspirate can be expressed into a preservative and submitted as a liquid-based specimen for processing by the ThinPrep or SurePath method.

Cell blocks are made from needle rinses and tissue fragments.[60,61] Particulate material should be quickly retrieved from the glass slides before staining for subsequent formalin-fixed, paraffin-embedded cell block preparation. Histological sections allow for architectural appraisal, special stains, and immunohistochemistry. Immunocytochemistry may be necessary if only smears are available.

Diagnostic Accuracy

The prerequisites for optimal results with FNAB are listed in Box 46.2. The sensitivity of FNAB varies according to the method used (i.e., blind vs. guided aspiration, number of passes, and operator skill), characteristics of the lesion (size, location, consistency, and heterogeneity), and standard of cytopathology service (e.g., quality of smears, combined cytohistological analysis, ancillary testing, reader expertise).[61-63] On-site cytology service may provide rapidly stained smears for evaluation of sample adequacy, retrieval of particulate material for cell block preparation, and triage of specimens for culture, flow cytometry, electron microscopy, and other ancillary tests, including molecular studies.[60,64,65] Imprint smears of core-needle biopsies should be thoroughly screened on-site and the corresponding material separately labeled per pass for subsequent correlation. In the absence of an on-site service, it is imperative that the aspirator learns how to make proper smears and that a tissue management protocol is clearly understood by the patient care team.

The sensitivity and specificity of percutaneous FNAB for detection of liver malignancy are about 90% (range, 67% to 100%) and 100%, respectively.[12,66,67] The positive and negative predictive values and overall accuracy of FNAB diagnosis for liver malignancy were reported in one large study to be 100%, 59.1%, and 92.4%, respectively.[12] EUS-FNA also has a high sensitivity (82% to 94%) and specificity (90% to 100%) for malignancy.[32,33,35,36] Similar to percutaneous FNAB, EUS-FNA leads to a better diagnostic yield with metastases compared with well-differentiated hepatocellular tumor nodules. False positives are rare. False-negative diagnoses are most often the result of a sampling error because of inexact needle localization related to small masses, large areas of necrosis, fibrosis, or a prominent inflammatory rim. The supplemental nature of FNAB and concomitant core-needle biopsy improves overall accuracy, especially for benign neoplasms and for heterogeneous carcinomas and poorly differentiated neoplasms that require ancillary studies.[63,68]

Liquid-based cytology of liver aspirates shows good correlation with conventional smears and reduces false-negative diagnoses.[69-71] Advantages include more representative sampling and better cell preservation. Disadvantages include no on-site assessment of adequacy or triage of specimens, no air-dried smears for Giemsa preparations, removal of background elements, high cost, and the need for familiarity with cytological artifacts and recognition of diagnostic pitfalls to avoid misinterpretation. In our experience (unpublished data) with the ThinPrep method, the cytological features of HCC appear to be rather nondifferentiated.[1] Cytoarchitectural features, such as arborizing trabecular structures, pseudoacinar rosettes, and peripheral or transgressing endothelium, are less evident or completely lost. Tumor aggregates tend to be tighter, three-dimensional, and smaller. Cells are usually smaller with nondescript shapes and denser cytoplasm, and they often have frayed borders.

DIAGNOSTIC ISSUES

Focal liver lesions range from cystic and inflammatory or infectious entities to benign or malignant primary and metastatic neoplasms. HCC is well known for its heterogeneity. Intrahepatic cholangiocarcinoma (CC) frequently shows nondescript features of adenocarcinoma. The phenotypic landscape is further muddied by the recently redefined combined hepatocellular-cholangiocarcinoma (cHCC-CCA), intermediate cell carcinoma, and cholangiolocarcinoma (CLC).[72,73] The liver is a common depository for metastases. Given these permutations, primary liver carcinomas can mimic many tumors and vice versa.[74,75] The diagnostic issues are listed in Box 46.3.

Integrative Approach to the Evaluation of Liver Aspirates

A stepwise algorithmic approach to evaluating liver aspirates includes full clinicopathological correlations[61,65,74,76] (Box 46.4):

1. *Evaluate clinical information.* A patient may be seen with one or more focal liver lesions in the following scenarios: routine medical checkup, screening or surveillance of chronic liver disease,[13,16] follow-up of a known cancer case, investigation of a symptomatic patient, or investigation of a pediatric lesion. Relevant clinical findings, liver function profile, serology, and tumor markers should be obtained.[21,55,56]

BOX 46.3 Diagnostic Issues in the Evaluation of Focal Liver Lesions

- Differentiating well-differentiated hepatocellular nodules from reactive hepatocytes
- Distinguishing various types of benign, well-differentiated hepatocellular nodules
- Differentiating early, well-differentiated hepatocellular carcinoma from benign hepatocellular nodules
- Recognizing hepatocellular carcinoma and its variants from their mimics
- Recognizing the components of combined hepatocellular-cholangiocarcinoma as part of a combination (not collision) tumor
- Differentiating poorly differentiated hepatocellular carcinoma from intrahepatic cholangiocarcinoma
- Differentiating intrahepatic cholangiocarcinoma from metastatic adenocarcinoma
- Differentiating poorly differentiated primary liver carcinomas from metastases
- Determining the histogenesis of nonhepatocellular tumors
- Determining the primary site of origin of malignant nonhepatocellular tumors
- Differentiating benign and malignant cystic lesions
- Recognizing inflammatory or infectious lesions that may mimic tumors

BOX 46.4 Integrative Approach to the Evaluation of Liver Aspirates

- Evaluate clinical information
- Evaluate radiological information
- Evaluate cytohistological findings
- Evaluate ancillary studies
- Correlate all previous steps

2. *Evaluate radiological information.* Focal liver lesions may be cystic or solid and single or multiple. The presence of preexisting or chronic hepatobiliary disease and associated radiological findings should be determined. Advances in dynamic contrast-enhanced imaging modalities have increased the sensitivity and specificity for detection of classic HCC.[3,8,10] The radiological recognition of combination tumors requires a high index of suspicion, especially when there is discordance between tumor markers and imaging appearances.[72] Siderotic nodules are readily detected on T2- or T2*-weighted MRI.[77,78]
3. *Evaluate cytohistological findings.* Smears are scanned at low power to establish the pattern and architecture before close inspection of cellular details as listed in Box 46.5. The operator should ascertain whether the lesion is (1) cystic (true cyst or pseudocyst) and benign or malignant or (2) solid (hepatocellular or nonhepatocellular) and benign or malignant. The diagnostic algorithms for evaluation of cystic and solid lesions of the liver are provided in Boxes 46.6 and 46.7, respectively.[74]
4. *Evaluate ancillary studies.* The initial cytomorphological impression is often crucial because the small amount of material may limit the utility of immunohistochemical and other ancillary tests.

BOX 46.5 Evaluation of Cytohistological Features of Aspirates of Focal Liver Lesions

PATTERN RECOGNITION (LOW POWER)
- Cellularity
- Architectural features
- Cellular composition
- Background

CELLULAR RECOGNITION (MEDIUM TO HIGH POWER)
- Size of cells
- Shape of cells
- Spatial relationship (e.g., degree of cohesion, crowding, polarity)
- Cytoplasm, nucleus, nucleus-to-cytoplasm ratio
- Inclusions, intracytoplasmic and intranuclear
- Pigments
- Vasculature
- Background

BOX 46.6 Algorithm for Diagnosing Cystic Lesions of the Liver

I. Cystic lesion with epithelial lining
   A. Cuboidal or low columnar epithelium: solitary bile duct cyst, fibropolycystic disease, and obstructive dilation of bile duct
   B. Ciliated epithelium: ciliated foregut cyst
   C. Biliary, mucinous, or oncocytic (with or without papillae)
      1. With ovarian-like stroma
         a. Mucinous cystic neoplasm with low-, intermediate-, or high-grade intraepithelial neoplasia
         b. Mucinous cystic neoplasm with associated invasive carcinoma
      2. Without ovarian-like stroma
         a. Biliary intraductal papillary neoplasm with low-, intermediate-, or high-grade intraepithelial neoplasia
         b. Biliary intraductal papillary neoplasm with an associated invasive carcinoma
   D. Intrahepatic cholangiocarcinoma associated with cystic change, arising from malignant transformation of preexisting cystic disease, or associated with cystically dilated bile ducts
   E. Metastases
II. Cystic lesion without epithelial lining
   A. Neoplastic (including tumor-like lesions)
      1. Cavernous hemangioma
      2. Mesenchymal hamartoma
      3. Cystic degeneration in benign or malignant tumors
      4. Undifferentiated embryonal sarcoma
   B. Nonneoplastic
      1. Laminated wall: hydatid cyst
      2. Inflammation and necrosis: pyogenic, fungal, or amebic abscess, granulomas, necrotizing eosinophilic granuloma, hydatid cyst
      3. Hemorrhagic cyst: cystic hematoma

5. *Correlate all previous steps.* Clinicopathological correlation is mandatory to arrive at a final definitive diagnosis. An "indeterminate" diagnosis may be rendered for very-well-differentiated hepatocellular nodules. Information obtained from all of the previous steps, including a complete immunohistochemical workup, may help establish a generic morphological diagnosis for nonhepatocellular lesions but cannot provide the specific organ of origin.

BOX 46.7 Algorithm for Diagnosing Solid Lesions of the Liver

HEPATOCELLULAR APPEARANCE

- Focal fatty change
- Large regenerative nodule
- Dysplastic nodule (low or high grade)
- Siderotic nodule (regenerative, dysplastic)
- Focal nodular hyperplasia
- Hepatocellular adenoma
- Hepatocellular carcinoma, variants and special types
- Hepatoblastoma

HEPATOCELLULAR AND GLANDULAR APPEARANCE

- Combined hepatocellular-cholangiocarcinoma

NONHEPATOCELLULAR APPEARANCE

- Glandular pattern: bile duct hamartoma, bile duct adenoma (peribiliary gland hamartoma), intrahepatic cholangiocarcinoma, combined hepatocellular-cholangiocarcinoma, cholangiolocarcinoma, metastases
- Squamous, including adenosquamous, pattern: Intrahepatic cholangiocarcinoma, metastases
- Mucinous pattern: mucinous cystic neoplasm, intrahepatic cholangiocarcinoma, metastases
- Papillary pattern: intraductal papillary neoplasm, intrahepatic cholangiocarcinoma, metastases
- Clear cell pattern: angiomyolipoma, metastases (renal cell carcinoma, adrenocortical carcinoma)
- Oncocytic cell pattern: angiomyolipoma, metastases (renal cell carcinoma, adrenocortical carcinoma), melanoma
- Small cell pattern: neuroendocrine tumor, lymphoma, metastases (small cell carcinoma, lobular carcinoma of breast, melanoma), inflammatory pseudotumor
- Large cell pattern: neuroendocrine carcinoma, metastases (undifferentiated carcinoma)
- Spindle cell pattern: cavernous hemangioma, infantile hemangioma, solitary fibrous tumor, inflammatory pseudotumor, angiomyolipoma, gastrointestinal stromal tumor, sarcomatoid carcinoma (including primary liver carcinomas and metastatic sarcomatoid renal cell carcinoma), sarcoma (primary and metastatic, including angiosarcoma, Kaposi's sarcoma, carcinosarcoma, hepatobiliary rhabdomyosarcoma, synovial sarcoma, and leiomyosarcoma)
- Giant cell pattern: sarcomatoid or giant cell carcinoma (primary liver carcinomas and metastases), sarcoma (primary and metastases)
- Others: nodular hematopoiesis, epithelioid hemangioendothelioma, germ cell tumors (teratoma, yolk sac tumor)

Cytohistology of the Liver

Normal Morphology

Aspirate smears of normal liver typically show a polymorphous cell population dominated by hepatocytes, occurring singly in short rows or small clusters and intermingling with scattered bile duct epithelial cells and sparse sinusoidal endothelial cells and Kupffer cells (Fig. 46.1A). Normal hepatocytes are large, polygonal cells with abundant granular cytoplasm and a centrally placed, round nucleus with a well-delineated nuclear membrane, granular chromatin pattern, and distinct nucleolus. Hepatocytes normally exhibit variations in cell and nuclear size (i.e., sibling polymorphism). The nucleus-to-cytoplasm ratio (N:C ratio) is approximately 1:3. Bile duct epithelial cells are smaller than hepatocytes and appear as flat, monolayered, honeycomb sheets of glandular epithelium (see Fig. 46.1B). They may also reveal an on-edge picket-fence arrangement or small acinar structures. The cells have minimal pale cytoplasm and equidistant, round to oval, bland nuclei without nucleoli. Bile duct epithelium can be differentiated from bile ductular epithelium.

Elongated endothelial cells and comma-shaped Kupffer cells are almost indistinguishable from each other, especially when they appear as nuclear streaks. The thickness of liver cords can be appreciated in large sheets of cells and in fragments of liver parenchyma by focusing on the nuclear streaks in different planes of magnification (Fig. 46.2).

Pigments

Lipofuscin is a fine, golden, granular, relatively nonrefractile pigment with Papanicolaou stain and appears black with Giemsa stain (Fig. 46.3). This predominantly perinuclear pigment is common in aspirates of adult livers, and its absence in the context of a mass lesion is considered suspicious for a hepatocellular neoplasm. One potential diagnostic pitfall is that lipofuscin stains similar to melanin with Fontana-Masson stain, and the sample may be mistaken for metastatic melanoma.[79]

Bile pigment varies in color, texture, size, and density, but it is best recognized by its coarse, irregular, rather amorphous, nonrefractile appearance. In Giemsa-stained preparations, bile appears as a purplish-black pigment within the cytoplasm of hepatocytes or as ropey strands within bile canaliculi (Fig. 46.4). Hall stain may be used to confirm the pigment as bile.

Iron or hemosiderin may be present in hepatocytes, bile duct epithelial cells, and Kupffer cells and appears as a coarse, golden-brown, refractile pigment with Papanicolaou stain and brown-black with Giemsa stain (Fig. 46.5). Malignant hepatocytes typically lose their ability to retain iron. In the setting of hemochromatosis, Perl (Prussian blue) stain is a helpful ancillary tool to highlight nonstaining tumor cells.[80,81]

Steatosis

Steatosis is common in the liver, and the examiner should be aware of focal fatty changes.[82,83] Cytologically, fat may be a single, large, intracytoplasmic vacuole in a cell with an eccentric nucleus (i.e., macrovesicular steatosis) (Fig. 46.6) or multiple, small vacuoles in a cell with a central nucleus (i.e., microvesicular steatosis). Fat is best appreciated in Giemsa-stained preparations, which often reveal abundant oil globules in the background as a result of ruptured hepatocytes.

Infections

Liver abscess formations are suspected radiologically by the characteristic double target sign on CT scan.[84] The most common is pyogenic abscess, in which case aspiration is performed for tissue confirmation, culture, and drainage.[85,86] Smears are dominated by acute inflammatory cells and cellular debris (Fig. 46.7). Cultures are helpful for identification of bacterial organisms. Special stains, such as Gram stain, are not usually helpful, but uniquely characteristic organisms may be readily identified on smears. For example, *Actinomyces* has sulfur granules (Fig. 46.8).

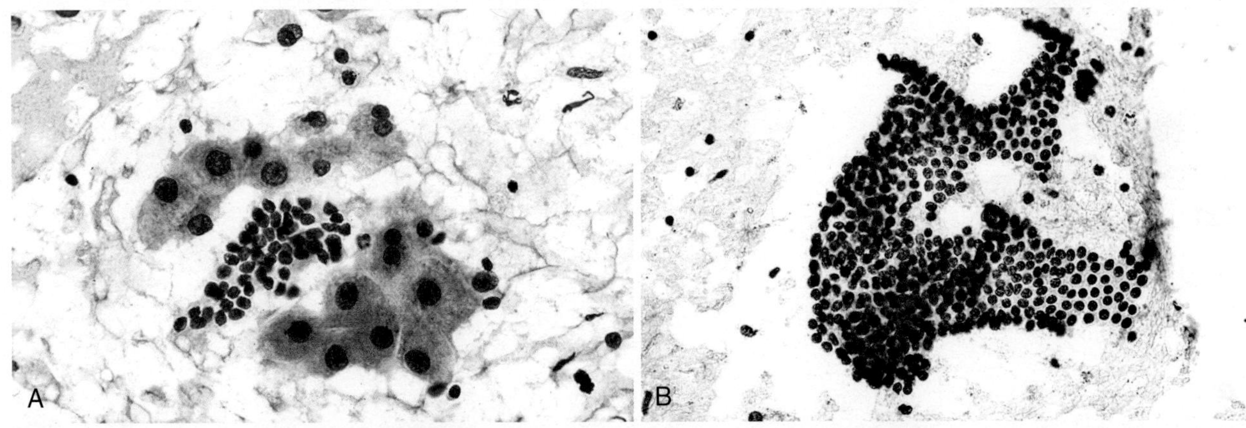

FIGURE 46.1 Normal hepatocytes and bile duct epithelium. A, The polygonal hepatocytes occur in narrow cords and exhibit mild polymorphism with ample granular cytoplasm; a central, round nucleus; well-delineated nuclear membrane; granular chromatin; and a distinct nucleolus. The nucleus-to-cytoplasm ratio is about 1:3. The small bile duct epithelial cluster consists of uniform cells with oval nuclei and indistinct cytoplasm (Papanicolaou stain). **B,** Bile duct epithelium from a larger duct displays a flat, monolayered, honeycomb sheet of glandular cells with nuclear palisading. The cells have minimal, pale cytoplasm and evenly spaced, regular, oval, bland nuclei without nucleoli (Papanicolaou stain).

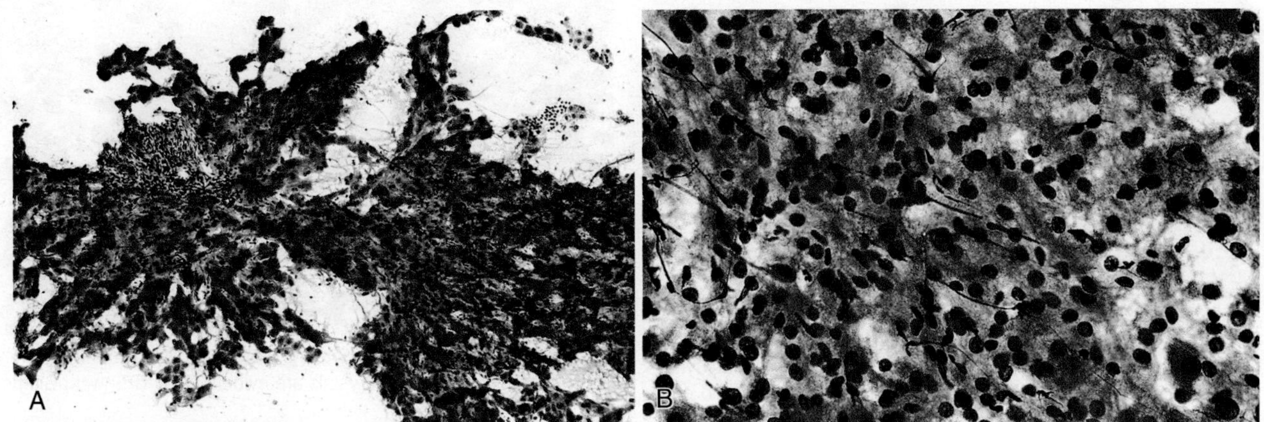

FIGURE 46.2 Normal liver parenchyma. A, Fragment of liver parenchyma with jagged edges shows narrow cords of hepatocytes, nuclear streaks, and a portal tract (Papanicolaou stain). **B,** Nuclear streaks represent Kupffer or endothelial cells sandwiched between hepatocytes and highlighting the narrow width of the cell cords (Papanicolaou stain).

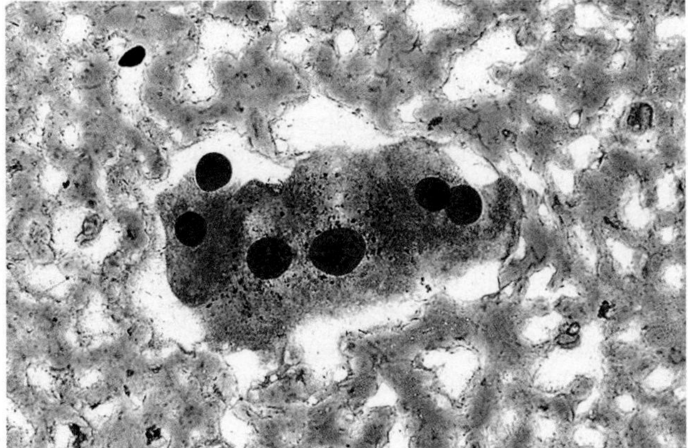

FIGURE 46.3 Lipofuscin pigment appears as nonrefractile, black granules located in the perinuclear cytoplasm of nonneoplastic hepatocytes (May-Grünwald-Giemsa stain).

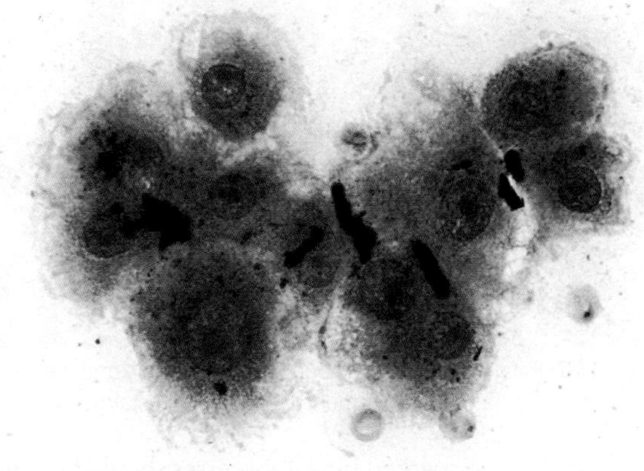

FIGURE 46.4 Bile pigment is seen as purplish-black, ropey strands within bile canaliculi and a few black droplets within the cytoplasm of nonneoplastic hepatocytes in a patient with cholestasis (May-Grünwald-Giemsa stain).

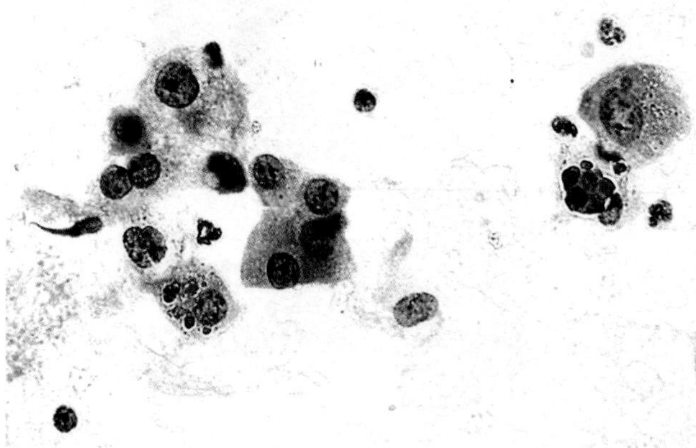

FIGURE 46.5 Hemosiderin (iron) pigment appears as coarse, golden-brown, refractile granules within the cytoplasm of nonneoplastic hepatocytes (Papanicolaou stain).

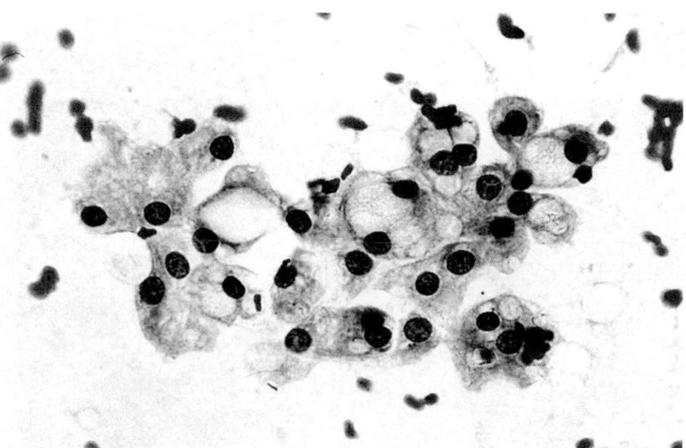

FIGURE 46.6 Macrovesicular steatosis. Nonneoplastic hepatocytes show large, intracytoplasmic fat vacuoles pushing the nucleus to one side of the cell cytoplasm (Papanicolaou stain).

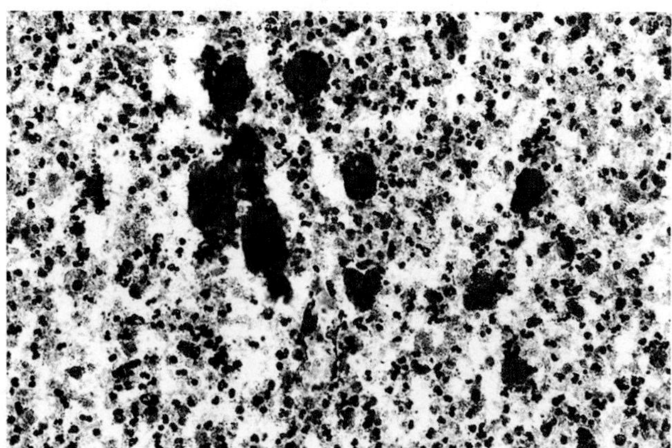

FIGURE 46.7 Pyogenic abscess. Abundant neutrophils and cellular debris show golden-brown bile pigment (Papanicolaou stain).

Smears from suspected fungal abscesses should be stained with Gomori methenamine silver and periodic acid–Schiff (PAS) stains. Amebic abscesses tend to be paucicellular with abundant amorphous granular debris, and trophozoites are rare. Necrotizing eosinophilic granulomas contain abundant eosinophils and possibly Charcot-Leyden crystals. Parasitic or fungal organisms should be sought (Fig. 46.9).

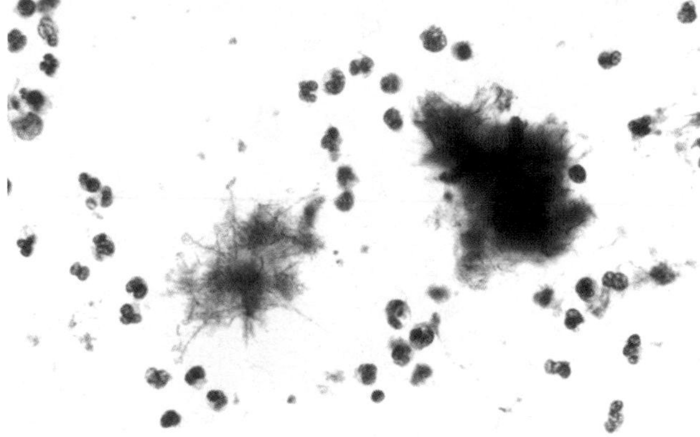

FIGURE 46.8 Abscess caused by *Actinomyces*. The fibrillar, star-shaped sulfur granules are characteristic of this organism (Papanicolaou stain).

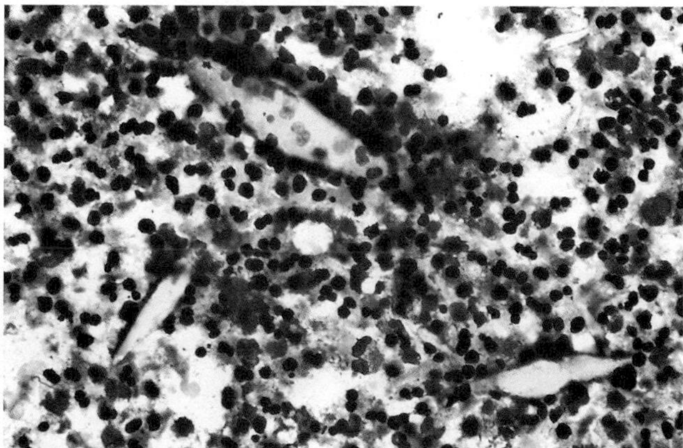

FIGURE 46.9 Necrotizing eosinophilic granuloma. Neutrophils, eosinophils, and Charcot-Leyden crystals are evident (May-Grünwald-Giemsa stain).

A potential diagnostic pitfall is that necrotic tumors may be associated with fever, simulating abscesses clinically and radiologically,[87] or they may become secondarily infected. If clinically warranted, aspiration cytology is recommended to avoid delay in instituting appropriate therapy.

Hydatid disease leads to cyst formation, which may become secondarily infected (see Cystic Lesions of the Liver). Echinococcosis is usually ruled out with clinical and imaging studies and the findings of a negative test result for specific echinococcal antibodies by serum enzyme immunosorbent assay performed before percutaneous needle aspiration.[88,89] In the event that a hydatid cyst is aspirated, the pathologist should search for protoscolices or hooklets of *Echinococcus granulosus* in the fluid or pus (Fig. 46.10).

Granulomatous inflammation may be caused by fungal or acid-fast organisms, but the presence of granulomas is not necessarily diagnostic of an infection. Cytologically, granulomas are composed of clusters of epithelioid histiocytes that have oval to elongated, sometimes twisted nuclei and visible but indistinct cytoplasm. Multinucleated giant cells may be present (Fig. 46.11). The characteristics of the necrotic background should also be evaluated. Gomori methenamine silver, PAS, and Ziehl-Neelsen staining may be performed on smears but are easier to perform on tissue sections.

Inflammatory pseudotumors are potential clinical, radiological, and cytohistological pitfalls because they mimic tumors. They may be lymphoplasmacytic, fibrohistiocytic, xanthogranulomatous, or granulomatous in nature (Fig. 46.12).[90-93]

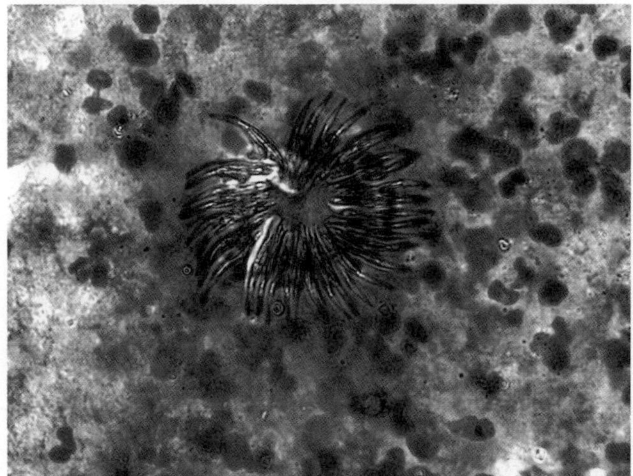

FIGURE 46.10 Hydatid cyst. The fluid contains single refractile hooklets or, rarely, intact echinococcal protoscolices (May-Grünwald-Giemsa stain).

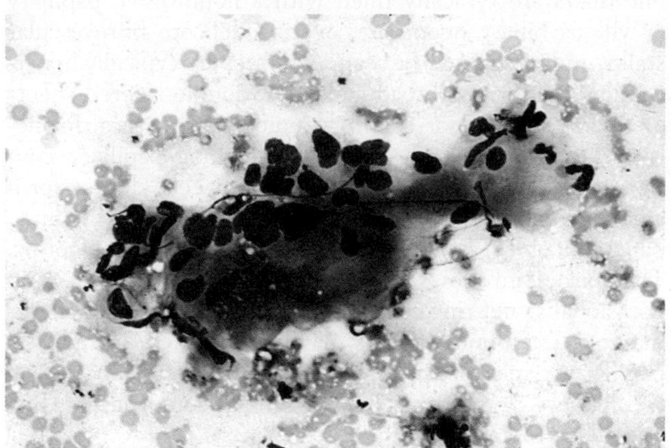

FIGURE 46.11 Tuberculous granuloma. A multinucleated Langhans giant cell has a horseshoe-shaped arrangement of the nuclei (May-Grünwald-Giemsa stain).

Activated lymphoid cells may be mistaken for lymphomas, atypical reactive hepatocytes for HCC, atypical reactive biliary epithelium for adenocarcinoma, atypical reactive stroma for sarcoma, and foamy histiocytes for amebic trophozoites. Immunoglobulin G4 (IgG4)–related disease may rarely manifest as a fibroblastic mass with lymphoplasmacytic infiltrates, eosinophils, IgG4-positive plasma cells, dense fibrosis of large bile ducts, and obliterative phlebitis.[94]

Nodular hematopoiesis is a rare diagnostic pitfall. Hematopoietic cells (especially megakaryocytes) may mimic inflammatory or malignant cells when perceived out of context.[95,96]

CYSTIC LESIONS OF THE LIVER

The type of cyst contents should be evaluated because the presence of mucin is a helpful diagnostic clue. The next step is to establish the presence and type of epithelial lining and whether it is neoplastic or malignant.[97] Box 46.6 provides a diagnostic algorithm for cystic lesions of the liver.

Cystic Lesions with an Epithelial Lining

Bile Duct Cyst, Simple Hepatic Cyst, and Fibropolycystic Disease

In cases of bile duct cyst, simple hepatic cyst, and fibropolycystic disease, the fluid may contain isolated cells or scant strips or sheets of cuboidal to low columnar epithelium without cytological atypia (Fig. 46.13).

Ciliated Foregut Cyst

Aspirates of foregut cysts are characterized by ciliated columnar cells and detached ciliated tufts.[98-100] The background usually contains amorphous debris and rare macrophages. The differential diagnosis includes cystic neoplasms.

Mucinous Cystic Neoplasm and Intraductal Papillary Neoplasm

Mucinous cystic neoplasms and intraductal papillary neoplasms have overlapping cytomorphological features. The cytodiagnosis may indicate a benign cyst, papillary neoplasm, or adenocarcinoma. FNAB alone cannot differentiate the various types of hepatobiliary cysts.[97,101] Generic

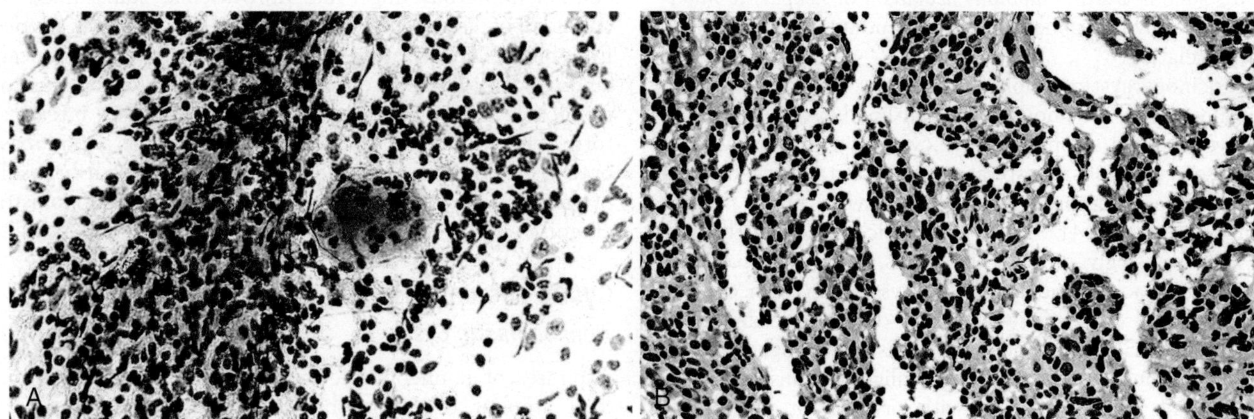

FIGURE 46.12 Lymphoplasmacytic-type inflammatory pseudotumor. A, Aspirate smears are dominated by lymphocytes and plasma cells, with occasional spindle-shaped fibroblasts and multinucleated foreign body giant cells (Papanicolaou stain). **B,** Cell block shows a heavy lymphoplasmacytic infiltrate with a granulation tissue background (hematoxylin and eosin stain).

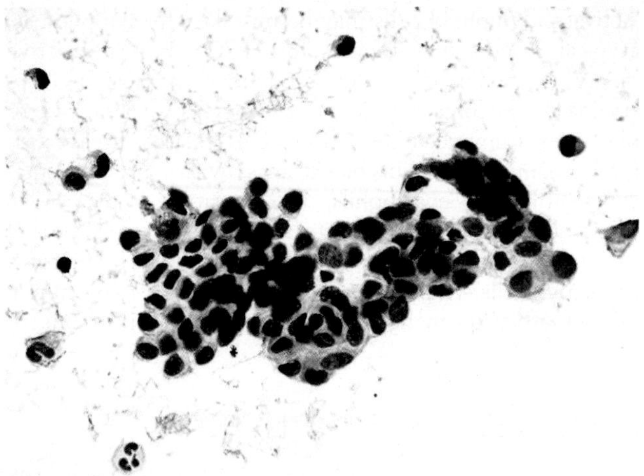

FIGURE 46.13 Solitary bile duct cyst. Flat honeycomb sheet of cuboidal epithelium with no cytological atypia (Papanicolaou stain).

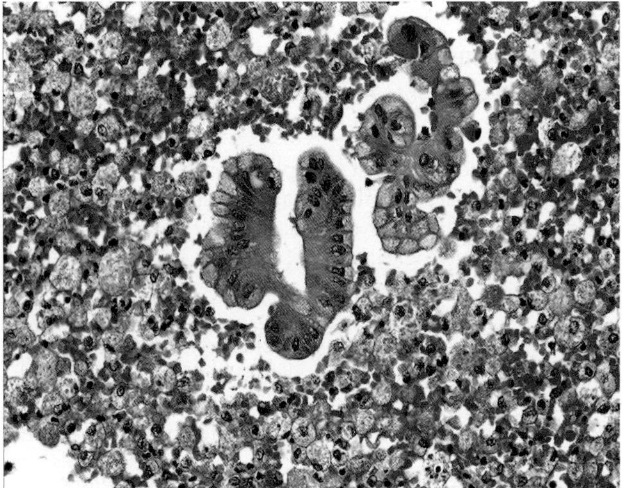

FIGURE 46.14 Mucinous cystic neoplasm. Mucinous glandular epithelium and foamy histiocytes predominate the contents of this benign hepatic cyst (cell block, hematoxylin and eosin stain). *(From Sidawy MK, Syed ZA. The Liver in Fine Needle Aspiration Cytology: A Volume in the Foundations in Diagnostic Pathology. Edinburgh: Churchill Livingstone; 2007.)*

terms such as *cystic mucinous neoplasm* or *neoplastic mucinous cyst* may be applied if imaging studies are not available for correlation.

Mucinous cystic neoplasms typically occur as single or multiloculated, mucinous, epithelial-lined cysts surrounded by ovarian-type stroma.[102] The cyst fluid may be watery or viscous. Diagnostic aspirates likely contain degenerated cuboidal to columnar epithelial cells with bland nuclear features (Fig. 46.14).[103] The neoplastic epithelial cells may be arranged singly, on edge, in sheets, or as small papillary tufts. The background usually shows mucin with chronic inflammatory cells, histiocytes, and debris. The degree of cellularity varies and tends to increase with higher grades of intraepithelial neoplasia. With malignant transformation, features of adenocarcinoma with or without mucin and cellular debris are often evident.[104] The definitive diagnosis requires correlation with clinical information, imaging studies, and histopathological confirmation of ovarian-type stroma surrounding the cyst.[97] Stromal components are not usually present with cyst content aspiration, but forceps biopsy of the cyst wall may sample the stroma, which can be confirmed with immunohistochemical stain for the estrogen receptor. The cyst fluid may be assayed for carcinoembryonic antigen and CA 19-9 to distinguish neoplastic from nonneoplastic liver cysts (Box 46.8).[101,105,106]

BOX 46.8 Mucinous Cystic Neoplasm

- Degenerated mucin-secreting cuboidal to columnar epithelium with bland nuclear features; arranged singly, on edge, in sheets, or as small papillary tufts
- Background usually shows mucin with chronic inflammatory cells, histiocytes, and debris
- Mesenchymal stromal components are usually absent
- Variable cellularity, depending on grades of intraepithelial neoplasia
- Features of adenocarcinoma seen with malignant transformation
- Assay of cyst fluid for carcinoembryonic antigen and CA 19-9

Biliary intraductal papillary neoplasm is a fusiform or cystic (unilocular or multilocular) luminal dilation in communication with the biliary tract. The affected intrahepatic bile ducts are typically filled with a noninvasive papillary or villous biliary neoplasm covering delicate fibrovascular stalks, and mucin may be seen. Aspirates are typically hypercellular, comprising broad and often double-layered sheets of ductal cuboidal or columnar epithelium with a distinctive three-dimensional, complex-branching papillary configuration (Fig. 46.15).[107] The sheets of cells do not form a honeycomb pattern but are crowded. Phenotypes include pancreaticobiliary, intestinal, gastric, and oncocytic forms. The epithelium shows intracytoplasmic mucin vacuoles and occasional signet ring cells. The nuclei show variable abnormalities. Psammoma bodies may be identified. Intraductal papillary neoplasms with associated invasive carcinoma have the highest degree of cellularity and pleomorphism (Box 46.9) (see Metastases).

Metastases

Metastatic papillary carcinomas of the pancreas and ovary can simulate intraductal papillary neoplasms. Smears may contain numerous finger-like fibrovascular stalks lined by cuboidal or columnar epithelium with cytological atypia. Endobiliary cancerization by metastatic colorectal adenocarcinomas without apparent stromal invasion is notorious for mimicking biliary intraductal papillary neoplasm, intestinal form. The intraductal metastasis may present as a solid mass or as a cystic luminal dilation of the biliary tree as a result of an associated fibroinflammatory process. Immunohistochemistry is necessary to delineate the two phenotypes.[108]

Cystic Lesions Without an Epithelial Lining

Nonneoplastic Cysts

Aspirates of nonneoplastic cysts typically reveal an abundant amount of turbid, brown fluid with inflammatory cells, macrophages, fibrin, debris, and bile or hematoidin pigment. The fluid lacks a lining of epithelial cells but may contain benign cells from surrounding liver parenchyma.

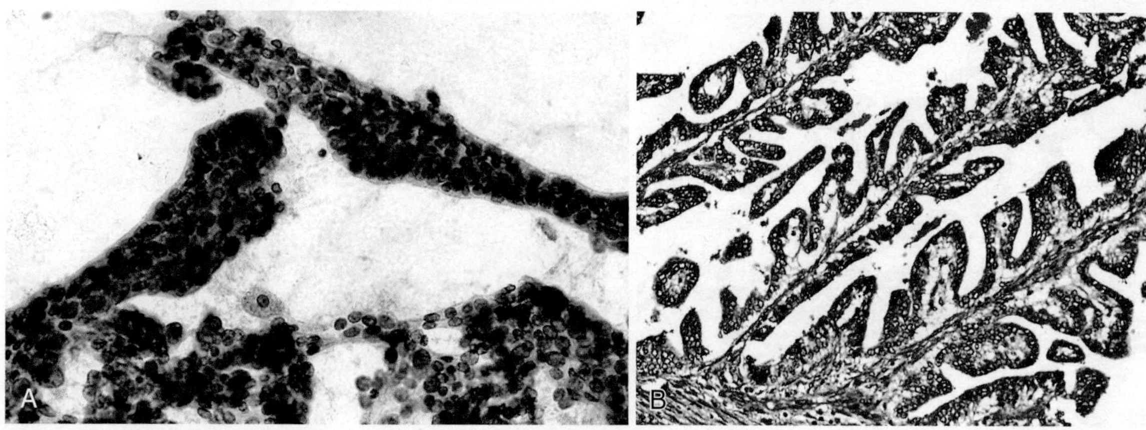

FIGURE 46.15 Biliary intraductal papillary neoplasm. A, Delicate, branching, finger-like fibrovascular stalks are lined by three-dimensional, double-layered (crowded) sheets of cuboidal epithelium (Papanicolaou stain). **B,** Histological section shows a complex branching papillary tumor, which would have been located within a cystically dilated duct (hematoxylin and eosin stain).

BOX 46.9 Biliary Intraductal Papillary Neoplasm

- Hypercellular smears
- Broad, double-layered sheets of ductal columnar epithelium with three-dimensional, complex-branching papillae
- Pancreaticobiliary, intestinal, gastric and oncocytic phenotypes
- Crowded sheets of cells with variable nuclear atypia
- Intracytoplasmic mucin vacuoles, including few signet ring cells
- Psammoma bodies
- Features of adenocarcinoma seen with malignant transformation
- Pitfall: Endobiliary cancerization by metastatic colorectal adenocarcinoma

The differential diagnosis includes inflammatory/infectious cysts, cystic hematomas, as well as true cysts and cystic neoplasms. A secondary bacterial infection may produce cyst fluid that contains abundant neutrophils and proteinaceous background debris. However, the presence of a neoplastic epithelial lining or background mucin excludes the diagnosis of a nonneoplastic cyst.

Neoplastic Cysts and Tumor-Like Lesions

Cavernous Hemangioma

Cavernous hemangiomas are usually asymptomatic and diagnosed incidentally during a workup for other conditions, such as during the process of staging a malignancy, and they can be difficult to distinguish from metastasis radiologically.[109-112] Hemorrhagic aspirates are often considered unsatisfactory. The nondiagnostic appearance of blood with loose rather than dense fibrous connective tissue and few or no background hepatocytes raises the possibility of a hemangioma in the proper clinical setting (Fig. 46.16). Histological material is crucial in establishing a specific diagnosis (Box 46.10).

Mesenchymal Hamartoma

Aspirates of mesenchymal hamartomas are obtained mainly in the pediatric population, with rare exceptions, and they usually show clusters of epithelial and mesenchymal or spindle-shaped cells with bland-appearing nuclei admixed with loose connective tissue (Fig. 46.17).[113-116] However, aspiration cytology rarely enables a definitive diagnosis, and cytology is of limited value because hepatoblastomas or malignant mesenchymal tumors are difficult to exclude confidently (Box 46.11).

Cystic Degeneration in a Benign or Malignant Tumor

Solid tumors may undergo central necrosis and cavitation, simulating cysts radiologically. If postablational therapeutic status has been excluded, a necrosis-associated tumor should raise suspicion of an abscess.[87] Necrosis is more likely to occur in malignant lesions, such as squamous cell carcinomas, neuroendocrine tumors, and metastases from colorectal adenocarcinomas and nonkeratinizing undifferentiated carcinomas in the nasopharynx. The diagnostic cells may be obscured by the process.

Undifferentiated Embryonal Sarcoma

Although most undifferentiated embryonal sarcomas appear on ultrasound imaging as solid lesions, CT and MRI imaging may detect a low-attenuation mass with a cystic appearance. Most cystic structures result from liquefactive necrosis and blood clots; however, true cystic spaces may also occur.[73] Aspirates recapitulate the histological pattern of the tumor.[117-121] Smears are usually composed of spindle cells and myxoid tissue, intermixed with pleomorphic cells ranging from small, round cells to large, multinucleated giant cells. Giant cells have bizarre nuclei and a massively deranged chromatin structure. They contain intracytoplasmic vacuoles and are AFP negative, PAS positive, but diastase-resistant hyaline globules (Fig. 46.18); extracellular globules may also be present. Immunostaining for α_1-antitrypsin, α_1-antichymotrypsin, and carcinoembryonic antigen is positive in tumor cells. The cytological differential diagnoses include rhabdomyosarcoma, hepatoblastoma, undifferentiated pleomorphic sarcoma, NOS (so-called malignant fibrous histiocytoma), and poorly differentiated HCC (Box 46.12).

SOLID LESIONS OF THE LIVER

Hepatocellular Appearance

Benign Hepatocellular Nodules

Benign hepatocellular nodules, such as focal fatty changes, large regenerative nodules, dysplastic nodules, focal

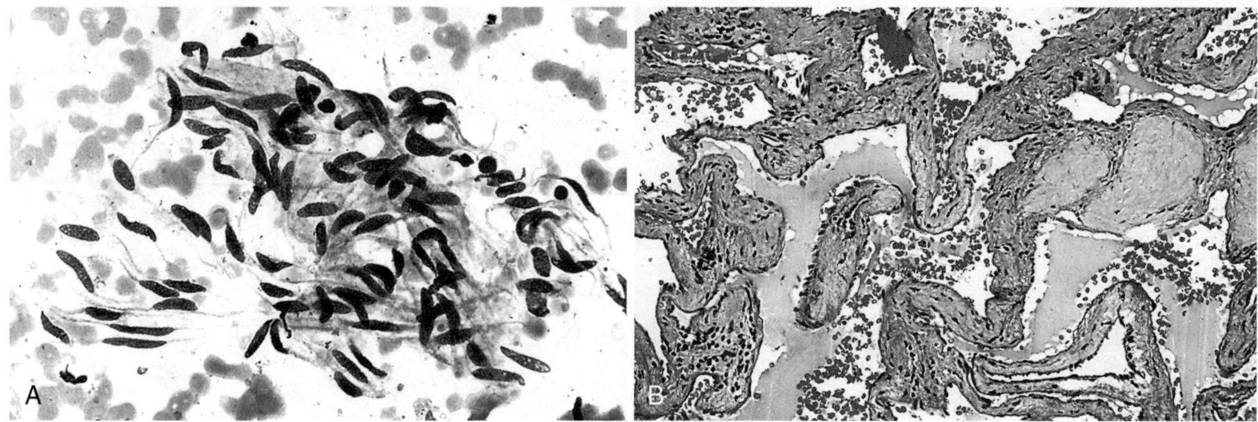

FIGURE 46.16 Cavernous hemangioma. A, Scanty clumps of loose fibrous connective tissue are seen in the blood (May-Grünwald-Giemsa stain). **B,** Histological section shows large, irregular, interconnecting endothelial-lined vascular spaces separated by loose connective tissue septa (hematoxylin and eosin stain).

BOX 46.10 Cavernous Hemangioma

- Bloody with scant cellularity on smears
- Loose connective tissue; usually few to no hepatocytes
- Smears commonly nondiagnostic; specific diagnosis depends more on cell block pattern

nodular hyperplasia, and hepatocellular adenomas, can be nonneoplastic or neoplastic and are discussed together because they share common cytological features, including fatty changes (Box 46.13).[22,122,123] Unfortunately, it is not always possible to distinguish these entities on the basis of smear cytology alone. They all can mimic well-differentiated HCC.

A focal fatty change may simulate a mass lesion radiologically.[82,83] Aspirates are composed of a polymorphous population of enlarged, fat-laden, nonneoplastic hepatocytes intermingled with bile duct epithelial clusters. Oil globules may be seen in the background on air-dried smears.

Aspirates from large regenerative nodules are similar to those from cirrhosis, in which a polymorphous liver parenchymal population shows evidence of hyperplasia and hepatocellular-interface restoration (i.e., bile ductular epithelium and stromal fragments).[63,76] Hyperplastic hepatocytes occur in two-cell-thick cords and exhibit slight polymorphism and binucleated forms. Normal bile duct epithelial clusters should be differentiated from bile ductular epithelial cells, which appear as curved, narrow, double-stranded rows of cells with overlapping, dark, oval nuclei; scant or absent cytoplasm; and a high N:C ratio. Nuclear disarray may be disconcerting. Ductules can be seen emanating from the jagged edges of sizeable parenchymal fragments (Fig. 46.19). Stroma may be seen in the background. The presence of ductules should raise the diagnostic threshold for a malignant process.

Hepatocellular atypia, such as large cell and small cell changes (e.g., dysplasia), are considered neoplastic precursor lesions and may be detected in aspirates from cirrhotic livers.[73,81,123-129] Hepatocytes with large cell changes show corresponding cellular and nuclear enlargement and mild nuclear atypia; but the normal N:C ratio (i.e., one to three or less) is maintained (Fig. 46.20). Hepatocytes with small cell changes are small and monotonous, with a subtle increase in the N:C ratio. The nuclear size is similar to that of normal hepatocytes, but there is less cytoplasm, imparting an impression of nuclear crowding (Fig. 46.21).[130]

Aspirates of low-grade dysplastic nodules show hepatocytes that exhibit large cell changes, whereas those from high-grade dysplastic nodules show hepatocytes with small cell changes. Dysplastic hepatocytes tend to occur singly or in narrow cords, usually one to two cells thick. Transgressing endothelium is not a feature. It is almost impossible to distinguish a small cell change from a well-differentiated or early HCC.[130,131] The key to recognizing a large cell change as benign is the sporadic placement of these cells in a background of otherwise reactive-appearing hepatocytes and accompanied by bile ductal or ductular epithelium and stroma. Availability of histological material for immunohistochemistry is invaluable.

Patients with cirrhosis without iron overload can accumulate iron within regenerative or dysplastic nodules, which are called *siderotic nodules*. Siderotic dysplastic nodules are considered to be premalignant, whereas siderotic regenerative nodules are a marker for severe viral or alcoholic cirrhosis.[76,77] Iron-free foci in patients with genetic hemochromatosis are likely to be malignant.[80,81]

Focal nodular hyperplasia is characterized by a proliferation of hepatocytes surrounding a central scar containing blood vessels and bile ducts. A brisk ductular reaction is often seen at the hepatocellular-stromal interface.[132] Aspirates typically contain a polymorphous population of cells, but this varies.[133] Hyperplastic hepatocytes abound in one- to two-cell-thick cords. Bile duct epithelium is usually evident (Fig. 46.22). The presence of ductular epithelium supports the benign nature of this lesion, but this feature can be mistaken for adenocarcinoma if it is the dominant component of the aspirate. A possible diagnostic pitfall is mistaking reactive stroma for a spindle cell neoplasm.[134] A characteristic geographic immunostaining pattern is seen with the use of glutamine synthetase.[135] Without radiological demonstration of a central scar, it may not be possible to differentiate focal nodular hyperplasia from large regenerative nodules on smear cytology because both show features of regeneration.

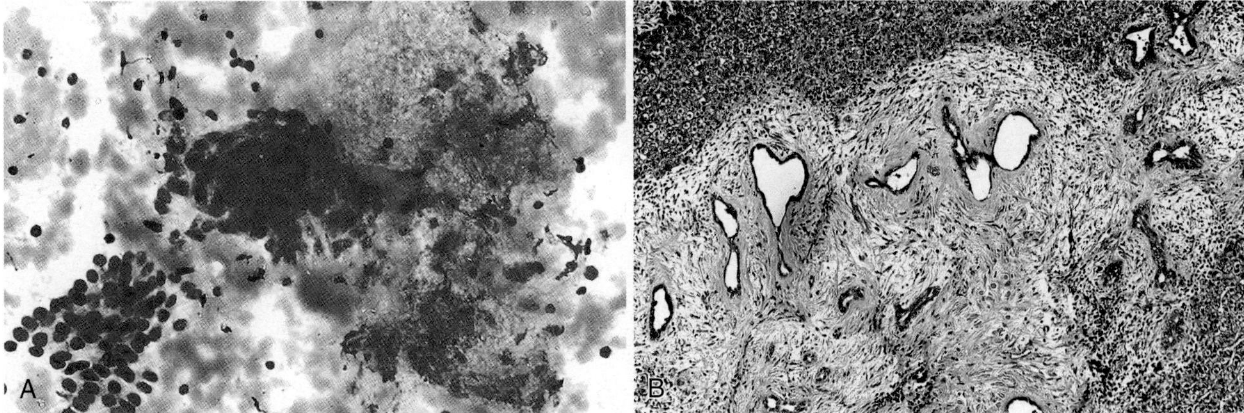

FIGURE 46.17 Mesenchymal hamartoma. A, Clusters of epithelial and spindle-shaped mesenchymal cells with bland nuclei are held together by myxoid matrix material (May-Grünwald-Giemsa stain). **B,** Histological section shows lobulated islands of loose myxoid matrix containing misshapen ductal structures and mesenchymal cells (Masson trichrome stain).

BOX 46.11 Mesenchymal Hamartoma

- Hypocellular smears
- Spindle-shaped cells with bland nuclei
- Loose myxoid matrix with bile duct–like epithelial clusters
- Cytology of limited value in establishing a definitive diagnosis

Aspirates of a hepatocellular adenoma are hypercellular and typically contain well-differentiated hepatocytes occurring in one- to two-cell-thick cords (Fig. 46.23). There is no significant atypia. Transgressing endothelium is common, but peripheral endothelium is lacking. The tumor cells are polygonal and have moderate granular cytoplasm. Some cells display fatty or clear cell changes and bile or lipofuscin pigment. Bile duct epithelium is absent. The reticulin framework is usually well preserved. CD34, which highlights capillarization of the sinusoids in HCC, can also positively stain adenomas, particularly in the periseptal areas. This may be a diagnostic pitfall in assessing small, fragmented liver core specimens and cell block preparations. Glypican 3 staining should be focal and weak at best.[136-138] The overall perspective on hepatocellular adenomas has evolved. There are currently six subtypes based on histological characteristics, immunohistochemical phenotypes, and molecular characterization.[73,139-141] The major impact of the molecular classification is to identify subjects who are at higher risk of bleeding and malignant transformation for appropriate management. The diagnosis requires clinical correlation. Chapter 56 provides more information on immunohistochemical markers and molecular subtyping of adenomas in tissue sections.[142] A note of caution is that immunostains used to subtype hepatocellular adenomas do not distinguish them from HCC. That said, taking into consideration the background liver disease (i.e., cirrhosis), the distinction can be made. For example, strong and diffuse nuclear staining with β-catenin supports a diagnosis of hepatocellular carcinoma over β-catenin–activated adenoma when there is a background of cirrhosis.[143]

A nodule-in-nodule lesion occurs when an HCC subnodule develops within a parent dysplastic or regenerative nodule.[144] Representative FNAB samples may be a problem because of the focality of proliferative clones within these nodules. Classic aspirates reveal more than one population of lesional hepatocytes, including malignant hepatocytes and dysplastic or hyperplastic hepatocytes in the background (Fig. 46.24). The presence of biliary epithelial cells varies.

Primary Malignant Hepatocellular Neoplasms

Hepatocellular Carcinoma

HCCs exhibit marked heterogeneity in differentiation, histological pattern (i.e., trabecular-sinusoidal, pseudoacinar, and solid types), and cell morphology. The World Health Organization (WHO) classification of HCC lists the classic type, several variants, and special types.[73] Sampling limitations of the FNAB technique and cytohistological challenges in the face of this diversity are recognized. Most tumors show relatively good hepatic preservation and obvious malignant features. However, diagnostic dilemmas exist at both ends of the spectrum—cytological features of malignancy are lacking at the well-differentiated end, and resemblance to hepatocytes is lacking at the poorly differentiated end.[145] The cytomorphological features of HCC are summarized in Box 46.14.[61,63,146-153] The cytological nuclear grading of HCC into well-, moderately, and poorly differentiated types is outlined in Boxes 46.15 to 46.17.[74,76]

Cellularity

Aspirates are typically hypercellular. Low-power scanning usually shows a granular smear pattern composed of trails of irregular tumor clusters, which reflects the prominent trabecular-sinusoidal pattern (Fig. 46.25).

Epithelial Cohesiveness

Cohesion is the rule for HCC. However, a strong tendency to dissociation is observed in very-well-differentiated and very-poorly differentiated tumors. Dispersed, small clusters or single cells are seen in smears of very-well-differentiated HCC with cords that are one or two cells thick and in poorly differentiated HCC with deficient reticulin.

Vascular Patterns

Arborizing tongues and nests of cohesive tumor cells more than two cells thick are wrapped peripherally by endothelium

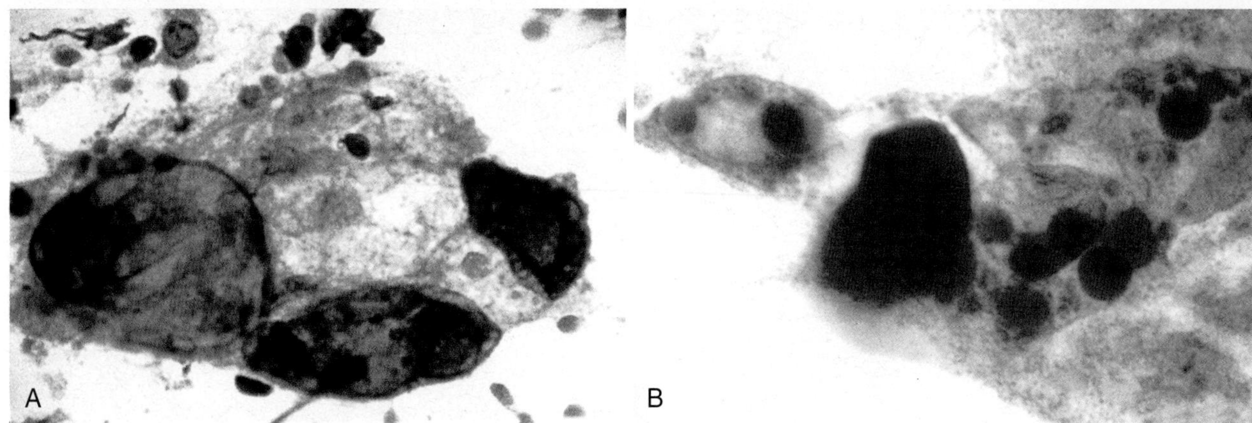

FIGURE 46.18 Undifferentiated embryonal sarcoma. A, Smears are composed of anaplastic and multinucleated giant tumor cells displaying bizarre nuclei and a deranged chromatin structure (Papanicolaou stain). **B,** Tumor cells may also contain periodic acid–Schiff (PAS)–positive, diastase-resistant intracytoplasmic globules (PAS with diastase digestion).

BOX 46.12 Undifferentiated Embryonal Sarcoma

- Hypercellular smears
- Large, pleomorphic anaplastic cells with multinucleated giant cells and atypical spindle cells
- Intracytoplasmic globules: periodic acid–Schiff positive, diastase resistant

BOX 46.13 Regenerative, Dysplastic, and Benign Neoplastic Hepatocellular Nodules

- Hepatocytes arranged in jagged irregular clusters, small clusters, short rows, and singly (depending on regenerative, dysplastic, or neoplastic nature)
- No peripheral endothelium
- Clusters rarely have transgressing endothelium (except for neoplastic aspirates)
- Reactive hepatocytes show sibling polymorphism with normal nucleus-to-cytoplasm (N:C) ratio (1:3) and frequent binucleation
- Sporadically placed large, atypical cells with mild nuclear pleomorphism of nuclear size but normal N:C ratio (in dysplastic hepatocytes with large cell change)
- Small, uniformly monotonous hepatocytes with increased N:C ratio and nuclear crowding (in dysplastic hepatocytes with small cell change)
- Variably prominent nucleoli but without macroeosinophilic nucleoli
- Cytoplasm usually abundant (except in small cell change) and granular but may show a fatty change, lipofuscin pigment, or iron deposition
- Bile duct epithelium present (except in neoplastic aspirates)
- Bile ductular epithelium and stromal fragments, indicative of hepatocellular-interface restoration, may be present (except in neoplastic aspirates)
- Reticulin stain shows retention of one- to two-cell-thick hepatic cords on cell block

(Fig. 46.26).[146,150,154] Although the trabecular-sinusoidal pattern is cytologically identified in less than one-half of tumors, it is specific for HCC and is one of the most important diagnostic clues for separating reactive and benign neoplastic proliferations from well-differentiated HCC.[51,146,150,155] More often, the pathologist encounters loosely cohesive sheets of tumor cells with transgressing, arborizing, or central endothelial proliferations (Fig. 46.27). Basement membranes are best appreciated in Giemsa-stained preparations as pink tram-lines.[61] Although this vascular appearance is not specific for HCC, it is rarely seen in nonneoplastic hepatocellular nodules, cirrhosis, and hepatitis.[150]

A pseudoacinar pattern is common. The cystically dilated canalicular spaces contain bile or pale secretions and are surrounded by polygonal cells with central nuclei similar to the adjacent sibling cells. The subtle rosette-like pattern is best appreciated by examining several planes in the tissue (Fig. 46.28). In some cases, the surrounding cells may assume a more columnar shape with basal nuclei simulating true acini. The concomitant presence of malignant acini may imply the presence of a cHCC-CCA.

Cellular Characteristics

A monomorphous population of atypical hepatocytes usually prevails. Tumor cells may be smaller, larger, or the same size as nonneoplastic hepatocytes. Better-differentiated HCCs are characterized by polygonal cells with well-defined cell borders; ample, dense granular cytoplasm; a uniformly elevated N:C ratio; a central, round nucleus; well-delineated nuclear membranes; macroeosinophilic nucleoli; and fine, irregularly granular chromatin (Fig. 46.29).[51,150] Mitoses increase in number with nuclear grade. Well-differentiated HCC cells tend to be conspicuous by their small size, striking monotony, subtle increase in N:C ratio, and nuclear crowding (Fig. 46.30). Poorly differentiated HCC cells tend to be highly pleomorphic with overlapping nuclei, thin nuclear membranes, irregular nuclear contours with convoluted forms, hyperchromasia, and numerous mitoses (Fig. 46.31).

Atypical naked hepatocytic nuclei may be plentiful in all grades of HCC (Fig. 46.32). This finding is a more reliable feature for separating primary from metastatic tumors than it is for differentiating benign from malignant tumors.[148]

Multinucleated tumor giant cells may be osteoclastic or pleomorphic (Fig. 46.33). The former type shows nuclear features that are similar to those of sibling cells. Although rare, tumor giant cells may be present, even in lower grades of HCC. Their presence does not necessarily indicate a higher-grade tumor.

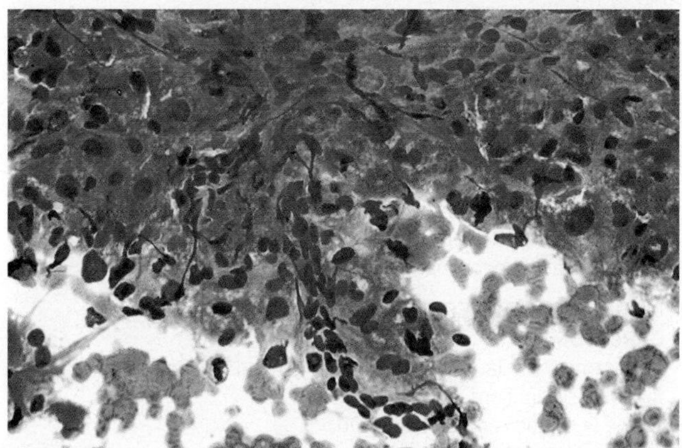

FIGURE 46.19 Large regenerative nodule. Reactive hepatocytes in irregularly shaped clusters are associated with a curved bile ductule emanating from the hepatocellular-stromal interface. The ductule consists of a double row of closely apposed, overlapping, small, darkly stained, oval nuclei with absent cytoplasm (May-Grünwald-Giemsa stain).

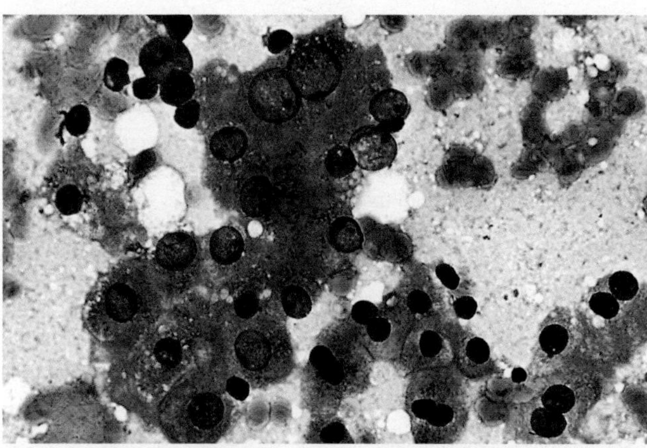

FIGURE 46.20 Hepatocytes with large cell changes. There is cell and nuclear enlargement. The nucleus-to-cytoplasm ratio is maintained at about 1:3. Compare with normal hepatocytes *(bottom right)* (May-Grünwald-Giemsa stain).

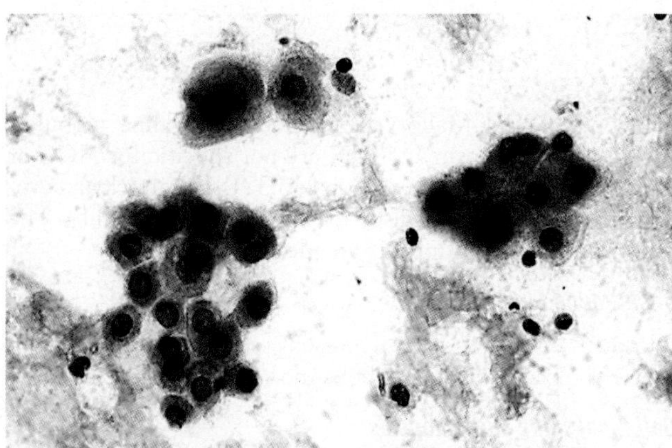

FIGURE 46.21 Hepatocytes with small cell changes. Monotonous, small hepatocytes exhibit decreased cytoplasm, an increased nucleus-to-cytoplasm ratio, and an impression of nuclear crowding. Compare with two clusters of normal hepatocytes in the vicinity (Papanicolaou stain).

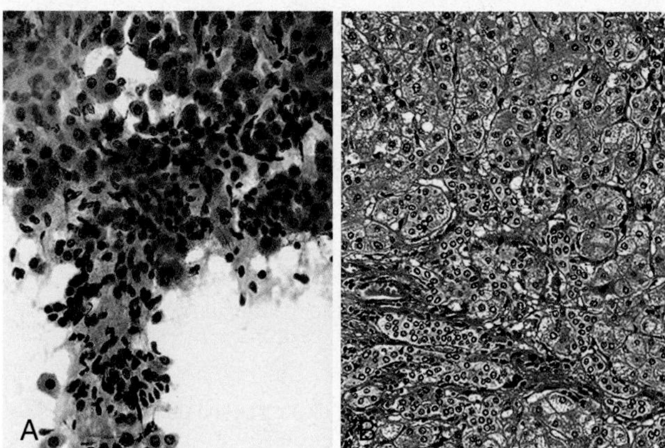

FIGURE 46.22 Focal nodular hyperplasia. A, Hyperplastic hepatocytes are present with ductules, which are represented by small, darkly stained, oval nuclei emanating from the hepatocellular-stromal interface (Papanicolaou stain). **B,** Histological section shows a brisk ductular reaction at the hepatocellular-stromal interface from the edge of a central scar (hematoxylin and eosin stain).

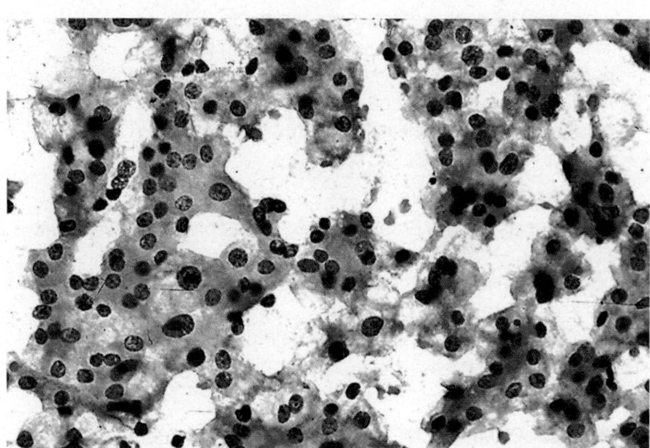

FIGURE 46.23 Hepatocellular adenoma. The hypercellular smear contains narrow cords (as many as three cells thick) of hepatocytes displaying mild sibling polymorphism but without significant cytological atypia (Papanicolaou stain).

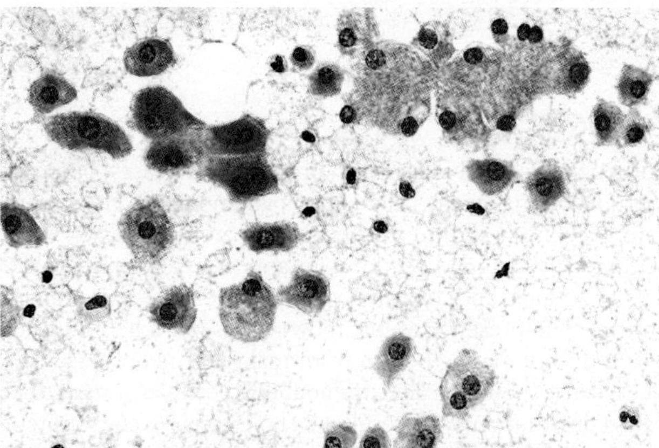

FIGURE 46.24 The nodule-in-nodule lesion is composed of a well-differentiated hepatocellular carcinoma arising within a large regenerative nodule. Notice the two populations of hepatocytes. Well-defined malignant hepatocytes from the subnodule exhibit mild pleomorphism, dense cytoplasm, and an increased nucleus-to-cytoplasm ratio. They are located among pale, hyperplastic hepatocytes with a normal nucleus-to-cytoplasm ratio from the parent nodule (Papanicolaou stain).

BOX 46.14 Cytological Findings of Fine-Needle Aspiration Biopsy for Hepatocellular Carcinoma

CELLULARITY
- Hypercellular
- Uniformly granular smear pattern

EPITHELIAL COHESIVENESS
- Cellular cohesion is the rule (tendency to dispersion at ends of cytomorphological spectrum)
- Arborizing tonguelike projections or balls of tumor cells with peripheral endothelium

PATTERNS
- Trabecular-sinusoidal pattern (indicated by the peripheral endothelium)
- Pseudoacinar pattern (implied by the rosette-like gaps in cellular aggregates)

CELLULAR CHARACTERISTICS
- Monomorphous population of abnormal hepatocytes
- Better-differentiated tumors are characterized by polygonal cells with well-defined cell borders, ample granular cytoplasm, round central nuclei with well-delineated nuclear membrane, prominent nucleoli, and granular chromatin.
- The nucleus-to-cytoplasm ratio increases in proportion to the nuclear grade.
- Nuclear pleomorphism correlates with irregular nuclear contours, mitoses, and multinucleated giant tumor cells.
- Atypical naked hepatocytic nuclei

CELLULAR INCLUSIONS
- Intracytoplasmic bile droplets or canalicular or pseudoacinar bile plugs
- Intracytoplasmic fat vacuoles
- Intracytoplasmic glycogen
- Intracytoplasmic hyaline globules, pale bodies, and Mallory-Denk bodies
- Intranuclear (cytoplasmic) inclusions

VASCULAR COMPONENT
- Peripheral endothelium
- Transgressing, arborizing, and central endothelium

BACKGROUND ELEMENTS
- Normal or reactive hepatocytes
- Bile duct epithelial clusters
- Hemorrhagic, necrotic background

BOX 46.15 Cytological Findings of Fine-Needle Aspiration Biopsy for Well-, Moderately, and Poorly Differentiated Hepatocellular Carcinoma

WELL-DIFFERENTIATED HEPATOCELLULAR CARCINOMA
- Tumor cells resemble hepatocytes in size, shape, and nuclear and nucleolar appearances.
- The nucleus-to-cytoplasm (N:C) ratio is slightly higher.
- Mitoses are exceptional.

MODERATELY DIFFERENTIATED HEPATOCELLULAR CARCINOMA

Cells remain similar to hepatocytes in general appearance, with the following distinctions.
- The N:C ratio is moderately high.
- Round to ovoid nuclei show a moderate degree of pleomorphism.
- Nucleoli are prominent, and mitoses are easily identifiable.

POORLY DIFFERENTIATED HEPATOCELLULAR CARCINOMA
- Resemblance to hepatocytes is lacking.
- Tumor cells exhibit marked pleomorphism, less cytoplasm, very high N:C ratio, thin nuclear membranes with irregular nuclear contours, hyperchromasia, and numerous mitoses.
- Multinucleated giant tumor cells are easily identifiable.

BOX 46.16 Well-Differentiated Hepatocellular Carcinoma

- On low-power microscopy, the smear pattern shows trails of smooth-edged, arborizing clusters of thickened trabeculae with peripheral endothelium (pathognomonic)
- On low power, the smear pattern shows many loosely cohesive sheets of hepatocytes with transgressing vessels (highly suspect finding)
- Monotonous, uniform hepatocytic cell population with subtle malignant features
- Pseudoacinar formation in cell clusters
- Nucleus-to-cytoplasm ratio higher than in normal hepatocytes (>1:3)
- Macroeosinophilic nucleoli
- Reduced number of binucleated cells
- Background free from bile duct epithelial cells
- Reticulin stain demonstrates loss of the normal one- to two-cell-thick hepatic cord architecture
- Iron stain fails to stain tumor cells in hemochromatosis
- α-Fetoprotein is helpful if positive but often is not
- Novel markers, such as glypican 3, glutamine synthetase, and heat shock protein 70, are helpful if two of three show positivity

Pigments

Although observed in less than one-half of all cases, bile production by malignant cells is pathognomonic of HCC with rare exception, and no further studies are necessary.[146] Bile within canaliculi and pseudoacini appears as greenish-black, ropey strands and blobs, respectively, on Giemsa-stained smears. The presence of bile, however, is not a helpful finding in differentiating benign from malignant neoplasms. The pathologist should be alert for nonhepatocellular tumors that cause obstruction with resultant cholestasis. A concomitant absence of lipofuscin pigment or iron-free hepatocytes in patients with iron overload supports a malignant diagnosis.

Cellular Inclusions

Intracytoplasmic fat and glycogen vacuoles are common in HCC (see the section Variants of Hepatocellular Carcinoma). Intracytoplasmic inclusions include hyaline globules, pale bodies, and Mallory-Denk bodies. Hyaline globules, such as α_1-antitrypsin and AFP, are not specific for HCC or malignancy in general (see Fig. 46.32). Intranuclear cytoplasmic inclusions are also not specific (Fig. 46.34). The presence of mucin supports an adenocarcinoma.

Background Elements

Bile duct epithelial cells, if present, should be few and far apart. The background may be hemorrhagic, necrotic, or both.

Cell Blocks and Microbiopsies

Cell blocks and microbiopsies may provide additional architectural and morphological clues to the diagnosis. It is not uncommon for hepatocytic features to be more apparent in histological sections than on smear cytology, potentially

BOX 46.17 Moderately to Poorly Differentiated Hepatocellular Carcinoma

- Low-power smear pattern usually resembles well-differentiated tumors; however, there is a dyshesive tendency in poorly differentiated tumors.
- Peripheral endothelium is virtually pathognomonic.
- Transgressing vessels are suggestive but cannot distinguish hepatocellular from renal cell carcinoma.
- Presence of intracytoplasmic bile is pathognomonic.
- Polygonal cells with central nuclei and prominent nucleoli have visible granular to clear cytoplasm in moderately differentiated tumors.
- Scant to no cytoplasm with a greater degree of pleomorphism and mitotic activity is seen in poorly differentiated tumors.
- Immunophenotype: positive for low-molecular-weight cytokeratins (CK) (e.g., Cam 5.2 antibody to CK8), polyclonal carcinoembryonic antigen and CD10 (canalicular), hepatocyte paraffin 1 (Hep Par 1), arginase-1, and thyroid transcription factor 1 (TTF-1); α-fetoprotein variable; negative for high-molecular-weight CK (e.g., AE1 antibody to CKs 10, 14, 15, and 16).

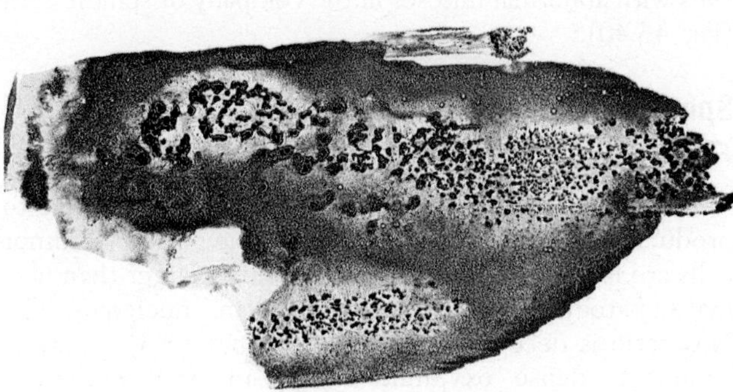

FIGURE 46.25 Hepatocellular carcinoma. Low-power view shows granular trails of tumor aggregates (May-Grünwald-Giemsa stain).

precluding the need for further confirmatory studies. Cords that are three or more cells thick are one of the most pathognomonic features of well-differentiated HCC. The use of Gomori silver stain for reticulin fibers on smears or cell blocks can prove diagnostically helpful.[51,155-157] The presence of an abnormal pattern of reticulin supports a diagnosis of HCC (Fig. 46.35). Perls (Prussian blue) iron stain is positive in hemosiderin-laden hepatocytes in hemochromatosis, but malignant hepatocytes typically remain unstained.[80,81]

Variants of Hepatocellular Carcinoma

Adequate representative sampling of hepatocellular carcinoma, a notoriously heterogeneous malignancy, will become even more crucial in the future, when molecular subclassification of HCC is implemented for the purpose of personalized, molecularly targeted therapy.[23]

Hepatocellular Carcinoma with Fatty Changes

Fatty changes may occur in all sizes and grades of HCC, independent of the steatosis present in nonneoplastic liver tissues (Fig. 46.36). The differential diagnosis includes

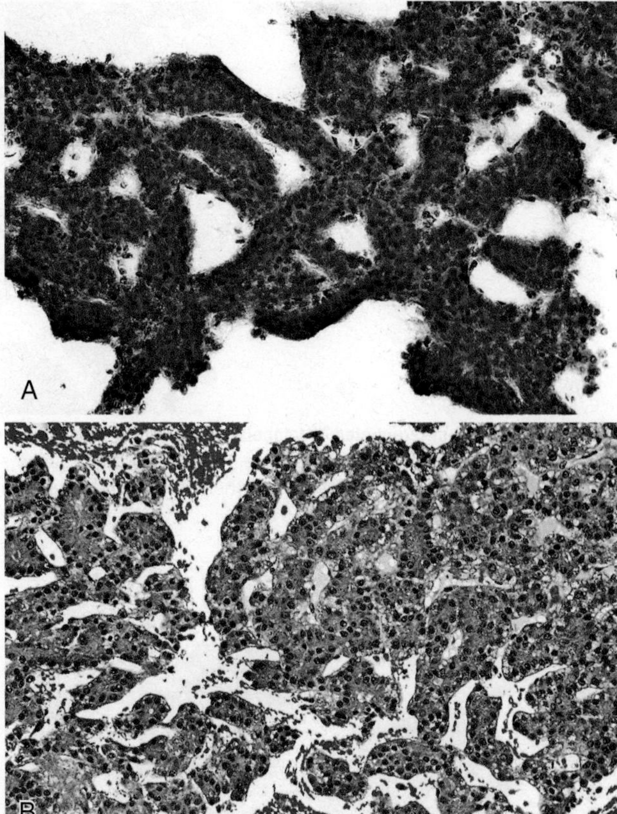

FIGURE 46.26 Well-differentiated hepatocellular carcinoma in a trabecular-sinusoidal pattern. A, Arborizing trabeculae of cohesive tumor cells, three to five cells thick, are wrapped peripherally by endothelium (Papanicolaou stain). **B,** The cell block shows a corresponding trabecular-sinusoidal pattern (hematoxylin and eosin stain).

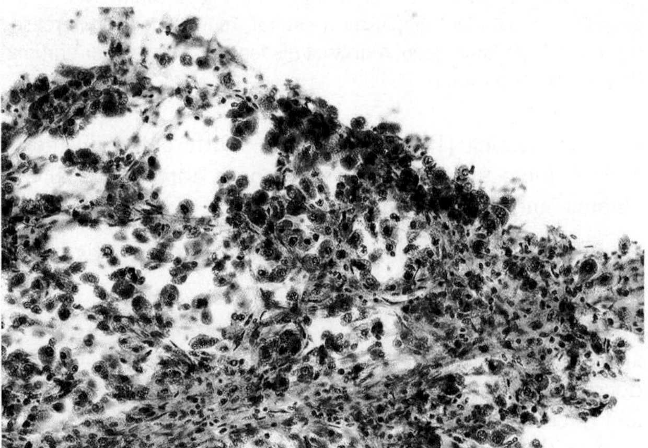

FIGURE 46.27 The transgressing endothelial pattern demonstrates an arborizing, proliferating, or transgressing meshwork of capillaries in a loosely cohesive sheet or aggregate of neoplastic hepatocytes (Papanicolaou stain).

well-differentiated hepatocellular nodules with fatty metamorphosis.[158] Poorly differentiated HCC cells may simulate malignant lipoblasts or signet ring cells.

Hepatocellular Carcinoma with Clear Cell Changes

Malignant hepatocytes may display clear, vacuolated, glycogen-laden cytoplasm that is best appreciated with

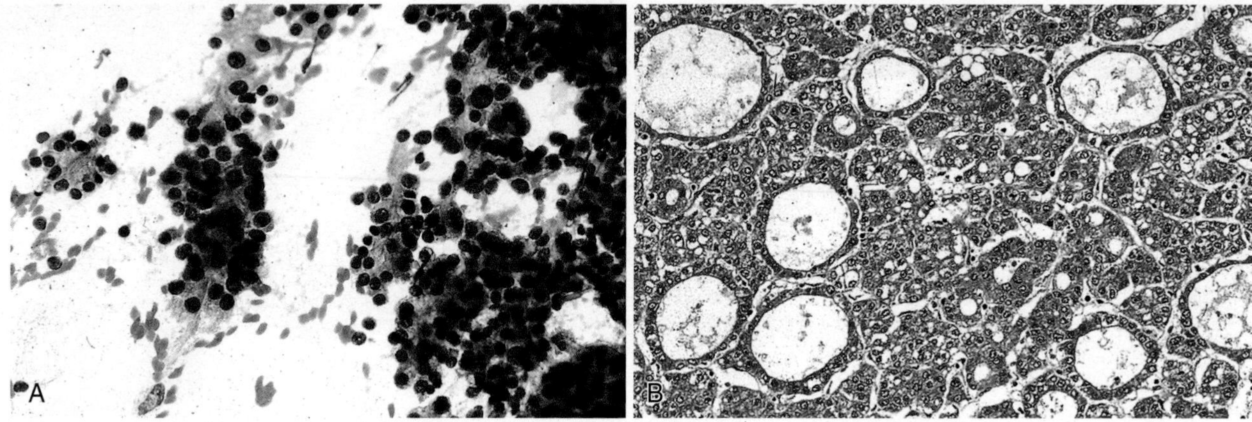

FIGURE 46.28 Well-differentiated hepatocellular carcinoma with a pseudoacinar pattern. A, Pale, rosette-like configuration of tumor cells indicates the presence of pseudoacini (Papanicolaou stain). **B,** Histological section shows trabecular-sinusoidal and pseudoacinar patterns. Notice the cystically dilated bile canaliculi containing secretions (hematoxylin and eosin stain).

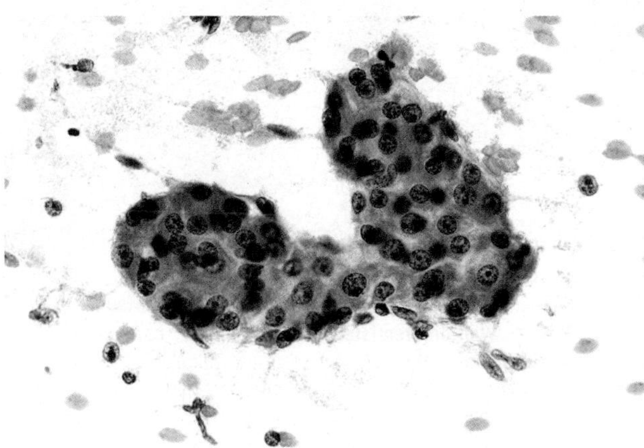

FIGURE 46.29 Moderately differentiated hepatocellular carcinoma. A broad cord of tumor cells is wrapped by endothelium. Notice the presence of granular cytoplasm; a central, round nucleus; increased nucleus-to-cytoplasm ratio; a distinct nucleolus; and granular chromatin (Papanicolaou stain).

Giemsa staining (Fig. 46.37).[159-161] Differential diagnoses include metastatic renal cell carcinoma, adrenocortical carcinoma, and angiomyolipoma.[162,163]

Hepatocellular Carcinoma with Small Cell Changes

Loosely cohesive small tumor cells may show scant cytoplasm, round nuclei, a high N:C ratio, granular chromatin, and a small nucleolus (Fig. 46.38). They mimic neuroendocrine tumors and have a similar tendency to dispersion and microacinar formation.[155,164-167] However, the salt-and-pepper chromatin pattern of endocrine tumor cells is typically lacking. Closer scrutiny of the smears may reveal more classic-looking HCC in other areas.

Hepatocellular Carcinoma with Pleomorphic Features

HCC cells with pleomorphic features are poorly differentiated and have a dyshesive tendency (Fig. 46.39). Multinucleated giant tumor cells and necrosis may be present.

Hepatocellular Carcinoma with Spindle Cell Features

Pleomorphic, spindle-shaped cells are indistinguishable cytologically from sarcoma cells (see Sarcomatoid Hepatocellular Carcinoma).[168]

Hepatocellular Carcinoma with Giant Cell Features

A pure giant cell variant is rare, and it should be differentiated from other giant cell carcinomas and sarcomas. The pathologist often encounters bizarre multinucleated giant cells with abnormal mitoses in the company of spindle cells (Fig. 46.40).

Special Types of Hepatocellular Carcinoma

Fibrolamellar Variant of Hepatocellular Carcinoma

The fibrolamellar variant of HCC is particularly prone to producing a dispersed smear pattern. The polygonal tumor cells are large (approximately three times larger than normal hepatocytes), as are the nucleus and nucleolus. The N:C ratio is deceptively low (less than 1 to 3). There is abundant, dense oxyphilic cytoplasm with numerous intranuclear inclusions, intracytoplasmic hyaline globules, and pale bodies (Fig. 46.41).[169,170] Peripheral and transgressing endothelium is usually lacking. The dense lamellar fibrosis is more likely to be seen in histological material (Box 46.18).

Scirrhous Type of Hepatocellular Carcinoma

The scirrhous type of HCC is rare. It should not be confused with the fibrolamellar variant of HCC and CC.

Undifferentiated Hepatocellular Carcinoma

Undifferentiated HCC cells may be loosely cohesive or show a tendency to dissociate. They are pleomorphic and nondescript, often without cytohistological or immunohistochemical clues to their histogenesis.[73]

Lymphoepithelioma-like Carcinoma

The small, pleomorphic cells of lymphoepithelioma-like carcinoma are admixed with prominent lymphocytes. Tumor cells may test positive for Epstein-Barr virus.[73]

Sarcomatoid Hepatocellular Carcinoma

The purely sarcomatoid variant of HCC is rare. It is more often seen in conjunction with tumor giant cells (Fig. 46.42). Extensive sampling may reveal areas of conventional HCC.[168] This variant should be differentiated from true sarcomas.

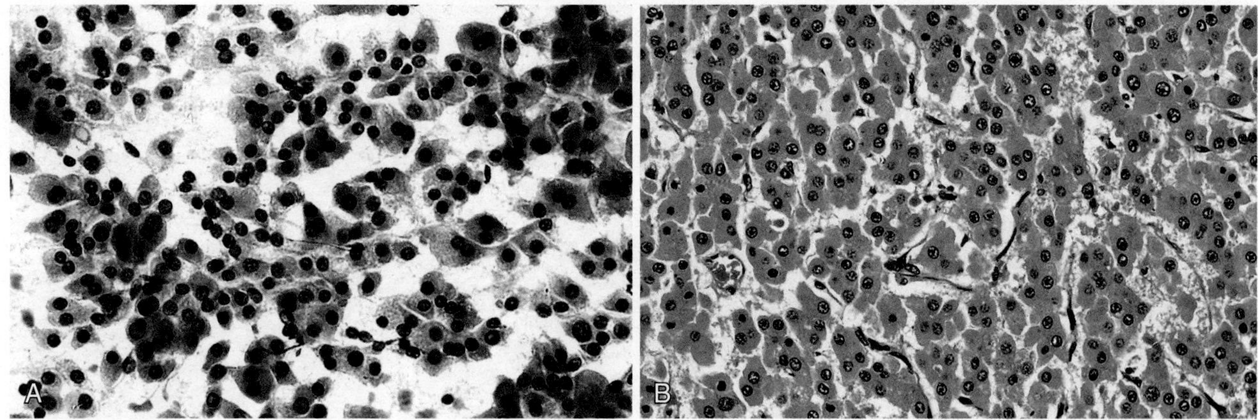

FIGURE 46.30 Well-differentiated hepatocellular carcinoma. A, Tumor cells are well defined, with dense granular cytoplasm, a round nucleus, and increased nucleus-to-cytoplasm ratio. Notice the dyshesive tendency among the cells (Papanicolaou stain). **B,** Histological section shows narrow cords of tumor cells separated by sinusoidal endothelium (hematoxylin and eosin stain).

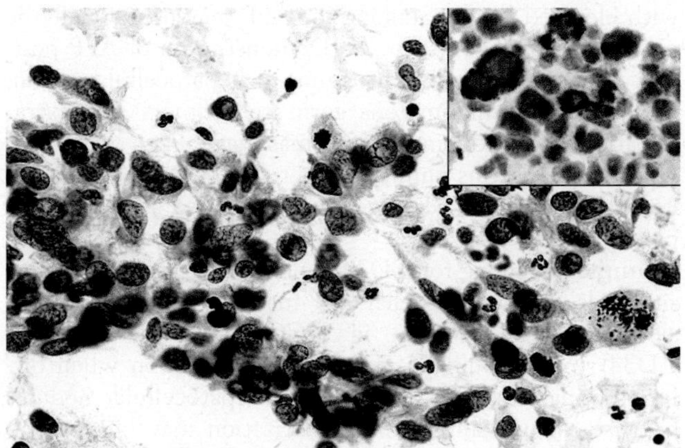

FIGURE 46.31 Poorly differentiated hepatocellular carcinoma. Highly pleomorphic tumor cells have frayed cytoplasm, hyperchromatic nuclei with irregular nuclear contours but without nucleoli, a high nucleus-to-cytoplasm ratio, and a mitosis. These cells do not resemble normal hepatocytes. Notice the dyshesive tendency of the cells (Papanicolaou stain). *Inset,* Tumor cells show strong positivity with Hep Par 1 antigen.

Very-Well-Differentiated Hepatocellular Carcinoma

Very-well-differentiated HCC is a tumor that looks hepatocytic but does not appear obviously malignant. Aspirates from small, early HCCs are nearly impossible to differentiate from high-grade dysplastic nodules because they are both composed of hepatocytes with small cell changes. The smear pattern may not be useful because there is a tendency to dispersion of the cells.

Cytological features indicating HCC include small cell size, an increased N:C ratio, cellular monomorphism, nuclear crowding, cords that are more than two cells thick, atypical naked nuclei, and lack of bile ducts.[51,63,138,171,172] Cytological parameters that distinguish very-well-differentiated HCC from cirrhosis include well-defined cell borders, scant cytoplasm, monotonous cytoplasm, thick cytoplasm, eccentric nuclei, and an increased N:C ratio (Fig. 46.43).[173] Vascular patterns may be subtle on direct smears, and the hepatocytic phenotype may be attenuated in liquid-based cytology (Fig. 46.44). Availability of cell blocks or microbiopsy material is helpful for assessing the architectural details and for ancillary stains.[174]

Diagnostic accuracy remains a challenge. Indeterminate reports are often rendered and include statements such as, "Features are those of a well-differentiated hepatocellular nodule. A well-differentiated HCC cannot be excluded."

Immunohistochemistry

An armamentarium of antibodies is available for comparative immunohistochemical analysis of primary and metastatic tumors of the liver.[175-178] A panel of immunostains has more discriminant value than individual stains. Immunohistochemistry is performed on cell blocks and microbiopsies rather than on smears, cytospins, and liquid-based preparations. Careful light microscopic assessment of the histological sections is crucial, and judicious use of immunostains is imperative when material is limited.[1] Double-staining protocols may help optimize tissue use.[179,180] Immunohistochemical results should always be interpreted within the broader clinical context of the case.

Stepwise logistic regression analysis has shown that an immunostain panel consisting of glypican 3,[175] hepatocyte paraffin 1 (Hep Par 1),[181-186] MOC-31 monoclonal antibody,[187-189] and cytokeratins CK20 and CK7/CK19[189-191] is most useful in diagnosing and differentiating HCC from metastatic adenocarcinoma on FNAB material, with accuracy rates of 90.5% and 91.7%, respectively.[188] In the HCC group, glypican 3 is the most sensitive (81%), followed by Hep Par 1 (71.4%) and polyclonal carcinoembryonic antigen (pCEA) (50%). In the metastatic adenocarcinoma group, MOC-31 is most sensitive (79.2%), followed by CK7 (41.7%).[189,192]

For hepatocellular nodules, the objectives of immunohistochemistry are twofold: to prove hepatocellular histogenesis and to demonstrate the malignant status of hepatocytes.[193] For investigation of hepatocellular histogenesis, the panel should include Hep Par 1,[181,182,185] thyroid transcription factor 1 (TTF-1),[194] and pCEA or CD10 to demonstrate canalicular formation.[184,189,192,195-198] Arginase-1 has joined the ranks of Hep Par 1.[199] However, Hep Par 1 and arginase-1 do not distinguish benign from malignant hepatocytes.[193] For determining malignancy, the panel

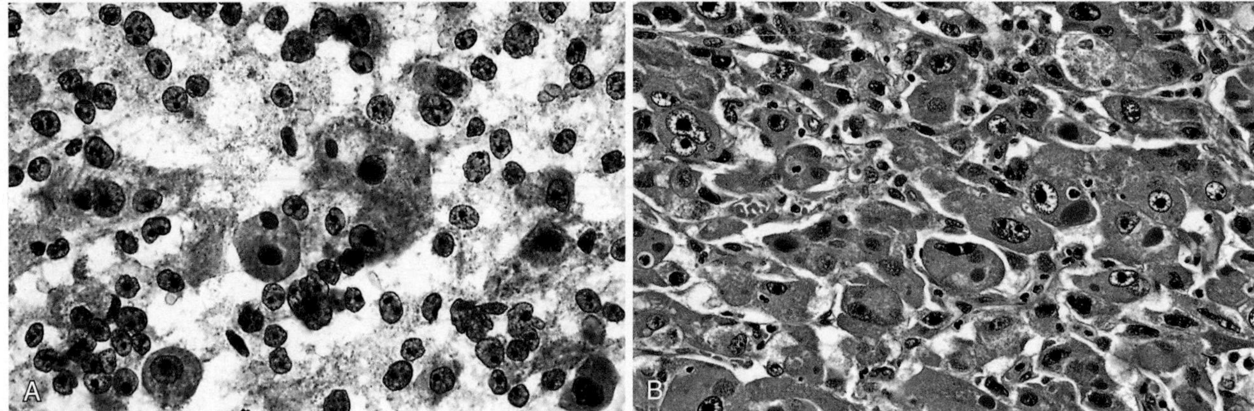

FIGURE 46.32 Moderately differentiated hepatocellular carcinoma. A, Atypical naked nuclei with well-delineated nuclear membranes, irregular nuclear contours, distinct nucleoli, and granular chromatin. Hyaline bodies are present in the cytoplasm of a few tumor cells (Papanicolaou stain). **B,** Histological section shows pleomorphic tumor cells containing intracytoplasmic hyaline bodies (hematoxylin and eosin stain).

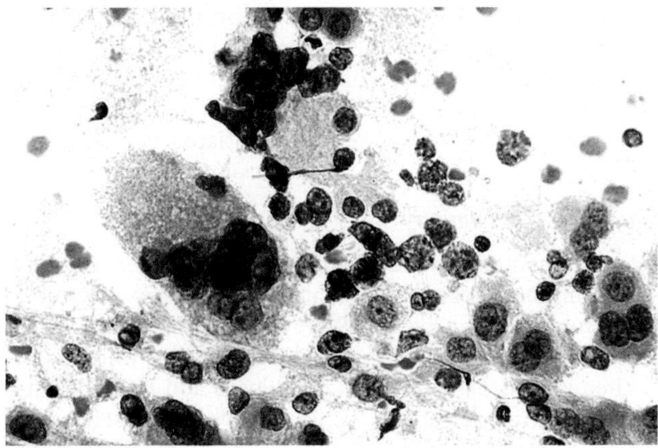

FIGURE 46.33 Hepatocellular carcinoma. Highly pleomorphic, multinucleated giant tumor cells have hyperchromatic nuclei with irregular nuclear contours and distinct nucleoli (Papanicolaou stain).

should include glypican 3,[200-205] glutamine synthetase,[206] and heat shock protein 70.[207] Positivity for two of three of these biomarkers indicates HCC.[208] Strong glypican 3 staining distinguishes benign from malignant hepatocytic proliferations, but a negative stain result does not exclude a malignant diagnosis because of the heterogeneity in staining patterns.[209] Glutamine synthetase shows a geographic, maplike staining pattern in focal nodular hyperplasia, but appreciation of this pattern can be difficult to appreciate in small, fragmented biopsies.[135]

Glypican 3, a heparin sulfate proteoglycan anchored to the plasma membrane, is an oncofetal protein that is overexpressed in HCC at the mRNA and protein levels. This marker may be detected in the serum and tissue of patients with HCC but not in benign hepatic lesions, and it has a higher specificity than AFP.[200,210] Immunohistochemistry studies have indicated great promise for glypican 3 in the distinction between benign and malignant hepatocytes on histological sections and on cytology material.[202,211]

A positive AFP result is helpful, but a negative result does not rule out malignancy.[73] Serum levels of AFP greater than 500 μg/L are highly associated with HCC, but not all tumors, particularly the fibrolamellar variant, are associated with elevated levels. Staining for AFP may occasionally be positive in reactive processes. Demonstration of AFP positivity points to a malignant tumor of hepatocellular origin, provided nonseminomatous germ cell tumors and extrahepatic AFP-producing carcinomas have been excluded. Unfortunately, this tumor marker has such low sensitivity (40%) that it is no longer recommended as part of the panel.[183,196]

Immunostaining for CD34 is negative in normal hepatic sinusoids. This endothelial cell marker highlights diffuse sinusoidal capillarization in HCC.[136,212] However, the CD34 result should be evaluated with caution when differentiating benign from malignant hepatocellular nodules because diffuse sinusoidal capillarization may be encountered in hepatocellular adenomas and focal nodular hyperplasia.[213] It demarcates cord thickness and is very helpful in cases of poorly differentiated HCC in which there is virtually no reticulin.[51,156,157]

In addition to highlighting lesions of a pure biliary immunophenotype, CK7/CK19 is also part of a panel of immunostains often used to elucidate a possible hepatic progenitor cell origin of certain primary liver carcinomas. The immunostain can also be used to demonstrate the absence of a ductular reaction at the invasive border of a small HCC, separating it from a high-grade dysplastic nodule.[214] The prognostic significance of CK7/19 expression in HCC is still being evaluated.[191]

Hepatoblastoma

Aspirates of hepatoblastoma can have a heterogeneous appearance, depending on the cell types in the tumor.[215,216] Smears of the epithelial or mixed epithelial and mesenchymal tumor type are dominated by epithelial cells, which may be fetal, embryonal, or anaplastic (Fig. 46.45). Fetal cells resemble normal hepatocytes, but they are usually smaller. The nuclei are central, round, and bland, and the cytoplasm may contain fat and glycogen.[217,218] The embryonal cell type is more primitive and undifferentiated, showing hyperchromatic nuclei and scant cytoplasm. These cells may form rosettes and trabeculae.[217,219] The anaplastic cell type resembles other small, round, blue cell tumors

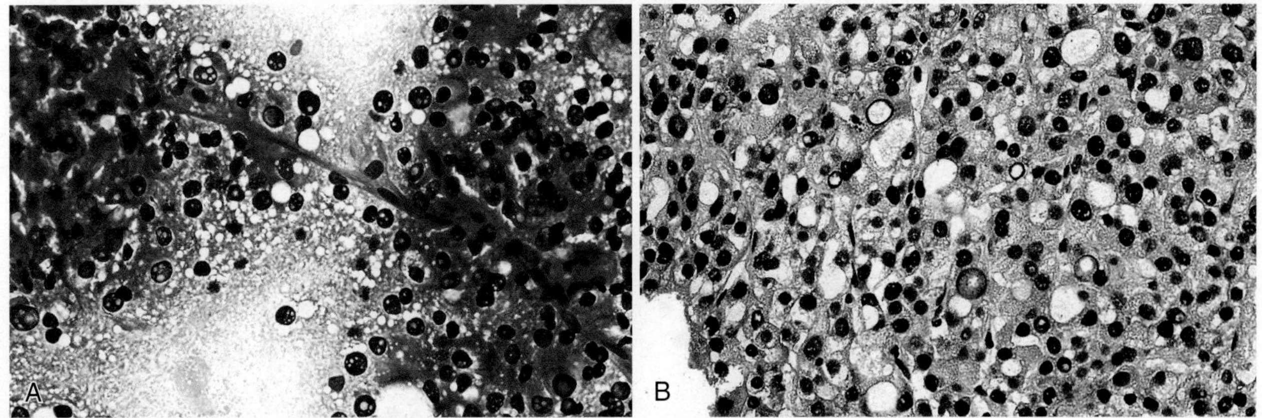

FIGURE 46.34 Hepatocellular carcinoma with fatty changes. A, Some tumor cells contain intracytoplasmic fat vacuoles and pale intranuclear inclusions. Notice the transgressing endothelium and leaked fat globules in the background (May-Grünwald-Giemsa stain). **B,** Cell block shows a corresponding macrovesicular fatty change and intranuclear inclusions (hematoxylin and eosin stain).

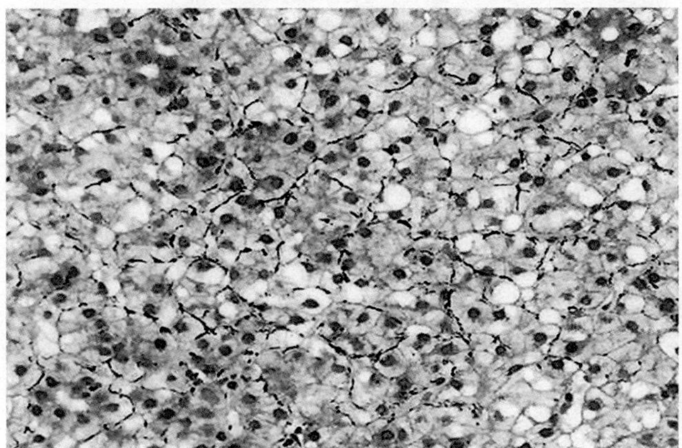

FIGURE 46.35 Hepatocellular carcinoma. Cell block shows an abnormal and deficient reticulin framework (Gomori reticulin stain).

of childhood and is impossible to distinguish from neuroblastoma or Wilms' tumor on morphology alone.[220,221] The mesenchymal component, if present, is a cellular spindle cell proliferation, but heterologous elements may also be evident, including osteoid, cartilage, skeletal muscle, and extramedullary hematopoiesis.[217-219] A myxoid matrix has been described.[222]

The primary differential diagnosis includes fetal-type hepatoblastoma, HCC, embryonal or anaplastic hepatoblastoma, and other pediatric small, round, blue cell tumors.[219,220] Cytomorphological features alone cannot help narrow the differential diagnosis; it requires ancillary studies and clinicopathological correlation. Hep Par 1 positivity supports a hepatic primary tumor over other small, round, blue cell tumors of nonhepatic origin,[223] but this stain cannot help separate hepatoblastoma from HCC. Cytokeratin (CK) staining can be helpful because most hepatoblastoma cells stain positively with high-molecular-weight CKs,[224] whereas most HCCs do not. Both tumors stain with low-molecular-weight CKs (e.g., Cam 5.2).[224] Polyclonal CEA stains hepatoblastomas with a variable and inconsistent canalicular or cytoplasmic pattern, depending on the type of hepatoblastoma.[223] This stain cannot help distinguish hepatoblastoma from HCC, but it can help differentiate primary from metastatic tumors (Box 46.19).

COMBINED HEPATOCELLULAR-GLANDULAR APPEARANCE

Combined Hepatocellular-Cholangiocarcinoma

Primary liver carcinomas show an array of differentiative states from hepatocytic through combined types to cholangiocytic. A recent consensus terminology addressed primary liver carcinomas with both hepatocytic and cholangiocytic differentiation.[72,73] There are three subcategories comprising cHCC-CCA, intermediate cell carcinoma, and CLC. They are discussed together in this section as they can occur with each other in various combinations and permutations. Hepatic stem progenitor cells (HSPC) may accompany all of them. Sampling error is to be expected in this highly heterogeneous landscape, even with multiple passes under imaging guidance. Acquisition of representative tumor tissue for diagnosis, molecular profiling, prognostication, and therapeutic options in this era of precision medicine with personalized targeted molecular therapy is the biggest challenge.

With greater awareness, cHCC-CCA will become less rare. The diagnosis is based on routine morphology with hematoxylin and eosin (H&E) staining; immunohistochemistry is supportive but not essential. An optimal FNAB specimen contains an intimate admixture of HCC, adenocarcinoma, and "transitional epithelium" (Fig. 46.46).[225-228] The HCC component may be obscured by other, more plentiful elements. The adenocarcinoma component may be highly variable in appearance. The transitional cells, which often predominate, often display hybrid features that are difficult to categorize. They may resemble malignant hepatocytes with a trabecular arrangement, but they may also exhibit acini with nuclear palisading. In contrast, they may display irregular nuclear contours, indistinct nucleoli, and less granular cytoplasm. Differentiating pseudoacini from true acini may be difficult. Mucin may not be present. Sampling issues may cause one cell population to predominate. The various cellular components may not always exhibit their expected immunophenotypes. Immunohistochemical confirmation of the presence of HSPC is difficult on limited tissue samples.[191,229] Useful immunostains include CK19, epithelial cell adhesion molecule (EpCAM), CD56 (NCAM), and ckit (CD117).

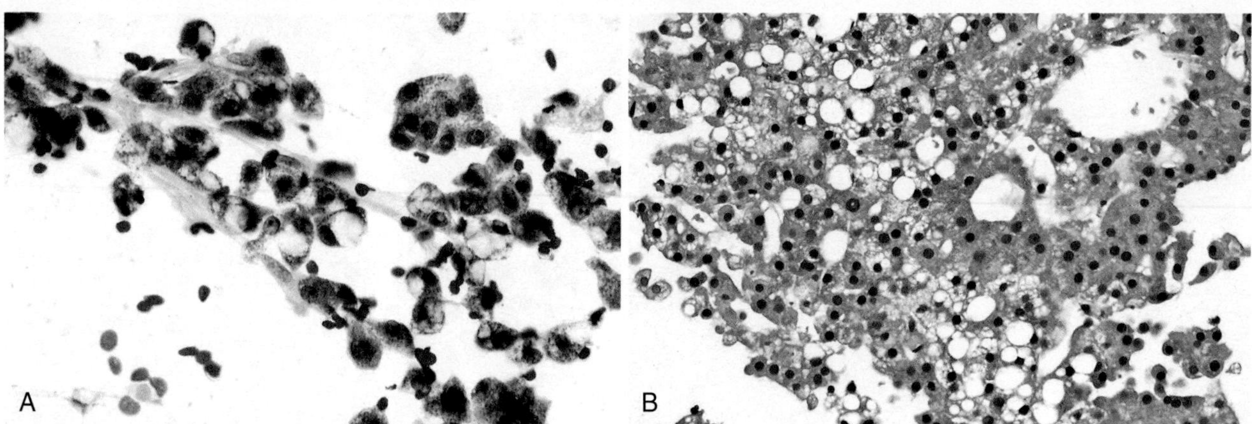

FIGURE 46.36 Hepatocellular carcinoma with fatty changes. A, Tumor cells with the intracytoplasmic fat vacuoles and eccentric nuclei mimic signet ring cells. Notice the transgressing endothelium (Papanicolaou stain). **B,** Cell block shows a trabecular-sinusoidal pattern and fatty changes (hematoxylin and eosin stain).

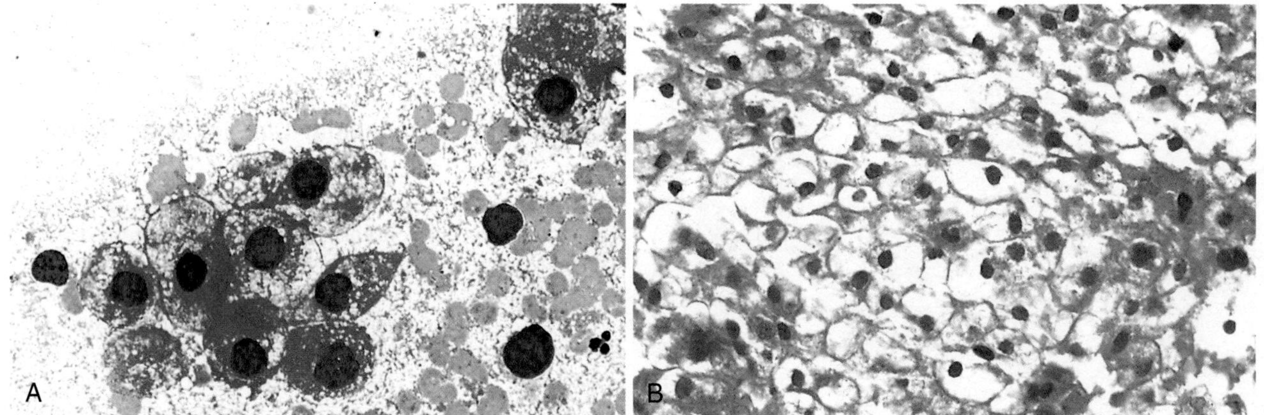

FIGURE 46.37 Hepatocellular carcinoma with clear cell changes. A, Tumor cells show ample pale, vacuolated cytoplasm and central round nuclei (May-Grünwald-Giemsa stain). **B,** Cell block shows well-differentiated tumor cells with central nuclei surrounded by clear cytoplasm; the nucleus-to-cytoplasm ratio is not increased (hematoxylin and eosin stain).

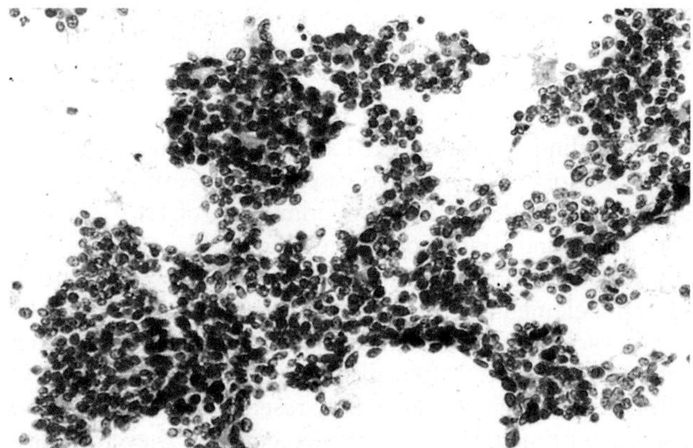

FIGURE 46.38 Hepatocellular carcinoma with small cell changes. Loosely cohesive small tumor cells have scant cytoplasm, round nuclei, indistinct nucleoli, and a high nucleus-to-cytoplasm ratio (Papanicolaou stain).

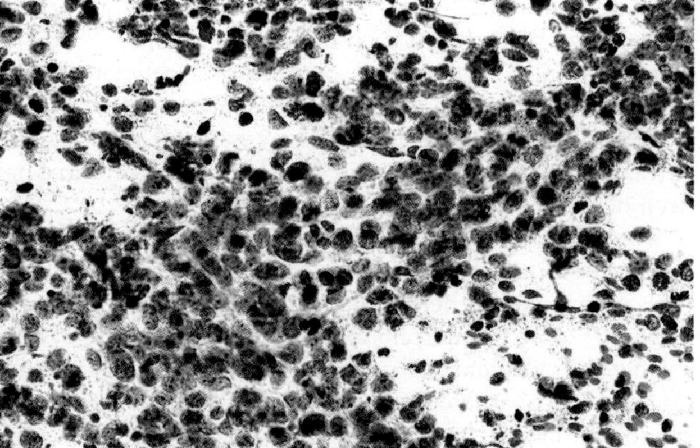

FIGURE 46.39 Hepatocellular carcinoma with pleomorphic features. Loosely cohesive, high-grade, poorly differentiated carcinoma cells have no resemblance to normal hepatocytes (Papanicolaou stain).

Intermediate cell carcinoma is characterized by a monomorphic population of tumor cells that are smaller than hepatocytes but larger than HSPC.[230] The rather nondescript cells are arranged in trabeculae, cords, solid nests, or strands against a desmoplastic stroma. The cells may have elongated, ill-defined glandlike structures, but there is no well-defined lumen or mucin production. The main histological differential diagnosis is poorly differentiated CC. FNAB diagnosis of this entity is only possible if cell block or microcore material is available for the immunohistochemical demonstration of both hepatocytic and cholangiocytic lineage within individual cells.

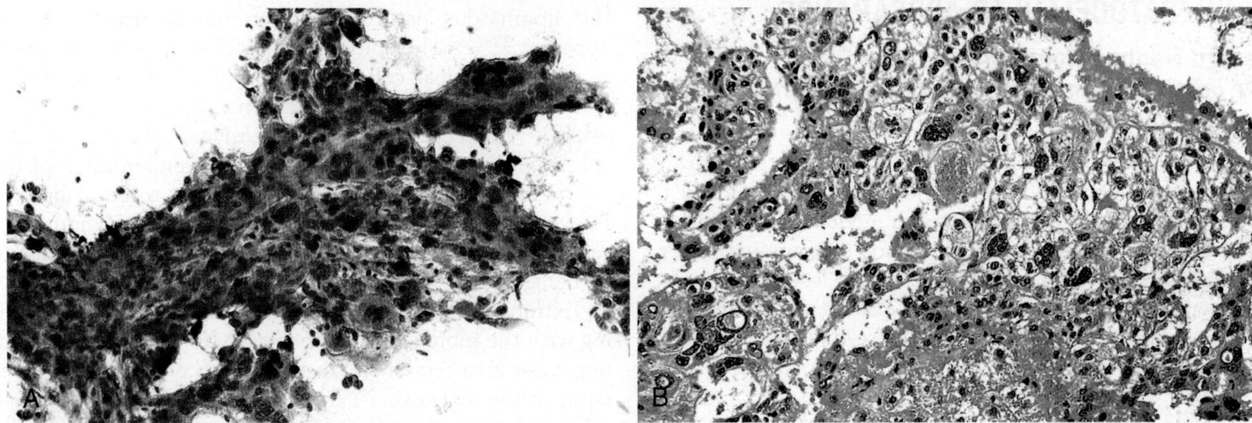

FIGURE 46.40 Hepatocellular carcinoma with spindle cell and giant cell features. A, High-grade tumor cells with bizarre hyperchromatic nuclei and multinucleated giant cells show an arborizing tonguelike configuration of cells, reminiscent of trabeculae (Papanicolaou stain). **B,** Cell block highlights the resemblance to hepatocytes, with focal retention of a trabecular-sinusoidal growth pattern (hematoxylin and eosin stain).

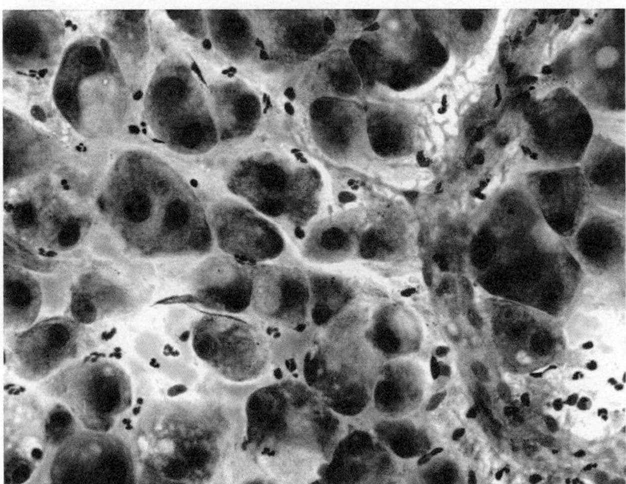

FIGURE 46.41 Fibrolamellar variant of hepatocellular carcinoma. Dispersed, large tumor cells have abundant cytoplasm, a low nucleus-to-cytoplasm ratio, and intracytoplasmic pale bodies (May-Grünwald-Giemsa stain).

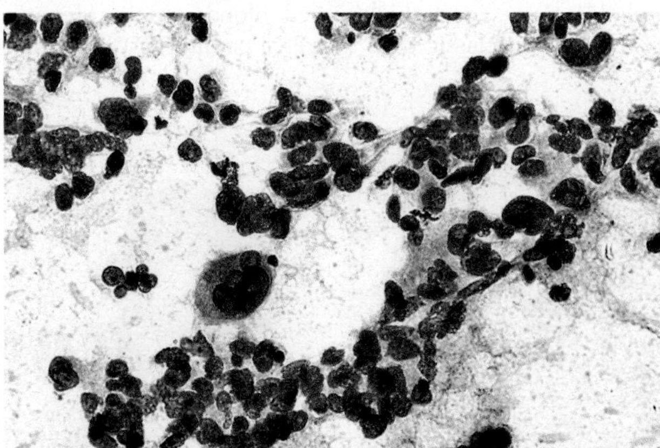

FIGURE 46.42 Sarcomatoid hepatocellular carcinoma. High-grade tumor cells with scant cytoplasm, ovoid hyperchromatic nuclei, a high nucleus-to-cytoplasm ratio, and a giant tumor cell (Papanicolaou stain).

BOX 46.18 Fibrolamellar Variant of Hepatocellular Carcinoma

- Usually dyshesive, large hepatocytes arranged singly and in loose clusters
- Smears may be paucicellular as a result of fibrosis.
- Transgressing vessels may be seen.
- Large, variably atypical nuclei with prominent nucleoli and frequent intranuclear inclusions
- Cytoplasm is characteristically abundant and oncocytic-appearing with hyaline and pale bodies.
- Deceptively low nucleus-to-cytoplasm ratio

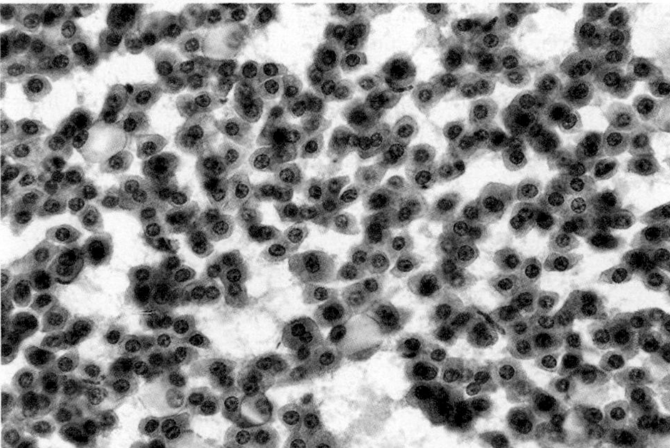

FIGURE 46.43 Very-well-differentiated hepatocellular carcinoma. Dispersed, small, monotonous tumor cells exhibit well-defined cell borders, dense eosinophilic cytoplasm, central round nuclei, distinct nucleoli, an increased nucleus-to-cytoplasm ratio, and nuclear crowding (Papanicolaou stain).

CLC closely resembles ductular reaction.[231,232] The tumor is characterized by an antler-like pattern of angulated, anastomosing, cordlike, slender malignant tubules in dense stroma. This histological picture translates to branching tramlines of cohesive small, overlapping atypical hyperchromatic nuclei with a high N:C ratio and scant cytoplasm. This is in contrast with the honeycomb sheets of glandular epithelium with possible mucin secretion in well-differentiated CCs. Immunohistochemical study shows luminal reactivity with epithelial membrane antigen (EMA) and polyclonal CEA as opposed to cytoplasmic CEA positivity in intrahepatic CC.

NONHEPATOCELLULAR APPEARANCE

Benign Nonhepatocellular Lesions

Bile Duct Hamartoma, Bile Duct Adenoma (Peribiliary Gland Hamartoma)

Bile duct hamartomas, also called *von Meyenburg complexes*, are small incidental subcapsular developmental anomalies. Bile duct adenoma is considered a nodular proliferative response to injury of peribiliary glands surrounding major bile ducts. Both may manifest as mass lesions mimicking neoplasms.[233] Aspirates show a glandular pattern (Fig. 46.47). Cell blocks may be helpful (Box 46.20).

Angiomyolipoma

Hepatic angiomyolipoma is regarded as a tumor of perivascular epithelioid cells (PEComa) that exhibits dual myomatous and lipomatous differentiation and melanogenesis.[234] Its protean morphological appearances result from a combination of adipose tissue, smooth muscle (spindled or epithelioid) tissue, and thick-walled blood vessels. Hepatic lesions are less classic than the renal counterpart, in which the lipomatous nature of the tumor is usually grossly apparent.[235-239] The epithelioid myoid elements may appear as oncocytic, clear cell, or pleomorphic, which can mimic HCC, renal cell carcinoma, sarcoma, and melanoma (Fig. 46.48).[240] Large, epithelioid, clear, myoid cells with a spider cell appearance (caused by perinuclear condensation of the cytoplasm and bizarre nuclei) may appear to be malignant. However, the absence of nuclear hyperchromasia and mitoses in the face of such an aggressive-looking lesion lends to its benignity.

Extramedullary hematopoiesis is common. Positive staining with the monoclonal antibody HMB-45 and other melanogenesis markers such as melan-A (i.e., MART1) helps confirm the diagnosis.[241] S100 protein, CD117, actin, desmin, and vimentin expression varies. Diagnostic difficulty arises when the fatty component is scant or focal or is not sampled, which may suggest a spindle cell lesion of the liver. In some cases, this lesion may be mistaken for a liposarcoma because of the presence of lipoblast-like cells (Box 46.21).

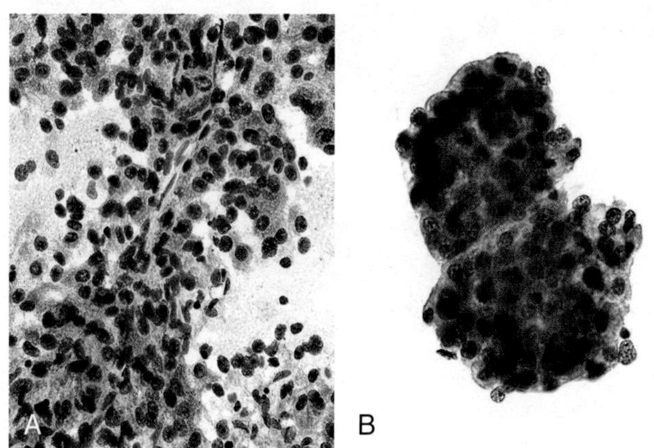

FIGURE 46.44 Hepatocellular carcinoma. A, Conventional smear shows a hypercellular aggregate of tumor cells with characteristic hepatocytic features and a subtle transgressing endothelial pattern (Papanicolaou stain). **B,** ThinPrep liquid-based smear shows a tightly cohesive, three-dimensional aggregate of tumor cells in a clean background. Hepatocytic features are less distinctive (Papanicolaou stain).

Primary Malignant Nonhepatocellular Lesions

Intrahepatic Cholangiocarcinoma

The most common histological appearance of mass-forming, intrahepatic CCs is a well- to moderately differentiated adenocarcinoma forming tubules and infiltrating sclerotic

BOX 46.19 Hepatoblastoma

- Epithelial-dominant smears; may see some mesenchymal (spindle cell) component and/or heterologous elements, especially extramedullary hematopoiesis
- Epithelial cells may be small hepatocytic (fetal type), small pleomorphic (embryonal type), or small undifferentiated (anaplastic type)
- Epithelial cells may be present in cohesive, crowded clusters, cords, ribbons, or rosettes
- Immunophenotype: positive for α-fetoprotein, low- and high-molecular-weight cytokeratins (Cam 5.2 and AE1 antibodies), polyclonal carcinoembryonic antigen with variably positive canalicular or cytoplasmic staining, and hepatocyte paraffin 1 (Hep Par 1)

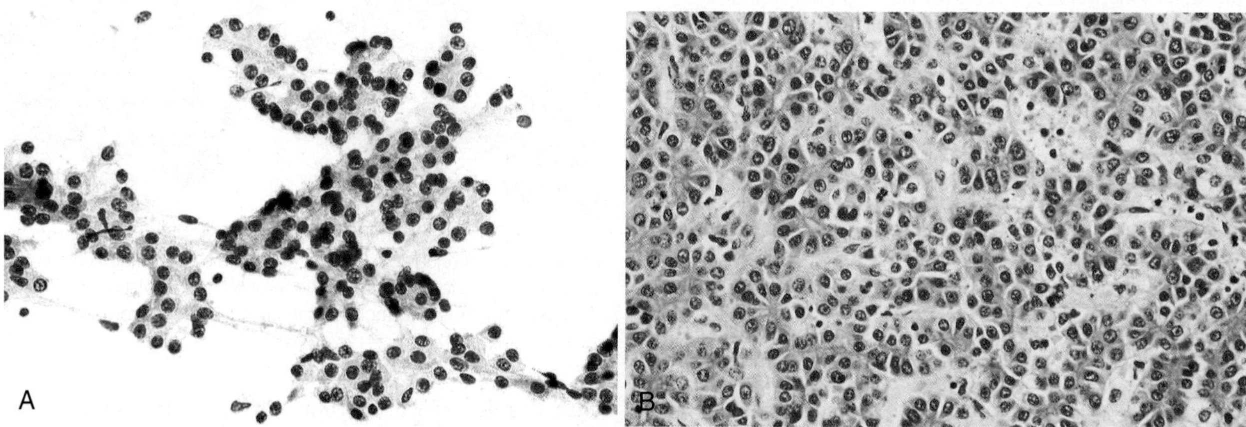

FIGURE 46.45 Hepatoblastoma, epithelial type. A, The fetal cell type resembles hepatocytes but consists of smaller cells with bland, round, central nuclei. There is rosette-like pseudoacinar formation (Papanicolaou stain). **B,** Histological section shows the resemblance of tumor cells to immature hepatocytes (hematoxylin and eosin stain).

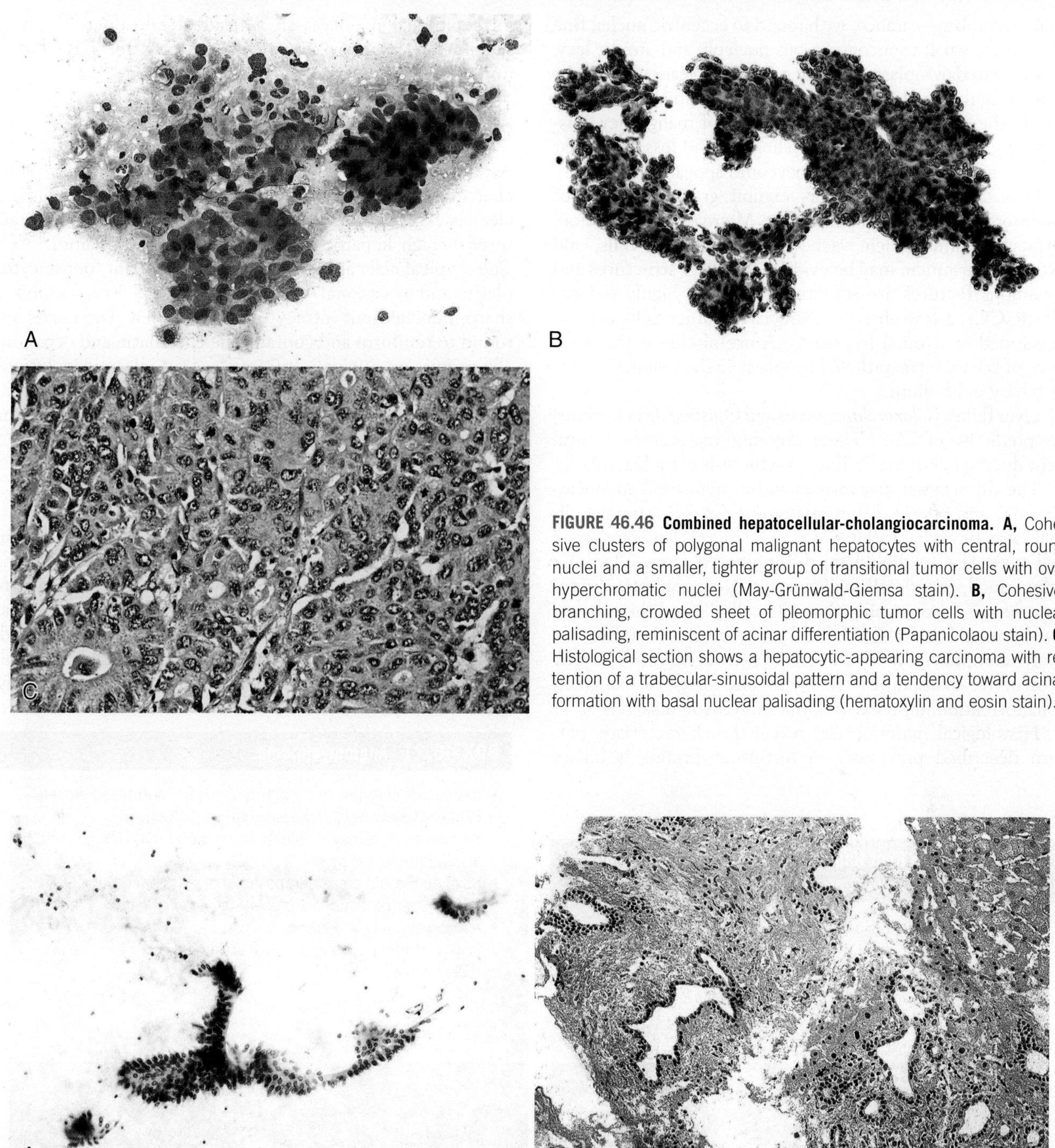

FIGURE 46.46 Combined hepatocellular-cholangiocarcinoma. A, Cohesive clusters of polygonal malignant hepatocytes with central, round nuclei and a smaller, tighter group of transitional tumor cells with oval hyperchromatic nuclei (May-Grünwald-Giemsa stain). **B,** Cohesive, branching, crowded sheet of pleomorphic tumor cells with nuclear palisading, reminiscent of acinar differentiation (Papanicolaou stain). **C,** Histological section shows a hepatocytic-appearing carcinoma with retention of a trabecular-sinusoidal pattern and a tendency toward acinar formation with basal nuclear palisading (hematoxylin and eosin stain).

FIGURE 46.47 Bile duct adenoma. A, Aspirate smears are dominated by benign-appearing bile duct epithelial cells, with uncharacteristically scant numbers of associated hepatocytes (Papanicolaou stain). **B,** Cell block preparations of core-needle biopsies show the characteristic angulated proliferation of variably dilated bile ductules in a fibrotic background, allowing a specific diagnosis.

stroma.[73,242] However, phenotypic diversity does exist.[243] EUS-FNA may be used to procure tumor tissue.[244,245] The degree of cellularity and desmoplasia determines whether aspirates are scanty or produce a readily recognizable adenocarcinoma with nonspecific features.[76] A low-power smear pattern demonstrating irregular, variously sized sheets of atypical to malignant glandular cells with peripheral palisading nuclei and branching, tapered columns is highly reminiscent of bile duct epithelium and suggests a primary adenocarcinoma (Fig. 46.49). CLC may occur in conjunction with classic CC, giving an additional feature of malignant ductular epithelial cells.[72]

Well-differentiated CC resembles normal bile duct epithelium. Sheets of cuboidal or columnar epithelial cells have a honeycomb appearance, with round to eccentric nuclei, fine chromatin, small to inconspicuous nucleoli, and ample, lacy, or vacuolated cytoplasm. Abrupt cell and nuclear enlargement with irregular nuclear membranes and prominent nucleoli within the same group are an indication of malignancy. Disorderly growth with crowding, piling up, and loss of nuclear polarity impart a "drunken" honeycomb appearance.

Less differentiated tumors exhibit greater degrees of pleomorphism and mitotic activity. Microacinar formation, intracytoplasmic mucin vacuoles in signet ring cells, and extracellular mucin may be evident. Papillary structures and squamous features are sometimes seen. In highly desmoplastic CCs, a few obscure, dissociated tumor cells may be entrapped in stromal fragments. A useful clue is the presence of biliary intraepithelial neoplasia in the residual sheets of biliary epithelium.

Liver flukes (*Clonorchis sinensis* and *Opisthorchis viverrini*) are predictive of CC.[73] The background may contain prominent ductular clusters.[246] Tumor diathesis is not a feature.

The differential diagnosis includes metastatic adenocarcinomas and poorly differentiated HCCs. The tumor cells may also be part of cHCC-CCA.[158,225-228] The rare small cell type of CC should be differentiated from CLC and other small, round cell malignancies. Nonneoplastic ductular cells are much smaller than CC cells,[246] and they should not be mistaken for CC.[231] CCs may be associated with a cystic component when there is cystic degeneration, cystic obstructive dilation of intrahepatic bile ducts, or malignant transformation in preexisting fibropolycystic disease.[73]

Histological material may reveal the characteristic pattern described previously. A fortuitous finding is biliary intraepithelial neoplasia in a residual bile duct.[247] These specimens also provide accessible tissue for CK7/CK19 immunostaining (Box 46.22).

Epithelioid Hemangioendothelioma

Aspirates from this low-grade malignant vascular tumor are characterized by a dyshesive population of atypical cells in a clean background, fragments of metachromatic stroma, scattered benign hepatocytes, and bile duct epithelium.[248-252] The atypical cells are polygonal with abundant, dense cytoplasm and occasional trailing. Some cells may exhibit a sharp, punched-out intracytoplasmic lumen. The nuclei are round to reniform and contain fine chromatin and occasionally prominent nucleoli. Intranuclear cytoplasmic inclusions and binucleated and multinucleated cells can also be seen. Diagnostic pitfalls include confusion with adenocarcinoma and angiosarcoma (Box 46.23).

Angiosarcoma

Aspirates of angiosarcoma are bloody and often paucicellular.[253] Malignant endothelial cells can be seen interdigitating among reactive hepatocytes. They are easier to appreciate in small clusters than in large clusters, in which they tend to blend with hepatocytes. The tumor cells have elongated, spindle-shaped, hyperchromatic nuclei with a distinct, prominent eosinophilic nucleus and ample cytoplasm. Frequently,

BOX 46.20 Bile Duct Hamartoma and Bile Duct Adenoma (Peribiliary Gland Hamartoma)

- High number of sheets of benign-appearing bile duct epithelium (BDH)/tubules and acini (BDA)
- Unusually few hepatocytes in the background

BOX 46.21 Angiomyolipoma

- Interlacing complex of smooth muscle, fat, and blood vessels; extramedullary hematopoiesis may be present.
- Smooth muscle may dominate smears and may demonstrate atypia (a potential pitfall).
- Solid epithelioid areas composed of clear to oncocytic cells with large spider cells may be present (a potential pitfall).
- Adipocytes may be lacking in aspirates.
- Immunohistochemistry: positive staining with HMB-45 and melan-A (i.e., MART1)

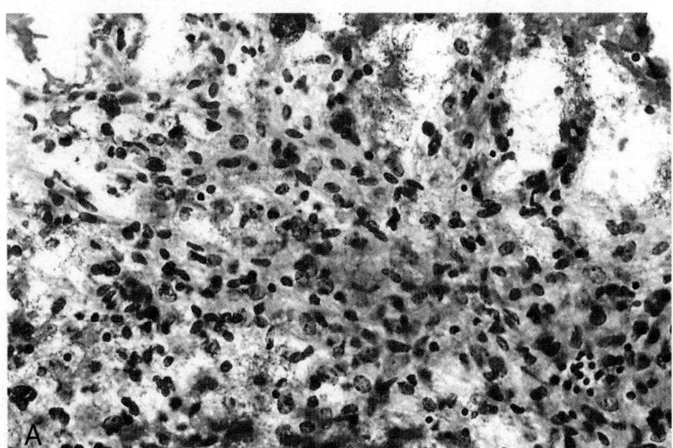

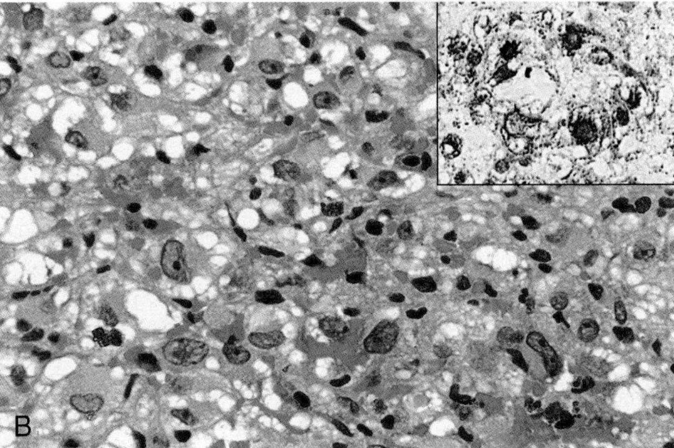

FIGURE 46.48 Angiomyolipoma. A, Hemorrhagic smear shows epithelioid myoid cells with clear cytoplasm and bland nuclei and scattered, larger "spider cells" with enlarged nuclei. Notice the presence of extramedullary hematopoietic cells (i.e., nucleated erythrocytes) and a prominent vascular network (Papanicolaou stain). **B,** Cell block preparation shows myoid cells with epithelioid features. The cytoplasm is eosinophilic, or vacuolated, with large spider cells displaying reniform bland nuclei, distinct nucleoli, and a perinuclear condensation of the cytoplasm, leaving a lacelike, vacuolated rim at the periphery. Hemosiderin pigment can be seen (hematoxylin and eosin stain). *Inset,* Tumor cells exhibit positivity with HMB-45.

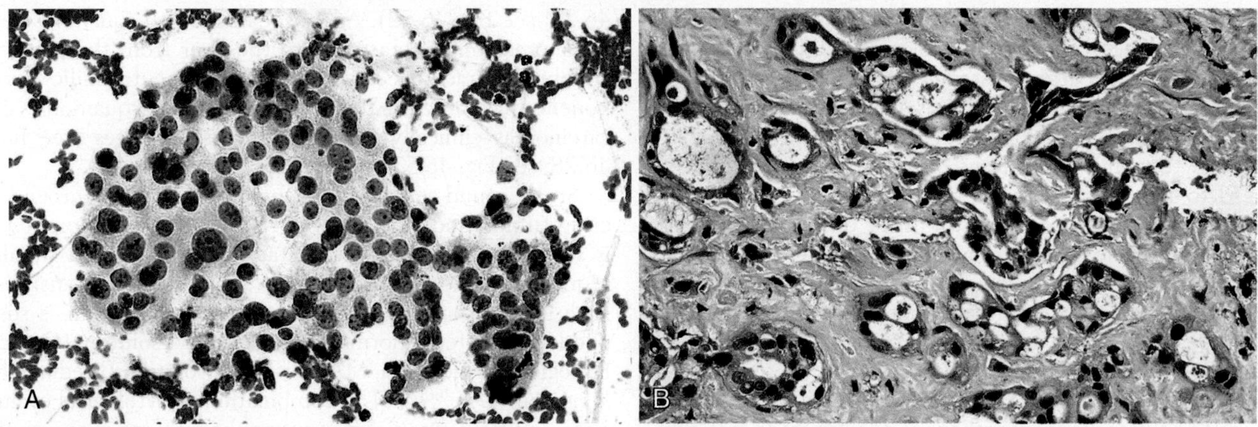

FIGURE 46.49 Intrahepatic cholangiocarcinoma. A, Sheet of bile ductal epithelium shows a drunken honeycomb appearance, overlapping nuclei, distinct nucleoli, and abrupt nuclear enlargement (Papanicolaou stain). **B,** Histological section from a biopsy shows an adenocarcinoma with desmoplasia (hematoxylin and eosin stain).

BOX 46.22 Intrahepatic Cholangiocarcinoma

- Glandular cells are arranged in flat, angulated sheets.
- Exaggerated honeycomb pattern results from mucinous cytoplasm.
- Nuclei are variably atypical depending on grade, but most are relatively low grade and not very atypical.
- Abrupt nuclear enlargement in a sheet and nuclear overlapping with a "drunken" honeycomb appearance favor a biliary origin.
- Atypia ranges from borderline to obviously malignant.
- Impossible to distinguish from other adenocarcinomas on the basis of morphology alone
- Cell blocks may help by demonstrating sclerotic stroma and portal tracts with biliary intraepithelial neoplasia
- Immunohistochemistry: positive for cytokeratin 7 (CK7) and CK19; CK20 staining usually negative, except for some hilar tumors

BOX 46.23 Epithelioid Hemangioendothelioma

- Dyshesive, atypical cells on a clean background with metachromatic stromal fragments, scattered benign hepatocytes, and bile duct epithelium
- Polygonal cells with abundant, dense cytoplasm, round to reniform nuclei with fine chromatin, and prominent nucleoli
- Some cells exhibit a sharp, punched-out intracytoplasmic lumen resembling signet ring cells.
- Binucleated or multinucleated giant cells
- Immunohistochemistry: positive for factor VIII, CD31, CD34, ERG, and CAMTA1

huge intracytoplasmic vacuoles, similar to those of signet ring cells, are identified (Fig. 46.50). Sometimes the tumor cells have a more epithelioid appearance. The differential diagnosis includes spindle cell sarcomas and poorly differentiated carcinomas. Immunostains for endothelial markers such as CD31, CD34, and ERG are almost always positive (Box 46.24).[254-256]

METASTATIC MALIGNANT NONHEPATOCELLULAR LESIONS

Most liver tumors are metastases.[73,75,257] Metastatic tumors tend to recapitulate the appearance of the primary tumor.

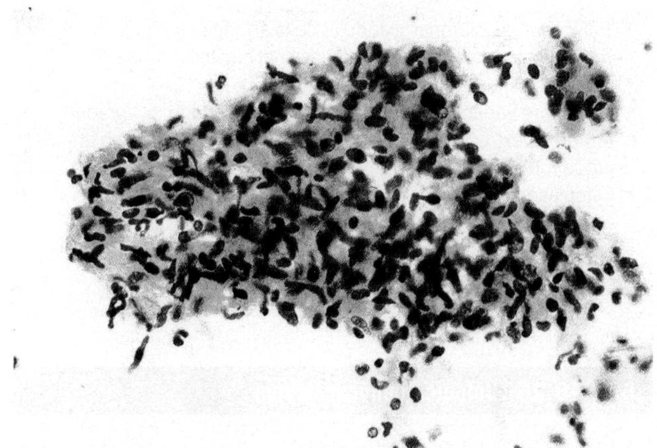

FIGURE 46.50 Angiosarcoma. Larger cell clusters appear to be hypercellular, and the individual malignant endothelial cells are more difficult to separate from the reactive hepatocytes (Papanicolaou stain).

BOX 46.24 Angiosarcoma

- Atypical to overtly malignant endothelial cells interspersed with hepatocyte clusters
- Spindle cell sarcoma, possibly with blood lakes
- May have epithelioid features, mimicking carcinomas
- Immunohistochemistry: positive for factor VIII, CD31, CD34 and ERG

Some nonhepatocellular malignancies may be de novo lesions in the liver. Distinction between a primary and metastatic malignancy has therapeutic and prognostic significance.

Metastatic tumors commonly encountered in FNAB of the liver include those from the colorectum (i.e., adenocarcinoma), pancreas (i.e., adenocarcinoma and neuroendocrine tumors), stomach (i.e., adenocarcinoma and gastrointestinal stromal tumors), breast, lung (i.e., adenocarcinoma, small cell carcinoma, and less commonly, squamous cell carcinoma), skin (i.e., melanoma), and bladder (e.g., transitional cell carcinoma). Lymphoma may be identified. Less common but diagnostically more challenging are metastases from the kidney and adrenal gland because of the morphological overlap with HCC. Sarcomas are rare; the most common type is metastatic uterine leiomyosarcoma.

A practical approach to the interpretation of these aspirates is to categorize the cytohistological findings according to the cytological patterns listed in Box 46.7.[74] The cytological features helpful in the diagnosis of a variety of metastatic tumors are reviewed along with accompanying supportive ancillary tests and illustrations (Boxes 46.25 to 46.28; Figs. 46.51 to 46.61).

Adenocarcinomas present the most difficulty in establishing a specific site of origin. Primary liver carcinomas that must be excluded include CC, cHCC-CCA, and cystic mucinous neoplasms with associated invasive carcinoma. The presence of an adenocarcinoma with dirty necrosis likely indicates a colonic primary tumor (see Boxes 46.25 and 46.26; see Fig. 46.51). Ductal carcinoma of the breast tends to be more monomorphous and lower grade (see Box 46.27; see Fig. 46.52). Adenosquamous and squamous cell carcinomas may metastasize to the liver from the pancreaticobiliary tract. Necrosis and a heavy neutrophilic component may obscure tumor cells in some squamous cell carcinomas clinically masquerading as abscesses (see Box 46.28; see Fig. 46.53).

Small, round cell tumors include lymphoma, neuroendocrine tumor, and small cell carcinoma.[258,259] If lymphoma is suspected on rapid interpretation, the physician should request a dedicated aspirate for flow-cytometry analysis, such as one that is not expressed onto a slide but is suspended in buffered normal saline, CytoLyt solution (Cytyc/Hologic, Marlborough, MA), or RPMI solution (Mediatech, Herndon, VA).[260-262] The combination of cytological evaluation and flow-cytometry immunophenotyping is often sufficient to help subclassify non-Hodgkin's lymphomas (Box

BOX 46.25 General Adenocarcinoma

- Polygonal to columnar glandular cells arranged in flat monolayered sheets, three-dimensional clusters, or singly
- Lumens in clusters in some cases
- Nuclei are variably atypical, ranging from bland in low-grade tumors to extremely atypical and obviously malignant in high-grade tumors
- Cytoplasm is delicate, frequently vacuolated, and sometimes wispy.
- Intracytoplasmic mucin may be present; mucicarmine or other mucin stains can help identify focal mucin production.

BOX 46.26 Colonic Adenocarcinoma

- Cigar-shaped, often palisading nuclei
- Variably prominent nucleoli; no macroeosinophilic nucleoli
- Dirty necrosis in the background (key identification point) (see Fig. 46.51)
- Immunohistochemistry: positive for cytokeratin 20 (CK20); negative for CK7 and CK19; and positive for carcinoembryonic antigen, MOC-31 monoclonal antibody, CDX2, and epithelial membrane antigen (EMA)

BOX 46.27 Ductal Type Breast Carcinoma

- Often low grade with a monomorphous cell population (see Fig. 46.52)
- Flat, angulated groups
- Single flame or cone-shaped cells
- Target cells (i.e., cells with intracytoplasmic lumen)
- Cell-in-cell arrangement
- Immunohistochemistry: positive or negative for estrogen/progesterone, but not specific; GATA-3 positivity is helpful; gross cystic disease protein 15 is supportive if positive.

BOX 46.28 Squamous Cell Carcinoma

- Large, polygonal cells arranged singly and in clusters (see Fig. 46.53)
- Usually high grade with large, hyperchromatic nuclei with irregular nuclear membranes
- Cytoplasm is dense and more nonvacuolated than in adenocarcinoma.
- Keratinizing squamous cells stain orangeophilic with Papanicolaou stain, but this feature may not be present.
- Background may be necrotic with abundant neutrophils.

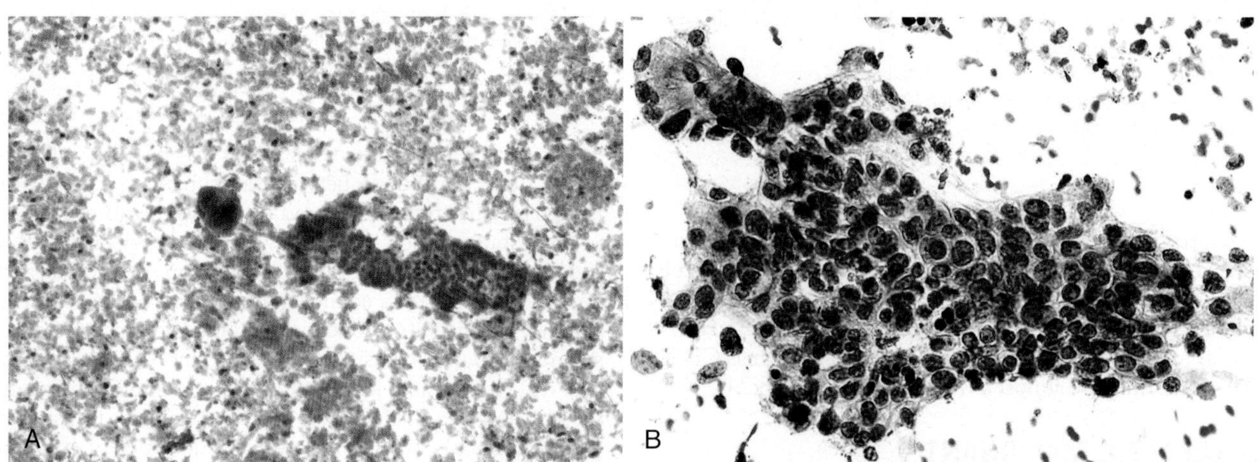

FIGURE 46.51 Metastatic colorectal adenocarcinoma. A, Tumor diathesis, which often is referred to as *dirty necrosis,* is commonly prominent in the background of metastatic colon cancer, and its presence should suggest a primary colon tumor in cases of metastatic carcinoma of unknown origin (Papanicolaou stain). **B,** Cohesive columnar cells are pleomorphic, with cigar-shaped, palisading nuclei (Papanicolaou stain).

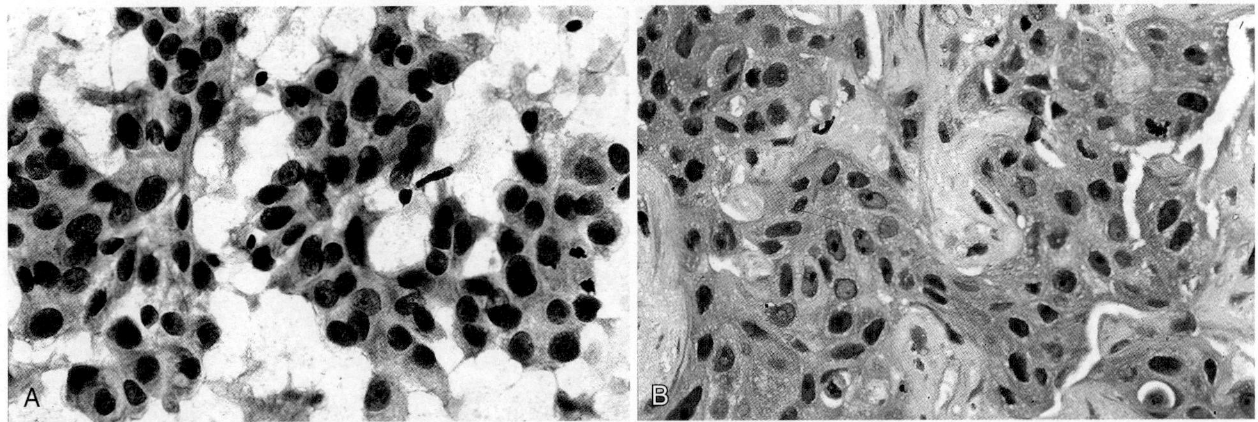

FIGURE 46.52 Metastatic ductal carcinoma of the breast. A, Monomorphous cohesive tumor cells show acinar features (Papanicolaou stain). **B,** Histological section shows an intermediate-grade ductal carcinoma with desmoplasia (hematoxylin and eosin stain).

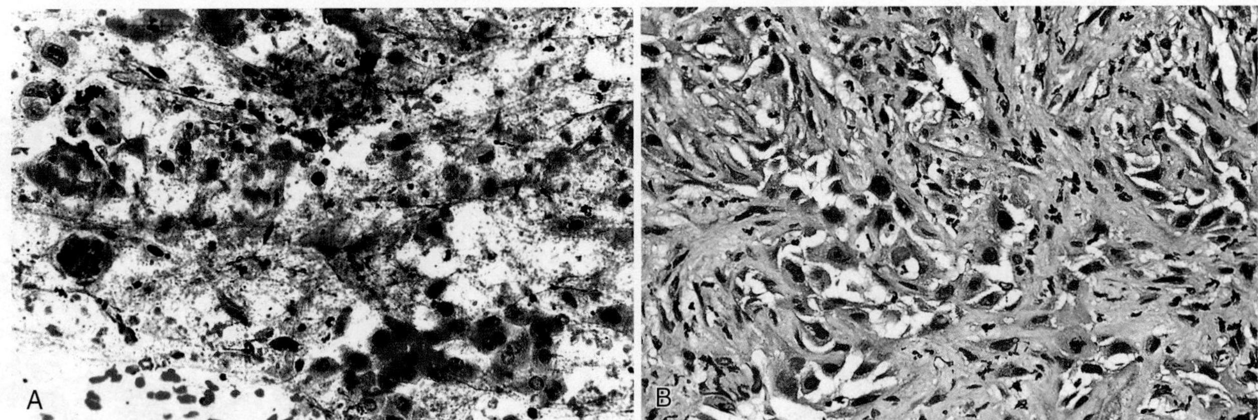

FIGURE 46.53 Metastatic squamous cell carcinoma. A, Large, pleomorphic, polygonal, and occasionally elongated shaped cells with a high nucleus-to-cytoplasm ratio, hyperchromatic nuclei, and orangeophilic keratinizing cytoplasm occur singly and in small clusters. Notice the dirty background (Papanicolaou stain). **B,** Histological section shows poorly differentiated squamous cell carcinoma with desmoplasia (hematoxylin and eosin stain).

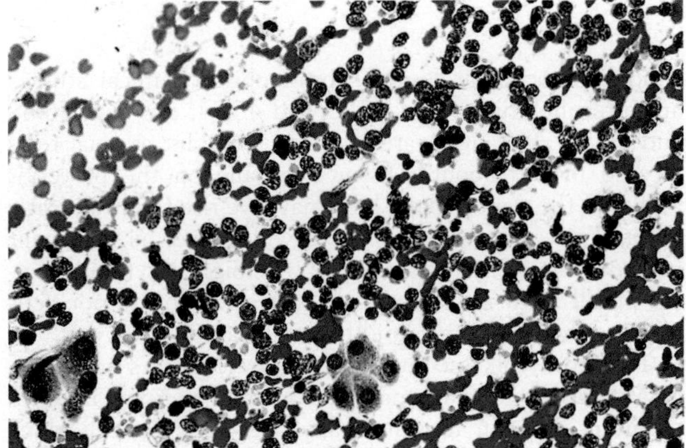

FIGURE 46.54 Non-Hodgkin's lymphoma. Single population of dyshesive, small, round tumor cells with scant cytoplasm, a high nucleus-to-cytoplasm ratio, a round nucleus with irregular nuclear contours, and coarse chromatin. Notice the presence of normal hepatocytes in the vicinity (Papanicolaou stain).

46.29; see Fig. 46.54). Inflammatory pseudotumors, particularly the lymphoplasmacytic type, should not be mistaken for lymphoma. Neuroendocrine tumors typically show a salt-and-pepper pattern of chromatin with immunopositivity for chromogranin and synaptophysin (Box 46.30; see Fig. 46.55).[263] Nuclear molding and streaking may be discernible in small cell carcinomas (Box 46.31; see Fig. 46.56). Metastatic melanomas often mimic other tumors and are potential diagnostic pitfalls, particularly when the primary site is inconspicuous or the tumor cells are amelanotic (Box 46.32; see Fig. 46.57).

Renal cell and adrenocortical carcinomas are characterized by polygonal cells with clear or oncocytic cytoplasm. Naked round nuclei with distinct nucleoli may be found in the latter. Transgressing endothelium is common in renal cell carcinomas, whereas peripheral endothelium is encountered in adrenocortical carcinomas. The presence of more prominent, complex central and branching vascular tufts should alert the pathologist to the possibility of

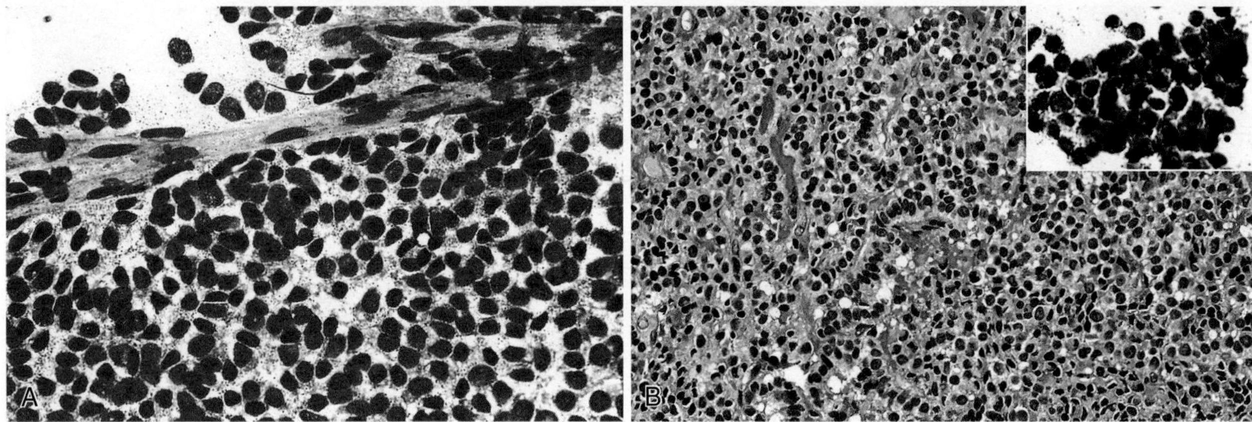

FIGURE 46.55 Neuroendocrine tumor. A, Dispersed, small, round tumor cells with visible granular cytoplasm and round nuclei have a salt-and-pepper chromatin pattern. Transgressing endothelium can be seen (May-Grünwald-Giemsa stain). **B,** Histological section shows small, round tumor cells arranged in nests and festoons with prominent (capillary) vascularity (hematoxylin and eosin stain). *Inset,* Tumor cells reacted positively with synaptophysin.

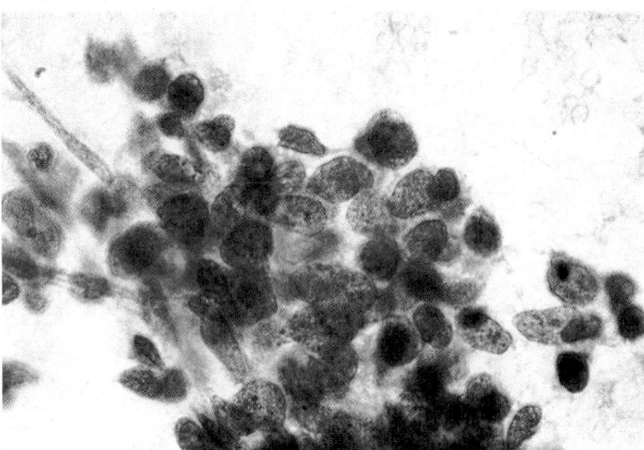

FIGURE 46.56 Metastatic small cell carcinoma. Small blue pleomorphic cells with little or no cytoplasm are present in clusters and have hyperchromatic, often molded nuclei with stippled chromatin (Papanicolaou stain).

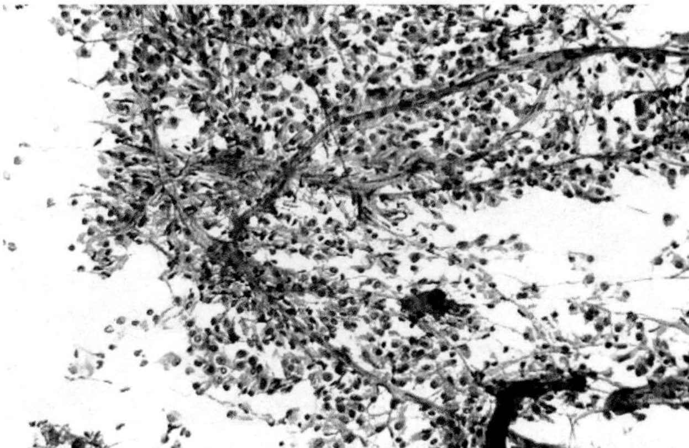

FIGURE 46.58 Metastatic renal cell carcinoma. Classic large polygonal cells show clear to granular cytoplasm, central nuclei, and nucleoli. The transgressing endothelial pattern is the most common vascular pattern of renal cell carcinoma and cannot be used to discriminate from hepatocellular carcinoma (Papanicolaou stain).

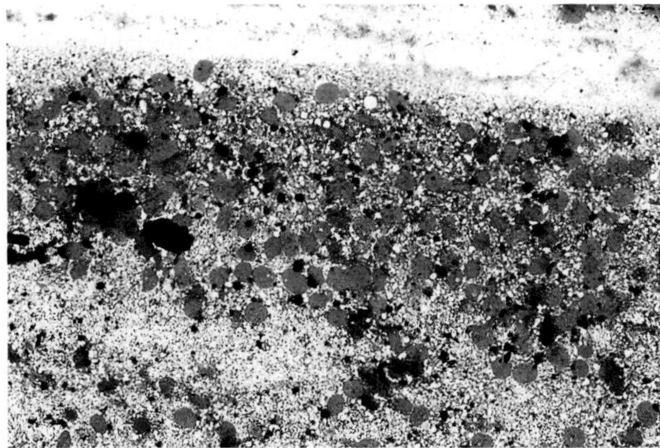

FIGURE 46.57 Metastatic melanoma. Dispersed, large cells with central nuclei and abundant black melanin pigment (May-Grünwald-Giemsa stain).

a nonhepatocellular lesion. Immunohistochemical studies are often helpful (Boxes 46.33 and 46.34; see Figs. 46.58 and 46.59).[264,265] On rare occasion, aberrant adrenal rests located in and about Glisson's capsule on the posterior aspect of the right hepatic lobe may give rise to intrahepatic adrenal rest neoplasms, some of which may be malignant but not necessarily metastatic.[266] The biggest cytohistological pitfall is to mistake the hepatoid-looking tumor cells laden with cytoplasmic lipid for malignant hepatocytes.

Hepatoid yolk sac tumors, similar to HCCs and adrenocortical carcinomas, may demonstrate peripheral endothelium, although it is normally seen only on cell block preparations. Tumor cells can be stained for placental alkaline phosphatase, and the result is negative for primary hepatic tumors.[267]

Spindle cell tumors in the liver are relatively uncommon.[268] Metastatic gastrointestinal stromal tumors (GISTs)

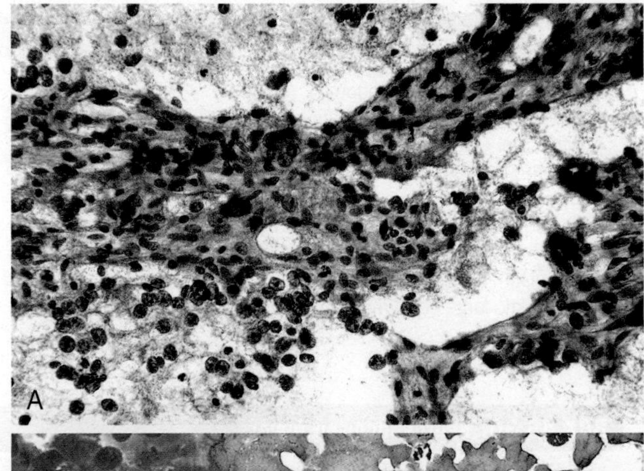

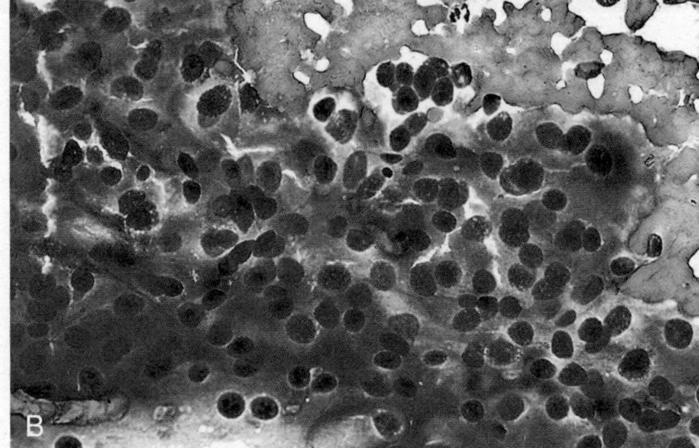

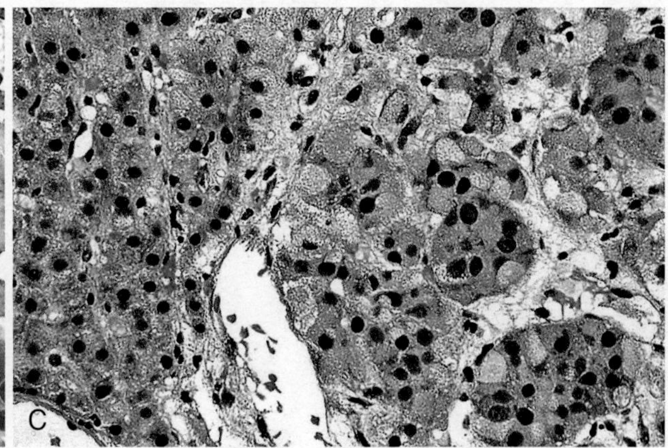

FIGURE 46.59 Metastatic adrenocortical carcinoma. A, Naked, round nuclei with distinct nucleoli and prominent branching vasculature (Papanicolaou stain). **B,** Polygonal cells with ample, nongranular cytoplasm; central, round nuclei; and prominent nucleoli (May-Grünwald-Giemsa stain). **C,** Histological section from a biopsy shows nests of tumor cells with a suggestion of rosette formation and sinusoidal growth. The cells exhibit eosinophilic cytoplasm; central, round nuclei; and intracytoplasmic pale bodies. These features are highly reminiscent of hepatocellular carcinoma (hematoxylin and eosin stain).

and leiomyosarcomas are the most important malignancies to recognize for therapeutic purposes. Epithelioid variants of GIST may be confused with hepatocellular and neuroendocrine tumors (Boxes 46.35 and 46.36; see Figs. 46.60 and 46.61).[269-274]

Not all AFP-producing carcinomas, hepatoid or nonhepatoid in appearance, arise in the liver. Rarely, the tumor can arise in an extrahepatic site such as an adenocarcinoma of the stomach.[275,276] These lesions are aggressive, have a proclivity for vascular invasion, and readily metastasize to the liver.

The full reference list may be accessed online *at Elsevier eBooks for Practicing Clinicians.*

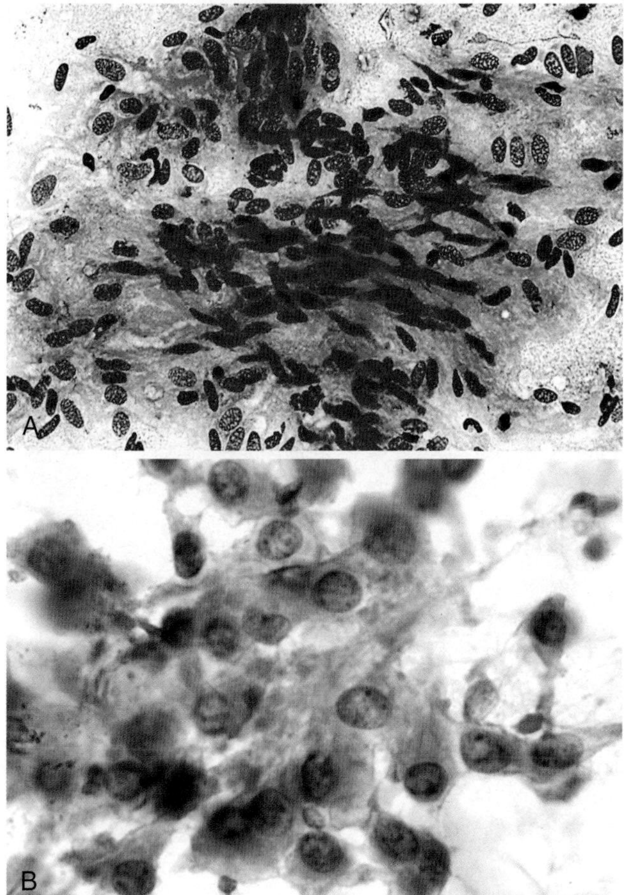

FIGURE 46.60 Metastatic gastrointestinal stromal tumor. A, Sheaves of monomorphic spindle cells with bland, cigar-shaped nuclei and cytoplasmic processes (May-Grünwald-Giemsa stain). **B,** An epithelioid phenotype may be difficult to distinguish from hepatocellular and neuroendocrine tumors (Papanicolaou stain).

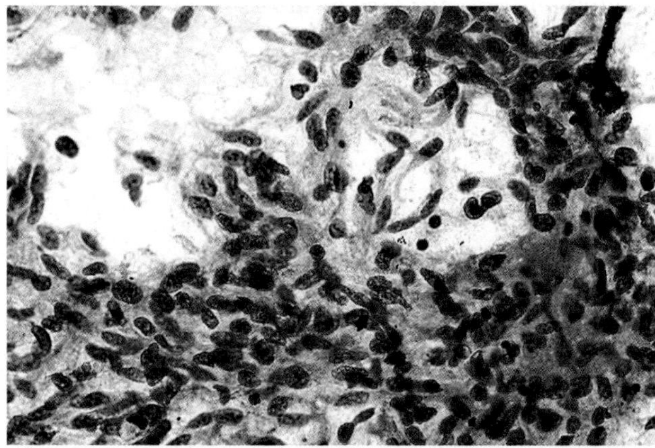

FIGURE 46.61 Metastatic leiomyosarcoma. Pleomorphic, spindle-shaped cells arranged in cohesive, three-dimensional groups with hyperchromatic, cigar-shaped nuclei and wiry cytoplasmic processes (Papanicolaou stain).

BOX 46.29 Non-Hodgkin's Lymphoma

- Mostly large B-cell lymphoma
- Dyshesive, single-cell population; may have pseudogroups (i.e., artifactual clustering)
- Lymphoglandular bodies (i.e., clumps of stripped-off cytoplasm) in the background
- Coarse, often peripherally clumped chromatin (see Fig. 46.54)
- Nucleoli may be present.
- Cytoplasm is scant to invisible but may be abundant in anaplastic large cell lymphoma.

BOX 46.30 Neuroendocrine Tumors

- Small, uniform, round cells with visible cytoplasm that tends to be scant and more evenly perinuclear in carcinoid tumors and more abundant and eccentric in pancreatic endocrine tumors (PETs) (see Fig. 46.55)
- Nuclei with coarse, stippled, salt-and-pepper chromatin that is more obvious in carcinoids than in PETs
- Nucleoli usually not present in carcinoid tumors but visible in PETs
- No nuclear molding, much less crush artifact, and no significant necrosis or apoptosis compared with small cell undifferentiated carcinoma
- Immunohistochemistry: positive for synaptophysin and chromogranin

BOX 46.31 Small Cell Carcinoma

- Small, pleomorphic round cells with little or no cytoplasm are arranged in clusters and singly (see Fig. 46.56).
- Nuclei are hyperchromatic with coarse, stippled chromatin.
- Nuclear molding is common and characteristic.
- Necrosis and apoptosis are common.
- Smear or crush artifact is invariably present because of the fragile nature of the cells.

BOX 46.32 Metastatic Melanoma

- Large, polygonal cells arranged singly and in clusters; may also be spindle cells or small round cells with scant cytoplasm (see Fig. 46.57)
- Central to eccentric nuclei with large nucleoli
- Intranuclear inclusions are common.
- Cytoplasm is commonly abundant, nongranular, and frequently nonpigmented.
- Fontana-Masson stain turns cytoplasmic melanin pigment black but also stains lipofuscin (possible diagnostic pitfall).
- Immunohistochemistry: positive for S100, HMB-45, and melan-A (i.e., MLANA or MART1); negative for keratin

BOX 46.33 Renal Cell Carcinoma

- Large, polygonal cells are arranged singly and in clusters (see Fig. 46.58).
- Transgressing endothelial pattern is the most common vascular pattern; peripheral endothelium is not a feature.
- Round, central nuclei with prominent macronucleoli (owl's eye) are typical in clear or granular cell type; papillary renal cell carcinoma (RCC) type does not demonstrate prominent nucleoli.
- Intranuclear inclusions can be seen and are common in the chromophobe type.
- Cytoplasm is commonly abundant and clear or granular; excessive and balloon-like in chromophobe RCC; and scant, often with hemosiderin, in papillary RCC.
- Immunohistochemistry: positive for keratin, vimentin, and epithelial membrane antigen; negative for carcinoembryonic antigen

BOX 46.34 Adrenocortical Carcinoma

- Medium-sized, polygonal cells are arranged singly and in clusters (see Fig. 46.59).
- No transgressing endothelial pattern, but peripheral endothelium may be seen on cell block.
- Nuclei are variably atypical with hyperchromasia and pleomorphism; nucleoli do not tend to be macroeosinophilic, as in hepatocellular carcinoma.
- Immunohistochemistry: positive for inhibin and melan-A (i.e., MLANA or MART1); vimentin and synaptophysin variable; negative for keratin, epithelial membrane antigen, and carcinoembryonic antigen.

BOX 46.35 Gastrointestinal Stromal Tumor

- Monomorphic spindle cells arranged in loose groups and singly; occasional epithelioid features
- Prominent vascular pattern (see Fig. 46.60)
- Relatively bland nuclei without overt hyperchromasia or pleomorphism
- Delicate cytoplasmic processes
- Little to no crush artifact
- Immunohistochemistry: positive for KIT, ANO1 (DOG1), and CD34; variably positive for smooth muscle actin; negative for desmin

BOX 46.36 Leiomyosarcoma

- Pleomorphic, spindle-shaped cells in tightly cohesive, three-dimensional groups and syncytia; occasional epithelioid features (see Fig. 46.61)
- Absence of a prominent vascular pattern
- Hyperchromatic, pleomorphic nuclei with crush artifact are common
- Wiry, refractile cytoplasmic processes or stroma, or both
- Immunohistochemistry: positive for desmin and smooth muscle actin; negative for KIT

CHAPTER 47

Acute and Chronic Infectious Hepatitis

Maria Westerhoff, Laura W. Lamps

Contents

INTRODUCTION

A wide variety of infectious agents can involve the liver. The most common are the "hepatotropic" viruses—those that preferentially involve the liver—including hepatitis A, B, C, D, and E. Many other viruses, such as cytomegalovirus (CMV) and Epstein-Barr virus (EBV), may produce hepatic injury as part of systemic infection. Although some infectious agents produce characteristic morphological patterns of injury, in many cases, the findings are relatively nonspecific. Therefore proper interpretation of liver biopsies requires adequate clinical information, including the patient's immunological status, travel history, clinical signs and symptoms, medications used, and serological test results.

VIRAL HEPATITIS

Viral hepatitis is defined by the presence of hepatocyte necrosis and inflammation resulting from a viral infection, which leads to a characteristic constellation of clinical and morphological features. Most cases are caused by one of four well-known hepatotropic viruses: hepatitis A (HAV), B (HBV), C (HCV), and E (HEV). HBV infection may be further complicated by co-infection, or superinfection, with hepatitis D virus (HDV). As mentioned earlier, other viruses, such as CMV and EBV, can cause hepatic injury and inflammation as part of a systemic illness, but the hepatitis in those cases is often overshadowed by the clinical manifestations of involvement of other organ systems. Other, unidentified types of viral hepatitis may also exist, based on the rare occurrence of posttransfusion hepatitis despite adequate screening of blood donors for known infectious agents.

Viral hepatitis is generally divided into acute and chronic forms, based primarily on clinical evidence of chronicity. The term *chronic hepatitis* is used when there is evidence of persistent hepatic necrosis and inflammation. Traditionally, particularly for HBV-infected patients, chronic hepatitis has been defined clinically by the presence of aminotransferase elevations lasting at least 6 months in duration. Histologically, however, chronic hepatitis refers to an ongoing necroinflammatory process that affects hepatocytes and is associated with portal-based chronic inflammation and fibrosis.

Acute Viral Hepatitis

Clinical Features

Acute viral hepatitis is often asymptomatic, and in many patients, it is recognized only in retrospect after serological tests reveal evidence of prior infection. In symptomatic patients, presenting symptoms often are only mild and nonspecific and include malaise, fatigue, low-grade fever, and flulike complaints. Asymptomatic or mild acute viral hepatitis is more common in children; adults are more likely to be symptomatic.

Symptomatic acute viral hepatitis is usually preceded by a prodrome phase that lasts from a few days to several weeks and is characterized by nonspecific symptoms such as nausea, vomiting, myalgia, anorexia, and malaise. Once jaundice develops, constitutional symptoms typically begin to wane. Physical examination is often notable only for jaundice and hepatomegaly. In addition, the liver may be tender to palpation. Serum aminotransferases, which are the key indicators of hepatocellular injury, are commonly elevated 10-fold above normal and often exceed 1000 units/L. In contrast, alkaline phosphatase is typically only mildly elevated; conjugated hyperbilirubinemia is present in some, but not all, patients. In most cases, full recovery occurs within a few weeks. In some, low-grade symptoms or signs persist for months. The treatment of acute viral hepatitis is generally supportive.

Fulminant hepatic failure develops in <1% of acute viral hepatitis cases. This is characterized by the rapid development of liver decompensation. Although acute liver failure may result from a variety of other causes, including exposure to drugs or toxins, autoimmune liver disease, or ischemia, 12% of cases in the United States are caused by acute viral hepatitis.[1] The clinical course of acute hepatic failure is characterized by coagulopathy, encephalopathy, and a high mortality rate in patients who do not undergo liver transplantation. For both acute HAV and acute HEV infection, patients with a background of chronic liver disease have a higher risk of a poor outcome.

Pathological Features

Table 47.1 summarizes the pathological features of acute and chronic hepatitis.

Patients with acute viral hepatitis seldom undergo liver biopsy because the diagnosis is usually easily established by noninvasive serological tests. On low-power microscopic examination, acute cases show a necroinflammatory process that involves all areas of the hepatic lobules, and hence it is not confined to the portal tracts. The combination of hepatocyte injury, loss, and regeneration with the presence of a mononuclear inflammatory infiltrate leads to a pattern termed *lobular disarray*, which reflects a disruption of the normal orderly architecture of the liver cell plates (Fig. 47.1).

Lobular hepatocellular changes include hepatocyte swelling, in which the affected cells are pale stained and show irregular, wispy cytoplasm and clumping of cytoplasm around the nucleus. Other forms of hepatocyte necrosis occur as well (described later). Swollen hepatocytes often undergo "lytic necrosis," marked by the presence of small foci of stromal collapse associated with small clusters of mononuclear inflammatory cells. In addition, hepatocytes may undergo acidophilic changes, in which the cell becomes shrunken, angular, and hypereosinophilic and contains a densely stained pyknotic nucleus. This type of necrosis leads to acidophil bodies (apoptotic bodies), which are small, mummified, rounded cell remnants that may also extrude fragments of degenerated nuclei. Apoptotic bodies may be phagocytosed by Kupffer cells, resulting in Kupffer cell hyperplasia. Individual or small clusters of necrotic hepatocytes are collectively referred to as "spotty" hepatocyte necrosis. Regeneration of hepatocytes contributes to the "busy" appearance of the hepatic lobules, because the liver cell plates are typically irregular and thickened. Nonspecific steatosis may also occur in cases of acute hepatitis.

TABLE 47.1 Histopathological Features of Acute and Chronic Hepatitis

Acute	Chronic
Predominantly lobular inflammation	Predominantly portal tract inflammation
Lobular regeneration and disarray	Lobular acidophil bodies
Hepatocyte swelling	Mononuclear inflammatory cells, occasional plasma cells
Kupffer cell aggregates, particularly highlighted in periodic acid–Schiff with diastase digestion	Portal-based lymphoid aggregates and lymphoid follicle formation
Apoptotic hepatocytes (acidophil bodies)	Progressive fibrosis with eventual cirrhosis
Mononuclear inflammatory cells, with occasional eosinophils and neutrophils	Interface hepatitis
Canalicular cholestasis	Bile ductular proliferation
Hepatocyte dropout, necrosis	

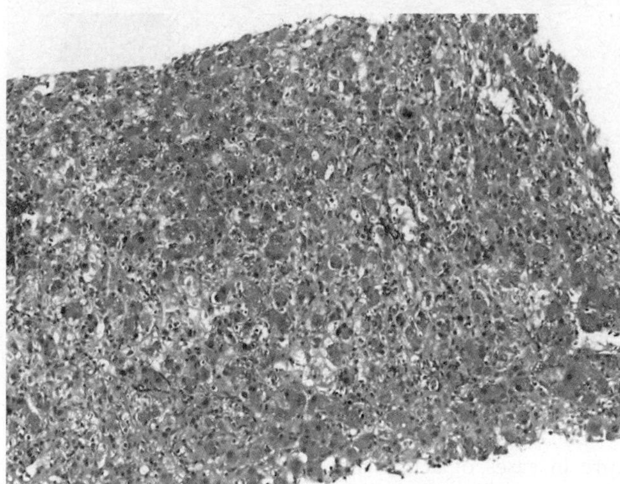

FIGURE 47.1 Acute viral hepatitis. Lobular disarray is caused by hepatocyte necrosis, hepatocellular regeneration, Kupffer cell hyperplasia and hypertrophy, and a diffuse, predominantly mononuclear inflammatory infiltrate.

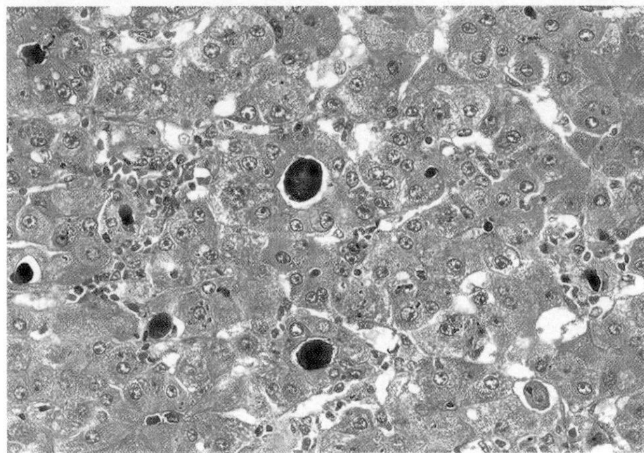

FIGURE 47.2 Acute viral hepatitis. Hepatocyte regeneration is seen in the form of cholestatic rosettes, with hepatocytes surrounding a central bile plug.

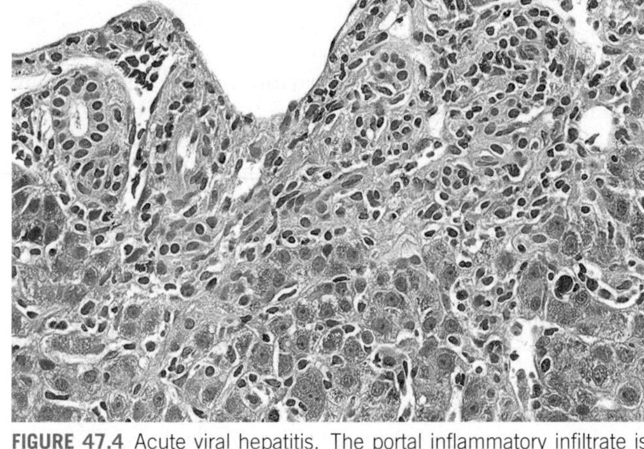

FIGURE 47.4 Acute viral hepatitis. The portal inflammatory infiltrate is primarily mononuclear cells, with scattered neutrophils and eosinophils. Inflammation spills into the adjacent parenchyma.

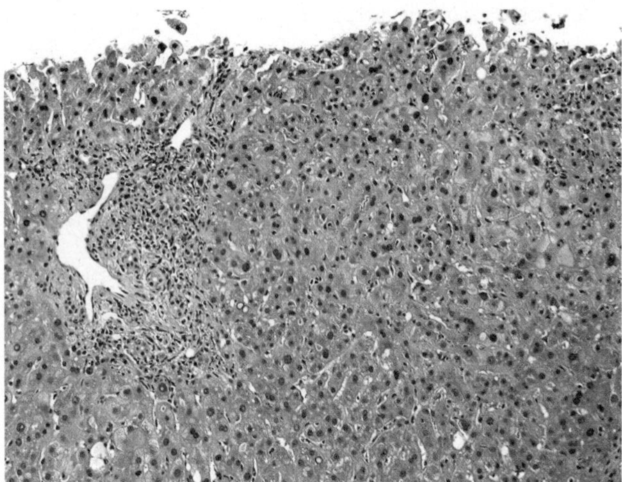

FIGURE 47.3 Cholestatic hepatitis. Portal and lobular inflammation is seen, as well as canalicular bile plugging and hepatocyte swelling.

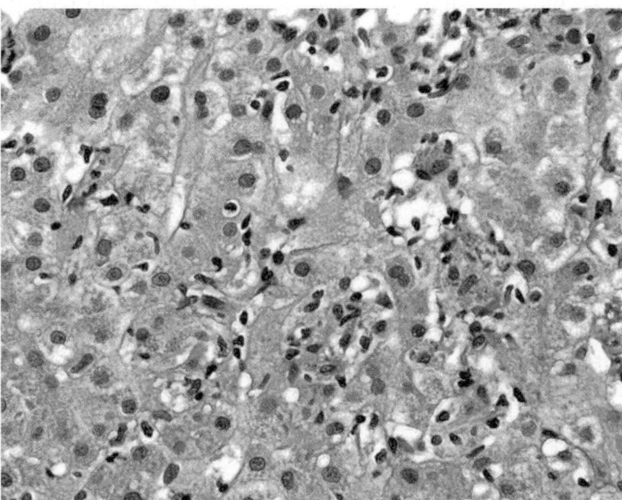

FIGURE 47.5 Periodic acid–Schiff staining after diastase digestion highlights Kupffer cell hyperplasia and the accumulation of phagocytized debris.

Canalicular cholestasis is not normally a prominent feature in cases of acute viral hepatitis. However, cholestasis may occasionally be so prominent that the histological changes mimic those of biliary obstruction. In this variant, termed *acute cholestatic hepatitis*, one sees marked lobular inflammation and hepatocanalicular cholestasis. There may also be bile accumulation within the lumina of bile ducts and ductules. The finding of a prominent bile ductular reaction associated with neutrophils (termed *cholangiolitis*) in the portal tracts may contribute to confusion with biliary obstruction. Marked hepatocyte swelling and regenerating cholestatic rosettes (hepatocyte "pseudoglands") may be present in the hepatic lobules (Figs. 47.2 and 47.3). Typically, cases of acute cholestatic hepatitis have a more prolonged clinical course.

The inflammatory infiltrate in cases of acute viral hepatitis is primarily mononuclear. It is composed of lymphocytes, macrophages, scattered eosinophils, and occasional plasma cells and neutrophils (Fig. 47.4). In contrast to chronic viral hepatitis, in which portal and periportal inflammation typically predominates, the inflammatory infiltrate in acute viral hepatitis usually is not concentrated to the portal tracts but is spread more evenly throughout the hepatic lobules. Sinusoidal mononuclear cells are often prominent. Kupffer cells are often more prominent and more numerous than usual; they are hypertrophic and may contain phagocytized cellular debris and abundant lipofuscin pigment, which is highlighted by staining with periodic acid–Schiff (PAS) stain after diastase digestion (Figs. 47.5 and 47.6).

Although the necroinflammatory process is typically panlobular, inflammation and necrosis in acute hepatitis may be more pronounced in the centrilobular areas. Bridging necrosis may develop in severe cases. This feature appears as a zone of necrosis that extends from the portal tracts to the central veins, and it is often associated with a more protracted clinical course (Fig. 47.7).

Immunohistochemistry for detection of viral antigens is generally not considered useful for evaluation of acute viral hepatitis because the virus is rapidly eliminated from liver cells and therefore is not detectable. Serological tests are the most reliable, and readily available, for diagnostic purposes.

Massive and Submassive Necrosis

In severe cases of acute viral hepatitis, large portions of the hepatocyte lobules (submassive necrosis) or entire contiguous lobules (massive necrosis) may undergo necrosis.

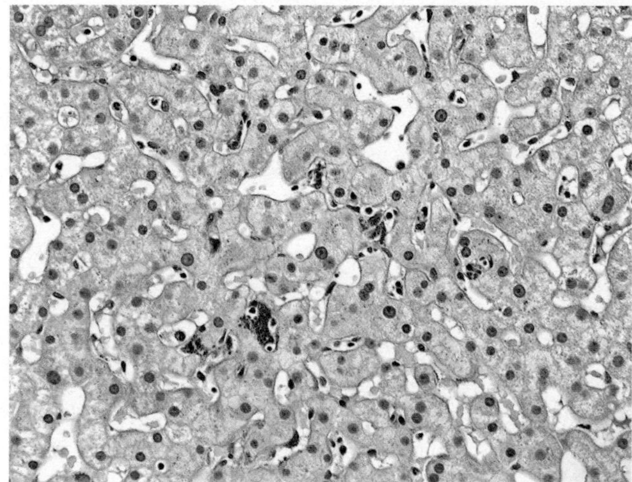

FIGURE 47.6 Periodic acid–Schiff staining after diastase digestion highlights Kupffer cells in deep magenta; they are in areas that used to be occupied by hepatocytes. The Kupffer cells have phagocytized cellular remnants of necrotic hepatocytes. As biopsies may be taken some time after the liver injury, biopsies accompanied by histories of recent markedly elevated liver chemistries may appear nearly normal but have these debris-laden Kupffer cells to indicate there is resolving acute hepatitis.

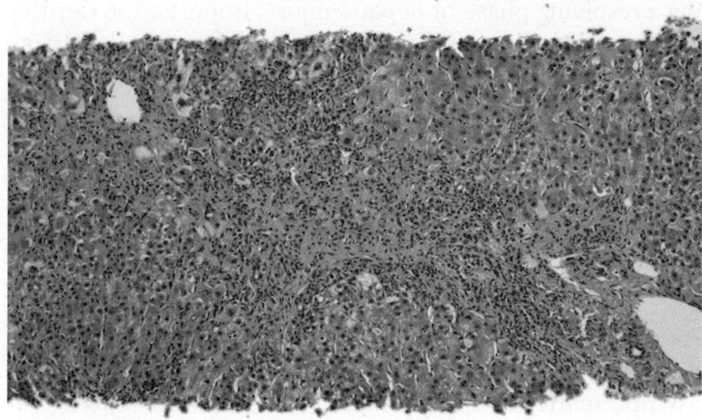

FIGURE 47.7 Bridging necrosis. An area without hepatocytes is seen spanning the portal tract on the bottom right to the central vein on the left top.

Submassive necrosis usually involves zone 3 hepatocytes initially, but it may extend to zone 2 regions with progression. Extensive destruction of hepatic parenchyma results in the clinical syndrome of "fulminant hepatic failure." On gross examination, livers with massive necrosis appear shrunken and flaccid, often showing wrinkling of the capsular surface and a mottled appearance of the liver parenchyma. Regenerating nodules of hepatocytes, which are often bile stained, may be irregularly distributed in the liver and may form nodular masses. The degree of necroinflammatory activity is variable, even among patients with a similar clinical course.[2] In fulminant cases, one often sees a prominent bile ductular reaction, with associated neutrophils (cholangiolitis), which is typically located in the peripheral region of the portal tracts (Fig. 47.8). However, the histological features of submassive or massive hepatic necrosis are not specific for acute viral hepatitis. This pattern of injury can develop

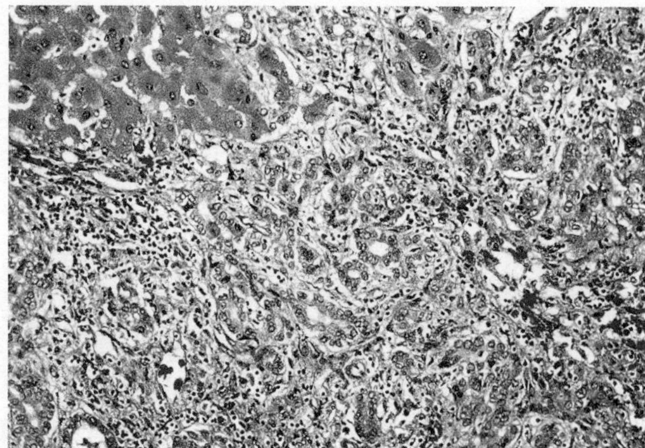

FIGURE 47.8 Acute viral hepatitis. Massive necrosis, defined as destruction of contiguous lobules, often exhibits marked bile ductular proliferation.

as a result of toxic injury, severe drug reaction, or Wilson's disease, among other causes. A trichrome stain to highlight connective tissue is useful to distinguish massive hepatic necrosis from cirrhosis, by demonstrating the lack of dense collagen deposition in the former. A reticulin stain is also helpful to demonstrate the presence of a collapsed reticulin framework (Fig. 47.9).

Prognostic Factors

Pathological features of acute viral hepatitis that are predictive of progression to chronicity are difficult to elucidate, in part because of the rarity of liver biopsies from patients with acute hepatitis. Furthermore, in patients with massive hepatic necrosis, an individual liver biopsy may not represent the overall status of the liver, because hepatocyte regeneration and necrosis can vary substantially from region to region.

Differential Diagnosis

Several major entities may be confused with acute viral hepatitis—in particular, chronic viral hepatitis, autoimmune hepatitis, and drug-induced hepatitis (Table 47.2). In cases in which the lobular inflammatory component is prominent, a markedly active chronic hepatitis may be confused with acute hepatitis. Some patients with autoimmune hepatitis exhibit an "acute" clinical picture and have a prominent lobular inflammatory infiltrate with extensive necrosis that may be difficult to distinguish from acute viral hepatitis. However, autoimmune hepatitis often reveals prominent plasma cell infiltrates. Even in the acute presentation of autoimmune hepatitis, plasma cell infiltration can be seen in the portal tracts and is associated with interface activity, albeit centrilobular necrosis and lobular plasma cell infiltration can be seen in this acute presentation as well. In addition, fibrosis often exists at the time of the initial biopsy in patients with autoimmune hepatitis, even with an acute clinical picture.[3] Of note, the Masson's trichrome stain used routinely to evaluate for fibrosis in livers must be evaluated with caution in fulminant hepatitis. Parenchymal collapse or areas of necrosis may mimic fibrosis but will have a paler blue color in comparison to the darker blue of true established fibrosis in chronic hepatitis (Fig. 47.10). To assist in this distinction, the trichrome staining pattern in suspected

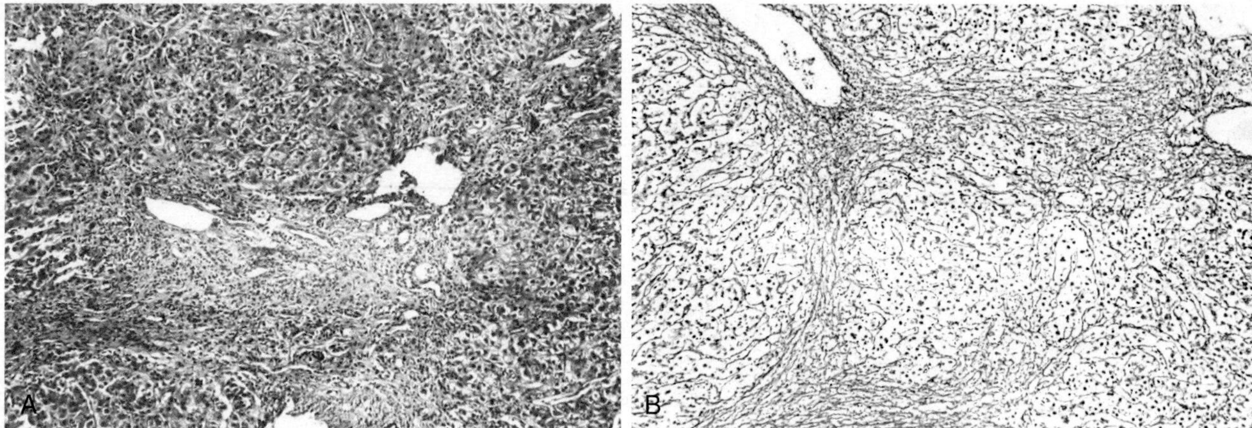

FIGURE 47.9 A, Hematoxylin and eosin section of an area of lobular necrosis from a patient with acute liver failure. **B,** Trichrome stain is pale blue in the areas of hepatocyte loss, compared with the darker blue of the collagen around the portal tract.

TABLE 47.2 Differential Diagnosis of Acute and Chronic Viral Hepatitis

Acute	Chronic
Autoimmune hepatitis	Autoimmune hepatitis
Drug-induced hepatitis	Primary biliary cholangitis
Toxins	Primary sclerosing cholangitis
Wilson's disease	Wilson's disease
Other infectious hepatitides (i.e., herpes simplex virus, Epstein-Barr virus)	α_1-Antitrypsin deficiency
Idiopathic	Drug-induced hepatitis
	Idiopathic

parenchymal collapse should be compared with the darker blue of the collagen surrounding portal structures. Reticulin stains can also help highlight areas of collapse and parenchymal extinction. Serological tests for autoimmune markers are usually helpful, although recent literature has shown that up to 20% of patients with clinical and histological features of autoimmune hepatitis have negative autoimmune serologies, particularly early in the course of disease. Viral serologies and molecular testing for DNA or RNA are of course helpful in confirming or excluding viral hepatitis.[3]

Drug-induced hepatitis can be indistinguishable from acute viral hepatitis (see Chapter 48 for more detail). The presence of prominent eosinophils, granulomas, sinusoidal dilation, prominent bile ductular reaction, cholestasis, and fatty change may suggest a drug reaction, but these are not considered pathognomonic features. Pericentral hepatocyte necrosis and dropout, as seen in classical Tylenol overdose, or overlapping findings of both cholestasis and lobular hepatitis suggest a drug reaction. Acute or chronic hepatitis that does not seem to fit into a discrete morphological category should raise the possibility of a drug reaction as well. Obtaining a complete history of drug and toxin exposures is critical to distinguish drug reactions from viral hepatitis. Furthermore, superimposed drug injury may develop in patients with acute viral hepatitis, so the two entities are not necessarily mutually exclusive.

A common clinical scenario that pathologists may encounter is a biopsy specimen obtained weeks after the appearance of clinical symptoms and elevated liver enzymes indicative of acute hepatitis. In this situation, a nearly normal liver with aggregates of Kupffer cells in areas of hepatocyte dropout may be the only finding. A PAS-D stain can highlight the debris-filled macrophages, suggesting a resolving phase of hepatic injury. Importantly, Kupffer cell aggregates should not be mistaken for nonnecrotizing granulomas.

Chronic Viral Hepatitis

Refer to Table 47.3 for a summary of the histopathological features of chronic viral hepatitis.

Clinical Features

As in acute hepatitis, patients with chronic hepatitis have a wide spectrum of clinical manifestations that range from asymptomatic to symptomatic and decompensated cirrhosis. Many patients are asymptomatic or have only mild, nonspecific complaints, such as fatigue. Findings on physical examination are typically few but include hepatomegaly and other stigmata of chronic liver disease, such as palmar erythema. Ascites and esophageal or cutaneous varices may also develop in patients with advanced cirrhosis. Serum aminotransferase levels fluctuate but are usually chronically elevated in the 2- to 10-fold range, although a substantial number of patients with mild chronic hepatitis C have persistently normal aminotransferase levels. Alkaline phosphatase and bilirubin levels are usually normal to only mildly elevated, unless hepatic decompensation has occurred, in which case high levels may be observed.

Pathological Features

As mentioned previously, chronic hepatitis is defined clinically as persistent necroinflammatory liver disease. Regardless of the specific etiology, chronic hepatitis is characterized by a combination of portal inflammation, interface (periportal) hepatitis, varying degrees of parenchymal inflammation and necrosis, and, in many cases, fibrosis. This histological pattern of injury is not specific for chronic viral hepatitis. It may also be seen in many other chronic conditions, such

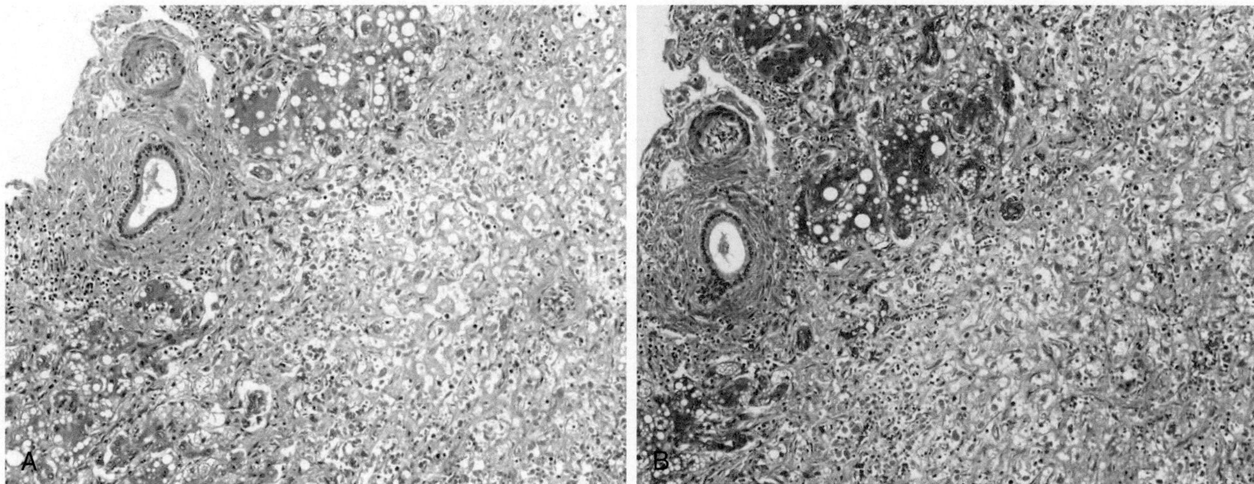

FIGURE 47.10 **A,** Area of hepatocyte dropout in acute hepatitis. **B,** Reticulin stain in an area of parenchymal collapse, highlighting absence of hepatocytes and compression of reticulin fibers to each other.

TABLE 47.3 Histopathological Features of Common Causes of Chronic Hepatitis

Feature	Chronic Viral Hepatitis	Autoimmune Hepatitis	Chronic Bile Duct Obstructive Disorders	Wilson's Disease
Portal tract inflammation	Yes, dense mononuclear cell	Yes, mononuclear; predominance of plasma cells at interface	Yes, neutrophils; mononuclear cells and eosinophils in autoimmune diseases	Yes, variable and mixed; mainly lymphocytes and plasma cells
Interface activity	Yes, mononuclear with hepatocyte apoptosis	Yes, plasma cells and hepatocyte apoptosis	Bile ductular reaction with associated neutrophils; hepatocyte feathery degeneration	Yes, variable; mononuclear cells with hepatocyte apoptosis and feathery degeneration
Lobular inflammation	Yes, mononuclear and macrophage aggregates	Yes, predominantly plasma cells and lymphocytes	Yes, predominantly periportal, as above	Yes, variable; predominantly mononuclear
Hepatocyte necrosis	Yes, hepatocyte apoptosis	Yes, hepatocyte apoptosis; bridging necrosis may be present	No; feathery degeneration	Yes, variable; hepatocyte apoptosis and feathery degeneration, with Mallory bodies
Fibrosis	Variable; usually periportal, may be perivenular	Yes; bridging necrosis leads to cirrhosis	Yes; periportal, may progress to cirrhosis	Yes, variable; periportal, with progression to cirrhosis
Other	Ground-glass cells (hepatitis B)	Giant syncytial multinucleated hepatocytes	Intracellular and canalicular cholestasis	Periportal glycogenated nuclei; steatosis; intracytoplasmic copper

as autoimmune hepatitis, metabolic disorders such as Wilson's disease and α_1-antitrypsin deficiency, chronic biliary disorders also exhibiting portal inflammation and fibrosis, and various types of drug reactions. Table 47.3 summarizes the histopathological features of chronic hepatitis (see also Table 47.1).

Portal Inflammation

Chronic hepatitis is characterized by the presence of an inflammatory infiltrate that involves the portal tracts, which may range from mild and patchy to prominent and diffuse. The infiltrates consist primarily of lymphocytes, often associated with a variable number of plasma cells. Scattered macrophages, neutrophils, and eosinophils may be found in some cases, but they are typically a minor component of the infiltrate in chronic viral hepatitis. Lymphoid follicles may be present, particularly in hepatitis C, and germinal centers may also be present (Fig. 47.11). A bile ductular reaction may be seen at the periphery of portal tracts, but this feature is not specific and usually is not very prominent in viral hepatitis. As with any type of bile ductular reaction, neutrophils are usually associated with the proliferating ductular epithelium as a result of cytokines released by biliary epithelium, and this should not be interpreted as evidence of biliary obstruction or acute cholangitis. Mild bile duct injury can also be seen, but this is not a prominent feature of chronic viral hepatitis.

Typically, the majority of portal tracts are equally involved by the inflammatory process. Interface hepatitis, also known as *interface activity* or *piecemeal necrosis*, is

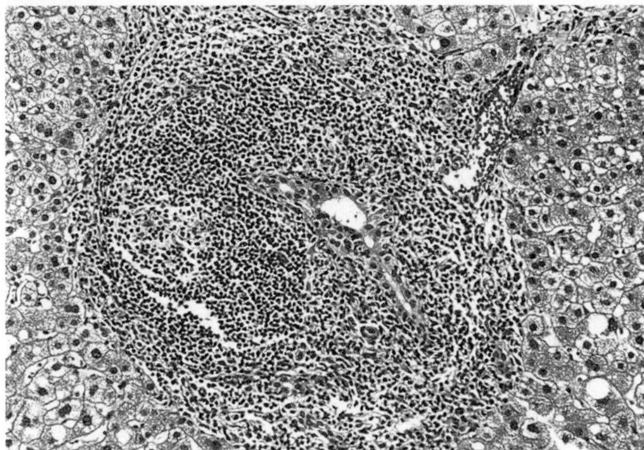

FIGURE 47.11 Chronic viral hepatitis. Mononuclear portal inflammation is variable; lymphoid aggregates, sometimes with germinal centers, are common in hepatitis C.

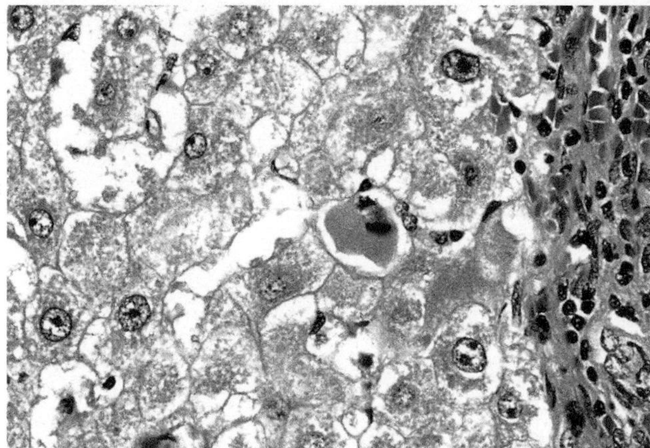

FIGURE 47.13 Chronic viral hepatitis. An acidophilic body with a partially extruded nucleus is present in the sinusoid.

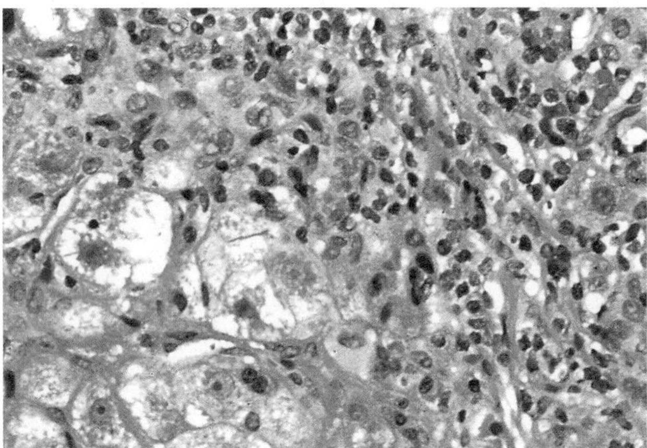

FIGURE 47.12 Chronic viral hepatitis. Interface hepatitis produces a ragged limiting plate, with (in this example) hepatocellular swelling.

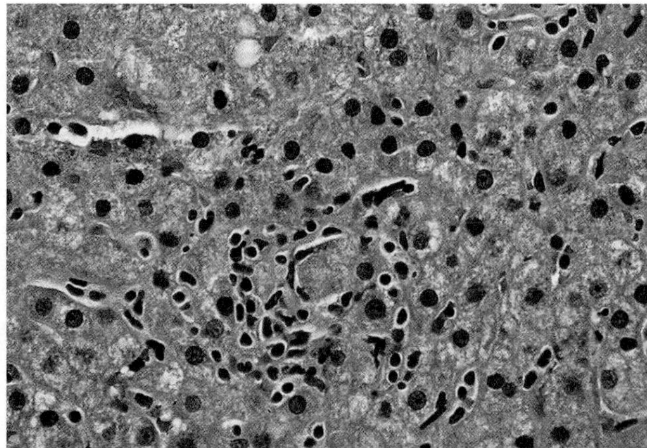

FIGURE 47.14 Chronic viral hepatitis. A cluster of mononuclear inflammatory cells is indicative of lytic hepatocyte necrosis.

characterized by inflammation and injury of the adjacent hepatocytes immediately surrounding the portal tracts. It is an important and common feature of chronic viral hepatitis, although it may be focal, or even absent, in cases with minimal or mild necroinflammatory activity. Lymphocytes and plasma cells in the periportal infiltrate are closely associated with degenerating hepatocytes (Fig. 47.12), such that indentation of the cytoplasm of the hepatocytes occurs, and one might even see engulfment of inflammatory cells by hepatocytes. Hepatocytes in areas of interface hepatitis–associated necrosis often appear pale or swollen and show clumping of cytoplasm. Apoptotic bodies (acidophil bodies) may be present as well.

Lobular Necroinflammatory Activity

In chronic viral hepatitis, hepatocyte necrosis is usually variable in severity and spotty in distribution. Lobular disarray, a feature characteristic of acute hepatitis, is not often prominent in chronic hepatitis unless there is marked activity. Acidophil bodies, which are usually more numerous in the periportal areas, may also be scattered in the hepatic lobules (Fig. 47.13). Mononuclear inflammatory cells tend to cluster around injured or dying hepatocytes (Fig. 47.14). Kupffer cells, in areas of spotty hepatocyte necrosis, may contain phagocytosed cellular debris. Hepatocyte swelling may be present in exacerbations of chronic viral hepatitis and may also be associated with zone 3 cholestasis. Regeneration of hepatocytes is recognized by the formation of liver cell plates that are two cells thick and by the formation of regenerating hepatocyte rosettes, as well as mitotically active hepatocytes.

Fibrosis

Progressive fibrosis of the limiting plate, as a result of continued necroinflammatory activity, leads to enlargement of the portal tracts and stellate periportal fibrous extensions (Fig. 47.15). Deposition of collagen and other extracellular matrix materials in the space of Disse at the leading edge of periportal fibrosis also results in capillarization of the sinusoids. Portal-portal fibrous septa represent the fibrous linkage of adjacent fibrotic portal tracts (Fig. 47.16). Portal-central fibrous bridges may also develop from superimposed episodes of severe lobular necroinflammatory activity involving zone 3 of the hepatic lobules. Central-central bridges form by the same mechanism but are far less common in chronic viral hepatitis. The end result of bridging fibrosis is cirrhosis, which is usually macronodular or of a mixed micronodular and macronodular type.

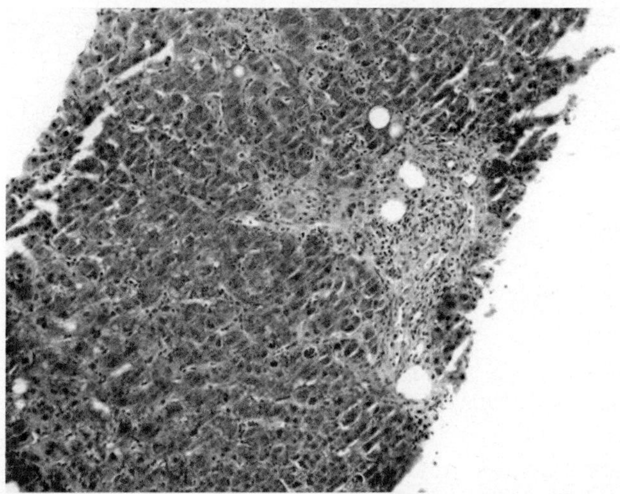

FIGURE 47.15 Chronic viral hepatitis. Portal fibrous expansion with periportal fibrous extension is seen in a patient with chronic hepatitis C.

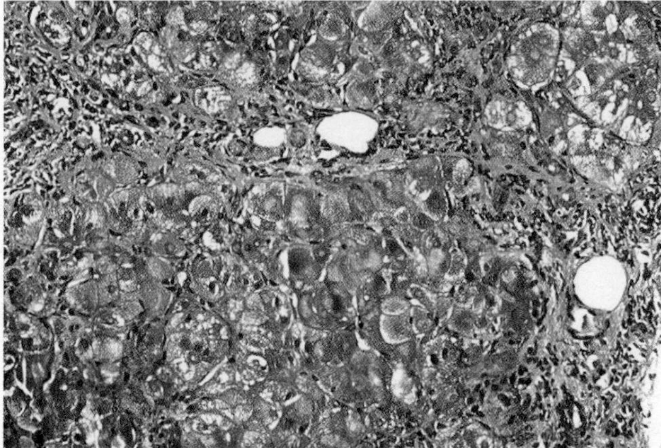

FIGURE 47.16 Chronic viral hepatitis. Portal-portal bridging fibrosis is seen in long-standing chronic hepatitis C. Focally, interface hepatitis involves the fibrous septa.

Nomenclature and Scoring

In the past, the term *chronic active hepatitis* was used to describe liver biopsies with interface hepatitis, and the term *chronic persistent hepatitis* was used for biopsies with portal inflammation but without significant periportal/piecemeal necrosis. This distinction was thought to be clinically important, because chronic persistent hepatitis was considered a relatively benign process without a high risk of progression to significant chronic liver disease. However, on identification of hepatitis C, and on recognition of the waxing and waning nature of the disease and the prolonged time to progression to cirrhosis in many cases, this nomenclature has been abandoned. Currently, the recommended practice is to use the term *chronic hepatitis*[4] and include a statement in the pathology report regarding the severity of necroinflammatory activity (grade), extent of fibrosis (stage), and etiology.[5] Prognostic factors should also be noted in the report (see later discussion).

Several different systems for scoring necroinflammatory activity and fibrosis have been developed (Table 47.4). The original Knodell system, first published in 1981, served as the prototype semiquantitative liver inflammation and fibrosis scoring system.[6] With modifications—such as the one proposed by Ishak and coworkers, which separates the grade of inflammation and necrosis from fibrosis—this system is still widely used, particularly in therapeutic trials in which the necroinflammatory activity in pretreatment and posttreatment liver biopsy specimens are compared.[7,8] In the original Knodell system, periportal necrosis (with or without bridging necrosis, intralobular necrosis, and inflammation), portal inflammation, and fibrosis are all assigned numeric values, which are then added to obtain a hepatitis activity index (HAI) that ranges from 0 to 22. One major criticism of this system is the inclusion of fibrosis (stage) as a determinant of activity (grade). In practice, the HAI is often modified so that bridging necrosis is dissociated from interface hepatitis, and only the elements that relate to grade are added together to produce the modified HAI (mHAI), with scores that range from 0 to 18; the stage, which indicates degree of fibrosis, is reported separately[9] (see Table 47.4). An alternative grading system used by the French METAVIR Cooperative Study Group evaluates only two features (periportal necrosis and lobular necroinflammatory activity) instead of three; portal inflammation is excluded because it is considered a prerequisite for the diagnosis of chronic hepatitis, even in cases without parenchymal activity.[10]

The various semiquantitative grading schemes, although useful for evaluating the effects of a particular treatment regimen in clinical trials, are typically not necessary or clinically relevant for routine pathology reporting of liver biopsies. For everyday diagnostic purposes, simpler schemes are sufficient. For instance, the Batts-Ludwig scoring system (Table 47.5) uses 5 categories (0 through 4) separately for both grade and stage[11] (Figs. 47.17 and 47.18). In the Batts-Ludwig system, grade is determined by evaluation of the degree of interface activity (lymphocytic piecemeal necrosis), lobular inflammation, and necrosis. Stage is scored from 0 to 4. A zero score refers to normal connective tissue (no fibrosis). Stage 1 indicates fibrous expansion of portal tracts; stage 2, periportal fibrosis; stage 3, portal-portal bridging fibrous septa; and stage 4, cirrhosis (see Fig. 47.18). Pathological stage is best evaluated with the use of a Masson trichrome stain, because delicate periportal or early bridging fibrous septa may not be easily apparent on hematoxylin and eosin (H&E) stain.

Prognostic Factors

Factors associated with progression of chronic viral hepatitis to cirrhosis may be divided into those related to specific viruses, host-related factors (see Treatment of Chronic Hepatitis C), and extraneous factors (e.g., alcohol use). For hepatitis C, development of chronic hepatitis is not related to the amount of virus at initial exposure. Viral genotype may be important in the progression of HCV infection. For instance, genotype 1 is associated with more severe disease than genotype 2.[12,13] However, other studies have not confirmed this association.[14] Host-related factors for disease severity are incompletely defined, but age at infection and gender appear to be relevant. Males and older individuals are more likely to show progression of fibrosis.[14,15] Alcohol consumption increases replication of hepatitis C and is

TABLE 47.4 Ishak Modified Hepatitis Activity Index (HAI) Grading and Staging of Chronic Hepatitis

Necroinflammatory Score	Portal Inflammation	Interface Hepatitis	Confluent Necrosis	Focal (Spotty) Lytic Necrosis, Apoptosis, and Focal Inflammation	Modified Staging	Descriptive
0	None	Absent	Absent	Absent	0	No fibrosis
1	Mild (some or all portal areas)	Mild (focal, few portal areas)	Focal confluent necrosis	One focus or less per 10× objective	1	Fibrous expansion of some portal areas, with or without short fibrous septa
2	Moderate (some or all portal areas)	Mild to moderate (focal, most portal areas)	Zone 3 necrosis in some areas	Two to four foci per 10× objective	2	Fibrous expansion of most portal areas, with or without short fibrous septa
3	Moderate to marked (all portal areas)	Moderate (continuous around <50% of tracts or septa)	Zone 3 necrosis in most areas	Five to 10 foci per 10× objective	3	Fibrous expansion of most portal areas with occasional P-P bridging
4	Marked (all portal areas)	Severe (continuous around >50% of tracts or septa)	Zone 3 necrosis + occasional P-C bridging	More than 10 foci per 10× objective	4	Fibrous expansion of portal areas with marked bridging (P-P and P-C)
5			Zone 3 necrosis + multiple P-C bridging		5	Marked bridging (P-P or P-C) with occasional nodules (incomplete cirrhosis)
6			Panacinar or multiacinar necrosis		6	Cirrhosis, probable or definite

From Ishak K, Baptista A, Bianchi L, et al. Histologic grading and staging of chronic hepatitis. J Hepatol. *1995;22:696-699.*
P-C, *Portal-central;* P-P, *portal-portal.*

associated with more severe disease.[16] In general, the grade of hepatic necroinflammatory activity in liver biopsy specimens correlates with the serum HCV RNA level,[17] and the rate of progression to cirrhosis correlates with high-grade activity and advanced stage in initial liver biopsies.[18] Hepatic steatosis is also associated with increased disease severity and is more commonly seen in infections with genotype 3b, as previously discussed.[15,19] Accumulation of iron in hepatocytes and Kupffer cells in hepatitis C may influence the disease course and response to therapy adversely.[15,20] However, many patients with chronic viral hepatitis, including hepatitis C, have abnormal results on serum iron studies but normal or only scant iron accumulation within the liver tissue.

Differential Diagnosis

The morphological patterns of chronic viral hepatitis are not specific to viral infection (see Table 47.4). The initial distinction should include distinguishing acute from chronic viral hepatitis, followed by differentiating chronic viral hepatitis from other forms of chronic hepatitis, such as autoimmune hepatitis. Distinction from acute hepatitis rests primarily on the pattern of lobular inflammation and necrosis in acute hepatitis, whereas chronic hepatitis shows predominantly portal inflammatory changes; fibrosis, in particular, is a cardinal sign of disease chronicity. However, in some cases, identification of acute versus chronic hepatitis may not be possible on morphological grounds alone; clinical evidence of chronic disease is usually very helpful.

Other conditions that may resemble chronic viral hepatitis can include primary sclerosing cholangitis (PSC), primary biliary cholangitis (PBC), metabolic disorders, and drug reactions.

PBC is a particularly important mimic of chronic viral hepatitis, because early in the course of disease, portal lymphocytic infiltrates in patients with PBC may resemble chronic viral hepatitis, particularly hepatitis C. The patchy nature of the portal inflammation in PBC, presence of florid-duct lesions, and loss of interlobular bile ducts are

TABLE 47.5 Batts-Ludwig Grading and Staging of Chronic Hepatitis

Grading Terminology				Staging Terminology		
Semiquantitative	**Descriptive**	**Interface Activity**	**Lobular Activity**	**Semiquantitative**	**Descriptive**	**Criteria**
0	Portal inflammation only; no activity	None	None	0	No fibrosis	Normal connective tissue
1	Minimal	Minimal; patchy	Minimal; occasional hepatocyte apoptosis	1	Portal fibrosis	Fibrous portal expansion
2	Mild	Mild; involving some or all portal tracts	Mild; little hepatocellular damage	2	Periportal fibrosis	Periportal or rare portal-portal septa
3	Moderate	Moderate; involving all portal tracts	Moderate; with noticeable hepatocellular damage	3	Septal fibrosis	Fibrous septa with architectural distortion; no obvious cirrhosis
4	Severe	Severe; may have bridging necrosis	Severe; with prominent diffuse hepatocellular damage	4	Cirrhosis	Cirrhosis

From Batts KP, Ludwig J. Chronic hepatitis: an update on terminology and reporting. Am J Surg Pathol. *1995;19:1409-1417.*

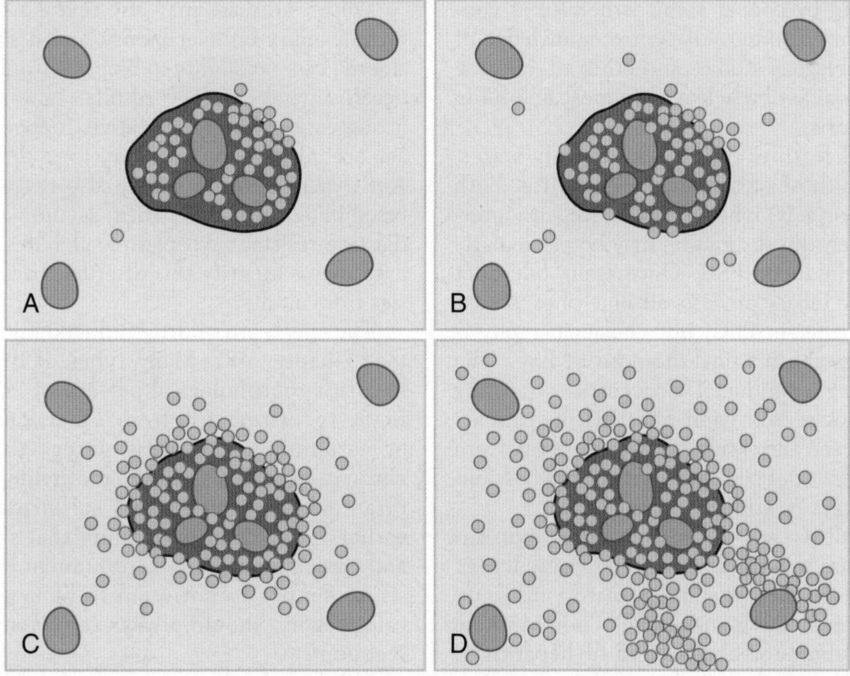

FIGURE 47.17 Grading scheme for increasing severity of portal and lobular necroinflammatory activity in chronic hepatitis (see Table 47.4). A, Minimal activity. **B,** Mild activity. **C,** Moderate activity. **D,** Severe activity. (*From Batts KP, Ludwig J. Chronic hepatitis: an update on terminology and reporting. Am J Surg Pathol. 1995;19:1409-1417.*)

helpful distinguishing features because these lesions occur in PBC but not in chronic viral hepatitis. Bile ducts may be infiltrated mildly by lymphocytes in chronic hepatitis C, but the degree of inflammation and duct destruction is not nearly as severe as in PBC. Furthermore, portal granulomas, especially those associated with injured bile ducts, are not a feature of viral hepatitis. In addition, chronic cholestasis is not a feature of precirrhotic chronic viral hepatitis and, by definition, indicates a chronic cholestatic condition. Furthermore, demonstration of increased copper or

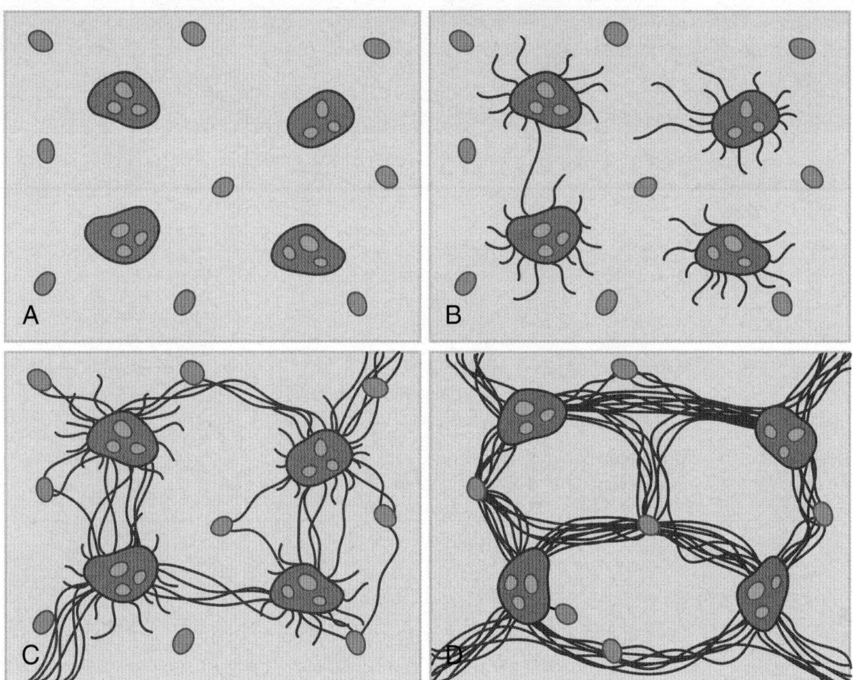

FIGURE 47.18 Staging scheme for assessment of progression of fibrosis in chronic hepatitis[38] (see Table 47.4). **A,** Portal fibrosis. **B,** Periportal fibrosis. **C,** Septal fibrosis. **D,** Cirrhosis. (*From Batts KP, Ludwig J. Chronic hepatitis: an update on terminology and reporting. Am J Surg Pathol. 1995;19:1409-1417.*)

copper-binding protein by copper stains is helpful in confirming a chronic biliary disorder. Of course, knowledge of the status of viral serological studies and other titers, such as the antimitochondrial antibody level, are most helpful in this differential diagnosis.

The morphological features of PSC, in its early stages, may also overlap with those of chronic viral hepatitis. Both may show a marked portal lymphocytic infiltrate with interface hepatitis; however, this distinction may be particularly difficult in cases of childhood PSC. Once again, bile duct loss suggests a chronic biliary process; alkaline phosphatase levels are typically higher in PSC, but cholangiography is usually necessary to establish a final diagnosis of PSC. The classic "onion-skinning" periductal concentric sclerosing lesions of PSC are not seen in viral hepatitis. In patients with ulcerative colitis and a liver biopsy that shows a pattern of inflammation suggestive of chronic hepatitis, the possibility of PSC should always be strongly considered.

Chronic viral hepatitis may be histologically indistinguishable from autoimmune hepatitis. The presence of numerous plasma cells in the portal inflammatory infiltrate and plasma cells in the lobules is suggestive of autoimmune hepatitis, but an autoimmune-like pattern of hepatitis C has also been described, and clinical correlation is often necessary to reliably distinguish these entities. Even in true cases of autoimmune hepatitis–like hepatitis C, treatment of the HCV addresses the overlap-like condition without the need for immunosuppression, which could exacerbate the infection. Bile duct infiltration by lymphocytes is also seen in autoimmune hepatitis, and therefore, it cannot be used to distinguish this condition from hepatitis C. Once again, serological studies are usually helpful and often diagnostic.

Wilson's disease may also reveal a chronic hepatitis pattern of injury on liver biopsy, and it should always be considered as a possibility in biopsies from young patients with negative viral serology results. Low serum ceruloplasmin is suggestive, but quantitative copper studies on liver tissue are, ultimately, necessary for a definitive diagnosis. α_1-Antitrypsin deficiency may also reveal a pattern of injury resembling chronic hepatitis; accumulation of PAS-positive, diastase-resistant cytoplasmic globules in periportal hepatocytes helps identify this disorder, particularly in liver biopsies from adults.

The spectrum of drug-induced injury in the liver is vast (see Chapter 48). Many types of drugs cause a chronic hepatitis morphological pattern of injury that can be difficult to distinguish from other causes, including viral or autoimmune hepatitis. Drugs that commonly cause chronic hepatitis include methyldopa, isoniazid, nitrofurantoin, dantrolene, and sulfonamides. As mentioned earlier, patterns of liver injury that show mixed hepatitic and cholestatic features, prominent eosinophils, cholestasis, or simply do not seem to fit in any discrete etiological category, should always raise consideration of a drug reaction.

Mild lobular hepatitis with spotty hepatocyte necrosis and a scant mononuclear inflammatory infiltrate may be seen as a nonspecific finding in a variety of systemic and immune-mediated disorders, as well as in patients with an intraabdominal inflammatory process. These changes may mimic mild acute or chronic hepatitis but are considered reactive in nature. In some cases, morphological changes of chronic hepatitis in a liver biopsy specimen are not associated with a specific etiology after extensive serological and clinical testing, and these cases may be labeled "cryptogenic" or "idiopathic." However, a drug reaction should always be considered in this setting. See Chapters 48 and 49 for more details on the differential diagnosis of hepatitis.

Specific Hepatitis Viruses

Hepatitis A

HAV is a small, 27-nm, nonenveloped, single-stranded RNA virus in the picornavirus family (Table 47.6). Although HAV remains the most common cause of acute viral hepatitis in the world, infection rates in the United States and other countries have declined progressively with increased use of hepatitis A vaccination.[21-23] Infection rates are higher in areas of poor sanitation or overcrowding, such as in developing countries and in institutions for people with developmental disabilities. Outbreaks in day care centers and residential institutions also occur, although proper handwashing and sewage disposal help reduce spread of the virus.[21]

The major route of transmission of HAV is oral ingestion of fecally excreted virus through person-to-person contact or ingestion of contaminated food or water. Approximately 50% of patients have no identifiable source of infection. Recent outbreaks in the United States have included illicit drug use and direct person-to-person spread as causes.[24] During infection, the virus is transported across intestinal epithelium and travels to the liver through the portal system, where it is taken up by hepatocytes. The virus replicates in hepatocytes and is then excreted into bile and shed into stool. HAV is not directly cytopathic; hepatocyte injury occurs via a cell-mediated immune mechanism. The virus is resistant to bile lysis and can be excreted into the intestine and feces or released into the systemic circulation. There are four genotypes, but only one serotype of the hepatitis A virus. The mean incubation period for HAV is 28 days (range, 15 to 40 days). The diagnosis is usually established by detection of immunoglobulin M (IgM) antibodies to HAV, which are usually detectable in serum within 1 to 2 weeks after exposure and may persist for 3 to 6 months.[25] However, serologies should be interpreted with caution. Antibodies to HAV may not always be indicative of clinical acute hepatitis, and in fact, a positive HAV antibody result is actually associated with a true clinical diagnosis of acute HAV in only a minority of cases. It is important to note that positive HAV-IgM may reflect a dormant infection or reflect a spurious result due to cross-reacting antibodies to another virus. Therefore a positive result may not be completely useful in the absence of symptoms, or outside the context of recognized outbreaks.[26] Anti-IgG antibody to HAV is detectable 5 to 6 weeks after exposure and persists for decades.

The clinical symptoms of HAV infection are usually mild, and many patients are completely asymptomatic. The most important factor that determines severity of disease is patient age: only 30% of children are symptomatic, compared with 70% of adults. The overall case-fatality rate resulting from fulminant hepatitis A is low (0.2%), but HAV infection may produce substantial morbidity in elderly patients and in those with preexisting chronic liver disease.[21] Hepatitis A accounts for 3% of fulminant liver failure overall in the United States. The onset of classic HAV infection is typically abrupt, characterized by the presence of fever, headache, malaise, and nonspecific gastrointestinal (GI) symptoms, followed by jaundice a week later. Symptoms usually resolve within 8 weeks.[27] A relapsing variant of hepatitis A has been recognized, and in as many as 10% of patients, the disease has a prolonged cholestatic course. However, chronic disease as a result of HAV virus infection is extremely rare. Acute hepatitis A is not commonly biopsied. Although histological features of acute HAV resemble those of acute hepatitis in general, plasma cells can be particularly prominent and portal inflammation can also be notable, making it challenging to distinguish from autoimmune hepatitis.[28] Pericentral cholestasis can also be present and it can resemble a biliary obstructive process.[29] Table 47.7 summarizes the clinical, laboratory, and histological features of hepatitis A as well as hepatitis B, C, D, and E.

Hepatitis B

HBV contains a partially double-stranded, circular DNA genome and is a member of the hepadnavirus family of viruses. The complete viral particle, referred to as the *Dane particle*, consists of an outer envelope that surrounds a core of DNA, the hepatitis B core antigen (HBcAg), the hepatitis B e antigen (HBeAg), and DNA-dependent polymerase. The outer envelope contains the hepatitis B surface antigen (HBsAg). Both complete and incomplete viral particles circulate in the blood of infected patients. In fact, HBsAg can circulate in large quantities as incomplete tubular or spherical structures that lack DNA. Viral DNA may become incorporated into host DNA within infected hepatocytes, particularly in young patients, and these patients are at high risk for subsequent development of hepatocellular carcinoma. The viral antigen load and subsequent antibody response may be used as serological markers to evaluate the time course of infection (Table 47.8).

TABLE 47.6 Viral Hepatitis

	Hepatitis A	Hepatitis B	Hepatitis C	Hepatitis D	Hepatitis E
Type of virus	RNA, picornavirus	DNA, hepadnavirus	RNA, flavivirus	RNA, defective virus	RNA, Hepevirus
Route of infection	Fecal-oral	Parenteral, perinatal, sexual	Parenteral, rarely sexual, sporadic	Parenteral	Fecal-oral
Chronic infection	No	10%	85%	5% in co-infection; as many as 70% in superinfection	Yes

TABLE 47.7 Summary of Clinical, Laboratory, and Pathological Features of Hepatitis A, B, C, D, and E

Type of Virus	Clinical	Laboratory	Pathology

Hepatitis A	• Symptomatic in 30% of children vs. 70% of adults
	• Abrupt onset, fever, headache, malaise, nonspecific GI symptoms, jaundice a week later
	• 3% of causes of acute liver failure
	• Relapsing
		HAV IgM
		Should be interpreted with caution in the absence of symptoms or outside context of recognized outbreaks due to potential for cross-reactivity with other viruses
			• Not biopsied frequently
			• In addition to **acute hepatitis** features (lobular disarray, random necrosis with acidophil bodies):
			  • Plasma cells may be prominent
			  • Portal inflammation may be prominent than the lobular hepatitis

Hepatitis B	• Most acute HBV hepatitis patients are asymptomatic, others have flulike symptoms
	• Chronic HBV hepatitis patients may be asymptomatic or have vague symptoms such as fatigue
		• Acute HBV: AST, ALT values in the 1000s with ALT>AST
		• Persistent elevation of ALT >6 months in patients that progress to chronic hepatitis
		Serologies in:
		  • Acute HBV infection: HBsAg, IgM anti-HBc, and HBeAg
		  • Recovery: IgG anti-HBc, anti-HBs, anti-HBe
		  • In chronic HBV: HBsAg does not subside and there is no anti-HBs; IgG anti-HBc (see Table 47.8 for more specific details)
			• Acute HBV: No ground-glass features, acute hepatitis features, lymphocytic portal inflammation
			• Chronic HBV: classic but not always identified: ground-glass inclusions in the cytoplasm and "sanded nuclei"
			  • Portal inflammation, interface activity, foci of lobular inflammation and necrosis
			  • High replicative, low inflammatory phase may have minimal necroinflammatory findings on biopsy but positive HBV immunohistochemistry

Hepatitis C	• Acute infection usually asymptomatic and only rarely recognized clinically • Chronic HCV patients have few or no symptoms	• PCR for detection of circulating viral RNA • Enzyme immunoassay for anti-HCV antibodies	• Acute HCV similar to other acute hepatitis, can also have lobular cholestasis in addition to the lobular inflammation • Chronic HCV: dense portal lymphocytic aggregates with mild interface activity, mild lobular inflammation, random distribution of steatosis
Hepatitis D	• Patient gets co-infected with HBV and HDV together as primary infection, or patient who already has chronic HBV gets infected with HDV • HBV+HDV coinfection →acute hepatitis indistinguishable from acute HBV hepatitis • Superinfection of a chronic HBV patient may present as severe acute hepatitis or exacerbation of chronic hep B; progression to chronic HDV in almost all superinfected patients	• Acute co-infection: short-lived HDAg is frequently missed; serum HDV RNA last longer than HDAg; anti-HDV late and low titer; patient has +HBsAg • Acute superinfection: +HBsAg patient, +HDV RNA, +Anti-HDV • Chronic HDV: Anti-HDV antibody in patient who has +HBsAg	• No distinctive feature for HBV+HDV primary co-infection but may have more pronounced necroinflammatory activity • Chronic HDV: more interface activity and lobular hepatitis • Nuclear +HDAg immunohistochemistry in acute HDV superinfection and in chronic HDV

Hepatitis E	• Acute
	• Asymptomatic if immunocompetent, or self-limited disease detected only by serological testing
	• Acute liver failure more likely in patients with underlying liver disease or pregnant women
	• Prolonged cholestasis (jaundice >3 months) in up to 60% of acute HEV that clears spontaneously
	• Chronic HEV: minimal nonspecific symptoms such as fatigue until decompensated cirrhosis
		• Acute HEV: Elevated AST, ALT, bilirubin, ALT in the thousands with symptoms
		• Chronic HEV: HEV RNA in stool or serum >6 months, almost exclusively in immunocompromised patients, usually genotype 3
			• HEV hepatitis has variable histological patterns
			• Acute HEV:
			  • In immunocompetent patient: similar histological features to other acute viral hepatitis; can also have cholestatic features such as pseudorosettes and canalicular bile plugs
			  • In patients with underlying liver disease: HEV infection can cause more pronounced necroinflammatory activity
			• Chronic HEV can look similar to other chronic viral hepatitis

ALT, *Alanine transaminase;* AST, *aspartate aminotransferase;* GI, *gastrointestinal;* HAV, HBV, HCV, HDV, HEV, *hepatitis A, B, C, and E;* HBc, *hepatitis B core antigen;* HBeAg, *hepatitis B envelope antigen;* HBsAg, *hepatitis B surface antigen;* HDAg, *HDV-encoded antigen;* IgM, *immunoglobulin M;* PCR, *polymerase chain reaction.*

TABLE 47.8 Serological Markers for Hepatitis B Infection in Acute and Chronic Disease*

	HBsAg	HBeAg	IgM Anti-HBc	IgG Anti-HBc	Anti-HBs	Anti-HBe
Acute						
Early phase	+	+	+			
Window phase		+				
Recovery phase				+	+	+
Chronic						
Replicative phase	+	+		+		
Low, nonreplicative phase	+			+		+
Flare of chronic hepatitis B	+	±	+	+		

Data from Lok ASF. Hepatitis B virus: screening and diagnosis. UpToDate (last updated August 22, 2018). Available at https://www.uptodate.com/contents/image?imageKey=GAST%2F60627&topicKey=ID%2F3680&source=outline_link

**Hepatitis B surface antigen* (HBsAg) *is present in the serum in both acute and chronic hepatitis and indicates an infectious state. Hepatitis B envelope antigen* (HBeAg) *is present in the serum in acute and chronic hepatitis and indicates a highly infectious state. Hepatitis B surface antibody* (anti-HBs) *is present in the serum in the recovery phase and in immunity (i.e., vaccination). Hepatitis B envelope antibody* (anti-HBe) *is present in the serum in the recovery phase. Total hepatitis B core antibody* (immunoglobulin [Ig] G anti-HBc) *is present in the serum in both acute and chronic hepatitis and indicates previous or ongoing infection. IgM antibody to hepatitis B core antigen* (IgM anti-HBc) *is present in the serum in acute hepatitis (as much as 6 months after infection).*

HBV is transmitted through exposure to infected body fluids and by intravenous drug use, sexual contact, and occupational activity. Perinatal transmission is common (90%) if the mother is HBeAg positive, which is indicative of highly infectious disease and active viral replication, but less common (10%) if the mother is HBsAg positive. In high-prevalence areas, HBV infection is often acquired by maternal–neonatal transmission, which results in a high rate of chronic disease. In areas of low prevalence, hepatitis B is mainly a disease of young adults, who acquire the virus through parenteral or sexual exposure. Posttransfusion hepatitis B is virtually nonexistent in the United States because of routine screening of blood donors.

HBV is responsible for as many as 40% of cases of acute hepatitis in the United States. Clinical symptoms of acute hepatitis develop in approximately 30% of infected adults but in only 10% of children younger than 4 years of age; they typically appear 45 to 180 days after exposure.[30] Fulminant hepatic failure occurs in approximately 1% of cases of acute hepatitis B; however, hepatitis B accounts for 7% of acute liver failure cases in the United States and up to 40% in Japan. Acute liver failure may also occur in patients with chronic hepatitis B in which mutations are present in the precore, or core promoter, regions of the viral DNA.[30] Chronic hepatitis develops in fewer than 10% of adult patients, but in as many as 90% of infected infants. The rate of progression to cirrhosis depends on the presence or absence of active viral replication and the severity of liver damage (evident histologically). For instance, 50% of patients with chronic hepatitis B and marked activity progress to cirrhosis within 4 years. The annual probability that cirrhosis will develop is estimated to be 12% for patients with chronic hepatitis B. Hepatocellular carcinoma develops in 2.4% of patients with chronic hepatitis B annually, as well as in 0.5% of patients with chronic hepatitis without cirrhosis.[30]

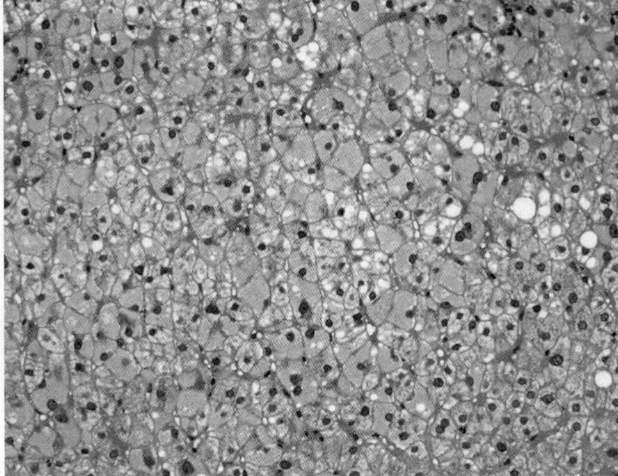

FIGURE 47.19 Ground-glass hepatocytes in chronic hepatitis B contain hepatitis B surface antigen.

Chronic Hepatitis B

Hepatitis B virus infection is characterized by the presence of varying degrees of portal inflammation, interface activity, spotty lobular inflammation, and necrosis. Patients with bridging or confluent necrosis are likely to have more advanced degrees of fibrosis (higher-stage disease).[31] Ground-glass cells containing abundant HBsAg within smooth endoplasmic reticulum may be recognized on H&E-stained tissue sections (Fig. 47.19). However, they are not present in all cases, and they are more likely to be numerous in biopsy samples that contain little necroinflammatory activity. When present, they denote active viral replication. Mimics or "pseudo-ground-glass" hepatocytes have been described in the absence of HBV infection.[32] HBcAg accumulation within hepatocyte nuclei produces a "sanded" appearance, but these changes are also seen in

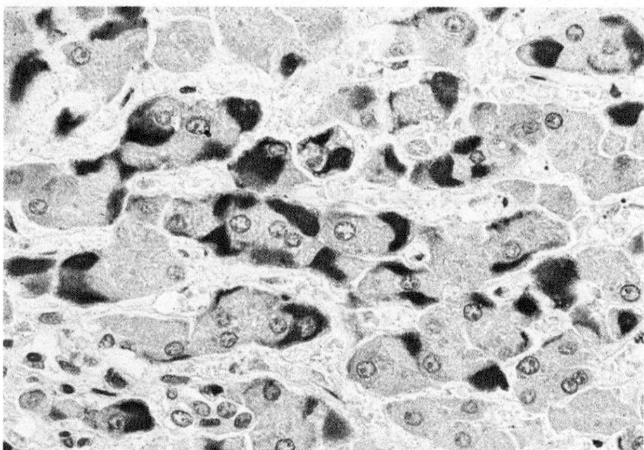

FIGURE 47.20 Positive cytoplasmic staining for hepatitis B surface antigen, with perinuclear cytoplasmic crescent-shaped staining (immunoperoxidase stain).

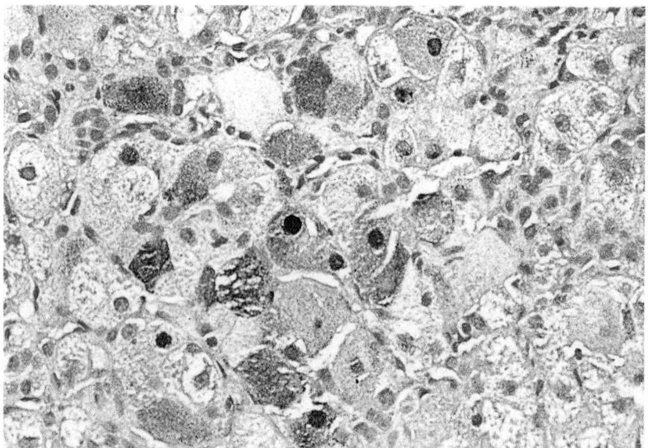

FIGURE 47.21 Positive nuclear and cytoplasmic staining for hepatitis B core antigen signifies active viral replication (immunoperoxidase stain).

HDV infection and are difficult to recognize on routine histological stains. Identification of cytoplasmic HBsAg may be facilitated by use of one of the Shikata stains, such as Victoria blue, orcein, or aldehyde fuchsin, or by immunohistochemistry (Fig. 47.20). HBcAg accumulation may also be identified with the use of immunohistochemical stains (Fig. 47.21). Cytoplasmic or membranous expression of this antigen correlates with higher levels of necroinflammatory activity.[33] Several phases with histological correlates are worth mentioning: in the "high replicative, low inflammatory" phase (previously known as "immune tolerant") that can be encountered in HBV chronic infections acquired at birth, the patient characteristically has high serum viral DNA and HBeAg+ status, normal or low serum ALT, and minimal or mild necroinflammatory findings on histology, but have immunohistochemical antigen positivity. These have no or only slow progression of fibrosis (Fig. 47.22). The "immune clearance" phase patient is characterized by oscillating levels of serum HBV DNA and alanine transaminase (ALT) levels that ultimately decrease and the patient loses HBeAg. Liver histology in this phase ranges from high necroinflammation with the episodes of hepatitis and minimal necroinflammation. The HBeAg-negative chronic phase shows moderate/high HBV DNA, high but oscillating ALT, low HGsAg levels, persistent necroinflammation, and

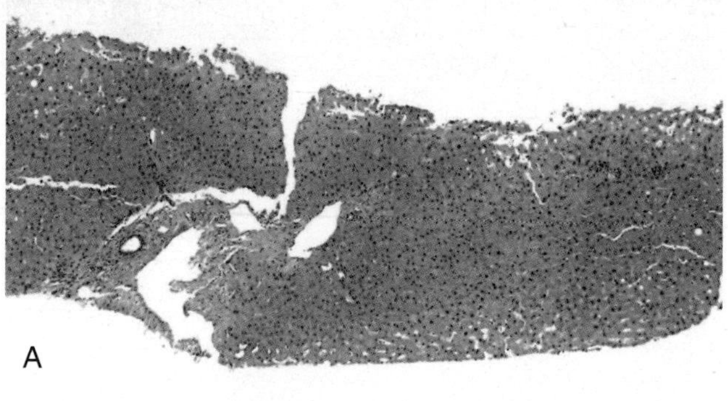

A

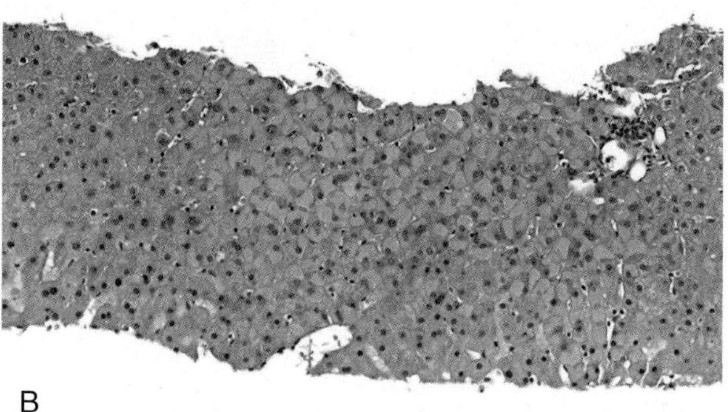

B

FIGURE 47.22 A, In this high replicative, low inflammatory phase of chronic hepatitis B, there is minimal parenchymal inflammation. **B,** Ground-glass hepatocytes are identified, but sometimes the hematoxylin and eosin stain will not show obvious findings of chronic hepatitis B; only the clinical and serological history and/or a positive immunohistochemical stain for hepatitis B will indicate that the patient has the infection.

progressive liver disease[34] (Fig. 47.23). Rarely, particularly in liver transplant or HIV patients, a rapidly progressive variant called "fibrosing cholestatic hepatitis" can occur; this has striking features of periportal fibrosis, bile ductular reaction, cholestasis, and swollen hepatocytes and may be accompanied by ground-glass change.[35]

Delta Virus Infection

Sanded hepatocyte nuclei may be seen in cases of hepatitis B with delta virus superinfection. Delta antigen may be demonstrated in nuclei of hepatocytes by immunohistochemical stains. Overall, the histopathological picture resembles that of hepatitis B without delta infection, but the degree of necroinflammatory activity is often more severe.

Hepatitis C

HCV is a spherical, enveloped, single-stranded RNA virus that measures approximately 50 mm in diameter. It is classified as a separate genus within the Flaviviridae family. The HCV genome is characterized by sequence heterogeneity as a result of pressure from the host immune system. This feature allows the virus to escape immune surveillance and establish chronic infection. Six major genotypes are recognized: the most common are 1a, 1b, 2a, and 2b.

HCV is transmitted primarily by parenteral exposure. Intravenous drug users and patients with hemophilia have a particularly high prevalence rate of infection. Intranasal cocaine use and sexual promiscuity are independent risk

High replicative, low inflammatory
- High HBV DNA
- Normal or low ALT
- HBeAg(+)
- High serum levels of HBeAg & HBsAg
- Mild or no necroinflammation
- No or slow fibrosis progression
- Decreased IL-10, IL-6, IL-8 & TNF-α
- No HBV DNA mutations

Immune clearance
- High changing to low or undetectable HBV DNA
- High decreasing to normal ALT
- Acute or intermittent hepatitis
- Declining HBeAg & HBsAg
- Eventual loss of HBeAg
- High changing to minimal necroinflammation
- Emergence of core and precore mutations

HBeAg(-) chronic
- Moderate to high HBV DNA
- High but fluctuating ALT
- Low HBsAg levels
- Persistent hepatitis
- Necroinflammation
- Progressive liver disease
- Immune clearance attempts ineffective

Non-replicative
- Low or undetectable HBV DNA
- HBeAg(-)
- Very low HBsAg levels
- Normal ALT

HBsAg loss/occult hepatitis B
- Serum HBV DNA phases, alternating undetectable and very low but detectable
- Detectable HBV DNA in the liver
- Intrahepatic replication-competent HBV genomes such as HBV cccDNA
- Integrated HBV DNA

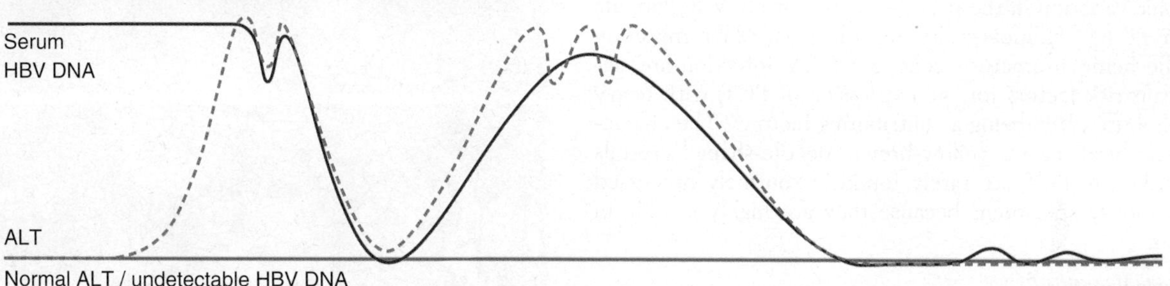

FIGURE 47.23 The major phases of chronic hepatitis B include the (1) high replicative, low inflammatory (previously known as immune tolerant) phase, (2) immune clearance, (3) HBeAg(−) chronic hepatitis, (4) nonreplicative (previously known as inactive carrier) phase, and (5) HBsAg loss/occult phase. The phases do not occur in all individuals and can occur nonconsecutively. (*From Chronic hepatitis B: virology, natural history, current management and a glimpse at future opportunities. Antiviral Res. 2015;121:47-58.*)

factors for infection,[36] although the risk associated with sexual transmission of HCV is low compared with that of the human immunodeficiency virus (HIV) or HBV.[37] Although this virus was initially identified as the etiological agent of transfusion-acquired "non-A, non-B" hepatitis, posttransfusion HCV has decreased dramatically because of widespread implementation of donor screening. The risk of infection with HCV is now estimated to be 0.01% to 0.001% for each unit of blood transfused.[37] Rates of perinatal transmission are estimated to be lower than 5%. Nevertheless, the current opiate crisis continues to make HCV infection a relevant health concern; between 2004 and 2014, there was a 400% increase in acute HCV among 18 to 29 year olds, paralleling the 600% increase in admissions for injected heroin.[38]

HCV accounts for approximately 15% of cases of acute hepatitis in the United States,[21] but acute infection is usually asymptomatic and only rarely recognized clinically. The incidence of acute HCV infection peaked in the late 1980s and early 1990s and has been steadily declining since, to fewer than 20 acute infections per 100,000 individuals per year.[39] The incubation period of hepatitis C is 7 weeks, with a range of 2 to 30 weeks based on studies of transfusion-acquired cases.[40] Fulminant hepatitis C is rare. Chronic infection is a far more common problem, occurring in up to 85% of infected patients. Most patients with chronic hepatitis C have either few, or no, symptoms. Serum aminotransferase levels are often only mildly elevated, fluctuating from 1.5 to 10 times the upper limit of normal, and as many as 30% of patients have normal aminotransferase levels.[41] Factors associated with progressive disease include patient age older than 40 years at the time of exposure, immunodeficiency, a high degree of viral heterogeneity, genotype 1, male gender, and long duration of infection.[39,41] Alcohol is known to potentiate viral replication and is associated with greater activity and fibrosis.[16] Although hepatic steatosis has been correlated with increased progression of fibrosis, it is unclear whether this result is confounded by associated metabolic abnormalities.[39] Diagnostic tests currently in use include polymerase chain reaction (PCR) for detection of circulating viral RNA and a third-generation enzyme immunoassay for detection of anti-HCV antibodies.

The natural history of HCV infection has proved challenging to study, in part because of the difficulty in determining onset of infection. In most patients, the disease is believed to have an indolent course for as long as 2 decades; cirrhosis has developed in 20% to 40% of patients in studies with at least 10 to 20 years of follow-up.[39,42] Currently, chronic hepatitis C is the reason for 30% of liver transplantations performed in the United States. The risk of hepatocellular carcinoma in HCV-related cirrhosis is estimated to be approximately 1% to 4% per year.[41]

Occult HCV infection is a more recently recognized entity that has two distinct types of clinical presentation. The first type occurs in patients with persistently elevated liver enzymes but negative serological test results for HCV.[43,44] The second type is seen in patients with positive anti-HCV serology, absence of serum HCV-RNA, and normal liver function test results. In an initial study of 100 patients with elevated liver function test results and negative HCV serology, more than half were found to have HCV-RNA in their livers by reverse transcriptase (RT)-PCR and in situ hybridization.[44] Preliminary studies have demonstrated that patients with occult HCV infection have higher triglyceride and cholesterol levels, decreased necroinflammatory scores and fibrosis, and fewer HCV-infected hepatocytes (by in situ hybridization).[43,45]

Patients with hepatitis C may also be co-infected with HIV, especially high-risk individuals such as intravenous drug users. As many as 25% of HIV-infected individuals in North America are also infected with HCV.[46,47] Effective use of highly active antiretroviral therapy (HAART) has decreased the morbidity and mortality rates from HIV infection and increased the risk of death from other causes, such as hepatitis C liver disease.

HCV infection is associated with a variety of extrahepatic manifestations and is now thought to be responsible for most cases of essential mixed cryoglobulinemia.[48] HCV is also strongly associated with porphyria cutanea tarda (PCT) in the United States, although there is marked geographic variation in the prevalence rate of HCV in patients with PCT.[49] Homozygosity for the Cys282Tyr mutation in the hemochromatosis gene and HCV infection are significant risk factors for the expression of PCT, with heavy alcohol use often being a contributing factor.[50] The characteristic birefringent, yellow-brown, needle-shaped crystals described in PCT are rarely found in routinely processed liver biopsy specimens because they are highly soluble in water.

Chronic Hepatitis C

Histologically, most cases of chronic hepatitis caused by HCV tend to be mild in terms of inflammatory activity. Dense aggregates of lymphocytes in the portal tracts are a distinctive, but not pathognomonic, feature of hepatitis C and one that is readily apparent on low-power examination (see Fig. 47.11). Focal interface activity, as opposed to the marked interface activity typically seen in autoimmune hepatitis, is typical of hepatitis C. Bile duct infiltration by lymphocytes and steatosis can also be seen. The degree of bile duct injury in hepatitis C is usually mild, and duct loss does not occur (Fig. 47.24). Steatosis in hepatitis C is usually macrovesicular; it is associated both with infection by HCV genotype 3, in which the virus is thought to be directly steatogenic, and with metabolic aberrations including insulin resistance in patients with chronic hepatitis C.[51] Steatosis and insulin resistance are associated with more severe fibrosis, poor treatment response, and increased risk of hepatocellular carcinoma in patients with chronic hepatitis C (Fig. 47.25).[52-55] Nonnecrotizing granulomas occur in a small percentage of cases, but other concurrent causes of granulomas should always be excluded.[56] The presence of scattered lobular acidophil bodies is a common feature of chronic hepatitis C. Mallory hyaline-like cytoplasmic inclusions have also been reported and have been associated with progression of fibrosis.[57] Immunoperoxidase staining for HCV has been reported in paraffin-embedded tissue, but these stains are difficult to interpret and therefore are not often used in routine clinical practice.[58]

Like hepatitis B, there is a rare variant of hepatitis C that can occur posttransplantation called *fibrosing cholestatic hepatitis* C. This rapidly progressive form is characterized by periportal sinusoidal fibrosis, bile ductular reaction, and hepatocyte swelling with lobular disarray. It can be difficult to distinguish from large bile duct obstruction. Fibrosing cholestatic hepatitis C is more likely to have more lobular disarray and periportal sinusoidal fibrosis. On the other hand, large duct obstruction is more likely to have periportal copper deposition that is usually seen in long-standing bile duct obstruction and have CK7+ intermediate hepatobiliary cells.[59]

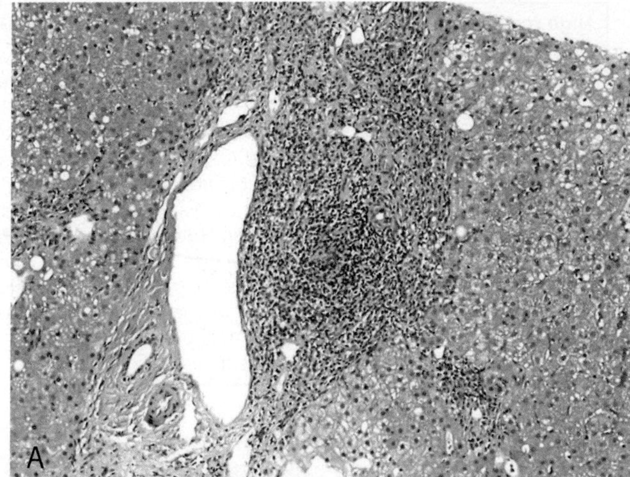

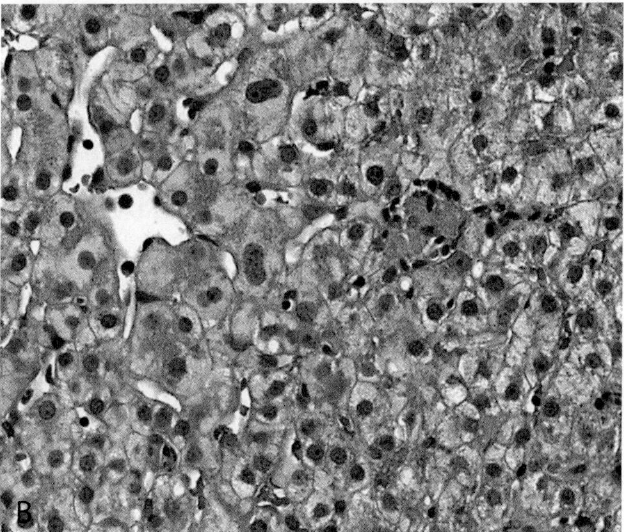

FIGURE 47.24 Chronic hepatitis C. **A,** There is a lymphoid aggregate centered on the portal tract with mild interface activity. **B,** The lobular parenchyma exhibits a few foci of necroinflammatory activity. There is a focus of lymphocytes and debris-filled macrophage in the place of a dead hepatocyte.

Treatment of Chronic Hepatitis C. Standard therapy for chronic HCV infection historically included the use of pegylated interferon and ribavirin,[60,61] but the advent of direct acting antiviral (DAA) therapies has revolutionized HCV treatment. In fact, HCV is no longer the most common cause of end-stage liver disease requiring liver transplant, decreasing from 24% of all adult liver transplant recipients in 2014 to just 12% in 2017.[62] DAAs directly act to inhibit the protein components of the HCV virus, with four main categories based on their target: NS3/4A protease inhibitors, nucleotide NS5B polymerase inhibitors, nonnucleoside NS5B polymerase inhibitors, and NS5A replication complex inhibitors.[63] The goal of treating HCV is now to cure the infection by achieving a sustained virological response (SVR), defined as undetectable HCV RNA 12 weeks (SVR12) or 24 weeks (SVR24) after completion of therapy. The cure rate demonstrated by the latest generation of DAAs approaches nearly 100% in treatment-naïve patients.

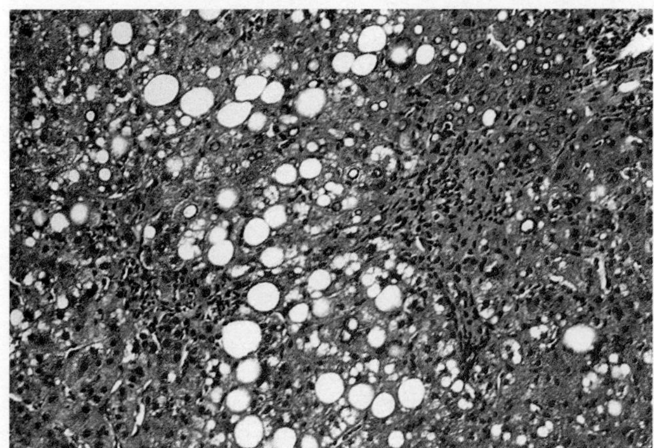

FIGURE 47.25 Chronic hepatitis C. Macrovesicular hepatic steatosis is a common feature in hepatitis C and often correlates with increased necroinflammatory activity.

Pathologists should be aware of several important clinical issues pertinent to the DAA era. First, in the context of transplant patients, persistent histological changes of active HCV identical to pretreatment biopsies can be seen even after completion of treatment and documented evidence of SVR.[64,65] Hence, pathologists should not automatically diagnose these histological findings as "recurrent hepatitis C" infection. Second, the risk of HCC still exists in DAA-treated patients with SVR, particularly in cirrhotic patients, where the risk of HCC is almost five-fold higher than similarly treated patients without cirrhosis.[66] Finally, liver biopsy for mere grading and staging HCV has become much less common and is more likely to be reserved for more complex clinical questions, such as whether or not there are concomitant diseases such as nonalcoholic steatohepatitis or autoimmune hepatitis.

Cirrhosis and Regression of Fibrosis in Chronic Hepatitis C

The potential for reversal of liver fibrosis has long been controversial (see Chapter 51 for details). For many years it was believed that, once established, scar tissue in the liver cannot be resorbed or replaced by healthy liver tissue. In the 1970s, several investigators questioned this assumption and investigated the potential reversibility of liver cirrhosis and the role of proteins such as collagenases in hepatic remodeling.[67] Some 40 years later, the idea of "regression" of hepatic fibrosis is more widely accepted and has been demonstrated in several rodent models and in human patients with autoimmune hepatitis, biliary obstruction, fatty liver disease, or viral hepatitis.[67-71] Basic science studies have also led to a better understanding of the pathogenesis of liver fibrosis through animal models, cell culture, and biochemical assays.[68,69] For instance, although hepatic stellate cells play a key role in hepatic wound healing and in matrix deposition and degradation, neutrophils and macrophages have also been shown to play a role in the degradation of matrix. Matrix metalloproteinases, which cleave collagen and other matrix components, may also be important in hepatic remodeling. Levels of tissue inhibitors of matrix metalloproteinases have been shown to decrease with fibrosis regression and clearance of activated hepatic stellate cells. The nuclear factor-κB (NF-κB) pathway, transforming growth factor-β, and nerve growth factor also play a role in the complicated orchestration of matrix generation and degradation.[67-72] (See Chapter 51.)

Although evaluation of liver biopsy specimens remains the gold standard for determination of the degree of fibrosis, much of the data on cirrhosis reversibility in DAA-treated HCV patients have largely been based on methods of fibrosis measurement that do not involve liver biopsy.[73] Studies performed when interferon and ribavirin regimens were the therapy of choice demonstrated histological regression of cirrhosis in 51% of patients who achieved SVR.[74] Another study during that time, evaluating cirrhotic HCV patients with at least 4 years follow-up subsequent to SVR, utilized paired biopsies along with liver stiffness measurements via transient elastography (TE). In that study, histological regression of cirrhosis occurred in 61% if patients, but TE overestimated fibrosis regression in that 21% of patients falling showing no cirrhosis on TE were shown to have cirrhosis on biopsy.[75] Regardless, in the current DAA-era, most studies of cirrhosis reversal are, in fact, based on TE. One report of 100 patients with advanced HCV fibrosis showed improvement of liver stiffness following treatment by TE in 55%. However, in patients with available liver biopsies, the reduction in liver stiffness was shown to be overestimated, with 4/9 patients in which TE indicated a less than F3 METAVIR stage actually showing F3 or F4 fibrosis on biopsy.[76] Hence, our knowledge of the actual reversibility of fibrosis and cirrhosis in the current DAA-related data is limited.

Combined Viral Infections

Combined infections with HBV and HCV are not uncommon, occurring in more than 10% of patients with hepatitis B.[77] In some patients, superinfection is associated with viral interference, which results in suppression of the preexisting virus by the more recently acquired virus. If coreplication of both HCV and HBV does occur, as evidenced by the presence of nucleic acids from both viruses, liver disease is likely to be more active and to show faster progression. The histological features of hepatitis C often predominate in liver biopsy specimens.

Co-infection with HCV or HBV (or both) and HIV is also common. Histological evaluation of liver biopsy specimens is complicated by the fact that HIV may directly affect the liver, and HAART also causes hepatotoxicity. Early studies of co-infected individuals showed an increased severity of liver disease, including necroinflammatory scores and fibrosis, compared with patients infected by HCV alone. However, subsequent studies showed that after stratification of patients by the status of their liver function test results, there were no significant differences in the degree of inflammation and fibrosis in co-infected versus solely HCV-infected individuals.[78-80] More recently, the severity of liver biopsy changes has been associated with HIV RNA levels at the time of biopsy.[81]

Hepatitis D

HDV, also known as the delta agent, is a small, defective RNA virus that requires HBsAg for packaging and transmission to cause infection and tissue injury. As such, HDV infection will always occur with HBV, either by co-infection or superinfection. It is spread by mechanisms similar to those that transmit HBV. HDV infection can cause acute or chronic hepatitis. Co-infection or superinfection can cause fulminant hepatic failure. HDV infection should be suspected in all patients with hepatitis B in whom severe exacerbation of disease activity develops. The finding of anti-HDV antibody in a patient who is seropositive for HBsAg is diagnostic. Three genotypes are recognized.[82] In general, the histological features of HDV infection are not distinctive, but HDV is associated with more pronounced necroinflammatory activity, and more rapid progression, than is seen in patients with isolated HBV infection. Microvesicular fat may be present in severe cases.[83] Delta antigen can be demonstrated by immunohistochemical means and is located primarily in hepatocyte nuclei.[83]

Hepatitis E

HEV is a small, quasi-enveloped, single-stranded RNA virus that was originally classified in the family Caliciviridae but subsequently placed in the family Hepeviridae.[84] Hepatitis E is endemic in parts of Africa, India, southeast and central Asia, and Mexico, but is also increasingly recognized in industrialized countries, where approximately 20% to 25% of the population of the United States and the United Kingdom are seropositive, with even higher rates in France (30% to 86%).[85-88] HEV infection with genotypes 1 and 2 primarily occurs via fecal-oral transmission through ingestion of contaminated water, with only sporadic cases associated with animal contact or consumption.[84] HEV transmission in industrialized countries, however, is largely through zoonotic means from consuming undercooked pork, game meat, oysters (genotypes 3 and 4), or camel meat and milk (genotype 7).[89]

The incubation period is generally 4 to 5 weeks. The patient's immune status determines the clinical course and histological features. The majority of immunocompetent patients are asymptomatic when infected with HEV, regardless of genotype. If patients present clinically, they have an acute self-limiting disease that is detected mainly with serological testing. Unless the patient has a preexisting liver disease, acute liver failure due to acute HEV is extremely rare in these immunocompetent individuals.[90] On the other hand, acute HEV infection in pregnant women is particularly severe. In this population it is associated with an increased risk of acute liver failure and a mortality rate as high as 25%.

In immunocompetent individuals in developing countries, the histological findings can be similar to other acute viral hepatitides, ranging from the typical morphological picture seen in acute viral hepatitis, to a cholestatic form with canalicular bile plugs and cholestatic pseudorosettes (Fig. 47.26).[91] Cases of autochthonous HEV in immunocompetent patients in industrialized countries have been described similarly. In a small series of patients with autochthonous infection, a severe form showing mixed portal and lobular inflammation with severe interface hepatitis and cholangiolitis was described.[92] Massive or submassive necrosis may occur in severe cases as well.

In patients with underlying liver disease, pronounced necroinflammatory activity on top of the findings of preexisting liver disease and fibrosis should provoke consideration of HEV. Although easy to overlook, HEV infection is important to consider, since these patients can benefit from therapy with antiviral medications such as ribavirin.

Although HEV infection has been considered a self-limited disease, persistent infection with evolution into a chronic course with liver fibrosis has been documented in immunocompromised patients and in patients with HIV infection.[93-96] HEV infection in this patient population can be readily missed, due to absent or nonspecific symptoms and only mild fluctuations in liver chemistries that linger and smolder, leading to a chronic course.[97,98] HEV RNA detection is useful for monitoring viremia in this situation. Chronic HEV infection in immunocompromised patients can result in significant morbidity and mortality, since untreated chronic HEV can result in rapid progression to cirrhosis. Histological findings of chronic active HEV hepatitis are similar to that seen in chronic hepatitis B or C (Fig. 47.27).

FIGURE 47.26 Acute hepatitis E infection in an immunocompetent individual. The histological features of acute HEV in this type of patient is similar to that seen in other acute viral hepatitis. In this case there is lobular inflammation, debris-filled macrophages in places of hepatocyte dropout, and a few acidophil bodies. (*Courtesy of Dr. Achim Weber, University of Zurich.*)

Clinically, several laboratory tests are used to establish a diagnosis.[99] This includes detection of HEV-specific IGM antibodies in the blood along with demonstrating a rise in IgG antibody levels over time. In immunocompromised patients, however, serological testing is less reliable than molecular testing for HEV RNA.[100] Molecular detection of HEV RNA is detectable in blood for a short, 3-week viremic period, but is present in stool samples for 5 weeks. As such, for pathologists faced with a biopsy, it is useful to know that a negative HEV RNA blood test does not exclude a relatively recent infection.

Other Hepatitis Viruses

GB virus type C (GBV-C), also known as the hepatitis G virus, was discovered in 1995 and is a flavivirus in the same family as HCV. This virus has been detected in 1.7% of the population and can be transmitted parenterally and by vertical transmission.[101] Viral replication occurs predominantly in lymphocytes, although the virus is also detectable in hepatocytes.

The single-stranded, nonenveloped DNA virus known as TT virus was originally suspected to cause transfusion-associated hepatitis, but later it was found in more than 90% of Japanese blood donors, casting doubt on its role in causing disease.[102] Similarly, the related single-stranded circular DNA virus, the SEN virus, has also been found in patients with transfusion-associated hepatitis, although direct causality has not been established.[103]

OTHER VIRAL INFECTIONS OF THE LIVER

A wide variety of nonhepatotropic viruses may affect the liver and cause a range of clinical manifestations, from mild, asymptomatic elevations in serum aminotransferases to dramatic and even fatal hepatic necrosis (Table 47.9). Nonhepatotropic viruses are often seen in neonates and in immunocompromised persons as part of disseminated infection.

SARS-CoV-2

A few cases of SARS-CoV-2 hepatitis have described severe acute hepatitis with bile duct injury. Specifically, lobular findings typical of acute hepatitis, such as lobular disarray with numerous acidophil bodies, were seen in conjunction with portal tract changes featuring mixed inflammation and prominent bile duct damage.[103a] In the autopsy setting, however, livers from patients dying of SARS-CoV-2 have not had bile duct damage reported; the main three features seen were mild lobular necroinflammatory activity, mild portal inflammation, as well as steatosis. Other infrequent histologic findings included lobular cholestasis, sinusoidal microthrombi, and non-necrotizing granulomas.[103b]

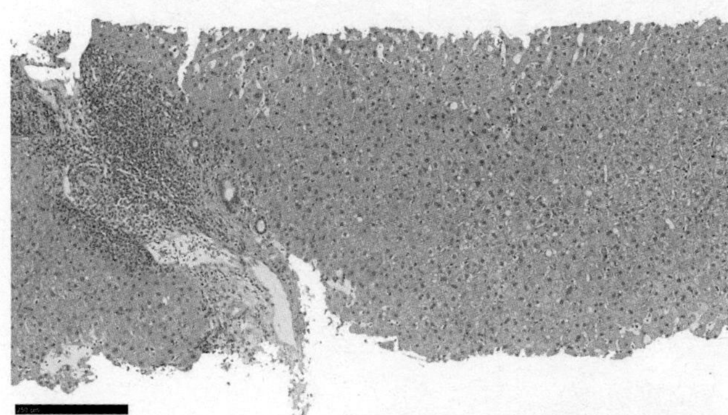

FIGURE 47.27 Chronic hepatitis E in immunocompromised individual. A dense portal lymphoid aggregate is seen, similar to that seen in other chronic viral hepatitis cases. However, immunohistochemical staining for pORF2 is positive, confirming hepatitis E. (*Courtesy of Dr. Achim Weber, University of Zurich.*)

Epstein-Barr Virus

The liver is affected in more than 90% of cases of EBV-related mononucleosis. Hepatic involvement is manifested by elevated aminotransferases,[104] and this is often accompanied by the other symptoms of mononucleosis. Jaundice occurs in only a minority of patients. Fulminant liver failure secondary to EBV infection has also been described, particularly in immunocompromised children[105] but also in healthy patients as well. Hepatitis (or fulminant hepatic failure) caused by EBV may not be accompanied by typical features of mononucleosis.[106] EBV hepatitis may also be associated with autoimmune phenomena, including autoimmune hemolytic anemia, thrombocytopenia, and positive autoimmune serologies.[107]

TABLE 47.9 Histological Comparison of Hepatic EBV, CMV, HSV, and Adenovirus Infection

Feature	EBV	CMV	HSV	Adenovirus
Inclusions	No	Yes	Yes	Yes
Sinusoidal lymphocytic infiltrate	Typical	Occasionally	No	No
Microabscess formation	No	Common	No	Rare
Zonal necrosis	Rare	Rare	Common	Common
Granulomas, including fibrin ring granulomas	Rare	Rare	No	Rare
Cholestasis	Rare	Rare (neonatal cases)	No	No
Giant cell change	No	Yes (neonatal cases)	No	No

CMV, *Cytomegalovirus;* EBV, *Epstein-Barr virus;* HSV, *herpes simplex virus.*

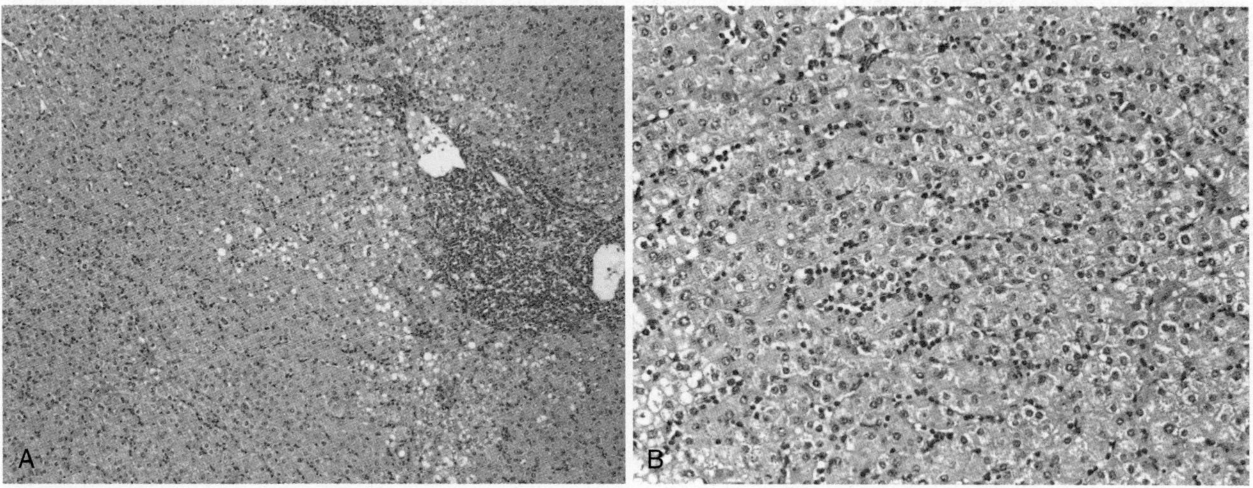

FIGURE 47.28 Lymphocytic portal inflammation **(A)** and a diffuse lymphocytic sinusoidal infiltrate arranged in a single-file, "string-of-beads" pattern **(A** and **B)** are characteristic of Epstein-Barr virus infection.

The most characteristic histological feature in otherwise healthy patients is the presence of a diffuse lymphocytic sinusoidal infiltrate arranged in a single-file, "string-of-beads" pattern, with occasional scattered atypical lymphocytes (Fig. 47.28). Focal apoptotic hepatocytes and steatosis may also be present. Cholestasis is not typical, but cholestatic hepatitis has been described in the context of EBV hepatitis.[104,108,109] Small Kupffer cell clusters and, rarely, discrete, noncaseating granulomas or fibrin ring granulomas may be present as well. Progression to chronic hepatitis or cirrhosis is rare. EBV hepatitis may also develop after solid organ transplantation, particularly after liver transplantation. The histological picture may be more severe in this context, showing a marked portal and periportal inflammatory infiltrate containing numerous atypical lymphocytes, immunoblasts, and plasma cells, as well as mild bile duct damage and prominent necrosis.[110]

Confirmatory tests include serological, immunohistochemical, in situ hybridization studies for EBV, and serum or tissue PCR.[111] However, serological studies may be unreliable in very young children and in immunocompromised patients. The differential diagnosis includes other types of viral infections (e.g., CMV). An EBV-like lobular sinusoidal lymphocytic infiltrate may be seen in transplant recipients with recurrent hepatitis C. Hepatic involvement by leukemia or lymphoma should also be excluded when atypical lymphocytes are present and especially when they are numerous. For a detailed discussion of EBV-related posttransplantation lymphoproliferative disorders, refer to Chapter 53.

Cytomegalovirus

Patients with CMV hepatitis may show an increase in aminotransferase levels, a cholestatic pattern of enzyme elevation, or both. The clinical and histological features of CMV hepatitis depend on the immune status of the host.

Cytomegalovirus Infection in Otherwise Healthy Patients

Primary CMV infection in otherwise healthy people is usually self-limited, although a mononucleosis-like syndrome may occur in some. CMV hepatitis in immunocompetent individuals is often part of a generalized multiorgan infectious process.[112] Rare cases of fulminant liver failure have been described, but chronic liver disease does not develop in this patient population. Liver biopsy findings resemble those of EBV infection. However, neither viral inclusions nor immunohistochemically demonstrable CMV antigen is typically evident in infected patients.[113]

Cytomegalovirus Infection in Immunocompromised Patients

CMV infection of the liver is more common in immunocompromised persons. CMV is the single most important pathogen in solid organ transplant recipients of all types.[112] CMV infection may be acquired by primary infection, reactivation, or superinfection by a new strain in a previously seropositive patient.[114] Infection typically occurs approximately 2 to 16 weeks after solid organ transplantation, when immunosuppression is most apparent. Symptoms range from mild to life-threatening. Knowledge of the time period in which a liver biopsy is taken with respect to the transplant date can therefore help guide pathologists to evaluate for the presence of CMV-infected cells. Although any organ may be involved, hepatic involvement often predominates. In liver transplant recipients, the allograft is the most common site of involvement[114,115] (see Chapter 52). In immunocompromised patients, CMV hepatitis is caused primarily by the direct cytopathic effects of the virus.[116,117]

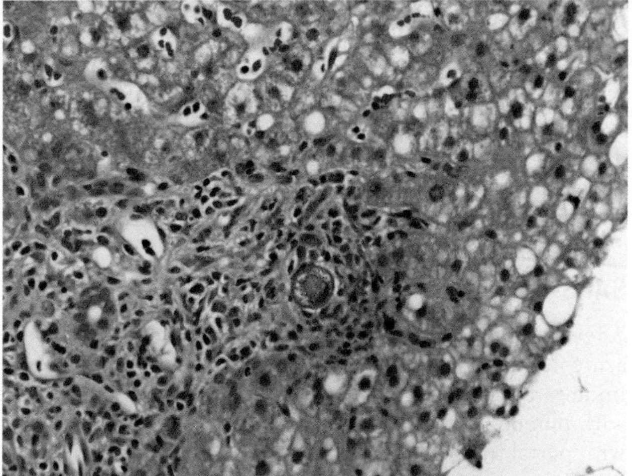

FIGURE 47.29 Characteristic nuclear and cytoplasmic inclusions of CMV seen in the portal tract. Cytomegalovirus inclusions cause enlargement of the entire cell.

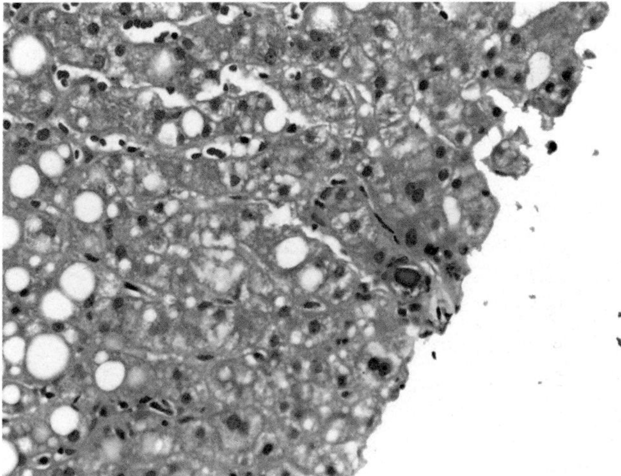

FIGURE 47.30 A large basophilic CMV inclusion is seen within the lobular parenchyma.

Infected cells show both nuclear and cytoplasmic enlargement (hence the name, "cytomegalovirus"). Characteristic "owl's eye" intranuclear viral inclusions (Fig. 47.29) and basophilic granular intracytoplasmic inclusions (Fig. 47.30) may be seen on routine H&E preparations. Inclusions may be present in the nucleus or cytoplasm of any liver cell type. Infected cells are often surrounded by a neutrophilic infiltrate (Fig. 47.31), either with or without admixed mononuclear cells. The number of viral inclusions may be extremely variable, and the diagnosis is easily missed when only a few inclusions are present. In addition, some infected cells may be associated with only a minimal amount of associated inflammation. However, the presence of typical neutrophilic microabscesses centered on injured and dying

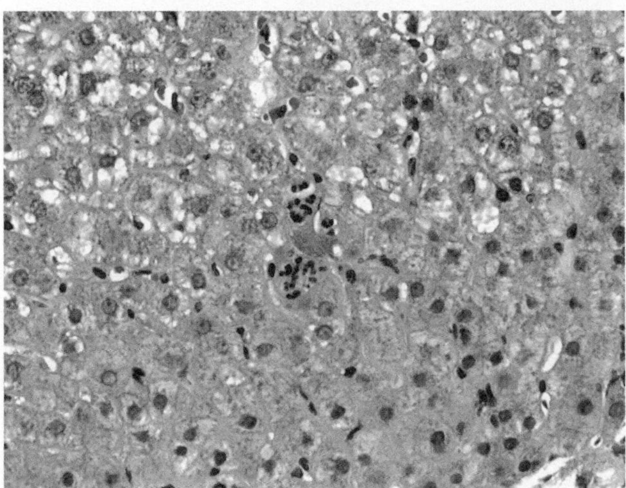

FIGURE 47.31 A neutrophilic microabscess surrounds a hepatocyte containing granular basophilic cytoplasmic cytomegalovirus inclusion in a liver transplant recipient.

hepatocytes in a transplant patient should always trigger suspicion of CMV infection. Other associated features include hepatocyte apoptosis and patchy necrosis, portal and lobular mononuclear inflammation, and rarely, granulomas, including those of the fibrin ring type.[118,119] Chronic liver disease does not occur in CMV-infected patients.

Cytomegalovirus Infection in Neonates

Liver involvement is a common feature of neonatal and perinatal CMV infection. Affected infants usually have hepatosplenomegaly and jaundice. Histologically, liver biopsy findings resemble opportunistic CMV infection, often showing a variable number of typical viral inclusions. A wide range of other pathological alterations also may be present, such as portal inflammation, cholestasis, giant cell transformation, necrosis, and prominent extramedullary hematopoiesis.[120] Bile duct damage and obliteration are rarely present, although CMV (as well as several other viruses) has been associated with biliary atresia and paucity of intrahepatic bile ducts. In rare cases, portal or sinusoidal fibrosis may develop as well.

Useful diagnostic aids include viral culture, PCR assays, in situ hybridization, and CMV serological studies and antigen tests.[114] However, isolation of CMV in culture does not imply active infection, because the virus may be excreted for months to years after the primary infection.[121]

The differential diagnosis in otherwise healthy persons includes other types of viral infections (e.g., EBV). The differential diagnosis in immunocompromised patients includes herpesvirus and adenovirus infection. Other causes of microabscesses, such as ischemia, should also be considered, particularly in transplant recipients.[122] In neonates, the differential diagnosis includes other causes of neonatal hepatitis and congenital disorders of bile ducts, as discussed previously.

Herpes Simplex Virus

Herpesvirus hepatitis is usually a disease of immunocompromised patients as part of disseminated infection, although it can rarely be seen in otherwise healthy persons.[123] However, hepatic manifestations may dominate the clinical picture. Neonates, children who are malnourished or recovering from other infections (particularly measles), pregnant women, and immunocompromised persons are also at significant risk of serious infection.[124]

Clinically, patients are typically febrile, and some have concomitant oral or mucosal herpetic lesions. Pharyngitis, headache, abdominal pain, or myalgias are also typical symptoms. Importantly, patients with herpes simplex virus (HSV) hepatitis may lack typical mucosal herpetic lesions.[125,126] Aminotransferases are typically quite elevated, and hepatomegaly is frequent. A rapidly progressive course associated with a high mortality rate is not uncommon. Therefore early liver biopsy is invaluable. However, both infants and adults with fulminant HSV infection may undergo liver transplantation successfully.[125,127]

Grossly, livers infected with HSV are enlarged and mottled and show multiple foci of necrosis, often surrounded by a zone of hemorrhage.[123,124] Histologically, randomly distributed ("geographic") zones of necrosis, ranging from microscopically focal to macroscopically visible with the naked eye, are characteristic. Portal tracts may be spared. The necrotic zones are often surrounded by congestion and extravasated red blood cells. However, inflammation is usually minimal.[123,124] Typical viral inclusions, both Cowdry type A and ground-glass cells, are usually present in hepatocyte nuclei, and these are particularly prominent at the periphery of necrotic areas (Fig. 47.32). Inclusions may be single or multiple.

Viral culture is a valuable diagnostic tool. Immunohistochemistry, in situ hybridization, and PCR assays can also be very useful. PCR may be performed on liver or blood, but detection of HSV in blood may lag behind detection of the virus in the liver in severely immunocompromised patients.[127]

The differential diagnosis includes mainly other types of viral infections, such as CMV and adenovirus. CMV does not cause the typical necrotic pattern of HSV, and adenovirus inclusions are usually more homogeneous in appearance. Although viral hemorrhagic fever can cause focal necrosis, widespread zonal necrosis and nuclear inclusions are typically absent. Varicella-zoster produces histological lesions identical to HSV, but varicella-infected patients typically also have a skin rash.[123,124] Ischemia or toxic (drug) injury (e.g., acetaminophen) can cause widespread necrosis, although the necrosis is usually more zonal in these conditions (particularly zone 3), and viral inclusions are absent.[123]

Human Herpesvirus 6

Human herpesvirus 6 (HHV-6) was originally isolated in the mid-1980s from patients with AIDS or lymphoproliferative disorders.[128] Primary infection by this lymphotropic virus affects mainly young children, who typically have benign and self-limited symptoms, including a viral exanthem. However, the virus may reactivate, typically in immunocompromised patients and transplant recipients. Based on serological tests and PCR assays performed on blood, HHV-6 is associated with hepatitis and fulminant liver failure, most notably in infants, children, and transplant recipients.[128-130] Most cases of HHV-6 in solid organ transplantation are likely related to reactivation of recipient virus, although primary HHV-6

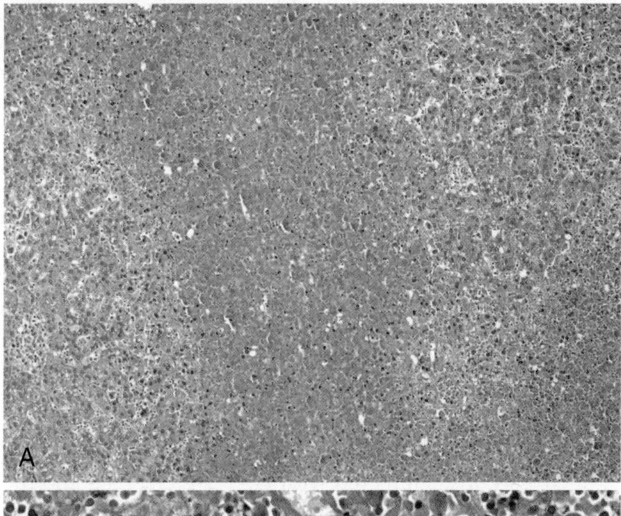

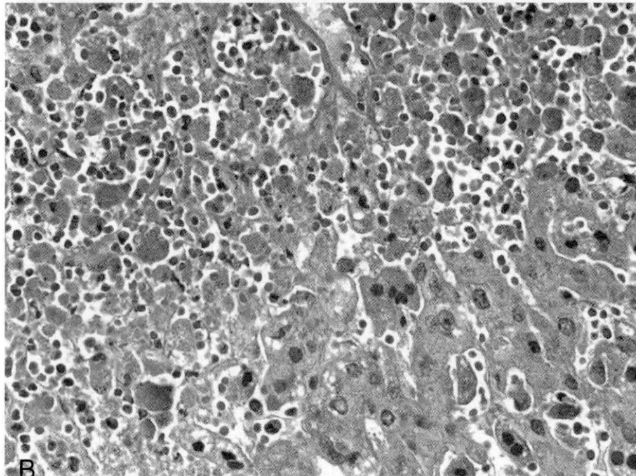

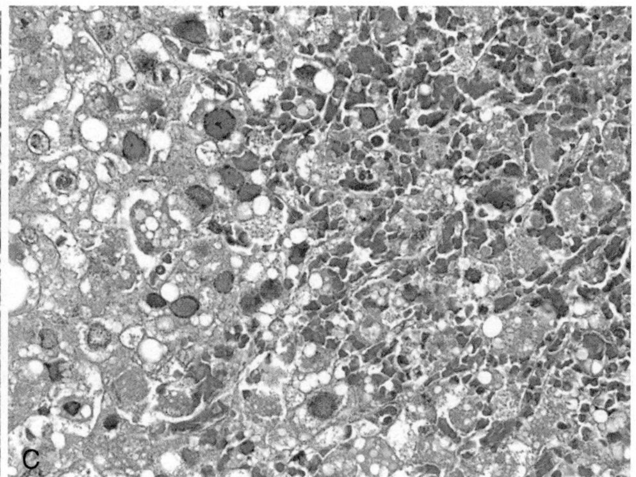

FIGURE 47.32 A, Herpes simplex hepatitis typically features geographic zones of necrosis, often surrounded by a zone of hemorrhage. **B,** Viral inclusions are visible in necrotic hepatocytes at the periphery of the necrotic areas. **C,** Typical inclusions are ground-glass cells with dark, smudgy nuclei and peripheral chromatin margination.

infections in naïve recipients have also been reported.[129,130] Infections are usually asymptomatic, although hepatitis has rarely been described in this population.[129,130] Fulminant liver failure has rarely been reported in immunocompetent adults.[131,132] The pathological findings in HHV-6 infection have not been well described, but they may resemble those of EBV infection in the liver.[131,132] Useful diagnostic tests include immunohistochemistry, serological assays, and PCR on blood or liver tissue.[130]

Enteric Viruses

The enteric group of viruses only rarely infect the liver, but when they do, fatal hepatic necrosis is often the end result. Adenovirus is most commonly implicated, usually in immunocompromised patients (particularly children). Clinically, the presenting symptoms include fever, hepatomegaly, and markedly elevated aminotransferase levels. Concomitant pneumonia and diarrhea reflect disseminated infection.[133]

Grossly, livers are enlarged and mottled, with foci of necrosis. Histological features resemble those of HSV infection, showing widespread zones of necrosis, typically with minimal associated inflammation. Intranuclear viral inclusions, known as "smudge cells," may be present. They may mimic the viral inclusions of HSV but are darker and more homogeneous in appearance (Fig. 47.33). Some cases feature randomly distributed, well-circumscribed inflammatory lesions consisting of mononuclear cells and granulocytes, with rare inclusions located at the periphery of the inflammatory infiltrate. Necrosis is usually much less prominent in these cases. Granulomas have been described as well.[134]

Useful diagnostic aids include immunohistochemistry, stool or tissue examination by electron microscopy, viral culture, and PCR. The differential diagnosis includes other types of viral infections, particularly HSV. Coxsackieviruses and echoviruses may induce a similar histological profile, but inclusions are seldom present.

Viral Hemorrhagic Fever

The geographic distribution, transmission, and clinical course of this diverse group of viruses are quite variable[135-138] (Table 47.10). Death from liver failure is rare in viral hemorrhagic fevers, with the exception of yellow fever. Liver pathology is similar regardless of the type of virus. Useful adjunctive tests include serological studies and immunohistochemistry, although these are not widely available. Patients usually experience a viral prodrome consisting of fever, headache, and myalgia, followed by hemorrhagic manifestations. Elevated aminotransferases and hepatomegaly are common. Histologically, viral hemorrhagic fever

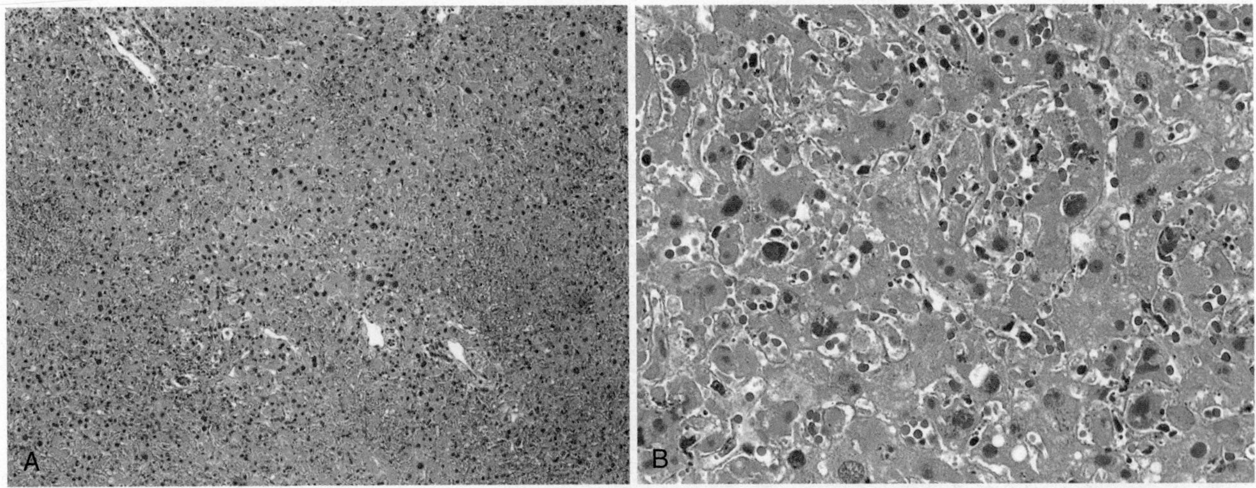

FIGURE 47.33 Adenovirus infection. A, Viral inclusions are typically detected in hepatocytes at the edge of large, randomly distributed areas of necrosis with minimal associated inflammation. **B,** Inclusions, known as "smudge cells," are dark and homogeneous.

TABLE 47.10 Viral Hemorrhagic Fevers

Disease	Geographic Distribution	Transmission or Reservoir	Selected Signs and Symptoms	Mortality Rate	Classic Histological Features
Dengue fever	Africa, Asia, tropical Americas, Caribbean	Mosquito/human	Viral prodrome and rash	<20%	Coagulative necrosis of midzonal and centrilobular hepatocytes Minimal lobular and portal inflammation, mostly macrophages
Yellow fever	Africa, South America	Mosquito/human	Viral prodrome with vomiting, jaundice; elevated bilirubin	10%-50%	Spares centrilobular hepatocytes (whereas dengue virus tends to intensely involve centrizonal region) Midzonal (zone 2) hemorrhagic hepatocyte necrosis with Councilman-Rocha Lima bodies within necrotic areas Immunohistochemical for yellow fever antigen; molecular studies for distinguishing different types of yellow fever strains
Lassa fever	West Africa	Person-to-person and body fluid/rat	Viral prodrome; vomiting, cough, abdominal pain	<25%	Random hepatocyte necrosis, macrophages surrounding necrotic hepatocytes
Marburg fever	Central/ southern Africa	Unknown	Viral prodrome, nausea, vomiting, diarrhea	Varies greatly: 25% in initial lab associated outbreak in 1967, >80% in outbreaks between 1998 and 2004	Similar to other viral hemorrhagic fevers: spotty to confluent coagulative hepatocyte necrosis, minimal inflammation Infrequent viral intracytoplasmic inclusions in hepatocytes, macrophages, and other cells
Ebola fever	Central Africa	Unknown	Similar to Marburg virus	>80%	Similar to other viral hemorrhagic fevers: spotty to confluent coagulative hepatocyte necrosis, minimal inflammation Microvesicular steatosis, Kupffer cell hyperplasia Intracytoplasmic viral inclusions in hepatocytes

shows foci of coagulative necrosis, but with only minimal inflammation. Necrosis is usually multifocal and randomly distributed, rather than massive. Yellow fever produces a midzonal pattern of injury characterized by hepatocyte necrosis and steatosis.[139] Some foci of necrosis may be surrounded by abundant macrophages.[136,140] Steatosis is variable, and cholestasis is not usually prominent. Adjacent intact hepatocytes may show regenerative changes and ballooning degeneration. Inclusions are not typically present. Of note, the original use of the term *Councilman body* for describing apoptotic hepatocytes was in the setting of yellow fever.

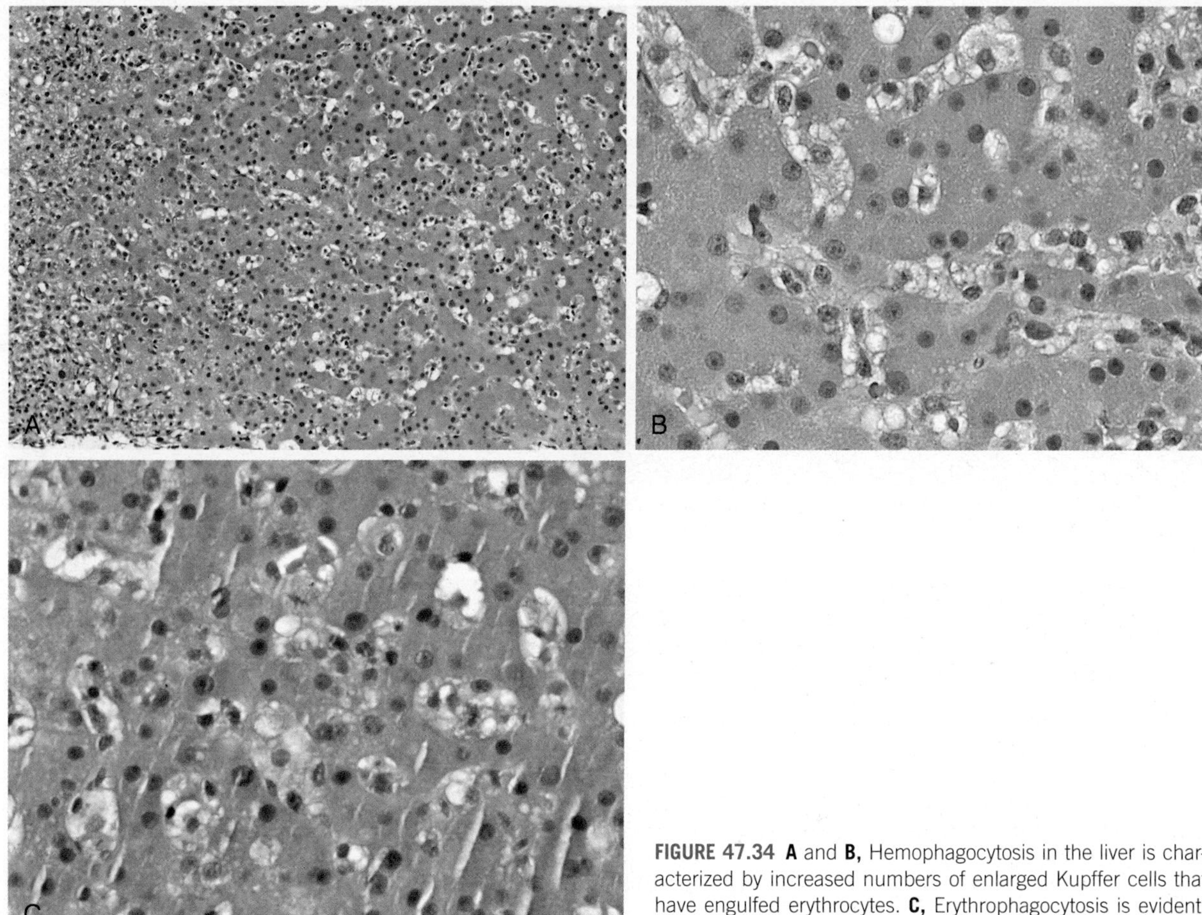

FIGURE 47.34 A and **B,** Hemophagocytosis in the liver is characterized by increased numbers of enlarged Kupffer cells that have engulfed erythrocytes. **C,** Erythrophagocytosis is evident, as there are red blood cells within the Kupffer cells.

Other viruses that cause hepatitis include measles (rubeola), rubella, and parvovirus, which may affect the liver in the context of hydrops fetalis. Primary HIV infection has been shown to cause liver involvement similar to EBV-related mononucleosis, as well as neonatal hepatitis.[141] Fulminant hepatic failure caused by varicella-zoster has been rarely reported as well, in both immunocompromised and apparently immunocompetent patients.[142-144]

The virus-associated (reactive) hemophagocytic syndrome (VAHS) is strongly associated with viral infection, particularly EBV, although other viruses have also been implicated.[145-148] The presenting symptoms include fever, hepatomegaly, splenomegaly, peripheral blood cytopenias, and lymphadenopathy. Many patients experience a viral-like prodrome. Adult patients are often immunocompromised; children with VAHS usually do not reveal an underlying immunodeficiency. Most patients recover spontaneously. Histological features include cytologically benign hemophagocytic histiocytes within both portal tracts and sinusoids. Kupffer cells may be hypertrophic and may show hemophagocytosis (Fig. 47.34) as well as siderosis.[149] Focal hepatocyte necrosis may be present.

BACTERIAL INFECTIONS OF THE LIVER

Suppurative Bacterial Infections

Suppurative hepatic inflammation is usually accompanied by hepatocyte necrosis. Lesions may range from microscopic microabscesses to macroscopic "pyogenic" abscesses. A general discussion of suppurative hepatic abscess is presented here, followed by a more detailed discussion of specific types of bacterial suppurative infections.

Pyogenic Bacterial Abscess

Pyogenic abscesses secondary to bacterial infection typically occur in older patients. Symptoms are usually nonspecific and include abdominal pain, hepatomegaly, malaise, and fever. Jaundice is rare.[150] Aminotransferases are usually elevated, but often with a disproportionately high alkaline phosphatase level. The mortality rate is high, especially if the abscess is associated with sepsis. In children, pyogenic liver abscesses may signal the presence of immunodeficiency (e.g., chronic granulomatous disease).[151]

In general, pyogenic abscesses are secondary infections that occur as a result of seeding from other sites, particularly the biliary tree and GI tract. They are often polymicrobial and are caused by a wide variety of organisms. The most commonly implicated organism in North America is *Klebsiella pneumoniae*.[152] Other common pathogens include *Escherichia coli*, *Staphylococcus aureus*, streptococci, *Proteus*, *Pseudomonas*, *Bacteroides*, and *Fusobacterium*. Less common, yet noteworthy, pathogens include *Aeromonas*, *Actinomycetes*, *Nocardia*, *Salmonella*, *Haemophilus influenzae*, and *Yersinia*.[150-154] Predisposing conditions include diabetes (particularly with *Klebsiella*-associated abscesses), intraabdominal malignancies, cholangitis, idiopathic inflammatory bowel disease, appendicitis, and diverticulosis.[155-158]

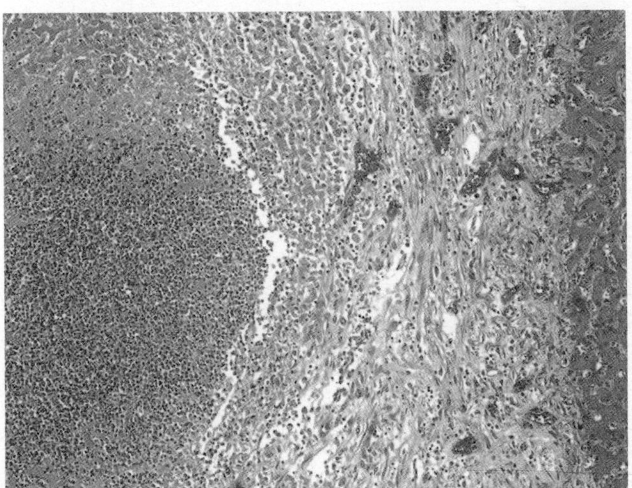

FIGURE 47.35 Hepatic abscess. A suppurative center is surrounded by granulation tissue and fibrosis in this *Staphylococcus*-related pyogenic abscess.

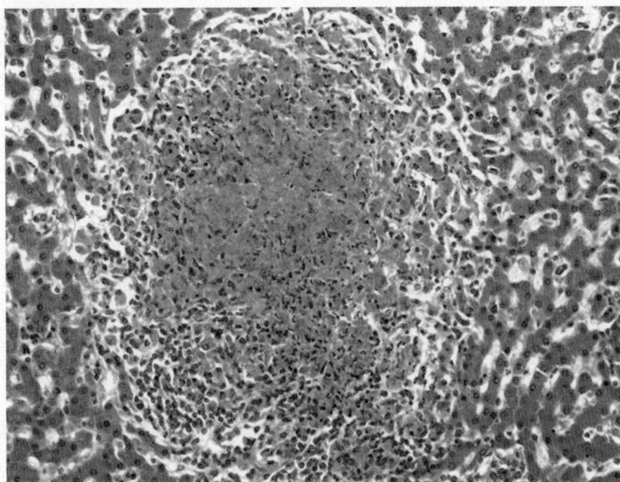

FIGURE 47.36 Suppurative microabscesses with surrounding macrophages are typical of tularemia in the liver.

Tumors, cysts, and infarctions may also become secondarily infected, leading to abscess formation.

Abscesses may be multiple or solitary, and they are more common in the right lobe of the liver.[155] Size ranges from microscopic to more than 3 cm in maximum diameter.[156] Similar to abscesses in other parts of the body, these consist of central suppurative inflammation and necrosis surrounded by organizing inflammation and fibrosis (Fig. 47.35). The fibrous ring may be quite prominent and may also contain bizarre, reactive fibroblasts and atypical reactive lymphocytes. Granulomatous reactions are occasionally present as well. Nonspecific reactive changes are usually present in the surrounding liver; examples are cholestasis, portal inflammation, ductular proliferation, and venulitis. If the primary site of infection is the biliary tract, changes of acute cholangitis may also be present. Organisms are occasionally detectable with special stains.

If a surgical drainage procedure or aspiration is undertaken, culture of the resultant purulent material is of paramount importance. Otherwise, blood cultures may be valuable in order to isolate the causative organism. The differential diagnosis primarily includes other causes of hepatic abscess such as amebic infection, hydatid disease, and necrotic tumors.

Tularemia

Francisella tularensis is a gram-negative coccobacillus that is endemic in many areas of North America. It is transmitted to humans from rodents and rabbits.[159] Hepatic involvement may be subclinical and is often a component of disseminated infection. Affected patients reveal elevated aminotransferases, hepatomegaly, and, rarely, jaundice. Histologically, suppurative microabscesses with surrounding macrophages are typically seen (Fig. 47.36). As the lesions evolve, they may become more granulomatous in appearance.[159,160] The organisms are only rarely evident on special stains. Therefore cultures, serological tests, and molecular tests are considered useful diagnostic modalities.[160]

Listeriosis

Listeria monocytogenes is a foodborne infection that may cause hepatitis. Hepatic listeriosis may occur in both neonates and adults; it is frequently a feature of disseminated infection in immunocompromised and diabetic patients. Histologically, scattered microabscesses are typical, and these are often associated with small granulomas. Occasionally, there is an exclusively microgranulomatous pattern, and in rare cases, true epithelioid granulomas are present.[161] Hepatic abscesses may also be associated with *Listeria*.[162] Short, pleomorphic, gram-positive rods may be identified by special stains. However, blood culture is the most important diagnostic test. DNA probes and immunohistochemistry may be useful but are not widely available.

Actinomycosis

Actinomycosis is a chronic, slowly progressive infection caused by the anaerobic gram-positive bacteria *Actinomyces israelii*. The majority of cases involving the liver are secondary to other sites of intraabdominal infection. However, outside this secondary context, primary hepatic actinomycosis can be unexpected clinically; it occurs in immunocompetent patients in 70% of cases and can closely mimic malignancies on imaging.[163] Patients may present with fever, right upper quadrant pain, and weight loss. On microscopy, one sees colonies of *Actinomyces* surrounded by neutrophils and large areas of hepatocyte necrosis. The radiating, filamentous, non–acid fast, gram-positive organisms can exhibit Splendore-Hoeppli reaction at the periphery of the inflammatory reaction (Fig. 47.37).[164]

Liver in Sepsis

Sepsis and bacteremia produce a wide spectrum of hepatic injuries. Both cholestatic and hepatitic patterns of enzyme elevation may be present. Histologically, some cases show predominantly neutrophilic inflammation (both portal and lobular) with microabscesses. Other cases reveal predominantly cholestatic features, with centrilobular canalicular cholestasis, ductular cholestasis–associated ductular proliferation (cholangiolitis), inspissated bile, and periductal neutrophilic inflammation (Fig. 47.38). The bile duct epithelium may be flattened and atrophic, showing vacuolation and necrosis. Focal necrosis of hepatocytes, mild portal inflammation, Kupffer cell hyperplasia, and fatty change

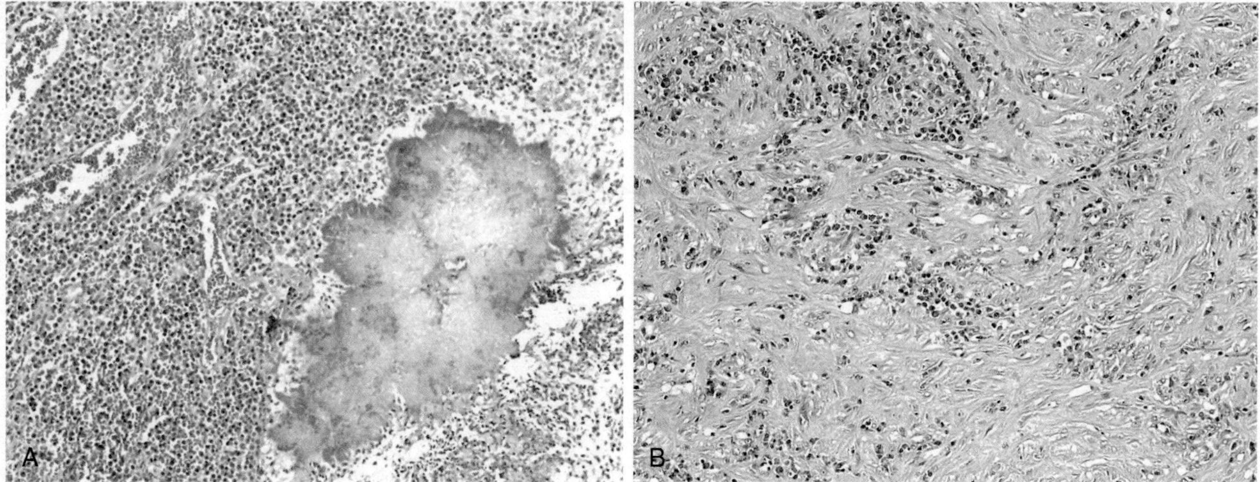

FIGURE 47.37 Actinomycosis. A, Colonies of filamentous *Actinomyces* organisms are seen, surrounded by plasma cells. **B,** Extensive fibrosis surrounds the chronic abscess; clinically, this lesion was concerning for a neoplasm because it was mass-forming.

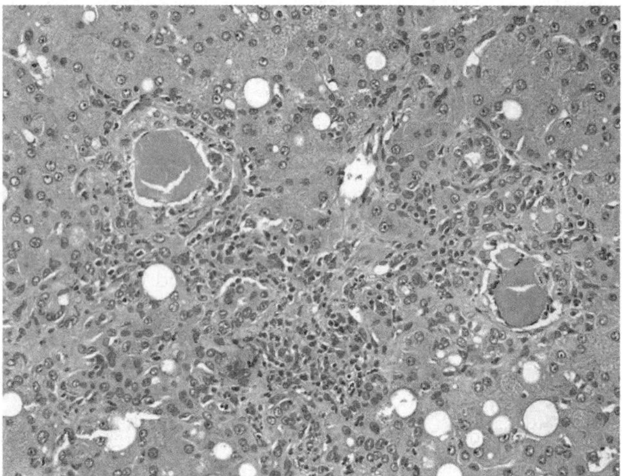

FIGURE 47.38 Sepsis. A portal neutrophilic infiltrate with ductular reaction, distended cholangioles with flattened epithelium, and dense inspissated bile are features often seen in patients with sepsis.

may also be present.[165-167] Venous congestion and ischemic necrosis may be prominent in cases of septic shock.

Granulomatous Bacterial Infections

Hepatic granulomas are reportedly present in 2% to 15% of all liver specimens examined in general practice.[168,169] The morphology of the granulomas often provides a clue to the specific diagnosis (Table 47.11). However, the etiology of most granulomas usually cannot be determined based on the histology. The discussion here focuses only on infectious causes of granulomas. Noninfectious causes of hepatic granulomas include sarcoidosis, PBC, adverse drug reaction, berylliosis, Hodgkin's disease, and foreign body reaction, among many others.[170,171] In addition, granulomas have been reported in a minority of patients with hepatitis C (in which case they may portend a favorable response to interferon therapy) and occasionally in patients with hepatitis B.[172,173]

Hepatic fibrin ring granulomas (Fig. 47.39) bear special mention. Although classically described in association with Q fever (discussed later), these lesions are essentially nonspecific. They have been observed in association with many diseases, including leishmaniasis, boutonneuse fever, Hodgkin's disease, allopurinol reaction, toxoplasmosis, CMV infection, mononucleosis, *Mycobacterium avium-intracellulare* (MAI) infection, immune checkpoint inhibitor-related hepatitis, and typhoid fever.[174]

Tuberculosis

Liver involvement is present in almost all cases of miliary tuberculosis, and it is common both in localized extrapulmonary tuberculosis and in association with pulmonary tuberculosis. Signs and symptoms of liver disease may be the dominant or presenting features of tubercular infection. Although liver involvement is often asymptomatic, hepatomegaly, right upper quadrant pain, and fever may be present. Ascites and jaundice are less frequent. Patients may reveal elevated bilirubin and aminotransferase levels and a disproportionately high alkaline phosphatase level.[175] Confluent granulomas may lead to the formation of hepatic masses (tuberculomas) and periportal lymphadenopathy.[175,176]

The histological hallmark of hepatic tuberculosis is the formation of epithelioid granulomas, often accompanied by caseation and giant cells (Fig. 47.40A). Similar changes can be seen within portal lymph nodes (see Fig. 47.40B). The granulomas are usually small, but they may coalesce to form large nodules or masses with central liquefactive necrosis.[176] Older lesions may show fibrosis, calcification, and occasionally amyloid.[177] Hepatic tuberculosis is often accompanied by reactive hepatitis. Because mycobacteria are usually difficult to detect on special stains (see Fig. 47.40C), culture and PCR assays are of significant value.

Mycobacterium Avium-Intracellulare

MAI infection is most commonly associated with, but is not limited to, patients with AIDS. The liver is involved in more than 50% of disseminated cases. Histologically, most liver biopsy specimens in immunocompromised patients show aggregates of foamy histiocytes in both the liver parenchyma and portal tracts (Fig. 47.41). Some patients, particularly those who are immunocompetent, reveal discrete epithelioid granulomas with associated neutrophils

TABLE 47.11 Classification of Granulomatous Lesions in the Liver by Histological Pattern

Fibrin Ring Granuloma	Microgranulomas	Stellate Microabscess with Granulomatous Inflammation	Foamy Macrophage Aggregates	Predominantly Suppurative, ± Granulomatous Inflammation	Epithelioid Granulomas, Infectious Causes	Epithelioid Granulomas, Other Causes
Infectious	Infectious	*Actinomyces*	*Rhodococcus equi*	Tularemia	Tuberculosis (*Mycobacterium tuberculosis*; usually caseating)	Drug reaction
Q fever	Listeriosis (rare)	*Nocardia*	Whipple disease	Listeriosis	Brucellosis	Foreign body reaction
Toxoplasmosis	Other	*Bartonella*	MAI (immunocompromised patients)	Melioidosis	MAI (immunocompetent patients)	Sarcoidosis
Salmonellosis	Usually a nonspecific reaction to liver injury	Tularemia	Lepromatous leprosy		Listeriosis (rare)	Autoimmune diseases
Cytomegalovirus		*Candida*	Histoplasmosis		Tuberculoid leprosy	Primary biliary cirrhosis
Epstein-Barr virus		Other fungi	Leishmaniasis		Tertiary syphilis	Hodgkin disease
Leishmaniasis					*Chlamydia*	Other paraneoplastic conditions
Other					Whipple disease (rare)	Chronic granulomatous disease of childhood
Drug reaction					Schistosomiasis	
Lupus					Fungal infections	
Metastases					Viral infections (rare)	

MAI, Mycobacterium avium-intracellulare.

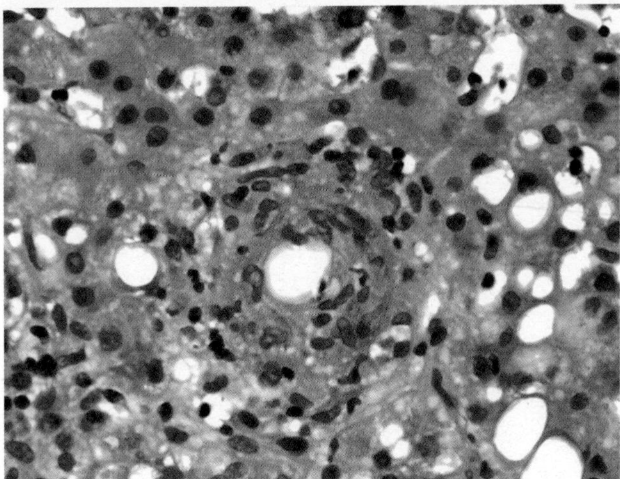

FIGURE 47.39 Fibrin ring granulomas typically consist of epithelioid cells with a central lipid vacuole surrounded by a fibrin ring.

and lymphocytes. Giant cells and necrosis are rare.[178,179] Organisms are usually abundant in immunocompromised patients, as revealed by acid-fast staining, but are rare in immunocompetent persons. Occasionally, and particularly in patients with AIDS, MAI forms pseudosarcomatous, spindle cell nodules that mimic a neoplastic process[180] (Fig. 47.42). Culture and PCR assays may be useful diagnostic adjuncts. The differential diagnosis includes other causes of foamy macrophage aggregates, such as *Rhodococcus equi* infection and Whipple's disease. Other atypical mycobacteria occasionally cause liver disease, including *Mycobacterium kansasii* and bacille Calmette-Guérin.

Recently, *Mycobacterium chimaera* (MC), a species within the *Mycobacterium avium* complex, has been associated with distinctive hepatitic features in a certain patient population.[181] Reports of MC outbreaks in open heart surgery patients undergoing valve replacements have been linked to contaminated heater-cooler water units that are associated with heart-lung machines.[182] The heater-cooler unit fans aerosolize the organism, and seed the surgical sites of these patients. MC infection can then have a latency period of months to years after the valve replacement procedure, but may ultimately affect the liver, manifesting as elevated alkaline phosphatase levels as well as mild increases in aspartate aminotransferase and alanine aminotransferase. Liver biopsy findings include small, ill-defined granulomas spread out in a sinusoidal distribution, and usually associated with background changes of venous outflow obstruction (sinusoidal dilatation, congestion, and hepatocyte plate atrophy) (Fig. 47.43). MC hepatitis is an aggressive disease and is associated with a high mortality rate.

Leprosy

More than 60% of patients with lepromatous leprosy and about 20% of those with tuberculoid leprosy (both caused by infection with *Mycobacterium leprae*) show hepatic involvement.[183,184] Liver disease is often subclinical.[161] Histologically, the findings depend on the type of leprosy. In lepromatous leprosy, aggregates of foamy histiocytes (lepra cells) in portal tracts and lobules, often containing numerous acid-fast bacilli, are characteristic. Giant cells and discrete granulomas are only rarely present, and the degree of inflammation is typically minimal. In tuberculoid leprosy, discrete, tuberculoid granulomas with associated giant cells are characteristic (Fig. 47.44). Bacilli are rare in this variant. Some patients manifest both lepromatous and tuberculoid granulomatous lesions.[185]

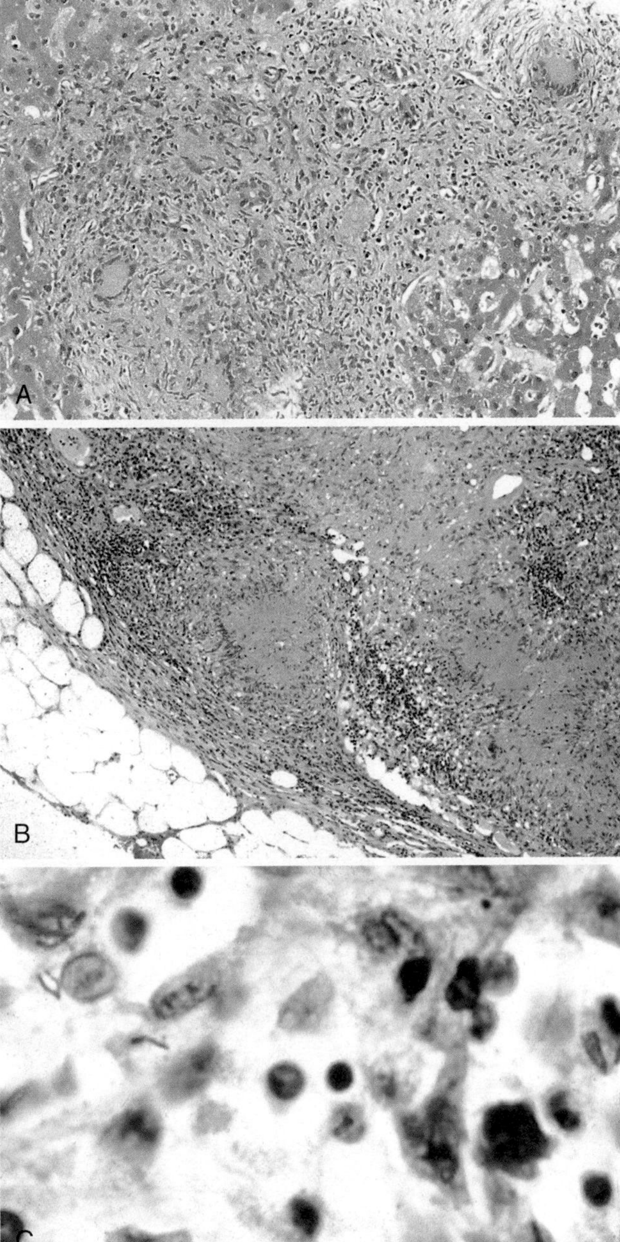

FIGURE 47.40 ***Mycobacterium tuberculosis* infection. A,** Coalescent epithelioid granulomas with numerous giant cells are present in the portal tracts. **B,** Similar changes are often seen in portal lymph nodes. **C,** Organisms may be seen with the use of acid-fast bacillus stains (Ziehl-Neelsen stain).

Bartonella Species

Bartonella henselae is the most common cause of cat scratch disease (CSD).[186] Patients usually have isolated lymphadenopathy in an area that drains the anatomic site of cat scratch inoculation, but a small percentage (1% to 2%) develop disseminated infection. These patients usually

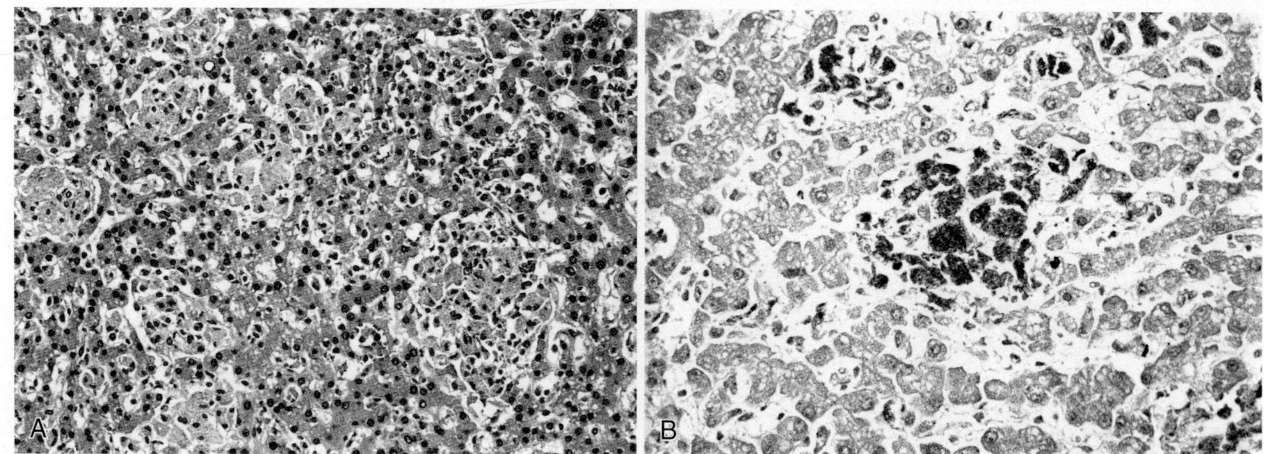

FIGURE 47.41 ***Mycobacterium avium-intracellulare*** **infection. A,** Aggregates of foamy macrophages are present in the liver parenchyma of an HIV-positive patient. **B,** Acid-fast bacillus stain highlights numerous organisms within macrophages (Ziehl-Neelsen stain). (*Courtesy of Dr. Lucas Campbell, Northwest Arkansas Pathology Associates.*)

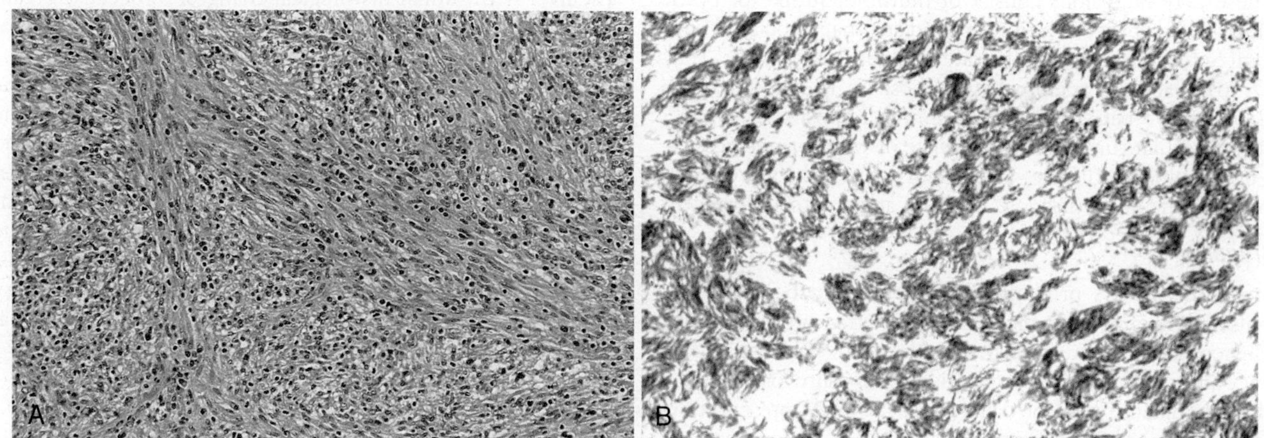

FIGURE 47.42 **A,** *Mycobacterium avium-intracellulare* can induce spindle-cell histiocytic nodules in the liver that can mimic spindle cell neoplasms. **B,** Acid-fast bacillus stains show that the histiocytes are filled with mycobacteria (Ziehl-Neelsen stain).

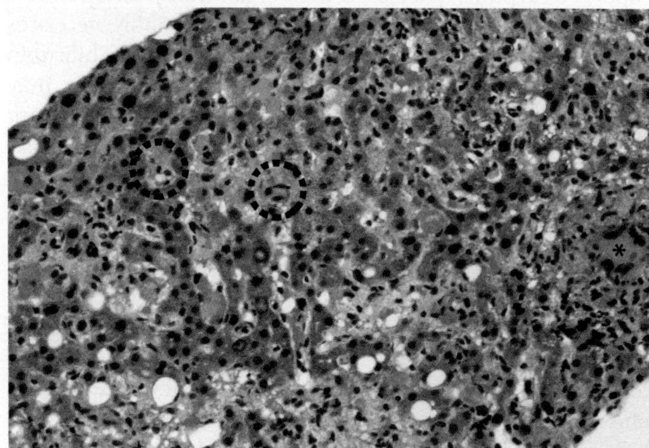

FIGURE 47.43 *Mycobacterium chimaera* (MC) hepatitis. Characteristic dual pattern of ill-formed sinusoidal histiocyte aggregates (circled) and venous obstructive like changes, including sinusoidal red blood cell congestion and hepatic plate compression. A multinucleated giant cell with granuloma (*) is seen in this case, but the main histological pattern of MC hepatitis is that of ill-formed sinusoidal granulomas. (*Courtesy of Dr. Nafis X. Shafizadeh, Kaiser Permanente, Woodland Hills Medical Center.*)

lack characteristic skin papules and superficial adenopathy, but have generalized symptoms such as weight loss, fever, and malaise. Liver lesions are usually multiple and are often associated with abdominal lymphadenopathy.[187] Patients with hepatic CSD are often younger than 10 years of age and are usually not immunocompromised. Patients typically respond well to antibiotic therapy.

The characteristic histological lesions of hepatic CSD consist of irregular, stellate microabscesses surrounded by an inner layer of palisading histiocytes, a rim of lymphocytes, and an outermost thick layer of fibrous tissue (Fig. 47.45). The outer fibrous zone is quite pronounced. The lesions often vary widely within the same specimen, ranging from early microabscesses to "old" lesions consisting of fibrosis and granulation tissue.[187] The differential diagnosis includes primarily other types of infections. A detailed patient history with specific questions pertaining to cat exposure is essential in establishing a correct diagnosis. Silver stains (Warthin-Starry or Steiner), molecular assays, and enzyme-linked immunosorbent assays are helpful diagnostic aids.

Both *Bartonella* species (*henselae* and *quintana*) are associated with hepatic bacillary angiomatosis-peliosis.[188]

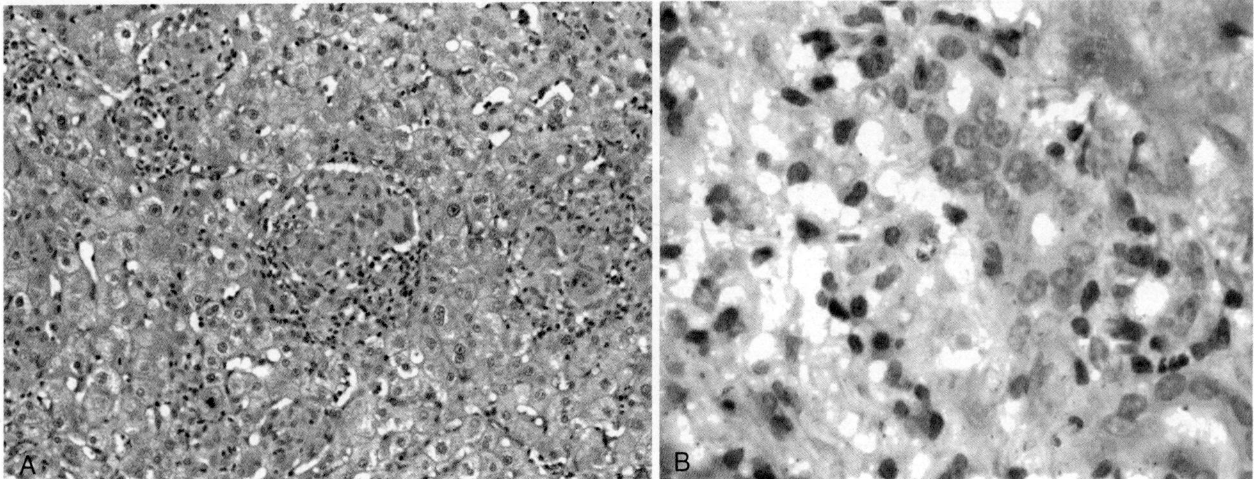

FIGURE 47.44 **A,** Discrete, epithelioid granulomas with associated giant cells and associated lymphocytes and giant cells are seen in this case of leprosy. **B,** Rare bacilli are found on acid-fast bacillus stain (Ziehl-Neelsen stain).

These peliotic lesions consist of multiple, slitlike or cystic blood-filled spaces in a fibromyxoid stroma, associated with a mixed inflammatory infiltrate and focal necrosis[189] (Fig. 47.46). Bacillary angiomatosis-peliosis is usually found in HIV-positive patients and may mimic Kaposi's sarcoma or other vascular tumors. The presence of well-formed vessels, a neutrophilic infiltrate, and organisms on silver precipitation staining helps diagnose bacillary angiomatosis correctly.

Brucellosis

Brucellosis occurs primarily in domestic and barnyard animals and is highly endemic in the Mediterranean basin, India, Mexico, and Central and South America.[190] Humans contract infection through occupational exposure or ingestion of contaminated food or dairy products.[190] At presentation, patients typically have fever, malaise, headache, and arthralgias. Lymphadenopathy and hepatosplenomegaly may also be present. Hepatic involvement is seen in approximately 50% of cases.[191] Liver biopsies often show noncaseating granulomatous inflammation, sometimes with giant cells.[191-193] Granulomas may be discrete and epithelioid or small and poorly formed (Fig. 47.47). Some patients manifest only a nonspecific reactive hepatitis pattern of injury.[192-194] Organisms are difficult to culture and are only rarely visible on special stains. Serological studies and an appropriate exposure history are most helpful in establishing a correct diagnosis.

Rickettsia *and Similar Species*

Most rickettsial illnesses affect the liver,[195] although involvement may be subclinical. *Coxiella burnetii* (causative agent of Q fever) is perhaps the most noteworthy because of its association with characteristic fibrin ring granulomas (Fig. 47.48).[196] True fibrin ring granulomas consist of a central lipid vacuole surrounded by a fibrin ring. However, some cases of Q fever have features intermediate between epithelioid and fibrin ring granulomas.[197,198] *Rickettsia conorii*, the causative agent of boutonneuse fever and South African tick bite fever, may cause either type of granulomas or a nongranulomatous reactive hepatitis.[199] *Rickettsia rickettsii* (Rocky Mountain spotted fever) induces a mixed portal inflammatory infiltrate, endotheliitis, cholestasis, and erythrophagocytosis.[200] *Rickettsia typhi* (murine typhus) may also involve the liver with similar histological changes.[201] Because organisms are difficult to detect in rickettsial illnesses, immunofluorescent stains and serological studies are quite helpful.

Human monocytic ehrlichiosis, a disease caused by the bacterium *Ehrlichia chaffeensis* and transmitted by the Lone Star tick found commonly in the south-central and southeastern United States, may also involve the liver. Histological findings include scattered lobular foci of lymphohistiocytic infiltrates and diffuse lymphohistiocytic infiltration of the sinusoids with increased phagocytosis. Cholestasis is often present as well. Immunohistochemistry and serological studies may be helpful because the ehrlichial morulae can be difficult to detect on H&E stain.[202]

Spirochete Infections

Syphilis

Both congenital and acquired syphilis (at any stage) may involve the liver. In addition, there are increasingly frequent reports of syphilis associated with organ transplantation and HIV infection.[203-205] In congenital hepatic syphilis, neonates show hepatomegaly, jaundice, and elevated serum bilirubin and aminotransferase levels.[179] Histological changes may be indistinguishable from neonatal hepatitis resulting from other causes and include prominent pericellular fibrosis with an associated mononuclear cell infiltrate, extramedullary hematopoiesis, and, rarely, small granulomas. Permanent liver damage rarely occurs in treated patients.[206-208]

The reported prevalence rate of liver involvement in early acquired syphilis varies widely, ranging from 1% to 50%. Usually, hepatic involvement is reflected only by the presence of abnormal laboratory test results, but jaundice, hepatomegaly, abdominal pain, and markedly elevated alkaline phosphatase levels have been reported as well.[209-211] The liver is typically involved in syphilis during the secondary or tertiary stages. Weeks to months following the primary chancre stage of syphilis, the secondary stage of syphilis is characterized by palmar rash, lymphadenopathy, and the systemic dissemination of the spirochetes. At this time the liver may be involved in the form of syphilitic hepatitis.[212] From 20% to 40% of HIV-positive patients with syphilis, in particular, have been reported to develop syphilitic

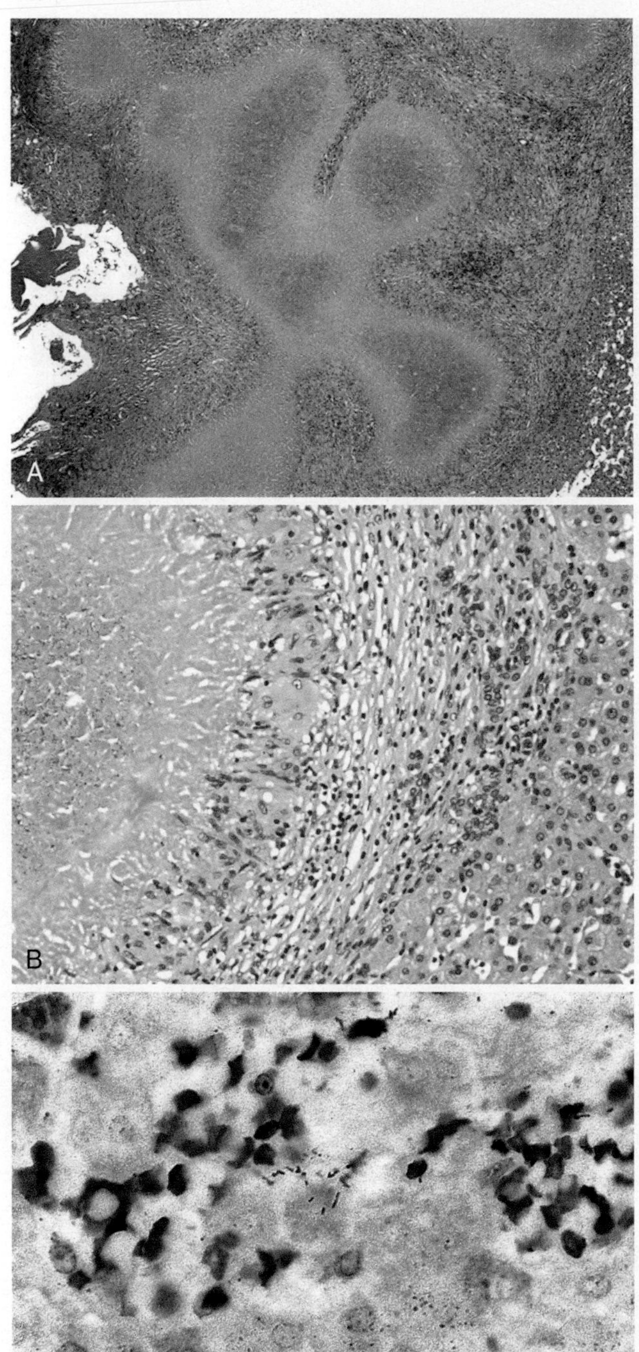

FIGURE 47.45 Cat scratch disease. The characteristic lesion of hepatic cat scratch disease resulting from *Bartonella henselae* consists of irregular, stellate microabscesses **(A)** surrounded by an inner layer of palisading histiocytes, an outer rim of mononuclear cells, and a thick layer of fibrous tissue **(B)**. **C,** Small, pleomorphic bacilli are occasionally detected within necrotic areas with the use of silver impregnation stains (Warthin-Starry stain).

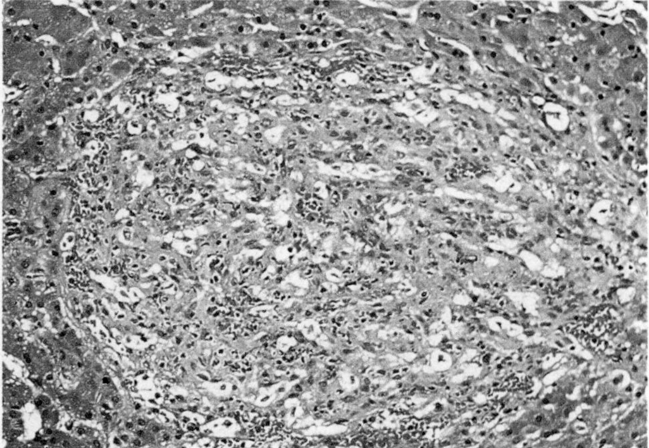

FIGURE 47.46 Hepatic bacillary angiomatosis consists of multiple, slit-like vascular spaces in a fibromyxoid stroma with an associated mixed inflammatory infiltrate.

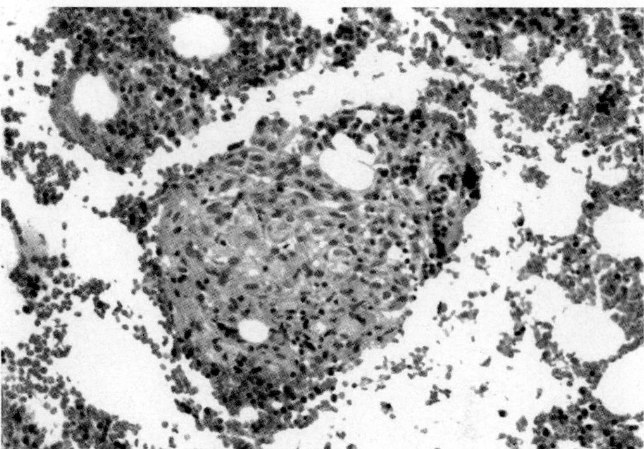

FIGURE 47.47 A small, epithelioid, noncaseating granuloma in a case of brucellosis. (*Courtesy of Dr. David Walker, University of Texas Medical Branch, Galveston.*)

hepatitis.[205] The histological findings of hepatic syphilis are variable, ranging from unremarkable, to nonspecific reactive changes, to more marked necroinflammatory changes (Fig. 47.49).[209,210] Portal inflammation in which bile ducts are surrounded by mononuclear cells or neutrophils can be seen. Rarely, granulomas, cholestasis, vasculitis, and bile duct damage have been described.[211] Sinusoidal fibrosis may be present, and it may persist after treatment. Spirochetes may be identifiable in some cases, particularly with use of immunohistochemistry. Serological tests are very useful diagnostic aids.

The rarely seen, but often discussed, pathological lesion of tertiary syphilis is termed the *gumma*. Gummas consist of a nodular focus of caseous necrosis surrounded by a fibrous inflamed wall, scattered granulomas, and associated endarteritis (Fig. 47.50).[213,214] Healing leads to a grossly distorted, scarred liver known as *hepar lobatum*. Clinically, nodular gummas may be confused with a neoplasm or with other types of infection.

Of note, both secondary and tertiary syphilis have been associated with mass-forming lesions. In particular, secondary syphilis-related inflammatory pseudotumors have been described in gay, bisexual, and other men who have sex with men (MSM), with innumerable organisms concentrated in the mass and associated blood vessels, but not in the background liver. In comparison to gummas, the inflammatory pseudotumors of secondary syphilis are more actively inflamed and are associated with a proliferating fibroblastic reaction, abscess formation, and many organisms, whereas

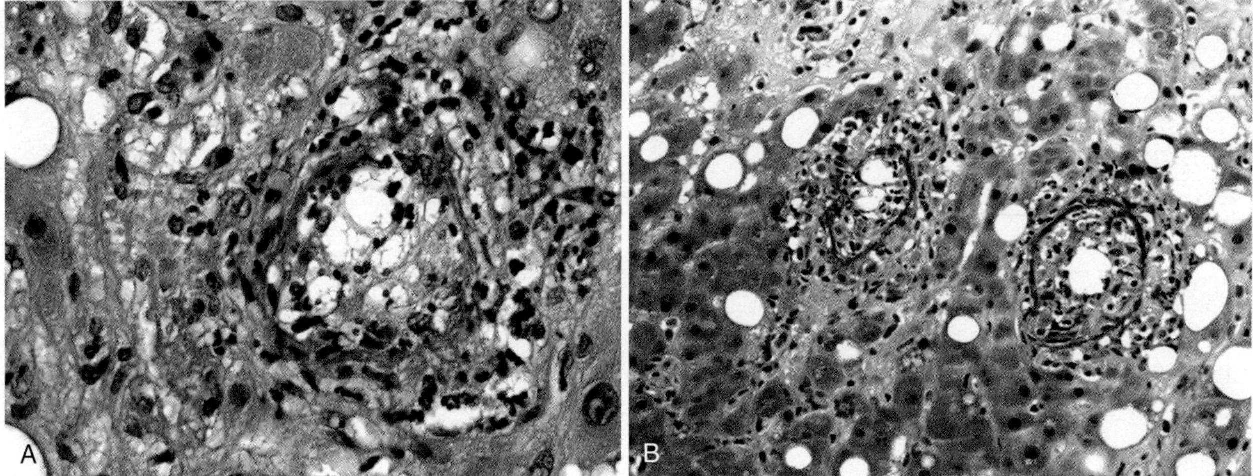

FIGURE 47.48 A, Fibrin ring granulomas in a case of Q fever. **B,** Trichrome stain highlights the fibrin ring. (*Courtesy of Dr. Dhanpat Jain, Yale University School of Medicine.*)

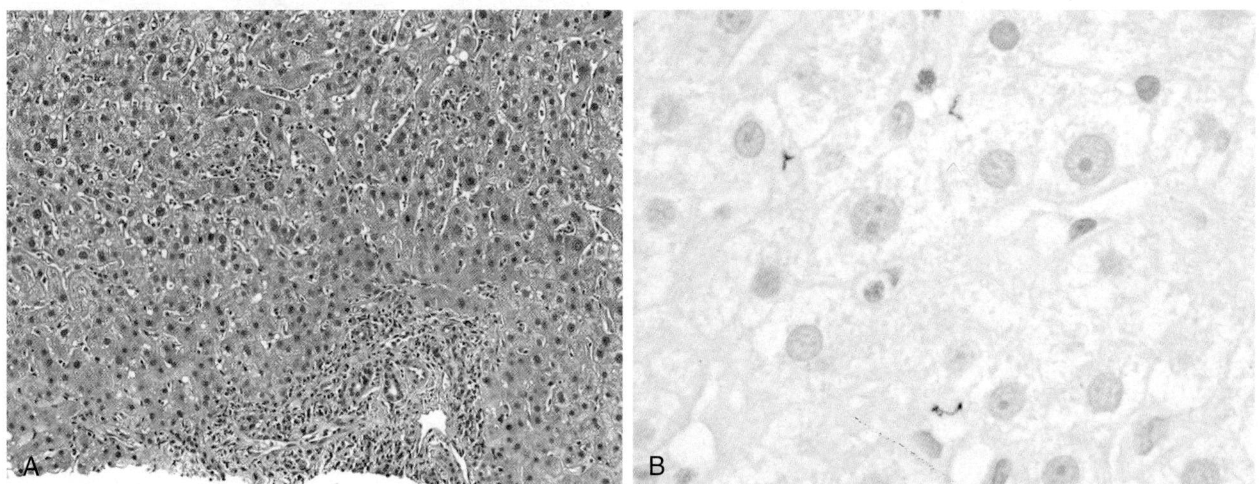

FIGURE 47.49 Syphilis shows variable histology. A, In this case, minimal and nonspecific findings are seen in the liver biopsy, such as mild portal and lobular lymphocytic inflammation as well as very mild bile ductular reaction. **B,** The immunostain for syphilis (antibody to *Treponema*) highlights multiple organisms within the sinusoids.

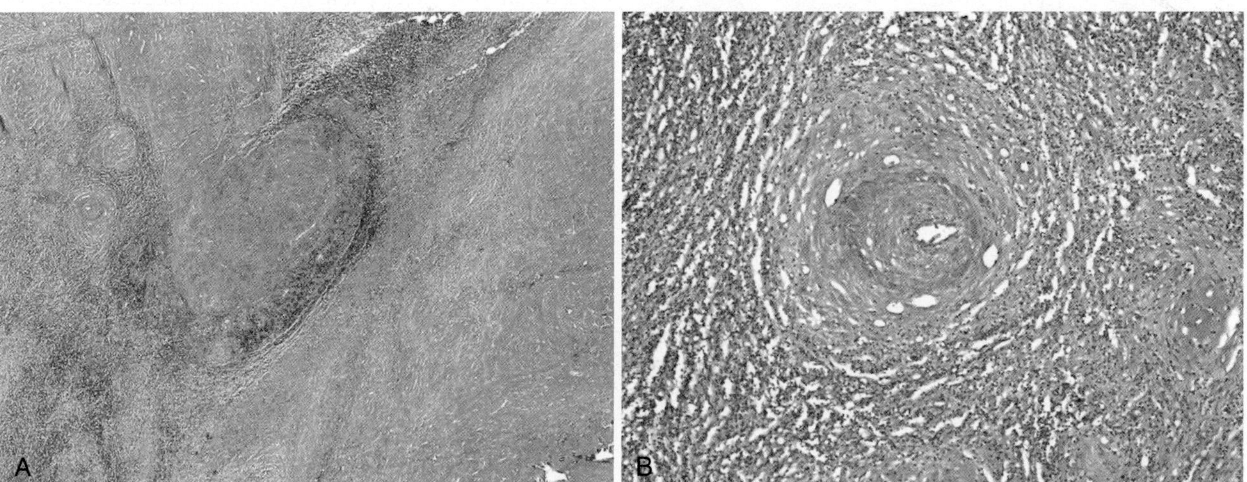

FIGURE 47.50 A, Syphilitic gummas consist of a nodular focus of caseous necrosis surrounded by an inflamed fibrous wall with chronic and granulomatous inflammation as well as endarteritis. Increased scarring occurs with healing. **B,** Scarred vessel in a field of chronic inflammation.

gummas are densely fibrotic lesions that may have central caseous necrosis but no active inflammation, and only rare or absent organisms.[212,215-217]

Other types of spirochetal infections that may involve the liver include infection with *Leptospira* (Weil's disease) and *Borrelia* species (causative agent of Lyme disease and other relapsing febrile illnesses). Infections with these agents usually cause a nonspecific reactive pattern of hepatitis. Silver impregnation stains may reveal organisms; serological studies and immunostains may also be of diagnostic value.

Miscellaneous Bacterial Infections

Salmonella *Species*

Acute systemic *Salmonella* infections, especially those associated with enteric fever, often involve the liver, and the mortality rate may be as high as 20%. The characteristic lesion is termed a *typhoid nodule* (even with nontyphoid *Salmonella* species); it consists of an aggregate of Kupffer cells admixed with scattered lymphocytes. Kupffer cell hyperplasia may be present.[218-220] Organisms are rarely detected in tissue sections.

Whipple's Disease

The Whipple bacillus *(Tropheryma whipplei)* can rarely infect the liver, even in the absence of small bowel involvement.[221,222] Histologically, PAS-positive bacilli are present in Kupffer cells. Often there is no significant inflammatory response, but epithelioid granulomas in association with Whipple's disease are well documented.[222] Electron microscopy and PCR assays may be useful diagnostic aids. The differential diagnosis includes infection by MAI or other intracellular organisms such as *Histoplasma capsulatum* and *R. equi*.

Other organisms that may infect the liver include *Chlamydia*, which can cause both perihepatitis (Fitz-Hugh–Curtis syndrome) and hepatitis; *R. equi*, which causes a granulomatous inflammatory pattern that mimics MAI infection; *Clostridium perfringens*, which can cause fulminant liver failure; and *Pseudomonas pseudomallei* (melioidosis), which can cause either small neutrophilic microabscesses or granulomas.

FUNGAL INFECTIONS OF THE LIVER

Hepatic fungal infections are typically seen as part of disseminated infection in immunocompromised patients, although rare cases have been described in otherwise healthy persons. The clinical features are similar, regardless of the type of fungus involved, and include hepatomegaly, abdominal pain, and elevated levels of aminotransferases and bilirubin.[223] Although fungi are often seen on routine H&E-stained sections in fulminant infection, Grocott methenamine–silver (GMS) and PAS stains are also invaluable diagnostic aids. Fungi can sometimes be correctly classified based on their morphological appearance in tissue sections. However, culture should always be relied upon as the gold standard for speciation, especially because antifungal therapy varies according to the type of fungus. A table describing the morphological features of fungal infections is provided in Chapter 4.

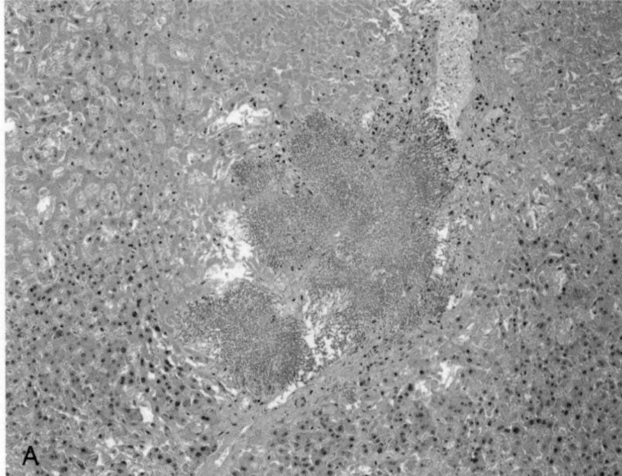

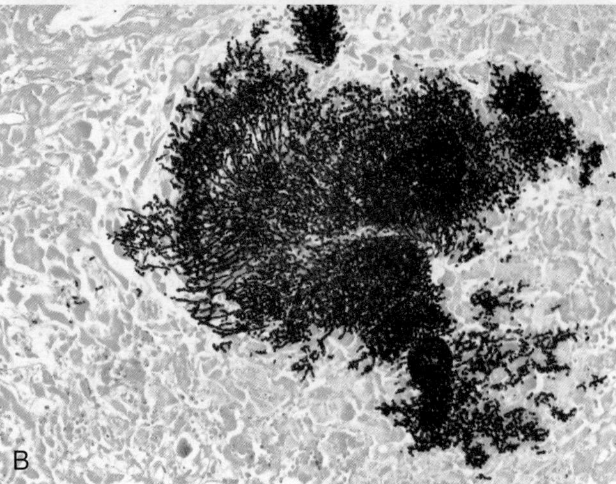

FIGURE 47.51 A, Large aggregate of *Candida albicans* present within the liver, with associated tissue necrosis. There is minimal associated inflammation in this severely immunocompromised patient. **B,** Grocott methenamine–silver stain shows the typical budding yeast and pseudohyphae of *C. albicans*. (*Courtesy Dr. Dan Milner, MD*)

Candidiasis

Candida is the most common cause of disseminated fungal infection in immunocompromised hosts, and liver involvement is frequent. Grossly, infected livers show multiple yellow-white nodules ranging in size from 1 mm to 2 cm.[224,225] The typical inflammatory reaction is granulomatous, often with central suppuration and a variable degree of necrosis (Fig. 47.51A). Giant cells are occasionally present. There may be surrounding palisading histiocytes and a fibrous scar, similar to hepatic CSD. Nonspecific findings such as cholestasis, portal inflammation, ductular proliferation, and sinusoidal dilation in areas of liver adjacent to the inflammatory lesion are often present.[224-226] Organisms are typically present in the center of the inflammatory lesion, but they may be few in number and only focally present. *Candida albicans* and *Candida tropicalis* both produce budding yeast, hyphae, and pseudohyphae (see Fig. 47.51B). *Candida (Torulopsis) glabrata* produces only tiny budding yeast, similar to *Histoplasma*.[226]

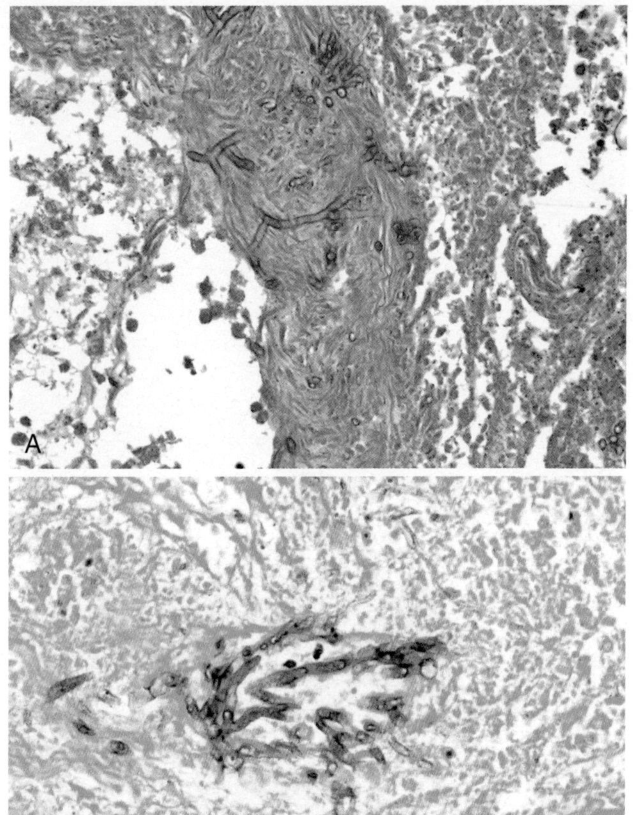

FIGURE 47.52 The typical lesion of aspergillosis consists of a nodular infarction centered on a blood vessel. **A,** This area of necrosis in the middle of an infarction contains *Aspergillus*. **B,** Grocott methenamine–silver stain highlights the septate hyphae that branch at acute angles.

Aspergillosis

Aspergillus infection usually begins in the lungs, and it occurs almost exclusively in immunocompromised patients. Grossly, affected livers show necrosis and the characteristic "target" lesion, consisting of a necrotic central zone of tissue with a hyperemic rim. The analogous histological lesion is a nodular infarct centered on a blood vessel that contains fungi (Fig. 47.52A). The inflammatory response ranges from minimal, to marked, and consists mainly of a neutrophilic response. Granulomatous inflammation is sometimes present as well.[223-226] *Aspergillus* hyphae are septate and branch at acute angles (see Fig. 47.52B).

The pathological picture of mucormycosis is similar to that of aspergillosis. However, mucor has broad, ribbon-like, pauciseptate hyphae that branch randomly at various angles.[226]

Histoplasmosis

Histoplasma capsulatum is endemic to the Mississippi and Ohio river valleys in the United States. Hepatic involvement occurs in more than 90% of patients with disseminated infection. Patients occasionally have signs of liver disease at presentation, and they do not always have symptoms of concomitant pulmonary involvement. Most biopsies show portal lymphohistiocytic inflammation and sinusoidal Kupffer cell hyperplasia (Fig. 47.53A,B). Discrete granulomas and giant cells are present in only a minority of cases. Organisms are usually present in both portal macrophages and Kupffer cells. In immunocompromised patients, large numbers of organisms may be present without a significant tissue reaction.[227] *Histoplasma* organisms are small, ovoid, usually intracellular yeast forms with small buds at the more pointed pole (see Fig. 47.53C). On an H&E-stained section, *Histoplasma* have a small "halo" around the organisms within macrophages (see Fig. 47.53D).

Talaromycosis (Formerly Penicilliosis)

Talaromyces marneffei, a dimorphic fungus endemic to Southeast Asia, resembles *H. capsulatum* but is more sausage-shaped and has a central crosswall rather than a bud. Infection is considered to be an AIDS-defining illness in endemic areas, although it can also be seen in other immunocompromised settings. Three patterns of hepatic talaromycosis have been described. The "diffuse" pattern is characterized by widespread macrophages in sinusoidal spaces with compression of the hepatocyte cords. The macrophages contain numerous organisms that can be highlighted by special stains (i.e., Grocott methenamine silver). The granulomatous pattern features multiple granulomas in the liver parenchyma and portal tracts, sparsely surrounded by other types of inflammatory cells. Organisms are seen in both intracellular and extracellular locations. Finally, a mix of both the "diffuse" and "granulomatous" patterns is seen in the majority of hepatic cases.[228] The size of the organisms may vary depending on where they are seen. Intracellularly, *T. marneffei* are 2 to 7 μm in diameter, round-to-oval yeast-like organisms. On the other hand, in an extracellular location, the organisms are commonly elongated and measure up to 15 μm in length (Fig. 47.54).

Cryptococcosis

Cryptococcus organisms are the most common cause of systemic mycosis in patients with AIDS.[229] The inflammatory reaction is variable and depends on the immune status of the host. It ranges from a suppurative, necrotizing inflammatory reaction with granulomatous features to virtually no reaction at all in immunocompromised hosts.[226,230,231] A pure granulomatous response is occasionally present. *Cryptococcus neoformans* is a round to oval-shaped yeast with narrow-based budding and often considerable variation in size (Fig. 47.55A). Due to the capsule, there may be a large soap bubble–like vacuole around the organisms on H&E-stained sections (see Fig. 47.55B). The mucopolysaccharide capsular material stains with Alcian blue, mucicarmine, Fontana-Masson stain, and colloidal iron; GMS stains are helpful as well. Some strains of *Cryptococcus* are only weakly mucicarmine positive (see Fig. 47.55C) or mucicarmine negative (capsule deficient). These capsule-deficient *Cryptococcus* strains will not be detected by antigen assays, as not enough capsular polysaccharide antigen is produced in order to be detected by the test. Despite these false-negative results, capsule-deficient *Cryptococcus* are positive on Fontana-Masson stain.[232,233] Finally, cryptococcosis may also involve the biliary tract.

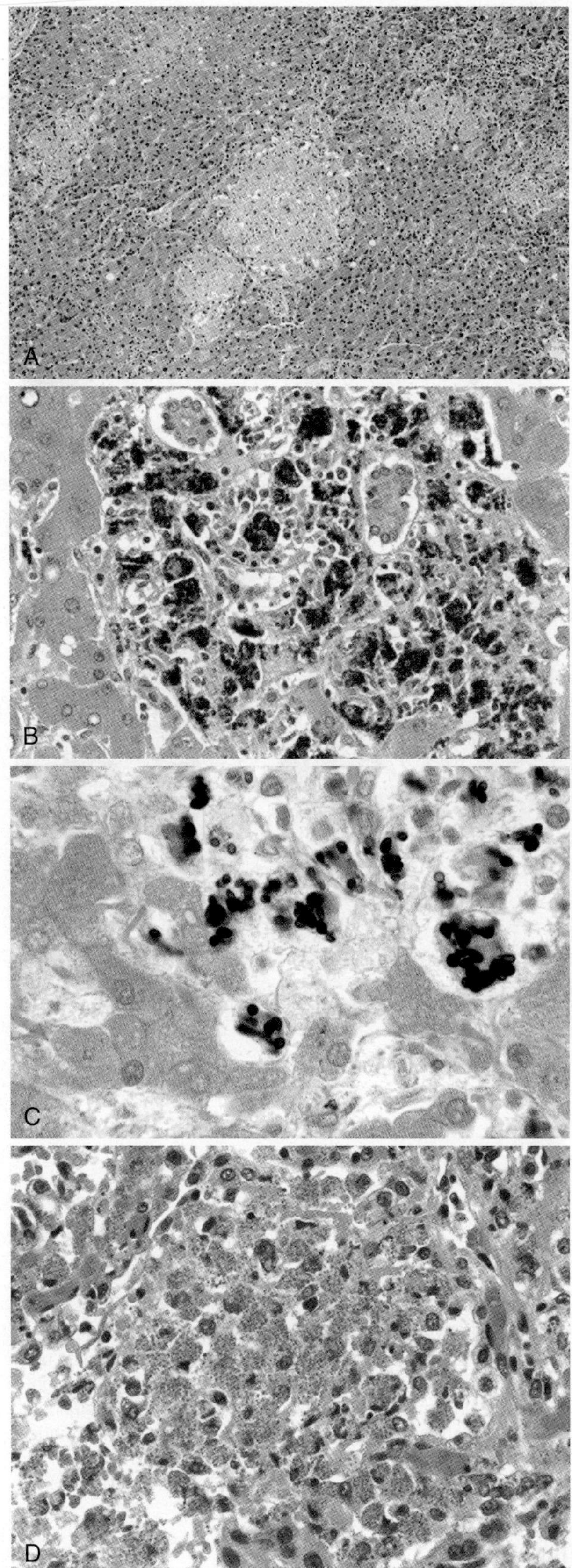

FIGURE 47.53 A, Nodular portal lymphohistiocytic inflammation is typical of hepatic histoplasmosis. **B,** Combined hematoxylin and eosin (H&E) and Grocott methenamine–silver (GMS) stain highlights the organisms within portal macrophages. **C,** GMS stain shows the typical histological features of histoplasma: uniformly small yeast with a bud at the more pointed pole. **D,** On an H&E-stained section, intracytoplasmic organisms have a pale "halo" around them.

Other fungal infections that occasionally involve the liver include those caused by *Pneumocystis jiroveci* (previously called *Pneumocystis carinii*), *Blastomyces dermatitidis*, *Paracoccidioides brasiliensis* (South American blastomycosis), and *Coccidioides immitis*.

The differential diagnosis includes other suppurative and granulomatous processes, especially bacterial and mycobacterial infections. Noninfectious causes of hepatic granulomas should always be considered, as well, although these are less likely if suppuration and necrosis are prominent. Helpful diagnostic aids, in addition to culture, include serological assays, antigen tests, and immunohistochemistry.

PARASITIC INFECTIONS OF THE LIVER

Protozoa

Malaria

Hepatic sequelae of malarial infection (jaundice, hepatomegaly, and elevated aminotransferases) are common, but hepatic failure usually does not occur. Grossly, affected livers are enlarged and congested and have a gray or dark brown appearance because of malarial pigment deposition. Concomitantly, the most striking microscopic feature is hemozoin pigment in macrophages along the sinusoids, in portal tracts, and in erythrocytes. The pigment forms dark brown clumps that do not react with an iron stain. Nonspecific associated changes include mild portal lymphocytosis, erythrophagocytosis, lipofuscin pigment, and Kupffer cell hyperplasia.[234,235] Parasites may be visible in erythrocytes.

Babesiosis is a tick-borne zoonotic illness that is clinically and pathologically similar to malaria; serological tests may be useful in distinguishing these organisms.[236]

Amebiasis

Hepatic amebiasis *(Entamoeba histolytica)* occurs when invasive colonic lesions seed the portal vein circulation. However, many patients do not have a history of GI complaints.[237] Clinically, patients come in because of fever, abdominal pain or tenderness, leukocytosis, and hepatomegaly; jaundice, weight loss, and malaise are also variably present.[237,238] Patients may show elevated alkaline phosphatase and aminotransferase levels.

Grossly, abscesses may be solitary or multiple.[239] Lesions range from pale, necrotic nodules to irregularly shaped abscesses with a fibrous capsule. The content of the abscesses reportedly resembles anchovy paste, and their size ranges from barely discernible to more than 20 cm in greatest diameter.[237,239] Occasionally, amebic abscesses can rupture through the liver capsule into the peritoneum or extend into the surrounding organs, including the skin.[239] Histologically, earlier lesions reveal the presence of amebic trophozoites in sinusoids, associated with focal necrosis and with a neutrophilic infiltrate. In more advanced cases, lesions consist predominantly of necrotic material containing nuclear debris and generally only a few intact inflammatory cells. Mononuclear cells and organisms may be present at the advancing edge (Fig. 47.56A). Eventually, peripheral granulation tissue and fibrosis develop. The amebae themselves resemble large macrophages (see Chapter 4). They contain foamy cytoplasm and a round, eccentrically placed nucleus; the presence of ingested red blood cells is pathognomonic of *E. histolytica* infection (see Fig. 47.56B).

The abscesses may mimic a neoplasm radiographically. Otherwise, the main differential diagnosis includes pyogenic

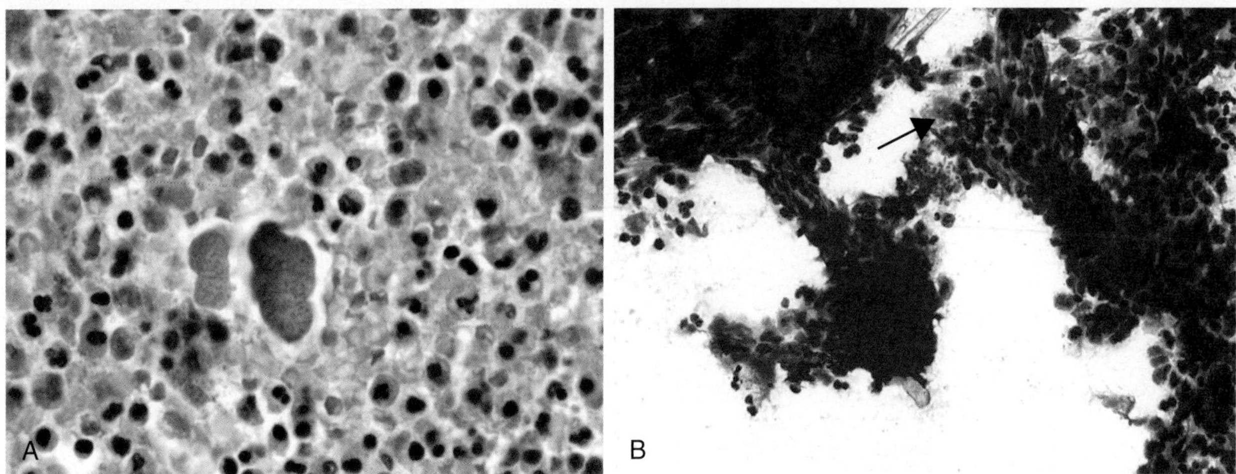

FIGURE 47.54 Talaromycosis. A, Numerous intracellular yeastlike organisms are seen within this macrophage, even without special stains. **B,** A Giemsa stain on this cytology specimen highlights a cluster of the oval organisms (in the center of the field), surrounded by the predominant groups of epithelial cells.

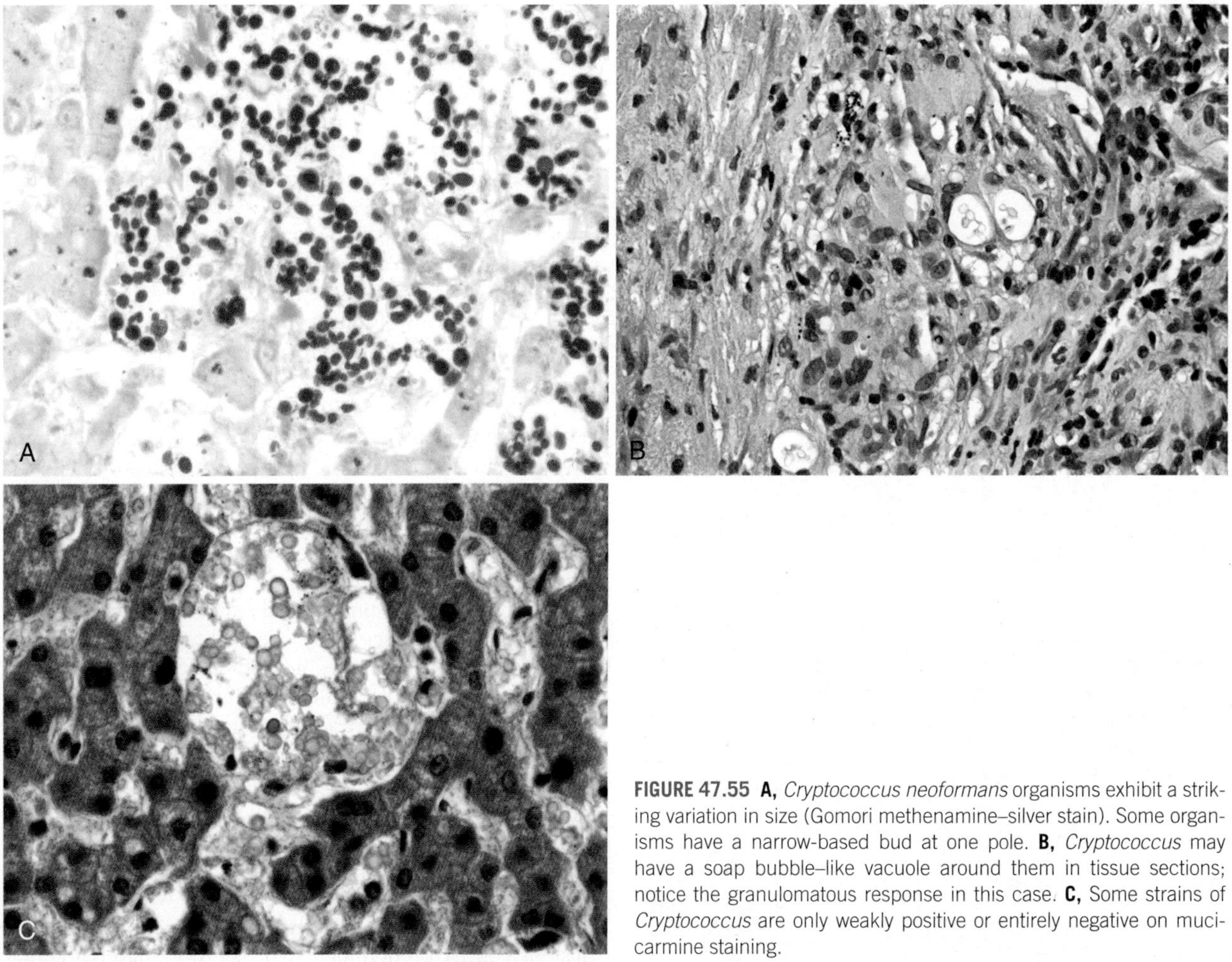

FIGURE 47.55 A, *Cryptococcus neoformans* organisms exhibit a striking variation in size (Gomori methenamine–silver stain). Some organisms have a narrow-based bud at one pole. **B,** *Cryptococcus* may have a soap bubble–like vacuole around them in tissue sections; notice the granulomatous response in this case. **C,** Some strains of *Cryptococcus* are only weakly positive or entirely negative on mucicarmine staining.

liver abscess; aspiration and culture are invaluable in resolving this differential, and sometimes amebae are even identifiable within the aspirate. The ciliate *Balantidium coli* can produce clinical and pathological changes similar to amebiasis.

Flagellates

Visceral Leishmaniasis (Kala-Azar)

Leishmaniasis is primarily caused by *Leishmania donovani,* an obligate intracellular protozoan transmitted by sandfly

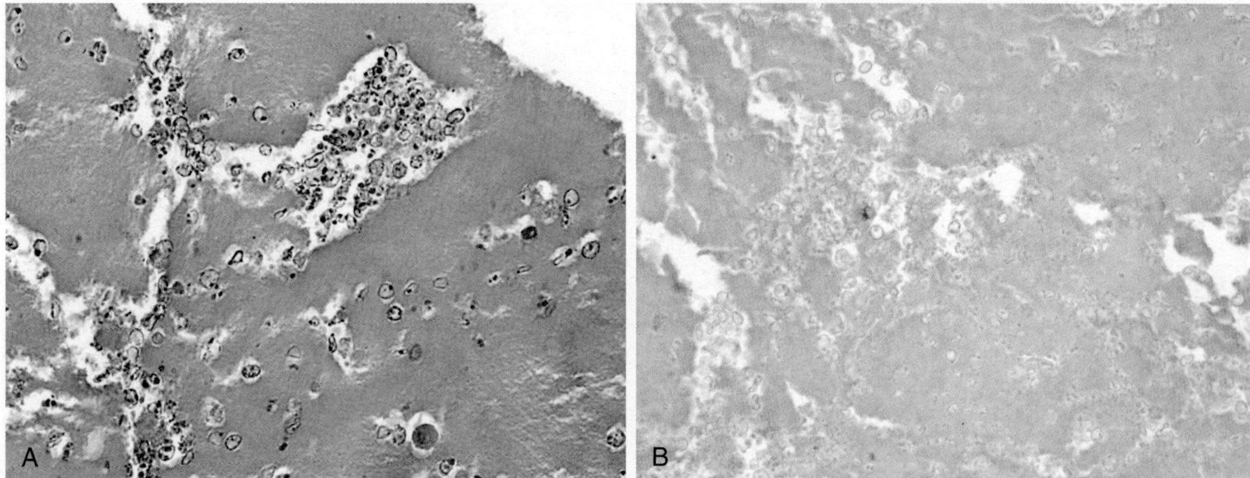

FIGURE 47.56 Amoebic abscesses consist predominantly of necrotic material with prominent nuclear debris and relatively few intact inflammatory cells. A, Organisms are often present at the advancing edge. Amebae have foamy cytoplasm and a round, eccentrically placed nucleus; they may mimic macrophages. The presence of ingested red blood cells is pathognomonic of *Entamoeba histolytica* infection. **B,** A CD163 stain is negative, confirming that these structures are not macrophages.

bites. It is endemic in more than 80 countries in Africa, Asia, South and Central America, and Europe. The infection may remain localized at the site of the bite, or it may disseminate widely via the reticuloendothelial system. Visceral leishmaniasis (kala-azar) is emerging as an important opportunistic infection among HIV-infected patients, particularly in southwestern Europe.[240-242] In endemic areas, it often affects children and young adults.

Most infections are asymptomatic. When progression to symptomatic visceral infection occurs, the average incubation period is 3 to 8 months but may extend for years. Patients often have hepatosplenomegaly, and laboratory abnormalities include pancytopenia, polyclonal hypergammaglobulinemia, hypoalbuminemia, and elevated erythrocyte sedimentation rate and C-reactive protein level.

The typical histological finding in the liver is hyperplastic Kupffer cells (and rarely hepatocytes) containing amastigotes (Fig. 47.57A,B). The amastigotes are rounded, 2- to 4-μm, basophilic organisms with a round to oval central nucleus and a thin external membrane. The kinetoplast lies tangentially or at right angles to the nucleus, producing a characteristic "double-knot" configuration. They are highlighted by Giemsa staining (see Fig. 47.57C). The organism-laden macrophages may form small nodules or loose granulomas. Fibrin ring and epithelioid granulomas have also been described.[243,244] *Leishmania* may be confused with other organisms, such as *Histoplasma*; *Leishmania* are GMS-negative, and *Histoplasma* lack a kinetoplast. The kinetoplast also distinguishes *Leishmania* from *Toxoplasma*. Serological studies and immunohistochemistry may aid in diagnosis.

Miscellaneous Flagellates

Granulomatous hepatitis and cholangitis associated with *Giardia lamblia* have rarely been reported.[245]

Coccidians

Coccidians can produce infection in both immunocompromised and healthy patients. Many infections are subclinical; although the most common manifestation is diarrhea, they also cause hepatobiliary disease. Although *Microsporidia* are now classified as fungi, and *Cryptosporidia* as Gregarines rather than coccidians, they are still considered together due to their similar clinical and morphological characteristics.

Hepatic toxoplasmosis *(Toxoplasma gondii)* is primarily a disease of immunocompromised patients. *Toxoplasma* hepatitis shows cholestasis, a mononuclear cell infiltrate, and focal hepatocyte necrosis; both crescent-shaped tachyzoites and tissue cysts containing bradyzoites may be present in hepatocytes.[246,247] Granulomatous hepatitis has been described as well. Giant cell hepatitis may be present in neonates. Immunohistochemistry, PCR assays, and serological tests provide useful diagnostic aids.

Cryptosporidium parvum and *Microsporidia* are the most common causes of AIDS-related cholangiopathy; these infections are discussed in detail in Chapters 4 and 38. They only rarely infect the liver.[248-250] Disseminated *Cystoisospora belli* infection has been rarely reported in the liver[251] and in mesenteric lymph nodes.

Helminths

Helminths (nematodes, trematodes, and cestodes) are more often a cause of serious disease in nations with deficient sanitation systems; poor socioeconomic status; and hot, humid climates. However, they are occasionally seen in developed countries as well. Hepatic helminthic infections manifest a wide range of clinicopathological findings. The differential diagnosis involves differentiation between the various types of worms. Other entities to consider include additional causes of granulomatous inflammation and hepatic abscesses.

Nematodes

Ascaris lumbricoides

The roundworm, *Ascaris lumbricoides*, is the most common source of human helminth infection. Clinical findings are variable and include hepatomegaly, cholecystitis,

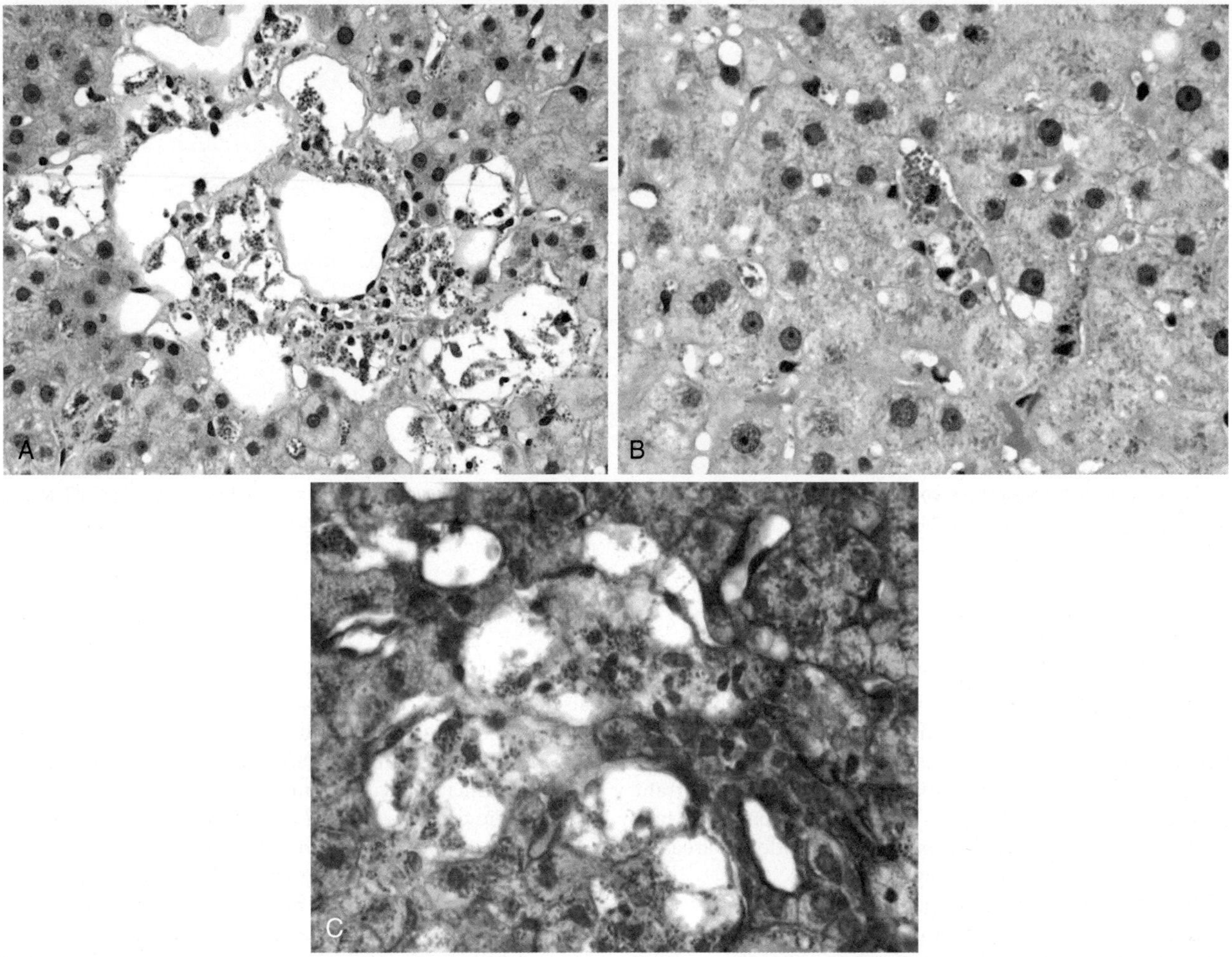

FIGURE 47.57 **A,** Macrophages and hepatocytes are distended by *Leishmania*, forming small nodules. **B,** The amastigotes are rounded, 2- to 4-μm, basophilic organisms with a round to oval central nucleus and a thin external membrane. **C,** *Leishmania* are positive on Giemsa staining. (*Courtesy of Dr. Rhonda Yantiss, Weill Cornell Medical College.*)

cholangitis, and hepatic abscess. Cholangitic superinfection by enteric bacteria is common. These are large worms (as great as 20 cm in length) and may be identified in the biliary tract, with accompanying reactive epithelial changes. Abscesses may contain worm remnants or, rarely, eggs with associated inflammation (often prominent eosinophils) and necrosis (Fig. 47.58).[252,253]

Toxocara canis

Toxocara canis is the most common cause of visceral larva migrans.[254] The usual presenting symptoms include hepatomegaly, fever, leukocytosis, eosinophilia, and pulmonary and central nervous system disturbances. Histologically, infected livers show central eosinophilic abscesses with Charcot-Leyden crystals and associated granulomatous inflammation.[255,256] Larval remnants are occasionally present and visible. On healing, fibrous scars develop. Many other helminths can cause visceral larva migrans, including *Toxocara catis*, *Capillaria*, *Ascaris*, and *Strongyloides stercoralis*.[255]

Enterobius vermicularis *(Pinworms)*

Pinworms *(Enterobius vermicularis)* are one of the most common human parasites. The rare "pinworm granuloma" is a hyalinized nodule with peripheral inflammation. Central necrosis with eggs and worm remnants may be present.[257,258]

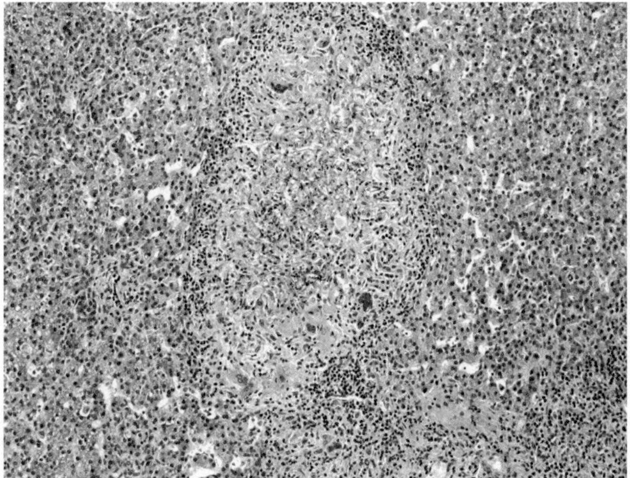

FIGURE 47.58 Abscess caused by *Ascaris* infection features a necrotic center with surrounding granulomatous inflammation and numerous eosinophils. No worm parts are visible. (*Courtesy Dr. Lucas Campbell, Northwest Arkansas Pathology Associates.*)

Strongyloides stercoralis

Many patients with *S. stercoralis* infection are asymptomatic, but the worm's capability for autoinfection allows it

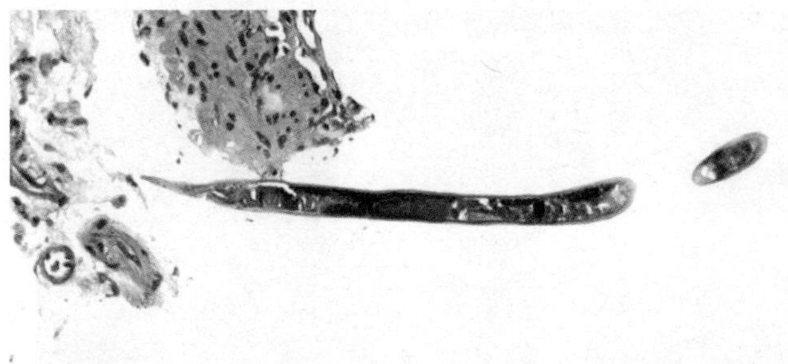

FIGURE 47.59 *Strongyloides stercoralis* worms are identifiable by the presence of sharply pointed tails.

to reside in the host and produce illness for 30 years or more. Hepatic involvement is typically part of disseminated disease (Fig. 47.59). Infected livers show larvae in portal vessels and sinusoids. Associated inflammation ranges from none to a nonspecific mixed inflammatory infiltrate. Granulomas are sometimes seen.[259]

Trematodes

Schistosomiasis

Schistosomiasis is the most common cause of portal hypertension in the world. Most hepatobiliary disease is caused by *Schistosoma mansoni*, *Schistosoma japonicum*, or *Schistosoma mekongi*, because the organisms prefer mesenteric and portal veins. Once settled in their vein of choice, adult worms copulate and produce thousands of eggs in their lifetime; approximately 50% of the eggs remain in the body.[260] Hypersensitivity to the eggs is the underlying cause of disease, and the resultant inflammation eventually leads to fibrosis and obstructive hepatobiliary disease.[260,261] Symptomatic patients have splenomegaly and signs of portal hypertension, particularly bleeding. Hepatic function is usually preserved.

Grossly, infected livers are enlarged and nodular. On cut surface, the typical pattern of portal fibrosis, known as pipestem or Symmers fibrosis, may be observed. Portal tracts are enlarged and stellate, but liver acinar architecture is usually unremarkable. Histological features vary with the duration of disease. Early schistosomiasis features portal inflammation with numerous eosinophils, Kupffer cell hyperplasia, and focal hepatocyte necrosis, but ova are rarely present. In chronic disease, there is typically a granulomatous reaction to the eggs, which are present in varying numbers in both granulomas and fibrotic areas (Fig. 47.60A–C). One usually sees associated mixed portal inflammation and giant cells. Ultimately, portal tracts become enlarged and densely sclerotic, with the development of fibrous septa that link the portal tracts together. Sinusoidal fibrosis may also develop. With progression of fibrosis, eggs may be difficult to detect. Schistosomal pigment, similar to malarial pigment, is often present in Kupffer cells and macrophages (see Fig. 47.60D).[177,260,261] Granulomas and fibrosis may also affect portal vein branches and lead to phlebitis, sclerosis, and thrombosis. Eventually, portal veins are obstructed and destroyed, with subsequent proliferation of hepatic arterial branches.[177]

The eggs are large. *S. mansoni* has an acid-fast shell (see Fig. 47.60E) and a prominent lateral spine, but exact speciation of schistosomes in the liver is difficult. The nematode *Capillaria* should always be considered in the differential diagnosis, because the eggs are similar in appearance.

Other trematodes that may infect the liver and biliary tract include flukes; *Clonorchis sinensis* and *Opisthorchis* species, which are associated with development of cholangiocarcinoma[262,263]; and *Fasciola hepatica*, which can cause calculi, cholangitis, obstructive jaundice, and granulomatous hepatitis.[264]

Cestodes

Echinococcus granulosus and Related Species

Hydatid disease is often subclinical, but some patients develop hepatomegaly, marked abdominal enlargement and distention, and ascites. Secondary infection of the cysts may also develop. Ultimately, some patients experience liver failure, portal hypertension, involvement of adjacent organs, and death.[265-267] Grossly, the cysts are large, unilocular, and round (Fig. 47.61A). The cyst fluid is strikingly antigenic and may lead to anaphylaxis on spillage. The inner layer of the cyst consists of a thin lining of epithelial cells that gives rise to the "brood" capsules from which scolices, or immature heads of adult worms, develop (see Fig. 47.61B). The outer cyst layers are composed of hyalinized, PAS-positive material surrounded by granulation tissue and fibrosis[268] (Fig. 47.62). Daughter cysts may develop in the main cyst. The differential diagnosis includes other types of cystic lesions. The scolex of the worm distinguishes hydatid disease from amebic abscess, pyogenic abscess, and noninfectious processes such as fibropolycystic liver disease.

The full reference list may be accessed online at *Elsevier eBooks for Practicing Clinicians.*

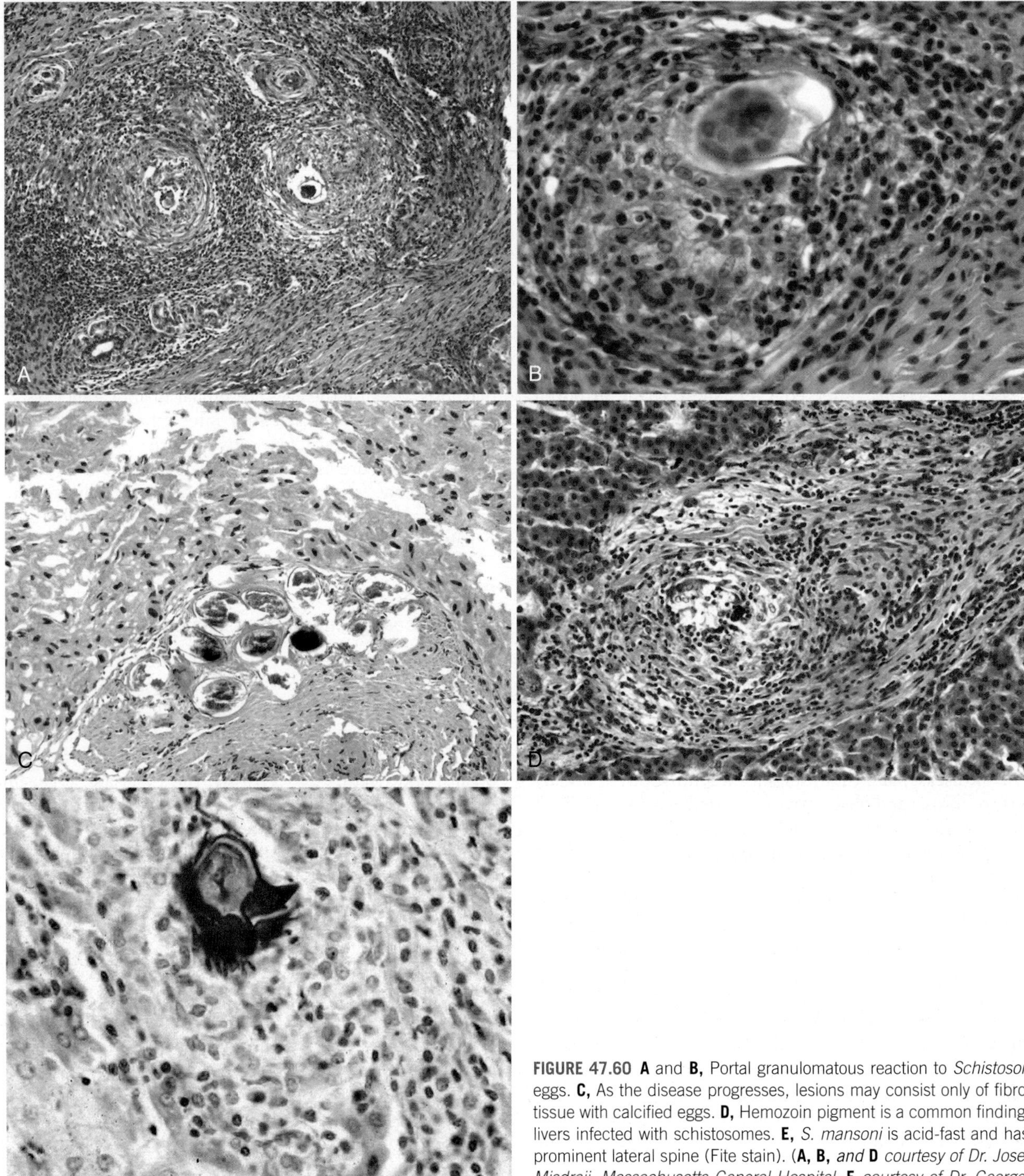

FIGURE 47.60 **A** and **B,** Portal granulomatous reaction to *Schistosoma* eggs. **C,** As the disease progresses, lesions may consist only of fibrous tissue with calcified eggs. **D,** Hemozoin pigment is a common finding in livers infected with schistosomes. **E,** *S. mansoni* is acid-fast and has a prominent lateral spine (Fite stain). (**A, B,** *and* **D** *courtesy of Dr. Joseph Misdraji, Massachusetts General Hospital;* **E** *courtesy of Dr. George F. Gray, Jr.*)

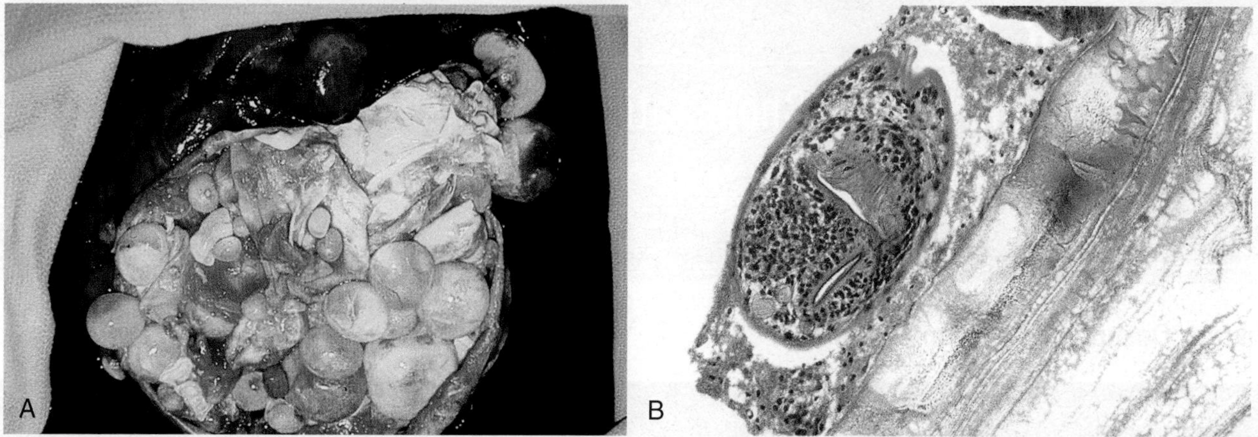

FIGURE 47.61 **A,** Grossly, echinococcal cysts are large, unilocular, and rounded. The inner lining of the echinococcal cyst consists of epithelial cells that give rise to brood capsules from which scolices develop. **B,** The outer cyst layers are composed of hyalinized, acellular, periodic acid–Schiff stain-positive material. (*Courtesy of Dr. George F. Gray, Jr.*)

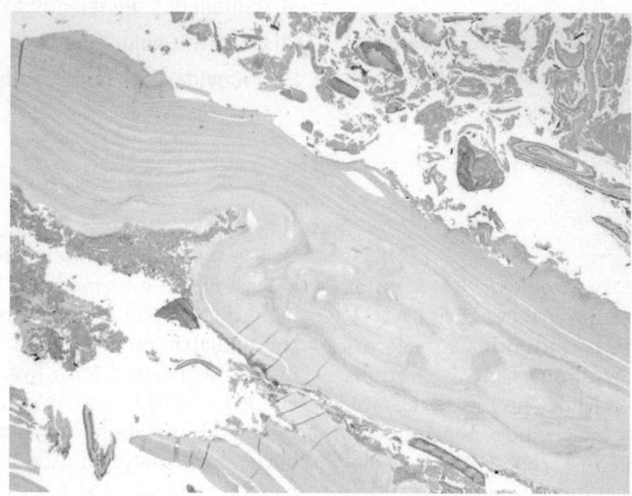

FIGURE 47.62 The histological section of the cyst shows a lamellated and highly fibrotic cyst wall.

CHAPTER 48

Autoimmune and Chronic Cholestatic Disorders of the Liver

Vikram Deshpande, Clifton G. Fulmer

Contents

INTRODUCTION

The three most common liver syndromes with a putative autoimmune cause are autoimmune hepatitis (AIH), primary biliary cholangitis (PBC), and primary sclerosing cholangitis (PSC). Overlap syndromes involve various combinations of these disorders. Other chronic cholestatic disorders discussed in this chapter include hepatobiliary involvement by immunoglobulin G4 (IgG4)-related disease. Some uncommon noncongenital chronic biliary diseases that can mimic PBC and PSC are reviewed as well as post–COVID-19 cholangiopathy. Pediatric cholestatic disorders (e.g., biliary atresia) are discussed in Chapter 54, and transplantation-related aspects of autoimmune liver disorders are covered in Chapter 52.

AUTOIMMUNE HEPATITIS

Autoimmune hepatitis (AIH) is an immune-mediated chronic hepatitis that primarily affects women and is associated with polyclonal hypergammaglobulinemia and a variety of circulating tissue-directed autoantibodies. There is a strong association with several common human leukocyte antigen (HLA) subtypes, including HLA DR3 (DRB1*0301), DR4 (DRB1*0401), and DR7 (DRB1*0701), as well as with other genetic disorders that lead to immune dysregulation.[1] Although a favorable response to corticosteroid-based immunosuppressive therapies is characteristic, AIH can progress to cirrhosis, and advanced fibrosis may, in fact, be present at the time of initial presentation (Box 48.1).[2]

AIH can be subclassified based on the specific complement of autoantibodies detected by serological testing (Table 48.1). AIH type 1 more commonly affects adults and is associated with circulating antinuclear antibodies (ANAs) and anti–smooth muscle antibodies (ASMAs) that target a variety of intermediate filaments and microfilaments, including F-actin.[3] In contrast, AIH type 2 primarily affects the pediatric population. It lacks ANAs and ASMAs and is instead associated with liver-kidney microsomal antibodies (LKM1, LKM3) and liver cytosol antibodies (LC-1) that target the metabolic machinery of hepatocytes.[4] The presence of circulating antibodies to soluble liver antigen/liver pancreas antigen (SLA/LP), which targets components of the transfer ribonucleoprotein complex SEPSECS, has been referred to as *AIH type 3* in the literature.[5] Although AIH type 3 affects a similar demographic as and clinically resembles AIH type 1, recognition of SLA/LP-positive patients may have clinical significance as this population is significantly more likely to relapse following the withdrawal of immunosuppressive therapy.[6]

The histological features of AIH are not specific and show significant overlap with a variety of different chronic liver diseases, including viral hepatitis, drug-induced liver injury (DILI), Wilson disease, toxic/metabolic injury, and chronic cholestatic liver disease. As such, knowledge of the patient's clinical history and previously performed laboratory studies is essential for appropriate interpretation of liver biopsy samples. At a minimum, attempts should be made to exclude the presence of viral hepatitis, recent exposure to hepatotoxic drugs, and significant alcohol intake before entertaining a diagnosis of AIH. A hepatitic pattern of elevated liver enzymes coupled with hypergammaglobulinemia and the presence of serum autoantibodies also supports a diagnosis of AIH, but again lacks specificity.[7,8]

Standardized diagnostic criteria for AIH were initially developed by the International Autoimmune Hepatitis Group in 1992 for therapeutic and research purposes. These

BOX 48.1 Key Features of Autoimmune Hepatitis

- Immune-mediated chronic hepatitis associated with circulating autoantibodies and hypergammaglobulinemia
- More common in women, with incidence peaks around 70 years of age and in young adulthood
- Considerably less common in children
- Associated with certain HLA haplotypes
- Associated with predominantly hepatitic pattern of liver injury
- Patients may be asymptomatic, but up to one-third present with established cirrhosis
- Diagnosis generally requires exclusion of infectious etiology, exposure to hepatotoxic medications, and significant alcohol intake
- Interface hepatitis, regenerative hepatocellular rosettes, and emperipolesis considered typical histological features
- Large numbers of plasma cells, plasma cell clusters, and Kupffer cell hyaline globules also frequently seen
- Generally very good clinical response to immunosuppressive medical therapy, including during disease relapse

TABLE 48.1 Subtypes of Autoimmune Hepatitis

Type of AIH	Autoantibody	Molecular Target
Type 1	ANA	Chromatin, ribonucleoproteins
	SMA	Cytoskeletal components, F-actin
Type 2	LKM1	CYP2D6
	LKM3	UGT
	LC-1	FTCD
Type 3	SLA/LP	SEPSECS
APAH	LM	CYP1A2

AIH, *Autoimmune hepatitis;* ANA, *antinuclear antibody;* CYP1A2, *cytochrome P-450 1A2;* CYP2D6, *cytochrome P-450 2D6;* FTCD, *anti-formiminotransferase cyclodeaminase;* LC-1, *liver cytosol 1 antibody;* LKM, *anti–liver-kidney microsomal antibody;* LM, *liver microsomal antibodies;* SEPSECS, *Sep (O-phosphoserine);* SLA/LP, *anti-soluble liver antigen/liver pancreas antigen;* SMA, *anti–smooth muscle antibody;* TRNA:Sec, *(selenocysteine),* UGT, *anti-uridine diphosphate glucuronosyltransferase.*

criteria incorporated patient demographic data, serum biochemical and serological studies, and histology to assign an aggregate score designed to predict a patient's likelihood of having AIH.[9] The scoring system was revised and modified by the same group in 1999 and has been demonstrated to have excellent diagnostic accuracy and effectively excludes AIH in patients with PBC and PSC (Table 48.2).[10] The system was further modified and simplified in 2008 with the development of a scoring system that was more applicable to routine clinical practice (Table 48.3).[11] Further modifications to the simplified criteria were published in 2021 that incorporated modern laboratory techniques like enzyme–linked immunosorbent assay (ELISA) and immunofluorescence testing for disease-associated autoantibodies in human epithelioma-2(HEp-2) cells rather than in frozen rodent tissue sections.[12]

Clinical Features and Epidemiology

Although there are significant regional differences, the worldwide incidence of AIH appears to be increasing.

TABLE 48.2 Diagnostic Criteria for Autoimmune Hepatitis: Minimum Required Parameters

Parameters	Score
History	
Sex	
Female	+2
Male	0
Alcohol average consumption	
<25 g/day	+2
>60 g/day	−2
History of hepatotoxic drug use	
Yes	−4
No	+1
Other autoimmune diseases	
Present	+2
Absent	0
Serum biochemical studies	
Serum ALP/ALT ratio	
<1.5	+2
>3.0	−2
Serum total globulin, γ-globulin, or IgG	
>2× normal	+3
1.5-2× normal	+2
1.0-1.5× normal	+1
Normal	0
Serology studies	
ANA, ASMA, or LKM1	
>1:80	+3
1:80	+2
1:40	+1
<1:40	0
AMA	
Negative	0
Positive	−4
Viral hepatitis markers	
Negative	+3
Positive	−4
Other autoantibodies	
Present	+2
Absent	0
HLA-DR3 or -DR4	
Present	+1
Absent	0
Treatment response	
Complete remission	+2
Remission with subsequent relapse	+3
Histology	
Interface hepatitis	+3
Lymphoplasmacytic infiltrate	+1
Hepatocyte rosetting	+1
None of the above	−5
Biliary changes	−3
Other changes	−3
Interpretation of aggregate scores	
Before therapy	
>15	Definite AIH
10-15	Probable AIH
After therapy	
>17	Definite AIH
12-17	Probable AIH

AIH, *Autoimmune hepatitis;* ALP, *alkaline phosphatase;* ALT, *alanine aminotransferase;* AMA, *antimitochondrial antibody;* ANA, *antinuclear antibody;* ASMA, *anti-smooth muscle antibody;* HLA, *human leukocyte antigen;* LKM1, *liver-kidney microsomal antibody 1.*

From Alvarez F, Berg PA, Bianchi FB, et al. International Autoimmune Hepatitis Group report: review of criteria for diagnosis of autoimmune hepatitis. J Hepatol. *1999;31:929-938.*

TABLE 48.3 Simplified Diagnostic Criteria for Autoimmune Hepatitis

Variable	Cutoff	Points
ANA or SMA	≥ 1:40	1
ANA or SMA	≥ 1:80	2
or LKM	≥ 1:40	
or SLA	Positive	
IgG	> Upper normal limit	1
	> 1.10 times upper normal limit	2
Liver histology (histological evidence of hepatitis is a necessary condition)	Compatible with AIH	1
	Typical AIH	2
Absence of viral hepatitis	Yes	2
Aggregate Score		
≥6	Probable AIH	
≥7	Definite AIH	

ANA, *Antinuclear antibody;* SMA, *smooth muscle antibody;* LKM, *liver-kidney microsomal antibody;* SLA, *soluble liver antigen antibody;* IgG, *immunoglobulin G;* AIH, *autoimmune hepatitis.*
From Hennes EM, Zeniya M, Czaja AJ, et al; International Autoimmune Hepatitis Group. Simplified criteria for the diagnosis of autoimmune hepatitis. Hepatology. *2008;48(1):169-176.*

A nationwide registry-based cohort study performed in Denmark between 1994 and 2012 showed an AIH incidence of 1.68 per 100,000 population per year, though it doubled over the course of the study period.[13] In Japan, the point prevalence of AIH increased from 8.7 per 100,000 in 2004 to 23.9 per 100,000 in 2016.[14] A similar registry-based cohort study in Finland reported an incidence of 1.1 per 100,000 person-years and showed an overall point prevalence of 14.3 per 100,000 at the end of 2015. In this work, 76% of AIH cases occurred in women, which is similar to the proportion described in other studies.[15] A population-based study from Korea showed a similar incidence rate of 1.07 per 100,000 persons, or a prevalence of 4.82 per 100,000 persons, while others performed in Alaskan Natives showed a point prevalence of 42.9 per 100,000, again highlighting marked regional variation in the incidence of AIH.[16,17]

Patients of any age may be affected by AIH. For AIH type 1, there appears to be an incidence peak at around 70 years of age, along with a smaller peak in young adults between 10 and 25 years of age.[13] Overall, AIH is rare in children, with an incidence of only 0.23 per 100,000. Nevertheless, in the juvenile population AIH type 1 is the most common form of AIH and is diagnosed 5.5 times more frequently than AIH type 2.[18] There are important differences between AIH type 1 and AIH type 2 with regard to patient demographics and clinical course. AIH type 2 patients with LKM1 antibodies are more likely to present at a younger age (median age 7.4 years) and frequently exhibit more aggressive, severely active disease than those with classical AIH type 1.[19] It is also extremely rare in adults in the United States, but fairly common in southern Europe and the United Kingdom, likely reflecting differences in genetic susceptibility as a result of regional variations in major histocompatibility complex (MHC) hapoltypes.[20,21]

Though not performed routinely for diagnostic purposes, AIH is strongly associated with certain HLA types. In northern European and North American populations HLA DRB1*0301 (DR3) appears to be the primary susceptibility haplotype, with DRB1*0401 (DR4) also showing a strong association with AIH type 1.[22] In a large Dutch cohort, 75% of AIH patients were HLA DR3 and DR4 positive. These patients had significantly higher serum IgG levels than those with other HLA haplotypes, and patients with HLA DR3 were more likely to require liver transplantation.[23] In addition to DR3, DRB1*1301 is frequently associated with AIH in some South American populations, while association with DRB1*0404 and DRB1*0405 has been reported in Mexican and Japanese populations.[24,25] A single-nucleotide polymorphism in the 3' untranslated region of HLA-DPB1 (rs9277534), which has been associated with the clearance of hepatitis B viral infection as well as the development of acute graft-versus-host disease following hematopoietic stem cell transplantation, may also contribute to AIH susceptibility, at least in Japanese populations.[26]

AIH type 2 is associated with somewhat different HLA haplotypes than AIH type 1. Like AIH type 1, HLA DR3 is significantly associated with susceptibility to AIH type 2 in one cohort (relative risk 4.25). However, the HLA DQB1*0201 allele appears to be the primary genetic determinant of AIH type, conferring the highest relative risk (6.40) of the HLA DR and DQ phenotypes in this study.[27]

Common polymorphisms in other non-MHC genes, including those coding for TNF-α and CTLA-4, have also been implicated as risk factors for the development of AIH. The *CTLA-4* gene includes a single base-exchange polymorphism at position 49 in exon 1. The G allele at this position is more common in patients with AIH type 1 than in controls, and the GG genotype may be associated with higher mean serum transaminase levels in patients with AIH.[28] Though not universal, this association appears to hold true across multiple ethnic backgrounds and may be related to deficient CTLA-4–mediated inhibition of T-lymphocyte proliferation in patients with the GG genotype.[29,30]

Autoimmune polyendocrinopathy-candidiasis-ectodermal dystrophy (APECED) is a monogenic disorder caused by biallelic point mutations in the autoimmune regulator gene *AIRE* that is characterized by chronic mucocutaneous candidiasis, hypoparathyroidism, and adrenal insufficiency related to loss of self-tolerance to endocrine organ tissue-specific antigens.[31] Historically, APECED-associated hepatitis (APAH) was thought to be a relatively rare manifestation of this disorder.[32] However, a recent study identified APAH in 42% of the APECED patients in their cohort, with about one-third showing histological and biochemical evidence of liver injury before exhibiting other features of systemic immune dysfunction.[33] In contrast with other forms of AIH, antinuclear and anti-smooth muscle antibodies are rare in the setting of APAH. Rather, liver microsomal antibodies (LMs) targeting CYP1A2 appear to be highly specific for APAH, but lack sensitivity, somewhat limiting their diagnostic utility.[34]

Despite difference with classic AIH, the majority of patients with APAH respond to typical immunosuppressive induction and maintenance regimens.[33]

The clinical presentation of AIH is remarkably protean and ranges from completely asymptomatic to fulminant hepatic failure.[35] Approximately 25% of patients present with nonspecific signs and symptoms that resemble acute viral hepatitis and include fatigue, abdominal pain, nausea, fever, and jaundiced mucus membranes and skin.[36] During periods of activity, serum transaminases are frequently markedly elevated and may exceed 1000 IU/mL.[37] In contrast, serum alkaline phosphatase levels usually fall within the normal range or are only mildly elevated. Hypergammaglobulinemia and elevated serum IgG are frequently present and are considered to be defining features of AIH, though this is not universal, even in cases presenting with fulminant hepatitis.[38]

Acute severe AIH resulting in massive hepatic necrosis and acute liver failure associated with coagulopathy and encephalopathy is a relatively rare manifestation of AIH. An immune-mediated process should, however, be considered in the differential diagnosis of all patients presenting with fulminant hepatic failure, as a dramatic response to immunosuppressive medical therapy is possible, and delay in the administration of corticosteroids has been associated with poor outcomes.[39] Histological features alone are, unfortunately, not sufficiently specific to diagnose this entity, though the presence of prominent zone 3 necroinflammatory activity and a plasma cell–rich inflammatory infiltrate is said to be characteristic.[35,39] Correlation of these histological features with the presence of circulating autoantibodies along with careful exclusion of infectious, toxic, and metabolic etiologies may improve diagnostic accuracy.[38]

At the other end of the spectrum, approximately one-third of patients with AIH are asymptomatic at the time of diagnosis.[40] Patients with asymptomatic AIH are more likely to be men and have significantly lower bilirubin and transaminase levels compared with their symptomatic counterparts, though histological changes including degree of necroinflammatory lobular activity and fibrosis are similar. Approximately 70% of asymptomatic AIH patients eventually develop clinical symptoms. Response to immunosuppression is excellent, slightly better than that seen in symptomatic populations, with no treatment failures observed, although relapse following cessation of therapy occurs at a similar rate.[41]

Approximately 34% of patients with AIH have established cirrhosis at the time of presentation, highlighting the chronic nature of this disease. The proportion of symptomatic and asymptomatic patients that have histologically confirmed cirrhosis during their initial workup is similar and is, perhaps not surprisingly, associated with poorer 10-year survival than those without advanced fibrosis.[42] A similar proportion of children with AIH have established cirrhosis at the time of presentation.[43,44]

Pathogenesis

AIH is chronic inflammatory syndrome associated with a defect in suppressor T-cell function that leads to loss of self-tolerance and the development of a T-cell–mediated immune response that primarily targets hepatocytes. Although most cases occur de novo without a clear triggering event, some medications and infections appear to be associated with development of AIH. Hepatitis A virus (HAV) infection, in particular, is strongly suspected to be a trigger for AIH. In genetically susceptible individuals, abnormal T-helper activation and the production of antibodies targeting the asialoglycoprotein receptor (ASGPR) continue to occur following viral clearance.[45] A similar association has been found with the Epstein-Barr virus (EBV).[46] Other possible hepatotropic and non-hepatotropic viral triggers have been suggested but have a less clear association with the development of subsequent immune-mediated liver injury.[47,48]

An ever-expanding list of drugs have been cited as proposed triggers of autoimmune liver disease. True drug-induced AIH (DI-AIH) is a self-perpetuating process that develops in patients not previously diagnosed with AIH.[49] In one large series, nitrofurantoin and minocycline were the most common medications associated with DI-AIH and produced a clinical syndrome virtually indistinguishable from de novo AIH.[50] DILI may also occur in the setting of methyldopa or hydralazine use, although only one-half of these cases show an immune-mediated phenotype resembling AIH with associated hypergammaglobulinemia and circulating autoantibodies.[51] More recently, DI-AIH has been linked with biological agents targeting TNF-α such as infliximab, adalimumab, and etanercept and was reported as a serious adverse event in a large international pharmacovigilance database.[52] Although drug discontinuation and the administration of corticosteroids frequently result in clinical improvement, as with de novo AIH, long-term immunosuppression may be required, and DI-AIH–related deaths have been reported.[52–54]

Numerous circulating autoantibodies have been identified in patients with AIH, but these lack specificity and play only a minor role in disease pathogenesis. ANAs targeting chromatin and ribonucleoprotein complexes are identified in nearly 80% of patients with AIH, but are also found in patients with other chronic liver diseases, including PBC, PSC, and NASH, dramatically limiting their diagnostic utility.[55] ASMAs show somewhat higher specificity for AIH than ANAs and are moderately sensitive in the diagnosis of AIH.[56] ASMAs target cytoskeletal components, including the microfilament F-actin, and are found in approximately 70% of AIH patients.[57] Higher autoantibody titers (greater than 1:40) have better diagnostic specificity, but the presence of ASMAs in otherwise asymptomatic patients with normal liver function tests generally does not portend the development of AIH.[58] As discussed earlier, the presence of ANAs and ASMAs defines AIH type 1.

In contrast, AIH type 2 is defined by the presence of anti-LKM1 antibodies, targeting CYP2D6; anti–LC-1 antibodies, targeting the folate-metabolizing enzyme formiminotransferase cyclodeaminase (FTCD); and LKM3, targeting uridine diphosphate glucuronosyltransferase (UGT), which is involved with drug and bilirubin metabolism.[59,60] Anti-LKM1 antibodies are generally found in children in the absence of other autoantibodies. As previously discussed, the HLA DQB1*0201 allele is the strongest genetic modifier conferring susceptibility to AIH type 2, although circulating LKM1 may also be associated with the DRB1*0701 allele.[19,27] Interestingly, DRB1*0701 is also associated with persistent HCV infection, at least in northern European Caucasian populations, and low titers of anti-LKM1 may be seen in individuals with chronic HCV, again suggesting the possibility of an infectious trigger in genetically susceptible individuals.[61] However, these antibodies appear to target a different epitope than those present in *de novo* AIH type 2.[7] Currently, the role of the humoral immune response as a mediator of hepatocellular injury in AIH is thought to be limited, at best.

Hepatic injury in AIH is, instead, believed to be primarily a T-cell–mediated process. Impairment of regulatory T-cell (T-reg) function results in a loss of immune tolerance to hepatocellular self antigens, leading to the initiation and propagation of an effector T-cell response.[62] Decreased activity and lower numbers of T-regs in patients with AIH result in an increase in the proliferation of effector T cells as well as their production of proinflammatory cytokines like interferon-gamma (IFN-γ) and IL-4.[63] Although the targeted self antigen is not known for most cases of de novo AIH, CYP2D6, SEPSECS, and FTCD have been well-characterized as the antigenic targets of both B cells and effector T cells in AIH type 2.[64,65] These observations have led some to hypothesize that molecular mimicry (i.e., when an immune response directed against pathogenic organisms or xenobiotics inadvertently targets structurally similar self antigen) may contribute to the development of AIH.[66,67] For example, there is significant sequence homology between CYP2D6 residues 193 to 212 and the HCV and CMV epitopes displayed by antigen-presenting cells, suggesting that viral infection is capable of initiating an inflammatory cascade that leads to a sustained immune response to self antigen.[64] Further work is needed to clarify the complex interplay among the genetic, environmental, and immunological factors that play a role in the pathogenesis of AIH.[68]

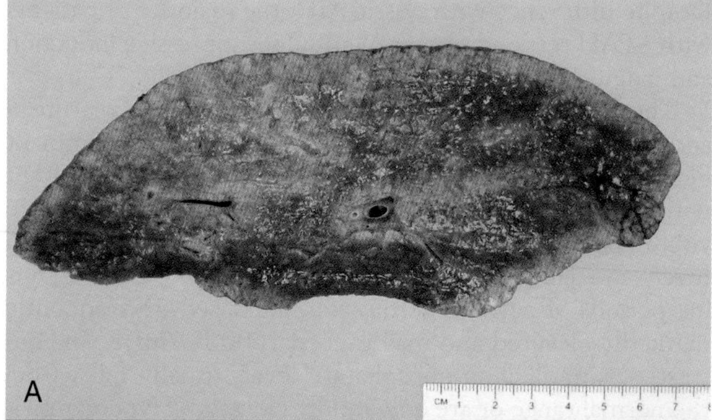

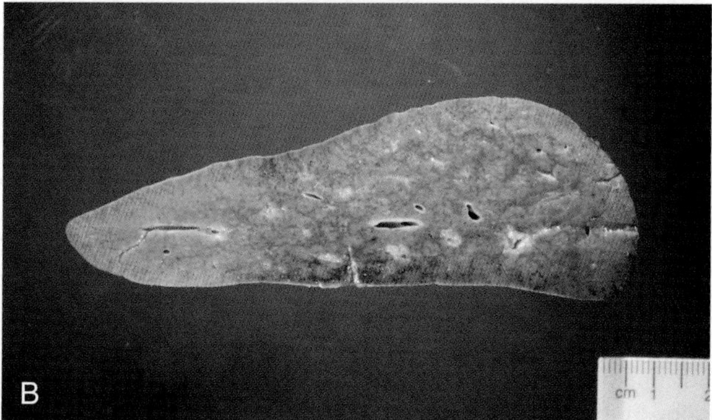

FIGURE 48.1 The liver in autoimmune hepatitis shows no specific gross features. A, In cirrhotic livers, the surface is shrunken and nodular. The cut surface is tan brown and nodular with abundant fibrous tissue. **B,** Livers explanted in the setting of fulminant hepatic failure are soft with large areas of necrosis. Islands of regenerating hepatocellular parenchyma may be identifiable.

Pathology

Gross Findings

Gross examination of the explanted liver for AIH is typically uninformative. Established cirrhosis is present in approximately one-third of AIH patients at the time of initial presentation and frequently shows a mixed micronodular/macronodular pattern that is indistinguishable from that seen in the setting of chronic viral hepatitis or burnt-out steatohepatitis.[69] The surface of the liver appears shrunken and nodular. Sectioning reveals tan-brown to bile-stained regenerative nodules that are enveloped by variably prominent, firm, gray-white fibrous tissues (Fig. 48.1A). The gross appearance of the liver in the setting of a fulminant clinical presentation is similarly nonspecific and is indistinguishable from toxic/drug-mediated injury and viral hepatitis. The hepatic capsule may appear contracted or shriveled. The cut surface frequently shows large areas of hemorrhage and soft necrosis. Islands of residual/regenerating hepatocellular parenchyma are occasionally identifiable in an otherwise necrotic liver (Fig. 48.1B).

Microscopic Findings

The histological appearance of the liver in AIH shows a great deal of variability with respect to grade and stage of the disease, but it tends to show a chronic hepatitis pattern of injury with elements of interface and lobular activity. The portal inflammatory infiltrate is typically rich in both lymphocytes and plasma cells, although variable numbers of histiocytes, eosinophils, and neutrophils may also be present. Plasma cells, in particular, are conspicuous in most cases, frequently forming clusters of greater than 5 cells and outnumbering the lymphocytic component of the inflammatory infiltrate.[70] These plasma cells tend to be immunoreactive for IgG. Although some authors have suggested that a preponderance of IgG-producing plasma cells supports a diagnosis of AIH over PBC, these observations are not specific to AIH, and interpretation of IgG:IgM ratios are challenging, limiting their practical application in routine clinical practice.[71,72] Importantly, the absence of a plasma cell–predominant infiltrate does not exclude a diagnosis of AIH and is occasionally encountered in otherwise typical cases of AIH.[69]

Bile duct inflammation may be seen as a component of AIH, but it does not necessarily imply the presence of an overlap syndrome (see later discussion). In one series, approximately 24% of patients with otherwise classical AIH showed biliary changes, including destructive cholangitis and ductopenia, but responded well to immunosuppression and lacked other histological and serological features of PBC.[73,74] Typically, bile duct changes in AIH are characterized by the presence of occasional mononuclear inflammatory cells with focal, if any, appreciable epithelial injury and the absence of florid duct lesions (Fig. 48.2). Cholestasis is generally not a feature of AIH , though it may be seen in severe cases with marked necroinflammatory activity.

In mildly active cases of AIH, there may be only a subtle, mild increase in portal lymphocytes and plasma cells associated with focal interface activity (Fig. 48.3).

With increasing disease activity, more portal inflammatory cells breech the limiting plate of hepatocytes to involve the periportal lobular parenchyma (Fig. 48.4A). In areas of interface hepatitis, evidence of hepatocellular injury, characterized by cellular swelling and ballooning degeneration, should be evident (Fig. 48.4B). Overt periportal

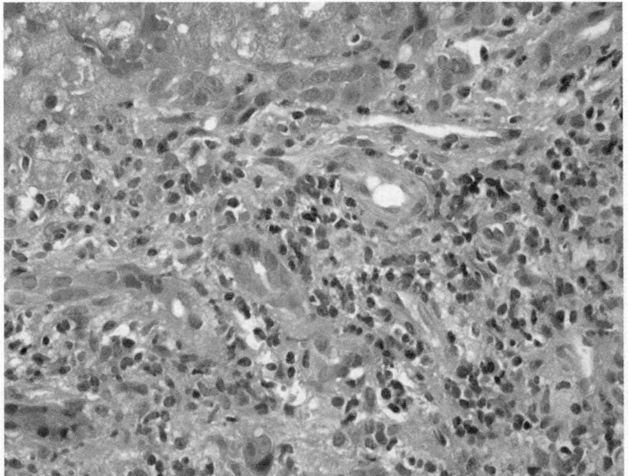

FIGURE 48.2 Native common bile duct branches may be infiltrated by occasional lymphocytes in otherwise typical autoimmune hepatitis. If present at all, bile duct injury is typically mild. Duct loss and florid duct lesions are not typical.

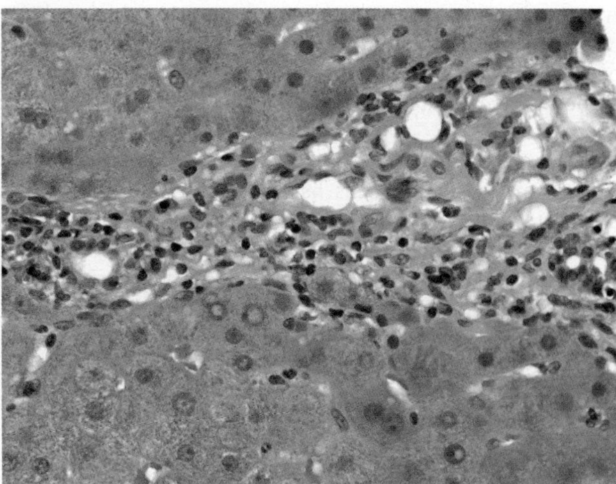

FIGURE 48.3 Autoimmune hepatitis with mild expansion of portal tract by lymphoplasmacytic inflammatory infiltrate and focal interface hepatitis.

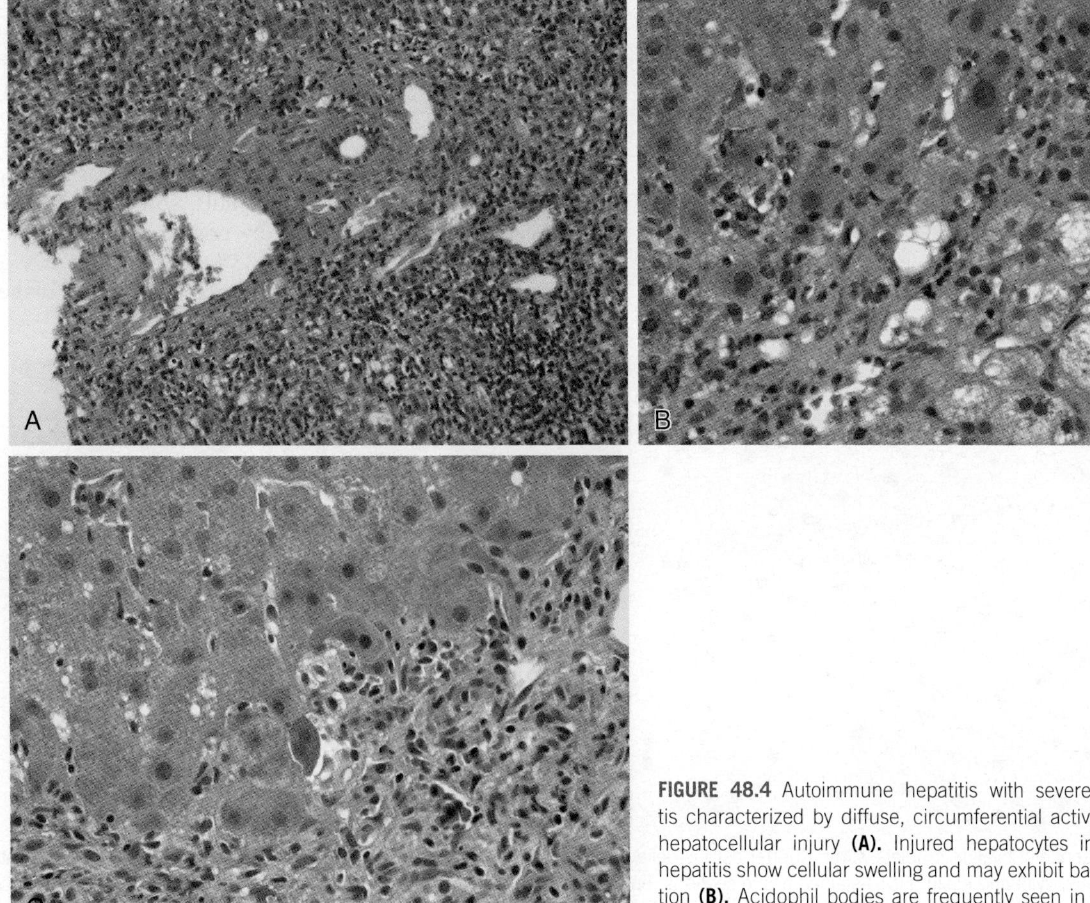

FIGURE 48.4 Autoimmune hepatitis with severe interface hepatitis characterized by diffuse, circumferential activity and associated hepatocellular injury **(A).** Injured hepatocytes in foci of interface hepatitis show cellular swelling and may exhibit ballooning degeneration **(B).** Acidophil bodies are frequently seen in foci with interface activity **(C).**

hepatocellular necrosis and acidophil bodies (Fig. 48.4C) may also be identified and has historically been referred to as *piecemeal necrosis*. Collectively, more than 80% of AIH cases show at least focal interface hepatitis involving most portal areas (Ishak grade A2). However, this histological finding alone is insufficiently specific to discriminate AIH from non-immune causes of acute hepatitis, which exhibit interface activity with a similar frequency. The presence of abundant plasma cells and plasma cell clusters appears to be a better indicator of immune-mediated injury (Fig. 48.5).[75]

More recently, the presence of hyaline droplets in the cytoplasm of Kupffer cells has been described as a novel diagnostic clue that is highly specific for the diagnosis of AIH. In the initial series, well-circumscribed bodies with a glassy appearance were identified in the cytoplasm of Kupffer cells in all of the AIH patients in their cohort and showed outstanding specificity.[76] These hyaline globules are periodic acid–Schiff (PAS) positive, diastase resistant (Fig. 48.6A), and immunoreactive for various immunoglobins, including IgG. Similar results have been reported by other groups, some of which advocate for the inclusion of Kupffer cell hyaline globules as a typical histological feature in the simplified diagnostic criteria for AIH.[11,70]

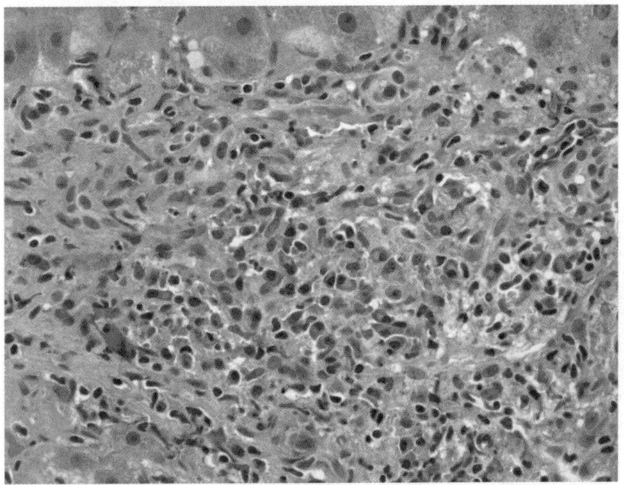

FIGURE 48.5 The presence of numerous plasma cells, including plasma cell clusters, is characteristic of autoimmune hepatitis.

The presence of intact lymphocytes and plasma cells within the cytoplasm of viable hepatocytes (emperipolesis) is identified in the majority of AIH cases (Fig. 48.6B). Data from some groups indicate that emperipolesis is significantly more common in the setting of AIH than it is in chronic viral hepatitis, going so far as to suggest that it is superior to the presence of plasma cells and interface hepatitis as a histological indicator of AIH.[77] Others contest that emperipolesis is difficult to reliably interpret in routine clinical practice and is, instead, correlated with inflammatory grade, regardless of etiology.[70,75] Nevertheless, emperipolesis is currently included with the presence of interface hepatitis and the formation of hepatocyte rosettes as “typical” histology for AIH in the simplified scoring system for AIH (discussed further later).

In addition to increased portal inflammation and interface hepatitis, AIH is typically associated with an element of lobular necroinflammatory activity as well. In cases with mild lobular activity, occasional aggregates of lymphocytes, plasma cells, and ceroid-laden Kupffer cells are identified in association with small foci of hepatocellular dropout (Fig. 48.7A). Acidophil bodies may also be encountered in the lobules, along with swollen hepatocytes with pale, rarefied cytoplasm and usually have no zonal predilection. In cases with severe lobular activity, more extensive lymphoplasmacytic inflammation is typically encountered and may be associated with large swaths of bridging or confluent hepatocellular necrosis (Fig. 48.7B). Regenerative hepatocellular rosettes may also be seen in cases with severe necroinflammatory lobular activity and are considered to be a typical histological feature of AIH that is purported to aid in its discrimination from chronic viral hepatitis (Fig. 48.8). The significance of hepatocellular rosettes has, however, been called into question by one group who identified unequivocal rosettes in only 33% of AIH cases as well as in a similar proportion of cases without AIH.[75] Further

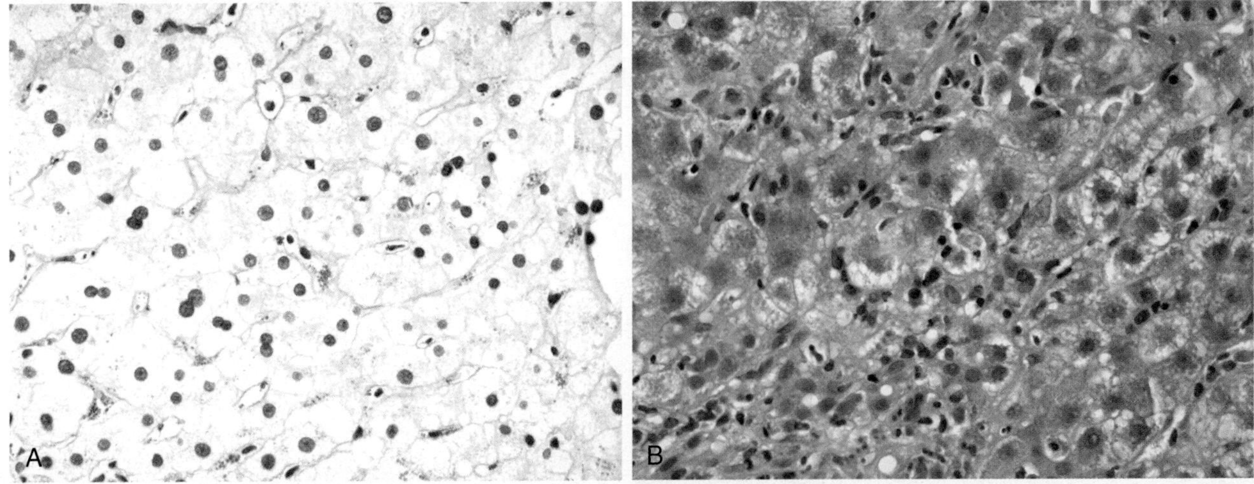

FIGURE 48.6 The presence of hyaline droplets within Kupffer cells is believed to be highly specific for autoimmune hepatitis. These hyaline droplets may be visible on hematoxylin and eosin (H&E)-stained tissue sections, but can be highlighted with a periodic acid-Schiff special stain with diastase digestion **(A).** Emperipolesis (intact lymphocytes and plasma cells within the cytoplasm of hepatocytes) is identified in most cases of autoimmune hepatitis, though it can be seen in other settings as well **(B).**

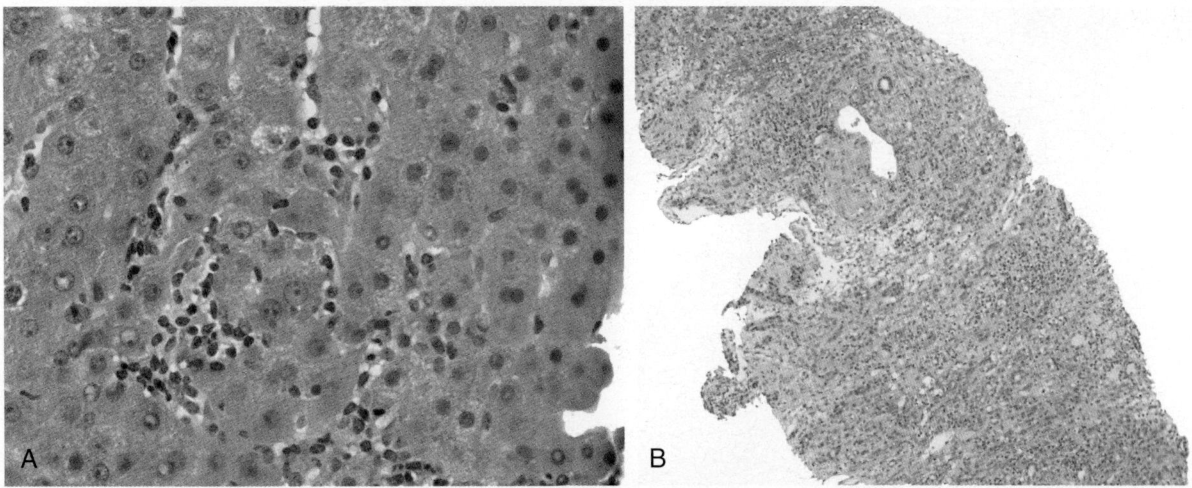

FIGURE 48.7 Lobular necroinflammatory activity is present in most cases of autoimmune hepatitis. A, Mild lobular activity is characterized by occasional aggregates of lymphocytes, plasma cells, and Kupffer cells with focal hepatocyte loss. **B,** Confluent necroinflammatory activity with parenchymal collapse can be seen in more severe cases.

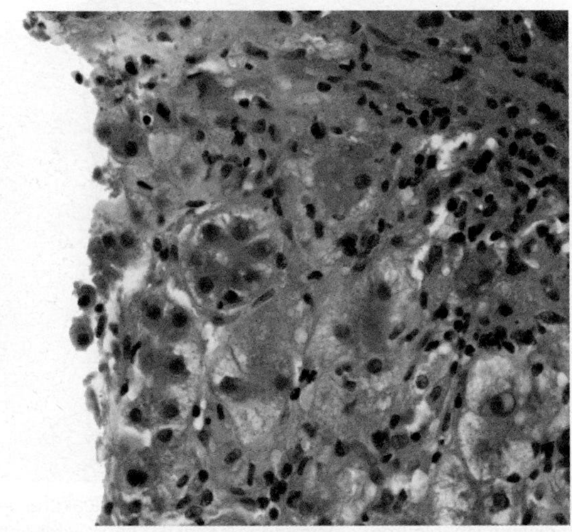

FIGURE 48.8 Regenerative hepatocellular rosettes are a typical histological feature of autoimmune hepatitis according to the simplified criteria. True hepatocellular rosettes have a clearly delineated central lumen.

FIGURE 48.9 Centrilobular necroinflammatory injury may also be present in autoimmune hepatitis. It can be seen in isolation or in addition to otherwise typical interface hepatitis. Perivenular necroinflammatory activity may also be seen in the setting of acute-onset autoimmune hepatitis.

refinement of the histological criteria considered to be typical or compatible with AIH will undoubtably occur in the future.

AIH occasionally presents with a centrilobular-predominant pattern of hepatocellular injury that may or may not be accompanied by increased lymphoplasmacytic portal inflammation and interface hepatitis, but responds well to immunosuppressive therapy (Fig. 48.9).[78] Some have hypothesized that this centrizonal pattern of injury represents an early form of the disease with the potential to progress to more classic AIH, although the recurrence of a predominantly centrizonal pattern of injury during periods of relapse suggests that it may be a distinct variant of immune-mediated liver injury.[79] Prominent centrilobular changes, namely the presence of a plasma cell–enriched inflammation and central perivenulitis, with massive hepatocellular necrosis may also be seen in the setting of AIH-associated acute liver failure.[35] Recognition of this pattern of injury is essential because initiating immunosuppressive therapy early dramatically improves prognosis.[38]

Although cases of acute-onset AIH undoubtably exist, AIH is generally considered to be a chronic disease, and fibrosis is often present at the time of initial clinical presentation.[80] The natural history liver fibrogenesis in AIH follows a similar pattern to that seen in chronic viral hepatitis, beginning with mild expansion of the portal tracts (Fig. 48.10A) and progressing to periportal and bridging fibrosis, and ultimately established cirrhosis (Fig. 48.10B). From a histological perspective, it is often not possible to differentiate cirrhosis that has developed in the setting of AIH from other etiologies, although interface hepatitis and a plasma cell–rich inflammatory infiltrate may occasionally persist. Attempts should, nevertheless, be made

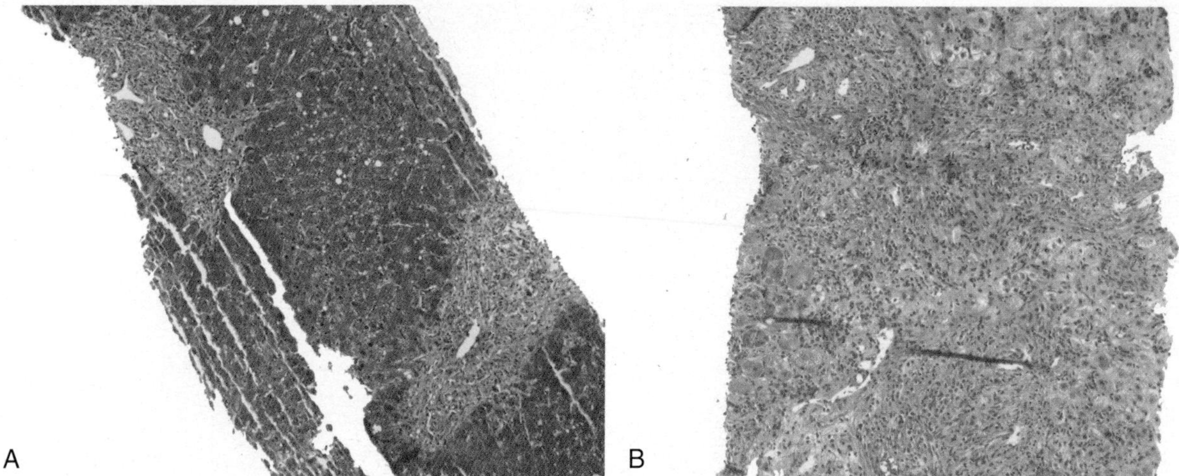

FIGURE 48.10 Autoimmune hepatitis is a chronic disease that leads to the development of liver fibrosis. Fibrosis progresses from a mild expansion of the portal tracts to periportal fibrosis **(A),** bridging fibrosis linking anatomically distinct structures, and ultimately, established cirrhosis **(B)** (Masson trichrome stains).

to accurately characterize the immune-mediated nature of the disease, as fibrogenesis is a dynamic process, and there is mounting evidence that immunosuppressive medical therapy can stabilize or reduce fibrosis stage in a subset of patients.[81,82]

The surgical pathologist's role in the diagnosis of AIH is relatively straightforward, as the histological pattern of injury is only one of the components used to predict a patient's likelihood of having the disease. According to the simplified diagnostic criteria for AIH, typical histological features of AIH include the presence of interface hepatitis, emperipolesis, and hepatocellular rosette formation, while features compatible with AIH are characterized by a chronic hepatitis pattern of injury, but fall short of that which is considered to be typical (see Table 48.3).[11] Correlating these histological findings with laboratory studies for circulating AIH-associated antibodies and serum IgG has excellent specificity for the diagnosis of AIH.[83] Other groups have proposed modified scoring systems that consider prominent plasma cells and Kupffer cell hyaline globules as typical features of AIH or require exclusion of biliary features using copper special stains and immunohistochemical stains for CK7, which purportedly identify cases of AIH that would have been misdiagnosed by applying the simplified score.[70,75] Further validation is, however, required, particularly in the setting of overlap syndromes in which features of biliary injury and chronic cholestasis coexist with typical features of AIH.

Differential Diagnosis

The pattern of injury seen in AIH is insufficiently specific to render a diagnosis based on histological findings alone. As such, the clinical exclusion of infectious, toxic, and metabolic etiologies is an essential component to the diagnostic workup of a patient with suspected AIH. Acute-onset AIH frequently shows extensive lobular and perivenular activity as well as perivenular necrosis.[35] The differential diagnosis for an acute hepatitis pattern of injury includes infectious etiologies, such as acute viral hepatitis A, B, and E, as well as infection with the Epstein-Barr virus and other nonhepatotropic viruses. Acute viral hepatitis A, in particular, may show a pronounced plasma cell–rich portal inflammatory infiltrate, along with interface activity and periportal necrosis (Fig. 48.11).[84] Acute viral hepatitis E is also characterized by an expansion of the portal tracts by a dense inflammatory infiltrate, although it is typically largely lymphocytic and associated with bile duct injury and cholestasis. The presence of centrizonal necrosis may also cause diagnostic confusion with acute-onset AIH.[85] Complicating matters further, patients previously diagnosed with AIH more frequently have antibodies to the hepatitis E virus than patients with other immune disorders and other forms of chronic viral hepatitis, and infection may contribute to severity of hepatocellular injury.[86] Although application of the modified and simplified International Hepatitis Group scoring systems can effectively discriminate AIH from acute viral hepatitis, this is rarely a diagnostic dilemma because serological studies for circulating antibodies and quantitative polymerase chain reaction (qPCR) testing for viral genetic material can reliably identify an active infection.[10,11,87]

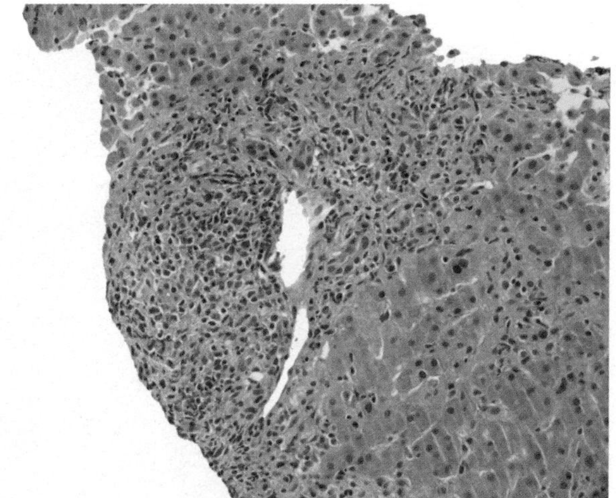

FIGURE 48.11 Viral infection can produce histological changes virtually indistinguishable from autoimmune hepatitis. Acute viral hepatitis A infection may show expansion of the portal tracts by a plasma cell–rich inflammatory infiltrate and interface hepatitis. The exclusion of an infectious etiology is essential to the diagnosis of autoimmune hepatitis.

Distinguishing AIH from DILI is complicated because some commonly prescribed medications have the potential to induce immune-mediated liver injury. DI-AIH can occur unpredictably, occasionally many months after initial exposure, and ongoing injury can be sustained following drug withdrawal.[88] Although some authors have proposed models that incorporate portal inflammation, portal plasma cells, intraacinar eosinophils, hepatocellular rosette formation, and cholestasis as a means to discriminate AIH from DILI, this may be challenging in routine clinical practice (Fig. 48.12).[89,90] The clinical exclusion of recent exposure to known or suspected hepatotoxic drugs and the application of the well-validated modified scoring system almost certainly have better performance characteristics than histological assessment alone.

The clinical differential for a patient with metabolic risk factors and increased transaminases will frequently include both nonalcoholic fatty liver disease (NAFLD) and AIH. This is, at least in part, caused by the fact that ANAs and ASMAs are significantly more common in patients with NAFLD than they are in the general population.[91] Autoantibody titers are, however, generally lower in patients with NAFLD than that seen in the setting of AIH, although there is significant overlap.[92] In situations in which there is diagnostic uncertainty, liver biopsy may be performed and shows good diagnostic accuracy.[93,94] The distinction between AIH and uncomplicated steatosis is typically straightforward because the presence of steatotic hepatocytes associated with minimal portal and lobular inflammation is not a typical feature of AIH. Discriminating AIH from nonalcoholic steatohepatitis (NASH) may be more challenging in some instances because portal inflammation is increased in progressive NAFLD and NASH, which may also show concurrent lobular inflammation and associated hepatocellular injury.[95] Interface hepatitis and plasma cell clusters would, however, be unusual in NASH. Conversely, the presence of hepatocellular ballooning and zone 3–predominant pericellular ("chicken wire") fibrosis is said to favor a diagnosis of NASH, as these findings are not typical for AIH.[69] Of course, given the prevalence of the metabolic syndrome in Western populations, AIH may coexist with NAFLD/NASH, which poses additional diagnostic challenges that are not adequately addressed by current scoring systems.[96,97]

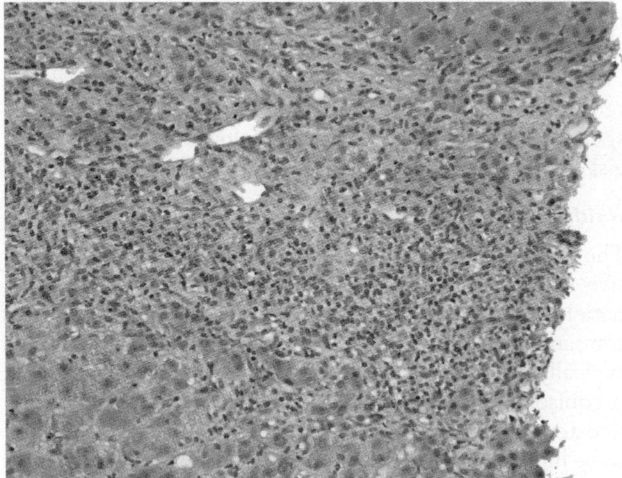

FIGURE 48.12 Distinguishing autoimmune hepatitis from drug-induced liver injury may be impossible. Nitrofurantoin, in particular, can induce an immune-mediated pattern of injury with numerous plasma cells and interface hepatitis.

Cases of AIH with prominent portal inflammation and less lobular activity may mimic chronic viral hepatitis. As discussed previously in the context of acute viral hepatitis, the exclusion of infection is easily accomplished with serological and PCR-based studies, so this is rarely a clinical question. Nevertheless, there are several morphological clues that may be helpful in suggesting the proper diagnosis if these studies have not been performed or are not yet available. The portal inflammatory infiltrate in chronic viral hepatitis C is typically rich in lymphocytes. Lymphoid aggregates are often particularly prominent and may have well-developed germinal centers.[98] Interface hepatitis is often present, but it is usually only mild and focal, and lobular injury is nearly always minimal (Fig. 48.13A). In contrast, lobular and

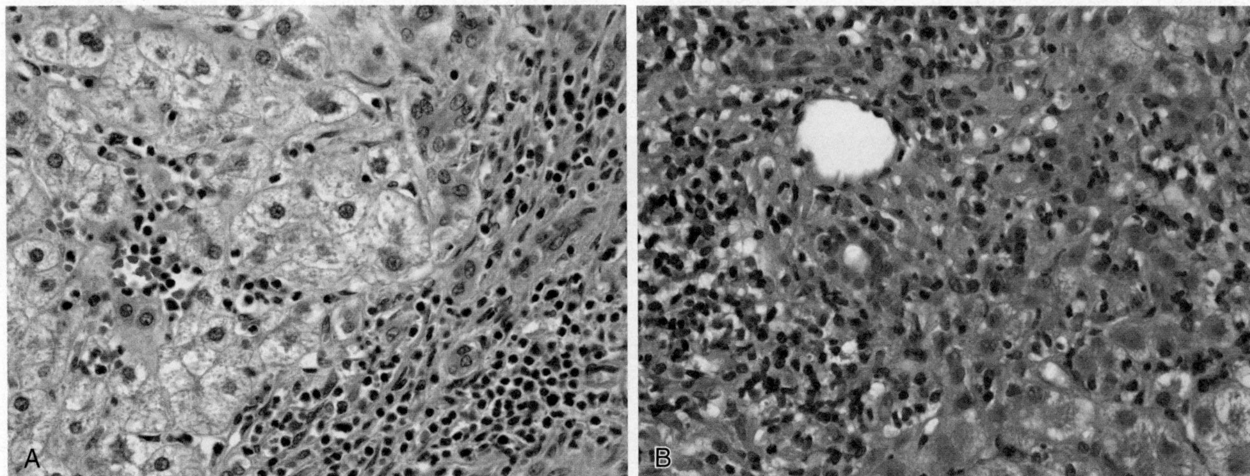

FIGURE 48.13 There is significant overlap between the histological features of chronic viral hepatitis and autoimmune hepatitis. **A,** In chronic viral hepatitis C, the portal inflammatory infiltrate is largely lymphocytic, and well-formed lymphoid aggregates may be prominent. Interface hepatitis is usually identifiable, but it is typically mild and focal. **B,** Plasma cells are usually more conspicuous in autoimmune hepatitis. Interface hepatitis is typically robust, and lobular necroinflammatory activity is more widespread and prominent.

interface activity is usually prominent in AIH (Fig. 48.13B). The presence of numerous or clustered plasma cells is also said to be relatively specific for AIH, although they may also be seen in the setting of chronic viral hepatitis C.[75,99]

In contrast with chronic viral hepatitis C, interface and lobular activity is often quite robust in chronic viral hepatitis B(HBV), particularly during the phase of immune clearance, or following the emergence of viral mutants or superinfection with the hepatitis D virus.[100,101] In these scenarios, periportal inflammation with interface hepatitis is often marked, and lobular necrosis can be extensive. Plasma cells are, again, thought to be uncommon in chronic viral hepatitis B compared with AIH, and viral surface and core antigen may be identifiable on H&E-stained tissue sections as cytoplasmic ground-glass inclusions and sanded nuclei, respectively.[102,103] These viral antigens can be identified with immunohistochemical stains performed on slides cut from formalin-fixed, paraffin-embedded tissue, but quantifying HBV DNA in a blood sample by qPCR is the most reliable means of detecting infection. Again, both the modified and simplified scoring systems are able to differentiate chronic viral hepatitis from AIH.

Given significant differences in treatment guidelines, AIH must be differentiated from PBC and PSC. From a biochemical standpoint, this is often not a challenge as AIH presents with a hepatitic pattern of liver injury, whereas PBC and PSC are characterized by cholestatic liver chemistries. The ratio of serum alkaline phosphatase (ALP) relative to transaminase levels is, in fact, a component of the modified scoring system, with lower AP levels favoring a diagnosis of AIH.[10] The absence of significant periportal copper deposition and large numbers of CK7-positive intermediate hepatobiliary cells also argue against a chronic cholestatic process in newer AIH scoring schemes.[75] Serum antimitochondrial antibodies (AMAs), particularly those targeting PDH-E2, are extremely sensitive and specific for PBC, although other AMAs may occasionally be detected in patients with AIH.[104] From a histological perspective, although focal bile duct inflammation is not infrequently encountered in AIH, destructive cholangitis with bile duct loss and florid duct lesions is not a feature of this disease and readily distinguishes it from PBC in most cases. Similarly, the presence of concentric fibrosis with obliterative bile duct scarring and loss is seen in PSC but not in AIH. Abnormal cholangiographic studies demonstrating bile duct strictures also strongly favor a diagnosis of PSC.

Variant forms of AIH with superimposed chronic cholestatic features (overlap syndromes) are discussed later in this chapter.

Grading and Staging

No grading and staging scheme has been developed for AIH. The system developed by Batts and Ludwig in 1995 is still routinely used in clinical practice to grade disease activity in chronic hepatitis, including AIH. The degree of interface hepatitis and lobular inflammation and necrosis are separately graded based on the intensity and distribution of necroinflammatory activity, with the more severe lesion determining the overall grade (Table 48.4). The degree of fibrosis is considered separately, with mild fibrous expansion of the portal tracts being characterized as stage 1, periportal fibrosis with fine strands of fibrosis in zone 1 as stage 2, septal fibrosis with connective tissue bridges linking anatomically distinct structures as stage 3, and established cirrhosis with nodular remodeling as stage 4.[105]

Other scoring systems such as the Scheuer system, French METAVIR system, Knodell system, and Ishak system may also be used with the choice being dictated by the specific needs of the treating hepatologist and the pathologist's experience with each system.[106-109]

Natural History and Treatment

The majority of cases of AIH respond to immunosuppressive medical therapy, which should be considered in all patients with active hepatic inflammation and elevated transaminases. Induction immunosuppression therapy is typically corticosteroid-based with either prednisone or prednisolone.[43] More recently, budesonide, a synthetic corticosteroid with high first-pass metabolism, has been shown to be highly efficacious at treating AIH while showing fewer steroid-specific side effects than prednisone.[110] The utility of budesonide is severely limited, however, in patients with significant portosystemic shunting, including those with established cirrhosis.[111]

Azathioprine may also be started at the initiation of induction therapy, although most centers delay administration for 2 weeks until steroid responsiveness is confirmed and testing for thiopurine methyltransferase activity

TABLE 48.4 Grading of Disease Activity in Chronic Hepatitis*

Grading Terminology		Criteria	
Semiquantitative Score	**Descriptive**	**Interface Hepatitis**	**Lobular Inflammation and Necrosis**
0	Portal inflammation only; no activity	None	None
1	Minimal	Minimal, patchy	Minimal; occasionally spotty necrosis
2	Mild	Mild; involving some or all portal tracts	Mild; little hepatocellular damage
3	Moderate	Moderate; involving all portal tracts	Moderate; with noticeable hepatocellular change
4	Severe	Severe; may have bridging necrosis	Severe; with prominent diffuse hepatocellular damage

**When a discrepancy exists between criteria, the more severe lesion should determine overall grade.*
From Batts KP, Ludwig J. Chronic hepatitis. An update on terminology and reporting. Am J Surg Pathol. *1995;19(12):1409-1417.*

excludes patients at high-risk for therapy-induced myelosuppression. Corticosteroids are gradually weened following normalization of serum aminotransferases and IgG. After 6 months, most patients can be maintained on azathioprine alone or another steroid-sparing agent like mycophenolate mofetil.[112,113]

Historically, AIH relapse following the withdrawal of immunosuppression was common. Patients with 2 years of sustained biochemical remission on monotherapy appear to have a greater likelihood of successfully discontinuing immunosuppression, although remission still occurs in approximately one-half of these patients. Higher serum transaminase levels during maintenance appears to be associated with a greater risk for relapse.[114] Most cases of relapse occur during the first 3 months following cessation of immunosuppression, although late relapses may also occur.[115] Biochemical response to further immunosuppressive therapy is typical following relapse.

The role of liver biopsy before the withdrawal of immunosuppressive therapy is somewhat controversial. Although the 2019 American Association for the Study of Liver Diseases (AASLD) practice guidelines acknowledge the utility of liver biopsy at excluding the presence of clinically unsuspected inflammation, histological examination is not mandatory in adults.[43] This is, at least in part, due to the fact that in one study, nearly one-half of patients with a sustained biochemical response on maintenance therapy and an absence of active inflammation at the time of biopsy experience disease relapse.[114] In contrast, prewithdrawal biopsy is still recommended in pediatric populations because the absence of inflammation appears to be associated with a greater likelihood of sustained remission.[116]

Treatment protocols for AIH continue to evolve but are effective at inducing remission in most instances. Nevertheless, approximately one-third of AIH patients have established cirrhosis at the time of initial presentation, and AIH is considered to be an appropriate indication for liver transplantation. Graft and patient survival in this population is generally very good.[117] However, AIH is reported to recur in 17% to 34% of allografts, but it can usually be managed with increased immunosuppression.[118,119]

PRIMARY BILIARY CHOLANGITIS

The term *primary biliary cirrhosis* was introduced by Ahrens and colleagues in 1950.[120] Most patients showed advanced fibrosis at diagnosis, hence for many decades the term *primary biliary cirrhosis* was accepted. In retrospect, this term is a misnomer because cirrhosis is not present in most patients at clinical presentation. This term *primary biliary cholangitis* has thus replaced the original term, and fortunately the acronym *PBC* stands unchanged.[121] PBC is a chronic bile duct–destructive disease that results in progressive cholestasis and cirrhosis. Although the precise pathogenesis remains uncertain, considerable evidence indicates that it is an autoimmune disease that occurs in genetically predisposed individuals after stimulation by an environmental factor. The diagnosis of PBC is based on cholestatic liver function tests, positive AMAs, and liver histology that is compatible with PBC. However, a biopsy is not an absolute requirement; the combination of abnormal liver chemistry and AMA has a sensitivity and specificity of >95%.

Clinical Features and Epidemiology

The incidence of the disease ranges from 0.9 to 5.8 per 100,000 people.[122] The key features of PBC are listed in Table 48.5 and compared with other cholestatic liver diseases. Approximately 90% of patients with PBC are female between 40 and 60 years of age (range, 20 to 80 years) (Box 48.2).[123] PBC occurs worldwide, and all races are susceptible.[123,124] There is some familial clustering of PBC, although less than 1% of first-degree relatives of patients with PBC develop the disorder.

Many patients with PBC are asymptomatic at presentation, detected primarily by the report of abnormal liver function tests. The early phase of disease is insidious, and symptomatic patients primarily report itching and fatigue. In later stages, the signs and symptoms of disease are either related to progressive cholestasis or cirrhosis. Among the former are pruritus, xanthomas, jaundice, and osteoporosis. The signs and symptoms of cirrhosis in PBC are the same as for other causes of cirrhosis: esophagogastric varices, ascites, spider angiomas, and splenomegaly.

PBC coexists with other autoimmune diseases; the strongest recognized associations are with connective tissue disorders such as rheumatoid arthritis, CREST syndrome (*c*alcinosis, *R*aynaud disease, *e*sophageal dysmotility, *s*clerodactyly, and *t*elangiectasia), systemic lupus erythematosus, Sjögren syndrome, dermatomyositis, interstitial lung disease, and autoimmune thyroid disease.[125,126]

Pathogenesis

The etiology of PBC is favored to be related to an interaction between genetic predisposition and environmental triggers.

Genetic Predisposition

Genetic predisposition is evidenced by a higher incidence in family members; 1.2% children of affected patients develop this disease, although the risk is highest among daughters of women with PBC.[127] A concordance rate of 60% in monozygotic twins has been described.[128] A strong linkage has been identified between HLA alleles and primary biliary cholangitis. DRB1*08, DR3, DPB1*0301, DRB1*08-DQA1*0401, and DQB1*04 are associated with susceptibility to the disorder, while DRB1*11 and DRB1*13 confers protection.[127] Genome-wide studies have identified associations between PBC and genes that involve myeloid cell differentiation and antigen presentation.[129] The evidence for environmental triggers comes in the form of geographic clustering; case clusters have been identified at sites of toxic waste disposal and low-income areas.

There is strong evidence that PBC represents an autoimmune attack directed toward autoantigens on biliary epithelium. PBC is thought to be initiated when tolerance to the 2-oxo-acid dehydrogenase complex (2-OADC), particularly the E2 subunit of pyruvate dehydrogenase complex (PDC-E2), is lost, resulting in development of these specific autoantibodies. The mechanisms underlying the development of these antibodies remains unknown. However, given that these mitochondrial proteins are highly conserved during evolution, molecular mimicry across bacterial organisms and loss of self tolerance resulting in autoantibody formation represents one plausible hypothesis

TABLE 48.5 Comparison of Key Clinical, Laboratory, and Radiological Features of Autoimmune Hepatitis, Primary Biliary Cholangitis, Primary Sclerosing Cholangitis, and IgG4-Related Sclerosing Cholangitis

	AIH	PBC	PSC	IgG4-RSC
Demographics	Female predominant (4:1) and all ages	Female predominant (9:1); usually >50 yr	Male predominant (7:3); classically diagnosed in 40s, associated with inflammatory bowel disease	Male predominant (4:1) Adults typically >40 yr
Symptoms	Commonly asymptomatic; symptomatic patients report jaundice, upper abdominal pain, and fatigue	Commonly asymptomatic; symptomatic patients report fatigue, pruritus, and occasionally xanthoma	Commonly asymptomatic; symptomatic patients report pruritus, abdominal pain, or jaundice	Painless jaundice
Liver function tests	Elevated ALT/AST	Elevated ALP, γ–GT	Elevated ALP, γ–GT	Elevated ALP, γ–GT
Dominant immunoglobulin	IgG	IgM	Mild IgG or IgM increase	IgG4
Autoantibodies	ANA, ASMAs (type 1 AIH) LKM1 (type 2 AIH), LC-1 (type 2 AIH), SLA/LP	AMA	No specific associations, frequently ANA/SMA positive	No specific associations, ANA may be positive
Cholangiogram	Normal	Normal	Strictures, beaded appearance	Strictures, beaded appearance
Key histology	Interface hepatitis, plasma cells	Florid duct lesion, lymphocytic cholangitis	Periductal onion-skin–like fibrosis	Portal-based inflammatory nodules, increased IgG4 cells
Therapy	Steroids and azathioprine as first line	UDCA	No proven therapy	Steroid and rituximab
Survival	Excellent	UDCA responders have normal life expectancy	Symptomatic patients ~50% chance of need for transplant over 15 years	Excellent

AIH, *Autoimmune hepatitis;* ALP, *alkaline phosphatase;* ALT, *alanine transaminase;* AMAs, *antimitochondrial antibodies;* ANAs, *antinuclear antibodies;* ASMAs, *anti–smooth muscle antibodies;* AST, *aspartate transaminase;* γ-GT, *γ–glutamyltransferase;* IgG4-RSC, *IgG4-related sclerosing cholangitis;* LC-1, *anti–liver cytosol 1;* LKM1, *anti–liver kidney microsomal 1;* PBC, *primary biliary cholangitis;* PSC, *primary sclerosing cholangitis;* SLA/LP, *soluble liver and pancreas antigen;* UDCA, *ursodeoxycholic acid.*

BOX 48.2 Key Features of Primary Biliary Cholangitis

- >90% of patients are women
- Positive antimitochondrial antibody is the key serological test positive in >95% of patients
- Cholestatic liver chemistry with elevated alkaline phosphatase and γ–glutamyltransferase
- Florid duct lesions represent key histological feature
- Differential diagnosis includes primary sclerosing cholangitis, drug-induced bile duct disease, and other causes of granulomatous hepatitis
- Ursodeoxycholic acid (UDCA) is first-line treatment

for the development of these antimitochondrial antibodies (AMA).[130]

The diagnosis of PBC typically requires a combination of positive AMA and elevated alkaline phosphatase in a patient without other causes of intrahepatic or extrahepatic cholestasis. A liver biopsy is not considered necessary to establish a diagnosis of PBC. Liver biopsy is considered essential only when the serology is atypical (i.e., negative AMA, a biochemical profile that shows a mixed cholestatic and hepatitic pattern) and when concurrent hepatic injury such as nonalcoholic steatohepatitis is considered.

A disproportionately elevated alkaline phosphatase relative to serum aminotransferases is a characteristic feature of PBC. All classes of serum immunoglobulins may be elevated, although a disproportionate increase in serum IgM is another characteristic feature of PBC. Total bilirubin is typically normal, elevated only in the end stage of disease. ANA positivity is seen in approximately one-third of patients.[131]

AMA constitutes the single most useful assay for the diagnosis of PBC at a titer of >1:40.[132] AMAs can be detected using either immunofluorescence or ELISA to the specific antigens.

AMA is identified in 95% of patients with PBC. AMA is also a highly specific test, identified in less than 1% of healthy individuals. Notably, a significant proportion of "healthy" patients with a positive AMA will eventually develop primary biliary cholangitis.[133] AMA targets the 2-oxo-acid dehydrogenase complexes (2-OADC), an enzyme complex present on the inner mitochondrial membrane. This complex includes pyruvate dehydrogenase (PDC-E2), branched chain 2-oxo-acid dehydrogenase (BCOADC-E2), and 2-oxo-glutaric acid dehydrogenase (OADC-E2).[134] Other antibodies that could be helpful in the context of PBC are anti-gp210 and anti-sp100, both ANAs. These are particularly helpful in the context of AMA-negative PBC.[134] ANAs are detected in a minority of patients, and their presence has been linked with a poor prognosis.[135]

Pathology

Gross Pathology

In early-stage PBC, the liver is often slightly enlarged and variably bile stained. In later stages, macronodular cirrhosis develops and is often associated with an intense green hue that reflects progressive cholestasis (Fig. 48.14). In contrast with PSC, cholangiectases and cholangitic abscesses are not seen.

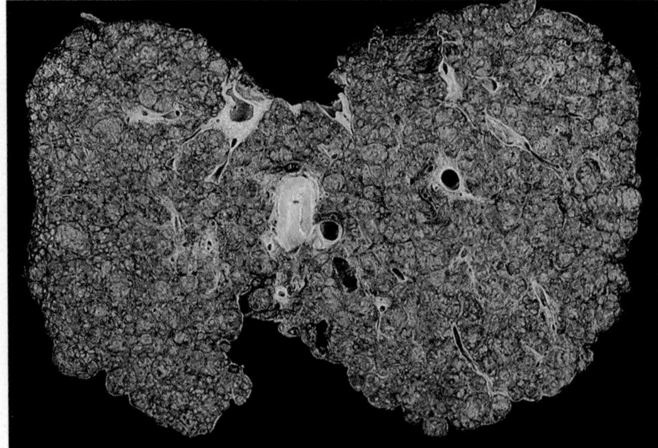

FIGURE 48.14 Gross appearance of stage 4 primary biliary cholangitis. A mixture of tan and green regenerative nodules is typical. (*Courtesy of Herschel Carpenter, MD, and Gerald Dayharsh, MD, Mayo Clinic, Rochester, MN.*)

Microscopic Pathology

Early and Intermediate Phase of Disease. The hallmark lesion of PBC is destructive cholangitis that affects interlobular and septal bile ducts (<70 to 80 μm in diameter) and ultimately results in duct loss. Unlike PSC, the large and extrahepatic ducts are spared. The term *nonsuppurative destructive cholangitis* accurately describes these lesions, but the more succinct term *florid duct lesion* is more commonly used (Figs. 48.15 to 48.18). Because these lesions are usually focal, they may be missed on liver biopsy. The florid duct lesion is characterized by an ill-defined cluster of epithelioid histiocytes (granuloma) accompanied by lymphocytes that are centered on septal and interlobular bile ducts, with histological evidence of bile duct damage and destruction. Well-formed sarcoidal-type granulomas are uncommon.

The bile duct damage in florid duct lesions is usually segmental in the longitudinal axis of the duct and in cross-section, with only a portion of the duct affected at one time. Granulomas are often poorly defined and tend to be associated with the bile duct in an eccentric fashion, although

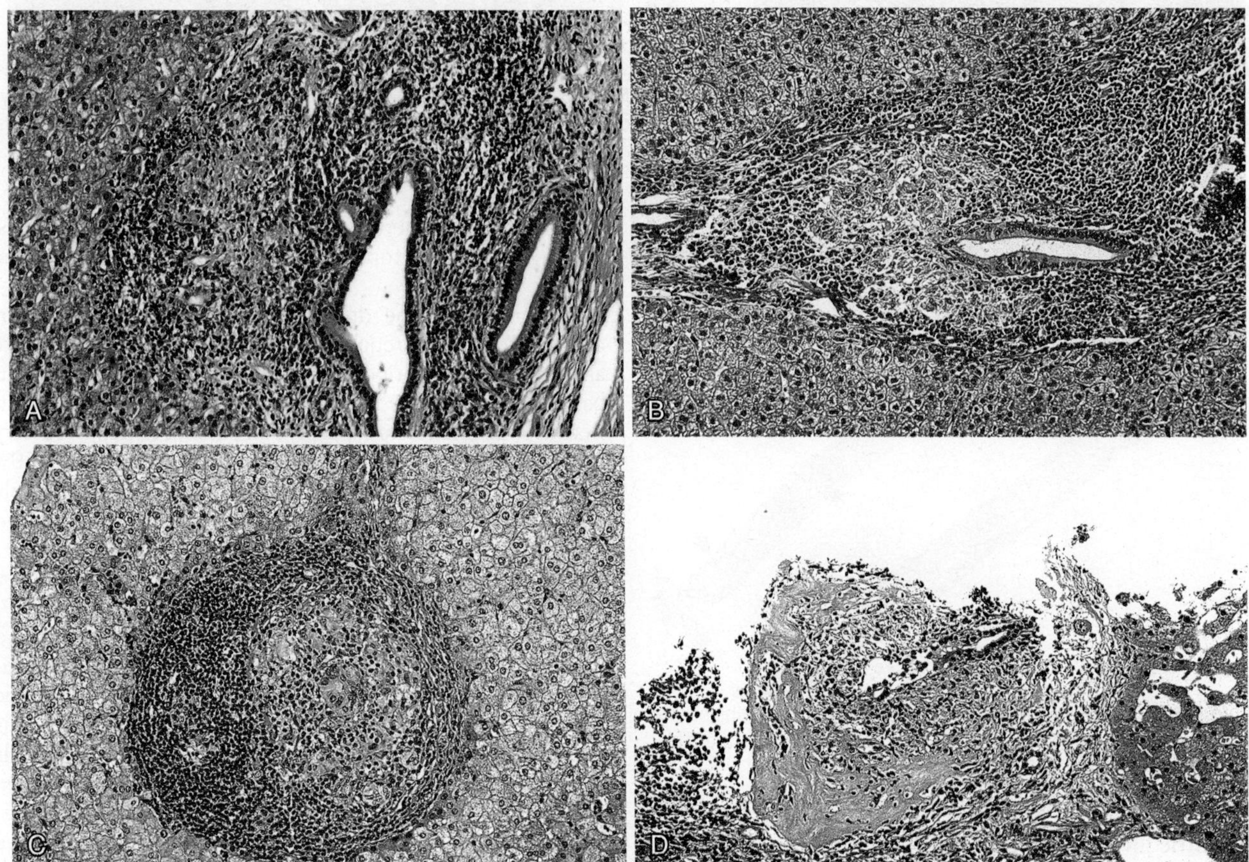

FIGURE 48.15 Granulomatous duct destruction in primary biliary cholangitis. Also referred to as *florid duct lesions,* they are characterized by granulomatous and lymphocytic cholangitis, which varies from ill-defined subtle lesions **(A)** to more obvious granulomas (**B** and **C**) to occasionally sclerotic granulomas **(D).** These lesions can involve ducts eccentrically or concentrically and are associated with breakdown of the basement membrane and eventual duct loss. Granulomatous duct destruction is often patchy, as evidenced by the sparing of some portal tracts, some portions of one bile duct **(B),** and some bile ducts within one portal tract **(A).**

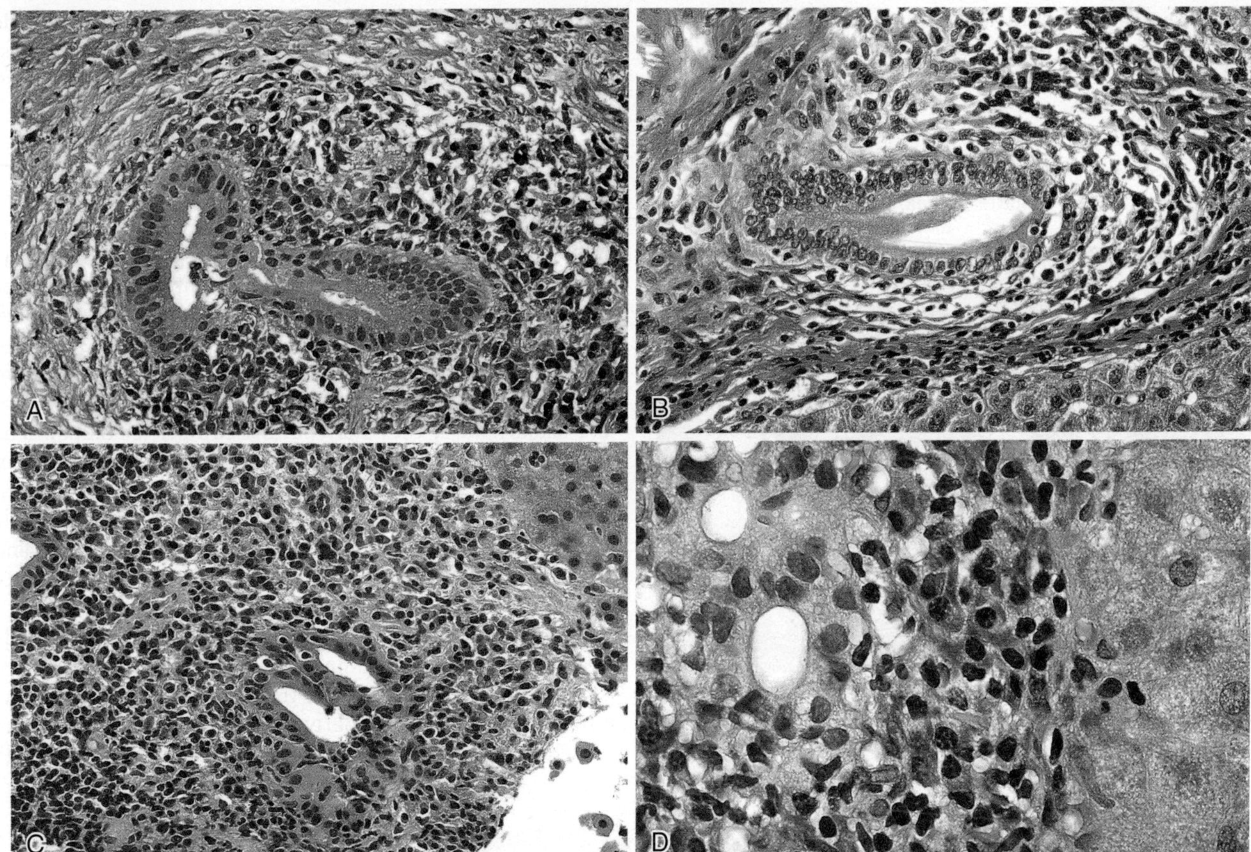

FIGURE 48.16 Lymphocytic cholangitis in primary biliary cholangitis (PBC). Intraepithelial lymphocytes are common in typical (i.e., antimitochondrial antibody [AMA]-positive) PBC **(A)** and in autoimmune cholangitis (i.e., AMA-negative PBC) **(B).** When associated with duct destruction, they have been referred to as *florid duct lesions* in typical PBC **(C)** and autoimmune cholangitis **(D),** but they can also be seen in primary sclerosing cholangitis, autoimmune hepatitis, and chronic viral- and drug-associated hepatitis.

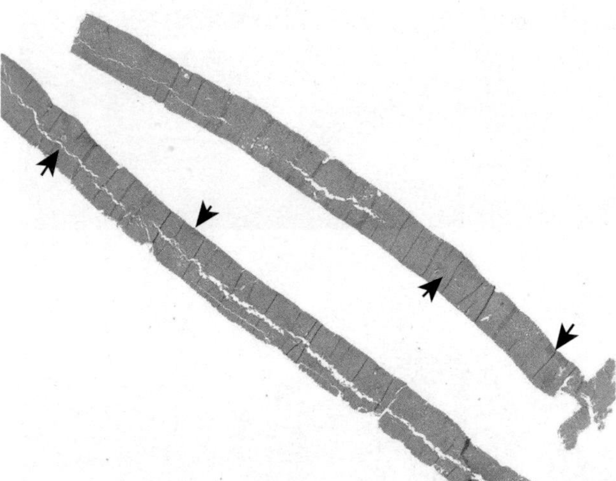

FIGURE 48.17 Primary biliary cholangitis. Low-power image highlights the patchy nature of the disease. The inflamed portal tracts are highlighted by the *arrows*.

concentric involvement may also be seen. Granulomas may also be found in portal structures without an obvious connection to a bile duct. Less commonly, they may be found in hepatic lobules. Additional characteristic features, but with a less dramatic form of bile duct injury, include disruption of the bile duct basement membrane (highlighted on a PAS/D stain), intraepithelial lymphocytes and plasma cells, biliary epithelial cytoplasmic vacuolization, and occasional mitotic figures.

The result of the destructive cholangitis is disappearance of the duct, frequently leaving a lymphoid aggregate and sometimes periodic acid Schiff–positive amorphous basement membrane material as remnants of the lost duct. Because the bile ducts typically run parallel to hepatic artery branches, the finding of an unaccompanied artery in >50% of portal tracts is presumptive evidence of a vanishing bile duct disease. All of these changes are typically accompanied by bile ductular proliferation.

Bile duct changes are also typically accompanied by a dense portal lymphoplasmacytic infiltrate (see Fig. 48.17; Fig. 48.19), which is typically patchy in early stages and may contain lymphoid aggregates and follicles, conspicuous plasma cells, and a few eosinophils. Plasma cells may be particularly conspicuous, mimicking AIH. Biliary damage is likely primarily caused by the T-cell infiltrates, but B cells appear to participate, primarily in the early stages. When comparing AIH and PBC in terms of plasma cell subsets, IgG-positive cells strongly predominate over IgM-positive cells in AIH, but in PBC, IgM-positive plasma cells are much more conspicuous and may predominate. However, subtyping of immunoglobulin subclasses is seldom performed in clinical practice. The portal lymphocytic infiltrate may spill over into the lobules, mimicking interface hepatitis, the so-called *biliary type piecemeal necrosis* (see Fig. 48.19). Unlike AIH, hepatocyte necrosis at the interface is exceptionally uncommon.

The hepatic lobules usually do not show significant histological changes. In some cases, clusters of lymphocytes and plasma cells may aggregate in the lobules, although acidophil bodies are absent or inconspicuous (Fig. 48.20A). Scattered, usually small, noncaseating, lobular granulomas may be seen as well on occasion (Fig. 48.20B).

A subtle form of nodular regenerative hyperplasia has been observed in almost 50% of patients with early-stage disease, and it may be prudent to perform a reticulin stain in select cases.[136] These changes may reflect portal venule damage by granulomas and contribute to the early development of portal hypertension. Portal hypertension may develop in noncirrhotic PBC patients, and some are associated with nodular regenerative hyperplasia.[136]

Late Phase of the Disease. Regenerative nodules in PBC and PSC are usually not as regular and round as in other forms of cirrhosis. The nodules often have a garland-shaped, irregular outline, not unlike pieces of a jigsaw puzzle. A progressive loss of ducts may occur early in the course of disease, with ductopenia usually being prominent in the later phase of the disease (Figs. 48.21 and 48.22). Florid duct lesions become less common with advancing stage, presumably reflecting loss of the target biliary epithelium.

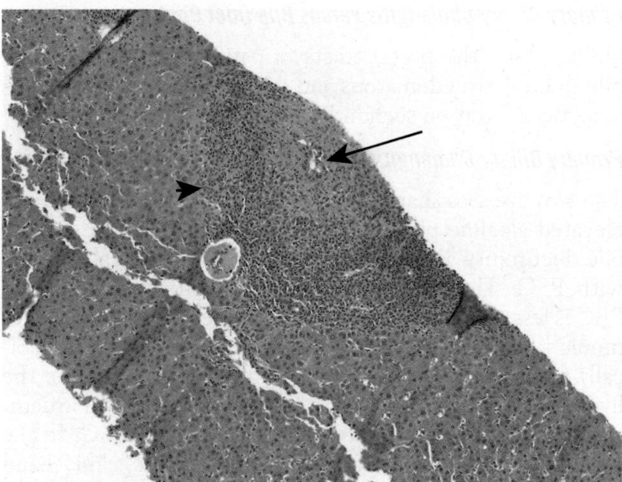

FIGURE 48.18 Primary biliary cholangitis. A florid duct lesion is shown. The bile duct *(arrow)* shows histological evidence of damage as evidenced by the irregular outline and cytoplasmic eosinophilia of biliary cells. The duct is surrounded by histiocyte-rich infiltrate. Also note the dense portal lymphoplasmacytic infiltrate *(arrowhead)*.

Periportal hepatocyte feathery degeneration, which is thought to reflect bile acid (cholate) stasis, helps distinguish PBC and PSC from chronic hepatitis resulting from autoimmune, viral, or drug causes. Additional changes associated with cholestatic liver include Mallory bodies and deposition of copper in periportal/periseptal hepatocytes (see Fig. 48.22C,D). The combined low-magnification effect of these features is a characteristic halo-like pattern surrounding regenerative nodules (see Fig. 48.22E).

Staging Primary Biliary Cholangitis

Although liver biopsy remains the gold standard for staging fibrosis, noninvasive methods such as transient elastography have emerged as viable alternatives because of the issues related to sampling errors and the risk of serious adverse effects, albeit rare, associated with liver biopsies. Clinically, patients are often characterized as early-, intermediate- (bridging fibrosis), and late-stage disease. There are several more complex staging systems that are less often used in the clinic and more often applied in the context of clinical trials. The three histological grading systems are illustrated in Table 48.6. The heterogeneity with regard to inflammation and fibrosis that is so characteristic of PBC compounded by sampling errors significantly limits the accuracy of these staging systems.[137]

Differential Diagnosis

PBC typically causes a chronic cholestatic disease with insidious onset, a long asymptomatic phase, and slow progression over the course of years. A patient presenting with acute onset of jaundice is unlikely to have PBC. One of the challenges associated with the histological diagnosis of PBC lies in the patchy nature of the disease; thus sampling error is always a consideration when PBC is considered clinically. A positive copper stain is often helpful in establishing the cholestatic nature of the disease, although it does

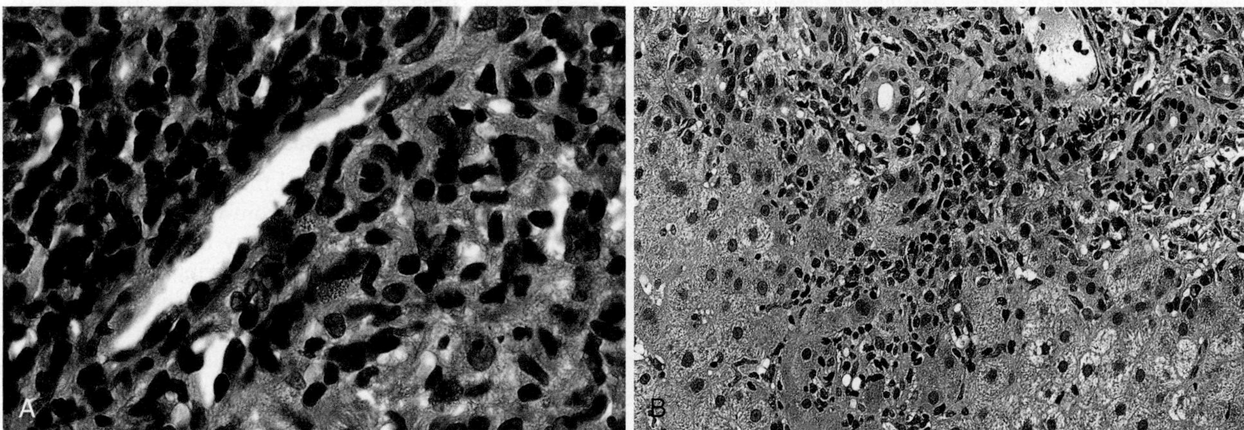

FIGURE 48.19 Portal inflammation in primary biliary cholangitis. A, Inflammation is typically dense but patchy in early-stage disease. Lymphocytes predominate, but plasma cells also may be conspicuous, and eosinophils may occur in small numbers. **B,** Some spillover into the periportal areas may be seen, but overt hepatocyte necrosis usually is not conspicuous.

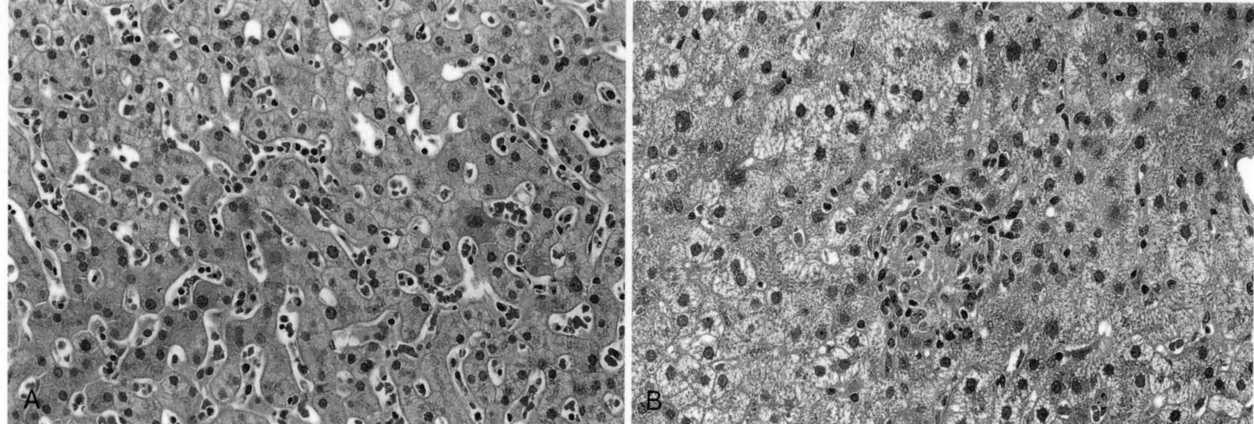

FIGURE 48.20 Hepatic lobule findings in primary biliary cholangitis (PBC).Although the hepatocytes usually are quiescent, some degree of sinusoidal lymphocytosis is common in PBC **(A),** and occasional granulomas may be seen **(B).**

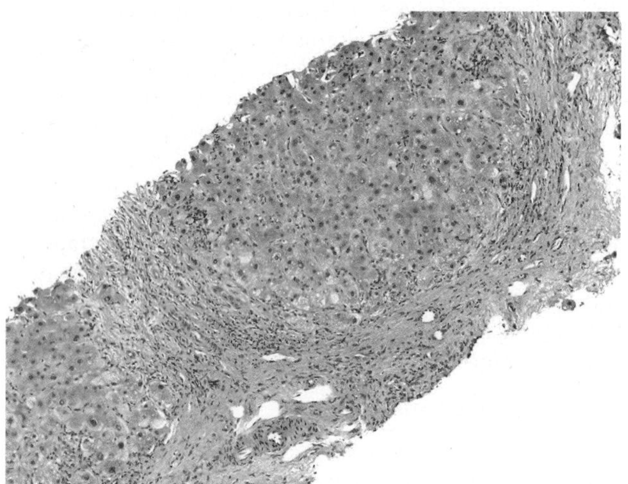

FIGURE 48.21 Primary biliary cholangitis with cirrhosis. Florid duct lesions are absent in the late phase of the disease. Bile ducts were essentially absent in this biopsy. Note the pale cytoplasm of periseptal hepatocytes, a finding secondary to the accumulation of bile salts, referred to as *cholate cholestasis.*

not distinguish PBC from other cholestatic diseases such as PSC.

Primary Biliary Cholangitis versus Autoimmune Hepatitis

Based solely on morphological grounds, the portal changes seen in AIH may overlap with those of PBC. However, the two diseases are invariably associated with distinctive clinical and serological findings. Although normal or mild elevation of transaminases and elevated alkaline phosphatase is characteristic of PBC, this pattern is reversed in AIH. The classic serology of AIH, ANA-positive, SMA-positive, and AMA-negative, is seen in the vast majority of cases. However, PBC may show ANA positivity, typically at low titers. Both diseases often feature a dense lymphocyte and plasma cell–rich infiltrate. Florid duct lesions are not seen in patients with isolated AIH. A copper stain could be helpful in this context, particularly in cases that lack bile duct injury. Copper within periportal hepatocytes would support a chronic cholestatic disease, and by extension, PBC. It should be emphasized that the diagnosis of PBC and its distinction from AIH must be based on a combination of clinical, biochemical, serological, and histological findings. This is also seen AIH/PBC overlap.

Primary Biliary Cholangitis versus Bile Duct Obstruction

Unlike PBC, the portal tracts in patients with obstructed bile duct(s) are edematous and lack the dense lymphoplasmacytic infiltration seen in PBC.

Primary Biliary Cholangitis versus Primary Sclerosing Cholangitis

The two diseases share in their often insidious presentation, elevated alkaline phosphatase, and histological evidence of bile duct injury. PBC thus shares many histological features with PSC. The pathognomonic florid bile duct lesion of PBC is less prevalent in late-stage disease, and the pathognomonic fibrous obliterative cholangitis lesion of PSC is typically focal and may not be sampled in needle biopsies of the liver (Table 48.7). However, it is notable that portal inflammation usually is more intense in PBC than in PSC. In the absence of pathognomonic histological features, clinical and serological findings often provide more reliable evidence in distinguishing the two diseases, with PBC characterized by antimitochondrial antibodies, while PSC shows a sclerosing and beaded appearance of cholangiogram (see Table 48.5).

Primary Biliary Cholangitis versus Drug-Induced Liver Injury

The cholestatic pattern of DILI may show features that overlap with PBC. Positive AMA and florid duct lesions would support a diagnosis of PBC. An acute onset with jaundice developing within weeks of starting the drug would favor DILI.

Primary Biliary Cholangitis versus Viral Hepatitis

In the early stages, histological manifestations of PBC and PSC may be indistinguishable from viral hepatitis (B or C) or AIH. All of these disorders may have a chronic active hepatitis pattern with portal and periportal inflammation (see Table 48.3). The presence of individual necrotic hepatocytes at the interface is not a hallmark feature of PBC or PSC. In contrast, hepatocyte necrosis with acidophil bodies, particularly at the interface, are a common feature of active chronic viral hepatitis or AIH. A duct-centric pattern of injury is exceptionally uncommon in viral hepatitis; rarely this is observed in patients with hepatitis C infection. A positive copper stain often provides compelling evidence

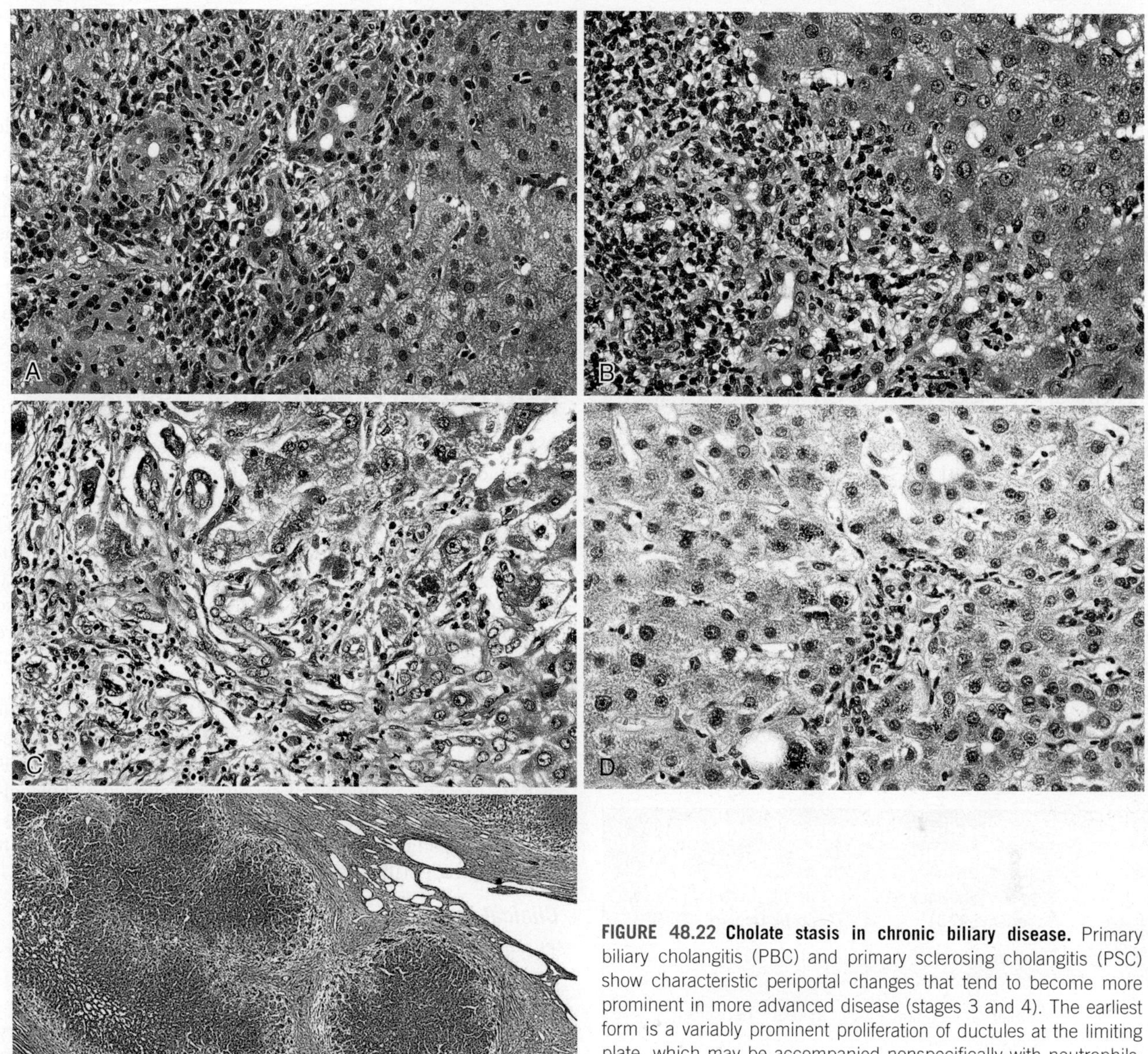

FIGURE 48.22 Cholate stasis in chronic biliary disease. Primary biliary cholangitis (PBC) and primary sclerosing cholangitis (PSC) show characteristic periportal changes that tend to become more prominent in more advanced disease (stages 3 and 4). The earliest form is a variably prominent proliferation of ductules at the limiting plate, which may be accompanied nonspecifically with neutrophils; examples of PBC **(A)** and PSC **(B)** are shown (H&E stain). In more advanced disease, progressive hepatocellular pseudoxanthomatous swelling with Mallory hyaline **(C; H&E stain)** and stainable copper **(D)** is evident. **E,** Swelling results in a halo-like pattern surrounding regenerative nodules in stage 4 disease (H&E stain).

of a chronic cholestatic disease; biopsies from patients with viral or autoimmune forms of chronic hepatitis are negative for copper.

Granulomatous Hepatitis

Hepatic granulomas, both with or without evidence of bile duct injury, should prompt a broad differential diagnosis. Sarcoidosis can mimic PBC because of duct loss and duct-centric granulomas. The granulomas in sarcoidosis are usually better developed, often confluent, and more numerous than in PBC. Granulomas are only randomly associated with bile ducts and are commonly located within the hepatic lobules in sarcoidosis. The degree of portal inflammation usually is more intense in PBC compared with sarcoidosis. Florid duct lesions have rarely been described in hepatitis C. Uncommonly, drugs may cause lesions that mimic the type of florid duct lesion seen in PBC. Carbamazepine may cause a granulomatous type of hepatitis and acute cholangitis.

Natural History

Asymptomatic patients with early-stage disease have a longer time to transplantation or disease-related death. Before widespread screening, the median survival of patients was 6 to 10 years. With most patients diagnosed early in the course of the disease and the introduction of ursodeoxycholic acid (UDCA), the overall median survival has significantly increased.[138]

Hepatocellular carcinoma develops in 6% of patients with PBC per year, although the risk is probably not as high as that seen in cirrhosis from other causes, such as viral hepatitis, hemochromatosis, or alcohol. Surveillance is recommended every 6 to 12 months. Older patients, male gender, advance histological stage, and inadequate response to UDCA are associated with an elevated risk for developing hepatocellular carcinoma.[139-141]

Treatment

The initial therapy of choice for PBC is long-term treatment with UDCA. Improvement in alkaline phosphatase is typically observed within 3 months of starting UDCA.[142,143] Approximately one-third of patients have an inadequate biochemical response.[142,143] UDCA is associated with a long-term survival benefit.[144] In a systematic review, of 4845 patients, UDCA was associated with higher rates of transplant-free survival at 5, 10, and 15 years compared with no treatment.[138]

The mechanisms underlying this favorable response with UDCA include (1) increased hydrophilic index of the circulating bile acid pool, (2) stimulation of hepatocellular and ductular secretions and thus elimination of bile acids, (3) protection against bile acid injury, and (4) immunomodulation and antiinflammatory effects of UDCA.[145] Obeticholic acid is used for patients with an inadequate biochemical response to UDCA. Obeticholic acid can be used in combination with UDCA.[144]

TABLE 48.6 Three Histological Staging Systems for Primary Biliary Cholangitis

Stage	Scheuer (Sherlock and Scheuer, 1973)	Ludwig (Ludwig, Dickson, and McDonald, 1978)
1	Florid duct lesions Portal inflammation	Portal inflammation
2	Ductular proliferation Portal expansion Interface hepatitis	Interface hepatitis
3	Scarring Paucity of bile ducts	Fibrous septa
4	Cirrhosis	Cirrhosis

From Ludwig J, Dickson ER, McDonald GS. Staging of chronic nonsuppurative destructive cholangitis (syndrome of primary biliary cirrhosis). Virchows Arch A Pathol Anat Histol. *1978;379(2):103-112; Sherlock S, Scheuer PJ. The presentation and diagnosis of 100 patients with primary biliary cirrhosis.* N Engl J Med. *1973;289(13):674-678.*

Of note, prior treatments included immunosuppressive drugs (e.g., azathioprine, D-penicillamine, corticosteroids, cyclosporine, methotrexate) and the antifibrotic agent colchicine, and they met with little success.

For patients with decompensated cirrhosis, orthotopic liver transplantation (OLT) has emerged as the most effective form of therapy. OLT is associated with excellent short- and long-term survival rates with 1-year survival rates of 90% to 95% (see Chapter 52).[146] PBC may recur in the allograft. In one study of 571 patients who had liver transplantation for PBC, the rates of recurrence at 5 and 10 years were 18% and 31%, respectively, and recurrence was associated with higher risk of graft loss.[147]

PRIMARY SCLEROSING CHOLANGITIS

PSC is a slowly progressive idiopathic cholestatic disease that is characterized by persistent and progressive biliary inflammation and fibrosis and variable outcomes. In some patients, end-stage liver disease necessitates liver transplantation. PSC typically involves both the intrahepatic and extrahepatic biliary system, although in 5% of cases the disease is confined to the small ducts, the so-called *small-duct PSC.*[148] The disease may overlap with AIH, although this syndrome is seen more often in children: 35% of children with PSC, but only 5% of adults show features of both PSC and AIH.[149]

The diagnosis of PSC is based on a combination of clinical features, a cholestatic biochemical pattern, and characteristic cholangiographic findings. By definition, a diagnosis of PSC requires exclusion of secondary sclerosing cholangitis (SSC), biliary diseases that often share clinical and radiological and sometimes morphological features of PSC, but features an identifiable underlying disease process.

Clinical Features

The median age at diagnosis is 41 years, with most patients being between 20 and 40 years of age (Box 48.3). Approximately 60% of patients with PSC are male.[150]

PSC occurs primarily in patients with inflammatory bowel disease (IBD); 70% to 80% of patients have both conditions. However, there are significant geographic variations with patients from Asia (35%) showing a lower incidence of IBD than those from the United States (80% have concomitant IBD).[151] Conversely, PSC develops in 2% to 8% of patients with ulcerative colitis and 2% to 3% of patients with Crohn disease.

The presentation is typically insidious, and abnormal liver function tests in otherwise asymptomatic individuals often lead to a diagnosis of PSC. Symptomatic patients at

TABLE 48.7 Histological Features of Primary Biliary Cholangitis and Primary Sclerosing Cholangitis

Feature	Primary Biliary Cholangitis	Primary Sclerosing Cholangitis
Bile duct damage	Present, interlobular ducts	Present, large and small ducts
Florid duct lesions	Present	Absent
Fibro-obliterative bile duct lesions	Absent	Present
Loss of bile ducts	Late stage of disease	Late stage of disease
Copper	Present, periportal hepatocytes	Present, periportal hepatocytes

BOX 48.3 Key Features of Primary Sclerosing Cholangitis

- Male predominance, fourth and fifth decade of life
- 80% of patients report inflammatory bowel disease
- Cholestatic liver chemistry with elevated alkaline phosphatase and γ–glutamyltransferase.
- Serology is unhelpful for diagnosis
- Cholangiographic abnormalities is gold standard for diagnosis, except for patients with small duct PSC
- Key histological features include periductal fibrosis and bile duct damage; may not be seen in needle biopsy specimens
- Medical treatment with ursodeoxycholic acid (UDCA) does not halt disease progression
- Most symptomatic patients require liver transplantation in 20 years

presentation report abdominal pain (20%), pruritus (10%), jaundice (6%), and fatigue (6%). An abrupt presentation with jaundice should raise the possibility of underlying cholangiocarcinoma. Hepatomegaly and/or splenomegaly may be observed at presentation.

Laboratory Investigation

The disease is characterized by a cholestatic enzymatic pattern with elevation of alkaline phosphatase (>4× the upper limit of normal) and gamma glutamyltransferase (GGT) levels seen in virtually all patients at presentation, although a normal level does not exclude PSC. Serum ALT and AST levels are often only mildly (two to three times the upper limit of normal) elevated or normal. Perinuclear antinuclear cytoplasmic antibodies (pANCAs) are identified in 80% of cases and ANAs and ASMAs in 20% to 50% of cases.[152] Unlike PBC, there is no diagnostically relevant serological assay for PSC. Serum IgG and IgM levels may be raised mildly in 50% of patients.

It should be noted that approximately 10% of patients with PSC have increased serum IgG4, a finding that should raise the possibility of IgG4-related sclerosing cholangitis (IgG4-RSC).

Pathogenesis

The pathogenesis of PSC involves a combination of hereditary and environmental factors. One possible scenario involves an unidentified environmental agent that triggers biliary damage but only in individuals susceptible to this disease.[153] Unlike most autoimmune diseases, PSC does not respond favorably to immunosuppressive therapy.

Genetic Predisposition

The relative risk among siblings with PSC is 9 to 39 times as high as the risk in the general population[154]; PSC is strongly associated with HLA class I and II regions (i.e., HLA-B*08, HLA-DRB1 alleles, and a locus near NOTCH4, respectively).[155-158] Genes of the interleukin-2 pathway (CD28, interleukin-2, and the alpha subunit of the interleukin-2 receptor) have also been associated with susceptibility to PSC.[155]

Environmental Triggers

An association with environmental triggers has been recognized. Notably, a history of smoking appears to be protective. Higher incidence of PSC has been reported in patients with exposure to farm animals, lower levels of fish consumption, and consumption of well-done steak or hamburgers.[159] These dietary habits could modulate the disease by altering the gut microbiome. The strong association of PSC with IBD also supports this "microbiota hypothesis."[160] One potential hypothesis involves the migration of intestinal microbial molecules through the portal system to initiate an aberrant immune response to cholangiocytes.

Aberrant Homing of Mucosal Lymphocytes to Primary Sclerosing Cholangitis Liver

Other theories for PSC revolve around the hepatic homing of activated intestinal T cells, the migration mediated by interaction of lymphoid cell surface receptor α4β7 and CCR9 and the anomalous expression in the liver of their associated ligands adhesion protein mucosal addressin–cell adhesion molecule 1 (MAdCAM-1) and the chemotactic protein CCL25; of note, the expression of these ligands is restricted to the liver.[161,162]

A Role for Cholangiocytes

Interestingly, the cholangiocytes may be actively involved in the cause and pathogenesis of PSC.[163] Cholangiocytes may express a number of proinflammatory cytokines such as tumor necrosis factor α, interleukin-6, and interleukin-8.[164] Cholangiocytes could thus aid in the recruitment and stimulation of T cells, macrophages, neutrophils, and natural killer cells.

Imaging

The hallmark of PSC is an abnormal cholangiogram as detected on either endoscopic retrograde cholangiopancreatography (ERCP) or magnetic resonance cholangiopancreatography (MRCP).[152] MRCP is now the recommended diagnostic investigation for PSC. Characteristic changes on cholangiogram include diffusely distributed, segmental, and multifocal strictures that lead to a beaded appearance (Fig. 48.23). These changes may not be seen in small-duct PSC. Less commonly, other conditions may show similar cholangiographic findings (see Differential Diagnosis).

Pathology

Apart from small-duct PSC and suspected cases of overlap syndrome, a liver biopsy is not necessary to establish a diagnosis of PSC. The diagnosis thus often relies on persistent (>6 months) increase in serum alkaline phosphatase and bile duct strictures on cholangiography.[148]

Gross Pathology

In early-stage disease, the liver is often slightly enlarged and variably bile stained. In later stages, similar to PBC, cirrhosis develops that may be intensely green, reflecting progressive cholestasis (Fig. 48.24A). In contrast with PBC, cholangiectases and cholangitic abscesses may develop. Cholangiectases are recognizable as cystic collections of bilious, sometimes calculous, dark green material that may be several centimeters in diameter, and they are usually located in the hilar region of the liver (Fig. 48.24B). Cholangitic abscesses, which presumably reflect superinfection of cholangiectases, have a more yellow appearance than cholangiectases (Fig.

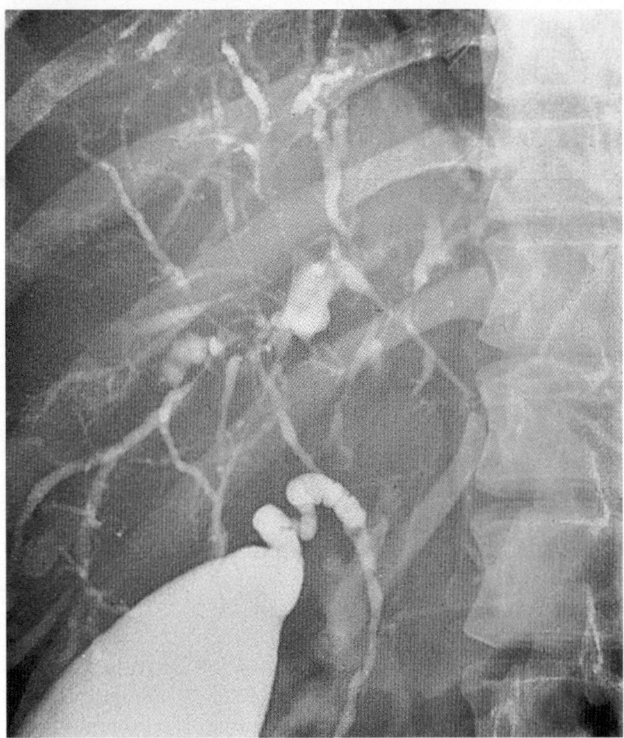

FIGURE 48.23 Abnormal cholangiogram in primary sclerosing cholangitis (PSC). The multiple beaded areas with intervening strictured areas are typical of PSC. Occasionally, infectious, eosinophilic, or ischemic cholangitis can have similar features. (*Courtesy of John Poterucha, MD, Mayo Clinic, Rochester, MN.*)

48.24C). The large intrahepatic and extrahepatic ducts may develop areas of gross stricture and concentric fibrosis. Cholangiocarcinoma and bile duct carcinoma are recognizable as firm, white, sclerotic lesions or masses.

Microscopic Pathology

The extrahepatic and intrahepatic large bile ducts appear thickened and fibrotic and infiltrated by small lymphocytes. Although, these alterations are nonspecific, they differ from changes seen in IgG4-RSC (see later). Histological examination of the explant specimen reveal cholangiectasis, duct dilation, epithelial atrophy with focal denudation, and mixed bilious material, neutrophils, and granulation tissue at the site of denudation (Figs. 48.25A and 48.26). Cholangitic abscesses are similar, but they tend to have a more exuberant neutrophilic infiltrate (see Fig. 48.25B).

The hallmark lesion of PSC on needle biopsies is periductal onion-skin type fibrosis and periductal inflammation involving interlobular ducts that range in size from 10 to 20 μm. Onion-skin type fibrosis is characterized by periductal collagen fibers that form concentric layers around interlobular bile ducts. The lumen of the duct is sometimes narrowed, narrower than the accompanying hepatic artery, which is typically the same diameter as the accompanying bile duct. The ductal cells may appear smaller than uninvolved bile ducts (Fig. 48.27A,B). The end stage of fibrous cholangitis, sometimes referred to as *fibrous-obliterative cholangitis,* is characterized by near-complete or complete loss of epithelium and the formation of fibrous scars; the latter may be the only evidence of a preexisting bile duct (Fig. 48.27C,D; Figs. 48.28 and 48.29). The fibrous scar is highlighted on a trichome and PAS/diastase stain (Fig. 48.30). A copper stain is a helpful ancillary test for the diagnosis of PSC (Fig 48.31). Periportal hepatocellular copper accumulation often indicates long-standing cholestatic process. However, copper is commonly found in patients with advanced fibrosis regardless of the underlying etiology, and thus a copper stain is of diagnostic value only in the early phases of the disease. These characteristic histological changes may not be seen on a liver biopsy, and the diagnosis often relies on a combination of subtle bile duct damage (Fig. 48.32) and demonstration of periportal copper accumulation.

Other changes commonly associated with PSC include portal expansion, portal edema, and bile ductular duplication. Characteristic changes of extrahepatic bile duct obstruction may be seen and consequent to the bile duct strictures. Portal tract from patients with PSC showed mild portal inflammation, and necro-inflammatory activity is generally not prominent. Marked portal and interface hepatitis should raise the possibility of an overlap syndrome with AIH, particularly in children. Cholestasis may be seen, particularly in the latter phase of the disease. Patients with advanced disease show bridging fibrosis or cirrhosis. The Ludwig system for staging fibrosis is illustrated in Table 48.8.

PSC is resistant to immunosuppressive therapy (also see later). Exceptional cases of PSC have been reported to be steroid responsive. A recent report alludes to the presence of portal-based inflammatory nodules in steroid-responsive examples of PSC (Fig. 48.33).[165,166]

Differential Diagnosis

Table 48.9 and Box 48.4.

Disease with Histological Evidence of Bile Duct Injury

The majority of these patients show a cholestatic pattern with elevation in alkaline phosphatase and GGT (see Table 48.9). Histologically, these diseases share some features of PSC, predominantly bile duct injury and/or loss.

The two closest mimics of PSC include PBC and IgG4-RSC. PBC is characterized by antimitochondrial antibodies and florid duct lesions. However, the focal nature of the inflammatory process implies that florid duct lesions may not be seen on needle biopsy. PBC is typically associated with a significantly higher density of portal lymphoplasmacytic infiltrate, and occasionally interface hepatitis, the so-called *biliary type interface hepatitis.*

Before the recognition of IgG4-related disease (IgG4-RD), IgG4-RSC was often mistaken for PSC. The significant clinical and histological overlap between these two diseases stresses the need for a thoughtful review of all available histological material including prior non-hepatic biopsies. The two features associated with IgG4-RD that hold the key to this distinction include (1) pancreatic involvement, and/or involvement of other organs, typically involved in IgG4-RD and (2) markedly elevated serum IgG4 levels, typically greater than four times the upper limit of normal (Tables 48.10 and 48.11).

Bile duct destruction with concentric periductal fibrosis, superficial epithelial necrosis, and biliary strictures

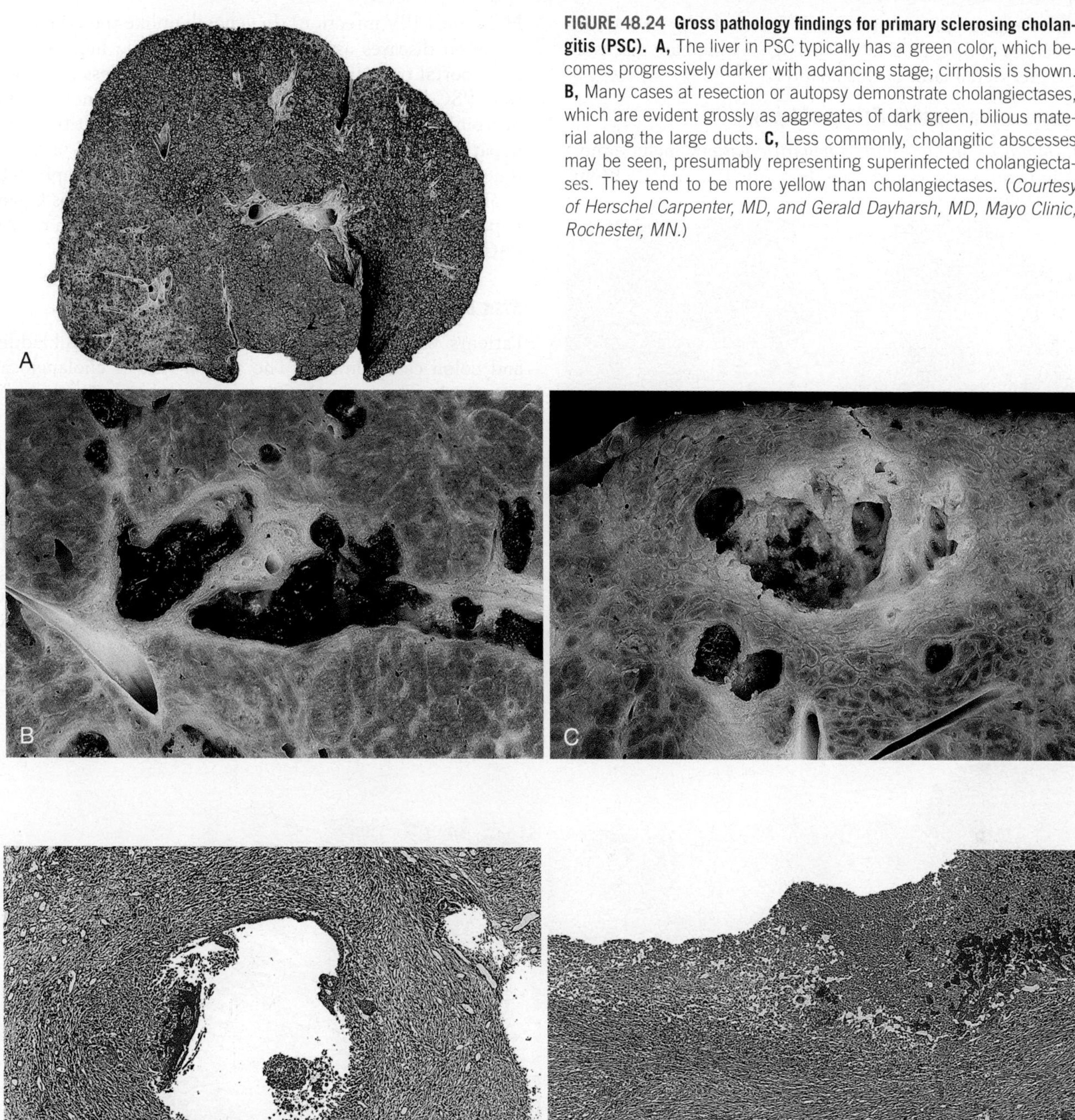

FIGURE 48.24 Gross pathology findings for primary sclerosing cholangitis (PSC). A, The liver in PSC typically has a green color, which becomes progressively darker with advancing stage; cirrhosis is shown. **B,** Many cases at resection or autopsy demonstrate cholangiectases, which are evident grossly as aggregates of dark green, bilious material along the large ducts. **C,** Less commonly, cholangitic abscesses may be seen, presumably representing superinfected cholangiectases. They tend to be more yellow than cholangiectases. (*Courtesy of Herschel Carpenter, MD, and Gerald Dayharsh, MD, Mayo Clinic, Rochester, MN.*)

FIGURE 48.25 Histopathology of cholangiectases and cholangitic abscesses in primary sclerosing cholangitis. Both lesions affect large intrahepatic and extrahepatic bile ducts. A, Cholangiectases show duct dilation, focal epithelial atrophy and loss, and a resulting mixture of bile, neutrophils, and granulation tissue along areas of denuded epithelium. **B,** Cholangitic abscesses likely reflect the same basic process with added bacterial superinfection, which results in a subjectively larger number of neutrophils.

indistinguishable from PSC can be seen in ischemic cholangitis (discussed later).[167,168] A chronic bile duct–destructive syndrome that may result in a biliary pattern of cirrhosis is associated with α_1-antitrypsin deficiency. This syndrome occurs more commonly in the pediatric population and in those with homozygous disease. It is less common in adults and patients with heterozygous disease.[169]

Idiopathic adulthood ductopenia (IAD) is a syndrome characterized by idiopathic, progressive duct loss without the cholangiographic or clinical features of PSC or idiopathic IBD. *Ductopenia* is defined as more than 50% loss of interlobular and septal bile ducts in 20 or more assessable portal tracts.[168] Morphologically, IAD can mimic small-duct PSC (see Miscellaneous Ductopenic Syndromes).

Cholangiographic mimics of PSC include any of the various causes of SSC (see Table 48.10),[170] which are discussed in greater detail later in this chapter.[171,172]

Diseases with a Hepatitic Pattern of Injury

Inflammatory mimics with a hepatitic pattern include most of the major causes of chronic hepatitis (i.e., AIH, chronic HCV and HBV infection). In general, unlike the other more common diseases associated with a chronic hepatitis pattern, portal tracts in PSC show significantly less inflammation. PSC lacks the interface activity and prominent lobular necroinflammatory activity typical of AIH, hepatitis B, and hepatitis C. The number of plasma cells in PSC usually is much lower than that seen in AIH and PBC. Lymphocytic cholangitis can be seen in PSC, PBC, AIH, hepatitis C, and hepatitis B, although destructive cholangitis is seen only in PSC and PBC (Fig. 48.34).

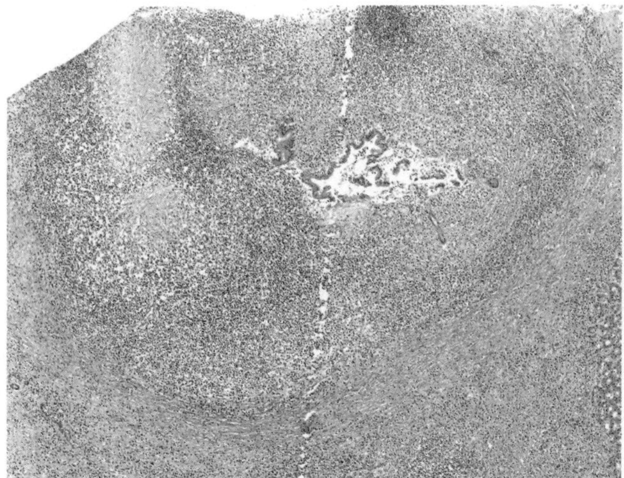

FIGURE 48.26 Primary sclerosing cholangitis. A large duct surrounded by a dense inflammatory infiltrate composed of lymphocytes, plasma cells, and neutrophils is shown. Note the extensive destruction of the bile duct.

Risk of Malignancy

Patients with PSC are at risk for bile duct, gallbladder, and colon carcinoma.[173] The annual risk of cholangiocarcinoma is 2%, and the 30-year cumulative incidence is 20%.[174,175] The adenocarcinoma typically arises within hilar or large intrahepatic bile ducts, but it can occur in the liver or in extrahepatic bile ducts. The invasive carcinoma arises in the background of biliary intraepithelial neoplasia (BilIN).[176] The tumors are typically advanced and thus associated with a poor prognosis.[177,178] Screening for cholangiocarcinoma has relied on conventional cytology, although morphological evaluation has a low sensitivity for the detection of cholangiocarcinoma; assessment of chromosomal abnormalities by FISH technique and mutation analysis using next-generation sequencing can increase the diagnostic sensitivity.[179,180]

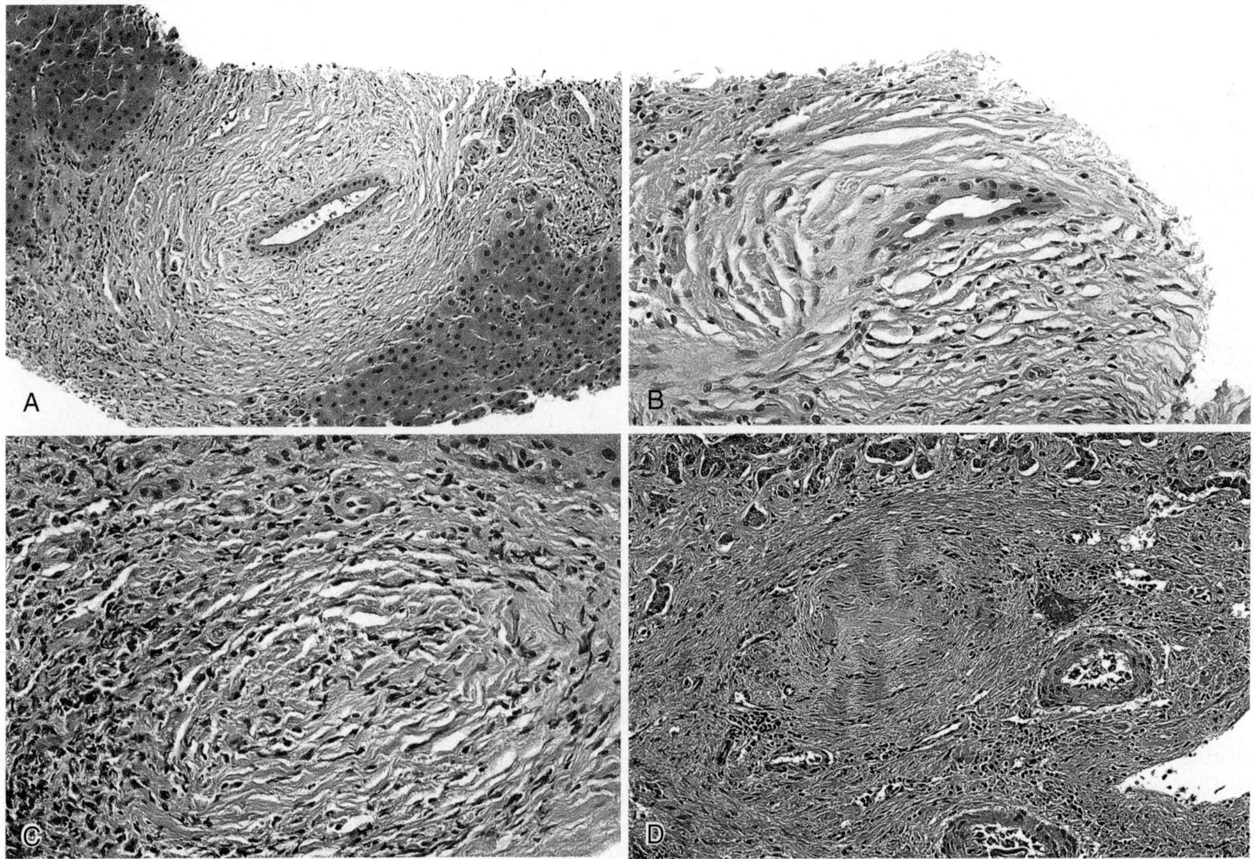

FIGURE 48.27 Small- to medium-sized, duct-destructive lesions in primary sclerosing cholangitis. A, Early phases of fibrous cholangitis show concentric periductal fibrosis with mild epithelial atrophy. **B,** Intermediate phases show a greater degree of fibrosis and epithelial atrophy. **C** and **D,** The end result is fibrous-obliterative cholangitis. It is a fibrous nodule without epithelium, typically adjacent to a hepatic artery, reflecting total obliteration of the duct.

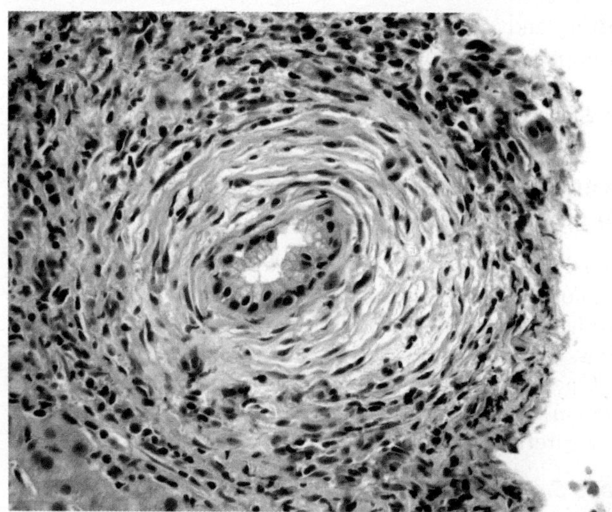

FIGURE 48.28 Primary sclerosing cholangitis. A patent bile duct with minimal injury surrounded by concentric onion-skin–type periductal fibrosis is shown. This appearance is highly characteristic of primary sclerosing cholangitis.

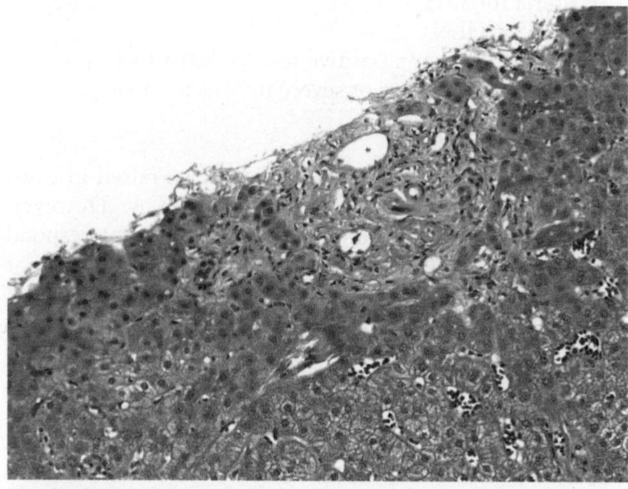

FIGURE 48.29 Primary sclerosing cholangitis. Expanded portal tracts with minimal inflammatory activity. Note the damaged bile duct. The bile duct lumen is narrowed, and the biliary cells lack the even distribution of nuclei seen in normal bile ducts.

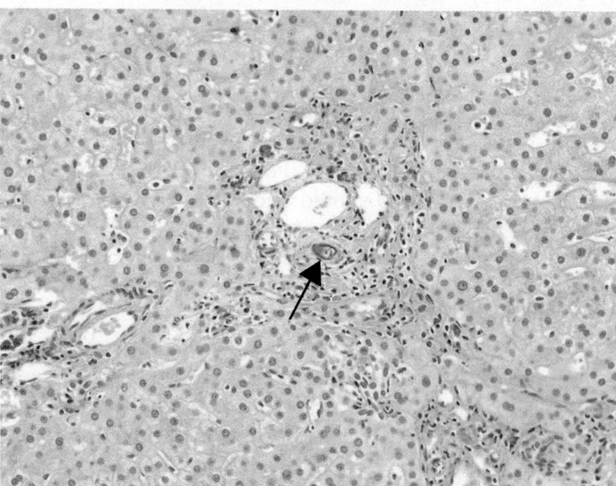

FIGURE 48.30 Primary sclerosing cholangitis. This periodic acid–Schiff (PAS)/diastase stain highlights the damaged bile duct *(arrow)*. Prominent basement membrane–like material is noted. The lumen is indistinct, and the epithelial cells are largely absent.

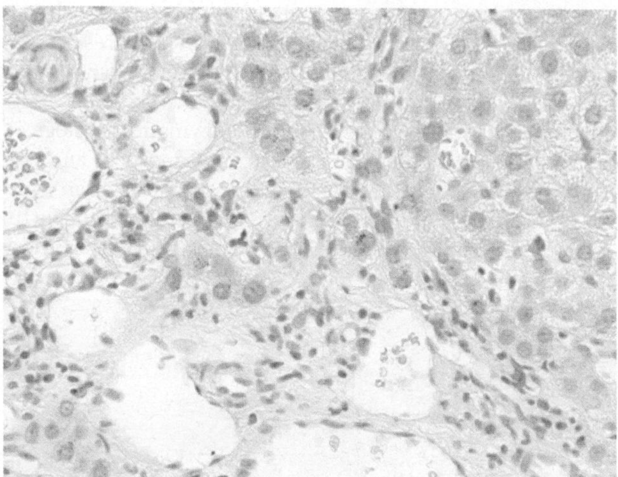

FIGURE 48.31 Primary sclerosing cholangitis. Copper stain shows the presence of reddish granules within periportal hepatocytes. The presence of copper in periportal hepatocytes indicates chronic cholestasis. Although this is not specific for primary sclerosing cholangitis, in the right clinical context, the presence of copper in a liver without significant fibrosis would support a diagnosis of primary sclerosing cholangitis.

Patients with concomitant IBD and PSC have a significantly higher risk of colon cancer than patients with only the former disease—four times as high.[181] Patients are also at a higher risk of gallbladder carcinoma; approximately 60% of mass lesions in the gallbladder are malignant. Furthermore, gallbladders from patients with PSC showed dysplasia in 37% of patients and adenocarcinoma in 14%.[182]

Natural History

Typical survival from the time of diagnosis to death or liver transplantation is 12 to 18 years. However, there is a considerable variation in clinical course, with some patients showing prolonged survival. Increasing age, low serum albumin levels, bilirubin elevation for >3 months, hepatomegaly, splenomegaly, and dominant bile duct stricture predict poor prognosis. Involvement of both intrahepatic and extrahepatic bile ducts at the time of diagnosis is another poor prognostic factor.[183] Of note, patients with small bile-duct disease generally have more favorable outcomes than those with classic disease.[178,184]

Treatment

Despite a plethora of clinical trials over several decades, there is no effective medical therapy for PSC. Patients are placed on ursodeoxycholic acid (UCDA), although there remains some controversy regarding the efficacy of this therapy. Although UCDA may improve alkaline phosphatase and GGT,[185] the drug does not improve survival.[186] Thus neither UCDA nor any other form of medical therapy has been shown to alter the natural history of PSC.[187] PSC patients are unresponsive to steroids and other forms of immunosuppression, although a small fraction of patients may appear steroid responsive.[165,188]

Liver transplantation has emerged as an effective therapy for these patients. After liver transplantation for PSC, the 1-year survival rate is approximately 85%, and the 5-year survival rate is approximately 72% (www.unos.org). Nevertheless, the disorder may recur in approximately 25% of patients after transplantation. Following liver transplantation, patients with IBD should undergo annual colonoscopy with surveillance biopsies.

OVERLAP SYNDROMES

An overlap syndrome refers to the concurrent presence of two autoimmune liver diseases that manifest either synchronously or metachronously.[189-192] The conceptual framework of overlap syndromes is presented in Fig. 48.35. The most common type of overlap syndrome is combined AIH/PBC. Combined AIH/PSC is the next most common,[193,194] and combined PBC/PSC is the least common and the most difficult to identify. In most cases, AIH constitutes one component of the overlap syndrome and is accompanied by either PSC or PBC. There is no single set of definitional features for a diagnosis of autoimmune liver diseases; instead, the diagnosis rests on a constellation of clinical, biochemical, imaging, serological, and histological features. It has thus proven difficult to precisely define overlap syndromes. In general, if an autoimmune hepatic disease shows significant deviation from key clinical, enzymatic, serological, radiological, or histological features, a diagnosis of an overlap syndrome should be considered. A diagnosis of an overlap syndrome should be considered only after a thoughtful clinical and histological deliberation in a multidisciplinary setting and after due attention to potential pitfalls. For example, mild lymphocytic interface activity in an otherwise typical example of PBC does not constitute sufficient evidence for an overlap with AIH.

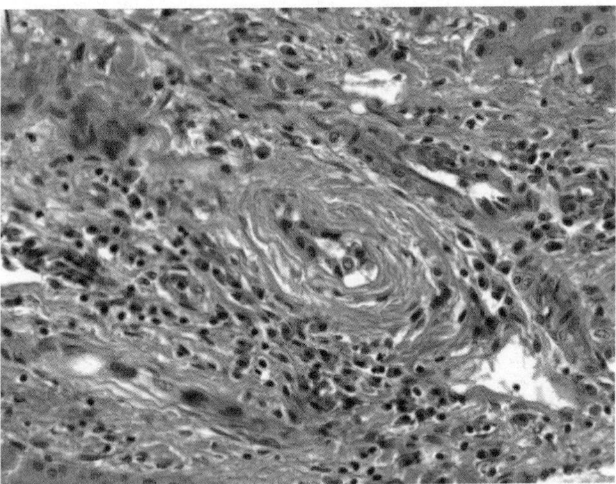

FIGURE 48.32 Primary sclerosing cholangitis. Note the damaged bile ducts with irregular distribution of biliary epithelial cells and vacuolated cells. Also note the periductal concentric fibrosis.

Overlap of Autoimmune Hepatitis with Primary Biliary Cholangitis

AIH/PBC overlap syndrome may be evident at initial diagnosis. In cases without synchronous involvement, the overlap syndrome typically resembles PBC at presentation (Figs. 48.36 and 48.37).

One of the proposed diagnostic criteria for AIH/PBC overlap requires the presence of two features of AIH and two criteria for PBC, as follows.[195]

Paris Criteria

Criteria for PBC

1. Alkaline phosphatase ≥2× upper limit of normal (ULN) or gamma-glutamyltransferase ≥5× ULN
2. Positive AMA
3. Liver biopsy with florid duct lesion

Criteria for AIH

1. ALT ≥5× ULN
2. IgG ≥2× ULN or a positive test for SMA (>1 in 80)
3. Liver with moderate or severe interface activity

Differential Diagnosis

Clinically, a diagnosis of AIH/PBC is often raised in cases that do not respond favorably with UDCA. However, given that a subset of patients with PBC do not respond adequately to UDCA, this feature, in isolation, should not be considered as evidence of overlap. Additionally, PBC may show a dense portal based lymphoid infiltrate with focal interface activity, the so-called *biliary-type interface activity*. The mere presence of interface activity should not prompt a diagnosis of overlap syndrome. Similarly, the mere presence of lymphocytic cholangitis in a liver biopsy from an otherwise typical case of AIH is not considered diagnostic of AIH/PBC or AIH/PSC overlap syndrome. The isolated presence of AMA in patients with AIH is insufficient for diagnosing an overlap syndrome with PBC. Application of the international AIH score is of limited value in addressing its putative context; the scoring system can effectively exclude a potential autoimmune component, but it lacks sensitivity in unmasking an AIH-associated overlap syndrome.[196]

Treatment

Treatment is typically initiated against the dominant disease: steroids for AIH and UCDA for PBC. Typically treatment is

TABLE 48.8 Ludwig System for Staging Primary Sclerosing Cholangitis

Stage		Histological Alterations
1	Changes limited to the portal tract	Portal edema, inflammation, and ductular proliferation
2	Involvement of the limiting plate	Periportal fibrosis and periportal hepatic inflammation
3	Portal-to-portal fibrosis	Fibrous septa extend between adjacent portal tracts, and ductopenia may be seen
4	Cirrhosis	Biliary-type cirrhosis with jigsaw puzzle–like appearance and paucity of bile ducts

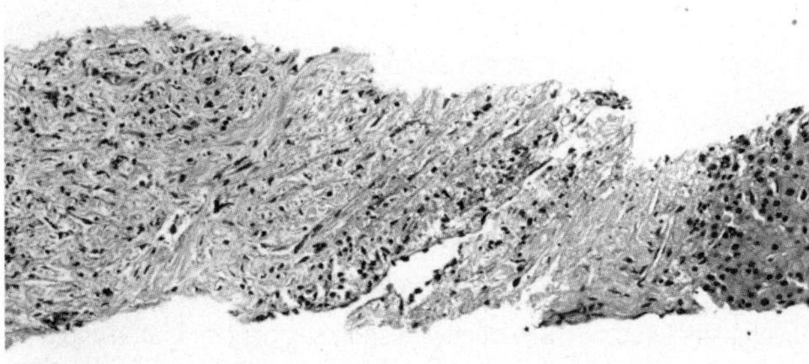

FIGURE 48.33 An example of primary sclerosing cholangitis responsive to steroids. The biopsy was characterized by these inflammatory nodules, an appearance resembling that seen in IgG4-related sclerosing cholangitis. The appearance on endoscopic retrograde cholangiopancreatography (ERCP) was typical of sclerosing cholangitis. This patient also reported a history of ulcerative colitis.

TABLE 48.9 Differential Diagnosis of Primary Sclerosing Cholangitis

Component	Possible Diagnosis
Hepatic pattern of injury	Autoimmune hepatitis Chronic hepatitis C Chronic hepatitis B Primary biliary cholangitis (less common)
Biliary pattern of injury *without* abnormal cholangiogram	Idiopathic adulthood ductopenia Ischemic cholangitis Childhood paucity of intrahepatic bile ducts (syndromic and nonsyndromic) α_1-Antitrypsin–associated duct loss Rare viral- or drug-associated loss Sarcoidosis Graft-versus-host disease ABCB4-associated cholangiopathy Surgical bile duct trauma Intraarterial chemotherapy Drug-induced sclerosing cholangitis Bacterial/parasitic cholangitis Recurrent pyogenic cholangitis
Biliary pattern of injury *with* abnormal cholangiogram	IgG4-related sclerosing cholangitis Langerhans cell histiocytosis Systemic mastocytosis Caroli disease Congenital hepatic fibrosis Other types of ductal plate abnormalities Hodgkin disease Metastatic disease Amyloidosis Hepatic allograft rejection Ischemic cholangitis Eosinophilic cholangitis Infection- or AIDS-related cholangitis Sclerosing cholangitis of critical illness COVID-19–related cholangiopathy

BOX 48.4 Major Causes of Secondary Sclerosing Cholangitis

IMMUNE DISORDERS
- IgG4-related sclerosing cholangitis
- Connective tissue disorders
- Vasculitis
- Idiopathic fibrosing disorders
- ABO incompatibility

ISCHEMIC DAMAGE
- Operative or blunt arterial trauma
- Thromboses
- After intraarterial chemotherapy
- Critically ill patients (CIPs)

INFECTIOUS OR IMMUNODEFICIENCY RELATED
- Bacterial cholangitis
- Recurrent pyogenic cholangitis
- Acquired or congenital immune deficiency
- Viral (cytomegalovirus) cholangitis
- Opportunistic or atypical bacteria or protozoans

INFILTRATIVE PROCESSES
- Eosinophilic cholangitis (gastroenteritis)
- Mast cell disease
- Langerhans cell histiocytosis

METASTASIS

initiated with UCDA, and steroids are added when there is a lack of adequate biochemical response.[197]

Autoimmune Hepatitis/Primary Sclerosing Cholangitis Overlap

In most patients, this overlap disease presents initially with features of AIH, and PSC is then diagnosed several years later. It is reported that using the modified AIH score leads to a diagnosis of an overlap syndrome in 8% to 10% of patients with PSC.[198]

Children have a higher incidence of AIH/PSC overlap syndrome.[199] Findings that raise suspicion of an overlap syndrome in patients with AIH include the presence of elevated serum alkaline phosphatase (above two-fold the upper limit of normal) or GGT, histological features of bile duct loss or injury, presence of concurrent IBD, and resistance to conventional steroid therapy.[200,201] There are no specific diagnostic criteria for a diagnosis of AIH/PSC overlap. However, it is generally believed that the diagnosis requires both typical imaging and biopsy features. This would include the presence of typical beading and stricturing of the biliary tree on imaging and/or onion-skin fibrosis/fibro-obliterative duct lesions on histology. Notably, given the overlapping serological feature between the two diseases, a diagnosis of overlap syndrome should not rely on this feature.

Differential Diagnosis

A thoughtful review of clinical and histological data is necessary before invoking a diagnosis of AIH/PSC overlap syndrome. It should be noted that the hepatic fibrosis may distort the intrahepatic biliary tree, and advanced fibrosis in AIH may mimic PSC.[202] Histologically, the isolated finding of nondestructive lymphocytic cholangitis is a not an

TABLE 48.10 Comparison of Immunoglobulin G4–Related Sclerosing Cholangitis and Primary Sclerosing Cholangitis

Characteristics	IgG4-Related Sclerosing Cholangitis	Primary Sclerosing Cholangitis
Clinical features		
Mean age at diagnosis	Usually adults (typically >40 years)	Children and adults
Gender (M:F)	4:1	2:1
Presentation	Painless jaundice	Pruritus Biochemical liver dysfunction
Associated coexisting conditions	Autoimmune pancreatitis Other manifestations of IgG4-related disease	Idiopathic inflammatory bowel disease Cholangiocarcinoma risk
Cholangiogram	Thickening of bile duct walls; long strictures with upstream dilation	Bile duct with short segment strictures and interspersed normal caliber or dilated segments (beads-on-a-string appearance)
Other features		
Serum IgG4 level >140 mg/dL	90%	15% (lower levels)
ANCA	Rare	70%-80%
Response to immunosuppressive therapy	Typical	None

ANCA, *Antineutrophil cytoplasmic antibody.*

TABLE 48.11 Comparison of Histological Features of Immunoglobulin G4–Related Sclerosing Cholangitis and Primary Sclerosing Cholangitis

	IgG4-Related Sclerosing Cholangitis	Primary Sclerosing Cholangitis
Small portal tracts		
Marked portal inflammation	Common	Rare
Ductular reaction	Common	Common
Fibrosis	Mild	Variable, may be advanced
IgG4-positive plasma cells (>10/HPF)	40%	10%
Fibroinflammatory nodule	Rare	None
Periductal concentric fibrosis	Less common	Common
Ductopenia	Less common	Common
Large bile ducts		
Distribution of inflammation	Transmural	Pronounced on the luminal side
IgG4-positive plasma cells (>50/HPF)	Common	Rare (~10%)
IgG4:IgG-positive plasma cell ratio	>40% (typically >70%)	<40%
Obliterative phlebitis	Common	Rare
Storiform fibrosis	Common	Rare
Erosion	Rare	Common
Xanthogranulomatous change	Rare	Common

HPF, *High-power field.*

uncommon finding in AIH and would not justify a diagnosis of overlap syndrome.

Treatment

Treatment is typically individualized and is based on clinical and histological features. UDCA is administered for the PSC component. A beneficial response to immunosuppressive therapy is reported in cases with a prominent hepatitis component on histology. Patients with overlap syndrome often report a poor outcome.

IMMUNOGLOBULIN G4–RELATED SCLEROSING CHOLANGITIS

IgG4-RD, a systemic fibroinflammatory disorder, commonly affects the pancreas and biliary tract.[165,203] Historically, these patients were misclassified as having PSC. Cases of sclerosing cholangitis associated with retroperitoneal fibrosis and Riedel's thyroiditis were reported as early as 1963.[204] In retrospect, these cases likely represent examples of IgG4-RSC. Most patients show involvement of both the biliary tract and pancreas; the former is now designated as IgG4-RSC and the latter as type 1 autoimmune pancreatitis (AIP). Rarely the disease spares the pancreas, and the involvement is restricted to the liver/biliary tract, a clinical scenario that poses a significant diagnostic challenge. In US and UK cohorts, isolated IgG4-RSC without AIP contributes to <10% of cases.[205,206]

Hepatic involvement is characterized by mass lesions and/or bile duct strictures. Before the recognition of IgG4-RD, IgG4-RSC was often misdiagnosed as PSC, while the mass-forming variant of the disease was mistaken for cholangiocarcinoma and/or pancreatic adenocarcinoma. On histology, the mass-forming lesions were diagnosed as *inflammatory pseudotumor.* The disease responds swiftly and dramatically to immunosuppressive agents, and such treatment can avert hepatic fibrosis and organ dysfunction.

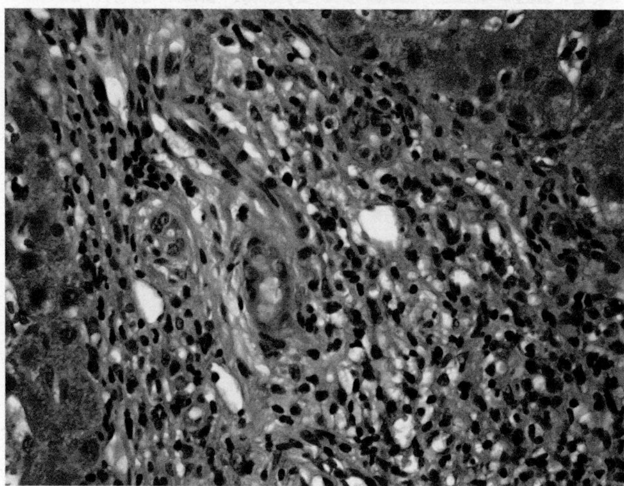

FIGURE 48.34 Hepatitis C infection. Note the damaged bile duct. There was no clinical or laboratory evidence of bile duct damage.

The diagnosis of IgG4-RSC is highly reliant on clinical, radiological, and serological features.[207-210] Notably, a single gold standard diagnostic test is lacking. The pathological changes of IgG4-RD are seldom specific in and of themselves, hence careful correlation with clinical and radiological features is paramount.

Clinical Features

At presentation, the majority of patients are in their 5th to 7th decades of life. Similar to other manifestations of IgG4-RD, IgG4-RSC shows a distinct male preponderance. Patients usually present with obstructive jaundice, weight loss, and dull abdominal pain. The symptoms are indistinguishable from other causes of obstructive jaundice, and malignancy is often the leading diagnosis. Symptoms related to other sites of disease may dominate the clinical presentation.

Pathogenesis

IgG4-RSC is the hepatic and biliary manifestation of IgG4-RD. The pathogenesis of IgG4-RD is covered in Chapter 40. Nevertheless, it is worth emphasizing the association between IgG4-RSC and the "blue-collar" workforce, suggesting an environmental agent as a causative factor.[211] Autoimmune diseases are identified in 10% of patients.[206]

Radiological Features

The disease is associated with characteristic radiological features. Nevertheless, like the clinical appearance, these features may be indistinguishable from PSC and/or cholangiocarcinoma.[212] The bile duct changes are best defined by cholangiography, either MRCP or ERCP. Radiological features of IgG4-RSC include long (>⅓ length) and multifocal bile duct strictures and mild upstream dilation. Concomitant diffuse pancreatic swelling and/or a thin, narrowed

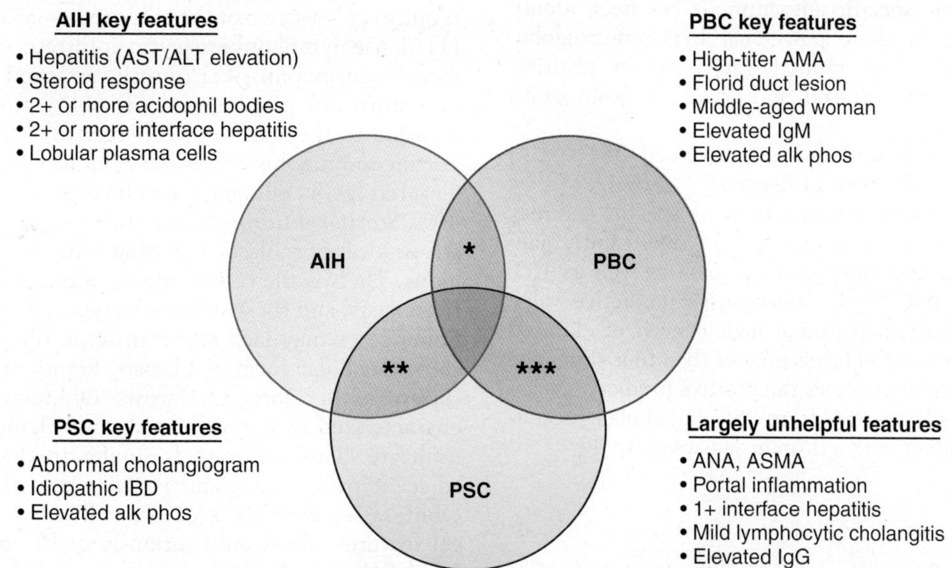

FIGURE 48.35 A conceptual framework for overlap autoimmune liver diseases. Ultimately, the diagnosis of overlap autoimmune liver disease must be individualized. This diagram highlights the major components of overlap autoimmune liver disease. Patients with overlap AIH/PBC *(*)* have features of AIH and PBC, and patients with overlap AIH/PSC *(**)* have features of AIH and PSC. Overlap PBC/PSC *(***)* is very uncommon but undoubtedly exists. Patients must have convincing features of both PBC and PSC. The features in the *bottom left* are common, nondiscriminatory features that are not useful in this context. *AIH,* Autoimmune hepatitis; *alk phos,* alkaline phosphatase; *ALT,* alanine aminotransferase; *AMA,* antimitochondrial antibody; *ANA,* antinuclear antibody; *ASMA,* anti–smooth muscle antibody; *AST,* aspartate aminotransferase; *IBD,* inflammatory bowel disease; *IgM,* immunoglobulin M; *PBC,* primary billary cholangitis; *PSC,* primary sclerosing cholangitis.

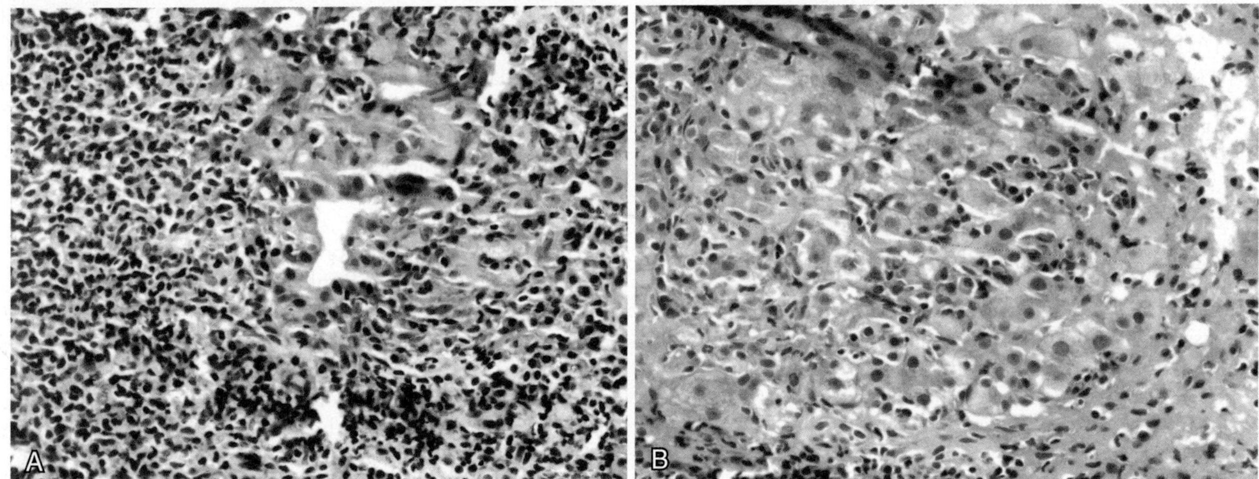

FIGURE 48.36 Overlap primary biliary cholangitis (PBC) and autoimmune hepatitis. A 63-year-old female patient with a history of autoimmune disease (lupus) had elevated serum liver test results, including elevated transaminases (AST, 233 IU/mL; ALT, 275 IU/mL) and alkaline phosphatase (217 IU/mL), with a normal serum globulin level. Viral serologies were negative. Needle biopsy revealed bridging fibrosis *(not shown)*, moderate portal inflammation with conspicuous plasma cells, and granulomatous cholangitis **(A)** with mild ductopenia, focally moderate interface hepatitis with numerous plasma cells **(B)**, and scattered apoptosis in zones 2 and 3 *(not shown)*. The combination of an autoimmune predisposition, negative viral serologies, no suspicious medications, and conspicuous plasma cells suggests autoimmune liver injury. The granulomatous duct destruction (strongly associated with PBC) and lobular injury out of proportion to that seen with pure PBC (i.e., moderate interface hepatitis, zone 2 and 3 acidophil bodies, and transaminases that were more than minimally elevated) indicate overlap PBC and autoimmune hepatitis. *ALT*, Alanine aminotransferase; *AST*, aspartate aminotransferase.

pancreatic duct often validates the diagnosis of IgG4-RSC. On cholangiography, four patterns of involvement are recognized.[213] Cross-sectional imaging may show thickened bile duct walls and a hepatic or perihilar mass. Radiological evidence of involvement of the kidney, lung, and salivary gland would strongly support a diagnosis of IgG4-RSC.

Laboratory and Serological Features

Although no single specific autoantibody has been identified, patients often show polyclonal hypergammaglobulinemia, and antinuclear antibody titers can be positive. Serum IgE levels are increased, and peripheral eosinophilia may be noted.

Serum IgG4 concentrations are increased (>1.4 g/L) in most patients at the time of diagnosis (>80%).[205,206,214] However, elevated serum IgG4 is far from specific and may be observed in a range of diseases, most significantly pancreatic carcinoma and cholangiocarcinoma as well as 15% of patients with PSC.[215,216] The positive predictive value of this test is greatly increased at higher levels of elevated serum IgG4. Serum IgG4 levels greater than four times the upper limit of normal increases the positive predictive value for differentiating IgG4-RSC from PSC and cholangiocarcinoma to 100%, albeit with a drop in sensitivity to 42%.[215]

Pathology

Gross Pathology

In patients with disease involving the bile duct, the wall is markedly thickened and fibrotic, with a pipestem-like quality (Fig. 48.38). A hilar mass mimicking a perihilar cholangiocarcinoma may be seen, and this lesion is occasionally associated with smaller millimeter–size lesions involving the hepatic parenchyma.[217] In some instances, the disease may present as a large intrahepatic mass (Fig. 48.39).[217,218]

Histological Features

The diagnosis relies on a combination of characteristic histological features and increased numbers of IgG4 plasma cells. Although similar histological features identified in the pancreas are also present in IgG4-RSC, the small and often fragmented biopsy specimens from this facet of the disease make this a diagnostic challenge.

General Histological Criteria. The diagnosis generally requires at least two of the three major criteria (Box 48.5): (1) dense lymphoplasmacytic infiltrate often accompanied by eosinophils, (2) fibrosis, arranged at least focally in a storiform pattern, and (3) obliterative phlebitis. In addition to these histological changes, two principal supporting immunohistochemistry findings are described: (1) elevated IgG4 cells and (2) an IgG4:IgG ratio greater than 40%. *Storiform fibrosis* refers to a cartwheel pattern with streams of fibroblasts radiating outward from a central nidus. The spindle cells comprise either myofibroblasts or fibroblasts, and these cells lack atypia and mitotic activity. Some cases may lack storiform-type fibrosis and instead show a cellular form of fibrosis. Biopsy samples may not capture either form of fibrosis. Obliterative phlebitis is characterized by a dense intraluminal lymphoplasmacytic infiltrate. This infiltrate is similar to that noted in the adjacent parenchyma and is accompanied by fibroblasts. Obliterative arteritis is occasionally observed. Histological features that would seriously question a diagnosis of IgG4-RD include necrosis, large numbers of giant cells, a predominantly histiocytic infiltrate, and necrotizing arteritis.

The IgG4:IgG ratio is often the single most useful parameter on biopsy specimens.[219] Pathologists should be aware that quantification of IgG and IgG4 on immunohistochemical staining can be problematic. The IgG staining in

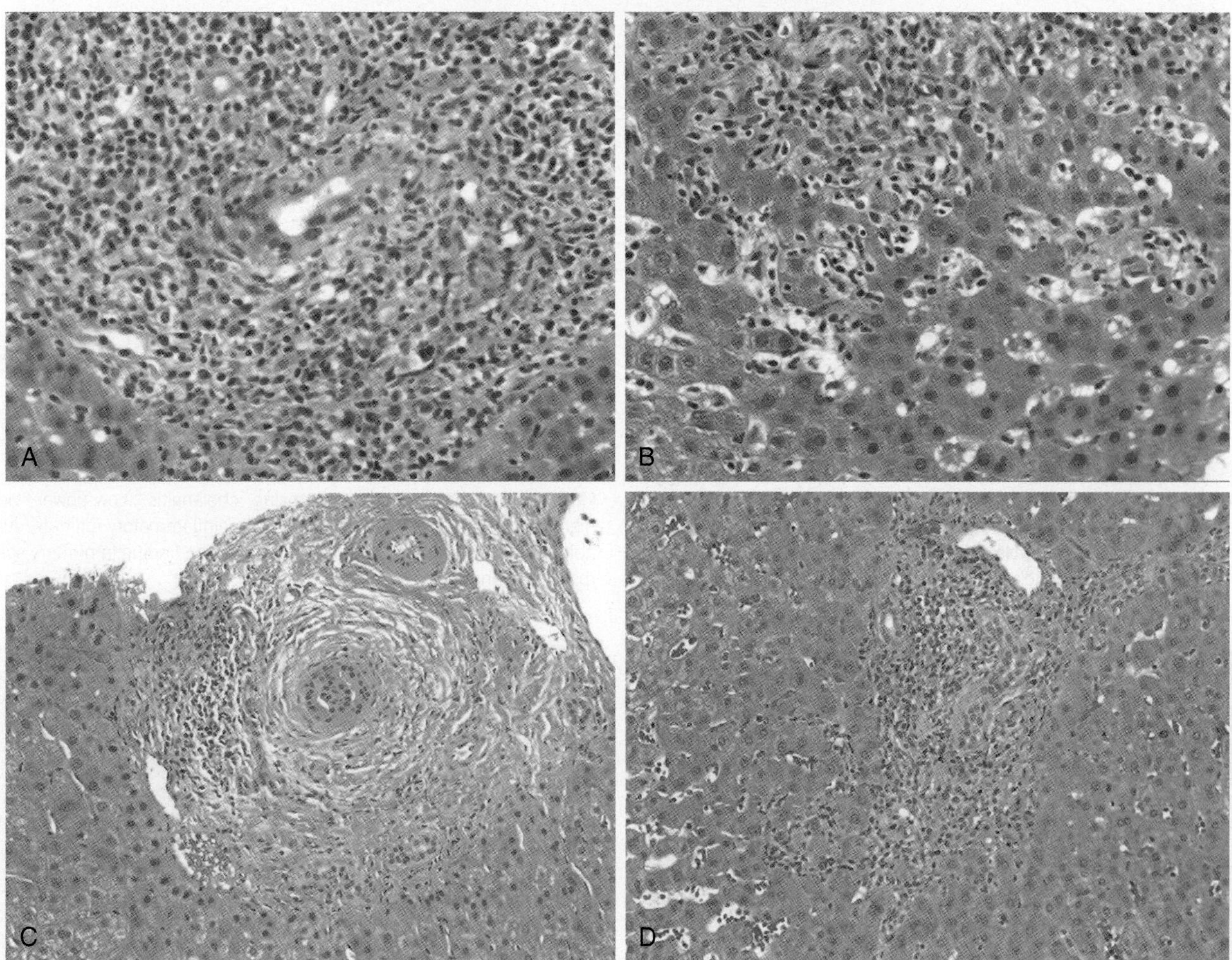

FIGURE 48.37 **A** and **B,** Overlap primary biliary cholangitis (PBC) and autoimmune hepatitis. This patient presented with elevated AST and ALT (3× ULN), elevated serum globulin levels, and a histological appearance consistent with autoimmune hepatitis. A positive AMA and alkaline phosphatase (4× ULN) was detected several years later. **A,** Biopsy shows lymphocytic cholangitis. **B,** The duct is surrounded by a lymphohistiocytic infiltrate, resembling a florid duct lesion. These features support PBC. In addition, several portal tracts showed severe interface activity, a finding that supports the diagnosis of autoimmune hepatitis. **C** and **D,** Overlap primary sclerosing cholangitis (PSC) and autoimmune hepatitis. This child presented with typical clinical, serological, and histological features of autoimmune hepatitis. An elevated alkaline phosphatase (5× ULN) and a cholangiographic appearance consistent with sclerosing cholangitis was noted 7 years following the original biopsy. Note the periductal onion-skin–type fibrosis **(C)** and interface activity **(D).** *ALT,* Alanine aminotransferase; *AST,* aspartate aminotransferase; and *ULN,* Upper limit of normal.

particular must be evaluated with caution because it may have high background signal.

It should be noted that near-exclusive reliance on elevated numbers of IgG4-positive cells is imprudent and correlation with other clinical and serological features is advisable (see the discussion on HISORt criteria in Diagnostic Algorithm).

Site-Specific Criteria

Bile Duct. The bile duct is thickened by a lymphoplasmacytic infiltrate, and unlike PSC, the disease involves the entire thickness of the duct (Fig. 48.40). Storiform-type fibrosis is generally seen in the outer half of the bile duct. These characteristic features of IgG4-RSC noted in resected samples are often not seen on biopsies. Forceps biopsies of the bile duct generally show a nonspecific lymphoplasmacytic infiltrate, and in this context, even the presence of >10 IgG4-positive cells is nonspecific and is seen in both PSC and cholangiocarcinoma.

An ampullary biopsy may aid in the diagnosis of IgG4-RSC. The histological features and pitfalls associated with ampullary biopsies is covered in Chapter 40.

Pseudotumoral Lesions. A targeted biopsy from a hepatic tumefactive lesion typically shows a dense lymphoplasmacytic infiltrate and storiform-type fibrosis (Fig. 48.41). Obliterative phlebitis may not be seen; an elastic stain may aid in uncovering partially or completely obliterated veins.[215] The mass lesions show increased numbers of IgG4-positive cells (Fig. 48.42). These lesions often show a prominent population of fibroblasts and myofibroblasts (Fig. 48.43). Notably, these cells do not show atypia.

Hepatic Nontumefactive Lesions. A nonfocal liver biopsy from a patient with suspected IgG4-RSC typically shows a portal lymphoplasmacytic infiltrate that mimics a chronic hepatitis pattern of injury. In addition, these biopsies often show changes related to downstream obstruction of bile ducts such as portal edema. Given the

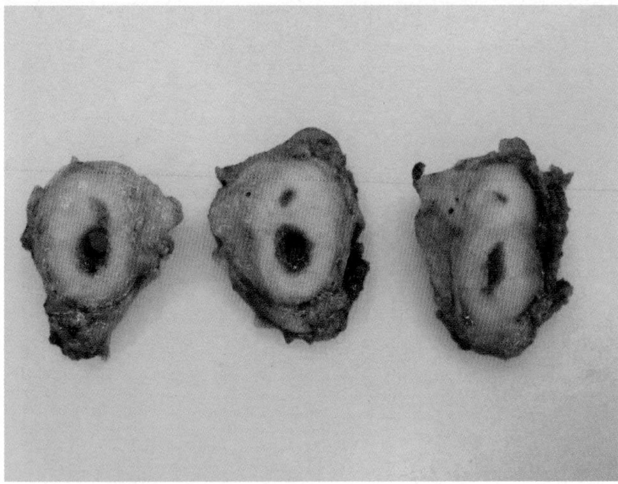

FIGURE 48.38 IgG4-related sclerosing cholangitis. The bile duct shown here in cross-section is markedly thickened and has a rigid "pipestem-like" quality. (From Zen Y, Nakanuma Y, Portmann B. Immunoglobulin G4-related sclerosing cholangitis: pathologic features and histological mimics. *Semin Diagn Pathol.* 2012;29(4):205-211.)

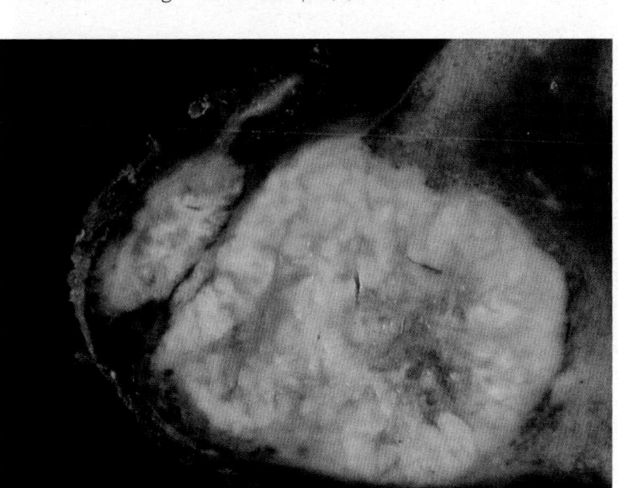

FIGURE 48.39 Tumefactive lesion in a patient with IgG4-related sclerosing cholangitis. Note the masslike lesion that mimics cholangiocarcinoma.

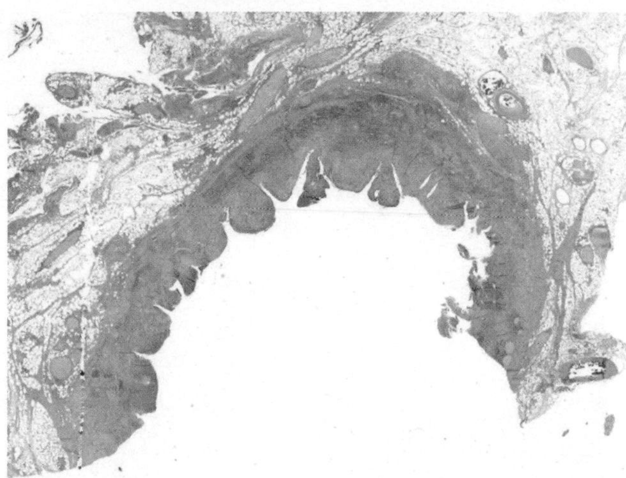

FIGURE 48.40 IgG4-related sclerosing cholangitis. Low-power view highlights the transmural nature of the fibroinflammatory infiltrate. Also note the intact biliary epithelium, an uncommon finding in primary sclerosing cholangitis.

FIGURE 48.41 IgG4-related sclerosing cholangitis. This tumefactive lesion shows a dense fibroinflammatory infiltrate with storiform-type fibrosis.

BOX 48.5 Histological Diagnosis of IgG4-Related Disease

Diagnosis requires BOTH histological (preferable 2) and immunohistochemical features

- **Histological features**
  - Dense lymphoplasmacytic infiltrate
  - Storiform-type fibrosis
  - Obliterative phlebitis
- **Immunohistochemical features**
  - Elevated numbers of IgG4-positive plasma cells
  - Elevated IgG4:IgG ratio >40%

otherwise nonspecific pattern of this infiltrate, the diagnosis of IgG4-RSC relies on (1) portal-based fibroinflammatory nodules (Fig. 48.44) and (2) >10 IgG4-positive cells (Figs. 48.45 and 48.46). The portal-based fibroinflammatory nodules show the classic plasma cell–rich fibroinflammatory infiltrate associated with IgG4-RD. These fibroinflammatory nodules are characteristic for IgG4-RSC; however, they are seen in only a minority of biopsies. Periductal fibrosis may also be seen, although less commonly than PSC (Fig. 48.47).

Diagnostic Algorithm

The diagnosis of IgG4-RSC should only be made in conjunction with the clinical, serological, and radiological appearance. The acronym *HISORt*, initially applied to the diagnosis of autoimmune pancreatitis, was subsequently adopted for IgG4-RSC. HISORt highlights the five cardinal diagnostic features of IgG4-RD: (1) *h*istology, (2) *i*maging, (3) *s*erology—specifically elevated serum IgG4, (4) *o*ther organ involvement, and (5) *r*esponse to immunosuppressive therapy.[205,220] Clinical, biochemical, and/or cholangiographic improvement is generally seen within 4 to 6 weeks after starting steroids. In instances in which there is uncertainty about the diagnosis, a trial of steroids is favored

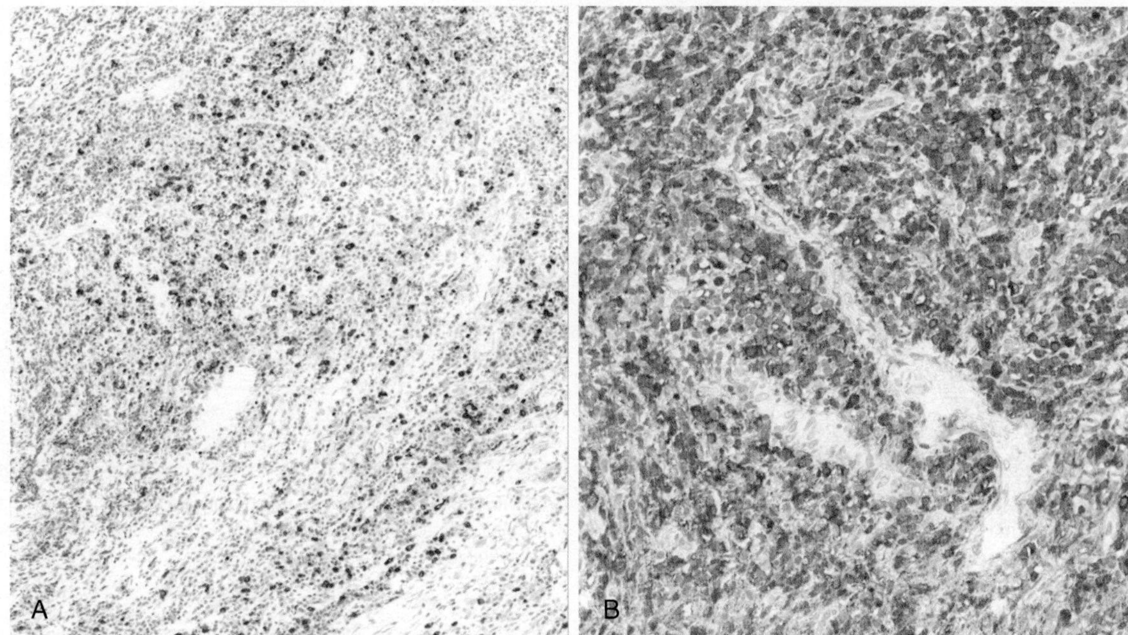

FIGURE 48.42 IgG4-related sclerosing cholangitis. Immunohistochemistry for IgG4 **(A)** and IgG **(B)** is performed on the example illustrated in Fig. 48.41. Note that the IgG4-positive cells are diffusely distributed throughout the lesion. The IgG preparation is difficult to enumerate because of the nonspecific background reactivity; however, the IgG4:IgG ratio was estimated at 42%.

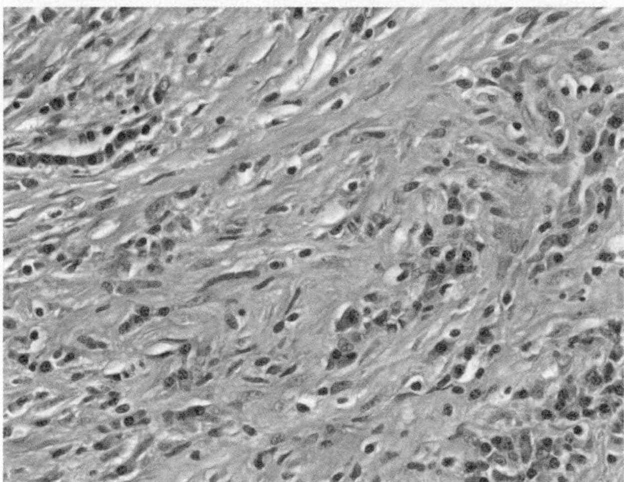

FIGURE 48.43 High-power view of IgG4-related sclerosing cholangitis. Note the prominent population of fibroblasts/myofibroblasts. Plasma cells are also prominent.

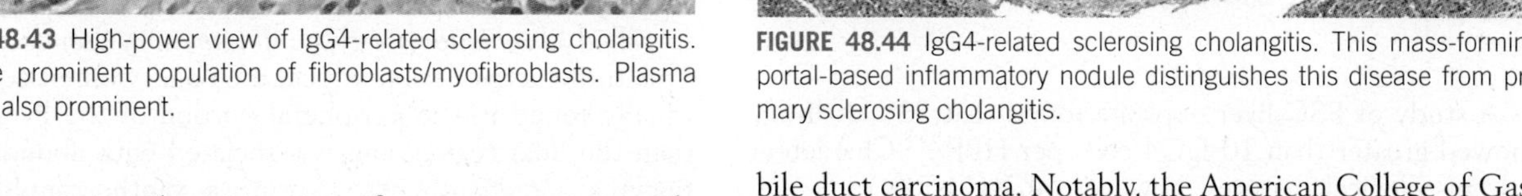

FIGURE 48.44 IgG4-related sclerosing cholangitis. This mass-forming portal-based inflammatory nodule distinguishes this disease from primary sclerosing cholangitis.

by many treating physicians. A swift response may provide an additional layer of reassurance but is not in and of itself diagnostic for IgG4-RSC. Bile duct carcinomas and pancreatic ductal adenocarcinomas may show limited but not sustained response to steroids.

Differential Diagnosis *(Box 48.6)*

Primary Sclerosing Cholangitis

The many overlapping features between PSC and IgG4-RSC make this distinction a difficult problem but one that is clinically significant given that IgG4-RD lesions resolve with immunosuppressive therapy. The two diseases are compared in Tables 48.10 and 48.11. PSC is also associated with a much poorer prognosis and a substantially increased risk of bile duct carcinoma. Notably, the American College of Gastroenterology recommends the measurement of serum IgG4 levels in all patients with possible PSC to exclude IgG4-RSC. However, it is important to note that serum IgG4 is elevated in up to 15% of patients with PSC.[221] The average age at presentation in PSC (44 years) is younger than in IgG4-RSC (63 years). A majority of cases of PSC come to light at laboratory evaluation for liver function tests, often in the context of IBD, whereas most cases of IgG4-RSC present with clinical and enzymatic changes of cholestasis. It should be noted that there is a small but significant association between IgG4-RD and IBD.[206] Histologically, inflammatory nodules, alluded to previously, are not seen in PSC. The loss of bile ducts may assist in the distinction, with paucity of bile ducts uncommon in IgG4-RSC.

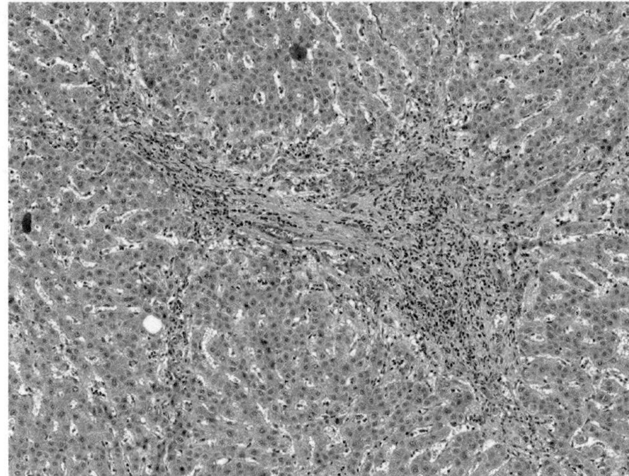

FIGURE 48.45 IgG4-related sclerosing cholangitis. The expanded portal tract is infiltrated by a mild lymphocytic infiltrate. Prominent bile ductal reduplication is also seen. This appearance is not specific for IgG4 related sclerosing cholangitis. Also see Fig. 48.46.

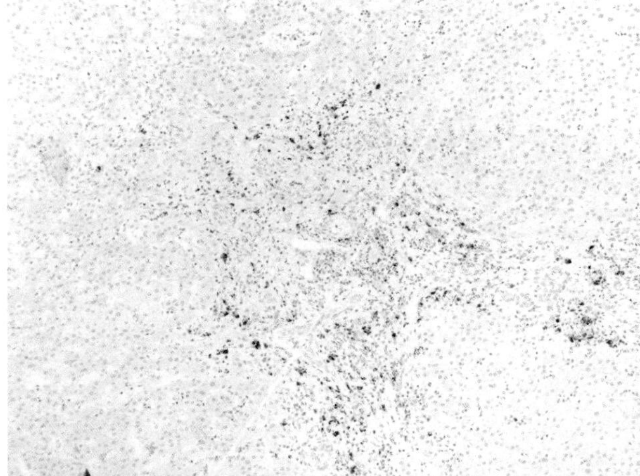

FIGURE 48.46 IgG4-related sclerosing cholangitis. Immunohistochemical stain for IgG4 performed on the case depicted in Fig. 48.45. Although the histological features are not specific, the presence of >10 IgG4-positive cells would support a diagnosis of IgG4-related sclerosing cholangitis.

A study of PSC liver explants found that 23% of livers showed greater than 10 IgG4 cells per HPF.[222] Characteristic histological features, however, of IgG4-RD were not identified in these patients.[222] Another study showed that 5% of 41 liver explants with PSC showed >100 IgG4-positive cells per HPF.[223] Thus the mere presence of elevated numbers of IgG4-positive cells does not distinguish PSC from IgG4-RSC.

Sclerosing Cholangitis with Granulocytic Epithelial Lesions

Sclerosing cholangitis with granulocytic epithelial lesions affects individuals in the first two decades of life and shows a cholangiographic appearance that resembles PSC. Histologically the disease is characterized by neutrophilic aggregates within bile ducts, the so-called *granulocytic epithelial lesions.*[224] IgG4 cells are not elevated, and serum IgG4 levels are normal. Unlike PSC, patients go into remission with prednisolone and/or ursodeoxycholic acid and do not relapse.[224]

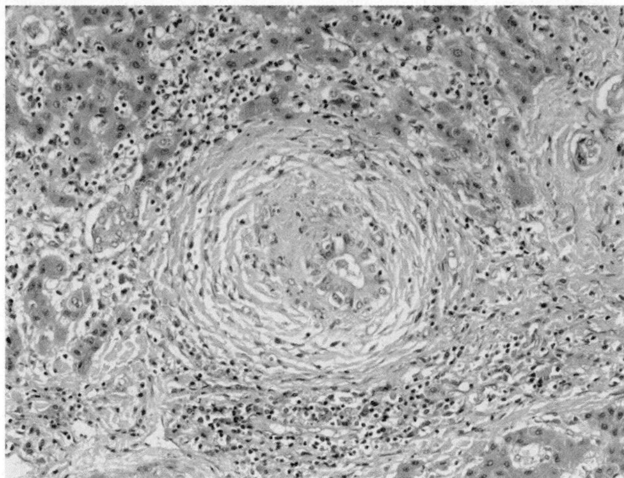

FIGURE 48.47 IgG4-related sclerosing cholangitis. Periductal onion-skin–type fibrosis is an uncommon finding in IgG4-related sclerosing cholangitis.

BOX 48.6 IgG4-Related Sclerosing Cholangitis: Clinical, Radiological, and Histological Differential Diagnosis

- Primary sclerosing cholangitis
- Bile duct carcinoma and intrahepatic cholangiocarcinoma
- Lymphoproliferative disorder
- Follicular cholangitis
- Sclerosing cholangitis with granulocytic epithelial lesions
- Fibrohistiocytic variant of inflammatory pseudotumor
- Cholangiocarcinoma

Hepatic Inflammatory Pseudotumor

Before the recognition of IgG4-RD, inflammatory mass-forming lesions were often referred to as *hepatic inflammatory pseudotumor.* In addition to IgG4-RD and inflammatory myofibroblastic tumors, a third category was recently teased out from this inflammatory pseudotumor cohort, the so-called *fibrohistiocytic-type inflammatory pseudotumor.*[218] This tumefactive lesion affects men and women equally, is usually found in the peripheral portion of the liver rather than the hilar region, and is associated with abundant histiocytes and giant cells creating a xanthogranulomatous inflammatory reaction. Storiform-type fibrosis may be seen, and the IgG4 stain is typically negative, or the numbers are fewer than 10 per HPF. The fibrohistiocytic variant of inflammatory pseudotumor appears to represent a reaction to bacterial infection, and many of these patients respond favorably to antibiotic therapy.[225]

Follicular Cholangitis

Follicular cholangitis typically affects elderly individuals and presents with obstructive jaundice (Fig. 48.48).[226] Histologically, the large bile ducts are surrounded by a dense lymphoid infiltrate, and germinal centers are prominent; plasma cells are either absent or sparse. The characteristic histopathological features of IgG4-RD are not identified.

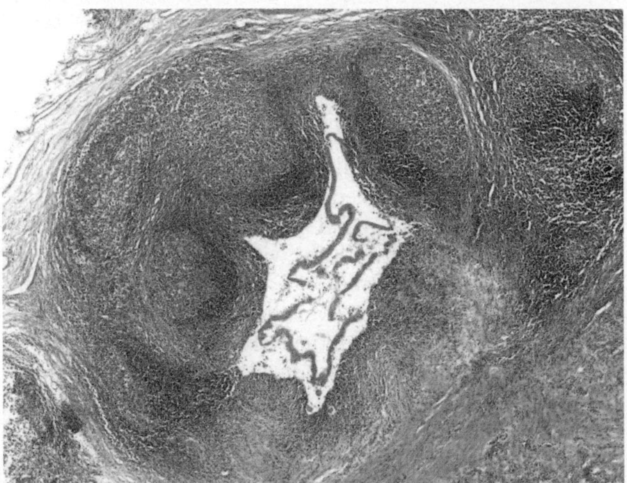

FIGURE 48.48 Follicular cholangitis. Note the large reactive germinal centers surrounding the bile duct. (From Zen Y, Nakanuma Y, Portmann B. Immunoglobulin G4-related sclerosing cholangitis: pathologic features and histological mimics. Semin Diagn Pathol. 2012;29(4):205-211).

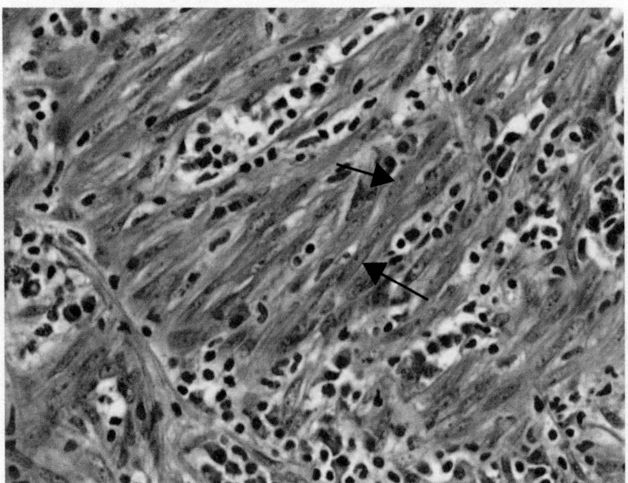

FIGURE 48.49 An inflammatory myofibroblastic tumor mimicking IgG4-related disease. The majority of plasma cells were positive for IgG4. However, unlike IgG4-related disease, note the significantly greater degree of cellular atypia *(arrows)* within the stromal compartment.

A disease similar to follicular cholangitis has also been recognized in the pancreas.[227]

Inflammatory Myofibroblastic Tumor

Inflammatory myofibroblastic tumor (IMT) is a mesenchymal neoplasm that is frequently accompanied by a dense inflammatory infiltrate composed of lymphocytes and plasma cells (Fig. 48.49).[228] Although high-grade IMTs are readily distinguished from IgG4-RD, low-grade examples may be indistinguishable from this entity, particularly on needle biopsies. IMTs may show bland spindle-shaped cells in an inflammatory background, thus mimicking tumefactive hepatic IgG4-related disease. Although obliterative phlebitis and storiform-type fibrosis are uncommon in IMTs, the authors' group has encountered both features in IgG4-RD, and some IMTs also show elevations of IgG4 cells at levels comparable with IgG4-RD.[228,229] The three most common genetic alterations in IMTs are *ALK*, *ROS1*, and *NTRK* fusions, and immunohistochemical assays serve as fairly robust surrogates for the translocation.

Other mesenchymal neoplasms such as the inflammatory variant of liposarcoma may also show elevated numbers of IgG4-positive plasma cells.

Cholangiocarcinoma

On imaging, there can be significant overlap between IgG4-RSC and cholangiocarcinoma. Cytological examination and next-generation sequencing analyses that identify common genetic alterations in bile duct carcinoma may be of great value.[180] However, these diagnostic techniques in and of themselves are imperfect. Genetic analyses, such as fluorescence in situ hybridization assays, may be falsely positive in IgG4-RSC. Aneuploidy in bile duct brushing specimens, a feature of malignancy, may also be detected in patients with IgG4-RD.[230]

Pathologists must keep in mind that bile duct carcinomas can also show elevated numbers of IgG4 cells. In studies of extrahepatic cholangiocarcinoma (bile duct carcinoma), greater than 10 IgG4 plasma cells per HPF were identified in 37% to 43% of cases, and greater than 50 IgG4 cells per HPF were counted in 6% of cases.[231,232] In another study of 16 cholangiocarcinomas, 4 (25%) cases showed ≥10 IgG4-positive plasma cells per HPF.[230] Thus an undersampled bile duct carcinoma may be misdiagnosed as IgG4-RSC if a pathologist is overreliant on the IgG4 cell count.

Treatment

IgG4-RD responds rapidly to immunosuppressive therapy.[233] A majority of patients relapse after withdrawal of immunosuppression. In an attempt to prevent flare-ups, patients are placed on low-dose corticosteroid therapy. Rituximab, an anti-CD20 antibody, is often used as a steroid-sparing agent.[234,235] Although the disease is responsive to immunosuppressive therapy, there is a risk of progressive fibrosis, and cases of cirrhosis have also been recognized.

IMMUNOGLOBULIN G4-RELATED AUTOIMMUNE HEPATITIS

IgG4-related AIH is characterized by clinical, serological, and histological features of AIH as well as increased numbers of IgG4-positive cells and an elevated IgG4:IgG ratio.[236-239] These patients also show elevated serum IgG4 and report the more characteristic features of IgG4-RD, including autoimmune pancreatitis and sclerosing cholangitis. Histologically, IgG4-related AIH resembles conventional AIH with marked portal lymphoplasmacytic inflammation and prominent interface activity. All three reported cases showed more than 30 IgG4-positive cells per HPF and an IgG4:IgG ratio that exceeded 40%. The hepatic manifestations responded favorably to steroid therapy. It is important to emphasize that this is an extremely uncommon manifestation of IgG4-RD, with only three well-documented cases of this entity.

It is important to distinguish IgG4-related AIH from cases of AIH with elevated numbers of IgG4-positive cells. These patients lack characteristic manifestations of IgG4-RD including an elevated serum IgG4 level and other organ involvement. The IgG4:IgG ratio is <40%. There is currently no unequivocal evidence that patients with AIH and increased numbers of IgG4-positive cells represent a distinct disease entity. Increased numbers of IgG4-positive cells have also been reported in transplant biopsies that show plasma cell hepatitis.[240] Collectively, the mere presence of increased numbers of IgG4-positive cells in AIH on a liver biopsy has no clinical significance, and these patients should not be diagnosed as having IgG4-RD.

Finally, liver biopsies from patients with IgG4-RSC may also show dense portal inflammation with increased numbers of IgG4-positive cells. However, the clinical picture in these patients is dominated by either sclerosing cholangitis or a hilar tumefactive lesion. These patients lack clinical or serological evidence of AIH.

SECONDARY SCLEROSING CHOLANGITIS

SSC is a syndrome characterized by intrahepatic or extrahepatic histological and cholangiographic evidence of sclerosing cholangitis in a patient without PSC. This disorder is a consequence of other disease processes.[172] SSC is not a distinct disease entity; it instead represents involvement of bile ducts by a variety of non-PSC diseases that result in a PSC-like syndrome. Potential causes include immune disorders, ischemia, toxic injury, infiltrative disorders, infections, and idiopathic fibrosis, as reviewed by Abdalian and Heathcote.[172]

Immune disorders other than PBC, PSC, and IgG4-related sclerosing cholangitis can cause intrahepatic duct loss and sclerosing cholangitis. Intrahepatic duct loss also can occur in alloimmune injury (e.g., allograft rejection, graft-versus-host-disease).

Ischemic cholangitis is another important cause of sclerosing cholangitis, occurring independently or as a component of other disorders that cause SSC. It is likely that at least some of the autoimmune, infectious, fibrosing, and infiltrative causes of sclerosing cholangitis have an element of ischemic injury as a result of microscopic vascular damage to the peribiliary vascular plexus (discussed later).

Infectious disorders (e.g., bacterial infection, recurrent pyogenic cholangitis) and immune deficiencies (e.g., AIDS cholangiopathy) occasionally complicated by superimposed viral or bacterial infections can cause SSC.[172] The patient's clinical features and culture results are usually considered more helpful for diagnostic purposes than liver biopsy, although *Cryptosporidium*, *Mycobacterium avium-intracellulare* complex, cytomegalovirus, or other opportunistic pathogens are rarely identified histologically.

Infiltrative processes can cause SSC through the tumefactive effect of tumor cells or secondary vascular damage. Eosinophilic cholangitis is characterized by a dense eosinophilic bile duct infiltrate. It may be isolated to the biliary system or represent a component of more generalized eosinophilic gastroenteritis. Peripheral blood eosinophilia, a clinical history of allergies or asthma, absence of evidence of parasitic infection, and a rapid response to corticosteroid therapy are clues to its diagnosis.[241] When the main biliary tract is affected, a PSC-like appearance may develop initially, with resolution expected after therapy. Peripheral liver biopsies often show a mechanical obstruction–like picture but without bile duct loss. Periductal eosinophilia is observed in some cases. Mast cell disease, Langerhans cell histiocytosis, and metastases are rare infiltrative causes of SSC.[172]

ISCHEMIC CHOLANGITIS

Ischemic damage to the biliary tract (i.e., ischemic cholangitis) is an underrecognized disorder. It may be one of the most common causes of SSC.[167] Patients at risk for ischemic cholangitis include those with prior biliary or upper abdominal surgery or trauma, thrombotic or vasculitic disorders, ABO-incompatible liver allografts, and hepatic intra-arterial chemotherapy (particularly floxuridine). Clinical manifestations depend on the severity of bile duct damage but usually mimic PSC with the formation of biliary strictures, secondary obstructive cholestasis, occasional intrahepatic bile duct loss, and superimposed infective cholangitis.

The condition is not considered reversible. Some cases are managed by stenting, whereas others require resection of the diseased portion of bile duct, which may necessitate liver transplantation.

An important distinction between hepatocytes and biliary epithelial cells (intrahepatic and extrahepatic) is that the former receive a dual blood supply (i.e., hepatic arterial and portal venous), whereas the latter depend only on hepatic arterial blood. Blood is supplied to the mid-extrahepatic bile duct through the 3-o'clock and 9-o'clock arteries, which are derived from the right hepatic artery superiorly and the retroduodenal artery inferiorly.[242] However, there are a variety of anatomical variations. For instance, the extrahepatic blood supply may be derived from the hepatic artery in some individuals or from the retroduodenal arteries in others. At the ultrastructural level, a rich anastomosing plexus of arterioles and venules surrounds the bile ducts.[243]

Ischemic cholangitis may be caused by a primary insult to the hepatic arteries, other major arteries, or the microscopic arteriolar vessels (i.e., peribiliary vascular plexus). The hepatic arteries may be compromised by surgical or traumatic interruption of the arteries (e.g., during liver transplantation) and thrombosis (e.g., spontaneous, secondary tumor, intraarterial chemotherapy). Smaller arteries may be involved in systemic vasculitides, ABO-incompatible transplantation, autoimmune disorders, and microthrombotic disease, such as hemolytic uremic syndrome,[244] which overlaps with immune-mediated SSC (see Table 48.10). One case of presumed ischemic cholangitis in a critically ill patient was thought to result from microthrombosis related to severe systemic illness with generalized hypotension and hypoxemia (i.e., shock cholangitis).[245]

Ischemic cholangitis initially manifests with atrophic-appearing biliary epithelium, followed in more severe cases by sloughing of the biliary epithelium (Fig. 48.50). This results in contact of bile with the underlying mesenchyme, which may cause an exuberant mixed neutrophilic, lymphocytic, and histiocytic reaction. This may result in bile duct dilation (i.e., cholangiectases), bile plugs, choledocholithiasis, and bacterial superinfection caused by bile stasis (i.e., cholangitic abscesses).

Fibrosis eventually occurs, causing a beaded cholangiographic appearance reminiscent of PSC. In needle biopsy specimens of peripheral liver, the dominant histological picture is typically that of large duct obstruction, with biliary atrophy or bile duct loss recognizable in more severe

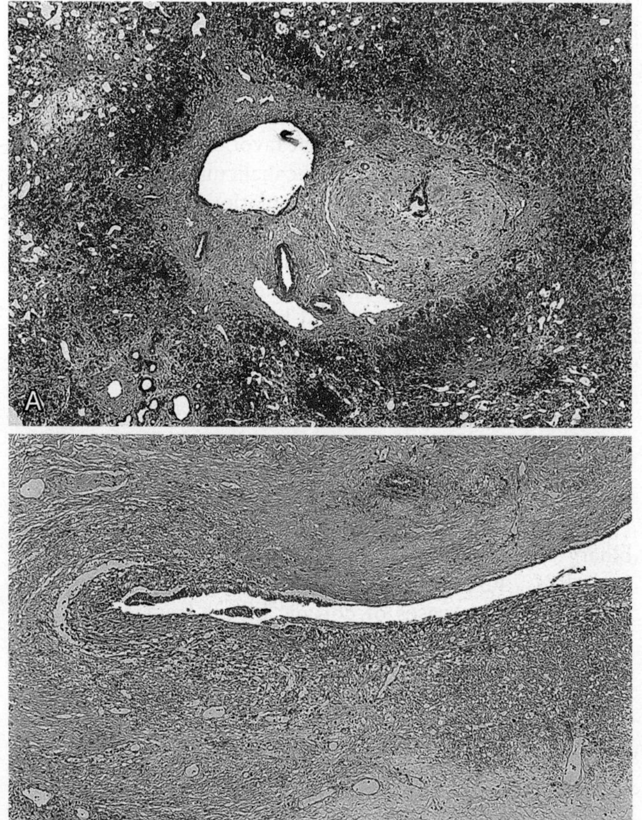

FIGURE 48.50 Bile duct damage in ischemic cholangitis mimics primary sclerosing cholangitis. A, In this case of ischemic biliary damage caused by hepatic vein thrombosis (i.e., Budd-Chiari syndrome) and presumed venous stasis affecting the biliary tree, the biliary epithelium is attenuated, and concentric periductal fibrosis occurs. **B,** Similar changes can be seen with disruption of the arterial blood supply to the bile ducts, which resulted from hepatic artery infusion of floxuridine chemotherapy (Masson trichrome stain).

cases. In long-standing cases, biliary-type fibrosis and cirrhosis may develop. In liver explants or autopsy specimens, the full spectrum of biliary damage is often apparent, with cholangiectases, cholangitic abscesses, strictures, and biliary sludge or stones, all of which mimic PSC.

MISCELLANEOUS DUCTOPENIC SYNDROMES

The mechanisms of bile duct loss remain poorly understood.[246] Ductopenia in the absence of an identifiable cause is called *idiopathic adulthood ductopenia*.[247] IAD is a syndrome characterized by progressive duct loss and its complications. It has no apparent cause (i.e., no morphological or serological features of PBC/AC, no abnormal cholangiogram or history of IBD to suggest PSC, and no other known bile duct–destructive condition).

Patients with IAD fall into two main categories: those with progressive disease that may ultimately lead to liver transplantation and those with a benign clinical course.[247] Rather than a distinct syndrome, IAD may represent a mixture of late-onset paucity of intrahepatic bile ducts, small duct PSC in the absence of IBD, and postviral duct destruction.[247]

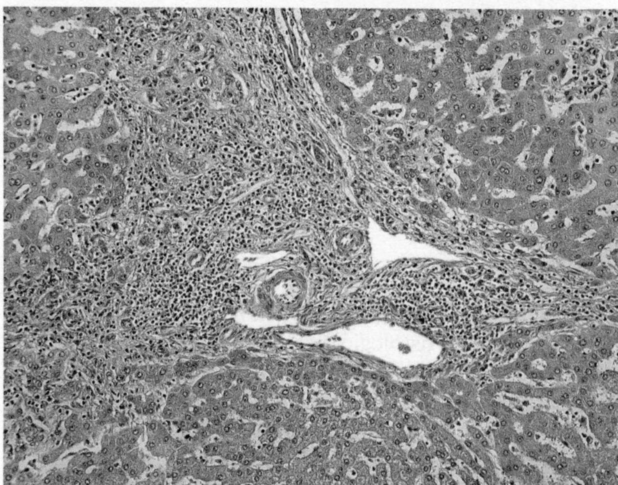

FIGURE 48.51 Idiopathic adulthood ductopenia. The portal tract lacks a bile duct and shows mild chronic inflammation; the lobules are quiescent. This 32-year-old male patient had a normal cholangiogram, no evidence of idiopathic inflammatory bowel disease, no serological evidence of primary biliary cirrhosis, and no other underlying risk factors for bile duct loss. He underwent liver transplantation for intractable pruritus.

The histological features in early-stage disease consist of focal bile duct dropout (>50% loss is the definition of *ductopenia*), with relatively minor nonspecific inflammation, absence of granulomas or other specific features, and perhaps mild ductular proliferation (Fig. 48.51). Late-stage disease shows progressive ductopenia, changes of cholestasis, and biliary-type fibrosis, as described earlier in PBC and PSC.

Ductopenia has rarely been associated with adverse drug reactions. Small intrahepatic ducts are affected most commonly. In these cases, duct regeneration may occur.[248] An unusual association between Hodgkin disease and ductopenia (i.e., vanishing bile duct syndrome) exists, although the mechanism is unclear.

OBSTRUCTIVE CHOLANGITIS

Clinical Features

In obstructive cholangitis (i.e., large duct obstruction), mechanical interruption of extrahepatic bile flow caused by biliary stones within large ducts or the bile duct, ampullary strictures, or masses may produce a clinical and histological picture that depends on the time frame (acute or chronic) and degree of stenosis (partial or complete obstruction). Nausea and vomiting are common early symptoms. Jaundice typically develops in cases of severe obstruction. Common duct obstruction with secondary (ascending) cholangitis may elicit the Charcot triad of symptoms (i.e., right upper quadrant pain, fever, and jaundice), with additional hypotension and mental status changes resulting in the Raynaud pentad, a poor prognostic sign. In patients with chronic, low-grade obstruction, progressive hepatic fibrosis and chronic biliary-type cirrhosis may evolve with the development of progressive pruritus and other consequences of established cirrhosis (e.g., portal hypertension, coagulopathies). Biochemically, acute bile duct obstruction is usually associated with a significant elevation in serum aminotransferase (alanine aminotransferase [ALT] and aspartate aminotransferase [AST]), alkaline phosphatase, and GGT levels, with hyperbilirubinemia in proportion to the degree of obstruction, but not often exceeding 25 mg/dL. In patients with chronic bile duct obstruction, serum aminotransferase levels tend to decrease, and alkaline phosphatase and GGT levels persist or slowly increase.

Pathology

Obstructive cholangitis does not have specific gross pathological features. Histologically, liver biopsies from patients with acute bile duct obstruction may show portal edema, ductular proliferation with neutrophils (i.e., cholangiolitis), tortuous bile ducts that may appear increased in number on histological sectioning, and, in some cases, intraluminal or intraepithelial bile duct neutrophils (i.e., cholangitis). Bile pigment may accumulate within the bile duct lumens and be visible on histological examination. Even in the acute stage of extrahepatic large duct obstruction, the pathologist often notices a temporal progression of histological changes. For instance, within the first 1 to 2 weeks of obstruction, cholestasis begins in the zone 3 (perivenular) region, which is often associated with portal edema and portal inflammation. In this early acute period, the pattern of cholestasis may mimic a drug effect, infectious hepatitis, or sepsis or shock.

Cholestasis in the early phase is often intracytoplasmic and canalicular with occasional large bile plugs. Thereafter, a marked marginal bile ductular reaction associated with neutrophils (i.e., cholangiolitis) develops in more than 80% of cases. In the following weeks and with continued obstruction, the parenchymal and portal changes become more developed, and cholestasis becomes more pronounced. Cholestasis extends to zone 2 and zone 1 (periportal) regions, the deposits become larger in size and number, and cholestatic liver cell rosettes associated with dense bile concretions may develop. Cholestatic feathery degeneration is common: hepatocytes are enlarged, rarefied, and degenerated. Lyses of liver cells and release of bile leads to the formation of bile lakes and bile infarcts, which are defined as clusters of confluent liver cells with feathery degeneration, bile stasis, and necrosis with or without macrophages. These features are virtually diagnostic of obstructive cholangitis. Bile infarcts are caused by the toxic action of bile salts. With repair, foreign-body giant cells and fibrous tissue become apparent.

If the obstructive cause is not reversed in the acute period, chronic changes develop, including further cholate stasis, copper accumulation, Mallory bodies, fibrosis, and cirrhosis. The bile ductular reaction may become extremely prominent. Eventually, a process resembling SSC develops. The small and large interlobular bile ducts show proliferation, branching, and increased tortuosity. The epithelium may appear degenerated or ulcerated, resulting in periductal fibrosis. Ductular proliferation is usually prominent. Canalicular cholestasis, often pericentral (zone 3) predominant, may be seen in severe cases (Fig. 48.52). Eventually, persistent chronic obstruction (Fig. 48.53) may result in a biliary cirrhosis–like histological appearance, except that the bile ducts usually persist.

Differential Diagnosis

The major differential diagnosis for acute bile duct obstruction is cholestatic drug injury. In some cases, knowledge of the clinical features is needed to establish a correct diagnosis. The histological features that favor bile duct obstruction include portal edema, zone 3 canalicular cholestasis, and acute cholangitis with bile accumulation within the lumens of the bile ducts. Drug reactions may also cause zonal cholestasis but not usually prominent edema. Cholestasis associated with systemic shock or sepsis (i.e., cholangitis lenta) tends to cause the formation of bile plugs in dilated zone 1 (periportal) cholangioles, which contrasts with drug reactions and acute bile duct obstruction. Nevertheless, all of these disorders may show brisk ductular proliferation with or without neutrophils.

For chronic biliary tract obstruction, the major differential diagnoses are chronic ductopenic syndromes (i.e., PBC, PSC, and SSC). All of these disorders show progressive biliary-type fibrosis and cholate stasis. However, in contrast with PBC, PSC, and SSC, bile ducts usually persist and remain viable in cases of chronic biliary tract obstruction. All of these disorders, including chronic bile duct destruction, may show some degree of ductular proliferation at the portal-parenchymal interface (i.e., limiting plate).

POST–COVID-19 CHOLANGIOPATHY

The novel coronavirus SARS-CoV-2 was identified as the cause of an epidemic of acute respiratory disease in the Hubei province of China in December 2019 and quickly developed into a worldwide pandemic.[249,250] Although coronavirus disease 2019 (COVID-19) primarily affects the respiratory system, digestive symptoms are also common and, according to one meta-analysis, approximately 19% of patients exhibit abnormal liver function tests at some point during their disease course. These abnormal biochemical studies typically reflect a hepatitic pattern of liver injury with only mild elevations in serum AST and ALT levels that rarely exceed one to two times the upper limit of normal.[251]

In contrast, a minority of patients recovering from severe COVID-19 develop a cholestatic pattern of liver injury characterized by marked elevations in serum alkaline phosphatase and total bilirubin that has been referred to in the literature as *post–COVID-19 cholangiopathy*. In one series of 12 patients, biliary tract abnormalities were universally identified by MRCP, with beading of the intrahepatic bile ducts, peribiliary enhancement, and thickening of the bile duct wall seen in most cases.[252] From a histological perspective, post–COVID-19 cholangiopathy shows features of large duct obstruction including portal tract edema associated with a brisk ductular reaction and an increased in periportal CK7-positive intermediate hepatobiliary cells (Fig. 48.54).[252] Paucity of interlobular bile ducts has been observed in some cases, but is not a universal feature of this disease process. Nevertheless, severe cholangiocyte injury associated with prominent vacuolization, apoptosis, and necrosis was seen in all cases in a single small study, as was portal/periportal fibrosis and microarteriopathy of hepatic artery branches and portal venous endothelial injury.[253]

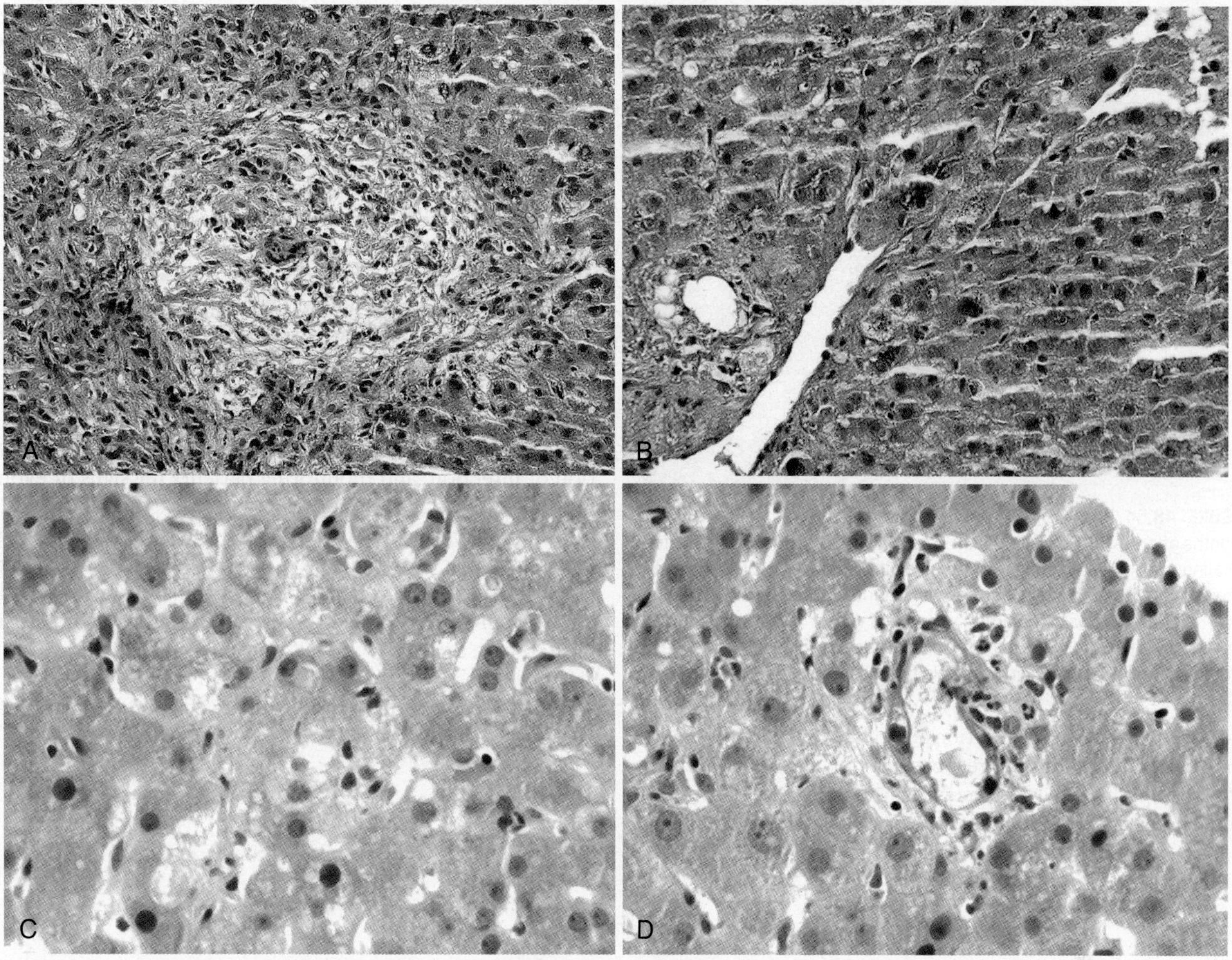

FIGURE 48.52 Liver changes of acute, high-grade mechanical bile flow impairment shown by needle biopsy. A, The portal tract shows prominent edema, leading to a rounded contour with some nonspecific ductular proliferation at the limiting plate. **B,** The central vein region from the same patient shows prominent pericentral (zone 3) canalicular cholestasis, the typical distribution of bile with high-grade mechanical obstruction. **C,** Centrilobular region shows canalicular and intracytoplasmic bile stasis associated with degenerating hepatocytes (i.e., cholestatic feathery degeneration). **D,** High-power view of a portal tract shows a degenerated and partially ruptured bile duct with bile in the lumen and extruding into the periductal space.

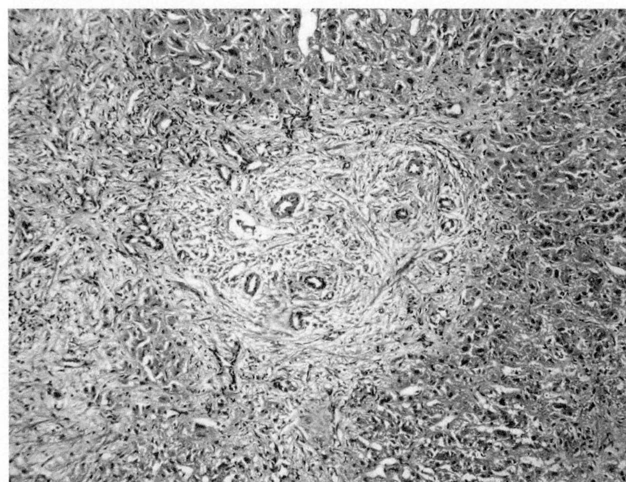

FIGURE 48.53 Liver changes of chronic, low-grade mechanical bile flow impairment shown by needle biopsy. The portal tract demonstrates abundant fibrosis (contrast with the edema of acute obstruction shown in Fig. 48.51), nonspecific ductular proliferation at the limiting plate, and fibrosis extending into periportal areas.

Some investigators hypothesize that COVID-19 cholangiopathy is a variant form of SSC given the similar radiographic and histological features of these disease entities. Roth and colleagues suggest that the microangiopathy and marked cholangiocyte injury seen in the setting of COVID-19 cholangiopathy warrants its distinction from SSC of the critically ill patient.[253] This hypothesis is supported by the fact that human cholangiocytes express the SARS-CoV receptor ACE2, which is essential for host cell entry, and SARS-COV-2 has been isolated from bile.[254,255] In addition, human organoid studies suggest that cholangiocytes are capable of supporting robust viral replication and that SARS-CoV-2 infection may upregulate the expression of pro-apoptotic genes in addition to interfering with bile acid exporter function.[256] SARS-CoV-2 in tissue can be detected on immunohistochemistry, although an in-situ hybridization platform is more specific and sensitive.[257,258]

This hypothesis is, however, not universally accepted, and some groups believe that ischemic-type bile duct injury resulting from a mechanical ventilation and

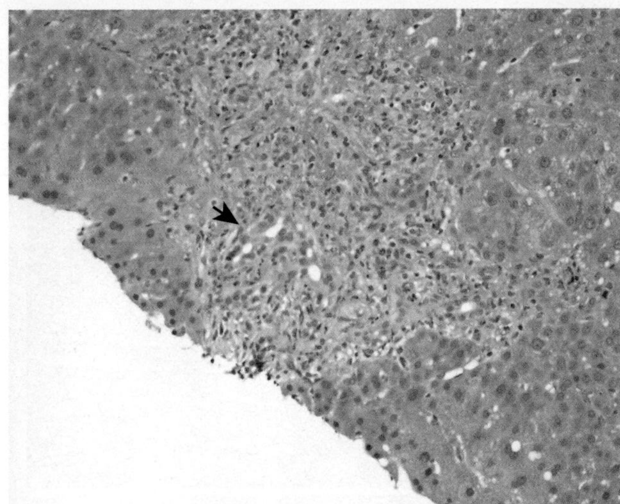

FIGURE 48.54 Post–COVID-19 liver. This biopsy was taken several months after SARS-CoV-2 infection. The patient presented with elevated alkaline phosphatase and gamma glutamyltransferase (GGT). The cholangiogram showed biliary strictures consistent with sclerosing cholangitis. The biopsy shows an enlarged portal tract with prominent bile ductular reduplication. Note the intact but damaged bile duct *(arrow)*. These changes are virtually indistinguishable from large bile duct obstruction.

vasopressor-induced reduction in splanchnic blood flow is the fundamental insult responsible for post–COVID-19 cholangiopathy.[259] Others suggest that the use of intravenous ketamine for maintenance sedation in mechanically ventilated patient may contribute to the development of COVID-19 cholangiopathy in a dose-dependent manner.[260] Further work is needed to better characterize the pathogenesis of biliary injury in the setting of COVID-19, which will facilitate the identification of patients at risk for developing post–COVID-19 cholangiopathy.

Regardless of the underlying pathogenesis, post–COVID-19 cholangiopathy is associated with significant morbidity and mortality. In one study, persistent or progressive biliary disease was identified by MRCP 6 to 12 months following the initial diagnosis of COVID-19 and after cardiopulmonary recovery. Several patients developed recurrent cholangitis and new-onset ascites and died following a protracted hospital course.[252] Despite the huge numbers of individuals infected with SARS-CoV-2 worldwide, post–COVID-19 cholangiopathy is likely an underrecognized late complication of infection, and monitoring patients for signs of evolving liver disease following recovery from severe COVID-19 may be warranted.[261] In patients who develop end-stage liver disease as a complication of post–COVID-19 cholangiopathy, referral for orthotopic liver transplantation should be considered and has led to favorable outcomes, at least in limited case series.[262]

The full reference list may be accessed online at *Elsevier eBooks for Practicing Clinicians*.

CHAPTER 49

Toxin- and Drug-Induced Disorders of the Liver

Brigitte Le Bail

Contents

INTRODUCTION

Because the liver is the major site of drug metabolism, it is also the major target of drug-induced injury. Despite rigorous preclinical and clinical toxicological studies and safety analyses in clinical trials, the frequency of drug hepatotoxicity has remained relatively unchanged during the years, and drug-induced liver injury (DILI) is still the main reason for removal of a drug from the market. Furthermore, adverse chemical reactions are not confined to pharmaceutical drugs (i.e., the drug itself and its excipients used for classic therapeutic purposes). Herbal medicines and dietary supplements (HDS), often used as self-medications, also represent potential hepatotoxins responsible for herb-induced liver injury (HILI). Various environmental toxins and recreational drugs, such as alcohol, illicit drugs (e.g., cocaine, heroin, ecstasy), criminal poisons, and industrial toxins (e.g., natural toxins, mushrooms, industrial chemicals, pesticides), can also give rise to hepatotoxicity. The list of putative offending drugs and toxins is extremely long and evolves with time. For instance, the recent development of immune checkpoint inhibitors (CPIs) has been accompanied by new cases of immune-mediated hepatitis and cholangitis (see later). Although all families of therapeutic agents can potentially be involved, a small group of drugs represent the most frequently incriminated molecules (Box 49.1). The circumstances of exposure to these various forms of liver toxins are listed in Box 49.2, with the exception of alcohol injury, which is discussed in Chapter 50.

Drug hepatotoxicity can be classified as either intrinsic or idiosyncratic. Intrinsic hepatotoxicity is predictable, dose dependent, and often characteristic of a particular agent when consumed in large quantities. Examples are ingestion of acetaminophen (paracetamol) and exposure to carbon tetrachloride or chloroform. Hepatotoxicity occurs in most of those who are exposed and starts shortly after some threshold for toxicity is reached. The mechanism of intrinsic injury can be direct, through damage to cells and organelles, or indirect, through conversion of a xenobiotic into an active toxin or through an immune-mediated mechanism. Idiosyncratic hepatotoxicity, by far the more frequent form of hepatotoxicity, involves unpredictable reactions that occur without warning and are unrelated to dose; they occur in particular hosts, depending on individual genetic variations in the metabolism of drugs and on environmental factors. Because the formation of reactive metabolites is a frequent mechanism of idiosyncratic reactions, the hepatotoxicity is highly dependent on the metabolic capacity of the host. In idiosyncratic toxicity, variable latency periods can be observed, from a few days to more than 1 year.

BOX 49.1 Some Drugs Frequently Implicated in Drug-Induced Liver Injury

Analgesics and antiinflammatory agents
- Acetaminophen (F)
- Diclofenac (F)
- Sulindac
- Ibuprofen
- Nimesulide

Anesthetics
- Halothane (F)

Antimicrobial agents
- Amoxicillin/clavulanic acid
- Azithromycin
- Erythromycin
- Clindamycin
- Minocycline
- Nitrofurantoin
- Levofloxacin
- Trovafloxacin (F)
- Trimethoprim/sulfamethoxazole (F)
- Antituberculosis drugs: INH + RFP + PZA (F)
- HAART and anti-HIV drugs (F)
- Dapsone
- Ketoconazole
- Thiabendazole

Anticonvulsants
- Carbamazepine
- Valproic acid (F)
- Phenytoin (F)
- Phenobarbital (F)
- Bentazepam

Psychotropic agents
- Paroxetine
- Disulfiram
- Atrium (combination of phenobarbital, febarbamate, and difebarbamate)
- Chlorpromazine

Anticancer agents
- Methotrexate (F)
- Oxaliplatin
- Cyclophosphamide (F)
- 5-Fluorodeoxyuridine (intraarterial)
- Infliximab and other antibodies

Lipid-lowering agents
- Atorvastatin and other statins
- Fenofibrate

Endocrine and metabolic agents
- Thiamazole
- Chlorpropamide
- Oral contraceptives
- Anabolic steroids
- Troglitazone
- Sulfonylureas

Cardiovascular agents
- Cordarone
- Captopril
- Verapamil
- Methyldopa

Others
- Medical herbs (germander, others) (F)
- Health supplements
- Vitamin A
- Illicit drugs: cocaine, ecstasy (F)
- Aflatoxin, *Amanita phalloides* (F), other natural poisons
- Paraquat herbicide (F)

F, *fatal outcome possible;* HAART, *highly active antiretroviral therapy;* HIV, *human immunodeficiency virus;* INH, *isoniazid;* PZA, *pyrazinamide;* RFP, *rifampicin.*

BOX 49.2 Circumstances of Exposure to Liver Toxins

DRUGS
- Treatment: prescription medications, self-prescription
- Self-poisoning, especially suicide attempts

DIETARY SUPPLEMENTS
- Vitamin cocktails
- Anabolic steroids

NATURAL TOXICANTS
- Food
- Food contaminants
- Alcohol abuse
- Folk and herbal medicine
- Bacterial infection
- Fungal, insect, and scorpion toxins

INDUSTRIAL CHEMICALS AND PESTICIDES
- Industrial accidents
- Household accidents with chemical products
- Self-poisoning with chemical products
- Low-level chronic exposure at the workplace
- Environmental pollution

Modified from Kahl R. Toxic liver injury. In: Bircher J, Benhamou J-P, McIntyre N, Rizzetto M, Rodés J, eds. Oxford Textbook of Clinical Hepatology. *2nd ed. Oxford: Oxford University Press; 1999:319 (Table 1). By permission of Oxford University Press.*

Diagnosis of a toxic liver injury or DILI is challenging, and it is often a diagnosis of exclusion and probability. Assessment of causality is difficult because almost all drugs and toxins are potentially hepatotoxic because of frequent idiosyncrasies and unpredictable toxicity, whereas predictable and dose-dependent liver toxins are rare. From a clinical or a pathological point of view, any pattern of hepatic injury may be encountered and may mimic other liver diseases, and a single drug can induce different lesions in different patients. The clinical presentation is usually acute and largely reversible, but chronic disease can occur. The time of onset of liver dysfunction varies depending on the drug and the patient and can be long after the first ingestion of the drug. Severe cases can occur and include mainly fulminant hepatitis: DILI/HILI is one of the major causes of acute liver failure with viral hepatitis. Significant fibrosis and cirrhosis may develop, and even hepatic tumors may occur. In addition, hepatocytes are usually the target in DILI, but some drugs may target endothelial cells, cholangiocytes, hepatic stellate cells, and/or Kupffer cells.

The Council for International Organizations of Medical Sciences (CIOMS) has proposed consensus criteria for terminology in DILI based on biological tests, chronology, and availability of liver biopsy. Six categories of DILI can be defined in this clinical system: hepatocellular injury, cholestatic injury, mixed injury, acute injury, chronic injury, and chronic liver disease (Table 49.1).

TABLE 49.1 CIOMS Consensus Criteria for Terminology in DILI

Terminology	Criteria
Hepatocellular injury	Isolated increase in ALT >2× normal, or ALT/ALP ≥5
Cholestatic injury	Isolated increase in ALP >2× normal, or ALT/ALP ≤2
Mixed injury	ALT and ALP increased and 2 < ALT/ ALP <5
Acute injury	Above changes present for <3 months
Chronic injury	Above changes present for >3 months
Chronic liver disease	This term is used only after histological confirmation

ALP, *Alkaline phosphatase;* ALT, *alanine aminotransferase;* CIOMS, *Council for International Organization of Medical Sciences;* DILI, *drug-induced liver injury.*

BOX 49.3 Value of Liver Biopsy When Hepatotoxicity Is Suspected

To determine the pattern or patterns of injury
To suggest mechanisms
To confirm or suggest a drug candidate
To assess the degree of injury (grade, stage)
To exclude or find other pathologies

The histological examination of a liver biopsy specimen is not always performed, either because the toxic episode may quickly resolve or because the information provided is disappointing. A delayed biopsy is often noncontributory. In addition, specific lesions are rare in this field. However, when analyzed by a specialist, the liver biopsy can often provide useful information for positive and differential diagnosis of DILI (Box 49.3). The lesions can be classified as to pattern of injury, an important topic that is discussed in detail later in this chapter.

DILI should be included in the differential diagnosis in cases with any hepatic laboratory abnormalities or hepatic dysfunction, but the assessment of causality of a drug in liver disease is often difficult. Discussion between clinicians and pathologists is especially important in this field of hepatology.

Current preclinical tests for hepatotoxicity are inadequate, reflecting our limited understanding of the mechanisms of drug toxicity. In particular, "hypersensitivity" and "idiosyncratic" reactions remain poorly understood and probably affect individuals possessing a rare combination of genetic and nongenetic factors that lead to drug toxicity in a given environmental setting. Many meetings on this topic have been organized by the Center for Drug Evaluation and Research (CDER) of the U.S. Food and Drug Administration (FDA) since 2001, and collection of data in regional or national registries (e.g., Spain, France, United States) or databanks has been encouraged. In the United States, the goal of the Drug-Induced Liver Injury Network (DILIN; https://dilin.org/) is to collect clinical data, genomic DNA, and liver tissues from patients who have experienced idiosyncratic drug reactions, in an effort to determine pathogeny and to offer a causality process and web application.[1] Recent studies from these groups have focused on the specific group of DILI cases with features of autoimmune hepatitis (AIH),[2] which could explain recurrent DILI with different drugs in the same patient.[3]

Despite much effort, hepatotoxicity remains a problem for many existing drugs, as well as those in development. This has a major economic impact because hepatotoxicity is the most frequent cause of postmarketing withdrawal of new medications.

This chapter reviews the main clinical features of toxin- and drug-induced disorders and describes the main pathological patterns attributed to drugs and toxins. In the last part, some frequently prescribed hepatotoxic drugs are described more extensively to illustrate the variety of clinicopathological presentations of liver injury.

For an extensive and detailed description of hepatotoxicity produced by a larger number of individual drugs, the reader is referred to a variety of specialized publications.[4-21] Synthetic and actualized data can also be obtained from specialized websites such as the complete and functional website from the DILIN group: LiverTox—NCBI Bookshelf (https://www.ncbi.nlm.nih.gov/books/NBK547852/). Finally, excellent clinical practice guidelines have been published from European and American scientific societies, including the role of liver biopsy in diagnostic evaluation.[22,23]

EPIDEMIOLOGY

DILI accounts for approximately 10% of cases of acute hepatitis in adults and more than 40% of cases in those older than 50 years of age.[13] In various series, it has accounted for 10% to 20% of cases of fulminant and subfulminant hepatitis[24] and for 2% to 5% of patients hospitalized for jaundice. The risk of a fulminant course is much greater for DILI (20%) than for viral acute hepatitis (1%). On the other hand, drugs are less often incriminated in chronic hepatitis or cirrhosis (<1% of cases).

However, it is probable that the real incidence of DILI is much higher because of unrecognized and benign presentations. In children, DILI is less frequent, but it is also an underrecognized cause of pediatric liver disease, and large series are rare. Children could represent 5% to 8.7% of DILI patients.[25]

A French study found an annual incidence of DILI of almost 14 cases per 100,000 population, a rate 16 times higher than that based on spontaneous reports.[26] The most common causes of DILI are the analgesic drug acetaminophen and several antiinfectious agents such as antibiotics from different families (e.g., amoxicillin/clavulanic acid [AMC; trade name Augmentin], erythromycin, minocycline) as well as antituberculosis drugs (especially isoniazid [INH]), psychotropic agents (e.g., chlorpromazine), anticonvulsants (e.g., valproic acid), anesthetics, oral contraceptives, lipid-lowering agents, antiinflammatory agents (e.g., diclofenac, disulfiram), and cardiovascular agents (e.g., amiodarone), as shown in large series[16,27,28] (see Box 49.1). In children, apart from acetaminophen, antimicrobial and central nervous system agents are the most commonly implicated drug classes, representing 50% and 40% of cases, respectively, as demonstrated in the recent DILIN series.[29] Another pediatric series from India emphasizes the role of antituberculosis drugs (e.g., INH, rifampicin [RFP], ethambutol) and anticonvulsants (phenytoin and carbamazepine),[25] pointing out the geographic specificity for certain drug toxicities. In this Indian pediatric population, hypersensitivity features such as skin rashes, eosinophilia, fever, lymphadenopathy, and Stevens-Johnson syndrome were frequently seen (41%) and were associated with a more favorable outcome.

The total number of drugs liable to be toxic to the liver exceeds 1100, and this long list must be frequently updated.[30] The highest frequency of hepatotoxicity for marketed drugs has been approximately 1% (for tacrine), but for most drugs, the risk is low (1/10,000 to 1/100,000) or extremely low (1/100,000 to 1/1,000,000 for antihistaminic compounds or penicillin). However, evaluation of the accurate incidence and risk factors as well as assessment of the causality of one or several toxic agents remains a major problem in DILI.[31]

In addition, overdoses of certain drugs are well known to be extremely toxic, not only in the context of a therapeutic misadventure (or with repeated doses, particularly in cases of excessive alcohol ingestion) but as a method of suicide. In the latter instance, acetaminophen is the drug most frequently used for suicidal overdose among adolescents and young adult women in the United States and Great Britain. When given in therapeutic doses for a period of 14 days, acetaminophen produced significant asymptomatic elevations in alanine aminotransferase (ALT) levels among healthy volunteers, suggesting that subclinical injury may be more common than previously believed. There was also a much lower incidence of acetaminophen toxicity as a cause of acute liver failure in children compared with adults, with almost half of all cases being indeterminate in origin.[32] Acetaminophen toxicity is reviewed more extensively later in this chapter.

The potential hepatotoxicity of herbal remedies commonly used for self-medication (i.e., alternative or "natural" treatments) and of other botanicals (e.g., the well-known mushroom poisoning from *Amanita phalloides*) should always be considered in the evaluation of pathology specimens. The list of confirmed or suspected hepatotoxic herbal components (e.g., Chinese herbs, germander[33]) is long, and the full extent of their toxicity remains unclear.[34] Many alimentary supplements, including vitamins, minerals, and botanical extracts, are also recognized as possible causes of DILI, as reviewed by Navarro in 2009.[21] For instance, many Herbalife products, used for nutrition or energy or to reduce stress, have been shown to commonly induce cytolysis, cholestasis, and even, in rare cases, acute liver failure.

Increased consumption of illicit drugs such as heroin, cocaine, and ecstasy, regardless of the route of administration (intranasally, intravenously, or by smoking), has increased the number of cases of hepatotoxicity[35] and potentiated other factors of liver disease. For example, daily cannabis smoking is significantly associated with progression of fibrosis in patients with chronic hepatitis C virus (HCV) infection.[36]

Frequently, hepatotoxicity is further potentiated by the use of other drugs in combination or by alcohol intake. Therefore, when prescribing a potentially hepatotoxic drug in a patient, it is particularly important to be aware of all additional risk factors for the liver in that patient, such as alcohol, diabetes, obesity, and chronic viral hepatitis. Otherwise, the risk of DILI will increase, and also the severity of the other liver diseases can worsen. During recent decades, for example, the evolving epidemic of nonalcoholic fatty liver disease caused by metabolic syndrome has potentiated the hepatotoxic properties of certain drugs such as methotrexate—and vice versa.[37]

Furthermore, a drug may be beneficial in the short term but harmful in the long term. For example, in individuals with human immunodeficiency virus (HIV) infection who also have hepatitis B virus (HBV) or HCV coinfection, alcohol abuse, or other hepatic risk factors, prolonged therapy with didanosine may induce chronic liver disease and may cause severe liver complications, such as variceal bleeding and portal thrombosis.[38]

CLINICAL ASSESSMENT AND PREDICTION OF HEPATOTOXICITY

Side effects attributed to drugs and toxins in the liver are numerous and variable. Although a slight acute hepatocellular or cholestatic/mixed hepatitis is the most common presentation, DILI can mimic all forms of acute or chronic hepatitis as well as biliary or vascular hepatopathy. In addition, some liver tumors (e.g., hepatocellular adenoma, angiosarcoma) may be attributed to the long-term exposure to various drugs or toxins. Therefore hepatologists and pathologists should consider possible drug-induced hepatotoxicity in the differential diagnosis of virtually any type of liver injury. Abnormal liver test results and nonspecific clinical signs may be present, including malaise, fatigue, abdominal discomfort, appetite loss, splenomegaly, icterus, or symptoms of acute liver failure. Signs of immunoallergic reaction, such as fever, rash, arthralgia, and eosinophilia, may be encountered but are infrequent and nonspecific. Chronological and clinical diagnostic criteria that are useful in making the diagnosis of DILI are provided in Box 49.4. Chronological criteria, although usually considered essential, require an accurate clinical history, which is not always possible. Many other difficulties are frequently encountered in making the diagnosis, as shown in Box 49.5. In some instances, clinical criteria[39] and laboratory data help eliminate other potential causes of hepatopathy and point to drug toxicity as the only possible differential diagnosis. Additional tests, such as seric dosage of the drug, can be helpful in some cases. Liver biopsy is not mandatory in the clinical survey, but it may provide substantial information regarding the positive and differential diagnosis of DILI (see later discussion), particularly if liver disease persists, provided that pertinent clinical information is provided and the pathologist is experienced.

Because of variability in both drug exposure and patient susceptibility, prediction of hepatotoxicity depends heavily on the specific type of drug used and patient characteristics (Box 49.6). Some acquired factors may enhance susceptibility to one type of drug but not another. Furthermore, various genetic factors, such as deficiency in certain isoforms of cytochrome P450 (CYP450) or in other enzymatic and metabolic pathways, may contribute to drug hepatotoxicity[13] (Table 49.2). In most instances, potentially fatal idiosyncratic reactions cannot be reliably predicted. For example, troglitazone, which was an approved drug for the treatment of diabetes mellitus, is an idiosyncratic, directly hepatotoxic

BOX 49.4 Diagnostic Criteria for Drug-Induced Liver Injury

CHRONOLOGICAL CRITERIA

Interval between beginning of treatment and onset of liver injury: 1 week to 3 months (shorter after readministration)
Regression of liver laboratory abnormalities after withdrawal of treatment (decrease of >50% in 1 week)
Relapse of liver laboratory abnormalities after accidental or intentional readministration of the offending drug

CLINICAL CRITERIA

Elimination of other causes (anamnesis, biological data, or imaging data)
- Previous hepatic or biliary disease
- Alcohol abuse
- Viral hepatitis (e.g., hepatitis A, B, C, D, or E virus; cytomegalovirus; Epstein-Barr virus; herpesvirus)
- Biliary obstruction
- Autoimmune hepatitis or cholangitis
- Liver ischemia
- Wilson disease
- Bacterial infection *(Listeria, Campylobacter, Salmonella)*

Positive clinical criteria
- Age >50 years
- Intake of many drugs
- Intake of a known hepatotoxic agent
- Specific serum autoantibodies: anti-M6, anti-LKM2, anti-CYP1A2, anti-CYP2E1
- Drug titration in blood: acetaminophen, vitamin A
- Hypersensitivity manifestations (fever, chills, skin rash, hypereosinophilia)

LIVER BIOPSY*

Eliminates other causes of liver injury
Shows lesions suggestive of drug-induced hepatotoxicity
Defines lesions for new drugs

** Not necessarily required but indicated for the purposes listed.*

BOX 49.5 Major Difficulties in the Diagnosis of Drug-Induced Liver Disease

Nonspecific clinical features
Treated disease itself is responsible for liver abnormalities (e.g., bacterial infection)
Intake of several hepatotoxic drugs (e.g., combined antituberculosis agents)
Comorbidities
Drug intake difficult to analyze
- Inaccurate history or chronology
- Self-medication
- Compounds considered safe (herbal remedies)
- Masked information
  - Illegal compounds
  - Offending agent not considered a "drug" by the patient
- Forgotten information (elderly)
- Patient in coma (fulminant hepatitis)

drug that led to an unacceptable rate of acute hepatic failure and was subsequently removed from the market.[40-42]

Causality can be assessed with more certainty if a clear chronological link can be demonstrated between drug intake and onset of the hepatotoxic event (Box 49.7). Components of the drug signature (e.g., pattern of liver test abnormalities, duration of latency before symptomatic presentation,

BOX 49.6 Assessing the Likelihood of Hepatotoxicity: Examples of Increased Probability

DRUG FACTORS

Drug is massively absorbed in the digestive tract
Drug is metabolized by the cytochrome P450 system
Drug belongs to a family with well-documented hepatotoxicity
Drug exhibits a molecular structure predisposing to the formation of reactive metabolites

PATIENT FACTORS (CONSTITUTIONAL AND ACQUIRED)

Age
- >60 years: isoniazid, nitrofurantoin
- Children: valproic acid, salicylates

Sex
- Women: methyldopa, nitrofurantoin
- Men: azathioprine

Nutrition
- Obesity: halothane
- Fasting/malnutrition: acetaminophen

Pregnancy: acetaminophen, tetracycline
Chronic alcohol abuse: acetaminophen
Intake of other drugs
- Enzyme induction: rifampicin, isoniazid
- Enzyme inhibition: troleandomycin, estrogens

Disease
- HIV infection: trimethoprim/sulfamethoxazole, sulfonamides

GENETIC FACTORS

See Table 49.2

presence or absence of immune-mediated hypersensitivity, response to drug withdrawal) in conjunction with certain genetic and environmental risk factors can be formulated into a clinically based scoring system that is predictive of the likelihood of liver injury. The best validated scoring system that takes into account all of these parameters is the CIOMS/Roussel-Uclaf Causality Assessment Method (RUCAM), which nonetheless has certain imperfections.[43] The Naranjo Adverse Drug Reactions Probability Scale (NADRPS) is another simple system based on similar items. Both systems produce a numerical score, indicating that the diagnosis of DILI is definite (or probable), possible, or unlikely. However, a review of 61 case reports of DILI in the PubMed database of the National Institutes of Health over the past decade indicates that in current practice, these scores are used in no more than 25% of published cases.[44]

Although it is difficult to provide definitive proof of responsibility for a particular offending drug, and readministration is ill advised, return to normal liver function after withdrawal of the drug is usually good supportive evidence of drug-induced toxicity. Additional tests may be performed on peripheral blood to identify a single causative agent. These may include drug dosing (e.g., acetaminophen), the double-locus sequence typing (DLST) method (which measures the patient's lymphoproliferative response to growing doses of the suspected causative drug), or the leukocyte migration test (LMT). However, these tests are not simple to perform and not feasible in routine practice.

PREVENTION OF DRUG HEPATOTOXICITY

Assessment of toxicity in human hosts is performed before and after marketing of all drugs. During the early stages of

TABLE 49.2 Genetic Factors Contributing to Drug Hepatotoxicity

Genetic Deficiency	Drugs	Comments
CYP2D6	Perhexiline	Enzyme deficiency: 6% of white population Perhexiline toxicity: 75% of patients are CYP2D6 deficient
CYP2C19	Atrium (combination of phenobarbital, febarbamate, and difebarbamate)	Enzyme deficiency: 3% to 5% of white population Atrium toxicity: all patients have a complete or partial deficiency
NAT2	Sulfonamides, dihydralazine	Transmitted as an autosomal recessive trait High frequency of the slow acetylation phenotype; this deficiency contributes to but is not sufficient for the toxicity
Sulfoxidation	Chlorpromazine	Not proven
Glutathione synthetase	Acetaminophen	Uncommon condition; deficient subjects are more susceptible to acetaminophen hepatotoxicity
Glutathione *S*-transferase type T	Tacrine	Needs to be confirmed
Hepatic detoxification capacity for reactive metabolites	Halothane, phenytoin, carbamazepine, amineptine, sulphonamides	Deficiencies observed in patients and some family members Precise defects are not identified
Genetic variations in the immune system	Halothane, tricyclic antidepressants, chlorpromazine, others	Association between several HLA haplotypes and some hepatotoxic drugs

CYP, *Cytochrome P450;* HLA, *human leukocyte antigen;* NAT2, N-*acetyltransferase 2.*

BOX 49.7 Causality Assessment

Very likely (rare): Drug overdose; relapse after accidental readministration; specific features of drug hepatitis
Compatible (many cases): No specific criteria; suggestive chronology; absence of other causes
Doubtful (frequent): Missing information (chronology, clinical data); no specific criteria; frequent in fulminant hepatitis
Incompatible: Demonstration of another cause; incompatible chronology; be aware that hepatitis can occur after discontinuation of treatment (e.g., halothane, amoxicillin/clavulanic acid)

drug development, preclinical studies in animals are mainly useful to detect dose-related predictable hepatotoxicity. Phase I safety studies in human volunteers test toxicity in few patients, after which more patients are exposed during efficacy testing in controlled clinical trials. However, almost 3000 patients must be included to demonstrate a 1/1000 incidence of DILI, and many drugs that may induce idiosyncratic hepatotoxicity escape detection during preclinical safety assessment and clinical trials.

From a pharmaceutical research perspective, metabolite profiling is essential to rational drug design.[45] This issue is addressed, at present, to eliminate molecules that are prone to metabolic bioactivation, based on the concept that formation of electrophilic metabolites triggers covalent protein modifications and subsequent organ toxicity. A cell-based approach for testing of cell viability, mitochondrial impairment, biliary transport, and CYP450 inhibition in the presence of a drug has become useful for the evaluation of putative hepatotoxicity.[46,47] The role of mitochondria in DILI, which may be altered through direct toxicity or through immune reaction, seems central, so new drug molecules should also be screened for possible mitochondrial effects. Although such an in vitro approach is pragmatic, it has its limitations because a linear correlation does not exist between toxicity and extent of bioactivation.

After marketing, surveillance and voluntary reporting of cases is necessary. Routine monitoring of liver enzymes does not seem useful to prevent clinically significant hepatotoxicity in the general population, but it may be interesting in high-risk patients who are taking well-known hepatotoxic drugs. At present, a few simple rules can be applied to help prevent drug hepatotoxicity (Box 49.8). In the future, advances in proteomics, metabolomics, genomics, and bioinformatics may pave the way to "personalized" pharmacotherapy in which the beneficial effect of a drug in an individual is maximized and the toxicity risk minimized.[48-50]

TREATMENT AND PROGNOSIS

In most cases, no specific treatment is available for DILI, and the main element of treatment is to stop administration of the offending agent, if possible. In most cases of DILI, liver injury is mild, and biological recovery occurs within days or weeks. However, recovery can take longer with certain drugs.

Because of the wide spectrum of manifestations (from asymptomatic liver test abnormalities to acute liver failure), the difficulties in evaluating the course of disease, and the possibility of spontaneous return to normal liver function because of patient metabolic adaptation, it is difficult to define criteria for cessation or for possible maintenance of the suspected causative drug.

The DILIN has developed a five-point system for grading severity based on liver tests, symptoms, jaundice, need for hospitalization, signs of hepatic failure, and death or need for liver transplantation (http://livertox.nih.gov/Severity.html).

BOX 49.8 Prevention of Drug Hepatotoxicity

BEFORE MARKETING

Detection of toxicity in animal or cellular models
Safety analysis in healthy volunteers and patients

AFTER MARKETING

Avoid readministration of the offending drug
Avoid readministration of drugs belonging to the same biochemical family
Avoid simultaneous administration of several drugs
- Cytochrome P450 inhibitors: cimetidine, ketoconazole, methoxsalen, and oleandomycin may be nonselective (e.g., cimetidine) or selective for a given CYP450 isoform
- Cytochrome P450 inducers: rifampicin, barbiturates, phenytoin; more selectively, omeprazole for CYP1A1 and CYP1A2

Control administration of drugs to patients with malnutrition (lack of defense against reactive metabolites) and to alcoholic patients
Be aware that older adult patients are more susceptible to drug hepatotoxicity
Be careful when administering drugs to patients with human immunodeficiency virus (HIV) infection
- Coadministration of many drugs
- Decreased ability to detoxify drugs (malnutrition)
- Higher susceptibility to some drugs (sulfonamides)

Genetic factors: genotyping and phenotyping tests are not widely available
Follow-up of blood liver tests may be useful for detecting hepatotoxicity

Various algorithms for management of DILI have been proposed, based on different biological thresholds. For instance, jaundice and bilirubin >3× upper limit of normal (ULN) or prothrombin time/international normalized ratio (PT-INR) >1.5× ULN should prompt discontinuation of a drug responsible for cholestatic-type injury. In hepatocellular or mixed disease, ALT >8× ULN at any one time, or ALT >5× ULN for >2 weeks, or ALT >3× ULN and either bilirubin >2× ULN or PT-INR >1.5× ULN would lead to drug withdrawal.[44]

The only example of a well-established specific treatment for drug-induced hepatotoxicity is prevention of severe hepatitis in patients with acetaminophen overdose by administration of *N*-acetylcysteine within the first 10 hours after consumption of the drug to detoxify reactive metabolites.[51]

The usefulness of corticosteroids in immunoallergic hepatitis has not been clearly demonstrated but could be tested. In autoimmune-like drug-induced hepatitis, corticosteroids are useful. Administration of ursodeoxycholic acid has been proposed for long-lasting chronic cholestasis and as symptomatic treatment for the relief of pruritus or as compensation for vitamin malabsorption.[13] In the worst-case scenario—drug- or toxin-induced fulminant hepatic failure—liver transplantation may be required.

The prognosis of drug-induced hepatotoxicity is usually excellent when the injury is acute, the cause is recognized, and the offending agent is withdrawn before the onset of severe acute or chronic injury. The term *Hy's law* refers to a method of assessing a drug's potential risk of causing serious hepatotoxicity and mortality. It is based on observations by Dr. Hy Zimmerman about the pejorative value of icteric cholestasis in DILI[52]: Drug-induced jaundice caused by hepatocellular injury without a significant obstructive component frequently leads to a poor outcome, with a 10% to 50% rate of mortality or transplantation. This fundamental observation is based on the fact that if there is enough hepatocellular damage to impair bilirubin excretion, then there is a potential threat to life.

Clinical elements for the assessment of prognosis include age (typically poorer for patients older than 50 years of age), sex (women being more susceptible to certain drugs), ethnicity and genetic background, nutritional status, multimedication association, and association of other general conditions (e.g., diabetes mellitus) or liver diseases (e.g., alcohol abuse, viral disease).

Because of heterogeneous reporting of biopsy findings in the literature, limited data exist on the impact of histology on the outcome of acute DILI. However, some data indicate that the extent of massive and submassive necrosis caused by toxic exposure is linked to a higher mortality rate (>85%), as also observed in other causes of acute liver failure. On the other hand, the presence of hepatic eosinophilia may be associated with a more favorable prognosis in DILI caused by disulfiram and other drugs.

In the setting of chronic hepatitis (as is possible with amiodarone, α-methyldopa, or methotrexate), progression to fibrosis and eventually cirrhosis may occur during an extended period. In these circumstances, withdrawal of the drug at a later date does minimize the risk of continued progression, but reversal of fibrosis is rare. An important caveat is the risk of alcohol-induced synergistic injury. Intake of alcohol in the setting of drug-induced chronic hepatitis may exacerbate the severity of injury and cause continued progression toward cirrhosis, even after the original offending drug has been withdrawn. Therefore exclusion of alcohol and other comorbidities is part of the treatment of chronic DILI.

Recently, attention has been paid to DILI and HILI with possible chronic evolution.[53] One year of abnormal liver tests are necessary for the diagnosis of chronic DILI, and 3 to 6 months for persistent hepatocellular and cholestatic damage, respectively. The prevalence of chronic DILI ranges from 5.7% to 39%. The patterns of chronic DILI include nonalcoholic fatty liver disease ("DASH"), AIH, cirrhosis, vanishing bile duct syndrome, nodular regenerative hyperplasia, peliosis, and adenomas, as described in the following sections.

PATHOLOGICAL PATTERNS OF TOXIC LIVER INJURY

Liver biopsy for adverse drug reaction is one of the most difficult and frustrating situations for the liver pathologist. Liver biopsy is not systematically done in cases of suspected DILI, and most of the time, the decision to perform a biopsy is made because of a complicated clinical situation, such as persistent abnormal liver test results after drug withdrawal, intercurrent medical conditions, multiple potential drug candidates, or a biological context suggestive of autoimmunity. The list of drugs associated with DILI is very long, but their association with liver injury may be tenuous, and pathological data are lacking in the literature. When available, histological features are often nonspecific and heterogeneous among different patients and studies.

An inadequate clinical history or incomplete reporting of drug intake (e.g., nature of the drug, timing) often seriously compounds the problem for the pathologist. Only rarely is an individual histological sign specific for a particular drug exposure; an example is fibrin-ring granuloma in allopurinol toxicity. Most of the time, a single lesion (e.g., steatosis) can be induced by various toxins. Conversely, one specific type of drug may give rise to different patterns of hepatotoxicity in different patients; for example, hepatitis, cholestasis, granulomas, or a combination of these tissue reactions can be related to phenylbutazone. Nonsteroidal antiinflammatory drugs (NSAIDs) can induce either severe hepatocellular or biliary damage, and amiodarone can produce both phospholipidosis and steatohepatitis, albeit by different mechanisms.

However, in the absence of other causes of liver disease, the association of a certain type of necrosis, the presence of a sparse or peculiar inflammatory infiltrate, and the concomitance of steatosis and cholestasis favor the diagnosis of DILI and suggest a mechanism of toxicity (Table 49.3).

Microscopic analysis of the liver benefits from knowledge of the clinical history and laboratory findings. It is based on a systematic, semiological analysis of all histological compartments of the liver. Adverse drug reactions affect mainly hepatocytes and bile duct epithelial cells but may also damage sinusoidal cells and vessels in the liver. The spatial organization of vessels, lobules, and sinusoids is illustrated in Fig. 49.1. Individual lesions must finally be grouped to define a general and overall pattern of liver injury. The most frequent patterns of DILI are acute hepatocellular injury, predominantly cholestatic injury (of hepatocellular or biliary origin), mixed hepatocellular-cholestatic injury (i.e., cholestatic hepatitis), steatosis pattern, vascular pattern, and neoplastic pattern. These patterns are detailed in Table 49.4, which also indicates examples of causative agents. The corresponding histology is described in the following sections. However, injury patterns are not mutually exclusive, and a mixed pattern of injury may occur in many instances of drug-related hepatotoxicity.[20]

TABLE 49.3 Histological Lesions Favoring DILI versus Other Liver Diseases and Suspected Mechanisms

Feature	Mechanism
Zone 3 necrosis	Susceptibility caused by CYP450 location
Massive necrosis	Intrinsic or idiosyncratic toxicity
Necrosis + little inflammation	Intrinsic toxicity
Minimal portal inflammation	Intrinsic or idiosyncratic toxicity
Many eosinophils	Hypersensitivity reaction
Many neutrophils	Inflammatory response of the innate immune system to drug-induced damage of hepatocytes
Granulomas	Hypersensitivity reaction
Microvesicular steatosis	Mitochondrial injury
Mixed patterns	Multiple targets
Cholestatic hepatitis	Idiosyncratic toxin
Steatosis + necrosis	Indirect toxin

CYP450, *Cytochrome P450;* DILI, *drug-induced liver injury.*

Hepatocellular Injury

Acute Hepatocellular Injury

Acute hepatitis accounts for 90% of drug-induced liver diseases. Essentially, this is clinically defined by ALT elevations at least 2× the ULN, which is a marker of hepatocyte injury (cytolysis). Elevated alkaline phosphatase (AP) is an enzymatic marker of cholestasis because this enzyme is present on the apical membranes of both hepatocytes and bile duct epithelial cells. Acute hepatocellular injury may be predominantly cytolytic (ALT/AP ratio ≥5) or cholestatic (ALT/AP ≤2), or it may occur in a combined form (ALT/AP between 2 and 5).

The mechanisms involved in the development of drug-induced acute hepatitis are complex.[5] They are rarely direct (e.g., lovastatin); usually, only massive doses of a foreign substance or extensive metabolism of a particular xenobiotic may lead to direct hepatotoxicity. Drug-induced acute hepatitis mainly results from the formation of hepatotoxic reactive metabolites, which often involve the CYP450 system. The CYP450 system, located mainly in the liver (hepatocytes) and predominantly in the centrilobular zone, metabolizes and eliminates essentially all liposoluble xenobiotics in the environment as well as most drugs used clinically. However, several xenobiotics are transformed by the CYP450 system into stable metabolites, and many others are oxidized into unstable, chemically reactive intermediates. Reactive metabolites can attack hepatic constituents (e.g., DNA, unsaturated lipids, proteins, glutathione). The end result of this in situ reaction may be either apoptosis or cytolytic necrosis. However, for many drugs, the formation of reactive metabolites is minimal and dose dependent, so a mild elevation of serum aminotransferases is often seen when the drug is used at therapeutic levels.

The CYP450 isoenzymes are under genetic control; therefore the hepatic level of a given isoenzyme varies considerably among different people. Furthermore, other agents can enhance the effect of certain drugs. For instance, chronic ethanol ingestion increases a particular isoenzyme of CYP450 (i.e., CYP2E1) that activates acetaminophen.

The binding of reactive metabolites to intracellular or circulating proteins leads to a structural modification that can "mislead" the immune system into mounting an immune attack against its own hepatocytes. Halothane hepatitis is a paradigm for immune-mediated drug hepatotoxicity[54,55] because of the presence of autoantibodies in the serum of affected patients. Toxic hepatitis caused only by activation of the host immune system (autoimmunity), without a contribution from direct hepatic metabolism of an exogenous drug, is uncommon. It is usually associated with hypersensitivity manifestations, such as fever, rash, and blood eosinophilia, also known as *DRESS* (drug rash with eosinophilia and systemic symptoms).

Genetic factors that affect hepatic drug metabolism and polymorphisms of major histocompatibility complex molecules may explain the particular susceptibility of some individuals to certain drug reactions. These factors have been clearly identified for some drugs (see Table 49.2 and the discussions of individual drugs in this chapter).

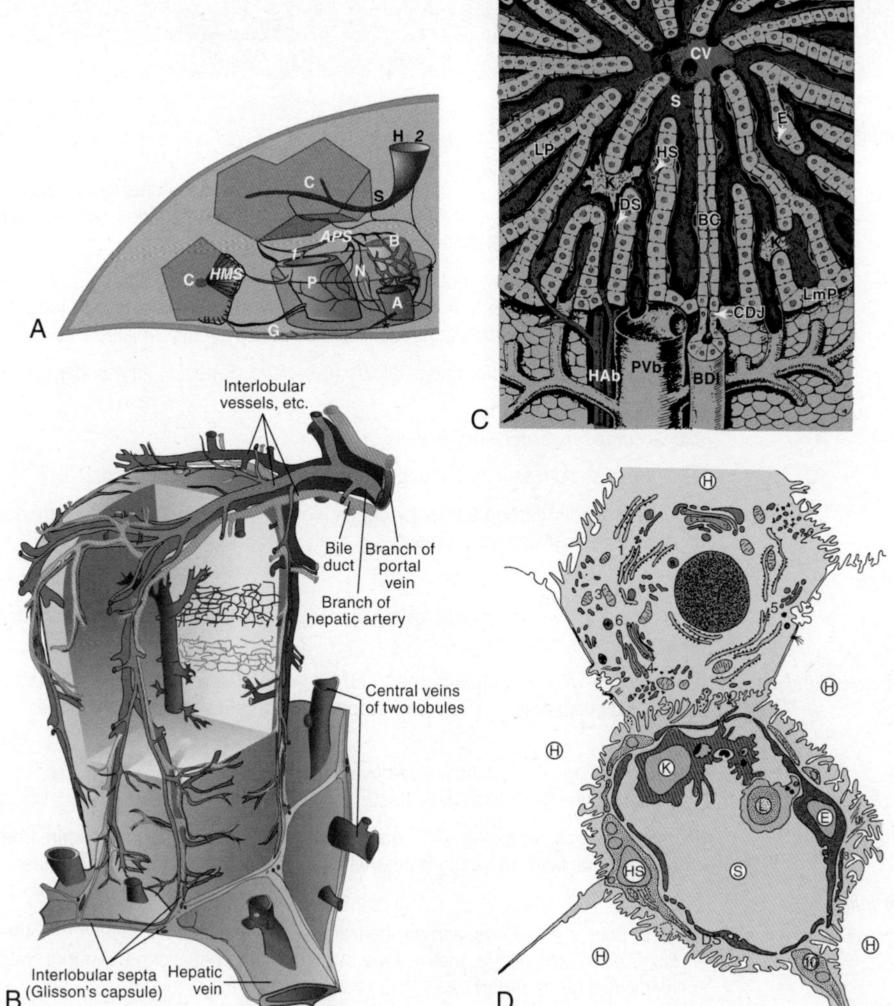

FIGURE 49.1 Schematic representations of liver architecture. A, Representation of hepatic artery compartmentalization reveals two distinct systems *(A)* within and outside of the portal tracts. Within the portal tract *(lower right)*, the artery feeds the bile duct *(B)* via the arterial peribiliary vascular plexus, the portal tract interstitium including nerve *(N)*, and the wall of the portal vein *(P)*. Drainage from the vascular beds is collected in a hepatic artery–derived portal system *(APS)*, which joins the portal vein *(1)* in the portal tract or at the level of the inlet venule on entering the hepatocytic lobule. Therefore the hepatic artery supplements the portal blood flow through the APS. Outside of the portal tract, the artery splits *(asterisks)* to supply the Glisson capsule *(G)*, which drains into the subcapsular lobules and the walls of the hepatic venous system, including the central *(C)*, sublobular *(S)*, and hepatic *(H)* veins. The latter represent pathways by which arterial blood may bypass the hepatic parenchyma and flow directly into the hepatic vein (*2*). Notice that within the lobule, inlet venules perfuse the lobular bed in conical sectors: the hepatic microcirculatory subunits *(HMS)*. **B,** Wax reconstruction (by A. Vierling, after Braus) of a hepatic lobule of a pig. A portion of the lobule has been dissected to show the bile capillaries and sinusoids. **C,** Diagram of a hepatic lobule. This figure summarizes the three-dimensional structure of the hepatic lobule revealed by scanning electron microscopy. *BC,* Bile canaliculus; *BDI,* bile ductule; *CDJ,* canaliculoductular junction; *CV,* central vein; *DS,* Disse space; *E,* sinusoidal endothelial cell; *HAb,* hepatic artery branch; *HS,* hepatic stellate cell; *K,* Kupffer cell; *LmP,* limiting plate; *LP,* liver plates; *PVb,* portal vein branch. **D,** Schematic representation of the hepatic parenchyma and sinusoids. *DS,* Disse space (located between the sinusoidal membrane of hepatocytes and the sinusoidal endothelial cells) containing the extracellular matrix; *E,* sinusoidal endothelial cell with fenestrae; *H,* hepatocyte; *HS,* hepatic stellate cell containing lipid droplets (vitamin A) and showing cytoplasmic processes in the Disse space; *K,* Kupffer cell; *L,* liver-associated lymphocyte; *S,* sinusoidal lumen; *1,* rough endoplasmic reticulum; *2,* smooth endoplasmic reticulum; *3,* mitochondria; *4,* Golgi apparatus; *5,* lysosomes; *6,* peroxisomes. (**A** from Ekataksin W, Kaneda K. Liver microvascular architecture: an insight into the pathophysiology of portal hypertension. *Semin Liver Dis.* 1999;19:359–382; **B** from Bloom W, Fawcett DW. Liver and gallbladder. In: Bloom W, Fawcett DW, eds. A Textbook of Histology. 10th ed. Philadelphia: WB Saunders; 1975:689; **C** modified from Muto M. A scanning electron microscopic study on endothelial cells and Kupffer cells in rat liver sinusoids. *Arch Histol Jpn.* 1975;37:369–386.)

Predominantly Cytolytic Injury

The predominantly cytolytic pattern of drug-induced acute hepatitis resembles acute viral hepatitis but without further specific features. Numerous drugs can cause this pattern of liver injury, including acetaminophen, NSAIDs, psychotropic drugs, a variety of herbal medicines, cocaine, and chemical agents such as carbon tetrachloride (see Table 49.4). Liver damage ranges from mild hepatitis, with rapid improvement after removal of the offending drug, to severe or even fatal liver failure. Hepatocyte death results from the necrotic process or apoptosis, or both. Marked lobular inflammation is typically present with toxicity from INH, monoamine oxidase inhibitors, anticonvulsants (phenytoin, valproate), and antimicrobials

TABLE 49.4 Pathological Effects of Drugs in the Liver

Pattern of Injury	Main Drugs
Hepatocellular injury	
Acute hepatocellular injury	
Predominantly cytolytic (spotty, submassive, massive)	*Conventional drugs* • Without hypersensitivity: acetaminophen, isoniazid, ketoconazole, valproic acid • With hypersensitivity: NSAIDs (almost all drugs), sulfonamides, almost all antidepressants (tricyclic, iproniazid), halothane, and derivatives *New causative drugs:* psychotropic and neurotropic drugs (e.g., tacrine), anti-HIV agents (e.g., didanosine, zidovudine), antimycotics (terbinafine), cytokines, growth factors (interleukins, granulocyte colony-stimulating factor), antidiabetic agents (troglitazone) *Herbal medicines:* pyrrolizidine alkaloids *(Crotalaria, Senecio)*, germander, Chinese herbal preparations *Illegal compounds:* cocaine, ecstasy *Excipients:* sodium saccharinate, polysorbate, propylene glycol *Chemical agents:* carbon tetrachloride, trichloroethylene, tetrachloroethylene, toluene, dimethylformamide, vinyl chloride
Predominantly cholestatic	
Pure cholestasis	Oral contraceptives, estrogens, estrogens + troleandomycin or erythromycin, androgens, tamoxifen, azathioprine, cytarabine
Cholestasis + mild cytolysis ("cholestatic hepatitis")	*Conventional drugs*: Phenothiazines, NSAIDs, macrolides, sulfonamides, β-lactam antibiotics, tricyclic antidepressants, carbamazepine, AMC, gold salts, propoxyphene *New drugs:* • Anti-HIV agents: didanosine, zidovudine, stavudine, ritonavir • Interleukins (ILs): IL-2, IL-6, IL-12
Mixed-pattern acute hepatitis	Numerous drugs, including AMC, aureomycin, azathioprine, cephalosporin, chemotherapeutic agents, lovastatin, meprobamate, methyldopa, nitrofurantoin, penicillamine
Chronic hepatocellular injury	
Chronic hepatitis (with risk of cirrhosis)	Valproic acid, amiodarone, aspirin, benzarone, diclofenac, flucloxacillin, halothane, iproniazid, isoniazid, methotrexate, methyldopa, nitrofurantoin, papaverine, ramipril, valproic acid; herbal medicines (germander)
Steatosis/steatohepatitis/phospholipidosis	
Predominantly microvesicular	Aspirin, tetracycline, valproic acid, alcohol, NSAIDs, anti-HIV drugs, fialuridine
Predominantly macrovesicular	Alcohol, methotrexate, corticosteroids
Nonalcoholic steatohepatitis (from steatosis to cirrhosis)	DEAEH, amiodarone, perhexiline maleate, anti-HIV and antiretroviral agents, corticosteroids, tamoxifen
Phospholipidosis	DEAEH, amiodarone, perhexiline maleate, total parenteral nutrition
Miscellaneous patterns	
Pigment accumulation	
Lipofuscin	Phenothiazines, aminopyrine
Hemosiderin	Excess dietary iron, alcoholism, total parenteral nutrition
Ground-glass changes	Phenobarbital, phenytoin, cyanamide
Anisonucleosis	Methotrexate
Increased mitoses	Colchicine, arsenic
Bile duct injury	
Acute cholangitis	
Cholestasis + bile duct degeneration with or without inflammation	Phenothiazines, ajmaline, carbamazepine, tricyclic antidepressants, macrolides, AMC, dextropropoxyphene
Chronic cholangitis ± ductopenia	
Primary biliary cholangitis–like	Phenothiazines, ajmaline, arsenic derivatives, tricyclic antidepressants; macrolides, thiabendazole, tetracycline, fenofibrate; herbal medicines (germander)
Primary sclerosing cholangitis–like	Arterial infusion with floxuridine, formol, and hypertonic saline injection into hydatid cyst; hepatic artery embolization

TABLE 49.4 Pathological Effects of Drugs in the Liver—cont'd

Pattern of Injury	Main Drugs
Vascular injury	
Portal vein lesions	
Hepatoportal sclerosis	Azathioprine, arsenic, Thorotrast, vinyl chloride
Nodular regenerative hyperplasia	Spanish toxic oil, oral contraceptives, azathioprine
Hepatic artery lesions	
Intimal hyperplasia	Oral contraceptives
Thrombosis	Transarterial chemoembolization
Hepatic vein lesions	
Hepatic vein thrombosis (Budd-Chiari)	Oral contraceptives, dacarbazine, irradiation, total parenteral nutrition
VOD/SOS	Pyrrolizidine alkaloids, azathioprine, antineoplastic agents, alcohol, heroin
Sinusoids	
Sinusoidal dilation/peliosis	Oral contraceptives, estrogens, anabolic steroids, azathioprine, vitamin A, tamoxifen, danazol, heroin
Sinusoidal cells	
Hepatic stellate cells	
Hypertrophy (lipid storage) ± perisinusoidal fibrosis	Vitamin A, methotrexate, azathioprine, 6-mercaptopurine
Kupffer cells/macrophages	
Storage	Talc, polyvinyl pyrrolidone, silicone, barium
Phospholipidosis	Amiodarone
Sinusoidal endothelial cells	(see Hepatic Vein Lesions)
Granulomatous reactions	
Epithelioid granulomas	Quinidine, hydralazine, phenytoin
Fibrin ring granulomas	Allopurinol
Granulomatous hepatitis (cytolytic ± cholestasis)	Phenylbutazone
Lipogranulomas	Mineral oil ingestion
Lipogranulomas with black pigments	Gold salts
Foreign body granulomas	Talc, surgical suture material
Hepatic tumors	
Benign	
Hepatocellular adenoma (± intratumoral hemorrhage, subcapsular hematoma, rupture)	Oral contraceptives, anabolic/androgenic steroids, estrogens
Malignant	
Angiosarcoma	Vinyl chloride, Thorotrast
Hepatocellular carcinoma	Oral contraceptives, anabolic/androgenic steroids, Thorotrast
Intrahepatic cholangiocarcinoma	Thorotrast

AMC, *Amoxicillin/clavulanic acid;* DEAEH, *diethylaminoethoxyhexestrol;* HIV, *human immunodeficiency virus;* NSAIDs, *nonsteroidal antiinflammatory drugs;* VOD/SOS, *venoocclusive disease/sinusoidal obstruction syndrome.*

(sulfonamides, trimethoprim/sulfamethoxazole [co-trimoxazole], ketoconazole) but is rare or absent with toxicity from acetaminophen, cocaine, ecstasy, or carbon tetrachloride. The differential diagnosis mainly includes viral hepatitis and AIH; some data may favor DILI and may suggest a mechanism of injury (Table 49.5; see Table 49.3).

Hepatitis with Spotty Necrosis/Apoptosis

When the mode of hepatocellular injury is predominantly cytolytic, necrosis/apoptosis can affect isolated hepatocytes in the lobule ("spotty" necrosis), resembling viral hepatitis; or, on occasion, it can take a mononucleosis-like appearance. In the former, ballooning or necrotic/apoptotic hepatocytes, scattered or in small foci, are distributed randomly in the lobule, with no or only a few inflammatory cells, leading to an acute hepatitis–like pattern or chronic lobular hepatitis (Fig. 49.2A,B). INH, sulfonamides, and diclofenac and other NSAIDs can cause this pattern of injury.

Neutrophils and eosinophils (see Fig. 49.2C) are often also present in the lobule and in some portal tracts. The presence of eosinophils favors a toxic rather than a viral cause of the hepatitis and suggests allergic mechanisms. The presence

TABLE 49.5 Possible Classification of DILI with AIH Features, Based on Clinical Characteristics and Histology

	Clinical Characteristics	Histology
AIH with DILI	Patients with known AIH; probably chance association	Usual AIH histology Often advanced fibrosis
Drug-induced AIH (e.g., anti–TNF-α, β-interferon)	Patients with unrecognized AIH or predisposition to AIH, in whom AIH is unmasked or induced by DILI; good response to steroids; relapse after withdrawal of immunosuppression with the need to continued immunosuppressive treatment; chance association of drug intake in a patient with first presentation of AIH cannot be ruled out	Usual AIH histology Centrilobular necrosis possible Prominent eosinophilic infiltrates (sometimes)
Immune-mediated DILI (e.g., nitrofurantoin, minocycline)	Clinical and biochemical signs similar to AIH; eosinophilia and rash may be present; good response to steroids; remission is maintained after successful withdrawal of steroids	Usual AIH histology Usually no advanced fibrosis Centrilobular necrosis possible

AIH, *Autoimmune hepatitis;* DILI, *drug-induced liver injury;* TNF, *tumor necrosis factor.*
Modified from Weiler-Norman C, Schramm C. Drug-induced injury and its relationship to autoimmune hepatitis. J Hepatol. *2011;55;747–749.*

of prominent neutrophils in portal tracts in a cytolytic hepatitis also favors DILI to other causes. Kupffer cells are often hypertrophied and contain pigments (lipofuscin, hemosiderin), which are best seen with periodic acid–Schiff (PAS) stain, with or without diastase digestion (d-PAS). Sometimes, and especially when the delay between the cytolytic peak and the time of biopsy is great, aggregates of pigmented d-PAS–positive macrophages without any necrosis or apoptosis are the only lesions seen *(resolving hepatitis)*. A prominent activation of Kupffer cells, associated with sinusoidal lymphocytosis showing lymphocytes in single files, characterizes the variant form of mononucleosis hepatitis–like injury, as typically observed in hepatotoxicity related to phenytoin (an anticonvulsant agent), paraaminosalicylate, or dapsone.

Hepatitis with Submassive Necrosis

In cases of hepatitis with submassive necrosis, liver necrosis (whether it appears as ballooning degeneration, apoptotic bodies, or coagulative necrosis) is usually zonal and occurs mainly in the centrilobular zones, leading to dropout and loss of hepatocytes, usually with preservation of periportal hepatocytes (Fig. 49.3). Extension of hepatocyte injury to the midzonal areas of the lobule may be strictly zonal and homogeneous, or it may be irregular, leading to the formation of well-demarcated, more or less confluent necrotic areas that contrast abruptly with surviving hepatocyte parenchymal regions. When necrosis is heterogeneous in distribution, it may lead to a maplike or geographic hepatitis (Fig. 49.4). In areas of severe hepatocyte necrosis and collapse, the reticulin framework and endothelial cells are often preserved and are mixed with variable numbers of inflammatory cells and hypertrophied Kupffer cells or macrophages that contain a brown ceroid pigment in their cytoplasm. Significant ductular proliferation may develop around portal tracts with time, as part of a regenerative and healing process. The collapse may lead to liver atrophy, Glisson capsule retraction, and approximation of portal tracts at the microscopic level. Lesions that are heterogeneous in distribution, with irregular regeneration and collapse, can be misleading if a biopsy (usually transjugular) is performed to assess the severity of the lesions and the extent of necrosis and regeneration.

Several types of drugs may lead to this type of necroinflammatory injury, with a generally zonal coagulative pattern affecting almost exclusively the centrilobular areas. Typical examples are acetaminophen and halothane.[52] In rare cases such as furosemide hepatotoxicity, one may see predominantly midzonal necrosis. Periportal necrosis is rare and should suggest other drugs such as cocaine[56,57] (Fig. 49.5), especially in combination with other toxins (e.g., halogenated hydrocarbons), as well as allylformate or albitocin.

Massive Necrosis

The term *massive necrosis* is used to describe necrosis of almost all of the normal hepatic lobule, which usually leads to clinically fulminant hepatitis requiring liver transplantation. This type of injury can occur with most of the drugs that cause submassive centrilobular necrosis. The most common example is suicidal or accidental overdose with acetaminophen[58,59] (Fig. 49.6) or halothane (Fig. 49.7), but other drugs also can cause this type of extensive, confluent coagulative necrosis (see Table 49.4). This same pattern of severe acute liver damage can result from mushroom poisoning with *A. phalloides* (Fig. 49.8) and other environmental or illicit drugs such as ecstasy.[60-63] This pattern of injury often leaves only a few remaining viable hepatocytes, usually in the periportal region, where surviving cells often exhibit microvesicular or macrovesicular steatosis (Fig. 49.8B). The collapsed parenchyma is often intermingled with a prominent bile ductular reaction or proliferation and a few inflammatory cells and Kupffer cells. As a general rule, a marked contrast between the severity of parenchymal necrosis and a poorly developed (mild) inflammatory portal reaction increases the likelihood that the liver injury was caused by a drug reaction as opposed to a viral infection. Liver atrophy is the rule.

Predominantly Cholestatic Injury

Cholestatic DILI may be caused by hepatocellular toxicity or, less frequently, by biliary lesions (see later discussion). Alterations of hepatobiliary transporters are often implicated in this type of DILI.[64] A mixed hepatocellular-cholestatic injury (cholestatic hepatitis) occurs more frequently with drugs than a pure cholestatic hepatocellular injury does, and this type of mixed disease is also discussed

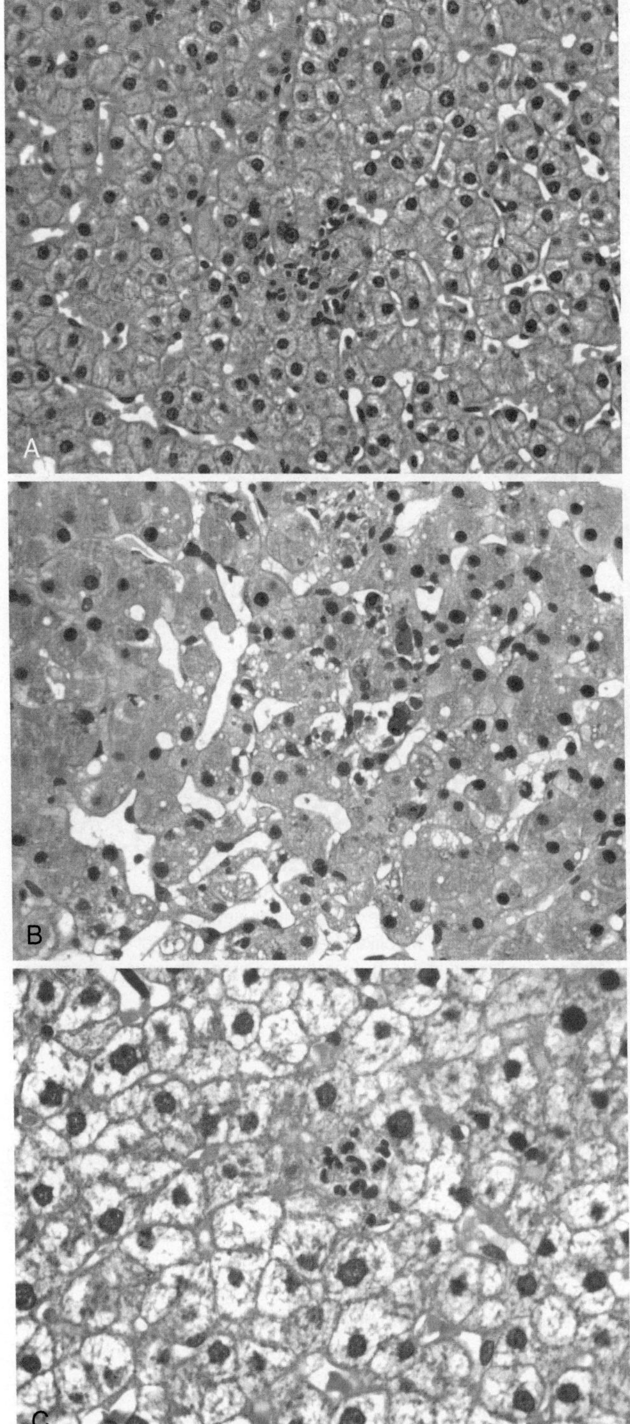

FIGURE 49.2 **Hepatitis with spotty necrosis/apoptosis. A,** Small lobular lymphohistiocytic inflammatory focus and rare acidophilic necrotic hepatocytes in a 30-year-old woman with mild cytolysis who was taking interferon-β for multiple sclerosis as well as oxcarbazepine. **B,** Focus of apoptotic hepatocytes without significant inflammation in a case of acute mixed hepatitis attributed to administration of naproxen (a nonsteroidal antiinflammatory drug) in a patient with metabolic cirrhosis. **C,** Lobular cluster of neutrophils and eosinophils and pale ballooned hepatocytes in a patient with chronic cytolysis and who was taking milnacipran (an antidepressant); other causes, including cytomegalovirus infection, were ruled out.

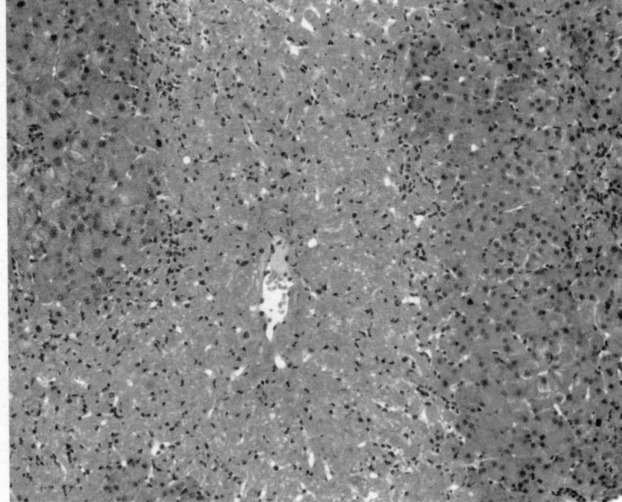

FIGURE 49.3 Acute hepatitis with zonal centrilobular necrosis in acetaminophen-induced subfulminant hepatitis. Coagulation necrosis and hepatocyte dropout are present around centrilobular veins.

later in this chapter. As mentioned earlier, severe cholestasis in DILI must be considered a pejorative prognostic factor.

Bland Cholestasis

The pattern of bland cholestasis is characteristic of anabolic or contraceptive steroid use. It is typified by the presence of prominent intrahepatic cholestasis, mainly in centrilobular hepatocytes, with the formation of canalicular plugs, corresponding to hepatocanalicular bilirubinostasis. On occasion, feathery degeneration of hepatocytes and liver cell rosettes may develop, especially in cases of prolonged cholestasis. Discontinuation of the offending drug is usually followed by complete recovery.

When cholestasis appears as isolated canalicular bilirubinostasis in a liver biopsy specimen with little or no inflammation, hepatocyte necrosis, or biliary lesions, the term *bland cholestasis* is used. In the absence of bile duct obstruction, it suggests DILI (Fig. 49.9; see Table 49.3).

Cholestatic Hepatitis

Mild hepatocyte ballooning/necrosis or apoptotic bodies and sometimes portal inflammation may be associated with cholestasis, in which case the injury is referred to as *cholestatic hepatitis* (Fig. 49.10; see Table 49.4).

Mixed hepatitis combines conspicuous cytolytic injury and cholestasis (Fig. 49.11) and is frequently associated with immunoallergic manifestations.[64] Many drugs can cause either pure cholestasis (mainly steroids) or a mixed pattern of cholestatic hepatitis, including psychotropic drugs,[65] antibiotics, antituberculosis drugs,[66] and the NSAID diclofenac[67] (see Table 49.4). In both instances, the prognosis is usually more favorable than for drug-induced acute hepatocellular hepatitis, as described previously.

A mixed pattern of hepatitis, in which features of both acute cytolytic and cholestatic hepatitis are present, is also considered highly suggestive of drug-induced hepatotoxicity (see Table 49.3).

In summary, regardless of the specific pattern of liver injury and the intensity of hepatocellular damage, the presence of predominantly centrilobular injury (particularly if

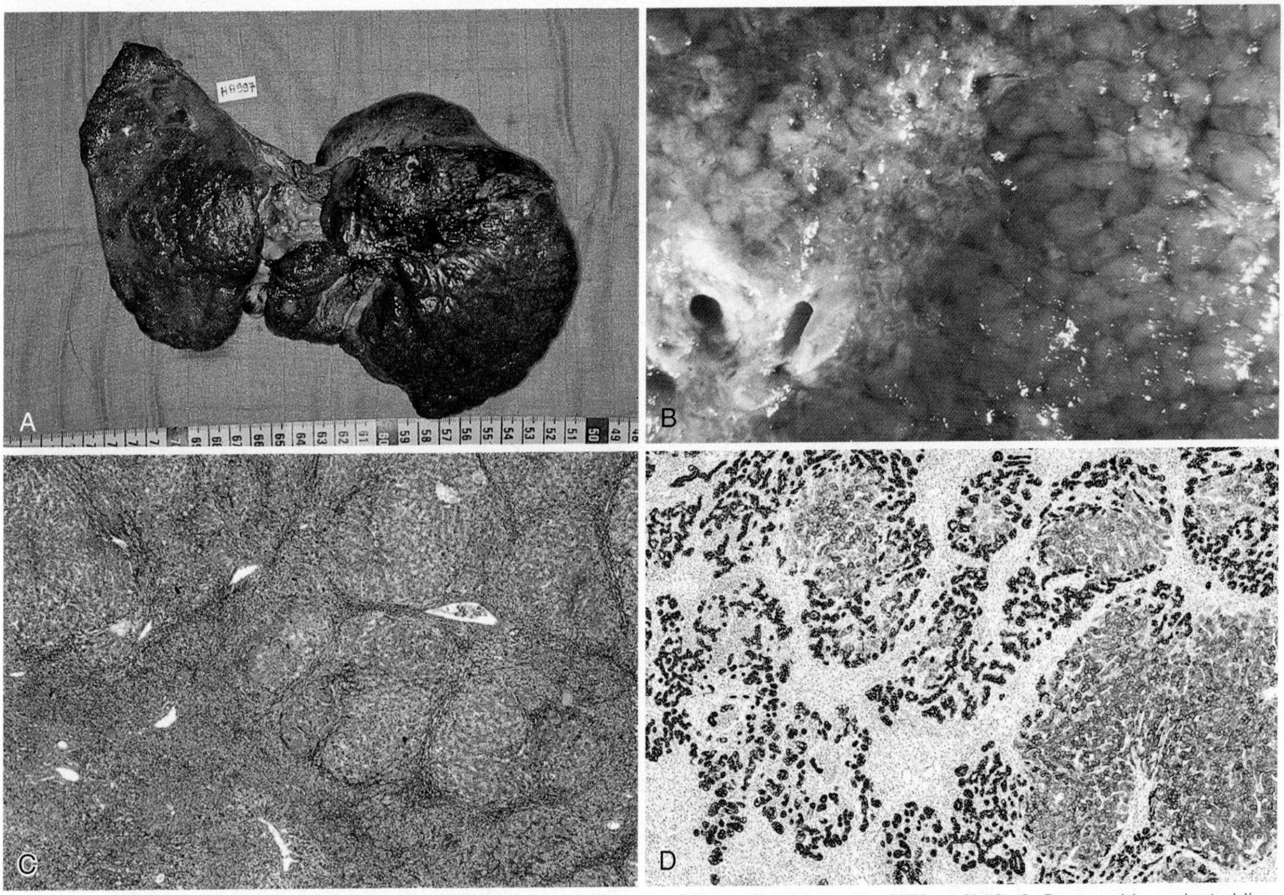

FIGURE 49.4 Subfulminant hepatitis in a 47-year-old woman who took alpidem (Ananxyl) for 6 months (150 mg/day). A, Dysmorphic explanted liver shows large atrophic areas located between nodular regenerative parenchymal areas. **B,** Fresh section of explanted liver viewed under a lens shows areas of collapse *(left)* contrasting with areas of persistent, viable, yellow-tan parenchyma *(right)*. **C,** "Maplike" hepatitis. Large areas of collapse *(left)* with loose connective tissue contrast with surviving parenchymal areas *(right)* (Masson trichrome stain). **D,** In collapsed areas, there is a prominent ductular proliferation mixed with inflammatory cells (pancytokeratin KL1 immunostain).

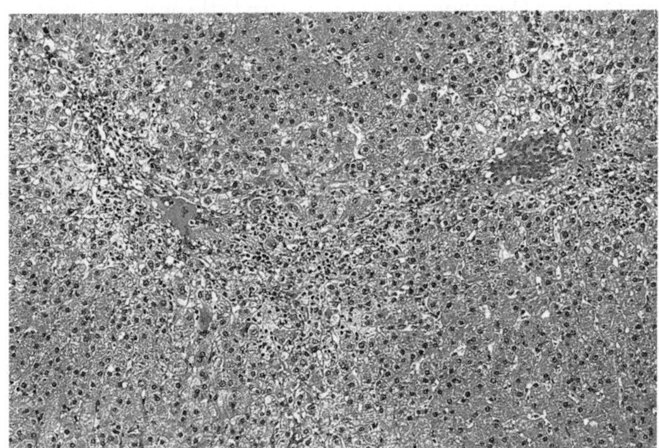

FIGURE 49.5 Submassive acute hepatitis caused by cocaine use in a 20-year-old man showing perivenular and bridging necrosis, mixed with an inflammatory reaction. (Courtesy Dr. M. Chevallier, Lyon, France.)

associated with scattered eosinophils) and portal neutrophils argues in favor of drug hepatotoxicity. In addition, mild lobular hepatitis with canalicular cholestasis and an absent or mild portal inflammatory reaction, sometimes unusually rich in neutrophils and eosinophils, may help differentiate DILI from viral hepatitis or AIH (Table 49.6 and Box 49.9; see Tables 49.3 and 49.5).

Chronic Hepatocellular Injury

The chronic hepatocellular pattern of liver injury is rarer than acute hepatitis and concerns fewer toxins. Approximately 10% to 15% of cases of acute DILI, either cytolytic or cholestatic, result in chronic disease. However, a histological pattern of chronic hepatitis does not necessarily imply that the injury has been going on for a long time or will persist. In the criteria from the CIOMS, chronicity of toxic liver *injury* is considered if abnormal liver tests are present for longer than 3 months, but the term *chronic liver disease* should be used only after histological confirmation (see Table 49.1).

Histological evaluation may reveal nonspecific features of chronic active hepatitis, resembling viral or autoimmune disease, with variable degrees of activity and fibrosis (Fig. 49.12). This chronic hepatitis–like histological pattern includes mixed inflammatory infiltrate (lymphocytes, macrophages, and possibly plasma cells and eosinophils) mainly located in portal and periportal areas, contrasting with the lobular-predominant infiltrate seen in an acute hepatitis–like pattern. Necrosis and apoptosis of hepatocytes is observed both as interface hepatitis and in the lobules. Some steatosis may be associated. Cholestasis, if associated, may suggest a toxic mechanism. A complete medical history is necessary to assess the respective role of toxins versus

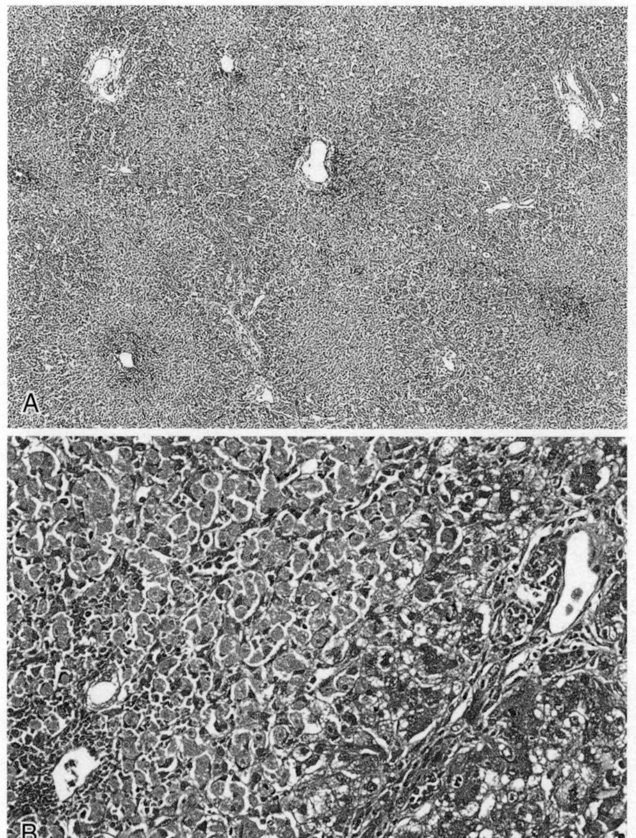

FIGURE 49.6 Fulminant liver failure in a 1-year-old child with a history of acetaminophen overdose (therapeutic misadventure: doses four times the normal daily dose for 4 days); section from liver explant. A, Submassive confluent centrilobular and midlobular necrosis with congestion around terminal hepatic veins. **B,** Centrilobular and midlobular necrosis of coagulative type (shrunken, eosinophilic hepatocytes, without nuclei), sparing only a rim of periportal hepatocytes, sometimes steatotic. (Courtesy Professor Linda D. Ferrell, University of California, San Francisco.)

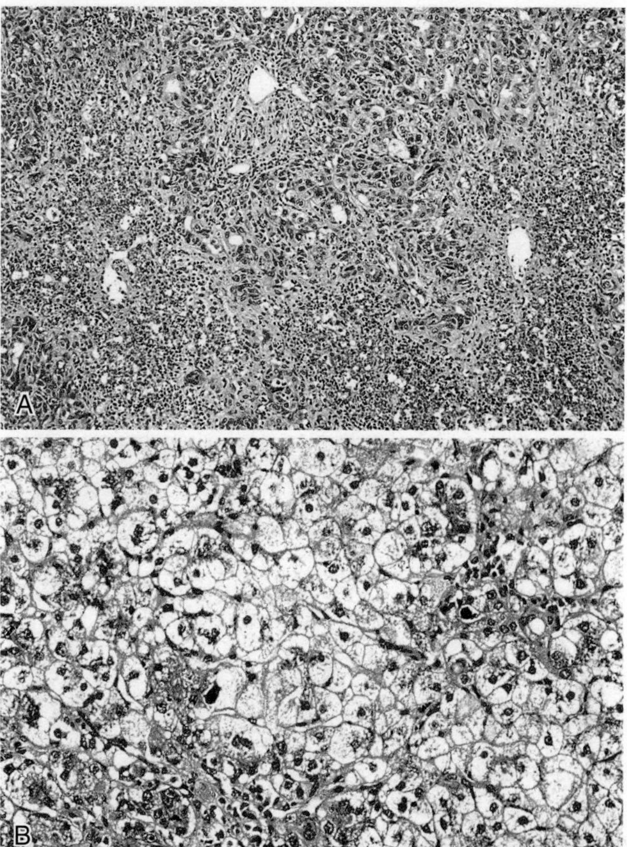

FIGURE 49.7 Halothane-induced hepatitis in a 6-year-old girl who underwent a second anesthesia 1 year after initial exposure; section from liver explant. A, Bridging, extensive collapse with severe centrilobular hemorrhagic necrosis, prominent ductular proliferation, mixed inflammation of the portal tracts, and parenchyma with a neutrophilic component. **B,** Foamy degeneration of hepatocytes and canalicular cholestasis. (Courtesy Bernard Portmann, King's College Hospital, London.)

other comorbidities such as alcohol intake and metabolic or viral disease.

Clinical and serological tests are usually necessary to eliminate the possibility of a viral hepatitis or AIH and to confirm the effect of a particular hepatotoxic agent (see Box 49.4).

The list of drugs that can induce a chronic hepatitis–like pattern (see Lewis and Kleiner[7] and Table 49.4) includes acetaminophen, acetylsalicylic acid, chlorpromazine, clometacin, dantrolene, erythromycin, haloperidol, infliximab, INH, methyldopa, nitrofurantoin, perhexiline maleate, phenytoin, propylthiouracil, tienilic acid (ticrynafen), various statins, and trazodone. Among numerous herbal medicines containing hepatotoxins, some, such as germander (a plant of the *Teucrium* genus used to treat obesity), may also lead to chronic hepatitis or even cirrhosis in addition to acute lesions.[68,69]

Drug-Induced Liver Injury with Features of Autoimmune Hepatitis

As reviewed by Czaja in 2011,[70] hepatitis induced by drugs or herbal medicines can, on occasion, look like AIH on histology and in the clinicobiological presentation. For example, drugs such as clometacin, methyldopa, minocycline, and nitrofurantoin can mimic type 1 AIH (see Chapter 48) because of histological lesions and the presence of antinuclear or anti–smooth muscle actin (anti-SMA) antibodies as well as hyperglobulinemia. Chronic hepatocellular injury caused by other drugs such as tienilic acid, iproniazid, and halothane can be accompanied by anti–liver-kidney microsomal type 2 antibodies (anti-LKM2), mimicking type 2 AIH (see Chapter 47), and the pathological features are usually less severe. Finally, in some cases, one may see morphological features suggestive of AIH but without autoantibodies (i.e., uracil, sulfonamides, etretinate); this condition is known as *autoimmune-like DILI*. As detailed later, statins, particularly simvastatin, atorvastatin, and lovastatin, can induce DILI on rare occasions. In fewer than 50% of cases, antinuclear and anti-SMA antibodies are observed. Histological analysis, when performed in these cases, shows features of chronic AIH with occasional eosinophilia.[71]

There have also been a few reports of AIH-like DILI caused by black cohosh, germander, and ma huang, which are herbal supplements.

As shown in Table 49.5, three situations can occur[2]: (1) some drugs may trigger real autoimmunity in predisposed patients (drug-induced AIH); (2) DILI with immune mechanisms may induce histological lesions very similar to those

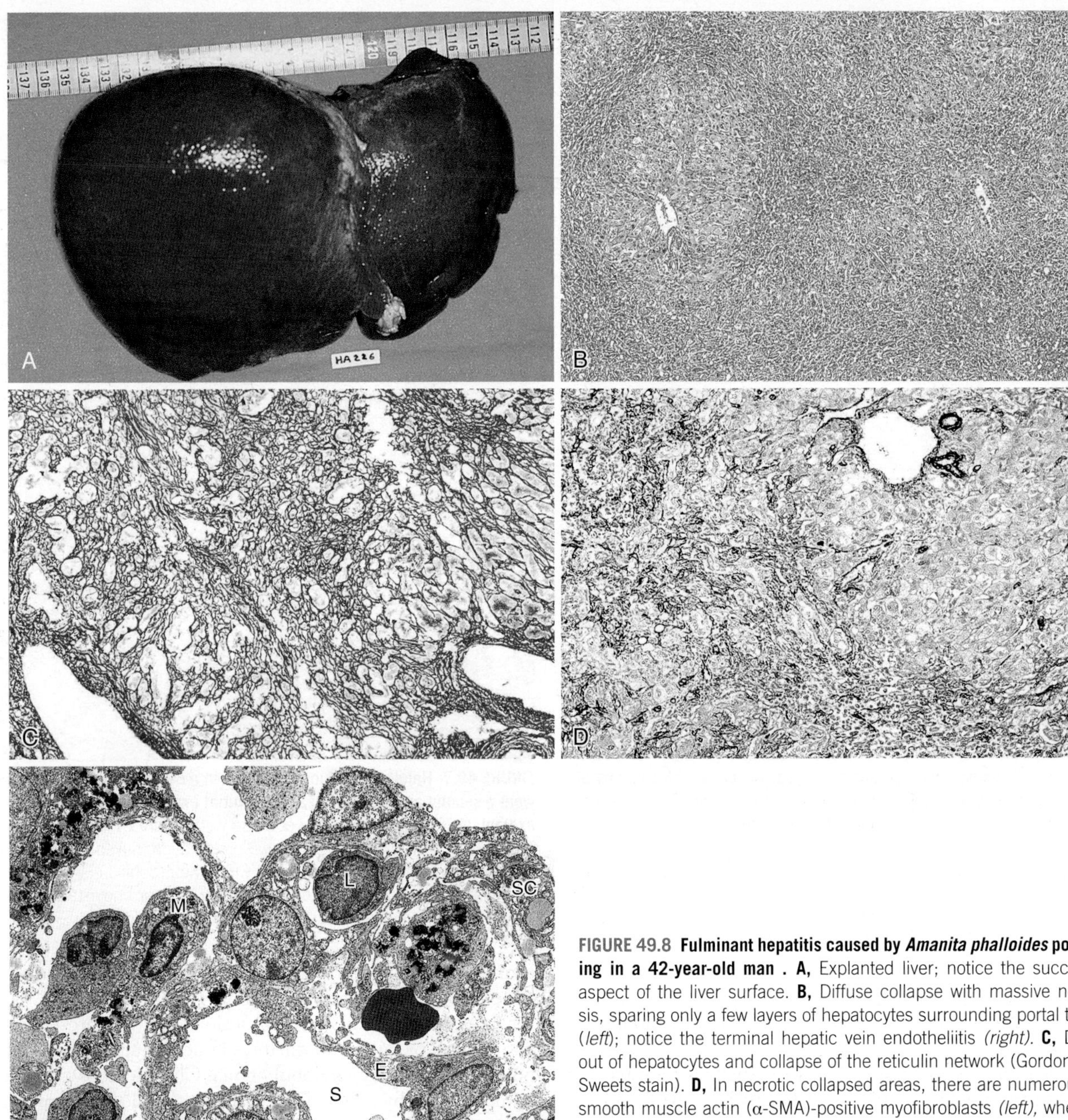

FIGURE 49.8 Fulminant hepatitis caused by *Amanita phalloides* poisoning in a 42-year-old man . A, Explanted liver; notice the succulent aspect of the liver surface. **B,** Diffuse collapse with massive necrosis, sparing only a few layers of hepatocytes surrounding portal tracts (*left*); notice the terminal hepatic vein endotheliitis *(right)*. **C,** Drop-out of hepatocytes and collapse of the reticulin network (Gordon and Sweets stain). **D,** In necrotic collapsed areas, there are numerous α-smooth muscle actin (α-SMA)-positive myofibroblasts *(left)*, whereas in the preserved portal zone, only vessel walls are positive *(right)* (α-SMA immunostain). **E,** Electron microscopy: general view of sinusoids *(S)* and remnants of necrotic hepatocytes *(H)*. Below a damaged, but still present, sinusoidal endothelial wall *(E)* are hepatic stellate cells *(SC)* containing dilated rough endoplasmic reticulum and some lipid vacuoles. Macrophages *(M)* and lymphocytes *(L)* are also present.

of AIH and may manifest with or without nonspecific autoantibodies (immune-mediated DILI); and (3) in some cases, DILI can occur in a patient with a preexisting typical AIH (AIH with DILI). However, classification between the first two groups remains uncertain and difficult.

It has been suggested that 9% of cases of AIH could be drug-induced AIH. Nitrofurantoin and minocycline would be responsible of 90% of these cases.

From a clinical point of view, cases of DILI with AIH features have an acute onset and develop mostly in females. They have a profile that is predominantly cytolytic or mixed (with minor cholestasis), but never a pure cholestatic profile. The course is characterized by the absence of relapse after corticoid withdrawal and the absence of cirrhotic evolution.[72]

Histologically, the hallmark of DILI with AIH features is the presence of a dense portal infiltrate with numerous plasma cells and eosinophils, associated with a moderate to severe interface hepatitis and possible fibrosis (Fig. 49.13). Whereas cytolytic and cholestatic forms of DILI could be distinguished from idiopathic AIH on the basis of combined histological features,[73] it seems impossible to clearly distinguish between drug-induced AIH and idiopathic AIH on the basis of histology alone.[72] In the largest series of 24 cases of

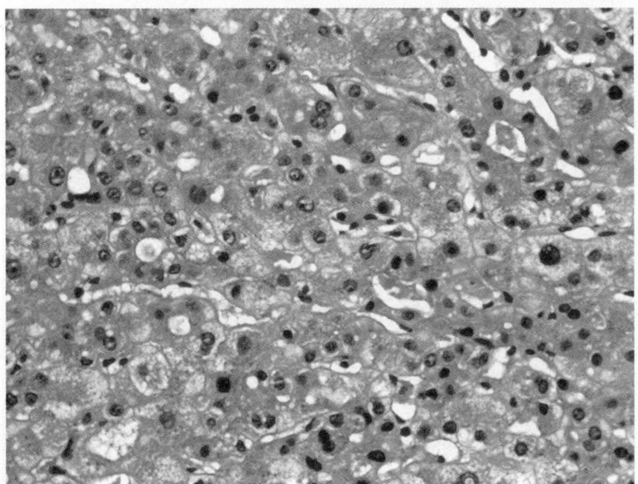

FIGURE 49.9 Bland cholestasis in drug-induced liver injury caused by ibuprofen (a nonsteroidal antiinflammatory drug). Notice the hepatocanalicular and Kupffer cell bilirubinostasis and hepatocytes forming cholestatic rosettes.

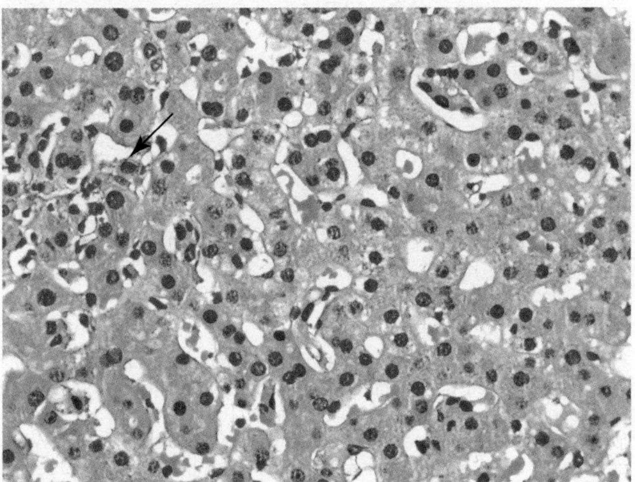

FIGURE 49.10 Cholestatic hepatitis caused by ketoprofen, a nonsteroidal antiinflammatory drug. Bilirubinostasis is prominent in hepatocytes and Kupffer cells, and there is also a mild mononuclear cell inflammatory infiltrate *(arrow)* in the lobules.

drug-induced AIH compared with idiopathic AIH, no differences were found concerning grade, stage (except that cirrhosis at baseline was more frequent in idiopathic AIH), portal inflammation, lymphoplasmacytic infiltrate, interface and lobular hepatitis, zone 3 and confluent necrosis, or rosette formation.[72] In a small subgroup of seven drug-induced AIH cases (diagnosis based on the international criteria of 1999 or the simplified criteria of 2008), no difference was found again for the severity of inflammation and for AIH-specific findings when comparing the biopsies with those of patients with idiopathic AIH.[73] However, in this small series, marked bridging fibrosis (Ishak score at least 4) and prominent intraacinar lymphocyte infiltration tended to be more observed in idiopathic AIH and DI-AIH, respectively ($P = .07$).

As mentioned previously, the main differential diagnoses of drug-induced hepatitis, whether acute or chronic, are viral hepatitis (e.g., HBV, HCV, Epstein-Barr virus [EBV]) and AIH. However, the inflammatory infiltrate, particularly

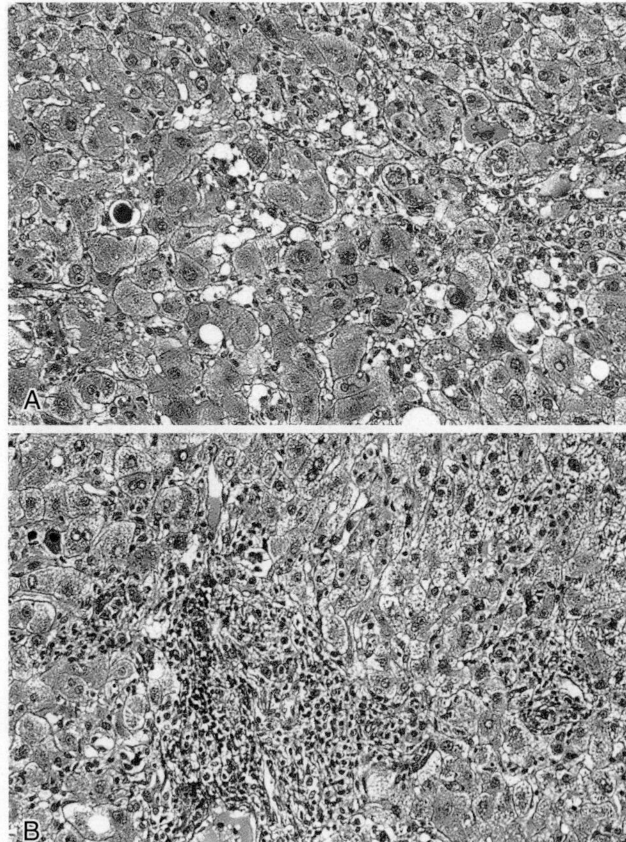

FIGURE 49.11 Mixed cytolytic and cholestatic hepatitis in a 64-year-old man taking several hepatotoxic drugs (oral hypoglycemics, hypolipidemic drugs, and omeprazole). A, Prominent centrilobular cholestasis with ballooning of hepatocytes *(right),* associated with spotty necrosis *(apoptotic body on the left).* **B,** There is also a moderate polymorphous portal infiltrate with ductular proliferation and interface hepatitis.

TABLE 49.6 Histological Features for the Diagnosis of Autoimmune Hepatitis versus Drug-Induced Liver Injury

Favoring AIH	Favoring DILI
Portal infiltrate more severe	Portal infiltrate mild or moderate
Significant portal fibrosis, cirrhosis	Minimal fibrosis a discovery
Prominent plasmacytic infiltrate in portal tracts	Prominent neutrophils in portal tracts (C)
Interface hepatitis more severe	Interface hepatitis mild or moderate
Hepatocyte rosette formation at the interface	Rosetting unusual
Prominent eosinophils in acini	Prominent lymphocytes in acini (H)
Prominent plasmacytes in acini	Canalicular cholestasis (H, C)
Severe lobular necrosis, bridging necrosis	Hepatocellular cholestasis (C)
Emperipolesis	

AIH, *Autoimmune hepatitis;* C, *cholestatic or mixed DILI;* DILI, *drug-induced liver injury;* H, *hepatocytic DILI.*

Modified from Suzuki A, Brunt EM, Kleiner DE, et al. The use of liver biopsy evaluation in discrimination of idiopathic autoimmune hepatitis versus drug-induced liver injury. Hepatology. *2011;54:931-939.*

BOX 49.9 Pathological Features That Help to Differentiate Drug-Induced Hepatitis from Viral or Autoimmune Hepatitis

ACUTE DRUG-INDUCED HEPATITIS
Well-demarcated, confluent centrilobular necrosis
Very mild lobular hepatitis with canalicular cholestasis
Absent or mild portal inflammatory reaction, sometimes rich in neutrophils and eosinophils
Epithelioid cell granulomas

CHRONIC DRUG-INDUCED HEPATITIS
No distinguishable features (inflammation, fibrosis/cirrhosis)

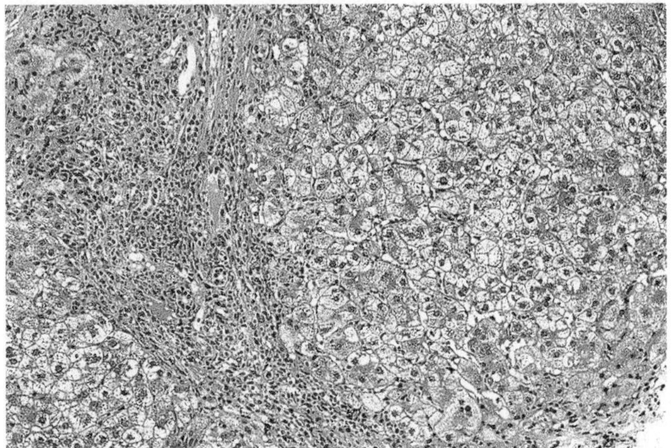

FIGURE 49.12 Active chronic hepatitis pattern of liver injury in diclofenac-induced hepatitis in a 74-year-old woman with rheumatoid arthritis. Shown are features of chronic hepatitis with portal fibrosis and moderate neutrophilic portal inflammation, with spillover into the periportal parenchyma and association with ballooned hepatocytes. (Courtesy Wilson Tsui, Caritas Medical Center, Kowloon, Hong Kong.)

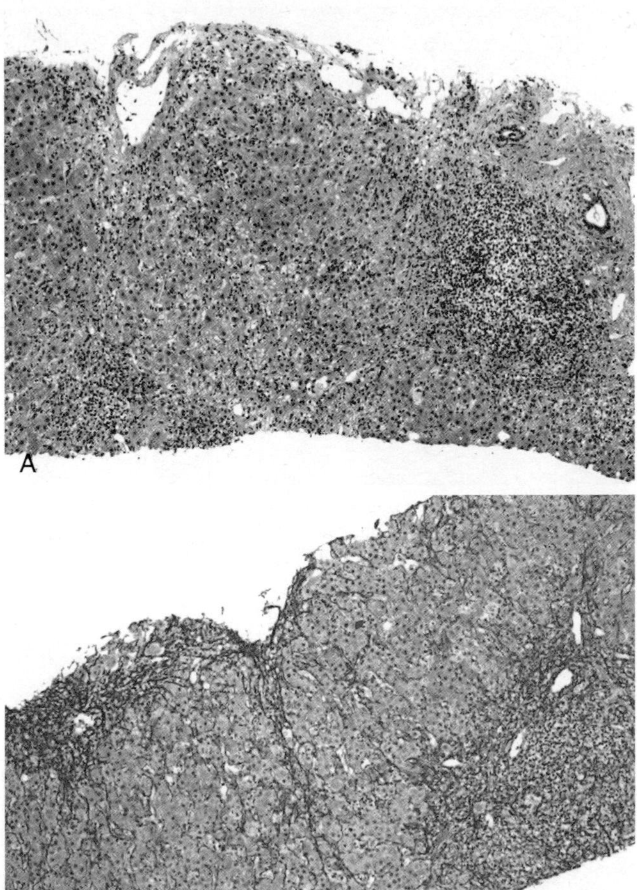

FIGURE 49.13 Active chronic hepatitis, thought to be an autoimmune hepatitis triggered by fenofibrate (Lipanthyl). This 54-year-old woman developed severe cytolysis (transaminases 10× ULN) and icteric cholestasis; both antinuclear and anti–smooth muscle antibodies were strongly positive. **A**, Note the massive follicular portal infiltrate, severe periportal and lobular activity, bridging necrosis, and centrilobular venulitis. **B**, Sirius red stain shows lobular disarray, hepatocyte collapse, and thin portal fibrous bridges.

in the portal tracts, is usually more prominent in viral etiologies, whereas the presence of eosinophils strongly suggests a drug toxicity. Serological data for viruses or for the presence of autoantibodies are of prime importance in this differential diagnosis (see Chapters 47 and 48). According to Suzuki and associates,[73] a combination of histological features could help first to discriminate DILI from idiopathic AIH (see Table 49.6). However, the concordance rate for the diagnosis among specialized pathologists is less than 30%, so the accuracy of histological diagnostic has been criticized.[11]

Steatofibrosis is another pattern for chronic DILI. The offending drugs are the same as those responsible for steatohepatitis, such as amiodarone and methotrexate (Fig. 49.14). These specific molecules are discussed later. Fibrosis is mainly pericellular and perisinusoidal, in zone 3. The respective roles of metabolic syndrome and alcohol abuse may be difficult to exclude before assessing the unique causality of the drug.

Steatosis/Steatohepatitis and Phospholipidosis

Steatosis (fatty liver), steatofibrosis (fatty liver and fibrosis, mostly pericellular in centrilobular areas), and steatohepatitis (fatty liver with inflammation or necrosis and fibrosis) are the three most frequent pathological manifestations of drug-induced hepatotoxicity. Of course, steatosis and steatohepatitis may be caused by alcohol ingestion or may be a manifestation of central obesity, diabetes, or hypertriglyceridemia with insulin resistance (see Chapter 50). However, drug reactions should always be considered as a potential cause of fatty liver disease. Specific drugs can also induce steatosis and other injury patterns.

Drug-Induced Steatosis and Steatohepatitis

Drugs may induce microvesicular or macrovesicular steatosis, mixed steatosis, steatohepatitis, or a combination of these conditions. Macrovesicular steatosis is a more indolent form of steatosis; it is characterized by the presence of one or more large intracytoplasmic fat droplets that displace the hepatocellular nucleus to the periphery of the cell, often indenting the nucleus. Microvesicular steatosis is clinically the more serious form and is often associated with severe hepatitic dysfunction and cytolysis. It appears as numerous small fat droplets that fill the cytoplasm of enlarged hepatocytes, but without peripheral displacement of the

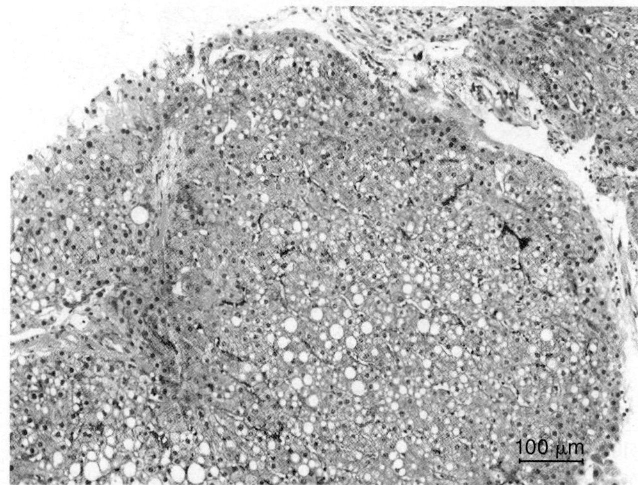

FIGURE 49.14 Chronic steatofibrosis pattern of liver damage attributed to methotrexate use in a 52-year-old woman treated for arthralgia related to systemic lupus erythematosus: periportal fibrous septa with mild inflammation, associated with microvesicular and macrovesicular steatosis.

cell nucleus. Special stains for lipid, such as Oil Red O or Sudan black on frozen sections, are sometimes necessary to differentiate microvesicular steatosis from clear cell degeneration; the degree of portal inflammation and cholestasis is usually minimal.

Microvesicular Steatosis

A large variety of drugs have been incriminated in the pathogenesis of steatosis (see Table 49.4). These include acetylsalicylic acid (aspirin) and valproic acid, which are more toxic in children and may lead to the development of Reye syndrome (Fig. 49.15). This severe condition is characterized clinically by the presence of vomiting and neurological signs with rapid coma, elevated aminotransferases, hyperammonemia, and coagulopathy. Histologically, there is diffuse and predominantly microvesicular steatosis, whereas inflammatory reaction and necrosis are strictly mild. In children, a clear association has been demonstrated with influenza and varicella infections. This association has led to the strong recommendation that salicylates be avoided in children with these viral diseases. In addition, inherited

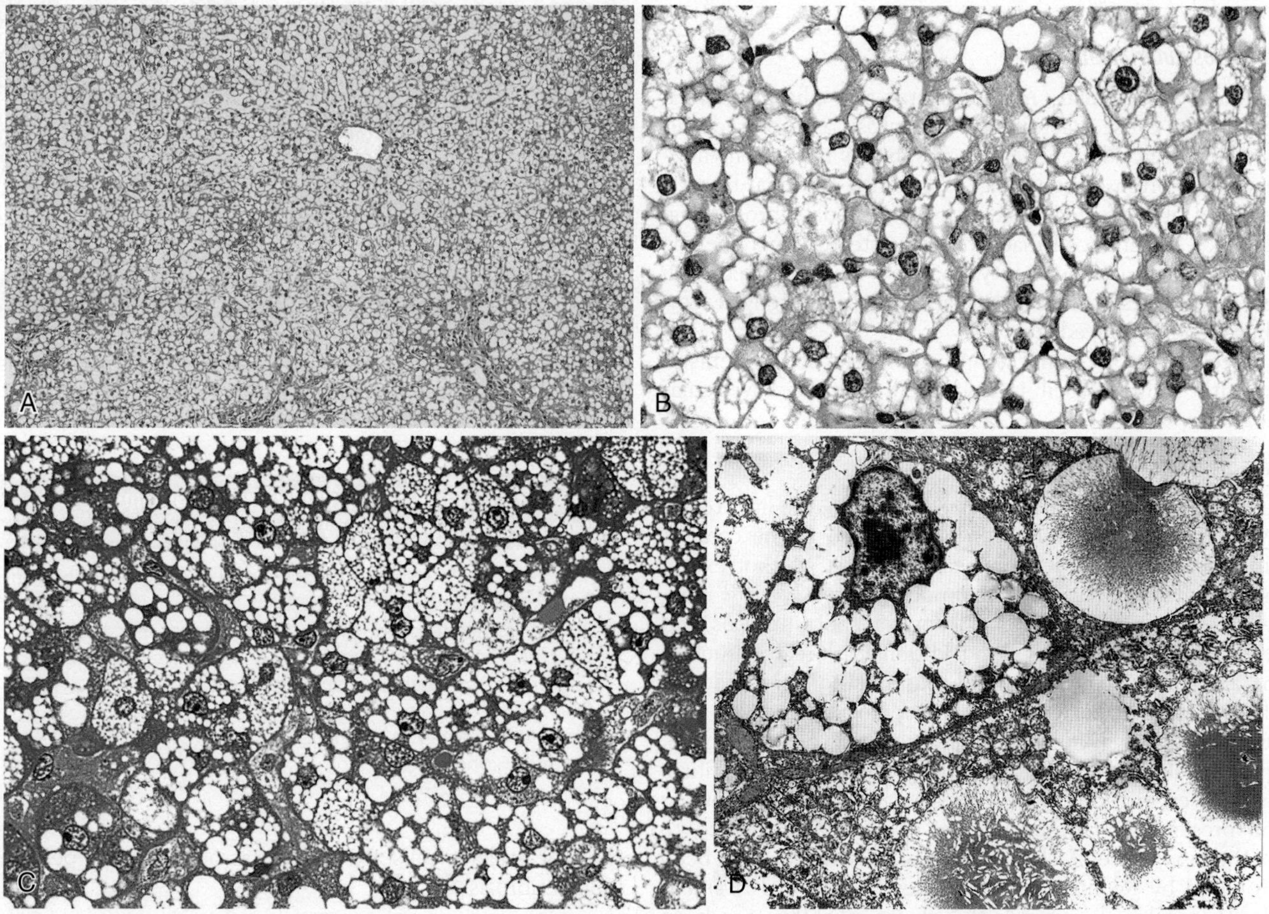

FIGURE 49.15 Predominantly microvesicular steatosis in a fatal case of Reye syndrome after intake of aspirin (acetylsalicylic acid; 600 mg/day for 3 days) in a 15-month-old girl. A, Panlobular, microvesicular steatosis. **B,** A few steatotic macrovacuoles are intermingled with microvesicular steatosis. **C,** Swollen hepatocytes are filled with lipidic microvacuoles surrounding the central nucleus (1-μm epon-embedded section; toluidine blue stain). **D,** In this electron microscopic view, lipidic microvacuoles fill the whole cytoplasm of one hepatocyte *(top),* indenting the nucleus, whereas a portion of another hepatocyte *(bottom)* contains macrovacuoles of lipids.

metabolic disorders should always be suspected and evaluated for in patients with a Reye-like syndrome. Other drugs that have been associated with steatosis include tetracycline (particularly in pregnant women); several antiviral nucleoside analogues,[74] such as fialuridine in hepatitis B[75]; a variety of anti-HIV drugs, such as didanosine, zidovudine,[76,77] and stavudine; and occupational or recreational toxins such as dimethylformamide and cocaine. In some severe cases, microvesicular steatosis may be associated with centrilobular cholestasis or necrosis, for example with valproic acid or anti-HIV retroviral agents (Fig. 49.16).

Because the underlying pathogenesis of drug-induced microvesicular steatosis is related to damage to the intracellular mitochondrial oxidative pathways, acute liver failure or chronic liver injury may ensue. In children, this condition may resemble inherited metabolic diseases, such as congenital enzymatic errors or mitochondrial cytopathic disorders of oxidative phosphorylation.[78] In patients with drug-induced microvesicular steatosis, in vitro or in vivo diagnostic studies can be conducted to assess the level of mitochondrial injury.[79] These studies include investigation of abnormal mitochondrial morphology, depletion of mitochondrial DNA, anomalies of respiratory chain enzymes and lactate production, and accumulation of drug (e.g., fialuridine) in association with both mitochondrial and chromosomal DNA.[46,79,80]

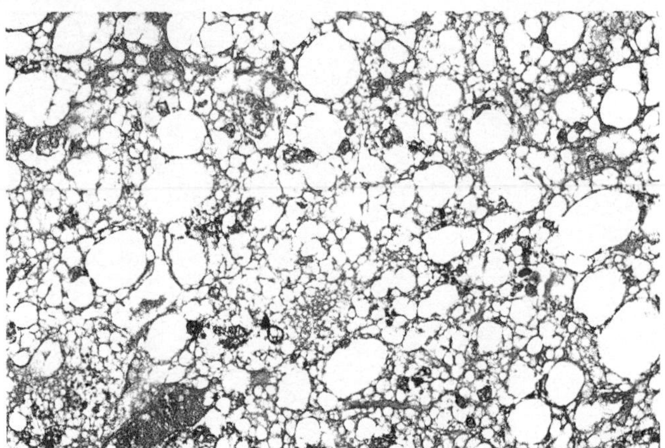

FIGURE 49.16 Predominantly microvesicular steatosis and cholestasis associated with administration of anti-human immunodeficiency virus (HIV) retroviral drugs. Fatal acute liver failure was observed in an HIV-infected patient treated with didanosine and zidovudine for 8 weeks: mixed massive steatosis, predominantly microvesicular with canalicular cholestasis.

Macrovesicular Steatosis

Glucocorticoids and methotrexate are pharmaceutical agents that cause macrovesicular steatosis as the predominant histological lesion. This occurs mainly in the centrilobular zone, often surrounding a thickened terminal hepatic vein and often associated with perisinusoidal fibrosis (Fig. 49.17). Drug-induced macrovesicular steatosis may be the only histological abnormality, or it may be associated with varying degrees of microvesicular steatosis, thereby resembling alcohol-induced steatosis.

Neoadjuvant chemotherapy for colorectal metastasis with 5-fluorouracil is associated with macrovesicular steatosis.

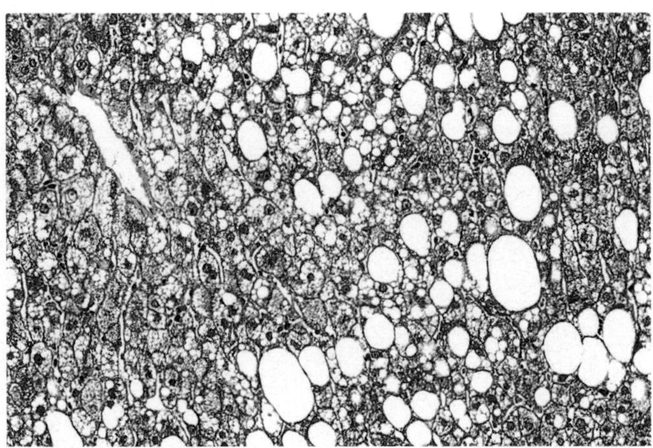

FIGURE 49.17 Macrovesicular steatosis associated with mild perisinusoidal and centrilobular fibrosis in a 54-year-old psoriatic patient treated with methotrexate for a long period (Masson trichrome stain). Note also the presence of anisonucleosis.

Steatofibrosis

As a form of chronic drug-induced hepatitis, the liver toxicity of methotrexate has been well studied in the context of treatment of both leukemia and psoriasis. Methotrexate-induced hepatotoxicity occurs more frequently after long-term treatment with daily small doses at short intervals, and particularly if associated with additional risk factors such as metabolic syndrome or alcohol abuse. Pathological features of methotrexate toxicity include hepatocytic changes (steatosis, ballooning, nuclear hyperchromasia, pleomorphism, and vacuolation) associated with various degrees of fibrosis or even cirrhosis. Liver biopsies are useful to monitor the presence and progression of liver changes related to methotrexate use. A classification of these lesions has been proposed by Roenigk and colleagues[81] (Box 49.10) and is often used by clinicians, although its reliability has been questioned.[82] The association of morbidities such as alcohol intake and metabolic syndrome should also be considered.

BOX 49.10 Roenigk Scoring System for Grading Methotrexate Hepatotoxicity

Grade I: Normal; mild fatty infiltration, mild nuclear variability, mild portal inflammation
Grade II: Moderate to severe fatty infiltration; moderate to severe nuclear variability; portal tract expansion, moderate to severe portal tract inflammation and piecemeal necrosis
Grade IIIa: Mild fibrosis
Grade IIIb: Moderate to severe fibrosis
Grade IV: Cirrhosis

Progression of fibrosis to cirrhosis can also occur after exposure to toxins such as arsenic or vinyl chloride or in cases of hypervitaminosis A, in which lipid-overloaded hepatic stellate cells are initially associated with perisinusoidal fibrosis.[83]

Nonalcoholic Steatohepatitis and Chemotherapy-Associated Steatohepatitis

As described in Chapter 50, *steatohepatitis* refers to the combination of steatosis and hepatocyte degeneration (especially ballooning degeneration and Mallory body formation)

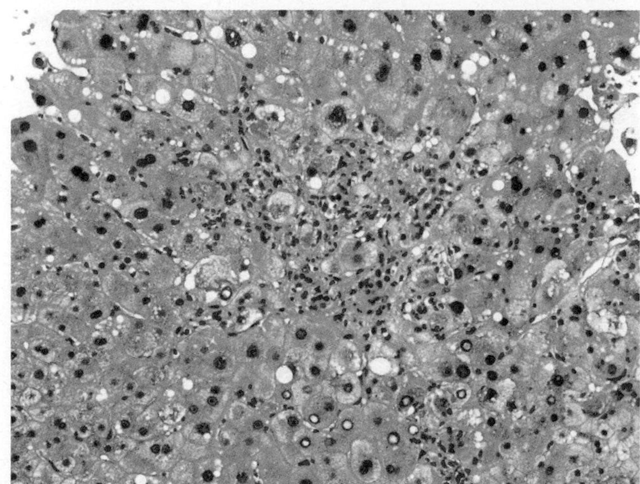
FIGURE 49.18 Nonalcoholic steatohepatitis (NASH) resulting from amiodarone use in an 87-year-old man with cardiac problems and without alcohol intake. Lesions are very similar to alcoholic hepatitis and include ballooned hepatocytes with Mallory-Denk bodies, neutrophils with satellitosis, and mild steatosis. Note the presence of some eosinophils.

combined with an inflammatory infiltrate (polymorphonuclear cells mixed with lymphocytes). Most cases are accompanied by some degree of pericellular fibrosis, which can progress to bridging fibrosis and cirrhosis.[84] Some drugs known to cause nonalcoholic steatohepatitis (NASH) are diethylaminoethoxyhexestrol (DEAEH), perhexiline maleate, amiodarone, and tamoxifen[85-90] (Fig. 49.18; see Table 49.4). These four cationic amphophilic compounds have a lipophilic moiety and an amine function that can become protonated. A high intramitochondrial concentration of protonated forms inhibits β-oxidation, which causes steatosis and leads to the mitochondrial formation of reactive oxygen species (ROS). ROS can trigger steatohepatitis by lipid peroxidation, cytokine release, and Fas ligand induction. All of these mechanisms can lead to hepatocyte death, fibrosis, and chemotaxis of neutrophils[91] (Fig. 49.19). Drug-induced steatohepatitis can coexist with other factors, such as obesity and diabetes.

Preoperative chemotherapy, particularly for colorectal liver metastases, induces regimen-specific hepatic changes that can affect patient outcome. Both response rate and toxicity should be considered when selecting preoperative chemotherapy. In addition to steatosis with 5-fluorouracil, a *chemotherapy-associated steatohepatitis* (CASH) can occur after treatment with irinotecan, especially in obese patients. Irinotecan-associated steatohepatitis can affect hepatic reserve and increase morbidity and mortality after hepatectomy.[92]

The single most important factor to aid in the diagnosis of steatotic liver disease is knowledge of the patient's clinical history. Intake of drugs known to cause hepatic steatosis or steatohepatitis and a thorough appreciation of the patient's alcohol intake are crucial, in addition to the presence or absence of a metabolic syndrome. Morphologically, differentiating drug-induced steatohepatitis from alcoholic steatohepatitis or from NASH is often difficult. Similar to NASH or alcohol-induced damage, drug-induced steatohepatitis shows Mallory bodies, mainly located in ballooned hepatocytes in zone 3 or randomly distributed in the lobule. However, some drugs, such as amiodarone, may lead to involvement of zone 1 hepatocytes.[93]

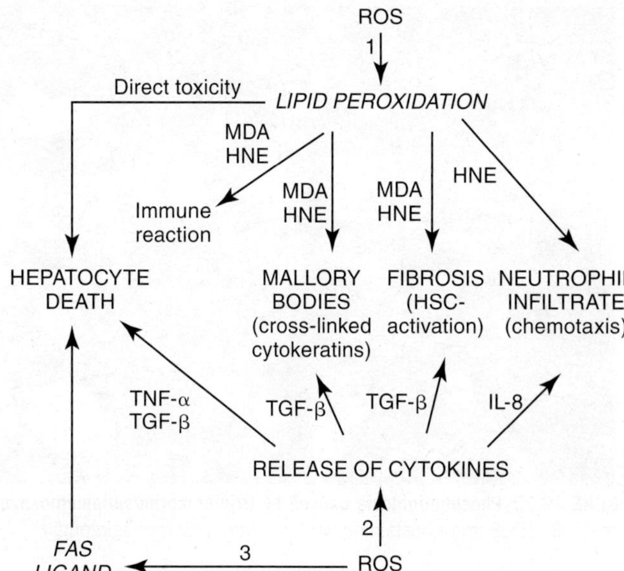

FIGURE 49.19 Mechanisms of induction of steatohepatitis from reactive oxygen species *(ROS)* through lipid peroxidation *(1)*, release of cytokines *(2)*, and Fas ligand induction *(3)*. *HNE*, 4-Hydroxynonenal; *HSC*, hepatic stellate cell; *IL*, interleukin; *MDA*, malondialdehyde; *TGF*, transforming growth factor; *TNF*, tumor necrosis factor. (From Pessayre D, Berson A, Fromenty B, et al. Mitochondria in steatohepatitis. *Semin Liver Dis*. 2001;21:57-69.)

Phospholipidosis

In humans, phospholipidosis has been observed mainly in association with three types of antianginal drugs—DEAEH, perhexiline maleate,[5] and amiodarone[94]—and rarely with some types of antibiotics (Fig. 49.20).[95] It can also be induced by parenteral nutrition.[96,97] In this particular type of injury (Fig. 49.21), hepatocytes and Kupffer cells are enlarged and appear foamy by light microscopy. On electron microscopy, the cytoplasm of affected cells is filled with characteristic lamellated and membrane-bound bodies, which correspond to phospholipids or gangliosides; the picture resembles the morphological appearance of Niemann-Pick disease. In contrast with NASH, phospholipidosis is a dose-related change.

The pathogenesis of injury is related to the fact that uncharged lipophilic drugs can easily cross the lysosomal membrane of cells. In the acidic intralysosomal milieu, the drug is protonated, becomes more water soluble, and accumulates inside the lysosomes. Protonated forms of the drug bind with phospholipids, hampering the action of intralysosomal phospholipases. The accumulation of drug-phospholipid complexes generates large lysosomes filled with pseudomyelinic figures. Because of the very slow dissociation of the drug-phospholipid complexes, the drug may be detectable in plasma, even several months after discontinuation of treatment.

Miscellaneous Patterns of Hepatocellular Injury

Pigment Accumulation

Lipofuscins accumulate in hepatocytes, particularly in the centrilobular zone (Fig. 49.22A), during the process of drug-induced damage, such as that caused by phenothiazine or aminopyrine. This pigment may be stained with Fontana

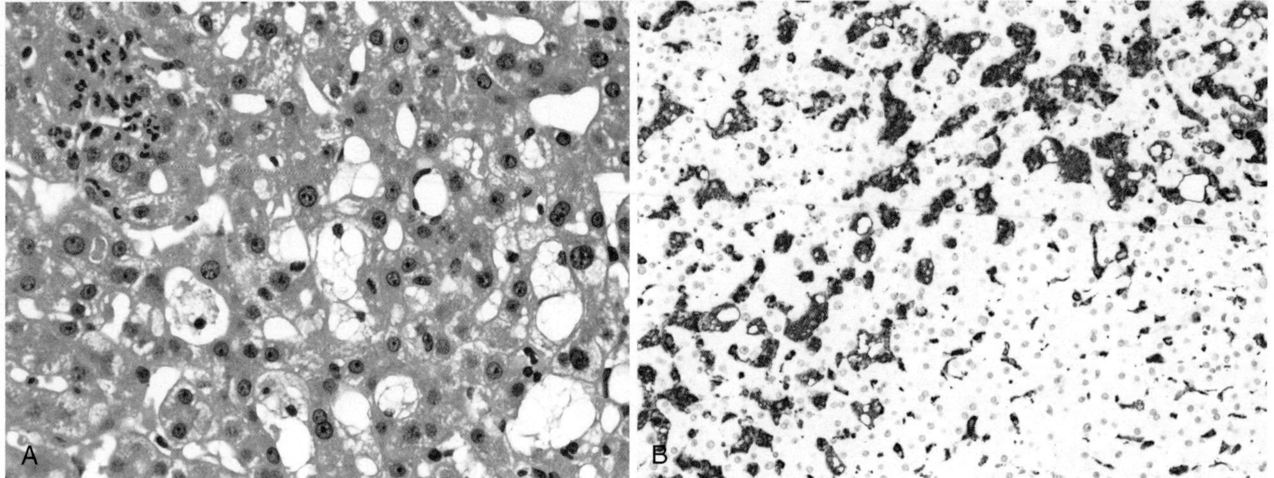

FIGURE 49.20 Phospholipidosis caused by (trimethoprim/sulfamethoxazole [Bactrim]). A, Swollen and vacuolated cells are visible in the sinusoidal lumina. **B**, CD68 immunostaining confirms their macrophagic origin.

stain for melanin (Fig. 49.22B) and should be differentiated from bile pigment, which often accumulates in bile canaliculi. In cases of excess dietary iron, alcoholism, parenteral nutrition, or transfusion, hemosiderin can also accumulate in hepatocytes, but it is predominantly observed in sinusoidal lining cells (e.g., Kupffer cells), and it is easily recognized with the use of Perls stain.

Adaptive Changes and Ground-Glass Hepatocytes

A frequent adaptive change of hepatocytes is the development of an abundant pale cytoplasm (Fig. 49.23) because of enlargement of the smooth endoplasmic reticulum induced by long-term treatment with anticonvulsant drugs such as phenobarbital or phenytoin. The terms *induced hepatocytes* and *induction cells* are often used for this lesion.

Ground-glass–like inclusions are much rarer in DILI. They appear as pale pink, intracytoplasmic globular structures, often surrounded by a clear halo. They are intensely positive on PAS staining, and the staining disappears with diastase pretreatment (Fig. 49.24). These inclusions correspond to complex material (e.g., glycogen, fragments of lysosomes and other organelles) that accumulates in periportal hepatocytes in patients who consume cyanamide, which is used in alcohol aversion therapy. Similar features have been observed with barbiturates, disulfiram, azathioprine, phenytoin, steroids, and immunosuppressive drugs used in organ transplantation.

Such hepatocytes resemble the ground-glass cells seen with chronic HBV infection, the presence of which is easily excluded by immunohistochemistry with anti–hepatitis B surface antigen (HBsAg) antibodies. This type of ground-glass inclusion may also be seen in Lafora disease (myoclonus epilepsy) and in type IV glycogenosis and fibrinogen storage disease; in some cases, none of these etiological factors is found. These inclusions resemble polyglucosan bodies described in humans, animals, and experimental models, suggesting a pathogenetic role of disturbed glycogen metabolism that is possibly related to polypharmacotherapy,[98] particularly with immunosuppressive agents and, more specifically, with mycophenolate mofetil (MMF).

Anisonucleosis and Increased Mitoses

Anisonucleosis (marked variability in hepatocyte nuclear size) is a consistent finding in biopsy specimens of patients who use methotrexate. Mitoses are strikingly increased (and sometimes rather atypical) in cases of colchicine therapy or acute arsenic intoxication, and this is often accompanied by hepatocyte ballooning, cholestasis, and mild inflammation.[99]

Bile Duct Injury

Acute Cholangitis

Acute cholestasis may be accompanied by bile duct degeneration with or without inflammation (cholangitis). Some hepatotoxins, such as Spanish toxic oil and the herbicide dipyridilium (Paraquat), can lead to isolated pure bile duct necrosis, as can transcatheter hepatic artery embolization (Fig. 49.25).

Acute cholangitis (with inflammation) has been reported with several drugs,[13,100] including AMC. It corresponds to a type of focal destructive cholangiopathy with influx of acute inflammation involving damaged bile ducts, and it is associated with a portal inflammatory infiltrate (Fig. 49.26). In addition, periportal hepatocytes are often ballooned and clarified because of cholate stasis. Cholestasis is usually easily evident and stands predominantly in the central zone, with accumulation of biliary pigment in hepatocytes as well as formation of bile plugs in the liver cell canaliculi (Fig. 49.27). Among antibiotics, Augmentin is the more frequently hepatotoxic drug, particularly in older men; its hepatotoxic potential is detailed later in this chapter. Recently, CPIs have been shown to induce cholangitis, often in association with lobular hepatitis. Acute cholangitis may be followed by prolonged cholestasis, and complications include vanishing bile duct and ductopenia in cases of severe acute injury to the bile ducts.[101,102]

Chronic Cholangitis

Most cases of drug-induced bile duct injury improve rapidly after withdrawal of the causative agent. However, approximately 10% of patients experience chronic cholestatic disease. A "delayed" cholestatic syndrome is defined

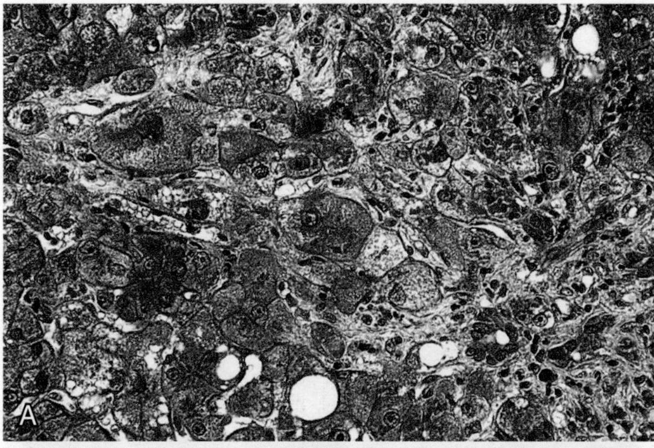

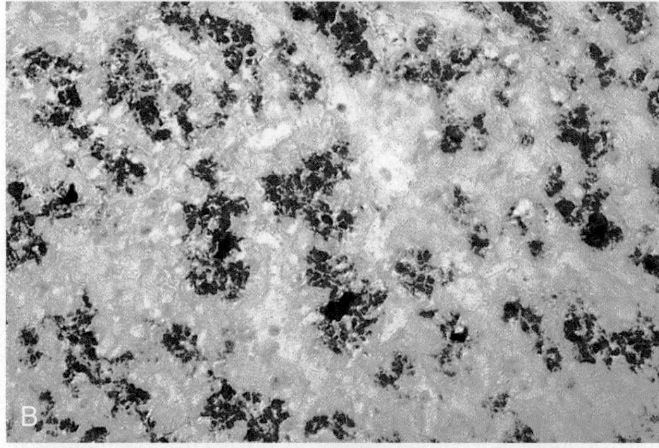

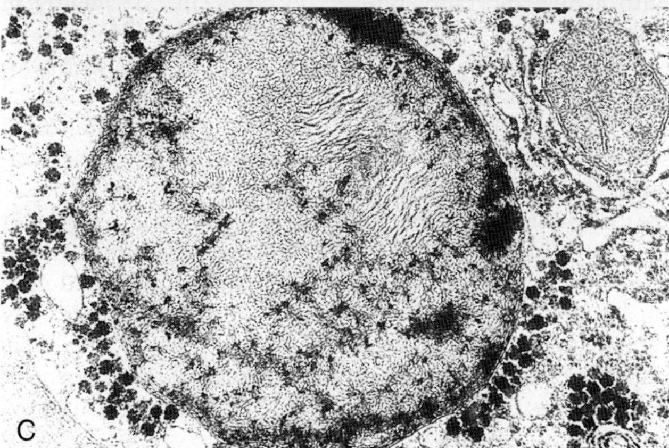

FIGURE 49.21 Perhexiline-induced phospholipidosis in a 59-year-old woman. A, Zone 1 foamy hepatocytes contain numerous Mallory bodies (Masson trichrome stain). **B,** Phospholipids are stained in blue on this frozen-section specimen (Nile blue sulfate stain). **C,** Electron micrograph of a membrane-bound liposomal inclusion in a hepatocyte shows some membranous arrays. (Courtesy P. Callard, Tenon Hospital, Paris.)

as persistence of jaundice for longer than 6 months or the presence of serological abnormalities (i.e., increased AP and γ-glutamyltranspeptidase) for longer than 1 year after cessation of the drug).

Mild alterations of the epithelium (vacuolization, nuclear disarray, mild lymphocytic exocytosis) have been described with chlorpropamide and phenytoin, and neutrophilic infiltration has been described with allopurinol, carbamazepine, and chlorpromazine. Destruction of the epithelium can develop with ajmaline barbiturate, carbamazepine, chlorpromazine, troleandomycin, flucloxacillin, and CPIs, particularly pembrolizumab.

In the chronic phase, the portal tracts show polymorphonuclear inflammation and ductular proliferation (cholangiolitis) associated with ductopenia of small biliary channels, which may mimic primary biliary cholangitis (PBC) or primary sclerosing cholangitis (PSC) (Fig. 49.28; Table 49.7).

Ductopenia

Some drugs can induce alterations of the small bile ducts, mimicking PBC or PSC (see Table 49.4) with cholestasis, portal fibrosis, inflammation, and bile duct damage culminating in marked ductopenia (called *vanishing bile duct syndrome*).[103] This has been reported to occur, for example, with chlorpromazine and various antimicrobial agents (Fig. 49.29). CPIs can also trigger ductopenia and the development of a form of sclerosing cholangitis (see Fig. 49.57).

Although the mechanism of drug-induced lesions of the small bile ducts remains largely unknown, it is thought that the initial destruction of bile ducts may be immunologically mediated. The causative drug or one of its metabolites may trigger an immune response directed against normal biliary epithelium. The differential diagnosis between DILI and idiopathic immune cholangiopathies relies on a set of clinicopathological criteria (see Table 49.7).

Injections of the hepatic artery with chemotherapeutic agents for treatment of metastatic colon cancer[104] can lead also to necrosis of larger ducts. When large bile ducts are involved (as with 5-fluorouracil), it has been suggested that damage may occur primarily to arteries leading to arterial fibrosis and stenosis; bile duct ischemia and loss may follow, with ensuing fibrosis. Histologically, the damage resembles PSC.

Parenteral nutrition may be associated with cholestasis and ductular proliferation, alone or with hepatocellular damage, fibrosis, and even cirrhosis[105,106] (Fig. 49.30). In a few cases, chronic cholangitis does not regress after withdrawal of the offending drug, and this can lead to end-stage biliary cirrhosis. The cellular mechanisms of drug-induced biliary lesions are various, often mixed, and depend on the causative drug.[107]

Vascular Injury

Drugs and chemicals can cause lesions at all levels of the hepatic vascular system (i.e., portal vein and branches, hepatic arteries, sinusoids, central veins, and hepatic veins). Often, the same drug can cause several types of vascular lesions; this suggests a basic common mechanism, such as toxicity to endothelial cells.[108] The molecular and cellular mechanisms remain essentially unknown, but impairment of sinusoidal endothelial cell glutathione and nitric oxide metabolic pathways appears to play an important role.[109]

Portal Vein Lesions

Hepatoportal Sclerosis

Lesions of hepatoportal sclerosis have been reported with some types of immunosuppressive agents and with chronic exposure to toxins such as arsenic, vinyl chloride, and copper sulfate. This lesion is characterized by sclerosis of small portal venules followed by periportal fibrosis, but without

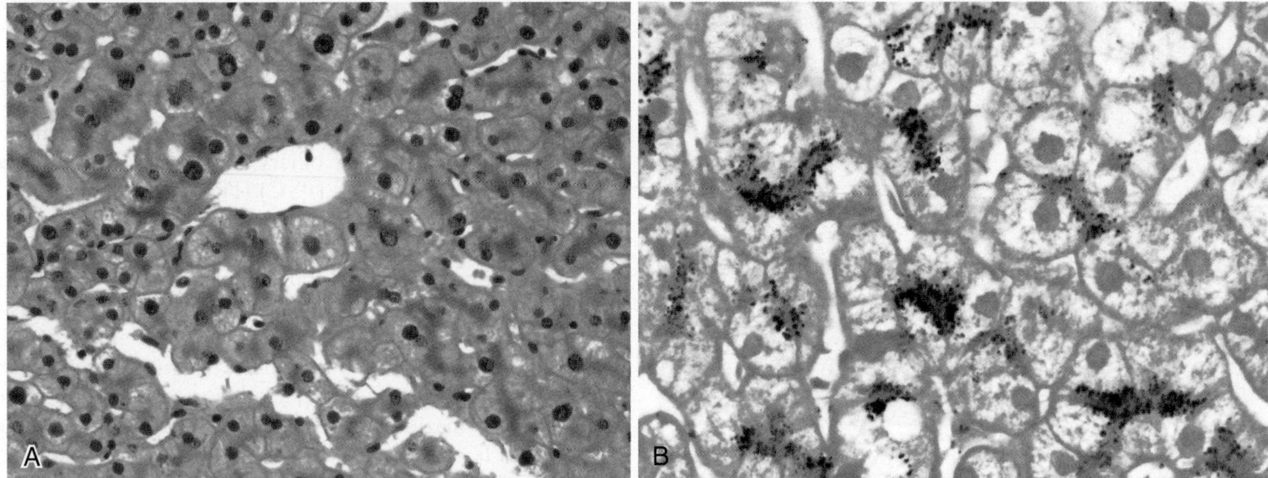

FIGURE 49.22 Lipofuscin accumulation in centrilobular hepatocytes in an older man who had taken many psychotropic drugs. A, The granular, fine and brown pigment stands in the canalicular pole of hepatocytes in zone 3. **B**, Lipofuscin composition is demonstrated by Fontana stain positivity.

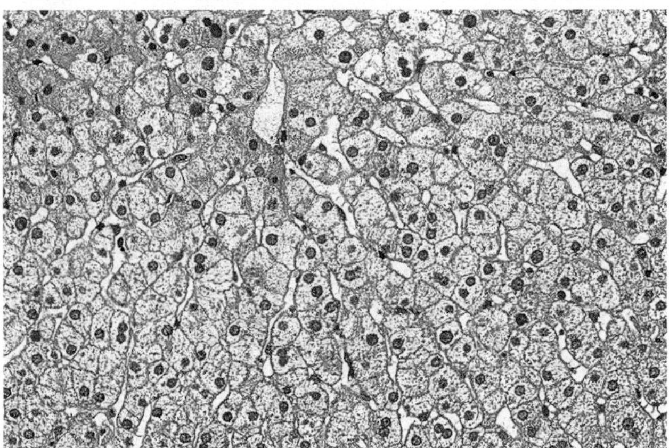

FIGURE 49.23 Adaptive changes of hepatocytes are visible in a biopsy specimen from a 39-year-old patient taking phenobarbital. Hepatocytes show enlarged and pale-staining cytoplasm.

development of cirrhosis, leading to noncirrhotic portal hypertension.

Nodular regenerative hyperplasia (NRH) may be associated with hepatoportal sclerosis or may be the consequence of sinusoidal dilation and peliosis (described later). Chemotherapeutic agents (e.g., azathioprine in transplantation, mercaptopurine, and 6-thioguanine in ulcerative colitis) as well as oral contraceptives can cause NRH.

Hepatic Artery Lesions

Intimal hyperplasia of the hepatic artery has been reported in association with the use of oral contraceptives. It usually is asymptomatic but rarely may lead to necrohemorrhagic lesions of the liver. Sclerosing and obliterative lesions of the hepatic artery branches caused by intraarterial drug infusions, which lead to bile duct injury, were discussed earlier in this chapter (see Fig. 49.25B).

Hepatic Vein Lesions

Venoocclusive disease (VOD) involves nonthrombotic obstruction of small terminal hepatic veins, which appear narrowed or occluded with loose subintimal mesenchyme and edematous fibrous tissue (Fig. 49.31). Because VOD is usually associated with sinusoidal endothelial cell injury, mainly in zone 3, followed by sinusoidal obstruction, it is now believed that VOD is part of the sinusoidal obstruction syndrome (SOS).[110] VOD/SOS may complicate treatment with anticancer drugs and also may result from intake of toxins such as alcohol, heroin, or herbal remedies containing pyrrolizidine alkaloids. Irradiation and chemotherapy used before bone marrow transplantation are another major cause of this lesion; in this context, it is frequently severe with a high mortality rate.[111] VOD occurs frequently in renal transplant recipients who are treated with immunosuppressive agents and corticoids; it is often associated with peliosis and may be followed by NRH.

VOD may be acute or chronic. In either instance, if severe enough, it may lead to massive parenchymal collapse (Fig. 49.32) and hepatic failure. The liver of a patient treated with radiation may also exhibit some aspects of chronic VOD (Fig. 49.33) or Budd-Chiari syndrome. Alkylating agents such as cyclophosphamide, busulfan, and melphalan are the main inducers of VOD, which is directly related to the formation of highly toxic metabolites. The unpredictable occurrence of VOD may be related to genetic polymorphisms in exporters that are responsible for removing toxic metabolites.

Budd-Chiari syndrome (see Chapter 52) is characterized by obstruction of large or small hepatic veins caused by thrombosis. This condition can lead to hepatic congestion and ischemic necrosis of the centrilobular hepatocytes, followed by an acute or chronic course. Alkaloids and irradiation, particularly when associated with oncological chemotherapy, can lead to Budd-Chiari syndrome. When it appears in women who have taken oral contraceptives, Budd-Chiari syndrome is almost always associated with coagulative abnormalities or a latent myeloproliferative disorder.[112]

Sinusoids

Sinusoidal Dilation

Sinusoidal dilation is a frequent incidental finding in patients who have taken oral contraceptives for a long period; it predominates in the periportal zone and is usually of no clinical consequence[113] (Fig. 49.34). On the other hand, sinusoidal

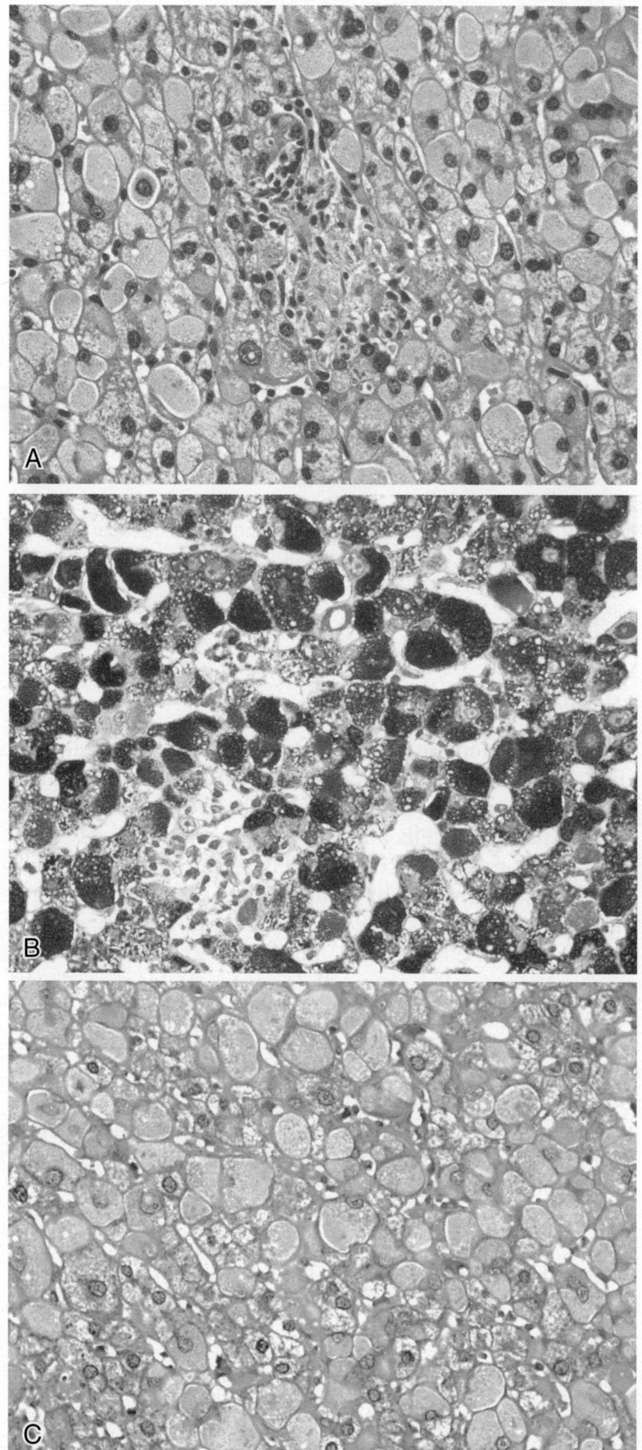

FIGURE 49.24 Ground-glass hepatocytes in drug-induced liver injury. A, On hematoxylin and eosin (H&E) stain, they appear as round and slightly eosinophilic, homogeneous cytoplasmic inclusions surrounded by a fine clear halo. **B**, They are strongly positive with periodic acid–Schiff (PAS) stain but negative after diastase reaction. **C**, Shikata stain is negative, eliminating hepatitis B surface antigen (HBsAg).

dilation induced by azathioprine may lead to fibrosis, and even cirrhosis, after several years; NRH may also be associated with this drug (Fig. 49.35). Microvascular alterations (e.g., sinusoidal dilation, perisinusoidal fibrosis), mainly in the centrilobular zone, have been described in abusers of

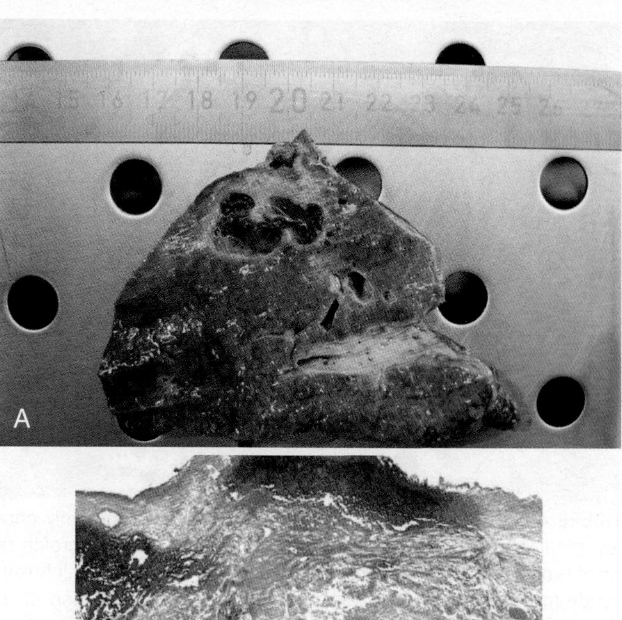

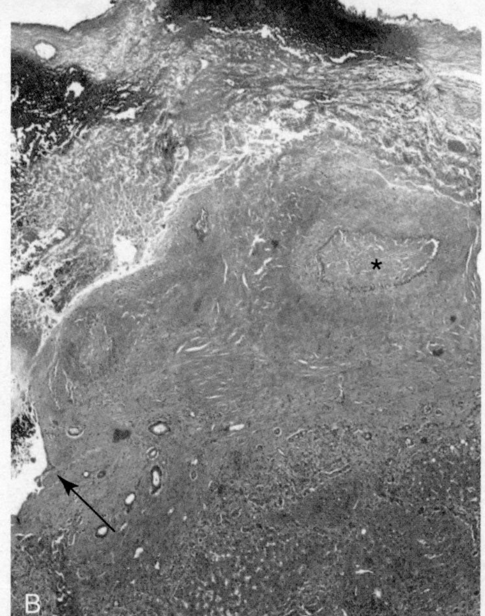

FIGURE 49.25 Ischemic cholangitis after transarterial chemotherapy for hepatocellular carcinoma on a cirrhotic liver. A, A large biliary lake containing bile and microlithiasis has developed in a dilated duct (explanted liver). **B,** The epithelial lining of the duct is totally destroyed *(arrow)*. The biliary wall is fibrosed, and obliterative arteriopathy is visible *(asterisk)*.

heroin. This agent is thought to have a direct vascular toxic effect that is potentially reversible if the drug is stopped.[114]

Systemic neoadjuvant chemotherapy for metastatic colorectal cancer frequently causes morphological lesions involving the hepatic microvasculature. Sinusoidal obstruction, complicated by perisinusoidal fibrosis and venoocclusive lesions of the nontumoral liver, should be included in the list of adverse side effects of colorectal systemic chemotherapy, particularly oxaliplatin use[115] (Fig. 49.36).

Peliosis

Peliosis associated with various drugs is much more rare than sinusoidal dilation (see Table 49.4). It is characterized by blood-filled spaces, haphazardly distributed in the lobule, that lack an endothelial lining. Most cases are asymptomatic, but long-standing peliosis (Fig. 49.37) may lead to perisinusoidal fibrosis or NRH. The main offending drugs are oral contraceptives; other potential agents include androgens, azathioprine, 6-thioguanine, and thiopurine.

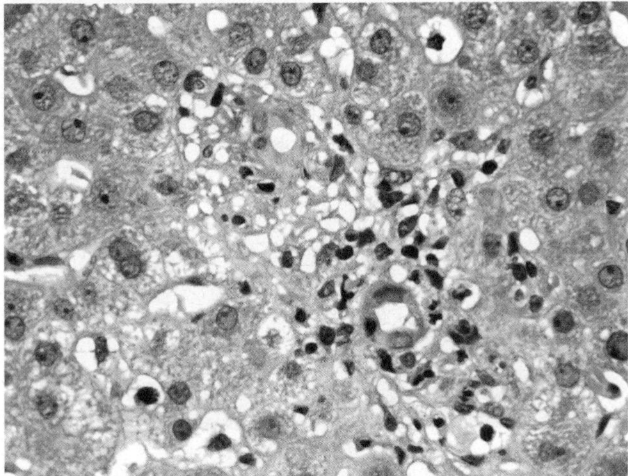

FIGURE 49.26 Acute cholangitis responsible for predominantly cholestatic liver disease in a 47-year-old woman who took ketoprofen (a nonsteroidal antiinflammatory drug) and in whom Stevens-Johnson syndrome developed. Note the dystrophic, ischemic-like aspect of the interlobular duct, the mild portal inflammatory infiltrate with mixed composition, cholestatic deposits in hepatocytes, and clarification of hepatocytes.

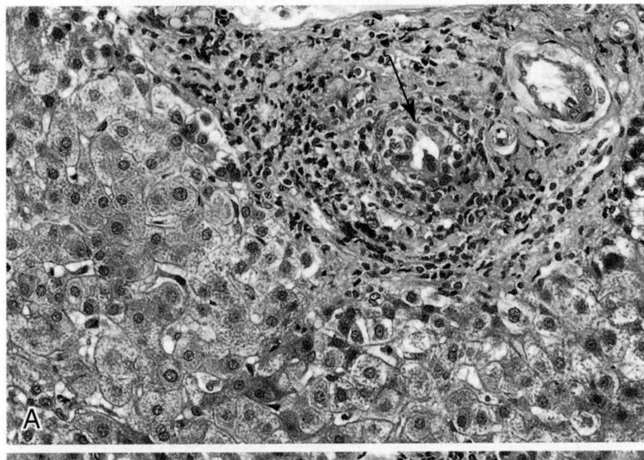

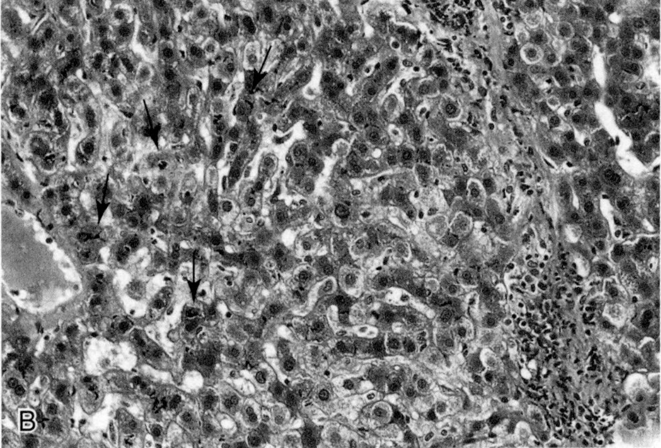

FIGURE 49.27 Focal destructive cholangiopathy induced by amoxicillin in a 65-year-old man (6 days after ingestion). A, Mixed portal inflammatory infiltrate surrounds a damaged bile duct *(arrow)*. **B,** There is centrilobular cholestasis with bile plugs in canaliculi and in the cytoplasm of hepatocytes *(arrows)*. (Courtesy Dr. M. Chevallier, Lyon, France.)

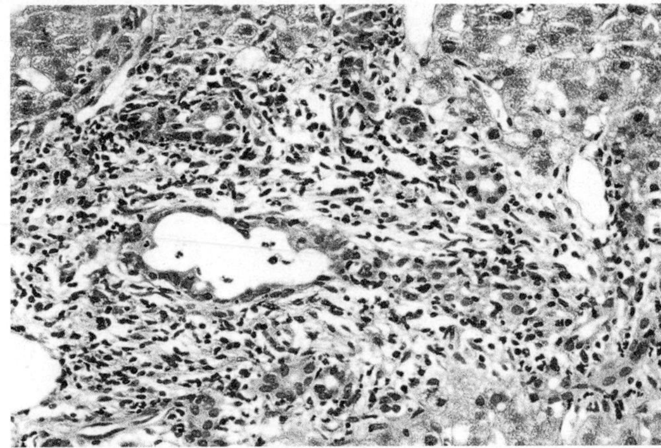

FIGURE 49.28 Chronic cholangitis resulting from flucloxacillin in a 72-year-old woman. Shown is a dilated interlobular bile duct with damaged epithelium penetrated by inflammatory cells in an enlarged portal tract with neutrophilic inflammation, eosinophils, and ductular proliferation. This appearance is reminiscent of primary biliary cholangitis–like chronic cholangitis. (Courtesy Jurgen Rode, Royal Darwin Hospital, Darwin, Australia.)

Sinusoidal Cells

Changes in Hepatic Stellate Cells. In hypervitaminosis A (Fig. 49.38), hypertrophied hepatic stellate cells that contain abundant lipid droplets are situated between the sinusoidal endothelial lining cells and the hepatocytes; typically, they are visible on light microscopy. Hypertrophic stellate cells are often accompanied by sinusoidal dilation and prominent perisinusoidal fibrosis. Lipid loading is better visualized with the use of epon-embedded 1-μm tissue sections and on electron microscopy. The extracellular matrix is deposited in the space of Disse, often with a more or less complete basement membrane and underneath the sinusoidal endothelial cells. This condition usually remains asymptomatic for a long time,[116] until large cumulative doses of vitamin A lead to fibrosis and even cirrhosis with portal hypertension. Perisinusoidal fibrosis is the result of myofibroblastic transformation of hepatic stellate cells (their "activated" phenotype). Expression of α-SMA (see Fig. 49.36E) is a characteristic feature of activated stellate cells, whereas immunostaining with cellular binding protein 1, which is a specific marker for quiescent stellate cells, allows easy visualization of these cells (see Fig. 49.36D), regardless of whether they are overloaded with lipids.[117]

Lesser degrees of stellate cell lipid storage, with or without perisinusoidal fibrosis (Fig. 49.39), are seen with drugs such as methotrexate and certain immunosuppressive agents. Methotrexate hepatotoxicity is enhanced by several intrinsic factors (e.g., psoriasis, diabetes, and obesity) and by concomitant alcohol exposure. Methotrexate-induced fibrosis develops insidiously but may lead to severe fibrosis and cirrhosis.

Changes in Kupffer Cells and Macrophages. Some drugs, toxins, and foreign materials are phagocytosed by Kupffer cells and other liver macrophages. Some of them, such as polyvinylpyrrolidone (stained with Congo red), talc, silicone (seen with phase contrast), gold, and the radiocontrast agent Thorotrast, exhibit characteristic features that are

TABLE 49.7 Main Differential Features of Drug-Induced Cholangitis versus Primary Biliary Cholangitis (PBC) and Primary Sclerosing Cholangitis (PSC)

	DIC	PBC	PSC
Age	Any age	Middle age	Middle age
Sex	M = F	M:F = 1:9	M:F = 2:1
Drug intake	Tolbutamide Phenothiazine		
Onset	Acute	Insidious	Insidious
Autoimmune antibodies		Anti-SMA (95%)	
Jaundice	Early	Late	Late
Histology	Possible ductopenia (nonsuppurative) Fibrosis ± cirrhosis	Fibro-obliterative Granulomatous Cholangitis Ductopenia Fibrosis ± cirrhosis	Cholangitis Fibrosis ± cirrhosis

F, *female;* M, *male;* SMA, *α-smooth muscle actin.*

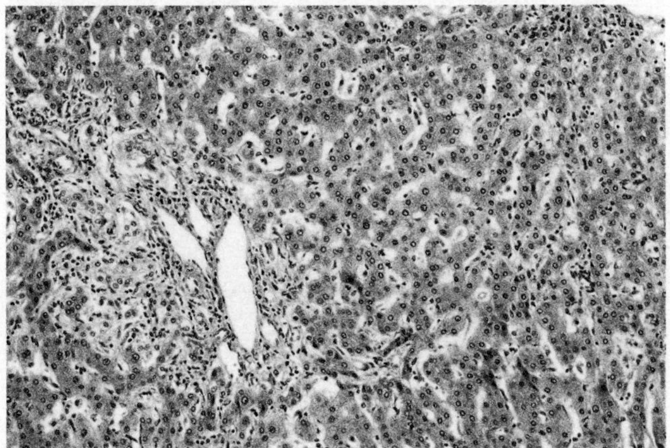

FIGURE 49.29 Vanishing bile duct syndrome linked with thiabendazole toxicity in a 27-year-old man who developed cholestatic liver disease after treatment of a presumed parasitic diarrheal infection. Ductopenia concerns interlobular ducts, and there is mild portal inflammation. (Courtesy Dr. Dale Snover, Fairview Southdale Hospital, Edina, MN.)

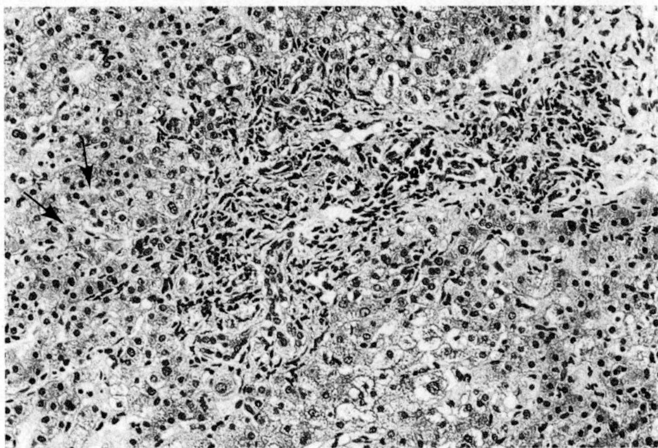

FIGURE 49.30 Biliary fibrosis secondary to total parenteral nutrition in a 43-year-old woman with life-threatening burns. Enlarged fibrotic portal tracts with ductular proliferation and mixed inflammation; hepatocytes appear ballooned. There is also moderate cholestasis *(arrows).*

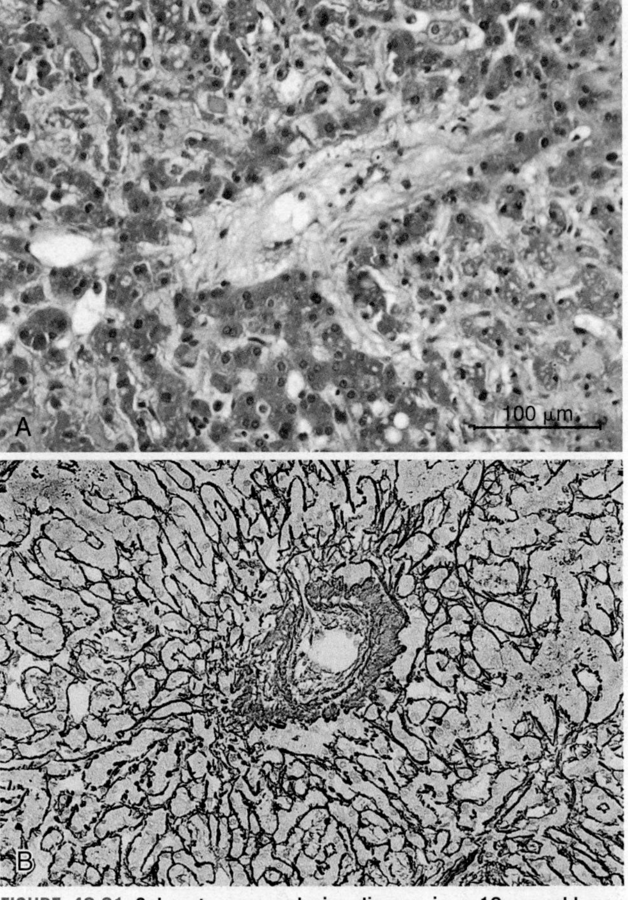

FIGURE 49.31 Subacute venoocclusive disease in a 19-year-old man treated with anticancer chemotherapy (actinomycin + vincristine [Oncovin]) for Ewing sarcoma. A, The wall of this hepatic vein is thickened, and the lumen is narrowed, by a subintimal deposition of loose connective tissue. **B,** In the lobule, the reticulin network is enhanced (Gordon and Sweets stain).

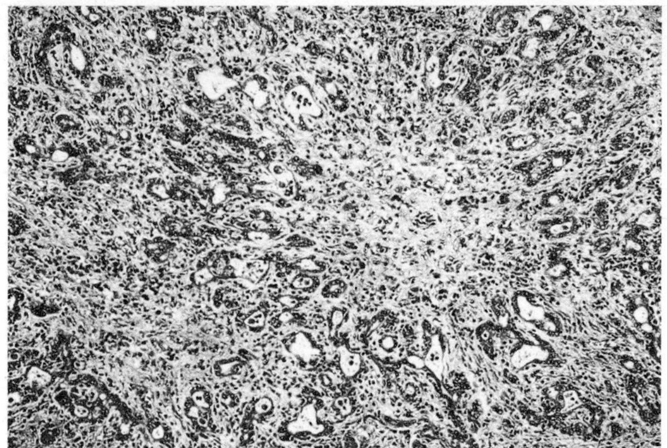

FIGURE 49.32 Chronic venoocclusive disease with massive collapse, confluent necrosis, cholangitis, and prominent ductular cholestasis manifesting as fatal subfulminant hepatitis attributable to use of herbal remedies in a 28-year-old man. (Courtesy James M. Crawford, University of Florida, Gainesville, FL.)

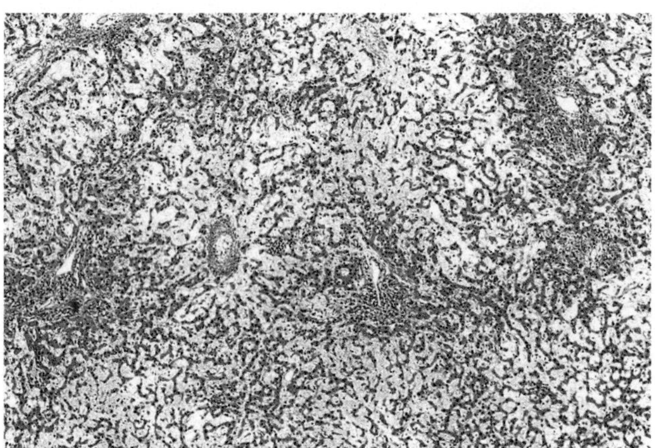

FIGURE 49.33 Chronic venoocclusive disease in a 50-year-old man , 1 year after radiation therapy for a retroperitoneal sarcoma, shows marked sinusoidal congestive dilation and atrophy of the rather disorganized hepatocytic plates.

visible with the use of standard or special techniques. Phospholipidosis (see Figs. 49.20 and 49.21), described earlier, can involve Kupffer cells as well.

Granulomatous Reactions

Numerous drugs (see Table 49.4) may lead to the development of a granulomatous reaction, which can be isolated or part of a cytolytic or a cholestatic hepatitis.

Most drugs cause noncaseating granulomas of variable size, located in the portal tracts or in the hepatic parenchyma. Some appear as clusters of nonepithelioid spumous macrophages (Fig. 49.40), but often these small granulomas are made of cells more or less typical of epithelioid cells (Fig. 49.41), mimicking sarcoidosis. Langerhans giant and multinucleated cells may be seen on occasion. A great number of drugs can induce this type of epithelioid reaction, including quinidine, hydralazine, and phenytoin but also carbamazepine, chlorpromazine, dapsone, INH, metaxalone, ranitidine, trimethoprim/sulphamethoxazole, and tolbutamide. An eosinophilic infiltrate may be associated and suggests hypersensitivity mechanisms.

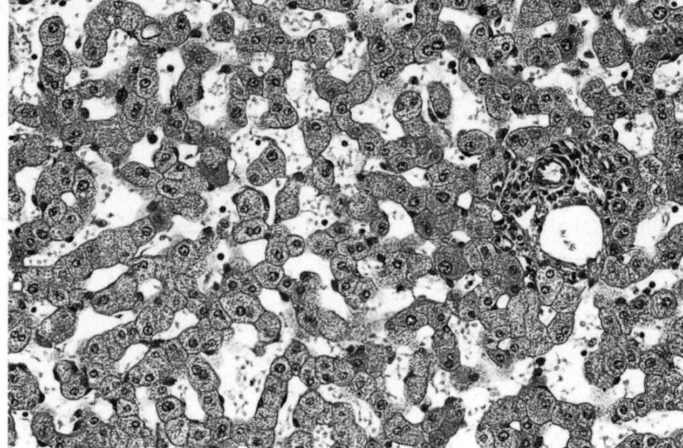

FIGURE 49.34 Sinusoidal dilation in a 45-year-old woman after long-term use of oral contraceptives.

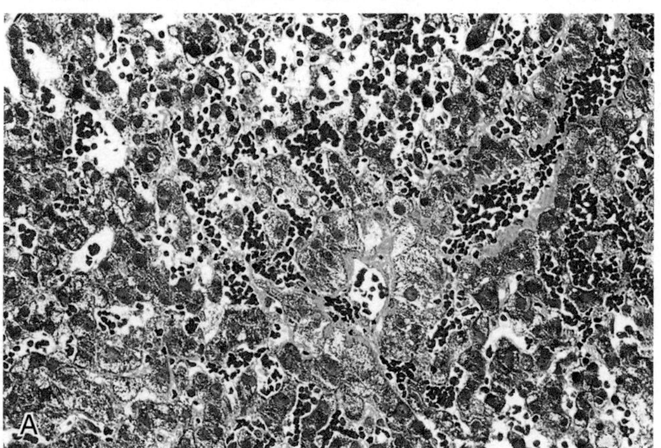

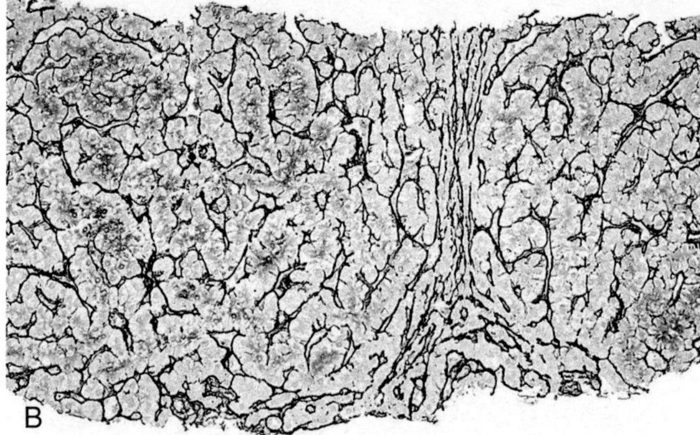

FIGURE 49.35 **Microvascular lesions in a renal transplant recipient who was taking azathioprine. A,** Prominent sinusoidal dilation is associated with perisinusoidal and central vein fibrosis (Masson trichrome stain). **B,** Typical appearance of nodular regenerative hyperplasia. Atrophic hepatocytic plates located in areas of enhanced reticulin network separate regenerative nodular areas (Gordon and Sweets stain).

Some drugs, such as phenylbutazone, can lead to granulomatous hepatitis with the formation of multiple granulomas, accompanied by some degree of hepatocytic degeneration or intrahepatic cholestasis. Granulomas with a fibrin ring appearance (Fig. 49.42), resembling Q fever, are rare but can occur with allopurinol and CPIs. *Lipogranulomas* may be induced by mineral oil ingestion or by gold salts[118]; macrophages contain fine, black or brown pigmented granules. Foreign body

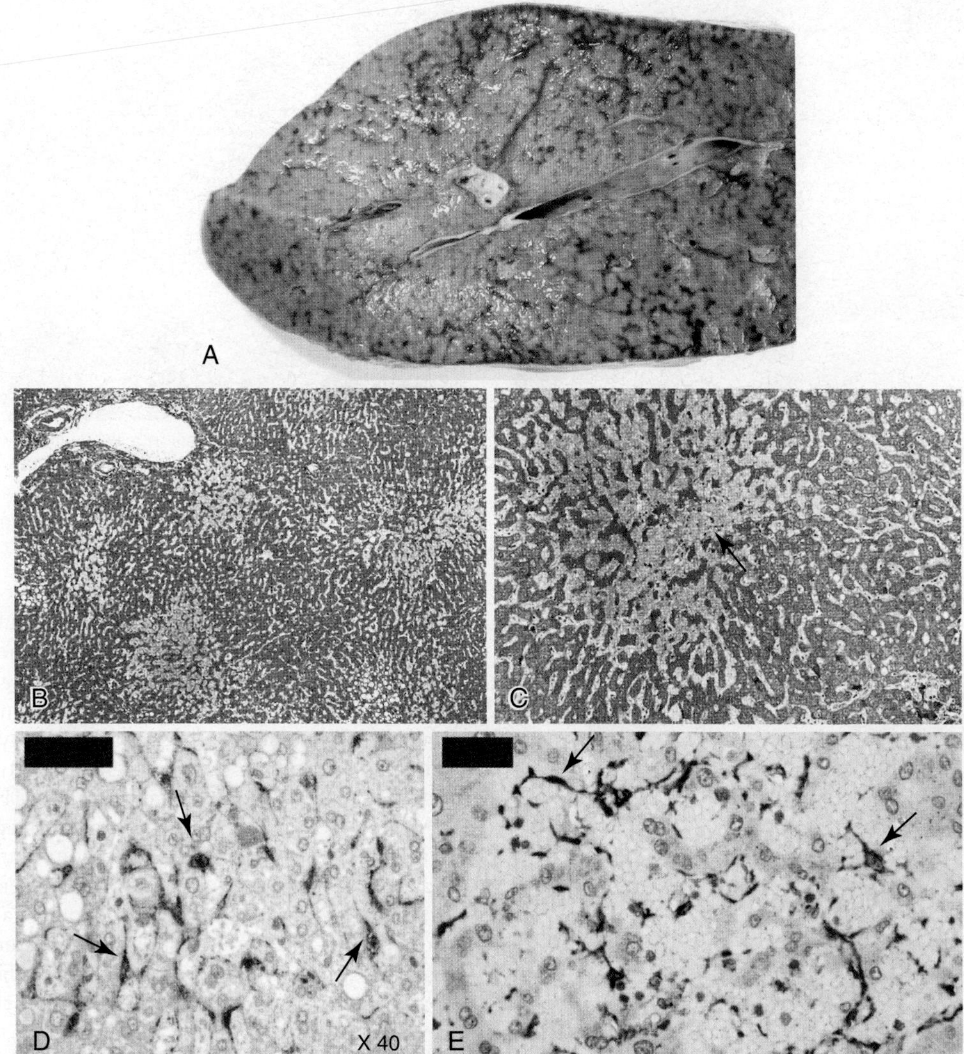

FIGURE 49.36 Left hepatectomy specimen from a 62-year-old man with metastatic rectal carcinoma after chemotherapy that included oxaliplatin. A, Abnormal-appearing nontumoral liver is nodular and shows congested areas. **B,** Sinusoidal dilation and congestion. **C,** Occlusion of central vein *(arrow)*. **D,** In areas of sinusoidal dilation, hepatic stellate cells are visible *(arrows)* with the use of cellular binding protein 1 (CRBP1) antibody immunostain. **E,** Hepatic stellate cells are activated and express α-smooth muscle actin *(arrows)*.

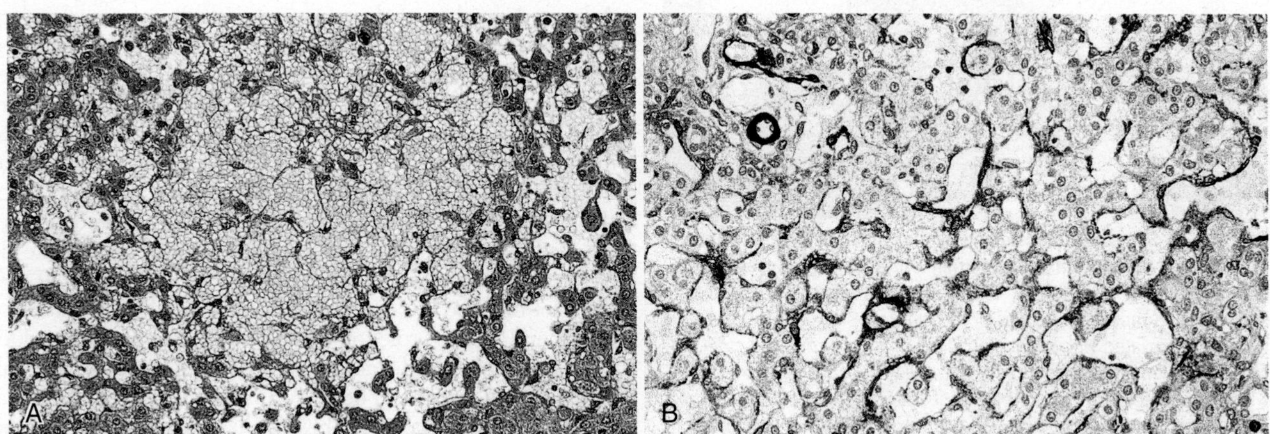

FIGURE 49.37 Microvascular lesions caused by anticancer chemotherapy in a 4-year-old boy before surgery for hepatoblastoma: nontumoral liver. A, Areas of peliosis and sinusoidal dilation. **B,** α-Smooth muscle actin (α-SMA)-positive hepatic stellate cells underlie dilated sinusoids (α-SMA immunostain).

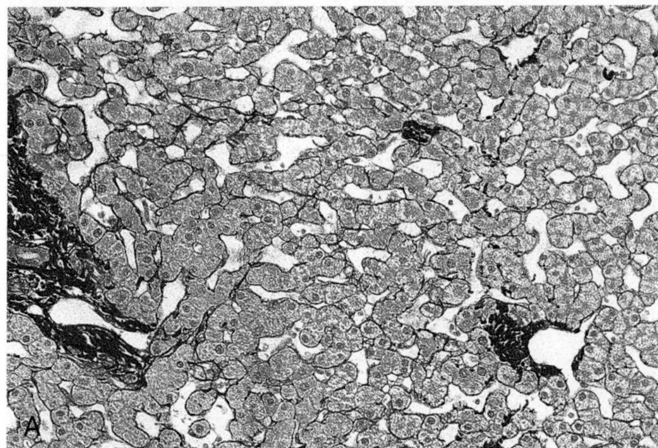

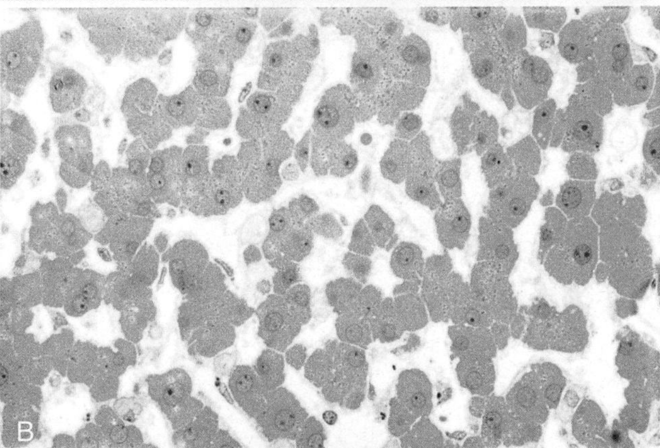

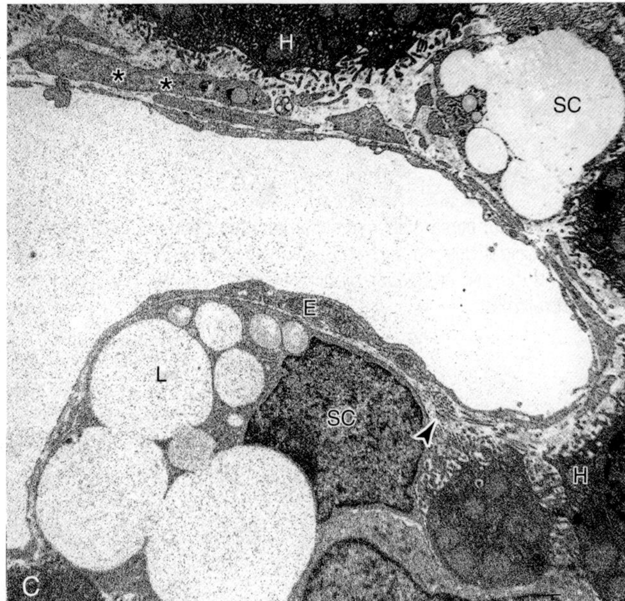

FIGURE 49.38 Sinusoidal fibrosis and lipid overload in hypervitaminosis A in a 50-year-old woman (a vegetarian who took high doses of vitamin A regularly for 4 years). A, The lobular architecture of the liver is preserved, with moderate fibrosis of the central vein, portal tracts, and sinusoids, associated with slight sinusoidal dilation (Sirius red stain). **B,** Large, lipid-overloaded hepatic stellate cells are bulging into sinusoidal lumina or intercalating in the recesses between hepatocytes (1-μm section, toluidine blue stain). **C,** On electron microscopy, two hepatic stellate cells (*SC*) and processes *(asterisks)* containing lipid droplets *(L)* are seen on each side of the sinusoidal lumen between the endothelial lining *(E)* and the hepatocytes *(H)*. Notice the collagen bundles *(arrowhead)* in the Disse space.

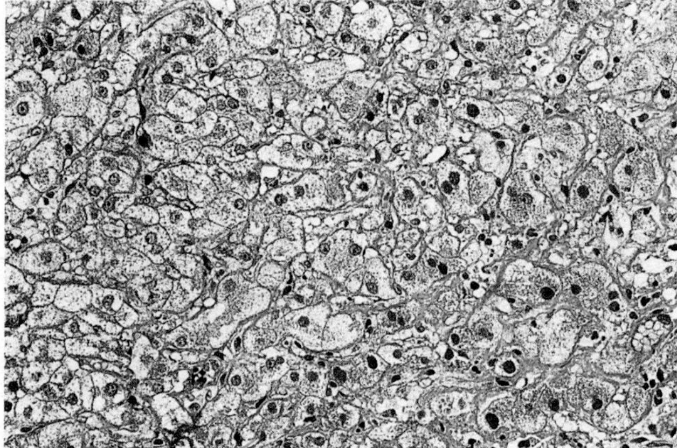

FIGURE 49.39 Sinusoidal fibrosis in a 62-year-old woman with polyarthritis treated with immunosuppressive agents. Prominent perisinusoidal fibrosis and hypertrophy of hepatic stellate cells *(middle of field)* was associated with nodular regenerative hyperplasia *(not shown).*

granulomas can develop as a response to talc, surgical suture material, or embolization material. Therapeutic embolization is performed either through a branch of the hepatic artery, for embolization of a tumor or for stopping hemorrhage of a ruptured liver tumor (Fig. 49.43), or through a portal vein branch, for generation of compensatory hypertrophy of a well-vascularized lobe before surgical resection of the other embolized, atrophic lobe containing tumor (Fig. 49.44).

Activated Kupffer cells and macrophages, as well as neutrophils, in the vicinity of granulomas are implicated as mediators of hepatotoxicity through the secretion of various cytokines and cytotoxic soluble factors[119] and through the production of reactive metabolites. Secreted inflammatory mediators can play both protective and pathological roles in hepatotoxicity, depending on the nature of the toxin and on individual susceptibility.

Although granulomas are classic features in liver toxicity, other causes such as sarcoidosis, infectious diseases (mainly bacterial or viral), or immunological diseases must also be considered.

Hepatic Tumors

A limited number of drugs are associated with the development of hepatic tumors. Hepatocellular adenoma (HCA) is most often associated with exposure to oral contraceptives and more rarely related to use of anabolic or androgenic steroids[120] (Fig. 49.45). HCAs may be complicated by intratumoral hemorrhage, rupture, and formation of a subcapsular hematoma. Their malignant transformation, particularly for the β-catenin–activated HCA subtype,[121,122] is much rarer but has been well documented (Fig. 49.46), as has the de novo occurrence of hepatocellular carcinoma (HCC).[123] Danazol-induced HCA or HCC may regress after cessation of treatment.[124-126] A role for oral contraceptives in the development and growth of focal nodular hyperplasia is controversial.

The development of other tumors, such as angiosarcoma, cholangiocarcinoma, and HCC, has been demonstrated after Thorotrast administration, following latency periods of several decades. With the discontinuation of Thorotrast use in 1955, the risk is now of historical interest only. The contrast agent is recognizable in Kupffer cells in liver tissue

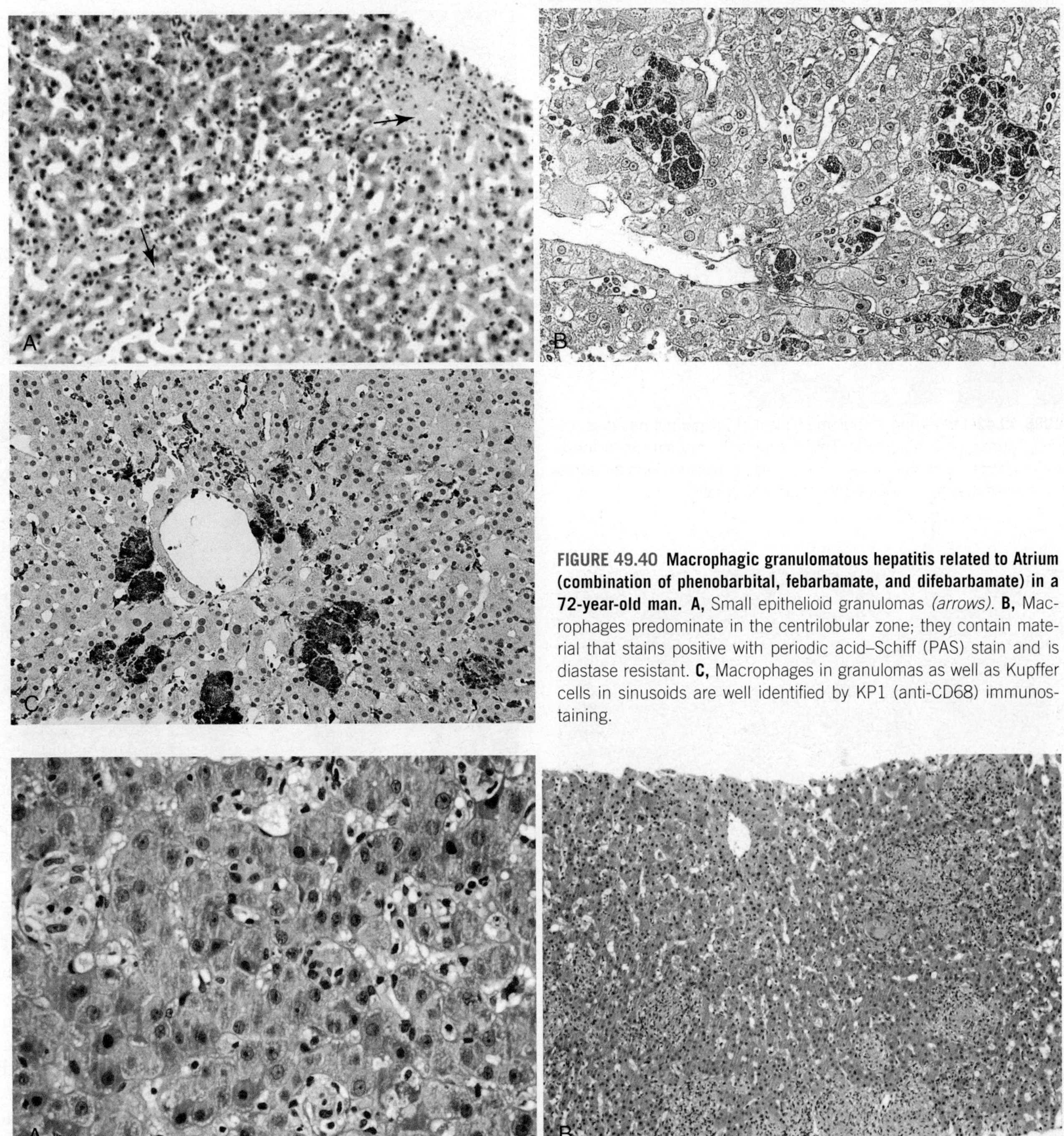

FIGURE 49.40 Macrophagic granulomatous hepatitis related to Atrium (combination of phenobarbital, febarbamate, and difebarbamate) in a 72-year-old man. A, Small epithelioid granulomas *(arrows).* **B,** Macrophages predominate in the centrilobular zone; they contain material that stains positive with periodic acid–Schiff (PAS) stain and is diastase resistant. **C,** Macrophages in granulomas as well as Kupffer cells in sinusoids are well identified by KP1 (anti-CD68) immunostaining.

FIGURE 49.41 Epithelioid granulomatous reactions in drug-induced liver injury. A, Granulomatoid inflammatory foci in glatiramer-associated hepatitis. **B,** Florid epithelio-gigantocellular hepatitis in a patient undergoing classic quadritherapy for tuberculosis. In the absence of active infection, granulomas were attributed to isoniazid toxicity.

surrounding the tumor (Fig. 49.47). As an occupational exposure, vinyl chloride also is associated with the occurrence of angiosarcoma.

EXAMPLES OF COMMON OFFENDING DRUGS

Analgesics

Acetaminophen

Acetaminophen, also called *paracetamol,* N-*acetyl*-p-*aminophenol,* or *APAP,* is one of the most popular and commonly used drugs since the 1960s. It is valued for its analgesic and antipyretic effects and is freely sold in developed countries. At therapeutic doses, it is a safe drug, even in alcoholic patients,[127] but large doses induce hepatic necrosis, resulting in acute cytolytic hepatitis and sometimes leading to acute liver failure. The mechanisms leading to liver necrosis comprise a complex sequence of events, including (1) CYP2E1 metabolism to a metabolite (*N*-acetyl-*p*-benzoquinone imine [NAPQI]), which depletes glutathione and covalently binds to tissue proteins; (2) loss of glutathione with increased formation of ROS and reactive

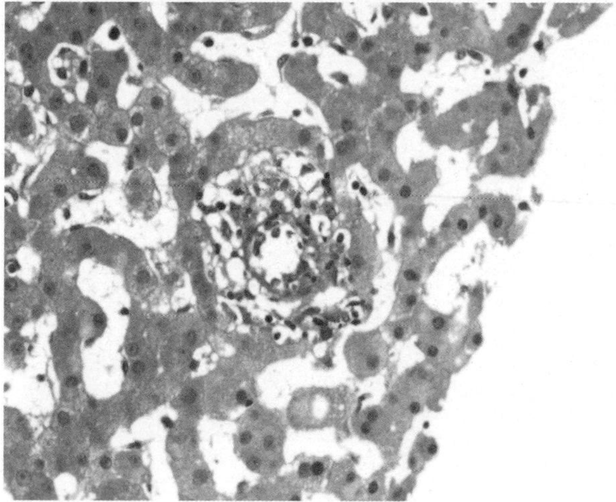

FIGURE 49.42 Fibrin-ring granuloma typical of allopurinol hepatitis occurring during gout treatment. This granuloma, very similar to those seen in Q fever, is characterized by a circular deposit of fibrin around a lipid vacuole that is in contact with inflammatory cells.

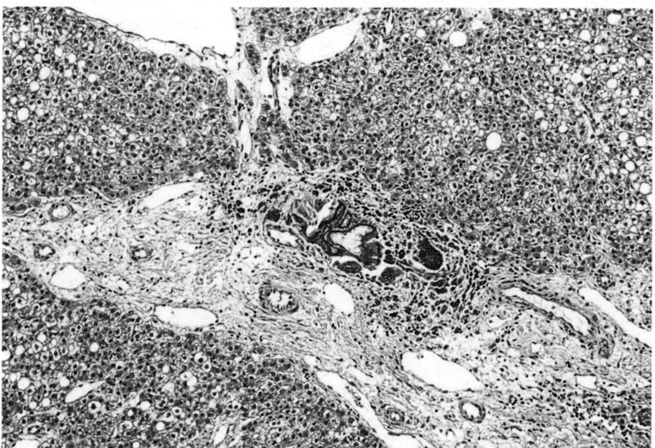

FIGURE 49.43 Foreign body granuloma surrounds a branch of the hepatic artery that was embolized with particles of polyvinyl alcohol to stop hemorrhage from a ruptured hepatocellular adenoma.

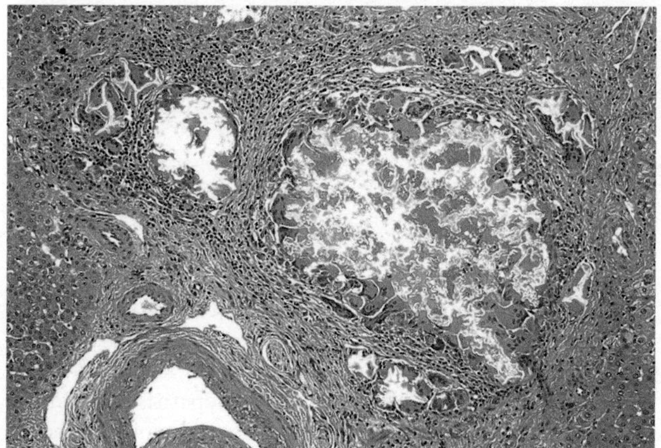

FIGURE 49.44 Foreign body granuloma surrounds a branch of the portal vein that was occluded by embolized material (mixture of histoacryl and Ethiodol [Lipiodol]) before resection of the atrophic lobe containing colon carcinoma metastasis.

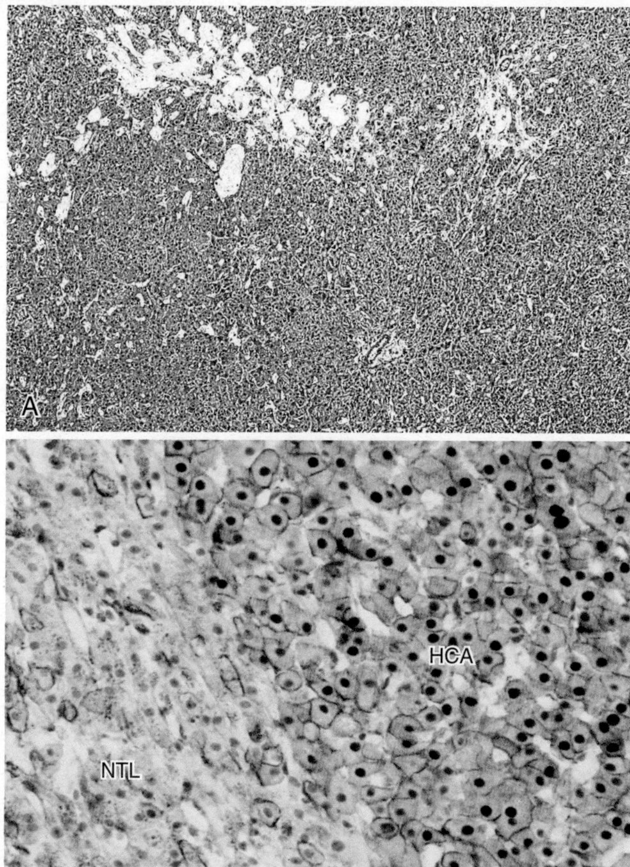

FIGURE 49.45 Hepatocellular adenoma (HCA) in a 14-year-old boy treated with androgens for aplastic anemia. A, Well-differentiated hepatocytic proliferation with areas of peliosis. **B,** Aberrant expression of β-catenin in nuclei and cytoplasm of hepatocytes *(HCA)*, contrasting with normal membranous staining of hepatocytes in nontumoral liver *(NTL)*.

nitrogen species in hepatocytes undergoing necrotic changes; (3) increased oxidative stress, associated with alterations in calcium homeostasis and initiation of signal transduction responses, causing mitochondrial permeability transition; (4) mitochondrial loss of membrane potential and dysfunction; and (5) loss of adenosine triphosphate (ATP), which leads to hepatocyte necrosis.[128] The mechanisms of toxicity are mainly intrinsic and indirect, through generation of the NAPQI metabolite; however, immunoallergy may also play a role.

In adults and adolescents, poisoning with acetaminophen usually results from attempted suicide or inadvertent acute overdose. In contrast, chronic overdosing of acetaminophen in children, especially infants, may result in hepatotoxicity.[129] Doses smaller than 2 g/day are safe in adults, but doses of 4 g/day over 14 days have been shown to increase ALT to three times the normal level. In reported cases of hepatotoxicity, the doses have varied from 7.5 to 70 g. Undoubtedly, there is individual susceptibility for this drug, and toxicity appears when a variable threshold is reached. Some risk factors for acetaminophen toxicity have been identified, including regular ingestion of alcohol, fasting or denutrition, and drug interactions with INH, RFP, anticonvulsants (phenobarbital), and

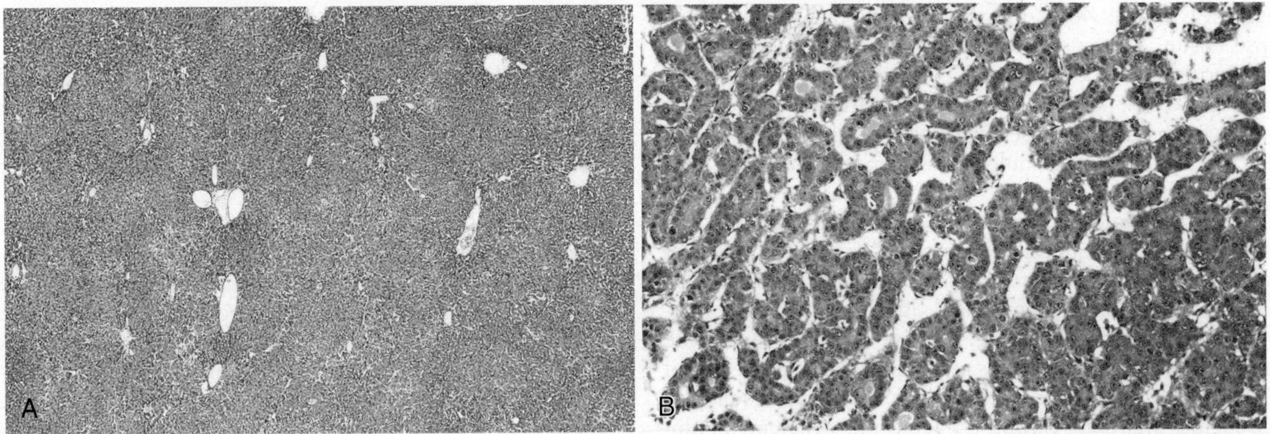

FIGURE 49.46 A, Large hepatocellular adenoma in a 24-year-old woman who took oral contraceptives for 4 years; incomplete resection. **B,** Section obtained 12 years later from the same patient (after two pregnancies followed by oral contraceptive intake) shows large, multifocal, trabecular and pseudoglandular hepatocellular carcinoma.

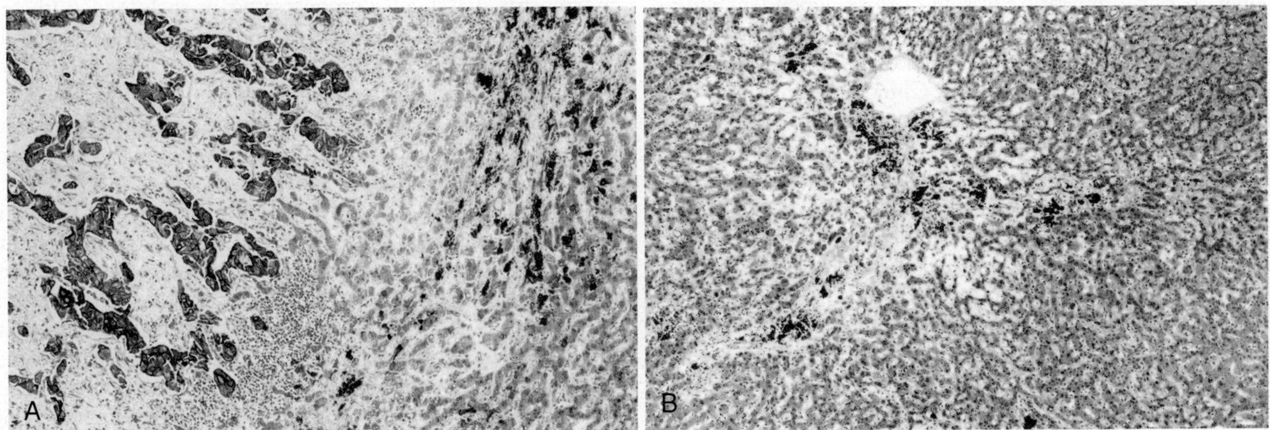

FIGURE 49.47 Cholangiocarcinoma in Thorotrast-induced liver injury. A, Thorotrast granules are deposited in macrophages *(right)* at the border of the cholangiocarcinoma *(left)* (cytokeratin 7 immunostain). **B,** Sinusoidal dilation, peliosis, and atrophy of hepatocytic plates, related to Thorotrast injury, are also seen in zones of Thorotrast deposits in nontumoral liver. (Courtesy A. Paul Dhillon, Royal Free Hospital, London.)

zidovudine. In patients with chronic alcohol abuse, doses as low as 4 g/day could induce severe liver injury.

About 10% of patients who have taken an overdose will develop acute liver failure. Patients may experience some asthenia, abdominal pain, and vomiting. Although most will recover, up to 25% of those who develop hepatic injury go on to acute liver failure with hepatic encephalopathy. Liver tests show cytolysis from 50 to 1000 times normal in the most severe cases. Lactic acidosis and hypothrombinemia may appear within a few days in severe cases. In various surveys of acute liver failure due to DILI performed in Western countries, acetaminophen is the top drug cause, accounting for 46% to 75% of these cases in the United States and the United Kingdom.

In the absence of treatment, mortality is the rule. Treatment involves both medical and surgical approaches. The antioxidant *N*-acetyl-cysteine, when administered during the first 12 to 15 hours after the toxic ingestion of acetaminophen, is an effective antidote that prevents progression to liver failure and globally decreases the mortality rate to 10%. In the absence of efficient medical therapy, severely affected patients will benefit from emergency orthotopic liver transplantation. In murine models, a novel therapeutic approach uses ARC (apoptosis repressor with caspase recruitment domain), which interacts with JNK (c-Jun *N*-terminal kinase) and ROS to block death from the caspase-dependent necrosis induced by acetaminophen.[130] Evaluation of prognosis and the decision for liver transplantation in cases of acute liver failure caused by acetaminophen are based mainly on the King's College Criteria[131]; additional prognostic factors such as radiological and histological findings and biological measurements (e.g., serum α-fetoprotein and phosphorus levels) could improve this evaluation.[132]

If a biopsy is performed, usually the transjugular route is used because of coagulation abnormalities. Histological injury starts with zonal hepatocyte necrosis affecting perivenular zone 3, the location of CYP2E1. Centrilobular hepatocytes undergo eosinophilic degeneration of cytoplasm, with pyknosis of nuclei, with no or only mild polymorphonuclear reaction (Fig. 49.48*A*). Lesions can extend to zone 2 (midlobular). Periportal hepatocytes may show only vacuolization and early degenerative changes, defining a submassive necrotic pattern (see Fig. 49.3). As time goes on, a ductular reaction may develop, and necrosis can become massive, affecting periportal hepatocytes (see

Figs. 49.6 and 49.48B). Hepatocyte dropout and liver collapse ensue. At transplantation, the liver capsule is found to be crumpled, and the parenchyma is collapsed and red.

In rare cases, patterns other than hepatic necrosis of liver have been described; these have included cholestatic hepatitis, chronic hepatitis, granulomatous hepatitis, steatosis, and cirrhosis.

Based on clinicobiological data, the differential diagnosis of acute acetaminophen hepatotoxicity first includes all other causes of acute cytolysis and acute liver failure (i.e., viral, autoimmune, ischemic, and other toxic causes). Biological tests and the serum level of acetaminophen provide useful data for the diagnosis. On biopsy, the presence of centrilobular acidophilic necrosis favors other drugs or toxins, such as aflatoxin, carbon tetrachloride, ethylene dichloride, or cocaine, but also circulatory failure.

Acetylsalicylic Acid

Aspirin is an old analgesic and antipyretic molecule that is known to cause, on rare occasion, a dose-dependent cytolytic hepatitis. The risk is increased in rheumatic patients and in children with lupus erythematosus, juvenile rheumatoid arthritis, or dermatomyositis. Clinical findings are typically mild, and the increase in transaminases is 5 to 40 times normal. These symptoms depend on both the dose and the blood concentration of the drug. Biopsy shows focal necrosis and mild portal inflammation. Case studies from the 1970s also suggest possible cholestasis, granulomatous reaction, steatosis, cirrhosis, and hypersensitivity syndrome (DRESS).[133]

As mentioned earlier, aspirin can also induce mitochondrial dysfunction responsible for severe metabolic disorders including metabolic acidosis, hepatic encephalopathy, hypoglycemia, azotemia, and acute and massive microvesicular steatosis (see Fig. 49.15). This condition is known as *Reye syndrome*, a peculiar disease that is epidemiologically associated with influenza or varicella in children taking aspirin.

Nonsteroidal Antiinflammatory Drugs

The family of NSAIDs includes carboxylic acids, oxicams, carboxamides, sulfonamides, and diaryl-substituted pyrazoles/furanones. It is one of the most frequently prescribed families of drugs around the world, and it also constitutes one of the main causes of DILI (roughly 10% of total cases). Although hepatotoxicity is uncommon, it is potentially lethal, especially in jaundiced patients (e.g., as much as 20% mortality in jaundiced patients with diclofenac). As described in several reviews,[134-136] the incidence of liver toxicity (ALT ≥3× ULN) caused by NSAIDS in population-based clinical studies varies from 0.29 to 9 per 100,000 patient-years, yet the risk of liver-related hospitalization is 3 to 23 per 100,000 patients. Diclofenac and sulindac are the NSAIDs most frequently concerned. Historically, several NSAIDs, such as benoxaprofen, bromfenac, and ibufenac, have been withdrawn from the market because of DILI.

The risk of liver toxicity appears to be six to nine times greater in patients who are taking other potentially hepatotoxic drugs (e.g., INH, AMC) or who have alcoholic or nonalcoholic fatty liver disease. Women older than 50 years of age who have an autoimmune disease are also at higher risk. Genetic susceptibility, implicating specific polymorphisms, has been demonstrated in diclofenac-induced DILI. Two main mechanisms of injury are possible and may be associated: hypersensitivity (idiosyncrasy) and metabolic aberration. Mechanisms have been well reviewed for diclofenac-induced liver injury, "a paradigm of idiosyncratic drug toxicity"[137] in which reactive metabolites, oxidative stress, and mitochondrial lesions play a role.

With NSAID use, patterns of acute and chronic hepatitis (Fig. 49.49), mixed hepatitis, cholestasis, and ductopenia may be encountered, even with the same molecule. Liver damage usually appears within 12 weeks after initiation of therapy. Analysis from various databases indicates that diclofenac and rofecoxib are associated with a higher level of transaminases compared with other NSAIDs or placebo. Massive hepatitis, requiring transplantation, can develop with diclofenac, sulindac, and oxicams. Diclofenac, ibuprofen, naproxen, oxicams, and nimesulide can cause pure cholestasis. Alterations of small bile ducts (Fig. 49.50A; see Fig. 49.26) can progressively lead to ductopenia, which has been reported mainly with ibuprofen and oxicams. After the causative drug is stopped, liver tests usually return to normal within 4 to 6 weeks in nonsevere cases.

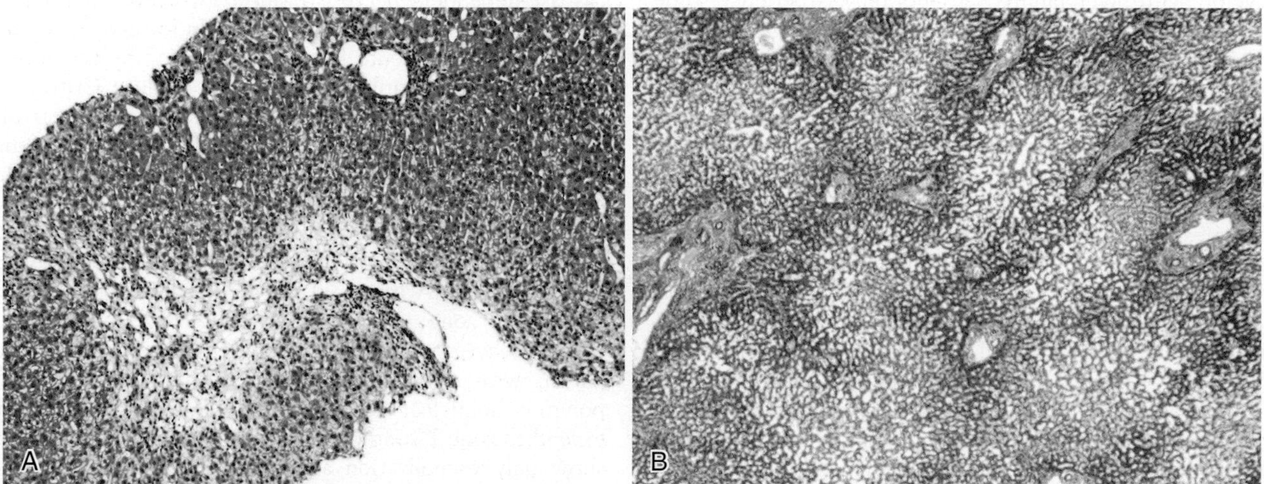

FIGURE 49.48 Two cases of acetaminophen-induced hepatitis of different severity. A, In the first case, there was loss of hepatocytes in centrilobular areas and a mild portal infiltrate; the patient had a spontaneous recovery. **B**, In the second case, extensive hemorrhagic and eosinophilic necrosis was submassive; the patient underwent liver transplantation.

Sulindac

The antiinflammatory effect of the sulindac molecule comes from its inhibition of cyclooxygenase (COX1 and COX2). The incidence of DILI with this drug is 5 to 10 times that observed with other NSAIDs. In the largest series of 91 cases documented by Tarazi and collaborators[138] from the FDA register, patients were usually older than 50 years of age, and a cholestatic pattern was predominant; hypersensitivity features were observed in 60% of cases. Mixed hepatitis was also frequent (see examples with ketoprofen and diclofenac in Figs. 49.10 and 49.12). In this series, 4 of 91 cases were fatal: 3 because of severe hypersensitivity and 1 because of fulminant hepatic failure. Cholestatic hepatitis, with irregular nuclei in hepatocytes, is possible. Acute cholangitis can develop in association with acute pancreatitis.

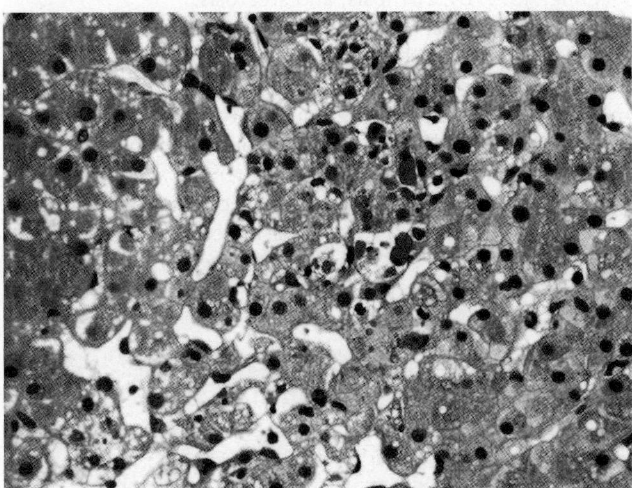

FIGURE 49.49 Acute hepatitis caused by ibuprofen. The lobule contains small necroinflammatory foci with apoptotic bodies and mild inflammatory infiltrate. The patient was a 48-year-old female with a biological profile indicating Stevens-Johnson syndrome and mixed hepatitis a few weeks after ibuprofen intake. Biliary lesions were also observed (see Fig. 49.50A).

Experimental data also suggest that sulindac, in association with lipopolysaccharide, can induce tissue hypoxemia via fibrin clot deposition in sinusoids. This could explain the immunoallergic idiosyncratic mechanism, in which the sulfide metabolite probably plays a role. The delay between introduction of the drug and the beginning of disease may be as long as 18 months.

Ibuprofen

Ibuprofen has antiinflammatory effects but also analgesic and antipyretic properties. It is globally a very safe drug, and since its introduction on the market in 1969, only a few cases of ibuprofen-related DILI have been published. The molecule can induce both hepatocellular and cholestatic liver disease (see Fig. 49.9). Some cholestatic cases have been associated on liver biopsy with ductopenia caused by a vanishing bile duct syndrome (see Fig. 49.50B).[139] Progressive cholestasis may lead to obstruction of large biliary ducts, PBC, PSC, end-stage cirrhosis, or other causes of chronic familial cholestasis. The discovery of ductopenia on biopsy should encourage the pathologist to look for inflammatory destructive lesions typical of PBC, ductular proliferation, bilirubinostasis, and onion-like periductular fibrosis for PSC or secondary sclerosing cholangitis.

An ischemic mechanism may occur after biliary surgery. In infants, Alagille syndrome and familial cholestatic syndromes must be checked. In the context of liver or bone marrow transplantation, chronic rejection and graft-versus-host disease should be considered.

Other drugs that may induce ductopenia include naproxen and tenoxicam (another NSAID), itraconazole, nitrosurea, Paraquat, sulpiride, terbinafine, and thiabendazole.

Antiinfectious Agents

Isoniazid and Antituberculosis Agents

Most of the time, antituberculosis drugs are used in combination to eradicate mycobacteria. Hepatotoxicity of the recommended regimen (usually INH + RFP + pyrazinamide

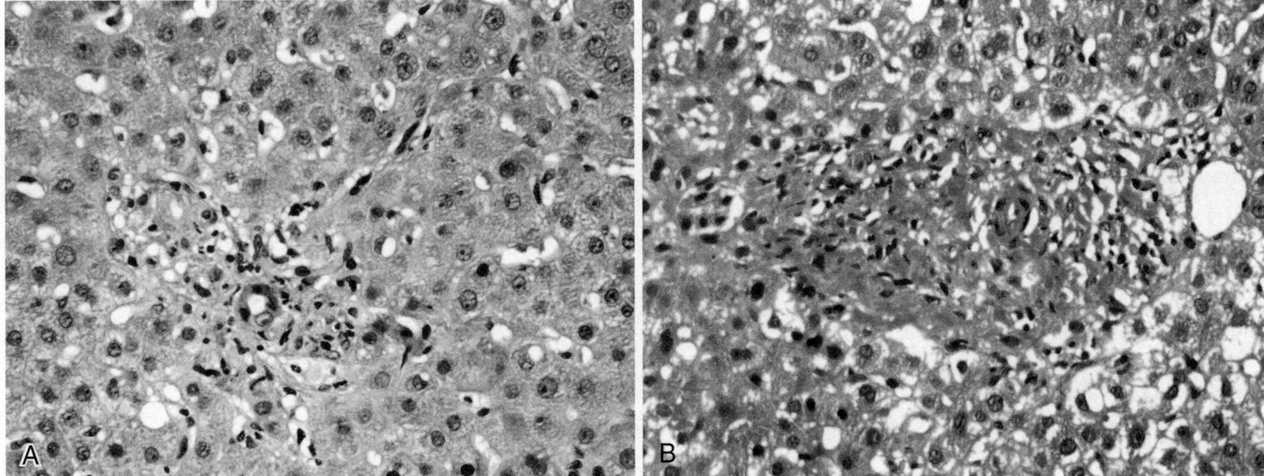

FIGURE 49.50 Severe biliary lesions associated with nonsteroidal antiinflammatory drug consumption. A, Interlobular bile duct alterations in a mixed (cytolytic and cholestatic) hepatitis induced by ketoprofen. This 48-year-old woman was diagnosed with Stevens-Johnson syndrome and severe cytolysis and cholestasis few weeks after taking ketoprofen. **B,** Toxic vanishing bile duct syndrome in a 57-year-old woman who developed Lyell syndrome after ibuprofen intake. There was concomitant cytolysis (10× the upper limit of normal), followed by progressively increasing icteric cholestasis. Interlobular bile ducts have disappeared from the portal tracts, where a mild inflammatory infiltrate persists.

+ ethambutol), ranging from simple enzyme elevations to potentially fatal hepatitis, has been reported in 2% to 27.7% of treated patients.[140] Based on a large meta-analysis of pediatric series, it appears that the risk of hepatotoxicity is considerably lower in children (jaundice, <1%; abnormal liver function tests, <10%) than in adults and concerns mainly children with disseminated forms of disease.[141] Antituberculosis agents remain the first cause of DILI in developing countries such as India, and they are the second cause of liver transplantation for DILI after acetaminophen toxicity.

Among these drugs, INH is the most dangerous, and the risk is greatly increased by association with RFP, a powerful enzyme inducer. In meta-analysis, INH alone is associated with hepatotoxicity in 1.1% of cases, compared with 2.6% for INH combined with RFP. RFP also reduces the delay before INH-associated hepatic injury: symptoms occur after 2 weeks with RFP, compared with 11 weeks without RFP.[142]

Immunogenetic factors also influence the risk of DILI, because there is acetylation phenotype polymorphism in the population, and higher transaminase levels are observed in slow acetylators. Among *N*-acetyltransferase 2 (NAT2) and CYP2E1 enzyme polymorphisms, NAT2 seems to play a major role.[143] Age, sex, ethnicity, malnutrition, alcoholism, HIV infection, chronic hepatitis B or C, and pregnancy also increase INH toxicity.

The mechanism of toxicity is thought to be mainly dose related; hypersensitivity or idiosyncrasy plays a minor role. Symptoms range from asymptomatic elevation of liver test results (10% to 20% of patients during the first months of treatment) to acute hepatitis (with anorexia, nausea, vomiting, epigastric discomfort, weakness, jaundice, and hepatomegaly) and even acute liver failure. Severe cases are more frequent in females and in children, and the fatality rate is 10% among patients who develop icterus. The risk of mortality is dose dependent: Death occurs in 43% of patients with a daily dose higher than 300 mg but in only 9% of those with a daily dose of 300 mg or less.[142] Clinical markers of poor prognosis are jaundice, hypoalbuminemia, ascites, and encephalopathy. Among 119 patients with acute liver disease, 86 had cytolytic hepatitis at presentation, 12 had cholestasis, and 46 had massive hepatitis. Other pathological presentations have been described on rare occasions, including chronic hepatitis (Fig. 49.51), granulomatous hepatitis (see Fig. 49.41B), cirrhosis, and steatosis.

The differential diagnosis mainly includes acute viral hepatitis (particularly hepatitis E in cholestatic cases), immunosuppression, and pregnancy. Tuberculous involvement of the liver with granulomatous hepatitis should also be considered. Close supervision is recommended for patients starting antituberculosis therapy. The consensus among professional authorities is to recommend the following: (1) monitor the presence of risk factors (especially liver diseases), (2) avoid the use of other potentially hepatotoxic drugs, (3) repeat liver function tests (particularly during the

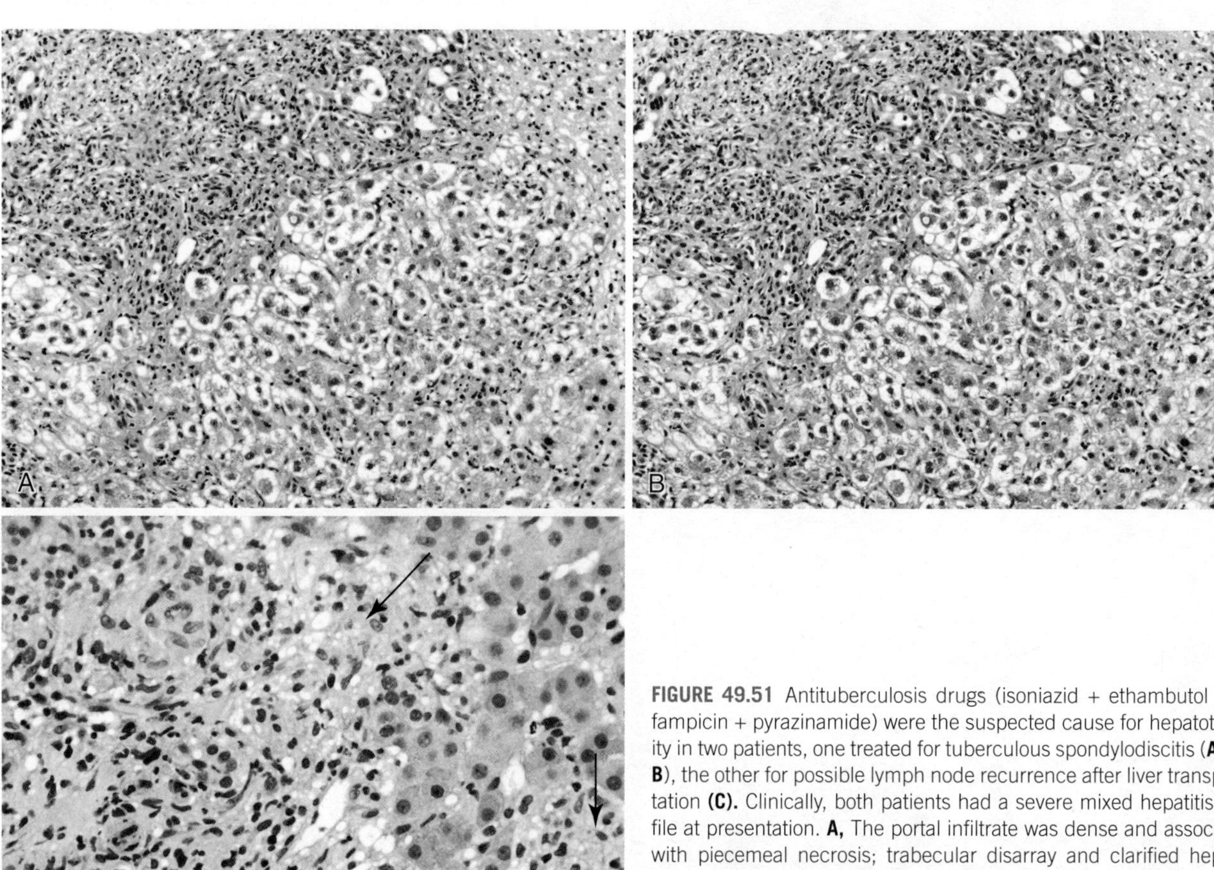

FIGURE 49.51 Antituberculosis drugs (isoniazid + ethambutol + rifampicin + pyrazinamide) were the suspected cause for hepatotoxicity in two patients, one treated for tuberculous spondylodiscitis (**A** and **B**), the other for possible lymph node recurrence after liver transplantation **(C)**. Clinically, both patients had a severe mixed hepatitis profile at presentation. **A,** The portal infiltrate was dense and associated with piecemeal necrosis; trabecular disarray and clarified hepatocytes were observed. At higher magnification (**B** and **C**), the infiltrate was shown to contain numerous neutrophils and eosinophils in both cases. Small epithelioid granulomas *(arrows),* without necrosis, were also observed in the second case **(C)** and could have been caused by isoniazid, in the absence of demonstrable mycobacteria in the liver.

first 2 months of treatment), and (4) withdraw antituberculosis drugs when the ALT is greater than 5 times normal or the bilirubin level is abnormal (or both) in an asymptomatic patient,[144] providing that the tuberculosis is of low severity in terms of radiographic extent, bacillary load, and infectiousness. Reintroduction of antituberculosis agents after recovery of liver function must be cautious and based on a less aggressive regimen. Specific guidelines for patients who are receiving other potentially hepatotoxic drugs, have a preexisting liver disease, are HIV positive, or are pregnant or within 3 months after delivery were published in 2006 by The American Thoracic Society.[145] Liver biopsy is not recommended in the flowchart for monitoring.

As with acetaminophen, *N*-acetylcysteine therapy is beneficial in acute liver failure caused by INH because of similar mechanisms of acetylation. Pyrazinamide (PZA) also carries a very elevated risk of hepatotoxicity, mostly dose related, and severe cases have occurred when the drug is used with RFP. Therefore caution is recommended in prophylactic therapy. Acute reversible AIH can occur after therapy with PZA + RFP. RFP alone can induce jaundice rarely, but RFP in association with INH increases the risk of cholestatic hepatitis. Ethambutol also can induce jaundice, and *p*-aminosalicylate can induce hypersensitivity syndrome and a pseudomononucleosis syndrome with atypical circulating lymphocytes. Streptomycin seems to be safe for the liver.

Amoxicillin/Clavulanic Acid

AMC is one of the most prescribed broad-spectrum oral antibiotics worldwide. It is used mainly for respiratory and sinusitis/otitis infections. Amoxicillin belongs to the penicillin group (β-lactams), and clavulanic acid is a β-lactamase inhibitor. The latter compound is considered hepatotoxic, and the risk of DILI with AMC is sixfold higher than with ampicillin alone. The AMC combination is well recognized as one of the most common causes of DILI, and it is preferentially responsible for a cholestatic or mixed type of liver disease. In Spain,[146] as in the United States, it is the first cause of nonacetaminophen DILI. Biological signs alone can be seen in as many as 15% of patients taking AMC, and the risk of liver injury is estimated to be between 1 and 17 per 100,000 in various registries. Some studies suggest that higher doses and longer duration of treatment favor AMC-associated hepatitis, whereas others consider age and male sex as major risk factors. In most instances, comorbidities and comedications do not play a major role. Extensive studies of single-nucleotide polymorphism markers have shown that class I and class II human leukocyte antigen genotypes affect susceptibility to AMC-DILI, indicating the importance of the adaptive immune response in pathogenesis[147]; however, these findings have limited utility as predictive or diagnostic biomarkers.

When symptomatic, patients usually exhibit nausea, vomiting, fatigue, malaise, abdominal pain, and jaundice after treatment of a respiratory, head and neck, or urinary tract infection.[148] Fever and pruritus, blood eosinophilia, and other symptoms of hypersensitivity such as Stevens-Johnson syndrome are associated in approximately 35% of cases, suggesting an immunoallergic mechanism of toxicity. Symptoms typically appear 20 days (±17 days) after the first ingestion[146] but can develop from 1 day up to 19 months after and persist for many weeks or months after stopping. Liver tests show increased levels of total bilirubin (reported range, 0.6 to 36.9 mg/dL) and AP and frequently an associated or isolated mild or moderate increase in transaminases. Etiological assessment includes ultrasound examination to exclude bile duct obstruction, serological markers for viral and bacterial infections (e.g., hepatitis A, B, C, or E; cytomegalovirus [CMV] or EBV infection; brucellosis; leptospirosis), titration of autoantibodies (antimitochondrial antibodies [AMA, AM2A], antinuclear antibodies [ANA], anti-LKM1, perinuclear antineutrophil cytoplasmic autoantibodies [pANCA]), and titration of immunoglobulins M and G for liver immune disease.

Histological studies, if performed, reveal centrilobular cholestatic hepatitis, which can rarely progress to hepatocellular damage. Various histological lesions can occur (Fig. 49.52). Canalicular cholestasis appears as bile plugs in dilated canaliculi and can be seen in isolation (bland cholestasis). Degenerative changes, hydropic degeneration, giant cell transformation, and necrosis of hepatocytes can be seen in centrilobular hepatocytes. Mild portal inflammation and lobular eosinophilia are frequently present. Granulomatous hepatitis has also been reported. In the most severe cases,[149,150] acute liver failure can appear; other possible adverse developments include chronic liver disease with bile duct damage, ductopenia, ductular proliferation, and portal fibrosis. In these cases, immune biliary disease (e.g., PBC) must be particularly addressed.

Treatment includes discontinuation of the therapy and possible corticotherapy for hypersentitivity.[151] Recovery is the rule, between 1 and 4 months after discontinuation; however, death or need for liver transplantation has been reported in 1% to 5% of cases of AMC-DILI and correlates with the level of bilirubin. Other patterns of AMC-induced DILI include cytolytic hepatitis (20% to 30% of reported series), massive hepatitis, steatosis, and granulomatous hepatitis (rare). It has been suggested that transaminases, AP, and bilirubin should be measured within 2 weeks and again 4 to 5 weeks after initiation of treatment, for timely recognition of undesired hepatic side effects.[150]

Immunosuppressive and Antineoplastic Drugs

Azathioprine (Imuran) is an immunosuppressive agent that was first used in kidney and liver transplantation and in graft-versus-host disease after bone marrow transplantation. It was the main antirejection treatment available before the introduction of calcineurin inhibitors, and it permits, if necessary, a lower dosing of these nephrotoxic drugs. It is also used in patients with autoimmune diseases, namely rheumatoid arthritis and inflammatory bowel disease.[152]

Azathioprine acts as an antiproliferative agent through inhibition of DNA synthesis. In addition to hepatocellular and cholestatic damage, it is well recognized that this drug can cause various types of vascular damage, resulting from different degrees of injury to the endothelial cells lining the sinusoids or the terminal hepatic venules. Azathioprine possibly causes a depletion of glutathione in these cells, followed by a subendothelial edema and a nonthrombotic congestion of sinusoids; after several months or years, fibrosis may develop.[153] Sinusoidal lesions induced by azathioprine can result in hypoperfusion of some areas, with regenerative

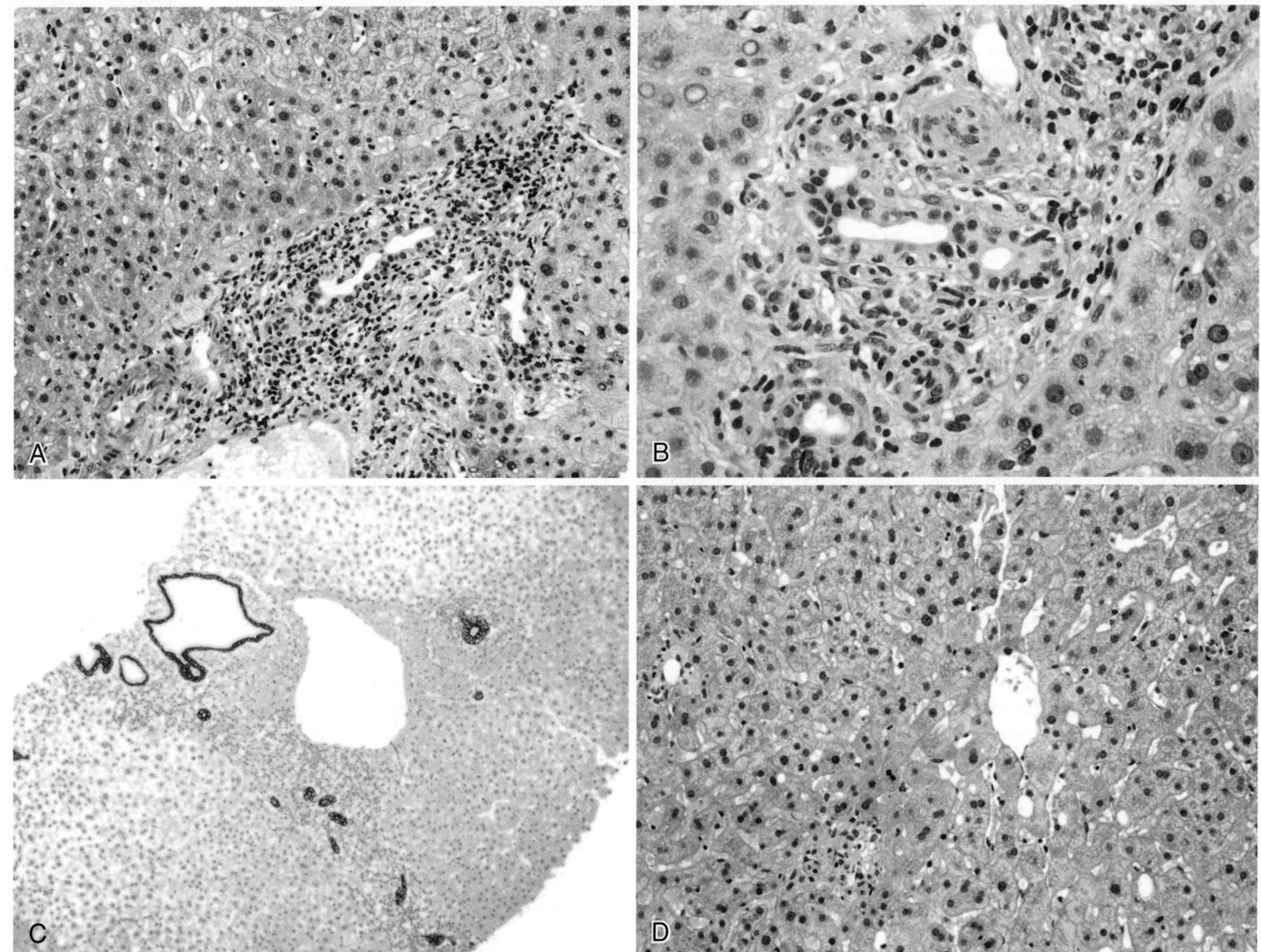

FIGURE 49.52 Amoxicillin/clavulanic acid (Augmentin) hepatotoxicity. This 82-year-old man developed icteric cholestasis and moderate cytolysis (5× the upper limit of normal), without fever or biliary obstruction, after Augmentin ingestion. **A**, Portal tracts are enlarged by a dense inflammatory infiltrate, and small biliary lumina are distorted. **B**, Cholangiocytes are dystrophic, and there is inflammatory exocytosis in the bile duct wall; neutrophils and eosinophils are visible in the portal infiltrate. **C**, Cytokeratin 19 staining shows abnormal caliber of the biliary tract. **D**, In the lobule, small inflammatory foci and mild steatosis are present.

hyperplasia in the normally perfused areas, leading to NRH (described earlier). The mechanism of azathioprine hepatotoxicity is immunoallergic and dose dependent.

The frequency and severity of hepatic side effects depend on dose and duration of treatment as well as the underlying disease and concomitant therapies. The incidence of azathioprine hepatotoxicity is relatively rare, reportedly in the range of 3% to 10%.[154] It usually occurs within the first 6 months of treatment and more often in transplant recipients than in patients treated for rheumatoid arthritis.

The side effects of this drug vary and lead to abnormal liver function test results. Injury can be predominantly hepatocellular or cholestatic, and various patterns can be observed. Mixed cholestatic hepatitis,[155] more often acute (10%) than chronic, can be observed, as can chronic cholestasis until destructive cholangiopathy or vanishing bile duct syndrome ensues. Vascular liver damage, primarily seen in male patients after renal transplantation, is well documented[156,157] and includes VOD/SOS, peliosis, sinusoidal dilation, perisinusoidal fibrosis, and NRH (Fig. 49.53; see earlier discussion and Fig. 49.35). Sinusoidal dilation is assumed to be an early and less severe form of VOD.

Clinical signs depend on the main target of the adverse features, from silent (detected only by abnormal blood liver tests, in approximately 30% of cases) to signs of more or less severe hepatitis/cholestasis, or portal hypertension in cases of severe vascular damage.

The differential diagnosis depends also on the main type of adverse effects. It comprises viral hepatitis, primary cholestatic diseases, cardiac failure, Budd-Chiari syndrome, VOD, and other drugs with endothelial toxicity (including many antineoplastic agents such as Adriamycin, carmustine, 5-fluorouracil, mitocin, and vinblastine).

Side effects are often reversible after withdrawal of the drug; however, permanent liver vascular damage, mainly VOD/SOS, has a poor prognosis and can be fatal, unlike NRH.[158] Therefore definitive discontinuation of azathioprine therapy is indicated if VOD/SOS is suspected. In all patients receiving long-term therapy with azathioprine, regular follow-up is indicated, and a liver biopsy is mandatory in case of clinical or biochemical liver abnormalities.

Oxaliplatin

Oxaliplatin is a third-generation platinum derivative that is commonly used to treat metastatic colorectal cancer before

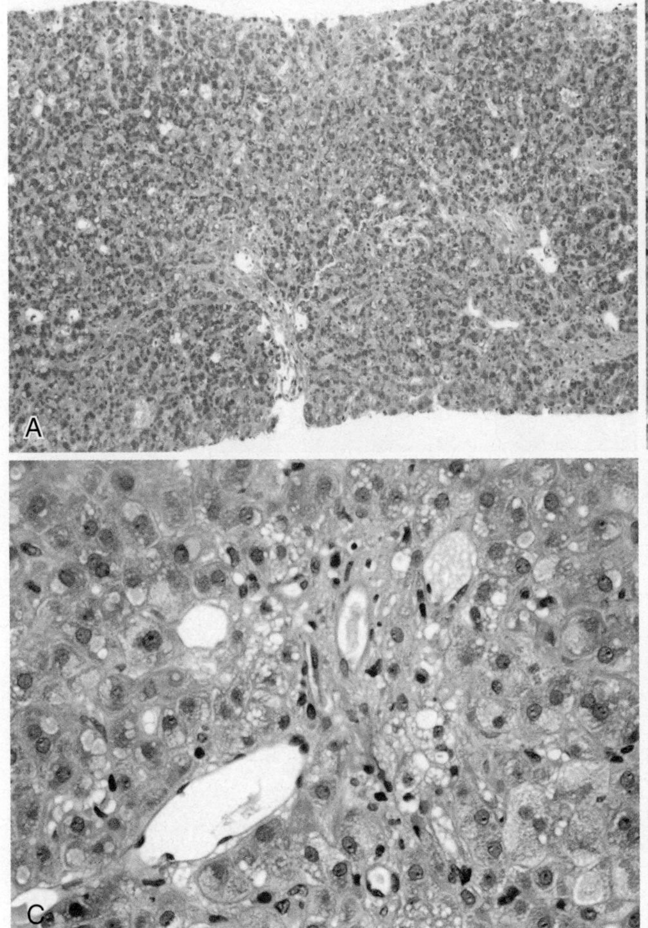

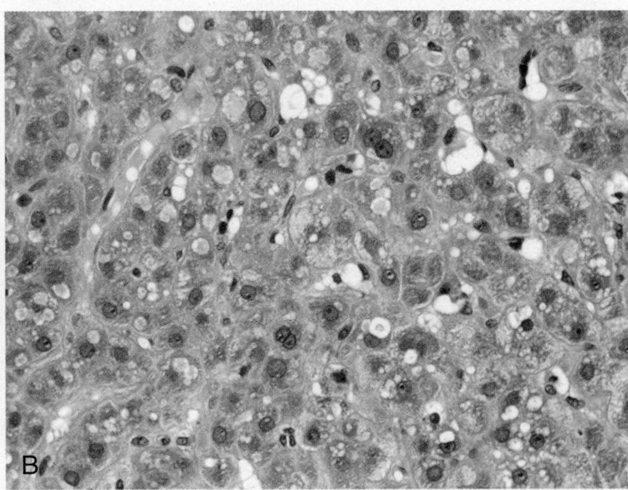

FIGURE 49.53 Azathioprine-induced toxicity. This 31-year-old man had undergone liver transplantation at 14 years of age for fulminant autoimmune hepatitis. He was taking azathioprine (Imurel), tacrolimus, and prednisolone when he developed progressive cholestasis, which was initially attributed to the irregular caliber of the biliary tract anastomosis. Histological analysis revealed a severe perisinusoidal fibrosis (**A**, Masson trichrome stain), hepatocanalicular cholestasis, pseudo–ground-glass inclusions in hepatocytes (**B**), mild cytolytic hepatitis with apoptotic bodies, and loss of interlobular ducts (**C**) in most portal tracts. All of these anomalies could have been caused by azathioprine.

liver resection and in patients with unresectable liver metastases. It is often used in combination with other cytotoxic chemotherapeutic agents, leading to a significant survival improvement.[159-161]

However, the hepatotoxicity of oxaliplatin is well recognized and dose dependent. It increases the postoperative morbidity, although adverse effects are most always reversible after treatment cessation.

It is well known that oxaliplatin is associated with microvascular injury, including sinusoidal dilation, VOD/SOS, and NRH (Fig. 49.54; see Fig. 49.36), all involving damage to the sinusoidal endothelial cell barrier and leading to portal hypertension. The incidence of sinusoidal injury ranges between 19% and 54%.[162,163]

The pathogenesis of oxaliplatin liver toxicity is thought to develop in several stages[160]: (1) damage of sinusoidal endothelial cells caused by increased ROS and depletion of glutathione transferase, (2) sinusoidal obstruction related to matrix deposition and bleb formation secondary to hepatocyte membrane injury, and (3) hepatic congestion and elevated portal pressure. Centrilobular fibrosis and NRH modify the intrahepatic blood flow, eventually causing portal hypertension.

Acute hepatitis, cholestasis, and hepatoportal sclerosis are rarer. Hepatoportal sclerosis can lead to acute portal hypertension, which can be successfully treated with transjugular intrahepatic portosystemic shunting.[160]

Methotrexate

Methotrexate, a folate analogue, has been used for more than two decades for its anticancer properties (e.g., against acute leukemias, lymphomas, osteosarcomas) and for treatment of autoimmune diseases such as rheumatoid arthritis and other rheumatic disorders, Crohn disease, psoriasis, and multiple sclerosis. The largest clinical series looking for methotrexate hepatotoxicity have come from dermatologists and rheumatologists. As documented in the Hepatox database, isolated biological abnormalities are very common, occurring in as many as 88% of cases in one series. Liver lesions are not infrequent and are variable. An acute hepatitis pattern ($n = 38$), mostly cytolytic ($n = 32$), was found in as many as 35% of treated patients; massive hepatitis also occurred ($n = 8$).

Numerous other presentations have been described, among which evolution to chronic hepatitis and even cirrhosis are the most frequent ($n = 49$ and $n = 43$, respectively). Methotrexate is one of the classic causes of presinusoidal fibrosis because of hepatic stellate cell activation (see Fig. 49.14). Liver fibrosis, increased collagen content, damage to the canals of Hering, and cirrhosis have been reported in patients receiving methotrexate therapy. This drug also induces dystrophic nuclei in hepatocytes (pleomorphism, hyperchromasia) and macrovesicular steatosis (see Fig. 49.17). Steatosis, steatofibrosis, and NASH are also possible (Fig. 49.55) and are frequently seen in patients with

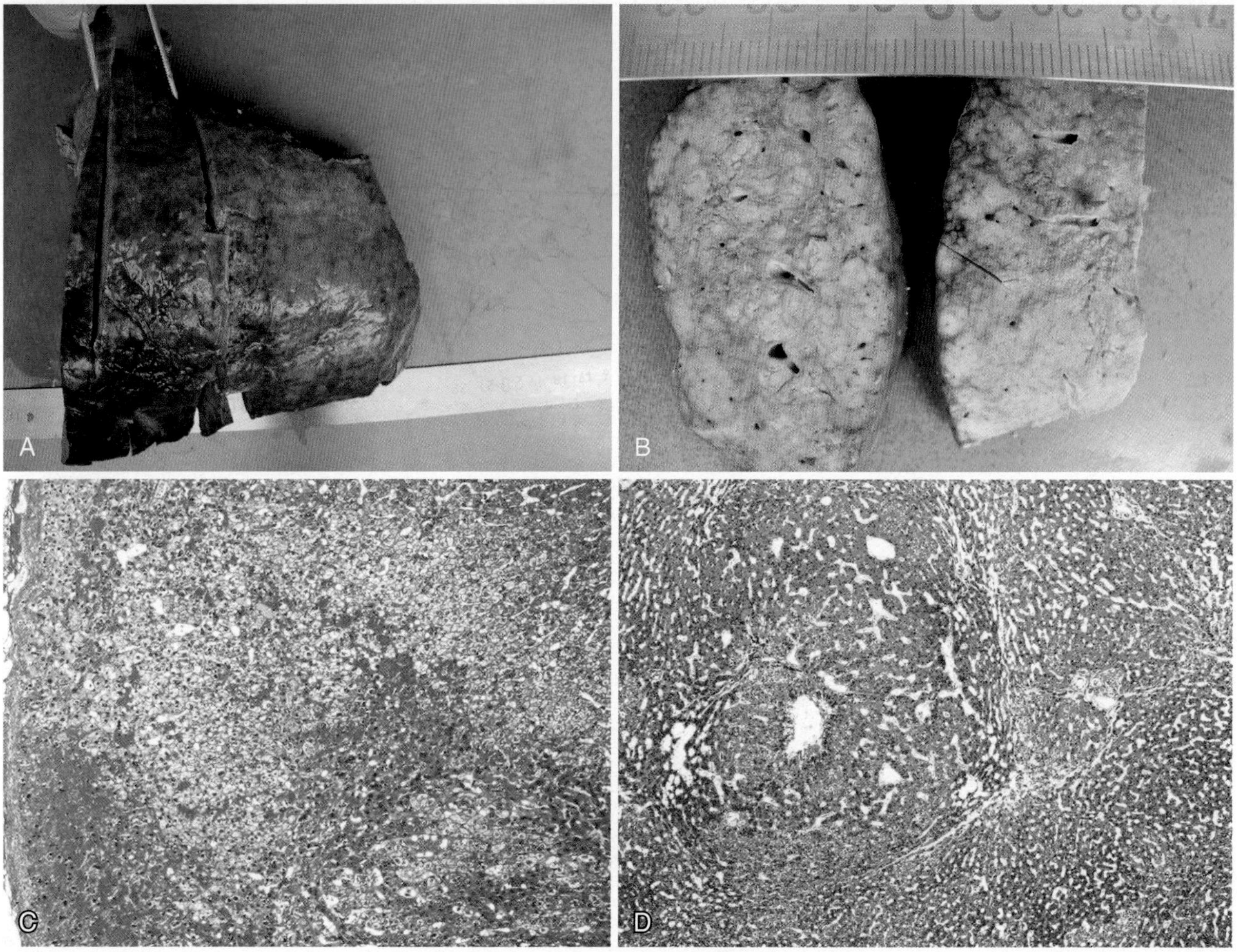

FIGURE 49.54 Vascular lesions attributed to oxaliplatin in a patient treated for colorectal metastasis. A, At gross examination, the liver appears irregularly congestive with an irregular surface. **B**, Sections show micronodular architecture of the parenchyma and hemorrhagic areas. **C**, This is confirmed on microscopy. Sinusoidal congestion is massive under the capsule, and hepatocellular rims are either atrophied or expansive, leading to nodular regenerative hyperplasia (NRH). **D**, NRH appears as a result of the irregular blood inflow.

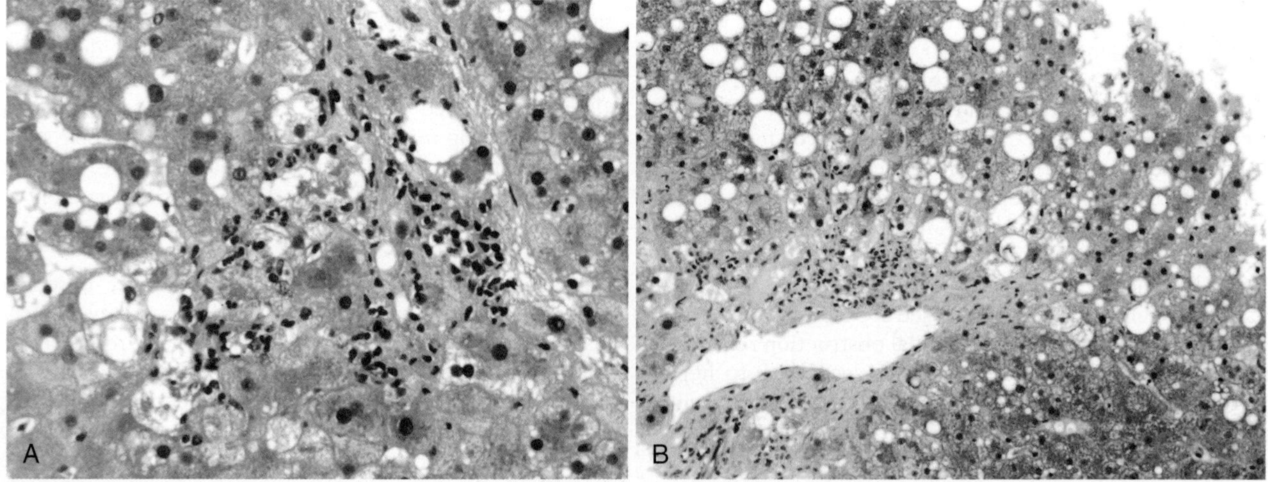

FIGURE 49.55 Methotrexate-induced liver injury. This 62-year-old man was treated with methotrexate for mycosis fungoides. He developed a nonalcoholic steatohepatitis (NASH) with steatosis, lobular inflammation, and hepatocyte ballooning **(A)** seen on biopsy and significant perisinusoidal fibrosis (**B,** Masson trichrome stain), which was classified IIIb in Roenigk system.

arthritis.[164] An AIH-like pattern can also be found on biopsy, with or without autoimmune markers, mostly in patients with rheumatoid arthritis and with the presence of the HLA-DR shared epitope. PBC has also been reported on occasion. However, old series may be criticized for not taking into account the roles of metabolic syndrome and HCV infection, two unrecognized and possibly associated conditions that are also responsible for fatty liver disease and development of fibrosis. Interaction with excess alcohol ingestion is also of great importance in the development of hepatopathy. However, intrinsic liver toxicity of methotrexate exists and can be demonstrated in animal models. Toxicity seems to be dose dependent, but there is interindividual variability in methotrexate pharmacokinetics, which is partially explained by transporter pharmacogenomics. Functional polymorphism at the *MTHFR* gene is thought to play an important role.

Progress in understanding the pharmacogenomics of methotrexate is continuing, and candidate genes are now individualized to better explain individual susceptibility to this drug.[165] It has been said that liver biopsy is necessary at the beginning of therapy (baseline biopsy) and regularly thereafter (at intervals of 1 year or longer) to monitor the development of liver fibrosis during the first 5 years of treatment. The pathologist may be asked to provide clues for the continuation or discontinuation of therapy, such as staging fibrosis and finding of comorbidities. A classification of the lesions has been proposed by Roenigk and colleagues (see Box 49.10) and is often used by clinicians,[81] although its reliability has been questioned.[82] Recently, noninvasive methods have been used with success to evaluate liver fibrosis in patients taking methotrexate and could be preferred to liver biopsy.[166]

Infliximab

Infliximab is a monoclonal antibody to human tumor necrosis factor alpha (TNF-α) used in the therapy of severe inflammatory bowel disease and rheumatoid arthritis. Side effects can affect the heart, bone marrow, kidneys, or skin. Reactivation of microbial infection, including hepatitis B, is also possible. Acute DILI of idiosyncratic type can develop and present differently[167-169]: (1) serum aminotransferase elevations with or without symptomatic hepatitis with jaundice; (2) hepatocellular injury associated with autoimmune markers (antinuclear and anti–smooth muscle antibodies), isolated or accompanied by frank clinical signs of AIH- or lupus-like syndrome and AIH features on liver biopsy (Fig. 49.56); or (3) cholestatic hepatitis. Most cases are mild, but on rare occasion severe disease can develop. AIH-like hepatitis may require corticosteroid therapy when infliximab discontinuation has no effect.

Floxuridine

Floxuridine, given by pump infusion via the hepatic artery for treatment of liver metastasis from colon carcinoma, has led to a high incidence of sclerosing cholangitis–like cholestasis. This effect is related to injury to the branches of the hepatic artery, explaining the use of the term *ischemic cholangiopathy*.

Interleukin 2

Interleukin 2, used to treat renal carcinoma, melanoma, and other malignancies, can induce mainly severe, acute intrahepatic cholestasis. Lobular hepatitis with sinusoidal lymphocytic infiltrates and focal necrosis, macrovesicular steatosis, and NRH have been also described.

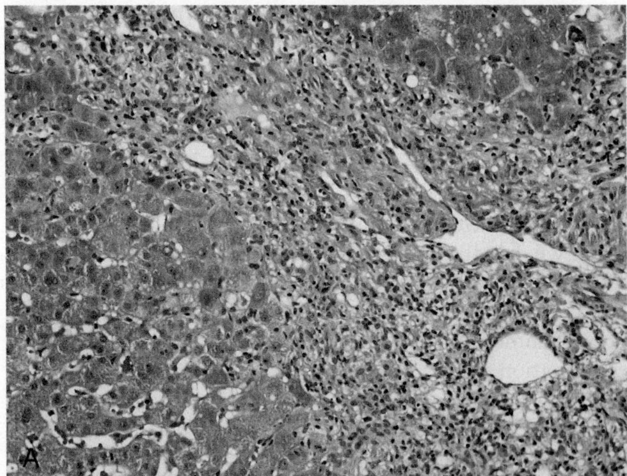

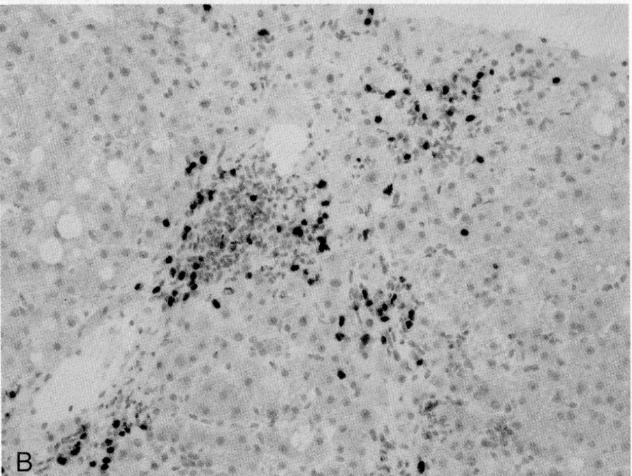

FIGURE 49.56 Infliximab-induced pseudo-autoimmune hepatitis. The biopsy revealed moderate portal inflammatory infiltrates, including mononuclear cells and eosinophils, moderate interface hepatitis, and lobular foci of activity **(A)**; MUM1 immunostains outlined many plasma cells **(B)**.

Immune Checkpoint Inhibitors

Immunotherapy for metastatic cancer using monoclonal antibodies (mAbs) directed against programmed death protein 1 (PD-1, a receptor expressed on CD8+ cytotoxic lymphocytes), or its ligand (PD-L1, present on cancer cells) or against cytotoxic T lymphocyte antigen 4 (CTLA-4, on lymphocytes) is a relatively new class of drugs that have revolutionized the prognosis of various advanced-stage malignancies. These antibodies increase anticancer effects of T lymphocytes by inhibiting the immune checkpoint receptor/ligand system at the surface of cells. First indications have been for metastatic melanoma, lung cancer, urothelial cancer, and head and neck cancers, but an increasing number of cancers may be treated with these drugs. First-generation drugs include ipilimumab (anti-PD1) and nivolumab (anti-CTLA4); pembrolizumab and atezolumab are successful drugs of the next generation designed to block the interaction between PD-1 and PD-L1, respectively. Unfortunately, aside from their usual spectacular antitumoral effect, these antibodies may also potentially induce immune-related adverse events (IRAEs) that most commonly affect the skin, luminal GI tract, endocrine organs, and, to a lesser degree, the liver. Immune-related acute hepatitis of all grades is estimated to affect 1% to 4% of patients treated with anti–PD-1 alone and 4% to 9% of patients treated with anti–CTLA-4; the combination of anti–PD-1 and anti–CTLA-4 mAbs raises this incidence up to 18%. Hepatitis most often becomes clinically evident 8 to 12 weeks after starting therapy, but it may occur at any time. Symptoms include fatigue, nausea, abdominal pain, and dark urine. Discontinuation of CPI therapy and addition of immunosuppression with steroids, either alone or in combination with MMF or 6-mercaptopurine, is usually followed by hepatitis resolution, but on occasion, cholestasis can persist. Acute liver failure was reported in 7% (2/28) of cases in a recent series.[170]

The severity of CPI therapy–induced hepatitis is classified using the National Cancer Institute's Common Terminology Criteria for Adverse Events (CTCAE), Version 4, from grade 1 to grade 5, based on modification of transaminases and bilirubin. The recommendation is to treat with steroids in grade 3 hepatitis, but a different algorithm for the assessment and management of patients with acute hepatitis during CPI treatment has been recently proposed[171] in which the severity of histological lesion (activity grade 3) also plays a role in the decision.

Since the introduction of these molecules, short series of patients with biopsies have been published.[172,173] They revealed various possible patterns of hepatic lesions, which can be found alone or in combination mainly revealing features of acute lobular hepatitis, some biliary changes, occasional granulomas, and steatosis (Fig. 49.57). One important point is that the hepatic lesions in CPI-induced hepatitis, although immune-induced, are not similar to those of idiopathic AIH. Noticeably, plasma cells are not usually present in large amounts. Evaluation of the CD8/CD4 ratio in the inflammatory infiltrate seems useful for the diagnosis because CPI favors the recruitment of CD8+ lymphocytes.[174]

Anti–CTLA-4 Monoclonal Antibodies

A panlobular hepatitis, with CD8 + rich T-lymphocyte infiltrates and numerous macrophages (CD68+) forming aggregates in the sinusoids is quite typical following therapy with anti–CTLA-4 monoclonal antibodies (e.g., ipilimumab). Scattered neutrophils and eosinophils are possible, whereas plasma cells are strikingly inconspicuous. Poorly defined epithelioid granulomas are frequent, and fibrin-ring granulomas may be seen.[171] Punctate or confluent necrosis and apoptosis are visible in the acute period, but if the biopsy is delayed, only PAS-diastase + pigmented macrophages may be visible, suggesting resolving hepatitis. Central vein endothelialitis and perivenular hepatocyte collapse is not uncommon. A second pattern shows centrilobular (zone 3) hepatitis, with perivenular necroinflammatory changes. A biliary pattern of injury is seen less frequently, consisting of a mild portal mononuclear infiltrate admixed with bile ductular proliferation, or a mixed neutrophilic/lymphocytic cholangitis. Cholangiocytes may become dystrophic. Steatosis or steatohepatitis has been described on occasion, and CPI could exacerbate preexisting lesions.

Anti–PD-1 Monoclonal Antibodies

Anti–PD-1 monoclonal antibodies (e.g., pembrolizumab) are associated with lobular hepatitis with mild portal inflammation. Necrosis and apoptosis of hepatocytes are typically mild. Biliary and cholestatic patterns may be encountered, with features of cholangiolitis, ductular proliferation, and marked cholangiocyte dystrophy. Progression to bile duct destruction and loss is possible. [174,175] Recent reports have also indicated that these drugs, particularly pembrolizumab, can induce a variant form of sclerosing cholangitis, with bile duct dilation without obstruction and diffuse hypertrophy of the extrahepatic bile duct wall.[176] A case of massive steatosis with steatohepatitis and Mallory bodies has also been reported.[175]

Anti–PD-L1 Monoclonal Antibodies

Anti PD-L1 monoclonal antibodies (e.g., atezolizumab) may cause lobular hepatitis. Portal inflammation granulomas are possible; bile duct injury, if any, seems mild.[174]

Combination of Ipilimumab and Nivolumab

The combination of ipilimumab and nivolumab may cause immune-induced hepatitis with lobular inflammation, macrophage aggregates, and endothelial injury. Steatosis is frequent, as are fibrin-ring granulomas.

The differential diagnosis of CPI immune-related hepatitis includes cryptogenic AIH, viral hepatitis, and other DILIs. In CPI hepatitis, inflammation is quite different from AIH; prominent plasma cell infiltrates are not present, sinusoidal macrophages are numerous, and CD8+ lymphocytes are dramatically increased.

Drugs Used in Cardiovascular Diseases

Amiodarone

Amiodarone has been widely used since the 1970s for its antiarrhythmic properties, and it is particularly efficient for the prevention of atrial fibrillation. It is metabolized by multiple CYP3A isoenzymes in the liver and is eliminated in the bile. Toxicity results from inhibition of fatty acid β-oxidation and from inhibition of phospholipase. Immunological mechanisms could contribute to liver fibrosis. Genetic susceptibility is also suspected. Amiodarone and desethylamiodarone (DEA, the main metabolite) are highly lipophilic molecules that are rich in iodine and are susceptible to accumulation in fatty liver and other tissues. Adverse effects can develop not only in the liver but also in the skin and the cornea (caused by ultraviolet light sensitivity), in the gut, in peripheral nerves, and in the cardiac conduction system.

The half-life of amiodarone is long (approximately 55 days), so 6 to 8 months is required to reach a steady state. There is clear evidence that the cumulative dose is an indicator of increased risk for toxicity, and the serum concentration-response relationship for effect, but there is also evidence of differing sensitivities to toxicity within the population. Symptoms can appear as long as 10 years after the first intake of the drug. In the 1980s, the use of higher doses was followed by several case reports of chronic liver toxicity (albeit <100 cases among >60 million people exposed worldwide); symptoms ranged from simple asymptomatic increase in transaminases to severe hepatitis and even cirrhosis.

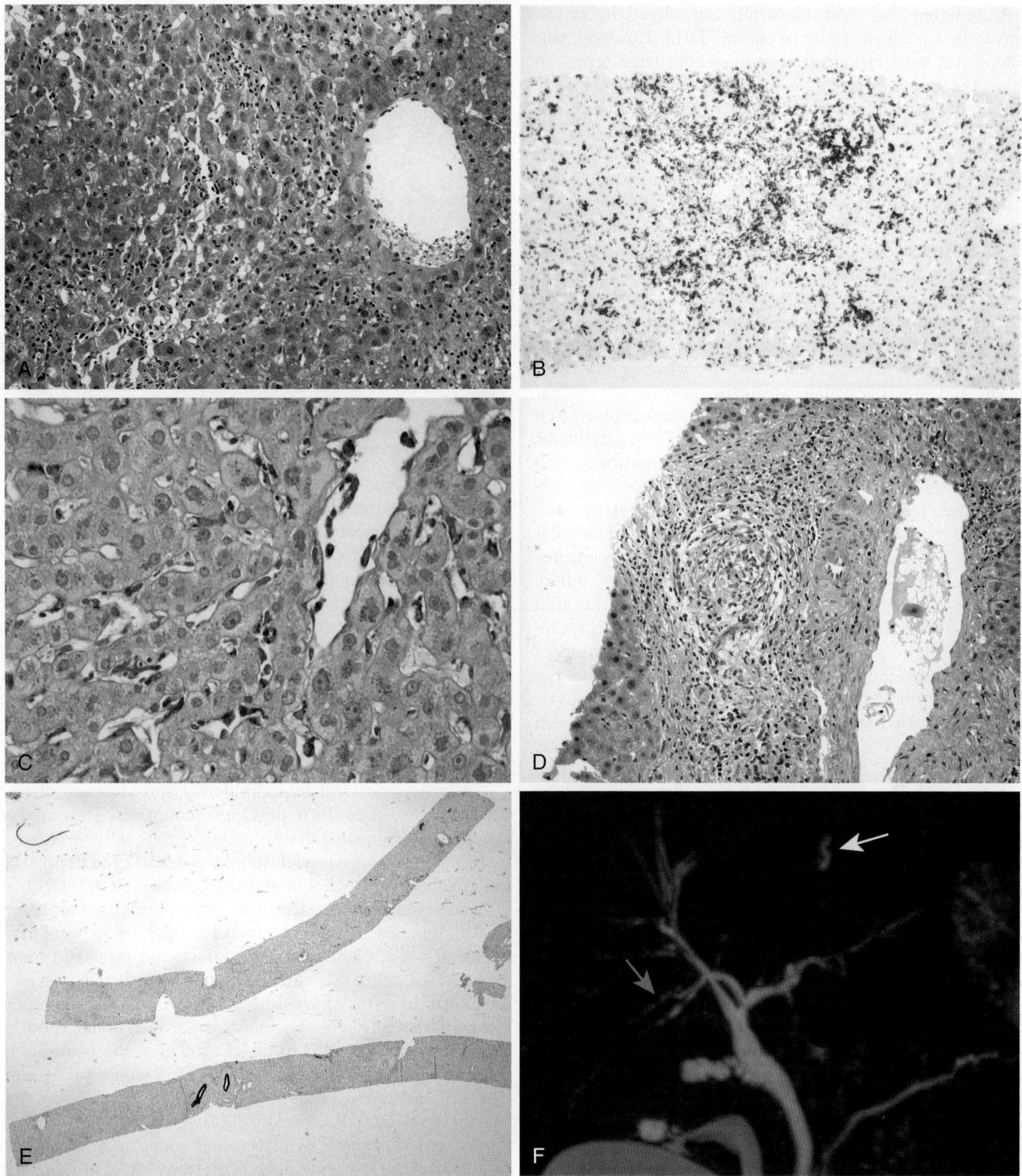

FIGURE 49.57 Immune checkpoint inhibitor–related lesions. Hepatitis pattern **(A to C):** lobular hepatitis is characterized by numerous lymphocytes and macrophages infiltrating the sinusoids, with spotty necrosis **(A);** all lymphocytes are CD8 positive by immunochemistry **(B).** PAS-diastase positive macrophages in sinusoids can be the only lesions in mild forms with delayed biopsy **(C).** Biliary pattern **(D to F):** inflammatory portal tracts can present severe lymphocytic cholangitis **(D)** and on occasion ductopenia may develop, as shown on CK19 staining **(E).** A form of sclerosing cholangitis is also possible and diagnosed on biliary MRI: segmental and smaller bile ducts are diffusely irregular in caliber *(orange arrow),* with suspended dilation *(yellow arrow),* whereas main ducts look normal **(F). A to D,** patients under pembrolizumab, predominantly cytolytic **(A to C)** or cholestatic **(D); E and F**, same patient under atezolizumab for lung carcinoma, presenting with icteric cholestasis.

Amiodarone has been classically considered by physicians to be a frequent cause of chronic DILI. However, this opinion has been criticized in more recent large series, in which the liver toxicity rate of amiodarone was typically estimated at approximately 2% to 4%. Indeed, asymptomatic elevation of transaminases, previously reported to occur in as many as 4% to 50% of cases, could have been induced in these patients by confounding variables such as alcohol intake, obesity, intake of other medications, or congestive/ischemic cardiac dysfunction, which were frequently present in the treated population. Clinically overt hepatic disease resulting from amiodarone seems to be relatively rarer (1% to 3%[177]) and is exclusively associated with an elevation of transaminases. In this classic presentation of amiodarone-induced DILI, liver histology reveals lesions very similar to those of alcohol-induced hepatitis,[178] including macrovesicular and microvesicular steatosis, polymorphonuclear leukocyte infiltration, satellitosis, ballooning degeneration of hepatocytes, and Mallory-Denk bodies with satellitosis (Fig. 49.58; see Fig. 49.18). Phospholipidosis may be seen in association or alone. Red inclusion bodies or foamy appearance of the cytoplasm may be seen on light microscopy. On electronic microscopy, they correspond to whorled lamellar lysosomal inclusions, which can be found in foamy macrophages (phospholipidosis) but also in hepatocytes, biliary endothelial cells, or Kupffer cells and are typical of this kind of DILI. These lamellar inclusions result from the inhibition of phospholipase A, which leads to the formation of complexes between the drug and the phospholipids of the lysosome membranes.

Rare cases of pseudoalcoholic cirrhosis have also been documented.[177,179] Cholestatic or granulomatous hepatitis is very uncommon. Some cases of fulminant hepatitis have been reported after intravenous infusion of the drug and are associated with centrilobular necrosis and microvesicular necrosis resembling Reye syndrome on histology. This could be linked to polysorbate 80, a component of the diluent used in the parenteral form, rather than amiodarone itself. Clinically, patients with classic amiodarone hepatitis may experience malaise, fatigue, anorexia, or vomiting, and hepatomegaly may develop. Usually, symptoms disappear within weeks after lowering of the dose or drug withdrawal, but improvement may not always be rapid because of the large diffusion capacity and storage of the molecule in the tissues.

The differential diagnosis includes preexisting cardiac hepatopathy, congestive or ischemic dysfunction, and other causes of chronic elevation of transaminases, particularly alcoholic and nonalcoholic fatty liver disease. When the disease is clinically silent, a control of transaminases is advised; an abnormal result may lead to a decrease in the dose or withdrawal of the drug. As reviewed in Babatin and colleagues,[178] it has been recommended that a complete liver chemistry profile is documented at baseline, followed by ALT checking after 1 month of therapy to rule out idiosyncratic sensitivity. ALT measurement at intervals of 3 months for the first year and semiannually thereafter should help detect late adverse effects. Antioxidants are useful in animal models but have not been validated in humans. Serial dosages could be useful to monitor the drug but are not possible in practice. Liver biopsy is invasive and is recommended only in selected cases, to assess the severity of the disease. The histological differential diagnosis includes alcoholic liver disease and NASH of metabolic or toxic origin. Similar lesions of steatohepatitis can be induced by perhexiline maleate, synthetic estrogens (4,4′-diethylaminoethoxyhex estrol), and other drugs such as methotrexate, tamoxifen, naproxen, irinotecan, raloxifene, and spironolactone. Computed tomography could be a good, noninvasive tool for the diagnosis of amiodarone DILI because the high iodine content of the molecule induces a hyperintense appearance, but this diagnostic tool must be validated.

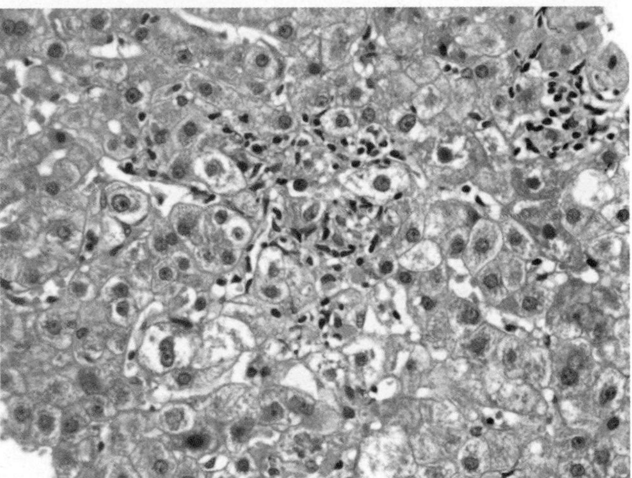

FIGURE 49.58 Amiodarone-induced acute hepatitis. This biopsy specimen shows lobular hepatitic foci with mild and mixed inflammatory infiltrate and ballooned or acidophilic necrotic hepatocytes.

Statins

Statins (also known as *HMG-CoA reductase inhibitors*) are widely used to treat hyperlipidemia and are prescribed to 10% to 20% of adults in developed countries. They are considered to be safe and very useful drugs. However, myalgia, increased creatine phosphokinase, and even myopathies mediated by mitochondrial disturbances are not infrequent. Concerning liver toxicity, an asymptomatic increase in transaminases is observed in 0.1% to 2.7% of patients in clinical trials. Clinical hepatic effects are rarer and mostly consist of acute hepatocellular injury, although mixed or cholestatic forms of DILI have also been observed on occasion. Although the pathogenesis is not well understood, the mechanism is thought to be idiosyncrasy. Lovastatin is the statin most often found to induce DILI, followed by simvastatin and atorvastatin.

In a review published in 2009,[71] a total of 40 cases of liver toxicity caused by statins was found in the literature. The affected patients had symptoms of acute hepatitis including anorexia, nausea, abdominal pain, fatigue, and jaundice (35%); two cases were fatal, and another resulted in liver transplantation. The duration of treatment before the appearance of symptoms varied from 5 days to 4 years (median, 4 months), and the resolution after withdrawal required several weeks to 6 months. A prior exposure to the same or another statin was frequently found (20%); a reintroduction test was positive in one case. Potential interactions with other drugs (e.g., nefazodone, amlodipine, ciprofloxacin) have been suspected and could result from inhibition or competition on the CYP450 isoenzyme CYP3A4.

ALT levels can rise as high as 1000 to 8000 IU/L (mean, 10 ULN), and bilirubin levels may become abnormal. Other causes of acute hepatitis must be checked in cytolytic patients taking statins, especially acute viral hepatitis due to hepatitis A (HAV), HBV, HCV, EBV, CMV, or herpes simplex virus (HSV), but also hepatitis E (HEV). Histology, when performed, usually shows a normal architecture, little or no fibrosis, a mixed portal infiltrate with lymphocytes and a variable number of neutrophils and eosinophils, canalicular and hepatocellular bilirubinostasis, some lobular necrosis and disarray, and mixed inflammation.

Nonspecific autoantibodies (e.g., ANA, anti-SMA, anti-LKM1) and other features of autoimmunity, including a hepatitis-like histological pattern, are present in approximately 25% of cases (Fig. 49.59); association with HLA-DR3 or -DR4 is possible in this group. On histology in autoimmune-like cases, portal fibrosis is more pronounced, there is piecemeal necrosis, and plasma cells are more conspicuous and mixed with lymphocytes, neutrophils, and eosinophils; cholangitis may rarely be present. These cases can benefit from corticoid therapy. Usually, autoantibodies and symptoms disappear (favoring the diagnosis of AIH-like DILI), but sometimes they persist after drug discontinuation, and it can be assessed that the emergence of a real AIH has been triggered by the use of the statin.

As mentioned earlier, certain histological patterns favor true AIH versus DILI (see Table 49.6). Because of the low frequency of DILI, follow-up assessment of transaminases in patients taking statins is not required nowadays, and recommendations from experts indicate that chronic liver disease, nonalcoholic fatty liver disease, and compensated cirrhosis are not contraindications to statin therapy. Because of the possibility of a severe outcome, liver function tests should be performed for patients taking statins who exhibit new symptoms such as nausea, lethargy, and abdominal pain, even if DILI is rare.[180]

Drugs Used in Transplantation

Changes in liver enzymes and histological abnormalities are so common in liver, kidney, heart, and bone marrow transplantation that identification of a drug as the cause is difficult.

Cyclosporine

Cyclosporine hepatotoxicity is predominantly cholestatic and is associated with mildly increased γ-glutamyltranspeptidase. Toxicity is possibly dose related. Hypertrophy of bile duct epithelial cells with cytoplasmic vacuoles and foamy material in sinusoids are the main abnormalities seen on liver biopsy. Biliary sludge or gallstone formation is reported in as many as 30% of transplant recipients. Acute hepatitis is described in as many as 25% of cases. Granulomatous hepatitis is rarely observed.

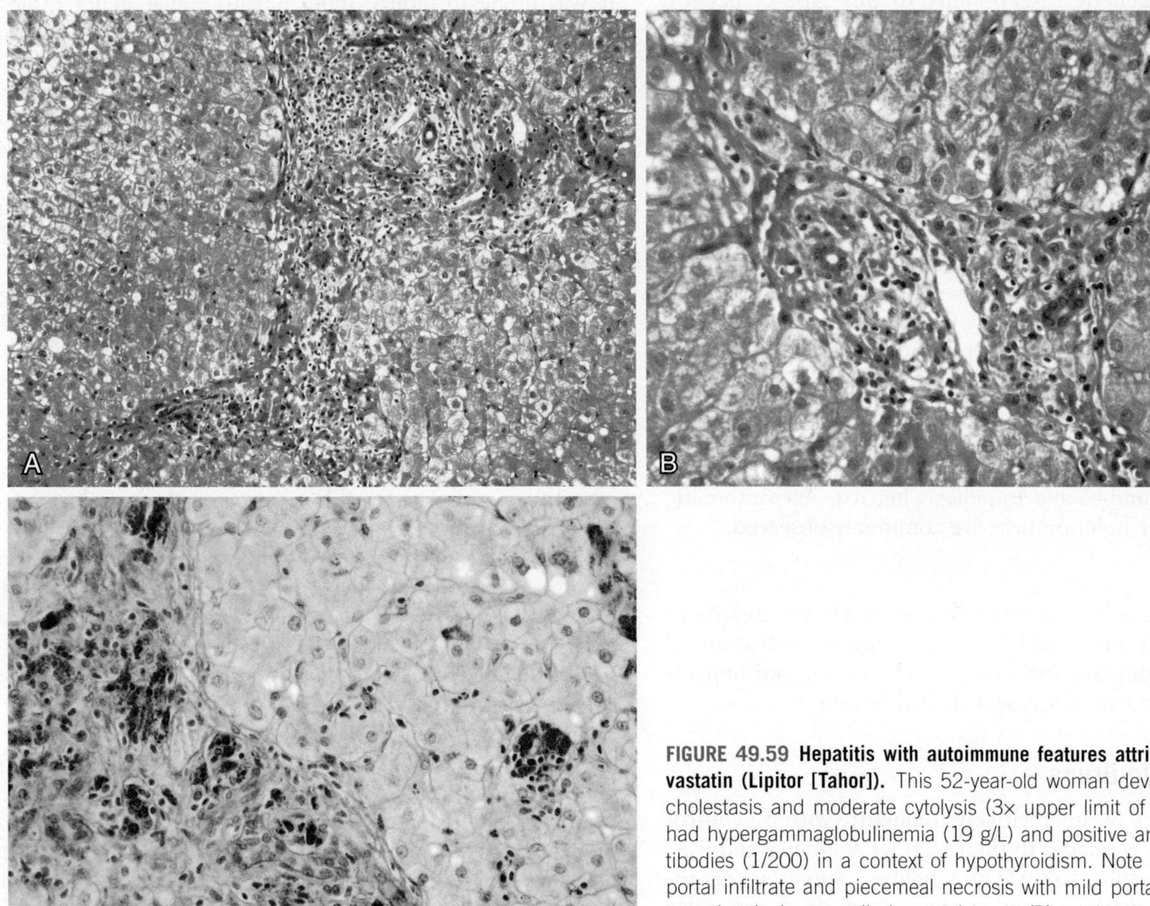

FIGURE 49.59 Hepatitis with autoimmune features attributed to atorvastatin (Lipitor [Tahor]). This 52-year-old woman developed icteric cholestasis and moderate cytolysis (3× upper limit of normal). She had hypergammaglobulinemia (19 g/L) and positive antinuclear antibodies (1/200) in a context of hypothyroidism. Note the moderate portal infiltrate and piecemeal necrosis with mild portal fibrosis **(A)**, occasional plasma cells in portal tracts **(B)**, and numerous macrophages that stain positive on periodic acid–Schiff staining with diastase digestion **(C)**.

Tacrolimus

Tacrolimus leads to elevated ALT and AP without clinical signs up to 37% of patients with liver transplants. Adverse effects occur after a period of latency lasting 2 to 24 weeks.[181]Acute hepatitis with perivenular hepatocellular necrosis on liver biopsy, cholestatic hepatitis, and vascular changes (VOD/SOS) are rarely reported.

Anabolic and Contraceptive Steroids and Estrogen Receptor Modulators

Contraceptive Pills

Contraceptive pills are implicated in the occurrence of acute cholestatic jaundice, peliosis hepatis, sinusoidal dilation (see Fig. 49.34), HCA, HCC, and Budd-Chiari syndrome, related to their thrombogenic effect. It was thought that HCA would disappear with the advent of new generations of contraceptive pills (second, third, and fourth generation), but this was not the case. New etiological factors, such as the metabolic syndrome linked to overweight and obesity, may play a role. Because of the rarity of this tumor in comparison with the high number of women taking oral contraceptives, other susceptibility factors could probably exist. HCAs (see Fig. 49.46), particularly those with β-catenin activation, can rarely and slowly transform into HCC.

Cholestatic jaundice is more frequent in women who have a personal or family history of jaundice of pregnancy, suggesting a genetic susceptibility to this type of hepatic injury.

C17-Alkylated Anabolic Steroids

These drugs are used in the treatment of aplastic anemia and by body builders. They lead to the same diseases as described for contraceptive pills.

Danazol

Danazol is an antihypophyseal drug related to the C17-anabolic steroids and can also lead to cholestatic jaundice, peliosis hepatis, HCA, and HCC. All of these side effects, even HCC, can disappear after withdrawal of the drug.

Tamoxifen

Tamoxifen is an antiestrogen that can cause or contribute to hepatic steatosis and NASH. It can lead to cholestatic and mixed jaundice and to peliosis hepatis. Asymptomatic abnormal liver function tests are commonly observed.

Flutamide

Flutamide is a synthetic antiandrogen used in the treatment of prostate cancer. It can lead to asymptomatic elevations of serum transaminases and to mixed cholestatic and hepatocellular injury, which occasionally can be severe.

Psychotropic Drugs

Hepatotoxicity occurs relatively frequently with psychotropic drugs and is related to their high fat solubility and liver metabolism leading to toxic metabolites. Numerous neuroleptics, anticonvulsants, and antidepressant drugs can cause hepatocellular, cholestatic, or mixed injury.

Carbamazepine

Carbamazepine is an anticonvulsant that can lead to all these types of toxicity of varying severity, with a fatal outcome in 10% to 15% of cases. Cholestatic injury may lead to severe ductopenia. Hepatic granulomas are reported in as many as 75% of liver biopsies. The high number of eosinophils, as well as a similar aspect of all the granulomas, suggests hepatotoxicity, rather than another cause of granulomas (e.g., sarcoidosis, tuberculosis). Rare observations of HCC have also been reported.[182]

Herbal and Dietary Supplements

Traditional/complimentary and dietary supplements are the main causes of DILI in Asia. Many Asian herbal traditional medicines, alone or in complex combinations, have been incriminated (for a detailed list, see the European Association for the Study of the Liver [EASL] clinical practice guidelines).[22] With these supplements, DILI usually presents as acute hepatitis. HDS represents up to 70% to 73% of DILI in Singapore and Korea.[183] In the United States, the DILIN has noted a tremendous increase in HDS-related liver injury: from 7% in 2004 to 2005 to 20% in 2013 to 2014[184,185]; data are quite similar in Spain, where they represent 13% of DILI cases.[183] In a recent meta-analysis[186] based on 31 studies (24 from Asia, 7 non-Asian) in which 7511 cases of HILI were included, HILI was found more frequently in females (69.8% vs. 30.2% male) compared with conventional DILI. It was prone to induce more hepatocellular injury (78.8% vs. 56.47%) and less cholestatic injury than DILI. The main herbs found to cause HILI were *Polygonum multiflorum* (root is traditionally used in Asia to prevent gray hair and to support liver and kidney function), *Psoralea corylifolia* (seeds are traditionally used in India and China for dermatitis), *Corydalis yanhusua* (used for inflammation and pain in Asia) and *Rheum officale* (used for intestinal transit trouble and for oral inflammation). Mechanisms of HDS-induced liver injury include direct hepatocyte toxicity induction of an immune response.

The symptoms of hepatitis occur 1 to 6 months after the beginning of treatment and stop with withdrawal. Aside from abnormal liver function tests (mostly transaminases) and nonspecific symptoms (abdominal pain, fatigue), some immunoallergic reaction symptoms, abnormal antibodies, and immune cell infiltration in liver biopsies are not uncommon.[187] The diagnosis of HILI is often difficult, and the causality may be impossible to prove; other etiologies for liver disease must always be excluded.

In the United States, body-building products are commonly associated with liver injury. Related DILI typically presents as prolonged cholestasis in a young male using anabolic androgenic steroids. These molecules can also induce a sinusoidal obstruction syndrome and may induce liver adenomas and HCCs.

In the West, *non–body-building HILI* is mostly observed in women taking HDS for weight loss, pain and inflammation, mood disorders, general health, or menopausal issues.[187] They range from mild transaminitis to liver failure requiring transplantation (11%). The causative agent may be a single ingredient or a multi-ingredient product. Among single-ingredient products, green tea extract (GTE or *Camellia sinensis*), used to support weight loss, is one of the most frequent causative agents in western countries, alone or in preparation (Exolise). It can induce acute hepatitis, acute cholestatic hepatitis, or acute liver failure. Another systematic review assessing liver injury using herbal medicine (in which European studies were overrepresented) indicated that greater celandine *(Chelidonium majus)* in Germany and germander *(Teucrium chamaedrys)* in France were the most common causative agents.[188]

Among other traditional/herbal products, khat (*Catha edulis,* chewing leaves is used in West Africa for stimulating effects), borage (*Borago officinalis,* used as a tisane for its draining, diuretic, and antitussive properties), chaparral (*Larrea tridentata,* used for flu syndrome, diarrhea, and rheumatisms), kava-kava (*Piper methysticum rhizoma,* used in the United States for relaxing and sedative properties), and extracts of black cohosh roots (*Actae racemosa,* containing phytooestrogens and used for menopausal syndrome) have been frequently reported (>70 cases) to induce acute cytolytic hepatitis, with occasional autoimmune presentation (black cohosh).

Pyrrolizide alkaloids (found in *Crotalaria, Senecio, Heliotrepium*) are specifically toxic to liver sinusoidal endothelium and can induce acute and chronic sinusoidal obstruction syndrome.

Among dietary preparations (often used for weight loss), some contain usnic acid (*LipoKinetx, UCP1, Oxy-Elite*), or linoleic acid (Plethoryl, Hydroxycut), both of which can induce liver toxicity.

Herbalife products may cause HILI, presenting as cytolytic or cholestatic hepatitis, with rare immunoallergic features.

ACKNOWLEDGMENTS

The author warmly thanks Prof. Paulette Bioulac-Sage and Prof. Charles Balabaud for their contribution to the writing of the first editions of this manuscript.

The full reference list may be accessed online at *Elsevier eBooks for Practicing Clinicians.*

CHAPTER 50

Fatty Liver Disease

David E. Kleiner

Contents

INTRODUCTION

Definitions

Steatosis, defined as the accumulation of triacylglycerides in hepatocytes, is a frequent finding in most liver biopsies.[1] Based on magnetic resonance measures of lipid signal in European normal-weight healthy adult volunteers, the normal liver contains approximately 3% to 5% lipid, with men having slightly more lipid than women.[2] By convention, histologically evident steatosis that occupies more than 5% of hepatocytes is considered pathological.[3]

Macrovesicular steatosis is an accumulation of lipid droplets of various sizes within hepatocytes (large and small droplet). Cell nuclei may be displaced peripherally when the droplets are large in size. It is common to observe a mixture of small- and large-sized droplets in the same cell and to find isolated droplets of lipid that do not fill the cell in its entirety.

Microvesicular steatosis has a different histological appearance, and clinical significance. The nuclei of affected hepatocytes are typically centrally located within abundant, foamy-appearing cytoplasm. Special stains, such as Oil Red O, may be necessary to confirm lipid accumulation, whereas in macrovesicular steatosis, the large- and small-sized lipid droplets are easily detectable on routine hematoxylin and eosin stain. Diseases associated with microvesicular steatosis are characterized by hepatic failure and lactic acidosis, rather than chronicity and potential fibrosis; the former features are the result of mitochondrial injury. The most common examples of purely microvesicular steatosis are acute fatty liver of pregnancy and Reye's syndrome. This process has also been reported in the setting of drug toxicity.[4] Drug-related entities are discussed specifically in Chapter 49.

Alcohol-induced liver disease (ALD) refers to the spectrum of liver disorders directly related to excessive alcohol use. This chapter focuses primarily on the pathological lesions of the ALD subset characterized by accumulation of lipid in the liver parenchyma.

Nonalcoholic fatty liver disease (NAFLD) occurs in patients without significant alcohol use. This clinicopathological entity is characterized by a variety of hepatic parenchymal injury patterns associated with more than 5% of the liver involved with macrovesicular steatosis.

The term *nonalcoholic steatohepatitis* (NASH) occurs in the same clinical setting as NAFLD, but NASH is a specific pattern of injury in the liver. In addition to revealing a variable amount of macrovesicular steatosis, there is also associated hepatocellular injury (most commonly seen as ballooning degeneration of hepatocytes), inflammation in the hepatic lobules or portal tracts, or both. These lesions and others that may be seen in steatohepatitis, are discussed in detail in this chapter.

Nomenclature

The term *ALD* refers to a spectrum of liver diseases and includes either large-droplet or a mixture of both large- and small-droplet macrovesicular steatosis, either with or without

TABLE 50.1 Symptoms, Signs, and Laboratory Abnormalities of Various Types of Alcohol-Induced Liver Disease

Symptoms and Signs	Fatty Liver	Alcoholic Hepatitis	Cirrhosis	Foamy Degeneration
Asymptomatic	+++	+	Portal hypertension	–
Right upper quadrant discomfort	+++	Pain, not mild	+ to ++	+
Hepatomegaly	++	++	+ to ++	+
Elevated AST, normal ALT	++	+	+ (normal if abstinent)	++
AST/ALT ratio	AST > ALT	AST/ALT >1-3 common	AST/ALT >1	AST > ALT
Marked AST elevation	<5 times normal	As much as 5 times normal	–	++
Marked alkaline phosphatase elevation	–	+/–	–	++
Bilirubin elevation	–	>10 mg/dL	– (unless advanced)	++
Jaundice	–	Cardinal sign	As above	++
Elevated white blood cell count	–	>10,000/mm^3	– (may be decreased)	–
Fever	–	+++	+ (with infection)	–
Ascites	–	+++	+ (advanced)	–

ALT, Alanine aminotransferase; *AST,* aspartate aminotransferase; –, does not occur; +, occurs uncommonly; ++, common; +++, very common.

lobular and portal inflammation; steatohepatitis with or without fibrosis; alcoholic hepatitis; alcoholic cirrhosis either with or without steatosis, steatohepatitis, or alcoholic hepatitis; and alcoholic foamy degeneration. Hepatocellular carcinoma (HCC) is a recognized consequence of ALD and cirrhosis.

NAFLD has a more limited pathological spectrum than ALD. NAFLD may manifest as either pure large droplet or a mixed large- and small-droplet macrovesicular steatosis, either with or without lobular or portal inflammation; steatohepatitis with or without fibrosis; and cirrhosis with or without steatosis or steatohepatitis. All of the features of NAFLD may be seen in ALD; therefore the term *nonalcoholic fatty liver disease* was introduced to distinguish these entities.[5,6] HCC may arise as a consequence of NAFLD-induced cirrhosis and is therefore also included within the spectrum of NAFLD lesions. HCC is increasingly recognized in patients with noncirrhotic NAFLD.[7,8] However, the true incidence of this neoplastic complication in cirrhotic or noncirrhotic livers is less certain than with ALD.

Although NASH and NAFLD are commonly used terms, neither truly represents the underlying pathophysiological disease process.[9,10] Although there are histological similarities with ALD, there are also differences. The relationship between NAFLD and alcohol use may not be as straightforward as originally believed because a few studies indicate that some patients may be at risk for liver disease from both causes simultaneously. Although modest alcohol use may have an effect on insulin resistance,[11,12] the presence of any potential benefits remains controversial.[13,14]

For pathologists, microscopically based diagnoses related to fatty liver diseases are descriptive (*steatosis* or *steatohepatitis*) because in most circumstances, only careful clinical evaluation can help determine the true underlying cause of the patient's illness. Different clinical situations may result in similar histological findings, and as with chronic hepatitis, knowledge of the patient's history is essential to establish an accurate etiology. Unlike chronic hepatitis, there are no serological tests available to diagnose NAFLD with complete certainty, although improvements continue to be made in methods of noninvasive evaluation.[15]

ALCOHOL-INDUCED LIVER DISEASE

Clinical Features

The clinical features of ALD vary considerably. Table 50.1 highlights the primary clinical manifestations of the four main clinicopathological subtypes of ALD: fatty liver, alcoholic hepatitis, alcoholic cirrhosis, and alcoholic foamy degeneration.

Patients with ALD and fatty liver may be asymptomatic or may have right upper quadrant discomfort at presentation (see Table 50.1). Patients with alcoholic hepatitis usually have abdominal pain and pancreatitis, whereas patients with cirrhosis and alcoholic foamy degeneration often experience only vague abdominal discomfort.[16-18] In all forms of ALD, the liver is typically enlarged. Fever, an elevated white blood cell count, and jaundice occur in various degrees with the different forms of ALD and may be related to ALD (e.g., alcoholic hepatitis) or to the presence of a secondary infection (e.g., peritonitis caused by alcoholic cirrhosis).

At clinical presentation, patients may have elevated serum levels of aminotransferases (i.e., aspartate aminotransferase [AST] and alanine aminotransferase [ALT]). A ratio of AST to ALT greater than 1 is useful in the evaluation of patients with ALD. AST levels are typically greater than ALT levels in all forms of ALD. Radiographic evaluation plays a role in screening for HCC in patients with cirrhosis and in the clinical care of critically ill patients with pancreatitis and suspected intestinal ileus.

Epidemiology and Prevalence

Worldwide, ALD has no social or ethnic barriers, but it is uncommon in very young and very elderly individuals. Both genders may be affected, although women are at higher risk. In the United States, 7.4% of the population meet the criteria for alcohol dependence or abuse. It is the leading cause of end-stage liver disease and liver-related mortality. It follows only heart disease and cancer as the major health issue in the United States.[19] The reported rates of per capita liters of alcohol consumed per year by individuals older than 15 years of age varies throughout the world: 13.9 in the Russian Federation; 12.9 in Germany, France, and the

United Kingdom; 8.5 to 9.3 in North America, Japan, and Australia; 5.0 in China, the Philippines, and Vietnam; 1.3 in Iran and Saudi Arabia; and 0.6 in Afghanistan and Pakistan.[19] Alcohol use may combine synergistically with other forms of chronic liver disease to generate progressive disease, malignancy, and morbidity.[20]

Familial Associations

Family, twin, and ethnic studies have confirmed genetic susceptibility to ALD.[19] Factors under investigation include gender, genes involved in the metabolism of alcohol, and other enzymes involved in the pathways of oxidative stress, various cytokines (e.g., tumor necrosis factor-α [TNF-α], interleukin-10 [IL-10]), genes involved in the oxidation of hepatic fat, mechanisms of matrix deposition and degradation in fibrosis, and immune reactions to endotoxin and toxic adducts.[21]

Risk Factors

Liver disease does not develop in all individuals who abuse alcohol. The risk for ALD, even among heavy drinkers, is less than 10% to 15%. Known risk factors include the amount of alcohol consumed during a 10- to 20-year period (>60 g/day for men; 20 to 30 g/day for women), gender (female > male), alcohol consumption at an early age (<14 years), central obesity, patterns of consumption (nonmealtime > mealtime; daily > weekend only; various types of beverages rather than one type), associated medications (acetaminophen), amount of coffee intake, and genes that regulate expression of proinflammatory cytokines and immune response mechanisms.[21,22] A sequence variation in the patatin-like phospholipase 3 *(PNPLA3)* gene, which encodes adiponutrin, is associated with the development of cirrhosis in patients with European or Native American ancestry.[21,23] Genome-wide association studies have also linked two other genes to risk of alcoholic cirrhosis: membrane bound O-acyltransferase domain-containing 7 *(MBOAT7)* and transmembrane 6 superfamily member 2 *(TM6SF2)*.[24] *PNPLA3* and *TM6SF2* have also been associated with features of progressive disease in NAFLD patients, suggesting shared pathways of injury.[25-27]

Pathogenesis

Alcohol-induced liver damage is a multifactorial process that involves alterations of the gut, gut microbiota, and hepatocellular metabolic pathways as well as activation of the innate and adaptive immune systems. Resultant outcomes are activation of proinflammatory and profibrogenic molecular mechanisms in specific liver cells.

The primary mechanism of alcohol-induced liver injury is hepatocellular oxidative stress.[28,29] Ethanol is metabolized to acetate in the liver mainly by two enzyme systems: alcohol and aldehyde dehydrogenases, which produce acetate by sequential oxidation of ethanol and the microsomal ethanol-oxidizing system (MEOS). The direct hepatotoxic effects of alcohol are caused primarily by acetaldehyde. Oxidative stress and free radical production result in mitochondrial damage, depletion of the antioxidants such as reduced glutathione, toxicity by free radicals, and induction of lipid peroxidation. Acetaldehyde-formed toxic adducts bind to proteins and lead to additional hepatocellular injury, serve as neoantigens for initiation of the adaptive immune response, and promote collagen production by hepatic stellate cells. The net effect of acetaldehyde production in hepatocytes is the accumulation of intracellular proteins, lipids, water, and electrolytes with the loss of the hepatocyte structural keratins 8 (K8) and 18 (K18). Histologically, there is cellular enlargement, ballooning, empty-appearing cells, steatosis, and loss of immunoreactivity for K8 and K18.[30]

The key enzyme of the MEOS is the ethanol-inducible CYP2E1, which is located primarily in the endoplasmic reticulum of acinar zone 3 hepatocytes. Activation of this enzyme system results in the production of reactive oxygen species, such as hydrogen peroxide (H_2O_2) and superoxide anions (O_2^-), which causes further lipid peroxidation of cell membranes. This enzyme system also metabolizes acetaminophen and produces the toxic metabolite *N*-acetyl-*p*-benzoquinone imine (NAPQI). Even small amounts of acetaminophen may augment depletion of the antioxidant capabilities of the liver in chronic alcoholism, which may relate to the increased risk of acute liver failure in this situation.[31]

Other sources of ethanol-induced oxidative stress include endotoxin-activated Kupffer cells, functionally impaired mitochondria, and ferric iron accumulation. Oxidative stress promotes hepatocellular injury, apoptosis, and necrosis; proinflammatory cytokine production (e.g., TNF-α, IL-1, IL-6, IL-17); and parenchymal inflammation with polymorphonuclear leukocytes (PMNs) and mononuclear cells and perisinusoidal fibrosis.[29,32,33]

Excessive alcohol intake leads to increased gut permeability and increased portal venous exposure to gut-derived endotoxins. This process results in Kupffer cell activation through the CD14/toll-like receptor 4 (TLR4) complex and activation of the innate immune response.[28,34] Alcohol consumption also leads to alterations in gut microbiota, reducing populations of beneficial bacteria and inducing dysbiosis.[35,36]

Increased lactate production, another downstream effect of ethanol metabolism, manifests as hyperuricemia and impaired carbohydrate metabolism. Hypoglycemia may occur. Chronic alcohol use impairs protein production and secretion. Multiple aberrations of lipid metabolism result in increased triglyceride production and subsequent accumulation (i.e., steatosis).

The mechanisms of fibrosis are under active scientific investigation. Ultimately, there is an imbalance between collagen deposition and degradation by activated hepatic stellate cells and portal myofibroblasts. Unique to ALD is the additional involvement of hepatocytes and sinusoidal endothelial cells in fibrogenesis through the production of transforming growth factor-β (TGF-β) and fibronectin isoforms.[37,38]

Pathology

Grossly, steatosis enlarges the liver and imparts a greasy appearance. Livers with advanced fibrosis or cirrhosis may be enlarged and firm, and they contain micronodules (≤3 mm in diameter) scattered throughout the parenchyma. In some cases, fibrotic livers may be small and firm. With time, the nodules may coalesce to form larger ones, at which point determination of the underlying cause may not be possible. HCCs often stand out on a background of cirrhosis as raised, green-tinged or darker nodules, typically larger than 8 mm in diameter.

The histological pattern of tissue injury in patients with alcohol-induced fatty liver disease initially involves acinar

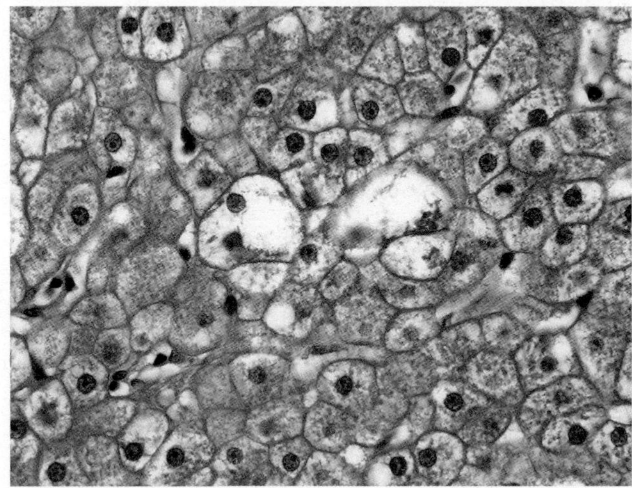

FIGURE 50.1 Ballooned hepatocytes are easily distinguished when surrounded by normal hepatocytes.

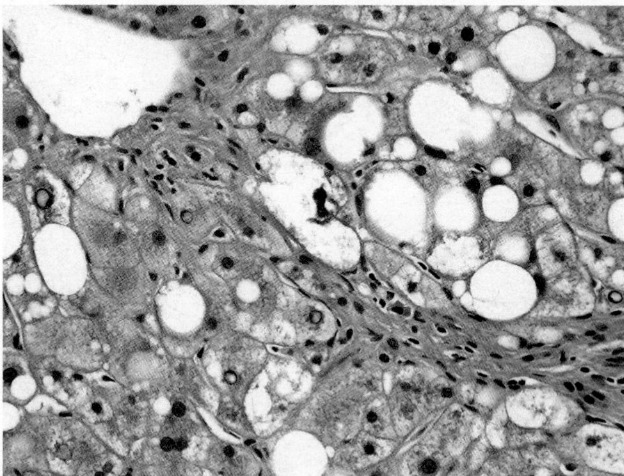

FIGURE 50.2 The ballooned hepatocyte in the center of the field is located among steatotic hepatocytes and is adjacent to fibrous tissue. There is a Mallory-Denk body in the ballooned hepatocyte.

zone 3 (roughly equivalent to perivenular) hepatocytes. In patients with cirrhosis, steatosis or steatohepatitis may or may not persist.[39]

Steatosis

Steatosis, the earliest pathological finding in ALD, is not consistently found in all forms of ALD.[40,41] Alcoholic steatosis is typically macrovesicular and is characterized by the presence of large intracellular droplets of lipid in hepatocytes (single or multiple) that displace the cell nucleus peripherally. A minor component of lobular chronic inflammation and/or mild portal inflammation may be present, but fibrosis is usually absent.

Steatohepatitis

Steatohepatitis is defined as the presence of both steatosis and hepatocyte injury. Injured hepatocytes may appear ballooned, apoptotic, or lytic. Confluent and bridging necrosis are rarely found in ALD.

Hepatocellular ballooning is considered an essential feature of steatohepatitis by most hepatopathologists.[42,43] Ballooned hepatocytes are enlarged cells with rarefied, reticulated cytoplasm (Fig. 50.1) that may or may not contain fat droplets and intracytoplasmic material referred to as *Mallory-Denk bodies* (MDBs) or *Mallory hyaline*. Ballooned hepatocytes are located predominantly in zone 3 and are commonly associated with some degree of perisinusoidal fibrosis (Fig. 50.2).[44]

Apoptotic hepatocytes, also called *acidophil bodies,* are common in patients with alcoholic steatohepatitis.[45] These round, eosinophilic fragments of cytoplasm located in the hepatic sinusoids may or may not retain nuclear pyknotic material. Lobular inflammation in patients with steatohepatitis is usually mild and consists of either mixed acute and chronic or mainly chronic inflammation. Scattered lobular microgranulomas and lipogranulomas are often present. Lobular lipogranulomas may consist of either multiple or single fat droplets surrounded by mononuclear cells and eosinophils (Fig. 50.3). Large portal lipogranulomas are frequently observed in ALD.[46] PMNs may be observed in small clusters adjacent to ballooned hepatocytes or shrunken eosinophilic (apoptotic) hepatocytes that contain MDBs. When PMNs are found next to hepatocytes that contain MDBs, the lesion is often referred to as *satellitosis* (Fig. 50.4).

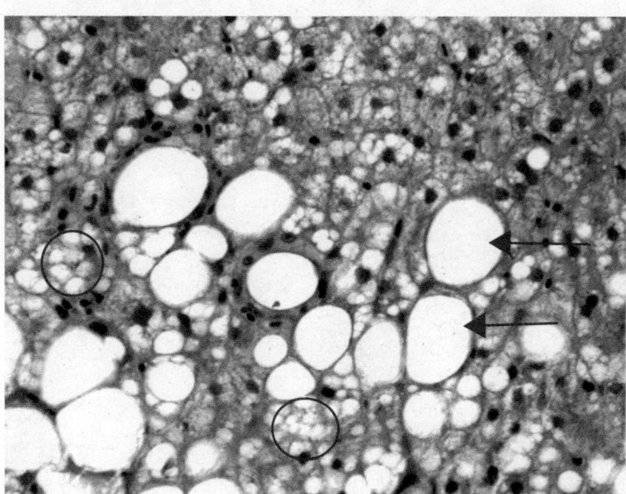

FIGURE 50.3 Mixed large (*arrows*)- and small (*circles*)-droplet macrovesicular steatosis. Each of the two lipogranulomas *(center)* consists of a single droplet of fat surrounded by pigmented Kupffer cells.

Although common, MDBs and satellitosis are not required for the diagnosis. MDBs are not specific to ALD; these inclusions are seen in NAFLD, chronic cholestatic liver disease, copper toxicity, and amiodarone toxicity. In steatohepatitis of any origin, MDBs are usually found in zone 3 hepatocytes (Fig. 50.5) and are more common in areas of perisinusoidal fibrosis, whereas in chronic cholestasis, copper toxicity, and amiodarone toxicity, MDBs are more common in periportal hepatocytes.[1,4] MDBs may also occur in focal nodular hyperplasia, hepatocellular adenoma, and HCC.[47] MDBs can sometimes be visualized by trichrome stains (Fig. 50.6) and confirmed by the use of immunohistochemistry for K8, K18, ubiquitin, or dynactin 4 (DCTN4, formerly designated p62).[48]

Some cases of ALD may show predominantly portal lymphocytic inflammation in the absence of serological evidence of chronic hepatitis B virus (HBV) or hepatitis C virus (HCV) infection. This feature may correlate with the degree of fibrosis[49] and may reflect an associated autoimmune component

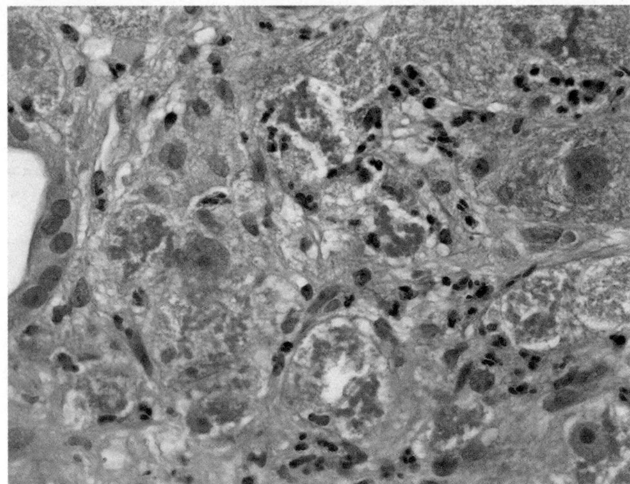

FIGURE 50.4 Multiple areas of satellitosis are evident in this field. Neutrophils surround hepatocytes harboring hyaline material.

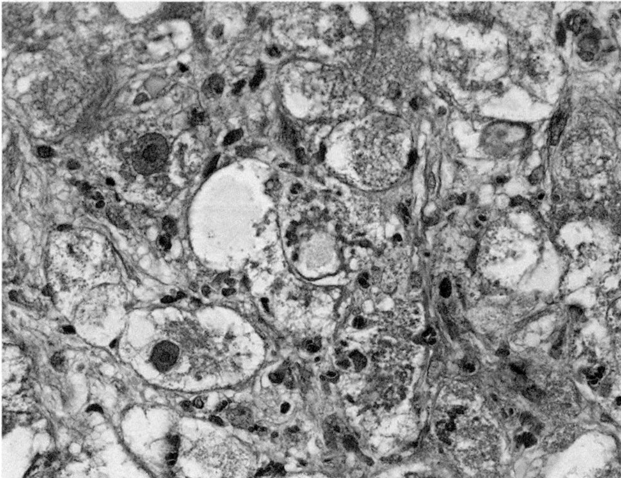

FIGURE 50.6 A large, ropy Mallory-Denk body is seen in the center of the field (trichrome stain).

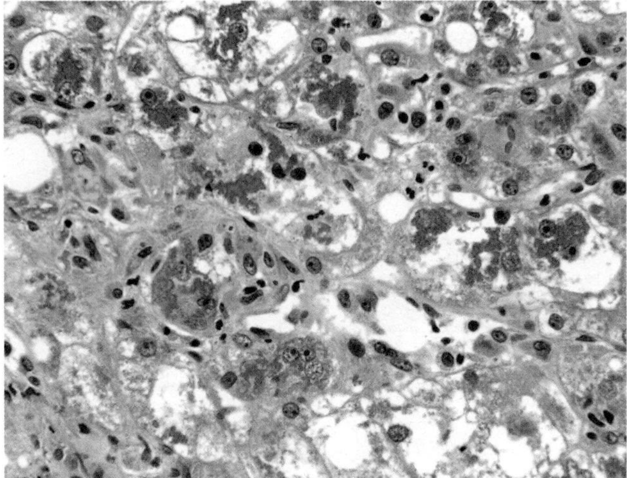

FIGURE 50.5 Numerous Mallory-Denk bodies are seen in a biopsy specimen from a patient with alcoholic steatohepatitis.

to the underlying liver disease.[50] Nevertheless, significant portal and periportal inflammation, particularly when lymphoid aggregates are present, should prompt consideration of concurrent chronic viral or autoimmune hepatitis. Ductular reaction associated with neutrophil infiltration may be related to the proinflammatory and neutrophil chemotactic character of the neo-ductules.[51] Sinusoidal macrophages (Kupffer cells) and possibly portal macrophages are activated by lipopolysaccharide leaking from a gut injured by exposure to ethanol.[52]

Alcoholic Hepatitis

Patients with alcoholic hepatitis may not necessarily have steatosis. Histological features of alcoholic hepatitis include hepatocyte ballooning, apoptotic bodies, MDBs with satellitosis, canalicular cholestasis, dense perisinusoidal fibrosis, and a perivenular lesion often referred to as *sclerosing hyaline necrosis* (i.e., MDBs, satellitosis, and obliterative fibrosis of the outflow vein).[39] Portal hypertension may occur with sclerosing hyaline necrosis. Bridging fibrosis and a ductular reaction may also be present. The absence of steatosis does not rule out alcohol-induced hepatitis.

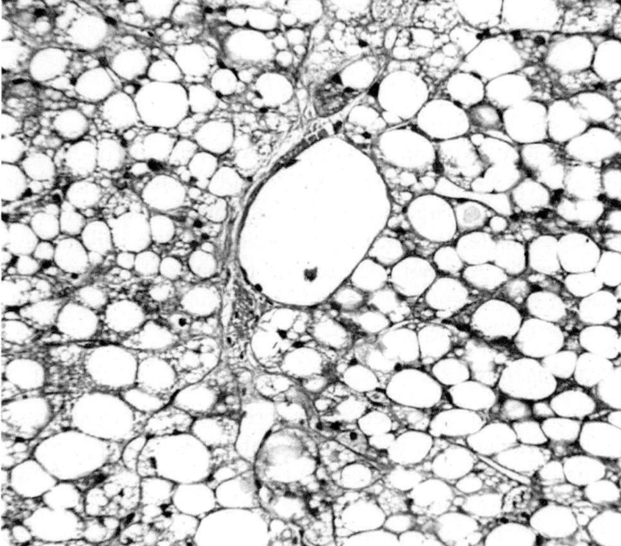

FIGURE 50.7 This biopsy was obtained from a patient with known alcoholism, hepatomegaly, and elevated aspartate aminotransferase and bilirubin values. It contains no inflammation, ballooning, or Mallory-Denk bodies and only a minor degree of fibrosis. Diffuse steatosis is evident, and a significant portion is microvesicular (trichrome stain).

Alcoholic Foamy Degeneration

Alcoholic foamy degeneration is an unusual and often serious type of ALD associated with marked elevations of aminotransferases, gammaglutamyltransferase (GGT), alkaline phosphatase, and bilirubin.[53,54] Histologically, it is characterized by diffuse, primarily microvesicular steatosis without inflammation or ballooning or by marked fibrosis, and it may be associated with canalicular cholestasis (Fig. 50.7). MDBs are uncommon. Perivenular and perisinusoidal fibrosis may be evident as well. Similar to other disorders that cause microvesicular steatosis, mitochondrial DNA shows evidence of injury.[55] Clinically, the disorder mimics extrahepatic biliary obstruction, but liver biopsy findings can be used to distinguish the two entities. Alcoholic foamy degeneration is reversible with abstinence from alcohol.

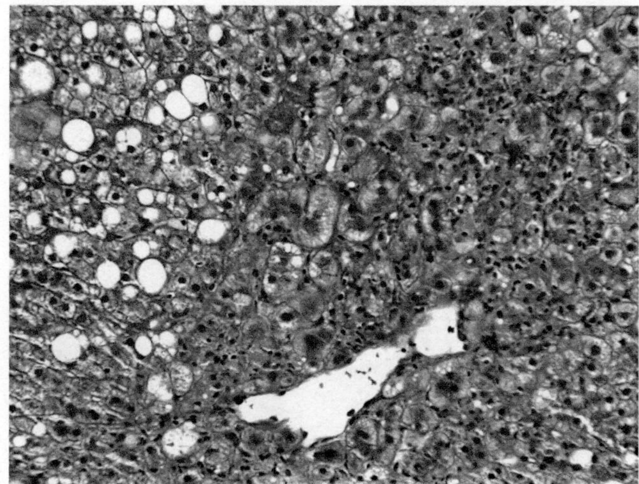

FIGURE 50.8 The dense zone 3 perisinusoidal fibrosis illustrates the characteristic "chicken wire" network of fibrosis (trichrome stain).

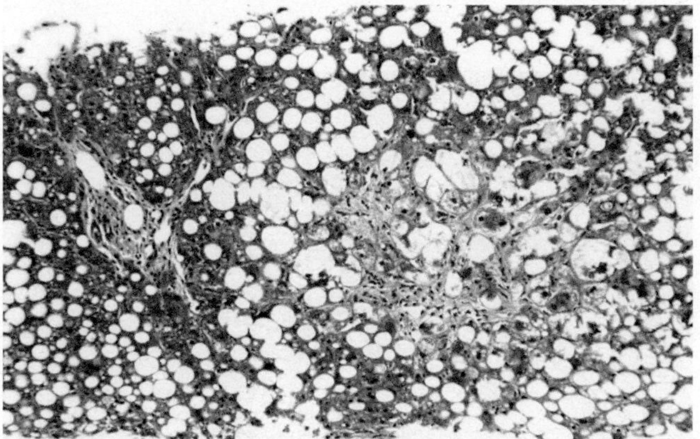

FIGURE 50.9 On low power, the zone 3 accentuation of steatohepatitis is best appreciated with a trichrome stain. Ballooning, steatosis, and perisinusoidal fibrosis can be seen.

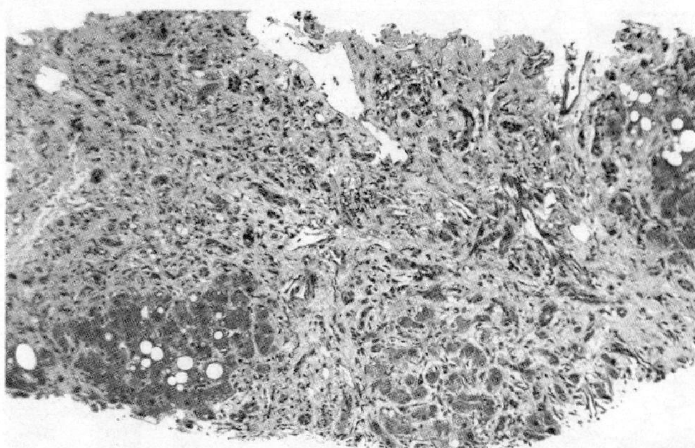

FIGURE 50.10 This biopsy from a patient with chronic alcoholism and portal hypertension shows dense perisinusoidal fibrosis and loss of hepatic architecture. This appearance is common in samples from patients with advanced alcohol-induced liver disease (trichrome stain).

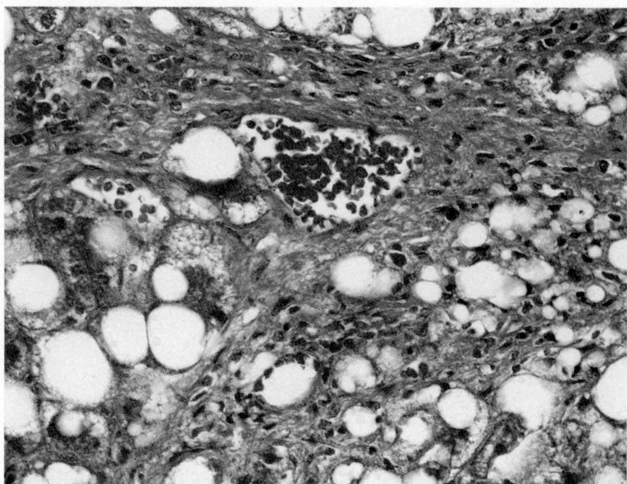

FIGURE 50.11 Dense perivenular fibrosis is seen more often in alcoholic liver disease than in nonalcoholic steatohepatitis (trichrome stain).

Fibrosis and Cirrhosis

The characteristic pattern of early fibrosis in patients with noncirrhotic alcoholic steatohepatitis or alcoholic hepatitis is pericellular or perisinusoidal. This pattern results from deposition of collagen in the space of Disse and is commonly referred to as *chicken wire fibrosis* (Fig. 50.8).

Fibrosis usually begins in zone 3 of the hepatic acini (Fig. 50.9). This type of fibrosis may be identified with or without steatohepatitis. However, when pericellular or perisinusoidal fibrosis occurs without steatohepatitis, it suggests that the patient had at least one prior episode of steatohepatitis in the past. In ALD, perisinusoidal fibrosis may involve large portions of the lobules and become quite dense in appearance (Fig. 50.10). In these cases, the patient may also have clinical evidence of portal hypertension in the absence of cirrhosis.

Perivenular fibrosis, a thickened sheath of collagen surrounding the outflow veins in the absence of perisinusoidal fibrosis, has been identified in patients with steatosis that subsequently progressed to cirrhosis (Fig. 50.11). This lesion is therefore considered a prognostic indicator of progression if alcohol exposure is continued.[56]

With disease progression, periportal fibrosis may develop (Fig. 50.12), followed in some cases by bridging fibrosis in a central-central, central-portal, or portal-portal pattern. In ALD, regions of parenchymal extinction (i.e., septa) may be quite broad (Fig. 50.13). After cirrhosis is established, areas of perisinusoidal fibrosis may not be evident. Periportal fibrosis and bridging fibrosis are often accompanied by a ductular reaction (Fig. 50.14). In ALD, isolated portal fibrosis in the absence of portal inflammation is uncommon and may be a manifestation of recurrent pancreatitis or biliary obstruction.[57] Itoh et al. observed a pattern of portal fibrosis characteristic of ALD known as *holly leaf* (Fig. 50.15).[58] This pattern of fibrosis, which is commonly associated with hemochromatosis, is characterized by portal expansion and nonbridging, small, fibrous extensions or spikes into the surrounding parenchyma that resemble the outline of the holly leaf.

In patients with ALD with bridging fibrosis, a periseptal ductular reaction may be prominent (see Fig 50.14). The ductular reaction, characterized by proliferation of K7- and/or K19-positive ovoid cells forming ductular structures in an inflammatory, stromal matrix,[59] is less likely to represent a cholestatic process in end-stage liver disease[60] and is more likely to represent the result of impaired regenerative activity of hepatocytes resulting from the antiregenerative effects of alcohol.[59,61]

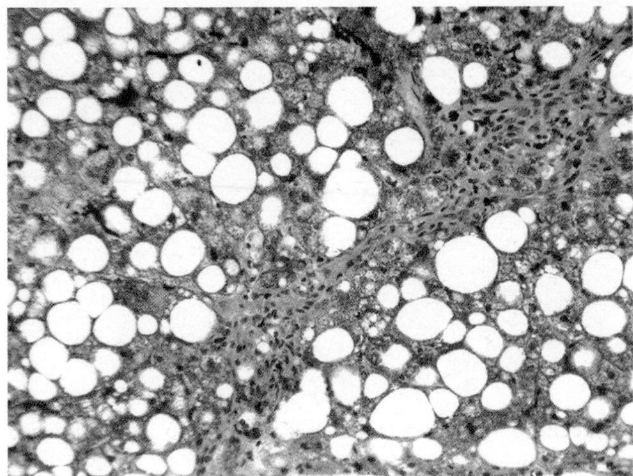

FIGURE 50.12 With progression of fibrosis in alcohol-induced liver disease, periportal fibrosis may be prominent (trichrome stain).

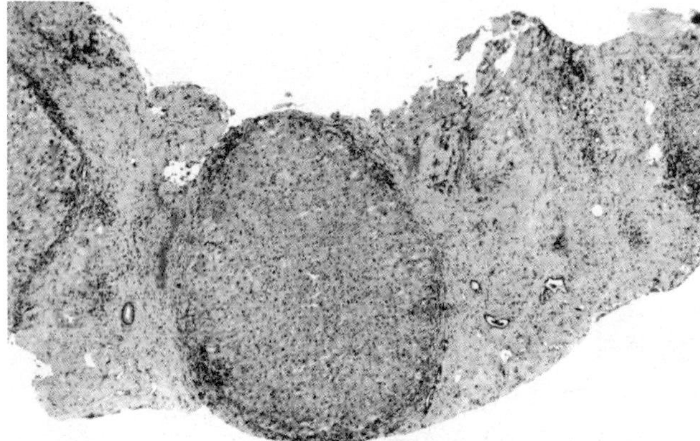

FIGURE 50.13 The small nodule is surrounded by broad regions of scar tissue (i.e., parenchymal extinction) in a patient with alcoholic cirrhosis.

ALD-associated cirrhosis may be macronodular, micronodular, or mixed. Micronodular nodules are typically less than 3 mm in diameter (Fig. 50.16). Larger nodules may develop when multiple nodules coalesce to form mixed micronodular and macronodular cirrhosis. Macronodular cirrhosis may be difficult to diagnose in liver biopsy specimens because of the large size of the nodules; clues to abnormal architecture can be sought by use of a reticulin stain (Fig. 50.17). Clusters of oncocytic hepatocytes suggest macronodular cirrhosis (see Chapter 51). Phlebosclerosis and occlusive disease of the terminal hepatic venules and sublobular veins occur frequently in patients with ALD-induced cirrhosis (Fig. 50.18).[56]

In ALD-associated cirrhosis, periseptal hepatocellular copper granules (Fig. 50.19) and, uncommonly, α_1-antitrypsin globules may be found. The role of heterozygosity for genes related to α_1-antitrypsin in promoting damage in patients with ALD is a subject of ongoing debate, but patients with MZ phenotype are overrepresented in transplant populations and present with more clinically advanced liver disease.[62] Increased iron levels in ALD are discussed later. Pseudotumoral nodules, which correspond to areas of active alcoholic hepatitis in cirrhotic livers, may be recognized on imaging studies and may be confused for HCC. These lesions may result from hypervascularity.[63]

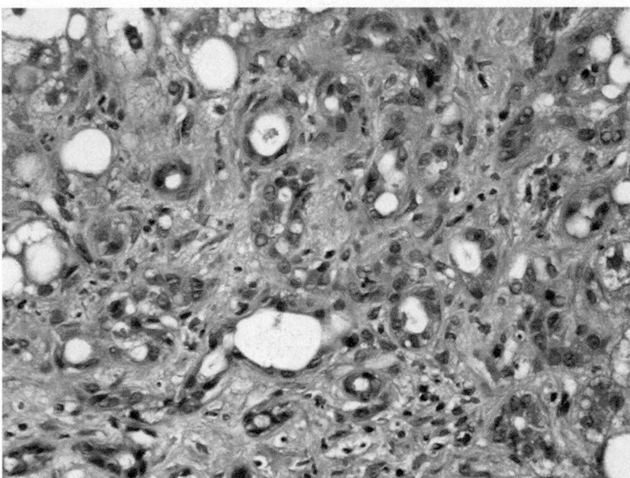

FIGURE 50.14 Prominent ductular reaction in a region of fibrosis in alcoholic liver disease. This finding may be periportal or may be seen within fibrotic bridges.

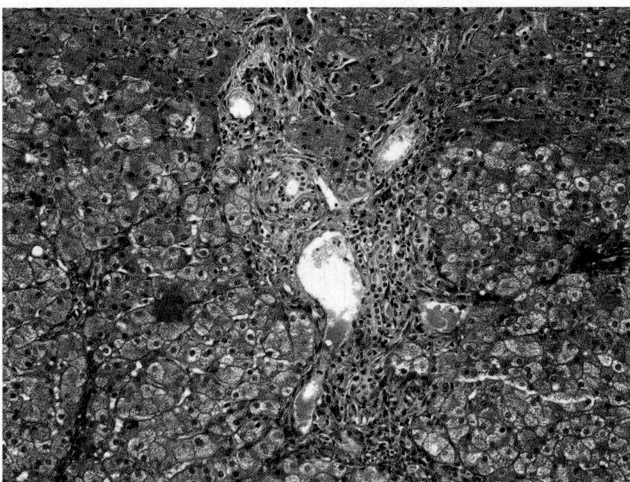

FIGURE 50.15 Periportal fibrosis with short septae can resemble a holly or maple leaf (trichrome stain).

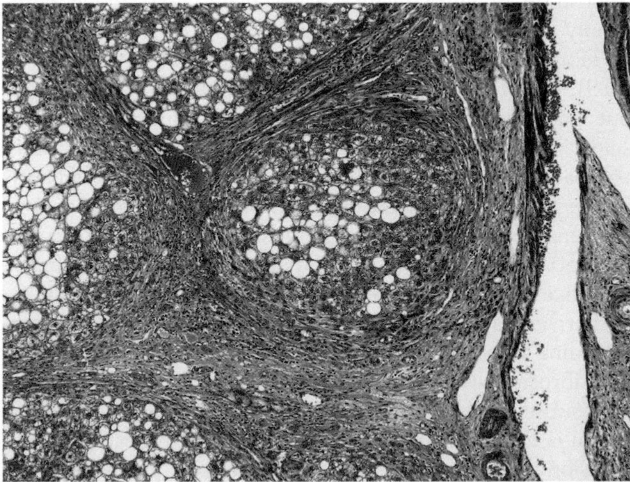

FIGURE 50.16 Micronodular cirrhosis showing a nodule about 1 mm in diameter (trichrome stain).

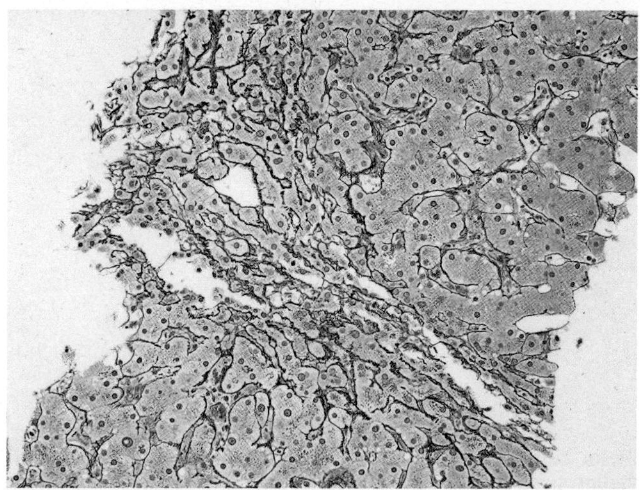

FIGURE 50.17 In this needle biopsy of macronodular cirrhosis, one can identify small regenerative nodules within the larger nodule on a reticulin stain. Although there is no fibrosis between the nodules, the liver cell plates are narrowed between regenerative nodules (reticulin stain).

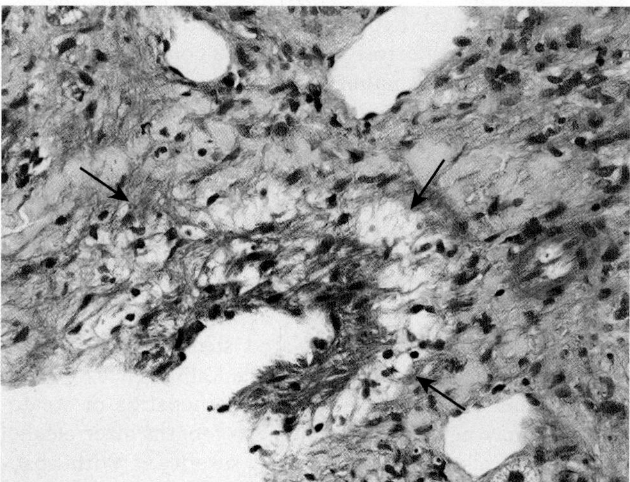

FIGURE 50.18 In this case of alcoholic hepatitis, one of the central veins show a veno-occlusive lesion. The approximate extent of the original vessel is indicated by *arrows* (trichrome stain).

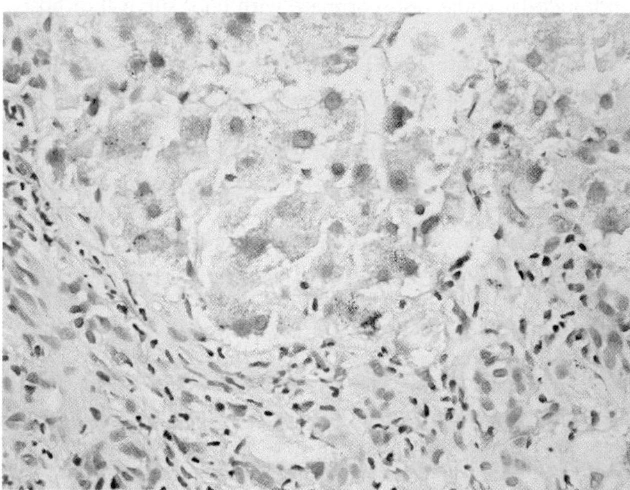

FIGURE 50.19 In both alcohol-related and nonalcoholic cirrhosis, copper may accumulate in periportal hepatocytes, here demonstrated as red cytoplasmic granules in a rhodamine stain.

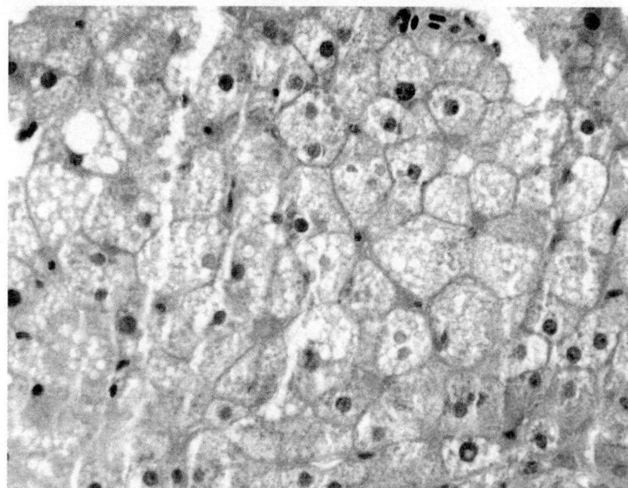

FIGURE 50.20 A nonzonal group of hepatocytes with tiny fat vacuoles is evident in the cytoplasm. Many of the hepatocytes also contain eosinophilic, round megamitochondria.

Other Pathological Features of Alcohol-Induced Liver Disease

Megamitochondria. Megamitochondria (i.e., giant mitochondria) are identified by light microscopy as intracytoplasmic, round or cigar-shaped, eosinophilic structures in hepatocytes, and they are most readily seen in hepatocytes that contain microvesicular steatosis (Fig. 50.20). They do not stain with periodic acid–Schiff (PAS) stain, allowing distinction from other round cytoplasmic inclusions such as α_1-antitrypsin globulin and serum inclusions. Megamitochondria may also occur in NASH, normal pregnancy, acute fatty liver of pregnancy, and Wilson's disease.

Iron Deposition. Mildly increased iron deposition is common in most forms of ALD. However, in a minority of cases, it may be moderate or severe.[64] Possible reasons for hemosiderosis in ALD include dysregulation of hepcidin production, intestinal iron absorption, the presence of iron in some types of alcoholic beverages, hemolysis related to spur cell anemia, and upregulation of the transferrin receptor.[64] With a modified Perls stain, iron deposition is usually in hepatocytes when mild, but eventually may accumulate in reticuloendothelial cells as well.[65] In ALD-related cirrhosis,[66] iron deposition may vary in quantity between individual regenerative nodules (Fig. 50.21).

Acute and Chronic Cholestasis. Several pathological processes related to ALD may result in intrahepatic cholestasis: both intrahepatic processes such as alcoholic foamy degeneration, alcoholic hepatitis, and alcoholic cirrhosis as well as extrahepatic processes such as alcoholic pancreatitis, gallstone obstruction, and sepsis. Intrahepatic cholestasis, characterized by canalicular bile thrombi, is observed in 15% to 32% of livers with ALD (Fig. 50.22).[67] Bile stasis in ALD may also be a manifestation of superimposed acute viral hepatitis or drug-induced cholestasis. In patients with established ALD-associated cirrhosis, a copper stain may show mild positivity, which represents chronic retention of bile salts caused by the cirrhotic remodeling.

In advanced cases of ALD, the cytoplasm of some hepatocytes may have a ground-glass appearance because of smooth endoplasmic reticulum proliferation, or it may be deeply eosinophilic, referred to as *oxyphil* or *oncocytic change*

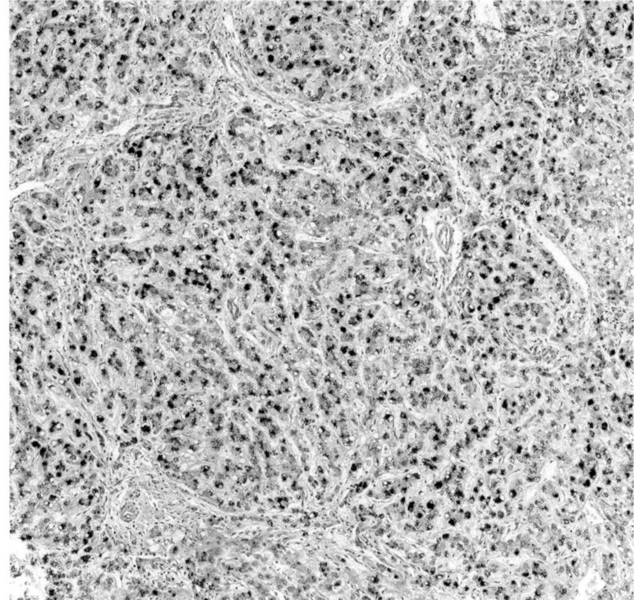

FIGURE 50.21 In a patient with alcoholic cirrhosis, the nodule in the center of the field shows prominent iron staining (modified Perls iron stain).

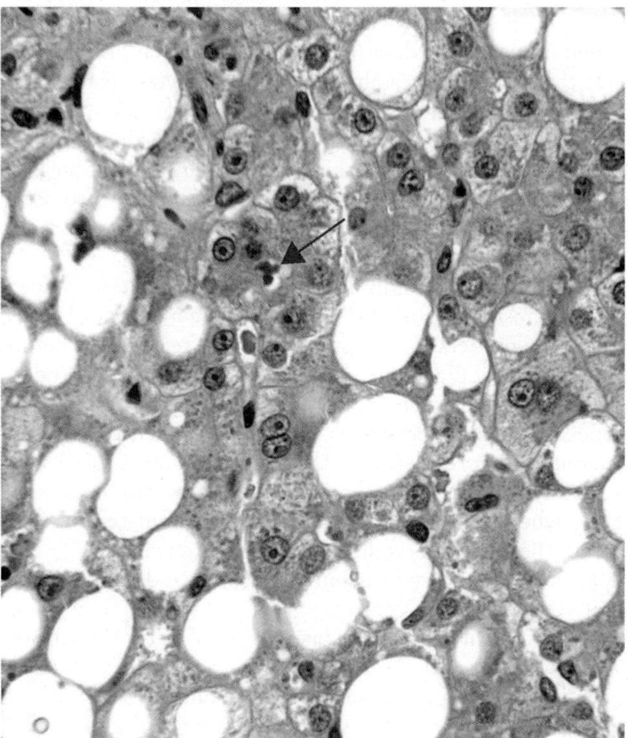

FIGURE 50.22 A cholestatic rosette with a central bile plug (*arrow*) and several surrounding hepatocytes containing intracellular bile are identified in a biopsy specimen from a patient with fatty liver disease resulting from alcohol-induced liver disease.

because of increased numbers of mitochondria.[68] Both changes are considered adaptive in nature. Historically, their presence was considered indicative of ongoing alcohol consumption, but one research group reported that they may also be observed after periods of prolonged abstinence.[69]

Vascular Lesions. Sclerosing hyaline necrosis, which is a marker of severe alcoholic hepatitis, and obliterative vein lesions may be responsible for the development of

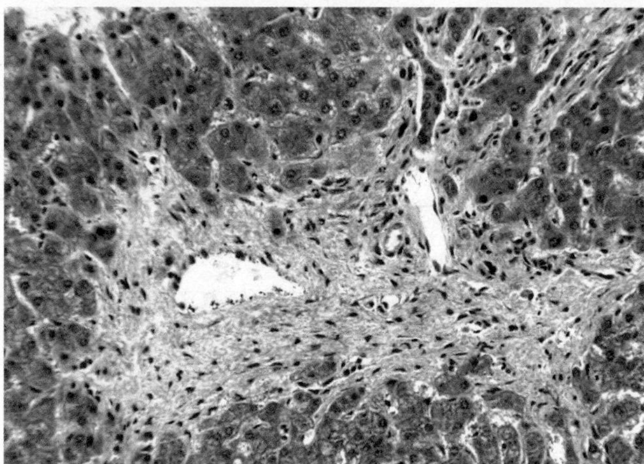

FIGURE 50.23 There is no evidence of steatosis or steatohepatitis in the biopsy specimen from a patient with alcohol-induced liver disease. The outflow vein is almost obliterated. A small artery branch lies close to the vein, and a ductular reaction is evident at the edge of the developing septum (trichrome stain).

noncirrhotic portal hypertension in patients with ALD. Sclerosing hyaline necrosis consists of a combination of acinar zone 3 lesions, including dense perivenular and perisinusoidal fibrosis (i.e., sclerosis), occlusion of terminal hepatic venules, MDBs, and liver cell necrosis and loss, resulting in the formation of large perivenular scars (see Figs. 50.11 and 50.18). Lesions of the terminal hepatic venules and sublobular veins include perivenular fibrosis, phlebosclerosis, and, less frequently, lymphocytic phlebitis (Fig. 50.23).[56] The number and severity of vascular lesions increases in proportion to the stage of fibrosis.

Treatment Effects. Alcohol-related steatosis may resolve completely within 4 weeks of alcohol abstinence.[69] However, lesions associated with alcoholic hepatitis or steatohepatitis may persist for as long as 6 months after alcohol withdrawal, albeit with decreased severity.[70] With abstinence, there is usually an increase in the degree of portal lymphocytic infiltration.[70]

Prognostic Lesions. The development of perivenular fibrosis is evidence of the potential to progress to cirrhosis. Canalicular and ductular cholestasis correlate with poor survival of hospitalized patients with ALD.[67] These patients have a reduced 5-year survival rate (22%) compared with patients with ALD who have no cholestasis or only mild cholestasis (54%).[71] The number of apoptotic bodies correlates positively with severe histological and clinical disease activity.[72,73] Alcoholic hepatitis, sclerosing hyaline necrosis, and severe steatosis represent poor-prognostic lesions in patients with ALD, particularly in patients with cirrhosis.[74] In noncirrhotic patients, mixed steatosis and the finding of megamitochondria in the initial liver biopsy of alcoholic patients without steatohepatitis correlate with an increased risk of subsequent fibrosis or cirrhosis on follow-up.[75] In acute-on-chronic liver failure caused by ALD, the finding of marked ductular bile stasis as well as many MDBs are significant predictors of in-hospital mortality.[76] A prognostic score based on the degree of fibrosis, neutrophil infiltration, cholestasis, and megamitochondria has been proposed for estimating 90-day mortality in alcoholic hepatitis.[67]

Lesions in the Allograft Liver. Any of the previously described lesions may manifest as either recurrent or de novo ALD in a liver allograft. Of course, care should also be taken to evaluate for the presence of other diseases of allograft, particularly acute and chronic rejection and recurrent hepatitis C, among others (see Chapter 53).

Natural History and Treatment

The financial and social burdens associated with ALD are quite significant.[19,77] Alcoholic hepatitis is associated with a significant risk of hospitalization and loss of time from work, morbidity and short-term mortality, and progression to cirrhosis within 5 years in up to 70% of individuals. Some affected individuals are able to reverse the disease process with complete abstinence.[19] A 12-year historical study from a national registry of Danish subjects comparing biopsy-proven ALD with the general population showed that the cirrhosis risk was higher for affected women than for men, and it was twice as high for patients with steatohepatitis compared with those with pure steatosis.[78]

Chronic alcohol abuse is responsible for as many as 45% of cases of HCC in Western countries.[79] In the United States, data from the SEER database suggest that the proportion of HCCs attributable to alcohol is 23.5% compared with 22.4% for HCVs.[80] Coexistent HCV infection has an additive effect on the risk of carcinoma.[19] Other comorbid factors, such as chronic hepatitis B, hemochromatosis, obesity, and cigarette smoking, contribute to an increased risk of HCC and mortality in patients with ALD.[81,82] Intrahepatic cholangiocarcinoma also has been linked to ALD.[83]

The mainstay of treatment for ALD is abstinence from alcohol. One of the pharmacological methods of treatment for alcoholism, cyanamide, may produce isolated, nonzonal eosinophilic globules in hepatocytes.[84] Treatment of hospitalized patients with alcoholic hepatitis includes steroids and nutritional support. The antioxidants pentoxifylline and *N*-acetyl-cysteine have potential efficacy.[16] Most institutions require 6 months of abstinence before listing alcoholic patients with cirrhosis for liver transplantation.[16] Liver transplantation for patients with acute alcoholic hepatitis is under study, but this remains controversial.[85,86]

NONALCOHOLIC FATTY LIVER DISEASE

Clinical Features

Individuals with NAFLD may be asymptomatic or may show mild, nonspecific symptoms such as fatigue and right upper quadrant discomfort or pain (Table 50.2). Fever is not a feature of uncomplicated NAFLD; when present, it suggests a different or concomitant liver disorder.

The most common clinical feature of NAFLD is central (truncal or abdominal) obesity, which is best assessed by measurement of waist circumference. For adult men, central obesity is a waist circumference greater than 102 cm, and for adult women, it is greater than 88 cm. Obesity is defined by body mass index (BMI), which is the weight in kilograms divided by the height in meters squared (kg/m^2). Compared with waist circumference, it is less specific and does not assess the anatomical location of the metabolically unique subcutaneous and visceral fat depots, or shape, of the body habitus. For non-Asian adults, the currently used terms are *overweight* (BMI >25 kg/m^2) and *obese* (BMI >30 kg/m^2). Because the Asian body habitus is deceptively thin and able to conceal visceral adiposity, lower BMI values for overweight and obese individuals have been recommended.[87]

Clinical evidence of hepatomegaly may be found in patients with an enlarged, fatty liver. Ascites and other features of portal hypertension may be identified in patients with NAFLD-associated cirrhosis. Obstructive sleep apnea, endocrine abnormalities (hypothyroidism, hypopituitarism, and hypogonadism), and acanthosis nigricans are also well-recognized associations of NAFLD.[88]

Laboratory values commonly assessed in patients with NAFLD include ALT, AST, and GGT. Patients also undergo tests for hyperglycemia (glycated hemoglobin [HbA_{1c}] is used to evaluate long-term glycemic control), tests for insulin resistance (based on calculations of fasting glucose and insulin levels by using quantitative insulin sensitivity check index [QUICKI] and homeostasis model assessment of

TABLE 50.2 Symptoms, Signs, and Laboratory Abnormalities of Nonalcoholic Fatty Liver Disease

Symptoms and Signs	Fatty Liver	Steatohepatitis	Cirrhosis
Asymptomatic	++	+	Portal hypertension
Right upper quadrant discomfort	++	++	+
Hepatomegaly	++	++	+
Elevated AST, normal ALT	–	–	–
AST/ALT ratio	AST/ALT < 1	AST/ALT < 1	AST/ALT ≥ 1
Marked AST elevation	–	–	–
Marked alkaline phosphatase elevation	–	–	–
Bilirubin elevation	–	–	–
Jaundice	–	–	–
Elevated white blood cell count	–	–	–
Fever	–	–	–
Ascites	–	–	+ (advanced)

ALT, Alanine aminotransferase; *AST*, aspartate aminotransferase; –, does not occur; +, occurs uncommonly; ++, common; +++, very common.

insulin resistance [HOMA-IR]), and tests of lipid parameters. Patients also need screening to exclude other types of chronic liver disease, including viral and autoimmune hepatitis, hemochromatosis, and chronic cholestatic liver diseases.[88]

The overall sensitivity of liver enzymes for detection of fatty liver disease is poor.[88,89] For instance, patients with normal ALT levels may have steatosis or advanced steatohepatitis[90,91] or they may have silent cirrhosis.[92,93] If elevated, the ALT value is usually greater than the AST value, and an ALT/AST ratio greater than 1 is often found in cases of precirrhotic NAFLD; the reverse situation occurs in ALD. Significant levels of autoantibodies, particularly antinuclear antibody, anti–smooth muscle antibody, and rarely, antimitochondrial antibody, have been reported in as many as 21% of individuals with NAFLD.[94] In some patients, only further detailed clinical testing or a liver biopsy can distinguish autoimmune hepatitis from concurrent autoimmune hepatitis with NAFLD, or NAFLD alone.[95] One possible association of autoantibodies with more severe disease has been suggested, but not confirmed.[94,96] In combination with the proven lack of reproducible gross evaluation of the liver by surgeons, authorities recommend a liver biopsy for all high-risk and bariatric patients,[97-99] especially when other causes of steatosis have been excluded.[88]

Abnormal iron studies are a common feature in patients with NAFLD. For instance, elevated serum levels of ferritin (but not transferrin saturation) may be found in patients with NAFLD and may cause clinical concern regarding an iron overload disorder.[100] The serum ferritin level in NAFLD patients has been reported as an independent predictor of the histological severity of the underlying liver disease.[101] An elevated serum ferritin level may indicate hepatocyte necrosis and systemic inflammation,[102] and it is a well-recognized feature of the metabolic syndrome (discussed later). The associations of iron dysregulation, *HFE* (hemochromatosis) mutations, and fibrosis with the metabolic syndrome remain subjects of debate.[100] One prior meta-analysis did not support an association between *HFE* genetic variants and NAFLD.[103]

The proinflammatory iron regulator hepcidin is expressed in the liver and adipose tissue of obese patients, and this finding correlates with low transferrin values in 68% of these individuals and anemia in 24%.[104] In NAFLD and NASH, hepcidin mRNA and protein are correlated with iron stores, but not the severity of the fatty liver disease.[105]

Laboratory tests are indicative of the complexity of this condition. Markers of systemic inflammation, such as elevated levels of C-reactive protein, fibrinogen, and plasminogen activator inhibitor 1, are found in the setting of NASH and fibrosis.[106] A depressed level of adiponectin, an antiinflammatory cytokine of visceral adipose tissue, is recognized as a characteristic feature of NAFLD or NASH.[107] Unlike ALD, leukocytosis, cholestasis, and jaundice are not typical features of noncirrhotic NASH.

By ultrasonography, computed tomography (CT), or magnetic resonance imaging (MRI), the characteristic finding in NAFLD is increased hepatic fat. The ultrasound finding is referred to as a *bright liver.* Magnetic resonance imaging proton density fat fraction (MRI PDFF) can separately identify the spin relation of hydrogen atoms on water and triglyceride to quantify the lipid content of the liver.[108] The controlled attenuation pattern (CAP) of sheer wave elastography is sensitive to lesser degrees of steatosis, but it is not accurate for distinguishing moderate from severe steatosis.[109] Imaging is also not an adequate replacement for tissue analysis for determination of the degree of disease activity or the stage of fibrosis in patients with precirrhotic NASH.[88]

Epidemiology and Prevalence

The epidemiology and prevalence of NAFLD are understood in terms of its relationship to obesity and its increased risk of stroke and heart disease, a group of associations referred to as *metabolic syndrome*. The common underlying feature of this syndrome is systemic insulin resistance. Studies have confirmed associations of NAFLD with hepatic insulin resistance, cardiovascular diseases,[110] and the metabolic syndrome in both adults[111] and children.[112] For the metabolic syndrome, a patient must have at least three of the following five conditions: elevated fasting glucose (>100 g/dL); obesity defined by country-specific waist circumference limits; arterial hypertension (>130 mm Hg systolic or >85 mm Hg diastolic); dyslipidemia as low levels of high-density lipoprotein (<40 mg/dL in men or <50 mg/dL in women); or hypertriglyceridemia (>150 mg/L).[113] Patients with NASH have a much higher likelihood of also having metabolic syndrome than those with fatty liver alone.[114]

NAFLD is a worldwide disorder, and it has been documented in almost all cultures. Prevalence rates vary from 13.5% in Africa to 31.8% in the Middle East, with a global prevalence estimated at 25.2%.[115] This global phenomenon is closely related to acquisition of a Western diet that is high in saturated fats and reduced physical activity.[116] Initially thought to be a disease predominantly of overweight women, the entire spectrum of NAFLD is now recognized as common among men of all ages, but severe NASH and advanced fibrosis remain more common among adult women.[88] Several studies have confirmed an underrepresentation of this disease in African Americans of all age groups and an overrepresentation in Hispanics,[88] but these differences may be explained by variation in the patatin-like phospholipase domain-containing protein 3 (PNPLA-3).[117]

Once referred to as a *disease of affluence*, NAFLD has become recognized as everyman's disease.[118] Type 2 diabetes and obesity present lifelong challenges to patients, and the social stigma surrounding obesity presents a challenge to developing a social health response.[119] Future projections of the rates of obesity, type 2 diabetes mellitus, and their complications in the developing world for the year 2030 are staggering. They range from 18.6% in sub-Saharan Africa to 79.4% in India. The projected percent positive change for type 2 diabetes mellitus incidence is 32% in Europe, 72% in the United States, 150% in India, 162% in sub-Saharan Africa, and 164% in the Middle East.[120]

Having considered the worldwide and multicultural nature of NAFLD, some studies have evaluated ethnic predisposition for this disease. An image-based study of hepatic steatosis from a large, urban, multiethnic population in the United States[108] found the following relative prevalence rates: Hispanic > white > African American. Subsequently, a clinic-based study that used liver tests and liver biopsy results differed only slightly,[99] showing the following ethnic prevalence rates: white > Hispanic > Asian. African Americans represented only 3% of patients in this cohort. Others have observed an apparent underrepresentation of African Americans in cohorts of patients with NAFLD.[121] A small biopsy series from an inner-city hospital in the United States that primarily serves African Americans confirmed the relative scarcity of the disease in this patient population. Less than 2% of 320 liver biopsies showed clinicopathological evidence of NAFLD, even though the BMI of the cohort was between 26.9 and 32.7.[122]

Unfortunately, most of the early prevalence studies were performed without a full understanding of the link between the metabolic syndrome and fatty liver disease. In later studies, surrogate markers, such as elevated ALT levels and a bright liver on ultrasonography, were used to examine study populations. However, as with pathological studies, the conclusions vary, which is partly related to the criteria used to define the positivity of test values. For example, in studies relying on elevated serum aminotransferase levels, recognized shortcomings included underrecognition of positive cases with normal test values, determination of criteria for normal values in an increasingly obese population in both adults and children,[123,124] determination of reliable ALT values from frozen sera, and ascertainment of the levels of alcohol intake.[125] Methods of assessment of body habitus (i.e., BMI, waist-to-hip ratio, midthigh measurements, and more sophisticated and expensive calculations) also vary.[126] Commonly cited studies[127-130] are listed in Table 50.3.

TABLE 50.3 Prevalence of Nonalcoholic Fatty Liver Disease Among US Adults Based on NHANES III Data*

Study	Criteria	Prevalence of NAFLD
Clark et al., 2002[127]	Any elevation of AST, ALT, GGT	23% of all U.S. adults 31% male 16% female 39% of obese men, 40% of obese women
Clark et al., 2003[128]	± patients with diabetes	AST >37 U/L, ALT >40 U/L (men) AST, ALT >31 U/L (women) 7.9% of all U.S. adults; 69% unexplained (5.5% of adults)
Ruhl and Everhart, 2003[129]	Elevated ALT only; excluded patients with diabetes	ALT >43 U/L (men and women) 2.8% elevated ALT, 65% explained by elevated body mass index
Lazo et al., 2013[130]	Ultrasound detection of fatty liver	19% of U.S. adults 24.1% Mexican-Americans 17.8% non-Hispanic Caucasian 13.5% non-Hispanic African American 20.2% men, 15.8% women

**Limitations of NHANES data: autoimmune hepatitis, primary biliary cirrhosis, Wilson's disease, and α_1-antitrypsin deficiency not excluded rigorously and absence of liver pathology for confirmation or exclusion.*

ALT, *Alanine aminotransferase;* AST, *aspartate aminotransferase;* GGT, *γ-glutamyltransferase;* NAFLD, *nonalcoholic fatty liver disease;* NHANES III, *Third National Health and Nutrition Examination Survey.*

Validation of the findings of the Third National Health and Nutrition Examination Survey (NHANES III) has emerged from subsequent studies. Using MRI PDFF to detect steatosis in a multiethnic population in the southwestern United States, one study found that 31% of 2287 unselected individuals had a greater than 5.5% rate of hepatic steatosis. Of these, 79% had normal ALT values.[108] One contemporaneous study from a large clinic population in California showed that of 742 individuals with newly diagnosed chronic liver disease, 21.4% had NAFLD.[131] NAFLD was found to be the most common cause of incidental liver function test abnormalities (26.4%) in a UK prospective primary care cohort of 1118 adults by a combination of ultrasound and biomarker assays; ALD was a close second (25.3%). Of the NAFLD cases, 7.6% had evidence of previously undetected advanced fibrosis.[132]

A U.S. biopsy-based prevalence study of asymptomatic adults found that 46% of 156 adult unselected patients who had steatosis on ultrasonography had NAFLD diagnosed on biopsy. Of these, 30% had diagnostic NASH, and 2.7% of those with NASH had advanced fibrosis (≥ stage 2). This led to an estimate that more than 2 million of the U.S. adult population was at risk for advanced fibrosis because of NASH. These findings led to the conclusion that the prevalence of NAFLD was greater than that of hepatitis C and posed a serious concern for the future of health care.[133]

A study in a predominantly nonaffluent, nonobese population in India represented by 1911 inhabitants of a rural community showed the prevalence of NAFLD diagnosed by ultrasonography and CT to be 8.7%. NASH was seen in 31% of 36 patients with potentially significant disease who underwent biopsy, 4 of whom had cirrhosis.[134,135]

The estimated prevalence rate of NAFLD in the United States is greater than that of ALD (Table 50.4). One study that examined changes in the prevalence of chronic liver

TABLE 50.4 Prevalence of Fatty Liver Disease Compared with Other Chronic Liver Diseases

Disorder	Prevalence
Nonalcoholic fatty liver disease	25%-75% of obese diabetic adults 16% of 15- to 19-year-old adolescents 38% of obese adolescents
Hepatitis C	1.3%-2.0%
Alcohol-induced liver disease	1%
Hepatitis B	0.3%-0.4%
Hereditary hemochromatosis	1/200-400 of northern European descent
Autoimmune hepatitis, primary biliary cirrhosis, primary sclerosing cholangitis	9-17/100,000
α_1-Antitrypsin deficiency	1/1500-7600
Wilson's disease	1/30,000

Data from McCullough AJ. Pathophysiology of nonalcoholic steatohepatitis. J Clin Gastroenterol. *2006;40(suppl 1):S17-S29; Yu AS, Keeffe EB. Elevated AST or ALT to non-alcoholic fatty liver disease: accurate predictor of disease prevalence?* Am J Gastroenterol. *2003;98:955-956.*

disease over time using the three NHANES studies suggested that the rate of NAFLD in the United States increased from 5.5% in 1988–1994 to 11% in 2005–2008. In contrast, the prevalence of ALD only changed from 1.4% to 2.1% in the same time frame.[136] Table 50.5 summarizes several published series focused on histological documentation of fatty liver in adult autopsies.[137-142] Correlations between body weight and diabetes were discussed in many of these studies long before the metabolic syndrome was identified as a specific entity. More than one investigator even suggested that steatosis was a normal consequence of aging (see Pathogenesis).

In summary, the true prevalence rate of NASH remains unknown, primarily because there are no reliable or specific noninvasive tests available that can establish an accurate diagnosis, or in fact, exclusion of this specific disease process. A review of noninvasive markers in NAFLD, NASH, and fibrosis suggests that serum tests and imaging tools have some value for assessing fatty liver disease.[15] Although liver biopsy evaluation is considered the "gold standard" of diagnostic tests, it cannot be used for screening. Results from biopsy studies reinforce the observations that not all obese individuals have hepatic steatosis[11,143,144] and that unexplained elevated ALT values cannot be assumed to indicate fatty liver disease. For example, Skelly and colleagues[145] showed that as many as one-third of 354 biopsies performed for unexplained elevated ALT levels were histologically normal or had abnormalities because of liver diseases other than NAFLD or NASH. Recommendations for the focused role of liver biopsy for patients with suspected NAFLD or NASH were discussed in the practice guidelines from the American Association for the Study of Liver Diseases[88] and in a consensus conference of the European Association for the Study of the Liver.[146]

Familial Associations and Risk Factors

The genetic predispositions found in patients with NAFLD are exemplified by differences in the incidence of other risk factors, such as obesity, diabetes, hypertension, and hyperlipidemia, among various ethnic populations. Studies have documented fatty liver disease and cirrhosis among kindreds.[147] One study of 20 patients showed a trend toward familial clustering and maternal linkage for insulin resistance among patients with NAFLD.[148] The NASH Clinical Research Network has identified family history of diabetes as an independent risk factor for NASH.[149]

Type 2 diabetes and obesity are risk factors for progressive disease in clinical[150] and histological studies.[11,89,149] Various possible environmental and genetic factors have been proposed for NAFLD,[151] including the type of diet,[152] exercise, smoking,[153] the gut microbiome,[154] endotoxin and related immune or cytokine responses, polymorphisms for genes that control fatty acid oxidation (e.g., microsomal transfer protein), and fibrosis (i.e., angiotensinogen and TGF-β).

Broad, nonexclusive categories of genes under investigation as potential risk factors for NAFLD[155] include those involved in the control of adiposity and insulin resistance (e.g., peroxisome proliferator–activated receptor-γ [PPAR-γ], central vs. peripheral fat depots); determinants of hepatic steatosis (i.e., free fatty acid delivery and de novo lipogenesis, processing, and egress); hepatic fatty acid oxidation pathways (e.g., mitochondrial, peroxisomal, microsomal); hepatic oxidative stress mechanisms (e.g., production, defense); cytokine effects (e.g., TNF-α, IL-6, adipokines); and determinants of progression of fibrosis. One genomic and proteomic study of 98 bariatric patients found downregulation of genes involved in defense against oxidative stress

TABLE 50.5 Prevalence of Fatty Liver Disease in Autopsy Studies

Study	Population Studied *(N)*	Prevalence of Fatty Liver	Associated Features
Hilden et al., 1977[137]	Motor vehicle accident victims; adults (503)	24% overall 0.5% had features of alcoholic hepatitis	*Age:* 1% <20 years 18% 20-40 years 39% >60 years *Overweight:* associated with steatosis, not age
Ground, 1982[138]	Aircrew, accidental deaths, all men (199)	15.6% overall 2.1% had features of alcoholic hepatitis	All healthy; none had overt alcoholism
Hornboll and Olsen, 1982[139]	678 Consecutive autopsies, all > 20 years of age (396 with alcohol and other exclusions)	54% overall 43% had <33% 11% had >33%	*Age:* no association after 40 years *Overweight:* strong association with degree of fatty change; diabetic people were more common in this group Diabetes not independently associated
Underwood Ground, 1984[140]	Aircraft, motor vehicle accidents, all men; all accidents associated with alcohol, other illnesses excluded (166)	21%	Questioned possible irregular use of alcohol as factor; discussed increased carbohydrate intake relationship to fatty liver disease
Wanless and Lentz, 1990[141]	Hospitalized, 207 obese patients, 144 matched nonobese controls; alcoholic patients excluded (351)	Steatosis: 36.3% overall, 29.2% obese, 7.1% lean Steatohepatitis: 18.5% obese, 2.7% lean	*Overweight:* prevalence and grade of steatosis and steatohepatitis correlated with grade of obesity *Diabetes:* increased the risk of steatohepatitis and fibrosis
Schwimmer et al., 2006[142]	Consecutive pediatric and adolescent autopsies in a single-county, nonselected (742)	Steatosis: 13% overall 2-4 years: 0.7% 15-19 years: 17.3%	*Age:* fatty liver incidence increased with age *Obesity:* 38% had fatty liver *Ethnicity:* Hispanic (11.8%), Asian (10.2%), white (8.6%), African American (1.5%)

in NAFLD cases and upregulation of genes associated with fibrogenesis and apoptosis in steatohepatitis cases.[156]

Genome-wide association and candidate gene studies have identified variants in several genes that have been associated with NAFLD and NASH.[151] The best studied is *PNPLA3*, which encodes adiponutrin, an insulin-responsive phospholipase involved in lipolysis and lipogenesis that correlates with accumulation of hepatic triglycerides and some histological features of severity of NASH with identical ethnic distributions in prevalence studies.[25,26,157-159] This association is not limited to adults.[160,161] Other variants that have been identified include transmembrane 6 superfamily 2 (TM6SF2),[27] membrane-bound O-acyltransferase domain-containing protein 7 (MBOAT7),[162] Kruppel-like factor 6 (KLF6),[163] and insulin receptor substrate-1 (IRS-1).[164]

Pathogenesis

Certain similarities (i.e., steatosis, oxidative damage, and cytokine response) and dissimilarities between the pathogenesis of NAFLD and ALD are highlighted in Fig. 50.24. The most commonly discussed driver of NAFLD is insulin resistance and associated lipotoxicity (i.e., fat in nonfat depots) and complex pathways of systemic and local inflammation.[165,166] The metabolic system of insulin involves signaling among skeletal muscle, adipose tissue, and liver.[167]

The manifestations of insulin resistance depend on the type of tissue involved. In visceral adipose tissue, there is unabated release of free fatty acids into portal venous blood. In peripheral muscle, insulin resistance manifests as an inability to use circulating glucose. In liver, continuation of glucose production (i.e., gluconeogenesis) combines with a lack of glycogen storage in the setting of hyperinsulinemia and hyperglycemia. Hepatic steatosis, which corresponds to an accumulation of triglycerides in hepatocytes, results from an imbalance between the delivery of free fatty acids and endogenous lipogenesis and fatty acid disposal, the latter via oxidation, and packaging of esterified fatty acids and triglycerides for export by apolipoproteins in the form of very-low-density lipoproteins. Each of these steps involves complex, genetically regulated pathways.

Current studies show that triglyceride accumulation is a mechanism of sequestration of potentially damaging free fatty acids and that nontriglyceride fatty acid metabolites likely drive subsequent necroinflammatory lesions recognized as NASH.[168] Our understanding of the pathogenesis of NAFLD and NASH also includes the roles of altered gut microbiota,[154] intestinal permeability and lipopolysaccharide (LPS) exposure,[169] differential macrophage activation in adipose tissue depots,[32,170] innate immunity,[171,172] and supporting activation by inflammasomes in obesity-related liver injury.[173]

Visceral (abdominal) adipose tissue is an energy storage depot and represents a source of highly active proteins, collectively referred to as adipokines or adipocytokines (Fig. 50.25). In NAFLD, adipokines such as TNF-α (elevated in NAFLD) and adiponectin (decreased in obesity and NAFLD), proinflammatory IL-6, proinflammatory and profibrogenic derivatives of the renin-angiotensin system, and resistin may be involved in the pathogenesis

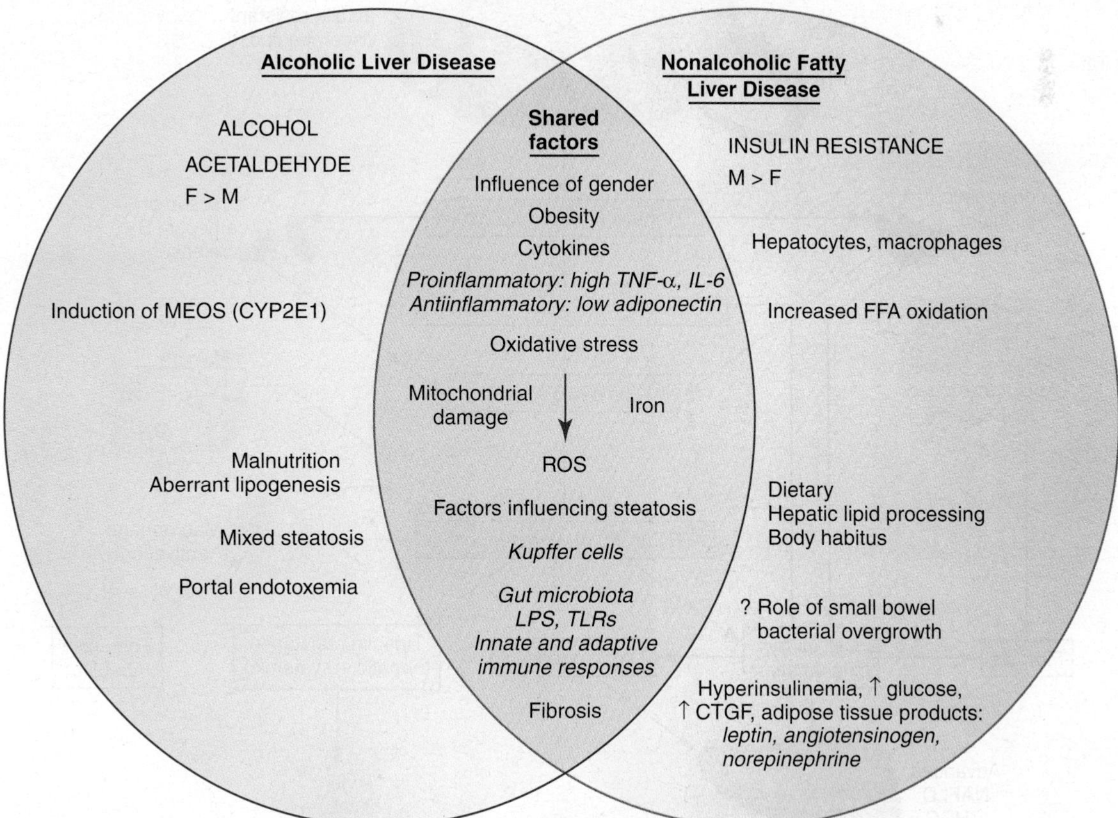

FIGURE 50.24 Alcohol-induced liver disease and nonalcoholic (obesity- and insulin resistance–related) fatty liver disease share several pathogenetic processes, which are shown in the overlapping portions of the Venn diagram. Conditions unique to each disease are highlighted in the nonoverlapping sections. *CTGF,* Connective tissue growth factor; *CYP2E1,* cytochrome P450 2E1; *F,* female; *FFA,* free fatty acids; *IL-6,* interleukin-6; *LPS,* lipopolysaccharides; *M,* male; *MEOS,* microsomal ethanol-oxidizing system; *ROS,* reactive oxygen species; *TLRs,* Toll-like receptors; *TNF-α,* tumor necrosis factor-α; ↑, increased levels.

of NAFLD.[174] Studies have demonstrated production of selected chemokines by the epithelial components of the ductular reaction in advanced NAFLD.[175] Leptin, another adipokine produced by peripheral adipose tissue, serves an important function in the control of satiety and appetite, and is essential for fibrogenesis. Disorders of leptin may result in severe insulin resistance and NASH, which may be partially countered by leptin replacement therapy.[176,177]

The amount of visceral adipose tissue increases with the age-related loss of estrogens and androgens in women and men. In men, this may be an early step in the alteration of insulin metabolism and progression to the metabolic syndrome.[178] In several autopsy studies, increasing patient age correlated with development of hepatic steatosis.

Pathology

On gross examination, livers from cases of NAFLD are similar to those with ALD. Noncirrhotic fatty livers are typically enlarged, yellow in color, and have a greasy consistency. Cirrhotic livers may be either small or enlarged in size. In cirrhosis, the fat may be irregularly distributed within the liver nodules, with yellow-colored nodules alternating with tan-colored nodules.

Features of NAFLD in morbidly obese and superobese (BMI ≥40 kg/m^2) individuals[144] may be different than in non–morbidly obese patients. However, most objective scientific studies are based on obese patients; thus the following discussion is based on this population of patients, unless stated otherwise.

The histological injury pattern of noncirrhotic fatty liver disease in adults, regardless of the cause, initially involves zone 3 hepatocytes (Fig. 50.26). In cirrhosis, steatosis and steatohepatitis may or may not persist. Table 50.6 outlines

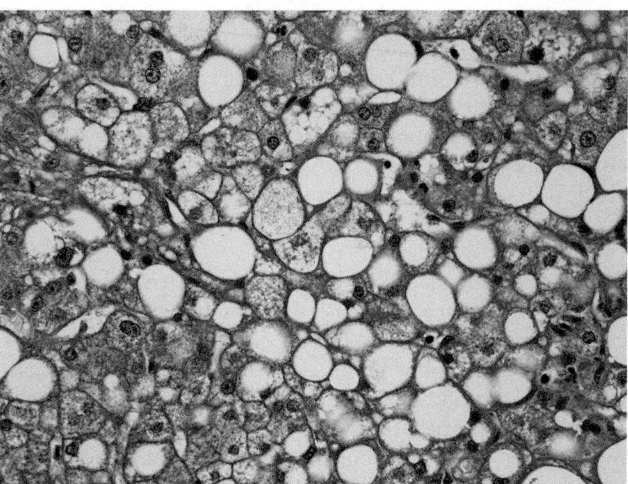

FIGURE 50.26 Mixed large- and small-droplet steatosis and mild ballooning are seen in zone 3 in a liver biopsy demonstrating steatohepatitis.

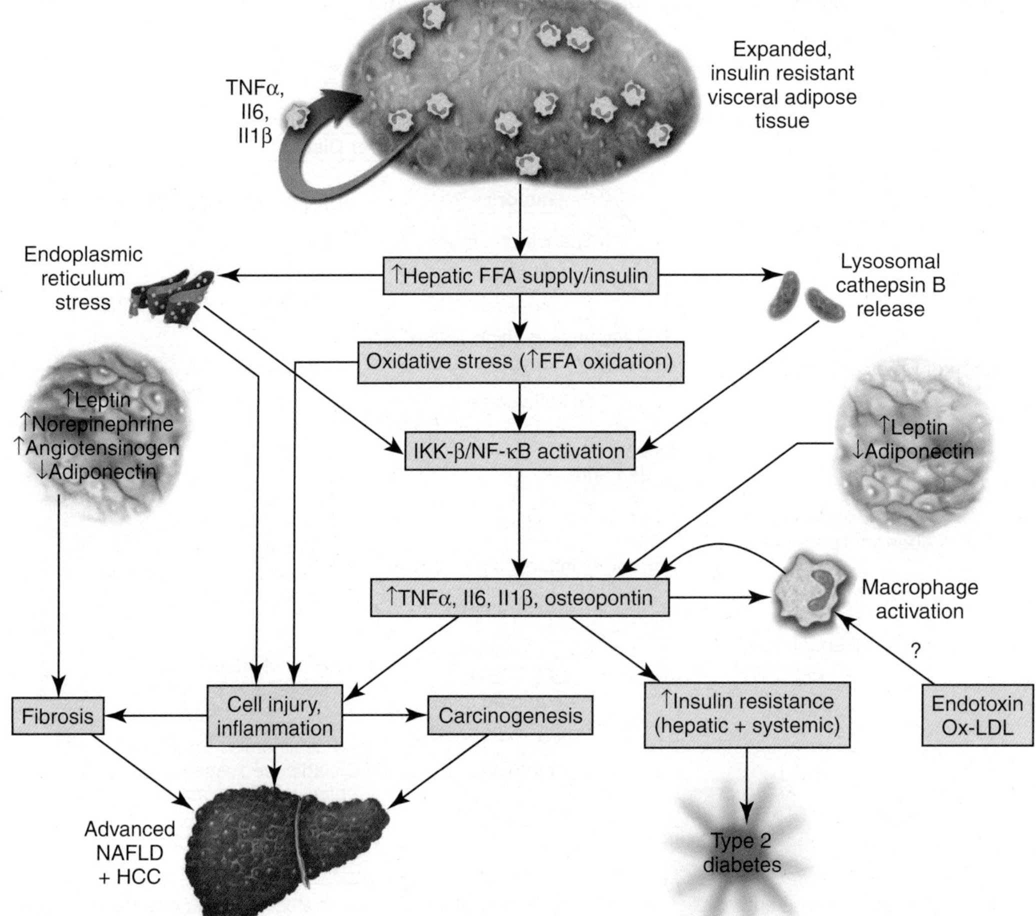

FIGURE 50.25 Possible pathways involved in the pathogenesis of nonalcoholic fatty liver disease. *FFA,* Free fatty acids; *HCC,* hepatocellular carcinoma; *IL,* interleukin; *NAFLD,* nonalcoholic fatty liver disease; *TNF-α,* tumor necrosis factor-α. (*From Day CP. From fat to inflammation. Gastroenterology. 2006;130:207-210.*)

TABLE 50.6 Clinical, Laboratory, Gross, and Histological Features of Alcoholic and Nonalcoholic Fatty Liver Disease		
Characteristics	**Alcoholic Fatty Liver Disease**	**Nonalcoholic Fatty Liver Disease**
Symptoms	Fatigue and anorexia with alcoholic hepatitis and cirrhosis	Usually none Abdominal discomfort or right upper quadrant pain with hepatomegaly
Signs	Fever and jaundice in alcoholic hepatitis	Acanthosis nigricans Hepatomegaly may not be palpable as a result of obesity
Aminotransferases	AST > ALT by a ratio of 2:1	ALT > AST, ratio may flip with cirrhosis
Bilirubin	Elevated in alcoholic hepatitis	Normal bilirubin until cirrhotic decompensation
Hematological changes	Leukocytosis common Erythrocyte mean corpuscular volume increases	Normal
Pathological Changes in Patients Without Cirrhosis		
Gross Features	Usually enlarged, soft, yellow, greasy liver	May be indistinguishable from noncirrhotic alcohol-induced liver disease
Histological Features		
Macrovesicular steatosis, zonal or diffuse	± (Zone 3 or diffuse)	*Required:* zone 3 or diffuse in adults; diffuse or zone 1 in children
Mixed large- and small- droplet steatosis	±	±
Nonzonal patches of true microvesicular steatosis	±	±
Steatohepatitis	±	±
Hepatocellular ballooning	±	±
Acidophil bodies	+	+
Megamitochondria	±	±
Mallory-Denk bodies, zone 3	±	±
Thick, ropy	More likely	Less likely
Thin, wispy	Less likely	More likely
With satellitosis	More likely	Less likely
Portal chronic inflammation	±	± (may be prominent in advanced stage)
Portal acute inflammation	± (accompanies ductular reaction, implies cholangiolitis, pancreatitis)	–
Lipogranulomas, portal or lobular	±	±
Glycogenated nuclei	±	±
Ductular reaction	Periportal, pericentral	Periportal at advanced stage
Iron: hepatocellular, zone 1 > zone 3	± (may be significant)	± (usually mild)
Iron: RES cells, punctate, panacinar	±	±
Fibrosis: zone 3 perisinusoidal	±	±
Dense, diffuse	More likely	Less likely
Delicate	Less likely	More likely
Dense perivenular fibrosis	+	–
Periportal stellate fibrosis	+ (with ductular reaction, acute inflammation)	–
Alcoholic foamy degeneration (pure microsteatosis)	+	–
Sclerosing hyaline necrosis, zone 3	+	–
Veno-occlusive lesions	+	–
Canalicular cholestasis, cholestatic rosettes	+	–
Pathological Changes in Patients with Cirrhosis		
Gross Features	Liver firm throughout; may be shrunken or quite large; may be cholestatic; grossly visible foci of parenchymal extinction	Not distinguishable from other hepatitic forms of cirrhosis
Histological Features		
May retain or lose active lesions of steatohepatitis	+	+
May be a cause of cryptogenic cirrhosis	+	+
Copper deposition, periseptal hepatocytes	±	Uncommon
Hepatocellular iron, RES cell iron (patients without *HFE* mutation)	Common	±
α_1-Antitrypsin globules; increased MZ phenotype (?)	±	–

HFE, Hemochromatosis gene; *MZ alleles,* reduce α_1-antitrypsin levels and impair liver function; *RES,* reticuloendothelial system; +, present; ±, present or absent; –, absent.

the key gross and microscopic features of NAFLD compared with ALD.

Steatosis

By definition, steatosis is present in 100% of NAFLD patients. The minimum criterion for NAFLD is a finding of at least 5% macrovesicular steatosis. In adults, steatosis commonly begins in zone 3 hepatocytes, which contrasts with predominantly zone 1 steatosis in hepatitis C (Fig. 50.27) and in pediatric NAFLD patients.

Assessment of the degree of steatosis is usually based on a semiquantitative scale, by evaluating the percentage involvement of the liver parenchyma. This may be accomplished by classifying the degree of involvement of the hepatic lobules using three grades (0% to 33%, 33% to 66%, and >66%)[179] or by using a four-grade system to account for a less than 5% "normal" category (<5%, 5% to 33%, 34% to 66%, and >66%).[180] Quantitative methods include digital image analysis,[181] morphometry,[182] and stereological point counting.[183] Although image analysis of whole-slide images may someday replace semiquantitation, this and other quantitative methods remain research techniques.

Rarely, NAFLD may occur without any inflammation; this condition is termed *isolated steatosis*. More often, there are rare, scattered microgranulomas (i.e., Kupffer cell aggregates) or mild degrees of portal and/or lobular inflammation, a pattern termed *steatosis with inflammation*.[6] The presence of inflammation and steatosis alone are insufficient for a diagnosis of steatohepatitis, which is discussed in the next section.

Steatohepatitis

The minimal criteria for steatohepatitis are steatosis, combined with hepatocellular ballooning degeneration, and lobular inflammation (Fig. 50.28). In the vast majority of cases, steatosis involves at least 5% of the liver parenchyma. However, in cirrhosis, steatosis may be quite minimal or irregularly

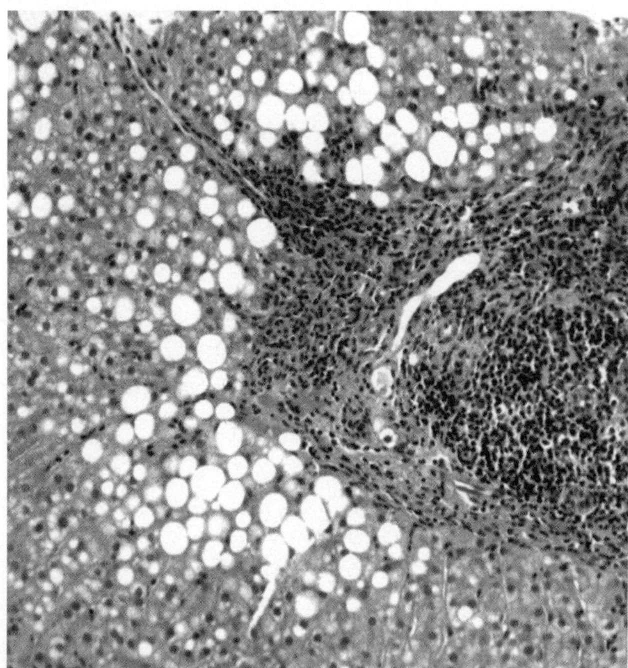

FIGURE 50.27 In a biopsy specimen from a patient with chronic hepatitis C, steatosis involves predominantly zone 1.

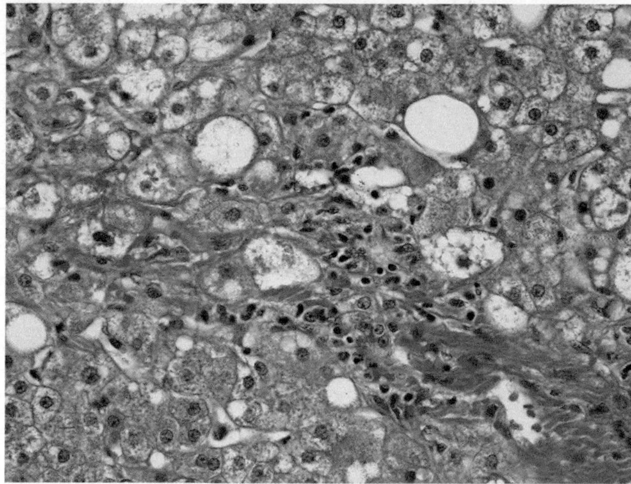

FIGURE 50.28 Photomicrograph shows the criteria for steatohepatitis: steatosis, ballooning, and mild lobular inflammation. However, the cause (alcoholic or nonalcoholic fatty liver disease) cannot be determined with certainty.

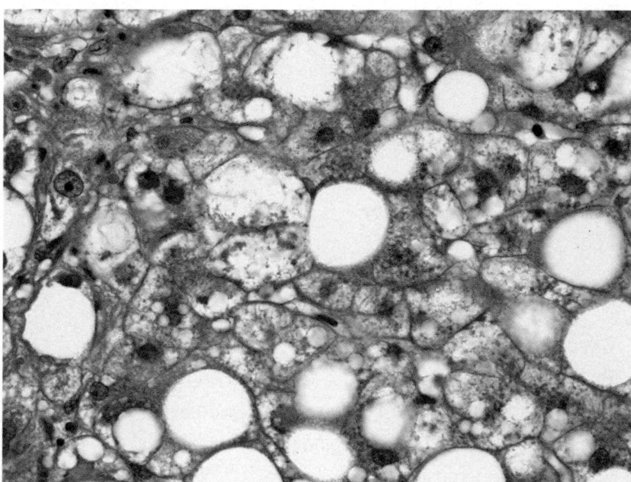

FIGURE 50.29 Ballooned cells in a background of steatosis. The ballooned cells have cytoplasmic clumps and irregular areas of cytoplasmic clearing.

distributed, although ballooning degeneration and inflammation are usually present. As with other forms of chronic liver disease, fibrosis is not required to establish a diagnosis of steatohepatitis. In the initial phases, steatosis is normally centered in zone 3. However, with progression, steatosis may involve the entire hepatic lobule. Nonzonal (irregularly distributed) steatosis may be seen in conjunction with advanced fibrosis.[184] Nonzonal patches of microvesicular steatosis may also occur in NAFLD (see Fig. 50.20), and this correlates with disease severity.[185] The degree and a pan-acinar distribution of steatosis is related to disease severity.[184]

Several histological types of hepatocellular injury may be seen in specimens from patients with NAFLD. These include ballooned hepatocytes (Figs. 50.29 and 50.30), apoptotic (acidophilic) bodies (Fig. 50.31), and foci of spotty necrosis (Fig. 50.32) formed of remnants of hepatocytes that have undergone lytic necrosis and surrounded by mononuclear cells and Kupffer cells. Areas of confluent and bridging necrosis are rare in NAFLD. The presence of submassive or

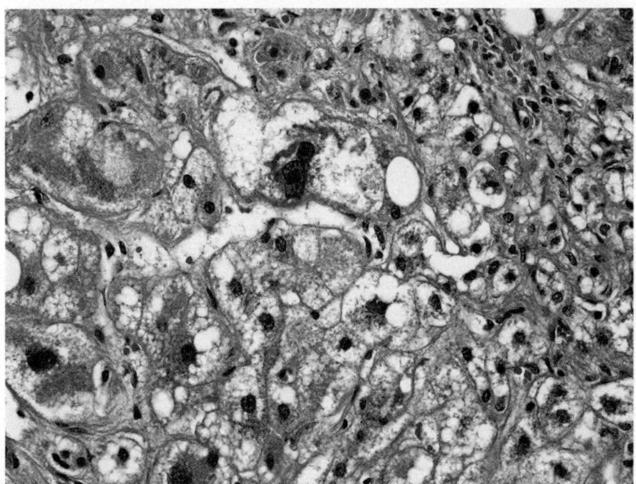

FIGURE 50.30 A large ballooned cell with a hyaline inclusion characteristic of a Mallory-Denk body dominates this part of acinar zone 3.

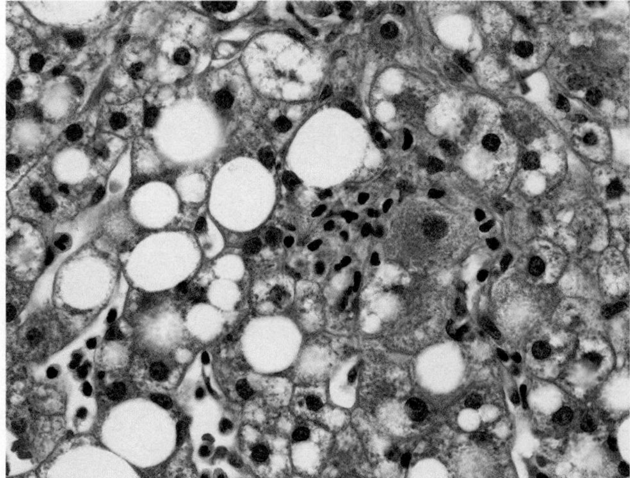

FIGURE 50.32 A cluster of lymphocytes and macrophages is in the center of the photomicrograph. Note the margination of inflammatory cells in nearby sinusoids.

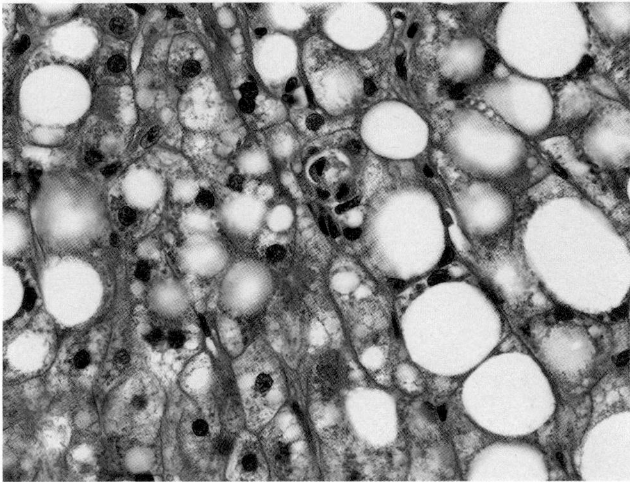

FIGURE 50.31 Apoptotic hepatocytes (acidophil bodies) may be seen occasionally in NAFLD and NASH.

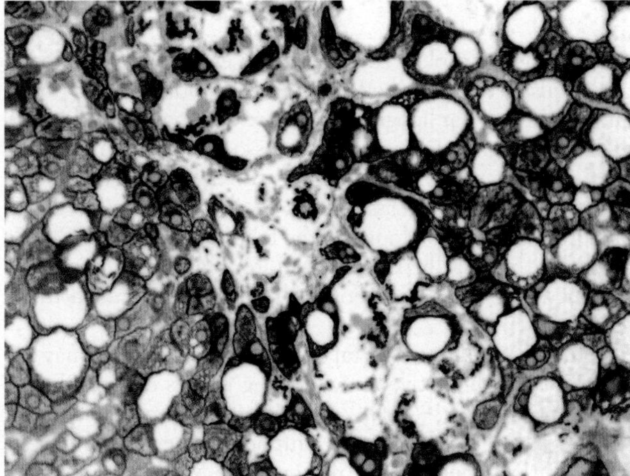

FIGURE 50.33 Keratin 8 and 18 (K8 and K18) immunohistochemistry highlights ballooned, empty-appearing hepatocytes in steatohepatitis caused by alcoholic or nonalcoholic liver disease, which contrasts with the normal, nonballooned hepatocytes that show cytoplasmic and membranous K8 and K18 immunoreactivity. Large fat droplets push parts of the cytoplasm aside in some steatotic hepatocytes, but the immunohistochemical pattern is not similar to that of ballooning. Mallory-Denk bodies, composed of the misfolded K8 and K18 filaments, stain positively within ballooned hepatocytes.

massive necrosis combined with features of steatohepatitis should always prompt a search for alternative etiologies.[4]

Hepatocyte ballooning is considered an essential, albeit sometimes challenging, histological feature of steatohepatitis.[43] Ballooned hepatocytes in NASH are similar to those seen in ALD (see Fig. 50.30). Ballooned cells are located predominantly in zone 3. They are commonly associated with perisinusoidal fibrosis[44] and secrete profibrogenic factors (see Fig. 50.2).[186] Loss of K8 or K18 immunoreactivity, either with or without ubiquitin staining, provides an objective histological marker for ballooned hepatocytes in steatohepatitis (Fig. 50.33).[30,44] PMNs may be associated with ballooned hepatocytes that contain MDBs *(satellitosis)*. Satellitosis (see Fig. 50.4) is less common in NAFLD than in ALD. In rare cases, hepatocyte ballooning may occur in the absence of significant steatosis or inflammation.[43] Specific immunophenotypes of activated lymphocytes correlate with disease activity.[187-189]

The number of apoptotic hepatocytes correlates with disease activity.[190] In fact, both serum and tissue markers of apoptosis are currently being evaluated as potential noninvasive diagnostic tools for fibrosis and NASH.[191,192] One study of NAFLD showed that positivity for the M30 antibody, which is directed against a caspase 3–cleaved K18 product, was identified in patients with steatohepatitis, but not in patients with steatosis or with a normal liver.[193]

The degree of lobular inflammation in NASH is usually mild. It can be either a mixture of both acute and chronic inflammation, or predominantly, or even exclusively, chronic. Inflammation results from innate and adaptive immune responses.[171] CD68-positive Kupffer cells are usually increased in zone 3.[188] Scattered lobular microgranulomas and lipogranulomas are commonly present. The former consists of clusters of Kupffer cells that are positive for periodic acid–Schiff stain with diastase digestion (d-PAS) and CD68. The latter

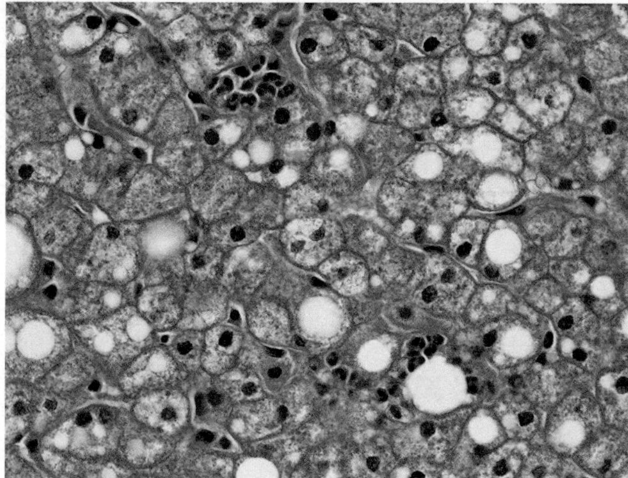

FIGURE 50.34 Clusters of neutrophils may be seen in liver resections and wedge biopsies taken during abdominal procedures. This is an artifact of the procedure rather than of any intrinsic liver disease and is known as *surgical hepatitis.*

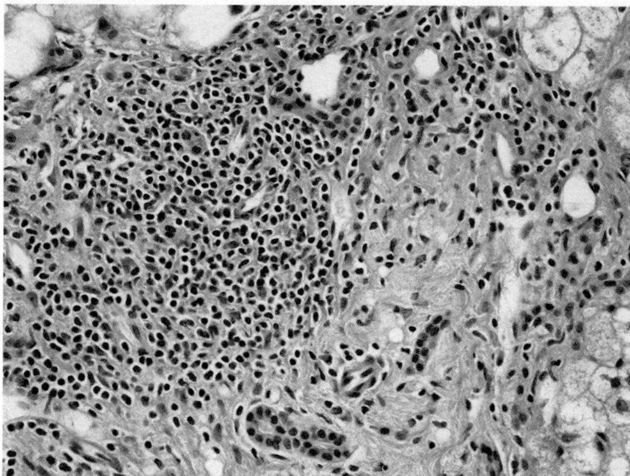

FIGURE 50.35 Prominent portal chronic inflammation can be seen in biopsies with advanced fibrosis.

consist of fat droplets surrounded or engulfed by mononuclear cells or eosinophilic PMNs (see Fig. 50.3). Large portal and/or perivenular lipogranulomas are common in NAFLD as well.[179] Lipogranulomas are often associated with a minimal amount of fibrosis. In this instance, the fibrosis should not be included in the overall assessment of disease stage (discussed later). PMNs may be found in the lobules. Clusters of PMNs near the terminal hepatic venule are common in surgically obtained biopsies, a condition referred to as *surgical hepatitis* (Fig. 50.34).[143]

Mild to moderate portal chronic inflammation may be seen in both the active and resolving phases of steatohepatitis (Fig. 50.35).[179,194,195] However, when portal chronic inflammation is marked or if lymphoid aggregates or extensive interface hepatitis is present, the pathologist should suspect the presence of a superimposed chronic liver disease, such as chronic viral hepatitis.[196] Increased portal inflammation in untreated patients with NAFLD correlates with increased histological activity and clinical severity. If the portal of inflammation is more than mild, it may be considered a marker of advanced disease.[195,197] However, moderate to severe portal chronic inflammation in NAFLD should always raise the possibility of a non-NAFLD concurrent disease. For instance, the finding of portal PMNs and cholangiolitis suggests alcohol-induced liver disease or biliary obstruction.[66]

Fibrosis and Cirrhosis

The characteristic pattern of early fibrosis in adult patients with noncirrhotic steatohepatitis is zone 3 pericellular (perisinusoidal) fibrosis, which results from deposition of collagen and extracellular matrix in the space of Disse (see Figs. 50.6 and 50.7). Ballooned cells may be seen in close relationship to areas of fibrosis. However, when isolated fibrosis is found, this is usually evidence of prior resolved steatohepatitis. Extensive dense perisinusoidal fibrosis associated with portal hypertension, as seen in some patients with ALD, has not been described in patients with NAFLD. The fibrosis pattern of diabetic hepatosclerosis, observed

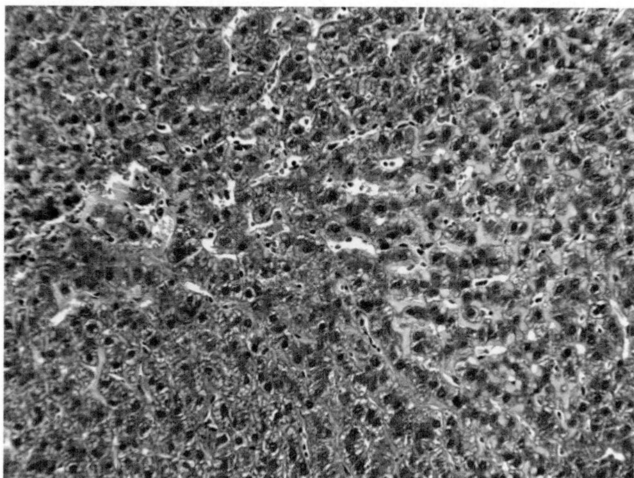

FIGURE 50.36 Diabetic hepatosclerosis. All reported cases are from patients with type 1 diabetes and end-organ damage from vascular complications. Note the lack of steatosis (trichrome stain).

in patients with type 1 diabetes who have severe microvascular injury, is also not normally seen in NASH. It is characterized by patchy, dense perisinusoidal collagen and basement membrane deposition in the absence of steatosis (Fig. 50.36).[198] With disease progression in NASH, fibrosis then usually develops in the periportal liver region (see Fig. 50.9). This may be followed by bridging fibrosis, which can be in a central-central, central-portal, or portal-portal pattern. Ultimately, cirrhosis develops (Fig. 50.37).

NAFLD-associated cirrhosis is most commonly macronodular or mixed macronodular and micronodular. After cirrhosis is established, active features of steatohepatitis, and even perisinusoidal fibrosis, may no longer be histologically apparent. This fact has been well documented in studies of serial liver biopsies and supports the theory that NAFLD is a major cause of cryptogenic cirrhosis.[199] Of course, active steatohepatitis may be observed in cases of established cirrhosis as well.[200]

Periportal and bridging fibrosis are often accompanied by a ductular reaction.[201,202] This consists of a proliferation of K7- and/or K19-positive hepatic progenitor cells, poorly formed

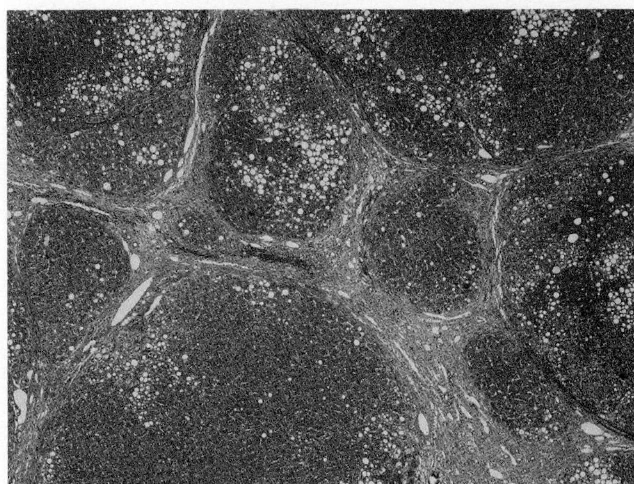

FIGURE 50.37 Irregular steatosis in a wedge biopsy showing cirrhosis and steatohepatitis (trichrome stain).

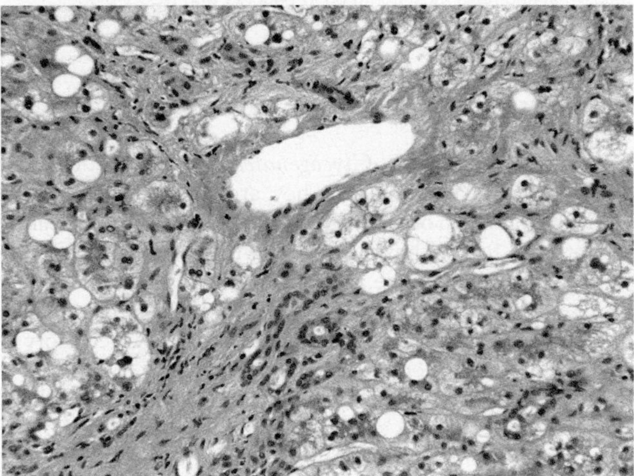

FIGURE 50.38 Projecting from the terminal hepatic venule in the center of the field is a septum with a ductular reaction. This is a common finding in alcohol-induced liver disease (ALD) and nonalcoholic fatty liver disease. The venule shows subendothelial thickening, which is a characteristic lesion of ALD. Even in this photomicrograph, dense perisinusoidal fibrosis is evident.

ductular structures, increased stromal matrix, and mild neutrophilic inflammation (Figs. 50.38 and 50.39).[203-205] A ductular reaction has also recently been reported near central veins as a marker of progressive fibrosis.[206] Because neo-angiogenesis may also develop near central veins as fibrosis develops (Fig. 50.40),[207] all of these findings may be linked to the process of anatomical remodeling of the liver acinus in NASH.

Isolated portal fibrosis (i.e., portal or periportal fibrosis without evidence of coexisting zone 3 perisinusoidal fibrosis) has been described in a subset of morbidly obese adults who have undergone bariatric surgery (Fig. 50.41).[143,208] However, it has not yet been clarified whether this finding represents a lesion within the spectrum of NAFLD common to nonmorbidly obese patients or whether it represents pathological resolution of injury in morbidly obese individuals.

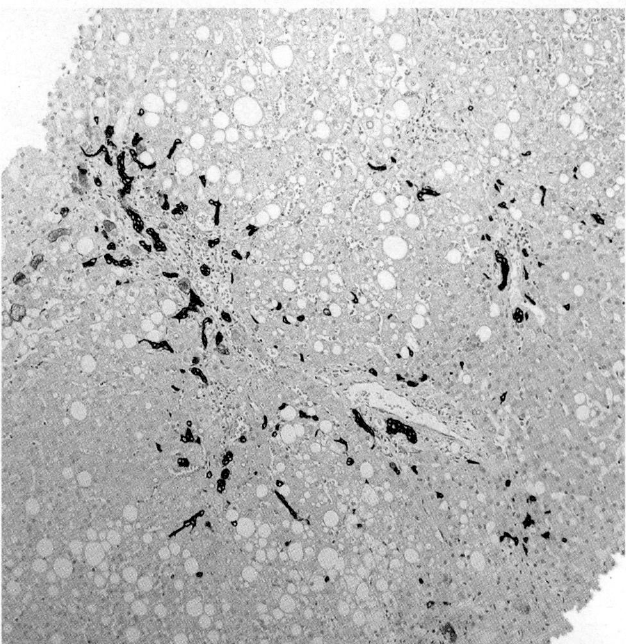

FIGURE 50.39 Keratin 7 immunohistochemistry highlights the ductular reaction adjacent to expanded portal tracts in the biopsy specimen of stage 2 steatohepatitis. Intermediate hepatocytes are occasionally seen. They are hepatocytes with submembranous keratin 7 positivity. (*Courtesy of A. Clouston.*)

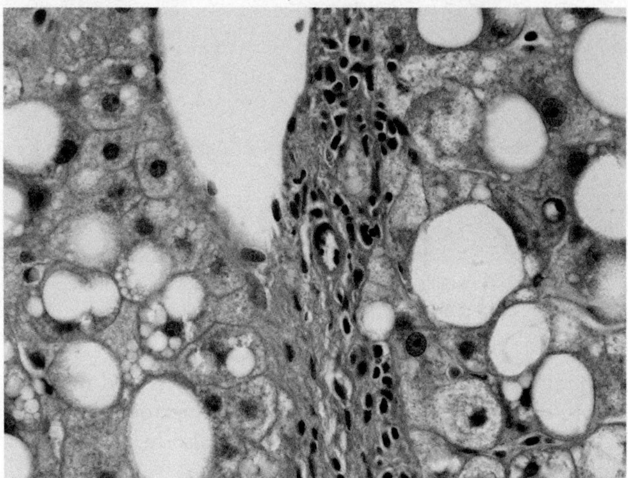

FIGURE 50.40 A small arteriole is seen near a central vein in a case of steatohepatitis with early bridging fibrosis.

Other Pathological Features of Nonalcoholic Fatty Liver Disease

Mallory-Denk Bodies. MDBs are aggregates of misfolded and hyperphosphorylated keratins 8 and 18.[209] Although MDBs are most often associated with ALD and NASH, they may also be seen in diseases in which copper accumulates in the liver and in patients with HCC.[210] In NAFLD, MDBs are most easily identified in ballooned hepatocytes, in which they may appear wispy and poorly formed or as more robust, ropy, and darkly eosinophilic globules. The Masson trichrome stain may be used to aid in the identification of MDBs (see Fig. 50.6). Immunohistochemical staining for K8 or K18 (see Fig. 50.33)

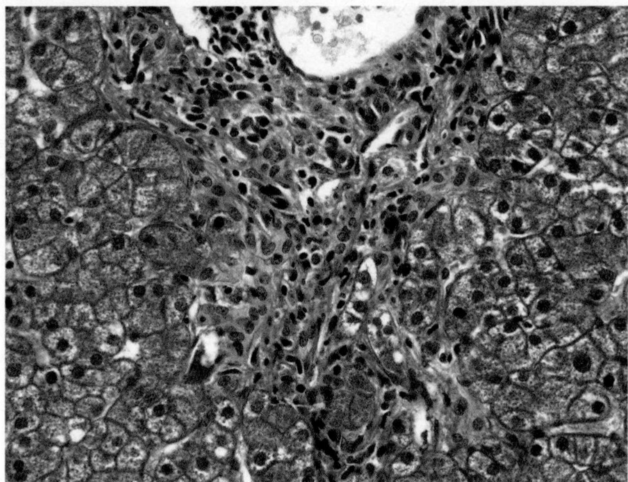

FIGURE 50.41 Periportal fibrotic expansion with ductular reaction and hepatocyte trapping in a wedge biopsy of liver with steatosis but no perisinusoidal or bridging fibrosis (trichrome stain).

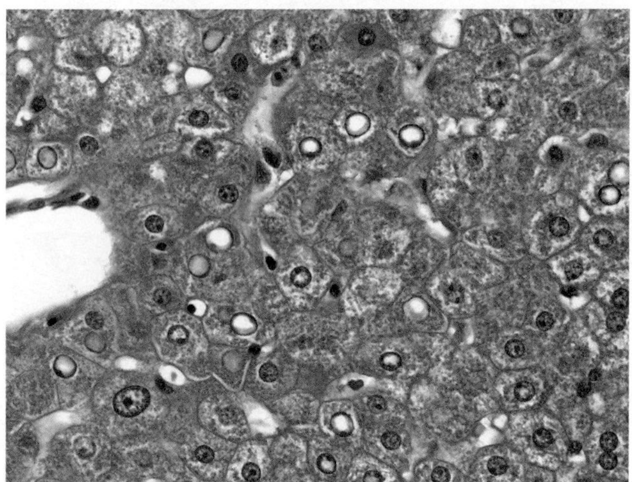

FIGURE 50.42 A small patch of hepatocytes with glycogen nuclei. Elsewhere the biopsy showed typical features of steatohepatitis.

ubiquitin may be positive in MDBs.[44,210] Increased numbers of MDBs correlate with higher degrees of necroinflammatory activity in patients with NAFLD[179] and also helps confirm a diagnosis of steatohepatitis.[89]

Megamitochondria. In NAFLD and NASH, megamitochondria are often apparent in hepatocytes that also contain microvesicular steatosis (see Fig. 50.20).[185] Ultrastructural studies of patients with NAFLD have shown that paracrystalline inclusions, loss of cristae, and nonzonality of megamitochondria are characteristic features of NAFLD.[211] Damaged mitochondria, including megamitochondria, accumulate in NASH, possibly as a result of impaired autophagy.[212] Megamitochondria are not unique to ALD or NAFLD and can be seen in drug and toxin injury, Wilson's disease, and pregnancy.

Iron Deposition. A mild degree of iron deposition in periportal, or periseptal, hepatocytes and punctate reticuloendothelial iron may be identified in up to 35% of NAFLD patients.[213] This feature may be related to disease severity.[213,214] Iron accumulation is likely the result

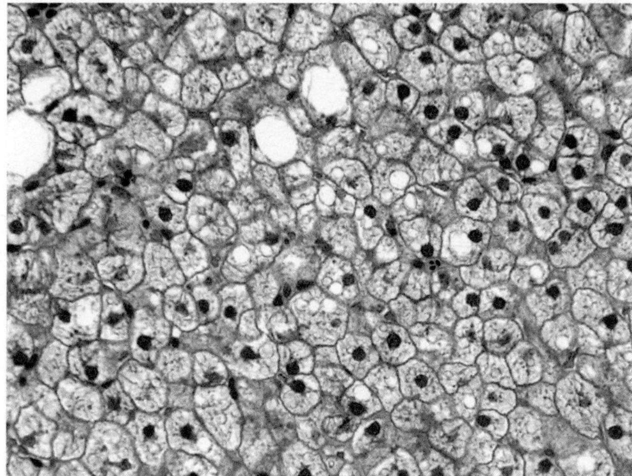

FIGURE 50.43 Glycogenic hepatopathy is characterized by diffuse involvement of hepatocytes with cytoplasmic glycogen deposition. There may be foci of macrovesicular steatosis, but this pattern is normally mild. This finding is most common in patients with type 1 diabetes.

of dysmetabolic iron overload from altered regulation of iron transport associated with steatosis and insulin resistance.[102]

Glycogenated Nuclei. *Glycogenated nuclei* are defined as clear, vacuolated nuclei. They are frequently found in NAFLD and often occur in clusters of cells in zone 1 liver or in scattered foci within the hepatocyte lobules (Fig. 50.42). Glycogenated nuclei are also common in diabetes, Wilson's disease, and in normal liver from children. Glycogenated nuclei are of uncertain clinical significance.[215] One theory is that they indicate hepatocyte senescence.[216]

Ductular Reaction. Ductular reaction occurs as a result of most forms of acute or chronic liver injury.[205] In NASH, this phenomenon correlates with the amount of portal-based fibrosis.[189] It has also been associated with insulin resistance and with hepatocellular[201] and ductular senescence.[202,204] The ductular reaction is a metabolically active process[202,204] that produces profibrogenic cytokines.[175] An extensive ductular reaction accompanied by other features of chronic cholestasis, such as pseudoxanthomatous changes of periportal hepatocytes, deposition of periportal copper, or bile duct injury, should alert the pathologist to the possibility of a superimposed chronic biliary disease such as chronic large duct obstruction, sclerosing cholangitis, or primary biliary cholangitis.

Hepatocellular Glycogen. Hepatocellular glycogen can accumulate in the cytoplasm of patients with NAFLD. Glycogen imparts a dull, grayish refractile appearance to the cytoplasm; this may occur in conjunction with steatosis or megamitochondria. In contrast with diffuse involvement by glycogenic hepatopathy, in patients with poorly controlled type 1 diabetes (Fig. 50.43),[217] this histological change in NAFLD may affect only patchy groups of hepatocytes. Because glycogen causes partial clearing of the cytoplasm, affected cells may mimic the appearance of ballooned hepatocytes. However, in glycogenated hepatocytes, the apparent clumping of cytoplasm is more regular compared with the usually more irregular cytoplasmic stranding and clumping characteristic of ballooned hepatocytes (Fig. 50.44).

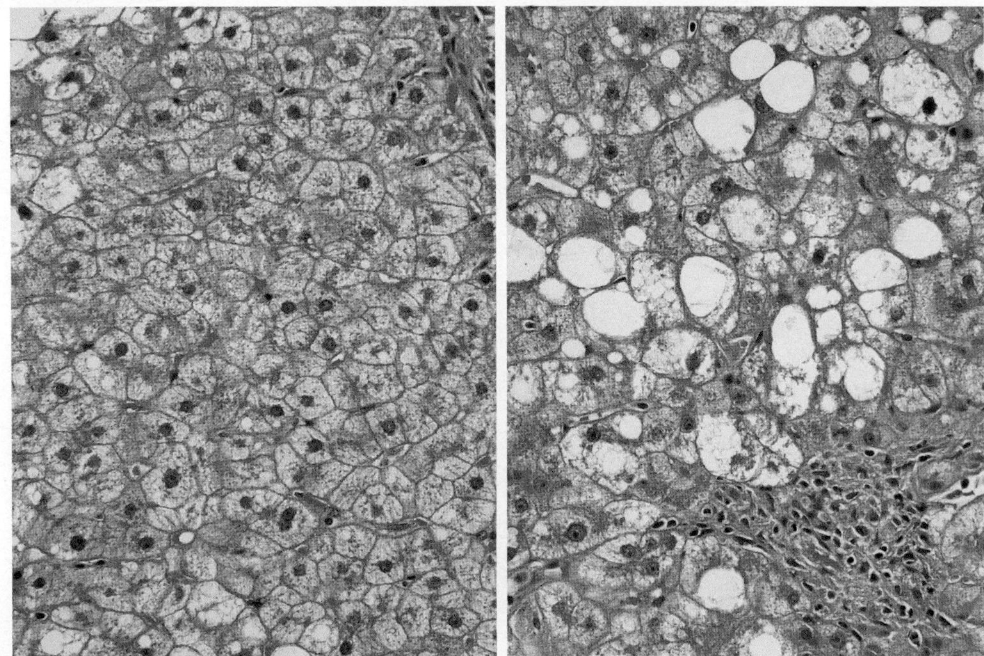

FIGURE 50.44 Comparison of glycogen accumulation and ballooned cells. A field of glycogenic hepatocytes *(left)* compared with the typical ballooned cells *(right)* in photomicrographs from the same case.

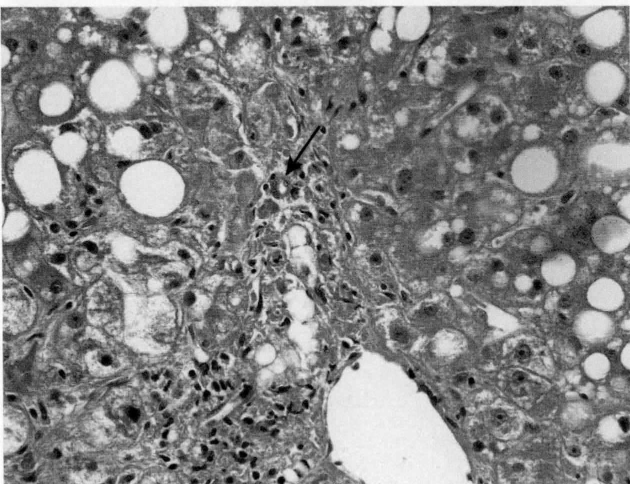

FIGURE 50.45 A small arteriole *(arrow)* is seen in the perivenular fibrosis in this case of NASH.

Vascular Alterations. Small intraacinar arteriolar branches can be seen in perivenular areas in patients with NAFLD, and it may occur with increased frequency as the degree of fibrosis increases (Fig. 50.45).[218] Since a ductular reaction has also been reported in NASH in perivenular regions,[206] care must be taken to avoid mistaking an area of perivenular fibrosis for a portal tract.

Treatment Effects. Resolution of steatosis, ballooning, lobular inflammation, steatohepatitis, fibrosis, and a decrease in the overall NAFLD activity score (NAS) have all been reported as potential positive effects of treatment (e.g., diet and exercise, medical, surgical) in various clinical trials that have been conducted in both adults and children.[219-222] Clinical trials have produced two additional observations. One is that resolution of the histological features of NAFLD may occur in placebo-treated patients,[222,223] and the second is that even after clinically successful treatment (Fig. 50.46), the relative degree of portal inflammation may actually increase in degree.[224] Laboratory values (rising aminotransferases)[194] and histological findings (recurrence of ballooning injury)[225] may provide evidence of recurrence after cessation of successful medical therapy.

Prognostic Lesions. Table 50.7 summarizes the results of clinicopathological studies that have correlated the histological features of NAFLD with fibrosis.[6,89,141,200,226-233] Using immunohistochemistry to demonstrate activated hepatic stellate cells, some studies have demonstrated correlation of this feature with advanced degrees of fibrosis in NAFLD.[234-236] One meta-analysis identified lobular inflammation as a predictive feature for fibrosis.[237] However, another subsequent meta-analysis that examined rates of fibrosis progression was not able to evaluate individual histological components as a result of a lack of consistent detail among the various studies.[238] Portal chronic inflammation is associated with advanced disease both histologically and clinically.[195,197] Infiltration of macrophages into portal areas was noted to precede the development of portal fibrosis in one study.[189] Steatosis has been shown to increase progressively with the degree of fibrosis up to the point of bridging fibrosis, but it later was shown to decrease with progression to cirrhosis.[89]

There is strong interest in the development of serum biomarkers and noninvasive imaging tests to diagnose NASH and the degree of fibrosis in NAFLD.[15] Calculated fibrosis indices, based on routine laboratory tests, can be used to estimate fibrosis, predict outcomes, and assess the fibrosis stage.[15,239,240] In patients with NAFLD, the presence of the metabolic syndrome clinically was identified as a marker of histological activity,[241] but not with the degree of fibrosis in one study.[89] Common features to many studies are older patient age, the presence of diabetes mellitus, the degree of insulin resistance, and the presence of

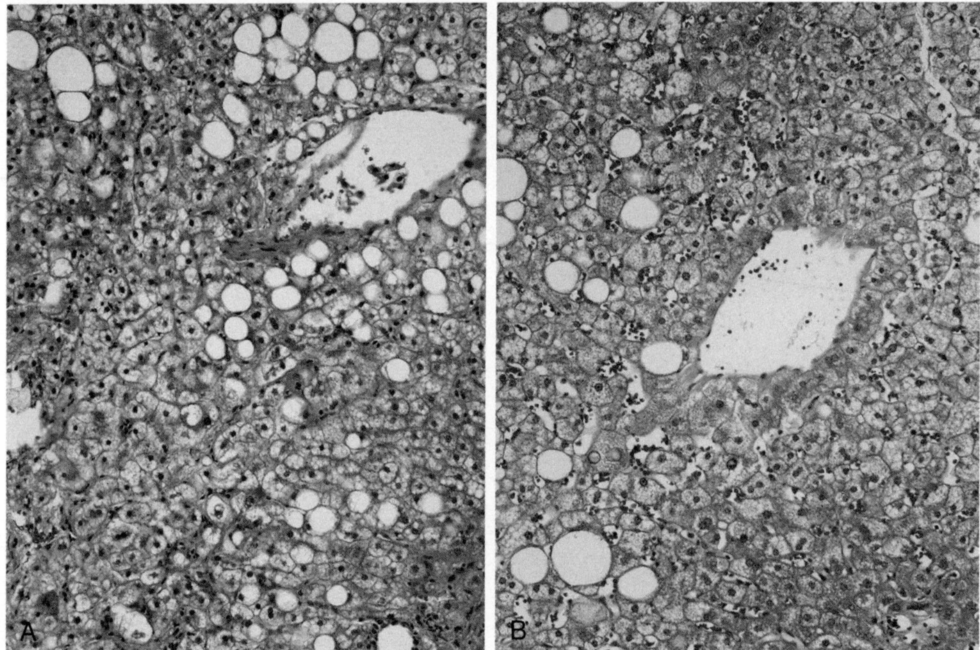

FIGURE 50.46 Improvement in histological injury after pioglitazone treatment. A, A field from the pretreatment biopsy with steatosis, ballooning, and inflammation. **B,** In the posttreatment biopsy the ballooning changes and inflammation have resolved, although steatosis remains.

TABLE 50.7 Histological Features of Nonalcoholic Fatty Liver Disease Associated with Fibrosis or Cirrhosis

Study	*N*	Steatosis	Lobular Inflammation	Ballooning/ Mallory-Denk Bodies	Other
Wanless and Lentz, 1990[141]	207	Yes	NA	NA/NA	
Matteoni et al., 1999[6]	98	Yes	Yes	Yes/yes	
Angulo et al., 1999[226]	144	No	No	Yes	
George et al., 1998[227]	51	Yes	Yes	NA	Stainable iron; C282Y *HFE* mutation
Shimada et al., 2002[200]	81	Yes	No	Yes	
Ratziu et al., 2000[228]	93/14*	Yes	Yes (with polymorphonuclear cells)	Yes	Four progressors: no evidence of portal fibrosis in first biopsy; necroinflammation in progressors only
Garcia-Monzon et al., 2000[231]	46	Yes	Yes	NA	
Gramlich et al., 2004[232]	132	Yes	Yes	Yes/yes	
Fassio et al., 2004[233]	106/22*	No	No	NA	Steatosis decreased or no change with fibrosis progression
Adams et al., 2005[229]	103/103*	No	No	No/no	Low initial fibrosis stage associated with higher rate of progression
Ekstedt et al., 2006[230]	129/68*	Yes (in first biopsy)	No	No/no	100% negative predictive value for progression when less than stage 2 in first biopsy
Neuschwander-Tetri et al., 2010[89]	693	Yes	Yes	Yes	Portal inflammation

**Repeat biopsies.*
HFE, Hemochromatosis gene; *NA,* not applicable.

elevated aminotransferase levels in both morbidly obese and non–morbidly obese populations.[11,89,228,237,242] The ratio of PMNs to lymphocytes has been shown to correlate with the degree of histological activity and with fibrosis in liver biopsies, but this has not been shown to be sufficiently predictive enough to be used in clinical practice.[243]

One proteomic approach has shown weight-dependent variations in NAFLD and NASH.[244] A meta-analysis of single-nucleotide polymorphism (SNP) studies has shown that the I148M variant of the *PNPLA3* gene is associated with increased histological severity as well as fibrosis in NAFLD.[245] This area of investigation will continue to grow because liver biopsies cannot be used to screen at-risk populations.

Natural History and Treatment

Long-term studies regarding the natural history of NAFLD, using paired biopsies, are challenging and few in number. Initially, there was general consensus that steatosis alone was nonprogressive.[246] It is now clear that up to 58% of patients with steatosis alone will eventually develop more disease activity and fibrosis over time.[247] In the presence of NASH, fibrosis progresses to cirrhosis in 31% to 42% of individuals during a period of 3.2 to 13.7 years.[248-250] Across the globe, the risk of HCC in patients with cirrhosis caused by NAFLD ranges from 2.4% to 12.8% over follow-up periods ranging from 3.2 to 7.2 years.[251] A recent meta-analysis of paired biopsy studies suggested that nonfibrotic NAFLD patients progress to fibrosis in about 14 years on average, while the average fibrosis patient progresses about one fibrosis stage every 7 years.[238] NASH and its associated fibrosis may also regress over time, as documented by observation of placebo-treated patients in various clinical trials.[220,221,223] In a recent long-term follow-up study, 21% of patients with steatosis alone progressed to definite steatohepatitis, and 44% progressed from no fibrosis to some fibrosis over an average of 4.9 years.[252] Because NASH has been demonstrated to respond to changes in lifestyle, disease activity and fibrosis may fluctuate with changes in weight and control of diabetes.[247,253] A post-hoc analysis of biopsy data from two phase III studies in the United States showed that improvement in fibrosis was associated with improvements in steatosis, ballooning, and portal inflammation regardless of whether the patient was in a placebo or treatment arm.[222] Similar findings were identified in a natural history study of 446 untreated patients.[252] Over the long term, disease fluctuations likely reduce the predictive power of baseline histological changes, but fibrosis stage remains a powerful and independent predictor of long-term outcome, even at the lowest detectable fibrosis stage.[254]

The literature is mixed in terms of the effect of NAFLD on overall survival. Some studies have shown no difference compared with the general population for individuals with cirrhosis caused by non-NAFLD forms of chronic liver disease.[230,255] In contrast, studies from multiple countries have shown that patients with NAFLD have a poorer overall survival rate.[229,248,256] Compared with patients with advanced chronic hepatitis C, NAFLD patients with advanced fibrosis or cirrhosis, have lower rates of liver-related complications and HCC[255] but similar overall mortality rates.[257] Obesity,[226] smoking,[254] increasing patient age,[226,228,254] and diabetes[11,226,254,258,259] are risk factors for progression of steatosis to steatohepatitis or cirrhosis. Caffeine consumption is protective against the development of fibrosis,[260-262] as is statin use.[254] The effect of alcohol on NASH is a subject of debate. Cross-sectional studies suggest that alcohol drinkers have less fibrosis than nondrinkers.[12] However, longitudinal studies have suggested that concurrent drinking is not beneficial in NASH.[14,263] Cardiovascular disease may be the leading cause of death of patients with advanced NAFLD.[230,254,264,265]

NASH-related cirrhosis, or liver failure, is the third most common indication for liver transplantation in the United States (over 20% in 2015) and has grown at an annual percentage change of 1.88% between 2012 and 2017.[266,266a] NAFLD and NASH accounted for 7.5% of deaths caused by chronic liver disease in the United States from 2007 to 2016. However, since 2013, deaths related to chronic hepatitis C have decreased, whereas deaths caused by NAFLD have increased at an annual percentage change of 11.3%.[267]

The risk of HCC among patients with NASH is not well known,[268] but it is a growing concern.[7,269-271] Patients with NAFLD are predicted to add 5800 cases of HCC per year in the United States, at an annual cost of $523 million.[272] Most cases are expected to develop in older patients.[272] Screening only patients with cirrhosis may not be adequate because several groups have reported HCC in noncirrhotic patients.[273-275] Benign liver tumors, such as adenomas and adenomatosis, have been reported in patients with various degrees of NAFLD,[276,277] and inflammatory hepatocellular adenomas are more common in patients with obesity.[278]

Trials of treatment for NAFLD have not been a great success, with the possible exception of weight-loss surgery.[279] Trials are aimed primarily at the presumed causes of disease and have included lifestyle interventions with weight loss and exercise, control of insulin sensitivity, and interventions broadly directed at reducing inflammation, hepatocyte injury, fibrosis, and hyperlipidemia.[165] Currently, there are no drug therapies approved by the U.S. Food and Drug Administration (FDA) for NAFLD or NASH. Clinical trials have evaluated the efficacy of several agents, including the insulin-sensitizing PPAR-γ agonist pioglitazone, either with or without antioxidants; antidiabetic drugs such as metformin and thiazolidinediones; the antioxidants betaine, ursodeoxycholic acid, and vitamins E and C; antifibrotic angiotensin-converting enzyme inhibitors and receptor blockers; bile acid receptor modulators; and the TNF-α antagonist pentoxifylline. Several reviews detail the trials and results.[280,281]

FATTY LIVER DISEASE IN VARIOUS PATIENT GROUPS

Concurrent Alcoholic and Nonalcoholic Fatty Liver Disease

Coexistence of NAFLD and ALD has been recognized as a significant risk factor for progression.[282] However, the contribution of each component cannot be determined histologically.

Alcohol use by individuals with NAFLD remains controversial. Modest alcohol intake protects against the effects of insulin resistance in morbidly obese individuals[11] and is associated with a decreased prevalence rate of steatohepatitis in non–morbidly obese patients with NAFLD.[12] However, moderate alcohol consumption correlates with progression of fibrosis in NAFLD.[14,263]

Fatty Liver Disease in Patients with Other Liver Disorders

Clinical complications of acute viral hepatitis A, B, and C, chronic hepatitis C, and acetaminophen toxicity are all seen occasionally in patients with alcoholism. These disorders require careful consideration by the pathologist when examining liver biopsy material with unusual findings.

The outcome of ALD with concurrent acute viral hepatitis depends on the stage of ALD. Patients with advanced-stage ALD may have a more severe course of acute viral hepatitis. Patients with chronic HCV infection and ALD show faster fibrotic progression than patients with only one of these conditions.[283] The histological features of superimposed hepatitis caused by HCV are similar to those seen in nonalcoholic patients (see Chapter 47), with more portal inflammation and portal-based fibrosis. Patients with alcohol dependency are also at risk for chronic pancreatitis and biliary obstruction separate from the changes of ALD, both of which may manifest histologically with cholangiolitis. The coexistence of ALD with hereditary hepatic iron overload and with α_1-antitrypsin deficiency results in findings typical of those specific disorders in addition to those of ALD.

The coexistence of NAFLD with other chronic liver diseases is of interest because of any number of factors, such as its possible influence on the progression of these other liver diseases, the high prevalence of chronic HCV infection, the increased incidence of diabetes among patients with HCV infection,[284] and the challenges of diagnosing NAFLD in the setting of other chronic liver disorders.[196,285] Several studies have shown a negative impact of steatosis and insulin resistance on the progression of disease in patients with either HCV infection or hereditary hemochromatosis.[286] In one series, 2.6% of more than 3000 nonallograft liver biopsies identified concurrent steatohepatitis (defined in this study as "steatosis combined with zone 3 perisinusoidal fibrosis") in patients with other types of chronic liver disease, such as hepatitis C, hemochromatosis, α_1-antitrypsin deficiency, or autoimmune hepatitis.[196]

Chronic hepatitis C is the most common chronic liver disease diagnosed with concurrent NASH (5% to 9% of chronic hepatitis C cases).[196,287] A diagnosis of NASH in the context of chronic viral hepatitis relies on the unique characteristics of NASH (zone 3 perisinusoidal fibrosis and hepatocyte ballooning), in addition to steatosis and lobular inflammation (Fig. 50.47).[196]

Rarely, clinical and histological features of either autoimmune hepatitis or primary biliary cirrhosis may be seen in patients with NAFLD.[196] Diagnosis of these concurrent liver disorders requires more than simply elevated levels of serum autoantibodies, and careful clinical-pathological correlation is required (Fig. 50.48).[94]

Fatty Liver Disease in Children

A variety of childhood genetic disorders are characterized by hyperinsulinemia, insulin resistance, and chronic liver injury. They include Bardet-Biedl, Alström, and Prader-Willi syndromes, lipodystrophy, and polycystic ovary syndrome.[288] Histological evaluation alone cannot define the cause of fatty liver disease in these cases. Other childhood disorders characterized by steatosis include HCV infection, rapid weight loss or starvation, and inborn errors of metabolism (e.g., urea cycle deficiency, fatty acid oxidation defects, organic acidemia, carnitine deficiency, cystic fibrosis, Wilson's disease).

The growing epidemic of childhood obesity has led to an increase in the prevalence of obesity-related conditions, such as the metabolic syndrome.[289] NAFLD, which strongly correlates with components of the metabolic syndrome such as visceral adiposity and insulin resistance,[112,290] is considered the most common cause of chronic liver disease in children throughout the world.[289] The prevalence of NAFLD among children increases with age and is higher among adolescent children.[291] Changes in sex hormones, insulin sensitivity, and adipose tissue distribution and function[292] during development; increased control over unhealthy food choices; and increased sedentary lifestyle with age are all considered

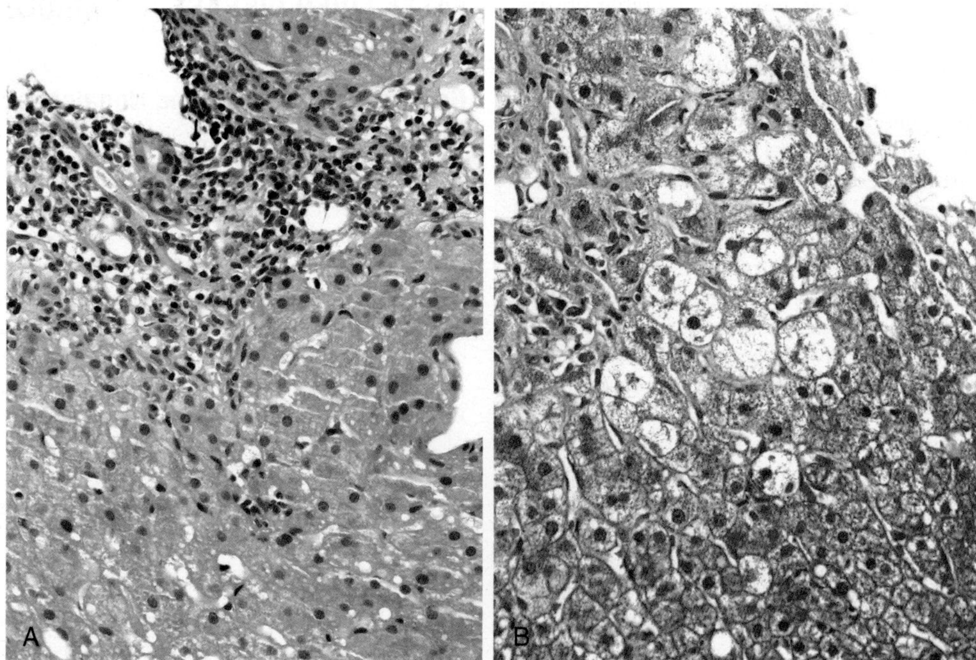

FIGURE 50.47 Chronic hepatitis C with steatohepatitis. A, The portal area shows dense lymphocytic inflammation and interface hepatitis. **B,** Perisinusoidal fibrosis, steatosis, and ballooned cells are shown around the central veins (trichrome stain).

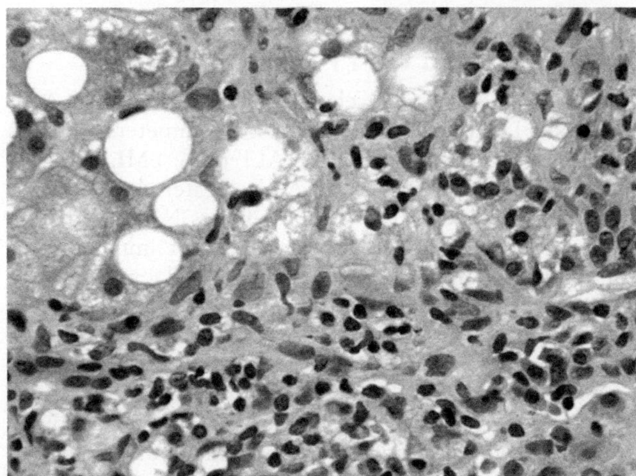

FIGURE 50.48 The abundance of plasma cells in the portal tracts and at the interface in conjunction with positive serology for antinuclear antibodies and an elevated value for total proteins confirms the diagnosis of autoimmune hepatitis in an obese woman. Other features of steatohepatitis and zone 3 perisinusoidal fibrosis were also seen, leading to a diagnosis of combined steatohepatitis and autoimmune hepatitis.

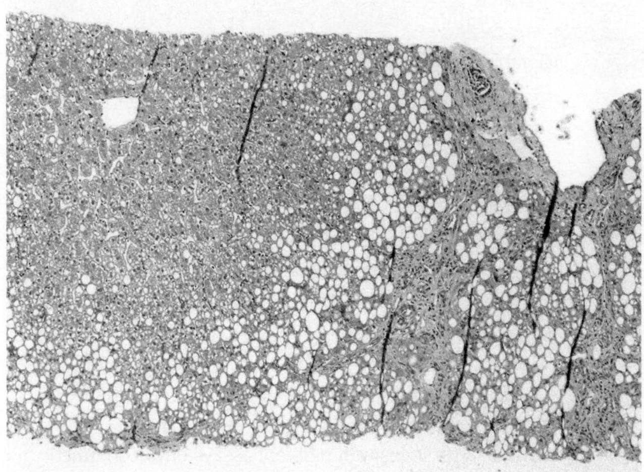

FIGURE 50.49 Fatty liver disease in a child is characterized by relative sparing of zone 3 and enlargement of the portal tract with mild portal inflammation. The steatosis is macrovesicular. No ballooning is seen.

influential factors. Equally disturbing for long-term liver disease is the convergence of binge alcohol drinking and adolescent obesity, both of which are on the increase.[293]

One retrospective histological study of autopsy livers from 742 unexplained deaths in individuals 2 to 19 years of age documented fatty liver disease in 13% overall, which corresponded to 17.3% of children in the 15- to 19-year age range, and 38% of all obese children.[142] The prevalence of fatty liver disease in children varied according to ethnicity: Hispanic (11.8%), Asian (10.2%), white (8.6%), and African American (1.5%).[142] This difference could be explained by the genetic background because a common variant of the *PNPLA3* gene associated with NAFLD in obese children is more common in Hispanics compared with African Americans.[142,161] NAFLD may result in cirrhosis in up to 5% of affected children. It is associated with shorter survival compared with age- and gender-matched control populations.[294]

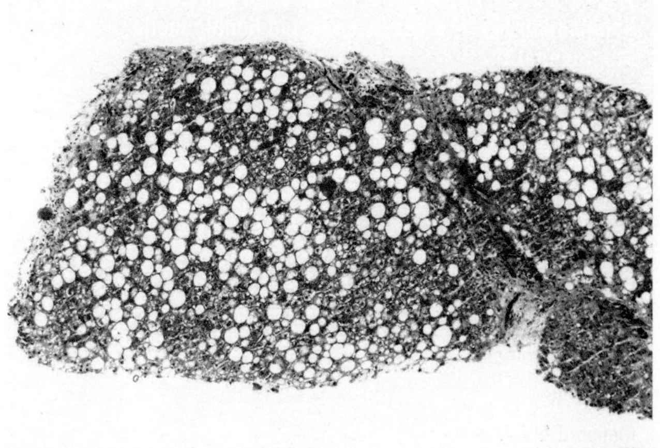

FIGURE 50.50 Portal-to-portal bridging fibrosis in a child with NAFLD (trichrome stain).

The histological features of pediatric NAFLD, especially in younger children, are different from those of adults (Fig. 50.49).[295,296] This has been documented repeatedly in studies from the United States,[295] Europe, [297] and Japan.[298] Liver biopsies from children with NAFLD show a predominance of portal-based chronic inflammation and fibrosis. The findings are usually more severe and often show zone 1 to panacinar steatosis, a lack of ballooning and MDBs, and a lack of zone 3 perisinusoidal fibrosis (Fig. 50.50) in contrast with typical adult NASH. This pattern of injury was identified in 51% of patients in a study by Schwimmer and colleagues,[295] and 27% of a multicenter cohort of patients seen by Patton et al.[290] This pattern is sometimes termed *type 2 (pediatric-type) NAFLD*,[295] while the NASH Clinical Research Network (CRN) uses the diagnostic term *borderline zone 1 fatty liver disease* in its publications to emphasize the zone 1 predominance of the injury and the lack of ballooning injury. [43] The typical zone 3 centric pattern of adult NASH was found in only 17% of cases in Schwimmer's study, but in 51% of the children in Patton's study.[290,295] Interestingly, the adult form of NASH was the predominant form of NAFLD observed in children and adolescents who underwent bariatric surgery in Saudi Arabia.[299] Table 50.8 compares the histological changes in adult and pediatric forms of NAFLD, whereas Table 50.9 compares the clinical findings. Cases with intermediate histological features have also been described in adolescents, with portal inflammation, periportal fibrosis, and a zone 3 distribution of steatosis.[295,300]

The type 2 pattern of NAFLD is more common among obese boys, younger individuals, and those of nonwhite ethnicity[295] and was confirmed by a later cohort.[290] The switch of the histological phenotype to an adult pattern in older children may reflect hormonal or endocrine changes related to puberty.[291] Further studies from Italy[297] and the United States[300] confirmed that only a minority of pediatric NAFLD biopsies (2.4% and 6.2%, respectively) showed a zone 3 pattern of steatosis. As prepubertal children become adolescents, there is a switch in steatosis from zone 1 to zone 3.[301] Although the data are only cross-sectional, the implication is that the predominant phenotype of NAFLD changes as children become adults.

TABLE 50.8 Histological Features of Adult and Pediatric Nonalcoholic Fatty Liver Disease and Nonalcoholic Steatohepatitis

Histological Feature	Adults	Children
Zone 3 predominance of histological lesions	+	–
Portal predominance of histological lesions	–	+
Steatosis	+ to +++	+++
Lobular inflammation	++	+
Portal inflammation	±	+ in most cases
Ballooning	±	–
Mallory-Denk bodies	+	–
Portal fibrosis	–*	+ in most cases
Zone 3 perisinusoidal fibrosis	+	–

**Isolated portal fibrosis occasionally is observed in morbidly obese adult patients with nonalcoholic fatty liver disease.*
+, Present; +++, present and usually severe; ±, present or absent; –, absent.

DIFFERENTIATING ALCOHOLIC FROM NONALCOHOLIC FATTY LIVER DISEASE

A clinical model was developed to help distinguish ALD from NAFLD based on a variety of parameters, such as mean corpuscular volume, AST/ALT ratio, BMI, and gender. An ALD/NAFLD index (ANI) greater than 0 favors ALD, whereas an ANI less than 0 favors NAFLD.[302] The same research group proposed the use of immunohistochemical markers. For instance, decreased expression of the insulin receptor and increased expression of protein tyrosine phosphatase 1B (PTPN1), a protein that acts as a negative regulator of insulin resistance, was demonstrated in patients with NAFLD compared with those with ALD.[303] This model has been tested successfully in a Korean cohort of patients, who showed improvement in the discrimination of the ANI by adding serum gamma-glutamyl transferase levels to the original ANI model.[304]

Table 50.6 highlights some of the clinical, laboratory, and pathological differences of ALD and NAFLD. Some data suggest that the degree of steatohepatitis is often more severe in ALD than in NAFLD, although this may

TABLE 50.9 Clinical Features of Nonalcoholic Fatty Liver Disease in Adults and Children

Feature	Adults	Children	Comments
Metabolic syndrome*	+	+	Sometimes called *insulin resistance syndrome* or *syndrome X*
Gender: M > F	Probably	+	Previously thought that F > M among adults
Central obesity	+	+	Central obesity is a greater risk because of various metabolic properties of visceral adipose tissue
Insulin resistance (calculated) or type 2 diabetes†	+	+	Linked to central obesity; in Asians, obesity measurements reflect different body habitus than in Westerners
Low adiponectin levels†	+	+	Nearly a universal association with NAFLD when assayed; adiponectin is lower in obese individuals with NAFLD compared with obese controls without NAFLD (adult and pediatric studies)
Ethnicity: Hispanic, Asian, white > African American	+	+	Several large series with different assays have confirmed these findings; poorly understood
Polycystic ovary syndrome†	+	+	Linked to insulin resistance
Lipodystrophy syndromes, acquired, congenital, and familial; generalized and partial†‡	+	+	Some forms of lipodystrophy because of leptin deficiency, some related to *PPAR-γ* mutations, and some acquired; all are characterized by different degrees and locations of subcutaneous fat loss, insulin resistance, acanthosis nigricans, polycystic ovary syndrome, and hepatic steatosis or steatohepatitis
Acanthosis nigricans†	Rare case reports	+ (common)	Skin condition directly linked to insulin resistance
Sleep apnea†	+	Possible but not studied	Studies link sleep apnea to obesity, hypoxic events, and insulin resistance
Pituitary or hypothalamic dysfunction†	+	+	Includes postsurgical or posttraumatic injury; adult-onset growth hormone deficiency
Petrochemical exposure	+		Well-documented case series from Brazil with biopsy evidence, rechallenge and long-term follow-up; insulin resistance in only 27% of cases
Autoantibodies (ANA, ASMA, AMA)§	±	Not reported	ANA is most commonly documented (6%-34%); AMA in 2% in only one series; ANA and ASMA in 0.4%-15%

**Metabolic syndrome as defined by the Adult Treatment Panel III.*
†Insulin resistance, type 2 diabetes mellitus, and obesity are associated features.
‡May occur in HIV-positive subjects treated with protease inhibitors. For review of lipodystrophies, see Walker UA, Schott M, Schebaum WA, et al. Acquired and inherited lipodystrophies. N Engl J Med. *2004;351:103-104.*
§Topic reviewed in Brunt EM. Pathology of fatty liver disease. Mod Pathol. *2007;20(suppl 1):S40-S48.*
AMA, Antimitochondrial antibody; *ANA,* antinuclear antibody; *ASMA,* anti–smooth muscle antibody; *F,* females; *M,* males; *NAFLD,* nonalcoholic fatty liver disease; *PPAR-γ,* peroxisome proliferator–activated receptor-γ; +, present; ±, present or absent; –, absent.

be a result of differences in clinical severity at the time of biopsy. Numerous MDBs, increased lobular infiltration by PMNs with satellitosis, and acute cholestasis are features more suggestive of ALD than NAFLD.[5,40] Reliable clinical information is, ultimately, essential in distinguishing ALD from NAFLD. Fig. 50.51 shows their shared and distinct histological features.

Features That Occur More Frequently in Alcoholic Liver Disease

Sclerosing hyaline necrosis, obliterative and inflammatory lesions of the hepatic outflow veins, alcoholic foamy degeneration, and acute cholestasis have all been described in noncirrhotic ALD, but not in patients with noncirrhotic NAFLD.[39,56] In contrast with NAFLD, alcoholic hepatitis may occur in the absence of steatosis in ALD.[39] Portal lipogranulomas are common in ALD.[69] In cirrhosis caused by ALD, regions of parenchymal extinction (septa) are often quite broad, in contrast with cirrhosis caused by NAFLD (see Fig. 50.10).

Features That Occur More Frequently in Nonalcoholic Fatty Liver Disease

In comparative histological studies, features that occur significantly more often in NAFLD than in ALD include marked steatosis, periportal hepatocellular glycogenated nuclei,[58,305] and lipogranulomas.[305] However, on an individual biopsy basis, the specificity of these histological features is questionable. There may also be qualitative differences in the type of collagen deposition in NAFLD or ALD. For instance, type I collagen is more common in NAFLD-associated steatohepatitis, whereas type III collagen is more common in ALD.[305]

GRADING AND STAGING OF FATTY LIVER DISEASE

Staging and grading systems for NAFLD have been modeled from chronic viral hepatitis. In general, in chronic liver disease, stage is represented by the degree of fibrosis. In contrast, the grade of liver disease consists of other features believed to be important in causing disease progression. In chronic hepatitis, grade is estimated by the degree of inflammation. In NAFLD, ballooning injury and steatosis are the main features of "grade," in addition to inflammation. In alcoholic hepatitis, the goal has been to link biopsy findings with short-term outcomes, usually survival. One such proposal for a novel histological score with prognostic value for alcoholic hepatitis is based on a semiquantitative assessment of histological parameters independently associated with short-term survival. These include lobular infiltration by PMNs, bile stasis, megamitochondria, and stage of fibrosis. The score has been validated in two independent cohorts from Europe and the United States.[67,306]

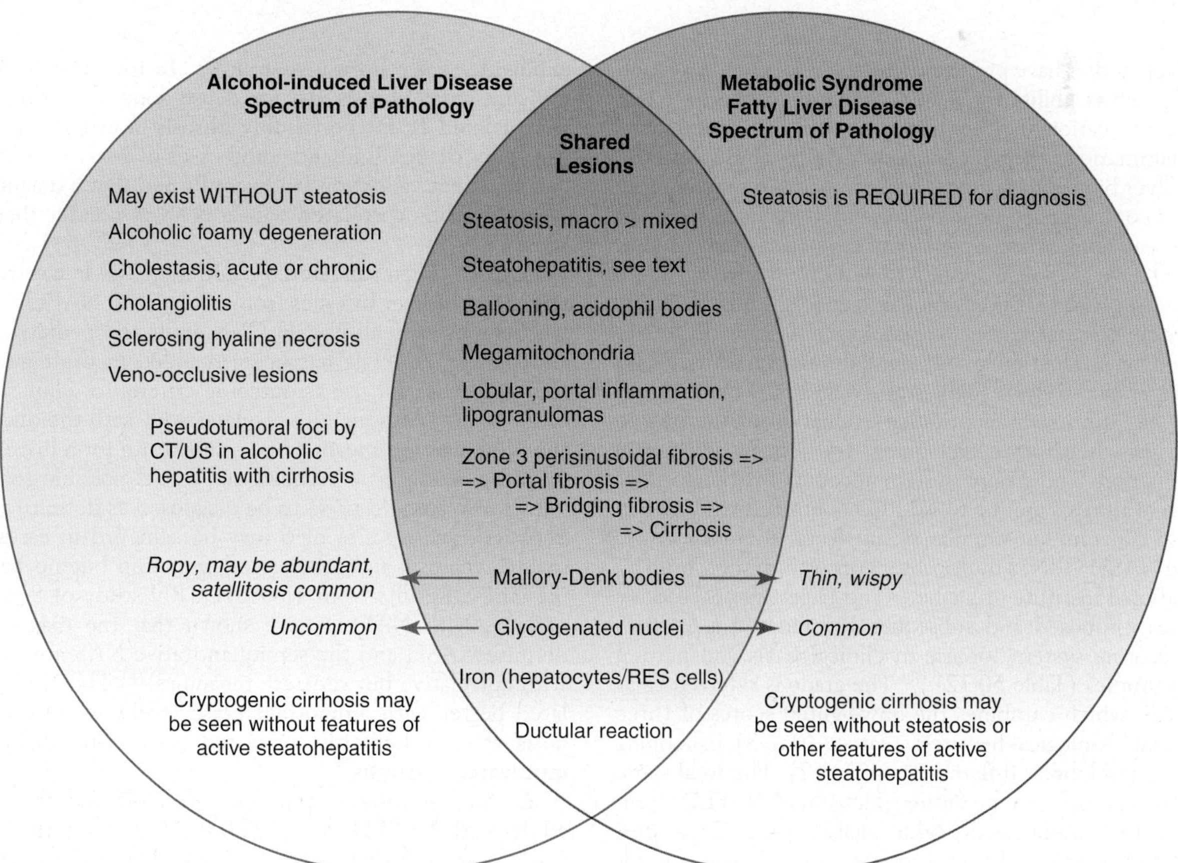

FIGURE 50.51 The Venn diagram highlights the shared *(overlapping)* and distinct *(nonoverlapping)* histological features of alcohol-induced liver disease and nonalcoholic fatty liver disease. *CT*, Computed tomography; *RES*, reticuloendothelial system; *US*, ultrasound.

TABLE 50.10 Brunt Grading System for Nonalcoholic Steatohepatitis

	Significant Histological Variables			
Lesion Grade	***Steatosis***	***Ballooning***	***Inflammation***	
Mild (grade 1)	1-2	Minimal	Lobular: 1-2	Portal: 0-1
Moderate (grade 2)	2-3	Mild	Lobular: 1-2	Portal: 1-2
Severe (grade 3)	2-3	Marked	Lobular: 3	Portal: 1-2
	Extent of Steatosis (1-3)	Extent of Lobular Inflammation (0-3)	Extent of Portal Inflammation (0-3)	
	1 ≤ 33%	0 None	0 None	
	2 33%-66%	1 <2 foci/20× field	1 Mild	
	3 ≥ 66%	2 2-4 foci/20× field	2 Moderate	
		3 >4 foci/20× field	3 Marked	

From Brunt EM, Janney CG, Di Bisceglie AM, Neuschwander-Tetri BA, Bacon BR. Nonalcoholic steatohepatitis: a proposal for grading and staging the histological lesions. Am J Gastroenterol. *1999;94:2467-2474.*

TABLE 50.11 Brunt Staging System for Nonalcoholic Steatohepatitis

Stage	Zone 3 Perisinusoidal Fibrosis	Periportal Fibrosis	Bridging Fibrosis	Cirrhosis
1	Focal or extensive	–	–	–
2	Focal or extensive	Focal or extensive	–	–
3	±	±	+	–
4	±	±	Extensive	+

+, Present; ±, present or absent; –, absent.

From Brunt EM, Janney CG, Di Bisceglie AM, Neuschwander-Tetri BA, Bacon BR. Nonalcoholic steatohepatitis: a proposal for grading and staging the histological lesions. Am J Gastroenterol. *1999;94:2467-2474.*

Other studies have proposed a histological grading system with predictive ability for alcoholic steatohepatitis based on semiquantification of either hepatocyte ballooning and lobular inflammation,[74] or ballooning and MDBs.[307] Because the use of liver biopsy to diagnose and predict outcome in ALD remains controversial, none of these systems have achieved widespread clinical use. Staging and grading systems used in NAFLD have also been applied to ALD.[40,265]

The first widely used semiquantitative grading and staging system for assessment of histological lesions in NASH is based on evaluation of necroinflammatory activity and fibrosis, respectively[179] (Tables 50.10 and 50.11). This system is based on semiquantitative evaluation of the degree of steatosis, hepatocyte ballooning, and lobular and portal inflammation. The staging system accounts for the specific pattern of fibrosis unique to NAFLD combined with assessment of concomitant vascular architectural alterations.

The NASH CRN, a multicenter consortium sponsored by the National Institute of Diabetes and Digestive and Kidney Diseases, proposed and subsequently validated a feature-based scoring system for use in clinical trials and natural history studies (Table 50.12).[180] The grade is referred to as the NAS, which combines the unweighted scores of three individual histological features: steatosis (0 to 3), ballooning (0 to 2), and lobular inflammation (0 to 2). The total score (0 to 8) encompasses the entire spectrum of NAFLD, from steatosis to steatohepatitis. Additional histological features, including the grade of portal inflammation[195] and recording of the zonal distribution of steatosis, make allowance for pediatric NAFLD. Staging follows the Brunt system, but subdivides early fibrosis as follows: 1a for delicate zone 3 perisinusoidal fibrosis, 1b for dense zone 3 perisinusoidal fibrosis, and 1c for portal-only fibrosis in order to account for pediatric NAFLD and some cases of bariatric NAFLD. A concurrent validation study confirmed that a diagnosis of steatohepatitis correlated with a NAS of greater than 5 in most cases.

NAS has been validated outside the CRN in a retrospective study of liver biopsies from adults with NAFLD[308] and has been used in all NASH CRN adult and pediatric clinical trials.[219-221,309] It has been included in draft guidance from the FDA for use as outcome criteria for clinical trials of NASH.[310] Although it correlates well with the diagnosis, the NAS was not meant to be a substitute for a histological diagnosis made by a pathologist.[180] It is possible for cases with a low NAS (3 or 4) to be diagnosed as definite steatohepatitis, and a score of 6 may be achieved in cases with severe steatosis and lobular inflammation but no ballooning injury. Results from a NASH CRN study of 976 adult patients with NAFLD have shown that the diagnoses of definite NASH and the semiquantitative NAS are distinct, with correlative but separate meanings.[311] The NAS correlated better with aminotransferase levels, while the diagnosis of steatohepatitis correlated better with diabetes in multivariate analysis.[311]

A third scoring system has been offered for use in adults with NAFLD and NASH. It differs from the NASH CRN system in that the score for lobular inflammation is graded as 0 to 2, and an activity score combines the ballooning score with lobular inflammation for a total that

TABLE 50.12 NASH Clinical Research Network Scoring System for Nonalcoholic Fatty Liver Disease

Steatosis Grade	Lobular Inflammation	Hepatocellular Ballooning
0 <5%	0 None	0 None
1 5%-33%	1 <2 foci/20x field	1 Few (mild, small)
2 33%-66%	2 2-4 foci/20x field	2 Many
3 >67%	3 >4 foci/20x field	
NAFLD Activity Score (NAS)		
0%-8 NAS = steatosis grade + inflammation grade + ballooning grade		
Fibrosis Stage		
0 None		
1a Mild (delicate) zone 3 perisinusoidal fibrosis, requires Masson trichrome stain to identify		
1b Moderate (dense) zone 3 perisinusoidal fibrosis		
1c Portal fibrosis only		
2 Zone 3 perisinusoidal fibrosis with periportal fibrosis		
3 Bridging fibrosis		
4 Cirrhosis		

NAFLD, *Nonalcoholic fatty liver disease;* NASH, *nonalcoholic steatohepatitis.*
From Kleiner DE, Brunt EM, Van Natta M, et al. Design and validation of a histological scoring system for nonalcoholic fatty liver disease. Hepatology. *2005;41:1313-1321.*

TABLE 50.13 Steatosis-Activity-Fibrosis (SAF) Scoring System for NAFLD

Steatosis Grade	Lobular Inflammation	Hepatocellular Ballooning
0 <5%	0 None	0 None: Only normal hepatocytes
1 5%-33%	1 <2 foci/20x field	1 Few: Clusters of hepatocytes with rounded shape and reticulated cytoplasm
2 33%-67%	2 >2 foci/20x field	2 Many: Enlarged hepatocytes (≥2x normal)
3 >67%		
Fibrosis Stage		
0 None		
1 Perisinusoidal or periportal fibrosis		
2 Perisinusoidal fibrosis and periportal fibrosis		
3 Bridging fibrosis		
4 Cirrhosis		

From Bedossa P, Poitou C, Veyrie N, et al. Histopathological algorithm and scoring system for evaluation of liver lesions in morbidly obese patients. Hepatology. *2012;56:1751-1759.*

TABLE 50.14 The SAF Diagnostic Algorithm for NAFLD and NASH

Steatosis	Ballooning	Lobular Inflammation	Diagnosis
0	0, 1, or 2	0, 1, or 2	Not NAFLD
1, 2, or 3	0	0	NAFL
		1	NAFL
		2	NAFL
	1	0	NAFL
		1	NASH
		2	NASH
	2	0	NAFL
		1	NASH
		2	NASH

From Bedossa P, Poitou C, Veyrie N, et al. Histopathological algorithm and scoring system for evaluation of liver lesions in morbidly obese patients. Hepatology *2012;56:1751-1759.*

varies from 0 to 4 (Table 50.13).[312] The steatosis grade (S), total activity (A), and fibrosis stage (F) are combined to provide a simple assessment of the pathology. In addition, the system includes an algorithm (FLIP algorithm) for classifying liver injury into diagnostic categories (Table 50.14).[312] This method has been demonstrated to be reproducible and useful for the stratification of adults with NAFLD.[313] It does not include a scale for evaluating portal inflammation.

Sampling error is an important issue in the histological diagnosis and semiquantitative assessment of NAFLD.[314,315] For example, studies that evaluated multiple biopsies from the right lobe[314] or from different lobes[316] showed excellent concordance for the grade of steatosis, moderate concordance for assessment of the degree of fibrosis, and fair agreement for the degree of necroinflammatory features. In NASH, as in chronic viral hepatitis,[317] the length of the tissue core affects the diagnostic yield. Definite NASH is more commonly diagnosed, and more extensive steatosis, lobular inflammation, and fibrosis is commonly observed in longer samples compared with shorter samples.[318] The needle diameter is also important.[315] Features of NAFLD, especially the degree of necroinflammation and fibrosis, may not be distributed uniformly throughout the liver parenchyma.

Thus pathologists should encourage clinical colleagues to obtain adequate cores of liver tissue, and preferably multiple cores. Caution is warranted in interpreting surgically obtained biopsies because inflammatory foci of PMNs (i.e., surgical hepatitis) render semiquantitative assessment of inflammation challenging.[143,319]

Four studies that assessed interobserver and intraobserver variability in NAFLD in adults have shown good to excellent kappa scores for evaluation of the extent of steatosis, the finding of perisinusoidal fibrosis, and the degree of fibrosis.[180,313,320,321] In all four studies, the degree of lobular inflammation showed the lowest levels of agreement, which is similar to the results of reproducibility studies of patients with chronic hepatitis.[322] One study evaluated interobserver and intraobserver variability between a community general pathologist and an experienced hepatopathologist by using the NASH CRN scoring system. Although there was good intraobserver agreement, there was only fair to good agreement for steatosis, lobular inflammation, and a definite diagnosis of NASH, and only poor agreement for ballooning and fibrosis staging.[323] Training sessions between experienced hepatopathologists and general pathologists can improve interobserver variability.[313]

OTHER FORMS OF FATTY LIVER DISEASE

Drug- and Toxin-Induced Fatty Liver Disease

In some instances, presumed drug-related steatohepatitis may be a manifestation of an underlying preexisting disorder. Table 50.15 lists some of the manifestations of fatty liver in non-ALD, non-NAFLD settings. Wilson's disease may result in some or all of the histopathological manifestations of NAFLD or NASH in any age group.

Less than 2% of cases of steatohepatitis are attributable to drug exposure.[324] Steatosis may result from injury that impairs fatty acid oxidation, decreases VLDL secretion, activates steatosis-related transcription factors, or by inducing obesity or lipodystrophy.[325] Direct hepatotoxicity or mitochondrial injury resulting in steatohepatitis or phospholipidosis has been reported with the use of cardiac medications such as Coralgil, amiodarone (Fig. 50.52), nifedipine, and diltiazem. Tamoxifen and related drugs for breast cancer, estrogens, and corticosteroids can aggravate obesity-related hyperinsulinemia or lipid abnormalities. Methotrexate-induced steatosis may be exacerbated by obesity, diabetes, and alcohol. The pattern of fibrosis caused by methotrexate is typically periportal, not pericentral, and other common features of steatohepatitis, such as ballooning and MDBs, are not usually associated with this agent. Toxins other than alcohol that may result in steatosis or steatohepatitis include industrial solvents (e.g., paint thinners), petrochemicals, aflatoxins, arsenic compounds, amanitin, rapeseed cooking oil, and cocaine.[326]

Fatty Liver Disease After Liver Transplantation

ALD and NAFLD may occur in allograft livers as a recurrence of the original disease or in the form of de novo liver disease. For patients with ALD who continue to drink alcohol after transplantation, the full range of symptoms and signs may occur.[327]

Determination of de novo or recurrent disease related to NAFLD is more complex. Steatosis may recur in 25% to 100% of patients who undergo liver transplantation for NASH-related cirrhosis, or cryptogenic cirrhosis. NASH recurs in 4% to 37% of these cases and progresses to advanced fibrosis and cirrhosis in some.[328-330] De novo steatohepatitis may occur in allograft livers, and in some affected patients, steatohepatitis may progress to advanced fibrosis and cirrhosis.[331,332] Risk factors are similar to those for patients without transplantation. In concert with decreased physical activity levels, obesity, diabetes, hypertension, and hypercholesterolemia all play a role in the development of fatty liver disease after liver transplantation.[328,332]

The risks associated with transplantation also include the effects of systemic immunosuppression. For instance, bolus treatment with corticosteroids is a well-recognized risk factor for fatty liver disease in transplant recipients. Other antirejection agents, such as cyclosporine, are diabetogenic and promote hypertension and hypercholesterolemia.[333] Recurrent HCV infection promotes insulin resistance and steatosis. The high frequency of steatosis (≤88%) and steatohepatitis among patients who undergo liver transplantation for cryptogenic cirrhosis favors NAFLD as a major cause of cryptogenic cirrhosis in the general population.[334,335]

Protein-Energy Malnutrition

Hepatic steatosis occurs in the most severe form of protein-calorie starvation, such as kwashiorkor, a disease that primarily affects the visceral protein compartments of the body. Marasmus affects the somatic (skeletal muscle) protein compartments, but the liver is not normally affected. In kwashiorkor, steatosis develops initially in periportal (zone 1) hepatocytes, and it may progress to involve the entire acinus in severe cases. Upon reintroduction of appropriate dietary protein, zone 3 steatosis is the first to resolve. Necroinflammatory lesions, fibrosis, and cirrhosis do not occur in the absence of concomitant liver disease. Steatohepatitis is also highly unusual in this disorder.[336]

Some types of dietary disorders, such as anorexia, bulimia, cachexia, massive (rapid) weight loss, and uncontrolled inflammatory bowel disease, have been associated with various degrees of hepatic steatosis as well. However, steatohepatitis and fibrosis are uncommon in these conditions.[1]

Parenteral Nutrition–Associated Liver Disease

Steatosis, steatohepatitis, and progressive fibrosis are well-recognized side effects of parenteral nutrition–associated liver disease (PNALD).[337] This more commonly manifests in older children and adults compared with infants or young children, in whom the features of cholestatic liver disease develop more often.[338,339] Steatosis, which is typically most prominent in zone 1 hepatocytes, develops in adults with PNALD. Zone 3 cholestasis and ductopenia also may be identified. Recent work has suggested that intestinal dysbiosis may play a significant role in the mechanism of PNALD.[340]

Celiac Disease

The association of celiac disease with the development of fatty liver disease is controversial. Some patients with

TABLE 50.15 Fatty Liver Cases Reported in Non-ALD, Non-NAFLD Clinical Settings

Clinical Setting and Medications	Mechanisms	Pathological Findings		
		*Steatosis**	*Steatohepatitis*	*Fibrosis/Cirrhosis*
Medications				
Nifedipine	Many patients also have features of MS	+	–	–
Diltiazem		+	–	–
Coralgil		+	–	–
Tamoxifen		+	+	+/+
Estrogens		+	–	–
Corticosteroids		+	–	–
Methotrexate		+	–	+ (periportal)/+
Highly active antiretroviral therapy in HIV-positive patients	Lipodystrophy and IR are common; drugs may also cause mitochondrial damage	++	+	
Amiodarone	Interference with mitochondrial respiration	+ (and phospholipidosis, cholestasis, zone 1)	± (Mallory-Denk bodies)	+ (periportal)
Toxins, industrial solvents	± IR and MS	+ (often zone 1)	±	+
Childhood syndromes (Bardet-Biedl, Alström, Prader-Willi)	Each includes insulin resistance and hyperinsulinemia	+	+	+/+
Allograft liver (de novo or recurrent disease)	Rejection therapy; inactivity; not well studied	+	+	+/+
Starvation, protein-calorie malnutrition (Kwashiorkor)	Complex pathophysiological process of lipids and carbohydrates	+ (zone 1)	–	–
Other nutritional disorders (anorexia, bulimia, cachexia, massive weight loss; pancreatic insufficiency)	± IR and MS	+	+	Possibly
Inflammatory bowel disease	Abnormal nutritional states	+	–	–
Celiac disease	Controversial	+	±	Portal fibrosis, cirrhosis
Lipoprotein disorders	Disorders of lipoprotein metabolism	+		
Liver Diseases				
HCV	May cause IR or hepatic steatosis; may be caused by host and/or viral factors	+ (as many as 70%; more common in genotype 3)	+ (as a concurrent disease process)	+/+ (as a concurrent disease superimposed on HCV)
HBV	Not known to cause IR or MS	±	–	–
HDV (Labrea hepatitis)		–		
Wilson's disease		++		
Tyrosinemia		+		
Galactosemia		+		
Metabolic or endocrine disorders	Complex mechanisms not necessarily related to IR	+	–	–
Hypothyroidism				
Hereditary fructose intolerance				
Cystinuria				
Miscellaneous (ischemia, hepatic regeneration, aging)	Not well known	+ (often zone 1)	–	–

**Steatohepatitis usually includes steatosis and inflammation and may include ballooning and fibrosis.*

ALD, Alcohol-induced liver disease; *HBV*, hepatitis B virus; *HCV*, hepatitis C virus, *HDV*, hepatitis D virus; *HIV*, human immunodeficiency virus; *IR*, insulin resistance; *NAFLD*, nonalcoholic fatty liver disease; *MS*, metabolic syndrome; –, does not occur; +, occurs uncommonly; ++, common; may or may not occur.

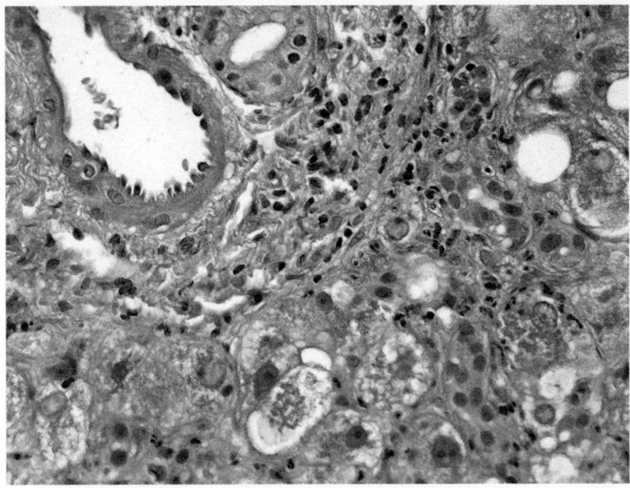

FIGURE 50.52 Liver injury associated with amiodarone shows a typical periportal distribution of ballooning with numerous Mallory-Denk bodies.

celiac disease may reveal elevated aminotransferase levels and hepatic steatosis, but these patients are typically underweight, not overweight. However, in a few reported cases of NAFLD with steatohepatitis, patients had concurrent celiac disease in which the liver disease responded positively to a gluten-free diet.[341] Increased intestinal permeability and small-intestinal bacterial overgrowth may be the underlying factors for the development of NAFLD in these cases.[342]

Viral Hepatitides

Viral hepatitides, particularly HCV infection, are often associated with a significant degree of hepatic steatosis. Many studies discuss the variables associated with steatosis in hepatitis C, such as the clinical status of the patient (e.g., BMI, metabolic syndrome), the role of HCV-induced insulin resistance, specific properties of certain HCV genotypes (particularly GT 3 and GT 1),[287,343] and possible coinfection with human immunodeficiency virus (HIV).[344] HCV has been strongly implicated in altered host lipid metabolism.[345] HIV infection is frequently associated with significant hepatic steatosis.[346] HBV-related steatosis may be as common as in the general population, and it is related mainly to nonviral host factors.[347]

Miscellaneous Causes of Fatty Liver Disease

Macrovesicular steatosis may be found in patients with inflammatory bowel disease, ischemia, heat stroke, liver regeneration, and aging. Tyrosinemia and galactosemia result in steatosis and fibrosis/cirrhosis in childhood. In these conditions, steatosis is primarily located in zone 1 hepatocytes. Lipoprotein metabolism disorders, such as abetalipoproteinemia, familial hypobetalipoproteinemia, Dorfman-Chanarin syndrome (i.e., abnormal lipid storage), and pseudoneonatal adrenoleukodystrophy, are all associated with the development of macrovesicular steatosis of the liver.[348,349]

The full reference list may be accessed online at Elsevier eBooks for Practicing Clinicians.

CHAPTER 51
Cirrhosis

Michael Torbenson

Contents

INTRODUCTION

Worldwide, cirrhosis leads to more than 1.3 million deaths per year and is the 14th leading cause of death.[1] Cirrhosis results from chronic liver injury and typically takes decades to develop and can be caused by numerous etiologies including metabolic disease, chronic viral hepatitis, autoimmune hepatitis, biliary disease, and fatty liver disease. The term *cirrhosis* derives from the Greek word κίρρος, meaning "tawny," and was used early in the 19th century to describe the gross appearance (tawny, nodular, and firm), and later the microscopic appearance, of livers with end-stage fibrosis.

Cirrhosis is a diffuse disease in which fibrosis leads to abnormal liver architecture with variably sized nodules. For many years, cirrhosis was thought to be irreversible, but seminal studies starting in the 1980s described the reversal of cirrhosis,[2,3] and there is now considerable evidence that effective treatment of the underlying liver disease can slow, halt, and sometimes reverse the fibrosis and even cirrhosis.[4,5] Currently, a clinical diagnosis of cirrhosis can be made with sufficient accuracy for patient management in most cases based on noninvasive tests or imaging findings.[1] Histology still plays an important role in fibrosis staging in difficult cases and can help elucidate the underlying cause of cirrhosis, evaluate the grade of disease activity, and examine for coexisting diseases.

CLINICAL COMPLICATIONS OF CIRRHOSIS

The consequences of cirrhosis can be broadly classified into mechanical, functional, or neoplastic. The *mechanical* effects result from obstruction of blood flow into or through the liver, which leads to increased pressure in the portal veins. Interestingly, in some cases, portal hypertension can be detected with bridging fibrosis, before there is histological cirrhosis.[6] The portal pressure increases gradually as cirrhosis develops but may worsen suddenly if there is thrombosis of the portal vein. Over time, the increased portal vein pressure leads to multiple intrahepatic and extrahepatic collaterals, which allow shunting of blood around the hepatic parenchyma via the splanchnic veins. This shunting can in turn lead to esophageal varices, which have a risk of rupture. Even with reversal of cirrhosis, most patients with portal hypertension do not see a complete remission of the elevated portal pressures[7] and are still at risk for variceal bleeding.[8] Cirrhosis also leads to systemic hemodynamic changes that can lead to renal and pulmonary failure.[9,10] *Functional* deficits result from decreased protein synthesis and decreased metabolic activity as a result of the loss of hepatocellular mass and intracellular retention of bile salts and other toxic substances. As examples, ascites develops in part because of low albumin levels[11] and hemorrhage may occur because of platelet dysfunction, platelet sequestration in the spleen, and decreased synthesis of proteins of the coagulation cascade because of fewer hepatocytes. *Neoplasia* is a late consequence of cirrhosis, with the 5-year cumulative risk of hepatocellular carcinoma reaching 30%.[12] Cirrhosis is also an important risk for cholangiocarcinoma.[13]

DEFINITION OF CIRRHOSIS

The core concepts that make up the current definition of cirrhosis have been well accepted for more than 100 years, with excellent microscopic and macroscopic descriptions extending back into the early 1900s. As one example, in 1911, Mallory described cirrhosis as "a chronic, progressive, destructive lesion of the liver combined with reparative activity and contraction on the part of the connective tissue."[14]

Cirrhosis is defined as diffuse nodularity of the liver caused by fibrosis (Fig. 51.1). Several features in this definition should be emphasized.

1. The entire liver must be involved. Of note, in some cases there can be increased fibrosis, and even parenchymal nodularity, in response to a focal injury, for example, adjacent to a mass lesion. Such changes, however, should not be equated with cirrhosis. In addition, terms such as *focal cirrhosis* should be avoided.
2. The fibrous bands can be of varying thickness and may connect portal tracts to portal tracts, portal tracts to central veins, or central veins to central veins. In many cirrhotic liver specimens, it is difficult to precisely classify fibrotic bands in this fashion, because of extensive tissue remodeling. Patchy areas of parenchymal loss can also occur, with replacement by large irregular areas of fibrosis.
3. The parenchymal nodules are created by islands of hepatic parenchyma surrounded by bands of fibrosis. The regenerative response of the hepatocytes typically produces nodules with a somewhat spherical conformation.
4. Although there are many different types of injuries to the liver, only those with certain characteristics result in cirrhosis. The injury must be both chronic and not too severe. Acute injury does not lead to fibrosis and if chronic injury is too severe, the liver will fail quickly, and the patient will die or undergo liver transplantation before there is sufficient development of fibrosis and architectural remodeling.
5. The time course for progression of chronic liver disease to cirrhosis is highly variable, even for the same type of disease.

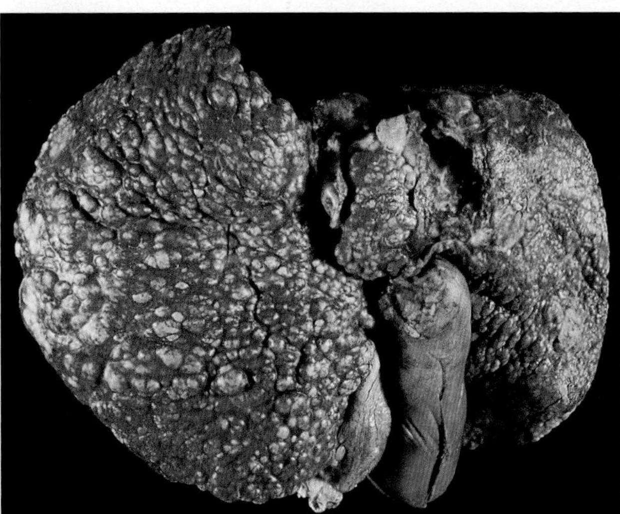

FIGURE 51.1 Macroscopic appearance of cirrhosis caused by hepatitis B virus. This view from the back shows a coarsely nodular capsular surface, shrinkage of the right lobe, and compensatory hypertrophy of the left lobe. The gallbladder has been inked blue.

COLLAGEN IN THE LIVER

Abnormal collagen deposition is the defining feature of fibrosis. The normal liver contains collagen, but this normal collagen is not classified as fibrosis. Thus there is no need for the term "no abnormal fibrosis" in a pathology report, as all fibrosis is abnormal by definition. In the normal liver, collagen types I and III are concentrated in the portal tracts and around terminal hepatic veins. Strands of type IV collagen (reticulin) are present in the space of Disse, where they form a delicate and uniform network that supports the liver cell plates. In cirrhosis, excessive amounts of types I and III collagen are deposited in the portal tracts, along individual liver cell plates in the space of Disse, and in regions of parenchymal collapse. A variety of noncollagenous matrix proteins are also deposited as part of liver fibrosis. In cirrhosis, the amounts of collagen, glycoproteins, and proteoglycans can increase severalfold.[15] On a percent area basis, total extracellular matrix components can increase from 5% in normal liver to 25% to 40% in cirrhosis.[16] Some of this is only an apparent increase, because of condensation of the normal structural collagen and other matrix components that occurs during parenchymal collapse and extinction.

The two main cell types that synthesize collagen in the liver are hepatic stellate cells[17,18] and portal fibroblasts.[19,20] Although typically not visible by hematoxylin and eosin (H&E) microscopy, quiescent hepatic stellate cells reside in the subendothelial space of Disse. They are an important reservoir of retinyl esters and other fat-soluble vitamins stored in tiny fat globules. During hepatic injury, stellate cells are stimulated by inflammatory mediators to become myofibroblasts, where they lose their fat globules, express α-smooth muscle actin in their cytoplasm, proliferate, and commence collagen synthesis.[18]

When stellate cells are activated in some chronic low-grade diseases such as fatty liver disease, collagen is deposited in the space of Disse, giving an appearance known as *pericellular fibrosis* or *sinusoidal fibrosis*. This type of delicate collagen is most easily appreciated in the areas around the central veins. Alternatively, widespread injury to hepatocytes, as in alcoholic hepatitis, may activate stellate cells throughout the liver, leading to extensive deposition of sinusoidal collagen. In either instance, the total matrix in the space of Disse increases and changes from one that contains delicate interspersed strands of fibrillar collagen (types III and IV) to one composed of a dense matrix of basement membrane–type matrix proteins, which closes the space of Disse to protein exchange between hepatocytes and plasma. In general, abnormal matrix deposition within the space of Disse occurs in those parts of the parenchyma where cell injury and inflammation are greatest.

Portal tract fibroblasts differ from stellate cells in location and physiology.[19,20] When activated and transformed into myofibroblasts, they are capable of rapid proliferation and deposition of collagen. The rapidity of fibrosis progression can vary considerably depending on the disease. For example, fibrosis arising from high-grade biliary tract obstruction can run an unusually aggressive course (e.g., biliary atresia) in which the liver can become cirrhotic within a few months. As an example of the opposite end of the spectrum, fibrosis progression in primary biliary cirrhosis is typically indolent and may extend for 20 or more years.

ANATOMICAL MODELS OF FIBROSIS AND CIRRHOSIS

3-D reconstruction of bridging fibrosis shows sheets or meshlike structures of fibrosis that begin at branch points in the portal tracts, extending into the parenchyma like webbing between the thumb and forefinger of a baseball mitt.[21-23] 3-D reconstruction of liver cirrhosis has consistently shown that cirrhotic nodules are organized along the portal veins, obtaining their blood flow directly from the portal veins, with blood passing through the sinusoids and into central veins that are located in the fibrous bands at the edge of the cirrhotic nodule.[23-27] As the liver remodels, new nodules of hepatocytes may start off as small buds of cells within the fibrous bands themselves[28] and larger nodules can be remodeled.[26]

MODELS OF CIRRHOSIS PATHOGENESIS

Liver cirrhosis is not, strictly speaking, the "end stage" of hepatic scarring because the process of liver remodeling is ongoing. The main anatomical elements in the pathophysiology of cirrhosis include deposition of collagen in the parenchyma and portal tracts, arterialization of parenchymal sinusoids, obliteration of small hepatic and portal veins with resultant loss of hepatocytes through a process termed *parenchymal extinction*, abnormal vascular physiology, and regeneration of hepatocytes (Box 51.1). There is, however, healthy debate concerning the role of each of these in the pathogenesis of cirrhosis. Understanding their relative contributions is important because the design of effective interventions to delay or reverse cirrhosis depends on understanding its pathogenesis.[29]

BOX 51.1 Pathobiology of Cirrhosis

- Deposition of collagen
  - Portal tract
  - Parenchymal (sinusoidal)
- Arterialization of parenchymal sinusoids
- Obliteration of portal veins and hepatic veins
  - Parenchymal extinction
- Vascular pathophysiology
  - Shunt formation
  - Congestive hepatopathy
  - Vascular thrombosis
- Hepatocyte regeneration
- Resorption of fibrous tissue
  - "Reversal" of cirrhosis

Hepatic Arterialization and Capillarization

Arterialization of the liver in cirrhosis has been known for more than a century. In 1907, Herrick perfused cadaver livers and demonstrated that resistance to flow in the hepatic artery of cirrhotic livers was markedly decreased.[30] This fact is documented daily by ultrasonographers when they examine patients with cirrhotic livers and find increased arterial flow in the liver, along with sluggish or even reversed flow in the portal vein. The histological manifestation is known as *capillarization* of the sinusoidal endothelial cells. Many years ago, using electron microscopy, studies showed that capillarization was associated with a constellation of ultrastructural changes, including a decrease in the number and size of sinusoidal endothelial fenestrations, loss of hepatocellular microvilli, and an increase in basement membrane material.[31,32] These studies found that sinusoidal endothelial cells in the normal liver lack a basement membrane and have fenestrations that are approximately 100 nm in diameter, occupying between 2% and 3% of the area of the endothelial cell. With the development of cirrhosis, however, deposition of extracellular matrix in the space of Disse is accompanied by a loss of fenestrations in the sinusoidal endothelial cells. In addition, whereas the diameter of the fenestrations only slightly decreases, the area occupancy (porosity) falls from 2% to 4% to less than 0.5%. This transformation of sinusoidal vascular channels is widely considered to explain the functional deficits in blood-hepatocyte solute exchange.[33] Rapid flow in sinusoids further decreases solute exchange.[34] Although these changes decrease exchange between hepatocytes and the blood, capillarization or arterialization may potentially be a protective form of adaptation that allows the hepatocytes to survive in a high-pressure, high-flow environment.

The sinusoidal endothelium in the cirrhotic liver may express CD34. Because this expression is a normal property of arterial endothelium, CD34 positivity is considered a marker of arterialization of the sinusoids. Sinusoidal arterialization is accompanied by α-smooth muscle actin staining in the sinusoidal wall (Fig. 51.2), reflecting the transformation of hepatic stellate cells into myofibroblasts. When severe, sinusoidal fibrosis in the perivenular region of the lobule may also partially obstruct vascular outflow, creating postsinusoidal vascular resistance.

Arterialization also occurs at the level of portal tracts, where an increased number (and size) of arterial profiles

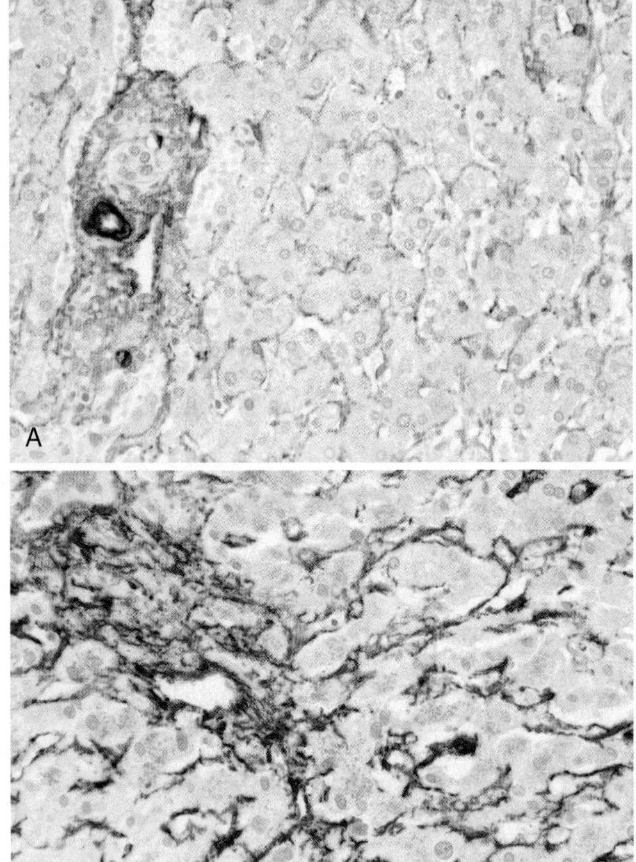

FIGURE 51.2 Immunohistochemistry for α-smooth muscle actin. A, Normal liver, showing smooth muscle surrounding the hepatic artery in a portal tract and little immunoreactivity elsewhere. **B,** Evolving cirrhosis, with extensive hepatic stellate cell activation, marked by α-smooth muscle actin immunoreactivity in the parenchymal sinusoids.

can be seen in cirrhosis. Arterialization of small portal tracts in cirrhosis can also be accompanied by obliteration of adjacent portal veins. Obliteration of small portal veins increases presinusoidal vascular resistance for blood inflow via the splanchnic system. In contrast, resistance to hepatic arterial blood flow decreases, owing to an increased arterial capacity. Hepatic arterial blood pressure is sufficient to supply blood to the liver, but the low pressure of the splanchnic system is not able to overcome the pressure impedance, leading to portal hypertension.

Parenchymal Extinction

Hepatocyte apoptosis and necrosis occurs in all types of liver diseases that progress to cirrhosis. Most of these injuries, when they are low grade, lead to local replacement of the injured hepatocytes and complete healing. Progressive disease leads to fibrosis, with subsequent increased sinusoidal vascular resistance and obstruction of blood flow. The convergence of these injuries (active liver injury plus vascular flow changes) leads to foci of contiguous loss of hepatocytes, called *parenchymal extinction lesions* (PEL) (Fig. 51.3). Detailed morphological studies suggest that parenchymal extinction plays a critical role in the pathogenesis of cirrhosis.[34-36] These extinction lesions typically involve a small portion of an acinus but rarely can involve larger units of one or more adjacent acini.

The concept of parenchymal extinction incorporates the following ideas: (1) parenchymal extinction is not directly caused by the initial hepatocellular injury but results from injury of the local vessels; (2) each parenchymal extinction lesion (PEL) has its own natural history and may be in an early or late stage of healing; (3) cirrhosis develops simultaneously with the accumulation of numerous independent and discrete PELs throughout the liver; and (4) parenchymal extinction may progress long after cirrhosis is already established, leading to slow conversion of a liver with compensated cirrhosis into a deeply cirrhotic organ incapable of sustaining life.

The pathogenesis of vascular obstruction depends on the size of the vessels and is outlined in Figure 51.4. In this model most small-vessel obliteration is secondary to local inflammation.[35] The hypothesis is that most PELs are produced by blockage of veins larger than 100 μm in diameter, because obstruction at this site cannot be easily circumvented by collateral flow within the sinusoids. Obstruction of several adjacent sinusoids is also difficult to circumvent. Tissue congestion occurs whenever blood entering the vasculature exceeds the ability of the outflow tract to carry that blood, a state known as *in-out imbalance*. If inflow is marked, congestion occurs even when the tissue has normal outflow capacity. Congestion is particularly severe when there is total obstruction of the outflow tract or when there is increased inflow in the presence of partial outflow obstruction. Congestive injury leads to reactive hyperemia, shunt formation, and angiogenesis. Therefore PELs are the result of local failure of the microvasculature, usually because of obstruction of hepatic veins or sinusoids. The mechanism for formation of PELs is detailed in Figure 51.5.

In early chronic liver disease, PELs are recognized by the close approximation of the terminal hepatic vein and the adjacent portal tract. They are often difficult to reliably identify because damaged small hepatic veins may appear only as a few collagen bundles lying adjacent to a portal tract. PELs become more evident as they aggregate and involve larger and more easily recognizable hepatic veins. PEL aggregates may be evident as two or more portal tracts that are bound together with a hepatic vein remnant apparent in the intervening space (see Fig. 51.2). With progression of disease, ongoing obstruction of hepatic veins and secondary arterial dilatation cause further congestive injury in the tissue located between the lesions. This creates a self-perpetuating pathophysiology that may eventually lead to interconnected portal tracts throughout the whole liver.

Shunt Formation

When PELS form, the close approximation of portal tracts and the adjacent terminal hepatic vein offers an opportunity for the artery in the portal tract to feed directly into the collapsed perivenous tissue. Occasionally, these arteries can be seen supplying a pool of blood surrounded by atrophic hepatocytes. In older lesions, a well-demarcated blood-filled channel may be visible; this suggests a stable, high-flow and high-pressure conduit connecting a small artery to a small

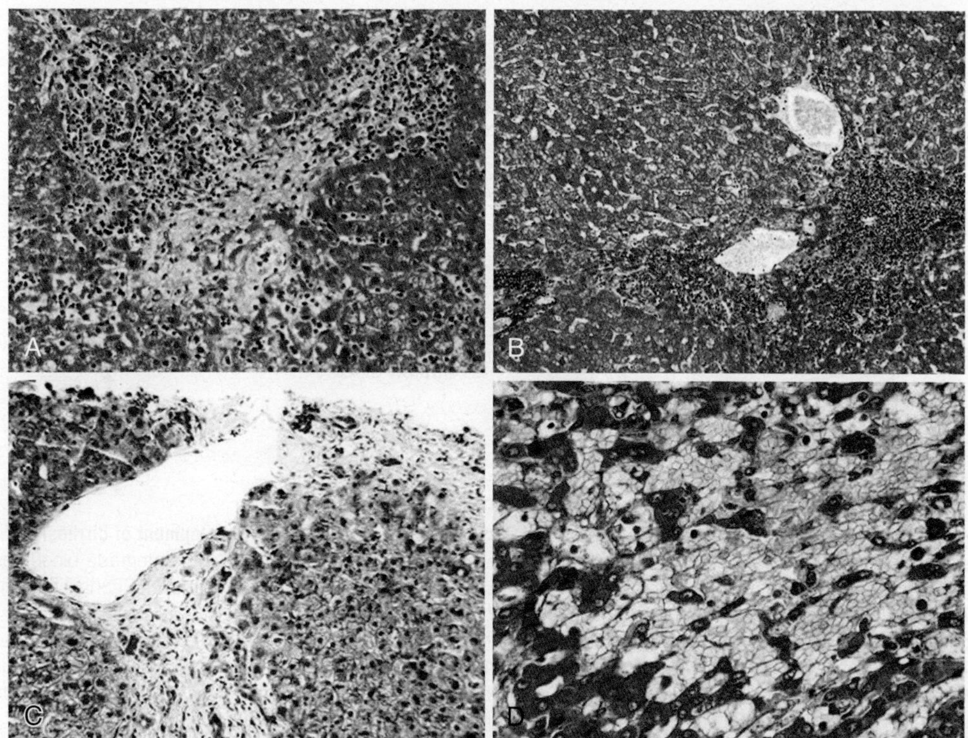

FIGURE 51.3 Photomicrographs of chronically diseased livers show various phases of the development of parenchymal extinction in chronic hepatitis C. A, Early-stage hepatitis C shows parenchyma in the process of extinction. There is loss of contiguous hepatocytes, atrophy of some adjacent hepatocytes, close approximation of portal tracts to the hepatic vein, thickening of the hepatic vein, and obliteration of the portal veins (elastic trichrome stain). **B,** Early-stage hepatitis C. After collapse, there is close approximation of portal tracts and hepatic veins, indicating the site of parenchymal extinction. In this example, an obliterated hepatic vein is present in the collapsed parenchyma to the right (elastic trichrome stain). **C,** Fibrous adhesions between two portal tracts *(top right* and *bottom left)* with intervening hepatic vein. The structures are closely approximated, indicating substantial loss of tissue volume. Notice the fibrous intimal thickening of the hepatic vein *(top right)* (Masson trichrome stain). **D,** In late-stage cirrhosis there is active congestive hepatopathy. This specimen exhibits congestive sinusoidal injury. In the center is a hepatic vein, showing the residual vein wall as a ring of thick collagen bundles.

hepatic vein. This appearance has been interpreted as an arteriovenous shunt. The formation of shunts between portal tracts and terminal hepatic veins enables portovenous and arteriovenous shunting through de novo vascular channels, effectively bypassing the parenchymal nodules. It is postulated that shunted blood flow through these "fast" vascular channels leaves the remainder of the hepatic parenchyma with significantly decreased blood flow.[34,35,37]

Congestive Changes

Venous and sinusoidal obstruction is caused by local inflammation occurring in the course of chronic hepatitis (Fig. 51.6).[35] The generation of soluble proinflammatory mediators in this setting is a powerful stimulus of fibrogenesis. However, organization of exudates is an additional possible stimulus of fibrogenesis, especially those exudates rich in fibrin. It is postulated that obstructed hepatic veins and PELs occur before fibrosis; therefore these lesions are thought to be at the leading edge of the pathogenesis of cirrhosis (Fig. 51.7).[38,39]

Collagen accumulation is determined by the rates of collagen synthesis and resorption (Fig. 51.8). The preexisting structural collagen of the liver condenses during the formation of PELs and is incorporated into septa. Although this is not true fibrosis per se, it can contribute to the scarring seen with cirrhosis.

Vascular Thrombosis

In angiographic and ultrasonographic studies, portal vein thrombosis has been detected in 0.6% to 16.6% of cirrhotic patients[40] and grossly visible portal vein fibrosis or thrombosis are found in 39% of cirrhotic livers at autopsy.[41,42] Venoocclusive lesions of hepatic veins smaller than 0.2 mm in diameter have been found in as many as 74% of cirrhotic livers examined at autopsy.[38,43,44] Obliterative lesions are found in 36% of portal veins and 70% of hepatic veins in livers removed at liver transplantation.[39] These data show that thrombosis of medium- and large-sized portal veins and hepatic veins is a common occurrence in cirrhosis and may represent a common pathway for the propagation of parenchymal extinction.

Regeneration

In the adult liver, hepatocytes, bile duct epithelial cells, and hepatic progenitor or stem cells maintain the potential to multiply during adult life.[45,46] In the normal liver, there is a slow turnover of hepatocytes. After injury or surgical reduction, however, the liver cells proliferate more rapidly and the liver can restore approximately three-fourths of its own mass within 6 months. Depending on the severity of the primary injury, liver regeneration may occur by at least two mechanisms.[47-49] In brief, with mild to moderate

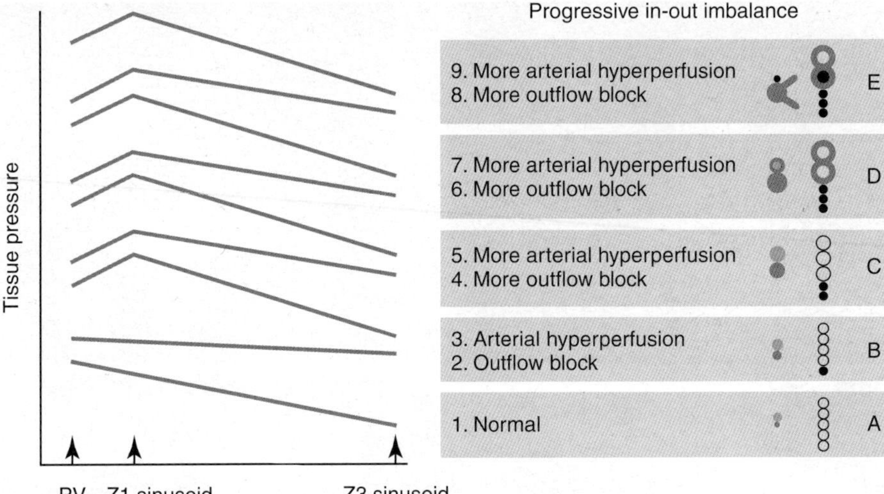

FIGURE 51.4 Schematic representation of the sequence of microvascular events that occur during the development of cirrhosis. *1,* The normal curve has a gentle pressure gradient from portal vein (*PV*) through zone 1 (*Z1*) to zone 3 (*Z3*) sinusoids, allowing antegrade blood flow in the sinusoids. *2,* The earliest important lesion is obliteration of terminal hepatic venules. This causes flattening of the curve with congestive changes. *3,* Reactive hyperemia (arterial dilatation) restores the pressure gradient but at a higher pressure and with more congestive changes. *4,* More outflow block occurs because of further hepatic venule obliteration. *5,* There is greater reactive hyperemia. *6* through *9,* Cycles of obstruction and increased arterial inflow lead to progressive intrahepatic hypertension. The diagrams on the right (*A–E*) show sequential changes in a microvascular domain composed of five terminal hepatic venules *(black circles)*, a portal vein *(blue dot)*, and an artery *(pink dot)*. *A,* Normal vessels. *B,* The primary chronic liver disease has caused obliteration of a hepatic venule. The artery has become enlarged, and the other hepatic venules and the portal vein have dilated to accommodate the increased flow. *C,* With more hepatic venule obliteration, the remaining hepatic venules, the portal vein, and the artery have dilated further. *D,* Rising flow has caused congestive injury to the remaining hepatic venules (congestive hepatic venopathy) *(open pink circles)* and the portal vein (congestive portal venopathy) *(blue dot with pink circle)*. There is further enlargement of the artery. *E,* An injured hepatic venule and the injured portal vein have become obstructed. The artery has undergone growth (angiogenesis) with arterialization of the sinusoids. The overall results of these changes are progressive obstruction of portal and hepatic veins, destruction of sinusoids, arterialization, and rising intrahepatic pressure. These changes are fueled by an imbalance of hepatic artery flow entering the liver and the capacity of the liver to drain that flow (hepatic artery flow > hepatic outflow capacity). The earliest injury was caused by the primary chronic liver disease that resulted in outflow block, but late events are caused by congestive injury resulting in progressive outflow block. (Diagram developed by IR Wanless, MD.)

hepatocellular loss, mature hepatocytes undergo replication. More extensive or massive hepatic necrosis stimulates proliferation of progenitor cells within the periportal region, particularly when necroinflammation occurs at the portal-parenchymal interface. Proliferation of these cells gives rise first to so-called ductular hepatocytes, in which ductular structures containing cuboidal cells and slightly larger cells with mitochondria-rich cytoplasm. With time, these cells mature into definitive hepatocytes or cholangiocytes and may repopulate damaged parenchymal regions and bile duct structures, respectively. In many cases of cirrhosis, a bile ductular proliferation within the fibrous septa coexists with the interspersed hepatocellular nodules. Thus these ductules may occur in cirrhosis of almost any cause and are not necessarily the result of biliary obstruction.

REVERSIBILITY OF CIRRHOSIS

Advances in medicine have led to many effective treatments for different liver diseases, such as chronic hepatitis C. With effective treatment, it has become clear that some cases of cirrhosis may reverse clinically and histologically.[50,51] This reversal of cirrhosis has now been documented in patients with many different liver diseases including hemochromatosis, autoimmune hepatitis, Wilson disease, primary biliary cirrhosis, extrahepatic biliary obstruction, alcoholic disease, and chronic viral hepatitis B. At the biochemical level, the mechanism for resorption of fibrosis involves activation of tissue metalloproteinases.[52] At the histological level, fibrosis is progressively removed and broad septa, which can become incomplete ("perforated") and eventually disappear. Other findings that can indicate cirrhosis/fibrosis regression include isolated thick bundles of collagen fibers, delicate periportal spikes of fibrosis, hepatic vein remnants, minute regenerative nodules, and isolated small clusters or cords of hepatocytes in fibrous bands (Fig. 51.9). The constellation of these findings has been called the hepatic repair complex.[3,53,54]

The hepatic repair complex represents an important model for understanding the basic biology of liver fibrosis, particularly the process of cirrhosis regression. The histological findings of cirrhosis regression, however, are not always easy to identify, their reproducibility has not been well defined, and experimental validation remains limited. Also, their clinical relevance for patient management has not been determined.

A recent study proposed a simplified and potentially useful method for assessing fibrosis regression/progression based on the thickness of the fibrotic bands in cirrhotic livers: if most fibrotic bands are thin on low power examination, then this is interpreted as a primarily regressive pattern of cirrhosis; if most bands are thick, then this is interpreted as a primarily progressive pattern of cirrhosis; if there is a relative equal mixture, then the findings are classified as indeterminate for progression versus regression.[55] This and other approaches have not been widely adopted by

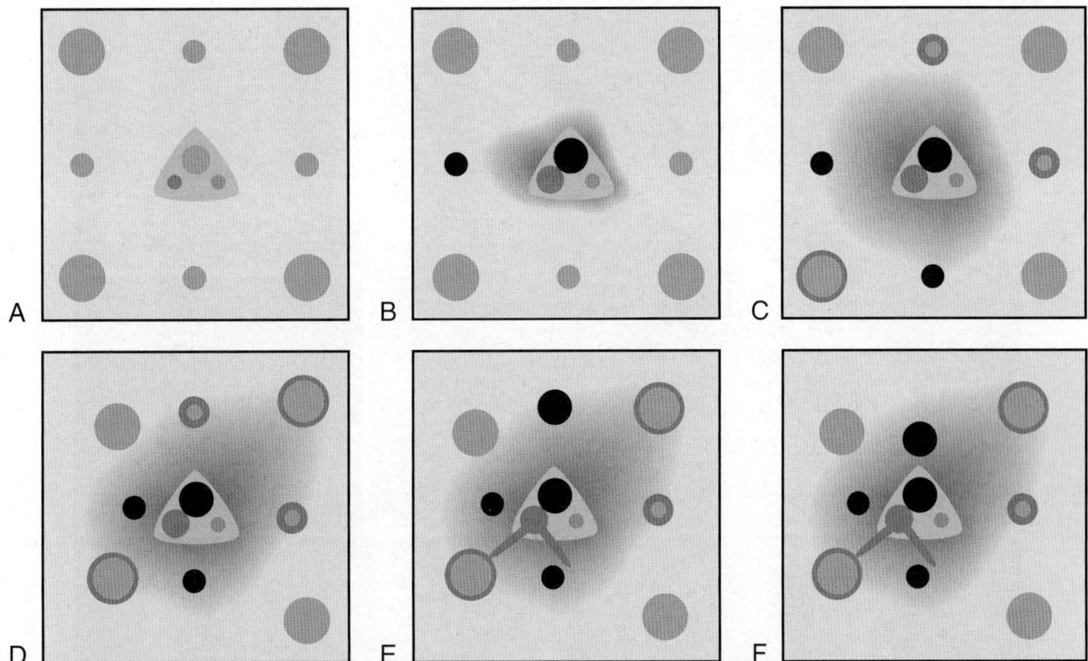

FIGURE 51.5 The microvasculature in chronic hepatitis with development of vascular lesions and secondary parenchymal extinction. Parenchymal extinction occurs when the microvasculature fails because the arterial blood flow is too great for a progressively diminishing outflow capacity. **A,** Normal portal tract and adjacent hepatic venules. **B,** Obliteration of one hepatic venule and the portal vein has occurred in response to hepatitis. Reactive hyperemia has occurred in response to the obstruction of veins. The remaining veins are able to carry the increased flow without congestive injury. **C,** An additional hepatic venule has become obstructed as part of the hepatitis, and the sinusoids and hepatic vein walls have become more congested. **D,** The sinusoids decompensate; hepatocytes become atrophic and die by apoptosis. This is recognizable as a parenchymal extinction lesion (PEL); the portal tract and hepatic venules become approximated. **E,** A congested hepatic venule has become obstructed with increased sinusoidal and hepatic venule congestion. Arterial twigs have grown into the congested tissue, leading to arteriovenous shunting. **F,** Further hepatocytes are lost, and the PEL becomes larger. (Diagrams developed by IR Wanless, MD.)

the pathology community, in part because there currently is no accepted relevance for patient management, even if a pathologist confidently identifies features that suggest regression in a liver biopsy with cirrhosis. After all is said and done, fibrosis staging is clinically important, and pathologists and radiologists put much effort into this endeavor, almost exclusively because it predicts clinical outcomes,[56-58] which can then be used to guide patient management. The histological findings of fibrosis regression have not yet reached this critical point, but it seems likely that ongoing studies will clarify this key question and help determine the clinical relevance of histological findings suggestive of fibrosis regression.

Of note, fibrosis progression/regression is an ongoing process, a back and forth between injury and repair. The previous description indicates that the equilibrium of injury and repair depends primarily on the continued presence (or absence) of the proinflammatory disease environment. Thus the degree of active liver injury also is relevant to fibrogenesis and can be assessed by histology and/or laboratory testing. Catastrophic events such as portal or hepatic venous obstruction by tumor or thrombosis can also quickly lead to significant shifts in the fibrosis progression/regression process.

Even with substantial resorption of fibrous septa, restoration of the hepatic architecture to a normal state does not always occur. Limiting factors can be the persistence of vascular abnormalities, that is, outflow obstruction and arterialization. If these vascular factors are sufficient to cause continued hepatocellular injury, fibrous septa will not resorb, and some degree of cirrhosis or incomplete septal cirrhosis will remain. Moreover, residual fibrosis may still lead to persistent presinusoidal resistance to portal blood flow, leading to continued clinical evidence of portal hypertension.

ANATOMICAL FINDINGS IN CIRRHOSIS

Historically, before most etiologies of cirrhosis were known, cirrhosis was commonly classified by its gross appearance into *micronodular* or *macronodular* cirrhosis, with micronodular cirrhosis showing nodules on average smaller than 3 mm in diameter and macronodular cirrhosis showing nodules mostly larger than 3 mm.[59] The term *mixed cirrhosis* describes livers in which nodules both larger and smaller than 3 mm coexisted, with no pattern predominating. These categories are not stable over time, as micronodular cirrhosis can transform to a macronodular pattern, in many cases presumably as part of cirrhosis regression (Figs. 51.10 and 51.11). This anatomical classification is of historical and biological interest, but is not relevant for clinical care, as cirrhosis is now classified by etiology and these antiquated classifications correlate poorly with etiology.

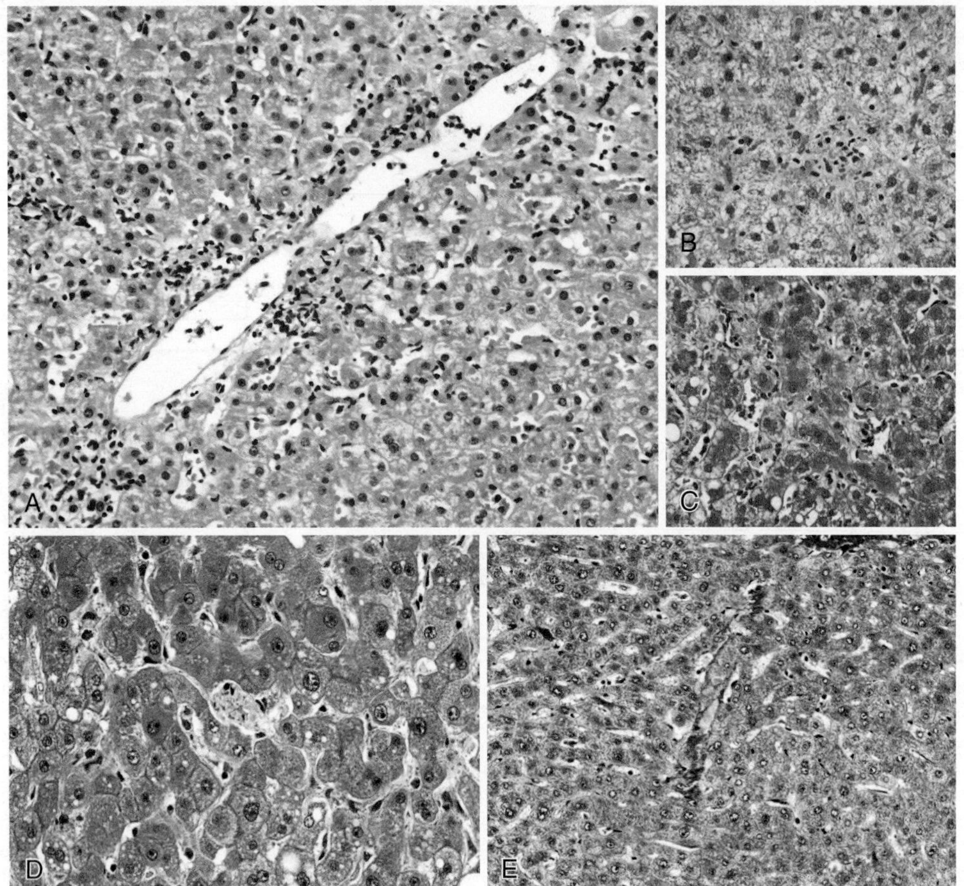

FIGURE 51.6 Small hepatic veins in chronic liver disease showing various degrees of injury. A, Chronic hepatitis B with diffuse mild parenchymal inflammation including hepatic vein phlebitis. **B,** Chronic hepatitis B with partial occlusion of the inflamed hepatic vein. **C,** Recurrent hepatitis C with partial occlusion of the hepatic vein. **D** and **E,** Alcoholic liver disease with postinflammatory occlusion of hepatic veins. In **E**, the hepatic vein lumen has filled with hepatocytes.

Macroscopic Features

The cirrhotic liver can be shrunken or enlarged, in particular with biliary patterns of cirrhosis. The capsular surface often shows nodularity. On cut sections, the liver parenchyma is typically firm and shows diffuse nodules of variable sizes and shape. The fibrotic septa surrounding the nodules are often visible. The color of the cirrhotic nodules will vary depending on their fat content (imparting a yellow color), amount of cholestasis (green color), and iron (in cases of severe iron overload, imparting a reddish brown color). In some cases, there may be areas of more extensive parenchymal collapse that involve an entire segment or subsegment of the liver, as a result of regional vascular compromise, a finding known as *regional parenchymal extinction* (or *confluent hepatic fibrosis*) (Fig. 51.12).[39]

Incomplete Septal Cirrhosis

Incomplete septal cirrhosis is a highly regressed form of cirrhosis that is often associated with portal hypertension but exhibits normal hepatocellular synthetic function.[3,8,60] Portal vein thrombosis can lead to portal hypertension in cases that might otherwise escape clinical attention. Macroscopically, the septa are usually invisible, but variation in the color of the parenchyma on cut section demonstrates the presence of nodules. The liver may be without significant distortion or may exhibit residual nodules. Because healed portal vein thrombosis is sometimes present, gross examination should include consideration of this possibility.

Microscopically, slender fibrovascular septa extend from portal tracts into the parenchyma but often do not connect with other portal tracts or hepatic veins. These septa demarcate large, rather inconspicuous nodules. Intrasinusoidal collagen away from the septa is not obviously increased, and there is little evidence of hepatocellular damage or inflammation. Portal tracts are variably attenuated, so that venous channels appear relatively increased. Other findings can include a variable mixture of thickened hepatocellular plates, dilated sinusoids, and compression of sinusoids between hyperplastic plates.[60] The plate pattern is disorganized, with irregular orientation of plates to portal tracts and terminal hepatic veins. Histological indicators of the original injurious process are usually absent.

The chief distinctions between incomplete septal cirrhosis and nodular regenerative hyperplasia are the fibrous septa. The nodules in incomplete septal cirrhosis are delineated by incomplete, delicate fibrous septa that lack obvious spherical features, whereas the nodules in nodular regenerative hyperplasia are associated with no or minimal portal fibrosis (no fibrous septa) and show distinctive curvilinear compression of hepatocyte plates, which can be highlighted by the reticulin stain.

Postnecrotic Cirrhosis

Postnecrotic cirrhosis is a historically interesting term[61] but is no longer commonly used in clinical practice. Even several decades ago, when its use was more common, the term's utility was hampered by inconsistent definitions and usage. Early on, the basic notion was to use this term for (1) cases that appeared cirrhotic and (2) followed clinically severe episodes of acute hepatitis. In retrospect, most of these cases represented acute on chronic liver disease with flares of autoimmune hepatitis or chronic hepatitis B. Also in retrospect, another subset of cases that were historically called postnecrotic cirrhosis did not have cirrhosis as we now define it, but instead the livers showed acute or subacute liver injury with massive necrosis, wherein the collapsed parenchyma stained light blue on trichrome, mimicking cirrhosis.

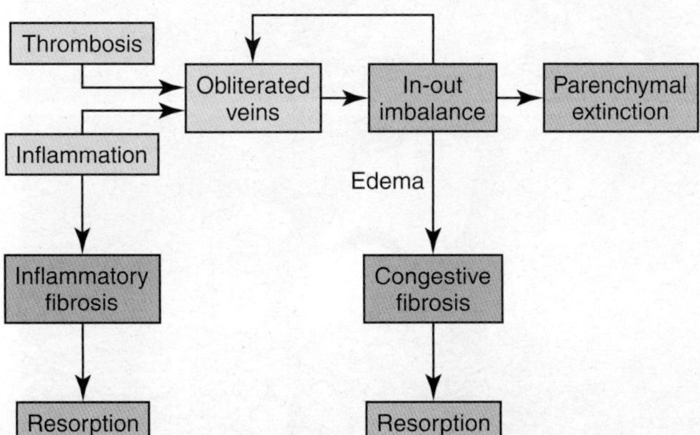

FIGURE 51.7 Diagram showing the main events in the formation of parenchymal extinction and fibrosis. Two mechanisms for venous obstruction are shown. Thrombosis is the initiating event in Budd-Chiari syndrome, whereas inflammation induces venous obstruction in most forms of chronic hepatitis. Venous obstruction and hyperemia lead to in-out imbalance and parenchymal extinction. Fibrosis may be induced by hepatitis-associated inflammation (inflammatory fibrosis) or by organization of congestive injury (congestive fibrosis). In the thrombotic pathway, the fibrosis (and complete cirrhosis) is caused by the congestive injury, and the inflammatory pathway is not important. In chronic hepatitis, fibrosis occurs initially by the inflammatory pathway, but as disease advances, congestive fibrosis becomes dominant. Fibrosis from both pathways can resorb, although congestive fibrosis is less likely to do so because of continuing congestive forces occurring in late cirrhosis.

In other settings, however, the term post necrotic cirrhosis was used for any cause of hepatitis-associated cirrhosis (e.g., viral or autoimmune), in particular if there was a macronodular pattern of cirrhosis, while in other settings the term was used essentially as a synonym for alcoholic liver disease. For these reasons, very careful reading is necessary to determine the context of usage when perusing the older literature where this term was used.

Episodes of massive hepatic necrosis often lead to large areas of necrosis (Fig. 51.13). Depending on the amount of time between injury and gross or histological examination of the liver, the necrosis can be either acute or subacute. In early disease, there is limited regeneration, while later there can be large nodules of regenerative hyperplasia, sometimes 5 cm or greater in size, occasionally being mistaken for malignancy by imaging studies or on gross examination. Because of the acute/subacute hepatic injury, these livers are usually severely cholestatic, even though the hepatitis activity may have largely resolved. Fibrosis evaluation can be challenging. There are cases with advanced fibrosis or cirrhosis that present with acute on chronic liver disease, but many cases of massive hepatic necrosis will show parenchymal collapse only and not true fibrosis. In those rare cases of patient survival without transplantation, the areas of parenchymal collapse can either be resorbed or sometimes become fibrotic.

Large Nodules in the Cirrhotic Liver

Occasionally, individual hepatocellular nodules can become substantially larger than those in the background liver. These may be large regenerative nodules, dysplastic nodules, or hepatocellular carcinoma.[62,63] Given that malignant transformation can occur in nodules smaller than 0.5 cm in diameter, sectioning at 0.3- to 0.5-cm intervals is important for adequate gross examination of the cirrhotic liver. The gross

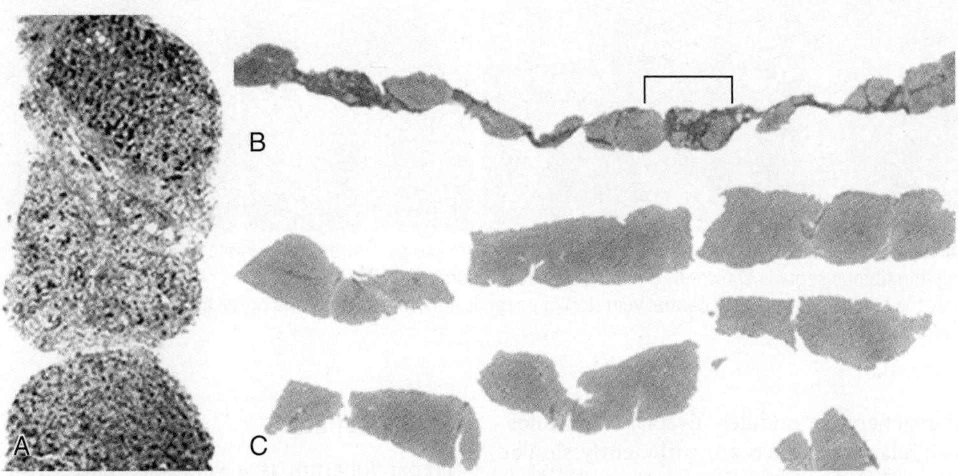

FIGURE 51.8 A and **B,** Fibrous septa regress and disappear with time, as illustrated in this patient with chronic hepatitis B and cirrhosis. **C,** 2½ years after successful treatment with lamivudine, a biopsy reveals marked reduction in fibrous septation. (*From Wanless IR, Nakashima E, Sherman M. Regression of human cirrhosis: morphologic features and the genesis of incomplete septal cirrhosis.* Arch Pathol Lab Med. *2000;124:1599-1607.*)

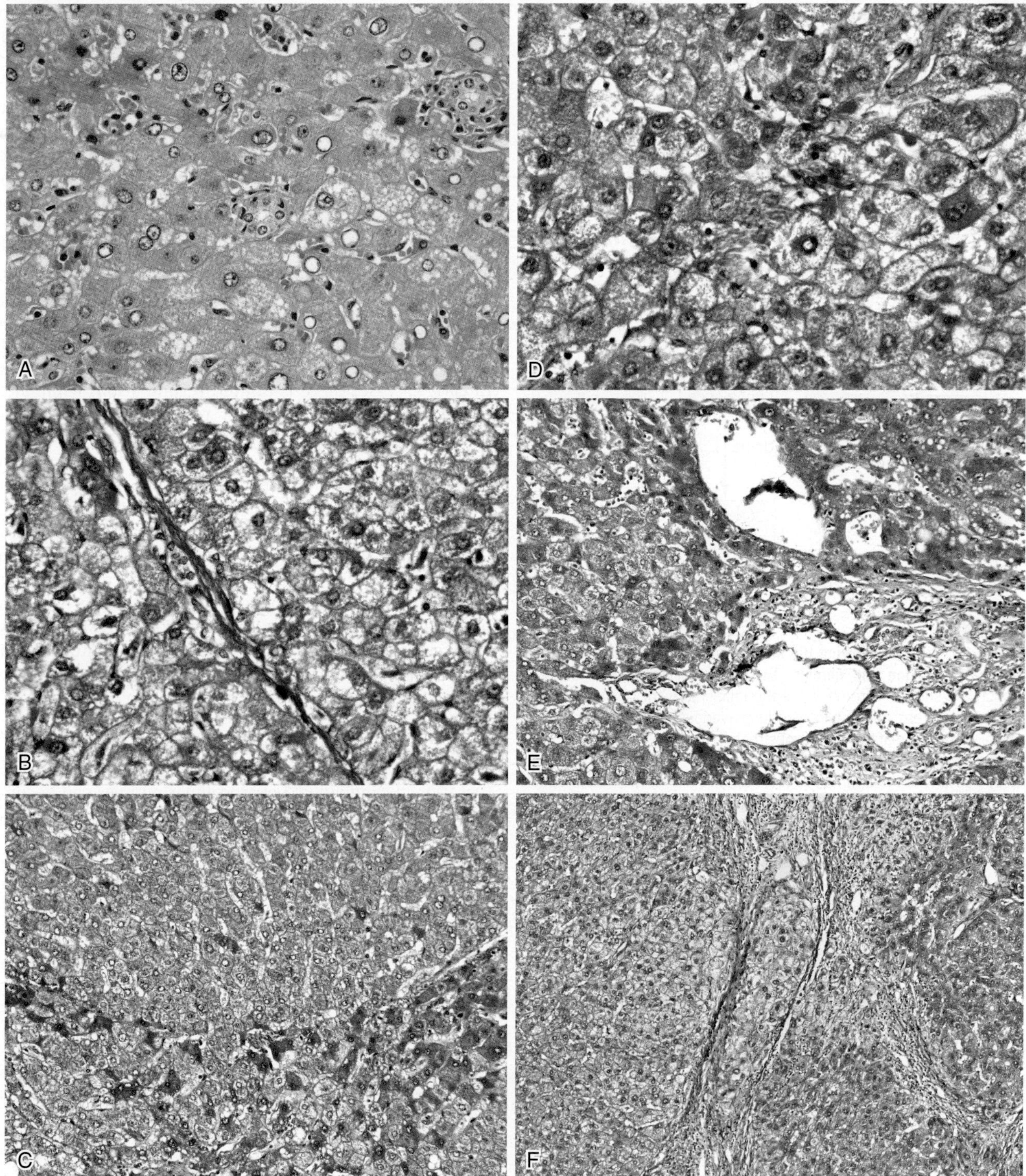

FIGURE 51.9 Hepatic repair complex.. A, In this cirrhotic nodule, remnants of two portal tracts are visible as isolated bile ducts, one with a thin collar of collagen. **B,** A long thin fibrous septa is shown. **C,** Because of partial resorption, this fibrotic band is perforated. **D,** A thick isolated bundle of collagen is highlighted by the trichrome stain. **E,** A central vein (top of image is adhered) to a fibrotic portal tract. **F,** A small, minute regenerative nodule is present within this fibrous band.

features of macroregenerative nodules, dysplastic nodules, and early hepatocellular carcinomas are sufficiently similar on gross examination that the distinction requires histological examination. In some cases, hepatocellular carcinomas arising within a dysplastic nodule can lead to a "nodule-in-nodule" appearance.

Hepar Lobatum

Hepar lobatum is a very rare pattern of injury in which deep linear clefts develop in the liver capsule giving the liver an irregular shape, also known as *potato liver* (Fig. 51.14). Hepar lobatum has been described in adults with syphilis,

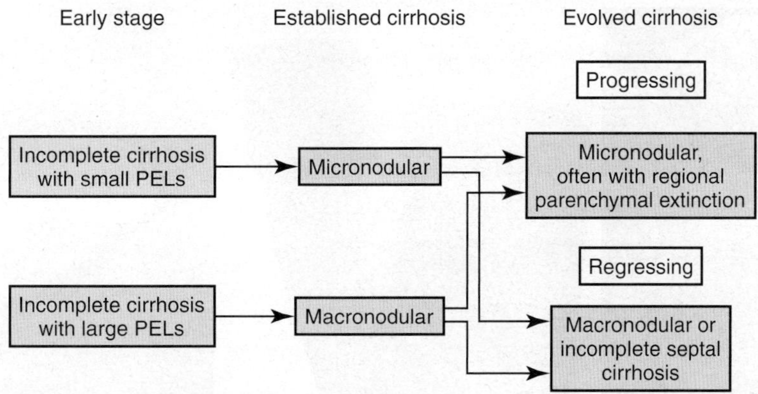

FIGURE 51.10 Anatomical classification of cirrhosis indicating transitions. Micronodular cirrhosis occurs when almost all portal tracts are linked by septa. Macronodular cirrhosis occurs when there are residual portal tracts not bound to septa within cirrhotic nodules. Progression or regression determines the evolution of these basic types. *PELs*, parenchymal extinction lesions.

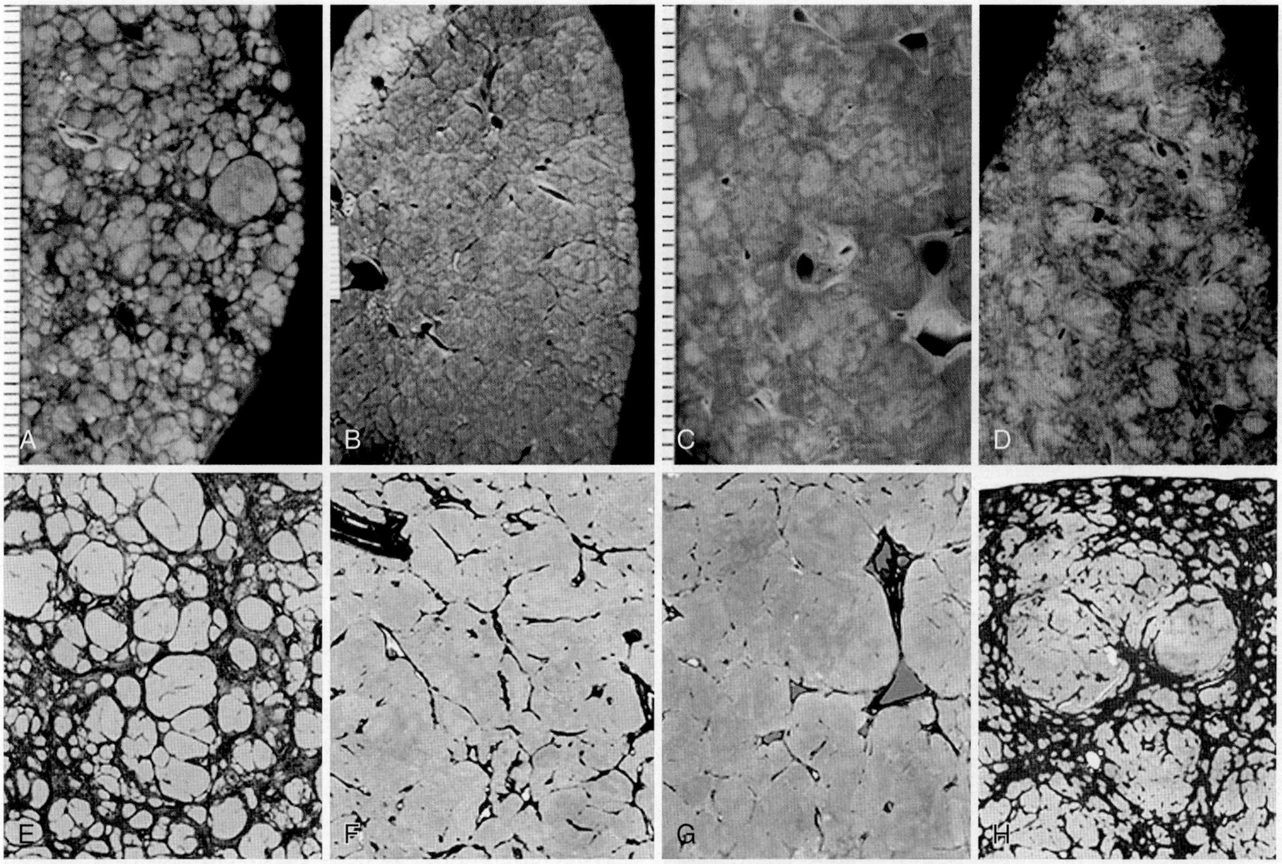

FIGURE 51.11 Examples of cirrhosis: photographs of the cut surface are matched with trichrome-stained, black and white images highlighting fibrosis. A and **E,** Micronodular cirrhosis caused by hepatitis C virus. Most nodules are smaller than 3 mm in diameter, and septa are fairly broad. **B** and **F,** Regressed incomplete cirrhosis caused by hepatitis B virus. The septa are delicate and often incomplete. **C** and **G,** Incomplete septal cirrhosis caused by hepatitis B virus. The nodules are more apparent grossly than histologically. Most septa are delicate and incomplete. **D** and **H,** Primary biliary cirrhosis with green parenchyma (after fixation) and mixed nodule size. The larger nodules are less cholestatic than the micronodules.

schistosomiasis, metastatic carcinoma (most commonly breast carcinoma), and Hodgkin disease.[64-66] This injury pattern is caused by areas of confluent parenchymal necrosis. This very rare and distinctive process is not true cirrhosis. Supernumerary hepatic lobes, a congenital defect, can have a similar appearance.

Infarction of Nodules versus Congestive Necrosis of Nodules

Necrosis of cirrhotic nodules may occur in association with systemic hypotension, typically after a variceal hemorrhage, or as a result of proximity to neoplasms that underwent

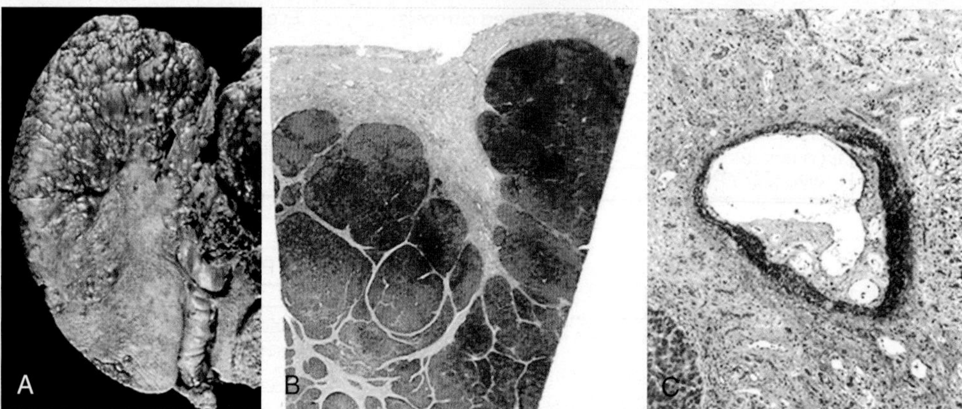

FIGURE 51.12 Regional parenchymal extinction, also known on imaging studies as confluent hepatic fibrosis, in a liver with cirrhosis caused by alcoholism plus hepatitis C. A, The left lobe has a large depressed region with a finely granular capsular surface. **B,** In this liver the regional extinction is largely subcapsular. In other livers, the extinct region extends deep toward the hilum. **C,** Such large regions of extinction are invariably associated with intimal thickening and luminal narrowing of medium-sized hepatic veins.

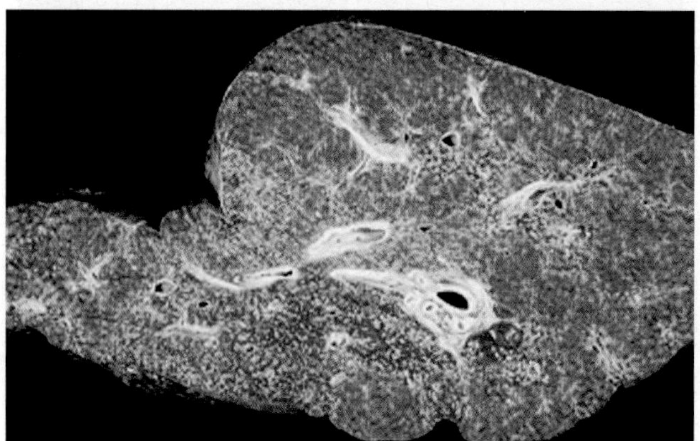

FIGURE 51.13 Fulminant hepatitis, idiopathic. The green regions contain regenerating hepatocytes. The brown regions are totally collapsed with no residual hepatocytes. Fibrosis in such livers is usually minimal.

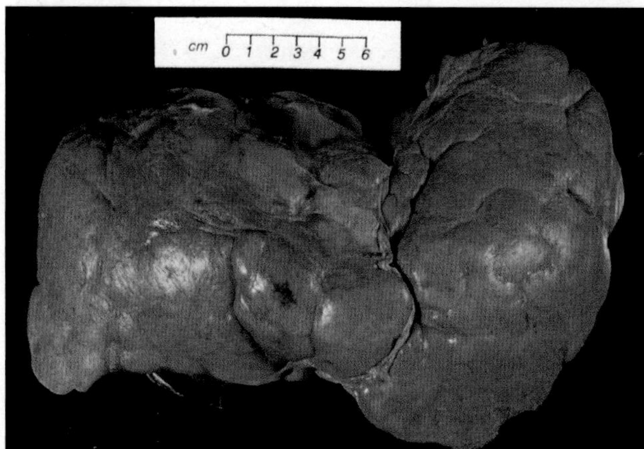

FIGURE 51.14 Hepar lobatum: "potato liver."

radiofrequency ablation or alcohol injection (Fig. 51.15). In some cases, the necrosis can be large enough to form a pseudotumor, which was called *anoxic pseudolobular necrosis* in the historical literature.[67]

Portal Vein Thrombosis

Portal vein thrombosis is a frequent complication of cirrhosis. One study found a cumulative 3-year incidence of 4% in patients with cirrhosis.[68] Portal vein thrombosis is occasionally seen when carcinoma invades the vascular tree.[69]

Patent Paraumbilical Veins

In patients with severe portal hypertension, there is often spontaneous opening of collateral veins within the round ligament.[70] These paraumbilical veins connect the umbilical portion of the left portal vein to the umbilicus, where caput medusae and a bruit may be detected on physical examination. Histological inspection of the round ligament can reveal these patent channels in cirrhotic livers.

Capsular Fibrosis

Capsular fibrous thickening of the splenic capsule can result from chronic exudation or transudation, especially in patients with cirrhosis or severe congestive heart failure. Although no longer in common usage, this condition historically has been called *sugar-coating (Zukerguss)*, as well as *perisplenitis cartilaginea*, which occasionally also affects the liver. The capsule may achieve a thickness of as much as several millimeters, with a tough, cartilage-like consistency. In some cases, the thickened capsule may be distinctly nodular, even though the liver parenchyma itself may not be.

ETIOLOGY

Many different diseases give rise to cirrhosis (Box 51.2). In the vast majority of cases the cause of cirrhosis is ultimately determined by correlation of histology with clinical, laboratory, and imaging findings. In fact, in most of the common liver diseases, the histological findings of active injury abate as the liver becomes cirrhotic, leaving behind only nonspecific changes. The next section reviews the histological findings seen in cirrhotic livers of various etiologies. Only very rare cases, however, are diagnosed solely by histological findings. Put another way, in general, it is unwise to be too dogmatic about histological findings as the sole criterion used to classify a cause of cirrhosis. On the other hand, histological evaluation is very helpful to establish broad patterns of injury (e.g., vascular disease, inflammatory disease, biliary disease) and to look for active injury. Histological evaluation is also very helpful to exclude specific diseases (e.g., an iron

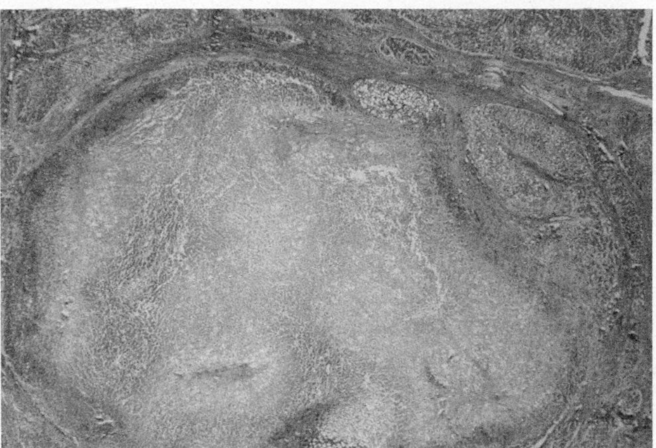

FIGURE 51.15 Infarcted cirrhotic nodule.

BOX 51.2 Major Causes of Cirrhosis

Chronic hepatitis
- Hepatitis B viral infection
- Hepatitis C viral infection
- Autoimmune hepatitis

Fatty liver disease
- Alcoholic liver disease
- Nonalcoholic fatty liver disease

Chronic biliary diseases
- Adults
  - Primary biliary cirrhosis
  - Primary sclerosing cholangitis
- Children
  - Biliary atresia
  - Cystic fibrosis

Inherited diseases
- Metal overload states
  - Hereditary hemochromatosis
  - Wilson disease

Storage disorders
- α_1-Antitrypsin storage disorder

Hepatic venous outflow obstruction (congestive cirrhosis)
- Budd-Chiari syndrome
- "Cardiac cirrhosis"
- Venoocclusive disease

Drug-induced cirrhosis

stain that shows minimal or mild iron excludes untreated genetic hemochromatosis as a cause of the cirrhosis).

Chronic Hepatitis

The most frequent forms of chronic hepatitis that lead to cirrhosis are hepatitis B, hepatitis C, and autoimmune hepatitis. These diseases are usually diagnosed by serological tests. Histologically, a subset of hepatitis B cases can show *ground-glass hepatocytes*, with distinctive cytoplasmic inclusions within hepatocytes. The orcein stain or immunohistochemical staining for hepatitis B surface and core antigens is more sensitive than H&E findings alone. Negative stains also do not exclude chronic hepatitis B, as the viral levels can be very low in cirrhotic livers.[71] Also of note, drug effects can sometimes show identical cytoplasmic inclusions.[72,73]

Plasma cell–rich portal inflammation is not specific but can suggest autoimmune hepatitis. Interface activity, however, is a nonspecific marker of active inflammation and does not help to distinguish autoimmune hepatitis from viral hepatitis or from any other inflammatory cause of cirrhosis. In any case, a final classification as autoimmune hepatitis requires positive serologies and exclusion of chronic viral hepatitis and other causes of cirrhosis.

Chronic hepatitis C as the cause of cirrhosis has sometimes been linked to portal lymphoid aggregates and/or lymphoid follicles, and fatty liver disease, but the associations are too weak to be clinically meaningful for any given case.

Fatty Liver Disease

Fatty liver disease is caused in most cases by alcohol use or by metabolic syndrome. Over time, steatohepatitis can become "burned out," losing both the fat and the findings of active injury (balloon cells, apoptotic bodies, lobular inflammation). In these cases, the final diagnosis rests on reasonably excluding other causes and having a compatible clinical history of either alcohol use or the metabolic syndrome. Of note, pericellular fibrosis is not specific for fatty liver disease and should not be the sole or even the primary reason for classifying a cirrhotic liver as being caused by fatty liver disease. Likewise, Mallory bodies are not specific for fatty liver disease because they are seen in chronic cholestasis and copper-overload states as well.

Chronic Biliary Diseases

Chronic biliary diseases are usually caused by duct obstruction or by primary biliary cirrhosis but may also be caused by hepatocellular defects in bile secretion, as seen with cholestatic drug reactions or familial transport defects. In adults, chronic duct obstruction is most often caused by primary sclerosing cholangitis. In primary sclerosing cholangitis, liver biopsies show obstructive type changes, with bile ductular proliferation and mixed inflammation. By the time the liver is cirrhotic, however, the findings can be relatively nonspecific. Helpful clues include loss of small bile ducts, concentric periductal fibrosis around medium- to large-sized intrahepatic bile ducts, and fibroobliterative duct lesions (Fig. 51.16). In cirrhotic livers from any cause, there are regenerative bile ductules at the margins of nodules and within septa (Fig. 51.17) and this pattern does not indicate chronic biliary obstruction.[74] A similar type of ductular proliferation occurs after massive hepatic necrosis, even if there is no fibrosis or cirrhosis, as part of the normal reparative process of the liver.[45,75]

In primary biliary cirrhosis, there is inflammatory destruction of medium-sized bile ducts. Although these lesions can easily be seen in needle biopsies, in many cases the typical florid duct lesion is not present because of sampling. Indeed, by the time the liver is cirrhotic, these lesions are mostly absent.

The presence of visible bile in a biopsy specimen is not necessary to diagnose chronic biliary disease. In fact, visible bile in tissue is almost never seen in primary biliary cirrhosis and primary sclerosing cholangitis until there is late cirrhosis with functional decompensation. Likewise, cirrhotic livers of any underlying etiology can become deeply cholestatic with clinical decompensation, sometimes triggered by drug-induced liver injury or systemic infections.

Cystic Fibrosis

In cystic fibrosis, thick, mucus-laden bile focally blocks bile flow, leading to elevated liver enzymes. Liver disease can be identified in infants, but the enzyme elevations tend to resolve, only to become evident again in teenage and early adult years.[76] Liver biopsies are now only rarely performed because of the availability of noninvasive measures of liver disease and fibrosis, but show biliary obstruction that manifests as bile ductular proliferation, mixed portal inflammation (neutrophils, lymphocytes), and portal fibrosis. Of note, these changes can be very patchy on biopsy. Inspissated secretions are occasionally found in the bile ducts, seen in about 1% to 5% of cases (Fig. 51.18).[77] There may be large duct strictures resembling primary sclerosing cholangitis. Steatosis (and less commonly steatohepatitis) is found in about 60% of specimens, with moderate or severe macrovesicular steatosis in about in 30%.[76,77] Patients with persistently elevated liver enzymes are at the highest risk for advanced fibrosis or cirrhosis, which develops in about 10%.[76,77]

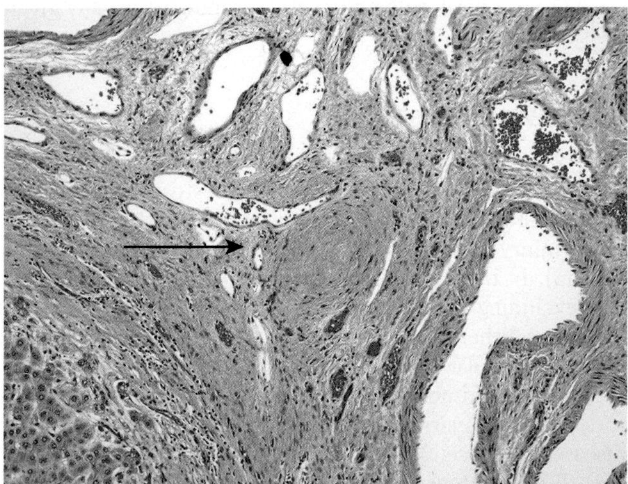

FIGURE 51.16 Primary sclerosing cholangitis. Near the artery is a fibrous cord, which is the only remnant of the bile duct.

Iron Overload

Genetic hemochromatosis is most often caused by homozygous C282Y mutations in *HFE*, but the clinical course of disease is influenced by gender, diet, and other genetic variables, so not all patients with mutations develop clinical disease. Marked iron overload also occurs in other medical conditions such as iron-deficient anemias (including inherited conditions such as thalassemia), hemolysis, transfusion, and portosystemic shunting. Iron overload is also a well-documented phenomenon in alcoholic cirrhosis.[78] The histological findings in marked iron overload from genetic and nongenetic causes both show sufficient overlap such that genetic testing is required to exclude inherited causes

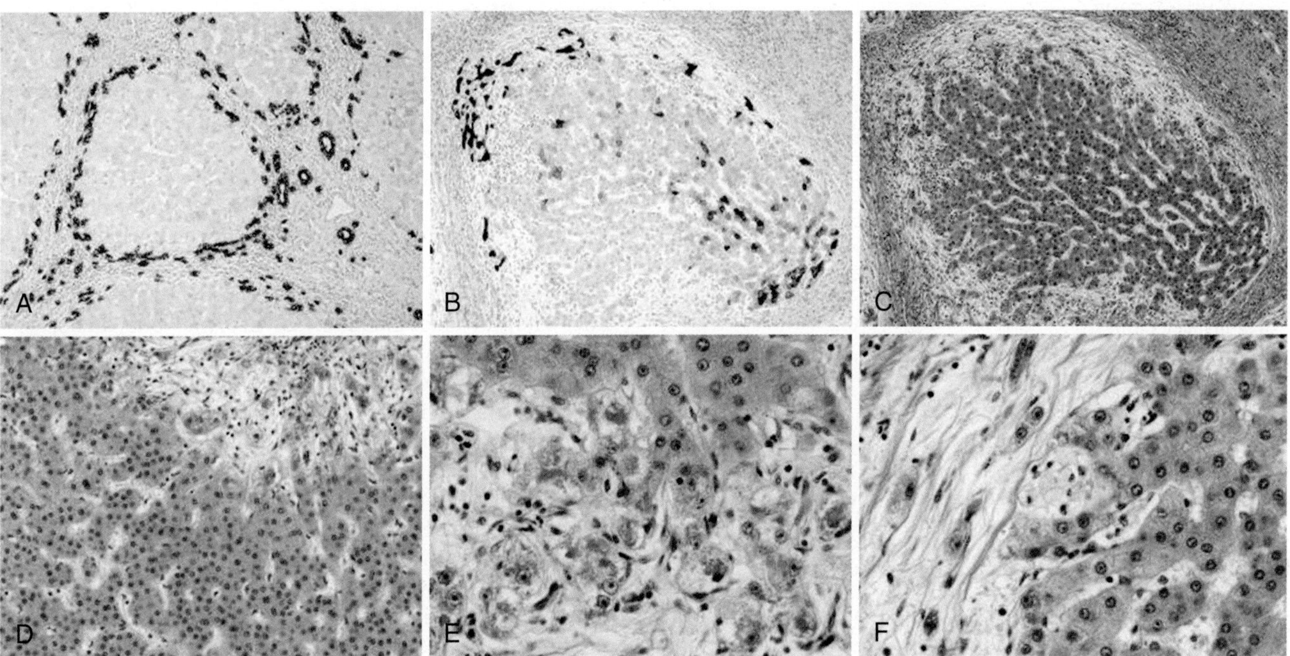

FIGURE 51.17 CK7 immunostain is useful to demonstrate ducts, ductules, and intermediate hepatobiliary cells. A, Cirrhosis caused by hepatitis C is an example of a nonbiliary type of cirrhosis. Cirrhotic nodules are surrounded by a rim of CK7-positive ductules. Ductules are usually found in cirrhosis and do not necessarily indicate cholestasis. **B,** CK7 staining of a cirrhotic nodule in a case of primary biliary cirrhosis reveals variable numbers of ductules at the margins of the nodule. The ductules may have been destroyed by cholestatic injury. There are occasional CK7-positive intermediate hepatobiliary cells within the nodule. **C,** Trichrome stain of the same nodule as in **B** shows a rim of fibrosis at the periphery of the nodule. Images **D** to **F** are from a patient in the cirrhotic stage of primary biliary cirrhosis. **D** and **E** show feathery degeneration of hepatocytes at the margin of a nodule, a feature also known as "cholate stasis." The pale hepatocytes are swollen and often contain Mallory bodies. In **D,** there are wide hepatocellular plates, a feature that may be mistaken for dysplasia or hepatocellular carcinoma. In **F,** there is a cluster of foamy macrophages *(center)*, a frequent finding in chronic cholestasis of any cause.

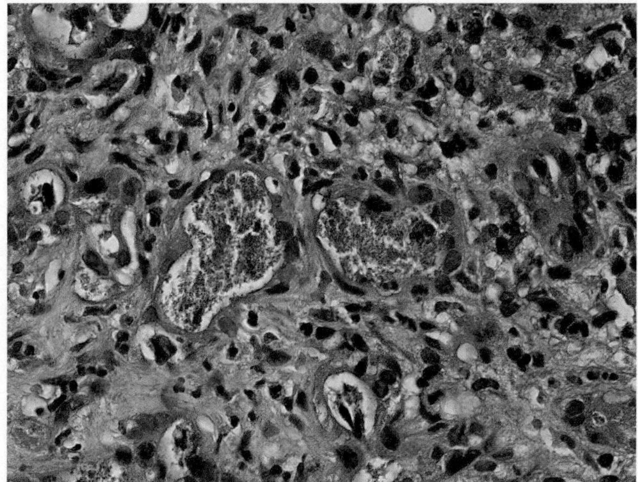

FIGURE 51.18 Cystic fibrosis. The ducts have a thick, eosinophilic, and granular material within their lumen.

with severe iron overload. In most cases, quantitative iron assays are not helpful for diagnostic purposes and the assay is performed for other reasons such as monitoring therapy. In general, mild nonspecific hemosiderosis is common in nonbiliary forms of cirrhosis, but less common in biliary forms of cirrhosis.

Iron accumulation is often heterogeneous in cirrhotic livers from any cause, both genetic and nongenetic. In particular, iron can be sparse in regenerating, dysplastic, or malignant hepatocytes that have had less time to accumulate intracellular iron.[79] Paradoxically, some dysplastic nodules selectively accumulate stainable iron in otherwise iron-free cirrhotic livers.[80]

Wilson Disease

The most common cause of severe copper overload is Wilson disease, in which copper deposition occurs in the liver, eyes, and basal ganglia. Copper in the cirrhotic liver does not always represent Wilson disease, however, as heavy copper deposition can occur in the paraseptal hepatocytes in biliary cirrhosis. On the other hand, not all cirrhotic nodules in Wilson disease will show copper deposition on copper stain. Quantitative copper analysis is an important test to consider if there is clinical concern for Wilson disease, as the copper stain is negative in about 15% of cirrhotic livers with a clinical diagnosis of Wilson diseae.[81] Other histological findings in Wilson disease are typically mild and nonspecific but commonly include steatosis, nuclear pleomorphism, Mallory bodies, ballooning degeneration, and glycogenated hepatocellular nuclei (Fig. 51.19).[81]

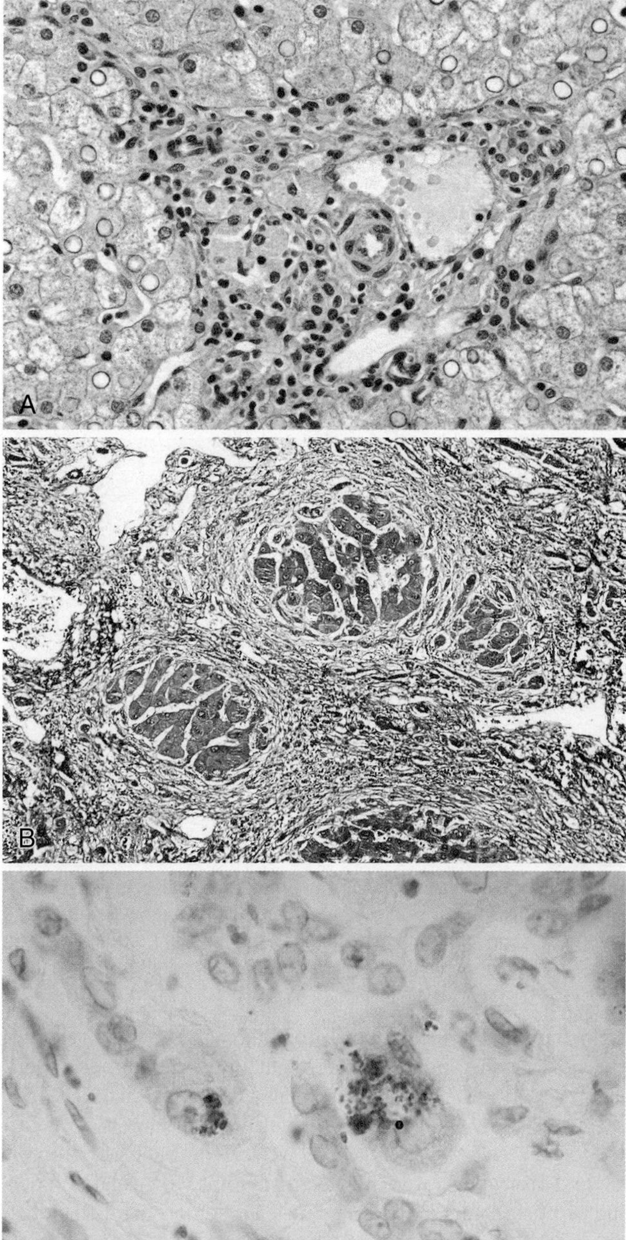

FIGURE 51.19 Wilson disease. A, Early Wilson disease shows portal tract inflammation and prominent glycogenated nuclei of hepatocytes. **B,** Cirrhotic stage of Wilson disease shows micronodular cirrhosis (Masson trichrome stain). **C,** Cirrhotic stage of Wilson disease shows accumulation of orange-hued copper within hepatocytes embedded in dense collagenous stroma (rhodanine stain for copper, hematoxylin counterstain).

Congestive Cirrhosis

The term *congestive cirrhosis* refers to cirrhosis caused by obstruction of medium- to large-sized hepatic veins, the vena cava, or the heart, as in hepatic vein thrombosis or congestive heart failure. Congestive cirrhosis is characterized by venocentric cirrhosis, sometimes called *reversed-nodularity cirrhosis* (Fig. 51.20).[82] This pattern is caused by dominant hepatic vein outflow obstruction with relatively intact portal veins that serve as outflow tracts. In this situation, hepatic vein to hepatic vein fibrosis results in nodules composed of portal tracts in the center and hepatic veins at the periphery within the fibrous septa.

With early or mild disease, congestive heart failure causes sinusoidal dilatation and mild parenchymal atrophy. With more severe or long-standing disease, fibrosis and cirrhosis can develop and appears to progress through obliteration of hepatic and portal veins leading to parenchymal extinction and then to fibrosis.[83] The fibrosis patterns tends to be dominated by irregular dense acinar fibrosis, often

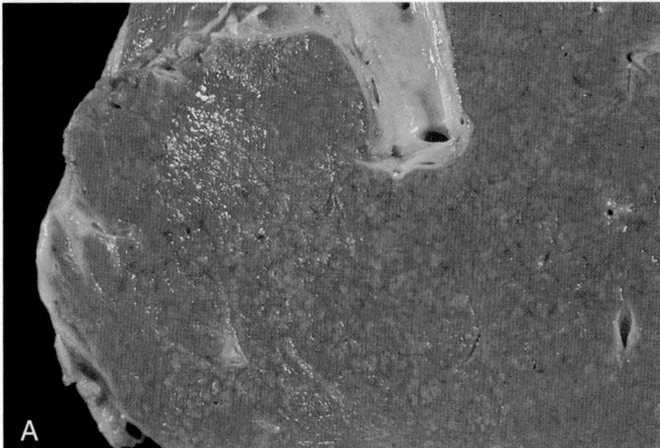

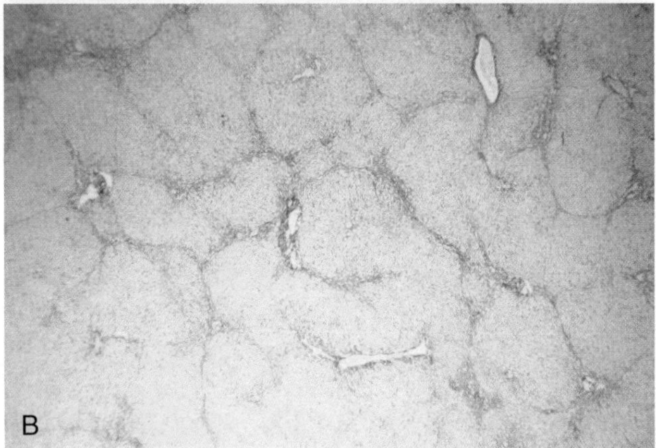

FIGURE 51.20 Cardiac cirrhosis. A, Gross image of cut liver surface shows nodular subdivision of liver parenchyma. **B,** Low-power image of reticulin stain shows bridging fibrous septa between terminal hepatic veins, with intact portal tracts within the center of parenchymal islands.

with haphazard and stellate fibrosis that is heavier around the portal veins, but only rarely with well-developed regenerative nodules.[84] In Budd-Chiari– induced cirrhosis, the liver can show well-developed nodularity, sometimes with the classic *reversed-lobulation*, where the bands of fibrosis extend from central vein to central vein, with relative sparing of portal tracts. However, at least some portal-to-portal and portal-to-central fibrous bands are seen.

Venoocclusive disease (synonym is *sinusoidal obstruction syndrome*) is a distinct cause of congestive hepatic damage that is accompanied by occlusion of the smallest tributaries of the hepatic venous system. It is most commonly associated with toxic induction therapy before bone marrow transplantation but may develop from other toxic causes, such as exposure to the alkaloids contained in certain herbal remedies. Ascites can develop because of increased resistance to blood flow in the sinusoids, but fibrosis is typically absent or mild.[85]

Drug-Induced Cirrhosis

Drugs only very rarely cause cirrhosis, and in most of these cases other known cofactors are present such as alcohol and/or nonalcoholic steatohepatitis. This is because most drugs cause clinically evident "acute" disease, so that drug exposure is terminated before cirrhosis can develop. A few drugs, however, such as amiodarone or methotrexate, can cause asymptomatic low-grade injury and have been linked to fibrosis and cirrhosis in case reports and small series.[86,87] Larger studies, however, have not consistently been able to document a relationship between amiodarone or methotrexate and an increased risk for fibrosis or cirrhosis, suggesting other risk factors are important drivers of cirrhosis.[88,89]

DIAGNOSIS OF CIRRHOSIS

The diagnosis of cirrhosis has undergone many changes over the past 200 years and continues to evolve. These changes may be divided into three eras, based on the dominant methodology used for diagnosis: (1) clinical, (2) histological, and (3) imaging/serological. Before the advent of needle liver biopsies, which became more widely used c. 1950, a diagnosis of cirrhosis was based on clinical criteria such as the presence of varices and ascites. Anatomical or histological confirmation was occasionally possible at surgery or autopsy. The introduction of the liver biopsy led to more sensitive and specific diagnoses of liver cirrhosis than clinical findings alone and was a mainstay of clinical management for several decades. Subsequently, the development of noninvasive techniques for assessing liver fibrosis has advanced to the point that they can provide sufficient information to manage patients in most cases. Biopsies are performed to rule out coexisting liver disease, help determine the cause of liver disease, or in cases in which noninvasive testing was technically inadequate or the imaging results were inconsistent with other clinical findings

Technical Issues

The four main types of liver biopsy procedures are wedge biopsy, cutting liver biopsy, fine-needle aspiration biopsy, and transvenous (transjugular or transfemoral) biopsy. Wedge biopsies provide the most liver tissue. They are obtained by incising the convexity of the liver surface or by resection of a small portion of the liver, often targeting the most inferior edge of the right lobe. The risk in histological evaluation of such specimens is misinterpretation of normal anatomy. In a subset of livers, there is a normal array of fibrous septa that penetrate from the Glisson capsule to a depth of approximately 0.5 cm into the liver parenchyma, partially ensheathing subcapsular portal tracts. If this is not understood, normal fibrous tissue may be erroneously diagnosed as portal or bridging fibrosis. In general, this staging pitfall is relatively easy to avoid because the large portal tracts look normal and the wedge biopsy, when evaluated properly, works well for determining fibrosis stage.

Percutaneous cutting needle biopsies are performed with a 16- to 20-gauge needle and can usually provide a diagnosis of cirrhosis on the first attempt; multiple needle passes are needed only if tissue is not obtained on the first pass. Many times, the biopsy tissue will be fragmented, but neither the presence nor the degree of fragmentation should be used as evidence of cirrhosis. On the other hand, specimen fragmentation alone is not sufficient reason to declare a biopsy as inadequate for fibrosis staging. Cirrhosis, for example, can still be recognized as rounded fragments of parenchyma surrounded by bands of fibrosis, as long as the fibrous bands are well formed. Thin wisps of fibrous tissue can also be seen in normal but fragmented biopsy specimens, representing normal portal structures.

Role of Biopsy

Liver biopsies obtained in the setting of clinical cirrhosis are usually performed for these reasons:

- Evaluation of abnormal laboratory or clinical findings that are inconsistent or unusual for the underlying liver disease
- Staging known chronic liver disease up to and including cirrhosis
- Searching for a cause of portal hypertension of unknown etiology
- Evaluation of a focal "mass" lesion

Histological Findings of Cirrhosis

Cirrhosis is defined as diffuse nodularity of the liver parenchyma caused by fibrous bands. In a small percent age of cases, usually with small biopsies, the liver specimen does not contain sufficient tissue for ready identification of these characteristics, in which case the best approach is to clearly convey in the surgical pathology report how much fibrosis is present as well as any challenges to fibrosis staging. Of course, connective tissue stains, such as Masson trichrome, are essential in making these histological determinations. As noted earlier, fragmentation of the tissue obtained from percutaneous liver biopsy is common and fragmentation per se is an unreliable indicator of cirrhosis.

Sampling error in small biopsies may be impossible to avoid entirely. As one example, cirrhosis composed of larger size nodules can rarely be about the only parenchyma sampled in a small sized liver biopsy, leading to understaging. Many authors recommend that needle biopsies should be at least 2.5 cm long in research studies to adequately stage and grade known diseases such as chronic hepatitis C,[90] as smaller sized biopsies have some risk for understaging liver disease. For clinical care, however, practical experience indicates that biopsies of approximately 1 cm in size or containing 10 portal tracts are typically sufficient to assess etiology, grade of activity, and fibrosis stage.

Staging Systems

Many publications describe methods for semiquantitative evaluation of fibrosis in chronic hepatitis and steatohepatitis. Common systems include the Ishak,[91] Metavir,[92] Batts-Ludwig,[93] NASH-CRN,[94] and SAF.[95]A system specific for vascular disease has also been proposed.[96] Regardless of the staging system, the stage must be estimated with the use of a connective tissue stain, such as Masson trichrome. The reticulin stain is a useful adjunct to detect nodular regenerative hyperplasia.

Pitfalls in Assessing Fibrosis

Assessing the degree of fibrosis is aided by knowledge of common artifacts and diagnostic pitfalls (Box 51.3). An overstained trichrome stain may easily be misinterpreted as showing pericellular fibrosis. One clue to overstaining is that the cytoplasm of hepatocytes should not stain the same color as collagen. If there is any doubt as to the quality of the trichrome stain, it is best to repeat it when possible. Large regions of parenchymal drop out from acute or

BOX 51.3 Pitfalls in Diagnosing Cirrhosis on Liver Biopsy

Misinterpretation of normal anatomy
- Large portal tracts and accompanying fibrous stroma
- Longitudinal sampling of portal tracts
- Fragmentation of normal liver tissue

Technical issues
- Overstained Masson trichrome stain

Misinterpretation of collapsed parenchyma
- Massive hepatic necrosis
- Submassive hepatic necrosis

Misinterpretation of tumor "mass effect" on adjacent parenchyma

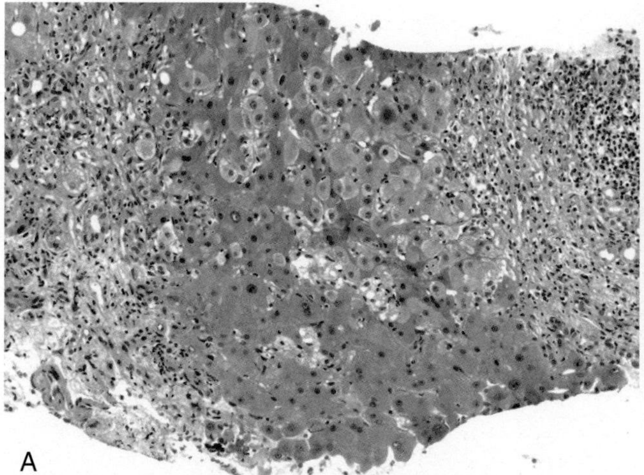

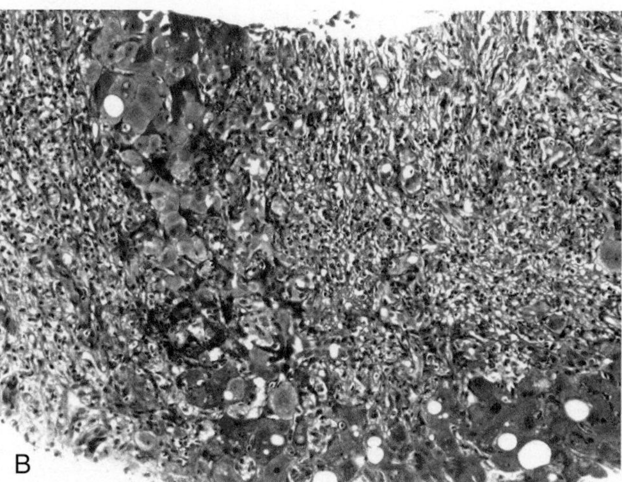

FIGURE 51.21 Massive hepatic necrosis illustrating collapse of connective tissue. A, Needle biopsy specimen from a patient with fulminant hepatic failure shows residual hepatocellular parenchyma between portal tract zones exhibiting ductular proliferation at the interface *(left)* and interface collapse of preexisting extracellular matrix *(right)*. The approximation of portal tracts and the narrow rim of residual hepatocellular parenchyma also indicate collapse. **B,** Adjacent tissue section, stained with Masson trichrome, shows even greater loss of hepatocellular parenchyma, extensive collapse of extracellular matrix, and entrapped proliferating ductules. Despite the prominent "blue" features of this tissue section, this is not cirrhosis.

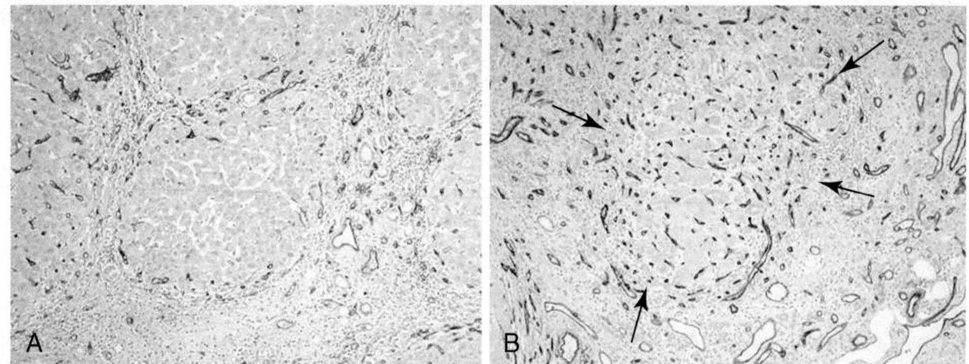

FIGURE 51.22 Angiogenesis in cirrhosis. The CD34 immunostain shows endothelium of arteries and veins. Normal sinusoidal endothelial cells are negative. In cirrhosis, there is a variable degree of arterialization of the sinusoids, seen as CD34 positivity. **A,** Mild cirrhosis. There is minimal CD34 positivity of sinusoidal endothelium at the periphery of the nodule. **B,** Severe cirrhosis. All sinusoidal endothelium is positive for CD34. Arrows show the margins of a cirrhotic nodule.

subacute injury can also be misinterpreted on liver biopsy as bridging fibrosis or cirrhosis (Fig. 51.21). On Masson trichrome stain, the lighter tinctural qualities of the type III and IV collagen in regions of parenchymal collapse can help distinguish massive hepatic necrosis from cirrhosis, which has strongly staining type I collagen fibers within bridging septa separating parenchymal nodules. Immunostain for CD34 may detect arterialized sinusoids that also indicate advanced disease (Fig. 51.22).

Mass lesions can show inflammation and parenchymal fibrosis at the margin. These parenchymal changes represent a mass effect and should not be overinterpreted as cirrhosis. Peritumoral parenchyma should not be used to stage chronic liver disease. In general, a section at least 1 cm away from the mass lesion is preferred.

ACKNOWLEDGMENT

The author is deeply indebted to Ian R. Wanless, MD, FRCPC and to James Crawford for their extensive work on this chapter in prior editions of this book.

The full reference list may be accessed online at Elsevier eBooks for Practicing Clinicians.

CHAPTER 52

Vascular Disorders of the Liver

Matthew M. Yeh, James M. Crawford

Contents

INTRODUCTION

Vascular diseases of the liver are less common than many other conditions, but they have assumed increasing importance in the differential diagnosis of liver disorders: in part because of improved ability to diagnose the more common chronic hepatitic and biliary liver diseases and in part because vascular damage can play a role in the pathophysiology of virtually all liver disorders. In most liver diseases, the primary injury affects hepatocytes or duct cells, and the vascular damage is secondary. However, there are many primary disorders of the hepatic vasculature, and these are the focus of this chapter. Hepatic vascular disease is classified according to the size and type of blood vessels involved because various etiological types of liver disease target different portions of the hepatic vasculature.

The vasculature of the liver is unique in that it has two afferent supplies: arterial and splanchnic. The hepatic artery accounts for 30% to 40%, and the portal vein accounts for 60% to 70% of the hepatic blood supply. The obligate pathophysiological outcome of disease affecting the afferent circulation is downstream ischemia. The degrees to which these two circulations are compromised account for the great variety of histological patterns produced by vascular disease. The patterns reflect the number and size of afferent vessels involved and whether obstruction is rapid onset or slow. Compromise of hepatic venous outflow also creates ischemic injury because blood flow through the liver is impeded. In this situation, however, localized or more general mechanical congestion may also contribute to hepatic damage, depending on the severity of the outflow obstruction. Indeed, isolated hepatic venous outflow obstruction may exhibit mixed features because thrombi can propagate in a retrograde fashion, and the sluggish intrahepatic blood flow can lead to secondary portal vein thrombosis.

As the predominant cell type in the liver, hepatocytes can manifest two levels of ischemic injury. Atrophy is a reduction of cell size that occurs in response to mild ischemia; it is typically seen in zone 3 of the parenchymal lobule in the setting of pure portal vein obstruction or isolated mild venous outflow obstruction. If portal vein compromise is accompanied by damage to the hepatic artery feeding the same region or to the regional hepatic vein, hepatocellular death occurs, again with a propensity toward zone 3. Primary obstruction of the hepatic veins, small or large, also leads to hepatocellular death. If, as a result of both upstream and downstream vascular compromise, all the hepatocytes in a lobule die, local collapse of the tissue leads to apposition of the portal tract and terminal hepatic vein with secondary fibrosis, creating a lesion referred to as *parenchymal extinction.* When parenchymal extinction is widespread, the accumulated lesions are recognized as cirrhosis (see Chapter 51 for greater detail). Considering that the pathology of hepatitis includes vascular damage, it may be a challenge to discern whether histological injury to the hepatic parenchyma is a result of primary vascular disease or part of a broader pattern of hepatitis that evolves to cirrhosis.

If primary vascular injury leads to zone 3 hepatocellular atrophy without fibrosis, the upstream hepatocytes in both zones 1 and 2 may hypertrophy, leading to thickened hepatocyte plates in these upstream zones. Other well-vascularized regions of the liver may regenerate and lead to the development of hepatocellular nodules, without the intervening fibrous septae that characterize cirrhosis. The combination of regional atrophy with nearby regeneration occurs in two major histological patterns. In nodular regenerative hyperplasia (NRH), the nodules are derived from individual lobules and are small, uniform, and diffusely distributed throughout the liver. If the nodule formation is across larger regions, larger regenerative nodules are formed, which are irregularly distributed. Focal nodular hyperplasia (FNH) constitutes a separate form of nodular hyperplasia, as discussed in the following sections.

Hepatic arterial compromise has a direct effect on bile duct epithelial cells because bile ducts derive their vascular supply exclusively from arteries. The most dramatic example is occlusion of the hepatic artery after liver transplantation, which leads to necrosis of the major bile ducts and loss of the organ. But other forms of vascular damage to the biliary tree may be more pernicious, including the recently described entity of secondary sclerosing cholangitis of critically ill patients (SSC-CIP, see later).

Agenesis of the portal vein and large spontaneous portosystemic shunts may be associated with other congenital anomalies.[1] In patients with cirrhosis, spontaneous large-caliber shunts are usually secondary to portal hypertension (see Arterioportal and Arteriovenous Shunts).

The clinical presentation of hepatic vascular disease depends on the location of the obstruction. Obstruction of portal veins is usually clinically silent initially, but severe and prolonged obstruction may lead to varices, usually without ascites or liver failure. Obstruction of hepatic arteries is usually silent, but it may result in necrosis of hepatocytes or bile ducts if combined with hypotension or with another vascular lesion, or if it occurs after organ transplantation. Obstruction of hepatic veins tends to cause increased formation of hepatic lymph, leading to ascites and, if severe, splanchnic varices and hepatic failure. The overarching conditions affecting these vascular compartments and their resultant hepatic disorders are provided in Tables 52.1 to 52.3.

The position of the liver, between the capillary bed of the intestines and the heart, accounts for the important clinical effects of portal hypertension caused by obstruction of blood vessels within the liver. Portal hypertension is commonly classified as either cirrhotic or noncirrhotic, according to the histology of the liver parenchyma. Before 1945, approximately 40% of patients with portal hypertension were thought to have noncirrhotic portal hypertension,[2] but in recent years, that percentage has decreased to less than 1%.[3] The decline in noncirrhotic portal hypertension is largely the result of recognition that although the fibrosis of cirrhosis is largely reversible after successful treatment of the primary liver disease, the abnormalities in vascular pathophysiology remain.[4-7] Specifically, patients with features of cirrhosis on biopsy specimens may subsequently have biopsy specimens that lack histological criteria of cirrhosis. However, these patients often continue to have portal hypertension because more normal portal and hepatic vein anatomy may never be completely restored. Therefore patients with "regressed" cirrhosis fall into the category of hepatic vascular disease and merit discussion in this chapter.

Alternatively, idiopathic noncirrhotic portal hypertension may develop as a result of three seemingly disparate conditions covered in this chapter, which nevertheless feature hepatic small vessel obliteration: hepato-portal sclerosis, incomplete septal cirrhosis, or nodular regenerative hyperplasia. The term *porto-sinusoidal vascular disease* (PSVD), often accompanied by liver biopsy to establish the histology, is now used to guide clinical diagnosis and management of patients with these conditions.[7a]

Although hepatic vessels have some unique properties, their response to stress is similar to that in other organs. Therefore the cause of hepatic vascular disease may be considered in terms of the elements of the Virchow triad: vascular injury, obstruction, and hypercoagulable states. Table 52.4 gives specific events and conditions under which hepatic vascular injury may occur. Table 52.5 lists the tumors and other conditions that can cause mechanical obstruction of the hepatic vasculature. Box 52.1 delineates the systemic conditions that can give rise to a hypercoagulable state affecting the liver.

Identification of normal vascular structures of the liver merits a brief discussion.[8] Portal veins divide dichotomously at acute angles and are accompanied by arteries and bile ducts. At the most terminal portions of the portal tree, portal veins disappear, leaving only the last traces of the hepatic artery/bile duct pairings. The smallest portal tracts, without or with portal veins, may be identified in Masson trichrome–stained sections on the basis of the delicate investment of connective tissue around the portal tract. Large hepatic veins also divide dichotomously, but the smallest hepatic veins enter larger branches at a right angle, similar to the bristles of a brush. There also is a slight preponderance of portal tracts versus hepatic veins within the hepatic parenchyma. In some disorders, portal veins are obliterated with local atrophy of the adjacent parenchyma, so hepatic veins often "migrate" toward the periportal region. When parenchymal extinction has occurred, a hepatic vein may be "tethered" to a portal tract by a short fibrous septum. For these reasons, identification of hepatic veins in some instances may be a challenge that can be solved by identifying elastic fibers in the wall of the vein or by tracing the vessel through multiple levels to a more recognizable centrilobular location within the parenchyma.

In the normal liver, lymphatic channels within portal tracts are difficult to identify because they have few or no muscle fibers and are not dilated on histological sections. Closer to the hepatic hilum, larger lymphatic channels may be identified and valves may be seen. When the hepatic vasculature is compromised, however, dilated lymphatic channels in the more distal portal tract distribution may become prominent. In cirrhosis, there may be an abundance of lymphatic channels within the fibrous septa, identified in part by the absence of erythrocytes in their lumina. Whether normal or abnormal, lymphatic endothelium stains positive with D2-40, whereas venous endothelium does not.

PORTAL VEIN DISEASE (PORTAL VEIN OBSTRUCTION)

Clinical Features

Obstruction of large portal veins most often occurs in adults with symptomatic cirrhosis, and the portal vein lesion is discovered during imaging studies. In the absence of cirrhosis,

TABLE 52.1 Differential Diagnosis of Portal Vein Obstruction

	Clinical Manifestations	Gross Features	Histopathological Features
Thrombosis of large portal vein	Hypercoagulable state (inherited or acquired, see Table 52.4); hepatomegaly; splenomegaly, tumor thrombus; injury to portal vein caused by hilar bile leak; iatrogenic	Mild thickening of intima; intraluminal fibrosis with racemose channels; or recanalization; formation of thin webs	Extramedullary hematopoiesis in myeloproliferative disease causing hypercoagulable state
Small portal veins	Portal hypertension (rare and mild)	Thrombosis in portal vein; vanishing of vein walls	Nonspecific obliteration of small portal veins; granulomas; thrombosis in portal vein; inflammation; vanishing of vein walls; paucity of majority of small portal veins; congestive portal venopathy; postthrombotic scarring; hepatoportal sclerosis
Schistosomiasis	Variceal bleeding; massive splenomegaly with normal liver tests and no ascites	Symmers' pipestem fibrosis	Eggs of *Schistosoma* species +/ granulomatous inflammation
Hepatoportal sclerosis	Idiopathic portal hypertension; normal or mildly elevated liver tests; hepatic venous pressure gradient typically not increased; static and slow progression without cirrhosis	Thromboemboli +/– recanalization, in large portal tracts	Portal vein intimal fibrosis and delicate septa; phlebosclerosis; atrophic liver parenchyma; distortion of distribution and distance between portal tracts and hepatic veins; NRH pattern may be seen; dilated and herniated portal vein into parenchyma; sinusoidal dilation near portal tracts; portal/periportal fibrosis +/–thin fibrous septa extending out +/– vague nodularity

TABLE 52.2 Differential Diagnosis of Hepatic Artery Obstruction

	Clinical Manifestations	Gross Features	Histopathological Features
Hepatic artery obstruction	Hepatic artery thrombosis after liver transplantation	Necrosis/rupture of perihilar parenchyma; bile leak; strictures; cysts;	Bile ductular reaction with associated neutrophilic infiltrates; ischemic cholangitis; *Candida* in necrotic debris; complete necrosis of the biliary tree with cholestasis; necrosis of perihilar parenchyma
Arteritis	Asymptomatic; portal hypertension; liver rupture (rare)	Infarction; hepatic rupture	Arteritis; giant cells in giant cell arteritis; granulomas in Wegener granulomatosis;
Arterioportal and arteriovenous shunts	Bruit, high-output congestive heart failure; ascites; diarrhea; weight loss; protein-losing enteropathy; hemobilia; portal hypertension	Dilated vessels; obliteration of portal veins	Numerous congested capillaries and arterioles, within or adjacent to portal tracts

TABLE 52.3 Differential Diagnosis of Hepatic Venous Outflow Obstruction

	Clinical Manifestations	Gross Features	Histopathological Features
Budd-Chiari syndrome	Hepatomegaly, ascites, fever, liver failure, gastrointestinal bleeding, jaundice, hepatic encephalopathy; hypercoagulable state/myeloproliferative disease	Massive hepatomegaly; affected lobes smaller over time; compensatory hypertrophy of unaffected regions (most commonly caudate lobe)	Sinusoidal congestion/dilation; hepatocyte atrophy/dropout; perivenular fibrosis; intimal fibrosis of large/medium-sized hepatic veins (many with recanalization); secondary thrombosis of small and large portal veins; extramedullary hematopoiesis
Congestive hepatopathy	Right-sided heart failure; constrictive pericarditis	Hepatomegaly; dark-red; mottled	Hepatocyte atrophy; sinusoidal dilation; degree of thrombosis usually less severe than Budd-Chiari syndrome; perivenular to bridging fibrosis; complete cirrhosis rare

TABLE 52.3 Differential Diagnosis of Hepatic Venous Outflow Obstruction—cont'd

	Clinical Manifestations	Gross Features	Histopathological Features
Sinusoidal obstruction syndrome (venoocclusive disease)	Tender hepatomegaly; ascites; rapid weight gain; hepatic failure; elevated serum bilirubin; hepatic venous pressure gradient greater than 10 mm Hg	Marked diffuse hemorrhage in early phase	Sinusoidal dilation, hepatocellular atrophy (+/−); hemorrhage, apoptosis/necrosis of sinusoidal endothelial cells and hepatocytes; collapse of hepatocytic plates; sinusoidal/pericellular fibrosis to advanced bridging fibrosis and cirrhosis
Oxaliplatin-based systemic neoadjuvant chemotherapy	Abnormal direct bilirubin, GGT, and platelet count; portal hypertension (caused by NRH); splenomegaly	Diffuse heterogenous hemorrhagic foci and parenchymal nodularity, outlined by congested areas	Congestion; sinusoidal dilation; NRH (+/−)

GGT, Gamma-glutamyl transpeptidase; *NRH,* nodular regenerative hyperplasia.

TABLE 52.4 Vascular Injury and Systemic Inflammatory Conditions Associated with Obstruction of Large Veins in the Liver

Condition	PV Thrombosis	HV Thrombosis
Catheterization		
Umbilical vein catheterization	+	−
Inferior vena cava catheterization	−	+
Trauma	+	+
Sarcoidosis	+	+
Umbilical sepsis	+	−
Cholecystitis	+	−
Pylephlebitis	+	−
Congenital hepatic fibrosis	+	−
Cytomegalovirus infection	+	−
Hematopoietic cell transplantation	+	−
Esophageal sclerotherapy	+	−
Schistosomiasis	+	−
Inflammatory bowel disease	+	−
Ventriculoatrial shunt	−	+
Sclerotherapy	−	+
Amyloidosis	−	+
Vasculitis or tissue inflammation	−	+
Tuberculosis	−	+
Fungal vasculitis	−	+
Idiopathic granulomatous venulitis	−	+
Filariasis	−	+
Inflammatory bowel disease	−	+
Mixed connective tissue disease	−	+
Protein-losing enteropathy	−	+
Celiac disease	−	+
5q deletion syndrome and hypereosinophilia	−	+

HV, Hepatic vein; *PV,* portal vein.

TABLE 52.5 Tumors and Other Stasis Lesions Associated with Obstruction of Large Veins in the Liver

	PV Thrombosis or Obstruction	HV Thrombosis
Hepatocellular carcinoma	+	+
Carcinoma of pancreas	+	−
Renal cell carcinoma	−	+
Adrenal carcinoma	−	+
Hodgkin disease	−	+
Epithelioid hemangioendothelioma	−	+
Wilms tumor	−	+
Leiomyosarcoma or leiomyoma	−	+
Metastatic neoplasm	−	+
Cirrhosis	+	+
Splenectomy	+	−
Retroperitoneal fibrosis	+	−
Congestive heart failure	−	+
Constrictive pericarditis	−	+
Membranous obstruction of inferior vena cava	−	+
Superior vena cava obstruction	−	+
Other congenital anomalies	−	+
Umbilical cord redundancy or placental thrombosis	−	+
Atrial myxoma	−	+
Sickle cell disease	−	+
Hydatid cyst	−	+
Hepatic abscess	−	+
Hematoma	−	+

HV, Hepatic vein; *PV,* portal vein; +, reported cases or case series; −, no reported examples.

large portal vein obstruction may develop as a primary event, often presenting as *idiopathic portal hypertension*, or secondary to inflammatory conditions involving the portal vein, such as schistosomiasis or sarcoidosis.[9] In these conditions, the portal vein thrombosis is typically silent until

BOX 52.1 Hypercoagulable States That Affect Hepatic Vasculature

MYELOPROLIFERATIVE DISEASE
Latent myeloproliferative disease
Polycythemia vera
Primary myelofibrosis
Paroxysmal nocturnal hemoglobinuria
Idiopathic thrombocytosis
Chronic myeloid leukemia
Promyelocytic leukemia
Multiple myeloma

GENETIC ANOMALIES
Protein C deficiency
Protein S deficiency
Antithrombin III deficiency
Factor II G20210A
Factor V Leiden
Heparin cofactor II deficiency
Plasminogen deficiency
Dysfibrinogenemia
Homocystinemia

OTHER HYPERCOAGULABLE STATES
Pregnancy
Oral contraceptive therapy
Lupus anticoagulant or antiphospholipid antibodies
Idiopathic thrombocytopenic purpura

the onset of bleeding varices; ascites is usually absent. During the asymptomatic period, clinical evidence of portal hypertension, especially splenomegaly or thrombocytopenia, often leads to the diagnosis through imaging studies. The portal vein may appear to be absent, and multiple hilar collaterals may result in an appearance termed *cavernous transformation.* Large collaterals develop in the round ligament in 5% of patients; rarely, this manifests as a bruit or an umbilical caput medusa. The round ligament collaterals are dilated paraumbilical veins that communicate with the left portal vein. Large collaterals between the extrahepatic portal vein and the renal or adrenal veins are frequently seen. Numerous smaller collaterals are often seen during imaging or abdominal surgery. Secondary aneurysmal dilation of the portal vein may also occur.

In contrast with this type of indolent natural history, acute portal vein obstruction accompanied by thrombosis of the mesenteric veins can be catastrophic and can lead to infarction of the intestines. This sequence often occurs in the setting of abdominal sepsis, trauma with vascular injury, cirrhosis, or growth of hepatocellular carcinoma into the main portal vein.

The portal vein branches are hypoplastic in patients with persistent ductus venosus or other congenital anomalies of the major vessels. Hepatic encephalopathy with hyperammonemia may be a presenting feature when portosystemic shunting is prominent.

Obstruction confined to the small portal veins is a rare cause of portal hypertension and tends to be milder than that seen in patients with large portal vein obstruction. Consideration is given at the end of this chapter to hepatoportal sclerosis, a condition that appears to arise from chronic damage to the large and small intrahepatic portal veins.

Pathogenesis

Large Portal Veins

Most often, portal vein obstruction occurs in the setting of another hepatic disease, particularly cirrhosis. Beyond that, thrombosis is the most frequent mechanism of large portal vein obstruction, again following the Virchow triad of thrombosis secondary to obstruction, venous inflammation, or a hypercoagulable state (see Tables 52.4 and 52.5 and Box 52.1). Hypercoagulable states causing portal vein obstruction may involve inherited abnormalities of the clotting cascade or acquired abnormalities of the platelets, as in polycythemia vera or other myeloproliferative diseases. Coincidental hypercoagulable states have also been documented to contribute to thrombosis, even when cirrhosis is present.[10]

Portal vein obstruction may also be related to inflammation of small portal veins in early primary biliary cholangitis with retrograde thrombosis. Injury to the portal vein vasculature may be caused by a hilar bile leak in primary sclerosing cholangitis or in biliary necrosis after transplantation, or by other events such as splanchnic sepsis, variceal sclerotherapy, or trauma. Trauma may result from blunt abdominal injury or from surgical interventions such as splenectomy, umbilical vein catheterization, portacaval shunt, insertion of a transjugular intrahepatic portosystemic shunt (TIPS), or a Kasai portoenterostomy procedure.

Small Portal Veins

Obliteration of small portal veins (obliterative portal venopathy) may develop secondary to local inflammation, thrombosis, congestive portal venopathy, or toxic injury. Local inflammation is important in any disease with portal inflammation, including chronic hepatitis, primary biliary cholangitis, primary sclerosing cholangitis, sarcoidosis, polyarteritis nodosa, and congenital hepatic fibrosis. Thrombosis may occur as a result of retrograde propagation of thrombi from hepatic veins or in response to sluggish and reversed blood flow, usually in cirrhotic livers. Also in cirrhotic livers, high intrahepatic pressure causes congestive venous injury. A variety of vasculotoxins, including azathioprine, cyclophosphamide, methotrexate, and arsenic, can cause endothelial injury and secondary luminal obliteration. In some geographic regions, schistosomiasis is the most frequent cause of portal vein disease and portal hypertension. The vascular changes in cirrhosis are discussed in Chapter 50.

Granulomas in sarcoidosis can cause phlebitis of small portal veins.[11] Medium-sized hepatic veins may also be affected. In most patients, granulomas in the portal tracts or associated portal fibrosis can cause presinusoidal resistance and portal hypertension, but not cirrhosis.[12,13] NRH and portal vein thrombosis may occur.[14]

Pathological Features

Portal vein thrombus is usually evident only in the healed state, after recanalization and fibrosis have already occurred. The healing process may be almost complete, so no residual changes or only slight pearly thickening of the intima is seen grossly. In other instances, residual high-grade obstruction causes marked intraluminal fibrosis containing numerous racemose channels, visible both at the time of initial opening of the portal vein (Fig. 52.1) and on fixation and

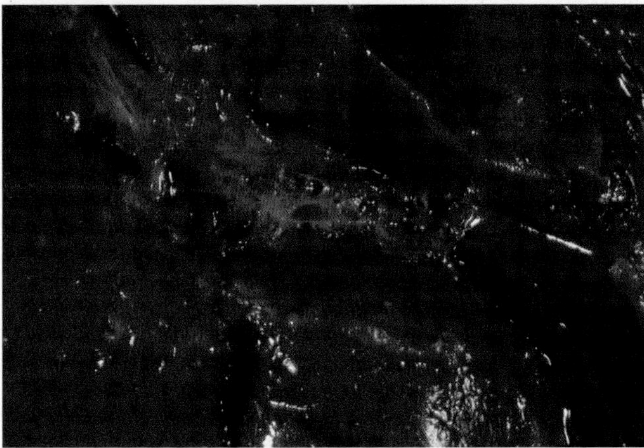

FIGURE 52.1 Portal vein at autopsy in a female patient who underwent umbilical vein catheterization as an infant with subclinical portal vein thrombosis, and splenectomy as a teenager owing to portal hypertension. Note the absence of the usual lumen and replacement by small recanalized channels within the portal vein bed. The patient succumbed to fulminant meningococcal sepsis at 21 years of age.

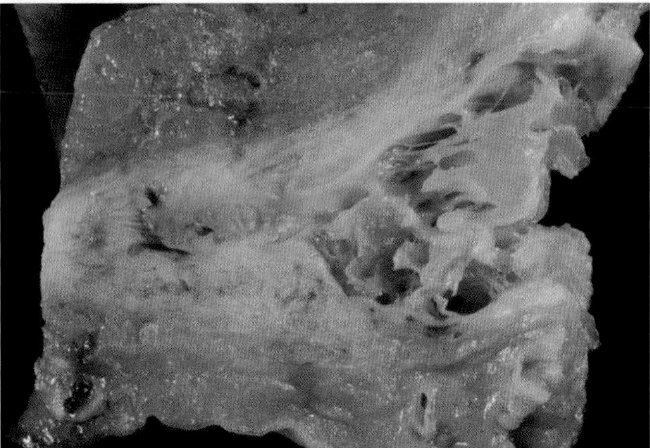

FIGURE 52.2 Organized portal vein thrombosis in the hilum of a formalin-fixed liver shows numerous recanalized channels and subtotal obstruction of the lumen.

cross-section (Fig. 52.2). Thrombi in large and medium-sized portal veins may recanalize almost completely, leaving a layer of residual intimal fibrosis (Fig. 52.3), or they may remain largely occluded (Fig. 52.4). Multiple layers of collagen indicate recurrent thrombosis. As thrombi heal with a granulation tissue response, small arteries are often seen within the neointima. When thrombosis or inflammatory injury involves small portal veins, the vein walls usually disappear completely within a few weeks after the inciting event. The elastic trichrome stain is better than Masson trichrome for identifying residua of vein walls, which are marked by the location of muscle bundles or variation in the elastic fibers (Fig. 52.5).

In the many conditions that may cause portal vein inflammation, thrombosis, and fibrous obliteration, several clues may indicate the originating cause. Portal granulomas may be seen in sarcoidosis and primary biliary cholangitis; bile duct paucity favors the latter (Fig. 52.6). Granulomas in sarcoidosis are usually numerous, but in inactive disease, they may resorb, making diagnosis difficult. Eggs of *Schistosoma* species may occur either with or without granulomatous inflammation (Fig. 52.7). Eggs are few in number with *Schistosoma mansoni* and numerous with *Schistosoma japonicum*. Irregular and dilated marginal ductules are found in most portal tracts in cases of congenital hepatic fibrosis (Fig. 52.8) and in occasional portal tracts in polycystic disease. Thorotrast deposits in portal macrophages may be associated with obliteration of small portal veins and noncirrhotic portal hypertension (Fig. 52.9). Marked parenchymal congestion or obstruction of hepatic veins may lead to portal vein thrombosis secondary to stasis; the congestion is a tip-off of the potential cause. As will be discussed in the chapter on cirrhosis (Chapter 50), thrombotic occlusion of portal veins and terminal hepatic veins within the same lobule lead to extinction of the intervening parenchyma; this process is common to virtually all progressive forms of hepatitis that lead to cirrhosis.[15]

Patients with noncirrhotic portal hypertension usually have delicate parenchymal septa, portal vein intimal fibrosis, and portal tracts with no evident portal vein (Fig. 52.10A–C), suggesting regressed cirrhosis and superimposed portal vein thrombosis or congestive portal venopathy.[16] After portal vein obliteration, the liver parenchyma becomes atrophic, with crowding of the portal tracts (see Fig. 52.10D). If the region of sinusoidal dilation is focal, it is called an *infarct of Zahn* (see Sinusoidal Dilation). Atrophy may be either uniform or mixed, with small regenerative nodules in a pattern referred to as NRH (discussed later).

Differential Diagnosis

Causes of portal hypertension in the absence of cirrhosis are variable. Worldwide, schistosomiasis is the most common cause. Alcohol-induced liver disease, inherited metabolic diseases, and autoimmune liver diseases can cause portal hypertension at the precirrhotic stage. However, the most important differential diagnosis is cirrhosis.

Exclusion of Cirrhosis and Regressed Cirrhosis

The diagnosis of portal vein disease does not rely on the histological appearance alone but requires consideration of clinical and imaging information. The most useful task in a patient with portal hypertension is to confirm the presence or absence of cirrhosis, including the possibility of regressed cirrhosis. This allows the investigation to be directed at the most likely cause of the cirrhosis.

Of course, biopsy specimen size is important in providing the pathologist with enough evidence to accurately exclude cirrhosis (see Chapter 50). Cirrhosis, particularly when highly regressed, is frequently missed when biopsy specimens are shorter than 2 cm in length. Regressed cirrhosis should be suspected when there is a reduction of both portal and hepatic veins, delicate remnants of fibrous septa are present, and lobular architecture is abnormal with an irregular arrangement of portal structures and hepatic veins, typically with hepatic veins in close approximation to portal tracts.

Irregularity of parenchymal architecture with atrophy and hyperplasia but without fibrosis, as may be seen in NRH, suggests small vessel disease, even if this is not represented in the biopsy specimen. Similar architectural changes may occur adjacent to mass lesions, including neoplasms

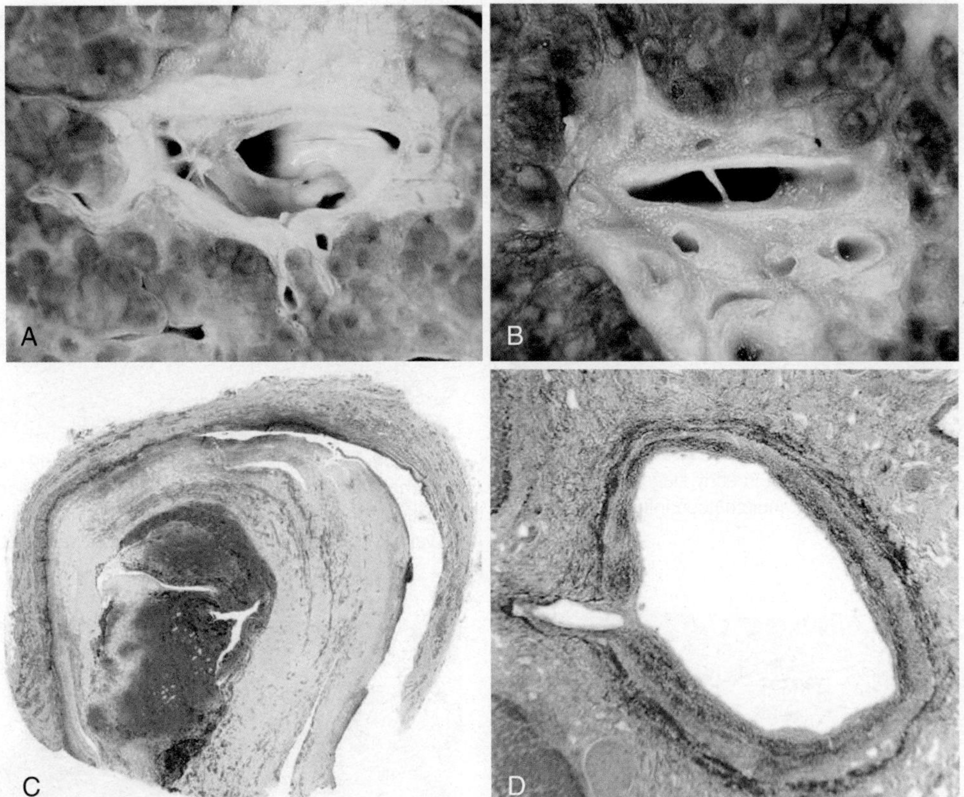

FIGURE 52.3 Portal vein thrombosis. A, Lobar portal vein with moderate stenosis caused by an organized thrombus. The liver is cirrhotic. **B,** Lobar portal vein with a delicate web as a result of an organized thrombus. **C,** Transverse section of the main portal vein shows several layers of organized thrombus, including a central region of recent thrombus (elastic trichrome stain). **D,** Medium-sized portal vein with concentric intimal fibrous thickening (Masson trichrome stain).

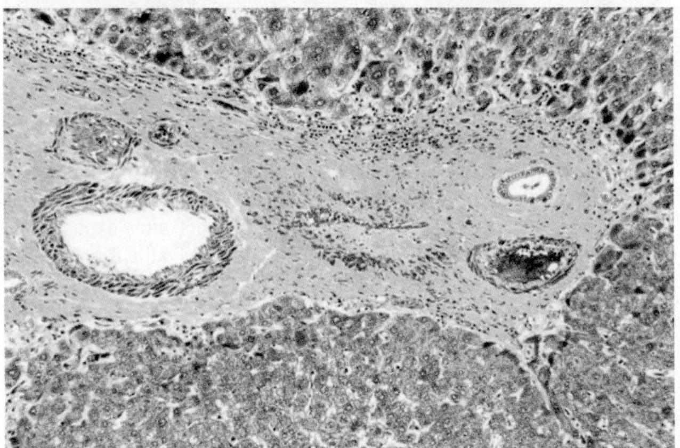

FIGURE 52.4 Portal vein obliteration in a noncirrhotic liver. The portal vein is obliterated by fibrosis (center of image). The original wall is identified by a row of muscle bundles (Masson trichrome stain).

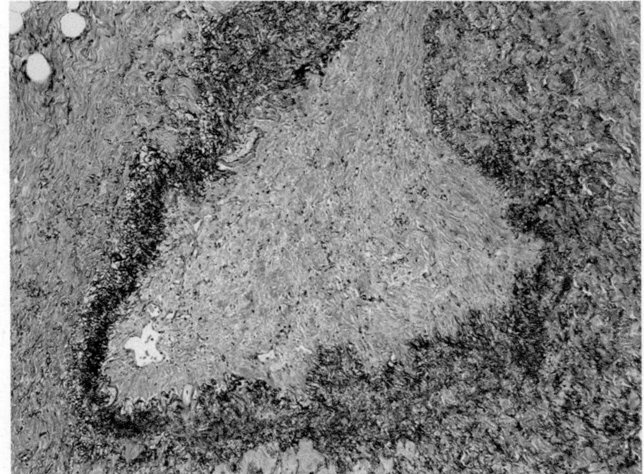

FIGURE 52.5 Portal vein post-thrombotic occlusion with minimal recanalization. The original portal vein wall is highlighted in this elastin stain (Verhoeff–Van Gieson elastin stain).

and abscesses, as a result of local mechanical derangement in blood flow.

Patients may be diagnosed with noncirrhotic portal hypertension on the basis of imaging studies (no identifiable alteration in hepatic features) or lack of biopsy evidence of cirrhosis. In the latter instance, the limited amount of tissue in liver biopsy specimens may make identification of regressed cirrhosis difficult. Alternatively, the histological manifestations of regressed cirrhosis may be termed *incomplete septal cirrhosis* or *hepatoportal sclerosis*, depending on the location of residual fibrous tissue (delicate parenchymal septa in the former, fibrotic portal tracts alone with obliteration of portal vein profiles in the latter).[17,18] Incomplete septal cirrhosis is discussed in Chapter 50; hepatoportal sclerosis is discussed later in this chapter. Last, *idiopathic portal hypertension* identified clinically may represent a mixture of diseases or one disease with various histological manifestations,[6] hence introduction of the new term *porto-sinusoidal vascular disease*.[7a]

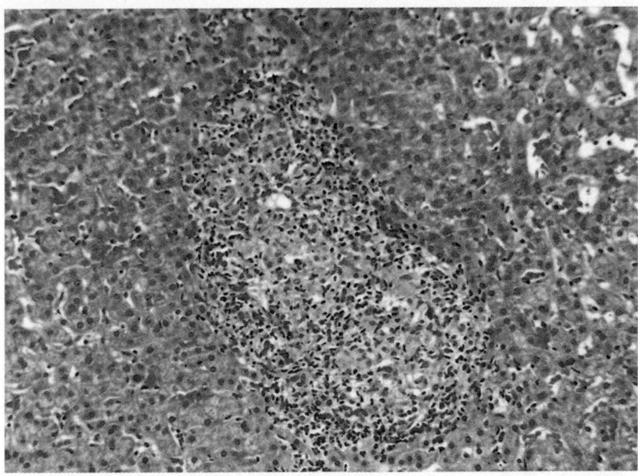

FIGURE 52.6 Obliterated small portal vein in early-stage primary biliary cholangitis. The vein is replaced by granulomatous inflammation, and the bile duct is absent.

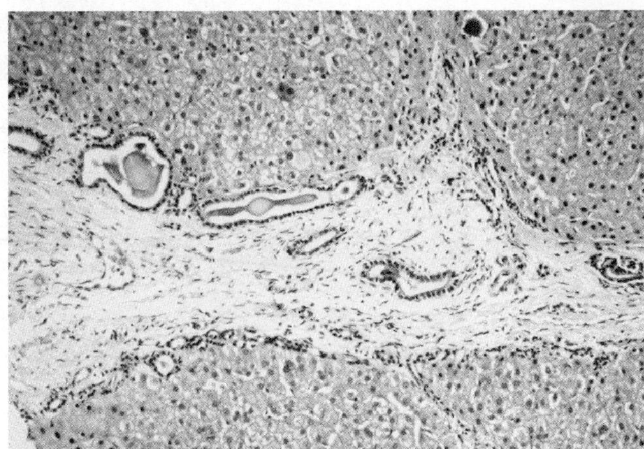

FIGURE 52.8 Congenital hepatic fibrosis, showing marginal dilated ductular channels with inspissated bile, retained interlobular bile duct, and hepatic artery profiles, but dense septal fibrosis with obliteration of portal veins; a residual portal vein profile is present on the left (H&E stain).

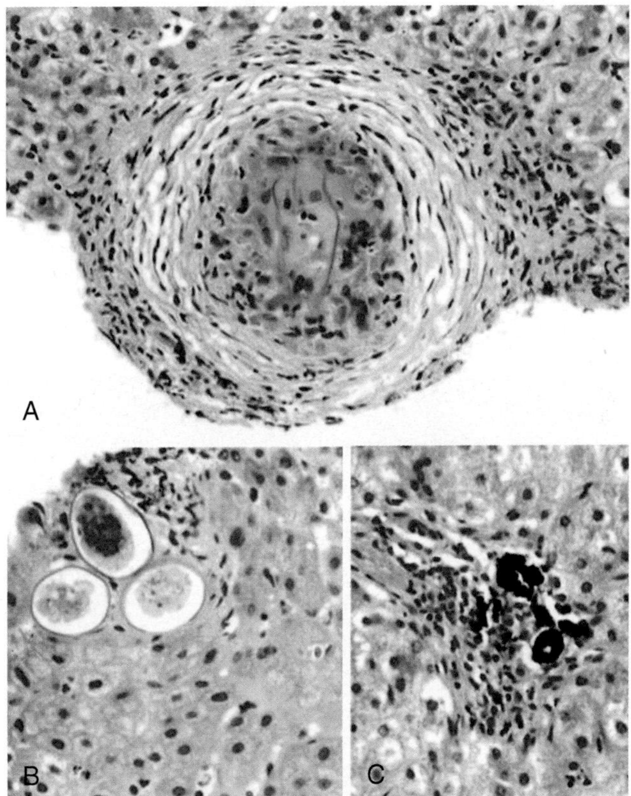

FIGURE 52.7 Schistosomiasis. A, *Schistosoma mansoni* egg surrounded by a fibrous granuloma. The large lateral spine is not visible in this tissue section. The portal vein is not seen and is presumably obliterated. **B,** *Schistosoma japonicum* is characterized by numerous small eggs, each with a small lateral spine that is rarely visible in histological sections. **C,** *Schistosoma* pigment in portal macrophages.

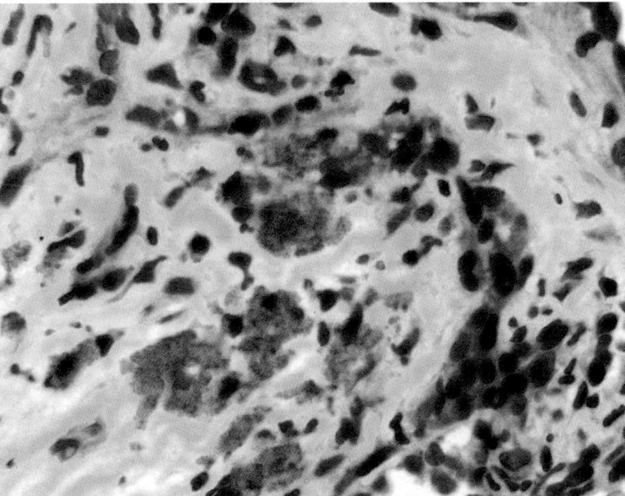

FIGURE 52.9 Thorotrast accumulates in macrophages as coarse granules within portal tracts as well as other organs (Masson trichrome stain). This patient had an angiosarcoma 42 years after exposure to Thorotrast. Thorotrast was visible on radiographs within the liver, spleen, and abdominal lymph nodes.

Exclusion of Portal Vein Thrombosis

Liver biopsy is seldom indicated for identification of large portal vein disease because peripheral biopsies do not sample these vessels. Recanalization of large portal vein thrombi make these lesions elusive from a clinical point of view. Prior thrombosis is suspected when there is prominent intimal fibrosis of portal veins, especially those larger than 200 μm in diameter. No specific histological features can be used to diagnose hypercoagulable states. Conversely, obliteration of small portal veins is nonspecific. Lesions associated with inflammatory obliteration of small portal veins should be sought, including duct lesions of primary biliary cholangitis, granulomas of sarcoidosis and schistosomiasis, and arteritis. Obliteration of subcapsular small portal veins is a common event among aged individuals.[19] However, the finding that the majority of small portal veins are missing is likely to be significant. Congestive portal venopathy and post-thrombotic scarring are often identical in appearance. Thrombosis, when present, involves many small- and medium-sized portal veins, whereas congestive lesions are usually patchy in distribution and confined to the small veins. This criterion is useful only when examining large samples, such as liver explant specimens. Congestive lesions are more likely to occur in cirrhotic livers, where high-grade hepatic vein outflow obstruction is characteristically present.

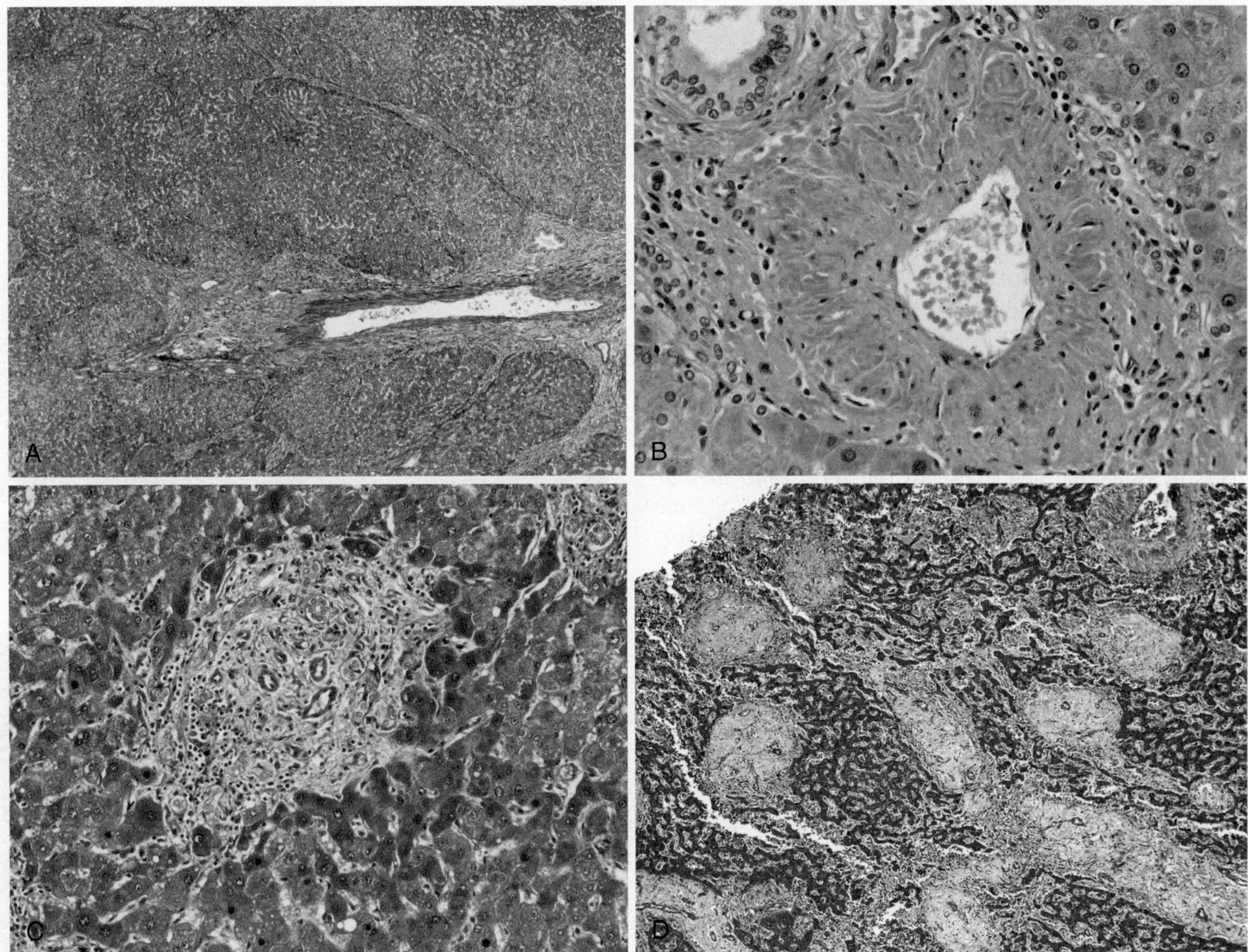

FIGURE 52.10 Portal tract and parenchymal changes in noncirrhotic portal hypertension. A, Regressed cirrhosis in a patient with former alcohol abuse who is now abstinent long-term. Low-power view showing a fibrosed sublobular portal tract with a delicate fibrous septa traversing the parenchyma (trichrome). **B,** Small portal vein from same liver showing medial thickening and intimal fibrosis (H&E stain). **C,** A different portal tract from the same liver showing hepatic artery, bile duct, and bile ductule profiles, with no evident portal vein (trichrome). **D,** Medium-power view of left hepatic lobe from a different patient, in which thrombosis of uncertain etiology affecting both lobar and smaller portal veins led to panlobar atrophy. Numerous fibrotic portal tracts, in which portal vein profiles are not evident, are closely approximated as a result of atrophy of the lobules (trichome).

Exclusion of Parasitic Disease

Schistosomes are trematode flukes. Some species may involve the liver, such as *S. japonicum* in Asia and *S. mansoni* in Africa and South America. Liver disease in schistosomiasis is attributed to the entrapment of parasitic ova in portal veins.[20] The secretion of ova induces a granulomatous reaction and collagen deposition. In an individual with severe infestation of schistosomes, marked portal fibrosis ensues; this condition is known as *Symmers' pipestem fibrosis*.[21] The clinical presentation of hepatic schistosomiasis mimics idiopathic portal hypertension in that variceal bleeding and massive splenomegaly with normal liver test results and no ascites are common manifestations.[9]

ARTERIAL DISEASE

The hepatic arterial system may be involved by systemic diseases such as amyloidosis or polyarteritis nodosa. Atherosclerosis may affect the extrahepatic arterial trunk, and the intrahepatic arteries may exhibit hyaline arteriosclerosis in older individuals. Atherosclerotic emboli may occasionally lodge in the hepatic arterial circulation. Regardless of cause, arterial disease in the liver is seldom symptomatic, mainly because of the smaller contribution of the hepatic artery to hepatic blood flow and compensation from portal veins. However, in patients with hypotension or congestive heart failure, infarcts or liver failure may occur as a result of regional arterial disease.[22,23] Moreover, as noted earlier, arterial compromise leading to ischemic damage to the biliary tree may lead to failure of the entire organ.

Liver Necrosis and Infarction

Forward-flow circulatory compromise to the liver may be the result of heart failure caused by acute myocardial infarction or circulatory shock resulting from hypovolemia, severe trauma, or sepsis.[24,25] Patients with circulatory shock have both low arterial blood pressure and reduced oxygen tension in the portal veins. Typically, a sharp rise in serum aminotransferases, with or without liver failure, develops in patients with shock. Enzymes typically normalize rapidly in those patients who survive.

Hepatic infarction has also been associated with antiphospholipid syndrome with or without associated Budd-Chiari syndrome,[26,27] hepatic trauma,[28] hepatic transplantation,[29] hepatic catheterization,[30] laparoscopic cholecystectomy,[31] TIPS insertion,[32] and alcohol injection.[33] A variety of hypercoagulable states and vascular injury syndromes may cause liver ischemia, including disseminated intravascular coagulation (DIC), sepsis, toxemia of pregnancy,[34] HELLP syndrome (i.e., hemolysis, elevated liver enzymes, and low platelet count),[35,36] arteritis,[37] sickle cell disease,[38] oral contraceptive use,[39] and acute pancreatitis.[40,41]

Pathological Features

Left-sided cardiac failure or shock may lead to the development of sharply demarcated zones of coagulative necrosis (Fig. 52.11). Zone 3 is usually most susceptible to the effects of ischemia, giving rise to the term *centrilobular necrosis*. Livers with marked zone 3 atrophy and/or zone 3 necrosis, combined with zone 3 hemorrhage from retrograde congestion (as from right-sided heart failure), often have a gross appearance that resembles the cut surface of a nutmeg and is termed *nutmeg liver* (Fig. 52.12). The combination on microscopy of centrilobular necrosis from forward-flow ischemia with centrilobular hemorrhage from retrograde congestion is termed *centrilobular hemorrhagic necrosis*.

Rarely, isolated zone 2 necrosis is seen.[42] Single-cell calcification may occur. Apoptotic bodies are usually observed in the zone between healthy and coagulated hepatocytes. Zone 1 necrosis is typical of diseases that produce intravascular fibrin deposition, such as toxemia of pregnancy and DIC (Fig. 52.13). The fibrin in these conditions may be present in arterioles, portal venules, and zone 1 sinusoids. Regardless of cause, a reticulin stain can help identify areas of architectural collapse resulting from loss of hepatocytes.

In the liver, an infarct is defined as ischemic necrosis involving two or more contiguous and complete acini; both zone 1 and zone 2 must be involved. Microscopic infarcts occur when at least two of the following vessels are involved in the same lobular unit of liver tissue: portal vein, hepatic vein, and hepatic artery (Fig. 52.14). In the presence of hypotension, lesser degrees of vascular obstruction are necessary to produce infarction. Often, no vascular obstruction can be identified.[22]

Differential Diagnosis

The differential diagnosis of zone 3 necrosis includes drug-induced injury, particularly with acetaminophen or cocaine. *Amanita phalloides* (mushroom) hepatotoxicity also shows zone 3 coagulative necrosis. Herpes virus infection results in geographic necrosis that resembles infarcts except that the margins of necrosis do not follow the normal hepatic acinar landmarks, and viral inclusions are usually visible at the rim of the necrotic area. Atrophy and sinusoidal dilation suggest underlying chronic passive congestion, as seen in patients with right-sided heart failure.[43] (see Hepatic Vein Disease).

Arteritis

Large- and medium-sized hepatic arteries may be affected in polyarteritis nodosa, Wegener granulomatosis, and rheumatoid arthritis. The arteritis is usually clinically silent, although hepatic rupture has been reported.[44,45] Small vessel arteritis, as in systemic lupus erythematosus (SLE) or rheumatoid arthritis, is also usually clinically silent but may result in obliteration of adjacent portal veins, leading to NRH and portal hypertension.[46-48] The histology of the various types of arteritis is the same in the liver as in other organs (Fig. 52.15).

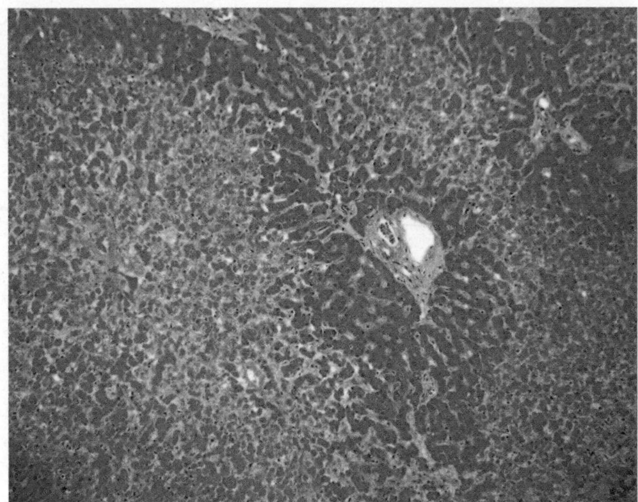

FIGURE 52.11 Ischemic necrosis. This postmortem liver shows preserved periportal parenchyma and necrosis of the entire zone 3 region near the terminal hepatic veins.

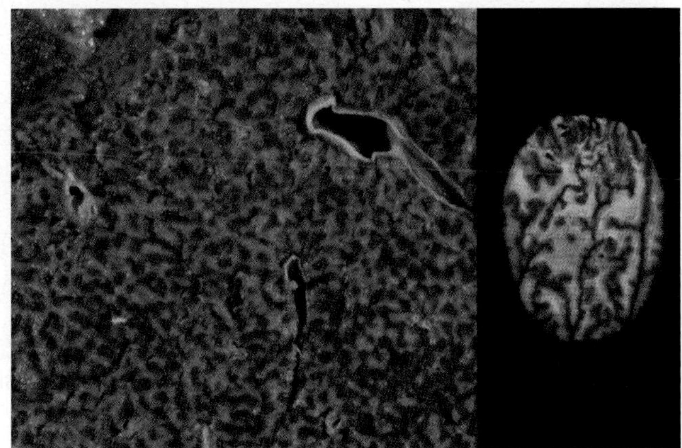

FIGURE 52.12 Centrilobular hemorrhagic necrosis. Cut section of formalin-fixed liver shows variegated pattern of hemorrhagic necrotic zone 3 parenchyma and preserved periportal parenchyma. This pattern is similar to that seen in a sliced nutmeg *(right)*.

Hepatic Artery Aneurysm and Rupture

Hepatic artery aneurysm (HAA) is infrequent and may involve intrahepatic arterial branches.[49] True HAAs are usually caused by atherosclerotic disease,[50] but trauma, infection, polyarteritis nodosa, Behçet's disease, and iatrogenic procedure–induced aneurysm may produce hepatic artery pseudoaneurysms.[51-53] This may include HAA following orthotopic liver transplantation.[54] Regardless, HAA may cause mechanical obstruction to biliary drainage,[54] or it may rupture outright.[49] Hemobilia[55] and fatal or near-fatal hemoperitoneum may result (Fig. 52.16).[56,57]

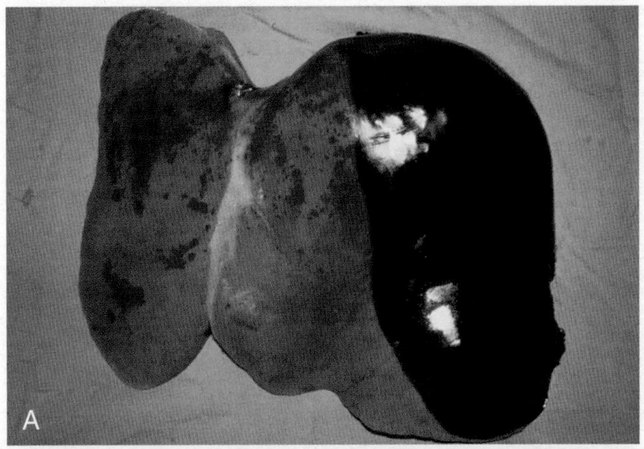

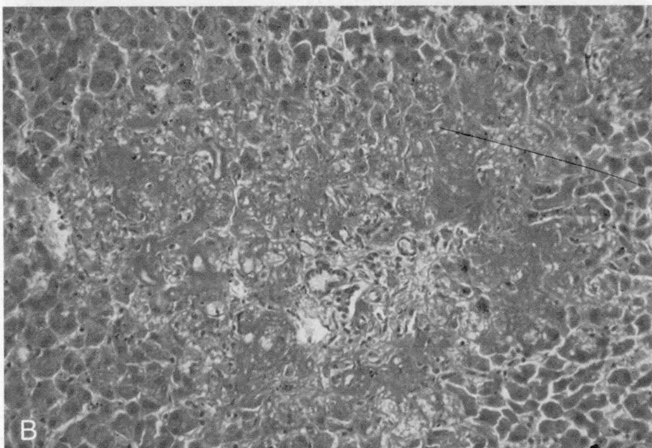

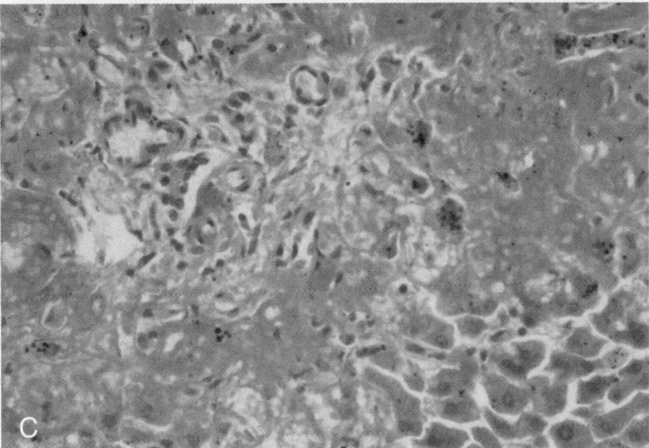

FIGURE 52.13 Fatal eclampsia. A, Postmortem liver showing extensive subcapsular hemorrhage and rupture into the abdominal cavity. **B,** Medium-power view showing a necrotic area around the portal tract (H&E stain). **C,** High-power view showing more clearly the periportal zone 1 necrosis (H&E stain).

Hepatic Artery Obstruction

Hepatic artery obstruction, caused by thrombosis, arteritis, or surgical ligation, is usually well tolerated unless hypotension or DIC is also present, in which case infarction may occur (Fig. 52.17). The hepatic artery also is susceptible to thrombosis following liver transplantation. Thrombosis of this vessel may be catastrophic because bile ducts of the implanted liver do not have the rich, anastomosing arterial bed that is present in the native liver and therefore are dependent on blood flow from an intact hepatic artery.

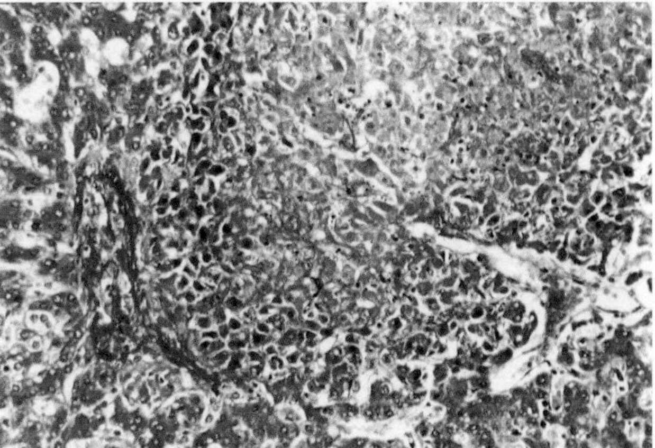

FIGURE 52.14 Infarct in a child with hypotension and sepsis. A recent thrombus is seen in the adjacent hepatic vein. The infarct was presumably a result of hypotension and superimposed local thrombosis.

This is caused not just by parenchymal necrosis, but also ischemia of the bile ducts, leakage of bile, and necrosis of the perihilar parenchyma[58] (Fig. 52.18A). The resulting necrotic debris often harbors *Candida* or other microorganisms. Necrotic debris accumulating in major bile ducts may also cause partial biliary obstruction (stricture or bile cast syndrome; see Fig. 52.18B). These dramatic events after liver transplantation often lead to liver failure, necessitating replacement of the organ.[59] Hepatic artery cannulation and infusion with floxuridine or other agents may also lead to biliary ischemia and eventually to large duct stenosis.[60,61]

Hepatic Complications in Critically Ill Patients

Secondary Sclerosing Cholangitis of Critically Ill Patients

Sclerosing cholangitis, both primary and secondary, is discussed in Chapter 48. Causes of secondary sclerosing cholangitis include autoimmune IgG_4-associated disease, drugs, infections, obstruction, and ischemia from hepatic artery compromise.[62] However, this section discusses specifically secondary sclerosing cholangitis in critically ill patients (SSC-CIP), first described by Scheppach et al. in 2001.[63] Occurring in approximately 1 of 2000 patients hospitalized in intensive care units,[64] cases are now increasingly reported, reflecting increased awareness of this condition. The presumed pathobiology is macro- and microcirculatory ischemic compromise with secondary ischemic cholangiopathy,[65,66] either without or with contribution from biliary infection or endotoxemia.[67-69] SSC-CIP may develop in the weeks to months following ICU admission for patients with conditions such as septic shock, trauma, and even electrical injury.[68,70,71] The ischemic and potentially immunological injury to small bile ducts may become self-aggravating, persisting well beyond the end of the intensive care stay, and manifesting only months later.[72]

Imaging of the biliary tree, either with endoscopic retrograde cholangiopancreatography (ERCP) or magnetic resonance cholangiopancreatography (MRCP) reveals segmental biliary dilation and stricture, either with or without biliary sludge. The pathology of SSC-CIP consists of cholangiocyte necrosis in both large and smaller bile ducts with ulceration of the biliary epithelium, bile cast formation, biliary obstruction, and irreversible destruction and obliteration

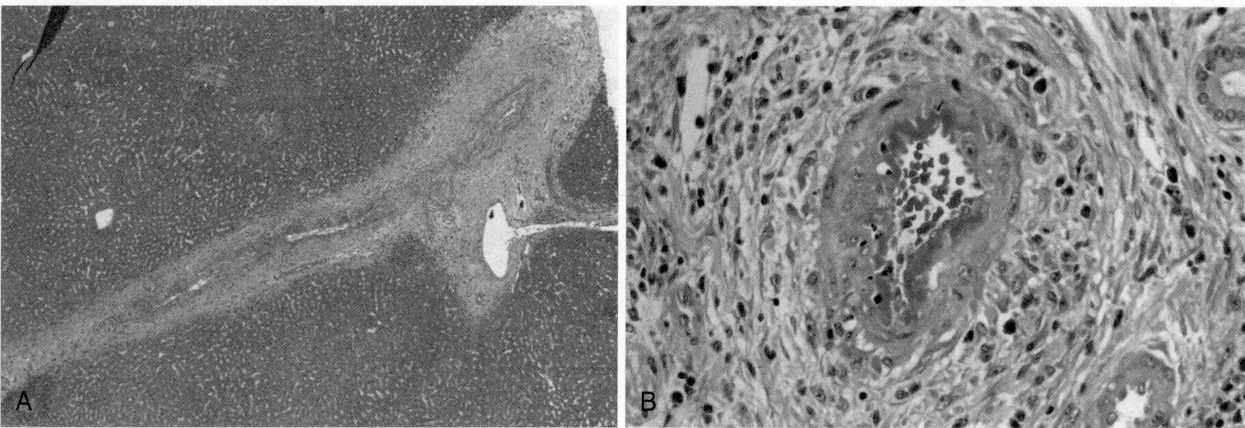

FIGURE 52.15 Polyarteritis nodosa in the liver. A, Longitudinal section of sublobular portal tract, showing a hepatic artery exhibiting coagulative necrosis along its entire length and an otherwise fibrotic portal tract. A sublobular portal vein with branching tributary is at the right of the image (H&E stain). **B,** Smaller portal tract exhibiting fibrinoid necrosis and leukocytoclasis in the wall of a hepatic artery (H&E stain).

of intrahepatic bile ducts, leading to secondary biliary cirrhosis.[68,70,71] Initial liver biopsy histology is consistent with chronic bile duct obstruction, with portal tract edema, inflammation, ductular reaction, and periductular fibrosis. With time, intrahepatic bile ducts are lost, and the liver progresses to secondary biliary cirrhosis. Perivenular necrosis and bile infarcts may develop in the parenchyma. Thrombosis of portal veins or hepatic arteries is absent, pointing toward antecedent systemic ischemia and underperfusion as the presumed etiology.[65]

COVID-19 and Post-COVID-19 Cholangiopathy

Separately, the disease caused by the SARS-CoV-2 virus, COVID-19, imparts its own pattern of damage to the liver. In autopsy series of patients who died with COVID-19 at the time of their acute illness, viral RNA is often detectable in liver tissue.[73,74] However prolonged the initial hospital admission might have been, the primary hepatic postmortem findings are sinusoidal congestion consistent with acute hepatic venous outflow obstruction,[73,75] and ischemic coagulative necrosis involving zone 3, sometimes including neutrophilic infiltrates similar to ischemia-reperfusion injury.[75] Lobular necroinflammation may be observed.[74] Importantly, in one series, early organizing thrombi involving portal venules were observed in 15 of 22 reported autopsies, with rare thrombi in hepatic arteries and arterioles.[75] In a separate series of 40 autopsies, although rare, phlebosclerosis of portal venules or terminal hepatic veins was observed, as was muscular hyperplasia of hepatic arteries, fibrinoid necrosis with endothelial cell apoptosis, or hyalinosis of the hepatic artery walls.[74] Selected hepatic arterial and terminal hepatic vein findings are illustrated in Figure 52.19. Lastly, Kupffer cell hemophagocytosis consistent with a hyperinflammatory syndrome has been noted.[75] Noting that obesity was a significant comorbidity in COVID-19 patients experiencing severe illness, steatosis indicative of nonalcoholic fatty liver disease (NAFLD) was frequently an accompanying finding at autopsy, sometimes with significant fibrosis.[74,75] Bile duct morphology at autopsy was essentially normal, although ductular cholestasis indicative of sepsis was sometimes present.[74]

It is therefore worrisome to encounter surviving COVID-19 patients who develop a severe SSC-CIP-like clinical syndrome in the months following prolonged hospitalization for severe illness.[76] Imaging findings are similar to SSC-CIP; serum elevations of alkaline phosphatase are prolonged and severe. On liver biopsy (Fig. 52.20), an extraordinary histology of extensive cholangiocyte vacuolization is accompanied by severe regenerative and degenerative changes of the bile duct and ductular epithelial layer. A microangiopathy is also observed, with hepatic artery muscular hypertrophy and endothelial swelling, portal vein endophlebitis, and focal features of sinusoidal obstructive syndrome (venoocclusive disease). Progressive bile duct paucity with severe hepatic fibrosis appears to develop, with potential progression to secondary biliary cirrhosis. In post-acute COVID-19 patients, viral protein or RNA was not detected in the liver biopsies. An ischemic etiology for the observed cholangiopathy may be the cause, similar to SSC-CIP. However, direct injury to the biliary epithelium from SARS-CoV-2 cannot be excluded, given the striking cholangiopathic changes that are beyond what has been described for SSC-CIP. Cholangiocytes express the receptor for viral entry into cells, angiotensin-converting enzyme 2 (ACE-2).[77] Hence, hepatologists and pathologists alike should consider post-COVID injury to the liver in postacute COVID patients who present with a cholestatic syndrome.

Arterioportal and Arteriovenous Shunts

Clinically relevant intrahepatic shunts between the splanchnic arterial system and the portal vein most commonly develop many months or years after penetrating trauma (e.g., gunshot wound, liver biopsy); arteriohepatic venous shunts may also occur but are much rarer.[78-80] Small shunts may close spontaneously over time, but medium- to large-sized shunts need endovascular or surgical management.[81] Large shunts may also occur as the result of a developmental anomaly such as fetal vascular abnormalities,[82] hepatic hemangioma,[83] or malignant tumors.[84] In some patients, shunts are found early in life; in others, especially with hereditary hemorrhagic telangiectasia, the shunts develop progressively during several decades. Increased arterial flow to the liver may be inapparent but can manifest with a bruit, high-output congestive heart

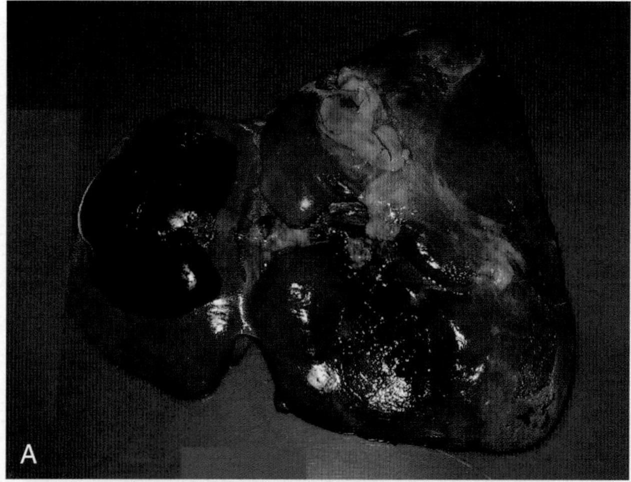

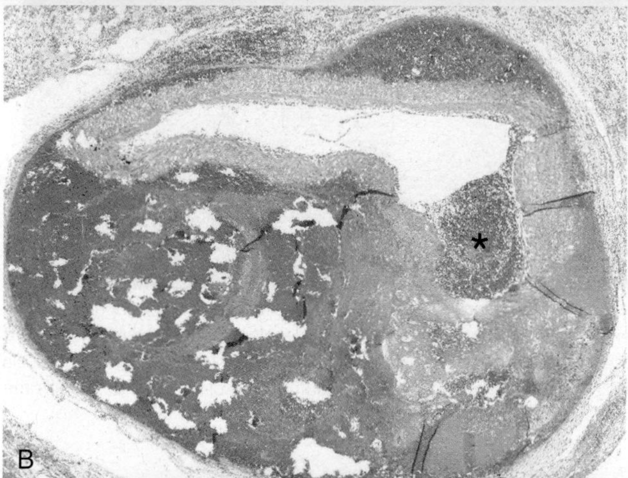

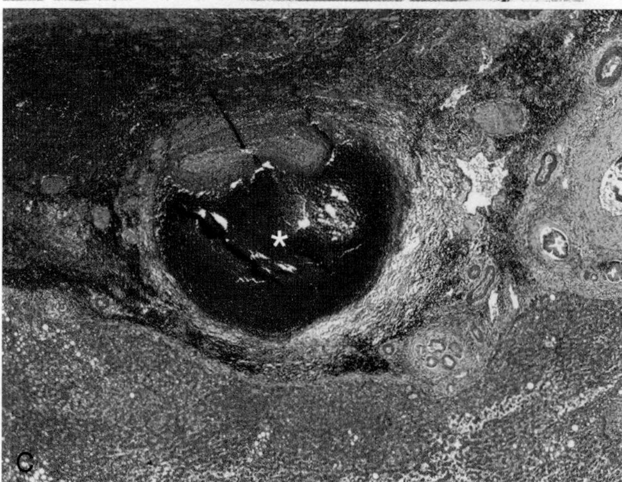

FIGURE 52.16 Fatal ruptured hepatic artery pseudoaneurysm from polyarteritis nodosa, with 2 L of free blood in the abdomen at time of death. A, Posterior view of a liver at autopsy showing subcapsular hematoma in the left lobe. **B,** Left main hepatic artery showing pseudoaneurysm on the right (asterisk), with dissection of blood within the adventitial space (H&E stain). **C,** More distal portion of the left main hepatic artery showing hemorrhage from the adventitial space (asterisk) into adjacent hepatic parenchyma (trichrome stain).

failure, ascites, diarrhea, weight loss, protein-losing enteropathy, or hemobilia.[85] When the shunt involves the portal vein, portal hypertension is the most important effect. The diagnosis depends on detecting a dilated high-flow channel by Doppler ultrasonography or other imaging studies. On arteriography, one may see an apparent doubling of the vascular tree, possibly because of early retrograde filling of the portal veins that run parallel to the arteries. The portal vein branches may be obliterated. The pathology depends on the underlying etiology. Systemic hemangiomatosis may create a honeycomb-like liver with a profound burden of arteriovenous malformations.[86] For cirrhotic arteriovenous shunts involving the portal venous system, numerous congested capillaries and arterioles, either within or adjacent to portal tracts, are characteristic.[87] The pathobiology and pathology of hereditary hemorrhagic telangiectasia is discussed further in Chapter 55.

SINUSOIDAL DISEASE

The sinusoids play a critical role as conduits of blood and nutrients to hepatocytes. The normal sinusoidal wall is composed of highly fenestrated endothelial cells and a delicate fibrillar matrix without a well-defined basement membrane or occlusive pericytes.[88] Stellate cells reside in the subendothelial space of Disse. These cells contain droplets of retinol esters and produce collagen in response to inflammation. They also have contractile properties that are activated by endothelin 1 and inhibited by nitric oxide.[89,90] The sinusoids must adapt to physiological and pathological alterations in arterial and venous blood flow. In chronic liver diseases, the stellate cells are activated and transformed into myofibroblasts, which lay down extracellular matrix causing hepatic fibrosis and, through their contractile activity, increase resistance to blood flow through the sinusoids. Many types of disorders involve histological changes of the sinusoids and small veins.

Sinusoidal Dilation

Sinusoidal diameter and hepatocyte size are fairly uniform within the normal liver, although there is a slight widening of sinusoidal diameter in zone 3. This uniformity is lost when there is local obstruction of portal or hepatic veins, which leads to hepatocellular atrophy and sinusoidal dilation and is often accompanied by a local compensatory increase in arterial blood flow. The resulting localized increase in the blood space is seen macroscopically as a darkened region of liver parenchyma, termed the *infarct of Zahn*.[91] When many adjacent obstructive portal vein lesions occur, hepatocyte atrophy causes the portal tracts to crowd together. Typically, these lesions are seen adjacent to neoplasms, which compromise regional blood flow because of their compressive mass effect, or with focal portal vein thrombosis.

In chronic congestive heart failure and constrictive pericarditis with retrograde impediment to hepatic venous outflow, a diffuse increase in sinusoidal pressure leads to zone 3 hepatocellular atrophy and sinusoidal dilation (Fig. 52.21). With time, pericellular fibrosis develops, obliterating small hepatic veins; rarely, cirrhosis that features a pericentral pattern of fibrous septation develops.

Sinusoidal dilation is also seen in patients with chronic wasting illnesses[92] such as tuberculosis or acquired immunodeficiency syndrome (AIDS)[92,93]; with malignancies, notably Hodgkin disease[94] or renal cell carcinoma[95,96]; and

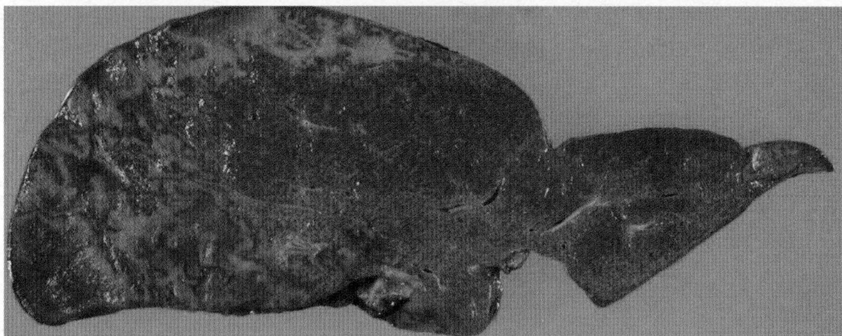

FIGURE 52.17 Gross specimen of a liver with hepatic artery thrombosis showing global ischemia with a geographical pattern of infarction (left). The noninfarcted portion of the liver exhibits the zonal pattern of ischemic centrilobular necrosis (right).

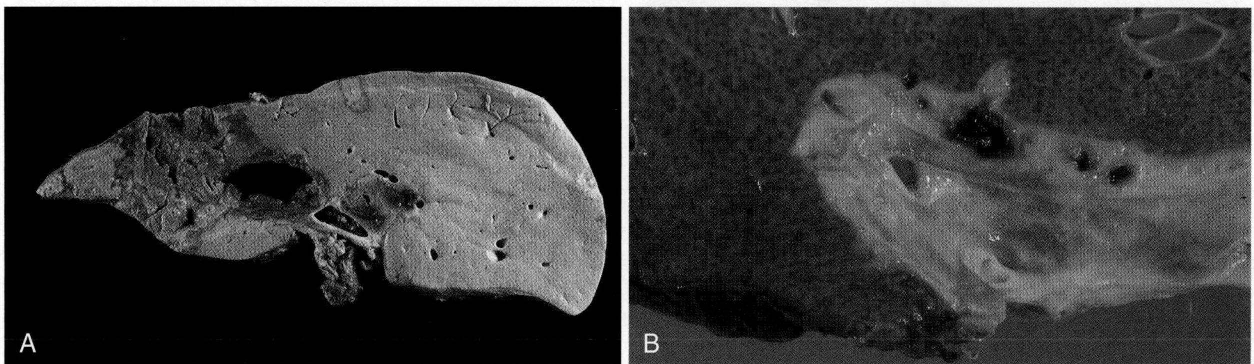

FIGURE 52.18 Failed liver grafts following hepatic artery thrombosis after liver transplantation. **A.** Hepatic artery thrombosis was diagnosed early after transplantation, before the onset of progressive cholestasis. Despite attempts to save the organ, liver failure developed after several months. At retransplantation, the hilar region is necrotic, with extension of necrosis into the left lobe. The regional necrosis also has led to retrograde thrombosis in the sublobar portal vein *(center of image)*. **B.** A separate failed graft requiring retransplantation, in which accumulation of necrotic debris fills the bile duct lumen; the liver parenchyma also shows zonal ischemia with a nutmeg appearance.

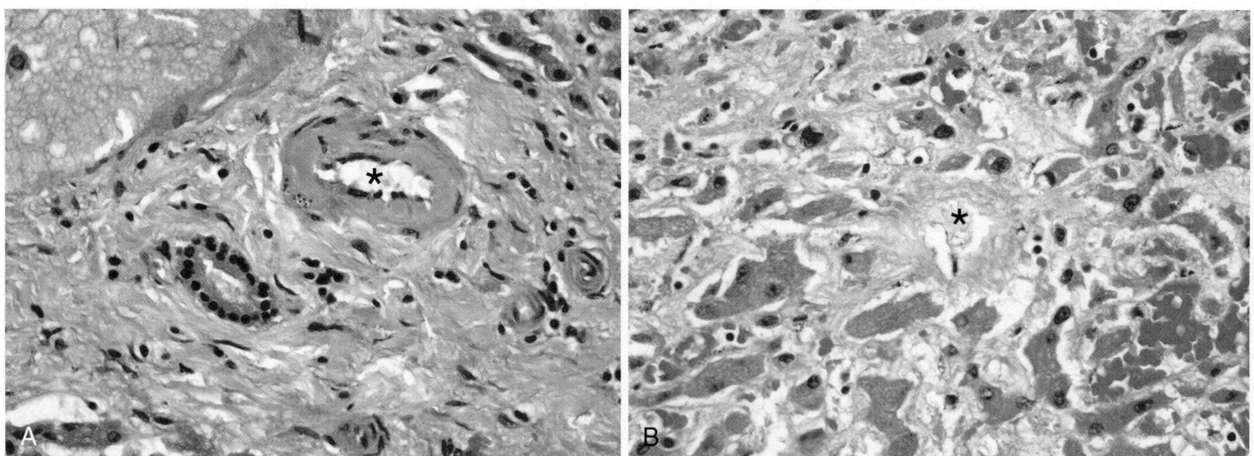

FIGURE 52.19 Hepatic microvascular findings in autopsies of COVID-19 patients. **A,** Hepatic artery *(asterisk)* exhibiting hyaline thickening of the media with focal nuclear dust. The interlobular bile duct is unremarkable (H&E stain). **B,** Terminal hepatic vein *(asterisk)* and congested perivenular zone 3, showing changes of sinusoidal obstruction syndrome (venoocclusive disease) (H&E stain).

within nodules of severe cirrhosis. Dilation of zone 1 and 2 sinusoids occurs during pregnancy and in women taking oral contraceptives.[97,98] The mechanism of this effect may be related to mild diffuse angiogenesis and increased arterial blood flow. Sickle cell disease characteristically shows small clumps of sickled red blood cells within sinusoids (Fig. 52.22). In this disease, sinusoidal fibrosis is often seen. Cirrhosis is rare; when present, it is caused by coincidental viral or other liver disease.

A sharp delineation between well-preserved zone 1 hepatocyte plates and atrophic zone 2 and zone 3 plates, with sinusoidal dilation, may result, not from retrograde obstruction to blood flow but from forward-flow underperfusion. This underperfusion may be caused by vascular disease affecting the portal veins and hepatic arteries (discussed earlier) or may occur in the setting of modest compromise of the vascular anastomoses in a hepatic transplantation graft.[99] Finally, parenchymal lesions that

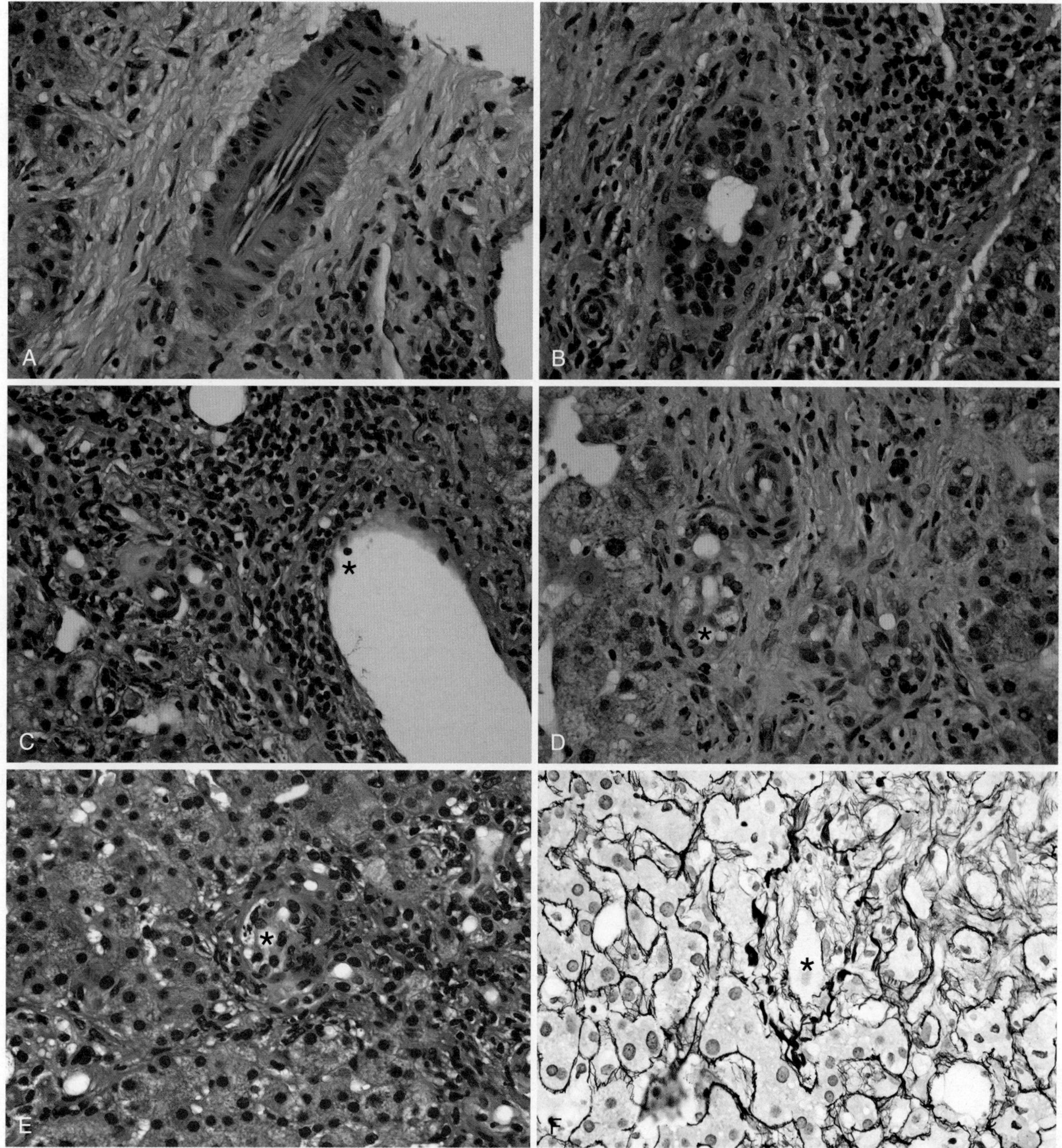

FIGURE 52.20 Post-COVID cholangiopathy in liver biopsies of post-acute patients following severe COVID-19. A, Hepatic artery showing smooth muscle hypertrophy of the media, and obliteration of lumen by endothelial vacuolization (H&E stain). **B,** Interlobular bile duct showing marked regenerative change and focal cholangiocyte apoptosis; there is marked portal tract predominantly mononuclear inflammation (H&E stain). **C,** Inflamed portal tract with portal vein endophlebitis (*asterisk,* H&E stain). **D,** Bile ductule with marked cholangiocyte cytoplasmic vacuolization; an adjacent hepatic artery shows smooth muscle hypertrophy of the media and endothelial vacuolization (H&E stain). **E,** Bile ductules showing cholangiocyte swelling and apoptosis (*asterisk,* H&E stain). **F,** Terminal hepatic vein (asterisk) showing features of sinusoidal obstruction syndrome (venoocclusive disease; reticulin stain).

create local scarring and "traction" on adjacent regions of the liver may create secondary sinusoidal dilation unrelated to the physiology of blood flow. The most dramatic features of "traction dilation" are seen in tertiary syphilis, in which gummatous lesions create a characteristic hepar lobatum macroscopically, with interspersed fibrotic scars and dilated sinusoidal spaces in the hepatic parenchyma surrounding the gummata (Fig. 52.23). More limited examples may be seen adjacent to other mass lesions of the liver if there is scarring of the surrounding parenchyma.

Peliosis Hepatis

Peliosis hepatis is defined as the presence of blood-filled spaces in the liver resulting from focal rupture of sinusoidal

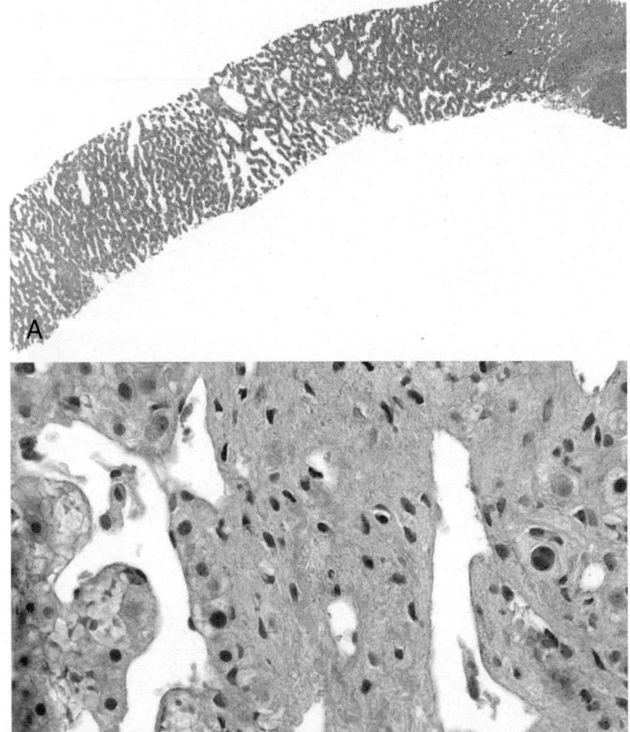

FIGURE 52.21 Congestive heart failure. A, Dilation of the sinusoidal spaces and atrophy (thinning) of the hepatocytic cords are visible in zone 3. **B,** When heart failure is persistent, collagen is deposited around the terminal hepatic veins and within the sinusoidal spaces.

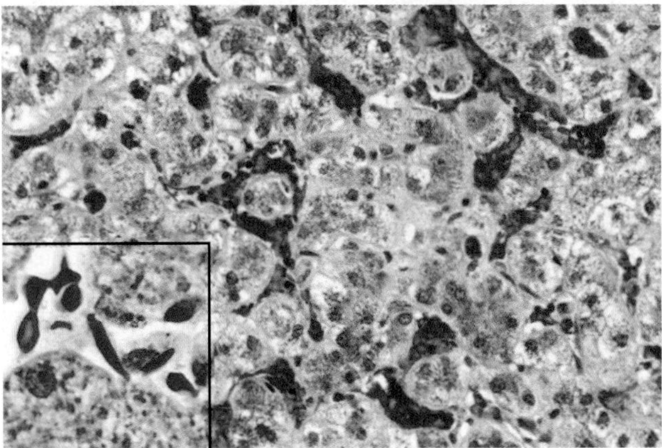

FIGURE 52.22 Sickle cell disease shows characteristic clumps of densely packed red blood cells blocking the liver sinusoids. *Inset* shows a sickled red cell (Masson trichrome stain).

walls.[100] The term was initially used to describe grossly visible lesions, but it is now also applied to microscopic lesions. Severe sinusoidal dilation may resemble peliosis. The difference, by definition, is that peliosis is caused by rupture of the sinusoidal walls, whereas these walls are intact in sinusoidal dilation.

Clinical Features

Peliosis may be minimal, asymptomatic, and grossly inapparent or severe in cases of cholestasis, liver failure, portal hypertension, development of a mass lesion, or spontaneous rupture. Calcifications may develop and can be seen radiologically.[101] Peliosis has been associated with exposure to a variety of drugs, including anabolic steroids, tamoxifen, corticosteroids, azathioprine, methotrexate, 6-thioguanine, 6-mercaptopurine, vinyl chloride, arsenic, and Thorotrast, and it may be seen in hairy cell leukemia[1,100,102,103] *Bartonella* infection can cause bacillary peliosis, which occurs mainly in immunosuppressed patients.

Pathological Features

The endothelial lining may be lost during lesion development, but it is usually regained in chronic lesions.[104] Severe peliosis is characterized by separation of the sinusoidal parenchyma from the portal tracts. The portal tracts appear similar to exfoliated branches of a tree in winter (Fig. 52.24). In *Bartonella* infection the organisms may be seen as a vague haze on hematoxylin and eosin (H&E)-stained sections but are well visualized with a Warthin-Starry stain.[105] Peliotic change to the sinusoidal vasculature may also be observed in various tumors, particularly hepatocellular adenoma, hepatocellular carcinoma, and angiosarcoma. Therefore it is important to examine the surrounding liver and the endothelial lining for these lesions.

Peliosis may be mistaken for hemangioma. However, in the latter condition, the blood-filled spaces are lined by a robust vascular wall, and the portal tracts do not extend into the blood-filled cavities, as they do in peliosis.

Bacillary Angiomatosis

Infection with *Bartonella* (formerly known as *Rochalimaea*) may manifest as vascular proliferative lesions in patients with HIV infection and other immunocompromised hosts.[106-108] Bacillary angiomatosis may affect the liver (called *bacillary peliosis hepatis*), spleen (bacillary splenitis), and skin. Necrotizing granulomatous disease is the other form of *Bartonella* infection. In patients with malignancy who are receiving chemotherapy or are immunocompromised as a result of HIV infection or organ transplantation, *Bartonella* infection should be considered in the differential diagnosis of a febrile illness.

Bacillary peliosis of the liver generates peliotic foci of necrosis within the parenchyma, characterized by multiple cystic blood-filled spaces or lakes.[109] Although peliosis has been described in patients receiving azathioprine and cyclosporine after organ transplantation and in those receiving anabolic androgenic and estrogenic steroids,[110-113] the finding of aggregates of *Bartonella* bacilli highlighted by a Warthin-Starry silver stain with a mixture of inflammatory cells in the background of fibromyxoid stroma helps support a diagnosis of infection caused by *Bartonella*.[105] Serological analysis, culture, and, ultimately, polymerase chain reaction (PCR) testing of peripheral blood or liver tissue may be confirmatory.[114]

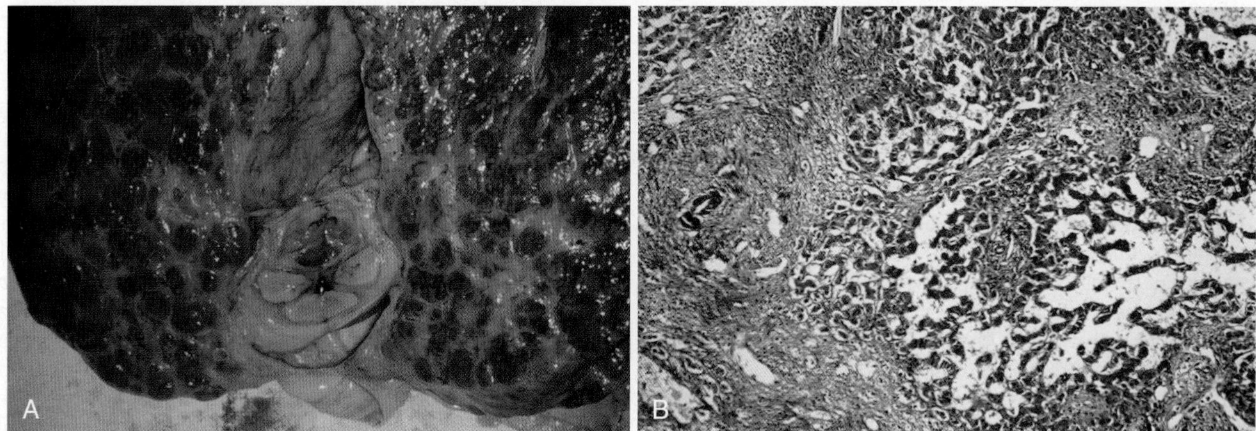

FIGURE 52.23 Syphilis affecting the liver. A, Cut-surface autopsy liver showing gummatous lesion in the porta hepatic, with surrounding morphology of "hepar lobatum." **B,** Low-power image showing dilation of sinusoids owing to traction of the bands of scar tissue (Masson trichrome stain).

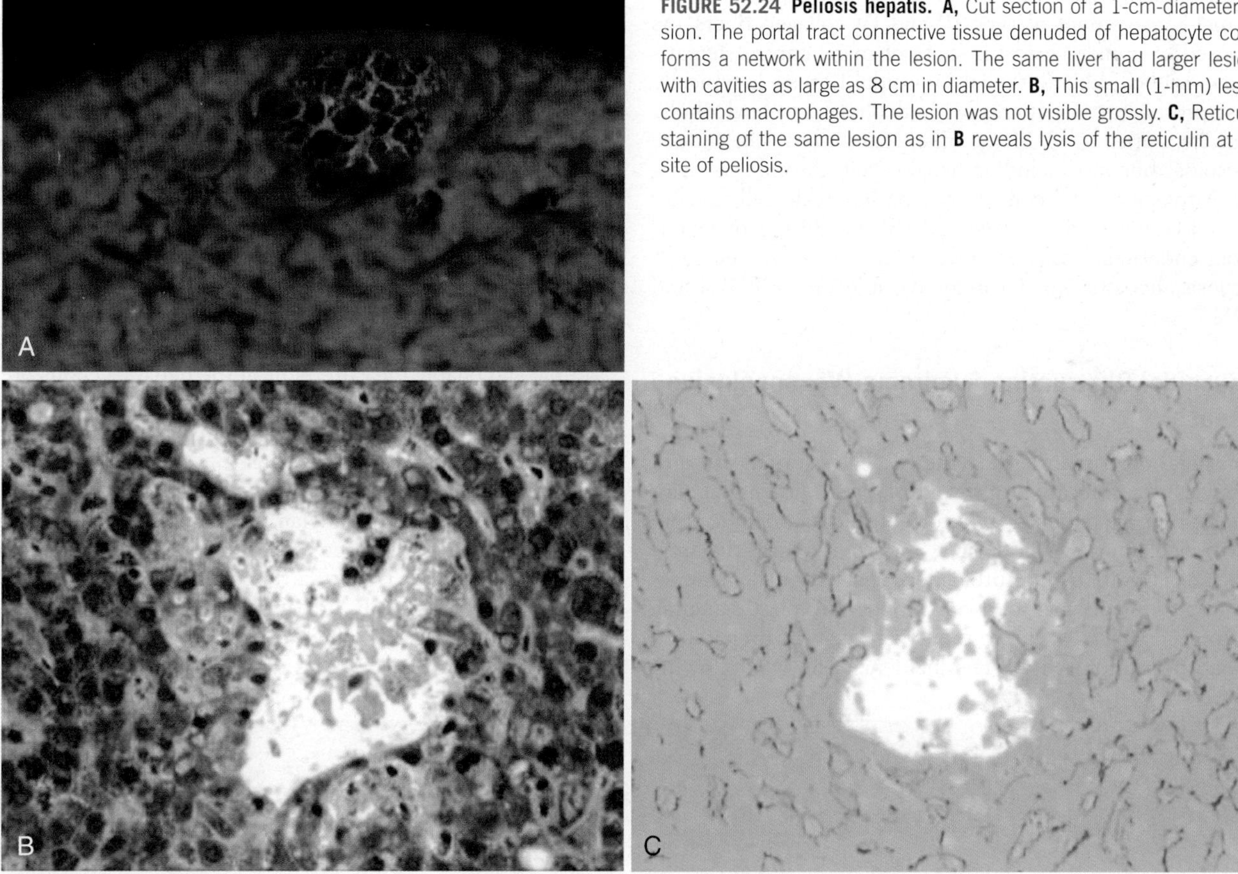

FIGURE 52.24 Peliosis hepatis. A, Cut section of a 1-cm-diameter lesion. The portal tract connective tissue denuded of hepatocyte cords forms a network within the lesion. The same liver had larger lesions with cavities as large as 8 cm in diameter. **B,** This small (1-mm) lesion contains macrophages. The lesion was not visible grossly. **C,** Reticulin staining of the same lesion as in **B** reveals lysis of the reticulin at the site of peliosis.

Sinusoidal Injury, Fibrosis, and Arterialization

Because of their close proximity to hepatocytes, sinusoids are injured in all forms of acute and chronic hepatitis. Hepatic parenchymal injury that leads to individual hepatocyte apoptosis does not disrupt the integrity of the sinusoids; necroinflammation of contiguous hepatocytes ("spotty necrosis") is more likely to do so. Hepatocyte necroinflammatory loss that spans across all acinar zones is termed *zonal* or *bridging necrosis* and risks further destruction of sinusoidal integrity. When necrotic regions collapse, the portal tracts and veins become closely approximated to each other. This is readily appreciated with a reticulin stain because collapse of the intervening parenchymal plates with complete loss of hepatocytes is evident. If hepatocyte necrosis involves only zone 3 hepatocytes, the liver cell plates may be "empty," but there may be little or no collapse of the reticulin framework, resulting in a lesion termed *evacuation of the liver cell plates*.[1] This lesion is most commonly seen in patients with allograft rejection, acetaminophen toxicity, or chronic hepatitis.

Sinusoids are normally lined by CD34-negative endothelial cells. In chronic liver disease, the endothelium becomes CD34 positive, first in endothelium near the portal tracts and later throughout the lobules (e.g., in cirrhosis). This is termed *capillarization* of the sinusoids, as more complete restructuring of the sinusoidal lining to a nonpermeable barrier takes place. Features of arterialization include decreased fenestration of the endothelial cells, increased collagen and other matrix proteins in the space of Disse, and loss of microvilli on the surface of hepatocytes.[115,116] Sinusoidal fibrosis is detected in early and active disease, usually in association with activated hepatic stellate cells, which stain positively for α-smooth muscle actin.

Sinusoidal fibrosis may be found in any type of chronic liver disease involving deposition of type 1 collagen fibers in the subendothelial space of Disse in addition to the normal complement of type III and IV collagen fibers. As opposed to broader bridging septa of many chronic hepatitis conditions, subendothelial sinusoidal fibrosis is typically most prominent in patients with alcoholic or nonalcoholic steatohepatitis.[117-119] Many other conditions can induce sinusoidal fibrosis, including hepatic vein thrombosis, vitamin A toxicity,[120,121] congenital syphilis, sickle cell disease, or even Gaucher disease (Fig. 52.25). CD34-positive sinusoidal endothelial cells are present to a variable degree in cirrhosis, hepatocellular carcinoma, adenomas, FNH, and NRH.

Sinusoidal Obstruction Syndrome (Venoocclusive Disease)

Sinusoidal obstruction syndrome (SOS) occurs most commonly as a complication of myeloablative regimens that are used to prepare patients for autologous hematopoietic stem cell transplantation (HSCT).[122] In recent years, the incidence of SOS following autologous HSCT for malignancy is 15%[123]; the incidence following HSCT for aplastic anemia is reported as 7%, owing to the lower levels of preparatory myoablation required.[124] The incidence of SOS following HSCT in the pediatric age group is reported as 2%,[125] although younger age is also reported to impart greater risk for developing SOS.[126]

SOS is defined by the presence of prominent obstructive, nonthrombotic lesions of the small hepatic veins in individuals exposed to either a hepatotoxin or radiation. The definition is based on the premise that the initial lesion is to the endothelium of sinusoids and small veins, leading to hemorrhage into the liver parenchyma and into the walls of terminal hepatic veins.[127,128] The former term, *venoocclusive disease* (VOD), reflects an important diagnostic feature, which is partial or complete occlusion of the lumen of the terminal hepatic vein (see later). Among survivors of SOS, the sinusoidal lesions become less apparent with time, and the major residual lesion is fibrous obliteration of small hepatic veins. This residual pattern of disease is the one that was characterized in the original description of VOD[129]; the acute sinusoidal lesions were not appreciated histologically or experimentally until many years later.[128,130]

Clinical Features

Patients with early disease exhibit tender hepatomegaly, ascites, rapid weight gain, and hepatic failure with elevated serum bilirubin.[127,131] The onset of this toxic syndrome can be diagnosed on clinical grounds, and percutaneous liver biopsy may be too risky a procedure given the potential of an evolving coagulopathy. Grading of severity is on the basis of these cardinal clinical signs; a multi-organ grading system has recently been proposed owing to the importance of multi-organ injury having a major impact on clinical outcomes.[132] If histological diagnosis is needed to exclude other conditions, transjugular biopsy can provide a tissue sample and enable measurement of the hepatic venous pressure gradient.[133,134] A gradient greater than 10 mm Hg is considered highly specific for SOS in patients undergoing hematopoietic cell transplantation.

Hepatic SOS is now classified as early and late-onset post HSCT: early occurring a median of 8 days (range 0 to 20 days) post-HSCT and late-onset with a reported median time to diagnosis of 46 days (range 22 to 93 days).[135] As noted, SOS occurs more commonly in patients undergoing autologous HSCT for malignancy, which requires higher doses of myeloablative therapy.[128,136] The drugs most often implicated

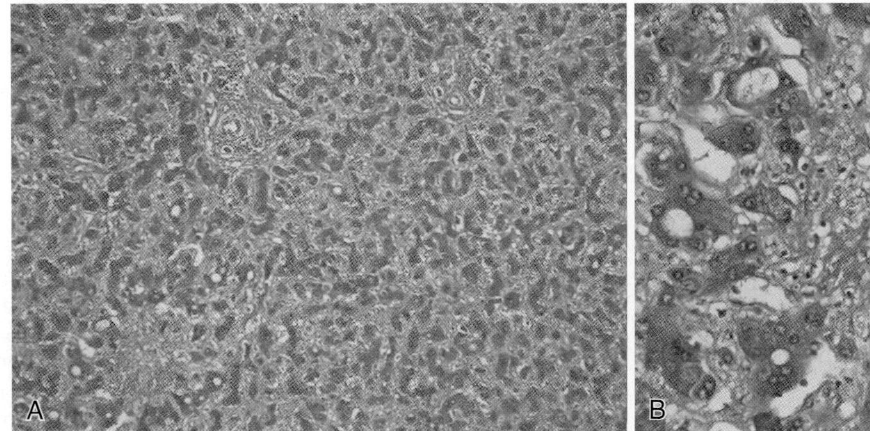

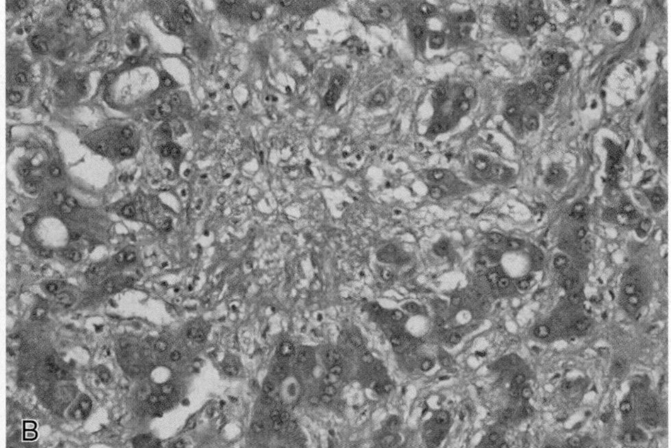

FIGURE 52.25 Congenital syphilis. A, Low-power view of hepatic parenchyma showing hepatocyte plates widely separated by sinusoidal material (H&E stain). **B,** High-power view showing extensive deposition of extracellular matrix within the sinusoids (H&E stain). Silver stain (not shown) would document a heavy burden of spirochetes.

are cyclophosphamide, busulfan, and gemtuzumab ozogamicin (Mylotarg[137]). Occasionally, SOS develops in patients given low doses of other drugs and toxins, such as azathioprine, cysteamine, dacarbazine, dactinomycin, carmustine (BCNU), 6-mercaptopurine, 6-thioguanine, dimethylbusulfan, cytosine arabinoside, indicine-*N*-oxide, mustine (mechlorethamine hydrochloride), doxorubicin, urethane, vincristine, mitomycin-C, oxaliplatin,[138] etoposide, arsenic, Thorotrast, and intraarterial flurodeoxyuridine.[139-141] Associated risk factors include HSCT with a mismatched HLA donor, a recipient history of liver disease or elevated serum transaminase levels, a prolonged time from initial diagnosis of cancer, and related to that delay, exposure to radiation, busulfan, and/or methotrexate before initiation of the myeloablative regime.[123] A pharmacogenetic susceptibility may also be operative.[142] SOS can also develop in patients who have not undergone HSCT but nevertheless have received radiation therapy[124] or cytotoxic medications: gemtuzumab ozogamycin,[143] neoadjuvant chemotherapy before resection of colorectal cancer metastatic to the liver, containing oxiplatinin, 5-fluorouracil, and leucovorin (FOLFOX) or irinotecan plus 5-fluorouracil and leucovorin (FOLFIRI)[131,138,144]; and even tacrolimus following liver transplantation.[145] Patients who survive acute SOS usually recover completely, but the residual lesions of VOD may remain in the liver for a long period. Portal hypertension or cirrhosis is rare. If cirrhosis becomes clinically manifest, it is usually associated with the presence of other disease (e.g., chronic hepatitis C).[146]

The initial description of VOD was in subjects exposed to pyrrolizidine alkaloids, and these compounds are still a significant cause of SOS in countries with high intake of herbal formulations containing these toxins.[147] These compounds are found in plants of the genera *Senecio, Heliotropium, Crotalaria,* and many others. Epidemics of pyrrolizidine alkaloid toxicity occur mainly in arid climates, where toxin-containing plants may overgrow crops during periods of drought. Livestock may be affected when grazing, and humans may be affected by eating bread derived from these crops. Herbal medicines created from toxic plants, commonly called *bush tea,* can cause severe disease, especially in young children. The reported mortality from pyrrolizidine-associated SOS varies from 16% to 40%, with the cause of death being liver failure.[148]

In the post-HSCT setting, the clinical diagnosis of SOS is based on the four cardinal signs noted earlier: hyperbilirubinemia, development of right upper-quadrant pain and tender hepatomegaly, ascites, and unexplained weight gain.[131] Because of an increased risk of bleeding, liver biopsy is usually transjugular. If performed, the indication for liver biopsy is multiple because exclusion of other etiologies such as graft-versus-host disease (GVHD) is critically important. Early identification of SOS is also important. Early treatment or even prophylactic, preemptive administration of the approved drug, defibrotide, has been shown to effective and reduce mortality.[149,150]

Pathological Features

Regardless of the cause, SOS has consistent morphological features. The lesions evolve with time, and the findings depend on the timing of the liver biopsy. Grossly, an affected liver has a bluish-red, marbled appearance that is especially prominent in the subcapsular region. This reflects marked diffuse hemorrhage.[151] Liver biopsies are almost never obtained during the acute stage. If so, the early histological changes, occurring as early as 1 week after cytoreductive or myeloablative therapy, include rounding and sloughing of sinusoidal endothelial cells and filling of the sinusoidal lumen with cytoplasmic blebs and erythrocytes. This debris embolizes downstream to the terminal hepatic venule, obstructing the lumen and associated with a widened and edematous subendothelial zone of the terminal hepatic venule that contains entrapped red blood cells, resulting in concentric narrowing of the venular lumina.[151] Clusters of debris from necrotic hepatocytes, dilated and destroyed sinusoids, and hemorrhage into the space of Disse can be seen surrounding the injured terminal hepatic venules (Fig. 52.26). The necrotic debris may also fill the venular lumina. In this early phase, the hepatic veins are often difficult to locate because of the degree of perivenous hemorrhage. Use of special stains, such as Masson trichrome or reticulin, may help demonstrate the presence and location of the hepatic veins. Examination of tissue under polarized light may also help identify the collagen bundles that surround the hepatic veins.

As SOS evolves and hepatic stellate cells are activated, liver biopsy will show that collagen fibers are deposited in the sinusoidal spaces and hepatic veins, typically of less than 200 μm in diameter; this constitutes the "VOD" lesion (Fig. 52.27). After several weeks, sinusoidal congestion and dropout (loss) of zone 3 hepatocytes develop, with sinusoidal fibrosis and intimal fibrosis of hepatic veins that are typically less than 200 μm in diameter (see Fig. 52.27); this constitutes the "VOD" lesion. Bridging fibrosis connecting hepatic veins can be seen in advanced stages.[134] The degree of sinusoidal sclerosis and venous luminal narrowing is associated with the severity of the clinical signs and symptoms.[151,152]

Differential Diagnosis

Although acute or chronic GVHD must be considered in patients who have undergone hematopoietic stem cell (bone marrow) transplantation, the histological patterns of injury are different from SOS. The injuries of GVHD center in the portal tracts, namely, bile duct damage and endotheliitis in acute GVHD and paucity of bile ducts in chronic GVHD.[152,153]

Sinusoidal Cellular Infiltration

Extramedullary hematopoiesis, characterized by the presence of megakaryocytes, normoblasts, and other hematopoietic cells, may be found in the liver of normal infants, in patients who have undergone cardiac bypass surgery, and in patients with myeloproliferative disorders.[154] Mast cells may be numerous in mastocytosis and, most likely because of obliterative hepatic venopathy, may be associated with portal hypertension.[155] Malignant neoplasms, including lymphoma and hairy cell leukemia, breast cancer, and malignant melanoma, may infiltrate the sinusoids and cause ischemia and hepatic failure (Fig. 52.28).[103,156-158] Inherited storage disorders, including especially Gaucher disease and Niemann-Pick disease (see Chapter 54), may also cause marked enlargement of Kupffer cells. However, these

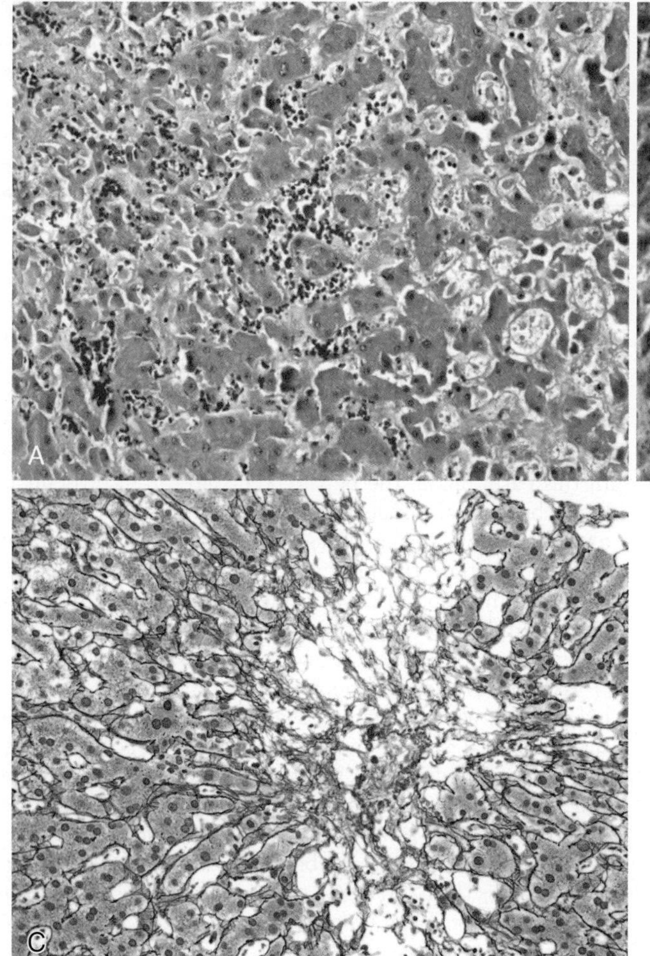

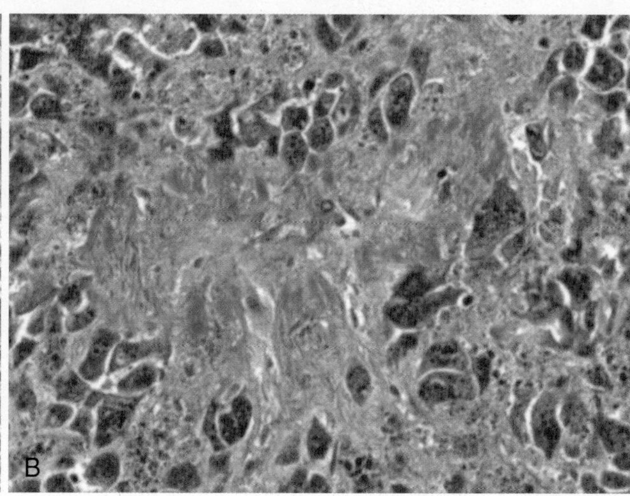

FIGURE 52.26 Sinusoidal obstruction syndrome. A, Dilated sinusoidal spaces in the early phase and clusters of debris from necrotic hepatocytes fill the hepatic venular lumina. **B,** Delicate collagen deposition within perivenular sinusoidal spaces is demonstrated by Masson trichrome stain. **C,** Collapsed hepatocytic cords surrounding the terminal hepatic venule are demonstrated by reticulin stain.

storage conditions do not readily cause portal hypertension, despite the hepatomegaly that develops. The splenomegaly and hypersplenism in these storage conditions is primary, rather than secondary to portal hypertension.

Amyloidosis and Light Chain Deposition Disease

Amyloidosis is a systemic infiltrative disease caused by tissue deposition of a wide variety of proteins, with over 28 precursor proteins having now been identified.[159] Although more than 90% of patients with amyloidosis have amyloid in the liver,[160,161] the most common form of hepatic amyloidosis in the United States is immunoglobulin light chain amyloidosis (AL) associated with plasma cell dyscrasia and reactive AA amyloidosis derived from serum amyloid A (SAA), typically seen with chronic inflammatory conditions. The next most common causes of hepatic amyloidosis are transthyretin (TTR) and leukocyte cell–derived chemotaxin-2 (LECT2).[162,163] TTR is a circulating protein mainly synthesized by the liver and the choroid plexus of the brain. Although TTR is an intrinsically amyloidogenic protein, patients with hereditary destabilizing missense variants in the *TTR* gene develop a systemic amyloidosis with particularly devastating effects on the peripheral and autonomic nervous system and cardiovascular system,[164] and the liver may be sufficiently unaffected as to be a potential donor organ for domino liver transplantation.[165]

Clinical Features

Patients with amyloidosis may have hepatomegaly, cholestasis, hepatic failure, ascites, or portal hypertension.[166,167] Other features include renal failure, nephrotic syndrome, and cardiomyopathy. Light chain deposition disease may also present with hepatomegaly, cholestasis, or hepatic failure.[168,169] Among patients with amyloidosis, those with hepatic involvement have significantly higher levels of alkaline phosphatase and C-reactive protein than those without hepatic amyloidosis.[170]

Pathological Features

With the exception of LECT2 amyloidosis, hepatic amyloid is deposited as a dense linear layer in the matrix space or connective tissue of the portal tracts, within thickened vascular walls of arteries or veins, or within the sinusoidal space of Disse. There is typically great variation in both the severity and the distribution of hepatic amyloid deposits (Fig. 52.29). Bile ducts and peribiliary glands may show subepithelial deposits.[171,172] The pattern of distribution does

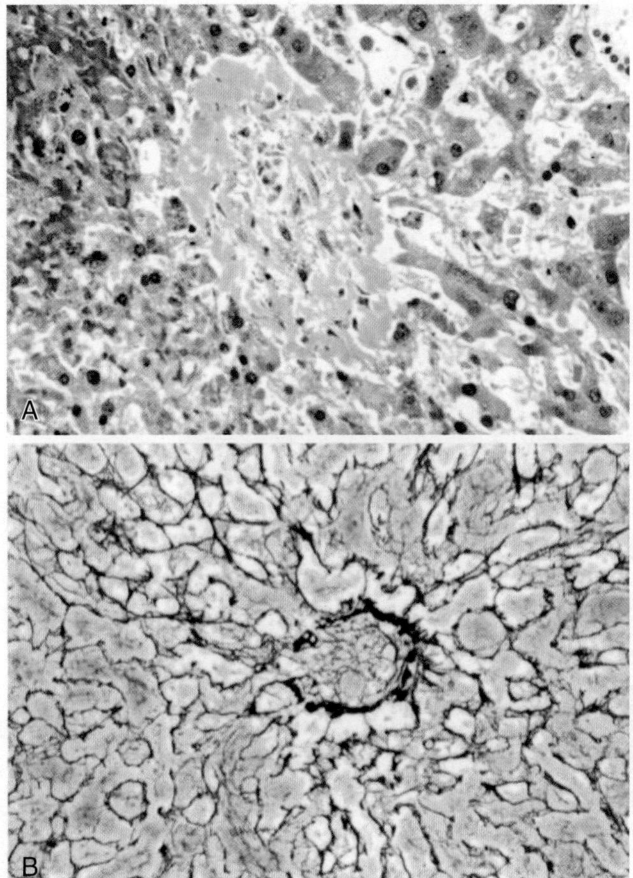

FIGURE 52.27 Venoocclusive disease after bone marrow transplantation (A) and after chemotherapy for a solid tumor (B) (Masson trichrome and reticulin stains).

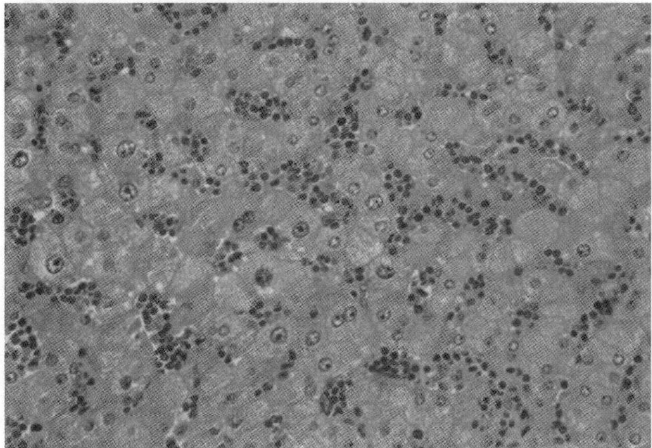

FIGURE 52.28 Leukemic infiltrate of hepatic sinusoids (H&E stain).

not distinguish between the different types of amyloid protein such as AA and AL amyloidosis,[160] although apolipoprotein A1 amyloidosis usually shows interstitial deposits in the portal tracts.[173] In TTR amyloidosis, hepatic deposition is largely confined to nerves, so that clinical evidence of liver disease is usually absent. The LECT2 variant of amyloidosis causes a distinctive deposition of globular deposits within portal tracts and sinusoids.[162,163,174] In advanced cases with massive infiltration, the liver is enlarged and has a rubbery elastic consistency. Severe sinusoidal involvement impedes hepatocellular nutrition, leading to atrophy and dropout of hepatocytes, especially in zone 1.[160] Venous involvement may lead to accentuation of hepatocyte loss and condensation of amyloid into a confluent mass (amyloidoma). NRH may occur in patients with amyloidosis.[175]

Amyloid deposits are usually easily recognized on routine staining. Amyloid deposits stain weakly with eosin and with periodic acid–Schiff (PAS) stain with diastase digestion (d-PAS); they are usually positive with Congo red stain. Minimal involvement may be visualized with Congo red staining followed by examination under polarized light to detect apple-green birefringence. Thioflavin-T stain and an immunostain for the P component are more sensitive than Congo red at detecting small amounts of amyloid. Congophilia of AA amyloid is abolished by permanganate treatment. With regard to the differential diagnosis, light chain deposition disease may involve the sinusoidal spaces in a manner that resembles amyloid on H&E and d-PAS stains.[168] However, these deposits have a granular ultrastructure, whereas amyloid deposits are fibrillar. Immunostains may be performed to subtype the protein deposits,[176,177] but may be suboptimal because of the difficulty of the reagents penetrating the dense beta-pleated sheets of amyloid protein. The one exception appears to be LECT2, which was reported to be positive by immunohistochemistry in all cases.[163] The definitive identification of protein requires mass spectrometry.[159]

The diagnosis of amyloidosis is often established in biopsy specimens of the rectum, abdominal fat pad, labial salivary glands, or liver. Injection of radiolabeled serum amyloid P component, followed by scintigraphy, is a sensitive and specific method for establishing a diagnosis of both AA and AL amyloidosis. This method avoids the need for biopsy and demonstrates the entire distribution of amyloid deposits within the human body.[172]

HEPATIC VEIN DISEASE

Hepatic venous outflow obstruction is the physiological event of impaired efflux of blood from the liver. *Congestive hepatopathy* is defined as histological lesions caused by hepatic venous outflow obstruction at sites including the sinusoids and hepatic veins of all sizes. The causes of hepatic venous outflow obstruction are many (see Tables 52.1 to 52.3). The term *congestive hepatopathy* has been used to describe the hepatic effects of congestive heart failure[178] but also applies to patients with primary intrahepatic venous outflow obstruction. The hepatic morphology is qualitatively identical regardless of whether the obstruction is primarily in the heart, the large hepatic veins (e.g., in Budd-Chiari syndrome), or in small hepatic veins (most forms of chronic liver disease).

The concept of congestive hepatopathy is useful because it distinguishes primary vascular pathophysiology from the diagnostically nonspecific vascular lesions observed in chronic liver disease. Another important feature of congestive hepatopathy is that congestive injury to the vascular bed leads to further outflow obstruction in a positive feedback loop. In the case of vascular pathophysiology secondary to chronic liver disease, the obstructive complications of vascular damage contribute to the irreversibility of late-stage cirrhosis (see Chapter 50).

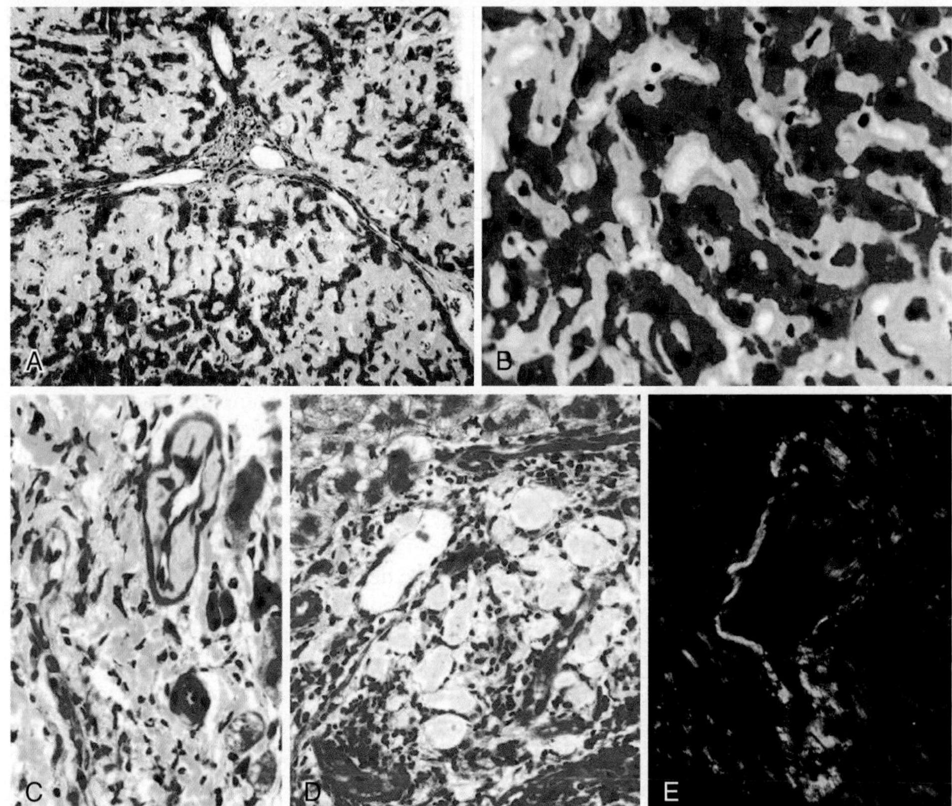

FIGURE 52.29 Amyloidosis. A, Linear type of amyloid deposition showing marked zone 1 perisinusoidal deposition with atrophy of hepatocytes (Masson trichrome stain). **B,** On higher magnification, there is marked expansion of the space of Disse with amorphous gray-blue amyloid material (Masson trichrome stain). **C,** Amyloid deposition is visible in an artery *(top right)* and in a portal vein wall (*lower left*) (Masson trichrome stain). **D,** LECT2 amyloidosis, with globular amyloid present in a portal tract (Masson trichrome stain). **E,** Linear arterial amyloid viewed under polarized light appears apple-green or orange (Congo red stain).

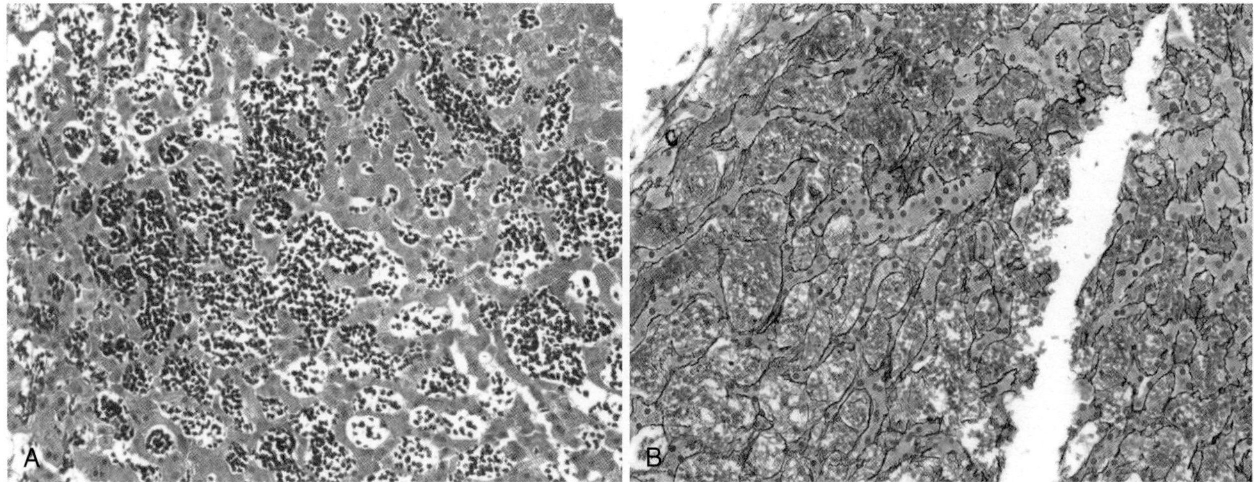

FIGURE 52.30 Sinusoidal dilation in congestive hepatopathy. A, The sinusoidal spaces are filled with red blood cells. **B,** Reticulin stain demonstrates that the hepatocytic cords are thinned and atrophic.

The histological features of congestive hepatopathy include congestive hepatic venopathy, congestive sinusoidal injury, congestive portal venopathy as a secondary complication, and interstitial edema. The histological appearance of these lesions varies in severity and chronicity. For congestive sinusoidal injury, the mildest form is sinusoidal dilation, with or without hepatocellular atrophy. More severe disease is marked by hemorrhage into the liver cell plates, apoptosis or frank necrosis of sinusoidal endothelial cells and hepatocytes, and collapse of the tissue (parenchymal extinction) (Fig. 52.30). In chronic congestive hepatopathy, sinusoidal fibrosis (pericellular fibrosis) develops. Portal fibrosis and then bridging fibrosis are markers of advanced disease.[179] Venous lesions also show a spectrum of changes, from

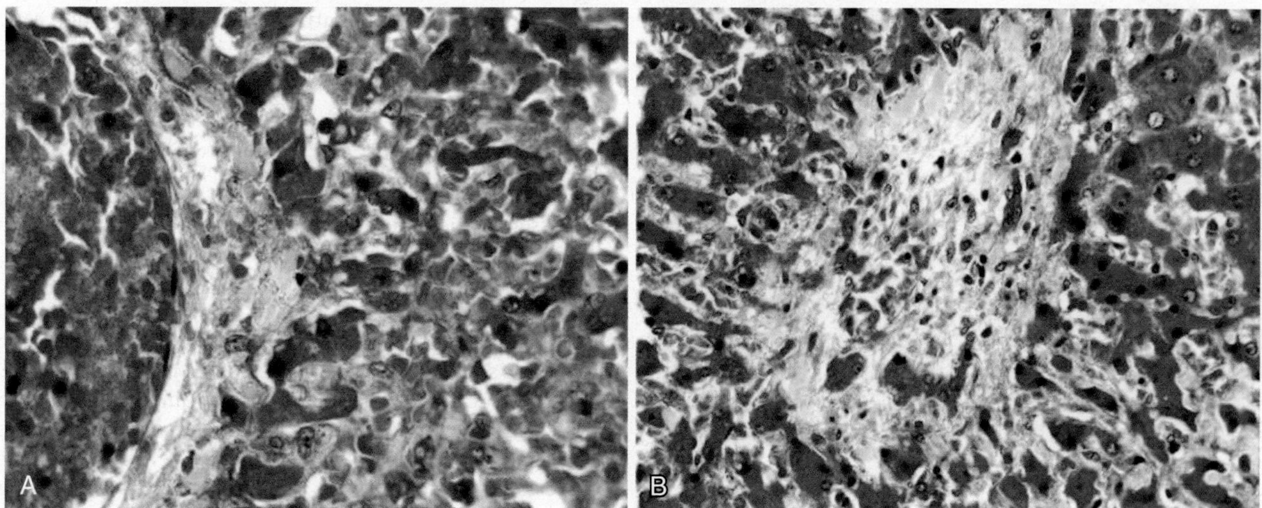

FIGURE 52.31 Intrahepatic congestive hepatopathy in a patient with schistosomiasis and noncirrhotic portal hypertension. A, The hepatic vein wall is thickened by edema, hemorrhage, and slight fibrosis (congestive hepatic venopathy). The adjacent sinusoids are markedly congested with atrophy of hepatocytes (congestive sinusoidal injury). **B,** The hepatic vein wall is markedly fibrotic with subtotal occlusion of the lumen. Hepatocytes have migrated into the neointima. Adjacent congestive sinusoidal injury includes hepatocellular atrophy and prominent apoptosis. See Figure 52.33 for more examples of congestive sinusoidal injury.

intimal edema and hemorrhage to intimal fibrosis with luminal obstruction. Figure 52.31 shows an example of chronic congestive hepatopathy in a patient with schistosomiasis.

When venous outflow obstruction is severe, the portal vein serves as an alternative outflow tract, and outflow obstruction may worsen when there is pathology in the portal vein (e.g., thrombosis). Dilation of the hepatic arteries and angiogenesis are other responses to venous outflow obstruction. In severe and advanced venous outflow obstruction, cirrhosis may develop as an end point.[179,180]

Thrombosis of Large Hepatic Veins (Budd-Chiari Syndrome)

Although *Budd-Chiari syndrome* originally referred to obstruction of the hepatic venous outflow tract at the level of the inferior vena cava,[181] the term now applies to hepatic venous outflow tract obstruction irrespective of the level or etiology of the obstruction.[182,184] Obstruction of the hepatic venous outflow tract can occur in the small hepatic veins, in large hepatic veins, in the inferior vena cava, or in a combination of large hepatic veins and inferior vena cava.[185] The predominant form of Budd-Chiari syndrome in certain regions of Asia is pure obstruction of the inferior vena cava or a combination of obstruction of the inferior vena cava and the hepatic vein.[186] Pure obstruction of the hepatic vein is the prevalent form of thrombosis in Western countries.[187]

Budd-Chiari syndrome occurs in the setting of prothrombotic conditions or risk factors underlying venous thrombosis. Myeloproliferative disorders account for as many as one-half of cases[188-191] and include such conditions as polycythemia vera, essential thrombocythemia, and idiopathic myelofibrosis.[192] There is a significant association between myeloproliferative disorders and a somatic point mutation of the JAK2 tyrosine kinase (i.e., *JAK2* V617F).[193-197] The prevalence of *JAK2* mutation is approximately 9% in Budd-Chiari syndrome.[198] Factor V Leiden mutation, antiphospholipid syndrome, and the *G20210A* prothrombin gene mutation are the next most common prothrombotic factors.[199] Other risk factors associated with Budd-Chiari syndrome include Behçet's disease,[200] hypereosinophilic syndrome,[201] granulomatous venulitis,[202] and pregnancy.[203] Amoebic abscess is an important cause of hepatic vein disease in developing countries. Sarcoidosis may involve medium- and large-sized hepatic veins.[204]

Clinical Features

Symptomatic obstruction of all three hepatic veins (Budd-Chiari syndrome) typically manifests with painful hepatomegaly, ascites, fever, and liver failure. Gastrointestinal bleeding, jaundice, and hepatic encephalopathy are uncommon. Portal venous obstruction is a common manifestation when the disease is severe.[205-207] Increasingly, patients are discovered with minimal symptoms and with imaging studies that reveal involvement of only one or two of the main hepatic veins.[208] Thrombi in large hepatic veins often recanalize early in the course of the Budd-Chiari syndrome, so some patients have cryptogenic cirrhosis and patent large hepatic veins on imaging studies at presentation. Obstruction of the vena cava is associated with dilated veins in the abdominal wall and chest and edema of the legs.[209] Serum transaminases, alkaline phosphatase, bilirubin, albumin, and prothrombin can be normal or increased. The protein level in ascitic fluid varies, but if it is higher than 3.0 g/dL, Budd-Chiari syndrome should be considered. However, the protein level can also be elevated in cardiac or pericardiac disease. Imaging studies such as ultrasonography with Doppler flow provide initial evidence of Budd-Chiari syndrome in most cases. Other imaging modalities include hepatic scintigraphy, computed tomography, and magnetic resonance imaging.[199] These modalities are most optimally used when the obstruction occurs in large hepatic veins.

The disease course is typically chronic, with less severe hepatic dysfunction compared with isolated hepatic vein disease.[210] Thrombosis typically recurs, leading to episodic worsening of disease, and this creates an acute-on-chronic

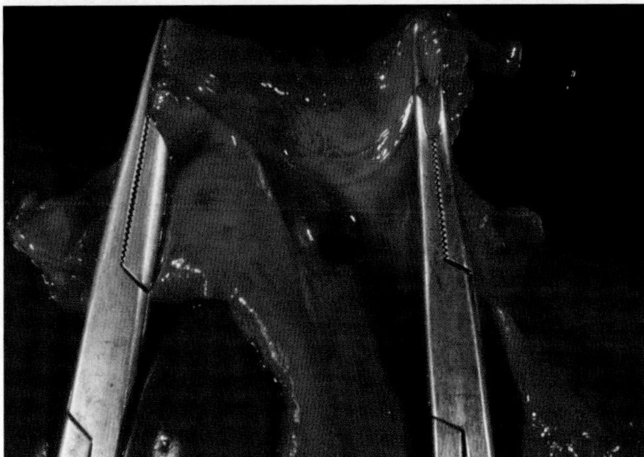

FIGURE 52.32 Eustachian valve in the inferior vena cava *(IVC)* at autopsy. The forceps are clamped at the level of the diaphragm; the superior transection of the IVC is at its entry point into the right atrium of the heart. A thin membranous valve in the IVC is present at the level of the diaphragm, just above the ostia of the hepatic veins. The corpus of a normal liver is visible in the background of the lower portion of the image.

condition of liver failure,[211,212] potentially causing cirrhosis.[213] As a result of either sluggish blood flow or reversal of blood flow in the portal veins, thrombosis of the large portal veins occurs in 10% to 20% of patients with hepatic vein obstruction. Blood from the caudate lobe drains directly into the inferior vena cava via the inferior right hepatic vein. If this vein is spared from the thrombotic process, the caudate lobe may undergo hyperplasia.[214] Caudate lobe hyperplasia or large regenerative nodules elsewhere in the liver may resemble a neoplasm clinically.[205] Long-standing Budd-Chiari syndrome has been shown to be a cause both of regenerative nodules [215] and hepatocellular carcinoma, especially in patients who have thrombotic involvement of the inferior vena cava.[210,216]

Pathogenesis

Thrombosis is the most common cause of large hepatic vein obstruction. This condition may occur in an otherwise normal liver or in a liver with an obstructing lesion such as a neoplasm or cirrhosis. As indicated in Table 52.1, hypercoagulable states are often associated with hepatic vein thrombosis. Oral contraceptives and pregnancy are important stimuli of the coagulation cascade. Other predisposing factors include paroxysmal nocturnal hemoglobinuria, factor V Leiden, prothrombin G20210A, and protein C deficiency. Frequently, patients may have more than one risk factor, typically an underlying hypercoagulable state with an acute initiating event such as commencement of oral contraceptive use, pregnancy, trauma, or infection.[217]

Membranous Obstruction of the Vena Cava

The term *membranous obstruction of the vena cava* refers to a short or long segmental narrowing that is believed to represent organized thrombus that has undergone partial resorption.[218] It is not to be confused with the eustachian valve, which is a normal vein valve that in some individuals is encountered in the inferior vena cava, just proximal to the effluence of the hepatic veins at or below the diaphragm (Fig. 52.32). Although membranous obstruction of the vena cava is rare in Western countries, it is a more common cause of Budd-Chiari syndrome in Asian countries.[188,219] These patients do not usually have a recognizable hypercoagulable state. Recurrent infections or other environmental factors probably initiate caval injury; hepatic outflow obstruction occurs only after thrombi extend to the ostia of the hepatic veins.[219] In this subgroup of patients, hepatocellular carcinoma is a frequent complication and results from their otherwise chronic liver disease.

Pathological Features

The gross and microscopic features of Budd-Chiari syndrome are shown in Figure 52.33. At the macroscopic level, acute obstruction of all three hepatic veins causes massive hepatomegaly with prominent engorgement of the liver parenchyma. With time, the affected lobes become smaller, whereas unaffected regions undergo compensatory hypertrophy, a phenomenon that most frequently affects the caudate lobe.

At the microscopic level, centrizonal sinusoidal congestion and dilation, atrophy and dropout of hepatocytes, and perivenular fibrosis are seen. Large- and medium-sized hepatic veins show intimal fibrosis, often in the form of multiple layers, suggesting recurrent thrombosis. Most veins achieve some degree of recanalization with the formation of multiple luminal channels or delicate webs. Secondary thrombosis of small and large portal veins may be observed as well. The type of parenchymal injury that occurs in cases of pure hepatic vein obstruction typically leads to a characteristic venocentric pattern of septation, termed *reverse nodularity*. The reason is that hepatocyte necrosis occurs mainly near the obstructed hepatic veins, which results in a central vein–to–central vein pattern of necrosis and, subsequently, fibrosis. The portal tracts are seldom incorporated into the fibrous septa.

When secondary portal vein thrombosis occurs, venoportal septa may develop, leading ultimately to a "venoportal" pattern of cirrhosis. By way of context, venoportal cirrhosis is the type seen in the cirrhosis that develops in the setting of chronic hepatitis.

Regions of liver only mildly affected by venous outflow obstruction may develop a pattern of atrophy and compensatory hyperplasia that can be mistaken for NRH. Indeed, large regenerative nodules in better-vascularized areas of the liver are detected in more than 50% of cases of hepatic vein thrombosis. Although the nodules are usually few in number and typically 1 to 2 cm in diameter, in some livers they may be numerous and can reach several centimeters in maximum diameter. Clinically and radiologically, these nodules may be misinterpreted as neoplasms or as FNH.

Liver biopsies are helpful for diagnosing hepatic vein outflow obstruction. A wedged hepatic venous pressure measurement may also be obtained.[134] A biopsy is sometimes used to determine the severity of the disease, including the presence of necrosis and fibrosis.[185] Biopsies obtained via the transvenous route may detect thrombotic material sampled from the lumen of the hepatic vein, consisting usually of thrombus organized with fibrous connective tissue.[219] Regional variation in pathological features may lead to spurious conclusions. Therefore biopsies taken for this purpose should be obtained from two sites.

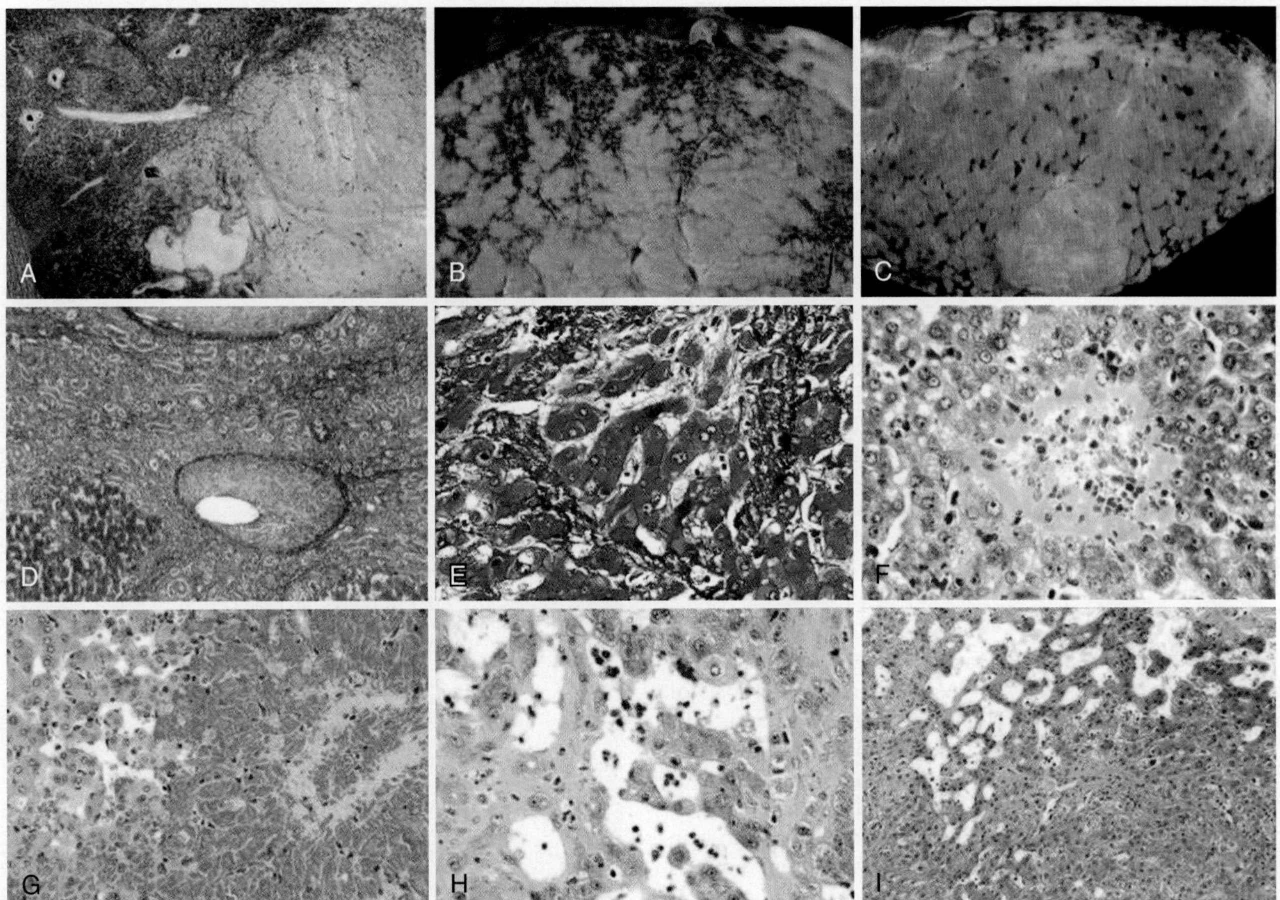

FIGURE 52.33 Budd-Chiari syndrome showing marked intrahepatic congestive hepatopathy with various degrees of congestive sinusoidal injury. A, Cut liver surface. There is marked variation in severity, from mild *(right)* to severe *(left)*. There is a recent infarct *(bottom, center)*. The patient had chronic disease with an episode of marked serum aminotransferase elevation shortly before transplantation. **B,** Moderately severe but heterogeneous disease with nodular regeneration in regions near patent hepatic veins. **C,** Moderate disease with a large regenerative nodule. **D,** Elastic trichrome stain demonstrates the original vein wall and highlights the area of intimal fibrosis. Surrounding parenchyma is extinct. **E,** This liver with hepatic vein thrombosis was resected more than 20 years after onset of clinical liver disease. Many medium hepatic veins are remodeled with hepatocytes residing in the former lumen (elastic trichrome stain). **F,** Small hepatic vein shows congestive hepatic venopathy. The lumen is replaced by fibroinflammatory tissue. This lesion is almost identical to venoocclusive disease shown in Figure 52.27 (Masson trichrome stain). **G,** Congestive sinusoidal injury. Recent venous obstruction is present with marked zone 3 dropout, hemorrhage into the cell plates, atrophy of surviving hepatocytes, and early organization of the hepatic vein. **H,** Congestive sinusoidal injury in chronic Budd-Chiari syndrome with marked sinusoidal dilation and sinusoidal fibrosis and atrophy of the few surviving hepatocytes (Masson trichrome stain). **I,** Congestive sinusoidal injury in chronic Budd-Chiari syndrome with a region showing sinusoidal dilation and hepatocellular atrophy, but without fibrosis.

Differential Diagnosis

Budd-Chiari syndrome should be suspected when one sees severe congestion or hemorrhage within the liver cell plates, recent thrombi within hepatic veins of any size, or intimal fibrous thickening of hepatic veins larger than 100 μm in diameter. Integration of the clinical history and imaging studies with the histological findings is important to establish a correct diagnosis.

In settings of acute or chronic obstruction to hepatic venous outflow, the differential diagnosis for Budd-Chiari syndrome includes SOS (after bone marrow transplantation or after exposure to pyrrolizidine alkaloids), pericarditis, and congestive heart disease. The pathological features of congestive heart failure, constrictive pericarditis, and chronic SOS may be quite similar to those caused by large hepatic vein thrombosis. Oxaliplatin-based systemic neoadjuvant chemotherapy in patients with metastatic colorectal cancer can cause injury to the hepatic microvasculature that leads to sinusoidal obstruction; this injury is manifested by perisinusoidal fibrosis that may mimic Budd-Chiari syndrome.[138,220] Some other forms of drug-induced injury manifest with thrombi within small-sized hepatic veins.[221]

Care must be taken to examine whether any of the following are present: vasculitis, neoplasm, granulomas (Fig. 52.34), sickled red cells, intraparenchymal abscess, or infectious agents, such as amebae or fungi. The presence of extramedullary hematopoiesis may suggest a myeloproliferative disease. Most hypercoagulable states require laboratory tests for diagnosis. Bone marrow culture may reveal the presence of a subclinical myeloproliferative disease if red blood cell colonies form, in vitro, without exogenous erythropoietin stimulation. Protein S and C deficiencies are difficult to diagnose because hepatic failure may result in a decrease of the serum levels of these proteins. Genetic tests are available for some types of anomalies of the coagulation cascade.

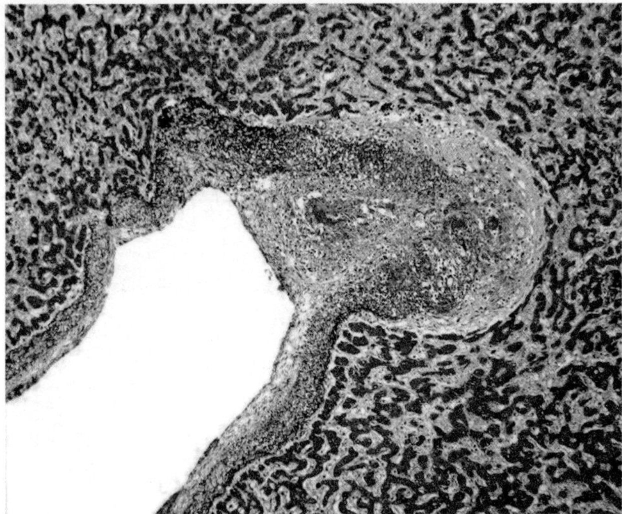

FIGURE 52.34 Sarcoidosis. This 1.5-mm-diameter hepatic vein has granulomas involving the intima, media, and adventitia (elastic trichrome stain).

Obliteration of small hepatic veins and congestion of the liver parenchyma are frequent findings in cirrhosis of any cause. Ironically, the long-standing venocentric cirrhosis caused by hepatic vein thrombosis may show little or no congestion, possibly because of the perivenous scarring or the parenchymal regeneration that occurs. As a result, accurate histological differentiation of hepatic vein thrombosis from other types of cirrhosis often requires large enough tissue samples to allow for an evaluation of the large hepatic veins. In any case, histological evaluation can be difficult because a liver with severe cirrhosis of any etiology often shows intimal thickening of medium- and large-sized hepatic veins caused by congestive venopathy or thrombosis.[222]

Long-standing obstruction to hepatic venous outflow, as in right-sided heart failure or constrictive pericarditis, can cause all of the features of congestive hepatopathy described earlier in patients with hepatic vein thrombosis, including formation of thrombi in intrahepatic veins. The degree of thrombosis is usually less severe than in patients with hepatic vein thrombosis without cardiac disease.[223] Typical microscopic changes include mild hepatocyte atrophy and sinusoidal dilation. In specimens with evidence of obliteration of hepatic veins, fibrous septation is often present as well. However, nodules completely surrounded only by fibrous septa rarely occur.[224] Therefore only cardiac sclerosis may develop (Fig. 52.35), as opposed to cardiac cirrhosis when portal vein thrombosis is superimposed (see Chapter 50).

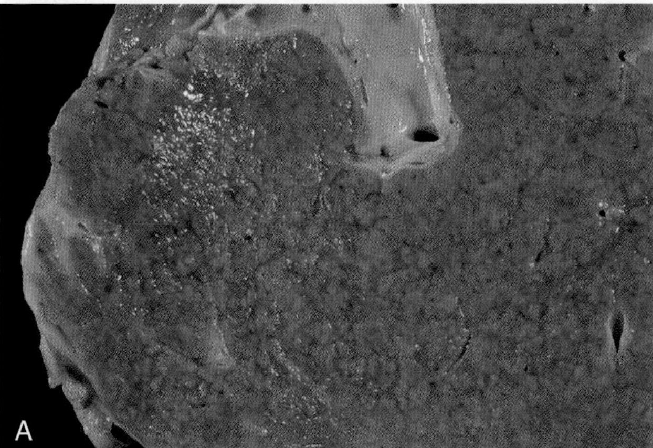

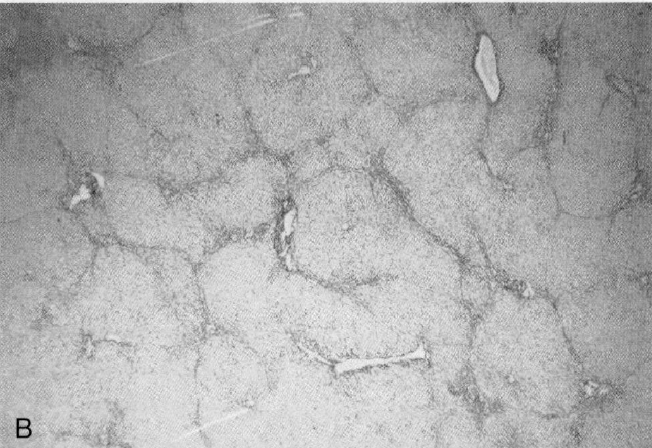

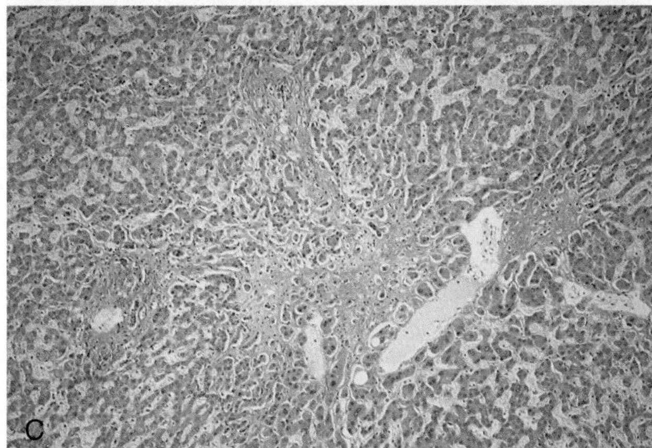

FIGURE 52.35 Cardiac sclerosis at autopsy, in the setting of chronic congestive heart failure. A, Cut surface of postmortem liver, showing finely subdivided hepatic parenchyma. **B,** Low-power image showing bridging fibrous bands in a vaguely hexagonal pattern. **C,** Medium-power image showing dilated sinusoids and bridging fibrous bands, predominantly linking terminal hepatic veins. **B,** Reticulin stain, 40×. **C,** Trichrome stain, 100×.

Small Hepatic Vein Disease (Obliterative Hepatic Venopathy)

Distinct from Budd-Chiari syndrome, which directly affects large to small intrahepatic veins, secondary injury to small hepatic veins may be caused by phlebitis, thrombosis, or luminal obstruction, and it may result in complete disappearance of the vessels. Indeed, small hepatic vein obstruction constitutes a fundamental component of the general evolution of cirrhosis.[225] Thus obliterative hepatic venopathy may occur in patients with many types of disorders, such as chronic viral hepatitis, steatohepatitis,[225] hepatic vein thrombosis,[205] congestive heart failure,[223] toxin- or radiation-induced injury,[226] mast cell disease,[155] sarcoidosis,[11] granulomatous phlebitis,[227] chronic granulomatous disease,[228] and inflammatory pseudotumor.[228] Identical lesions may also occur adjacent to hepatic neoplasms and abscesses. Recurring fibro-obliterative venopathy is a rare form of diffuse small hepatic vein occlusion that was reported in liver transplants in two published cases.[229,230]

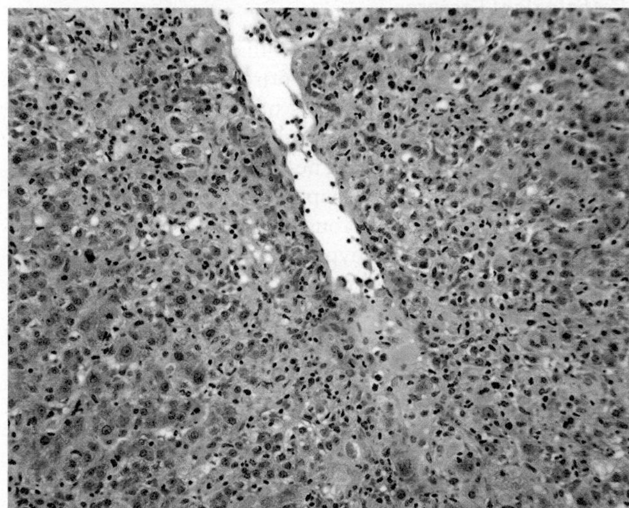

FIGURE 52.36 Active phlebitis of a small hepatic vein in autoimmune hepatitis.

The pathogenesis of obliterative hepatic venopathy varies according to the specific etiology and includes the effects of local inflammation, thrombosis, and congestive hepatic venopathy. Local inflammation is the cause in most cases of chronic hepatitis, steatohepatitis, and hepatic abscesses (Fig. 52.36). The vessel lesions that occur in patients with chronic hepatitis and cirrhosis are discussed in Chapter 50. The specific etiology may be indicated by the histological milieu in which the venopathy occurs, such as steatohepatitis, chronic viral or autoimmune hepatitis, sarcoidosis-related granulomas, or vascular thrombosis.

NODULAR HYPERPLASIA AND OTHER TUMOR-LIKE CONDITIONS

Nodular hyperplasia is a family of lesions in which benign, apparently regenerative, hepatocytes form nodules as a response to parenchymal injury or vascular compromise in the liver. The lesions are classified according to their size, distribution, and histological appearance.[231,232] Clinically and pathologically, they should be distinguished from neoplastic liver nodules, which are discussed more fully in Chapter 56.

Large Regenerative Nodules

Large regenerative nodules measure from 1 cm to many centimeters in diameter.[231] They may develop in patients with massive hepatic necrosis, cirrhosis, Budd-Chiari syndrome (see Fig. 52.33C), hereditary hemorrhagic telangiectasia, portal vein absence, or portal vein thrombosis. *Partial nodular transformation* is an obsolete term that was originally applied to noncirrhotic livers with a large perihilar nodule in patients with portal hypertension. It is now believed that this condition represents the presence of large regenerative nodules in response to portal vein thrombosis.

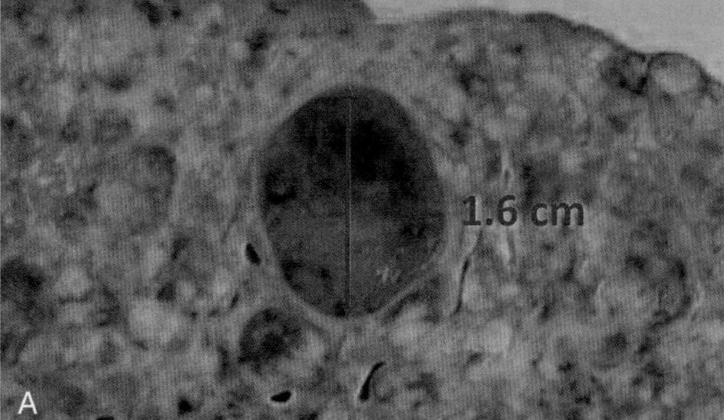

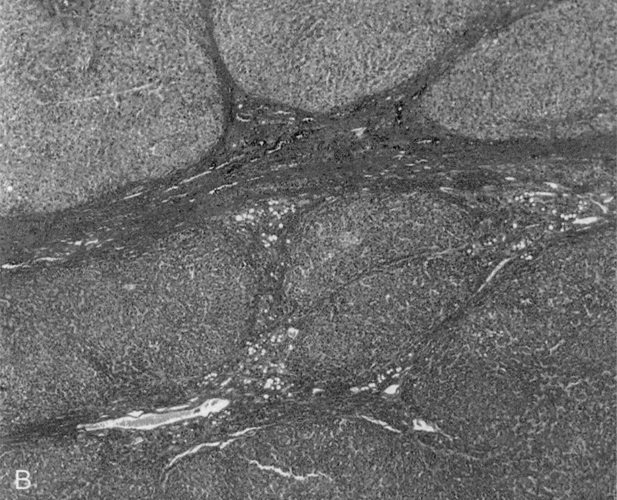

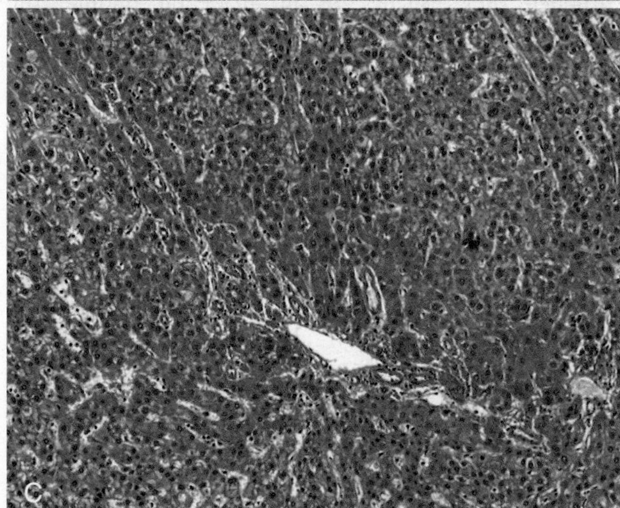

FIGURE 52.37 Large regenerative nodule. A, Liver at explant showing cirrhosis and a 1.6 cm maximum diameter large regenerative nodule on cut surface. **B,** Low-power image showing fibrous septae interior a large regenerative nodule in a different explant liver (H&E stain). **C,** Medium-power image of the nodule in **B** showing a disorganized parenchyma surrounding a central vascular arterial supply in which an interlobular bile duct also is present. The parenchymal hepatocytes retain a normal nuclear-to-cytoplasmic ratio, and hepatocyte plates remain in the range of two cells thick (H&E stain). *(**A** courtesy Dr. Linda Ferrell.)*

Pathological Features

Large regenerative nodules are evident macroscopically, either on the external surface of the liver (Fig. 52.37A) or on a cut surface. Especially in cirrhotic livers, a key distinguishing feature of large regenerative nodules is that they are the same color as the surrounding liver, and they do not bulge from the cut surface of the liver. This must be distinguished from neoplastic nodules, especially hepatocellular carcinoma, which are likely to be of a different color and usually bulge on the cut surface. Microscopically, large regenerative nodules reveal penetrating major portal tracts with normal anatomic structures (portal vein, hepatic artery, bile duct), usually in incomplete fibrous septae (see Fig. 52.37B), and also curvilinear hepatocyte plates that are one to two hepatocytes thick. The hepatocytes exhibit low nucleus-to-cytoplasm ratio, absence of mitotic figures, and absence of atypia (see Fig. 52.37C).[233] Lobar hyperplasia in Budd-Chiari syndrome, adjacent to actual liver neoplasms, and in biliary conditions such as primary sclerosing cholangitis and biliary atresia is physiologically similar to large regenerative nodules. However, hepatocyte regenerative activity, particularly in the presence of cholestasis, may impart an appearance of atypia difficult to distinguish from dysplasia. Regenerative nodules that occur in the absence of an identifiable portal vein may be confused with FNH.

Focal Nodular Hyperplasia

FNH is, essentially, a large regenerative nodule with characteristic clinical and histological features. This lesion is discussed more fully in Chapter 56.

Clinical Features

FNH is the most frequent type of large regenerative nodule, and it is the most common benign solid liver lesion, occurring in approximately 3% of the adult population. Ninety percent of patients are women of childbearing age, two-thirds of whom have a history of oral contraceptive use. FNH also occurs in children and in the elderly. Although they usually are an incidental finding, the lesions can cause pain and in rare instances can hemorrhage. Hepatic hemangioma coexists in 20% of patients. A variety of systemic vascular anomalies have been found in association with FNH, including absence of portal vein, dystrophic systemic arteries (often with spontaneous rupture), and vascular anomalies in the brain.[234] Astrocytoma and meningioma have also been reported in patients with FNH. Hepatic imaging studies characteristically show increased arterial flow involving a large artery, centripetal flow, and prolonged opacification.

Pathogenesis

The nodularity of FNH is thought to be a manifestation of hepatocellular hyperplasia in response to increased arterial blood flow.[235,236] The cells in FNH have been shown to be polyclonal.[237] The consistent presence of a single large feeding artery led to the suggestion that FNH may represent a hyperplastic response to the effects of altered blood flow from a large anomalous artery.[238] However, the presence of arteriovenous shunts in FNH indicates that the artery may be a secondary phenomenon. Instead, a hypothesis has been advanced that it reflects injury to the portal vein, which results in secondary large arterioportal venous shunts, leading to arterialization of the portal vein with irregular intimal thickening resembling a dystrophic artery.[239] The actual injury to the portal vein may, ironically, be arterial in origin, with focal ischemic damage to portal and hepatic veins and to bile ducts, leading to the inflammation, ductular reaction, and focal bridging fibrosis.[240] This hypothesis would also explain the occurrence of FNH in syndromes of arteriovenous malformations.

Pathological Features

FNH nodules range from a few millimeters to larger than 5 cm, occasionally occupying an entire lobe of the liver (Fig. 52.38). Although in most cases of FNH they are solitary, approximately 20% occur as multiple lesions. Grossly, the lesion is well demarcated and not encapsulated. The cut surface shows a central, star-shaped scar with radiating septa. Microscopically, thick fibrous septa are invariably present within a nodule of hyperplasic hepatocytes arranged in cords as much as two cells thick; they are revealed by a reticulin stain. A bile ductular reaction is present on the border between the fibrous septa and parenchyma; this is demonstrated by a cytokeratin 7 (CK7) stain. Many thick-walled arteries are present within the fibrous septa. Inflammatory infiltrates of mononuclear cells are also present in the fibrous septa. Changes of chronic cholestasis with cholate stasis and accumulation of copper (demonstrated by rhodanine stain) or copper-binding protein (demonstrated by Victoria blue stain) are also very common.[241] In equivocal cases when the typical features such as fibrous septa, ductular reaction, and thick-walled arteries are lacking, glutamine synthetase stain showing characteristic broad and anastomosing regions mimicking a "maplike" pattern is diagnostic.[242] FNH-like nodules that contain portal veins or bile ducts may represent large regenerative nodules as a precursor to FNH.[243]

Differential Diagnosis

Clinically and pathologically, FNH should be distinguished from hepatic adenoma (see Chapter 56). This is not usually difficult, unless one is evaluating only biopsy specimens. Adenomas are more uniform in appearance, without alternating areas of hepatocyte hyperplasia and atrophy. Adenomas also have less periarterial collagen than FNH. FNH exhibits neither hemorrhage nor malignant transformation, unlike hepatocellular adenoma.

Most adenomas do not contain bile ducts or ductules. However, "inflammatory" hepatocellular adenoma can show overlapping histological features with FNH, including ductular reaction and perivascular and/or patchy glutamine synthetase staining. Hence, care must be taken to distinguish between the nodularity, fibrous stroma, dystrophic blood vessels, and ductular reaction of FNH versus the telangiectasia, hemorrhage, and steatosis observed in inflammatory hepatocellular adenomas.[244]

Nodular Regenerative Hyperplasia

NRH is defined by the presence of multiple 1- to 2-mm nodules separated by regions of hepatocyte atrophy with little or no fibrous septation (Fig. 52.39). NRH develops in circumstances in which the intrahepatic circulation is heterogeneous, particularly when small portal veins are obliterated and the hepatic circulation is replaced by arterial flow. Most cases are associated with systemic disorders involving endothelial damage of vasculature. This includes inflammatory, rheumatological, and autoimmune disorders as well myeloproliferative disorders,[245] infections such as HIV,[246] and treatment with immune checkpoint inhibitors.[247] NRH also can develop in the years following solid organ transplantation (including liver transplantation) or following bone marrow transplantation.[248] Other associated conditions include polyarteritis nodosa, systemic sclerosis,

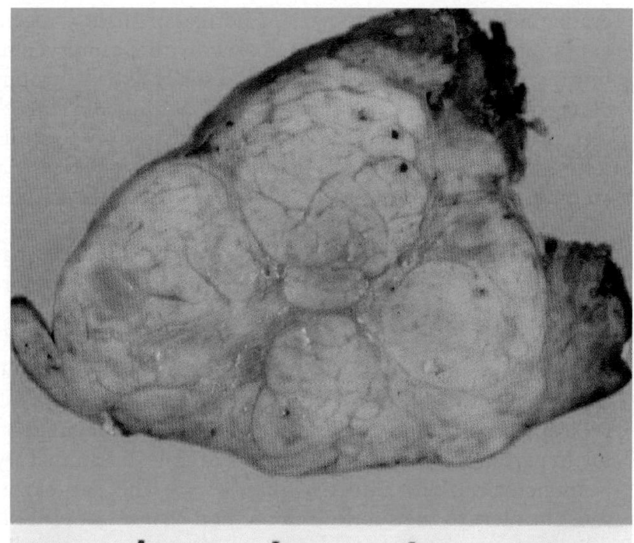

FIGURE 52.38 Focal nodular hyperplasia (FNH). A, Cut surface shows central scar containing large vessels and fibrous septa resembling cirrhosis. **B,** Masson trichrome stain reveals the typical central stellate scar and radiating septa separating nodular parenchyma. **C,** H&E stain shows prominent hepatic arteries within the central stellate scar. **D,** H&E stain shows inflammatory cell infiltrate, especially mononuclear cells, and ductular reaction, with absence of normal bile ducts. **E,** Immunohistochemistry for glutamine synthetase shows the characteristic broad and anastomosing regions mimicking a "maplike" pattern. In most instances, this is a useful feature to distinguish this lesion from a hepatic adenoma.

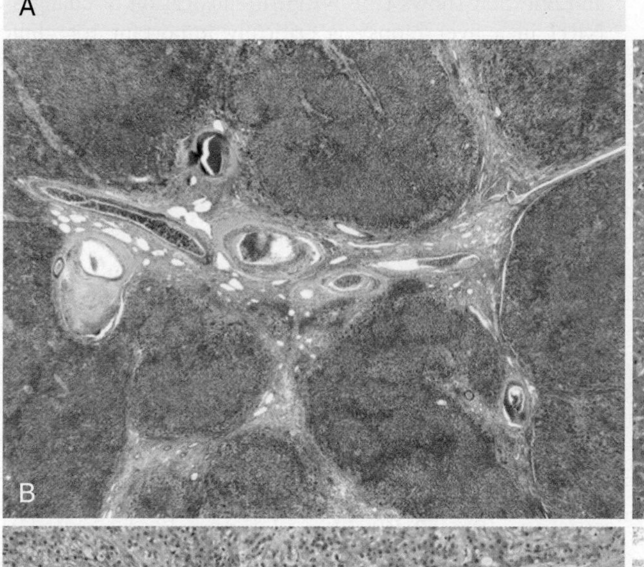

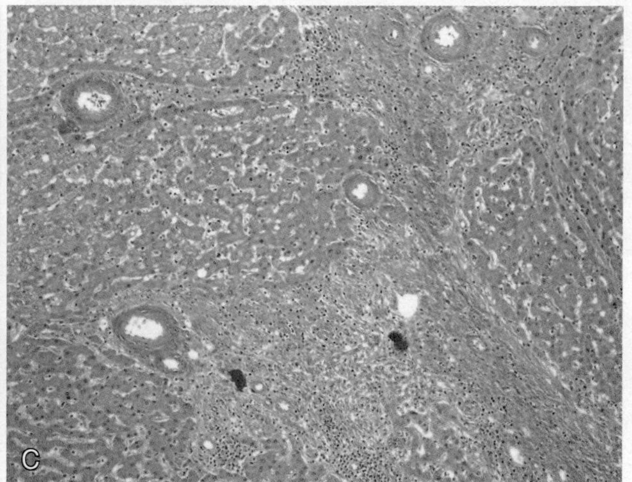

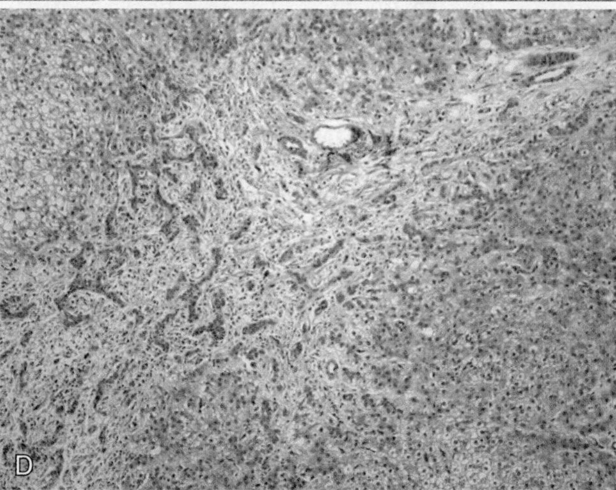

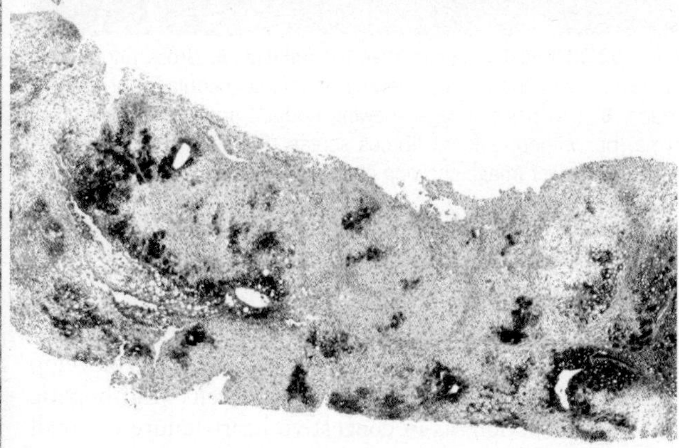

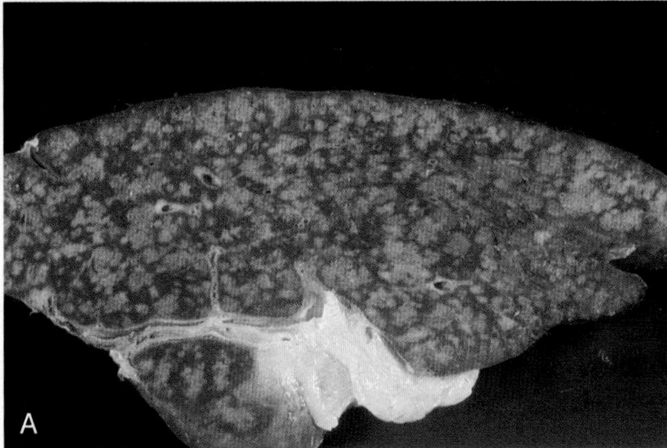

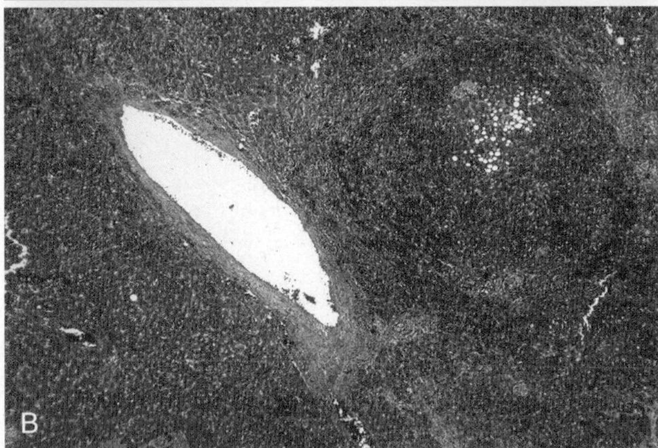

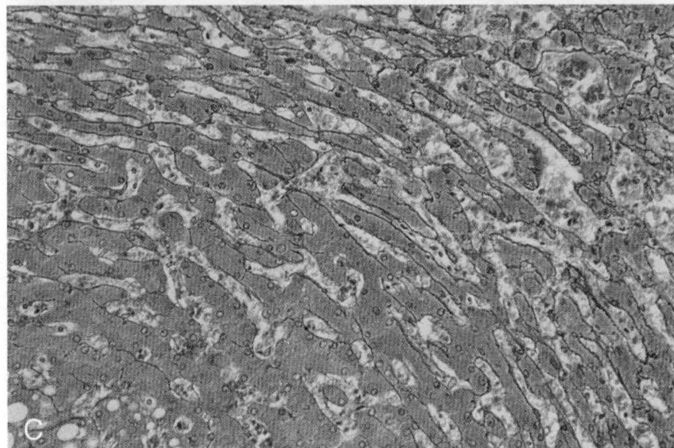

FIGURE 52.39 Nodular regenerative hyperplasia. A, Gross photograph of a fixed postmortem liver showing ill-defined nodularity of the cut surface. **B,** Low-power image showing nodular appearance of parenchyma, but without evident fibrous septae (Masson trichrome stain). **C,** Medium-power image showing characteristic curvilinear thinned hepatocyte plates *(top right)* adjacent to a nodule region with modestly thickened hepatocyte plates (*bottom left;* reticulin stain).

systemic lupus erythematosus, chronic granulomatous disease, cystinosis, and mastocytosis.[249,250] NRH may develop adjacent to intrahepatic mass lesions as well. Mild hepatic outflow obstruction, as in congestive heart failure or small hepatic vein obstruction, may contribute to the development of NRH. However, major outflow obstruction causes more severe degrees of hepatocyte loss, which leads to cirrhosis rather than NRH. The prevalence of NRH ranges from 0.72% to 2.6% in autopsy series.[249,251,252] The risk for NRH increases with age.[249]

Pathologically, the capsular surface of the liver often reveals minimal shallow irregularities that may be mistaken for cirrhosis. Microscopically, NRH is composed of regenerating nodules of hepatocytes of normal or slightly regenerative appearance that abut each other without intervening fibrosis. The area between nodules usually shows atrophy of the hepatocytes and condensation of reticulin, which can impart a false impression of fibrous tissue. A reticulin stain may help delineate the nodular contours as well as the compressed and atrophic hepatocytic cords; Masson trichrome stain demonstrates absence of fibrous septa. Portal structures are usually present, but small portal veins may be obliterated. Sinusoids may be arterialized, and therefore may show positivity with CD34 stain.

Clinically, NRH is best viewed as a perfusion disorder.[253] It may be asymptomatic, or it may be associated with portal hypertension, usually without ascites. Liver biopsy is typically obtained as part of evaluation of unexplained portal hypertension in patients with systemic inflammatory, immunological, and infective diseases.[245] The pathologist must be alert to the subtle architectural changes of NRH in a limited sample obtained by liver biopsy because the distinction can be difficult between an "almost normal" liver[254] and one that shows true NRH. Identification of changes of NRH in a liver biopsy is critically important for clinical management because an explanation can be provided for the patient's idiopathic portal hypertension.[255] Only rarely is the portal hypertension of sufficient severity as to raise an issue of liver transplantation.[256] There are extremely rare instances of the development of a primary liver malignancy in the setting of NRH.[257,258]

Hepar Lobatum

Hepar lobatum is a condition in which the presence of deep furrows in the liver capsule causes the lobes to be segmented. This gross anatomic finding is usually accompanied by almost normal-appearing liver parenchyma. Hepar lobatum may result from any disease that causes focal obstruction of adjacent large portal and hepatic veins, most often Hodgkin disease, metastatic breast carcinoma, or syphilitic gummata (Fig. 52.40). Hepar lobatum develops when the primary lesion causes obstruction of vessels while tumor growth remains slow and minimal.

FIBROTIC CONDITIONS WITH VASCULAR PATHOPHYSIOLOGY

Cirrhosis is the most important fibrotic condition of the liver associated with impaired blood flow. However, two noncirrhotic conditions are also associated with impaired blood flow in which fibrosis is prominent and portal hypertension occurs.

Congenital Hepatic Fibrosis

The occurrence of splenomegaly and portal hypertension in an otherwise healthy child or adolescent may prompt evaluation for the presence of clinically undetected cirrhosis or inherited conditions. Congenital hepatic fibrosis is a condition in which dense portal tract–based bridging fibrous septa develop during the course of childhood and adolescence

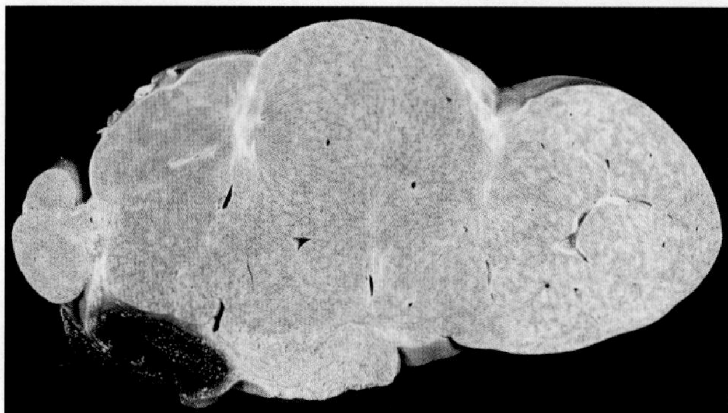

FIGURE 52.40 Hepar lobatum from a patient with Hodgkin disease in remission. The liver is subdivided by dense fibrous septa that result in the formation of deep clefts in the capsule. The left lobe is hypertrophic *(right)*, and the right lobe is atrophic, as demonstrated by marked displacement of the gallbladder.

(see Fig. 52.37; see Chapter 55). Sclerosis of portal tracts impairs the flow of portal vein blood into the liver. However, this condition is not considered true cirrhosis. The parenchyma of the liver is not damaged, and regenerative nodules do not develop.

Hepatoportal Sclerosis

In the period 1884 to 1910, Banti proposed the term *morbus Banti* for a condition characterized by the presence of primary cryptogenic splenomegaly and anemia not associated with hematological disease.[259] In the first half of the 20th century, the association of portal hypertension and splenomegaly with "Banti disease" was expanded to include patients with cirrhosis or portal vein thrombosis.[260,261] In the 1960s, investigators in India established a disease entity termed *noncirrhotic portal hypertension*,[262] which is characterized histologically by "obliterative portovenopathy." A similar type of noncirrhotic sclerosis of intrahepatic portal veins is termed *hepatoportal sclerosis*.[17] Working in Calcutta, Basu and colleagues established that patients with noncirrhotic intrahepatic portal vein sclerosis had a more favorable prognosis than patients with cirrhosis,[263] and they termed this condition *idiopathic portal hypertension*. Ultimately, the diagnostic names given to this condition included *Banti disease, hepatoportal sclerosis, noncirrhotic portal fibrosis, obliterative portal venopathy, noncirrhotic intrahepatic portal hypertension, benign intrahepatic portal hypertension,* and *idiopathic presinusoidal portal hypertension*,[261,264-266] and now porto-sinusoidal vascular disease.[7a]

The geographic distribution of IPH is not homogeneous throughout the world. It is rare in the West, and most series have been reported from Asian countries including India and Japan. However, the prevalence appears to have significantly decreased in Japan after 1970.[261]

Definition

Hepatoportal sclerosis denotes a condition consisting of portal hypertension, splenomegaly, and anemia (caused by hypersplenism) in a patient without cirrhosis but with dense portal tract fibrosis and obliteration of portal veins.[261] By definition, parasites, myeloproliferative disease, and radiographic evidence of occlusion of the major hepatic and portal veins are excluded. However, some studies also describe IPH as a condition that results from thrombosis of the intrahepatic portal veins[267] and hepatoportal sclerosis as an "abnormality of intrahepatic portal veins with portal fibrosis and nodular regeneration."[268] Thus confusion persists regarding the definition of this condition. To create further confusion, dense portal tract fibrosis also may be the residuum of regressed cirrhosis (discussed in Chapter 50) or a remnant lesion of intrahepatic portal vein thrombosis (discussed earlier in this chapter).

The underlying etiology of hepatoportal sclerosis remains unclear. Factors such as infection, autoimmunity, and hypercoagulopathy have been suggested based on epidemiological or experimental studies.[269-275] The key issue remains whether portal tract sclerosis can arise de novo and generate "true" hepatoportal sclerosis. Chronic exposure to arsenic, which may occur after years of arsenic ingestion at concentrations of 0.01 mg/kg/day, does, in fact, result in a "true" hepatoportal sclerosis.[276] For example, Nevens and coworkers[277] described eight patients who had been treated for psoriasis and had received arsenic-containing Fowler solution. The total arsenic intake varied from 4 to 16 g, and the interval between treatment and the onset of portal hypertension ranged from 2 to 16 years. Datta and colleagues[278] reported the development of noncirrhotic portal hypertension in nine patients from northern India, all of whom had consumed high levels of arsenic from contaminated drinking water, adulterated opium, or indigenous medicines. The hypothesis has been advanced that arsenic can cause hepatoportal sclerosis by inducing chronic damage to the intrahepatic portal veins; whether this involves bone fide thrombosis of these veins is not known.

Other direct hepatotoxic causes of hepatoportal sclerosis have been more difficult to substantiate.[279] Rather, conditions associated with noncirrhotic portal hypertension in which the reported histological lesion is "hepatoportal sclerosis" include latent or overt myeloproliferative syndromes,[280] a variety of prothrombotic states,[278] HIV infection,[281] and the rare Adams-Oliver syndrome.[268] In Japan, a role for immunological abnormalities has also been suggested.[261] Cases of hepatoportal sclerosis reported in children include association with Adams-Oliver syndrome and Turner syndrome, although most cases do not have a clearly identifiable etiology.[282,283]

Clinical Features

Clinically, hepatoportal sclerosis is manifested by portal hypertension, splenomegaly, and pancytopenia resulting from hypersplenism. Aside from splenomegaly, anemia, and noncirrhotic portal hypertension,[261] patients usually have normal or near-normal serum transaminases, bilirubin, and alkaline phosphatase levels. Hepatic function is intact. Esophageal varices are often demonstrable by endoscopy or radiography, and the hepatic veins are patent. The extrahepatic portal vein is patent, usually with the formation of collateral vessels. There may be normal or slightly elevated wedge hepatic venous pressure. Not all of these radiographic studies need to be performed to invoke the diagnosis, nor is a liver biopsy (percutaneous or transjugular) always necessary. Nevertheless, by definition, associated clinical evidence of portal hypertension should be unequivocal.

Assuming that other conditions are excluded, the prognosis for patients with hepatoportal sclerosis is generally

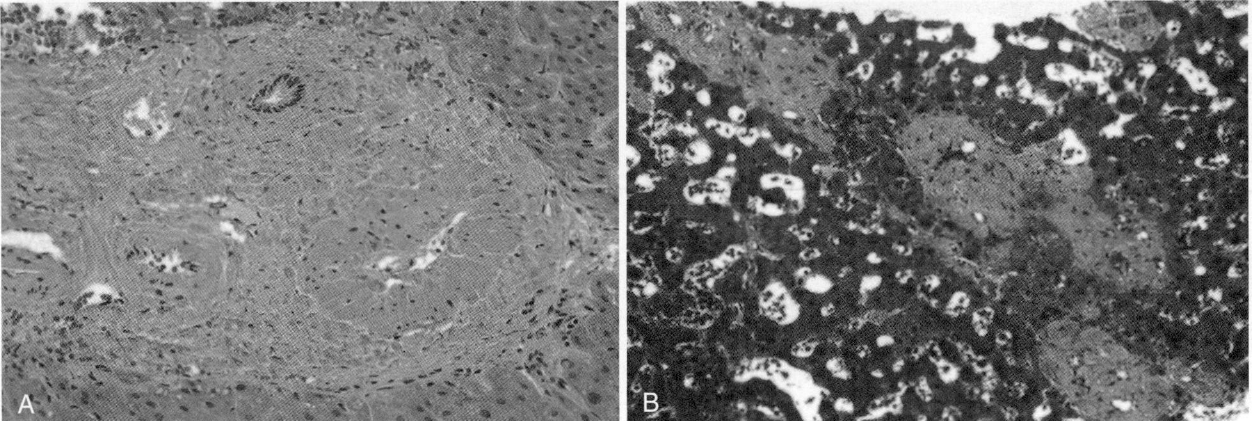

FIGURE 52.41 Hepatoportal sclerosis, showing sclerosis of portal tracts with obliteration of portal vein lumina on H&E staining **(A)** and Masson trichrome staining **(B).**

good. In general, hepatic synthetic function is preserved, and treatment is directed at relief of portal hypertension. Massive bleeding caused by varices is the most common cause of death. Therefore in severe cases, mitigation of variceal bleeding is critical, either endoscopically or surgically. On occasion, hepatic synthetic dysfunction may necessitate liver transplantation.[284]

Pathological Features

The pathological changes of hepatoportal sclerosis are attributable to persistent circulatory insufficiency of the portal venous system.[285] Macroscopically, the liver may be normal in size or mildly atrophic, with an irregular undulating and finely wrinkled surface contour.[261] Surface features of atrophy are not uniformly distributed, and there may be distinct disproportionality in the sizes of the liver lobes. Definite nodule formation is uncommon. On cut surface of a resected or autopsied liver, the trunk of the portal vein and major intrahepatic portal vein branches may be dilated and may show thickening of the muscular wall. Fibrosis of portal tracts may extend throughout the corpus of the liver, commonly forming spikes or wedges. Conspicuous phlebosclerosis and perivascular fibrosis in the portal tracts may be present, along with newly formed thrombi. The distribution of hepatic veins may be irregular, and they may be sclerosed or obliterated in atrophic regions.

The cardinal pathological features of IPH are attributed to compromise of the intrahepatic terminal portal radicles with significant fibrosis of the portal tracts and atrophy of the hepatic parenchyma resulting from insufficient perfusion from the portal system.[261] Microscopically, the primary features are marked portal fibrosis, obliteration of intrahepatic terminal portal vein radicles, and a variable degree of parenchymal atrophy (Fig. 52.41). The lobular architecture is maintained, but occasional portal-to-portal or portal-to-central bridging septa may be present.[194,281] Some cases show extensive ischemic changes in the parenchyma. Portal veins, when identified, exhibit thickening and sclerosis of the wall, with a reduction in luminal diameter and muscular hypertrophy or fibrosis. In many portal tracts, portal vein radicles are completely obliterated by fibroelastosis. These changes are best demonstrated with an elastin stain. In other portal tracts, organized thrombi with recanalization may be present. The bile ducts may show concentric periductal fibrosis. Marked dilation of the sinusoids may also be present, resulting in "megasinusoids," which are believed to result from portal hypertension. When one is examining the portal tracts of livers with this condition, hepatic arteries and bile ducts serve as valuable anatomic landmarks. Portal veins usually exhibit much larger diameter than the hepatic arteries. However, in hepatoportal sclerosis, the calibers of affected portal veins are similar to those of the hepatic arteries or even smaller. Although thrombosis of the portal veins is a known phenomenon, it is very rare, accounting for only as much as 3% in reported series.[286]

The hepatic parenchyma between affected portal tracts is atrophic, with shrunken hepatocytes and dilated sinusoids. Abnormally dilated blood vessels may be seen connecting residual portal veins to sinusoids. It is thought that increased portal pressure may aggravate the formation of these abnormal vessels,[286] which appear to serve as collaterals formed in response to the blockage of the portal blood flow.[287] In affected regions, phlebosclerosis and occlusion of the terminal hepatic venules or major branches of the hepatic veins may also be present; this condition is considered to be a result of the persistent insufficiency of the portal blood supply. The hepatic parenchyma commonly shows vague nodularity with hyperplasia but without surrounding fibrous septa. Collagen deposition within the sinusoidal spaces that surround the hepatocytes in a patchy fashion may occasionally be seen. However, hepatoportal sclerosis does not evolve to cirrhosis.

Differential Diagnosis

To establish a diagnosis of hepatoportal sclerosis, cirrhosis, especially highly regressed cirrhosis, should be excluded, along with overt extrahepatic portal vein thrombosis, hepatic vein thrombosis, and the presence of intrabiliary parasites and schistosomiasis. This disorder remains a diagnosis of exclusion. Only then can reassurance of a benign clinical course be conveyed to the patient.

ACKNOWLEDGMENT

We are indebted to Ian R. Wanless, MD, FRCPC, for his extensive work on this chapter in prior editions of this book.

The full reference list may be accessed online at *Elsevier eBooks for Practicing Clinicians.*

CHAPTER 53

Pathology of Liver and Hematopoietic Stem Cell Transplantation

Mohamed I. El Hag, James M. Crawford, Anthony J. Demetris

Contents

INTRODUCTION

Liver transplantation is used worldwide to treat a broad spectrum of end-stage liver diseases. Nonalcoholic fatty liver disease–induced cirrhosis, alcohol-induced liver disease, and hepatitis C virus (HCV) infection are the leading indications in North America, Europe, and South America. In Asia, hepatitis B virus (HBV)–induced cirrhosis is responsible for most liver transplantation, followed by the previously listed causes. Recurrence of the original disease is common after transplantation, and liver allografts are susceptible to a variety of technical complications that cause dysfunction and produce morphological manifestations.

This chapter focuses on aspects of common diseases in the transplantation setting and on conditions unique to allografts, such as infection, rejection, small-for-size syndrome, preservation/reperfusion injury, and minimization of immunosuppression. We will also introduce the reader to machine perfusion for extended-criteria donors and suboptimal organs, and current advances in immune-tolerance and weaning protocols. Most disorders are discussed in the order in which specimens are received, from donor and then recipient, after transplantation. The terminology and acronyms used in liver transplantation are listed in Table 53.1. The material in this chapter is

TABLE 53.1 Acronyms Used in Liver Transplantation

Acronym	Definition
ACR	Acute cellular rejection
AHR	Acute humoral rejection
AMR	Antibody-mediated rejection
ASTS	American Society of Transplant Surgeons
CIT	Cold ischemia time
DAA	Direct-acting antiviral
DCD	Donation after cardiac death
DDLT	Deceased donor liver transplantation
DSA	Donor-specific antibodies
ECD	Extended-criteria donors
FCH	Fibrosing cholestatic hepatitis
FDA	Food and Drug Administration
GVHD	Graft-versus-host disease
HAT	Hepatic artery thrombosis
HSC(T)	Hematopoietic stem cell (transplantation)
IPTH	Idiopathic posttransplantation hepatitis
IS	Immunosuppression
LDLT	Living donor liver transplantation
NRH	Nodular regenerative hyperplasia
PHP	Portal hyperperfusion
PTLD	Posttransplantation lymphoproliferative disorder
SFSS	Small-for-size (graft) syndrome
SOS	Sinusoidal obstruction syndrome
TCMR	T cell–mediated rejection
VOD	Venoocclusive disease

based on multiple previous publications and book chapters from our group. Therefore redundancy is difficult to avoid.[1-6]

DONOR EVALUATION

Cadavers

Gross and frozen-section examination can assist in evaluation of nonideal or extended criteria donors (ECDs) as defined by various characteristics.[7-9] Included are advanced donor age (>60 years), large-droplet macrovesicular steatosis (>40%), cold ischemia time (>12 hours), partial liver allografts, donation after cardiac death (DCD), hemodynamic instability, use of vasopressors, hypernatremia, HBV or HCV infection or hepatitis B core antibody (anti-HBc) positivity, history of cancer, or finding of a liver mass, fibrosis, or other focal lesions.

Feng and colleagues[10] introduced the concept of a *donor risk score* based on a study of more than 20,000 transplants; the scores inversely correlate with 1- and 3-year recipient survival times. The overall score is the sum of component scores for the following parameters: donor age > 60 years, anoxic and cerebrovascular causes of death, black race, short height, DCD, split or partial grafts, regional or national sharing, and cold ischemic time.

Evaluation of donor livers by a pathologist is most often requested because of the gross appearance, texture, or color of the donor liver, known pre-existing donor disease (e.g., HCV infection), and the clinical history or circumstances of the donor's death or harvesting procedure. The opioid crisis has greatly expanded the donor pool. Goldberg et al.[11] analyzed the Organ Procurement and Transplantation Network (OPTN) data and showed that the largest relative growth in deceased organs comes from donors suffering from drug overdose. This subset of donors brings in unique challenges and perceptions of increased disease transmission risk (e.g., HCV, HIV). In our experience, the circumstances surrounding their death and hypotension results in organ hypoperfusion and variable ischemic changes involving abdominal organs, especially watershed areas such as the terminal ileum and cecum. Patients and doctors alike may be hesitant to use these organs because of perceptions of increased risk of infection transmission (e.g., HCV, HIV), which are usually covered by donor screening serology and ischemic damage.[12] In reality, these donors tend to be younger and more likely to be Caucasian when compared with donors who die from stroke and cardiovascular disease, and livers donated by those who die from drug overdose are associated with longer graft survival when compared with donors who die from cardiovascular disease.[11] Patients and physicians must weigh the benefits of utilizing these organs against the risk of dying or severe morbidity while on a waitlist. Intraoperative evaluation of organs for evidence of ischemia and necrosis helps in the decision-making process.

Considering the importance of gross examination, the tissue for frozen-section evaluation should be fresh, preferably obtained in the presence of a pathologist, who should also inspect the organ to ensure that the tissue sample represents the liver as a whole. Three tissue samples should be collected if the gross appearance is uniform: two 2.0-cm, 16-gauge needle cores, one each from the right and left lobes, and one 2.0-cm^2 subcapsular right lobe wedge biopsy. The wounds are closed by sutures. Core biopsies are useful for staging the degree of fibrosis, and wedge biopsies are used to evaluate arterial or arteriolar disease, steatosis, and extent of hepatocellular necrosis if present.

A few suggestions can help pathologists avoid introduction of artifacts during sample preparation. Fresh liver tissue should be immediately transported to the frozen-section room on a paper towel moistened with preservation solution or in a plastic specimen container. Storage in physiological saline, air drying, and placement of the tissue sample on an absorbent substrate should be avoided. Air-drying and storage in physiological saline can cause hepatocytes to appear shrunken or necrotic, which can lead to overestimation of ischemic injury. Absorbent substrates also blot fat out of the tissue, resulting in underestimation of the extent of fatty infiltration.

Difficulty cutting the frozen section should alert the pathologist to the possibility of a steatotic donor liver, and fragmentation of sections should also alert the pathologist to the possibility of advanced fibrosis. Recognition of hepatocytes in various stages of injury or necroapoptosis caused by ischemic damage can be enhanced by staining several sections with eosin for increasing lengths of time.

This enhances the contrast between viable and damaged or nonviable hepatocytes; the latter are hypereosinophilic and often show early nuclear karyorrhexis.

Histopathological findings should be correlated with the donor's history and laboratory values. Because partial or fragmented clinical histories can be misleading, the pathologist should aggressively request additional information if the biopsy findings do not correlate with the known history or histopathological findings. However, donor evaluation by biopsy is only one laboratory test. Pathologists are unable to predict the adequacy of organ function after transplantation based solely on the absence of significant histopathological findings on frozen-section evaluation of the donor organ.

Generally, organs are disqualified for transplantation if the donor is positive for certain serologically confirmed infections (e.g., human immunodeficiency virus [HIV], rabies) or has had a history of malignancy with a high transmission risk.[13,14] Biopsy findings that usually disqualify organs include diffuse necrosis involving more than 10% of hepatocytes, severe large-droplet macrovesicular steatosis involving 50% or more hepatocytes, moderate or severe atherosclerosis of intrahepatic artery branches, and definite evidence of bridging fibrosis.[15-18] Large-droplet macrovesicular steatosis is defined as a single fat droplet that distends the involved hepatocyte to a size that is obviously larger than adjacent nonsteatotic hepatocytes.[18a] In our experience, polarized light microscopy at the time of frozen-section examination offers a rapid, easy, and accurate estimate of liver fibrosis without the need for a trichrome stain.

Some ECD factors that may have histopathological manifestations are advanced donor age (>60 years), large-droplet macrovesicular steatosis (>40%), HCV infection, cardiovascular instability or ischemic injury, and occasionally DCD. Other ECD factors are not reliably associated with specific histopathological findings and do not justify biopsy evaluation: black race, short stature, cerebrovascular cause of death, hypernatremia (>155 mEq/L), cold ischemia time exceeding 12 hours, and partial-liver allografts.

DCDs represent approximately 4% to 5% of the total donor pool,[19] but their use is fraught with potential pitfalls. Reich and colleagues reviewed the American Society of Transplant Surgeons (ASTS) best practice guidelines.[19] DCD livers are exposed to significant warm ischemia, which optimally should be limited to less than 20 minutes. Even under ideal circumstances, DCDs are still susceptible to ischemic cholangiopathy that can develop several weeks to months after transplantation. It is thought that suboptimal flushing of the peribiliary capillary plexus leads to microvascular thrombosis and subsequently to poor reperfusion and ischemic injury to the biliary tree. Various extracorporeal machine perfusion approaches have the potential to change this outlook.[20,21]

A grossly fatty appearance of the organ is the most common reason for requesting frozen-section evaluation of a cadaveric donor liver (Fig. 53.1). Experienced donor surgeons are usually able to accurately estimate the severity of steatosis before biopsy evaluation, except for donors with small-droplet macrovesicular steatosis. Digital imaging photosharing to estimate steatosis can be hampered by lighting conditions in operating rooms that significantly influence the gross appearance of donor livers and can lead to inaccurate estimation of the degree of steatosis.

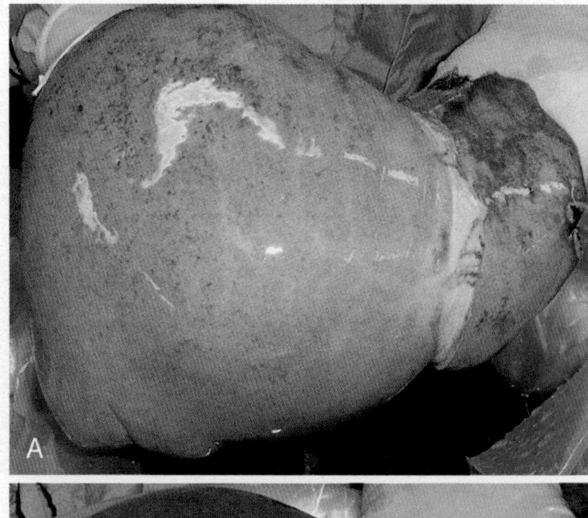

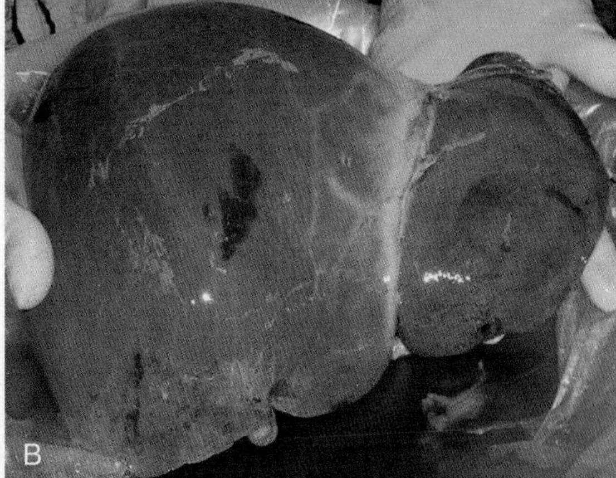

FIGURE 53.1 Gross appearance of a fatty donor liver **(A)** compared with a normal, nonfatty donor liver **(B)**.

Large vacuolar macrovesicular steatosis is now defined as fat globules that distend the involved hepatocytes to a size that is larger than typical nonsteatotic nearby hepatocytes with peripheral nuclear displacement. Small-droplet steatosis (previously known as *microvesicular steatosis*) is defined as all non–large-droplet steatosis. Moderate large-droplet steatosis (>30%) increases susceptibility to preservation/reperfusion injury, impairs regeneration, and is associated with decreased graft survival.[8,9,22] Small-droplet steatosis is often found after a short period of warm ischemia or other insults and usually does not adversely affect outcome. One study, however, associated high-grade, small vacuolar steatosis with delayed graft function.[23] In our opinion, the severity of large-droplet steatosis can be roughly estimated on hematoxylin and eosin (H&E)–stained slides alone. Fat stains are unnecessary.

Most studies confirm the reproducibility of identifying donor macrovesicular steatosis of 50% or more of affected hepatocytes by frozen-section evaluation before transplantation,[24,25] but reproducibility is decreased at the lower cutoff value of 30%.[24,25] One study recommended that pathological evaluation be abandoned[26] because of poor intrapathologist and interpathologist reproducibility for microvesicular and macrovesicular steatosis, inflammation, and hepatocyte ballooning and because of poor correlation between pathologists and computerized morphometric fat assessment.[27] Use of guideline images as a tool to improve assessment of hepatic steatosis can be very useful, particularly in centers

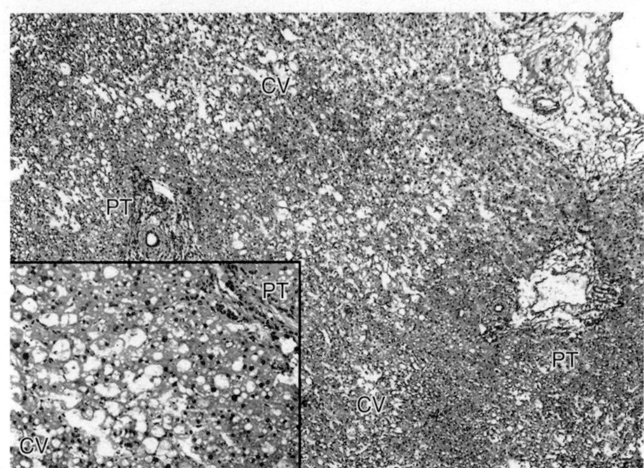

FIGURE 53.2 Microscopic frozen section of a fatty liver shows macrovesicular steatosis involving approximately 50% of the hepatocyte volume. *Inset,* The portal tract and centrilobular region at higher magnification. *CV,* Central vein; *PT,* portal tract.

with low volumes.[28] Other modalities used to assess steatosis include clinical and biochemical parameters[29] and hepatic computed tomography (CT) in conjunction with other noninvasive clinical data,[30] and magnetic resonance imaging (MRI).[31]

The use of donor livers with >30% large-droplet steatosis is controversial and varies among transplantation centers. The objective measure for assessing risk (Donor Risk Index) incorporates multiple variables such as donor age, DCD, split grafts, and ischemia time, but not steatosis.[10] The extent of large-droplet macrovesicular steatosis might even be more important than DRI in evaluating outcomes.[32] Most disqualify donor livers when large-droplet steatosis exceeds an estimate of 50% (Fig. 53.2) because it has been reliably associated with an increased risk of early graft dysfunction and failure.[8,9,22,32,33] This practice, however, has been questioned,[23,33,34] particularly if other risk factors (e.g., cold ischemia time) or complications are absent or have been mitigated and with careful selection of recipients (donor recipient algorithm).[34-37]

Utilizing data from United Network for Organ Sharing (UNOS) and the European Liver Transplant Registry databases, Dutkowski and colleagues[38] analyzed outcome of liver transplants with biopsy proven steatosis utilizing the Balance of Risk (BAR) stratification.[39] The BAR score ranges from 0 to 27 and factors in donor and recipient data to define three risk groups; low morbidity/mortality group, increased morbidity but low mortality group, and high mortality/morbidity group. They showed that use of allografts with >30% macrovesicular steatosis is only acceptable in the low morbidity/mortality group. This approach probably explains the acceptable outcomes of utilizing severely steatotic livers at some centers. Importantly, methods of estimating steatosis in various studies are not necessarily similar.

Some studies have applied an evenly distributed range for scoring large-droplet macrovesicular steatosis (mild <30%, moderate = 30% to 60%, and severe >60%),[40] but we and others[9,41] use a scale that more closely reflects the triage algorithm for ECD at our center. Mild donor large-droplet macrovesicular steatosis (<10%) does not influence the decision-making process; moderate large-droplet macrovesicular steatosis (10% to 30%) is typically used for transplantation, but other criteria (e.g., ECD characteristics) are also taken into consideration. Livers with more than 30% (severe) large-droplet steatosis are used only in special circumstances, such as when the cold ischemic time is kept to a minimum (<9 hours) and there are few or no other ECD risk factors. Outcomes in these situations are comparable to those for nonsteatotic donor livers.[34,35] A sample donor liver evaluation form from our center is shown in Fig. 53.3.

Necrosis in donor biopsies has negatively affected recipient outcomes in some[40,42] but not all studies.[23,25] An algorithmic and reproducible method of quantifying the necrosis has not been defined, which may account for differences in observations. In our experience, the liver is usually disqualified if more than 10% of nonsubcapsular hepatocytes are necrotic, and the necrosis diffusely involves the wedge and needle cores. However, assessment should not be based on necrosis limited only to subcapsular areas because this finding is quite common, especially when the harvesting operation is associated with vigorous manipulation. Correlation with serial preharvest donor serum liver injury test profiles can be used as an additional gauge of the extent of necrosis. A rising transaminase trend at the time of harvesting should trigger additional caution.

Many centers use mildly diseased HCV-positive donors to prolong the life of an HCV-positive recipient with end-stage HCV-induced liver failure and in HCV-negative patients with fulminant hepatic failure.[43,44] Graft and patient outcomes have been minimally affected by donor HCV status,[43,44] but more rapid progression of fibrosis can occur.[45] All HCV-positive donors at our institution are subjected to frozen-section biopsy analysis. Those with nonbridging fibrosis (<3 of 6 on the Ishak scale) are offered to potential recipients after informed consent is obtained. Other groups report a fibrosis cutoff value of one lower stage (<2 of 6).[45] Efforts to expand the donor pool by transplanting HCV-infected donor organs to uninfected recipients (HCV-mismatched transplantation) is being investigated and is gaining acceptance by some programs.[46-50] This is in part caused by long organ waiting lists, the presence of effective direct-acting antiviral (DAA) therapy, and possibly cost-effectiveness, particularly for kidney recipients.[51,52] Although early results are encouraging, few data are available on liver transplantation from infected donors to uninfected recipients. Further studies and trials are underway. Further discussion of use of HCV-infected organs is available here.[53]

Anti–HBc-positive donors can transmit HBV to naïve and unvaccinated recipients.[54] The risk is lower in vaccinated and anti–HBc-positive recipients and can be further reduced by anti-HBV medications and passive antibodies.[55] Donor biopsy evaluation usually is not helpful in this circumstance because most biopsies are normal in the absence of other diseases.

Neoplastic, infectious, and metabolic diseases have been inadvertently transferred from donors to recipients.[14] Examples that may be detectable by pathologists include various cancers, amyloidosis (often subtle histopathological manifestations), hemochromatosis, and fungal, viral, and parasitic diseases. [14] Metabolic diseases such as familial amyloid polyneuropathy,[56] oxalosis,[57] and possibly α_1-antitrypsin

Type of specimen (check all that apply) ☐ Needle ☐ Wedge ☐ Other

Large-droplet macrovesicular steatosis ☐ %

Small-droplet macrovesicular steatosis ☐ None ☐ Mild ☐ Moderate ☐ Severe

Fibrosis ☐ None ☐ Portal ☐ Portal and periportal ☐ Bridging ☐ Cirrhosis

Necrosis ☐ None ☐ Centrilobular ☐ Periportal ☐ Midzonal ☐ Random

Percent of biopsy involved by necrosis ☐ %

mHAI							
Periportal or interface hepatitis	0 ☐	1 ☐	2 ☐	3 ☐	4 ☐		
Confluent necrosis	0 ☐	1 ☐	2 ☐	3 ☐	4 ☐	5 ☐	6 ☐
Spotty lobular necrosis	0 ☐	1 ☐	2 ☐	3 ☐	4 ☐		
Portal inflammation	0 ☐	1 ☐	2 ☐	3 ☐	4 ☐		

Hepatic artery intimal sclerosis/hyalinosis No ☐ Yes ☐

Any evidence of neoplasia No ☐ Yes ☐

FIGURE 53.3 Sample donor liver evaluation form. A pathologist should indicate the type of liver biopsy being evaluated (needle core vs wedge biopsy). Percentage of large-droplet macrovesicular steatosis should be estimated and recorded. We record small-droplet macrovesicular steatosis (formerly microvesicular steatosis) semiquantitatively as none, mild, moderate or severe. Fibrosis stage should also be indicated prominently, as potential allografts with bridging fibrosis are generally not used for transplantation. Extent of necrosis if present is also recorded. Any ancillary findings that might be of interest to the transplant team are also mentioned in a comment.

deficiency[58] can be transferred with the donor organ in so-called *domino transplants*. The rationalization for this approach is the expectation that the latency period between transplantation and onset of disease in the recipient constitutes a gain in life span (years to decades). Post hoc analysis of donor data for recipients with unexpected complications may provide valuable insight.

Efforts to expand the donor pool by using ECD, DCD, marginal, and severely steatotic livers led to advances in liver preservation techniques. Dynamic machine perfusion is the latest in organ protective/preservation strategies, promising to decrease preservation/reperfusion injury, extend organ viability, and promote regeneration.[59-62] Techniques at various temperatures (hypothermic oxygenated machine perfusion, subnormothermic machine perfusion, and normothermic machine perfusion) for preservation of abdominal organs have been developed and have been well reviewed by Weissenbacher et al. and Linares et al.[20,21] Normothermic machine perfusion, however, is the technique that has attracted the most attention. A recent randomized trial of normothermic preservation in liver transplantation showed a 50% lower rate of organ discard, lower graft injury as assessed by hepatocellular enzymes, and no significant difference in bile duct complications.[63]

Living Donors

Living donor liver operations account for approximately 5% of all livers transplanted in North America and Europe but represent most transplantations performed in Asia.[64] According to OPTN data, the number of these operations has been steadily growing in the United States with 401 living donor liver transplantations out of 8250 total liver transplants in 2018. Living donor liver transplantation can address donor organ shortage and decrease wait times. In experienced centers, this has been reported to be associated with better long-term outcome and decreased resource utilization.[65,66] Because major liver resection is risky (mortality rate of approximately 2 deaths per 700 patients),[67] most centers routinely subject potential living donors to a rigorous screening protocol. Liver biopsy evaluation is included at some centers to further minimize donor risk, but the popularity of this practice is decreasing.[68-71]

A thorough stepwise medical and surgical donor evaluation screen is performed for any major medical diseases, obesity, previous major abdominal surgery, anatomical compatibility between the donor and recipient, infectious diseases that could be transmitted to the recipient, psychosocial issues, and any liver function abnormality or disease that may put the donor at risk.[67,71] Abnormalities detected during the workup can disqualify a potential donor, signal the need for a liver biopsy, or require further observation and follow-up evaluation (e.g., weight loss in the potential donor).

Several groups have reported histopathological findings for likely living donors.[71] Most are normal or show mild steatosis, but 20% to 50% show mostly minimal or mild abnormalities. Large-droplet macrovesicular steatosis of varying severity is identified in 14% to 53% of potential donors and is the most common reason for donor disqualification.[68-73]

Disqualification rates based on biopsy findings alone vary from 3% to 21%.[71] Most programs try to limit the severity of macrovesicular steatosis in living donors to less than 30% because this level does not adversely affect the postoperative course of the donor or recipient.[70] Candidates with biopsies showing more than 30% of macrovesicular steatosis undergo diet modification and other treatments to reduce hepatic steatosis. Some programs limit macrovesicular steatosis to less than 10% or 20%.[73,74]

Other biopsy findings include low-grade chronic hepatitis of undetermined origin, nonnecrotizing granulomas, and a variety of unexpected findings (e.g., early-stage primary biliary cholangitis [PBC]).[71] Mild (1+ to 2+ on a scale of 0 to 4+) periportal hepatocellular iron deposits occur in approximately 17% of mostly male potential donors. Hepatocyte iron deposits probably represent a normal finding in men that does not preclude transplantation. Unexplained portal tract eosinophilia may be seen, and in two cases, it did not adversely affect the postoperative clinical course of the donor or recipient.[71] A frozen-section examination initiated by the surgeon because of a black-appearing liver usually correlates with the presence of hepatocellular lipofuscin pigmentation; this finding alone should not deter the surgeon from moving forward with the transplant.

SOURCES OF GRAFT DYSFUNCTION

Graft Dysfunction after Transplantation

Influence of Donor Type, Operative Approach, and Timing of Causes of Dysfunction

Accurate biopsy interpretation requires familiarity with the type of donor and operation because many causes of dysfunction are attributable to agonal events in the donor and to complications during harvesting and implantation of the donor organ. In Western countries, orthotopic liver transplantation with a whole cadaveric donor liver is the most common procedure. The native liver is replaced in an anatomically correct fashion after resection of the donor gallbladder. End-to-end anastomoses connect the recipient and donor portal vein, hepatic artery, bile duct (except for those with primary sclerosing cholangitis [PSC]), and vena cava.[75] Donor and recipient are usually matched for size and ABO blood group, unless the recipient is critically ill, or the donor pool is limited by blood type.

Operative variations include the use of live donors, split livers (single, usually adult liver divided into two portions for two recipients), Roux-en-Y hepaticojejunostomy biliary reconstruction, and alternate vena caval anastomoses.[76,77] For example, living donor operations are common in Asia. Because the operative approach can lead to complications that cause graft dysfunction, it is important for the pathologist to understand the histopathological effects of transplantation and the methods used for all vascular and biliary anastomoses.

Regardless of the type of donor or operative approach, technically demanding operations that deviate from reconstruction of normal anatomy increase the risk of complications (e.g., biliary tract issues, suboptimal venous drainage). Reduced-size liver (splits and living donor) transplantations increase the risk of both vascular and biliary tract complications.[76,78] Accurate biopsy interpretation requires an understanding of the characteristic periods during which certain causes of allograft dysfunction occur (Table 53.2). The pathologist should be aware of the original disease, time from transplantation, type of graft (whole liver or reduced-size graft), and liver injury test profile, which often provides enough information to generate a reasonably accurate diagnosis, even without biopsy evaluation. Because liver injury often has more than one cause, all clinical parameters should be explored before the final histopathological diagnosis is given.

Posttransplantation Needle Biopsies of Allografts

Allograft biopsies are used to: (1) determine the cause of dysfunction, (2) assess the effect of therapy or progression of disease, and (3) document the immunological and architectural tissue status to help guide immunosuppressive therapy. Tissue triage depends on the reason for the biopsy, the clinical differential diagnosis, and the time after transplantation. Allograft needle biopsy should follow the American Association for the Study of Liver Diseases recommendations for liver biopsies, in general: two passes with a 16-gauge needle for assessment of fibrosis. Fibrosis staging is subject to sampling error for small biopsies (<20 mm long), and those containing fewer than 11 portal tracts may not be representative.[79]

Most diagnostically important histopathological studies can be completed on routinely processed, formalin-fixed, paraffin-embedded (FFPE) sections. A clinical differential that incorporates antibody-mediated rejection (AMR) optimally includes fresh-frozen tissue for C4d staining.[80,81] FFPE samples can also be used for C4d immunohistochemistry staining, but is less sensitive than frozen tissue.[81-83] Typically two H&E-stained slides, each containing two- to four-step sections, a C4d immunohistochemical stain performed on FFPE, one trichrome, and a cytokeratin 7 (CK7)-stained slide are reviewed. The most frequently used special stains, which are ordered only after review of the H&E slides, include trichrome, iron, and copper to detect chronic cholestasis. CK7 is especially useful for programs with a high rate of reduced-size and ECD grafts because it nicely detects ductular metaplasia of periportal hepatocytes in cases with suboptimal biliary drainage, ductopenia, and chronic rejection.[84] Periportal hepatocyte copper deposition helps distinguish chronically suboptimal biliary drainage because of a biliary stricture (usually positive) from chronic ductopenic rejection (usually negative). Perivenular hepatocytes show similar changes with suboptimal venous drainage and with steatohepatitis. Sign-out stations should have access to the electronic medical records, serial laboratory results, immunosuppression drug levels, and donor-specific antibody (DSA) data.

Optimal information needed for interpretation of posttransplantation allograft biopsies includes the original disease, ABO compatibility, DSA status, time after transplantation, and type of donor and transplant operation (e.g., standard whole-organ cadaveric, DCD, reduced-size cadaveric, living related). These variables influence susceptibility to specific complications and consequently affect the morphological differential diagnosis.

A clinical differential diagnosis is valuable, but complete clinical information can bias biopsy interpretation; therefore the slide review should be completed before the pathologist

TABLE 53.2 Timing of Common Allograft Syndromes

Syndrome	Clinical Associations and Observations	Peak Period
Preservation/reperfusion injury	Long cold (>12 hours) or warm (>120 minutes) ischemic time; older donor age (>60 years), hemodynamically unstable, DCD, repeat anastomosis; poor bile production; prolonged cholestatic phase predisposes to biliary sludge syndrome	Recognized primarily in postreperfusion biopsies and biopsies obtained during the first few weeks after OLT; changes may persist for several months, depending on severity of the initial injury
Early acute antibody-mediated rejection	ABO-incompatible donor; high-titer (>1:32) lymphocytotoxic crossmatch DSAs; persistently low platelet counts and complement levels during first several weeks after transplantation	First several weeks to months after transplantation; later onset with de novo DSA can occur, usually with less pronounced features
T cell–mediated rejection	Younger, healthier female and inadequately immunosuppressed recipients, long cold ischemic times, and disorders of dysregulated immunity (e.g., PSC, AIH, PBC)	Peak depends on IS regimen; usually 3-40 days; later onset usually associated with inadequate IS
Chronic rejection	Usually occurs in inadequately immunosuppressed patients (e.g., infections, tumors, PTLD); patients have a history of moderate or severe or persistent TCMR episodes or are noncompliant	Bimodal distribution; early peak during first year and later increase in noncompliant and inadequately immunosuppressed patients
Hepatic artery thrombosis	Suboptimal anastomosis; pediatric or small-caliber vessels; donor and/or recipient atherosclerosis; suboptimal or difficult arterial anastomosis; large difference in vessel caliber across anastomosis; hypercoagulopathy; suboptimal arterial flow (vasospasm caused by small-for-size syndrome)	Bimodal distribution; early peak at 0-4 weeks and later peak at 18-36 months
Biliary tract obstruction or stricturing	Arterial insufficiency or thrombosis; long cold ischemia, DCD, difficult biliary anastomosis; AMR; original disease of PSC	Varies, but timing can be used to determine cause: <6 months, usually mechanical, preservation/reperfusion injury (ischemic cholangiopathy), or AMR; >6 months, recurrent disease or mechanical
Venous outflow obstruction	Difficult piggyback hepatic vein reconstruction; cardiac failure	Usually during the first several months
Opportunistic viral (e.g., CMV, EBV, adenovirus) and fungal infections	Seropositive donors to seronegative recipients (often pediatric); excessive IS	0-8 weeks; much less common thereafter, except for EBV-related PTLDs and other EBV-related tumors
Recurrent or new-onset viral hepatitis (e.g., HBV, HCV, HEV)	Original disease HBV, HCV, or acquired HEV-induced hepatitis in patients with contact with animals or culinary exposures	Usually first becomes apparent 4-6 weeks after transplantation and persists thereafter; earlier onset (<2 weeks) in aggressive cases
Recurrent AIH, PBC, and PSC	Original disease of AIH, PBC, or PSC	Usually >6 months after transplantation; incidence of recurrence increases with time after transplantation
Alcohol abuse	Recipient psychiatric comorbidity or social instability; noncompliance with treatment protocols; GGT/ALP ratio >1.4	Usually >6 months
NASH	Original disease of NASH or cryptogenic cirrhosis; persistent or worsening risk factors for NASH in the general population	Usually 3-4 weeks and increases with time if risk factors persist

ABO, *Blood group system;* AIH, *autoimmune hepatitis;* ALP, *alkaline phosphatase;* AMR, *antibody-mediated rejection;* CMV, *cytomegalovirus;* DCD, *donation after cardiac death;* DSAs, *donor-specific antibodies;* EBV, *Epstein-Barr virus;* GGT, *γ-glutamyltransferase;* HBV, *hepatitis B virus;* HCV, *hepatitis C virus;* HEV, *hepatitis E virus;* HLA, *human leukocyte antigen;* HSV, *herpes simplex virus;* IS, *immunosuppression;* NASH, *nonalcoholic steatohepatitis;* OLT, *orthotopic liver transplantation;* PBC, *primary biliary cholangitis;* PTLD, *posttransplantation lymphoproliferative disorder;* PSC, *primary sclerosing cholangitis.*

Modified from Demetris AJ, Nalesnik M, Randhawa P, et al. Histologic patterns of rejection and other causes of liver dysfunction. In: Busuttil RW, Klintmalm GB, eds. Transplantation of the Liver. *Philadelphia: Saunders; 2005:1057–1128.*

correlates the findings with the clinical history and laboratory results to generate the differential diagnosis. We routinely also evaluate any previous biopsy slides, which greatly assists with interpretation of the current biopsy, and specifically comment in our reports on the effects of therapeutic intervention and disease progression or response. Post hoc multidisciplinary conference review of all liver allograft biopsies is an essential quality assessment tool to track outcomes of clinical interventions based on liver biopsy interpretations, providing feedback to the clinicians and pathologists.

Evaluation of the Failed Allograft

Gross examination of failed allografts should use an approach similar to that for native hepatectomy specimens.[85] Special attention should be paid to dissection and inspection of the biliary, hepatic artery, portal vein, and hepatic vein patency and integrity of anastomotic sites. A thorough examination may require assistance of the operative surgeon. Routine tissue sampling for microscopy should include anastomoses included with the resected specimen, superficial and deep sections of the right and left lobe, at least one deep hilar section with cross-sections of medium-sized bile ducts and arteries, and any grossly obvious defects.

The most common causes of allograft failure vary according to the time after transplantation. Preservation/reperfusion injury or primary dysfunction (currently becoming less common), vascular thrombosis, and death of the patient are the leading causes of allograft failure within the first several weeks after transplantation.[86,87] Allograft failure resulting from T cell–mediated rejection (TCMR) or acute AMR has become rare.[83,88] Recurrent disease (PSC and autoimmune hepatitis [AIH]), delayed manifestations of technical complications (e.g., vascular thrombosis, biliary sludge syndrome), and patient death are most commonly responsible for late graft failures (>1 year after transplantation).[89,90] Typical chronic rejection (see the "Chronic Rejection" section later in this chapter) has become an uncommon cause of graft failure, and its incidence continues to decrease.[89,91] Recurrent HCV-induced cirrhosis has historically been the leading cause of allograft failure and retransplantation,[92] and it has been responsible for about 30% of retransplantation procedures in the United States.[93] However, since the introduction of DAA agents, the rates of retransplantation for recurrent HCV have steadily declined from 20.4% in 2005 to 1.25% in 2014, particularly at 1 year posttransplantation.[94] There has also been significant improvement in 1-year graft and patient survival.[94] Figure 53.4 provides a flowchart to simplify diagnosis of early allograft dysfunction.

Reduced-Size and Living Related Allografts

Normal liver structure and function depends on optimal portal venous and hepatic artery inflow and adequate venous outflow and biliary drainage. Transplantation of a portion of the liver (e.g., living donors, cadaveric splits) necessarily compromises at least one of these vascular or biliary conduits, especially near the cut edge of the residual liver fragment. The pathologist should be aware of operative technical details and the exact origin of the posttransplantation biopsy because sampling errors in reduced-size allografts can be quite misleading. The clinical and laboratory context is important to determine whether there is a sampling artifact.

For example, infarcted parenchyma or morphological features of high-grade biliary or venous outflow obstruction can be localized to biopsies when obtained near the cut surface in otherwise well recipients with normal or near-normal liver injury test results. The histopathological changes are attributable to localized defects of blood or bile flow and are not representative of the entire organ. If the patient has more than one biliary anastomosis, biopsies from one lobe may show obstructive cholangiopathic changes, whereas the other lobe may be normal.

Early after transplantation, reduced-size/living donor allografts usually undergo rapid growth and may be more susceptible to damage from needle biopsies[95] and AMR.[96] Biliary leaks and biloma are also recognized early posttransplantation complications in living donor liver transplants.[78] Late after transplantation, portal venopathy, low-grade ductular reactions, bile duct stricture, and nodular regenerative hyperplasia (NRH) are fairly common.[97]

Preservation/Reperfusion Injury

The term *preservation/reperfusion injury* refers to organ damage that occurs during agonal events in the donor, graft preservation, sanguineous reperfusion in the recipient, and perioperative events.[98,99] *Cold ischemia* refers to damage that occurs when the donor organ is stored in preservation fluid and immersed in an ice bath. It preferentially damages sinusoidal endothelial cells, causing them to lift from the underlying matrix. In general, optimal cold ischemic time should be less than 12 hours. *Warm ischemia* refers to

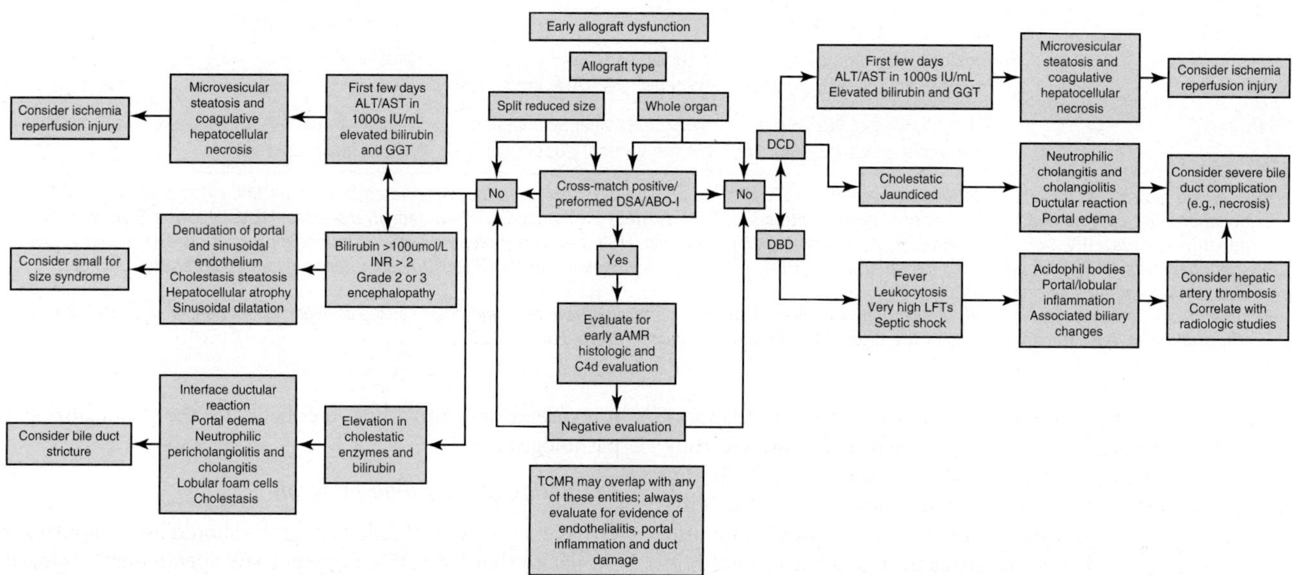

FIGURE 53.4 Flow chart showing causes of early allograft dysfunction and associated biochemical markers and key clinical features. Reduced size grafts from split cadaveric or living donors are specially susceptible to biliary complications and AMR. Allografts obtained from DCD donors are also susceptible to ischemia-reperfusion injury and ischemic cholangiopathy (due to blood component sludging and damage to the peribiliary plexus).

the time the organ is exposed to blood but is suboptimally perfused because of hypotension or death of the patient. Pathophysiological mechanisms of warm and cold ischemia and preservation/reperfusion injury have been reviewed elsewhere.[98,99] Preexisting steatosis increases susceptibility to warm and cold ischemic injury.[98,99]

DCD donors merit special mention because these organs suffer from a different type of warm ischemia insult. Instead of a relatively smooth transition from adequate blood perfusion to cold preservation solution, blood flow stops completely in the DCD donor. Ideally, the time from pronouncement of cardiac death to infusion with preservation solution should be less than 20 minutes. But even in the best of circumstances, considerable blood component sludging and subsequent damage can occur in the peribiliary plexus, which often results in ischemic cholangiopathy,[100-102] the bane of DCD donor livers.

Dysfunction attributable to preservation/reperfusion injury usually occurs shortly after transplantation. Technical or vascular insults, such as arterial or venous thrombosis, alloimmunological or adverse drug reactions, toxin exposure, and infections, must be excluded. Donor and recipient hypotension, warm ischemia, metabolic abnormalities, cold ischemia during organ preservation, and reperfusion injury contribute to the syndrome of preservation/reperfusion injury.

Clinical Features

Reliable early (during the first week) signs of significant preservation/reperfusion injury after complete revascularization include poor bile production and markedly (>2500 IU/mL) elevated serum aminotransferases that persist for several days and elevated serum lactate levels[17] followed by a rapid normalization of the ALT/AST ratio during the first week. This is typically followed by a prolonged cholestatic phase characterized by persistent elevation of total bilirubin and GTP values. Grafts that recover from early significant injury have gradual resolution of abnormal liver injury test results, but they are also at risk for ischemic cholangiopathy and the biliary sludge syndrome.[103,104]

Pathological Features

Postreperfusion needle biopsies obtained within several hours of complete revascularization can reliably gauge the extent of preservation/reperfusion injury.[17,105,106]

Mild damage that occurs in many liver allografts includes microvesicular steatosis, which is usually attributable to warm ischemia, hepatocellular cytoaggregation (i.e., detachment and "rounding up" of individual hepatocytes from each other), and hepatocellular swelling.[17,85] Severe injury is characterized by confluent, often zonal, coagulative necrosis, particularly if it is periportal or bridging, and severe neutrophilic inflammation.[17,105] Surgical hepatitis or manipulation injury, characterized by perivenular sinusoidal neutrophilia without nearby hepatocyte necrosis, and necrosis and neutrophilia in the immediate subcapsular parenchyma in wedge biopsies, should not be included in the assessment of preservation/reperfusion injury.

Repair responses usually begin 1 to 2 days after injury and are directly proportional to the severity of the hepatocyte damage and necrosis. Mild injury is usually followed by hepatocellular mitosis and hepatocyte plate thickening. The "cholestatic" phase includes mild centrilobular hepatocellular swelling, and hepatocanalicular cholestasis often coexists and persists for several weeks (Fig. 53.5). Severe preservation/

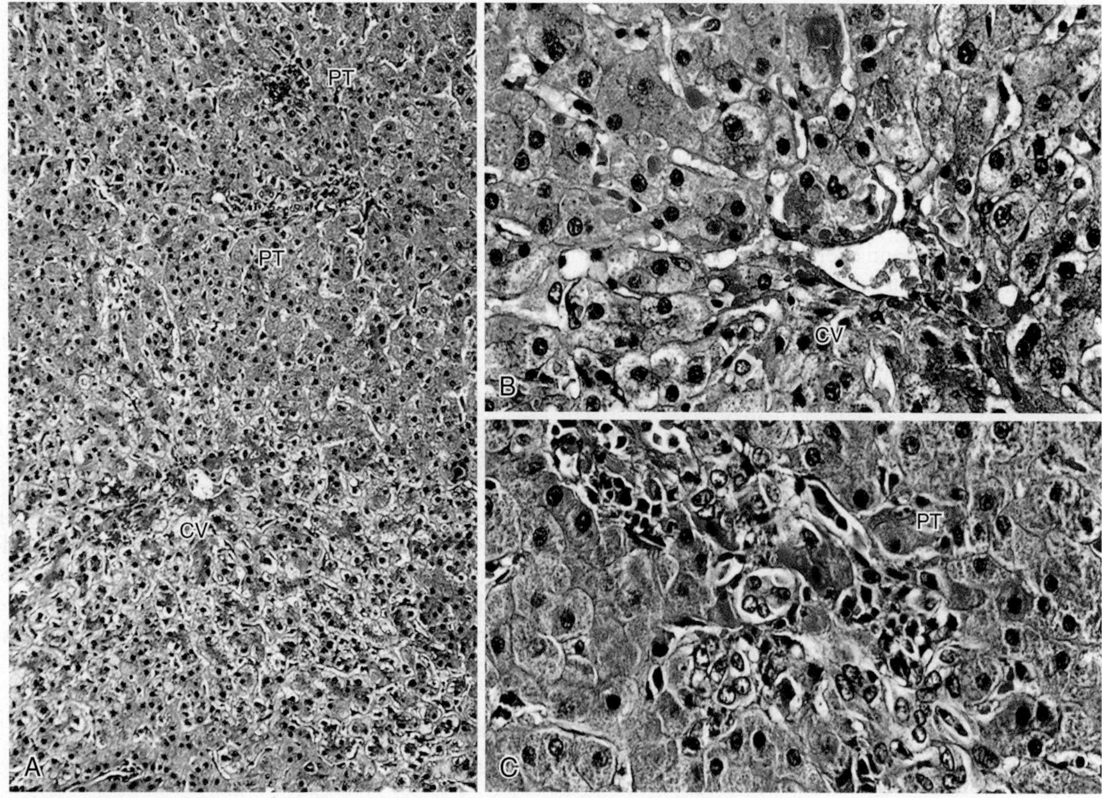

FIGURE 53.5 Mild preservation/reperfusion injury is characterized by centrilobular hepatocyte swelling **(A)** and mild canalicular cholestasis **(B).** Note the minimal ductular reaction with no portal edema or inflammation **(C).** *CV,* Central vein; *PT,* portal tract.

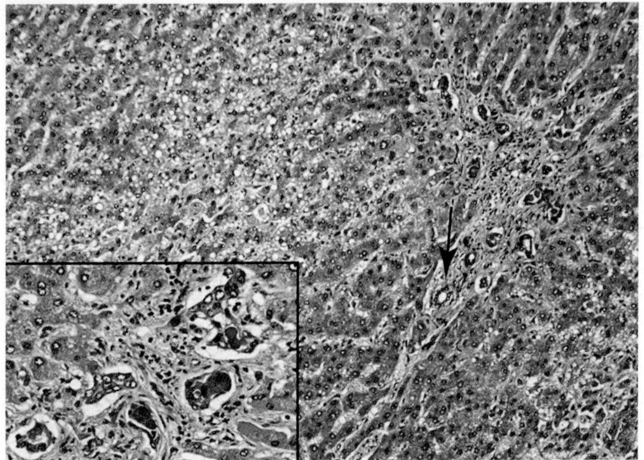

FIGURE 53.6 Severe preservation/reperfusion injury is characterized by centrilobular hepatocyte swelling, canalicular cholestasis, portal tract expansion, and cholangiolar proliferation. It is often accompanied by mild, nonspecific inflammation and cholangiolar bile plugs *(inset)*. Note the absence of edema around the true bile duct *(arrow)* and the inflammation around the cholangioles at the interface zone. These features help distinguish preservation injury from biliary obstruction.

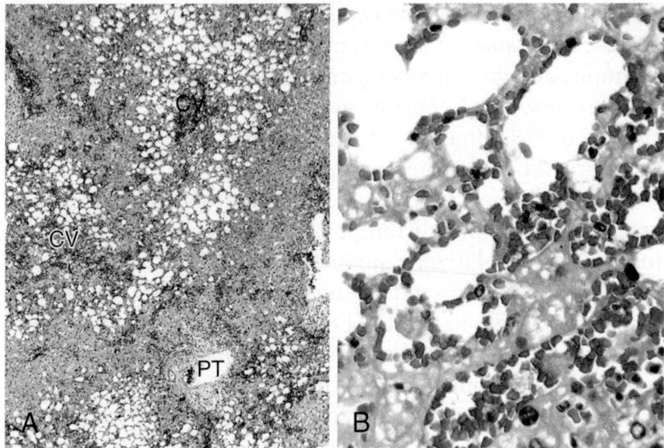

FIGURE 53.7 A–B, Reperfusion of a donor liver with severe macrovesicular steatosis results in release of fat globules into the sinusoids resulting from hepatocyte injury during preservation and reperfusion. Fat globules coalesce and form large, bubble-shaped, open spaces within the sinusoids. They cause focal fibrin deposition, congestion, and mild neutrophilia **(B).** *CV,* Central vein; *PT,* portal tract.

reperfusion injury is usually accompanied by marked centrilobular hepatocellular swelling and hepatocanalicular and cholangiolar cholestasis.[17,85] These features often persist for 1 or 2 months (Fig. 53.6). Cholangiolar proliferation is usually triggered by severe injury (e.g., periportal and confluent bridging necrosis).[17,85] Coexistent sepsis (common during this period) can also contribute to the pattern of injury. If the graft recovers, normal architecture can be restored, but patients are at risk for ischemic cholangiopathy.

Preservation/reperfusion injury of steatotic (>20% large-droplet macrovesicular steatosis) donor livers causes death of some fat-containing hepatocytes. This causes release of large lipid droplets into the sinusoids that coalesce into even larger globules, which trigger local fibrin deposition, neutrophilia, red blood cell congestion, and local obstruction of sinusoidal blood flow, referred to as *lipopeliosis* (Fig. 53.7).[15] If the liver recovers, the large fat globules become surrounded by macrophages and eventually resolve over several weeks.[107] Because normal hepatocytes require only 4 to 6 hours to undergo the entire apoptotic cycle, recognition of apoptotic hepatocytes or coagulative necrosis in a biopsy obtained more than several days after transplantation should arouse suspicion of another, usually ischemic, insult.[108]

Differential Diagnosis

Suboptimal biliary drainage, pancreatitis, sepsis, acute AMR, and cholestatic hepatitis can produce histopathological changes that resemble preservation/reperfusion injury. Detailed donor information, including age and organ type (e.g., ECD, DCD), cold and warm ischemic times, operative difficulties, recipient's clinical profile, blood culture, blood crossmatch, and results for DSAs and C4d staining help determine the likely source or sources of injury.[83] However, preservation/reperfusion injury and operative technical difficulties most often are the causes of liver injury early after transplantation.

Examination of true bile ducts (not cholangioles) contained within the true portal tract stroma and cholangioles at the interface zone provide useful clues for distinguishing preservation/reperfusion injury from suboptimal biliary drainage. The latter usually cause at least some degree of periductal lamellar edema or produce stellate-shaped septal bile duct lumens with neutrophils in the lumen or infiltrating between biliary epithelial cells. Preservation/reperfusion injury does not usually show true bile duct changes unless it is associated with or leads to ischemic cholangiopathy. Instead, neutrophils surround the interface zone cholangioles. Centrilobular hepatocanalicular, cholangiolar cholestasis and intralobular neutrophil clusters are common to both disorders. The clinical context, history, and laboratory results are often needed to distinguish sepsis from preservation/reperfusion injury.

TCMR superimposed on preservation injury is recognized by the typical TCMR-type inflammatory infiltrate in portal and perivenular regions (blastic and smaller lymphocytes and occasional eosinophils), which are an excellent early marker of an emerging rejection reaction, especially when associated with lymphocytic cholangitis and lymphohistiocytic central perivenulitis. Distinguishing preservation injury from AMR is discussed later (see Antibody-Mediated Rejection).

Drug- and/or viral-induced cholestatic hepatitis can be difficult to distinguish from preservation injury without knowledge of the clinical history, but the typical periods of onset differ substantially. Viral-associated cholestatic hepatitis has been reported only for patients infected with HBV or HCV and is currently rare because of effective DAA agents. In this context, cholestatic hepatitis usually worsens with time unless the patient is treated with decreased immunosuppression or antiviral therapy, whereas the trend is gradual improvement for patients with preservation/reperfusion injury. Drug-induced cholestatic hepatitis early after transplantation is rare.

Small-for-Size Syndrome

Pathophysiology

Normal liver structure, function, and growth depend on finely balanced portal and hepatic artery inflow and hepatic venous outflow and biliary tract drainage. It is difficult for surgeons to divide reduced-size donor livers (e.g., living donor, splits) with sufficient precision such that all of these requirements are satisfied in the donor and recipient. This is especially true when a reduced-size or living donor allograft (<30% of the expected recipient's liver volume or <0.8% of the recipient's body weight) is placed into the hyperdynamic and hypertensive portal circulation characteristic of a cirrhotic recipient. The donor liver fragment may be unable to accommodate the increased portal inflow, especially if hepatic venous drainage is compromised.[109,110] Too much portal venous inflow can injure portal venous and periportal sinusoidal endothelium[97,111] and contribute to allograft dysfunction. This is referred to as *portal hyperperfusion/small-for-size syndrome* (PHP/SFSS).

The arterial buffer response, which refers to reciprocal regulation of portal venous and hepatic artery hepatic blood flow, is an important aspect of PHP/SFSS.[112,113] Increased portal venous flow, as occurs in SFSS, causes arterial constriction and diminishes hepatic arterial flow, which results in suboptimal oxygenation. This predisposes the patient to arterial thrombosis and ischemic cholangitis, particularly if the arterial anastomosis is imperfect. Conversely, decreased portal venous flow, as occurs in cases of portal venopathy, causes hepatic arterial dilation and increased arterial flow.

The arterial buffer response is thought to be mediated by portal venous flow and the relative washout rate of adenosine,[112,113] an arterial vasodilator produced in the portal tracts. Other compounds, such as adenosine triphosphate (ATP) and hydrogen sulfide (H_2S), and sensory innervation are likely to be involved.[113] Temporarily reducing portal venous flow by transient portal-caval shunting, banding, splenic artery ligation, and pharmacological manipulation can ameliorate some PHP/SFSS manifestations.[109,113-115] Conversely, low portal inflow can impair liver regeneration and cause graft steatosis because the hepatic parenchyma depends on portal venous blood.[116,117] Primary alterations in hepatic artery flow do not cause flow changes in the portal circulation. Reduced-size or living donor allografts are usually required to grow after transplantation and are likely to experience PHP/SFSS to some extent, although it may not be clinically evident. Portal hyperperfusion is an important physiological stimulus of liver regeneration.[97] Portal pressure elevation after partial hepatectomy inversely depends on the size of the graft.[118] The rate of subsequent hepatocyte regeneration is directly proportional to increased portal pressure and flow.[119,120] Failure of liver regeneration is usually not the major clinical problem associated with PHP/SFSS, although regeneration can be impeded by suboptimal hepatic venous drainage in severe cases.[121] Instead, PHP/SFSS becomes clinically significant when the structural integrity of the hepatic vasculature is compromised by the arterial buffer response, in which hepatic arterial flow counteracts changes in portal venous flow. Decreased arterial flow causes parenchymal or biliary ischemia and infarction. Splanchnic venous stasis and perfusion of the liver with endotoxin-rich blood may contribute to the evolving cholestasis.[97]

The optimal approach to avoid this complication is to gradually titrate venous inflow and have adequate venous drainage, which can be achieved surgically or pharmacologically.[122] This creates venous inflow high enough to trigger and sustain regeneration but not high enough to directly cause sheer stress injury or indirectly compromise arterial flow because of sustained spasm as part of the arterial buffer response.

Clinical Features

Dahm and colleagues defined PHP/SFSS as at least two of the following complications occurring on 3 consecutive days in the first several weeks after transplantation: elevated bilirubin (>100 μmol/L), international normalized ratio (INR) higher than 2, and grade 3 or 4 encephalopathy after exclusion of technical, immunologic, or infectious complications.[123] Surgeons are usually aware of the potential for PHP/SFSS, but the diagnosis can be difficult to establish with certainty. Clinical manifestations are not specific and may be caused by other insults (e.g., portal vein thrombosis).

It is often difficult to determine whether PHP/SFSS contributes to complications that may otherwise be deemed technical, especially because the latter are encountered with increased frequency in reduced-size allografts. For example, a strong arterial buffer response can lead to significant arterial vasospasm and predispose to thrombosis, especially if blood vessels are a smaller caliber than normal.[97] This event may be misinterpreted as a technical complication. Risk factors for PHP/SFSS in living donor liver transplants include recipients of the left lobe (compared with the right lobe), higher portal reperfusion pressure, high preoperative bilirubin, older donor age, and higher donor BMI.[124] Recognition and amelioration of these factors using a variety of proper planning and surgical and pharmacological approaches has decreased the incidence and severity of this complication.[122]

Pathological Features

PHP/SFSS has been observed reliably in experimental animal models[111,119,125,126] and occasionally in postreperfusion or early posttransplantation allograft biopsies obtained within the first several days in humans. Sheer stress resulting in portal vein and periportal sinusoidal endothelium denudation occurs as early as 5 minutes after transplantation.[97,111,119,125,126] In severe cases, microvascular rupture at the portal vein–sinusoidal junction can result in hemorrhage into the portal and periportal connective tissue and dissect into hepatic parenchyma.[127,128]

If the allograft survives the initial crisis, reparative changes occur, including endothelial cell hypertrophy and subendothelial edema accompanied by growth of myofibroblasts and endothelial cells into the subendothelial space. Eventually, this process leads to fibrointimal hyperplasia or intimal thickening and luminal obliteration or recanalization of thrombi (Fig. 53.8). Venous findings typical of PHP/SFSS are uncommon in peripheral core-needle biopsies. Instead, a constellation of nonspecific findings can be seen including centrilobular hepatocanalicular cholestasis, centrilobular hepatocyte steatosis or hepatocyte atrophy with sinusoidal dilation, centrilobular hepatocyte necrosis, and a low-grade ductular reaction (Fig. 53.9).

Review of operative and radiographic reports and clinical history followed by a discussion with the surgeon will help determine whether PHP/SFSS is contributing to biopsy findings. Hilar sections of allografts that fail because of PHP/SFSS frequently show changes of traumatic injury to large portal vein endothelium, focal fibrointimal hyperplasia of vein branches, evidence of arterial vasospasm, and, in

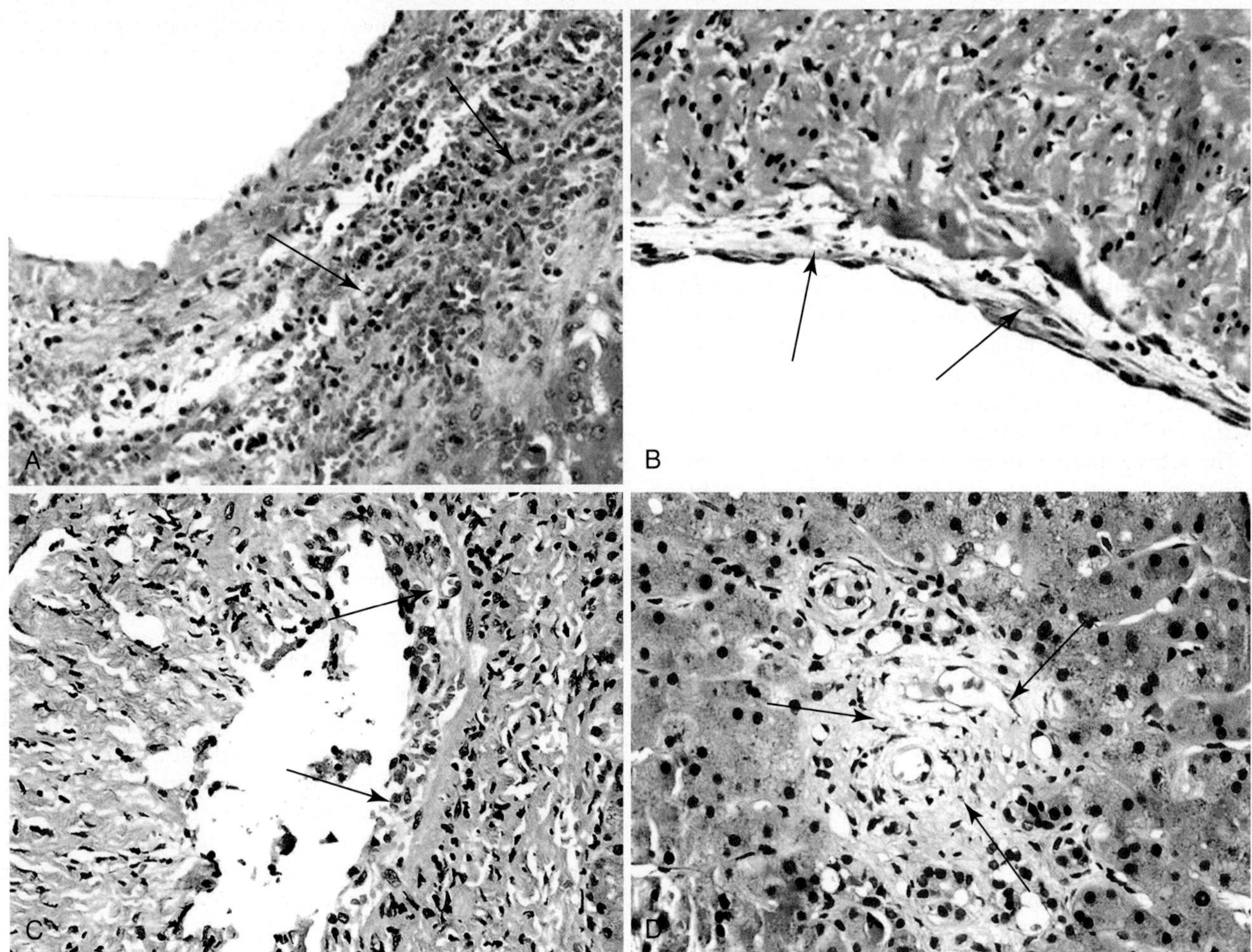

FIGURE 53.8 A, In the section from a failed liver allograft with portal hyperperfusion and small-for-size syndrome, note the hemorrhage in the portal tract and periportal connective tissue *(arrows)*. This usually occurs within days after transplantation. **B,** The main portal vein in the liver hilum shows endothelial cell hypertrophy, subendothelial edema, early influx (activation) of subendothelial myofibroblasts *(arrows)*, and focal hemorrhage into the connective tissue around the mural myocytes. **C,** The intermediate healing phase of traumatic injury to portal veins is characterized by activated endothelial cells and ingrowth and organization of myofibroblasts into the subendothelial space *(arrows)*. **D,** Late changes in the small portal vein branches include thrombosis and recanalization *(arrows)*. Obliterative portal venopathy and nodular regenerative hyperplasia occur later after transplantation. (From Demetris AJ, Kelly DM, Eghtesad B, et al. Pathophysiological observations and histopathological recognition of the portal hyperperfusion or small-for-size syndrome. *Am J Surg Pathol.* 2006;30:986–993.)

some cases, ischemic cholangitis, particularly if the hepatic artery has thrombosed.[97]

If the graft recovers, portal hypertension and ascites resolve over a period of several weeks. Although a near-normal architecture usually occurs, NRH as a result of portal venopathy from the initial injury can occur.[97]

Differential Diagnosis

Suboptimal arterial flow resulting from arterial thrombosis or stricturing, sepsis, hypotension, suboptimal biliary tract drainage from a variety of causes, or ischemic cholangitis can cause pathological changes similar to those of PHP/SFSS. However, arterial vasospasm is usually detectable microscopically only in failed allografts and only when severe primarily in medium-sized perihilar arteries.

Preservation/reperfusion injury is a differential diagnostic consideration, but living donor grafts are usually not affected significantly. Because portal hyperperfusion can lead to diminished arterial flow and thrombosis, it is not surprising that more than one complication may occur. Suboptimal biliary tract drainage alone is usually not accompanied by portal tract connective tissue hemorrhage, centrilobular hepatocyte ischemic changes, or significant NRH. When these changes are found, PHP/SFSS should be considered.

COMPLICATIONS OF TRANSPLANTATION

Vascular Complications

Most vascular complications occur within the first several months after transplantation; they are related to anastomotic imperfections (e.g., narrowing, flaps, dramatic caliber reductions), preexisting donor atherosclerotic disease, vascular tree trauma, creation of kinks or abnormal tortuosity, metabolic or physiological abnormalities that predispose to thrombosis, or a combination of these factors. Potential problems often manifest because of factors that increase the technical difficulty of the vascular anastomoses (e.g., small-caliber vessels in pediatric recipients,

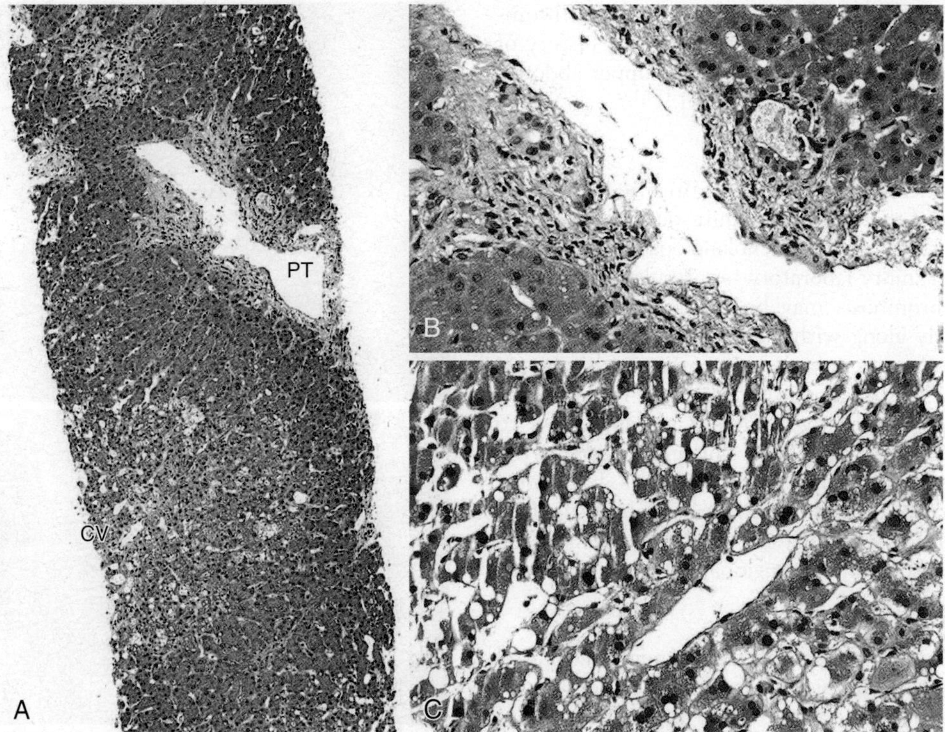

FIGURE 53.9 **A,** Typical findings of small-for-size syndrome include centrilobular canalicular cholestasis, centrilobular steatosis or atrophy, hemorrhage, and bile ductular proliferation at the portal-periportal interface. **B,** At higher magnification, the interface zone shows a low-grade bile ductular reaction and focal cholangiolar cholestasis. **C,** High magnification of the centrilobular region shows microvesicular steatosis and cholestasis. Centrilobular hepatocyte atrophy, congestion, and necrosis may also be seen. These features are not specific for small-for-size syndrome. *CV,* Central vein; *PT,* portal tract. (From Demetris AJ, Kelly DM, Eghtesad B, et al. Pathophysiological observations and histopathological recognition of the portal hyperperfusion or small-for-size syndrome. *Am J Surg Pathol.* 2006;30:986-993.)

reduced-size grafts, abnormal anatomy such as piggyback venal caval anastomosis). Physiological or metabolic abnormalities that decrease hepatic blood flow or promote coagulation, such as cardiac failure, clotting abnormalities, TCMR, and infections, also increase the risk of vascular complications.

Vascular interposition arterial grafts or small venous segments, which are used to link the donor and recipient arteries or veins, respectively, can be a significant source of problems. Vascular grafts increase the need for sutured anastomoses; some vessel segments might have been cryopreserved or stored in preservation fluid for one to several days before implantation and may be marginally viable. These factors increase the risk of thrombosis, stimulate atherogenesis, and serve as a nidus of infection.

Hepatic Artery Thrombosis

Pathophysiology

Hepatic artery thrombosis is the most common major vascular complication and an important cause of early allograft damage, failure, and retransplantation.[129] It occurs in 2% to 20% of transplants, usually within 30 days of transplantation.[130,131] Early hepatic artery thrombosis maybe detected by routine use of Doppler ultrasonography in the early postoperative period, allowing for timely intervention and decreasing complications associated with hepatic artery thrombosis. Allografts are more susceptible to arterial ischemia than native livers because they are devoid of a collateral arterial circulation early after transplantation.

The hepatic artery exclusively supplies the extrahepatic and intrahepatic bile ducts, hilar and portal tract connective tissue, and hilar lymph nodes. These structures are preferentially damaged by inadequate arterial flow or by arterial thrombosis, often resulting in *ischemic cholangitis*[85,103] or *ischemic cholangiopathy,*[104] terms that denote ischemic damage to the biliary tract. Ischemic cholangiopathy manifests as frank necrosis, poor anastomotic healing, biliary leaks, and cholangitic abscesses, resulting in biliary sludge syndrome and recurrent bacteremia.[130-132]

A second, smaller wave of technically related arterial thromboses occurs 1 to 3 years after transplantation.[131,133] Suboptimal arterial anastomoses can cause turbulent arterial flow downstream from the suture line, which eventually leads to arterial fibrointimal hyperplasia, luminal narrowing, and thrombosis. Fibrointimal hyperplasia often develops more quickly in arterial interposition grafts and predisposes to thrombosis.

Reported risk factors for early hepatic artery thrombosis include cytomegalovirus (CMV) mismatch (i.e., seropositive donor liver in a seronegative recipient), low weight of a pediatric recipient, procoagulant activity, retransplantation, use of arterial conduits, prolonged operation time, variant arterial anatomy, and low-volume transplantation centers.[130] Late hepatic artery thrombosis is not uncommon, with an estimated incidence of 4.8%. [134] Risk factors for late hepatic artery thrombosis include prior episode of thrombosis, small donor size, split/reduced-size grafts, history of TCMR, prolonged operation time, previous upper abdominal surgery, and possibly retransplantation.[134,135]

Clinical Features

Most early hepatic artery thromboses manifest clinically with one or more of the following manifestations: fever, leukocytosis, septic shock, ischemic cholangiopathy, and severe elevations of liver injury laboratory test results. [130,131] Late hepatic artery thrombosis may be asymptomatic or may present insidiously along with cholangitis, relapsing fever, sepsis (related to hepatic infarcts), abscesses, and ischemic cholangiopathy with subsequent impaired bile flow.[130,131]

Ultrasonography is mostly used as a screening tool to inspect hepatic arterial blood flow, but angiography is the most reliable method of establishing a diagnosis. Early after transplantation, urgent surgical revascularization is often attempted to salvage the graft, but even if successful, the graft can develop ischemic cholangiopathy.

Pathological Features

Hepatic artery thrombosis can be uncommonly diagnosed on peripheral core-needle biopsies because needle biopsies sample subcapsular parenchyma, which is only sometimes affected.[85,136] Structures more susceptible to ischemic injury include the perihilar tissue and large bile ducts, which are not routinely sampled by biopsy.

Peripheral core-needle biopsies can show a variety of changes; included are frank centrilobular coagulative necrosis, marked centrilobular hepatocyte swelling, acidophil bodies, "ischemic hepatitis" (similar to that seen in viral hepatitis), lobular and portal inflammation, biliary tract complications such as cholestasis, cholangiolar proliferation, acute cholangiolitis, and obstruction or stricturing.[137] The peripheral biopsy may be unremarkable because arterial collaterals render the thrombosis inconsequential or the necrosis of bile ducts and biliary sludging have not developed in the peripheral liver parenchyma. Chronic suboptimal arterial flow can cause centrilobular hepatocellular atrophy and sinusoidal widening.

Examination of failed allografts with hepatic artery thrombosis (Fig. 53.10) often reveals necrosis of the hilar or perihilar bile ducts (Fig. 53.11) with leakage of bile into the surrounding connective tissue and veins. [137] Biliary sludge, biliary abscesses seeded with fungi and bacteria, infarction of hepatic hilar lymph nodes, and patchy parenchymal infarction may also be seen.

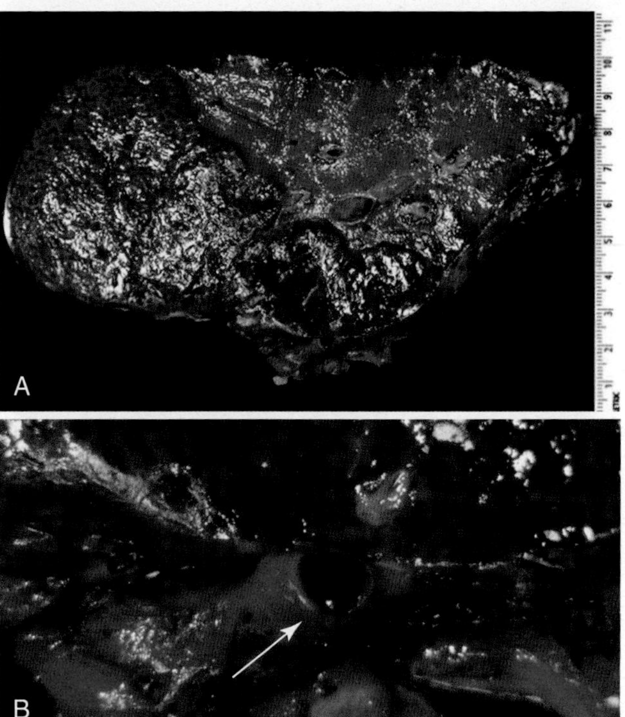

FIGURE 53.10 Failed liver allograft from a 56-year-old female patient 57 days after transplantation of the right lobe from a living related donor.**A,** The liver shows a large segmental area of parenchymal extinction and collapse. The hepatic parenchyma in other areas shows diffuse, severe cholestasis. **B,** A large perihilar hepatic artery had total luminal occlusion resulting from an organizing thrombus *(arrow).*

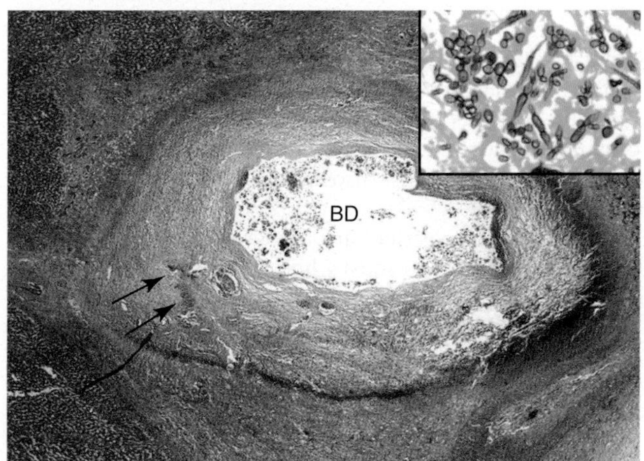

FIGURE 53.11 Typical microscopic appearance of a liver allograft that failed because of hepatic artery thrombosis. Note the necrosis of the large bile duct wall and leakage of bile into the surrounding connective tissue. *Inset,* Necrotic tissue should be stained with Gram and Grocott stains to detect microorganisms. In this case, *Candida* was identified with Grocott stain in the area indicated *(arrows)* in the larger view.

Differential Diagnosis

Because hepatic artery thrombosis or arterial narrowing can mimic almost every type of liver allograft syndrome, uncommon manifestations can easily be overlooked or misdiagnosed. Centrilobular ischemic necrosis most reliably indicates hepatic artery thrombosis (HAT), but HAT can also result in centrilobular hepatocyte swelling and biliary tract obstruction or cholangitis. Chronic suboptimal arterial flow can cause biliary epithelial cell senescence that resembles chronic rejection and centrilobular hepatocyte atrophy and sinusoidal widening. Ischemic hepatitis can appear similar to the lobular phase of acute or recurrent viral hepatitis (e.g., HCV infection, which is now rare). However, Liu and colleagues suggest that a combination of apoptosis and mitosis (i.e., low ratio of apoptosis to mitosis) without inflammation is more common in ischemic hepatitis than in recurrent hepatitis C, in which apoptosis predominates.[138] The relationship between arterial thrombosis and biliary tract complications is common; therefore examination of hepatic arterial patency should be performed when biliary tract complications are encountered.

Portal Vein Thrombosis

Pathophysiology

Portal vein complications, which affect 1% to 2% of liver allograft recipients, are less common than hepatic artery complications.[139,140] Early complications include thrombosis, strictures, and poor flow because of persistent collateral circulation or hypotension. The incidence is increased in reduced-size grafts and when cryopreserved venous interposition grafts are used.[141] Risk factors include problems with the portal venous anastomosis, small portal vein diameter, pediatric recipients, previous portal vein thrombosis, surgical shunting before transplantation, and splenectomy. Similar to native livers, long-surviving liver allografts with cirrhosis are also susceptible to portal vein thrombosis.[139]

Clinical Features

Portal vein thrombosis in a noncirrhotic allograft can cause widespread necrosis with massive elevation of liver injury tests and lactic acidosis (Fig. 53.12A). Clinical manifestations can include bleeding varices, fulminant hepatic failure, and portal hypertension with massive ascites and edema.[139] If the thrombus is partial, small infarcts can develop, or the liver can become seeded by intestinal bacteria, which may cause relapsing fever. The clinical presentation of portal vein thrombosis in a cirrhotic allograft is the same as that in a native liver with cirrhosis: variceal hemorrhage, splenomegaly, and ascites.

Pathological Features

Findings depend on the severity of portal vein flow compromise, time after transplantation, and the structural integrity of the allograft. Complete portal vein obstruction early after transplantation in a noncirrhotic allograft often causes massive coagulative necrosis. Suboptimal portal vein flow because of strictures, kinks, or persistent collateral circulation can result in periportal or midzonal linear-shaped zones of hepatocyte atrophy and/or necrosis (Fig. 53.12B),[142] focal confluent coagulative necrosis, unexplained zonal or panlobular macrovesicular steatosis, and NRH. In fact, when macrovesicular steatosis rapidly appears early (within several weeks) in a nonsteatotic donor liver after transplantation, persistent venous collaterals that have failed to close or have reopened after transplantation should be suspected as an underlying cause. Bacterial or fungal infection of a partial portal vein thrombus can result in miliary hepatic abscesses.

Differential Diagnosis

Suboptimal portal vein blood flow can be difficult to distinguish from suboptimal hepatic venous drainage. Linear-shaped zones of ischemic necrosis or hepatocellular atrophy favor the former, whereas red blood cell congestion in and around central veins and centrilobular sinusoids and obliterative central venopathy suggest suboptimal hepatic venous drainage. Ultrasonography and angiography often are needed to specify the cause of the vascular abnormality. Cases of suboptimal portal vein flow that manifest with intrahepatic steatosis must be distinguished from recurrent or de novo steatosis and steatohepatitis.

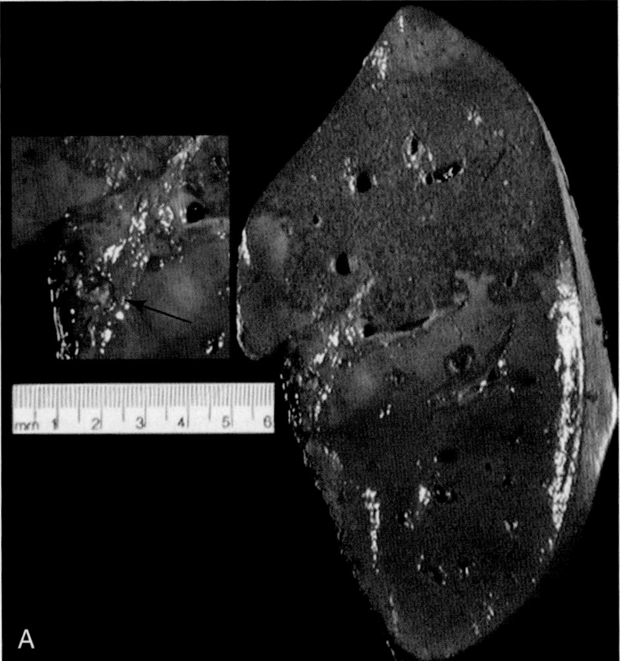

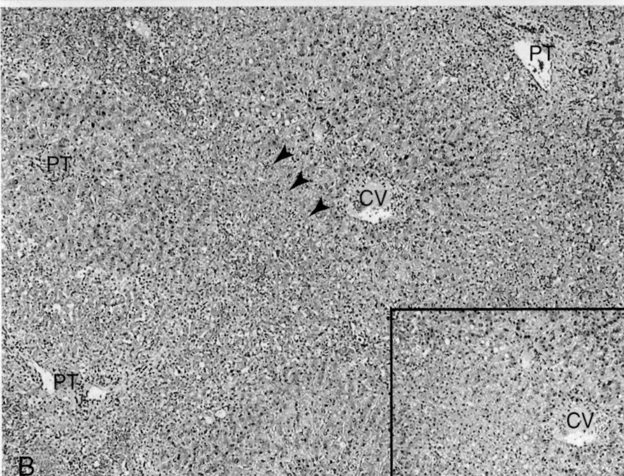

FIGURE 53.12 **A,** The recent but partially organized *(arrow)* portal vein thrombus resulted in liver allograft failure. **B,** In the peripheral parenchyma at higher magnification, note the linear midzonal area of hepatocyte atrophy, congestion, hemorrhage *(arrowheads),* and ductular reaction at the interface zone. *CV,* Central vein; *PT,* portal tract. *Inset,* The same area *(arrowheads)* is shown at higher magnification. (From Ruiz R, Tomiyama K, Campsen J, et al. Implications of a positive crossmatch in liver transplantation: a 20-year review. *Liver Transpl.* 2012;18:455-460.)

Hepatic Vein and Vena Cava Complications

Pathophysiology

Suboptimal hepatic venous outflow, including the hepatic veins and vena cava, are relatively uncommon. Risk factors include reduced-size or living donor allografts without inclusion of the middle hepatic vein,[109] difficulties with reconstruction of the venous outflow tract, and alternative anastomoses such as the piggyback approach.[76] Late hepatic vein stenosis at the anastomotic site can be seen as a result of extrinsic compression by an enlarging liver, fibrosis, and fibrointimal hyperplasia.[143] Significant stenosis or thrombosis of the outflow tract is associated with significant clinical and pathological manifestations.

Clinical Features

The clinical presentation depends on the severity of outflow tract compromise. Severe stenosis or thrombosis can lead to Budd-Chiari syndrome, with hepatic enlargement, tenderness, ascites, and edema. Less severe stenosis may cause only histopathological manifestations or an increase in the portal vein–vena cava pressure gradient. In less severe cases, it is often difficult to determine whether surgical intervention is required.

Pathological Features

Congestion and hemorrhage involving the perivenular sinusoids are the most reliable histopathological findings of suboptimal hepatic venous drainage (Fig. 53.13). Bland centrilobular hepatocyte necrosis and dropout are also usually present. Chronically suboptimal hepatic venous drainage can include perivenular fibrosis and central vein occlusion with venocentric cirrhosis, particularly if outflow obstruction is severe or of long duration. Chronic changes can also be accompanied by NRH changes, and a ductular reaction at the interface and/or centrilobular areas; this can make it difficult to recognize architectural landmarks and to exclude suboptimal biliary drainage.

Differential Diagnosis

If any of the previously described perivenular changes are not accompanied by noticeable inflammation, suboptimal hepatic venous drainage should be suspected. A major differential consideration is chronic AMR, which can also contribute to noninflammatory perivenular subsinusoidal fibrosis.[144-148] Recognition of an immune-mediated cause may be aided by the finding of interface activity, portal collagenization and portal vein and capillary uptake of C4d staining, and detection of serum DSAs of relatively high MFI (>10,000 mean fluorescence intensity [MFI])[3,144-146] (see the Chronic Rejection section). If acute or chronic centrilobular vascular changes are accompanied by significant lymphocytic, histiocytic, or lymphoplasmacytic inflammation, an immunologically mediated cause of injury such as acute or chronic TCMR, plasma cell–rich rejection or AIH, or an adverse drug reaction should be suspected.

Perivenular inflammation can be transient in some cases of immune-mediated centrilobular injury and later manifest as bland perivenular fibrosis, when it might be indistinguishable from mechanical venous outflow obstruction.[149] Finally, pathologists should not cavalierly recommend invasive radiographic studies of vena caval patency in their reports.

Biliary Tract Issues

Pathophysiology

Despite improvements in surgical techniques, the biliary tree continues to be the "Achilles heel" of liver transplantation. Biliary complication rates have been declining in recent years but continue to represent a major source of postoperative mortality and morbidity. Complications vary by center and occur in approximately 20% of recipients in whole-organ cadaveric donors, and an even higher incidence is observed for living and reduced-size allografts, but center-specific effects are seen.[78,150,151] Biliary tract reconstruction

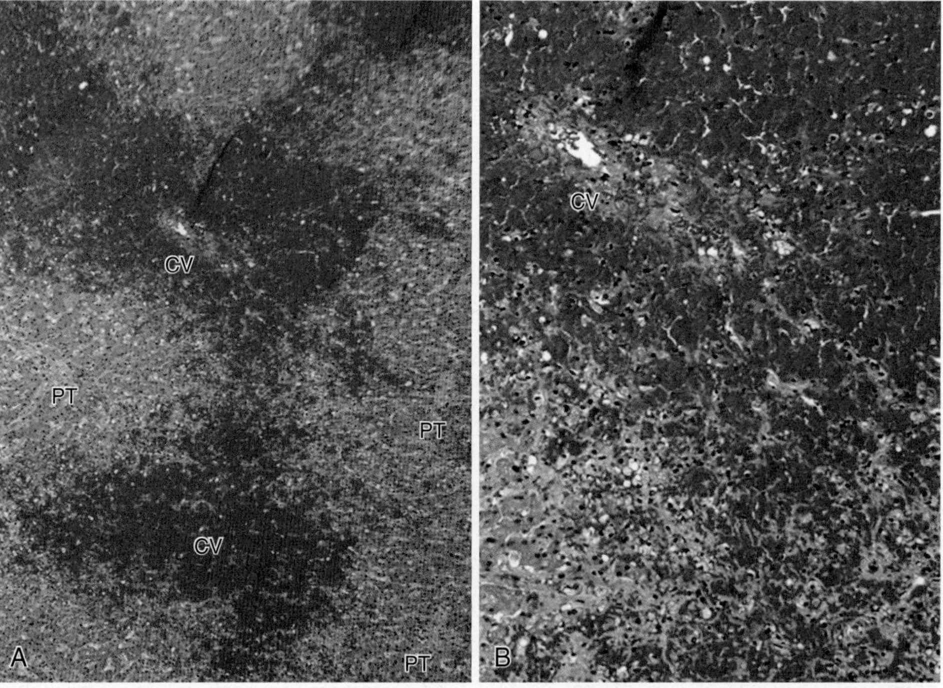

FIGURE 53.13 Suboptimal hepatic venous outflow caused by hepatic vein or vena caval stricturing or thrombosis frequently shows bland centrilobular sinusoidal dilation, hepatocyte atrophy, congestion, and hemorrhage. Note the absence of significant perivenular inflammation, which helps distinguish suboptimal venous outflow from centrilobular-based rejection. The area indicated by *CV* in the low-power image **(A)** is illustrated at higher magnification in **B.** *CV,* Central vein; *PT,* portal tract.

approaches vary considerably among surgeons and depend on primary liver disease, graft type, and previous transplants/biliary surgery.

The most common biliary anastomosis used for cadaveric whole organs are end-to-end, duct-to-duct, and donor biliary–recipient enteric anastomoses. Duct-to-duct anastomoses are fairly common because of ease of surgical anastomosis and presentation of the sphincter of Oddi, and it allows for postoperative diagnostic and therapeutic instrumentation (e.g., endoscopic retrograde cholangiopancreatography [ERCP], stent placement). A more time-consuming choledochojejunostomy anastomosis (donor biliary–to–recipient enteric anastomosis) is usually performed on recipients with a history of PSC or other biliary tract abnormalities. Most biliary tract complications are attributable to ischemic or traumatic injury, immunological injury, surgically introduced abnormal anatomy, or a combination of these factors. All predispose to poor biliary tract wound healing, suboptimal drainage, and/or reflux, occurring singly or often in combination.[150,152]

The extrahepatic donor bile duct immediately adjacent to the anastomosis is particularly vulnerable to ischemic injury. To ascertain adequate arterial flow and duct viability after completion of the hepatic arterial anastomosis, the terminal end of the donor extrahepatic bile duct is progressively trimmed back toward the liver until bleeding occurs from the cut surface to assure adequate arterial flow.

The peribiliary arterial plexus is particularly vulnerable to preservation/reperfusion injury during operative manipulation.[153] In DCD donors, blood component sludging or use of the more viscous University of Wisconsin solution[154,155] can promote clogging of the peribiliary capillary plexus and prevent adequate reperfusion after transplantation.[150] Machine perfusion (still in its infancy) might offer improved outcomes, particularly when DCD and ECD organs are utilized for transplantation.[156,157]

Other causes of biliary tract ischemia resulting from arterial or peribiliary plexus injury include small-for-size syndrome and severe arterial vasospasm,[97] prolonged cold ischemia, hepatic artery thrombosis/stenosis, older donors with atherosclerotic disease, and preformed or de novo donor anti-antibodies (e.g., ABO isoagglutinin, anti–human leukocyte antigen [HLA] antibodies).[150,158,159] Once the myriad of other causes of biliary tract complications have been excluded, recurrent primary disorders such as recurrent PSC or primary biliary cholangitis (PBC) should be considered, but recurrent disease usually occurs more than 6 months after transplantation.

Biliary tract complications, the majority of which start within 3 months after transplantation, include anastomotic dehiscence, transmural necrosis, bile leakage, cholangitic abscesses, ascending cholangitis, bile casts (Fig. 53.14), strictures, ampullary dysfunction, and biliary-vascular fistulas.[150,160-164] These complications occur in approximately 15% of whole cadaveric allografts and as many as 30% of reduced-size or living donor allografts, but the incidence is decreasing as surgical approaches impr ove.[78,150,165,166]

Bile leaks mostly occur at anastomotic sites. The former are more common and are likely caused by technical issues or ischemia at the anastomosis. Nonanastomotic leaks may occur at the site of cystic duct, T-tube, or as a complication of acute hepatic artery thrombosis.[151,164-168] Another source of bile leaks is from small transected bile ducts at the hepatic resection surface in recipients of living or reduced-size grafts.[169]

Strictures are the most common biliary complication.[151,170] They are categorized according to location and the time after transplantation as *intrahepatic* or *extrahepatic*, *nonanastomotic* or *anastomotic*, and *early* or *late* (>30 days postoperative).[160-165] Intrahepatic strictures are further categorized as *perihilar* or *peripheral*. Peripheral intrahepatic strictures are less common and tend to occur later after transplantation.[151]

Anastomotic strictures usually appear within the first several months after transplantation, but they appear at a reduced rate for many years.[160,165] Risk factors for anastomotic strictures include postoperative bile leaks, female donor–male recipient combinations, and a more recent year of transplantation.[150,160,165] Compared with nonanastomotic strictures, anastomotic strictures are more amenable to correction either by surgical or radiological intervention; anastomotic strictures also have less of a negative impact on long-term graft and patient survival.[150,160,165]

Nonanastomotic strictures usually (1) occur later after transplantation (>1 year), (2) are less amenable to treatment, (3) are generally progressive, and (4) negatively affect graft and patient survival.[160-165] These usually occur in the more peripheral biliary tree and are associated with vascular/microvascular and immunological risk factors, alone or in combination. The major vascular risk factor is hepatic artery thrombosis/stenosis.[167] Immunological damage at the microvascular level induces ischemia by disruption of the microvascular circulation at the peribiliary capillary plexus level by circulating donor-specific antibodies (DSA) and isoagglutinin and direct cytotoxic lymphocytic damage.[159,171-173] Immunological risk factors also include PSC and AIH as the original disease.[164] Other risk factors for nonanastomotic strictures include use of high-viscosity preservation solution, Roux-en-Y biliary anastomoses, and CMV infection.[150,161-163]

Nonanastomotic strictures occurring earlier (<1 year) are often associated with preservation-related injury[163,174] and are usually located in perihilar bile ducts. Similar to the nonanastomotic strictures that occur later, risk factors for early stricture include long cold and warm ischemic times, high-viscosity preservation solution, older recipient age, a duct-to-duct biliary anastomosis, and bile leaks.[163]

Clinical Features

Liver injury tests that show relatively selective elevation of γ-glutamyl transferase (GGT)/alkaline phosphatase (ALP) versus ALT/AST levels is the usual method of detecting early or minor biliary tract complications such as strictures and stones. Clinical signs and symptoms are uncommon unless the patient develops jaundice or acute cholangitis. Biliary tract problems are also often first suspected on routine or protocol biopsy evaluation, especially with the use of routine CK7 staining (see later). However, cholangiography (e.g., magnetic resonance cholangiopancreatography [MRCP], duct-to-duct ERCP, percutaneous transhepatic cholangiography [PTC]) is often used to confirm the diagnosis and localize the defects.[160,165,175]

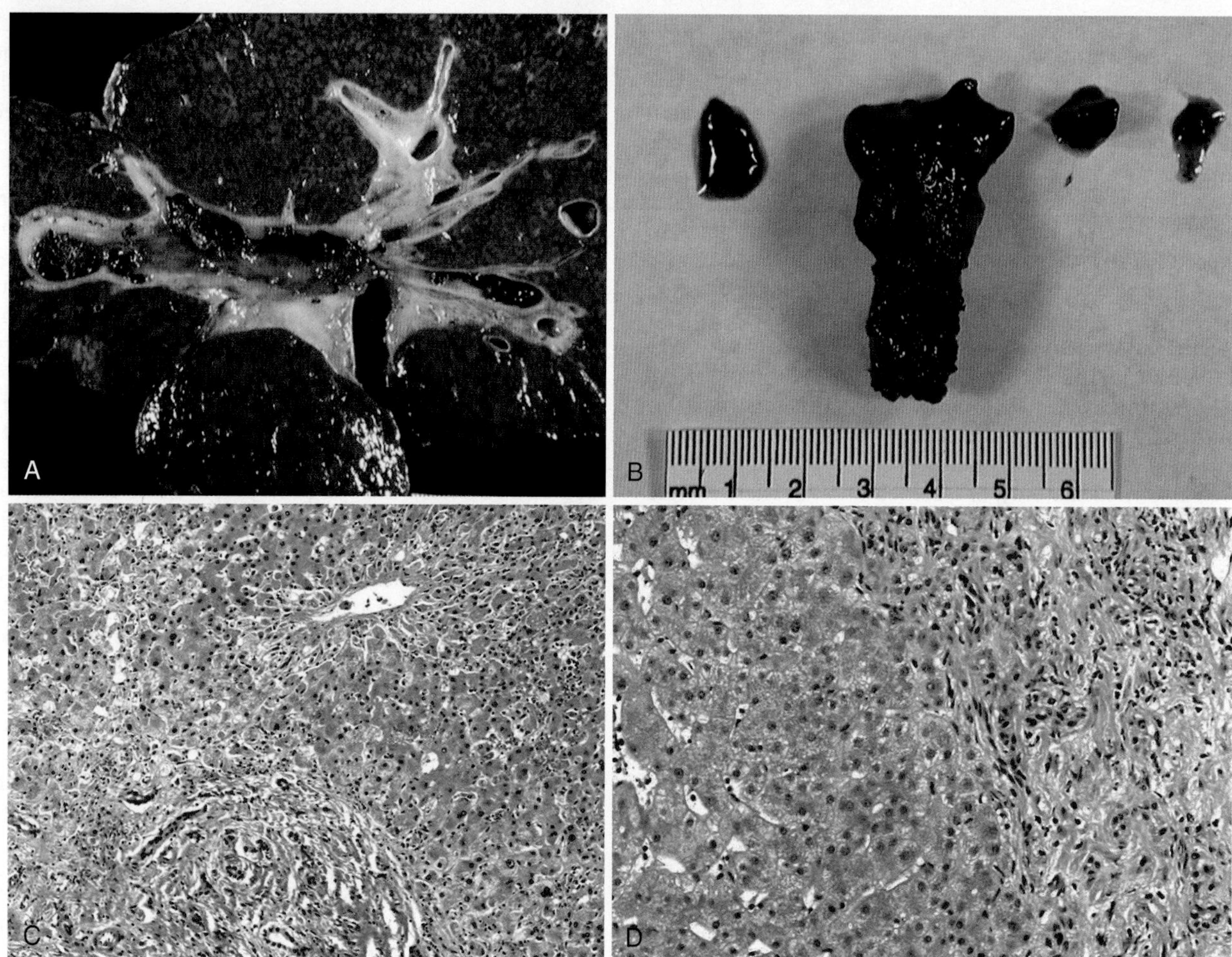

FIGURE 53.14 Bile duct complications after liver transplantation. A, This failed liver allograft had large bile casts and fibrous obliteration of the hilar hepatic artery caused by organized thrombus. Note the multiple bile casts and sludge in the right and left hepatic ducts. **B,** A large bile cast was occluding the common hepatic duct. Hepatic arterial ischemia is often responsible for bile duct damage and sloughing, leading to biliary cast syndrome. **C,** Liver biopsy shows ischemic cholangiopathy, which occurred several weeks after liver transplantation and ischemic compromise of the intrahepatic biliary tree. The medium-power view of an expanded portal tract shows bile ductular proliferation, a hepatic lobule with clusters of ceroid-laden macrophages, and apoptotic hepatocytes. **D,** The high-power view of the portal tract–hepatic lobule interface shows a ductular reaction typical of biliary strictures or sludge, which is often accompanied by neutrophilic portal or periportal inflammation and periductal edema.

More serious biliary tract complications, such as obstruction, cholangitic abscesses, and ascending cholangitis, usually manifest with fever, jaundice, right upper quadrant pain, and intermittent bacteremia. During the first several months after transplantation, T-tube stents provide access for cholangiograms, which are routinely performed before clamping at 1 week postoperatively and again at the time of T-tube removal.[160]

Histopathological Features

Allograft biliary tract complications are histopathologically identical to those seen in native livers. Portal, periportal, periductal, and pericholangiolar edema; predominantly neutrophilic portal inflammation; intraepithelial and intraluminal neutrophils in true bile ducts; stellate-shaped lumens in small septal ducts, an interface ductular reaction; centrilobular hepatocanalicular cholestasis; and small clusters of neutrophils and foam cells throughout the lobules are typical findings of stricturing or obstructive cholangiopathy (see Fig. 53.14). With time, chronic biliary tract strictures are often associated with mixed or predominantly chronic portal inflammation, biliary epithelial cell senescence changes, and low-grade ductopenia involving small bile ducts. More than 1 year after transplantation, in addition to the classic features described previously, biliary strictures are a relatively common cause of portal eosinophilia.

Ancillary stains are extremely helpful and a very sensitive method of pointing toward suboptimal biliary drainage. We routinely perform CK7 staining on all allograft biopsies because of our frequent use of living donor allografts at our centers; if positive, we follow up with a copper stain. CK7 immunostaining is used to detect ductular metaplasia of periportal hepatocytes when there is suboptimal biliary drainage, either at the lobular level or at larger branches of the biliary tree (supralobular). Rhodamine copper stain highlights periportal hepatocellular copper deposition that mostly occurs after chronically (more than several months) suboptimal biliary drainage. We usually perform CK7 and copper stains in tandem with the following interpretation: (1) CK7+/copper–: recent biliary tract stricture and/or intrahepatic ductopenia (usually chronic rejection); (2) CK7+/copper+: supralobular biliary stricture/suboptimal biliary drainage; and (3) CK7–/copper+: recently decompressed biliary stricture.

Biliary-vascular fistulas are recognized by red blood cells in the lumen of bile ducts or by bile concretions in blood vessels. Occasionally, an inordinate elevation of the serum bilirubin level is associated with a fistula. In contrast, periductal hemorrhage surrounding small interlobular bile ducts is an inconsequential finding in asymptomatic patients when a biopsy is obtained within 1 or 2 days after transhepatic cholangiography.[176]

Differential Diagnosis

The differential diagnosis is influenced by the time after transplantation, the patient's original disease, previous operative and complication history, rejection history, and DSA analyses. Within the first several weeks after transplantation, suboptimal biliary drainage with or without cholangitis can be difficult to distinguish from preservation/reperfusion injury, TCMR, and acute AMR, particularly if the patient was treated with increased immunosuppression before the biopsy was obtained.

Features that favor suboptimal biliary drainage over TCMR include neutrophilic-predominant portal inflammation, periductal edema, retention of the normal nucleus-to-cytoplasm ratio in biliary epithelial cells, and an absence of perivenular mononuclear inflammation and endothelialitis. TCMR is favored when the mixed portal inflammation is composed of blastic and small lymphocytes, plasma cells, and eosinophils. Lymphocytic cholangitis, an increased nucleus-to-cytoplasm ratio in biliary epithelial cells, and perivenular inflammation also are usually seen. Portal eosinophilia in early TCMR and AMR can be quite striking, especially in patients treated with steroid-sparing immunosuppressive regimens.[177] In acute AMR, portal capillary dilation, capillaritis, and importantly, strong and diffuse portal capillary C4d staining can be used to distinguish acute AMR from suboptimal biliary drainage/cholangitis (see Antibody-Mediated Rejection section). Late-onset chronic biliary tract complications occasionally manifest with predominantly mononuclear portal inflammation, biliary epithelial cell senescence changes, and low-grade ductopenia.[178] Late-onset chronic biliary strictures can also cause portal eosinophilia and mimic acute TCMR and chronic rejection, viral hepatitis, and recurrent autoimmune disorders.

It can be difficult to differentiate chronic rejection from biliary strictures/suboptimal drainage from other causes, especially recurrent PSC, in peripheral core-needle biopsies.[179] The at-risk populations are similar. Both conditions can cause intrahepatic cholestasis, biliary epithelial cell senescence changes, and small bile duct loss. Careful examination of the clinical history, evaluation of serial biopsies, and analysis of the histopathology are needed to distinguish between biliary strictures and chronic rejection.[179]

In our experience, features that favor biliary strictures and/or recurrent PSC over chronic rejection include a history of biliary tract complications, PSC as the original disease, periductal lamellar edema involving true bile ducts, stellate portal expansion, portal neutrophilia, a ductular reaction affecting at least some portal tracts, and deposition of copper or copper-associated protein in periportal hepatocytes. Features that favor mixed TCMR with chronic rejection over suboptimal biliary drainage include: a previous history of rejection; inadequate immunosuppression; lymphoplasmacytic portal inflammation; small portal tracts; absence of a ductular reaction; ductular metaplasia of periportal hepatocytes on CK7 staining, but negative copper staining; and active central perivenulitis with or without perivenular fibrosis.

Findings in failed allografts that can be used to favor biliary strictures or recurrent PSC over chronic rejection include significant enlargement/increased weight; bile-pigmented sinus histiocytosis in hilar lymph nodes, if present; mild focal eccentric fibrointimal hyperplasia in perihilar hepatic artery branches versus foam cell arteriopathy; and significant concentric fibrointimal hyperplasia.[179] In addition, suboptimally draining extrahepatic or large intrahepatic bile ducts in recurrent PSC/biliary strictures often show focal ulceration, periductal lymphoplasmacytic inflammation, and fibrosis. In chronic rejection, large-duct inflammation and ulceration are unusual. When the infiltrate shows plasma cell–rich infiltrates, the possibility of recurrent or de novo immunoglobulin G4 (IgG4)-associated sclerosing disease should be considered.[180]

Angiography and cholangiography (e.g., ERCP) are also useful in making the distinction between obstructive cholangiopathy and chronic rejection. Pruning of peripheral arterial and biliary trees and poor peripheral filling are seen in chronic rejection. Suboptimal biliary drainage, however, usually shows some intrahepatic duct dilation on cholangiography, but arterial changes are not seen or are insignificant.

Clinicopathological correlation can also help distinguish late-onset biliary tract complications from late-onset acute rejection. Adequate immunosuppressive drug levels with preferential elevation of GGT and alkaline phosphatase levels[181] favor suboptimal biliary drainage because late-onset acute rejection is unusual in this circumstance. Finally, in our experience, it is not possible to reliably distinguish recurrent PSC from other causes of biliary tract obstruction or stricturing on the basis of peripheral core needle biopsy evaluation alone.

Allograft Rejection

Liver allograft rejection has been traditionally categorized as follows: *hyperacute* (occurring immediately after revascularization), *acute* (onset of graft dysfunction over a period of days), and *chronic* (evolves over weeks to months). Rejection is also broadly categorized on the predominant pathophysiological mechanism of injury: *AMR, TCMR, mixed AMR and TCMR,* and *chronic rejection,* which also often shows a mixed pattern of antibody and T cell–mediated injury. AMR can be further subcategorized into *hyperacute, acute (aAMR),* and *chronic active AMR (cAMR).* TCMR can occur early or late in the allograft age, and corresponding histological features are also different. These different types of rejection occur as a continuum and often show overlapping features.

This section will reflect recent advances in pathophysiology and diagnostic criteria of acute and chronic AMR as well as changes in rejection terminology (Table 53.3). Discouraged terminology includes *humoral rejection, acute cellular rejection, de novo AIH,* and *plasma cell hepatitis* in favor of *AMR, TCMR,* and *plasma cell rich–rejection.*[3] It is also clear now that many cases that were previously labeled as

TABLE 53.3 Old versus New Banff Recommended Terminology

Older Discouraged Terminology	Newer Encouraged Terminology
Acute cellular rejection	T cell–mediated rejection
Humoral rejection	Antibody-mediated rejection
De novo autoimmune or plasma cell-rich hepatitis	Plasma cell–rich rejection
Idiopathic posttransplant hepatitis	More specific terminology when possible • Late-onset TCMR • Chronic active AMR • Chronic hepatitis of known cause (e.g., hepatitis E)

AMR, *Antibody-mediated rejection;* TCMR, *T cell–mediated rejection.*
Modified from Demetris AJ, Bellamy C, Hübscher SG, et al. 2016 Comprehensive Update of the Banff Working Group on Liver Allograft Pathology: Introduction of antibody-mediated rejection. Am J Transplant. *2016;16(10):2816–2835.*

idiopathic posttransplantation hepatitis can now be categorized as *late-onset TCMR* and/or *chronic AMR.*[147,148,182,183]

Antibody-Mediated Rejection

Crossing ABO blood group barriers predictably causes severe liver allograft injury, unless plasmapheresis is used to lower isoagglutinin titers to below 1:16.[80] Without these efforts, crossing ABO barriers leads to an approximately 60% incidence of significant AMR and graft failure.[158] It should be noted that ABO-incompatible liver allografts are routinely used in Asian programs in which the donor pool is limited.

Advances in antibody and complement depletion and desensitization protocols utilizing rituximab, intravenous immunoglobulins, plasmapheresis techniques, local graft infusion, splenectomy, and vigorous antirejection and microcirculatory protective therapy have shown acceptable results, in some cases comparable to ABO-compatible transplants.[184-189] Short- and long-term outcomes in pediatric cases (particularly children younger than 2 years of age) undergoing ABO-incompatible liver transplantation are identical to those with ABO-compatible allografts.[190,191] Despite improvement, ABO-incompatible recipients are still at risk for biliary tract complications.[192]

Liver allografts are much less susceptible than other solid organ allografts to damage from anti-HLA AMR as a result of many heterogenous tolerance mechanisms.[3,158,193-196] However, depending on the circumstances, the liver is not completely spared from injury by these and other non-HLA antibodies.[197] Although DSAs do not routinely influence organ triage or recipient selection at most centers,[157,159,198] there are short- and long-term implications to preformed and de-novo DSAs.[199-201] They are associated with decreased 5-year patient and graft survival, increased incidence of TCMR and AMR, graft fibrosis and chronic rejection, and late-onset T cell–mediated rejection and plasma cell–rich rejection (probably mixed T cell–mediated and antibody-mediated rejection).[146,202-207]

Two distinct patterns of AMR are increasingly being recognized in liver allografts: (1) acute AMR, and (2) chronic AMR.[3,146-148,182,194,208] Hyperacute rejection is now exceedingly rare as ABO barriers are not crossed without desensitization protocols and complement depletion.[189,209] Acute AMR can present early with pronounced manifestations or late with more subtle morphological and clinical presentation (Fig. 53.15). Early acute AMR is increasingly being recognized as a cause of allograft dysfunction in about 5% of allografts.[83] It generally occurs in highly sensitized recipients within the first several weeks after transplantation and is characterized by DSA that persists after transplantation, refractory thrombocytopenia, hypocomplementemia, and allograft dysfunction.[198,210] Initial evidence of acute AMR in humans was shown in ABO-incompatible transplants and in recipients with preformed lymphocytotoxic antibodies.[80,198] Infrequently, late-onset acute AMR with more attenuated features can occur months to years after transplantation in patients who do not adhere to prescribed immunosuppression therapy and is associated with de-novo as well as preformed DSA.[202,204,207] Criteria and categories for diagnosis of acute AMR have been defined by the Banff Working Group based on a combination of clinical, histopathological, and serological findings(Box 53.1).[3]

Improvements in immunosuppression, surgical techniques, and control of original disease recurrence have resulted in frequent long-term (beyond 10 years) survival and increasing concern regarding allograft structural integrity and function, particularly in pediatric transplant recipients.[183] Greater understanding of chronic AMR emerged from long-term follow-up of pediatric liver transplant recipients, immunosuppression weaning trials, study of DSA and chronic rejection, and outcomes of suboptimal immune suppression,[3,146,183,205,211-217] with incidence of class II DSA in long-term allograft survivors ranging from 38% to over 50% in recent studies.[183,218] Multiple studies have linked progressive allograft fibrosis to anti–class II DSA, angiotensin II type 1 receptor (AT1R), and portal inflammation, providing further evidence of chronic long-term consequences of immunological injury.[146,182,214,217-220]

The exact incidence of cAMR is not entirely clear yet, but it is believed to be around 8% at 10-year post transplantation.[218] Risk factors for development of de novo DSA include retransplantation,[207] young age,[207,221] cyclosporine as opposed to tacrolimus, low calcineurin inhibitor levels, and Model for End-Stage Liver Disease (MELD) scores.[202,222] The effect of immunosuppression on de novo DSA is reviewed here.[222] A recent study describing the histopathology of 460 liver allografts identified chronic fibrosing hepatitis as the leading cause of retransplantation >10 years posttransplantation in pediatric recipients and the second leading cause (after original disease recurrence) in adults.[129] cAMR is thought to occur in a small percentage of recipients with persistent de novo DSA, especially those directed at DQ.[202,204] The 2016 Banff Working Group proposed criteria for the diagnosis of probable cAMR (Box 53.2).[3,147,148,218] (In the presence of only minimal or absent C4d staining, cases are classified as *possible cAMR*).

Given our expanding knowledge of AMR and its short- and long-term implications on liver allografts, more granular diagnostic criteria and diagnostic categories similar to those available for renal allograft pathology are likely forthcoming.

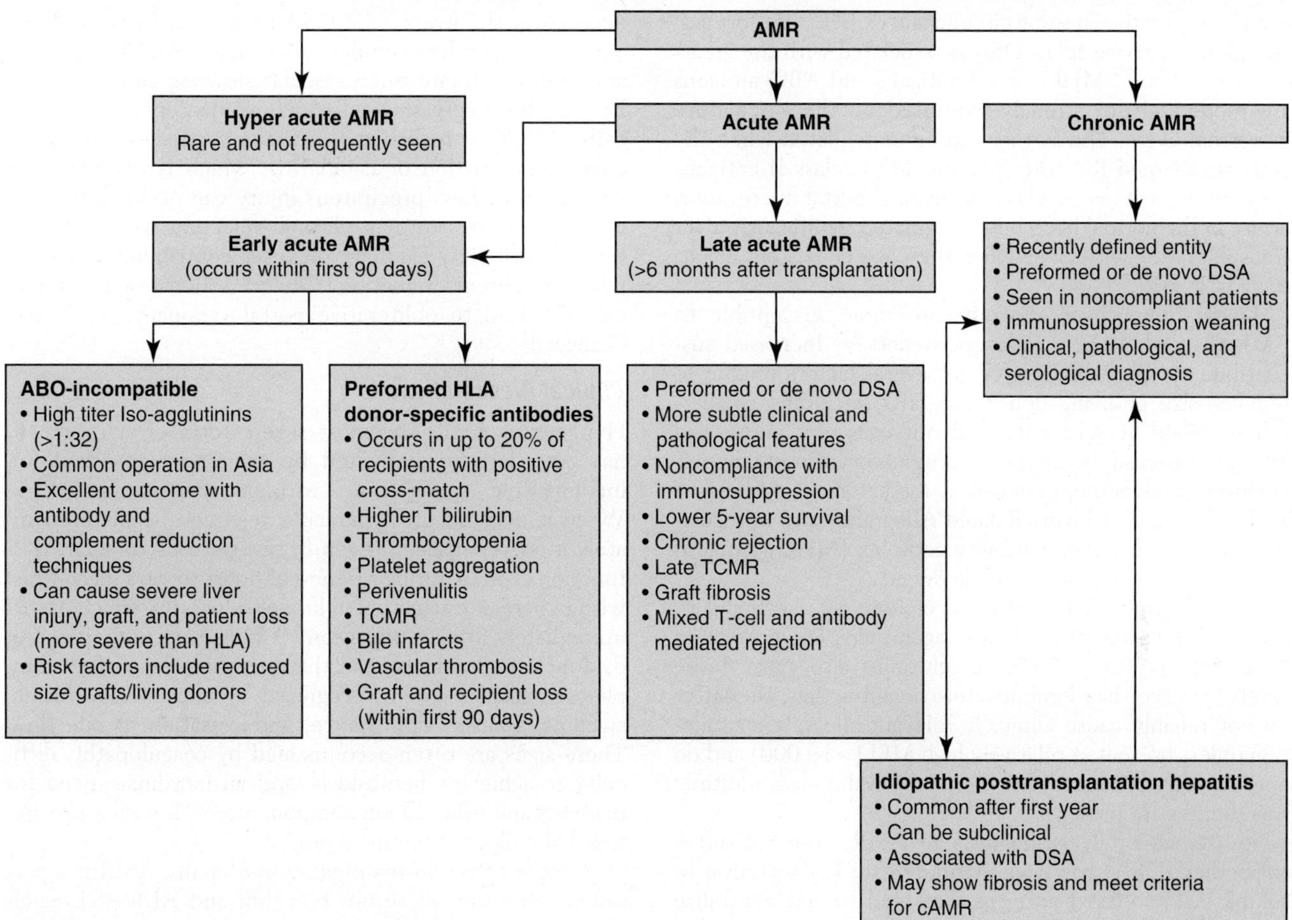

FIGURE 53.15 Chart depicting current understanding of AMR. Depending on time of onset, risk factors, and clinical and pathological manifestations, AMR can be subcategorized into *hyperacute* (rarely seen), *early aAMR* (usually seen in ABO incompatible allografts and severely sensitized recipients), *late-onset aAMR* (generally seen more than 6 months after transplantation and associated with immunosuppression noncompliance, milder clinical and pathological manifestations, and overall lower 5-year graft survival), and *chronic active AMR* (likely the leading cause of pediatric re-transplantation).

BOX 53.1 Diagnosis of Acute AMR

1. Definitive for acute/active AMR (all four criteria required):
   a. Histopathological pattern of injury consistent with acute AMR, usually including portal microvascular endothelial cell hypertrophy, portal capillary and inlet venule dilation, monocytic eosinophilic and neutrophilic portal microvasculitis, portal edema ductular reaction, and cholestasis (see Pathological Features for h-scoring and other associated pathological features).
   b. Positive serum DSA (MFI usually >5000)
   c. Diffuse microvascular endothelial C4d deposition (C4d score = 3) on formalin-fixed or frozen tissue in ABO-compatible allografts and/or portal stromal C4d in ABO-incompatible allografts (see Pathological Features for C4d scoring)
   d. Reasonable exclusion of other insults that may cause a similar pattern of injury (see Differential Diagnosis)
2. Suspicious for AMR (both criteria required)
   a. DSA is positive
   b. Nonzero h-score with (C4d-score + h-score = 3 or 4)
3. Indeterminate for AMR (requires a + b and c or d)
   a. C4d-score + h-score = >2
   b. DSA not available, equivocal, or negative
   c. C4d staining not available, equivocal, or negative
   d. Coexisting insult may be contributing to the injury

BOX 53.2 Diagnosis of Probable cAMR

1. Histopathological pattern of injury consistent with chronic AMR (both a and b required):
   a. Otherwise unexplained pattern of injury and at least mild mononuclear portal and/or perivenular inflammation with interface and/or perivenular necro-inflammatory activity
   b. At least moderate portal/periportal, sinusoidal, and/or perivenular fibrosis
2. Recent circulating HLA DSA in serum samples (MFI usually >5000)
3. At least focal C4d positivity (involving >10% of portal tract microvascular endothelia)
4. Reasonable exclusion of other insults that may cause a similar pattern of injury

Pathophysiology

The consequences of preexisting and/or de novo antidonor antibodies depend on the class, subclass, specificity, titer, C1q binding characteristics, and timing of the antibody response, and, importantly, on the density and distribution of target antigens in the liver tissue.[211,223,224] Antibodies can cause various degrees of damage and can even be protective in some circumstances.[225-227] Preformed, complement-fixing IgG3 DSA is associated with the greatest risk.[223,228,229] MHC class I antigens and ABO antigens are moderately to strongly expressed on the vasculature in normal livers. The former can be upregulated when the graft is inflamed for other reasons. MHC class II antigens are expressed at low levels in the hepatic portal microvasculature in the normal liver, but upregulated significantly after transplantation, especially when there is a coexistent insult, such as TCMR.[230-232]

Living donor liver allografts are more susceptible to AMR than whole-liver cadaveric donors.[233] Increased susceptibility is probably related to several factors unique to reduced-size or living donor allografts, including smaller-caliber blood vessels; enhanced microvascular injury and arterial vasospasm because of a combination of portal hyperperfusion and pathophysiological mediators of AMR (see Reduced-Size and Living Related Allografts) and upregulation of major histocompatibility complex (MHC) antigens on the microvasculature and bile ducts.

ABO incompatibility places recipients at risk for early acute AMR, especially when isoagglutinins are present in high titers (>1:32).[198,209] Isoagglutinins also cause more severe damage than lymphocytotoxic antibodies; the latter do not reliably cause clinically relevant allograft dysfunction unless present at relatively high MFI (>10,000) and do not routinely influence short-term survival, unless multiple specificities are present.[83,88,234,235]

Resistance of liver allografts to AMR from anti-HLA antibodies (DSA) has been attributed to: (1) secretion of soluble MHC class I antigens that bind to and neutralize anti–class I HLA[236]; (2) phagocytic properties of Kupffer and liver sinusoidal endothelial cells (LSECs), which express abundant Fcγ receptors that enable them to clear different immune complexes, complement-fixing donor-specific HLA antibodies, and platelet aggregates; (3) a dual afferent hepatic blood supply and a large microvascular surface area effectively diluting antigen-antibody complexes; (4) unique regenerative ability of the liver; and (5) low level of MHC II expression.[3,158,193-196]

Preformed DSA are encountered in about 8% to 12% of mostly female recipients.[83,88,234,235] Only 5% to 20% of recipients with a positive crossmatch have strong enough sensitization to cause clinically significant liver injury.[83,198]

The patient population at risk for severe AMR because of anti-HLA antibodies is small; therefore acute AMR is rare (occurring in approximately 5% among patients harboring anti-HLA antibodies[237]) and often overlooked as a cause of early liver dysfunction or failure. Many programs do not routinely conduct pretransplantation crossmatching or DSA determinations. Even if crossmatches or DSA assays are performed, further studies (e.g., dilution runs, C1q binding) and posttransplantation monitoring for DSA persistence are not routinely carried out.

Antibodies cause damage by binding to allograft endothelium and fixing complement. In severe cases, antibody-complement binding triggers the complement cascade with direct endothelial damage, deposition of platelet-fibrin thrombi, and initiation of the clotting and fibrinolytic cascades. In rapidly evolving cases, this leads to microvascular thrombosis, arterial vasospasm, and coagulopathy that act in concert to impair blood flow and cause hemorrhagic necrosis of the liver.[225,226] DSA binding can also facilitate antibody-dependent cellular cytotoxicity (ADCC) in which antibodies facilitate microvascular sludging and binding of Fc-receptor–expressing cells such as macrophages and NK cells. ADCC is recognized in tissue sections as microvascular inflammation or capillaritis, which is distinct from endotheliitis. Less precipitous injury can occur during the transition from acute to chronic rejection when destruction of peribiliary capillary plexuses contributes to ductopenic or chronic rejection.[228,238-240] Microvascular injury can also lead to obliterative portal venopathy and NRH changes.[159,241]

Clinical Presentation

Hyperacute AMR, the most severe form of acute AMR, has been largely eliminated by avoiding high-risk ABO-incompatible transplants without pretreatment.[189,209] When it does occur, hyperacute rejection begins immediately after reperfusion. Even in severe cases, allograft dysfunction evolves during a period of hours to days, in contrast with hyperacute rejection in kidney allografts, which occurs immediately after reperfusion.[158] However, initial signs of dysfunction can develop in the operating room after complete revascularization, recognized by uneven reperfusion, swelling, a dusky appearance, and cessation of bile flow. These signs are often accompanied by coagulopathy, difficulty in achieving hemostasis, and an inordinate need for platelets and other blood components.[80] However, precipitous liver allograft failure is rare.

A more common manifestation of acute AMR is a persistent elevation of serum bilirubin and ALT/AST levels (depending on whether the antibodies are isoagglutinin or anti-HLA) during the first several days to weeks after transplantation. This is often accompanied by persistence of circulating DSA, the presence of multiple DSA specificities, unexplained and often refractory thrombocytopenia, and low serum complement activity levels.[81,198,237,242] In severe cases, hepatic angiograms, obtained to exclude an arterial thrombosis, usually show segmental narrowing (indicative of immunologically mediated arterial vasospasm) and diffuse luminal narrowing with poor peripheral blood flow leading to bile duct loss and chronic rejection.[158,243]

Pathological Features

Histopathological manifestations of AMR depend on the timing of the biopsy; the subclass, titer or DSA MFI, and specificity of the anti-donor antibodies (HLA, ABO); and whether TCMR coexists.[158] Isoagglutinins usually cause more red blood cell congestion and necrosis than anti-HLA or lymphocytotoxic antibodies (Fig. 53.16).

Hyperacute Rejection and Early Acute Antibody-Mediated Rejection (ABO-Incompatible Transplants, ABO-Compatible with Preformed Antibodies)

Hyperacute rejection is rare and largely limited to the era of ABO-incompatible transplants without pretreatment[189,209]; therefore the next few paragraphs are largely of historical importance. However, hyperacute rejection can reappear in the current era if isoagglutinin titers rebound after transplantation. Despite its rarity, early morphological evidence of AMR and its complications comes from studies of liver

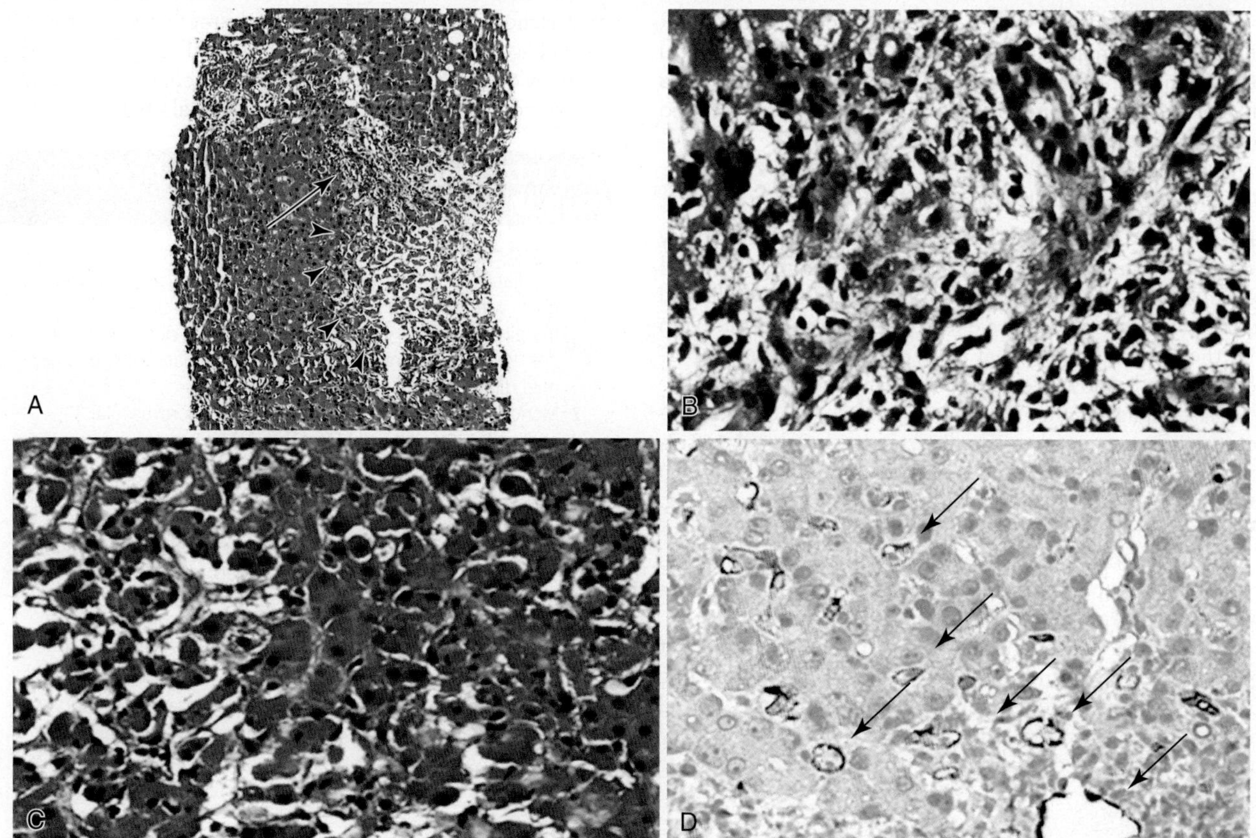

FIGURE 53.16 Composite images for a patient with antibody-mediated rejection were obtained 5 days after transplantation of an ABO-incompatible organ. A, Portal tract with neutrophilic cholangiolitis and a small periportal infarct *(arrowheads)*. **B,** The portal or periportal region indicated by the *arrow* in **A** is shown at higher magnification. **C,** Focal sinusoidal congestion adjacent to a small infarct. **D,** C4d immunostaining highlights the endothelium of portal veins, capillaries, and sinusoidal cells *(arrows)*.

transplantation across ABO barriers.[80,208,244] High-titer isoagglutinin (>1:64) often causes prominent red blood cell and focal neutrophil sludging in the sinusoids and platelet-fibrin thrombi in periportal sinusoids, portal veins, and central veins.[80,245,246] Acidophilic hepatocyte necrosis develops within 2 to 6 hours after reperfusion in untreated recipients. This is often quickly followed by portal or periportal edema, necrosis, focal hemorrhage, C4d deposits in portal stroma,[245] and diffuse endothelial C4d deposits in portal veins, capillaries, and sinusoids.[83,245]

In severe untreated cases, confluent coagulative necrosis, prominent sinusoidal and venous congestion, and edema and hemorrhage into the portal tracts appear within 1 to 5 days.[80,83,245] Portal veins often show fibrin deposition. If sampled, medium-sized arteries show endothelial cell hypertrophy and evidence of arterial vasospasm, such as mural myocyte vacuolization, wrinkling of the elastic lamina, and thickening of the wall with narrowing of the lumen. Neutrophilic or necrotizing arteritis is only occasionally observed. Portal neutrophilia, cholangiolar proliferation, and small areas of confluent hepatic necrosis begin to appear at 2 to 3 days after transplantation. If untreated, progressive hemorrhagic infarction occurs in ABO-incompatible organs during the next 1 to 2 weeks.

ABO-incompatible allografts that fail because of untreated AMR are often grossly enlarged, cyanotic, and mottled, and they show areas of geographic necrosis. Capsular ruptures, hepatic artery, or portal vein thrombosis can develop in extreme cases. Microscopically, changes in the hilum or perihilar region can be particularly helpful in recognizing that acute AMR caused or contributed to allograft failure. Included are congestion and leukocyte margination in the peribiliary vascular plexus (e.g., evidence of ADCC), partially organized thrombi in arterial branches, focal mural necrosis of large septal bile ducts, and inflammatory and necrotizing arteritis. Late sequelae of acute AMR include biliary sludge and stricturing caused by obstructive cholangiopathy, obliterative arteriopathy, loss of small bile ducts, and chronic rejection.[80,189,247-249]

Reperfusion biopsies from patients with high-MFI multispecificity DSA can show platelet aggregates in the portal and terminal hepatic veins more often than crossmatch-negative controls.[17,198] In those destined for dysfunction, diffuse portal microvascular C4d positivity is seen in postreperfusion biopsies.[210] Other findings, such as portal microvascular endothelial cell hypertrophy, eosinophilic and histiocytic portal microvasculitis, inlet venulitis, portal edema, ductular reaction, and diffuse portal microvascular C4d staining, combined with spotty acidophilic necrosis of hepatocytes and centrilobular hepatocellular swelling, accompanied by cholangiolar proliferation and hepatocanalicular cholestasis, often occur during the first week after transplantation in patients with high MFI and multispecific DSA. [210] Inflammatory and necrotizing arteritis is rare, but it is almost diagnostic when detected. Coexistent TCMR with portal eosinophilia is common.[237] Clinicopathological correlation with exclusion of other causes of dysfunction and staining for C4d and other immune deposits are needed to confirm the diagnosis.[81-83,240]

Late-Onset Acute Antibody-Mediated Rejection

Late-onset (>6 months) acute AMR is characterized by microvascular injury, similar to aAMR in other organs.[250,251] Examination of the portal microvasculature shows dilated capillaries and inlet venules extending from the portal vein into the lobule. Endothelial cells are enlarged or "hypertrophic" and show eosinophilic transformation of the cytoplasm causing a hob-nailing appearance.[210] This is associated with margination of leukocytes in the portal vessels or "capillaritis." The dilated capillaries may be filled with eosinophils, neutrophils, monocytes, and macrophages (Fig. 53.17).[210,252] Banff stresses the importance of these microvascular changes as signature lesions of acute AMR[3] and proposed a histopathology score (h score) based on them as part of the criteria for diagnosing aAMR[3] (Box 53.3).

Some portal-based changes associated with late-onset acute AMR may mimic impaired biliary flow, including ductular reaction, neutrophilic pericholangiolitis, portal eosinophilia, and portal edema.[194,195,198,210] The biliary changes encountered with aAMR may be related to bile duct ischemia secondary to antibody-mediated microvascular damage involving the peribiliary capillary plexus, and an element of direct cytotoxic biliary epithelial damage cannot be excluded.[159] Lobular and parenchymal changes that can

BOX 53.3 Histopathology Score of Lesions for Diagnosis of Acute AMR

1 Portal microvascular endothelial cell enlargement (portal veins, capillaries, and inlet venules) involving a majority of portal tracts with sparse microvasculitis defined as three to four marginated and/or intraluminal monocytes, neutrophils, or eosinophils in the maximally involved capillary with generally mild dilation.

2 Monocytic, eosinophilic, or neutrophilic microvasculitis/capillaritis, defined as at least 5 to 10 leukocytes marginated and/or intraluminal in the maximally involved capillary, prominent portal and/or sinusoidal microvascular endothelial cell enlargement involving a majority of portal tracts or sinusoids, with variable but noticeable portal capillary and inlet venule dilation and variable portal edema.

3 As above, with marked capillary dilation, marked microvascular inflammation (10 or more marginated and/or intraluminal leukocytes in the most severely affected vessels), at least focal microvascular disruption with fibrin deposition, and extravasation of red blood cells into the portal stroma and/or the space of Disse (subsinusoidal space).

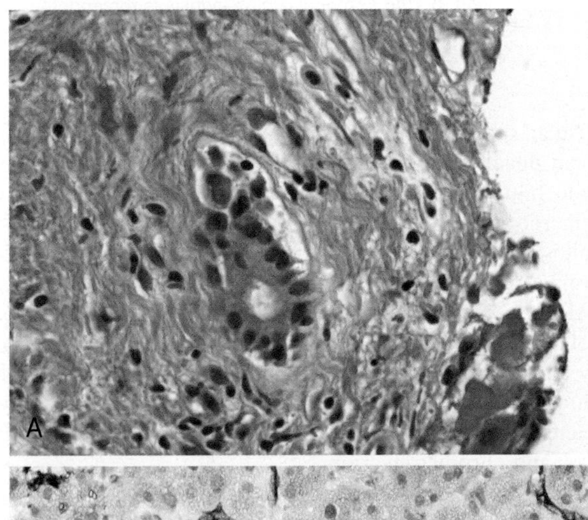

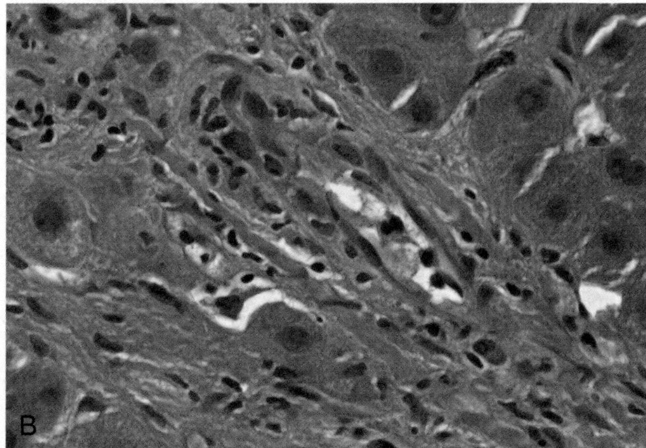

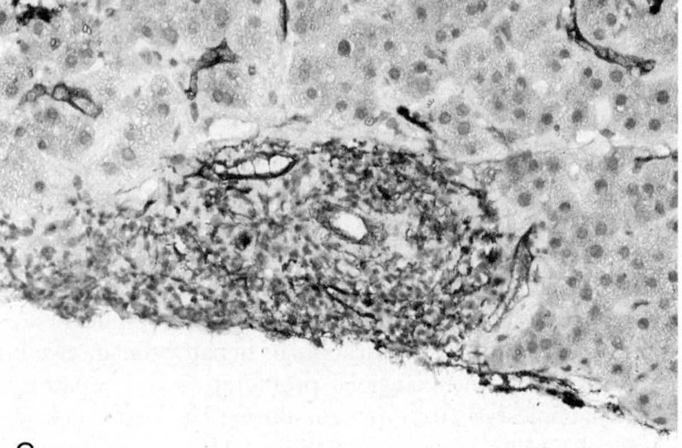

FIGURE 53.17 Images from a young male transplant recipient presenting with mixed TCMR and aAMR. The patient suffered from allograft loss due to severe AMR and was retransplanted. **A,** At high magnification, portal capillaries are dilated and filled with monocytes and leukocytes. **B,** Also at high magnification, dilated capillaries are seen with enlarged and swollen endothelial cells. **C,** C4d immunohistochemistry demonstrates diffuse uptake by portal capillaries and veins in the majority of portal tracts. C4d uptake is also seen in inlet venules and sinusoids.

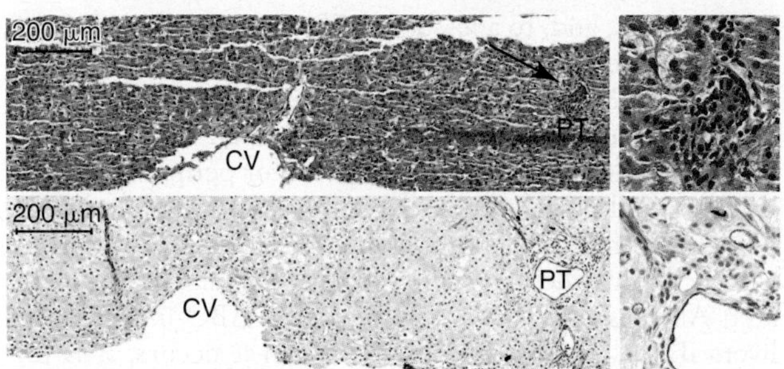

FIGURE 53.18 Liver allograft from a lymphocytotoxic crossmatch-positive recipient obtained 10 days after transplantation for primary biliary cholangitis. The patient developed unexplained hyperbilirubinemia and had a significant decrease in platelet counts. Other causes of allograft injury had been excluded. Compare the H&E-stained *(top)* and C4d-stained *(bottom)* specimens. The portal tracts *(PT)* from each are shown at higher magnification in the *insets (right)*. Note the positive C4d staining in the portal vein, portal capillaries, and central vein *(CV)*. The sinusoids were weakly stained or negative in this case. The low-grade ductular reaction and area of mild acute cholangiolitis *(arrow in top panel)* are seen at higher magnification *(inset)*, revealing mild hepatocyte swelling and hepatocanalicular cholestasis.

be seen with aAMR include hepatocanalicular cholestasis, hepatocyte ballooning, and central venulitis.[252]

Macrophages along with NK cells play an important role in AMR as they are responsible for antibody-dependent cell-mediated cytotoxicity by interaction of Fcγ receptors on their surfaces and IgG molecules.[253] Dankof et al. showed higher CD68-positive cell counts in C4d-positive liver allografts.[254] The macrophage marker CD68 is also successfully used as an adjunct in the diagnosis of pathological AMR in cardiac allografts.[255,256] In our experience, macrophage markers (CD163 and CD68) to assess sinusoidal macrophage aggregates are very helpful in the diagnosis of aAMR in select cases. We also observed higher macrophage counts in DSA-positive allografts with plasma cell–rich rejection.

Banff criteria for definitive aAMR is based on a biopsy showing changes consistent with an AMR-related pattern of injury (histopathology criteria), clinicopathological exclusion of causes of a similar pattern of injury, serological evidence of DSAs, and evidence of strong and diffuse antibody or complement (C4d) deposition within the injured allograft (Fig. 53.18).[3]

The latter is defined by strong portal vein, capillary, and usually periportal sinusoidal endothelial staining involving most portal tracts.[82,194,204,210,237,252,257,258] In an effort to standardize C4d interpretation, the 2016 Banff Working Group established criteria for C4d-(immune) scoring based on immunohistochemistry performed on formalin-fixed paraffin-embedded tissue (Box 53.4)[3]

Difficulties can be encountered in establishing a correct diagnosis because liver allografts are large and able to absorb high antibody loads (especially anti–class I HLA antibodies)[236] and are therefore resistant to AMR-related damage.[17,158,198,259,260] In some cases, the immune deposits are ephemeral[80,198] or can be associated with other insults.[81] Clinicopathological similarities exist between AMR and preservation injury, sepsis, and biliary or vascular complications.[80,198]

Intrahepatic immune deposits are ephemeral in AMR, even when evaluated by immunofluorescence in frozen tissue sections.[80-82,194,198] In severe cases, selective deposits of

BOX 53.4 Criteria for C4d-(Immune) Scoring

- **0** No C4d deposition in portal microvasculature.
- **1** Minimal (<10% portal tracts): C4d deposition in >50% of the circumference of portal microvascular endothelia (portal veins and capillaries)
- **2** Focal (10% to 50% portal tracts): C4d deposition in >50% of the circumference of portal microvascular endothelia (portal veins and capillaries), usually without extension into the periportal sinusoids
- **3** Diffuse (>50% portal tracts): C4d deposition in >50% of the circumference of portal microvascular endothelia (portal veins and capillaries), often with extension into the inlet venules or periportal sinusoids

IgG, IgM, C3, or C4 are usually detectable in the sinusoids and in the perihilar arteries, portal veins, and peribiliary plexus.[80,81,198] However, recognition that C4d persists for several days can be detected in FFPE tissues and correlates with circulating DSAs makes an AMR diagnosis easier to establish in kidney allografts.[261,262]

Bellamy[82] and Hubscher[194] reviewed the literature on C4d immunohistochemistry in liver allografts. Normal liver and allograft biopsies are usually negative for C4d staining. Portal vein, arterial, and capillary C4d and sinusoidal endothelial C4d have been detected in crossmatch-positive recipients more often than in crossmatch-negative controls[263] and in patients with isolated AMR.[81,237,264] Endothelial cell C4d staining is most specific for AMR, but portal vein C4d stromal staining has also been described in cases of ABO-incompatible AMR,[245] TCMR,[263] and chronic rejection.[240,265] Kozlowski and coworkers[81] suggested that C4d staining of FFPE tissue sections is nonspecific and that linear sinusoidal C4d deposits in frozen tissue specimens are needed to establish AMR. We found that C4d staining in FFPE tissue is reliable and that portal microvascular endothelial cell deposits are most specific. However, clinicopathological correlation is needed to establish a diagnosis of AMR with certainty. In contrast, portal and perivenular stromal staining is commonly observed and difficult to interpret. In nonliver allografts, interstitial or peritubular capillary microvascular endothelial C4d staining is used mainly to determine whether antibodies contribute to allograft injury.

As in other allografts, C4d deposits are often accompanied by TCMR.[83,240,245,254,264,266-270] In some studies, the burden of C4d deposits is directly proportional to the Banff grade.[245,254,264,266-270] Necrotic and steatotic hepatocytes can show nonspecific C4d staining.

Portal vein and capillary C4d deposits can occasionally be detected when other insults are thought to be the underlying cause of allograft dysfunction, including biliary obstruction,[266] recurrent HBV infection,[267] and recurrent HCV infection.[268] C4d staining has also been described in portal vein and capillary, sinusoidal, central vein, and arterial endothelial cells; in lymphoid nodules; and in periductal and portal stromal cells in native pediatric livers with hepatitis B, hepatitis C, AIH, and overlap syndromes that include AIH and PSC.[271] Endothelial C4d deposits in non–rejection-related allograft disorders are less widespread than in severe AMR or TCMR. Similar to kidney and heart allografts, liver C4d deposits have been associated with macrophage and plasma cell infiltrates.[254] It should be noted, however, that coexistent insults (e.g., recurrent AIH) do not preclude DSA binding to the tissue and contributing to the damage. In fact, the two-hit hypothesis speculates that any insult that contributes to MHC II upregulation increases susceptibility to DSA-related damage.[272]

Chronic Antibody-Mediated Rejection

The possibility that chronic or low grade, persistent AMR (cAMR) may contribute to indolent but progressive fibrosis has received increased attention, particularly for pediatric recipients.[144-146,182,183,216] Evidence supporting this association includes increased prevalence and titer of DSAs associated with tissue C4d deposits and suboptimal immunosuppression.[144-146] Histological criteria for cAMR was first reported and validated by O'Leary et al.[147,148] and elegantly reappraised by Dao et al.[218] Microvascular disruption characteristic of acute AMR is not the predominant feature of chronic AMR, but it can occur when superimposed late-onset acute AMR is seen.

Characteristic features include mononuclear portal inflammation associated with interface hepatitis, lobular/perivenular inflammation, subsinusoidal fibrosis, and dense acellular portal collagen deposition "portal collagenization" (Fig. 53.19).[147] Obliteration of portal veins "obliterative portal venopathy" likely leads to NRH changes.[241] In cases with double-positive DSA and C4d, Dao et al.[218] demonstrated that perivenular fibrosis, portal inflammation, and lobular inflammation are significant histological findings. Other histological features associated with cAMR include perivenulitis and isolated vascular lesions.[148,171] The inflammatory infiltrate is an admixture of macrophages and lymphocytes with some plasma cells. Biliary epithelial senescence and ductopenia can be seen in chronic AMR but at lower rates. Another histological feature is focal nodular hyperplasia like nodules in explanted allografts.

C4d is an integral element in evaluating biopsies for chronic AMR. C4d positivity is associated with posttransplant DSA, graft fibrosis, and graft loss.[147,171] At least focal C4d uptake (mostly in portal capillaries in inlet venules) is needed for a diagnosis of probable cAMR.[3]

Differential Diagnosis

Distinguishing AMR from preservation/reperfusion injury and suboptimal biliary drainage early after transplantation can be difficult. The presensitization state, persistence of circulating antibodies, diffuse C4d staining,[83] and posttransplantation clinical and laboratory profile can provide discriminating information. AMR should be suspected in female liver allograft recipients (often with autoimmune disorders) with high-MFI, multispecific DSAs who have received a liver with a short cold ischemic time but who show persistent DSAs after transplantation and develop graft dysfunction, refractory and otherwise unexplained thrombocytopenia, and circulating low complement levels in the first several weeks after transplantation.[81,83,198,242]

Alloantibody-mediated acute AMR should be favored instead of preservation/reperfusion injury when any of the following histopathological findings are detected: (1) diffuse endothelial cell enlargement combined with macrophage, eosinophil, and neutrophil margination on the luminal aspect of portal vein branches, portal capillaries, inlet venules, and, to a lessor extent, central veins; (2) occasional blastic lymphocytes and eosinophils and other features of TCMR in the portal or perivenular areas; and (3) diffuse portal microvascular endothelial cell C4d staining.[83] Similar findings associated with portal or periportal edema, necrosis, and portal interstitial hemorrhage should raise the possibility of ABO incompatibility–associated acute AMR.

Precipitous allograft failure from severe anti-HLA–mediated AMR is rare, but rarely occurs in ABO-incompatible livers if not adequately treated. When it occurs, it is difficult to distinguish from hemorrhagic liver necrosis caused by hypotension, poor perfusion, sepsis, or vascular thrombosis. Unless unequivocal evidence of AMR is detected, such as inflammatory or necrotizing arteritis or diffuse complement (C4d) deposition combined with serological evidence of antidonor antibodies, the cause of allograft failure can be extremely difficult to determine with certainty.

T Cell–Mediated Rejection

TCMR manifests by predominantly lymphocytic infiltrates involving primarily portal areas with associated lymphocytic bile duct and vascular damage. The Banff Working Group now recognizes that TCMR can occur early (within 6 months), likely secondary to direct alloantigen presentation, or late (>6 months), likely secondary to indirect alloantigen presentation.[3] Most episodes of TCMR occur early (within 30 days after transplantation) because the reaction is precipitated by mass migration of donor cells into recipient lymphoid tissues.[274-276] Early TCMR rarely leads to allograft failure or permanent allograft damage because it usually is easily controlled by increased immunosuppression.[91,277] Late TCMR, however, has a different clinical, serological, and histopathological appearance. It is more often subclinical, with minimally elevated liver injury tests, and the histopathology more closely resembles chronic hepatitis. It is also more difficult to completely control with increased immunosuppression. TCMR occurring later also more often indolently produces permanent allograft damage, possibly resulting from a delay in treatment.[4,276,278,279]

Clinical Features

Early acute TCMR usually manifests clinically between 5 and 30 days after transplantation, depending on the immunosuppressive regimen. It currently affects approximately 30% of liver transplant recipients.[280] Presensitized patients or patients who receive less-than-optimal baseline immunosuppression are at increased risk.

Early after transplantation, when biliary T-tubes are in place, decreased bile flow and thin, pale bile are commonly seen and do not necessarily denote acute rejection. Likewise, ascites may develop because of increased intrahepatic hydrostatic pressure that results in liver swelling and increased lymph production.[281] These clinical findings alone are not sufficient to implicate acute rejection.

TCMR usually manifests as nonselective elevation of liver injury test values. Leukocytosis and eosinophilia are frequently identified.[281] The levels of a variety of proteins (e.g., interleukins, neopterin, amyloid A protein) are increased in the peripheral blood, but none of the proteins is routinely assayed to monitor recipients. Instead, TCMR

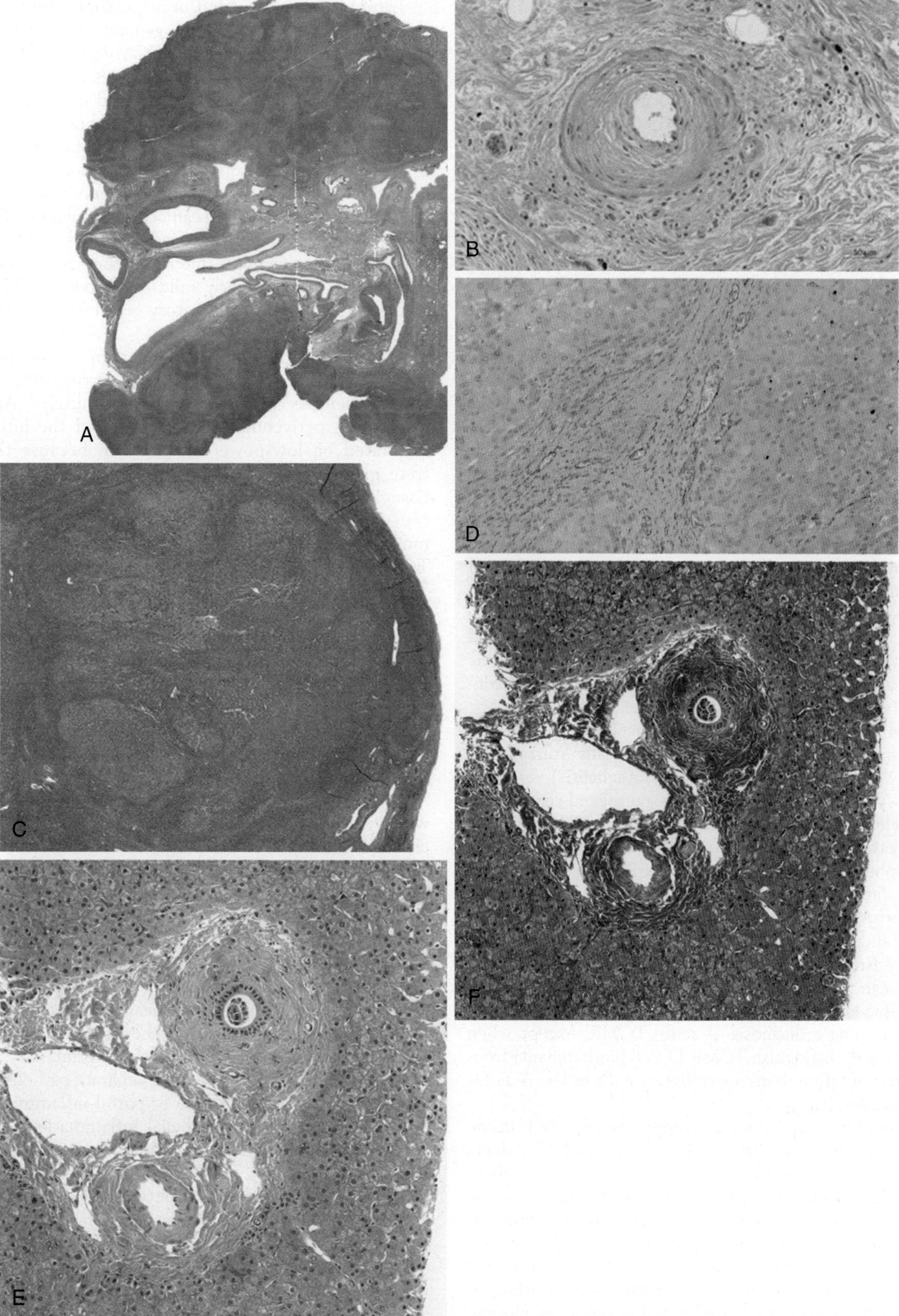

FIGURE 53.19 A, Low-power image from an allograft explanted at time of retransplantation for cAMR in a patient with strong C1q positive DSA showing altered architecture and fibrosis. **B,** Higher-magnification view of inset demonstrating an artery with fibrointimal hyperplasia. This arterial lesion can occur with or without inflammation as an isolated finding, which points toward cAMR. **C,** Focal-nodular hyperplasia-like lesion is identified in the explanted allograft. **D,** C4d by immunohistochemistry performed on the explanted liver demonstrating diffuse uptake by portal veins and microvasculature. **E** and **F,** H&E and trichrome-stained sections from a portal tract seen at higher magnification in a biopsy from a different patient with cAMR demonstrating thickened collagen fibers deposition, a finding referred to as *portal collagenization.*

is usually suspected on clinical grounds and then confirmed by core needle biopsy or reflexively treated.

Risk factors for the development of early acute TCMR include the immunosuppressive regimen; young and "relatively healthy" recipients (e.g., normal serum creatinine level, low Child-Pugh classification); advanced-age donors; recipients of deceased donor allografts; donor-recipient HLA-DR mismatch; patients with immune dysregulated syndromes (e.g., PSC, AIH, PBC) and acute liver failure; long cold ischemic times; and *HLA*-C genotype.[276,280,282] As mentioned earlier, late-onset TCMR occurring more than 1 year after transplantation often has a different histopathological appearance resembling chronic hepatitis.[278,280,282-284]

Pathological Features and Grading

Most typical episodes of acute TCMR are characterized by (1) predominantly mononuclear but mixed portal inflammation containing blastic or activated lymphocytes, neutrophils, and eosinophils; (2) subendothelial inflammation of portal and/or central veins; and (3) lymphocytic bile duct damage.[6,281] Minimal diagnostic criteria needed to establish a diagnosis of acute TCMR include at least two of the aforementioned pathological findings. A TCMR diagnosis is further substantiated if more than 50% of the ducts or central veins are damaged or if unequivocal endothelialitis of portal or central vein branches is identified. Histopathological evidence of severe injury includes perivenular inflammation accompanied by centrilobular hepatocyte necrosis and dropout, inflammatory and/or necrotizing or lymphocytic intimal arteritis, and inflammatory features such as central-to-central, bridging inflammation and necrosis.[277,281]

TCMR-associated infiltrates are encountered predominantly in portal tracts but also occasionally surrounding central veins. *Endotheliitis* (i.e., endothelialitis) refers to lymphocytes located underneath the portal and central vein endothelium. This characteristic feature of TCMR may be seen in other types of allograft dysfunction.[285]

Lymphocytes participating in TCMR are predominantly T cells (as expected), including CD8-positive cells that often surround and invade damaged bile ducts.[286,287] CD20-positive B cells usually account for only a minor proportion of the infiltrate. Macrophages and other leukocytes are present and can predominate in severe TCMR.[286-288] Immunophenotypic analysis is not prognostically or clinically useful for establishing a diagnosis of acute TCMR, except when attempting to distinguish TCMR (T cell predominant) from posttransplantation lymphoproliferative disorder (PTLD) (B cell predominant).

Lymphocytic cholangitis (lymphocytes located inside ductal basement membranes) involving small bile ducts (<30 μm in diameter) associated with evidence of biliary epithelial cell injury (e.g., paranuclear vacuolization, apoptotic bodies, increased nucleus-to-cytoplasm ratio, mitoses, and prominent nucleoli) are typical acute TCMR features. Breaks in the basement membrane indicate severe bile duct damage. Cytoplasmic eosinophilia and multinucleation usually signal senescence-related changes and chronic injury.[178] Portal or peribiliary granulomas are not a feature of acute or chronic rejection; if granulomas are present, a non–rejection-related cause of duct injury, such as recurrent PBC, a coexistent mycobacterial or fungal infection, or sarcoidosis, should be suspected.

Lymphocytic intimal and/or necrotizing arteritis is a very specific feature of rejection, in general, and a defining feature of severe TCMR or mixed TCMR/AMR.[273] However, it is rarely detected in needle biopsies because the most commonly affected arteries are located in the liver hilum. Because recognition of arteritis in peripheral needle biopsies is a poorly reproducible finding,[289] it is not usually included in grading schemes. Isolated vascular lesions characterized by intimal thickening, and luminal stenosis with or without inflammatory infiltrate can occur in isolation of TCMR; they may indicate chronic active TCMR or cAMR.[123] The portal tract–parenchyma interface zone is usually unremarkable in cases of early mild and moderate TCMR. In severe cases, portal inflammatory cells involve the periportal parenchyma.[4]

TCMR-type infiltrates can be seen in the perivenular sinusoids and connective tissue surrounding terminal hepatic venules (i.e., central perivenulitis).[4] Appreciation of the perivenular predominance of the infiltrate is facilitated on low-power examination because the infiltrate might not be located in the perivenular connective tissue, but extend a distance of 3 to 5 hepatocytes from the central vein edge. Perivenulitis occurs more commonly later (>100 days) after transplantation. Severe TCMR is diagnosed when typical portal changes of acute TCMR are accompanied by perivenular inflammation and zonal centrilobular congestion, hemorrhage, and hepatocyte necrosis and dropout, which is usually accompanied by a lymphohistiocytic inflammatory infiltrate, including pigment-laden macrophages.

The Banff grading scheme for acute and chronic TCMR was constructed on data generated by recognized experts in liver transplant pathology, hepatology, and surgery from many of the major hepatic transplantation centers in North America, Europe, and Asia (Tables 53.4 and 53.5).[3] It is widely used[290] easy to apply, and reproducible.[291] It is scientifically correct and has prognostic significance, but currently, graft failure from otherwise typical acute TCMR or chronic rejection is relatively uncommon.[277,292]

The Banff system uses descriptive grades of *indeterminate, mild* (Fig. 53.20), *moderate* (Fig. 53.21), and *severe* TCMR (Fig. 53.22; see Table 53.4). It also uses a semiquantitative rejection activity index (RAI) (see Table 53.5),[3] which is a remnant of the European grading system[293] and the conceptual equivalent to the hepatitis activity index.[294] RAI semiquantitatively scores the extent of structure involvement and severity of three separate pathological features, each on a scale of 0 to 3: portal inflammation, bile duct damage, and subendothelial inflammation. The individual components are then summed to determine a total RAI score.

There is direct correlation between the total RAI score and rejection grade and correlation with increased risk of persistent or recurrent acute TCMR, chronic rejection, and graft failure[277]: indeterminate (1 to 2), mild (3 to 4), moderate (5 to 6), and severe (>6). The maximum possible total RAI score is 9, but biopsies rarely achieve this score.[277] Instead, most episodes are mild, have a total RAI score of less than 6, and promptly respond to increased immunosuppression, unless there are coexistent acute AMR changes. Isolated TCMR episodes, even if severe, do not lead to significant fibrosis, bile duct loss, or arteriopathy as determined in subsequent or follow-up biopsies.[277] Graft failure from TCMR is unusual.

Treating with increased immunosuppression can diminish some characteristic findings needed to establish the diagnosis; it can also lead to centrilobular hepatocyte swelling and hepatocanalicular cholestasis, causing further confusion. One week or longer is usually required for rejection-related changes to completely resolve after therapy.

Most instances of late rejection (>100 days) are characterized by features found in early TCMR, described earlier. However, other features become more noticeable.[4] Included are fewer blastic lymphocytes, more prevalent necro-inflammatory interface activity, less venous subendothelial inflammation, more frequent central perivenulitis, and low-grade lobular necro-inflammatory activity. This slight transformation of late-onset TCMR causes it to more closely resemble chronic hepatitis in some cases.[4]

Late TCMR can present as prominent central perivenular inflammation and hepatocyte dropout with minimal or

TABLE 53.4 Banff Working Group Criteria for Liver Allograft T Cell–Mediated Rejection

Global Assessment*	Criteria
Indeterminate	Portal and/or perivenular inflammatory infiltrate that fails to meet the criteria for mild acute rejection
Mild	Rejection infiltrate in a minority of portal tracts or perivenular areas that is usually mild and confined within the portal spaces and absence of hepatocellular dropout for those presenting with isolated perivenular infiltrates
Moderate	Rejection infiltrate expanding most or all portal tracts and/or perivenular areas with confluent necrosis/hepatocellular dropout limited to a minority of perivenular areas
Severe	Similar to moderate, with spillover into periportal areas and moderate to severe perivenular inflammation that extends into the hepatic parenchyma and is associated with perivenular hepatocyte necrosis involving a majority of perivenular areas

Global assessment of rejection grade is made on review of the entire biopsy specimen and only after a diagnosis of rejection has been established. It is inappropriate to provide a rejection grade when the diagnosis of rejection is uncertain.

Modified from Demetris AJ, Nalesnik M, Randhawa P, et al. Histologic patterns of rejection and other causes of liver dysfunction. In: Busuttil RW, Klintmalm GB, eds. Transplantation of the Liver. *Philadelphia: Saunders; 2005:1057–1128.*

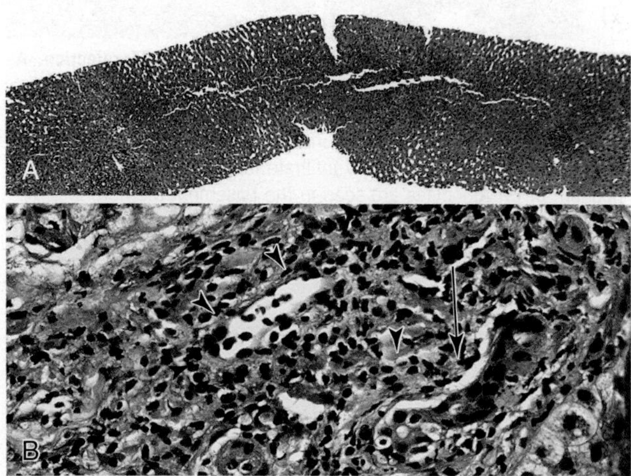

FIGURE 53.20 A, Typical low-power appearance of mild acute rejection. Notice the mild portal inflammation, which expands a few portal tracts in this biopsy. **B,** At higher magnification, the three typical features of classic acute cellular rejection can be seen. The infiltrate contains blastic and smaller lymphocytes, eosinophils, and occasional neutrophils and macrophages. Inflammatory bile duct damage *(arrow)* and subendothelial infiltration of the portal vein branches *(arrowheads)* are evident.

TABLE 53.5 Rejection Activity Index

Category	Criteria	Score*
Portal inflammation	Mostly lymphocytic inflammation involving but not noticeably expanding a minority of portal tracts	1
	Expansion of most or all portal tracts by a mixed infiltrate containing lymphocytes with occasional blasts, neutrophils, and eosinophils	2
	Marked expansion of most or all portal tracts by a mixed infiltrate containing numerous blasts and eosinophils, with inflammatory spillover into the periportal parenchyma	3
Bile duct inflammation damage	A minority of ducts are cuffed and infiltrated by inflammatory cells and show only mild reactive changes, such as increased nucleus-to-cytoplasm ratio of the epithelial cells	1
	Most or all ducts are infiltrated by inflammatory cells. Some ducts show degenerative changes, such as nuclear pleomorphism, disordered polarity, or cytoplasmic vacuolization of the epithelium.	2
	As above, with most or all ducts showing degenerative changes or focal luminal disruption	3
Venous endothelial inflammation	Subendothelial lymphocytic infiltration involving some portal and/or hepatic venules	1
	Subendothelial infiltration involving most or all portal and/or hepatic venules	2
	As above, with moderate or severe perivenular inflammation that extends into the perivenular parenchyma and association with perivenular hepatocyte necrosis	3

**Total rejection activity index (RAI) score = sum of all component scores for portal inflammation, bile duct inflammation or damage, and venous endothelial inflammation.*

Modified from Demetris AJ, Nalesnik M, Randhawa P, et al. Histologic patterns of rejection and other causes of liver dysfunction. In: Busuttil RW, Klintmalm GB, eds. Transplantation of the Liver. *Philadelphia: Saunders; 2005:1057–1128.*

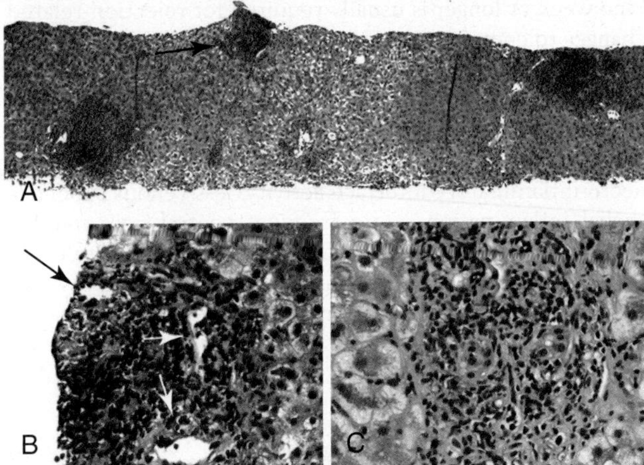

FIGURE 53.21 Composite images of moderate acute cellular rejection. A, Low magnification shows that all of the portal tracts are expanded by a rejection-type infiltrate. The indicated field *(arrow)* is magnified in **B. B,** Subendothelial infiltration of the portal vein branches *(arrows)* and the composition of the inflammatory infiltrate indicate a moderate level of rejection. **C,** Lymphocytes are seen in the basement membrane of the small bile duct *(center)*. Note the perinuclear vacuolization of the biliary epithelial cells.

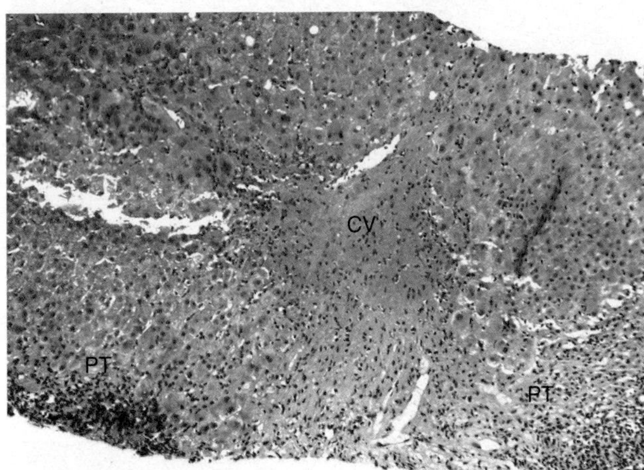

FIGURE 53.22 Severe acute rejection is characterized by marked portal and perivenular inflammation combined with perivenular hepatocyte necrosis or dropout and at least focal central-to-central bridging. Central perivenulitis in this biopsy specimen corresponds to a score of 3 (i.e., severe central perivenulitis). *CV,* central vein; *PT,* portal tract.

no portal tract changes (i.e., isolated central perivenulitis) (Fig. 53.23).[295-298] These cases may wax and wane, resolve spontaneously,[297] or evolve into typical chronic rejection with ductopenia and perivenular fibrosis. Some of the variation is likely related to sampling issues. Subendothelial inflammation of the portal or central veins is not a required finding. Extensive and severe perivenular fibrosis resembling Budd-Chiari syndrome or a sinusoidal obstruction-type syndrome can develop as a consequence of severe and/or persistent central perivenulitis.[149,299] cAMR can also contribute to or cause perivenular and subsinusoidal fibrosis.[147,148,218] The Banff Working Group proposal for grading isolated central perivenulitis rejection is described in Table 53.6. However, the Banff Working Group is working on an update to reflect current knowledge and understanding.

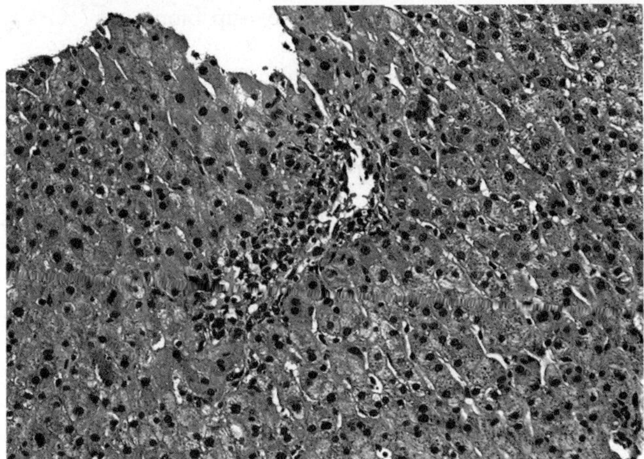

FIGURE 53.23 Some cases of acute cellular rejection, especially those that occur late after transplantation, show perivenular inflammation but have little or no portal inflammation or bile duct damage. This example would be graded as mild central perivenulitis. Isolated central perivenulitis is graded as *minimal/indeterminate, mild, moderate,* and *severe.* (Banff Working Group, Demetris AJ, Adeyi O, Bellamy CO, et al. Liver biopsy interpretation for causes of late liver allograft dysfunction. Hepatology. 2006;44:489-501.)

TABLE 53.6 Banff Working Group: Biopsy Findings for Late Allograft Dysfunction*

Description	Biopsy Findings
Minimal or indeterminate	Perivenular inflammation involving a minority of terminal hepatic veins, with patchy perivenular hepatocyte loss but without confluent perivenular necrosis
Mild	As above, but involving most terminal hepatic veins
Moderate	As above, with focal confluent perivenular hepatocyte dropout and mild or moderate inflammation, but without bridging necrosis
Severe	As above, with confluent perivenular hepatocyte dropout and inflammation involving most hepatic venules and with central-to-central bridging necrosis

**Grading descriptors of late-onset T cell–mediated rejection presenting as isolated central perivenulitis. Data from Banff Working Group, Demetris AJ, Adeyi O, et al. Liver biopsy interpretation for causes of late liver allograft dysfunction.* Hepatology. *2006;44(2):489–501.*

Differential Diagnosis

The differential diagnosis of TCMR depends on the time since transplantation. Early-onset TCMR should be distinguished from preservation injury from obstructive cholangiopathy/cholangitis during the first several months after transplantation (discussed previously). Late-onset TCMR must be differentiated from recurrent hepatitis B or C and AIH.

Hepatitis and TCMR show predominantly mononuclear portal inflammation, bile duct damage, and acidophilic necrosis of hepatocytes. The severity and prevalence of lymphocytic cholangitis, interface activity, lobular changes, and perivenular inflammation and hepatocyte dropout should be carefully assessed.[300] Features that favor TCMR include lymphocytic cholangitis and perivenular inflammation involving a majority of bile ducts and central veins, respectively, and low-grade or absent lobular and interface necro-inflammatory activity. Conversely, recurrent or new-onset viral hepatitis or AIH is favored when interface and lobular necro-inflammatory activity predominate over bile duct and perivenular changes. Regardless, correlation with serum viral nucleic acid and autoantibody studies is essential.

Alloimmune hepatitis[301] resembles viral hepatitis in most aspects, except the former shows conspicuous plasma cells and aggressive interface activity. Because many of these patients also harbor DSA, a *plasma cell–rich rejection* diagnosis is preferred over the term *de novo AIH*.[3]

Plasma Cell–Rich Rejection

Plasma cell–rich rejection (previously known as *de-novo AIH/plasma cell–rich hepatitis*) is an uncommon and incompletely understood cause of late graft dysfunction.[3] It occurs in approximately 3% to 5% of recipients, usually more than 1 year after transplantation. It resembles native AIH to a great extent and is associated with serological and histological features reminiscent of AIH in patients transplanted for disorders other than AIH. Plasma cell–rich rejection as a concept has been recognized for a while in renal transplantation but has only recently been included in the Banff classification as an atypical presentation of rejection, likely representing a mixed TCMR and AMR etiology.[3,302-304] Criteria for diagnosis of plasma cell–rich rejection are listed in Table 53.7.

Pathophysiology

Plasma cell hepatitis or de-novo AIH was initially described in pediatric recipients as a cause of late graft dysfunction with autoimmunity and poor prognosis.[305] Subsequent reports in adults showed that it often arises in interferon-treated HCV recipients,[3,302-304,306-310] and it was more recently described in HCV-positive recipients treated with DAAs.[311,312] Other reported immune-mediated graft effects of interferon and DAA treatment include acute and chronic rejection and ductopenia.[313,314]

An atypical liver-kidney microsomal (LKM) autoantibody pattern directed against the cytosolic enzyme glutathione S-transferase (GST) T1 polymorphism (GSST1) has also been described as a risk factor for plasma cell–rich rejection/hepatitis.[315-320] Null-GSTT1 genotype recipients of a GSTT1-positive donor liver generate donor-specific antibodies as well as a T cell response against allografts that contribute to the development of hepatitis.[321] Microvascular C4d deposits are described, although this finding is not uniformly reported.[315,317-319] Other autoantibodies detected in this setting include those directed against CK8 and CK18,[322] atypical anti-LKMs (i.e., isoforms of carbonic anhydrase III), subunit β1 of the proteasome, and members of different GST families.[323] These associations with antibody mechanisms and evidence of complement activation support that plasma cell hepatitis is an atypical form of mixed TCMR and AMR rather than a de-novo AIH. In pediatric patients, however, there are calls to separate de-novo AIH in pediatrics from plasma cell–rich rejection in adults, evidence that this change in terminology has not been widely accepted.[324]

Further evidence supporting a rejection-related classification is the presence of HLA donor-specific antibodies in about 60% of cases and evidence of microvascular complement activation demonstrated by C4d deposition.[206,315] Subgroups of plasma cell–rich rejection can show overexpression of IgG4-positive cells, more prominent lymphocytic cholangitis, central perivenulitis, and respond to immunosuppression.[325]

Clinical Presentation

A diagnosis of plasma cell–rich rejection is currently limited to recipients transplanted for causes other than AIH. Most patients are detected initially because of elevated liver function test values. This usually occurs when an attempt is made to routinely discontinue corticosteroids from the immunosuppression regimen. A diagnosis is established on the basis of a liver needle biopsy and correlated with clinicopathological and serological profiles. Risk factors include acute rejection, steroid dependence, tacrolimus-based immunosuppression, female donor, young recipients, and HLA-DR3 and DR4.[326,327] Most patients respond to immunosuppressive therapy; however, the relapse rate can be up to 37%.[326] The same study showed a rate of 30% progression to cirrhosis in a median of 37 months and death or retransplantation in about 33% of patients. In the current era, patients treated with DAA who develop immune-mediated graft dysfunction show elevated ALT, bilirubin, and alkaline phosphatase. The median time to develop rejection after discontinuing treatment is over 2 months (76 days).[311]

Pathological Features

Morphological features show similarities to those seen in AIH: prominent plasma cell–rich portal and interface

TABLE 53.7 Criteria for Diagnosis of Plasma Cell–Rich Rejection*

	Criteria 1 and 3 must be fulfilled; criterion 2 is desirable but not absolutely required
1	Portal and perivenular plasma cell–rich inflammation (estimated >30%) with easily recognizable periportal/interface and/or perivenular necro-inflammatory activity involving a majority of portal tracts and/or central areas. Banff component score for endothelial injury is usually 3 because of the severe perivenular activity.
2	Lymphocytic cholangitis is usually present and a desirable feature, but not absolutely required (Banff component score for bile duct injury is usually 1 or more).
3	Original disease other than autoimmune hepatitis

**Banff component scores are from the Rejection Activity Index (see Table 53.5), which is usually 5 or more in cases of plasma cell–rich rejection.*

Modified from Demetris AJ, Bellamy C, Hübscher SG, et al. 2016 comprehensive Update of the Banff Working Group on Liver Allograft Pathology: Introduction of antibody-mediated rejection. Am J Transplant. *2016;16(10):2816–2835.*

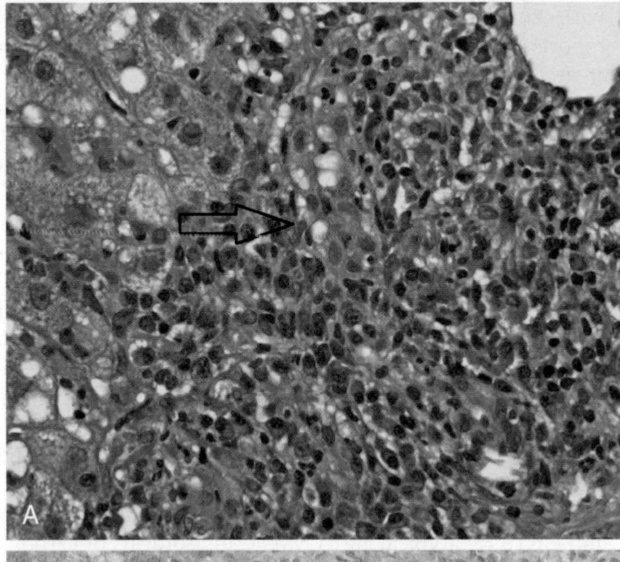

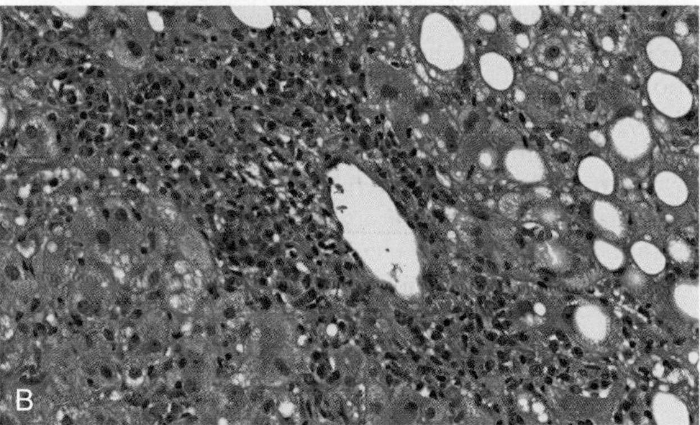

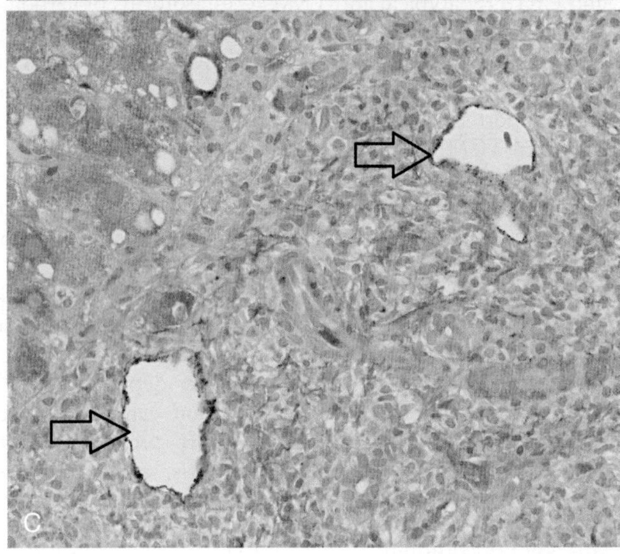

FIGURE 53.24 Liver allograft biopsy from a patient transplanted for PSC who developed DSA against DQ6 and DQ7 and is also positive for AT1R auto-antibodies. Biopsy shows plasma cell-rich rejection, with a RAI of 8/9. **A,** Higher magnification of a H&E- stained section showing a portal tract with damaged bile duct (*arrow*) and clusters of plasma cells. **B,** Higher magnification of a central vein with perivenulitis and clusters or plasma cells. **C,** C4d immunohistochemistry performed on paraffin tissue demonstrating uptake by portal vein branches (*arrows*) and adjacent microvaculature.

inflammation involving the majority of portal areas. Perivenular necro-inflammatory activity with plasma cell–rich infiltrate, hepatocellular dropout, and hemorrhage is usually present and involves the majority of central areas (Fig. 53.24). By definition, the plasma cell component should be greater than 30%.[3] Bile duct damage "lymphocytic cholangitis" is usually present but not a required feature for diagnosis. Most cases will show moderate to severe rejection grade with an RAI ≥5/9. In our experience, ancillary studies demonstrating C4d uptake by portal microvasculature and demonstration of increased sinusoidal macrophage aggregates by CD163 or CD68 can be helpful in establishing the diagnosis. Demonstration of increased IgG4-positive plasma cells is also a helpful feature.

Differential Diagnosis

Major differential considerations would include recurrent HCV (currently rare because of DAA) and AIH, both of which can demonstrate a significant plasma cell component. C4d deposition and prominent central perivenular inflammation help differentiate plasma cell–rich rejection from recurrent HCV.[302,328] HCV RNA quantification is needed to rule out recurrent HCV. This differential will become less common as transplantation for HCV is declining and recipients who are HCV positive are treated with DAA. According to Banff recommendations, a diagnosis of plasma cell–rich rejection should not be made in recipients with original disease of AIH unless there is also clear evidence of alloimmunity. Recurrence of other diseases of dysregulated immunity such as PSC and PBC are also included in the differential diagnosis. Both tend to show a "biliary-gestalt" with evidence of impaired biliary flow, ductular metaplasia of hepatocytes on CK7, and copper deposition in periportal hepatocytes. PBC is also patchy in nature and does not usually demonstrate the diffuse portal involvement seen in plasma cell–rich rejection and TCMR.

Chronic Rejection

The clinical and histopathological presentations of chronic rejection is evolving. Traditionally, chronic rejection has been defined as "immunologic injury that evolves from severe or persistent acute rejection and results in potentially irreversible damage to bile ducts, arteries, and veins."[5]

Historically, chronic rejection typically occurred within the first year after transplantation.[5] More recently, with the advent of better immunosuppression and more prevalent long-term survival, chronic rejection can present indolently as a low-grade chronic hepatitis with or without perivenular fibrosis and evolve toward typical cirrhosis over a period of many years to decades after transplantation.

Traditionally defined chronic rejection (e.g., ductopenia, obliterative arteriopathy, perivenular fibrosis) affects approximately 3% to 5% of liver allograft recipients 5 years after transplantation, which is a dramatic decrease in incidence since the 1980s, when the incidence was 15% to 20%.[5] Better recognition and control of TCMR, reversibility of the early phases of chronic rejection, the unique immunological properties of liver allografts, and the ability of the liver to regenerate without fibrosis after recovery from acute rejection have contributed to the decreased incidence of chronic rejection. Robust data do not exist on whether or not the rate of chronic rejection increases with time after transplantation because it is currently recognized that changes including idiopathic posttransplantation hepatitis (IPTH), obliterative portal venopathy,[241] and perivenular subsinusoidal, portal, or periportal fibrosis are now included in this category.

Nevertheless, chronic rejection is an important cause of late liver allograft dysfunction and failure, particularly in patients who show chronic hepatitic-type changes with low-grade necro-inflammatory–type interface activity[183] and otherwise unexplained fibrosis.[146] Clinically, chronic rejection is seen mostly in patients with suboptimal immunosuppression therapy, either electively or because of adverse consequences such as renal insufficiency or immunosuppression-related neoplastic disorders.[329]

Risk factors for chronic rejection are divided into alloantigen-dependent and non–alloantigen-dependent categories. Alloantigen-dependent, immunologic, or rejection-related factors are the most important, especially the number and severity of acute rejection episodes.[5,282] In cyclosporine-treated cohorts, risk factors for late-onset acute rejection include younger recipient age; male-to-female sex mismatch; a primary diagnosis of AIH or biliary disease; baseline immunosuppression; interactions between HLA-DR3, tumor necrosis factor status, and CMV infection[330]; and non-white recipients.[5] Use of interferon-α to treat recurrent HCV infection is a risk factor of historical interest.[314,331] Prospective studies suggest that persistent, strong DSAs, particularly the IgG3 subclass, are associated with late graft loss and chronic rejection.[171,211,223,228,237,238,332] In a large tacrolimus-treated cohort, matching factors described for the cyclosporine-treated patients were eliminated as significant risk factors, but the influence of the number and severity of TCMR episodes remained.[329] Non–alloantigen-dependent or nonimmunological risk factors include donor age older than 40 years.[329]

Pathophysiology

Immunological mechanisms of injury that contribute to allograft damage during early and late TCMR and AMR likely also contribute to the development of chronic rejection,[5,277,329,333-336] including an antibody-associated injury.[243,228,238,332] Bile duct loss in chronic rejection has been attributed to a combination of direct immunological and indirect ischemic damage resulting from obliterative arteriopathy, small artery or arteriolar loss, and destruction of the peribiliary capillary plexus,[239,337] with a possible contribution from alloantibodies.[159,198,238,243] Cumulative damage triggers biliary epithelial cell senescence.[178] Several studies have shown that the early phase of chronic rejection is potentially reversible,[178,335,338,339] provided that ductules and surrounding microvasculature are preserved.[340]

Clinical Features

Chronic rejection usually emerges in patients with a history of suboptimal immunosuppression, episodes of recurrent acute TCMR, and/or acute and/or chronic AMR episodes who develop a progressive cholestatic liver enzyme profile that is suboptimally responsive to increased immunosuppression.[281] Two clinical settings are typical: (1) after multiple or unresolved episodes of TCMR and/or acute and/or chronic AMR and (2) indolently without preceding clinically recognizable episodes of rejection. Both scenarios are relatively common, but the latter presentation is receiving increased attention and importance. Late-onset TCMR (>1 year after transplantation) typically occurs in inadequately immunosuppressed and/or inadequately monitored patients as a result of noncompliance or because of infectious, neoplastic, or toxic complications of chronic immunosuppression.[329]

Traditionally defined chronic rejection usually manifests as "cholestatic" liver injury test results (GGT/ALP > ALT/AST).[181,281,341] Persistent elevation of ALT and total bilirubin levels usually marks the transition from acute to chronic rejection and can presage allograft failure.[295,329,335] Clinical symptoms become apparent with the appearance of jaundice; biliary strictures and sludging and loss of hepatic synthetic function are other late findings that often occur immediately before allograft failure.[281] Hepatic angiograms show pruning of the intrahepatic arteries with poor peripheral filling and segmental narrowing, reflecting the obliterative arteriopathy of chronic rejection.[281,342]

Pathological Features and Staging

Traditionally defined chronic rejection primarily affects portal and perivenular areas (Fig. 53.25). It is divided into early (Fig. 53.26) and late (Fig. 53.27) stages according to the most recent Banff scheme (Table 53.8), which also suggests scoring fibrosis based on Venturi et al.[3,343] Traditionally defined early-stage chronic rejection is characterized by mild portal inflammation, lymphocytic cholangitis, biliary epithelial cell senescence changes involving most small bile ducts, and some degree of small bile duct loss (usually involving less than 50% of portal tracts). Compared with acute TCMR, chronic rejection usually shows less severe portal inflammation and fewer eosinophils, but more evident plasma cells, macrophages, and mast cells.[344] Ductular reactions are not a prominent feature of early-stage chronic rejection.

Recognition of biliary epithelial cell senescence-related changes is critical to the diagnosis of early chronic rejection.[178] Typical features include nuclear enlargement, hyperchromasia, and uneven spacing resembling cytological dysplasia; syncytia formation; eosinophilic transformation of the cytoplasm; and bile ducts only partially lined by biliary epithelial cells (see Figs. 53.25 and 53.26). The appearance

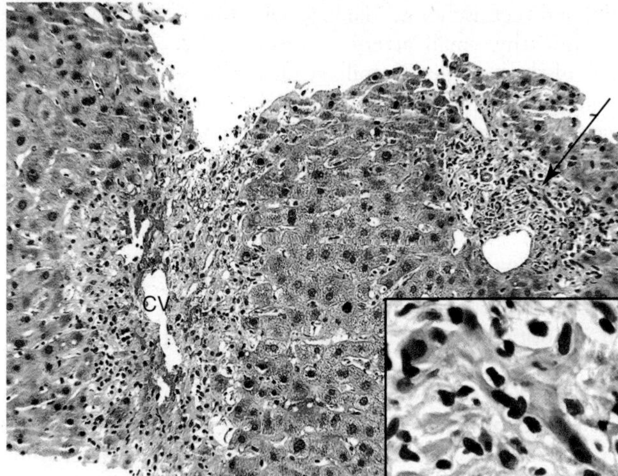

FIGURE 53.25 Transition from acute to chronic rejection. *CV,* Central vein. Note the mild degree of portal inflammation, bile duct damage *(arrow),* and early epithelial senescence changes *(inset).* The degenerated bile duct *(arrow)* is shown at higher magnification in the *inset.* Note the perivenular inflammation, hepatocyte dropout, and fibrosis.

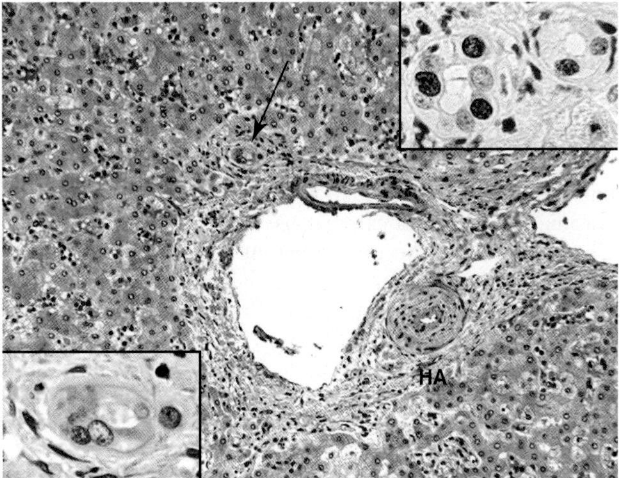

FIGURE 53.26 Early chronic rejection is characterized by senescence changes of the biliary epithelium (*arrow* and *bottom inset*), such as cytoplasmic eosinophilia, syncytial formation, ducts partially lined by epithelial cells, and expression of CDKN1A *(top inset)* without simultaneous expression of Ki67. Note the fibrointimal hyperplasia and luminal narrowing of a branch of the hepatic artery (HA).

is quite similar to active graft-versus-host disease (GVHD), which is covered later. Immunohistochemical markers of senescence and downregulated cell cycle progression, such as CDKN2A (p16) and CDKN1A (p21), are expressed in biliary epithelial cells under severe stress.[178,345] Downregulation of epithelial junctional proteins combined with upregulation of mesenchymal proteins may occur in response to injury.[346,347]

Traditionally defined late-stage chronic rejection is characterized by bile duct loss involving more than 50% of portal tracts. Arteriolar loss can also be seen.

Crawford and colleagues[348] defined a portal tract as "a focus within the parenchyma containing connective tissue (by Masson trichrome stain) and at least two luminal structures, each with a continuous connective tissue circumference." In normal liver sampled by percutaneous liver biopsy, bile ducts

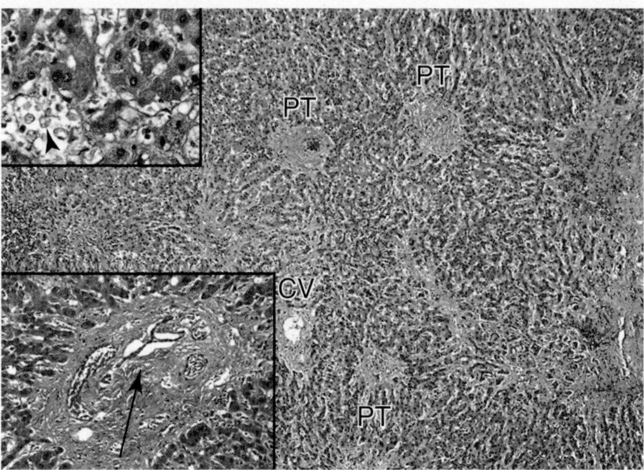

FIGURE 53.27 Late-stage chronic rejection within the lobule is characterized by severe perivenular fibrosis and at least focal central-to-central bridging fibrosis. It is almost invariably accompanied by centrilobular hepatocanalicular cholestasis and intrasinusoidal foam cell clusters (*top inset, arrowhead*). In the portal tracts, the late stage of chronic rejection is characterized by loss of small hepatic artery branches and small bile ducts, although an occasional biliary epithelial cell can be detected in portal tracts *(bottom inset, arrow). CV,* Central vein; *PT,* portal tract.

and hepatic artery branches are seen in 93% ± 6% and 91% ± 7% of portal tracts, respectively.[348] These percentages may be lower in larger tissue samples.[239] With two standard deviations from the normal as a cutoff, bile duct loss is more confidently diagnosed when less than 80% of portal tracts contain bile ducts. Arterial loss is diagnosed when less than 75% of portal tracts contain hepatic artery branches.

A similar approach uses the concept of bile duct–artery parallelism. Ductopenia can be defined by at least one unpaired artery in more than 10% of all portal tracts or two unpaired arteries in different portal tracts.[349] Unpaired arteries were defined as arteries without an accompanying bile duct within a distance of 10 hepatic artery diameters from the edge of the artery.[349]

Late chronic rejection can cause bile duct and arterial loss,[239,337] which can present difficulties when trying to apply these diagnostic algorithms. Portal tract recognition should be based primarily on the parenchymal location of the putative structure; cholestasis in chronic rejection is centrilobular.

A ductular reaction at the interface zone is unusual in chronic rejection unless the liver is in a recovery phase.[335,338,339] Staining with CK19 and CK7 can help document bile duct loss in chronic rejection, and the latter detects ductular metaplasia of periportal hepatocytes.[84] When a ductular reaction is easily noticeable by routine light microscopy, it usually signals either regrowth of bile ducts[335,338,339] or a downstream biliary stricture. The latter can be more confidently suggested by identifying periportal hepatocyte copper deposits, which are unusual in chronic rejection.

Early chronic rejection in perivenular areas is characterized primarily by lymphoplasmacytic and histiocytic inflammation (see Fig. 53.25),[200,209] often accompanied by hepatocyte dropout and mild perivenular fibrosis.[5,336] Spotty acidophilic hepatocytes elsewhere in the parenchyma can be seen during evolution from early to late chronic rejection.[350]

TABLE 53.8 Features of Early and Late Chronic Liver Allograft Rejection

Structure	Early Chronic Rejection	Late Chronic Rejection
Small bile ducts (<60 μm)	Bile duct loss in <50% of portal tracts	Loss in ≥50% of portal tracts
	Senescence-related changes involving most ducts: eosinophilic transformation of the cytoplasm; nuclear hyperchromasia; uneven nuclear spacing; ducts only partially lined by biliary epithelial cells	Degenerative changes in remaining bile ducts
Terminal hepatic venules and zone 3 hepatocytes	Intimal or luminal inflammation	Focal obliteration
	Lytic zone 3 necrosis and inflammation	Inflammation varies
	Mild perivenular fibrosis	Severe perivenular fibrosis, defined as central-to-central bridging fibrosis
Portal tract hepatic arterioles	Occasional loss involving <25% of portal tracts	Loss involving >25% of portal tracts
Large perihilar hepatic artery branches	Intimal inflammation, focal foam cell deposition without luminal compromise	Luminal narrowing by subintimal foam cells; fibrointimal proliferation
Large perihilar bile ducts	Inflammation, damage, and focal foam cell deposition	Mural fibrosis
Other	Transitional hepatitis* with spotty necrosis of hepatocytes	Sinusoidal foam cell accumulation; marked cholestasis

**Transitional hepatitis is characterized by mild lobular disarray and spotty, acidophilic necrosis of hepatocytes that can occur during evolution from early to late stages of chronic rejection.*

Modified from Demetris A, Adams D, Bellamy C, et al. Update of the International Banff Schema for Liver Allograft Rejection: working recommendations for the histopathologic staging and reporting of chronic rejection. An International Panel. Hepatology. *2000;31:792–799.*

Perivenular changes in late, traditionally defined, chronic rejection include moderate to severe (bridging) perivenular fibrosis and occasionally obliteration of terminal hepatic venules, similar to sinusoidal obstruction syndrome/veno-occlusive disease (see Fig. 53.27).[5] Well-developed cirrhosis arising from traditionally defined chronic rejection is unusual until the very late stages, when venous obliteration can lead to parenchymal extinction and venocentric cirrhosis.[333] True regenerative nodules are uncommon, possibly because coexistent obliterative arteriopathy blunts any regenerative response.[351] Perivenular hepatocyte ballooning and dropout, centrilobular hepatocanalicular cholestasis, obliterative portal venopathy with NRH, and intrasinusoidal foam cell clusters (rarely bile infarcts) are other common findings in late chronic rejection.

A final diagnosis of chronic rejection should be based on a combination of clinical, radiologic, laboratory, and pathological findings. Minimal histological diagnostic criteria are defined by the Banff consensus document[3] (see Table 53.8); early chronic rejection must include at least two of the following findings: (1) biliary epithelial senescent changes affecting most bile ducts and bile duct loss involving <50% of portal tracts, (2) occasional loss of <25% of portal tract hepatic arterioles, (3) at least mild perivenular fibrosis with or without centrizonal necrosis and inflammation, (4) foam cell arteriopathy and/or intimal inflammation without luminal compromise, (5) large perihilar bile ducts with inflammation and foam cell deposition, and (6) hepatitis with spotty necrosis of hepatocytes ("transition hepatitis"). Minimal diagnostic criteria for late chronic rejection must also include at least two of the following findings: (1) bile duct loss in >50% of portal tracts, (2) loss of >25% of portal tract hepatic arterioles, (3) central vein with at least moderate fibrosis with fibrous bridge formation and focal obliteration, (4) hepatic artery branch with foam cell arteriopathy with luminal compromise and fibrointimal hyperplasia, (5) perihilar bile duct mural fibrosis, and (6) sinusoidal foam cell accumulation and cholestasis.[3]

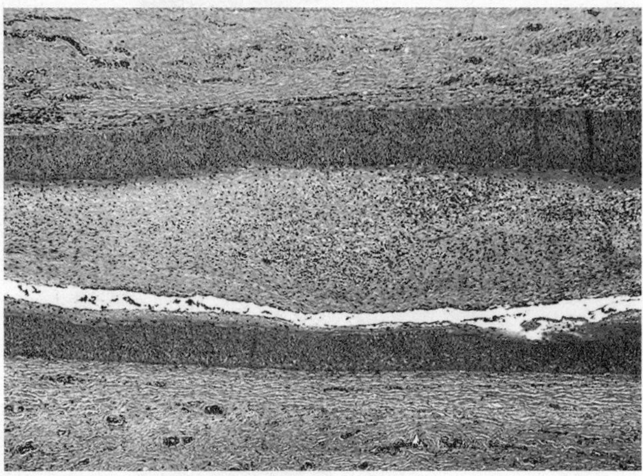

FIGURE 53.28 The obliterative arteriopathy characteristic of chronic rejection usually preferentially involves the first- and second-order branches of the hilar hepatic artery, although it may also involve the peripheral branches. It is characterized by intimal thickening and narrowing of the lumen. Intimal thickening is related to deposition of foamy macrophages and proliferation of myofibroblasts, which are intermixed with lymphocytes and foamy macrophages.

Not all of the aforementioned features can be reliably recognized on peripheral needle biopsy. Illustration of these features is much easier in explanted failed allograft specimens at the time of retransplantation because diagnostic findings can be seen in first-, second-, and third-order branches of the hepatic artery (Fig. 53.28). Obliterative arteriopathy is usually found in at least some of the perihilar arteries, except in cases characterized by bile duct loss and perivenular fibrosis alone. Accumulation of foamy macrophages usually occurs initially in the intima, which triggers proliferation of intimal and migration of medial donor-derived myofibroblasts. This causes intimal thickening, luminal narrowing, and medial thinning as arteries attempt to dilate and compensate for reduced arterial flow. Eventually, compensatory mechanisms fail, and the entire arterial wall may be replaced by foam cells. The artery may undergo thrombosis, causing necrosis of large bile ducts and ischemic cholangiopathy.

Foamy macrophages may also be seen around bile ducts and veins and within the connective tissue. Large perihilar bile ducts can show sloughing of the epithelium, biliary sludge, mural fibrosis, and acute and chronic inflammation in and around the ducts.

Chronic rejection staging assumes that the diagnosis has already been established with certainty.[3,5] According to Banff criteria, [3] *early chronic rejection* implies that a potential for recovery exists if the immunological insult can be mitigated, whereas *late chronic rejection* implies that the potential for recovery is limited and retransplantation should be considered. However, the clinical course after establishing a diagnosis varies considerably. Biopsy findings provide only one rough prognostic indicator of potential reversibility that should be correlated with other clinical and laboratory parameters.

A dedicated system for liver allograft fibrosis scoring has been proposed and validated by Venturi et al.[343,352] The 2016 comprehensive update of the Banff Working Group suggests adoption of this fibrosis scoring system. The fibrosis is assessed in three different compartments on a scale from 0 to 3 for a total score of 9 (Table 53.9).

TABLE 53.9 Liver Allograft Fibrosis Score*

Compartment/ Score	0	1	2	3
Portal tracts	No fibrosis	Nonexpanding fibrosis in less than 50% of portal tracts 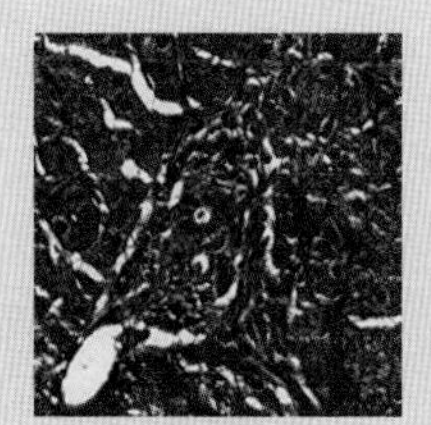	Fibrosis in more than 50% of portal tracts and/or expansion into short fibrous septa into periportal parenchyma 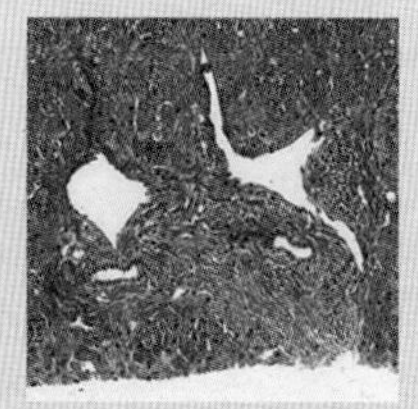	Marked expansion of most or all portal tracts with portal to portal or portal to central bridging fibrosis with or without occasional nodules 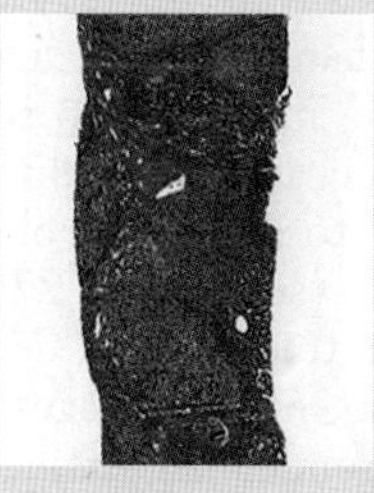
Sinusoids (zones 1 and 2)	No fibrosis	Little fibrosis with thin focal collagen deposits involving less than 50% of sinusoids 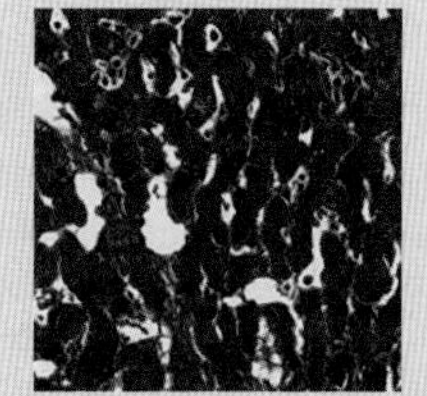	Little fibrosis with thin diffuse collage deposits involving more than 50% of sinusoids, or thicker but focal fibrosis in less than 50% of sinusoids 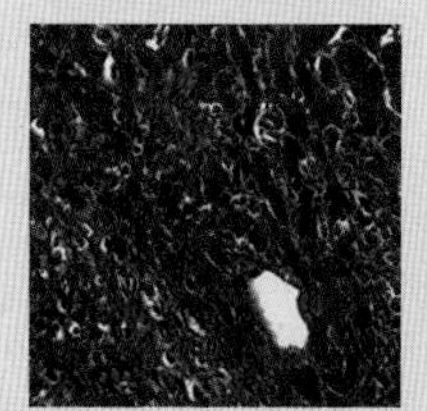	Thick, marked, and diffuse sinusoidal fibrosis 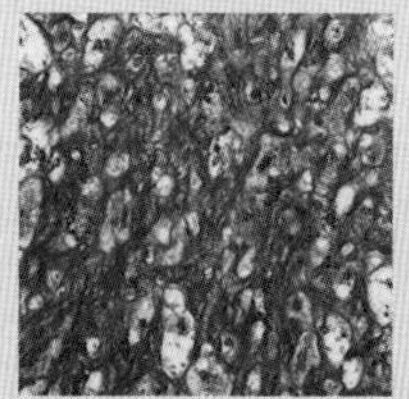
Centrilobular vein	No fibrosis	Circular perivenular fibrosis involving less than 50% of central veins without invasion into the perivenular parenchyma 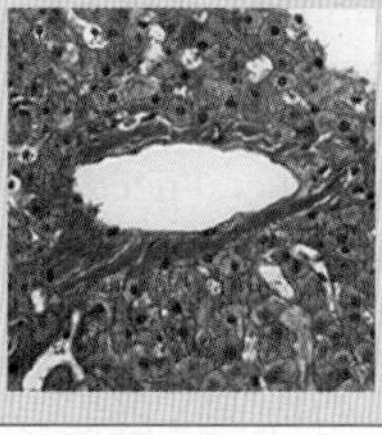	Circular perivenular fibrosis in more than 50% of central areas and/or expansion into short fibrous septa into perivenular parenchyma 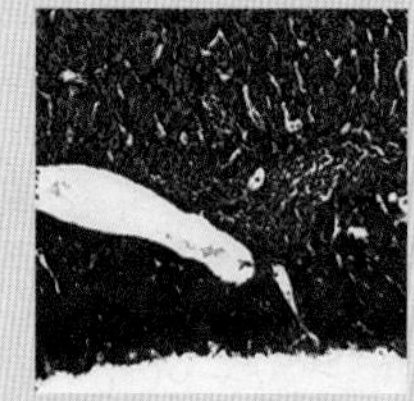	Marked centrilobular fibrosis with bridging to other central or portal areas 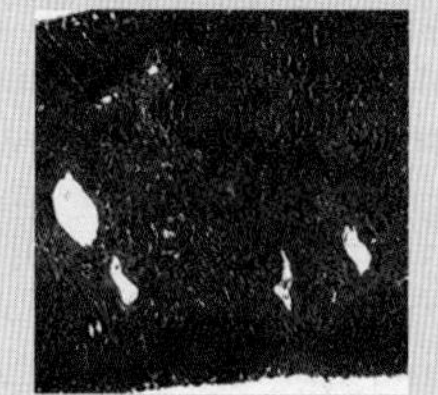

**Scoring is performed on three different compartments. The final score is calculated by adding the scores of the three components for a possible final score of 9.*

Modified from Venturi C, Sempoux C, Bueno J, et al. Novel histologic scoring system for long-term allograft fibrosis after liver transplantation in children. Am J Transplant. *2012;12(11):2986–2996.*

Differential Diagnosis

A diagnosis of traditionally defined chronic rejection is primarily based on damage and loss of small bile ducts and perivenular fibrosis in peripheral core needle biopsies; arteries with pathognomonic changes are only rarely seen.[5] Duct injury and ductopenia can also occur because of non–rejection-related complications, such as obstructive cholangiopathy, hepatic artery stricturing or thrombosis, cholangitic drug-induced liver injury (DILI), and CMV infection. Perivenular fibrosis can also be caused by suboptimal hepatic venous drainage and cAMR as well as other causes of perivenular injury. Therefore a diagnosis of chronic rejection based on biliary epithelial senescence or loss with or without perivenular fibrosis should first exclude other non–rejection-related causes of ductal injury and perivenular fibrosis.

Chronic rejection is probably most difficult to distinguish from suboptimal biliary drainage including recurrent PSC.[179] Histopathological features that can be seen in both disorders include biliary epithelial cell senescence-related changes, hepatocanalicular cholestasis, widespread ductular metaplasia of periportal hepatocytes on CK7 staining, and focal bile infarcts. Findings that favor suboptimal biliary drainage include bile duct loss in some portal tracts, accompanied by a ductular reaction in others; neutrophil clusters within the lobules; bile infarcts; deposition of copper or copper-associated protein in periportal hepatocytes; and hepatocanalicular cholestasis out of proportion to the prevalence of ductopenia (<50%). Features that favor chronic rejection include central perivenulitis or fibrosis and an absence of changes typical of suboptimal biliary drainage, described earlier, especially including negative staining for periportal hepatocyte copper deposits in chronic rejection. The clinical course of events can also provide important information; persistent TCMR or suboptimal immunosuppression favor chronic rejection, whereas a history of biliary strictures or ischemic cholangiopathy risk factors favors suboptimal biliary drainage. Cholangiography or angiography may be required to distinguish chronic rejection from biliary obstruction. Studies usually show pruning and poor peripheral filling in patients with chronic rejection.

Isolated ductopenia involving less than 50% of portal tracts can be seen without significant elevations of liver function tests. Whether these uncommon cases represent an early phase of chronic rejection or a sampling issue remains uncertain. Isolated perivenular fibrosis can be caused by mechanical outflow obstruction, DILI, cAMR,[3,144-147] and nonrejection causes of hepatic outflow obstruction. C4d staining and evaluation of DSA can help exclude cAMR.[3,148]

The most reliable approach to diagnosing chronic rejection is to review all prior biopsies, conduct copper, C4d, and CK7 staining, evaluate DSA, and closely correlate the histopathological findings with the clinical course.

Posttransplantation Infections

The pathologist should always consider the possibility of an infection when reviewing tissue specimens from liver allograft recipients. Stress and operation-related tissue damage combined with immunosuppression needed to prevent rejection in the first 2 months after transplantation places the recipient at high risk for serious opportunistic fungal and viral infections. Bacterial infections usually occur more than 6 months after transplantation. Fever, anastomotic or wound dehiscence, retransplantation, persistent abdominal pain, leukocytosis, and vascular thrombosis are clinical signs, symptoms, or circumstances that should arouse further suspicion of infection.

Because bacterial and fungal infections often arise in nonviable tissue, when encountered, necrotic tissue should be routinely subjected to special stains for microorganisms. Granulomas with or without coexistent acute and chronic inflammation are surrogate markers of infection, but they may not occur because of immunosuppression. Histopathological manifestations of deep fungal and bacterial infections are familiar to most pathologists and are beyond the scope of this chapter.

In general, infections resulting from opportunistic viral infections such as CMV, Epstein-Barr virus (EBV), herpes simplex virus (HSV), varicella-zoster virus (VZV), or adenovirus do not usually cause clinically significant acute hepatitis in immunocompetent individuals. However, their manifestations in immunosuppressed liver allograft recipients depend on the clinical setting. Reactivation infections usually develop in adult patients carrying latent infections, whereas more severe primary infections usually develop in naïve, mostly pediatric populations. An important aspect of all infections, however, is that viral shedding into the peripheral circulation can be monitored by measuring viral antigens or nucleic acids. When viral markers surpass certain empirically set thresholds, preemptive lowering of immunosuppression and treatment with specific antiviral agents can prevent active disease.[353] Therefore monitoring and preemptive therapy has dramatically reduced the incidence of diseases (histopathological manifestations) caused by these viruses. A tissue diagnosis of CMV, EBV, HSV, adenovirus, or VZV hepatitis is becoming rare for routine adult cases and uncommon for pediatric cases.

Cytomegalovirus Hepatitis

Effective prophylactic and preemptive therapy has greatly decreased the incidence of CMV hepatitis, but among seronegative recipients, prophylaxis has also been associated with suboptimal long-term outcomes.[354,355] Even though clinically significant CMV disease is uncommon or rare, it has been associated with an increased risk of TCMR and chronic rejection, biliary strictures, vascular thrombosis, accelerated HCV disease recurrence (currently irrelevant), other opportunistic infections, and decreased patient and graft survival.[354,355]

Risk factors for CMV hepatitis include seronegativity before transplantation, TCMR, enhanced viral replication (usually associated with overimmunosuppression), mycophenolate mofetil and/or antileukocyte antibody therapy, human herpesvirus 6 (HHV-6) and HHV-7 co-infections, gene polymorphisms for toll-like receptors, mannose-binding lectin deficiency, chemokine and cytokine defects (e.g., interleukin-10 [IL-10], CC2 [formerly MCP1], CCR5), and deficiency of viral-specific T cells.[354,355] An emerging challenge is compartmentalized disease, in which CMV is detectable in tissue biopsies but not in serological or molecular assays.[354,355]

Clinical Features

Depending on the extent of viral dissemination, any organ system can be involved. The most common signs and symptoms of active CMV infection are gastrointestinal in origin. Fever, diarrhea, mucosal ulcers, leukopenia, and low-grade hepatitis can be seen; the latter usually manifests as modestly elevated liver function tests.[354,355] Respiratory insufficiency and retinitis are signs of severe disseminated disease.[354,355]

Pathological Features

CMV hepatitis is most commonly characterized by spotty hepatocyte necrosis, Kupffer cell hypertrophy, mild lobular disarray, neutrophilic and/or histiocytic microabscesses and/or microgranulomas, and patchy lobular inflammation. Under current pharmacological therapies, infected hepatocytes rarely contain diagnostic nuclear or cytoplasmic inclusions. Instead, inclusions are usually limited to patients who are over-immunosuppressed and not adequately monitored or treated. Any cell type can be infected. Diagnostic features include large eosinophilic intranuclear inclusions surrounded by a clear halo and accompanied by small basophilic or amphophilic cytoplasmic inclusions. In severe cases (largely of historical significance), numerous cells containing CMV inclusions can be found throughout the liver. CMV infection alone does not cause submassive or massive necrosis.[356]

Infected cells are often surrounded by neutrophils, microabscesses, or clusters of macrophages and lymphocytes, or *microgranulomas*. CMV hepatitis can be associated with mild lymphoplasmacytic portal inflammation with bile duct infiltration and damage that can resemble TCMR or early chronic rejection (Fig. 53.29). Bile duct loss and chronic rejection have been associated with persistent CMV infection in allografts.[354,355]

Viral inclusions are currently rare because of effective therapy; therefore vigilance is required to suspect the diagnosis on H&E findings. Occasional cases may contain fragmented nuclear CMV inclusions but are difficult to recognize without immunoperoxidase staining or in situ hybridization. Rapidly dividing tissues such as young granulation tissue, proliferating cholangioles, the edges of infarcts, abscesses, or other intraparenchymal defects are fertile soil for CMV growth.[85] Immunoperoxidase stain for an epitope of the CMV matrix phosphoprotein 65 (pp65) may be more sensitive, but it requires frozen tissue. It is used less frequently than the monoclonal antibody against CMV p52, an early nuclear protein that works better in FFPE specimens.[354]

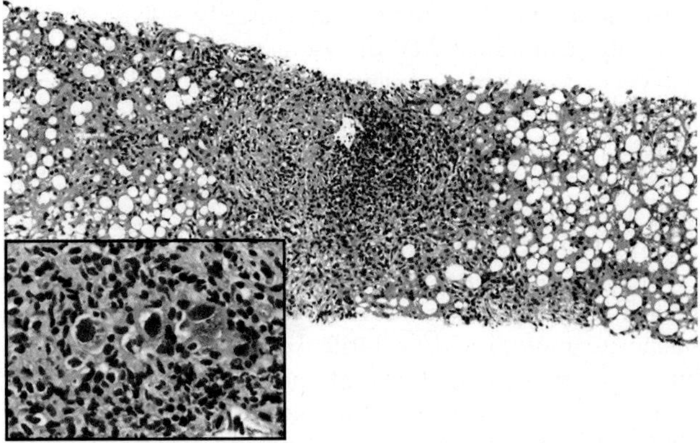

FIGURE 53.29 Cytomegalovirus (CMV) hepatitis can show mononuclear or mixed portal inflammation, focal bile duct damage, and small clusters of neutrophils or macrophages (i.e., microgranulomas) scattered randomly throughout the hepatic lobules. *Inset,* Characteristic nuclear and cytoplasmic CMV inclusions are seen in an inflamed portal tract.

Differential Diagnosis

CMV hepatitis can be difficult to distinguish from the early phase of HBV or HCV recurrence (currently both are rare because of effective DAA) and EBV hepatitis. CMV can also be difficult to distinguish from HSV hepatitis because both disorders can cause multinucleation and intranuclear eosinophilic inclusions surrounded by halos. However, CMV inclusion–containing cells can also show small basophilic or amphophilic cytoplasmic inclusions that are not seen in HSV-infected cells. Conversely, circumscribed foci of coagulative necrosis characteristic of HSV is not a feature of CMV hepatitis.

In CMV cases presenting without inclusions, subtle clues that enable distinction from early acute HBV or HCV hepatitis include less lobular disarray and hepatocyte swelling in the former. Microabscesses and microgranulomas are not usually seen in the early lobular phase of HBV or HCV infection. A definitive diagnosis of CMV hepatitis requires characteristic inclusions or demonstration of viral antigens or nucleic acids with immunostaining or in situ hybridization.

CMV hepatitis can resemble EBV hepatitis because both may show mild lymphoplasmacytic portal and lobular inflammation and occasionally contain blastic and atypical lymphocytes. However, EBV hepatitis usually causes more substantial sinusoidal lymphocytosis and mild cytological atypia of lymphocytes, whereas CMV hepatitis causes more intralobular foci of inflammation (e.g., microgranulomas, microabscesses). Deeper sections, staining for EBV and CMV viral antigens, and in situ hybridization for EBV nucleic acid are usually required to make the correct diagnosis.

CMV hepatitis most commonly develops in patients who have recently completed an augmented immunosuppressive regimen for rejection. In some cases, it is difficult to determine whether the liver injury is attributable to residual CMV hepatitis, relapse of TCMR, or development of chronic rejection. O'Grady and colleagues showed an association between CMV infection and chronic rejection,[357,358] further complicating the issue. Others have not found this association.[359] Priority should be given to the CMV diagnosis followed by augmented anti-CMV therapy and follow-up biopsy after 1 to 2 weeks if liver function abnormalities persist.

Herpes Simplex and Varicella-Zoster Viral Hepatitis

Type 1 and 2 HSV and VZV hepatitis may occur any time after transplantation.[356] Patients often present with fever, vesicular rashes, fatigue, body pain, and elevated liver injury tests. Undetected HSV hepatitis can rapidly lead to submassive or massive hepatic necrosis, hypotension, disseminated intravascular coagulation, metabolic acidosis, and death.[360] Fulminant cases are more common with primary infections. VZV-induced hepatitis is rare because of effective vaccines and anti-VZV hepatitis immunoglobulin.[361]

Pathological Features

Recognition and prompt reporting of HSV and VZV hepatitis is essential because of the availability of effective pharmacological therapy. Without treatment, the infection can be rapidly fatal. Localized and diffuse patterns of HSV hepatitis have been described.[360] Both histopathological patterns cause circumscribed areas of coagulative-type necrosis (Fig. 53.30).[356,360] The necrotic centers are typically occupied by ghosts of hepatocytes intermixed with neutrophils and nuclear debris. Viable hepatocytes rim the periphery and usually contain HSV or VZV hepatitis inclusions. Infected cells are usually slightly enlarged and contain ground-glass nuclei or characteristic Cowdry type A eosinophilic inclusions. Multinucleate smudgy cells are occasionally seen. However, diagnostic inclusions of HSV or VZV hepatitis may be absent on H&E-stained slides.

Immunoperoxidase stains for HSV antigens are confirmatory. In our experience, antibody preparations used to detect HSV 1 and 2 can show cross-reactivity with each other and with VZV hepatitis, making it difficult to distinguish these viruses. In our experience, antibodies used to detect the VZV hepatitis precursor and mature glycoprotein are more discriminating. If a histopathological diagnosis of HSV or VZV hepatitis is being considered on the basis of H&E staining, the physicians should be immediately notified.[362] This will prompt effective antiviral therapy that can be discontinued if the diagnosis is not confirmed on immunostaining.

Human Herpesvirus 6

HHV-6, a member of the β-*Herpesviridae* subfamily of human herpesviruses, is a ubiquitous virus that usually infects humans during the first 2 years of life and then remains dormant in more than 90% of adults.[363] Reactivation infection occurs in 15% to 80% of liver allograft recipients, usually during the first 2 to 8 weeks after transplantation; it is often precipitated by over-immunosuppression.[363]

HHV-6 clinical manifestations include fever with or without rash, myelosuppression, hepatitis with allograft dysfunction, pneumonitis, and neurological dysfunction. Indirect effects attributed to HHV-6 include exacerbation of CMV disease, increased severity of HCV recurrence (of historical significance), and increased manifestations from other opportunistic infections.[363]

Liver allograft biopsy findings include lymphocytic portal inflammation and patchy lobular inflammation, including microabscesses,[364,365] confluent periportal "targetoid" hepatocellular necrosis,[366] and syncytial giant cell hepatitis.[367] TCMR can also reportedly coexist.[364,365] Syncytial giant cell transformation of biliary epithelium was reported in the setting of heart transplantation.[368] Immunoperoxidase stains for HHV-6 localize viral antigens primarily to mononuclear inflammatory cells[364] and hepatocyte syncytial giant cells.[367]

Human Herpesvirus 8

HHV-8 is a lymphotropic γ-*Herpesviridae* family member that contributes to the development of Kaposi sarcoma, multicentric Castleman disease, and primary effusion lymphoma in the general population and among liver allograft recipients.[369-371] HHV-8 infection is prevalent in sub-Saharan Africa and in southern Italy, but is less prevalent elsewhere.[369-371] As with other opportunistic viral infections, primary HHV-8 is often more severe and can result in liver dysfunction, multiorgan failure, multicentric Castleman disease, and Kaposi sarcoma.[369-371] Liver biopsy findings resemble those of acute viral hepatitis (Fig. 53.31), showing lobular disarray, ballooning, hepatocyte swelling and apoptosis, and a ductular reaction.[369-371]

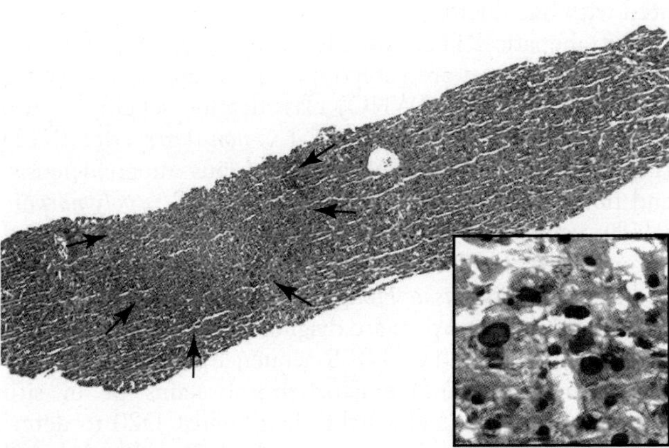

FIGURE 53.30 Herpes simplex virus (HSV) hepatitis and varicella-zoster virus (VZV) hepatitis are characterized by maplike areas of necrosis that do not show any particular geographic distribution *(arrows)*. *Inset,* At high magnification, a characteristic eosinophilic intranuclear inclusion of HSV infection can be seen.

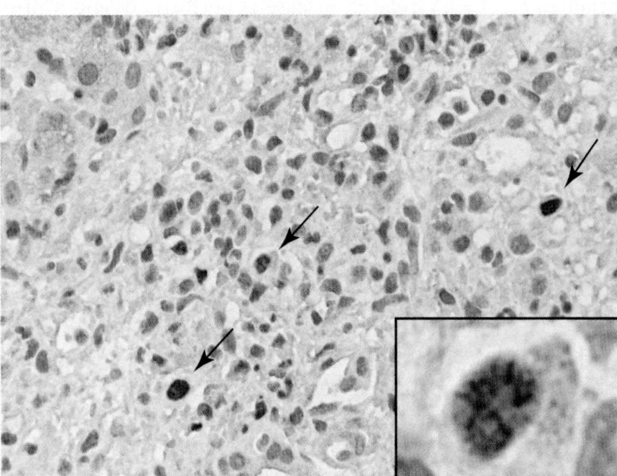

FIGURE 53.31 Liver allograft biopsy from a 53-year-old man 4 months after liver transplantation for alcohol-related cirrhosis shows marked lobular reactivity, with clusters of apoptotic hepatocytes, Kupffer cell hypertrophy, and sinusoidal lymphocytosis. Immunohistochemical staining for human herpesvirus 8 with the LANA2 antibody was positive in scattered cells *(arrows)* with a homogeneous or speckled nuclear staining pattern *(inset)*.

Epstein-Barr Virus

EBV infection immortalizes B lymphocytes in vitro but lies dormant in B lymphocytes and some epithelial cells in vivo because the immune system effectively controls viral replication.[372-374] Potent immunosuppression depresses the T cell–immune surveillance that normally keeps EBV replication and B cell proliferation in check. Immunosuppression can enhance EBV replication and increase the risk of clinically manifested EBV infection, ranging from self-limited EBV-like syndromes to aggressive PTLDs.[372-374] Similar to other opportunistic viruses, disease incidence and severity is higher among seronegative, usually pediatric recipients. The likelihood of infection increases with time after transplantation and is strongly associated with high-dose immunosuppression.[372-374]

Clinical Features

EBV-related complications include hepatitis; gastroenteritis; lymphoproliferative disorders (B cell, T cell, natural killer [NK] cell, and Hodgkin-like); smooth muscle tumors; and a variety of cancers (e.g., nasopharyngeal, gastric).[372-376] Signs and symptoms often resemble infectious mononucleosis, including fever, lymphadenopathy, pharyngitis, and elevated liver injury tests. Atypical presentations include bone pain, arthralgia, joint effusions, encephalitis, pneumonitis, and ascites. Liver allograft hepatitis or posttransplantation lymphoproliferative disease (PTLD) involvement usually produces mildly elevated ALT and AST values; pancytopenia is occasionally found.[377-379]

Risk factors for more serious EBV-associated disease include primary infection, over-immunosuppression, underlying Langerhans cell histiocytosis, and coexistent CMV disease. Late-onset PTLD does not appear to be influenced by the type of immunosuppressive agents but instead the overall immunosuppression duration and intensity.[372,373,380]

Peripheral blood monitoring for EBV nucleic acid is effectively used to monitor viral replication[372]; when elevated, physical examination for lymphadenopathy and other signs of EBV-related disease is performed, and a preemptive immunosuppression reduction is usually made.[381] Treatment for EBV-related disorders depends on the clinicopathological presentation and clonality of the proliferating lymphocytes. Polyclonal infectious mononucleosis-like syndromes usually respond to a reduction of immunosuppression, whereas monomorphic PTLD resembling clonal lymphomas often require more aggressive immunotherapy or chemotherapy, or both.[372-374,376]

Pathological Features

EBV-related hepatic histopathology ranges from mild sinusoidal lymphocytosis to low-grade acute hepatitis characterized by portal expansion because of atypical monomorphic lymphocytes (resembling diffuse large B cell lymphomas) signaling PTLD (Fig. 53.32) involvement.[377-379,382] Patients with enhanced EBV replication and viremia can show increased intragraft T cells and B cells,[383] with the latter occasionally containing EBV-encoded small RNA (EBER) sequences. Rare EBER-positive cells may be admixed with other inflammatory cells associated with other causes of allograft dysfunction, even in patients without EBV-related disorders.[382] The assertion that EBV causes chronic hepatitis or recurrent acute relapses is controversial.[384]

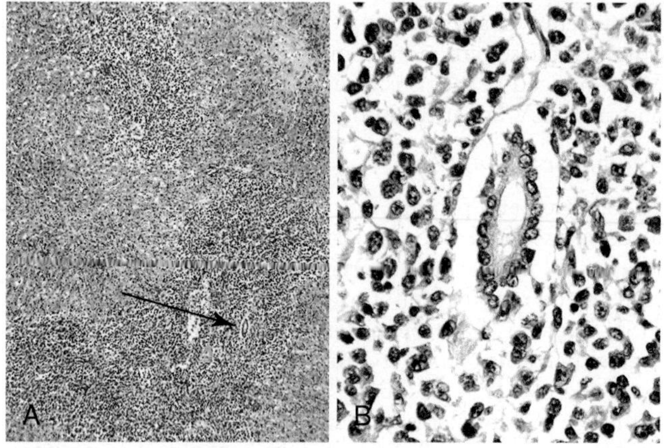

FIGURE 53.32 A, Liver allograft involvement by posttransplantation lymphoproliferative disease produces a maplike expansion of the portal tracts with atypical lymphoblasts and cells with plasmacytoid differentiation. **B,** At higher magnification, note the absence of overt bile duct damage despite a marked inflammatory infiltrate.

Low-grade EBV "hepatitis" usually manifests as mild portal lymphoplasmacytic inflammation and mild sinusoidal lymphocytosis composed of small or mildly atypical lymphocytes, similar to EBV hepatitis seen in native livers. Other lobular changes include focal mild hepatocellular swelling and disarray, occasional apoptotic hepatocytes, and regenerative activity (plate thickening and mitotic activity).

Hepatic PTLDs manifest as cytologically atypical often monomorphic lymphoplasmacytic portal infiltrates; subendothelial localization of lymphocytes in portal and central veins can mimic TCMR. Atypical cells are usually intermixed with small and blastic lymphocytes, plasmacytoid lymphocytes, and plasma cells in early or polymorphic lesions. In monomorphic lesions, atypical cells predominate and manifest as maplike enlargement of portal tracts resulting from sheets of atypical immunoblastic cells that can obscure the normal portal anatomic landmarks. Atypical cells can also be seen in the sinusoids. Rare cases can develop confluent necrosis. Hodgkin lymphoma–like PTLDs with classic Reed-Sternberg cells can also occur, and they may be associated with bile duct loss.

Extrahepatic PTLDs usually occur in the lymph nodes and intestines and are categorized according to the World Health Organization (WHO) classification scheme[385] into four major categories: Category 1 is *non-destructive PTLD* (i.e., plasmacytic hyperplasia, infectious mononucleosis, and florid follicular hyperplasia); category 2 is *polymorphic PTLD;* category 3 is *monomorphic PTLD* (subcategorized according to the B cell or T cell lymphoma it resembles); and category 4 is *classic Hodgkin lymphoma PTLD.*

EBV-related disorders are diagnosed by in situ hybridization for EBV RNA (i.e., EBER sequence). Routine workup should include immunohistochemical stains or in situ hybridization for κ and λ light chains and CD20 to determine possible responsiveness to anti-CD20 antibodies and other lymphocyte phenotype markers when PTLD resembles conventional lymphomas.[374] If fresh tissue is available, a portion may be submitted for flow cytometry and molecular analyses, which enables a more detailed phenotypic characterization and study of immunoglobulin gene rearrangement, respectively.

Differential Diagnosis

EBV hepatitis and PTLD can be difficult to distinguish from severe TCMR on cursory examination. Features that favor TCMR include pleomorphic, rejection-type portal or perivenular inflammatory infiltrates, conspicuous eosinophils, and severe bile duct damage that is proportional to the severity of inflammation. Features favoring EBV include a relatively monomorphic portal infiltrate consisting primarily of activated and immunoblastic mononuclear cells (predominantly B cells).[386] Many infiltrative cells show plasmacytic differentiation, and some show atypical cytological features. Patchy and lymphocytic cholangitis is less severe than would be expected based on the severity of the portal inflammatory infiltrate, whereas eosinophils are usually less conspicuous.

Low-grade EBV hepatitis can be difficult to distinguish from nonspecific "reactive hepatitis" and acute HBV, HCV, or CMV hepatitis. HCV and EBV hepatitis can both show sinusoidal lymphocytosis, but EBV-related disorders usually contain atypical cells. In contrast, lymphocytes associated with HCV hepatitis are usually small, round, and inactive appearing, and they form nodular aggregates in the portal tracts.[377-379,382] Clinical suspicion and increased peripheral blood EBV levels also point to the correct diagnosis.

The final diagnosis of any type of EBV-related disorder depends on in situ hybridization for EBV RNA (i.e., EBER probe). However, results should be interpreted with caution[387] because rare EBER-positive cells are found in lymphoid tissues from the general population. These cells are found with slightly increased frequency in allograft recipients, the significance of which is controversial.[387] However, clustering of EBER-positive cells or the presence of EBER-positive cells in tissues that show other pathological features of EBV-associated disease indicates enhanced EBV replication. These patients are at increased risk for EBV-related diseases.

Adenovirus Hepatitis

Pathophysiology

Adenovirus is a double-stranded DNA virus with 51 serotypes. It causes a substantial number of respiratory infections in children younger than 5 years of age and manifests as conjunctivitis, pharyngitis, croup, bronchiolitis, bronchitis, and pneumonia; diarrhea can also occur. Adenoviral allograft hepatitis is largely restricted to primary infections in pediatric recipients,[388-391] although adult cases have been reported[392,393] and mimic those seen in the general population.[394]

Adenovirus hepatitis usually first presents 50 to 100 days after transplantation.[394] Symptoms include fever, respiratory distress, elevated liver function tests, diarrhea, and leukocytosis; the diagnosis is confirmed by liver biopsy examination.[390-393] Adenovirus subtypes 1, 2, and 5 have been isolated from the lung and gastrointestinal tract.[390,391,395] Allograft hepatitis is most often caused by viral subtype 5, but in the general population, hepatitis has also been caused by subtypes 2, 11, and 16.[390,391]

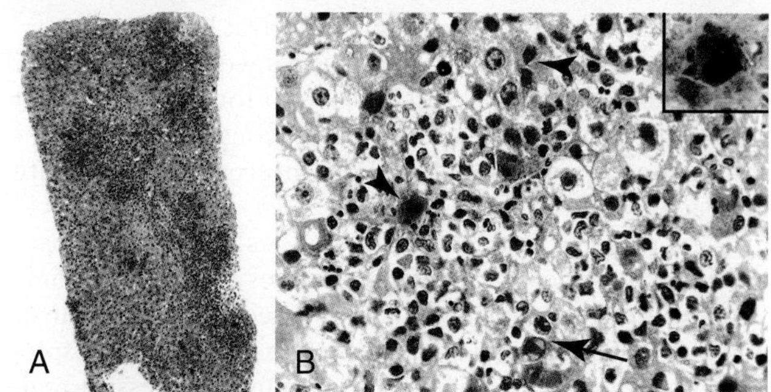

FIGURE 53.33 A, Specimen of adenovirus hepatitis shows aggregates of macrophages with few lymphocytes and hepatocellular necrosis. Some cases may have a pattern of necrosis similar to herpes simplex virus or varicella-zoster virus infection. **B,** Characteristic smudgy cells *(arrowheads)* and intranuclear inclusions *(arrow)* of adenovirus infection are positive with immunoperoxidase staining *(inset)*.

Histopathological Features

Adenovirus hepatitis is uncommon but is suspected by suspicious nuclear inclusions that are difficult to recognize with certainty. The extent of associated necrosis ranges from spotty to submassive or massive necrosis.[388] Typical cases show "poxlike" granulomas that consist of macrophages with or without neutrophils spread randomly throughout the liver parenchyma (Fig. 53.33). Alternatively, the granulomas can surround small, maplike areas of necrosis.[390-392] Viral inclusions are usually found in nuclei of viable hepatocytes near the edge of necrotic zones or granulomas. Infected cells have a smudgy appearance with crowding of chromatin near the nuclear membrane, which makes the nucleus appear like a "baked muffin." Immunohistochemical staining is usually required to confirm the diagnosis. Given that there are 51 serotypes, it is prudent to use antibodies reactive with the hexon protein common to all serotypes (e.g., MAB805, blend of clones 20/11 and 2/6, Chemicon International, Temecula, CA).[393]

Differential Diagnosis

Other causes of focal hepatocyte necrosis and hepatic granulomas include HSV or VZV, infarcts, and deep fungal and mycobacterial infections. Adenovirus usually causes less necrosis than HSV or VZV hepatitis. Multinucleated giant cells are rare in adenoviral hepatitis. Adenovirus-associated granulomas are usually much larger than the small necrogranulomas of CMV hepatitis. CMV causes cytomegaly and produces eosinophilic intranuclear inclusions surrounded by a clear halo and basophilic or amphophilic small cytoplasmic inclusions. Adenovirus does not cause cytomegaly; adenovirus causes a "smudgy" nuclear appearance, and cytoplasmic inclusions are not seen. Immunostaining or in situ hybridization for adenovirus antigens is usually needed to confirm the diagnosis. Stains are used to exclude HSV, VZV, and CMV viral antigens or nucleic acids.

LATE LIVER ALLOGRAFT DYSFUNCTION

Determining the cause or causes of late dysfunction from liver allograft biopsies and consequences of any findings has become simultaneously more challenging and increasingly important. Excellent short-term survival, effective control of recurrent diseases (e.g., HBV, HCV, and PBC), and steadily improving long-term survival limits the spectrum of potential insults. These issues were addressed by members of the Banff Working Group for Liver Allograft Pathology, who spent several years constructing a consensus document to help guide interpretation of late biopsies.[4]

Late protocol liver allograft biopsies have been abandoned at most centers. Instead, biopsies are obtained only when there is unexplained and sustained elevation of liver injury tests above baseline values for that patient.[4] Despite differences in the recipient pool, immunosuppressive regimens, and study designs, the structural integrity, biopsies findings, and causes of late liver allograft dysfunction (>1 year) are remarkably similar among various centers and over time.[181,317]

Leading causes of late liver allograft dysfunction include recurrence of the original disease, (especially nonalcoholic steatohepatitis, NASH), suboptimal biliary drainage,[181,317] and classically defined acute and/or chronic TCMR (4% to 38% of late biopsies). Hepatic steatosis and chronic steatohepatitis has gradually become the "new normal" and is especially common as recurrent and de novo disease late after transplantation. A complete clinical and laboratory profile including results of therapeutic interventions or diagnostic tests, original disease, immunosuppression levels, and any previous biopsy findings should be incorporated into a final interpretation.[4,181,317]

Many programs have abandoned protocol biopsies in asymptomatic, long-term survivors with normal or near-normal liver test values, which is controversial.[4,317,396-398] Arguments against obtaining biopsies in such patients include unpleasant patient experience, biopsy costs and risks, and the potential for precipitation of unnecessary therapy, and these should be weighed against early detection of clinically silent de novo and recurrent disease (late-onset TCMR, AIH, alcoholic steatohepatitis/NASH) and identification of recipients who may safely benefit from lower immunosuppression.[4,181,317,399]

Most biopsies (>70%) obtained after more than 1 year from recipients with elevated liver injury tests show significant abnormalities.[4,181,317,399] Recurrent disease, suboptimal biliary tract drainage, late-onset subclinical rejection (TCMR and/or cAMR), and chronic steatosis/steatohepatitis are common findings. A minority of biopsies from asymptomatic recipients (~25%) with normal liver function test results also show significant abnormalities, especially if the original disease is one that commonly recurs (e.g., NASH, alcohol, PBC, AIH, and TCMR). [4,181,317,399]

Minor pathological abnormalities are also common (~70%), even in the absence of recurrent disease. Included are mild portal venopathy and NRH, thickening and hyalinization of small hepatic artery branches, fibrosis, steatosis, and nonspecific portal inflammation with or without interface activity[4] and lobular inflammation. As recurrent disease becomes less common, it is becoming apparent that many of these seemingly minor changes are attributable to indolent rejection reactions.[183]

Laboratory tests used to establish a specific disease diagnosis before transplantation should be interpreted with caution after transplantation.[4] For example, autoantibodies (e.g., AMA, ANA) can reappear after transplantation in patients with PBC or AIH, regardless of whether or not histopathological evidence of disease recurrence is detected.

Because more than one insult can contribute to late post-transplantation allograft injury, a complete clinical and serological correlation, including DSA determinations, greatly assists in the final interpretation.[4,399] For example, late-onset TCMR and de novo DSA appearance is often precipitated by inadequate immunosuppression, as is recurrent AIH.[4,317]

Criteria used to diagnose the various causes of late liver allograft dysfunction[4] should be supported by positive serological, molecular, immunological, or radiographical evidence, whereas other insults with similar morphological manifestations should be reasonably excluded (Tables 53.10 and 53.11). Monitoring progressive fibrosis is an important aspect of long-term follow-up, particularly in pediatric recipients [146,216] and in patients with diseases that commonly recur (e.g., AIH, NASH, alcohol, PBC, PSC). More recent recognition of active chronic AMR may contribute to progressive perivenular, sinusoidal, and other patterns of fibrosis.[3,147,148] Noninvasive assays (e.g., elastrography) have been proposed to replace biopsies, but they provide suboptimal information and do not enable further elucidation of underlying pathophysiological mechanisms.[400,401]

In adults, recurrence of the patient's original disease is quite common and a significant cause of late liver allograft injury, whereas TCMR is most common in pediatric recipients.[183] However, many diseases that used to recur (e.g., HBV, HCV, PBC) now have effective therapies that either diminish the need for transplantation or prevent or greatly ameliorate the severity and impact of disease recurrence. Therefore rejection (TCMR and chronic AMR) is playing an increasingly common role in late graft injury along with recurrent hepatocellular and cholangiocarcinomas, toxic insults, and metabolic conditions (e.g., alcohol abuse, adverse drug reactions, metabolic syndrome).

Eligibility for transplantation in patients with cirrhosis complicated by hepatocellular carcinoma is based on the stage of the disease at the time of transplantation. Candidates who fulfill the Milan criteria (i.e., one lesion ≤5 cm or two or three lesions ≤3 cm) with a serum AFP ≤ 1000 ng/mL are given added MELD priority, but data suggest that these criteria are too stringent.[402,403] Highly selected, early-stage (I and II), localized, node-negative cholangiocarcinomas in patients who have received neoadjuvant chemoradiation may be treated by transplantation, particularly those with PSC.[404]

Numerous other diseases of uncertain origin can recur after liver transplantation. They include sarcoidosis,[405,406] idiopathic granulomatous hepatitis,[181] postinfantile giant cell hepatitis,[407] and Budd-Chiari syndrome, although Budd-Chiari syndrome is associated with coagulation abnormalities.[408] Liver transplantation can also purposely transmit diseases from donor to recipient; examples include familial amyloidosis polyneuropathy[56] and oxalosis.[57] In these situations, genetically abnormal but morphologically normal livers are used as "domino" transplants in which the life-prolonging therapeutic effects of a disease-producing liver are thought to outweigh the long-term consequences of disease transmission.

TABLE 53.10 Common Histopathological Features of Late Liver Allograft Dysfunction*

Histopathological Features	AIH	Acute Rejection	Chronic Rejection	Chronic Viral Hepatitis B and C	PBC	PSC or BD Strictures
Distribution, severity, and composition of portal inflammation	Usually diffuse; predominantly mononuclear, intensity varies; often a prominent plasma cell component	Usually diffuse; intensity varies; mixed, rejection-type infiltrate	Patchy; usually minimal or mild lympho-plasmacytic	Patchy; intensity varies, predominantly mononuclear; nodular aggregates	Noticeably patchy; intensity varies, predominantly mononuclear; nodular aggregates and granulomas	Usually patchy to diffuse, depending on stage; mild neutrophilic, eosinophilic, or occasionally mononuclear predominant
Presence and type of interface activity	Usually prominent and defining feature: necro-inflammatory type; often plasma cell rich	Focally present and mild necro-inflammatory type	Minimal or absent	Variable, usually not prominent, necro-inflammatory and ductular types	Important feature later in disease process: ductular and necro-inflammatory types with copper deposition	Prominent and defining feature: ductular type with portal and periportal edema
BD inflammation and damage	Varies; involves a minority of BDs	Usually involves most BDs	Focal, ongoing lymphocytic BD damage; inflammation wanes with duct loss	Variable; if present, involves a minority of BDs	Granulomatous or focally severe lymphocytic cholangitis is diagnostic in proper setting	Periductal lamellar edema, fibrous cholangitis, acute cholangitis, multiple intraportal ductal profiles
Biliary epithelial senescence changes and small bile loss	Absent or involves a minority of BDs or portal tracts, but may be focally severe	Absent or involves a minority of BDs	Senescence or atrophy and atypia involves most remaining BDs	Absent or involves a minority of BDs	Small BD loss associated with ductular reaction	Small BD loss associated with ductular reaction
Perivenular mononuclear inflammation and/or hepatocyte dropout	Varies; can involve most perivenular regions, similar to rejection; may be plasma cell rich	Varies; if defining feature, should involve most perivenular regions; may show subendothelial inflammation of veins	Usually present but varies	Variable, but usually mild; involves a minority of perivenular regions	Variable, but usually mild; involves a minority of perivenular regions	Absent
Lobular findings and necro-inflammatory activity	Severity varies; rosettes may be present and prominent	Variable; if present, concentrated in perivenular regions	Variable; if present, concentrated in perivenular regions	Disarray and severity vary Necro-inflammatory activity	Mild disarray, parenchymal granulomas; periportal copper deposition and cholestasis are late features	Disarray unusual; neutrophil clusters with or without cholestasis
Pattern of fibrosis during progression to cirrhosis	Usually macronodular, posthepatitic pattern	Rare	Uncommon; usually a venocentric pattern; may evolve to biliary pattern with time	Usually macronodular, hepatitic pattern; may be micronodular	Biliary pattern	Biliary pattern

AIH, *Autoimmune hepatitis;* BD, *bile duct;* PBC, *primary biliary cirrhosis;* PSC, *primary sclerosing cholangitis.*

**Histopathological findings should be combined with clinical, serological, radiographic, and important exclusionary criteria listed in Table 53.11 to arrive at a final diagnosis. The same findings apply to recurrent AIH and plasma cell–rich rejection.*

Modified from Banff Working Group, Demetris AJ, Adeyi O, et al. Liver biopsy interpretation for causes of late liver allograft dysfunction. Hepatology. *2006;44(2):489–501.*

TABLE 53.11 Inclusion and Exclusion Criteria for Diagnosis of Recurrent and New-Onset Chronic Necro-inflammatory Diseases After Liver Transplantation and Timing and Pattern of Liver Test Elevations

Diagnosis	Original Disease	Serology and Molecular Testing*	Timing† and Liver Injury Test Profile‡	Important Exclusion Criteria
Recurrent AIH	AIH	Autoantibodies (ANA, ASMA, ALKM) usually in high titers (>1:80); raised serum IgG	>6 months Hepatocellular	Acute and chronic rejection, HBV, HCV, HEV infection, as determined by third-generation ELISA assay and/or serum or tissue PCR
Recurrent HBV or HCV	HBV- or HCV-induced cirrhosis	HBV or HCV infection with standard, third-generation serological criteria and/or positive molecular testing for HBV or HCV nucleic acids	Usually 6-8 weeks, but as early as 10 days Usually hepatocellular, but may be cholestatic	Acute and chronic rojection AIH
Recurrent PBC	PBC	Positive for AMA but little additional benefit because AMA level remains elevated in most patients after transplantation	>1 year Cholestatic	Biliary tract obstruction or strictures
Recurrent PSC	PSC	NA	Usually >1 year Cholestatic	HA thrombosis or stenosis, chronic (ductopenic) rejection, abnormal surgical anatomy, anastomotic strictures alone, nonanastomotic strictures occurring <90 days after OLT, and ABO incompatibility
TCMR	NA	NA	Any time Usually hepatocellular; may be mixed if superimposed on chronic rejection	Inadequate IS usually but not always present Important exclusions: biliary tract obstruction or strictures, HBV, HCV, AIH
Plasma cell–rich rejection	HCV, PBC; associated with interferon and DAA treatment of HCV	ALKM, HLA-DSA, GST1	Usually >1 year; usually hepatocellular pattern of liver injury	Original disease of AIH
Chronic rejection	NA	NA	Any time, but usually <1 year Cholestatic; rarely hepatocellular in venoocclusive variant	Usually inadequate IS Important exclusions: biliary tract obstruction or strictures, HBV, HCV, AIH
Chronic active AMR	NA	De novo DSA usually directed at HLA class II DQ	>1 year May be subclinical	Usually suboptimal IS. Important exclusions: biliary tract obstruction or strictures, chronic portal vein thrombosis, causes of altered vascular flow, HCV, HBV, AIH
Idiopathic posttransplantation hepatitis	Nonviral and non-AIH	Testing negative for HBV, HCV, and HEV infection and autoantibodies	>1 year Usually hepatocellular	Late-onset TCMR, chronic active AMR, all other causes of chronic hepatitis (e.g., HEV), and biliary tract obstruction or strictures reasonably excluded; all attempts should be made to determine a cause before establishing this diagnosis

AIH, *Autoimmune hepatitis;* ALP, *alkaline phosphatase;* AMA, *antimitochondrial antibody;* AMR, *antibody-mediated rejection;* ANA, *antinuclear antibodies;* ALKM, *anti–liver-kidney microsomal antibodies;* ASMA, *anti–smooth muscle antibodies;* AST, *aspartate aminotransferase;* ELISA, *enzyme-linked immunosorbent assay;* GGT, *γ-glutamyltransferase;* GST1, *glutathione S-transferase T1;* HA, *hepatic artery;* HBV, *hepatitis B virus;* HCV, *hepatitis C virus;* HEV, *hepatitis E virus;* IgG, *immunoglobulin G;* IS, *immunosuppression;* NA, *not applicable;* OLT, *orthotopic liver transplantation;* PBC, *primary biliary cirrhosis;* PCR, *polymerase chain reaction;* PSC, *primary sclerosing cholangitis;* TCMR, *T cell–mediated rejection.*

**See Table 53.10 for compatible histopathological findings.*

†Usual timing of first onset.

‡Sustained elevation of levels for more than 1 month: hepatocellular pattern = ALT and/or AST > ALP and/or GGT; cholestatic pattern = ALP and/or GGT > AST and/or ALT.

Modified from Banff Working Group, Demetris AJ, Adeyi O, et al. Liver biopsy interpretation for causes of late liver allograft dysfunction. Hepatology. *2006;44:489–501.*

Recurrent Hepatitis Virus Infections

Historically, HBV and HCV infections have accounted for most liver transplantations worldwide, with HBV-induced cirrhosis continuing to predominate in Asia[409]; HCV-induced cirrhosis has been superseded by alcohol-induced liver disease and NASH as the leading indications for liver transplantation in the United States.[410,411] This is related to the introduction of safe and effective DAAs that are approved by the U.S. Food and Drug Administration (FDA).[412,413] Hence discussion of HCV recurrence in this chapter is largely for its historic significance and rare untreated cases that appear. Similar to the opportunistic viruses, HBV and HCV can remain in the circulation and infect extrahepatic tissues. If HBV or HCV are capable of replication, they will universally reinfect the new liver. Effective screening of blood products and organ donors has dramatically decreased acquisition of new infections during the transplantation period, but newly acquired infections can occur after transplantation.[414]

Highly effective DAAs have nearly completely eliminated clinical and histopathological presentations and evolution of HBV- and HCV-induced hepatitis in liver allograft recipients, except for the rare untreated recipients that appear. Hepatitis E virus (HEV) has also been identified as a cause of chronic hepatitis in liver allograft recipients[415-417] and reportedly may mimic rejection.[418]

Hepatitis A Virus

Hepatitis A (HAV)-induced fulminant hepatic failure is a rare indication for liver transplantation in developed countries and uncommonly in Asia.[419]

Several reports show that HAV infection can persist and recur after transplantation, as demonstrated by detection of HAV RNA by reverse transcription–polymerase chain reaction (RT-PCR) in liver tissue, serum, and stool at the time of transient graft dysfunction.[420,421] Biopsy findings at the time of posttransplantation liver dysfunction show active hepatitis, including mild portal inflammation, focal lymphocytic cholangitis, ductular cholestasis, hepatocyte apoptosis, and hepatocyte swelling and disarray with cholestasis.[420,421] However, HAV RNA has been reported in liver allograft tissue from patients with otherwise typical TCMR or chronic rejection.[420-423] Therefore a diagnosis of recurrent or persistent HAV infection after transplantation should be based on detailed clinicopathological and serological correlations in recipients showing a "hepatitic" pattern of liver injury.

Hepatitis B and D Viruses

The incidence of HBV-induced cirrhosis and liver transplantation for this condition is decreasing dramatically in Western countries because of mandatory HBV vaccination programs and effective DAAs that arrest disease progression and potentially reverse preexisting fibrosis. However, HBV infection remains the leading indication for liver transplantation in China.[409] Active viral replication before transplantation, recognized by hepatitis B e antigen (HBeAg) seropositivity or detection of HBV DNA in the circulation, causes allograft reinfection in most cases. Reinfection and recurrent disease are less predictable in patients who had HBV-induced fulminant liver failure or those co-infected with hepatitis D virus (HDV) who become anti-HBe positive and serum HBV DNA and HBeAg negative before transplantation.[424-426]

Rare naïve recipients can acquire HBV infection during or after transplantation.[425,426] Hepatitis B core antibody (anti-HBc)–positive donors are one possible source of infection; they can effectively transmit HBV to naïve, unvaccinated recipients. HBV transmission from anti-HBc–positive donors is largely prevented in vaccinated recipients, in those made immune by previous HBV infection (anti-HBc positive), or in recipients treated prophylactically.[55]

Pharmacological treatment of HBV after transplantation cannot entirely prevent allograft reinfection, but significantly diminishes the clinical and histopathological manifestations of HBV-induced allograft dysfunction.[425,426] Therapies include polyclonal and monoclonal hepatitis B immune globulins, interferon-α, and antiviral drugs such as lamivudine and other nucleoside analogues such as adefovir, entecavir, and tenofovir.[427,428] These agents effectively control viral replication and limit recurrent disease incidence to less than 10%, particularly when anti-HBsAg is combined with lamivudine or other nucleoside analogues.[425,426]

Clinical Features

Untreated recipients, who are largely of historic interest, manifest clinical signs and symptoms approximately 6 to 8 weeks after transplantation. The same might be true of individuals who acquire de novo HBV infection after transplantation. The most common sign in monitored recipients is elevation of liver ALT and AST levels.[429,430] More significant disease is similar to presentations in the general population with nausea, vomiting, jaundice, and, in rare cases, fulminant hepatic failure. Severe disease associated with fibrosing cholestatic hepatitis (FCH; currently rare because of DAA therapy) on biopsy (see later) can develop in recipients treated with high-dose immunosuppression. Once diagnosed, rapid tapering and withdrawal of immunosuppression should be avoided in HBV-infected recipients who have evidence of active viral replication to avoid re-arming the immune system and causing severe immunologically-mediated liver injury and fulminant hepatic failure.

Pathological Features

The histopathological manifestations of HBV infection of hepatic allografts are similar to those seen in native livers, except for the rare occurrence of the fibrosing cholestatic variant.[430,431] However, recurrent HBV disease has been largely eliminated because of effective DAA therapy; therefore the number of posttransplantation liver biopsies obtained for evaluation and the severity of recurrent acute and chronic HBV hepatitis have practically disappeared.[425,426] However, it is important to recognize the various HBV posttransplantation manifestations because they can reappear in inadequately treated recipients, in patients who harbor drug-resistant viral mutants, and the rare unvaccinated recipient who acquires de novo HBV after transplantation.

HBV-related disease typically manifests as acute hepatitis beginning 4 to 6 weeks after transplantation, accompanied by hepatocyte cytoplasmic hepatitis core antigen expression[429,430] followed by surface antigen expression,[429,430] spotty hepatocyte apoptosis, lobular inflammation, Kupffer

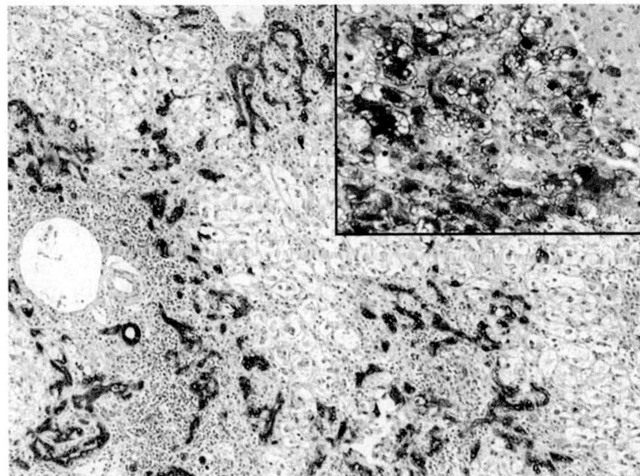

FIGURE 53.34 Cytokeratin 19–stained fibrosing cholestatic hepatitis is characterized by marked cholangiolar proliferation and hepatocyte swelling. Swollen and degenerated hepatocytes often show overproduction of hepatitis B core antigen, which is usually nuclear but may also be cytoplasmic in cases of massive viral replication *(inset)*.

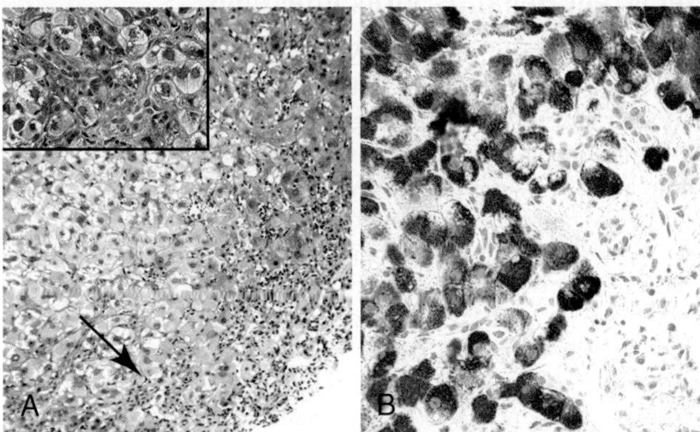

FIGURE 53.35 A, Overproduction of hepatitis B surface antigen can lead to degeneration of hepatocytes and cholangiolar proliferation. Cholangiolar proliferation *(arrow, inset)* is often associated with pericholangiolar fibrosis. **B,** Note the immunohistochemical staining pattern for hepatitis B surface antigen.

cell hypertrophy, and lobular disarray, combined with variable portal inflammation. Confluent, bridging, and even submassive necrosis develops in a small percentage of untreated HBV-positive recipients, especially if immunosuppression is rapidly lowered or withdrawn completely after establishing the diagnosis.[429]

Delta agent (HDV) co-infection of HBV-positive recipients usually results in a lower incidence of recurrent disease compared with HBV-positive, HDV-negative recipients, particularly in pharmacologically treated recipients.[432] The effects of HDV on HBV-related pathology in untreated recipients is similar to that seen in the general population.[433]

Delta agent co-infection can be detected by immunohistochemical staining.[434] Anti-HBV pharmacological therapy effectively controls HDV replication and disease.[432]

Spontaneous resolution of HBV hepatitis in untreated liver allograft recipients is rare, but instead evolves toward chronic hepatitis with variable, but mostly more aggressive necro-inflammatory activity. Cirrhosis can develop 12 to 18 months after transplantation. [429,430] Evolution from acute to chronic HBV hepatitis in untreated patients is characterized by portal lymphoplasmacytic inflammation with necro-inflammatory–type interface activity, but with relative sparing of the bile ducts, portal vein, and hepatic veins. Lobular findings in the chronic phase are usually less conspicuous; included are mild lobular disarray, low-grade necro-inflammatory activity, and hepatocytes with ground-glass cytoplasm (HBsAg) of sanded nuclei (HBcAg) that stain positively for hepatitis B surface antigen and core antigen, respectively.

Massive HBV replication in the setting of strong immunosuppression and MHC nonidentity between the liver and recipient can lead to the development of FCH (Figs. 53.34 and 53.35). This condition can also result from emergence of viral mutants.[430,435] Findings include marked hepatocyte swelling, lobular disarray, cholestasis, and prominent ductular and fibrotic-type interface activity, often with minimal or mild portal and lobular inflammation. Swollen and degenerating hepatocytes usually show massive hepatocellular expression of HBV core and surface antigens, which suggests that HBV is directly cytopathic in these circumstances.[430,436]

Differential Diagnosis

Acute HBV should be distinguished from other causes of acute hepatitis, such as CMV, HCV, and EBV infection, and other causes of spotty hepatocyte apoptosis, such as "ischemic hepatitis." The most reliable approach to distinguish acute HBV hepatitis from other disorders is to review the clinical, histopathological, immunohistochemical, and serological patient profile.

The routine histopathological appearance of chronic HBV hepatitis can be quite similar to HCV, AIH, and adverse drug reactions. An active periportal and lobular hepatitis combined with detection of ground-glass hepatocytes or viral antigens and nucleic acids in blood or tissues and an absence of other causes of chronic hepatitis and late-onset TCMR favor recurrent or de novo chronic HBV infection[430] Serological evidence of viral infection or detection of viral antigens or nucleic acids in the liver should be correlated with the histological pattern of injury. Patients with HBsAg positivity in the absence of detectable HBV DNA usually do not show biopsy features of HBV-related hepatitis.[427] Features used to distinguish TCMR from acute or chronic hepatitis are discussed earlier in this chapter.

Hepatitis C Virus

Superseded by alcoholic liver disease (ALD) and NASH, HCV-induced cirrhosis is no longer the leading indication for liver transplant listing in the United States.[410,411] This is related to the introduction of safe and effective FDA-approved DAA agents.[412,413] that are transforming the care and outcome of patients with HCV, both before and after transplantation. Data from multiple centers comparing the pre-DAA to DAA era show a decline in the percentage of patients who undergo transplantation for HCV, decreased listing of HCV-positive patients, improved patient and graft survival in recipients, culling of waiting lists, and an overall decrease in rate of retransplantation.[93,94,413,437-440] The effectiveness of these medications has also enabled confident use of HCV-positive donors without bridging fibrosis.

The advances in treating HCV before and after transplantation will reflect on the range of pathological changes observed by pathologists in native liver explants and subsequent allograft biopsies. Soon, the following discussion will be of historic value, with the exception of immune-mediated graft dysfunction associated with DAAs and interferon therapy.[309,311,312]

In untreated patients, reinfection and subsequent viremia occur within days after transplantation in most HCV-positive recipients. New-onset HCV infection after transplantation usually is similar to that seen in the general population. Chronic hepatitis, which usually evolves slowly, develops in most untreated patients. In the pre-DAA era, fibrosis progression was substantially faster than in native livers, producing cirrhosis in as many as 20% of patients 5 years after transplantation. Aggressive disease progression is often attributable to a combination of immunosuppression and MHC mismatching between the donor and recipient, which leads to alloimmunological injury and impaired immunological control of viral replication.[441-443]

New antiviral therapies have been successful in inducing sustained virological response (SVR) in transplant recipients as well as high rates of SVR in previously untreated recipients with early HCV recurrence after liver transplantation.[444,445] The rate of biopsy-proven rejection is low after treatment with DAA.[444] DAA therapy can significantly decrease very aggressive forms of recurrence in the form of FCH, which develops in a few untreated recipients.

The genotypes of HCV after transplantation usually reflect those of the recipient population. Type 1b is the most prevalent type in European centers[446,447] and in some large North American sites where it accounts for 25% to 60% of the affected patients.[448] In another North American study, type 1a was predominant.[448] This type is the least responsive to therapy.[449]

Liver damage from recurrent HCV is mediated by a combination of viral replication and immune-mediated damage in recipients untreated with DAA.[450] As with HBV, rapid tapering of immunosuppression can precipitate rapidly progressive disease.[451-453] This is likely related to re-arming of the immune system at a time of high HCV replication, thereby triggering a more aggressive form of immune-mediated hepatitis. [451-453] Instead, slow tapering of immunosuppression, particularly in long-surviving recipients, is advisable[451-453] unless DAA is available. Although of decreasing relevance, heavy immunosuppression increases viral replication and promotes liver damage from HCV infection.[450] Similar to nontransplantation patients,[454] nucleotide polymorphisms of IL28B and HCV RNA mutations in liver allograft recipients predict more aggressive disease.[455,456]

The rate of fibrosis progression increases with time after transplantation in untreated recipients, which again is largely only of historical interest.[441,443,457,458] In keeping with fibrogenesis models,[450] a combination of insults, such as coexistent steatosis, high viral replication, oxidative stress, iron deposits, or coexistent damage from preservation/reperfusion injury, biliary structuring, or TCMR, can accelerate disease progression. This may explain why extended criteria donor use in HCV-positive recipients counterbalances some improvements in HCV medical management.[441,443,450]

The complex interplay between the immune system, HCV, and immunosuppression[459] leads to distinct pathological variants of recurrent HCV and rejection, including atypical presentations and variants, FCH, overlap with acute and chronic rejection, and susceptibility to a distinct form of plasma cell–rich rejection that likely represents a mixed T cell–mediated and antibody-mediated injury (comprehensively discussed earlier).

Clinical Features

Clinical features of recurrent HCV hepatitis usually become apparent 3 to 6 weeks after transplantation, mimicking those seen in the general population: elevations of ALT and AST are fourfold to eightfold above baseline levels.[450]

Jaundice at initial presentation is unusual unless the recipient is at risk for FCH. Fulminant liver failure is not seen outside of the FCH setting, which has been clearly associated with over-immunosuppression that usually occurs during the first year after transplantation. It is characterized clinically by malaise, jaundice, and marked elevations of bilirubin, alkaline phosphatase, and GGT levels and evolves subacutely during a period of weeks to months. Later-onset FCH most commonly occurs when recurrent HCV is misdiagnosed as TCMR, and the patient is treated vigorously with increased immunosuppression. Early recognition of FCH relies on a high index of suspicion, an understanding of the clinical circumstances of its emergence, and the finding of markedly elevated HCV RNA levels.

Pathological Features

Usual Variant

The usual appearance of HCV infection in DAA-untreated liver allograft recipients is similar to that seen in native livers. However, in allografts, the acute phase usually shows less portal and lobular inflammation, the chronic phase shows less nodular aggregates of portal-based lymphocytes, and there is more ductular-type interface activity.[450,460]

The acute lobular phase of recurrent HCV infection usually appears between 4 and 12 weeks, but it can be detected as early as 10 to 14 days after transplantation. Lobular disarray, Kupffer cell hypertrophy, hepatocyte apoptosis, mild sinusoidal lymphocytosis, mild mononuclear portal inflammation, and macrovesicular steatosis involving periportal and midzonal hepatocytes are typical findings (Fig. 53.36). Lymphocytic cholangitis and reactive changes of the biliary epithelium, if present, involve only a minority of bile ducts.[450] The transition from acute to chronic recurrent HCV infection is accompanied by waning of the lobular changes, increased portal inflammation, variable portal-based nodular lymphoid aggregates, and emergence of necro-inflammatory and ductular-type interface activity.[450] The latter feature can occasionally be prominent, making it difficult to distinguish from cholangiopathic disorders (Fig. 53.37).

Chronic recurrent HCV infection is usually evident in 6 to 12 months after transplantation. It is usually dominated by portal and periportal changes such as portal lymphocytic inflammation, occasional portal-based lymphoid aggregates, and necro-inflammatory and ductular-type interface activity with various degrees of severity. Focal lymphocytic cholangitis can be seen, but it is neither

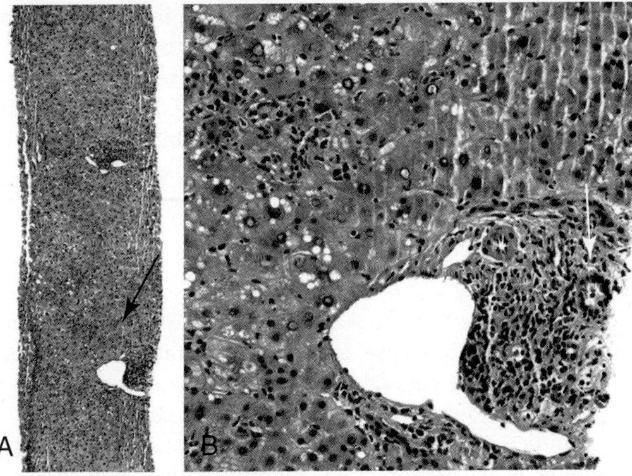

FIGURE 53.36 A–B, The early stage of recurrent hepatitis C virus (HCV) infection is characterized by changes that primarily occur in the lobules, but mild, predominantly mononuclear portal inflammation also can be seen at low magnification **(A).** The portal tract and nearby lobule *(arrow)* can be seen at higher magnification **(B).** Note the mild mononuclear portal inflammation but absence of inflammatory bile duct damage *(arrow).* The specimen also has a prominent lobular disarray, Kupffer cell hypertrophy, and acidophilic or apoptotic hepatocytes, which are the most characteristic features of early recurrent HCV infection.

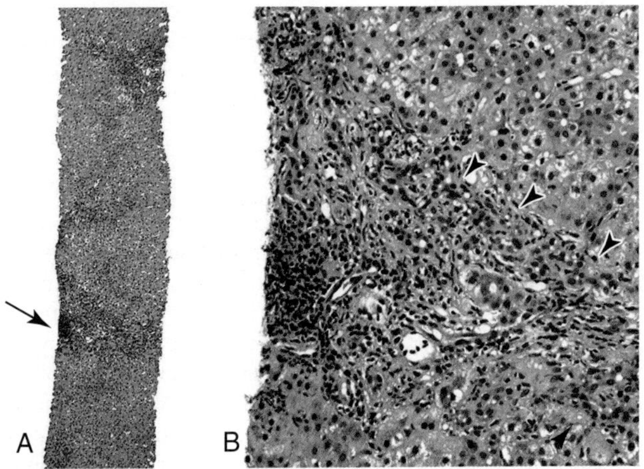

FIGURE 53.37 The chronic stage of recurrent hepatitis C virus (HCV) infection is often similar to that seen in native livers. **A,** It is predominantly characterized by mononuclear inflammation, consisting of small lymphocytes that are occasionally arranged into nodular aggregates *(arrow).* The aggregates, however, are less commonly encountered when compared with native livers. The portal tract *(arrow)* in **A** is shown at higher magnification in **B. B,** The portal inflammation in recurrent HCV infection is not ductulocentric *(bottom arrowhead).* Instead, the interface zone shows various degrees of necro-inflammatory and ductular-type activity that can be prominent, sometimes making it difficult to distinguish it from biliary tract disease *(top arrowheads).*

severe nor widespread, involving a minority of bile ducts, and duct loss does not occur. Mild noncircumferential lymphohistiocytic inflammation surrounding central veins (i.e., central perivenulitis) can be identified in a minority of central veins, but is neither severe nor widespread in recurrent HCV infection.

Data regarding morphological changes seen in recurrent HCV treated with DAA are still limited. Patients with recurrent HCV treated with DAA show decreased inflammation and fibrosis at a pace faster than that seen with interferon therapy.[461,462] In addition, posttreatment biopsies also show a decrease in fat content, but others show continued liver inflammation and fibrosis progression in a minority despite apparent viral clearance.[463] Pathologists and clinicians must remain vigilant for post-DAA treatment rejection in patients, particularly those treated with sofosbuvir and ledipasvir.[311] Reported rejection types include plasma cell–rich, TCMR, and chronic rejection. HCV is believed to have an immune suppressive effect in liver allografts; therefore rapid virus clearance decreases level of immune suppression and frees up the immune system from targeting HCV to recognizing and targeting the graft.

Fibrosing Cholestatic Hepatitis

This section, again, is largely of historical interest and for the rare patient that might still be encountered. HCV-induced FCH usually occurs in the first year after transplantation in over-immunosuppressed recipients. It is usually characterized by markedly elevated HCV RNA levels, reflecting the homogeneous viral quasispecies in the peripheral circulation (usually 30 to 50 million IU/mL). Liver damage in FCH is likely caused by direct viral cytopathic effects on hepatocytes. The intrahepatic immune response in FCH related to HCV infection is typically a type 2 helper T cell (Th2) response, in contrast with the type 1 (Th1)-predominant response in conventional recurrent HCV infection.[464]

The most common features of "classical" FCH include cholestasis, hepatocyte ballooning degeneration, paucity of mononuclear portal inflammation, fibrosis (i.e., periportal, portal, and bridging), and a ductular reaction (Fig. 53.38).[465] Spotty apoptosis or necrosis and mild mixed or neutrophilic-predominant portal inflammation are also often seen. However, HCV-associated FCH can show a spectrum of severity; mild cases show only mild hepatocyte swelling, slightly more mononuclear portal inflammation, and minimal ductular reaction.

Overlap of Recurrent Hepatitis C with Acute and Chronic Rejection

Establishing a histopathological diagnosis of acute TCMR and/or late-onset TCMR and chronic rejection in the context of recurrent HCV infection can be difficult. In untreated recipients, the most frequent mistake is to overdiagnose TCMR, which leads to unnecessary additional immunosuppressive therapy.[300,450] Features associated with TCMR and chronic rejection include mononuclear lymphocytic cholangitis and biliary epithelial senescence changes, respectively, and central perivenulitis and fibrosis involving most portal tracts or terminal hepatic veins, respectively. Recurrent or new-onset HCV changes include lobular and interface necro-inflammatory along with ductular-type interface activity. The key to establishing a final diagnosis and the predominant insult is to determine which constellations of findings predominate.

Most clinically significant TCMR episodes that occur in patients with recurrent HCV infection are graded as moderate according to the Banff criteria.[3,6] Biliary epithelial cell senescence involving most bile ducts leads to a diagnosis of chronic rejection, which is often associated with a reduction in immunosuppression or treatment with an immune stimulator such as interferon-α.[310,450] When TCMR or chronic

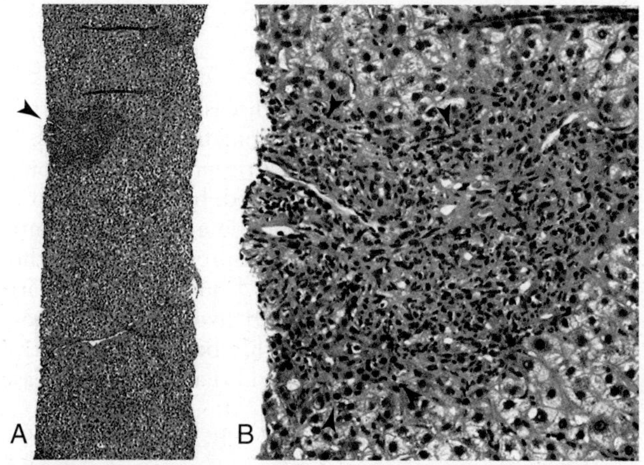

FIGURE 53.38 Fibrosing, cholestatic hepatitis C virus (HCV) infection is a relatively uncommon and atypical manifestation of recurrent HCV infection that usually occurs during the first year after transplantation in heavily or overly immunosuppressed recipients. It is invariably associated with marked viral replication as measured by viral nucleic acids in the serum; typical values are more than 30 million U/mL. **A,** The histology is characterized by relatively modest portal inflammation *(arrowhead),* degenerative swelling or ballooning of hepatocytes, lobular disarray, and cholestasis. The portal tract *(arrow)* in **A** is shown at higher magnification in **B. B,** Fibrotic and ductular-type interface activity *(arrowheads)* also can be seen.

rejection is the predominant process, the pathological changes should be obvious. Clinically significant rejection episodes occurring in the context of recurrent HCV infection are usually associated with relatively low peripheral blood HCV RNA levels (<1 to 5 million IU/mL), which suggests that immunological mechanisms associated with rejection also contribute to virus clearance.[300,443]

Differential Diagnosis

The differential diagnosis for acute and chronic recurrent HCV infection includes TCMR and chronic rejection; recurrent non-HCV viral hepatitis (e.g., HBV, CMV, EBV); recurrent or new-onset AIH, PBC, or PSC; and suboptimal biliary tract drainage.[450,460] C4d deposits, HCV protein, and nucleic acid expression have been used as adjunctive techniques to assist with the differential diagnosis, although with limited success.[450,460]

The timing of the liver biopsy is important in untreated recipients. HCV infection is an uncommon cause of allograft dysfunction during the first several weeks after transplantation, except for rare cases that begin as early as 10 to 14 days. Instead, most cases of recurrent HCV infection occur between 3 and 8 weeks after transplantation. Most TCMR episodes, in contrast, occur in the first 30 days.[466]

Distinguishing recurrent HCV infection from other causes of chronic hepatitis, such as HBV infection, AIH, and drug-induced hepatitis, requires evaluation of the patient's clinical, biochemical, and serological profile. A detailed histopathological examination can then be extremely helpful. Detection of HBV viral antigens or circulating nucleic acids or ground-glass cells or sanded nuclei can distinguish HBV from HCV infection. Confluent necrosis is rarely seen in HCV infection alone. Typical recurrent AIH is recognized by sheets (>30% of infiltrate) of plasma cells in portal and perivenular areas of necro-inflammatory activity. In contrast, low-grade periportal and midzonal steatosis and portal lymphoid aggregates favor recurrent HCV infection.

FCH caused by recurrent HCV infection can be difficult to distinguish from suboptimal biliary drainage and hepatic artery thrombosis. Portal edema, ductular metaplasia of periportal hepatocytes on CK7 staining, portal or periportal neutrophilia, and bile infarcts are helpful features associated with suboptimal biliary drainage/acute cholangitis. A prominent ductular reaction and acute cholangiolitis without portal edema is more characteristic of cholestatic hepatitis. Lobular disarray and marked hepatocellular swelling are typical of viral hepatitis but uncommon in obstructive cholangiopathy alone.

Hepatitis E Virus

Pathophysiology and Clinical Features

HEV is a single-stranded, quasi-enveloped, hepatotropic RNA virus that is endemic in southern Asia and Africa. It has at least five different genotypes that can infect humans (genotypes 1, 2, 3, 4, and 7). HEV genotypes 3, 4, and 7 are frequently associated with zoonotic infections, whereas HEV genotypes 1 and 2 primarily infect humans as waterborne illnesses. HEV is most often transmitted by the fecal-oral route, but transmission by blood transfusion, contact with pigs and other animals, and consumption of infected and undercooked meat has also been repo rted.[415,416,467,468-473]

HEV is an endemic cause of self-limited acute hepatitis in developing countries and an emerging disease in industrialized countries. Severe acute disease occurs predominantly in pregnant women. Rarely, fulminant hepatic failure can be seen in immunocompetent patients, with reports of both progressive disease requiring liver transplantation and spontaneous recovery.[474,475] Chronic infection can occur in immunosuppressed individuals.[476] As with other hepatitic viruses, acute infection is diagnosed by HEV RNA detection and anti-HEV IgM seroconversion; convalescence is mostly marked by HEV nucleic acid clearance.[471,477]

The prevalence of HEV infection in liver allograft recipients varies by region and study, ranging from 1% to 28%.[478] Hepatitis E infection occurs at a higher rate in liver allograft recipients than other organ recipients and is associated with acute and chronic hepatitis in children and adults.[415,416,469-473,479-481] Genotype 3, perhaps acquired through contact with pigs or other animals or by eating insufficiently cooked meat, is suspected in some cases, particularly in developed countries. Transmission through blood transfusion has also been reported in the setting of liver transplantation.[482]

Acute illness is characterized by elevated liver injury tests, fatigue, arthralgias, weight loss, and myalgias during a period of 1 to 2 weeks. Chronic or relapsing disease occurs more commonly in patients who acquire primary infection after transplantation.[415,416,469-473,481] Chronic infection is usually confirmed by HEV RNA PCR because anti-HEV IgM and later anti-HEV IgG seroconversion is often delayed for weeks or months. Some cases spontaneously resolve, but chronic hepatitis develops in as many as 60% who fail to clear the virus, and up to 15% show progression to cirrhosis.[471] In solid organ transplant recipients, chronicity should be considered when there is active HEV replication persisting over 3 months rather than the usual definition of chronic hepatitis (viral replication of more than 6 months).[483] Risk factors for the development of chronic hepatitis include tacrolimus immunosuppression and low platelet counts.[471] Lowering immunosuppression and ribavirin treatment may lead to resolution of the HEV infection and favorably influences the course of the chronic hepatitis.[471,484,485]

Pathological Features and Differential Diagnosis

The acute and chronic phases of HEV infection in the transplanted liver are similar to those of HBV and HCV infections.[415,469,472,481] The acute phase is characterized predominantly by spotty hepatocyte necrosis or apoptosis and lobular inflammation with variable portal inflammation. Portal tracts may show mild to moderate expansion by inflammation composed mainly of lymphocytes and variable necro-inflammatory–type interface activity. [415,486] Focal ductular reaction and ceroid-laden macrophages can also be seen. In contrast with immunocompetent patients, cholestasis and lobular disarray are not prominent features.[486-488]

Chronic HEV hepatitis is usually characterized by some degree of lymphocytic and lymphoplasmacytic portal inflammation, necro-inflammatory–type interface activity, and fibrosis.[415,469,472,481,486] The same criteria used to distinguish chronic recurrent HBV and HCV infections from acute and chronic rejection can be used for chronic HEV-associated hepatitis. Detection of HEV RNA on FFPE tissue can be performed by in-situ hybridization, immunohistochemistry for ORF2, and PCR.[486,488,489] Serological and molecular studies for HEV RNA are needed to make a definitive diagnosis.[476]

Disorders of Dysregulated Immunity

Disorders of immune regulation, including PBC, PSC, AIH, sarcoidosis, and overlap syndromes, commonly recur after liver transplantation. The incidence is roughly 25% at 5 years after transplantation, with a progressive increase in the incidence of recurrent disease over time. Higher rates of recurrence are reported in patients transplanted with ESLD secondary to overlap syndrome between AIH, PBC, and/or PSC.[490] The severity and rate of progression of recurrent disease may be less aggressive than in nontransplantation patients.[491,492] Recurrence of these diseases negatively affects long-term morbidity and mortality, but successful treatment with ursodeoxycholic acid and other newer agents may prevent disease progression before and after transplantation.[493,494]

Establishing a diagnosis of disease recurrence can be complicated because clinical, serological, histopathological, and radiographical findings potentially suggestive of recurrent disease can occur in other disorders. For example, there are numerous causes of non–PSC-related intrahepatic biliary strictures. Serological studies used to establish a diagnosis of AIH, PBC, or overlap syndromes before transplantation (e.g., ANAs, AMA-M2, elevated IgG levels) often disappear transiently shortly after transplantation then reappear (usually at lower titers), even without clinical or histopathological evidence of recurrent disease. Specific consensus criteria were proposed by the Banff Working Group to suggest a standardized approach to recurrent diseases.[4]

Primary Biliary Cholangitis

Pathophysiology

PBC is a rare, chronic cholestatic disease that is characterized by destructive lymphogranulomatous cholangitis.[495] Pathophysiological mechanisms triggering the autoimmune response are poorly understood, but are believed to result from a combination of genetic and environmental factors.[496-499] Left untreated, PBC progresses to cirrhosis over a period of 10 to 30 years.[495,500] In recent years, fewer PBC patients have required liver transplantation, and the need is occurring later in life because of effective treatment with ursodeoxycholic acid that can slow disease progression.[495,500,501]

Prevalence rates for recurrent PBC range from 9% to 35%, with an average time to recurrence of 3 to 5.5 years.[495,500] Reported recurrence rates among centers depend on whether liver biopsies are done by indication or protocol, sampling error, and the histopathological criteria used to establish the diagnosis. [495,500] We are unaware of case reports of de novo PBC.

For the recipient, reported risk factors for recurrent PBC vary among studies, particularly between North American/European and Japanese studies, possibly resulting from immunogenetic differences.[502] In general, recent work shows that risk factors include younger age at transplantation and/or PBC diagnosis, male gender, HLA status, high IgM levels, sex mismatch, severe elevation in markers of cholestasis within first year posttransplantation, and immunosuppression with tacrolimus.[502-506] Cyclosporine is reported to be protective from recurrent PBC by some studies.[502,506] The donor age, gender, and ischemic time also influence the risk of recurrence. [495,500]

Clinical Features

Signs and symptoms of recurrent PBC depend on the type of surveillance program: those that perform protocol biopsies detect recurrent disease in mainly asymptomatic patients who often have near-normal liver function test values.[500] Other symptoms, such as fatigue and metabolic bone disease, can be multifactorial and nonspecific. In a large Mayo Clinic study, only 12% of patients with recurrent PBC reported disease-related symptoms, with fatigue and pruritus being the most common.[500] Programs that perform biopsies only by indication usually detect recurrent PBC because of a preferentially increased alkaline phosphatase and/or GGT level as part of routine serological monitoring.

Recurrent PBC may progress after liver transplantation. Although the need for retransplantation after recurrent PBC is rare, recent data show recurrent PBC impairs long-term graft survival.[506] AMA-M2 detection is of little additional benefit in establishing the diagnosis because AMA levels decline transiently after transplantation but then recur in most patients, even in those without recurrent disease. Allograft biopsies are needed to establish a diagnosis with certainty. Treatment with ursodeoxycholic acid after transplantation may result in biochemical improvement; some studies have not shown a significant impact on patient or allograft survival,[500] but a more recent meta-analysis suggested a beneficial effect in delaying the onset and/or reducing the incidence of recurrent disease.[507]

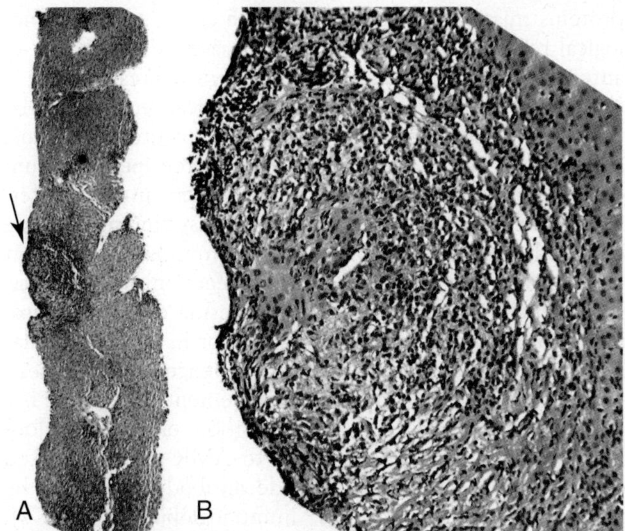

FIGURE 53.39 The pathological manifestations of recurrent primary biliary cholangitis in allografts are similar to those in native livers. **A,** Note the patchy but prominent portal mononuclear inflammation. **B,** Lymphohistiocytic destructive cholangitis. The portal tract *(arrow)* in **A** is shown at higher magnification in **B.**

Pathological Features

The morphological features of recurrent PBC are the same as in native livers. Diagnostic features include noninfectious, noncaseating, granulomatous, and lymphocytic cholangitis producing breaks in the ductal basement membranes, which are referred to as *florid duct lesions* (Fig. 53.39).[500] Patchy, dense portal lymphoplasmacytic infiltrates 1 year after transplantation may herald the development of recurrent disease.[508]

Diagnostic bile duct lesions are not always found.[509] Instead, cases may have patchy, mononuclear portal inflammation, focal lymphocytic cholangitis, and portal lymphoid nodules. A biliary cause is further indicated by a prominent ductular reaction at the interface zone, periportal edema, cholestasis, ductular metaplasia of periportal hepatocytes on CK7 staining, accumulation of copper or copper-associated pigment in periportal hepatocytes, and patchy loss of small bile ducts. The latter findings are referred to as a *biliary gestalt*. Collectively, these features strongly suggest recurrent PBC if they occur in the proper clinical context.

A diagnosis of recurrent PBC is difficult in biopsies with only mild lymphocytic cholangitis and no other histological features suggesting a biliary cause of disease. For example, recurrent PBC may manifest initially as chronic hepatitis.[181,510] Liver biopsy sampling may be inadequate, or the clinical and histological features may represent an overlap syndrome with AIH.[510,511]

As in native livers, lobular findings in recurrent PBC are usually mild and nonspecific. Included are mild spotty hepatocyte apoptosis, mildly increased sinusoidal lymphocytes, changes of mild NRH and portal venopathy, and small Kupffer cell granulomas. More significant lobular findings usually indicate another or coexistent disorder. Recurrent PBC progression is also characterized by the development of biliary-type fibrosis, cholestasis, deposition of copper and copper-associated proteins at the edge of hepatic lobules, and portal-to-portal bridging fibrosis. We routinely conduct CK7 stains on all liver allograft biopsies, which is very helpful in detecting the early stages of cholangiopathic processes.

Differential Diagnosis

The differential diagnosis of recurrent PBC depends on the stage of disease. Included are acute TCMR and chronic rejection; suboptimal biliary drainage; chronic viral, autoimmune, or idiopathic hepatitis; and DILI. These disorders can coexist with recurrent PBC. Other causes of granulomatous cholangitis, such as fungal, acid-fast bacterial, sarcoidosis, PSC, or HCV with portal granulomas,[512] should be excluded.

A biliary gestalt is one of the most helpful constellations of findings that can be used to distinguish biliary tract pathology from other causes of dysfunction. Neither acute nor chronic TCMR shows significant ductular reaction or leads to biliary-type fibrosis or cirrhosis. Rejection-associated portal inflammation and lymphocytic cholangitis usually involve most portal tracts and preferentially involve the small bile ducts (<20 μm in diameter). PBC-associated portal inflammation and lymphocytic cholangitis, in contrast, is typically patchy in distribution and preferentially involves medium-sized bile ducts (40 to 50 μm in diameter).

Recurrent PBC can also be difficult to distinguish from obstructive cholangiopathy. A history of biliary tract pathology or radiographic evidence of stricturing favors obstructive cholangiopathy. Histopathological features that favor suboptimal biliary drainage over recurrent PBC include portal and periportal edema and neutrophilic inflammation in and around true bile ducts, centrilobular hepatocanalicular cholestasis, bile infarcts, and intralobular neutrophil clusters.

PBC can be difficult to distinguish from chronic viral hepatitis and AIH, particularly because some manifestations of recurrent HCV may show a prominent ductular reaction. In these cases, the bile ducts should be examined for evidence of lymphocytic or granulomatous duct damage and small bile duct loss. Most cases of chronic hepatitis do not produce the biliary gestalt. Portal granulomas, without damage to bile ducts, have been reported in patients with recurrent chronic HCV.[513] CK7 and copper stains can be used to distinguish ductular reactions associated with chronic cholestasis from those related to other disorders.

Given the broad differential diagnosis and sometimes difficult to appreciate classic features of recurrent PBC, ancillary studies can be very helpful in identifying recurrent disease. In our experience, as in native disease, screening for reduced Hering canals by CK19, increased dendritic cells on CD1a and/or S100 protein, ductular metaplasia of periportal hepatocytes visualized by CK7, and periportal copper deposition are all very useful features when trying to distinguish recurrent PBC from other differential diagnoses or trying to establish a diagnosis of early PBC recurrence.[514-519]

Recurrent Autoimmune Hepatitis

Clinical Features and Pathophysiology

AIH is a typically waxing and waning chronic necroinflammatory liver disease that (untreated) has the potential to progress to cirrhosis. The diagnosis is based on a combination of serological findings (e.g., elevated ANA, SMA, and serum IgG levels), appropriate histopathological findings, and steroid responsiveness combined with the exclusion of other causes of liver injury.[318,319] Establishing a diagnosis of recurrent AIH after liver transplantation is more difficult than before transplantation because serological abnormalities used to establish the diagnosis before transplantation persist or transiently decline and then reappear in most AIH-afflicted recipients. Risk factors for recurrent AIH include suboptimal immunosuppression, recipient HLA-DR3 and DR4, type 1 AIH versus type 2 AIH before transplantation, high IgG before transplantation, severe inflammation in the explanted donor liver, and long follow-up.[318,319,520,521]

Most patients with recurrent AIH are detected initially because of elevated liver injury tests, often first detected when attempting to routinely discontinue corticosteroids from the immunosuppression regimen. A diagnosis is established on evaluation of a liver needle biopsy and correlated with clinicopathological and serological profiles.

Pathological Features and Differential Diagnosis

Histopathological features typically associated with AIH can be seen with other causes of allograft dysfunction.[319] For example, histopathological findings used to support a diagnosis of AIH, such as plasma cell–rich (>30% of infiltrate) periportal and perivenular necro-inflammatory activity, can be seen in other disorders such as recurrent HCV infection and plasma cell–rich TCMR.

Therefore the Banff Working Group advocated relatively strict criteria to establish a diagnosis of recurrent AIH after liver transplantation[4] and recently further refined specifically by establishing separate diagnostic criteria for plasma cell–rich rejection (formerly *de-novo AIH*).[3] Native liver AIH, plasma cell–rich TCMR after transplantation, and recurrent AIH can be virtually indistinguishable in an individual case. All can show prominent, plasma cell–rich, necro-inflammatory interface activity and some degree of perivenular necro-inflammatory activity. This constellation of features is an excellent but not infallible marker of autoimmunity.[522,523] Distinguishing centrilobular-based and late-onset TCMR from AIH can be quite challenging, particularly given the increased risk of late-onset rejection occurrence in patients transplanted for autoimmune diseases.[283] Inflammatory bile duct damage or biliary epithelial senescence changes involving a majority of bile ducts, more prominent central perivenulitis and perivenular fibrosis, and higher RAI scores favor TCMR.[325]

After a hepatic pattern of injury is established histopathologically, the clinical and serological profiles are needed to support an autoimmune cause (e.g., ANA, ASMA, LKM, serum γ-globulins) and exclude other causes of chronic hepatitis, such as HBV, HCV, HEV, PBC, and obstructive cholangiopathy.[317-319]

Bile Salt Export Pump Deficiency

De novo immunoglobulin G antibodies directed against bile salt export pump (BSEP) proteins (expressed on the canalicular membrane of hepatocytes) can develop in pediatric patients who underwent transplantation for end-stage liver disease secondary to progressive familial intrahepatic cholestasis type 2 (PFIC-2).[524] These children are deficient for this protein before transplantation.[524] This non-HLA DSA-related injury results in cholestatic graft dysfunction similar to the original PFIC-2 disease. It has been proposed that proteins missing in recipients at birth can trigger immunological reactions after transplantation as a result of lack of autotolerance.[525-527] The histopathological presentation in these cases is different from that of typical recurrent AIH, plasma cell–rich rejection, and typical acute or chronic AMR. The clinical presentation most often includes jaundice, pruritus, and elevated bilirubin and aminotransferases, but normal GGT levels.[525-527] Biopsy findings include canalicular cholestasis, hepatocyte multinucleate giant cells, prominent interface ductular reaction, and fibrosis. In patients with BSEP antibodies, plasma cell–rich necro-inflammatory activity at the interface or in the perivenular region and inflammatory bile duct damage have not been described.[525-527] Evidence of complement activation has been demonstrated by C4d deposition on immunofluorescence examination.[528] Similar to AMR in transplanted organs, treatment options include antibody reduction by plasmapheresis, intravenous immunoglobulins (IVIGs), and rituximab.[529] The presence of alloantibodies against graft antigens, evidence of complement activation and clinical improvement by antibody reduction, are all features of AMR; hence this cause of dysfunction may be better classified as a form of AMR rather than *recurrent or autoimmune BSEP.* BSEP disease after liver transplantation is reviewed by Kubitz and colleagues here.[530]

Recurrent Primary Sclerosing Cholangitis

Clinical Features

PSC is a disease of dysregulated immunity, but the underlying cause is unknown. It usually occurs in young men (60% to 70% of cases) with coexistent ulcerative colitis.[531] It is the most common indication for liver transplantation in Scandinavian countries.[532] The recurrence rate is approximately 20% at 5 years, and it increases with time after transplantation. Data suggest that recurrent disease adversely affects long-term patient and allograft survival.[521,533] Recurrent PSC can be quite difficult to diagnose with certainty and distinguish from other causes of biliary strictures, even when strict criteria are used.[534] Many other disorders, such as ischemic injury from prolonged preservation or non–beating heart donors, imperfect biliary anastomoses, inadequate hepatic arterial flow, and AMR, may cause nonanastomotic intrahepatic biliary strictures that mimic recurrent PSC.

The early stage of recurrent PSC usually comes to clinical attention more than 6 to 9 months after transplantation as selective elevation of alkaline phosphatase and GGT levels attributable to the development of nonanastomotic intrahepatic biliary strictures. Occasionally, inadequately followed patients have jaundice or signs and symptoms of ascending cholangitis. Nonanastomotic intrahepatic biliary strictures that develop before 90 days after transplantation are usually not attributable to recurrent disease, and other potential causes should be investigated.[134,164,169,172]

Risk factors for the development of recurrent PSC include donor or recipient HLA-DRB1*08, absence of donor HLA-DR52, gender mismatch, advanced donor age, male recipient, older and younger recipient age, an intact colon, related donors or ECDs, duct-to-duct anastomosis, ABO incompatibility, acute rejection, maintenance steroid therapy for ulcerative colitis for more than 3 months, coexistent cholangiocarcinoma, concurrent CMV infection, ulcerative colitis, presence of active colitis posttransplant, and INR at transplantation.[521,533,535,536] Several studies have shown that colectomy before or after transplantation is protective, but the utility of pretransplant colectomy has been questioned. A recent systematic review by a group from Birmingham and the Netherlands summarizes relevant literature.[537] Explants from patients with PSC showing increased IgG4-positive cells (10 or more per high-power field) are associated with a more aggressive course and PSC recurrence.[538] Patients with PSC are also at greater risk for antibody-mediated and steroid-resistant rejection.

As in native livers, recurrent PSC progresses during a period of years and eventually results in biliary-type cirrhosis. Studies suggest that recurrent disease adversely affects long-term patient and allograft survival and leads to higher retransplantation rates.[539] Cholangiographic findings that help distinguish recurrent PSC from other causes of biliary strictures include time after transplantation (>90 days), mural irregularity, diverticulum-like outpouchings, and features resembling PSC in native livers.[540] These findings, however, are not specific. Percutaneous transhepatic cholangiography and ERCP may be more sensitive than MRCP in detecting early abnormalities.

Pathological Features

Morphological features of recurrent PSC are identical to native livers and cannot be reliably distinguished from other causes of biliary tract obstruction or stricturing in peripheral core needle biopsies (Fig. 53.40). Findings typical of early-stage recurrent PSC include mild, nonspecific acute and chronic pericholangitis and low-grade ductular-type interface activity; eventually "biliary gestalt" gradually appears. Included are irregular, stellate-shaped fibrous expansion of portal tracts, accompanied by some degree of portal/periportal edema, periductal lamellar edema, stellate-shaped lumina of septal bile ducts, intraepithelial and/or intraluminal neutrophils within bile ducts, fibrous cholangitis, small bile duct loss, pigmented macrophages in portal connective tissue, ductular-type interface activity surrounded by edema, and periportal ductular metaplasia of periportal hepatocytes on CK7 staining, accompanied later by deposition of copper and copper-associated protein on special stains. As is typical for biliary diseases, the spatial relationship between the expanded portal tracts and the central veins remains intact until well-developed cirrhosis appears.

Lobular findings in early recurrent PSC include cholestasis, lobular neutrophil clusters, and changes of mild NRH. Late-stage recurrent PSC is characterized by biliary fibrosis/cirrhosis, cholestasis, intralobular foam cell clusters, deposition of copper and copper-associated protein, and Mallory-Denk bodies at the edge of the nodules. Occasionally, eccentric intimal hyperplasia of arteries adjacent to damaged bile ducts may be observed.

Differential Diagnosis

We routinely first recognize recurrent PSC in protocol liver biopsies that show ductular metaplasia of periportal hepatocytes on CK7 staining and preferential elevation of the ALP/GGTP > AST/ALT, followed later by development of a biliary gestalt, described earlier. However, extensive clinicopathological and radiographic correlations are needed to determine whether recurrent PSC or one of the many other causes of biliary tract strictures is responsible for the biopsy changes. This distinction is not possible based on needle biopsy findings alone.

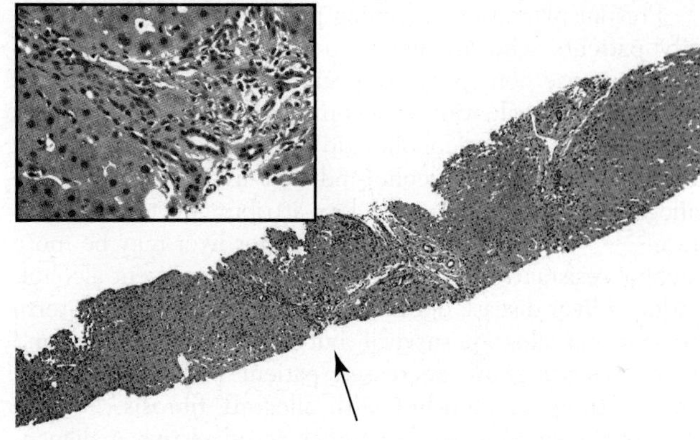

FIGURE 53.40 The pathological findings in recurrent primary sclerosing cholangitis are the same as those seen in many other causes of biliary tract strictures. Mild portal expansion of the true bile ducts is caused by edema, and a ductular reaction at the interface zone and stellate portal fibrosis can be seen. The portal tract *(arrow)* is shown at higher magnification in the *inset*.

Recurrent Alcohol-Induced Liver Disease

End-stage alcohol-induced liver disease is now a leading indication for liver transplantation and has superseded HCV as one of the most common indications for transplant wait listing.[410] Alcoholic hepatitis is also an increasingly, albeit controversial popular indication.[541,542] Altogether, all forms of alcoholic liver disease are often combined with other conditions such as HCV infection, hepatocellular carcinoma, and metabolic disorders (e.g., hemochromatosis, α_1-antitrypsin deficiency).[543] The incidence of recurrent alcohol use or abuse after transplantation is difficult to determine with certainty. The reported recurrence rate ranges from 15% to 50% at 5 years after transplantation.[544] Most incidences of recidivism tend to occur within the first 2 to 3 years posttransplantation.[543,545] Recurrent alcohol abuse can directly damage allografts or indirectly contribute to allograft dysfunction as a result of rejection-related injury related to noncompliance with immunosuppression therapy.[544,546]

Clinical Features

Problems with alcohol recidivism are usually detected because of elevation of liver injury tests,[546] missed medical appointments,[547] inappropriate social behavior,[181] and noncompliance with immunosuppression therapy. [544,546] A variety of more recently introduced biomarkers that point toward alcohol use (e.g., urinary ethyl glucuronide and/or ethyl sulfate, serum carbohydrate-deficient transferrin, whole-blood phosphatidylethanol) have gained acceptance in monitoring.[548] Older traditional methods, such as high GGT/alkaline phosphatase ratio can also provide evidence suggestive of alcohol recurrence.[181,546] A small minority of patients experience a rapid downhill course after transplantation because of recidivism and recurrent alcoholic steatohepatitis.[549-551]

Pretransplantation screening programs attempt to identify patients who are likely to relapse after transplantation. Because none is entirely successful, a comprehensive psychosocial evaluation is recommended.[545,546,552] Studies suggest that most alcoholics do not relapse badly enough to cause significant alcohol-induced liver disease in the allografts, and that allograft loss attributable to alcohol is rare.[553,554] Alternatively, the new donor liver may be more alcohol resistant. Most studies show that recurrent alcohol-induced liver disease does not significantly affect long-term patient and allograft survival, but more recent studies and meta-analyses show decreased patient and graft survival and a strong relationship with allograft fibrosis.[543,555,556] Cardiovascular disease and upper aerodigestive malignancies related to long-term alcohol and tobacco abuse are a significant source of morbidity and mortality in this patient population.[544,546]

Pathological Features

Histopathological features of alcohol abuse in allograft livers are identical to those in native livers. Graft biopsies from recidivists show more steatosis, steatohepatitis, and pericellular fibrosis.[555] Both small- and large-droplet steatosis involving primarily centrilobular hepatocytes is common. The zonal distribution of steatosis is distinctive (Fig. 53.41). More significant abuse can lead to "foamy" degeneration of centrilobular hepatocytes, followed by fully developed alcoholic hepatitis with Mallory-Denk bodies, ballooning degeneration of hepatocytes, and lobular inflammation with satellitosis. However, steatosis and steatohepatitis including Mallory-Denk bodies can also be observed in abstinent patients, and they are not specific markers for recurrence, possibly because of other metabolic fatty liver risk factors.

Severe alcoholic relapse eventually leads to perivenular and subsinusoidal fibrosis and recurrent alcoholic cirrhosis 5 to 6 years after transplantation and about 4 years post-relapse.[546,549,556-558] In our experience, relapse can also present with increased iron deposition in periportal hepatocytes and reticuloendothelial cells. Hepatocytes may not show significant steatosis.[181] As in native livers, alcoholic steatohepatitis can coexist with HCV infection and any other cause of allograft dysfunction. Combined insults lead to more rapid development of fibrosis.[546,549]

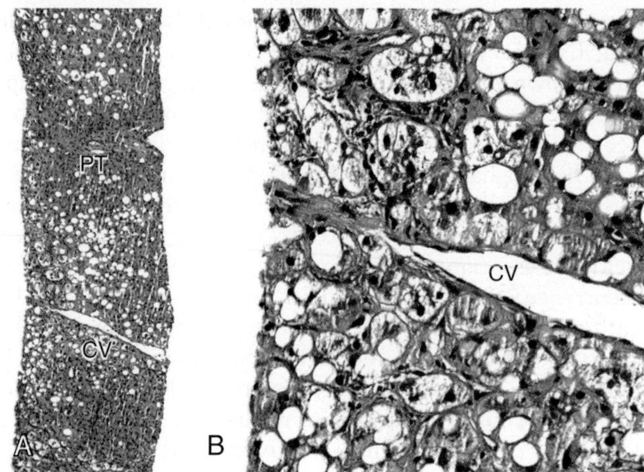

FIGURE 53.41 A, Recurrent alcohol abuse is characterized by centrilobular, mixed macrovesicular and microvesicular steatosis. **B,** Frank alcoholic hepatitis with Mallory hyaline and foamy degeneration of hepatocytes is seen in the perivenular area. Severe recidivism can lead to perivenular fibrosis. *CV,* Central vein; *PT,* portal tract.

Recurrent Nonalcoholic Steatohepatitis

Clinical Features

Nonalcoholic fatty liver disease (NAFLD) is now the leading indication for liver transplant waitlist registration in the United States, followed by alcoholic liver disease and HCV.[410] Hepatocellular carcinoma complicating NASH has also been noticeably increasing, particularly in women.[559-561]

Recurrent disease risk factors include posttransplant BMI, female gender, alcohol consumption, dyslipidemia, diabetes, and metabolic syndrome with insulin resistance that persists after transplantation.[562-566] Persistence of some of these factors is at least partially attributable to immunosuppressive medications. Recurrent steatosis is detected in over 50% at 1 year and 70% to 100% at 3 to 5 years.[567] Steatohepatitis develops in 5% to 25% of patients, and less than 5% of patients develop progressive fibrosis and cirrhosis, which may be influenced by dietary habits.[561-566,568]

A significant proportion of patients who undergo liver transplantation for cryptogenic cirrhosis develop NAFLD after transplantation.[561,563,569-571] Presumably, these patients had undetected NAFLD before transplantation, but the pathological features were not detected in the explanted cirrhotic liver.

Recurrent NAFLD is frequently detected in allograft biopsies in asymptomatic patients. A minority of otherwise healthy recipients develop unexplained NAFLD after transplantation (de novo NAFLD). In these patients, metabolic testing for insulin resistance and a search for more esoteric causes of NAFLD are warranted.

Histopathological Features

Detailed descriptions of the histopathology of hepatic steatosis and steatohepatitis are given in Chapter 50, and these conditions are not known to be different in allografts.[572] NAFLD refers to biopsies in which more than 5% of hepatocytes show steatosis. A diagnosis of NASH requires evidence of hepatocyte injury (e.g., ballooning, apoptosis, lytic necrosis) and lobular inflammation. Fibrosis is not required.[572] Fibrosis typically begins in the perivenular sinusoids.

Differential Diagnosis

The differential diagnosis of recurrent alcoholism and NAFLD is extensive and includes all of the disorders known to cause small- and large-droplet macrovesicular steatosis and steatohepatitis in the general population. True microvesicular steatosis is not covered given the rarity of its occurrence in allografts. The histopathological changes of recurrent alcohol-induced liver disease is difficult to distinguish from NAFLD. Findings that favor alcohol-induced injury include more severe steatohepatitis overall, including numerous Mallory-Denk bodies, neutrophilic satellitosis, and cholestasis.

Determination of the underlying cause of steatohepatitis in allografts can be difficult. As in native livers, steatohepatitis occurs most commonly in patients with risk factors such as obesity, diabetes, hyperlipidemia, excessive alcohol use, and polycystic ovary syndrome. However, it can also be associated with nutritional causes (e.g., malnutrition, starvation, rapid weight loss, and intestinal surgical interventions to promote weight loss). Hepatic steatosis and steatohepatitis can be caused by numerous medications such as glucocorticoids, amiodarone (usually associated with Mallory-Denk bodies out of proportion to the severity of steatosis), perhexiline maleate, synthetic estrogens (e.g., tamoxifen), calcium channel blockers, methotrexate, valproic acid, and cocaine.

Steatosis and steatohepatitis can be caused by a variety of genetically-based metabolic disorders reviewed here.[573] Other, less common causes include inflammatory bowel disease, intestinal bacterial overgrowth, and exposure to environmental toxins (e.g., phosphorous, petrochemicals, toxic mushrooms, and organic solvents). Abnormalities of hepatic blood flow are an important cause of hepatic steatosis and steatohepatitis,[142] especially when they appear in allografts early (within several months after transplantation). Examples include portosystemic shunting because of collaterals that persist after transplantation, prehepatic portal hypertension, and patent ductus venosus.

Idiopathic Posttransplantation Hepatitis

Clinical Features and Pathophysiology

IPTH is a diagnostic term originally coined by Hubscher[574] to describe allograft biopsies with typical "chronic hepatitis" changes, but without clinical or serological evidence of viral hepatitis (especially chronic untreated HBV, HCV and chronic HEV), autoimmunity, or DILI.[178,265] According to the definition, features used to diagnose TCMR, such as bile duct damage and venous endothelial inflammation, are neither severe nor widespread, but can be focally present.[4,399,574] Most recipients are diagnosed by analysis of protocol allograft biopsies. They are usually asymptomatic, with normal or near-normal liver function test values. The incidence and prevalence are higher in centers that use protocol biopsies. Lack of a consensus definition, different immunosuppressive regimens, undiscovered viruses (e.g., HEV),[415] or a combination of these factors probably explains the reported variations in the frequency of IPTH.[575]

Studies including late allograft changes in pediatric liver transplant recipients (not significantly affected by disease recurrence), greater understanding of the role of HLA and donor-specific antibodies, and analysis of biopsies from immunosuppression-weaning trials has improved our understanding of IPTH.[3,146,183,200,206,213,216,219,283,343,352] Indeed, accumulating evidence points toward an alloimmune etiology such as late-onset TCMR with or without associated chronic AMR. Therefore use of the term *IPTH* is being replaced in many cases by *late-onset TCMR associated with chronic AMR*.

Evans et al. demonstrated progressive chronic hepatitis in pediatric liver recipients undergoing protocol biopsies at 1, 5, and 10 years, with incidence increasing over time (22% at 1 year, 43% at 5 years, and 64% at 10 years). They also showed that the incidence and severity of fibrosis also increases over time (52%, 81%, and 91% at 1, 5, and 10 years, respectively) with about 15% progressing to cirrhosis.[182] A clear nonalloimmune cause for the hepatitis has not been identified in most cases, but autoantibody positivity was detected in a higher frequency. Subsequent studies also identified a high incidence of histological abnormalities on protocol biopsies performed ≥1 year post–liver transplant exceeding 70% at 20 years posttransplantation, and an association between cholestatic hepatitis (inflammation), HLA class II DSA, non-HLA antibodies, no steroids, prior episodes of TCMR, chronic rejection, and progressive graft fibrosis.[147,215,216,219,220,576-578] The area has been succinctly reviewed by Kelly et al.[216] Two recent studies documenting chronic allograft changes in pediatric and adult recipients showed similar results.[183,579]

Feng et al. reported on 157 highly selected pediatric liver recipients screened for enrollment into an immunosuppression-weaning trial.[183] Clustering analysis based on protocol predetermined histopathological findings resulted in three distinct clusters: cluster 1 was characterized by interface hepatitis (n = 34); cluster 2 showed more than mild fibrosis with or without interface hepatitis (n = 45); and cluster 3 (the remainder of cases) showed neither (near normal). Molecular whole-genomics mRNA expression profiling showed overexpression of TCMR-related genes in cluster 1 but not clusters 2 or 3. Cluster 1 patients also showed a higher incidence of class II DSA, association with higher mean fluorescence intensity sum (MFI sum >20,000), and higher ALT levels.

Londoño et al. studied 67 adult liver transplant recipients >10 years posttransplantation without disease recurrence or other posttransplant complication.[579] However, 76% showed histological abnormalities: 67% showed portal inflammation, 27% showed interface hepatitis, and 43% showed fibrosis. Patients with portal inflammation also showed a transcriptional profile resembling TCMR. All of this evidence points toward an alloimmune nature for IPTH and that it is likely a form of late rejection with or without associated chronic AMR.

Pathological Features and Differential Diagnosis

Idiopathic posttransplant chronic hepatitis is characterized by portal tract lymphocytic inflammation and some degree of mostly interface and with lesser severity lobular necroinflammatory activity without prominent bile duct damage. Central inflammation can be seen. Significant plasma cell inflammation composing more than 30% of the infiltrate is uncommon and suggests recurrent AIH or plasma cell–rich rejection.[3] The differential diagnosis for chronic allograft hepatitis includes hepatitis virus infection (A, B, C, D, and E), DILI, so-called autoimmune hepatitis, "hepatitic" manifestation of hematological disorders, and TCMR. A thorough clinical, serological, and molecular evaluation is needed to confidently sort among these possibilities. However, in the current era, late-onset TCMR is most common and frequently associated with de novo DSA.

Immunosuppression Optimization

Liver allograft biopsy evaluation plays a critical role in immunosuppression optimization, including the possibility of complete withdrawal of immunosuppression from a small number of highly selected recipients.[4,317,399,580] Liver allografts suffer less permanent damage from TCMR than other solid organs.[276] If TCMR does occur during or after weaning, it is usually rapidly reversible with readministration of immunosuppression. Importantly, affected allografts usually heal without significant fibrosis or loss of function.[4,276,317,399,580-582]

Clinical/demographic characteristics associated with successful weaning in some (but not all) studies include a longer period between transplantation and weaning[583,584] (preferably more than 3 years), a tendency for less DSA production,[583,585] a low incidence of previous TCMR episodes, nonautoimmune primary liver disease, already minimized immunosuppression,[584] and lower recipient age at the time of transplantation.[586,587]

Histopathological Features and Differential Diagnosis

Formal immunosuppression minimization is usually conducted in the context of an organized clinical trial that mandates preweaning biopsies.[399] The histopathological findings in these biopsies are typical of protocol biopsies obtained from asymptomatic, long-surviving recipients with normal or near-normal liver function test values who did not suffer from diseases that typically recur after transplantation (e.g., HCV, AIH, PBC, PSC), except for those who required liver transplantation for alcoholic steatohepatitis and NASH.[4,317,399] Baseline preweaning biopsies document baseline inflammatory and structural changes to avoid confusion introduced with findings on postweaning biopsies. They also serve to exclude patients with advanced fibrosis and architectural distortion and other disorders that may be confused with changes precipitated by immunosuppression weaning.[399]

Most current immunosuppression minimization protocols exclude patients with advanced fibrosis (i.e., ≥3 on the Ishak scale or any Venturi subcomponent score of 3: severe portal/periportal, sinusoidal, or perivenular). The rationale for excluding those with advanced fibrosis is the fear of decompensation introduced by accelerated immunological injury on a compromised liver. It may also make subtle increases in the severity of fibrosis more difficult to detect. One study of HCV-positive recipients questioned the validity of this approach, positing that the fibrosis may have been the result of prior suboptimal viral control,[588] but this concern is largely of historical interest.

Preweaning biopsy findings associated with subsequent successful weaning include less portal inflammation[581,583,589]; fewer CD3-positive and lobular CD8-positive lymphocytes but more CD45RO-positive lymphocytes within the lobules[581,589]; less recent monocyte immigrants into the liver as identified by Mac387 staining[581]; less intralobular lymphocyte-APC pairings as identified by automated image analysis[581]; portal fibrosis only in HCV-positive recipients[588]; and less prevalent microvascular C4d deposits.[583] Conversely, portal inflammation in HCV-negative patients, more intralobular CD3-positive CD8-positive and CD45-MHCII-positive (lymphocyte-APC pairs), and tissue C4d deposits in patients with circulating DSAs likely represents a latent form of rejection that manifests clinically after reduction or removal of immunosuppression.[399]

Follow-up biopsies are usually obtained in response to an elevation in liver function test values. This usually occurs in the first several months after drug withdrawal has exceeded 70% of starting immunosuppression and is preceded or accompanied by development of de novo DSA in patients who ultimately experience rejection.[399,580,581,590] However, increases in liver function test results can be nonspecific and spontaneously return to baseline without intervention. An elevated GGT level is a sensitive indicator of TCMR after weaning.[591,592] Weaning of immunosuppression can also accelerate original disease recurrence.[399,580]

TCMR episodes during or after weaning from immunosuppression usually exhibit typical features of acute TCMR, but presentation as an active chronic hepatitis and/or central perivenulitis is not uncommon. TCMR occurring more than 1 year after transplantation may differ biologically and histologically from that occurring in the first several months after transplantation because the host-graft immune relationship is different in the early and late periods after transplantation. TCMR can evolve more slowly late after transplantation and be subclinical. The immunosuppressive regimens used before weaning, such as lymphocyte-depleting antibodies, can alter the histopathological appearance of TCMR after weaning.[4,399,580]

Histopathological differences between TCMR that occur during or after weaning and early allograft TCMR include less prevalent and severe inflammatory bile duct damage, more prevalent and severe interface and perivenular necroinflammatory activity, and less portal venous subendothelial inflammation. Therefore a resemblance to low-grade chronic hepatitis is often seen,[399,580] but since most causes of chronic viral hepatitis are effectively treated, sorting among differential diagnostic possibilities in the current era is less problematic than in years past.

Although mostly of historical interest, early and rapid weaning of immunosuppression from HCV-positive[453] and some HCV-negative recipients[593] treated with lymphocyte-depleting antibodies can re-arm the immune system (i.e., *immune reconstitution syndrome*),[453] which manifests pathologically as severe hepatitis with rapid progression of fibrosis.[453] Formerly stable patients in whom HCV infection progression is accelerated in the course of weaning without histological signs of TCMR constitute a significant challenge. These patients may require more gradual weaning or more effective treatment aimed at inhibiting HCV replication.

More data are becoming available about protocol follow-up biopsies in patients after lowering or complete withdrawal of immunosuppression.[4,399,580,594] Development of progressive, rejection-related fibrosis is a particular concern,[4,399] although this has also occurred in patients who are maintained on immunosuppression.[4,399] Studies suggest that perivenular fibrosis in particular is associated with DSAs and tissue deposits of C4d.[144-146] However, in two distinct pediatric cohorts who were completely weaned from all immunosuppression, there was no systemically increased inflammation or fibrosis in a follow-up period of 4[581] or 5[594] immunosuppression-free years, despite the appearance of DSA in some of the cohort.

To effectively monitor fibrosis status, the Banff Working Group encouraged two adequate passes with a 16-gauge needle that is more than 20 mm long and protocol biopsies of more than 11 portal tracts[79] in patients who do not develop symptoms or have biochemical evidence of liver injury at 1, 3, 5, and 10 years after a major decrease or total withdrawal of immunosuppression.[399] Current protocols have even lessened the number of biopsy timepoints, but a fear of subclinical injury exists in patients maintained on little or no immunosuppression.

Biopsy findings that should prompt close follow-up and that may indicate worsening immunological damage include increased inflammation associated with tissue damage (e.g., interface and/or perivenular or biliary epithelial cell necroinflammatory activity, clearly advancing fibrosis (usually >1 change in any Venturi subcomponent score), or appearance of obliterative arteriopathy. An algorithm for evaluating and following these patients was proposed by the Banff Working Group (Fig. 53.42).

Long-Term Histopathological Changes Not Caused by Recurrent Disease

Some histopathological changes in long-surviving allografts cannot be attributed to recurrent disease and/or rejection. Some may represent DILI or supplement-induced liver injury or consequences of long-term engraftment and abnormal graft physiology.[4,181,317] Included are portal venopathy and NRH (Fig. 53.43), thickening and hyalinization of small hepatic artery branches,[181,595] subsinusoidal fibrosis, and nonspecific portal and lobular inflammation.[4,181,317] More recently, however, some of these changes are being attributed to chronic AMR-related injury. Livers from older patients transplanted into younger recipients (e.g., parent-to-child living donation) continue to age at the same or an accelerated rate.[596] If NRH is detected less than 4 years after transplantation, progression to portal hypertension may occur.[597]

Adverse Drug Reactions and Toxic Injury

Hepatic allograft manifestations of DILI are usually similar to those that occur in native livers. One exception is drugs that elicit immunoallergic reactions, which may be attenuated because of immunosuppression. It can be difficult to distinguish DILI from TCMR, recurrent disease, and other complications. Complaints of DILI after liver transplantation are uncommon to rare.[598]

Azathioprine has been associated with centrilobular necrosis and with central vein and subsinusoidal fibrosis, but similar changes are seen with TCMR.[599] NRH has been attributed to chronic toxicity,[595] but it is also frequently seen in recipients who have not been treated with this medication.

Pseudo–ground-glass cells (i.e., hepatocytes with ground-glass cytoplasm that are HBsAg negative) can be seen in liver allografts. A commonly encountered inclusion in liver allografts consists of abnormal glycogen resembling polyglucosan bodies,[600] which are probably related to disturbances in glycogen metabolism as a result of multiple medications.

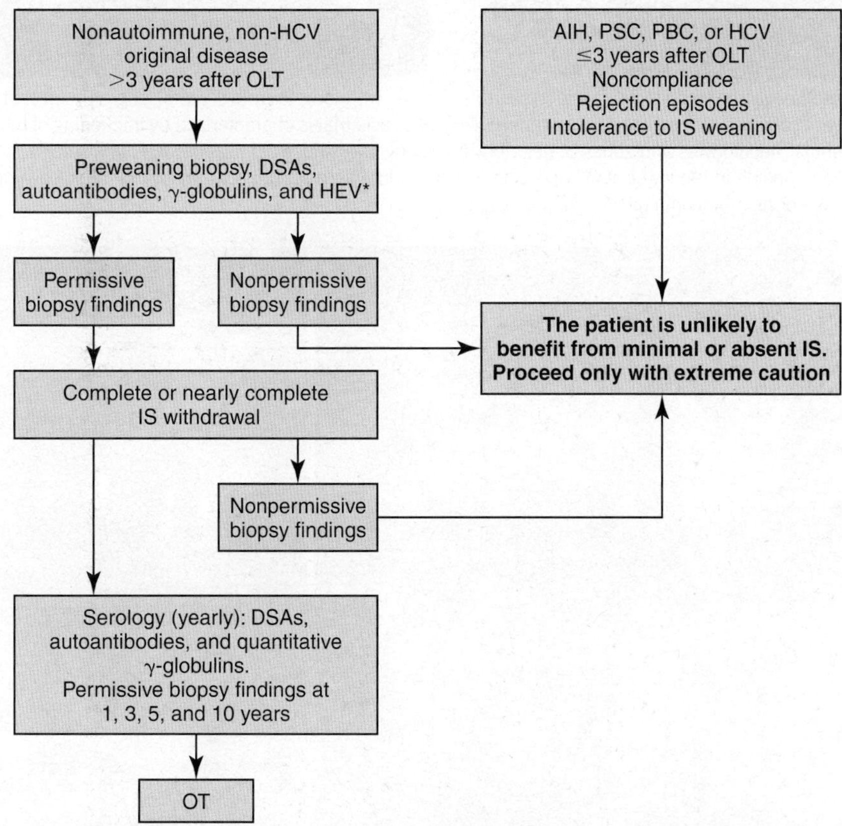

FIGURE 53.42 Banff algorithm to evaluate and monitor patients being considered for withdrawal of immunosuppression. *AIH,* Autoimmune hepatitis; *DSA,* donor-specific antibody; *HCV,* hepatitis C virus; *HEV,* hepatitis E virus; *IS,* immunosuppression; *OLT,* orthotopic liver transplantation; *OT,* operational tolerance; *PBC,* primary biliary cirrhosis; *PSC,* primary sclerosing cholangitis. Hepatitis E virus (HEV) testing *(asterisk)* should be considered for patients with preweaning biopsy samples that show idiopathic posttransplantation hepatitis. (From Banff Working Group on Liver Allograft Pathology. Importance of liver biopsy findings in immunosuppression management: biopsy monitoring and working criteria for patients with operational tolerance. *Liver Transpl.* 2012;18:1154–1170.)

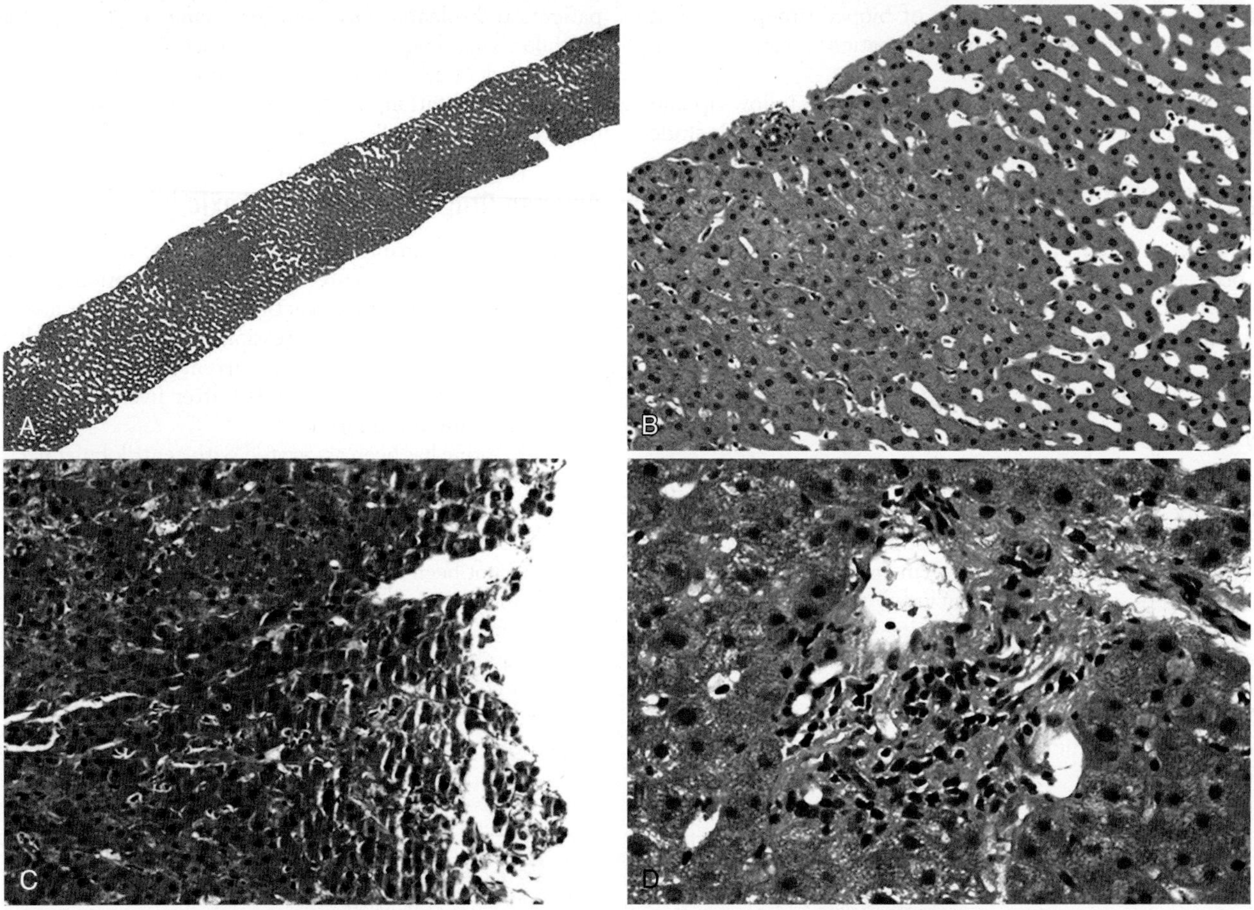

FIGURE 53.43 The composite image shows changes typically seen in patients with long-term (>5 years) engraftment that are not attributable to a specific disease. **A,** Low magnification shows mild nodular, regenerative hyperplasia that is characterized by thickening of the periportal hepatic plates *(more solid areas)* of perivenular hepatocytes and zones of hepatocyte atrophy and sinusoidal dilation. **B,** Higher magnification of **A.** Note the focal sinusoidal dilation and a vague nodule in the lower-right aspect. **C,** Subsinusoidal fibrosis. **D,** Focal, mild, mononuclear portal inflammation without inflammatory bile duct damage or necro-inflammatory interface activity.

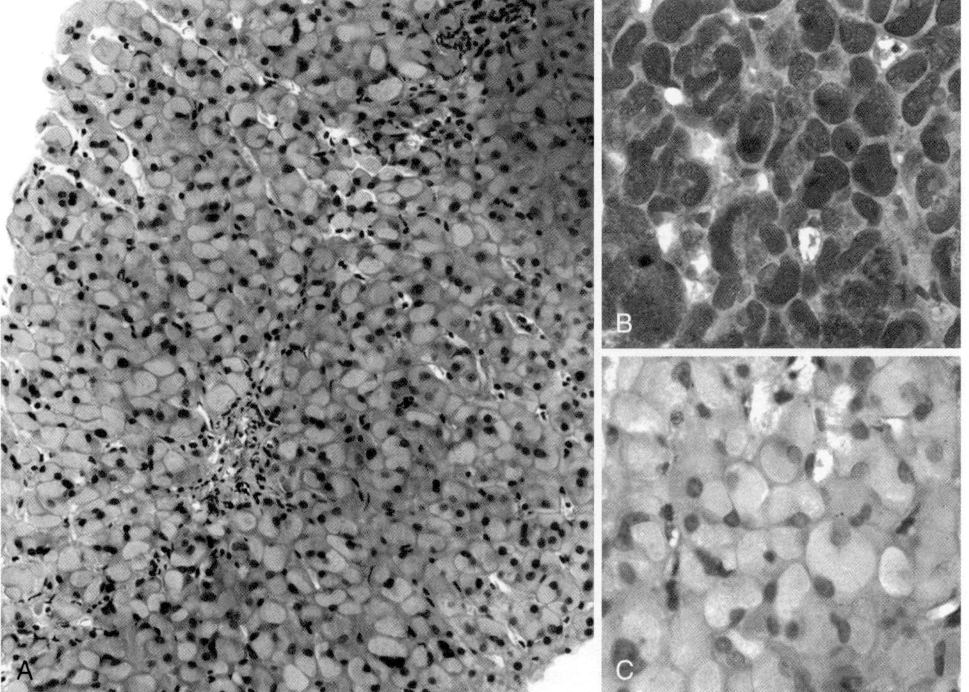

FIGURE 53.44 Ground-glass–like hepatocellular inclusions without a singularly defined cause are more common in liver allograft biopsy specimens than in native livers. The differential diagnosis includes hepatitis B surface antigen, cyanamide aversion therapy for alcohol abuse, Lafora disease, type IV glycogenosis, and fibrinogen storage disease. **A,** H&E stain. **B,** Periodic acid–Schiff (PAS) stain. **C,** PAS stain with diastase digestion (d-PAS). PAS-positive inclusions help characterize the type of inclusion.

These inclusions are PAS positive/diastase sensitive (Fig. 53.44) and resemble non–membrane-bound glycogen deposits on ultrastructural examination. Similar deposits can be seen in Lafora disease, type IV glycogenosis, adult-onset polyglucosan disease, and inclusions associated with cyanamide therapy. Another type of inclusion is referred to as *acquired endoplasmic reticulum storage disease* (e.g., fibrinogen storage disease) in which deposits are PAS-negative and segregated from the remainder of the cytoplasm by membrane inclusions on ultrastructural examination.

Hematopoietic Stem Cell Transplantation

Liver disease occurs in most patients before or after hematopoietic stem cell transplantation (HSCT) and can range from mild and reversible disease to hepatic failure.[601,602] Indeed, clinically overt liver disease presenting early after HSCT plays a significant role in adverse outcomes and is often considered to be the primary cause of death. [603] Patterns of damage fall into the broad categories of pretransplantation disease, toxic injury caused by medications, recurrence of the primary disease, immunologically mediated injury (i.e., GVHD), and a combination of these insults.[602,604]

Pretransplantation liver diseases that increase the risk of liver disease after transplantation include hepatic fungal infections, untreated viral hepatitis in the donor, all causes of chronic liver disease in the general population (e.g., HBV or HCV infection, cholestatic diseases, alcohol, NAFLD), biliary tract stones, and iron overload. Significant hepatic fibrosis and architectural distortion before transplantation increase the risk of mortality after transplantation.[602]

The most common and feared type of liver toxicity usually results from the cytoreductive therapy used during induction. It may take the form of a generalized impairment of liver function in the immediate posttransplantation period, sinusoidal obstruction syndrome (SOS), or NRH months later.[605-607] HSCT recipients are not spared from other potential adverse drug reactions. Systemic infections that involve the liver or infection by opportunistic viruses (e.g., HSV, VZV, CMV, adenovirus) or hepatotropic viruses (e.g., HAV, HBV, HEV) are always considerations. GVHD is always a potential cause of liver dysfunction.[608]

Given the risks of percutaneous, transjugular, or operative liver biopsy in the immediate posttransplantation period, a liver biopsy is not normally obtained at that early time. However, with the passage of time after transplantation, a liver biopsy may become increasingly necessary to sort out the diagnostic possibilities for these patients. Moreover, the availability of targeted therapies and the need to choose an optimal management strategy constitute potentially strong reasons for performing a liver biopsy, even in the pediatric patient.[609]

Sinusoidal Obstruction Syndrome

SOS, previously called *venoocclusive disease* (VOD), is a manifestation of induction cytotoxicity, especially cyclophosphamide and total body irradiation.[601,602,605] It directly damages the hepatic sinusoidal endothelium.[602,605] It occurs in approximately 15% of HSCT recipients, but the incidence varies by center and treatment regimen.[610] The pathology of this condition is presented in Chapter 52.

For the purposes of this chapter, the key discussion pertains to clinical context. Sudden weight gain, hepatomegaly, and abdominal tenderness are the initial signs of the liver toxicity of SOS. These symptoms typically occur 10 to 20 days after the initiation of cytoreductive therapy.[602] Hyperbilirubinemia usually occurs 4 to 10 days later. Clinical criteria are used to establish a diagnosis, and liver biopsies usually are unnecessary.[610] The Seattle criteria include the finding of two or more of the following symptoms within 30 days after transplantation: bilirubin level of 2 mg/dL (34 μmol/L) or higher, hepatomegaly, right upper quadrant pain, and ascites with or without unexplained weight gain of more than 2% higher than baseline. The new Seattle criteria require manifestation of the clinical features by day 20 after transplantation. The Baltimore criteria require a bilirubin level of 2 mg/dL or higher by day 21 after transplantation and at least two of the following: hepatomegaly (usually painful), ascites, and weight gain of more than 5% higher than baseline.

The mortality rate associated with SOS varies with the severity of disease, although the criteria for severity have not been uniformly defined.[602,610] The overall mortality rate is less than 30%, but it can be as high as 80% for severely affected individuals. In addition to the cardinal clinical signs of SOS, manifestations of severe disease include multiorgan failure, defined as an oxygen requirement (i.e., oxygen saturation ≤90% in room air or ventilator dependence), renal dysfunction (i.e., doubling of the baseline creatinine level or dialysis dependence), or encephalopathy in addition to liver failure. [602,610] Although persistent severe liver dysfunction is a harbinger of a fatal outcome, the liver disease is not usually the direct cause of death. Most patients succumb to renal, cardiopulmonary, and multiorgan failure.[602,610]

Risk factors for SOS fall into two general categories.[611] Some factors predate transplantation and are related to preexisting liver injury or global inflammation. Included are viral or alcoholic steatohepatitis, elevated liver enzyme levels, heavy pretreatment (especially with hepatotoxic agents), a history of infection and long antibiotic exposure, and reduced diffusing capacity of the lung for carbon monoxide. Other risk factors are related to transplantation therapy. They include total body irradiation, cyclophosphamide exposure and dosage, oral busulfan use, and injuries related to hepatotoxic medications.[602,610,611]

As noted, liver biopsy during the acute phase of SOS is unusual. However, as the initial days after HSCT become weeks, the differential diagnosis for liver dysfunction broadens, and liver biopsy may be indicated. Even if other causes of liver injury are dominant, careful examination of post-HSCT liver biopsies reveals a high incidence of subtle lesions within terminal hepatic veins. [612] For a definitive diagnosis of SOS, obvious centrilobular congestion without readily identifiable terminal hepatic veins on H&E staining should prompt evaluation of connective tissue stains to exclude SOS. In the chronic stage of SOS, collagen deposition in and around affected terminal hepatic venules leads to their progressive obliteration (Fig. 53.45). Persistence of lesions during weeks to months results in the development of dense perivenular fibrosis, which often radiates into the liver parenchyma. The scar tissue often contains hemosiderin-laden macrophages, and congestion can subside. The terminal hepatic vein lumina are usually difficult to identify. There may be severe destruction of lobular parenchyma and, rarely, evolution to cirrhosis.[605,607]

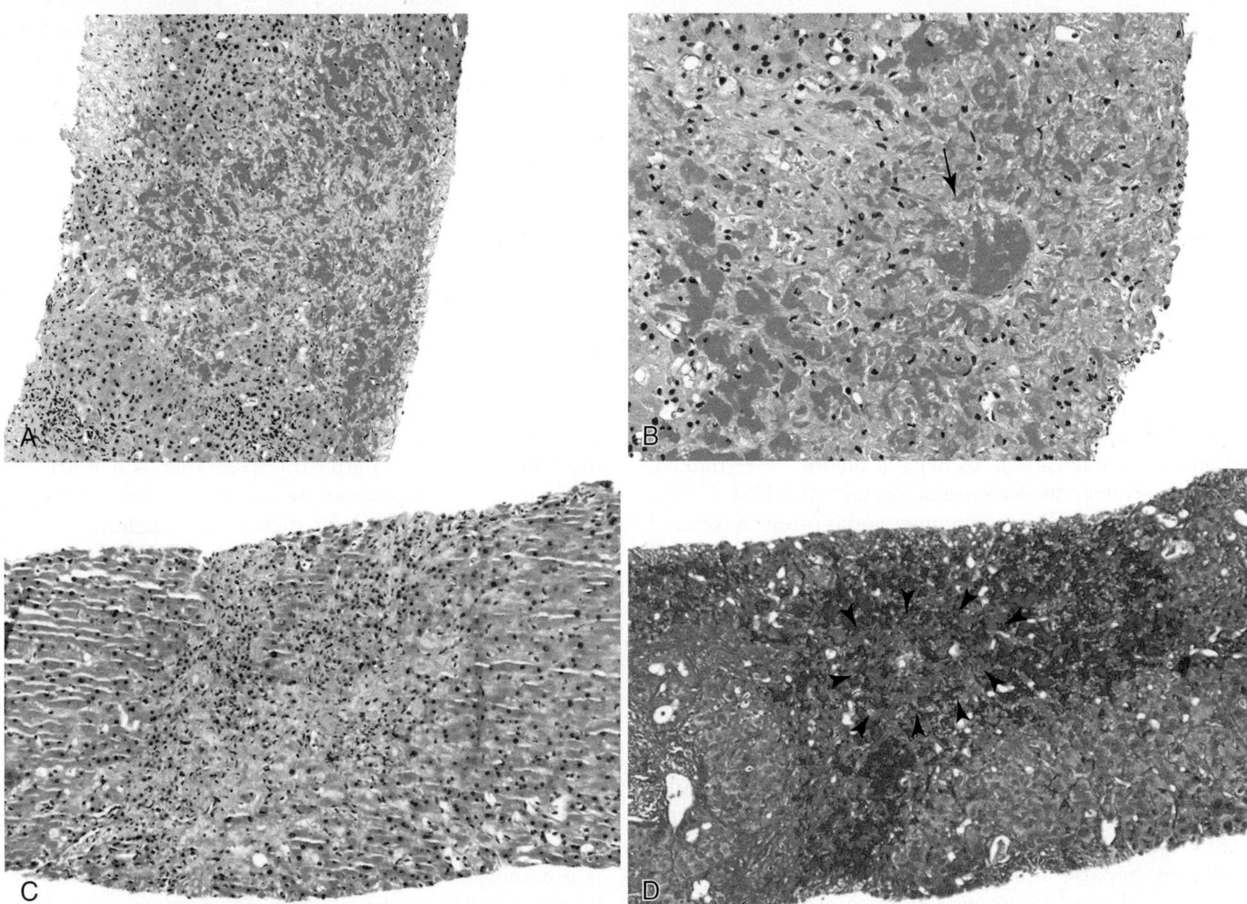

FIGURE 53.45 Sinusoidal obstruction syndrome (i.e., venoocclusive disease). A, Acute stage. Medium-power magnification shows pericentral hemorrhage and necrosis without a terminal hepatic vein. **B,** Acute stage. Medium-power view shows occlusion of the terminal hepatic vein *(arrow)*. **C,** Later stage. Low-power view shows fibrous septa radiating out from the central region without a terminal hepatic vein. **D,** Later stage. Low-power view shows a preexisting rim of terminal hepatic vein *(arrowheads)* and almost complete obliteration of the lumen. The intraluminal stroma contains type III and IV collagen and does not stain as intensely with Masson trichrome stain.

Differential Diagnosis

Diagnoses to be excluded include GVHD, other causes of venous outflow obstruction (e.g., Budd-Chiari syndrome, congestive heart failure), drug reactions (e.g., toxic effects of hyperalimentation), and infections (e.g., viral hepatitis, fungi, and sepsis). Budd-Chiari syndrome features centrilobular congestion and potentially parenchymal destruction but without occlusion of the terminal hepatic veins. Drug reactions usually exhibit parenchymal damage with hepatocellular apoptosis, cholestasis, and inflammation. Although severe SOS can produce similar histology, identification of terminal hepatic vein lesions is a key finding. The clinical features of posttransplantation drug toxicity and SOS are similar. There is less need to make a specific diagnosis of SOS by liver biopsy for these unstable patients than to exclude other potential causes of hepatic dysfunction.

OTHER TRANSPLANTATION EFFECTS

Graft-versus-Host Disease

HSC transplantation involves grafting of stem cells obtained from mobilized peripheral blood or donor bone marrow into an immunosuppressed patient whose marrow has been abrogated by cytoreductive therapy. The process confers disease-free survival advantages but carries an increased risk of chronic GVHD.[613] Three conditions are necessary for the development of GVHD: infusion of immunocompetent cells, histocompatibility differences between the donor and recipient, and inability of the recipient to destroy donor cells.

GVHD usually arises in the setting of allogeneic bone marrow transplantation for myeloproliferative disorders, although it may also occur following HSCT for solid tumors.[614] The likelihood that GVHD will develop increases with the degree of histoincompatibility between donor and recipient, but it also has occurred after autologous and syngeneic bone marrow transplantation and occasionally after solid organ transplantation (especially liver) because of the resident lymphocytes that are transplanted with the organ. GVHD develops in three sequential phases: activation of antigen-presenting cells; donor T cell activation, proliferation, differentiation, and migration; and target tissue destruction.[615] A role for intestinal microbiota in the early development of GVHD has been proposed as a result of the compromise to intestinal integrity during the myeloablative induction regime, release of endotoxin and potentially intact bacteria into the splanchnic circulation, and promotion of a pro-inflammatory milieu.[616] Acute and chronic GVHD are related, but sufficient clinical and histological differences indicate that they may represent distinct disease processes.[615]

Clinical symptoms of GVHD consist of skin changes, diarrhea, and weight loss, reflecting involvement of the epithelium of the skin, alimentary tract, liver, and other tissues such as mucous membranes, bronchial epithelium, and muscles. Despite HLA identity between patient and donor, the incidence of acute GVHD is 26% to 32% among recipients of sibling donor grafts and 42% to 52% among recipients of unrelated donor grafts.[615]

The three main organs involved in acute GVHD are the skin, liver, and gastrointestinal tract. Historically, acute and chronic forms were arbitrarily defined based on the time after transplantation (less or more than 100 days, respectively). The overall severity of disease is based on the extent and severity of target organ involvement.[615,617,618] The current consensus is that clinical manifestations determine whether signs and symptoms of GVHD are acute, chronic, or overlapping (i.e., diagnostic features of acute and chronic GVHD appear together),[615,617,618] noting that clear morphological distinction between acute and chronic GVHD may not be possible.[619] The clinical manifestations of acute, chronic, and overlapping GVHD are discussed elsewhere.[615,617,618]

Acute Graft-versus-Host Disease

In acute GVHD, liver dysfunction may develop within days, but it more commonly manifests 2 to 4 weeks after transplantation. Laboratory tests show a gradual rise in serum levels of direct and indirect bilirubin, alkaline phosphatase, and transaminases. Hepatomegaly may occur, although usually without pain. The syndrome of acute GVHD includes the appearance of a red, maculopapular rash on the trunk, soles, palms, and ears (which may progress to total body involvement), with bullae formation and desquamation in severe cases. Intestinal symptoms include crampy abdominal pain, anorexia, nausea, vomiting, watery or bloody diarrhea, and paralytic ileus.

With progression to severe disease, coagulopathy and bleeding diatheses may develop, along with hepatic failure, ascites, and encephalopathy. Full-scale destruction of the epithelium of the alimentary tract in advanced cases leads to fatal sepsis. The incidence of acute GVHD ranges from 10% to more than 80% among bone marrow recipients, depending on the degree of histoincompatibility, number of T cells in the graft, patient age (incidence increases with age), and the type of immunoprophylactic regimen.

The certainty of a diagnosis of acute GVHD is based on the extent of clinical findings and on exclusion of drug toxicity and infection. Unlike SOS, weight gain and right upper quadrant pain are rare. The pathological features of acute GVHD in liver biopsies result from selective damage of the epithelium of small bile ducts. Rigorous adherence to morphological diagnostic criteria is essential to avoid overdiagnosis of GVHD and potentially disastrous immunosuppression.

Chronic Graft-versus-Host Disease

Historically, chronic GVHD is a syndrome that develops 100 days or more after transplantation. It is currently defined mostly by disease characteristics and presentation.[615] It most often arises as an extension of acute GVHD, but it can also occur after a long disease-free interval or de novo, without previous episodes of acute GVHD. Unlike the acute form, chronic GVHD is a heterogeneous disease that involves a much broader range of organ systems, including the skin, gastrointestinal tract, liver, minor salivary glands, lymph nodes, mouth, eyes, lungs, and musculoskeletal system. Involvement culminates in a blend of autoimmune syndromes that feature target organ atrophy, fibrosis, and loss of secretions and exocrine function.[615]

The incidence of chronic GVHD ranges from 30% among recipients of fully histocompatible sibling donor transplants to 60% to 70% among recipients of mismatched HSCs or cells from an unrelated donor.[620] Other factors that increase the likelihood of chronic GVHD include a prior episode of acute GVHD, older recipient age, female donor (especially multiparous) with a male recipient, and use of peripheral blood stem cells.[615] Severe chronic GVHD imparts a grave prognosis.[620,621]

A limited form of chronic GVHD consists of localized skin disease and mild liver dysfunction. Severe chronic GVHD consists of generalized or localized skin involvement or liver dysfunction with one of the following: severe chronic liver damage; eye, mucosalivary, or mucosal involvement; or disease involvement of other target organs.[615] Chronic GVHD can significantly affect the quality of life of long-term survivors and lead to death. The overall incidence of chronic GVHD among bone marrow transplant recipients ranges from 33% for HLA-identical sibling transplants to 64% for matched unrelated donor transplants.

Chronic GVHD is the most common cause of cholestatic liver disease in long-term survivors of HSCT. Elevations of liver indices (e.g., serum bilirubin, alkaline phosphatase, transaminases) are nonspecific. Elevated levels can result from cholestatic drug injury, sepsis, hepatic infection with hepatotropic viruses or opportunistic microorganisms, recurrence of malignancy, development of PTLD, and from extrahepatic biliary disease (e.g., stones, infection). Chronic GVHD and viral hepatitis may coexist in the same patient, and elevated serum levels of transaminases cannot distinguish these diseases. As with acute GVHD, rigorous adherence to the criteria for diagnosing chronic GVHD in liver biopsies is essential for guiding clinical management.

Pathology of Graft-versus-Host Disease

Pathological interpretation relies on the clinical context and on the pathologist's assessment of the probability that the observed histology is attributable to GVHD. One of four liver biopsy interpretations can be used: negative for features of GVHD, features suggestive of GVHD, findings consistent with GVHD, and unequivocal features of GVHD.[618] Histological findings in a liver biopsy cannot readily distinguish between acute and chronic GVHD, and they are not specific for GVHD.[622] Hence great care must be taken in establishing the clinicopathological diagnosis of GVHD.

Acute Graft-versus-Host Disease

Nonspecific features of acute GVHD include hepatitic changes such as cholestatic and ballooning hepatocytes, apoptotic hepatocytes, and lymphocytic lobular infiltration, all features that resemble drug- or virus-induced hepatitis. More characteristic of acute GVHD is mild portal tract

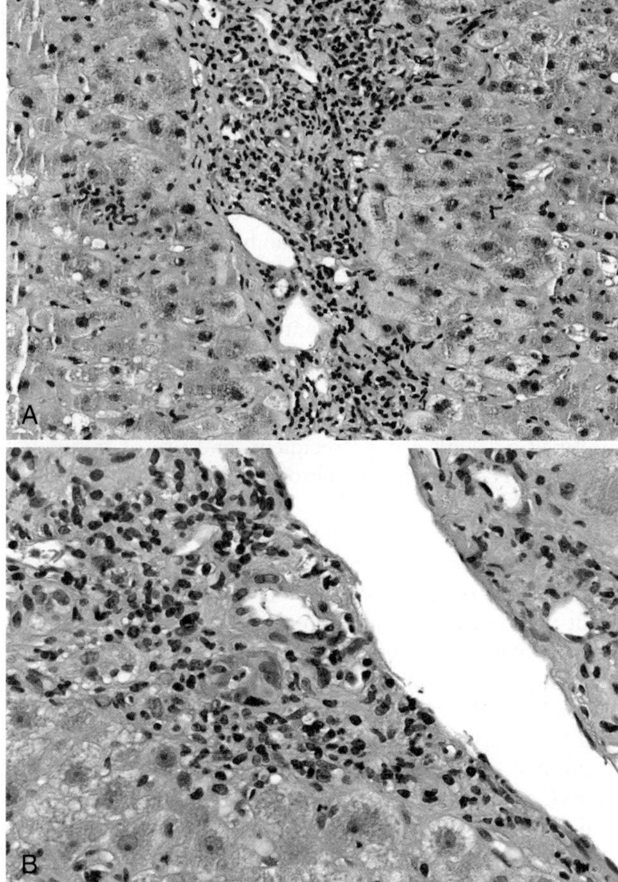

FIGURE 53.46 Acute graft-versus-host disease. A, Medium-power magnification shows a portal tract containing an activated, mixed inflammatory infiltrate, portal vein endotheliitis, and a difficult to discern interlobular bile duct *(center)*. **B,** High-power magnification shows a damaged bile duct surrounded and infiltrated by mononuclear inflammatory cells. Note the dysmorphic-appearing biliary epithelium.

inflammation, with infiltration of lymphocytes into the biliary epithelium causing vacuolization and necrosis of interlobular bile ducts. Unlike acute rejection in the liver graft, endothelial injury, which manifests as endotheliitis, is an uncommon finding in hepatic GVHD.[623]

Characteristic morphological changes resulting from GVHD may not be obvious in the early stage of disease.[618] For example, bile duct damage is identified only rarely in the first 35 days after bone marrow transplantation.[624] Clinical improvements in grafting regimens, widespread use of prophylaxis, and improved clinical management have reduced the incidence and severity of hepatic GVHD but have also rendered the histological diagnosis of GVHD more difficult.

Acute hepatic GVHD results from a direct attack of donor lymphocytes on recipient biliary epithelium of small bile ducts, and this morphological feature must be identified (Fig. 53.46).[604,624-627] Lymphocytic infiltrates surround, invade, and disrupt the walls of interlobular bile ducts, causing cholangiocyte cytoplasmic vacuolization, nuclear pleomorphism, loss of nuclei, and sloughing of epithelial cells into the bile duct lumen. Residual bile duct epithelial cells may appear attenuated ("withering" of the bile duct epithelium). Portal tract inflammation may be minimal despite damage to bile ducts because patients with acute GVHD are usually pancytopenic.

Chronic Graft-versus-Host Disease

Chronic GVHD is characterized mainly by portal lymphocytic infiltration with or without plasma cells or eosinophils and by damage to small (<45 μm in diameter) interlobular bile ducts.[628] Although there is no clear distinction between the morphological features of acute and chronic hepatic GVHD, long-term injury increases the amount of portal tract fibrosis.[618] Biliary epithelial cell degeneration resembling acute GVHD may be seen, but more commonly, damaged bile duct cells show cytoplasmic eosinophilia and other senescence-related changes similar to those of liver allograft rejection. Similar to acute GVHD, lymphocytes are in close contact with bile duct cells. Bile duct loss is usually a relatively late phenomenon in chronic GVHD, although it has been observed as early as 1 month after bone marrow transplantation.[629,630] The extent of ductopenia is not associated with the occurrence of extrahepatic GVHD in the skin and gut.[631] Ductular reaction is not a prominent feature of either acute or chronic GVHD.[622]

Most cases of cirrhosis occurring after HSCT have been attributed to HCV infection rather than GVHD,[618] but rare GVHD-related cases have been reported.[632-634] Unlike acute GVHD, hepatocellular damage is minimal in most cases of chronic GVHD, except that the loss of interlobular bile ducts gives rise to progressive hepatocellular cholestasis. In the more advanced stages of chronic GVHD, cholestasis may be so severe that it leads to degeneration of hepatocytes, particularly at the portal tract margins. Venous endotheliitis is not a prominent feature of chronic GVHD.

An unusual form of hepatitic GVHD has been reported.[602] Patients with chronic GVHD of the liver may have significantly elevated levels of transaminases and parenchymal damage resembling that of acute viral hepatitis. This is considered to be akin to AIH[635] and possibly related to tapering or withdrawal of immunosuppression. However, characteristic bile duct destructive features are also seen (Fig. 53.47). Liver biopsy plays an important role in evaluating long-term survivors of bone marrow transplantation with a hepatitic syndrome.[636]

Features of GVHD vary in severity from one portal tract to another, and this variability makes interpretation of liver biopsies difficult. The damage to interlobular and septal bile ducts is usually segmental. A diagnosis of GVHD may be confirmed by demonstrating inflammatory cells in the liver of donor origin by molecular techniques, but testing is not commonly performed. In experienced hands, a biopsy diagnosis of hepatic GVHD has a sensitivity of 66%, specificity of 91%, and a predictive value of 86%.[624]

Differential Diagnosis

Although viral hepatitis, cholangitis lenta (from sepsis), SOS, and disease recurrence (of either myeloproliferative or solid malignancy) are in the differential diagnosis, the primary distinction usually to be made on liver biopsy post-HSCT is between GVHD and DILI (Table 53.12).[631,637] The key histological features to observe are percent bile duct loss in portal tracts, bile duct damage, ductular reaction, cholestasis, and parenchymal hepatocyte apoptosis.[637]

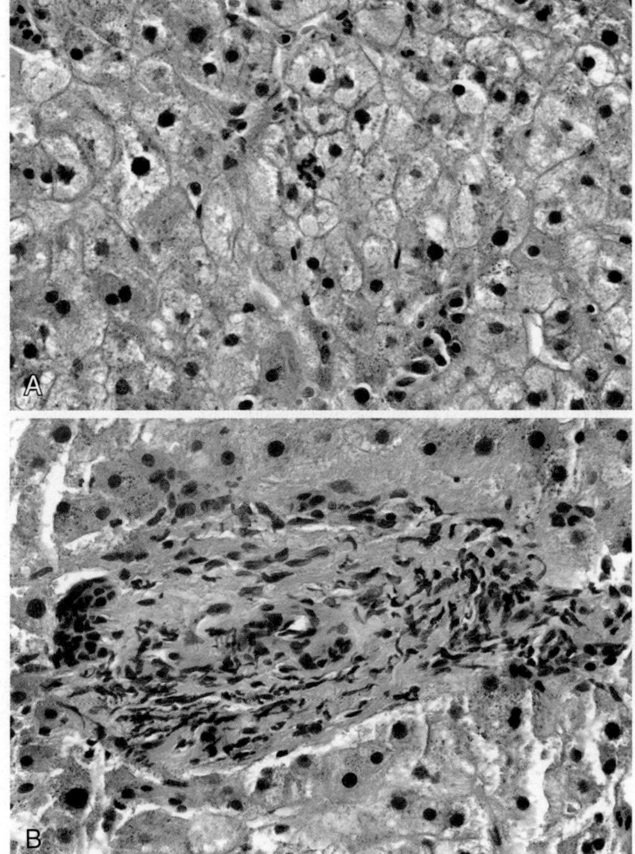

FIGURE 53.47 Acute graft-versus-host disease resembling acute viral hepatitis. A, Medium-power magnification of the parenchyma shows spotty inflammation. **B,** Medium-power magnification shows portal tract inflammation. Note the bile duct damage in these cases, which is relied on to make the diagnosis with certainty.

Patients with GVHD are more likely to have bile duct loss, bile duct damage, cholestasis, and hepatocyte apoptosis. Ductular reaction is more likely to be observed in DILI. The degrees of portal tract or lobular inflammation, bile duct intraepithelial lymphocytes, or endotheliitis (when observed) do not distinguish between GVHD and DILI.

To create further difficulty, distinguishing hepatic GVHD from a vanishing bile duct syndrome pattern of DILI is difficult and a potential cause of misinterpretation. Interestingly, the latter may have a greater extent of bile duct loss, accompanied by ductular reaction, hepatocellular injury, an autoimmune-like hepatitis, and potentially venous outflow obstruction.[631] In addition, although hepatic GVHD shows variable but diffuse involvement of most portal tracts, a vanishing bile duct syndrome of DILI tends to show a mixture of completely uninvolved portal tracts interspersed with affected ones.[637] This issue is reflected in a consensus report that ductopenia, portal fibrosis, and chronic cholestasis reflect chronicity in the post-HSCT setting, but are not specific for chronic hepatic GVHD.[638]

Being cautious in interpreting bile duct loss therefore is appropriate because ductopenia after HSCT is likely to be, at least in part, drug induced in association with previous chemotherapy. [631] Specifically, ductopenia may not entirely be related to a graft-versus-host immune reaction. The implication is that ductopenia after HSCT is not a cardinal indication for treatment with immunosuppressive (and potentially hepatotoxic) drugs, and it must be placed in the broader context of the morphological and clinical picture and the need to maintain graft-versus-tumor effects and immune defenses against infectious pathogens.[639]

A further consideration is the development of second malignancies, with a cumulative incidence of 1% at 10 years after HSCT[640] and causing 5% to 10% of late deaths after HSCT.[641] Total body irradiation is associated with development of solid tumors elsewhere in the body, but also posttransplant lymphoproliferative disease that is donor-derived and may be present in the liver. Particularly worrisome is EBV-associated PTLD, which may mimic acute GVHD,[641] and possibly even coexist with the GVHD in the same liver biopsy. The pathologist must be alert to the potential presence of polymorphic and atypical lymphocytes in the post-HSCT liver biopsy, as the treatment of PTLD and GVHD are divergent regarding immunosuppression.

Nodular Regenerative Hyperplasia

NRH has been reported after solid organ (primarily renal) and bone marrow transplantation.[642-644] NRH is also common in long-term survivors of HSCT.[181] The presumed common event is vascular injury as the result of abnormal activation of the immune system. The clinical syndrome of NRH, hepatomegaly, and ascites may be confused with SOS. This entity must be considered in patients exhibiting liver dysfunction after HSCT.

The diagnosis can be established only by histological examination of liver tissue. Pathological diagnosis of NRH can be difficult in small biopsies, and a reticulin stain helps evaluate nodularity and interposed liver cell plate compression in the liver parenchyma. Although fibrous septa are not part of the spectrum of NRH changes, thin, fibrous septa may develop with time in a few cases.

Systemic Infection After Stem Cell Transplantation

Systemic infection with hepatic involvement is always a possibility in the HSC recipient. Liver biopsy assists in assessment of fungal and opportunistic viral infections. Hepatotropic viral infection occurs in patients with hematopoietic disorders, and it may recur in the posttransplantation period.[645,646] Even in the absence of direct hepatic infection, endotoxemia or sepsis may induce severe cholestasis.[647]

Iron Overload

HSC transplant patients are at risk for developing iron overload as a result of repeated transfusions,[648] with deposition of hemosiderin in the liver and other organs such as spleen, heart, and endocrine tissue. In transfusion-related iron overload, hemosiderin accumulates first in Kupffer cells and later within hepatocytes. Iron accumulation is almost always an incidental finding. However, in patients with known GVHD, elevated serum transaminases after HSCT may reflect hepatic iron toxicity rather than exacerbation of the GVHD, even in patients who are wild-type

TABLE 53.12 Differential Diagnosis of Graft-versus-Host Disease versus Drug-Induced Liver Injury*

Feature	Graft-versus-Host Disease	Drug-Induced Liver Injury
Bile duct loss	Characteristic: ductopenia defined as bile ducts:portal tracts ratio <0.5	May occur in DILI, usually less than GVHD but may occasionally be more severe than seen in GVHD
Bile duct damage	Characteristic, with cholangiocyte squamatization, eosinophilia, vacuolization and apoptosis; nuclear hyperchromasia and disarray; cholangiocyte necrosis with denuding of basement membrane and cellular debris in bile duct lumen, but without cholangiocyte regenerative changes	Variable, with cholangiocyte regenerative changes and/or cholangiocyte necrosis and shedding of cellular debris into bile duct lumen
Bile duct intraepithelial lymphocytes	May be present, nonspecific	May be present, nonspecific
Ductular reaction	May be present, but limited	More prominent in DILI
Portal tract inflammation	May be present, but portal tracts tend to be paucicellular, with predominantly mononuclear inflammation	Variable inflammation, mononuclear or mixed (with neutrophils and eosinophils)
Endotheliitis (portal vein or terminal hepatic vein)	May be present, helpful but not specifically diagnostic	May be present in DILI
Lobular inflammation	May be present (a "hepatitic" pattern)	May have an autoimmune-like hepatitis
Hepatocyte apoptosis	Usually more frequent than in DILI	May be present
Hepatocanalicular cholestasis	Usually more prominent than in DILI	May be present, and is prominent in cholestatic pattern of DILI
Venous outflow obstruction	Not likely to be present	May occur in DILI

Based on Maximova[631] and Stueck[637]. Histologic features of acute liver graft-versus-host disease defined as presence of dysmorphic or destroyed small bile ducts with or without cholestasis and lobular and/or portal inflammation (Shulman[638]). Acute GVHD defined as <100 days post-transplant; chronic GVHD defined as >100 days post-transplant.

for C282Y and H63D; iron-reduction therapy may be indicated rather than intensification of immunosuppressive therapy.[649]

Liver Pathology Before Transplantation of Other Organs

Pretransplantation liver biopsies are often used to assess the presence of chronic liver disease in patients who are being evaluated for transplantation. Candidates for renal allografts may undergo liver biopsy evaluation to assess architectural integrity related to HCV infection. Significant iron overload also may be detected in these patients with chronic kidney disease. Potential small-intestinal allograft recipients frequently undergo screening liver biopsies to assess the structural integrity and long-term effects of total parenteral nutrition–induced injury or to assess for the presence of intestinal failure–associated liver disease (IFALD).[650]

Of increasing interest is evaluation of the liver before heart or heart-lung transplantation. The starting point is that heart transplantation is the best option for irreversible and critically advanced heart failure. [651] In turn, pulmonary hypertension is frequently observed in advanced heart failure as a result of reactive vasoconstriction and remodeling of the pulmonary vasculature, with right ventricular failure being a critical risk factor for posttransplant mortality.[652] The concern is that the liver is already damaged as a result of circulatory compromise (see Chapter 52), with ascites and hyperbilirubinemia before transplantation serving as independent risk factors for poor outcomes following heart transplantation.[653] Serum liver enzymes (transaminases reflecting hepatocellular injury; alkaline phosphatase and γ-glutamyl transpeptidase reflecting bile duct injury) and serum bilirubin are frequently elevated in advanced heart failure as a result of hepatic congestion and potentially superimposed ischemic injury.[654] Patients with high MELD scores are poorer candidates for cardiac transplantation. [655] As noninvasive tests may be misleading, liver biopsy may therefore be performed to assess the level of hepatic fibrosis as a histological diagnosis of cirrhosis is considered a contraindication for heart transplantation or may lead to consideration of combined heart-liver transplantation. [656] The potential for pretransplantation liver damage is further complicated by use of left-ventricular assist devices (LVADs) in end-stage patients with heart failure, extending the time that the liver is subjected to circulatory compromise.[657,658] As guidelines remain unclear, decision making for ultimately proceeding to heart transplantation in the setting of liver compromise is on a case-by-case basis. A high MELD score may help in donor stratification[659] and is considered to be a prognostic indicator of potential difficulties after heart transplantation rather than an absolute contraindication for such transplantation.[660] Pretransplant liver biopsy improves risk stratification of patients with advanced heart failure and suspected irreversible liver dysfunction.[661,662]

Liver Pathology After Transplantation of Other Organs

Exacerbation of the metabolic syndrome and NAFLD[663]; chronic viral hepatitis B, C, and E[664]; and opportunistic infections (e.g., CMV, EBV, HSV, VZV, adenovirus) occur in recipients of nonliver solid organs such as kidney, heart, lung, small intestine, or pancreas.[664,665] Viruses (e.g., CMV, EBV) that do not usually cause hepatitis in the general population can cause hepatitis in immunosuppressed recipients of liver allografts and other solid organs. For instance, the progression of chronic HBV and HCV infection can be accelerated in immunosuppressed solid organ transplant recipients. SARS-CoV-2 infection also has emerged as a concern in the posttransplantation setting.[666]

The high prevalence of HCV infection among recipients of renal transplants reflects the necessity of long-term hemodialysis,[667] and infection can progress rapidly to cirrhosis.[668] Cholestatic HCV hepatitis has been described in cardiac and renal allograft recipients.[669,670] Severe FCH may occur in patients serologically negative for HBV and HCV infection. This is attributed to the combined effects of CMV infection and azathioprine toxicity.[671] GVHD affecting the liver may also occur after nonliver organ transplantation because of the donor lymphoid tissue transplanted with the organs,[672-674] as can atypical malignancies such as PTLD.[675]

In keeping with the congestive hepatopathy that can precede heart transplantation, hepatic dysfunction after heart transplantation may remain, but posttransplant liver biopsy is unusual.[676] Cardiogenic liver fibrosis may persist long after heart transplantation, as demonstrated in patients who have undergone a Fontan procedure in early childhood to treat tricuspid atresia and then undergo heart transplantation later in adolescence. Because there is a virtual universal presence of advanced hepatic fibrosis by adolescence, post–heart transplantation liver biopsies do not show further evolution of the liver fibrosis, but they also do not show perceptible regression of the fibrosis.[677]

ACKNOWLEDGMENT

We are grateful to our surgical colleagues and mentors who provided the specimens and environment in which to study them.

The complete reference list may be accessed online at *Elsevier eBooks for Practicing Clinicians.*

CHAPTER 54

Liver Pathology in Pregnancy

Kamran Badizadegan

Contents

INTRODUCTION

Pregnancy is an altered physiological state designed to support the developing fetus, and gastrointestinal complaints are common during pregnancy. Although de novo abnormalities of the liver occur infrequently, they require prompt diagnosis and treatment to avoid the potentially high rates of maternal and fetal morbidity and mortality associated with them.

This chapter focuses on the pathophysiology and diagnosis of liver diseases that are unique to pregnancy. In most cases, the panoply of diseases discussed constitutes the differential diagnosis. In practice, some of the most frequent causes of liver disease in pregnancy are common disorders such as viral hepatitis and gallstone disease (Table 54.1), and the differential diagnosis of liver pathology in pregnancy must always be broadened to include these abnormalities.

LABORATORY AND HISTOLOGICAL CHANGES OF THE LIVER IN PREGNANCY

Hepatic histopathology in pregnancy is often nonspecific, and knowledge of the clinical history and physical signs and symptoms is essential for the diagnosis of liver disease. Evaluation of liver disease is further complicated by normal physiological changes in liver function test (LFT) results as a function of gestational age. Despite these well-known physiological alterations, most clinical laboratories use data from a normal adult population as reference ranges, leaving the correct evaluation of liver function abnormalities in the pregnant patient to the subjective judgment of clinicians and pathologists. A few important physiological changes in LFTs as a function of gestational age are depicted in Fig. 54.1 and discussed later to demonstrate the complexity of physiological changes in laboratory values during pregnancy. Given significant variability in technique and patient populations, the original literature[1-5] and locally developed reference ranges must be consulted for appropriate interpretation of patient-specific laboratory results during pregnancy.

Compared with age-matched, nonpregnant women, the total serum protein and albumin levels are lower during all three trimesters (Fig. 54.1A), and the concentration of serum albumin can decrease by as much as 60% by the second trimester. The physiological basis of this change is a subject of debate, although hemodilution during pregnancy is thought to play a role. Among other serum proteins, the levels of coagulation factors VII to X are higher during pregnancy, and fibrinogen levels may increase. Concentrations of α- and β-globulins are also slightly higher than normal, although γ-globulin levels may decrease.

Serum alkaline phosphatase activity increases during pregnancy and is significantly higher during the third trimester (Fig. 54.1B), although most of this activity is thought to originate from the placenta. Serum levels of alanine aminotransferase (ALT), aspartate aminotransferase (AST), γ-glutamyltranspeptidase (GGT), 5′-nucleotidase, bilirubin, and total bile acids and the prothrombin time remain within typical reference ranges during normal pregnancy, although each of these analytes may be subject to various increasing or decreasing trends during pregnancy (Fig. 54.1C–D).[3,5] Total, free, and conjugated bilirubin levels in all trimesters may be lower than in nonpregnant control patients, with the most significant changes (as much as 50%) occurring in total bilirubin (Fig 54.1D) and free bilirubin levels in the second and third trimesters. Serum triglyceride levels are higher in pregnancy, and cholesterol levels may increase by as much as 200% during the third trimester.

TABLE 54.1 Common Causes of Abnormal Liver Function Tests in Pregnancy

Condition*	1st Trimester	2nd Trimester	3rd Trimester
Hyperemesis gravidarum	X	X	
Gallstones	X	X	X
Hepatitis (various etiologies)	X	X	X
Intrahepatic cholestasis of pregnancy (ICP)	X	X	X
Preeclampsia/eclampsia		X	X
Hemolysis, elevated liver enzymes, and low platelets (HELLP) syndrome		X	X†
Acute fatty liver of pregnancy (AFLP)			X†
Budd-Chiari syndrome			X†
Hepatic rupture			X

*Conditions are ordered by the typical time of presentation during pregnancy.
†Extending into the postpartum period.

The histological appearance of the liver in uncomplicated pregnancy is essentially normal based on limited available evidence. Minor nonspecific changes have been described, including mild nuclear pleomorphism, increased glycogen, mild steatosis, mild portal inflammation, and reactive Kupffer cells, none with a specific diagnostic significance.[6-10]

The onset of maternal symptoms in relation to the trimester of pregnancy can help in the differential diagnosis of hepatic pathology (see Table 54.1). Severe nausea and vomiting during the first trimester are key clinical signs of hyperemesis gravidarum (HG), a disease with a relatively benign course and outcome. Later onset of nausea and vomiting suggests preeclampsia when accompanied by headache and peripheral edema or hepatic rupture when accompanied by abdominal pain with or without systemic hypotension. Pruritus in the third trimester, particularly of the palms and soles, is characteristic of intrahepatic cholestasis of pregnancy (ICP) and typically precedes the clinical manifestation of jaundice. Right upper quadrant and midabdominal pain in the third trimester may indicate acute fatty liver of pregnancy or hepatic rupture, both of which require immediate clinical intervention. Signs and symptoms of acute and chronic viral hepatitis and extrahepatic biliary disease are the same in pregnant women as in nonpregnant women, and their onset is not generally correlated with the gestational age.

INTRAHEPATIC CHOLESTASIS OF PREGNANCY

With an estimated average incidence of 0.1% to 2% in all pregnancies, ICP is one of the most important pregnancy-associated hepatic diseases.[11-14] Geographic, ethnic, and familial clustering is well described in ICP and must be considered in the diagnostic evaluation. The average incidence of ICP in Europe and the United States varies from 0.1% to 1.5%, whereas the estimated incidence in South America is up to 4%. However, the declining incidence of ICP in countries such as Chile and Bolivia, as well as the seasonal variations in incidence, suggest an environmental contribution to the disease.[13,15,16]

Specific geographic regions also show significant ethnic variations, suggesting a genetic linkage. For instance, the

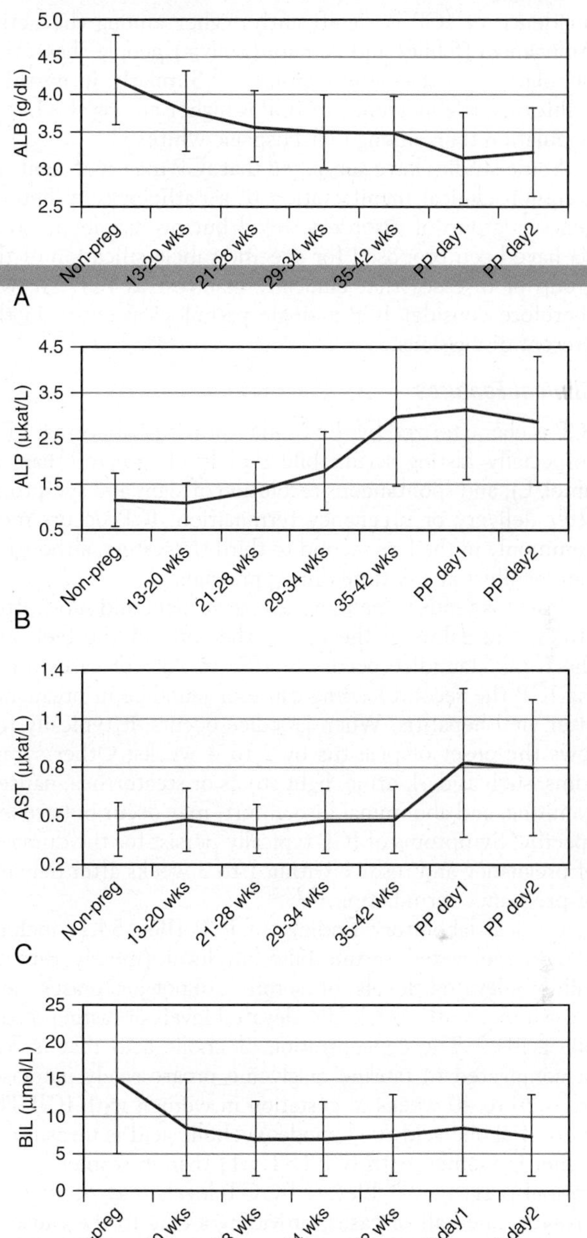

FIGURE 54.1 Liver function reference ranges can change as a function of gestational age during normal pregnancy and the postpartum (PP) period. Data shown here represent center lines (50th percentile) for **(A)** serum albumin (ALB), **(B)** alkaline phosphatase (ALP), **(C)** aspartate aminotransferase (AST), and **(D)** total bilirubin (BIL), assuming normal distribution of results reported by Klajnbard et al. (2010).[3] Error bars represent the 2.5th and 97.5th percentiles reported in the same study.[3] These data highlight potentially significant changes in liver function test results during normal pregnancy. (Note: The values shown here are for demonstration purposes. Readers must refer to laboratory-specific reference intervals and the original literature for appropriate evaluation of test results in individual patients.)

incidence of ICP is significantly higher among the native Araucanian (Chile) and Aimara (Bolivia) people than other populations in the same regions.[17,18] Similarly, in northern California, the incidence of ICP is higher among the Latina population than among non-Hispanic whites.[19]

Some studies have suggested that ICP may represent the common clinical manifestation of a pathologically heterogeneous group of disorders,[11,20,21] but no diagnostic criteria have been proposed for specific subclassification of the group of diseases that clinically manifest as ICP. We will therefore consider ICP a single pathological entity in the present discussions.

Clinical Features

ICP is characterized by the triad of pruritus, abnormal LFTs (especially fasting serum bile acid levels greater than 10 μmol/L), and spontaneous resolution of signs and symptoms after delivery or pregnancy termination. ICP occurs most commonly in the late second to third trimesters, although it can manifest at any time during pregnancy.

Pruritus tends to be more severe at night and most often affects the palms of the hands, the soles of the feet, and the trunk. Jaundice occurs in 10% to 25% of cases, making ICP the second leading cause of jaundice in pregnancy after viral hepatitis. When jaundice occurs, it typically follows the onset of pruritus by 2 to 4 weeks. Other symptoms, such as dark urine, light stools or steatorrhea, nausea, vomiting, and abdominal discomfort, may occur but are less specific. Symptoms of ICP typically persist for the duration of pregnancy and resolve within 1 to 3 weeks after delivery or pregnancy termination.[13,22-26]

Clinical laboratory findings in ICP (Box 54.1) include a mildly elevated serum bilirubin level (mostly direct), mildly elevated levels of serum aminotransferases, and most importantly, markedly elevated levels of fasting serum bile acids.[27] The concentration of cholic acid that is free or conjugated to taurine or glycine progressively increases from 20 to 40 weeks of gestation in women with ICP. The ratio of cholic acid to chenodeoxycholic acid is measurably higher in women with ICP (>1.5:1) than in women with a normal pregnancy.[28] Elevated GGT levels may occur in as many as one-half of cases, providing a clue to the cause of the condition.[29,30] Dyslipidemia with elevated levels of total cholesterol, low-density lipoprotein cholesterol, and apolipoprotein B-100 has also been observed.[31] Increased serum autotaxin levels have been proposed to represent a sensitive and specific marker for ICP, distinguishing it from other pruritic disorders that may occur during pregnancy, but the commercial availability of this test is currently limited.[32]

The maternal outcome in ICP is generally favorable,[12,26,33-35] although recent studies have suggested an association with chronic liver disease and cirrhosis.[21,36] Women with severe ICP may be at increased risk of preterm delivery relative to a healthy pregnancy comparison group (25% vs. 6.5%).[37] The fetal complications of ICP are more serious and consist of prematurity (19% to 60%), fetal distress (22% to 33%), meconium staining (9% to 24%), and perinatal death (1% to 2%).[19,34,35]

There is evidence for a direct link between maternal fasting bile acid levels and maternal-fetal complications of ICP. In a prospective cohort study of almost 45,000 pregnancies with 693 cases of ICP, no increase in fetal risk was detected when maternal serum bile acid levels were less than 40 μmol/L,[38,39] suggesting the appropriateness of expectant management in mild ICP. Ursodeoxycholic acid (UDCA) is otherwise the treatment of choice for management of pruritus and normalization of liver function.[40,41] Delivery as early as the fetal lung maturity allows is the definitive treatment for ICP, and dexamethasone may be used to promote fetal lung maturity.[41]

BOX 54.1 Major Clinical and Laboratory Features of Intrahepatic Cholestasis of Pregnancy

Characteristic time of onset: second to third trimester
Clinical features: pruritus with or without jaundice
  Occurs in: <5%
Blood and serum assay results
  ↑ Serum bile acids (>10 μmol/L)
  ↑ Aminotransferases (1 to 4 times normal)
  ↑ Alkaline phosphatase (1 to 2 times normal)
  ↑ Bilirubin (<6 mg/dL)
  ↑ Cholesterol and triglycerides
Pathology: intrahepatic cholestasis, predominantly in a pericentral distribution
Pathophysiology: defects in transport across the canalicular membrane

Pathological Features

Because a diagnosis of ICP is typically made according to clinical criteria, liver histopathology in ICP has not been extensively reported. Findings are thought to be subtle and consist primarily of hepatocellular bile and canalicular bile plugs, occurring predominantly in a pericentral distribution with minimal or no hepatocellular necrosis and minimal portal inflammation (see Fig. 54.1).[42-44] The histological differential diagnosis of ICP is broad and includes other common entities such as drug-induced hepatocellular injury and early extrahepatic biliary obstruction. Nevertheless, the combination of intrahepatic cholestasis with clinical features (i.e., pruritus and elevated levels of serum bile acids) virtually limits the diagnosis to ICP.

One study showed an association of ICP with abnormalities of the placenta, including syncytial knots, focally thickened amniotic basement membranes, small chorionic villi for gestational age with dense fibrotic stroma, and crowding and congestion of the villi.[45] These abnormalities were proposed to be associated with fetal complications of ICP, but subsequent case-control studies found no significant difference between placental histopathology in ICP versus controls.[46]

Pathogenesis

The pathogenesis of ICP has been gradually characterized over the past two decades and supports the concept of heterogenous but related abnormalities. Several lines of evidence point to altered metabolism of steroid hormones and bile acids, and various mechanistic roles for disruption of bile acid transport into and out of the hepatocyte by estriol, progesterone, and their intrahepatocellular conjugates have been proposed.[13,23,24,47,48] Familial clustering, increased incidence in first-degree relatives of patients with ICP,[49-51] and linkage to human leukocyte antigens indicate one or more genetic factors.[18,50,52] Furthermore, it has been suggested that immune dysregulation plays a role in disturbed placental bile acid and serum lipid transportation.[47,53,54]

Association with dietary factors such as selenium[55,56] and temporal/seasonal variations in incidence[13,15,16] suggest one or more environmental factors in the pathogenesis of ICP. Demonstration of increased intestinal permeability in patients with ICP during and after pregnancy[20] provides further evidence that the hepatic pathogenesis of ICP may be under the control or influence of extrahepatic factors. Collectively, these somewhat disjointed observations and hypotheses about the pathogenesis of ICP and its associated risk factors suggest that ICP may represent the end result of a heterogeneous group of pregnancy-associated hepatic insults rather than a unique pathophysiological entity.

The genetic basis of ICP began to emerge from studies of patients with ICP and elevated serum GGT activity. Two pedigrees were initially reported, with ICP in the mothers of children who were born with the autosomal recessive form of progressive familial intrahepatic cholestasis (PFIC) and elevated serum GGT activity, a disease commonly referred to as type 3 PFIC.[57,58] The affected children had homozygous mutations in the hepatocellular phospholipid transporter *ABCB4* gene (also known as *multidrug resistance 3 [MDR3]*), whereas ICP developed during pregnancy in mothers who were heterozygous for *ABCB4*. ABCB4 is a class III multidrug-resistant P-glycoprotein that mediates translocation ("flipping") of phosphatidylcholine (lecithin) across the bile canalicular membrane of hepatocytes.

To better characterize the pathogenic role of ABCB4 in the development of ICP, Dixon and associates investigated eight women with ICP and increased serum GGT activity who had no personal or family history of PFIC.[59] DNA sequence analysis revealed a heterozygous missense mutation in *ABCB4*, resulting in the expression of a nonfunctional protein at the cell surface in one of eight patients. Several subsequent reports on the association between ABCB4 and ICP provide further evidence for a defect in this canalicular transporter protein in the pathogenesis of ICP.[30,60-68] As many as 1 in 5 patients with ICP may have a mutation in the *ABCB4* gene, and many different mutations of the gene have now been reported.

In addition to the compelling data regarding the role of ABCB4 in the pathogenesis of a subset of ICP cases, other cases have been associated with benign, recurrent intrahepatic cholestasis (BRIC; Fig. 54.2).[69,70] BRIC, which is genetically associated with a mutation in the same region of chromosome 18 as type 1 PFIC (Byler disease), is an intrahepatic cholestatic disease in which affected patients have normal serum GGT activity. This sharp biochemical contrast with ABCB4-associated cases of ICP points to alternative mechanistic pathways for another subset of women with ICP. Lastly, the *ABCB11* gene, which is associated with PFIC type 2, may also contribute to ICP. Mutations in the bile salt export pump (BSEP), which is the product of the *ABCB11* gene, as well as transcription factors driving *ABCB11* expression, have been identified in subsets of patients with ICP.[30,66,68,71-73]

It is not surprising that different defects in transport across the hepatocyte canalicular membrane can lead to similar clinical phenotypes, which are collectively recognized as ICP. Fundamentally, the phenotype of ICP can

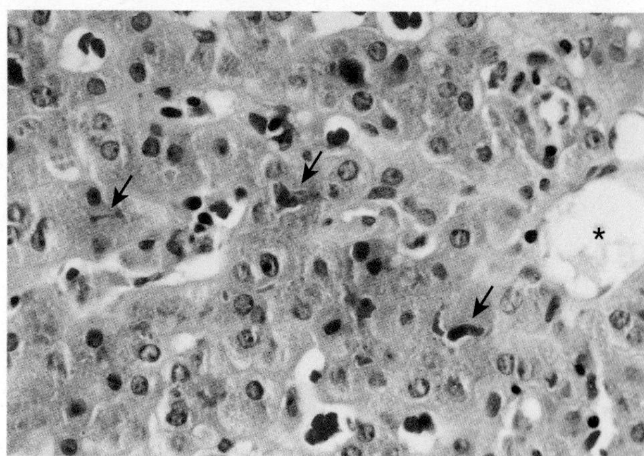

FIGURE 54.2 Liver biopsy specimen from a 19-year-old woman with benign, recurrent, intrahepatic cholestasis who had jaundice early in the second trimester. High-power view of hepatic parenchyma in the vicinity of a central vein *(asterisk)* shows moderate cholestasis with prominent canalicular bile plugs *(arrows)*. A minimal mononuclear infiltrate is identified in the portal tracts, and occasional acidophilic bodies can be seen *(not shown)*.

result from any disruption in the steady state between the uptake of bile salts into the hepatocytes and transport of bile salts across the canalicular membrane into bile. Estrogens, progesterone, and their conjugates disrupt the steady state by interfering with bile acid transporters at the basolateral membrane and inhibiting efficient bile acid transport across the canalicular membrane. In compromised hosts, such as heterozygous mothers with *ABCB4* mutations, the added insult from pregnancy-associated hormones is sufficient to tilt the balance toward a cholestatic disease. Future research will undoubtedly reveal other molecular pathways and canalicular transporters that can result in ICP through similar or related pathways.

ACUTE FATTY LIVER OF PREGNANCY

Acute fatty liver of pregnancy (AFLP) is a serious and potentially fatal complication for the pregnant mother and fetus. AFLP occurs in an estimated 1 to 3 of 10,000 pregnancies, and the disease is classically associated with first pregnancies, multiple gestations, low body mass index, and a male fetus.[74-83] AFLP usually occurs late in the third trimester (>30 weeks of gestation) or in the immediate postpartum period. Rare exceptions manifesting as early as 22 weeks of gestation have been reported.[84-86]

Clinical Features

The initial clinical presentation of AFLP is often vague and includes headache, abdominal pain, nausea, vomiting, and a variety of other nonspecific "prodromal" symptoms.[41,78,79,87,88] Prodromal symptoms are typically followed by jaundice as the disease progresses. Progressive and severe hepatic failure accompanied by coagulopathy and encephalopathy ensues, typically within 1 to 2 weeks of the onset of jaundice. If untreated, patients may rapidly deteriorate, with gastrointestinal bleeding, seizures, coma, and renal failure with acute tubular necrosis.

AFLP may be associated with preeclampsia in 20% to 40% of patients.[74,89,90] In these circumstances, the presenting

BOX 54.2 Major Clinical and Laboratory Features of Acute Fatty Liver of Pregnancy

Characteristic time of onset: third trimester
Clinical features
- Abdominal pain
- Nausea and vomiting
- Jaundice
- ±Coagulopathy
- ±Encephalopathy

Blood and serum assay results
- ↑ Aminotransferases (1 to 5 times normal)
- ↑ Alkaline phosphatase (1 to 2 times normal)
- ↑ Bilirubin (<10 mg/dL)
- ↑ Uric acid
- ±↑ Prothrombin time and partial thromboplastin time
- ±↑ Platelets
- ±↑ White blood cells

Pathology: microvesicular steatosis, centrilobular to diffuse
Pathophysiology: mitochondrial fatty acid β-oxidation defects

BOX 54.3 Swansea Criteria for the Diagnosis of Acute Fatty Liver of Pregnancy*

Vomiting
Abdominal pain
Polydipsia and polyuria
Encephalopathy
Elevated bilirubin (>14 μmol/L)
Hypoglycemia (<4 mmol/L)
Elevated urea (>340 μmol/L)
Leucocytosis ($>11 \times 10^9$/L)
Ascites or bright liver on ultrasound scan
Elevated transaminases (AST or ALT >42 IU/L)
Elevated ammonia (>47 μmol/L)
Renal impairment (creatinine >150 μmol/L)
Coagulopathy (PT >14 seconds or aPTT >34 seconds)
Microvesicular steatosis on liver biopsy

**A minimum of six criteria is required to support the diagnosis. Values in parentheses were suggested by Knight and colleagues.*[83]
aPTT, *Activated partial thromboplastin time;* ALT, *alanine aminotransferase;* AST, *aspartate aminotransferase;* IU, *international units;* PT, *prothrombin time.*

signs and symptoms include those of pregnancy-induced hypertensive disorders (discussed later). A rare association between AFLP and ICP has been reported in which the patient had pruritus at presentation, which is more common for ICP than AFLP,[91] although the significance of this association remains unclear. Other concomitant disorders such as neoplastic lesions and sepsis have been reported,[92-95] but there is no proof of a definitive association at this time.

Because early diagnosis and prompt treatment of AFLP are essential to maternal and fetal well-being, LFT parameters must be measured promptly in any pregnant woman past 22 weeks of gestation who has any of the aforementioned prodromal symptoms or signs of AFLP. The LFT results for AFLP typically suggest mild to moderate hepatocellular damage with mild cholestasis (Box 54.2). Serum aminotransferase levels usually are elevated in AFLP, although rarely to the extent observed in acute viral hepatitis. The bilirubin level is normal early in the course, but it increases if the pregnancy is not terminated. Alkaline phosphatase levels are also elevated, but distinguishing hepatic from placental isoenzymes may not be practical or fruitful. The peripheral blood analysis may show leukocytosis and thrombocytopenia,[96] and disseminated intravascular coagulation may be present.[97,98] Blood urea nitrogen and serum creatinine levels may be elevated, but uric acid levels are disproportionately high, making them diagnostically valuable. Blood glucose levels are typically low, and clinically significant hypoglycemia may occur.

Historically, liver biopsy has been the gold standard for the diagnosis of AFLP, but coagulopathy often prevents liver biopsy in the acute clinical setting. Fatty infiltration of the liver can also be easily assessed by noninvasive imaging methods such as ultrasonography or magnetic resonance imaging. The Swansea criteria, which use the clinical symptoms and laboratory findings of women with liver disease in pregnancy, constitute a reliable indicator of AFLP, with or without a liver biopsy (Box 54.3).[83,99-103] In one study, application of the Swansea criteria resulted in 100% sensitivity, 57% specificity, an 85% positive predictive value, and a 100% negative predictive value for diffuse or perivenular microvesicular steatosis on liver biopsy.[100]

Regardless of the cause or type of presentation, the mainstay of therapy for AFLP is immediate delivery and supportive care. Liver transplantation, artificial liver support, and plasma exchange have been tried as alternative therapies with various levels of success,[104-108] and transplantation is the option of last resort in fulminant hepatic failure caused by AFLP. Despite all clinical efforts, AFLP continues to be a serious complication of pregnancy, with maternal or fetal death occurring in 1% to 20% of all cases, depending on the availability and level of care.[76,80,83]

Pathological Features

Microvesicular steatosis of hepatocytes is the pathological hallmark of AFLP. Classically, steatosis involves the pericentral zone and spares the periportal hepatocytes, although panlobular and periportal involvement may be seen.[82,96] In most cases, the fat droplets are large enough and their location well enough preserved to produce readily recognizable vacuolar change on routine sections with hematoxylin and eosin (H&E) staining (Fig. 54.3A). Occasionally, individual fat droplets may be too small to be resolved by routine light microscopy or too poorly preserved to result in a classic vacuolar pattern on H&E-stained sections (Fig. 54.3B). In these circumstances, hepatocytes may look essentially normal, be somewhat dilated, or exhibit diffuse cytoplasmic ballooning not readily distinguishable from ballooning degeneration or other forms of acute hepatocellular damage. Therefore a portion of any liver biopsy specimen obtained for clinical suspicion of AFLP during pregnancy or in the immediate postpartum period must be processed as a frozen section for oil red O or Sudan black staining, or be processed for electron microscopy (Fig. 54.3C).

Although fatty change is considered the diagnostic histological hallmark of AFLP, a host of other microscopic abnormalities were reported in a detailed study of 35 cases by Rolfes and Ishak.[82] Hypertrophied Kupffer cells containing lipid or lipofuscin were prominent in areas of fatty change in

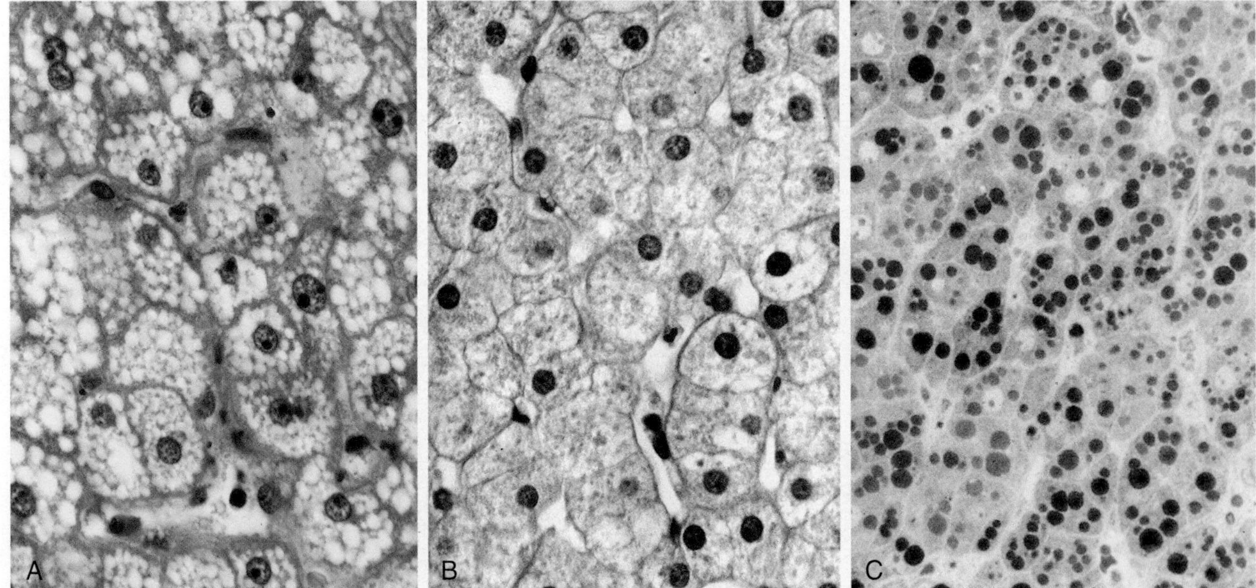

FIGURE 54.3 **A,** Microvesicular steatosis can be identified by numerous, optically clear vacuoles on routine hematoxylin and eosin (H&E) staining, as shown in this liver biopsy specimen from a 32-year-old woman at 34 weeks' gestation who had mildly increased levels of aminotransferases and a "giant fatty liver" seen on ultrasonography. **B,** Microvesicular steatosis in metabolic fatty liver disease may not always be apparent on routine H&E staining, as demonstrated in this biopsy specimen from a patient with liver failure and suspected long-chain 3-hydroxyacyl-CoA dehydrogenase deficiency. **C,** Toluidine blue–stained plastic sections of an adjacent piece of the biopsy specimen shown in B demonstrates numerous hepatocellular fat droplets.

most cases. Evidence of intrahepatic cholestasis, including bile canalicular plugs and acute cholangiolitis, was seen in two-thirds of cases. Significant mononuclear lobular inflammation (comparable with acute viral hepatitis) and inflammation of the central veins were identified in 25% of cases, and 75% showed evidence of extramedullary hematopoiesis with prominent megakaryocytes and cells of erythroid lineage. Most notable by its absence in this large series of cases was sinusoidal fibrin deposition. Despite frequent clinical signs and symptoms of pregnancy-induced hypertensive disorders in patients with AFLP, the absence of fibrin deposition was considered evidence of a lack of histological overlap between these two entities.[82]

Although fatty infiltration of the liver is an extremely sensitive diagnostic marker for AFLP, it is nonspecific. The histopathological differential diagnosis of AFLP is therefore broad and includes various other forms of fatty liver disease, including essentially all toxic, metabolic, and drug-induced conditions that may lead to microvesicular steatosis of hepatocytes. A definitive diagnosis of AFLP can therefore be made only in conjunction with the appropriate clinical signs and symptoms.

Pathogenesis

Significant progress has been made in understanding the pathogenesis of AFLP. Most importantly, a strong association between fetal fatty acid oxidation disorders and maternal AFLP has been established,[109-119] suggesting that AFLP is fundamentally a disorder of mitochondrial fatty acid β-oxidation (FAO).

Mitochondrial β-oxidation of fatty acids is a critical step in intermediary metabolism in hepatocytes. FAO is a source of energy for hepatocytes under physiological stress and results in production of various metabolic intermediates that can be used as a source of energy by other vital organs such as the brain. One of the key enzymes in mitochondrial FAO is long-chain 3-hydroxyacyl-CoA dehydrogenase (LCHAD), which catalyzes the third step in β-oxidation of long-chain fatty acids on the inner mitochondrial membrane. LCHAD activity occurs on the C-terminal portion of the α subunit of the microsomal triglyceride transfer protein (MTTP, also known as *trifunctional protein* [TFP]). MTTP also contains the active sites of long-chain 2,3-enoyl-CoA hydratase and long-chain 3-ketoacyl-CoA thiolase, catalyzing the second and fourth steps in fatty acid β-oxidation, respectively.

A recessively inherited defect in LCHAD in the infant is responsible for most of the occurrences of AFLP in the mother. A significant number of reported cases result from a 1528G→C mutation in exon 15 of the α subunit of *MTTP*, which results in the exchange of glutamic acid for glutamine at amino acid position #474. Although various MTTP deficiencies have emerged as important causes of metabolic disease in children, only limited mutations that typically result in abnormal LCHAD activity have been associated with maternal liver disease in pregnancy.[112,117,119-124]

In addition to *MTTP* mutations with LCHAD deficiency, other components of mitochondrial FAO have been associated with maternal disease in pregnancy. Fetal short-chain acyl-CoA dehydrogenase (SCAD) deficiency and fetal carnitine palmitoyltransferase deficiency were each reported in association with maternal AFLP several years ago (Fig. 54.4).[125,126] Santos and colleagues provided the first description of a normal fetus with a maternal FAO defect in medium-chain acyl-CoA dehydrogenase (MCAD) resulting in AFLP in the late third trimester.[116] In a case-control study comparing fetal oxidation defects with the occurrence of maternal liver disease during pregnancy, two cases of medium chain acyl-CoA dehydrogenase deficiency were associated with AFLP.[109] Remarkably, the maternal liver disease occurring with FAO in the children

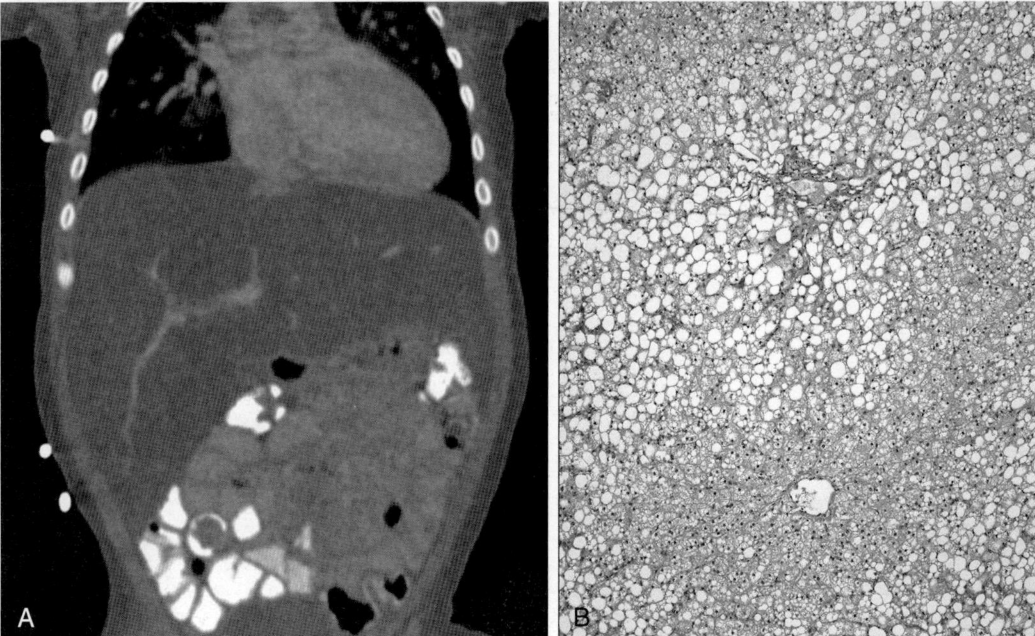

FIGURE 54.4 A, Newborn infant had massive hepatomegaly that was seen as a homogenously enlarged liver on computed tomography. The liver occupies more than one-half of the abdominal cavity and displaces the intestines to the left. **B,** Wedge biopsy of the liver shown at low magnification shows diffuse microvesicular and macrovesicular steatosis that is most prominent in the periportal zone. Subsequent biochemical studies confirmed a carnitine palmitoyltransferase 1 deficiency. The mother, who met the Swansea criteria for the diagnosis of acute fatty liver of pregnancy, was managed expectantly, and no biopsy was performed.

also included preeclampsia and HELLP syndrome (*h*emolysis, *e*levated *l*iver enzymes, and *l*ow *p*latelets). The risk of liver disease developing in a mother in pregnancy if the child had LCHAD or short- and medium-chain defects was, respectively, 50 times or 12 times more likely than in control patients.

The precise mechanisms through which LCHAD or other FAO deficiencies result in fatty liver or hepatic failure are unknown. It has been postulated that the increasing metabolic demands of the third trimester in a compromised host result in excessive metabolic stress that cannot be handled by the heterozygous mother's deficient metabolism.[122] The placenta may also be an important factor in the pathophysiology. The genetic makeup of the placenta is identical to that of the fetus. Natarajan and colleagues found that the placentas at birth in mothers with AFLP showed oxidative stress in the mitochondria and peroxisomes and had compromised mitochondrial function compared with controls.[115] The patient's serum showed elevation of oxidative and nitrosative stress markers with decreased antioxidant levels. The placentas and sera showed increased levels of arachidonic acid, which caused mitochondrial damage in the Chang liver cell line and increased lipid accumulation as identified by Nile red staining.[115] This proposed mechanism is reminiscent of ICP in which normally masked (subclinical) cellular deficiencies present themselves as a disease during the altered physiological state of pregnancy.

PREECLAMPSIA AND ECLAMPSIA

Preeclampsia occurs in 2% to 8% of all pregnancies and is classically defined as (1) new-onset hypertension of at least 140 mm Hg systolic or 90 mm Hg diastolic and (2) proteinuria of greater than 0.3 g/24 hours after 20 weeks of gestation.[41,127,128] Recent international consensus guidelines, however,[129] broaden the definition to de novo hypertension after 20 weeks of gestation accompanied by proteinuria and/or evidence of maternal acute kidney injury, liver dysfunction, neurological features, hemolysis or thrombocytopenia, and/or fetal growth restriction (FGR). When accompanied by new-onset grand mal seizure in a patient without a preexisting brain abnormality, the condition is known as *eclampsia,* although the fundamental disease and pathophysiology remain the same.[41,127,128] Progression to eclampsia is rare, occurring in only 0.1% to 0.2% of all pregnancies, but when it happens, it is associated with significant maternal and fetal morbidity and mortality. In addition to a first pregnancy, which is the most common risk factor for preeclampsia (4.1% for first vs. 1.7% for later pregnancies),[130] many other clinical and social conditions have been associated with the risk of preeclampsia (Box 54.4).

Clinical Features

Preeclampsia can be diagnosed as early as 20 weeks of gestation (by definition), but is most common near term. Severe cases may be clinically defined as blood pressure of 160/110 mm Hg or higher and proteinuria of greater than 5 g/24 hours, with or without multiorgan involvement and severe central nervous system symptoms, although recent international guidelines emphasize the spectrum of disease and do not recommend subclassification as "severe" preeclampsia.[129] The liver is a nonspecific target organ, and LFT results may include increased levels of aminotransferases, which may be accompanied by a mild increase in serum bilirubin, alkaline phosphatase, and uric acid levels (Box 54.5). Systemic inflammatory markers such as extracellular serum heat shock proteins, C-reactive protein, and tumor necrosis factor alpha levels show significant correlation with

BOX 54.4 Conditions Associated with Increased Risk of Preeclampsia or Eclampsia

First pregnancy
Limited period of cohabitation with the conceiving father
Family history
Multiple gestation
Obesity
Pregestational diabetes
Preexisting hypertension
Extreme maternal age (<20 or >45 years)
History of low-birth-weight infants
Poor prenatal care
Infection (e.g., urinary tract infection, periodontal disease, chlamydial or cytomegalovirus infection)
Autoimmune disease
Preexisting thrombophilia
Hydramnios
Molar pregnancy
Low maternal serum vitamin D levels
Hydrops fetalis
Large placenta

BOX 54.5 Major Clinical and Laboratory Features of Preeclampsia or Eclampsia

Characteristic time of onset: late second to third trimester
Clinical features
- Hypertension
- Edema
- Nonspecific symptoms
- Disseminated intravascular coagulation

Blood and serum assay results
- ↑ Aminotransferases (1 to 100 times normal)
- ↑ Alkaline phosphatase (1 to 2 times normal)
- ↑ Bilirubin (<5 mg/dL)
- ↑ Uric acid
- ↑ Prothrombin time and partial thromboplastin time
- ↓ Platelets (typically >70,000/mm^3)

Pathology
- Parenchymal and subcapsular hemorrhage
- Periportal fibrin, hemorrhage, and necrosis

Pathophysiology: endothelial dysfunction caused by placenta-derived soluble factors

markers of liver damage such as serum AST and lactate dehydrogenase.[131-135] Clinical and laboratory findings often include evidence of systemic vascular activation and damage such as moderate thrombocytopenia and disseminated intravascular coagulation with evidence of microangiopathic hemolysis.

Untreated preeclampsia can progress to hypertensive crisis with life-threatening renal failure. Progression to eclampsia is heralded by seizures, and coma eventually ensues. Maternal and fetal morbidity and mortality correlate with the severity of disease, the time of onset of the condition during the pregnancy, multiple gestations, preexisting maternal disease, and clinical management. The overall maternal mortality rate in developed countries is as high as 1.8%, with more than 80% of cases caused by complications of the central nervous system and the remainder resulting from catastrophic hepatic complications such as hepatic rupture and fulminant hepatic failure. The highest risk of death is among older women, women without prenatal care, and women with onset of hypertension before 28 weeks of gestation. Patients with severe preeclampsia or eclampsia have similar risks of developing intravascular coagulation (8%), HELLP syndrome (10% to 15%), and liver hematoma (1%).[136]

Fetal complications are common and include increased risk of abruptio placentae, intrauterine FGR, and prematurity.[136] Reduced risk of preeclampsia has been achieved in some studies with low-dose aspirin treatment and low-molecular-weight heparin started early in pregnancy,[137,138] and various nutritional supplements and modifications have been suggested.[128,139-141] Delivery is the treatment of choice for mild preeclampsia after 36 weeks of gestation, and women with severe preeclampsia should be delivered as early as clinically possible.[41,136]

The long-term sequelae of preeclampsia affect both the mother and infant. Women with pregnancy complicated by preeclampsia have a subsequent increased risk of preeclampsia in future pregnancies,[142] as well as hypertension, type 2 diabetes mellitus, and stroke.[143-148] Offspring of women with preeclampsia also have increased blood pressure and double the risk of stroke in later life.[149] Male children born to mothers with preeclampsia may have alterations in neonatal microvascular adaptation after birth.[150] Being born preterm or with FGR because of preeclampsia or other causes is associated with an increased risk for gestational diabetes and preeclampsia in adulthood.[151]

Pathological Features

Hepatic involvement in preeclampsia and eclampsia is primarily characterized by patchy parenchymal and subcapsular hemorrhage. Microscopically, the periportal zone is preferentially affected and may reveal a combination of fibrin deposition, hemorrhage, and hepatocellular necrosis (Fig. 54.5).[14,43,152,153] Thrombi and evidence of endothelial damage may be seen in the branches of the hepatic arteries and less commonly in the portal veins. In practice, the diagnosis of preeclampsia or eclampsia is always made clinically, and the classic pathological changes are seen only in rare instances of maternal death resulting from severe disease.

Liver biopsies may be done (but rarely are) for patients with mild or clinically indeterminate liver disease. In these circumstances, the histological finding may be nonspecific and limited to mild and focal portal or periportal abnormalities. Because of the focal nature of the hepatic involvement, the absence of specific findings on a liver biopsy should not be used to exclude a diagnosis of preeclampsia. These findings are not specific to hypertensive disorders, and an almost identical morphology may be seen in other conditions of altered hemostasis, such as a hypercoagulable state of any etiology.

Pathogenesis

The placenta plays a key role in the pathogenesis of preeclampsia and related hypertensive disorders. Occurrence of the disease in molar pregnancies in which there is no fetal development suggests a required and sufficient role for the placenta in the pathogenesis of preeclampsia, and rapid disappearance of the disease after delivery provides further

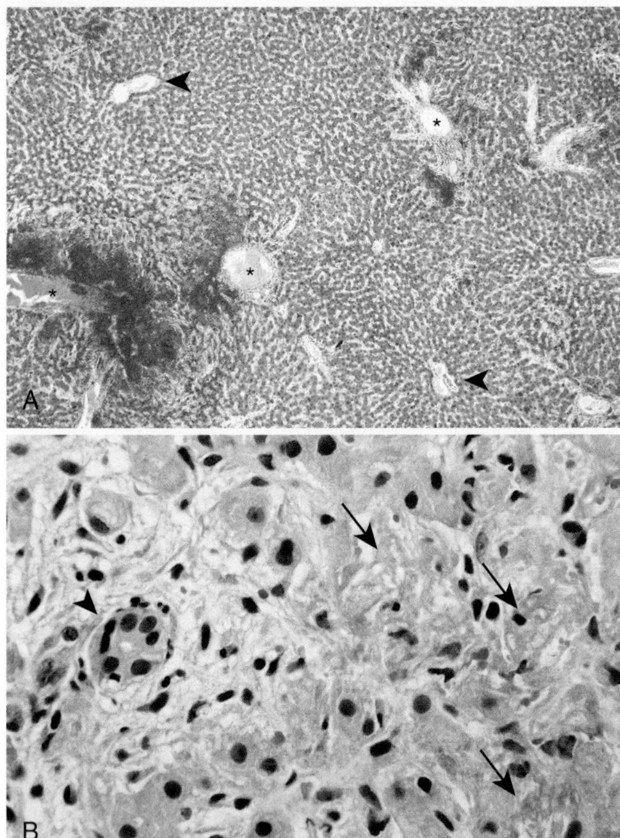

FIGURE 54.5 **A,** Classic histopathology of eclampsia is characterized by patchy areas of hemorrhage, fibrin deposition, and hepatocellular necrosis in the vicinity of the portal tracts *(asterisks).* The pericentral areas *(arrowheads)* are virtually free from disease, and no significant inflammatory infiltrate is seen. **B,** The liver biopsy specimen also shows fibrin in the vicinity of a portal tract (*arrowhead* points to the bile duct), with obliteration of sinusoids and damaged periportal hepatocytes *(arrows).* This biopsy specimen, which came from a 30-year-old pregnant woman with abnormal liver function test results, can be distinguished from a pregnancy-induced hypertensive disorder only on the basis of clinical data (i.e., first-trimester pregnancy and a hypercoagulable state with antiphospholipid antibodies).

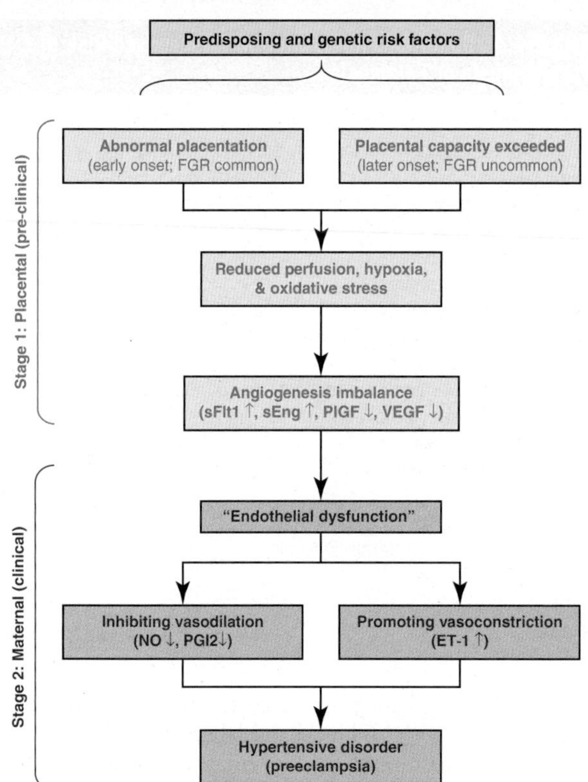

FIGURE 54.6 **The two-stage model of preeclampsia pathogenesis.** The placental (preclinical) stage begins either as a result of abnormal placentation or physiological circumstances such as multiple gestation in which perfusion demands on the placenta exceed its capacity. The ensuing placental hypoxia and oxidative stress result in angiogenic dysregulation through the expression of soluble fms-related tyrosine kinase 1 *(sFlt1)* and soluble endoglin *(sEng),* resulting in the deactivation of circulating angiogenic factors such as vascular endothelial growth factor *(VEGF)* and placental growth factor *(PlGF).* These changes trigger the maternal (clinical) stage of the disease, which is characterized by systemic endothelial dysfunction. Key features of the maternal stage are inhibition of vasodilation through a decrease in nitric oxide *(NO)* and prostacyclin *(PGI2),* and promotion of vasoconstriction through an increase in endothelin-1 *(ET-1).* The cumulative effect is a systemic vascular dysfunction that clinically presents in the form of a placenta-driven hypertensive disorder.

support for a placenta-derived factor in the maintenance of maternal symptoms. Significant progress in elucidating the pathogenesis of preeclampsia has been detailed in multiple recent reviews.[154-157]

The pathogenesis of preeclampsia is thought to constitute a two-stage model in which placental factors and maternal factors each play a critical role (Fig. 54.6). In the early-onset presentation of the disease, the first stage (preclinical) is characterized by abnormal placentation resulting from insufficient cytotrophoblastic invasion of the spiral arteries. Predisposing factors are numerous (see Box 54.4) and include genetic, immunological, and environmental risks. FGR is common because of placental insufficiency, and the vascular abnormalities eventually result in placental hypoxia and oxidative stress.

In the late-onset forms of preeclampsia, the prevailing hypothesis is that placental hypoxia and oxidative stress ensue when the placental capacity exceeds demand, such as multiple gestations or postterm pregnancy. Under these circumstances, placentation is not necessarily abnormal, and FGR is often absent. Because physiological demands exceed placental capacity, however, hypoxia and oxidative stress ensue and result in progression of the disease.

Regardless of the inciting event (abnormal placentation or excess physiological demand), oxidative stress results in the release of placenta-derived, soluble fms-related tyrosine kinase 1 (sFlt1) through unknown mechanisms. sFlt1 is a splice variant of vascular endothelial growth factor receptor 1 (VEGFR1) that binds and deactivates circulating angiogenic factors including vascular endothelial growth factor (VEGF) and placental growth factor (PlGF). Decreased levels of VEGF and PlGF lead to systemic maternal endothelial dysfunction, including a decrease in vasodilators such as nitric oxide (NO) and prostacyclin (also known as *prostaglandin I2* [PGI2]) and an increase in vasoconstrictors including endothelin-1 (ET-1).

Working in concert with the effects of sFLT1, other angiogenic signaling molecules including soluble endoglin (sEng) as well as adhesion molecules sICAM-1 (soluble forms of

BOX 54.6 Major Clinical and Laboratory Features of HELLP Syndrome

Characteristic time of onset: late second to third trimester
Clinical features
- Epigastric or right upper quadrant pain
- Nausea and vomiting
- Headache
- Edema
- Hypertension

Blood and serum assay results
- ↑Aminotransferases (1 to 100 times normal)
- ↑Alkaline phosphatase (1 to 2 times normal)
- ↑Bilirubin (<5 mg/dL)
- ↑Uric acid
- ↑Prothrombin time and partial thromboplastin time
- ↓Platelets (<100,000/mm^3)
- Hemolysis

Pathology
- Same as preeclampsia
- Acute fatty liver (?)

Pathophysiology
- Endothelial dysfunction caused by placenta-derived soluble factors
- Mitochondrial fatty acid oxidation defects (?)

HELLP, *Hemolysis, elevated liver enzymes, and low platelets;* ↑, *increased;* ↓, *decreased.*

intercellular adhesion molecule-1) and sVCAM-1 (soluble forms of vascular cell adhesion molecule-1) are altered early in the course of these hypertensive disorders.[158,159] The cumulative effect of these circulating signaling molecules as well as other contributing factors beyond the scope of this chapter is the initiation of the systemic hypertensive disorder that is the hallmark of preeclampsia and related disorders.

Collectively, these findings support the hypothesis that placenta-derived circulating factors that alter maternal endothelial function play a central role in disease development in maternal preeclampsia and related hypertensive disorders such as HELLP syndrome (discussed later). Future research will undoubtedly result in translation of these fundamental discoveries into targeted therapies and monitoring strategies for these disorders.[157]

HELLP SYNDROME

HELLP syndrome is a severe complication that occurs in an estimated 0.5% of all pregnancies and is characterized by the triad of *h*emolytic anemia, *e*levated *l*iver enzymes, and *l*ow *p*latelets (Box 54.6).[129,160,161] HELLP syndrome is closely associated with preeclampsia, and the most recent international classification of hypertensive disorders in pregnancy considers HELLP syndrome a manifestation of preeclampsia and not an independent entity.[129]

Clinical Features

Despite the well-known association between HELLP syndrome and preeclampsia, these entities exhibit distinct clinical differences. The peak period of clinical onset for HELLP is between 27 and 36 weeks of gestation, but unlike preeclampsia, as many as one-third of cases are diagnosed in the immediate postpartum period.[160] The most common presenting symptoms of HELLP syndrome are abdominal pain (40% to 100% of cases), nausea and vomiting (29% to 100%), and headache (29% to 84%), and most patients have peripheral edema (50% to 70%) and proteinuria (85% to 100%).[160,162,163]

Hypertension may be absent in as many as 12% to 18% of HELLP cases based on current diagnostic criteria, making a prompt diagnosis of a hypertensive disorder difficult.[129,162] This may be further complicated by the fact that the differential diagnosis of thrombocytopenia in pregnancy is often broad and includes gestational thrombocytopenia, immune thrombocytopenia, thrombotic thrombocytopenic purpura, and hemolytic-uremic syndrome. These entities account for the majority of pregnancy-associated thrombocytopenia cases and do not necessarily progress to HELLP syndrome.[164,165]

HELLP syndrome is associated with significant maternal and fetal complications, and the disease may recur in up to 27% of subsequent pregnancies or be associated with preeclampsia in subsequent pregnancies.[160,166-170] The maternal mortality rate is up to 1%, and the most serious maternal morbidities are disseminated intravascular coagulation, abruptio placentae, acute renal failure, and pulmonary edema.[162,171] Infants born to mothers with HELLP syndrome are at significantly increased risk for low birth weight and prematurity,[166,167] and infants born at a very early gestational age are at the highest risk for perinatal death.[162] The mortality rate and the rate of other neonatal complications, however, do not appear to be significantly different from those of matched neonates born to mothers without HELLP syndrome and who were treated in a neonatal intensive care unit.[167]

Definitive treatment of rapidly progressing thrombocytopenia or fetal distress is delivery.[41] Expectant management and various medical treatment options with steroids and plasma exchange may be considered, but consensus guidelines are lacking. Evidence suggests that corticosteroids administered to women with HELLP syndrome or preeclampsia early in the course of the disease may improve perinatal and maternal outcomes.[172,173]

Pathological Features and Pathogenesis

The pathological features of HELLP syndrome depend on the underlying pathophysiological processes. In classic form of HELLP syndrome associated with pregnancy-associated hypertensive disease, the pathological features are within the spectrum of changes described for preeclampsia and eclampsia.[174]

The underlying pathophysiology of classic HELLP syndrome is shared with preeclampsia and is fundamentally related to maternal endothelial dysfunction as detailed earlier in this chapter. However, animals treated with sFLT1 develop hypertension and proteinuria but not hemolysis and thrombocytopenia, suggesting that additional cofactors may be required for the phenotype of HELLP in the setting of preeclampsia.[175] In a subset of patients, this cofactor appears to be sEng, which synergistically works with sFLT1 to induce severe preeclampsia, hemolysis, thrombocytopenia, and elevated liver functions in animal models.[176] sEng is a placenta-derived TGF-beta coreceptor that is typically elevated in the sera of patients with preeclampsia (Fig. 54.6). sEng inhibits the formation of capillary tubes in vitro and induces vascular permeability and hypertension in vivo.[176] sEng may be a biomarker for severity of preeclampsia,[158,159] but it remains unclear whether it is a specific biomarker for HELLP syndrome in pregnant women with preeclampsia.

In spite of known associations between HELLP syndrome and preeclampsia, the incomplete biological and clinical overlap between these entities remains an area of active investigation. An intriguing alternative hypothesis for the pathogenesis of HELLP syndrome (or a subset of patients with HELLP syndrome) is suggested by an observed association between HELLP syndrome and LCHAD deficiency, SCAD deficiency, and MTTP deficiency, as reported in several studies.[109,112,118,119,124,177] In these cases, the liver pathology closely resembles that of AFLP. These associations link two seemingly divergent pathological mechanisms (one of endothelial dysfunction and one of mitochondrial FAO deficiency), and in the face of other contradictory resu lts,[120,178,179] leave many questions unanswered at this time.

Lastly, the alternative pathway of complement fixation has been proposed to contribute to the pathogenesis of HELLP syndrome,[180-184] but the mechanistic role of the complement system in the pathophysiology of pregnancy induced hypertensive disorders is not fully described. Despite uncertainties about pathophysiology, the pathological distinction between AFLP and vascular abnormalities associated with hypertensive disorders is straightforward and poses no diagnostic challenge.

HEPATIC RUPTURE

Clinical Features

Hepatic rupture is a potentially catastrophic complication of pregnancy, with an overall reported incidence of up to 4 cases per 100,000 deliveries.[185-190] Large subcapsular hematomas, the pathological background in which most cases of hepatic rupture occur, have been reported in 0.9% of pregnant women with HELLP syndrome.[160] Although HELLP syndrome is the primary risk factor for rupture, hepatic rupture has been reported in a variety of other conditions including uncomplicated pregnancies,[191] and in patients with AFLP,[192] as well as multiple other conditions.[193-198]

Regardless of the underlying cause, hepatic rupture typically manifests with acute abdominal pain associated with nausea and vomiting, followed by abdominal distention and hypovolemic shock. Diagnosis is readily made by abdominal imaging, and emergent surgical and medical treatment is required to prevent maternal and fetal mortality. Maternal mortality rates of 30% to 75% have been reported, commonly as a result of massive abdominal hemorrhage.[199,200] Fetal mortality rates are also high (60% to 80%) and often related to a combination of maternal hypotension, abruptio placentae, and prematurity.[199,200] Recurrence of rupture in subsequent pregnancies has been reported.[201,202]

Pathological Features and Pathogenesis

The pathological processes that lead to hepatic rupture are poorly understood, and they are most likely as varied as the underlying causes of rupture. In hypertensive disorders, the most likely sequence of events is intrahepatic or intracapsular hemorrhage with tissue disruption leading to hematoma formation, followed by distention and rupture of the capsule (Fig. 54.7). The events initiating intrahepatic hemorrhage in hypertensive disorders are unknown, but they are most likely related to parenchymal ischemia that results from fibrin thrombi or reduced blood flow caused by endothelial dysfunction.

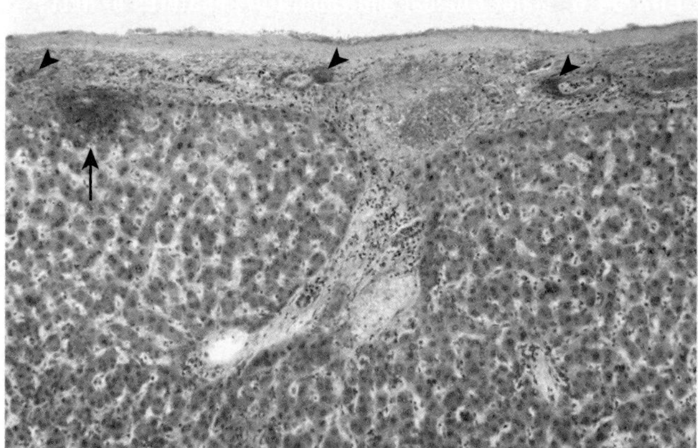

FIGURE 54.7 Multiple subcapsular hematomas *(arrow)* and multifocal intracapsular hemorrhages *(arrowheads)* were identified in this fatal case of eclampsia. The vascular branches of the portal tracts are in direct continuity with the Glisson capsule, and periportal hemorrhage extends into and beneath the liver capsule, which may cause rupture.

Hepatic rupture is most commonly associated with hematomas that occur on the superior and anterior aspects of the right lobe of the liver. The gross and microscopic pathology is otherwise that of the underlying condition leading to hematoma, tissue disruption, and rupture.

HYPEREMESIS GRAVIDARUM

Clinical Features

Nausea and vomiting are common during pregnancy, occurring in up to 70% of pregnant women.[203-205] Nausea and vomiting most commonly begin at 4 to 7 weeks of gestation, and they typically regress by the 16th week. HG is defined as a severe, intractable form of nausea and vomiting that causes secondary abnormalities such as dehydration and electrolyte imbalance.[203-205] HG is diagnosed in up to 10% of all pregnancies and may be associated with mildly elevated bilirubin (<5 mg/dL, all unconjugated), aminotransferases (usually less than two times normal), and alkaline phosphatase (less than two times normal) levels.[206-212] HG occurs more commonly in young women in their first pregnancy, and the incidence may depend on ethnicity.[213,214]

Maternal abnormalities promptly return to normal with supportive treatment, and more aggressive treatment regimens do not appear to improve outcome. Perinatal outcomes for patients with HG have been the subject of debate. Infants born to mothers with HG have been reported to have lower gestational age, lower birth weight, evidence of mild intrauterine FGR, evidence of neurodevelopmental abnormalities, and various other conditions, but multiple recent aggregate analyses have failed to reach a definitive conclusion about any of these associations.[215-219]

Pathological Features and Pathogenesis

The pathophysiology of HG remains unknown. A causative link between *Helicobacter pylori* infection and HG has been proposed, but most studies have methodological limitations, and the suggested association has not been definitively confirmed in recent aggregate analyses.[205,220,221] Liver histology in HG is typically normal, but a variety of nonspecific findings including mild steatosis, mild cholestasis, and occasional necrotic hepatocytes have been described.[206,222] Rare cases of severe liver damage have been reported,[212] but it is unlikely that such unusual cases represent the pathology of otherwise uncomplicated hyperemesis. No specific mechanisms of liver damage have been described, and the mild hepatic abnormalities are thought to result from dehydration and other systemic changes associated with hyperemesis or pregnancy in general.

VIRAL HEPATITIS E INFECTION

Clinical Features

Viral hepatitis is the leading cause of jaundice in pregnancy. Hepatitis C infection is thought to have an association with ICP,[223] but with the exception of hepatitis E virus (HEV) infection, the clinical course of viral hepatitis does not seem to be significantly affected by pregnancy. Needless to say, treatment of viral hepatitis in pregnancy requires special consideration as the mother and child are both at risk of complications caused by these viral infections,[224-231] especially in the setting of fulminant viral hepatitis.[232,233]

HEV is relatively uncommon in the United States, but various serotypes are globally distributed, with an estimated 14 million symptomatic cases and 300,000 deaths annually.[234] HEV is primarily transmitted via the fecal-oral route, although zoonotic and foodborne transmission have also been described. HEV is responsible for a large number of epidemic and sporadic forms of acute hepatitis in underserved and disadvantaged geographic regions.[234-238]

HEV infection manifests in patients after an incubation period of 2 to 10 weeks with a clinical illness resembling other forms of acute viral hepatitis. In pregnant women, the illness can be particularly severe, with mortality rates as high as 27%.[233,239-243] HEV is also a major cause of fulminant hepatic failure in pregnancy, with HEV seropositivity in 76% of the pregnant women versus 30% of controls.[233,244-246] The mortality rate is also significantly higher among pregnant HEV-positive women (65%) compared with nonpregnant patients (23%).[245] In addition to maternal disease, there is a significant risk of vertical transmission to the infants born to mothers with HEV infection and an increased risk of poor fetal outcomes in general.[240,242,247]

HEV infection is typically diagnosed by serological markers and by quantitative measurement of HEV RNA titers. Serological assays show anti-HEV immunoglobulin M (IgM) antibody early during clinical illness, although the IgM antibody disappears rapidly within a few months. Anti-HEV IgG antibody appears later and persists for at least a few years. Although potentially efficacious anti-HEV vaccines are available, none is currently approved for clinical use in the United States.[248-250]

Pathological Features and Pathogenesis

Histopathology of HEV infection in pregnancy has been rarely described. The pathology appears to be that of an acute cholestatic hepatitis (Fig. 54.8) with some resemblance to

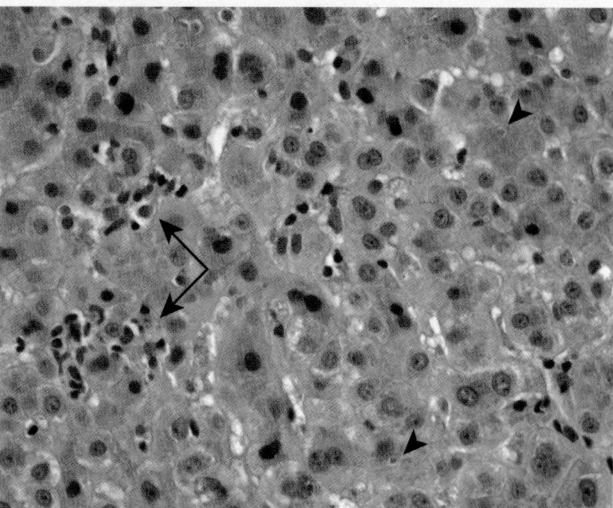

FIGURE 54.8 At clinical presentation, a patient with hepatitis E infection had mild, acute cholestatic hepatitis characterized by focal lobular inflammation *(arrows)* and prominent hepatocellular and canalicular cholestasis *(arrowheads).*

acute hepatitis A infection.[244,251-253] Findings commonly include a dense portal inflammatory infiltrate associated with various forms of bile duct damage, including acute or lymphocytic cholangitis and interface hepatitis. Lobular hepatocellular damage is often prominent and may include canalicular bile stasis, cholestatic hepatocellular rosettes, ballooning degeneration of hepatocytes, acidophilic bodies, and focal or confluent hepatocellular necrosis. The main histological differential diagnosis in pregnancy is ICP. Markedly elevated levels of aminotransferases may be helpful in distinguishing viral hepatitis from ICP, in which aminotransferase levels are typically only mildly elevated.

HEV is a nonenveloped, single-stranded RNA virus that belongs to the genus *Hepevirus* of the family Hepeviridae.[254,255] The HEV genome has been cloned and the infectious nature of the viral replicons experimentally confirmed. There are four genotypes with specific geographic distribution. Genotypes 1 and 2 are common in most of Asia, Africa, and Mexico. Genotype 3 is the predominant genotype in North and South America, Australia, and Europe. Genotype 4 is found mainly in far east Asia. Questions remain about the clinical differences between different genotypes as well as the specific nature of virus interaction with hepatocytes and their pathogenic mechanisms. The most likely etiology of liver damage is indirect hepatocyte injury as a result of the immune response to HEV infection.[238]

HERPESVIRUS INFECTION

Clinical Features

Clinically significant liver disease resulting from nonhepatitic viral infection is uncommon, but it can be devastating in pregnancy. With the exception of herpesviruses, these viral infections are neither more common nor more severe in pregnancy. Among the different serotypes, herpes simplex virus (HSV) infections are the most common, with a seropositivity rate of as much as 30% for HSV type 2 in a large cohort of pregnant women.[256]

Dissemination of HSV from the primary site of infection is often associated with primary or secondary immunodeficiency states, but on rare occasions, it may occur in otherwise healthy individuals. A disproportionate number of disseminated infections in otherwise healthy individuals appears to be associated with pregnancy, particularly during the third trimester.[257-262] Suspicion of the disease and prompt diagnosis with liver biopsy, culture, and serological tests are important because treatment with antiviral agents may be successful in controlling a disease that otherwise has extremely high maternal and fetal mortality rates.

Clinical presentation is somewhat nonspecific and includes nausea, vomiting, fever, and abdominal pain, and LFTs often show markedly increased levels of aminotransferases. Timely liver biopsy for tissue diagnosis in clinically suspected cases is important because there is significant maternal and fetal morbidity and mortality, classic mucocutaneous vesicular lesions may be absent in the majority of cases, and viral cultures may be negative in some.[259,260,262] Infection with other members of the Herpesviridae family, including cytomegalovirus, Epstein-Barr virus, and varicella-zoster virus, can also occur and result in hepatic disease in pregnancy.[258] With the exception of potential fetal transmission, these infections are not specifically different in the background of pregnancy than in nonpregnant patients.

Pathological Features and Pathogenesis

The underlying factors predisposing some pregnant women to more severe herpesvirus infections are unknown, but altered immunity during the course of pregnancy likely plays a role. Liver pathology in cases of HSV infection is similar to that in the nonpregnant state. It is characterized by irregular areas of hemorrhage and necrosis without significant inflammation but with classic viral inclusions in the surrounding hepatocytes (Fig. 54.9). In a questionable case, immunohistochemical stains and molecular assays for viral markers can provide a definitive diagnosis.

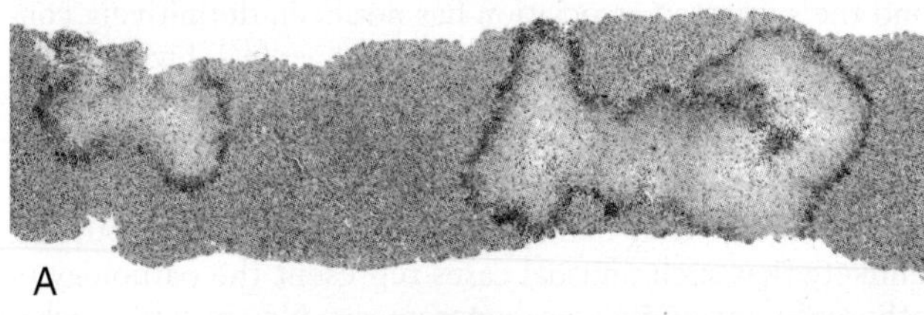

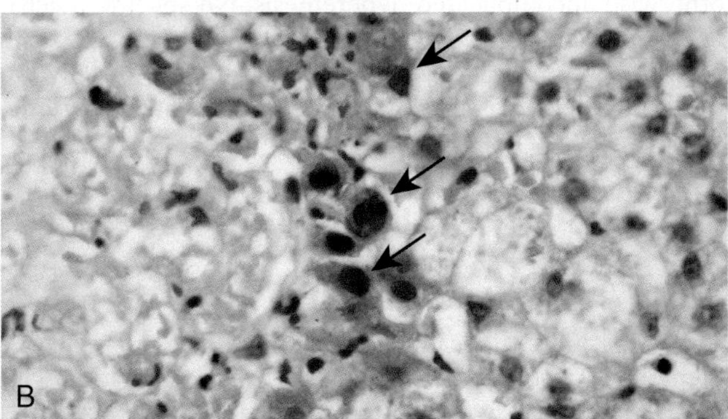

FIGURE 54.9 A, Low-power examination of the liver of a patient with herpesvirus hepatitis shows multifocal zones of geographic necrosis. **B,** High-power examination of the hepatocytes at the periphery of the zones of necrosis shows multiple cells with eosinophilic, amorphous, intranuclear inclusions *(arrows)* that are diagnostic of herpesvirus infection.

BUDD-CHIARI SYNDROME

Clinical Features

Budd-Chiari syndrome is the clinical manifestation of hepatic venous outflow obstruction and is classically caused by thrombotic occlusion of hepatic vein branches or the inferior vena cava. Pregnancy, including the early postpartum period, accounts for approximately 5% to 15% of documented cases.[263-265]

Clinical presentation with abdominal pain, hepatomegaly, and ascites is often insidious, although a disproportionate number of pregnancy-related cases have an acute onset and are associated with massive ischemic damage.[263,264] Proper diagnosis requires clinical imaging studies, including Doppler ultrasonography and possibly MRI.[87] Treatment with anticoagulants and thrombolytic agents may be sufficient for management of less severe cases, but surgical options such as portacaval shunt or transplantation may be necessary. Conversely, patients with Budd-Chiari syndrome are known to be at risk of various complications during pregnancy.[266-269]

Pathological Features and Pathogenesis

Pregnancy is a hypercoagulable state, and it is likely that the increased incidence of Budd-Chiari syndrome is an unintended consequence of this physiological change. However, some studies have suggested that factor V Leiden deficiency may be responsible for the atypical presentation of Budd-Chiari syndrome during pregnancy.[263,270,271] In a study of 63 cases, Budd-Chiari syndrome with massive ischemic necrosis was encountered only in carriers of factor V Leiden mutation, three (75%) of whom were pregnant; the fourth was on oral contraceptives.[263]

In addition to factor V, other components of the coagulation system have been implicated. Rautou and associates reported that among seven pregnant or postpartum women with Budd-Chiari syndrome, two had factor V Leiden mutation, one of whom had a myeloproliferative disease; two had protein S deficiency, one of whom had a myeloproliferative disease; one had antiphospholipid syndrome and a myeloproliferative disease; one had myeloproliferative disease alone; and one had no identified predisposing factor.[271] These observations have led to the hypothesis that a physiological decrease in the level of protein S during pregnancy may be a predisposing factor for Budd-Chiari syndrome.[272] The liver histopathology, differential diagnosis, and pathogenesis of Budd-Chiari syndrome in pregnancy are otherwise identical to those in nonpregnant patients.

CONCLUSIONS

Liver pathobiology is normally affected by the pathophysiological alterations and hormonal effects of pregnancy. Although many of the hepatic disorders encountered during pregnancy are similar to those that occur in the nonpregnant population, recognition of liver diseases specific to pregnancy is critical because they have a profound impact on maternal and fetal outcomes. Despite significant advances in understanding the underlying molecular and cellular mechanisms, histopathology of the liver in pregnancy-related disorders is often nonspecific.

The primary role of the pathologist in evaluation of liver disease in pregnancy is to provide confirmatory evidence for a clinically suspected diagnosis or to guide the clinical team toward an alternative diagnosis. For these goals to be accomplished, a clear dialogue must take place between clinicians and pathologists to convey clinically relevant data and to ensure proper handling and triage of biopsy material.

The full reference list may be accessed online at Elsevier eBooks for Practicing Clinicians.

ACKNOWLEDGMENT

We appreciate the contributions of Dr. Jacqueline Wolf to the previous editions of this chapter.

CHAPTER 55

Inherited Metabolic and Developmental Disorders of the Pediatric and Adult Liver

Sarangarajan Ranganathan, James M. Crawford, Milton J. Finegold

Contents

INTRODUCTION

Jaundice, which is observed in almost every newborn, is termed *physiological* because it clears within a few days, after hepatic activation of bilirubin conjugation. This phenomenon reflects a unique feature of prenatal life: Many functions of the liver that are required after birth for nutrition, metabolic balance, and detoxification and excretion of endogenous chemicals are provided to the developing fetus by the placenta and the mother. "Pathological" jaundice (i.e., extending beyond the usual "physiological" time frame) is the most frequent indication for liver biopsy in children, especially infants because functional immaturity is not limited to glucuronidation; intrinsic defects in many processes and structures lead to cholestasis. This is even more evident in premature infants. Not only do the first challenges to hepatobiliary function account for liver diseases that "adult" pathologists encounter very rarely, but maternal–fetal interactions are not always beneficial. Certain infections and immunologically mediated injuries are observed only in infants.

This chapter focuses on constitutional deficiencies of the liver that necessitate examination of tissue for diagnosis and treatment. Myriad chromosomal imbalances and heritable mutations that manifest with dysmorphism and multisystem disease, such as Down syndrome, may affect the liver but can be diagnosed clinically; they are included in this chapter only if they offer a challenge to diagnosis. Anatomical and synthetic defects, such as clotting factor deficiencies that do not lead to hepatobiliary dysfunction, are covered in other publications.[1,2] Against the roster of inherited conditions described in this chapter, it is worth noting the conditions included in United States recommended uniform screening panel for newborns (Table 55.1)[3]; only a subset of this chapter's disorders are included. Hence evaluation of hepatic disease in the pediatric population extends well beyond information obtained from the routine constitutional screening performed at the time of birth.

We have incorporated a practical approach to liver biopsy that is derived from Jevon and Dimmick's classification of the histological pattern of pediatric liver biopsies, which identify six dominant patterns.[4] Additionally, we emphasize the progress made during the past two decades with regard to decoding the genetic basis of disease that has resulted in improved therapeutics as well as reclassification and renaming of disease entities, genes, and proteins. In the preparation of this chapter, we have benefited from Online Mendelian Inheritance in Man (OMIM; www.omim.org), an online compendium of human genes and phenotypes maintained by the Johns Hopkins University and developed by the National Center for Biotechnology Information (NCBI). This searchable database provides a unique accession number for each entity and incorporates all alternative disease names and gene nomenclature. Throughout the text and in the tables, we have provided OMIM numbers for heritable conditions to assist readers.

PEDIATRIC LIVER BIOPSIES

Indications for Liver Biopsy in Children

In addition to prior liver or bone marrow transplantation (see Chapter 43), the most common indications for liver biopsy in the pediatric age group are conjugated hyperbilirubinemia in young infants (Table 55.2); tumor diagnosis (see Chapter 56); and assessment of liver injury, inflammation, and fibrosis. Metabolic diseases may manifest with fetal demise immediately after birth or at any age thereafter (Table 55.3).

For young infants with conjugated hyperbilirubinemia, biliary atresia is the most important and common condition that is amenable to surgical treatment. Choledochal cysts and other rare causes of duct obstruction that lead to jaundice shortly after birth are rare and are typically diagnosed by imaging studies rather than liver biopsy. Biliary atresia must be recognized quickly if surgical hepatic portoenterostomy is to be successful in reestablishing biliary drainage. Biopsy specimens from these patients are often obtained before the results of noninvasive studies, such as protease inhibitor typing, are available. Even in infants with probable biliary atresia, a liver biopsy may be performed to exclude other potential causes of jaundice. Therefore clinical management decisions rely heavily on morphological assessment of liver biopsy specimens (Table 55.4). After exclusion of biliary atresia and infections, consideration should be given to the possibility of an inherited disease as the cause of the patient's illness.

In older children, hepatomegaly, liver tumors, or chronic liver disease may prompt a liver biopsy. When liver disease appears after the neonatal period, clinical studies are typically used to identify the specific cause of the disease. Clinically diagnosed disorders include hepatitis B virus (HBV) and hepatitis C virus (HCV) infection, Wilson disease, reticuloendothelial storage disorders, steatosis, drug-induced hepatitis, autoimmune hepatitis, and cholangiopathy. Unusual causes include Alagille syndrome and metabolic storage disorders. On occasion, liver tissue may be obtained from a child with portal hypertension in whom none of these conditions is suspected. In such cases, congenital vascular anomalies (see Chapter 52) and congenital hepatic fibrosis should be considered. Liver biopsies are used to assess the severity of disease and the response to treatment in all of these disorders.

TABLE 55.1 Uniform Screening for the Newborn

Recommended Uniform Screening Panel: Core Conditions	Recommended Uniform Screening Panel: Secondary Conditions
Organic Acid Conditions	**Organic Acid Conditions**
Propionic academia (PROP)	Methylmalonic academia with homocystinuria (Cbl C,D)
Methylmalonic academia (MUT)	Malonic academia (MAL)
Methylmalonic academia (Cbl A,B)	Isobutrylglycinuria (IBG)
Isovaleric academia (IVA)	2-Methylbutyrylglycinuria (2MBG)
3-Methylcrotonyl-CoA carboxylase deficiency (3MCC)	3-Methylglutaconic aciduria (3MGA)
Glutaric academia type I (GA1)	2-Methyl-3-hydroxybutyric aciduria (2M3HBA)
3-Hydroxy-3-methylglutaric aciduria deficiency (HMG)	**Fatty Acid Oxidation Disorders**
β-Ketothiolase deficiency (BKT)	Short-chain acyl-CoA dehydrogenase deficiency (SCAD)
Holocarboxylase synthetase (multiple carboxylase) deficiency (MCD)	Medium/short-chain L-3-hydroxyacyl-CoA dehydrogenase deficiency (M/SCHAD)
Fatty Acid Oxidation Disorders	Glutaric academia type II (GA2)
Carnitine uptake defect/carnitine transport defect (CUD)	Medium-chain ketoacyl-CoA thiolase deficiency (MCAT)
Medium-chain acyl-CoA dehydrogenase deficiency (MCAD)	2,4 Dienoyl-CoA reductase deficiency (DE RED)
Very-long-chain acyl-CaA dehydrogenase deficiency (VLCAD)	Carnitine palmitoyltransferase type I deficiency (CPT-1A)
Long-chain L-3 hydroxyacyl-CoA dehydrogenase deficiency (LCHAD)	Carnitine palmitoyltransferase type II deficiency (CPT II)
Trifunctional protein deficiency (TFP)	Carnitine acylcarnitine translocase deficiency (CACT)
Amino Acid Disorders	**Amino Acid Disorders**
Classic phenylketonuria (PKU)	Argininemia (ARG)
Maple syrup urine disease (MSUD)	Citrullinemia type II (CIT II)
Homocystinuria (HCY)	Hypermethioninemia (MET)
Tyrosinemia type I (TYR)	Benign hyperphenylalaninemia (H-PHE)
Arginosuccinic academia (ASA)	Biopterin defect in cofactor biosynthesis (BIOPT BS)
Citrullinemia type I (CIT)	Biopterin defect in cofactor regeneration (BIOPT REG)
Endocrine Disorders	Tyrosinemia type II (TYR II)
Primary congenital hypothyroidism (CH)	Tyrosinemia type III (TYR III)
Congenital adrenal hyperplasia (CAH)	**Hemoglobin Disorders**
Hemoglobin Disorders	Various other hemoglobinopathies (Var Hb)
S,S disease (sickle cell anemia) (Hb SS)	**Other Disorders**
S, β-thalassemia (Hb S/bTh)	Galactoepimerase deficiency (GALE)
S,C disease (Hb S/C)	Galactokinase deficiency (GALK)
Other Disorders	T-cell–related lymphocyte deficiencies
Critical congenital heart disease (CCHD)	
Cystic fibrosis (CF)	
Classic galactosemia (GALT)	
Hearing loss (HEAR)	
Severe combined immunodeficiency (SCID)	

 From Urv TK, Parisi MA. Newborn screening: beyond the spot. Adv Exp Med Biol. *2017;1031:323–346; Advisory Committee on Heritable Disorders in Newborns and Children. Recommended uniform screening panel. US Department of Health and Human Services. https://www.hrsa.gov/advisory-committees/heritable-disorders/recommendations-reports/reports/index.html.*

Pediatric Liver Biopsy Specimen

Because of the broad range of diseases in children, evaluation of liver biopsies in these patients is distinct from that in adults. To perform all potentially necessary tests on a liver biopsy specimen, prior arrangements should be in place to ensure adequate specimen processing (Table 55.5).

Formalin-fixed specimens should be processed for routine light microscopy. Serial sections should be obtained. For example, a ribbon of 20 sections may be placed on 10 slides, with two tissue sections per slide. The first and last slides should be stained with hematoxylin and eosin (H&E) stain. Periodic acid–Schiff (PAS) stain with and without diastase digestion, trichrome stain, Perls iron stain, and reticulin techniques may be used on intervening slides. The remaining unstained slides may be held for possible future use.

Normal and Potentially Misleading Features of the Liver in Infants and Children

Some key features in the liver of infants and children differ from those in the adult liver (Table 55.6). Variations occur in architecture, specific cell populations, content of hepatocytes, and response to injury.

Architecture

The liver undergoes substantial growth after birth. It normally doubles in weight within the first month of life, doubles again during the first year of life, and does not reach its mature size until late adolescence. The portal tract system grows in parallel with the liver. Therefore the most peripheral aspects of the liver may exhibit developmental residua of fetal histology. For instance, residual bile duct plates may

TABLE 55.2 Liver Disease in Infants

Bile duct stricture	Peroxisomal disorders
Biliary atresia	Zellweger syndrome
Choledochal cyst	Mitochondrial cytopathies, Reye syndrome
Caroli syndrome	Urea cycle disorders
Alagille syndrome	Hereditary disorders of bilirubin metabolism
Neonatal infection	Crigler-Najjar syndrome
Cytomegalovirus	Gilbert syndrome
Herpesvirus	Dubin-Johnson syndrome and Rotor syndrome
Hepatotropic viruses (hepatitis E)	Hereditary disorders of bile formation and transport
Human immunodeficiency virus	Progressive familial intrahepatic cholestasis, types 1 to 5
Parvovirus B19	Disorders of bile acid biosynthesis
Paramyxovirus	Disorders of protein biosynthesis and targeting
Enteric viruses (echoviruses, coxsackieviruses, adenoviruses)	α_1-Antitrypsin deficiency
Rubella (congenital)	Cystic fibrosis
Bacterial sepsis	Miscellaneous inherited disorders
Urinary tract infection	Trisomy 21
Listeriosis	Aagenaes syndrome
Toxoplasmosis *(Toxoplasma gondii)*	Citrullinemia, type II
Syphilis (congenital)	X-linked adrenoleukodystrophy
Neonatal hemochromatosis	Miscellaneous nonneoplastic conditions
Disorders of carbohydrate metabolism	Shock/hypoperfusion (as from congestive heart failure in congenital heart disease)
Glycogen storage disease, types I and IV	Parenteral nutrition
Galactosemia	Fetal alcohol syndrome
Fructosemia	Drugs
Disorders of amino acid metabolism	Budd-Chiari syndrome
Tyrosinemia	Multiple hemangiomas (with high-output cardiac failure)
Disorders of glycolipid and lipid metabolism	Idiopathic neonatal hepatitis/syncytial giant cell hepatitis
Niemann-Pick disease types A, B, and C	Neonatal sclerosing cholangitis with ichthyosis
Gaucher disease	Neonatal lupus
Hurler disease	Neoplasia
Wolman disease	Neonatal leukemia
Disorders of glycoprotein metabolism	Neuroblastoma
Congenital disorder of glycosylation type Ib	Hepatoblastoma
	Langerhans cell histiocytosis
	Hemophagocytic lymphohistiocytosis

rim the portal tracts, and the latter contain a more cellular mesenchyme and a centrally placed portal vein (Fig. 55.1).[5] The dimensions of hepatic lobules remain constant with growth. However, hepatocyte cords may remain two cells thick well into the fourth postnatal year. This should not be misinterpreted as regenerative hyperplasia in response to tissue injury.

Cell Populations

Hematopoietic elements are commonly present in liver biopsy specimens obtained during the postnatal months. Granulopoiesis predominates in portal tracts, whereas erythropoiesis is common in the parenchyma.

Hepatocyte Content

Until a postnatal age of approximately 3 months, hepatocytes normally contain copper-binding protein and copper (demonstrable by orcein and rhodanine techniques, respectively) and granules of hemosiderin, particularly in periportal hepatocytes. These deposits are considered to be physiological and disperse with time. Conversely, hepatocyte alterations characteristic of various storage disorders may be inconspicuous in early infancy because of the time required to accumulate abnormal substances, such as α_1-antitrypsin (A1AT). One dramatic exception to the concept of physiological iron deposition occurs in newborns who exhibit liver failure at birth, which is usually attributable to severe liver injury in utero. In this scenario, marked iron deposits may be present in hepatocytes at birth, giving rise to the term *neonatal iron storage disease* or *perinatal hemochromatosis*.[6] A severe degree of necrosis and fibrosis is also present in patients with this condition. The extrahepatic reticuloendothelial system does not exhibit iron accumulation, highlighting the primacy of the liver injury.[7] The finding of severe perinatal hepatic siderosis is nonspecific and indicates the development of liver injury during gestation.[8] A lesser degree of hemosiderosis, with reticuloendothelial system deposits, may be seen in cases of maternal–fetal blood group incompatibility with significant hemolysis.

Response to Injury

Giant multinucleated hepatocytes, with or without bile pigment, are often present in infants with liver disease, regardless of the etiology. This change is considered nonspecific and reactive. Multinucleated hepatocytes are formed by syncytial breakdown of cell-to-cell borders, but with partial preservation of the canalicular aspects of the cell membrane.[9] Canalicular remnants with retained bile may be observed within the cytoplasm. Giant cells exhibit multiple

TABLE 55.3 Presentation of Metabolic Diseases That Involve the Liver

Age	Hepatic Failure Encephalopathy (±Bleeding)	Jaundice (Hepatitis)	Failure to Thrive and/or Hepatomegaly (Hypoglycemia)	Failure to Thrive and/or Hepatomegaly (Normal Sugar)	Portal Hypertension (Ascites, Bleeding, Splenomegaly)
Newborn	Galactosemia, mitochondriopathies, urea cycle defects, glutaric aciduria II	Crigler-Najjar syndrome type I	Leprechaunism, fructose 1.6 diphosphatase deficiency		
First 2 months	Wolman disease, tyrosinemia, perinatal hemochromatosis	α_1-Antitrypsin deficiency, NPD type C	GSD 1a, Ib	Zellweger syndrome	GSD IV
First 6 months	Hereditary fructose intolerance, LCAD deficiency, carnitine deficiency, propionic acidemia	Byler disease, Alagille syndrome, THCA, 3β-HSD, isomerase deficiency	GSD III	Lysinuric protein intolerance, MPS, other storage diseases	
First 2 years	MCAD deficiency, mitochondriopathies	Cystic fibrosis, Rotor syndrome		GSD VI and IX, congenital disorder of glycosylation type Ib, glycoprotein	
Up to 6 years				Cholesterol ester storage, NPD types A and B, cystinosis, hereditary fructose intolerance	
Puberty/and adolescence	Wilson disease, erythropoietic porphyria	Gilbert syndrome, Wilson disease, Dubin-Johnson syndrome			α_1-Antitrypsin deficiency, Wilson disease, lipoatrophic diabetes
Adults					Gaucher disease, citrullinemia, hemochromatosis

GSD, *Glycogen storage disorder;* 3β-HSD, *3β-hydroxysteroid dehydrogenase;* LCAD, *long-chain acyl-coenzyme A dehydrogenase;* MCAD, *medium chain acyl-coenzyme A dehydrogenase;* MPS, *mucopolysaccharidoses;* NPD, *Niemann-Pick disease;* THCA, *trihydroxycholestanoic acid.*

TABLE 55.4 Pathologist's Role in Infantile Cholestasis

Action	Examples
Find treatable condition	Large duct obstruction, especially biliary atresia
	Galactosemia
Prevent inappropriate treatment	α_1-Antitrypsin deficiency mimics BA
	No surgery for Alagille syndrome; must recognize lack of large duct obstruction pattern in Alagille syndrome
Secure samples for diagnosis	Urine for FAB-GC/MS for bile acids
	Frozen liver for enzymes and molecular studies
	PCR for virus
Provide data for the family	Hereditable conditions
Monitor course of treatment and prognosis	After Kasai portoenterostomy or transplantation, biopsies and serial α-fetoprotein levels
Elucidate pathogenesis (with a goal of prevention)	Role of fasting versus TPN

BA, *Biliary atresia;* FAB-GC/MS, *fast atom bombardment gas chromatography/mass spectrometry;* PCR, *polymerase chain reaction;* TPN, *total parenteral nutrition.*

TABLE 55.5 Bedside Processing of Pediatric Liver Biopsy Specimens

Snap-freezing	Use liquid nitrogen; core tissue 2 cm in length; air-sealed specimen vial
Electron microscopy	Use electron microscopy fixative; core tissue 0.3 cm in length
Formalin fixation	Use neutral-buffered formalin; core tissue at least 1 cm (1-2 cm) in length

Do not use a biopsy sponge.
Do not place tissue in saline or transport media.
Do not let the specimen sit exposed to air.

nuclei, either scattered throughout the cytoplasm or clustered toward one pole of the cell. This reaction may persist well into childhood if the inciting disorder is not resolved. Multinucleated giant cell change is unusual in older children and adults, but it may occur in some disorders such as autoimmune hepatitis and paramyxovirus hepatitis.[10,11]

The histological spectrum of neonatal hepatitis includes giant cell change in hepatocytes, intralobular cholestasis, necrosis of hepatocytes, and intrahepatic hematopoiesis. All of these features are nonspecific events in infancy and can be observed in biliary atresia, A1AT storage disorder, and many other conditions (Table 55.7). With advances in

TABLE 55.6 Normal and Potentially Misleading Features of Pediatric Liver Tissue

Architecture	Physiological hyperplasia: liver cell plates two cells thick
	Residual ductal plate architecture, particularly at periphery of liver
Absence of bile ducts	Recognize apparent paucity in early biopsies of extreme preterm infants
Extramedullary hematopoiesis	Portal tracts: granulocytic extramedullary hematopoiesis
	Parenchyma: erythropoietic extramedullary hematopoiesis
Hepatocyte contents	Hemosiderin granules Copper deposits

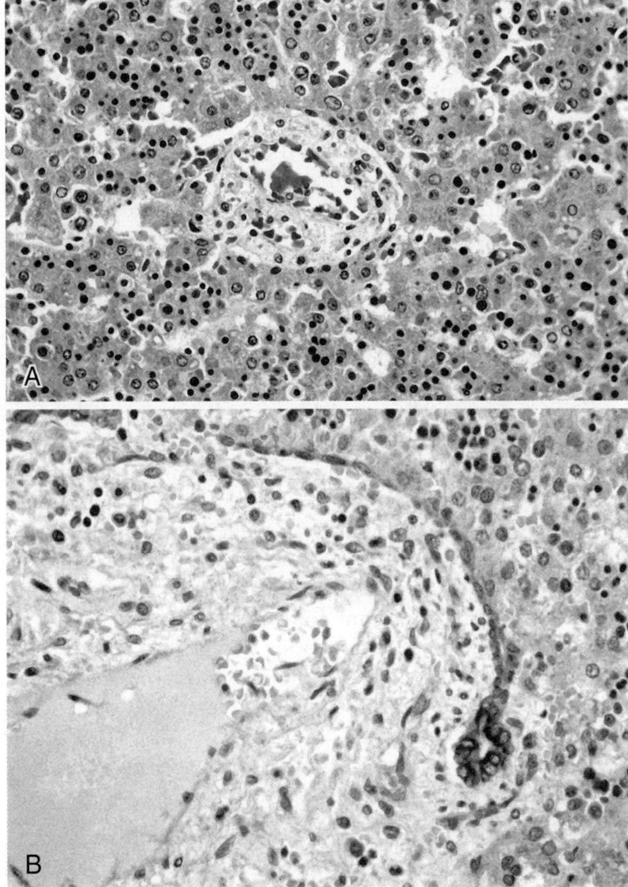

FIGURE 55.1 Histology of the perinatal liver. A, Tissue near the hilum of the liver exhibits residual erythropoietic extramedullary hematopoiesis in parenchymal sinusoids, evident as focal collections of normoblasts. **B,** Tissue near the capsule is stained for cytokeratin 19. An immature portal tract contains a rim of biliary epithelium (termed the *ductal plate*) but without a mature terminal bile duct. Such immature portal tracts may be sampled by percutaneous liver biopsy.

biochemistry and molecular genetics, many conditions formerly grouped within the category of *neonatal giant cell hepatitis* can now be specifically diagnosed, including progressive familial cholestasis types 2 and 3 and various bile salt synthetic defects.

TABLE 55.7 Etiology and Differential Diagnosis of Neonatal Hepatitis

Infantile Cholestasis with Giant Cells	
Normal or Low GGT	***Elevated GGT***
PFIC type 2 (BSEP disease)* PFIC 4 (TJP2 defect) PFIC 5 (FXR defect) MYO5B defect Bile salt synthetic defects* ARC syndrome Familial hypercholanemia CALFAN syndrome	PFIC type 3 (ABCB4/MDR3 disease)* Niemann-Pick disease type C Alagille syndrome Perinatal hemochromatosis Rubella, cytomegalovirus, herpesvirus type 6, parainfluenza α_1-Antitrypsin deficiency McCune-Albright syndrome Navajo neurohepatopathy Biliary atresia Hemophagocytosis syndromes
Infantile Cholestasis without Giant Cells (±Bile Duct Damage)	
PFIC type 1 (Byler disease, Greenland cholestasis)† Alagille syndrome Cytomegalovirus Hypopituitarism* Cystic fibrosis Citrullinemia type II Smith-Lemli-Opitz syndrome Prematurity, fasting, total parenteral nutrition* North American Indian childhood cirrhosis Jeune syndrome Trisomy 21 (Down syndrome) Trisomy 18 Neonatal lupus Septo-optic dysplasia	
Infantile Cholestasis Plus Necrosis (±Steatosis)	
Galactosemia Hereditary fructose intolerance Tyrosinemia type I Pearson mitochondrial DNA deficiency Perinatal hemochromatosis Bacterial (i.e., gram-negative) sepsis Hepatitis B virus Cytomegalovirus Echovirus Herpes simplex virus types 1 and 2 Hemophagocytic syndrome Bile salt synthetic defects	

ARC, *Arthrogryposis, renal dysfunction, and cholestasis;* BSEP, *bile salt export pump;* GGT, *γ-glutamyltransferase;* PFIC, *progressive familial intrahepatic cholestasis.*
**Prompt medical intervention is possible and can be lifesaving, protect the central nervous system, and avert transplantation.*
†Medical intervention is possible.

APPROACH TO THE DIAGNOSIS OF PEDIATRIC LIVER DISORDERS IN LIVER BIOPSIES

When evaluating pediatric liver biopsy specimens, a careful review of patient age at disease onset (see Table 55.3), clinical manifestations, and routine laboratory workup findings is essential (Table 55.8). If the presentation includes hepatomegaly, awareness of extrahepatic involvement is also helpful (Table 55.9). It is useful to initially classify the histological pattern of disease into one of the six patterns of injury described initially by Jevon and Dimmick.[4] Although these patterns often overlap, it is usually possible to define the predominant pattern in an individual case.[12,13] This section describes an algorithmic approach to the diagnosis of liver disorders, beginning with the histological patterns of tissue injury (see Boxes 55.1 to 55.6). A detailed description of the major entities is found later in this chapter.

Cholestatic Pattern

The differential diagnosis of cholestatic disease in childhood is extremely broad and includes extrahepatic biliary obstruction (biliary atresia, choledochal cyst), infections, immune regulatory defects such as Langerhans cell histiocytosis, genetic disorders, metabolic disorders, total parenteral nutrition (TPN), and toxin exposures (see Table 55.2). Liver biopsies to determine the cause of cholestasis should be performed only after completion of a thorough radiological and laboratory workup, including ultrasound, hepatobiliary scintigraphy, viral serology, Pi typing for A1AT deficiency, and sweat chloride testing to rule out the more common causes of cholestasis in this age group.[14]

TABLE 55.8 Workup of Neonatal Cholestasis*

Soon After Birth	Short Delay	Insidious Onset
Bacterial cultures TORCH antibodies CBC differential, platelets Reticulocyte count Coombs test Urine sediment for inclusions Radiography of skull, bones	Variable symptoms Syphilis serology Urinary reducing sugars, $FeCl_3$, amino acids Sweat test Ophthalmic examination Skin examination for hemangiomas Abdominal radiographs for free air, ascites Upper gastrointestinal radiographs	Darkening of diaper Pale stool Feeding off Slow growth Prematurity or small for dates Many cases with GCT have this history Abnormal feeding history, intravenous amino acids

CBC differential, *Complete blood cell count with differential;* GCT, *giant cell transformation;* TORCH, *toxoplasmosis, other agents, rubella, cytomegalovirus, and herpes simplex.*
**Acute presentation: bleeding, seizures, and vomiting.*

When confronted with a predominantly cholestatic pattern of liver injury in a biopsy specimen, a useful starting point is the serum level of γ-glutamyltransferase (GGT) (Box 55.1). Serum levels of GGT, a canalicular membrane protein, are usually low in disorders of defective bile acid synthesis or bile salt secretion. These entities (Table 55.10) are discussed later in this chapter. Although the histological features differ among some of these entities (e.g., lack of giant cells in progressive familial intrahepatic cholestasis type 1 [PFIC1] compared with PFIC2 and PFIC3), ultrastructural examination, specialized enzymatic assays, and genetic testing are crucial in diagnosing these disorders. Among the cholestatic disorders with normal or low serum GGT, congenital defects in bile acid synthesis are commonly diagnosed by urinary mass spectrometry. Peroxisomal biogenesis disorders, such as Zellweger syndrome, neonatal adrenoleukodystrophy, and infantile Refsum disease, typically manifest with cholestasis, necrosis, and siderosis. These disorders are caused by mutations in multiple peroxin *(PEX)* genes.[15] Biochemical diagnosis involves measurement of very-long-chain fatty acids in plasma and erythrocyte plasmalogen.[16] Whole-genome sequencing is providing novel mechanistic and diagnostic insights for peroxisomal disorders.[17]

Congenital hepatic fibrosis and Caroli disease are two rare disorders of ductal plate malformation that deserve mention here. Both manifest with cholestasis and cholangitis and often with portal hypertension.[18] Both are associated with autosomal recessive polycystic kidney disease (ARPKD), and both carry mutations in *PKHD1* (fibrocystin). The gene is defective in up to 30% of cases of ARPKD.[19]

The current approach to diagnosis of neonatal cholestatic infants is by genetic testing using several comprehensive commercially available panels performed using next-generation sequencing techniques.[20,21] This includes most genes that have been identified in various childhood and adult genetic diseases and includes all genes for PFICs including *TJP2* and *MYO5B*, as well as genes in Alagille syndrome and peroxisomal disorders, to name a few. For the desperately ill neonate, rapid whole-genome sequencing may be critically important for clinical decision making.[22] Thus the advent of genetic testing has facilitated interpretations of liver biopsies, and the latter is now used more often to stage the degree of parenchymal involvement by

TABLE 55.9 Hepatomegaly with Extrahepatic Associations—Diagnostic Studies

Hepatomegaly	Splenomegaly	Mental Retardation	Neurodegeneration
Steatohepatitis (liver biopsy)	Biliary cirrhosis (liver biopsy)	Sly (fibroblast culture; β-galactosidase)	GSD type IV (liver; branching enzyme)
Budd-Chiari syndrome (MRI)	NPD type C (fibroblast culture; cholesterol esterification)	Wolman disease (fibroblast culture; acid lipase)	GSD type VIII (liver; phosphorylase B)
GSD type VI (liver; phosphorylase)	Cholesteryl-ester storage disease (fibroblast culture; acid lipase)	NPD type C (fibroblast culture; cholesterol esterification)	Sialidosis (fibroblast culture; neuraminidase)
GSD type IX (liver; phosphorylase kinase)	NPD type B (leukocyte; acid sphingomyelinase)	Mannosidosis (fibroblast culture; α-mannosidase)	
GSD type X (liver; complement C3 and C5, AMP-dependent kinase)		Fucosidosis (fibroblast culture; α-fucosidase)	
Congenital disorder of glycosylation type Ib (serum transferrin)		NPD type A (leukocyte; acid sphingomyelinase)	

AMP, *Adenosine monophosphate;* GSD, *glycogen storage disorder;* NPD, *Niemann-Pick disease.*

BOX 55.1 Diagnostic Algorithm for Cholestatic Pattern

NORMAL-GGT CHOLESTASIS

1. Giant cell hepatitis
   - Consider **progressive familial intrahepatic cholestasis type 2 (PFIC2)** → EM: amorphous canalicular bile → confirm with *ABCB11* gene sequencing
   - Consider PFIC4, PFIC5, and MYO5B disease → confirm with cholestatic gene panel
2. Dilated canaliculi with pale bile
   - Centrilobular fibrosis → **progressive familial intrahepatic cholestasis type 1 (PFIC1)** → EM: coarse granular canalicular bile → *ATP8B1* gene sequencing (30%-40% positive)
   - No fibrosis → **benign recurrent intrahepatic cholestasis** → confirm with *ATP8B1* or *ABCB11* gene sequencing
3. EM: dense amorphous canalicular bile
   - **PFIC2** → as above
   - **Arthrogryposis, renal dysfunction, and cholestasis (ARC) syndrome** → in the setting of arthrogryposis, perform *VPS33B* and *VIPAR* gene sequencing
   - **Familial hypercholanemia (FHCA)** → *TJP2* and *BAAT* and *EPHX1* gene sequencing

HIGH-GGT CHOLESTASIS

1. Bile duct/portal tract ratio > 0.9
   - Giant cell change ± cirrhosis → consider **progressive familial intrahepatic cholestasis type 3 (PFIC3)** → confirm with *ABCB4* gene sequencing
   - Cirrhosis with prominent bile ductular proliferation → **North American Indian childhood cirrhosis (NAIC)** → confirm with *CIRH1A* gene sequencing
   - Hepatocellular siderosis → confirm with iron stain → **GRACILE syndrome** → confirm with *BCS1L* gene sequencing
   - Giant cell hepatitis ± cirrhosis → PAS-positive diastase-resistant hepatocyte inclusions → A1AT staining by immunohistochemistry → **α_1-Antitrypsin (A1AT) deficiency** → EM: homogeneous inclusions within RER → confirm with Pi typing
   - Giant cell hepatitis ± cirrhosis → PAS negative → consider **Niemann-Pick disease type C** → EM: membrane-bound laminated structures and dense osmiophilic bodies → confirm with filipin staining in cultured fibroblasts and cholesterol esterification assays or with *NPC1* and *NPC2* gene sequencing
   - Neonatal sclerosing cholangitis with ichthyosis caused by claudin-1 (*CLDN1*) mutation
2. Bile duct/portal tract ratio < 0.9 (ductopenia)
   - Giant cell hepatitis and cirrhosis → consider **Alagille syndrome (AGS)** → confirm with *JAG1* (and *NOTCH2*) gene sequencing
   - Giant cell hepatitis with bridging fibrosis or cirrhosis → PAS-positive diastase-resistant hepatocyte inclusions → A1AT staining by immunohistochemistry → **A1AT deficiency** → as above

EM, *Electron microscopy;* GGT, *γ-glutamyltransferase;* GRACILE, *growth retardation, amino aciduria, cholestasis, iron overload, lactic acidosis, and early death;* PAS, *periodic acid–Schiff;* RER, *rough endoplasmic reticulum.*

respective diseases rather than to diagnose specific entities. Liver biopsies, however, continue to help in diagnosis of extrahepatic biliary atresia (EHBA) and to differentiate from paucity of bile ducts.

Steatotic Pattern

A steatotic pattern of injury is present when there is a prominent and diffuse distribution of fat vacuoles within hepatocytes. Steatosis is a common histopathological finding in several types of inherited disorders that affect the liver; those in which other histological features predominate are discussed separately. When one is considering the differential diagnosis of a primary steatotic pattern of liver injury, the most useful feature is the type of fat accumulation: microvesicular, macrovesicular, or mixed microvesicular and macrovesicular (Box 55.2).

Microvesicular steatosis results from perturbation of mitochondrial metabolism, fatty acid β-oxidation (FAO), or electron transport chain function, through either a genetic defect or drug-induced[23] inhibition of the pathways. The latter mechanism may result from a variety of drugs, including aspirin, ibuprofen, valproate, and zidovudine (see Chapter 49 for details on Reye syndrome). The diagnostic workup of genetic defects in FAO or electron transport chain function is often based on the clinical presentation and relies on specialized biochemical and metabolic testing of plasma, urine, and biopsied muscle tissue.[4,24,25] Pathological features in liver biopsy specimens, such as microvesicular steatosis, cholestasis, fibrosis, cirrhosis, abnormal mitochondrial ultrastructure, and immunohistochemical demonstration of mitochondrial enzyme deficiency, support the diagnosis.[4] Fresh-frozen liver is essential for specialized biochemical and genetic assays, particularly for analysis of the ratio of mitochondrial DNA (mtDNA) to nuclear DNA by Southern blotting (used for diagnosis of mtDNA depletion syndrome). Whole-exome sequencing is also making inroads in diagnosis of these disorders.[26] Also, histological examination of the liver is highly relevant in the postmortem examination of patients with suspected mitochondrial disorders.

Diffuse macrovesicular steatosis or mixed microvesicular and macrovesicular steatosis can develop in several inherited and acquired conditions (Table 55.11). Two inborn errors of carbohydrate metabolism, galactosemia and hereditary fructose intolerance, are classically associated with steatosis in newborns and infants. Galactosemia is diagnosed through urine biochemical testing and red cell enzyme assays.[27] Liver biopsy, if performed, shows macrovesicular steatosis with fibrosis and cirrhosis. A liver biopsy is indicated in hereditary fructose intolerance for confirmatory aldolase B enzyme assays on fresh-frozen tissue,[27] although molecular assays to detect *ALDOB* mutations are now available.[28] The pathological features mimic those of galactosemia, except that cirrhosis is usually absent.[29] Steatosis, with or without biliary cirrhosis, is common in cystic fibrosis (CF). Liver disease is relatively uncommon in young patients with CF but can lead to significant morbidity. In patients in whom the diagnosis was confirmed by positive sweat chloride testing and mutations in the CF transmembrane conductance regulator gene (*CFTR*), the diagnosis is suspected when eosinophilic material is present within bile ducts in liver biopsies (see later).[4]

TABLE 55.10 Genetic Defects and Available Testing for Inherited Disorders That Manifest with a Cholestatic Pattern

Disorder	Gene	Protein	Inheritance	Secondary Pattern	Confirmatory Testing
Progressive Familial Intrahepatic Cholestasis (PFIC) Syndrome					
PFIC1 (allelic disorder: BRIC)	*ATP8B1*	ATPase, class I, type 8B, member 1	AR	Cirrhotic	Gene sequencing
PFIC2	*ABCB11*	ATP-binding cassette, subfamily B, member 11	AR	Hepatitic Cirrhotic	Gene sequencing
PFIC3	*ABCB4 (MDR3)*	ATP-binding cassette, subfamily B, member 4	AR	Cirrhotic	Serum LPX, genotyping
PFIC4	*TJP2*	Tight junction protein 2	AR	Hepatitic	Gene sequencing
PFIC5	*NR1H4 (FXR)*	Nuclear receptor subfamily 1, group H, member 4	AR	Hepatitic Cirrhotic	Gene sequencing
CALFAN syndrome	*SCYL1*	Homolog of *Saccharomyces cerevisiae*	?AR	Acute liver failure, neuropathy, cerebellar atrophy	
Congenital Bile Acid Synthetic (CBAS) Defects					
CBAS1	*HSD3B7*	3β-Hydroxy-Δ5-C_{27}-steroid dehydrogenase	AR	Hepatitic	Blood spot ESI-MS or urine MS
CBAS2	*AKR1D1*	Δ4-3-Oxosteroid 5β-reductase	AR	Hepatitic Steatotic	Blood spot ESI-MS or urine MS
Peroxisomal Biogenesis Disorders					
Zellweger syndrome	*PEX* genes	Peroxisomal biogenesis factors	AR	Hepatitic Cirrhotic Steatotic	↑ Plasma VLCFA by GC
Neonatal adrenoleukodystrophy	*PEX*	Peroxisomal biogenesis factors	AR	—	↑ Plasma VLCFA by GC
Infantile Refsum disease	*PEX*	Peroxisomal biogenesis factors	AR	—	↑ Plasma VLCFA by GC
Others					
North American Indian childhood cirrhosis	*CIRH1A*	Cirhin	AR	Cirrhotic	R565W (c.1741C→T) genotyping
Alagille syndrome	*JAG1; NOTCH2*	Jagged1; Notch-2	AD	Cirrhotic Hepatitic	Gene sequencing
Niemann-Pick disease type C	*NPC1; NPC2*	Niemann-Pick disease types C1 and C2	AR	Hepatitic Storage	Filipin staining in fibroblasts

AD, *Autosomal dominant;* AR, *autosomal recessive;* ATP, *adenosine triphosphate;* ATPase, *adenosine triphosphatase;* BRIC, *benign recurrent intrahepatic cholestasis;* ESI, *electrospray ionization;* GC, *gas chromatography;* LPX, *lipoprotein X;* MS, *mass spectrometry;* OMIM, *Online Mendelian Inheritance in Man (www.omim.org);* VLCFA, *very-long-chain fatty acids.*

BOX 55.2 Diagnostic Algorithm for Steatotic Pattern

MICROVESICULAR STEATOSIS

1. Cholestasis
   - Consider mitochondrial **electron transport chain (ETC) disorders** → confirm with specialized testing (enzymatic activity of ETC complexes; mtDNA analyses)
   - Oncocytic transformation → Consider **mtDNA depletion syndrome (MDS)** → EM: enlarged pleomorphic mitochondria with unusual cristae → confirm with specialized testing including genotyping *dGUOK, POLG,* and so on
   - EM: enlarged mitochondria with increased cristae → consider **fatty acid oxidation (FAO) disorders** → hypoketotic hypoglycemia → confirm with specialized testing including gene sequencing for *ACADM, ACADL,* and so on (see Table 55.11)

MACROVESICULAR STEATOSIS

1. Cirrhosis
   - Hepatocyte vacuolation, foamy Kupffer cells, macrophages with positive lipid stains → consider **Wolman disease** → see Box 55.3
   - Hepatocyte stainable copper → consider **Wilson disease** → see Box 55.4
   - Inspissated material within bile ducts → consider **cystic fibrosis (CF)** → confirm with *CFTR* gene sequencing, sweat chloride testing
2. Cholestasis without cirrhosis
   - Consider **hereditary fructose intolerance (HFI)** → confirm with fructose-1-phosphate aldolase assay on liver tissue and *ALDOB* sequencing
3. Hepatocyte cytoplasmic storage
   - Consider **glycogen storage disease (GSD)** types I, III (see Box 55.3), VI, and IX
   - Consider Chanarin-Dorfman syndrome (ABHD5 mutation)—mixed steatosis with skin disease
   - Consider lysosomal lipase deficiency diseases (Wolman disease and CESD)

CESD, *cholesteryl-ester storage disease;* EM, *Electron microscopy;* mtDNA, *mitochondrial DNA.*

TABLE 55.11 Genetic Defects and Available Testing for Inherited Disorders That Manifest with a Steatotic Pattern

Disorder	Gene(s)	Protein(s)	Inheritance	Secondary Pattern	Confirmatory Testing
Mitochondrial Disorders					
FAO disorders, ETC disorders, mtDNA depletion syndrome, etc.	Multiple *ACADM*, *ACADL*, etc.	Multiple	Mostly AR		Plasma acylcarnitine and gene sequencing
Inborn Errors of Carbohydrate Metabolism					
Hereditary fructose intolerance	*ALDOB*	Aldolase B	AR	Cholestatic	Liver enzyme activity and sequencing
Galactosemia	*GALT*	Galactose-1-phosphate uridyltransferase	AR	Cirrhotic	RBC GALT assay
Cystic fibrosis	*CFTR*	Cystic fibrosis transmembrane conductance regulator	AR	Hepatitic Cholestatic	Sweat chloride, gene sequencing

AR, *Autosomal recessive;* ETC, *electron transport chain;* FAO, *fatty acid oxidation;* mtDNA, *mitochondrial DNA;* RBC, *red blood cell.*

Organic acidurias and urea cycle disorders may occasionally demonstrate steatosis or focal glycogenosis,[4] but these disorders are diagnosed through urine chromatographic analyses.[30] In some cases, progression to fibrosis and even cirrhosis may occur. Other disorders may demonstrate steatosis as a secondary feature. Biopsies of glycogen storage disease (GSD) types I and III often reveal steatosis. The liver in Wilson disease may be steatotic, but the predominant pattern is hepatitic or cirrhotic or both, with positive staining of copper using rhodanine to confirm.

Storage Pattern

A storage pattern is characterized by the presence of enlarged, swollen, and pale hepatocytes and/or reticuloendothelial cells, including sinusoidal Kupffer cells and portal macrophages. The stored material results from specific enzyme deficiencies in various metabolic pathways. A diverse group of disorders (>30) result in the development of a storage pattern within the liver, most of which cause hepatomegaly (see Table 55.9). Most, but not all (e.g., not the X-linked disorders, Fabry disease, or Hunter disease), are inherited in an autosomal recessive fashion. These disorders often demonstrate variable penetrance and expressivity, with different clinical and histological manifestations among family members with the same genetic defect. For a comprehensive discussion of these disorders, readers are referred to several excellent review articles.[4,27,31]

For pathologists confronted with biopsy specimens revealing a storage pattern, the most efficient approach involves a pediatric geneticist and a clinical biochemist because the patient's clinical presentation and laboratory findings often suggest the most likely diagnosis. The storage pattern can be subclassified as either *lysosomal* or *cytoplasmic*. Because reticuloendothelial cells are rich in lysosomes, Kupffer cells and histiocytes are typically more involved in lysosomal storage diseases than in disorders with cytoplasmic storage (e.g., GSD types I, III, and IV). However, this distinction is not absolute because diffuse hepatic and extrahepatic involvement of the reticuloendothelial system is a well-documented feature in some GSDs, particularly GSD type IV.[32] Distinguishing lysosomal (membrane-bound) from cytoplasmic storage disorders by electron microscopy is therefore quite useful.

Hepatic involvement in Pompe disease (GSD type II) is variable.[33] The liver architecture is usually intact. PAS-positive diastase-sensitive inclusions are present within histiocytes and hepatocytes (Box 55.3). Diagnostic confirmation is usually established by measurement of acid α-glucosidase activity in muscle or fibroblasts. Additional confirmation can be done by *GAA* gene sequencing.

The differential diagnosis of cytoplasmic storage disorders includes GSD types I, III, IV, VI, and IX (Table 55.12). These disorders are discussed later in this chapter.

The differential diagnosis of lysosomal storage disorders with foamy histiocytes includes lipidoses (Table 55.13), chiefly Gaucher disease, Farber disease, Niemann-Pick disease (NPD) types A and B, GSD type II, mucopolysaccharidoses, and GM1 gangliosidosis. In Gaucher disease, the most common lysosomal storage disorder, there is a characteristic diffuse infiltration by engorged histiocytes (Gaucher cells) containing PAS-negative cytoplasmic ("crinkled-paper") inclusions of glucosylceramide.[4] Hepatocytes are typically spared. On demonstration of tubular structures by electron microscopy, one should, for confirmation, measure the level of leukocytic or fibroblastic acid β-glucosidase activity and sequence the *GBA* gene for mutations.[31]

Hepatitic Pattern

The hepatitic pattern, in infants, reveals hepatocellular unrest (variability in cell and nuclear size and shape) with or without necrosis, diffuse giant cell transformation of hepatocytes, extramedullary hematopoiesis, and prominent cholestasis[4] (see Table 55.7). In older children, portal, interface, or lobular inflammation (or some combination of these) is typically present, but usually without cholestasis. Chief among the inherited disorders that manifest with a hepatitic pattern are A1AT deficiency and Wilson disease. A number of other inherited disorders with characteristic histological patterns of injury (e.g., NPD type C, Alagille syndrome with cholestasis) can also manifest with a superimposed hepatitic pattern on liver biopsies. These entities are discussed later in this chapter.

BOX 55.3 Diagnostic Algorithm for Storage Pattern

MEMBRANE-BOUND (LYSOSOMAL) INCLUSIONS BY ELECTRON MICROSCOPY

1. Hepatocyte microvesicular steatosis
   - Lipid stains positive → **Wolman disease/cholesterol-ester storage disease (CESD)** → EM: cholesterol crystals → confirm with enzyme activity and *LIPA* gene sequencing
2. Predominantly RES involvement with hepatocyte sparing
   - Histiocytes, Kupffer cells with "crinkled-paper" inclusions → **Gaucher disease** → EM: tubular structures → confirm with enzyme activity and *GBA* gene sequencing
   - Foamy histiocytes and lipogranulomas → **Farber disease** → EM: curvilinear structures → confirm with enzyme activity and *ASAH1* gene sequencing
3. Foamy histiocytes and hepatocytes
   - PAS negative → Lipid stains positive → **Niemann-Pick disease type A** → EM: myelin-like figures → confirm with enzyme activity and *SMPD1* gene sequencing
   - PAS positive → EM: monoparticulate glycogen (**Pompe disease [GSD type II]**); fibrillogranular material or empty vacuoles (**mucopolysaccharidoses** or **GM1 gangliosidosis**) → confirm with enzyme activity and gene sequencing
4. Cirrhosis
   - Wolman disease or Gaucher disease → as above

EXCLUSIVELY CYTOPLASMIC STORAGE BY ELECTRON MICROSCOPY

1. Hepatic adenomas
   - PAS positive, diastase sensitive → **von Gierke disease (GSD type I)** → confirm with enzyme activity on fresh liver tissue
2. Cirrhosis
   - PAS positive, diastase resistant → colloidal iron positive → EM: amylopectin-like fibrillary structures → **Andersen disease (GSD type IV)** → confirm with enzyme activity and *GBE1* gene sequencing
   - PAS positive, diastase sensitive → **GSD type III** → confirm with enzyme activity
   - PAS positive, diastase resistant → **α_1-antitrypsin**—EM: endoplasmic reticulum
   - Cytoplasmic eosinophilic globules → **Fibrinogen defect**—EM: endoplasmic reticulum
   - Fingerprint inclusions

EM, *Electron microscopy;* GSD, *glycogen storage disease;* PAS, *periodic acid–Schiff;* RES, *reticuloendothelial system.*

When investigating biopsy specimens with a hepatitic pattern for a suspected inherited disorder, it is crucial to rule out acquired causes of hepatitis (e.g., infection, toxin or drug exposure, TPN) that are far more common in this age group. It is also important to evaluate the clinical presentation and laboratory results. For example, A1AT deficiency liver disease can manifest either in the neonatal period with hepatitis or later in childhood with cirrhosis, but clinical manifestations of Wilson disease are rare before 5 years of age[34] (see Table 55.3). On biopsy, the presence of PAS-positive, diastase-resistant inclusions within zone 1 hepatocytes is characteristic of A1AT deficiency, but immunostaining is more sensitive and specific. Importantly, the neonate with A1AT-associated hepatitis may not exhibit hepatocyte inclusions on liver biopsy; serum A1AT phenotyping by isoelectric focusing (Pi typing) is the confirmatory assay for diagnosis of A1AT deficiency in cases of suspected neonatal hepatitis, and it is particularly valuable in cases that mimic EHBA (i.e., bile duct proliferation, no biliary excretion on scintigraphy).[35] Diagnosis of Wilson disease is less straightforward; screening for decreased serum ceruloplasmin levels (<20 mg/dL) can be problematic because both decreased (hypoceruloplasminemia or aceruloplasminemia) and elevated levels (acute-phase reaction) may be seen in other conditions (Box 55.4). A low serum alkaline phosphatase level may be a useful clue to the etiology, as well as increased unconjugated bilirubin, which reflects hemolysis in children with acute liver decompensation.

Cirrhotic Pattern

Cirrhosis, an end-stage response to chronic liver injury, is common to several different types of inherited disorders. Therefore the differential diagnosis of liver biopsies with a cirrhotic pattern rests largely on the presence or absence of other characteristic microscopic findings (Box 55.5). Metabolic disorders that lead to cirrhosis also carry an increased risk of neoplasia (Box 55.6). Advanced stages of congenital hepatic fibrosis (discussed earlier) may be confused with cirrhosis; however, bile duct ectasia is a characteristic feature of the former.[36] Although mitochondrial hepatopathies may lead to several different patterns of liver injury, it is most often steatosis. Less often, these disorders may manifest with hepatitis and cirrhosis.

Tyrosinemia, caused by a deficiency of fumarylacetoacetate hydrolase,[37] can lead to cirrhosis in early life (infancy), hepatic failure, hepatocellular necrosis, or giant cell hepatitis.

Hereditary hemochromatosis (HH) is caused by mutations in the hemochromatosis *(HFE)* gene[38] and leads to cirrhosis and hepatocellular carcinoma (HCC). Although the defect in iron metabolism is present at birth, the clinical manifestations of HH are rarely apparent before adulthood, when long-term effects of chronic iron overload typically manifest[39] (see later discussion).

Neoplastic Pattern

Several types of inherited disorders predispose the child to the development of focal nodular hyperplasia, hepatic adenoma, and HCC.[40] In contrast, hepatoblastoma, the most common malignancy in the liver of children, is infrequently associated with inherited metabolic disorders, although trisomy 18, neurofibromatosis, and congenital hepatic fibrosis have been linked to hepatoblastoma. The increased risk for HCC is chiefly caused by the development of cirrhosis, but HCC can arise in noncirrhotic patients with A1AT deficiency, hemochromatosis, or GSD type I.[2,41] The histological features and biological behavior of HCC and adenomas arising in patients with a metabolic disorder are similar to those of neoplasms that arise in cirrhosis resulting from other causes. Cirrhosis and neoplasms that arise in inherited

TABLE 55.12 Features of Important Glycogen Storage Disorders That Affect the Liver

Disorder	Inheritance	Gene	Protein	Storage Material	Liver Histology		Other Features	Ultrastructure	Diagnostic Testing
					Parenchyma	RES			
GSD Ia (von Gierke disease)	AR	*G6PC*	Glucose-6-phosphate, catalytic subunit	Glycogen	PAS+, diastase-sensitive cytoplasmic glycogen	–	Steatosis, adenomas, HCC	–	Fresh liver enzyme activity, genetic testing
GSD Ib	AR	*SLC37A4*	Glucose-6-phosphate transporter						
GSD II (Pompe disease)	AR	*GAA*	Acid α-glucosidase	Glycogen	PAS+ vacuoles	–	–	Membrane-bound monoparticulate glycogen	Fibroblast and/or muscle enzyme activity, genetic testing
GSD III	AR	*AGL*	Glycogen debranching enzyme	Glycogen	PAS+, diastase-sensitive cytoplasmic glycogen	–	Steatosis, cirrhosis, HCC	–	Fresh liver or muscle enzyme activity, genetic testing
GSD IV (Andersen disease)	AR	*GBE1*	Glycogen debranching enzyme	Glycogen	PAS+, diastase-sensitive cytoplasmic glycogen	Kupffer cell inclusions±	Cirrhosis, HCC	Amylopectin-like cytoplasmic glycogen	Fresh liver or fibroblast enzyme activity, genetic testing

AR, *Autosomal recessive;* GSD, *glycogen storage disorder;* HCC, *hepatocellular carcinoma;* PAS, *periodic acid–Schiff stain;* RES, *reticuloendothelial system.*

TABLE 55.13 Major Disorders of Lipid Metabolism That Affect the Liver

Disorder	Inheritance	Gene	Protein	Storage Material	Liver Histology		Other Features	Ultrastructure	Diagnostic Testing
					Parenchyma	RES			
Gaucher disease	AR	*GBA*	Acid β-glucosidase	Glycosylceramide	–	Gaucher cells (20-100 μm): eosinophilic corrugated "crinkled-paper" cytoplasm	Fibrosis, rarely cirrhosis	Spindled tubular structures	Enzymes activity (l, f) ± *GBA* mutations
Niemann-Pick disease types A and B	AR	*SMPD1*	Acid sphingomyelinase	Sphingomyelin	Vacuolated hepatocytes	Niemann-Pick cells (25-75 μm): foamy histiocytes, lipofuscin+	ORO+, LXB+, PAS–	Laminated myelin-like figures	Enzymes activity (l, f)
Niemann-Pick disease type C	AR	*NPC1* *NPC2*	NPC1, NPC2	Cholesterol	Cholestasis, giant cell transformation	Sea-blue histiocytes	Cirrhosis	Whorled aggregates	Filipin staining (f) + *NPC1, NPC2* mutations
Farber disease	AR	*ASAH1*	Acid ceramidase	Ceramide	–	Lipogranulomas, foamy histiocytes	Fibrosis	Curvilinear Farber bodies	Enzymes activity (l, f, p)
GM1 gangliosidosis	AR	*GLB1*	β-galactosidase 1	Glycosphingolipids	Vacuolated hepatocytes	Finely vacuolated		Fibrillogranular material	Enzymes activity (l, f, p)
Wolman disease CESD	AR	*LIPA*	Acid liposomal lipase	Cholesterol esters	Microvesicular droplets	Enlarged vacuolated, periportal foamy histiocytes	ORO+, cirrhosis, (Wolman disease)	Cholesterol crystal profiles	Enzymes activity (l, f) + *LIPA* mutations

AR, *Autosomal recessive;* CESD, *cholesteryl-ester storage disease;* f, *fibroblast enzyme activity;* l, *leukocyte enzyme activity;* LXB, *luxol-fast blue;* ORO, *oil red O;* p, *plasma enzyme activity;* PAS, *periodic acid–Schiff;* RES, *reticuloendothelial system.*

BOX 55.4 Diagnostic Algorithm for Hepatitic Pattern

1. Giant cell hepatitis
   - PAS-positive diastase-resistant hepatocyte inclusions → A1AT staining by immunohistochemistry → consider α_1-**Antitrypsin (A1AT) deficiency** → see Box 55.1
2. Cholestasis, steatosis
   - Consider mitochondrial hepatopathies → see Box 55.2
3. Increased hepatocyte stainable copper
   - Consider **Wilson disease** → EM: pleomorphic dilated mitochondria → confirm with hepatic copper content >250 µg/g dry weight; urinary copper excretion after penicillamine challenge >25 µmol/24 hour → DNA haplotype analysis and/or *ATP7B* gene sequencing in affected families

EM, *Electron microscopy;* PAS, *periodic acid–Schiff.*

BOX 55.5 Diagnostic Algorithm for Cirrhotic Pattern

STEATOSIS

1. Hepatocyte vacuolation and foamy Kupffer cells, macrophages
   - Lipid stains positive → consider **Wolman disease** → EM: cholesterol crystals → confirm with enzyme activity and *LIPA* gene sequencing
2. Increased hepatocyte stainable copper
   - Consider **Wilson disease** → see Box 55.4
3. Increased hepatocyte iron
   - Consider **hereditary hemochromatosis (HH)** → measure hepatic iron (hepatic iron index > 2) → confirm with *HFE* testing
4. Giant cell hepatitis
   - PAS-positive diastase-resistant hepatocyte inclusions → A1AT staining by immunohistochemistry → consider α_1-**Antitrypsin (A1AT) deficiency** → see Box 55.1
   - PAS negative → consider **tyrosinemia** → confirm with elevated blood/urine succinylacetone levels
   - Cholestasis, steatosis → consider mitochondrial hepatopathies → see Box 55.2

HEPATOCYTE AND/OR RES INCLUSIONS

1. Exclusively cytoplasmic inclusions on EM
   - PAS positive, diastase resistant, colloidal iron positive → EM: amylopectin-like fibrillary structures → **Andersen disease (GSD type IV)** → see Box 55.3 and Fig. 55.23
   - PAS positive, diastase sensitive → **GSD type III** → see Box 55.3
2. Membrane-bound (lysosomal) inclusions on EM
   - Histiocytes, Kupffer cells with "crinkled-paper" inclusions → **Gaucher disease** → see Box 55.3
   - PAS-positive inclusions → EM: fibrillogranular material or empty vacuoles **(mucopolysaccharidoses)** → see Box 55.3

CHOLESTASIS

1. Normal GGT cholestasis
   - Consider **progressive familial intrahepatic cholestasis type 2 (PFIC2) or PFIC1** (also consider PFIC4, PFIC5, and MYO5B disease) → see Box 55.1
2. High GGT cholestasis
   - Consider PFIC3, North American Indian childhood cirrhosis (NAIC), and Alagille syndrome → see Box 55.1
   - Giant cell hepatitis → PAS negative → consider **Niemann-Pick disease type C** → see Box 55.1

EM, *Electron microscopy;* GGT, *γ-glutamyltransferase;* PAS, *periodic acid–Schiff;* RES, *reticuloendothelial system.*

BOX 55.6 Diagnostic Algorithm for Metabolic Diseases Predisposing to Hepatocellular Neoplasms

HEPATIC ADENOMA

1. Consider glycogen storage disease (GSD) type I → see Box 55.3
2. Alagille syndrome

HEPATOCELLULAR CARCINOMA

1. Noncirrhotic
   - Storage pattern → consider **GSD type I** → see Box 55.3
   - Consider α_1-**Antitrypsin (A1AT) deficiency** → see Box 55.1
   - Increased hepatic iron → consider **hereditary hemochromatosis (HH)** → see Box 55.5
2. Cirrhotic liver with cholestasis
   - Consider progressive familial intrahepatic cholestasis (PFIC), especially types 2, 3, and 4; Wilson disease; Alagille syndrome; and A1AT deficiency → see Box 55.1
3. Cirrhotic liver without cholestasis
   - Consider **GSD type III** and **GSD type IV** → see Box 55.3
   - Consider **HH** → as above
   - Consider tyrosinemia

metabolic disorders are indicative of advanced disease (not necessarily advanced age), and the diagnostic features of the underlying disorder can usually be identified in nonneoplastic areas of the liver tissue (see Box 55.6).

Most patients with GSD type I have hepatic adenomas by 15 years of age, although adenomas may be present in early childhood. Dysplastic changes and HCC within individual adenomatous nodules have also been reported in this condition.[42,43]

Among all of the metabolic disorders of the liver, hereditary tyrosinemia (discussed later) carries the highest risk for development of HCC (13% to 15% incidence).[37,44] Typically, hepatocellular dysplasia and foci of HCC develop in a background of mixed micronodular and macronodular cirrhosis, but treatment should begin in infancy as soon as succinyl acetone is detected in the urine to abort the mutagenic process.[45] Not all infants manifest overt liver dysfunction with time.[37]

The incidence of HCC in patients with HH (discussed later) is approximately 10%. Most cases develop in a background of cirrhosis.[41] Because of the widespread availability of testing for the *HFE* gene mutations C282Y and H63D and sensitive transferrin-iron screening tests, a biopsy diagnosis is required only in cases with a negative genotype or high ferritin levels.

Other inherited disorders that are less commonly associated with HCC include A1AT deficiency, PFIC2, PFIC3, PFIC4 (TJP2 defect), Wilson disease, Alagille syndrome, and GSD types I, III, and IV. The characteristic biopsy features were described earlier. A1AT deficiency is a precursor to HCC.[46] In some cases, PiZ heterozygotes were found to have HCC (and cholangiocarcinoma) in noncirrhotic livers.[47] Fanconi anemia, familial adenomatous polyposis, and Beckwith-Weidemann syndrome are other syndromes that predispose to cancer. Three percent of patients with Fanconi anemia develop adenomas or HCC,[48] and hepatoblastoma has a well-known association with both familial adenomatous polyposis and Beckwith-Weidemann syndrome.[49-51] Finally, cholangiocarcinoma is a rare complication of Wilson disease and congenital hepatic fibrosis.[52,53] This tumor was

BOX 55.7 Most Common Inborn Errors of Metabolism Associated with Acute Life-Threatening Illness

Organic acidurias
Congenital lactic acidurias
- Pyruvate oxidation defects
- Gluconeogenesis defects
- Krebs cycle defects
- Respiratory chain defects

Mitochondrial fatty acid β-oxidation disorders
- Defects of membrane-bound enzymes
- Defects of matrix enzymes

Urea cycle defects
Amino acid disorders
- Maple syrup urine disease
- Nonketotic hyperglycinemia

Molybdenum cofactor deficiency

recently described in two children with PFIC2.[54] Cases of HCC in an MDR3 explant liver and association with a TJP2 defect have also been recently reported.[55,56]

LIVER DISEASES OF INFANCY

Acute Life-Threatening Illness and Sudden Death

Although sudden death within 2 to 3 days after birth is usually caused by nonmetabolic conditions such as sepsis or congenital heart disease,[57] some inborn errors of metabolism are also associated with acute life-threatening illness (Box 55.7). As mentioned earlier, decision making on behalf of a desperately ill neonate may be critically informed by rapid whole-exome sequencing,[22] including the decision to provide comfort measures only.

FAO defects lead to cardiac arrhythmias and can cause sudden death (see Mitochondrial Cytopathies).[58] At autopsy, excess droplets of fat may be present in the liver and heart of patients with an FAO defect. If an FAO disorder is suspected, tissue specimens should be obtained as soon as possible after death, before autopsy, for metabolic testing[59,60] (Table 55.14). Both liver and muscle tissue should be obtained for analysis. In addition, urine and cerebrospinal fluid should be snap-frozen and stored for further analysis. Blood spots should be obtained for analysis of acylcarnitines. Whole-blood specimens should be placed in an ethylenediaminetetraacetic acid (EDTA) tube for DNA extraction and in a lithium heparin tube (spun and separated within 20 minutes of collection) for metabolite analysis. A full-thickness skin biopsy should be performed under sterile conditions within 12 hours of death for fibroblast culture and archiving.

Sudden and unexplained death in an infant or young child is often the first manifestation of medium chain acyl-coenzyme A dehydrogenase (MCAD) deficiency, the most common FAO disorder.[61] MCAD deficiency manifests with hepatomegaly and steatosis and may be confused with Reye syndrome. A particular Lys304Glu mutation in the *ACADM* gene is highly prevalent in some populations. Since the institution of newborn screening, early diagnosis has led to prospective management of acute episodes of hypoketotic hypoglycemia.

TABLE 55.14 Investigation of Acute Life-Threatening Disease and Sudden Death

Collect	Blood, urine, CSF, vitreous humor (dodecanoic acid = MCAD deficiency) Bile (carnitine and acylcarnitines = FAO disorders)
Freeze	Liver, skeletal, cardiac muscle
Sample for cell culture	Skin fibroblasts (DNA and enzyme analyses)

CSF, *Cerebrospinal fluid;* FAO, *fatty acid oxidation;* MCAD, *medium chain acyl-coenzyme A dehydrogenase.*

Neonatal Hemochromatosis

Clinical Features

Neonatal hemochromatosis (NH), also termed *neonatal iron storage disease,* is a rare syndrome that is characterized by the presence of congenital cirrhosis and fulminant liver failure. This condition exhibits abundant iron deposition in the liver and in other organs, but not in the reticuloendothelial system (spleen or bone marrow).[7] Clinically, patients with NH, either before birth or shortly thereafter, exhibit liver failure, including hypoglycemia, coagulopathy, hypoalbuminemia, ascites, and hyperbilirubinemia. Although some infants recover with exchange transfusion and some survive to transplantation, most die of their disease. Most cases of NH belong to the group of gestational alloimmune liver disease (GALD).[62]

Pathogenesis

NH has been described in association with various conditions, including metabolic disorders (tyrosinemia, Δ4-3-oxosteroid 5β-reductase deficiency, mtDNA mutations, and Zellweger syndrome); infections (echovirus 9, cytomegalovirus [CMV], herpes simplex virus, rubella, and parvovirus B19); and karyotypic disorders (Down syndrome).[63,64] As a result, some authors regard NH as a final common phenotype of any gestational insult that culminates in abnormal iron metabolism.[65,66] At least three patterns of disease transmission have been described: transmission of maternal alloantibodies, autosomal recessive inheritance, and matrilineal inheritance.[67] In the last instance, several reports have documented women with more than one affected child, but the children were fathered by different men. Although gonadal mosaicism in these mothers has not formally been excluded, the possibility of mitochondrial inheritance also has not been excluded. NH is not associated with mutations in the *HFE* gene, which is involved in most cases of HH (see later discussion).

In 2004, Whitington and Hibbard first reported giving high-dose intravenous γ-globulin to pregnant women with a history of a previously affected infant, and this treatment prevented recurrence in a small series.[68] Their findings have since been confirmed in many centers, and it is now imperative to determine the etiology of all perinatal forms of acute liver injury.[69] Mimicry of hemochromatosis has been seen in cases of mtDNA depletion[63] and other circumstances, which presumably do not benefit from intravenous immunoglobulin therapy.

The antibody responsible for NH has yet to be determined. Complement fixation induced by immunoglobulin G of maternal origin is detected by immunofluorescence for the membrane attack complex on hepatocytes. One patient with cirrhosis at birth did not have hemosiderosis and survived without specific therapy.[70] However, the usual scenario is fatal necrosis with extensive parenchymal siderosis without reticuloendothelial iron, suggesting dysfunction of macrophages. This has been observed even prenatally: Three of eight stillborn or very premature infants had no extrahepatic siderosis.[71,72] Recently, Whitington and colleagues have provided insight into the severe degree of parenchymal siderosis that accompanies the hepatocellular injury.[72] The injured livers have significantly reduced hepcidin, hemojuvelin, and transferrin gene expression compared with normal livers.

Antibodies to mitochondrial proteins are responsible for primary biliary cirrhosis, a disease that affects women disproportionately. Two patients transmitted this disease transplacentally to their infants, producing transient liver injury. One infant was born with ascites and conjugated hyperbilirubinemia. In the other infant, the presentation was more insidious. His biopsy, at 5 weeks, showed portal inflammation involving bile ducts and ductules, mild portal fibrosis, and multinucleated giant hepatocytes typical of neonatal hepatitis. Immunofluorescence was able to detect immunoglobulin G deposits surrounding hepatocytes. Within 3 months, both infants showed no evidence of liver dysfunction, and the antibodies were undetectable.[73]

NH resembles neonatal hepatitis in infants with systemic lupus erythematosus, in which the mother has high titers of antinuclear anti Ro (SSA) and anti La antibodies.[74]

Pathological Features

The liver in patients with NH (usually seen at postmortem examination) reveals cirrhosis and cholestasis (Fig. 55.2). Confluent areas of hepatocellular loss and a variable degree of hepatocyte regeneration are typical. Residual hepatocytes may demonstrate giant cell or pseudoacinar transformation. Iron deposition is typically coarsely granular and located predominantly within hepatocytes, sparing Kupffer cells. Extrahepatic sites of siderosis include the parenchymal cells of the heart, thyroid, pancreas, adrenal glands, kidneys, and the submucosal glands of the gastrointestinal and upper respiratory tracts. It has now been shown that examples of GALD exist without evidence of hepatic siderosis. While the diagnosis of this entity has been a challenge, the recognition of the deposition of the C5b-9 complex by immunohistochemistry on necrotic hepatocytes in 2010 has led to an increase in recognition of this entity.[75] Dubruc et al. showed 100% expression in GALD though only 26% of their cases showed staining in more than 75% of hepatocytes.[76] This has improved the outcome of future pregnancies because of the ability to administer IV-IG in the prenatal period of subsequent pregnancies.[77] Having said this, there are issues with this staining technique because recent literature suggests overlap of staining in necrotic livers as a result of viral or other etiology, as well as suspected cases of GALD with negative C5b-9 staining.[78] It is therefore important to exclude other causes, especially viral causes, of neonatal acute liver failure.

Natural History

NH carries a high risk of death, and a high index of suspicion is required to diagnose this disorder at first presentation, as this has impact on management of subsequent pregnancies for the mother.[79] NH remains in the differential diagnosis of severely ill neonates who survive beyond the first days of life. Demonstration of siderosis in biopsy samples from oral submucosal glands is a rapid diagnostic method. T2-weighted magnetic resonance imaging (MRI) can be used to assess the presence of iron in various tissues. Siderosis of the liver and extrahepatic organs may also accompany other conditions, such as erythropoietic disorders, sickle cell disease, thalassemia, and erythroblastosis from blood group incompatibility. However, hemosiderosis affects the reticuloendothelial system primarily. These other diseases need to be excluded by other clinical and laboratory studies.

Neonatal Jaundice

Heritable disorders of bilirubin conjugation can rarely produce liver dysfunction (see later discussion). Liver diseases of infancy most often manifest with jaundice owing to conjugated hyperbilirubinemia. This occurs because of the relative immaturity of hepatic secretory and excretory functions in early life. Some of the disorders that cause neonatal jaundice are listed in Table 55.2. In all cases of neonatal jaundice, the possibility of biliary atresia or hepatic damage caused by drug exposure (including inadvertent drug overdose) should be excluded. Infants requiring TPN are at risk for cholestatic liver disease (see Chapter 49). Infectious causes of liver disease in infancy include enterovirus, parvovirus B19, and adenovirus, which cause direct cytopathic cell death, as well as bacterial sepsis, urinary tract infection, and intrauterine exposure to maternal infections (of the "TORCH" acronym), all of which cause liver damage to neonates and infants (see Chapter 47). Acquired syphilis is an exceedingly uncommon cause of perinatal liver disease.

Inherited metabolic disorders of carbohydrate, amino acid, and lipid and glycolipid metabolism, along with disorders of the biosynthetic and secretory pathways for bile acids, should always be considered in the differential diagnosis of neonatal jaundice (see Table 55.7). Storage of abnormal A1AT and abnormal function of the CFTR compromise hepatic formation of bile. Defects in the transporters responsible for bile formation give rise to progressive familial intrahepatic cholestasis. Inherited defects of peroxisomal and mitochondrial function can cause neonatal jaundice. Shock may cause cholestatic liver damage in neonates. Alagille syndrome may manifest in early infancy as "giant cell hepatitis"; it can mimic biliary atresia[80] and may lead to Kasai portoenterostomy (KPE). The nonspecific designation of "neonatal hepatitis/giant cell hepatitis" applies to the 25% of patients in which a specific etiology for neonatal jaundice remains undetermined.

Biliary Atresia

Biliary atresia manifests as a fibrosing destruction of extrahepatic and intrahepatic bile ducts of unknown etiology, presenting usually in the initial weeks after birth. Biliary

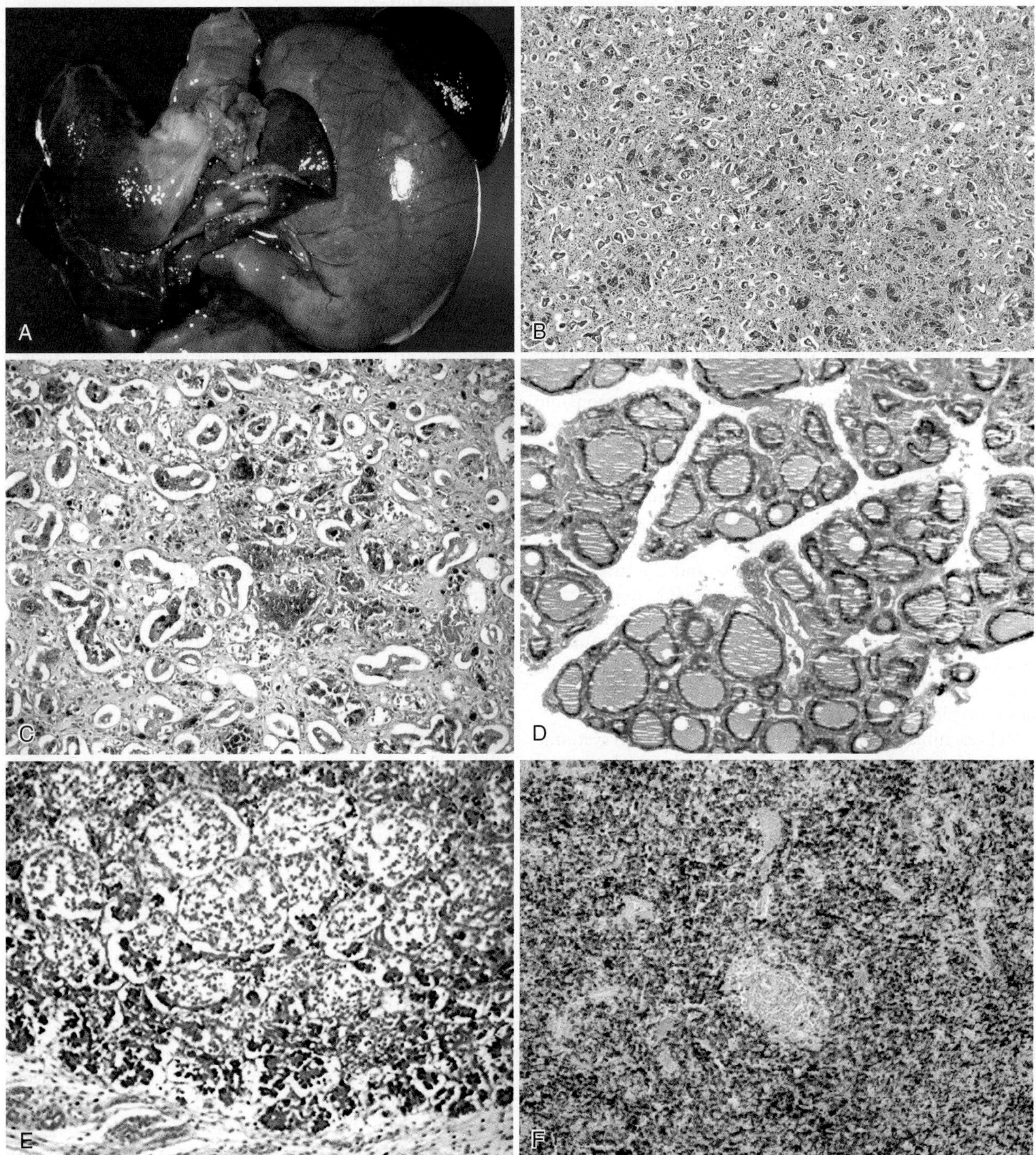

FIGURE 55.2 Perinatal hemochromatosis. A, Abdominal viscera at autopsy of a 19-day-old infant. The liver is small, and the spleen is enlarged. **B,** Advanced hepatocellular necrosis with collapse and ductular proliferation (H&E stain). **C,** Perls iron stain reveals four or more instances of hemosiderosis of hepatocytes, in the midst of the surrounding ductular proliferation. **D,** The thyroid follicular epithelium contains abundant hemosiderin. **E,** Pancreatic acini contain abundant hemosiderin. No hemosiderin was found in the reticuloendothelial cells of spleen **(F)**, lymph nodes, or bone marrow.

atresia has long been classified as extrahepatic on the basis of involvement of that portion of the biliary tree. However, this concept is imprecise because the anatomy of abnormal bile ducts in affected patients varies markedly. A recommended terminology is *obliterative cholangiopathy,* with two major types: noncystic and cystic.[81] The cystic disorders include different types of choledochal cysts (described later in this chapter) and *cystic biliary atresia.* The noncystic forms include the different variants and presentations of *noncystic biliary atresia* (the predominant form of biliary atresia) and neonatal sclerosing cholangitis.

The widespread use of screening fetal ultrasound performed during pregnancy has resulted in increased detection of cystic lesions in the hilum of the fetal liver, with the differential diagnosis of cystic biliary atresia versus choledochal cyst.[82] As many as 10% of infants ultimately diagnosed with biliary atresia have prior fetal ultrasound indicating this cystic form of biliary atresia. The postnatal pathology of the extrahepatic biliary tract in these cases is not notably different than in other patients with EHBA.[83,84] The proximal biliary remnants of these patients with cystic biliary atresia exhibit cysts which lack epithelium and inflammation and exhibit myofibroblastic hyperplasia interposed with atretic segments of the biliary tree, especially caudad to the cyst. This is in contrast with choledochal cysts, which have preserved uninjured epithelium and no subepithelial cicatrix.[85] That being said, the frequency of biliary atresia in infants with choledochal cysts is 13% to 44%; choledochal cyst (with preserved epithelium) is found in 8% to 11% of infants with biliary atresia, suggesting a shared pathogenesis[86] with a proposed continuum between the two entities.[87] Moreover, prenatal nonvisualization of the fetal gallbladder during the second trimester in neonates subsequently diagnosed with biliary atresia provides further support for the premise that some cases of biliary atresia are of fetal rather than perinatal onset.[88] Indeed, in an infant suspected of having biliary atresia, preoperative ultrasound demonstrating a cyst >5 mm in the hilum with no patent gallbladder is associated with favorable postoperative outcomes following portoenterostomy.[89] Persistent nonvisualization of the fetal gallbladder on second-trimester ultrasound requires consideration of other conditions as well, including CF, Alagille syndrome, and chromosomal anomalies.[90,91]

Clinical Features

Biliary atresia accounts for more than 30% of all cases of cholestasis in neonates. This disorder has an incidence of 1 in 5000 to 19,000 live births, occurring more frequently in Asian countries such as Taiwan and Japan when compared with North America and Europe.[92] Most cases are sporadic and do not reveal a positive family history of neonatal cholestasis. A series of 30 sets of twins revealed only 2 sets with both infants affected by EHBA, and both pairs were dizygotic.[93] There are reports of a 20-year-old mother who underwent a portoenterostomy for EHBA at 64 days of age and subsequently gave birth to a daughter with EHBA[94] and of a family cluster of 5 children in which 2 dizygotic twin sisters and a third sibling all had EHBA.[95] Variation in epigenetic modifications of genomic DNA has been suggested for these occasional familial presentations.[96] Genes related to bile duct dysmorphogenesis (including ciliopathies) overlapping with features of biliary atresia in both humans and nonhuman model systems have been proposed, sparking continued interest in identifying potential causative and modifying genes relevant to patients with biliary atresia.[97]

Infants presenting with biliary atresia are usually of normal gestational age and birth weight. Cholestatic jaundice is the main clinical presentation. It typically develops in the first few weeks of life and does not remit, unlike the mild physiological jaundice of early infancy. Furthermore, in physiological jaundice, the mildly elevated serum bilirubin is primarily unconjugated, and the serum levels of alanine aminotransferase (ALT) and aspartate aminotransferase (AST) are normal. The progressive biliary obstruction that characterizes biliary atresia leads to a progressive increase in serum bilirubin levels in which conjugated bilirubin represents 50% to 80% of the total. A recent study of conjugated or direct-reacting bilirubin in the first 48 hours of life revealed significant elevations in all infants with biliary atresia compared with aged-matched controls, even though the total bilirubin level was not increased.[98] Serum levels of GGT are increased several times above normal. Liver biosynthetic function, as indicated by serum albumin levels and prothrombin time, is usually normal at initial presentation.

In keeping with the aforementioned discussion, ultrasound should be performed in suspected cases of biliary atresia to exclude the presence of an extrahepatic biliary tract anomaly, such as a choledochal cyst. Hepatobiliary scintigraphy is also useful to assess the status of biliary tract function, but in many hepatocellular diseases of infants, there also is an absence of excretion of the labeled molecule into the intestine. Ultrasound shear wave elastography has also been shown to be discriminatory for biliary atresia.[99]

Percutaneous liver biopsy is used to determine whether there is histological evidence of large bile duct obstruction. Biopsy features of atresia may also occur with other extrahepatic forms of biliary obstruction (Box 55.8). The overall accuracy rate of percutaneous liver biopsy for diagnosis of biliary atresia has recently been shown to be around 90.1%, with a sensitivity of 88.4% and a specificity of 92.7%.[100] The decision to proceed with a biliary tract exploratory surgical procedure does not rest solely on the pathological findings in a liver biopsy specimen. The presence of acholic stools, an undetectable or irregular contour of the gallbladder on sonographic studies, and failure to excrete into the intestine the radioactive tracer iminodiacetic acid by hepatobiliary scintography (HIDA scan) are findings that lend support to a diagnosis of biliary atresia,[101] but may not be sufficiently discriminating.[102] Magnetic resonance cholangiopancreatography (MRCP) is not optimal for visualization of the extrahepatic biliary tract in children younger than 3 months of age.[103] Intraoperative cholangiography, whether laparoscopic or during open laparotomy, is a confirmatory procedure before actual performance of KPE portoenterostomy.[104]

BOX 55.8 Biliary Tract Obstruction

EXTRAHEPATIC BILIARY OBSTRUCTION WITHOUT ATRESIA—RARE EVENTS IN INFANCY

Choledochal cyst
Spontaneous perforation of bile duct
Bile plug syndrome
Segmental cystic dilation of biliary ducts
Duodenal atresia (more common in Down syndrome)
Peptic ulceration secondary to duplication of intestine
Compression by enlarged lymph node
Hemangioendothelioma and other neoplasms of head of pancreas

EXTRAHEPATIC OBSTRUCTION—LIVER HISTOLOGY

Portal tract and periportal fibrosis
Bile duct and ductular proliferation
Bile duct "thrombi" or plugs
±Giant cell transformation
±Portal inflammation, mixed
±Persistent extramedullary hematopoiesis
Beware of α_1-antitrypsin, timing of biopsy

TABLE 55.15 Biliary Atresia: Pathogenesis

Proposed Mechanisms	Syndromic vs. Nonsyndromic	Associated Malformations
Genetic or epigenetic susceptibility, involving abnormal development of maturing biliary tract[94,108,122-124,145-147] Defect in fetal circulation[120] Occult viral infection[94,108,109] Rubella Cytomegalovirus Retrovirus Reovirus type 3 Rotavirus Toxin exposure *in utero* Disorder of immunologic-inflammatory system (including maternal chimerism)[94,116-118]	15% are syndromic, having associated malformations[94,115,131,139] 85% are nonsyndromic with no malformations	Polysplenia or asplenia Intestinal malrotation or atresia, anomalies of the portal vein and hepatic artery, abdominal situs inversus Congenital cardiovascular disease including absence of the vena cava Genitourinary anomalies

Pathogenesis

Biliary atresia is not a single disease with a defined etiology.[105] An all-encompassing hypothesis is that a genetically susceptible individual undergoes inflammatory destruction of the extrahepatic biliary system in response to as yet undetermined environmental factors. Potential pathogenetic mechanisms include a genetic defect in morphogenesis with or without defective prenatal hepatic circulation, environmental triggers such as intrauterine or perinatal viral infection or toxin exposure, and immunological dysregulation in the perinatal period (Table 55.15).[105] These hypotheses have been put forth on the basis of epidemiological studies and molecular analyses of tissue specimens from human patients. Mouse models of biliary atresia have provided some additional clues.[106-108]

Morphogenesis and Genetics

Systemic dysregulation of morphogenesis in patients with biliary atresia is well-documented,[109] such as the coexistence of nonhepatic embryological abnormalities, evidence for abnormal development of the ductal plate of the maturing intrahepatic biliary tract, and overexpression of certain regulatory genes in children who have an early form of biliary atresia.[110,111] Developmental abnormalities with which biliary atresia is associated include polysplenia or asplenia (biliary atresia splenic malformation syndrome); cardiovascular defects including absence of the inferior vena cava, abdominal situs inversus, intestinal malrotation, or atresias (duodenal atresia, esophageal atresia with tracheoesophageal fistula); and anomalies of the portal vein and hepatic artery (see Table 55.15).[112,113] In a large multi-institutional North American study, biliary atresia occurred in a syndromic fashion with laterality defects and spleen anomalies in ~10% of cases, with at least one malformation but without laterality defects in ~5%, and as nonsyndromic biliary atresia in the remaining ~85% of cases .[114]

Mutations in *CFC1* and *ZIC3* lead to laterality defects and biliary atresia in some patients. The *Inv* mouse that develops situs inversus also develops biliary obstruction. The *JAG1* gene has also been implicated in the pathogenesis of biliary atresia because affected patients with a poor outcome also show a high frequency of *JAG1* single-nucleotide polymorphisms.[115] The persistent expression of HES1 protein in the nuclei of biliary epithelial cells specimens of biliary atresia obtained up to 3 months after birth offers more evidence for disorderly Notch signaling in this disease. In normal development, such expression is silenced by 16 weeks of gestation.[116] Genome-wide association studies in Chinese children have identified variants of the *ADD3* gene, and its knockdown in zebrafish has shown biliary abnormalities.[117,118] *ADD3* is expressed in hepatocytes and biliary epithelia and is involved in the assembly of spectri-actin membrane protein networks at sites of cell-to-cell contact. Defective *ADD3* could lead to excessive deposition of actin and myosin, leading to biliary fibrosis.[105] Biliary atresia also has been reported in a premature neonate with 1p36 deletion syndrome; a chromosome with no prior reports of genes linked to biliary atresia but with associated gastrointestinal abnormalities including intestinal malrotation and anomalies in pancreatobiliary anatomy.[119]

The ciliopathies responsible for polycystic disease and congenital hepatic fibrosis (discussed later) may have a new and potentially meaningful relationship to biliary atresia. Other ciliary dysfunction contributes to laterality defects in embryonic development, including syndromic biliary atresia. Hartley and colleagues[120] used immunohistochemistry and found that expression of fibrocystin was missing in the biliary epithelium of the biliary atresia patients, suggesting a role for *PKHD1* or genes involved in primary ciliogenesis in this disease. More recently, a variant in the primary cilia protein PKD1L1 has been reported.[121] Chu and associates[122] initially and Karjoo et al.[123] showed that the cilia in biliary epithelium of five affected children were fewer, shorter, and abnormally oriented. Two other patients with biliary atresia who had no other malformations displayed alterations similar to those in epithelium of patients with other cholestatic diseases. Therefore the defects may be secondary and nonspecific. Hence tantalizing evidence continues to accumulate regarding genetic and epigenetic influences on the development of biliary atresia.

Environmental Triggers

The concept of a hepatotropic virus capable of causing cholangiolar and structural damage as a common factor causing "infantile obstructive cholangiopathy" was introduced in the 1970s.[124] Identification in 1992 of higher titers of antibodies against reovirus type 3 in jaundiced infants with biliary atresia compared with those without biliary atresia[125] and in 1998 of reovirus RNA in liver and/or biliary tissues of infants with biliary atresia and choledochal cysts[126] sparked further interest in a potential infectious etiology. No evidence for reovirus as an associated agent has been found in subsequent studies.[127,128] However, rhesus reovirus inoculated intraperitoneally within 12 hours of birth in the mouse is now an established experimental model of a biliary atresia-like condition.[129] Other viral agents (CMV, rotavirus) also are able to cause inflammatory destruction of bile ducts when introduced into neonatal mice.[130] The weakness of the viral hypothesis is that viral genomic material can be found in a substantial minority of infants diagnosed with biliary atresia, without clear evidence that such transient infections can incite the powerful inflammatory response characteristic of this disorder.[92]

An outbreak of ovine biliary atresia in New South Wales, Australia, in 1964 born to dams that had grazed on weeds of the genus *dysphania glomulifera* (red crumweed or pigweed) raised the possibility that *in utero* fetal exposure to an environmental toxin might cause biliary atresia.[131] Recently, four potentially toxic isoflavonoids isolated from extracts of *dysphania spp.* have been tested in a zebrafish system model of early bile duct development. One, now named *biliatresone,* caused fish biliary maldevelopment.[132] Work with a neonatal mouse model shows that this effect is not species specific, raising the possibility that even human biliary atresia could arise as a result of maternal exposure to this or other toxins.[133]

Inflammation

The most striking feature of biliary atresia is the inflammatory and fibrotic destruction of bile ducts, definitional for an obliterative cholangiopathy. Hypotheses about exposure of neoantigens on the biliary epithelium as a result of exposure to cholangiopathic toxins or viruses have abounded.[133] The occurrence of biliary atresia in the child with progressive familial intrahepatic cholestasis 3 (PFIC 3) in which bile salts are secreted into bile without accompanying secretion of phosphatidylcholine and cholesterol[134] suggest that biliary atresia may be an extreme outcome of exposure of the biliary tree to toxic biophysical properties of an abnormal bile.

Abnormal expression of intercellular adhesion molecular 1 (ICAM-1), vascular cell adhesion molecular 1 (VCAM-1), E-selectin, and P-selectin on endothelial cells and biliary epithelium in livers of infants with biliary atresia[135,136] indicate triggering of a strong inflammatory reaction in biliary atresia. Prevention of experimental inflammatory destruction of bile ducts occurs in mice that are deficient in interferon-γ.[109] Studies of human liver specimens at different phases of disease progression point to the presence of a proinflammatory commitment of lymphocytes with a predominant type 1 helper T cell (Th1) phenotype. Molecular profiling of liver tissue from children with biliary atresia has revealed a unique proinflammatory footprint related to activation of lymphocytes, particularly natural killer cells.[96] Further work has shown that the T-cell infiltrate is oligoclonal in nature, suggestive of a specific provocation.[137] CD8+ T cells are the predominant cell line in the infiltrate, with the suggestion from murine studies that there is a limited time window for an imbalance between cytotoxic T cells and an absence of regulatory T cells (T-regs, which suppress and inhibit natural killer cell expansion) to render the liver susceptible to biliary tract damage.[92] In the mouse model of reovirus-induced biliary atresia, prevention of proliferation of T lymphocytes and the activation of NK cells through depletion of dendritic cells prevented the development of biliary atresia.[138] Collectively, these findings support the premise that triggering of the cellular immune response is critical for development of biliary atresia.

Biliary atresia may thus represent a final common pathway of perinatal inflammatory destruction of the extrahepatic and potentially intrahepatic biliary tree. Indeed, neonatal systemic lupus can mimic biliary atresia.[139,140] It is not surprising that analysis of the initial biopsies of 47 infants with biliary atresia showed overexpression of genes associated with inflammation or fibrosis or both.[141] The patients with a fibrosis signature were older and had decreased duration of transplant-free survival following KPE. When serum samples collected at the same time from 19 infants with biliary atresia and 19 with other forms of neonatal cholestasis were subjected to gel electrophoresis and tandem mass spectrometry, a combination of 11 proteins was able to discriminate between the two groups.[142,143] Among them were apolipoproteins CII and E, whose genes on chromosome 19 are regulated by farnesoid X receptor, which in turn is responsive to bile acids. Proinflammatory "positive" acute phase reactants, such as complement C3, were upregulated, and there was a relatively reduced level of "negative" acute-phase proteins such as prealbumin. The humoral response also may be activated, based on evidence from the murine model of biliary atresia for increased levels of antibodies to alpha-enolase, an enzyme ubiquitously expressed on a variety of cells, including biliary epithelial cells and hepatocytes.[144]

Prompted by the similarities between biliary duct inflammation and graft-versus-host disease (GVHD), in 1992 Suskind and colleagues were first to describe maternal "microchimerism" in the livers of infants with biliary atresia.[145] Human leukocyte antigen (HLA) class I matching was significantly more prevalent in 57 maternal-child pairs with biliary atresia than in 50 control pairs (odds ratio, 2.46), possibly providing for greater survival of the chimeric lymphocytes.[146] This has led to the hypothesis that a "first hit" for biliary atresia is a GVHD-like interaction of maternal effector chimeric T lymphocytes engrafted within the fetus, with target fetal tissues.[147] This hypothesis has been challenged by the absence of maternal microchimerism in regional lymph nodes of children with nonsyndromic biliary atresia.[148] Regardless, the concept of some form of autoimmunity being active in biliary atresia remains of interest, supported by the occurrence of autoimmune disorders in 44% of family members of patients with biliary atresia.[114]

Pathological Features

A diagnosis of biliary atresia is favored if a liver biopsy specimen exhibits bile ductular proliferation (neocholangioles), portal edema, and fibrosis but lacks sinusoidal fibrosis.[100] Neutrophilic cholangitis and pericholangitis may or may not be present. The presence of bile plugs within bile duct lumina (which are distinct from the lumina of neocholangioles at the margins of portal tracts), portal edema, and increased numbers of bile duct profiles are helpful diagnostic findings with the largest odds ratio for predicting biliary

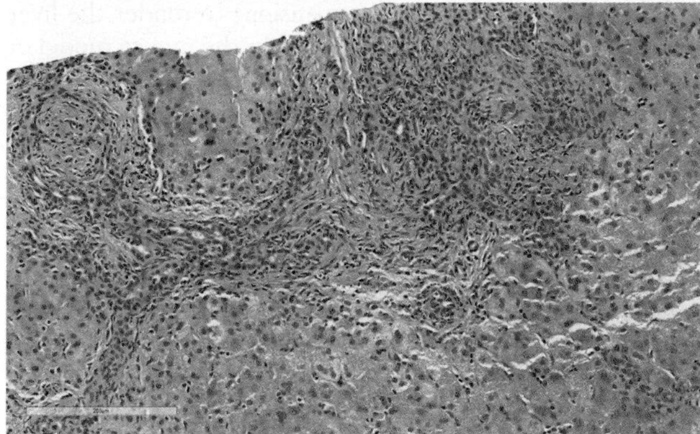

FIGURE 55.3 The portal region in an advanced case of extrahepatic biliary atresia demonstrates extensive ductular reaction with inflammation as well as severe cholestasis in the periportal parenchyma.

atresia versus nonbiliary atresia[100] (Fig. 55.3). In fact, the extent of ductular reaction in wedge liver biopsies of children with biliary atresia, obtained at the time of portoenterostomy, is positively associated with improved 1-year survival of the native liver following KPE.[149] Fifteen percent of biliary atresia cases show giant cell transformation of hepatocytes (Fig. 55.4). The progressive fibrosis observed in biliary atresia may be abetted in part by epithelial-mesenchymal transition.[150,151]

The classic "obstructive" findings of bile duct proliferation and inspissated bile plugs are not always the result of atresia (see Box 55.8). Conversely, some cases of biliary atresia may show nonclassic features such as prominent portal tract arteries with medial hypertrophy, associated with disappearance of interlobular bile ducts and an absence of bile duct proliferation (Fig. 55.5A,B).[152,153] In keeping with the developmental theory of biliary atresia, a subset of affected patients exhibit ductal plate malformation (see Fig. 55.5C). Recapitulating immature fetal portal tracts, this latter entity consists of portal tracts without an interlobular bile duct but with a centrally located hypertrophic hepatic artery and a peripheral rim of bile ductular structures. However, this phenomenon is not limited to the 20% to 25% of patients with a laterality defect (biliary atresia splenic malformation). As a result, biliary atresia can be difficult to diagnose at the time of percutaneous liver biopsy, even for the most experienced pediatric hepatopathologist (see Fig. 55.5D). The age of the child at biopsy does not help resolve this difficulty.[100] Nevertheless, the pathologist must advise the clinical team whether the histology of the liver biopsy justifies the patient being subjected to surgical intervention, with or without the performance of confirmatory intraoperative cholecystographic imaging before performance of the KPE. The alternative is that the pathologist advises the clinical team that the differential diagnosis of nonsurgical cholestatic disorders is of sufficient concern as to justify further noninvasive studies, rather than moving quickly to surgical intervention.

On performance of a KPE, the bile duct remnant is submitted for pathological examination.[154] Typical findings in the remnant include fibrosis and obstruction of the lumen, a variable degree of periductal inflammation, and apoptotic degeneration of residual bile duct epithelium (Fig. 55.6). These findings do not differ in syndromic cases of biliary atresia, cases discovered by prenatal ultrasound, and nonsyndromic postnatal biliary atresia, supporting the concept of a shared pathogenetic pathway.[109,155]

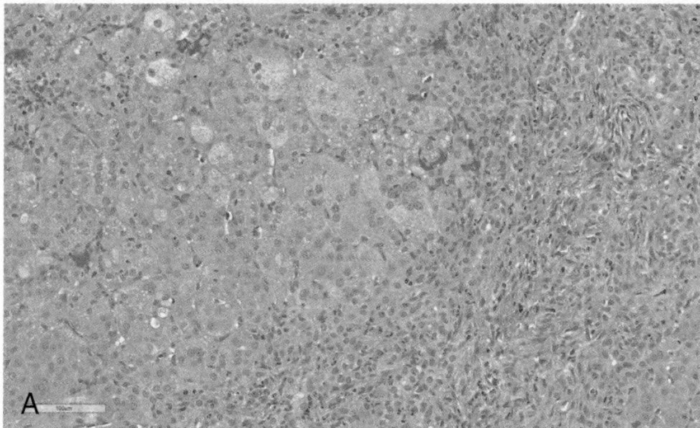

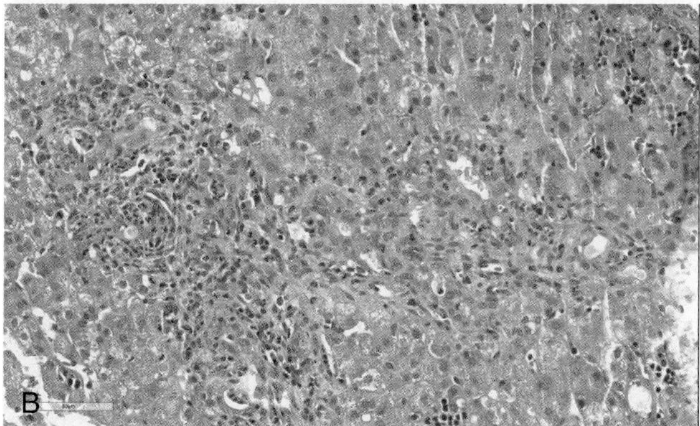

FIGURE 55.4 Lobular changes of "neonatal hepatitis" in extrahepatic biliary atresia. A, Marked lobular disarray with giant cell transformation and marked ductular proliferation with inflammation and edema. **B,** Portal tract in the same patient showing prominent bile plugs within ducts, inflammation, and proliferated ductules.

Natural History and Treatment

Before 1959, when the KPE procedure was introduced, biliary atresia was considered to be uniformly fatal by 2 years of age, with a median age at death of 10 months. The best survival rate in KPE patients with a native liver is 53% at 10 years, although reported native liver survival rates at 10 years are more commonly in the 35% range.[156,157] In the first report of the U.S. Biliary Atresia Research Consortium in 2006, a decline in total bilirubin at 3 months after KPE to less than 2 mg/dL was seen in 36.5% of children, and a favorable response (to <6 mg/dL) was seen in another 29%. Most patients in the excellent bilirubin response group had more favorable outcomes (as measured by "native liver survival"), a finding confirmed in more recent reports.[158,159] The 25% of children with a laterality defect fared more poorly, even if treated earlier.[160,161] Atresia of the common hepatic duct or ducts at the liver hilum (Ohi types 2 and 3)[162] had a poorer prognosis than an atretic common bile duct (Ohi type 1), similar to the prognosis in biliary atresia patients with other malformations, ascites at surgery, or delay in surgery beyond day 75.[161] Children operated on within the first 30 days had a 2-year 74% native liver survival rate.[163] At King's College Hospital in London, 56% of infants with EHBA cleared jaundice, and the 2-year survival rate in patients with their native liver was 65%. The 51

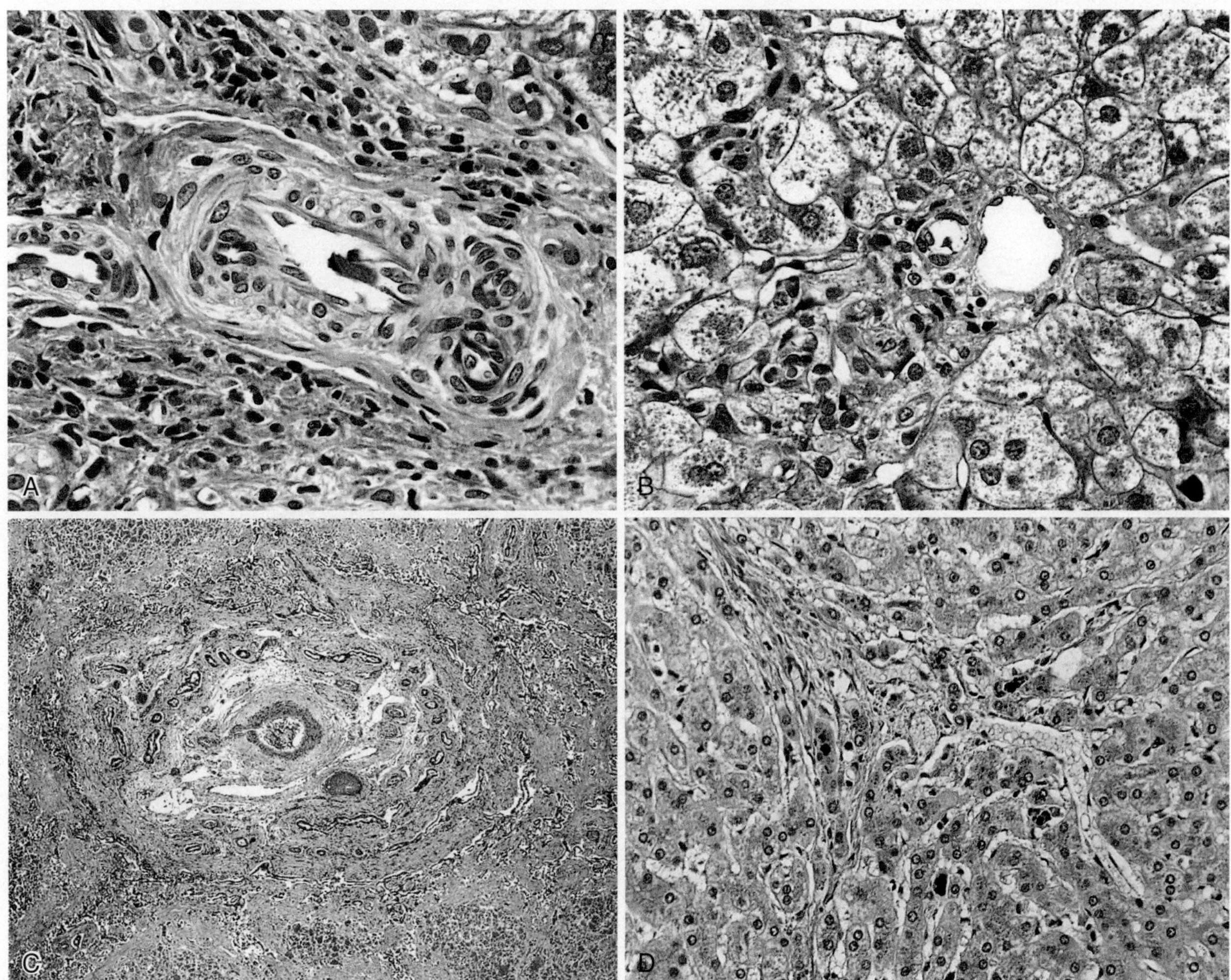

FIGURE 55.5 Nonclassic features of portal tracts in extrahepatic biliary atresia. A, Arterial medial hypertrophy without an accompanying interlobular bile duct. **B,** Portal tract without an interlobular bile duct but otherwise unremarkable. **C,** Ductal plate malformation with fibrosed portal tract, centrally located hepatic arteries, and a peripheral rim of ductular structures. **D,** Lack of bile plugs and lack of proliferating bile ducts. This was a second biopsy specimen, which was obtained from an 8-week-old infant because findings on initial biopsy (at 6½ weeks of age) did not suggest the disease; exploratory laparotomy and intraoperative cholangiography were required for a definitive diagnosis.

patients with biliary atresia splenic malformation or biliary cysts tended to be operated on earlier had poorer outcomes if the procedure was delayed.[164] Nevertheless, the same group reported that even when surgery was performed on day 100 or even later, 45% of patients were alive with their native liver at 5 years, and 40% at 10 years, suggesting that patients may postpone transplantation by the KPE.[165] In a report of native liver histology in 23 patients after a clinically successful KPE with an average follow-up of 4.2 years, resolution in histological cholestasis occurred in a majority of patients (83%), but fibrosis and bile duct proliferation persisted. In these "native liver survivors," fibrosis had progressed to cirrhosis (stage 4 METAVIR) in 52% of patients, associated with the presence of portal hypertension.[166]

Infants who do not respond to the KPE suffer from recurrent episodes of ascending cholangitis or sepsis caused by the immediate proximity of a bowel segment to the porta hepatis of the residual biliary tree. Regardless of the presence or absence of ascending cholangitis, the liver has a higher likelihood of progression cirrhosis with portal hypertension.[166] Large bile lakes may form at the hilum, indicating a persistent effort at bile secretion by hepatocytes (Fig. 55.7). The pathogenesis of progressive fibrosis in chronic cholestatic diseases, including biliary atresia, PFIC, and Alagille syndrome, has been linked to persistence of Hedgehog (Hh) signaling, which normally promotes embryonal duct differentiation and then shuts off as the liver matures.[167] Immunohistochemical colocalization of the Hh transcription factor Gli2 and the mesenchymal markers vimentin and FSP1 in some of the reactive ductular epithelial cells in these diseases is evidence of reversal of mesenchymal-epithelial transition. Similar colocalization of FSP1 and cytokeratin 7 was shown in ductular epithelium, and this ductal cell derangement may lead to fibroplasia.[167] Growth failure, malnutrition, deficiencies of lipid-soluble vitamins, and altered protein–energy and nutrient utilization are expected complications.

A failed KPE in a patient with biliary atresia is the most frequent indication for liver transplantation in infants and young children, accounting for 32.3% of all pediatric liver transplants in 2016. In such instances, prior performance of a KPE does not adversely affect outcomes of liver

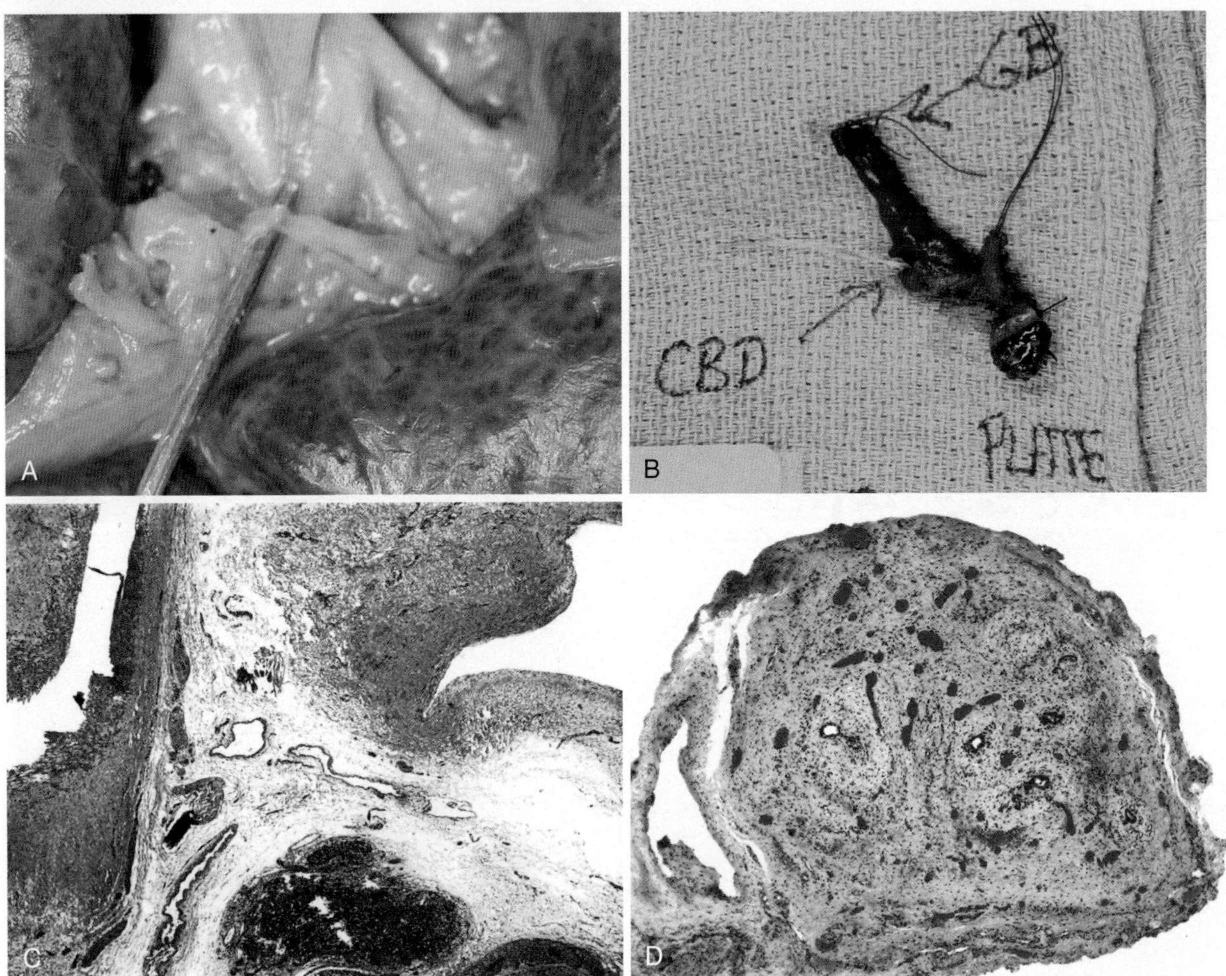

FIGURE 55.6 Biliary atresia at surgery. A, The common hepatic duct is a fibrous cord in a syndromic 9-week-old infant. **B,** This specimen was oriented by the surgeon for the pathologist and shows the hypoplastic gallbladder *(GB)*. The hilar resection includes some liver parenchyma *(PLATE)*, and the junction with the cystic duct is also marked *(CBD)*. **C,** This histological liver hilum specimen shows portal vein *(right)*, hepatic artery *(left)*, a lymphoid aggregate, and some lymphatic channels, but neither a duct nor inflammation. **D,** Cross-section of common hepatic duct reveals multiple small residual bile duct profiles with intact epithelium embedded in loose fibrous tissue with minimal lymphocytic infiltration and scattered venules.

transplantation in children with biliary atresia,[168] although patients subjected to laparoscopic KPE are less likely to have adhesions at the time of liver transplantation, when compared with those whose KPE was by open laparotomy.[157] Patient survival after orthotopic transplantation for biliary atresia in the U.S. United Network for Organ Sharing from 1988 to 2003 was 85.8% at 10 years, with graft survival of 72.7%. The decision to transplant a patient with biliary atresia who has progressed to end-stage liver disease is critical; entry of a patient into the "intent-to-transplant" pathway is associated with excellent overall outcomes, with 97% survival at 5 years in one published series.[169] Pathological examination of explanted livers for occult malignancy is crucial for all forms of chronic liver disease in children.

Neonatal Sclerosing Cholangitis

In addition to neonatal sclerosing cholangitis associated with ichthyosis (OMIM 607626) caused by *CLDN1* mutations, several infants of consanguineous matings have been described with progressive sclerosing cholangitis from infancy.[170,171] An 8-month-old Arab boy reported by Bar Meir and associates[172] had elevated immunoglobulins and anti–smooth muscle titers, but there were no such abnormalities in his mother. These few patients serve to highlight the concept of an intrahepatic form of biliary "atresia," but they also manifest extrahepatic ductal lesions by imaging, similar to older patients with progressive sclerosing cholangitis.[173,174] Langerhans cell histiocytosis can lead to sclerosing cholangitis as part of a systemic process in young children (see Paucity of Intrahepatic Bile Ducts) (Fig. 55.8). Therefore it may be most useful to consider that there is a continuum of inflammatory and sclerosing processes that may have a heritable basis in susceptibility[175] and that show a variable degree of ductal obliteration.[176] More recently *DCDC2* mutations, a gene located on the cilia, has been shown as a cause of neonatal sclerosing cholangitis.[177,178]

Neonatal Hepatitis Syndrome

A neonatal hepatitis syndrome resembling biliary atresia was first described by Burns in 1817. By the mid-1950s, two distinct disease categories of cholestasis of infancy were established: *biliary atresia*, an inflammatory sclerosing syndrome

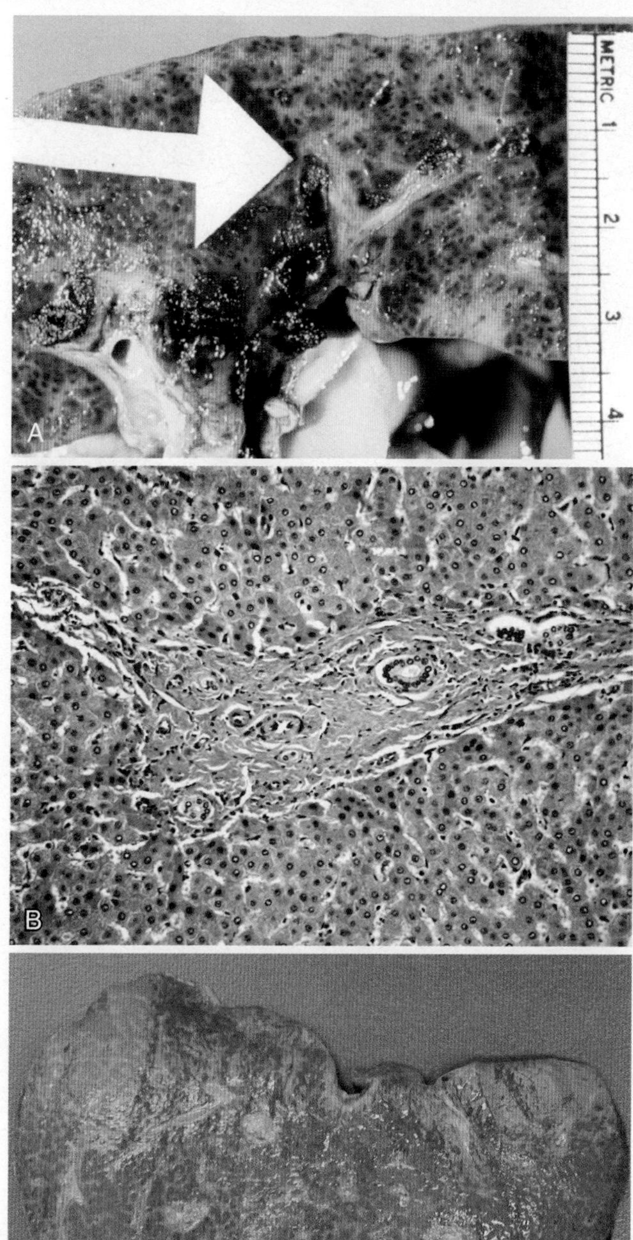

FIGURE 55.7 Liver specimens after Kasai portoenterostomy (KPE). A, Bile lakes *(large arrow)* reflect the persistent secretion of bile from hepatocytes despite complete duct obliteration. **B,** When the KPE is successful, bile will drain and histological cholestasis will resolve (liver biopsy). **C,** Explanted liver at age 4 years in KPE patient showing progression to cirrhosis.

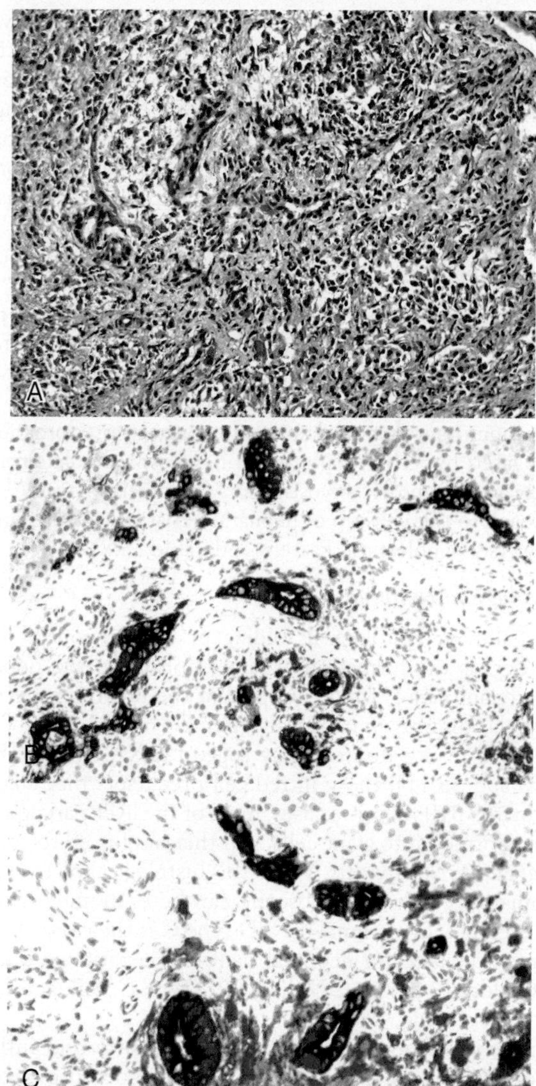

FIGURE 55.8 Langerhans cell histiocytosis in a 6-week-old infant with rash and jaundice. A, A dense infiltrate of eosinophils and histiocytes is concentrated around the portal bile ducts. **B,** The infiltrating histiocytes *(red)* are strongly positive for CD207. Duct epithelium is cytokeratin 19 positive *(brown)*. **C,** CD1a-positive Langerhans cells *(red)* with Birbeck granules are usually rare in the liver, but not in this example.

of the extrahepatic biliary tract with hepatic features of bile duct obstruction, and *neonatal hepatitis*, a nonobstructive type of neonatal cholestatic syndrome with characteristic hepatitic features. At the time, neonatal cholestasis resulting from disorders of bile formation and transport was not yet recognized. In subsequent decades, enormous progress was made in the molecular characterization of neonatal cholestatic disorders. This entity is now best considered a clinicopathological syndrome in which there are many potential etiologies, including infections, anatomical or structural defects, metabolic and inherited disorders, hormonal insufficiency, and vascular, toxic, and immune causes (see Table 55.7).

A review of all biopsies designated *neonatal giant cell hepatitis* at the Johns Hopkins and University of Chicago tertiary hospitals from 1984 to 2007 found 62 cases (75% boys; average age, 2 months).[179] Of the cases with clinical follow-up, half proved to be idiopathic. Ultimately, 8% of patients were found to have biliary atresia, 6% Alagille syndrome, 6% bile salt synthetic defects, and 16% hypopituitarism. At the Texas Children's Hospital in Houston, 151 infants up to 3 months of age had a biopsy performed because of persistent conjugated hyperbilirubinemia. Fifty-nine percent were boys. However, among the 80 patients (53%) who were found to have extrahepatic biliary obstruction, 60%

were girls. Forty-eight patients had neonatal hepatitis, with or without giant cells, one of whom proved to have CMV infection. One infant had A1AT deficiency, one hypopituitarism, one McCune-Albright syndrome, and one Langerhans cell histiocytosis. Sixteen had paucity of intrahepatic bile ducts, but none was syndromic (i.e., Alagille syndrome) at this early age. Disorders without a specific identifiable etiology now account for about 25% of the total.[14]

Clinical Features

Persistent unconjugated hyperbilirubinemia raises the possibility of an inherited defect in bilirubin conjugation or hemolysis. Diagnostic assessment and therapeutic intervention is then critically important to avoid kernicterus and permanent neurological damage. In contrast, predominantly conjugated hyperbilirubinemia in newborns should prompt a rigorous diagnostic investigation for biliary atresia.[95] An approach to the workup of neonatal hepatitis was presented earlier (see Cholestatic Pattern and Table 55.8).

Pathological Features

The hallmark histological finding of many neonatal liver disorders is the formation of large multinucleated hepatocytes (giant cells), which are part of the broader spectrum of lobular disarray in neonatal hepatitis (Fig. 55.9). Nuclear inclusions in hepatocytes may suggest DNA viruses (Figs. 55.10 and 55.11); those in red cell precursors may suggest parvovirus B19. In some cases, most of the liver parenchyma is transformed into giant cells, and this is referred to as *syncytial giant cell hepatitis*. When this histological picture predominates, electron microscopy can be extremely helpful and even pathognomonic if NPD type C is the cause. Of 40 infants evaluated for neonatal giant cell hepatitis in a Denver Children's Series, 27% had NPD type C. Splenomegaly was a useful clue.[180]

In neonatal hepatitis, the relative proportion of inflammatory cells is not considered informative because ongoing apoptosis may lead to extensive hepatocyte destruction and accumulation of residual lymphocytes and macrophages.[13] In some cases, parenchymal inflammation is minimal or absent. In addition, parenchymal neutrophils are an uncommon finding. Occasional islands of erythropoiesis are a normal finding. In all instances, the biopsy should be examined carefully for evidence of viral cytopathic change.

Portal tracts may be inconspicuous, whether normal or abnormal. In general, at least five to seven portal tracts are required to consider the tissue sample adequate for histological evaluation. Ten or more portal tracts are preferred. Bile duct hypoplasia was more common among infants with hypopituitarism, compared with other conditions, in the Johns Hopkins/University of Chicago series.[179] No other biopsy finding was helpful in distinguishing possible etiologies in that series. Exclusion of biliary atresia or A1AT storage disorder requires verification that most, if not all, portal tracts contain a terminal bile duct, a companion hepatic artery, and a portal vein and that bile ductular proliferation, edema, neutrophilic inflammation, and fibrosis are absent. Although the portal tracts in patients with neonatal hepatitis may be expanded by a mixed inflammatory infiltrate, this should not be confused with normal granulocytic hematopoiesis occasionally found within portal tracts.

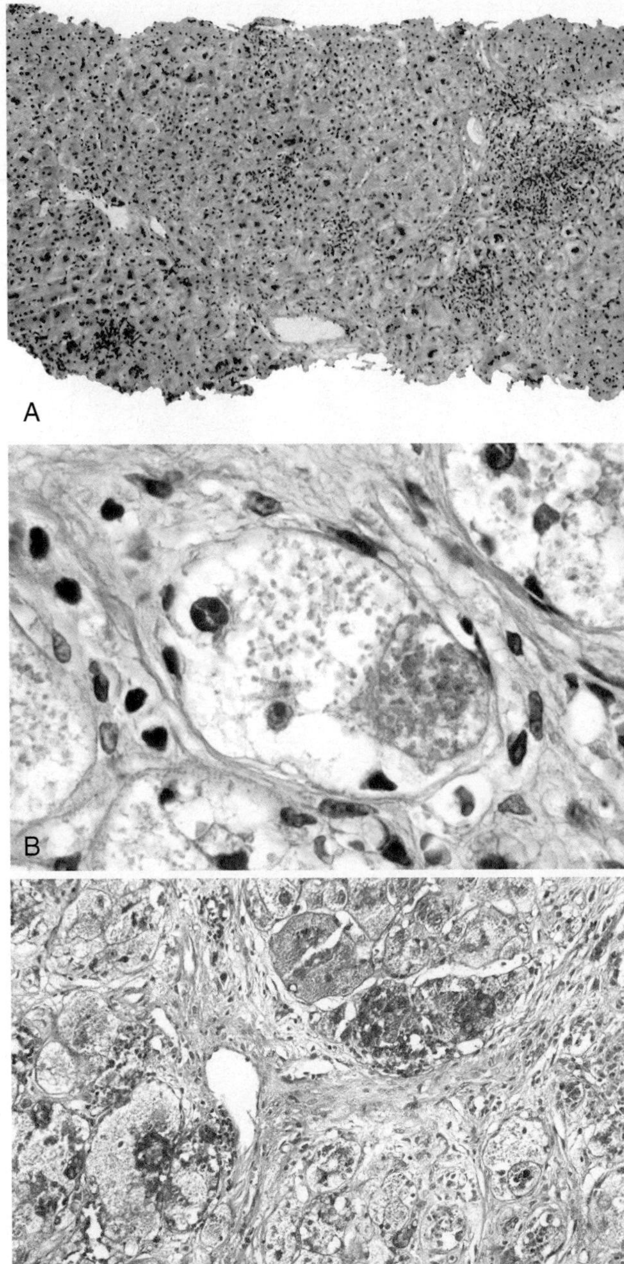

FIGURE 55.9 Neonatal hepatitis. A, Biopsy specimen shows inflamed portal tracts, patchy inflammation of the parenchyma, extensive lobular disarray, and abundant prominently enlarged nuclei. **B,** Enlarged hepatocyte with retained bile pigment, multiple nuclei, and surrounding sinusoidal inflammatory cells and collagen fibers. **C,** Masson trichrome-stained tissue section shows evolving fibrosis of a portal tract with periportal fibrous septa, extensive giant cell transformation of the parenchyma, and retained bile pigment within hepatocytes.

Occasionally, massive hepatic necrosis, with marked accumulation of parenchymal iron, may be observed in patients with Down syndrome. One infant in the Texas Children's Hospital series had an exceptional degree of hepatocellular necrosis, and the cause was pyruvate kinase deficiency.[14] The observation of massive necrosis should also prompt consideration of NH (discussed earlier; see Table 55.7).

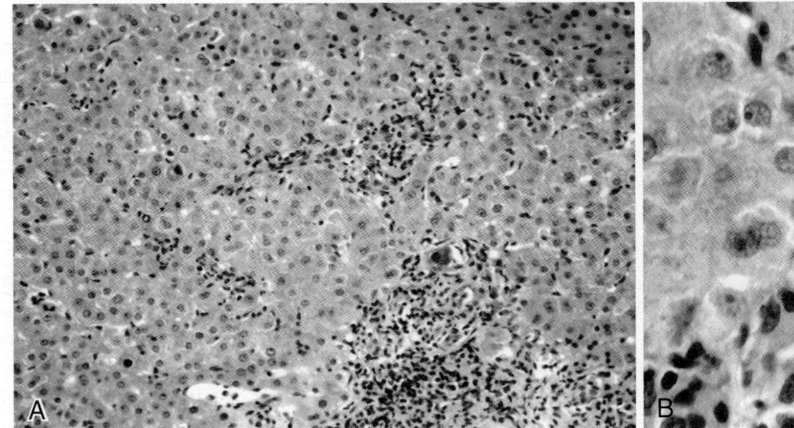

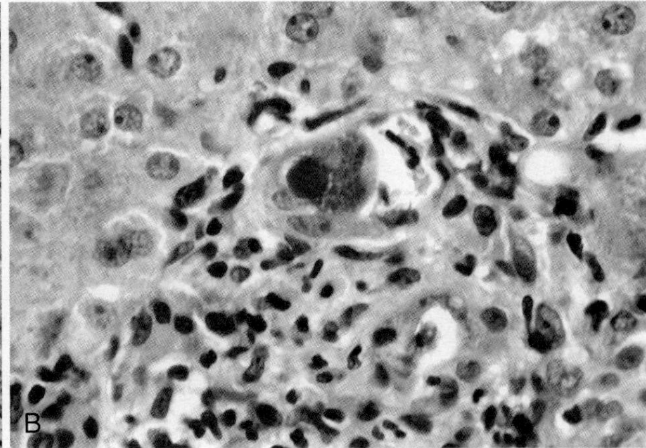

FIGURE 55.10 Cytomegalovirus (CMV) hepatitis. A, Portal and lobular inflammation with lobular disarray. A prominent hepatocyte with viral cytopathic effect is evident toward the *lower right.* **B,** High-power image of an infected hepatocyte shows the characteristic CMV nuclear and cytoplasmic inclusions.

Differential Diagnosis

Once biliary atresia and *A1AT* mutations have been excluded on the basis of both clinical findings and percutaneous liver biopsy, then the differential diagnosis of neonatal hepatitis syndrome must be pursued. Infections of the newborn have been mentioned, and Chapter 47 addresses some of these disorders. Extensive lobular disease, with or without giant cells, may be seen in patients with biliary atresia (see Fig. 55.4). Therefore lobular changes should not divert attention from the features in the portal tracts. Second, nonclassic features of biliary obstruction may be observed in biopsy specimens from patients with biliary atresia, in which ductular reaction has not yet occurred and hepatic arteries exhibit hypertrophy of the media smooth muscle (see Fig. 55.5A,B).[153] Sometimes, alert detection of acholic stools prompts an early biopsy, but the time of onset and rate of progression can vary greatly.[181] (For a detailed discussion of the differential diagnosis, see Cholestatic Pattern and Table 55.7.)

Natural History and Treatment

The natural history of neonatal hepatitis depends heavily on the specific etiology (Table 55.16). For instance, pharmacological intervention is imperative for many of the infectious disorders. Many of the other disorders, including hypopituitarism, tyrosinemia, and bile salt synthetic defects, benefit dramatically from prompt intervention.[182] In about a quarter of all infants, no cause is found.[183] The prognosis for "idiopathic" neonatal hepatitis syndrome is considered favorable; the mortality rate is 13% to 25%.[184] Predictors of a poor clinical outcome include severe or prolonged (>6 months) jaundice, acholic stools, familial occurrence, and persistent hepatomegaly. Peak bilirubin level is not predictive of outcome. Sepsis is a devastating complication and is associated with a poor outcome. For infants whose liver disease resolves, the prognosis is quite favorable; most have no residual liver dysfunction. Many children benefit from a cholestatic gene panel evaluation that may pinpoint the exact defect (see Box 55.1).

The management of idiopathic neonatal hepatitis syndrome is supportive and includes adequate nutrition. Dietary measures, such as use of lactose-free, low-protein formulas, may mitigate further liver damage until the results of tests for galactosemia, hereditary tyrosinemia type I, and hypopituitarism, for example, become known. Elemental formulas containing medium-chain triglycerides help maintain caloric intake in severely ill patients. Infants with chronic cholestasis require fat-soluble vitamin supplementation. Pruritus associated with chronic cholestasis is difficult to treat in many patients.[2]

Syncytial Giant Cell Hepatitis

In 1991, a putative novel form of hepatitis was first described in patients 5 months to 41 years of age.[185] Clinical features of a severe type of hepatitis required liver transplantation in five patients; five others died of their liver disease. Liver histology revealed replacement of the parenchyma with abundant large syncytial multinucleated (giant) hepatocytes that contained up to 30 nuclei per cell. Electron microscopy revealed intracytoplasmic structures consistent with paramyxovirus nucleocapsids (Fig. 55.12). Injection of liver homogenate from an affected patient into two chimpanzees led to an increase in the titer of paramyxovirus antibodies in one.

One year later, a separate report concluded that syncytial giant cell hepatitis may have a variety of causes, such as autoimmune hepatitis, hepatitis A virus (HAV) or HBV infection, Epstein-Barr virus infection, or, potentially, HCV infection.[186] Three of the patients had fulminant hepatic failure; two others developed severe chronic hepatitis. However, a further seven patients fared quite well. Therefore syncytial giant cell hepatitis represents a tissue reaction pattern that may develop as a result of multiple causes and does not always imply an ominous prognosis. This interpretation has been supported by subsequent reports in which generalized bacterial sepsis, viral infection, toxoplasmosis, syphilis, listeriosis, and even tuberculosis were shown to induce a similar histological pattern of injury. Viral causes include CMV, rubella, herpes simplex virus, human herpesvirus 6, varicella, coxsackievirus, echovirus, reovirus 3, parvovirus B19, human immunodeficiency virus (HIV), enteroviruses, paramyxovirus, HAV, HBV, or (rarely) HCV; some adult patients were coinfected with HIV and HCV.[187]

The *Paramyxoviridae* are divided into the subfamily Paramyxovirinae, containing *Paramyxovirus* (Sendai virus, parainfluenza virus type 3), rubella, mumps, parainfluenza

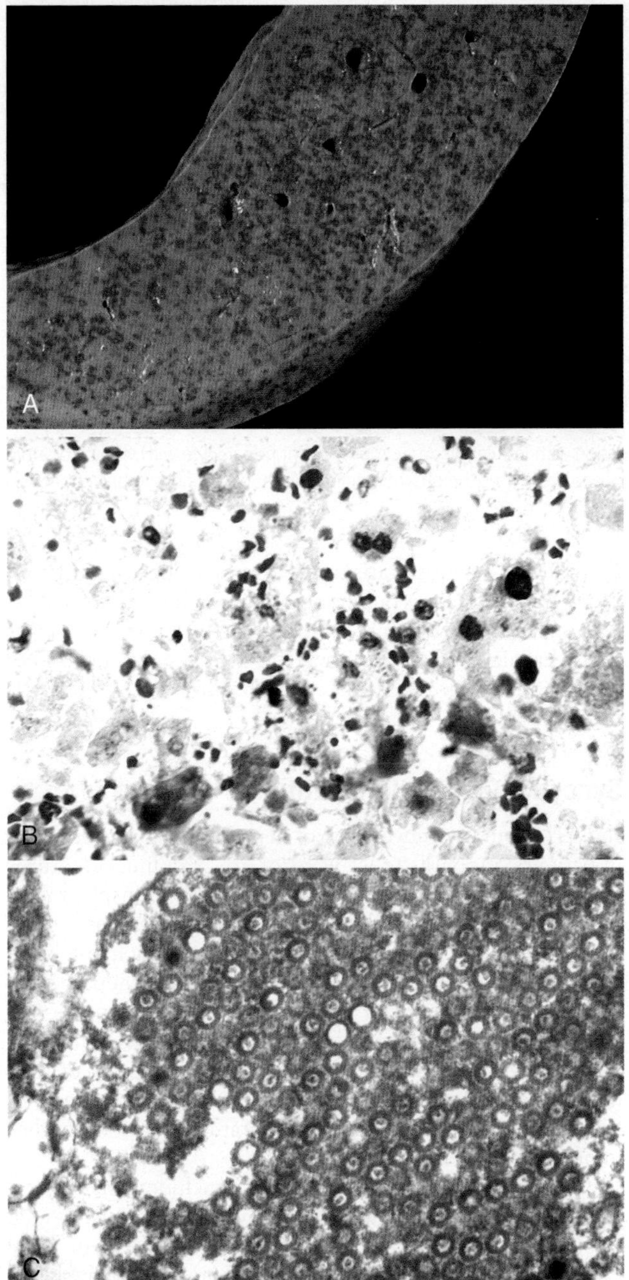

FIGURE 55.11 Herpes simplex virus infection. A, Gross image of a postmortem liver shows overall pallor and numerous hemorrhagic foci of necrosis. **B,** The edge of a necrotic focus shows hepatocytes with nuclear inclusions characteristic of herpesvirus infection and other pyknotic hepatocyte nuclei. **C,** Ultrastructural image of herpesvirus virions in the nucleus of a hepatocyte.

virus type 2, and *Morbillivirus* (measles), and the subfamily Pneumovirinae, containing the *Pneumovirus* genus (respiratory syncytial virus). Therefore, even by ultrastructural examination, the differential diagnosis for syncytial giant cell hepatitis is quite broad.

PAUCITY OF INTRAHEPATIC BILE DUCTS

Neonates with conjugated hyperbilirubinemia may exhibit paucity of small intrahepatic (interlobular) bile ducts. A variety of disorders can cause nonsyndromic duct paucity (Table 55.17), including A1AT storage disorder and hypopituitarism. Langerhans cell histiocytosis may cause severe cholangitis with a dense infiltrate of eosinophils as well as CD207-positive and CD1a-positive histiocytes (see Fig. 55.8). In patients who survive infancy, duct loss can be severe. Sclerosing cholangitis caused by Langerhans cell histiocytosis has been reported in an adult.[188] Some cases of paucity are idiopathic.[183] Among congenital infections, CMV infection is the most important; viral inclusions may be found within bile duct epithelial cells (see Fig. 55.10). In severe neonatal hepatitis, paucity of bile ducts may be evident on liver biopsy specimens. Clinical presentation of severe cholestasis, either early in life or later in childhood, should always raise the possibility of syndromic paucity of bile ducts (Alagille syndrome).

α_1-Antitrypsin Deficiency

A1AT is a hepatic storage disorder that mostly manifests later in life (see later discussion). However, 11% of individuals with PiZZ mutations in *SERPINA1*, the *A1AT* gene, may develop conjugated hyperbilirubinemia in infancy.

A1AT storage disorder can mimic the histological appearance of biliary atresia, with portal tract changes that include edema, scant acute inflammation, proliferating bile ductules, and bile plugs within bile duct lumina (Fig. 55.13). Characteristic globular inclusions of staining material (PAS) with diastase digestion (d-PAS) in periportal hepatocytes are typically not present for weeks or months, but immunohistochemistry for the protein is more sensitive, as is electron microscopy for demonstration of the protein within endoplasmic reticulum. Bile pigment, hemosiderin, and copper-binding protein may be present within periportal hepatocytes, all of which are highlighted as fine granules in tissue sections stained with d-PAS. Protease inhibitor typing by serum immunoelectrophoresis is required for diagnosis.

Syndromic Paucity of Bile Ducts: Alagille Syndrome

Clinical Features

Some infants and young children with conjugated hyperbilirubinemia have associated facial dysmorphism and cardiovascular, vertebral, and ocular malformations. The combination of extrahepatic abnormalities and deficiency of interlobular bile ducts is termed *Alagille syndrome*.[189] Alagille syndrome is an autosomal dominant disorder with an estimated frequency of 1 in 70,000 live births, increased to an incidence of 1 in 30,000 live births in the molecular era.[190] Sporadic cases account for 45% to 50%. The mortality rate is 15% to 20%. Deaths are mostly caused by hepatic or cardiovascular complications.

Before the advent of genetic testing, a diagnosis of Alagille syndrome required demonstration of paucity of interlobular bile ducts and clinical evidence of at least three major of the following abnormalities: characteristic facies, posterior embryotoxon, butterfly vertebrae, renal disease, and cardiac anomalies. However, bile duct paucity is evident in only 60% of infants who undergo biopsy before 6 months of age.[191] Furthermore, there is wide phenotypic variability in patients with this disorder, ranging from mild subclinical findings to complete liver failure and complex congenital

TABLE 55.16 Natural History of Common Causes of Neonatal Jaundice

Etiology	Natural History
Biliary atresia	Death by 1 to 2 years of age without Kasai procedure or liver transplantation
α_1-Antitrypsin storage disorder	Progressive chronic liver disease with risk of cirrhosis
Neonatal infection	Resolution of infection required for survival
Disorders of Carbohydrate Metabolism	
Glycogen storage disease	Maintenance of blood sugar levels enables survival Risk of chronic renal disease High probability of hepatic adenomatosis Liver transplantation is curative in some forms
Galactosemia	Dietary galactose restriction enables survival Neurodevelopmental complications may persist
Fructosemia	Avoidance of dietary fructose enables survival Lifelong risk of metabolic crises on fructose exposure
Disorders of Amino Acid Metabolism	
Tyrosinemia	Pharmacological treatment enables survival High lifetime risk of hepatocellular carcinoma
Disorders of Glycolipid and Lipid Metabolism	
Niemann-Pick disease types A and C	Type A: fatal outcome of progressive neurological disease Type C: survival into adulthood possible; neurological compromise may occur
Hereditary Disorders of Bile Formation	
Progressive familial intrahepatic cholestasis	Biliary diversion may ameliorate; liver transplantation for cirrhosis, neoplasia; persistent diarrhea in type 1
Disorders of bile acid biosynthesis	Dietary treatment with bile acids can ameliorate effects of disease
Idiopathic neonatal hepatitis	Highly variable, most likely representing undiscovered genetic abnormalities Cholestatic liver disease may persist into later childhood

heart disease.[192,193] Most patients with hepatic involvement are seen clinically within the first 6 months with jaundice, hepatomegaly, pruritus, and failure to thrive. Laboratory studies reveal conjugated hyperbilirubinemia and increased serum levels of GGT, alkaline phosphatase, bile acids, and cholesterol. Serum ALT and AST levels may be normal or mildly elevated. Currently, genetic testing is almost always conclusive and is included as part of the cholestatic gene panel.

Pathogenesis

Mutations in Jagged1 (*JAG1*), a ligand in the Notch signaling pathway, have been identified in 94% of patients with Alagille syndrome.[194-196] Mutations in the *NOTCH2* gene, which encodes a receptor for Jagged1, have been identified in some *JAG1* mutation–negative patients.[196,197] It is hypothesized that defects in *JAG1* result in an arrest of branching and elongation of bile ducts during postnatal liver growth.[191] In support of this theory, Libbrecht and associates reported a case in which an explanted liver from a 16-year-old patient with Alagille syndrome demonstrated paucity of bile ducts in peripheral liver parenchyma but normally developed bile ducts in the perihilar areas.[198] Deletions in a single *JAG1* allele are sufficient to cause ALGS, suggesting haploinsufficiency as the disease-causing mechanism. Recent mouse models with mutant *JAG1* that have been developed by Andersson et al.[199] and Adams et al.[200] will help better define the mechanism of ALGS as it showed binding of NOTCH2 rather than NOTCH1 by JAG 1^{Ndr} in these mice. The interaction of the NOTCH and WNT pathways in biliary epithelial development is of great interest for aberrant organogenesis and response to injury.[201-203]

Pathological Features

To diagnose paucity of bile ducts, the liver biopsy specimen should contain at least 7 portal tracts, and preferably at least 10. Normally, on routinely stained tissue sections (H&E or Masson trichrome) of mature liver tissue, approximately 90% of portal tracts contain an interlobular bile duct, either as a single duct or as multiple duct profiles,[5] paired in close apposition to branches of the hepatic artery of similar outside diameter. The presence of multiple portal tracts containing arteries and veins but not bile ducts should prompt consideration of bile duct paucity, which is defined by an absence of, or marked reduction in, the number of interlobular bile ducts within portal tracts. In pediatric patients, a bile duct-to-portal tract ratio of less than 0.8 is often used as a cutoff point between normal and abnormal, although the number of bile ducts may be normally (physiologically) low in preterm infants. However, in any age group, a ratio of less than 0.4 is strongly suggestive of bile duct paucity. When making this assessment, large portal tracts should not be considered in the equation. Furthermore, incomplete portal tracts that are partially transected by the biopsy should be excluded from the analysis because absence of a bile duct may simply represent a sampling artifact. Specimens from patients with Alagille syndrome are conspicuous for their lack of portal tracts and parenchymal inflammation, but they may have abundant giant cells, as in neonatal hepatitis (Fig. 55.14).

Immunohistochemical staining for cytokeratin 7 or 19 is useful to highlight bile duct epithelium. Because hepatocytes in cholestatic livers often acquire cytokeratin 7 immunoreactivity (see Fig. 55.14D), cytokeratin 19 is preferred for quantitating bile ducts.[204] Immunoreactive ductular profiles at the margins of portal tracts should not be confused with true interlobular bile ducts (see Fig. 55.1). A persistent lack of canalicular CD10 immunopositivity, although physiological in infants younger than 2 years of age, is a characteristic finding in Alagille syndrome.[205] The Masson trichrome stain is also helpful in identifying small portal tracts because of its ability to detect delicate amounts of connective tissue.[206] These small portal tracts should be included in the portal tract count when one is assessing bile ducts.

In the evaluation of a liver biopsy specimen for potential paucity of bile ducts, the pathology report should indicate how many portal tracts and bile ducts were identified. The staining method should also be reported. Paucity of

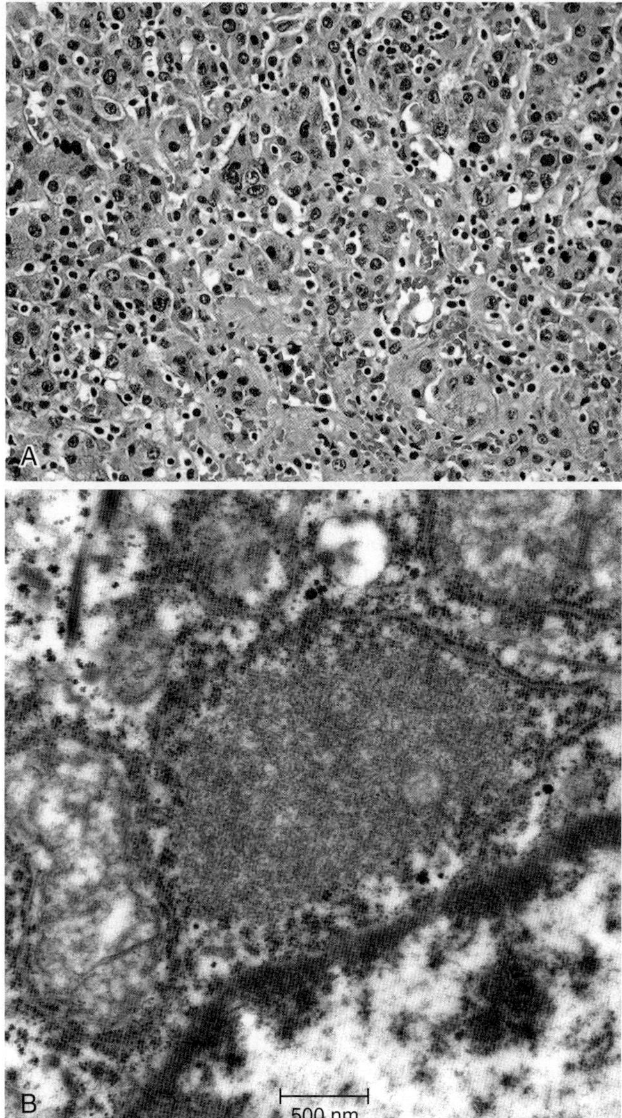

FIGURE 55.12 Paramyxovirus hepatitis in 4-year-old with 8 days of jaundice progressing to fulminant hepatic failure. A, Diffuse hepatocellular necrosis and mixed inflammation. Some cells have smudged nuclear chromatin, and others have very prominent nucleoli. There is fibrin in some sinusoids. **B,** Ultrastructurally, cytoplasmic filamentous inclusions measuring 10 to 20 nm are characteristic of paramyxovirus; this finding was confirmed by polymerase chain reaction.

interlobular bile ducts is not a specific disorder; instead, it represents a pathological feature that may have a variety of causes.

Differential Diagnosis

When Alagille syndrome cannot be distinguished from biliary obstruction on liver biopsy, and the clinical and radiological features fail to detect the extrahepatic manifestations in an infant with Alagille syndrome, patients have at times still been treated by KPE. Even at a major center with extensive experience with these diseases, 4.4% of patients were mistakenly operated on, and afterward their liver disease progressed more rapidly to end-stage cirrhosis.[80] Alagille histology may show an overlap with EHBA with marked ductular proliferation and fibrosis but shows absence of

TABLE 55.17 Causes of Nonsyndromic Paucity of Bile Ducts

Infants	Adolescents and Adults
Prematurity	Immune-mediated causes
Infection	Primary biliary cirrhosis
Cytomegalovirus	Primary sclerosing cholangitis
Rubella	Liver allograft rejection
Syphilis	Graft-versus-host disease
Hepatitis B virus	Metabolic
Metabolic disorders	Cystic fibrosis
α_1-Antitrypsin storage disorder	Toxic insults
Niemann-Pick disease type C	
Cystic fibrosis	
Zellweger syndrome	
Mitochondrial cytopathies	
Byler syndrome	
Prune-belly syndrome	
Hypopituitarism	
MYO5B liver disease	
Genetic: chromosomal disorders	
Trisomy 18, trisomy 21	
Partial trisomy 11	
Monosomy X	
Neonatal sclerosing cholangitis-ichthyosis	
Immune-mediated causes	
Liver allograft rejection	
Graft-versus-host disease	
Severe idiopathic neonatal hepatitis	
End-stage extrahepatic atresia	

Modified from Roberts EA. Neonatal hepatitis syndrome. Semin Neonatol. *2003;8:357–374.*

interlobular bile ducts. Because Alagille disease progression is highly variable, every effort must be made to avoid surgery.

Caution is also required in the interpretation of hepatobiliary scintigraphy and cholangiographic studies. Typically, both extrahepatic and intrahepatic bile ducts in patients with Alagille syndrome are markedly hypoplastic; therefore on hepatobiliary scanning, one may not see excretion of radioisotope into the intestines (mimicking biliary atresia).[191] Similarly, intraoperative cholangiography may not necessarily demonstrate opacification of the proximal extrahepatic ducts. These diagnostic pitfalls underscore the importance of a careful and full physical examination and radiological evaluation in patients with suspected Alagille syndrome.

No genotype-phenotype correlation with severity for *JAGGED1* mutations was found among 33 patients with Alagille syndrome who were older than 10 years of age.[207]

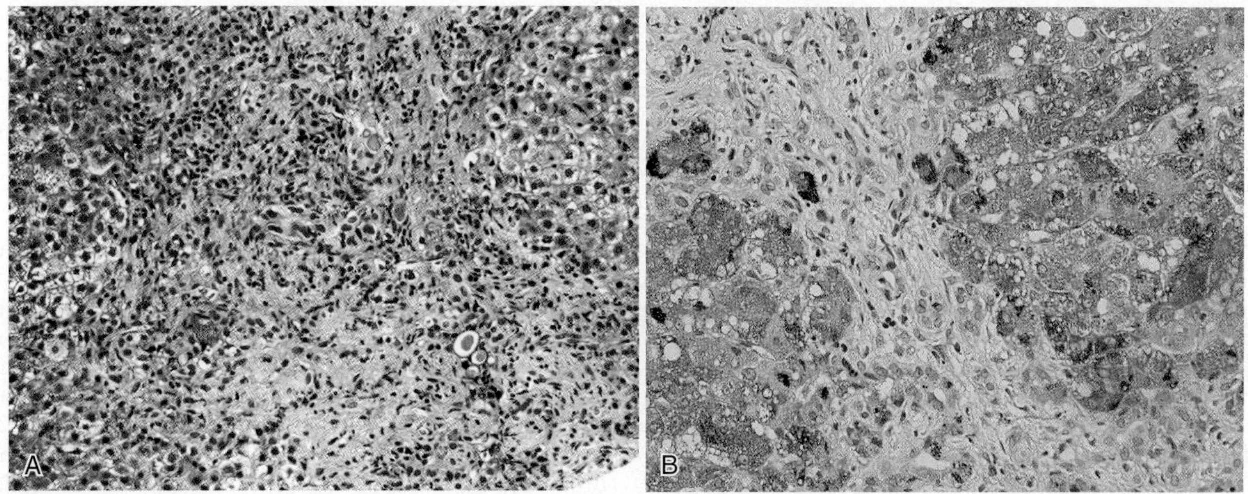

FIGURE 55.13 **α_1-Antitrypsin storage disease, acute. A,** Biopsy at 11 weeks of age in an infant with the *PiZZ* genotype is indistinguishable from extrahepatic obstruction. A widely expanded portal tract displays abundant bile in the ducts, mixed inflammation, and fibrosis. **B,** Immunostaining reveals the protein in periportal hepatocytes.

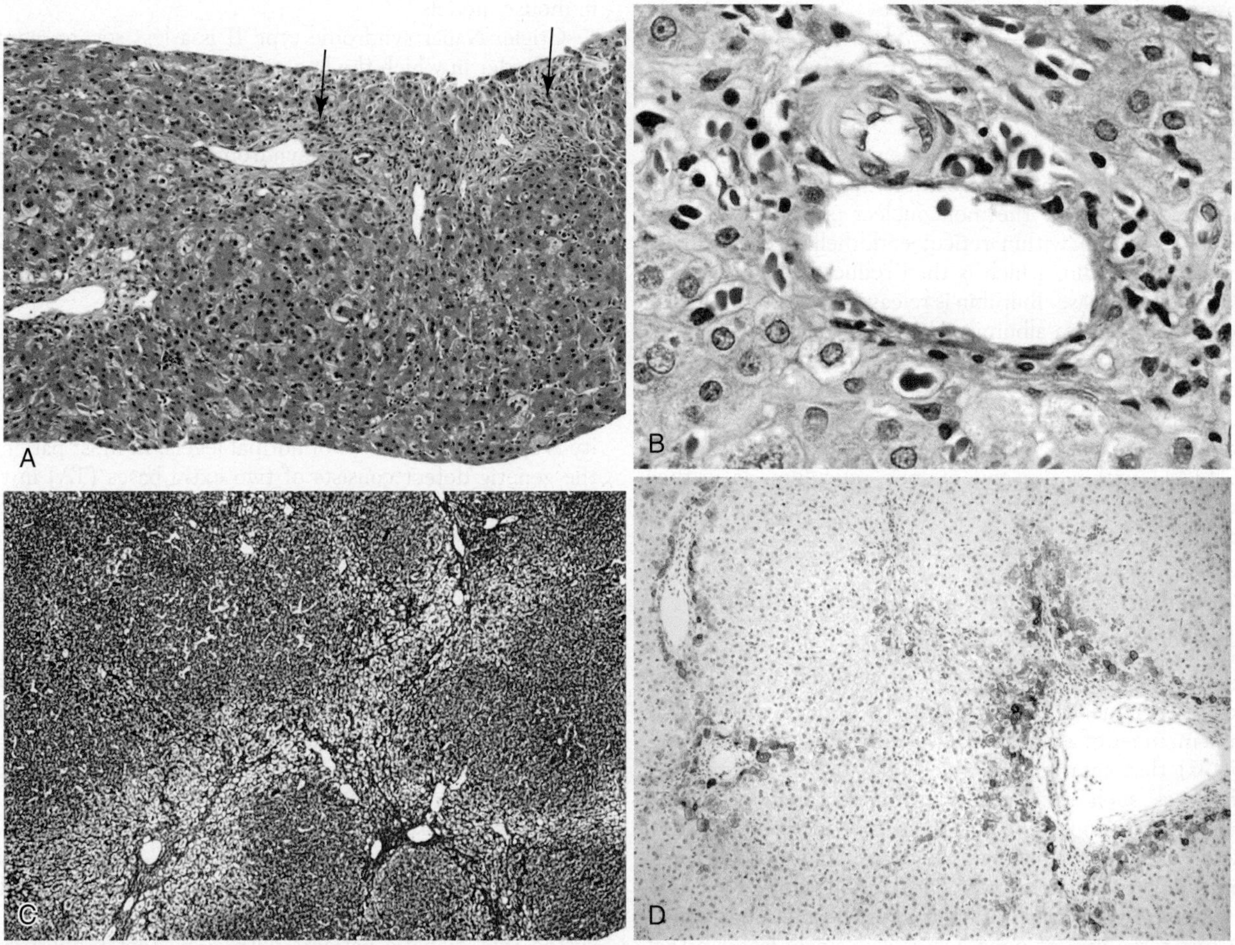

FIGURE 55.14 **Alagille syndrome. A,** Initial biopsy of a 2-month-old infant shows small collapsed bile ducts *(arrows)* and mild canalicular cholestasis with giant cells. **B,** Biopsy collected from patient at 5 years of age is lacking portal bile ducts and is not inflamed. Canalicular cholestasis is evident in the parenchyma. **C,** Progressive fibrosis with bridging in an 8-year-old patient. **D,** Cytokeratin 7 is expressed in ductular hepatocytes in response to complete duct absence. (*From Ernst LM, Spinner NB, Piccoli DA, et al. Interlobular bile duct loss in pediatric cholestatic disease is associated with aberrant cytokeratin 7 expression by hepatocytes. Pediatr Dev Pathol. 2007;10:383–390.*)

Those children with elevated total bilirubin (>6.5 mg/dL), conjugated bilirubin (>4.5 mg/dL), and cholesterol (>520 mg/dL) before 5 years of age had significantly worse liver disease later. Sequencing of the entire coding region of *JAG1* is now available and should be used in patients in whom there is a strong clinical suspicion and in family members of probands with mutations.

Natural History

Alagille syndrome is a benign illness in many children. However, young children with protracted severe jaundice usually have a poorer prognosis. Between 10% and 50% of patients with Alagille syndrome eventually progress to cirrhosis and liver failure.[208] Cases of HCC in Alagille syndrome have been described, as in every chronic cholestatic disease of infants.[209] The overall mortality rate from Alagille syndrome is estimated to be 20% to 25%; death occurs mainly from cardiac disease, intercurrent infection, or progressive liver disease. Liver transplantation is warranted for patients with severe hepatic disease. Because of the presence of multiple organ defects in Alagille syndrome, the outcomes of liver transplantation are poorer than for patients with EHBA, especially with regard to death during the first 30 postoperative days. No pretransplant factors were identified among the 87% of patients who survived to 1 year, compared with those who did not.[210]

HEREDITARY DISORDERS OF BILIRUBIN METABOLISM

Bilirubin is the end product of heme degradation, which is derived predominantly from the breakdown of senescent erythrocytes by the mononuclear phagocytic system. Heme oxygenase within reticuloendothelial cells oxidizes heme to biliverdin, which is then reduced to bilirubin by biliverdin reductase. Bilirubin is released into the circulation and binds to serum albumin. Uptake of bilirubin by hepatocytes occurs via a carrier-mediated system at the level of the sinusoidal membrane. Bilirubin is then conjugated with either one or two molecules of glucuronic acid by bilirubin uridine diphosphate (UDP)-glucuronosyltransferase (i.e., UGT1A1) within the endoplasmic reticulum. It is then excreted as water-soluble, nontoxic bilirubin glucuronides into bile.

Crigler-Najjar Syndrome and Gilbert Syndrome

Classification and Pathogenesis

The hepatic conjugating enzyme UGT1A1 is a product of the *UGT1A1* gene, which is located on chromosome 2q37. It is a member of a family of UDP-glucuronosyltransferases (UGTs) that catalyze the glucuronidation of an array of substrates such as steroid hormones, carcinogens, and drugs. The various types of UGTs are distributed within a wide range of tissues, including liver, kidney, intestines, skin, lung, olfactory epithelium, and testis. UGT1A1 is located primarily within the smooth and rough endoplasmic reticulum of hepatocytes as a single isoform that catalyzes the glucuronidation of bilirubin to form its monoglucuronidated and diglucuronidated forms. In humans, two members of the UGT1 family possess the capability to glucuronidate bilirubin in vitro, but only one isoform is physiologically relevant in vivo. The bilirubin glucuronidating isoform is termed *UGT1A1* because it is generated from the exon 1A of the *UGT1* gene locus. Multiple mutations in *UGT1A1* cause hereditary unconjugated hyperbilirubinemia: Crigler-Najjar syndrome types I and II and Gilbert syndrome.[211]

Clinical and Pathological Features

In Crigler-Najjar syndrome type I, the liver UGT1A1 enzyme is completely absent. Colorless bile contains only trace amounts of unconjugated bilirubin. Serum unconjugated bilirubin reaches very high levels, leading to severe jaundice and icterus. Without liver transplantation, this condition is invariably fatal (because of kernicterus), usually within 18 months of birth. In a recent review of 22 patients undergoing liver transplant for Crigler-Najjar syndrome type I, the pathological features showed canalicular cholestasis and significant pericentral sinusoidal, periportal, and mixed patterns of fibrosis in almost 41% of the patients. The fibrosis appeared to be progressive and more in older children at the time of transplant. This suggests the need for early recognition of this disease and intervention to arrest progression of fibrosis and need for earlier liver transplantation.[212,213] This has led to attempts to use AAV8 gene therapy to ameliorate the changes with preliminary success in mouse models.[214]

Crigler-Najjar syndrome type II is a less severe, nonfatal disorder in which the hepatic level of UGT1A1 enzyme activity is greatly reduced but not absent, and the enzyme is capable of forming only monoglucuronidated bilirubin. In contrast with the type I syndrome, the only major clinical consequence is the presence of extraordinarily yellow skin caused by moderate to high levels of circulating unconjugated bilirubin. Phenobarbital treatment may improve bilirubin glucuronidation by inducing hypertrophy of the hepatocellular endoplasmic reticulum.

Gilbert syndrome is a relatively common benign, inherited condition.[215] Affected patients have mild, fluctuating hyperbilirubinemia in the absence of hemolysis or liver disease. Typically, hepatic bilirubin glucuronidating activity is approximately 30% of normal levels. In most patients, the genetic defect consists of two extra bases (TA) in the TATAA element (TATA box) in the promoter region of the *UGT1A1* gene. This creates an $A(TA)_7TAA$ element, rather than the normal $A(TA)_6TAA$ of the *UGT1A1* gene ("an extra TA in the TATA box"), and results in reduced expression of UGT1A1. In some cases, patients are heterozygous for missense mutations in the *UGT1A1* gene. Gilbert syndrome affects 3% to 10% of the population. Mild hyperbilirubinemia may go unrecognized for many years and is not associated with functional derangements of the liver. When detected in adolescents or adults, it is typically in association with an unrelated stress, such as intercurrent illness, strenuous exercise, or fasting, that reduces hepatic levels of the obligate cofactor for UGT1A1, UDP-glucuronic acid. Gilbert syndrome has no clinical consequence except for anxiety related to persistent jaundice. A 2007 study suggested that diabetic patients with coexistent Gilbert syndrome have a lower incidence of vascular complications and a reduction in serum markers of oxidase stress and inflammation, possibly because of the antioxidant effect of bilirubin.[216]

In all disorders of bilirubin conjugation other than Crigler-Najjar type I, the liver is morphologically normal by both light and electron microscopy.

Dubin-Johnson Syndrome

Dubin-Johnson syndrome is an autosomal recessive disorder characterized by the presence of conjugated hyperbilirubinemia caused by mutations in the *ABCC2* gene. *ABCC2* encodes the hepatocyte canalicular multispecific organic anion transporter (cMOAT), the transport protein responsible for secretion of bilirubin conjugates into bile.[217,218] There are many different mutations in the protein that cause functional defects in protein maturation and localization to the canalicular plasma membrane.[219,220] The key consequence is profound conjugated hyperbilirubinemia. Patients affected with this disorder show profound jaundice but are otherwise normal. Presentation may be at any age until the sixth decade of life. Rarely, neonatal hepatitis has been reported in patients with Dubin-Johnson syndrome.[221]

Affected livers reveal deep discoloration, not from retained bilirubin pigment but from accumulation of a chemical polymer in lysosomes that resembles epinephrine.[222] On liver biopsy, the liver tissue core appears dark. By light microscopy, prominent globular pigmented inclusions are present within hepatocytes (Fig. 55.15). Pigmented inclusions may be inconspicuous in infants but become more prominent during childhood. In a recent review of neonatal cases of Dubin-Johnson syndrome, pigment was seen in only 3 of 8 infants with the syndrome.[221] Immunohistochemistry for MRP2 (cMOAT) shows complete absence of the protein along the canaliculi.

The conjugated hyperbilirubinemia of Dubin-Johnson syndrome is not toxic to the central nervous system or other tissues. Treatment with ursodeoxycholic acid may be beneficial for the rare infants who develop neonatal hepatitis.[221]

Rotor Syndrome

Rotor syndrome resembles Dubin-Johnson syndrome in that it produces a benign type of conjugated hyperbilirubinemia. The jaundice is more often evident in infancy. It is a rare autosomal recessive disorder (frequency, 1 in 10^6) that is caused by the simultaneous deficiency of two hepatocyte sinusoidal membrane organic anion transporters (OATP1B1 and OATP1B3), which are encoded by *SLCO1B1* and *SLCO1B3* on chromosome 12p.[223] In Rotor syndrome, loss of these two proteins impairs hepatocyte uptake of conjugated bilirubin. In contrast with Dubin-Johnson syndrome, no pigment accumulates in hepatocytes, but urinary coproporphyrin 1 excretion is similarly very abundant. Although there is no clinical dysfunction, the defect may contribute to hepatotoxicity from drugs that require conjugation for excretion.

HEREDITARY DISORDERS OF BILE ACID METABOLISM AND BILE FORMATION

Bile is a complex mixture of bile salts, phosphatidylcholine, cholesterol, bilirubin, glutathione, and electrolytes combined with pigments and metabolites of drugs. Approximately 50% of the dry weight of bile consists of bile salts—conjugates of bile acids and glycine or taurine. The two primary bile acids in humans, cholic acid and chenodeoxycholic acid, are synthesized within hepatocytes, where they become conjugated to the amido groups of glycine or taurine to form bile salts. Bile salts are exported through the hepatocyte canalicular membranes into the canaliculus, where they are admixed with other components of bile, and flow through the biliary tree. Defects in the synthesis of bile acids or in the export of bile salts to the canaliculus lead to cholestatic disorders in humans and deficiency of fat-soluble vitamins and steatorrhea in the liver (see Table 55.10).

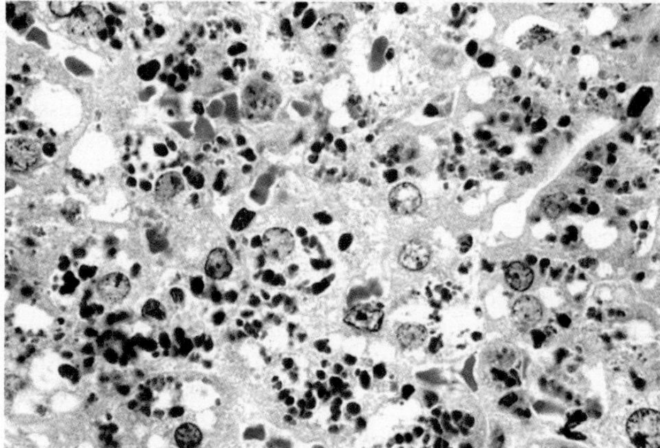

FIGURE 55.15 Dubin-Johnson syndrome. Large, nonrefractile globular inclusions are present within hepatocytes.

Inborn Errors of Bile Acid Synthesis

Inborn errors of bile acid synthesis are rare inherited disorders in which the bile acid biosynthetic pathway is severely impaired. This condition results in buildup of toxic biosynthetic intermediates and manifests clinically as neonatal hepatitis syndrome or in childhood as chronic cholestasis. These diseases are extremely rare, with a projected incidence of about 1 in 50,000 to 100,000 and an increased incidence in inbred populations. All defects are inherited as autosomal recessive mutations of genes coding for various enzyme defects.[224] Patients can be screened for these disorders by mass spectrometric analyses of urinary bile acids and bile alcohols.[225]

3β-Hydroxy-Δ5-C_{27}-Steroid Oxidoreductase Deficiency

3β-Hydroxy-Δ5-C_{27}-steroid oxidoreductase, the second enzyme in bile acid biosynthesis, is a microsomal oxidoreductase that removes hydrogen atoms from the steroid nucleus. Mutations in the *HSD3B7* gene that encodes the enzyme have been reported in 15 patients in 13 families studied.[226] In another 18 patients,[227] the majority had neonatal conjugated hyperbilirubinemia, rickets, and hepatomegaly. Liver biopsy revealed giant cell transformation and hepatocyte disarray with cholestasis, bridging fibrosis, and, rarely, cirrhosis. These infants typically have normal serum levels of GGT and low serum total bile acid concentrations. Dietary administration of cholic acid, with or without ursodeoxycholic acid, inhibits endogenous biosynthesis of bile acids and markedly reduces accumulation of aberrant bile acid precursors. With this regimen, infants can develop normally.

Δ4-3-Oxosteroid 5β-Reductase Deficiency

Δ4-3-Oxosteroid 5β-reductase is a cytosolic enzyme that is responsible for 5β reduction of the nucleus of the steroid molecule. Infants affected by an autosomal recessive disorder in which the enzyme is inactive produce excessive amounts of Δ4-3-oxo bile acids, which are toxic at high levels. Mutations in the *AKRID1* gene,[228] which encodes the enzyme, have been reported in patients with severe neonatal cholestasis and coagulopathy. Serum GGT levels are usually normal in this disorder. Liver biopsy may reveal giant cell hepatitis and hepatic scarring resembling NH.[229] Treatment with cholic acid, with or without ursodeoxycholic acid, is beneficial.

Other Bile Acid Biosynthetic Disorders

Neonatal jaundice with hepatosplenomegaly develops in patients who have a deficiency in the 24,25-dihydroxycholanoic cleavage enzyme.[224] Because this enzyme is important for the alternative pathway of bile acid biosynthesis, which produces chenodeoxycholic acid, dietary treatment with chenodeoxycholic acid plus cholic acid is beneficial.

Other inborn errors of bile acid metabolism have been described in patients with neonatal liver disease.[224,230,231]

Progressive Familial Intrahepatic Cholestasis and other Defects in Bile Secretion or Transport

Several disorders manifest in neonates or children with cholestasis resulting from defective bile secretion or transport. Chief among them are the progressive familial intrahepatic cholestatic (PFIC) disorders, originally comprising three autosomal recessive disorders (PFIC1, PFIC2, and PFIC3; see Table 55.10) caused by mutations in three canalicular proteins, respectively: familial intrahepatic cholestasis type 1 (FIC1) encoded by *ATP8B1*; bile salt export pump (BSEP) encoded by *ABCB11*; and multidrug-resistance protein 3 (MDR3) encoded by *ABCB4*.[232] All three disorders typically manifest in early childhood with conjugated hyperbilirubinemia and are characterized by the presence of elevated plasma bile acids and defective bile secretion. PFIC2 and PFIC3 are caused by defective transport of bile components, whereas PFIC1 results from a failure to maintain canalicular membrane lipid asymmetry and fluidity.[232] Genetic mutations causing PFIC4 (tight junction protein 2 [TJP2] defect) and PFIC5 (farnesoid receptor [NR1H4] defect) have been described in the past decade.[233-235] More recently, the MYO5B defect causing cholestatic liver disease in children with microvillous inclusion disease (MID) has also been recognized,[236] and newer defects (e.g., cholestasis, acute liver failure, and neurodegeneration [CALFAN]) continue to be discovered.[237] The advent of a comprehensive neonatal cholestatic gene panel has helped in identification of many new novel genetic defects and has considerably eased the ability to diagnose a large proportion of these cases, which were idiopathic until 5 years ago.[238,239]

When PFIC is suspected, measurements of serum GGT, another canalicular protein, provides the major clue. Only PFIC3 is characterized by high GGT levels, whereas PFIC1 and PFIC2, along with TJP2, FXR, and MYO5B defects, are referred to as *low* (normal) GGT cholestatic disorders (see Table 55.7). Liver biopsy played a critical role in the diagnosis of PFIC disorders until the recent past and is now more useful to assess the extent of liver injury in these disorders. Molecular genetic testing for all of these genes is currently the gold standard for diagnosis.[238,240] Gene sequencing of the individual genes causing PFIC 1, 2, or 3 has in fact revealed over 154 different variants of mutations, suggesting that additional variants remain to be detected.[241]

Progressive Familial Intrahepatic Cholestasis Type 1

PFIC1 (also known as *ATP8B1 disease, FIC1 disease*, or *Byler disease*) is a multisystemic disease caused by mutations in the *ATP8B1* gene located on chromosome 18q21.[242] The *ATP8B1* gene product, FIC1, is a P-type adenosine triphosphatase that acts as a lipid "flippase," internalizing phosphatidylserine from the outer to the inner leaflet of the canalicular membrane. This activity has been found to be crucial in maintaining lipid asymmetry of the membrane. Before identification of the causative gene and its mutations, PFIC1 was referred to as *Byler disease,* named after the Amish kindred in whom the disease was first described. Patients with PFIC1 typically develop jaundice, extreme pruritus, coagulopathy, and growth failure within the first several months of life. Laboratory studies usually reveal elevated levels of ALT, AST, alkaline phosphatase, and bile acids. However, the serum level of GGT is normal or low, despite the presence of cholestasis. Liver disease caused by PFIC1 is progressive and leads to the development of cirrhosis by 20 years of age.

Other entities caused by mutations in *ATP8B1* include the allelic disorder benign recurrent intrahepatic cholestasis 1 (BRIC1; OMIM 243300),[242,243] which is a milder, nonprogressive form that manifests with recurrent bouts of cholestasis and pruritus, and Greenland familial cholestasis, which is a form of PFIC1 seen in the Inuit population.

Histologically, PFIC1 is characterized by the presence of bland intracanalicular cholestasis, small uniform-appearing hepatocytes, canalicular bile plugs, and minimal or no inflammation (Fig. 55.16A). Ultimately, a micronodular pattern of fibrosis and cirrhosis develops with disease progression. Transmission electron microscopy is useful in distinguishing PFIC1 from other causes of cholestasis. In PFIC1, the canalicular bile is coarse and granular, commonly referred to as *Byler bile*[244] (see Fig. 55.16B).

The *ATP8B1* gene is expressed in several nonhepatic tissues (e.g., acinar cells of the pancreas and ileal and colonic enterocytes). Consequently, patients with PFIC1 may also show a variety of extrahepatic manifestations, including chronic diarrhea, pancreatic insufficiency, pancreatitis, and elevated sweat chloride levels.[245] Chronic diarrhea and pancreatitis persist, and they are even exacerbated after liver transplantation. This is because of restoration of normal hepatic secretion of bile salts into bile and an impaired ability of intestinal epithelium to reabsorb bile salts for return to the enterohepatic circulation. Histologically, no definite abnormality was noted in a case report with preserved brush border staining in the ileum.[246] Therefore the recommended treatment of choice is surgical interruption of the enterohepatic circulation of bile acids by either partial external biliary diversion or partial ileal exclusion.[247]

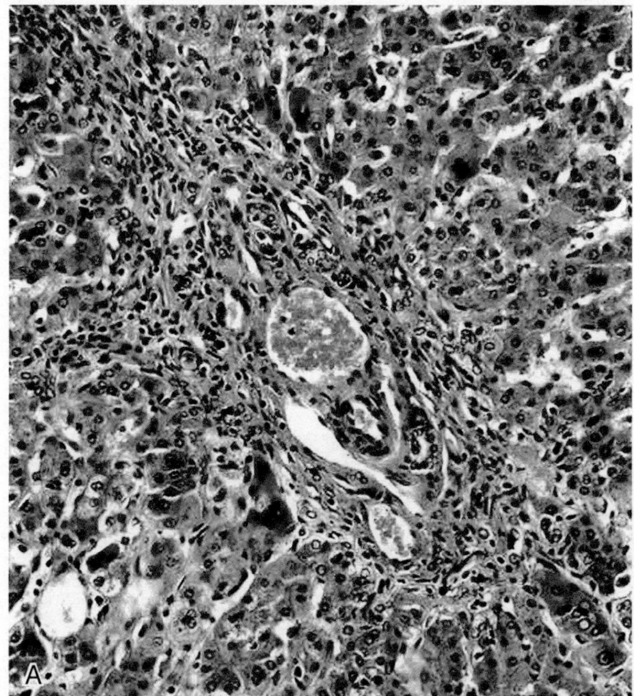

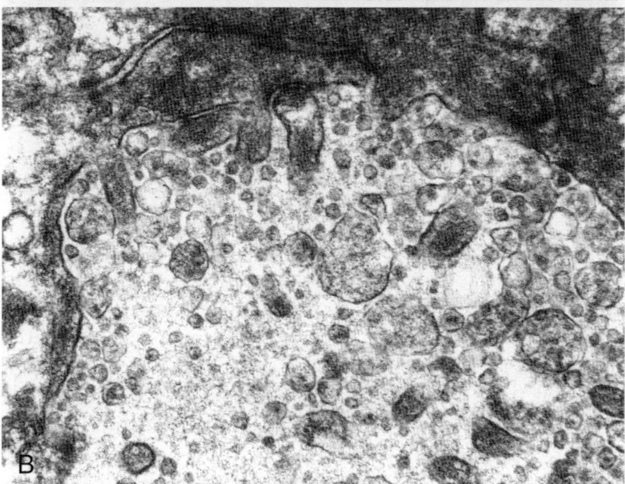

FIGURE 55.16 Progressive familial intrahepatic cholestasis type 1. A, Severe parenchymal cholestasis, lobular disarray, and portal tract expansion with evolving fibrosis are seen. All portal tract structures are present (i.e., portal vein, hepatic artery, interlobular bile duct). There are no giant cells. **B,** Electron microscopy shows dilated canaliculus filled with coarse, granular biliary material. Canalicular microvilli are reduced in number, and the pericanalicular ectoplasm is thickened. Intercellular tight junctions are intact. (*Courtesy Dr. Alberto Quaglia, King's College, London.*)

Progressive Familial Intrahepatic Cholestasis Type 2

PFIC2 (also called *ABCB11 disease* or *BSEP disease*) is caused by mutations in the *ABCB11* gene,[248] in which more than 100 different mutations have been described.[249] The *ABCB11* gene encodes for the major canalicular bile salt transporter, BSEP. Like PFIC1, PFIC2 manifests in infancy as severe cholestasis, pruritus, jaundice, malabsorption of fats and fat-soluble vitamins, and failure to thrive. Laboratory studies show elevated serum levels of ALT and AST and normal or low serum GGT levels. Liver disease in patients with PFIC2 is more severe than in patients with PFIC1. Rapid progression to end-stage cirrhosis typically occurs within the first decade of life. Liver biopsies from patients with PFIC2 reveal neonatal hepatitis with hepatocellular disarray, edema, inflammation, giant cell transformation, and, ultimately, portal fibrosis (Fig. 55.17).[250] Several cases of HCC and cholangiocarcinoma have been reported as well.[54] Ultrastructurally, the bile in PFIC2 is amorphous or filamentous.

van Mil and colleagues[251] identified eight distinct mutations in *ABCB11* in eight different families whose members had recurrent bouts of cholestasis similar to BRIC1 but without *ATP8B1* mutations. This disorder has now been termed *BRIC2* (OMIM 605479) (Table 55.18). It is more often associated with cholelithiasis compared with BRIC1. Liver biopsies typically show cholestasis with hepatocyte swelling.

Progressive Familial Intrahepatic Cholestasis Type 3

PFIC3 (also called *ABCB4 disease* or *MDR3 disease*) is caused by mutations in the *ABCB4* gene located on chromosome 7q21, which codes for MDR3.[252] Mutations in *ABCB4* have also been linked to intrahepatic cholestasis of pregnancy.[253] MDR3 is a "floppase" in the canalicular membrane of hepatocytes that translocates phosphatidylcholine to the outer leaflet of the membrane, from which it is extruded by bile salts. Under normal conditions, extruded phosphatidylcholine complexes with bile salts to form mixed micelles, thereby protecting the biliary epithelium from the detergent action of secreted bile salts and constituting the fundamental mechanism by which phospholipid (and with it, cholesterol) are secreted into bile.[254] In the absence of secreted phosphatidylcholine, the biliary epithelium becomes damaged, and GGT is released into the systemic circulation. Markedly elevated serum GGT levels distinguish PFIC3 from PFIC1 and PFIC2, both of which exhibit normal serum levels of GGT.[255]

Similar to PFIC1 and PFIC2, PFIC3 manifests clinically as jaundice, pruritus, hepatomegaly, and elevated serum liver enzymes. Unlike PFIC1 and PFIC2, the age at onset is variable, ranging from 1 month to 20 years. The liver disease is progressive and eventually leads to the development of fibrosis and cirrhosis.[256]

The liver in PFIC3 exhibits extensive bile ductular proliferation, portal inflammation, and fibrosis[257] (Fig. 55.18). These findings are nonspecific and may be confused with extrahepatic biliary obstruction. Bile duct paucity has also been reported by the same group.[258] Hepatocellular carcinomas are reported to develop in PFIC 3 patients.[55]

Progressive Familial Cholestasis Type 4 (Tight Junction Protein Defect)

Defects in TJP2 protein were identified in 2014 in a group of children with low GGT cholestasis without mutations in *ATP8B1* or *ABCB11* genes.[233] They have a homozygous mutation in *TJP2* located on 9q21.11. The children presented in the first 3 months of life with normal/low GGT, and there was a high incidence of consanguinity. Extrahepatic manifestations involving neurological and respiratory systems have been reported. Liver biopsy studies are limited but show a bland cholestasis with progressive fibrosis (Fig. 55.19A–D). Immunohistochemistry for TJP2 shows complete absence of staining, and there is also reduced staining

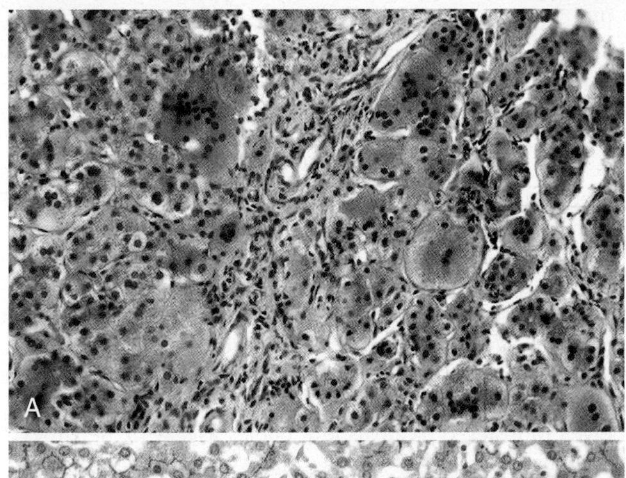

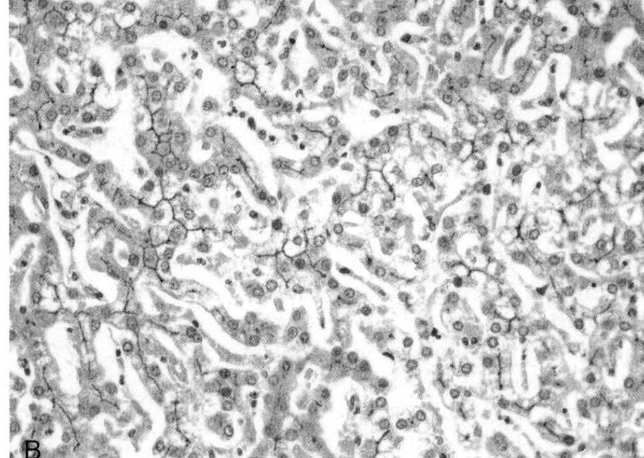

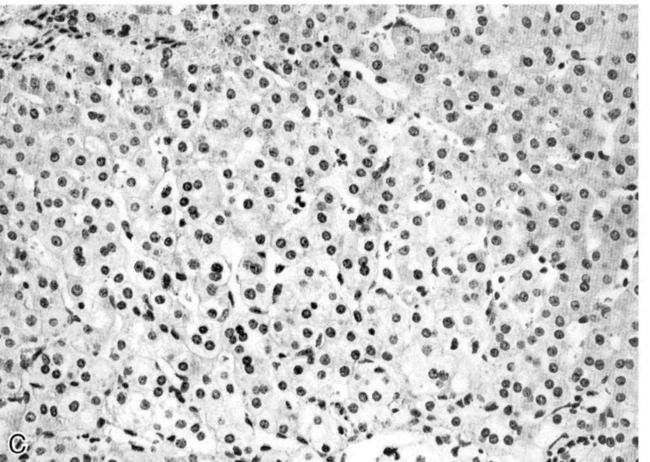

FIGURE 55.17 Progressive familial intrahepatic cholestasis type 2. A, Neonatal hepatitis with prominent giant cell transformation, portal tract expansion, and lobular inflammation. **B,** Bile salt export protein in normal liver decorates all canalicular membranes. **C,** No bile salt export protein is found in an affected 3-month-old patient.

for claudin-1 in canaliculi. HCC has been documented in these livers.[56] Liver transplantation appears to be the only treatment at this time.

Progressive Familial Intrahepatic Cholestasis Type 5 (Farnesoid X Receptor Deficiency, NR1H4 Defect)

The farnesoid X receptor (FXR) is a nuclear receptor and transcription factor encoded by the *NR1H4* gene located on 12q23.1.[259] The FXR plays an important role in the regulation of bile acids and is involved in regulation of other cholestatic genes such as ABCB11 and ABCB4. Children present at an early age with low to normal GGT cholestasis with elevated AST and ALT. There is marked elevation of serum α-fetoprotein (AFP). Liver failure develops in the first 2 years of life and warrants liver transplantation. Liver biopsies show ductular reaction, diffuse giant cell transformation, and ballooning of hepatocytes and intralobular cholestasis, progressing to cirrhosis over time. Liver immunohistochemistry has shown absence of BSEP protein expression with preserved MDR3 expression in the canaliculi.

Cholestatic Liver Disease of Microvillous Inclusion Disease (MYO5B Defect)

MID is a cause of intractable diarrhea in children resulting from *MYO5B* mutations, and it necessitates intestinal transplantation. A subgroup of these patients develops a neonatal cholestatic disease first reported by Girard et al. in 2014.[236] The cholestasis may precede or follow intestinal transplantation. It was characterized by intermittent jaundice, intractable pruritus, increased serum bile acids, and normal GGT levels. Liver histology shows canalicular cholestasis with varying degrees of fibrosis and markedly decreased to absent BSEP staining (Fig 55.19E–F). A subgroup of these patients develops progressive paucity of bile ducts. Ultrastructural abnormalities in canalicular microvilli are reported.[236] A subsequent report also mentioned cholestasis in *MYO5b* mutations with normal GGT levels but without associated MID.[260] Biliary diversion appears to be helpful in treating the symptoms of cholestasis, though liver-intestinal transplantation may be necessary in severe cases.

Differential Diagnosis

Clinically, PFIC1, 2, 4, or 5 should be suspected in any neonate or infant who develops progressive symptomatic cholestasis and has elevated serum bile acid levels and low to normal serum GGT levels. On liver biopsy, bland intracanalicular cholestasis is more often seen in PFIC1 than in the other types of PFIC; the latter more commonly reveal a neonatal hepatitis pattern. Ultrastructural analysis will show coarse Byler bile in PFIC1. Several rare disorders, including inborn errors of bile acid synthesis (described earlier), familial hypercholanemia, and ARC syndrome (*a*rthrogryposis, *r*enal dysfunction, and *c*holestasis, discussed in the next section) also manifest with low-GGT cholestasis and should be considered in the differential diagnosis. PFIC3 is characterized by elevated serum levels of GGT. PFIC4 and PFIC5 still do not have specific histological features

TABLE 55.18 Inherited Disorders of Bile Acid Synthesis and Transport*

Common Names	Gene	Chromosome	Function	Location	Diseases
FIC1	*ATP8B1*	18q21.3	Phosphatidylserine "flippase"	Hepatocyte canalicular (apical) membrane; cholangiocytes, enterocytes	PFIC1, BRIC1, Byler disease, Byler syndrome
BSEP	*ABCB11*	2q31	Bile salts exporter	Hepatocyte canalicular (apical) membrane	PFIC2, BRIC2
MDR3	*ABCB4*	7q21	Phosphatidylcholine "flippase"	Hepatocyte canalicular (apical) membrane	PFIC3, ICP
TJP2 defect	*TJP2*	9q21.11	Maintain junctional integrity	Hepatocyte canalicular membrane	PFIC4
FXR	*NR1H4*	12q23.1	Bile acid homeostasis	Nuclear receptor	PFIC5
MRP2 (cMOAT)	*ABCC2*	10q24	Anionic transporter	Hepatocyte, enterocyte, kidney tubular epithelium: apical membranes	Dubin-Johnson syndrome
OATP1B1 and OATP1B3	*SLCO1B1* and *SLCO1B3*	12p	Organic anion (bilirubin glucuronide) transporter	Hepatocyte sinusoidal membrane	Rotor syndrome
CFTR	*CFTR*	7q31.2	Chloride ion transporter	Bronchial epithelium, enterocyte, bile duct epithelium, pancreatic ductal epithelium: apical membranes	Cystic fibrosis
IBST	*SLC10A2*	13q33	Bile salt/sodium transporter	Cholangiocytes, intestine: apical membranes	PBAM
ATP7B	*ATP7B*	13q14.3	Copper transporter	Hepatocyte endoplasmic reticulum	Wilson disease

ATP7B, *ATPase, Cu++ transporting, beta polypeptide;* BRIC, *benign recurrent intrahepatic cholestasis;* BSEP, *bile salt export pump;* CFTR, *cystic fibrosis transmembrane conductance regulator;* cMOAT, *canalicular multispecific organic anion transporter;* FIC, *familial intrahepatic cholestasis;* IBST, *intestinal bile salt transporter;* ICP, *intrahepatic cholestasis of pregnancy;* MRP, *multidrug-resistance protein;* OATP, *organic anion transporter protein B;* PBAM, *primary bile acid malabsorption;* PFIC, *progressive familial intrahepatic cholestasis.*

**Also refer to Table 55.10.*

to distinguish and should be suspected in any low/normal GGT neonatal cholestasis in which PFIC1 and PFIC2 have been excluded. Immunohistochemistry is very useful, and genetic analysis will provide the correct diagnosis in most cases.

Natural History

Patients with PFIC1 or PFIC2 develop cholestasis as neonates or infants. Liver damage is progressive and leads to cirrhosis during the course of several years. Death caused by liver failure is common within the first or second decade of life. PFIC3 has a more variable time of presentation but eventually results in cirrhosis. The development of HCC and cholangiocarcinoma has been well-documented in patients with PFIC2. It appears that protein-truncating mutations have a greater risk of leading to malignancy than missense mutations.[249] As mentioned earlier, HCC has also been reported associated with MDR3 and TJP2 defects.[55,56]

Liver transplantation resolves the cholestatic phenotype in these disorders, but extrahepatic symptoms, such as diarrhea and failure to thrive, remain.[261] At least four patients with BSEP deficiency have been reported to develop autoantibodies to BSEP after liver transplantation, presumably because of lack of immune tolerance mediated by self-antigen exposure during development. Such antibodies have caused recurrence of cholestasis by targeting BSEP protein in the graft. Although several such patients with recurrent BSEP disease after transplantation have undergone repeat transplantation, it appears that the antibody response may be effectively controlled by altering the immunosuppressive regimen.[262,263] Patients with PFIC1 develop severe steatosis in the allograft liver as a manifestation of disease recurrence.[264]

Patients with BRIC2 usually have a milder course of disease characterized by intervening periods of normal liver function. However, some patients have developed permanent cholestasis later in life.[251]

Arthrogryposis, Renal Dysfunction, and Cholestasis Syndrome

ARC syndrome is a rare, autosomal recessive, multisystemic disorder characterized by germline mutations in two endosomal vesicular trafficking proteins: VPS33B and VIPAS39 (also called *VIPAR*).[265,266] Affected individuals have low-GGT cholestatic jaundice in the newborn period. Liver biopsy shows bland canalicular and hepatocyte cholestasis with multinucleated hepatocytes. Biopsy in these individuals is associated with a significant risk of

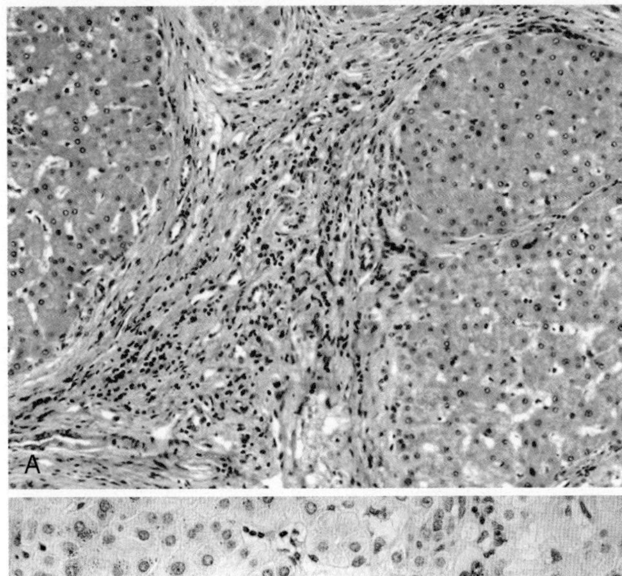

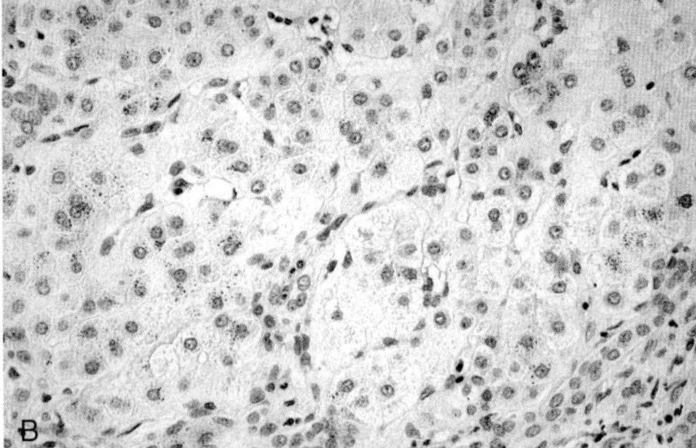

FIGURE 55.18 Progressive familial intrahepatic cholestasis type 3. A, Cirrhotic liver with bile ductular proliferation and cholangitis. **B,** Rhodanine stain reveals abundant copper *(red granules),* as in all chronic cholestatic diseases.

hemorrhage, presumably because of an associated platelet storage pool defect.[265] Therefore molecular analyses are extremely important to confirm the diagnosis. Recognition of this syndrome in the absence of arthrogryposis is challenging.[267]

Familial Hypercholanemia

Familial hypercholanemia (FHCA) is a low-GGT cholestatic disorder that is characterized by elevated serum bile acids and fat malabsorption. FHCA is caused by mutations in three genes: *TJP2*, *BAAT*, and *EPHX1*.[268] *BAAT* mutations lead to failure of conjugation of bile acids to glycine or taurine. The inheritance pattern can be oligogenic, with genotypes of both *BAAT* and *TJP2* influencing the phenotype.[269] Liver biopsy findings may reveal only mild cholestasis. Patients usually respond to treatment with ursodeoxycholic acid.

Other extremely rare disorders that lead to defective bile acid transport and secretion and cause neonatal cholestasis include the syndrome of ichthyosis, leukocyte vacuoles, alopecia, and sclerosing cholangitis (ILVASC), which is caused by mutations in the claudin-1 gene *(CLDN1)*.[270] Readers are referred to other publications for details on these disorders.[2]

Cystic Fibrosis

CF is the most common lethal genetic disease in Caucasians, with an incidence of 1 in 2500 live births.[271] This autosomal recessive disease is caused by mutations in the cystic fibrosis transmembrane conductance regulator *(CFTR)* gene; the CFTR protein is important in the maintenance of fluid balance across epithelial cells.[272] The basic defect lies in the production of thickened secretions in the airways and glandular ducts, which results from abnormal electrolyte transport. Organs affected in CF include the lungs, pancreas, salivary and sweat glands, biliary tree, liver, and intestines.

Clinical Features

Phenotypic expression of CF is extremely heterogeneous. Meconium ileus and failure to thrive are key features in infants. The diagnosis relies on a combination of clinical features, biochemical testing, and radiological assessment. Chronic liver disease is one of the major complications of CF. In infants, the most common hepatic features are cholestasis and hepatomegaly. Laboratory studies in infants with liver involvement reveal elevated serum levels of AST, ALT, alkaline phosphatase, and GGT.

Pathogenesis

The genetic defect in CF resides in the gene responsible for the CFTR protein, which maintains fluid balance across epithelial cells. This cyclic adenosine monophosphate (AMP)-dependent chloride channel is responsible for transmembrane efflux of chloride ions (Cl^-). Under physiological conditions, cyclic AMP-stimulated chloride secretion through the low-conductance CFTR channels imposes a negative luminal potential and an osmotic gradient that triggers passive secretion of sodium ions (Na^+) and water. The apical chloride gradient also facilitates extrusion of bicarbonate (HCO_3^-) into the lumen via Cl^-/HCO_3^- exchange. In the biliary tract, this causes biliary alkalinization, which is required for proper digestive function.

Because chloride exchange is critical for transepithelial fluid transport, all epithelia involved in the movement of water are potentially affected by defective CFTR function. In particular, the epithelia of the bronchopulmonary tree, the pancreatic ducts, the hepatobiliary duct system, and the intestines are unable to maintain proper fluid secretion. Hence a tenacious, mucus-rich substance accumulates in the respiratory passages and in the ducts of the pancreas and liver. This results from a failure to secrete the fluid that is needed to mobilize proteinaceous secretions away from these passageways.

The CFTR protein undergoes a "life cycle"[273] with several stages:

1. Biosynthesis, conformational maturation in the endoplasmic reticulum, and trafficking from the endoplasmic reticulum to the plasma membrane
2. Endocytic retrieval from the plasma membrane to early or sorting endosomes
3. Recycling of endocytosed CFTR back to the cell surface
4. Targeting of endocytosed CFTR for degradation

More than 900 mutations of the *CFTR* gene on chromosome 7 have been described.[273] The predominant, but by no means the only, clinically significant mutation is *ΔF508*,

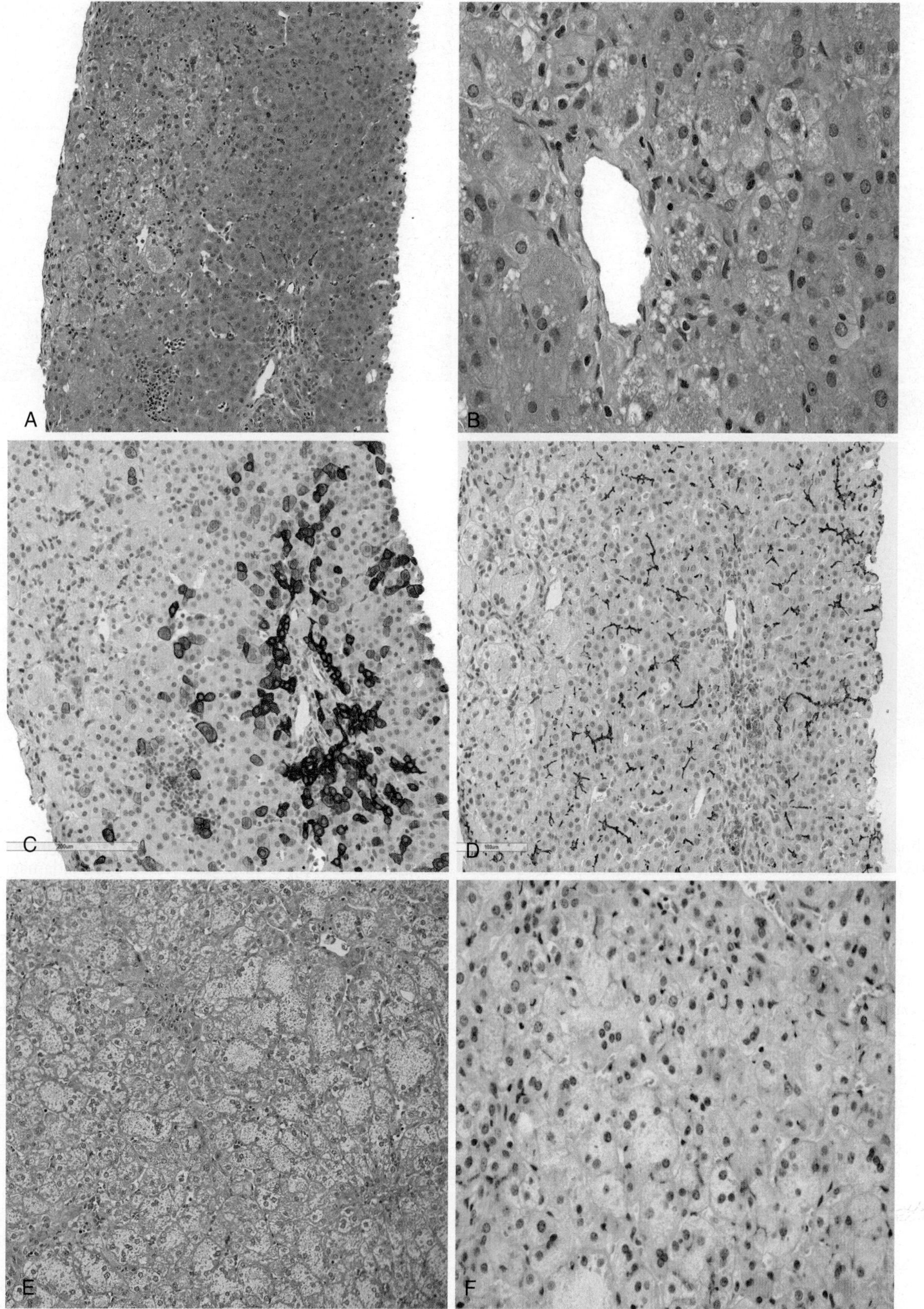

FIGURE 55.19 Progressive familial intrahepatic cholestasis type 4 (TJP2 defect) and MYO5B defect. A, H&E stain showing variable giant cell hepatitis pattern. **B,** Closer view of giant cells with cholestasis. **C,** CK7 stain highlighting periportal ectopic staining with ductular reaction and inconspicuous bile duct. **D,** BSEP stain showing decreased staining in giant cell areas only. **E,** H&E-stained section of MYO5B defect–associated liver biopsy with giant cell hepatitis pattern. **F,** BSEP stain showing decreased canalicular staining.

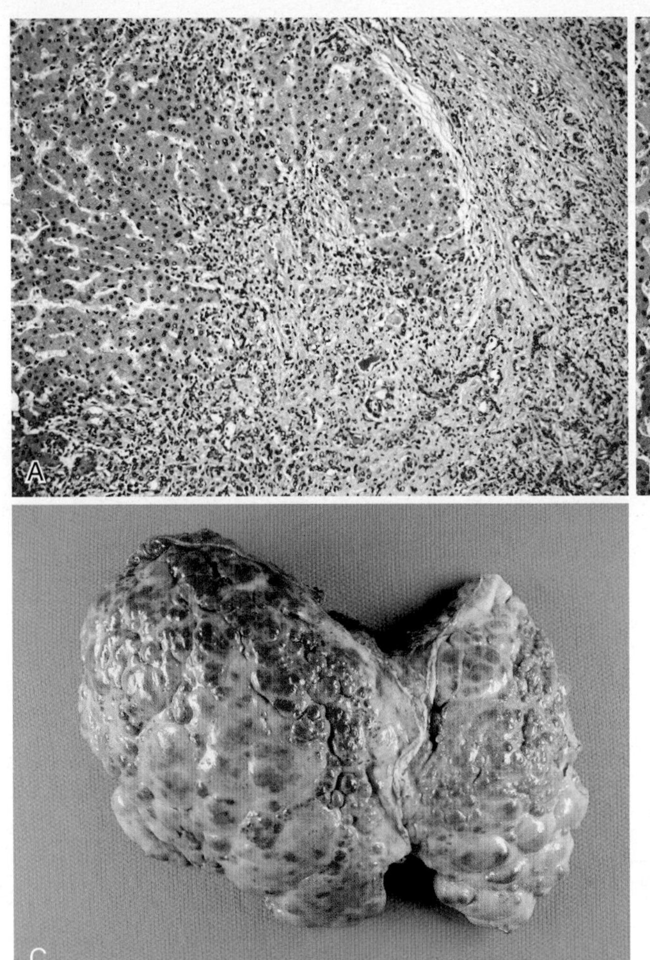
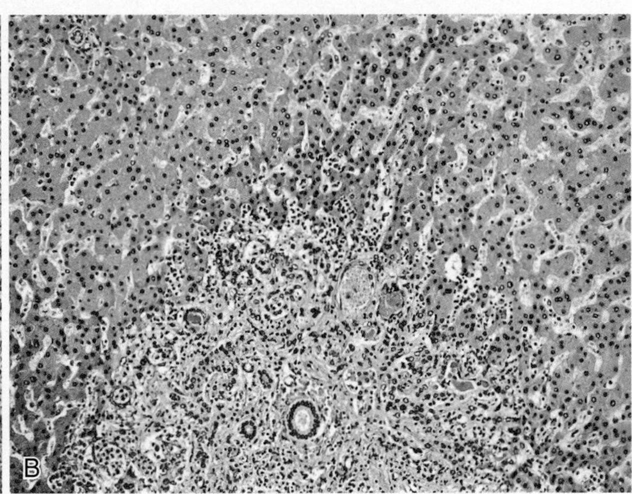

FIGURE 55.20 Cystic fibrosis. A, Severe portal inflammation and duct proliferation. **B,** Bile plugs in ducts are often pink as well as yellow. There is no bile seen in the canaliculi, and there are no hepatocytes retaining bile, despite the "obstructive" pattern in the tracts, reflecting the focal nature of the process. **C,** Explant of cirrhotic liver with macronodularity and no obvious bile.

which is found in 70% of patients with CF. The mutation in *ΔF508* causes deletion of a phenylalanine at position 508, which results in the development of an immature protein that is not fully glycosylated. Instead, the translated peptide misfolds within the endoplasmic reticulum and is recognized by the quality control machinery of the endoplasmic reticulum. It is ubiquitinated and targeted for proteasomal degradation. Although CFTR is not the only cellular mechanism for chloride transport, failed delivery of ΔF508-CFTR to the plasma membrane leads to impaired epithelial fluid transport and, thus to the clinical manifestations of CF. A newly described *CFTR* mutation (c.3871G > T) was discovered in a 2-month-old infant in whom all signs pointed to EHBA.[274] More recent data suggest interactions between CFTR and the Src family of tyrosine kinases in cholangiocytes as a mechanism to maintain toll-like receptor proteins, especially TLR4 in an inactive state. Defects in this interaction caused by *CFTR* mutations lead to phosphorylation of TLR4 and its activation, resulting in activation of downstream signaling pathways in response to lipopolysaccharide recognition and subsequent inflammation in response to gut microbiota.[275]

Pathological Features

Liver involvement occurs in 20% to 50% of patients with CF, and the prevalence increases with age. Rarely, infants develop giant cell hepatitis.[276] More often (in a third of infants with CF), a chronic form of biliary damage develops because of failure to adequately secrete bile. Viscous, glycoprotein-rich bile plugs the intrahepatic biliary tree; this is the source of the historical term *mucoviscidosis* (Fig. 55.20). In neonates and infants, the histological findings are typically nonspecific and include portal edema, bile ductular proliferation, inflammation, and early fibrosis. Neonatal hepatitis, paucity of intrahepatic bile ducts, and steatosis can also be present.

Hypoplasia of the extrahepatic bile ducts has been described in CF, which, together with the presence of bile ductular proliferation, may be confused with EHBA. With time, chronic biliary plugging leads to inflammation and portal tract scarring. Expanded portal tracts contain bile ducts filled with inspissated granular eosinophilic material, bile ductular proliferation, cholangitis, fibrosis, and chronic inflammation. Focal biliary fibrosis, the classic lesion of CF, may develop by adolescence.[271] Ultrasound shows evidence of nodularity within the liver in children without significant alterations in liver enzymes and is now a recommended method for following children older than 6 years of age with CF liver disease.[277] Obliterative portal venopathy is now being increasingly recognized in children with portal hypertension in CF patients.[278]

Natural History

The median survival time in patients with CF now exceeds 30 years. With improvement in therapy and long-term care of these patients, liver complications have emerged as a significant medical issue.[279,280] Liver disease is now considered the third most common cause of death after cardiorespiratory and lung transplantation complications. It accounts for approximately 2% of the overall mortality rate in CF. Oral administration of ursodeoxycholic acid stimulates secretion of bile and is free from serious side effects. Gene therapy and drugs that correct the CFTR protein are therapeutic approaches currently in the experimental phase.[281]

Aagenaes Syndrome

Aagenaes syndrome, also referred to as *cholestasis-lymphedema syndrome*, is a rare autosomal recessive disorder that clinically manifests as intermittent cholestasis and lower-limb edema.[282] The genetic locus has been mapped to chromosome 15q, but the molecular defect is unknown.[283] It was reported initially in a Norwegian kindred but has also been described in other ethnic groups. A neonatal hepatitis syndrome that evolves slowly into a chronic cholestatic condition is characteristic. There may be localized lower limb lymphedema or more subtle generalized edema despite normal serum albumin levels. These lymphatic abnormalities manifest clinically later than in neonatal jaundice. This cholestatic condition also shows clinical features of pruritus and deficiencies in fat-soluble vitamins.

DISORDERS OF CARBOHYDRATE METABOLISM

Glycogen Storage Diseases

Classification and Clinical Features

GSDs are mostly inherited in an autosomal recessive manner. They include disorders with a wide variety of enzymatic defects (see Table 55.12),[284,285] all of which lead to hepatomegaly caused by massive retention of glycogen within the liver. Three types, GSD Ia, Ib, and III, manifest with hypoglycemia in infancy because of the inability of infants to maintain steady blood glucose levels between feedings. GSD type I has an overall incidence of approximately 1 in 100,000 births.[286] In addition to hypoglycemia, hyperlipidemia, hyperuricemia, and neutropenia (in type Ib) are well-known manifestations of GSD type I. Hepatomegaly and hypoglycemia are also common manifestations of GSD type III, although typically the onset of fasting-induced hypoglycemia is gradual compared with type I. GSD type IV does not manifest clinically with hypoglycemia; more commonly, there is progressive liver cirrhosis in infancy or early childhood. This disorder may be suspected prenatally based on polyhydramnios, decreased fetal movement, and dilated cardiomyopathy. Early perinatal death may also occur.[287] Hypoglycemia is rare unless the patient develops liver failure. Clinical presentation later in life includes congestive cardiac failure, skeletal muscle weakness, and sensorineural hearing loss.

In all types of GSD, the diagnosis is established by biochemical demonstration of the specific enzyme defect and aided by identification of mutations in the genes. GSD types Ia, Ib, III, and IV primarily cause cytosolic accumulation of glycogen within hepatocytes, and hepatic involvement is the predominant manifestation. GSD types II, VI, and IX are not discussed in this chapter; type II, a lysosomal storage disease, manifests primarily with cardiac and skeletal myopathy, and types VI and IX are very rare causes of hepatomegaly in children.[288]

Pathogenesis

GSD type I (von Gierke disease) is caused by failure of terminal dephosphorylation of glucose-6-phosphate (G6P) by the enzyme glucose-6-phosphatase (G6Pase).[289] The action of G6Pase enables release of glucose, which is derived from glycogen breakdown and gluconeogenesis, into the circulation. It is responsible for 80% of hepatic glucose production. GSD type Ia is caused by mutations in the *G6PC* gene, which encodes for the catalytic subunit of G6Pase. GSD type Ib is caused by mutations in the *SLC37A4* gene, which encodes for the G6P transporter. The catalytic subunit is active on the luminal aspect of the endoplasmic reticulum, and the transporter normally delivers the substrate (G6P) from the cytoplasm into the endoplasmic reticulum (Fig. 55.21). Therefore deficiency in either the catalytic subunit or the transporter leads to an inability of the liver to convert G6P into glucose.

GSD type III (also called *Forbes disease* or *limit dextrinosis*) is caused by a defect in amylo-1,6-glucosidase, the glycogen debranching enzyme encoded by the *AGL* gene. Both Type IIIa (muscle and liver) and IIIb (only liver) are associated with distinct variants of the *AGL* gene.[290] The abnormal glycogen stored in cells has short outer chains. Most mutations in *AGL* are inconsequential, with only a handful accounting for disease.[27]

GSD type IV (Andersen disease) arises from a defect in 1,4-α-glucan branching enzyme 1, which is encoded by the *GBE1* gene. A deficiency in this glycogen branching enzyme leads to marked accumulation of amylopectin-like polysaccharides within tissues. Multiple mutations have been described, with variable degrees of clinical severity.[291-293]

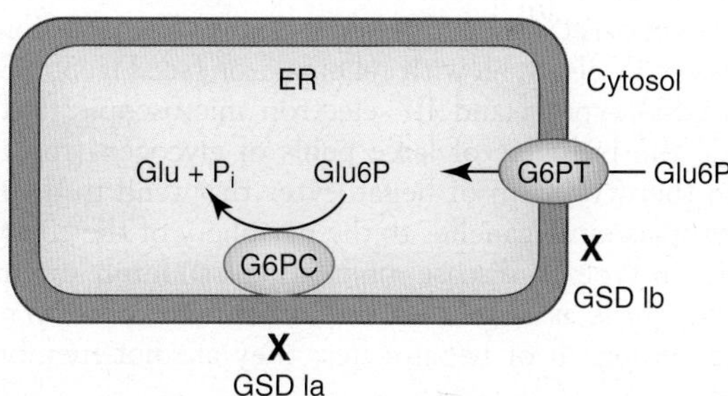

FIGURE 55.21 Subcellular location and function of glucose-6-phosphate translocase *(G6PT)* and glucose-6-phosphatase, catalytic subunit *(G6PC)*, the two proteins affected in glycogen storage disease *(GSD)* type I. G6PC is located within the lumen of the endoplasmic reticulum *(ER)*, where it catalyzes the terminal step in gluconeogenesis and glycogenolysis to release free glucose. Mutations in the *G6PC* gene cause GSD type Ia. G6PT, encoded by the *SLC37A4* gene, is an ER membrane transporter that regulates the rate-limiting step of glucose-6-phosphate transport into the ER lumen. Mutations in *SLC37A4* lead to GSD type Ib. P_i, inorganic phosphate.

Pathological Features

On gross inspection, the liver in patients with GSD is typically enlarged, smooth, and pale in appearance. A fine reticular pattern of fibrosis is often present, and this feature may be prominent in GSD types III and IV. Types III and IV may exhibit frank micronodular cirrhosis or mixed micronodular and macronodular cirrhosis. Hepatic adenomas, and even HCC, can develop in patients with GSD type I or III.[40] Steatosis is a notable feature in both types I and III.

Histologically, GSDs are characterized by the presence of enlarged hepatocytes (≥2× normal size) with wispy, pink, rarified cytoplasm and a centrally placed nucleus[284] (Fig. 55.22). The hepatocyte cell membranes are thickened because of displacement of intracellular organelles to the periphery of the cytoplasm as a result of excess stored glycogen. As such, the hepatocytes appear similar to plant cells. Intracellular lipid vacuoles are often present as well, particularly in GSD types I and III. Glycogenated nuclei may be evident in periportal hepatocytes. Perivenular Mallory bodies and peliosis hepatis may be observed in GSD type Ia.[294] Fibrosis and cirrhosis occur most commonly in GSD type IV but may also occur in type III.

Excess cytoplasmic glycogen stains brightly with PAS stain (see Fig. 55.22). However, washout of glycogen that occurs during formalin fixation may result in less intense staining. Glycogen is better preserved in alcohol-fixed tissues. Regardless of the type of fixative used, the glycogen is digested by diastase in GSD types I and III.

As mentioned earlier, a distinctive feature of GSD type I is the development of hepatic adenomas.[295] Abnormalities of chromosome 6 have been described only in GSD type 1a adenomas, with reduced insulin-like growth factor 2 receptor (IGF2R) and large tumor suppressor kinase 1 (LATS1) in more than 50% of tumors.[296] A distinctive feature of GSD type IV disease is the presence of pale, or lightly eosinophilic, ground-glass inclusions within hepatocytes (Fig. 55.23). Inclusions are usually most notable in the periportal zone but may be present anywhere in the hepatic lobule. In both formalin- and alcohol-fixed tissue, inclusions stain intensely positive with the PAS stain. Because GSD type IV is caused by a defect in a branching enzyme that results in long, insoluble polymerized strands of glycogen, the inclusions are resistant to diastase digestion and remain positive on d-PAS–stained tissue sections. The inclusions in GSD type IV also stain with colloidal iron (see Fig. 55.23D).

In GSD types I and III, electron microscopic findings include the presence of large pools of glycogen (rosettes) within the cytoplasm of hepatocytes that tend to displace the cytoplasmic organelles to the periphery of the cell (Fig. 55.24). In type IV disease, undulating, randomly oriented, delicate fibrils as large as 5 nm in diameter occupy most of the cytoplasm of hepatocytes; they are not membrane bound.

Natural History

Patients with GSD type I or III may survive into adulthood if they do not die in infancy. The primary goal of therapy is to maintain blood glucose levels higher than 70 g/dL. This may be achieved by infusion of glucose-containing solutions into the stomach or by constant administration of uncooked cornstarch, or both. Surviving patients manifest metabolic and systemic derangements throughout childhood and into adulthood. Liver fibrosis may progress to cirrhosis in GSD III. Progressive myopathy and cardiomyopathy may cause morbidity in adults.[290]

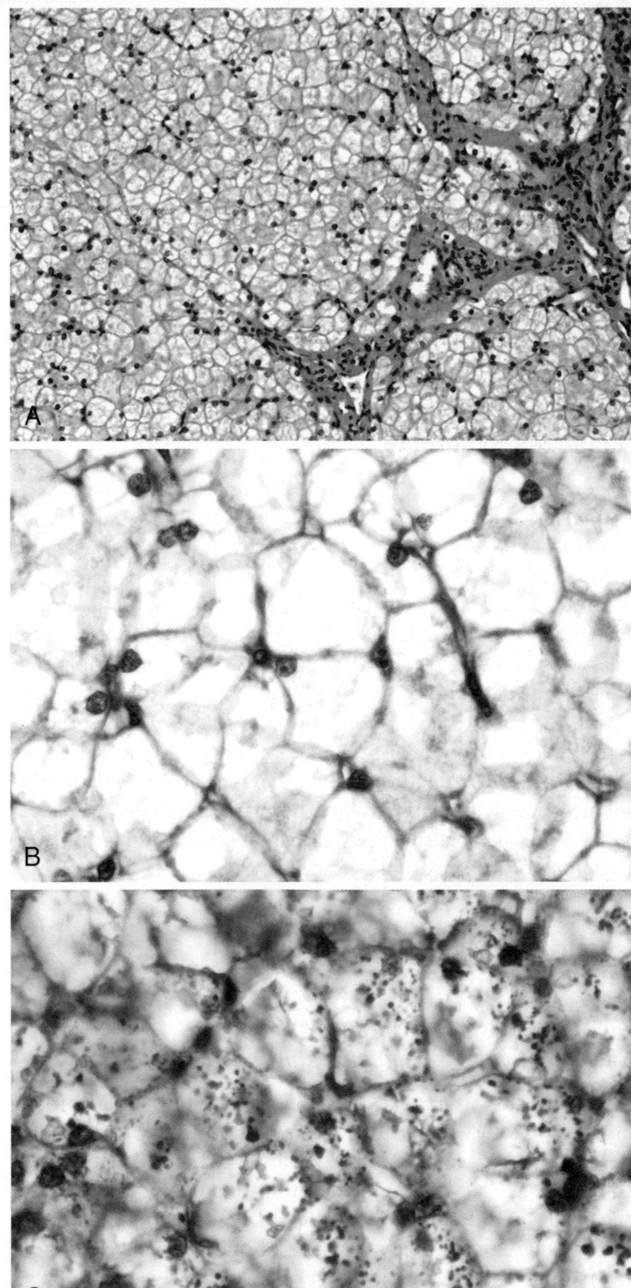

FIGURE 55.22 Glycogen storage disease type I. A, Minimal inflammation, portal and periportal septal fibrosis, and enlarged hepatocytes with flocculent cytoplasm is present. **B,** Hepatocytes have prominent plasma membranes, displaced nuclei, and flocculent cytoplasm. **C,** PAS-stained tissue section shows scattered glycogen deposits throughout the cytoplasm.

Liver transplantation is curative, although renal damage is common in patients with type I disease and persists after liver transplantation. Liver failure related to end-stage GSD type IV is treated by liver transplantation. However, transplantation may not mitigate disease progression in other viscera, notably the heart. In one study, 9 of 14 patients undergoing liver transplantation survived at least 10 years,

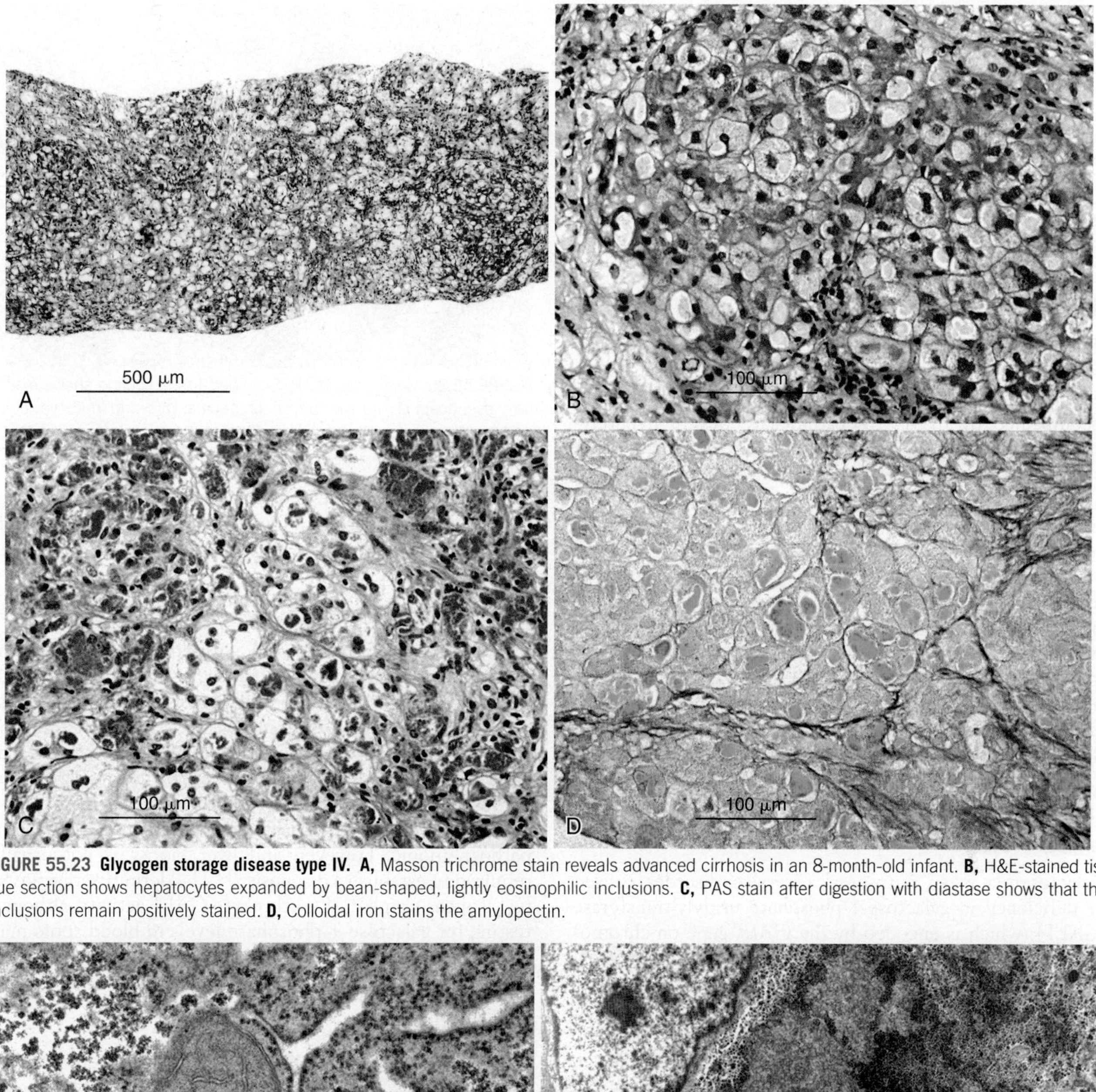

FIGURE 55.23 Glycogen storage disease type IV. A, Masson trichrome stain reveals advanced cirrhosis in an 8-month-old infant. **B,** H&E-stained tissue section shows hepatocytes expanded by bean-shaped, lightly eosinophilic inclusions. **C,** PAS stain after digestion with diastase shows that the inclusions remain positively stained. **D,** Colloidal iron stains the amylopectin.

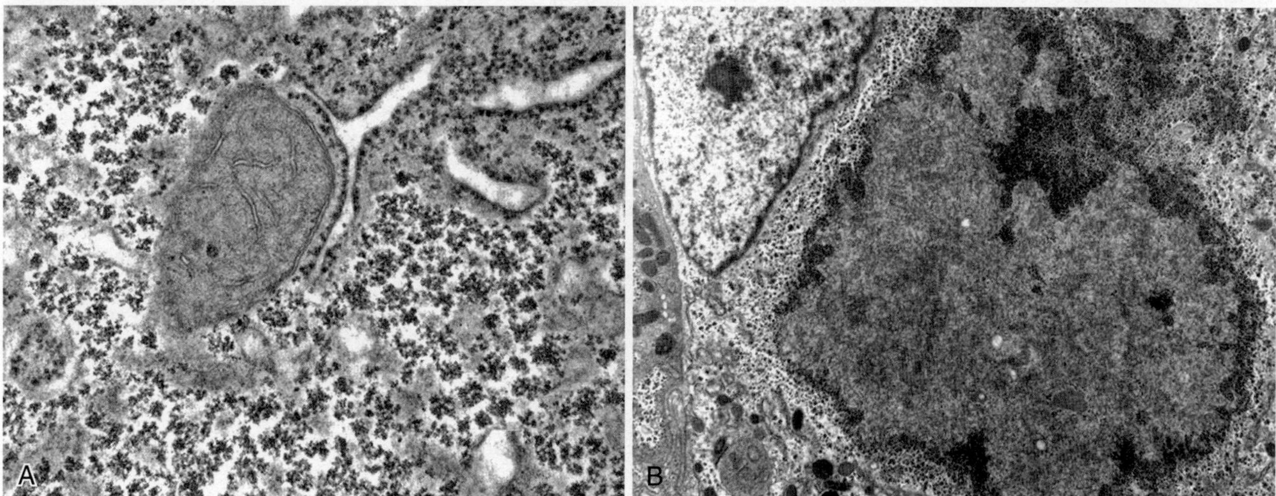

FIGURE 55.24 Glycogen storage disease *(GSD).* A, Electron microscopy in GSD type Ia shows retention of abundant glycogen rosettes within the hepatocyte cytoplasm. **B,** In GSD type IV, the retained amylopectin is fibrillar and not membrane limited.

whereas 2 died as a result of heavy cardiac amylopectinosis after transplantation.[297] At least two other patients have been reported with a similar outcome.[298] Unfortunately, there are no clinical, morphologic, or molecular predictors of posttransplantation outcome.

Current attempts at gene therapy for GSD type Ia are in progress in animal models. Preliminary results demonstrate correction of metabolic abnormalities and prevention of adenoma development but no effect on myeloid derangements or renal function.[299,300]

Hepatic adenomas related to GSD type I develop as early as 3 years of age but are more common in the second decade of life. Type I is highly prone to the formation of multiple adenomas (adenomatosis), which occurs in 22% to 75% of affected patients by puberty.[42,301-303] Adenomas also occur in as many as 25% of patients with GSD type III. Patients with both type I and type III disease have an increased risk of HCC.[42,304,305] Other forms of GSD have also been reported to be associated with HCC, including GSD VI.[306]

Mauriac Syndrome

Mauriac syndrome is characterized by severe growth retardation in patients who have poorly controlled type 1 diabetes mellitus. Delayed puberty and cushingoid features are accompanied by massive hepatomegaly. Severe hyperglycogenosis is responsible for the effects. Possible causes are marked fluctuations in available insulin, decreased levels of insulin-like growth factor 1 (IGF1) and growth hormone, circulating hormone inhibitor, or defective hormone receptors. A mutation in the catalytic subunit of liver glycogen phosphorylase kinase has been shown to cause Mauriac syndrome.[307] The availability of long-acting insulin and monitoring of glycated hemoglobin (HbA_{1c}) have dramatically reduced the incidence of Mauriac syndrome.[308] The syndrome occurs in males and females equally and is most common in adolescents, although it may occur in young toddlers and in adults. Patients may undergo biopsy because of the presence of an autoimmune serology profile.[309]

Galactosemia

Clinical Features

Galactosemia is an autosomal recessive disorder caused by deficiency in galactose-1-phosphate uridylyltransferase (GALT), which is encoded by the *GALT* gene on chromosome 9p13. The incidence of galactosemia is approximately 1 in 16,000 to 160,000 live births.[310] Currently, over 300 variations in the *GALT* gene are reported. The clinical features are highly variable and include vomiting, diarrhea, malnutrition, progressive liver disease, mental retardation, cataracts, and, eventually, ovarian failure. Galactosemia can cause both acute and chronic liver disease, either of which can result in liver failure. Newborns may be prone to *Escherichia coli* septicemia.[311] Two other forms of galactosemia, caused by deficiencies of the galactokinase (GALK) enzyme and the galactose epimerase (GALE) enzyme, represent extremely rare distinct entities with limited or no liver involvement and therefore are not discussed here.

Pathogenesis

The GALT enzyme is responsible for the generation of UDP-galactose from galactose-1-phosphate and UDP glucose, which enables metabolic processing of galactose. Absence of this enzyme leads to systemic accumulation of galactose. Multiple allelic variants in the *GALT* gene may result in diminished to absent enzymatic activity. Mutational analysis reveals that c.563A>G (p.Glin188Arg) homozygosity is the most common genotype seen in 57% of patients in the GalNet registry.[310] The Duarte variant is associated with diminished enzyme production and a milder form of disease. The pathogenesis of disease in patients with galactosemia remains unclear. However, toxicity seems to result from accumulation of the metabolic byproducts galactose-1-phosphate and galactitol.

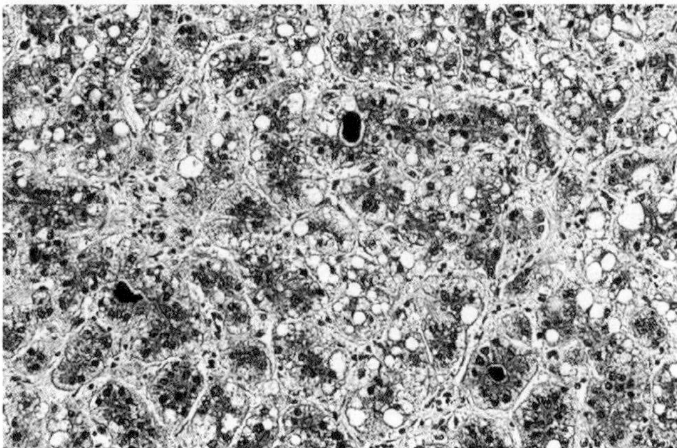

FIGURE 55.25 Galactosemia. PAS-stained tissue section shows extensive pseudoacinar transformation of hepatocytes and microvesicular and macrovesicular steatosis. Hereditary fructose intolerance is similar.

Pathological Features

Liver disease is typically severe, with diffuse macrovesicular and microvesicular steatosis, cholestasis, ductular proliferation, intralobular fibrosis, portal fibrosis, and cirrhosis (Fig. 55.25). Within 4 to 6 weeks of age, pseudoacinar transformation of hepatocytes surrounding dilated and empty canaliculi may be present; fibrosis followed by cirrhosis develops in the later stages. The early changes can be reversed by dietary restriction of galactose. These findings are not pathognomonic, however, and liver biopsy is not usually required to establish a diagnosis.[312] The definitive diagnostic test is measurement of erythrocyte GALT activity, although testing for galactose-1-phosphate levels in blood spots may be sufficient to establish a diagnosis. Analysis of mutations in the *GALT* gene confirms the diagnosis.

Natural History

Galactosemia is treated by dietary galactose restriction, which reverses early hepatic dysfunction. Screening for galactosemia is included in most newborn screening programs in the United States. Early detection undoubtedly reduces mortality rates from this disease. However, even in long-term survivors, late complications, including speech abnormalities, ataxia, cognitive impairment, and ovarian failure, often persist.[313]

Hereditary Fructose Intolerance

Clinical Features

Hereditary fructose intolerance is an autosomal recessive disorder caused by deficiency of fructose-1,6-bisphosphate aldolase B enzyme in the liver, kidney, and intestines.[314] The overall disease frequency is estimated to be 1 in 20,000 births. The usual clinical presentation is vomiting, hepatomegaly, and failure to thrive after fructose or sucrose is introduced into the diet of an infant. Jaundice is present in almost half of all affected children. Dietary fructose leads to fructosemia and fructosuria, hypophosphatemia, and metabolic acidosis. Serum levels of tyrosine and methionine may also be elevated, so hereditary tyrosinemia is included in the differential diagnosis (see later discussion).

Pathogenesis

About 65 mutations in the *ALDOB* gene, located on chromosome 9q22.3, have been reported in patients with hereditary fructose intolerance.[315] This enzyme converts fructose-bisphosphate to glyceraldehyde and dihydroxyacetone phosphate as part of normal fructose metabolism. Levels of fructose-1-phosphate accumulate in patients and result in inhibition of gluconeogenesis and glycogenolysis.

Pathological Features

Liver biopsies obtained during the first weeks of life typically reveal macrovesicular steatosis and cholestasis. Giant cell transformation occurs as well, along with other characteristic histological manifestations of neonatal hepatitis, including a periportal ductular reaction and pseudoacinar transformation of hepatocytes. Fibrosis develops early in life and may progress to cirrhosis. Ultrastructural analysis reveals prominent smooth endoplasmic reticulum and the formation of concentric and irregularly placed arrays of membranous material.[316] The diagnosis is established by enzymatic analysis of aldolase B activity within liver or intestinal tissue. More than 90% of patients are diagnosed with the use of a panel of allele-specific oligonucleotides that detect the most common mutations in the *ALDOB* gene.

Natural History

Hereditary fructosemia may result in acute liver failure or cirrhosis. Dietary restriction of fructose, sorbitol, and sucrose leads to clinical recovery, with normal health, growth, and development, provided that severe liver or renal disease has not developed.[315] In the latter instance, persistent renal tubular defects may lead to rickets and metabolic acidosis. Actuarial survival figures have not been reported. The risk of life-threatening metabolic derangement remains when fructose-rich foods are consumed. At any age, accidental exposure to very small quantities of harmful sugars, even in a single meal, can precipitate symptoms and severe metabolic disturbances.

CONGENITAL DISORDERS OF GLYCOSYLATION

Congenital disorders of glycosylation (CDGs), formerly referred to as *carbohydrate-deficient glycoprotein syndromes*, comprise a rare but rapidly growing group of inherited disorders characterized by defective *N*-linked conjugation of glycan moieties to proteins.[317] The CDG syndromes are typically multisystemic, consisting of dysmorphic facies, developmental delay, and, in several subtypes, liver dysfunction. CDG type Ia and type Ib are two of the best characterized subtypes. They are caused by mutations in the genes for phosphomannomutase 2 *(PMM2)* and mannosephosphate isomerase *(MPI)*, respectively. CDG type Ib, in particular, can manifest with only liver disease consisting of periportal fibrosis and ductal plate malformations that mimic congenital hepatic fibrosis (Fig. 55.26). Diagnosis of CDG syndromes is established by isoelectric focusing of serum transferrin and is confirmed by molecular analyses. A CDG gene panel is also available.[318] Hypoglycosylation of intercellular adhesion molecule 1 (ICAM1) is also useful diagnostically.[319]

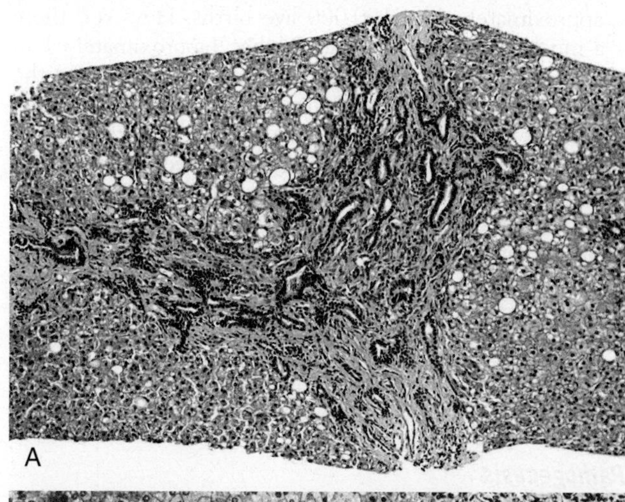

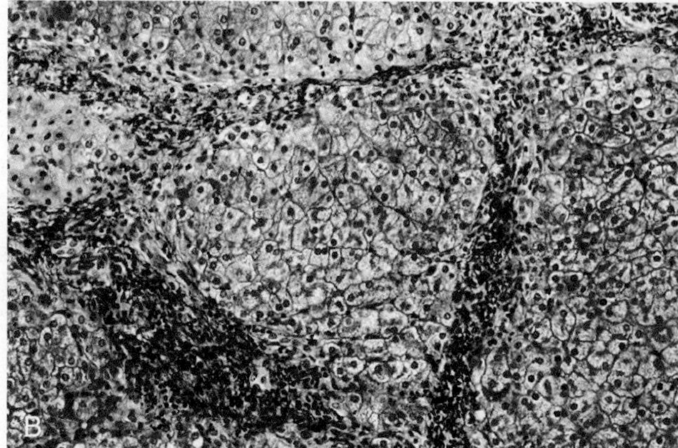

FIGURE 55.26 Congenital disorder of glycosylation type Ib in a 1-year-old infant with hyperinsulinemic hypoglycemia and hepatomegaly. A, The ectatic bile ducts in expanded but uninflamed portal tracts are identical to those in congenital hepatic fibrosis associated with autosomal recessive polycystic kidney disease (see Fig. 55.43). **B,** A 5-year-old patient with this defect has diffuse bridging portal fibrosis without duct ectasia (trichrome stain).

Mucopolysaccharidoses

Mucopolysaccharidoses (MPSs) comprise a rare group of lysosomal storage disorders in which degradation of glycosaminoglycans (mucopolysaccharides) is impaired. All of these disorders are autosomal recessive except for Hunter disease (MPS type II), which is X-linked. MPSs are clinically heterogeneous disorders with variable systemic manifestations. Hepatosplenomegaly develops in several types, but hepatic dysfunction is not a common manifestation of MPS. A diagnosis is usually established by a combination of enzyme activity measurements and molecular analyses. For more information, readers are referred to other comprehensive reviews on this topic.[31,320]

DISORDERS OF AMINO ACID METABOLISM

Hereditary Tyrosinemia

Clinical Features

Hereditary tyrosinemia type I is an autosomal recessive disorder that is caused by a deficiency of fumarylacetoacetate hydrolase (FAH),[37] the last enzyme in the tyrosine degradation pathway. Worldwide, the incidence of this disorder is approximately 1 in 100,000 live births. However, there is a much higher incidence in Quebec (approximately 1 in 17,000 live births) because of a founder effect. Among the various potential causes of elevated serum levels of tyrosine, hereditary tyrosinemia type I is the only one that causes liver disease. Other causes of elevated tyrosine levels include transient tyrosinemia of the newborn, liver disease of any etiology, and enzyme deficiencies in other steps of the tyrosine catabolic pathway. The presence of elevated levels of serum and urine succinylacetone in a patient with liver disease is pathognomonic for hereditary tyrosinemia type I. The diagnosis can be confirmed by measurement of FAH enzyme activity in cultured skin fibroblasts or in liver biopsy specimens. Prenatal diagnosis is possible by culture of amniocytes or by measurement of succinylacetone in amniotic fluid.

Pathogenesis

Deficiency of the FAH enzyme results in elevated serum levels of tyrosine fumarylacetoacetate and its metabolites, succinylacetoacetate and succinylacetone. Evidence suggests that neurological crises, liver disease, and even risk of malignant transformation are at least partially caused by the presence of these metabolites. The *FAH* gene is located on chromosome 15q25.1. More than 90 disease-causing variants in this gene have been reported.[37]

Pathological Features

Liver tissue in the acute stage of hereditary tyrosinemia typically shows a hepatitic pattern of injury and inflammation with necrosis, steatosis, cholestasis, and, occasionally, giant cell transformation[4] (Fig. 55.27). In the chronic stage, there is usually a mixed micronodular and macronodular cirrhosis with bile duct proliferation and, most significantly, foci of dysplasia or HCC, or both[321] (Fig. 55.28). Foci of nodular regeneration, with liver cell dysplasia, may be difficult to distinguish from carcinoma. Cirrhotic livers show a "reversion" pattern, which was first reported by Kvittingen and colleagues.[322,323] This pattern is characterized by rare discrete regenerative nodules immunoreactive for FAH protein interspersed with FAH-negative nodules. DNA analyses of these nodules have revealed that they are heterozygous for the *FAH* gene sequence of at least three separate mutations in different populations.[323,324] There is an inverse correlation between the extent of the mutant nodules and clinical severity.[324]

Natural History

Treatment consists of administration of nitisinone [2-(2-nitro-4-trifluoromethylbenzoyl)-1, 3-cyclohexanedione] (NTBC), which is an inhibitor of the second enzymatic step in the tyrosine catabolic pathway. Before the introduction of nitisinone therapy, the mortality rate was 75% by 2 years of age. Between 10% and 20% of patients developed HCC as early as 12 months of age,[37,44] making hereditary tyrosinemia the form of liver disease with the highest risk of HCC. Even in the NTBC era, however, long-term monitoring for the development of HCC is still required. NTBC therapy reduces but does not eliminate the risk of HCC,[325] and the treatment must be started in infancy to abort the mutagenic process.[326] Patients who develop nodules despite therapy require liver transplantation. Biopsy is not recommended in this scenario because of the risk of seeding.[312]

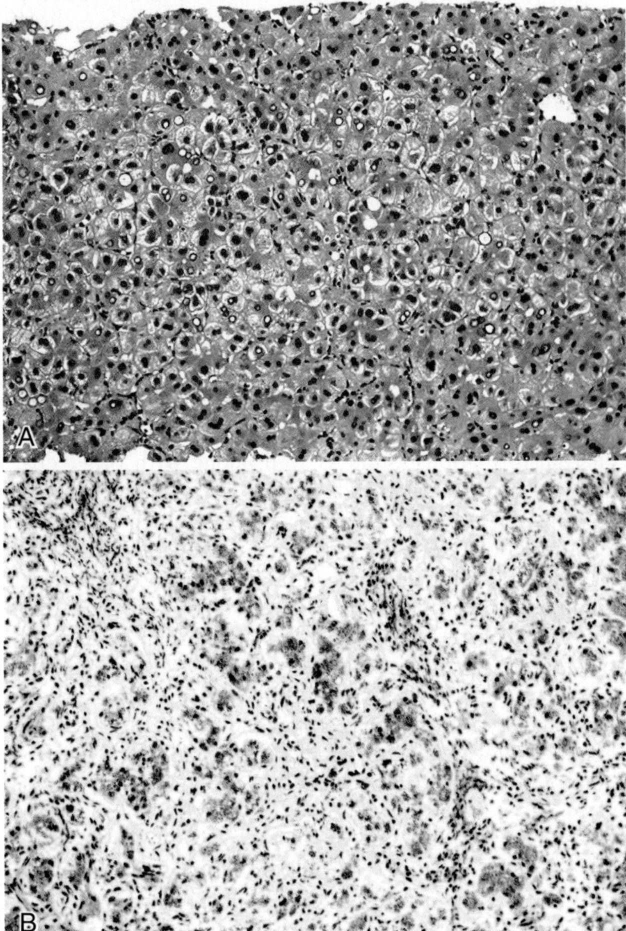

FIGURE 55.27 Tyrosinemia, acute. A, Biopsy specimen from 15-week-old infant shows hepatocellular pleomorphism. **B,** α-fetoprotein expression denotes early dysregulation of gene expression because of toxic metabolites.

DISORDERS OF LIPID METABOLISM

Disorders of lipid metabolism that significantly involve the liver are listed in Table 55.13. All are autosomal recessive lysosomal storage disorders caused by enzyme or transporter deficiencies that impair lysosomal degradation of substrate material. Hepatosplenomegaly in infancy or in preschool children is a common presentation. Chanarin-Dorfman syndrome also comes into the differential diagnosis in children with nonbullous congenital ichthyosiform erythroderma and is associated with steatosis.[327] Not discussed here are those rare disorders that do not significantly affect hepatic function or in which hepatic involvement is of little clinical significance, such as Fabry disease, mucolipidoses, and metachromatic leukodystrophy.

Gaucher Disease

Clinical Features

Gaucher disease is an autosomal recessive lysosomal storage disorder that is characterized by accumulation of glucocerebroside (or glucosylceramide) in tissues as a result of a deficiency in the enzyme β-glucosidase. Gaucher disease is the most common genetic lysosomal storage disorder.

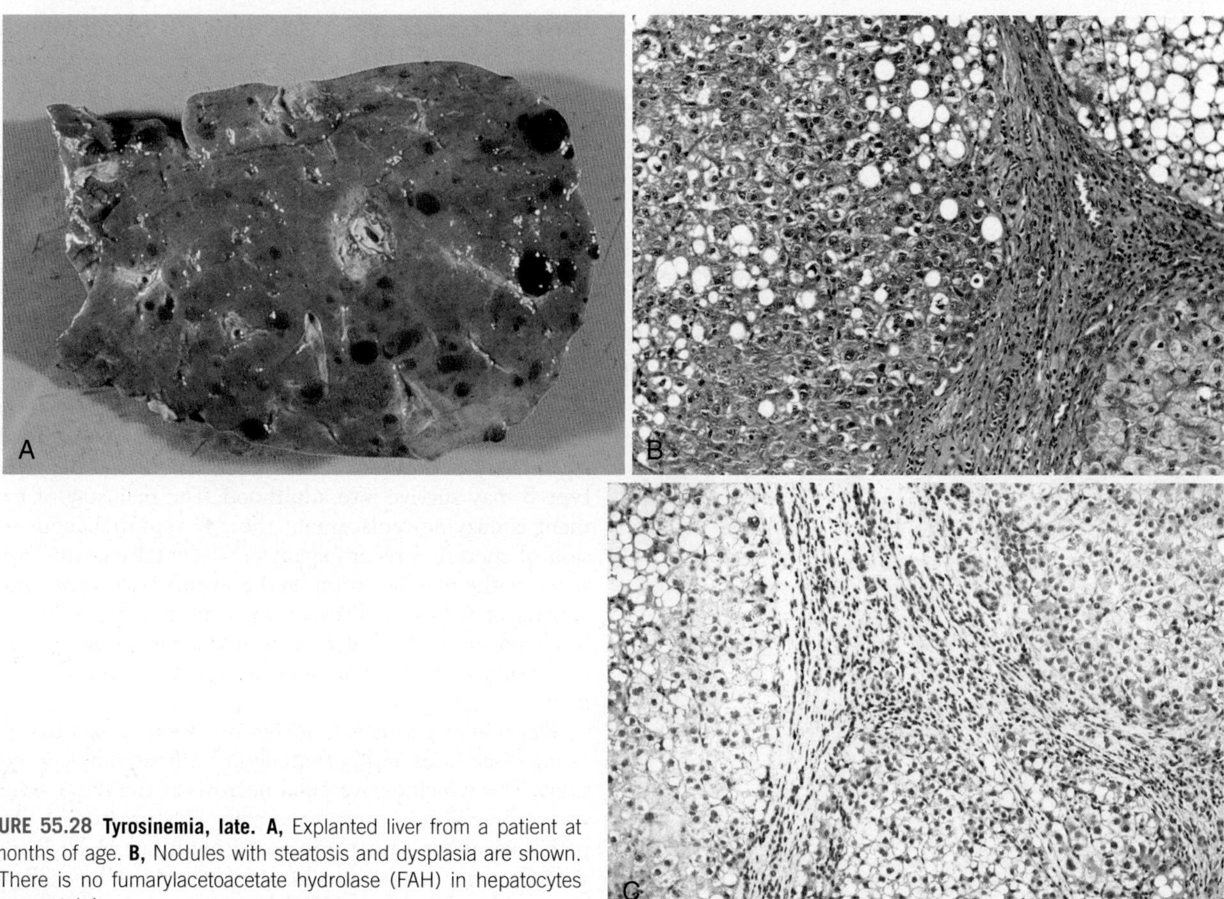

FIGURE 55.28 Tyrosinemia, late. A, Explanted liver from a patient at 8 months of age. **B,** Nodules with steatosis and dysplasia are shown. **C,** There is no fumarylacetoacetate hydrolase (FAH) in hepatocytes (immunostain).

Worldwide, its incidence has been estimated to be 1 in 50,000 to 100,000 live births,[328,329] but the disease is much more common in Ashkenazi Jews (as high as 1 in 855 live births).[330] Based on the degree and severity of nervous system involvement, three clinical forms are recognized. Approximately 90% of Gaucher disease patients have the type 1, or nonneuronopathic, variant. This form usually manifests with widespread visceral involvement characterized by splenomegaly, hepatomegaly, and bone marrow infiltration, which leads to infarction or fracture.[330] Other common clinical manifestations are anemia and bleeding secondary to thrombocytopenia. Type 2 and type 3 Gaucher disease are the neuronopathic forms. In addition to visceral involvement, neurological deterioration, developmental delay, horizontal gaze palsies, and hydrops fetalis are reported manifestations.

Gaucher disease is usually diagnosed based on histology (identifying so-called *Gaucher cells*) and documentation of a low level of acid β-glucosidase activity in peripheral blood leukocytes or cultured fibroblasts. DNA sequencing analysis of the *GBA* gene, which encodes β-glucosidase, is commercially available and is very helpful in atypical cases, prenatal diagnosis, and carrier screening.

Pathogenesis

Glucocerebroside is a major component of cell membranes. While senescent cells degrade and are engulfed by macrophages, the absence of lysosomal acid β-glucosidase activity results in accumulation of glucocerebroside within macrophage lysosomes. In types 2 and 3 Gaucher disease, neuronal accumulation of glucocerebroside and its derivative, glucosylsphingosine, is probably caused by deregulation of endogenous synthesis and turnover of these molecules. Although the pathogenesis of organ dysfunction is not well understood, it is believed that the macrophage-derived proinflammatory cytokines interleukin 8 (IL-8) and macrophage colony-stimulating factor (M-CSF) have an important role.

More than 200 mutations have been reported in the *GBA* gene. The common mutations *N370S, L444P, c.84dupG,* and *c.155 + 1G> A (IVS2 + 1)* account for 96.5% of mutations in Ashkenazi Jews.[331]

Pathological Features

The glycolipid is stored in elongated lysosomes that fill the cytoplasm of macrophages, imparting a characteristic fibrillar or striated appearance similar to crinkled paper. The engorged macrophages, referred to as *Gaucher cells,* are 20 to 100 μm in diameter and are one of the most characteristic histopathological features of this disorder. Major organ systems involved include the bone marrow, spleen, lymph nodes, liver, and lung, as well as the brain in the variant forms.

In the liver, Kupffer cells and portal tract macrophages are affected. The Gaucher cells are lightly eosinophilic and have a faintly striated ("crinkled-paper") cytoplasmic appearance (Fig. 55.29). PAS or Masson trichrome stain helps to highlight the striations. There may also be intrahepatic

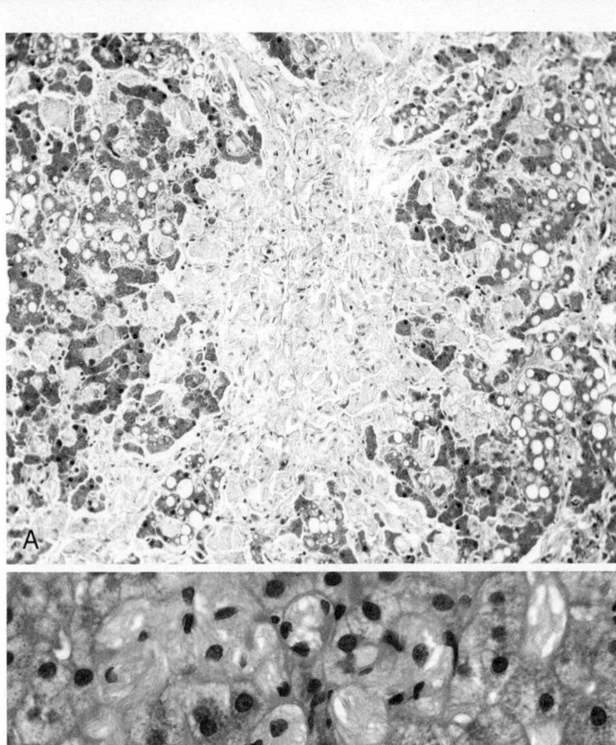

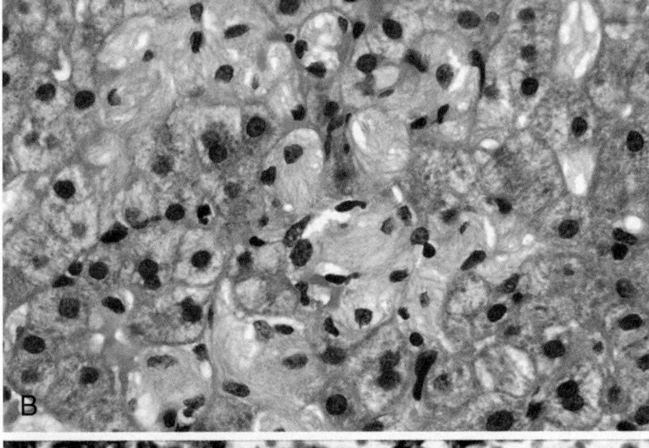

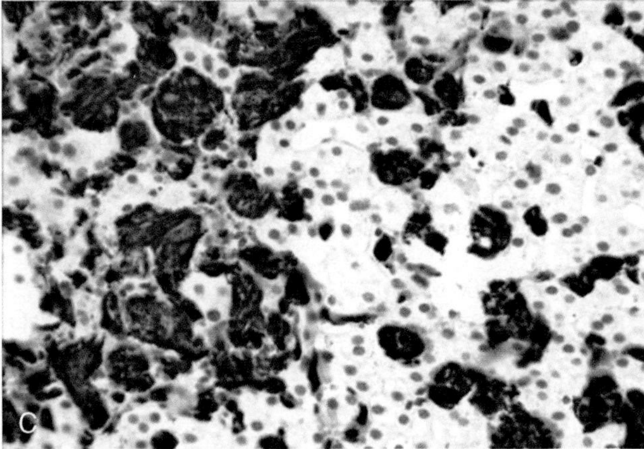

FIGURE 55.29 Gaucher disease. A, Low-power image of this liver shows a portal tract region massively expanded by enlarged macrophages. The surrounding sinusoids also contain abundant macrophages, and hepatocytes exhibit macrovesicular steatosis and lobular disarray. **B,** High-power image of parenchyma reveals sinusoidal macrophages that are slightly basophilic and have a fibrillar appearance to their cytoplasm. **C,** Immunostaining for CD26 demonstrates positive immunoreactivity of the sinusoidal macrophages. (*Courtesy Dr. Antonio Perez-Atayde, Children's Hospital Medical Center, Boston.*)

accumulation of iron caused by ingestion of erythrocytes. Gaucher cells may completely block the sinusoidal spaces and compress hepatocytes, leading to disruption and atrophy of the hepatocyte plates. Reticulin and collagen fibers increase in the space of Disse. Eventually, severe sinusoidal fibrosis, formation of bridging septa, and micronodular cirrhosis may develop.

Differential Diagnosis

Hepatosplenomegaly, thrombocytopenia, and bone pain in children raise the differential diagnosis of other metabolic storage diseases and malignancy. In tissue samples, a key differential is NPD. In this disorder, the large sinusoidal histiocytes have foamy cytoplasm with round vacuoles, in contrast with Gaucher cells, which exhibit characteristic fibrillar or striated cytoplasm.

Natural History

The natural history of Gaucher disease is variable. Type 1 manifests in childhood or adulthood. Type 2 manifests during infancy or in utero and is fatal, whereas patients with type 3 may survive into adulthood. The mainstay of treatment is enzyme replacement therapy via intravenous infusion of modified recombinant or placental enzyme, which reverses the manifestations and prevents long-term complications of Gaucher disease. Bone marrow transplantation has been successful but may be accompanied by significant posttransplantation morbidity. Rarely, liver transplantation may be required.

Delay in diagnosis of Gaucher disease may lead to debilitating disabilities and potentially life-threatening complications. These include avascular necrosis of the femoral head, severe bleeding, chronic bone pain, life-threatening sepsis, pathological bone fractures, and growth failure.[332] Patients with Gaucher disease are also at increased risk for malignant hematological tumors. HCC has been reported in several affected patients at all ages irrespective of whether or not the liver showed cirrhosis.[333] There is an increased incidence of HCC in patients with an intact spleen. It is also important to remember that almost three-fourths of patients with liver nodules in Gaucher disease turn out to have benign *gaucheromas*, an important differential for hepatic nodules in Gaucher disease.[334] Monitoring of liver fibrosis by transient elastography is now recommended.[334]

Niemann-Pick Disease Types A and B

Clinical Features

NPD types A and B are allelic variants of a lysosomal sphingolipid storage disorder caused by deficiency of lysosomal acid sphingomyelinase. It is characterized by widespread deposition of undegraded sphingomyelin in cells, particularly in those of the reticuloendothelial system. NPD type A (the neurovisceral form) usually manifests in infancy and runs a fatal course during the first few years of life. This type is particularly common in the Ashkenazi Jewish population, with a carrier frequency of 1 in 80.[335] Patients with NPD type B (the nonneuronopathic form) typically have a less severe course and often reach adulthood. The highest incidence of NPD type B is among individuals of Turkish, Arabic, and North African ancestry.[336]

Pathogenesis

NPD types A and B are both caused by mutations in the *SMPD1* gene that encodes for acid sphingomyelinase.[335] Fewer than 20 mutations are known, of which three (R496L, L302P, and fsP330) account for 92% of

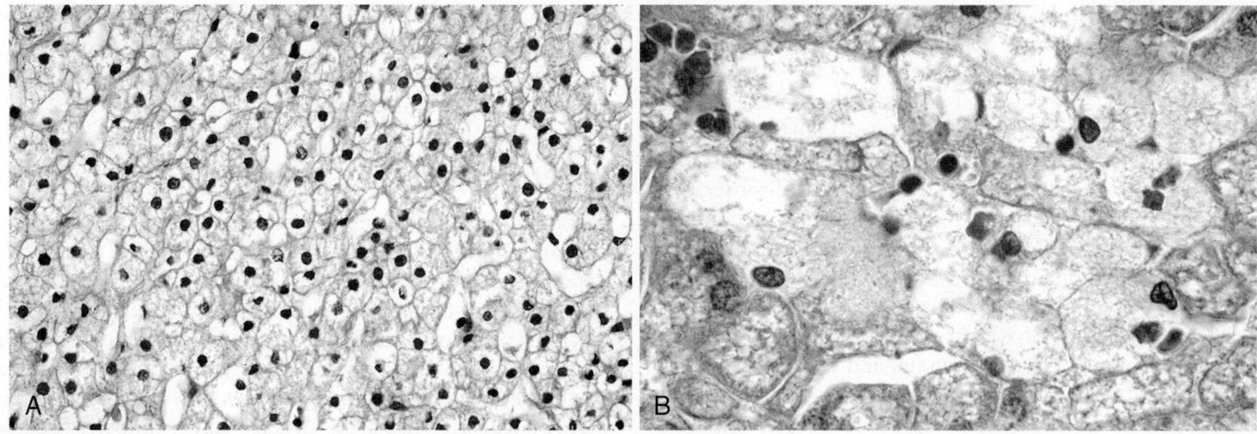

FIGURE 55.30 Niemann-Pick disease type A. A, Low-power image of liver parenchyma shows enlarged, pale hepatocytes. Sinusoidal macrophages are also enlarged but difficult to identify at this magnification. **B,** High-power image of liver parenchyma shows the center of the field filled with enlarged sinusoidal macrophages. Hepatocytes are at the periphery of this image.

mutant alleles in Ashkenazi Jewish patients with NPD type A. The R496L mutation is also found in NPD type B patients, along with compound heterozygosity for other, less deleterious mutations. Therefore it is typical for patients with NPD type B to have some residual enzyme activity. However, NPD types A and B cannot be reliably distinguished based on residual enzyme activity alone. Both are characterized by massive accumulation of sphingomyelin, as well as cholesterol and other lipids, in lysosomes of cells throughout the body, especially monocytes/macrophages. In type A, but not type B, an increase in lysosphingomyelin (sphingosylphosphorylcholine) is found in the brain and may contribute to neurological manifestations.

Pathological Features

As indicated earlier, prominent accumulation of large macrophages with foamy cytoplasm within the spleen, bone marrow, brain (in NPD type A), liver, and lymph nodes is the characteristic finding. Niemann-Pick cells are large (25 to 75 μm), lipid-laden, foamy cells that stain negative for PAS but positive with lipid stains on frozen sections. Occasionally, Kupffer cells contain lipofuscin. The liver is grossly smooth and firm. On sections, foamy Kupffer cells fill the sinusoids (Fig. 55.30). Hepatocytes may also be vacuolated. However, cirrhosis and liver failure are uncommon consequences. Electron microscopy demonstrates dense lipid inclusions, which are typically spherical and range from 1 to 5 μm in diameter. The inclusions consist of concentric lamellae of myelin-like figures, with a periodicity of roughly 5 nm (Fig. 55.31B). The diagnosis is confirmed by measurement of leukocytic acid sphingomyelinase activity. Identification of pathogenic alleles of *SMPD1* by genetic analysis can also be helpful and is currently available in the neonatal cholestasis gene panel.

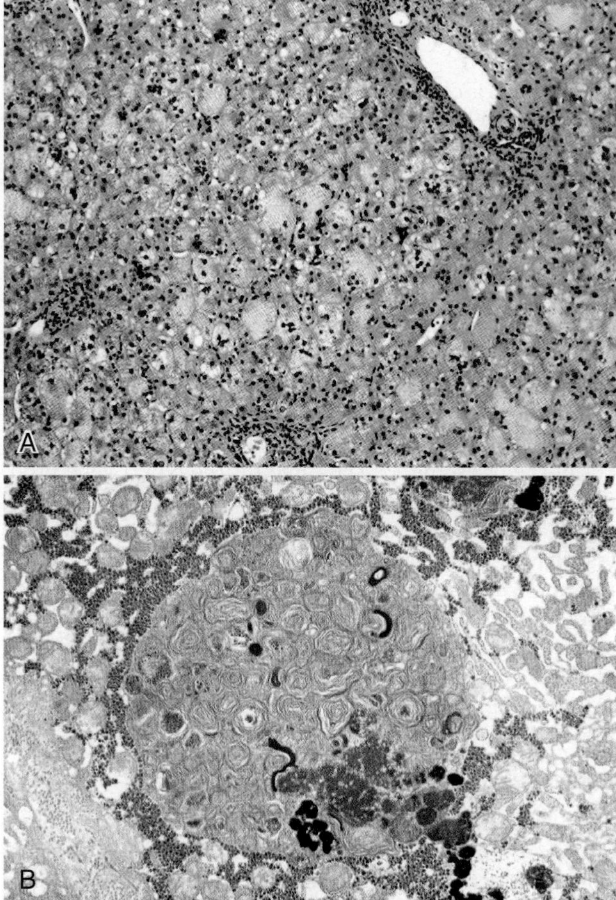

FIGURE 55.31 Niemann-Pick disease type C. A, Diffuse hepatocyte swelling caused by cytoplasmic lipid other than usual triglycerides steatosis is present in almost all hepatocytes in a 5-week-old infant. **B,** Phospholipid forms myelin figures in hepatocyte cytoplasm.

Natural History

Patients with NPD type A suffer from progressive neurodegenerative changes in infancy that lead to severe developmental impairment and death within the first 1 to 2 years of life. In NPD type B, nervous system involvement is less evident, and survival into adulthood is possible. Neurological involvement in type B has been linked to the presence of a cherry-red macula in many patients. At present, no specific treatment options exist, although bone marrow transplantation has been tried in some patients with NPD type B. The development of enzyme replacement therapies is promising.

Niemann-Pick Disease Type C

Clinical Features

NPD type C is an autosomal recessive lysosomal storage disorder that results from defective intracellular trafficking of endocytosed cholesterol. In this respect, NPD type C is different from most other lysosomal storage disorders, in which deficiency of lysosomal hydrolases leads to accumulation of substrates. NPD type C is more common than type A and type B combined, with a worldwide prevalence of 1 in 150,000.[337] Clinically, it is an extremely heterogeneous disorder, with progressive neurological disease manifesting as vertical supranuclear palsy, ataxia, and dystonia. Splenomegaly is another common finding. Hepatic involvement is frequent; neonatal cholestasis is present in approximately half of patients. Therefore NPD type C is one of the leading inherited metabolic causes of neonatal cholestasis.[180] In some cases, fulminant hepatic failure and death during early infancy have been reported.[338] Prenatal disease may manifest as hydrops.

Pathogenesis

NPD type C is caused by mutations in two genes, *NPC1* and *NPC2*. In 1997, *NPC1* was identified by positional cloning as the gene responsible for NPD type C.[339] Approximately 95% of patients have mutations in this gene. *NPC1* encodes for a transmembrane protein that has been localized to the late endosomes/lysosomes. Approximately 4% of patients have mutations in *NPC2*,[340] a gene that encodes a lysosomal cholesterol-binding protein. Based on biochemical studies and crystallographic evidence, a model has been proposed in which cholesterol is de-esterified within the lysosome by lysosomal acid lipase (the enzyme that is defective in Wolman disease) and then transferred to NPC2; NPC2 transfers the cholesterol moiety to NPC1, which aids in its efflux out of the lysosome.[341] The cargo for the NPC1 gene product includes not only cholesterol but also other glycolipids, which explains the intracellular accumulation of glycolipids such as GM2 ganglioside in neurons and fibroblasts of patients with type C disease.[342] Demonstration of impaired intracellular cholesterol transport by filipin staining of cultured skin fibroblasts is the diagnostic method of choice; however, recent guidelines recommend simultaneous use of both filipin staining and genetic analysis of *NPC1* and *NPC2* now available in the gene panel.[343]

Pathological Features

Liver biopsies in NPD type C reveal severe neonatal hepatitis with pericellular fibrosis and pseudoacinar formation. Portal tract features that suggest extrahepatic biliary obstruction may be present[344] (see Fig. 55.31). In contrast with NPD type A, storage cells typical of NPD are often not detected in neonatal livers affected by type C disease. However, electron microscopy reveals the typical ultrastructural changes of lamellar cytoplasmic inclusions.

Natural History

Almost all patients with NPD type C die within 10 to 25 years of age.[343] The prognosis depends on the age at onset of neurological symptoms. Patients with neurological involvement in infancy have a poorer prognosis. A subset of patients die in early infancy from hepatic failure or pulmonary failure. At present, there is no cure for NPD type C, but therapy with miglustat (approved in the United States only to treat Gaucher disease) has reportedly led to stabilization of clinical symptoms and an improved quality of life.[343]

Farber disease

Farber disease is caused by deficiency of lysosomal acid ceramidase, which is encoded by the *ASAH1* gene. The disease is characterized by widespread subcutaneous, soft tissue, and visceral lipogranulomas. On liver biopsy, collections of foamy histiocytes and multinucleated cells, combined with the presence of characteristic curvilinear structures (Farber bodies) on electron microscopy, are highly suggestive of Farber disease. Liver biopsies are particularly crucial in the neonatal-visceral subtype of this disorder, which can manifest with isolated liver involvement in infancy or as hydrops fetalis.[345,346] Confirmatory tests include acid ceramidase activity measurements in leukocytes, cultured skin fibroblasts, plasma, or amniocytes, where it usually measures less than 6% of control values.[347] Molecular evaluation of the *ASAH1* gene is also helpful.

GM1 Gangliosidosis

GM1 gangliosidosis is caused by deficiency of the enzyme β-galactosidase, which is encoded by the *GLB1* gene. Hepatosplenomegaly is prominent, particularly in the neonatal-onset form of disease. Liver biopsy findings in GM1 gangliosidosis are characterized by the presence of foamy histiocytes and enlarged hepatocytes with PAS-positive inclusions.[31] Decreased activity of β-galactosidase in leukocytes is confirmatory. *GLB1* gene sequencing can be performed in difficult cases. Ultrastructurally, cells exhibit either empty vacuoles or membrane-bound fibrillogranular material, characteristic findings that are also seen in various mucopolysaccharidoses.

Lysosomal Acid Lipase Deficiency

Two allelic disorders, Wolman disease and cholesteryl-ester storage disease (CESD), represent two variant phenotypes of lysosomal acid lipase deficiency. Severe (null) mutations in the lysosomal acid lipase *(LIPA)* gene lead to the former, whereas less deleterious mutations that result in residual enzyme activity lead to CESD. Diffuse microvesicular steatosis, with or without cirrhosis, is characteristic of Wolman disease and CESD. In both disorders, demonstration of lipid (cholesteryl-esters and triglycerides) by Oil red O and Sudan black stains on frozen sections (Fig. 55.32) and ultrastructural demonstration of membrane-bound lipids should lead to evaluation of lysosomal acid lipase activity in leukocytes and skin fibroblasts.[31] The *LIPA* gene can also be sequenced for mutations.[348]

PEROXISOMAL DISORDERS

Zellweger Syndrome

Zellweger syndrome is the prototypical peroxisomal disorder, exhibiting multiple abnormalities of peroxisome

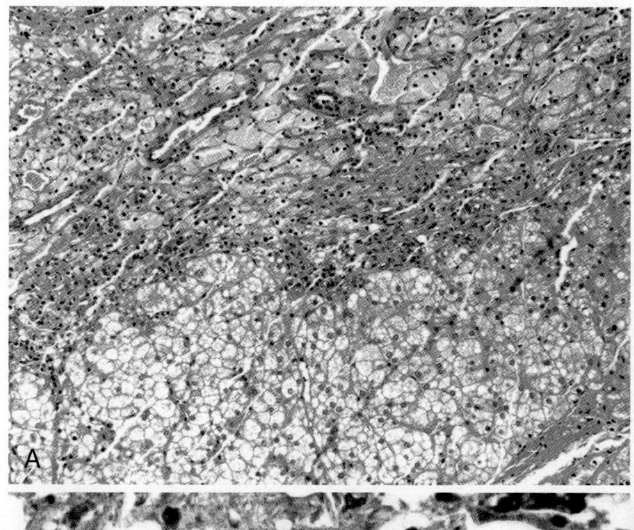

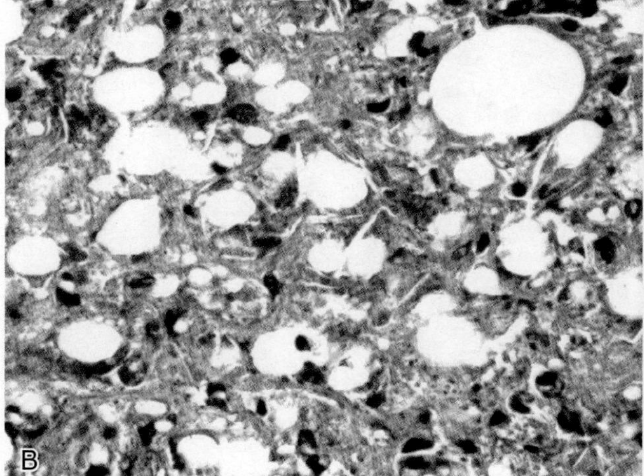

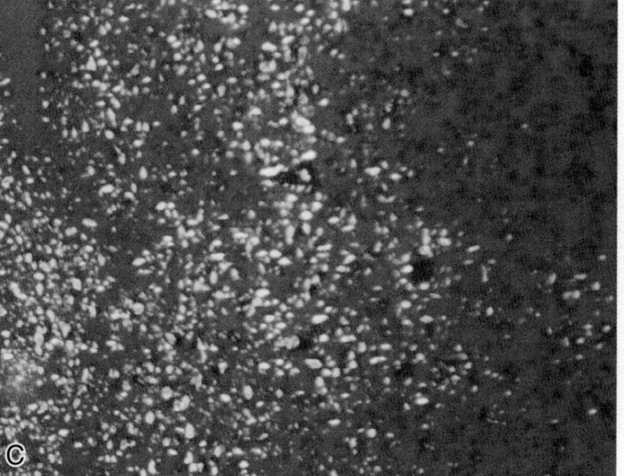

FIGURE 55.32 Cholesterol-ester storage disease. A, Microsteatosis is present in hepatocytes and Kupffer cells. The portal tract is expanded by foamy macrophages and bile duct proliferation (H&E stain). **B,** Cholesterol-ester crystals are dissolved during the processing of fixed tissue (trichrome stain). **C,** Polarized light demonstrates the cholesterol-esters in frozen sections.

function.[349] This autosomal recessive disorder is rare, occurring in only 1 in 100,000 births. Among the several peroxisomal genes, Zellweger syndrome is most often associated with mutations in *PEX1* and *PEX6*.[350] Clinical features of the syndrome include profound muscular hypotonia, facial dysmorphism with a high forehead and large fontanelles, developmental delay, seizures, bony abnormalities including epiphyseal calcifications, and cystic malformations of the brain and kidneys.

Hepatic involvement may not be prominent in the perinatal period, although some infants show persistent conjugated hyperbilirubinemia. Even in patients without jaundice, hepatosplenomegaly and evidence of impaired hepatic biosynthetic function may be present (Table 55.19). Histologically, the liver often shows paucity of the small intrahepatic bile ducts and fibrosis (Fig. 55.33). Hemosiderin is usually excessive initially but declines with age. Other changes noted include prominent glycogenated nuclei and abnormal bile duct epithelium.[351] Electron microscopy reveals an absence of peroxisomes within hepatocytes; mitochondria may also appear abnormal. A particularly interesting and novel observation, evident by electron microscopy and by light microscopy and highlighted by immunostaining of canalicular proteins, is the focal loss of tight junction integrity (see Fig. 55.33E), which permits bile to regurgitate into the bloodstream. This implies a defect in claudins, which has yet to be demonstrated and is not obviously related to peroxisomal deficiency. Although affected infants may develop cirrhosis, the extrahepatic features of the syndrome usually dominate the clinical picture. A rare case of HCC has been reported in adulthood.[351]

TABLE 55.19 Liver in Zellweger Syndrome

Feature	% of Cases
Enlargement	78
Fibrosis	76
Cholestasis	59
Micronodular cirrhosis	37

Data from Heymans HSA, Bosch H, Schutgens RBH, et al. Deficiency of plasmalogens in the cerebro-hepato-renal (Zellweger) syndrome. Eur J Pediatr. *1984;142:10–15.*

Mitochondrial Cytopathies

Clinical Features

Mitochondrial disorders are an extraordinarily diverse group of diseases that can progress rapidly from apparent normality at birth to overt liver failure.[352,353] Included in this category are respiratory chain complex mutations[354,355] and defects of long-chain fatty acid transport and FAO[356,357] (Table 55.20). Liver failure can also complicate Pearson marrow-pancreas syndrome (which is caused by mtDNA deletions),

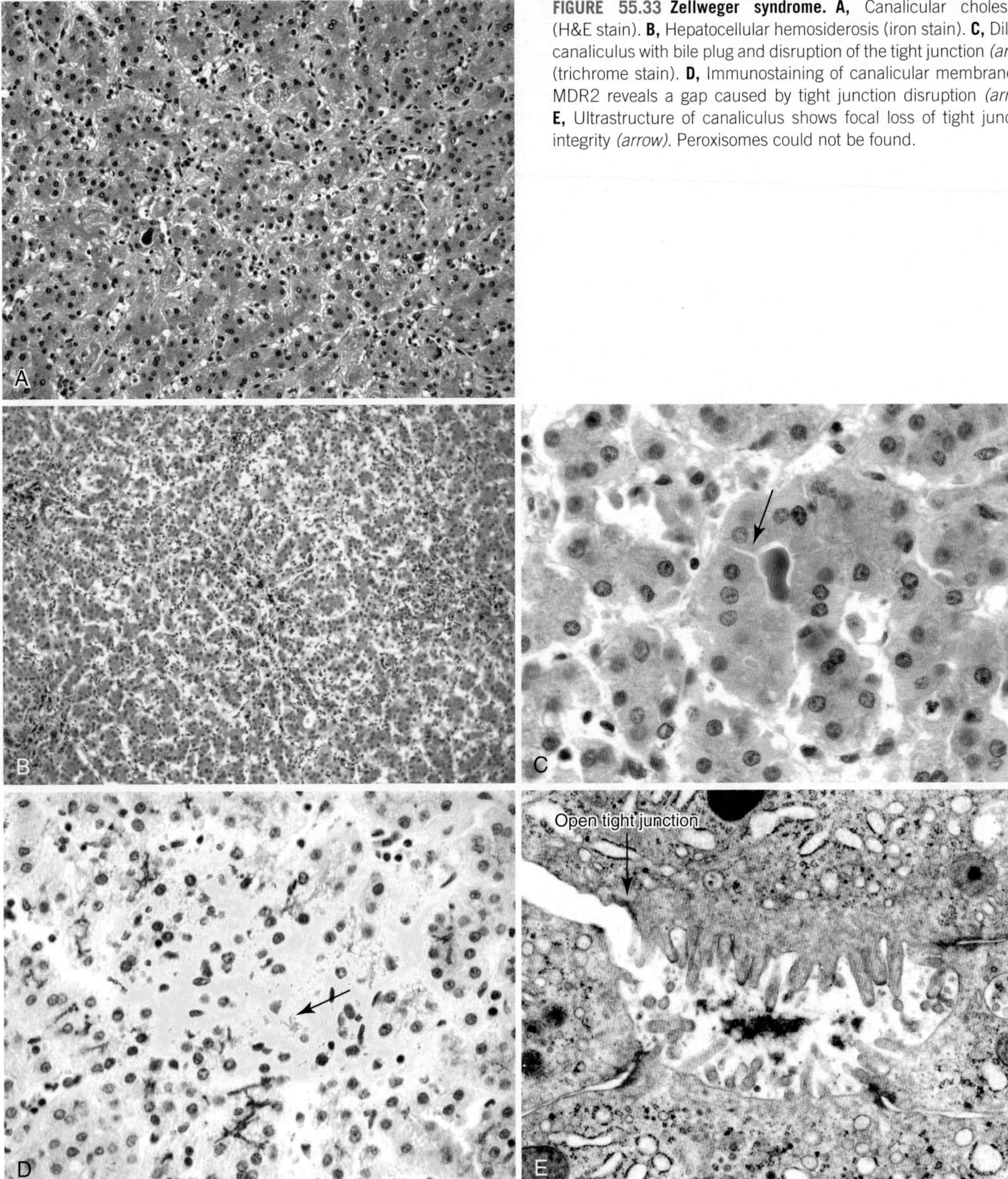

FIGURE 55.33 Zellweger syndrome. A, Canalicular cholestasis (H&E stain). **B,** Hepatocellular hemosiderosis (iron stain). **C,** Dilated canaliculus with bile plug and disruption of the tight junction *(arrow)* (trichrome stain). **D,** Immunostaining of canalicular membrane for MDR2 reveals a gap caused by tight junction disruption *(arrow).* **E,** Ultrastructure of canaliculus shows focal loss of tight junction integrity *(arrow).* Peroxisomes could not be found.

and Alpers' progressive poliodystrophy.[358] Defects that arise from mutations in nuclear genes are inherited as an autosomal trait, whereas defects in genes that are encoded by mtDNA are inherited maternally. Targeted array comparative genomic hybridization (CGH) can be very helpful for diagnosis.[359]

The general functional defect of mitochondrial disorders occurs in mitochondrial production of adenosine triphosphate (ATP). Other biochemical abnormalities may also occur, such as increased intracellular production of reactive oxygen species or defective β-oxidation, related to the specific underlying genetic mutation. Liver disease may present clinically during the first week of life. In this setting, sudden death may be wrongly attributed to sepsis. Alternatively, patients may have transient hypoglycemia, lactic acidosis, severe neurological impairment with hypotonia, myoclonic seizures, developmental delay, and cardiomyopathy, which can lead to a rapidly fatal course.[360] In a second group of patients, the onset of symptoms is delayed from 2 to 18 months, and liver disease and neurological impairment are initially less severe.[312] Liver failure may still occur, but in its absence, some patients survive into adulthood. Because many infants with mitochondrial disorders exhibit

TABLE 55.20 Mitochondrial Hepatopathies

Primary Disorders	Secondary Disorders
Electron transport protein complex deficiency	Reye syndrome
Cytochrome C oxidase deficiency	Copper overload (Wilson disease, North American Indian childhood cirrhosis, ?cholestasis)
Mitochondrial DNA depletion syndrome	Iron overload (primary hemochromatosis, perinatal hemochromatosis, tyrosinemia type I, Zellweger syndrome, other causes)
Alpers' disease	Drugs/toxins (valproic acid, iron, salicylic acid, ethanol, cyanide, antimycin A, amobarbital, rotenone, nucleoside analogues, and others)
Pearson marrow-pancreas syndrome	Conditions causing mitochondrial lipid peroxidation (e.g., cholestasis, hydrophobic bile acid toxicity)
Navajo neurohepatopathy	
Urea cycle enzyme deficiencies	
Carnitine palmitoyltransferase I and II deficiencies	
Carnitine acylcarnitine translocase deficiency	
ETF and ETF dehydrogenase deficiencies	
PEPCK deficiency (mitochondrial)	
Acyl-CoA dehydrogenase deficiency (long, medium, and short chain) and other fatty acid oxidation defects	
Nonketotic hyperglycinemia (glycine cleavage enzyme)	

CoA, *Coenzyme A;* ETF, *electron transfer flavoprotein;* PEPCK, *phosphoenolpyruvate carboxykinase.*

abnormalities before birth, prenatal diagnosis may be possible. Drug toxicity producing mitochondrial dysfunction, microsteatosis, and encephalopathy was described by Reye (see Chapter 49).

Pathological Features

Given the vast number and variety of genetic defects that cause mitochondrial cytopathies, specific pathological features have not been defined. Defects in FAO (Box 55.9) result in microvesicular steatosis, ballooning degeneration, and even cholestasis[361] (Fig. 55.34A). Respiratory chain disorders also exhibit microvesicular steatosis, a variable degree of cholestasis and ductular proliferation, variable and sometimes progressive fibrosis, and even cirrhosis.[312] Hepatocytes may show hemosiderosis[362] and an oncocytic appearance because of the presence of increased mitochondria.[363] Ultrastructural findings include pleomorphic mitochondria with decreased or absent cristae and a granular, fluffy matrix[58,362] (see Fig. 55.34B).

UREA CYCLE DISORDERS

Urea cycle disorders comprise a group of metabolic disorders that classically manifest early in life; they are usually diagnosed clinically and confirmed with biochemical and molecular genetic testing.[364] Except for the X-linked disorder ornithine transcarbamylase deficiency, all are autosomal recessive conditions. Although liver biopsy is not a common diagnostic procedure in these disorders, those that are associated with hepatic pathology are discussed here.[365] Urea cycle disorders are now the most frequent cause of liver transplantation in children with metabolic diseases.[366]

BOX 55.9 Laboratory Findings Common to Disorders of Fatty Acid Oxidation

Hypoglycemia
- Hypoketosis (negative or 1+ urine ketones)
- Elevated plasma free fatty acids (FFA)
- Plasma FFA > β-hydroxybutyrate

Acidosis
- Mild to moderate
- Increased lactate (especially in LCAD deficiency)

Mild to moderate increases in AST and ALT, usually without hyperbilirubinemia

PT, PTT normal or mildly elevated

Elevated creatine kinase (CPK)
- Cardiac and skeletal muscle
- Marked with episodic muscle weakness, rhabdomyolysis, and myoglobinuria

Mild elevation of ammonia

Marked hyperuricemia

Low plasma carnitine (except in CPT 1 deficiency)
- Elevated acylcarnitine (except in CPT 1 deficiency)
- Specific accumulating acylcarnitines

ALT, *Alanine aminotransferase;* AST, *aspartate aminotransferase;* CPT, *carnitine palmitoyltransferase;* LCAD, *long-chain acyl-coenzyme A dehydrogenase;* PT, *prothrombin time;* PTT, *partial thromboplastin time.*

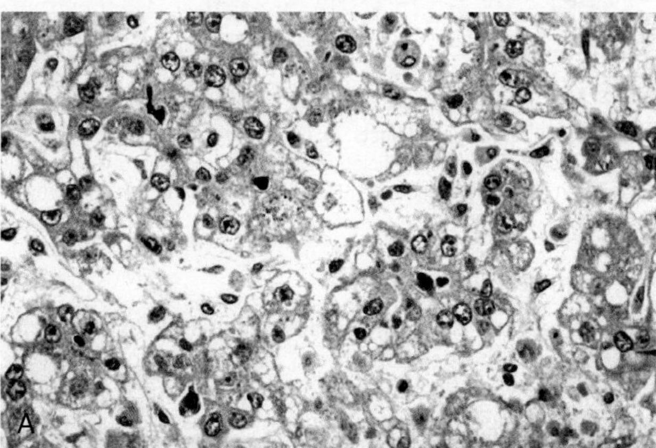

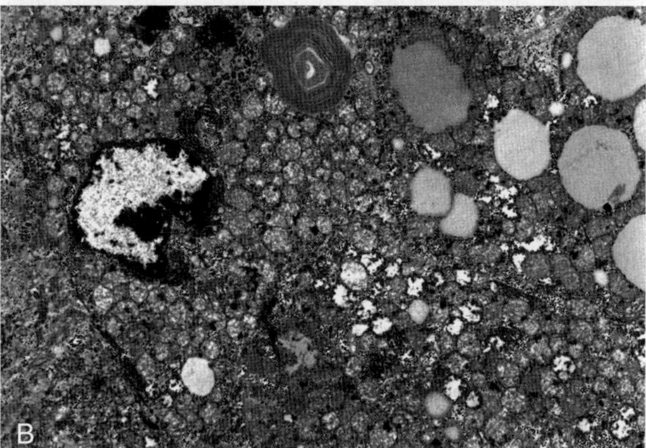

FIGURE 55.34 Mitochondriopathy in mitochondrial DNA depletion syndrome caused by mutations in the mitochondrial inner membrane protein MPV17 (Navajo neurohepatopathy). A, Diffuse hepatocellular steatosis is accompanied by canalicular cholestasis in a 1-month-old infant with lactic acidosis, hypoglycemia, and failure to thrive. Muscle weakness was also evident. **B,** Electron microscopy reveals an abundance of pleomorphic mitochondria in addition to the steatosis.

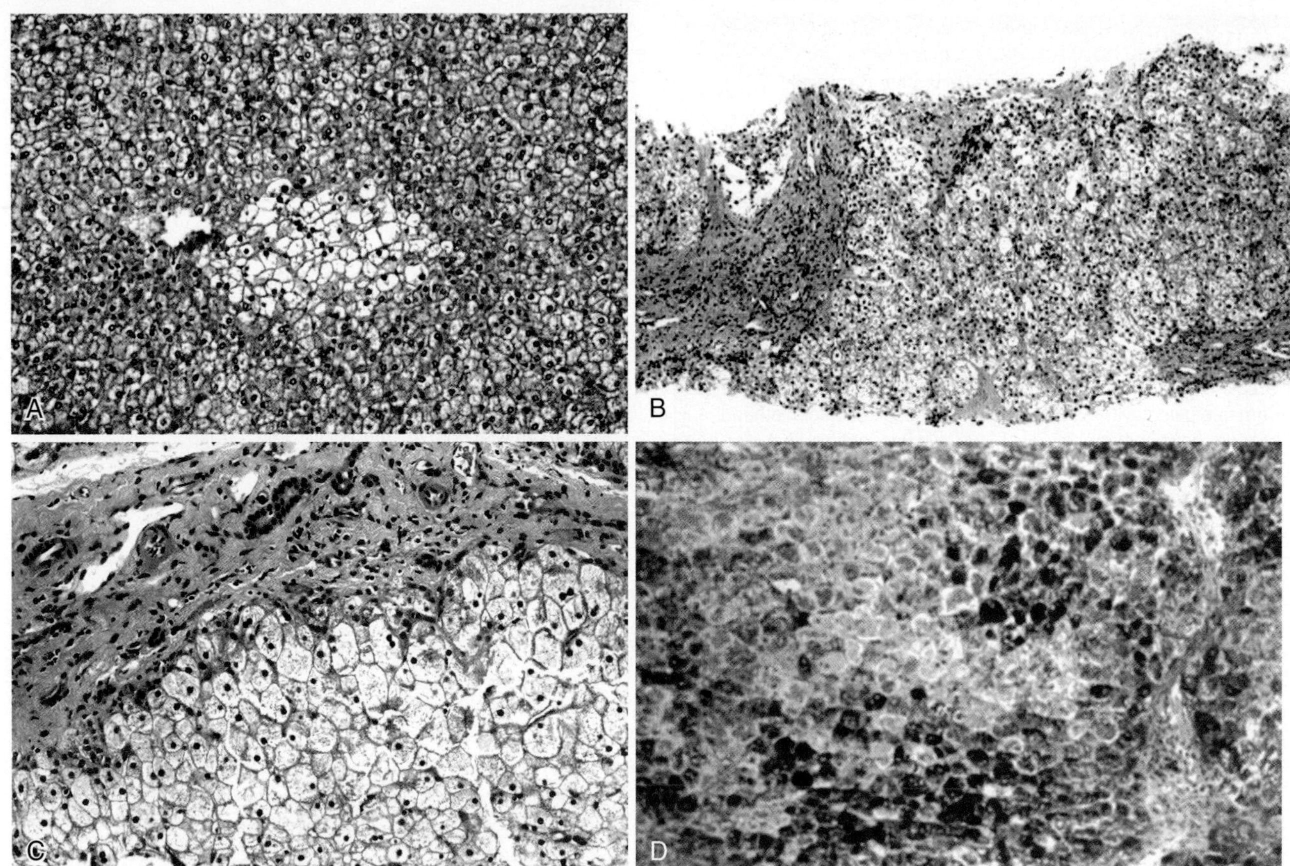

FIGURE 55.35 Urea cycle defects. A, Ornithine transcarbamylase deficiency in this 8-month-old patient shows in focal hepatocellular glycogenosis. **B,** Argininosuccinate lyase deficiency causing cirrhosis in 6-year-old child (trichrome). **C,** Hepatocellular glycogenosis resembles the amylopectinosis of glycogen storage disease type IV (see Fig. 55.23). **D,** PAS stain reveals abundant glycogen.

Argininosuccinic Aciduria

Argininosuccinic aciduria is caused by deficiency of the enzyme argininosuccinate lyase, a urea cycle enzyme encoded by the *ASL* gene on chromosome 7q11. Although rapid-onset hyperammonemia in newborns is a classic presentation, some patients have a milder course and later onset characterized by hepatomegaly. Liver biopsy reveals enlarged hepatocytes with clear cytoplasm because of glycogen accumulation, portal fibrosis, and, rarely, cirrhosis (Fig. 55.35B). Ultrastructural examination reveals abundant mitochondria, sometimes with swollen cristae. Diagnosis is confirmed by plasma amino acid analyses.[367]

Ornithine Transcarbamylase Deficiency

Ornithine transcarbamylase deficiency is caused by mutations in the *OTC* gene on chromosome Xp11. Males are severely affected in the neonatal period, but female carriers may present with liver enlargement and focal glycogenosis (see Fig. 55.35A).

Citrin Deficiency (Citrullinemia Type II)

Type II citrullinemia is caused by mutations in the *SLC25A13* gene, which encodes the transporter protein citrin. Although citrin is not an actual urea cycle enzyme, deficiency of this mitochondrial membrane aspartate transporter limits the cytoplasmic availability of aspartate, which is necessary for the third step of the urea cycle catalyzed by argininosuccinate synthetase. Hence citrin deficiency is considered to be part of the spectrum of urea cycle disorders.[368] Type I citrullinemia is caused by argininosuccinate synthetase deficiency, a classic urea cycle disorder.

Citrin deficiency (type II citrullinemia) manifests in at least two distinct entities, an early-onset form that causes neonatal intrahepatic cholestasis or childhood dyslipidemia,[369] and an adult-onset form that results in sudden neuropsychiatric abnormalities.[370] On biopsy, both forms are characterized by the presence of diffuse fatty liver with fibrosis.[370,371] Some patients progress to cirrhosis. Confirmatory testing with molecular genetic analysis is available.

INHERITED AND METABOLIC DISEASES OF ADOLESCENTS AND ADULTS

Hereditary Hemochromatosis

The total body iron pool ranges from 3 to 4 g in normal adults. HH is a group of inherited iron overload disorders that are characterized by defective regulation of iron homeostasis and excessive iron accumulation. The molecular pathogenesis and pathological features of HH have been characterized to a great extent during the past decade and are briefly described here.

Pathogenesis

The primary regulator of body iron stores is hepcidin, a 25–amino-acid peptide encoded by the *HAMP* gene that is secreted exclusively by hepatocytes.[372] Hepcidin lowers plasma iron levels by negatively regulating ferroportin, the iron-exporting protein located within duodenal enterocytes and macrophages. Hepcidin levels are, in turn, regulated by plasma iron levels in a classic negative feedback loop: Increased iron levels upregulate hepcidin, leading to decreased intestinal iron absorption and reduced export from the reticuloendothelial system iron store.

Several proteins act as iron sensors and are critical in upregulating hepcidin levels in response to increased iron. Chief among these are HFE, the transferrin receptor TfR2, and hemojuvelin. HFE is a major histocompatibility complex (MHC) class I–like transmembrane protein encoded by the *HFE* gene on chromosome 6p21.3. On hepatocyte membranes, HFE forms a complex with the transferrin receptors TfR2 and TfR1 to act as an iron sensor by binding iron-bound transferrin (holotransferrin). On binding, holotransferrin, HFE, and TfR2 are believed to upregulate hepcidin production, probably through bone morphogenetic protein 6 (BMP6)-dependent signaling. The *HJV* gene encodes hemojuvelin, a BMP6 coreceptor expressed in hepatocytes that also plays an important role in hepcidin production.

The various forms of HH are caused by mutations in these key regulators that disrupt the hepcidin-ferroportin axis. Genetic aberrations that attenuate hepcidin production or lead to hepcidin resistance cause excessive absorption of iron from the duodenum and release of iron stored in macrophages. The result is an increase in plasma levels of iron, which is then deposited in hepatocytes, cardiac myocytes, the pancreas, and other body sites. Thus hepatocytes, by virtue of being the source of hepcidin as well as the principal storage site of excess iron, are both the cause and the effect in HH.

Specific Types of Iron Storage Diseases

Patients with inherited iron overload disorders are now categorized as having either *HFE*-associated HH or non–*HFE*-associated HH (Table 55.21); the latter category includes juvenile HH, *TFR2*-associated HH, and ferroportin disease.

HFE-Associated Hereditary Hemochromatosis. *HFE*-associated HH (*HFE*-HH) is the most common type of HH, accounting for 85% to 90% of patients with HH. It is one of the most common autosomal recessive genetic disorders among people of Northern European ancestry. The most common genotypes (approximately 1 in 250 Caucasians) are homozygous for the *C282Y* mutation and, less commonly, compound heterozygous for the *C282Y/H63D* mutations (called *type Ib*). However, *HFE*-HH is a disorder with incomplete penetrance; only approximately 10% of *C282Y* homozygotes progress to full clinical disease with end-organ manifestations.[373] A third HFE genotype known as *type Ic* is related to mutation S65C but does not cause clinical disease.[374] Therefore although genotyping for *HFE* mutations is an excellent test to identify at-risk presymptomatic individuals, to screen for carriers, and confirm the diagnosis in individuals with clinical disease, by itself it is not deemed sufficient for diagnosing HH. *HFE*-HH is characterized by low levels of serum hepcidin because of the mechanisms described earlier.

HFE-HH may manifest as abnormal serum iron indices or as frank clinical disease characterized by hepatic, cardiac, pancreatic, and pituitary involvement. End-organ dysfunction caused by progressive iron accumulation is not usually evident before the fifth or sixth decade of life. Males and females are equally affected, although clinical disease develops at a later age in females, most likely because of physiological menstrual blood loss. The range of clinical manifestations of overt disease includes cirrhosis and portal hypertension, cardiac myopathy, pancreatic endocrine failure and diabetes, pituitary dysfunction leading to skin pigmentation ("bronze diabetes"), and decreased libido. Because the relative risk for HCC is 20 in patients with advanced fibrosis or cirrhosis, HCC surveillance is important in affected patients and is recommended for fibrosis above stage 3.[374]

The American Association for the Study of Liver Diseases (AASLD) guidelines on diagnosis and management of HH[373] recommend assessment of serum iron indices (transferrin saturation and ferritin) as the first step for both symptomatic individuals and asymptomatic first-degree adult relatives of an affected individual. *HFE* genotyping should be performed if the transferrin saturation is 45% or higher

TABLE 55.21 Classification, Molecular Genetics, and Diagnostic Features of Hereditary Hemochromatosis

HH Type	Alternate Names	Gene	Inheritance	Protein	Normal Function	Serum Indices	Liver Iron Deposition
Type 1	*HFE*-associated HH	*HFE*	AR	HFE	Upregulates hepcidin	TS++, ferritin+, hepcidin–	Hepatocyte+++, Kupffer+/–
Type 2A	Juvenile hemochromatosis	*HJV*	AR	Hemojuvelin	Upregulates hepcidin	TS++, ferritin+, hepcidin–	Hepatocyte++, Kupffer+/–
Type 2B	Juvenile hemochromatosis	*HAMP*	AR	Hepcidin	Iron regulator	TS++, ferritin+, hepcidin–	Hepatocyte+++, Kupffer+/–
Type 3	*TFR2*-associated HH	*TFR2*	AR	Transferrin receptor 2	Upregulates hepcidin	TS++, ferritin+, hepcidin–	Hepatocyte+++, Kupffer+/–
Type 4	Ferroportin disease	*SLC40A1*	AD	Ferroportin	Major iron exporter	Variable	*Kupffer+++

AD, *Autosomal dominant;* AR, *autosomal recessive;* HH, *hereditary hemochromatosis;* TS, *transferrin saturation.*
**For ferroportin disease caused by hepcidin resistance (see text), liver iron deposition patterns are similar to HH types 1 to 3.*

or the ferritin level is increased. Iron-overloaded individuals who are *C282Y* homozygotes or *C282Y/H63D* compound heterozygotes should be further triaged for liver biopsy if ferritin levels are higher than 1000 μg/L or liver enzymes are elevated because these patients have the highest risk for cirrhosis. Liver biopsy may also be beneficial in non-*C282Y* homozygotes to rule out other causes of hepatic dysfunction. Although liver biopsies and measurements of hepatic iron content[375] and hepatic iron index (HII) have been the historical gold standard for diagnosis of HH (see later discussion), these measures have been supplanted by widespread *HFE* genotyping combined with serum iron studies. Therefore a biopsy is now recommended to stage the degree of liver disease in patients with *HFE* mutations. Note has been made that there is considerable variation between different countries in recommended guidelines for management of HH.[376]

Juvenile Hereditary Hemochromatosis. Juvenile HH is a rare, but highly penetrant, autosomal recessive form of HH that is characterized by an aggressive course and an earlier age at onset, in the teens and early adulthood. Most individuals have mutations in the *HJV* gene that encodes the BMP6 coreceptor hemojuvelin,[377] whereas a small percentage of patients have mutations in the *HAMP* gene that encodes for hepcidin. The G320V mutation in *HJV* is the most common mutation reported worldwide. Serum levels of hepcidin are undetectable,[378] and endocrinopathies, liver failure, and cardiac myopathies are prominent manifestations.

***TFR2*-Associated Hereditary Hemochromatosis.** A third autosomal recessive form of HH is caused by mutations in the *TFR2* gene, which encodes for the TfR2 transferrin receptor. This rare form is clinically similar to *HFE*-HH. Hepcidin levels are decreased.[379]

Ferroportin Disease. Ferroportin disease is an autosomal dominant form of hemochromatosis. It is unique in that hepcidin levels can be normal. In one of two variant forms, mutations in the *SLC40A1* gene lead to defective function of ferroportin and trapping of iron within macrophages. Serum ferritin levels are very high, and transferrin saturation is low. Liver biopsy shows iron accumulation within Kupffer cells, a feature that is distinct from the parenchymal iron accumulation that characterizes other forms of HH.

An alternative form, in which ferroportin function is retained but the protein is resistant to hepcidin-mediated downregulation, has also been identified. The pattern of iron accumulation in hepcidin-resistant ferroportin disease is similar to that of classic hemochromatosis, with parenchymal storage of excess iron. Therefore different pathogenic mechanisms underlie the variable clinical and histological findings in this disease.[379]

Pathological Features

Within the liver, iron first becomes evident as golden-yellow hemosiderin granules in the cytoplasm of periportal hepatocytes (Fig. 55.36A). Hepatocytes initially take up and store iron as hemosiderin dispersed evenly within the cytoplasm and then, ultimately, in the form of hemosiderin granules within lysosomes. Because lysosomes are distributed predominantly in the subapical region of hepatocytes, a pericanalicular pattern of iron staining (with Prussian blue) is typical. A chicken-wire–like distribution of Prussian blue–positive granules within periportal hepatocytes is usually the first histological indication of the possibility of HH (see Fig. 55.36B). With increasing iron accumulation, one sees progressive involvement of the remainder of the lobule and, eventually, accumulation of hemosiderin granules within bile duct epithelium and Kupffer cells.

With widespread use of genotyping and serum iron indices, the role of liver biopsy in HH has evolved from the gold standard procedure for iron quantitation and diagnosis to a highly useful adjunct for staging the degree of fibrosis. Semiquantitative grading scales based on iron stains have been used to grade the intensity of stainable iron deposits in hepatocytes, sinusoidal cells, and portal tracts,[379] but the procedures are tedious and are not routinely used. Because iron is a direct hepatotoxin, inflammation is characteristically absent in affected patients. Fibrous septa develop slowly during the course of many years, leading, ultimately, to a micronodular pattern of cirrhosis. The presence of inflammation, such as mononuclear inflammation in portal tracts or hepatocellular steatosis, should prompt serious consideration of a coexistent, non–iron-related liver disease.

Hepatic iron content measured by atomic absorption spectrometry is the standard method for iron quantitation. Levels lower than 400 μg of iron per gram dry weight of liver (<30 μmol/g) are considered to be normal.[379] Adults with HH exhibit levels greater than 10,000 μg/g dry weight of liver. Because iron accumulation is a lifelong process, the

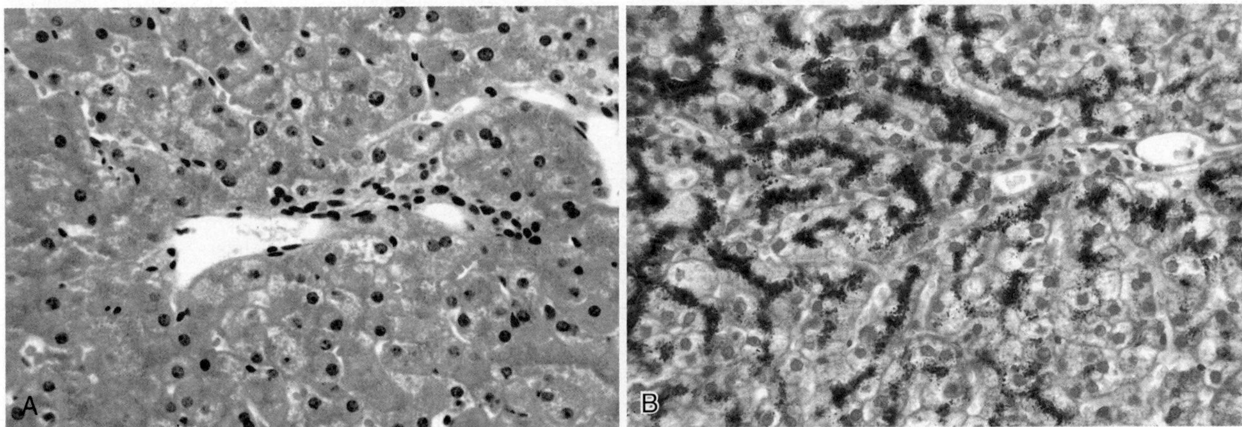

FIGURE 55.36 Hereditary hemochromatosis. A, Pericanalicular brown granules are seen in periportal hepatocytes (H&E stain). **B,** Same specimen as in **A** is stained with Prussian blue, demonstrating pericanalicular hemosiderin deposits.

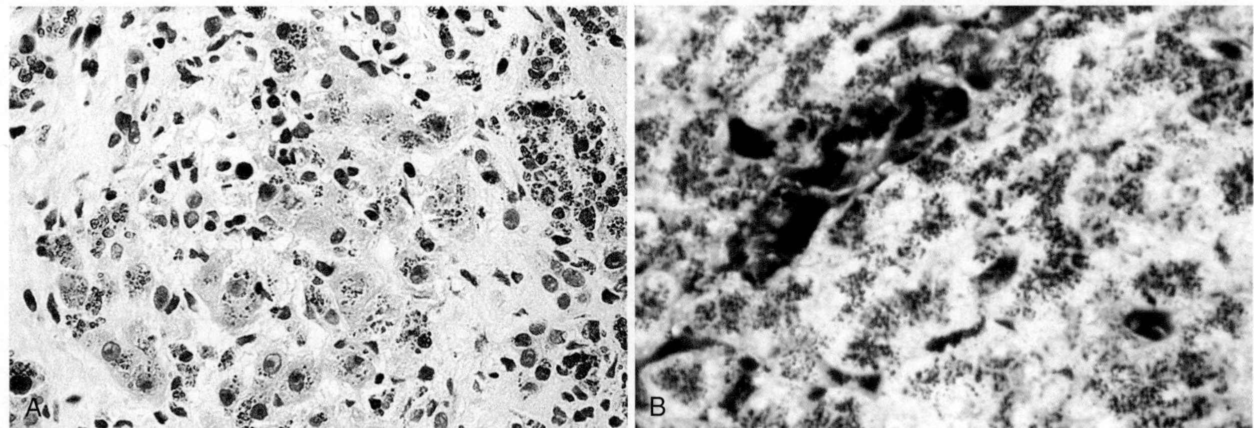

FIGURE 55.37 Liver in secondary iron overload. A, Large, dense, brown granules of hemosiderin are present in Kupffer cells, with smaller granules present in hepatocytes (H&E stain). **B,** There is dense Kupffer cell iron deposition along with hepatocellular deposition; this is the "reticuloendothelial" pattern of iron deposition (Prussian blue stain).

hepatic iron index (HII), calculated as μmol/g dry weight of liver divided by the patient's age, has been historically used as a guide to the probability that a patient has HH.[379] Levels greater than 1.9 have a 93% sensitivity for diagnosis of HH and a specificity of 93%. However, widespread genotyping has revealed that phenotypic expression can occur at lower HII levels. Therefore an elevated HII is currently not a required criterion for diagnosis. Current American College of Gastroenterology guidelines recommend non–contrast-enhanced MRI in conjunction with software used to estimate HIC (MRI T2) to noninvasively measure liver iron concentration in non-*C282Y* homozygotes with suspected iron overload.[374]

In the absence of liver injury resulting from other causes, individuals who are heterozygous for an *HFE* mutation are not at risk for iron overload or liver disease, although their hepatic iron levels are intermediate between those of normal and homozygous individuals during the course of a lifetime. The presence of increased iron may also exacerbate liver injury from other causes, such as HCV infection or alcohol abuse, but it does not appear to worsen the severity of nonalcoholic steatohepatitis.[380]

Differential Diagnosis

Given the recommendation for combined use of serum iron indices and genotyping studies, the differential diagnosis in symptomatic individuals is often restricted to iron overload conditions at the time of liver biopsy.

An important differential diagnosis involves distinguishing HH from secondary iron overload, in which Kupffer cells are typically the first cells to show iron accumulation, only later showing accumulation of iron in hepatocytes (Fig. 55.37). A predominantly reticuloendothelial pattern of iron accumulation reliably predicts the absence of homozygosity for the *C282Y* mutation.[375] The most common cause of secondary hemochromatosis is hemolytic anemia associated with ineffective erythropoiesis. In this disorder, excess iron accumulates as a result of transfusions and increased intestinal iron absorption. Transfusion-related systemic siderosis, as in aplastic anemia, leads to parenchymal injury only in extreme cases. Alcohol-induced cirrhosis is often associated with a modest increase in stainable iron within Kupffer cells and in periportal hepatocytes; occasionally, the levels parallel those seen in HH.

A rather unusual form of iron overload that resembles HH occurs in sub-Saharan Africa. This results from ingestion of alcoholic beverages that are fermented within iron containers (Bantu siderosis). A genetic susceptibility to iron accumulation has been identified in this population as well.[381] NH was discussed earlier in this chapter.

Finally, as mentioned earlier, hepatic inflammation or necrosis (or both) in a patient with liver siderosis should always suggest the possibility of a coexistent alternative cause of liver injury.

Natural History and Treatment

The clinical manifestations of HH are typically first apparent in the fifth decade of life, with men seen earlier than women. Clinical symptoms are usually secondary to end-stage parenchymal disease. Death may result from cirrhosis or cardiac failure. The risk of HCC is 20-fold greater than in the general population.[373] However, treatment of the iron overload state has not been shown to decrease the risk of carcinoma. HCC occurs in patients who have been successfully treated by phlebotomy with normalization of their systemic iron levels and also in noncirrhotic livers.[382]

The mainstay of therapy consists of early detection and phlebotomy. Genetic testing for *HFE* mutations is widely available and is recommended for parents and siblings of an affected proband. The potential coexistence of Wilson disease and hemochromatosis in the same patient or family is intriguing with respect to the role of ceruloplasmin in iron transport.[383,384]

Wilson Disease

Clinical Features

Wilson disease, also known as *hepatolenticular degeneration,* is an autosomal recessive disorder that is marked by accumulation of toxic levels of copper in the liver, brain, kidney, and cornea.[385] The worldwide prevalence is 1 in 30,000 to 40,000 individuals. Both the age at onset and the clinical presentation are extremely variable. The disorder rarely manifests before 5 years of age. There is no gender preference.

Wilson disease may manifest clinically with liver disease, a progressive neurological disorder, or a psychiatric illness.

In older patients, neuropsychiatric manifestations include tremor, motor incoordination, behavioral changes, and even frank psychosis. Hepatic involvement as the initial presentation is more common in children and young adults. However, the spectrum of hepatic involvement is very broad, ranging from asymptomatic disease to hepatomegaly with mild biochemical derangement to features of autoimmune hepatitis or chronic hepatitis progressing to cirrhosis, and even to acute liver failure with Coombs-negative hemolytic anemia. Almost half of patients with liver disease lack Kayser-Fleischer (K-F) rings, the characteristic corneal lesion signifying extrahepatic copper deposition, or any concomitant neurological symptoms, and these cases are diagnostically challenging.

Pathogenesis

Ingested copper is normally absorbed in the duodenum and transported to the liver bound to albumin. Free copper atoms dissociate from the complex within hepatocytes and are added to apoceruloplasmin, the predominant copper transporter in plasma, to form holoceruloplasmin. Excess hepatic copper is secreted into bile. This hepatic excretion pathway represents the primary route of elimination of copper from the human body.

Wilson disease is caused by mutations in *ATP7B*, a gene on chromosome 13 that encodes a hepatocyte canalicular membrane ATP-dependent metal transporter.[386-388] More than 300 mutations in *ATP7B* have been identified in affected individuals, mostly in compound heterozygotes, and genotype-phenotype correlations are incomplete.

Clinically significant mutations in *ATP7B* disable hepatocyte canalicular-membrane export of copper into bile, which leads to accumulation of copper within hepatocytes. When the capacity of the liver to segregate copper is exceeded, spillover occurs into extrahepatic sites, including the cornea, where distinctive K-F rings are seen, or into the basal ganglia. Loss of *ATP7B* function also impairs the incorporation of copper into apoceruloplasmin. The subnormal level of ceruloplasmin seen in patients with Wilson disease is a result of the shorter half-life of apoceruloplasmin. Recent interest in abnormal lipid metabolism in Wilson disease[389] has emerged from Lutsenko's molecular analyses of the *ATP7B* knockout mouse.[390]

Pathological Features

Hepatic changes in Wilson disease range from relatively minor to massive, culminating with liver failure.[312] Biopsy is only rarely performed on patients who have acute hepatitis at presentation. At this stage, the liver typically exhibits ballooning of hepatocytes, cholestasis, and apoptosis and contains only a limited lymphocytic (portal) infiltrate. More typical are liver biopsies from patients already in the precirrhotic or cirrhotic state. Characteristic features include mild to moderate macrovesicular steatosis, vacuolization of hepatocyte nuclei (which represents either glycogen or water accumulation), and variable degrees of hepatocyte necrosis (Fig. 55.38). Mallory bodies are occasionally present as well. Moderate to severe parenchymal and portal tract mononuclear inflammation is typically found in patients who are acutely ill at presentation. The degree of mononuclear inflammation is more variable and may actually subside in patients with chronic disease. The liver may be completely cirrhotic at the time of biopsy. Cirrhosis is usually of the macronodular type. Mixed or micronodular cirrhosis may also develop on occasion. Rare patients may have fulminant liver failure at presentation and show massive liver necrosis on biopsy.

Hepatic copper deposits can be demonstrated by special stains. The copper component of the protein complexes appears as red-orange flecks in rhodanine-stained tissue sections (see Fig. 55.38D). The sulfhydryl-rich copper-binding proteins appear as black-brown flecks with the use of an orcein stain. Both the copper-binding proteins and the copper component of the protein complexes appear within periportal hepatocytes in the early stages of disease and then involve the entire lobule with time. Because copper deposition can be highly variable within or between cirrhotic nodules, histological examination of copper deposition in biopsy specimens is prone to sampling error.

Because histology alone cannot reliably distinguish Wilson disease from viral- or drug-induced hepatitis, quantitative demonstration of hepatic copper content in excess of 250 μg per gram of dry weight is helpful in establishing a correct diagnosis. Assessment of hepatic copper levels is best performed on fresh liver tissue obtained with a needle that has been rinsed with a chelating solution before use to remove trace copper levels. Excavation of paraffin-embedded tissue blocks is an option, but this method may yield an artifactually low level of measurable copper.

Differential Diagnosis

Wilson disease should be included in the differential diagnosis of unexplained liver disease that develops between childhood and middle adulthood. A low serum alkaline phosphatase level in a child with acute liver failure is a clue to Wilson disease. Unconjugated bilirubinemia reflecting hemolysis is another important clue.[391] In the second decade of life, Wilson disease may manifest with moderate to severe chronic hepatitis or even cirrhosis. In the third decade of life, the most common histological finding is severe liver fibrosis and cirrhosis. Therefore Wilson disease should be included in the differential diagnosis of almost all types of chronic hepatitis that manifest in the second to fourth decades of life. Histological identification of steatosis and Mallory bodies in a patient with chronic hepatitis and fibrosis should prompt consideration of Wilson disease, even though alcohol is a more common cause of these histological findings.

Because biliary excretion is the normal mechanism of copper elimination from the body, copper also accumulates in patients with chronic obstructive cholestasis. The distribution of stainable copper deposits is periportal. When cirrhosis develops, as in primary biliary cirrhosis or primary sclerosing cholangitis, stainable copper deposits are periseptal.

Ceruloplasmin levels provide a useful screening test for Wilson disease because most patients have subnormal levels of this protein. However, ceruloplasmin is an acute-phase reactant, so hepatic inflammation of any cause may lead to an elevation of serum ceruloplasmin. Conversely, ceruloplasmin levels may be diminished in liver failure, Menkes' disease, or aceruloplasminemia. The AASLD[392] recommends a combination of serum ceruloplasmin level, 24-hour urinary copper excretion, and slit-lamp examination of corneal K-F

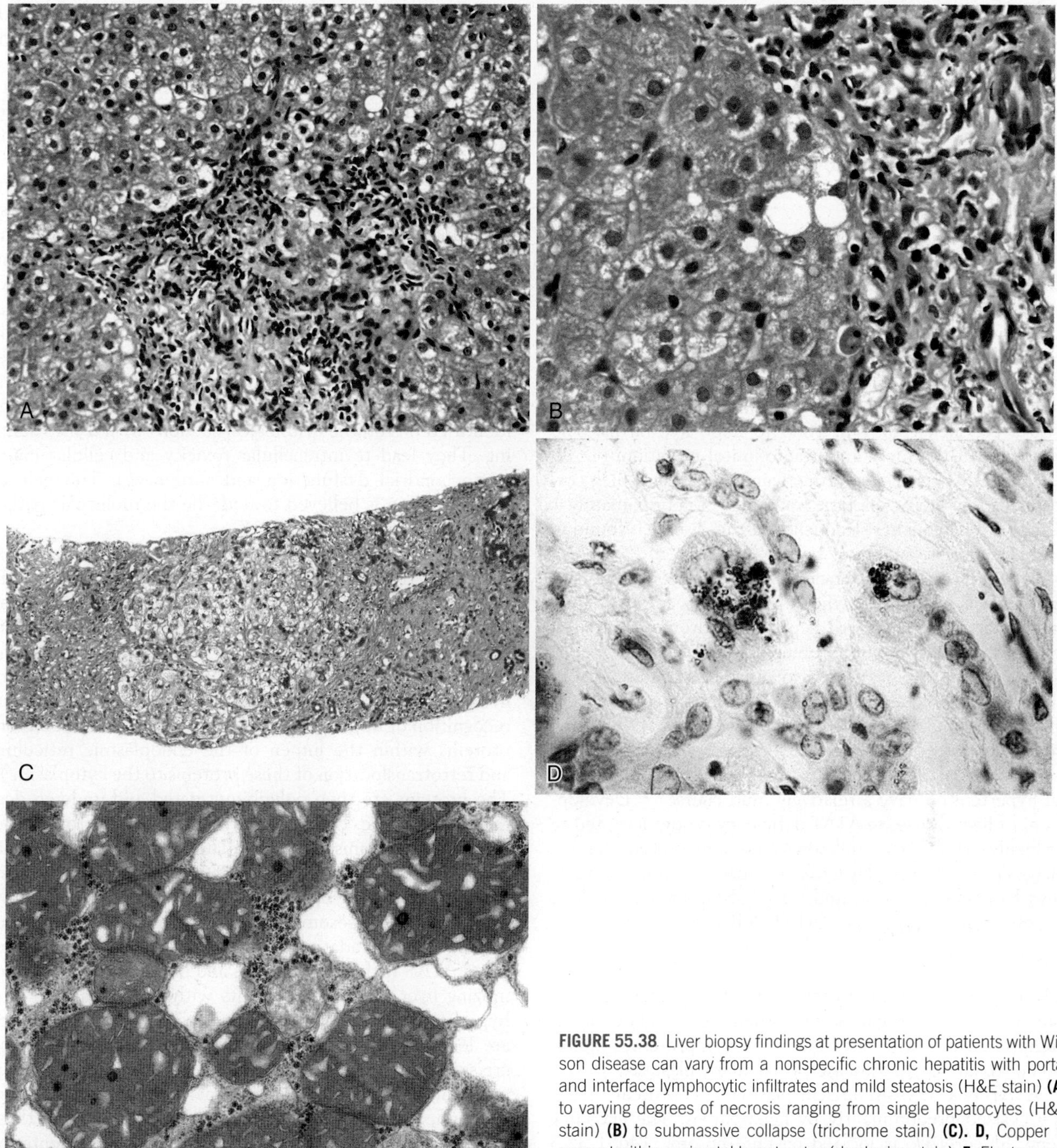

FIGURE 55.38 Liver biopsy findings at presentation of patients with Wilson disease can vary from a nonspecific chronic hepatitis with portal and interface lymphocytic infiltrates and mild steatosis (H&E stain) **(A)** to varying degrees of necrosis ranging from single hepatocytes (H&E stain) **(B)** to submassive collapse (trichrome stain) **(C)**. **D,** Copper is present within periportal hepatocytes (rhodanine stain). **E,** Electron microscopy shows mitochondria with dense matrices, increased dense (calcium phosphate) granules, and dilated cristae.

rings as the initial screening tests of choice. Hepatic copper content greater than 250 μg per gram dry weight of liver is the single most sensitive and accurate biochemical test for Wilson disease. However, recent studies suggest that reducing the threshold to 70 μg/g improves sensitivity.[312] Mutation analysis of *ATP7B* by direct sequencing should be performed if the diagnosis is difficult. Recently, serum zinc levels have been shown to be extremely low in children with acute liver failure as compared with those with WD without ALF and hence a marker of severity of disease.[393]

Natural History and Treatment

Untreated Wilson disease runs an invariably fatal course because of the development of cirrhosis and neuropsychiatric complications. Treatment typically consists of copper chelation therapy accomplished by oral administration of penicillamine or trientine hydrochloride.[312,394] Zinc interferes with copper absorption and is an alternative. The treatment is palliative, with the goal to restore and maintain systemic copper balance. Early diagnosis of Wilson disease is important because pharmacological chelation of copper to facilitate its urinary excretion can halt or even reverse liver damage in affected patients. Limiting intake of dietary copper is an ineffective strategy. Liver transplantation may be required in some instances. On rare occasions, HCC or cholangiocarcinoma may develop in patients affected by Wilson disease.[209]

α_1-Antitrypsin Deficiency Liver Disease

Clinical Features

A1AT deficiency liver disease is the most common inherited metabolic disorder that leads to liver transplantation in childhood.[395] Low levels of this important protease inhibitor result in obstructive lung disease in adulthood, the most common manifestation of A1AT deficiency. However, the pathogenesis of liver disease in A1AT deficiency is entirely different from the one that causes pulmonary manifestations. A1AT deficiency is an autosomal recessive disorder with a prevalence of 1 in 1600 to 2000 live births. The frequency of the most important clinical mutation, PiZ, is 0.0122 in the white North American population, which corresponds to a PiZZ genotype frequency of approximately 1 in 6700.[396] The highest frequency of this disease is found in Swedish and Latvian populations.[397]

Patients with A1AT deficiency are at risk for pulmonary emphysema and liver cirrhosis. The most common liver manifestation is a neonatal hepatitis syndrome, associated with conjugated hyperbilirubinemia and acholic stools. Therefore it is important to distinguish this condition from biliary atresia[398] (see Fig. 55.13). However, in a prospective study done in Sweden, only approximately 17% of PiZ infants demonstrated signs of liver disease during the first two decades of life.[399] Some patients with cirrhosis and portal hypertension have a relatively mild course.[400] Development of liver disease in A1AT deficiency is now accepted to be highly variable, with unknown environmental and genetic factors postulated to play a role. Prospective population surveys have not demonstrated a risk of either liver or lung disease in heterozygotes for A1AT deficiency.

Pathogenesis

A1AT is a major serum protein that suffuses interstitial tissues at times of inflammation, when vascular integrity is compromised. The major function of this protein is inhibition of tissue serine proteases, particularly elastase.

A1AT is a 394–amino-acid plasma glycoprotein that is synthesized predominantly by hepatocytes. The encoding gene, *SERPINA1*, is located on chromosome 14q31-32.3 and is highly polymorphic. At least 75 A1AT alleles have been identified; they are denoted alphabetically by their migration pattern on an isoelectric gel. The general notation *Pi* stands for "protease inhibitor." An alphabetic letter corresponds to the polypeptide's migration position on an electrophoretic gel, and two letters denote the individual's genotype. Because circulating levels of A1AT reflect a contribution from both alleles, heterozygous states typically produce circulating levels of A1AT that are intermediate between those expected for the homozygous state and those in individuals without A1AT deficiency.

The most common genotype is PiMM, which occurs in 90% of individuals and is considered to be the wild type. Most allelic variants exhibit a relatively conservative substitution within the polypeptide chain and produce normal circulating levels of functional A1AT. Some variants, including the *PiS* allele, result in a reduction of serum A1AT levels when homozygous (PiSS) but without clinical manifestations. Rare variants, termed *Pi-null*, result in a complete absence of detectable serum A1AT in the homozygous state.

Clinically, the most common relevant genetic mutation is *PiZ*, which causes a Glu342Lys missense change in the protein.[401] Homozygotes for the *PiZZ* genotype have circulating A1AT levels approximately 10% of normal. These individuals are at high risk for pulmonary disease. The pathophysiology of liver disease is different from that of pulmonary disease. Although the liver synthesizes A1AT for release into plasma, A1AT is not required for liver function. The PiZ-mutant protein produces a conformationally altered unstable protein that is prone to homomeric aggregation. Such aggregates are retained within the endoplasmic reticulum (hence the deficiency in the plasma) and can be identified on routine histological sections with d-PAS staining. They lead to intracellular toxicity and cellular injury (mitochondrial dysfunction and autophagy). This gain of toxic function is believed to underlie the molecular pathogenesis of liver disease.

All individuals with the PiZZ genotype accumulate misfolded A1AT polypeptide within the endoplasmic reticulum of hepatocytes. However, not all PiZZ individuals develop liver disease. Only patients who have additional defects in the degradation mechanisms for retained proteins in the endoplasmic reticulum are at risk for clinically significant liver disease.[401] The normal degradative machinery requires recognition of misfolded, unassembled, or mutant secretory proteins within the lumen of the endoplasmic reticulum and retrotranslocation of these proteins to the cytoplasm.[402] The proteins are then polyubiquitinated and undergo degradation by the cytoplasmic multicatalytic proteasome. The other mechanism for degradation of retained abnormal A1AT is autophagy, in which intracellular organelles are sequestered within newly formed autophagosomes, which then fuse with lysosomes so all components are degraded. This second degradation pathway is activated by the aggregated A1AT within hepatocytes and plays a key role in minimizing liver damage in patients with this disease.[403] It is hypothesized that some individuals with the PiZZ genotype are less able to eliminate misfolded A1AT and therefore are subject to progressive liver damage. Investigation of the mechanisms involved in proteasomal and autophagic system function, and whether changes in the functionality of these systems account for differences in the clinical presentation and natural history of A1AT storage disease, represents an important area for future research.[402] In animal models, bile duct ligation has been shown to increase autophagy in A1AT livers by accumulation of bile acids with subsequent clearance of the globules.[404] Coinheritance of additional defects in hepatocellular protein processing may be involved.

Individuals who are homozygous for null alleles of the *SERPINA1* gene develop pulmonary disease. However, because no A1AT polypeptide is synthesized, these patients are not at risk for liver disease.

Pathological Features

In approximately 11% of individuals with the PiZZ genotype, a cholestatic form of hepatitis develops in infancy. As discussed earlier, this condition resembles neonatal hepatitis

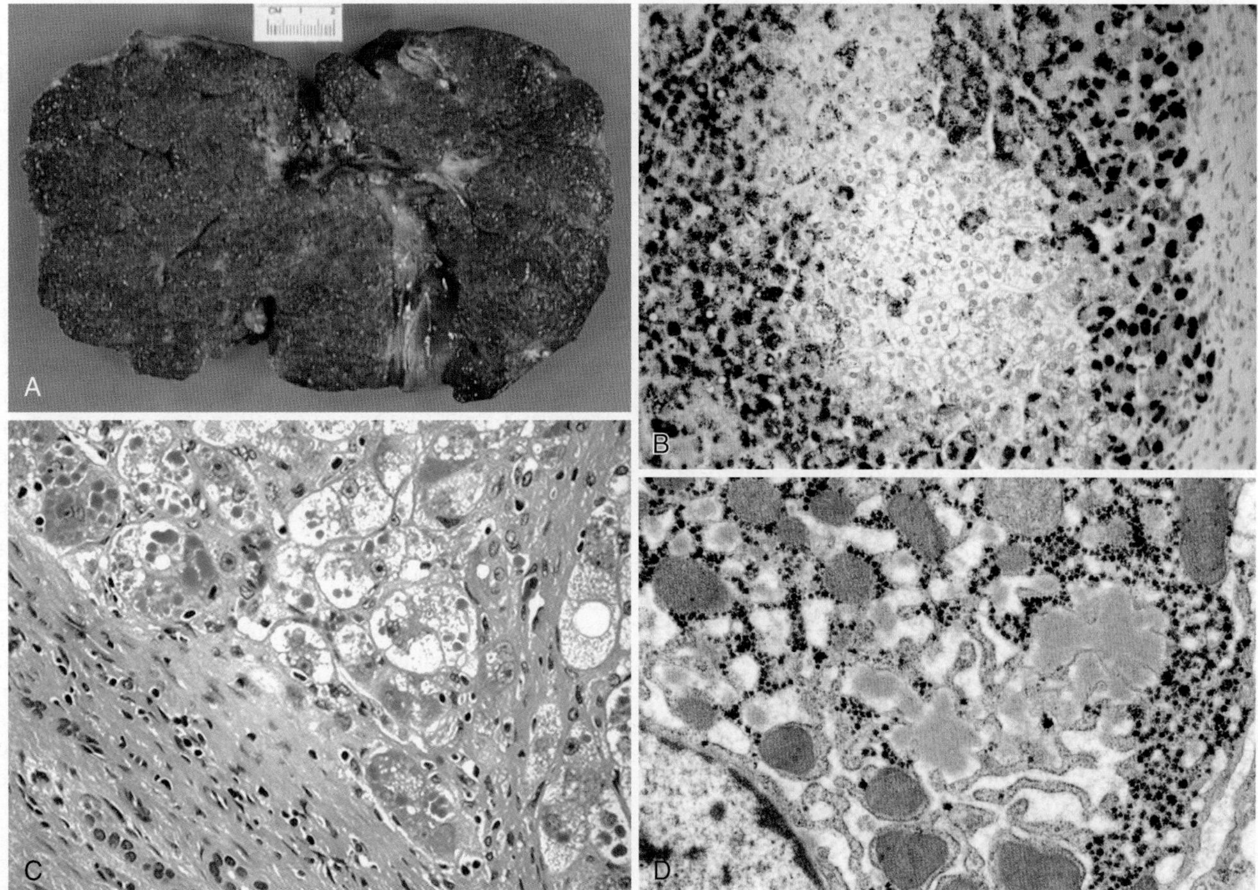

FIGURE 55.39 α_1**-Antitrypsin storage disease. A,** Micronodular cirrhosis in an explant from a 6-year-old patient. **B,** Markedly prominent accumulation of A1AT protein in hepatocytes of an older individual, as detected by immunohistochemistry. **C,** Abundant glycoprotein is present in periportal hepatocytes. **D,** The protein distends the endoplasmic reticulum in this electron photomicrograph.

or biliary atresia. Characteristic features include paucity of interlobular bile ducts, proliferation of bile ductules at the margins of portal tracts, panlobular hepatocellular and canalicular cholestasis, and, occasionally, giant cell transformation of hepatocytes and hepatocyte rosetting[4] (see Fig. 55.13). Inflammation tends to be minimal. Cholangiography may reveal a patent but narrowed extrahepatic biliary tract. Hepatocellular inclusions of A1AT are not prominent in young children. Immunohistochemistry can be used to confirm the presence of A1AT in globular inclusions (see Fig. 55.13).

The 80% to 90% of individuals with the PiZZ genotype who do not become ill as infants may develop chronic liver disease, typically in the fourth or fifth decade of life. Liver biopsies reveal a severely fibrotic or cirrhotic liver, usually with intracellular globules of A1AT easily evident within periportal hepatocytes. These intracellular globules are eosinophilic on H&E-stained tissue sections (Fig. 55.39) and stain magenta with d-PAS.

Demonstration of A1AT inclusions within hepatocytes does not establish with certainty that the patient is homozygous for *PiZZ*. A1AT inclusions can develop in patients who are heterozygous for the *PiZ* mutation (i.e., the *PiMZ* genotype).[405] In the latter instance, d-PAS–positive globules within hepatocytes are typically identified as an incidental finding on liver biopsy performed for other reasons. Serotyping is required to determine whether the individual is of a *PiMZ* or *PiZZ* genotype.

Natural History and Treatment

Neonatal cholestasis related to A1AT storage disease resolves by 6 months of age without treatment in approximately 25% of affected children. An additional 25% of patients show persistently abnormal AST and ALT levels, prolonged cholestasis, and pruritus. In another 25%, the patient's jaundice resolves, but the raised ALT and AST levels often persist, along with an enlarged liver and spleen. The remaining 25% of patients either die of cirrhosis or require liver transplantation at ages ranging from 6 months to 17 years.[406]

Pulmonary emphysema and cirrhosis are the most common underlying causes of death (72% and 10%, respectively).[407] Death from liver disease usually occurs within 2 years of the clinical diagnosis of cirrhosis. An additional 3% of affected individuals die of HCC or cholangiocarcinoma, usually, but not always, in the setting of cirrhosis. Treatment of lung disease is similar to that used for chronic obstructive pulmonary disease. The treatment, and cure, for severe hepatic disease at any age is orthotopic liver transplantation. Although gene therapy has been experimentally attempted in A1AT-deficient individuals, perhaps the most exciting finding has come from Perlmutter and colleagues, who showed that the common antiepileptic drug, carbamazepine, can be used successfully to enhance autophagy in mouse models of A1AT liver disease, thereby reducing hepatic load and fibrosis.[408] It remains to be seen whether similar effects can be achieved in humans with A1AT deficiency liver disease.

Hereditary Transthyretin Amyloidosis

This section on hereditary disorders of hepatic metabolism bears mention of hereditary transthyretin amyloidosis (hereditary ATTR). This rare fatal autosomal disorder is characterized by progressive buildup of amyloid fibrils in organs and tissues of mutated transthyretin (TTR), with more than 130 *TTR* gene mutations identified thus far.[409] Wild-type TTR can also become amyloidogenic by mechanisms not yet understood. Hereditary ATTR manifests as sensorimotor neuropathy, autonomic neuropathy, cardiomyopathy, and nephropathy, especially in men older than 60 years of age.[410] Because the liver is the main biosynthetic source of either wild-type or mutated TTR, this disease qualifies as an inherited disorder of hepatic metabolism. Importantly, the liver itself remains undamaged, and it manifests no morphological or other physiological impairment.

Pending the outcome of clinical studies for recent potential pharmaceutical and gene therapies,[410] the standard therapeutic option remains orthotopic liver transplantation, which can lead to improvement in sensory and motor impairment as well as long-term overall survival.[411,412] A key curiosity of this disorder is that, in the performance of orthotopic liver transplantation to cure patients of hereditary ATTR, their explanted livers can be used as a donor organ for select liver transplant recipients (e.g., with liver tumors or acute liver failure).[413] Overall experience with "domino liver transplantation" is favorable, although a limited subset of recipients of a hereditary ATTR liver may require retransplantation.[414]

ABNORMAL DEVELOPMENT OF LIVER ANATOMY

In both pediatric and adult patients, aberrant liver anatomy can be difficult for surgeons and pathologists to assess.[415,416] Often, detailed imaging studies are required before the surgeon embarks on major hepatic surgery.[417,418]

The embryological origin of the liver involves formation of a dorsal bud from the primitive foregut, growth and invasion of tissue into the mesenchymal septum transversum, and separation of the growing liver from the nascent diaphragm. This forms a predominantly epithelial organ that lies free within the abdominal cavity and is invested within the Glisson capsule on its convex surface. Hepatic macroanatomy is divided into right and left lobes, delineated by the ventral midline falciform ligament, the caudate lobe as the dorsal bulge of the liver between the groove of the inferior vena cava and the dorsal midline, and the quadrate lobe in the right lateroinferior region located between the falciform ligament and the gallbladder fossa. For surgeons, the liver is divided into eight segments on the basis of vascular anatomy. Termed the *Couinaud system*,[419] this is the basis for the PRETEXT system used by radiologists and surgeons for determining resectability of liver tumors.

Agenesis and Hypogenesis

Agenesis or hypogenesis of the right hepatic lobe is a rare congenital anomaly that is usually identified radiographically.[420] It is typically accompanied by compensatory enlargement of the left hepatic lobe, posterior interposition of the hepatic flexure of the colon, retrohepatic or suprahepatic position of the gallbladder, absence of the right hepatic artery and portal vein, and absence of the right intrahepatic bile ducts. There may also be partial or complete absence of the right side of the diaphragm as well as intestinal malrotation. Agenesis of the left lobe of the liver can lead to gastric volvulus.

Because agenesis or hypogenesis of a hepatic lobe is usually clinically silent, most cases are identified incidentally in adulthood. The differential diagnosis includes severe hepatic lobe atrophy secondary to liver cirrhosis or other conditions such as cholangiocarcinoma, choledocholithiasis, prior fulminant hepatitis, Caroli disease, or prior surgical resection.[421] Patients with right hepatic lobe agenesis may have portal hypertension. Some patients exhibit symptoms of atypical cholecystitis, choledocholithiasis, or portal hypertension. Radiographic criteria for diagnosing agenesis of the right hepatic lobe are absence of the right hepatic vein, the right portal vein and its branches, and the right hepatic ducts. In contrast, in severe lobar atrophy, the hilar vascular and ductal structures are present. The pathogenesis of lobar agenesis is unclear, but it presumably involves abnormal embryological growth and development of the vasculature, or possibly localized thrombosis. Agenesis of the right hepatic lobe has been described in association with absence of the infrarenal segment of the inferior vena cava,[421] raising the possibility that vascular compromise, in multiple vascular channels, may occur in utero.

Anomalies of Position

Anomalies of position include situs inversus, accessory lobes, and ectopic hepatic tissue. Situs inversus is part of a spectrum of laterality disorders with an autosomal recessive genetic predisposition. The incidence of situs inversus totalis is 1 in 5000 to 20,000 births.[422] Accessory or ectopic liver has an incidence of between 0.47% and 0.7% in laparoscopic studies.[423] It is classified either as an accessory liver, when it is connected to the main liver, or as true ectopia, when no connection is present.[424] An estimated 20 million people in the United States have cholelithiasis, and approximately 300,000 cholecystectomies are performed annually.[425] Therefore both surgeons and pathologists are likely to encounter cases of anomalous or ectopic liver during the course of their career.

Situs Inversus

Situs inversus totalis represents anatomy that is a perfect mirror image of the normal positions of visceral organs. The normal anteroposterior relationships are preserved, and this can occur with either dextrocardia or levocardia.[426] Patients with situs inversus totalis and dextrocardia can be completely asymptomatic. However, Kartagener syndrome occurs in approximately 20% of these patients. Kartagener syndrome is situs inversus totalis and dextrocardia combined with impaired ciliary movement resulting in sinusitis and bronchiectasis. Workup of a child with unexplained neonatal respiratory distress, recurrent otitis media, chronic nasal drainage and sinusitis, and chronic bronchitis for primary ciliary dyskinesia may reveal situs inversus totalis or other laterality defects in 50% of cases.[427]

Partial rotations of visceral organs ("situs ambiguous" or "situs inversus partialis") and levocardia are often associated with congenital heart diseases and other organ anomalies. In these situations, the organ anomalies can be a major life-limiting condition. Although the liver is otherwise anatomically normal in situs inversus totalis (Fig. 55.40), there is an increased likelihood of biliary tract and vascular anomalies in patients with situs inversus partialis. These include duodenal atresia, biliary atresia, gastroschisis with malrotation, congenital hepatic fibrosis, tracheoesophageal fistula, Currarino's triad, and pheochromocytoma.[428]

Liver transplantation may be needed for patients with situs inversus or other hepatic anomalies[429,430]; biliary atresia occurs in 10% to 20% of children with situs inversus,[431] and children with biliary atresia may have other visceral anomalies.[130,432] Liver transplantation of adults with situs inversus is rare.[433]

Accessory Lobe

An accessory lobe or liver arises from a normally situated liver and is usually attached to the liver by a broad-based or a narrow stalk containing afferent and efferent vasculature and bile ducts. The accessory lobe may be located in an infrahepatic position, and it extends into the thoracic cavity in some patients.[434] The size of accessory lobes may be substantial, equaling, or, in some cases, exceeding 15% of the total liver mass.[435] Accessory lobes may manifest as a mass lesion and be misinterpreted as a malignant tumor,[434] or they may obstruct other vessels, such as the inferior vena cava.[436] When the accessory lobe has a narrow pedicle, it may be subjected to torsion, leading eventually to infarction, liver failure, sepsis, and death.

Ectopic Liver

Ectopic liver tissue may occur in various subdiaphragmatic sites, usually in the vicinity of the native liver, such as on the gallbladder, hepatic ligaments, omentum, or retroperitoneum.[437] It usually ranges in diameter from a few millimeters to several centimeters. Occasionally, ectopias are present in the small intestine or pancreas.[437] Intrathoracic heterotopic liver may occur as a separate mass lesion in the presence of an intact diaphragm and without connection to the native liver.[438] Ectopic liver has also been reported in the mediastinum,[439] umbilical cord,[440,441] and stomach.[442] The cause of ectopic liver is attributed to aberrant migration of hepatocytes during embryogenesis[443] or, in the case of thoracic heterotopia, to anomalous extension of hepatic tissue into the developing thorax before fusion of the septum transversum.[438]

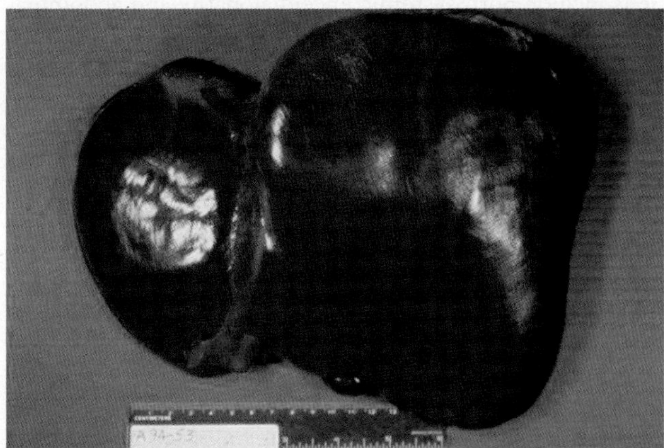

FIGURE 55.40 An otherwise unremarkable liver from a patient with situs inversus totalis who died of heart disease. The *ruler* attests to the correct orientation of this photograph.

Although ectopic liver is usually silent, it can cause clinical symptoms such as abdominal pain resulting from recurrent torsion, compression of adjacent organs, intraperitoneal bleeding, or obstruction of the esophagus or portal vein.[424] Histologically, the ectopic liver tissue is usually normal in appearance but may exhibit histological features similar to those of the native liver in conditions such as alcohol-induced liver disease.[444] Ectopic or heterotopic liver may be a site of tumor formation (including HCC[445,446] and mesenchymal hamartoma[438]), or it may be a site of metastasis from HCC of the native liver.[447] HCC is observed in approximately 30% of ectopic livers.[448] Ectopic liver does not have normal vascular and ductal anatomy and may be metabolically impaired; therefore it may have a propensity for hepatocarcinogenesis that is not shared with the native liver.[444,445] Fortunately, most cancers that arise in ectopic liver have a favorable prognosis because the likelihood of complete resection is high.[449-452]

Ectopic liver is also susceptible to A1AT retention.[424] Supradiaphragmatic heterotopic liver is usually associated with cardiac anomalies and other congenital anomalies such as diaphragmatic hernia, and, occasionally, pectus excavatum or intralobar pulmonary sequestration.[438,453,454] Ectopic liver may be misinterpreted clinically and radiographically as a malignant tumor.

Pancreatic Heterotopia

Pancreatic heterotopia within liver tissue is a metaplastic process involving multipotential cells within the ductular compartment of the liver. This view is based on a detailed study of 382 liver explants from patients with end-stage liver disease, 16 (4.2%) of which contained pancreatic exocrine tissue.[455] The pancreatic tissue was located in close proximity to reactive bile ductules and also exhibited a transitional immunophenotype similar to both bile ductules and pancreatic acinar tissue. Adenocarcinoma has been found to arise within intrahepatic pancreatic tissue.[456,457]

Ciliated Hepatic Foregut Cyst

Simple biliary cysts are usually an incidental finding in adults. When multiple, they are viewed as a component of polycystic liver disease (discussed later). In contrast, ciliated hepatic foregut cysts (CHFC) are a rare form of cystic liver disease, with over 100 cases reported[458,459] since the original description in 1857. With increased awareness of this condition, particularly by imaging, most of the cases have been reported within the past 15 years.

Cysts range from 1 to 13 cm in diameter. Histologically, CHFC exhibits four layers: a lining of pseudostratified ciliated columnar epithelium, a subepithelial layer of loose connective tissue, a smooth muscle layer, and an outer rind of tough fibrous tissue. By immunohistochemistry, the epithelial layer is positive for epithelial membrane antigen (EMA) and carcinoembryonic antigen (CEA).[460] The cilia are immunoreactive for actin and desmin. Endocrine cells are present within the epithelial layer, similar to respiratory epithelium, and show immunoreactivity to chromogranin, synaptophysin, bombesin, and calcitonin.[461] Because these lesions are usually identified by imaging studies, fine-needle aspiration cytology is very helpful in confirming the diagnosis.[462] The characteristic cytological feature is the presence of ciliated, pseudostratified, tall columnar epithelial cells suspended within a mucoid background. Additional findings include goblet cells, macrophages, and hepatocytes.

This cystic condition usually manifests in adulthood,[459] but can appear at any age including prenatally. There is no predilection for males or females. Although right upper quadrant pain and obstructive jaundice are common at presentation, most patients are asymptomatic. The cysts are usually discovered incidentally by imaging or during surgical exploration. Cysts occur most commonly in segment IV of the left lobe of the liver. Most are simple cysts, but multiloculation can occur. CHFCs are almost always benign. On occasion, squamous metaplasia is present in the epithelial lining. Squamous cell carcinoma has been reported in three patients with large cysts.[459]

The presence of ciliated epithelium favors a foregut origin of these cysts. Wheeler and Edmondson[463] proposed that CHFCs develop as a result of detachment and migration of buds from the esophageal and bronchial regions of the foregut and their subsequent entrapment in the liver. Bronchial cysts (with their attendant cartilaginous elements) and esophageal cysts share a common embryological origin with CHFC. One possible explanation for the occurrence of ciliated cysts in intraabdominal locations (including liver) and in the retroperitoneum is the presence of two patent pleuroperitoneal canals spanning the septum transversum, which close by the eighth week of embryogenesis.[464] It is therefore relevant that the left lobe of the liver, and in particular, segment IV, where most CHFCs are found, constitute the bulk of the entire liver during the fourth to sixth weeks of development.[459] Despite the embryological origin of these cysts, they enlarge gradually during life and therefore are usually detected in adulthood. Surgery remains the mainstay of treatment, and complete resection is recommended.[465]

Hereditary Hemorrhagic Telangiectasia (Osler-Weber-Rendu Syndrome)

An arteriovenous malformation (AVM) represents a disruption of the normal vascular pattern of an interposed capillary network located between the arterial and venous circulations. An artery or arteriole connects directly to a vein or venule, bypassing nutrient exchange and shunting blood directly to the venous system.[466] The usual anatomical configuration is a nidus of dilated feeding arteries or arterioles connecting to a draining vein or system of veins. Although AVMs can affect any vascular bed, the mature liver is generally free from AVMs except in cases of hereditary hemorrhagic telangiectasia (HHT). This is a rare inherited vascular disorder that is also known as Osler-Weber-Rendu syndrome, after initial case reports by Henri Rendu in 1896, Sir William Osler in 1900, and Frederick Parkes Weber in 1907.[466] HHT is characterized by spontaneous epistaxis, mucocutaneous telangiectasias, and visceral AVMs in patients with a family history of this syndrome. Three of these four findings are diagnostic of HHT, according to the Curaçao criteria.[467] Solid organs (lungs, brain, liver) may exhibit large AVMs.

HHT is a genetically heterogeneous autosomal dominant disorder, with more than 80% of patients having heterozygous mutations in two genes.[468] HHT type 1 is caused by mutations in the endoglin gene (*ENG*, chromosomal locus 9q34), and HHT type 2 is caused by mutations in the gene that encodes activin A receptor type II–like 1 (*ACVRL1*, chromosomal locus 12q13). Both ENG and ACVRL1 (previously called ALK-1) modulate endothelial response to the transforming growth factor-β superfamily of ligands, are present on endothelial cells, and are involved in angiogenesis.[469] Mutations in *SMAD4 (MADH4)* have been identified in patients with features of both juvenile polyposis and HHT (known as *JPHT syndrome*). There are possibly two additional HHT disease–causing genes on chromosomes 5q and 7p. There are hundreds of individual mutations, and almost every family with HHT has been found to have a unique mutation. Heterozygous mosaicism has also been described.[470] The estimated genetic frequency of this disorder is about 1 in 5000 individuals.[471]

The most common clinical manifestations are spontaneous and recurrent epistaxis and multiple telangiectasias, the latter of which occur on the lips, face, tongue, or hands in adulthood.[471] One third of affected individuals exhibit symptoms by 10 years of age, and 80% to 90% by 21 years of age. Symptomatic gastrointestinal bleeding, usually low grade, occurs in 20% to 25% of affected individuals, usually after 50 years of age. However, the clinical phenotype of HHT is heterogeneous, showing extremely varied presentations, even among members of a family with the same mutation.[471] Rarely, brain and lung AVMs cause symptoms, and complications of bleeding or shunting can be sudden and catastrophic. Hepatic AVMs are relatively common in HHT, being identified in 40% to more than 80% of patients screened by Doppler ultrasound or computed tomography.[472] Only 5% to 8% of these patients are symptomatic, as a consequence of either shunting (including heart failure), biliary ischemia, or portal hypertension.[473] Biliary and hepatic necrosis, when severe, can lead to acute liver failure. Hemorrhage is rare. Other uncommon manifestations include portosystemic encephalopathy and abdominal angina. Hepatic shunting can usually be treated medically. Embolization of the hepatic artery has had unpredictable results, with a postprocedure mortality rate of 20% caused by necrosis of the biliary tree.[474]

Because liver biopsy can cause serious complications, the diagnosis should be made by imaging.[472] Liver transplantation is currently the only therapeutic option for severe hepatic involvement in patients with HHT.[475]

Liver pathology in HHT consists of microscopic telangiectasias and direct arteriovenous and portovenous shunts, as evidenced by patent channels between portal arterioles or veins and ectatic sinusoids or between portal arteries and veins (Fig. 55.41).[472] Progressive enlargement of these vascular lesions results in the formation of large, confluent vascular masses and macroscopic AVMs that are detectable by imaging. Most commonly, these AVMs connect hepatic artery to portal vein, followed by hepatic artery to hepatic vein and portal vein to hepatic vein. Blood supply derangements lead to secondary pathological changes, including increased fibrous tissue deposition in portal and periportal locations. Liver cirrhosis does not occur unless there are other cofactors, such as chronic viral infection or iron overload.[476] The deranged vascular supply of the liver leads to parenchymal perfusion abnormalities that incite hepatocellular regenerative activity, either diffusely or focally, giving rise to nodular regenerative hyperplasia or focal nodular hyperplasia, respectively.[472,477] When nodular regenerative hyperplasia coexists with HHT-induced fibrotic tissue around abnormal intrahepatic blood vessels, an erroneous diagnosis of cirrhosis may be made. Last, the intrahepatic arteriovenous shunting may result in injury to the intrahepatic biliary tree, which is fed exclusively by the hepatic artery. This may result in chronic cholestasis, or, rarely, liver failure from necrotizing cholangitis.[478,479] Rupture of telangiectatic lesions and ischemic necrosis of intrahepatic bile ducts can occur and may precipitate regional loss of hepatic integrity.[479]

ABNORMAL DEVELOPMENT OF THE BILIARY TRACT

The intrahepatic biliary tract is subject to a striking set of developmental abnormalities, collectively termed *ductal plate malformations* (DPMs) based on the theory that embryological arrest of ductal plate development is the underlying cause (Table 55.22).[111,114,480] Distinctions among these various conditions are not sharp because a spectrum of abnormalities may be present in a single individual. In addition, different family members of a proband may exhibit different abnormalities of the intrahepatic biliary tree.

Von Meyenburg Complex (Biliary Hamartoma)

Von Meyenburg complex (biliary hamartoma) consists of a variable number of dilated and/or tortuous bile ducts embedded within dense fibrous, sometimes hyalinized, stroma (Fig. 55.42A).[481,482] The complexes are typically found within expanded portal tracts. The lumina of the dilated ducts often contain inspissated bile and may connect to each other. Von Meyenburg complexes are found incidentally in 5% to 6% of adult autopsies and only rarely in children. They are usually small, are multiple, and may occur anywhere in the liver.[483]

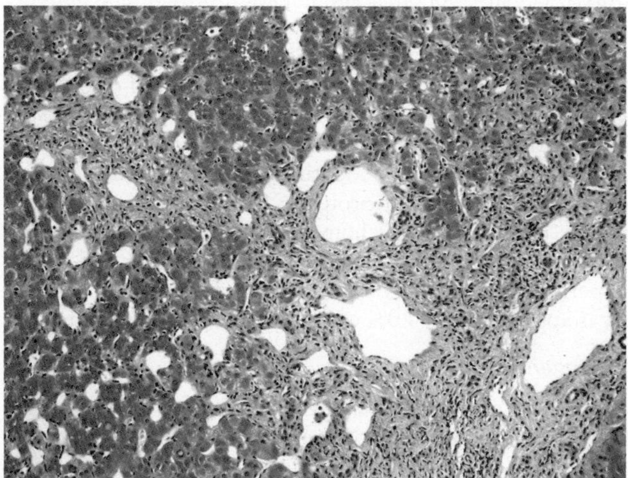

FIGURE 55.41 Hereditary hemorrhagic telangiectasia (Osler-Weber-Rendu syndrome). The portal tract is expanded by dilated vascular spaces and a cellular mesenchyme. Numerous dilated sinusoidal channels are evident in the periportal region.

Desmet[481] hypothesized that von Meyenburg complexes arise as a result of arrest or perturbation of the remodeling of the ductal plates that occurs in the late phase of embryological development of the intrahepatic biliary tree. Von Meyenburg complexes are common in patients with congenital hepatic fibrosis or polycystic liver disease, supporting Desmet's hypothesis. Polycystic kidney and hepatic disease 1 gene mutations have been reported in a family cohort of von Meyenburg complexes.[484] Cholangiocarcinoma arising within von Meyenburg complexes has been reported.[485]

Autosomal Recessive Polycystic Kidney Disease

Clinical Features

ARPKD typically manifests in neonates or infants with massive bilateral nephromegaly caused by diffuse dilation of the collecting ducts, sufficient to compromise lung growth in utero. Affected neonates may die of pulmonary insufficiency. ARPKD arises from mutations in the polycystic kidney and hepatic disease 1 gene *(PKHD1)*, located on chromosome 6p21.[486,487] The encoded protein, fibrocystin, is one of many that are normally present on the primary cilia of the renal tubules and intrahepatic bile ducts.[488] Although the exact function of fibrocystin is unknown, it is believed to play a vital role in maintenance of the structural integrity of organs such as the kidney and liver through modulation of a variety of cellular functions such as cell proliferation, secretion, apoptosis, and terminal differentiation.[120,489]

Pathological Features

Macroscopically, visible liver cysts are seldom evident in patients with ARPKD.[481] Rather, portal tracts may be enlarged by connective tissue and rimmed by numerous dilated bile duct profiles; this is the characteristic feature of congenital hepatic fibrosis in children with less severe renal disease who survive infancy (Fig. 55.43). Normal interlobular bile ducts within the center of portal tracts

TABLE 55.22 Developmental Abnormalities of the Intrahepatic Biliary Tree (Including Alagille Syndrome)

Abnormality	Genetic Mutations (If Known)
Alagille syndrome	*JAG1* (also *NOTCH2*)
Von Meyenburg complex	No specific genetic associations; may be present in polycystic liver disease and congenital hepatic fibrosis
Congenital hepatic fibrosis	May coexist with autosomal recessive polycystic kidney disease; fibrocystin gene
Polycystic liver disease	Usually coexists with autosomal dominant polycystic kidney disease; polycystin-1 and polycystin-2 genes *(PKD1, PKD2)*
Caroli disease/ syndrome	Reported autosomal recessive and autosomal dominant associations

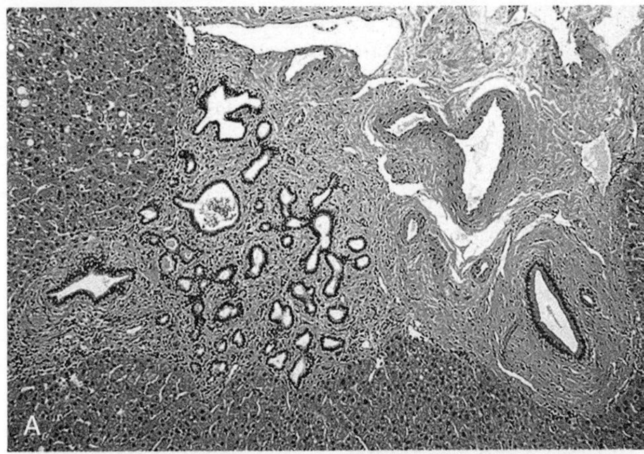

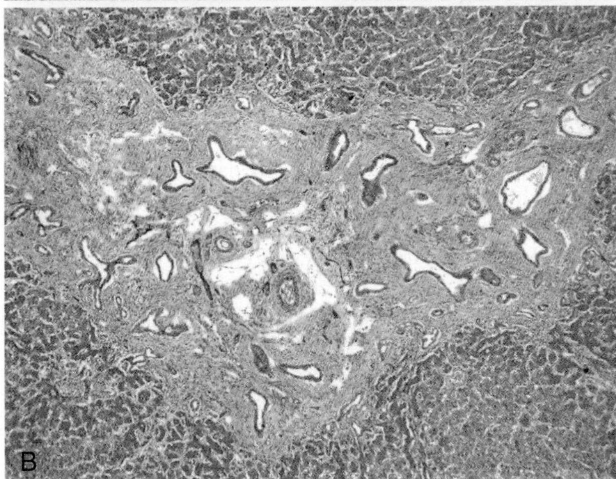

FIGURE 55.42 A, Von Meyenburg complex in an adult liver (H&E stain). **B,** Liver from a 4-month-old patient with classic Joubert syndrome has multiple ectatic portal ducts within widely expanded and fibrotic portal tracts throughout the liver. No ductal plate features at the interface are evident (trichrome stain).

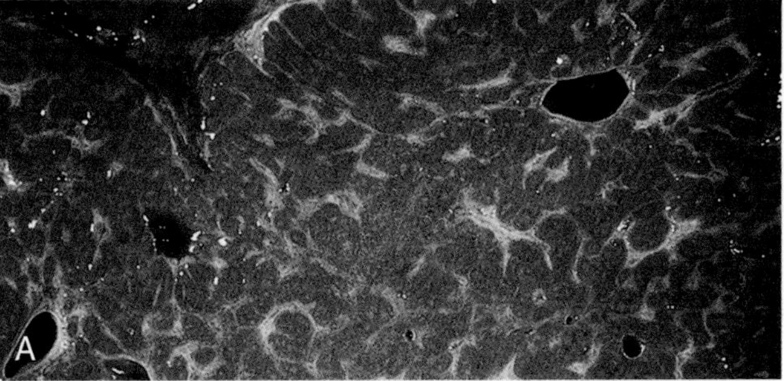

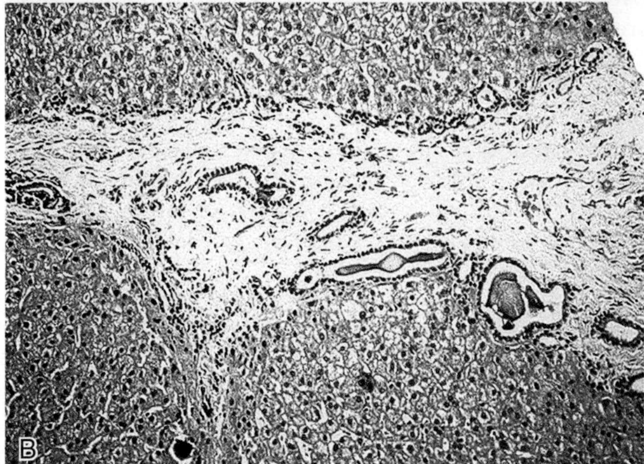

FIGURE 55.43 Congenital hepatic fibrosis. A, Gross specimen shows dense fibrous bands subdividing the liver but without definitive formation of nodules. **B,** Low-power photomicrograph shows diagnostic dense fibrosis of portal tracts with numerous marginal dilated bile ductular profiles. Bile retention may lead to cholangitis, but none is evident here.

are often absent. This histological picture corresponds to incompletely remodeled ductal plates. In keeping with the normal development of the biliary tree, these malformed bile ducts are continuous with the rest of the biliary system.

Natural History

Seventy-nine percent of children who have undergone kidney transplantation for ARPKD develop complications of congenital hepatic fibrosis.[490]

Congenital Hepatic Fibrosis

Clinical Features

Congenital hepatic fibrosis is a condition in which progressive fibrosis of the portal tract system leads to hepatomegaly and portal hypertension. Affected individuals may become symptomatic because of abdominal distention related to hepatosplenomegaly, respiratory distress from visceromegaly and ascites, or rupture of an unsuspected esophageal varix. Cholangitis also may be a presenting symptom. Congenital hepatic fibrosis should be suspected in children who have symptoms of portal hypertension. Congenital hepatic fibrosis may also be accompanied by isolated anomalies of the gallbladder or common bile duct or by dilation of the large intrahepatic bile ducts, referred to as *Caroli syndrome.*[481] A congenital hepatic fibrosis–like histological pattern of disease is also a major feature of the rare autosomal recessive disorder known as *Meckel syndrome*[491] and several other maldevelopment syndromes, including asphyxiating thoracic dystrophy, Ivemark syndrome, COACH syndrome (*c*erebellar vermis hypo/aplasia, *o*ligophrenia, congenital *a*taxia, ocular *c*oloboma, and *h*epatic fibrosis), and Joubert syndrome (see Fig. 55.42B).

Congenital hepatic fibrosis is also a feature of the rare CDG type Ib, an autosomal recessive inherited disorder of glycosylation[492] (see earlier discussion and Fig. 55.26). MPI enzyme deficiency accounts for the majority of cases.[493] This disorder is detected by identification of altered *N*-linked glycosylation of serum proteins. Clinical features include severe mental and psychomotor retardation, dysmorphic features, retinitis pigmentosa, failure to thrive, and portal hypertension caused by congenital hepatic fibrosis. Mortality is approximately 20% within the first 2 years of life.

Pathogenesis

Congenital hepatic fibrosis is considered to be an autosomal recessive disorder because most children have coexistent ARPKD or dilation of the intrahepatic or extrahepatic biliary tree, characteristic of Caroli syndrome. There are also reports of congenital hepatic fibrosis occurring in families with autosomal dominant polycystic kidney disease (ADPKD).[494-496]

Pathological Features

The liver in patients with congenital hepatic fibrosis is typically of normal size. On gross examination, irregular whitish areas of fibrosis are typically evident (see Fig. 55.43A). Histologically, the portal tracts show expansion by connective tissue, with wide areas of septal bridging fibrosis connecting portal tracts to each other (see Fig. 55.43B). Persistent ductal remnants are usually evident along the margins of portal tracts and fibrous septa (see Fig. 55.43B). Interlobular bile ducts may be present, but their epithelium is usually intact, and bile is usually not retained. Portal veins may be hypoplastic or completely absent.[497] Intercurrent bouts of cholangitis may lead to destruction of large bile ducts.

Natural History

With advancing age, there is a decrease in the number of bile duct profiles and an increase in the degree of fibrosis within portal tracts. Similarly, renal cysts become less prominent, and there is an increasing degree of interstitial fibrosis.[498] The clinical consequences are based on portal hypertension. Primary hepatic malignancies, both cholangiocarcinoma and HCC, have been reported in patients with congenital hepatic fibrosis,[499] although the lifetime risk of malignancy is unknown.[500,501]

"Adult" Polycystic Liver Disease

Clinical Features

Polycystic diseases of the liver are a variable group of clinical conditions; they are almost always associated with ADPKD, which is one of the more common hereditary diseases in humans, occurring in 1 in 1000 individuals. It is characterized by the progressive development and enlargement of multiple fluid-filled cysts in the kidneys that may ultimately lead to end-stage renal disease. There is an age-dependent increase in the prevalence of hepatic cysts in patients with ADPKD. Very rarely, the disease may manifest in an infant.[502] Twenty percent of patients with ADPKD in their third decade of life have liver cysts, as do 75% by the seventh decade. At any phase of disease, women are likely to have more numerous and larger cysts than men. Nulliparous women who have never used estrogens are less likely to have cysts than women who have been pregnant or have used hormone replacement therapy.[503]

Polycystic liver disease usually manifests clinically as asymptomatic liver enlargement. The number and size of cysts increases with age, and the disease typically becomes apparent in the fourth decade of life. Significant symptoms occur in as many as 20% of affected individuals and may include abdominal pain, orthopnea, dyspnea, early satiety, and abdominal distention. These are usually considered to be mechanical symptoms caused by massive liver enlargement. In women, the disease typically manifests earlier in life and exhibits a more severe clinical phenotype. Pregnancy causes even further discomfort.

Pathogenesis

Most cases of ADPKD (80% to 85%) develop from mutations in the *PKD1* gene, which is located on chromosome 16q13.3.[504,505] The encoded protein is polycystin-1 (PC1), a large receptor-like integral membrane protein that is important for cell–cell and cell–matrix interactions. In the remainder of ADPKD cases (15% to 20%), the disease is milder and is caused by mutational changes in another gene *(PKD2)*, located on chromosome 4q21-23, which encodes polycystin-2 (PC2). This latter molecule is a transmembrane protein that acts as a nonspecific calcium-permeable channel. Both polycystins function together in a nonredundant fashion for regulation of cellular proliferation, migration, differentiation, and morphogenesis. PC1 and PC2 are thought to inhibit cystogenesis in a dose-dependent way, with cystogenesis occurring when the concentration of PC1 or PC2 falls below a certain threshold.[506] More than 1500 different mutations of *PKD1* and *PKD2* have been identified; this high degree of genetic complexity remains an obstacle to routine genetic testing in patients with ADPKD. Fibrocystin (mutations of which also cause ARPKD) probably works in conjunction with cellular proteins involved in ADPKD, namely polycystin-1 and polycystin-2.[489]

Patients with ADPKD carry a germline mutation in *PKD1* or *PKD2*. A second somatic mutation leads to loss of both normal alleles and thus loss of polycystin function. The affected cells lose their normal terminally differentiated state, revert to a less differentiated phenotype, and undergo proliferation. In the kidney tubule epithelium, these events lead to renal cyst formation; in the hepatic biliary epithelium, they lead to biliary cyst formation.[507]

A small subset of patients with liver cysts do not have kidney cysts. This constitutes autosomal dominant polycystic liver disease (ADPLD), which may occur independently of ADPKD, as documented by a large retrospective study of autopsies in Finland.[508] Two proteins are implicated in the pathogenesis of polycystic liver disease.[509] The first is hepatocystin, the noncatalytic β-subunit of glucosidase IIa that is involved in folding and quality control of glycoproteins synthesized in the endoplasmic reticulum. The second protein is Sec63p, which is an integral endoplasmic reticulum membrane protein thought to be involved in the protein translocation machinery of the endoplasmic reticulum. Sec63p is also implicated in the endoplasmic reticulum–associated degradation pathway (discussed earlier with regard to A1AT storage disease). Hepatic cysts are thought to develop from ductal plate malformations at the level of the intralobular bile ductules.[510]

Pathological Features

Hepatic involvement in patients with polycystic liver disease may be completely incidental. Alternatively, the liver itself may show massive involvement (Fig. 55.44A,B), not unlike renal disease. The cysts are lined by a simple biliary epithelium (Fig. 55.44C). There is a strong positive correlation between the density of von Meyenburg complexes and the clinical severity of polycystic liver disease.[511]

Natural History

Liver enlargement in patients with polycystic liver disease can cause compression of the inferior vena cava, leading to edema of the lower extremities, cyst infection, hemorrhage, or rupture. There may be mechanical compromise of thoracoabdominal visceral function necessitating liver transplantation.[512] The percentage of patients with lifetime clinical complications of liver cysts is approximately 26%, regardless of whether or not the cysts are associated with polycystic kidney disease. Fatal hepatic failure, with venous compression

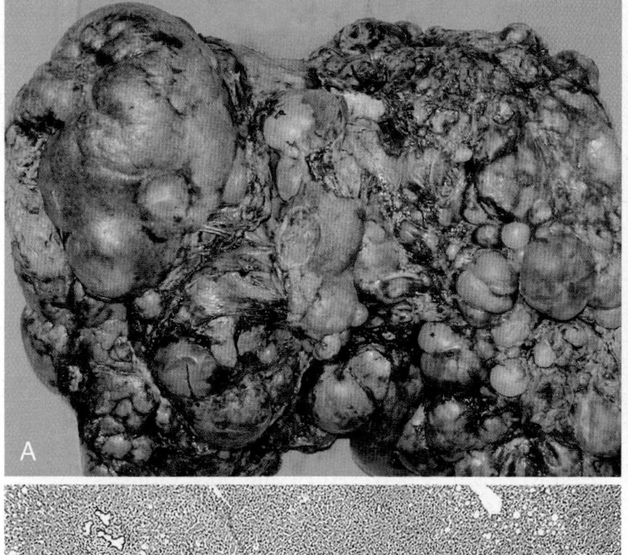

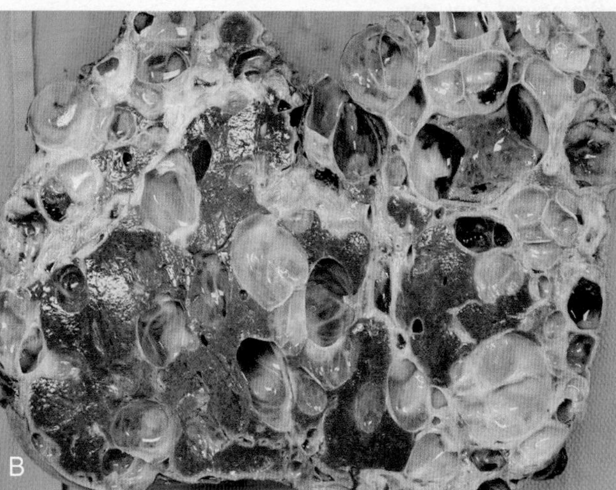

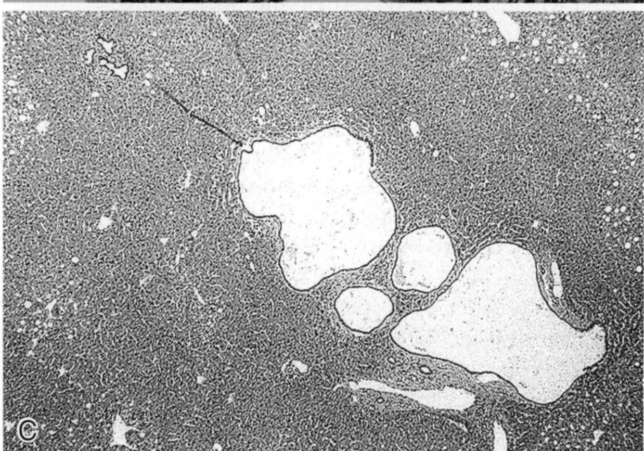

FIGURE 55.44 Polycystic liver disease. A, Massive involvement of the liver by polycystic liver disease. **B,** Cut section from the liver of a 56-year-old patient. **C,** Photomicrograph shows a liver cyst lined by simple biliary epithelium.

and ascites, is distinctly uncommon.[513] Approximately 10% of patients will develop cerebral aneurysms.

To date, no curative form of therapy has been developed for patients with polycystic liver disease. Surgical cyst decompression or partial hepatectomy are alternatives to liver transplantation, and they are more likely options in patients with isolated polycystic liver disease.[512] Liver transplantation is used mainly for patients with ADPKD. Death from liver disease is unusual. Renal failure constitutes the primary life-limiting complication of ADPKD.

Recent advances in treatment of ADPKD focus on reducing the growth of cysts so as to shift care from beyond supportive care for the disease complication to potentially disease-modifying therapies.[506] Unresolved questions in the midst of ongoing clinical trials include the development of early disease biomarkers to facilitate intervention, and understanding the role of modifier genes in predicting disease progression.

Caroli Disease and Caroli Syndrome

Congenital dilation of the large intrahepatic bile ducts can involve the left and right hepatic ducts, the segmental ducts, and the area branches. A pure type, characterized by ectasia of the intrahepatic bile ducts without further histological abnormalities, is referred to as *Caroli disease*. A combined type, in which the ductal ectasia is associated with histological lesions of congenital hepatic fibrosis, is referred to as *Caroli syndrome*.[481]

In Caroli disease, bile duct abnormalities may be confined to only one part of the liver. Caroli disease may be associated with choledochal cysts. In contrast, Caroli syndrome (with accompanying congenital hepatic fibrosis) affects the whole liver and is transmitted as an inherited trait. It is described as autosomal recessive in some reports[335] and autosomal dominant in others, either with or without an association with ADPKD.[514]

The proposed pathogenesis of Caroli disease is total or partial arrest of remodeling of the ductal plate of the larger intrahepatic bile ducts (dysgenic bile ducts).[350,351] This hypothesis is supported by the persistence of vascular bridges across the cystically dilated bile duct lumina, an anatomical feature that is readily identifiable by radiographic imaging techniques.[515]

In Caroli disease, there are focal dilations of the intrahepatic bile ducts, predominantly the segmental ducts. Characteristically, enlarged ducts wrap around neighboring hepatic arteries in a crescent-like fashion (Fig. 55.45A)[516] and are in continuity with the remainder of the biliary system. Multiple adjacent dilated biliary structures may be present (see Fig. 55.45B). In Caroli syndrome, the major ducts of the entire intrahepatic biliary tree, including those of the hepatic hilum, are dilated, and histological features of congenital hepatic fibrosis are present. Large duct ectasias predispose to repeated attacks of cholangitis, and there is also risk of portal hypertension, intrahepatic lithiasis, amyloidosis, and cholangiocarcinoma. Recurrent cholangitis may

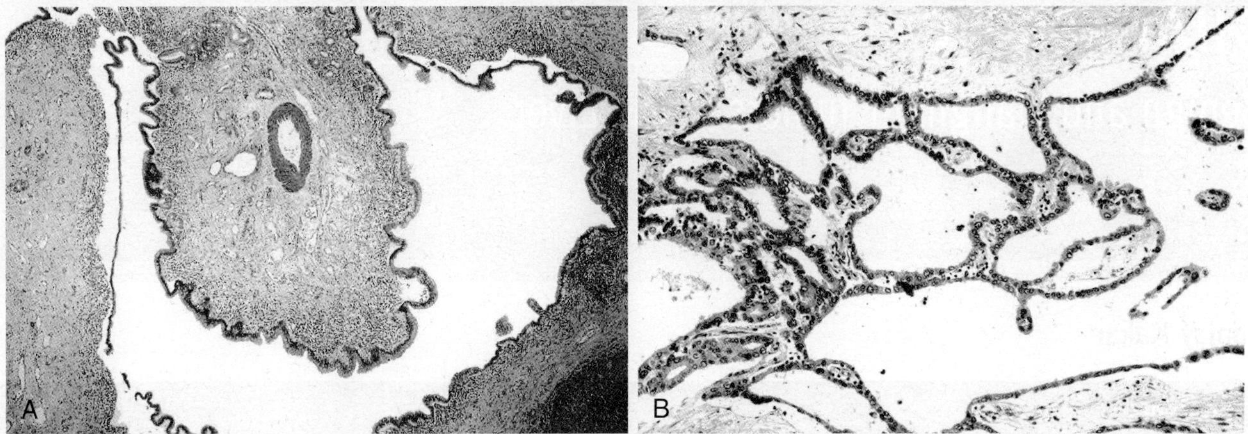

FIGURE 55.45 Caroli disease. A, Cross-section of a massively dilated intrahepatic bile duct, with a hepatic artery profile visible in residual portal tract tissue. **B,** In a different case, contiguous dilated biliary profiles are present within an expanded portal tract mesenchyme. (**A** *courtesy Dr. Bernard Portmann, King's College, London.*)

be difficult to control clinically and may lead to death of the patient from uncontrolled biliary infection within 5 to 10 years after the onset of the recurrent cholangitis. Cholangiocarcinoma occurs in as many as 7% of patients with Caroli syndrome.[36,517]

CONCLUSION

The role of the pathologist in pediatric liver diseases is evolving rapidly in relation to the immense and ongoing advances in molecular genetics. Explanations of disease mechanisms and genetic pathways are beginning to provide for targeted therapies and interventions using various viral vectors. The role of the pathologist now includes disease assessments and need for therapeutic interventions in addition to diagnosis, and, as in the past, to anticipate and identify possible untoward consequences.

***The full reference list may be accessed online at** Elsevier eBooks for Practicing Clinicians.*

CHAPTER 56

Benign and Malignant Tumors of the Liver

Sanjay Kakar

Contents

PROCESSING TECHNIQUES

Specimen analysis should include information important for tumor staging, and mandatory cancer synoptic features should be noted in the gross description. This includes tumor size (size and location of the five largest nodules in cases with multiple tumors, and range of size for others), extent of necrosis of each nodule, local extrahepatic extension, gross vascular invasion of portal/hepatic veins, and distance from resection margin(s). A tumor-free margin of at least 1 cm has been associated with a more favorable prognosis for some types of malignant tumors.

Microscopic evaluation should involve an adequate number of tissue sections relative to tumor size. Sections from the edge of the tumor are recommended for detection of vascular invasion and for examining viable tumor in cases with necrosis. Sections from nonneoplastic liver should always be included for assessment of the underlying chronic liver disease, if any.

Biopsy methods using small-core and fine-needle aspiration techniques (preferably with cell block) are most often used for acquiring biopsy specimens.

HEPATOCELLULAR TUMORS

Hepatocellular Adenoma

Clinical Features

Hepatocellular adenomas (HCAs) are rare tumors that constitute less than 2% of all liver tumors, with an incidence of 2 to 3 per 1 million per year in the Western world.[1] Young women in the reproductive age group are most commonly affected, while occurrence in men and children is rare. The incidence is increasing, mostly because of the obesity epidemic. Tumors in older women (>50 years of age) and men are being increasingly encountered.[2]

The tumor may come to attention incidentally on imaging, or due to signs such as abdominal pain, mass demonstrate variable echogenicity in HCAs, and is not helpful in diagnosis. HCAs typically show arterial enhancement on CT with contrast, with persistent enhancement in the delayed phase. MRI with liver-specific contrast agents can often distinguish areas of fat and telangiectasia, and it can help determine the subtype of HCA[3]; however, a definitive diagnosis of HCA based on imaging is often not possible.

The serum alkaline phosphatase level may be elevated in HCA, but serum α-fetoprotein (AFP) levels are typically either normal or only minimally elevated.

Pathogenesis and Risk Factors

Oral contraceptive and anabolic steroid use are well-known risk factors for HCA. HCAs may regress with cessation of oral contraceptive use.

Other risk factors include obesity, metabolic syndrome, and inherited metabolic disorders such as glycogen storage diseases I and IV, galactosemia, tyrosinemia, and familial diabetes mellitus.[4,5] The genetic basis is briefly discussed with each subtype in the following sections and in further detail in Chapter 45.

Pathological Features

Adenomas may be single or multiple. They are rather arbitrarily designated as *adenomatosis* when >10 tumors are present.[6] HCAs are unencapsulated tumors most often with an irregular, ill-defined border. They occur mostly in noncirrhotic livers. However, rare cases of inflammatory HCA have been described in patients with cirrhosis.[7] The tumors are usually soft, tend to bulge on cut section, and are lighter in color than the surrounding liver parenchyma. However, the appearance can vary with the degree of necrosis or hemorrhage. Inflammatory HCAs can be particularly ill-defined. In some cases, they may impart a congestive appearance, or bogginess to the parenchyma. HCAs usually lack significant fibrosis or nodularity, but these features can be present, especially in inflammatory HCA.[8,9] Rarely, HCAs may have a slate gray to black color caused by a large amount of lipofuscin pigment *(black adenoma)*.

Microscopically, HCAs are composed of a relatively uniform population of hepatocytes arranged in cell plates that are most typically one to three cells thick (Fig. 56.1). The reticulin framework of the cell plates is usually largely intact (Fig. 56.2). However, the sinusoids may appear compressed, resulting in a uniform and solid appearance. The tumor cells can be slightly smaller or larger than normal hepatocytes, but the nucleus-to-cytoplasm ratio is usually normal. The cytoplasm of tumor cells may be eosinophilic or clear, or it may contain fat, bile, lipofuscin pigment, or Mallory hyaline (rare). Multinucleated tumor cells or rare hepatocytes with large atypical nuclei may be present. Mitotic figures are typically absent. Unpaired arterioles (without accompanying bile ducts) are a characteristic feature of HCA. Kupffer cells may be present in adenomas, but are fewer than in normal liver. Rarely, a partial capsule surrounds the tumor, showing foci of tumor cells that merge with adjacent liver parenchyma at sites where the capsule is absent. A bile ductular reaction is typically absent, but can be seen especially in inflammatory HCA, and this feature may simulate normal portal tracts (see Fig. 56.1). Portal tracts are occasionally found within HCAs at the border of the tumor. Areas of infarction and hemorrhage are frequent findings, especially in larger tumors. Peliosis-like changes can be seen in *HNF1A*-inactivated and inflammatory subtypes.

The WHO recognizes four subtypes of HCA based largely on genetic analysis: (1) hepatocyte nuclear factor 1α *(HNF1A)*-inactivated HCA (H-HCA), (2) inflammatory HCA (previously termed *telangiectatic HCA*), (3) β-catenin–activated HCA, and (4) unclassified HCA. These subtypes can be identified by immunohistochemistry (Tables 56.1 and 56.2).[10,11]

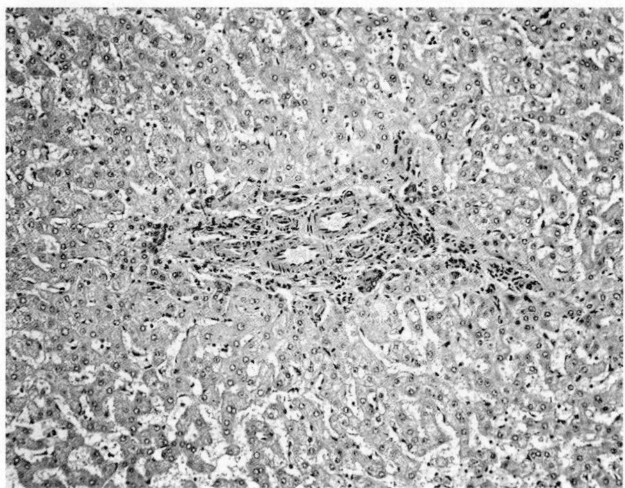

FIGURE 56.1 Inflammatory hepatocellular adenoma characterized by thin cell plates, sinusoidal dilation clusters of small arteries in fibrous stromal area *(center)*, mild mixed inflammatory infiltrate, and ductular reaction at the periphery. This zone can be mistaken for normal portal zones.

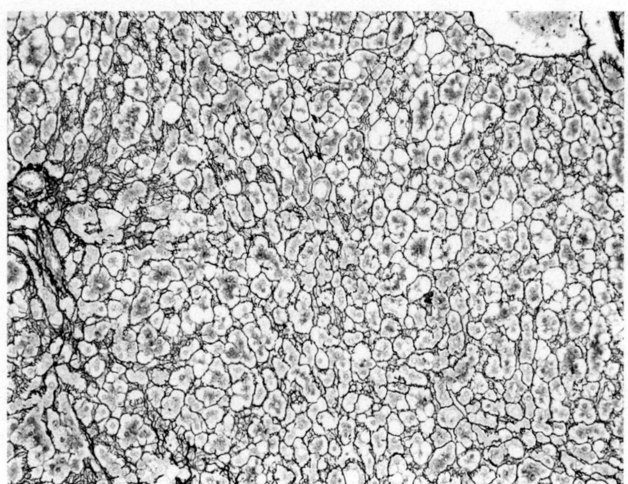

FIGURE 56.2 Intact reticulin framework in hepatocellular adenoma.

H-HCAs are characterized by somatic or germline *HNF1A* mutations. Germline mutations can be associated with maturity onset diabetes of the young (MODY3). These tumors often show marked steatosis, lack cytological atypia, and have a low association with hepatocellular carcinoma (HCC; Fig. 56.3A). In some of these tumors, foci with pseudoacinar architecture can be prominent. These HCAs show loss of cytoplasmic liver fatty acid binding protein (LFABP) on immunohistochemistry (Fig. 56.3B). Transformation to HCC can occur but is uncommon. It likely occurs in less than 5% of cases.

Inflammatory HCAs (previously termed *telangiectatic HCAs*) are characterized by activation of the interleukin (IL)-6 signaling pathway, most commonly caused by mutations in the *IL6ST* gene.[11,12] The typical morphological features of this subtype are sinusoidal dilation and lymphocytic inflammation (Fig. 56.4A). A variable degree of ductular reaction and fibrous septa can be present in these tumors,

TABLE 56.1 Subtypes of Hepatocellular Adenoma

HCA Subtype	Histological Features	Immunohistochemistry	Clinical Associations
HNF1A inactivated	• Diffuse fatty change • Pseudoacinar change and peliosis, especially in nonfatty lesions	LFABP1 negative	• Maturity-onset diabetes of the young type 3 (if familial) • Can be multiple • Risk for HCC low
Inflammatory	• Dilated sinusoids • Inflammation • Prominent fat in some cases • Ductular reaction often present	Cytoplasmic staining with CRP and SAA 10% may have β-catenin mutations	• Obesity very typical association • Adenomatosis can occur
β-catenin activated (best considered as atypical neoplasms, not adenoma)	• Focal atypical features • Pseudoacini • Small cell change • Cytological atypia	β-catenin nuclear staining and diffuse GS staining	• Affects both men and women • Associated with anabolic steroids • High risk for HCC

CRP, *C-reactive protein;* GS, *glutamine synthetase;* HCA, *hepatocellular adenoma;* HCC, *hepatocellular carcinoma;* HNF1A, *hepatocyte nuclear factor 1α;* LFABP, *liver-type fatty acid binding protein;* SAA, *serum amyloid A.*

TABLE 56.2 Immunohistochemistry of Hepatocellular Adenoma and Focal Nodular Hyperplasia

	HNF1A-Inactivated HCA	Inflammatory HCA	β-catenin-Activated Tumors	Focal Nodular Hyperplasia
LFABP (cytoplasmic)	Lost	Intact	Intact	Intact
SAA	Negative	Positive (80%-90%)	Can be positive (10%)	Typically negative
CRP	Negative	Positive (~100%)	Can be positive (10%)	Periseptal staining; typically not diffuse
β-catenin (nuclear)	Negative	Negative	Positive (<50% of cases), can be focal	Negative
GS	Patchy	Patchy	Diffuse	Maplike
CD34	Patchy to diffuse sinusoidal staining	Patchy to diffuse sinusoidal staining	Patchy to diffuse sinusoidal staining	Patchy to diffuse sinusoidal staining
CK7	Can be positive in patchy small hepatocytes	Can be positive in patchy small hepatocytes	Can be positive in patchy small hepatocytes	Highlights ductular reaction

CRP, *C-reactive protein;* GS, *glutamine synthetase;* HCA, *hepatocellular adenoma;* HNF1A, *hepatocyte nuclear factor 1α;* LFABP, *liver-type fatty acid binding protein;* SAA, *serum amyloid A.*

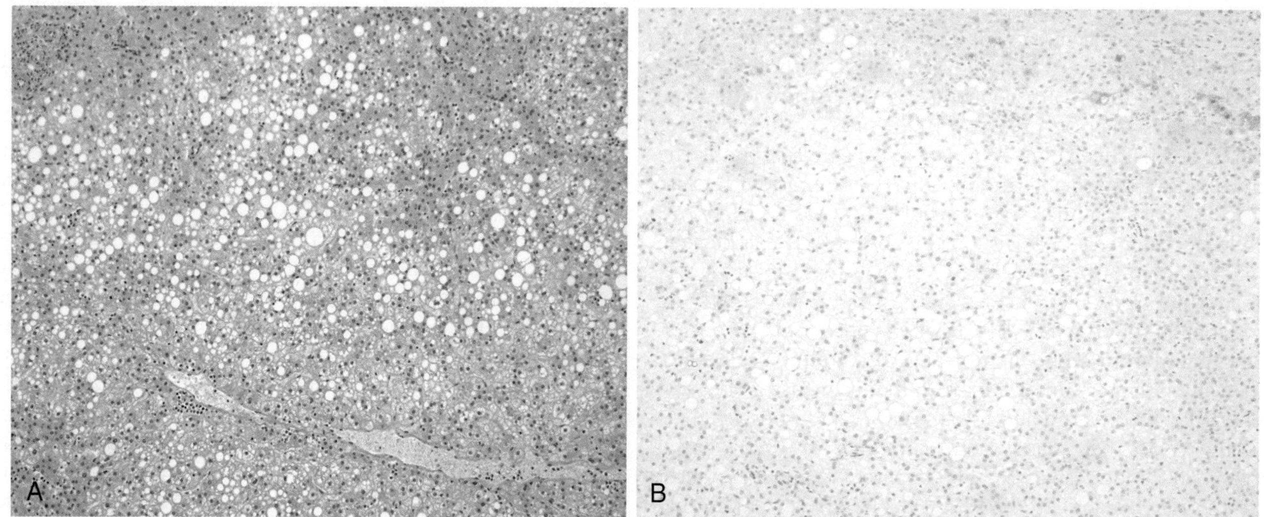

FIGURE 56.3 *HNF1α*–inactivated HCA (H-HCA) characterized by prominent intralesional steatosis. A, The tumor cells without fat have a highly eosinophilic or cleared-out cytoplasm. **B,** Loss of cytoplasmic liver fatty acid binding protein (LFABP) in H-HCA; a few normal hepatocytes are positive.

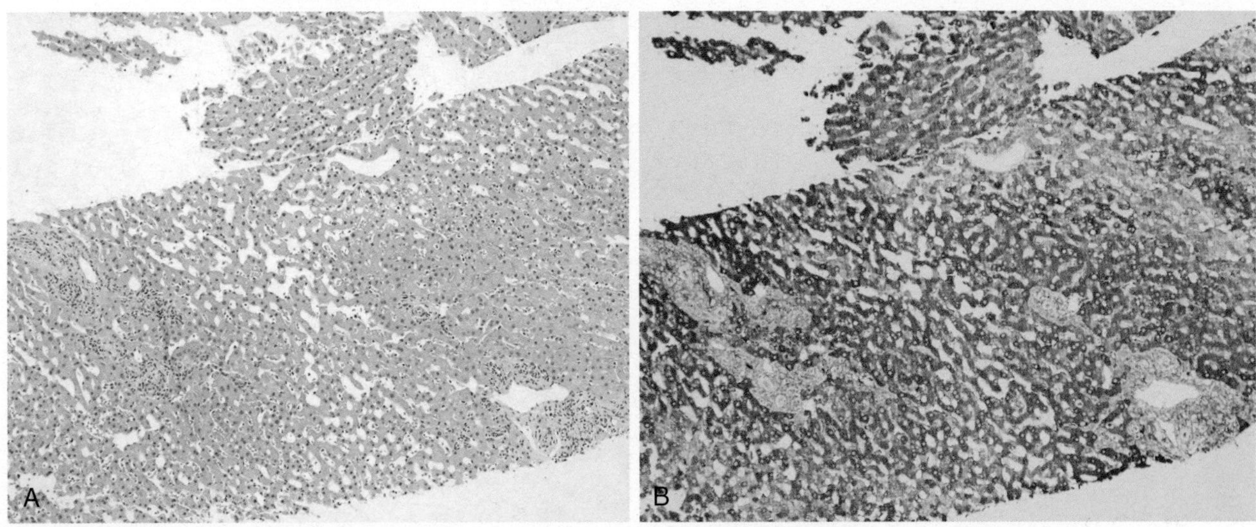

FIGURE 56.4 Inflammatory hepatocellular adenoma characterized by sinusoidal dilation and mild ductular reaction **(A).** The lesional hepatocytes show diffuse staining with C-reactive protein **(B).**

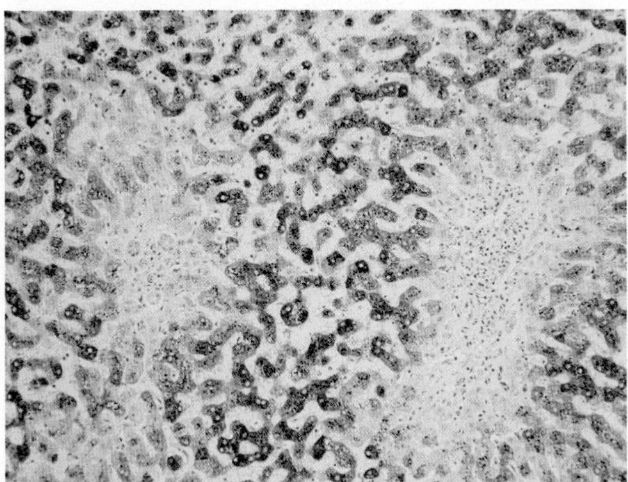

FIGURE 56.5 Diffuse granular cytoplasmic staining with serum amyloid A in inflammatory HCA.

which closely mimic focal nodular hyperplasia (FNH). Immunohistochemistry for inflammatory markers such as serum amyloid A (SAA) and C-reactive protein (CRP) show granular cytoplasmic staining and helps confirm the diagnosis (Fig. 56.4B; Fig. 56.5). CRP is more sensitive and is positive in nearly 100% of cases, while SAA is more specific with a sensitivity of 80% to 90%. Transformation to HCC can occur, usually through β-catenin activation, which is observed in 10% of cases.

β-catenin–activated tumors frequently exhibit atypical cytological features and have a high association (40% to 50%) with concurrent or subsequent HCC. Hence these tumors are best placed in a separate *atypical* category, rather than as a subtype of HCA. The designation of *atypical hepatocellular neoplasm*[12] (AHN) and *borderline tumor*[13] has been used in the WHO 2019 scheme. The term *hepatocellular neoplasm of uncertain malignant potential* (HUMP)[14] has been proposed by an international group of liver pathologists, but it is not included in the WHO scheme. There is lack of consensus on the use of terminology for these tumors, and all three terms are appropriate as long as the significance is properly discussed in a comment. These tumors often occur in men (~40%). They are characterized by activation of the Wnt signaling pathway, most commonly resulting from a *CTNNB1* (β-catenin) exon 3 mutation. In a small minority of cases, mutations in other components of the Wnt signaling pathway *(APC, AXIN)* may be involved.[15] Cytological atypia, prominent nucleoli, small cell change, a pseudoacinar pattern, and bile plugs may be present (Fig. 56.6A).[11-13,16] Nuclear staining with β-catenin occurs in a subset of cases (<50%), but it is not sensitive for the diagnosis of this subtype (especially on biopsy) as the staining may be focal or even negative despite the presence of an exon 3 β-catenin mutation (Fig. 56.7). Nuclear β-catenin leads to overexpression of glutamine synthetase (GS). Diffuse GS staining (moderate to strong cytoplasmic staining in ≥50% of tumor cells) is a better marker of β-catenin activation (Fig. 56.6B). Diffuse GS staining can be diffuse homogeneous (>90% of tumor cells) or diffuse heterogeneous (50% to 90% of tumor cells) (Fig. 56.8).[9,11] A diffuse homogeneous pattern is nearly always related to mutations associated with a high level of β-catenin activation, while a diffuse heterogeneous pattern is more common with mutations associated with an intermediate level of β-catenin activation (such as S45); however, the correlation of the pattern of staining and type of mutation is not perfect.[16] For practical purposes, diffuse GS staining irrespective of whether it is diffuse homogeneous or heterogeneous is currently regarded as evidence of β-catenin activation.

The unclassified group of tumors lack typical features of the other subtypes. For instance, HCAs with a *CTNNB1* (β-catenin) exon 7 or 8 mutation show weaker β-catenin activation, generally lack diffuse GS, and thus typically fall into this category based on morphology and immunohistochemistry.[17] A sonic hedgehog–activated subtype (shHCA) has been recently described, which is associated with a high risk of bleeding. [18] Immunohistochemistry for prostaglandin D synthase may help identify this variant, but it has not been widely tested.[19] Argininosuccinate synthetase 1 (ASS1) has been proposed as a marker of shHCA,[20] but it is also positive in other subtypes like inflammatory HCA. Thus its diagnostic use in this setting has not yet been well established.

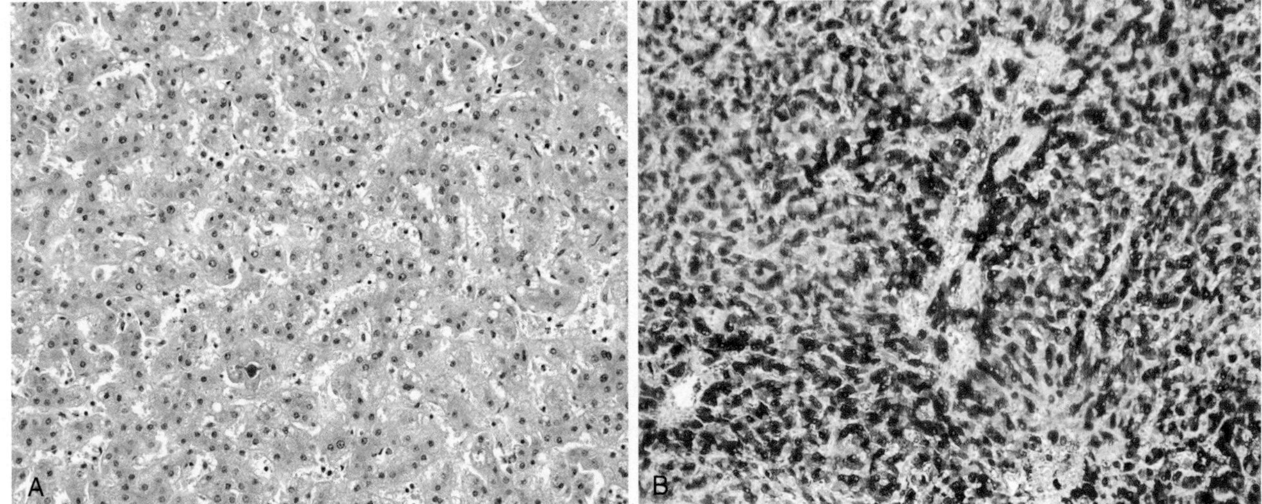

FIGURE 56.6 Well-differentiated hepatocellular neoplasm with β-catenin activation. A, Cytological atypia is mild in this case, but can focally be more prominent. Bile plugs can be present**. B,** Diffuse homogeneous staining with glutamine synthetase is a typical feature and is commonly used to identify β-catenin activation.

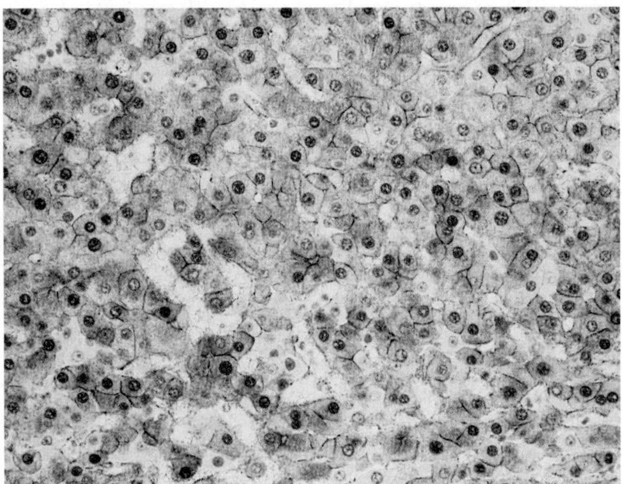

FIGURE 56.7 Positive nuclear staining with β-catenin immunohistochemistry indicates the presence of β-catenin activation.

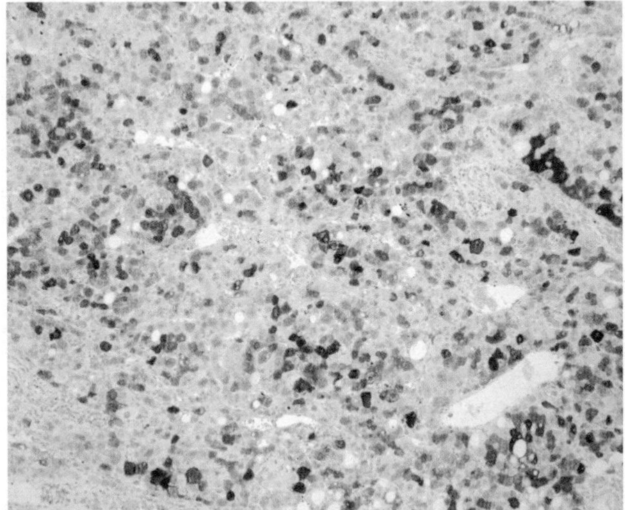

FIGURE 56.8 Diffuse heterogeneous staining with glutamine synthetase is characterized by moderate to strong staining in more than half but less than 90% of tumor cells and is a result of β-catenin activation in most cases.

Differential Diagnosis

The main differential diagnosis of HCA includes FNH and well-differentiated HCC (Table 56.3 and Table 56.4). The presence of nodular architecture, a central scar, fibrous septa, a prominent ductular reaction, and large arteries within fibrous stroma favor FNH, but these findings overlap with HCA, especially the inflammatory subtype. A map-like GS pattern (FNH), SAA/CRP (inflammatory HCA), and LFABP (*HNF1A*-inactivated HCA) help in confirming a diagnosis of HCA.

Lack of cytological atypia, thin cell plates, absence of prominent small cell change or pseudoacini, and an intact reticulin framework help distinguish HCC from HCA. Tumors with β-catenin activation and/or focal or mild cyto-architectural atypia that is insufficient for a diagnosis of HCC are best categorized as *atypical hepatocellular neoplasm.*[13,14] It is important to note that LFABP loss, positive SAA, and/or CRP can be observed in HCC. Hence these stains should not be used to distinguish HCA and HCC, but they should be used to subclassify HCA after the diagnosis of HCA has been made based on a combination of morphology and a reticulin stain.

Increased sinusoidal staining with CD34 is common in HCA and is not helpful for distinction from HCC. Positivity with glypican 3 (GPC3), an oncofetal protein, favors HCC but is positive in less than 50% of well-differentiated HCCs.

In small biopsies, distinction between HCA and normal liver may also be difficult. Diffuse staining with CD34 and patchy GS staining in regions distant from the perivenous region of the liver help favor HCA. SAA and CRP should be interpreted with caution because these stains can also be positive in adjacent nonlesional liver.[9]

Treatment

HCAs >5 cm in size are at a higher risk for hemorrhagic complications and HCC. Thus surgical excision is recommended for tumors of this size and those with high-risk features such as male gender and β-catenin activation.[21] Because resection is recommended for HCAs >5 cm and

TABLE 56.3 Immunohistochemical Analysis of Liver Tumors

Clinical and Morphological Situation	Immunohistochemistry
"Hepatoid" tumor in noncirrhotic liver	Two hepatocellular markers (Arg-1, Hep Par 1, GPC-3) CK7/CK19/MOC31: any two markers for neuroendocrine tumors, adrenocortical carcinoma, angiomyolipoma, melanoma, depending on setting Site-related markers if necessary (e.g., TTF-1, CDX-2, SATB2, GATA3)
Clear cell tumors, such as HCC, renal cell carcinoma, and melanoma	Hepatocellular markers (HCC) PAX2/PAX-8 (RCC) SOX10/S-100 (melanoma) SF-1 (adrenocortical carcinoma) Synaptophysin, chromogranin (clear cell neuroendocrine tumors) CK7/CK19/MOC31 (clear cell adenocarcinoma)
HCC versus well-differentiated NET	Hepatocellular markers (HCC) Synaptophysin, chromogranin (NET)
Nonepithelial tumors mimicking carcinoma	SOX-10, S100 (melanoma) HMB-45 (epithelioid AML, melanoma) SMA, desmin (epithelioid AML) KIT, DOG1 (GIST) ERG, CD31 (vascular tumors)
Adenocarcinoma	Albumin ISH, BAP1 (intrahepatic cholangiocarcinoma) CK7, CK19 (upper GI, pancreas, intrahepatic cholangiocarcinoma) CK20, CDX2, SATB2 (colorectal) TTF-1, napsin-A (lung) GATA3, ER, PR (breast) NKX3.1, PSA (prostate)

AML, *Acute myeloid leukemia;* HCC, *hepatocellular carcinoma;* NET, *neuroendocrine tumor;* RCC, *renal cell carcinoma.*

in males (any size), it can be argued that subtyping and risk subtyping is not necessary for patient management. For smaller tumors in women, the decision to perform a resection may rest on pathological risk factors including β-catenin activation. Accurate assessment of GS and β-catenin immunohistochemistry is crucial in these cases. If the staining pattern with GS and β-catenin immunohistochemical results are unclear based on the biopsy, sequencing assays can be used to confirm mutations in the Wnt signaling pathway. For patients with multiple HCAs, the management is guided by the size and risk factors of the individual nodules. Nodules with a higher risk are resected, whereas others may be followed up by imaging.

Focal Nodular Hyperplasia

Clinical Features

FNH is a benign, nonneoplastic lesion that is most commonly encountered in young women. The estimated incidence is 0.9% to 3%.[22] Most are asymptomatic and are thus discovered incidentally. However, large ones can be symptomatic. FNH is difficult to characterize on ultrasonography, but it is well visualized on contrast-enhanced CT imaging with hyperattenuation in the arterial phase and isoattenuation in the delayed phase. A central scar with a hypoattenuated appearance in the arterial phase can be seen in 70% of cases.[23] On MRI, FNH gives an isointense to hypointense signal on T1-weighted images and appears hyperintense or isointense on T2-weighted images.

FNH may increase in size with oral contraceptive use, but this is not thought to be a risk factor in its development. Multiple FNH has been described in association with hepatic hemangioma, vascular malformation, meningioma, and astrocytoma.[24] FNH has no known malignant potential. It is not considered a precursor of fibrolamellar HCC despite its rare association with this malignant tumor.

TABLE 56.4 Comparison of Hepatocellular Adenoma, Focal Nodular Hyperplasia, and Hepatocellular Carcinoma

Morphological Feature	Hepatocellular Adenoma	Focal Nodular Hyperplasia	Hepatocellular Carcinoma
Bile ductular reaction	Usually absent, can be prominent in inflammatory HCA	Present in fibrous septa in most cases	Usually absent
Aberrant arterioles	Often present, usually without prominent surrounding connective tissue	Arteries with thick walls often present in fibrous stroma	Often present
Sinusoidal dilation	Typically present	Typically absent (can be present in a small subset of cases)	Typically absent (can be present in a small subset of cases)
Connective tissue component	Occasional fibrous septa	Central scar with prominent fibrous septa in most but not all cases	Stroma typically scant (can be prominent in scirrhous variant)
Cell plate architecture	1-3 cells wide	1-3 cells wide; foci of plates >3 cells wide may be seen at periphery	Typically >3 cells wide
Reticulin stain	No significant loss of reticulin framework	No significant loss of reticulin framework; focally wide plates can be highlighted	Multifocal loss
Immunohistochemistry			
GS	Patchy (diffuse if β-catenin activated)	Maplike staining	Diffuse staining in 30%-40%
β-catenin	Membranous staining	Membranous staining	Nuclear staining in 20%-30% of cases
SAA, CRP	Positive in inflammatory HCA	SAA typically negative; CRP shows periseptal staining	Both can be positive
LFABP	Lost in H-HCA	Intact	Lost in rare cases
CD34	Patchy or diffuse sinusoidal	Patchy or diffuse sinusoidal	Patchy or diffuse sinusoidal
Glypican-3	Negative	Negative	Positive in <50% of well-differentiated cases

CRP, *C-reactive protein;* GS, *glutamine synthetase;* HCA, *hepatocellular adenoma;* LFABP1, *liver-type fatty acid binding protein;* SAA, *serum amyloid A.*

Pathogenesis

The pathogenesis of FNH has not been well established, but it is thought to result from a hyperplastic or altered growth response to alterations in parenchymal blood flow.[22] The presence of numerous abnormal muscular vessels in FNH and the occurrence of similar nodules (*FNH-like lesions*) in association with hemangiomas, vascular abnormalities, and adjacent to other mass lesions lend support to this theory. FNH can also develop in association with vascular disorders (heart disease, Budd-Chiari syndrome)[22] and hereditary conditions such as hereditary hemorrhagic telangiectasia (Osler-Weber-Rendu disease). The terms *FNH-like regenerative nodules* and *FNH-like lesions* have been used in these clinical settings, but the morphology in most of these cases is similar to sporadic FNH.

Most cases that were previously designated as *telangiectatic FNH* were likely inflammatory HCA. However, sinusoidal dilation (telangiectasia) can be seen in FNH as well.[25]

Pathological Features

FNH is usually a solitary lesion, but it can be multifocal in about 20% of cases.[22,26] The multinodular appearance can simulate cirrhosis in some cases. FNH tends to be lighter in color than the surrounding liver parenchyma. Occasionally, FNH may be pedunculated. FNH is normally well demarcated from the adjacent normal liver parenchyma, but a fibrous capsule is usually absent. FNH may vary considerably in size, ranging from 1 mm to 19 cm.[26] FNH has a central fibrous scar in 60% to 70% of cases, which consists of fibrovascular tissue, not dense scar tissue.

Microscopically, FNH is composed of normal-appearing benign hepatocytes arranged in incomplete nodules and partially separated by fibrous tissue that extends outward from the central fibrous zone of the tumor. A ductular reaction is normally present in the fibrous septa in most cases, but FNH does not contain interlobular bile ducts. Atypia of the hepatocytes is not typically present. However, in some cases, wider cell plates (3 to 4 cells thick), focal pseudoacinar structures, and focal reticulin loss may be seen, especially at the periphery of the lesion. The hepatocytes may demonstrate increased glycogen, fat, ballooning degeneration, Mallory hyaline, bile, lipofuscin, iron, and copper or copper-associated protein.[24] Occasional atypical hepatocytes containing larger-sized nuclei and mild hyperchromasia, either with or without conspicuous nucleoli, may be seen.

Medium- to large-sized, thick-walled, muscular vessels that often exhibit myointimal myxoid or fibromuscular hyperplastic changes are characteristic of FNH and are normally present in the central scar and fibrous septa (Figs. 56.9 and 56.10). Portal tracts are absent in FNH, except at the periphery of the lesion, although a bile duct of intermediate or large caliber may be found in the central fibrous zone in rare cases.[26] The sinusoids may be dilated, and Kupffer cells may be evident. Inflammatory cell infiltrates are relatively common and consist mainly of lymphocytes, although neutrophils and eosinophils may be present, particularly surrounding bile ductular structures. Rarely, granulomas are present as well.

The reticulin framework is largely intact in FNH; focal loss can be seen at the periphery of tumors and encircling

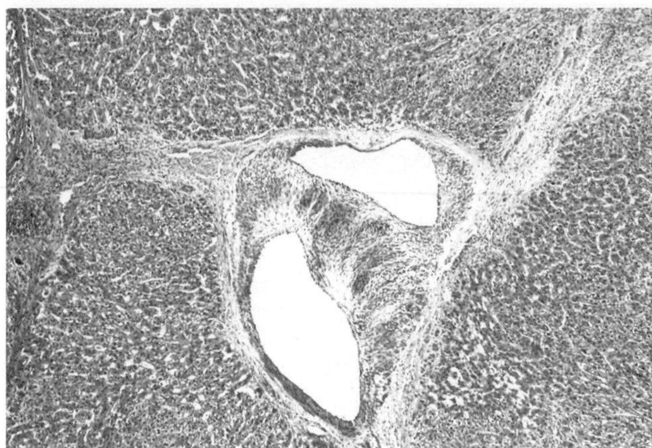

FIGURE 56.9 Focal nodular hyperplasia with aberrant arteries without accompanying bile ducts of similar size.

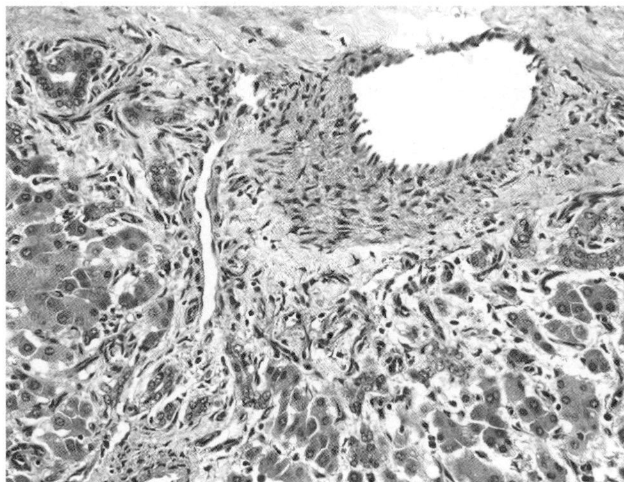

FIGURE 56.10 Focal nodular hyperplasia with aberrant thick-walled artery and ductular reaction that typically occurs at the junction of the stroma and parenchymal nodules.

small groups of hepatocytes in some cases. Immunohistochemistry with GS demonstrates intense staining of broad interconnected groups of hepatocytes, creating a maplike (geographical) pattern of staining (Fig. 56.11).[27] However, small areas in the periseptal region are often negative. A maplike pattern may not be clearly apparent around the central scar.

Differential Diagnosis

Nodular architecture, fibrous septa, ductular reaction, and large, thick-walled arterioles in fibrous stroma favor FNH over HCA, but there is overlap in the morphological features of FNH and inflammatory HCA (see Table 56.3). Immunohistochemistry with GS and SAA/CRP plays an important role in diagnosis on needle biopsy. SAA can be positive in 10% to 20% of FNH cases, while CRP typically shows periseptal staining that fades in areas away from the septa. Although focal plate thickening and focal reticulin loss can mimic HCC, these changes are confined to small areas of FNH (typically the periphery). The focality of these changes as well as a maplike GS pattern helps in its distinction from HCC.

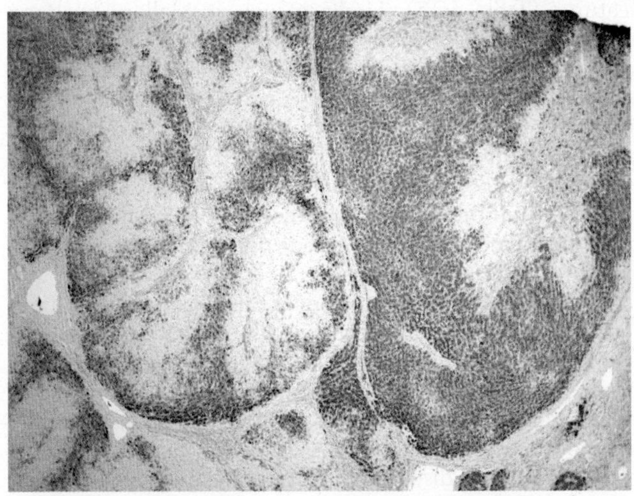

FIGURE 56.11 Glutamine synthetase immunostain demonstrates a map-like staining pattern in focal nodular hyperplasia.

Treatment

Surgical resection is usually not necessary for FNH unless the lesion is pedunculated, large, or symptomatic. Of course, excision of FNH is justified if the lesion cannot be differentiated from HCC or HCA on biopsy.

Benign and Dysplastic Lesions in Cirrhosis

Cirrhotic nodules frequently contain scattered, enlarged hepatocytes with abundant cytoplasm and atypical, enlarged nuclei but with a preserved nucleus-to-cytoplasm ratio (Fig. 56.12). This cytological feature was previously designated *large cell dysplasia,* but the term *large cell change* is now recommended because this is likely a degenerative change.[24]

Cirrhotic nodules may also contain small-sized hepatocytes with normal, slightly smaller, or slightly larger nuclei and scant cytoplasm, both of which result in an overall increase in the nucleus-to-cytoplasm ratio (Fig. 56.13). This cytological feature was previously designated *small cell dysplasia,* but the term *small cell change* is now recommended because this may represent either a regenerative or dysplastic process.[24] Dysplasia in cirrhotic livers may manifest as *dysplastic foci* (<1 mm) or *dysplastic nodules* (>1 mm).[24]

Dysplastic foci consist of clusters of small cells with a variable degree of atypia, and they show a high prevalence in chronic hepatitis B and C, α_1-antitrypsin deficiency, and tyrosinemia. Cytoplasmic fat or glycogen may be different from that seen in the surrounding liver. In the setting of marked hepatocellular siderosis (as in hereditary hemochromatosis), areas of hepatocytes without iron *(iron-free foci)* are observed in around 8% of cases.[28] These foci have preneoplastic potential, and this finding should be noted in the liver biopsy.

Macroregenerative and Low-Grade Dysplastic Nodules

In cirrhosis, benign nodules without significant atypia larger than 1 cm in size are referred to as *large regenerative nodules* or *macroregenerative nodules.*[24] These are otherwise similar to conventional regenerative cirrhotic nodules, and they lack cytoarchitectural atypia or reticulin abnormalities. Portal tracts can be present within these nodules

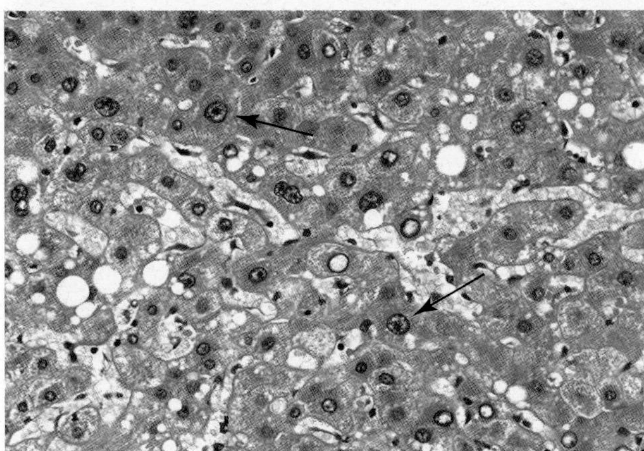

FIGURE 56.12 Large cell change. Hepatocytes with markedly enlarged nuclei and more abundant cytoplasm (*arrows*) are scattered rather than clustered together.

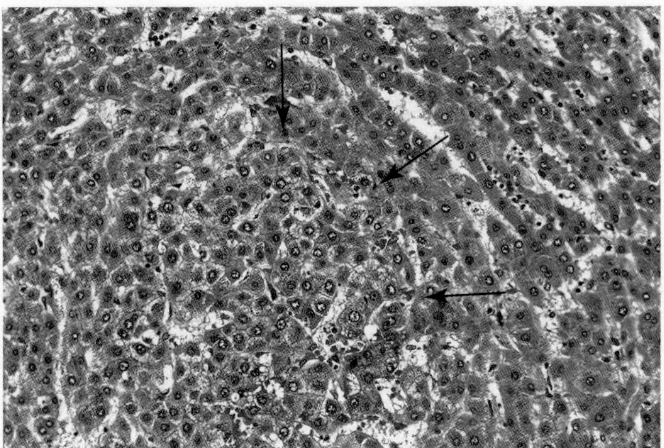

FIGURE 56.13 High-grade dysplastic focus with small cell change. Notice the nodule of small cells with a high nucleus-to-cytoplasm ratio and thickening of cell plates (arrows).

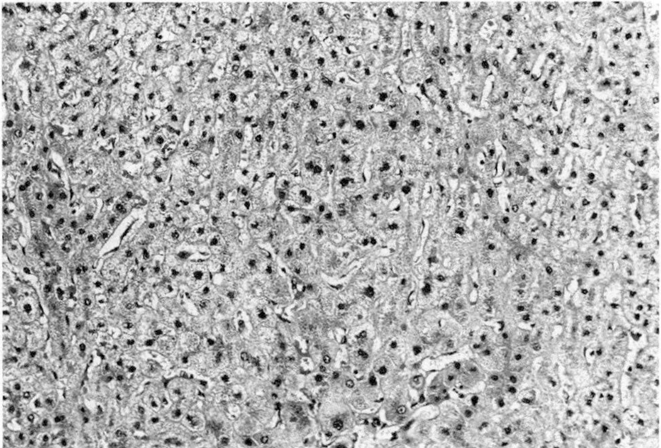

FIGURE 56.14 The morphology and cell plate architecture in large and low-grade dysplastic nodules is similar to normal liver.

(Figs. 56.14 and 56.15). Fibrous septa can extend into the nodule and may have a few scattered arterioles without accompanying bile ducts. Increased sinusoidal CD34 staining may be seen, but diffuse staining is typically absent. Low-grade dysplastic nodules are believed to represent a clonal proliferation of hepatocytes that lack high-grade

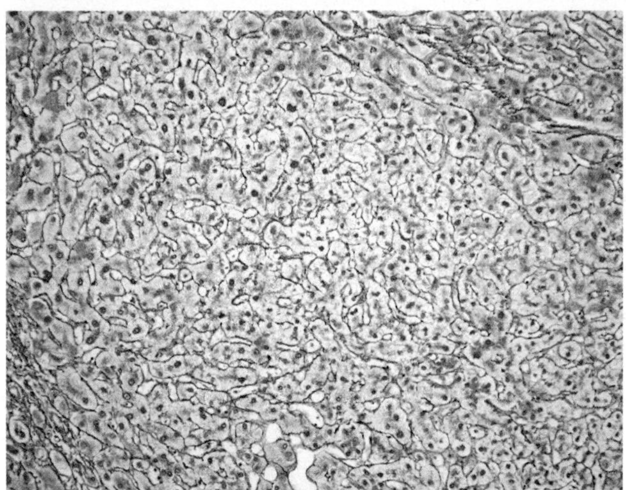

FIGURE 56.15 Reticulin stain demonstrates intact cell plate architecture in a large regenerative nodule.

features (Table 56.5). Findings such as Mallory hyaline, bile stasis, clear cytoplasm, iron or copper deposits, a slight decrease in cell size, and focal or diffuse fatty changes may be present in these nodules. Low-grade dysplastic nodules are often indistinguishable from large regenerative nodules unless clonality analysis is performed. Low-grade dysplastic nodules lack a strong association with HCC and do not require specific treatment. Hence the distinction of large regenerative nodule and low-grade dysplastic nodules is not clinically relevant.

Regenerative nodules may occur in a noncirrhotic liver in a variety of clinical settings, such as nodular regenerative hyperplasia, vascular diseases such as Budd-Chiari syndrome, congenital heart disease and portal vein thrombosis, or as sequela of hepatocyte necrosis. These nodular proliferations can have a morphological appearance of an HCA or FNH, and the distinction is based on the overall clinical setting.

TABLE 56.5 Differentiating Features of Nodular Lesions in Cirrhosis

Morphological Feature	Macroregenerative (Large Regenerative) Nodule	Low-Grade Dysplastic Nodule	High-Grade Dysplastic Nodule	Well-Differentiated Hepatocellular Carcinoma
Hepatocyte size	Similar to cirrhotic nodules	Uniform population of hepatocytes without atypia (suggesting clonal proliferation)	Normal or small	Often smaller than normal hepatocytes
Nuclear density more than twice normal	Absent or focal	Absent or focal	Can be focally present	Common
Large cell change	Absent or focal	Absent or focal	Absent or focal	Can be present
Cell plates ≥3 cells thick	Absent	Absent	Absent or focal	Common
Reticulin framework	Intact	Intact	Intact or focal loss	More than focal loss in most cases
Increased iron	Can be present	No definite data	Typically absent	Typically absent, even in siderotic liver
Periphery of nodule	Well circumscribed	Well circumscribed	Well-circumscribed in most cases	Can have infiltrative border with parenchymal or stromal invasion
Portal tracts or fibrous tissue zones	Typically present; often with bile ductular reaction	Typically present	Can be present	Often absent; can be present in early HCC or entrapped at edge of tumor
Mitoses	Typically absent	Typically absent	Typically absent or rare	Can be present
Ductular reaction at periphery	Typically present, circumferential	Typically present, circumferential	Present in most cases, may be focally absent	Absent in areas of stromal or parenchymal invasion (can be highlighted with CK7 stain)
CD34	No or minimal increase in sinusoidal staining	No or minimal increase in sinusoidal staining	Patchy increase in sinusoidal staining in most cases, often at periphery	Patchy to diffuse increase in sinusoidal staining in most cases
Glutamine synthetase (GS)	No diffuse staining	No diffuse staining	Diffuse staining uncommon	Diffuse staining in 30%-40%
Glypican-3 (GPC3)	Negative	Negative	Negative in most cases	Can be positive
Heat shock protein 70 (HSP70)	Negative	Negative	Negative in most cases	Can be positive
At least two markers positive: GS, GPC3, HSP70	No	No	No	Positive in 50%-70%

High-Grade Dysplastic Nodules

High-grade dysplastic nodules,[24] previously referred to as *borderline nodules*, are preneoplastic lesions that can arise in cirrhosis of any etiology. These come to clinical attention on imaging, or they may be encountered by the pathologist in resections or explants. The reported prevalence in cirrhosis varies widely with numbers ranging from 11% to 40%.[2]

Pathological Features

The nodules do not have any distinctive gross features, but they may stand out because of their larger size or different appearance from surrounding nodules. The size is typically <2 cm, and most are between 0.5 and 1.5 cm.[29] High-grade dysplasia may involve an entire visible nodule, in which case it is considered a *high-grade dysplastic nodule* or as *high-grade dysplastic foci* (typically ≤1 mm) within a large regenerative nodule (see Fig. 56.13). Sampling by core needle biopsy may miss the area of diagnosis of HCC, which may occur focally in high-grade dysplastic nodules.

By definition, cytoarchitectural atypia is present but is insufficient for a definitive diagnosis of HCC. The typical morphological features are of small cell change (see Fig. 56.13), high nucleus-to-cytoplasm ratio, and increased nuclear density (defined as an increased number of hepatocyte nuclei in a given field compared with normal liver). Portal tracts are often present in dysplastic nodules. Unpaired arterioles can be present but are typically not numerous. CD34 staining is often increased at the periphery, while diffuse sinusoidal staining is uncommon.

Other common features include focally thick cell plates (three cells or more), focal decrease in the reticulin framework, and focal pseudoacinar (pseudoglandular) architecture. Foci of Mallory bodies, fat, clear cell change, cytoplasmic basophilia, rare mitoses, and bile can be present. High-grade dysplastic lesions tend to lack iron deposits, which can be seen in regenerative nodules.

Differential Diagnosis

The distinction of a large regenerative nodule from HCC is based primarily on morphology and the features on reticulin staining (see Table 56.5). Cell plates greater than three cells thick, nuclear density more than twice normal, prominent pseudoacinar architecture, multifocal loss of reticulin framework, and numerous unpaired arteries favor HCC. Diffuse GS (evidence of β-catenin activation), positive glypican-3, and positive HSP70 are features that favor HCC, hence a combination of these stains has been advocated for routine diagnosis. Based on initial studies, positive results with two or more of these markers have 100% specificity for HCC, with a sensitivity of 70% in resections and 50% in biopsies.[30,31] However, GPC3 has low sensitivity for well-differentiated HCC, and HSP70 is helpful in only a small minority of cases. The value of this panel of markers is limited in most cases,[32] whereas GS, and less commonly GPC3, can help contribute to the diagnosis in some circumstances (personal observation).

Treatment

These lesions are treated with ablation and, less commonly, with resection.

Hepatocellular Carcinoma and Its Variants

Clinical Features

HCC is the most common primary malignant tumor in the liver. The presenting signs and symptoms include abdominal pain, weight loss, and hepatomegaly. In some cases, a palpable mass may be clinically apparent. Features of cirrhosis or underlying liver disease can be present. Rare cases can be associated with paraneoplastic syndromes such as hypoglycemia, erythrocytosis, hypercholesterolemia, hypercalcemia, precocious puberty, gynecomastia, hypertrophic pulmonary osteoarthropathy, hyperthyroidism, dysfibrinogenemias, and skin manifestations.

In the United States, approximately 85% of HCCs occur in patients with cirrhosis. The incidence is low in Europe and North America (2 to 7 cases per 100,000 persons) and high in eastern Asia and southern Africa (30 cases per 100,000 persons). The mean age of occurrence depends on the specific geographical location, being approximately 60 years of age in North America, approximately 35 years in Africa, and 40 to 60 years in Taiwan. HCC is three times more common among men than women, and it is the fifth most common malignancy in men and the eighth most common in women worldwide.

AFP, an oncofetal protein, is synthesized by the yolk sac and fetal hepatocytes, but it is very low or undetectable in healthy adults. Elevated serum AFP is observed in 70% to 80% of patients with HCC, with levels of >400 ng/mL in about 50% of cases.[33] Large tumor size, poor differentiation, and advanced stage correlate with higher AFP levels. However, AFP may be normal in tumors <2 cm, nearly 40% of early cases, and even 10% to 15% of advanced cases.[33] On the other hand, mild to moderate elevations (typically <400 ng/mL) are often observed in benign conditions such as tyrosinemia, steatosis, chronic hepatitis, and cirrhosis. Elevated AFP levels can also occur in nonhepatocellular tumors such as gastric/colonic adenocarcinomas, ovarian tumors, and germ cell tumors. Patients with cirrhosis are screened every 6 months by ultrasound and serum AFP level.[34]

Imaging

HCC may be more echogenic or less echogenic than adjacent liver parenchyma. Contrast-enhanced CT or MRI has high sensitivity for the diagnosis, but lesions smaller than 2 cm may not show the characteristic enhancement in the arterial phase and washout in the venous phase. The Liver Imaging Reporting and Data System (LI-RADS) is used to classify liver lesions into five categories based on radiological features: *LR-1* (definitely benign), *LR-2* (probably benign), *LR-3* (moderate probability of benign or malignant), LR-4 (probably malignant), and LR-5 (definitely malignant).[35] Liver biopsy is recommended for diagnosis for mass lesions in noncirrhotic liver and in smaller (<2 cm) and radiologically indeterminate lesions in cirrhotic liver.

Risk Factors

The major etiological association is cirrhosis, which is present in more than 80% of cases. Cirrhosis related to alcohol use and viral hepatitis accounts for most of the HCC cases in the United States. There is also a high risk of HCC in the setting of cirrhosis resulting from hemochromatosis or α_1-antitrypsin deficiency. HCC can also develop with chronic viral hepatitis (B and C) in the absence of cirrhosis. Diabetes, obesity, and metabolic syndrome have been increasingly linked to higher risk for HCC.[36,37] Other risk factors include exposure to thorium dioxide (Thorotrast), aflatoxins, and estrogenic steroids.

Pathogenesis

HCC results from a multistep process that often occurs in the setting of various risk factors (e.g., chronic hepatitis), exposure to certain toxic or viral agents, and genetic alterations (see Chapter 44 for details).

Pathological Features

On gross examination, HCC may form a solitary mass or multiple scattered discrete nodules. Rarely, the entire lesion is composed of multiple nodules similar in size to typical cirrhotic nodules (Fig. 56.16), and this has been referred to as *cirrhosis-like* or *cirrhotomimetic variant.* [38] Most tumors have a circumscribed border and are well delineated from the surrounding liver, while a minority of tumors have an infiltrative appearance. A fibrous capsule can be present. Most HCCs lack abundant stroma and hence are soft, with variable necrosis. In contrast, abundant stroma is present in fibrolamellar and scirrhous variants, which tend to be firm and gray-white. HCC nodules may have a yellow hue if rich in fat, while a green color can result from bile.

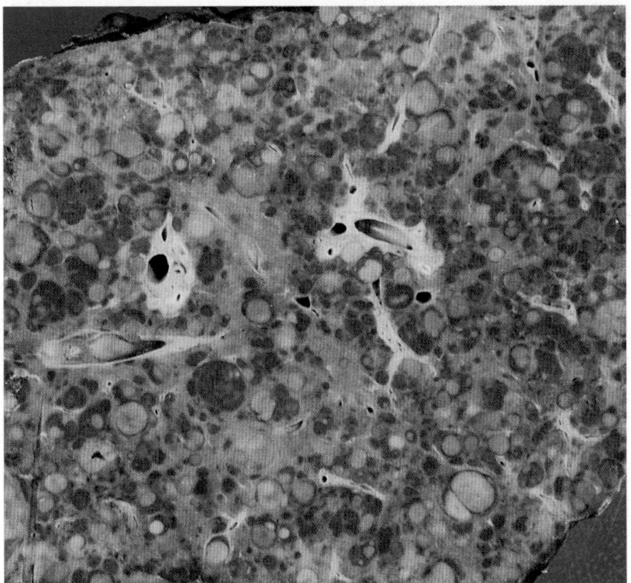

FIGURE 56.16 Cirrhosis-like hepatocellular carcinoma with yellow tumor foci and green cirrhotic nodules.

Invasion of the portal or hepatic vein or their large branches can be seen, particularly in association with large tumors. Small HCCs (<2 cm in diameter) usually lack vascular invasion, necrosis, and hemorrhage. The nonneoplastic liver often shows cirrhosis.

The tumor manifests a variety of growth patterns: *trabecular, pseudoacinar,* and *compact.* The *trabecular (plate-like) pattern* is the most common (Figs. 56.17 and 56.18) and mimics the cell plate architecture of normal liver. However, the cell plates are typically three or more cells thick and are lined by endothelial cells. Occasionally, the tumor cell plates or trabeculae may be separated by fibrous tissue instead of endothelial cells (Fig. 56.19). The *pseudoacinar (pseudoglandular) pattern* is characterized by glandlike or pseudoacinar spaces lined by tumor cells (Fig. 56.20) and can lead to a misdiagnosis of adenocarcinoma when prominent. The spaces represent dilated canaliculi and may contain bile or proteinaceous material. The spaces can also develop as a result of central necrosis within trabeculae and contain protein, cellular debris, or macrophages. The pseudoacinar pattern is frequently admixed with the trabecular pattern (Fig. 56.21). The *compact (solid) pattern* of HCC is characterized by sheets of tumor cells that lack clearly identifiable endothelial cell–lined trabeculae or cell plates (Fig. 56.22). It is more common in poorly differentiated HCCs. Compressed trabeculae may be highlighted with endothelial cell markers in some cases.

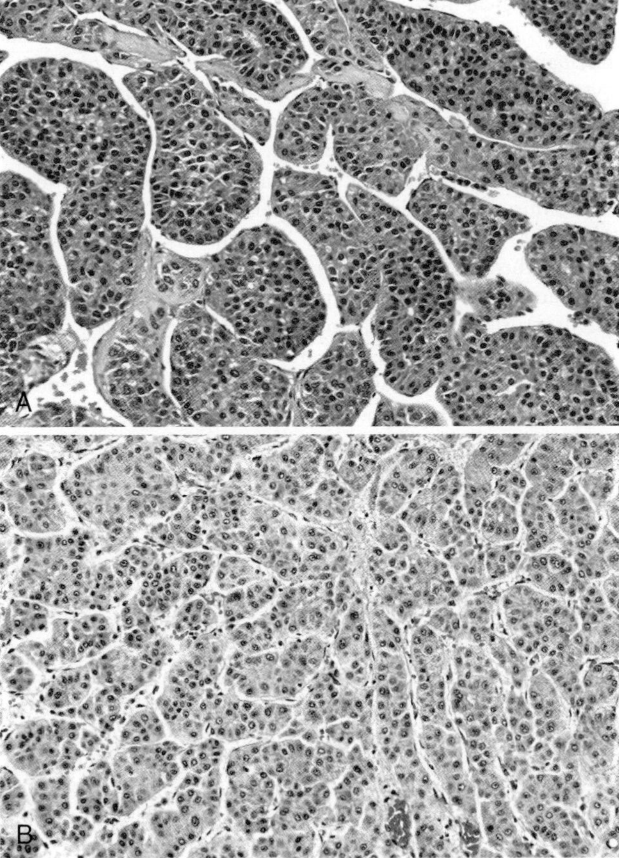

FIGURE 56.17 A, HCC with a trabecular growth pattern. The trabeculae are lined by endothelial cells. Bile stasis and small-cell change are evident. **B,** The cell plates are three cells or wider in most of the tumor. Small cell change is present.

The tumor cells often show small cell change (see Figs. 56.17 and 56.18). Large cell change is less frequent, except in high-grade tumors. Admixed foci of small and large cell change can occur. Kupffer cells are typically absent in HCC.

The tumor cells in HCC tend to be polygonal with some resemblance to normal hepatocytes, at least in well-differentiated and moderately differentiated cases. Most tumors reveal a variable degree of atypia in the form of nuclear pleomorphism and prominent nucleoli. Intranuclear vacuoles (composed of cytoplasmic invaginations) and

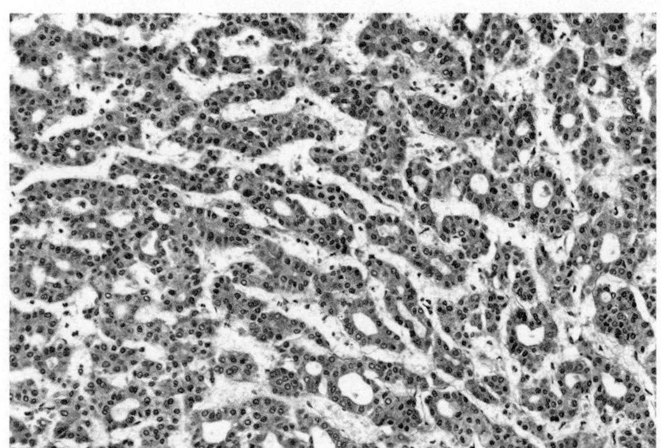

FIGURE 56.18 Reticulin stain shows extensive loss of the reticulin framework, which is normally visible as black strands of subendothelial connective tissue. The cell plates are relatively thin, and pseudoglands (i.e., acinar structures) are evident.

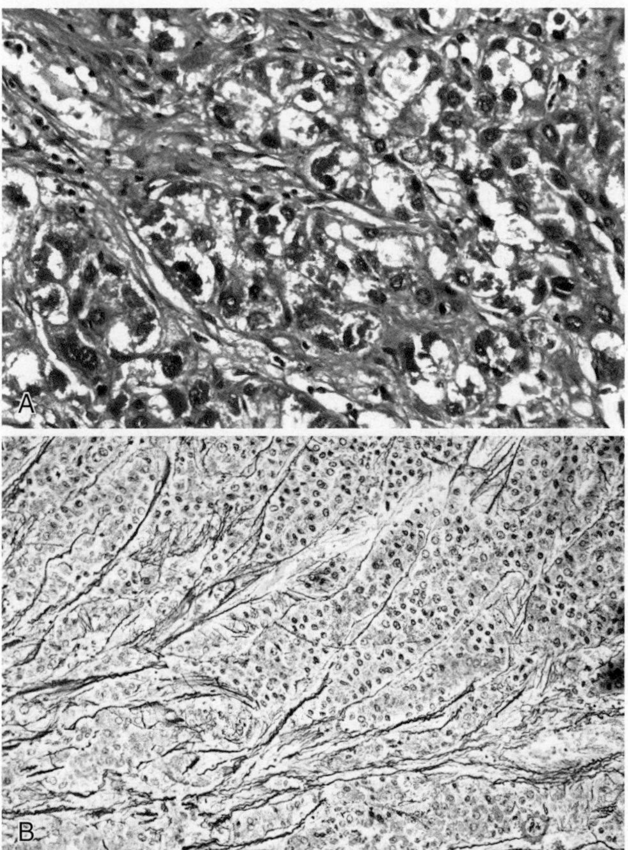

FIGURE 56.19 **A,** Hepatocellular carcinoma with trabeculae separated by relatively thin fibrous bands. Mallory hyaline is seen in many of the tumor cells. **B,** Reticulin stain shows increased staining along the thin, fibrous septa that separate the tumor trabeculae. The tumor cell plates tend to line up in a side-by-side (ribbon-like) pattern.

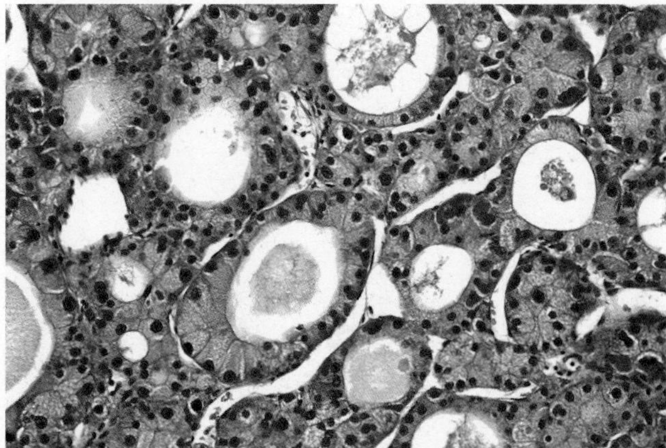

FIGURE 56.20 Hepatocellular carcinoma with pseudoacinar (pseudoglandular) architecture and proteinaceous debris. Bile can also be present *(not shown)*.

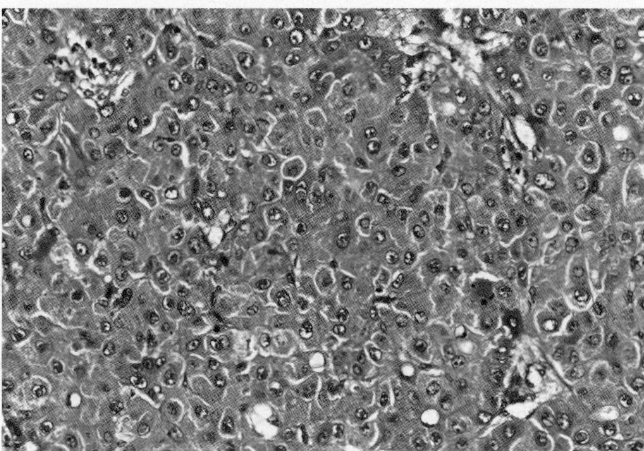

FIGURE 56.21 Hepatocellular carcinoma with a solid growth pattern and tumor cells arranged in sheets without definable cell plates or trabeculae.

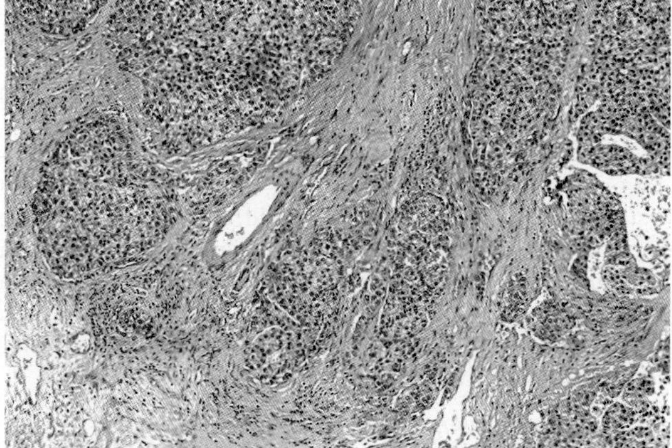

FIGURE 56.22 The scirrhous variant of hepatocellular carcinoma with tumor nests separated by abundant fibrous tissue.

glycogenation of nuclei are common (Fig. 56.23). The cytoplasm may be more basophilic compared with normal hepatocytes, may have a granular appearance, or may be brightly eosinophilic as a result of a large number of mitochondria. Mallory hyaline, globular acidophilic bodies, or cytoplasmic inclusions (related to proteins such as albumin, fibrinogen, α_1-antitrypsin, or ferritin) may be seen (see Fig. 56.23).

Fat (Fig. 56.24) or glycogen may be prominent in some HCCs, leading to a clear cell appearance. Other less frequent cytoplasmic changes include pale bodies, which are round to oval, lightly eosinophilic or clear cytoplasmic structures most frequently seen in fibrolamellar HCCs. Ground-glass cells containing hepatitis B surface antigen are found

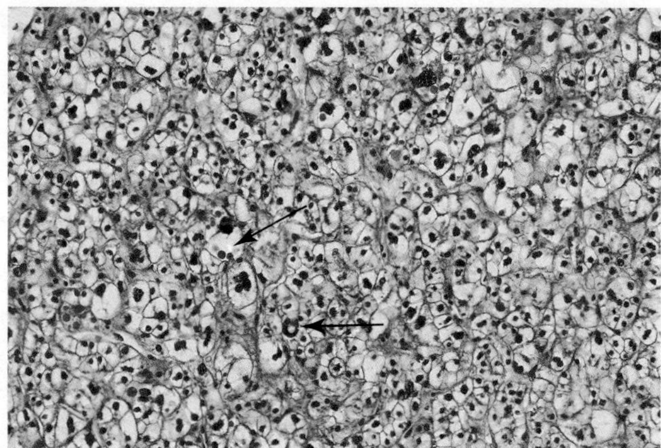

FIGURE 56.23 The clear cell variant of hepatocellular carcinoma with prominent cytoplasmic clear cell change. An occasional intranuclear vacuole *(bottom arrow)*, focally enlarged pleomorphic nuclei, and eosinophilic cytoplasmic globules (*top arrow*) can be seen.

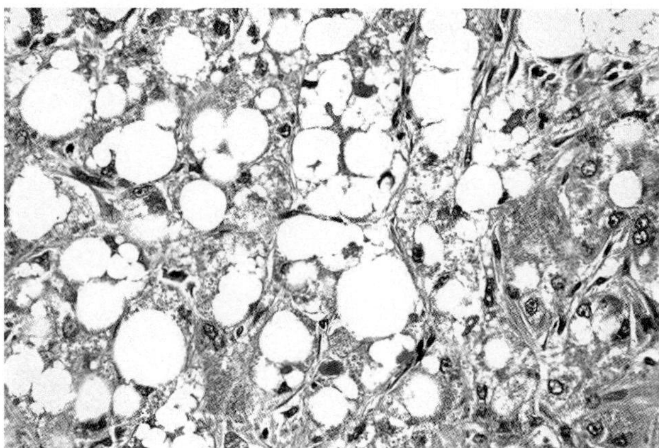

FIGURE 56.24 Hepatocellular carcinoma with prominent fatty change shows fat droplets in the cytoplasm.

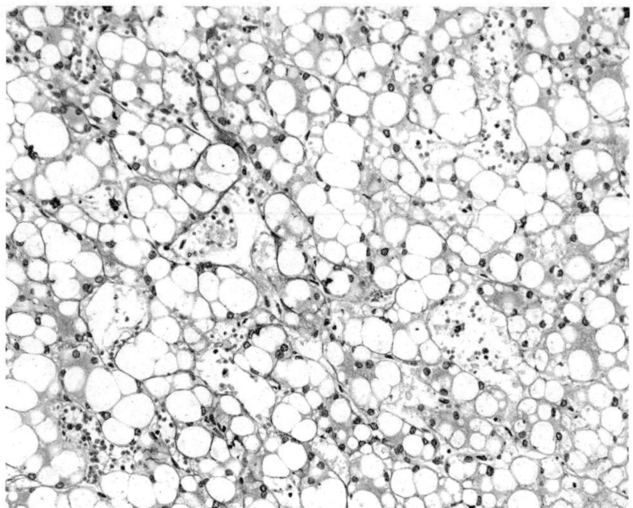

FIGURE 56.25 A disrupted reticulin network in a hepatocellular adenoma with fat. This is a common finding in benign liver with fat and should not be mistaken for hepatocellular carcinoma.

in some patients with HBV infection, and dark brown to black pigment similar to that seen in the Dubin-Johnson syndrome can be present.

In HCC, reticulin stain typically shows loss or fragmentation of the reticulin framework, although the reticulin pattern can be intact in very-well-differentiated cases (see Fig. 56.18). Reticulin stain is not helpful for HCC with prominent fat because reticulin loss can also be present in nonneoplastic liver with steatosis (Fig. 56.25).[39] Areas with no or less prominent steatosis should be sought in the tumor to evaluate the reticulin framework.

Histological Grading of Hepatocellular Carcinoma

The original system developed by Edmondson and Steiner in 1954 had four grades.[40] However, the WHO 2019 scheme categorizes HCC into three grades[2]: *well-differentiated, moderately differentiated*, and *poorly differentiated*.

1. Well-differentiated tumor cells resemble mature hepatocytes, with minimal to mild nuclear atypia. The cytoplasm ranges from abundant and eosinophilic to moderate and basophilic.
2. Moderately differentiated tumor cells resemble hepatocytes and show moderate nuclear atypia. Multinucleated cells occasionally can be present. The cytoplasm ranges from abundant and eosinophilic to moderate and basophilic.
3. Poorly differentiated tumor cells may or may not appear hepatocellular on morphology, and they show marked nuclear pleomorphism. Anaplastic giant cells can be present, and cytoplasm is scant to moderate and usually basophilic.

"Small" (Early and Progressed) Hepatocellular Carcinoma

By definition, small HCCs are tumors that measure 2 cm or less in diameter. These are divided into *early HCC* and *progressed HCC*.[2] Early HCCs are very-well-differentiated tumors with indistinct margins and no capsule. Microscopically, these tumors often show fat, pseudoacinar architecture, few intratumoral portal zones, thin cell plates (<3 cells thick), few unpaired arteries, and sparse sinusoidal staining with CD34. These HCCs closely resemble high-grade dysplastic nodules, but they are distinguished by the hallmark feature of stromal invasion.[41] The latter is characterized by invasion of tumor cells into adjacent septa, hepatic parenchyma, or portal tracts. Invasion into intratumoral portal tracts can also be present. Unlike regenerative nodules in cirrhosis, areas of stromal invasion lack a ductular reaction at the tumor-stroma interface, a feature that can be highlighted by CK7 staining.[42] In contrast, small *progressed* HCCs have distinct outlines and often show a capsule. Microscopically, these tumors are indistinguishable from larger HCCs with clearly evident cytoarchitectural atypia, lack of portal tracts, more unpaired arterioles, and increased sinusoidal staining with CD34.

Histological Variants of Hepatocellular Carcinoma

Several histological variants of HCC are recognized in the WHO 2019 classification and together account for a third of all HCCs (Table 56.6). These include scirrhous, fibrolamellar, steatohepatitic, clear cell, lymphocyte-rich, neutrophil-rich, macrotrabecular massive, chromophobe, and sarcomatoid variants. The importance of recognizing these histological variants is primarily to avoid errors in diagnosis. Apart from fibrolamellar HCCs, there are no treatment differences based on histological variants of HCC.

TABLE 56.6 Histological Variants of Hepatocellular Carcinoma

Histological Variant	Definition	Key Features
Scirrhous	>50% of tumor comprises fibrous stroma	• Hep Par 1 has low sensitivity, often positive for Arg-1 and GPC-3 • Variable prognosis, different outcomes in different studies
Fibrolamellar	• Abundant oncocytic cytoplasm • Prominent nucleoli • Lamellar fibrosis	• Young, noncirrhotic liver • Normal AFP • *DNAJB1-PRKACA* fusion • Prognosis similar to HCC in noncirrhotic liver
Steatohepatitic	• Ballooned tumor cells with fat and Mallory hyaline • Pericellular fibrosis may be present	• Often occur in fatty liver disease but can occur in other settings • Reticulin stain may not be helpful because of prominent fat • GS and GPC-3 can help in diagnosis of well-differentiated cases
Lymphocyte-rich	More lymphocytes than tumor cells in most areas	• Can be mistaken for lymphoma or benign inflammatory process • Subset may have lymphoepithelioma-like morphology; EBV positivity is rare
Neutrophil-rich	• Prominent neutrophilic infiltrate in the tumor	• Often associated with fever and leukocytosis • Can be mistaken for an infectious process • Related to granulocyte-colony stimulating factor (G-CSF) production by tumor cells
Macrotrabecular	• Cell plates ≥10 cells thick in at least 50% of the tumor	• Defined as >6 cell thick in some studies • Frequent *TP53* mutation and *FGF19* amplification • Poor prognosis
Chromophobe	• Clear to lightly stained cytoplasm • Low grade with focal striking nuclear atypia • Pseudocysts	• Recently described subtype • Associated with alternative lengthening of telomeres

The *scirrhous variant* (4% of all HCCs) is characterized by abundant fibrous stroma composing more than 50% of the tumor (see Fig. 56.22) and can be mistaken for cholangiocarcinoma or metastatic adenocarcinoma. Atypical radiological features, low sensitivity of Hep Par 1 and pCEA, as well as frequent staining with CK7/CK19/MOC31, can add to the diagnostic confusion. Arginase-1 and glypican-3 are positive in most cases.[43] The term *sclerosing hepatic carcinoma* was used in older literature and likely included both HCCs and cholangiocarcinomas associated with hypercalcemia; it is not a recognized variant, and this term should be avoided.

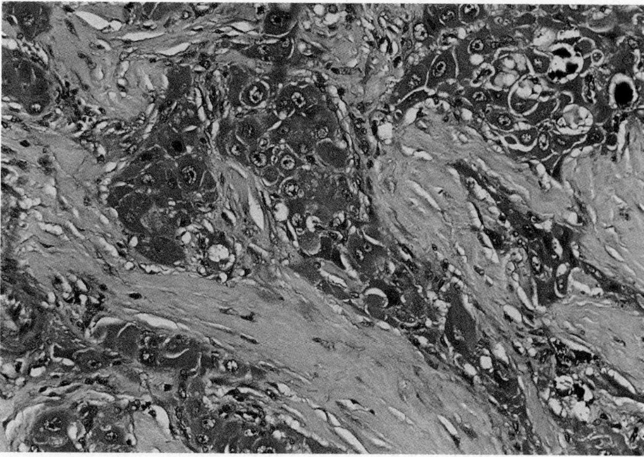

FIGURE 56.26 The tumor cells in fibrolamellar hepatocellular carcinoma have abundant eosinophilic granular cytoplasm, polygonal shape, and large, round nuclei with prominent nucleoli. The tumor cells are arranged in small groups and are separated by dense lamellar collagen.

The *fibrolamellar variant* (1% of all HCCs) occurs mainly in young adults without cirrhosis (mean age, 26 years) and shows a higher incidence in women than in men.[44-46] The most common clinical symptoms include abdominal pain or swelling, anorexia, weight loss, jaundice, and hemoperitoneum (rare). No definite risk factors have been identified in patients with this tumor type. FNH-like changes have been observed adjacent to fibrolamellar HCC in some cases,[47,48] but this is likely secondary to vascular changes adjacent to the tumor, and not a true precursor lesion. Except in rare cases, serum AFP levels are usually normal.[44,45]

Fibrolamellar HCCs are typically well-circumscribed, nodular, yellow- to brown-colored tumors with extensive fibrosis. A prominent central fibrous zone, as seen with FNH, may be identified in some cases. Larger tumors may show foci of hemorrhage and necrosis. Satellite lesions are rare. A triad of microscopic features is essential to establish an accurate diagnosis: dense bands of lamellar fibrosis (Fig. 56.26), polygonal-shaped tumor cells with eosinophilic granular cytoplasm, and large vesicular nuclei with prominent nucleoli. Cytoplasmic pale bodies, which may contain fibrinogen and albumin can be present, but they are not specific because they can occur in conventional HCC as well. Other features that may be present include acinar structures, bile, mucin (rare), eosinophilic globules, multinucleated tumor cells, copper, fat, epithelioid granulomas, and peliosis hepatis.

Fibrolamellar HCCs are typically positive for hepatocellular markers by immunohistochemistry. In addition, most tumors are positive for CK7 and CD68;[49] negative results with these markers should raise doubt regarding the diagnosis, but positive results are not diagnostic because they can also be positive in conventional HCCs. Staining for CK19 and epithelial cell adhesion molecule (EpCAM) is positive in up to 30% of cases.[50] Neuroendocrine markers may be focally positive as well.

In classic cases of fibrolamellar HCC, it is not difficult to differentiate it from benign lesions such as FNH and adenomas. Strict reliance on the characteristic triad of microscopic features is essential to distinguish it from conventional HCCs and other variants such as scirrhous HCC.

Fibrolamellar HCC is characterized by deletion of 400 kb on chromosome 19 that leads to fusion of the promoter and first exon of *DNAJB1*, a heat shock protein, with nine exons of *PRKACA*, the catalytic domain of protein kinase. The resulting fusion transcript codes for a chimeric protein that likely plays a role in the pathogenesis of the tumor.[51] This deletion has been reported in nearly all fibrolamellar HCCs, but not in other liver tumors including conventional HCC, hepatoblastoma, or intrahepatic cholangiocarcinoma.[52] This fusion can be demonstrated by fluorescence in situ hybridization (FISH) and can help in the diagnosis of morphologically ambiguous cases. The same fusion was recently described in oncocytic pancreatic and biliary neoplasms.[53,54]

Fibrolamellar HCCs, in general, have a more favorable prognosis when compared with HCC as a whole, but the outcome is similar when compared with stage-matched conventional HCCs in patients without cirrhosis.[55] Complete resection of the involved lobe is the preferred form of therapy. When tumor location precludes surgical resection, liver transplantation is an option.

Steatohepatitic variant (5% to 20% of all HCCs) shows features of steatohepatitis in the tumor cells in the form of steatosis, ballooning, Mallory hyaline, inflammation, and pericellular fibrosis (Fig. 56.27).[56,57] It has been suggested that at least three of these features should be present for a diagnosis of this variant and that changes should involve at least 50% of the tumor[57]; however, these cutoffs are not included in the WHO classification. This variant typically occurs in the setting of metabolic risk factors for fatty liver disease, and the nonneoplastic liver may show steatohepatitis. A minority of cases can occur in other settings such as hepatitis C.

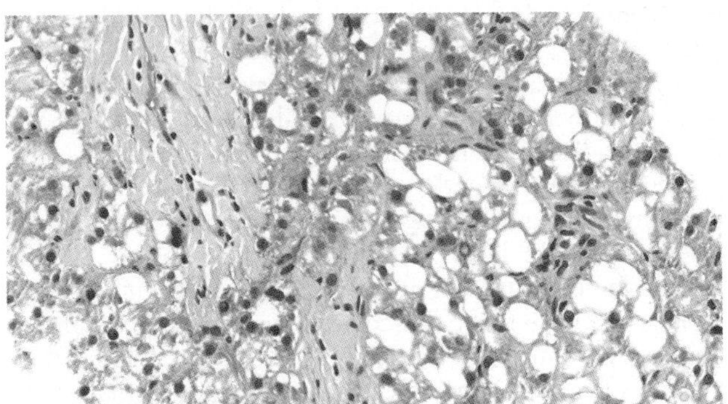

FIGURE 56.27 Steatohepatitic hepatocellular carcinoma with fat and ballooned tumor cells with Mallory hyaline.

Clear cell variant (<10% of all HCCs) is characterized by cytoplasmic glycogen accumulation in the tumor cells imparting a clear appearance involving at least 80% of the tumor cells.[2,58,59] Occasional fat vacuoles can be present. This variant is thought to have a more favorable prognosis based on a limited number of cases. The main importance of this variant is its morphological resemblance to other clear cell neoplasms such as renal cell carcinoma. The distinction is usually straightforward on immunohistochemistry as clear cell HCCs are positive for hepatocellular markers and yield negative results with renal markers like PAX8.

Lymphocyte-rich variant (<1% of all HCCs) refers to HCCs with a prominent lymphoid infiltrate in which the lymphocytes outnumber the tumor cells in most fields (Fig. 56.28).[2] The prominent lymphoid infiltrate can mimic a lymphoma. A syncytial growth pattern similar to nasopharyngeal carcinoma can be seen. Epstein-Barr virus (EBV) is typically negative in the tumor cells,[60] although rare positive cases have been described.[61] Microsatellite instability is not observed in these tumors. These tumors have a more favorable prognosis and may have high PDL-1 expression with a potential for immunotherapy.[62]

Neutrophil-rich variant (<1% of all HCCs) refers to HCCs with marked diffuse neutrophilic infiltrate in the tumor (Fig. 56.29), usually as a result of granulocyte colony-stimulating factor production by the tumor cells.[1,63] The patient may have systemic symptoms like fever and leukocytosis, which along with the histological picture dominated by neutrophils, can be mistaken for an infectious process. A poorer prognosis has been ascribed to these tumors.

Macrotrabecular massive variant (5% of all HCCs) is a recently described variant characterized by thick trabeculae (≥10 cells thick per the WHO classification, ≥6 cells thick in

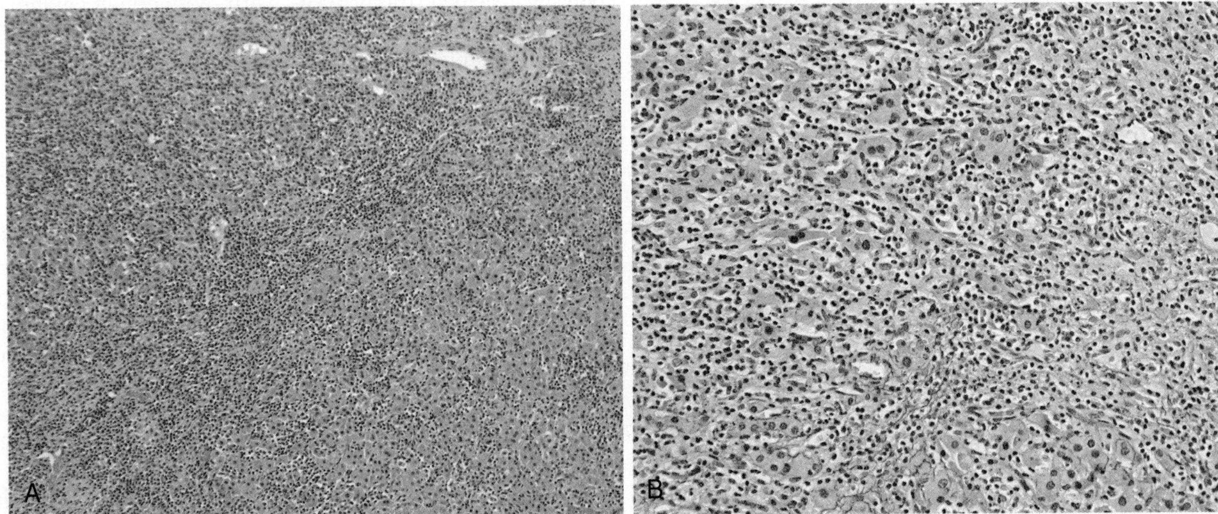

FIGURE 56.28 A, Lymphocyte-rich hepatocellular carcinoma characterized by a prominent lymphocytic infiltrate that obscures the neoplastic hepatocytes and can be mistaken for lymphoma. **B,** Extensive loss of reticulin confirms the diagnosis of hepatocellular carcinoma.

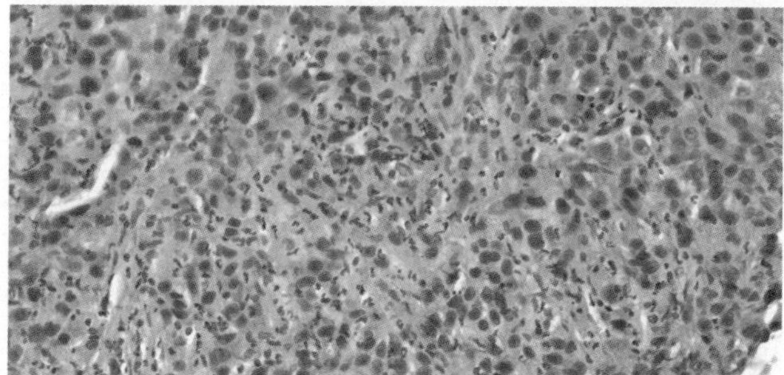

FIGURE 56.29 Poorly differentiated hepatocellular carcinoma with marked neutrophilic infiltrate.

some studies) composing more than 50% of the tumor.[2,64,65] This variant has been associated with high serum AFP, *TP53* mutations, *FGF19* amplification, and a poor prognosis.[64-66]

Chromophobe variant (<5% of all HCCs) is a recently described and not yet fully characterized variant that shows light staining cytoplasm *(chromophobe)*, mostly bland tumor nuclei, and focal areas of marked nuclear atypia.[67] Scattered pseudocysts can be present. This variant has been associated with alternative lengthening of telomeres but has no known prognostic significance.[67]

Sarcomatoid variant (<5% of all HCCs) was recognized as a variant of HCC in the prior WHO scheme, but it is not mentioned as a variant in the WHO 2019 scheme and is regarded as an example of poorly differentiated HCC.[2] Other terms like *spindle cell carcinoma* and *carcinosarcoma* have also been used synonymously, while the latter has been employed by some for cases with heterologous elements.[68] The sarcomatoid component may show malignant spindle, epithelioid, or pleomorphic cells; areas of conventional HCC are necessary to make the diagnosis (Fig. 56.30). Heterologous differentiation along the lines of leiomyosarcoma, rhabdomyosarcoma, chondrosarcoma, and osteosarcoma can occur in classical HCC following chemotherapy or transarterial chemoembolization.[68-70] Immunohistochemistry for pancytokeratin is positive in the sarcomatous area in a majority of cases,[70] while hepatocellular markers are usually negative. The diagnosis cannot be established with certainty in the absence of conventional HCC areas. The clinical setting of cirrhosis and positive keratin may help favor sarcomatoid HCC in these cases. The prognosis is poorer compared with classical HCC.[68,70]

Immunohistochemical Markers in Hepatocellular Carcinoma

Hepatocellular Markers

Arginase-1 (Arg-1) is a urea cycle enzyme that is produced only in hepatocytes. Cytoplasmic staining, either with or without nuclear staining with Arg-1, has high sensitivity and specificity for HCC (both >80%). Staining is also present in 70% to 80% of poorly differentiated and scirrhous cases.[71,72] Arg-1 can be negative in 5% of well-differentiated cases. [73] Most nonhepatocellular tumors are negative for Arg-1, but focal staining has been described in various adenocarcinomas in rare cases. Furthermore, hepatoid adenocarcinomas in the gastrointestinal tract, pancreas, and in other sites are typically positive for Arg-1.

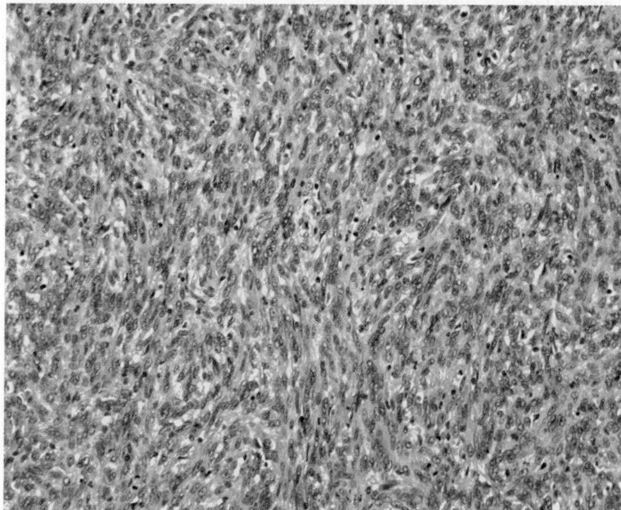

FIGURE 56.30 Malignant spindle cell neoplasm in the liver. The diagnosis of sarcomatoid hepatocellular carcinoma was established based on typical features of hepatocellular carcinoma in other portions of the tumor.

Hepatocyte antibody (i.e., clone OCH1E5.2.10 or Hep Par-1 antibody) demonstrates a granular cytoplasmic pattern in most HCCs, but it may be negative in approximately half of poorly differentiated HCCs and scirrhous HCCs.[74-76] Aberrant staining is present in many adenocarcinomas, including those from the stomach and lung, and less commonly cholangiocarcinomas and neuroendocrine neoplasms.

Glypican-3 (GPC-3) is an oncofetal antigen that has a high degree of sensitivity for poorly differentiated and scirrhous HCC, while more than 50% of well-differentiated HCCs as well as benign hepatocytes are typically negative (Fig. 56.31).[77-80] Occasional cirrhotic nodules and high-grade dysplastic nodules may also show patchy GPC-3 staining. Many nonhepatocellular tumors, such as squamous cell carcinoma, melanoma, nonseminomatous germ cell tumors, and rare cases of cholangiocarcinoma can also be GPC-3 positive.

Polyclonal antibody to carcinoembryonic antigen (pCEA) yields a canalicular pattern of staining in most HCCs. It cross-reacts with biliary glycoprotein in the bile canaliculus.[81] Cytoplasmic and/or luminal staining is usually present in most adenocarcinomas. However, the sensitivity of pCEA is low in poorly differentiated HCC and scirrhous HCC. Occasionally, it can be difficult to distinguish a canalicular pattern of staining from a membranous or luminal staining pattern commonly seen in adenocarcinomas.

Albumin in situ hybridization (not immunohistochemistry) is a useful marker of primary hepatic origin, as it is positive in both HCC (80% to 90%) and intrahepatic cholangiocarcinomas (iCCAs; 60% to 70%), but is negative in most other carcinomas.[82-85] Pancreatic acinar cell carcinomas can be strongly positive,[86] while focal staining can occur in carcinomas from a variety of sites such as gallbladder, breast, and lung.[85]

Other hepatocellular markers include CD10, bile salt export pump (BSEP), and villin, which show a canalicular pattern similar to pCEA in HCCs. AFP has a low sensitivity (30%) and is usually negative in well-differentiated cases.

Low-Molecular-Weight Cytokeratins

Low-molecular-weight cytokeratins (CK8 and CK18) are expressed in HCCs similar to normal benign hepatocytes. Hence most HCCs are positive with CAM5.2 and in pan-keratin cocktails such as AE1/AE3.

CK7, CK19, and/or MOC31 (antibody directed against EpCAM) are positive in 10% to 20% of HCCs, and they tend to be more common in scirrhous and poorly differentiated cases.[87-90] CK20 staining has been described in a small proportion of HCCs.[91]

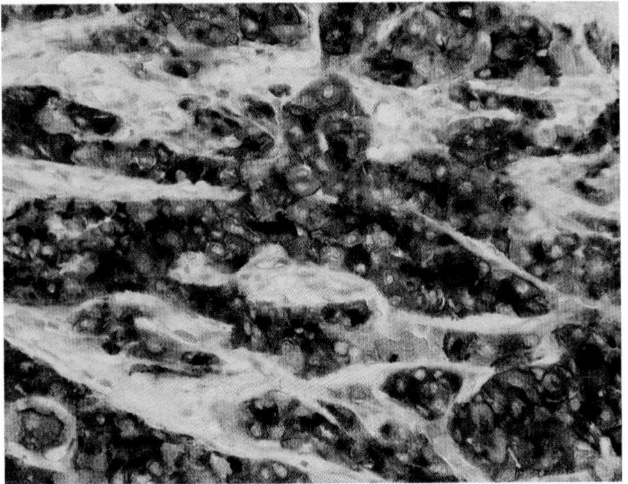

FIGURE 56.31 Hepatocellular carcinoma with focal glypican 3 immunostaining in a moderately differentiated portion of the tumor.

CD34 shows an increase in sinusoidal staining in HCCs as a result of arterialization of the blood supply, but it is of limited diagnostic value because of overlap with benign lesions, such as FNH and adenomas.

Differential Diagnosis

HCC must be distinguished from FNH, adenoma, and high-grade dysplastic nodules at the well-differentiated end of the spectrum (see earlier sections) and from cholangiocarcinoma and nonhepatocellular tumors for moderate or poorly differentiated cases (Tables 56.7 to 56.9).

Hepatocellular Carcinoma versus Adenocarcinoma

Because of significant overlap of staining patterns in these two types of tumor, at least two hepatocellular markers (arginase-1, Hep Par 1, glypican-3) and at least two markers more commonly positive in adenocarcinoma (CK7, C19, MOC31) are recommended (see Table 56.7).[88] Histochemical stains for epithelial mucins, such as mucicarmine or PAS-diastase, can also help in confirming an adenocarcinoma because HCCs are typically negative (except some fibrolamellar carcinomas).

The most common adenocarcinomas that must be distinguished from HCCs are intrahepatic cholangiocarcinoma, extrahepatic biliary, pancreatic, gastroesophageal, and colorectal. Upper GI and pancreaticobiliary adenocarcinomas

TABLE 56.7 Differentiating Features of Hepatocellular Carcinoma, Cholangiocarcinoma, and Metastatic Adenocarcinoma

Pathological Feature	Hepatocellular Carcinoma	Cholangiocarcinoma	Metastatic Adenocarcinoma
Acinar pattern	Pseudoglands: tumor cells have hepatocytic appearance; lumen contains bile, pink material, or debris	Glands have nuclei with side-by-side, low columnar arrangement or apical nuclei; mucin in lumina	Glands have nuclei with side-by-side, columnar arrangement or apical nuclei; mucin in lumina
Solid pattern	No intracellular mucin but possible intracellular fat droplets	May have intracellular vacuoles containing mucin	May have intracellular vacuoles containing mucin
Prominent fibrous stroma	Uncommon, except in scirrhous variant	Common	Common
MOC-31, CK7, CK19	Positive in 10%-20%	At least one marker positive in nearly all cases	At least one marker positive in nearly all cases (pancreas, upper GI sites)
CK20	Positive in 5%-10%	Positive in 5%-10%	Positive in 5%-10% (upper GI/ pancreas), >80% (colorectal)
Arginase-1	Positive	Negative	Negative (rare hepatoid carcinomas are positive)
Hepatocyte antibody (Hep Par1)	Positive (low sensitivity in poorly differentiated and scirrhous HCC)	Positive in <5%	Positive in <5% (rare hepatoid carcinomas are positive)
Glypican-3	Positive (low sensitivity in well differentiated HCC)	Negative (can be positive in ~5%)	Typically negative
Polyclonal CEA	Positive with canalicular pattern (low sensitivity in poorly differentiated and scirrhous HCC)	Positive with cytoplasmic, luminal, or membranous pattern	Positive for cytoplasmic, luminal, or membranous pattern
Albumin ISH	Positive (80%-90%)	Positive (60%-70%)	Negative (pancreatic acinar cell carcinomas can be positive)
BAP1 immunohistochemistry	Lost in ~5%	Lost in 10%-20%	Intact in most cases

ARG1, *Arginase 1;* BAP1, *BRCA-associated protein 1;* GI, *gastrointestinal;* GPC3, *glypican 3;* HCC, *hepatocellular carcinoma;* Hep Par 1, *hepatocyte paraffin 1 antigen;* ISH, *albumin in situ hybridization;* MOC-31, *monoclonal antibody.*

TABLE 56.8 Comparison of Hepatocellular Carcinoma and Neuroendocrine Tumors

Pathological Feature	Hepatocellular Carcinoma	Well-Differentiated Neuroendocrine Tumor
Solid, trabecular, and/or acinar patterns	Common	Common
Small, uniform cells	Common in well-differentiated tumors	Common
Pleomorphic or large tumor cells with variable nuclear features	Common in moderately to poorly differentiated HCCs	Uncommon
Arginase, Hep Par 1	Positive	Typically negative (Hep Par 1 can be positive in rare cases)
Chromogranin, synaptophysin	Negative (can be focally positive); rare cases can have more than focal staining, often with synaptophysin	One or both positive
CK7, CK19, and/or MOC-31	Positive in 10%-20% of cases	At least one marker positive in most cases

HCC, *Hepatocellular carcinoma;* MOC, *monoclonal antibody.*

TABLE 56.9 Differentiation of Hepatocellular Carcinoma from Other Tumors with "Hepatoid" Appearance

Pathological Feature	Hepatocellular Carcinoma	Renal Cell Carcinoma, Clear Cell Type*	Adrenal Cortical Carcinoma	Melanoma	Angiomyolipoma
Clear cell change	Present in clear cell variant	Present	Common	Present in clear cell melanoma	Uncommon
Pancytokeratin	Positive	Positive	Negative or focal	Negative	Negative
Hepatocellular markers	Positive	Negative	Negative	Negative	Negative
PAX-2/PAX-8	Negative	Positive	Negative	Negative	Negative
S100, HMB-45	Negative	Negative	Negative	Usually positive for one or both	HMB-45 positive
SMA/desmin	Negative	Negative	Negative	Negative	Usually positive
SF-1, Inhibin	Negative	Negative	Usually positive	Negative	Negative

SF-1, *steroidogenic factor-1.*
**Other markers like RCC antigen, epithelial membrane antigen, and carbonic anhydrase IX can be used to support clear cell RCC if necessary.*

are typically positive for CK7, CK19, and/or MOC31. Because a subset of HCCs can be positive for these markers, positive mucin stains and/or negative results with hepatocellular markers are crucial for diagnosis. Aberrant Hep Par 1 can be seen in adenocarcinomas; arginase-1 and albumin ISH can help in establishing the diagnosis in these cases, with the caveat that albumin ISH is positive in intrahepatic cholangiocarcinoma. Site-specific markers, such as TTF-1 and napsin A (lung), GATA 3 (breast, urinary bladder), PAX8 (renal, gynecologic), CDX2 and SATB2 (intestinal), and NKX3.1 (prostate), may be obtained depending on the clinical setting.

Hepatocellular Carcinoma versus Neuroendocrine Neoplasms

HCCs can closely resemble neuroendocrine neoplasms morphologically because both can show solid, pseudoacinar, and trabecular growth patterns (see Table 56.9). A prominent vascular or capillary network and stromal hyalinization favor a neuroendocrine tumor. Similar to other GI/pancreatic sites, these tumors are categorized into well-differentiated neuroendocrine tumors (NETs) and poorly differentiated neuroendocrine carcinomas (large cell or small cell) based on the morphology and further assessment with Ki-67 proliferation index. Loss of Rb and diffuse p53 staining on immunohistochemistry can help distinguish a neuroendocrine carcinoma from a grade 3 NET in morphologically challenging cases.[92,93] Primary neuroendocrine neoplasms are extremely rare in the liver.[94]

Immunohistochemistry is very helpful for distinguishing these tumors. Pitfalls in diagnosis include rare staining of HCC with neuroendocrine markers. In fact, rare cases can show diffuse synaptophysin staining. Focal positivity with neuroendocrine markers is well known in fibrolamellar HCC. Furthermore, rare cases of neuroendocrine neoplasms may show aberrant staining with Hep Par 1; CK7, CK9, and/or MOC31 are positive in the majority of neuroendocrine tumors. Recently described neuroendocrine markers, such as insulinoma-associated protein 1 (INSM1), may have a higher sensitivity for NET, but additional studies are needed to confirm this.[95] Because treatment for metastatic NETs varies according to the site of origin, immunohistochemistry with TTF-1 (lung), CDX-2 (intestinal), polyclonal PAX-8 (pancreatic), ATRX/DAXX (lost in a subset of pancreatic NETs), PDX-1 (pancreatic), and prostatic acid phosphatase (rectum) can help in determining site of origin of a NET.[96] There is significant overlap in the staining patterns of NETs from different anatomical sites; thus confirmation of the primary site is based also on correlation with clinical and radiological findings.

Hepatocellular Carcinoma versus Other Tumor Types

Metastatic clear cell renal cell carcinoma (RCC) may be difficult to distinguish from the clear cell variant of HCC (see Table 56.9).[97,98] Hepatocellular markers (Arg-1 or Hep Par 1) and PAX2/PAX8 can help distinguish these entities in most cases. Additional markers that are often positive in RCC, such as EMA, carbonic anhydrase IX, and RCC antigen, can also be used if necessary.

Melanoma can mimic HCC, but this tumor is easily distinguished based on positive staining with SOX-10 or S100 and negative staining with hepatocellular markers. Additional melanocytic markers such as HMB-45, melan-A, and tyrosinase can also be helpful (see Table 56.9). The solid and trabecular architecture common in metastatic adrenocortical carcinomas can be difficult to distinguish from HCC. Positive staining with steroidogenic factor 1(SF-1) and absence of negative results with hepatocellular markers can help confirm the diagnosis of adrenocortical carcinoma.[99] These tumors are also generally negative or only focally positive for pancytokeratin, and they are also positive for inhibin, synaptophysin, and melan-A.

Prognosis and Treatment

The 5-year survival is 18% overall and 2% for metastatic disease based on the SEER data. The outcome improves to 60% to 70% for early-stage cancers that can be treated with resection or transplantation. The key prognostic factors are pathological stage, adequacy of the surgical resection margins (at least 1 cm), and the presence or absence of cirrhosis. Pathological stage includes size and the number of tumor nodules, vascular invasion, and lymph node and distant metastases. The impact of histological tumor grade and subtype on prognosis is considered less important. However, almost all small, early HCCs are well differentiated and have a favorable prognosis, whereas poorly differentiated HCCs and those with CK19 positivity have a poorer outcome.[100-102] HCCs that arise in a noncirrhotic liver are associated with a more favorable outcome.

Liver transplantation is effective therapy for HCC in patients with cirrhosis who meet certain criteria (Milan criteria: solitary or multiple tumors with cumulative tumor size <5 cm and no evidence of large vessel invasion). If aggressive tumors are excluded based on poor tumor differentiation established on liver biopsy, favorable results have been reported for tumors that exceed Milan criteria, [103,104] but this practice is not widely used. Alternative therapies, such as cryoablation, percutaneous ethanol injection, transarterial chemoembolization, kinase inhibitors like sorafenib, and, more recently, PDL-1 inhibitors, are used in inoperable cases and may help improve survival.

Combined Hepatocellular Carcinoma-Cholangiocarcinoma

Combined (mixed) HCC-cholangiocarcinoma (cHCC-CCA) accounts for approximately 5% of all primary liver carcinomas. The risk factors are similar to those for HCC, as evidenced by its frequent association with HCV or HBV infection and cirrhosis.[105,106] The pathogenesis is uncertain; progenitor or stem cell origin as well as transdifferentiation have been proposed as underlying mechanisms of bidirectional tumor differentiation.[107,108]

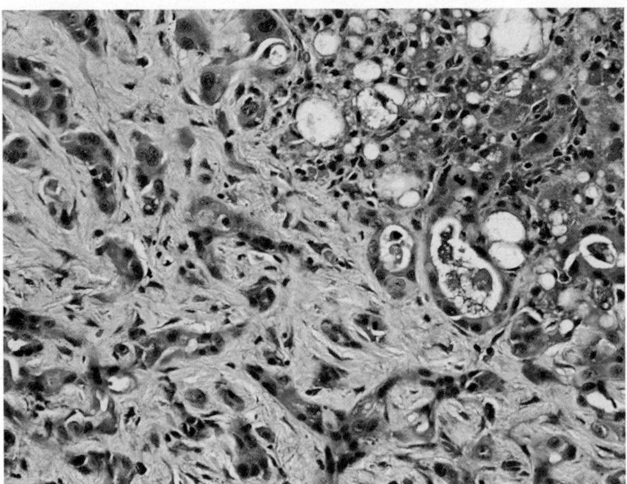

FIGURE 56.32 Combined hepatocellular-cholangiocarcinoma shows bile in the hepatocellular carcinoma component with a pseudoacinar pattern and blue mucin in the small glands in the cholangiocarcinoma component.

By definition, cHCC-CCA demonstrates morphological evidence of both components of the tumor that is supported by immunohistochemistry (Fig. 56.32).[2] Polygonal-shaped tumor cells with a "hepatoid" appearance provide morphological evidence for HCC, which is then further supported by showing the presence of bile, cytoplasmic fat, and/or Mallory hyaline. Confirmation by one or more hepatocellular markers, such as Arg-1, Hep Par 1, and GPC-3, is further evidence of an HCC component. If these markers are not informative and the suspicion for HCC is high, one or more of the less sensitive markers, such as AFP, polyclonal CEA, CD10, and BSEP, should be considered.

The cholangiocarcinoma component shows discrete glands morphologically typically in a prominent fibrous stroma, either with or without mucin. Positivity for CK7, CK19, and/or MOC-31 can help confirm a cholangiocarcinoma component. However, positive staining with these markers without supportive morphological features should not be considered as evidence for cholangiocarcinoma because these markers can be positive in 10% to 20% of HCCs as well. Collision tumors, in which these elements are completely separate or situated adjacent to each other, are not considered cHCC-CCA.[2]

Several subtypes of combined cHCC-CCA, with stem cell features, were noted in the WHO 2010 classification, but these have been eliminated in the 2019 classification because of lack of specific morphological or immunohistochemical markers for stem cells. The term *intermediate carcinoma* has been used when tumor cells show both morphological and immunohistochemical features that are intermediate between HCC and CCA.[109] However, the diagnostic criteria for this tumor are not clearly defined. As per the WHO 2019 classification, this term should be used only for rare tumors that are almost exclusively composed of tumor cells with intermediate characteristics.[2] It is imperative to use stringent criteria because the diagnosis of a cholangiocarcinoma component has important treatment implications; for instance, a lymph node dissection is indicated if the tumor is resected, 5FU- or oxaliplatin-based treatment is indicated if chemotherapy is needed, and denial of liver transplant is indicated in most centers.[110] In challenging cases, sequencing analysis may help favor a cholangiocarcinoma component if typical changes such as *IDH1* or *PBRM1* mutation or *FGFR* translocation are identified.

BILIARY TUMORS

Bile Duct Hamartoma

Bile duct hamartoma, also called *von Meyenburg complex*, is considered a remnant of the ductal plate. These lesions often occur sporadically; when multiple and located adjacent to cysts, they may be part of the spectrum of polycystic liver disease or ductal plate malformation disorders.

Bile duct hamartomas are usually small (<0.5 cm), gray to white, irregularly shaped lesions that are usually located in and at the periphery of portal tracts. Multifocality is common. Microscopically, bile duct hamartomas consist of numerous, small- to medium-sized ductules that are embedded in dense collagen (Fig. 56.33). The ductules are often dilated and can form cystic spaces with intraluminal eosinophilic debris or inspissated bile. The ductules are lined by small cuboidal or flattened cells with round to oval nuclei. Bile duct hamartomas are benign lesions with no malignant potential.

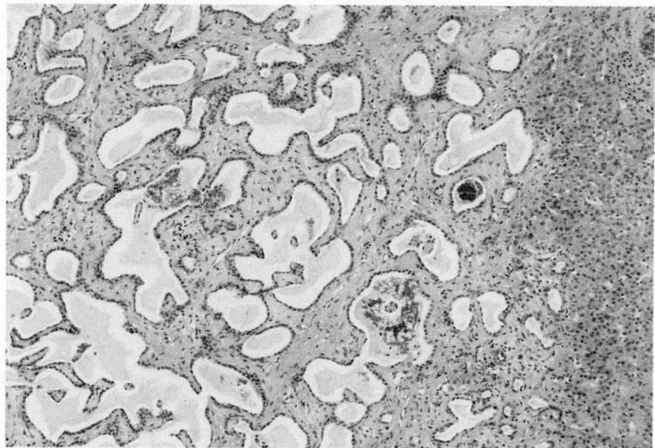

FIGURE 56.33 Dilated ductular structures in a bile duct hamartoma lined by cuboidal to flattened epithelium, focally containing bile.

Bile Duct Adenoma

Clinical Features

Bile duct adenomas are benign biliary neoplasms that are typically discovered incidentally at laparotomy, and a biopsy is usually performed to exclude a metastatic carcinoma. These can occur in patients of any age group, but they are more common after 20 years of age and in men than in women. They can occur in patients with cirrhosis. Originally, it was believed that bile duct adenomas are not true neoplasms and may instead represent a localized ductular reaction as a result of prior injury,[111] or a type of peribiliary gland hamartoma.[112] However, the neoplastic nature of bile duct adenomas is supported by the finding of *BRAF* V600E mutations in 53% to 87% of cases.[113,114]

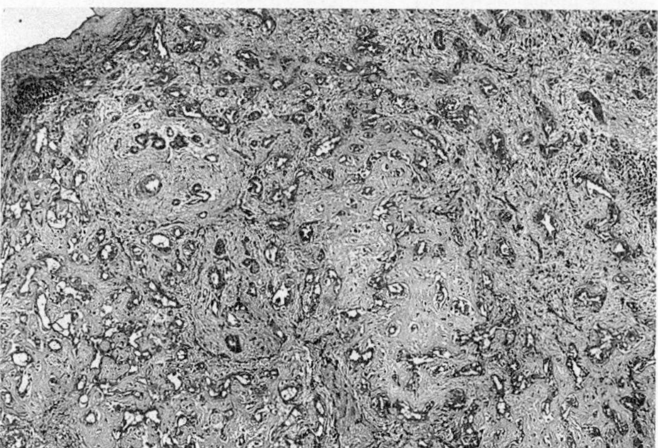

FIGURE 56.34 Subcapsular bile duct adenoma comprising evenly spaced ductules in fibrous tissue. Inflammation is scant, and there is no cytological atypia.

Pathological Features

Bile duct adenomas are small (<2 cm in diameter), firm, white to gray-tan, well-circumscribed lesions. They are usually located directly underneath the liver capsule, but they may develop deep in the liver parenchyma, particularly in the setting of cirrhosis. They may be single or multiple.

Histologically, the ductules are usually uniform in size, nondilated, and contain less intervening fibrous stroma than bile duct hamartomas (Figs. 56.34 and 56.35). However, abundant dense collagen may be seen in the center of larger or longstanding lesions. The ductules have a tubular shape and are cuboidal cells with bland, round- to oval-shaped nuclei and without mitotic activity. Mucinous metaplasia α_1-antitrypsin globules and focal staining with neuroendocrine markers can be seen in the ductal cells in some cases.

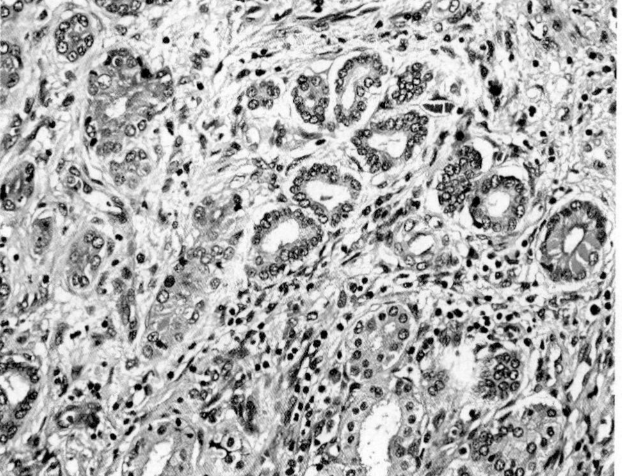

FIGURE 56.35 Higher magnification of a bile duct adenoma shows round and uniform nuclei of the ductular cells.

Residual portal tracts are often preserved either within or at the periphery of the lesion. Small aggregates of lymphocytes may be present as well, most often at the periphery of the lesion. The biliary epithelium is positive for CK7 and CK19; immunohistochemistry for the *BRAF* V600E mutant protein can help confirm the diagnosis.[113,114]

TABLE 56.10 Bile Duct Adenoma Compared with Cholangiocarcinoma and Metastatic Adenocarcinoma

Pathological Feature	Bile Duct Adenoma	Cholangiocarcinoma	Metastatic Adenocarcinoma
Size	Most are <2 cm	Most are >3 cm	Variable
Underlying cirrhosis	Can be present	Can be present	Rare
Glandular pattern	Curvilinear or tubular glands, uniform size; uniform spacing	Variation in glandular shapes and sizes; irregular spacing	Variation in glandular shapes and sizes; irregular spacing
Cytological atypia	Minimal atypia	Variable, moderate atypia at least focally present in most cases	Variable, moderate atypia at least focally present in most cases
Mitotic activity	Typically absent	May be seen	May be seen
Mucinous epithelium	May be present	May be present	May be present
Portal tracts in lesion	Common	Uncommon except at invasive edge	Uncommon except at invasive edge
Dense fibrosis	Common	Common	Common
α_1-Antitrypsin globules	May be seen	Absent	Absent
Ki-67 proliferation index	<10% in most cases	Most cases >10%	Most cases >10%
p53	Patchy mild to moderate staining	Subset shows diffuse strong staining or total absence ("null pattern")	Subset shows diffuse strong staining or total absence ("null pattern")
BAP1	Nuclear (normal pattern)	Loss of nuclear staining in 10%-20%	Nuclear (normal pattern)
BRAF V600E	Positive in majority	Usually negative (positive in 3%-5%)	Usually negative
DPC4	Nuclear (normal pattern)	Loss of nuclear staining in 5%-10%	Loss of nuclear staining in 50%-60%

Differential Diagnosis

Bile duct adenomas may be difficult to distinguish from metastatic adenocarcinomas, particularly on frozen-section analysis. The finding of complex architecture with fused/cribriform/papillary growth pattern, more than mild cytological atypia, infiltrative borders, a destructive growth pattern, necrosis, and mitotic activity all strongly favor adenocarcinoma, whereas bland cytological features, uniform ductules, and lack of significant atypia without mitosis favor a bile duct adenoma (Table 56.10).

A high Ki-67 proliferative index (>10%) and diffuse strong p53 staining can help support adenocarcinoma. Because some bile duct adenomas may show a higher proliferation rate and moderate p53 staining, the utility of these stains is limited.[115] Immunostaining for *BRAF* V600E and positive results with albumin in situ hybridization would favor bile duct adenoma, whereas loss of DPC4 (50% to 60% of pancreatic adenocarcinomas) favors metastatic adenocarcinoma.[116,117] If bile duct adenoma versus intrahepatic cholangiocarcinoma is being considered, loss of BAP1 can help support the latter (10% to 20% of cases).[117]

Mucinous Cystic Neoplasms

Clinical Features

Mucinous cystic neoplasms (MCNs), formerly known as *hepatobiliary cystadenomas,* are rare lesions that can present as a palpable mass, abdominal pain or discomfort, and, less commonly, jaundice, complications of tumor rupture, and infection. MCNs occur almost exclusively in women and are similar to their pancreatic counterpart.[2]

The mean ages of patients with MCN, either with and without adenocarcinoma, are 45 and 59 years, respectively. Some patients have elevated serum levels of CA 19-9.

Pathological Features

MCNs typically are multilocular tumors and contain either a smooth or somewhat trabeculated epithelial lining. The cysts may contain serous, mucinous, gelatinous, and bloody or purulent material. MCNs do not communicate with the biliary tract. Large, polypoid projections or dense masses in the wall of the cysts often indicate areas of malignant transformation. Thorough examination of MCNs is necessary as malignant transformation can be focal.

Microscopically, the cysts are typically lined by a single layer of epithelial cells, usually of the mucinous type, and contain an immunoprofile similar to biliary-type epithelium (CK7 and CK19 positive). The cells may be flat, cuboidal, or columnar (Fig. 56.36). Small papillary tufts may be present. The nuclei in most cases are small, bland, basally located, and have no mitotic activity. Subclassification into low- and high-grade intraepithelial neoplasia (dysplasia) is similar to pancreatic MCN. High-grade dysplasia, evidenced by marked nuclear pleomorphism, loss of polarity, mitotic figures, and multilayering of the epithelium, warrants careful and extensive examination for invasive adenocarcinoma, which is rare and occurs in <10% of cases. Unequivocal stromal invasion is considered necessary to establish a diagnosis of invasive adenocarcinoma. Adenocarcinomas can arise in MCN with low-grade dysplasia as well. The invasive component often shows tubulopapillary histology and prominent desmoplastic response typical of invasive adenocarcinomas of the pancreatobiliary tree.[118]

Rarely, gastric, intestinal, or squamous metaplasia can be present in MCNs. In addition, half of these lesions show scattered chromogranin- or synaptophysin-positive endocrine cells.[2] The cyst wall may be lined focally by macrophages and other secondary changes such as fibrosis, hyalinization, and calcification. Similar to pancreatic MCN,

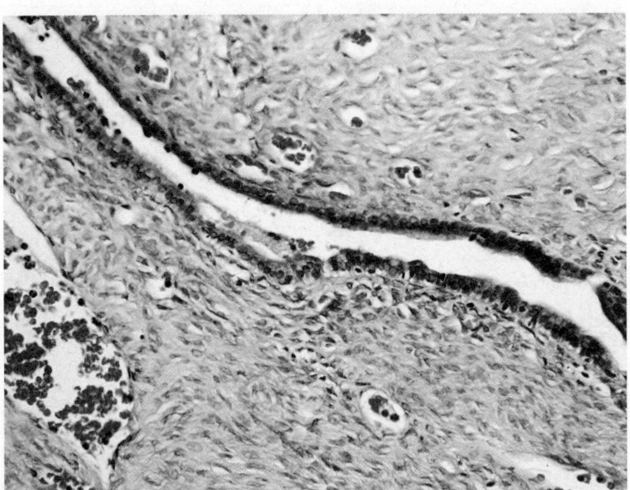

FIGURE 56.36 Low-grade mucinous cystic neoplasm with cysts lined by bland, cuboidal to columnar, ductal-type epithelium. The underlying stroma has a hypercellular spindle cell appearance similar to ovarian stroma.

the characteristic ovarian-like stroma is considered necessary for diagnosis, but it may be focal, especially in cases with secondary changes in the cyst wall. Immunohistochemistry for ER, PR, inhibin, and FOXL2 can help highlight the stroma.[119,120] The lining epithelial cells are positive for CK7 and CK19, as expected in biliary epithelium.

Differential Diagnosis

Other cystic lesions in the differential diagnosis are simple biliary cysts, polycystic liver disease, and intraductal papillary neoplasm of bile ducts. Simple cysts are usually not multiloculated, but they can be multifocal. Mucinous epithelium and ovarian-like stroma are not present in these lesions. Multiple von Meyenburg complexes in the cyst wall and a history of cystic kidney disease can help in the diagnosis of polycystic liver disease. Prominent papillary proliferation and communication with the biliary tree indicate an intraductal papillary neoplasm, which lacks an ovarian-type stroma and typically comprises biliary-type epithelium without prominent mucinous features. Other rare disorders in the differential include endometriosis with cystic change, which typically shows a combination of endometrial glands, endometrial stroma, and evidence of hemorrhage such as hemosiderin-laden macrophages. Microcystic (serous) adenoma is more common in the pancreas, but it can rarely occur in the liver. The presence of a cuboidal nonmucinous lining epithelium, clear cytoplasm (glycogen-laden, PAS-positive, diastase sensitive), GLUT1 positivity, and absence of ovarian-like stroma distinguishes this entity from MCN.

Treatment and Outcome

Noninvasive MCNs have an excellent outcome when treated by surgical resection. Invasive MCNs are prone to recurrence, but the outcome is thought to be more favorable than intrahepatic cholangiocarcinoma.[2]

Simple (Biliary) Cysts

Simple cysts are dilated biliary radicles that are usually asymptomatic and discovered as an incidental finding. They

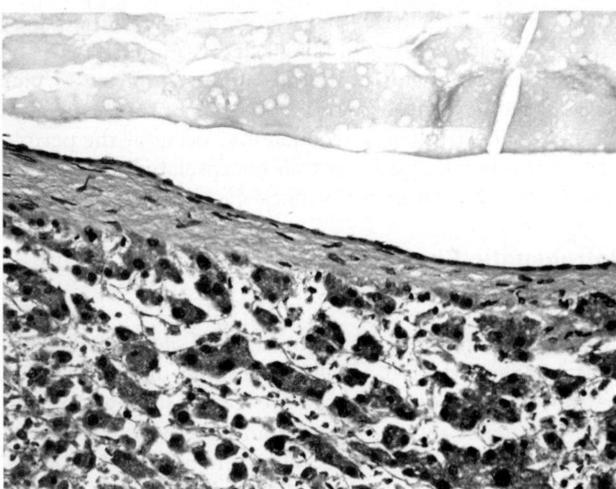

FIGURE 56.37 A simple cyst lined by flattened epithelium that rests on relatively acellular, fibrous stroma.

typically occur in patients older than 40 years of age. Simple cysts have no premalignant potential.

Pathology

These cysts are usually located directly underneath the liver capsule, but they may occur deep in the liver parenchyma as well. They typically contain clear, light yellow-colored fluid. These cysts are lined by cuboidal to low columnar epithelium with a fibrous wall (Fig. 56.37). The epithelium may be focally disrupted or flattened. Evidence of reactive stromal changes and recent or remote hemorrhage may be evident in the cyst wall. The epithelium expresses CK7 and CK19, similar to normal biliary epithelium. When multiple von Meyenburg complexes (i.e., biliary hamartomas) are present in association with the cysts, the possibility of polycystic liver disease should be considered.

Other Benign Biliary Tumors or Lesions

Biliary adenofibroma is a rare entity that consists of ductular and stromal elements with both solid and microcystic regions.[121] The ductular components may be similar to those in bile duct adenomas, but they often have tortuous or branching configurations, they may be dilated, and they may form microcysts. The cuboidal or low columnar epithelium lining the ducts is often flattened in microcysts. Foci of apocrine change, epithelial tufts, and mitotic figures may be present. These lesions do not produce mucin, but some cysts may contain eosinophilic fluid. The stroma is composed of spindle-shaped fibroblasts and may have patchy chronic inflammation.

Microcystic adenomas, which are grossly and microscopically similar to microcystic adenomas (i.e., serous cystadenoma) of the pancreas, are rare in the liver. Similar to its pancreatic counterpart, this tumor consists of numerous microcysts lined by cuboidal epithelial cells that contain abundant cytoplasmic glycogen (PAS positive), as discussed earlier.

The term *biloma* describes a large collection of bile located outside the bile ducts and often found in perihepatic tissues related spatially to the gallbladder or large hepatic ducts. A biloma can result from trauma, iatrogenic injury, ischemic damage, or severe infection of the biliary tree. The lesion consists of bilious debris admixed with and surrounded by inflammatory cells and macrophages, which often have a xanthomatous appearance. An exuberant fibrous connective tissue reaction may occur at the periphery of the lesion and impart an encapsulated appearance. The preferred treatment is surgical excision.

Intrahepatic Cholangiocarcinoma

Clinical Features

iCCAs are primarily malignant tumors of older adults, with both genders affected equally. The tumor usually remains asymptomatic until it reaches a late stage in its development. The prevalence rate is high in Southeast Asia, where liver fluke infestation is endemic. The incidence in the United States has increased from 0.44 to 1.12 per 100,000 over a 40-year period.[122] The majority of cases afflict patients between their fifth and seventh decades, with a slight male predominance.

Serum levels of CA 19-9 can be elevated but have limited utility in diagnosis because of limited sensitivity and specificity (both approximately 60%).[123]

On noncontrast CT , iCCA has a hypoattenuated appearance with irregular margins, while it shows peripheral rim enhancement in the arterial phase and progressive hyperattenuation on venous and delayed phases on contrast-enhanced CT. On MRI, it shows low signal intensity on T1-weighted MRI, and high signal intensity on T2-weighted imaging, with an enhancement pattern similar to CT findings on contrast MRI.[124]

The major risk factors are infections by liver flukes (*Clonorchis* and *Opisthorchis* species), hepatolithiasis, and primary sclerosing cholangitis.[125-127] Other risk factors include congenital anomalies of the biliary tree (such as congenital hepatic fibrosis, Caroli disease)[128-130] and exposure to chemicals like asbestos and Thorotrast.[131] Chronic viral hepatitis B and C as well as cirrhosis of any etiology are well-established risk factors for iCCA.[132]

Pathological Features

iCCAs most commonly appear as firm, white-tan lesions because of the abundant fibrous stroma ("mass forming"). Tumors involving the larger ducts may lead to strictures or thickening of bile ducts with varying involvement of the adjacent liver parenchyma; this has been referred to as the *periductal-infiltrating type*. Tumors can also show mixed *mass-forming and periductal-infiltrating* patterns.[133]

Microscopically, the tumor shows features of adenocarcinoma composed of infiltrative tubules/glands or cords of tumor cells in abundant fibrous stroma. Papillary, micropapillary, cystic, and solid growth patterns can be seen. Based on the extent of gland formation, the tumors can be well-differentiated (>95%), moderately differentiated (50% to 95%), or poorly differentiated (<50%). The cytological atypia can be mild in well-differentiated cases and can be difficult to distinguish from benign biliary lesions. Foci of cells with higher cytological atypia, increased nucleus-to-cytoplasm ratio, prominent nucleoli, increased variation in nuclear size, and loss of polarity are often seen, at least focally (Fig. 56.38). Other features that favor a malignant

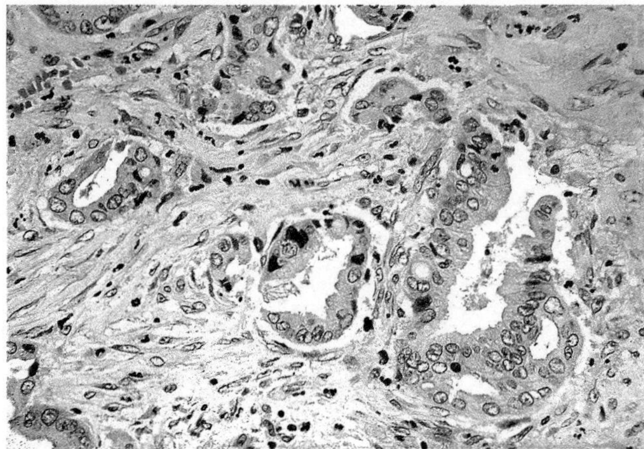

FIGURE 56.38 An intrahepatic cholangiocarcinoma with malignant glands embedded in an inflamed fibrous stroma. The cuboidal epithelium shows considerable variability in cytological features.

diagnosis include intracytoplasmic lumina, a cribriform pattern, multilayering of nuclei, intraluminal cellular debris, perineural/lymphovascular invasion, and destructive infiltration of portal tracts or hepatic parenchyma. Some cholangiocarcinomas spread in a pagetoid fashion along the biliary mucosa. This type of spread may be difficult to differentiate from high-grade intraepithelial neoplasia (BilIN-3).[134] Metastatic adenocarcinomas can also show intraductal spread mimicking BilIN-3.

iCCAs have been divided into *small-duct* and *large-duct* types.[2,135,136] These types have distinct clinical, pathological, and mutational profiles (Table 56.11). The small-duct type (also called *peripheral* or *cholangiolar type*) is composed of cuboidal to low columnar tumor cells that contain scanty cytoplasm, while the large-duct type (also called *hilar* or *bile duct type*) comprises intermediate to large glands with tall columnar tumor cells. The large-duct type has a higher propensity for lymph node involvement and a relatively poorer outcome. Two subtypes of small-duct iCCA have been recognized: the *cholangiolocellular* (CLC) and *ductal plate malformation* (DPM) pattern. The CLC pattern is characterized by anastomosing cords and glands of tumor cells with low-grade nuclei and an "antler horn–like" branching pattern mimicking a ductular reaction. These tumors were categorized in the WHO 2010 classification as *combined hepatocellular cholangiocarcinomas with stem cell features*. However, based on morphologic, immunohistochemical, and molecular similarities, this is now considered a subtype of small-duct iCCA. [1,137] The DPM subtype is characterized by dilated curvilinear glands, low-grade nuclei, and inspissated bile reminiscent of ductal plate malformation (Fig. 56.39).[138] A variety of less common histological subtypes like mucinous, signet ring cell, clear cell, adenosquamous, clear cell, mucoepidermoid, lymphoepithelioma-like, adenosquamous, and sarcomatoid (spindle cell) have been described.

Precursor Lesions

Two types of precursor lesions are recognized: flat/micropapillary lesions referred to as *biliary intraepithelial neoplasia (BilIN)/dysplasia* and papillary lesions *(intraductal papillary neoplasm)*. Both are usually associated with the large-duct type of iCCA.

TABLE 56.11 Comparison of Small-Duct and Large-Duct Subtypes of Intrahepatic Cholangiocarcinoma

Feature	Small-Duct Type	Large-Duct Type
Risk factors	Chronic viral hepatitis, cirrhosis	Primary sclerosing cholangitis, liver flukes, hepatolithiasis
Location	Periphery	Close to hilar region
Precursor lesions	Not known	Biliary intraepithelial neoplasia or intraductal papillary neoplasm
Gross appearance	Mass forming	Mass forming, periductal-infiltrative, or both
Microscopic features	• Small glands/tubules in fibrotic stroma • Cuboidal or low columnar tumor cells • Mucin often present	• Larger glands in fibrotic stroma • Columnar to cuboidal tumor cells • Typically mucin negative
Perineural invasion	Can be present	Common
Immunohistochemistry	• CK7, CK19 positive • CD56, luminal EMA positive	• CK7, CK19 positive • CD56 negative, membranous EMA positive
Mutational profile	*IDH1*, *IDH2* mutations, *FGFR2* fusions	*KRAS* mutations
Outcome	5-year survival 35%-40%	5-year survival 20%-25%

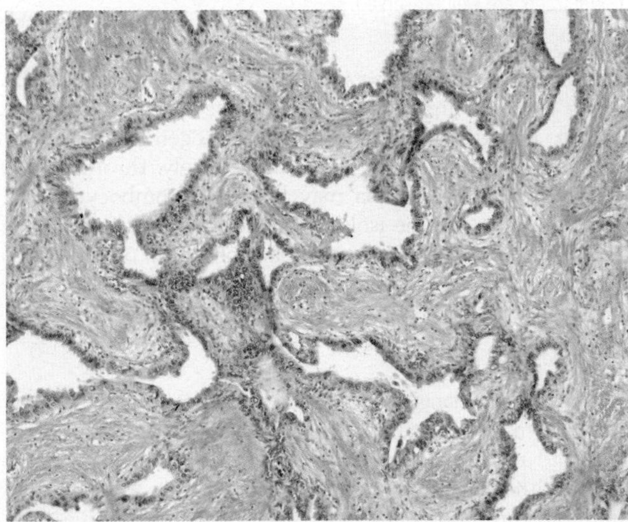

FIGURE 56.39 Intrahepatic cholangiocarcinoma with a ductal plate malformation–like pattern with branching variably dilated glands showing curvilinear outlines (100×).

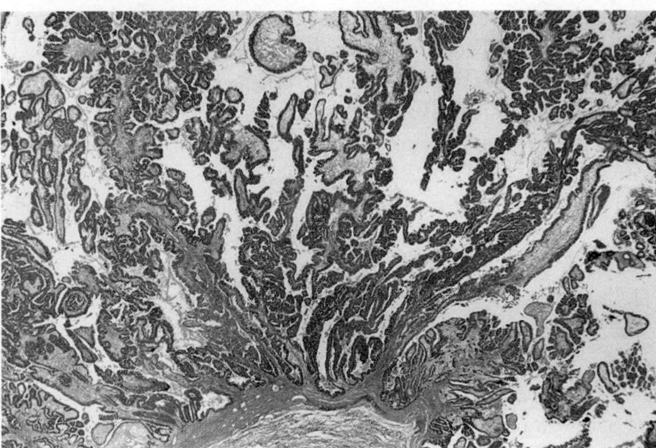

FIGURE 56.40 A papillary growth pattern in cholangiocarcinoma with tumor cells arranged in thin, delicate fronds. Invasion was evident in other parts of the tumor.

Biliary intraepithelial neoplasia (BilIN) is characterized by flat or micropapillary proliferations indicated by dysplasia and is divided into *low grade* (includes former categories of BilIN1 and BilIN2) and *high grade* (formerly BilIN3).[139] Low-grade changes are defined by nuclear stratification, crowding, hyperchromasia, increase in nucleus-to-cytoplasm ratio, and variably prominent nucleoli. A micropapillary pattern can be seen, but architectural atypia is minimal, and there is no loss of polarity. High-grade changes are defined by moderate to marked cytological atypia, loss of polarity, and complex architecture (glandular fusion, cribriform pattern). A "clinging" pattern in the setting of predominantly denuded epithelium may be seen. BilIN may show biliary, intestinal, or gastric phenotypes.

Intraductal papillary neoplasm of bile ducts (IPNB) (also known as *biliary papilloma* and *biliary papillomatosis*) is an intraductal proliferation with a papillary and/or tubular growth pattern. Men are affected more than women (about 2.4 to 1), and patients are usually middle-aged or older (mean age, 60 years). A mass lesion can be identified in the dilated bile ducts on imaging and is better visualized on MRI than CT. Its communication to the biliary tree can be demonstrated by MRCP.[139] IPNB is typically multifocal and forms a soft and polypoid or cauliflower-like intraductal mass distending the duct. The papillae are lined by columnar epithelial cells and supported by a delicate fibrovascular stroma (Fig. 56.40). It is classified into *low grade* and *high grade*, similar to BilIN.[140] The lining cells resemble biliary epithelium in most cases, but clear or oncocytic differentiation and intestinal metaplasia can be seen. Frank invasion of the stalk and/or periductal tissue is a requisite for a diagnosis of invasive adenocarcinoma. Intraductal papillary neoplasms must be differentiated from MCNs and other cystic lesions (discussed earlier).

Differential Diagnosis

Benign biliary proliferations, metastatic adenocarcinoma, and hepatocellular carcinoma must be distinguished from iCCA. It can be challenging to distinguish well-differentiated iCCA cholangiocarcinoma from benign biliary lesions, such as bile duct adenomas (see Bile Duct Adenomas section and Table 56.10), extensive ductular reaction related to parenchymal loss, and fibrosis following ischemic injury or ablation in cirrhotic livers (Fig. 56.41). In the latter situation, the ductular reaction often maintains the background architecture of cirrhotic nodules, and a somewhat nodular grouping of ductules can usually be identified at low magnification.

Immunohistochemistry and mucin stain can help differentiate intrahepatic cholangiocarcinoma from HCC (see Table 56.7). Differentiation from metastatic adenocarcinomas, especially from those from the pancreas, biliary tree, and gastroesophageal location, may be difficult because of overlapping morphological and immunohistochemical features. Loss of BAP1 (10% to 20% of intrahepatic cholangiocarcinomas) and positive albumin in situ hybridization (60% to 70% of intrahepatic cholangiocarcinomas) can be helpful because these changes are absent or rare in other primary abdominal adenocarcinomas.[117,140-143] Sequencing analysis can help if characteristic genetic changes seen in intrahepatic cholangiocarcinoma such as *IDH1* and *BAP1* mutations or *FGFR2* fusions are present. These mutations are rare or absent in other adenocarcinomas.[144] A colonic origin of a tumor is suggested by the presence of tall columnar cells with prominent luminal necrosis and can be confirmed by positivity for CK20, CDX-2, and SATB2, whereas CK7 is typically negative or only focally positive. CK19 can be positive in iCCA as well as colonic adenocarcinoma, whereas CK20 can be positive in a subset of CCAs. CDX2 is typically patchy in CCA compared with diffuse strong staining in most colonic adenocarcinomas.

Prognosis and Treatment

The prognosis for iCCA is extremely poor because the disease is usually advanced at the time of diagnosis, rendering surgical removal either very difficult or impossible. The estimated 5-year survival is 30% to 40% for resectable cases and less than 10% for unresectable ones. Multiple tumors, vascular invasion, perineural invasion, lymph node involvement, and positive resection margin are well-established adverse prognostic factors.[145] Chemotherapy or chemoradiation is used for unresectable cases as well as in cases with high-risk features after resection (such as positive margin, lymph node involvement). Precision medicine holds promise for iCCA, and the U.S. Food and Drug Administration (FDA) has recently approved targeted therapy for iCCA with *FGFR2* fusion.

Intraductal papillary neoplasms are regarded clinically as borderline or low-grade malignant tumors because of multicentricity, tendency to recur, and ability to undergo malignant transformation.[146-148] The tumor is associated with significant morbidity and mortality. Morbidity most often results from recurrent bouts of cholangitis, obstructive jaundice, sepsis, and hemobilia. Although most intraductal papillary neoplasms with an associated invasive carcinoma have a low incidence of metastasis, the probability of achieving cure without liver transplantation is low because of multicentricity.

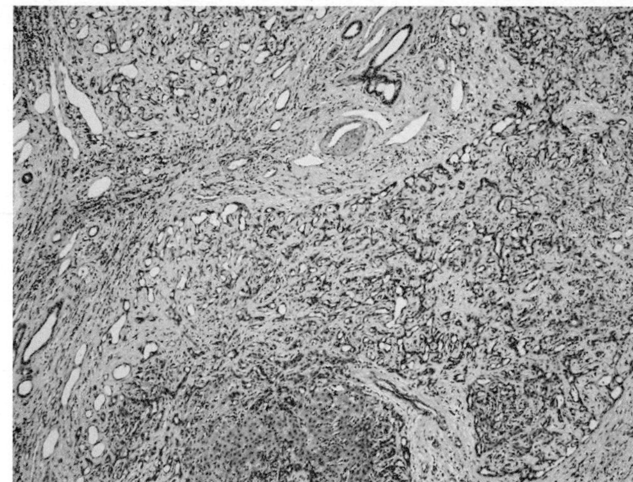

FIGURE 56.41 Bile ductular reaction resulted from ischemic injury following ablation of the tumor by embolization. The ductular reaction occurs in areas with preexisting acini indicating metaplastic reaction. The portal tracts are well preserved.

MESENCHYMAL TUMORS

Hemangioma

Clinical Features

Cavernous hemangioma is the most common primary tumor of the liver. This benign vascular neoplasm is usually asymptomatic and most often discovered as an incidental finding at the time of surgery or autopsy. Cavernous hemangiomas often require surgical excision because of their large size and/or intratumoral hemorrhage. Estrogen therapy may result in enlargement of the tumor. Rarely, thrombosis in a cavernous hemangioma may lead to thrombocytopenia. These tumors may be isolated or multiple, or they may be associated with cavernous hemangiomas in other organs as part of von Hippel–Lindau disease or skeletal-systemic hemangiomatosis syndrome.

Pathological Features

Cavernous hemangiomas are well-circumscribed, red- or red/brown-colored tumors. They usually have a spongy texture and a honeycombed surface, which is mainly an expression of the cavernous vascular component. Many lesions undergo thrombosis and sclerosis, which results in a firm, white-tan appearance. Larger lesions may also contain small satellite foci in the liver parenchyma adjacent to the main tumor mass.[149]

The hallmark of this tumor is the presence of thin-walled cavernous vascular channels lined by a single layer of flattened endothelial cells without cytological atypia or mitotic activity (Fig. 56.42). Sclerotic zones may be extensive, and vascular channels may be thrombosed. Sclerosed hemangiomas may have only a few remaining vascular channels and thus mimic a localized scar. Multiple dilated vascular channels (with morphological features identical to those of hemangioma) may be seen in the liver parenchyma adjacent to primary cavernous hemangiomas.[149]

Hepatic small-vessel neoplasm is an uncommon vascular tumor that has been recently described and is composed of small anastomosing thin-walled vessels with an infiltrative border. The vascular spaces may be compressed in some areas, imparting a cellular appearance and masking the vascular nature of the tumor. The anastomosing vascular pattern can be mistaken for angiosarcoma, but the bland endothelial cell morphology, low proliferation index, and absence of diffuse p53 staining point toward a benign tumor. This tumor is likely benign and is probably similar to the entity described as anastomosing hemangioma.[150,151]

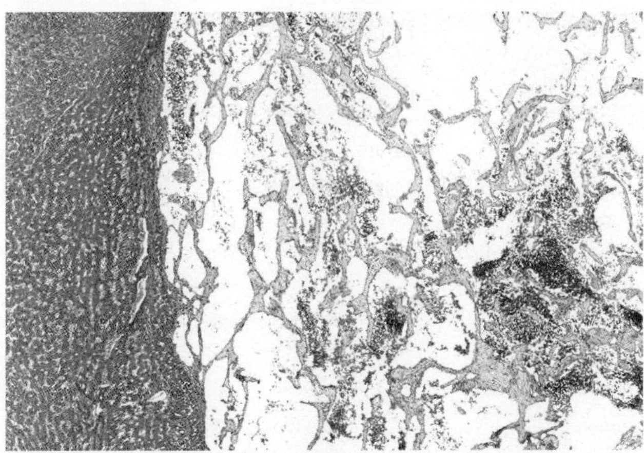

FIGURE 56.42 A cavernous hemangioma composed of large vascular channels in which flattened endothelial line a fibrous stroma.

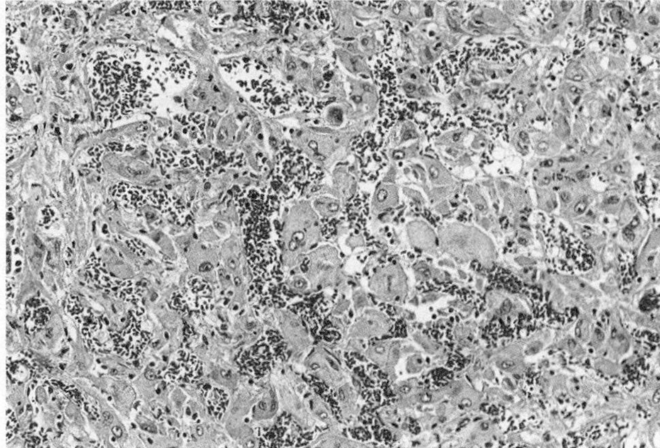

FIGURE 56.43 An angiomyolipoma consists of epithelioid cells with abundant eosinophilic cytoplasm, nuclei with prominent nucleoli, and dilated vascular channels.

Angiomyolipoma

Clinical Features

Angiomyolipomas belong to the family of perivascular epithelioid tumors (PEComas) and rarely occur in the liver. Patients are usually 30 to 40 years of age, and they occur equally between the genders. Most angiomyolipomas are sporadic, but 5% to 15% occur in association with tuberous sclerosis.[152,153] The sporadic tumors often harbor a *TSC2* mutation;[153] a small subset may harbor a *TFE3* translocation or amplification without a *TSC2* mutation.[154-157] Many cases are asymptomatic, being identified incidentally on imaging studies. The imaging features are strikingly similar to HCC with arterial enhancement and venous washout. Thus these tumors are generally indistinguishable on radiological grounds.[154]

Pathological Features

The gross appearance of these tumors may be firm white to yellow to soft and hemorrhagic depending on the extent of fat, vascular component, and necrosis.[152,153] Typically, the tumor is composed of three elements that are admixed with each other: fat, smooth muscle (spindle and/or epithelioid), and thick-walled blood vessels. Some tumors may be monotypic and compose only the smooth muscle component, which can be largely or exclusively epithelioid. Epithelioid cells have a round or polygonal shape with abundant eosinophilic cytoplasm and prominent nucleoli, and they can be arranged in a trabecular pattern (Fig. 56.43). The cytoplasmic contents can be oncocytic in appearance and are often condensed around the nucleus, leaving a clear zone directly underneath the cell membrane, resulting in an appearance akin to a spider web (Fig. 56.44).[152]

The vascular component is typically composed of thick-walled arterial or venous-like channels mixed with thin-walled, venous-like spaces. Adipose tissue consists of mature fat cells scattered throughout the tumor, either singly or in clusters or sheets of cells. The fat component of angiomyolipomas may be scant or absent. Foamy macrophages containing fine droplets of lipid are often present. Peliotic spaces closely associated with areas of hemorrhage are common. These spaces typically lack an endothelial lining. Hematopoietic elements, including megakaryocytes as well as erythroid and myeloid precursors, are often scattered

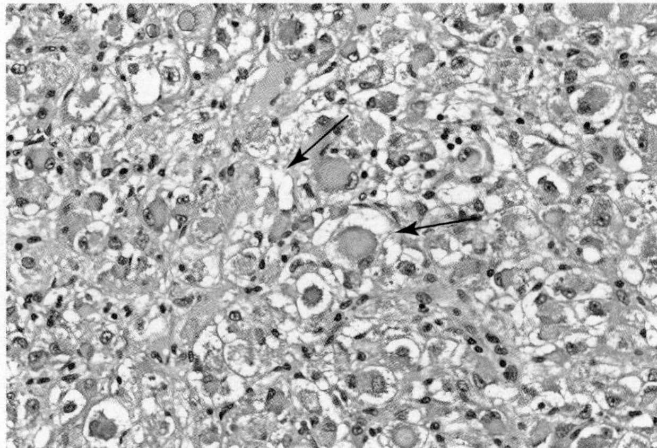

FIGURE 56.44 An angiomyolipoma has epithelioid cells with abundant cytoplasm. Some tumor cells show cytoplasm concentrated in the center of the cell with peripheral clearing near the cell membrane *(arrows)*, imparting a spider web appearance.

within the tumor. An inflammatory component, typically composed of lymphocytes, can be prominent in some cases (inflammatory variant of angiomyolipoma). Hemosiderin and melanin pigments are rare.

The tumors show characteristic myomelanocytic differentiation that can be demonstrated by expression of myoid (desmin, smooth muscle actin) and melanocytic (HMB-45, melan A) markers.[152,153] At least one melanocytic and one smooth muscle marker is positive in 80% to 90% of cases.[155,156] Keratin is typically negative, whereas S100 is either negative or focally positive. Positive staining for TFE3 may be seen in cases that harbor a *TFE3* translocation or amplification.[156]

Differential Diagnosis

Most diagnostic issues arise in monotypic angiomyolipomas in which a predominance of the epithelioid component is present and there is a lack of fat, all of which lead to a close resemblance to hepatocellular neoplasms (Table 56.12). The distinction is mostly straightforward with immunohistochemistry because angiomyolipomas show positive staining for myomelanocytic markers and are negative for keratin and hepatocellular markers.

TABLE 56.12 Epithelioid Angiomyolipoma Compared with Hepatocellular Carcinoma and Hepatocellular Adenoma

Pathological Feature	Epithelioid Angiomyolipoma	Hepatocellular Carcinoma	Hepatocellular Adenoma
Cirrhosis	Not present	80%-85%	Rare
Cell outlines	Indistinct	Usually distinct	Usually distinct
Cytoplasm	Eosinophilic or oncocytic cytoplasm; condensation around nucleus (spider web pattern)	Eosinophilic or oncocytic cytoplasm, fat may be present	Eosinophilic cytoplasm, fat may be present
Nuclei	Round/oval to plump spindle variable size; nucleoli can be prominent	Variable	Typically uniform without large prominent nucleoli
Mitotic activity	Absent	Can be present	Absent
Trabecular pattern	Can be present	Common	Cell plates typically 1-2 cells thick
Foamy macrophage clusters	Can be present	Absent	Absent
Reticulin stain	Reticulin-poor stroma	Loss or fragmentation of reticulin framework	Largely intact reticulin framework
Pancytokeratin	Negative	Positive	Positive
Hepatocellular markers	Negative	Positive	Positive
Myomelanocytic markers	Positive	Negative	Negative
Glutamine synthetase	Can be diffuse	Can be diffuse	Patchy (diffuse if β-catenin activated)

TABLE 56.13 Differentiating Histological and Clinical Features of Mesenchymal Tumors in Adults

Morphological Feature or Immunostain	Angiomyolipoma	Epithelioid Hemangioendothelioma	Angiosarcoma
Risk factors	Tuberous sclerosis, around 10%	Unknown	Vinyl chloride, Thorotrast
Gross appearance	Yellow-tan; hemorrhage and necrosis common	Firm, white to tan; calcifications may be present	Dark red to brown, hemorrhagic, with irregular, spongy texture; may be cystic and necrotic
Satellite nodules	Absent	May be present	Common
Vascular invasion	May be present	Common	May be present
Cellular morphology	Spindle and/or epithelioid myoid component, fat (may be absent in monotypic cases)	Spindle (dendritic), epithelioid cells common	Spindle and/or epithelioid
Growth pattern	Solid or trabecular; necrosis may be present	Small nests, cords, or single cells in myxoid or fibrous stroma; papillary tufts in vascular spaces	Anastomosing vascular channels or sinusoidal growth (scaffolding pattern); solid and papillary patterns can be present, cystic areas in larger tumors
Immunostains	Positive: SMA, desmin, HMB-45, melan A; TFE3 (small subset)	Positive for vascular markers (ERG, CD31, factor VIII, FLI1); CAMTA1, TFE3	Positive for vascular markers (ERG, CD31, factor VIII, FLI1); p53 and Myc often diffuse

Rare cases with a prominent inflammatory component can mimic an inflammatory pseudotumor. Features of angiomyolipoma do not overlap with other mesenchymal tumors, such as epithelioid hemangioendotheliomas and angiosarcomas (Table 56.13).

Treatment and Outcome

Most angiomyolipomas behave in a benign fashion, but recurrence and metastasis can occur in rare cases. Size >10 cm, marked nuclear pleomorphism, diffuse nuclear atypia, and mitoses >2 per 10 high-power fields have been associated with malignant behavior, but morphological features are not reliable in predicting outcome.[153,155]

Inflammatory Pseudotumor

Clinical Features

Inflammatory pseudotumors are not a distinct entity, but a diagnostic term that is used for nonneoplastic mass lesions that can result from a variety of infectious and inflammatory processes.[157-160] Patients may have abdominal pain, fever, chills, jaundice, vomiting, and weight loss. An infectious etiology is suggested by the positive response to antibiotics in some cases, even though organisms are often not demonstrable. Ascending biliary infections and systemic infections like mycobacterial, Q fever, and syphilis infections have been implicated. An inflammatory pseudotumor can result from infectious and noninfectious etiologies. If neutrophils are prominent, it raises the possibility of an organizing abscess, which can be related to biliary tract infection. These tumors may mimic cholangiocarcinoma when they occur in the hilar region of the liver.

Pathological Features

The gross appearance of inflammatory pseudotumors varies considerably, especially if the lesion is large and contains foci of fibrosis, hemorrhage, and necrosis.[155] These lesions vary considerably in size, and they may be solitary or multiple. They can develop anywhere in the liver parenchyma.

Microscopically, inflammatory pseudotumors consist of a mixture of inflammatory and fibrous stroma, but the relative amounts of these components vary considerably (Fig. 56.45). The stromal component often comprises myofibroblasts, and these cysts are positive for smooth muscle actin. A varying amount of dense fibrous stroma, either with or without hyalinization, can be present.

The inflammatory component usually contains a variable mix of lymphocytes and a polyclonal population of plasma cells,[157-160] neutrophils, and eosinophils. Macrophages (often xanthomatous) can be numerous and ill-formed, or they may be present as well-formed granulomas, which can be necrotizing. Immunohistochemistry for *Treponema* can help evaluate syphilis, and AFB and GMS stains can be obtained for cases that show granulomas and/or necrosis. Phlebitis and IgG4-positive plasma cells along with serum IgG4 level can help evaluate IgG4-sclerosing disease. The ratio of IgG4 to IgG-positive plasma cells (0.4 or higher) is more reliable than the number of IgG4-positive cells alone.[161]

Differential Diagnosis

Inflammatory pseudotumors must be distinguished from neoplastic entities that can have a prominent inflammatory component, such as inflammatory myofibroblastic tumors (IMTs), inflammatory fibrosarcomas, hematopoietic neoplasms, histiocytic tumors, follicular dendritic cell tumors, and angiomyolipomas. ALK immunohistochemistry and/or *ALK* FISH can help evaluate IMT. Clonality of plasma cells can be evaluated by kappa and lambda light-chain immunohistochemistry or in situ hybridization. Follicular dendritic cell tumors can mimic an inflammatory pseudotumor; immunohistochemistry for CD21, CD23, and/or CD35 can help identify this rare neoplasm. The inflammatory form of angiomyolipoma may mimic an inflammatory pseudotumor and can be identified with melanocytic markers such as HMB-45. Other mesenchymal tumors such as angiosarcomas, metastatic gastrointestinal stromal tumors (GISTS), and spindle cell sarcomas generally lack a prominent inflammatory component and often have more pronounced cytological atypia and mitotic activity. Inflammatory pseudotumor-like changes may be seen at the edge of another neoplasm; correlation with radiological findings can confirm that the biopsy is representative of the lesion.

Treatment and Outcome

The optimal treatment for inflammatory pseudotumors is not established. Some cases may regress after use of antibiotics or corticosteroids; spontaneous regression has also been reported.[159] The uncertainty about the diagnosis or underlying etiology may result in resection of the lesion.

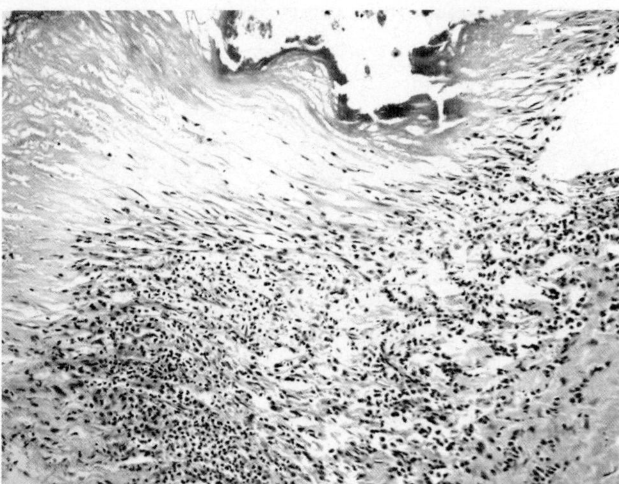

FIGURE 56.45 An inflammatory pseudotumor adjacent to a damaged hilar bile duct in a case of primary sclerosing cholangitis. The lesion is composed of mixed inflammation and fibrous tissue that forms a mass lesion.

Angiosarcoma

Clinical Features

Angiosarcoma is a rare primary malignant vascular tumor that usually occurs in middle-aged adults but can rarely occur in children.[162,163] Presenting signs include hepatomegaly, ascites, jaundice, thrombocytopenia, hemoperitoneum, and liver failure. Risk factors include Thorotrast and vinyl chloride exposure, but most angiosarcomas occur in the absence of known risk factors.

On noncontrast CT and MRI, angiosarcomas have a heterogeneous appearance because of areas of hemorrhage and necrosis. On contrast-enhanced imaging, there is early arterial enhancement followed by progressive filling of contrast in the tumor, which is in contrast to the venous washout typical of HCC.[164] Angiosarcomas can be multifocal, and a distinct mass lesion may not be appreciated on imaging in up to 20% of cases.[164,165]

Pathological Features

On gross examination, angiosarcomas are typically large, hemorrhagic tumors with indistinct borders and often contain both solid and cystic areas; the latter usually contains blood. Satellite nodules may be present in some cases. Histologically, these tumors typically have a mixed histological pattern, showing sinusoidal, solid, papillary, and cavernous patterns of growth. The sinusoidal pattern is the most distinctive pattern in the liver, in which the neoplastic endothelial cells line both sides of the hepatic cell plates in a scaffold-like arrangement that dissects the plates, often resulting in sinusoidal dilation (Fig. 56.46). The tumor cells that line the cell plates are more numerous, hyperchromatic, and larger compared with normal endothelial cells. The sinusoidal pattern is more likely to be identified at the periphery of the tumor. Tumors with a dominant sinusoidal pattern may not form a distinct mass on imaging. The tumor can be composed of anastomosing vascular channels lined by

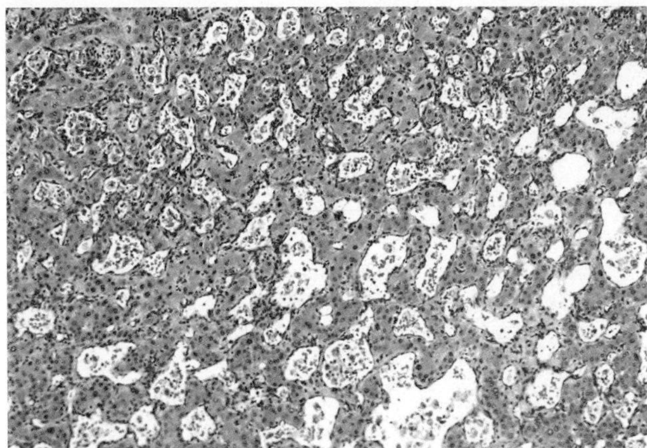

FIGURE 56.46 This angiosarcoma shows atypical cytological features, dilation of sinusoids, and lining of hepatocyte cell plates in a scaffold-like pattern.

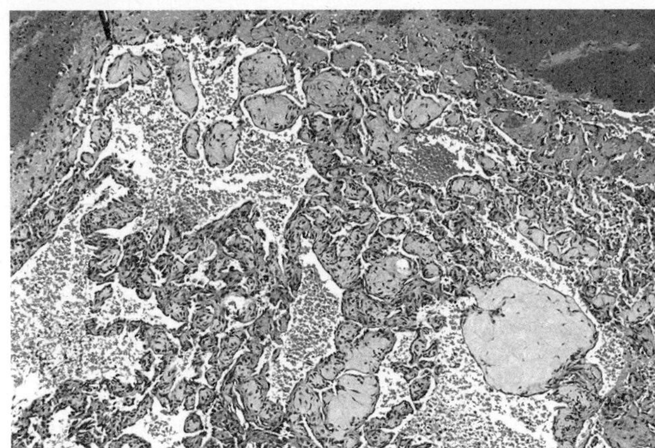

FIGURE 56.48 An angiosarcoma forming focal vascular spaces with necrosis and a focal papillary growth pattern comprising nodules of stroma lined by the tumor cells protruding into a lumen.

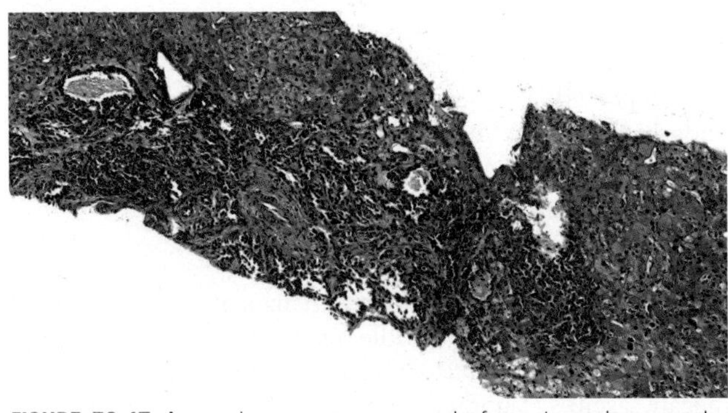

FIGURE 56.47 An angiosarcoma composed of anastomosing vascular channels lined by neoplastic endothelial cells exhibiting a hobnail pattern.

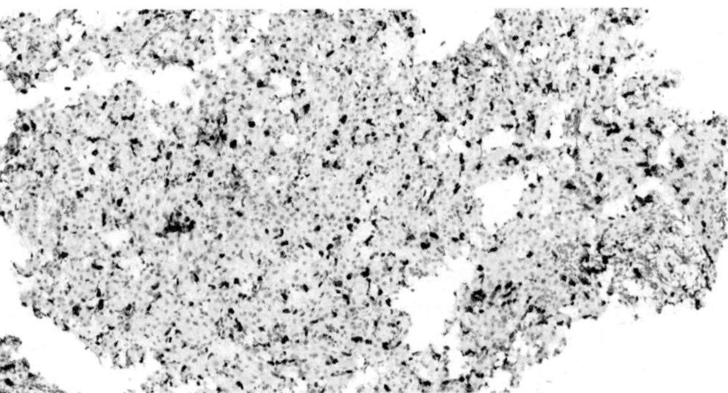

FIGURE 56.49 A high Ki-67 proliferation index in the neoplastic endothelial cells in the sinusoidal pattern of angiosarcoma helps establish the diagnosis.

atypical cells with hobnailing (Fig. 56.47). The solid pattern may have a fascicular, or whorled, appearance and can be similar to other spindle cell sarcomas. The papillary pattern consists of nodules of stroma lined by tumor cells that protrude into a lumen (Fig. 56.48). The cavernous pattern consists of large, blood-filled spaces and is most commonly seen in combination with the other patterns. Unusual patterns with an epithelioid appearance, multiple spindle cell nodules, and hemangioma-like features have been described.[165] Endothelial markers, such as CD31, ERG, and FLI1, are typically positive in tumor cells; factor VIII and CD34 are also positive, but less often used. Immunostaining for Ki-67 and p53 can help in the diagnosis, especially for cases with a sinusoidal pattern (Fig. 56.49).[166]

Differential Diagnosis

Other vascular tumors like hepatic small-vessel neoplasms (HSVNs; Fig. 56.50), epithelioid hemangioendotheliomas (EHEs), and Kaposi sarcoma may enter in the differential diagnosis. A destructive growth pattern with obliteration of underlying liver architecture, marked atypia, and diffuse p53 staining helps in distinction of HSVN from EHE. Unlike EHE, angiosarcomas lack zonation and are negative for CAMT1 (see Table 56.13). HHV-8 immunostaining in Kaposi sarcoma can help in the distinction if necessary. Distinction from other sarcomas is based on positive staining with endothelial markers. Keratin can be positive in angiosarcomas, and this can lead to confusion with a poorly differentiated carcinoma in cases with an epithelioid morphology.

Treatment and Outcome

Most patients are unresectable at presentation. The overall mean survival is less than 6 months.[163] Spontaneous rupture leading to peritoneal hemorrhage can occur in one fourth of cases.[164]

Epithelioid Hemangioendothelioma

Clinical Features

EHE is a rare, low-grade vascular malignancy that occurs in adults of any age, but tends to be more common among females.[167] Most lesions are discovered as an incidental finding, but presenting symptoms and signs may include upper abdominal discomfort or a mass lesion.[168] Serum alkaline phosphatase levels may be elevated in some cases.

On noncontrast imaging, EHE appears as low-density lesions and shows centripetal enhancement in the arterial phase with homogeneous enhancement in the venous phase. Peripheral rim enhancement is seen on MRI with contrast with a central low signal intensity ("black target-like" sign).[168]

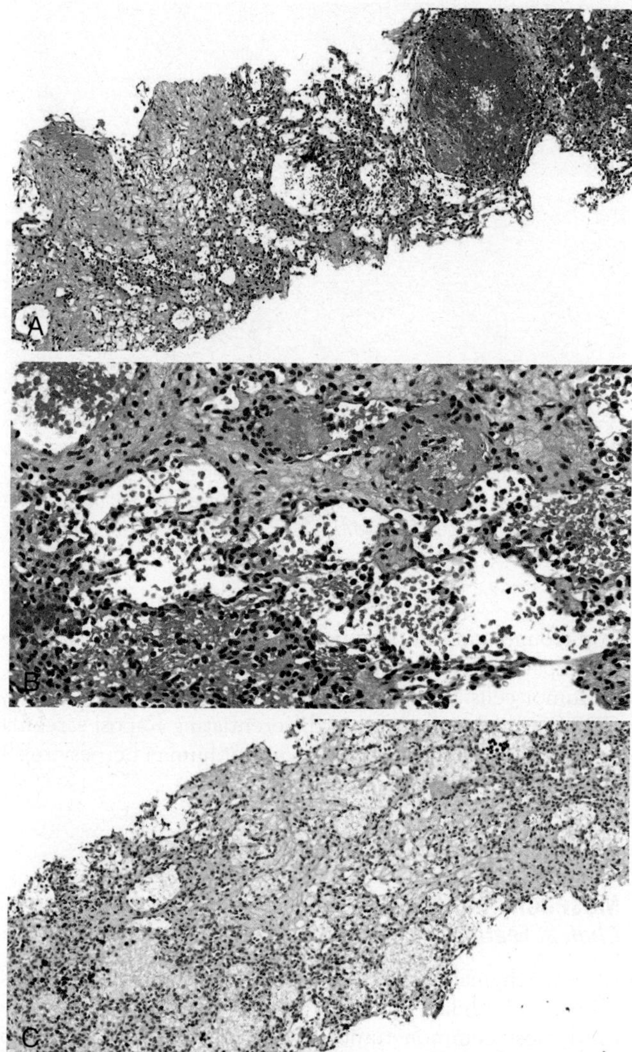

FIGURE 56.50 A, A hepatic small-vessel neoplasm characterized by anastomosing vascular channels (×80) that can be mistaken for angiosarcoma. **B,** The neoplastic endothelial cells often show hobnailing but lack significant cytological atypia (×200). **C,** The low Ki-67 proliferation index (×100) helps in the distinction from angiosarcoma. This entity may be similar to anastomosing hemangioma.

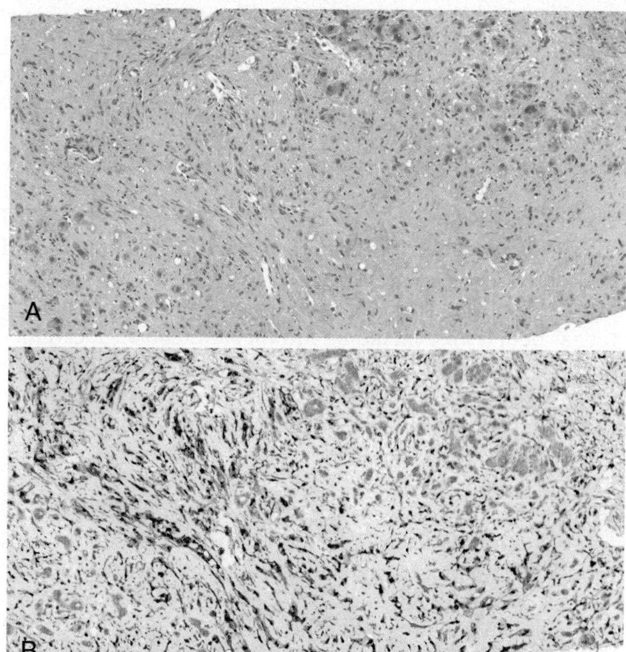

FIGURE 56.51 Epithelioid hemangioendothelioma cells may be dendritic and epithelioid, and they are embedded in myxoid to fibrous stroma. Cells with intracytoplasmic lumina are often present. **A,** The tumor cells characteristically spread between the hepatic cords. **B,** Immunohistochemistry for CAMTA1 shows nuclear staining and helps confirm the diagnosis.

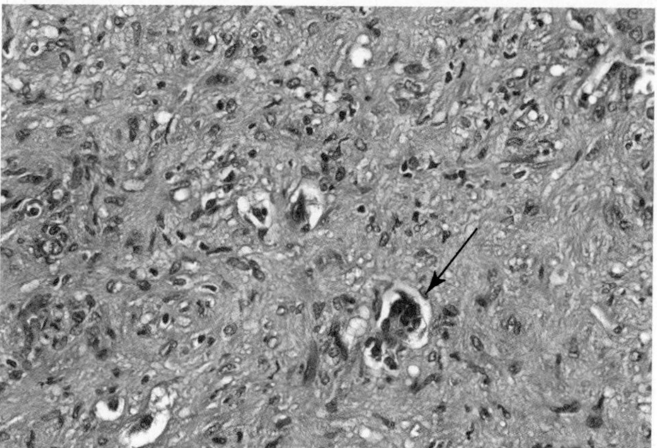

FIGURE 56.52 The tumor cells in epithelioid hemangioendotheliomas may form small tufts in capillary lumens *(arrow)*.

Pathological Features

On gross examination, epithelioid hemangioendotheliomas are firm, white- to yellow-colored tumors that often have ill-defined borders. The tumor is usually multifocal, with involvement of both lobes of the liver. Calcifications may add a gritty consistency to the tumor.

Microscopically, the tumor shows characteristic zonation with a myxoid to sclerotic hypocellular center, infiltrating tumor cells in myxoid stroma in the mid-portion and a cellular periphery with infiltration of hepatic sinusoids. The tumor cells may be dendritic or epithelioid in appearance. The former are irregularly shaped, elongated, or stellate cells with long, branching processes. The cytoplasm may contain a vacuole that represents an intracellular luminal space. Epithelioid tumor cells are rounder and contain more abundant cytoplasm than dendritic cells (Fig. 56.51). These cells often form small papillations, or tufts, in thin-walled vascular spaces (Fig. 56.52). Both cell types are typically surrounded by a myxoid or fibrous stroma, and the dense stroma may be calcified.

The tumor tends to grow around, and leave intact, preexisting structures, such as portal tracts and residual hepatocytes. Bile ducts may be present in the tumor, particularly at the periphery of the lesion. The tumor also has a predilection for invading large vascular structures, such as portal and central veins, mimicking the appearance of vascular thrombosis. Scattered inflammatory cells, such as lymphocytes and neutrophils, are often present. Endothelial markers, such as CD31, ERG, and FLI1, are positive in tumor cells; factor VIII and CD34 are also positive. WWTR1-CAMTA1 fusion has been identified in nearly 90% of epithelioid hemangioendotheliomas; this leads to nuclear overexpression of

CAMTA1, which can be identified by immunohistochemistry, and is very useful for diagnosis (see Fig. 56.51).[169] A subset of cases is characterized by YAP-TFE3 translocation and is positive for TFE3 immunohistochemistry, whereas CAMTA1 is negative.[170]

Differential Diagnosis

The most important differential diagnoses are epithelial tumors (especially intrahepatic cholangiocarcinoma) and angiosarcoma. The epithelioid morphology and positive staining for keratin (rare cases) can mimic malignant epithelial neoplasms, including intrahepatic cholangiocarcinomas and HCCs (see Table 56.13). Intracellular lumina can lead to a mistaken impression of abortive gland formation. Keratin positivity within trapped hepatocytes or bile ducts can also be mistaken as evidence of a carcinoma. Keratin may stain some tumor cells.[171] Tumor growth in large vessels may mimic an organizing thrombus, and a small biopsy from a myxoid/sclerotic center with an inconspicuous cellular component may not be recognized as neoplastic. CAMTA1 and TFE3 immunohistochemistry can help distinguish angiosarcoma and other mesenchymal tumors (see Table 56.13).

Prognosis and Treatment

The prognosis is more favorable compared with angiosarcomas, even if excision is incomplete or extrahepatic metastases are identified. Liver transplantation has been performed for unresectable cases with localized disease.

Kaposi Sarcoma

Clinical Features

Kaposi sarcoma is a low grade malignant vascular neoplasm that occurs most often in the setting of acquired immunodeficiency syndrome (AIDS) and rarely in immunosuppressed patients in the absence of AIDS, or in immunocompetent older adult patients (more commonly in Europe and Africa). Liver involvement has been noted on one third of cases in autopsy series of AIDS patients.[172] Human herpesvirus 8, which occurs in the semen of infected patients and is transmitted through sexual contact, is thought to play a causative role. The tumor appears as hyperechoic nodules on ultrasound. A hypoattenuated appearance is typical on contrast-enhanced CT, and most of the lesions will enhance in the venous phase.[173]

Pathological Features

The pathological features in the liver are similar to those that occur at other sites in the body. On gross examination, the tumor may be fibrous, hemorrhagic, and multifocal, and it often centers on portal tracts. Microscopically, the tumor consists of a spindle cell proliferation that forms slit-like spaces or, in larger lesions, a fibrosarcomatous growth pattern (Fig. 56.53). Cellular pleomorphism and mitotic activity are minimal, and extravasation of erythrocytes, hemosiderin deposits, and small eosinophilic globules are common. Growth of tumor cells into sinusoidal spaces, usually at the periphery of tumor nodules, is a typical pattern observed in the liver. This results in dilated channels containing erythrocytes that replace normal sinusoids imparting a peliotic appearance (see Fig. 56.53). The tumor also tends to surround and infiltrate portal tracts but does not involve the hepatic artery or interlobular bile ducts.

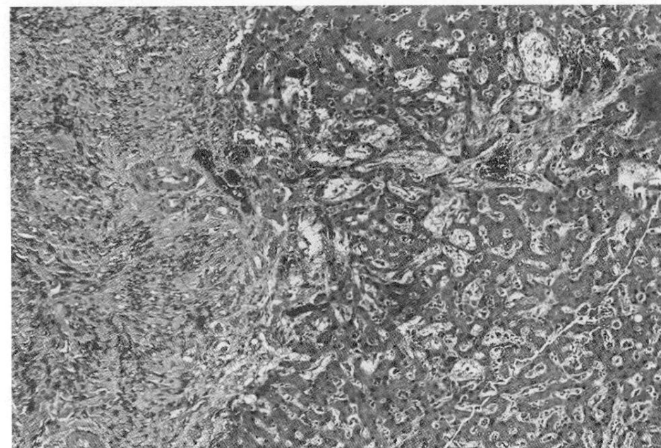

FIGURE 56.53 Kaposi sarcoma tends to involve the portal zones as a solid proliferation of spindle cells *(left)*, but when the tumor cells extend into the lobule, they grow along the sinusoidal spaces, resulting in sinusoidal dilation and peliosis *(right)*.

Tumor cells are positive for endothelial markers (CD31, CD34), which are useful in differentiating Kaposi sarcoma from fibroblastic tumors. Positivity for human herpesvirus 8 is pathognomonic.[174]

PEDIATRIC NEOPLASMS (TABLE 56.14)

Mesenchymal Hamartoma

Clinical Features

A mesenchymal hamartoma is a benign tumor that occurs primarily in children younger than 2 years of age. It is the third most common tumor of the liver in this age group (after hepatoblastoma and infantile hemangioma).[175,176] At presentation, patients often have a palpable liver mass, abdominal enlargement, or respiratory distress; the latter is caused by tumor compression. As in hepatoblastoma, serum AFP levels can be high. The tumor can also arise in Beckwith-Wiedemann syndrome.[177] Mesenchymal hamartomas can have translocations affecting 19q and may be capable of transforming into undifferentiated (embryonal) sarcomas (discussed later).[178]

Pathological Features

Mesenchymal hamartomas may be solid or cystic. Cysts may contain translucent fluid or gelatinous material[175,176] and probably develop from degeneration of loose tumor mesenchymal tissue. The tumors may enlarge through progressive accumulation of fluid in the cysts.

Histologically, mesenchymal hamartomas contain a mixture of epithelial and stromal components. The former consists of relatively normal-appearing hepatocytes and bile ducts, both of which are usually surrounded by myxoid or fibrous stroma (Fig. 56.54). The hepatocytes are often arranged in small clusters or larger groups but retain the normal plate architecture (Fig. 56.55). Bile duct structures are typically arranged in a branching pattern and are associated with an acute inflammatory infiltrate. Cystic spaces, when present, may be lined by flattened to

TABLE 56.14 Histological Features of Pediatric Tumors

Tumor Type	Clinical Features	Major Histological Features	Differential Diagnosis
Mesenchymal hamartoma	Tends to become cystic; no risk of malignancy	Mixture of hepatocytes, cystic change, myxoid to fibrous stroma, ductules	Hepatoblastoma: fetal and embryonal component, higher degree of atypia in cellular hepatocellular and stromal components; small samples may be mistaken for normal liver
Infantile hemangioma	Association with cardiac failure	Vascular channels of various sizes; infiltrative edges entrap ducts and hepatocytes	Angiosarcoma: rare in children; higher degree of cytoarchitectural atypia, necrosis
Hepatoblastoma	Malignant; occurs at <5 years of age and mostly in noncirrhotic liver; AFP elevated	Fetal and/or embryonal hepatocellular components in most cases; mesenchymal component can be present; multinodularity common	HCC: often associated with cirrhosis or underlying metabolic or storage disorder in older age group; more atypical cytological features
Embryonal (undifferentiated) sarcoma	Malignant; aggressive tumor; poor prognosis; occurs in 6- to 10-year age group	Anaplastic and pleomorphic tumor cells, necrosis, eosinophilic globules	Any poorly differentiated carcinoma or sarcoma

AFP, *α-Fetoprotein*; HCC, *hepatocellular carcinoma.*

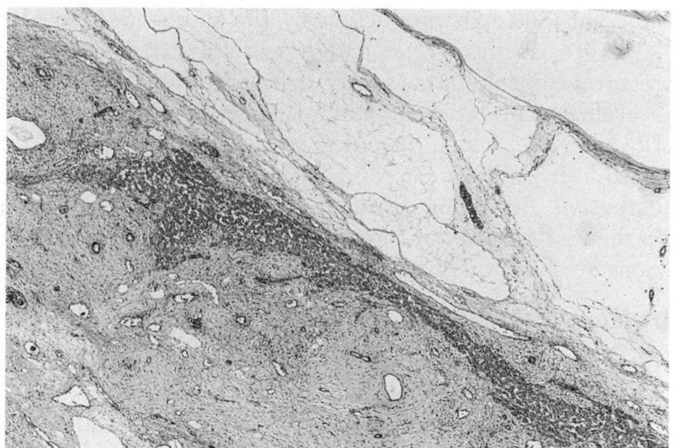

FIGURE 56.54 Mesenchymal hamartoma has multiple, thin-walled cysts *(top right)*. The hepatocyte clusters are separated by myxoid stroma that contains ductular elements.

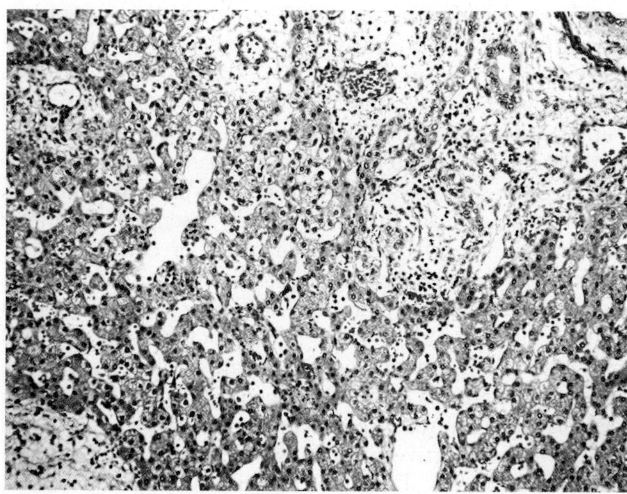

FIGURE 56.55 The solid component of a mesenchymal hamartoma consists of cytologically unremarkable hepatocytes arranged in groups that have a preserved cell plate architecture.

cuboidal epithelial cells surrounded by fibrous tissue (see Fig. 56.54). Occasionally, the cysts lack a distinct epithelial lining. The stroma contains small vascular structures, spindle cells, and inflammatory cells. Normal portal tracts are typically absent. Extramedullary hematopoiesis is often observed. There are no diagnostic immunohistochemical findings. The ductal elements are positive for CK7 and CK19, while the stromal elements express vimentin and smooth muscle actin.

Prognosis and Treatment

Mesenchymal hamartomas are benign tumors with a favorable outcome after complete resection. Rare cases of transformation to embryonal sarcoma have been reported.[179]

Infantile Hemangioma

Clinical Features

Infantile hemangiomas, formerly known as *infantile hemangioendotheliomas,* is the second most common tumor (after hepatoblastoma) in children younger than 3 years of age. Most reported cases have been in infants younger than 6 months of age. The tumor is twice as common among females.

The tumor is often multifocal, and can involve other organs in approximately 10% of patients. The tumors may be associated with other congenital anomalies, such as bilateral renal agenesis, Beckwith-Wiedemann syndrome, hemihypertrophy, and meningomyelocele.[180,181]

Patients usually present with an abdominal mass or distention (with hepatomegaly), jaundice, diarrhea, constipation, vomiting, congestive heart failure, or failure to thrive. Other, less common presentations include thrombocytopenia resulting from sequestration of platelets in the tumor and rupture with hemoperitoneum.

Pathological Findings

Infantile hemangiomas are poorly circumscribed lesions. They may be solid and cystic with hemorrhage. Hemorrhagic foci usually alternate with fibrotic (solid) areas. The tumors are typically multifocal.

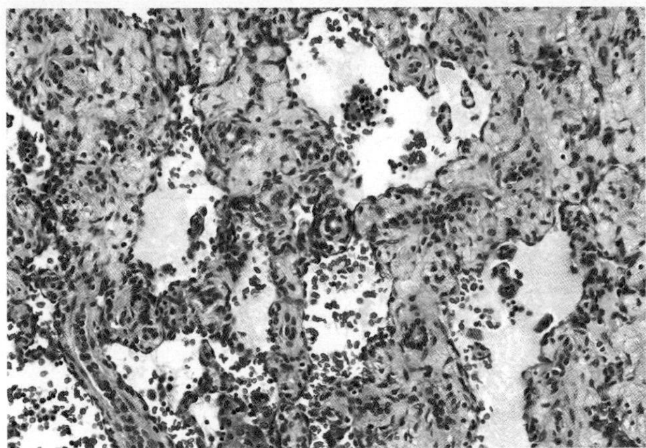

FIGURE 56.56 An infantile hemangioma with the vascular channels lined by endothelial cells. Occasional residual bile duct elements are present in the fibrous stroma.

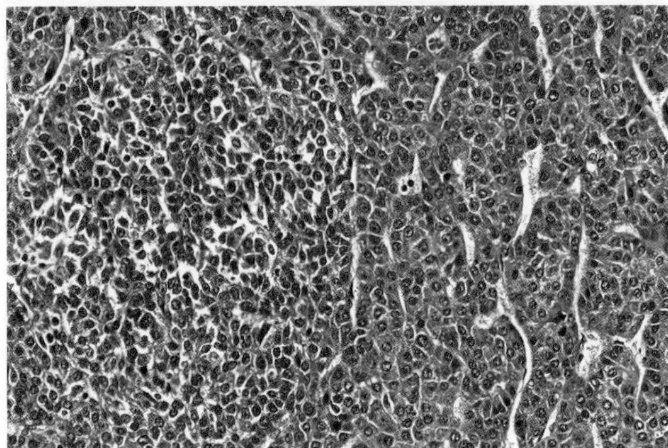

FIGURE 56.57 Epithelial patterns of hepatoblastoma. The embryonal component *(left)* has small, somewhat undifferentiated tumor cells arranged in a ribbon-like pattern. The fetal component *(right)* has better-differentiated tumor cells with pink cytoplasm and round nuclei that are arranged in thick trabeculae.

The tumor shows a mixture of small vascular channels and irregularly shaped cavernous spaces (Fig. 56.56). Both types of vascular channels are lined by a single layer of endothelial cells. The vascular spaces are separated by a poorly developed stroma containing scattered collagen or reticulin fibers. Small bile ducts and hepatocytes may be identified in the stroma and are often accentuated near the periphery of the tumor (see Fig. 56.56). Focal areas of necrosis, hemorrhage, fibrosis, and calcifications are often seen. Tumor endothelial cells stain with typical vascular endothelial markers. The tumor formerly designated as *infantile hemangioma/hemangioendothelioma* has cytological and architectural atypia and is now classified as *angiosarcoma*. The morphological findings in infantile hemangioma overlap with vascular malformation. Large thick-walled blood vessels and absence of GLUT1 by immunohistochemistry point toward the latter entity.[182]

Prognosis and Treatment

Infantile hemangiomas are histologically benign, but the mortality rate is high because of multifocality and large size, which often leads to cardiac or hepatic failure.[180] The tumors may regress, but more often, surgical resection, embolization, hepatic arterial ligation, or chemotherapy or irradiation (or both) are used to prolong patient survival. Angiosarcomas may rarely arise in these tumors.

Hepatoblastoma

Clinical Features

Hepatoblastomas are the most common malignant liver neoplasm in children.[183] Approximately 66% occur in children younger than 2 years of age, and 90% occur before 5 years of age. Rarely, it occurs in adults. Males are affected twice as often as females. Hepatoblastomas are associated with other congenital conditions, such as Beckwith-Wiedemann syndrome, Down syndrome, familial polyposis coli, hemihypertrophy, renal malformation, and other chromosomal abnormalities in as many as one third of cases.[183]

Presenting symptoms, such as abdominal mass, failure to thrive, and weight loss, are common. Less common features include vomiting, diarrhea, and jaundice. Rarely, affected patients may have signs of precocious puberty, such as virilization, which is associated with human chorionic gonadotropin production by the tumor. Serum AFP levels are usually elevated and are a useful marker for tumor recurrence or metastasis after therapy. Tumor resectability is evaluated by "*Pre*treatment assessment of disease *ext*ent" (PRETEXT), which includes radiological assessment of zonal liver involvement, vascular invasion, and extrahepatic extension. Activation of the Wnt signaling pathway is seen in the vast majority of tumors and is often related to mutations involving *CTNNB1* (β-catenin) or *APC*.[184]

Pathological Features

Hepatoblastomas typically occur as a large single mass in patients with a noncirrhotic liver. The tumor is often multinodular and usually contains areas of hemorrhage and necrosis. Because distinct tumor nodules may contain different histological components, generous tissue sampling is recommended. After chemotherapy, tumors often become quite necrotic, but the mesenchymal components, especially osteoid, remain prominent.[185]

Microscopically, the two main subtypes are *epithelial and mixed epithelial-mesenchymal*. The epithelial type is composed of embryonal and/or fetal patterns (Fig. 56.57 and Fig. 56.58). In the epithelial subtype, the embryonal pattern represents the more immature form. It consists of small tumor cells with round to oval nuclei and scant basophilic cytoplasm. The cells tend to form tubular, acinar, or ribbon-like structures (see Fig. 56.57). The fetal pattern represents a more mature form that more closely resembles fetal liver and has tumor cells arranged in plates or cords (see Fig. 56.57). Fetal tumor cells are typically smaller than normal hepatocytes, but they are slightly larger than embryonal tumor cells. Fetal cells resemble hepatocytes with a moderate amount of eosinophilic cytoplasm or clear cytoplasm, the latter related to lipid or glycogen. Eosinophilic and clear cytoplasmic features often occur in the same tumor, which results in a distinctive alternating pattern of pink and white areas (Fig. 56.59). Fetal cell nuclei are small and round, similar to normal fetal liver cells. In the embryonal and fetal patterns, mitotic figures are rare. Extramedullary hematopoiesis is often associated with the fetal component. Fetal

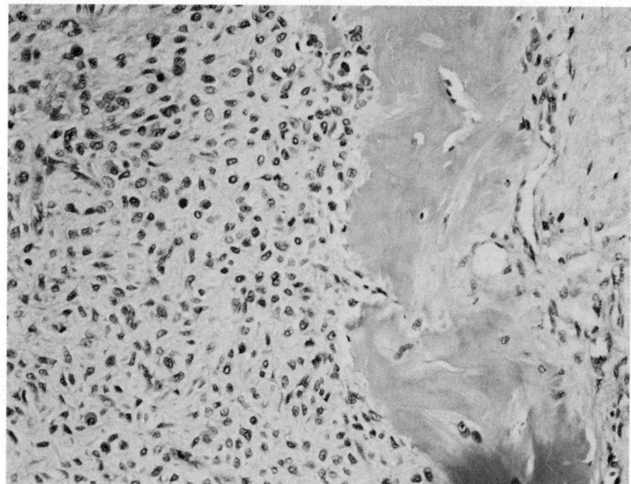

FIGURE 56.58 Mesenchymal patterns of hepatoblastoma. Notice the osteoid *(right)* and adjacent undifferentiated mesenchyme *(left)*.

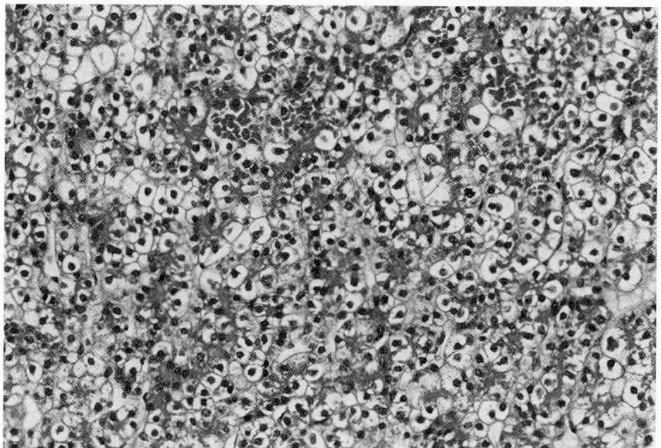

FIGURE 56.59 The fetal component of a hepatoblastoma has an alternating white and pink pattern of staining of the cytoplasm.

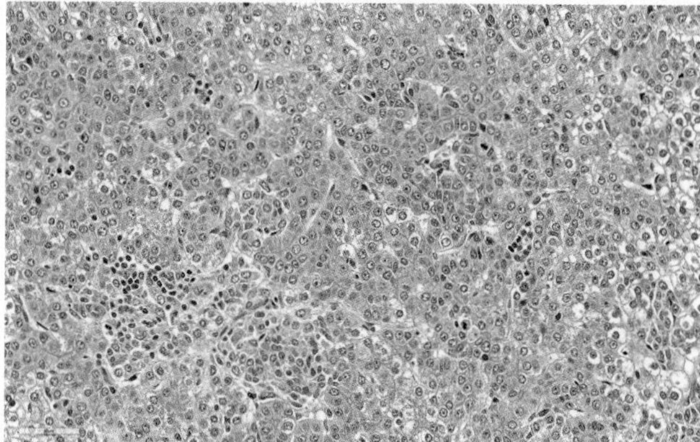

FIGURE 56.60 The crowded fetal pattern of hepatoblastoma with larger and more closely packed nuclei compared with the fetal pattern. *(Courtesy Dr. Cho, UCSF Pediatric Pathology).*

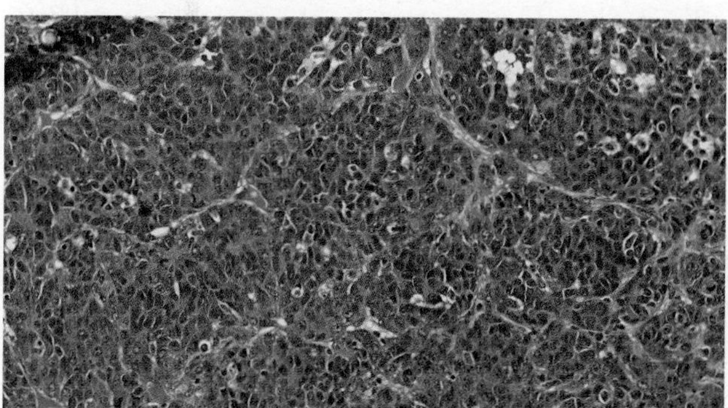

FIGURE 56.61 Macrotrabecular pattern of hepatoblastoma with more than 10 cell thick plates, which can closely mimic hepatocellular carcinoma *(Courtesy Dr. Cho, UCSF Pediatric Pathology).*

areas with higher mitotic activity (>2 per high-power field) and larger, more pleomorphic closely packed nuclei are categorized as *crowded fetal pattern* (Fig. 56.60). Hepatoblastomas composed only of the fetal areas without crowded fetal features are categorized as *pure fetal hepatoblastomas*.

Less common epithelial subtypes include *small-cell undifferentiated* and *macrotrabecular*. The small-cell type consists of sheets of small tumor cells with scant cytoplasm and with no evidence of hepatocellular differentiation. Other patterns of hepatoblastoma are necessary to distinguish this from other small round cells tumors, such as neuroblastomas.

The macrotrabecular type consists of trabeculae more than 10 cells thick (Fig. 56.61). Fetal and embryonal tumor cells form the trabeculae, but a much less common pattern consists of large cells with abundant cytoplasm, which can closely mimic HCC. Other patterns of hepatoblastoma help distinguish the macrotrabecular variant of hepatoblastoma from HCC. Tumors with a minor macrotrabecular component should be classified according to the most predominant patterns. The term *cholangioblastic HB* has been used for tumors that contain ductular differentiation at the periphery of epithelial HBs. This should not be confused with a ductular reaction at the tumor periphery that is commonly observed after chemotherapy.[186]

The mixed epithelial and mesenchymal subtype is usually composed of epithelial patterns admixed with spindle cell mesenchyme. Osteoid is a common finding (see Fig. 56.58). A rare subtype is mixed hepatoblastoma with teratoid features, which contains epithelial and mesenchymal components along with other tissue types, such as intestinal-type glands, squamous epithelium, melanin pigment, and other mesenchymal elements, including cartilage, skeletal muscle, and neural tissue (Fig. 56.62).

The epithelial component of hepatoblastomas is positive for hepatocellular markers, such as Hep Par 1, arginase-1, and glypican-3. AFP can be positive in the embryonal component. Diffuse glutamine synthetase staining and nuclear β-catenin is observed in most cases.[183,184]

Differential Diagnosis

Pure fetal hepatoblastomas may resemble HCAs. Alternating pink and clear areas along with identification of other patterns helps confirm the diagnosis. Age, clinical setting, and AFP level can also help in the diagnosis. Similarly, the clinicopathological setting and identification of other patterns can help distinguish the macrotrabecular variant of hepatoblastoma from HCC.

Prognosis and Treatment

The treatment of choice is complete surgical resection. Chemotherapy is used preoperatively, except for the *pure fetal* subtype, which is treated with surgical resection alone.

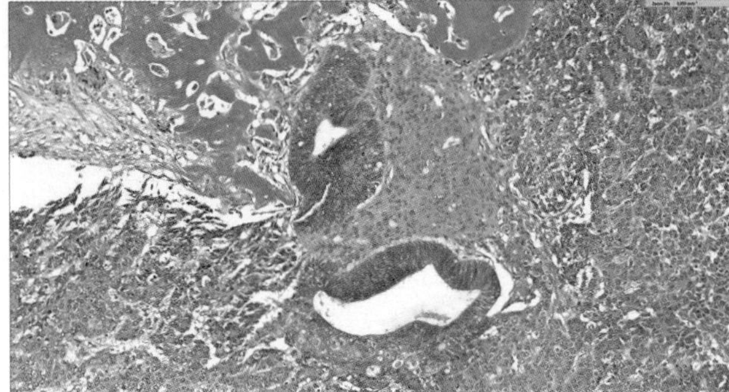

FIGURE 56.62 Mixed hepatoblastoma with teratoid features characterized by epithelial *(right)*, mesenchymal *(top left)*, and neuroepithelial *(center)* elements. *(Courtesy Dr. Cho, UCSF Pediatric Pathology).*

Certain histological subtypes such as *small cell* and *macrotrabecular* have been associated with poorer outcome.[183]

Prognosis is related to completeness of surgical excision, tumor stage, and response to chemotherapy.[183] Additional potential indicators of poor prognosis are young age at presentation (<1 year), large tumor size, vascular invasion, and involvement of adjacent vital organs.

Embryonal (Undifferentiated) Sarcoma

Clinical Features

Embryonal sarcomas are rare liver tumors that typically occur in children between 6 and 10 years of age. Rarely, older children, teenagers (<20 years),[187] and adults may be affected.[188] Common presenting features include a mass lesion and abdominal pain.[187,189]

The histogenesis of this tumor is unknown. Risk factors have not been reliably identified. Rare cases have been reported to arise from mesenchymal hamartomas.[190] Molecular studies have suggested a possible relationship between these two tumors because both lesions have 19q chromosomal abnormalities.[190,191]

Pathological Features

Embryonal sarcomas are usually large, soft tumors with cystic (often multicystic) and solid areas and a white, shiny, or gelatinous mucoid surface. Areas of necrosis and hemorrhage are often observed.

Microscopically, embryonal sarcomas contain a mixture of stellate and spindle-shaped cells embedded in a myxoid stroma. The tumor cells have a granular or bubbly appearance and light pink cytoplasm and contain cytoplasmic globules that are d-PAS positive (Fig. 56.63). Globules may also be seen in the extracellular stroma. Other features include large, atypical tumor cells with hyperchromatic nuclei and multinucleation, dense collagen deposits, and numerous mitotic figures. Extramedullary hematopoiesis is often identified, and entrapped hepatocytes and ductules may be observed at the periphery of the tumor.

Embryonal sarcomas stain with vimentin, α_1-antitrypsin, and α_1-antichymotrypsin.[189,192] Staining for GPC3 expression is positive in this tumor, including the giant tumor cells.[193] The differential diagnosis includes angiosarcoma and rhabdomyosarcoma, but immunostaining for CD34 and myogenin is negative in embryonal sarcomas and helps exclude these possibilities.[192]

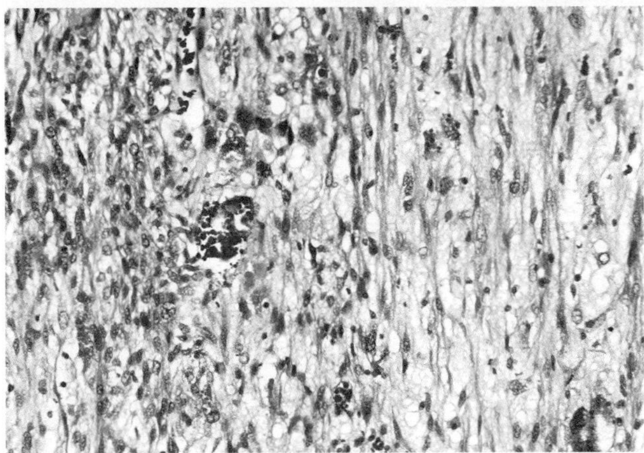

FIGURE 56.63 Embryonal (undifferentiated) sarcoma with spindle to stellate shape and myxoid stroma.

Prognosis and Treatment

The prognosis has been considered poor,[189] with complete surgical excision usually offering the most favorable outcome. However, newer therapeutic modalities have contributed to improvements in survival.

Other Pediatric Liver Tumors

Hepatocellular neoplasms, not otherwise specified (HCN-NOS) are tumors with overlapping features of both hepatoblastomas and HCCs (previously termed *transitional cell liver tumors*).[183,194] These tumors occur in older children (typically older than 8 years of age), have very high AFP levels, and are associated with an aggressive course. Both *CTNNB1* mutations similar to hepatoblastoma and *TERT* promoter mutations similar to HCC can occur, supporting the hybrid nature of the tumor.

Calcifying nested stromal-epithelial tumors are rare, low-grade, malignant tumors that occur in young children and are composed of nested spindle to epithelioid cells surrounded by cellular stroma (Fig. 56.64).[195] The epithelioid cells resemble hepatocytes. Calcification and bone formation can occur.

HEMATOPOIETIC MALIGNANCIES

Leukemias and lymphomas may secondarily involve the liver (see Chapter 31).[196] Leukemic involvement of the liver typically exhibits a diffuse pattern of infiltration of the sinusoids by malignant cells, except chronic lymphocytic and acute lymphoblastic leukemias, which often involve the portal tracts, a pattern that is more typical of lymphoma. Hairy cell leukemia may be associated with the formation of a peliosis hepatis–like lesion consisting of dilated sinusoids lined by tumor cells. Immunostains for various types of hematopoietic cells are helpful in determining a diagnosis in these cases.

Hodgkin lymphoma usually involves the liver as nodular masses in the portal tracts. Occasionally, epithelioid granulomas may be found in the parenchyma or in the portal tracts, but they should be accompanied by a typical Hodgkin infiltrate to confirm liver involvement. Rarely, intrahepatic cholestasis and paucity of bile ducts may be seen.[197]

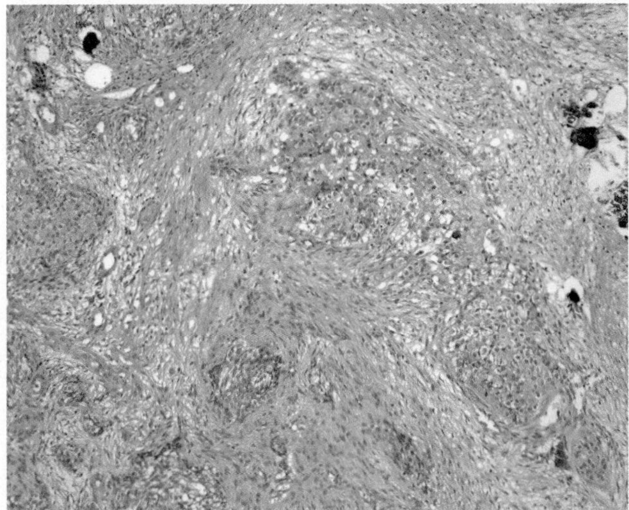

FIGURE 56.64 Nests of spindle to epithelioid cells in a fibrotic stroma with calcifications in a calcified nested stromal epithelial tumor.

Low-grade B-cell lymphomas often form nodular masses in the portal tracts (Fig. 56.65), while high-grade B-cell lymphomas often form large, destructive lesions. T-cell/NK-cell lymphomas typically show sinusoidal infiltration, which is similar to leukemia and reactive conditions such as EBV hepatitis.[196] Hepatosplenic T-cell lymphoma characteristically shows involvement of liver, spleen, and bone marrow without clinically evident nodal disease. Widening of sinusoids, cytological atypia, and abnormal immunophenotype (CD3 positive with loss of pan T-cell markers such as CD5 or CD7) help in distinguishing a neoplastic from a reactive infiltrate. Intrahepatic cholestasis, rarely with ductopenia[198] and epithelioid granulomas similar to those seen in Hodgkin lymphoma, has been seen. Primary hepatic non-Hodgkin lymphoma is rare, but can occur in the setting of AIDS or as posttransplantation lymphoproliferative disorder related to EBV infection in liver allografts.

OTHER LESIONS INVOLVING THE LIVER

Benign Neoplasms

Other benign neoplasms that may involve the liver include chondroma,[199] fibroma, leiomyoma, lipoma, lymphangioma, myxoma, schwannoma,[200] solitary fibrous tumor,[201] and adrenal and pancreatic rests. Granular cell tumors may involve the biliary tract.[202]

Focal fatty change is a localized zone of hepatocytes that contains abundant fat. This finding is often subcapsular and may be confused grossly or radiographically with a neoplasm, but this lesion should not be confused with the fatty nodules seen in adenomatosis, particularly of the *HNF1A*-inactivated type. Focal fatty change may also be associated with diabetes or alcoholic hepatitis.[203]

Solitary necrotic nodules are rare nonneoplastic lesions that consist of a central zone of amorphous, eosinophilic debris rimmed by a hyalinized fibrotic capsule containing prominent elastic fibers. These lesions may be clinically mistaken for metastatic disease and can rarely be associated with a parasitic infection.[204]

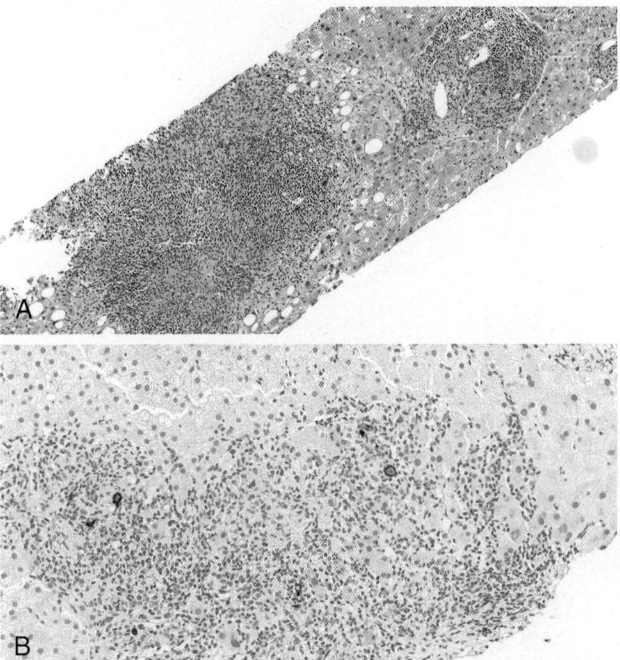

FIGURE 56.65 A, Marked expansion of the portal tracts by lymphoid infiltrate predominantly comprising small lymphocytes and a few large lymphocytes with prominent nucleoli in T-cell–rich histiocyte-rich large B-cell lymphoma. **B,** CD20 immunohistochemistry highlights the large lymphocytes.

Segmental atrophy of the liver (nodular elastosis) can mimic a neoplasm.[205] These atrophic liver lesions likely result from remote vascular injury and are characterized by hepatocellular atrophy, sclerotic vessels, and a varying degree of elastosis, depending on the age of the lesion (Fig. 56.66).

Malignant Tumors

Neuroendocrine tumor, fibrosarcoma, malignant fibrous histiocytoma, follicular dendritic cell tumor, leiomyosarcoma, liposarcoma, malignant mesenchymoma, malignant mixed tumor, osteosarcoma, pheochromocytoma, plasmacytoma, malignant rhabdoid tumor, rhabdomyosarcoma, malignant schwannoma, squamous carcinoma, malignant trophoblastic tumor, teratoma, and yolk sac tumor have been described as primary malignancies in the liver.[206-214]

METASTATIC NEOPLASMS

Metastatic neoplasms are the most common type of malignant tumor in noncirrhotic livers, while metastasis to cirrhotic liver is rare. Tumors with polygonal "hepatoid" cells, such as neuroendocrine neoplasms, renal cell carcinomas, adrenocortical carcinomas, epithelioid soft tissue tumors (angiomyolipomas, GISTs), and melanomas must be distinguished from HCC, while metastatic glandular tumors must be distinguished from bile duct adenomas and intrahepatic cholangiocarcinomas (see Tables 56.7 to 56.12). For spindle cell and sarcomatoid tumors, the differential diagnosis

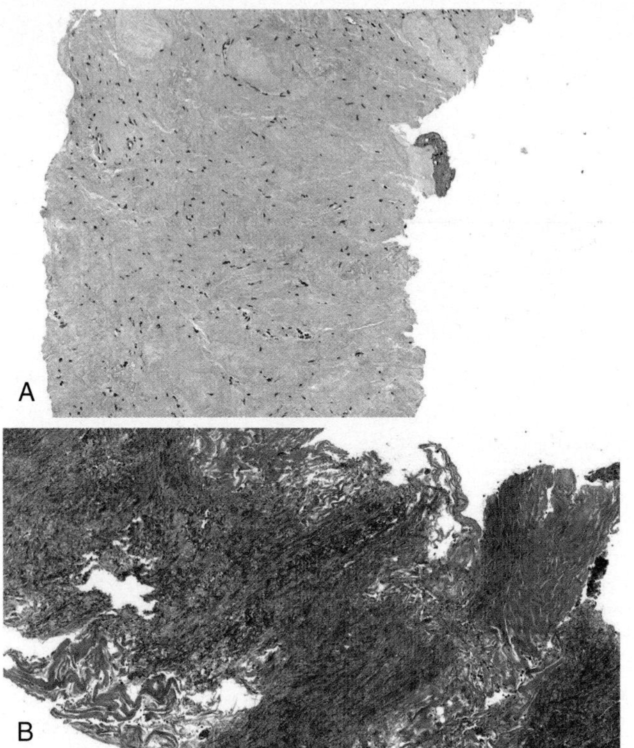

FIGURE 56.66 A, Late stage of nodular elastosis characterized by loose hypocellular stroma, which is rich in elastic fibers and can radiologically mimic a neoplasm. **B,** The elastic fibers can be highlighted by elastic van Gieson stain.

includes sarcomatoid carcinoma (HCC or cholangiocarcinoma) and sarcoma. Most sarcomas in the liver other than angiosarcomas are metastatic. Both GISTs and melanomas merit consideration in this setting.

FROZEN-SECTION TECHNIQUE FOR LIVER TUMORS AND SPECIAL CONSIDERATIONS

Frozen sections of liver tumors are often submitted to evaluate the possibility of metastatic adenocarcinoma when liver lesions are noted intraoperatively. FNH, bile duct adenoma, and biliary hamartoma are the most common incidental benign lesions that must be distinguished from primary or metastatic carcinomas (see Table 56.10). An artificially increased width of the liver cell plates in a thick section should not be interpreted as well-differentiated HCC.

As FNH can be easily mistaken for cirrhosis, it is wise to obtain a biopsy sample of the noninvolved liver adjacent to the tumor mass to help exclude cirrhosis. The features of bile duct adenoma that help differentiate primary from metastatic adenocarcinoma have been discussed. Frozen sections can also be requested to evaluate liver parenchymal or bile duct margins. Evaluation of liver margins usually is not challenging, but portal and central veins should be carefully examined for vascular involvement. Examination of bile duct margins in the hilum or the hepatic and common ducts can be challenging because of exuberant hyperplastic, atrophic, reactive, and/or inflammatory changes involving surface epithelium or peribiliary glands. Retention of overall lobular contour helps in pointing toward a benign process, while a frankly infiltrative architecture and perineural invasion would indicate malignancy. Embolization or ablation of a neoplasm before the biopsy can result in ischemic changes in the liver parenchyma (e.g., necrosis, fibrosis) and marked ductular reaction with epithelial atypia. These changes can mimic cholangiocarcinoma.

The full reference list may be accessed online at Elsevier eBooks for Practicing Clinicians.

INDEX

Page numbers followed by "f " indicate figures, "t" indicate tables, and "b" indicate boxes.

A

C

D

F

G

H

J

K

L

M

N

O

P

Q

R

S

T

U

V

W

X

Y

Z